Angelina S. Yeou, M.D.

Endocrinology and Metabolism

Endocrinology and Metabolism

Second Edition

EDITORS

Philip Felig, M.D.
Chief Executive Officer, Sandoz Pharmaceuticals Corporation
Group Vice President, Sandoz Corporation, and
President, Sandoz Research Institute
East Hanover, New Jersey
Clinical Professor of Medicine
Yale University School of Medicine

John D. Baxter, M.D.
Director, Metabolic Research Unit
Chief, Division of Endocrinology, Moffitt Hospital
Professor of Medicine and Biochemistry and Biophysics
University of California, San Francisco

Arthur E. Broadus, M.D., Ph.D.
Associate Professor of Medicine
Chief, Division of Endocrinology
Yale University School of Medicine

Lawrence A. Frohman, M.D.
Professor of Medicine
Director, Division of Endocrinology and Metabolism
and General Clinical Research Center
University of Cincinnati College of Medicine

McGraw-Hill Book Company

New York St. Louis San Francisco Auckland Bogotá Hamburg
Lisbon London Madrid Mexico Milan Montreal New Delhi Panama Paris
San Juan São Paulo Singapore Sydney Tokyo Toronto

NOTICE

Medicine is an ever-changing science. As new research and clinical experience broaden our knowledge, changes in treatment and drug therapy are required. The editors and the publisher of this work have checked with sources believed to be reliable in their efforts to provide drug dosage schedules that are complete and in accord with the standards accepted at the time of publication. However, readers are advised to check the product information sheet included in the package of each drug they plan to administer to be certain that the information contained in these schedules is accurate and that changes have not been made in the recommended dose or in the contraindications for administration. This recommendation is of particular importance in connection with new or infrequently used drugs.

Endocrinology and Metabolism

3 4 5 6 7 8 9 0 HALHAL 8 9 4 3 2 1 0 9 8

ISBN 0-07-020390-3

This book was set in Goudy Old Style by McFarland Graphics and Design; the editors were J. Dereck Jeffers and Mariapaz Ramos-Englis; the production supervisor was Thomas J. LoPinto.
The cover was designed by Edward R. Schultheis.
Arcata Graphics/Halliday was printer and binder.

Library of Congress Cataloging-in-Publication Data

Endocrinology and metabolism.

Includes bibliographies and index.
1. Endocrine glands—Diseases. 2. Metabolism—Disorders. I. Felig, Philip, date. [DNLM:
1. Endocrine Diseases—metabolism. WK 100 E536]
RC648.E464 1986 616.4 86-20932
ISBN 0-07-020390-3

To our wives
and
children

Florence, Clifford, David, and Elliot
PF

Lee, Leslie, and Gillian
JDB

Carole, Courtney, and Elizabeth
AEB

Barbara, Michael, Marc, Erica, and Rena
LAF

Contents

Contributors **xlv**
Preface **xlvii**

Part I GENERAL ENDOCRINOLOGY

1 Introduction to the Endocrine System 3

John D. Baxter, Lawrence A. Frohman, Arthur E. Broadus, and Philip Felig

Definitions and Scope of Endocrinology 3
Types of Hormones and Their Synthesis and Release 5
Circulation of Hormones 6
Hormone Metabolism 6
Regulation of Hormone Levels 7
Hormone Uptake and Internalization 7
Mechanisms of Hormone Action 8
Regulation of Hormone Responsiveness 8
Classification of Hormone Action 8
Evolution of the Endocrine System 9
    Origin of Hormones and Other Regulatory Ligands 9
    Origin of Receptors and Other Mediators of Regulatory Ligand Actions 10
    Diversification of Families of Hormones 11
Evolution of the Endocrine Glands 11
Integration of the Endocrine System 12
    Integrated Actions of a Given Class of Hormone 12
    Hormone Synergisms: Recruitment of Multiple Hormones for Coordinate Responses 13
    Hormone Antagonisms: Fine Tuning of Metabolism 13
    Mechanisms for Attenuating or Terminating the Response 13
Actions of Hormones 13
    Intermediary Metabolism and Growth 14
    Highly Specific Functions 14
        Tropic actions 14
        Mineral and water metabolism 14
        Cardiovascular functions 14
        Reproductive functions 14
        Developmental actions 15
Disorders of the Endocrine System 15
    Hormone Deficiency Syndromes 15
        Hypofunction of endocrine glands 15
        Hormone deficiency secondary to extraglandular disorders 16

1 (*Continued*)

Hyporesponsiveness to hormones 16
Abnormal production or administration of antagonists 17
Hormone Excess Syndromes 17
Hyperfunction of endocrine glands 17
Ectopic hormone production 17
Iatrogenic causes 17
Tissue hypersensitivity 18
Autoimmune disease 18
Hormone biosynthetic defects 18
Secondary hormone hypersecretion 18
Multiple Endocrine Syndrome 18
Abnormalities of Endocrine Glands Not Associated with Hormonal Imbalance 18
Clinical Assessment of Endocrine Status 19
History and Physical Examination 19
Laboratory Testing 19
Hormone levels 19
Dynamic testing 21
Tests that provide indirect information 21
Evaluation of the sensitivity of target cells to hormones 22
Treatment of Endocrine Diseases 22
Hormone Therapy 22
References 22

2 The Clinical Manifestations of Endocrine Disease **23**

Lawrence A. Frohman, Philip Felig, Arthur E. Broadus, and John D. Baxter

Generalized Symptoms 24
Weakness and Fatigue 24
Weight Loss 24
Weight Gain 25
Body Temperature 25
Skin 25
Nose, Voice, and Tongue 26
Gastrointestinal System 27
Hematopoietic System 27
Cardiovascular System 28
Urinary Tract 29
Sexual Function 29
Bones and Joints 31
Central Nervous System 31
Neuromuscular Abnormalities 32
Ophthalmic Abnormalities 33

3 Gene Expression and Recombinant DNA in Endocrinology and Metabolism **35**

Barry J. Gertz and John D. Baxter

Genes and Their Expression 35
DNA structure and replication 35
Chromatin 37
RNA structure and function 38
Gene Expression 39
Regulation of Gene Expression 41
Gene Evolution 43
Mechanisms of Genetic Disease 44
Recombinant DNA Technology 44
Hybridization 45
DNA Sequencing 46

Sources of DNA for Molecular Cloning 47
DNA synthesis 47
Reverse transcription of mRNA 48
Chromosomal genes 49
Transfer of Cloned Genes into Mammalian Cells 49
Production of Medically Important Proteins by Recombinant DNA Techniques 50
Products of recombinant DNA technology 52
New drug delivery systems 52
Use of DNA in the diagnosis of genetic disease 53
Potential for gene therapy 54
Ethical and Biosafety Considerations 54
Impact of Molecular Biology in Medicine 55
References 55

4 Biosynthesis, Secretion, and Metabolism of Hormones **59**
Gordon N. Gill

Peptide Hormones 59
Biosynthesis of Messenger RNA 59
Biosynthesis of Peptide Hormones 63
Secretion, Transport, and Metabolism of Peptide Hormones 66
Steroid Hormones 68
Cholesterol Substrate for Steroid Hormone Formation 68
The Rate-Controlling Steps in Steroid Hormone Synthesis 69
Pathway of Steroid Hormone Biosynthesis 71
Tropic Regulation of Steroid Hormone Synthesis 74
Transport and Metabolism of Steroid Hormones 75
Thyroid Hormone 75
Iodine Metabolism 76
Anatomy of a Distinctive Biosynthetic Pathway 77
Transport and Metabolism 78
References 79

5 Molecular Mechanisms of Hormone Action: Control of Target Cell Function by Peptide, Steroid, and Thyroid Hormones **82**
Kevin J. Catt

General Aspects of Hormone Action 82
Classes of Hormone Action and Domains of Hormonal Control 83
Local Hormonal Regulation: Paracrine and Autocrine Secretion 84
Peptide Hormone Receptors 85
General Aspects of Cell Surface Receptors for Peptide Hormones 85
Binding Characteristics of Peptide Hormone Receptors 87
The Nature of Hormone-Receptor Interaction 88
Chemical and Physical Properties of Peptide Hormone Receptors 89
Receptor Structure and Function 91
The acetylcholine receptor 91
The EGF receptor 92
The insulin receptor 93
The β-adrenergic receptor 94
Peptide Hormone Receptors and Membrane Components 95
Receptor Mobility and Hormone Action 96
Hormone Receptors and Target Cell Desensitization 97
Receptor Occupancy and Activation of Target Cell Responses 99
Receptor Phosphorylation and Hormone Action 101
Synthesis and Regulation of Peptide Hormone Receptors 102
Biosynthesis and turnover of receptors 102
Receptor regulation in endocrine target cells 104
Effects of receptor regulation on cell responses 104

5 (*Continued*)

Fate of the hormone-receptor complex 106
Functional Classes of Membrane Receptors 109
Intracellular Mediators of Peptide Hormone Action 110
The Second Messenger Hypothesis 110
Adenylate Cyclase, Cyclic AMP, and cAMP-Dependent Protein Kinase 111
Regulation of adenylate cyclase activity 112
The dual control of hormone-sensitive adenylate cyclase 113
Cyclic AMP-dependent protein kinases 115
Mechanisms of glycogenolysis and lipolysis 118
The general role of protein phosphorylation in cAMP action 120
Hormones that use cyclic AMP as a second messenger 121
Guanylate Cyclase, Cyclic GMP, and cGMP-Dependent Protein Kinase 122
Calcium and Calcium-Dependent Enzyme Systems 123
Regulation of intracellular calcium concentration 123
Mechanisms of calcium's action as a second messenger 123
Interactions between calcium and cyclic nucleotides 127
Hormone Action and Phospholipid Metabolism 128
Phospholipids: Structure, metabolism, and functions 128
Hormonal effects on phospholipid metabolism 129
Steroid Hormones 134
Classes of Steroid Action 134
Plasma Binding and Steroid Action 135
Steroid Uptake by Target Cells 137
Steroid Hormone Receptors 137
Steroid Hormone Receptors: Activation and Nuclear Binding 141
Steroid Hormone Agonists and Antagonists 141
Estrogen antagonists 141
Androgen antagonists 142
Progesterone antagonists 142
Glucocorticoid antagonists 142
Mineralocorticoid antagonists 142
DNA Structure and Organization 143
Nuclear Binding of Steroid Receptors 143
Role of the Nuclear Matrix in Steroid Hormone Action 144
Control of Gene Transcription by Steroid Hormones 145
Effects of hormone-receptor complexes on chromatin 145
Receptor interactions with genetic control elements 146
Gene Structure and Processing of mRNA Transcripts 147
Thyroid Hormones 148
Cellular Receptors for Thyroid Hormone 149
Nuclear Actions of Thyroid Hormones 150
Oncogenes and Cellular Regulation 150
Nuclear Oncogenes 151
Cytoplasmic Oncogenes 152
Disorders of Receptor Function 154
References 158

6 Hormone Assays 165

Judith L. Vaitukaitis

Bioassays 166
In Vivo Assays 166
In Vitro Assays 167
Cytochemical Assays 168
Ligand Assays 168
Radioimmunoassay 168
Iodination 171
Generation of Antisera 171

Assay Sensitivity 172
Assay Specificity 173
Effect of Serum Proteins 174
Separation of Bound and Free Hormone 174
Circulating Endogenous Antibody 175
Steroid Assays 175
Further Assay Validation 176
Radioreceptor Assays 176
Immunoradiometric Assays 176
Enzyme-Linked Immunoassays 177
Characterization of Hormone-Receptor Binding 178
Hormone Receptors and Disease States 179
Practical Considerations 179
Assay Variation 179
Hormone Stability 180
References 180

Part II NEUROENDOCRINOLOGY AND THE PITUITARY

7 Neuroendocrine Physiology and Disease **185**
Lawrence A. Frohman and Dorothy T. Krieger

General Concepts of Neuroendocrinology 185
Feedback 185
Hypophysiotropic Concept 187
Anatomic Aspect 190
Hypothalamus 190
Median Eminence-Portal System 191
Pituitary 192
Neurotransmitters, Neuropeptides, and Neuropharmacological Regulation 193
Neurotransmitter Regulation of Hypophysiotropic Neurosecretory Cells 193
Neurotransmitter Synthesis and Metabolism 194
Neuropharmacological Effects 195
Neuropeptides and Pituitary Hormone Release 197
The Hypophysiotropic Hormones: Chemistry, Distribution, Effects 199
Thyrotropin Releasing Hormone 201
Gonadotropin Releasing Hormone 202
Somatostatin 204
Corticotropin Releasing Factor 205
Growth Hormone Releasing Hormone 206
Prolactin Inhibiting Factor 207
Prolactin Releasing Factor 207
Melanocyte Stimulating Hormone–Inhibiting Factor 207
Neuropeptides 207
Substance P 208
Neurotensin 209
Angiotensin 209
Endorphins and Enkephalins 209
Effect of Hormones on Brain 211
Peptide Hormone–Nervous System Interactions 211
Effects of Target Gland Hormones on Central Nervous System Function 213
Effects of Hormones on Sexual Dimorphism of the Brain 215
The Pineal Gland 216
Synthesis of Pineal Principles 216

7 (*Continued*)

CNS Rhythms and Neuroendocrine Function 218
Endocrine Disorders Due to Central Nervous System Disease 221
Diseases of the Hypothalamus 221
Etiology of hypothalamic disease 222
Disturbances of pituitary function due to hypothalamic disease 225
Nonpituitary disorders due to hypothalamic disease 231
Other CNS Disorders 236
Diseases of the pineal gland 236
Pseudotumor cerebri 237
Cerebral gigantism 237
Huntington's chorea 237
Behavioral Disorders 237
Psychiatric illness 237
Emotional deprivation 239
References 239

8 Diseases of the Anterior Pituitary **247**

Lawrence A. Frohman

Pituitary Gland 247
Anatomy 247
Blood and Nerve Supply 248
Embryology 249
Cell Types 250
Anterior Pituitary Hormones 252
Corticotropin-Related Peptides 252
ACTH 254
β-LPH, MSH, and related peptides 256
Endorphins and enkephalins 256
Extrapituitary ACTH and related peptides 257
Glycoprotein Hormones 257
TSH 257
Gonadotropins: LH and FSH 260
Other glycoprotein hormones 263
Somatomammotropic Hormones 263
Growth hormone 264
Prolactin 270
Hypopituitarism 273
Etiology 274
Primary hypopituitarism 273
Secondary hypopituitarism 276
Clinical Features 277
Differential Diagnosis 279
Diagnostic Procedures 279
Treatment 284
Pituitary Tumors 287
Classification 287
Signs and Symptoms 288
Diagnostic Procedures 290
Differential Diagnosis 295
Therapy 298
Pituitary Tumors Associated with Hormone Hypersecretion 300
Growth Hormone–Secreting Pituitary Tumors: Acromegaly 300
Prolactin-Secreting Tumors: Amenorrhea-Galactorrhea Syndrome 306
ACTH-Secreting Tumors: Cushing's Disease 315
TSH-Secreting Tumors 320
Gonadotropin-Secreting Pituitary Tumors 320
α-Subunit-Secreting Pituitary Tumors 321

Details of Hypothalamic-Pituitary Testing 321
ACTH 321
TSH 323
LH and FSH 323
Growth Hormone 324
Prolactin 326
References 327

9 **Posterior Pituitary** 338
Gary L. Robertson

Posterior Pituitary Hormones 338
Anatomy 338
Chemistry 338
Biosynthesis and Release 339
Regulation of Secretion 341
Vasopressin 341
Oxytocin 349
Distribution and Clearance 350
Extrahypophyseal pathways 350
Biologic Action 351
Thirst 353
Maintenance of Salt and Water Balance 354
Pathologic Hypofunction 357
Etiology 357
Pathophysiology 359
Diagnosis 363
Therapy 365
Pathologic Hyperfunction 368
Etiology and Pathophysiology 368
Diagnosis 373
Therapy 374
Tests Used in Diagnosis 375
Hypofunction 375
Hyperfunction 376
General Considerations 376
References 377

Part III THYROID DISEASE

10 **The Thyroid: Physiology, Hyperthyroidism, Hypothyroidism, and the Painful Thyroid** 389
Robert D. Utiger

Physiology and Anatomy 389
Clinical Anatomy 389
Physical examination 390
Histology 390
Chemistry of Thyroid Hormones 391
Thyroid Hormone Biosynthesis 392
Iodide economy 392
Thyroidal hormonogenesis 393
Extrathyroidal hormonogenesis 394
Thyroid hormone production and metabolism 394
Transport and Cellular Binding of Thyroid Hormones 395
Serum binding proteins 395
Cellular hormone entry and binding 397
Actions of Thyroid Hormones 398

10 *(Continued)*

Molecular mechanisms of thyroid hormone action 398
Thermogenic actions 398
Thyroid hormone-catecholamine interactions 399
Effects on protein synthesis 399
Effects on carbohydrate and lipid metabolism 399
Regulation of Thyroid Hormone Production 400
Control of thyroid secretion 400
Thyrotropin and regulation of thyroid secretion 402
Regulation of thyroid secretion by iodide 403
Regulation of extrathyroidal triiodothyronine production 403
Evaluation of Thyroid Function 404
Serum thyroxine concentration 404
Serum T_4 binding capacity (T_3-resin uptake) and free thyroxine index 405
Serum free thyroxine concentration 406
Serum triiodothyronine concentration 406
Serum reverse triiodothyronine concentration 407
Serum TSH and TRH testing 407
Serum thyroglobulin concentration 408
Antithyroglobulin and antithyroid microsomal antibodies 408
Radionuclide and other tests 408
Tests of thyroid hormone action in tissue 409
Physiological Variables Affecting Pituitary-Thyroid Function and Tests 409
Pregnancy 409
Fetal thyroid function 409
Infants and children 410
Sex 410
Aging 410
Environmental factors 410
Alterations in Serum Thyroid Hormone Binding 410
Increased serum binding 411
Decreased serum binding 411
Nonthyroidal Illness 412
Decreased extrathyroidal T_3 production 414
Decreased serum thyroxine concentrations 414
Increased serum thyroxine concentrations 415
Effects of Various Drugs on Thryoid Function 415
Glucocorticoids 415
Adrenergic antagonists 416
Propylthiouracil and methimazole 416
Iodine 416
Iodinated radiographic contrast agents 416
Amiodarone 416
Lithium 416
Phenytoin 416
Hyperthyroidism 417
Pathophysiology of Hyperthyroidism 417
Causes of Hyperthyroidism 418
Graves' disease 418
Thyroiditis 421
Exogenous hyperthyroidism 422
Toxic multinodular goiter 422
Toxic uninodular goiter (thyroid adenoma) 423
Ectopic hyperthyroidism (struma ovarii) 423
Thyroid carcinoma 423
Thyroid-stimulating hormone excess 423
Clinical Manifestations of Hyperthyroidism 424

General appearance 425
Skin and appendages 425
Eyes 425
Thyroid gland 425
Cardiovascular system 426
Respiratory function 426
Gastrointestinal system 426
Hematopoietic system 426
Renal function 427
Nervous system and muscle 427
Energy and intermediary metabolism 428
Endocrine system 428
Laboratory Diagnosis of Hyperthyroidism 429
Serum thyroid hormone concentrations 429
Thyroid radioiodine uptake and scanning 430
Serum TSH and other thyroid stimulators 430
Tests of pituitary-thyroid regulation 430
Summary: Diagnosis of hyperthyroidism 431
Other laboratory manifestations of hyperthyroidism or diseases causing it 432
Treatment of Hyperthyroidism 432
Treatment of hyperthyroidism due to Graves' disease 432
Thyroiditis 437
Toxic multinodular goiter 437
Thyroid adenoma 438
Special Situations 438
Thyroid storm 438
Hyperthyroidism during pregnancy 438
Neonatal hyperthyroidism 440
Postpartum hyperthyroidism 440
Extrathyroidal Manifestations of Graves' Disease 440
Infiltrative ophthalmopathy 440
Localized myxedema and thyroid acropachy 443
Hypothyroidism 444
Causes of Hypothyroidism 445
Chronic autoimmune thyroiditis 445
Transient autoimmune thyroiditis 446
Hypothyroidism following radioiodine therapy 446
Postoperative hypothyroidism 446
Transient hypothyroidism 447
Thyroid dysgenesis (sporadic nongoitrous cretinism) 447
Hypothyroidism due to thyroid injury from other causes 447
Biosynthetic defects in thyroid hormonogenesis 447
Hypothyrotropic hypothyroidism 449
Generalized resistance to thyroid hormones 450
Clinical Manifestations of Hypothyroidism 450
General appearance 451
Skin and appendages 451
Thyroid gland 452
Nervous system 452
Musculoskeletal system 452
Cardiovascular-pulmonary system 453
Fluid and electrolyte metabolism 453
Gastrointestinal system 454
Intermediary metabolism 454
Hematopoietic system 454
Endocrine system 455
Illness and surgery in hypothyroid patients 456
Laboratory Diagnosis of Hypothyroidism 456
Serum thyroid hormone and TSH concentrations 456
Summary: Diagnosis of hypothyroidism 457
Other laboratory procedures 457

10 (*Continued*)

Treatment of Hypothyroidism 458
Special Clinical Situations 459
Thyroid hormone withdrawal 459
Hypothyroidism in newborn infants and children 460
Myxedema coma 460
The Painful Thyroid 461
Subacute Thyroiditis . 461
Hemorrhage in a Thyroid Nodule 462
Radiation Thyroiditis 462
Suppurative Thyroiditis 462
References 462

11 The Thyroid: Nodules and Neoplasia **473**
Gerard N. Burrow

Goiter 473
Classification of Goiter and Thyroid Neoplasia 473
Historical Overview 473
Etiology of Goiter 474
TSH secretion 474
TSH stimulation of the thyroid gland 474
Endemic Goiter 476
Geography, diet, and iodine abundance 476
Development of endemic goiter 477
Clinical findings in endemic goiter 477
Cretinism 478
Prophylaxis of endemic goiter 479
Sporadic Goiter 479
Sex and age in relation to goiter 480
Genetic influences on goiter formation 480
Specific inherited defects in thyroid hormone biosynthesis 480
Specific goitrogens 481
Nontoxic goiter 482
Incidence 482
Presentation and complications 483
Risk of carcinoma in multinodular goiter 483
Laboratory evaluation 484
Therapy 484
Solitary Thyroid Nodules 486
Factors Predisposing to Thyroid Cancer 486
Gender 486
Age 487
Previous irradiation of the head and neck 487
Physical characteristics 487
Laboratory Diagnosis 488
Radioisotopic scan of the thyroid 488
Ultrasound 489
Other imaging techniques 490
Thyroid biopsy 490
Management of the Solitary Thyroid Nodule 492
Thyroid hormone suppression 493
Thyroid Carcinoma 494
Classification 494
Incidence of Thyroid Carcinoma 495
The Effects of Radiation on the Development of Thyroid Carcinoma 495
Natural History of Thyroid Carcinoma 496
Papillary carcinoma 496
Follicular carcinoma 497
Anaplastic carcinoma 497

Therapy of Thyroid Carcinoma 497
Therapy of papillary carcinoma 498
Therapy of follicular carcinoma 499
Therapy of anaplastic carcinoma 500
Subsequent Follow-up 500
Thyroglobulin determinations 500
Medullary Carcinoma of the Thyroid 501
Natural History 501
Clinical Course 501
Diagnosis 502
Therapy of Medullary Carcinoma 503
References 504

Part IV ADRENAL DISEASE

12 The Adrenal Cortex 511

John D. Baxter and J. Blake Tyrrell

History of Study of the Adrenal Cortex 511
Structure of the Adrenal Cortex 513
Development of the Adrenal Cortex 515
Chemistry of the Adrenal Steroids 515
Steroid Biosynthesis 517
Cholesterol Uptake and Synthesis 517
Pregnenolone Formation 518
Modifications of Pregnenolone 518
Cortisol Synthesis 518
Synthesis of Aldosterone, DOC, and Other Mineralocorticoids 519
Synthesis of Adrenal Androgens 519
Synthesis of Estrogens 519
The Fetal Adrenal 520
Quantities of Steroids Produced 520
Inhibitors of Adrenal Steroid Biosynthesis 521
Regulation of Adrenal Steroid Biosynthesis 522
Regulation of Glucocorticoid Production 522
The hypothalamic-pituitary-adrenal axis 522
Regulation of ACTH release 523
ACTH and related peptides 524
Actions of ACTH on the adrenal 525
Actions of glucocorticoids on the adrenal 527
Actions of other factors on the adrenal 527
Spontaneous patterns of ACTH and cortisol release 527
Changes in the spontaneous rhythm 529
Feedback inhibition of ACTH release 530
Regulation of Mineralocorticoid Production 531
Angiotensin II 532
Potassium ion 532
Pituitary gland 533
Sodium ion 533
Other factors 533
Spontaneous patterns of aldosterone release 534
Interruption of the spontaneous patterns of aldosterone release 534
Regulation of Adrenal Androgen Production 535
Regulation of Adrenal Estrogen Production 536
Physical State of Steroids in Plasma 536
Cortisol and Other Glucocorticoids 536
Corticosteroid-binding globulin 537
Albumin and other cortisol-binding proteins 538

12 (*Continued*)

Physiological role of plasma binding 538
Aldosterone 539
Deoxycorticosterone 540
Adrenal Androgens and Estrogens 540
Metabolism of Adrenocortical Steroids 540
Cortisol 540
Corticosterone, 11-Deoxycortisol, and 11-Deoxycorticosterone 542
Aldosterone 542
Androgens and Estrogens 542
Variations in Steroid Metabolism 543
Actions of Glucocorticoids 544
Intermediary Metabolism 544
Carbohydrate metabolism 544
Glycogen metabolism 546
Lipid metabolism 547
Protein and nucleic acid metabolism 548
Liver 548
Muscle 548
Immunological and Inflammatory Responses 548
Effects on vasoactive and other inflammatory agents 549
Leukocyte movement 549
Leukocyte function 550
Erythroid Cells and Thrombocytes 551
Fibroblastic and Epithelial Tissues 551
Cardiovascular system and fluid and electrolyte balance 552
Bone and Calcium Metabolism 554
Central Nervous System 555
Adrenal Medulla 556
Eye 556
Gastrointestinal Tract 556
Growth and Development 557
Production and Clearance of Other Hormones 558
Reproductive Function 558
Synergistic and Antagonistic Interrelationships between Glucocorticoids and Other Hormones 558
Glucocorticoids and Stress 559
Molecular Mechanisms of Glucocorticoid Hormone Action 559
Glucocorticoid Agonists and Antagonists 561
Structure-Activity Relations of Glucocorticoids: Basis for Biological Activity 562
Definition of a Glucocorticoid 563
Physiological Actions of Mineralocorticoids 563
Kidney 563
Extrarenal Tissues 565
Molecular Mechanisms of Mineralocorticoid Action 565
Mineralocorticoid Agonists and Antagonists 567
Definition of a Mineralocorticoid 568
Actions of Adrenal Androgens and Estrogens 568
Laboratory Evaluation of Adrenocortical Function 568
Plasma Cortisol and Related Steroids 569
Cortisol 569
Determination of other plasma steroids 571
Plasma ACTH and Related Peptides 571
Urinary Corticosteroids 572
Free cortisol 572
17-Hydroxycorticosteroids and 17-ketogenic steroids 572
Cortisol Production Rate 573
Dexamethasone Suppression Tests 573
Low-dose tests 573

High-dose tests 574
Tests of Pituitary-Adrenal Reserve 576
ACTH stimulation tests 577
Insulin-induced hypoglycemia, pyrogen, and vasopressin stimulation tests 578
Metyrapone testing 578
CRF testing 579
Mineralocorticoids 579
Androgens 579
Plasma androgens 580
Urinary androgens 580
Clinical utility 580
Adrenocortical Insufficiency 581
Primary Adrenocortical Insufficiency (Addison's Disease) 581
Idiopathic adrenocortical insufficiency 582
Primary adrenocortical insufficiency due to invasive or hemorrhagic disorders 585
Familial glucocorticoid deficiency 586
Pathophysiology 586
Clinical features 586
Laboratory features of primary adrenocortical insufficiency 589
Secondary Adrenocortical Insufficiency 590
Etiology 590
Pathophysiology 590
Clinical features 591
Laboratory features 592
Diagnosis 592
Treatment 594
Acute addisonian crisis 594
Chronic adrenal insufficiency 595
Steroid coverage for illness, surgery, or trauma 596
Prognosis and Survival 597
Hypoaldosteronism 597
Hyporeninemic hypoaldosteronism 597
Normoreninemic or hyperreninemic hypoaldosteronism 598
Pseudohypoaldosteronism unresponsive to aldosterone 599
Adrenocortical Hyperfunction 599
Cushing's syndrome 599
Classification, occurrence, and age and sex distributions 600
Pathology 600
Etiology and pathogenesis 602
Pathophysiology 604
Clinical and laboratory features 606
Features suggesting a specific etiology 608
Diagnosis and differential diagnosis 609
Treatment of Cushing's syndrome 615
Nelson's syndrome 619
Prognosis 619
Hyperaldosteronism 620
Primary hyperaldosteronism 620
Secondary hyperaldosteronism 620
Hirsutism and Virilism 622
Congenital Defects in Adrenal Steroid Biosynthesis 624
21-Hydroxylase Deficiency 624
Incidence, genetics, and biochemical defect 624
Pathology, pathophysiology, and steroid secretion 626
Clinical features 626
Diagnosis 627
Treatment 627
11β-Hydroxylase Deficiency 628

12 (*Continued*)
17α-Hydroxylase Deficiency 628
Cholesterol Side Chain Cleavage Enzyme Deficiency 629
3β-Hydroxysteroid Dehydrogenase Defect 629
Corticosterone Methyloxidase Deficiency Types 1 and 2 (18-Hydroxylation Defect) 630
References 631

13 Diseases of the Sympathochromaffin System **651**
Philip E. Cryer

Sympathochromaffin Physiology 652
Biochemistry of the Catecholamines 652
Catecholamine biosynthesis 652
Catecholamine degradation 653
Physiology of Adrenergic Axon Terminals and Chromaffin Cells 653
Organization of the sympathochromaffin system 653
Catecholamine formation, storage, and release 655
Biologic inactivation of catecholamines 655
Mechanisms of catecholamine action 656
Biologic Effects of the Catecholamines 659
Integrated Physiology of the Sympathochromaffin System 662
Measurement of catecholamines and catecholamine kinetics 662
Patterns during physiologic adaptation 664
The Biologic Roles of Epinephrine and Norepinephrine: Hormones and Neurotransmitters 664
Sympathochromaffin Pathophysiology 667
Pheochromocytoma 667
Origin and distribution 667
Clinical manifestations 668
Diagnosis 668
Screening 671
Treatment 671
Other sympathochromaffin tumors 672
Autonomic Dysfunction 672
Hypoglycemia 677
Other Disorders 678
Endocrine-metabolic disorders 678
Cardiovascular disorders 680
Pulmonary disorders 681
Central nervous system disorders 681
Behavioral disorders 681
Gastrointestinal disorders 681
Renal disorders 682
Miscellaneous disorders 682
Diagnostic Testing 682
Measurement of Catecholamines and Their Metabolites 682
Indirect Tests of Autonomic Function 685
References 686

14 The Endocrinology of Hypertension **693**
John D. Baxter, Dorothee Perloff, Willa Hsueh, and Edward G. Biglieri

General Features of Hypertension 694
The Epidemiology of Hypertension 694
Genetic and Environmental Influences 697
The Physiology of Blood Pressure Control 697
The Autonomic Nervous System 697
The Hemodynamics of Hypertension 698

Borderline hypertension 698
Established hypertension 698
The Complications of Sustained Hypertension 698
Cardiac effects of hypertension 699
Vascular structural changes in hypertension 699
Acceleration of atherosclerosis in hypertension 699
The effect of hypertension on the brain 700
Renal effects of hypertension 700
Hormonal Modifiers of Blood Pressure 701
The Renin-Angiotensin System 701
Components of the Renin-Angiotensin System 702
Renin 702
Angiotensinogen (renin substrate) 705
Angiotensin-converting enzyme 705
Angiotensins I, II, and III 706
Role of the Renin-Angiotensin System in Hypertension 707
Experimental hypertension 707
Renin-secreting tumors 708
Renovascular hypertension 708
Other forms of secondary hypertension 708
Accelerated hypertension 709
Essential hypertension 709
Ions and Blood Pressure 711
Actions of Individuals Ions 711
Sodium chloride 711
Calcium 712
Magnesium 714
Potassium 714
Sodium Transport and Blood Pressure 715
Cellular elements involved in sodium transport 715
Circulating inhibitors of sodium transport 717
Possible role of sodium transport abnormalities in hypertension 718
Atrial Natriuretic Factor 718
Synthesis and Release 719
Sites of Synthesis 719
Circulation 720
Regulation of ANF Release and Synthesis 720
Actions of ANF 720
Renal actions 720
Effects on renin 722
Effects on aldosterone 722
AVP Release 722
Actions on the vasculature 722
Intracellular fluid volume 722
Cardiac actions 722
Effects on blood pressure 723
Effects on water intake 723
Integrated effects on physiology 723
Structure-Activity Considerations for ANF 723
Molecular Mechanisms of Action 723
ANF receptors 723
Postreceptor actions 723
Role of ANF in Physiology and Disease 724
Adrenal Steroids and Hypertension 724
Mineralocorticoids 724
Aldosterone 725
Deoxycorticosterone 725
18-Hydroxydeoxycorticosterone 725
18-Hydroxycorticosterone 725
16α,18-dihydroxy-DOC, 19-hydroxyandrostenedione, and 19-oxoandrostenedione 725

14 *(Continued)*

19-NOR-DOC 726
Other steroids 726
Glucocorticoids 726
Laboratory Tests for the Evaluation of Hypertension 727
Renin 727
Angiotensin II 728
Aldosterone 728
Deoxycorticosterone 730
18-Hydroxycorticosterone 730
Sodium and Potassium 730
Evaluation of the Hypertensive Patient 732
Physical Examination 732
Laboratory Tests 734
Renovascular Hypertension 735
Historical Background 735
Pathologic Etiology of Renovascular Hypertension 735
Atherosclerosis 735
Fibromuscular dysplasia 737
Other causes of renovascular hypertension 738
Renin-secreting tumors 738
Natural History of Renal Artery Lesions 738
Clinical Characteristics of Patients with Renovascular Hypertension 739
Specific Diagnostic Studies for Renovascular Hypertension 740
Intravenous urogram 740
Radionuclide renal imaging (renal scintigraphy) 742
Dynamic computer tomography of the kidneys 742
Ultrasonic duplex scanning 742
Renal arteriography 742
Digital subtraction angiography 743
Divided renal function tests 744
Bilateral renal biopsy 744
Plasma renin determination 744
Sequencing of Diagnostic Tests for Renovascular Hypertension 746
Medical Therapy for Renovascular Hypertension 746
Revascularization Approaches to Renovascular Hypertension 748
Surgical techniques 749
Transluminal angioplasty 750
Results of revascularization procedures 750
Aldosterone Excess (Primary Aldosteronism) 751
Occurrence and Classification 751
Adenoma 752
Hyperplasia 753
History and Physical Findings 755
Hypertension 755
Initial Diagnosis 755
Determination of the Etiology of Primary Aldosteronism 759
18-OHB 759
CT scanning 759
Bilateral adrenal vein catheterization 760
Iodocholesterol scanning technique 760
Circadian and postural changes in plasma aldosterone level 761
Saline infusion test 761
Glucocorticoid treatment 762
Diagnosis of surgically remediable hyperplasia (primary hyperplasia) 762
Treatment 762
Pathologic Findings 764
Carcinoma 764

Deoxycorticosterone Excess Hypertension 764
Hypertension and Congenital Adrenal Hyperplasia 765
Deoxycorticosterone-Producing Adrenocortical Adenoma 766
Cushing's Syndrome and Adrenal Malignancies 766
Other Low-Renin Hypertension Syndromes Associated with Hypokalemia 768
Iatrogenic Syndromes: Licorice, Carbenoxolone, or Steroid Ingestion 768
Low-Aldosterone Hypertension Unresponsive to Dexamethasone 768
Spironolactone-responsive subgroup 768
Spironolactone-unresponsive subgroup 769
Dexamethasone-responsive 769
Syndrome of probable insensitivity to glucocorticoids 769
Possible existence of an as yet unidentified mineralocorticoid 769
Pseudohypoaldosteronism Type 2 Low-Renin Hypertension with Hyperkalemia 770
Low-Renin Essential Hypertension 770
References 772

15 Glucocorticoid Therapy **788**

J. Blake Tyrell and John D. Baxter

Physiological and Pharmacological Actions of Glucocorticoids in Relation to Steroid Therapy 790
Therapeutic Influences 790
Adverse Influences 791
Molecular Mechanisms for Glucocorticoid-Mediated Therapeutic Influences 791
Kinetic Considerations 792
Manifestations of Iatrogenic Cushing's Syndrome 792
Comparisons with Spontaneous Cushing's Syndrome 792
Ocular Changes 793
Ischemic Necrosis of Bone 793
Osteoporosis 793
Infections 795
Myopathy 795
Atherosclerosis 796
Dose and Time Dependency and Reversibility 796
Diagnosis of Iatrogenic Cushing's Syndrome 796
Determinants of Glucocorticoid Potency 796
Bioavailability 796
Distribution 797
Metabolism and Clearance 797
Concentration at Sites of Action 799
Agonist Activity 799
Overall Estimation of Glucocorticoid Potency 799
Variations in Sensitivity to Glucocorticoids: Glucocorticoid Resistance 799
Glucocorticoid Preparations 800
Steroids with Glucocorticoid Activity Available for Therapy 800
Orally and Parenterally Active Preparations 800
Intraarticular Preparations 801
Topical Preparations 802
Corticosteroid Aerosols 802
ACTH 802
Some General Principles 803
Selection of Patients 803
Need for empirical data 803
Short-term versus long-term 803
Testing the sensitivity 803
Dose-Response Considerations 804

15 (*Continued*)

The Use of Adjunctive Therapy 805
Specific Measures to Reduce Side Effects 805
Cognizance of Objective Criteria 805
The Circadian Rhythm 805
Adjusting the Dose 806
Alternate-Day Therapy 806
Special Situations 807
Pregnancy 807
Diabetes 808
Surgery 808
Psychiatry 808
Peptic Ulcer 808
Pediatrics 808
Kaposi's Sarcoma 809
Withdrawal of Glucocorticoids and Suppression of the Hypothalamic-Pituitary-Adrenal Axis 809
Kinetics and Dosage Required for Suppression 809
Kinetics of Return to Normal Axis Function 810
Steroid Withdrawal Syndromes 812
Evaluation of Axis Function 813
Withdrawal Protocols and Indications for Steroid Coverage 813
References 814

Part V GONADAL DISEASE

16 The Testis **821**

Richard J. Santen

Anatomy 821
Central Nervous System and Hypothalamic-Pituitary Axis 821
Peptidergic system 821
Aminergic system 823
Steroid receptor neurons 823
Tanacytes 823
Portal venous system 824
Anterior pituitary 825
Testes 825
Interstitial cell compartment 825
Seminiferous tubular compartment 825
Sertoli cells 826
Germinal epithelia 826
Physiology 832
Hypothalamic-Pituitary-Leydig Cell Axis 832
Overview 832
Hypothalamus 832
Pituitary 836
Testis 837
Feedback interaction 844
Hypothalamic-Pituitary-Germ Cell Axis 848
Overview 848
Hypothalamus 848
Pituitary 848
Testis 849
Feedback control of FSH release 850
Interactions between the LH-Leydig Cell and FSH-Germ Cell Axes 850
Hypothalamus and pituitary 850
Testis 851

Prolactin Effects on Male Reproduction 851
Clinical Evaluation of the Hypothalamic-Pituitary-Testicular Axis 852
Anatomic and Histologic Assessment 852
Pituitary and hypothalamus 852
Testis and surrounding structures 852
Spermatozoa 853
Assessment of Hormonal Status 854
Basal levels 854
Dynamic tests 855
Biologic Effects of Sex Steroids on Target Organs 857
Genetic Tests 857
Age-Dependent Physiologic Changes in Testicular Function 858
Prepuberty 858
Puberty 858
Postpuberty 860
Clinical Disorders 861
Introduction 861
Hypogonadotropic Syndromes 861
Organic causes 861
Physiologic delayed puberty (constitutional delay) 869
Hypergonadotropic Hypogonadism 870
Overview 870
Genetic disorders 870
Functional prepubertal castrate syndrome (anorchia) 873
Gonadal toxins 874
Enzyme defects 874
Viral mumps orchitis 874
Male climacteric 874
Hormone resistance 875
Treatment 875
Delayed adolescence 875
Adult hypogonadotropic hypogonadism 877
Hypergonadotropic hypogonadism 877
Germinal Cell Failure 878
Overview 878
Hypergonadotropic Syndromes 878
Sertoli-cell-only syndrome 879
Idiopathic seminiferous tubular failure with hyalinization 879
Eugonadotropic Germinal Cell Failure 879
Idiopathic 879
Varicocele 880
Infections 880
Sinopulmonary-Infertility Syndrome 880
Genetic Syndromes 881
Autoimmunity 881
Approach to the Infertile Male 881
Disorders Associated with Nonphysiologic Secretion of Gonadotropins 882
Gonadotropin-Producing Tumors 882
Precocious Puberty 882
Cryptorchism 883
Pathophysiology 883
Rationale for Treatment 885
Treatment 886
Gynecomastia 886
Overview 886
Physiologic Forms of Gynecomastia 887
Pathologic Forms of Gynecomastia 887
Evaluation 889
Treatment 889
Impotence 889
Male Contraception 890

16 (*Continued*)

Androgen-Dependent Neoplasia 891
Testicular Tumors 892
References 892

17 The Ovary: Basic Principles and Concepts
A. Physiology **905**

Gregory F. Erickson

Anatomy 905
Morphology 905
Blood Vessels 906
Innervation 907
Histology 908
Ovarian Follicles 908
Primordial follicle 908
Primary follicle 908
Secondary follicle 908
Tertiary follicle 912
Graafian follicle 913
Atretic follicles 915
Ovarian Interstitial Cells 916
Primary interstitial cells 916
Theca interstitial cells 916
Secondary interstitial cells 917
Hilus cells 920
Corpora Lutea 921
Biogenesis of Ovarian Hormones 924
Steroids 924
Cholesterol substrate 924
Intracellular cholesterol transport 925
Cholesterol side chain cleavage 925
Metabolism of steroid hormones 925
Gonadotropin control 926
Protein 926
Ovarian Cytodifferentiation: Underlying Control Mechanisms 927
The Granulosa Cell 927
The interstitial cells 929
The corpus luteum 929
The oocyte 932
Follicle Development: Control Mechanisms 934
Recruitment 934
Atresia 935
Selection 936
Ovulation 939
Physiological Correlates of Ovarian Activity with Aging 940
The Fetal Period 940
Premenarche 941
Menarche 941
Postmenarche: The Normal Menstrual Cycle 941
Menopause 944
References 944

B. Clinical **951**

Robert I. McLachlan, David L. Healy, and Henry G. Burger

Ovarian Disorders in Teenagers 951
Primary Amenorrhea 951
Short stature and no pubertal development 951

Normal stature and no or minimal pubertal development 953
Normal stature with normal pubertal development 954
Virilization and/or anomalous genitalia 954
Menarcheal Menorrhagia 955
Ovarian Disorders in Young Adults 955
Secondary Amenorrhea 955
Premature ovarian failure 956
Hyperprolactinemia and galactorrhea 958
Nutritional amenorrhea 960
Polycystic ovary syndrome 961
Clinical features 961
Pathophysiology 962
Management of polycystic ovary syndrome 963
Virilization and Hirsutism 964
Clinical assessment and investigation 964
Management 965
Female Infertility: Management by Ovulation Induction 966
Gonadotropic ovulation induction 967
Pulsatile administration of GNRH 969
Menorrhagia and Dysmenorrhea 970
Premenstrual Syndrome 974
Ovarian Disorders in Middle Age 974
Endocrinology of the Menopause 974
Climacteric Symptoms 976
Postmenopausal Problems 977
Osteoporosis 977
Atherosclerotic cardiovascular disease 977
Long-Term Hormone Replacement Therapy 978
Modes of administration 978
Benefits and risks 979
Postmenopausal Bleeding 980
References 980

18 Sexual Differentiation 983

Jeremy S.D. Winter

Normal Sex Determination and Sexual Differentiation 984
Genetic Sex 985
Chromosomal errors 985
Properties and functions of the sex chromosomes 987
Gonadal Sex 989
Testicular differentiation 989
Ovarian differentiation 992
Differentiation of the Genital Ducts 992
Female internal genital development 992
Male internal genital development 992
Differentiation of the urogenital sinus and external genitalia 994
Feminization of the external genitalia 994
Masculinization of the external genitalia 994
Hormonal Sex: Differentiation of the Hypothalamic-Pituitary-Gonadal Axis 994
Gonadal steroid production 994
Sex steroids in the fetal circulation 994
Actions of sex steroids on the genitalia 995
Control of fetal gonadal function 996
Perinatal Adaptations of the Reproductive Endocrine System 997
Gender Role and Psychosexual Differentiation 999
Abnormal Sexual Differentiation 1000
Errors of Primary Sex Determination 1000

18 (*Continued*)

Sex chromosome anomalies associated with functional testes and male phenotype 1000
Sex chromosome anomalies associated with ovaries and female phenotype 1003
Sex chromosome anomalies associated with bisexual gonadal development 1003
Sex chromosome anomalies associated with dysgenetic gonads 1004
Anomalies of gonadogenesis without chromosomal abnormality 1009
Errors of Sexual Differentiation 1011
Persistent paramesonephric ducts 1011
Defective genital virilization (male pseudohermaphroditism) 1011
Virilization of a genetic female (female pseudohermaphroditism) 1020
Clinical Approach to Disorders of Sexual Differentiation 1031
The Newborn with Abnormal Genitalia 1031
Virilization during Childhood or Adolescence 1033
Delayed Puberty, Amenorrhea, and Infertility 1033
References 1033

Part VI FUEL METABOLISM

19 **The Endocrine Pancreas: Diabetes Mellitus** **1043**
Eleazar Shafrir, Michael Bergman, and Philip Felig

Physiology of Fuel Metabolism 1043
Carbohydrate Metabolism 1045
Glycogenesis and glycogenolysis 1045
Glycolysis 1047
Gluconeogenesis 1049
Integration of glycolysis and gluconeogenesis: The lactate (Cori) and alanine cycles 1051
Tricarboxylic acid cycle 1052
Other pathways of glucose metabolism 1053
Fat Metabolism 1055
Synthesis of fatty acids and triglycerides 1055
Mobilization of fatty acids 1056
Oxidation of fatty acids 1057
Ketogenesis and ketone utilization 1059
Interactions of Fat and Carbohydrate Metabolism 1061
Amino Acid Metabolism 1062
The glucose-alanine cycle 1062
Protein repletion and feeding 1064
Insulin 1064
History 1064
Chemistry 1064
Biosynthesis 1065
Insulin secretion 1067
Insulin action 1073
Insulin receptors 1077
Postreceptor events 1080
Insulin resistance 1080
Insulin degradation 1082
Glucagon 1082
Chemistry and biosynthesis 1082
Circulating glucagon 1082
Secretion 1083

Action 1083
Degradation 1085
Catecholamines 1085
Glucocorticoids 1086
Growth Hormone 1086
Insulin-like Growth Factors 1086
Pancreatic Polypeptide 1087
Regulatory and Counterregulatory Hormones 1087
Fuel-Hormone Interactions 1088
Body composition 1088
The basal state 1089
Fuel availability: The fed state 1090
Fuel need 1091
Fuel-hormone imbalance 1092
Diabetes Mellitus 1092
History 1092
Definition and Classification 1093
Etiology 1094
Genetics 1094
Viral infections and other environmental factors in type I diabetes 1096
Autoimmunity in type I diabetes 1097
Obesity and nutrition in type II diabetes 1098
Summary of etiologic factors 1098
Pathogenesis 1099
Insulin secretion 1099
Insulin resistance 1101
Glucagon secretion 1103
Other hormones 1103
Pathophysiology 1104
Carbohydrate metabolism 1104
Protein and amino acid metabolism 1104
Protein-carbohydrate interactions 1105
Fat metabolism and diabetic hyperlipidemia 1105
Summary 1107
Diagnosis 1108
Fasting plasma glucose concentration 1108
Oral glucose tolerance testing 1108
The intravenous glucose tolerance test 1111
Insulin determination 1111
Urinary glucose determination 1111
Glycohemoglobin 1112
Summary of diagnostic criteria and diagnostic terms 1112
Prevalence 1112
Pathology 1113
Islets of Langerhans 1113
Blood vessels 1114
The kidney 1114
The eye 1115
Nervous system 1115
Other tissues 1115
Clinical Manifestations 1115
Symptoms of hyperglycemia 1116
Diabetic retinopathy 1116
Diabetic nephropathy 1119
Diabetic neuropathy 1121
Coronary artery disease 1123
Peripheral vascular disease: The diabetic foot 1123
The skin 1124
Infectious complications 1125
Pathogenesis of Diabetic Complications 1125
Biopsy studies 1126
Metabolic studies 1126

19 (*Continued*)

Effect of treatment 1129
Summary 1130
Mortality 1130
Treatment 1130
Insulin therapy 1131
Diet therapy 1139
Oral hypoglycemic agents 1140
Exercise 1144
Future treatment 1147
Hyperglycemic-Ketoacidotic Emergencies 1149
Diabetic ketoacidosis 1149
Hyperosmolar nonketotic coma 1154
Lactic acidosis 1155
Pregnancy and Diabetes 1155
Maternal and fetal fuel metabolism 1156
Diagnosis 1158
Classification 1158
Effect of pregnancy on the course of diabetes 1159
Effect of diabetes on the outcome of pregnancy 1159
Lipoatrophic Diabetes 1163
Secondary Diabetes 1163
Pancreoprival diabetes 1163
Endocrine-associated diabetes 1164
Glucose intolerance in nonendocrine disease 1165
References 1165

20 Hypoglycemia **1179**

Robert S. Sherwin and Philip Felig

Definition 1179
Signs and Symptoms 1180
Nonhypoglycemia 1181
Classification 1182
Fasting Hypoglycemia 1182
Starvation in normal humans 1182
Mechanisms and classification of fasting hypoglycemia 1184
Insulin-producing islet cell tumors 1184
Extrapancreatic tumor hypoglycemia 1187
Hypoglycemia in endocrine-deficiency states 1187
Hypoglycemic hepatic disease 1187
Hypoglycemia due to substrate deficiency 1188
Insulin autoimmune hypoglycemia 1188
Postprandial Hypoglycemia 1188
Definition 1189
Symptoms 1189
Prevalence and diagnosis 1189
Pathophysiology 1190
Classification 1191
Treatment 1192
Induced Hypoglycemia 1193
Insulin-induced hypoglycemia 1193
Sulfonylurea-induced hypoglycemia 1194
Factitious hypoglycemia 1194
Alcohol-induced hypoglycemia 1195
Leucine sensitivity 1196
Hereditary fructose intolerance 1197
Hypoglycin 1198
Diagnostic Evaluation 1199
History and Physical Examination 1199

Laboratory Tests 1199
References 1201

21 The Obesities 1203

Lester B. Salans

Definition 1203
Metropolitan Life Insurance Company Weight Tables 1204
The Fogarty Conference Tables 1205
National Center for Health Statistics Tables 1205
Body Mass Index 1206
Summary 1206
Prevalence and General Characteristics 1206
Prevalence of Obesity in Adults 1207
Prevalence of Obesity in Children 1207
Socioeconomic Aspects of Occurrence 1207
Health Consequences 1207
Resistance to Weight Loss 1208
Growth and Development of Adipose Tissue 1208
Etiology and Pathogenesis 1210
Genetic Factors 1211
Central Nervous System Factors 1212
Endocrine Factors 1215
Adrenal cortical hormones 1215
Thyroid hormones 1215
Growth hormone 1215
Other hormones 1215
Insulin 1215
Metabolic Factors 1216
Metabolic defects in laboratory animals 1216
Metabolic defects in humans 1217
Nutritional Factors 1219
Maternal nutrition 1220
Nutrition during infancy 1220
Childhood nutrition 1220
Adult nutrition 1221
Physical Activity 1221
Adipose Cell Hypothesis 1221
Psychological Factors 1222
Other Nonphysiological Factors 1223
Classification of Obesity 1224
Health Consequences of Obesity 1224
Mortality 1224
Diabetes Mellitus 1226
Plasma insulin levels in obesity 1227
Insulin resistance 1228
Mechanisms responsible for insulin resistance 1229
Overeating 1230
Fat distribution 1230
Insulin secretion 1231
Hyperlipoproteinemia 1231
Cardiovascular Consequences 1232
Hypertension 1232
Endocrine Consequences 1232
Sex steroid abnormalities 1232
Thyroid function 1233
Adrenal function 1233
Pulmonary Consequences 1233
Miscellaneous Consequences 1234
Treatment of Obesity 1234
Diet 1235

21 *(Continued)*

Exercise 1237
Behavior Modification 1237
Psychotherapy 1238
Drug Therapy 1238
Gastrointestinal Surgery 1239
Community Involvement 1239
Management of Associated Problems 1240
References 1240

22 Disorders of Lipid Metabolism 1244

D. Roger Illingworth and William E. Connor

The Plasma Lipoproteins 1245
Lipoprotein Classification 1245
Lipoprotein Composition 1246
Chylomicrons 1246
Very-low-density lipoproteins 1247
Low-density lipoproteins 1247
High-density lipoproteins 1247
Abnormal lipoproteins 1247
The Apoproteins 1247
Structure 1247
Function 1248
Lipoprotein Structure 1249
Synthesis and Catabolism of Lipids and Lipoproteins 1249
Lipids 1249
Cholesterol 1249
Triglyceride 1250
Phospholipids 1250
Enzymes Active in Lipoprotein Metabolism 1251
Lecithin cholesterol acyltransferase 1251
Lipoprotein lipase and hepatic lipase 1251
Lipoprotein Metabolism 1251
Chylomicrons 1251
Very-low-density lipoproteins 1252
Low-density lipoproteins 1252
High-density lipoproteins 1253
Free fatty acids 1254
Atherogenicity of Individual Lipoprotein Particles 1254
The Hyperlipidemias 1255
Classification of Hyperlipidemias 1255
Criteria for the Diagnosis of Hyperlipoproteinemia 1255
Secondary Hyperlipidemias 1256
Dietary 1256
Diabetes 1257
Hypothyroidism 1258
Renal disease 1258
Bile duct obstruction, $alpha_1$ antitrypsin deficiency 1259
Alcohol 1259
Drug-induced hyperlipoproteinemia 1259
Hypercholesterolemia 1260
Familial hypercholesterolemia 1260
Familial combined hyperlipidemia 1264
Thresholds for the drug treatment of hypercholesterolemia 1265
Combined Hypercholesterolemia and Hypertriglyceridemia 1266
Primary type III hyperlipoproteinemia 1267
Hepatic lipase deficiency 1270
Hypertriglyceridemia 1270
Hyperchylomicronemia: Types I and V hyperlipoproteinemia, familial apoprotein C-II deficiency 1270

Diagnostic laboratory features 1271
Type IV hyperlipoproteinemia 1272
Disorders of High-Density Lipoproteins 1274
Familial Apolipoprotein A-I and C-III Deficiency 1275
HDL Deficiency with Planar Xanthomas 1275
Fish Eye Disease 1275
Apo A-I Milano 1276
Familial Hypoalphalipoproteinemia 1276
Tangier Disease 1276
Definition 1276
Clinical features 1276
Genetics 1277
Diagnostic laboratory features 1277
Pathophysiology 1277
Treatment 1277
Familial Hyperalphalipoproteinemia 1277
Other Lipoprotein Disorders 1277
Abetalipoproteinemia 1277
Definition 1277
Clinical characteristics 1278
Genetics 1278
Laboratory findings 1279
Pathophysiology 1279
Treatment 1279
Hypobetalipoproteinemia 1279
Familial Lecithin Cholesterol Acyltransferase Deficiency 1280
Clinical features 1280
Genetics 1280
Diagnostic laboratory features 1280
Pathophysiology 1280
Treatment 1280
Sterol Storage Diseases 1280
Atherosclerosis 1280
Xanthomas 1282
Acid Cholesterol Ester Hydrolase Deficiency 1283
Wolman's disease 1283
Cholesterol ester storage disease 1283
Familial Diseases with Storage of Sterols other than Cholesterol 1283
Cerebrotendinous Xanthomatosis 1283
Clinical manifestations 1283
Laboratory and pathological findings 1284
Pathophysiology 1284
Treatment 1284
Sitosterolemia and Xanthomatosis 1285
Clinical features 1285
Chemistry, absorption, and metabolism of plant sterols in humans 1285
Laboratory abnormalities 1285
Pathophysiology 1285
Diagnosis 1286
Treatment 1286
Dietary Treatment of Hyperlipidemia 1286
The Effects of Specific Nutrients on the Plasma Lipids and Lipoproteins 1287
Cholesterol 1287
Dietary fat, amount and saturation, kinds of polyunsaturation 1288
Calories and obesity 1290
Carbohydrate 1291
Fiber 1291
Alcohol 1291
Protein 1292
Lecithin 1292

22 (*Continued*)

Minerals and vitamins 1292
Implementation of the Single-Diet Concept for the Treatment of Hyperlipidemia 1292
The cholesterol–saturated fat index of foods 1294
The Alternative Diet: A Phased Approach to the Dietary Treatment of Hyperlipidemia 1296
The chemical composition of the alternative diet 1297
Predicted plasma cholesterol lowering from the three phases of the alternative diet 1297
The use of the alternative diet in diabetic patients, pregnant patients, children, and hypertensive patients 1297
Pharmaceutical Agents for the Treatment of Hyperlipoproteinemia 1298
Bile Acid Sequestrants 1298
Mechanism of action 1298
Side effects 1298
Indications and dosage 1299
Nicotinic Acid 1299
Mechanism of action 1300
Side effects 1300
Indications and dosage 1300
Probucol 1300
Mechanism of action 1301
Side effects 1301
Indications and dosage 1301
Clofibrate 1301
Mechanism of action 1301
Side effects 1301
Indications and dosages 1301
Gemfibrozil 1302
Mechanism of action 1302
Side effects 1302
Indications and dosage 1302
Neomycin 1302
Mechanism of action 1302
Side effects 1303
Indications and dosage 1303
Dextrothyroxine 1303
Mechanism of action 1303
Side effects 1303
Indications and dosage 1303
Miscellaneous Agents 1303
Anabolic steroids 1303
Progestational agents 1303
Estrogens 1304
Future Advances 1304
Fibric acid derivatives 1304
HMG CoA Reductase Inhibitors: Lovastatin (Mevinolin) and Related Compounds 1304
The Surgical Treatment of Hyperlipoproteinemia 1305
Surgical Procedures in Homozygous Familial Hypercholesterolemia 1306
Laboratory Tests in the Diagnosis of Hyperlipidemias 1306
Collection and handling of the sample 1306
Lipid determinations 1306
Lipoprotein Separations 1306
Indications 1306
Available methods 1307
Additional Laboratory Tests 1307
References 1308

Part VII CALCIUM AND BONE METABOLISM

23 Mineral Metabolism 1317

Andrew F. Stewart and Arthur E. Broadus

Cellular and Extracelllar Mineral Metabolism 1317
General Considerations 1317
Cellular Mineral Metabolism 1318
Cellular calcium metabolism 1318
Cellular phosphorous and magnesium metabolism 1320
Extracellular Mineral Metabolism 1320
Calcium 1320
Phosphorus 1321
Magnesium 1321
Parathyroid Hormone 1321
Embryology, Anatomy, and Histology of the Parathyroid Glands 1321
Biosynthesis and Secretion of PTH 1322
Sequence and biosynthesis of parathyroid hormone 1322
Control and mechanism of parathyroid hormone secretion 1324
Circulating Fragments and Metabolism of Parathyroid Hormone 1326
Biological Effects and Mechanism of Action of Parathyroid Hormone 1328
History 1329
Effects of parathyroid hormone on bone 1329
Effects of parathyroid hormone on the kidney 1332
Effects of parathyroid hormone on other tissues 1337
Calcitonin 1337
Historical Introduction 1337
Embryology, Anatomy, and Histology 1338
Chemistry and Biosynthesis of Calcitonin 1338
Secretion and Metabolism of Calcitonin 1340
Biological Effects and Mechanisms of Action of Calcitonin 1342
Effects of calcitonin on bone 1342
Effects of calcitonin on the kidney 1343
Physiological Significance of Calcitonin 1343
Vitamin D 1344
Historical Introduction 1344
Chemistry 1344
Formation, Transport, Metabolic Sequence of Activation, and Metabolism of Vitamin D 1346
Biological Effects and Mechanism of Action of Vitamin D 1351
Intestinal absorption of calcium and phosphorus 1351
Effects of vitamin D in the intestine 1354
Effects of vitamin D on bone 1355
Effects of vitamin D on the kidney 1356
Effects of vitamin D on other tissues 1357
Integrated Control of Mineral Homeostasis 1357
Normal Mineral Homeostasis and Balance 1357
Systemic Calcium Homeostasis 1358
Maintenance of a normal serum calcium 1358
Defense against hypocalcemia 1358
Defense against hypercalcemia 1359
Systemic Phosphorus Homeostasis 1360
Maintenance of a normal serum phosphorus 1360
Defense against hypophosphatemia 1360
Defense against hyperphosphatemia 1361

23 (*Continued*)

Systemic Magnesium Homeostasis 1361
Intestinal absorption of magnesium 1362
Renal tubular handling of magnesium 1362
Intracellular fluid and the skeleton 1362
Influence of Other Hormones on Mineral Homeostasis 1363
Chemical and Biochemical Analyses Related to Mineral Metabolism 1363
Routine Chemical Determinations in Serum 1363
Calcium 1363
Phosphorus 1365
Magnesium 1365
Alkaline phosphatase 1365
Routine Chemical Determinations in Urine 1366
Calcium 1366
Phosphorus 1367
Magnesium 1368
Intestinal Calcium Absorption 1368
Mineral Balance 1369
Hormonal Measurements 1369
Parathyroid hormone 1369
Calcitonin 1374
Vitamin D 1375
Assessment of Bone Metabolism and Skeletal Homeostasis 1376
Hypercalcemia 1376
Primary Hyperparathyroidism 1377
History 1377
Incidence and natural history 1377
Pathology and etiology 1378
Clinical presentation and pathophysiology 1379
Primary hyperparathyroidism and renal stones 1381
Hyperparathyroid bone disease 1384
Nonspecific features of primary hyperparathyroidism 1388
Clinical variants of primary hyperparathyroidism 1391
Familial endocrine neoplasia and familial hypocalciuric hypercalcemia 1392
Physical findings 1395
Laboratory findings and definitive diagnosis 1395
Preoperative localization studies 1398
Parathyroid exploration and perioperative management 1400
Medical management of primary hyperparathyroidism 1401
Malignancy-Associated Hypercalcemia 1403
Introduction 1403
Local osteolytic hypercalcemia 1403
Humoral hypercalcemia of malignancy 1404
Lymphoma-associated hypercalcemia 1409
Uncommon variants of malignancy-associated hypercalcemia 1410
Pathophysiology and diagnosis 1410
Treatment 1411
Endocrinopathies 1411
Thyrotoxicosis 1411
Adrenal insufficiency 1412
Pheochromocytoma 1412
VIP-OMA syndrome 1412
Medications 1413
Thiazide diuretics 1413
Vitamins A and D 1413
Milk-alkali syndrome 1414
Lithium 1414
Estrogens and antiestrogens 1415
Sarcoidosis and Other Granulomatous Diseases 1415
Miscellaneous Conditions 1416
Immobilization 1416

Acute renal failure 1417
Idiopathic hypercalcemia of infancy 1417
Serum protein abnormalities 1417
Differential Diagnosis of Hypercalcemia 1417
Medical Therapy 1420
General measures 1420
Calciuretic measures 1420
Measures which inhibit bone resorption 1420
Hypocalcemia 1422
Clinical Manifestations of Hypocalcemia 1422
Hypoparathyroidism 1424
Postoperative hypocalcemia and hypoparathyroidism 1424
Idiopathic hypoparathyroidism 1425
Other acquired forms of functional hypoparathyroidism 1425
Pseudohypoparathyroidism 1426
Neonatal hypocalcemic syndromes 1430
Other Hypocalcemic Conditions and Tetanic Syndromes 1431
Differential Diagnosis 1432
Treatment 1433
Acute hypocalcemia 1433
Chronic hypocalcemia 1433
Hypophosphatemia and Hyperphosphatemia 1435
Hypophosphatemia 1435
Pathogenesis 1435
Pathophysiological consequences of hypophosphatemia 1438
Treatment 1438
Hyperphosphatemia 1438
Hypomagnesemia and Hypermagnesemia 1439
Hypomagnesemia and Magnesium Depletion 1439
Pathogenesis 1439
Symptoms 1441
Diagnosis and treatment 1441
Hypermagnesemia 1442
Testing 1442
Serum Chemistries 1442
Urine Determinations 1443
Biochemical and Immunoassay Determinations 1443
Testing for Pseudohypoparathyroidism 1444
Miscellaneous Determinations 1445
References 1445

24 Metabolic Bone Disease 1454

Frederick R. Singer

Clinical Evaluation of Metabolic Bone Disease 1454
History and Physical Examination 1454
Clinical Chemistry 1454
Radiology and Nuclear Medicine 1456
Bone Biopsy 1456
Osteomalacia and Rickets 1458
Clinical Presentation 1458
Bone Pathology 1460
Classification and Pathogenesis 1461
Vitamin D Abnormalities 1461
Hypophosphatemia 1464
Miscellaneous 1465
Treatment 1466
Osteoporosis 1468
Clinical Presentation 1468
Bone Pathology 1470
Classification and Pathogenesis 1471
Treatment 1474
Osteopetrosis 1477

24 (*Continued*)

Renal Osteodystrophy 1478
- Clinical Presentation 1478
- Bone Pathology 1479
- Pathogenesis 1479
- Treatment 1480

Hereditary Hyperphosphatasia 1481
Fibrous Dysplasia 1482
Paget's Disease of Bone 1483
- Clinical Presentation 1484
- Bone Pathology 1486
- Pathogenesis 1487
- Treatment 1488

New Concepts in Local Regulation of Bone Metabolism 1491
- Cell-Cell Interactions 1491
- Bone Cell and Matrix Factors 1491

References 1491

25 Nephrolithiasis 1500

Karl L. Insogna and Arthur E. Broadus

General Considerations 1500
Theories and Physical Chemical Aspects of Renal Stone Pathogenesis 1503
- Theories of Stone Pathogenesis 1504
- Physical Chemical Aspects of Stone Formation 1504
  - Cystine stones 1506
  - Uric acid stones 1506
  - Magnesium ammonium phosphate stones 1506
  - Calcium phosphate stones 1507
  - Calcium oxalate and mixed calcium stones 1507

Anatomical Considerations 1508
Medullary Sponge Kidney 1509
Cystinuria 1510
- Genetics and Occurrence 1512
- Pathophysiology and Clinical Manifestations 1512
- Diagnosis 1514
- Treatment 1515

Uric Acid Calculi 1517
- Purine Metabolism and Uric Acid Excretion 1517
- Pathogenesis of Uric Acid Stones and Clinical Populations at Risk 1518
- Diagnosis 1520
- Therapy 1521

Magnesium Ammonium Phosphate Stones 1521
- Pathogenesis 1522
- Populations at Risk 1522
- Clinical Manifestations 1522
- Diagnosis 1523
- Treatment 1523

Calcium Phosphate Stones 1524
- Pathogenesis 1524
- Patient Populations at Risk 1525
- Diagnosis and Treatment 1526

Calcium Oxalate and Mixed Calcium Stones 1527
- General Considerations 1527
- Family History 1529
- Medications 1530
- Urinary pH 1530
- Diet 1531
- Low Urine Volume 1531

Hypercalciuria 1531
Definition, detection, and incidence of hypercalciuria 1532
Physiology of normal and abnormal calcium excretion 1535
Classification of hypercalciuria 1536
Diagnosis 1551
Treatment 1553
Hyperoxaluria 1556
Absorption, production, and renal clearance of oxalate 1556
Classification of hyperoxaluric states 1557
Diagnosis 1559
Treatment 1560
Hyperuricosuria 1561
Uric acid metabolism and definition of hyperuricosuria 1561
Pathogenesis 1562
Diagnosis 1563
Treatment 1563
Hypocitraturia 1564
Renal metabolism of citrate 1564
Acid-base status and citrate excretion 1565
Hypocitraturia and nephrolithiasis in patients with acid-base abnormalities 1565
Hypocitraturia and nephrolithiasis in patients without acid-base disturbances 1566
Idiopathic Calcium Stones 1566
Testing and General Principles of Therapy 1567
General Considerations 1567
Testing 1567
Initial evaluation 1568
Subsequent evaluation 1568
Evaluation of the patient with a single stone event 1569
Oral calcium tolerance test 1569
General Principles of Therapy 1570
Recent Advances in the Surgical Treatment of Nephrolithiasis 1571
References 1572

Part VIII MISCELLANEOUS DISORDERS

26 Disorders of Growth and Development 1581

Margaret H. MacGillivray

Biologic Stages of Growth 1581
Control of Growth Processes 1582
Genetic Factors 1582
Tissue-Specific Factors 1582
Hormonal Regulation 1583
Growth hormone 1584
Thyroid hormone 1589
Gonadal steroids: androgens, estrogens, and the pubertal growth spurt 1589
Nutrition 1591
Physiology of Skeletal Growth 1591
Developmental Stages 1591
Intrauterine Life 1591
Infancy: Birth to 2 Years of Age 1592
Childhood 1593
Adolescence 1593

26 (*Continued*)

Short Stature 1595
Clinical Approach to Short Stature 1595
History 1595
Physical examination 1597
Radiographic studies 1598
Laboratory studies 1598
Causes of Short Stature 1598
Introduction 1598
Causes of normal short stature 1599
Pathologic short stature (Table 26-6) 1601
Growth Excess 1613
Normal Variants 1613
Familial, genetic, or constitutional tall stature 1613
Familial early maturation 1614
Pathologic Overgrowth 1614
Congenital virilizing adrenal hyperplasia 1614
Precocious sexual maturation 1616
Acromegaly and gigantism 1618
Hyperthyroidism 1619
Chromosome abnormalities 1619
Miscellaneous syndromes 1619
Appendix: Details of Testing Procedures in Children 1621
Pituitary-Hypothalamic Evaluation 1621
Growth hormone 1621
FSH and LH concentrations 1621
Prolactin concentration 1623
Vasopressin 1623
Adrenal Function Tests 1623
Basal hormone levels 1623
ACTH suppression tests 1623
ACTH stimulation tests 1624
References 1624

27 Gastrointestinal Hormones and Carcinoid Tumors and Syndrome 1629

Guenther Boden and John J. Shelmet

The Gut as an Endocrine Organ 1629
Gut Hormones and Hormone-like Peptides 1630
Gastrin 1630
Cholecystokinin 1636
Vasoactive Intestinal Polypeptide 1638
Gastric Inhibitory Polypeptide 1641
Secretin 1643
Gastrointestinal Glucagon 1644
Gut Glucagon-like Immunoreactants 1644
Pancreatic Polypeptide 1645
Somatostatin 1647
Bombesin and Gastrin-Releasing Peptide 1650
Substance P 1651
Neurotensin 1651
Motilin 1652
Carcinoid 1652
Historical Background 1652
References 1659

28 Multiglandular Endocrine Disorders 1662

Leonard J. Deftos, Bayard D. Catherwood, and Henry G. Bone III

Multiple Endocrine Neoplasia Type 1 1662

Definition and History 1662
Components of the Syndrome 1663
Primary hyperparathyroidism 1664
Pancreatic tumors 1664
Pituitary tumors 1665
Other associations 1665
Clinical Evaluation 1666
Patient evaluation 1666
Family evaluation 1666
Epidemiology 1667
MEN in Other Species 1667
Pathogenesis 1667
Theories of pathogenesis 1667
Management 1668
Parathyroid 1668
Pituitary 1668
Gastrinoma 1669
Insulinoma 1669
Multiple Endocrine Neoplasia Type 2 (MEN 2) 1669
Medullary Thyroid Carcinoma 1670
Embryology 1670
Pathology 1670
Occurrence 1671
Natural history 1671
Secretory products 1671
Pheochromocytoma 1675
Occurrence 1675
Adrenal medullary hyperplasia 1675
Hyperparathyroidism 1676
Occurrence 1676
Pathology 1676
Relationship to MTC 1676
Multiple Mucosal Neuromas 1677
Mucosal neuromas 1677
Gastrointestinal abnormalities 1677
Marfanoid habitus 1677
Pluriglandular Endocrine Insufficiency Syndromes 1678
Pluriglandular Autoimmunity with Addison's Disease 1678
Addison's disease with hypoparathyroidism 1680
Hypoparathyroidism without Addison's disease 1682
Isolated Addison's disease 1682
Schmidt's syndrome 1682
Addison's disease with other endocrinopathies 1683
Thyroid Disease and Diabetes Mellitus without Addison's Disease 1684
Other Disorders 1684
Diagnosis, Complications, and Surveillance 1685
Genetics of Pluriglandular Endocrine Insufficiency Syndromes 1686
Nonautoimmune Pluriglandular Dysfunction 1686
References 1687

29 Ectopic Hormone Production 1692
David N. Orth

Criteria for Diagnosis of Ectopic Hormone Secretion 1693
Incidence of Ectopic Hormonal Syndromes 1696
Hypotheses Concerning the Mechanism of Ectopic Hormone Secretion 1698
Hypercalcemia of Malignancy 1702
Clinical Presentation 1702
Tumor Osteolytic Factors 1703
Treatment 1705
Ectopic ACTH Syndrome 1706
Clinical Presentation 1706

29 (*Continued*)

Tumor Peptide Products 1708
Treatment 1710
Ectopic Secretion of Antidiuretic Hormone 1711
Clinical Presentation 1711
Tumor Peptide Products 1711
Treatment 1712
Ectopic Secretion of Gonadotropins 1713
Clinical Presentation 1713
Tumor Peptide Products 1714
Treatment 1715
Hyperthyroidism Associated with Nonpituitary Tumors 1715
Clinical Presentation 1715
Tumor Peptide Product 1715
Treatment 1715
Hypoglycemia Associated with Non-Islet-Cell Tumors 1716
Clinical Presentation 1716
Tumor Hypoglycemic Factors 1716
Treatment 1717
Tumor-Associated Osteomalacia 1717
Clinical Presentation 1717
Tumor Hyperphosphaturic Factor 1717
Treatment 1718
Ectopic Secretion of Other Hormones 1718
Calcitonin 1718
Growth Hormone 1718
Hypothalamic Hormones 1719
Gastrin Releasing Peptide 1720
Erythropoietin 1721
Placental Lactogen 1722
Prolactin 1722
Renin 1722
Gut-Brain Peptides 1723
Other Humoral Factors 1724
Other Paraneoplastic Syndromes 1724
Multiple Ectopic Hormones 1724
Ectopic Hormones as Tumor Markers 1724
General Characteristics 1724
Screening 1725
Localization 1725
Evaluation of Therapy 1726
References 1726

30 Hormone-Responsive Tumors 1736

Jean-Claude Heuson and André Coune

Breast Cancer 1736
Incidence and Mortality in Western Countries 1736
Risk Factors and Etiology 1737
Sex 1737
Geographic distribution and age 1737
Age as a prognostic factor 1739
Reproductive experience 1739
Role of individual hormones 1740
Familial aggregation 1741
Viruses 1741

Hormonal Regulation of Tumor Growth 1742
Murine mammary tumors 1742
Human breast cancer 1744
Therapy of breast cancer 1746
Primary breast cancer 1746
Advanced breast cancer 1746
Laboratory Procedure: Assay for Estrogen Receptors 1752
Adenocarcinoma of the Prostate 1753
Incidence 1753
Clinically manifest cancer 1753
Incidental cancer 1753
Risk Factors and Etiology 1753
Geographic distribution 1753
Socioeconomic factors 1753
Familial and genetic factors 1753
Occupational factors 1754
Diet 1754
Relation to benign hypertrophy 1754
Endocrine factors 1754
Possible role of viruses 1754
Information from animal tumor models 1755
Hormonal Regulation of Tumor Growth 1755
Animal tumors 1755
Human tumors 1755
Role of hormones 1756
Steroid hormone receptors 1756
Clinical evidence 1756
Natural History 1756
Pathology 1756
Local extension and dissemination 1756
Clinical Staging and Diagnosis 1757
Classification systems 1757
Staging procedure 1757
Diagnosis of pathology 1758
Tumor Markers 1758
Acid phosphatase 1758
Other tumor markers 1758
Steroid receptors 1758
Criteria for Prognosis 1758
Clinical variables 1758
Histologic and endocrine variables 1759
Evaluation of Response to Treatment 1759
Treatment 1759
Treatment of stages A and B 1759
Treatment of stages C and D 1760
Endocrine treatment of resistant or relapsing tumors 1761
Chemotherapy 1761
Adjuvant hormone treatment and chemotherapy 1761
Steroid Receptor Assay 1762
Therapeutic Prospects 1762
Adenocarcinoma of the Endometrium 1762
Incidence 1762
Risk Factors and Etiology 1762
Endogenous endocrine factors 1762
Exogenous factors 1763
Steroid receptors 1763
Treatment 1763
Endocrine treatment 1763
Chemotherapy 1764
References 1764

31 Prostaglandins, Kallikreins and Kinins, and Bartter's Syndrome 1768
Harry S. Margolius, Perry V. Halushka, and Jürgen C. Frolich

Prostaglandins 1768
Historical background 1768
Nomenclature 1769
Prostaglandins as tissue hormones 1769
Actions of leukotrienes 1771
Biochemistry 1771
Prostaglandin synthesis and metabolism 1771
Synthesis and metabolism of leukotrienes 1772
Inhibition of prostaglandin biosynthesis 1773
Organ Systems 1773
Reproduction 1773
Renal prostaglandins 1774
Gastrointestinal tract 1776
Cardiovascular system 1777
Circulating prostaglandins 1777
Circulatory shock 1777
Blood pressure 1777
Clinically important cardiovascular functions of prostaglandins 1778
Lungs 1779
Metabolic effects 1779
Kallikreins and Kinins 1780
Biochemistry of the Systems 1781
Localization of System Components 1784
Relations of Kallikreins and Kinins to Renin and Prostaglandins 1784
Kallikrein-kinin and renin-angiotensin relationships 1785
Kallikrein-kinin and prostaglandins 1785
The Roles of Kallikreins and Kinins 1785
Renal function 1785
Hypertension 1786
Other renal, circulatory, and metabolic disorders 1786
Bartter's Syndrome 1787
Introduction 1787
Clinical Presentation 1787
Biochemical, Histological, and Anatomical Findings 1787
Pathogenesis 1788
Treatment 1789
References 1789

Index ***1795***

Contributors

JOHN D. BAXTER, M.D.
Director, Metabolic Research Unit; Chief, Division of Endocrinology, Moffitt Hospital; Professor of Medicine and Biochemistry and Biophysics, University of California, San Francisco, San Francisco, California [1,2,3,12,14,15]

MICHAEL BERGMAN, M.D.
Associate Professor of Medicine and Director of Rachmiel Levine Diabetes Center, New York Medical College, Valhalla, New York; Associate Attending Physician and Director of Diabetes Clinic, Westchester County Medical Center, Valhalla, New York [19]

EDWARD G. BIGLIERI, M.D.
Professor of Medicine, University of California, San Francisco, San Francisco, California [14]

GUENTHER BODEN, M.D.
Professor of Medicine, Department of Medicine, Temple University Health Science Center, Philadelphia, Pennsylvania [27]

HENRY G. BONE III, M.D.
Director, Clinical Research, CIBA–GEIGY Corporation, Summit, New Jersey [28]

ARTHUR E. BROADUS, M.D., Ph.D.
Associate Professor of Medicine and Chief, Division of Endocrinology, Yale University School of Medicine, New Haven, Connecticut [1,2,23,25]

HENRY G. BURGER, M.D., F.R.A.C.P.
Director, Medical Research Centre and Department of Endocrinology, Prince Henry's Hospital, Melbourne, Australia [17B]

GERARD N. BURROW, M.D.
Sir John and Lady Eaton Professor of Medicine, University of Toronto, Toronto, Ontario, Canada [11]

BAYARD D. CATHERWOOD, M.D.
Clinical Investigator, San Diego Veterans Medical Center, La Jolla, California; Chief, Endocrinology/Metabolism Section, Medical Service, Atlanta Veterans Medical Center, Decatur, Georgia; and Associate Professor of Medicine, Emory University School of Medicine, Atlanta, Georgia [28]

KEVIN J. CATT, M.D., Ph.D.
Chief, Endocrinology and Reproduction Research Branch, National Institute of Child Health and Human Development, National Institutes of Health, Bethesda, Maryland [5]

WILLIAM E. CONNOR, M.D.
Professor of Medicine; Head, Division of Endocrinology, Metabolism, and Clinical Nutrition, Department of Medicine, Oregon Health Sciences University, Portland, Oregon [22]

ANDRÉ COUNE, M.D.
Institut J. Bordet, Polyclinique a. Claude, Boulevard de Waterloo 125, Brussels, Belgium [30]

PHILIP E. CRYER, M.D.
Professor of Medicine and Director, Metabolism Division, Washington University School of Medicine; Associate Physician, Barnes Hospital, St. Louis, Missouri [13]

LEONARD J. DEFTOS, M.D.
Professor of Medicine and Chief of Endocrinology, Department of Medicine (Endocrine Section), University of California and San Diego Veterans Administration Medical Center, La Jolla, California [28]

GREGORY F. ERICKSON, Ph.D.
Associate Professor, Research Center, School of Medicine, University of California, San Diego, La Jolla, California [17A]

PHILIP FELIG, M.D.
Chief Executive Officer, Sandoz Pharmaceuticals Corporation; Group Vice President, Sandoz Corporation; and President, Sandoz Research Institute, East Hanover, New Jersey; Clinical Professor of Medicine, Yale University School of Medicine, New Haven, Connecticut [1,2,19,20]

LAWRENCE A. FROHMAN, M.D.
Professor of Medicine; Director, Division of Endocrinology and Metabolism; and Director, General Clinical Research Center, University of Cincinnati College of Medicine, Cincinnati, Ohio [1,2,7,8]

JÜRGEN C. FROLICH, M.D.
Head, Department of Clinical Pharmacology, Fischer-Bosch Institute of Clinical Pharmacology, Stuttgart, West Germany [31]

BARRY J. GERTZ, M.D., Ph.D.
Clinical Pharmacology, Merck, Sharp, and Dohme Research Laboratories, Rahway, New Jersey [3]

GORDON N. GILL, M.D.
Professor of Medicine, University of California, San Diego Medical School, La Jolla, California [4]

PERRY V. HALUSHKA, M.D.
Professor of Pharmacology and Medicine, Medical University of South Carolina, Charleston, South Carolina [31]

DAVID L. HEALY, B.Med.Sci., Ph.D., F.R.A.C.O.G.
Wellcome Senior Clinical Research Fellow, Medical Research Centre, Prince Henry's Hospital; Department of Obstetrics and Gynecology, Monash University, Melbourne, Australia [17B]

Numbers in brackets refer to chapter numbers.

JEAN-CLAUDE HEUSON, M.D.†
Professor of Medical Oncology, Service de Médecine et Laboratoire d'Investigation, Clinique H. Tagnon, Institut J. Bordet, Brussels, Belgium [30]

WILLA HSUEH, M.D.
Associate Professor of Medicine and Endocrinology, University of Southern California Medical Center, Los Angeles, California [14]

D. ROGER ILLINGWORTH, M.D., Ph.D.
Associate Professor of Medicine, Division of Endocrinology, Metabolism, and Clinical Nutrition, Oregon Health Sciences University, Portland, Oregon [22]

KARL L. INSOGNA, M.D.
Assistant Professor of Medicine, Division of Endocrinology, Yale University School of Medicine; Research Associate, West Haven Veterans Administration Medical Center, West Haven, Connecticut [25]

DOROTHY T. KRIEGER, M.D.†
Professor of Medicine and Director, Division of Endocrinology, Mt. Sinai School of Medicine, New York, New York [7]

MARGARET H. MacGILLIVRAY, M.D.
Professor of Pediatrics, State University of New York at Buffalo; Co-Director, Division of Endocrinology, Buffalo Children's Hospital, Buffalo, New York [26]

HARRY S. MARGOLIUS, M.D., Ph.D.
Professor of Pharmacology and Medicine, Medical University of South Carolina, Charleston, South Carolina [31]

ROBERT I. McLACHLAN, F.R.A.C.P.
Clinical Research Fellow, Medical Research Centre, Prince Henry's Hospital; Department of Anatomy, Monash University, Melbourne, Australia [17B]

DAVID N. ORTH, M.D.
Professor of Medicine and Director, Division of Endocrinology, Vanderbilt University, Nashville, Tennessee [29]

DOROTHEE PERLOFF, M.D.
Clinical Professor of Medicine and Director, Hypertension Clinic, University of California, San Francisco, San Francisco, California [14]

GARY L. ROBERTSON, M.D.
Professor, Department of Medicine and Director, General Clinical Research Center, The University of Chicago, Chicago, Illinois [9]

†Deceased

LESTER B. SALANS, M.D.
Vice President, Preclinical Research, Sandoz Research Institute, East Hanover, New Jersey [21]

RICHARD J. SANTEN, M.D.
Professor of Medicine and Chief, Division of Endocrinology, The Milton S. Hershey Medical Center, Pennsylvania State University, Hershey, Pennsylvania [16]

ELEAZAR SHAFRIR, Ph.D.
Chairman, Department of Biochemistry, Hadassah University Hospital, Jerusalem, Israel [19]

JOHN J. SHELMET, M.D.
Fellow, Section of Metabolism/Diabetes, Department of Medicine, Temple University, Philadelphia, Pennsylvania [27]

ROBERT S. SHERWIN, M.D.
Professor of Medicine, Department of Internal Medicine, Division of Endocrinology, Yale University School of Medicine, New Haven, Connecticut [20]

FREDERICK R. SINGER, M.D.
Professor, Department of Medicine, Section of Endocrinology, Clinical Research Center, University of Southern California, Los Angeles, California [24]

ANDREW F. STEWART, M.D.
Associate Professor of Medicine, Division of Endocrinology, Yale University School of Medicine; Chief, Section of Endocrinology, West Haven Veterans Administration Medical Center, West Haven, Connecticut [23]

J. BLAKE TYRRELL, M.D.
Clinical Professor of Medicine, Metabolic Research Unit, Department of Medicine, University of California, San Francisco, San Francisco, California [12,15]

ROBERT D. UTIGER, M.D.
Professor of Medicine and Director, Clinical Research Unit, The University of North Carolina at Chapel Hill, Chapel Hill, North Carolina [10]

JUDITH L. VAITUKAITIS, M.D.
Director, General Clinical Research Center Program Branch, Division of Research Resources, National Institutes of Health, Bethesda, Maryland [6]

JEREMY S.D. WINTER, M.D., F.R.C.P.
Professor, Department of Pediatrics; Head, Section of Endocrinology and Metabolism, Children's Hospital, Winnipeg, Manitoba, Canada [18]

Preface

The purpose of this book, as in its previous edition, is to provide the reader a blending of physiologic and pathophysiologic principles with specific details of practical management of endocrine and metabolic disorders. In attempting to cover the broad spectrum of endocrine and metabolic disease, attention has been paid to common clinical entities as well as more esoteric diseases. While basic biologic concepts are presented, the clinical orientation is maintained by focusing on the steps necessary to establish a diagnosis and the details of instituting and maintaining a therapeutic regimen once a diagnosis has been established. To facilitate a rational approach to diagnoses, flow diagrams are presented.

The burst of new knowledge in endocrinology and metabolism over the last 5 to 6 years has necessitated that the second edition contain extensive rewriting and, in some instances, totally new chapters, rather than merely minor revisions of the first edition. A new chapter has been added to provide coverage of the fundamental concepts of gene expression and recombinant DNA technology as they relate to the endocrine system. Special attention has been provided to include up-to-date references in all chapters.

The overall effort required of contributors as well as editors has been at least as great as with the first edition. We are grateful to our contributors for the excellence with which they have met their commitments. We thank our secretaries Madeline Wizorek, Carmel DiPaolo, Susan Corke, Nancy Canetti, and Vivian Martin for their efforts as well as their understanding and patience. Finally we are indebted to the Health Professions Division of McGraw-Hill Book Company for providing the support and encouragement necessary for the success of this project.

PART I

GENERAL ENDOCRINOLOGY

1

Introduction to the Endocrine System

John D. Baxter
Lawrence A. Frohman
Arthur E. Broadus
Philip Felig

DEFINITIONS AND SCOPE OF ENDOCRINOLOGY

The endocrine system, along with the nervous system, has evolved to provide mechanisms for communication between cells and organs. Such systems have been critical for the development and function of multicellular organisms that, in higher species such as humans, have rather sophisticated control systems. These systems regulate and thereby permit growth and development, reproduction, homeostasis, and responses to changes in the environment such as provocative stimuli and stress.

The term *endocrine* refers to the process of secretion of biologically active substances into the body. This contrasts with the term *exocrine*, which refers to external secretion, generally via anatomically identifiable ducts such as into the gastrointestinal tract. As the term is ordinarily used, an endocrine gland or cell is one that secretes substances referred to as *hormones* that exert regulatory functions, typically in cells other than those in which they are produced. The term *hormone* is derived from a Greek verb meaning "to set in motion." Strictly speaking, then, a hormone is a substance that is secreted by one cell and travels through the circulation, where it exerts actions on other cells.

In order to act, hormones must interact with other loci on or in the target cell. These sites are termed *receptors* (Chap. 5). Thus, a receptor is a locus where the hormone is bound. A receptor has two functions. First, it must be able to distinguish the hormone from all the other chemicals present in the circulation and to bind it. Thus, a receptor must be capable of binding the hormone tightly enough and also must not bind extraneous substances. The hormone binding sites on receptors have evolved to have unique configurations that are complementary to the hormones they bind. In general, these hormone-receptor interactions are noncovalent in nature and are reversible. Second, the receptor must be able to transmit the information gained from the binding to trigger the intracellular response. Thus, substances that bind hormones, even tightly, but do not trigger subsequent responses are not receptors; examples include *transport proteins* (discussed below) and enzymes involved in hormone biosynthesis or metabolism (see Chap. 4).

These simple distinctions serve to define endocrinology, receptors, and hormones in most cases. Thus, for example, insulin (Chap. 19) is secreted from an endocrine gland, the pancreatic islets, travels in the circulation, and associates with insulin receptors present on most tissues, where the hormone-receptor interaction triggers numerous responses involved in regulating the metabolism of carbohydrates and other substances. Parathyroid hormone (PTH) (Chap. 23) is synthesized in and released from the parathyroid glands, travels through the circulation, and binds to several target tissues, where it regulates calcium homeostasis. In addition to these clear examples, there are numerous others in which the distinctions may appear to be fuzzy and imprecise. In most cases these seeming discrepancies are more apparent than real.

A major area of overlap in terms of the function of regulatory molecules involves the nervous system, and an entire discipline, neuroendocrinology, has evolved to address the relation between the nervous and endocrine systems. This is discussed in detail in Chap. 7. Overall, the nervous system has evolved to release regulatory substances from nerve cells or their axons to act across synaptic junctions on adjacent cells. Sometimes these substances, or *neurotransmitters*, travel considerable distances to act, but when they do so, they in general travel along the axons. Acetylcholine, catecholamines, and dopamine are examples of well-known neurotransmitters.

The brain is also an endocrine gland (Chap. 7). It is the major source for some hormones. The hypothalamic releasing hormones or factors include thyrotropin releasing hormone (TRH), corticotropin releasing factor (CRF), growth hormone releasing hormone (GRH), gonadotropin releasing hormone (GnRH), somatostatin, and dopamine; all are produced in the hypothalamus, whence they travel through the hypophyseal portal system to stimulate or inhibit the synthesis and release of pituitary hormones. Some of the hormones of the anterior pituitary (Chap. 8) and all those of the posterior pituitary (Chap. 9) are also synthesized in the hypothalamus.

Since both the nervous and the endocrine systems gradually came to use various ligands to serve their regulatory functions, it is not surprising that the same or related ligands can be used both as neurotransmitters and as hormones. Thus, both norepinephrine, secreted from nerve endings, and epinephrine, secreted from the adrenal medulla, act through adrenergic receptors (Chap. 13). Dopamine is a well-established neurotransmitter that is also active after it travels through the circulation. The brain produces a number of other hormones (Chap. 7). Prolactin, growth hormone, pro-opiomelanocortin (POMC), renin, and atrial natriuretic factor are examples of these brain hormones, but brain production probably contributes negligibly to the circulating levels of these substances. Therefore, if they exhibit biologic activity (something not yet established), it is probably a local role in regulation. If this is true, then they may be neurotransmitters. How can these overlaps be resolved in terms of definition? For the most part, the answers are simple. If a given ligand is released into the circulation to act, it is a hormone; if it is released from a nerve terminal to act locally, it is a neurotransmitter. The same substance can be both a neurotransmitter and a hormone.

The nervous and endocrine systems are also related in other ways. Thus, in many cases the function of endocrine tissues is controlled by the autonomic nervous system. Endocrine glands such as the pituitary, pancreatic islets, renal juxtaglomerular cells, and adrenal gland respond to neural stimulation. Again, while the overlaps are obvious, the definitions can still be simple, and it is possible that the same cell can function as both an endocrine cell and a nerve cell.

The designation of endocrine tissue has of necessity broadened with recent advances in the understanding of endocrinology: some tissues are specialized specifically as endocrine glands, while other endocrine glands also serve other functions. Examples of the first are the thyroid, pituitary, parathyroid, and adrenal glands and the pancreatic islets. The central nervous system, on the other hand, serves other functions, and the ovaries and testes, in addition to producing hormones, also produce oocytes and sperm, respectively. The atrium of the heart produces atrial natriuretic factor (Chap. 14), the liver, somatomedin (Chap. 26), the kidney, erythropoietin,[1] and the gastrointestinal tract, numerous hormones such as gastrin, somatostatin, and cholecystokinin (Chap. 27). Although some of these molecules have not generally been officially recognized as hormones, in the strict sense they should be.

Do hormones need to travel through the circulation to act? No. It is likely that local release of hormones to act on cells in the immediate vicinity is important. The release of growth factors in tissues such as bone may be an example of such a phenomenon (Chap. 24). The release of somatostatin by the pancreatic delta cells with the potential to suppress insulin release by the beta cells and glucagon release by the alpha cells may provide an additional example (Chap. 19). In addition, substances such as the prostaglandins and prostacyclins are in all likelihood released to act on cells in their immediate vicinity (Chap. 31). This type of intracellular communication has been termed *paraendocrine* or *paracrine* and thereby incorporated into the general discipline of endocrinology.

Hormones can also act on cells that produce them, although the overall importance of this is not yet established. This type of communication has been termed *autocrine.* One instance in which this is probably important is the cancer cell. Certain oncogenes act by encoding or stimulating the production of growth factors that are critical for progression of the malignant state.[2-4] Insulin has an inhibitory effect on its own secretion, independent of changes in blood glucose levels (Chap. 19).

Still other examples can be cited in which semantic distinctions become fuzzy and overlaps occur between endocrinology and other disciplines. For instance, renin of renal origin is ordinarily considered a hormone, but rather than acting on other cell types, it functions as an enzyme in the bloodstream to release angiotensin I from its substrate, angiotensinogen (Chap. 14). The regulators of the immune response, such as the interleukins,[5,6] the growth factors (Chap. 26), erthyropoietin,[1] and other factors, function as hormones or in paracrine or autocrine regulation but are ordinarily not considered hormones even though they should be.

Endocrinology needs to be considered in quantitative as well as qualitative terms. Excesses or deficiencies of hormones result in disease. Classically, the endocrine status was signal-oriented, with the dominant consideration being how much or how little of the hormone was present. These considerations remain important, and the signal consideration has been expanded to include reserve. For example, the diagnosis of adrenal insufficiency is made not on the basis of a random measurement of the plasma cortisol but on the extent to which cortisol can be released in response to provocative stimuli (Chap. 12). More recently, attention has been focused as well on the response limb of the endocrine system. In interpreting the significance of a given hormone concentration in the blood, it is equally critical to know how sensitive the target cells are to that hormone. Syndromes of frank hormone unresponsiveness have been known for years; pseudohypoparathyroidism (Chap. 23) and testicular feminization (Chap. 16) are examples. However, it is now clear that responsiveness to hormones is extensively regulated by the homologous hormone, by other hormones, and by nonhormonal mechanisms (Chap. 5) and that quantitatively abnormal responsiveness to hormones can contribute to disease. Type II diabetes with elevated insulin levels and impaired cellular sensitivity to insulin is a well-studied example (Chap. 19), and other problems, such as some cases of hypercholesterolemia (Chap. 22), thyroid hormone resistance (Chap. 10), and hypertension (Chap. 14), are also candidates for the abnormal responsiveness category.

TYPES OF HORMONES AND THEIR SYNTHESIS AND RELEASE

As hormone evolution has proceeded, a number of types of molecules have been recruited to regulate body processes: peptides, lipids, and amino acid analogues all serve as hormones. Sophisticated mechanisms have also evolved to synthesize these hormones. The types of hormones that exist and the mechanisms by which they are synthesized are discussed in detail in Chap. 4. Additional details of the biosynthetic steps in the production of individual hormones are provided in the individual chapters. These hormones and mechanisms of synthesis are discussed here only in outline form to provide perspective.

Peptide hormones vary in size, composition, number of chains, modification of groups, and mechanisms of production. Thus, whereas growth hormone is a single chain of 191 amino acids (Chaps. 8 and 26), TRH is a cyclized tripeptide with modified amino groups (Chaps. 7 and 10). The glycoprotein hormones, thyroid stimulating hormone (TSH), luteinizing hormone (LH), follicle stimulating hormone (FSH), and chorionic gonadotropin (CG), all have two peptide chains, one of which (α chain) is common to all, while the other (β chain) is unique for each member of the set (Chap. 8). Insulin, on the other hand, consists of two chains that are derived from a single gene product (preproinsulin) (Chap. 19). Many hormones, such as corticotropin (ACTH; 39 amino acids), β-endorphin (29 amino acids), and insulin, are proteolytic products of a larger precursor protein (Chaps. 7 and 8). Some hormones (e.g., FSH) are glycosylated, whereas others (e.g., ACTH in humans) are not.

The steroid hormones and prostaglandins are derived from the lipids cholesterol and arachidonic acid, respectively (Chap. 4). They are synthesized through a series of reactions that modify their parent compounds.

The amino acid analogues include epinephrine, norepinephrine, dopamine (Chap. 13), and thyroid hormones (Chap. 10) that are all derived from tyrosine, and 5-hydroxytryptamine, derived from tryptophan.

A variety of control mechanisms regulate hormone synthesis, release, and removal. In general, the fine tuning of hormone levels involves influences on production and release, with the removal mechanisms showing less variation. There are marked variations in terms of the regulation of production and release. For example, with insulin, the pancreatic beta cells can store several days' supply of the hormones; the stimuli to insulin release (e.g., hyperglycemia) result in an early release that reflects the discharge of stored insulin, followed by a slower release associated with an increase in insulin production (Chap. 19). With steroids, on the other hand, there is little storage of the hormone, and the stimuli to release increase the production of new hormone that is relatively rapidly released (Chap. 4).

In general, the endocrine glands secrete the form of the hormone that is active in the target tissue. However, in a few cases, metabolic conversion in peripheral tissues results in the final active form of the hormone. For instance, testosterone, the major product of the testis, is converted to dihydrotestosterone in peripheral tissues (Chap. 16). The latter steroid is responsible for many (but not all) androgenic actions. Vitamin D, originating from the skin or diet, undergoes sequential hydroxylations in liver and kidney before the final active hormone, 1,25-dihydroxycholecalciferol, is formed (Chap. 23). The major active thyroid hormone is triiodothyronine (T_3); the thyroid gland produces some T_3, but most of it comes from monodeiodination of thyroxine (T_4) to T_3 in the peripheral tissues (Chap. 10).

CIRCULATION OF HORMONES

The released hormone may circulate free or bound (Chap. 4). The peptide hormones circulate predominantly free or loosely associated with other proteins, while the small-molecule hormones circulate mostly bound to proteins. In many cases there are transport proteins that have a high affinity for the specific hormone. Examples are thyroxine-binding globulin (TBG), which binds thyroxine (Chap. 10), and corticosteroid-binding globulin (CBG, or transcortin), which binds cortisol (Chap. 12). These result generally in over 90 percent of the hormones in the circulation being present in the bound form. Aldosterone represents an exception (Chap. 12). In this case, there is no specific transport protein that binds tightly much of the hormone, and about 50 percent of it is free in the circulation; the remainder is mostly loosely bound to albumin. The levels of the transport proteins can change under a variety of circumstances. For example, both TBG and CBG levels can be increased by estrogens. These changes can affect the total hormone levels, with important consequences for the clinical interpretation of measured hormone levels.

In most cases, the free rather than the plasma-bound hormones are biologically active. Further, control systems that regulate hormone levels do so by adjusting the free hormone, with only secondary effects on the plasma-bound hormone. The actual role of the plasma binders in fact is not known. They appear to be extensively present in animals, so it is conceivable that they have some role. They appear not to be essential for transport of the hormones, which are sufficiently soluble at physiologically active concentrations. Since they sequester the hormones, they may serve a reservoir function. For example, when hormone levels drop, dissociation of plasma-bound hormone occurs, thereby providing additional free hormone. In this way, and conversely by protein sequestration of hormones when levels rise, the plasma transport proteins also serve to blunt rapid changes in hormone levels. These proteins, through binding of the hormones, also affect their clearance. It has been proposed that CBG sequesters cortisol in the kidney and decreases its ability to occupy mineralocorticoid receptors (Chap. 12); this leaves these receptors free to be occupied by the main mineralocorticoid hormone, aldosterone. Transport proteins in other cases are important for carrying regulatory molecules. The lipoproteins are important for carrying cholesterol that regulates its own biosynthesis (see Chap. 22), and the vitamin B_{12}-binding protein is important for carrying this vitamin to its sites of action.[7] However, these molecules are not generally considered hormones.

HORMONE METABOLISM

If the levels of hormones are to be regulated in response to various needs, there must be mechanisms for hormones to be cleared from the circulation once they are released. Details of hormone metabolism are given in Chap. 4 and in the sections on individual hormones. The rate of clearance of different hormones varies enormously, with half-lives ranging from a few minutes for many polypeptide hormones such as angiotensin or ACTH (Chap. 12) to days for thyroxine (Chap. 10). Thyroxine is involved in more long-term responses, whereas angiotensin II and ACTH are needed for shorter-term responses such as those to shock. Therefore, it is efficient for thyroid hormone to be cleared slowly, but such a mechanism would not allow ACTH or angiotensin levels to vary rapidly. The time required for reaching a new steady state in response to changes in hormone release is dependent on the half-life of the hormone in the circulation. The peptide hormones are mostly cleared by proteolytic destruction on the surface of tissues or after their uptake by cells through internalization mechanisms (Chap. 4). Thyroid hormones, steroids, and catecholamines are metabolically altered inside tissues in which the products are recycled into general metabolic pathways (thyroid and catecholamine hormones) or excreted by the kidneys or the gastrointestinal tract (steroid hormones). Although a variety of factors can affect hormone metabolism, these in general are not regulated extensively as compared with those that regulate hormone synthesis and release. Nevertheless, there are special circumstances in which such perturbations in hormone metabolism are clinically important. For example, the administration of drugs such as barbiturates that enhance steroid metabolism can influence the dose of administered glucocorticoid (Chap. 12); and the administration of thyroid hormone, which increases steroid clearance, can precipitate latent adrenal insufficiency (Chap. 12).

REGULATION OF HORMONE LEVELS

A variety of mechanisms regulate circulating hormone levels (Fig. 1-1), as discussed in the individual sections on specific hormones. Thus, there are mechanisms for (1) spontaneous, or basal, hormone release; (2) feedback inhibition by hormones of their synthesis and/or release; (3) hormone release stimulated or inhibited by particular levels of substances that either are or are not regulated by the same hormones; (4) establishment of circadian rhythms for hormone release by systems such as the brain; and (5) brain-mediated stimulation or inhibition of hormone release in response to anxiety, anticipation of specific activity, or other sensory input.

In some cases complex regulatory networks are present, whereas in other cases the endocrine cells are more independent. The first situation is illustrated by the axis comprising the hypothalamus, the anterior pituitary or adenohypophysis, and the target endocrine gland (Chaps. 8 and 12). Thus, the hypothalamus produces CRF, which travels down the portal vessels through the hypothalamic stalk to the anterior pituitary, where it stimulates ACTH release. ACTH then travels to the adrenal gland, where it stimulates the release of cortisol. The latter in turn inhibits both CRF and ACTH release (feedback inhibition). The brain establishes circadian rhythms and can trigger increased CRF release in response to stress. The pancreatic islets are an example of a more independent system (Chap. 19). Insulin release is regulated primarily by the levels of blood glucose, decreasing with hypoglycemia and increasing with glucose ingestion. However, hormones such as gastric inhibiting peptide and other substances such as specific amino acids (e.g., arginine) can also affect insulin release, as can stress and trauma via signals from the autonomic nervous system.

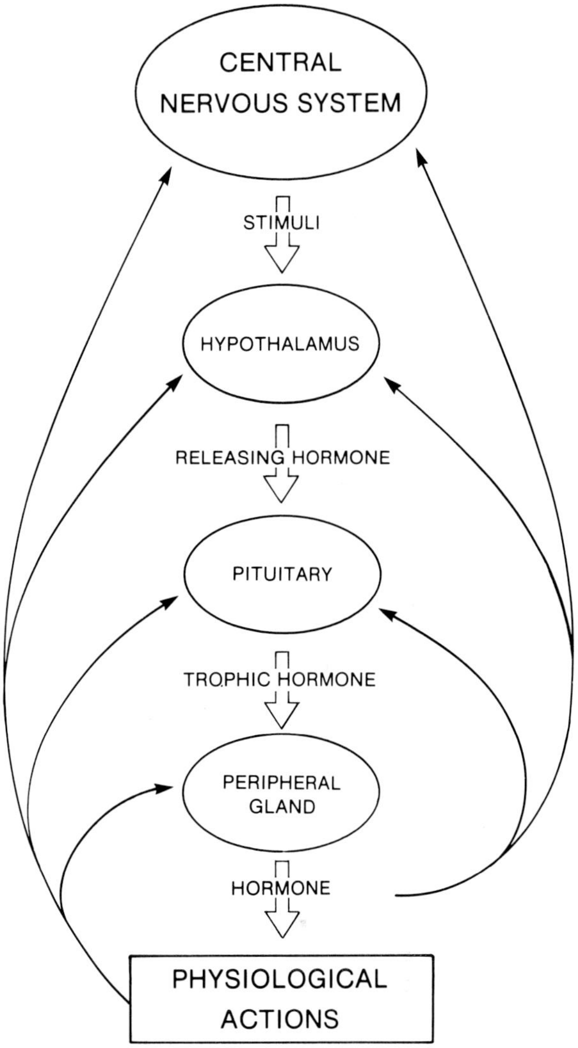

FIGURE 1-1 Organization of a set of endocrine glands, with interrelated regulatory elements. Shown is the flow of information from the central nervous system through the hypothalamus to the pituitary and then to the peripheral glands. Also indicated is that either the hormone product of the peripheral gland or the physiologic actions induced by the hormone can produce feedback inhibition of the stimuli to hormone release at any of several loci. As a rule, all the potential regulatory influences do not operate with respect to a given set of glands, nor do all of the components shown operate for all endocrine glands. (*From Baxter JD, in Wyngaarden JB, Smith LH Jr (eds): Cecil's Textbook of Medicine. Philadelphia, Saunders, 1985, p 1221.*)

HORMONE UPTAKE AND INTERNALIZATION

Various mechanisms account for the uptake of the different hormones by peripheral tissues. These are discussed extensively in Chap. 5 and in the sections on individual hormones. The polypeptide and catecholamine hormones and the prostaglandins bind to receptors on the cell surface and are internalized (Chap. 5). The cell surface receptor-hormone interactions initiate actions of these hormones (Chap. 5). These interactions also result in the subsequent internalization of the hormone-receptor complex. Hormones can also be internalized by bulk fluid endocytosis (Chap. 5), but this pathway is probably of minor significance.

The internalization mechanism also serves to deliver some regulatory ligands into the cell for intracellular actions. Cholesterol is transported into the cell bound to lipoproteins and there inhibits cholesterol uptake (Chap. 22). Thyroid hormones also bind to surface sites and are internalized (Chaps. 5 and 10). Once inside the cell, the hormone binds to nuclear receptors and affects the transcription of particular genes. However, it is not known whether the internalization accounts for most or all of the uptake of thyroid hormones. The question of whether polypeptide hormones are internalized to act inside the cell is a subject of active inquiry, and proof that this is the case has not yet been provided (Chap. 5). Steroid hormones that act inside the cell appear to be capable of readily penetrating cells and do not require a specific internalization mechanism; the hydrophobic nature of these molecules may allow them essentially to dissolve in the cell membrane and reappear in the internal milieu of the cell.

MECHANISMS OF HORMONE ACTION

The mechanisms of hormone action are discussed in detail in Chap. 5. In brief, the actions of peptide and catecholamine hormones and the prostaglandins that bind to receptors on the cell surface are due to influences of the hormone-receptor interactions on intracellular mediators, or *second messengers.* The most extensively studied mechanism is the activation of the enzyme adenylate cyclase by hormones such as beta-adrenergic agonists, ACTH, glucagon, and PTH. This enzyme catalyzes the conversion of ATP to adenosine 3′,5′-monophosphate (cyclic AMP, or cAMP), which activates a particular serine and threonine kinase. Phosphorylations induced by this molecule then alter the conformations of a diverse number of molecules, with consequent metabolic effects on cells. For example, such phosphorylations activate glycogenolysis. Other hormone-receptor interactions, such as those involving insulin, alpha-adrenergic agents, and β-endorphin, can inhibit adenylate cyclase. Tyrosine kinase can be activated by the action of hormones such as epidermal growth factor (EGF) and insulin. Many hormones promote an increase in intracellular calcium. This occurs with alpha-adrenergic agonists and angiotensin II. The calcium comes either from the extracellular fluid or from intracellular stores in organelles such as mitochondria or the sarcoplasmic reticulum. The calcium so released binds to calmodulin and other calcium-binding proteins, thereby activating them to induce other metabolic effects, as on glycogenolysis, transport processes, steroidogenesis, and muscle contraction. In many cases, hormones stimulate the production and/or turnover of phospholipids. These effects can influence and cause increased calcium influx into the cytosol and can activate another serine and threonine kinase, termed C *kinase.* Thus, these hormones utilize a variety of intracellular mediators, and a given hormone may utilize more than one of these (and other) pathways.

As indicated earlier, steroid and thyroid hormones act for the most part by binding to intracellular receptors. The thyroid hormone receptors are associated with chromatin in the presence or absence of the hormone; the hormone-receptor interaction induces changes in the transcription of specific genes. The steroid receptors are either loosely associated or unassociated with chromatin in the absence of the hormone; steroid binding induces the receptor-steroid complexes to bind to specific sites on the DNA, where they affect the initiation of transcription of specific genes. The translation products of the steroid- or thyroid hormone–regulated mRNAs in turn have or represent metabolic effects on the cells. For example, thyroid hormones can increase the levels of beta-adrenergic receptors, with consequent effects on beta-adrenergic sensitivity, and glucocorticoids increase the levels of gluconeogenic enzymes, with subsequent increases in glucose production.

REGULATION OF HORMONE RESPONSIVENESS

Hormone responsiveness is regulated extensively (Chap. 5). A common pattern is down regulation due to the homologous hormone's induction of a decrease in the levels of its own receptors; this occurs with most polypeptide hormones, catecholamine-responsive systems, and prostaglandin responses, and it occasionally occurs with steroid and thyroid hormones. Less commonly, hormones may increase responsiveness to themselves by increasing their receptors (angiotensin II and its adrenal receptors). Hormones also regulate responsiveness by influencing postreceptor aspects of the response; and there are numerous situations in which hormones antagonize or enhance the responses to other hormones by affecting receptors or postreceptor responses. For example, estrogens increase progesterone receptors; glucocorticoids in the liver affect the actions of epinephrine and glucagon at postreceptor loci. Thus, in the clinical assessment of a given state, not only hormone levels but also hormone responsiveness must be considered.

CLASSIFICATION OF HORMONE ACTION

Considered superficially, it might seem simple to classify hormone action. Glucocorticoid action would include all actions of glucocorticoids; insulin action would include all actions of insulin, etc. However, using these hormones as examples, it will be seen that the situation is not so simple. Many glucocorticoid actions *are* typical of glucocorticoids, such as induction of gluconeogenesis and glycogen deposition in liver, but in other cases glucocorticoids can affect sodium transport in a manner similar to aldosterone (Chap. 12). Similarly, many of the actions of insulin are typical for insulin, such as those which lower the blood sugar, but in other cases insulin can act analogously to somatomedin (Chaps. 5 and 19). These apparent paradoxes occur because cortisol can bind to the mineralocorticoid receptors that have a higher affinity for aldosterone and more typically mediate aldosterone action, and insulin can bind to somatomedin receptors that have a higher affinity for somatomedin.

Fortunately, pharmacologists have dealt with this problem and have developed a simple basis for classifying drugs that is also applicable to hormones. This classification is based on the receptors rather than the hormone. A given class of action is defined as that class mediated through a given type of receptor. Thus, epinephrine action, rather than including all actions mediated by epinephrine, is defined by the type of receptor that mediates the effect. Epinephrine can have actions through β_1- or β_2-adrenergic receptors or through α_1 or α_2 receptors (Chaps. 5 and 13). Similarly, cortisol can have actions mediated through glucocorticoid or mineralocorticoid receptors, and insulin can have actions mediated through insulin or somatomedin receptors.

Currently, various receptors are defined through the use of binding studies. For example, glucocorticoid receptors bind steroids in the order dexamethasone > prednisolone > cortisol > aldosterone >> testosterone, whereas mineralocorticoid receptors bind aldosterone = deoxycorticosterone > cortisol (Chap. 12). The various receptors are now being isolated and their structures determined either directly or indirectly through an examination of their genes (see Chap. 3). Thus, it should be possible soon to characterize and define hormone action even more precisely.

EVOLUTION OF THE ENDOCRINE SYSTEM

The evolution of each of the various endocrine systems has involved the assimilation of a number of individual components whose functioning is coordinated in an effective manner. These components include the hormone itself and means for regulating its concentrations and responding to it. It is likely that the roots of these systems are found in simpler regulatory systems that preceded them. The discussions that follow, although they are speculations on how these steps might have occurred, nonetheless provide a conceptual framework for further thinking on the subject.

Simple and Complex Regulation

Tomkins classified regulation within cells as simple or complex.[8] With simple regulation, chemicals involved in a metabolic pathway, such as the reactants or products, regulate enzymatic or other processes important for the pathway. Such regulation is illustrated by feedback inhibition of an enzyme by products of the reaction. If regulation were limited to simple mechanisms, survival might be tenuous, since the regulatory ligands themselves are important intermediaries, and large changes in their concentrations might imperil the organism. Thus there was a need for more sophisticated mechanisms for metabolic control. This more complex regulation involves the use by cells of regulatory ligands that are neither reactants nor products of the processes which they regulate. Such ligands, therefore, may not have any obvious relation to the chemicals involved in the pathway. For example, cAMP regulates the metabolism of glucose and glycogen (Chaps. 5 and 19), but it differs chemically from these carbohydrates.

Origin of Hormones and Other Regulatory Ligands

Regulatory ligands of the endocrine system include not only hormones but also second-messenger mediators of hormone-receptor interactions (Chap. 5). For a ligand to assume a role in complex regulation, its concentration should change in response to conditions that would benefit from its actions. Tomkins further proposed that the concentrations of regulatory ligands such as cAMP could be varied in response to such conditions because they were by-products rather than important intermediates.[8] As such, their production rates could vary when other factors affected the major pathways. ATP is ordinarily converted to ADP or AMP. This reaction is frequently linked to other reactions such as the conversion of glucose to glucose 6-phosphate. Tomkins speculated that glucose deprivation might therefore diminish both phosphorylation of glucose and conversion of ATP to ADP. In this circumstance, more ATP might be degraded by alternative pathways, as by conversion to cAMP. As a consequence, cAMP could become a "symbol" of insufficient glucose availability, in that it would accumulate when levels of the sugar decreased.

The production of molecules that are now known as hormones may also have been first regulated in response to changes in cellular conditions.[9] For example, steroid hormone production may have been affected when cellular events altered the synthesis, metabolism, or utilization of cholesterol, which is a precursor to all the steroid hormones.[9] Incorporation of cholesterol into membranes is associated with cell growth. When growth is affected, there is altered utilization of cholesterol and potential changes in its conversion to other molecular species such as the steroid hormones. Thus steroids might have evolved into symbols for regulating cell growth. Other factors might also have increased steroid production. For instance (Fig. 1-2), it is possible that with decreased carbohydrate utilization and consequent decreased generation of pyruvate, there would be impaired utilization of acetyl CoA for oxidation through the citric acid cycle and for lipogenesis.[9] This might affect the pathway acetyl CoA → cholesterol → steroids. Such events might explain how glucocorticoids came to symbolize glucose deprivation and to take on such roles as enhancing the production and availability of glucose (Chap. 12).

Analogous speculations can be extended to the other hormones. Thyroid and catecholamine hormones are by-products of tyrosine, and their production may have first been regulated by circumstances that affected the metabolism of this amino acid. Many of the polypeptide hormones are derived from the cleavage of large proteins, and variations in their production may have had their origins in events that affected the metabolism of the precursor proteins. The genes for these precursor proteins may have evolved from genes that encoded proteins critical for cellular structure or metabolism. Similarly, the genes encoding polypeptide hormones that make up an entire gene may have been derived from an evolutionary precursor gene that served an essential cellular function.

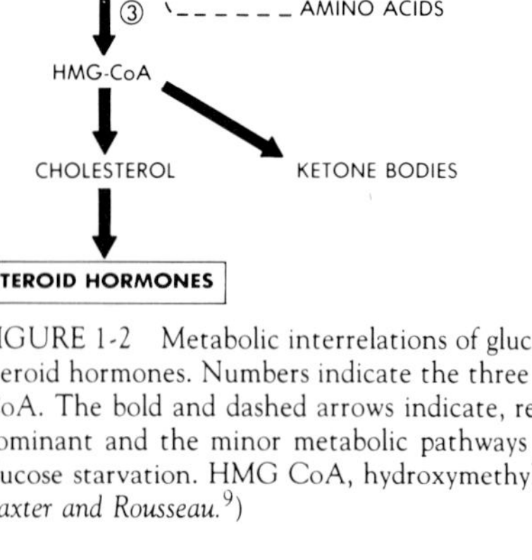

FIGURE 1-2 Metabolic interrelations of glucose, acetyl CoA, and steroid hormones. Numbers indicate the three major fates of acetyl CoA. The bold and dashed arrows indicate, respectively, the more dominant and the minor metabolic pathways under conditions of glucose starvation. HMG CoA, hydroxymethylglutaryl CoA. (*From Baxter and Rousseau.*[9])

Of course, not all symbols for metabolic control are regulated by simply increasing their synthesis. Ions such as Ca^{2+}, Mg^{2+}, K^{+}, and Cl^{-} are extensively used in the regulation of homeostasis (Chap. 5). In these cases, rather than creating the ions, changes in metabolism could alter their concentrations in specific cellular compartments (cytosol, mitochondria, sarcoplasmic reticulum, etc.). For instance, lack of glucose or other substrate could result in a lack of ATP or other substances which would affect the activity of transport systems involved in the maintenance of ion-concentration gradients across membranes. The ions could then take on regulatory functions by interacting with proteins that evolved as described above.

Origin of Receptors and Other Mediators of Regulatory Ligand Actions

Once mechanisms were established to regulate the concentrations of a ligand by appropriate stimuli, there was a need for the ligand to develop means to affect the appropriate metabolic pathway(s). To do this, the ligand must interact with other molecules in the cell. Binding proteins for products such as cAMP were probably already present by the time these ligands appeared, since enzymes that bound their precursors had to be present to form the ligand.[8] If these proteins could be modified to have activities that affected the metabolic pathway and if these were stimulated by binding of the ligand, elements for the complex regulation would be established. Genetic events such as mutation, deletion of gene sequences, or insertion of additional gene sequences would allow the genes for such proteins ultimately to produce a molecule with the needed regulatory properties. These mechanisms are described in more detail in Chap. 3. There would be a selective advantage for any cells containing such regulatory proteins, as these would help the cell to respond in a way that would overcome the original problem (e.g., glucose deprivation) that stimulated the production of the regulatory ligand. For example, in *Escherichia coli* cAMP accumulates when there is a low concentration of glucose.[8] The nucleotide binds to a regulatory protein (Fig. 1-3), and the complex then stimulates the production of enzymes that metabolize other carbohydrates such as galactose and lactose. These actions, therefore, provide an alternative carbohydrate source that can be utilized by the organism in the absence of glucose. Thus cAMP, a key mediator in hormone action and neurotransmission in humans, developed as a regulator of metabolism in much lower species.

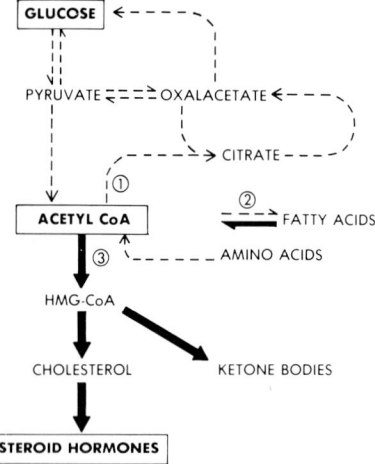

In mammals, the protein to which cAMP binds specifically is a regulatory subunit whose association with a specific protein kinase inhibits its activity (Fig. 1-3 and Chap. 5). The binding of cAMP promotes a dissociation of the regulatory subunit from the catalytic subunit, which, its inhibition by the regulatory subunit removed, is then active.

Regulatory proteins, or receptors in this case, have also evolved to bind hormones specifically and to transmit this information into postreceptor events. For example, the binding of steroid hormones to their receptors induces conformational changes that stimulate the receptors to bind to specific DNA sequences and to influence the transcription of specific genes (Chap. 5).

To gain such specialized and highly specific functions, proteins have had to develop the structures they now have by evolution of the genes that dictate their amino acid sequences (Chap. 3). In some cases, other genes evolved to express products that modify these proteins (e.g., through glycosylation). Since the evolution of genes has apparently occurred by mechanisms such as mutation of preexisting genes and recombination of pieces from different genes (mentioned above), some constraints are placed on the way the proteins can evolve. Therefore, it has probably been simpler evolutionarily to modify preexisting structures than to create entirely new genes. It may not then be surprising that there is some homology in the amino acid sequences of diverse proteins, because their genes may have arisen by evolution from common precursor genes. Since, as pointed out earlier, binding sites on proteins for regulatory ligands such as cAMP and steroids or their analogues must have existed by the time these ligands appeared, it is easy to see how modification of the genes for these proteins could result in other proteins with high binding specificity for the regulatory ligand.

Figure 1-3 shows one hypothetical scheme for the evolution from a primitive glucotransferase of three types of regulatory protein that are known to exist: (1) the bacterial cAMP-binding protein (CAP or CRP protein) that regulates transcription of several genes, such as those which code for the enzymes involved in the metabolism of lactose; (2) the mammalian cAMP-binding protein, which regulates the cAMP-dependent protein kinase that mediates cAMP action in humans (Chap. 5); and (3) adenylate cyclase (Chap. 5). For the bacterial protein and the kinase, the ATP-binding site of the primitive glucokinase evolved to have a greater specificity for binding cAMP. With the bacterial protein, a polynucleotide (DNA)-binding function was also added. With the kinase, the glucophosphotransferase function evolved to have a protein phosphorylation activity. Finally, adenylate cyclase itself may have

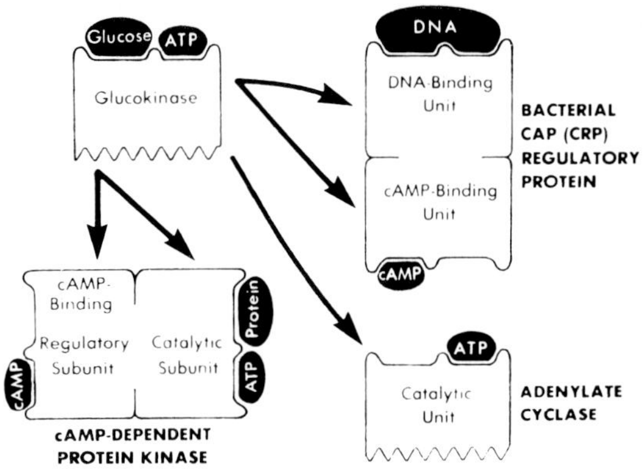

FIGURE 1-3 Speculations on the origin of cAMP-dependent protein kinase, adenylate cyclase, and the bacterial cAMP regulatory protein. (*From Baxter JD, MacLeod KM, in Bondy PK, Rosenberg LE (eds): Metabolic Control and Disease. Philadelphia, Saunders, 1980, p 106.*)

evolved from the glucokinase to have a predominantly cAMP-generating rather than ADP-generating function. These formulations, although speculative, nevertheless illustrate how molecular evolution of such regulatory proteins could have occurred.

Diversification of Families of Hormones

Once a given regulatory molecule became established, there was probably evolutionary pressure to preserve it. There might also be an opportunity for the molecule to extend its domain. For example, a hormone that increased in concentration in response to stress might be recruited to elicit additional responses that would relieve the stress. These responses would be recruited by mechanisms similar to those described in the preceding sections. Thus, angiotensin II stimulates not only vascular constriction but also aldosterone release, with consequent effects to conserve sodium (Chap. 12). Conversely, variants of the initial hormone might be produced, and with time these might take on one set of the responses while leaving other responses to the original hormone. Thus, cortisol and aldosterone are both released in response to stress, yet they elicit different sets of responses that help in the adjustment to stress (Chap. 12). These influences would therefore result in diversification of hormones and of their responses.

EVOLUTION OF THE ENDOCRINE GLANDS

As multicellular organisms evolved, cells began to secrete proteins and other ligands that could act on other cells. In many circumstances communication between cells in close proximity was adequate. However, as more complex forms of life evolved, it became necessary to have the more elaborate diversification that now exists for the specialized cells of the nervous and endocrine systems; these cells release regulatory signals that act at more distant sites.

The central nervous system (CNS) has emerged as dominant in regulating and coordinating bodily functions. With its development, many processes came to be regulated by direct nerve-to-cell contact. In simpler forms of life (invertebrates) the CNS communicates directly with all peripheral cells, and the neurotransmitter or messenger can be released in the immediate vicinity of the target cell.[10] This mechanism is preserved in higher forms of life in the autonomic nervous system but is inadequate for survival of the more complex and highly developed species.

The next step in complexity, the release of regulatory molecules to act at more distant loci, apparently became necessary as direct nerve-to-cell contact became impractical. The first process to evolve was direct neurosecretion of hormones from the CNS or from specialized effectors developed as outgrowths of nerve endings. The former is represented by the direct release of neurosecretory granules from invertebrate nerve cells as described by Ernst Scharrer[11] and the latter by cells of the posterior pituitary which secrete vasopressin (Chap. 9) and cells of the adrenal medulla that secrete epinephrine (Chap. 13). In a parallel manner, cells of neural crest origin with neurosecretory elements migrated to various other parts of the body, generally in association with the foregut and midgut and their outpouchings, resulting in CNS-like cells secreting the same neurotransmitters or peptides.[12,13] This provides an explanation of the presence of somatostatin, vasoactive intestinal peptide (VIP), neurotensin, substance P, etc., in the gut and pancreas (Chap. 27); for the neurosecretory granule–containing Kultschitzsky cells in the bronchi; and for the paraendocrine amine precursor uptake and decarboxylation (APUD) cells (Chap 7).[12] Hormone-producing tumors of the lung, gut, and pancreas (Chap. 29) may also have had their origin in this process.

The possible need for higher concentrations of many hormones at particular locations—cortisol acting on phenylepinephrine *N*-methyl transferase (PNMT) in the adrenal medulla (Chap. 13), testosterone acting on spermatogenesis in the testis (Chap. 16), estrogen acting on corpus luteum formation (Chap. 17), and insulin and glucagon regulating hepatic glucose regulation (Chap. 19)—may have required the location of glands that secrete them in areas distant from the CNS. An additional means for the control of these glands evolved with those intermediary hormones which could be produced near the CNS and be more readily under its control. Thus the anterior pituitary developed in close proximity to the CNS, so that its hormones could be under the control of the releasing-factor hormones synthesized in the brain (Chaps. 7 and 8).

Two other evolutionary processes occurred which helped to integrate the endocrine system. First, the appearance of portal vascular systems, hepatic (Chap. 27) and hypophyseal (Chaps. 7 and 8), permitted the localization of hormone action on the basis of concentration as well as the specificity of tissue receptors. Second, varying degrees of susceptibility of hormones to degradation by plasma served an important role in limiting the duration of their effects (discussed above).

INTEGRATION OF THE ENDOCRINE SYSTEM

The maintenance of homeostasis in multicellular organisms requires simultaneous monitoring of a number of functions in a coordinated manner. For instance, a fright response that may involve muscular activity requires the recruitment of the musculoskeletal system. To support this, the pulmonary and cardiovascular systems must also be prepared. For all this, energy sources must be mobilized in a manner that does not compromise critical functions of the organism. Thus, mechanisms have evolved to release glucose from glycogen, and other mechanisms are recruited to keep the blood glucose level at an acceptable concentration by increasing glucose production, stimulating alternative pathways to obtain energy (e.g., through mobilization of stored fat), and decreasing glucose consumption by tissues that are not in immediate need of the substrate. The contributions of the endocrine system to these types of control involve (1) an integrated set of responses to each hormone, (2) coordination of simultaneous responses by several hormones, (3) counterbalancing influences by other hormones, and (4) mechanisms for terminating or attenuating the response.

Integrated Actions of a Given Class of Hormone

As discussed earlier, there may be a selective advantage in the ability of hormones to regulate simultaneously several different processes that together lead to a given result. Thus, hormones typically stimulate integrated sets of responses: several simultaneous responses can be stimulated within a given cell, and responses can be stimulated in multiple organs, as described above for angiotensin II. Glucocorticoids are also illustrative in terms of their fuel-metabolizing and catabolic effects. These steroids enhance gluconeogenesis and glucose production in liver, decrease glucose uptake in peripheral tissues, enhance protein breakdown, and decrease protein synthesis in, for example, fat, muscle, and lymphoid and fibroblastic tissues (Chap. 12). They also stimulate lipolysis (Chap. 12). These actions together serve to increase the blood glucose concentration at the expense of substrate in certain tissues. This glucose is made available, however, for immediate use by other tissues and in particular the brain, whose continuous function is crucial for survival and is dependent specifically on glucose as a substrate; the brain is not a target for the catabolic actions of the glucocorticoids (Chap. 12).

Hormone Synergisms: Recruitment of Multiple Hormones for Coordinate Responses

The endocrine system has evolved in such a way that particular stimuli can affect simultaneously more than one hormone. The actions of these hormones may be complementary in achieving an overall response. For example, several classes of hormone (e.g., epinephrine, glucagon, glucocorticoids, growth hormone) are involved in glucose conservation (Chaps. 8, 12, 13, and 19). They act to increase blood glucose levels by stimulating increases in glucose synthesis, decreases in glucose utilization in certain tissues, and mobilization of substrates that serve as precursors for glucose synthesis (e.g., glycerol and lactate) and as alternative sources of energy (e.g., free fatty acids). The overall effects of these hormones in concert are greater than those of any single hormone. The plasma concentrations of all these hormones are increased with severe hypoglycemia (although in ordinary physiologic circumstances the blood glucose concentration is not the major control of epinephrine, growth hormone, and glucocorticoid production). Catecholamines (Chap. 13), vasopressin (Chap. 9), angiotensin II (Chaps. 12 and 14), glucocorticoids (Chap. 12), mineralocorticoids (Chap. 12), and other hormones are released in response to shock. These hormones increase vascular reactivity, conserve sodium, stimulate cardiac function, and elicit other actions that are useful in compensating for the insult.

Hormone Antagonisms: Fine Tuning of Metabolism

In many cases responses to hormones are countered by other hormones. This provides capabilities in addition to those derived from removal of a hormone. For instance, insulin opposes the glucose-elevating properties of epinephrine, glucagon, glucocorticoids, alpha-adrenergic agonists, and growth hormone (Chap. 19). It stimulates glucose uptake in fat and glycogen synthesis. It inhibits glucose synthesis, lipolysis, and glycogenolysis. Further, it stimulates protein synthesis and inhibits protein breakdown. Progesterone inhibits some actions of estrogens (Chap. 17). Thyrocalcitonin tends to lower the serum [Ca^{2+}], whereas PTH tends to elevate concentrations of the ion (Chap. 23).

The antagonisms do not always extend to all responses. For instance, although insulin actions are mostly antagonistic to the actions of the glucocorticoids, both classes of hormones tend to enhance glycogen accumulation (Chaps. 12 and 19). The alpha- and beta-adrenergic agonists both increase glycogenolysis and gluconeogenesis, although the two classes of hormones can have opposing influences on vascular (Chap. 13), muscular (Chap. 13), and hormonal (e.g., insulin) (Chap. 19) secretory responses. The fact that two classes of hormones can be synergistic for some responses and antagonistic for others can occasionally be explained in terms of the individual needs they serve.

Mechanisms for Attenuating or Terminating the Response

The responses are attenuated or terminated by a variety of mechanisms. First, most hormones, particularly stress hormones, are cleared rapidly from the circulation such that when secretion ceases the response rapidly disappears. Second, many hormones exert feedback inhibition of their own release. These inhibitory actions occur typically through actions of other hormones secreted in response to the initial hormone (e.g., blockage of TSH release by thyroid hormone, Chap. 10), or through sequelae of the hormone's action (e.g., PTH-induced increases in Ca^{2+} levels block PTH release). Third, as already discussed, hormones can induce a decrease in sensitivity to their actions. Finally, other hormones secreted simultaneously can blunt the responses; for example, a role of glucocorticoids released in stress may be to blunt the actions or secretions of other hormones (Chap. 12).

ACTIONS OF HORMONES

Hormones affect essentially all types of body processes. Several of the more prominent types of influence among the numerous actions deserve particular emphasis.

Intermediary Metabolism and Growth

A number of different hormones regulate intermediary metabolism and growth. Thus glucocorticoids, catecholamines, prostaglandin E_1, and glucagon tend to promote availability and/or mobilization of glucose and other fuels and in some cases tissue catabolism and antianabolism (Chap. 19). Glucocorticoids (in excess) also inhibit growth (Chap. 12). Insulin and certain growth factors, including the somatomedins, tend to have opposite effects, with varying degrees of growth-promoting and fuel-storing actions (Chap. 19). Androgens, progestins, and estrogens tend to be growth factors (Chaps. 16 and 17), although progesterone at a physiologic level can antagonize the effects of estrogens (Chap. 17). Growth hormone, prolactin, and placental lactogen tend to be growth-promoting, although the growth responses may be due solely or in part to stimulation of the production of growth factors such as somatomedin (Chaps. 8 and 26). In addition, many of the actions of growth hormone and chorionic somatomammotropin, independent of the ones mediated secondarily by the somatomedin(s), are more of the fuel-mobilizing type, with a tendency to stimulation of hyperglycemia, increased lipolysis, etc. (Chap. 19). Interestingly, many of the surface-active hormones of the fuel-mobilizing group activate adenylate cyclase, whereas those of the growth-stimulating fuel-storage group commonly do not do this (Chap. 5). Thus, as in bacteria, cAMP is used by a number of hormones for mobilization of carbohydrate.

Highly Specific Functions

TROPIC ACTIONS

The integration of the endocrine system has required the evolution of hormones whose functions are specifically designed to regulate glands specialized in the production of other hormones. This is the case with TSH, which regulates thyroid hormone production (Chaps. 8 and 10); CG, which regulates progesterone production (Chap. 17); FSH, important for follicular and Sertoli cell maturation (Chaps. 16 and 17); LH, which regulates progesterone production in the female (Chap. 17) and testosterone production in the male (Chap. 16); ACTH, which regulates glucocorticoid production (Chaps. 7, 8, and 12); angiotensin, which regulates aldosterone production (Chaps. 12 and 14); and renin, which stimulates angiotensin production (Chaps. 12 and 14). In some cases, hormones with highly specialized functions not primarily involving hormone production have evolved. This is the case with the pigment-regulating melanocyte stimulating hormone (MSH) (Chap. 8), the prolactin stimulation of milk production, and the oxytocin involvement in uterine contraction (Chap. 17). Although these hormones may have additional roles (e.g., angiotensin II), for the most part the number of target tissues for these classes of hormones is restricted. In many cases, these tropic hormones activate adenylate cyclase, but some of them (angiotensin II, oxytocin) apparently do not (Chap. 5).

MINERAL AND WATER METABOLISM

Aldosterone, vasopressin, PTH, calcitonin, and vitamin D are hormones that have the specialized functions of regulating ion and water concentrations (Chaps. 9, 12, 14, and 23). There is diversity in their mechanisms of action, and the target tissue distribution for each class of these hormones is rather restricted. However, these are not the only hormones that affect fluid and electrolyte metabolism, which is also influenced by insulin, glucagon, glucocorticoids, and catecholamines (Chaps. 12–14 and 19).

CARDIOVASCULAR FUNCTIONS

The atrium of the heart devotes more of its synthetic efforts to producing a hormone, atrial natriuretic factor, than to producing any other protein, and this hormone has extensive effects on the cardiovascular system (Chap. 14). In addition, numerous other hormones affect cardiovascular function and blood pressure. These include the catecholamines (Chaps. 13 and 14), thyroid hormone (Chaps. 10 and 14), angiotensin II (Chaps. 12 and 14), mineralocorticoids (Chaps. 12 and 14), bradykinin (Chaps. 14 and 31), and the sex steroids (Chaps. 16 and 17). Most of these hormones also have other important metabolic actions for which they are predominantly known (e.g., glucocorticoids, sex steroids). The fact that they also regulate cardiovascular responses underscores the importance of this system in responding to numerous physiologic and pathologic perturbations. Further, many elements of these systems are predominantly under CNS control by catecholamines and acetylcholine released at nerve endings.

REPRODUCTIVE FUNCTIONS

Hormones are dominant in the control of reproductive functions, as is evidenced by the lack of reproductive capacity in their absence (Chaps. 16–18). Thus, the gonadotropins of pituitary origin (LH, FSH; Chaps. 8, 16, and 17) or placental origin (CG; Chaps. 8 and 17) play important roles in regulating reproductive organs such as the ovary and testes, which in turn produce hormones such as the sex steroids, androgens, estrogens, and progestins. These steroids control functions critical for pregnancy and for sexual differentiation and development and influence secondary sexual characteristics such as voice, hair, and muscular development, as well as sexual behavior to some extent.

DEVELOPMENTAL ACTIONS

Hormones play a crucial role in extrauterine growth and development. The sex steroids (Chaps. 16 and 17), insulin (Chap. 19), other growth factors and hormones (Chap. 26), thyroid hormone (Chap. 10), and glucocorticoids (Chap. 12) are all important in this respect. Sometimes the effects are predominantly on growth, as illustrated by the dwarfism due to growth hormone deficiency or gigantism due to growth hormone excess (Chaps. 8 and 26). In other cases the influences are on development, as illustrated by the pseudohermaphroditism associated with insensitivity to androgens (Chap. 18). In yet others the effects are on growth and development, as illustrated by the lack of growth and brain development in cretinism (Chaps. 10 and 26). In fact, most of the hormones mentioned are important at some stage for development. In some cases (e.g., growth hormone), it is not clear that the hormone is even needed in the adult, even though its metabolic effects can be classified with those hormones affecting intermediary metabolism.

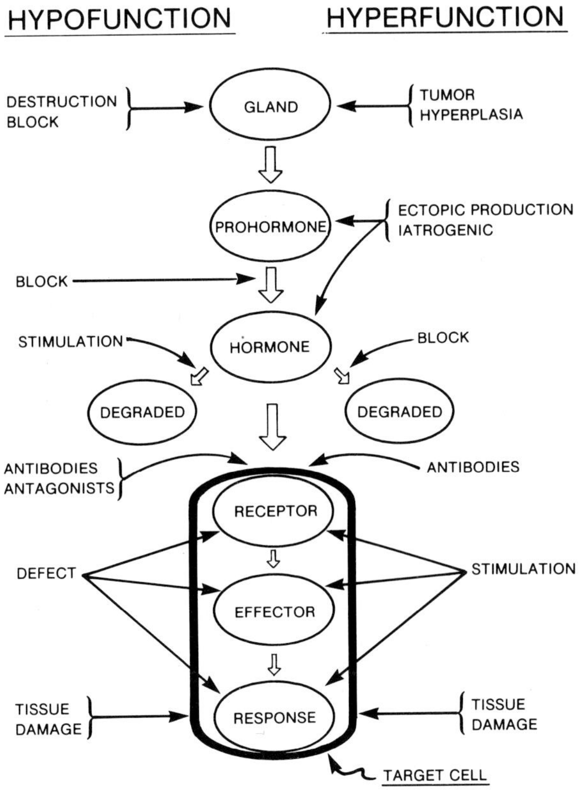

FIGURE 1-4 Causes of hypofunction or hyperfunction of the endocrine system. (*From Baxter JD, in Wyngaarden JB, Smith LH Jr (eds): Cecil's Textbook of Medicine. Philadelphia, Saunders, 1985, p. 1229.*)

DISORDERS OF THE ENDOCRINE SYSTEM

Endocrinology has traditionally been signal-oriented, concerning itself largely with whether hormones are secreted appropriately or inappropriately (i.e., in excess or deficiency). Most recognizable disorders of the endocrine system are indeed due to an excess or a deficiency of particular hormones, whether caused by abnormalities of endocrine glands, ectopic production of hormones, abnormal conversion of prohormones to their active forms, or iatrogenic factors. But endocrine abnormalities may also be due to changes in the responses (either enhanced or diminished) of target tissues to hormones. These disorders can occur by a variety of mechanisms (Fig. 1-4).

Hormone Deficiency Syndromes

HYPOFUNCTION OF ENDOCRINE GLANDS

Endocrine glands may be injured or destroyed by neoplasia, infections, hemorrhage, autoimmune disorders, and other causes. The destruction may be acute but is commonly chronic, with normal basal hormone production until late in the disease. The gland is usually compromised in its reserve capacity before the basal level of secretion falls and it cannot respond normally in circumstances in which an increase in hormone production is needed. Such partial defects may therefore not be detected by measurement of basal hormone levels and may require other testing of the reserve function of the gland. Since many manifestations of endocrine disease require weeks or even months to develop, the clinical presentation may vary over a considerable range, depending on the rapidity of glandular destruction.

As would be expected, a deficiency of a hormone that controls the synthesis and release of another hormone may result in a syndrome which simulates a primary deficiency of that target organ. Thus, hypothalamic lesions resulting in impaired secretion of releasing hormones may be manifested by pituitary dysfunction, and the latter may result in abnormalities in the function of its various target organs (gonads, thyroid, adrenals) (Chaps. 7 and 8).

Genetic defects can cause endocrine hypofunction, usually because of abnormalities in hormone synthesis and rarely because of the production of an abnormal hormone (as documented for insulin in rare forms of diabetes mellitus) (Chap. 19). These genetic defects in hormone synthesis may be partial or complete. For example, a rare form of growth hormone deficiency is due to deletion of the growth hormone gene (Chap. 26). A partial defect may be somewhat analogous to incomplete destruction of the gland—i.e., basal hormone production may be normal but reserve may be inadequate. In fact, sometimes genetic defects present not with the problems of hormone deficiency but with manifestations of a compensatory adaptation. For example, partial blocks in thyroid hormone biosynthesis may result in an enlarged thyroid gland (goiter) that is due to the TSH hypersecretion resulting from low levels of thyroid hormone (Chaps. 10 and 11). In the 17α-hydroxylase deficiency syndrome there is defective cortisol production and consequent ACTH hypersecretion, with excessive production of adrenocorticosteroids that are not 17α-hydroxylated (Chap. 12). One of these, corticosterone, substitutes for cortisol, so manifestations of cortisol deficiency are not observed. On the other hand, excessive compensatory synthesis of corticosterone and deoxycorticosterone leads to a mineralocorticoid excess syndrome with hypertension and hypokalemia.

HORMONE DEFICIENCY SECONDARY TO EXTRAGLANDULAR DISORDERS

In principle, a number of types of extraglandular disorders may result in hormone deficiency. These may involve defective conversion of prohormones to active forms, enhanced degradation of hormones, or the production of substances (antibodies, hormone antagonists) that block the actions of hormones. Impaired conversion of a prohormone to a hormone occurs in chronic renal failure and in vitamin D-dependent rickets type 1, in which there is defective conversion of 25-hydroxycholecalciferol to 1,25-dihydroxycholecalciferol (Chap. 23). A rare form of androgen deficiency is due to an abnormality in 5α-reductase, which converts testosterone to dihydrotestosterone (Chap. 18). In this condition there is only partial loss of androgenic effects, since testosterone itself is weakly active in some target tissues. Rare forms of diabetes mellitus result from antibodies to the insulin receptor that block insulin action (Chap. 19). Antibodies to insulin develop during insulin therapy of diabetes and may affect the availability of insulin (Chap. 19). Although no primary disorders are known to be due to enhanced hormone degradation, this may vary with other factors or disease states and may affect the response to exogenously administered hormones; for example, phenytoin and thyroid hormone increase the metabolism of certain glucocorticoids (Chap. 12). Also, such influences may unmask or aggravate a partial hormonal deficiency; for example, administration of thyroid hormones may unmask latent Addison's disease (Chap. 12).

HYPORESPONSIVENESS TO HORMONES

Hormone levels may be normal or even elevated in the presence of manifestations of endocrine deficiency. These conditions may be due to some of the problems listed above—e.g., antibodies to the insulin receptor (Chap. 19) and abnormal conversion of testosterone to dihydrotestosterone (Chap. 18). They may also be due to decreased ability of the endocrine target gland to respond to the hormone. Such disorders may be acquired or genetic, and they may be due to abnormalities at any step in the cascade of the hormone response from the receptor to the effect generated.

Several syndromes are associated with receptor abnormalities. The most commonly recognized abnormality of this type occurs in obese patients with type II diabetes mellitus (Chap. 19). In this case, chronic hyperinsulinemia induced by increased food intake induces insulin resistance, in part by down regulating the concentration of insulin receptors. Recognition of this problem also affects the therapy, since treatment is directed not only at correcting the hyperglycemia with insulin or other drugs but also at decreasing insulin need by dietary maneuvers that secondarily decrease insulin levels and thereby restore tissue sensitivity to the hormones. This form of diabetes also exhibits the additional abnormality whereby the pancreatic islets do not release insulin normally in response to glucose. In the testicular feminization syndrome there is unresponsiveness to androgens (Chap. 18). As a consequence, a female phenotype occurs in a person with a male genotype. Most persons with this X-linked disorder have a defect in the androgen receptor.

At least one disorder is due to an abnormality in the coupling of hormone-receptor complexes to effector mechanisms. In pseudohypoparathyroidism there are symptoms and chemical derangements of hypoparathyroidism associated with elevated PTH levels and insensitivity to this hormone (Chap. 23). In some of the patients this insensitivity is due to decreased levels of the guanyl nucleotide–binding regulatory protein that couples the PTH receptor complex to adenylate cyclase.

Overall damage to the hormone target tissue may result in insensitivity to hormones. For instance, renal disease may lead to insensitivity to vasopressin (Chap. 9), and liver disease may lead to insensitivity to glucagon (Chap. 19).

There are several forms of target organ insensitivity in which the molecular mechanisms have not been elucidated. One form of dwarfism is due to an impaired responsiveness to growth hormone, resulting in failure to generate somatomedin (Chap. 26). Vasopressin-resistant diabetes insipidus is not associated with frank renal disease (Chap. 9). There is a syndrome of hypercortisolism with decreased sensitivity to glucocorticoids (Chap. 12). In this case, the hypercortisolism compensates for the hyposensitivity, but the mineralocorticoid actions of the steroid also cause hypertension with hypokalemia.

ABNORMAL PRODUCTION OR ADMINISTRATION OF ANTAGONISTS

Rarely, endogenously produced or exogenously administered substances may produce a hormone-deficient state. Antibodies to the insulin receptor may produce insulin resistance with functional insulinopenia (Chap. 19). Cimetidine given for peptic ulcer disease[14] and spironolactone for hypertension (Chap. 14) may act as androgen antagonists and produce an androgen-deficient state.

Hormone Excess Syndromes

Hormone excess syndromes may result from hyperfunctioning endocrine glands, from ectopic hormone production by tumors, less commonly from influences on target tissues that enhance hormone sensitivity, from autoimmune disease in which antibodies cause hypersecretion of hormones or act as hormone agonists, from defects in hormone biosynthesis in which precursor hormones produced in excess have deleterious consequences, and from iatrogenic or therapeutic administration of hormones or substances that act like hormones.

HYPERFUNCTION OF ENDOCRINE GLANDS

The most common cause of hormone excess syndromes is hyperfunction of endocrine glands secondary to tumors of the glands or hyperplasia of several causes. Hyperfunctioning tumors of endocrine glands are usually well-differentiated adenomas (although carcinomas also occur), so the prognosis is usually favorable with early diagnosis. In addition to the manifestations of hormone excess, local extension of the tumor may produce symptoms.

Hyperplasia is a cause of hyperfunction of several of the endocrine glands (thyroid, adrenals, parathyroids). The most common form of thyroid hyperplasia appears to be due to an immunologic abnormality in which antibodies stimulate the gland in a manner similar to TSH (Chap. 10). Hyperplasia of the zona fasciculata and zona reticularis of the adrenal with consequent cortisol hypersecretion is usually due to ACTH hypersecretion by a pituitary tumor or an ectopic hormone–secreting tumor (Chaps. 12 and 29). The cause in other cases of endocrine gland hyperplasia is less clear, as with hyperplasia of the adrenal zona glomerulosa resulting in excessive aldosterone production (Chap. 14) or chief cell hyperplasia of parathyroid glands with PTH hypersecretion (Chap. 23).

ECTOPIC HORMONE PRODUCTION

Sometimes hormones are produced in excess by cells of endocrine or nonendocrine origin that are not normally the primary source of the hormone (Chap. 29). In most cases, hormones produced ectopically by tumors are those which arise from a single gene (e.g., ACTH, growth hormone, prolactin, PTH, calcitonin, gastrin, erythropoietin) or two genes (human chorionic gonadotropin, hCG). This may be due to the fact that the synthesis of other hormones (e.g., steroids, thyroid hormones, catecholamines) requires a large number of genes not ordinarily expressed by the tumor which would need to be activated to produce the hormone. Although a large number of different types of tumor can produce hormones, specific cell types are more commonly involved in this process (Chap. 29). For instance, APUD cells are commonly associated with ectopic hormone production. These cells are found in small-cell carcinoma of the lung, carcinoid tumors, thymomas, and other tumors. Although a number of molecular mechanisms are now understood that could explain how genes that are ordinarily not expressed are activated in tumors, those actually causing ectopic hormone production are not well understood.

IATROGENIC CAUSES

When hormones are used to treat nonendocrine diseases, when hormone replacement therapy is excessive, and sometimes when patients self-administer hormones (or their analogues), iatrogenic endocrine disease may occur. Patients will sometimes take excessive doses of glucocorticoids (Chap. 12) or thyroxine (Chap. 10) because these hormones produce a feeling of well-being. Rarely, administration of nonhormonal substances can cause hormonelike effects. Licorice ingestion can produce a syndrome mimicking primary aldosteronism, for example (Chap. 14).

TISSUE HYPERSENSITIVITY

Endocrine excess syndromes caused by hypersensitivity of target tissues are uncommon. Thyroid hormones increase the catecholamine receptors in certain tissues and thereby lead to excessive beta-adrenergic stimulation (Chap. 10). In this case, the hyperresponsiveness is actually part of the syndrome of hyperthyroidism. Many of the manifestations of primary aldosteronism are simulated in a rare syndrome with low plasma renin and aldosterone levels in which the kidney responds as if excessively stimulated by aldosterone (Chap. 14). Finally, disease of the target tissue itself can render it excessively sensitive to a hormone. For instance, cardiac arrhythmias, such as atrial fibrillation in thyrotoxicosis, probably occur most frequently in an already damaged heart (Chap. 10).

A lingering question is whether subtle abnormalities in the sensitivity to hormones contribute to the pathogenesis of disease more often than is generally perceived. With more refined methods for measuring alterations in sensitivity to hormones it may be possible to detect more subtle abnormalities. For instance, are some forms of essential hypertension due to increased sensitivity to pressor substances or decreased sensitivity to vasodilator substances (Chap. 14)? Are some forms of osteoporosis due to abnormalities in sensitivity to estrogens or to calcium-regulating hormones (Chap. 24)? Why do glucocorticoids increase the intraocular pressure (and even precipitate glaucoma) in some persons but not in others (Chap. 12)?

AUTOIMMUNE DISEASE

In addition to endocrine deficiency states which may be precipitated by autoimmune mechanisms (e.g., Schmidt's syndrome, discussed below and in Chap. 12), autoimmune disease can result in the production of antibodies that act as hormones. The most frequent situation in which this occurs is thyrotoxicosis (Graves' disease, Chap. 10). Rarely, antibodies to the insulin receptor are formed that have insulin-like actions (Chap. 19).

HORMONE BIOSYNTHETIC DEFECTS

Certain adrenal steroid biosynthetic defects (the 21α-and 11β-hydroxylase syndromes) result in overproduction of hormones proximal to the block; these syndromes are discussed in Chap. 12.

SECONDARY HORMONE HYPERSECRETION

Hypersecretion of hormones may be due to excessive physiologic stimulation of glands that are basically normal. The secondary hyperaldosteronism of hepatic disease and ascites, congestive heart failure, the nephrotic syndrome, and other conditions is illustrative (Chap. 12). The excess aldosterone aggravates the tendency to edema in these conditions. Secondary hyperparathyroidism occurs in azotemia (Chap. 24).

Multiple Endocrine Syndromes

Simultaneous involvement of more than one endocrine gland may result in syndromes of hyper- or hypofunction. The most common syndrome of multiple endocrine deficiences may involve the pancreatic islets, thyroid, adrenals, and gonads (Chap. 28). The disease appears to be caused by immunologic destruction of the glands. This may result from common antigenic determinants, caused possibly by a common developmental origin of the glands.

At least three syndromes of multiple endocrine hyperfunction result from hyperplasia, adenomas, or carcinomas of endocrine tissues, termed *multiple endocrine neoplasia* (MEN) types 1, 2, and 3 (Chap. 28). Type 1 is associated with hyperfunction of the parathyroids, pancreatic islets, and pituitary. In some cases more than one hormone may be produced by the tumor; islet cell tumors can produce insulin, glucagon, gastrin, vasoactive intestinal peptide (VIP), prostaglandins, ACTH, vasopressin, somatostatin, and serotonin. MEN type 2 is associated with pheochromocytoma (sometimes bilateral and extraadrenal), medullary carcinoma of the thyroid, and parathyroid hyperplasia. MEN type 3 is associated with medullary thyroid carcinoma, pheochromocytoma, and other features such as neuromas. These syndromes are often familial, with a dominant transmission, but the basic pathogenesis is unknown. In at least one of these types (MEN 1), hypersecretion of one hormone by a gland may produce hyperfunction and tumor formation in another gland: thus GRH hypersecretion by a pancreatic islet tumor leads to acromegaly and pituitary tumors.

Abnormalities of Endocrine Glands Not Associated with Hormonal Imbalance

Tumors, nodules, cysts, infiltrative diseases, and other abnormalities may involve endocrine glands without significantly impairing their secretory functions. For instance, nodules of the thyroid gland are common but usually nonfunctioning (Chap. 11). The major problem is that they may become malignant. Sometimes particular processes have a propensity for affecting an endocrine tissue; this is the case with tuberculosis and the adrenals (Chap. 12).

CLINICAL ASSESSMENT OF ENDOCRINE STATUS

The assessment of the endocrine status of a patient relies on findings from the history and physical examination and on laboratory testing. The latter may involve measurements of levels of hormones or their metabolites in plasma or urine, either in the basal state or in response to provocative testing. Laboratory tests may also be used to measure abnormalities that result from derangements in hormonal secretion and to evaluate the patient's sensitivity to hormones.

History and Physical Examination

Many syndromes of hormonal excess or deficiency display manifestations that are readily apparent at the time of initial presentation, e.g., severe thyrotoxicosis (Chap. 10) or Cushing's syndrome (Chap. 12). In other instances, the clinical presentation is more subtle and the physician must rely on laboratory testing to establish a diagnosis. This is especially true in the early stages of most endocrine problems, in elderly persons (e.g., with thyrotoxicosis or myxedema) (Chap. 10), or when the disease presents acutely and has not been present long enough for chronic manifestations to develop. Since it is beneficial to treat these diseases early, it is important for the physician to consider endocrine diseases in patients without full-blown manifestations, despite the fact that in the early stages of many of these disorders—e.g., adrenal insufficiency (Chap. 12), hypothyroidism (Chap. 10), Cushing's syndrome (Chap. 12), hyperparathyroidism (Chap. 23)—the presenting symptoms and signs are sufficiently vague to suggest more common problems. Thus, endocrine diseases should be considered in the differential diagnosis of many common problems, such as weakness, tiredness, vague gastrointestinal discomfort, hypertension, or weight loss or gain (Chap. 2). Once the diagnosis is considered, it is usually relatively easy to establish whether or not the disorder is present. Since endocrine diseases may be caused by primary processes external to the endocrine systems, the physician should consider these in taking the history and performing the physical examination. Sometimes the primary process (e.g., carcinoma of the lung producing ACTH, tuberculosis causing adrenal insufficiency) will so dominate the clinical presentation that hormonal abnormalities are more difficult to detect clinically.

Laboratory Testing

HORMONE LEVELS

Over the past few decades, assays have been developed to measure the levels of most of the hormones in body fluids. These assays vary in the ease with which they can be performed and their overall reliability; some assays are generally available, while others are performed only in certain research institutions. These latter are described in detail in Chap. 6.

Radioimmunoassay

The advent of radioimmunoassay, first developed for measuring plasma insulin levels, was a major breakthrough in endocrinology. Antibodies that are relatively specific for certain chemical groups or conformations of the hormone can be developed for the polypeptide hormones and also for the smaller ligands such as thyroid and steroid hormones. The success of the assay depends on the specificity of the antibody as well as its affinity for the hormone.

In most cases, radioimmunoassay yields extremely accurate information. However, there are problems the physician should consider in interpreting the results. The antibody may cross-react with related hormones or with precursors or metabolites of the hormone. If these compounds are present in sufficient concentration, they can give spuriously high values. For instance, some antibodies are specific for the carboxy-terminal portion of PTH (Chap. 23). This part of the molecule is present in certain circulating fragments of PTH that are biologically inactive. This is especially true in chronic renal disease, in which PTH levels by radioimmunoassay are extremely high. This problem can be avoided by the use of antibodies that are specific for other parts of the PTH molecule.

Competitive Protein-Binding and Radioreceptor Assays

These assays depend on the availability of a protein that binds the hormone with high affinity and specificity. The protein may be the normal receptor for the hormone or it may be another protein, usually a plasma hormone–binding protein such as CBG, TBG, or sex hormone–binding globulin (SHBG). The assay is performed in a manner analogous to the radioimmunoassay.

These assays provide an indication of summed products of the affinities times the concentrations of all compounds in the sample that bind to the protein. Typically, however, only one hormone accounts for most or all of the activity that is present. Radioreceptor assays are not widely used currently, in part because it is difficult to work with receptor preparations, but several competitive protein-binding assays were for a time in general use. Noteworthy are the CBG-isotope and TBG assays for cortisol and thyroxine, respectively, which depend on the fact that the major chemical substance in plasma that binds to CBG is cortisol and the major substance that binds to TBG is thyroxine.

Chemical Assay

Many hormones can be assayed by chemical means. For example, the fluorimetric assay for cortisol depends on the fluorescence of steroids with Δ^4-3-ketone, 20-ketone, and 11β-and 21-hydroxyl groups. Ordinarily, cortisol is the only steroid present in the circulation at sufficient concentration to react significantly in this way, although in certain congenital adrenal biosynthetic defects and adrenal carcinomas other steroids can contribute substantially to the assay results.

High-Performance Liquid Chromatography

The development of more sophisticated high-performance liquid chromatography (HPLC) techniques has increased the capability of the methods for routine measurements. Although these methods are not commonly used for hormone measurements, they will probably be used increasingly for the measurement of smaller molecules such as steroids, catecholamines, and small peptides.

Levels of Free Hormone

Free hormone, rather than that which is protein-bound, is usually the best index of the effective concentration of the hormone in plasma. The problems with assessment of total hormone concentrations caused by potential variations in the concentrations of plasma steroid and thyroid hormone–binding proteins have been emphasized earlier in this chapter.

Levels of free hormone can be assessed in several ways. (1) The free hormone can be physically separated from that which is plasma-bound and measured directly, although this method has not yet come into general use. (2) The plasma concentration of the binding protein can be measured directly. Again, this approach has not been applied widely. (3) The saturation of the binding protein can be assessed. When plasma levels of binding proteins are high, the protein will be undersaturated and less of the total hormone will be free, whereas the converse occurs when plasma levels are low. This approach is now used in the case of thyroid hormone (Chap. 10). Thus, the T_3 uptake assay measures the capacity of plasma for T_3 binding, which reflects the extent of saturation of thyroid hormone–binding proteins. By combining knowledge of the total T_4 levels and the extent of saturation of the proteins, a reasonable estimate of the effective free plasma hormone concentration can be obtained (Chap. 10). The same reasoning is applied to the measurement of free testosterone, used in the evaluation of hirsutism (Chap. 17). (4) An index of the free hormone concentration can sometimes be obtained by measuring the urinary excretion of the free hormone (or that of one of its metabolites). For instance, a small fraction (less than 1 percent) of the secreted cortisol is excreted unchanged into the urine (Chap. 12). A measurement of the 24-h urine free cortisol usually provides a reasonable estimate of the integrated levels of free plasma hormone. In essence this method uses the glomerular basement membrane to separate hormone that is bound from that which is free.

Secretion and Production Rates

Hormone production can be assessed by more complicated assays that involve either the injection of radioactive tracers or a combined assessment of plasma levels and hormone excretion. These techniques can circumvent many of the problems in interpretation associated with measurements of plasma or urinary hormones alone. Unfortunately, these procedures are cumbersome and not generally available.

Selective Sampling

Sometimes more accurate indications of a hormone excess state and the site of hormone hypersecretion can be obtained by assaying the venous effluent from a given gland or organ. For example, in renovascular hypertension, peripheral renin levels may be normal, but sampling from a catheter inserted into the renal veins may reveal renin hypersecretion from one side and hyposecretion from the other side (Chap. 14). Pituitary venous effluent sampling from the petrosal sinuses can be useful to determine whether ACTH hypersecretion results from a pituitary adenoma or from an ectopic site (Chap. 12).

Clinical Interpretation

With marked hormone excess or deficiency states, plasma or urinary hormone measurements commonly provide a clear indication of the abnormality. Nevertheless, it is important to be aware of the limitations of such tests. Hormone levels increase and decrease with physiologic stimuli, the presence of which must be considered when evaluating the significance of a hormone determination. For instance, plasma insulin levels should be evaluated in relation to the plasma glucose concentration (Chap. 19), and PTH levels should be considered in relation to the serum calcium levels (Chap. 23). Basal hormone secretion may not reflect the functional capacity of the gland, as considered in more detail under Dynamic Testing, below. Hormone levels should be evaluated in relation to target cell sensitivity. For example, in type I diabetes mellitus plasma insulin levels are often elevated but may still be inappropriately low in view of the associated hyperglycemia and insulin resistance (Chap. 19). Since the release of many hormones is not constant, random readings can be particularly misleading. Cortisol, for example, is released episodically (Chap. 12). In Cushing's syndrome, the number of these episodic releases may be increased. Although this commonly results in an elevation of the plasma cortisol throughout the day, the morning plasma levels of this steroid may be normal. Since cortisol production integrated over a 24-h period is increased in Cushing's syndrome, the 24-h urinary free cortisol provides a more accurate index of cortisol hypersecretion.

Although urinary measurements can sometimes be more useful than plasma assays for obtaining an integrated assessment of the production of certain hormones (especially steroids), they cannot be used in this way for other hormones (e.g., thyroid hormones) whose metabolites are not predominantly secreted into the urine. Further, urinary metabolites of steroids can sometimes be derived from several sources (e.g., 17-ketosteroids from the adrenals and gonads), and hormone excretion can be influenced by changes in renal function. There are also circumstances in which the quantities of metabolites (e.g., of aldosterone) can be primarily affected by factors that do not affect the production of the hormone.

Sometimes the significance of hormone levels can be evaluated only by the simultaneous measurement of more than one hormone. For instance, with progressive damage to the thyroid gland and impaired release of thyroid hormones, secretion of TSH increases in a compensatory fashion so that normal plasma levels of the thyroid hormones may be maintained (Chap. 10). By simultaneously measuring thyroid hormone levels and TSH, an indication of the compensatory response can be obtained. Such a simultaneous assessment of linked hormones can also provide an indication of the site of a primary defect. Plasma estrogens are low in ovarian failure (Chap. 17). If ovarian failure is due to disease of the ovary, plasma gonadotropins will be elevated. If ovarian failure is secondary to pituitary or hypothalamic disease, plasma gonadotropin levels will be normal or decreased.

DYNAMIC TESTING

Provocative testing assesses the ability of a gland to respond to stimuli as an index of its reserve capacity. This is especially useful when plasma or urinary hormone measurements are borderline. It can also yield information about the site of the endocrine defect. In some cases, a hormone is administered that stimulates the release of one or more other hormones. For example, the administration of GnRH stimulates LH and FSH release (Chap. 8), and TRH stimulates TSH and prolactin release (Chap. 8). In other cases, hormone production is blocked to interrupt normal feedback inhibition. Metyrapone blocks cortisol production by inhibiting 11β hydroxylation, thereby stimulating ACTH release (Chap. 12). The elevated ACTH levels increase the release of adrenal steroids proximal to the block (e.g., 11-deoxycortisol). Sometimes a physiologic stimulus to hormone release is given. Insulin-induced hypoglycemia is used to assess the secretory ability of cells that produce ACTH and growth hormone (Chap. 8). With endocrine hyperfunction, provocative tests can assess the extent to which the normal physiologic mechanisms that control hormone release are suppressed or the degree of autonomy of the hormone-producing tumor or hyperplastic gland. In primary aldosteronism resulting from an aldosterone-producing adenoma, the plasma renin levels are suppressed by excessive sodium retention and will not rise with acute postural, salt restriction, or diuretic stimuli (Chap. 14). In Cushing's syndrome resulting from ectopic secretion of ACTH by a tumor, the glucocorticoid dexamethasone will not ordinarily suppress the elevated ACTH levels (Chap. 12).

TESTS THAT PROVIDE INDIRECT INFORMATION

Useful information can frequently be obtained from laboratory tests that provide an index of the actions of the hormones (or a lack of them) or else an indication of the primary process causing the endocrine disease. Thus, in the case of diabetes mellitus, diagnosis and assessment of therapy depend on measurement of plasma glucose rather than insulin levels (Chap. 19). In like manner, it is helpful to follow the serum calcium levels in hyperparathyroidism (Chap. 23) and the serum potassium levels in primary aldosteronism (Chap. 14). Such tests often provide indices of the severity of the condition that are even more important than the hormone level. In conditions in which immunologic processes are important, assessment of antibody levels can be helpful. Other tests provide information that is more corroborative in nature but which nonetheless can be useful. For instance, the serum sodium is almost always greater than 139 meq/liter in patients with an aldosterone-producing adenoma (Chap. 14); the plasma cholesterol tends to be high in hypothyroidism and low in hyperthyroidism (Chap. 10); the serum potassium tends to be high in Addison's disease (Chap. 12); the alkaline phosphatase tends to be elevated in osteomalacia (Chap. 24); and the serum phosphate level tends to be elevated in acromegaly (Chap. 8).

EVALUATION OF THE SENSITIVITY OF TARGET CELLS TO HORMONES

Suspicion of hyposensitivity to a hormone is raised when manifestations of deficiency of the hormone occur in the presence of elevated hormone levels. In type 2 diabetes mellitus there is hyperglycemia with hyperinsulinism (Chap. 19); in pseudohypoparathyroidism, hypocalcemia is observed in the face of elevated PTH levels (Chap. 23), and pseudohermaphroditism caused by the testicular feminization syndrome is characterized by decreased androgenization with elevated plasma testosterone levels (Chap. 18). The existence of hyposensitivity can be confirmed by administering the hormone in question and determining the presence or extent of response, although commonly it is not necessary to do this. In some cases, as with insulin or androgen resistance, it is possible to obtain further confirmation of the hyposensitivity state by isolating cells from the patient and measuring receptors or responses, although the techniques for this are not generally available. Conversely, hypersensitivity to hormones is characterized by low hormone levels relative to the response. In low-renin essential hypertension the adrenal glomerulosa is excessively sensitive to angiotensin II (Chap. 14). This is reflected by normal to elevated plasma aldosterone levels in the presence of low angiotensin II levels. This sensitivity can be documented by measuring the plasma aldosterone levels following an infusion of angiotensin.

TREATMENT OF ENDOCRINE DISEASES

For endocrine deficiency syndromes, hormones are generally administered to replace the deficiency. In general, the hormone that is deficient is replaced. In some cases this is not possible or expedient, and other hormones are given that help compensate for the defect. For instance, vitamin D is given instead of PTH to treat hypoparathyroidism, since it can increase the extracellular Ca^{2+} (Chap. 23). In cases in which hormone resistance is present, steps are taken when possible to alleviate this, as through diet restriction in type II diabetes (Chap. 19).

In hormone-excess syndromes, a variety of approaches are used. Hyperfunctioning tumors are removed when possible, and sometimes hyperplastic glands are removed. In other cases drugs are given to block hormone production, such as propylthiouracil in thyrotoxicosis (Chap. 10) and bromocriptine for prolactin-producing adenomas (Chap. 8). Antagonists such as spironolactone can sometimes be useful in primary aldosteronism due to hyperplasia (Chap. 14).

For both excess and deficiency syndromes adjunctive therapy is frequently important. Thus multiple measures are used to treat the complications of diabetes mellitus, and patients with Addison's disease are cautioned to avoid stress (Chap. 12).

HORMONE THERAPY

Finally, it should be remembered that hormones, which affect so many processes, are also used extensively to treat diseases that do not have a primary endocrine basis. For example, glucocorticoids are used to treat a large number of conditions (Chap. 15), releasing factors such as GnRH are used to block gonadotropin release (Chap. 17), steroid antagonists are used to treat hormone-responsive tumors (Chap. 30), and catecholamines are used to treat shock and other cardiovascular problems (Chap. 13).

REFERENCES

1. Dexter TM, Heyworth C, Whepton AD: The role of growth factors in hemopoiesis. *Bioassays* 2:154, 1984.
2. Bishop JM: Cellular oncogenes and retroviruses. *Annu Rev Biochem* 52:301, 1983.
3. Bishop JM: Viral oncogenes. *Cell* 42:23, 1985.
4. Kingston RE, Baldwin AS, Sharp PA: Transcriptional control by oncogenes. *Cell* 41:3, 1985.
5. Feldman M: Lymphokines and interleukins emerge from the primeval soup. *Nature* 313:351, 1985.
6. Duff G: Many roles for interleukin-I. *Nature* 313:352, 1985.
7. Rosenberg LE: Disorders of propionate and methylmalonate metabolism, in Stanbury JB, Wyngaarden JB, Frederickson DA, Goldstein JL, Brown MS (eds): *The Metabolic Basis of Inherited Disease.* New York, McGraw-Hill, 1983, pp 474–479.
8. Tomkins GM: The metabolic code. *Science* 189:760, 1975.
9. Baxter JD, Rousseau GG: Glucocorticoids and the metabolic code, in Baxter JD, Rousseau GG (eds): *Glucocorticoid Hormone Action.* Heidelberg, Springer-Verlag, 1979, pp 613–627.
10. Bern HA, Knowles FGW: Neurosecretion, in Martini L, Ganong WF (eds): *Neuroendocrinology*, vol 1. New York, Academic, 1966, pp 139–186.

11. Scharrer E: Principles of neuroendocrine regulation. Endocrines and the central nervous system. *Assoc Res Nerv Ment Dis* 43:1, 1966.
12. Pearse AGE: The cytochemistry and ultrastructure of polypeptide hormone-producing cells of the APUD series and the embryologic, physiologic and pathologic implications of the concept. *J Histochem Cytochem* 47:303, 1969.
13. Pearse AGE: The diffuse neuroendocrine system and the APUD concept: Related "endocrine" peptides in brain, intestine, pituitary placenta and anuran cutaneous glands. *Med Biol* 55:115, 1977.
14. Funder JW, Mercer J: Cimetidine, a histamine H_2-receptor antagonist, occupies androgen receptors. *J Clin Endocrinol* 48:189, 1979.

2

The Clinical Manifestations of Endocrine Disease

Lawrence A. Frohman
Philip Felig
Arthur E. Broadus
John D. Baxter

Diseases of the endocrine-metabolic system account for some of the most common disorders encountered in humans—diabetes, obesity, and thyroid abnormalities. In recent years, a host of newer laboratory techniques, including radioimmunoassay, receptor methodology, recombinant DNA techniques, hormone stimulative and suppressive procedures, and advances in diagnostic imaging have markedly enhanced diagnosis and clarified the pathophysiology of such diseases. Nevertheless, in many instances the disorder remains unrecognized until relatively late in its course; symptoms may be attributed to some other disease process, and laboratory results may be confusing rather than helpful. Some of the difficulties relate to the complex clinical presentation and the multiplicity of organ systems which may be affected by a given disease process (e.g., thyrotoxicosis may masquerade as an intractable cardiac arrhythmia in an apathetic patient). A second problem concerns the nonspecific nature of some symptoms (e.g., weakness may be the major complaint in Addison's disease).

A further difficulty may arise from the laboratory tests. The striking biochemical and physiological disturbances which occur in endocrine disease, often with only minimal anatomic changes or physical findings (e.g., diabetes, hyperparathyroidism), tend to focus the physician's attention on the laboratory results, frequently without consideration of the total clinical picture. For the patient with asymptomatic hypercalcemia due to hyperparathyroidism, early diagnosis and treatment based on an elevated serum calcium level obtained during routine multiphasic laboratory screening may prevent subsequent development of bone disease or renal stones. On the other hand, an elevation in the serum thyroxine level of a euthyroid patient may lead to inappropriate use of antithyroid drugs if the physician fails to obtain a history of estrogen use. Similarly, the finding of a small adrenal nodule on abdominal computed tomographic evaluation for some specific but unrelated complaint (e.g., abdominal pain) may also lead to confusion and unnecessary diagnostic or therapeutic procedures.

Consequently, the clinical approach which is most successful in diagnosis and management is that which combines a high index of suspicion with knowledge of the various clinical constellations in which endocrine-metabolic disorders may appear, plus an understanding of the indications, interpretation, and inherent weaknesses of various testing procedures. In this chapter the major clinical signs and symptoms which may call attention to a variety of endocrine-metabolic disorders are reviewed. Various testing procedures are considered in Chap. 6.

GENERALIZED SYMPTOMS

Hormones affect the function of all tissues and organ systems. Consequently the symptoms and signs of endocrine disease are extremely diverse. They may vary from generalized, such as fatigue, to localized, such as weakness of the extraocular muscles. The variable nature of the clinical presentations of many endocrine disorders may result in their going unrecognized for prolonged periods (e.g., the failure to recognize, particularly in the elderly, recurrent supraventricular tachycardia or heart failure as a manifestation of hyperthyroidism). On the other hand, there is a tendency (both in the lay population and in the medical community) to attribute an endocrine basis to common complaints even when evidence is lacking. For example, hypoglycemia is often invoked to explain weakness and depression, obesity is frequently attributed to a "slow metabolism," and baldness is often ascribed to "glandular dysfunction." While each of these symptoms may in fact be due to an endocrine-metabolic disorder, the diagnosis should rest not on the nature of the symptom but on rigorous clinical and laboratory evaluation.

Weakness and Fatigue

Weakness generally refers to an overall lack of strength (easy fatigability, "loss of pep") which may be persistent or episodic in nature. Persistent weakness may reflect altered muscle function, as in some types of endocrine myopathy, or electrolyte disturbance, dehydration, or the effects of hormonal lack or excess through mechanisms which are poorly understood.

Generalized weakness is a common complaint in patients with Addison's disease or panhypopituitarism. In spontaneous or iatrogenic Cushing's syndrome weakness secondary to steroid-induced myopathy may be observed. Both hypothyroidism and hyperthyroidism may result in fatigue even when there is hyperactivity and nervousness in the hyperthyroid state.

Hypokalemia accompanying hyperaldosteronism, other mineralocorticoid-excess states, or Bartter's syndrome and hypercalcemia of hyperparathyroidism or malignant disease may result in a generalized decrease in strength. In the poorly controlled diabetic or in a patient with Addison's disease dehydration may result in or worsen weakness. Furthermore, in some diabetics even in the absence of severe hyperglycemia, postprandial fatigue and somnolence may be reversed by improved regulation of the blood glucose.

Patients with depression, which is common in many endocrine dysfunctions, frequently complain of fatigue or weakness. A distinction between weakness due to organic dysfunction and a feeling of fatigue due to depression can often be made. Patients with depression commonly feel "too weak" to initiate physical activity, whereas those with true weakness generally notice difficulty in the process of exertion or attempted exercise.

Episodic weakness may be caused by hypoglycemia in patients with an insulinoma. Since a marked fall in blood glucose results either in a counterregulatory response which restores the blood glucose to normal or in impairment in brain function (syncope or seizures), persistent generalized weakness lasting for days to weeks cannot be ascribed to hypoglycemia. Episodic weakness may also be observed in patients with pheochromocytoma or the carcinoid syndrome as a manifestation of paroxysmal hormonal release and in thyrotoxicosis complicated by periodic paralysis.

Weight Loss

A decrease in body weight in the absence of voluntary or involuntary caloric restriction or a marked increase in exercise generally indicates the presence of an underlying disease process. From a diagnostic standpoint it is useful to differentiate weight loss associated with anorexia from that occurring in association with hyperphagia or a normal appetite. In the absence of anorexia or diuresis, an increase in metabolic rate, abnormal losses of calorie-containing substrates in urine (e.g., glycosuria or ketonuria), or failure of gastrointestinal absorption must be present in the patient with weight loss. In hyperthyroidism and in decompensated diabetes (in which there is marked glycosuria) weight loss in the presence of hyperphagia is frequently observed. Weight loss due to increased caloric expenditure may also be observed in pheochromocytoma. In patients with severe diabetic neuropathy involving the autonomic nervous system, digestive and absorptive processes may be impaired, resulting in severe cachexia despite seemingly adequate caloric consumption.

Weight loss associated with anorexia is observed in Addison's disease, hyperparathyroidism, and other hypercalcemic states. In hypothyroidism weight loss may occur in the presence of hypometabolism because of accompanying anorexia. In anorexia nervosa a severe disturbance of appetite (reflecting a psychologic and/or hypothalamic disturbance) results in weight loss to the point of cachexia.

Weight Gain

An increase in body weight may reflect an accumulation of interstitial fluid (edema) or an increase in body fat (adiposity). Weight gain due to fluid retention can generally be recognized by palpable edema or rapidity of the increment in weight. A gain in weight of 1 kg or more per day invariably indicates fluid retention.

Weight gain due to an increase in adipose tissue is observed in Cushing's syndrome, where there is a characteristic truncal (rather than peripheral) distribution, a "buffalo hump" (increased fat over the lower part of the back of neck), and large supraclavicular fat pads. In patients with insulin-producing islet-cell tumors a weight gain of 10 to 15 kg may be observed because of repeated bouts of hypoglycemia resulting in appetite stimulation and increased food intake. Hypometabolism due to hypothyroidism may also result in an increase in body fat. However, fluid retention may also contribute to weight gain in hypothyroidism, as reflected by fluid excess in myxedematous tissues or the presence of ascites or pleural or pericardial effusions.

Obesity is commonly observed in association with type 2 diabetes. However, it is the obesity which is the predisposing factor to the development of diabetes rather than the reverse. In rare circumstances, disturbances of hypothalamic satiety centers result in weight gain; this may be observed in patients with central nervous system disease (trauma, encephalitis, or tumors) or pituitary tumors with sufficient suprasellar extension to compress the ventral hypothalamus.

It should be noted that primary endocrine-metabolic disorders account for less than 5 percent of all cases of obesity (body weight 30 percent or more above ideal). Furthermore, extreme degrees of weight gain—body weight in excess of 115 to 135 kg (250 to 300 lb)—are almost never due to a primary endocrine disturbance. On the other hand, obesity may *secondarily* result in a variety of alterations in endocrine and metabolic processes.

Edema may be observed in association with cardiac failure accompanying thyrotoxicosis, myxedema, or acromegaly. In severe anorexia nervosa or in diabetic nephropathy resulting in proteinuria, edema may develop as a consequence of hypoalbuminemia. Edema is generally not observed in patients with primary hyperaldosteronism. On the other hand, corticosteroids exhibiting a mineralocorticoid effect may precipitate or exacerbate fluid accumulation when administered to patients with underlying cardiac disease. Mineralocorticoids used in the treatment of Addison's disease rarely cause edema when given in excess in the absence of manifest cardiac disease.

Body Temperature

A mild increase in body temperature may be observed in thyrotoxicosis. In thyroid storm (an acute exacerbation of hyperthyroidism), a fever of 101°F or more is characteristic. Hyperpyrexia may occur in primary hypothalamic disease, in secondary disturbances of hypothalamic function following pituitary surgery, or in severely decompensated Addison's disease. Cerebral edema, a rare complication of diabetic ketoacidosis, may also result in high fever. Mild increases in temperature may also be seen in untreated Addison's disease. However, caution must be exercised in attributing fever in Addison's disease or diabetic ketoacidosis to the endocrine problem, since infections may be responsible for aggravating these conditions.

Hypothermia is common in hypoglycemia, particularly when induced by alcohol. Severe hypothyroidism (myxedema coma) may also be complicated by hypothermia. Hypothermia may be missed on routine physical examination unless care is taken to "shake down" the thermometer to below 96°F (35.5°C) prior to its insertion.

SKIN

Hyperpigmentation of the skin is a characteristic finding in Addison's disease. It is accentuated in the exposed parts of the body. The knuckles, elbows, knees, areolae, genitalia, buccal mucosa, palmar creases, and recent scars are the sites of maximum pigmentation. Similar pigment changes may occur in 15 to 60 percent of patients who undergo bilateral adrenalectomy as treatment for Cushing's disease (bilateral adrenal hyperplasia) and are usually indicative of the presence of an ACTH (adrenocorticotropic hormone)-producing pituitary tumor (Nelson's syndrome). Ectopic production of ACTH by various neoplasms (e.g., lung, pancreas) may also lead to hyperpigmentation. In acromegaly an increase in pigmentation is observed in as many as 40 percent of cases.

Acanthosis nigricans is a syndrome in which there are localized areas of gray-brown hyperpigmentation in the posterior region of the neck and axillae. It is frequently encountered in uncomplicated obesity but may also be seen in patients with polycystic ovaries, Cushing's syndrome, and acromegaly. Acanthosis nigricans has also been identified in rare diabetic patients with severe insulin resistance associated with a decrease in insulin receptors or the presence of a circulating antibody to the insulin receptor.

A generalized decrease in pigmentation occurs in panhypopituitarism. Focal areas of depigmentation (*vitiligo*) are observed in Addison's disease, thyrotoxicosis, and hypoparathyroidism.

Hirsutism, which is defined as an increase in facial hair in women beyond that which is cosmetically acceptable, is observed in a variety of androgen-excess states, including Cushing's syndrome, congenital adrenal hyperplasia, polycystic ovary syndrome, and virilizing ovarian or adrenal tumors. An increase in facial hair may also occur in acromegaly.

A decrease in body hair accompanying endocrine disease may be generalized (scalp, axillary and pubic areas, and extremities), localized to the scalp (*alopecia*), or restricted to the lateral third of the eyebrow. In hypopituitarism and hypothyroidism any of these patterns may be noted. In Cushing's syndrome and virilizing ovarian or adrenal tumors frontal baldness may occur. Hair loss may also be observed in thyrotoxicosis and hypoparathyroidism. Most patients with severe alopecia, however, do not have an endocrine disease.

Coarse, dry skin is found in myxedema and in hypoparathyroidism. In the former the changes may be so marked as to resemble ichthyosis. In acromegaly the skin is also coarse and has a leathery texture with enlargement of the sweat glands and a true thickening of the various skin layers.

Excessive sweating occurs in thyrotoxicosis and acromegaly. Acute paroxysms of sweating accompanying adrenergic discharge are observed in pheochromocytoma and during hypoglycemic episodes in patients with insulinomas, also in insulin-treated diabetics experiencing an insulin reaction.

Acne is observed in men and women with Cushing's syndrome or androgen-producing tumors of the adrenal and in women with congenital adrenal hyperplasia, polycystic ovaries (idiopathic hirsutism, persistent estrus syndrome), and virilizing tumors of the ovary.

Striae, plethora, thinning of the skin, easy bruisability, and ecchymoses may be observed in spontaneous Cushing's syndrome or after glucocorticoid therapy in pharmacologic doses.

NOSE, VOICE, AND TONGUE

The hypertrophy of mucous membranes which occurs in acromegaly results in pale, boggy nasal mucosa, frequently associated with symptoms of nasal and sinus obstruction. Hyperplasia of the membranes of the eustachian tube often results in intermittent middle-ear blockage and recurrent episodes of serous otitis media. Pituitary tumors may erode the floor of the sella and extend into the floor of the sphenoid sinus and even into the nose. With rupture of the dura, cerebrospinal rhinorrhea may occur. The latter can be diagnosed by the presence of glucose in the nasal discharge, which is detected by use of a glucose oxidase–impregnated dip stick.

Loss of olfaction can be due to a tumor in the region of the hypothalamus which destroys the olfactory nerve. It can also be seen with Kallman's syndrome, a congenital form of hypothalamic hypogonadism.

The tongue is increased in size and frequently furrowed in acromegaly. In more severe cases difficulty in articulation can be noted. The tongue, palate, and buccal and gingival mucosa are often hyperpigmented in Addison's disease and with ACTH-producing pituitary tumors, particularly after adrenalectomy (Nelson's syndrome). There are discrete patches of hyperpigmentation in each of these locations, which at times may be confluent. Tongue pigmentation may be present normally in blacks and is therefore of less diagnostic significance.

In hypothyroidism the tongue is enlarged because of myxedematous infiltration, often resulting in slurred speech. In hyperthyroidism a fine rhythmic tremor which is evident in the outstretched fingers is also present in the tongue. Fine fascicular movements of the tongue may occur in hyperparathyroidism.

In acromegaly, hypertrophy of the larynx leads to a huskiness of the voice; an increase in the paranasal sinuses tends to give the voice more resonance. Myxedematous infiltration of the larynx in hypothyroidism results in deepening of the voice and, occasionally, severe hoarseness. Laryngeal examination reveals dullness, thickening, and flabbiness of the free margins of the true vocal cords. With advanced myxedema, smooth edematous polyps may form on the vocal cords. Deepening of the voice frequently occurs in women in the presence of increased androgen secretion, as in Cushing's syndrome, congenital adrenal hyperplasia, or virilizing adrenal or ovarian tumors. In men the influence of excess androgens on the voice cannot be detected clinically unless it occurs during the prepubertal period, as in congenital adrenal hyperplasia. The voice changes do not always completely disappear upon removal of the excess androgen. Large goiters and invasive thyroid carcinomas can also produce hoarseness.

In males in whom pubertal changes fail to occur as a result of androgen deficiency due to a hypothalamic, pituitary, or gonadal disturbance, the voice remains high-pitched. However, once the voice has acquired the typical characteristics of an adult male, loss of androgen does not cause any change in quality.

GASTROINTESTINAL SYSTEM

Anorexia is often observed in primary hyperparathyroidism and other hypercalcemic conditions, Addison's disease, and diabetic ketoacidosis. A reduction in appetite may also occur in hypothyroidism, panhypopituitarism, and apathetic hyperthyroidism. Anorexia nervosa is characterized by abnormal ideation regarding body weight and food intake in addition to loss of appetite. Nausea and vomiting are often seen in diabetic ketoacidosis, in hyperparathyroidism and other disorders with significant hypercalcemia, and in Addison's disease.

An increase in appetite commonly accompanies hyperthyroidism, diabetes mellitus with moderate hyperglycemia, glucocorticoid therapy, and Cushing's syndrome and is seen in about 15 percent of patients with an insulinoma.

Oropharyngeal dysphagia may be caused by a large goiter or by a locally invasive thyroid carcinoma.

Abdominal pain occurs in a variety of endocrine disorders. Nonspecific, diffuse abdominal pain occurs frequently in children with diabetic ketoacidosis; if the pain is unresolved with control of the ketoacidosis, a primary intraabdominal event should be suspected. Ileus with gaseous and colicky pain may be observed in myxedema. Patients with addisonian crisis often present with diffuse abdominal pain. Less severe pain is a frequent complaint with chronic adrenal insufficiency. In thyroid storm abdominal pain may be a major complaint. Both acute and chronic patterns of abdominal pain occur in patients with the carcinoid syndrome. In primary hyperparathyroidism abdominal pain may be due to peptic ulcer disease or to pancreatitis. In addition, a minority of patients with this disease present with a diffuse and poorly described abdominal pain of uncertain cause which resolves with surgical correction of the hyperparathyroidism. Symptoms of severe or recurrent peptic ulcer are the most characteristic features of the Zollinger-Ellison syndrome. Gastrointestinal bleeding may complicate peptic ulceration in primary hyperparathyroidism and in the Zollinger-Ellison syndrome. Gastrointestinal bleeding may also occur in Turner's syndrome because of associated intestinal telangiectasia.

Constipation occurs frequently in hypothyroidism and in patients with marked hypercalcemia or hypokalemia. Constipation may also occur with pheochromocytoma. Patients with diabetic autonomic neuropathy may complain of constipation alternating with diarrhea; often the diarrhea is nocturnal in these patients and is accompanied by fecal incontinence.

Diarrhea may be prominent in patients with metastatic medullary carcinoma of the thyroid and in patients with a metastatic carcinoid tumor. Approximately one-third of those with the Zollinger-Ellison syndrome present with diarrhea; frank steatorrhea may be seen in both the Zollinger-Ellison and carcinoid syndromes. Hyperthyroidism is associated with an increased frequency of somewhat poorly formed stools rather than actual diarrhea. Explosive and life-threatening diarrhea dominates the clinical picture in patients with pancreatic cholera due to tumors of the islets that produce vasoactive intestinal polypeptide or other gastrointestinal neuroendocrine tumors.

Significant hepatic abnormalities are uncommon in endocrine disorders, but liver function tests may be abnormal in both severe thyrotoxicosis and myxedema and also in patients with far-advanced carcinoid tumors. In poorly controlled diabetics hepatomegaly due to fatty infiltration may be observed.

HEMATOPOIETIC SYSTEM

Anemia occurs frequently in a wide variety of endocrine disorders. The anemia may be a direct consequence of the specific endocrine deficiency or hypersecretion or may result from a complication of endocrine disease such as acute blood loss anemia or iron-deficiency anemia due to peptic ulcer disease in primary hyperparathyroidism or the Zollinger-Ellison syndrome.

A mild normocytic normochromic anemia with hypoplastic bone marrow regularly accompanies panhypopituitarism and is corrected by replacement therapy with thyroid, adrenal, and gonadal hormones. Growth-hormone deficiency, therefore, appears not to play a major role in the development of this anemia.

The anemia may be partially masked by a coincident contraction in plasma volume.

A mild to moderate anemia is commonly noted in hypothyroidism. The type of anemia that results specifically from deficiency of the thyroid hormones is a normocytic normochromic anemia with hypoplastic bone marrow. A decrease in erythropoietin production may explain the anemia in this condition; it is readily reversed by thyroid replacement therapy. The anemia most frequently encountered in hypothyroidism, however, is the microcytic hypochromic anemia of iron deficiency. Several mechanisms are responsible for this frequency of iron deficiency, including the high incidence of menorrhagia in female patients and the approximately 50 percent incidence of achlorhydria and iron malabsorption in patients of both sexes. A macrocytic hyperchromic anemia occurs in about 10 percent of patients with hypothyroidism and may be due to deficiency of vitamin B_{12} or folic acid or both. Although decreased gastric acid production, poor vitamin B_{12} absorption, and reduced serum levels of vitamin B_{12} are seen with considerable frequency in these patients, classic pernicious anemia occurs in only about 5 percent of hypothyroid patients. Patients with both antithyroid and antiparietal cell antibodies are of considerable interest but are quite uncommon.

Hyperthyroidism is usually not accompanied by anemia, although severely thyrotoxic patients may display a mild normocytic normochromic or hypochromic anemia. Pernicious anemia with antiparietal cell antibodies occurs in approximately 3 percent of patients with Graves' disease.

Patients with adrenal insufficiency have a mild normocytic normochromic anemia which is often not readily apparent because of the concomitant decrease in plasma volume. Patients with Cushing's disease display a mild erythrocytosis with hemoglobin levels 1 to 2 g/100 ml higher than normal; this is less often observed with the administration of pharmacologic doses of exogenous steroids.

Androgens have a well-known erythropoietic effect, and pharmacologic doses are employed in treating a variety of refractory anemias. This effect accounts for the higher hemoglobin values seen in sexually mature males than in females and prepubertal males.

A normocytic normochromic anemia occurring in about 20 percent of patients with primary hyperparathyroidism, particularly in patients with severe hypercalcemia, resolves following surgical correction of the disease. Iron-deficiency anemia may occur in hyperparathyroidism complicated by peptic ulcer disease and gastrointestinal bleeding.

Patients with a pheochromocytoma may display a slight increase in hemoglobin values because of the concomitant contraction in plasma volume. There may also be a direct catecholamine influence on erythropoietin production.

A relative leukopenia is frequently noted in panhypopituitarism. Approximately 10 percent of patients with thyrotoxicosis present with leukopenia and/or granulocytopenia. Failure to recognize leukopenia prior to instituting treatment with antithyroid drugs may lead to confusion, since these drugs (e.g., propylthiouracil) may suppress the granulocyte count. The lymphocyte number is normal or slightly increased in hyperthyroid patients, leading to a relative lymphocytosis. Lymphadenopathy occurs commonly in Graves' disease, and splenomegaly can be detected in about 10 percent of patients; these findings do not occur in patients with Hashimoto's thyroiditis. No consistent abnormalities in leukocyte values are noted in hypothyroidism. In Cushing's syndrome, mild granulocytosis, lymphopenia, and eosinopenia are commonly observed. The latter finding was for many years considered a diagnostic clue to the disorder. A lymphocytosis observed in Addison's disease in rare instances may be high enough to suggest leukemia. A leukocytosis of 15,000 to 30,000 cells per cubic millimeter regularly occurs in diabetic ketoacidosis, so a leukocyte count is of little value in suggesting infection as the initiating event leading to the ketoacidosis. A marked leukocytosis is also routinely observed in hyperosmolar nonketotic coma. A minority of patients with pheochromocytoma display a mild leukocytosis.

Glucocorticoids may acutely promote a rise in platelets; thrombocytosis may also be observed with chronic glucocorticoid excess.

CARDIOVASCULAR SYSTEM

Tachycardia almost always accompanies hyperthyroidism and pheochromocytoma. Ordinarily this is of sinus origin, but occasionally there may be paroxysmal atrial tachycardia or atrial fibrillation with a rapid ventricular response. (An ectopic arrhythmia with these conditions usually signifies underlying heart disease.) The tachycardia may give rise to palpitations. Tachycardia also occurs when there is dehydration, as with adrenocortical insufficiency due to destruction of the gland or 11β-hydroxylase deficiency, and in uncontrolled diabetes. There is ordinarily a bradycardia in hypothyroidism.

An increased incidence of myocardial infarction and stroke can be observed with any of the syndromes that result in hypercholesterolemia or hypertension. Hypercholesterolemia may be present with hypothyroidism and diabetes. Hypertension is associated with primary aldosteronism, pheochromocytoma, Cushing's syndrome, glucocorticoid therapy (occasionally), and renal disease (as in diabetes or hypercalcemia). It is likely that differences in endocrine secretions explain the greater incidence of myocardial infarction in men than in women before the menopause. An increased incidence of myocardial infarction and stroke is reportedly associated with the use of contraceptive steroids. Although these drugs affect lipid metabolism and can cause hypertension, the reasons for the increase in cardiovascular problems with their use are not established. The incidence of myocardial infarction, stroke, and peripheral vascular disease is increased with diabetes.

Typically, heart size is smaller than usual in Addison's disease, hypopituitarism, and hyperthyroidism. With hypothyroidism and any conditions associated with hypertension, the heart size may be increased and congestive heart failure may be present. Cardiac failure may accompany hyperthyroidism or pheochromocytoma, presumably because of the excessive demands on the heart due to the excessive beta-adrenergic stimulation associated with thyroid hormone or catecholamine excess. In younger people this rarely leads to congestive failure, but in the elderly, with underlying atherosclerotic disease, these conditions can lead to serious cardiac decompensation. Heart size is increased in acromegaly, though function may not be impaired.

Edema may accompany any circumstance in which there is congestive failure. It may accompany hypoproteinemia associated with diabetic nephropathy or severe anorexia nervosa. Surprisingly, it is uncommon in primary aldosteronism in spite of an increase in total body sodium.

Occasionally toxic reactions or resistance to the drugs used in the treatment of cardiovascular disease may signify endocrine disease. For instance, digitalis toxicity may be precipitated more rapidly in hyperthyroidism and pheochromocytoma and with hypokalemia, as in primary aldosteronism. Insensitivity to the bradycardia and antianginal effects of beta-adrenergic blockers may occur with hyperthyroidism.

URINARY TRACT

Frequency, polyuria, and nocturia (or enuresis in children) are classically observed in diabetes mellitus and in central or nephrogenic diabetes insipidus. Severe hypercalcemia or hypokalemia may impair renal tubular concentrating ability, so these symptoms may also be seen in patients with primary hyperparathyroidism and other hypercalcemic disorders and in patients with primary aldosteronism and Bartter's syndrome. Patients with diabetic autonomic neuropathy may complain of frequency, incontinence, or urinary retention.

Diabetes mellitus is associated with an increased incidence of urinary tract and mycotic vaginal and vulvar infections. Patients with diabetes are also prone to the development of papillary necrosis as a complication of pyelonephritis. A number of glomerular lesions occur in diabetes mellitus that are associated with proteinuria and progressive renal impairment. The most specific and important of these is nodular glomerulosclerosis. Mild proteinuria may also be observed in myxedema.

Nephrolithiasis and/or nephrocalcinosis occur in a variety of endocrine disorders. Renal stones are the most common specific complication of primary hyperparathyroidism. An increased incidence of stones is also observed in a number of other hypercalcemic or hypercalciuric conditions, including sarcoidosis, vitamin D intoxication, idiopathic hypercalciuria, and thyrotoxicosis, and possibly in patients with longstanding Cushing's disease and acromegaly. Nephrocalcinosis, with or without a history of stone or renal impairment, occurs in primary hyperparathyroidism, vitamin D intoxication, and the milk-alkali syndrome.

Turner's syndrome may be accompanied by a number of congenital renal abnormalities.

SEXUAL FUNCTION

Endocrine disease must be considered when there is impotence or a change in libido but accounts for only a small proportion of these problems. Changes in libido irregularly accompany hypo- and hyperfunctioning of the adrenal cortex and the thyroid gland, hypokalemia with primary aldosteronism or Bartter's syndrome, hypercalcemia, anorexia nervosa, gonadal failure (ovarian or testicular), poorly controlled diabetes, and hypopituitarism. Impotence can be observed with gonadal failure (primary or secondary), diabetes with autonomic neuropathy, drug therapy of hypertension (especially with methyldopa), and hypothyroidism. Hyperprolactinemia of any etiology but particularly that associated with pituitary tumors results in decreased libido in both sexes and, frequently, impotence. Any severe illness, including endocrine disease, may be associated with decreased libido, although in such illness it is unusual for this to be a prominent complaint.

Amenorrhea or oligomenorrhea can be observed in gonadal dysgenesis (e.g., Turner's syndrome), primary ovarian failure, the testicular feminizing and pseudohermaphroditic syndromes, Kallman's syndrome (gonadotropin deficiency associated with anosmia), the adrenogenital syndrome, or menopause. Menstrual disturbances generally occur in hypopituitarism, as in Sheehan's syndrome (panhypopituitarism secondary to pituitary necrosis in women who have suffered postpartum hemorrhagic shock), in patients with prolactin-secreting pituitary tumors, and in Chiari-Frommel syndrome (hyperprolactinemia associated with prolonged lactation and amenorrhea following delivery). Amenorrhea or oligomenorrhea may appear in women following discontinuation of oral contraceptives, especially if they have a history of prior menstrual irregularities. These problems may also occur in Cushing's syndrome, hyperthyroidism, hypothyroidism, anorexia nervosa, or polycystic ovaries (with increased estrogen and androgen production). When amenorrhea is associated with diabetes, adrenal insufficiency, or hypothyroidism, the syndrome of multiple endocrine deficiency (Schmidt's syndrome) should be considered. Most endocrinopathies in severe form can result in secondary amenorrhea.

Metrorrhagia, or bleeding between menstrual periods, can be present in hyperestrogen states resulting from a number of causes, including high-dose estrogen therapy. Spontaneous causes include anovulation secondary to diverse disorders and excess estrogen production due to tumors. For example, with anovulation associated with polycystic ovarian disease or the period just prior to and following the menarche, continued gonadotropin secretion results in the formation of a number of estrogen-producing nonovulatory graafian follicles. Tumors causing metrorrhagia may be of ovarian origin (e.g., thecoma, granulosa cell tumor) or of adrenal or pituitary origin. Ectopic production of trophic factors (e.g., ACTH) by tumors may secondarily stimulate estrogen production leading to metrorrhagia.

Infertility can result from any of the causes of amenorrhea or oligomenorrhea listed above. With oligomenorrhea there may be either oligoovulation or anovulation—the distinction is important, since pregnancy can occur in the former case. Infertility may result from a restricted luteal phase leading to defective support of the implantation of the fertilized egg. This situation results from deficient progesterone production due to either defective responsiveness to luteinizing hormone (LH) or inadequate LH production. The latter may result from pituitary disease or from defective hypothalamic function due to psychogenic or neurogenic problems.

In the male, endocrine problems resulting in hypothalamic-pituitary or testicular failure account for only a small proportion of cases of infertility or subfertility. Prolactin-producing pituitary tumors have been implicated in some cases of male infertility.

In the female, changes due to androgen excess are termed *virilization*. These include hirsutism (discussed above), male pattern baldness, deepened voice, acne, and clitoral enlargement. The excess androgens may be of ovarian or adrenal origin or may result from exogenous androgen administration. Excess androgen production of ovarian etiology may result from hyperplasia (as in polycystic ovaries or ovarian androgenic dysplasia) or tumor (e.g., arrhenoblastoma, hilar cell tumor, adrenal rest tumor, or gynandroblastoma). Excess adrenal androgen production may be due to Cushing's syndrome, enzyme defects (e.g., 11- or 21-hydroxylase deficiency), or neoplasia and in the absence of glucocorticoid excess may account for some cases of idiopathic hirsutism.

Precocious puberty may be due to a hormone-secreting tumor (most commonly ovarian but less commonly adrenal) or to constitutional, physiological, or organic disturbances (e.g., postencephalitis, postmeningitis, postcerebral trauma, hypothalamic lesions, pinealoma or other tumors of the central nervous system). It is characterized by early breast development, axillary and pubic hair, onset of menstrual periods, and, in true precocious puberty, fertility. True cyclic menses and fertility are not, however, seen with adrenal or ovarian tumors which suppress gonadotropin secretion and cause precocious pseudopuberty. Sometimes there may be isolated precocious breast development or appearance of pubic hair. A major problem with this syndrome is that there is premature closure of the epiphyses, and as a consequence many of the subjects are of short stature.

Gynecomastia, or abnormal breast enlargement, occurs physiologically in normal males at puberty, subsiding ordinarily during adolescence. It should be differentiated from breast enlargement due to excess fat tissue rather than ductal tissue (e.g., obesity and lipoma) and from breast tumors.

Gynecomastia may be caused by estrogen-producing tumors that are usually of adrenal origin (usually carcinomas) but may rarely be of chorionic, testicular granulosa cell or interstitial cell origin. It may also be seen in cirrhosis, presumably because of a decrease in the metabolic clearance of circulating estrogens.

Gynecomastia may occur after estrogen, androgen, digitalis, reserpine, hydralazine, meprobamate, phenothiazine, chorionic gonadotropin, or spironolactone therapy or marijuana use; and it may be seen in hypergonadotropic hypogonadism such as Klinefelter's syndrome or Reifenstein's syndrome. Gynecomastia may signify a pituitary or ectopic tumor (usually of pulmonary origin) producing prolactin (occasionally) or gonadotropins (rarely). Gynecomastia is sometimes seen after chronic hemodialysis, in hyperthyroidism, and during recovery from severe malnutrition.

Nonpuerperal lactation (galactorrhea) may occur as a consequence of several types of pituitary disturbance. Commonly, these are associated with increased prolactin production. Galactorrhea may occur after anesthesia, thoracic surgery, exercise, nipple stimulation, sexual intercourse, chest wall trauma, infection (herpes zoster), spinal cord lesions, and several drugs (phenothiazines, reserpine, methyldopa, and dopaminergic blockade). Galactorrhea is frequently associated with pituitary microadenoma. Galactorrhea is sometimes observed with acromegaly, other pituitary tumors, and destructive lesions of the hypothalamus and pituitary stalk. It may also be seen with hypothyroidism or estrogen therapy and is commonly observed in women with chronic renal failure.

BONES AND JOINTS

Decreased linear growth, dysgenetic epiphyseal centers, and ultimate dwarfing are observed in hypothyroidism occurring in childhood. Abnormalities in linear growth are also observed in poorly controlled diabetes mellitus, panhypopituitarism, isolated growth-hormone deficiency, and endogenous or exogenous glucocorticoid excess. Androgen excess produces an increased *rate* of linear growth, but premature closure of the epiphyseal centers ultimately leads to short stature. Short stature is also observed in Turner's syndrome.

Primary or secondary androgen insufficiency is associated with the development of eunuchoidal skeletal proportions. An unusual pattern of disproportionate growth of the lower extremities occurs in Klinefelter's syndrome.

Increased periosteal bone formation leads to typical facial and acral bone abnormalities in acromegaly. If the disease begins prior to epiphyseal closure, increase in linear growth leading to gigantism occurs as well. The various forms of rickets are associated with a number of bone deformities, including bowing of the limbs, frontal bossing, and beading of the ribs. Shortened fourth metacarpals occur regularly in pseudohypoparathyroidism and Turner's syndrome.

Osteoporosis is a feature of a variety of endocrine disorders. Osteoporosis occurs in endogenous and exogenous hyperadrenocorticism, adult hypophosphatasia and other metabolic bone diseases, and hypogonadism, as well as after premature ovarian failure. It is particularly severe in Turner's syndrome. Osteopenia is regularly observed in patients with longstanding hyperthyroidism or hyperprolactinemia; bone biopsies in these patients reveal a variable admixture of osteoporosis, osteomalacia, and osteitis fibrosa cystica. Osteoporosis is reported occasionally in acromegaly. Severe calcium deficiency may result in osteoporosis, but there is scant evidence to suggest that calcium deficiency plays a primary role in the osteoporosis commonly encountered in the United States. Mild osteopenia has been reported in both children and adults with diabetes mellitus.

Osteomalacia with diffuse bone pain and tenderness and muscular weakness occurs in simple vitamin D deficiency and in vitamin D and calcium malabsorption due to a number of gastrointestinal diseases. A variety of renal tubular disorders are associated with rickets in children and osteomalacia in adults. Tumor-associated osteomalacia is an unusual and particularly severe form of the disorder which occurs in association with mesenchymal neoplasms.

The factors responsible for anticonvulsant-associated osteomalacia are complex, and significant osteopenia is not commonly observed in patients receiving anticonvulsant therapy in the United States. Clinically significant osteitis fibrosa cystica may occur with severe primary hyperparathyroidism; mild clinical or subclinical osteopenia in patients with less severe hyperparathyroidism may be due to osteoporosis, osteomalacia, or mild osteitis. The pathogenesis of renal osteodystrophy is complex, and the predominant bone lesion in individual patients may be osteoporosis, osteomalacia, or osteitis fibrosa cystica. In the majority of patients with advanced renal insufficiency, several of these lesions coexist.

In acromegaly, bone overgrowth with distortion of the articular plate leads to degenerative arthritis, which may be severe and disabling. Chronic chondrocalcinosis (pseudogout) may occur in primary hyperparathyroidism; there are questionable associations between acute episodes of pseudogout and diabetes mellitus and between primary gout and primary hyperparathyroidism.

Increased levels of serum uric acid have been reported in primary hyperparathyroidism, myxedema, nephrogenic diabetes insipidus, Bartter's syndrome, and Paget's disease. Some reports suggest that episodes of acute gouty arthritis occur with increased frequency in several of these disorders. Marked elevations in serum uric acid may accompany diabetic ketoacidosis but resolve rapidly with control of the ketoacidosis.

CENTRAL NERVOUS SYSTEM

Headache is a common finding in pituitary tumors and is caused by pressure of the expanding tumor on the dura. With rupture of the dura, the headache frequently disappears. Headache is characteristically present in pituitary apoplexy and may be present as well in tumors of the hypothalamus or the parasellar region. Headache also occurs in pseudotumor cerebri, in hypertensive episodes associated with pheochromocytoma, and in insulinomas in relation to episodes of hypoglycemia. Headache may also be a prominent symptom in patients with the "empty sella" syndrome. Although the headaches remain constant in individual patients, no characteristics are specific to the individual disease entities.

Depression, lethargy, apathy, and impaired mentation (disorientation and confusion) are seen in hyperparathyroidism and in other hypercalcemic states. They also occur in hypothyroidism, in hypoglycemia irrespective of cause, in Cushing's syndrome, and in severe hyperglycemia associated with diabetic ketoacidosis and nonketotic hyperosmolar states. Marked changes (either increases or decreases) in serum osmolality such as are seen in severe diabetes insipidus (hypernatremia) and in hyponatremic states due to vasopressin-secreting tumors, Addison's disease, or myxedema also lead to a decreased sensorium. In each of these disorders, if the hormonal or metabolic disturbance is left untreated, a comatose state will develop.

Focal as well as generalized convulsions may occur in patients with severe hypocalcemia associated with hypoparathyroidism. Tetany generally precedes the onset of convulsions by a variable period of time, ranging from days to years. Hypoglycemic convulsions may similarly be focal or generalized, as may those associated with nonketotic hyperglycemic states. In contrast, diabetic ketoacidosis is not accompanied by convulsions, probably because of the anticonvulsive effect of acidosis and/or ketosis. Convulsions have been reported in severe myxedema, in Addison's disease and hypopituitarism, and in states of water intoxication, usually associated with excess vasopressin secretion.

Central nervous system effects, either direct or indirect, have been demonstrated for virtually every hormone studied. It is therefore not surprising that many abnormalities in endocrine function cause profound behavioral disorders. In hypopituitarism depression is common and psychoses are occasionally seen. In hypothyroidism, psychoses (myxedema madness) manifested by hallucinations, paranoid behavior, dementia, and even classic schizophrenic reactions can occur. The premorbid personality as well as age are important determinants of the type of behavioral changes produced. In general, older patients are more prone than younger ones to develop a typical organic brain syndrome. The response to treatment is usually excellent. However, in elderly patients behavioral aberrations may persist. Hypothyroid patients are generally less aware of exteroceptive stimuli. Consequently during the initial period of replacement therapy, behavioral problems may worsen until the patient readjusts to the new level of recognizable environmental input signals. Patients with hyperthyroidism show mood fluctuations which may progress to delirium and, as thyroid storm approaches, a florid psychosis. Patients with insulinomas causing repeated and undiagnosed hypoglycemic episodes may develop bizarre behavioral disturbances due to impaired central nervous system metabolism. The diagnosis of a toxic psychosis is not infrequently made in such patients. In Addison's disease a depressive psychosis can occur. In Cushing's syndrome (spontaneous and iatrogenic) one may see either depression or, more commonly, euphoria and emotional lability, and rarely, true psychotic behavior.

NEUROMUSCULAR ABNORMALITIES

Neuropathy is one of the commonly recognized long-term complications of diabetes mellitus. In about 15 percent of diabetic patients symptoms of neuropathy are present, while abnormalities of nerve conduction are demonstrable in as many as 50 percent of patients. The clinical spectrum of diabetic neuropathy includes (1) acute mononeuropathy which may involve cranial or peripheral nerves, (2) mononeuropathy multiplex, (3) distal polyneuropathy, and (4) autonomic neuropathy.

In mononeuritis multiplex there is involvement of a mixed sensorimotor nerve or group of nerves, resulting in pain and focal weakness. Frequently the sites of involvement are the hip, knee, and thigh areas, with resultant pain on walking.

In diabetic polyneuropathy there is distal, symmetric involvement primarily of sensory fibers. The feet and legs are affected to a greater extent than the hands. Numbness and paresthesias are the major complaints. There is loss of the ankle jerk and of various sensory modalities (vibration, position, light touch).

Autonomic neuropathy generally appears in patients who already have severe peripheral neuropathy. The symptoms include lack of sweat secretion, diarrhea which is particularly severe at night and is accompanied by fecal incontinence, orthostatic hypotension, impotence, and an atonic bladder.

Polyneuropathy involving primarily sensory nerves is also occasionally observed in patients with hyperparathyroidism.

A mononeuropathy involving the distal median nerve and due to compression at the wrist (*carpal tunnel syndrome*) is observed in acromegaly and hypothyroidism. Thickening of connective tissue in acromegaly or increased deposition of mucinous material between connective tissue fibers in myxedema results in pressure on the median nerve in its passage through the carpal tunnel. The symptoms consist of numbness, tingling, and pain in the radial two-thirds of the palmar surface of the hand and fingers. Weakness of abduction and apposition of the thumb may also occur.

A prolongation of the reflex relaxation time ("hung-up reflexes") in the absence of other evidence of neuropathy is a characteristic finding in hypothyroidism. Similar findings may occur in hyponatremic states such as Addison's disease and the syndrome of inappropriate secretion of antidiuretic hormone (ADH).

Impaired motor function due to myopathic changes may be observed in hyperthyroidism, hypothyroidism, spontaneous or iatrogenic Cushing's syndrome, and disorders of calcium and phosphorus metabolism.

In hyperthyroidism weakness is most marked in the pelvic girdle and thigh muscles and is accompanied by muscle atrophy. The shoulder and hand muscles may also show atrophy. However, tremor rather than weakness is the more prominent symptom in the upper extremities.

Myopathy may also occur in myxedema, in which patients may complain of stiffness and aching in addition to weakness. The muscles may appear hypertrophic because of infiltration with mucinous material.

Corticosteroid myopathy is characterized by weakness that is more prominent in the proximal limb and girdle musculature, resulting in difficulty in arising from a sitting position and in raising the arms.

In hypophosphatemic rickets and osteomalacia, muscle weakness and atrophy are common. In Klinefelter's disease, the weakness that commonly occurs is due to androgen deficiency.

Episodic weakness accompanied by hypokalemia is observed in patients with primary hyperaldosteronism or Bartter's syndrome and occasionally in patients with thyrotoxicosis. In the latter the attacks simulate those observed in familial periodic paralysis, but a family history of episodic paralysis is lacking.

In diabetic amyotrophy, involvement of a peripheral motor nerve or nerve end plate in the neuropathic process results in focal weakness and atrophy in the absence of sensory loss, thereby simulating primary myopathic disease.

Acromegalic neuromyopathy is occasionally seen in patients with long-standing disease. Extreme weakness, primarily of proximal musculature, is the predominant finding.

OPHTHALMIC ABNORMALITIES

Diminished vision occurs with several endocrine diseases as a consequence of pressure on the optic nerve or tract, retinal degeneration, or vascular disease. In patients with pituitary tumors exhibiting suprasellar extension, pressure on the optic chiasm typically results in a bitemporal hemianopsia, although other specific and often asymmetrical field defects can occur. The visual impairment can progress to complete blindness and optic atrophy. The blindness may occur suddenly in association with hemorrhage into the tumor.

Pigmentary optic atrophy has been reported in association with several hereditary syndromes in which obesity, diabetes, mental retardation, and hypogonadism are components. Severe to total visual loss is frequently present. Visual loss may also occur in severe thyroid ophthalmopathy (Graves' disease) as a result of increased orbital pressure leading to compression and ischemia of the optic nerve.

Cataracts and lenticular opacities that can impair vision are seen in hypothyroidism, hypoparathyroidism, and diabetes. Transient impairment of vision with symptoms of myopia developing over days to weeks accompanies severe hyperglycemic symptoms in approximately one-third of patients with newly discovered or poorly regulated type I diabetes. Hyperopic changes are less frequent but more dramatic in onset, often appearing several days after the onset of insulin treatment. Both symptoms disappear after several weeks of therapy. Blurring of both near and distant vision may develop rapidly during episodes of hyperglycemia in diabetics receiving insulin therapy; the visual impairment resolves as the blood glucose concentration returns to normal. These rapid changes in visual acuity due to marked fluctuations in blood glucose must be differentiated from the more permanent and serious visual loss which may occur in diabetic retinopathy. Diabetic retinopathy in its most severe form results in decreased vision by fibrous scar tissue formation in the macular area in association with neovascularization and by hemorrhage into the subhyaloid space or the vitreous humor. Acute, reversible blurring of vision may also occur during attacks of hypoglycemia.

Pain in or about the eye can occur in Graves' ophthalmopathy because of increased intraorbital pressure. It is also seen in diabetes associated with ophthalmoplegia or with rubeosis iridis, a form of neovascularization of the iris which can cause a painful hemorrhagic glaucoma.

Swelling around the eyes or periorbital edema is commonly seen in patients with myxedema, in whom the eyelids and surrounding skin exhibit a nonpitting, puffy swelling which appears boggy. Chemosis and swelling of the lids and periorbital tissue are prominent features of progressive Graves' ophthalmopathy and serve to distinguish the disease from retroorbital tumors, in which these changes are not seen. Increases in lacrimal gland size as well as soft-tissue swelling in the periorbital area are frequently seen in acromegaly. Periorbital edema may also occur in diabetics with severe renal disease and the nephrotic syndrome.

Loss of the lateral third of the eyebrow is seen in hypothyroidism and in hypopituitarism but is not diagnostic of these diseases. In long-standing hypoparathyroidism, the hair of the eyebrows and eyelids becomes thin and patchy.

Ophthalmoplegia or eye muscle weakness leading to diplopia may be seen with pituitary tumors which extend laterally into the cavernous sinus and impinge on the oculomotor nerves. Slight to moderate impairment of eye movements is extremely common in thyrotoxicosis. In its mildest form, asymptomatic symmetrical impairment of elevation of the eyes without diplopia is frequently missed. Unilateral weakness of the superior rectus muscle leading to upper lid retraction may be the first manifestation of Graves' disease. With increasing ophthalmoplegia, diplopia may occur on lateral or superior gaze. Myasthenia gravis can also cause ophthalmoplegia, but ptosis is a more common finding. Diabetic ophthalmoplegia involves the third and sixth nerves with equal frequency, has a rapid onset associated with pain on the ipsilateral side of the face, and, if the third nerve is involved, characteristically spares the pupil. Improvement occurs spontaneously in a few days or weeks, and complete recovery is almost invariable.

Severe protrusion of the eye in Graves' exophthalmos can impair total closure of the lids (*lagophthalmos*), resulting in corneal exposure during sleep and potentially dangerous exposure keratitis. In hypothyroidism discrete gray-colored spots may occur in the central portion of the cornea but do not generally interfere with vision.

In hyperparathyroidism and other hypercalcemic states of long duration, deposit of calcium phosphate crystals, a condition referred to as *band keratopathy*, may be observed at the medial and lateral margins of the cornea close to, but separate from, the cornea-sclera junction. Slit-lamp examination is frequently required to demonstrate the presence of keratopathy. In hypoparathyroidism there may be severe keratoconjunctivitis. Dilatation of conjunctival venules is seen in patients with diabetes, in parallel with the changes in retinal vessels. The dilatation, which is initially reversible, eventually becomes fixed and exhibits sacculations and even exudation.

Loss of pupillary reflexes may occur with pituitary tumors which invade the cavernous sinus. In diabetic ophthalmoplegia, the pupil is generally spared.

Both flaky and crystalline lenticular opacities are occasionally seen in hypothyroidism, but they generally do not interfere with vision. In contrast, cataracts and lenticular opacities are the most common of the eye findings in hypoparathyroidism. They may appear as diffuse white opacities separated by fluid clefts or as small and discrete punctate opacities in the lens cortex seen only on slit-lamp examination. The opacities are usually bilateral and frequently do not interfere with vision, though in some cases mature cataracts develop and require extraction. In younger diabetics cataracts are classically of the "snowflake" type and appear as bilateral dense bands of white spots situated in the subcapsular region of the lens. In older diabetics cataracts are morphologically indistinguishable from the senile cataracts in nondiabetics. Although cataracts are no more frequent in diabetics than in nondiabetics, they mature more rapidly and require extraction at an earlier age. Long-term treatment with high-dose glucocorticoids has been associated with posterior capsular cataracts.

Retinal changes characteristic of hypertension can be seen in acromegaly, primary aldosteronism, Cushing's syndrome, pheochromocytoma, and diabetes. Diabetics also exhibit a specific retinopathy consisting of capillary, arteriole, and venule microaneurysms appearing as small punctate red dots along the course of small vessels. These lesions may be confused with small hemorrhages but can be differentiated by fluorescein angiography. They are almost always bilateral and tend to be most frequent in the perimacular area. Microaneurysms are seen less frequently with other diseases such as malignant hypertension, chronic anemias, and central retinal venous thromboses. Coalescence and rupture of microaneurysms lead to hemorrhages; the leakage of protein leads to exudation.

Papilledema is seen in patients with benign intracranial hypertension (pseudotumor cerebri), often associated with the use of oral contraceptives. It also occurs in severe Graves' exophthalmos, hypoparathyroidism, the empty sella syndrome, neuroblastoma, and severe hypertension due to pheochromocytoma. It is observed less frequently in Cushing's syndrome and pituitary tumors, and in rare instances in primary aldosteronism.

Glaucoma can be precipitated or aggravated by spontaneous or iatrogenic hypercorticism. Glaucoma is also observed with increased frequency in diabetes mellitus.

3

Gene Expression and Recombinant DNA in Endocrinology and Metabolism

Barry J. Gertz
John D. Baxter

The past few decades have seen the generation of a tremendous amount of new information concerning the structure and function of genes. This information is now being used to devise more sophisticated and direct means to diagnose, prevent, and treat disease. The technology that has been developed, particularly recombinant DNA methodology, is also providing new approaches to understanding human physiology and the pathogenesis of disease. Particularly exciting is the capacity to produce large quantities of purified proteins which were previously of limited availability or essentially unobtainable.

Human insulin[1,2] and growth hormone[3-5] produced by recombinant DNA techniques are currently in clinical use. Many new drugs and vaccines will be developed, the ability to diagnose disease and predict susceptibility to disease will be greatly expanded, and new types of therapy (including gene transfer) may become available. The physician will therefore have to achieve some understanding of this new technology in order to assess its strengths and weaknesses and apply it to the management of endocrine and metabolic diseases. The rapid development of the technology also raises ethical issues whose consideration requires a basic knowledge of gene expression and regulation and their manipulation by recombinant DNA techniques. The purpose of this chapter is to provide a conceptual framework for understanding the essential aspects of gene expression and the application of recombinant DNA methodology in endocrinology. Reviews are cited where appropriate.

GENES AND THEIR EXPRESSION

The modern era of molecular biology received its greatest impetus in 1953 when Watson and Crick reported the structure of deoxyribonucleic acid (DNA).[6] This finding provided at once an insight into how, through complementary base pairing, DNA replication might occur and thus how the genetic profile of an organism could be maintained from generation to generation.[7-9] Subsequent breakthroughs have yielded a considerable body of information including (1) how the DNA of a cell evolves and replicates;[7,8] (2) the means by which the DNA is *expressed*,[7-10] i.e., how it is transcribed into ribonucleic acid (RNA) and how these transcripts may be either translated into protein—e.g., for messenger RNA (mRNA)—or utilized in other ways—as transfer RNA (tRNA) or ribosomal RNA (rRNA); and (3) how gene expression is controlled.[7-11] Knowledge in these areas continues to accumulate at an unprecedented pace. A few critical aspects of the structure and function of DNA are described below for purposes of orientation. The references cited offer more detailed information.

DNA STRUCTURE AND REPLICATION

The structure of DNA is shown in Figs. 3-1 and 3-2. DNA contains a "backbone" made up of deoxyribose molecules linked by connecting phosphate groups. These connections occur through the 3′ hydroxyl moiety of the first sugar and the 5′ hydroxyl moiety of the next sugar. Since the 5′ moiety of the first sugar is free and the 3′ moiety of the last sugar is free, the direction of the molecule is described as 5′ to 3′. These designations serve as a reference for orientation. Genes are described as being transcribed from 5′ to 3′, since the sugars in the RNA molecule are linked in a 5′ to 3′ orientation. The first nucleotide of the initial RNA product has a free 5′ triphosphate group (which may subsequently be modified). The 5′ end of a gene ordinarily refers to the position where transcription is initiated. The portion of the gene farther along in the 5′ direction is designated the *upstream*

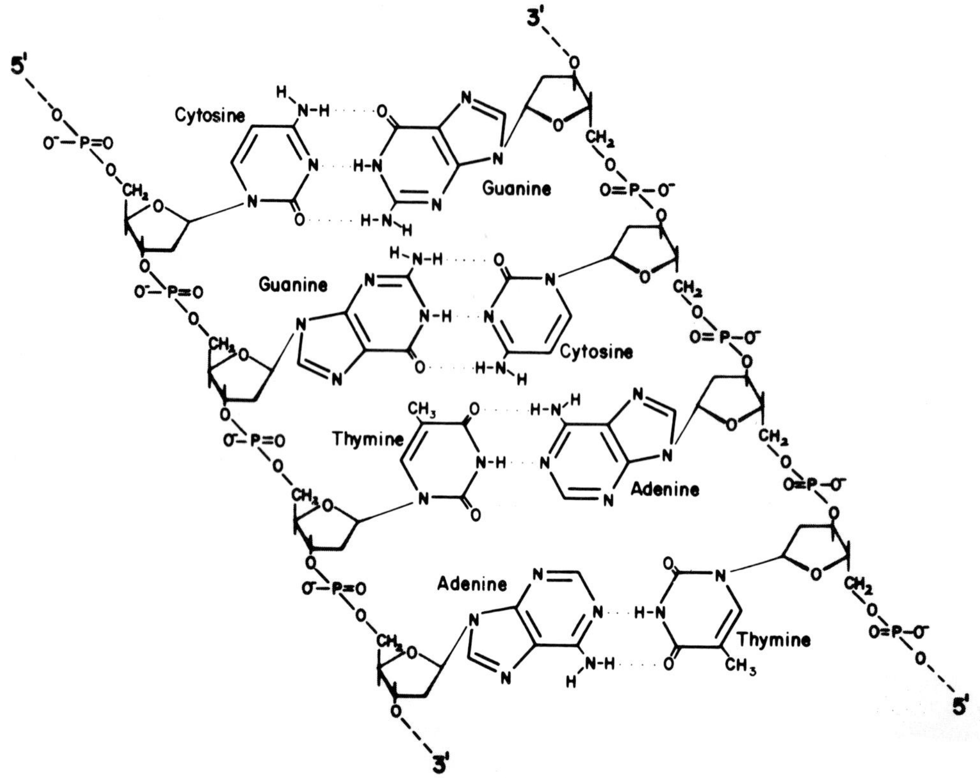

FIGURE 3-1 Structure of DNA. Several structural features of a short stretch of double-stranded DNA are shown. The sugar-phosphate backbones are shown on the outside, running antiparallel to one another; that on the left running 5′ to 3′, and that on the right from 3′ to 5′. The purines adenine and guanine are shown on the inside hydrogen-bonded to the pyrimidines thymine and cytosine, respectively.

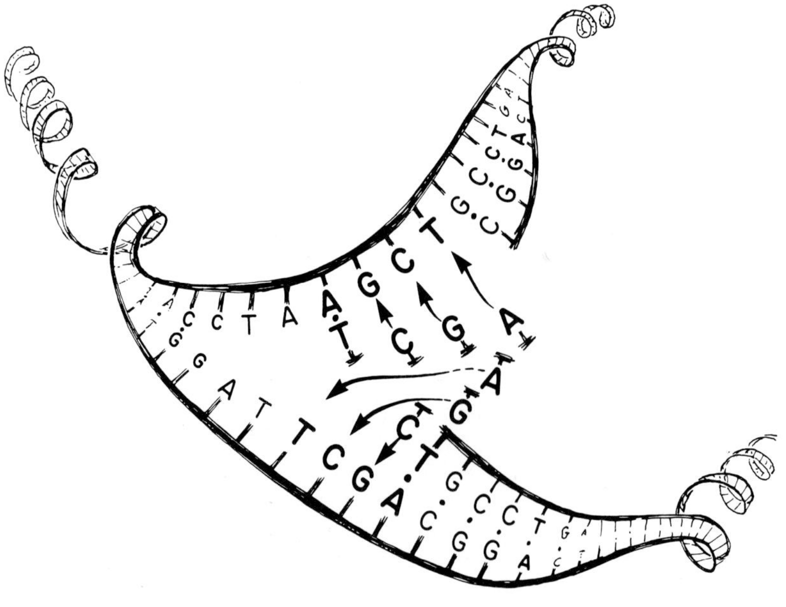

FIGURE 3-2 Highly simplified schematic representation of the essential features of DNA replication. The double helix unwinds and two daughter strands of DNA are synthesized. Each of the resulting DNA molecules contains one strand of the original parent DNA molecule (semiconservative replication). Complementary base pairing directs the sequence of addition of nucleoside triphosphates by DNA polymerase (not shown). Each daughter strand of DNA is synthesized in the 5′ to 3′ direction, requiring one strand to be synthesized in a discontinuous fashion. A, adenine; G, guanine; T, thymine; C, cytosine.

portion, and the 3′ end is the *downstream* portion of the gene, where transcription terminates.

Connected to each sugar of the DNA backbone is one of four bases, adenine (A), guanine (G), cytosine (C), or thymine (T). Adenine and guanine are purines, and cytosine and thymine are pyrimidines. *Nucleosides* are bases bound only to the sugar moiety. When the base is coupled to a sugar and a phosphate group it is termed a *nucleotide.* As an example, adenine (a base) bound to ribose is termed *adenosine* (a nucleoside); adenosine coupled to a phosphate group is designated *adenylic acid* (a nucleotide). Several nucleotides linked together in a polymer generate a *nucleic acid.*

DNA is composed of two strands of nucleic acid that run antiparallel to each other (i.e., the two strands of nucleotides run in opposite directions); the purine bases of one strand are hydrogen-bonded to the pyrimidine bases of the complementary strand: A base-pairs with T, and G base-pairs with C. This complementary base pairing means that the order of the bases along one strand of the DNA dictates that along the other strand. This feature is critical in DNA replication and transcription for determining the precise structure of, respectively, the DNA progeny and the RNA products of genes. These two strands are wound around each other, generating the well-known *double helix.* The DNA exists within the cell complexed with proteins in a highly ordered, compacted configuration referred to as *chromatin.* As described later, these associated chromatin proteins play an important role in determining gene expression.

It is the order of the bases along the DNA strand, along with the feature of precise base pairing, which allows "like to replicate like" and permits information storage. It can be thought of as the body's computer program, transmitting a replicate of itself to progeny, directing the developing embryo to differentiate properly into an adult organism, and organizing the enzymatic and other machinery necessary for all the complex metabolic functions of the cell.

When DNA replicates (Fig. 3-2), the individual strands are separated and nucleoside triphosphates are aligned along the sugar-phosphate backbones, the order determined by complementary base pairing. The sugar moieties are then connected via phosphodiester linkages enzymatically, resulting in complementary DNA strands. Each daughter strand of DNA is synthesized in the 5′ to 3′ direction, which necessitates the synthesis of one of the daughter strands in a discontinuous fashion. The actual mechanics of this process are highly complex and outside the scope of this chapter (for review, see Refs. 7 and 8), but the result is two molecules of DNA that are identical to the original DNA. One strand of each daughter DNA molecule is derived from the parent DNA and the other is newly synthesized—a process referred to as *semiconservative replication.*

CHROMATIN

The chromosomal DNA in the nucleus of the cell, as indicated above, is packaged into a configuration termed *chromatin.*[7,8,12] This material contains substantial quantities of protein that serve as a matrix to fold the DNA and participate in replication and transcriptional control activities. The major chromatin proteins are histones, of which there are five major classes. The DNA is wound twice around a histone octamer (consisting of two copies each of H2A, H2B, H3, and H4) to form structures called *nucleosomes* (Fig. 3-3). On

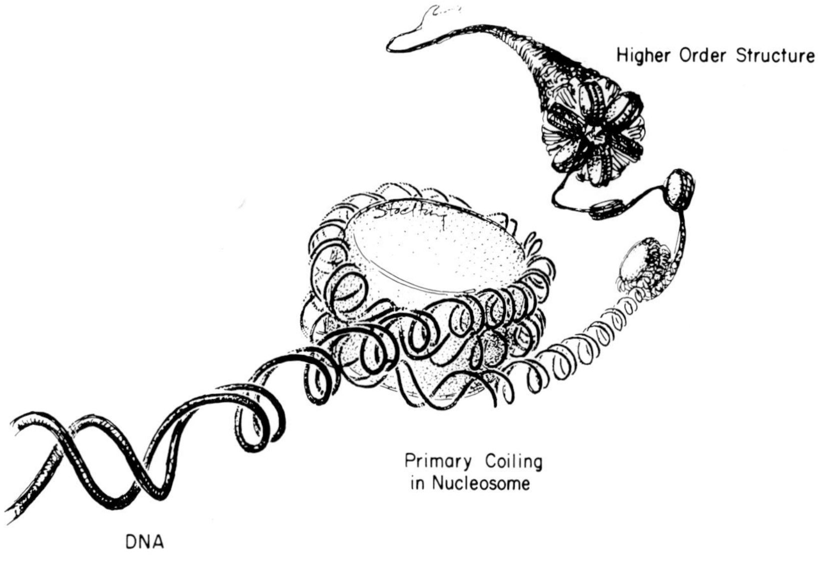

FIGURE 3-3 The fundamental unit of chromatin, the nucleosome, represents two turns of the DNA double helix around a core of histone molecules. The nucleosomes are separated by linker DNA and, under appropriate salt conditions in the presence of H1 histone, will form higher-order structures such as the 30-nm fiber. One possible orientation of the nucleosomes in the 30-nm fiber is depicted here.

electron microscopy this structure, along with the "linker" DNA, appears like beads on a string. The nucleosomes are further organized into a 30 nm chromatin fiber. The exact nature of the packaging is not known, but H1 histones appear to be actively involved. These coils of DNA undergo additional folding which allows the rather long strands of DNA to be packaged efficiently.[12–14] The second major class of proteins in chromatin are the nonhistone proteins; these include enzymes (e.g., RNA polymerase) and other proteins that participate in gene transcription, DNA replication, the mediation of the actions of hormones and other regulatory factors, and tissue-specific expression. A well-defined subgroup is the high-mobility group proteins. These may participate, by as yet undefined mechanisms, in tissue-specific gene expression.[14]

Using a variety of techniques, including the in vitro sensitivity of certain regions of DNA to the nonspecific DNA cleavage enzyme DNase I as a probe of chromatin structure, it has been demonstrated that not all regions of chromatin are alike. Regions of chromatin which are transcriptionally active are found to be more sensitive to this reagent and thus may be in a more open (i.e., accessible) configuration[15]—e.g., the ovalbumin gene region in nuclei from the estrogen-stimulated oviduct is more sensitive to DNase cleavage than the same gene region in nuclei from tissues in which it is not expressed.[16] As another example, glucocorticoid activation of gene expression may be associated with an increase in the DNase sensitivity of the stimulated gene.[17] This suggests that one result of the interaction of the steroid-receptor complex with DNA is an alteration in chromatin configuration.

Other proteins are contained within a structure, termed the *nuclear matrix*, that serves as an overall scaffolding for the nucleus.[18–20] DNA which is transcriptionally active or undergoing replication appears to be selectively associated with this matrix.[20] Interestingly, estrogen stimulation of the ovalbumin gene in the chicken oviduct results in a reversible association of the ovalbumin gene region with the nuclear matrix.[20]

RNA STRUCTURE AND FUNCTION

The first step in gene expression is the transcription of DNA into RNA (Figs. 3-4 and 3-5). RNA is similar in overall structure to DNA except that in RNA the sugar moiety is ribose instead of deoxyribose, and the pyrimidine uracil (U) replaces T and U then base-pairs with A. Moreover, RNA in mammalian cells is ordinarily not double-stranded, although there may be folding of the RNA on itself (*secondary structure*) that results in portions of it being double-stranded. Some of the RNA viruses, however, are double-stranded.[7,8]

The three major classes of RNA are mRNA, tRNA, and rRNA. Minor RNA species appear to play important roles in several cellular processes, although a precise function has not yet been assigned to each of them[21]—e.g., (1) the small RNA molecules involved in the processing events necessary for the production of a mature mRNA (see below)[22,23] and (2) the RNA component of the *signal recognition particle* involved in the translocation of proteins across the endoplasmic reticulum.[24,25] mRNA contains sequences that are translated into protein (see below). tRNA is involved in protein synthesis, transferring amino acids onto a

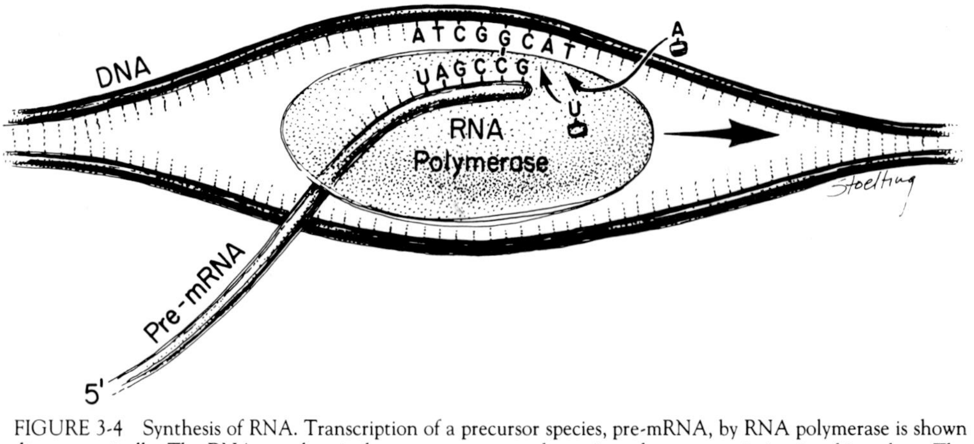

FIGURE 3-4 Synthesis of RNA. Transcription of a precursor species, pre-mRNA, by RNA polymerase is shown diagrammatically. The DNA template is shown to open over the region where transcription is taking place. The enzyme RNA polymerase directs the addition of ribonucleoside triphosphates into the growing pre-mRNA, with the actual sequence determined by complementary base pairing of purines and pyrimidines. The pyrimidine (U) found in RNA is shown as base-pairing with A. Even before transcription of the pre-mRNA is completed, the cap (a methylated guanine nucleotide) will be added to the 5′ end.

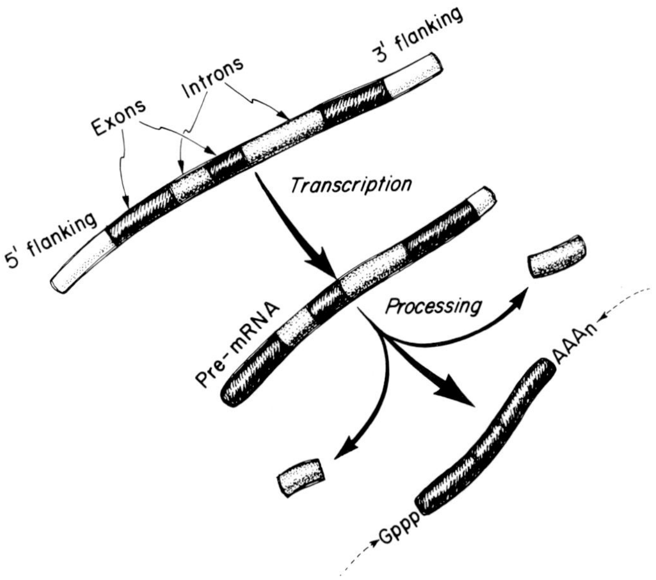

FIGURE 3-5 The initial steps in gene expression of a typical eukaryotic gene encoding a polypeptide. Exons, those regions present in the mature transcript, and introns, those segments destined to be excised from the primary transcript, are distinguished in the parent gene by shading. Both exons and introns are transcribed into the primary gene product, or pre-mRNA. This precursor species then undergoes several processing steps, which include the splicing of the exons associated with removal of the introns, addition of a cap at the 5′ end, and cleavage and polyadenylation at the 3′ end. This mature transcript is then transported into the cytoplasm.

nascent peptide. Ribosomal RNA, along with proteins, forms a structure termed the *ribosome* that is also involved in protein synthesis. The mRNA and tRNA molecules bind to the ribosome during translation, as discussed in Chap. 4. A series of tRNA molecules exists, each of which covalently binds a specific amino acid. Such "charged" tRNA molecules participate in the addition of amino acids onto a protein through the formation of peptide bonds.

Gene Expression

In addition to the regions of DNA that are transcribed into RNA, other segments critical for accurate gene expression are present on the DNA.[7,8] These DNA segments direct where the enzymes involved in transcription will start and how efficiently the gene will be transcribed.[26,27] Other regions of the DNA (control or regulatory sequences) are involved in receiving regulatory signals, such as hormone-receptor complexes, that either inhibit or facilitate gene transcription. Still other sequences may function to determine the tissue-specific expression of a gene, possibly through interaction with factors (e.g., proteins) of limited tissue distribution.[28–30]

Transcription is carried out by enzymes termed *RNA polymerases* (Fig. 3-4). The region of DNA which determines the basal level of expression and directs where RNA polymerase initiates transcription is termed the *promoter;* the promoter region for mRNA transcription is primarily located just upstream, i.e., farther along in the 5′ direction, from the start of transcription,[7,8,27,28] whereas the promoters for tRNA and rRNA genes may be located in part within the gene.[7,8,31,32] For transcription to proceed the DNA strands are separated and RNA polymerase facilitates base pairing along one of the strands and subsequent polymerization from individual ribonucleoside triphosphates that serve as building blocks (Fig. 3-4). Transcription termination in eukaryotes is not well understood but appears to occur over a limited region of DNA rather than at a discrete site,[33] the 3′ end of an mRNA being defined by cleavage and processing of a larger precursor (see below).

The structure of a mammalian gene encoding an mRNA is shown in Fig. 3-5. The DNA upstream from the start of transcription is called the *5′-flanking DNA;* that downstream from the site directing the addition of the poly A tail (see below) in the pre-mRNA is called the *3′-flanking DNA.* The transcribed portion of a gene is composed of exons interrupted by introns, or intervening sequences. The primary transcript, or pre-mRNA, contains both exon and intron sequences; however, the intron sequences are removed from this precursor and the exon sequences are spliced together in the process of formation of the mature RNA product that contains only exon sequences.[10] These processing events, which are just beginning to be understood from in vitro studies, involve large RNA-protein complexes which have been termed *spliceosomes.*[34a,34b,35] These entities, along with specific processing signals present in the sequence of the primary RNA transcript, direct the precise excision of the introns and exon ligation.[36] Such splicing signals, present in the sequence of the pre-mRNA, include a GT pair at the 5′ end of an intervening sequence and an AG at the 3′ end.[26,37] Mutations at these locations can result in aberrant splicing and an altered gene product.[38] Introns are present in most genes encoding mRNA molecules,[39] and their number can vary considerably—e.g., there are 2 for the human insulin gene,[40] 9 for the human renin gene,[41] and 17 for the low-density lipoprotein (LDL) receptor gene.[42]

The mRNA transcript can also be modified in other ways. A chain of A residues added to the 3′ end of most (but not all) mRNA molecules is termed the *poly A tail.*[10,33] This modification involves the sequence AAUAAA (or minor variants) at the 3′ end, which directs, to a major extent, cleavage of the primary transcript approximately 10 to 30 nucleotides downstream.[43] This is followed by the addition of a stretch of A residues, catalyzed by the enzyme polyadenylate polymerase. Also a "cap" is added to the 5′ end of the mRNA that is a methylated nucleotide in the reverse orientation.[7,8,10,44] Thus the term *cap site* refers to the first nucleotide of the mRNA, i.e., the site of the start of transcription. The precise function of these structures is unknown, though they appear to play a role in determining the stability of eukaryotic mRNA molecules.[45a,45b] The primary transcripts of tRNA and rRNA genes also undergo processing to yield functional RNA molecules.[7,8]

Introns may serve a number of functions: Their presence is sometimes required for mRNA formation in eukaryotes,[46] and DNA structures important for regulating gene expression may, on occasion, be found within introns. For example, a structure that binds the glucocorticoid receptor and probably mediates responsiveness to these steroids is found in an intron of the human growth hormone gene,[47a,47b] and a region important in regulating expression of the immunoglobulin heavy chain gene is also located within an intron.[28]

The fact that genes are split into introns and exons has in all likelihood facilitated the process of evolution of genes.[48,49] It is now thought that one mechanism critical for gene evolution involves the movement of DNA segments into existing genes.[39,50,51] Such insertions can result in the addition of amino acid segments which significantly modify the function of the original gene product. One of the best known examples in which the functional domains of the protein product can be traced back to separate exon regions of the gene is the LDL receptor.[42] For example, the highly negatively charged region of the LDL receptor which appears to be responsible for binding lipoproteins is composed of seven 40-amino acid repeat segments, four of which are encoded by separate exons while the remaining three are all on a single exon. The first exon encodes the signal sequence of the protein, while exons 16 and 17 encode the transmembrane domain, and exons 17 and 18 the cytoplasmic domain of the receptor. Insertions may also bring in domains that contain regulatory structures, conferring on the modified gene new possibilities for control of its expression. The advantage of introns for such rearrangements of DNA lies in the fact that the genetic events can be somewhat imprecise. For example, a recombination event might bring a DNA segment comprising an exon, flanked by intervening sequences, into an existing gene. If this segment is inserted into an intron of the existing gene with the proper splicing signals, a new exon would be added to the gene that would be expressed in an altered mRNA product. The protein translated from this modified mRNA would then have an additional segment of amino acids. For this evolutionary event to occur, all that is needed are breaks within the intron in segments that do not contain critical control structures such as those which affect RNA processing; if introns and their removal by processing did not occur, such insertions would need to be much more precise to avoid compromising the coding sequence of the original gene.

The requirement for the removal of intervening sequences from the primary transcript engendered the possibility that differential processing of a pre-mRNA could result in more than one mature mRNA species being derived from a single gene. Although this mechanism appears uncommon, one prominent example in the endocrine system involves the pre-mRNA of the calcitonin gene, which can undergo differential processing to yield two distinct mRNA species.[52,53] In the brain the result is an mRNA encoding the calcitonin gene–related peptide (CGRP). In the parafollicular cells of the thyroid gland the result is predominantly the mRNA for calcitonin. Both these mRNA species share three exons at the 5′ end which encode the amino-terminal portion common to both the calcitonin and CGRP precursor peptides. However, the mRNA molecules have distinct 3′ ends because of the splicing of different downstream exons and the use of different polyadenylation sites. It is this region of the mRNA which codes for the distinct carboxy-terminal portions of the respective precursor peptides. The distinct precursor peptides can then be proteolytically cleaved to release either calcitonin or CGRP.

After the mRNA is synthesized in the cell nucleus, it is transported to the cytoplasm, where it can be translated into protein. The amino acid sequence of the protein is dictated by the sequence of bases along the mRNA, with each set of three nucleotides (a *codon*) specifying an amino acid according to the genetic code. The 5′ end of the mRNA usually includes a region, of variable length, termed the *5′-untranslated region,* which ends at the first codon for the polypeptide. The first codon of the mRNA that is translated is always AUG, which codes for methionine, although this methionine is sometimes removed from the nascent peptide. Individual amino acids are covalently linked to tRNA molecules specific for each amino acid. These tRNA molecules bind to the mRNA through an *anticodon loop,* which is a loop of the tRNA containing three nucleotides that are complementary to those of the mRNA codon. For example, a methionine tRNA would contain UAC in its anticodon loop that would base-pair with the AUG on the mRNA. Although each codon is unambiguous in terms of its amino acid specificity, the code is redundant in that for all amino acids except tryptophan and methionine, more than one codon specifies a given amino acid. Thus if the nucleic acid sequence of an mRNA is known, the amino acid sequence of its translation product will be known with certainty. If the amino acid sequence of a protein is known, however, the nucleic acid sequence of the mRNA and the gene from which it is transcribed can be only partially known. The ribosome moves along the mRNA in the process of protein synthesis until it reaches a "stop," or termination, codon. At this point translation ceases and the ribosome dissociates from the mRNA. From the stop codon to the polyadenylation signal (AAUAAA) is a region of highly variable length referred to as the *3′-untranslated region.*

As discussed in Chap. 4, the primary translation product, or precursor protein, may undergo extensive modification. For example, a signal peptide sequence which can serve to target a protein for secretion may be removed from a preprotein during the process of entry of the protein into the secretory apparatus (as with preproinsulin) (Chaps. 4 and 19). Another role for such proteolytic processing is the release of one or more peptides from a larger protein precursor. Corticotropin (ACTH) is a 39-amino acid protein that is contained in the middle of a much larger protein, proopiomelanocortin (POMC), and is released from POMC by specific proteolytic cleavage events (Chaps. 7, 8, and 12). Also, sugars or other chemical groups may be added after translation (Chap. 4).

Regulation of Gene Expression

During development of an organism, cells must differentiate in order to perform numerous specialized functions. This involves the expression of selective regions of the genome. Furthermore, hormones, neurotransmitters, and other regulatory signals must be capable of controlling the expression of DNA in various tissues in different ways. The molecular mechanisms involved in the regulation of gene expression are just beginning to be understood.[16,29,30,54–57b] The principal control appears to be at the level of transcription of the DNA into pre-mRNA, although other steps involved in gene expression are also regulated.

The structure of most genes in the germ line cells (i.e., the reproductive cells) is essentially identical to that in the various differentiated or somatic cells. However, there are exceptions. The DNA may be modified by methylation of cytosine residues. When this occurs the methylation patterns can be inherited. The effect of such methylation generally is an inhibition of gene expression.[58a,58b] This mechanism appears to be involved in the inactivation of one of the X chromosomes in cells that contain two X chromosomes. The result is transcriptional activity of only one of each pair of X chromosomes in a given cell.[59] In other cases DNA can undergo rearrangement and/or mutation. During the development of antibody-producing cells there is both rearrangement and mutation of immunoglobulin gene regions to generate the expressed immunoglobulin genes. This permits a vast number of different immunoglobulin genes to be formed from a relatively small number of genes present in the progenitor cells of the immune system.[60,61]

As stated above, the predominant control of gene expression appears to be at the level of transcription. The promoter structures for different genes (discussed in the previous section) may vary in their capacity to facilitate the initiation of transcription. This affects the basal level of activity of the gene. Control or regulatory sequences can, in concert with the proteins that interact with them, affect the efficiency of the promoter in initiating transcription. A few examples illustrate this point.

The insulin gene contains structures in the 5′-flanking DNA that are critical for efficient transcription initiation.[29,29a] However, these structures function only in pancreatic endocrine cells (specifically the β cells). Presumably another gene (or genes) in the β cells encodes a protein (or proteins) that acts on the insulin gene regulatory elements to facilitate initiation of transcription.

A second example of such a control structure is the DNA element that mediates glucocorticoid hormone action (Fig. 3-6). As described in Chap. 5, glucocorticoids bind to intracellular receptors and the steroid-receptor complex binds to DNA. The site on DNA where these receptors bind has been termed the *glucocorticoid regulatory element* (GRE).[57b,62–65] The steroid-receptor complex binds to the GRE more tightly than to random DNA. This binding, in some unknown way, then facilitates RNA polymerase action at the promoter located near the GRE. This enhance-

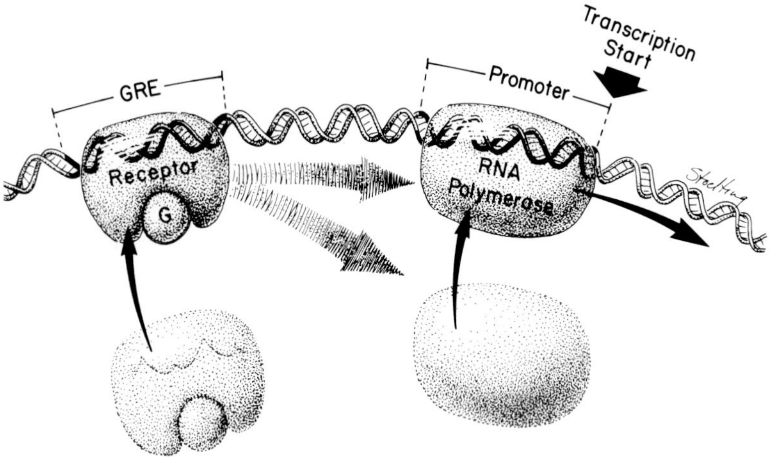

FIGURE 3-6 Binding of the glucocorticoid-receptor complex at the GRE. The steroid-receptor complex binds to specific DNA sequences (the GRE). This binding event, in some unknown fashion, enhances (or in some cases inhibits) the interaction of RNA polymerase with the promoter of the glucocorticoid-regulated gene. The result is a stimulation (or inhibition) of transcription of the gene.

ment, or in some cases inhibition, of promoter activity probably involves some alteration in chromatin structure, as suggested previously.[17] For several glucocorticoid-regulated genes (metallothionein,[64] human growth hormone[47a,47b]), the putative GRE has been defined by both binding studies and functional assays. The latter type of study involves splicing the sequence of DNA proposed to have the properties of a GRE to a gene which is normally not inducible by glucocorticoid and demonstrating that the new hybrid gene, when transferred to a glucocorticoid-responsive cell, can then be regulated by the steroid (see Transfer of Cloned Genes into Mammalian Cells, later in this chapter, and Fig. 3-13).[57b,62-65] Glucocorticoid regulatory elements have been found in glucocorticoid-responsive genes predominantly in the 5′-flanking DNA at a distance of a few to over a thousand nucleotides away from the promoter.[57b,62-66] However, a putative GRE for the human growth hormone gene appears to be located downstream within an intron.[47a,47b] In some cases the result of interaction of the glucocorticoid-receptor complex with the gene is an inhibition of transcription. For example, this is the case for the POMC gene.[67,68] Analogous structures appear to mediate the actions of other classes of steroid hormones, including estrogens, progestins, and androgens, each acting through its respective receptor.[69-71]

The mechanism(s) by which such GRE segments, or hormone response elements, actually affect transcriptional activity have not been precisely defined. However, these elements belong to a larger class of DNA structures termed *enhancers*[28,54,72-75] that were described initially in DNA tumor viruses. They have the capacity to augment (or enhance) transcriptional activity even if located several thousand nucleotides away from a promoter, in either orientation relative to the promoter, and whether located upstream or downstream from the gene.[72-75] These control or regulatory DNA sequences are in effect "cassettes" of information that have been inserted into the DNA in the vicinity of a promoter and which affect promoter function, in some cases in response to regulatory proteins. A gene may contain several different such cassettes that may allow for control of expression by a variety of factors, including those involved in tissue-specific expression or regulation by extrinsic factors such as hormones or neurotransmitters.

It should be noted that other classes of hormones also regulate gene activity, although the molecular details are sparse compared to the steroid-regulated systems. As examples, these include (1) thyroid hormone, which regulates levels of growth hormone[76-78] and malic enzyme mRNA levels;[79] and (2) the peptide hormones such as insulin, which inhibits phosphoenolpyruvate carboxykinase gene activity,[80] epidermal growth factor, which induces prolactin mRNA,[81] and glucagon, which, via its effects on cAMP accumulation, activates transcription of the hepatic tyrosine aminotransferase gene.[82]

Gene expression can also be regulated at the level of RNA processing or turnover, although this is probably less common than transcriptional control. As discussed above, the pre-mRNA from the calcitonin gene can be processed in two ways such that in brain and certain other tissues the mRNA for CGRP is produced and in the parafollicular cells of the thyroid gland calcitonin mRNA is primarily made.[52,53] Presumably, tissue-specific factors regulate this differential RNA processing. Variable RNA processing has been described for transcripts of the growth hormone gene, although the differences in the resulting mRNA molecules are less striking.[83] Hormones and other factors can also regulate mRNA (and consequently protein) levels by affecting mRNA stability. Part of the mechanism by which prolactin stimulates an accumulation of casein in the mouse mammary gland is a prolactin-mediated decrease in the rate of casein mRNA breakdown, with a consequent increase in casein mRNA.[84] In addition, estrogen stimulates accumulation of ovalbumin mRNA in the chicken oviduct by decreasing the rate of turnover, as well as stimulating synthesis, of the mRNA.[85,86] The means by which hormones accomplish such selective stabilization of mRNA molecules is unknown. Potentially, hormones could also regulate the efficiency of processing or the stability of a pre-mRNA in the nucleus to alter gene expression.[87]

There are examples in which gene expression is also regulated at posttranslational loci and through effects on the efficiency of mRNA translation.[88] For peptides that are cleaved from larger precursor molecules, tissue-specific factors may direct which peptides are released. Consider that, in the rat anterior pituitary, ACTH and β-lipotropin (β-LPH) are released from POMC, whereas in the intermediate lobe proteolytic cleavage of POMC results largely in α-melanocyte stimulating hormone (α-MSH) and corticotropin-like intermediate lobe peptide.[89] The extensive control of enzyme activity through the actions of hormones and other regulatory substances is described in Chap. 5.

Gene Evolution

Genes are generated during evolution through rearrangements, additions, or deletions of DNA segments, through mutations of nucleotides, and through duplications. The products of such duplication events can then evolve independently. This is the probable origin of the so-called gene families, which can vary from a few to many genes. Gene families are usually identified through comparisons of their members' overall organization in the genome and homologies (similarities) in their nucleotide sequences.[48,51,83] Examples of gene families include growth hormone, prolactin, and placental lactogen (chorionic somatomammotropin); insulin and the somatomedins; and the glycoprotein hormones (thyroid stimulating hormone, chorionic gonadotropin, luteinizing hormone, and follicle stimulating hormone).

A current model for the evolution of the growth hormone gene family is illustrative (Fig. 3-7).[49,90] Initially there was a primitive gene with a promoter and one exon. This exon segment was ultimately duplicated four times to yield the present-day exons 2, 4, and 5, with two of the segments present in exon 5. Apparently an intron was removed from between the two duplicated segments constituting exon 5. Two additional DNA segments were inserted, one encoding what is now exon 3 and another contributing sequences of the 5′-flanking DNA, exon 1, and part of the first intron. The latter insertion brought in a new promoter as well as the putative GRE of the human growth hormone gene; this left a primitive promoter upstream from the current promoter that is still weakly active. This precursor gene underwent mutation and several duplications to evolve into the genes coding for growth hormone, prolactin, and placental lactogen. Thus the genes for these three hormones have a similar overall structure, with five exons separated by four introns. When the exons are aligned to maximize homology (sequence similarity) between them, the introns are found to interrupt the coding

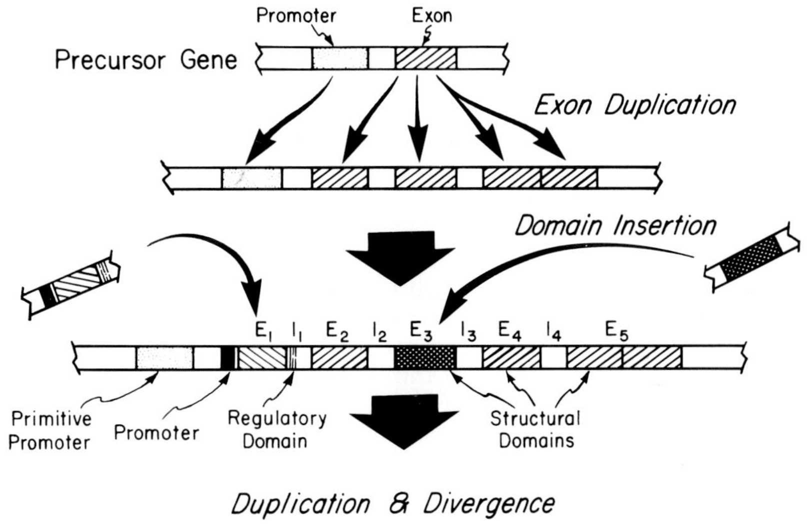

FIGURE 3-7 Evolution of the growth hormone gene family. The ancestral gene with its promoter and single exon undergoes several modifications as a result of exon duplication and DNA insertion events. Finally, as a result of gene duplication and mutation, the members of the growth hormone gene family emerge (growth hormone, prolactin, human placental lactogen). See text for details.

sequence at similar locations. Finally, upstream from each gene's dominant promoter is a weakly active promoter element.

Mechanisms of Genetic Disease

The precise molecular mechanism for most of the genetic diseases encountered in endocrinology and metabolism are not known. Examples of such diseases with some genetic basis are pseudohypoparathyroidism (Chap. 24), certain forms of dwarfism (Chap. 26), congenital adrenal hyperplasia (Chap. 12), diabetes mellitus (Chap. 19), and the disorders of lipoprotein metabolism (Chap. 22). In other circumstances an increased susceptibility to disease is inherited, as with type 1 diabetes.

A number of molecular mechanisms can account for genetic disease, and these have been most clearly elucidated for nonendocrine diseases such as the thalassemias.[91] There may be base change (point) mutations that result in an altered codon (a mis-sense mutation). If the subsequent amino acid change in the protein is deleterious, an altered protein that is deficient in its function will result. This type of mutation has been found to be a rare cause of diabetes mellitus.[92,93] Alternatively, a mutation may result in the generation of a translation stop codon (a nonsense mutation), which can result in the absence of functional protein.[94] In some cases such mutations result in an RNA product which is unstable and does not accumulate normally.[95] Proper processing of pre-mRNA to mature mRNA may be interrupted by a point mutation in a processing site.[38,96] In addition, there may be a deletion of a DNA segment that disrupts gene function[96a] or that results in an abnormal RNA product. These types of mutations could also affect the processing of pre-mRNA into mRNA. Finally, the entire gene may be deleted, as has been reported to occur in a rare form of growth hormone deficiency.[97]

RECOMBINANT DNA TECHNOLOGY

The essence of recombinant DNA technology is that pieces of DNA can be cut or ligated together outside of living cells.[7,8,98,99] This *recombinant DNA* can then be inserted back into a living cell, such as a prokaryote (a nonnucleated cell such as a bacterium) or eukaryote (a nucleated cell such as a yeast or a mammalian cell), in which it can be replicated. In this way, starting from a single molecule, many new molecules can be obtained. These molecules can be isolated and used to promote greater understanding of basic biological processes such as how cells regulate gene expression. Alternatively they can be put to practical use, as in the production of hormones or other proteins that cannot be obtained in adequate quantity by other methods.

One of the major developments that led to this new technology was derived from studies of the process of restriction and modification in bacteria.[7,8] This is the process whereby these organisms can destroy DNA they recognize as foreign and yet protect their own genetic information by appropriate modifications. These studies led to the discovery of a set of enzymes, termed *restriction enzymes,* or *restriction endonucleases,* that bind to DNA at specific sequences and cleave it precisely at these loci. The enzymes are named for the bacteria from which the enzyme is derived. The first restriction enzyme discovered, termed *Eco*RI, was isolated from *Escherichia coli;* its action is depicted in Fig. 3-8. The availability and use of these enzymes has allowed scientists to cleave DNA at specific sites. For example, if a DNA fragment is incubated under appropriate conditions with *Eco*RI, the DNA will be cleaved at all sites containing the sequence shown in Fig. 3-8. In this case the cleavage yields short, single-stranded, overhanging ends that are complementary to one another (*sticky ends*). If one of the resulting pieces is isolated and incubated with a DNA fragment from another source that has been cut with the same enzyme, the complementary ends of each DNA fragment will base-pair (Figs. 3-8 and 3-9). The resulting hybrid DNA molecules can then be ligated together enzymatically, to form a new recombinant DNA molecule (Fig. 3-9). Some restriction enzymes yield blunt-ended fragments rather than overhanging or sticky ends; blunt-ended fragments can also be ligated to other blunt-ended fragments, although this is somewhat less efficient.

Several steps in the cloning of a gene are shown in Fig. 3-10. Plasmids are frequently the starting material for constructing recombinant DNA molecules. These are circular pieces of double-stranded DNA which replicate in bacteria as episomes, i.e., extrachromosomally (Fig. 3-9). They frequently transmit antibiotic resistance; for example, they may contain the gene for β-lactamase, which cleaves the β-lactam ring of ampicillin and thus confers ampicillin resistance. A recombinant plasmid containing inserted foreign DNA (such as that encoding a human gene) may be constructed as depicted in Fig. 3-9. The plasmid is then transfected into bacteria, usually *E. coli*, by a process which makes them more permeable and thus able to take up foreign DNA. These bacteria can then be grown in culture, and the plasmid that has been taken up can replicate within the bacterial cell. The inserted DNA will be replicated along with the other genes resident on the plasmid. In practice, when bac-

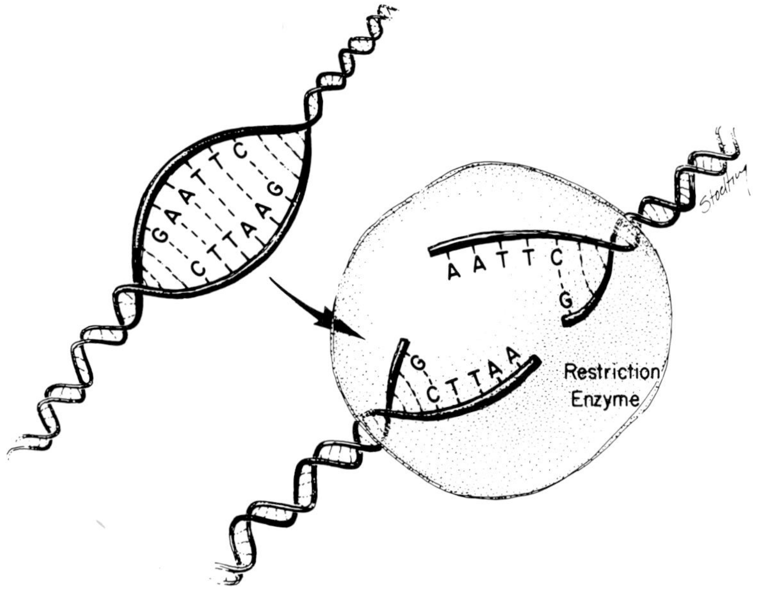

FIGURE 3-8 Endonucleolytic cleavage of DNA by the restriction enzyme *Eco*RI. The six-base-pair sequence recognized by the restriction endonuclease is enlarged for illustration purposes. The result of cleavage is two single-stranded sticky ends, i.e., overhanging, four-nucleotide complementary DNA segments.

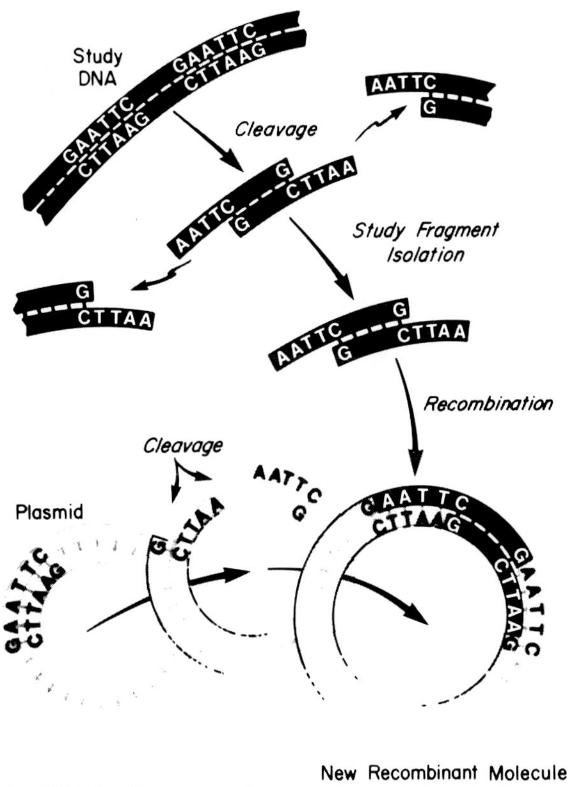

FIGURE 3-9 Generation of a recombinant DNA molecule. The study DNA is cleaved with a restriction enzyme (in this case *Eco*RI), and the released fragment is purified (i.e., separated from the parent DNA on the basis of size by agarose gel electrophoresis). A suitable plasmid containing a unique site for the same enzyme is prepared by cleavage with the enzyme, then mixed together with the purified fragment. The complementary overhanging ends anneal to one another and are then ligated together enzymatically (by DNA ligase) to yield a new recombinant molecule.

teria are transfected with plasmid DNA, only a small percentage of the microorganisms will actually take up the plasmid DNA, and on a probability basis only a single plasmid enters per bacterium. If a plasmid containing an antibiotic-resistance gene is used, one can select for those bacteria harboring these recombinant plasmids by culturing them in the presence of the appropriate antibiotic. Bacteria lacking plasmid DNA will then succumb to the antibiotic. That population of cells derived from a single parent cell harboring the foreign DNA is said to represent a *clone* of cells, and the DNA insert of the plasmid is said to be cloned (Fig. 3-10). Once a clone is obtained, the bacteria can be grown in mass quantity, the plasmid DNA isolated from other bacterial constituents, and the DNA insert released from the plasmid by cleaving it with the same restriction enzyme as was utilized for its initial isolation. This DNA can then be separated from the plasmid DNA by electrophoretic techniques and characterized. In this fashion large quantities of homogeneous DNA fragments can be produced for study purposes. One common use for such homogeneous pieces of DNA is to prepare radiolabeled probes for hybridizations.

Hybridization

A fundamental property of single-stranded DNA or RNA is its propensity to anneal through base pairing, i.e., to hybridize, to a strand of DNA or RNA containing complementary sequences (Fig. 3-11). This very precise process is based on the AT (or AU), GC hydrogen bonding discussed earlier, which permits a

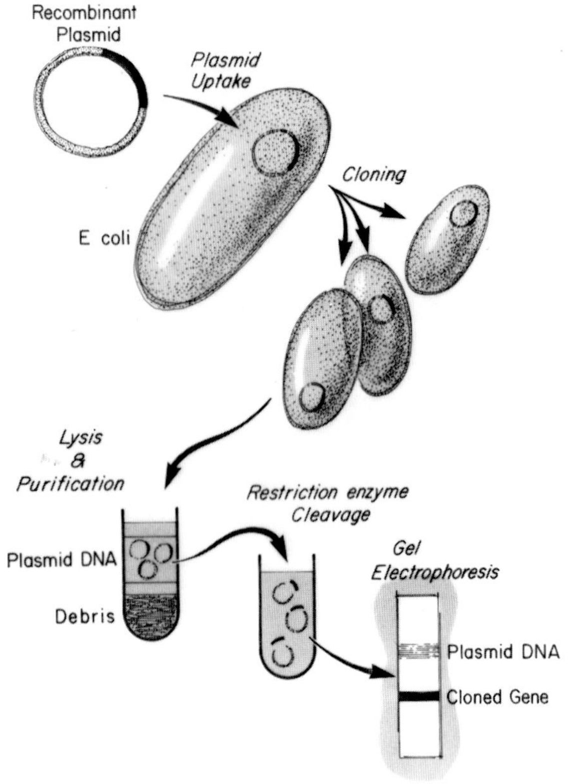

FIGURE 3-10 Cloning of DNA. Bacteria are treated to facilitate the uptake of DNA, often using recombinant plasmids containing a DNA insert of interest. Culturing in the presence of an antibiotic selects for those bacteria harboring a plasmid containing an appropriate antibiotic-resistance gene along with the DNA insert. Those bacteria which have failed to take up the plasmid will succumb to the antibiotic. Single colonies (a clone) of the now resistant bacteria are selected for mass culture and are then lysed and the cloned plasmid DNA purified. Cleavage with the appropriate restriction enzyme will release the DNA insert, yielding quantities of homogeneous DNA suitable for further experimentation (e.g., sequencing or preparation of specific radiolabeled DNA probes).

single-stranded nucleic acid to find its complement from among millions of noncomplementary competing molecules. Recombinant DNA technology makes extensive use of this property in virtually all its applications. For example, after radiolabeling, a homogeneous population of DNA molecules can be used as a probe to identify a complementary DNA or RNA fragment which has been size-fractionated on a gel or to localize a single colony of bacteria containing a plasmid with complementary DNA sequences from among thousands of bacterial clones, each harboring a different plasmid. One approach involves gel electrophoresis of the sample; the DNA or RNA in the gel then is transferred ("blotted") onto nitrocellulose filter paper, affixed to the paper, and then exposed to the radiolabeled probe. Originally described for the transfer of DNA molecules (*Southern blotting*),[100,101] RNA can be similarly transferred if properly treated (commonly referred to as *northern blotting*).[101] Radiolabeled probes can also be used to quantify levels of a specific mRNA by allowing the probe to hybridize to a mixture of RNA molecules either in solution or on a piece of filter paper, eliminating the nonhybridized probe, and determining the strength of the signal from the radiolabeled hybrids. The amount of radioactivity in the hybrid is proportional to the amount of specific mRNA (Fig. 3-11).

DNA Sequencing

Another breakthrough that has facilitated the development of recombinant DNA technology is the design of methods to rapidly sequence DNA. Two methods

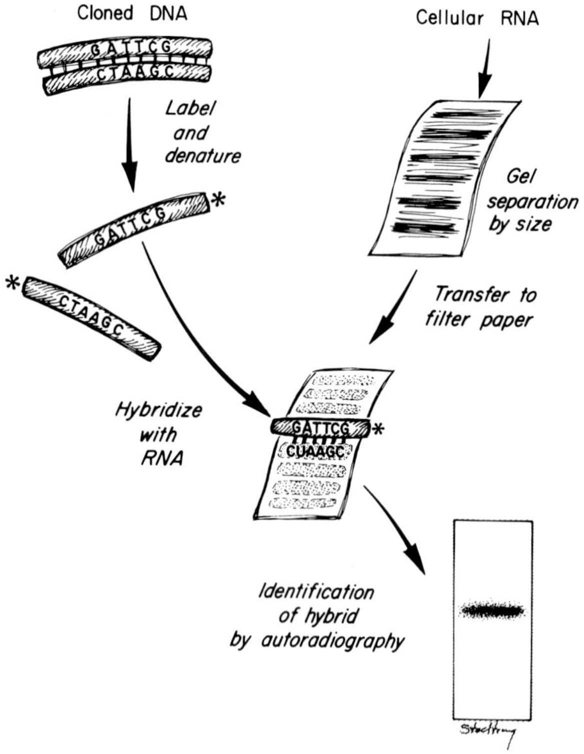

FIGURE 3-11 Use of hybridization to identify specific RNA sequences. A cloned piece of DNA is radiolabeled with ^{32}P nucleoside triphosphates and denatured. Cellular RNA is separated on the basis of size by agarose gel electrophoresis. The RNA is transferred by diffusion blotting onto nitrocellulose filter paper and fixed to the paper. The radiolabeled cDNA probe is incubated with the filter paper. Hybridization with complementary RNA sequences takes place and the nonhybridized probe is eliminated by washing. Autoradiography of the filter reveals the location (size) of the RNA species, and the strength of the signal is used for quantification.

are available (for review see Refs. 102 and 103). The chemical degradation technique of Maxam and Gilbert[102] relies on the systematic cleavage of homogeneous DNA fragments radiolabeled at one end. Reaction conditions are so chosen that the cleavage process in a given reaction occurs at only one (or two) of the four nucleotides (G residues, for instance) and that each susceptible position in a DNA molecule is cleaved at a low frequency. The result is a series of radiolabeled DNA fragments extending from the labeled end to each location of the given nucleotide (i.e., at each G) in the original DNA fragment. These can be visualized after size fractionation of the DNA and radioautography; the size of each band corresponds to the position of the base in the starting DNA (Fig. 3-12).

The chain termination technique of Sanger[103] uses a homogeneous population of single-stranded DNA molecules as templates for complementary DNA synthesis. DNA synthesis is initiated at a particular site with the use of a small "primer" oligonucleotide that hybridizes to a specific sequence. DNA synthesis then proceeds in the presence of radiolabeled nucleotide triphosphate precursors. In addition, the reaction is performed in the presence of an analogue of one of

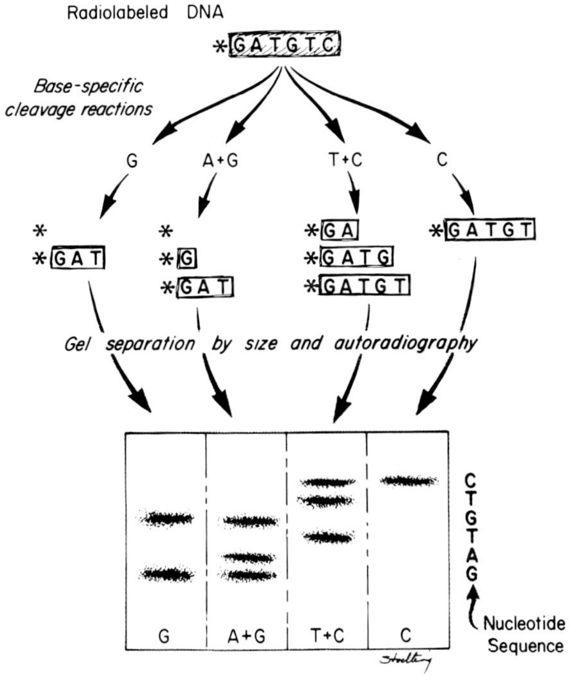

FIGURE 3-12 DNA sequencing by the chemical degradation technique. The radiolabeled DNA is subjected to four separate cleavage reactions, each of which is specific for one (or two) nucleotides. The resulting fragments from each reaction are separated on a gel, and the sequence is read from the autoradiogram. See text for details.

the nucleotides, which has a 3′-OH group so modified that when it is incorporated into a growing DNA chain, further elongation cannot proceed past that nucleotide. Four separate reactions are utilized, each reaction including one modified nucleotide (dideoxy-ATP for example) in addition to the four unmodified nucleotides. Conditions are so chosen that termination of synthesis of the complementary DNA molecule occurs infrequently at each occurrence of a given base (A in this example). The result is a series of radiolabeled fragments for each reaction that extend from the start site of synthesis to each occurrence of the base analyzed. These are then size-fractionated on gels; the size of each band corresponds to a position of the complementary base in the original template DNA.

By use of these methods, even genes that are several thousand nucleotides in length can be sequenced in a reasonable period of time. Thus, once a gene is obtained in pure form, its primary structure, or nucleotide sequence, can be determined rapidly and accurately.

Sources of DNA for Molecular Cloning

In order to obtain DNA elements for molecular cloning, three different sources are ordinarily utilized to procure the DNA of interest: DNA produced by chemical synthesis, cellular mRNA which can be reverse-transcribed into DNA, and chromosomal DNA.

DNA SYNTHESIS

Methods have recently been developed by which DNA molecules can be synthesized rather easily.[104] For example, DNA molecules composed of as many as 70 nucleotides can now be synthesized within a reasonable time using currently available mechanical synthesizers. By combining a number of oligonucleotides produced in this fashion, it is possible to synthesize an entire gene, provided its structure or that of the protein it encodes is known. This approach was used for the first synthesis of human insulin by recombinant DNA techniques.[1] At the time this was done the human insulin gene had not been isolated. However, the amino acid sequence of human insulin was known, and this information was used to select the nucleotide sequence of the synthetic gene. DNA fragments which would encode the amino acids of the A and B chains of human insulin were inserted into separate plasmids. In each case the synthetic gene segments were cloned in phase into the middle of a bacterial gene. When these plasmids were transfected into (separate) bacteria, the microorganisms synthesized a *fusion protein* containing the amino acids encoded by the bacterial gene linked to the human insulin A or B chain sequences. The A and B chains of human insulin were later cleaved from their respective fusion proteins, purified, and then joined together chemically through the disulfide bonds that ordinarily connect these two chains.

More commonly, however, smaller DNA segments are produced to facilitate the construction of genes or recombinant DNA molecules. For example, small DNA segments containing desired restriction enzyme sites (*linkers*) are frequently added to the ends of DNA fragments to aid in the production of recombinant molecules. Other chemically synthesized fragments are used commonly as probes to detect complementary DNA pieces in genes or in clones of bacteria. Finally, as discussed above and also in a subsequent section, synthetic DNA may be used to prepare hybrid genes that are combinations of different mammalian or bacterial genes. These may be used for protein production in the appropriate host cell.

REVERSE TRANSCRIPTION OF mRNA

Cellular mRNA encoding a particular protein can be isolated from cells that produce the protein product of interest. DNA strands complementary to this mRNA (i.e., cDNA) can be produced from the mRNA template, using deoxyribonucleoside triphosphates and the enzyme reverse transcriptase.[7,8,98,99] This enzyme is isolated from retrovirus-infected cells. *Retroviruses* are RNA viruses that have the ability to copy their RNA into DNA (*reverse transcription*). To initiate reverse transcription, the reaction must be primed by an oligonucleotide that hybridizes to the RNA being copied. As described earlier, most mRNA molecules have a polyadenylate, or poly A, tail. Oligomers of polydeoxythymidylate can hybridize to this poly A tail and serve to prime the reaction. Following formation of this cDNA, the RNA is destroyed and the single-stranded cDNA is then copied into a double-stranded DNA molecule, using either reverse transcriptase which can also copy DNA into DNA, or else DNA polymerase.

To insert the cDNA into a plasmid, several different methods can be utilized. For example, chemically synthesized double-stranded DNA linker molecules containing an appropriate restriction site may be ligated to the ends. The entire fragment may then be inserted into a plasmid at the same restriction enzyme site (see Fig. 3-9).

Since any given cell contains thousands of different mRNA molecules, reverse transcription of total cellular mRNA will yield thousands of different cDNA molecules. Thus, in order to obtain a given cDNA the investigator must either isolate the mRNA of interest prior to cDNA synthesis or else generate a large number of clones from the mixture of starting cDNA molecules and identify those clones containing the cDNA of interest. In most cases, the specific mRNA cannot be obtained in homogeneous form prior to cloning, therefore some reliance must be placed on the latter technique. However, mixtures of mRNA molecules are sometimes greatly enriched for an mRNA of interest prior to molecular cloning. This can be accomplished in several ways, including (1) starting with a tissue containing a high concentration of the mRNA, (2) isolation of a limited size range of mRNA molecules by physical separation techniques, and (3) immunoprecipitation of polysomes (collections of ribosomes containing mRNA and attached nascent protein chains) by the use of antisera that recognize the nascent peptide product of the mRNA.

In any case, all the mRNA molecules present at the time of reverse transcription will serve as templates for cDNA synthesis. This will yield, after cloning into the appropriate host cell, a so-called cDNA library representing from a few clones up to millions of clones, each harboring the same parent plasmid but a different cDNA insert. This cDNA library must then be screened for the clone containing the plasmid with the cDNA insert of interest.

A cDNA library may be screened in several ways.[98,99] If even a portion of the amino acid sequence of the protein encoded by the mRNA is known, this information can be used, through knowledge of the genetic code, to predict a partial DNA sequence for the cDNA. Small oligonucleotide DNA molecules complementary to a portion of the nucleotide sequence of the cDNA can be synthesized. Usually a group of such oligonucleotides are made to include all possible sequences in that portion of the cDNA, as determined by the degeneracy in the genetic code; this will compensate for a lack of knowledge of the exact codons in the cDNA. If a large stretch of amino acids is known, oligonucleotides are synthesized complementary to that region of the cDNA with the minimum number of possible codon choices. Alternatively, a single large oligonucleotide (50 to 70 nucleotides in length) may be utilized, with the codon choices determined by their probability of use.[105] These oligonucleotides can be radioactively labeled and hybridized to the DNA of the clones comprising the cDNA library after transfer of the DNA to filter paper. Only the DNA from those clones of cells carrying plasmids with the correct cDNA should hybridize to these oligonucleotide probes, and these can be identified by radioautography. The clones can then be isolated for further analysis of the cDNA insert. In some circumstances one may already have available a specific cDNA but desire to isolate the gene or the homologous cDNA of a different species. In this case the cDNA itself can be radiolabeled and used to probe the appropriate library to identify the clones of interest.

Another approach for screening a cDNA library is to clone the cDNA into a site in the plasmid that is somewhere in the middle of a bacterial gene.[106] In this case, approximately one out of six recombinant molecules will contain a cDNA insert that is in the correct orientation, with the codons of the cDNA in phase with respect to the coding sequence of the bacterial gene. The bacteria will express this cDNA as part of a fusion protein containing bacterial and cDNA-encoded amino acid sequences. This is analogous to the situation described above for the synthesis of human insulin. Screening this cDNA expression library with an antibody against the protein product of interest will permit identification of that clone producing the appropriate fusion protein and thus harboring the correct cDNA-containing plasmid. Bacteriophage vectors can also be utilized in this fashion.[107]

An additional method for screening a cDNA library relies on the ability of a cDNA to hybridize specifically to the mRNA from which it was derived and thereby block the ability of that mRNA to be translated in a cell-free reaction.[98,99] Translation of the mRNA of interest is identified through the production of its protein product in the reaction, detected, for instance, by immunoprecipitation. Plasmid DNA is isolated from each of the clones to be screened and allowed to hybridize to an RNA sample containing the mRNA of interest. If the group of plasmids being screened contains the desired cDNA, then the mRNA sequestered in the hybrid cDNA-mRNA molecule will not be able to direct the synthesis of protein in the cell-free translation reaction. This is referred to as *hybrid arrest*. The converse operation uses filter-bound cDNA-containing plasmids to "pull out" a specific mRNA from a mixture of mRNA molecules. The hybridized mRNA is then eluted from the filter and identified by translating it in the cell-free system. This is referred to as *hybrid-selected* or *hybrid release* translation. These techniques may also be used to confirm that a cDNA identified by another method is indeed the correct one.

To establish rigorously that the cDNA isolated is in fact the correct one, the nucleotide sequence of the cDNA is ordinarily determined. This is then compared with the amino acid sequence of the protein, if known.

CHROMOSOMAL GENES

Using techniques analogous to those used for cDNA cloning, described above, it is possible to clone chromosomal genes, i.e., the portions of a chromosome which ultimately code for a protein. Chromosomal DNA isolated from cell nuclei can be cleaved into fragments by use of a restriction enzyme and the resultant fragments ligated into the appropriate restriction site of bacterial virus (bacteriophage) DNA.[98,99,108] The use of bacteriophage to carry the chromosomal DNA inserts is necessitated by their large size (often several thousand nucleotides). Certain classes of such viruses can also be used to clone cDNA. The recombinant bacteriophage is used to infect a bacterial host in which its DNA is replicated.

A radiolabeled cDNA or chemically synthesized oligonucleotides may then be used to screen the bacteria for that clone containing the bacteriophage with the chromosomal insert of interest. This is done by transferring the DNA of the phage that has infected the bacteria to a filter paper and then hybridizing the filter to radioactive cDNA. The specificity of this hybridization allows one to identify the correct clone or plaque where the bacteria are lysed with the desired chromosomal insert. One can then produce this particular bacteriophage in large quantities to obtain sufficient chromosomal DNA for analysis.

Genes can also be cloned into yeasts.[98,99] These organisms have plasmids similar to bacteria, and they can be used in an analogous fashion. Yeasts have been used to study the mechanisms of regulation of eukaryotic gene expression and to produce medically useful proteins.

Transfer of Cloned Genes into Mammalian Cells

Another major advance in molecular biology is the development of methods to transfer cloned genes into mammalian cells where the genes can be expressed. This methodology has had its greatest impact by providing a means to understand gene function, but it is also being used to produce proteins which may be important therapeutically.

DNA can be transferred into mammalian cells in several ways: (1) DNA can be microinjected into the nucleus of a cell;[109] (2) calcium-phosphate precipitates of DNA can be prepared which will be phagocytosed by cells;[110] (3) protoplasts, i.e., bacteria stripped of their cell walls, can be prepared from bacteria which harbor plasmids with mammalian gene inserts and then fused to mammalian cells, thereby delivering the DNA inside the cell.[111] Additional methods include direct electroporation of plasmid DNA into recipient cells[112] and the use of viral vectors to deliver DNA to specific cell types.[113]

If an experiment requires only a relatively brief examination of the function of the transferred DNA, this can be studied a short time (usually 48 to 60 h) after the transfer (transient expression assay).[29,114] Most of the transfected DNA will not integrate into the host chromosome and will be destroyed after a few days; it will, however, integrate into the host chromosome at low frequency, replicate along with it, and be stably expressed. The relatively small number of cells in which this has occurred can be isolated in several ways. For example, the DNA of interest can be cotransfected with DNA containing a selectable gene—i.e., a gene whose product confers on the cell some new property allowing for its selective survival, such as the gene encoding resistance to neomycin.[115] In this case, when the cells are cultured in the presence of neomycin (actually an analogue of it that ordinarily kills the cells), only those cells that both integrate and express the neomycin-resistance gene will survive and propagate. Most of the time, these cells will also have integrated the study gene.

These gene transfer techniques have been utilized to study, among other questions, the mechanisms of hormonal regulation of gene expression. The first breakthrough in this area occurred when the cloned $\alpha_{2\mu}$-globulin gene was transferred into mouse fibroblasts and its expression was found to be glucocorticoid-regulated.[116] This experiment indicated that all the information necessary for a response to glucocorticoids was present on the cloned gene fragment that was transferred. Additional studies (Fig. 3-13) have involved deleting successive portions of a gene (e.g., progressively deleting increasing amounts of the 5′-flanking DNA), transferring the truncated gene, and assaying for loss of steroid responsiveness. This type of analysis permits a more refined identification of those DNA segments required for the hormonal effect.[64,65,117] Other experiments involved isolating the DNA segment whose deletion resulted in extinction of the hormonal response and testing its ability to confer on a normally nonhormonally regulated gene the capacity for hormonal responsiveness. For example, glucocorticoid response elements (glucocorticoid regulatory elements, or GREs, discussed earlier and illustrated in Fig. 3-5) were identified in this way. The GRE was initially spliced upstream from a heterologous promoter that ordinarily is not responsive to glucocorticoids; after transfer of the hybrid gene, glucocorticoid responsiveness of this promoter was demonstrable.[47b, 65, 118]

Production of Medically Important Proteins by Recombinant DNA Techniques

A major use of recombinant DNA technology is the production of medically useful proteins. Once a gene has been cloned, conditions can often be so chosen that it can be used to produce the protein it encodes. To date, this is the only means available for producing moderate- to large-size proteins in quantity. Although the methods for synthesizing peptides through chemical techniques have improved considerably in recent years, these have not progressed to the point where large proteins (e.g., of over 100 amino acids) can be made efficiently. Although some proteins, insulin for

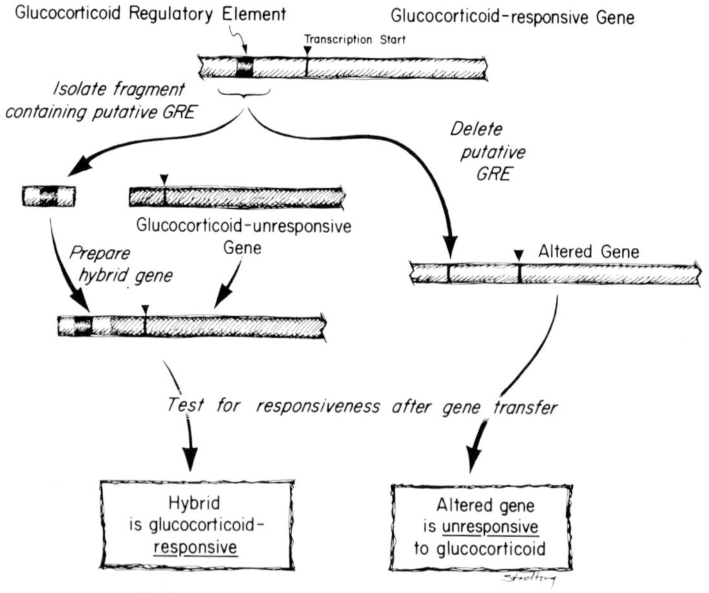

FIGURE 3-13 Identification of DNA sequences required for glucocorticoid responsiveness. Two separate types of experiments are illustrated. In one experiment (on the left), the DNA containing the GRE is isolated and tested for its ability to confer glucocorticoid responsiveness on a normally nonregulated gene after gene transfer. In the other experiment (on the right), the putative GRE is deleted from the 5′-flanking DNA and the gene is no longer steroid-responsive after gene transfer.

example, can be obtained by isolating them from animals, this approach has its limitations. It is not practical when large quantities of proteins naturally produced in minute amounts are needed, such as interferon or erythropoietin.

As discussed earlier, genes require control sequences in order to be expressed. Therefore, mammalian DNA sequences inserted randomly into bacterial DNA will commonly not be expressed efficiently. In order to obtain efficient expression, the sequences that encode the medically relevant protein are inserted into plasmids in such a way that they are placed downstream from bacterial control sequences. Such sequences would include a promoter, the sequences encoding a ribosomal binding site, and an AUG (methionine) codon that is necessary in the mRNA to initiate translation. Ordinarily, a promoter that is highly active in bacteria is chosen to enhance the yields. In this way bacterial control sequences direct the synthesis of the foreign protein. Utilizing this method of direct expression, the synthesized protein can frequently be obtained in yields that are several percent of the total bacterial proteins.[3,4] These proteins are then purified from the bacteria. This approach was utilized to express initially methionine–human growth hormone.[3]

The major drawbacks of this approach are that (1) the protein product may be unstable in the bacterial environment, (2) it may be necessary to have the protein without the initiating methionine, and (3) sometimes the protein needs to be modified (for example, by glycosylation) to be active. The first two of these drawbacks may be bypassed by synthesizing a *fusion*, or *hybrid protein* from which the desired protein can be cleaved (Fig. 3-14). This was described earlier for the example of human insulin, in which the DNA sequences encoding the chains of human insulin were so inserted into the coding sequence of a bacterial gene that they were in phase. In this way the bacteria synthesize a hybrid protein containing bacterial and mammalian amino acids. These genes are so constructed that a proteolytic or chemically susceptible cleavage site occurs at the junction of the bacterial and mammalian amino acid sequences. This approach was also used for the first bacterial synthesis of human somatostatin, the first mammalian protein to be made by recombinant DNA techniques,[119] and β-endorphin.[120]

Some proteins are produced more efficiently in yeasts.[121] The approaches are typically similar to those used in bacteria. One useful feature is that yeasts can be programmed to secrete their expressed proteins, a feature that aids in purification of the protein. In addition, the amino-terminal methionine of these secreted proteins may be removed, eliminating a possibly unwanted amino acid.

Mammalian cells are being used increasingly for the production of recombinant DNA–derived proteins. Increased production and the use of more refined media devoid of expensive animal serum have stimulated the use of this approach. The mammalian gene coding sequences are commonly inserted downstream from a highly active promoter to facilitate yields.[122,122a,122b] Use of mammalian cells also has the

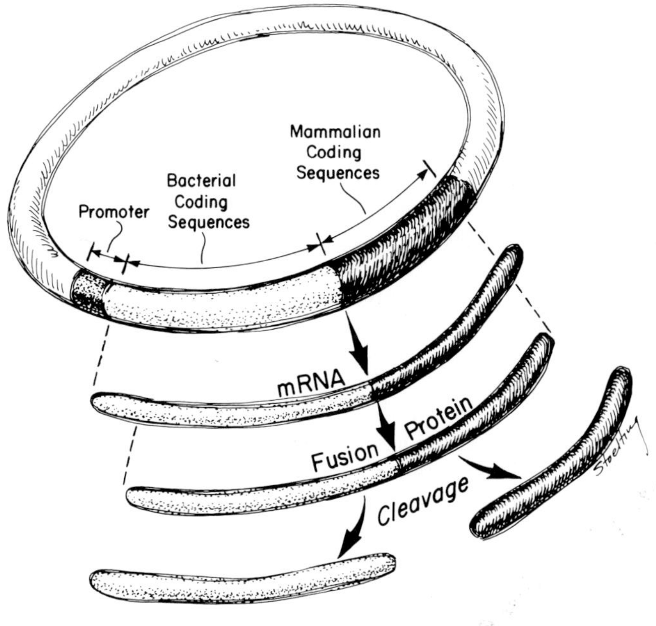

FIGURE 3-14 Expression of a mammalian protein as a fusion protein in bacteria. Sequences coding for a mammalian protein are linked, in phase with respect to the genetic code, to sequences coding for a bacterial protein. The hybrid protein gene is expressed under the control of the bacterial promoter. If engineered properly, the fusion protein can be cleaved (chemically or enzymatically) to release the mammalian protein, which can then be further purified.

advantage that these cells can add important carbohydrate groups to the proteins when this is necessary for full activity; this may not be done correctly by yeasts and is not performed at all by bacteria. Plasminogen activators, now in clinical trials, are being produced by mammalian cells.[123,123a] More complex proteins such as factor VIII can also be expressed in cultured mammalian cells.[122a,122b]

PRODUCTS OF RECOMBINANT DNA TECHNOLOGY

The human body produces thousands of different proteins, including those which function as hormones or enzymes. A deficiency or excess of many of these proteins is well recognized as contributing to human disease. Recombinant DNA technology, by the means outlined above, will make possible the production of many of these proteins in pure form to allow testing of their clinical utility. In addition to providing the natural proteins, the technology should facilitate the production of derivatives which may prove useful either as antagonists or as more specific agonists. For example, derivatives which possess a more limited, and thus clinically more specific, range of activities compared to the parent protein might be produced. A comprehensive review of progress in this area is outside the scope of this chapter, but a few examples relevant to endocrinology are cited.

Human insulin prepared by recombinant techniques is now available.[1,2] This ensures an unlimited supply of this hormone. Growth hormone has recently become available to replace cadaver-derived human growth hormone, which may in some cases have been contaminated with the Creutzfeldt-Jakob virus.[3-5] Erythropoietin is being developed.[124] This hormone may be useful in a number of anemias, and it is hoped that in certain situations it may decrease the need for transfusion with its associated problems. Atrial natriuretic factor is being tested in humans for the treatment of hypertension, edema, and related states.[125,126] This hormone increases the glomerular filtration rate directly and antagonizes the renin-angiotensin system, thereby promoting hypotension and natriuresis with relative potassium sparing.[127] It is also a vasodilator. Other potentially useful hormones include growth factors such as epidermal growth factor, somatomedins, and nerve growth factors.

A protein (or proteins) termed *macrocortin* or *lipocortin* is of particular interest to the endocrinologist.[128,128a] This protein inhibits phospholipase A_2, a key enzyme in the generation of arachidonic acid and thus in the formation of prostaglandins, prostacyclins, and leukotrienes. This inhibitor is induced by glucocorticoids and is thought to mediate some of the anti-inflammatory actions of these steroids.[128] Conceivably such peptides could be used instead of glucocorticoids in certain circumstances and might be associated with fewer side effects than these steroids. Another peptide that may replace glucocorticoids in neonatology is pulmonary surfactant protein.[129] This protein is induced by these steroids and is deficient in the neonatal respiratory distress syndrome.

Recombinant DNA technology lends itself ideally to vaccine production, and a number of different approaches are being used. Individual genes encoding important antigens can be cloned and expressed; this bypasses the need to give inactivated organisms and may be safer and more specific. Indeed, recent studies have demonstrated that several viral antigens can be inserted into a single benign viral vector to be used for immunization. In early animal studies these polyvalent vaccines have resulted in antibodies to all the viral antigens.[130] It is possible that these vaccines could have an impact greater than merely preventing the target disease. For example, it has been postulated that the prevention of certain viral diseases might decrease the incidence of type 1 diabetes.[131]

As stated previously, protein derivatives with specific advantages may be produced. In addition, hybrid molecules composed of two (or more) different molecules could theoretically be produced by linking together portions of different genes. Already there is a major effort to test the activity of hybrid and variant immunoglobulin molecules.[132] Molecules with antagonist activity can also be produced. For example, parathyroid hormone (PTH) antagonists result when a few of the PTH amino-terminal amino acids are deleted;[133] conceivably these could be useful in treating certain hypercalcemic states associated with excess PTH or PTH-like activity.

NEW DRUG DELIVERY SYSTEMS

The products of recombinant DNA technology are largely proteins. They are generally unstable in and poorly absorbed from the gastrointestinal tract. This necessitates their administration by injection, which limits their utility. However, this problem is being bypassed in several ways. As more information is accumulated, it may be possible to determine the critically active structures of these proteins and design orally active drugs that contain these essential elements.

In addition, a number of systems are being developed to facilitate delivery of these drugs. Microemulsions may be used which encapsulate and facilitate movement of a drug through cell membranes and into the cell.[134] Implantable devices that release a drug over a prolonged period are being developed. Another approach involves mixing the protein with a bile salt analogue and spraying the mixture into the nose.[135,136] This has now been shown to be effective, at least over short periods of time, for delivering insulin to diabetics.[137] The insulin in this case is absorbed rapidly into the circulation, mimicking intravenous delivery. This feature makes the route of administration advantageous in that postprandial hyperglycemia can be more easily controlled because of the rapidity of onset of insulin action.

USE OF DNA IN THE DIAGNOSIS OF GENETIC DISEASE

In addition to the classic genetic diseases, in which individual enzyme deficiencies are often responsible,[138] more subtle, and in most cases undefined, genetic defects contribute to the development of many common diseases, e.g., diabetes mellitus and hypertension, and a tendency to premature atherosclerosis. The ability to analyze genes in detail may permit detection of appropriate DNA segments which could provide a means to diagnose these conditions as well as contribute to our understanding of their pathogenesis. Rapid tests utilizing recombinant DNA probes are now available for diagnosing genetic diseases such as some types of thalassemias,[139] sickle cell anemia,[140,140a] and phenylketonuria.[141]

Although in principle one could isolate from a patient a gene presumed to be responsible for disease and determine its primary structure, this procedure is cumbersome and not practical for general clinical use. However, other techniques are available. In many cases, it should be possible to isolate DNA from biopsy specimens, blood cells, or amniotic fluid cells, for example, cleave it with restriction enzymes, fractionate it on gels, and transfer it to filter paper. The genetic defect might then be detected by hybridizing with particular DNA probes, thus providing a new means of diagnosis.

This methodology relies heavily on analysis of genetic polymorphisms (Fig. 3-15). *Polymorphisms* are differences in the primary structure of a given gene; these can be observed between the two alleles of a given gene in the same person or between the genes of two different persons. Most commonly the polymorphism reflects single nucleotide differences, but in some cases it can involve inserted or deleted segments of DNA. These differences can occur in the sequences of the gene that are transcribed or in the flanking DNA. In the process of replication, mutations in the DNA occur at a low frequency. Most of these are silent, in that they have no effect on the function of the gene or on its products. Nevertheless, once these mutations occur, they are inherited and can be used as genetic markers.

Assume, for instance, that a given person develops a single base mutation that results in a genetic trait, for example, a tendency to develop hypertension. Even if one knew which gene was involved, it might be difficult to detect the change without sequencing the entire gene. However, this person is likely to have additional differences from other people

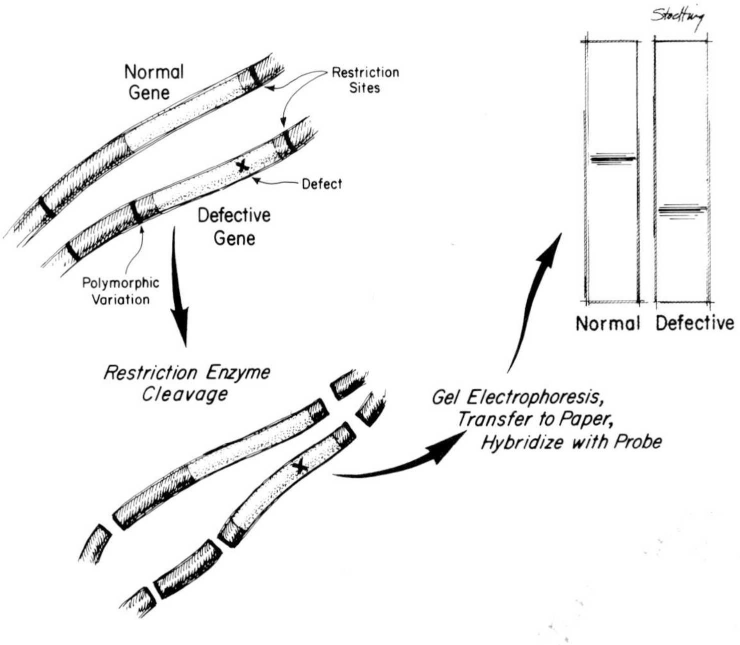

FIGURE 3-15 Use of restriction fragment length polymorphisms as genetic markers of disease. In the case illustrated, a mutation resulting in a defective gene is associated with a polymorphic variation in the 5′-flanking DNA which results in the presence of a restriction site not present in unafflicted individuals. Cleavage with the appropriate restriction enzyme will yield a smaller fragment for the defective gene than for the normal gene. Subjecting the various fragments to size fractionation on a gel and to hybridization to the radiolabeled gene (or its cDNA) as a probe will allow identification of the aberrant fragment. This obviates the need for isolation and cloning of the genomic DNA to identify the mutation within the gene.

somewhere in or around the affected gene. Occasionally these differences result in the generation or loss of a restriction endonuclease cleavage site (Fig. 3-15). In this case, cleavage of that person's DNA with the restriction enzyme will result in DNA fragments of a different size from that of another person. This aberrent fragment can be identified after size fractionation of the fragments on a gel, transfer of the DNA to filter paper, and hybridization to a radiolabeled probe from the gene. If the restriction site polymorphism is inherited along with the mutation that results in disease susceptibility, this polymorphism can be used as a genetic marker for the disease. All that is required for this type of analysis is (1) an established linkage between a restriction fragment length polymorphism and a disease and (2) an appropriate probe. It is not necessary to know anything about the gene product.

A similar application of such methods within endocrinology has involved study of the association of certain structural features of genes with certain metabolic diseases, e.g., diabetes mellitus. The insulin gene has been cloned and sequenced.[40] When the DNA including the insulin gene from several unrelated persons was cleaved with restriction enzymes, it was discovered that a region close to the insulin gene was of variable size.[142] The polymorphic region near the insulin gene is actually the result of different-size insertions located about 300 base pairs upstream from the start site of transcription. Several studies have identified different alleles as being associated with an increased risk of specific types of diabetes mellitus.[143,144] The exact nature of this association is unclear, but certain alleles may be linked to genes which confer a susceptibility to the disease, an association analogous to that of many human leukocyte antigens (HLA).

POTENTIAL FOR GENE THERAPY

Since genes can be transferred into mammalian cells and function after such transfer, it follows that there is a potential for inserting genes into the cells of patients. The advantages of such an approach are obvious. For example, if the insulin gene could be appropriately transferred to a patient with type 1 diabetes, the gene might be capable of delivering insulin to the patient on a continuous basis, thereby obviating insulin injection. Similar considerations apply to other diseases, such as the thalassemias, sickle cell anemia, hypoparathyroidism, and other deficiency states. Conversely, gene transfer therapy could also be used to treat hypercholesterolemia or hypertension by transferring genes whose products would act to lower cholesterol levels or blood pressure. However, the initial application of this therapeutic technique will probably involve attempts to correct certain immunodeficiency states.[145]

Although most researchers now agree that this therapy will ultimately be possible, it is also true that a number of problems need to be solved before it becomes generally applicable. The gene needs to be delivered to the right tissue, for example, globin genes to erythroid cells. The gene needs to function adequately but not excessively; for example, one must ensure that the insulin gene would function in a cellular environment capable of responding appropriately to blood glucose levels. Stably integrated genes are now obtained in the laboratory by applying gene transfer techniques to dividing cells, whereas many targets for gene transfer therapy are nondividing cells. Since the integration of genes into the chromosome results in an interruption of the cellular DNA at the site of integration, there is a potential for mutation and consequently malignant transformation or even death of the cell.[145]

Although these problems are substantial, one can conceive of approaches to circumvent them. For example, it might be possible to isolate and propagate in culture the relevant cells, transfer the gene to these cells and document its proper functioning, and demonstrate that the cells are not malignantly transformed. At that point they could be delivered back to appropriate locations in the body. These cells might, for instance, be so inserted in a capsule that they could be removed if it is desired to terminate treatment or if other problems develop.

This technology should provide a powerful means to approach a number of diseases. Such methods will also raise a number of ethical and related issues that physicians will need to face.[146]

Ethical and Biosafety Considerations

Recombinant DNA technology, like most other technologies, has the potential for misuse, either accidental or deliberate. When it first emerged in the early to mid-1970s, great concern was raised about its overall safety. It was feared, for example, that *Escherichia coli* harboring potentially toxic genes, if accidently leaked into the environment, would propagate and cause great damage. Fortunately, most of these concerns have now been allayed; the laboratory strains of *E. coli* used do not multiply well outside the laboratory or in the human intestine, and in general there is no environmental pressure to favor the growth of those organisms harboring cloned genes. Nevertheless, the potential does exist for inserting genes in other organisms in ways that could be harmful. For these and other reasons, most agree that there should be guidelines for conducting such research.

Impact of Molecular Biology on Medicine

While there have been important practical applications of recombinant DNA technology, its greatest impact has been in the basic information provided about genes—their function, regulation, and products. In addition, the production of medically useful products has provided the means to further investigate more basic questions. For example, now that erythropoietin is available in substantial quantity, it will be possible to learn much more about its actions, biological roles, and therapeutic uses.

Recent progress in cancer research is illustrative both of the impact of molecular biology on medicine and on the interplay of the endocrine system in growth control. The study of retrovirus genes capable of inducing neoplastic transformation (*oncogenes*) has generated an enormous body of information.[147–149] Several potential mechanisms by which normal cellular proliferation may become neoplastic have been identified. In some cases, the tumor-promoting genes of these viruses encode proteins related to growth factors. The v-sis gene product of one class of such viruses is similar to one of the two subunits of platelet-derived growth factor.[150,151] These oncogens are generally named for the virus harboring that gene; in this case, sis refers to simian sarcoma virus, and v refers to the viral gene. In other cases, these viral oncogenes encode proteins that are analogues of growth factor receptors; the v-erb B oncogene encodes a protein similar to the epidermal growth factor receptor.[152] In addition, this group of viruses, through their insertion in the DNA, might also activate cellular genes with growth-stimulating activity.[153] Of tremendous importance was the finding that these viral oncogenes were actually acquired from the DNA of vertebrates (the normal cellular loci referred to as *proto-oncogenes*).[147] These proto-oncogenes may serve either as the origin of certain retrovirus oncogenes or undergo alterations to function themselves as active oncogenes. The gene referred to as c-Ha-ras (c because of its cellular origin, and Ha-ra because of its homology to the viral v-Ha-ras gene) was isolated from a bladder carcinoma and found to encode a protein that appears to be a version of a guanyl nucleotide–binding protein that may regulate adenylate cyclase.[147,154] This gene may be involved in a significant number of human cancers.[155]

There is much evidence to suggest that cancer is not a one-step process.[156] For example, some genes may perform the function of converting the cell to a state that allows for continued replication; cancer would not ensue until a second gene is activated that stimulates cell growth. The requirements of a multistep process might explain why certain endocrine malignant diseases (postradiation thyroid cancer, the tumors of the multiple endocrine neoplasia syndromes) require years to develop. Other aspects of malignant transformation may involve processes that result in inability of the tumor to be suppressed by the body's immune system. The recent availability of recombinant DNA–produced proteins such as tumor necrosis factor will greatly facilitate studies of these aspects.[157,158]

With the emergence of an understanding of the fundamental molecular aspects of cancer, as well as the control of normal cell growth, scientists can begin to design new approaches to cancer prevention, diagnosis, and treatment. For example, if growth factor activation is involved, novel means to block the effects of that activation or to terminate it could be designed. Endocrinology will benefit particularly from these approaches as a better appreciation is developed of the molecular mechanisms of hormone action and the role of hormones in normal and neoplastic cell growth.

REFERENCES

1. Goeddel DV, Kleid DG, Bolivar F, et al: Expression in Escherichia coli of chemically synthesized genes for human insulin. *Proc Natl Acad Sci USA* 76:106, 1979.
2. Keen H, Glynne A, Pickup JC, et al: Human insulin produced by recombinant DNA technology: Safety and hypoglycemic potency in healthy men. *Lancet* 2:398, 1980.
3. Goeddel DV, Heyneker HL, Hozumi T, et al: Direct expression in *E. coli* of a DNA sequence for human growth hormone. *Nature* 281:544, 1979.
4. Martial JA, Hallewell RA, Baxter JD, Goodman HM: Human growth hormone: Complementary DNA cloning and expression in bacteria. *Science* 205:602, 1979.
5. Hintz RL, Rosenfeld RG, Wilson DM, et al: Biosynthetic methionyl human growth hormone is biologically active in adult man. *Lancet* 1:1276, 1982.
6. Watson JD, Crick FHC: Molecular structure of nucleic acids: A structure for deoxyribose nucleic acid. *Nature* 171:737, 1953.
7. Alberts B, Bray D, Lewis J, et al: *Molecular Biology of the Cell.* New York, Garland, 1983.
8. Lewin B: *Genes II.* New York, Wiley, 1985.
9. Wolpert L: DNA and its message. *Lancet* 2:853, 1984.
10. Nevins JR: The pathway of eukaryotic mRNA formation. *Annu Rev Biochem* 52:441, 1983.
11. Gehring WJ: The molecular basis of development. *Sci Am* 253:152B, 1985.
12. Igo-Kemenes T, Horz W, Zachau HG: Chromatin. *Annu Rev Biochem* 51:89, 1982.
13. McGhee JD, Felsenfeld G: Nucleosome structure. *Annu Rev Biochem* 49:1115, 1980.
14. Weisbrod S: Active chromatin. *Nature* 297:289, 1982.
15. Weintraub H, Groudine M: Chromosomal subunits in active genes have an altered conformation. *Science* 193:848, 1976.
16. O'Malley BW: Steroid hormone action in eucaryotic cells. *J Clin Invest* 74:307, 1984.
17. Zaret KS, Yamamoto KR: Reversible and persistent changes in chromatin structure accompanying activation of a glucocorticoid-dependent enhancer element. *Cell* 38:29, 1984.
18. Pardoll D, Vogelstein B, Coffey DS: A fixed site of DNA replication in eucaryotic cells. *Cell* 19:527, 1980.
19. Robinson SI, Nolkin BD, Vogelstein B: The ovalbumin gene is associated with the nuclear matrix of chicken oviduct cells. *Cell* 28:99, 1982.

20. Ciejek EM, Tsai MJ, O'Malley BW: Actively transcribed genes are associated with the nuclear matrix. *Nature* 306:607, 1983.
21. Lerner MR, Steitz JA: Snurps and scyrps. *Cell* 25:298, 1981.
22. Padgett RA, Mount SM, Steitz JA, Sharp PA: Splicing of messenger RNA precursors is inhibited by antisera to small nuclear ribonucleoprotein. *Cell* 35:101, 1983.
23. Moore CL, Sharp PA: Site-specific polyadenylation in a cell-free reaction. *Cell* 36:581, 1984.
24. Walter P, Blobel G: Signal recognition particle contains a 7S RNA essential for protein translocation across the endoplasmic reticulum. *Nature* 299:691, 1982.
25. Walter P, Gilmore R, Blobel G: Protein translocation across the endoplasmic reticulum. *Cell* 38:5, 1984.
26. Breathnach R, Chambon P: Organization and expression of eucaryotic split genes coding for proteins. *Annu Rev Biochem* 50:349, 1981.
27. McKnight SL, Kingsbury R: Transcriptional control signals of a eukaryotic protein coding gene. *Science* 217:316, 1982.
28. Gillies SD, Morrison SL, Oi VT, Tonegawa S: A tissue-specific transcriptional enhancer element is located in the major intron of a rearranged immunoglobulin heavy chain gene. *Cell* 33:717, 1983.
29. Walker MD, Edlund T, Boulet AM, Rutter WJ: Cell specific expression controlled by the 5'-flanking region of insulin and chymotrypsin genes. *Nature* 306:557, 1983.
29a. Edlund T, Walker MD, Barr PJ, Rutter WJ: Cell-specific expression of the rat insulin gene: Evidence for role of two distinct 5' flanking elements. *Science* 230:912, 1985.
30. Dynan WS, Tjian R: Control of eukaryotic messenger RNA synthesis by sequence-specific DNA-binding proteins. *Nature* 316:774, 1985.
31. Brown DD: The role of stable complexes that repress and activate eucaryotic genes. *Cell* 37:359, 1984.
32. Grummt I, Skinner JA: Efficient transcription of a protein-coding gene from the RNA polmerase I promoter in transfected cells. *Proc Natl Acad Sci USA* 82:722, 1985.
33. Birnstiel ML, Busslinger M, Strub K: Transcription termination and 3' processing: The end is in site! *Cell* 41:349, 1985.
34a. Hernandez N, Keller W: Splicing of in vitro synthesized messenger RNA precursors in HeLa cell extracts. *Cell* 35:89, 1983.
34b. Padgett RA, Hardy SF, Sharp PA: Splicing of adenovirus RNA in a cell-free transcription system. *Proc Natl Acad Sci USA* 80:5230, 1983.
35. Grabowski PJ, Seiler SR, Sharp PA: A multicomponent complex is involved in the splicing of messenger RNA precursors. *Cell* 42:345, 1985.
36. Keller W: The RNA lariat: A new ring to the splicing of mRNA precursors. *Cell* 39:423, 1984.
37. Mount SM: A catalogue of splice junction sequences. *Nucleic Acids Res* 10:459, 1982.
38. Treisman R, Proudfoot NJ, Shander M, Maniatis T: A single-base change at a splice site in a β-thalassemic gene causes abnormal RNA splicing. *Cell* 29:903, 1982.
39. Gilbert W: Genes in pieces revisited. *Science* 228:823, 1985.
40. Bell GI, Pictet RL, Rutter WJ, et al: Sequence of the human insulin gene. *Nature* 284:26, 1980.
41. Hardman JA, Hort YJ, Catanzaro DF, et al: Primary structure of the human renin gene. *DNA* 3:457, 1984.
42. Sudhof TC, Godstein JL, Brown MS, Russell DW: The LDL-receptor gene: A mosaic of exons shared with different proteins. *Science* 228:815, 1985.
43. Proudfoot NJ, Brownlee GG: 3' Non-coding region sequences in eukaryotic mRNA. *Nature* 263:211, 1976.
44. Shatkin AJ: Capping of eukaryotic mRNAs. *Cell* 9:645, 1976.
45a. Furuichi Y, LaFiandra A, Shatkin AJ: 5'-Terminal structure and mRNA stability. *Nature* 266:235, 1977.
45b. Darnell JE, Nevins JR, Zeevi MY: The role of poly(A) in mammalian gene expression, in O'Malley B (ed): *Gene Regulation.* UCLA Symposium 26, 1982, p 161.
46. Hamer DH, Smith KD, Boyer SH, Leder P: SV40 recombinants carrying rabbit β-globin gene coding sequences. *Cell* 17:725, 1979.
47a. Moore DD, Marks AR, Buckley DI, et al: The first intron of the human growth hormone gene contains a binding site for glucocorticoid receptor. *Proc Natl Acad Sci USA* 82:699, 1985.
47b. Slater EP, Rabenau O, Karin M, et al: Glucocorticoid receptor binding and activation of a heterologous promoter by dexamethasone by the first intron of the human growth hormone gene. *Mol Cell Biol* 5:2984, 1985.
48. O'Malley BW, Means AR, Stein JP: Gene structure and evolution, in Roy AK, Clark JN (eds): *Gene Regulation by Steroid Hormones II.* New York, Springer-Verlag, 1983, p 1.
49. Miller WL, Baxter JD, Eberhardt NL: Peptide hormone genes: Structure and evolution, in Krieger D, Brownstein N, Martin T (eds): *Brain Peptides.* New York, Wiley, 1983, p 15.
50. Doolittle WF: Genes in pieces: Were they ever together? *Nature* 272:581, 1978.
51. Miller WL, Eberhardt NL: Structure and evolution of the growth hormone gene family. *Endocr Rev* 4:97, 1983.
52. Amara SG, Jonas V, Rosenfeld M, et al: Alternative RNA processing in calcitonin gene expression generates mRNAs encoding different polypeptide products. *Nature* 298:240, 1982.
53. Jonas V, Lin CR, Kawashima E, et al: Alternative RNA processing events in human calcitonin/calcitonin gene-related peptide gene expression. *Proc Natl Acad Sci USA* 82:1994, 1985.
54. Goodbourn S, Zinn K, Maniatis T: Human β-interferon gene expression is regulated by an inducible enhancer element. *Cell* 41:509, 1985.
55. Wright S, Rosenthal A, Flavell R, et al: DNA sequences required for regulated expression of β-globin genes in murine erythroleukemia cells. *Cell* 38:265, 1984.
56. Gehring WJ: The homeo box: A key to the understanding of development? *Cell* 40:3, 1985.
57a. Darnell JE: Variety in the level of gene control in eukaryotic cells. *Nature* 297:365, 1982.
57b. Lan NC, Karin M, Nguyen T, et al: Mechanisms of glucocorticoid hormone action. *J Steroid Biochem* 20:77, 1984.
58a. Bird AP: DNA methylation—how important in gene control? *Nature* 307:503, 1984.
58b. Ehrlich M, Wang R: 5-Methylcytosine in eukaryotic DNA. *Science* 212:1350, 1981.
59. Chapman VM, Kratzer PG, Siracusa LD, et al: Evidence for DNA modification in the maintenance of X-chromosome inactivation of adult mouse tissues. *Proc Natl Acad Sci USA* 79:5357, 1982.
60. Tonegawa S: The molecules of the immune system. *Sci Am* 253:122, 1985.
61. Robberts TH: DNA juggling in the immune system. *Lancet* 2:1086, 1984.
62. Payvar F, DeFranco D, Firestone GL, Edgar B, Wrange O, Okiet S, Gustafsson J, Yamamoto KR: Sequence-specific binding of the glucocorticoid receptor to MTV DNA at sites within and upstream of the transcribed region. *Cell* 35:381, 1983.
63. Scheidereit C, Geisse S, Westphal HM, Beato M: The glucocorticoid receptor binds to defined nucleotide sequences near the promoter of mouse mammary tumor virus. *Nature* 304:749, 1983.
64. Karin M, Haslinger A, Holtgreve H, Richards R, Kravter P, et al: Characterization of DNA sequences through which cadmium and glucocorticoid hormone induce human metallothionein IIA gene. *Nature* 308:513, 1984.
65. Chandler VL, Maler BA, Yamamoto KR: DNA sequences bound specifically by glucocorticoid receptor *in vitro* render a heterologous promoter hormone responsive *in vivo.* *Cell* 33:489, 1983.
66. Ponta H, Kennedy N, Skroch P, Hynes NE, Groner B:

Hormonal response regions in the mouse mammary tumor virus long terminal repeat can be dissociated from the proviral promoter and has enhancer properties. *Proc Natl Acad Sci USA* 82:1020, 1985.

67. Eberwine JK, Roberts JL: Glucocorticoid regulation of pro-opiomelanocortin gene transcription in the rat pituitary. *J Biol Chem* 259:2166, 1984.

68. Israel A, Cohen SN: Hormonally mediated negative regulation of human pro-opiomelanocortin gene expression after transfection into mouse L cells. *Mol Cell Biol* 5:2443, 1985.

69. Moen RC, Palmiter RD: Changes in hormone responsiveness of chick oviduct during primary stimulation with estrogen. *Dev Biol* 78:450, 1980.

70. Renkowitz R, Schutz G, von der Ahe D, Beato M: Sequences in the promoter region of the chicken lysozyme gene required for steroid regulation and receptor binding. *Cell* 37:503, 1984.

71. von der Ahe D, Janich S, Scheidereit C, Renkawitz R, Schutz G, Beato M: Glucocorticoid and progesterone receptors bind to the same sites in two hormonally regulated promoters. *Nature* 313:706, 1985.

72. Khoury G, Gruss P: Enhancer elements. *Cell* 33:313, 1983.

73. Parker M. Enhancer elements activated by steroid hormones? *Nature* 304:687, 1983.

74. Banerji J, Olson L, Schaffner W: A lymphocyte-specific cellular enhancer is located downstream of the joining region in immunoglobulin heavy chain genes. *Cell* 33:729, 1983.

75. Gruss P: Magic enhancers? *DNA* 3:1, 1984.

76. Martial JA, Baxter JD, Goodman HM, Seeburg PH: Regulation of growth hormone messenger RNA by thyroid and glucocorticoid hormones. *Proc Natl Acad Sci USA* 74:1816, 1977.

77. Spindler SR, Mellon SH, Baxter JD: Growth hormone gene transcription is regulated by thyroid and glucocorticoid hormones in cultured rat pituitary tumor cells. *J Biol Chem* 257:11627, 1982.

78. Evans RM, Binberg NC, Rosenfeld MG: Glucocorticoid and thyroid hormones transcriptionally regulate growth hormone gene expression. *Proc Natl Acad Sci USA* 79:7659, 1982.

79. Oppenheimer JH: Thyroid hormone action at the nuclear level. *Ann Intern Med* 102:374, 1985.

80. Granner D, Andreone T, Sasaki K, Beale E: Inhibition of transcription of the phosphoenolpyruvate carboxykinase gene by insulin. *Nature* 305:549, 1983.

81. Murdoch GH, Potter E, Nicolaisen AK, Evans RM, Rosenfeld MG: Epidermal growth factor rapidly stimulates prolactin gene transcription. *Nature* 300:192, 1982.

82. Hashimoto S, Schmid W, Schutz G: Transcriptional activation of the rat liver tyrosine aminotransferase gene by cAMP. *Proc Natl Acad Sci USA* 81:6637, 1984.

83. Moore DD, Conkling MA, Goodman HM: Human growth hormone: A multigene family. *Cell* 29:285, 1982.

84. Guyette WA, Matusik RJ, Rosen JM: Prolactin-mediated transcriptional and post-transcriptional control of casein gene expression. *Cell* 17:1013, 1979.

85. Cell RF: Estrogen withdrawal in chick oviduct: Selective loss of high abundance classes of polyadenylated messenger RNA. *Biochemistry* 16:3433, 1975.

86. McKnight GS, Palmiter RD: Transcriptional regulation of the ovalbumin and conalbumin genes by steroid hormones in chick oviduct. *J Biol Chem* 254:9050, 1979.

87. Vannice JC, Taylor JM, Ringold GM: Glucocorticoid-mediated induction of α_1-acid glycoprotein: Evidence of hormone-regulated RNA processing. *Proc Natl Acad Sci USA* 81:4241, 1984.

88. Itoh N, Okamoto H: Translation control of proinsulin synthesis by glucose. *Nature* 283:100, 1980.

89. Eberwine JH, Roberts JL: Analysis of pro-opiomelanocortin gene structure and function. *DNA* 2:1, 1983.

90. Slater EP, Baxter JD, Eberhardt NL: Evolution of the growth hormone gene family. *Am Zool* (in press).

91. Orkin SH, Kazaziain HH: The mutation and polymorphism of the human β-globin gene and its surrounding DNA. *Annu Rev Genet* 18:131, 1984.

92. Shoelson S, Haneda M, Blix P, et al: Three mutant insulins in man. *Nature* 302:540, 1983.

93. Haneda M, Polonsky KS, Bergenstal RM, et al: Familial hyperinsulinemia due to a structurally abnormal insulin. *N Engl J Med* 310:1288, 1984.

94. Chang JC, Kan YW: β^0 Thalassemia, a nonsense mutation in man. *Proc Natl Acad Sci USA* 76:2886, 1979.

95. Marquat LE, Kinniburgh AJ, Rachmileintz EA, Ron J: Unstable β-globin mRNA in mRNA-deficient β^0 thalassemia. *Cell* 27:543, 1981.

96. Treisman R, Orkin SH, Maniatis T: Specific transcription and RNA splicing defects in five cloned β-thalassemia genes. *Nature* 302:591, 1983.

96a. Antonarakis SE, Waber PG, Kittur SD, et al: Hemophilia A. Detection of molecular defects and of carriers by DNA analysis. *N Engl J Med* 313:842, 1985.

97. Phillips JA, Hjelle BL, Seeburg PH, Zachmann M: Molecular basis for isolated growth hormone deficiency. *Proc Natl Acad Sci USA* 78:6372, 1981.

98. Glover DM (ed): *DNA Cloning*, vols I and II. Oxford, IRL Press, 1985.

99. Old RW, Primrose SB: *Principles of Gene Manipulation*, 3d ed. Oxford, Blackwell, 1985.

100. Southern E: Detection of specific sequences among DNA fragments separated by gel electrophoresis. *J Mol Biol* 98:503, 1975.

101. Thomas PS: Hybridization of denatured RNA and small DNA fragments transferred to nitrocellulose. *Proc Natl Acad Sci USA* 77:5201, 1980.

102. Gilbert W: DNA sequencing and gene structure. *Science* 214:1305, 1982.

103. Sanger F: Determination of nucleotide sequences in DNA. *Science* 214:1205, 1981.

104. Caruthers MH: Gene synthesis machines: DNA chemistry and its uses. *Science* 230:281, 1985.

105. Ullrich A, Bell JR, Chen EY, et al: Human insulin receptor and its relationship to the tyrosine kinase family of oncogenes. *Nature* 313:756, 1985.

106. Kemp DJ, Cowman AF: Direct immunoassay for detecting *Escherichia coli* colonies that contain polypeptides encoded by cloned DNA segments. *Proc Natl Acad Sci USA* 78:4520, 1981.

107. Young RA, Davis RW: Efficient isolation of genes by using antibody probes. *Proc Natl Acad Sci USA* 80:1194, 1983.

108. Lawn RM, Fritsch EF, Parker RC, et al: The isolation and characterization of linked δ- and β-globin genes from a cloned library of human DNA. *Cell* 15:1157, 1978.

109. Capecchi MR: High efficiency transformation by direct microinjection of DNA into cultured mammalian cells. *Cell* 22:479, 1980.

110. Pellicer A, Wigler M, Axel R, Silverstein S: The transfer and stable integration of the HSV thymidine kinase gene into mouse cells. *Cell* 14:133, 1978.

111. Sandri-Goldin RM, Goldin A, Levine M, Glorioso JC: High frequency transfer of cloned herpes simplex virus type I sequences to mammalian cells by protoplast fusion. *Mol Cell Biol* 1:743, 1981.

112. Potter H, Weir L, Leder P: Enhancer dependent expression of human K immunoglobulin genes introduced into mouse pre-B lymphocytes by electroporation. *Proc Natl Acad Sci USA* 81:7161, 1984.

113. Doehmer J, Barinaga M, Vale W, et al: Introduction of rat growth hormone gene into mouse fibroblasts via a retroviral DNA vector: Expression and regulation. *Proc Natl Acad Sci USA* 79:2268, 1982.

114. Banerji J, Rusconi S, Schaffner W: Expression of a β-globin

gene is enhanced by remote SV40 DNA sequences. *Cell* 27:299, 1981.

115. Southern PJ, Berg P: Transformation of mammalian cells to antibiotic resistance with a bacterial gene under control of the SV40 early promoter. *J Mol Appl Gen* 1:327, 1982.

116. Kurtz DT: Hormone inducibility of rat $\alpha 2\mu$-globulin genes in transfected mouse cells. *Nature* 291:629, 1981.

117. Dean DC, Knoll BJ, Riser ME, O'Malley BW: A 5'-flanking sequence essential for progesterone regulation of an ovalbumin fusion gene. *Nature* 305:551, 1983.

118. Karin M, Haslinger A, Holtgreve H, Cathala G, Slater E, Baxter JD: Activation of a heterologous promoter in response to dexamethasone and cadmium by metallothionein gene 5'-flanking DNA. *Cell* 36:371, 1984.

119. Itakura K, Hirose T, Crea R, et al: Expression in *Escherichia coli* of a chemically synthesized gene for the hormone somatostatin. *Science* 198:1056, 1977.

120. Shine J, Fettes I, Lan NC, et al: Expression of cloned β-endorphin gene sequences by *E. coli*. *Nature* 285:456, 1980.

121. Smith RA, Duncan MJ, Moin DT: Heterologous protein secretion from yeast. *Science* 229:1219, 1985.

122a. Wood WI, Capon DJ, Simonsen CC, et al: Expression of active human factor VIII from recombinant DNA clones. *Nature* 312:330, 1984.

122b. Toole JJ, Knopf JL, Wozney JM, et al: Molecular cloning of a cDNA encoding human antihaemophilic factor. *Nature* 312:342, 1984.

123. Flameng W, Van de Werf F, Vanhaecke J, et al: Coronary thrombolysis and infarct size reduction after intravenous infusion of recombinant tissue-type plasminogen activator in nonhuman primates. *J Clin Invest* 75:84, 1985.

123a. Collen D, Topol EJ, Tietebrunn AJ, et al: Coronary thrombolysis with recombinant human tissue-type plasminogen activator: A prospective, randomized, placebo-controlled trial. *Circulation* 70:1012, 1985.

124. Lee-Huang S: Cloning and expression of human erythropoietin cDNA in *Escherichia coli*. *Proc Natl Acad Sci USA* 81:2708, 1984.

125. Richards AM, Ikram H, Yandle TG, et al: Renal haemodynamic and hormonal effects of human alpha atrial natriuretic peptide in healthy volunteers. *Lancet* 1:545, 1985.

126. Richards AM, Nicholls MG, Espiner EA, et al: Effects of α-human atrial natriuretic peptide in essential hypertension. *Hypertension* 7:812, 1985.

127. Needleman P, Adams SP, Cole BR: Atriopeptins as cardiac hormones. *Hypertension* 7:469, 1985.

128. Blackwell GJ, Carnuccio R, DiRosa M, et al: Macrocortin: A polypeptide causing the antiphospholipase effect of glucocorticoids. *Nature* 287:147, 1980.

128a. Wallner BP, Mattaliano RJ, Hession C, et al: Cloning and expression of human lipocortin, a phospholipase A_2 inhibitor with potential anti-inflammatory activity. *Nature* 320:77, 1986.

129. White RT, Damn D, Miller J, et al: Isolation and characterization of the human pulmonary surfactant apoprotein gene. *Nature* 317:361, 1985.

130. Perkus ME, Piccini A, Lipinskas BR, Paoletti E: Recombinant vaccinia virus: Immunization against multiple pathogens. *Science* 229:981, 1985.

131. Albin J, Rifkin H: Etiologies of diabetes mellitus. *Med Clin North Am* 66:1204, 1982.

132. Morrison SL: Transfectomas provide novel chimeric antibodies. *Science* 229:1201, 1985.

133. Horiuchi N, Holick MF, Potts JT, Rosenblatt M: A parathyroid hormone inhibitor *in vivo:* Design and biological evaluation of a hormone analog. *Science* 220:1053, 1983.

134. Davies SF, Walker IM: Multiple emulsions as targetable delivery systems: Drug and enzyme targeting, in Green R, Widdler KJ (eds): *Methods in Enzymology*. New York, Academic, 1984.

135. Gordon GC, Moses AC, Silver RD, et al: Nasal absorption of insulin: Enhancement by hydrophobic bile salts. *Proc Natl Acad Sci USA* 82:7419, 1985.

136. Moses AC, Gordon GC, Carey ML, et al: Insulin administered intranasally as an insulin-bile salt aerosol: Effectiveness and reproducibility in normal and diabetic subjects. *Diabetes* 32:1040, 1983.

137. Salzman R, Manson JE, Griffing GT, et al: Intranasal aerosolized insulin: Mixed meal and long term use in type I diabetes. *N Engl J Med* 312:1078, 1985.

138. Stanbury JB, Wyngaarden JB, Fredrickson DS, Goldstein JL, Brown MS (eds): *The Metabolic Basis of Inherited Disease*, 5th ed. New York, McGraw-Hill, 1983.

139. Pirastu M, Kan YW, Cao A, et al: Prenatal diagnosis of β-thalassemia: Detection of a single nucleotide mutation in DNA. *N Engl J Med* 309:284, 1983.

140. Chang JC, Kan YW: A sensitive new prenatal test for sickle cell anemia. *N Engl J Med* 307:30, 1982.

140a. Saiki RK, Scharf S, Faloona F, et al: Enzymatic amplification of β-globin genomic sequences and restriction site analysis for diagnosis of sickle cell anemia. *Science* 230:1350, 1985.

141. Woo SLC, Lidsky AS, Guttler F, et al: Cloned human phenylalanine hydroxylase gene allows prenatal diagnosis and carrier detection of classical phenylketonuria. *Nature* 306:151, 1983.

142. Bell GI, Karam JH, Rutter WJ: Polymorphic DNA region adjacent to the 5' end of the human insulin gene. *Proc Natl Acad Sci USA* 78:5759, 1981.

143. Rotwein PS, Chirqwin J, Province M, et al: Polymorphism in the 5'-flanking region of the human insulin gene: A genetic marker for non-insulin-dependent diabetes. *N Engl J Med* 308:65, 1983.

144. Bell GI, Horita S, Karam JH: A polymorphic locus near the human insulin gene is associated with insulin-dependent diabetes mellitus. *Diabetes* 33:176, 1984.

145. Anderson WF: Prospects for human gene therapy. *Science* 226:401, 1984.

146. Anderson WF, Fletcher JC: Gene therapy in human beings. When is it ethical to begin? *N Engl J Med* 303:1293, 1980.

147. Bishop JM: Viral oncogenes. *Cell* 42:23, 1985.

148. Heldin CH, Westermark B. Growth factors: Mechanisms of action and relation to oncogenes. *Cell* 37:9, 1984.

149. Kingston RE, Baldwin AS, Sharp RA: Transcriptional control by oncogenes. *Cell* 41:3, 1985.

150. Doolittle RF, Hunhapiller NW, Hood LE, et al: Simian sarcoma virus oncogene, v-sis, is derived from the gene (or genes) encoding a platelet-derived growth factor. *Science* 221:275, 1983.

151. Waterfield MD, Scrace GT, Whittle N, et al: Platelet-derived growth factor is structurally related to the putative transforming protein p28sis of simian sarcoma virus. *Nature* 304:35, 1983.

152. Downward L, Yarden Y, Mayes E, et al: Close similarity of epidermal growth factor receptor and v-erb B oncogene protein sequences. *Nature* 307:521, 1984.

153. Bishop JM: Cellular oncogenes and retroviruses. *Annu Rev Biochem* 52:301, 1983.

154. Shih C, Weinberg RA: Isolation of a transforming sequence from a human bladder carcinoma cell line. *Cell* 29:161, 1982.

155. Yoakum GH, Lechner JF, Gabrielson EW, et al: Transformation of a human bronchial epithelial cells transfected with Harvey ras oncogene. *Science* 227:1174, 1985.

156. Lano H, Parada LF, Weinberg RA: Tumorigenic conversion of primary embryo fibroblasts requires at least two cooperating oncogenes. *Nature* 304:596, 1983.

157. Shirai T, Hiroshi Y, Ito H, et al: Cloning and expression in *Escherichia coli* of the gene for human tumor necrosis factor. *Nature* 313:803, 1985.

158. Sikora K: Cancer toxin genes cloned. *Nature* 312:699, 1984.

4

Biosynthesis, Secretion, and Metabolism of Hormones

Gordon N. Gill

Endocrinology is the study of hormones, which are allosteric effectors; hormone receptors, which are the allosteric proteins to which they bind; and biological consequences of this interaction. Although the kinetics of interaction between hormone and receptor protein are complex, the interaction can be represented overall as a bimolecular reaction:

$$\underset{[H]}{\text{Hormone}} + \underset{[R]}{\text{Receptor}} \underset{k_2}{\overset{k_1}{\rightleftharpoons}} \underset{[HR]}{\text{Hormone}\cdot\text{Receptor}}$$

The binding of hormone to receptor protein involves primarily hydrophobic interactions with hydrogen bonds, van der Waals forces, and salt bridges but not covalent linkages. Allosteric regulation can thus be quickly terminated once the allosteric effector is reduced in concentration. In the mass action equation shown, formation of the active [HR] complex depends on the concentration of both the hormone and the receptor protein as well as on the intrinsic affinity of the receptor for the hormone. Genetic and acquired endocrine diseases are ultimately expressed as an alteration from normal in one term of this equation.

Extensive control systems regulate all components of these basic ingredients of the hormone-response system. Synthesis, secretion, transport, and metabolism of hormones determine the hormone concentration term, while synthesis, modification, and metabolism of receptor protein determine the receptor concentration term in this equation. The present chapter is concerned with biosynthetic and metabolic pathways which determine the concentration of hormone available to receptors; factors determining receptor concentration, which are equally important, are discussed in Chap. 5.

Hormones have one of two major chemical structures: peptide or steroid. Although different hormones have distinct biological effects, all hormones of the peptide class and all hormones of the steroid class share common features of biosynthesis, secretion, transport, and mechanism of action with others of the same class. These common features provide a framework in which unique characteristics of a particular hormone can be understood and in which comparisons between hormones can be made. Because thyroid hormone and catecholamines, which have the amino acid tyrosine as a central structural nucleus, are synthesized and metabolized via pathways which are unique and distinct from peptide or steroid hormones and from each other, these are considered separately. Thyroid hormone is summarized in this chapter and catecholamines in Chap. 13.

PEPTIDE HORMONES

Biosynthesis of Messenger RNA

Because peptide hormones are small secretory proteins, their biosynthesis and secretion occur via the same processes as larger nonhormonal secretory proteins such as immunoglobulins, albumin, pancreatic enzymes, and egg white proteins. The biosynthetic steps are general ones for all proteins, although there are a number of interesting variations such as multigene families, derivation of different hormones from a common RNA precursor by differential splicing, generation of multiple hormones from a common protein precursor, and synthesis of multisubunit hormones.

In eukaryotes, genes encoding proteins are organized with the general scheme shown in Fig. 4-1. DNA sequences whose transcripts appear in mature messenger RNA (*exons*) are interrupted by intervening sequences (*introns*) which are transcribed into messenger RNA precursors but removed during the process of messenger RNA maturation before delivery of the exon-containing messenger RNA to the cytoplasm, where translation into protein occurs. Genes coding for proteins are transcribed by RNA polymerase II, a large multisubunit enzyme[1] which begins transcription at the initiation site upstream from the first ATG sequence for the messenger RNA. The site of initiation, where capping occurs,[2] is followed by a nontranslated leader sequence of variable length[3] before the ATG which codes for AUG, the messenger RNA translation start signal.

Capping, which occurs at the site of initiation, begins early during the process of transcription by RNA polymerase II. In the capping reaction guanylyl transferase adds a 5′-terminal GTP to form a 5′—5′ bond GpppX, and the guanosine is methylated at N_7 by N_7 methylase.[2] Capping facilitates binding of ribosomes and translation initiation factors to mark the AUG codon used for initiation and stabilizes messenger RNA against degradation.

Important regulatory regions of DNA are commonly located on the 5′ side of the initiation site.[4] A region rich in A + T, the Goldberg-Hogness box, with the sequence TATAAAA, is located about 30 base pairs before the start site.[5,6] RNA polymerase II binds to this region and initiates RNA synthesis 30 base pairs downstream. This ATA box is analogous to the Pribnow box in prokaryotes, a promoter region of RNA polymerase binding. Deletions or mutations in the ATA box result in loss of specificity of initiation, indicating that this sequence dictates the correct start site.[5-7] The efficiency of initiation is determined by DNA sequences which generally lie about 200 to 400 base pairs before the first coding region at the 5′ end of the gene. At least two such regions have been identified where deletions or mutations reduce the efficiency of initiation 10- to 20-fold.[5,7] One such site has the sequence CCAAT.[4,5] These control elements may facilitate the initial entry of RNA polymerase II.

Although the gene organization shown in Fig. 4-1 is common, several well-transcribed genes lack both ATA and CCAAT sequences. The epidermal growth factor receptor and *ras* genes lack such sequences;

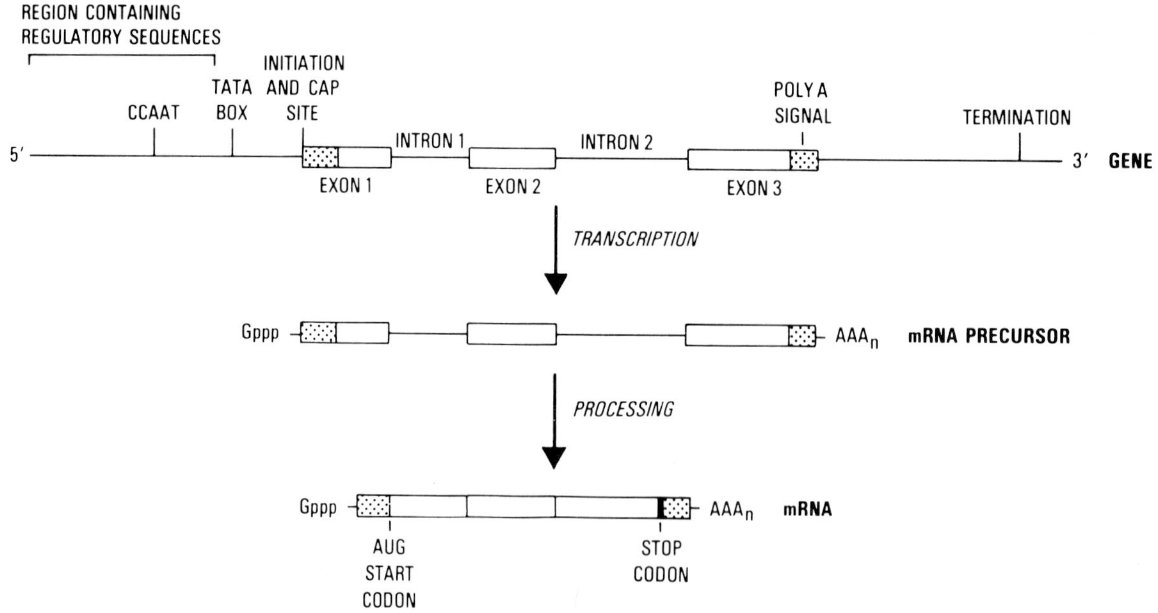

FIGURE 4-1 Messenger RNA synthesis. Exons are indicated by boxes with untranslated regions shaded and introns by single lines. The primary transcript, which is cleaved before polyadenylation, is not shown. Enhancer sequences may be located in the 5′ region, within the coding portion of the gene, or 3′ to the coding region.

instead, these important growth-regulating genes contain CCGCCC as well as TCC repeats 5′ to the transcription start site.[8,9]

DNA sequences which enhance transcription (*enhancers*) have also been identified. These sequences function independently of position and orientation to the gene, i.e., they may occur 5′ to, or within, or 3′ to the coding sequences. Such sequences may provide bidirectional entry sites for RNA polymerase II and are sites of hypersensitivity to DNAse.[10] Such enhancers appear to be cell-specific and increase transscription 10- to 100-fold.[11,12]

The biosynthesis of many peptide hormones is regulated at the level of transcription of their genes by heterologous hormones. The sites of action of regulatory hormones are partly at the 5′ end of target genes. Several models which provide insight into the regulation of transcription have been studied. Glucocorticoids, which regulate synthesis of several peptide hormones, including growth hormone and adrenocorticotropin (ACTH), exert their effects on transcription through direct interaction with the 5′ regions flanking these genes. The mouse mammary tumor virus (MTV), which is endogenous to many mouse genomes, is also regulated by glucocorticoids. The MTV genome is flanked by 5′ and 3′ long terminal repeats. Fusion of the 3′ long terminal repeat to other genes such as thymidine kinase confers glucocorticoid regulation on those genes.[13] Deletion mutations map two such responsive regions within 200 base pairs 5′ to the initiation site, and there is evidence that glucocorticoid receptors specifically bind to DNA sequences in these regions.[14,15] A consensus DNA sequence, recognized by glucocorticoid hormone receptor complexes and required for regulation of gene expression, has been identified 5′ to several responsive genes, including metallothionein, growth hormone, and MTV.[16] The progesterone receptor similarly binds specifically to sequences on the 5′ end of regulated genes.[17] A model to explain coordinate induction of different structural genes suggests that repetitive cis-acting sequences located 5′ to several induced genes function as *receptor* sequences to bind proteins such as activated steroid hormone receptors.[18] The receptor sequences for steroid hormone receptors are proposed to be enhancer sequences which are active as enhancers only when the receptor protein is bound there. These activated enhancer sequences may be associated with DNA sequences capable of forming a Z structure[19] and may act to alter DNA structure distal to the regulatory region. This model of the regulation of transcription by steroid hormones is covered fully in Chap. 5.

Peptide hormones also regulate transcription of peptide hormone genes via control regions 5′ to the initiation site. Prolactin, but not growth hormone, synthesis is increased by thyrotropin releasing hormone (TRH) and epidermal growth factor (EGF). When the 5′ sequences of the prolactin gene were fused to the coding region of the growth hormone gene and transfected into A431 cells, EGF enhanced growth hormone transcription.[20] EGF had no effect on transcription of transfected growth hormone DNA containing its own 5′ sequences, indicating that specific responsiveness to peptide and steroid hormones resides partly in the sequences located 5′ to the site of initiation of transcription.

The rate of transcription of genes thus depends on specific sequences usually located 5′ to the beginning of the coding sequence. These DNA sequences are the sites for binding of specific proteins such as steroid hormone receptors and other regulatory proteins.[21–23] Some of these proteins are activated via hormone binding or covalent modification. The presence and arrangement of DNA regulatory sequences determine which proteins can bind; some of these proteins are activated in response to environmental signals and others may be constitutively expressed. The molecular mechanisms through which bound proteins control the rate of transcription are incompletely defined. DNA binding appears to direct the regulatory proteins to specific genes, but the active region of the protein appears distinct from its DNA-binding region.[24]

Regulation occurs not only during the process of transcription but also during RNA processing.[25] The initial RNA polymerase II transcript is a large nuclear RNA which contains both exons and introns. Unlike translation in prokaryotes, which may occur during transcription, translation in eukaryotes occurs only after maturation and transport of messenger RNA to the cytoplasm. Maturation requires excision of introns and splicing together of exons. This process follows the general GT-AG rule that introns begin with GT and end with AG.[3,26] The donor sequence for exon-intron boundaries[27] is

C A
AAG/GTGAGT

and the acceptor sequence for intron-exon junctions[27] is

T C
Cn NTAG/G

This sequence is complementary to the sequence of the abundant small nuclear U1 RNA which is found in ribonuclear protein particles.[28,29] The U1 RNA is thought to form the recognition component of the splicing enzyme complex to bind the 5′ donor site during intron excision and splicing reactions.[28–32]

Termination of transcription occurs 3′ to the final coding exon, in some cases many bases downstream. Poly(A) addition (tailing) occurs near points of cleavage in messenger RNA precursors and is dictated by the sequence AAUAAA, which is located 14 to 30 base pairs upstream of the poly(A) tail.[4] The sequence at the start of the poly(A) tail is also similar in many genes.[33,34] Poly(A) addition is catalyzed by a poly(A) polymerase enzyme.[35]

More than one peptide hormone may be encoded in a single gene. As detailed subsequently, several peptides may be derived by proteolytic processing from a common precursor protein. Alternative RNA processing may also yield different peptide hormones. Many genes are simple transcription units with a single poly(A) addition site and a constant pattern of RNA splicing, but there are also complex transcription units with multiple poly(A) addition sites and alternative RNA splicing sites which can generate multiple messenger RNA species from a single gene.[36] The organization of the calcitonin gene is shown in Fig. 4-2. In C cells of the thyroid a polyadenylation signal at the end of the calcitonin exon is used.[37] In nervous tissue a second polyadenylation signal at the end of a downstream exon is used, and during processing, the calcitonin exon is removed,[38] so that mature messenger RNA encodes a carboxy-terminal region different from that of the messenger RNA encoding calcitonin. The two precursor protein products have a common amino-terminal region but different carboxy-terminal sequences. In C cells of the thyroid, calcitonin is processed from the precursor protein to function in

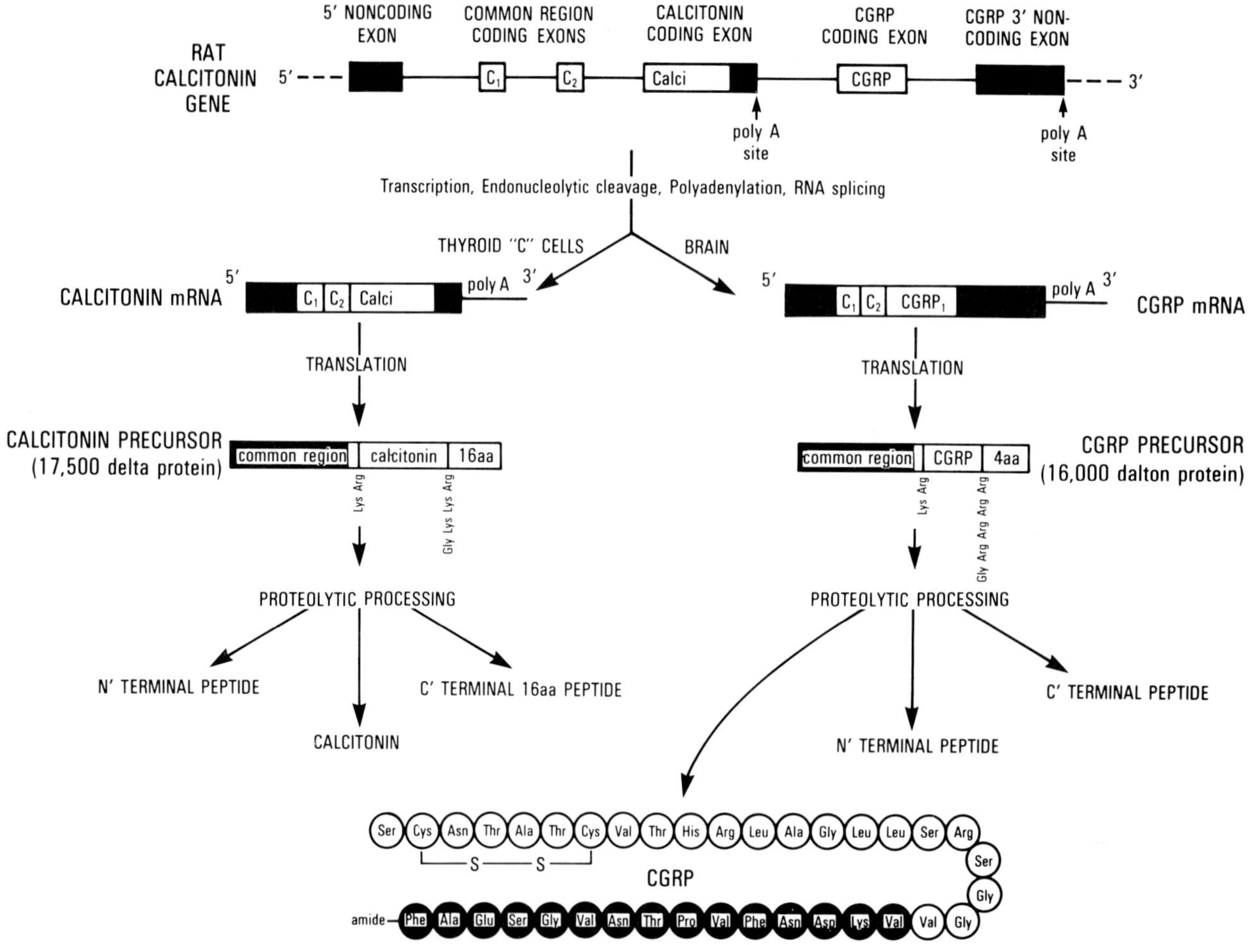

FIGURE 4-2 Generation of peptide hormone diversity by alternative RNA splicing. The rat calcitonin gene contains two common coding exons, a calcitonin exon and a calcitonin gene–related protein (CGRP) exon. Calcitonin is formed when a poly(A) site at the 3′ end of the calcitonin exon is used; CGRP is formed when a poly(A) site in an exon 3′ to CGRP is used. The resulting messenger RNAs have a common 5′ end but divergent 3′ ends. Proteolytic processing results in N-terminal peptides, calcitonin or CGRP, and C-terminal peptides. Calcitonin and CGRP have different biological activities. (*From Rosenfeld et al.*[38])

regulation of calcium metabolism, whereas in nervous tissue a calcitonin gene-related peptide (CGRP) is processed from its precursor protein to function in nociception, ingestive behavior, and modulation of autonomic responses. Alternative RNA processing thus creates diversity in peptide hormone formation similar to the alternative RNA processing which occurs in immunoglobulin gene expression as well as in several other proteins.[36] Alternative protein processing may also create diversity, as with the ACTH precursor in intermediate and anterior lobe pituitary cells.[39]

Biosynthesis of Peptide Hormones

Because peptide hormones are small proteins, their mature messenger RNAs frequently encode information for initial translation products which are larger than the secretory form of the peptide; that is, messenger RNA is translated into larger protein precursors, which are then processed by a series of proteolytic cleavages to yield the final secreted peptide products.

Messenger RNA translation begins at the AUG codon, specifying methionine, which lies downstream from the cap site. Because peptide hormones are secretory proteins, synthesis is on endoplasmic reticulum-bound polyribosomes, with vectorial movement of the growing peptide into the endoplasmic reticulum space (Fig. 4-3). A leader sequence of 15 to 25 largely hydrophobic amino acids is located at the amino terminus of the protein. When this "pre" portion emerges from the ribosome it binds a signal recognition particle consisting of six proteins and a 7-S RNA.[40] In the absence of endoplasmic reticulum membranes, the signal recognition particle prevents further synthesis of these proteins so that presecretory proteins are not made in the cytoplasm.[41] When the signal recognition particle–arrested ribosome complex binds with high affinity to a specific integral membrane protein, termed the *signal recognition particle receptor*, or *docking protein*,[42,43] the signal recognition particle is displaced from the nascent protein chain and its amino-terminal signal sequence.[44] The ribosome, with its growing peptide chain, is now bound to the rough endoplasmic reticulum via membrane proteins, termed *ribophorins*, which probably bind the signal sequence and ribosome. Protein synthesis then resumes, and the

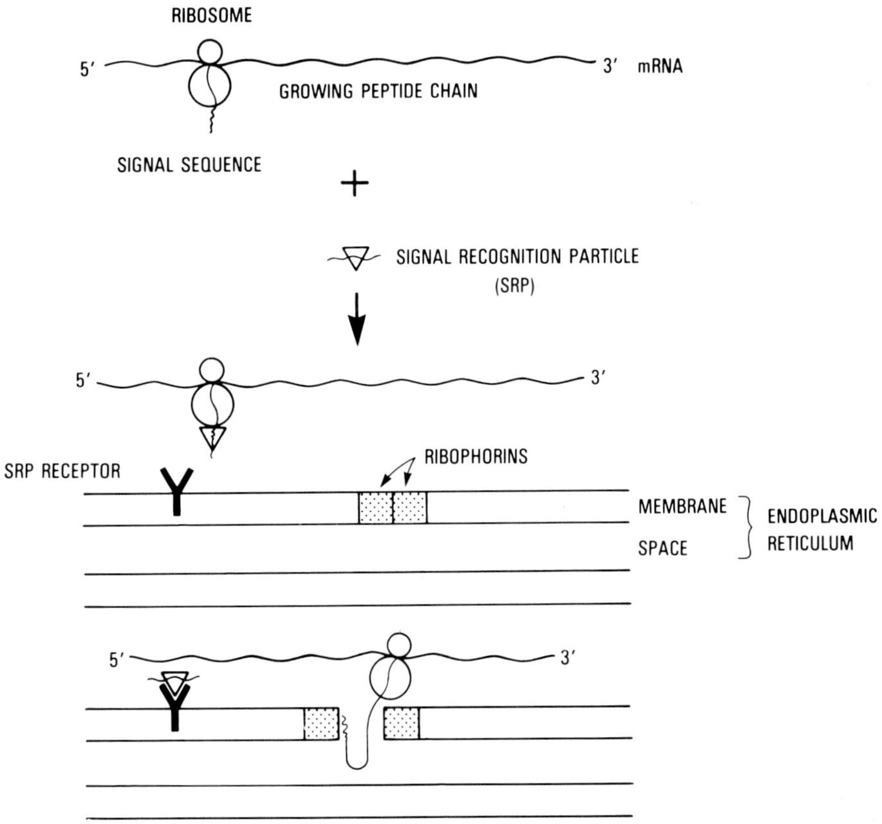

FIGURE 4-3 Synthesis of secretory proteins. The signal sequence at the amino terminus is bound by the signal recognition particle (SRP), which arrests cytoplasmic translation and delivers the complex to a recognition protein intrinsic to the endoplasmic reticulum (ER) membrane. This SRP receptor binds and displaces SRP so that the ribosome and signal sequence can bind to neighboring ribophorins in the ER. Protein synthesis then resumes and vectorially delivers the growing peptide chain to the lumen of the ER, where the signal sequence is removed and additional modifications occur.

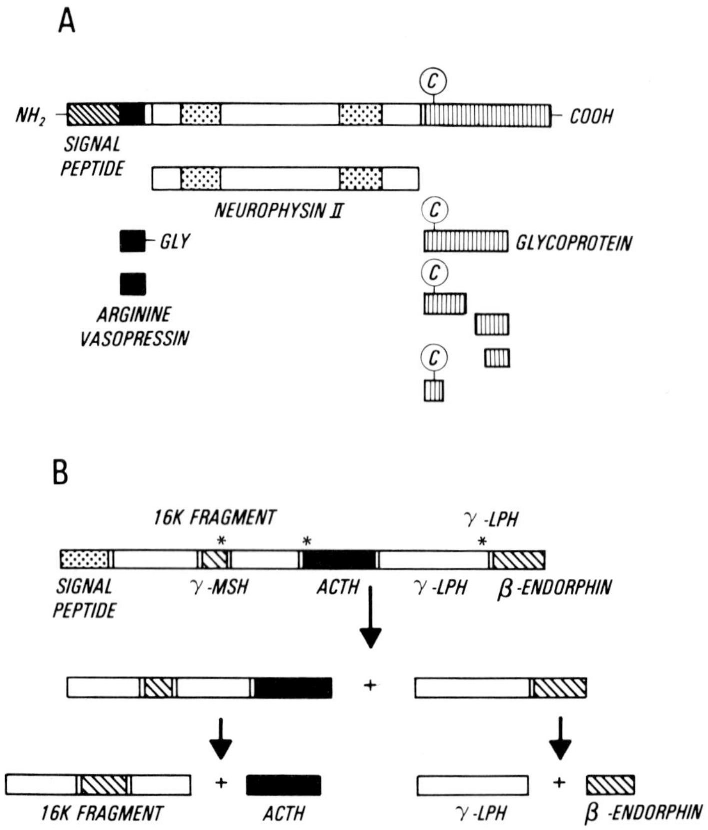

FIGURE 4-4 Proteolytic processing of precursor proteins within the endoplasmic reticulum. (A) Structure of the bovine antidiuretic hormone (ADH)–neurophysin II precursor and its proteolytic processing. The 19-amino acid signal peptide is followed by ADH (residues 1 to 9). Neurophysin II begins after processing signals at residue 13 and extends to residue 107; its internal homology is shown by hatched area. The glycoprotein portion of the precursor is located at the carboxyl terminus. (*From Land et al.*[47]) (B) Structure of the bovine ACTH precursor and its proteolytic processing in the anterior pituitary. Reiterated MSH core sequences are indicated by an asterisk. Dibasic amino acid residues, which serve as the recognition signal for proteolytic processing, are indicated by open spaces in the bars. (*From Nakanishi et al.*[48])

nascent chain is translocated to inside the endoplasmic reticulum space. For secretory proteins such as peptide hormones, the completed peptide will ultimately be located completely within the endoplasmic reticulum space, whereas membrane-bound proteins such as hormone receptors will have their amino termini within this space (ultimately to face the outside of the cell), with a portion of the carboxyl terminus of the protein remaining in the membrane and cytoplasm. Some peptide hormones are generated by proteolytic processing from receptor-like precursors.[45,46]

Within the endoplasmic reticulum the precursor protein is cleaved, covalently modified, and folded into the form which will ultimately be secreted. A signal peptidase first removes the "pre," or leader sequence, portion of the hormone. Larger precursor "pro" hormones are then further processed within this membrane-enclosed space by proteolytic enzymes. Most processing involves trypsin-like activity which recognizes dibasic amino acid residues. For carboxy-terminal amidation, glycine serves as the donor at the cleavage site.

Peptides generated during processing of protein precursors may have a variety of functions. The precursor of antidiuretic hormone and oxytocin contains the specific neurophysins which serve as carriers for these two peptides from their site of synthesis in the magnicellular nuclei in the hypothalamus to storage sites in the posterior pituitary (Fig. 4-4A).[47] The ACTH precursor contains information for several peptides, which may all be involved in stress responses. Figure 4-4*B* shows the structure of the ACTH precursor molecule predicted from the DNA sequence.[48] The core sequence for melanocyte stimulating hormone (MSH) is reiterated within the structure of the precursor, suggesting that it arose during evolution by gene duplication. A 16,000 M_r fragment is located on the amino-terminal side, and β-lipotropin is located on the carboxy-terminal side of the ACTH sequence. Dibasic amino acids serve as recognition signals for proteolytic enzymes which cleave the precursor protein into the final hormonal products. In addition, both glycosylation and phosphorylation of the ACTH precursor occurs within the endoplasmic reticulum.[39] There is evidence for different processing of the same precursor in different cells. In the intermediate lobe of the pituitary ACTH is processed to α-MSH, in which the amino-terminal serine is acetylated and the carboxy-terminal valine is amidated from the adjacent glycine, and to corticotropin-like intermediate peptide (CLIP; $ACTH_{18-39}$).[39] In the anterior pituitary, the ACTH precursor is processed as shown in Fig. 4-4*B*.

The connecting peptide (C peptide) present in the insulin precursor serves another function—to provide correct folding and alignment of the A and B chains of insulin. The insulin precursor has the structure: Hydrophobic leader sequence·B chain · C peptide · A chain.[49] The leader sequence is rapidly removed, and the C peptide serves to fold and align the A and B chains of insulin (Fig. 4-5). The disulfide bonds between cysteines A7 and B7, A20 and B19, and A6 and A11 are required for biological activity of insulin. If the disulfide bonds between the A and B chains of insulin and the intra-A chain disulfide bond are chemically reduced and reoxidized in vitro, random coupling of half-cysteine residues occurs and only a small fraction of biological activity is restored. However, reduced and reoxidized proinsulin (B chain · C peptide · A chain) can generate almost full biological activity.[50] The specific configuration of the proinsulin molecule presumably brings the correct pairs of half-cysteine residues into close approximation for formation of the mature disulfide-bonded insulin. During maturation in the endoplasmic reticulum space and Golgi complex, the C peptide, which is flanked by dibasic residues, is removed and mature insulin is secreted by the β cell with about equimolar amounts of inactive C peptide. Proinsulin has only a small fraction of the activity of insulin, so removal of C peptide is necessary. An interesting genetic variant proinsulin resistant to proteolytic processing results in the secretion of unprocessed proinsulin.[51]

Some examples of the functions which are served by additional information contained in the precursor prohormone proteins include (1) correct folding and disulfide bond formation (insulin), (2) cosynthesis of transport protein with hormone (ADH · neurophysin), (3) formation of two or more peptides with similar activities (enkephalins),[53] and (4) formation of several peptides which regulate components of a physiological response (ACTH · 16,000 M_r peptide · β-endorphin). Additional information about precursor protein sequences will probably reveal new functions and provide more insight into the evolution of this class of signaling molecules.

Active hormones may also be generated outside cells by processing from circulating precursors. The precursor for angiotensin II is a glycoprotein synthesized mainly in the liver. Renin, a proteolytic enzyme made in juxtaglomerular cells of the kidney, cleaves a decapeptide from the circulating angiotensin precursor glycoprotein. This decapeptide is then further processed to the octapeptide angiotensin II by removal of two carboxy-terminal amino acids by a converting enzyme found in endothelial cells of vascular beds, especially those of the lung.

The cellular pathway followed by secretory proteins and peptides is shown in Fig. 4-6. The newly synthesized protein located within the luminal space is carried within transport vesicles, which bud from the endoplasmic reticulum, to the Golgi complex. These transport vesicles fuse with the Golgi complex in such a manner that the protein always remains within a membrane-bound space. Vesicles bud from the Golgi complex and ultimately fuse with the plasma membrane to discharge the mature protein or peptide to the exterior of the cell during the process of secretion.

Several covalent modifications may occur during this intracellular journey. Glycosylation is the major modification affecting peptide hormones such as thyroid stimulating hormone (TSH), luteinizing hormone (LH), follicle stimulating hormone (FSH), and human chorionic gonadotropin (hCG). Initial addition of core oligosaccharide occurs within the endoplasmic reticulum. The predominant glycosylation via nitrogen link-

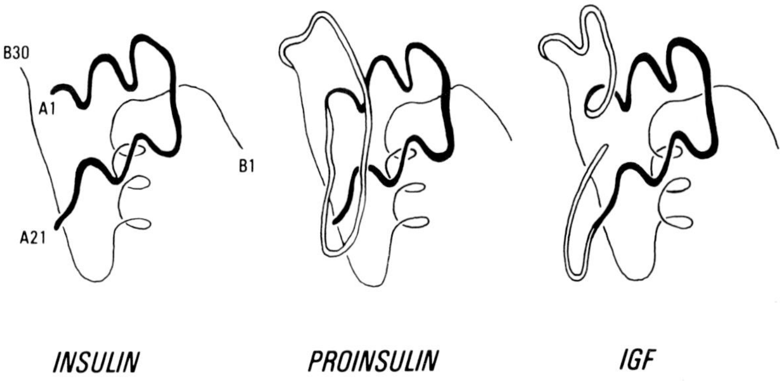

FIGURE 4-5 Schematic representation of three-dimensional structures based on x-ray analysis of insulin and on model building of proinsulin and of insulin-like growth factor 1. The A chain of insulin is shown by the thickened line, the B chain by the solid line, and the connecting peptide by a broken line. Disulfide bridge locations are indicated in the text. (*Modified from Blundell et al.*[52])

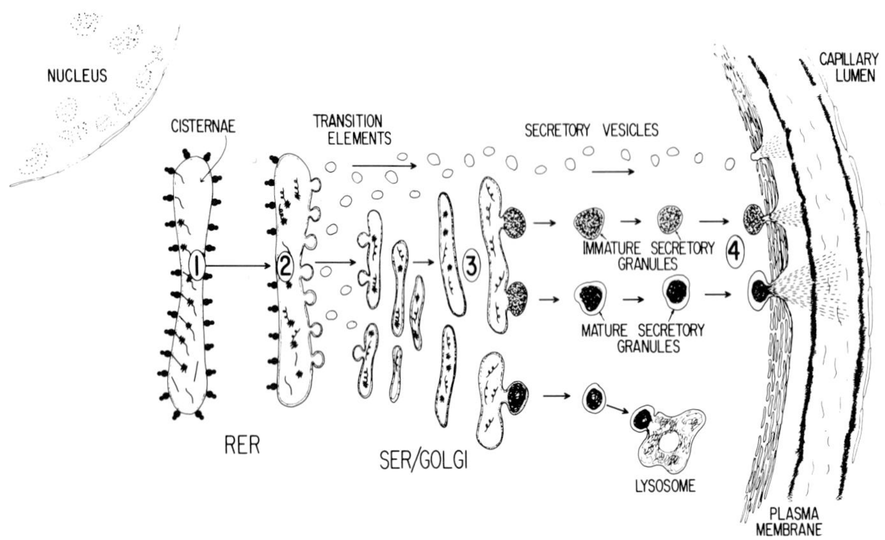

FIGURE 4-6 Schema of subcellular transport and secretory pathway in a protein-secreting cell. RER, rough endoplasmic reticulum; SER, smooth endoplasmic reticulum; Golgi, Golgi complex. (1) Synthesis of proteins on polyribosomes attached to the endoplasmic reticulum and vectorial discharge through the membrane into the cisternal space. (2) Formation of shuttling vesicles (transition elements) from the endoplasmic reticulum followed by their transport to and incorporation by the Golgi complex. (3) Formation of secretory granules in the Golgi complex. (4) Transport of secretory granules to the plasma membrane, fusion with the plasma membrane, and exocytosis resulting in release of granule contents into extracellular space. Note that secretion may occur via transport of secretory vesicles and immature granules as well as mature granules. Some granules are taken up by lysosomes and destroyed (crinophagy).

age occurs on asparagine residues found within the sequence asn-x-ser or -thr. This sequence occurs in proteins which are synthesized in the endoplasmic reticulum space but is rare in cytoplasmic proteins, so that glycosylation of intracellular proteins is avoided. Less commonly, oligosaccharides are oxygen-linked via the hydroxyl side-chain group of serine, threonine, or hydroxylysine. The core *N*-linked oligosaccharide contains two *N*-acetylglucosamine and three mannose residues (Fig. 4-7). The core oligosaccharide is first formed in the endoplasmic reticulum on an activated lipid molecule, dolichol, via a pyrophosphate bridge and is then transferred intact to the growing polypeptide chain.[54] Complex oligosaccharides are formed within the Golgi complex, where variable numbers of glucosamine-galactose-sialic acid residues are added to the mannose core, through the action of galactosyl transferase enzymes. High-mannose oligosaccharides, which contain additional mannose residues attached to the core, are donated via the dolichol pathway and are trimmed to various degrees by mannosidase enzymes present in the Golgi complex.

The α subunits of the glycoprotein hormones LH, FSH, TSH, and hCG contain two oligosaccharides of the *N*-linked complex type; β subunits contain either one or two similar oligosaccharides.[55] hCG β, which has a carboxy-terminal amino acid extension, contains three additional oligosaccharides O-linked to serine residues in this extension.[56,57] In addition to the usual oligosaccharide structures, the pituitary hormones TSH and LH contain peripheral sulfate groups.[58]

Glycosylation of secretory proteins may serve many functions. Glycosylation may favor the protein conformation necessary for optimal intracellular combination of the two subunits which are synthesized on separate messenger RNAs for hormones such as TSH, LH, FSH, and hCG.[59] Glycosylation may also stabilize the hormones in the circulation. Glycoprotein hormones have circulating half-lives considerably longer than nonglycosylated peptide hormones, and desialylation results in a markedly reduced circulating half-life,[60] presumably owing to accelerated clearance via the hepatic asialoglycoprotein receptor.[61] Glycosylation may also be important in receptor recognition, either via effects on hormone conformation or via interaction with cellular recognition sites.

Secretion, Transport, and Metabolism of Peptide Hormones

Within the Golgi apparatus, proteins which are destined for secretion undergo additional maturation. Modification of carbohydrate, added initially in the rough endoplasmic reticulum, is carried out. Newly synthesized and matured secretory peptides and proteins are then accumulated into condensing vacuoles,

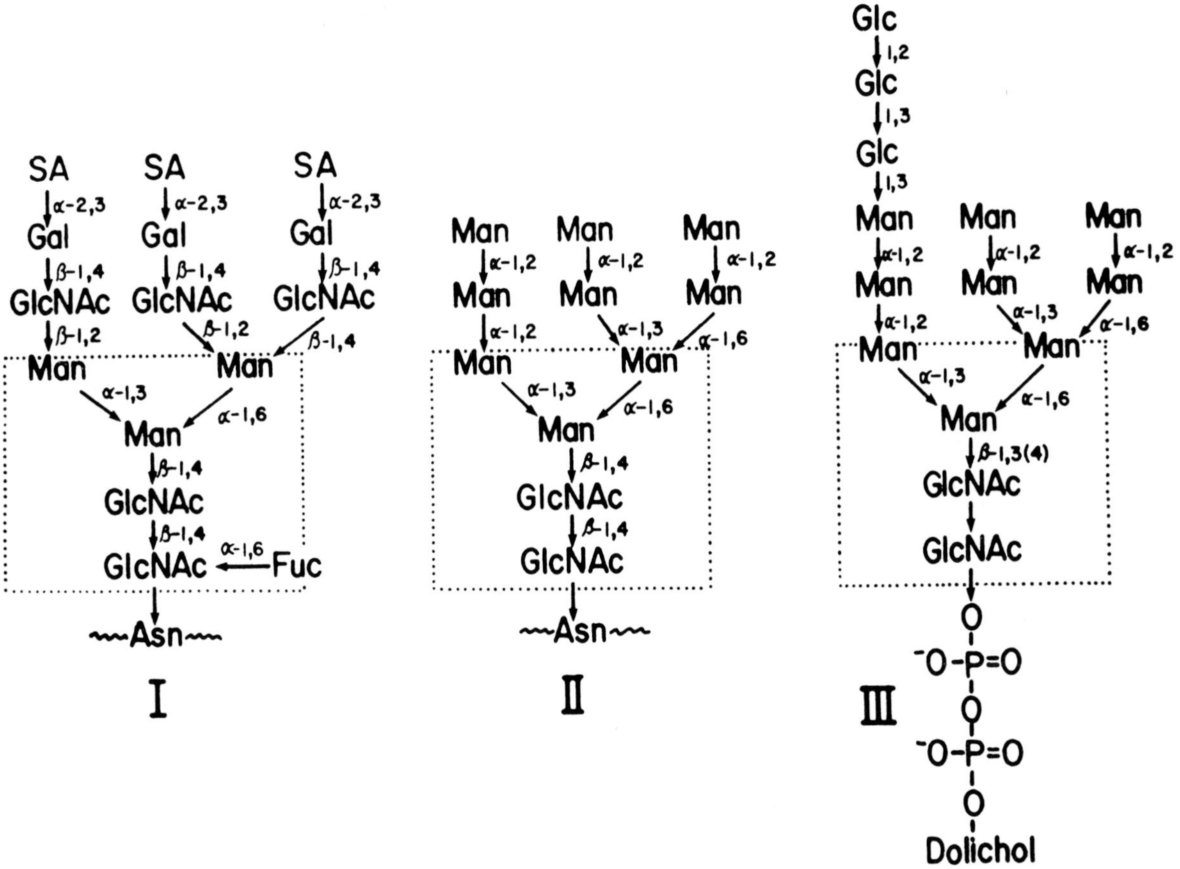

FIGURE 4-7 Structure of asparagine-linked oligosaccharides. The dolichol-linked precursor is shown on the right (III); protein-linked complex (I) and high-mannose (II) oligosaccharides are shown on the left and center, respectively. (*From Hubbard and Ivatt.*[54])

which lose water and form mature secretory granules. Mature secretory granules contain large amounts of stored hormone, which can be readily identified by specific immunostaining. In the absence of a secretory stimulus such granules accumulate; conversely, intensely secreting cells have few secretory granules. In response to a secretory stimulus, the stored peptides are discharged by exocytosis, in which the membrane of the secretory granule fuses with the cell membrane (Fig. 4-6). Secretion is directed, occurring at the apical part of the cell, so that the peptide hormone is discharged into the circulation. The membrane of the secretory granule is then reabsorbed into the cell by endocytosis and reutilized.

Secretion is regulated by specific signals, many of them hormonal, which couple the rate of secretion to the metabolic needs of the organism. A fundamental action of many hormones is to control secretion, and the mechanisms through which this occurs are detailed in Chap. 5. Biosynthesis of peptide hormones is coupled to secretion, although the precise biochemical basis of this coupling is poorly defined. Kinetically, two "pools" of hormone have been described, one a rapidly releasable one which reflects hormone stored in secretory granules as well as that being synthesized and the other a slowly releasable one which reflects predominantly newly synthesized hormone.

Once secreted, peptide hormones have a short half-life in the circulation. Most peptide hormones, such as ACTH, parathyroid hormone (PTH), insulin, glucagon, ADH, TRH, gonadotropin releasing hormone (GnRH), and corticotropin releasing hormone (CRH), act rapidly and are degraded rapidly, having circulating half-lives of 3 to 7 min. Metabolic clearance studies must be interpreted with some caution because of the complexity of degrading systems for different hormones in different tissues, but several general principles appear to operate for most peptide hormones. Although peptide hormones may be cleaved by circulating proteases, the initial step leading to the major pathway for peptide hormone degradation is binding to receptors in target cells. The receptor does not itself degrade the hormone but delivers it to degradative enzymes located both in the cell membrane and in the interior of target cells. Insulin degradation, for example, is directly related to receptor binding in liver cells, quantitatively the most important site of insulin clearance.[62,63] Peptide hormone degradation is catalyzed by cellular proteases which appear somewhat specific. Lysosomal enzymes may contribute to degradation of hormone delivered via absorptive endocytosis, but specific enzymes such as an insulin protease which cleaves insulin and glucagon,[64,65] a postproline cleaving enzyme which cleaves ADH and TRH,[66] a pyroglutamyl aminopeptidase which cleaves TRH and GnRH,[67] and others appear to first inactivate peptide hormones, which are then further degraded by other cellular proteases (Fig. 4-8). Reduction of disulfide bonds may also be important for inactivation of certain hormones such as insulin and ADH.[64,66]

The glycoprotein hormones have significantly longer circulating half-lives than unmodified peptide hormones. hCG, the most heavily glycosylated peptide hormone, has a circulating half-life of about 4 h. Removal of terminal sialic acid markedly shortens the half-life of circulating glycoprotein hormones,[69] because the modified proteins are now recognized and cleaved by the asialoglycoprotein receptor present principally in liver.[61] Although most peptide hormones circulate at low concentrations as unbound species, some hormones such as the insulin-like growth factors are bound to carrier proteins in serum.[70] Such binding provides a circulating reservoir and an extended half-life. Platelet-derived growth factor and epidermal growth factor are present in platelet granules and are presumably released in high concentrations when platelet activation and release reactions are triggered.[71,72]

The short circulating half-life of most peptide hormones provides for rapid termination of their biological actions. In normal physiology, synthesis and secretion are regulated to deliver appropriate concentrations of hormone to target tissues. Inactivation of both hormone and receptor buffers tissues against excessive responses. These buffering systems are a barrier to clinical use of peptide hormones and, with the notable exception of insulin, have limited widespread therapeutic use of most peptide hormones.

STEROID HORMONES

The pathways for biosynthesis of steroid hormones by adrenal cortex, ovary, and testis are similar. Many of the biosynthetic enzymes are identical, with specialized enzymes providing modifications which give the final unique steroid structure recognized by target tissue hormone receptors. The rate-limiting step subject to acute hormone regulation is the same in adrenocortical and gonadal tissues; subcellular organization of biosynthetic enzyme pathways is also the same. Enzymes synthesizing the active form of vitamin D are similar to other steroid hydroxylases but are located in different organs (liver and kidney) rather than within a single gland.

Cholesterol Substrate for Steroid Hormone Formation

All steroid hormones are derived from cholesterol, which is provided by de novo synthesis from acetate or by uptake of circulating cholesterol synthesized in the liver and carried in low-density lipoprotein (LDL) particles. In either case, cholesterol may be used

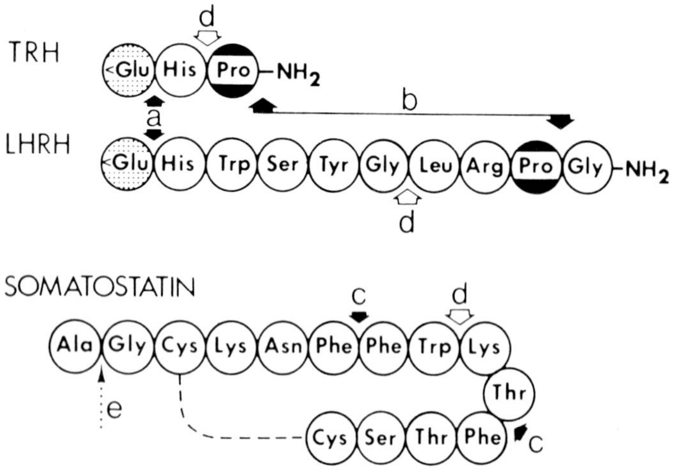

FIGURE 4-8 Sites of proteolytic degradation of three neurohormones. The major sites of cleavage are indicated by arrows. (a) Pyroglutamyl peptidase. (b) Postproline cleaving enzyme. (c) Carboxyl (acid) proteinase. (d) Neutral endopeptidase. (e) Aminopeptidase. (*From Chertow.*[68])

immediately for hormone biosynthesis or stored in the gland in lipid droplets as cholesterol esters. The number of LDL receptors in steroidogenic cells is higher than in non-steroid-secreting cells,[73,74] and up to 70 percent of cholesterol utilized for steroid hormone production in the human adrenal cortex is provided from LDL cholesterol.[75] LDL receptors are increased in steroidogenic cells in response to tropic hormones.[76,77] This increase in LDL receptors results from increased steroid hormone synthesis, which utilizes and reduces cellular cholesterol. A reduction in cellular cholesterol increases LDL receptors to facilitate cholesterol uptake; reduced cellular cholesterol also enhances the activity of 3-hydroxy-3-methylglutaryl coenzyme A synthase (HMG-CoA synthase) and HMG-CoA reductase, the two rate-controlling enzymes of cholesterol synthesis.[78,79] Cholesterol availability is thus tightly coupled to the metabolic requirements of steroidogenic cells (Fig. 4-9).

Steroidogenic cells contain abundant lipid droplets in which cholesterol esters are stored. In response to tropic hormones, cholesterol esterase is activated via cAMP-dependent phosphorylation[80] to provide free cholesterol as substrate for steroid hormone synthesis. With prolonged stimulation lipid droplets are depleted of cholesterol, but they are subsequently replenished when stimuli are removed. With prolonged stimulation most of the cholesterol substrate for steroidogenesis is provided by facilitated uptake of LDL cholesterol. Facilitated uptake from LDL, release from cholesterol ester storage depots, and de novo synthesis provide sufficient cholesterol to sustain the 10-fold increase in adrenal cortisol production which occurs in response to severe stress; when basal conditions are reestablished, regulatory mechanisms reduce uptake and synthesis to levels appropriate to lower cortisol production rates (Fig. 4-9). Similar changes occur in ovarian and testicular cells stimulated by tropic hormones to produce estrogen, progesterone, and testosterone.

The Rate-Controlling Step in Steroid Hormone Synthesis

The rate-limiting step in total steroid synthesis in steroidogenic tissues is cleavage of the side chain of cholesterol to yield pregnenolone (Fig. 4-10).[81] Cholesterol transformation and subsequent steroid hormone biosynthesis are catalyzed by cytochrome P450 enzymes and dehydrogenases. Stimulation of steroidogenesis in adrenal cortex, ovary, and testis results from accelerated formation of pregnenolone because subsequent enzyme activities are present in relative excess.

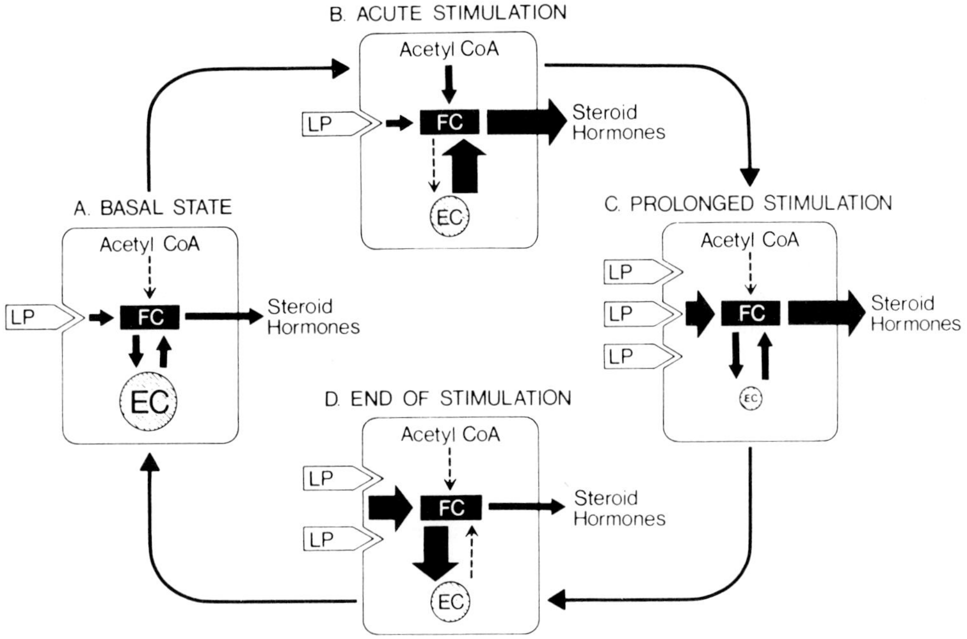

FIGURE 4-9 Provision of cholesterol for steroid hormone formation. The small metabolically active pool of free cholesterol (FC) which is the precursor of steroid hormone formation is maintained in response to stimuli by hydrolysis of cholesterol esters (EC), by de novo synthesis from acetyl CoA, and by facilitated uptake from circulating lipoproteins (LP). See text for details. (*From Brown et al.*[73])

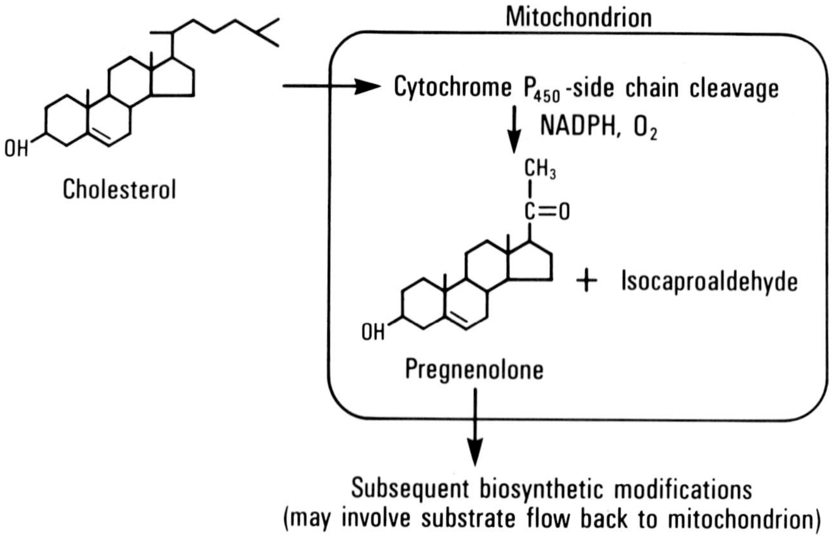

FIGURE 4-10 The rate-limiting step of steroid hormone biosynthesis.

The cholesterol side-chain cleavage enzyme cytochrome $P450_{scc}$ is located in the inner mitochondrial membrane,[82] and stimulation of steroid hormone formation results from increased interaction of cholesterol with this enzyme.[83,84] Although hormones such as ACTH, FSH, LH, and hCG increase general cholesterol availability (Fig. 4-9), regulation of the rate of steroidogenesis depends on facilitated interaction of free cholesterol with mitochondrial cytochrome $P450_{scc}$, probably by transfer of cholesterol from the outer to the inner mitochondrial membrane.[82] Because adequate active cytochrome $P450_{scc}$ and fully reduced adrenodoxin are present, the major limitation appears to be transfer of cholesterol to the enzyme.[84,85] The detailed mechanism through which ACTH, FSH, LH, and hCG, via their intracellular mediator cAMP, increase interaction of cholesterol with cytochrome $P450_{scc}$ is not fully understood, but it appears to involve synthesis of an activator protein[86] and polyphosphoinositides.[87,88] Both the activator protein and the polyphosphoinositides are increased in response to elevated concentrations of cAMP, and both increase pregnenolone formation when added to isolated mitochondria. These mediators are envisioned as facilitating delivery of cholesterol to $P450_{scc}$ located in the inner mitochondrial membrane.

The side-chain cleavage reaction catalyzed by cytochrome $P450_{scc}$ resembles other monoxygenations of cytochrome P450, but three sequential monoxygenations are involved in the scission of the carbon-carbon bond.[89] Mitochondrial cytochrome P450 enzymes such as $P450_{scc}$, involved in synthesis of adrenal and gonadal steroid hormones, $P450_{11\beta}$, involved in cortisol synthesis, $P450_{CMO}$, involved in aldosterone synthesis, and $P450_{1\alpha}$, involved in $1,25(OH)_2$ vitamin D synthesis, utilize a flavoprotein (adrenodoxin reductase) and an iron-sulfur protein (adrenodoxin, a form of ferrodoxin), NADPH (reduced form of nicotinamide adenine dinucleotide phosphate), and molecular oxygen.[90] Microsomal cytochrome P450 enzymes such as 17- and 21-hydroxylases and C17,20-lyase in adrenal cortex and gonads and vitamin D 25-hydroxylase in liver utilize a different flavoprotein, cytochrome P450 reductase, for electron transfer.[91] Cholesterol is first hydroxylated at C22, then it is hydroxylated at C20, and the resulting glycol is cleaved to yield the 20-ketone plus isocapraldehyde. Evidence for dihydroxylation at C22 rather than hydroxylation at C20 has been presented.[92] As in other cytochrome P450 enzymes, the active site region consists of a substrate-binding site and a heme-iron catalytic site.[93] A general model of the reaction cycle of cytochrome P450 includes substrate binding, heme reduction, and oxygen binding (Fig. 4-11).[94] Substrate binding occurs first, then the iron-oxo hydroxylating complex is formed, followed by product formation. The introduction of activated oxygen into the substrate yields the hydroxylated steroid product which is released along with a molecule of water. Abortive cycles induced by binding of a pseudosubstrate can result in the production of oxygen-derived radicals which destroy the enzyme.[95] The large antioxidant armamentarium of steroidogenic cells probably evolved as a protective mechanism against such abortive cytochrome P450 cycles.

Steroidogenic tissues contain large numbers of specialized mitochondria and an extensive network of smooth endoplasmic reticulum. The enzymes which progressively modify the cholesterol molecule are located in these two compartments, and substrate

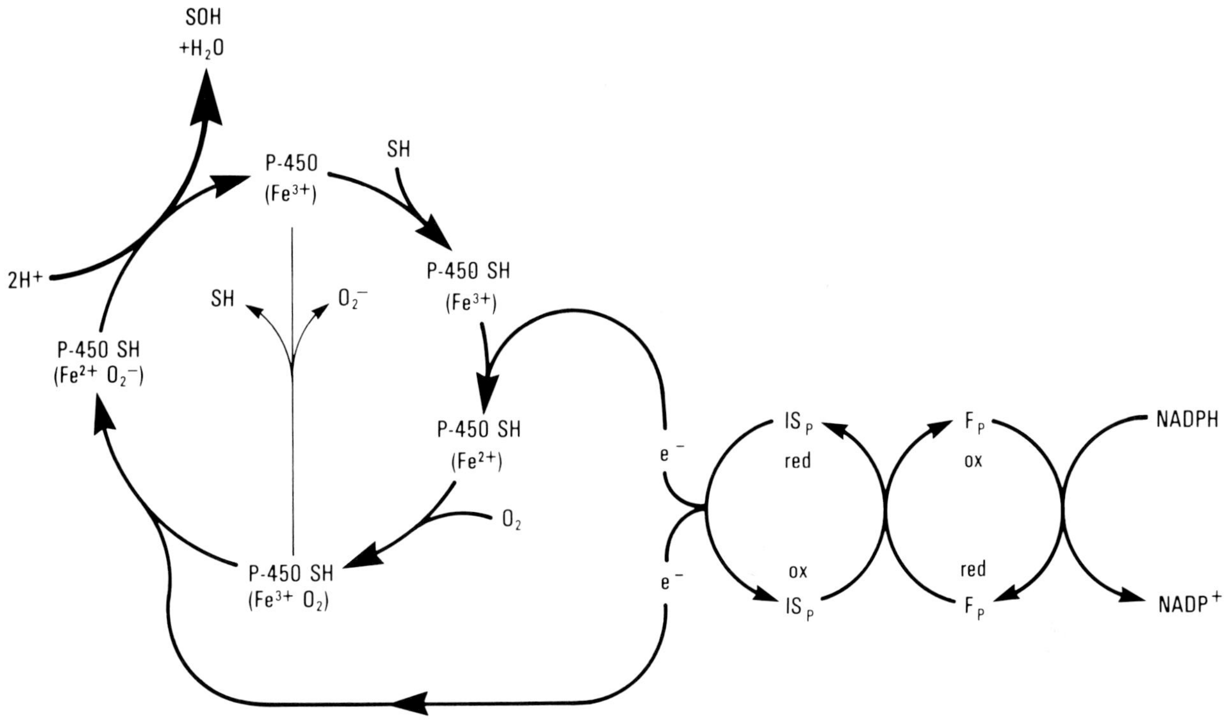

FIGURE 4-11 Model of cytochrome P450 reaction cycle. Electrons are transferred from NADPH via flavoprotein adrenodoxin reductase (Fp) and the iron-sulfur protein adrenodoxin (IS). Substrate (SH) binding to the enzyme brings the portion of the molecule to be modified close to the active center containing porphyrin-bound iron-oxo complex. The cycle is completed with production of product (SOH) and water. When a pseudo substrate is bound, the complex breaks down to form ferric P450 and superoxide (O_2^-) (center).

flows from mitochondria to endoplasmic reticulum and back to mitochondria as it is progressively modified.

Pathway of Steroid Hormone Biosynthesis

Figure 4-12 shows the pathway for steroid hormone synthesis in the adrenal cortex. After cholesterol side-chain cleavage, pregnenolone flows out of mitochondria to the endoplasmic reticulum, where it is sequentially modified. In human adrenal cortex cells, pregnenolone is converted to 17α-OH pregnenolone by cytochrome $P450_{17}$.[96] 17α-OH pregnenolone is converted to progesterone by a 3β-hydroxysteroid dehydrogenase–$\Delta^{4,5}$-isomerase enzyme complex, which converts the 5,6 double bond of cholesterol to a 4,5 double bond and the 3-OH group to a ketone.[97] Cytochrome $P450_{21}$ then adds a hydroxyl group to C21 of 17α-OH progesterone. The product, 11-deoxycortisol, flows back to mitochondria, where cytochrome $P450_{11\beta}$ catalyzes hydroxylation at C11 to yield cortisol, the final active product.

Zona glomerulosa cells contain a specialized mitochondrial cytochrome P450, corticosterone methyl oxidase, which hydroxylates corticosterone at C18 in a double hydroxylation, followed by loss of water to give the aldehyde.[98] Because glomerulosa cells lack cytochrome $P450_{17}$, progesterone is hydroxylated at C21 to yield 11-deoxycorticosterone and then at C11 to yield corticosterone. Mitochondrial cytochrome $P450_{CMO}$ then catalyzes formation of aldosterone, the active mineralocorticoid.

To produce androgens and estrogens, the C20,21 side chain must be removed. This reaction is catalyzed by C17,20-lyase, an activity associated with cytochrome $P450_{17}$.[99] This enzyme converts 17α-OH pregnenolone to dehydroepiandrosterone (DHA) and 17α-OH progesterone to androstenedione. In the human fetal zone of the fetal adrenal cortex, 3β-hydroxysteroid dehydrogenase–$\Delta^{4,5}$-isomerase activity is low, so pregnenolone flows primarily to DHA, which is then sulfated and transported to the placenta. The human definitive zone of the fetal adrenal cortex and also the adult adrenal cortex have increased, though still low, 3β-hydroxysteroid dehydrogenase–$\Delta^{4,5}$-isomerase activity, so C17,20-lyase competes with this enzyme for precursor, and significant amounts of the androgen precursors DHA and androstenedione are made in addition to cortisol. About

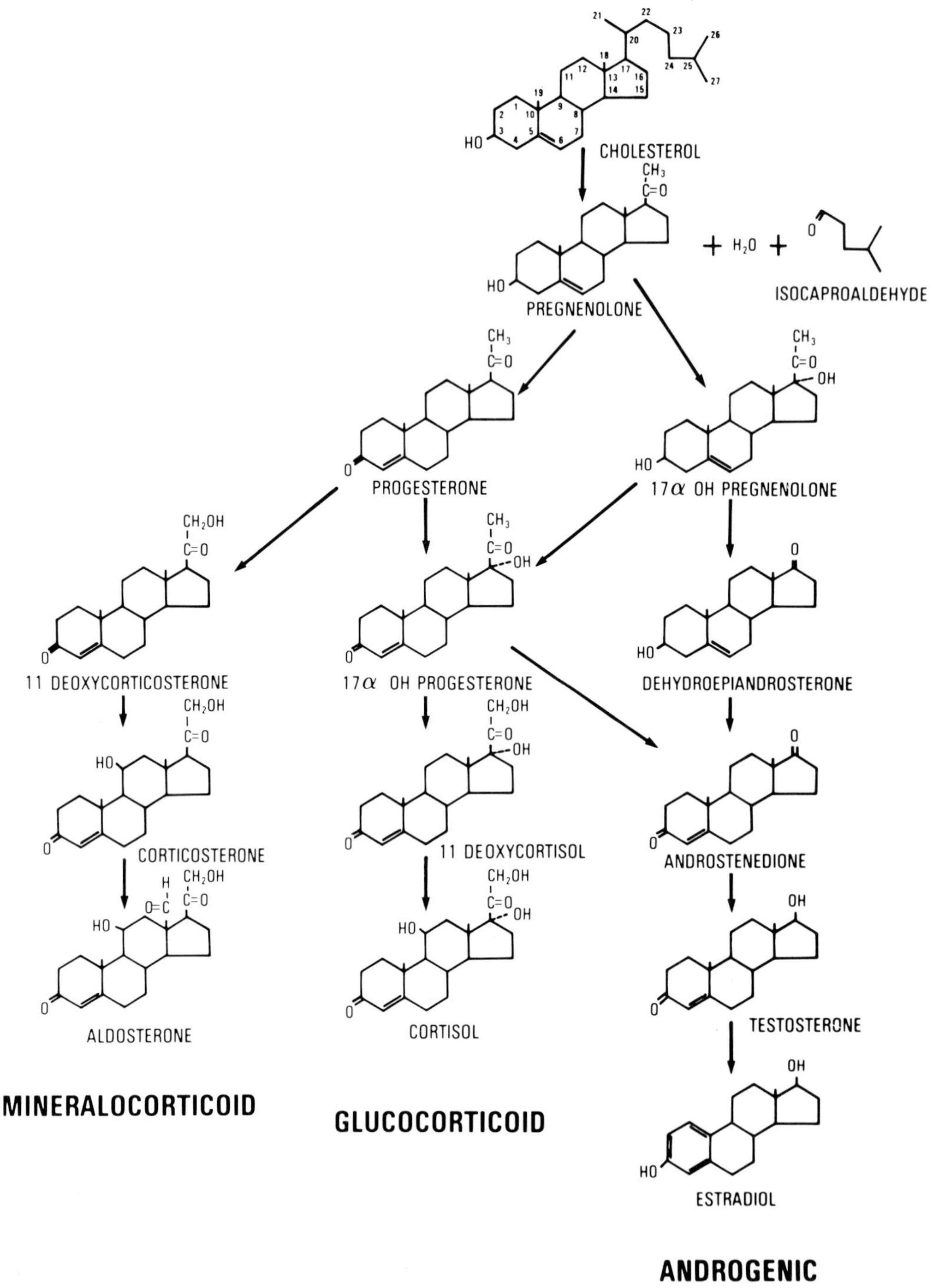

FIGURE 4-12 Pathway for biosynthesis of steroid hormones. The relative concentrations of the various enzymes determines the flow of reactants through the pathway and the final steroid hormone products.

half the pregnenolone formed in the human adrenal cortex is metabolized to DHA.

Leydig cells of the testis lack cytochrome $P450_{21}$ and $P450_{11\beta}$ activity. The androgen pathway shown on the right in Fig. 4-12 thus predominates, and androstenedione is converted to the active androgen, testosterone.

Estrogen and progesterone are the principal steroid products of the ovary. Granulosa cells which are converted to luteal cells during the second half of the menstrual cycle contain low levels of cytochrome $P450_{17}$ and C17,20-lyase and thus convert little pregnenolone or progesterone to androgens. Because these cells also lack cytochrome $P450_{21}$ and $P450_{11\beta}$ activities, progesterone is their major steroid product. Given these enzyme deficiencies, estrogen synthesis must depend on the participation of theca cells with granulosa cells (Fig. 4-13).[100] Theca cells produce androstenedione, which is converted to estrogen by granulosa cells.[101] In granulosa cells, androstenedione is converted to estrone by aromatase, which catalyzes formation of two additional double bonds in the A ring; aromatase similarly converts testosterone to estradiol. Ovarian steroidogenesis thus depends on cooperation between two cell types, theca and granulosa, and two tropic hormones, LH and FSH.[102]

The active steroid hormone $1,25(OH)_2$ vitamin D, or $1,25(OH)_2D$, is also synthesized from cholesterol, but the biosynthetic enzymes are located in three separate organs: skin, liver, and kidney. Initially vitamin D_3 is formed by ultraviolet irradiation of precursor 7-dehydrocholesterol present in skin (Fig. 4-14). Formation of vitamin D_3 proceeds via a 6,7 cis isomer intermediate, previtamin D.[103] Adequate exposure to ultraviolet light is necessary for this initial step in $1,25(OH)_2D$ formation, with more exposure being required for darker-skinned races. A dietary precursor, ergocalciferol or vitamin D_2, which differs from vitamin D_3 by a double bond between C22 and C23 and a methyl group at C24, is formed in plants from ergosterol. Although most foods have only low amounts of vitamins D_2 and D_3, irradiation can convert precursors to vitamins D_2 and D_3. Intestinal absorption occurs principally in the ileum and requires bile salts.

Vitamins D_3 and D_2 are transported in plasma to liver via a vitamin D transport protein. This transport protein has a greater affinity for vitamin D_3 than previtamin D, so the latter remains in skin depots.

In the liver, vitamin D_3 is hydroxylated at C25 by a microsomal enzyme, cytochrome $P450_{25}$; 25(OH)D, which is the major circulating form of vitamin D, is then transported via the α-globulin vitamin D transport protein to proximal tubule cells of the kidney, where the final modification to produce the active species occurs. In the kidney, 1α-hydroxylation of 25(OH)D is catalyzed by mitochondrial cytochrome $P450_{1\alpha}$, a cytochrome P450 enzyme with the properties shown in Fig. 4-12.[104] Biologically active $1,25(OH)_2D$ is secreted and transported to its site of action.

In this unusual endocrine system with large amounts of precursor present in skin (previtamin D) and circulation [25(OH)D], the major site for synthetic regulation is at the final biosynthetic step in kidney proximal tubule cells. Elevated PTH and decreased serum phosphorus are the major factors known to stimulate cytochrome $P450_{1\alpha}$ activity to increase formation of $1,25(OH)_2D$.[105]

Several additional modifications of the 25(OH)D nucleus occur. Hydroxylation at C24 is favored when hydroxylation at C1 is low, whereas hydroxylation at C24 is low when hydroxylation at C1 is high, suggesting that the formation of $24,25(OH)_2D$ represents a

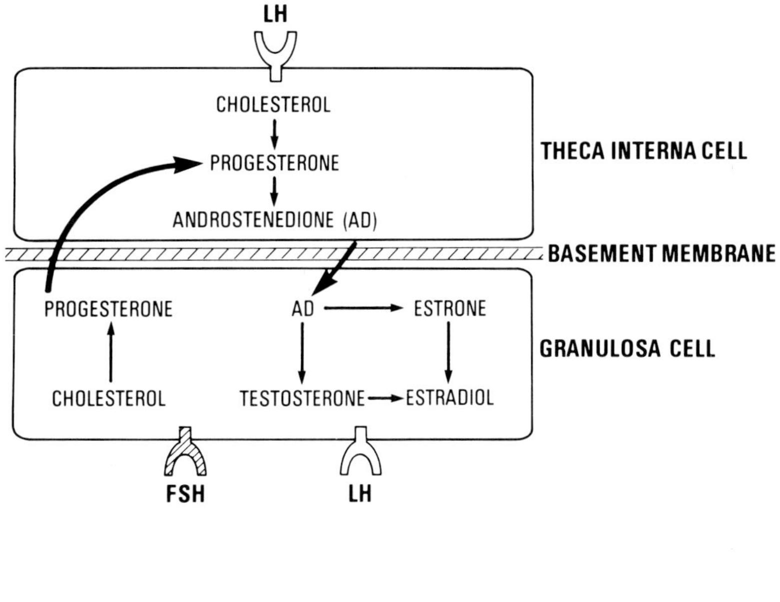

FIGURE 4-13 Two-cell, two-gonadotropin model of ovarian steroid hormone synthesis. Granulosa cells produce principally progesterone but contain aromatase, which converts androstenedione and testosterone to estrone and estradiol, respectively. Androstenedione is synthesized in theca interna cells and transported to adjacent granulosa cells.

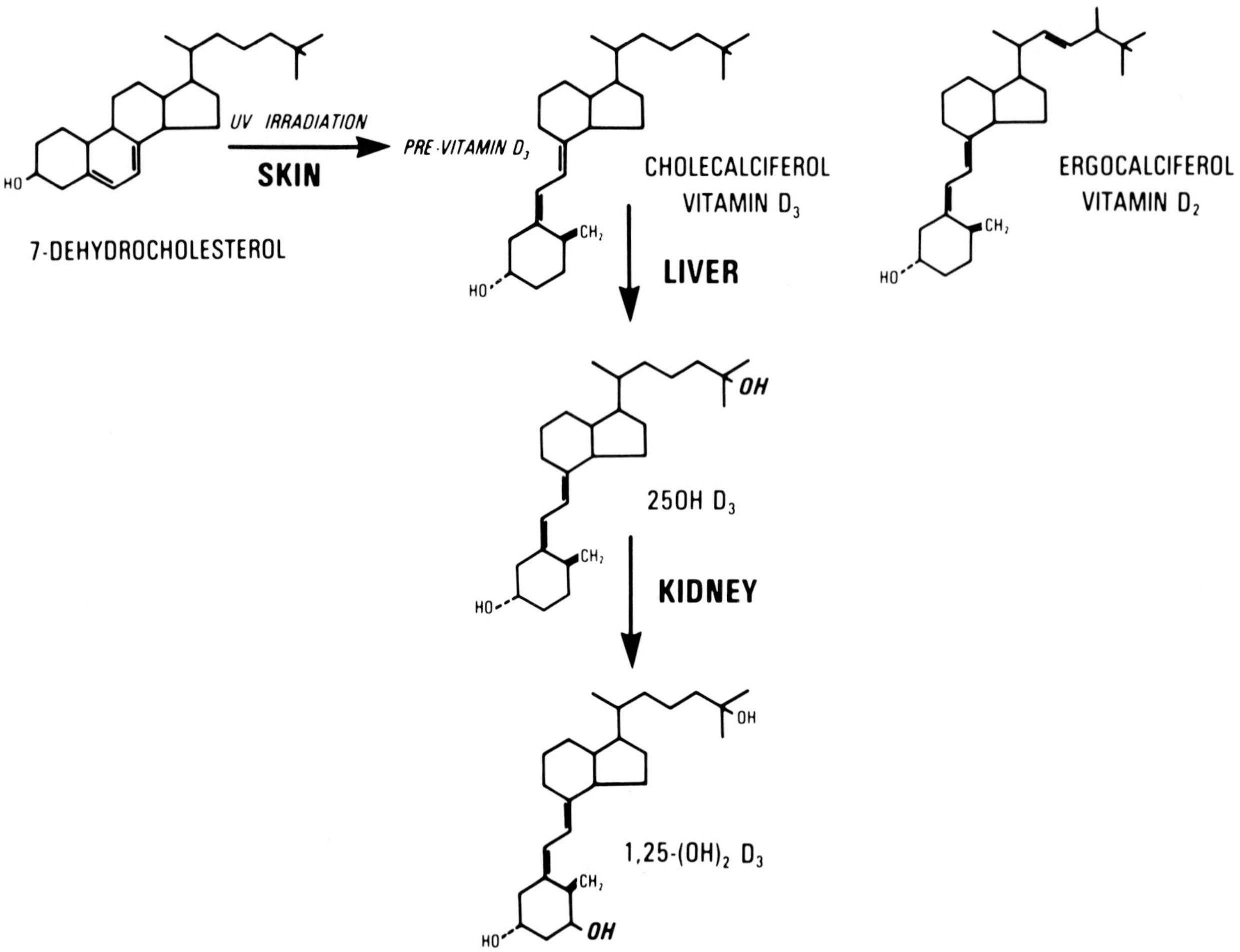

FIGURE 4-14 Biosynthesis of metabolically active $1,25(OH)_2D$.

pathway for inactivation of the steroid.[106] Hydroxylation at C26 may also occur, with or without hydroxylation at C24 and C1.

Tropic Regulation of Steroid Hormone Synthesis

Hormones such as ACTH, FSH, LH, and hCG not only acutely stimulate steroid hormone production but also chronically increase the synthetic capacity of their target glands by inducing synthesis of the enzymes of the biosynthetic pathway. Historically, these tropic effects were recognized from target gland atrophy with hypophysectomy before there was knowledge of the regulation of steroid hormone formation.[107] After hypophysectomy all the steroid-synthesizing enzymes decrease; administration of tropic hormones restores these to normal by increasing specific messenger RNAs and consequent enzyme protein biosynthesis.[84,108–110] In adrenocortical cells, ACTH coordinately increases synthesis of cytochromes $P450_{scc}$ and $P450_{11\beta}$, adrenodoxin, and adrenodoxin reductase;[110,111] in granulosa cells, FSH induces aromatase,[112,113] and increases in most other enzymes also occur.[84,102]

These tropic effects increase the capacity of the adrenal cortex to produce steroids during chronic stress and of the ovary to produce steroids during the menstrual cycle. Optimal enzyme induction requires increased protein biosynthetic capacity, which is achieved by the coordinate action of growth-promoting factors. The coordinate effects of ACTH and growth factors result in hypertrophied, hyperfunctional adrenocortical cells. The growth factors stimulate cell hypertrophy so that specific inductive effects of ACTH are maximal.[114] ACTH does not directly stimulate cell growth; rather, it blocks cell replication.[115] This coordinate action by two types of signal (ACTH, which induces differentiated function but inhibits replication, and growth factors such as fibroblast growth factor and insulin, which increase cell growth and biosynthetic capacity) provides amplification in response to need and a return to baseline when that need is over. This method of response is well suited to hormone biosynthetic cells, which must frequently change their production capacity, because it permits large changes in this capacity without cell replication or cell death.[116]

Transport and Metabolism of Steroid Hormones

In contrast to peptide hormones, steroid hormones are not stored but are secreted as synthesized. Increased secretion therefore directly reflects increased synthesis. Following secretion into the circulation, steroid hormones are bound to transport glycoproteins which are made in the liver. Evidence that transport proteins are not essential for the activity of steroid hormones comes from patients with genetic deficiencies of binding protein who have normal endocrine function and from the observation that some synthetic analogues (e.g., dexamethasone) which are highly active bind poorly to transport proteins. The plasma binding proteins provide a reservoir of hormone, protected from metabolism and renal clearance, which can be released to cells. This reservoir significantly prolongs the circulating half-life of steroid hormones, buffers increases in hormone production, and provides a source of hormone when production decreases. The concentration of binding proteins is regulated and affects the concentration of free active hormone.

There are three main steroid hormone transport proteins: corticosteroid binding globulin (CBG), which binds cortisol and progesterone, sex hormone binding globulin (SHBG), and vitamin D binding globulin (DBG). CBG is a 52,000 M_r glycoprotein which binds cortisol and progesterone with about equal affinity (K_d = 30 nM).[117] CBG contains one high-affinity binding site and is normally present in concentrations sufficient to bind about 250 ng of cortisol per milliliter. When cortisol concentrations exceed this, the hormone is weakly bound by albumin, and metabolism and excretion of the free hormone increase. Except in the third trimester of pregnancy, when high levels of progesterone occur, cortisol concentrations exceed those of progesterone about 10-fold, so most binding sites on CBG are filled by cortisol. CBG production is increased by estrogens, so by the third trimester of pregnancy CBG concentrations are twice those of the nonpregnant state; CBG production is also increased by thyroid hormone.

The affinity of SHBG for testosterone is significantly greater than its affinity for estradiol.[118] Under most conditions, the single binding site on the molecule is occupied by testosterone and estradiol is weakly bound to albumin. The concentration of SHBG is increased 5- to 10-fold by estrogens and is decreased twofold by androgens; thyroid hormone also increases SHBG.

DBG, a 56,000 M_r glycoprotein, has a single binding site with a higher affinity for 25(OH)D than for 1,25$(OH)_2$D or previtamin D_3.[119] The relative binding affinities provide a reservoir of circulating 25(OH)D, as well as ready release of active 1,25$(OH)_2$D to target tissues. Like other steroid hormone transport proteins, DBG is also synthesized in increased amounts in response to estrogen.

The small fraction of free steroid hormone, which is in equilibrium with that bound to transport protein, binds to intracellular hormone receptors to induce biological responses. The free fraction is also metabolized, principally in the liver, to inactive, water-soluble derivatives. Cortisol, for example, is inactivated by reduction of the 4,5 double bond of the A ring. Less polar ketone groups such as those at C3 and C20 are converted to hydroxyl groups. Hydroxyl groups, especially at carbon 3, are conjugated with glucuronide and sulfate to render them more water-soluble for effective renal clearance. Hydroxylations of other steroids are also important for increasing solubility and for conjugation with glucuronic acid or sulfate. Estradiol is hydroxylated at either C2 or C16 and can be conjugated at either position, aldosterone can be conjugated via hydroxyls at either C3 or C18, and cortisol can be hydroxylated at C6. More than 50 steroid metabolites, reflecting various combinations or substitutions, have been identified, though most are produced in only small amounts.[120]

Although most metabolic alterations of steroid hormones result in inactivation, there are several which enhance or alter biological activity. The biological activity of testosterone is increased by 5α-reductase, which converts testosterone to 5α-dihydrotestosterone, the active species in the male reproductive tract and skin.[121] 5α-Reductase is localized in target tissues such as the prostate, so that activation of precursor testosterone occurs at the site of action. Circulating androstenedione, produced in adrenal cortex and gonads, can be converted to testosterone. Aromatase, the cytochrome P450 required for estrogen production, is located in peripheral tissue cells and in producer granulosa cells in the ovary. Significant quantities of estradiol are produced in both men and women by conversion of circulating androstenedione and testosterone to estrone and estradiol.[122]

THYROID HORMONE

In contrast to many hormones whose concentrations fluctuate rapidly in response to environmental signals, thyroid hormone is remarkably stable. It is synthesized

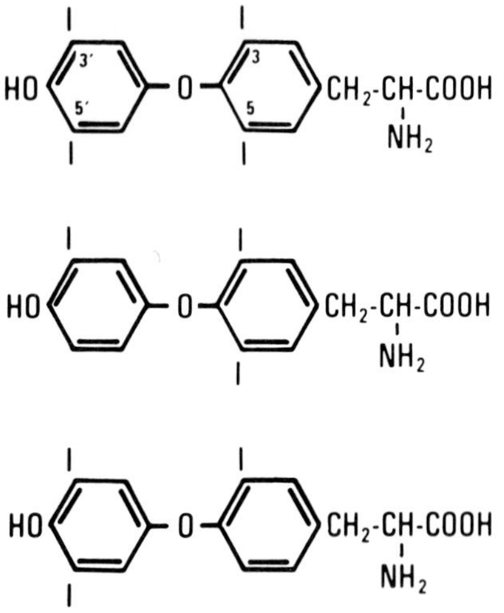

THYROXINE (T_4)

3,5,3′ TRIIODOTHYRONINE (T_3)

3,3′,5′- TRIIODOTHYRONINE (reverse T_3)

FIGURE 4-15 The major circulating thyroid hormones.

in the largest endocrine gland, stored in large quantities in thyroid follicles as part of the structure of a protein molecule, secreted as a prohormone, transported in the circulation bound to carrier proteins, and converted to its most active form in peripheral tissues.

Iodine Metabolism

Thyroid hormones are iodinated derivatives of the amino acid tyrosine (Fig. 4-15). Thyroxine (T_4), the major secretory product of the thyroid gland, consists of two phenyl rings linked via an ether bridge with an alanine side chain on the inner ring. Thyroxine contains four iodine atoms attached to carbons 3 and 5 of the inner ring and 3′ and 5′ of the outer ring. These substitutions impose a three-dimensional structure on the molecule so that the planes of the aromatic rings are perpendicular to each other.[123] 3,5,3′-Triiodothyronine (T_3), the most active form of the hormone, is principally derived from T_4 by removal of one iodine from the outer ring, whereas 3,3′,5′-triiodothyronine (reverse T_3), the major inactive metabolite of T_4, results from removal of iodine from C5 of the inner ring.

Because iodine is an essential structural component, biosynthesis of thyroid hormone depends on iodine metabolism. Dietary iodine intake in western cultures is normally about 250 μg per day but may be greater because of the use of iodized salt and of iodates in bread and processed foods. In inland mountainous areas of the world iodine intake may be less than 60 μg per day. In these areas, growth of the thyroid gland and enhanced trapping of iodide maintain a euthyroid state. Although the adaptive capacity of the gland is great, when iodine intake falls below 20 μg per day thyroid gland compensation may be inadequate, and endemic hypothyroidism and cretinism occur.

Under basal conditions, the thyroid uses about 60 μg of iodide daily for thyroid hormone biosynthesis (Fig. 4-16). Of this, 50 μg is of dietary origin and 10 μg is from hormone turnover. Iodide is concentrated from the circulation by active transport via an iodide pump or trap located at the basal surface of the thyroid cell. The concentrating mechanism requires metabolic energy from ATP and Na^+, K^+-ATPase–mediated sodium transport.[125] The transport process effectively extracts iodide from the circulation and can concentrate it more than 100-fold within the thyroid cell. Other anions such as perchlorate and pertechnetate are also concentrated, and these ions have been used for thyroid function tests and for imaging.

Cellular uptake of iodide is regulated by TSH and by local control mechanisms. The local autoregulatory mechanisms help provide adequate iodide for hormone synthesis when circulating levels are low and

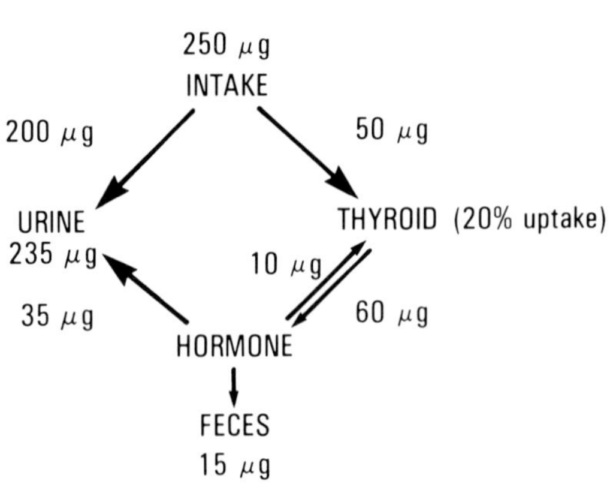

FIGURE 4-16 Average human daily iodine balance in the United States. (*From Robbins.*[124])

prevent excessive hormone synthesis when circulating iodide concentrations are high. In response to large quantities of iodine (2 mg or more), there is a sharp decrease in iodination of tyrosine residues in thyroglobulin.[126] The decreased organification (Wolff-Chaikoff effect) is an acute adaptive response to high intracellular concentrations of iodide. When high iodide concentrations persist, thyroid cells adapt by decreasing active transport of iodide into the cell.[127] Increased cellular concentrations of unbound iodide are then dissipated and the block to organification is removed. Ingestion of large amounts of iodine thus does not normally affect thyroid hormone synthesis. When these autoregulatory mechanisms are defective, dietary iodine can have marked effects on thyroid hormone synthesis. When inhibition of organification does not occur in response to increased cellular iodide, increased thyroid hormone synthesis and hyperthyroidism may occur (iod-Basedow effect). If organification is inhibited but transport of iodide does not adaptively decrease, high cellular concentrations of iodide will result in decreased thyroid hormone synthesis (iodide goiter and hypothyroidism).

Anatomy of a Distinctive Biosynthetic Pathway

Thyroid cells are organized into follicles with their basal surfaces exposed to the circulation and their apical surfaces facing the lumen of the central follicle, which is filled with thyroglobulin. Iodide is taken up at the basal surface and is rapidly oxidized and incorporated into tyrosine residues in thyroglobulin molecules. In the biosynthetic pathway outlined in Fig. 4-17, both the organification and coupling reactions shown occur at the apical surface of the cell, in microvilli which extend into the colloid space. Thyroid peroxidase is a membrane-bound heme-protein enzyme complex which catalyzes both organification and coupling reactions.[128–130] The proposed reaction scheme for thyroid peroxidase (E) is

(1) Organification:

$$E + H_2O_2 \xrightarrow{\;-H_2O\;} EO \longrightarrow [EOI]^- \xrightarrow{+\text{ tyrosine}} \text{iodotyrosine} + OH^- + E$$

(2) Coupling:

$$E + H_2O_2 \xrightarrow{\;-H_2O\;} EO \xrightarrow{+\text{ DIT (thyroglobulin)}} T_4 + E$$

The antithyroid drugs (thioureylene compounds) inhibit organification and coupling reactions by inactivating both EO and $[EOI]^-$.[128,131]

Tyrosines which are iodinated are present in thyroglobulin, a large multisubunit glycoprotein of 660,000 M_r.[132,133] Thyroglobulin, which accounts for about 50 percent of the total protein made by thyroid cells, has only an average content of tyrosine, but these tyrosines appear to be available for iodination both because of their location in the primary structure and because of the tertiary structure of the mature glycosylated protein. Thyroglobulin is trans-

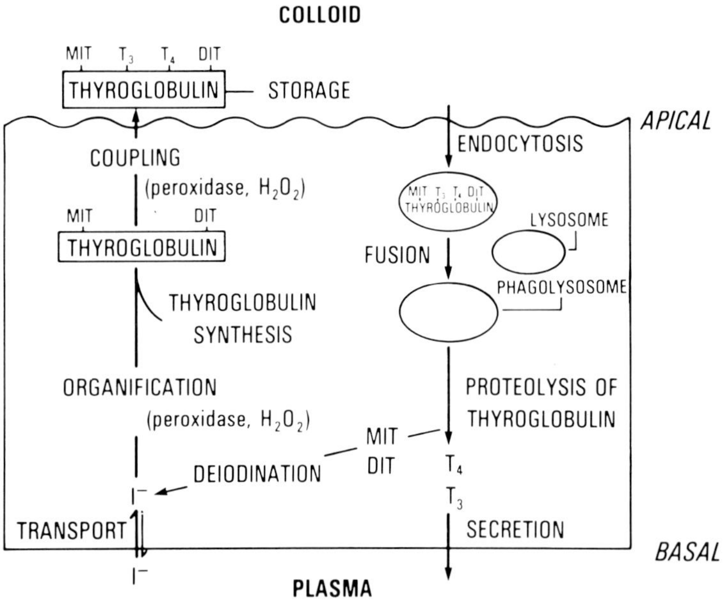

FIGURE 4-17 Pathway for biosynthesis of thyroid hormones.

ported in vesicles to the microvilli at the apical surface, where iodination, coupling, and secretion into the follicular lumen occur. Normally iodinated thyroglobulin present in lumen colloid contains about 26 atoms of iodine with 3 to 4 T_4 and 0.2 T_3 residues as well as 6 residues of monoiodotyrosine and 4 residues of diiodotyrosine.[134] Iodide availability affects the proportions of T_3 and T_4, with more T_3 being present when iodide is low.[135]

Large amounts of thyroglobulin are stored as colloid in the lumen of thyroid follicles. Formation of active thyroid hormone requires readsorption of colloid by endocytosis and breakdown of thyroglobulin to T_4 and T_3. Thyroglobulin may be broken down via lysosomal hydrolases, but there is also evidence for cleavage by halogens and peroxidases.[136,137] If the latter hypothesis is correct, the steps in thyroid hormone synthesis (organification, coupling, and proteolysis) all use one substrate, thyroglobulin, and one enzyme, thyroid peroxidase, and the cellular organization shown in Fig. 4-17 serves to segregate these various reactions.

T_4 and T_3 are secreted in a ratio of about 10:1. The iodine in mono- and diiodotyrosine is reclaimed for hormone biosynthesis by a thyroid deiodinase enzyme. This deiodination pathway reclaims about 50 percent of the iodine of thyroglobulin and is quantitatively important in thyroid gland economy, as demonstrated by the fact that congenital defects in deiodinase result in goitrous hypothyroidism.

TSH, which is the major regulator of thyroid gland function, is reported to increase each step of the biosynthetic pathway. A rate-limiting step analogous to that for steroid hormone synthesis has not been identified, but increased availability of iodide via active transport is among the most rapid responses to TSH.

Transport and Metabolism

T_4, the major secretory product of the thyroid, circulates bound to serum proteins. The binding proteins, like those which transport steroid hormones, are made in the liver, and their synthesis is increased by estrogens and decreased by androgens. More than 99 percent of T_4 is bound to three proteins: thyroid binding globulin (TBG), thyroid binding prealbumin (TBPA), and serum albumin. TBG, a 63,000 M_r glycoprotein, which binds about 75 percent of circulating T_4, has the highest affinity,[138] TBPA has a lesser affinity, and serum albumin has the least affinity but highest capacity. Protein binding provides a large protected reservoir of hormone. Because of extensive protein binding, T_4 has a circulating half-life of about 1 week, while T_3, which is bound less tightly to protein, has a half-life of 1.3 days.

Thyroxine is a prohormone and requires activation in target tissues via 5′-deiodination to metabolically active T_3. 5′-Deiodination is catalyzed by a microsomal enzyme which requires reduced thiols for activity.[139] This enzyme, which is especially prominent in liver and kidney, accounts for more than 80 percent of T_3 production under normal conditions. Its activity and thus the production of T_3 is influenced by many factors. The first site of control of thyroid hormone synthesis is the thyroid gland, where TSH regulates T_4 production. Under most conditions, conversion of T_4 to T_3 in the periphery is proportional to the concentration of substrate T_4, but a second point of control is present in target organs such as liver and kidney, where under several conditions conversion of T_4 to T_3 is decreased. Fasting, illness, cortisol, propylthiouracil, and other drugs all reduce 5′-deiodinase activity.[140] During fasting there is a 20 percent decrease in plasma T_3 by the end of the first day and a 50 percent decrease at the end of 3 days.[141] This decrease in T_3 production is thought to be an adaptive response contributing to a decreased metabolic rate and to conservation of body tissues when substrate is unavailable. Use of the circulating pool of prohormone T_4 is thus coupled to metabolic needs.

5′-Deiodinase found in the pituitary and central nervous system differs from that in liver and kidney. It has a lower K_m for T_4, it is not inhibited by propylthiouracil, and its activity increases rather than decreases in hypothyroidism.[142] This enzyme is important in feedback effects of T_4 on TSH secretion, as well as in biological effects on the nervous system. This second 5′-deiodinase converts T_4 to T_3 in the pituitary to provide a normal hypothalamic-pituitary-thyroid axis under conditions such as fasting where circulating T_3 concentrations are low because of inhibition of liver and kidney 5′-deiodinase. If circulating T_3 were the major feedback regulator of TSH, the reduced circulating concentrations of T_3 in fasting and in systemic illness would remove feedback inhibition to increase TSH and thus thyroid hormone production. The second 5′-deiodinase of the pituitary allows feedback control via circulating T_4 rather than T_3 and serves to maintain normal thyroid gland production, preventing the thyroid from inappropriately compensating for the physiologically important reduction in circulating T_3 concentrations.

Deiodination of the inner ring of T_4 by 5-deiodinase yields reverse T_3 (rT_3), an inactive metabolite.[140] About equal amounts of T_3 and rT_3 are formed from T_4, but rT_3 is cleared more rapidly, so circulating concentrations are lower. When 5′-deiodinase activity is reduced, as in fasting, greater amounts of T_4 are metabolized to rT_3.

Inactivation of T_3 occurs by additional deiodinations to give $3,3'-T_2$ and $3,5-T_2$ and by deamination and decarboxylation of the alanine side chain and conjugation with glucuronic acid and sulfate.

REFERENCES

1. Roeder RG: Eukaryotic nuclear RNA polymerases, in Losick R, Chamberlin M (eds): *RNA Polymerase.* Cold Spring Harbor Laboratory, 1976, pp 285–329.
2. Shatkin AJ: Capping of eukaryotic mRNAs. *Cell* 9:645, 1976.
3. Breathnach R, Benoist C, O'Hare K, Gannon F, Chambon P: Ovalbumin gene: Evidence for a leader sequence in mRNA and DNA sequences at the exon-intron boundaries. *Proc Natl Acad Sci USA* 75:4853, 1978.
4. Benoist C, O'Hare K, Breathnach R, Chambon P: The ovalbumin gene-sequence of putative control regions. *Nucleic Acids Res* 8:127, 1980.
5. Grosveld GC, deBoer E, Shewmaker CK, Flavell RA: DNA sequences necessary for transcription of the rabbit β-globin gene in vivo. *Nature* 295:120, 1982.
6. Wasylyk B, Derbyshire R, Guy A, Molko D, Roget A, Teoule R, Chambon P: Specific in vitro transcription of conalbumin gene is drastically decreased by single-point mutation in T-A-T-A box homology sequence. *Proc Natl Acad Sci USA* 77:7024, 1980.
7. McKnight SL, Kingsbury R: Transcriptional control signals of a eukaryotic protein-coding gene. *Science* 217:316, 1982.
8. Ishii S, Xu Y-H, Stratton RH, Roe BA, Marlino GT, Pastan I: Characterization and sequence of the promoter region of the human epidermal growth factor receptor gene. *Proc Natl Acad Sci USA* 82:4920, 1985.
9. Ishii S, Merlino GT, Pastan I: Promoter region of the human Harvey *ras* proto-oncogene: Similarity to the EGF receptor proto-oncogene promoter. *Science* 230:1378, 1985.
10. Khoury G, Gruss P: Enhancer elements. *Cell* 33:313, 1983.
11. Gillies SD, Morrison SL, Oi VT, Tonegawa S: A tissue-specific transcription enhancer element is located in the major intron of a rearranged immunoglobulin heavy chain gene. *Cell* 33:717, 1983.
12. Banerji J, Olson L, Schaffner W: A lymphocyte-specific cellular enhancer is located downstream of the joining region in immunoglobulin heavy chain genes. *Cell* 33:729, 1983.
13. Groner B, Ponta H, Beato M, Hynes NE: The proviral DNA of mouse mammary tumor virus: Its use in the study of the molecular details of steroid hormone action. *Mol Cell Endocrinol* 32:101, 1983.
14. Govindan MV, Spiess E, Majors J: Purified glucocorticoid receptor-hormone complex from rat liver cytosol binds specifically to cloned mouse mammary tumor virus long terminal repeats in vitro. *Proc Natl Acad Sci USA* 79:5157, 1982.
15. Chandler VL, Maler BA, Yamamoto KR: DNA sequences bound specifically by glucocorticoid receptor in vitro render a heterologous promoter hormone responsive in vivo. *Cell* 33:489, 1983.
16. Karin M, Haslinger A, Holtgreve H, Richards RI, Krauter P, Westphal HM, Beato M: Characterization of DNA sequences through which cadmium and glucocorticoid hormones induce human metallothionein-II_A gene. *Nature* 308:513, 1984.
17. Compton JG, Schrader WT, O'Malley BW: DNA sequence preference of the progesterone receptor. *Proc Natl Acad Sci USA* 80:16, 1983.
18. Davidson EH, Jacobs HT, Britten RJ: Very short repeats and coordinate induction of genes. *Nature* 301:468, 1983.
19. Nordheim A, Rich A: Negatively supercoiled simian virus 40 DNA containing Z-DNA segments within transcriptional enhancer sequences. *Nature* 303:674, 1983.
20. Supowit SC, Potter E, Evans RM, Rosenfeld MG: Polypeptide hormone regulation of gene transcription: Specific 5′ genomic sequences are responsible for epidermal growth factor regulation of prolactin gene expression. *Proc Natl Acad Sci USA* 81:2975, 1984.
21. Hollenberg SM, Weinberger C, Ong ES, Cerelli G, Oro A, Lebo R, Thompson EB, Rosenfeld MG, Evans, RM: Primary structure and expression of a functional human glucocorticoid receptor cDNA. *Nature* 318:635, 1985.
22. Greene GL, Gilna P, Waterfield M, Baker A, Hort Y, Shine J: Sequence and expression of human estrogen receptor complementary DNA. *Science* 231:1150, 1986.
23. Dynan WS, Tjian R: Control of eukaryotic messenger RNA synthesis by sequence-specific DNA-binding proteins. *Nature* 316: 774, 1985.
24. Keegan L, Gill G, Ptashne M: Separation of DNA binding from the transcription-activating function of a eukaryotic regulatory protein. *Science* 231:699, 1986.
25. Nevins JR: The pathway of eukaryotic mRNA formation. *Annu Rev Biochem* 52:441, 1983.
26. Breathnach R, Chambon P: Organization and expression of eukaryotic split genes coding for proteins. *Annu Rev Biochem* 50:349, 1981.
27. Mount SM: A catalogue of splice junction sequences. *Nucleic Acids Res* 10:459, 1982.
28. Rogers J, Wall R: A mechanism for RNA splicing. *Proc Natl Acad Sci USA* 77:1877, 1980.
29. Lerner MR, Boyle JA, Mount SM, Wolin SL, Steitz JA: Are snRNPs involved in splicing? *Nature* 283:220, 1980.
30. Mount SM, Pettersson I, Hinterberger M, Karmas A, Steitz JA: The U I small nuclear RNA-protein complex selectively binds a 5′ splice site in vitro. *Cell* 33:509, 1983.
31. Lerner MR, Steitz JA: Snurps and scyrps. *Cell* 25:298, 1981.
32. Busch H, Reddy R, Rothblum L, Choi YC: SnRNAs, SnRNPs and RNA processing. *Annu Rev Biochem* 51:617, 1982.
33. Proudfoot NJ, Brownlee GG: 3′ non-coding region sequences in eukaryotic messenger RNA. *Nature* 263:211, 1976.
34. Fitzgerald M, Schenck T: The sequence 5′-AAUAAA-3′ forms part of the recognition site for polyadenylation of late SV40 in RNAs. *Cell* 24:251, 1981.
35. Brawerman G: The role of poly(A) sequence in mammalian messenger RNA. *CRC Crit Rev Biochem* 10:1, 1981.
36. Wall R: Biosynthesis and regulation of immunoglobulins. *Annu Rev Immunol* 1:393, 1983.
37. Amara SG, Jonas V, Rosenfeld MG, Ong ES, Evans RM: Alternate RNA processing in calcitonin gene expression generates mRNAs encoding different polypeptide products. *Nature* 240:240, 1982.
38. Rosenfeld MG, Mermod J-J, Amara SG, Swanson LW, Sawchenko PE, Rivier J, Vale WW, Evans RW: Production of a novel neuropeptide encoded by the calcitonin gene via tissue-specific RNA processing. *Nature* 304:129, 1983.
39. Eipper BA, Mains RE: Structure and biosynthesis of pro-ACTH/endorphin and related peptides. *Endocrinol Rev* 1:1, 1980.
40. Walter P, Blobel G: Signal recognition particle contains a 7S RNA essential for protein translocation across the endoplasmic reticulum. *Nature* 299:691, 1982.
41. Walter P, Blobel G: Translocation of proteins across the endoplasmic reticulum: III. Signal recognition protein (SRP) causes signal sequence-dependent and site-specific arrest of chain elongation that is released by microsomal membranes. *J Cell Biol* 91:557, 1981.
42. Gilmore R, Walter P, Blobel G: Protein translocation across the endoplasmic reticulum: II. Isolation and characterization of the signal recognition particle receptor. *J Cell Biol* 96:470, 1982.

43. Meyer DI, Krause E, Dobberstein B: Secretory protein translocation across membranes—the role of the "docking protein." *Nature* 297:503, 1982.
44. Gilmore R, Blobel G: Transient involvement of signal recognition particle and its receptor in the microsomal membrane prior to protein translocation. *Cell* 35:677, 1983.
45. Gray A, Dull TJ, Ullrich A: Nucleotide sequence of epidermal growth factor cDNA predicts a 128,000-molecular weight protein precursor. *Nature* 303:722, 1983.
46. Lee DC, Rose TM, Webb NR, Todaro GJ: Cloning and sequence analysis of a cDNA for rat transforming growth factor-α. *Nature* 313:489, 1985.
47. Land H, Schutz G, Schmale H, Richter D: Nucleotide sequence of cloned cDNA encoding bovine arginine vasopressin-neurophysin II precursor. *Nature* 295:299, 1982.
48. Nakanishi S, Inoue A, Kita T, Nakamura M, Chang ACY, Cohen SN, Numa S: Nucleotide sequence of cloned cDNA for bovine corticotropin β-lipotropin precursor. *Nature* 278:423, 1979.
49. Steiner DR: Insulin today. *Diabetes* 26:322, 1977.
50. Steiner DS, Clark JL: The spontaneous reoxidation of reduced beef and rat proinsulins. *Proc Natl Acad Sci USA* 60:622, 1968.
51. Gabbay KH, DeLuca K, Fisher JN Jr, Mako ME, Rubenstein AH: Familial hyperproinsulinemia: An autosomal dominant defect. *N Engl J Med* 294:911, 1976.
52. Blundell TL, Bedarkar S, Rinderknecht E, Humbel RE: Insulin-like growth factor: A model for tertiary structure accounting for immunoreactivity and receptor binding. *Proc Natl Acad Sci USA* 75:180, 1978.
53. Noda M, Furutani Y, Takahashi H, Toyosato M, Hirose T, Inayama S, Nakanishi S, Numa S: Cloning and sequence analysis of cDNA for bovine adrenal preproenkephalin. *Nature* 295:202, 1982.
54. Hubbard SC, Ivatt RJ: Synthesis and processing of asparagine-linked oligosaccharides. *Annu Rev Biochem* 50:555, 1981.
55. Pierce JG, Parsons TF: Glycoprotein hormones: Structure and function. *Annu Rev Biochem* 50:465, 1981.
56. Kessler MJ, Reddy MS, Shah RH, Bahl OP: Structures of *N*-glycosidic carbohydrate units of human chorionic gonadotropin. *J Biol Chem* 254:7901, 1979.
57. Kessler MJ, Mise T, Ghai RD, Bahl OP: Structure and location of the O-glycosidic carbohydrate units of human chorionic gonadotropin. *J Biol Chem* 254:7909, 1979.
58. Parsons TF, Pierce JG: Oligosaccharide moieties of glycoprotein hormones: Bovine luteotropin resists enzymatic deglycosylation because of terminal O-sulfated *N*-acetylhexosamines. *Proc Natl Acad Sci USA* 77:7089, 1980.
59. Weintraub BD, Stannard BS, Meyers L: Glycosylation of thyroid stimulating hormone in pituitary tumor cells: Influence of high mannose oligosaccharide units on subunit aggregation, combination and intracellular degradation. *Endocrinology* 112:1331, 1983.
60. Ashwell G, Morell AG: The role of surface carbohydrates in hepatic recognition of circulating glycoproteins. *Adv Enzymol* 4:99, 1974.
61. Ashwell G, Harford J: Carbohydrate-specific receptors of the liver. *Annu Rev Biochem* 51:531, 1982.
62. Terris S, Steiner DF: Binding and degradation of ^{125}I-insulin by rat hepatocytes. *J Biol Chem* 250:8389, 1975.
63. Baldwin D Jr, Terris S, Steiner DF: Characterization of insulin-like actions of anti-insulin receptor antibodies. *J Biol Chem* 255:4028, 1980.
64. Duckworth WC, Kitabchi AE: Insulin metabolism and degradation. *Endocrinol Rev* 2:210, 1981.
65. Duckworth WC, Heinemann MA, Kitabchi AE: Purification of insulin specific protease by affinity chromatography. *Proc Natl Acad Sci USA* 69:3698, 1972.
66. Walter R, Simmons WH, Yoshimoto T: Proline specific endo- and exopeptidases. *Mol Cell Biochem* 30:111, 1980.
67. Griffiths EC, McDermott JR: Enzymatic inactivation of hypothalamic regulatory hormones. *Mol Cell Endocrinol* 33:1, 1983.
68. Chertow BS: The role of lysosomes and proteases in hormone secretion and degradation. *Endocrinol Rev* 2:137, 1981.
69. Morell AG, Greboriadis G, Scheinberg IH, Hickman J, Ashwell G: The role of sialic acid in determining the survival of glycoproteins in the circulation. *J Biol Chem* 246:1461, 1971.
70. Smith GL: Somatomedin carrier proteins. *Mol Cell Endocrinol* 34:83, 1984.
71. Ross R, Vogel A, Davies P, Raines E, Kariya B, Rivest MJ, Gustafson C, Glomset J: The platelet-derived growth factor and plasma control cell proliferation. *Cold Spring Harbor Conf Cell Proliferation* 6:3, 1979.
72. Oka Y, Orth DN: Human plasma epidermal gorwth factor/β-urogastrone is associated with blood platelets. *J Clin Invest* 72:249, 1983.
73. Brown MS, Kovanen PT, Goldstein JL: Receptor-mediated uptake of lipoprotein cholesterol and its utilization for steroid synthesis in the adrenal cortex. *Recent Prog Horm Res* 35:215, 1979.
74. Kovanen PT, Basu SK, Goldstein JL, Brown MS: Low density lipoprotein receptors in bovine adrenal cortex. *Endocrinology* 104:610, 1979.
75. Carr BR, Simpson ER: De novo synthesis of cholesterol by the human fetal adrenal gland. *Endocrinology* 108:2154, 1981.
76. Kovanen PT, Goldstein JL, Chappell DA, Brown MS: Regulation of low density lipoprotein receptors by adrenocorticotropin in the adrenal gland of mice and rats in vivo. *J Biol Chem* 255:5591, 1980.
77. Kovanen PT, Faust JR, Brown MS, Goldstein JL: Low density lipoprotein receptors in bovine adrenal cortex: I. Receptor-mediated uptake of low density lipoprotein and utilization of its cholesterol for steroid synthesis in cultured adrenocortical cells. *Endocrinology* 104:599, 1979.
78. Brown MS, Goldstein JL: Receptor-mediated endocytosis: Insights from the lipoprotein receptor system. *Proc Natl Acad Sci USA* 76:3330, 1979.
79. Brown MS, Anderson RGW, Goldstein JL: Recycling receptors: The round trip itinerary of migrant membrane proteins. *Cell* 32:663, 1983.
80. Beckett GJ, Boyd GS: Purification and control of bovine adrenal cortical cholesterol ester hydrolase and evidence for the activation of the enzyme by a phosphorylation. *Eur J Biochem* 72:223, 1977.
81. Stone D, Hechter O: Studies on ACTH action in perfused bovine adrenals: The site of action of ACTH in corticosteroidogenesis. *Arch Biochem Biophys* 51:457, 1954.
82. Privalle CT, Crivello JF, Jefcoate CR: Regulation of intramitochondrial cholesterol transfer to side-chain cleavage cytochrome P-450 in rat adrenal gland. *Proc Natl Acad Sci USA* 80:702, 1983.
83. Gill GN: ACTH regulation of the adrenal cortex. *Pharmacol Ther* (B) 2:313, 1976.
84. Simpson ER, Waterman MR: Regulation by ACTH of steroid hormone biosynthesis in the adrenal cortex. *Can J Biochem Cell Biol* 61:692, 1983.
85. Simpson ER, McCarthy JL, Peterson JA: Evidence that the cycloheximide-sensitive site of adrenocorticotropic hormone action is in the mitochondrion. *J Biol Chem* 253:3135, 1978.
86. Pedersen RC, Brownie AC: Cholesterol side-chain cleavage in the rat adrenal cortex: Isolation of a cycloheximide-sensitive activator protein. *Proc Natl Acad Sci USA* 80:1882, 1983.
87. Farese RV: Phosphoinositide metabolism and hormone action. *Endocrinol Rev* 4:78, 1983.
88. Farese RV: Phospholipids as intermediates in hormone action. *Mol Cell Endocrinol* 35:1, 1984.
89. Hall PF, Lewes JL, Lipson ED: The role of mitochondrial cytochrome P-450 from bovine adrenal cortex in side chain cleavage of 20S,22*R*-dihydroxycholesterol. *J Biol Chem* 250:2283, 1975.
90. Gustafsson J-A, Carlstedt-Duke J, Mode A, Rafter J: *Biochemistry, Biophysics and Regulation of Cytochrome P-450.* New

York, Elsevier-Holland Biomedical, 1980.

91. Mannering GJ: Hepatic cytochrome P-450-linked drug metabolizing enzymes, in Jenner P, Testa B (eds): *Concepts in Drug Metabolism,* part B. New York, Marcel Dekker, 1981, pp 53–166.

92. Burstein S, Dinh T, Co N, Gut M, Schleyer H, Cooper DY, Rosenthal O: Kinetic studies on substrate-enzyme interaction in the adrenal cholesterol side-chain cleavage system. *Biochemistry* 11:2883, 1972.

93. Sheets JJ, Vickery LE: Proximity of the substrate binding site and the heme-iron catalytic site in cytochrome P-450_{scc}. *Proc Natl Acad Sci USA* 79:5773, 1982.

94. Coon MJ, White RE: Cytochrome P-450, a versatile catalyst in monooxygenation reactions, in Spiro TG (ed): *Metal Ion Activation of Dioxygen.* New York, Wiley, 1980, pp 73–123.

95. Hornsby PJ, Crivello JF: The role of lipid peroxidation and biological antioxidants in the function of the adrenal cortex. *Mol Cell Endocrinol* 30:1, 1983.

96. Hornsby PJ, Aldern KA: Steroidogenic enzyme activities in cultured human definitive zone adrenocortical cells: Comparison with bovine adrenocortical cells and resultant differences in adrenal androgen synthesis. *J Clin Endocrinol Metab* 58:121, 1984.

97. Finkelstein M, Shaefer JM: Inborn errors of steroid biosynthesis. *Physiol Rev* 59:353, 1979.

98. Ulick S, Kusch K: A new C-18 oxygenated corticosteroid from bullfrog adrenals. *J Am Chem Soc* 82:6421, 1960.

99. Nakajin S, Hall PF: Microsomal cytochrome P-450 from neonatal pig testis: Purification and properties of a C21 steroid side chain cleavage system (17α-hydroxylase-C17,20 lyase) *J Biol Chem* 256:3871, 1981.

100. Short RV: Steroids in the follicular fluid and in the corpus luteum of the mare: A "two cell type" theory of ovarian steroid synthesis. *J Endocrinol* 24:59, 1962.

101. Ryan KJ: Granulosa-thecal cell interaction in ovarian steroidogenesis. *J Steroid Biochem* 11:799, 1979.

102. Hseuh AJW, Adashi EY, Jones PBC, Welsh TH Jr: Hormonal regulation of the differentiation of cultured ovarian granulosa cells. *Endocrinol Rev* 5:76, 1984.

103. Holick MF, Clark MB: The photobiogenesis and metabolism of vitamin D. *Fed Proc* 37:2567, 1978.

104. Frazer DR, Kodicek E: Unique biosynthesis by kidney of a biologically active vitamin D metabolite. *Nature* 228:764, 1970.

105. Haussler MR, McCain RA: Basic and clinical concepts related to vitamin D metabolism and action. *N Engl J Med* 297:974, 1977.

106. DeLuca HF, Schnoes HK: Vitamin D: Recent advances. *Annu Rev Biochem* 52:411, 1983.

107. Smith PE: Hypophysectomy and a replacement therapy in the rat. *Am J Anat* 45:205, 1930.

108. Ney RL, Dexter RN, Davis WW, Garren LD: A study of the mechanism by which adrenocorticotropic hormone maintains adrenal steroidogenic responsiveness. *J Clin Invest* 46:1916, 1967.

109. Purvis JL, Canick JS, Mason JI, Estabrook RW, McCarthy JL: Lifetime of adrenal cytochrome P-450 as influenced by ACTH. *Ann NY Acad Sci* 212:319, 1973.

110. DuBois RN, Simpson ER, Kramer RE, Waterman MR: Induction of synthesis of cholesterol side chain cleavage cytochrome P-450 by adrenocorticotropin in cultured bovine adrenocortical cells. *J Biol Chem* 256:7000, 1981.

111. Kramer RE, Anderson CM, Peterson JA, Simpson ER, Waterman MR: Adrenodoxin biosynthesis by bovine adrenal cells in monolayer culture. *J Biol Chem* 257:14921, 1982.

112. Dorrington JH, Armstrong DT: Effect of FSH on gonadal functions. *Recent Prog Horm Res* 35:301, 1979.

113. Erickson GF, Hseuh AJW: Stimulation of aromatase activity by follicle-stimulating hormone in rat granulosa cells in vivo and in vitro. *Endocrinology* 102:1275, 1978.

114. Gill GN, Hornsby PJ, Simonian MH: Hormonal regulation of the adrenocortical cell. *J Supramol Structure* 14:353, 1980.

115. Masui H, Garren LD: Inhibition of replication in functional mouse adrenal tumor cells by adrenocorticotropin mediated by adenosine 3′:5′-cyclic monophosphate. *Proc Natl Acad Sci USA* 68:3206, 1971.

116. Gill GN, Crivello JF, Hornsby PJ, Simonian MH: Growth, function and development of the adrenal cortex: Insights from cell culture. *Cold Spring Harbor Conf Cell Proliferation* 9:461, 1982.

117. Burton RM, Westphal U: Steroid hormone-binding proteins and blood plasma. *Metabolism* 21:253, 1972.

118. Bardin CW, Musto N, Gunsalus G, Kotite N, Cheng SL, Larrea F, Becker R: Extracellular androgen binding proteins. *Annu Rev Physiol* 43:189, 1981.

119. Norman AW, Roth J, Orci L: The vitamin D endocrine system: Steroid metabolism, hormone receptors and biological response (calcium binding proteins). *Endrocrinol Rev* 3:331, 1982.

120. Monder C, Bradlow LH: Cortolic acids: Explorations at the frontier of corticosteroid metabolism. *Recent Prog Horm Res* 36:345, 1980.

121. Wilson JD, Walker JD: The conversion of testosterone to 5α-androstan-17β-ol-3-one (dihydrotestosterone) by skin slices of man. *J Clin Invest* 48:371, 1969.

122. Siiteri PK, MacDonald PC: Role of extraglandular estrogen in human endocrinology, in Greep RO, Astwood EB (eds): *Handbook of Physiology.* Baltimore, Williams & Wilkins, 1973, sec 7, vol 2, pt 2, p 615.

123. Cody V: Thyroid hormones: Crystal structure, molecular conformation, binding and structure-function relationship. *Recent Prog Horm Res* 34:437, 1978.

124. Robbins J: Iodine deficiency, iodine excess and the use of iodine for protection against radioactive iodine. *Thyroid Today* 3 (8):1, 1980.

125. DeGroot LJ, Niepomniszcze H: Biosynthesis of thyroid hormone: Basic and clinical aspects. *Metabolism* 26:665, 1977.

126. Wolff J, Chaikoff IL: The inhibitory action of iodide upon organic binding of iodine by the normal thyroid gland. *J Biol Chem* 172:855, 1948.

127. Braverman LE, Ingbar SH: Changes in thyroidal function during adaptation to large doses of iodide. *J Clin Invest* 42:1216, 1963.

128. Magnusson RP, Taurog A, Dorris ML: Mechanism of iodide-dependent catalytic activity of thyroid peroxidase and lactoperoxidase. *J Biol Chem* 259:197, 1984.

129. Nakamura M, Yamazaki I, Nakagawa H, Ohtaki S: Steady state kinetics and regulation of thyroid peroxidase–catalyzed iodination. *J Biol Chem* 258:3837, 1983.

130. Morrison M, Schonbaum GR: Peroxidase-catalyzed halogenation. *Annu Rev Biochem* 45:861, 1976.

131. Edelhoch H, Irace G, Johnson ML, Michot JL, Nunez J: The effects of thioureylene compounds (goitrogens) on lactoperoxidase activity. *J Biol Chem* 254:11822, 1979.

132. Ui N: Synthesis and chemistry of iodoproteins, in Greer MA, Solomon DH (eds): *Handbook of Physiology: III. Thyroid.* Washington, American Physiological Society, pp 55–75.

133. Vassart G, Bacolla A, Brocas H, Christophe D, de Martynoff G, Leriche A, Mercken L, Parma J, Pohl V, Targovnik H, Van Heuverswyn G: Structure, expression and regulation of thyroglobulin gene. *Mol Cell Endocrinol* 40:89, 1985.

134. Izumi M, Larsen PR: Triiodothyronine, thyroxine and iodine in purified thyroglobulin from patients with Graves' disease. *J Clin Invest* 59:1105, 1977.

135. Greer MA, Grimm Y, Studer H: Qualitative changes in the secretion of thyroid hormones induced by iodine deficiency. *Endocrinology* 83:1193, 1968.

136. Alexander NM: Oxidative cleavage of tryptophanyl peptide bonds during chemical- and peroxidase-catalyzed iodinations. *J Biol Chem* 249:1946, 1974.

137. Dunn JT, Kim PS, Dunn AD, Heppner DJ Jr, Moore RC: The

role of iodination in the formation of hormone-peptides from thyroglobulin. *J Biol Chem* 258:9093, 1983.
138. Robbins J, Cheng S-Y, Gershengorn MC, Glinoer D, Cahnmann HJ, Edelhoch H: Thyroxine transport proteins of plasma: Molecular properties and biosynthesis. *Recent Prog Horm Res* 34:477, 1978.
139. Larsen PR, Silva JE, Kaplan MM: Relationships between circulating and intracellular thyroid hormones: Physiological and clinical implications. *Endocrinol Rev* 2:87, 1982.
140. Chopra IJ, Solomon DH, Chopra U, Wu S-Y, Fisher DA, Nakamura Y: Pathways of metabolism of thyroid hormones. *Recent Prog Horm Res* 34:521, 1978.
141. Wartofsky L, Burman KD: Alterations in thyroid function in patients with systemic illness: The "euthyroid sick syndrome." *Endocrinol Rev* 3:164, 1982.
142. Silva JE, Leonard JL, Crantz FR: Evidence for two tissue specific pathways for in vivo thyroxine 5′-deiodination in the rat. *J Clin Invest* 69:1176, 1982.

5

Molecular Mechanisms of Hormone Action: Control of Target Cell Function by Peptide, Steroid, and Thyroid Hormones

Kevin J. Catt

GENERAL ASPECTS OF HORMONE ACTION

Hormones were originally regarded as blood-borne factors of peptide or steroid nature that serve to communicate between central and peripheral endocrine organs, or within major functional systems such as the gut and kidney. Recently, the traditional view of hormones as endocrine regulators has been broadened by a more general appreciation of the common features that are shared by hormones, neurotransmitters, and growth factors. All hormones and related chemical messengers that are responsible for communication between cells are characterized by their ability to interact with specific recognition sites, or receptors, that activate biochemical signaling mechanisms within their respective target cells.

In the endocrine system, hormones secreted into the bloodstream by the several endocrine organs are recognized and bound by specific receptors located on or in their individual target cells. Communication between the nervous system and nonneuronal endocrine cells (the *neuroendocrine* system) is usually mediated by neuropeptides that serve as local peptide hormones; these are often identical with peptides of the peripheral endocrine system. Between and within neuronal systems, and between neurons and muscle cells, communication is achieved by small neurotransmitter molecules such as acetylcholine (ACh), norepinephrine, serotonin, amino acids, and other biogenic amines.

All forms of biological regulation are based upon specific interactions between complementary molecules, based on their three-dimensional shapes or conformations, that cause changes in the properties and function of one or both members of the ligand pair. This type of molecular information transfer is highly developed in hormone receptors and regulatory enzymes, systems with many features in common. Indeed, most receptors for hormones and transmitters are directly or indirectly coupled to enzymatic proteins which amplify the effect of ligand binding on subsequent metabolic and biosynthetic processes. In the simplest sense, hemoglobin acts as a "receptor" for oxygen while serving as one of the many binding and transport proteins responsible for distribution of small molecules within the organism. Plasma contains numerous binding proteins for circulating ligands such as steroid and thyroid hormones as well as metals, lipids, and vitamins. However, the binding of hormones to such plasma proteins does not usually alter the activity of the carrier molecules, which serve largely as reservoirs and/or transport systems for hormones and other ligands. Also, although such binding proteins are analogous to hormone receptors in their ability to interact with the circulating ligand, they are often selective for the native hormone and may not bind hormone analogues which possess high affinity for the cellular receptor sites.

The characteristic features of peptide and steroid receptors include their location and abundance in hormone-responsive tissues, their high specificity and affinity for agonist and antagonist ligands, and their ability to elicit a specific cellular response when activated by the homologous hormone or its agonist analogues. Endocrine target cells exhibit a wide variety of specific metabolic responses to hormonal stimulation, but these are mediated by a relatively small group of intracellular signaling mechanisms that are initiated by receptor activation. In this way, the diverse cellular responses that are genetically determined by the intrinsic enzymatic pathways of each target tissue can be elicited through the mediation of a few hormone-activated effector systems that are common to many cell types.

The dual properties of hormone *recognition* and target cell *activation* imply that at least two separate regions or structural domains of the receptor molecule are involved in the transduction of environmental stimuli into target cell responses. Recently, specific domains that are responsible for ligand binding and cellular activation have been demonstrated in several receptor molecules located on the plasma membrane or within the cytoplasm of endocrine target cells.

Classes of Hormone Action and Domains of Hormonal Control

The evolution of hormonal control mechanisms in multicellular organisms has led to the development of two major regulatory systems which integrate the functions of endocrine organs and their target cells. The blood-borne hormones or chemical messengers secreted by the hypothalamus, pituitary, gut, and peripheral endocrine tissues can be broadly subdivided into "peptide"- and "steroid"-type hormones (Fig. 5-1). The former group includes neurotransmitters, catecholamines, and growth factors, as well as the traditional peptide and protein hormones. The latter group includes thyroid hormones and vitamin D in addition to the typical steroid hormones.

The more general system is that controlled by steroid hormones, which are responsible for the regulation of enzymes controlling the metabolic and secretory activities of numerous peripheral tissues. These relatively apolar and hydrophobic molecules are secreted by the adrenal and gonads and usually circulate in association with plasma binding proteins, which serve as a reservoir and maintain an effective concentration of free steroid in the extracellular fluid. The free steroids diffuse readily into cells, but exert their metabolic effects only upon target tissues that contain their specific receptor proteins. These intracellular

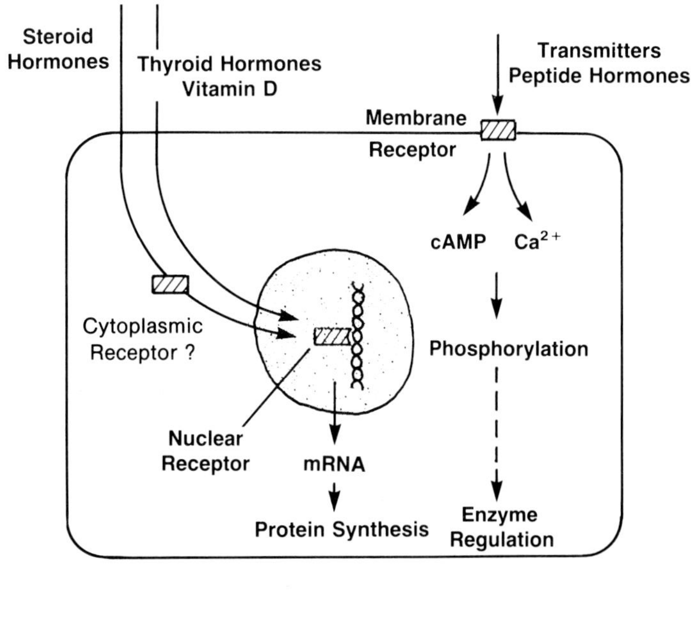

FIGURE 5-1 General mechanisms of target cell activation by hormones acting on plasma membrane receptors (R) and those acting via cytoplasmic and nuclear receptors (L). Membrane receptors for peptide hormones and transmitters produce a signal, usually cyclic AMP or calcium, for activation of the subsequent phosphorylation steps through which their actions are expressed. The steroid-type hormones, including thyroxine and vitamin D, cause activation of intracellular receptors followed by chromatin binding and regulation of gene transcription, with increased (or sometimes decreased) production of specific mRNAs.

receptors in turn mediate the effects of steroid hormones upon nuclear processes that regulate gene expression and the synthesis of specific proteins. In some cells, steroid hormone actions are expressed through the synthesis of regulatory enzymes that control metabolic reactions, as exemplified by the effects of corticosteroids on carbohydrate and protein metabolism. In more specialized tissues, steroid hormones induce cellular differentiation and stimulate the formation of specific proteins that are released from the cell to be used locally or transported in the circulation. Such effects are prominent features of the hormonal control of reproductive tissues by gonadal steroids, which stimulate the synthesis of several proteins with local actions in the reproductive tract. In general, adrenal steroids control the synthesis of enzymes that regulate intracellular metabolic activity, whereas gonadal steroids also stimulate the production of proteins that are secreted by the target cell and participate in the mechanisms of reproduction. There is considerable overlap between these two extremes, and many of the effects of gonadal steroids are expressed through regulation of intracellular metabolic events in their peripheral target tissues. The actions of gonadal steroids upon synthesis of reproductive proteins, such as ovalbumin and avidin in the avian oviduct, are prominent and previously were more readily amenable to analysis than the more subtle effects of steroids on intracellular enzymes. For this reason, studies on the mechanisms of action of estrogen and progesterone on the synthesis of oviduct proteins have led to major advances in the molecular biology of steroid hormone action.[1,2] However, recent advances in DNA technology, and gene transfer in particular, have facilitated the study of more complex regulatory mechanisms, including the definition of steroid control elements in the DNA.[2a,2b]

The properties and actions of thyroid hormones are in many ways analogous to those of steroids, despite their chemical similarity to peptide hormones and amino acid transmitters. For example, the lipophilic properties of thyroid hormones are more similar to those of steroids than peptide ligands, which are generally hydrophilic in nature. Also, circulating thyroid hormones are largely bound to specific plasma proteins, and diffuse readily into their target cells via a small pool of free extracellular hormone to interact with nuclear receptor sites. Finally, their rapid stimulation of mRNA and protein synthesis indicates that thyroid hormones, like steroids, exert most of their actions in the nucleus, by regulating genomic processes that control the biosynthetic and metabolic activities of the target cell.[3]

The actions of peptide hormones, in contrast to the predominantly nuclear effects of steroid and thyroid hormones, are expressed through their interaction with highly selective cell surface receptors that regulate plasma membrane and cytoplasmic enzyme systems in specific groups of target cells.[4,5] This feature is characteristic of the numerous peptide, protein, and glycoprotein ligands which function as hormones and growth factors, as well as transmitters such as catecholamines and ACh.[6] The specific binding of hormonal ligands alters the molecular conformation of their receptor sites and changes the activities of plasma membrane enzyme systems that produce signals with transient or long-term effects on target cell function. In certain target tissues, such as the pituitary-dependent peripheral endocrine organs (adrenal, thyroid, and gonads), the maintenance of cellular differentiation and function is completely dependent upon peptide hormone action. In this sense, the trophic hormones of the pituitary gland (adrenocorticotropic hormone, ACTH; thyroid stimulating hormone, TSH; luteinizing hormone, LH; and follicle stimulating hormone, FSH) share certain functional similarities with gonadal steroids such as estradiol in maintaining the differentiated state and secretory activity of their hormone-dependent target cells. Other peptide hormones, including insulin, prolactin, and growth hormone (GH), are functionally analogous to adrenal steroid hormones in exerting their major actions on metabolic processes rather than maintenance of target cell differentiation.

Such generalizations about the major metabolic effects of steroid, thyroid, and peptide hormones are convenient for the broad functional classification of hormone action. However, the domains of action of the individual hormones are by no means exclusive, and the major classes of ligands sometimes overlap in their sites and modes of action. Thus, it is convenient to regard steroid and thyroid hormones as regulators of *nuclear* events and peptide hormones as controlling *plasma membrane* and *cytoplasmic* processes when defining the primary cellular actions of these ligands. Nevertheless, steroid and thyroid hormones exert several extranuclear actions,[7] and many peptide hormones influence gene expression as well as eliciting rapid target cell responses. For these reasons, there is no absolute distinction between the two major classes of hormonal ligands in terms of their abilities to regulate both metabolic and functional responses to hormonal stimulation. All types of hormones are essentially similar in eliciting programmed biochemical responses from their target cells when recognized and bound by the appropriate plasma membrane or intracellular receptors.

Local Hormonal Regulation: Paracrine and Autocrine Secretion

The systemic actions of blood-borne hormones in controlling peripheral target cell function are often supplemented by the regulatory effects of locally formed messengers that exert precise functional adjustments in response to the prevailing tissue requirements. Such local actions are exerted by the products of endocrine/paracrine cells (Fig. 5-2) and local neurons, which release amines and peptide hormones that act upon adjacent target cells. Paracrine cells are abundant in epithelial structures in the thyroid, respiratory, gastrointestinal, and genitourinary tracts; local neurons have a similarly wide distribution in many organs and tissues. These central and local regulatory mechanisms are integrated by the neuroendocrine system, which is composed of neurons and endocrine cells that share common pathways of peptide synthesis, processing, and secretion. These include the coproduction of amine transmitters and peptides, the processing of large precursors to give biologically active peptides, the costorage of amines and peptides in secretory granules, and the secretion of such stored products in response to synaptic or hormonal stimulation.[8] While the role of locally released amines in tissue regulation is not yet clear, the accompanying peptides are believed to exert local hormonal actions and to serve as neuropeptides by binding to receptors in regional target cells (such as smooth muscle in the gut and airways) and in the adjacent intramural neuronal systems.

An additional form of local hormonal regulation, which appears to be of major importance in the normal and aberrant control of cell proliferation by growth factors, is that of *autocrine* stimulation of cellular growth and differentiation (Fig. 5-2). Many normal and transformed cells secrete peptides such as transforming growth factors (TGF-α and TGF-β), and peptides related to platelet-derived growth factor (PDGF), which act via receptors in the cells of origin to stimulate or inhibit their proliferation. Such autocrine mechanisms of self-stimulation are probably of major importance in physiological processes such as wound healing and rapid embryonic growth, and their inappropriate expression in conditions such as atherosclerosis and neoplasia could be related to the pathogenesis of these disorders.[9] Other autocrine mechanisms include changes in the number or affinity of receptors for growth factors and the expression of proteins that subvert the normal pathways of hormone action. For example, the *erbB* oncogene promotes cell transformation by expressing truncated EGF receptors with unregulated growth activity (see Oncogenes and Cellular Regulation, below), and several other oncogenes are known to encode major regulatory components of the intracellular signaling pathways that mediate the normal growth response.[10]

PEPTIDE HORMONE RECEPTORS

General Aspects of Cell Surface Receptors for Peptide Hormones

All peptide hormones and transmitter molecules exert their primary regulatory effects by binding to specific high-affinity receptor sites in the plasma membrane of their respective target cells. Such receptors have been demonstrated in numerous target cells for peptide hormones and neurotransmitters by direct binding studies with radioactive ligands.[4-6] In many tissues, correlations between specific binding of radiolabeled hormones and activation of target cell responses have shown that such sites are the biologically relevant hormone receptors that mediate cellular responses to the circulating hormone. In some tissues, peptide receptors have been provisionally identified by their high affinity and specificity for biologically active forms of the homologous hormone and its agonist and antagonist analogues. The use of competitive inhibitors to block both hormone binding and the consequent target cell response provides additional validation of those hormone receptors for which antagonists are available. Certain receptor sites, such as those for ACh and catecholamines, have been largely characterized by radioligand-binding studies with labeled antagonists of high specificity and affinity.

The site of action of peptide hormones upon cell membranes was suggested by Sutherland and Robi-

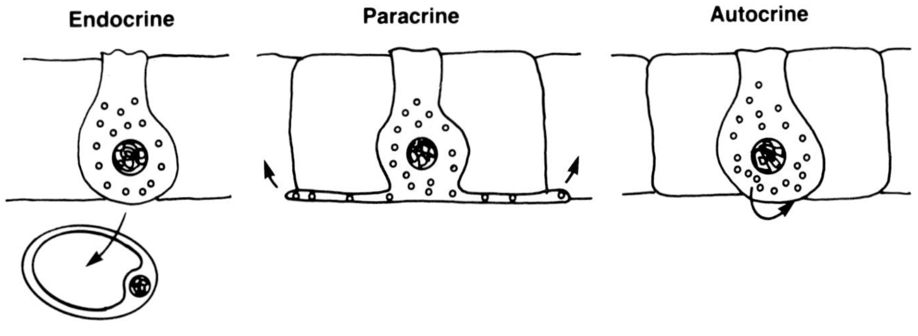

FIGURE 5-2 The major modes of intercellular communication. The hormonal products of endocrine cells are released into the bloodstream to be carried to distant target cells. Paracrine cells release their products in proximity to neighboring cells, often from long processes with bulbous terminals. Autocrine cells release products which act on their own external receptors to regulate cell growth. (*Adapted from Hakanson and Sundler.*[8])

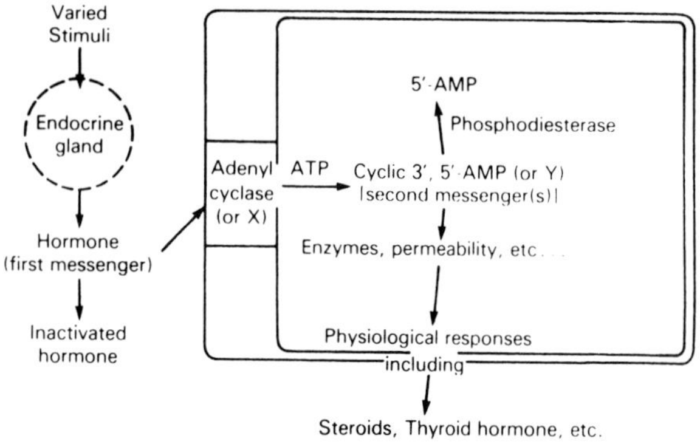

FIGURE 5-3 Sutherland's concept of the hormone as first messenger and cyclic AMP (or other mediators) as the second (intracellular) messenger through which peptide hormone action is expressed. (*From Sutherland and Robison.*[11])

son's observation that interaction of catecholamines with the plasma membrane of pigeon erythrocytes led to activation of adenylate cyclase.[11] Since then, numerous peptide hormones have been shown to interact with cell surface receptors and to influence plasma membrane–associated enzymes and ion transport mechanisms (Fig. 5-3). The surface location of peptide hormone receptors was further indicated by the ability of brief exposure to hormone to elicit a prolonged target cell response, attributable to bound hormone, and by the rapidity with which specific antisera can terminate the actions of peptide hormones in vitro. Also, enzymes and other agents acting on membrane proteins and lipids can modify or abolish the ability of peptide hormones to stimulate adenylate cyclase activity. Direct evidence for the plasma membrane location of peptide hormone receptors has also come from autoradiographic and direct binding studies with cells or membranes and radiolabeled hormone preparations. These approaches have defined the location and binding characteristics of peptide hormone receptors, as well as their functional relationship to target cell responses.

The ability of peptide hormones to regulate their target cells depends on their interaction with specific plasma membrane binding sites (receptors) which take up the information-bearing molecule from the extracellular fluid. For example, the responsiveness of adrenal fasciculata cells to pituitary regulation is conferred by their specific cell surface receptors which sense the circulating concentration and secretory profile of ACTH. The extremely low concentrations (about 10^{-10} M) of peptide hormones in the circulation, in the presence of a million fold excess of other proteins, requires that target cell receptors possess both high specificity (to recognize the hormone) and high affinity (to bind the hormone present at low concentrations). The well-defined class of receptors for "conventional" peptide hormones (such as pituitary trophic peptides and gut hormones) is supplemented by analogous sites for local and peripheral transmitter molecules (such as ACh, catecholamines, and prostaglandins), and a growing group of 50 or so neuropeptides that regulate peripheral and central neural function.[12] These numerous peptide hormones are characterized by their ionic charge and intrinsically hydrophilic nature, with little or no significant binding to plasma proteins, and by their ability to bind to highly specific recognition sites on the exposed region of receptor molecules. The manner in which receptors and other intrinsic membrane proteins are embedded in the lipid bilayer of the target cell plasma membrane is illustrated in Fig. 5-4.[13]

Another specialized region of peptide hormone receptors, located on the membrane-associated portion of the binding molecule, interacts with the regulatory components of effector enzymes such as adenylate cyclase, whose catalytic domain is exposed on

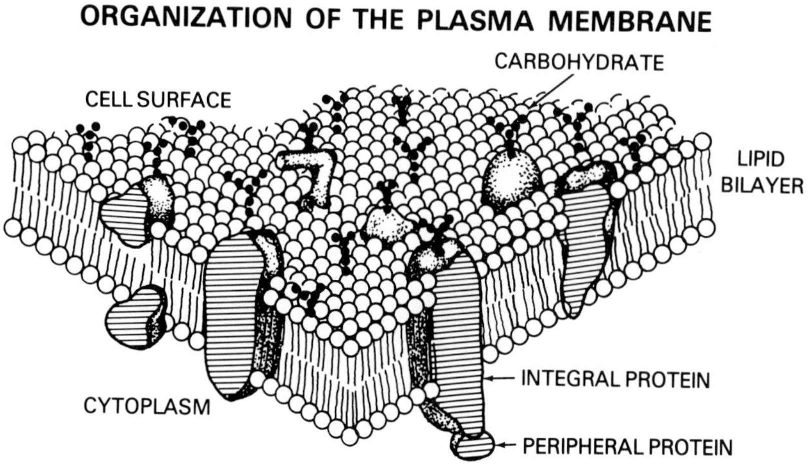

FIGURE 5-4 A general view of the structure of the plasma membrane. The proteins of the plasma membrane are visualized as floating within the phospholipid matrix, some spanning the lipid bilayer and others embedded in the inner or outer surface of the membrane. Proteins protruding on the external surface of the cell are predominantly glycoproteins, as indicated by the numerous carbohydrate residues. Many of these external proteins function as receptors for ligands and viruses in the extracellular environment, and in turn interact with other membrane proteins during the transmission of hormonal signals to the interior of the cell. (*Based on the model proposed by Singer and Nicholson.*[13])

the inner, cytoplasmic surface of the cell membrane. Although many peptide hormones are known to be internalized by the target cell after binding to their surface receptors, it is the initial interaction with the plasma membrane receptors that elicits the acute target cell response. The intracellular application of peptide hormones does not evoke the characteristic cellular response,[14] reflecting the need for hormone-receptor interaction at the cell surface. The binding of hormones and agonist ligands to their plasma membrane receptors triggers the activation of one or more effector enzymes which in turn control cyclic nucleotide production, phospholipid breakdown, ion fluxes, and membrane transport mechanisms. These immediate consequences of agonist-receptor interaction are followed by modulation (stimulatory or inhibitory) of cytoplasmic and nuclear processes that regulate target cell function. Many of these regulatory steps involve phosphorylation of membrane or cytoplasmic proteins, with subsequent changes in the activities of enzymes responsible for synthesis, transport, or metabolism of molecules that are essential for cellular activity.

The best-defined plasma membrane enzyme system that is regulated by peptide hormones is adenylate cyclase, which catalyzes the transformation of ATP to cyclic AMP. Once formed during receptor activation, the cyclic nucleotide stimulates *cAMP-dependent protein kinase,* a widely distributed cytoplasmic phosphokinase that initiates many of the phosphorylation-dependent events involved in target cell regulation.[15] Other membrane-bound enzymes influenced by peptide hormone–receptor interactions include those concerned in ion transport and calcium pumping, methyltransferases involved in phospholipid methylation, and phospholipases responsible for cleavage and deacylation of membrane phospholipids. These last processes are responsible for phosphoinositide turnover and calcium gating, and also provide precursors such as arachidonic acid for conversion to prostaglandins (PGs), thromboxanes, prostacyclins, leukotrienes, and other active metabolites. Hormonal effects on Na^+,K^+-ATPase, membrane-bound protein kinases, and catechol-O-methyltransferase have also been observed. Thus, multiple receptor-mediated events occur at the plasma membrane level and participate in the integrated responses of target cells to receptor activation by the homologous hormone (Table 5-1).

Binding Characteristics of Peptide Hormone Receptors

Binding studies with radioisotopically labeled peptide hormones have defined several characteristic properties that apply to the majority of peptide hormone receptors. The universal feature of such receptors is their ability to bind the corresponding chemical messenger or hormone in the presence of a vast excess of other molecular species. This property is readily demonstrable with labeled hormone as a selective high-affinity binding reaction which leads to the formation of a specific hormone-receptor complex. Such interactions have been observed in numerous hormone-responsive tissues, and are regarded as obligatory properties of a putative receptor site. The presence of such high-affinity binding sites, together with appropriate ligand specificity for agonist and antagonist analogues, is compelling evidence for the presence of hormone receptors in endocrine target tissues.[4] Specific binding sites are also present in cells other than those of recognized target tissues, e.g., insulin

Table 5-1. Plasma Membrane Receptors and Target Cell Effector Systems

Receptors	Effector system
CRF, GRF, ACTH, TSH, MSH, LH, FSH, glucagon, PTH, calcitonin, β-adrenergic, vasopressin V_2, dopamine D_1, serotonin 5-HT_2	Adenylate cyclase: activation
α_2-Adrenergic, somatostatin, opiate, muscarinic acetylcholine, adenosine A_1	Adenylate cyclase: inhibition
α_1-Adrenergic, muscarinic, histamine H_1, vasopressin V_1, TRH, GnRH, angiotensin II, serotonin 5-HT_1, PDGF, thrombin	Phospholipase C activation, calcium mobilization, and protein kinase C activation
EGF, insulin, IGF 1, PDGF	Tyrosine phosphorylation
Nicotinic acetylcholine	Sodium channel activation
GABA, glycine	Chloride channel activation

Abbreviations: ACTH, adrenocorticotropin; CRF, corticotropin releasing factor; EGF, epidermal growth factor; FSH, follicle stimulating hormone; GABA, gamma aminobutyric acid; GnRH, gonadotropin releasing hormone; GRH, growth hormone releasing hormone; 5-HT, 5-hydroxytryptamine, IGF, insulin-like growth factor; LH, luteinizing hormone; MSH, melanocyte stimulating hormone; PDGF, platelet-derived growth factor; PTH, parathyroid hormone; TRH, thyrotropin releasing hormone; TSH, thyrotropin.

and GH receptors in lymphocytes and prolactin receptors in liver, adrenal gland, and kidney. The physiological view of receptors embodies a cellular response as well as the recognition site, but such a definition would exclude receptors for which the functional response is not yet determined, and those which are isolated, solubilized, or situated on an unresponsive cellular component. Thus, receptors can also be characterized by their specific binding of the hormonal ligand and its structural analogues, plus the potential to transmit a regulatory signal even if the effector elements are lacking or unidentified.

The most comprehensive view of a peptide hormone receptor embodies the dual functional properties of surface recognition (binding) plus transduction of the hormone-receptor interaction into a specific biological response (activation). Whether the cellular response is peptide secretion, steroidogenesis, contraction, or ion transport, the mechanisms which mediate hormone action usually include changes in calcium and phospholipid turnover, calcium shifts, and altered cyclic nucleotide production and/or metabolism. In many target tissues there is a close relationship between hormone binding and biochemical responses at the plasma membrane level. For example, receptor occupancy and activation of adenylate cyclase in plasma membrane fractions are closely correlated during the actions of ACTH in the adrenal, glucagon in the liver, vasopressin in the kidney, catecholamines in the avian erythrocyte, FSH in the seminiferous tubule, and LH in the testis and ovary. Hormone binding to specific receptors is also associated with increased synthesis and release of cAMP in many intact target tissues and cells.[16] Correlations of hormone binding with other characteristic cellular responses include those of insulin with glucose oxidation in fat cells or amino acid transport in thymocytes, catecholamines with sodium transport in erythrocytes, LH with testicular androgen production, and angiotensin II with aldosterone production in adrenal glomerulosa cells.

It is sometimes suggested that the definition of hormone receptors should be restricted to tissue binding sites that are associated with a defined biochemical or cellular response. However, the demonstration of specific and high-affinity binding sites with radiolabeled agonist or antagonist ligands can provide a valid index of hormone receptors when appropriate requirements of the binding technique are observed. These include the use of labeled hormone of demonstrated biological activity (prepared by monoiodination or tritiation), accurate determination of nonspecific binding, and exclusion of binding to degradative or other enzymatic activities in tissue fractions. The majority of peptide hormone receptors exhibit high specificity for biologically active hormones and their agonist or antagonist derivatives; high binding affinity, with equilibrium association constants of 10^9 to 10^{11} M^{-1}; and saturability at relatively low hormone concentrations. These properties are consistent with the high selectivity and low concentration of hormone receptors, which usually number about several thousand sites per cell in most target tissues.

Specific binding of peptide hormones to their receptors is highly temperature-dependent and usually proceeds rapidly at 37°C in a diffusion-limited manner. In contrast, the rate of dissociation of the hormone-receptor complex varies widely for individual ligand-receptor pairs. In intact cells, there is often a tightly associated and poorly reversible component of the bound hormone, and even covalent binding to a small proportion of the receptors for insulin, thrombin, and EGF has been described.[17] In vitro studies of binding constants and thermodynamic properties are often complicated by degradation of hormone and/or receptor molecules when analyses are performed at 37°C. For this reason, receptor-binding studies are usually performed at lower temperatures (4 to 24°C) to minimize the effects of degradation. Consequently, relatively little is known about the kinetic and equilibrium binding properties of hormone receptors under physiological conditions. The rates of ligand binding and dissociation, and the turnover of hormone molecules and receptor sites under in vivo conditions of temperature and tissue perfusion, need further study to define the physiological aspects of hormone-receptor interactions at the target cell level.

The Nature of Hormone-Receptor Interaction

The binding of peptide hormones to their plasma membrane receptors depends upon both hydrophobic and electrostatic interactions. The importance of hydrophobic effects in peptide-receptor binding is indicated by the effects of temperature and agents such as urea on the binding process. For certain peptides, such as ACTH and angiotensin II, electrostatic interactions are also involved in the interaction with receptor sites. A basic region of the ACTH molecule is important for binding to adrenal receptors, and binding of angiotensin II to adrenal receptors is markedly influenced by the basicity of the amino-terminal residue. The activation processes which result from hormone binding can also be influenced by electrostatic effects, as shown by the ability of charged compounds such as polylysine to stimulate adenylate cyclase activity and steroidogenesis in adrenal and Leydig cells.

The role of hydrophobic interactions in receptor binding has been indicated by x-ray diffraction studies on the three-dimensional structures of insulin and glucagon.[18] In the insulin molecule, the relatively constant surface region which determines biological activity includes many hydrophobic residues. Binding of insulin to its receptor has been proposed to occur by a process analogous to dimerization, and to depend upon the additive effects of hydrophobic interactions and hydrogen bonds. Also, the effects of modification of specific amino acid residues upon biological activity and receptor binding can be correlated with changes in the conformation of the insulin molecule.

In contrast to the relatively rigid structure of insulin, which appears necessary to achieve the spatial arrangement of amino acids necessary for receptor binding, the glucagon molecule has an elongated and fairly flexible structure. Like insulin, glucagon molecules readily aggregate by hydrophobic bonding, in this case to form a trimeric structure. At the low concentrations present in the circulation, glucagon probably circulates as a monomer with random conformation. It has been suggested that the biologically active conformation is a helical structure which interacts with the receptor through two hydrophobic regions at each end of the helix, and that the extended amino-terminal domain is important for activation of adenylate cyclase.[19]

These observations indicate that both insulin and glucagon molecules become associated via their hydrophobic regions during storage as granules, and also bind to receptor sites by predominantly hydrophobic interactions. The presence of two hydrophobic regions, first observed in the glucagon monomer, has also been noted in secretin and vasoactive intestinal peptide. Certain smaller molecules such as thyrotropin releasing hormone (TRH), gonadotropin releasing hormone (GnRH), angiotensin II, and bradykinin also exhibit twofold symmetry. This has led to the suggestion that symmetrical features of peptide sequences are reflected in the receptor structure and that such peptides bind to two similar or identical subunits in the receptor. The presence of two subunits has been described for the LH, insulin, and angiotensin II receptors. Such subunit structure in hormone receptors could reflect a general property that is relevant to the evolution of symmetry and internal homologies in peptide hormones, as well as to the occurrence of cooperative interactions during receptor binding.[20]

In contrast to the well-defined mechanisms involved in receptor binding and activation, the processes that terminate hormone-receptor interaction are poorly understood. While reversal of the binding reaction can certainly occur, it appears that mechanisms other than simple dissociation according to the law of mass action can determine the duration of receptor activation in the intact cell. Although a degradative mechanism for hormone release has been considered, hormone degradation by isolated target cells is largely unrelated to receptor binding sites. Also, hormones which are specifically bound to target tissues usually retain full biological activity after elution from the receptor sites. This feature can be used to advantage in the preparation of radiolabeled hormones for receptor analysis, by affinity purification on particulate receptor sites to select the most biologically active molecules. In many endocrine target cells, some of the hormone-receptor complexes are inactivated or degraded by processes including internalization and lysosomal catabolism. However, one of the most important mechanisms favoring termination of specific hormone binding may be the fall in receptor affinity that occurs when the agonist-receptor complex interacts with regulatory proteins that bind GTP. This process is particularly well-defined for hormones involved in the modulation of adenylate cyclase activity (see below).

Chemical and Physical Properties of Peptide Hormone Receptors

The protein nature of plasma membrane receptors for polypeptide hormones is indicated by their susceptibility to digestion by proteolytic enzymes and peptidases. Many cell surface receptors are also affected by phospholipases, suggesting that they contain a functionally significant phospholipid component, or that binding activity is influenced by their association with phospholipids in the plasma membrane. Recently, several cell surface proteins have been found to be attached to the plasma membrane by glycophospholipid residues. The lipid component in such protein-membrane linkages is phosphatidylinositol (PI), which is covalently attached to the membrane proteins, usually at their carboxy-terminal regions (Fig. 5-5). The phosphatidylinositol-specific enzyme phospholipase C, which cleaves between the glyceride backbone and inositol phosphate, releases several proteins from the cell surface. These include enzymes such as alkaline phosphatase, 5′-nucleotidase, and acetylcholinesterase and other superficial proteins such as the variable surface glycoprotein of trypanosomes and the thy-1 protein of brain and lymphocytes.[21] This mode of attachment may facilitate the release of surface molecules in response to environmental stimuli and signals, and could be relevant to the deactivation of certain plasma membrane receptor sites. Carbohydrate moieties are also present in many peptide receptors, including those for insulin, LH, FSH, prolactin, angiotensin,

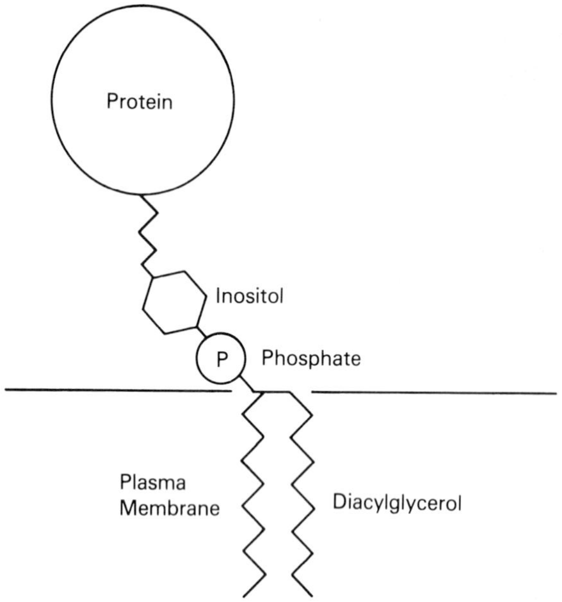

FIGURE 5-5 Membrane anchoring of cell surface proteins by phosphatidylinositol. (*Modified from Low and Kincade.*[21])

and GnRH, and are probably a general feature of cell surface recognition sites. Certain receptors, such as those for ACh, insulin, LH, and FSH depend on disulfide groups for the maintenance of their biologically active conformation.

The physicochemical characterization of peptide hormone receptors has been complicated by their relative insolubility in aqueous solutions, reflecting the characteristic hydrophobicity of many intrinsic membrane proteins. In some tissues, receptors can be released from the cell membrane by limited enzyme digestion or by incubation under hypotonic conditions that favor shedding of surface receptors. However, solubilization of hormone receptors for physicochemical analysis usually requires their extraction from tissue homogenates and membrane fractions with mild nonionic detergents such as Triton X-100 and polidocanol (Lubrol), or zwitterionic detergents such as Chaps. Dissolution of plasma membranes by such detergents usually leads to loss of the functional coupling between hormone-binding sites and their membrane-associated effector systems. However, partial restoration of hormone-stimulated adenylate cyclase activity has been observed after removal of detergent, and hormone responsiveness of solubilized adenylate cyclase is sometimes retained after extraction from tissue fractions with nonionic detergents. The many receptor sites that have been solubilized by detergent extraction from target cell membranes include those for ACh, catecholamines, insulin, GnRH, angiotensin II, glucagon, LH/human chorionic gonadotropin (hCG), FSH, TSH, prolactin, and GH. In several cases, the detergent-extracted soluble receptors have been purified and reconstituted into artificial lipid bilayers with their effector systems, or into host cell membranes, for studies of their activation mechanisms under defined conditions.[22]

In some tissues, the preformed hormone-receptor complexes produced by saturation of target cells with labeled hormone can also be extracted with nonionic detergents. Such soluble hormone-receptor complexes are usually more stable than the free or unoccupied soluble receptors, and have certain advantages for physical characterization. In the ovary, LH receptors prelabeled in vivo by injection of ^{125}I-hCG exhibit the same physical characteristics as the hormone-receptor complexes formed by labeling ovarian membranes in vitro prior to solubilization. Several free receptors and hormone-receptor complexes have been shown by gel filtration and density gradient centrifugation to have molecular weights ranging from 130,000 to 400,000 and to exhibit subunit structure on SDS/polyacrylamide gel-analysis.

Many detergent-solubilized receptors behave during physical analysis as elongated molecules with relatively large hydrodynamic radii (6 to 7 nm) in relation to their sedimentation constants of 6.5 to 9.0 S. These properties are largely due to the glycoprotein nature and marked asymmetry of the receptor molecule, but are sometimes accentuated by binding of detergent to the solubilized protein. Purification of detergent-solubilized hormone receptors has been performed by conventional fractionation procedures and also by affinity chromatography on gel-ligand complexes. Such purifications have usually been performed on a relatively small scale, the major exception being the cholinergic receptor protein from the electric tissue of certain fish. Affinity chromatography has also been applied to the isolation of receptors for insulin, EGF, catecholamines, LH/hCG, and prolactin. Although usually obtained in relatively small yield, the purified receptors are often quite stable, and retain high affinity and specificity for the hormonal ligand. Recently, several plasma-membrane receptors have been isolated and completely characterized, and others have been highly purified. LH receptors of mol wt 160,000 have been purified about 30,000-fold, equivalent to near-homogeneity of the receptor sites. The purified LH receptor migrates as an 80,000 M_r component during SDS gel electrophoresis, suggesting that the native holoreceptor is a dimer composed of two similar subunits.[16] Prolactin and GH receptors have been isolated from mammary tissue, ovary, and liver by affinity chromatography, and antibodies to the purified prolactin receptor have been shown to inhibit the biological actions of prolactin upon its target tissues.[23] The purification of sufficient quantities of receptor sites from target tissues and/or the preparation of antibodies to the receptor molecule are prerequisites for the cloning and identification of receptor cDNA and deduction of the amino acid sequence of the receptor. As described below, such approaches have begun to clarify the structural features that determine the hormone-binding sites, and the domains responsible for activation of the intrinsic or membrane-associated enzyme systems that mediate peptide hormone action.

Receptor Structure and Function

Major progress has been made in the purification and structural characterization of several plasma membrane receptor sites for polypeptide hormones and neurotransmitters. This has been achieved by two main approaches, one based on the preparation of synthetic DNA probes (from partial amino acid sequence information) for hybridization screening of DNA libraries to identify cDNA clones, and the other on the use of receptor antibodies to screen cDNA libraries constructed in expression vectors such as λ-gt11. By these methods, the primary structures of receptors for acetylcholine, EGF, insulin, and interleukin 2, the related receptors for light (rhodopsin) and β-adrenergic catecholamines, the antigen receptor of T lymphocytes, and the low-density lipoprotein (LDL) receptor have been deduced and analyzed in terms of receptor organization and function. The structural analysis of cell membrane receptors for transmitters and peptide hormones has revealed several new aspects of receptor design and has begun to clarify the manner in which structural features of receptors are related to their ligand-binding and signal-generating functions. The structural and functional properties of some of the major receptors for hormonal ligands are described below.

THE ACETYLCHOLINE RECEPTOR

Due to its abundance in the electric organ of certain fish, the nicotinic ACh receptor was the first cell surface receptor to be extensively analyzed and characterized. In addition to subunit isolation and partial amino acid sequencing, in vitro translation of the receptor mRNA has been performed[24] and the cDNA sequences coding for the major molecular components of the receptor have been determined.[25] The ACh receptor of the electric fish *Torpedo californica* is a complex protein composed of four peptide chains, α, β, γ, and δ, with molecular weights, respectively, of 40,000, 50,000, 60,000, and 65,000. There is considerable amino acid homology between the four subunits, suggesting that they have evolved through gene reduplication.[26] The subunits are combined in the ratio $\alpha_2\beta\gamma\delta$ to form a pentameric receptor of mol wt 250,000; the receptor binds cholinergic ligands and serves as a ligand-regulated channel through which sodium ions pass in the 1 ms or so that the pore remains open during receptor activation. The α subunits are responsible for binding ACh, and the other three subunits are involved in the formation and function of the ion channel.[27]

The holoreceptor molecule is about 8 nm in diameter and extends across the plasma membrane to protrude by about 5 nm above the cell surface. The outer face of the ACh receptor bears a 2.5-nm pit which leads to the 0.65-nm ion translocation pore, through which sodium can pass during the ligand-induced gating process. The native form of the membrane receptor may be a large dimer formed of two mol wt 250,000 multisubunit channels linked by a disulfide bond.[28] Like most cell membrane receptors, the outer surface of the molecule is glycosylated, and probably contains hydrophobic regions for interaction with corresponding domains of the activating ligand molecule. All four subunits are synthesized with leader sequences and are exposed on both sides of the plasma membrane; each subunit also has four hydrophobic α-helical transmembrane domains. There is also a fifth, amphipathic domain that places the carboxyl terminus of each subunit on the cytoplasmic side of the plasma membrane, and forms a hydrophilic lining of the cation channel to accommodate the high rate of flow of hydrated cations through the channel.[29] The 250,000 M_r pentamer contains the acetylcholine-binding site, the ion channel, and the structural elements involved in the regulation of channel opening by ACh (Fig. 5-6).

Cloning and sequencing of the complementary or genomic DNAs has revealed the complete amino acid sequence of all four subunits of the *Torpedo* receptor and the calf muscle receptor, and of human muscle α and γ subunits. A further subunit, ε, has been found in calf muscle, and has sequence homologies with the γ subunits of *Torpedo* and mammals.[30] The detergent-solubilized pentameric receptor, when inserted into artificial membranes, regulates cation flux in a similar manner to that found in the subsynaptic membrane receptor in situ. Furthermore, the cloned cDNAs of the *Torpedo* subunits can be expressed in *Xenopus* oocytes to produce a functional ACh receptor. In this system, analysis of both mutant receptors bearing subunits altered by mutagenesis of the cDNA and hybrid receptors composed of subunits from fish and mammal can be performed to identify regions of the individual

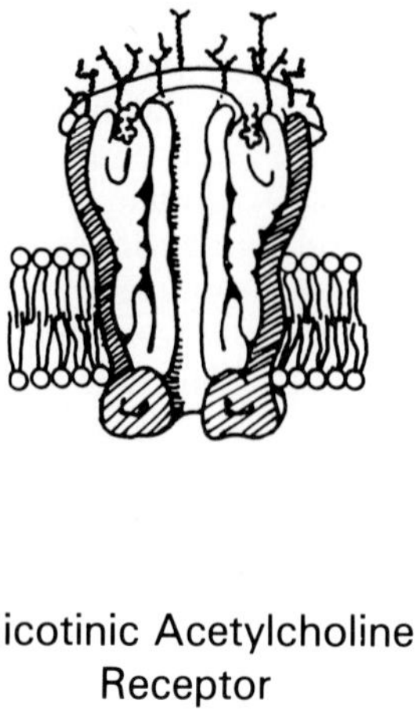

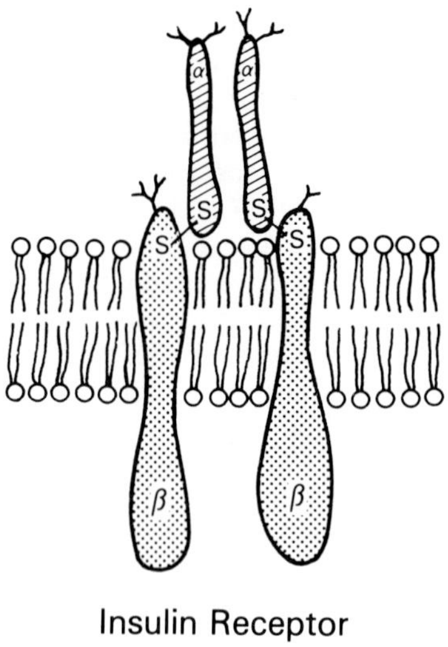

FIGURE 5-6 Comparison of the dimeric arrangement of the nicotinic acetylcholine receptor of *Torpedo* electric tissue (left) and the subunit structure of the insulin receptor. The immunoglobulin-like structure of the insulin receptor may prove to be a general feature of certain classes of peptide hormone receptor sites. (Modified from Lindstrom J: Autoimmune response to acetylcholine receptors in myasthenia gravis and its animal model, in *Advances in Immunology*. New York, Academic, 1979, vol 27, pp 1–50.)

subunit molecules which mediate the conductance and gating behavior of the channel.[31]

THE EGF RECEPTOR

The EGF receptor is a mol wt 170,000 glycoprotein that mediates the mitogenic action of EGF in numerous target cells. Binding of EGF to the plasma membrane receptor stimulates receptor clustering and endocytosis, and subsequently initiates DNA replication.[32] The EGF receptor has a protein core of mol wt ~140,000 which possesses intrinsic tyrosine kinase activity that is stimulated by ligand binding. Thus, interaction of EGF with its receptor leads to tyrosine phosphorylation of the receptor molecule as well as other cellular proteins. The autophosphorylation sites on the EGF receptor are located within its cytoplasmic domain, near the carboxyl terminus of the molecule.[33] The receptor is also phosphorylated at threonine residues by protein kinase C in cells treated with tumor-promoting phorbol esters, which prevent the effects of EGF on tyrosine phosphorylation and cause loss of high-affinity EGF-binding sites.[34] Proteolytic cleavage of the EGF receptor separates the kinase domain from the EGF-binding domain, giving an active catalytic fragment of M_r 42,000 that can phosphorylate its own tyrosine residues and those of other proteins. The EGF tyrosine kinase fragment is similar to those derived from $pp60^{src}$ and other oncogene kinases; if generated during processing of the EGF receptor, it could serve as an intracellular signaling mechanism to transmit the message derived from activation at the plasma membrane level.[35]

The primary amino acid sequence of the EGF receptor was determined from the nucleotide sequences of cDNA clones of receptor mRNA, derived from the A431 human epidermoid carcinoma cell line.[36,37] The receptor precursor consists of a 24-amino-acid signal peptide followed by a 1186-amino-acid receptor protein containing regions responsible for hormone binding, membrane attachment, protein kinase activity, and autophosphorylation (Fig. 5-7). The extracellular amino-terminal region of the receptor (621 amino acids) contains the EGF-binding domain and is rich in cysteine residues (for disulfide bond formation)

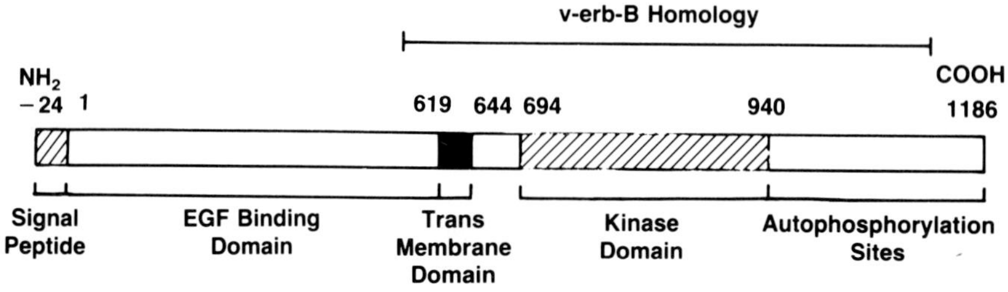

FIGURE 5-7 Linear structure of the EGF receptor protein. The external EGF-binding domain is on the left and the cytoplasmic phosphorylation domain is on the right. The region of sequence homology with the *erbB* oncogene product is shown above. (*Modified from Hunter.*[38])

and glycosylation sites. The arrangement of the cysteines suggests that the receptor surface may be bifurcated to form an EGF-binding cleft.[38] The external binding region is followed by a hydrophobic, membrane-spanning domain of 26 amino acids, bounded on its cytoplasmic side by a highly basic segment of the 542-residue COOH-terminal portion of the molecule. One site at which protein kinase C phosphorylates the EGF receptor is a threonine residue within this basic sequence, nine residues from the plasma membrane in the 50-residue segment prior to the protein kinase domain. Since protein kinase C is membrane-associated when activated by phorbol esters or endogenous diacylglycerol (DAG), it could readily phosphorylate such threonine residues within the cytoplasmic domain of the receptor molecule and modulate its binding and signaling functions.[39]

The carboxy-terminal region of the EGF receptor has marked sequence homology with the *erbB* gene product, and with the catalytic domains of other protein kinases including the tyrosine kinase products of the *src* gene family. The *c-erbB* gene and the gene for EGF are situated in the same region of human chromosome 7. Their common genomic localization, with the 85 percent sequence homology between the relevant regions of the two gene products, suggests that the *v-erbB* oncogene is derived from the EGF receptor gene, i.e., that the EGF receptor gene *is* the *c-erbB* gene.[38]

The *v-erbB* gene product is a truncated EGF receptor with no external binding site; it has been proposed to be constitutively active in cells transformed by the avian erythroblastosis virus. Its similarity to the EGF receptor is so close that a *v-erbB* cDNA probe could be used to identify a *Drosophila* EGF receptor which shares many structural features with the human EGF receptor. These include the extracellular ligand-binding domain with two cysteine-rich regions, a hydrophobic transmembrane region, and a cytoplasmic kinase domain. The presence of these domains in the *Drosophila* receptor (for which the endogenous ligand has not yet been identified as a *Drosophila* EGF homologue) indicates that the coding sequences of the extracellular binding and intracellular kinase domains must have arisen over 800 million years ago.[40] Although the physiological role of EGF in specific target cells has yet to be defined, the EGF receptor has recently been found to serve as a receptor for vaccinia virus. In this regard the EGF receptor resembles other ligand receptors that serve as receptors for certain viruses, including the ACh receptor (rabies virus), the β-adrenergic receptor (reovirus), the complement receptor CR2 (Epstein-Barr virus), and the T4 lymphocyte antigen (HLTV-III).[41]

THE INSULIN RECEPTOR

The structure of the insulin receptor has been analyzed in binding sites purified by affinity chromatography and by SDS gel electrophoresis after precursor incorporation, cross-linking, and precipitation with anti-receptor antibodies. These approaches have shown that the receptor is composed of two α subunits (mol wt 130,000) and two β subunits (mol wt 90,000), which are joined by disulfide bonds to form the cross-linked heterotetramer $(\alpha\beta)_2$ of mol wt 350,000 to 400,000.[42] As shown in Fig. 5-6, the receptor has a symmetrical immunoglobulin-like structure (β-S-S-α)-S-S-(α-S-S-β) and probably binds more than one molecule of insulin. Both subunits are accessible on the outer surface of the cell membrane, and although insulin binds predominantly to the α subunit, the β subunit may also participate in the binding site. An important feature of the β subunit is its intrinsic protein kinase activity, which can catalyze the autophosphorylation of a tyrosine residue within its own structure when activated by insulin.[43]

The multivalent nature of the insulin receptor is relevant to the occurrence of negative cooperativity, manifested by concave Scatchard plots, during the binding of insulin to its receptor sites in many tissues.[44] The apparent presence of negative cooperativity could also be related to factors such as dissociation of the mol wt 350,000 receptor sites into smaller components with reduced affinity for insulin, possibly associated with proteolytic nicking of the receptor and partial reduction of the binding complex.[42] Biosynthetic studies have revealed that the insulin receptor is derived from a single glycosylated precursor in which disulfide bonds link the future α and β subunit regions. The precursor is further glycosylated in the Golgi apparatus and cleaved, then inserted into the plasma membrane with both subunits exposed on the cell surface. The β subunit spans the membrane bilayer and contains the protein kinase domain in its cytoplasmic portion. The receptor for the GH-dependent peptide termed *somatomedin* C (or insulin-like growth factor 1, IGF 1) appears to be similar in subunit composition to the insulin receptor,[45] though different in fine structure, as shown by its peptide-binding specificity and immunological distinction from the insulin receptor.

The complete amino acid sequence of the human insulin receptor has been determined from a human placental cDNA library cloned in the vector λ-gt10 and screened by hybridization with synthetic oligonucleotide probes for portions of the α and β subunits. By this approach a single cDNA clone containing the entire sequence of the receptor was isolated and analyzed.[46] The receptor precursor deduced from the nucleotide sequence of the cDNA contains 1370 amino acids, arranged as a 27-residue signal sequence followed by the α subunit, a precursor processing enzyme cleavage site, and then the β subunit. A single 23-amino-acid transmembrane region is present in the β subunit, which also contains sequence homologies with the EGF receptor and products of the *src* oncogene family. The absence of a membrane-spanning region in the α subunit is consistent with its location on the outer surface of the cell, together with 194 residues of the β chain. Glycosylation sites are correspondingly more abundant in the α subunit, which is also rich in cysteine residues by comparison with the β subunit. The presence of sequence homology between the α chain and the external domain of the EGF receptor could be relevant to a common feature of the ligand-binding sites, or to the mechanisms of receptor turnover and intracellular processing.

Comparison of the structures of the insulin and EGF receptors shows several analogies, in that both receptors cross the membrane bilayer only once, and both have tyrosine-specific protein kinase domains commencing 50 residues from the end of the transmembrane region (Fig. 5-8). However, no common sequences assignable to intracellular signaling have been identified, apart from the protein kinase domain, and the mechanisms of signal transmission await further exploration by modification of the molecular structure of the receptor.

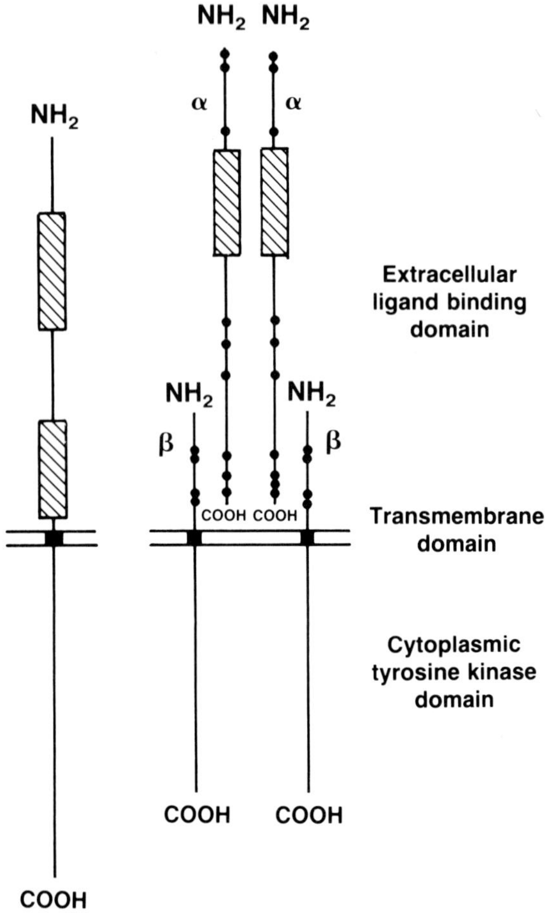

FIGURE 5-8 Schematic comparison of the insulin receptor (right) and the EGF receptor (left). Regions of high cysteine content are shown as hatched areas. The single cysteine residues (black circles) may be involved in formation of the $\alpha_2\beta_2$ insulin receptor complex. Note that the α subunits are completely extracellular, whereas the β subunits, which possess tyrosine kinase activity, are predominantly intracellular. (*From Ullrich et al.*[37])

THE β-ADRENERGIC RECEPTOR

The β-adrenergic receptor, which mediates the physiological actions of adrenaline and other catecholamines that exert their effects through activation of adenylate cyclase via the guanyl nucleotide regulatory protein (Ns), has been purified from mammalian lung[47] and turkey erythrocytes.[48] Partial amino acid sequence information was used to isolate cDNA clones encoding the receptor, which was found to contain seven membrane-spanning regions and a long intracellular carboxyterminal domain. The receptor resembles rhodopsin in its structural and functional properties, since both have sequence homologies and seven transmembrane regions, and act by regulating GTP-binding proteins, either Ns (β-receptor) or transducin (rhodopsin). When rhodopsin is stimulated by light it couples to transducin, which binds GTP and activates a phosphodiesterase that hydrolyses cyclic GMP and causes closure of ion channels on the rod cell membrane to mediate the visual response. Of additional interest is the absence of introns from the β-adrenergic receptor gene, similar to histones and interferons but in contrast to the rhodopsin gene and those for other cell-surface receptors. The presence of several membrane-spanning regions is also a feature of glucose and anion transporter systems, and of the sodium pump and enzymes such as HMG CoA reductase, but has not been observed in other cell-surface receptors. Whether this structural feature is relevant to the interaction of the receptor with Ns within the plasma membrane or on its cytoplasmic surface is not yet known, and it remains to be seen whether other receptors that act through nucleotide regulatory proteins possess similar trans-membrane domains. The sequence and three-dimensional homologies between the β-adrenergic receptor and rhodopsin are accompanied by several functional similarities in addition to their interaction with nucleotide regulatory proteins. These include homologous desensitization and light adaptation, both of which involve receptor phosphorylation that is mediated by β-adrenergic receptor kinase (which phosphorylates only the agonist-occupied form of the receptor) and rhodopsin kinase (which phosphorylates only the light-bleached form of rhodopsin). These findings indicate that the mechanisms of regulation of the individual trans-membrane signaling systems are basically similar in nature and may represent a general process for controlling the coupling of receptors to guanine nucleotide regulatory proteins within the lipid bilayer of the cell membrane.

Peptide Hormone Receptors and Membrane Components

Several possibilities have been suggested to explain the mechanisms by which hormone-receptor interactions lead to modification of specific membrane-associated enzymes. The original view that hormone receptors are structurally coupled to adenylate cyclase and serve as regulatory subunits of the enzyme has been replaced by more complex models that are consistent with the fluid and dynamic nature of the cell membrane. The most widely accepted model is the *mobile receptor* hypothesis, which was originally proposed to explain the mechanism by which adenylate cyclase is modulated within the cell membrane by hormone-receptor interaction;[49] it is based upon the assumption that the receptor and enzyme units are separate and discrete molecules (Fig. 5-9). In this model, hormone binding causes a conformational change in the receptor and increases its affinity for membrane components that are involved in the activation of adenylate cyclase and other effector enzymes.

Although hormone receptor sites are physically distinct from signal-generating enzymes such as adenylate cyclase, there is a close functional connection between the receptor and effector molecules. The dependence of hormonal activation of adenylate cyclase in certain membranes and solubilized preparations upon phospholipids indicates that a coupling component of lipid nature is necessary for the association of the two activities. Studies on the relationship between specific hormone receptors and adenylate cyclase activity under a variety of developmental and physiological conditions have also shown a close correlation between the two activities.

Subsequent models have taken into account the functional complexity of the adenylate cyclase system, which contains at least three sites at which individual ligands act to modify the activity of the enzyme. These include the hormone receptor site, the catalytic site, which reacts with MgATP, and an intermediate regulatory site which reacts preferentially with guanyl nucleotides. The ability of guanyl nucleotides to enhance the activation of hepatic adenylate cyclase by glucagon suggested that active and inactive forms of adenylate cyclase complex could be interconverted by the concordant actions of the hormone and guanyl nucleotide.[50] Such effects of GTP and its synthetic analogues have been observed in numerous hormone-responsive target tissues, where guanyl nucleotides function as allosteric activators of adenylate cyclase. Synthetic GTP analogues that are resistant to enzymatic hydrolysis, such as Gpp(NH)p and GTP-γ-S, activate adenylate cyclase through the same nucleotide site as GTP. Guanyl nucleotides enhance the basal as well as hormone-stimulated cyclase activity, and the combination of hormone treatment and Gpp(NH)p causes prolonged activation of adenylate cyclase. In some tissues, binding of radiolabeled Gpp(NH)p to cell membranes can be corre-

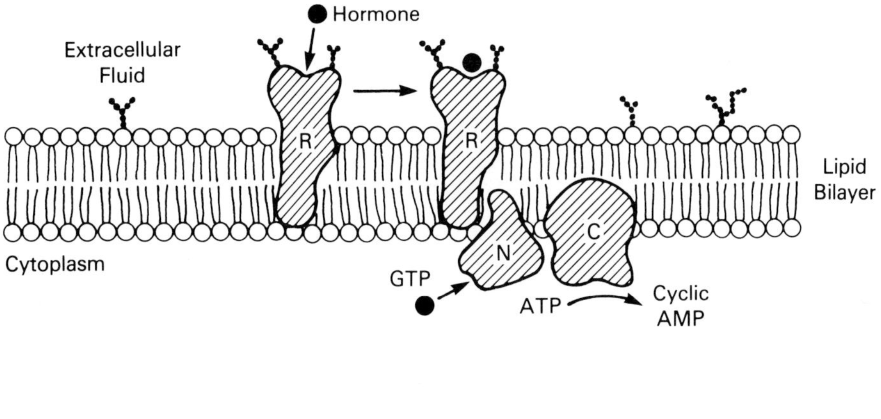

FIGURE 5-9 The "floating receptor" two-step model of peptide hormone–receptor interaction and activation of adenylate cyclase within the cell membrane.

lated with the hormonal activation of adenylate cyclase. The interaction between guanyl nucleotides and adenylate cyclase activity exemplifies a general feature of peptide hormone action,[51] and reflects the major role of nucleotide regulatory proteins in transmembrane signaling mechanisms (Fig. 5-10).

The actions of guanyl nucleotides upon adenylate cyclase and other effector enzymes are often accompanied by decreased affinity of the corresponding hormone receptor sites. Both GTP and Gpp(NH)p reduce the affinity of receptors for hormones such as glucagon, angiotensin II, and catecholamines by increasing the dissociation rate constant of the hormone-receptor complex. These effects of guanyl nucleotides are exerted through a group of guanyl nucleotide–dependent regulatory proteins, which both control the activities of plasma membrane effector enzymes and influence the binding properties of the receptor sites to which they are coupled.

Receptor Mobility and Hormone Action

Recognition of the dynamic and fluid state of the cell membrane, and of the ability of several hormone-receptor systems to interact with the same adenylate cyclase system in certain cells, stimulated interest in the role of receptor mobility within the plasma membrane as an essential feature of hormone action. The mobile receptor hypothesis postulates a conformational change in the receptor after hormone binding, with the acquisition of special ability to bind to and perturb other membrane proteins such as adenylate cyclase. This two-step activation mechanism permits the hormone-receptor complexes to interact sequentially with other membrane components, such as nucleotide regulatory proteins, and to be influenced themselves by such interactions. For example, stabilization of the final ternary complex could increase the apparent binding affinity, as is now recognized to occur in several hormone-receptor systems. Also, the ability of GTP to decrease receptor affinity in several systems, now known to involve the nucleotide regulatory proteins and their interaction with the receptor, provides a mechanism by which the high receptor affinities necessary for hormonal regulation can be maintained without compromising the rapidity of control by unduly slow dissociation rates.[48]

The conformational change caused by hormone binding can be regarded as a highly specific response of the receptor to its interaction with homologous ligand. This change is triggered by agonist ligands (but not antagonists); it leads to the expression of the information encoded within the receptor via activation of its membrane effector systems. Other maneuvers which perturb cell surface receptors, in particular their interaction with both lectins and receptor antibodies which cross-link the sites, can also lead to receptor activation and stimulation of the cellular response (Fig. 5-11). Thus, as indicated in Table 5-2, a number of receptor antibodies, including those to receptors for TSH,[52] insulin,[53] EGF,[54] and prolactin,[55] can exert agonist-like effects on their respective target cells. An interesting variant of the cross-linking effect is the acquisition of agonist activity by receptor-bound GnRH antagonist analogues after cross-linking by specific antibody which stimulates LH release from pituitary cells, presumably via receptor microaggregation and activation of the gonadotroph.[56] An analogous effect is seen with deglycosylated hCG derivatives, which act as receptor-blocking antagonists

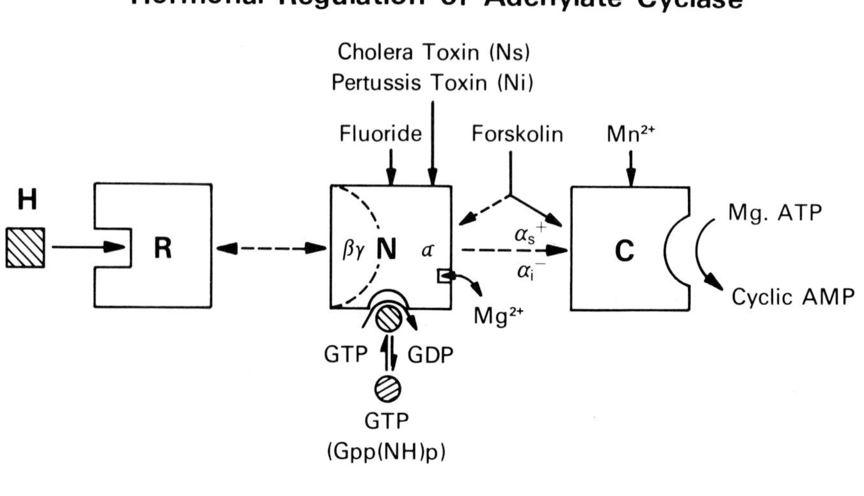

FIGURE 5-10 A three-component model of the hormone-receptor-adenylate cyclase system. The hormone-receptor (H·R) complex modulates the GTP-binding activity of the guanyl nucleotide regulatory subunit (N), which in turn activates (or inhibits) adenylate cyclase (C). The hormone-induced activation of the GTP·N complex is terminated by hydrolysis of GTP at or near the regulatory site.

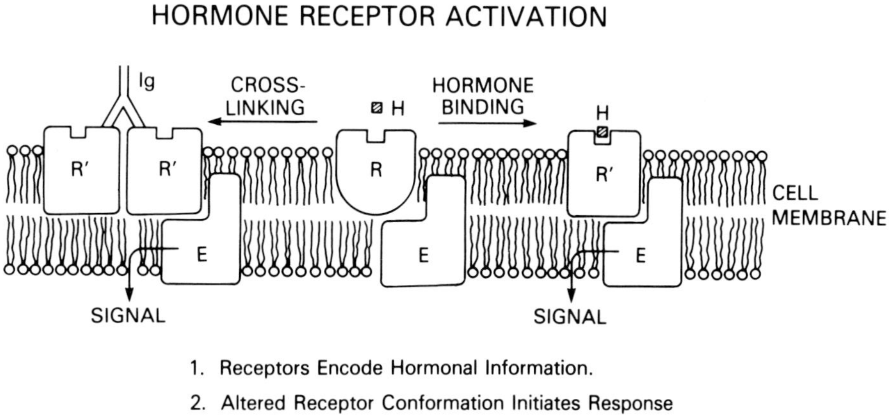

FIGURE 5-11 Peptide hormone receptor mobility and altered receptor comformation during specific hormonal activation (*right*) and nonspecific activation by perturbation induced by cross-linking with antibodies and lectins (*left*).

but cause target cell activation after cross-linking by anti-hCG antibodies.

The processes of cell growth, movement, and recognition are coordinated by a supramolecular complex of cell surface receptors and submembranous fibrillar structures, by which changes (surface modulation) in receptor conformation, mobility, and distribution lead to changes in the associated cytoplasmic components. These structural interactions are probably responsible for the aggregation (clustering, patching, and capping) of receptors that is induced by cross-linking agents such as divalent antibodies and multivalent lectins. Monovalent ligands such as hormones can also lead to receptor redistribution in the cell membrane, with clustering of sites to form aggregates on the cell surface. Such clustering is probably an important prelude to internalization of hormone-receptor complexes, but may also be important in the early phase of hormone action (Fig. 5-12). Thus, certain bivalent antibodies to the insulin receptor bind to receptors and exert insulin-like actions in isolated adipocytes, whereas monovalent Fab′ antibody fragments bind to the receptor but do not evoke a biological response. Addition of anti-F(ab′)$_2$ antiserum to cross-link the Fab′-receptor complexes can restore the insulin-like action of the antibody.[57] These effects indicate that receptor cross-linking or microaggregation is important in the agonist actions of anti-receptor antibodies, and perhaps in the actions of insulin itself. This proposal is consistent with the mobility of insulin receptors and their ability to form clusters in the cell membrane, and with the insulin-like effects of certain lectins. However, the extent to which insulin and other hormonal ligands exert their specific cellular actions via receptor cross-linking and microaggregation is still uncertain, and the ability of cross-linking maneuvers to mimic hormonal activation does not necessarily reflect the physiological mechanism by which specific ligand binding elicits the characteristic target cell response.

Table 5-2. Biological Activity of Receptor Antibodies

Receptors	Biological responses
TSH	Thyroid hormone secretion
Insulin	Glucose uptake, hypoglycemia
Catecholamine	Adenylate cyclase activation
Prolactin	Casein synthesis
EGF	DNA synthesis

Hormone Receptors and Target Cell Densensitization

As noted above, peptide hormone receptors exist in a dynamic and mobile state in the plasma membrane. The receptors are not only able to diffuse freely in the plane of the membrane to interact with effector systems or to form clusters, but are also distributed between the cell surface and intracellular sites of recycling, synthesis, and degradation, in a dynamic equilibrium that is readily perturbed by hormonal activation. With this knowledge it is not difficult to understand the marked change in attitude about hormonal activation mechanisms, from the simple

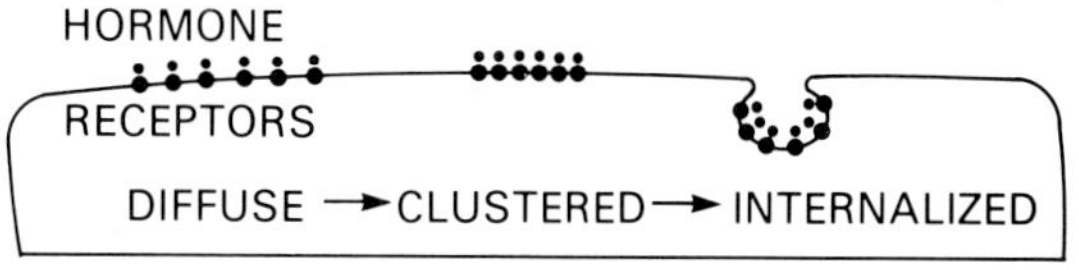

FIGURE 5-12 Distribution of receptors and hormone-receptor complexes within the target cell membrane during peptide hormone action.

concept of cell stimulation as an on/off type of event with prompt release of the ligand to one in which complex conformational and metabolic changes occur in the hormone-receptor complexes and the associated membrane components. Many peptide hormones have been shown to "down-regulate" their homologous receptors,[58] a phenomenon analogous to the process of antigenic modulation in lymphocytes.[59] The mechanisms by which hormones decrease the numbers of their specific receptors are discussed in more detail below. The process of down-regulation can be an important determinant of cell responsiveness to hormone treatment, and in particular of the changes seen during hormonal desensitization.

Decreased responsiveness of target cells during continuous or repeated exposure to the stimulatory ligand has been noted in many tissues, and has been described by terms such as tachyphylaxis, refractoriness, or desensitization. This is a common characteristic of hormone-stimulated adenylate cyclase responses,[60] but also occurs in other effector enzyme systems. In many cells, exposure to stimulatory hormones causes a rapid initial burst of cyclic AMP formation, followed by a fall to near the basal level and a loss of responsiveness to further hormonal stimulation. The mechanism of this transient response to hormonal action can involve several of the components of the enzyme systems responsible for cAMP synthesis and degradation, as described below. From the functional standpoint, such responses could permit rapid cellular activation by the regulatory ligand, while protecting against excessively large or sustained rises in hormone concentration. Most peptide hormones are secreted episodically, and often exhibit short-lived pulses in the circulation, while the secretion and actions of neurotransmitters are also characteristically transient. The corresponding ligand-responsive membrane effector systems have developed in such a manner as to be optimally activated by intermittent stimulation, and may thus exhibit a complementary relationship with the mode of presentation of their hormonal regulators.

The process of desensitization, or hormone-induced attenuation of cellular responsiveness, is the result of several contributory mechanisms.[61] A general distinction can be made between *heterologous* desensitization, in which exposure to one hormone impairs the subsequent responses to other ligands, and *homologous* desensitization, in which the attenuation is hormone-specific and limited to the ligand itself. Heterologous desensitization appears to be caused by the inhibitory effect of one of the products of the activation process, such as cyclic AMP, which temporarily impairs the ability of the effector system to respond to other hormonal and nonhormonal stimuli. One such mechanism involves modification of the receptor or the nucleotide regulatory protein, possibly via phosphorylation by cAMP-dependent protein kinase or protein kinase C. Such events may occur normally as a mechanism to limit the cellular response to hormonal activation. During excessive stimulation of any one hormone receptor system, the overproduction of cyclic AMP or DAG could modify other receptor systems via phosphorylation of a proportion of the available regulatory sites within the plasma membrane. Another potential factor in heterologous desensitization is increased phosphodiesterase activity, which could cause a general increase in cAMP degradation and thus impair the ability of other cAMP-dependent hormones to elicit their responses.

The more selective form of hormonal refractoriness, homologous desensitization, is primarily attributable to hormone-induced changes at the receptor level. These include events such as persistent occupancy by bound hormone, structural modification or inactivation of the receptors, and internalization with recycling or degradation of the sites.[62] Such changes occur in many states of excessive hormone secretion, and serve to buffer the cell response to abnormally high or persistent levels of hormonal stimulation. In most cases the system continues to respond to the elevated level of hormonal stimulation, albeit to a less extreme degree than would be expected in the absence of desensitization. In at least one situation, during treatment with GnRH and its superagonist analogues, target cell desensitization is so marked that gonadotroph function is selectively inhibited[63] and gonadotropin secretion is suppressed in the face of continued administration of the releasing hormone agonist.[64]

Following the initial hormonal activation of adenylate cyclase, the hormone-receptor complex undergoes a further conformational change that terminates its coupling to the cyclase system and leaves the sites refractory to further stimulation. Then, depending upon the rate at which the hormone dissociates from the receptor, the sites become resensitized over a period of minutes or hours. In some cases, as exemplified by the β-adrenergic receptor, loss of accessible binding sites during desensitization is also related to the formation of a high-affinity state during association with the nucleotide regulatory protein. In this system, the return of the receptors to their low-affinity active state is hastened by the binding of guanyl nucleotides to the regulatory protein.[60]

There is also evidence for covalent and structural changes in β-adrenergic receptors during prolonged desensitization, which correlates with increased phosphorylation of the receptor protein.[65] In addition, phosphorylation of receptors occurs very rapidly during homologous desensitization by β-adrenergic agonists, and may account for the early uncoupling process that precedes sequestration (and presumably dephosphorylation) of the sites within endocytic vesicles. This rapid form of receptor phosphorylation is mediated by a distinct β-adrenergic receptor kinase (βAR kinase) with specificity for the agonist-occupied sites[65a] and differs from the more slowly developing impairment of receptor function that occurs during prolonged exposure to agonists. βAR kinase appears to be closely similar to rhodopsin kinase and, like the latter, can phosphorylate a specific region of light-bleached rhodopsin. Also, just as phosphorylation of bleached rhodopsin by rhodopsin kinase reduces its interaction with transducin, phosphorylation if the β-adrenergic receptor by βAR kinase causes uncoupling of the receptor from the stimulating guanine nucleotide regulatory protein.[65b]

In more slowly binding and dissociating hormone-receptor systems, such as the interaction of gonadotropins with testicular and ovarian target cells (Fig. 5-13), the phases of desensitization and internalization become merged and the initial period of refractoriness due to homologous desensitization is followed by a pronounced loss of LH receptors due to internalization and degradation of the hormone-receptor complexes.[66] Endocytic processing may also occur to some extent during the desensitization of β-adrenergic and other receptors, such that a proportion of the sites could undergo transient occlusion in a perimembranous pool prior to being reactivated and once more available at the cell surface.

Receptor Occupancy and Activation of Target Cell Responses

In most endocrine target cells, activation of adenylate cyclase and target cells by agonist ligands is proportional to the degree of receptor occupancy. However, the receptor binding affinity (K_d) measured by radioligand assays is often less than the hormone concentration required for half-maximal biological response (ED_{50}), and maximal cellular responses are evoked by occupancy of only a small proportion of the available receptors. Even when increasing receptor occupancy is accompanied by increasing responses over a wide range of hormone binding, the response is usually not directly proportional to the number of occupied receptors. Also, it is well recognized that many hormones can stimulate the production of much more cAMP than is necessary to evoke a maximum biological response in the target cell. Such observations have suggested that many hormone-responsive tissues contain *spare* or excess receptors, as originally recognized during studies on drug-responsive tissues.[67] Even when present in great excess over the number needed to elicit the maximal cell response, such spare sites are by no means superfluous. Spare receptors could serve as a reservoir of surface recep-

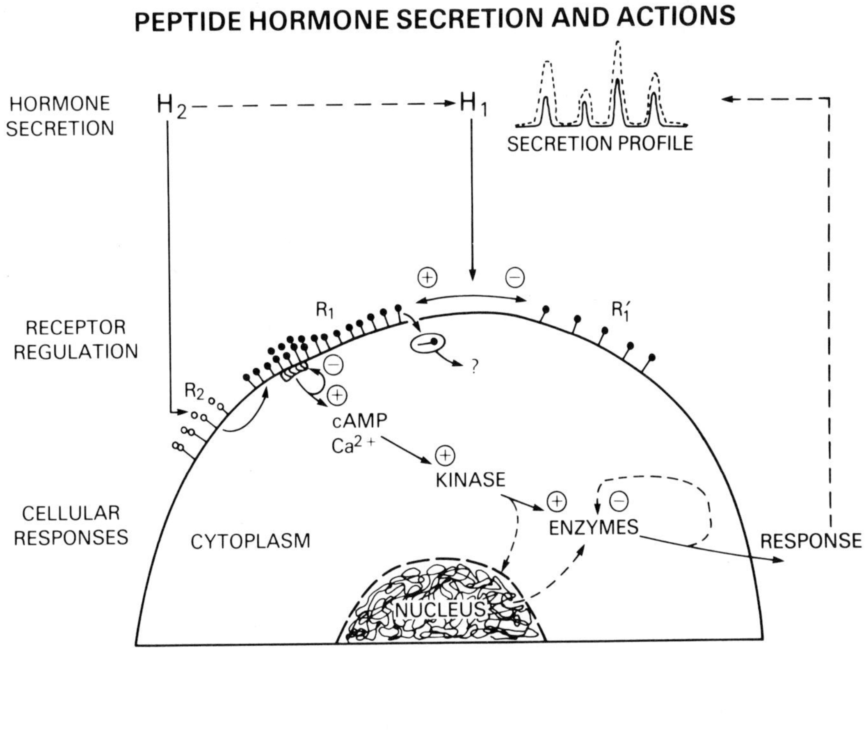

FIGURE 5-13 Receptor regulation and desensitization in endocrine target cells. Receptors for a given hormone (R_1) are down-regulated by the homologous hormone (H_1) and by other hormones (H_2) through their separate receptor sites (R_2). Postreceptor desensitization of plasma membrane effector systems and of subsequent metabolic steps can significantly alter the target cell response in the presence or absence of receptor down-regulation.

tors, and also to increase the sensitivity of the target cell to activation by low hormone concentrations. Thus, the presence of a high density of plasma membrane receptors would favor rapid ligand association to attain the critical level of occupancy that causes target cell activation.

The term "spare receptors" is used in a relative sense, and the degree of receptor excess may differ according to the biological response that is measured.[68] For example, hormone receptors are rarely "spare" for adenylate cyclase. Thus, good correlations are commonly observed between ligand binding and adenylate cyclase activation, even though nonlinear coupling often occurs between receptor occupancy and enzyme responses. Likewise, hormone binding to intact target cells is usually accompanied by serial increases in cAMP production, and most tissues do not contain excess receptors that are not coupled to adenylate cyclase. In contrast, measurements of more distal responses, such as muscle contraction, steroidogenesis, glucose oxidation, lipolysis, and ion transport, often show that the maximum biological response is evoked by occupany of only a small fraction of the receptor population (Fig. 5-14). This phenomenon is probably related to the marked amplification of hormonal activation that occurs during the subsequent steps that lead to the final cell response. It is clear that hormonal activation of the small number of receptors needed to elicit the cellular response would be facilitated by the presence of a relatively large pool of receptors at the target cell surface. An additional role for spare receptors is to serve as a reservoir of available sites during the continuous processing and degradation of receptors that occurs during the course of hormonal activation and regulation of target cell function.

The presence of excess receptors has been clearly established by direct binding studies with labeled hormones in certain cells and target tissues. This effect is particularly marked in the interstitial cells of the testis, where LH binding to 5 to 10 sites per cell initiates androgen secretion and occupany of only 1 percent of the LH receptor population is sufficient to elicit maximum testosterone production.[69] However, further binding of gonadotropin causes a progressive increase in the production and release of cAMP, indicating that most of the binding sites identified with radioactive hormone are functionally active receptors with the capacity to stimulate adenylate cyclase activity.

In certain tissues, hormone binding and the subsequent biological response are closely related over the entire range of receptor occupancy. Thus, the binding of angiotensin II to its adrenal receptors is not linearly correlated with increasing aldosterone production, but the progressive steroid response to increasing receptor occupancy indicates that there are few if any spare angiotensin receptors in the zona glomerulosa cell.[70] Similarly, there is a close correlation between insulin binding and stimulation of amino acid transport in isolated thymocytes. The relationship between receptor occupancy and specific cellular responses varies widely among individual target tissues, from the extreme case of the Leydig cell with full activation by minimal receptor occupancy, to the almost continuous relationship between receptor occupancy and response in the glomerulosa cell and the thymocyte. Within a single cell type, such as the fat cell during exposure to insulin, increasing degrees of receptor occupancy can elicit sequential biological responses. In fat cells, occupancy of only a few insulin receptors is sufficient to inhibit lipolysis, whereas glucose metabolism is maximally stimulated when only 2 to 3 percent of the

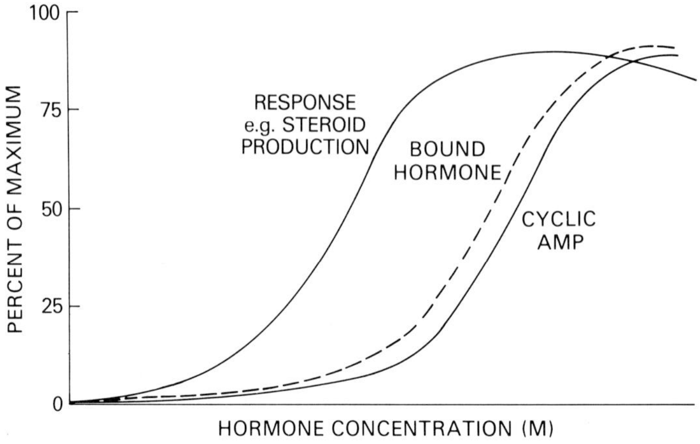

FIGURE 5-14 Concentration-response curves for hormone binding, cyclic AMP formation, and steroid production during stimulation of gonadal and adrenal cells by gonadotropins and ACTH, respectively.

receptors are occupied, and amino acid transport and protein synthesis are stimulated at higher degrees of receptor occupancy.[71]

In general, when hormone binding and biological responses are closely related the receptors are limiting in terms of target cell activation. When abundant or spare receptors are present, the more distal elements are limiting; in the case of adenylate cyclase–mediated responses, the limiting step is often beyond the formation of cyclic AMP, which can be produced in much greater amounts than necessary to elicit the target cell response. In many tissues, hormonal stimulation is accompanied by release of cAMP into the extracellular fluid, with elevation of blood and/or urinary levels of the cyclic nucleotide.

Receptor Phosphorylation and Hormone Action

Within the accepted framework of peptide hormone action, with primary binding to specific receptors and secondary activation of plasma membrane effector enzymes, many questions remain to be clarified about the intermediate steps that are involved in the activation process. It is clear that protein-phospholipid and protein-protein interactions are crucial components of the activation mechanism, but the nature and sequence of these processes are only now being elucidated. In addition to the phosphorylation of cytosolic proteins that mediates cellular responses to many forms of hormone action via cAMP-, calcium-, or phospholipid-dependent protein kinases, plasma membrane proteins are also phosphorylated during receptor activation. These include the receptors themselves and their transducing proteins, which thus become targets for local regulatory mechanisms in the course of subserving their primary function of transmembrane signaling. The phosphorylation of the β-adrenergic receptor by a specific kinase during catecholamine-induced desensitization, as discussed above, may represent a general feature of receptor desensitization by homologous hormones. An additional form of receptor phosphorylation of major potential significance is determined by the protein kinase activity of the receptor itself. Several of the peptide hormones and growth factors that do not act through the known kinase systems possess tyrosine kinase activity, and undergo autophosphorylation after activation by agonist ligands (Table 5-3). Such peptides rapidly induce phosphorylation of tyrosine residues in their own receptors by stimulating the intrinsic kinase activity of the receptor itself. Thus, the β subunit of the insulin receptor acts as an insulin-dependent protein kinase,[72] and tyrosine residues (as well as serine and threonine) are phosphorylated during activation of receptors for EGF, insulin, and other mitogenic peptides.[73]

In addition to the frequent occurrence of tyrosine phosphorylation during the regulation of cell growth and metabolism by peptide hormones and growth factors, cell transformation by oncogenic retroviruses (typified by the Rous sarcoma virus, RSV) is also associated with protein phosphorylation at tyrosine residues.[74] Several of the transforming proteins of oncogenic viruses possess tyrosine-specific protein kinase activity, as exemplified by the protein product ($pp60^{src}$) encoded by the RSV *src* gene that mediates cellular transformation. Furthermore, the RSV tyrosine kinase also stimulates phosphorylation of one of the cellular proteins in which EGF promotes tyrosine phosphorylation.[75] These findings have important implications about the role of peptide hormones in the normal control of cellular growth, via processes related to tyrosine phosphorylation, and also about the manner in which such events may contribute to the loss of growth control in transformed and neoplastic cells. The ability of transforming growth factors to bind to the EGF receptor and induce phosphorylation at specific tyrosine sites in the receptor raises the possibility that EGF receptor phosphorylation may be involved in cell transformation.[76]

Of particular relevance to hormonal regulation is the occurrence of tyrosine phosphorylation during the interaction of certain hormones with their plasma membrane receptors (Table 5-3). Such hormone-dependent phosphorylations involve tyrosine residues of the receptors themselves, as well as other membrane proteins and exogenous peptide substrates. This applies to insulin, EGF, and other peptides that exert growth and mitogenic actions and do not operate through adenylate cyclase and cAMP-dependent pro-

Table 5-3. Receptor Phosphorylation

Ligand-activated (tyrosine):
EGF receptor (and v-erbB protein)
Insulin receptor (β subunit)
PDGF receptor
IGF 1 (somatomedin C) receptor
Ligand-activated (serine, threonine):
β-Adrenergic receptor
Rhodopsin
Constitutive (serine, threonine):
Nicotinic acetylcholine receptor
IgE receptor
Sodium channel

tein kinase. Such a control mechanism operating via tyrosine phosphorylation at the plasma membrane level could be analogous to the control of cytoplasmic processes via phosphorylation of serine and threonine residues by cAMP- and calcium-dependent protein kinases.[73]

Insulin-stimulated autophosphorylation of the insulin receptor β subunit in the intact cell involves serine and threonine as well as tyrosine residues, whereas tyrosine residues in the receptor and other proteins are preferentially phosphorylated in cell-free systems and solubilized or purified receptors. In partially purified insulin receptors from hepatoma cells, insulin causes autophosphorylation of the β subunit with incorporation of two phosphate residues per receptor site. Insulin greatly increases the V_{max} for autophosphorylation of the receptor kinase, and Mn^{2+} decreases the K_m of the enzyme for ATP.[77]

Tyrosine phosphorylation is relatively minor in most cells, and although the tyrosine kinase activity of receptors and proteins that modify cell growth and metabolism may reflect a major role in regulation, the endogenous substrates and consequences of tyrosine phosphorylation are not clear. A potential role of tyrosine phosphorylation during insulin action has been suggested by the finding of impaired kinase activity and receptor phosphorylation in fibroblasts and mononuclear cells of patients with severe insulin resistance and normal insulin-binding characteristics.[78,79] However, some of the insulin receptor antibodies that mimic the effects of insulin on cellular responses including glucose transport, lipogenesis, and receptor internalization do not cause phosphorylation of the insulin receptor β subunit.[80] Such findings suggest that activation of tyrosine-specific protein kinase might not be an obligatory step in coupling receptor binding to insulin action.[81]

Two other important examples of ligand-dependent receptor phosphorylation are provided by rhodopsin and the EGF receptor. As noted earlier, rhodopsin serves as the receptor for photons in retinal rod cells, and acts via a guanyl nucleotide regulatory protein (transducin) to stimulate cyclic GMP breakdown and closure of sodium channels.[82] The activated form of rhodopsin is immediately phosphorylated at serine and threonine residues by a cAMP-independent rhodopsin kinase, a reaction which terminates the retinal processes that decrease cGMP levels and modulate sodium flux in the light-sensitive rod cells. In the case of the EGF receptor, ligand binding stimulates the intrinsic kinase activity of the receptor itself, which becomes autophosphorylated at a tyrosine residue during EGF-induced cell activation. The purified EGF receptor, which has a molecular weight of 150,000 to 170,000, contains specific domains for hormone binding and tyrosine kinase activity. The ligand-binding domain of the receptor is displayed on the outer surface of the plasma membrane, and the kinase and substrate domains are located in the cytoplasmic region of the receptor. The interaction of EGF with its external binding site apparently causes a conformational change in the transmembrane receptor molecule. This leads to enhanced kinase activity and autophosphorylation of the cytoplasmic domains of the receptor, which are adjacent to intracellular proteins that participate in the mechanism of cell activation.[83]

It should be noted that the EGF-stimulated protein kinase phosphorylates adjacent membrane proteins as well as the EGF receptor itself. The ability of the receptor kinase to phosphorylate other membrane proteins does not depend upon its autophosphorylation, and both activities of the receptor are catalyzed by the same enzymatic site on the receptor protein.[84] The manner in which receptor phosphorylation is related to the mitogenic action of EGF is not known with certainty, but the ability of a cyanogen bromide–cleaved, biologically inactive EGF derivative to promote receptor phosphorylation suggests that such phosphorylation is not a prerequisite for the mitogenic action of the peptide. However, EGF-induced phosphorylation could be related to the early effects of EGF, including activation of Na^+,K^+-ATPase and ornithine decarboxylase, that are not required or are not alone sufficient to initiate DNA synthesis.[85] Probably of more importance are the aggregation of the EGF-receptor complexes into clusters, a process that is not stimulated by the CNBr-treated EGF derivative, and the phosphorylation of tyrosine residues in other cellular substrates, of which vinculin and progesterone receptors are but two examples.

Synthesis and Regulation of Peptide Hormone Receptors

BIOSYNTHESIS AND TURNOVER OF RECEPTORS

Plasma membrane receptors are generally similar to other membrane proteins in their biosynthetic sequence, being assembled on ribosomes bound to the endoplasmic reticulum (ER) and translocated into the lumen of the ER for transfer to the Golgi apparatus and thence to the plasma membrane.[85a] Like secretory and lysosomal proteins, plasma membrane proteins carry a 15- to 20-amino-acid leader sequence that determines their translocation and passage through the ER-Golgi system.[85a] Such signal sequences have a basic amino terminus and an apolar central domain, and are usually located at the amino-terminal end of the molecule. They are transiently present in most proteins and are cleaved after insertion into the ER membranes. The insertion of nascent peptide chains into the ER membrane is mediated by RNA-protein signal recognition particles, which "dock" the ribosomal complexes at the ER membrane so that protein synthesis continues only on ribosomes attached to the ER.

The transported proteins from the ER enter the Golgi compartments and undergo extensive glycosylation and remodeling of asparagine-linked oligosaccharide chains, followed by addition of galactose residues prior to their emergence and sorting for delivery to plasma membrane, lysosomes, and secretory granules.[85b] The signals that determine the destination of each type of protein are currently being elucidated by biochemical, genetic, and recombinant DNA approaches. In the case of lysosomal proteins, it is the presence of terminal mannose 6-phosphate residues on the oligosaccharides of lysosomal protein precursors that determines their segregation and delivery to lysosomes. At least some of the sorting of membrane proteins is performed by clathrin-coated vesicles in the Golgi system, which also participate in the recycling of internalized plasma membrane receptors following their dissociation from bound ligands in endosomes (Fig. 5-15). In some cases, the receptor proteins are associated with secretory granules, which may serve as a route for recruitment of intracellular receptors to the plasma membrane during ligand-induced exocytosis. This form of receptor recruitment occurs with various ligands in pituitary cells, pancreatic islets, neutrophils, and fibroblasts, and is a feature of somatostatin receptor regulation in pituitary and pancreatic cells. Other pathways for the migration of cell surface receptors to the plasma membrane must operate in nonsecretory cells, again presumably converging on those involved in the recycling of internalized receptors back to the plasma membrane. The biochemical routing signals of cell surface receptors, which may include their characteristic membrane-spanning hydrophobic domains, have yet to be established. It is of interest that the amino acid sequences of membrane transport systems and ion channels, in contrast to the single membrane-anchoring hydrophobic region of many cell surface receptors, contain several membrane-spanning regions that presumably subserve their functional activities as transporters of small molecules such as glucose, sodium, and anions.[86]

An almost universal feature of hormone-regulated target cells is their ability to respond to changes in ambient ligand concentration by changing the number and/or affinity of their surface receptors.[87] Such regulation of plasma membrane receptors by the homologous ligand commonly occurs in cells exposed to neu-

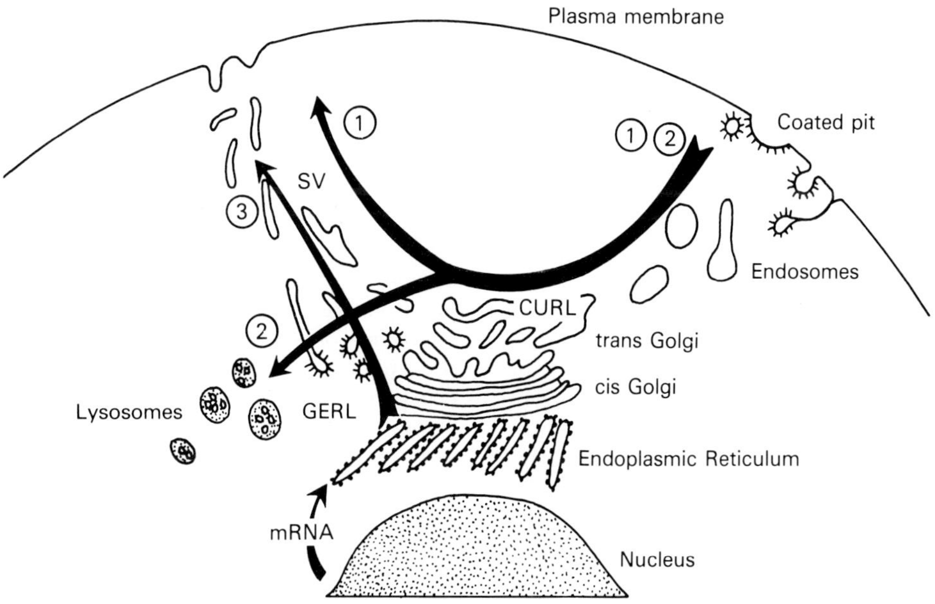

FIGURE 5-15 Biosynthesis and recycling of hormone receptors. The major pathways for polypeptide receptor formation and endocytosis are: (1) endocytosis and recycling (many receptors and receptor-transferrin and receptor-immunoglobulin complexes); (2) endocytosis-lysosome pathway (some receptors, most ligands); (3) biosynthesis-secretion pathway (receptors). Abbreviations: GERL, Golgi–endoplasmic reticulum–lysosome region; CURL, compartment of uncoupling of ligand and receptor. (*Modified from Dickson.*[85b])

rotransmitters, peptides, protein and glycoprotein hormones, and surface-modulating factors such as lectins and immunoglobulins. As noted above, desensitization of cellular responses by agonist ligands is often accompanied by temporary loss of receptor sites. However, hormone-stimulated cells may show decreases in receptor number in the absence of desensitization or refractoriness, or even in the presence of enhanced responsiveness. The mechanism of receptor regulation by homologous ligands depends on the mobility of the hormone-receptor complexes within the lipid bilayer and their endocytosis at specialized regions of the plasma membrane. Thus, stimulation of target cells by hormonal ligands initiates a complex sequence of regulatory changes that accompany or follow the characteristic cellular response. These include changes in the amount of (or accessibility) and activity of the molecular components of the signaling pathway, as well as alterations in cellular biosynthetic responses to further hormonal stimulation.

RECEPTOR REGULATION IN ENDOCRINE TARGET CELLS

Peptide hormone receptors are not only regulated by the homologous hormone, but are sometimes influenced by other hormones that act on the same target cell (Fig. 5-13). Homologous receptor regulation, in which increased hormone concentrations usually cause a decrease in the number of their specific receptors, was first observed for the insulin receptors of liver and cultured lymphocytes.[19] Such down-regulation of insulin receptors also occurs in human obesity and in genetic or induced obesity in rodents, and seems to be a general consequence of the raised blood insulin levels associated with insulin-resistant states. The converse effect, increased insulin receptors in states of reduced insulin secretion, has been observed in the livers of diabetic hamsters and rats. Many other receptors are down-regulated by the homologous hormones, including those for catecholamines, opiates, corticotropin releasing factor (CRF), TRH, GH, gonadotropins, and glucagon. A few receptors, notably those for insulin, exhibit negative cooperativity on exposure to increasing concentrations of the homologous hormone. If operative under physiological conditions, this could provide a mechanism whereby partial receptor occupany leads to decreased affinity of the residual sites, with reduction of target cell sensitivity in the presence of increased insulin concentration.

Certain hormone receptors, such as those for angiotensin II, prolactin, and GnRH, are increased in number by exposure to moderately elevated hormone concentrations. However, the more usual response, with loss of accessible receptors from the cell surface, probably affects all receptors when hormone levels are sufficiently elevated. In the testis and ovary, an increase in total LH receptor number precedes the receptor loss caused by high-dose gonadotropin treatment, suggesting that hormonal stimulation causes new sites to be exposed prior to the more prominent phase of receptor down-regulation.[88] The manner in which testicular gonadotropin receptors are regulated by LH or hCG changes markedly during development. Thus, fetal-neonatal Leydig cells show an increase of LH receptors after hCG treatment, in contrast to the prominent receptor loss and desensitization that occurs in the adult testis after gonadotropin administration.[89]

An important factor in receptor regulation is the rate and extent of the reversibility of formation of the hormone-receptor complex. Peptide hormone binding to cell surface receptors has been assumed to be freely reversible, and indeed the hormone-receptor complex usually shows an early phase of rapid dissociation. However, this is often followed by a prolonged phase of slow and incomplete dissociation, particularly in the intact cell. In many cases the initial binding reaction is followed by a conformational change in the receptor that results in tighter binding of the ligand. This can be represented by the sequence

$$H + R \rightleftharpoons H{\cdot}R \longrightarrow H{\cdot}R'$$

in which the primary hormone-receptor complex ($H{\cdot}R$) is converted to a poorly reversible form, $H{\cdot}R'$. One form of higher-affinity binding is brought about by interaction of occupied receptors with components of the adenylate cyclase system, and can be reversed by guanyl nucleotides. This high-affinity state is seen after receptor binding of catecholamines, glucagon, prostaglandin E, dopamine, and muscarinic ligands.[90] Another form of tight binding, which becomes progressively resistant to dissociation, occurs with insulin, EGF, prolactin, and LH, and is probably a preliminary step to the process of internalization of the hormone-receptor complex. In either case, prolonged occupancy by undissociated ligand is always a potential cause of functional receptor loss, and should be evaluated during studies of receptor regulation. As well as reducing the number of available binding sites, continued occupancy by ligand favors the probability that hormone-receptor complexes will be degraded or otherwise processed and destroyed. This could involve occlusion within the cell membrane or shedding from the cell surface, but current evidence favors the process of endocytosis and subsequent lysosomal breakdown of the internalized hormone-receptor complexes.

EFFECTS OF RECEPTOR REGULATION ON CELL RESPONSES

Implicit in the interpretation of receptor regulation is the assumption that end-organ responsiveness will be altered by changes in receptor concentration. If no other changes occurred, a reduction in membrane receptors would be expected to decrease target cell sensitivity in tissues containing abundant spare receptors and decrease the magnitude of the target cell response when receptor concentration becomes the limiting factor in the ability to elicit a hormonal response (Fig. 5-16). The general function of receptor regulation as a mechanism to decrease target cell sensitivity in the face of high hormone concentrations could have certain biological advantages. An obvious example is blood glucose homeostasis, in which decreased numbers of insulin receptors and reduced sensitivity of peripheral tissues to insulin would blunt the effect of hyperinsulinemia on the circulating glucose concentration. Receptor regulation could also minimize or buffer the cardiovascular responses to excessive levels of angiotensin II and catecholamines. This could contribute to the marked resistance to angiotensin II that occurs in many clinical states of increased renin secretion. However, the biological function of receptor regulation is less evident for other stimulators, such as GH, and gonadotropins, which exert long-term biological effects on the target cells.

The effects of receptor regulation on cellular responses to hormones have been studied in several tissues, particularly those in which hormone action is mediated by the adenylate cyclase–protein kinase system. An important distinction to be made in such hormone-treated tissues is between acute desensitization of the effector system (usually adenylate cyclase) and the development of true receptor loss, often as a delayed and more slowly reversible consequence of hormone-receptor interaction.

Analysis of the level at which regulation of surface receptors causes altered metabolic responses depends on the ability to measure changes in the hormone-activated pathway that is triggered by receptor binding. For several peptide hormones, such as insulin, GH, and prolactin, the immediate mechanism of action on target cells is not clearly defined. Although insulin modulates the activity of several membrane enzymes, including adenylate cyclase, phosphodiesterase, and ATPase, the relation of these effects to its actions on membrane transport systems and anabolic responses remains unclear. Where early events in hormone action have not been identified, the effect of receptor regulation on cell responses can be examined by measuring changes in transport systems and biosynthetic processes. This approach has been used to analyze the effects of insulin receptor regulation in adipocytes and hepatocytes on glucose or amino acid transport and lipid synthesis.

The consequences of receptor regulation on target cell function have been extensively studied in steroidogenic cells of the adrenal and gonads, which respond to trophic hormones with specific steroid secretion via an adenylate cyclase–dependent mechanism. In these cells it is possible to analyze several levels of response, from receptor occupancy, through cyclic AMP production and kinase activation, to stimulation of pregnenolone production and subsequent biosynthetic steps leading to steroid secretion. Cells obtained from animals given desensitizing doses of trophic hormone show marked changes in receptor content and metabolic responses to hormone stimulation in vitro. Such desensitized cells provide evidence for several consequences of receptor regulation induced by hormone treatment in the intact target tissue, including decreased cAMP formation and lesions in the steroid biosynthetic pathway.[47]

It has been noted already that protracted down-regulation of peptide hormone receptors also occurs in target cells during prolonged hormonal stimulation and hypertrophy of postreceptor response mechanisms, as observed in the CRF receptors of the pitui-

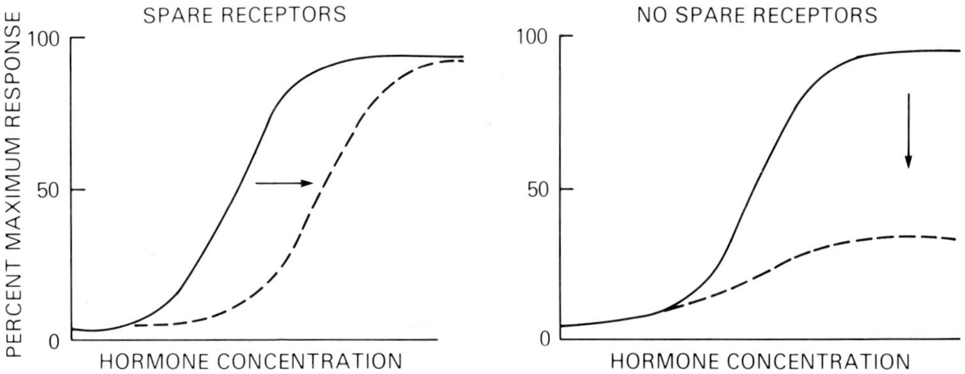

FIGURE 5-16 Effects of receptor loss on biological responses (e.g., steroidogenesis) in target cells with or without "spare" receptors.

tary gland after adrenalectomy. Under these circumstances, the ACTH response to receptor activation is enhanced despite the decreased number of plasma membrane receptors, due to increased efficiency of transduction of the hormonal stimulus via the enzymatic and secretory pathways of the chronically stimulated target cell.

FATE OF THE HORMONE-RECEPTOR COMPLEX

Until recently, most studies of peptide hormone action were focused on the immediate and short-term effects of hormone binding and activation of the cell surface receptor sites. Relatively little is known about the termination of hormone action, and the important long-term actions of hormones on cell growth and differentiation. All of these processes may be related to the fate of the hormone-receptor complex, in which the initial reversible interaction is often followed by the formation of a higher-affinity binding state that dissociates slowly and favors prolonged occupancy of the receptor sites.[87] This process may be a prelude to endocytosis of the complex, since the widespread occurrence of peptide hormones and binding sites within target cells suggests that processing and internalization of the complex is a frequent consequence of hormone-receptor interaction.

The role of receptor-mediated endocytosis and turnover of receptors has been clearly shown for cholinergic receptors,[91] LDL-receptor complexes,[92] and EGF receptors,[93] and is of major importance in the processing of hormone-receptor complexes in endocrine tissues. Studies of gonadotropin receptors in the Leydig cell have suggested that each receptor site might be occupied only once, then processed and degraded rather than reused for further hormone binding.[47] The extent to which this sequence occurs in different tissues may vary according to the ligand affinity and rate of receptor turnover, but such a mechanism appears to operate in the testis and ovary after hCG stimulation, and may apply to many receptor systems. The internalization mechanism for peptide hormones has many features in common with the processes of surface modulation in lymphocytes[59] and the coated pit system responsible for receptor-mediated endocytosis of macromolecules such as LDL (Fig. 5-17). The converse effect of certain peptide hormones, with an increase in receptor number, is probably caused by changes in membrane conformation and receptor recruitment from intracellular sites, followed by increased receptor synthesis. The long-term increases in receptors caused by certain

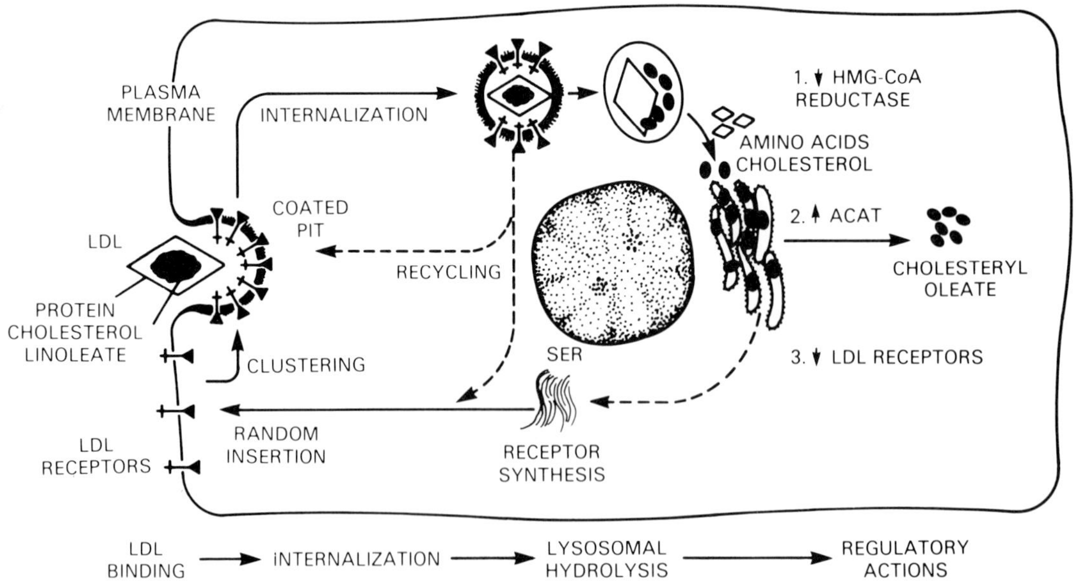

FIGURE 5-17 The LDL uptake pathway in cultured fibroblasts. The LDL receptors synthesized in polyribosomes insert randomly into the cell membrane and undergo clustering into coated pits followed by internalization within endocytic vesicles. After depositing the LDL in lysosomes, the receptors are recycled and return to the cell surface, where they again cluster in coated pits. The incoming cholesterol suppresses formation of the microsomal enzyme (HMG-CoA reductase) that is rate-limiting for cholesterol biosynthesis, stimulates the enzyme responsible for cholesterol ester synthesis, and inhibits synthesis of the LDL receptors. (*Modified from Brown and Goldstein.*[91])

hormones, such as angiotensin II in the adrenal glomerulosa cell[94] and GnRH in the pituitary gonadotroph,[95] could be components of the general cell response to trophic hormone action.

In several cell types, cytoplasmic contractile elements are involved in receptor mobility and regulation. Thus, ligand-receptor interaction in lymphoid cells is followed by patch formation, then by aggregation into a few larger patches or a single cap, and finally by internalization or shedding of the cross-linked receptors. Although receptor patching and capping commonly occur in cells exposed to multivalent ligands, such as immunoglobulins and lectins, similar changes have been observed in endocrine target cells when receptors are occupied by univalent ligands such as hormones and transmitters. The processes leading to aggregation and internalization of multivalent ligands are relevant to the turnover and fate of peptide hormone receptors, particularly during receptor regulation in response to increased concentrations of hormonal ligands. While the progression to patching and capping may not apply in vivo, redistribution and clustering of receptors for hormones and other univalent ligands is believed to precede the internalization and subsequent processing of the hormone-receptor complexes.

A typical example of the role of hormone internalization in ligand-induced receptor loss is the processing of EGF in human fibroblasts.[24] The cell-bound mitogen is rapidly degraded in a manner consistent with internalization and lysosomal breakdown, and surface receptors for EGF simultaneously disappear from the cells. Degradation of EGF receptors after peptide binding is also demonstrable by affinity labeling, which shows rapid proteolytic processing of the covalent receptor-hormone complexes durng the loss of membrane receptor sites. Both receptor processing and DNA synthesis are half-maximally stimulated when only 10 percent of the receptors are occupied by the mitogen. Direct visualization of the internalization of fluorescent derivatives of peptides, including EGF, insulin, and GnRH, has shown that the hormone-receptor complexes are initially distributed uniformly on the cell membrane, then rapidly undergo aggregation into patches that are internalized to form endocytic vesicles within the cytoplasm.[96]

Insulin is also rapidly internalized by target cells, including hepatocytes, adipocytes, fibroblasts, and lymphocytes, and the concomitant uptake of receptor sites probably accounts for the "down regulation" of plasma membrane receptors in insulin-treated cells.[97] Like many other ligands, the receptor-bound insulin is initially located on microvilli and in coated pits on the cell surface. Whether such internalized hormone and receptors play a role in the cellular actions of insulin is not yet clear. In vivo, the uptake of insulin by liver cells is very rapid; internalization of up to 90 percent of the bound hormone occurs within 10 min, followed by association of the hormone with intracellular vesicles and ER.[98] The hormone-receptor complexes are subsequently taken up in endocytic vesicles, which undergo conversion into vacuoles called *endosomes* or *receptosomes*[99] prior to further processing of the internalized complexes. The final fate of the hormone-receptor complex may vary in different cell types, but could involve lysosomal degradation of the ligand and a proportion of the internalized receptor sites. In addition, some of the receptors may be recycled to the cell surface via a system of vesicles and exocytic evaginations.

In many cells, there is considerable recycling of plasma membrane proteins following the formation of endocytic vesicles during the processes of both receptor-mediated and fluid-phase pinocytosis. The plasma membrane that is internalized during the formation of endocytic vesicles often undergoes sorting to separate the vacuolar membrane from its contents, such that the endocytosed material is accumulated or metabolized within the cell, while the membrane components recycle to and from the surface after fusion events with other endocytic vesicles, lysosomes, or Golgi apparatus.[100] Many proteins, hormones, toxins, and viruses enter cells by receptor-mediated endocytosis and find their way to various destinations via defined intracellular pathways. The occupied peptide hormone receptors usually become concentrated in clathrin-coated pits on the cell surface prior to internalization, a route shared by numerous ligands and viruses. The ability of coated pits to distinguish between occupied and unoccupied receptors implies that hormone binding causes a conformational change in the receptor site that is recognized by the trapping mechanism of the pit.[101] However, receptors that capture macromolecular nutrients, including those for LDL and transferrin, as well as for asialoglycoproteins and α_2-macroglobulin, are already clustered in coated pits in the absence of the ligands. Such receptors undergo continuous endocytosis and recycling to the plasma membrane even in the absence of ligand, in contrast to the triggering of endocytosis that appears to result from the binding of hormonal ligands to their receptor sites.

The receptor-bound ligand rapidly enters the cells through coated pits and passes into adjacent vesicles, the endosomes (or endocytic vesicles or receptosomes) (Fig. 5-18). These appear to form from the base of the coated pit or from perimembranous coated vesicles, possibly under the driving force of an osmotic gradient. The endosomes move by saltatory motion to the Golgi region of the cell within about 20 min,

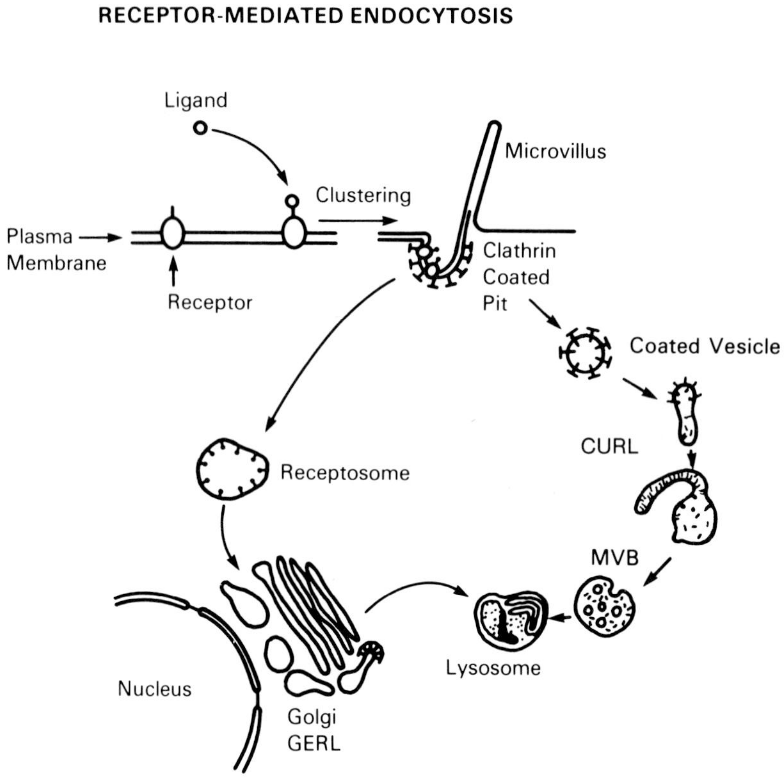

FIGURE 5-18 Receptor-mediated endocytosis of peptide hormone–receptor complexes via coated vesicles and/or endosomes (receptosomes). Most of the internalized ligand is degraded in lysosomes; a variable and probably small fraction of receptors is recycled to the plasma membrane.

apparently along the tracks of microtubules connecting the Golgi apparatus to the cell surface. Endosomes or receptosomes are 2 to 4 μm in diameter and do not contain hydrolytic enzymes, but their internal pH is acidic, similar to that of lysosomes. Endosomes do not appear to fuse directly with lysosomes, but probably pass on their contents via secondary endosomes or coated pits present in the reticular portion of the Golgi apparatus.[102] In either case, the endosome provides an acid environment through which the internalized receptor-ligand complexes must pass, and is also the site from which membrane recycling occurs to the cell surface. Since many hormones and other ligands are rapidly dissociated from their receptors at pH 5 to 6, the acidic environment of the endosome favors release of the bound hormone from its internalized receptor sites. Whereas the ligand is usually delivered to lysosomes for degradation, the receptors are often returned to the cell membrane to engage in further cycles of ligand binding and internalization. These processes are major features of the cellular processing of macromolecules, toxins, and viruses. In the case of transferrin, it is the bound iron that is released within the endosome, while the receptor-transferrin complex is returned to the cell surface.[103] One route by which receptors reach the plasma membrane is via the exocytic pathway after fusion of receptosomes with Golgi elements, especially in cells that are rich in secretory granules.

The extent to which various peptide hormones and their receptors are internalized and then recycled or degraded is still under study. Most peptide ligands enter their target cells to some degree by receptor-mediated endocytosis; this would account for the occurrence of down regulation in many agonist-stimulated cells and tissues. However, the prevalence of receptor recycling to the plasma membrane is less clear. Minor degrees of recycling of receptors for insulin and a few other peptides has been observed, and may be a general consequence of the internalization process. In most cells the internalized hormone is rapidly degraded after its transfer to lysosomes, but in some cases the ligand is recycled and released from the cell. This has been observed with enkephalin and EGF, and also occurs during the transit of ligands across specialized mural cells, as in the receptor-mediated transport of insulin and possibly other hormones across vascular endothelial cells.[104]

Further evidence for hormone internalization has come from studies on the uptake and metabolism of gonadotropins in cells of the testis and ovary. The presence of gonadotropin-binding sites in the cytoplasm of ovarian cells has been demonstrated by immunocytochemistry and autoradiography. After in vivo treatment with hCG, localization of the hormone is demonstrable in the cytoplasm and in membrane and perinuclear sites. In the corpus luteum, significant amounts of ^{125}I-hCG are taken up into endocytic vesicles and incorporated into dense bodies, presumably lysosomes. Lysosomal degradation of gonadotropins also occurs in Leydig tumor cells, in which the binding and metabolism of ^{125}I-hCG is not affected by agents which alter microfilaments and microtubules.[105] The loss of gonadotropin receptors induced by hCG in the ovary is accompanied by progressive internalization of receptor-bound ^{125}I-hCG, and a proportion of the translocated radioactivity can be identified as the hormone-receptor complex after solubilization and density gradient centrifugation.

In ovarian granulosa cells and testicular Leydig cells, gonadotropin binding is prominent over microvilli and is followed by receptor aggregation and internalization of the bound hormone, which occurs only occasionally via coated pits and vesicles. The internalized complexes are partly incorporated into lysosomes and degraded, and some are localized over Golgi elements, whence recycling to the plasma membrane could occur.[106] Such findings have indicated that internalization is a common sequel to hormone-receptor interaction and is probably responsible for down regulation of surface receptors after exposure to elevated concentrations of the homologous hormone.[87] In many endocrine target cells, agonist-induced phosphorylation of receptor sites may be an important factor in the initiation of receptor internalization, as well as in the modulation of receptor function.

A recent and important development in the understanding of receptor processing has been the finding that certain integral membrane proteins undergo rapid turnover between the plasma membrane and a microvesicular pool that regulates cellular membrane transport and appears to be derived from the Golgi complex. This mechanism participates in insulin stimulation of glucose transport, histamine stimulation of gastric acid secretion, and vasopressin stimulation of water permeability in bladder and kidney cells.[107] In the glucose transporter system, recruitment of transporter elements from a light membrane (presumably Golgi) fraction to the plasma membrane occurs during insulin action in fat cells.[108] This change in glucose transporter sites, measured by binding studies with cytochalasin B, occurs simultaneously with the insulin-stimulated increase in glucose uptake, and is presumed to be responsible for the action of insulin on glucose transport.[109] A similar form of turnover between plasma membrane and adjacent residues has been observed for plasma membrane receptors, including those for IGF 2, transferrin, LDL, and insulin, and may be a general feature of the regulation of cell surface receptors for peptide hormones. This type of translocation has been well demonstrated for β-adrenergic receptors, which undergo sequestration into a vesicular membrane fraction after occupancy by agonist ligands in several tissues. In this location the receptors are segregated from their membrane effector systems, and are no longer coupled to the guanyl nucleotide regulatory and catalytic subunits of adenylate cyclase.[109a]

Functional Classes of Membrane Receptors

Peptide hormones and other cell surface ligands are internalized and degraded at widely differing rates after binding to their plasma membrane receptors. The two extremes of ligand-receptor activation and processing are associated with two general classes of receptors,[110] according to the extent to which the ligand-receptor system primarily subserves information transfer, as in the case of hormone receptors, or mediates ligand uptake and metabolism, as exemplified LDL receptors (Table 5-4). By these criteria, one

Table 5-4. Classification of Plasma Membrane Receptors

Class I Receptors: Hormones and Growth Factors
Major function is information transfer and rapid metabolic regulation.
Internalization is not required but often occurs.
Occupancy by ligand alters receptor conformation and elicits typical cellular response.
Receptor activation by ligand (or antibody or lectin) releases encoded signal.
Ligand-receptor complexes are subsequently metabolized; receptors usually are not reused.
All show down regulation and/or desensitization.
Disordered function leads to under- or overstimulation of target cell.
Class II Receptors: Nutrients and Ligands for Clearance
Major function is internalization of macromolecules.
Binding only mediates ligand uptake; has no signal function.
Metabolism of ligand may alter cell activity.
No change in surface receptors (except LDL, secondarily).
Internalized receptors are not catabolized, but are recycled and reused.
Rarely show down regulation.
Disordered function leads to inadequate or excessive ligand internalization.

major class of receptors (class I) is responsible for binding traditional hormones, neurotransmitters, and other hormonal agents such as IgE and chemotactic peptides. This class of receptors often shows down-regulation and/or desensitization after binding their agonist ligands; their major function is target cell stimulation and rapid regulation of metabolic processes. Internalization of the hormone-receptor complex often occurs, but is not an essential step in the target cell activation mechanism. In contrast, class II receptors are mainly concerned with the uptake and internalization of macromolecules, and are recycled to the cell surface after endocytosis. They do not usually undergo down-regulation, except as a secondary response to altered cellular metabolism, as in the case of LDL receptors.

Disordered function of class I receptors is manifested by under- or overstimulation of cellular activity, whereas abnormalities of class II receptors give rise to inadequate or excessive internalization of the macromolecular ligand. This functional classification of plasma membrane receptors provides a useful basis for comparing the biochemical and functional properties of individual receptor systems, and for relating their physiological features to the clinical consequences of abnormalities in receptor structure and function.

Table 5-5. Formation and Disposition of Intracellular Messengers

1. Derived from abundant precursors
   - ATP, GTP
   - Membrane phospholipids
   - Extracellular Ca^{2+} and internal Ca^{2+} stores
2. Rapidly generated during hormone action
   - cAMP, cGMP
   - IP_3, DG
   - Elevated cystolic Ca^{2+} concentration
3. Usually formed in small amounts
   - cAMP, cGMP
   - IP_3, DG
   - Ca/calmodulin
4. Rapidly decreased by available enzymatic mechanisms
   - Phosphodiesterase
     - cAMP → AMP
     - cGMP → GMP
   - Inositol and lipid metabolism
     - $IP_3 \rightarrow IP_2 \rightarrow IP \rightarrow$ inositol
     - DG → PA
   - Calcium pumps

Abbreviations: DG, diacylglycerol; IP_3, inositol trisphosphate; PA, phosphatidic acid.

INTRACELLULAR MEDIATORS OF PEPTIDE HORMONE ACTION

The Second Messenger Hypothesis

The transfer of incoming hormonal signals to the cell interior is performed by a group of "second messengers" that are generated at the plasma membrane level as a consequence of receptor activation (Table 5-5). The original formulation of this concept by Sutherland and Robison (Fig. 5-3) envisaged a general transduction mechanism by which peptide hormones act upon the cell surface to stimulate the formation of second messengers such as cyclic AMP. This general scheme of peptide hormone action on membrane receptors and adenylate cyclase was based upon studies with catecholamines, vasopressin, glucagon, and ACTH. It has since been extended to other hormones and transmitters that influence adenylate cyclase activity either positively or negatively to increase or decrease intracellular cAMP levels. In addition, many hormones and neurotransmitters stimulate a calcium-dependent signaling system that involves the production of two recently identified messengers, inositol trisphosphate (IP_3) and diacylglycerol, from the phospholipids of the plasma membrane. However, for several peptide hormones, including insulin, GH, and prolactin, the exact mechanisms of target cell activation have not been clarified. Several growth factors have recently been found to promote phosphorylation of their homologous receptors via an intrinsic kinase domain of the cytoplasmic region of the receptor molecule, but the signaling process initiated by such autophosphorylation is not yet known.

For tissues in which cyclic AMP is the major second messenger of peptide hormone action, the manner in which a single effector system is translated into a spectrum of individual target cell responses is not completely clear. This question is complicated by the dual nature of many peptide and protein hormones, which function both as trophic factors with long-term effects on cell growth and differentiation, and as regulators of rapid target cell responses such as steroidogenesis and hormone secretion. An outline of these slow and rapid actions of hormones that exert both long-term growth effects and short-term metabolic effects[111] is shown in Fig. 5-19. The relationship between these two aspects of peptide hormone action is not well understood, and current knowledge about cellular responses to hormone-receptor interaction is largely based on studies of the early actions of peptide hormones upon their target cells. There is now evidence for the participation of several messenger systems in target cells that were previously thought to be under the control of a predominant signal pathway,

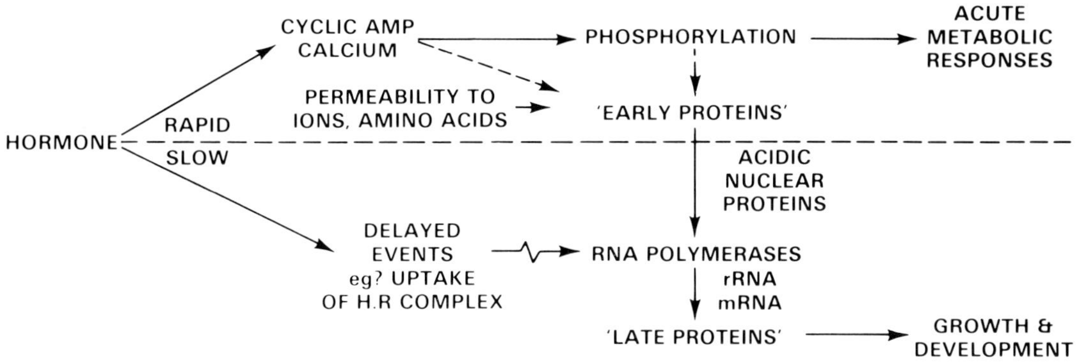

FIGURE 5-19 General scheme of the integration of early and late responses to hormones causing both acute metabolic responses and long-term growth and development. (*After Tata.*[111])

such as cAMP/protein kinase A, calcium/calmodulin, and DAG/protein kinase C. The interacting effects of these multiple activation systems could account for many of the immediate and long-term effects of hormones on target cell function. Internalization and processing of the hormone-receptor complex, while not involved in the immediate cell response, could also generate signals responsible for the maintenance of cell differentiation.

The intracellular signal molecules generated by hormone-receptor interaction subsequently act upon membrane and cytoplasmic proteins to alter rate-limiting steps in effector systems that control target cell responses. The best-characterized mediators are calcium and cyclic AMP, which act as intracellular transmitters to adjust target cell metabolism in response to external regulatory factors such as hormones and other ligands. The calcium stimulus is provided by an increase in cytosolic calcium concentration, both by uptake of calcium from the extracellular fluid and redistribution of intracellular calcium stores; the cyclic nucleotides, however, are generated from ATP and GTP by activation of nucleotide triphosphate cyclizing enzymes situated in the plasma membrane and cytosol, respectively. The formation of cAMP is directly linked to cell surface receptor occupancy and activation of adenylate cyclase bound to the inner surface of the plasma membrane. In contrast, guanylate cyclase is located predominantly in the cytosol, and is not activated directly by hormonal stimuli. Calcium has important effects on both adenylate and guanylate cyclase activity and on cyclic nucleotide breakdown by phosphodiesterases. Thus, changes in the intracellular calcium concentration can exert significant effects upon cellular cyclic AMP and cyclic GMP levels.[112] Conversely, in several tissues, including nerve, muscle, and secretory cells, the cyclic AMP pathway appears to act by modulating the intracellular level of calcium.

Although the essential role of calcium in stimulus-response coupling during activation of contractile and secretory processes is well established, the manifold actions of cyclic AMP as a second messenger have tended to overshadow the importance of calcium as an intracellular regulator. More recently, the significance of regulatory interactions between cyclic nucleotides and calcium has been recognized,[113] and the primacy of calcium as a cytosolic mediator has been demonstrated in numerous hormone-dependent target tissues.[114]

Adenylate Cyclase, Cyclic AMP, and cAMP-Dependent Protein Kinase

Since hormonal stimulation of target cells is usually intermittent and transient, intracellular second messengers must be subject to rapid turnover (by decay or recycling) so that repetitive and graded external stimuli can be faithfully converted into quantitative cellular responses (Table 5-5). The dynamic equilibrium between formation and removal of cyclic nucleotides controls their intracellular levels in basal and hormone-activated states, and permits rapid responses to changes in extracellular regulators. This regulation is largely exerted through activation or inhibition of adenylate cyclase within the cell membrane, leading to changes in the production and intracellular concentration of cyclic AMP. In some cells, the rate of breakdown of cAMP by specific phosphodiesterases is also under hormonal regulation, and can influence the intracellular concentration and actions of the nucleotide (Fig. 5-3). In all eukaryotic cells, the actions of cAMP are expressed through the activation of cAMP-dependent phosphokinases (protein kinases) that catalyze the phosphorylation of specific protein substrates in the target cell. The elucidation of this major pathway of peptide hormone action includes clarification of the hormonal regulation of adenylate cyclase and phosphodiesterase, and of the activation and functions of cAMP-dependent protein kinase.

REGULATION OF ADENYLATE CYCLASE ACTIVITY

Cyclic AMP and adenylate cyclase were discovered during studies on the control of hepatic glycogenolysis exerted by adrenaline and glucagon,[11] which stimulate the activity of glycogen phosphorylase and promote the breakdown of glycogen to glucose phosphates. The activation of glycogen phosphorylase by these hyperglycemic hormones was found to require an intermediate step (later shown to be phosphorylation by protein kinase) that was stimulated by a heat-stable factor generated by the interaction of hormone with the particulate fraction of the liver cell. The latter reaction was found to require ATP, which in the presence of hormone and magnesium ion was converted to cAMP and inorganic phosphate. The enzyme responsible for this step was shown to be situated on the inner surface of the plasma membrane, and to be activated by a wide variety of peptide hormones (Fig. 5-3). Originally referred to as *adenyl cyclase,* the plasma membrane enzyme has since been termed *adenylate cyclase* or *adenylyl cyclase* to more precisely describe its specific cyclizing action on ATP.

The identification of adenylate cyclase as a membrane-bound enzyme that is regulated by catecholamines and peptide hormones was followed by numerous studies on the involvement of cAMP in hormone-dependent processes. It soon became evident that only hormones such as peptides and transmitters, which are bound to the cell surface, activate adenylate cyclase. In contrast, hormones such as thyroxine and steroids, which act via intracellular receptors, have no consistent effects upon the adenylate cyclase–cAMP system. The cyclizing enzyme was at first envisaged as a receptor subunit (the recognition site for peptide hormones) and a catalytic subunit (to convert ATP to cyclic AMP). Later, these subunits were proposed to exist as separate entities, floating in the lipid bilayer of the cell membrane, which become associated into an active unit upon hormonal occupancy of the receptor site.[48] This concept led to a two-step theory of enzyme activation, in which the hormone-receptor complex diffuses laterally within the cell membrane to interact with (and activate) the catalytic subunits situated on the cytoplasmic surface of the plasma membrane (Fig. 5-9).

This relatively simple model of the adenylate cyclase system was further elaborated by the recognition that an intermediate process (transduction) intervenes between hormone-receptor interaction and activation of the catalytic subunit. This intermediate coupling step was discovered in the hepatic adenylate cyclase system, where guanyl nucleotides were found to enhance the activation of adenylate cyclase by glucagon and to promote dissociation of the hormone from its receptors. These findings suggested that glucagon does not directly stimulate adenylate cyclase, but facilitates its activation by guanyl nucleotides. Regulatory effects of guanyl nucleotides upon adenylate cyclase have been observed in a wide variety of eukaryotic tissues, where they act as obligatory cofactors in the actions of many peptide hormones and transmitters.[50] The general dependence of peptide hormones on guanyl nucleotides for both activation and inhibition of adenylate cyclase has led to the recognition of several nucleotide regulatory proteins that mediate peptide hormone action on adenylate cyclase and other membrane enzymes.

The current view of hormonal activation of adenylate cyclase incorporates ligand-dependent introduction of GTP to the regulatory site as the primary step in peptide hormone action (Fig. 5-10). Binding of GTP to an adjacent regulatory protein (N) converts the inactive catalytic unit (C) to its active enzymatic cyclizing form; this activation process is terminated by hydrolysis of the bound GTP to GDP, which returns the enzyme to its basal state. This mechanism has been supported by the finding that hormone-stimulated GTPase activity is associated with the guanyl nucleotide regulatory site. The ability of nonhydrolyzable GTP analogues [such as Gpp(NH)p and GTP-γ-S] to cause marked and prolonged activation of adenylate cyclase is further evidence for this mechanism. The resistance of such synthetic analogues to hydrolysis by GTPase causes persistent occupancy of the regulatory site by an active nucleotide instead of the usual transient effect of bound GTP, which is rapidly degraded to GDP. This mechanism also accounts for the ability of cholera toxin to "lock" the adenylate cyclase system into a persistently activated state. This phenomenon is dependent upon the availability of GTP, and reflects the inhibition of hormone-stimulated GTPase activity by the toxin.[116] The effect of cholera toxin is exerted through stimulation of ADP-ribose transfer (from NAD^+) to the GTP-binding protein,[117] with consequent inhibition of its GTPase activity and prolonged activation of adenylate cyclase.

These findings have led to the view that adenylate cyclase activity is "turned on" by hormone-stimulated GTP binding in the presence of ATP substrate, and turned off by GTP hydrolysis at the regulatory site, as shown in Fig. 5-20. The turn-off reaction is inhibited by nonphysiological agents such as Gpp(NH)p and cholera toxin, and may also serve as a control point for regulation of adenylate cyclase activity by other intracellular signals.

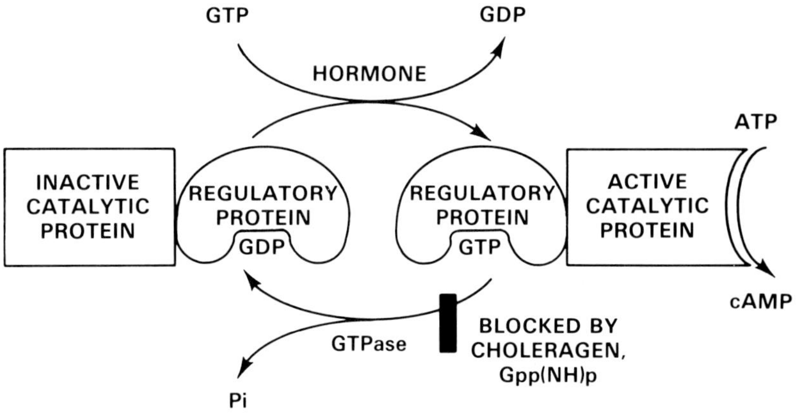

FIGURE 5-20 Role of guanyl nucleotides in the hormonal regulation of adenylate cyclase. Hormone-receptor interaction leads to binding of GTP to the regulatory site and activation of adenylate cyclase. Hydrolysis of GTP to GDP by an associated GTPase restores the enzyme to its inactive form. Cholera toxin irreversibly inactivates the enzyme by blocking GTPase activity. Occupancy of the GTP regulatory site by nonhydrolyzable analogues such as Gpp(NH)p also causes prolonged activation of the enzyme. (*After Cassell et al.*[116])

The importance of the regulatory site has also been shown by studies on reconstitution of hormone-sensitive adenylate cyclase, employing both cell fusion and addition of soluble cell extracts to complementary membranes. In fusion experiments, heterokaryons formed between erythroleukemia cells (without β receptors) and turkey erythrocytes (containing β receptors and chemically inactivated adenylate cyclase) showed catecholamine-responsive cyclase activity that was absent from the donor cells.[118] Also, receptors for LH have been transferred in lipid-rich ovarian extracts to adrenal fasciculata cells, where they mediate effects of gonadotropins on cAMP and corticosteroid production.[16] Such findings suggest that a general coupling mechanism occurs between hormone receptors and the components of the adenylate cyclase system, manifested by the interaction between heterotopic receptors and adenylate cyclase of the host cell. In reconstitution experiments, plasma membranes of mutant lymphoma cells that possess β-adrenergic receptors and adenylate cyclase which are uncoupled (i.e., not responsive to catecholamines) have shown return of catecholamine-stimulated cyclase activity after addition of extracts from wild-type cells.[118] This reflects the incorporation of a coupling factor into the mutant cell membrane, and has led to the discovery of the nucleotide regulatory proteins that are described below. Like the cell fusion studies noted above, this result emphasizes the physical independence of hormone receptors and adenylate cyclase, and demonstrates the ability of receptors to undergo lateral movement and interact with the nucleotide regulatory units within the cell membrane. This implies that regions of conformational similarity are present in many hormone receptors, in addition to the unique conformations that exist in the region of the specific hormone-binding site.[119] More detailed structural analysis of peptide hormone receptors should reveal the nature of the common domain that is responsible for interaction with the regulatory components of membrane effector enzymes.

THE DUAL CONTROL OF HORMONE-SENSITIVE ADENYLATE CYCLASE

During the last 5 years, notable advances have been made in the analysis of adenylate cyclase systems and their control by hormones, transmitters, and drugs. Following the realization that hormones can exert inhibitory as well as stimulatory effects on adenylate cyclase, these two opposing forms of control were found to be mediated by specific guanyl nucleotide–binding regulatory proteins in the plasma membrane.[120] The receptors that cause activation of adenylate cyclase include those for stimulatory hormones and ligands, as listed in Table 5-1 and exemplified by β-adrenergic agonists, and hypothalamic and pituitary hormones, including CRF, growth hormone releasing factor, ACTH, LH, FSH, and TSH. Those causing inhibition of adenylate cyclase include receptors for α_2-adrenergic and muscarinic agonists, opiates, angiotensin II, and somatostatin. With the exception of somatostatin, the physiological significance of most such inhibitory effects is not yet clear.

The nucleotide regulatory proteins that mediate the stimulatory and inhibitory control of adenylate cyclase by hormone receptors are termed *Ns* and *Ni* (or Gs and Gi) to indicate the importance of guanyl nucleotides in this process.[121] Both Ns and Ni are $\alpha\beta\gamma$ heterotrimers that are structurally and functionally related to transducin, the regulatory protein that couples rhodopsin, the photon receptor, to a cGMP-specific phosphodiesterase in the rod outer segment. The three proteins are composed of dissimilar subunits, with individual differences in the α subunits (mol wt 39,000 to 42,000), similar β subunits of mol wt 35,000, and γ subunits of mol wt 5000 to 8000. The α subunits of Ns and Ni are specifically ADP-ribosylated by cholera toxin (Ns-α) or *Bordetella pertussis* toxin (Ni-α), which respectively stimulate adenylate cyclase or block its inhibition by hormones such as somatostatin. The α subunits also contain binding sites for guanyl nucleotides and magnesium. Occupancy of the former sites by GTP induces an active state of the N protein that can either stimulate or inhibit the catalytic (C) unit of adenylate cyclase; this process is normally terminated by the intrinsic GTPase activity of the regulatory protein. In the presence of Mg^{2+}, nonhydrolyzable GTP analogues such as Gpp(NH)p induce an irreversible form of the active state that persists after removal of the nucleotide and is associated with prolonged activation of adenylate cyclase activity by the bound analogue.

Each of the nucleotide regulatory proteins is activated by the dissociation of their subunits under the influence of hormonal ligands or added guanyl nucleotides, with release of the activated α subunits from the inhibitory influence of the common $\beta\gamma$ subunits (Fig. 5-21). Thus, in the case of the stimulatory Ns protein, hormones promote the sequence: $\alpha \cdot \beta \cdot \gamma$ + GTP $\rightleftharpoons$ $\alpha \cdot$GTP + $\beta \cdot \gamma$. The free guanyl nucleotide–activated α subunit interacts with and stimulates the enzymatic activity of the C unit of adenylate cyclase. In contrast, the $\beta\gamma$ subunit pair serves to inhibit activation, and may also terminate the activation process by recombining with the free α subunit to form the inactive $\alpha\beta\gamma$ Ns trimer. The manner in which the activated α subunit stimulates the enzymatic activity of the C unit is not yet known, but may involve an increase in enzyme affinity for free Mg^{2+}, which appears to be rate-limiting for cyclase activity in the intact cell.[122]

The primary structure of the α subunit of Ns, the GTP-binding stimulatory protein of adenylate cyclase, has been deduced from the sequence of a bovine adrenal cDNA clone that encodes the entire sequence of Ns.[123] The Ns α subunit shows striking homologies with the α subunit of transducin, which regulates phosphodiesterase activity in the visual transduction system. However, there is very little homology between the Ns α subunit and the oncogene *ras*–encoded proteins that modulate adenylate cyclase activity, except in short regions that may be involved in GTP binding and hydrolysis. The regions of homology between Ns-α and transducin-α are such that more than one-half of the Ns-α sequence shows at least 30 percent identity with the corresponding half of transducin-α. Such homology must reflect common properties of the two α subunits, including binding and hydrolysis of guanyl nucleotides, interaction with the $\beta \cdot \gamma$ subunit pairs, and ADP-ribosylation by bacterial toxins.

The mechanism by which Ni causes inhibition of adenylate cyclase activity is also not completely clear, since both the GTP-activated α subunit of Ni and the free β subunit (or $\beta\gamma$) can exert inhibitory effects on enzyme activity.[124] It is possible that the $\beta\gamma$ subunits generated by activation and dissociation of Ni (which is present in considerable excess over Ns in the plasma membrane) could complex with activated Ns α subunits and thus diminish adenylate cyclase activity.[121]

In conjunction with their effects upon adenylate

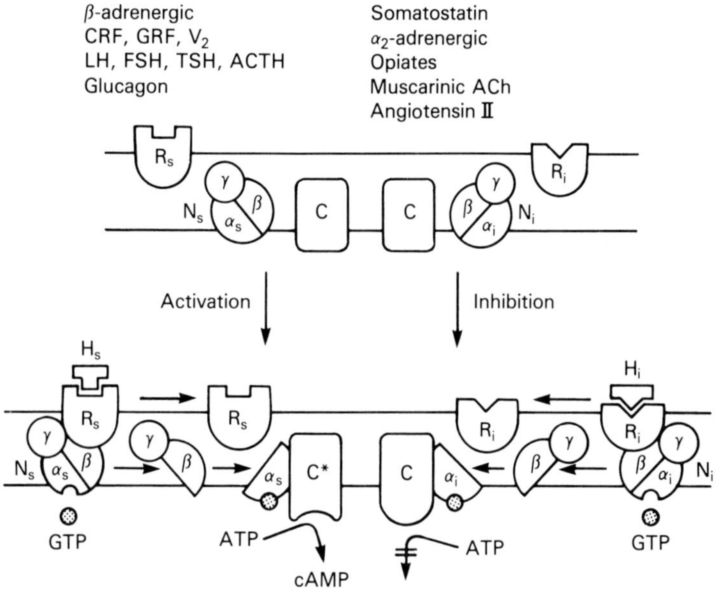

FIGURE 5-21 Regulation of adenylate cyclase activity by stimulatory and inhibitory hormones via specific receptors (Rs, Ri) and guanine nucleotide stimulatory (Ns) and inhibitory (Ni) regulatory proteins. (*Modified from Helmreich and Pfeuffer.*[120])

cyclase activation, guanyl nucleotides frequently influence the binding kinetics and affinity of the hormone-receptor interaction. An important effect of GTP on receptor affinity is its ability to reduce the "tightness" of hormone binding, from that of high affinity (almost irreversible in some cases) to a much lower affinity state. This was first observed for the binding of glucagon and β-adrenergic agonists to their receptors and is a frequent feature of the binding of agonist ligands that stimulate adenylate cyclase. In contrast, binding of β-adrenergic antagonists is not altered by guanyl nucleotides, indicating that coupling of the receptor-ligand complex to adenylate cyclase is necessary for guanyl nucleotides to enhance the dissociation of receptor-bound agonist.[90] While the evidence from studies on the glucagon system favors the existence of distinct nucleotide sites involved in the regulation of receptor binding and adenylate cyclase activity, the role of these sites in hormonal activation and receptor-enzyme coupling is still uncertain. The low-affinity receptor state induced by GTP has been considered to be the favored precursor state for the coupling process, and the uncoupled high-affinity form of the receptor may be associated with the inactive state of the enzyme, as seen in desensitization of adenylate cyclase by increasing hormone concentrations.[90]

CYCLIC AMP–DEPENDENT PROTEIN KINASES

The discovery of cyclic AMP and its role in mediating the hormonal stimulation of hepatic glycogenolysis led to the recognition that the cyclic nucleotide is involved in a wide variety of metabolic functions. This was indicated by the universal presence of cAMP in prokaryotes and eukaryotes and its involvement in reactions other than those concerned with hormone action.[11] Cystic AMP–dependent phosphorylation and activation of regulatory enzymes, first observed for phosphorylase kinase in liver cells, proved to be a general mechanism in eukaryotic cells, in which all the actions of cAMP are expressed through phosphorylation of protein substrates. Cyclic AMP–dependent protein kinases are present in all eukaryotic cells, where they serve to mediate the effects of cAMP on cellular metabolism.[125] In prokaryotes, the actions of cAMP are expressed through another mechanism, by interaction of cyclic AMP–binding proteins with regulatory regions of the genome. Several other types of protein phosphokinase, in addition to the cAMP-dependent enzymes, are present in most cells and participate in metabolic control mechanisms.

In animal tissues, cAMP-dependent protein kinases catalyze the transfer of phosphate from ATP to specific serine (and sometimes threonine) residues of many protein substrates. These include enzymes such as phosphorylase kinase, glycogen synthase, and hormone-sensitive lipase, as well as nonenzymatic cellular proteins such as histones, nuclear nonhistone proteins, ribosomal proteins, microtubules, and membranes.[126] Most of the enzyme substrates exist in either phosphorylated or dephosphorylated forms, and are interconverted between their active and inactive states by the concerted actions of protein phosphokinase and phosphoprotein phosphatase. Protein phosphokinases, including cyclic AMP–dependent protein kinase, transfer the γ phosphate group from ATP to protein substrates, while phosphoprotein phosphatases catalyze the hydrolysis of phosphate groups from phosphoproteins. This cycle of phosphorylation and dephosphorylation is a ubiquitous mechanism of cellular regulation, not only for metabolic enzymes but also for control of contractile mechanisms, membrane activities, and nuclear processes. At the functional level, such effects are expressed as the physiological processes of muscle contraction, secretion, and neuronal function.

The recognition that all animal cells contain cAMP-dependent protein kinase led to the concept that the diverse effects of cAMP are expressed through this single class of enzymes.[15] In this view, the specificity of cAMP-mediated responses depends on the actions of the protein kinase and particularly on the nature of the protein substrates present in specific cell types.

A multitude of protein kinases might be expected to catalyze the phosphorylation of individual protein substrates during mediation of the many actions of cAMP. However, only two major forms of the cAMP-dependent enzyme have been identified in animal cells, so the specificity of each phosphorylation reaction must also depend on the location and nature of the protein substrate. Each protein substrate is believed to control a specific metabolic or physiological process, the rate of which is increased or decreased by phosphorylation of the regulatory protein. The manner in which protein phosphorylation mediates the biological actions of hormones and transmitters that operate through cyclic AMP is shown in Fig. 5-22.

The several forms of protein kinase can be broadly divided according to their nucleotide dependence or independence (Table 5-6). Cyclic nucleotide–independent protein kinases are present in all regions of the cell and are presumably regulated by other intracellular signals. More recently discovered classes of protein kinase depend on calcium-calmodulin or calcium and phospholipid components for activation, and are intimately involved in transmembrane control systems that are regulated by calcium. Many of the hormonally controlled protein kinases in endocrine

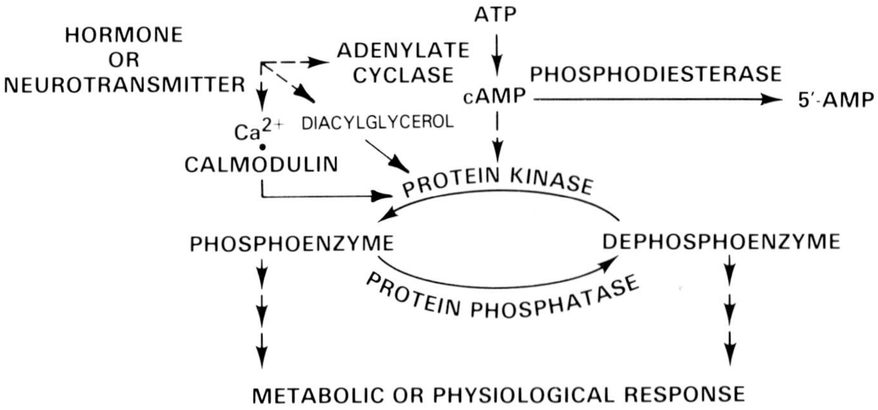

FIGURE 5-22 Stimulation of metabolic responses in an endocrine target cell by hormones which regulate protein phosphorylation via activation of protein kinases by cyclic AMP, calcium-calmodulin, and diacylglycerol (protein kinase C).

target cells are dependent on cyclic AMP or, less often, cyclic GMP. Such cyclic nucleotide–dependent protein kinases are abundant in the cytosol, but also occur in plasma membranes and other cell organelles. They are activated by micromolar concentrations of cyclic purine nucleotides (cAMP and cGMP), and are rapidly stimulated by the rises in cyclic nucleotide production that follow hormone action on the cell membrane. Both types of cyclic nucleotide–dependent protein kinase are activated by binding of the nucleotide to a specific site on the enzyme.

Cyclic AMP–dependent protein kinase exists in the inactive form as a tetramer composed of two types of subunits, one for binding cAMP and the other for catalysis of phosphate transfer to the protein substrate. The inactive tetramer consists of two binding or regulatory (R) subunits and two enzymatic or catalytic (C) subunits. Binding of cAMP to the R subunits causes the $R_2 \cdot C_2$ tetramer to dissociate, with release of the active C subunits responsible for phosphotransferase activity.[127] This sequence can be represented by the equation:

$$\underset{\text{(inactive)}}{R_2 \cdot C_2} + 4\text{cAMP} \rightleftharpoons R_2 \cdot \text{cAMP}_4 + \underset{\text{(active)}}{2C}$$

Once formed, the free C subunit is functionally similar to a cyclic AMP–independent protein kinase, but can be distinguished by its characteristic size (mol wt 38,000) and reactivity with a heat-stable inhibitory protein which blocks its catalytic activity and prevents recombination with the regulatory subunit. The catalytic subunit is common to both major forms of cAMP-dependent protein kinase, whereas the regulatory subunits show several differences. The regulatory subunits released on dissociation of protein kinase are believed to remain as an R_2 dimer, and later undergo reassociation with free catalytic subunits. In the absence of cAMP, the regulatory and catalytic subunits bind to each other with high affinity, and at physiological concentrations are mainly present as the inactive holoenzyme.[128]

The mammalian cAMP-dependent protein kinase holoenzymes can be fractionated into two major types by ion exchange chromatography (Table 5-7). The type I protein kinase is less acidic, and is eluted from DEAE-cellulose by salt concentrations below 100 mM. It is readily dissociated by substrate (histone) or high salt concentration (0.5 M NaCl), and re-forms slowly after dissociation by cAMP. The type II enzyme is more acidic and elutes from DEAE-cellulose at salt concentrations above 100 mM; it is slowly dissociated by histone and salt, but reassociates rapidly to form the inactive holoenzyme. The two forms of protein kinase are present in most tissues but their proportions vary in each cell type. Thus, the type I enzyme predominates in rabbit skeletal muscle, whereas the type II enzyme is present in bovine cardiac muscle. The two holoenzymes are generally sim-

Table 5-6. Classification of Protein Kinases

Cyclic nucleotide–dependent kinases
cAMP-dependent protein kinases, types I and II
cGMP-dependent protein kinases
Calcium-dependent kinases
Calcium/calmodulin-dependent protein kinases, types I, II, and III
Calcium/phospholipid-dependent protein kinase (protein kinase C)
Cyclic nucleotide– and calcium-independent kinases
Casein kinases
Pyruvate dehydrogenase kinase
Glycogen synthase kinase 3
Rhodopsin kinase; β-adrenergic receptor kinase
Tyrosine-specific kinases
Growth factor receptors
Oncogene products

Table 5-7. Properties of cAMP-Dependent Protein Kinases

	Type I	Type II
Tissue source	Rabbit skeletal muscle Cardiac muscle	Cardiac muscle Bovine brain Rat adipose tissue
Subunit structure	R_2C_2	R_2C_2
Molecular weight:		
Holoenzyme	~170,000	~185,000
R subunit	49,000	51,000–56,000
C subunit	39,000	39,000
Elution from DEAE-cellulose	< 0.1 M NaCl	0.2 M NaCl
Autophosphorylation	No	Yes
Reassociation after removal of cAMP	Slow	Rapid
Dissociation by salt and histone	Rapid	Slow

ilar in subunit composition ($R_2 \cdot C_2$) and molecular weight (about 170,000), and their catalytic subunits are identical (M_r 39,000). The regulatory subunits differ in their molecular weights, R1 being smaller (mol wt 49,000) and more uniform in size than R2 (52,000 to 56,000). Functionally, the main distinguishing features are that the type I enzyme binds MgATP, whereas the type II enzyme catalyzes the phosphorylation of its own regulatory subunit by ATP. Binding of ATP by the type I enzyme reduces its affinity for cAMP, and presumably favors the inactive state of the enzyme. The type I subunit, while binding ATP, is not phosphorylated by either enzyme, in contrast to the autophosphorylation shown by the type II enzyme.[129] This difference reflects the replacement of the serine residue that is autophosphorylated in the type II regulatory subunit by an alanine residue in the type I subunit.[130] The role of autophosphorylation of cAMP-dependent and other protein kinases is summarized in Table 5-8.

The functional significance of these two effects upon the R subunits is not clear, though the phosphorylation of type II enzymes could represent a more evolved form of the substrate (ATP) binding that occurs in the type I enzyme. The phosphorylation of type II protein kinase is accompanied by a decrease in the rate of reassociation of the dissociated R and C subunits. Thus, phosphorylation may serve to control the activity of the dissociated enzyme by regulating its rate of return to the inactive form. Increased dephosphorylation of R would favor recombination to the $R_2 \cdot C_2$ holoenzyme, followed by release and degradation of cAMP. In this way, the proportions of active and inactive enzyme could be regulated in the absence of changes in cAMP concentration. Another possibility is that type II enzymes concerned with rapid cycling of metabolic processes, as in cardiac and nerve tissue, have acquired the capacity for more highly regulated inactivation by the ultrashort feedback effect of a phosphorylation/dephosphorylation step on the regulatory subunit.

In addition to its role in the phosphorylation of defined enzymes such as phosphorylase kinase, cAMP-dependent protein kinase phosphorylates numerous basic proteins (including histones, casein, and protamine), as well as many denatured proteins (such as egg white lysozyme and bovine serum albumin) that are not substrates in their native states. Small basic peptides are also phosphorylated by the enzyme, as are

Table 5-8. Autophosphorylation and Protein Kinase Activity

Autophosphorylated Protein Kinases
Regulatory (R) subunit of cAMP-dependent protein kinase
Tyrosine kinase: EGF, insulin receptors
Protein kinase C
Ca^{2+}/calmodulin-dependent protein kinase type II
Effects of Autophosphorylation on Enzyme Activity
Diminished reassociation with holoenzyme
Activation of enzyme
Regulation of membrane association (?)
Decreased affinity for calmodulin, increased substrate phosphorylation

synthetic peptide sequences similar to the phosphorylated regions of native and denatured protein substrates. Although the phosphorylation reaction performed by protein kinase is not particularly selective for individual protein sequences, it has relatively high specificity for serine residues in defined regions of the primary sequence of many proteins. The structural requirements for phosphorylation of peptide substrates by protein kinase include the presence of two adjacent basic amino acids, one of which is arginine; the pair is situated two to five residues to the amino-terminal side of the target serine residue.[131]

In physiologically important protein substrates for cAMP-dependent protein kinase, two forms of amino acid sequence at the phosphorylation site have been defined:

1. -Lys-Arg-X-X-Ser-X-X
2. -Arg-Arg-X-Ser-X

In these sequences, X stands for any amino acid, though residues immediately adjacent to the serine usually have hydrophobic side chains. The first type of phosphorylation site, in which the basic amino acids are separated from serine by two residues, occurs in the β subunit of phosphorylase kinase and in glycogen synthase. The second type, with one intervening residue, occurs in pyruvate kinase and the regulatory subunit of type II cAMP-dependent protein kinase. Because the rate of phosphorylation depends on a relatively common primary sequence around the phosphorylated site, the substrate specificity of individual proteins must depend upon their secondary and tertiary (i.e., three-dimensional) conformations to restrict the accessibility of potentially phosphorylated regions to the catalytic enzyme units. A proposed role for secondary structure in substrate specificity is the location of the phosphorylated serine at the hydrophilic surface of substrate proteins, in a hydrogen-bonded β-bend structure that may be recognized by the protein kinase.[132]

Recently, the R^{II} subunit was found to be more heterogeneous than formerly realized, and subclasses of R^{II} were observed in various species and tissues, according to their antigenicity and apparent molecular weights, which range from 52,000 to 56,000.[133] Whether these isoforms of R^{II} represent different gene products is not yet known, but their selective regulation during differentiation and hormonal stimulation could provide an avenue for specific actions mediated via the cAMP-kinase pathway. In some tissues, free R^{I} and R^{II} subunits are present in considerable excess over the catalytic subunit, raising the possibility that R subunits may interact with other cellular proteins or structures. A selective increase in R^{II} subunit is stimulated by cAMP-mediated ligands in several cells and tissues in association with the induction of differentiation, as in the maturing rat granulosa cell under the influence of FSH.[134] It is possible that much of the type II holoenzyme exists in the autophosphorylated form in situ, and that R^{II} becomes dephosphorylated after dissociation of the enzymes by cAMP.

MECHANISMS OF GLYCOGENOLYSIS AND LIPOLYSIS

The hormonal control of intermediary metabolism and energy production has been one of the best-studied areas of peptide hormone action. The general aspects of hormonal regulation of glucose homeostasis are relatively well defined, but the cellular mechanisms are more complex than formerly believed. During fasting, the liver is the main source of circulating glucose, which is released at a rate dependent on the blood glucose level and the actions of catabolic hormones such as glucagon and catecholamines. Insulin is the major inhibitor of glucose release under physiological conditions, and opposes the actions of the catabolic hormones when secreted after feeding. The glucose released from the liver during fasting is derived from glycogenolysis until glycogen stores are depleted, and then by gluconeogenesis from lactate and amino acids. The neural and hormonal control of glycogen metabolism in skeletal muscle and liver is mediated by changes in the phosphorylation states of phosphorylase kinase, glycogen phosphorylase, and glycogen synthase.

Early studies on hepatic glycogenolysis in dog liver revealed that cAMP, formed by adenylate cyclase in response to glucagon and epinephrine, caused activation of glycogen phosphorylase.[135] This reaction depends on the conversion of phosphorylase kinase from its inactive (dephosphorylated) form to the active phosphorylated enzyme, which then catalyzes the activation of glycogen phosphorylase by a further phosphorylation step. The active glycogen phosphorylase breaks down glycogen to glucose 1-phosphate, which is converted to glucose 6-phosphate and then to free glucose to be released into the circulation. The cAMP-dependent enzyme responsible for activation of phosphorylase kinase, originally termed "phosphorylase kinase kinase," was found to be widely distributed in nature and capable of catalyzing the phosphorylation of many protein substrates other than phosphorylase kinase. This led to the view that all the actions of cAMP in higher organisms are mediated by protein phosphorylation reactions performed by cAMP-dependent protein kinase, which acts as the intracellular receptor for cyclic AMP.[15]

Phosphorylase kinase is activated by calcium ions as well as by cAMP, and thus serves as a target of the two major intracellular messenger systems. The enzyme is quite large (mol wt 1,300,000) and is a complex of four subunits with the structure $\alpha\beta\gamma\delta_4$. The α and β subunits contain phosphorylation sites for cAMP-dependent protein kinase, the γ subunit is the catalytic domain, and the δ subunit is calmodulin that is complexed to the γ subunit. Phosphorylation of the α and β subunits by cAMP-dependent protein kinase increases phosphorylase kinase activity about 20-fold and substantially increases its affinity for calcium. In this manner, phosphorylation both enhances catalytic activity and also promotes activation in the absence of a rise in calcium concentration. The activity of the dephosphorylated form of phosphorylase kinase is also increased by the binding of a second molecule of calmodulin (the δ subunit) to the α and β subunits of the enzyme in the presence of calcium. In skeletal muscle, troponin C can substitute for calmodulin and increases the activity of the dephosphorylated enzyme 20-fold, so it is probably the major activator of phosphorylase kinase in vivo. Thus, the activity of phosphorylase kinase is controlled by two similar calcium-binding proteins whose relative importance depends on the phosphorylation state of the enzyme. Whereas calmodulin determines the calcium sensitivity of the phosphorylated enzyme, troponin C acts as the dominant regulator of the dephosphorylated enzyme.[136]

The general scheme of glycogen metabolism in the liver, illustrated in Fig. 5-23, depends on the activation of protein kinase by catabolic hormones, followed by phosphorylation of phosphorylase kinase and glycogen synthase. Phosphorylation activates the kinase and deactivates the synthase, causing accelerated phosphorolytic breakdown of glycogen and reduced synthesis of glycogen from UDP-glucose. Protein kinase was also found to mediate the effects of cAMP on glycogen breakdown in skeletal muscle during the provision of glucose 1-phosphate for glycolysis. In addition to stimulating the breakdown of glycogen to glucose and inhibiting glycogen synthesis, cAMP also stimulates gluconeogenesis from precursors such as alanine, lactate, and pyruvate in the liver.

Although glucagon is regarded as the primary regulator of rapid hepatic glucose release, catecholamines also appear to be important in humans and other species. Originally, the glycogenolytic actions of both glucagon and catecholamines were believed to be mediated by cAMP; calcium was believed to play an additional role in the stimulation of phosphorylase kinase. Currently, the actions of glucagon on hepatic glycogenolysis (and gluconeogenesis) are clearly attributable to cAMP, though probably at concentrations far below those produced during experimental stimulation of hepatic cells with glucagon. In contrast to the actions of glucagon, the stress hormones, such as catecholamines, vasopressin, and angiotensin II, stimulate glycogenolysis and gluconeogenesis through mechanisms other than cAMP. Although epinephrine can activate adenylate cyclase via hepatic β-adrenergic receptors to enhance cyclic AMP formation, the effects of catecholamines on hepatic glycogenolysis are primarily mediated by α-adrenergic receptors, and are independent of cAMP. Instead, the catecholaminergic activation of phosphorylase depends upon the α_1-adrenergic stimulation of calcium-dependent mechanisms in the hepatocyte.[137]

Vasopressin and angiotensin II also stimulate liver phosphorylase by a cAMP-independent mechanism that depends on the calcium status of the hepatocyte; this provides a common mode of action of the three stress hormones. These peptides activate hepatic phosphorylase by mobilizing intracellular calcium stores, leading to a rise in cytoplasmic calcium concentration which stimulates phosphorylase b kinase.[138] The intracellular source of the calcium mobilized during hormone action has been variously attributed to the mitochondria, ER, and plasma membrane. Current evidence favors the ER as the source from which catecholamines (and vasopressin and angiotensin II) release calcium to the cytoplasm and extracellular fluid. This implies that a second messenger formed by hormone-receptor interaction at the plasma membrane leads to elevation of cytosolic calcium concentration by increasing the mobilization of calcium from intracellular stores.[47] This messenger is now believed to be inositol 1,4,5-trisphosphate formed during the ligand-stimulated breakdown of phosphatidylinositol 4,5-bisphosphate in the cell membrane.[139] Cyclic GMP production is also elevated during α-adrenergic stimulation of liver cells, but this probably reflects changes in free intracellular calcium concentration and consequent stimulation of guanylate cyclase. The functional importance of the effects of this group of hormones on glycogenolysis may lie in their relationship to acute stress, since they stimulate phosphorylase activity at concentrations present in blood during shock and dehydration.[140]

In addition to its action on glycogen breakdown to provide glucose as an energy source, cAMP has a major role in the mobilization of free fatty acids from adipose tissue. This depends on the phosphorylation and activation of hormone-sensitive lipase, which regulates the rate-limiting step of ester bond hydrolysis during degradation of triglycerides. Rapidly acting hormones, including glucagon, epinephrine, and ACTH, increase hormone-sensitive lipase activity by phosphorylation effected by cAMP-dependent protein kinase. Since adipose tissue also contains phosphorylase and glycogen synthase, the presence of three enzyme systems controlled by cAMP-dependent protein ki-

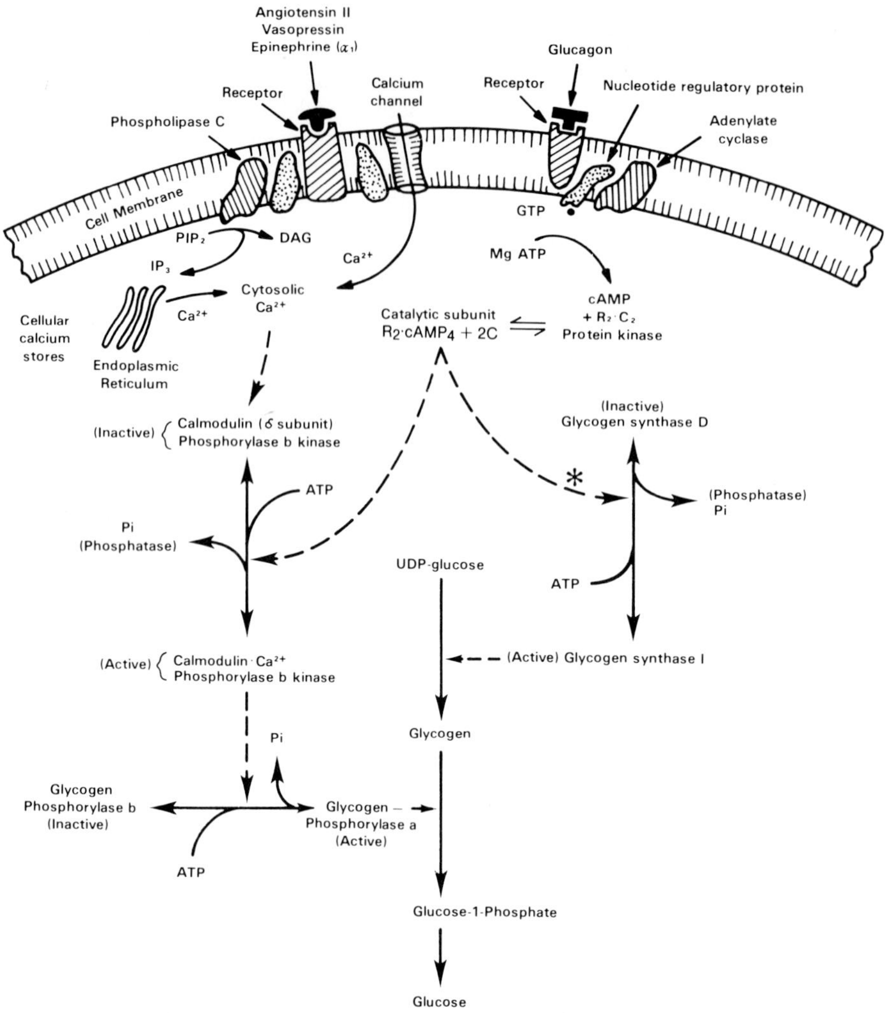

FIGURE 5-23 Control of hepatic glycogenolysis by hormones acting through cAMP-dependent protein kinase and calcium-dependent processes. The catalytic (C) subunit released from the protein kinase holoenzyme by cAMP phosphorylates and activates glycogen phosphorylase (via phosphorylase kinase) and causes phosphorylation and inactivation of glycogen synthase (*, probably via the same enzyme), leading to glycogen breakdown and increased glucose production. Increased cytosolic calcium caused by uptake or mobilization of calcium stores acts to mediate the action of α agonists (and vasopressin and angiotensin II) on activation of phosphorylase kinase, by combining with calmodulin, the δ subunit of phosphorylase b kinase.

nase raises the need for post-cAMP mechanisms to regulate and integrate the several enzymatic processes initiated by protein kinase.[141]

THE GENERAL ROLE OF PROTEIN PHOSPHORYLATION IN cAMP ACTION

The recognition that many hormones raise cAMP levels in their target tissues, and that similar levels of cAMP-dependent protein kinase activity are present in most mammalian cells, led to the idea that the actions of cAMP in eukaryotic tissues are expressed through phosphorylation of enzymes and other regulatory proteins. This mechanism of action differs radically from that operating in prokaryotes, where cAMP acts through a "steroid-like" mechanism in which the cAMP receptor protein (CAP or CRP) activates gene expression after binding to the promoter sites of catabolite-sensitive genes in the bacterial DNA.[142] As noted in Chap. 1, it is conceivable that the bacterial cAMP-binding protein and the regulatory cAMP-binding subunit evolved from a primitive glucotransferase system. The two proteins share structural similarities: each is a dimer of two identical subunits and each binds two molecules of cAMP. Amino acid sequence homologies between CRP and the regulatory subunit of cAMP-dependent protein kinase suggest that a cAMP-binding domain has been conserved in both proteins.[143] In bacteria, the cAMP-binding domain is coupled to a DNA-binding domain which it influences via allosteric conformational changes. In eukaryotes, the cAMP-binding domain influences the interactions between the regulatory (binding) and catalytic (phosphokinase) subunits of cAMP-dependent protein kinase. In eukaryotic organisms, high-affinity binding of cAMP is virtually confined to the regulatory subunit of protein kinase, which acts in conjunction with adenylate cyclase to express the actions of many different hormones. Since the number of individual cAMP-dependent protein kinases is limited to two major types, the functional diversity of hormone actions must depend upon the specificity of the enzymes and their accessibility to specific substrates, or to specific *regions* of protein substrates.

Although other cAMP-binding proteins have been identified in certain mammalian tissues, these do not show the high affinity and specificity of the regulatory subunit of protein kinase. As a substrate, cAMP also binds to phosphodiesterases that are present in most cells, but again without the high specificity and affinity of the protein kinase regulatory subunit. Thus, the present view that cyclic AMP acts only through activation of protein kinase is probably correct, as is the notion that phosphorylation of serine or threonine residues in proteins or peptides is always involved in cAMP action. The possibility that the R·cAMP complex undergoes migration to the nucleus or other sites to exert regulatory actions has been raised, though translocation of the holoenzyme or free C subunits to nuclei has been more frequently proposed. Some of these redistributions of binding or enzymatic subunits between cytoplasmic and particulate sites may be overestimated by the experimental conditions, but others appear likely to represent true translocation of phosphokinase activity to the nucleus. Since most of the acute responses to protein hormones are initiated within seconds or minutes and do not depend upon alterations in RNA or protein synthesis, nuclear actions of cAMP would not be anticipated during the rapid regulatory effects of the cyclic nucleotide. However, cAMP-dependent protein kinase may have a role in the phosphorylation of nuclear proteins and the control of transcription and RNA synthesis. Thus, in rat pituitary tumor cells, cAMP stimulates GH gene transcription and nuclear protein phosphorylation through cAMP-dependent protein kinase, and stimulates prolactin gene transcription through a calcium-dependent mechanism.[144]

HORMONES THAT USE CYCLIC AMP AS A SECOND MESSENGER

Although many peptide hormones have been shown to operate through receptor-mediated activation of adenylate cyclase and cAMP formation, in other cases it has not been possible to demonstrate a role for cAMP in the mechanism of peptide action. Other suggested intracellular mediators of peptide hormone action include calcium, cyclic GMP, potassium, prostaglandins, and changes in membrane potential or intracellular redox potential. In fact, there is little definitive evidence for the contribution of most of these factors to peptide hormone action, though a great deal of recent evidence has implicated calcium as a major intracellular regulator in hormone-stimulated cells. Changes in ion concentrations within intracellular compartments are very difficult to measure, and this has caused difficulty in ascribing specific effector properties to calcium and potassium signals during hormone action. In contrast, hormone-induced cAMP production can be relatively large in comparison to the basal intracellular level of the nucleotide, and significant amounts of cAMP are often released into the extracellular fluid during target cell stimulation by peptide hormones. Such extracellular cAMP has been shown to have a biological role in lower organisms (e.g., slime mold), but is not thought to act as an intercellular messenger in higher animals. In mammalian tissues, extracellular cAMP levels are elevated only during high or excessive hormone stimulation, as in the kidney during infusion or hypersecretion of parathyroid hormone.

However, the changes in cAMP production in response to physiological concentrations of peptide hormones are usually quite small, sometimes causing apparent dissociations between target cell responses and degree of cAMP production. Such apparent discrepancies have been resolved by careful measurements of cAMP concentration in specific cellular compartments (e.g., bound to the regulatory subunit of protein kinase). By this approach, excellent correlations have been found between R·cAMP levels and the steroidogenic responses of testis, ovary, and adrenal to their respective trophic hormones.[16] However, the application of similar approaches to other peptide hormones, such as angiotensin II and GnRH, has shown no relationship between cAMP and hormone-induced cell responses (i.e., aldosterone secretion and LH release), indicating that other factors (such as calcium) must act as the second messenger for such ligands. The role of calcium as an intracellular regulator of hormone action is described in more detail below.

A summary of the peptide hormones and their known mediation by cAMP is given in Table 5-1.

Several peptides and proteins are primarily dependent on cAMP as second messenger (e.g., ACTH, LH, FSH, TSH, glucagon), while some are clearly more calcium-dependent (e.g., angiotensin II, GnRH) and others are definitely not mediated by the cyclic nucleotide (e.g., GH, prolactin, insulin, and other growth factors). Even when the actions of a peptide hormone on specific cell responses are attributed to cAMP as the second messenger, this does not exclude the existence of other actions (e.g., on cell growth and maintenance of differentiated functions) that may not be mediated by cyclic nucleotides.

Guanylate Cyclase, Cyclic GMP, and cGMP-Dependent Protein Kinase

While the second messenger concept of hormone action has been extensively validated for cyclic AMP, there is relatively little evidence for a role of cyclic GMP in target cell regulation by hormones. The soluble and membrane-bound forms of guanylate cyclase are not subject to receptor-mediated regulation, and cGMP elicits only a few physiological responses within the cell.[145] The actions of hormones that increase phospholipid turnover are often accompanied by a rise in cGMP level, probably reflecting activation of guanylate cyclase by protein kinase C and/or in association with stimulation of phospholipase A_2 and the formation of arachidonic acid metabolites. Recently, a major physiological role of cGMP has been defined in vascular smooth muscle during the action of atrial natriuretic factor (or atriopeptin), which activates particulate guanylate cyclase and causes dramatic increases in cGMP concentrations in smooth muscle, kidney, endothelial cells, and adrenal glands. Such increases in cGMP concentration are responsible for smooth muscle relaxation and vasodilation, changes that are presumably mediated by activation of cGMP-dependent protein kinase and phosphorylation of specific proteins involved in the contractile mechanism.

Cyclic GMP also has an important messenger role in visual transduction, by modulating a cation channel in the rod photoreceptors of the retina. This action depends on the binding of cGMP to a regulatory protein on the plasma membrane, a process that is terminated briefly when photon-activated rhodopsin stimulates cGMP phosphodiesterase via the guanyl nucleotide regulatory protein transducin. The resulting increase in cGMP concentration and the related change in cytosolic calcium level are involved in the control of the light-sensitive sodium current across the rod plasma membrane.

Cyclic GMP–dependent protein kinases are abundant in insects and arthropods, but have a more limited distribution in mammalian tissues, where they function in a different manner from the cAMP-dependent enzyme. Their affinity for cAMP is much lower than for cGMP, and their enzyme activity is usually less than that of the cAMP-dependent form. Whereas the cAMP-dependent kinases mediate the regulation of major metabolic pathways including lipolysis, glycogenolysis, and steroidogenesis, the cGMP-dependent enzyme is involved in the actions of cGMP on processes including gene expression and neuronal function. The cGMP-dependent kinase is activated by binding of cGMP to a regulatory site on the enzyme, without the subunit dissociation that is characteristic of the cAMP-dependent enzyme. Marked amino acid sequence homologies exist between cGMP- and cAMP-dependent protein kinases, suggesting a common evolutionary origin of the enzymes from a primitive ancestral phosphotransferase.[146] The homology between the two forms of cyclic nucleotide–dependent protein kinase has been supported by studies on their phosphorylation sites and their most stable structural elements, the location of disulfide bonds and positions of the least mutable amino acids, cysteine and tryptophan.[147]

Calcium and Calcium-Dependent Enzyme Systems

The importance of calcium as an activator of cell function has been evident for almost a century, since Ringer's demonstration of its contribution to the contractility of frog heart muscle. In addition to its central role in muscle contraction and neuromuscular transmission, calcium plays an essential part in secretory processes and is involved in many aspects of intracellular regulation.[148] The general function of calcium as an intracellular messenger was predicted by the *stimulus-secretion* hypothesis, which proposed that calcium ions serve as the primary link between stimulus and secretion.[149] More recent evidence has emphasized the importance of both positive and negative interactions between calcium and cyclic nucleotides[113] in their roles as the major components of an intracellular signaling system that regulates target cell function in response to external stimuli.[114] These messengers undergo rapid changes in hormone-stimulated cells and their intracellular concentrations represent the dynamic equilibrium between production and removal of the signal. The extremely rapid turnover of messenger molecules permits swift cellular responses to hormone activation and prompt termination of the response on withdrawal of the stimulus. During hormone action, the intracellular levels of second messengers are usually controlled by changes in rates of signal generation, as when adenylate cyclase activity or calcium influx is stimulated or inhibited by extracellular ligands. However, changes in rates of signal removal are also important determinants of their intracellular levels, as when cAMP and cGMP are regulated by altered phosphodiesterase activity and calcium by membrane-bound calcium pumps. The interactions between calcium and cyclic nucleotide generation and metabolism are particularly important in this regard, since the enzymes reponsible for both synthesis and degradation of cAMP and cGMP are influenced by calcium-dependent feedback mechanisms that integrate the activities of the second messengers during hormonal stimulation.[114]

REGULATION OF INTRACELLULAR CALCIUM CONCENTRATION

During peptide hormone action, the messenger function of calcium depends upon its rapid changes in concentration at specific intracellular sites for the control of calcium-dependent metabolic processes. These effects usually involve the activation or inhibition of rate-limiting regulatory enzymes by calcium-dependent protein kinases. Of major importance during hormone action are the effects of calcium on adenylate and guanylate cyclase and phosphodiesterase, critical enzymes in the dynamic control of intracellular cyclic nucleotide levels. Many of the regulatory actions of calcium on intracellular enzyme systems are mediated by calmodulin, a low-molecular-weight calcium-binding protein that is present in most eukaryotic cells. This acidic protein was discovered as a regulator of brain phosphodiesterase[150] and has since been recognized as an essential intermediate in the control of numerous calcium-regulated enzymes. In many cases, calmodulin is closely associated with the regulated enzyme, and the Ca^{2+}-calmodulin complex serves as the regulatory ligand which mediates the effects of free Ca^{2+} upon enzyme activation or inhibition.

The primary event in the expression of calcium-mediated cellular responses to external stimuli is the movement of calcium ions into the cell cytoplasm. The calcium involved in such movements is derived from two major sources, the extracellular fluid, in which the free calcium concentration is about 1200 μM, and intracellular stores in microsomes, mitochondria, and plasma membrane. The cytosolic free calcium concentration is very low (about 0.1 μM) and does not usually exceed 1 μM during hormonal stimulation. Plasma membranes contain an appreciable amount of bound calcium, both on the inner surface and in the glycocalyx of the external surface of the cell. In addition to the large extracellular to intracellular calcium concentration gradient, the transmembrane electrical gradient also favors calcium entry; yet the rate of calcium influx is usually low in the absence of external stimuli. Such restricted membrane permeability, and the presence of an external perimembranous pool of bound calcium, render many cells relatively unresponsive to changes in ambient calcium concentration, particularly in the basal state. However, the increased sensitivity to calcium that frequently accompanies hormonal stimulation suggests that altered membrane permeability is an essential step in cell activation.[114] Although redistribution of internal calcium stores often causes rapid increases in cytosolic calcium levels during cell activation by hormonal ligands, increased entry of calcium through the plasma membrane is the more general source of the calcium signal in excitable tissues.

The influx of calcium through the plasma membrane can result from a stimulus-induced change in membrane permeability, via either receptor-operated calcium channels during hormone action or voltage-sensitive calcium channels during changes in membrane potential. The latter mechanism is not usually involved in peptide hormone action, but is responsible for the stimulatory effect of high potassium concentrations on secretory cells in vitro, since depolarization of the plasma membrane causes increased calcium entry through voltage-sensitive channels. Elevations of intracellular calcium concentration, whether due to influx or mobilization of calcium, are rapidly corrected by increases in calcium efflux. This is achieved by active extrusion of excess cytosolic calcium from neuromuscular cells by exchange with sodium and from nonexcitable cells by the plasma membrane calcium pump, Ca^{2+},Mg^{2+}-ATPase. For this reason, hormonal stimuli that cause redistribution of intracellular calcium are usually accompanied by increased calcium efflux, due to activation of the plasma membrane calcium pump by calcium-calmodulin during restoration of the normal cytosolic calcium concentration.

MECHANISMS OF CALCIUM'S ACTION AS A SECOND MESSENGER

Calcium-Calmodulin and Enzyme Activation

The biological actions of calcium are largely mediated by its interaction with binding proteins such as calmodulin (Table 5-9), and are expressed through three major mechanisms in neuromuscular, secretory, and other tissues. In addition to interacting with cellular contractile elements, calcium-calmodulin participates in the regulation of metabolic enzyme activity and the control of membrane permeability. In many cells, the effects of calcium on adenylate cyclase, guanylate cyclase, and phosphodiesterase are important in regulating the cytosolic levels of both cyclic nucleotides and in linking the intracellular messenger systems by feedback mechanisms that integrate their biological activities. Many of these actions are expressed through the interaction of calcium with specific cellular binding proteins, as summarized in Table 5-9.

A major advance in the understanding of calcium's actions came with the discovery of the calcium-dependent regulatory protein calmodulin and the recognition that it is structurally and functionally similar to troponin C and other calcium-binding proteins.[150] During muscle contraction, calcium is bound by troponin C to form a complex which facilitates the interaction between actin and myosin and activates the myosin ATPase necessary for repetition of the actin-myosin reaction. The presence of actin in noncontractile cells suggested that similar contractile elements participate in cell mobility and movement of organelles, granule release, and endocytosis.

Many cells have extensive arrays of actin and myosin-like filament proteins attached to the inner surface of the plasma membrane, and often to the membranes of secretory granules. Such actin-containing microfilaments could mediate the effects of calcium on cell motility, membrane fluidity, and rearrangements or internalization of membrane-associated proteins and their bound extrinsic ligands.

Although the troponin component of muscle was not initially detected in noncontractile cells, the later discovery of troponin-like calcium-binding proteins in many cell types led to the recognition of calmodulin as a general calcium-dependent regulatory protein. Calmodulin is one of a family of small, acidic calcium-binding proteins which have evolved from a single ancestral calcium-binding protein. Several of these proteins (parvalbumin, troponin C, intestinal calcium-binding protein) are restricted to certain tissues and carry out specific functions in one or another metabolic process or pathway. In contrast, calmodulin is present in all eukaryotic cells and subserves numerous metabolic functions that are often dependent on changes in protein phosphorylation or dephosphorylation and enzyme activation. Calmodulin-like proteins are widely distributed in animal and plant tissues and mediate many of the physiological actions of calcium by controlling the activities of specific enzymes.[151]

The functional role of calmodulin in noncontractile tissues is thus analogous to that of troponin C in muscle, i.e., to mediate calcium's actions on regulatory enzyme systems. Calmodulin is sometimes associated with the array of microfilaments, and in other cases is intimately associated with calcium-regulated enzymes as a tightly bound subunit or congener. By serving as an intracellular calcium receptor, calmodulin modifies calcium transport, the calcium-dependent regulation of cyclic nucleotide and glycogen metabolism, and such processes as secretion and cell motility. Calmodulin is also a dynamic component of the mitotic apparatus, where it may regulate microtubule polymerization, actomyosin, and membrane-bound calcium pumps. Many of the effects of calmodulin on cellular processes are mediated through the regulation of enzymes involved in protein phosphorylation and dephosphorylation.[152]

Following its identification as a calcium-dependent regulator of cyclic nucleotide phosphodiesterase, calmodulin was purified from several tissues and characterized as a receptor protein of mol wt 17,000 with high specificity and affinity for Ca^{2+}. Each calmodulin molecule contains four calcium-binding sites, occupancy of which leads to a conformational change that causes calmodulin to activate its dependent enzyme systems. The protein contains 148 amino acids with a high content of phenylalanine and acidic residues, and shows considerable sequence homology with troponin C from skeletal and cardiac muscle. The calmodulin molecule has been highly conserved throughout evolution, and shows significant α-helicity that is markedly

Table 5-9. Some Major Calcium-Binding Proteins

Protein	Function	Location
Calmodulin	Activation of many enzymes in animal and plant tissues Cyclic nucleotide metabolism Metabolic pathways Calcium fluxes Neuronal phosphorylation Cell motility and division	All eukaryotic cells
Troponin C	Triggers contractile systems	Skeletal and cardiac muscle
Intestinal calcium-binding proteins	Calcium transport in gut	Intestinal tract
Parvalbumin	Calcium buffering and muscle relaxation	Vertebrate skeletal muscle

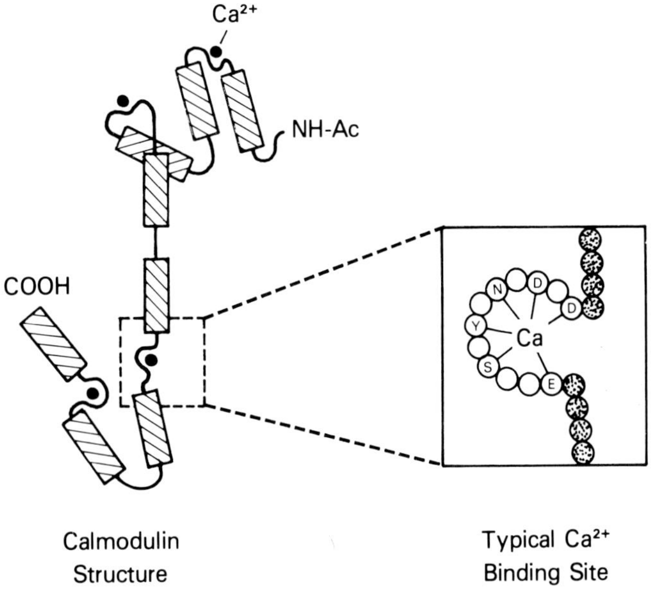

FIGURE 5-24 Conformation and Ca^{2+}-binding domains of the calmodulin molecule. *Left:* The molecule is composed of α helices (shaded regions) linked by calcium-binding loops, arranged as a bilobar structure with two calcium (C)-binding domains at each end. *Right:* The amino acids of the connecting loops (light circles) between those forming the α helices (dark circles) contain calcium-binding amino acid residues (D, Asp; N, Asn; Y, Tyr; S, Ser; E, Glu) and sequences (shaded) that favor the formation of β turns. (*Modified from Klee et al.*[152] and *Babu et al.*[153])

increased by calcium binding. The resulting conformational change in the calmodulin molecule favors its binding to enzymes and other regulatory proteins and to drugs such as phenothiazines. Crystallographic analysis of the three-dimensional structure of calmodulin shows it to consist of two linked globular regions, each of which binds two calcium ions.[153] The two calcium-binding domains are connected by an eight-turn stretch of α helix that is probably buried in the absence of calcium and becomes exposed when calcium is bound (Fig. 5-24). This long exposed region of α helix is involved in the calcium-dependent interaction of calmodulin with various proteins and drugs. The chicken calmodulin gene has been cloned and its DNA sequence has been found to contain eight exons and seven introns. Three of the four calcium-binding domains are interrupted by introns, consistent with the view that introns separate regions to be displayed on the surface of the protein molecule.

The importance of calmodulin as the mediator of calcium's actions was first recognized in brain tissue, in which the activation of a calcium-dependent phosphodiesterase was found to require its presence as a modulator protein. The enzymes now recognized to depend on calmodulin for calcium activation include brain adenylate cyclase and phosphodiesterase, erythrocyte membrane Ca^{2+},Mg^{2+}-ATPase, and a series of calcium-calmodulin (CaM)-dependent protein kinases (Table 5-10). The latter enzymes include protein kinases of strict or limited substrate specificity, such as phosphorylase kinase and myosin light chain kinase, and a multifunctional enzyme (CaM kinase II) that is abundant in brain and phosphorylates a variety of substrates (synapsin 1, glycogen synthase, microtubule-associated protein 2, and tyrosine hydroxylase). Others include CaM kinase I, with specificity for synapsin

Table 5-10. Calcium- and Calmodulin-Regulated Enzymes

Cyclic nucleotide metabolism
Adenylate cyclase
Cyclic nucleotide phosphodiesterase
Protein phosphorylation
Myosin light chain kinase: smooth muscle, nonmuscle tissue
Phosphorylase kinase: phosphorylase; glycogen synthase
CaM-dependent protein kinase I: synapsin I, site I
CaM-dependent protein kinase II: synapsin I, site II glycogen synthase, MAP 2, tryptophan monooxygenase
CaM-dependent protein kinase III: 100,000-Mr protein in many tissues
Protein dephosphorylation
Calcineurin: multifunctional phosphoprotein phosphatase; acts on many brain and other phosphoproteins, including tyrosylphosphoproteins
Calcium transport
Ca^{2+}, Mg^{2+}-dependent ATPase (plasma membrane Ca^{2+} pump)
Sarcoplasmic (Ca^{2+}) ATPase (sarcoplasmic Ca^{2+} transport)
Other
NAD kinase (plants)

Abbreviations: CaM, calmodulin; MAP, microtubule-associated protein.

1, and CaM kinase III, which phosphorylates a mol wt 100,000 protein of unknown function that is present in many mammalian tissues.[154]

Enzyme activation by calmodulin and binding of calmodulin to the enzyme are both dependent on the presence of calcium. As calcium concentration is increased, the calmodulin binds Ca^{2+} and becomes conformationally changed to its active state, which then associates with the enzyme to enhance catalytic activity. It is possible that the degree of occupancy of the four calcium-binding sites varies for the systems regulated by calmodulin, and may help to explain its diverse biological actions. The role of calmodulin in phosphorylation of the myosin light chain kinase may be related to the regulation of smooth muscle contraction, by determining the balance of activity between phosphorylated (inactive) and dephosphorylated (potentially active) myosin kinase. Occupancy of β receptors by epinephrine and stimulation of cAMP formation leads to activation of protein kinase and phosphorylation of myosin kinase. The phosphorylated kinase binds calmodulin with lower affinity than the unphosphorylated enzyme. At low levels of calcium-calmodulin, the myosin kinase is less active and phosphatase activity may predominate, causing fewer myosin molecules to be in the phosphorylated state. Then, actin-myosin interaction would not occur, resulting in relaxation of smooth muscle.[155]

Several proteins have been found to bind calmodulin in various tissues, and were initially regarded as potential modulators of calmodulin activity. However, they have mostly proved to be calmodulin-regulated enzymes such as calcineurin, which binds calmodulin in the nervous system. Calcineurin was first discovered as an inhibitor of phosphodiesterase in the brain[152] and is now known to be a multifunctional phosphoprotein phosphatase with broad specificity for neuronal and other phosphoproteins, including tyrosyl phosphoproteins such as the EGF receptor.

Calcium-Dependent Regulatory Enzymes: Protein Kinase C

In addition to true calcium receptor proteins such as calmodulin and troponin C, which serve to regulate metabolic pathways by binding to enzyme proteins, calcium is also bound directly to several calcium-regulated enzymes without the intervention of calmodulin or other receptor proteins. Perhaps the most important enzyme in this category is the phospholipid-dependent multifunctional phosphokinase termed *protein kinase* C. This enzyme is dependent for its activity on calcium and the phospholipid moiety phosphatidylserine. Protein kinase C is activated by DAG, which is produced from inositol phospholipids in response to extracellular stimuli.[156] Free DAG is present in extremely low concentrations in membranes of unstimulated cells; its concentration rises rapidly during receptor-activated hydrolysis of phosphoinositides by phospholipase C. Small amounts of DAG markedly increase the affinity of protein kinase C for calcium, and activate the enzyme in the absence of a change in cytosolic calcium concentration (Fig. 5-25).

Protein kinase C was first detected in brain, and was later shown to be activated by thrombin in platelets in the absence of a rise in cytosolic calcium concentration. The calcium- and phospholipid-dependent enzyme has since been found in numerous tissues and organisms, and its activity in many tissues exceeds that of cAMP-dependent protein kinase. Protein kinase C is activated in response to receptor binding of many extracellular signals; it is also activated by tumor promoters such as tetradecanoylphorbol acetate (TPA), which bind to the enzyme and substitute for DAG in causing its activation.[157] Most of the protein kinase C in unstimulated cells is located in the cytoplasm, but the enzyme undergoes redistribution to the plasma membrane during treatment with phorbol esters and certain hormonal ligands. Activation of protein kinase C by TPA differs from the effect of DAG mainly in terms of potency and duration, since the endogenous lipid is metabolized by DAG kinase and diglyceride lipase in ligand-stimulated cells. Certain synthetic diglycerides such as dioctanoyl glycerol, which penetrate the cell membrane, are also potent stimuli of protein kinase C in intact cells.

Protein kinase C is a single polypeptide chain of mol wt 77,000; it contains two functional regions, a hydrophobic membrane-binding domain and a hydrophilic catalytic domain, that are cleaved by calcium-dependent proteases. The hydrophilic segment is enzymatically active in the absence of calcium, phospholipid, and DAG, and is sometimes termed *M-kinase.* Once activated by DAG or phorbol esters, protein kinase C causes phosphorylation of serine and threonine residues in numerous tissue proteins. The primary structure of the enzyme, determined from brain cDNA clones, contains an amino terminal cysteine-rich domain, followed by a calcium-binding domain and a carboxy-terminal region, with homology to other protein kinases, that represents the 50 kD catalytic fragment released by proteolysis.[158]

Many of the receptors which activate protein kinase C also elevate the cytosolic calcium level, which in some cases can potentiate the effects of kinase C activation. Thus, platelets exposed to individually ineffective concentrations of both calcium ionophore and synthetic DAG are stimulated to the maximal extent seen with thrombin and platelet-activating factor, as a result of synergism between

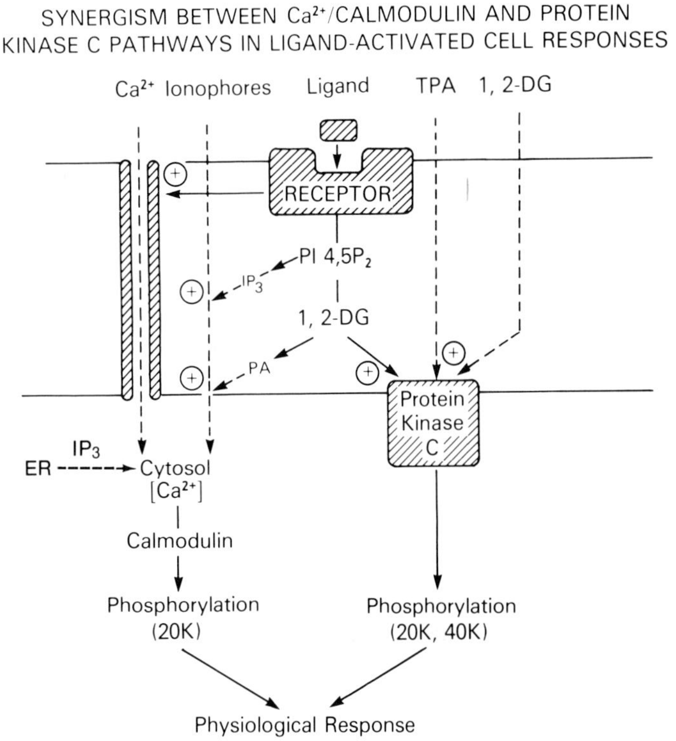

FIGURE 5-25 Ligand-induced activation of calmodulin-dependent phosphorylation by Ca^{2+} and of protein kinase C by diacylglycerol. The actions of calcium-mobilizing messengers can be mimicked by Ca^{2+} ionophores and those of diacylglycerol by phorbol esters and synthetic diacylglycerol.

elevated cytosolic calcium and protein kinase C. It is probable that hormonal responses in some cells are largely controlled by calcium changes, but in others are dominated by activation of protein kinase C, and in others require both mechanisms for maximum activation (Fig. 5-25). It is also likely that the two pathways control different phases or processes of the response to hormonal stimulation in certain cells. Since the calcium response is relatively small and transient in many cells, due to the compensatory increase in calcium efflux, the sustained activation of protein kinase C by DAG may serve to prolong the cellular response during continued stimulation by hormonal ligands.[159] This could involve factors such as secondary activation of phospholipase A_2, via phosphorylation of lipocortin and suppression of its inhibitory action on the enzyme, with increased production of arachidonic acid.

There are also situations in which protein kinase C acts as a negative feedback regulator of target cell responses.[160] One such effect of protein kinase C is to attenuate the agonist-induced elevations of cytosolic calcium concentration in several cell types. This is caused by (1) inhibition of phosphoinositide hydrolysis and IP_3 formation, perhaps with accelerated breakdown of IP_3, leading to reduced calcium mobilization; and (2) stimulation of calcium extrusion by activation of plasma membrane calcium pumps. Such effects are probably responsible both for the decreasing duration of the calcium signal and the diminution of secretory responses that sometimes occur during exposure of target cells to high hormone concentrations.

Another way in which protein kinase C attenuates signal transduction is through inhibitory effects on the receptor site itself. Thus, phorbol esters promote kinase C–dependent phosphorylation of several peptide hormone receptors, including those for EGF and insulin. In the EGF receptor, phosphorylation of a cytoplasmic threonine residue by protein kinase C causes a decrease in tyrosine kinase activity, and also a decrease in receptor affinity. More long-term effects of phorbol esters include loss of receptors and, in some cases, impairment of the coupling between receptors and adenylate cyclase, possibly via an action on the guanyl nucleotide regulatory protein. The extent to which various hormonal agonists can elicit these inhibitory consequences of kinase C activation is not yet clear, but there is abundant evidence that protein kinase C has a bidirectional role in cellular regulation and may participate in the termination as well as the prolongation of agonist-induced responses.

INTERACTIONS BETWEEN CALCIUM AND CYCLIC NUCLEOTIDES

The interactions between calcium and cyclic nucleotides are frequently reciprocal in nature and are integrated into a network of feedback reactions through which the two signaling systems regulate each other's activities. The relationships between cAMP and calcium can be divided into two general types according to their participation in monodirectional or bidirectional control systems within individual target tissues.[114]

Monodirectional systems are those found in cells regulated by a single stimulus, in which a simple on/off type of control, depending upon the presence or absence of the stimulus, operates. Either calcium or cAMP may act as the second messenger, according to cell type; if cAMP is formed, it augments the calcium signal. Tissues in which such monodirectional controls operate include the nervous system, adrenal medulla, anterior pituitary, endocrine and exocrine pancreas, adrenal cortex, bladder, salivary glands, and photoreceptors. In all of these tissues, cell activation is regulated in only one direction (off vs. on), and activity is terminated by removal of the stimulus. In most cases, calcium appears to serve as the second messenger and cAMP has an indirect action on or augments the effects of calcium. In tissues controlled by the pituitary trophic hormones, i.e., adrenal, testis, ovary, and thyroid, cAMP has a more prominent role as second messenger, but again acts in close liaison with calcium in the regulation of steroidogenic enzymes and thyroxine secretion.

Bidirectional control systems operate in cells regulated by two independent stimuli, such that one stimulus initiates cell activity and the other terminates the response, usually by opposing the action of the first stimulus. In such tissues, calcium is usually the primary signal for the first stimulus, and cAMP mediates the inhibitory effect of the second stimulus by decreasing the intracellular level of calcium. Thus, in contrast to the synergism between cAMP and calcium in monodirectional systems, the effects of cAMP and calcium are antagonistic in bidirectional systems. Tissues in which bidirectional control is operative include smooth muscle, cardiac muscle, melanophores, platelets, and mast cells. In these cell types, ligand-induced activation is mediated by increased calcium mobilization or influx, and inhibitory agonists lower cytoplasmic calcium concentration via the actions of cAMP.[161] Liver and adipose tissue exhibit some of the features of unidirectional systems, since cAMP increases intracellular calcium concentration and favors the unidirectional glycogenolytic effects of epinephrine and glucagon. However, insulin antagonizes the effects of those catabolic hormones, perhaps through an inhibitory effect on intracellular levels of cAMP, which operates as the major second messenger in this tissue. In the more general case of bidirectional systems, the opposing roles of calcium and cAMP are clearly defined, and may involve both inhibition of phospholipase C by cAMP and other inhibitory effects on the stimulus-response coupling pathway. The control of phospholipase C by cAMP would regulate both IP_3-dependent calcium mobilization and DAG-mediated activation of protein kinase C.[160] Cyclic GMP has been reported to exert both inhibitory and synergistic effects on calcium-dependent responses in various cell types. However, it seems that cGMP levels are often regulated by the intracellular calcium concentration, and thus serve as a reflection of calcium's actions rather than as the primary antagonist of cAMP. A summary of the relationships between receptor activation and the subsequent changes in calcium mobilization and cAMP formation is shown in Fig. 5-26.

Hormone Action and Phospholipid Metabolism

Recent work on peptide hormone action has shown that membrane phospholipids and their metabolic products play an important part in the target cell response to hormonal stimulation. There are at least three major ways in which phospholipids participate in hormone action.

1. As a source of arachidonic acid precursors for synthesis of PGs and related compounds with secondary target tissue effects.
2. By increased turnover of inositol phospholipids and formation of polyphosphoinositides and their products that influence target cell responses (e.g., secretion, steroidogenesis).
3. By increased phospholipid methylation, with formation of phosphatidylcholine from phosphatidylethanolamine, and consequent changes in membrane fluidity and receptor mobility within the plasma membrane.

PHOSPHOLIPIDS: STRUCTURE, METABOLISM, AND FUNCTIONS

Naturally occurring phospholipids are derivatives of glycerol phosphate or sphingosine phosphate, containing two fatty acids and a hydrophilic substituent such as choline, ethanolamine, inositol, or serine. They are major constituents of lipoproteins and cell membranes, and are abundant in nerve tissue and brain. The phosphoglycerides have the general structure shown in Fig. 5-27, formed by esterification of glycerol phosphate with two long-chain fatty acids and a hydrophilic component. An important feature of phospholipids is their ability to interact with both hydrophobic and hydrophilic domains and to occupy

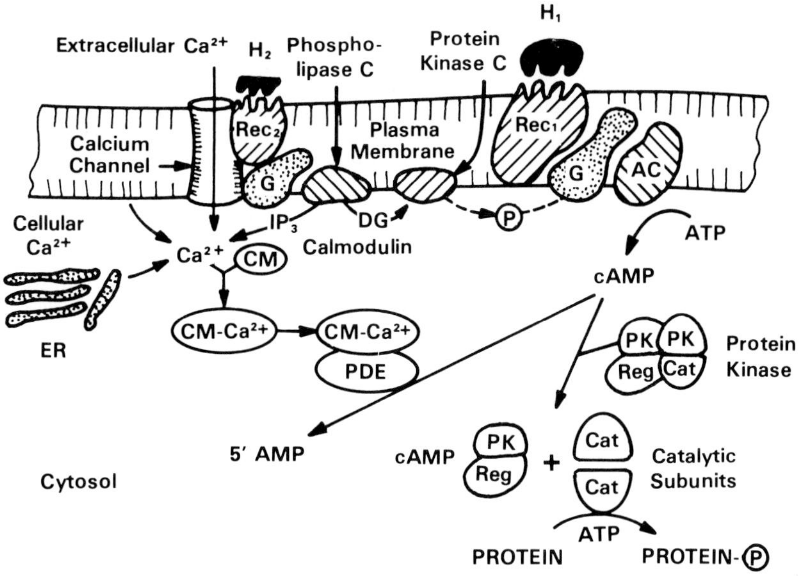

FIGURE 5-26 Peptide-receptor mediated interrelationships between calcium mobilization and cAMP formation and degradation.

the interface between organic and aqueous environments. Thus, in lipoproteins they serve as the bond between the protein fraction and the transported neutral lipid, and in the cell membrane they form the characteristic lipid bilayer that defines the intracellular space.

In the plasma membrane, about 60 percent of the phospholipid is phosphatidylcholine, which is partly synthesized within the membrane by methylation of phosphatidylinositol (PI). Lesser quantities of PI and phosphatidylserine are present, and the fatty acid constituents vary in length and degree of saturation in various tissues. Phosphatidylcholines, or *lecithins*, are synthesized by three pathways in animal tissues. In the major pathway, analogous to that of PI synthesis, choline is phosphorylated by ATP to give phosphocholine. This combines with CTP to form CDP-choline, which reacts with DAG in the presence of phosphocholine transferase to give phosphatidylcholine. The second pathway of phosphatidylcholine synthesis is by acylation of lysophosphatidylcholine (formed by hydrolysis of lecithin by phospholipase A). The third pathway, which is particularly relevant to the effects of hormonal stimulation on membrane phospholipids,

is via sequential methylation of phosphatidylethanolamine molecules within the cell membrane.

HORMONAL EFFECTS ON PHOSPHOLIPID METABOLISM

Stimulation of Release and Metabolism of Arachidonic Acid

Most peptide hormones stimulate the production of arachidonic acid and its oxygenated metabolites by their target tissues, often with secondary effects on vascular and cellular responses during hormone action. Although PGs rarely act as mediators of peptide hormone action, stimulation of these locally formed tissue hormones during target cell activation is an important component of the cellular response to peptide hormone-receptor interaction. Prostaglandins and the related prostacyclins and thromboxanes are rapidly synthesized from polyunsaturated fatty acid precursors, in particular arachidonic acid, during target cell stimulation. The unsaturated fatty acids in cells are present as phosphoglyceride, which must be deacylated by phospholipases to provide the substrate for

$$
\begin{array}{c}
 \begin{array}{c} O \\ \| \end{array} \\
 CH_2-O-C-R_1 \\
\begin{array}{c} O \\ \| \end{array} | \\
R_2-C-O-CH \begin{array}{c} O \\ \| \end{array} \\
 | \\
 CH_2-O-P-O-R_3 \\
 | \\
 O
\end{array}
$$

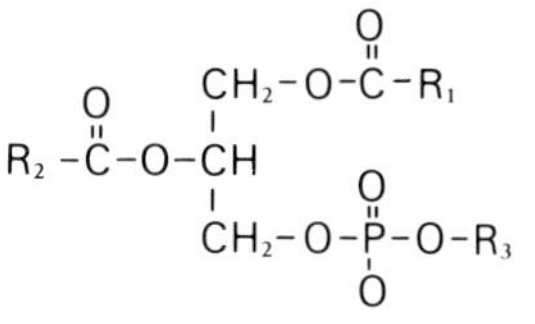

R_1, R_2 = FATTY ACIDS
R_3 = CHOLINE, ETHANOLAMINE, INOSITOL, SERINE.

FIGURE 5-27 General structures of the major phospholipids.

GENERAL STRUCTURE OF PHOSPHOLIPIDS

metabolism to PGs and other active intermediates. Arachidonic acid is the most abundant unsaturated fatty acid in tissue phospholipids, and undergoes metabolism by two major routes, the *cyclooxygenase* and *lipooxygenase* pathways. The immediate products of the cyclooxygenase pathway are endoperoxides (PGG_2 and PGH_2), which are converted to prostaglandins (PGE_2, $PGF_{2\alpha}$, and PGD_2) by enzymes termed "prostaglandin synthetase," as well as to thromboxanes (TXA_2 and TXB_2) and prostacyclins (PGI_2) by corresponding synthetases (Fig. 5-28). The classification of these endoperoxidase metabolites depends on the degree of unsaturation of their precursor fatty acids: eicosatetraenoic acid is converted to class 1 products (PGE_1, $PGF_{1\alpha}$, TXA_1, etc.) and arachidonic acid to class 2 products, including PGE_2, $PGF_{2\alpha}$, TXA_2, TXB_2, and PGI_2.[162]

The thromboxanes and prostacyclins, which are also formed by further metabolism of the endoperoxides produced by the cyclooxygenase pathway, serve as important regulators of platelet and vessel-wall interactions. PGI_2 is produced in large amounts by vascular endothelium and smooth muscle cells, where its formation is modulated by hydroperoxide metabolites of the lipooxygenase pathway.[163] PGI_2 is a highly potent inhibitor of platelet aggregation, and its production in endothelial cells is stimulated by thrombin and inhibited by LDLs. There is also evidence to suggest that decreased capacity of vascular smooth muscle cells to produce PGI_2 may contribute to the development of atherosclerosis.

The more recently defined lipooxygenase pathway converts arachidonic acid to hydroxy fatty acids, including hydroperoxyeicosatetraenoic acids (HPETEs), which are then metabolized to hydroxyeicosatetraenoic acids (HETEs). The HETEs and their leukotriene metabolites are important mediators of inflammatory responses, including neutrophil chemotaxis and other consequences of platelet cyclooxygenase and PGI_2 production in vascular tissue. There is considerable evidence that lipooxygenated metabolites of arachidonic acid participate in GnRH-induced release of LH from pituitary gonadotrophs,[164] and also in the secretory responses to several other ligands and peptide hormones. A recently discovered pathway leading to the formation of epoxide derivatives of arachidonic acid has also been implicated in ligand-stimulated secretion in several tissues.

Each of the above pathways for production of active arachidonic acid metabolites depends on an adequate supply of the unsaturated fatty acid precursor from membrane phospholipids. Many forms of receptor-mediated cell activation involve membrane-bound phospholipases which catalyze the hydrolysis of

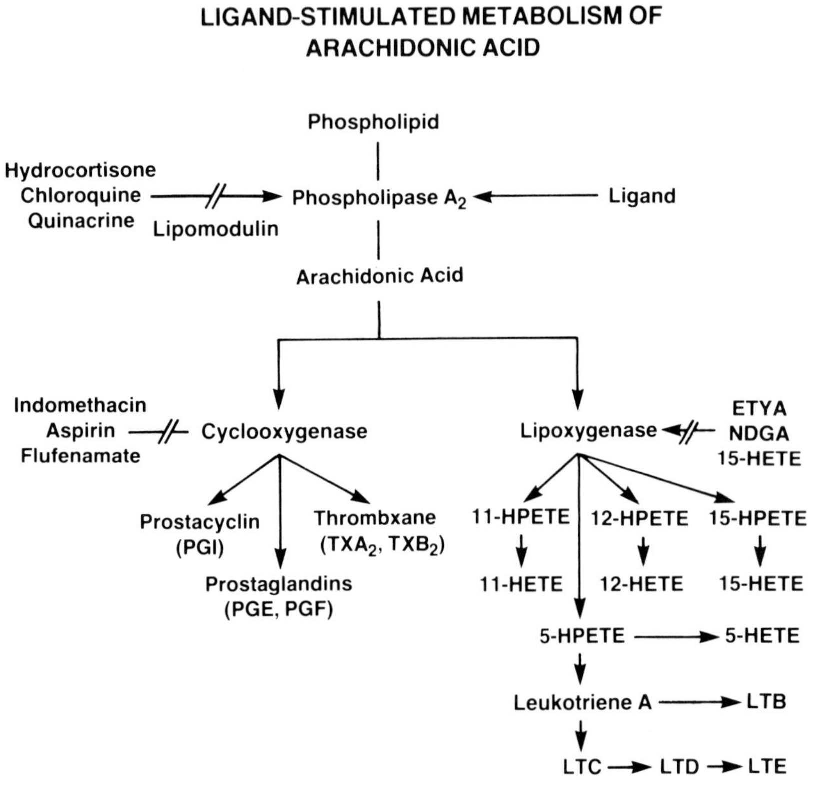

FIGURE 5-28 Pathways of formation and metabolism of arachidonic acid. The unsaturated fatty acid is released from membrane phospholipids by phospholipase C and diacylglyceride lipase and is converted to active derivatives by the enzymes of the lipoxygenase, cyclooxygenase, and prostaglandin synthase pathways.

ester linkages in glycerophospholipids. Phospholipase A_2, which cleaves fatty acids at position 2 of diacylglycerophospholipids to yield the lysophospholipid and an unsaturated fatty acid, commonly arachidonic acid, is particularly important in this regard. The deacylated phospholipid is rapidly reacylated by transfer of a coenzyme A–activated fatty acid. Arachidonic acid is also produced by the action of diglyceride lipase upon the diacylglycerol released during hydrolysis of phosphoinositides by phospholipase C. This source of the fatty acid may be especially important in hormone-regulated secretory cells, such as those responsible for production of gonadotropins and prolactin. Ligand-stimulated turnover of membrane phospholipids provides arachidonic acid for metabolism by the cyclo- and lipooxygenase pathways (Fig. 5-28), and may influence membrane permeability and the activities of other membrane-bound enzymes.[165]

The activation of phospholipase A_2 is calcium-dependent, and the enzyme is normally inhibited by lipocortin (or lipomodulin), a 40-kD protein whose inhibitory activity is suppressed by protein kinase C-dependent phosphorylation. In this way, activation of kinase C synergizes with raised cytosolic calcium to stimulate phospholipase A_2 and to enhance the release of arachidonic acid and its metabolic products.[166]

In the adrenal, the actions of ACTH on steroidogenesis are dependent on calcium as well as cAMP formation, and at least a part of the calcium requirement may be related to the phospholipase-mediated turnover of membrane phospholipids during activation of the adrenal cortex. While this mechanism may reflect a general property of hormone-regulated secretory cells, other sites in the pathway of phospholipid metabolism are also modulated during hormonal stimulation of specific target cells. Thus, in ovarian granulosa cells, LH does not increase arachidonic acid formation, but increases PG production by acting later in the pathway to enhance PG synthetase activity.[167] The stimulatory effect of LH on PG synthesis in the graafian follicle does not mediate the steroidogenic actions of the gonadotropin, but seems to be essential for ovulation to occur.[168]

Stimulation of Phosphoinositide Turnover

Inositol phospholipids make up a minor but important proportion of the plasma membrane phospholipids in eukaryotic cells. The major inositol lipid in most cells is PI, in which myoinositol phosphate is attached by

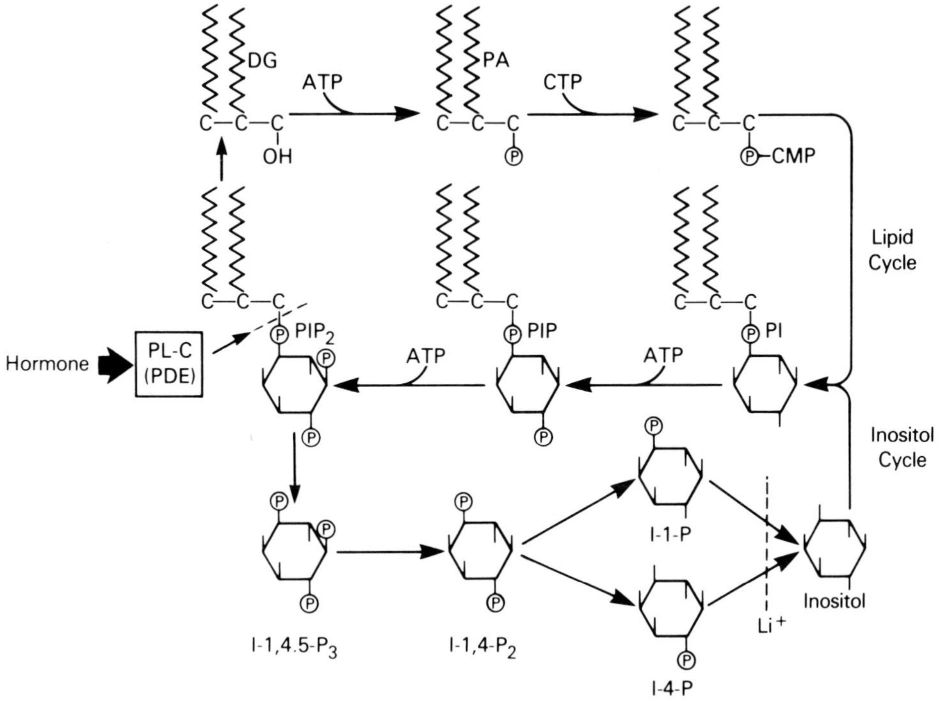

FIGURE 5-29 Hormone-stimulated breakdown of inositol phospholipids and the subsequent metabolism of inositol phosphates and lipids prior to the resynthesis of polyphosphoinositides in the plasma membrane.

a diester linkage to the DAG moiety. Much smaller amounts of the polyphosphoinositides (di- and triphosphatidylinositols), bearing one or two phosphates on the inositol hydroxyl groups, are present in the plasma membrane. The inositol phospholipids are interconverted by ATP-dependent kinases and phosphomonoesterases, and are cleaved by phosphodiesterases to inositol phosphates and DAG. The cyclic pathways involved in breakdown and resynthesis of polyphosphoinositides in agonist-stimulated cells are shown in Fig. 5-29.

The metabolism of inositol phospholipids has been known for several years to be enhanced during stimulation of many secretory cells, with increased incorporation of radioactive phosphate and inositol into PI and its precursor, phosphatidic acid.[169] This so-called PI response, which is now known to reflect phosphoinositide breakdown and resynthesis, has since proved to be a general and characteristic feature of agonist binding to cell surface receptors whose activation causes elevation of the intracellular calcium concentration.[170] The PI response is independent of the extracellular calcium concentration; its frequent association with receptor-mediated increases in cytosolic calcium concentration led to the recognition that PI breakdown participates in a common mechanism whereby receptor activation controls the intracellular calcium concentration.[170] Ligand-induced elevations in cytoplasmic calcium concentration could result from increased plasma membrane permeability (calcium gating), but in secretory cells is frequently dependent on mobilization of calcium from intracellular stores. In general, there is a good correlation between increased inositol lipid turnover and calcium mobilization in hormone-stimulated tissues. Conversely, hormones that cause receptor-mediated increases in intracellular cyclic AMP concentration rather than calcium concentration usually have little or no effect on phosphoinositide metabolism. Thus, the PI response is not simply a general response of cells to activation of their surface receptors, but appears to be a specific feature of hormonal stimuli for which calcium mobilization is an essential component of the target cell response.[171]

An additional feature of receptor activation that accompanies increased phosphoinositide turnover is a rise in cGMP production, reflecting stimulation of guanylate cyclase activity. As noted above, this may be due to increased intracellular calcium mobilization, and is probably not an important factor in the genesis of specific target cell responses.

Although there is clearly a close relation between the PI response and calcium mobilization during activation of many cellular receptors, the nature of the link between these processes has only recently been clarified. This is now believed to be inositol 1,4,5-trisphosphate, which is formed during the hydrolysis of phosphatidylinositol 4,5-bisphosphate (PIP_2) by phospholipase C.[172] The cellular site of receptor-mediated phosphoinositide turnover is at the plasma membrane, where IP_3 is released and causes rapid mobilization of stored calcium into the cytoplasm (Fig. 5-30). Hormone-stimulated IP_3 production is an essential component of many receptor activation mechanisms, and may result in the opening of cell surface calcium channels, as well as promoting the release of calcium from microsomal stores into the cytoplasm.[173]

The most important aspect of phosphoinositide metabolism is the central role of polyphosphoinositides and their metabolites in the actions of peptide hormones and transmitters.[139] These highly charged lipids undergo extremely rapid metabolic turnover, and are broken down within a few seconds during cell stimulation by calcium-mobilizing ligands such as α-adrenergic and muscarinic agonists. The hydrolysis of PIP_2 to IP_3 and DAG forms a major signal transduction system for controlling diverse cellular responses, since the mobilization of calcium by IP_3 is integrated with the activation of protein kinase C within the plasma membrane by DAG.[39] Once released into the cell, IP_3 binds to microsomal and membrane receptors to mobilize calcium, and is rapidly degraded in a stepwise manner to inositol via inositol 1,4-bisphosphate and inositol monophosphate.[174] The breakdown of inositol monophosphate to inositol is inhibited by lithium, which is sometimes employed to amplify the agonist-induced accumulation of inositol phosphates during studies on hormone-dependent phosphoinositide metabolism.[175]

A close correlation between IP_3 production and secretagogue-induced calcium release has been observed in several cell types. In permeabilized pancreatic cells, cholecystokinin-induced IP_3 release is unchanged when the rise in calcium concentration is abolished by chelating agents, whereas reduction of IP_3 production by inhibition of phospholipase C prevents the rise in calcium release.[176] Such studies have supported the concept that agonist-induced calcium mobilization is mediated by IP_3 or other higher inositol phosphates produced during target cell activation.

Many peptide hormones have been shown to increase PIP_2 hydrolysis and to act through IP_3 to mobilize calcium from intracellular pools. These include TRH,[177] GnRH, and angiotensin II, all of which depend upon calcium-mediated mechanisms to stimulate target cell responses. Additional physiological actions of IP_3 as a calcium-mobilizing signal have been found in the visual system, where IP_3 acts in *Limulus* photoreceptor transduction, and in smooth muscle, where IP_3 increases cytosolic calcium level. In skeletal muscle, IP_3 may serve as the chemical media-

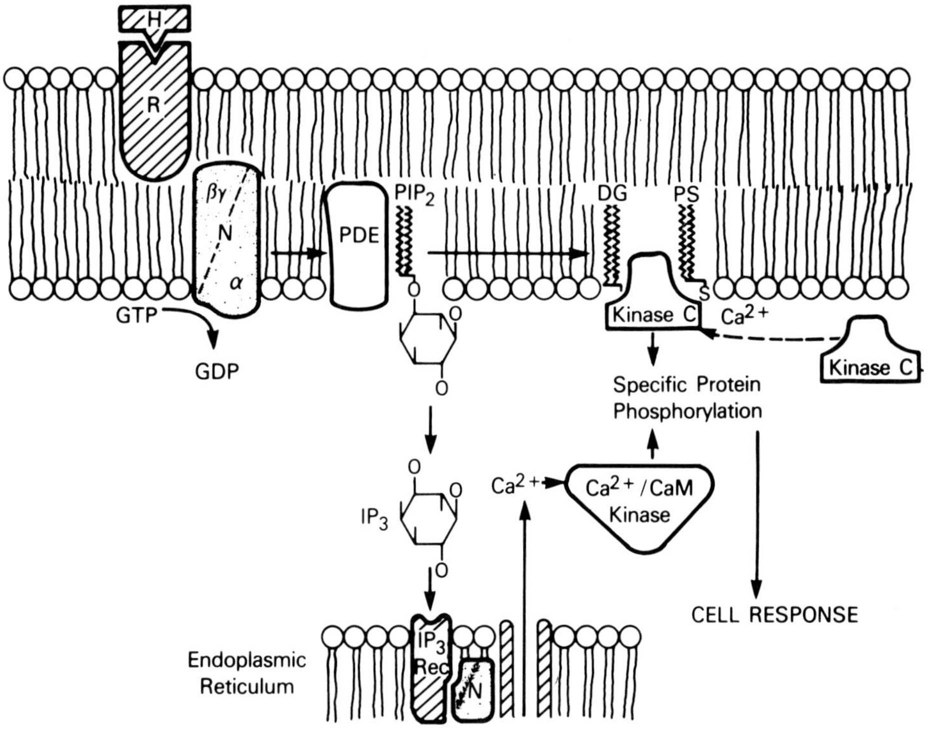

FIGURE 5-30 Receptor-mediated activation of phospholipase C in the target cell plasma membrane, with production of inositol 1,4,5-triphosphate and diacylglycerol and stimulation of calcium mobilization and protein kinase C activity.

tor in excitation-contraction coupling, to transmit the message from the plasma membrane to the sarcoplasmic reticulum to release calcium into the cytoplasm, and to initiate muscle contraction.[179]

The activation of phospholipase C–mediated generation of IP_3 and DAG is enhanced by the addition of guanyl nucleotides to permeabilized cells[179a] or membrane fractions. The coupling component between receptor activation and PIP_2 hydrolysis is a guanyl nucleotide regulatory protein, related to those involved in the regulation of adenylate cyclase by stimulatory and inhibitory hormones. In some cells the Ni unit has been implicated in phosphoinositide breakdown, but in most cases the nucleotide regulatory protein appears to be a distinct and as yet unidentified entity, sometimes termed *Nx*.

In addition to the potential synergistic actions of IP_3 and DAG formed during hormone-stimulated PIP_2 hydrolysis, there are several situations in which stimulation of protein kinase C by DAG or phorbol esters leads to inhibition of IP_3 formation. Such an effect is seen in the inhibition of α_2-adrenergic- and angiotensin II–stimulated smooth muscle responses by phorbol esters.[179b] This suggests that activation of protein kinase C may attenuate receptor coupling to phospholipase C by phosphorylation of the receptor or the nucleotide regulatory protein.

A potential role for polyphosphoinositides in hormone action has also been identified in the adrenal cortex, where ACTH rapidly increases the levels of diphospho- and triphosphoinositides. These effects are also produced by cAMP and are blocked by protein synthesis inhibitors, as are the effects of ACTH. Addition of diphosphoinositide to adrenal mitochondria or isolated cells increases production of pregnenolone and corticosterone, suggesting that the polyphosphoinositides could have a mediating role in the actions of ACTH and cAMP on steroidogenesis.[180]

Stimulation of Phospholipid Methylation

The synthesis of phosphatidylcholine from phosphatidylethanolamine in cell membranes occurs in two sequential methylation steps, by transfer of methyl groups from *S*-adenosylmethionine under the control of two enzymes, *phosphomethyltransferase* 1 and 2. The first enzyme transfers one methyl group to form phosphatidylmonomethylethanolamine; both the substrate, phosphatidylethanolamine, and the first methyltransferase enzyme are located on the cytoplasmic side of the plasma membrane. The second enzyme transfers two more methyl groups, again derived from S-adenosylmethionine, to form phosphatidylcholine. Both the phosphatidylcholine produced and the second methyltransferase are located on the exterior surface of the membrane. The topographical distribution of the enzymes and reactants facilitates the rapid transfer of phospholipids across the plasma membrane by successive methylations.[181] The intramembrane synthesis of the intermediate product, phosphatidylmonomethylethanolamine causes local changes in membrane fluidity and permits increased lateral mobility of intrinsic membrane proteins. β-Adrenergic stimulation of phospholipid methylation and decreased membrane viscosity in reticulocytes are accompanied by unmasking of cryptic β-adrenergic receptors, with increased lateral movement of the receptors and enhanced coupling between receptors and adenylate cyclase. Several hormone receptors, including those for prolactin and LH, are increased in number by methylation of membrane phospholipids. Other membrane events influenced by the synthesis and translocation of methylated phospholipid include calcium-dependent ATPase, leukocyte chemotaxis, mast cell histamine secretion, and lymphocyte mitogenesis. In cultured astrocytoma cells, stimulation of both β-adrenergic and benzodiazepine receptors causes increased phospholipid methylation in an additive manner, suggesting that methyltransferases located in separate domains near the respective receptors are independently stimulated by the two ligands.[182]

These ligand-induced changes in phospholipid methylation and membrane fluidity probably reflect a general phenomenon that influences membrane structure and function during many forms of cellular regulation by hormones and other ligands. They may also explain the short-lived increase in receptors for the homologous hormone and other hormones, which is observed after target cell stimulation. Thus, LH causes a transient increase in both LH and prolactin receptors in the rat testis, and ACTH causes an initial rise in adrenal prolactin sites. In each case, these elevations in receptor number precede the well-recognized process of receptor loss or "down-regulation" that begins several hours after occupancy in vivo. In the Leydig cell, activation of LH receptors is rapidly followed by a cAMP-dependent increase in phospholipid methyltransferase activity, which may be related to changes in receptor exposure and other membrane-associated events in gonadotropin action.[183] The extent to which increased membrane fluidity controls receptor-cyclase coupling in endocrine target cells is not yet known; this mechanism may be an important component in the regulation of cellular sensitivity and responsiveness to hormonal stimulation.

STEROID HORMONES

The major classes of steroid hormones secreted by the gonads and adrenal gland include the androgens, estrogens, progestins, glucocorticoids, and mineralocorticoids. The steps in biosynthesis of these steroids from cholesterol depend upon the complement of metabolic enzymes present in the individual steroidogenic target cells. The overall rates of steroid synthesis and secretion are regulated by pituitary trophic hormones such as LH, FSH, and ACTH in the gonads and adrenal fasciculata zone, and by angiotensin II and other factors in the zona glomerulosa (see Chap. 12). In their target tissues, steroid hormones elicit specific cell responses by stimulating the expression of genes which code for enzymes and other regulatory proteins that determine the specific metabolic and/or secretory activities of the target cell.

Classes of Steroid Action

Each of the specialized steroid-secreting tissues produces one major steroid with a relatively restricted class of action upon target tissues. Since the various steroid hormones are formed via a common biosynthetic pathway from cholesterol and their biological properties are determined by a limited number of structural differences, it is not surprising that the actions of certain steroid molecules show some degree of overlap. Such effects are usually manifested only at high concentrations of the hormone, but may occur under physiological conditions and during steroid therapy. An example of the former is the antimineralocorticoid action of progesterone during pregnancy; examples of the latter include the salt-retaining or mineralocorticoid effects of steroids that exert their primary actions through glucocorticoid receptors, and the antiglucocorticoid effects of progesterone antagonists (Chaps. 12, 14). Such effects are caused by interaction of the heterologous steroids with receptors that are normally occupied by the homologous ligand. Since the biological domain of action for each of the steroid subtypes depends primarily upon the receptors through which it acts and the associated activation pathway, hormone action could be classified according to the receptors through which each characteristic effect is mediated.[184] Each of the major steroid hormones interacts with specific receptors that are present in the respective target cell and not in other tissues. Formation of the specific hormone-receptor complex is followed by an activation step that increases the affinity of the complex for nuclear binding sites. Binding of the steroid-receptor complex to these nuclear elements controls the transcription of specific gene sequences coding for enzymes and regulatory proteins that mediate the characteristic target cell response. Such elements are composed of DNA and may be modulated by acceptor proteins on the DNA as well as on the nuclear membrane and the nuclear matrix.

The gonadal sex steroids, androgen, estrogen, and progesterone, are predominantly involved in the regulation of gene expression and growth in reproductive tissues. In contrast, the adrenal steroids serve mainly as metabolic regulators to control intermediary metabolism and electrolyte homeostasis (Table 5-11). Glucocorticoids are regarded as the original adrenal steroids in evolutionary development; mineralocorticoids are seen as more recently emerged hormones for the specific control of salt balance.[184]

The individual actions of each class of steroid hormones, expressed through their specific receptor sites, are primarily determined by their molecular conformations. As with all regulatory ligands, including drugs and hormones, the expression of agonist activity results from the ability to combine with and activate the specific receptor sites which control the subsequent metabolic step or sequence that is influenced by the ligand. In the steroid hormones, the basic ring structure is modified during biosynthesis by side chain cleavages, reductions, and hydroxylations, plus aromatization of the A ring in the case of estrogens (Chap. 4). The structures of natural steroids that are typical of the major classes are shown in Fig. 5-31, together with examples of synthetic compounds that have been developed for therapeutic use as steroid agonists and antagonists.[185]

Plasma Binding and Steroid Action

In the circulation, gonadal and adrenal steroids are present both free and bound, complexed to plasma proteins. Although the secreted steroids are water-soluble at the low concentrations occurring in plasma (about 10^{-9} M), most of the circulating hormones are transported as steroid-protein complexes. These are of two major types, involving both high-affinity, low-capacity binding to steroid-specific globulins such as testosterone-binding globulin (TeBG) or corticosteroid-binding globulin (CBG or transcortin) and low-affinity, high-capacity binding to albumin. More than 98 percent of the gonadal steroids are protein-bound, and about 95 percent of the circulating hydrocortisone and 50 percent of the aldosterone are bound to plasma protein (Chap. 12). Since it is the free hormone concentration that is active at the target cell, the role of plasma binding may be that of a reservoir or buffer that controls the access of hormone to target cell receptors. Although each of the steroid hormones can be bound by one or another of the plasma proteins, the extent and tightness of binding (i.e., affinity) varies considerably between steroids. Thus, about 40 percent of the circulating aldosterone is weakly bound to serum albumin, whereas over 90 percent of hydrocortisone and testosterone are bound to CBG and sex hormone–binding globulin, respectively. The latter protein also binds estradiol, though probably not to a major extent under physiological conditions.

For the traditional steroid hormones, and for related hormones such as vitamin D and thyroxine, there is no indication that plasma binding has an important role in the biological mechanism of steroid hormone action. As noted above, the free hormone is the biologically active fraction, and its concentration correlates well with the magnitude of the hormone response. Also, steroids are active in the absence of their binding proteins, and many synthetic steroid analogues that do not bind to transport proteins exert potent biological actions on the target tissue by interacting with the specific intracellular receptors. When the concentrations of binding proteins are elevated or decreased by disease or therapeutic measures, the free steroid concentrations remain relatively constant despite changes in the total level of circulating steroid.

Although plasma binding appears to have little if

Table 5-11. Classes of Steroid Hormone Action

Tissue	Steroid hormone	Actions
Testis	Androgens	Male secondary sexual characteristics Reproduction: spermatogenesis
Ovary:		
Follicle	Estrogens	Female secondary sexual characteristics
Corpus luteum	Progestin	Reproduction: pregnancy
Adrenal:		
Zona fasciculata	Glucocorticoids	Metabolic regulation
Zona glomerulosa	Aldosterone	Sodium homeostasis

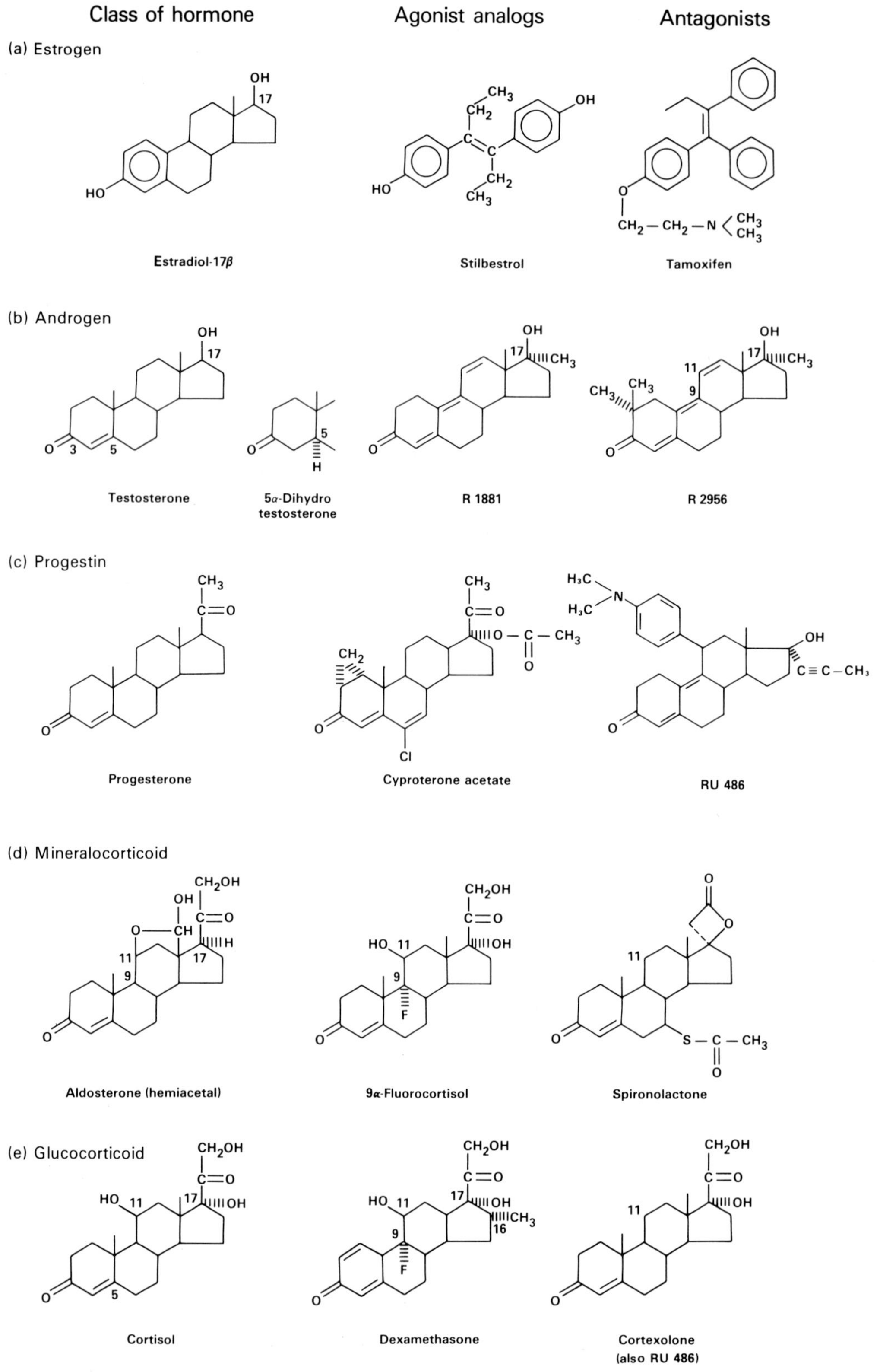

FIGURE 5-31 Structures of the major classes of steroid hormones. (*Modified from Mainwaring.*[185])

any direct role in hormone action other than to serve as a reservoir of circulating steroid, it can obviously influence the rate of clearance of secreted or administered hormones from the circulation. Binding to plasma proteins may also provide a buffer to minimize the influence of episodic hormone secretion on the free steroid concentration presented to the target cell. During treatment with steroid hormones, binding to the plasma transport protein could reduce the rate of metabolism of the administered steroid, and could provide a reservoir from which free hormone is subsequently released. The extent to which these effects of plasma binding influence the duration and magnitude of the individual steroid responses is not clear, but could obviously be relevant to the pharmacokinetics of steroid therapy.[186] Access of steroid hormones to the brain is not inhibited by binding to albumin, whereas globulin-bound hormone is not transported into brain. Thus, the hormone fraction in plasma that is available for transport into brain is not restricted to the free fraction, but includes also the larger albumin-bound moiety.[187] In rat plasma, this would comprise 60 percent of the progesterone, 40 percent of the testosterone, and 15 percent of the corticosteroid, in contrast to the 2 to 8 percent of total plasma hormone that is free.

Differential binding of steroids to plasma proteins also contributes to the action of aldosterone on its specific mineralocorticoid receptors in the kidney. The major aldosterone-binding sites also show high affinity for deoxycorticosterone (DOC) and low but detectable affinity for hydrocortisone. Since the circulating concentration of DOC is similar to that of aldosterone and circulating hydrocortisone concentration is orders of magnitude higher, these steroids should be able to occupy the renal mineralocorticoid receptor. However, both DOC and hydrocortisone are over 90 percent bound in the circulation to albumin and CBG, whereas only 40 percent of the circulating aldosterone is weakly bound to albumin. For these reasons, DOC and glucocorticoids are much less effective competitors for the aldosterone receptors in vivo than under plasma-free conditions in vitro: e.g., 1 to 5 percent vs. 80 percent for DOC. Without the selectivity conferred by the plasma binding of DOC and glucocorticoids, aldosterone could not occupy mineralocorticoid receptors and exert selective regulation on sodium homeostasis. In this manner, plasma binding serves to confer specificity in vivo by keeping "inappropriate" steroids (such as DOC, corticosterone, and hydrocortisone, which can act as mineralocorticoids but are secreted under ACTH control) from binding to high-affinity, low-capacity receptor sites in mineralocorticoid target cells.[188] Tissue-localized CBG-like proteins also contribute to modulation of steroid action, as in the case of renal proteins that sequester cortisol and render the mineralocorticoid receptor available for occupancy by aldosterone.

It should be noted that the circulating steroid-binding proteins differ in several aspects from the intracellular steroid receptors that mediate the target cell response. Physically, the binding proteins are relatively stable, soluble globular glycoproteins, whereas the receptors are asymmetric, relatively more hydrophobic, and much less stable. Functionally, the transport proteins usually bind preferentially with the natural steroid molecule, and poorly or not at all with more potent synthetic analogues. Conversely, the receptor molecule binds both the natural and synthetic steroids (or their metabolites) in proportion to their biological activities.

Steroid Uptake by Target Cells

Apart from the uptake of cholesterol, which is internalized by the receptor-mediated endocytosis of plasma lipoproteins,[92] there is little evidence to suggest that plasma membrane transport mechanisms are involved in the uptake of steroid hormones. Instead, steroids are believed to diffuse freely and rapidly through the cell membrane, which does not appear to limit their access to the intracellular receptor sites. Although steroid uptake does not in general seem to be limited by membrane barriers or transport processes, changes in membrane properties can affect steroid uptake.[188a] In addition, there are several examples of steroid action at the plasma membrane level. Thus, progesterone stimulates differentiation of the frog oocyte[189] by acting at the cell surface to initiate processes leading to the meiotic maturation response.[190] These include a drop in cAMP level and a decrease in protein kinase activity, followed by reinitiation of the first meiotic cell division. The ability of progesterone to interact with the oocyte plasma membrane and inhibit adenylate cyclase activity,[191] and other evidence for steroid hormone interaction at the target cell surface,[7] suggests that the plasma membrane could play a part in the cellular uptake and actions of steroid hormones.

Steroid Hormone Receptors

The ability of steroid hormones to regulate nuclear processes was originally shown by the discovery that estrogens and androgens increase RNA synthesis in the uterus and prostate, respectively.[192,193] Subsequently, tritium-labeled steroid hormones were found to accumulate in their respective target cells' nuclei after in vivo administration. Thus, radioactive estrogens were taken up by female reproductive tissues, which are characterized by their content of specific estrogen receptors that are not detectable in other tissues. Estrogen receptors were originally found to be located predominantly in the cytosol of estrogen-deprived and immature rat uteri, and appeared to undergo translocation to the nucleus after exposure to estrogen.[194] All classes of steroid hormones were subsequently shown to bind to specific receptors detected initially in the cytoplasm of their respective target tissues and to undergo activation and apparent translocation to the nucleus, as shown in Fig. 5-32.

The original two-step model of steroid hormone action (i.e., binding to cytoplasmic receptors followed by translocation to the nucleus) has been revised in the light of recent evidence that estrogen receptors are predominantly concentrated in the cell nucleus at all times. This was previously recognized for thyroid hormone and vitamin D receptors, and seems to apply to steroid hormone receptors as well. In estrogen target cells, studies on receptor distribution by immunocytochemical[195] and cell enucleation[196] methods have shown that most or all of the unfilled estrogen receptors are located in the nucleus. Although there is conflicting evidence regarding glucocorticoid receptor translocation, it is possible that both the traditional "cytosolic" and "nuclear" forms of the receptor normally reside in the nuclear compartment, and the more loosely associated unoccupied receptors escape into the cytosol during cell fractionation. The cytosolic receptor could thus be a preparation artifact, and the activated receptor may acquire its increased affinity for regulatory elements within the nucleus, rather than undergo physical translocation from cytoplasm to nucleus.[196]

The cytosolic estrogen receptor behaves as an 8-S protein during density gradient centrifugation in low-salt media, and as a 4-S form under conditions simulating intracellular ionic strength.[197] The ability of antiestrogens such as clomiphene and nafoxidine to reduce the specific uptake of estrogen and the associated uterine growth response indicate the importance of receptor binding as an early step in estrogen action. After exposure to estrogen and warming, the cytosolic 4-S receptor is converted to a 5-S form with marked affinity for isolated nuclei and chromatin. The nature of the 4-S to 5-S conversion is not clear, but may involve a conformational change or some form of hormone-induced dimerization.[198] The same cytoplasmic receptors and nuclear translocation process are observed in many estrogen-dependent tissues, including anterior pituitary and mammary tumors. Hormone-dependent human breast cancers take up more estrogen than autonomous tumors, and the estrogen receptor content of excised mammary cancers can be used to predict the clinical response to endocrine ablation or blockade in patients with advanced breast cancer.

Purification of the estrogen-receptor complexes has been difficult because of their instability and tendency to aggregate. However, the nuclear estradiol-receptor complex has been isolated as a 4.8-S protein

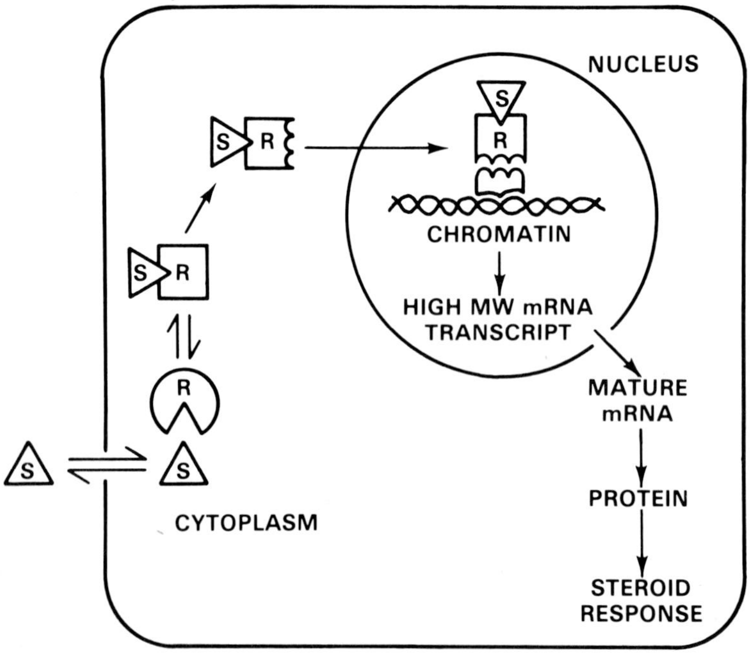

FIGURE 5-32 Diagram of the steps in steroid hormone action. Activation of the intracellular receptors by steroid hormones is followed by nuclear binding of the complex and stimulation of mRNA synthesis. (*From Baxter and McLeod,*[184] *by permission.*)

of mol wt 66,000 and monoclonal antibodies to the estrogen receptor have been generated by immunization with purified preparations of the nuclear estradiol receptor of calf uterus and MCF-7 breast cancer cells. Such antibodies cross-react with receptors from estrogen-sensitive tissues and tumors from several animal species.[199] One of the many possible applications of such antibodies is the development of immunochemical methods for the measurement of estrogen receptors in target tissues, including human breast cancers for evaluation of their estrogen dependence.

The structure of the human estrogen receptor has been determined by the analysis of cloned DNA corresponding to the estrogen receptor gene of MCF-7 breast cancer cells. Complementary DNA clones corresponding to the translated sequence of receptor mRNA from MCF-7 cells were identified in expression vector libraries by screening with monoclonal antibodies to the estrogen receptor and synthetic oligonucleotide probes corresponding to peptide sequences from the purified receptor.[200] After selection of a cDNA clone of appropriate length to contain the 65-kilodalton receptor, nucleotide sequencing revealed an open reading frame of 1785 nucleotides encoding the estrogen receptor. The receptor molecule was found to be composed of 595 amino acids and had a molecular weight of 66,200, similar to previously estimated values of 65,000 to 70,000 for the functional receptor. The cDNA clone containing the translated portion of the receptor mRNA was also expressed in Chinese hamster ovarian cells to give a functional estradiol-binding receptor protein that sedimented as a 4-S complex in the absence of salt.

The amino acid sequence of the estrogen receptor shows significant regions of homology with the human glucocorticoid receptor and the *v-erbA* oncogene product. The homologous region is rich in cysteine, lysine, and arginine residues, and may represent a DNA-binding domain of the steroid receptors and the *v-erbA* proteins. The glucocorticoid and estrogen receptors both contain a proline-rich region upstream from the cysteine-rich basic amino acid region and a carboxy-terminal hydrophobic region that may correspond to the steroid-binding domain. The sequence homologies between the two steroid receptors and the *erbA* oncogene protein suggest that all are derived from a common primordial gene, and are now related by their retention of shared coding sequences for a domain that is responsible for DNA recognition and binding.[201]

Progesterone receptors are present in female reproductive tissues, including the oviduct, uterus, and vagina; they have been characterized as 6.5- to 8-S "cytosolic" components that dissociate to a 4-S form in the presence of salt, analogous to the estrogen receptor. The nature and quantity of the progesterone receptor is markedly influenced by estrogen. The rat uterine progesterone-receptor complex from unstimulated animals sediments at 4- to 5-S in low-salt gradients, and is converted to a larger component (6.5- to 8-S) after treatment with estrogen.[202] Also, during the estrous cycle, the large cytosolic form (6.7-S) predominates at proestrus, and a smaller (4.5-S) form is present at diestrus, consistent with the effects of administered estrogen. The concentration of progesterone receptors in reproductive tissues is markedly increased by estrogen treatment. The number of uterine sites is maximum at proestrus in animals, and is higher in hyperplastic human endometrium than during the proliferative and secretory phases of the menstrual cycle.

The properties of progesterone receptors have been extensively studied in the immature chick oviduct; in this tissue estrogen promotes the differentiation of tubular gland cells which secrete the major egg white proteins ovalbumin, conalbumin, and lysozyme, and stimulate the formation of progesterone receptors. After estrogen withdrawal, ovalbumin synthesis ceases, but it can be reinitiated by treatment with either estrogen or progesterone. Treatment with progesterone also causes epithelial differentiation to form goblet cells that synthesize avidin, an oviduct protein with extremely high affinity for biotin. The oviduct "cytosolic" progesterone receptor sediments as a 3.8-S complex, and undergoes "translocation" to the nucleus by a temperature-dependent process in the presence of progesterone. The nuclear progesterone-receptor complex is a 4-S species similar to that present in the cytosol, and does not show the change in sedimentation properties that is characteristic of the nuclear estrogen receptor, which converts from a 4-S to a 5-S form during activation. The "cytosolic" 8-S progesterone receptor has been purified and separated into two 4-S components, A and B, with mol wts of 110,000 and 117,000. The B component appears to interact specifically with oviduct chromatin, and may be responsible for the tissue-binding specificity of the activated progesterone receptor.[203]

Androgen receptors have been identified in male genital and accessory sex tissues by binding studies with tritiated testosterone and dihydrotestosterone. The androgen receptors present in the cytosol of prostate, seminal vesicles, and other male tissues sediment as 8- to 9-S forms in low-salt gradients, and as a 4-S form in the presence of salt. Similar to the estrogen and progesterone receptors, the cytosolic androgen-receptor complex undergoes temperature-dependent activation and translocation to the nucleus, whence it can be extracted as a 3-S form.[204] An important feature of the androgen receptor system in male accessory sex tissues is the requirement for conversion of testosterone to dihydrotestosterone (DHT) prior to receptor binding and activation. Thus, the 3-S nuclear androgen-receptor complex in these tissues contains DHT, not testosterone, formed by the action of cytoplasmic 5α-reductase prior to binding to the receptors. The need for enzymatic conversion of androgenic hormones to DHT to achieve receptor activation in many male target tissues is relevant to certain forms of genetically determined androgen resistance. The testicular feminization syndrome, an extreme form of male pseudohermaphroditism, can arise from both defective synthesis of DHT and a receptor defect in androgen action. The comparable syndrome in rodents appears to result from a defect in the androgen receptor rather than an abnormality in the reduction of testosterone to DHT.[205]

Glucocorticoid receptors were originally identified in hepatic and lymphoid cells and are present in most mammalian tissues, in keeping with the widespread regulatory actions of hydrocortisone and related corticosteroids. The receptors are unstable in the absence of steroid, and exhibit high affinity and stereospecificity for natural glucocorticoids and potent synthetic analogues such as dexamethasone and triamcinolone. Like other steroid-receptor complexes, the cytosolic glucocorticoid-receptor complex rapidly undergoes temperature-dependent activation with acquisition of the ability to bind to nuclear chromatin. The glucocorticoid-receptor complex sediments as a 7-S species in low-salt gradients and converts to a 3- to 4-S form at high ionic strength. The activated steroid-receptor complex sediments as a 5- to 9-S form and has a lower isoelectric point, which leads to altered mobility on ion exchange media (phosphocellulose and DEAE-cellulose) as well as enhanced affinity for DNA and chromatin.[206] This change in ionic properties permits separation of the activated and nonactivated complexes on DEAE-cellulose. Analysis of thymus cell cytosol by this procedure has shown that the nonactivated complex is present only in the first minute after exposure to dexamethasone, and is rapidly converted to the activated complex within the next few minutes.[207]

The glucocorticoid receptor has been purified from rat and human tissues as a dimeric protein containing subunits of M_r 94,000. The receptor contains steroid- and DNA-binding regions, and also a major immunogenic region that is distinct from the two functional domains of the molecule. By the use of receptor antibodies as specific probes, receptor cDNA sequences have been cloned from lymphoid cells and fibroblasts, and the complete amino acid sequence of the human glucocorticoid receptor has been determined.[208] Two forms of the receptor, α and β, were found, consisting of 777 and 742 amino acids, respectively, with differences in the carboxy-terminal region. The two forms of the receptor diverge in sequence at amino acid 727 and contain additional open reading frames of 50 (α) and 15 (β) amino acids at their carboxyl termini. The α form of the receptor is predominant in human cells and cDNA libraries, and selectively binds glucocorticoids after expression in an in vitro translation system. The translation product programmed by α glucocorticoid receptor mRNA is functionally active, as shown by binding of tritiated triamcinolone. Corticosteroids and progesterone (consistent with its antiglucocorticoid activity) compete for binding to the protein, but estrogen and testosterone do not. The receptor sequence contains a cysteine-arginine-lysine-rich region that may be a part of the DNA-binding domain. Chromosome mapping indicates that the glucocorticoid receptor is encoded by a single gene on chromosome 5, and that another gene on chromosome 16 contains homology with the receptor. As noted elsewhere, a major feature of interest in the glucocorticoid receptor is its homology with the product of the oncogene *v-erbA*, suggesting that the DNA-binding domains of both the genes for both proteins are derived from a common primordial regulatory gene.[209]

Aldosterone receptors have been found in mineralocorticoid target tissues such as kidney, bladder, parotid gland, and gut. Such receptors in secretory epithelia are extremely labile and difficult to analyze, and their study has been complicated by the presence of other receptors for the structurally and biologically similar glucocorticoids in target tissues.[210] The relative affinities of the two classes of receptors for aldosterone and glucocorticoids are such that aldosterone binds primarily to the type 1 (mineralocorticoid) sites at low and physiological concentrations, and to increasing numbers of the glucocorticoid sites at higher concentrations. Conversely, glucocorticoids have low mineralocorticoid activity at physiological levels but bind to type 1 sites and exert sodium-retaining effects when present (or administered) at supraphysiological concentrations. When studied by techniques which correct for the interference by glucocorticoid sites, aldosterone receptors bind mineralocorticoids in proportion to their biological activity, and react with hydrocortisone (at sufficiently high concentrations) as well as the more active sodium-retaining steroids aldosterone and DOC. The principal cytoplasmic aldosterone-receptor complex sediments as an 8.5-S form in low-ionic-strength gradients and as a 4-S form at high ionic strength.[211] The nuclear receptors extracted by 0.3 M KCl also sediment at 4-S, and undergo maximum translocation from the cytosol (i.e., increased affinity for nuclear binding sites) within 10 min after injection of aldosterone.

Steroid Hormone Receptors: Activation and Nuclear Binding

Each of the major classes of steroid hormones, including estrogens, progestins, androgens, glucocorticoids, and mineralocorticoids, has been shown to act according to the general model described above. This involves specific binding to intracellular receptors, followed by activation, or transformation, of the complex to a form with high affinity for nuclear binding sites. Binding of the activated complex to nuclear acceptor sites on the target cell chromatin modulates the transcription of specific genes responsible for the synthesis of particular species of mRNA (Fig. 5-32).

The process of receptor activation is hormone-induced and temperature-dependent, and usually provokes a change in the apparent molecular weight, charge, and/or conformation of the complex. However, there is no constant change that characterizes the activation process for all classes of steroid hormone. Only the estrogen receptor shows an increase in sedimentation rate, from 4-S to 5-S. The androgen-receptor complex and some progesterone-receptor complexes show decreased sedimentation after activation, and the glucocorticoid receptors exhibit altered charge properties. Thus, although a general process of steroid hormone receptor activation is necessary for nuclear binding and action, the nature of this change varies for the individual steroid hormone receptors, and the general basis of the activation process remains unclear.[212]

Steroid Hormone Agonists and Antagonists

As for many other types of biologically active ligands, whether drugs, transmitters, or hormones, steroid hormones and their derivatives can be classified as agonists, antagonists, or inactive compounds. In general, agonist activity is proportional to the affinity of binding to receptors and the efficacy with which the hormone-receptor complex activates the biological response. Antagonists also show high receptor affinity, but do not bind and/or activate effectively in the nucleus. An allosteric model for the actions of steroid agonists and antagonists in altering receptor conformation and activity is shown in Fig. 5-33. The distinction between agonists and antagonists is rarely absolute, and many compounds act as partial agonists (or partial antagonists) by binding to receptors and eliciting a less than maximal response even at full occupancy of receptor sites. Pure agonists may be weak or strong, depending on their affinity for the receptors, but do not act as antagonists. Thus, weak agonists can elicit the same biological response as potent agonists when present at a concentration high enough to cause

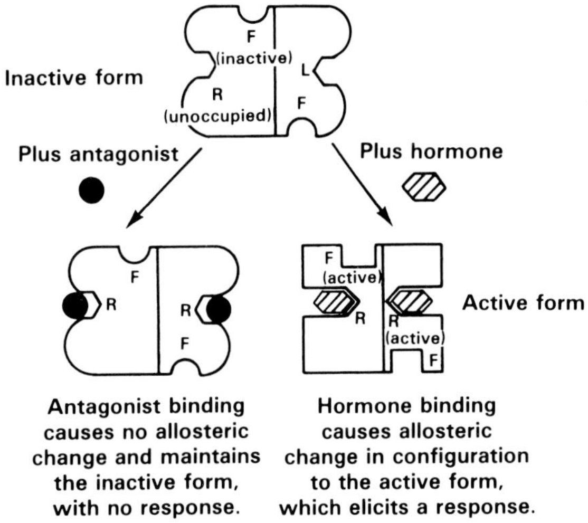

FIGURE 5-33 An allosteric model for steroid ligand–receptor interactions. The receptor contains both a steroid-binding site (L) and a functional site (F) necessary for biological activity, and can exist in either inactive or active configurations. (*From Mainwaring,*[185] *by permission.*)

occupancy of the same proportion of receptors. In contrast, partial agonists cannot elicit the full response even when occupying most or all of the receptors, and may then act to antagonize or block the effects of added agonist compounds. Partial agonists can be regarded as part of a spectrum of activity between pure agonists and pure antagonists. For most clinical and research purposes, pure agonists and antagonists are clearly preferable. However, many antagonists possess some degree of agonist activity, and this should be taken into account during their use in therapy and receptor-binding analysis. It should also be noted that, whereas the activity of given agonists is relatively constant in various tissues, partial agonists and antagonists can display variable degrees of agonist and antagonist activity in specific target tissues, or under different experimental conditions.

ESTROGEN ANTAGONISTS

Certain nonsteroidal antiestrogen derivatives, such as nafoxidine and tamoxifen, antagonize the estrogen-induced responses leading to uterine growth and target cell hyperplasia. Such compounds bind to the estrogen receptors and promote the apparent translocation of the antagonist-receptor complex. Within the nucleus, the complex binds to chromatin and is retained for a prolonged period, causing initial stimulation of RNA polymerase and cell hypertrophy. However, the binding of the antagonist-receptor complex is not followed by subsequent replenishment of the cytosol receptors, whether by recycling or resynthesis, as occurs after receptor translocation by estrogen agonists.[213] Estrogen antagonists decrease the rate of proliferation of breast cancer cells in vitro by inhibiting estrogen-dependent production of specific proteins and growth factors that exert autocrine effects on cell division. Progestins also act as estrogen antagonists, via effects mediated by the progesterone receptor, again to reduce the rate of estrogen-dependent protein synthesis.

ANDROGEN ANTAGONISTS

The most active naturally occurring antiandrogen is progesterone, and some of the most potent androgen antagonists are highly active progestin derivatives. Antiandrogens antagonize the effects of testosterone or DHT by competing for the androgen-binding sites on receptors present in androgen-dependent target tissues.[214] Such compounds are of potential value in the treatment of hirsutism and other masculinizing syndromes, and in the management of prostatic hyperplasia and carcinoma. The highly active progestin antiandrogens, such as cyproterone acetate, interact with progesterone receptors as well as with androgen receptors. However, not all progestins are androgen antagonists, and chlormadinone acetate has relatively low antiandrogenic activity despite its close structural resemblance to cyproterone acetate. The presence of a cyclopropane group on ring A of cyproterone acetate is the major structural difference between these two compounds, and may be important for antiandrogenic activity. Some of the antiandrogens also cause suppression of gonadotropin secretion, with consequent reduction of testosterone production as well as blockade of androgen action. Others, such as medroxyprogesterone, also inhibite 5α-reductase activity and thus impair DHT formation. It is important to note that certain progestin antiandrogens also possess other hormonal activities, e.g., cyproterone acetate is also androgenic, antiestrogenic, and antigonadotropic.[215] In addition, prolonged treatment with cyproterone to achieve antiandrogenic effects can also lead to suppression of adrenal function by inhibition of ACTH secretion. Spironolactone also interacts with estrogen and androgen receptors, as well as with aldosterone receptors, and can exert estrogenic and antiandrogenic effects, including gynecomastia and loss of libido. Nonsteroidal androgen antagonists include flutamide, which has no hormonal activity and is equipotent with cyproterone acetate as an antiandrogen. Like the progestins, flutamide inhibits androgen uptake and nuclear retention in target tissues by competing for binding to the intracellular androgen receptor.

PROGESTERONE ANTAGONISTS

An effective progesterone antagonist has been developed by the synthesis of a 19-nortestosterone derivative (RU 486) bearing a dimethylaminophenyl substitution at the C-11β position. This molecule resembles a derivative of the progestin norethindrone with an aromatic nucleus at the 11β position (which probably confers antagonist properties) and a 17α side chain that increases affinity for the progesterone receptor. This compound has very little progesterone activity, but binds with high affinity to the progesterone receptor and is a potent progestin antagonist. RU 486 has powerful antiprogesterone activity in animals and humans, and exerts antifertility effects in women at several points in the reproductive cycle and during early pregnancy.[215a] The prominent antiglucocorticoid effects of RU 486 (see below) have not been a significant problem in the clinical use of the drug in the doses and schedules required for its antifertility effects.

GLUCOCORTICOID ANTAGONISTS

The development of clinically useful glucocorticoid antagonists is complicated by the ability of increasing ACTH secretion to overcome the effect of glucocorticoid blockade via increased adrenal secretion of hydrocortisone. However, several steroids display partial, or tissue-dependent, competitive inhibition of the actions of hydrocortisone and related glucocorticoids.[216] Most glucocorticoids possess an axial 11β hydroxyl group which may be important for receptor-binding activity.[91] 11-Deoxysteroids such as cortisone, 11-desoxy-17-hydroxycorticosterone (also called cortexolone, 11-deoxycortisol, or compound S), and progesterone bind to glucocorticoid receptors and act as partial agonists or antagonists, at least in vitro, when they are not further metabolized to glucocorticoids. In vivo, the latter effect prevents these steroids from exerting significant antiglucocorticoid actions, with the exception of nonmetabolized compounds such as cyproterone acetate. The antiprogestin RU 486 is also a powerful glucocorticoid antagonist with high affinity for the glucocorticoid receptor; it causes significant elevations in plasma ACTH and cortisol levels due to blockade of the central and peripheral actions of adrenal corticosteroids, and should be of major value in the clinical management of patients with excessive cortisol secretion.

MINERALOCORTICOID ANTAGONISTS

Compounds such as spironolactone act as aldosterone antagonists by competitive inhibition of aldosterone binding to mineralocorticoid receptors, forming a receptor-antagonist complex that does not undergo translocation and nuclear binding. Such receptor-antagonist complexes show different sedimentation properties from those of the receptor-aldosterone complex; they may represent either inactive forms of the receptor or the effects of altered conformational properties induced by antagonist binding.[217] In addition to its other actions, described above, high doses of spironolactone also inhibit aldosterone biosynthesis, thus exerting an additional antimineralocorticoid effect (see Chap. 12).

Other compounds which interact with the mineralocorticoid receptors include nonsteroidal agents such as anti-inflammatory drugs (e.g., phenylbutazone) and glycerrhetic acid. These agents compete with aldosterone for binding to renal receptors and produce sodium retention and other steroidal effects. Thus, the interaction of such agonist compounds with the aldosterone receptors leads to activation of the target cell response, presumably via the same nuclear mechanism responsible for mediating the effects of endogenous mineralocorticoid on electrolyte transport.

DNA Structure and Organization

The hydrogen-bonded nucleotide polymers that compose the double helix of DNA contain the genetic information that directs the synthesis and composition of the protein molecules of the organism. The genetic message within DNA requires three forms of RNA to be translated into specific cellular proteins. The message is transcribed both constitutively and under the control of hormones and other regulatory molecules. In eukaryotic organisms, the DNA is composed of about 100,000 genes, only a minority (about 10 percent) of which are active within any one cell. The majority of the DNA, which is not required for individual cell function, is packaged into a series of higher-order structures in which the unwanted genes are not accessible to the proteins that control transcription.[218] Conversely, the genes that must be actively expressed to determine the differentiation and function of an individual cell are arranged in a readily accessible manner. Both of these structural arrangements depend on the interaction of DNA with histones, the five basic proteins that are responsible for the primary folding of DNA into the compact form termed *chromatin.* The basic unit of chromosome chromatin is the *nucleosome,* a small particle composed of histones and DNA in a highly organized structure. Each nucleosome is a discoid assembly (6 × 11 nm) of mol wt 200,000, composed of an octamer of four histone proteins (two each of H2a, H2b, H3, and H4) around which two turns of the DNA duplex are wrapped as a superhelix of about 150 base pairs.[219] The polynculeosome chain based on the 2-nm DNA fiber becomes condensed into 10-nm coils of about six nucleosomes per turn, which are further wound into spiral arrays to form a 30-nm solenoid structure in which each turn contains about 1200 base pairs of DNA.[220] This structural arrangement causes sequence elements that are spaced along the DNA chain to approximate in the higher-order chromatin structure. The solenoids of nucleosomes are probably further supercoiled to achieve an even more compact form in the interphase chromosomes.

Nuclear Binding of Steroid Receptors

Interaction of the activated cytoplasmic hormone-receptor complexes with the nucleus of target cells is necessary for the expression of biological effects of the steroid hormones. Once activated, the steroid-receptor complex acquires the ability to bind to chromatin as well as DNA and other polyanions, and becomes concentrated in the nuclear compartment. The finding of unoccupied estrogen receptors in nuclei as well as in cytoplasm of unstimulated cells suggests that the free receptor may be distributed throughout the target cell, even though its tight binding in the nucleus may depend on conversion to the activated chromatin-binding forms, with displacement of the equilibrium between nuclear and extranuclear distribution.

Within the nucleus the activated complex binds to acceptor sites on the chromatin and initiates the synthesis of specific mRNA and protein.[221] The sites that bind glucocorticoid-receptor complexes have been studied in the greatest detail. These sites, which are termed *glucocorticoid regulatory elements* (GREs), contain specific DNA sequences that have a much higher affinity than random DNA for the hormone-receptor complexes. An additional chromatin protein may also participate in the binding reaction. These DNA sequences have been best characterized in the mouse mammary tumor virus genome and human metallothionein-IIa gene, for which consensus sequences of 6 to 16 nucleotides have been proposed.[221a,221b,221c] Of these, the hexanucleotide TGTT/CCT occurs most consistently. However, DNA footprinting studies show that the receptor covers a broader span of DNA, and since this sequence also occurs commonly in genes that are not steroid-regulated, the hexanucleotide may be necessary but is not sufficient to confer receptor-binding specificity. The main points of contact between the glucocorticoid-receptor complex and the DNA are probably along the major groove, and the nucleotides at these loci may be more critical than the intervening nucleotides.[221d,221e] It appears that progesterone-receptor complexes bind to nuclear sites similar to those that bind glucocorticoid-receptor complexes, although the contact points differ somewhat.[221b,221e] Much less is known about the structures of the nuclear binding sites for estrogen, androgen, and vitamin D receptors. The DNA-binding site of the receptor molecule is thought to contain lysine, arginine, and histidine residues, and to be influenced by agents which affect sulfhydryl groups.

At least one receptor molecule, for progesterone, has been proposed to contain two subunits, one (A) with nonspecific affinity for DNA and another (B) with specific affinity for oviduct chromatin. The selective binding of progesterone-receptor complexes depends on interaction of the B subunit with a specific nonhistone protein fraction of chromatin, which may be responsible for the tissue specificity of progesterone action. Such a dual binding process might increase the template activity of chromatin by making initiation sites available for the synthesis of mRNAs for avidin and other oviduct proteins.[203]

The high capacity of the nucleus for hormone receptor binding probably indicates that these sites are in excess over the receptors and that the latter are limiting for the maximal steroid response.[2a,221f] It is possible that only a few of these nuclear receptor sites are responsible for regulation of specific genes. Thus, saturability of the nuclear sites by hormone-receptor complexes is not always observed, and up to 10,000 complexes can be translocated during stimulation by physiological hormone concentrations. Linear correlations between biological responses (such as mRNA synthesis) and receptor occupancy are demonstrable up to several thousand receptors per nucleus. Alternatively, it is possible that translocated hormone receptor complexes are bound to many low-affinity nuclear sites, masking the interaction with the small number of acceptor sites responsible for gene regulation.[198]

Role of the Nuclear Matrix in Steroid Hormone Action

Just as many of the structural and functional properties of the cell are determined by the cytoskeleton, with its specific arrays of structural proteins, the nucleus also contains a skeleton or matrix which has a fundamental role in nuclear function.[223] The nuclear matrix is composed of the residual 10 to 15 percent of nuclear protein and associated components that remain after detergent and salt extraction of nuclei to remove phospholipids, histones, and some nonhistone proteins. The residual protein matrix consists of a peripheral lamina derived from the nuclear envelope, with residual nuclear pore complexes surrounding an internal fibrous network containing residual ribonucleoprotein (RNP) particles and the nucleolus. Several fundamental nuclear processes, including DNA organization and replication as well as heterogeneous nuclear RNA (hnRNA) synthesis and processing, are associated with the nuclear matrix. The supercoiled loops of chromatin in interphase nuclei are anchored to the scaffold of the nuclear matrix, possibly by specific DNA sequences at the attachment site.[224] The anchorage points of the supercoiled loops to the nuclear matrix are the sites at which DNA replication takes place under the control of DNA polymerase, which is also associated with the matrix (Fig. 5-34).

Both estrogens and androgens, which influence these processes in their target cells, bind specifically to the nuclear matrices of steroid-responsive tissues after in vivo administration. In the uterus, estrogen-induced growth responses are correlated with the interaction of estradiol-receptor complexes with the nuclear matrix, at sites that may be involved in the replenishment and processing of receptors. In the prostate, the presence of DHT receptors in the nuclear matrix is associated with androgenic stimulation of the gland. Also, in vitro binding studies have shown that bound androgen-receptor complexes are present in salt-resistant chromatin fractions of rat prostate and testis, and bound progesterone-receptor complexes are present in corresponding fractions of the chick oviduct.[225]

Within the nuclear matrix, the residual deproteinized DNA is bound over short regions separated by free loops of DNA that can be digested by restriction endonucleases. The matrix-bound DNA contains actively transcribed genes, including constitutively expressed genes and those whose transcription is

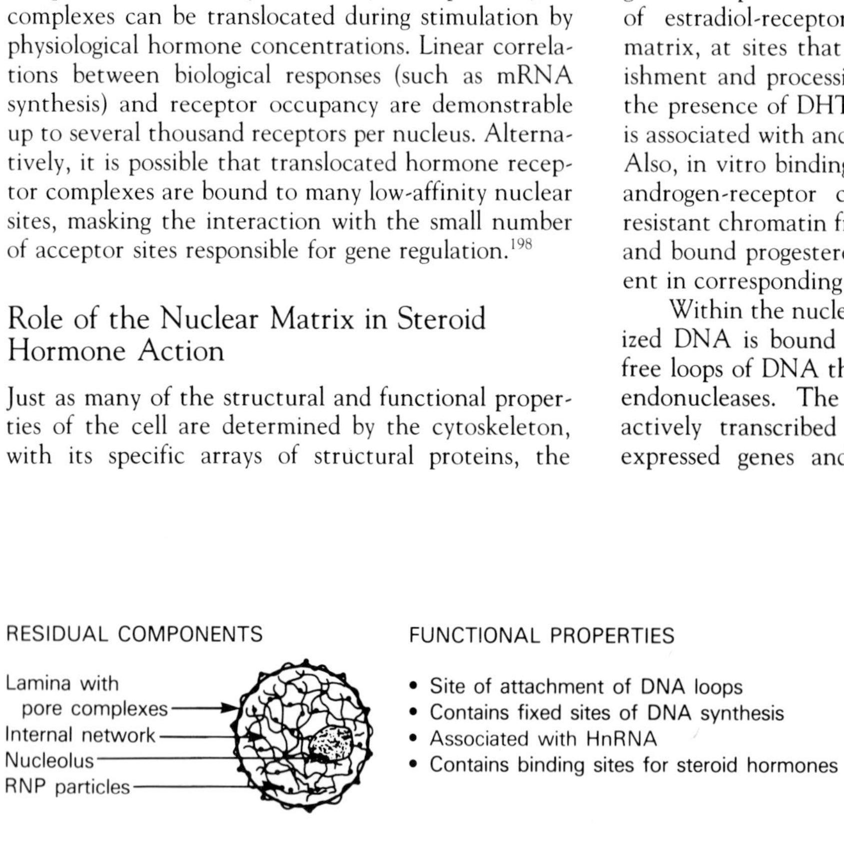

FIGURE 5-34 Organization and functions of the nuclear matrix. The salt-extracted, DNAse I–digested, detergent-treated nuclear framework is lipid-free and contains only 10 percent of the original nuclear proteins. It is involved in DNA synthesis, gene transcription, and RNA processing and contains receptor sites for estrogens, androgens, and glucocorticoids in the respective target cells and tissues. (*Modified from Barrack and Coffey.*[225])

induced by hormones and other regulators, such as the ovalbumin gene.[226] In the absence of hormone, with cessation of transcription the ovalbumin gene ceases to be bound to the matrix. It appears that gene transcription occurs mainly on the protein skeleton of the nuclear matrix, with which steroid hormone receptors also become associated during hormonal stimulation. It is not clear whether the attachment of inducible genes to the matrix is promoted by steroid hormones or is a general concomitant of gene transcription and reflects the accessibility of the steroid regulatory elements in this portion of the DNA to binding of steroid-hormone complexes.

Control of Gene Transcription by Steroid Hormones

EFFECTS OF HORMONE-RECEPTOR COMPLEXES ON CHROMATIN

After the interaction of steroid hormones with their specific intracellular receptor proteins, the activated hormone-receptor complexes bind rapidly to defined DNA sequences on the chromatin and influence the transcription of specific genes with consequent effects on synthesis of specific mRNAs and proteins. Several of the specific proteins whose production is regulated by steroid hormones acting on mRNA synthesis are listed in Table 5-12. The synthesis of many other steroid-induced proteins is known to be influenced by primary actions of the hormone-receptor complex on gene transcription and the rate of mRNA formation.

Much information has come from studies on the effects of sex steroids on both RNA and protein synthesis in hormone-deficient target tissues. For example, during primary stimulation of immature rat uterus and the chick oviduct by estrogen, all major forms of RNA and many proteins are synthesized throughout the phase of cellular growth and differentiation.[227] In the uterus, synthesis of mRNA for a characteristic "induced protein" is an early response to estrogen.[228] In the chick oviduct, tubular gland cell proliferation is accompanied by synthesis of several egg white proteins, of which ovalbumin is a major component. The oviduct, if allowed to regress after the primary response to estrogen, responds to further estrogen or progesterone treatment with a rapid increase in production of mRNAs controlling the synthesis of specific proteins for export, including ovalbumin and conalbumin. The rate of ovalbumin mRNA synthesis, measured either by in vitro translation or cDNA hybridization, increases rapidly after estrogen administration, and is closely correlated with the rate of ovalbumin synthesis. After withdrawal of estrogen, the concentration of ovalbumin mRNA molecules decreases rapidly to low levels, commensurate with the dependence of the ovalbumin gene upon the presence of estrogen for continued transcription of mRNA.

Table 5-12. Specific Proteins Regulated by Steroid Hormones via Control of mRNA Synthesis*

Steroid hormone	Protein
Estrogen	Ovalbumin
	Conalbumin
	Apo-VLDL
	Vitellogenin
	Prolactin
Progesterone	Avidin
	Uteroglobin
	α_2-microglobulin
	Aldolase
Glucocorticoids	Tyrosine aminotransferase
	Tryptophan oxygenase
	Glutamine synthetase
	Growth hormone
	Corticotropin
	Mammary tumor virus

*Many other steroid hormone-dependent proteins are known (e.g., renin substrate, thyroxine-binding globulin, corticosteroid-binding globulin), but the level at which their production is regulated has yet to be defined by direct assay of mRNA formation during hormone action.[1]

Even in circumstances in which steroids do not have a major effect on overall protein synthesis, as in certain glucocorticoid-responsive cells, the steroid still affects a significant subset (i.e., about 1 percent) of the expressed genes of the cell (Chap. 12). In some cases, the actions are more complex, and increased mRNA synthesis may be decreased by addition of a second hormone which inhibits the action of the first, such as antagonists of estrogen or androgen.

Although the effect of steroid hormones is usually to *increase* the rate of mRNA synthesis, on many occasions specific gene transcription is *decreased* by hormone treatment, as in the inhibitory effect of glucocorticoids on proopiomelanocortin (POMC) gene expression in anterior pituitary cells (Chap. 12). Pituitary levels of POMC mRNA rise progressively after adrenalectomy and are decreased by glucocorticoid treatment. The rate of transcription of the gene for POMC increases markedly within 1 h after adrenalectomy and is suppressed by glucocorticoid treatment.[229] Evidence that corticosteroids regulate the rate of formation of the precursor mRNA molecule has also been obtained in cultured pituitary tumor cells.[230] However, the acute suppression of ACTH release by glucocorticoids occurs too rapidly to be attributed to decreased mRNA synthesis, indicating that glucocorticoids also exert a rapid inhibitory effect at the level of ACTH secretion.

Inhibitory control at the level of mRNA synthesis is particularly relevant to the feedback effects of steroid and thyroid hormones upon the secretion of the respective trophic hormones; it also occurs during estrogen suppression of levels of mRNA for LH subunits in castrated animals. An example of the concurrent inhibitory and stimulatory actions of steroid hormones on protein synthesis is the stimulation of GH gene expression by dexamethasone during its suppression of POMC gene expression.[229] Steroid hormone–receptor complexes may also alter RNA processing or stability,[227a,227b] although the usual effect is to enhance RNA synthesis.[198]

RECEPTOR INTERACTIONS WITH GENETIC CONTROL ELEMENTS

The molecular mechanisms by which steroid hormones elicit genomic transcription appear to involve binding of the steroid-receptor complexes to regulatory DNA sequences in the vicinity of the induced genes. Direct studies on the interaction between steroid-receptor complexes and specific DNA sequences have been facilitated by molecular cloning of selected gene fragments of known structure, and by studies on the sequence requirements of cloned genes for expression after transfer to steroid-responsive cells. Analysis of the interaction between the glucocorticoid-receptor complex and DNA sequences has been facilitated by the sensitivity of the mouse mammary tumor virus genome and the human metallothionein-IIa gene to stimulation by dexamethasone in cultured cells. Expression of these genes within the host cells is enhanced by binding of the dexamethasone-receptor complex to a region in the 5′ flanking region of the genes, centered about 200 nucleotides upstream of the transcription start site. This glucocorticoid response element operates as an enhancer sequence to control the rate of initiation of transcription at the promoter site.[231] Thus, when the GRE is positioned by ligation upstream of a promoter that ordinarily is not steroid-regulated and the hybrid gene is transferred into a glucocorticoid-responsive cell, its expression can be regulated by dexamethasone. Unexpectedly, the GRE can function in either orientation and whether upstream from the promoter or downstream from it in an intron. The GRE can also function over considerable distances, in some cases over 1000 nucleotides away from the promoter.

Binding of the glucocorticoid receptor to other genes has also been observed, and these sites have been shown to participate in the control of transcription by glucocorticoids. In the case of the human growth hormone gene, a functional GRE is present in the first intron. The progesterone receptor binds at the 5′ flanking region of several oviduct protein genes to enhance their expression. In the case of the ovalbumin gene, the DNA sequence required for progesterone receptor binding and induction of transcription is located 100 to 200 base pairs upstream from the coding sequence.[232] During estrogen action in the oviduct, the stimulation of ovalbumin gene expression may result from removal of the inhibitory effect of a negative regulatory element located 300 to 400 bases upstream of the cap site, beyond the sequence at which progesterone acts to enhance the activity of the ovalbumin promoter site.[233]

The mechanisms by which binding of the hormone receptor complexes to DNA affect the initiation of transcription are not known. However, steroids cause local changes in chromatin structure that can be detected by differences in DNase-hypersensitive sites near the promoter.[231] Other changes in chromatin structure have been observed[2a,221g,231] and could be due to conformational alterations induced by DNA-receptor complex binding or to some catalytic function inherent in or modulated by the receptor complex or by its binding to DNA. Hormone-receptor complexes have also been found to alter RNA polymerase activity in isolated nuclei and the template function of target cell chromatin. Estrogens and androgens stimulate the activities of nucleolar and nucleoplasmic RNA polymerases (polymerases 1 and 2) in the respective target cells (uterus and prostate). Also, the progesterone-receptor complex enhances the template activity of chromatin from the chick oviduct but not from nontarget tissues, though this may be a secondary effect.

The accumulation of mRNA during steroid hormone action could result from both direct, rapid effects on transcription and secondary effects of protein formed during the initial stimulation of mRNA synthesis. Thus, the effect of ecdysone on insect chromatin leads to a temporal series of puffs; protein synthesis is required for the late but not the early puffs.[234] Removal of steroid causes regression of the early but not the late puffs, suggesting that the early effects of the steroid include synthesis of a protein that induces the later puffs.[235] Changes in the rate of degradation of mRNA could also mediate hormonal effects on mRNA accumulation, as exemplified by the much longer half-life of ovalbumin mRNA in oviducts of estrogen-treated chicks as compared to those from whom estrogen has been withdrawn.[236] Thus, the effects of the steroid-receptor complex could include induction of a protein that increases mRNA stability, as well as the primary action increasing mRNA synthesis.

Gene Structure and Processing of mRNA Transcripts

The synthesis of primary RNA transcripts on the DNA template is followed by several important processing steps that precede the appearance of translatable mRNA in the cytoplasm. As described in Chaps. 3 and 4, most of the eukaryotic genes are split into short coding sequences, or exons, of variable length that are interrupted by stretches of noncoding DNA, or introns, that do not appear in the complementary structure of the corresponding mRNA. Instead of being copied directly from the gene sequence, mRNA is initially transcribed as a much larger RNA product from which the intervening sequences are excised. The primary RNA transcript undergoes extensive processing or editing, including polyadenylation of the 3′ end and "capping" by methylated guanosine at the 5′ end of the mRNA molecule,[237] before entering the cytoplasm as the mature mRNA that directs translation and protein synthesis at the ribosomal level.[238]

A current view of the organization of the ovalbumin gene, shown in Fig. 5-35, is that the structural gene is interrupted by at least seven intervening sequences.[238] Stimulation by estrogen causes a coordinate increase in transcription of the structural and intervening sequences of the ovalbumin gene, with accumulation of both high-molecular-weight RNA containing ovalbumin sequences and cytoplasmic ovalbumin mRNA.[239] The large precursor mRNA molecules containing the intervening sequences are enzymatically processed by excision of the inserts and subsequent ligation to form the mature mRNA.

The function of the intervening sequences (i.e., the introns) in eukaryotic structural genes has not been resolved. One suggestion is that they flank regions of the gene that code for functional domains of the protein, and that the coding sequences have approximated during evolution by a process involving the introns.[240] This proposal is supported by the structural arrangement of genes coding for collagen and albumin, which corresponds to the modular repeated regions of the proteins, and those coding for immunoglobuins, in which the exons encode functional domains of the antibody molecule. The absence of introns in prokaryotes and lower eukaryotes may reflect the loss of intervening sequences from the primitive genome to facilitate rapid cell division, a

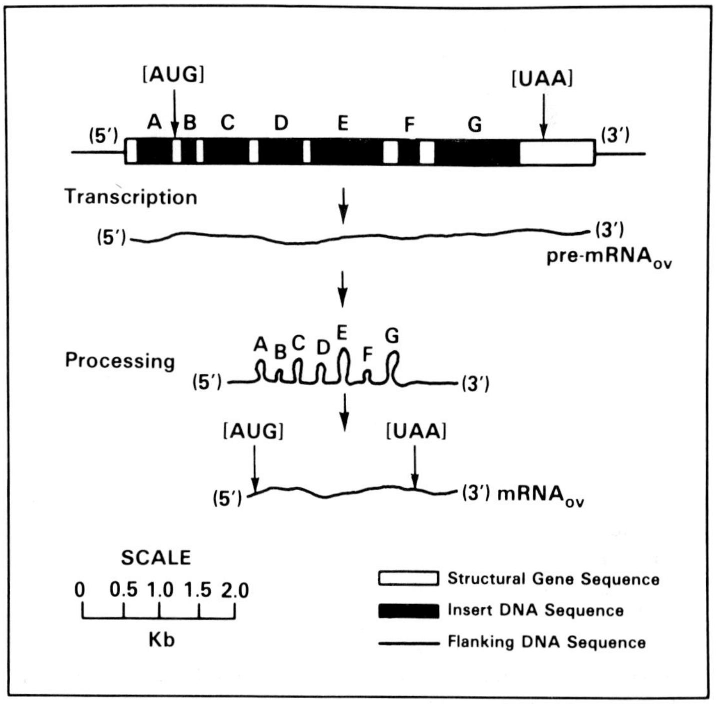

FIGURE 5-35 Structural organization and transcription of the ovalbumin gene, showing the structural and intervening sequences identified in the chick ovalbumin gene. The expression of the entire gene is stimulated by estrogen and the intervening sequences are subsequently processed away by excision and ligation to form the mature mRNA. (*Modified from Chan et al.*[1])

proposal supported by the structure of the pyruvate kinase gene of yeast and vertebrates. In the chicken pyruvate kinase gene, the 10 introns divide the coding sequences into sections that encode discrete elements of secondary structure, mainly between stretches of residues in α-helical or β-sheet arrangement.[241] Such a nonrandom placement of introns suggests that the split structure of the chicken pyruvate kinase gene is more ancient than that of the yeast gene. Whether a similar explanation applies to the ovalbumin gene is not clear, since the specific functions of this oviduct protein are not known.

Analysis of the genome in the vicinity of the ovalbumin gene has revealed the presence of two adjacent genes with sequence homologies with the ovalbumin gene.[242] The two additional genes also possess similar intron patterns to the ovalbumin gene and are expressed during estrogen stimulation, though to a much smaller degree than the ovalbumin gene. Such a cluster of ovalbumin-related genes could arise during evolution by parallel assembly from a mixture of closely related and unrelated regions, or by duplication of an ancestral gene in which the intronexon pattern was fixed from the outset.[243] Whether the different expression of the three genes during estrogen action reflects differences in the efficiency of transcription or the manner of subsequent processing and stabilization of mRNA has yet to be determined. The organization of the ovalbumin region is analogous to that of the globin genes, and the clustering of structurally and functionally related genes may be a common feature of eukaryotic genomes.[244]

The messenger RNA precursors of eukaryotic cells, the hnRNA transcripts, are packed into ribonucleoprotein particles (hnRNP) as soon as they are formed on the gene. The spherical particles are built up from a thick ribbon of newly synthesized ribonucleoprotein and contain 5 to 10 core protein components. The RNP ribbon is folded into an asymmetric ring-shaped or toroidal structure with a central hole and a narrow cleft through the periphery of the particle.[245] The surface of the RNP particle has four domains, the first containing the 5′ end of the transcript and the fourth containing the 3′ end. The distinctive structure of the RNP particle is probably relevant to the transport and processing of the pre-mRNA molecule. The individual domains of the particle may subserve recognition and binding functions when the particle associates with the fibrous elements of the nuclear matrix and when it migrates to the nuclear pore. Also, the change in shape from ringlike to rodlike configuration on passing through the pore could depend on the domain structure of the particle. It is also likely that processing of the pre-mRNA molecule, including polyadenylation and splicing, occurs in one or more of the domains of the particle. Whether regulation by steroids occurs at the level of the RNP particle has not yet been determined.

THYROID HORMONES

The thyroid hormones exert numerous and diverse effects upon differentiation, development, and metabolic homeostasis. These effects are produced by controlling the synthesis and activity of regulatory proteins, including key metabolic enzymes, hormones, and receptors. The prominent action of thyroid hormones exerted on thermogenesis and oxygen consumption is partly due to stimulation of the sodium pump by induction of the plasma membrane transport enzyme Na^+,K^+-ATPase.[246] This and other cellular responses to thyroid hormones are preceded by a latent period, and depend upon hormonal induction of RNA synthesis by regulation of specific gene expression at the nuclear level. Direct effects of thyroid hormones on cell membranes and mitochondria have also been reported, but most of the effects of thyroid hormones on metabolic processes are mediated by the activation of nuclear processes leading to increased formation of specific RNAs.

The major iodothyronine secreted by the thyroid gland is thyroxine (T_4); it is accompanied by a small amount of the highly active metabolite triiodothyronine (T_3). In the peripheral tissues, about 40 percent of the secreted T_4 is deiodinated to T_3, which reenters the bloodstream; this accounts for most of the production of circulating T_3, the major metabolically active thyroid hormone (Chap. 10). In certain tissues, the intracellular thyroid hormone is derived largely from locally formed T_3 rather than from the plasma hormone. This conversion occurs to a variable extent in the plasma membrane and ER of different tissues; it is high in the brain and anterior pituitary gland and less marked in liver and kidney. The greater dependence of the pituitary on T_3 conversion from circulating T_4 rather than from the plasma T_3 pool could reflect the need for a rapid pituitary TSH response to minor changes in secretion of T_4 by the thyroid gland.[247]

Most of the circulating thyroid hormone is bound to the plasma proteins TBG, thyroxine-binding prealbumin (TBPA), and albumin. All of these proteins bind T_4 more tightly than T_3. TBG carries about 70 percent of the bound T_4 in plasma; of the remainder, about 10 percent is bound to TBPA and 20 percent to albumin.[248] The free thyroid hormone in plasma and extracellular fluid is responsible for controlling target cell activity; the function of the binding proteins, apart from acting as a reservoir of the circulating precursor hormone, is not clear. An interesting feature of TBPA is its resemblance to certain aspects of the cellular thyroid hormone receptor, including the presence of a putative DNA-binding site rich in charged amino acids and tryptophan residues.

Cellular Receptors for Thyroid Hormone

Although cytoplasmic and mitochondrial binding proteins for T_3 have been identified, their binding of thyroid hormones does not show a close correlation with cellular responses and their affinity is low by comparison with the nuclear binding sites that represent the major receptors responsible for thyroid hormone action.[249] Unlike the steroid hormones, which were formerly believed to require interaction with cytosolic receptors prior to their translocation to the nucleus, thyroid hormones rapidly become associated with specific nuclear receptor sites without apparent need for an intermediate binding step in the cytoplasm (Fig. 5-36). The nuclear binding proteins for T_3 are of high affinity and low capacity, and are universally distributed in thyroid hormone–responsive tissues (liver, kidney, heart, pituitary, etc.); they are absent or low in nonresponsive tissues (testis, spleen) as well as from tissues of patients with familial thyroid hormone resistance.

The nuclear receptor for T_3 is an acidic nonhistone chromosomal protein with M_r of 50,000 and sedimentation coefficient of 3.5 S. Studies with micrococcal nuclease, which preferentially digests DNA regions amenable to transcription by RNA polymerase 2, have indicated that bound $[^{125}I]T_3$ in the nucleus is associated with a 5.5- to 6-S complex with M_r of 125,000, which contains the T_3-labeled 3.5-S receptor bound to an accessory protein. The preferential release of the receptor complex by endonuclease digestion is consistent with its location in readily accessible, or "open," DNA, probably in the linker region of DNA between adjacent nucleosomes. The nuclear affinities of T_3 analogues are highly correlated with their biological activities, and receptor occupancy is followed by increased RNA polymerase activity and mRNA formation, with accelerated synthesis of several cellular proteins.[3]

In addition to binding to the nuclear receptor sites that mediate their diverse physiological effects on cellular metabolism, T_3 also binds to sites in the plasma membrane of responsive target tissues. Such sites are present in erythrocytes, thymocytes, 3T3 fibroblasts, and GH_3 pituitary tumor cells, as well as human placenta and carcinoma cells. These sites are of M_r 55,000 on SDS gel electrophoresis.[251] After binding to the plasma membrane sites, T_3 is internalized via endocytic vesicles in a manner similar to peptide hormones and other ligands.[252] In the placenta, the T_3-binding protein of the plasma membrane appears to be a dimer with mol wt about 140,000.[253] Although the binding of T_3 to the plasma membrane sites can initiate its uptake by the cell, it is not yet known whether this mechanism quantitatively accounts for

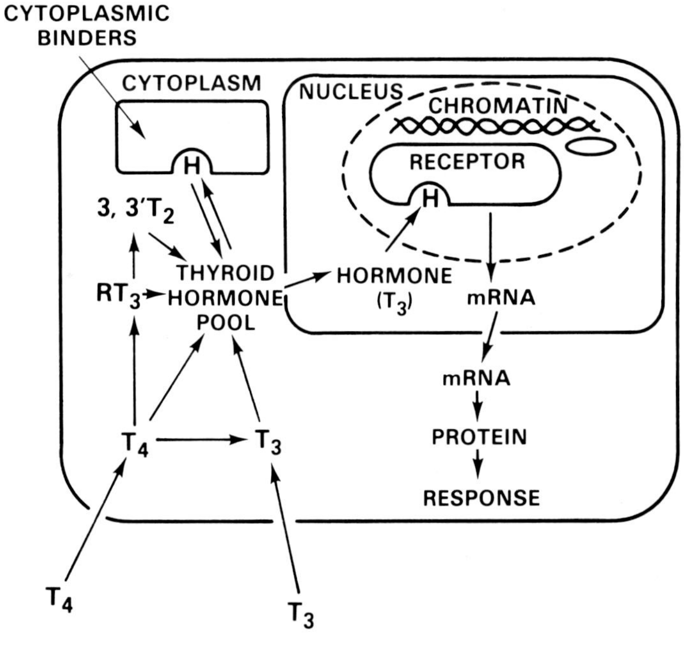

FIGURE 5-36 Actions and interconversion of T_4 and T_3 in thyroid hormone–responsive cells. The nuclear activation process depends on T_3 binding to nuclear receptors, analogous to the activation of steroid-responsive target cells. (*From Eberhardt et al.,*[248] *by permission.*)

thyroid hormone uptake. This binding may also mediate the stimulatory actions of thyroid hormone on transport of amino acids and sugars into the cell. In vivo studies show only a modest concentration gradient for L-T_3 from plasma to cytosol, but preferential uptake of D-T_3 in certain tissues (liver and kidney). However, there is selective uptake of L-T_3 by the cell nucleus,[254] via a stereospecific nuclear uptake system that accounts for the higher potency of the L form of T_3 in vivo.

Nuclear Actions of Thyroid Hormones

Stimulation of nuclear events by thyroid hormone has been shown to involve increased formation of high-molecular-weight nuclear RNA and mRNA, similar to the actions of steroid hormones.[255] These effects reflect the regulation by thyroid hormone of transcription of a specific subset of the expressed genes of the cell, an action that can be either stimulatory or inhibitory.[255a] In hypothyroid animals the rates of formation of both ribosomal RNA and mRNA are markedly reduced, and rapidly return to normal after treatment with T_3. The specific proteins regulated by thyroid hormone include TSH and GH in pituitary cells, α_2-microglobulin in the liver, the mitochondrial enzyme α-glycerophosphate dehydrogenase (α-GPD), and the cytoplasmic malic enzyme.[3] In the pituitary gland, T_3 acts at the nuclear level to regulate the synthesis and secretion of TSH by decreasing the rate of α and β subunit gene transcription. The inhibitory effect of T_3 on TSH subunit gene expression is concentration-dependent, being half maximal at plasma T_3 levels around 1 ng/ml, and is directly proportional to the occupancy of nuclear T_3 receptors.[257] These features suggest that the receptors are rate-limiting for such responses to thyroid hormone.

These general aspects of thyroid hormone action are not manifested by all target tissues to the same extent, because of the effects of species and tissue specificity and individual variations in the relationship between nuclear occupancy and biological response. Thus, the effects of T_3 on α-GPD and malic enzyme vary markedly in tissues and between species, and each tissue appears to respond to T_3 in an individual and characteristic fashion.[114] Another feature of T_3 action is its frequent participation in multihormonal regulation of mRNA synthesis. This is evident for α_2-microglobulin mRNA production, which is influenced by hydrocortisone, androgen, and GH, as well as T_3. In pituitary cells, both thyroid and glucocorticoid hormones influence the rate of GH production and exert synergistic effects on the synthesis of GH mRNA by influencing the rate of transcription of the GH gene by RNA polymerse II.[258] In pituitary tumor cells, the rate of GH gene transcription is directly proportional to T_3 receptor occupancy during the first hour of induction, suggesting that (1) gene activation by the receptor is rapid, and (2) the receptor is close to the gene regulatory sites.[259] However, even in these cloned cells the domain of thyroid hormone control differs from that of steroid hormone action in that some proteins are altered by both classes of hormone, whereas others are affected only by one class.[255a] The glucocorticoid-induced response requires the presence of T_3, suggesting that the two independent receptors may interact at adjacent regulatory sites on the gene. Another important action of thyroid and glucocorticoid hormones is stabilization of the mRNA for GH, a posttranscriptional effect that enhances the accumulation of GH mRNA and consequently the rate of GH production.[259]

Metabolic factors also modify the effects of T_3 on selective gene expression, in particular during fasting and after carbohydrate administration. Thus, the induction of malic enzyme by T_3 depends on carbohydrate intake, and does not occur during fasting. However, fasting does not impair the response of α-GPD to T_3, again illustrating the importance of local cellular factors in the expression of thyroid hormone action.[3] Obviously, much of the modulation of thyroid hormone action in specific tissues and under varied physiological conditions could be exerted at the post-receptor level, by modification of the rate of mRNA synthesis and processing in the nucleus and its subsequent translation to specific proteins within the cytoplasm. Recent gene transfer experiments indicate that a thyroid hormone–responsive element is located in the 5′ flanking DNA of the rat GH gene.[259a,b] This element has not been characterized as fully as the steroid-responsive elements, but it probably acts in an analogous manner.

ONCOGENES AND CELLULAR REGULATION

A major development in the understanding of cellular regulation by external and internal signals has been the discovery that many viral transforming genes, or *oncogenes*, exert pleiotropic actions that are expressed through the activation of nuclear or cytoplasmic mechanisms that normally participate in the control of cellular function by hormones and growth factors. The most prominent action of oncogenes is stimulation of mitosis, so their ability to code for proteins that generate mitotic signals is an appropriate characteristic. What is more surprising is the precision with which oncogenes have usurped the regulatory functions of proteins responsible for information transfer, signal transduction, and gene transcription and the extent to which oncogene research is beginning to illuminate new aspects of cell regulation.

Oncogenes were originally identified in tumorigenic retroviruses such as RSV; in this virus a single gene (*src*) is responsible for inducing sarcoma formation in chickens. Such transforming genes were initially thought to be introduced by the virus into the host cells and to transform them into malignant cells.[10] However, following the recognition that *src* is an almost-identical copy of a normal chicken gene, it was realized that most oncogenes are derived from the normal cell genome, where they originate from genes (proto-oncogenes) of which a small number of copies are present and which are highly conserved throughout the animal kingdom, from vertebrates to insects and yeast. Each retroviral oncogene has arisen by incorporation of a normal gene (i.e., proto-oncogene) from the host cell (*c-onc*) into the viral genome (*v-onc*). In this manner, the retrovirus acquires the capacity to act as a transforming or oncogenic retrovirus, and can transmit oncogenes both within and between species. The retroviral oncogenes have arisen from infrequent recombinational accidents in which up to 30 normal cellular proto-oncogenes are acquired by the retrovirus and function as viral oncogenes, becoming activated either by enhanced transcription or by mutation. The capture of proto-oncogenes by animal retroviruses usually involves trimming at either end of the gene; trimming may be essential for the enhanced expression that is typical of viral transformation. However, such activated proto-oncogenes do not alone cause transformation of primary cells, and probably act as either initiation or maintenance genes in multigene carcinogenesis.[260]

A smaller number of oncogenes have been found in the DNA of various tumor cells (derived by chemical transformation or from human tumors) by transfection experiments in which the tumor DNA induces transformation in cultured recipient cells, often 3T3 cells. These oncogenes have been isolated from human bladder and lung carcinomas, neuroblastomas, leukemias, and sarcomas (*ras*), and human and chicken lymphoma (*myc* and *B-lym*); all are closely related to a corresponding DNA sequence of the normal cellular genome.[261]

The normal function of proto-oncogenes is not well understood, but the proteins that they encode in normal cells, and which are gene products in transformed and tumor cells, are often related to normal proteins involved in cellular regulation. They include proteins that regulate nuclear transcriptional activity and cytoplasmic second messenger molecules, as well as cell membrane receptors and growth factors that influence cell multiplication and differentiation. Thus, the oncogene-encoded proteins initiate a relatively small number of mechanisms that operate through specific actions exerted on regulatory pathways in the nucleus, cytoplasm, and plasma membrane. It has become clear that many of these pathways are closely related to those which mediate the effects of hormones and other environmental signals on cell growth, differentiation, and secretion. Oncogenes can be classified according to their effects on cellular phenotype, and also by the nuclear or cytoplasmic localization and sites of action of their gene products.[262]

Nuclear Oncogenes

Nuclear oncogenes include oncogenes derived from cellular proto-oncogenes such as *myc*, *N-myc*, *myb*, *P53*, and *fos*, as well as those of DNA tumor viruses (*SV40 large T*, polyoma *large T*), whose products are located in the nucleus. The nuclear oncogenes of cellular origin are usually activated by processes that lead to deregulation of the production of their encoded proteins, rendering the gene constitutively active and unresponsive to its normal transcriptional regulators. This is exemplified by the deregulation of *myc* gene expression by chromosomal translocation. In this process, its promoter-enhancer regulation is replaced by sequences from immunoglobulin genes, often with loss of the initial noncoding exon of the *myc* sequence. The *myc* gene can also be deregulated by the acquisition of adjacent retroviral promoter-enhancer sequences that override its normal regulatory elements, and by amplification in certain tumors. In the case of the *P53* gene product, deregulation can occur via simple overproduction of the protein after attachment to a constitutive transcriptional promoter, and also by association with the SV40 large T antigen to form a protein-protein complex of greatly increased stability.[262]

Recently, the *erbA* oncogene of avian erythroblastosis virus, which potentiates the effects of *erbB* by blocking erythrocyte maturation at an early stage, has been found to share regions of homology with the genes of glucocorticoid, estrogen, and progesterone receptors.[200,208] This finding suggests that the *erbA* genes encode a group of regulatory molecules which, like the steroid receptors, bind to specific DNA sequences to regulate gene expression. The steroid receptor genes and the *erbA* proto-oncogene may have arisen from a common primordial gene during the evolution of such a family of transcriptional regulatory proteins, and the *v-erbA* gene could favor transformation by inappropriate regulation of gene expression in the erythroblast.[209] Since steroid hormone receptors are now believed to be normally resident within the cell nucleus (and to appear in the cytosol largely as a consequence of cell disruption) the *erbA* proto-oncogene is probably more correctly regarded as a nuclear oncogene, consistent with the presumed site at which its product acts on gene transcription.

Cytoplasmic Oncogenes

Many of the oncogenes which code for cytoplasmic protein products are derived from proto-oncogenes that are normally responsible for the regulation of cellular growth and metabolic activity (Fig. 5-37). This now widely accepted concept was first indicated by the finding that the *src* gene product of RSV is a tyrosine-specific protein kinase. The *src* gene family is now known to include at least seven viral oncogenes that code for tyrosine kinase; the best-studied gene product is $pp60^{src}$, a mol wt 60,000 phosphoprotein that phosphorylates a protein substrate of mol wt 34,000. The corresponding cellular proto-oncogene (*c-src*) codes for a protein that is similar to $pp60^{src}$ but is present at only 1 to 2 percent of the $pp60^{src}$ level in transformed cells. The normal cellular *src* protein product is also a tyrosine kinase, and phosphorylates a mol wt 34,000 protein substrate. Cyclic AMP causes enhanced phosphorylation of $pp60^{src}$ and also increases its tyrosine kinase activity, but is not required for the tyrosine phosphokinase reaction.

Increased expression of *c-src* does not cause neoplastic transformation, so the mutations in *v-src* must enable the viral gene to transform cells and cause tumors, perhaps via new substrate specificities conferred on $pp60^{v\text{-}src}$. Surprisingly, a form of $pp60^{c\text{-}src}$ is abundant in neurons, despite their fully differentiated and mitotically inactive state, and the expression of *v-src* in rat pheochromocytoma cells causes differentiation similar to that induced by nerve growth factor. These findings suggest that *c-src* may have an important role in cell differentiation, as opposed to the largely proliferative effects of its viral conterpart.[263]

Recently, both *src* and the related *ros* oncogene product have been found to phosphorylate phospholipids as well as proteins. These actions include the phosphorylation of PI to form disphosphatidylinositol (PIP) (*ros*) or both PIP and triphosphatidylinositol (PIP_2) (*src*). Both the *src* and *ros* gene products are present at the inner surface of the cell membrane, where their lipid kinase activities could convert PI to its higher phosphorylated forms.[264] The increased formation of polyphosphoinositides in the cell membrane would favor the production of the metabolically active second messenger molecules and DAG via cleavage by phospholipase C. The effects of these signals on mobilization of intracellular calcium and activation of protein kinase C, respectively, could account for many of the pleiotropic changes that occur during oncogene activation. Such findings also suggest that other tyrosine kinases, including other oncogene products and plasma membrane receptors for insulin, EGF, and PDGF, could also phosphorylate membrane phospholipids and promote the formation of IP_3 and DAG.

The *ras* gene family also gives rise to protein products (of mol wt ~21,000) that are located on the inner surface of the plasma membrane. The mammalian ras proteins bind GTP and have GTPase activity, and share sequence homologies with the guanyl nucleotide regulatory proteins, such as transducin, Ns, and Ni, that mediate signal transduction generated by ligand interaction with the cell surface receptors for

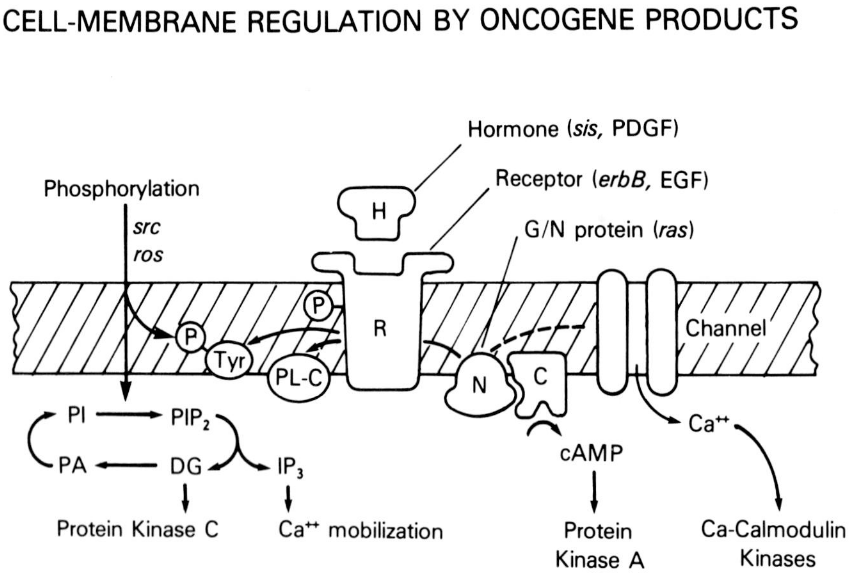

FIGURE 5-37 Cellular regulation by oncogene products that mimic the effects of ligands, receptors, and regulatory enzymes responsible for cell growth and the hormonal control of target cell responses.

hormones and transmitters.[265] Mutant *ras* genes that encode altered proteins are present in many tumor cells, and can cause malignant transformation when transfected into mammalian cell lines. The protein product of the *ras* oncogene also binds GTP, but has impaired GTPase activity. The mutant *ras* protein, like the normal nucleotide regulatory protein (Ns), can activate adenylate cyclase in yeast systems, but does so continuously. This has been attributed to its low GTPase activity and loss of the normal termination process via hydrolysis of the bound GTP that engenders the active state of the protein. Such a defect in GTPase activity would tend to disrupt the normal regulation of cell function by external hormones and signals, and could favor autonomous overactivity of membrane effector enzymes that are controlled by the state of activation of the nucleotide regulatory proteins.

The human genome contains three cellular *ras* genes (ras^H, ras^K, ras^N), and activated forms of each gene are demonstrable in many tumor cell DNAs by transfection of 3T3 cells. The transforming potential of the *ras* gene is activated by structural mutations involving various amino acid substitutions at positions 12 or 61 of the *ras* protein, or by overexpression of the normal ras^H protein.[266] The diverse amino acid substitutions at position 12 or 61 that confer transforming activity upon ras^H do not affect the localization or guanyl nucleotide–binding properties of the mutant proteins, but consistently reduce their rates of GTP hydrolysis. The many similarities between *ras* gene products and the plasma membrane guanyl nucleotide regulatory proteins that mediate receptor-induced second messenger formation (membrane localization, nucleotide binding, GTPase activity, and partial sequence homologies) suggest that mutational activation of *ras* genes depends on inadequate GTP hydrolysis and impairment of physiological deactivation of *ras* proteins. However, while reduced GTP hydrolysis is a characteristic feature of most mutant ras^H proteins, the absence of a quantitative correlation between the extents of GTPase inhibition and transforming activity indicates that reduced GTP hydrolysis is not sufficient to activate *ras* transforming potential.[266] Also, the high transforming activity of a Thr^{59} mutant *ras* gene product with normal GTPase activity indicates that transformation by ras proteins can occur by mechanisms that do not involve the effects of impaired GTPase activity.[267]

The *erbB* viral oncogene, originally identified in avian erythroblastosis virus, is a member of the *src* gene family and codes for a plasma membrane protein with an amino acid sequence that is similar to almost one-half of the EGF receptor.[37] The regions encoded by the *erbB* oncogene correspond to the cytoplasmic and transmembrane segments of the EGF receptor, giving a protein that represents a truncated EGF receptor which has lost its external EGF-binding domain. Since the *erbB* gene product contains the protein kinase (cytoplasmic) domain of the EGF receptor, it could be involved in signal transfer within the cell, but would not be regulated in the absence of the receptor-binding region of the receptor.[38] The *erbB* protein product has recently been shown to have tyrosine kinase activity, and its marked structural similarity to the kinase domain of the EGF receptor suggests that the protein could act as an unregulated source of intracellular phosphorylations, leading to persistent stimulation of cell division and acquisition of the transformed phenotype. Such a mechanism presumes that the *erbB* gene product could mimic the consequences of EGF receptor activation, but would not be turned off in the absence of the ligand-binding domain.

The marked similarity between the chicken *erbB* oncogene product and the human EGF receptor indicates that the transmembrane and cytosolic portions of the receptor are highly conserved and suggests that the EGF receptor gene gave rise to *erbB* in the course of infection by the erythroblastosis virus. Furthermore, both the *erbB* proto-oncogene and the EGF receptor gene are located on the long arm of human chromosome 7, consistent with the probability that the receptor gene gave rise to the viral oncogene, which encodes a truncated or otherwise altered protein that subverts the normal function of the receptor, and is constitutively active rather than ligand-regulated.[38] Recently, the *neu* oncogene, which encodes a mol wt 185,000 cell surface protein with similarities to the *v-erbB* product and the EGF receptor, has been identified as coding for a plasma membrane receptor related to but distinct from the EGF receptor, with tyrosine kinase activity.[268] The gene for this receptor is located on chromosome 17, coincident with the site of the *neu* oncogene and distinct from that of the EGF receptor. The ligand for this new receptor has not yet been identified. Some of the structural features of the tyrosine kinase family of receptors and oncogene products and of the largely extracellular LDL receptor are shown in Fig. 5-38.

A further link between genes for growth factors or their receptors and oncogenes was provided by the finding that the *fms* oncogene product of a feline sarcoma virus is similar to the receptor for the colony stimulating growth factor CSF 1, which stimulates the production of macrophages from their precursor cells. In this case, the *v-fms* gene product may act as a competent receptor that, when delivered by the tumor virus to cells such as fibroblasts, causes them to become aberrantly responsive to the CSF 1 which

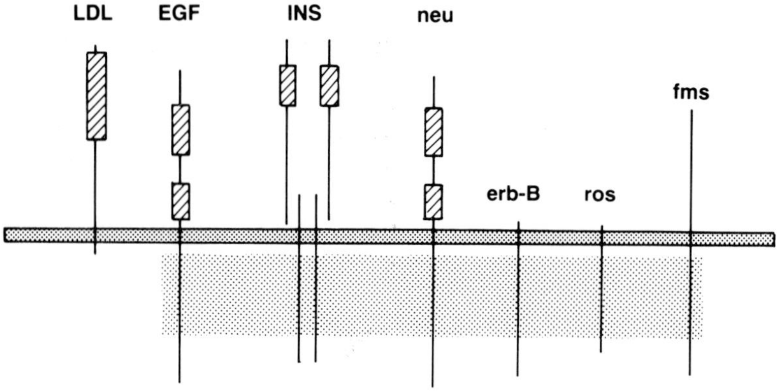

FIGURE 5-38 Structural features of peptide hormone receptors and oncogene products bearing tyrosine kinase domains (stippled area) within their cytoplasmic regions, and of the predominantly extracellular LDL receptor. The hatched boxes indicate the cysteine-rich regions that are believed to be involved in the formation of ligand-binding domains within the extracellular portions of the receptor molecules. (*Modified from Coussens et al.*[268])

they normally synthesize and secrete into the extracellular medium.[269]

An additional feature of the EGF receptor system is the presence of sequence similarities between EGF, TGF-α, and two proteins that are produced by the vaccinia virus. One of the vaccinia proteins (19 kilodaltons) appears to be a growth factor and contains an amino acid sequence that is similar to a disulfide loop present in both EGF and TGF-α. This region of EGF and TGF-α participates in their binding to the EGF receptor, suggesting that vaccinia virus could use this binding domain to interact with the EGF receptor in the course of infecting cells. Such a mechanism has been supported by the finding that occupancy of EGF receptors, whether by the EGF molecule or its synthetic decapeptide antagonist fragments, inhibits vaccinia virus infection.[41] The inhibitory actions of EGF and its fragments parallel their affinity for the EGF receptor, consistent with competitive blockade of virus binding to the growth factor receptor. Thus, the receptor for EGF, like those for several other cell-regulating ligands, may serve as a site of specific viral attachment prior to invasion of the host cell. A major 28-kilodalton vaccinia protein also has sequence similarities with the *v-erbB* transforming protein and the EGF receptor. Whether such similarities reflect a common ancestry or convergent evolution of proteins with similar functions is not yet known, but it seems to be advantageous for the virus to mimic specific host proteins concerned in growth factor activity and cellular binding sites.

A further class of oncogene products includes peptides or proteins that exert their actions after secretion from the transformed or neoplastic cell. In addition to their similarities to certain plasma membrane and nuclear receptors involved in normal mechanisms of growth control, oncogene products are sometimes related to polypeptide growth factors that act on cell surface receptors to initiate intracellular signals leading to DNA synthesis and cell division.[270] Thus, TGF-α is produced in many human cancer cells and binds to the EGF receptor, and its expression in transformed cells is influenced by oncogene products such as $p21^{ras}$. The most direct example of oncogene-dependent growth factor production is that of the simian sarcoma virus *v-sis* protein product, which is closely related to the B chain of human PDGF.[277] The extensive similarity between the two proteins, including almost complete identity over a region of 104 amino acids, suggests that the *c-sis* gene is the cellular gene encoding the B chain of PDGF. The dimeric structure of PDGF, which is necessary for its biological activity, depends on the disulfide linkage of the A and B subunit chains to form the AB heterodimer of mol wt 30,000. The *v-sis* gene product, $p28^{sis}$, is rapidly dimerized after synthesis and processed by proteolysis to give $p24^{sis}$, which resembles a PDGF BB homodimer. Cells transformed with simian sarcoma virus release an oncogene product that has PDGF activity in terms of receptor binding and stimulation of DNA synthesis, and which is neutralized by anti-PDGF antisera.[272] The production of such a major mitogen analogue in cells carrying PDGF receptors would initiate an autocrine loop leading to constitutive activation by the abnormally expressed growth factor. There may be other examples of oncogene products that express transforming activity by interacting with the normal mitogenic pathways of the cell.

DISORDERS OF RECEPTOR FUNCTION

Although clinical disorders attributable to aberrant structure or function of peptide hormone receptors are not common, there are several well-defined receptor abnormalities which are associated with distinct endocrine syndromes. The conceivable spectrum of receptor diseases could range from simple over- or underproduction of receptors to abnormalities of receptor structure and coupling mechanisms, with the additional and now well-recognized effects of autoantibodies to the receptors and their associated membrane proteins. Although the effects of nonlethal genetic defects in steroid receptor biosynthesis and function have been implicated in certain forms of human androgen resistance,[273] rickets,[274] and other forms of steroid hormone resistance (Chap. 12), comparable deficiencies in peptide hormone receptors have not yet been documented. Indeed, since many peptide hormones exert essential trophic actions on their target tissues, the absence of the corresponding receptors would be manifested by end-organ atrophy, and would therefore not be amenable to analysis and detection due to the absence of functioning target tissue. If such receptors were also present in more accessible locations, comparable to the insulin receptors of circulating monocytes and erythrocytes, it might be possible to detect their deficiency even after regression of the major target organ. However, with the possible exception of angiotensin II, receptors for peptide hormones other than insulin have not been detected in blood cells, and the potential role of receptor defects in atrophic end organs has remained a matter of speculation.

The converse situation, receptor overproduction, could also be involved as a possible contributory factor in several endocrine disorders. These include low-renin hypertension, with hyperplasia and increased sensitivity of the adrenal zona glomerulosa to angiotensin II; pituitary microadenomas responsible for Cushing's disease, with hypercortisolism as a result of inappropriate secretion of corticotropin by the pituitary; and other functioning pituitary and gut tumors presenting as hyperplastic endocrine lesions. Pituitary adenomas associated with Cushing's disease and acromegaly are sometimes attributed to the effects of prolonged overstimulation by the respective hypothalamic releasing hormones, which have been recently characterized as relatively large peptides of 41 amino acid residues (CRF) and 44 residues (GRF). However, it is also possible that such lesions develop as the result of abnormal target cell sensitivity to the respective hypothalamic hormones. This may be due either to increased number of receptors or excessive receptor-mediated responses to normal levels of the hypothalamic peptide in pituitary portal blood. The latter possibility is more consistent with the observation that resection of pituitary microadenomas in Cushing's disease is often followed by transient ACTH-cortisol deficiency and subsequent return to normal functioning of the hypothalamic-pituitary-adrenal axis, indicating that the primary disorder was intrinsic to the ACTH-secreting adenoma rather than due to hypersecretion of hypothalamic CRF.[275] The advent of radioimmunoassays for these hypothalamic regulators should permit the analysis of their secretory profiles and levels in patients with pituitary tumors, and may ultimately clarify the basis for at least some of these lesions.

Abnormal receptor affinity is another possible mechanism of receptor disease, but again there is no documented example of such a lesion in a peptide hormone receptor site. This is perhaps surprising, since defects in protein structure leading to reduced receptor affinity might be expected to occur more frequently than those in which the abnormality is so severe as to cause complete loss of binding affinity, a situation equivalent to the reduction in number or absence of receptor sites. On the other hand, a moderate decrease in receptor affinity could remain as an occult lesion if compensated by an increase in secretion of the regulatory hormone, and would be devoid of clinical manifestations other than those occasioned by the compensatory rise in hormone secretion. Such a disorder has recently been defined in a father and son with hypercortisolism associated with reduced glucocorticoid receptor affinity.[276] Both subjects had increased ACTH secretion that was resistant to dexamethasone suppression, and the father had hypokalemia and hypertension, attributable to the effects of increased adrenal secretion of cortisol and ACTH-dependent mineralocorticoids (DOC and corticosterone). It also appears likely that between-species differences in steroid receptor affinity could be responsible for the high blood hydrocortisone levels that are characteristic of certain primates.[277]

As a working classification of receptor disorders, pathological changes in receptor structure and function can be considered under three broad categories: altered receptor concentration or affinity, anti-receptor antibodies, and abnormal receptor-effector coupling. Decreases in receptor concentration (Table 5-13) are well documented for several forms of insulin resistance and in familial hypercholesterolemia with reduced LDL receptors. In the latter state, there is hope that the use of inhibitors of hydroxymethylglutaryl CoA reductase will lower circulating LDL levels and permit a rise in the down-regulated LDL receptors at least to the heterozygous level, with consequently improved handling of plasma LDL.[278] As noted above, the absence of receptors could be involved in various forms of idiopathic hypofunction of endocrine organs, though whether as cause or effect may be difficult to discern. Angiotensin II receptors are known to be dynamically regulated by sodium balance, with increased concentration in the adrenal zona glomerulosa and decreased concentration in smooth muscle during sodium restriction. These changes in receptor content contribute to the reciprocal alterations in adrenal and

Table 5-13. Conditions with Altered Receptor Concentration

- Insulin resistance
  - Obesity
    - Decreased insulin receptors, reversed by low-calorie diet
    - Secondary to hyperinsulinemia
  - Diabetes mellitus
    - Adult-onset diabetes: obesity and insulin-resistance
    - Inverse relationship between receptors and plasma insulin concentration
  - Other conditions with hyperinsulinemia
    - Insulinoma
    - Acromegaly
    - Exogenous insulin therapy
- Familial hypercholesterolemia
  - One functional gene for LDL receptor in heterozygotes
  - Reduced receptoprs compensated by increased plasma LDL concentrations
  - HMG-CoA reductase inhibitors lower LDL concentration, increase receptors
- Idiopathic hypofunction
  - Defective trophic hormone receptors
  - Cause or effect?
- Angiotensin II receptor alterations
  - Adrenal receptors increased by sodium restriction; low-renin hypertension (?)
  - Vascular receptors decreased by sodium restriction; high blood angiotensin II level

Abbreviations: HMG, hydroxymethylglutaryl; LDL, low-density lipoprotein.

vascular sensitivity that occur during sodium deprivation, via the effects of increased concentration of circulating angiotensin II.[279] In patients with low-renin hypertension, an increase in the number of adrenal receptors for angiotensin II could be a factor in the higher sensitivity of the adrenal to angiotensin, and the occurrence of normal blood aldosterone levels in the face of decreased plasma renin activity.[280]

Changes in receptor affinity are less common than changes in receptor number (Table 5-14), and have been most clearly defined for the insulin receptor, during functional decreases in affinity resulting from the competitive antagonist effects of anti-receptor antibodies. The adrenal angiotensin II receptor, like the insulin receptor, can show transiently increased affinity when exposed to increased ligand concentrations, as during the onset of sodium restriction. Increased angiotensin receptor affinity could also be implicated in the adrenal hypersensitivity of low-renin hypertension and the increased vascular responsiveness in essential hypertension.

Table 5-14. Altered Receptor Affinity

- Decreased insulin receptor affinity: most receptor antibodies
- Increased insulin receptor affinity
  - Fasted obese patients
  - Acromegaly
  - Insulinoma
  - Glucose loading
- Increased adrenal angiotensin II receptor affinity
  - Sodium restriction
  - Low-renin hypertension?

The best-defined group of disorders affecting peptide hormone receptors are those which result from the development of antibodies to the individual receptor sites (Table 5-15). Such antibodies may exert either blocking or destructive effects, as in the case of those to the acetylcholine receptor in myasthenia gravis, or persistent stimulation, as seen in Graves' disease due to the effects of thyroid-stimulating immunoglobulins.[52] Less commonly, antibodies to the insulin receptor have been detected in certain patients with marked insulin resistance, often in association with acanthosis nigricans and evidence of systemic immune disease.[281] Such antibodies can exert several biological actions in vitro after binding to the insulin receptor. These include insulin-like actions that are attributable to the consequences of receptor activation, inhibition of insulin binding to its receptor by acting as competitive antagonists and decreasing the apparent affinity of the receptors for insulin, and desensitization of the

Table 5-15. Anti-receptor Antibodies

- Graves' disease
  - Antibodies to TSH receptor stimulate thyroid function
- Myasthenia gravis
  - Antibodies to acetylcholine receptors present
  - Degradation of receptors increased
- Insulin receptor antibodies
  - Acanthosis nigricans:
    - Type A: younger, female, polycystic ovary syndrome
    - Type B: older, autoimmune disease
  - Ataxia telangiectasia
  - Usually competitive antagonists; decrease receptor affinity
  - Intrinsic insulin-like activity; depends on receptor aggregation (compare concanavalin A)
  - Insulin actions receptor-encoded
- β_2-Adrenergic receptor antibodies
  - Allergic rhinitis
  - Asthma

target cell to insulin action. The predominant effects of such antibodies in vivo are to cause insulin resistance and hyperglycemia in association with hyperinsulinemia. However, a few patients with antireceptor antibodies have developed hypoglycemia at some stage in their clinical course and in one patient fasting hypoglycemia was the only manifestation of autoantibodies to the insulin receptor.[53] Such insulin-mimetic actions of insulin receptor antibodies are analogous to the hyperthryoidism of Graves' disease, in which TSH receptor antibodies cause persistent activation of the thyrotropin receptor and excessive thyroid hormone secretion.

Another recently described and intriguing form of receptor autoantibodies are those to the β-adrenergic receptor. Such antibodies have been detected in certain patients with allergic rhinitis and asthma as specific autoantibodies to the β_2 receptor that is present in lung and human placenta. The occurrence of such autoantibodies to β-adrenergic receptors is associated with abnormal autonomic responsiveness, manifested by β-adrenergic hyposensitivity with α-adrenergic and cholinergic *hyper*sensitivity.[282] Such an imbalance between the latter factors, which promote bronchospasm and mast cell mediator release, and the former, which reduces these effects, may be of importance in the pathogenesis of bronchial asthma.

Abnormalities in coupling of receptors to their membrane effector systems are beginning to be recognized (Table 5-16), most clearly in patients with pseudohypoparathyroidism.[283] In this disorder, resistance to parathyroid hormone is related to impaired cAMP responses in the kidney, recently shown to result from partial deficiency of the nucleotide regulatory protein (Ns) involved in adenylate cyclase activation.[284] Such patients also exhibit defects in other endocrine systems that depend on adenylate cyclase, including partial gonadotropin resistance in several cases[285] as well as resistance to thyrotropin and glucagon.[286] A less well-defined defect may exist in the regulation of *lipomodulin*, a glucocorticoid-dependent protein modulator of phospholipase A_2 activity in the plasma membrane,[287] which may influence arachidonate-mediated inflammatory responses in connective tissues. The presence of antibodies to lipomodulin in sera from several patients with arthritis suggests that abnormalities in the control of the prostaglandin pathway and other routes of phospholipid metabolism may be important components of the inflammatory process in certain connective tissue diseases.[288]

One of the most interesting aspects of receptor-mediated cell regulation to achieve clinical relevance has been the recently recognized ability of GnRH agonists to desensitize the pituitary gonadotrophs and inhibit gonadotropin secretion. Early reports on the

Table 5-16. Abnormal Receptor-Effector Coupling (Early Post-receptor Defects)

Deficient receptor-cyclase coupling: pseudohypoparathyroidism, type 1
Deficiency of Ns protein
Genetic heterogeneity
Resistance to hormones stimulating adenylate cyclase
Other potential coupling defects
Cytosolic modulators of cyclase
Other modulators of membrane enzymes (e.g., lipomodulin)
Effectors of calcium-dependent hormones
Effectors of insulin and growth factors
Pituitary desensitization by GnRH agonists

physiological and pharmacological actions of GnRH stimulation were soon followed by the recognition that adverse or inhibitory effects on pituitary-gonadal function are common sequelae of treatment with GnRH or its potent superagonist analogues.[289] Such effects were also observed in numerous animal studies, and were shown to result from a combination of pituitary and gonadal desensitization; the former effect is the dominant factor in primates.

Studies in female monkeys have clearly demonstrated that normal pituitary-gonadal function is critically dependent on the temporal pattern of GnRH stimulation. In animals with hypothalamic lesions, excessively frequent or continuous exposure to GnRH is unable to maintain normal gonadotropin secretion, whereas hourly pulses of GnRH are fully effective.[64] At the same time, daily intranasal administration of a potent GnRH agonist was shown to inhibit gonadotropin secretion in postmenopausal and cycling women, and to be an effective contraceptive agent.[65] Such agents were also shown to cause luteal-phase defects in women[290] and inhibit pituitary-testicular function in normal men[291] and male monkeys.[292]

In addition to its potential for fertility control, receptor-mediated desensitization of the pituitary by GnRH agonists has been employed in several clinical situations in which suppression of gonadotropin secretion is of therapeutic value. These include the treatment of idiopathic precocious puberty,[293] metastatic breast cancer,[294] prostatic cancer,[295] and endometriosis.[296] The extreme susceptibility of the gonadotrophs to desensitization by GnRH agonists may be responsible for two interesting clinical features of disordered pituitary function. First, the extreme rarity of gonadotropin-secreting tumors may reflect the propensity of the gonadotroph to undergo regression rather than hyperplasia when exposed to excessive stimulation by GnRH. Second, the well-recognized association between hyperprolactinemia and impaired gonadotropin secretion could include a local element of desensitization of the gonadotroph, caused by stimulatory factors produced by the overactive lactotrophs, especially since the two cell types are often adjacent within the pituitary gland. While such a paracrine form of local regulation has yet to be demonstrated in the pituitary, its existence is implied by the ability of GnRH to stimulate prolactin release in cocultures of gonadotrophs and lactotrophs[297] and by the concomitant responses in serum LH and prolactin concentrations sometimes elicited by GnRH treatment.

The recognition that appropriately timed pulsatile stimulation with GnRH is necessary to optimally elevate gonadotropin secretion[298] has led to renewed interest in the use of GnRH therapy in hypopituitary hypogonadal states, with quite striking success. Intermittent treatment with GnRH has been established as a successful method for induction of ovulation in hypothalamic amenorrhea,[299] and more recently for the induction of puberty in men with idiopathic hypogonadotropic hypogonadism.[300] These recent developments have clearly demonstrated the importance of understanding the regulatory significance of episodic hormone secretion and the way in which appropriate modifications in the structure and mode of presentation of peptide agonists can lead to extraordinary changes in the receptor-mediated responses of the target cell.

REFERENCES

1. Chan L, Means AR, O'Malley BW: Steroid hormone regulation of specific gene expression. *Vitam Horm* 36:259, 1978.

2. Roy AK, Clark JH: *Gene Regulation by Steroid Hormones II.* New York, Springer-Verlag, 1983.

2a. Lan NC, Karin M, Nguyen T, Weisz A, Birnbaum MJ, Eberhardt NL, Baxter JD: Mechanisms of glucocorticoid hormone action. *J Steroid Biochem* 20:77, 1984.

2b. Yamamoto KR: Steroid receptor regulated transcription of specific genes and gene networks. *Ann Rev Genet* 19:209, 1985.

3. Oppenheimer JH: Thyroid hormone action at the cellular level. *Science* 203:971, 1979.

4. Roth J, Lesniak MA, Bar RS, et al: An introduction to receptors and receptor disorders. *Proc Soc Exp Biol Med* 162:3, 1979.

5. Catt KJ, Dufau ML: Peptide hormone receptors. *Annu Rev Physiol* 39:529, 1977.

6. Lefkowitz RJ, Michel T: Plasma membrane receptors. *J Clin Invest* 72:1185, 1983.

7. Szego C: Mechanisms of hormone action: Parallels in receptor-mediated signal propagation for steroid and peptide effectors. *Life Sci* 35:2383, 1984.

8. Hakanson R, Sundler F: The design of the neuroendocrine system: A unifying concept and its consequences. *Trends Pharmacol Sci* 4:41, 1985.

9. Sporn MB, Roberts AB: Autocrine growth factors and cancer. *Nature* 313:745, 1985.

10. Gordon H: Oncogenes. *Mayo Clin Proc* 60:697, 1985.

11. Sutherland EW, Robison GA: *Pharmacol Rev* 18:145, 1966.

12. Snyder SH: Drug and neurotransmitter receptors in the brain. *Science* 224:22, 1984.

13. Singer SJ, Nicholson G: The fluid mosaic theory of the structure of cell membranes. *Science* 175:721, 1972.

14. Philpott HG, Petersen OH: Extracellular but not intracellular application of peptide hormones activates pancreatic acinar cells. *Nature* 281:684, 1979.

15. Greengard P: *Cyclic Nucleotides. Phosphorylated Proteins and Neuronal Function.* New York, Raven, 1978.

16. Dufau ML, Catt KJ: Gonadotropin receptors and regulation of steroidogenesis in the testis and ovary. *Vitam Horm* 36:462, 1978.

17. Fox CF, Vale R, Peterson SW, Das M: The EGF receptor: Identification and functional modulation, in Sato GH, Ross R (eds): *Hormones and Cell Culture.* New York, Cold Spring Harbor Laboratory, 1978, p 143.

18. Pullen RA, Lindsay DG, Wood SP, Tickle IJ, Blundell TL, Wollmer A, Krail G, Brandenburg D, Zahn H, Gliemann J, Gammeltoft S: Receptor-binding region of insulin. *Nature* 259:369, 1976.

19. Blundell TL, Humbel RE: Hormone families: Pancreatic hormones and homologous growth factors. *Nature* 287:781, 1980.

20. Beddell CR, Shepley GC, Blundell TL, Sasaki K, Dockerill S, Goodford PJ: Symmetrical features in polypeptide hormone-receptor interactions. *Int J Pept Protein Res* 9:161, 1977.

21. Low MG, Kincade PW: Phosphatidylinositol is the membrane-anchoring domain of the thy-1 glycoprotein. *Nature* 318:62, 1985.

22. Levitski A: Reconstriction of membrane receptor systems. *Biochim Biophys Acta* 833:127, 1985.

23. Shiu RPC, Friesen HG: Blockade of prolactin action by an antiserum to its receptors. *Science* 192:259, 1976.

24. Sumikawa K, Houghton M, Emtage JS, Richards BM, Barnard EA: Active multi-subunit ACh receptor assembled by translation of heterologous mRNA in *Xenopus* oocytes. *Nature* 292:862, 1982.

25. Noda M, Takahashi H, Tanabe T, Toyosato M, Furutani Y, Hirose T, Asai M, Inayama S, Miyata T, Numa S: Primary structure of α-subunit precursor of *Torpedo californica* acetylcholine receptor deduced from cDNA sequence. *Nature* 299:793, 1982.

26. Raftery MA, Hunkapiller MW, Strader CD, Hood LE: Acetylcholine receptors: Complex of homologous subunits. *Science* 208:1541, 1980.

27. Stevens CF: The acetylcholine receptor. *Nature* 281:13, 1980.

28. Wise DW, Schoenborn BP, Karlin A: Structure of acetylcholine receptor dimer determined by neutron scattering and electron microscopy. *J Biol Chem* 256:4124, 1981.

29. Lindstrom J, Criado M, Hochschwender S, Fox JL, Sarin V: Immunochemical test of acetylcholine receptor subunit models. *Nature* 311:573, 1984.

30. Takai T, Noda M, Mishina M, Shimizu S, et al: Cloning, sequencing and expression of cDNA for a novel subunit of acetylcholine receptor from calf muscle. *Nature* 315:761, 1985.

31. Sakmann B, Methfessel C, Mishina M, Takahashi T, Takai T, Kurasaki M, Fukusa K, Numa S: Role of acetylcholine receptor subunits in gating of the channel. *Nature* 318:538, 1985.

32. Carpenter G, Cohen S: Peptide growth factors. *Trends Biochem Sci* 9:169, 1984.

33. Downard J, Parker P, Waterfield MD: Autophosphorylation sites on the epidermal growth factor receptor. *Nature* 311:483, 1984.

34. McCaffrey PG, Friedman BA, Rosner MR: Diacylglycerol modulated binding and phosphorylation of the epidermal growth factor receptor. *J Biol Chem* 259:12502, 1984.

35. Basu M, Biswas R, Das M: 42,000-molecular weight EGF receptor has protein kinase activity. *Nature* 311:477, 1984.

36. Lin CR, Chen WS, Kruiger W, Stolarsky LS, Weber W,

Evans RM et al: Expression cloning of human EGF receptor complementary DNA: Gene amplification and three related messenger RNA products in A431 cells. *Science* 224:843, 1984.

37. Ullrich A, Coussens L, Hayflick JS, Dull TJ, Gray A, Tan AW, et al: Human epidermal growth factor receptor cDNA sequence and aberrant expression of the amplified gene in A431 epidermoid carcinoma cells. *Nature* 309:418, 1984.

38. Hunter T: The epidermal growth factor receptor gene and its product. *Nature* 311:414, 1983.

39. Hunter T, Ling N, Cooper JA: Protein kinase C phosphorylation of the EGF receptor at a threonine residue close to the cytoplasmic face of the plasma membrane. *Nature* 311:480, 1984.

40. Livneh E, Glazer L, Segal D, Schlessinger J, Shilo B-Z: The *Drosophila* EGF receptor gene homolog: Conservation of both hormone binding and kinase domains. *Cell* 40:599, 1985.

41. Eppstein DA, Marsh YV, Schreiber AB, Newman SR, Todaro GJ, Nestor JJ: Epidermal growth factor receptor occupancy inhibits vaccinia virus infection. *Nature* 318:663, 1985.

42. Jacobs S, Cuatrecasas P: Insulin receptor: Structure and function. *Endocr Rev* 2:251, 1981.

43. Shia MA, Pilch PF: The β-subunit of the insulin receptor is an insulin-activated protein kinase. *Biochemistry* 22:717, 1983.

44. De Meyts P, Rousseau GG: Receptor concepts: A century of evolution. *Circ Res* 46(suppl 1):3, 1980.

45. Czech MP: Structural and functional homologies in the receptors for insulin and the insulin-like growth factors. *Cell* 31:7, 1982.

46. Ullrich A, Bell JR, Chen EY, Herrera R, Petruzzelli LM, Dull TJ et al: Human insulin receptor and its relationship to the tyrosine kinase family of oncogenes. *Nature* 313:756, 1985.

47. Dixon RAF, Kobilka BK, Strader DJ, Benovic JL et al: Cloning of the gene and cDNA for mammalian β-adrenergic receptor and homology with rhodopsin. *Nature* 321:75, 1986.

48. Yarden Y, Rodriguez H, Wong S K-F, Brandt DR, et al: The avian β-adrenergic receptor: Primary structure and membrane topology. *Proc Natl Acad Sci USA* 83:6795, 1986.

49. Cuatrecasas P, Hollenberg MD, Chang K-J, Bennett V: Hormone receptor complexes and their modulation of membrane function. *Recent Prog Horm Res* 31:37, 1975.

50. Rodbell M: The role of hormone receptors and GTP-regulatory proteins in membrane transduction. *Nature* 284:17, 1980.

51. Helmreich EJM, Pfeuffer T: Regulation of signal transduction by β-adrenergic hormone receptors. *Trends Pharmacol Sci* 6:438, 1985.

52. McKenzie JM, Zakarija M: LATS in Graves' disease. *Recent Prog Horm Res* 33:29, 1977.

53. Taylor SI, Grunberger G, Marcus-Samuels B, Underhill LH, Dons RF, Ryan J, Roddam RF, Rupe CE, Gorden P: Hypoglycemia associated with antibodies to the insulin receptor. *N Engl J Med* 307:1422, 1982.

54. Schreiber AB, Lax I, Yarden Y, Eshar Z, Schlessinger J: Monoclonal antibodies against receptor for epidermal growth factor induce early and delayed effects of epidermal growth factor. *Proc Natl Acad Sci USA* 78:7535, 1981.

55. Djiane J, Houdebine L-M, Kelly PA: Prolactin-like activity of anti-prolactin receptor antibodies on casein and DNA synthesis in the mammary gland. *Proc Natl Acad Sci USA* 78:7445, 1981.

56. Conn PM, Rogers DC, Stewart JM, Niedel J, Sheffield T: Conversion of a GnRF agonist to an antagonist: Implication for a receptor microaggregate as the functional unit for signal transduction. *Nature* 296:653, 1982.

57. Kahn CR, Baird KL, Jarret DB, Flier JS: Direct demonstration that receptor crosslinking or aggregation is important in insulin action. *Proc Natl Acad Sci USA* 75:4209, 1978.

58. Roth J, Kahn CR, Lesniak MA, Gorden P, De Meyts P, Megyesi K, Neville DM, Gavin JR, Soll AH, Freychet P, Goldfine ID, Bar RS, Archer JA: Receptors for insulin, NSILA-s and growth hormone: Applications to disease states in man. *Recent Prog Horm Res* 31:95, 1975.

59. Raff M: Self regulation of membrane receptors. *Nature* 259:265, 1976.

60. Lefkowitz RJ, Wessels MR, Stadel JM: Hormones, receptors, and cyclic AMP: Their role in target cell refractoriness. *Curr Top Cell Regul* 17:205, 1980.

61. Hertel C, Perkins JP: Receptor-specific mechanisms of desensitization of β-adrenergic receptor function. *Mol Cell Endocrinol* 37:245, 1984.

62. Strulovici B, Lefkowitz RJ: Activation, desensitization and recycling of frog erythrocyte β-adrenergic receptors. *J Biol Chem* 259:4389, 1984.

63. Belchetz PE, Plant TM, Nakai Y, Keogh EJ, Knobil E: Hypophyseal responses to continuous and intermittent delivery of hypothalamic gonadotropin-releasing hormone. *Science* 202:631, 1978.

64. Bergquist C, Nillius SJ, Wide L: Reduced gonadotropin secretion in postmenopausal women during treatment with a stimulatory LRH analogue. *J Clin Endocrinol Metab* 49:472, 1979.

65. Strulovici B, Cerione RA, Kilpatrick BF, Caron MG, Lefkowitz RJ: Direct demonstration of impaired functionality of a purified desensitized β-adrenergic receptor in a reconstituted system. *Science* 225:837, 1984.

65a. Benovic JL, Strasser RH, Caron MG, Lefkowitz RJ: β-Adrenergic kinase: Identification of a novel protein kinase that phosphorylates the agonist-occupied form of the receptor. *Proc Natl Acad Sci USA* 83:2797, 1986.

65b. Benovic JL, Mayor I, Somers RL, Caron MG, Lefkowitz RJ: Light-dependent phosphorylation of rhodopsin by β-adrenergic receptor kinase. *Nature* 321:869, 1986.

66. Harwood JP, Conti M, Conn PM, Dufau ML, Catt KJ: Receptor regulation and target cell responses: Studies in the ovarian luteal cell. *Mol Cell Endocrinol* 11:121, 1978.

67. Stephenson RP: A modification of receptor theory. *Br J Pharmacol* 11:379, 1956.

68. Goodford PJ: Receptors, spare receptors and other binding sites. *Trends Pharmacol Sci* 5:90, 1984.

69. Mendelson C, Dufau ML, Catt KJ: Gonadotropin binding and stimulation of cyclic adenosine 3',5'-monophosphate and testosterone production in isolated Leydig cells. *J Biol Chem* 250:8818, 1975.

70. Douglas J, Saltman S, Fredlund P, Kondo T, Catt KJ: Receptor binding of angiotensin II and antagonists: Correlation with aldosterone production by isolated adrenal glomerulosa cells. *Circ Res* 38(suppl 2):108, 1976.

71. Kono T, Barham FW: Effects of insulin on the levels of adenosine 3',5'-monophosphate and lipolysis in isolated rat epididymal fat cells.

72. Shia MA, Pilch PF: The β-subunit of the insulin receptor is an insulin-activated protein kinase. *Biochemistry* 22:717, 1983.

73. Hollenberg MD: Receptor-mediated phosphorylation reactions. *Trends Pharmacol Sci* 3:271, 1982.

74. Sefton BM, Hunter T, Beemon K, Eckhart W: Evidence that the phosphorylation of tyrosine is essential for cellular transformation by Rous sarcoma virus. *Cell* 20:807, 1980.

75. Erickson E, Shealy DJ, Erickson RL: Evidence that renal transforming gene products and epidermal growth factor stimulate phosphorylation of the same cellular protein with similar specificity. *J Biol Chem* 256:11381, 1981.

76. Reynolds FH, Todaro GJ, Fryling C, Stephenson JR: Human transforming growth factors induce tyrosine phosphorylation of EGF receptors. *Nature* 292:259, 1981.

77. White MF, Haring H-U, Kasuga M, Kahn CR: Kinetic properties and sites of autophosphorylation of the partially purified insulin receptor from hepatoma cells. *J Biol Chem* 259:255, 1984.

78. Grunberger G, Zick Y, Gorden P: Defect in phosphorylation

of insulin receptors in cells from an insulin-resistant patient with normal insulin binding. *Science* 223:932, 1984.

79. Grigorescu F, Flier JS, Kahn CR: Defect in insulin receptor phosphorylation in erythrocytes and fibroblasts associated with severe insulin resistance. *J Biol Chem* 259:15003, 1984.

80. Simpson IA, Hedo JA: Insulin receptor phosphorylation may not be a prerequisite for acute insulin action. *Science* 223:1301, 1984.

81. Zick Y, Rees-Jones RW, Taylor SI, Gorden P, Roth J: The role of antireceptor antibodies in stimulating phosphorylation of the insulin receptor. *J Biol Chem* 259:4396, 1984.

82. Liebman PA, Sitaramayya A, Parkes JH, Buzdygon B: Mechanisms of cGMP control in retinal rod outer segments. *Trends Pharmacol Sci* 5:293, 1984.

83. Maciag T: The human epidermal growth factor receptor-kinase complexes. *Trends Biochem Sci* 7:197, 1982.

84. Cassel D, Pike LJ, Grant GA, Krebs EG, Glaser L: Interaction of epidermal growth factor-dependent protein kinase with endogenous membrane proteins and soluble peptide substrate. *J Biol Chem* 258:2945, 1983.

85. Yarden Y, Schreiber AB, Schlessinger J: A nonmitogenic analogue of epidermal growth factor induces early responses mediated by epidermal growth factor. *J Cell Biol* 92:687, 1982.

85a. Rothman JE, Lenard J: Membrane traffic in animal cells. *Trends Biochem Sci* 10:176, 1985.

85b. Dickson RB: Endocytosis of polypeptides and their receptors. *Trends Biochem Sci* 10:164, 1985.

86. Wickner WT, Lodish HF: Multiple mechanisms of protein insertion into and across membranes. *Science* 230:400, 1985.

87. Catt KJ, Harwood JP, Aguilera G, Dufau ML: Hormonal regulation of peptide receptors and target cell responses. *Nature* 280:109, 1979.

88. Chan V, Katikineni M, Davies TF, Catt KJ: Hormonal regulation of testicular luteinizing hormone and prolactin receptors. *Endocrinology* 108:1607, 1981.

89. Huhtaniemi IT, Nozu K, Warren DW, Dufau ML, Catt KJ: Acquisition of regulatory mechanisms for gonadotropin receptors and steroidogenesis in the maturing rat testis. *Endocrinology* 111:1711, 1982.

90. Hoffman BB, Lefkowitz RJ: Radioligand binding sites of adrenergic receptors: New insights into molecular and physiological regulation. *Annu Rev Pharmacol Toxicol* 20:581, 1980.

91. Fambrough DM: Control of acetylcholine receptors in smooth muscle. *Physiol Rev* 59:165, 1979.

92. Brown MS, Goldstein JL: Receptor-mediated endocytosis: Insights from the lipoprotein receptor system. *Proc Natl Acad Sci USA* 76:3330, 1980.

93. Cohen S, Haigler HT, Carpenter G, King L, McKanna JA: Epidermal growth factor: Visualization of the binding and internalization of EGF in cultured cells, and enhancement of phosphorylation of EGF in membrane preparations in vitro, in Sato GH, Ross R (eds): *Hormones and Cell Culture.* New York, Cold Spring Harbor Laboratory, 1979, p 131.

94. Capponi AM, Aguilera G, Fakunding JL, Catt KJ: Angiotensin II: Receptors and mechanisms of action, in Sofer RL (ed): *Biochemical Regulation of Blood Pressure.* New York, Wiley, 1981, p 205.

95. Clayton RN, Catt KJ: Gonadotropin-releasing hormone receptors: Characterizations, physiological regulation and relationship to reproductive function. *Endocr Rev* 2:186, 1981.

96. Maxfield FR, Schlessinger J, Schechter Y, Pastan I, Willingham MC: Collection of insulin, EGF and α_2-macroglobuin in the same patches on the surface of cultured fibroblasts and common internalization. *Cell* 14:805, 1978.

97. Gorden P, Carpentier J-L, Freychet P, Orci L: Internalization of polypeptide hormones. *Diabetologia* 18:263, 1980.

98. Goldfine ID, Jones AL, Hradek GT, Wong KY: Electron microscope autoradiographic analysis of [^{125}I]iodoinsulin entry into adult rat hepatocytes *in vivo:* Evidence for multiple sites of hormone localization. *Endocrinology* 108:1821, 1981.

99. Pastan IH, Willingham MC: Journey to the center of the cell: Role of the receptosome. *Science* 214:504, 1981.

100. Steinman RM, Mellman IS, Muller WA, Cohn ZA: Endocytosis and the recycling of plasma membrane. *J Cell Biol* 96:1, 1983.

101. Pastan I, Willingham MC: Receptor-mediated endocytosis: Coated pits, receptosomes and the Golgi. *Trends Biochem Sci* 8:250, 1983.

102. Helenius A, Mellman I, Wall D, Hubbard A: Endosomes. *Trends Biochem Sci* 8:245, 1983.

103. Klausner RD, Ashwell G, Van Renswoude J, Harford JE, Bridges KR: Binding of apotransferrin to K562 cells: Explanation of the transferrin cycle. *Proc Natl Acad Sci USA* 80:2263, 1983.

104. King GL, Johnson SM: Receptor-mediated transport of insulin across endothelial cells. *Science* 227:1583, 1985.

105. Ascoli M, Puett D: Degradation of receptor-bound human choriogonadotropin by murine tumor Leydig cells. *J Biol Chem* 253:4892, 1978.

106. Amsterdam A, Naor Z, Knecht M, Dufau ML, Catt KJ: Hormone action and receptor distribution in endocrine target cells: Gonadotropins and gonadotropin-releasing hormone, in Middlebrook JL, Kohn LD (eds): *Receptor-Mediated Binding and Internalization of Toxins and Hormones.* New York, Academic, 1981, p 283.

107. Lienhard GE: Regulation of cellular membrane transport by the exocytotic insertion and endocytic retrieval of transporters. *Trends Biochem Sci* 8:107, 1983.

108. Kono T, Suzuki K Dansey LE, Robinson FW, Blevins TL: Energy-dependent and protein synthesis-independent recycling of the insulin-sensitive glucose transport mechanism in fat cells. *J Biol Chem* 256:6400, 1981.

109. Karnieli E, Zarnowski MJ, Hissin PJ, Simpson IA, Salans LB, Cushman SW: Insulin-stimulated translocation of glucose transport systems in the isolated rat adipose cell. *J Biol Chem* 256:4772, 1981.

109a. Strasser RH, Stiles GL, Lefkowitz RJ: Translocation and uncoupling of the β-adrenergic receptor in rat lung after catecholamine promoted desensitization *in vivo. Endocrinology* 115:1392, 1984.

110. Kaplan J: Polypeptide-binding membrane receptors: Analysis and classification. *Science* 212:14, 1981.

111. Tata JR: Thyroid hormone receptors, in Schulster D, Levitski A (eds): *Cellular Receptors for Hormones and Neurotransmitters.* New York, Wiley, 1980, p 127.

112. Goldberg ND, Haddox MC: Cyclic GMP metabolism and involvement in biological regulation. *Annu Rev Biochem* 46:823, 1977.

113. Rasmussen H, Jensen P, Lake W, Friedmann N, Goodman DBP: Cyclic nucleotides and cellular calcium metabolism. *Adv Cyclic Nucleotide Res* 5:375, 1974.

114. Berridge MJ: The interaction of cyclic nucleotides and calcium in the control of cellular activity. *Adv Cyclic Nucleotide Res* 6:1, 1975.

115. Rodbell M: The role of hormone receptors and GTP-regulatory proteins in membrane transduction. *Nature* 284:17, 1980.

116. Cassel D, Levkovitz H, Selinger Z: The regulatory GTPase cycle of turkey erythrocyte adenylate cyclase. *J Cyclic Nucleotide Res* 3:393, 1977.

117. Moss J, Vaughan M: Activation of adenylate cyclase by choleragen. *Annu Rev Biochem* 48:581, 1979.

118. Schramm M, Orly J, Eimerl S, Korner M: Coupling of hormone receptors to adenylate cyclase of different cells by fusion. *Nature* 268:310, 1977.

119. Ross EM, Gilman AG: Biochemical properties of hormone-sensitive adenylate cyclase. *Annu Rev Biochem* 49:533, 1980.

120. Helmreich EJM, Pfeuffer T: Regulation of signal transduction by β-adrenergic hormone receptors. *Trends Biochem Sci* 10:438, 1985.

121. Gilman AG: Guanine nucleotide-binding regulatory proteins and dual control of adenylate cyclase. *J Clin Invest* 73:1, 1984.

122. Maguire ME: Hormone-sensitive magnesium transport and magnesium regulation of adenylate cyclase. *Trends Biochem Sci* 9:73, 1984.

123. Robishaw JD, Russell DW, Harris BA, Smigel MD, Gilman AG: Deduced primary structure of the α subunit of the GTP-binding stimulatory protein of adenylate cyclase. *Proc Natl Acad Sci USA* 83:1251, 1986.

124. Houslay MD: A family of guanine nucleotide regulatory proteins. *Trends Biochem Sci* 9:39, 1984.

125. Greengard P: Phosphorylated proteins as physiological effectors. *Science* 199:146, 1978.

126. Krebs EG, Beavo JA: Phosphorylation-dephosphorylation of enzymes. *Annu Rev Biochem* 48:923, 1979.

127. Corbin JD, Sugden PH, West L, Flockhart DA, Lincoln TM, McCarthy D: Studies on the properties and mode of action of the purified regulatory subunit of bovine heart adenosine 3′:5′-monophosphate-dependent protein kinase. *J Biol Chem* 253:3997, 1978.

128. Hofmann F: Apparent constants for the interaction of regulatory and catalytic subunit of cAMP-dependent protein kinase I and II. *J Biol Chem* 255:1559, 1980.

129. Rosen OM, Rangel-Aldeo R, Erlichman J: Soluble cyclic AMP-dependent protein kinases: Review of the enzyme isolated from bovine cardiac muscle, in Horecker BL, Stadtman EF (eds): *Current Topics in Cellular Regulation.* New York, Academic, 1977, vol 12, p 39.

130. Hoppe J: cAMP-dependent protein kinases: Conformational changes during activation. *Trends Biochem Sci* 10:29, 1985.

131. Huang T-S, Feramisco JR, Glass DB, Krebs EG: Miami Winter Symposium. New York, Academic, 1979, vol. 16, p 449.

132. Feramisco JR, Glass DB, Krebs EG: Optimal spatial requirements for the location of basic residues in peptide substrates for the cyclic AMP-dependent protein kinase. *J Biol Chem* 255:4240, 1980.

133. Robinson-Steiner AM, Beebe SJ, Rennels SR, Corbin J: Microheterogeneity of type II cAMP-dependent protein kinase in various mammalian species and tissues. *J Biol Chem* 259:10596, 1984.

134. Darbon J-M, Knecht M, Ranta T, Dufau ML, Catt KJ: Hormonal regulation of cyclic AMP-dependent protein kinase in cultured ovarian granulosa cells. *J Biol Chem* 259:14778, 1984.

135. Rall TW, Sutherland EW, Berthet J: The relationship of epinephrine and glucose to liver phosphorylase. IV. *J Biol Chem* 244:463, 1957.

136. Cohen P: The role of protein phosphorylation in neural and hormonal control of cellular activity. *Nature* 296:613, 1982.

137. Blackmore PF, Brumley FT, Marks JL, Exton JH: Studies on α-adrenergic activation of hepatic glucose output. *J Biol Chem* 253:4851, 1978.

138. Garrison JC, Borland MK, Florio VA, Twible DA: The role of calcium ion as a mediator of the effects of angiotensin II, catecholamines, and vasopressin on the phosphorylation and activity of enzymes in isolated hepatocytes. *J Biol Chem* 254:7147, 1979.

139. Berridge MJ, Irvine RF: Inositol triphosphate, a novel second messenger in cellular signal transduction. *Nature* 312:315, 1984.

140. Hems DA, Rodrigues LM, Whitton PD: Rapid stimulation by vasopressin, oxytocin and angiotensin II of glycogen degradation in hepatocyte suspensions. *Biochem J* 172:311, 1978.

141. Steinberg D, Mayer SE, Khoo JC, Miller EA, Miller RE, Fredholm B, Eichner R: Hormonal regulation of lipase, phosphorylase and glycogen synthase in adipose tissue. *Adv Cyclic Nucleotide Res* 6:549, 1975.

142. de Crombrugghe B, Busby S, Buc H: Cyclic AMP receptor protein: Role in transcription activation. *Science* 224:831, 1984.

143. Weber I, Takio K, Titani K, Steitz T: The cAMP-binding domains of the regulatory subunit of cAMP-dependent protein kinase and the catabolite gene activator protein are homologous. *Proc Natl Acad Sci USA* 79:7679, 1982.

144. Waterman M, Murdoch GH, Evans RM, Rosenfeld MG: Cyclic AMP regulation of eukaryotic gene transcription by two discrete molecular mechanisms. *Science* 229:267, 1985.

145. Houslay MD: Renaissance for cyclic GMP? *Trends Biochem Sci* 10:465, 1985.

146. Monken CE, Gill GN: Structural analysis of cGMP-dependent protein kinase using limited proteolysis. *J Biol Chem* 255:7067, 1980.

147. Monken CE, Gill GN: A comparison of the cyclic nucleotide-dependent protein kinases using chemical cleavage at tryptophan and cysteine. *Arch Biochem Biophys* 240:888, 1985.

148. Gomperts BD: Calcium and cell activation, in Cuatrecasas P, Greaves MF (eds): *Receptors and Recognition.* London, Chapman & Hall, 1976, ser A, vol 2, p 43.

149. Rubin RP: The role of calcium in the release of neurotransmitter substances and hormones. *Pharmacol Rev* 22:389, 1970.

150. Cheung WY: Calmodulin plays a pivotal role in cellular regulation. *Science* 207:19, 1980.

151. Means AR, Dedman JR: Calmodulin—an intracellular calcium receptor. *Nature* 285:73, 1980.

152. Klee CB, Crouch TH, Richman PG: Calmodulin. *Annu Rev Biochem* 49:489, 1980.

153. Babu YS, Sack JS, Greenhough TJ, Bugg CE, Means AR, Cook WJ: Three-dimensional structure of calmodulin. *Nature* 315:37, 1985.

154. Nairn AC, Bhagat B, Palfrey HC: Identification of calmodulin-dependent protein kinase III and its major M_r 100,000 substrate in mammalian tissues. *Proc Natl Acad Sci USA* 82:7939, 1985.

155. Conti MA, Adelstein RS: Phosphorylation by cyclic adenosine 3′-5′-monophosphate-dependent protein kinase regulates myosin light chain kinase. *Fed Proc* 39:1569, 1980.

156. Michel B: Ca^{2+} and protein kinase C: Two synergistic cellular signals. *Trends Biochem Sci* 8:263, 1983.

157. Nishizuka Y: The role of protein kinase C in cell surface signal transduction and tumor promotion. *Nature* 308:693, 1984.

158. Parker PJ, Coussens L, Totty N, Rhee L, et al: The complete primary structure of protein kinase C—the major phorbol ester receptor. *Science* 233:853, 1986.

159. Rasmussen H, Barrett PQ: Calcium messenger system: An integrated view. *Physiol Rev* 64:938, 1984.

160. Drummond AH, Macintyre DE: Protein kinase C as a bidirectional regulator of cell function. *Trends Pharmacol Sci* 6:233, 1985.

161. Knight DE, Scrutton MC: Cyclic nucleotides control a system which regulates Ca^{2+} sensitivity of platelet secretion. *Nature* 309:66, 1984.

162. Levine L: Deacylation of cellular lipids and arachidonic acid metabolism in cultured cells, in Sato GH, Ross R (eds): *Hormones and Cell Culture.* New York, Cold Spring Harbor Laboratory, 1979, p 623.

163. Moncada S, Vane JR: Arachidonic acid metabolites and the interactions between platelets and blood-vessel walls. *N Engl J Med* 300:1142, 1979.

164. Naor Z, Catt KJ: Mechanism of action of gonadotropin-releasing hormone: Arachidonic acid as an intermediate in luteinizing hormone release. *J Biol Chem* 256:256, 1981.

165. Vogt W: Role of phospholipase A_2 in prostaglandin formation, in Galli C et al (eds): *Advances in Prostaglandin and Thromboxane Research.* New York, Raven, 1978, vol 3, p 89.

166. Tonqui L, Rothhut B, Shaw AM, et al: Platelet activation—a role for a 40K anti-phospholipase protein indistinguishable from lipocortin. *Nature* 321:177, 1986.

167. Clark MR, Marsh JM, LeMaire WJ: Mechanism of luteinizing hormone regulation of prostaglandin synthesis in rat granulosa cells. *J Biol Chem* 253:7757, 1978.

168. Lindner HR, Zor U, Kohen F, Bauminger S, Amsterdam A,

Lahav M, Salomon Y: Significance of prostaglandins in the regulation of cyclic events in the ovary and uterus, in Samuelsson B (ed): *Advances in Prostaglandin and Thromboxane Research.* New York, Raven, 1979, vol 6, p 1371.

169. Hokin MR, Hokin LE: Enzyme secretion and the incorporation of P^{32} into phospholipids of pancreas slices. *J Biol Chem* 203:967, 1953.

170. Michell RH: Inositol phospholipids and cell surface receptor functions. *Biochim Biophys Acta* 415:81, 1975.

171. Berridge MJ: Phosphatidylinositol hydrolysis: A multifunctional transducing mechanism. *Mol Cell Endocrinol* 24:115, 1981.

172. Berridge MJ, Dawson RMC, Downes CP, Heslop JP, Irvine RF: Changes in the levels of inositol phosphates after agonist-dependent hydrolysis of membrane phosphoinositides. *Biochem J* 212:473, 1983.

173. Burgess GM, Godfrey PP, McKinney JS, Berridge MJ, Irvine RF, Putney JW: The second messenger linking receptor activation to internal Ca release in liver. *Nature* 309:63, 1984.

174. Storey DJ, Shears SB, Kirk CJ, Michell RH: Stepwise enzymatic dephosphorylation of inositol 1,4,5-triphosphate to inositol in liver. *Nature* 312:374, 1984.

175. Berridge MJ, Downes CP, Hanley MR: Lithium amplifies agonist-dependent phosphatidylinositol responses in brain and salivary glands. *Biochem J* 206:587, 1982.

176. Streb H, Heslop JP, Irvine RF, Schulz I, Berridge MJ: Relationship between secretagogue-induced Ca^{2+} release and inositol polyphosphate production in permeabilized pancreatic acinar cells. *J Biol Chem* 260:7309, 1985.

177. Gershengorn MC, Geras E, Purrello VS, Rebecchi MJ: Inositol trisphosphate mediated thyrotropin-releasing hormone mobilization of nonmitochondrial calcium in rat mammotropic pituitary cells. *J Biol Chem* 259:10675, 1984.

178. Brown JE, Rubin LJ, Ghalayini AJ, Tarver AP, Irvine RF, Berridge MJ, Anderson RE: Myo-inositol polyphosphate may be a messenger for visual excitation in *Limulus* photoreceptors. *Nature* 311:160, 1984.

179. Volpe P, Salviati G, Di Virgilio F, Pozzan T: Inositol 1,4,5-trisphosphate induces calcium release from sarcoplasmic reticulum of skeletal muscle. *Nature* 316:347, 1985.

179a. Cockcroft S, Gomperts BD: Role of guanine nucleotide binding protein in the activation of polyphosphoinositide phosphodiesterase. *Nature* 314:531, 1985.

180. Farese RV: Phosphoinositide metabolism and hormone action. *Endocr Rev* 4:78, 1983.

181. Hirata F, Strittmayer WJ, Axelrod J: β-Adrenergic receptor agonists increase phospholipid methylation, membrane fluidity and β-adrenergic receptor-adenylate cyclase coupling. *Proc Natl Acad Sci USA* 75:368, 1979.

182. Hirata F, Axelrod J: Phospholipid methylation and transmission of biological signals through membranes. *Science* 209:1082, 1980.

183. Nieto A, Catt KJ: Hormonal activation of phospholipid methyltransferase in the Leydig cell. *Endocrinology* 113:758, 1983.

184. Baxter JD, McLeod KM: Molecular basis for hormone action, in Bondy PK, Rosenberg LE (eds): *Metabolic Control and Disease.* Philadelphia, Saunders, 1980, p 104.

185. Mainwaring WIP: Steroid hormone receptors, in Schulster D, Levitski A (eds): *Cellular Receptors for Hormones and Neurotransmitters.* New York, Wiley, 1980, p 91.

186. Westphal U: *Steroid-Protein Interactions.* New York, Springer-Verlag, 1971.

187. Perdridge WM, Mietus LJ: Transport of steroid hormones through the blood-brain barrier. Primary role of albumin-bound hormone. *J Clin Invest* 64:145, 1979.

188. Funder JW, Feldman D, Edelman IS: The roles of plasma binding and receptor specificity in the mineralocorticoid action of aldosterone. *Endocrinology* 92:994, 1973.

189. Smith LD, Ecker RE: The interaction of steroids with *Rana pipiens* oocytes in the induction of maturation. *Dev Biol* 25:232, 1971.

190. Baullieu E-E, Godeau F, Schorderet M, Schorderet-Slatkine S: Steroid-induced meiotic division in *Xenopus laevis* oocytes: Surface and calcium. *Nature* 275:593, 1978.

191. Sadler SE, Maller JL: Progesterone inhibits adenylate cyclase in *Xenopus* oocytes. *J Biol Chem* 56:6368, 1981.

192. Mueller GC, Herranen AM, Jervell KJ: Studies on the mechanism of action of estrogens. *Recent Prog Horm Res* 14:95, 1958.

193. Williams-Ashman HG, Reddi AH: Actions of vertebrate sex hormones. *Annu Rev Physiol* 33:31, 1971.

194. Jensen EV, Jacobson HI: Basic guides to the mechanism of estrogen action. *Recent Prog Horm Res* 18:387, 1962.

195. King WJ, Greene GL: Monoclonal antibodies localize oestrogen receptor in the nuclei of target cells. *Nature* 307:745, 1984.

196. Welshons WV, Lieberman ME, Gorski J: Nuclear localization of unoccupied oestrogen receptors. *Nature* 307:747, 1984.

197. Gorski J, Toft D, Shyamala S, Smith D, Notides A: Hormone receptors: Studies on the interaction of estrogen with the uterus. *Recent Prog Horm Res* 24:45, 1979.

198. Jensen EV: Interaction of steroid hormones with the nucleus. *Pharmacol Rev* 30:477, 1979.

199. Greene GL, Fitch PW, Jensen EV: Monoclonal antibodies to estrophilin: Probes for the study of estrogen receptors. *Proc Natl Acad Sci USA* 77:157, 1980.

200. Greene GL, Gilna P, Waterfield M, Baker A, Hort Y, Shine J: Sequence and expression of human estrogen receptor complementary DNA. *Science* 231:1150, 1985.

201. Green S, Walter P, Kumar V, Krust A, Bornert JM, Argos P, Chambon P: Human oestrogen receptor cDNA: Sequence, expression and homology to v-*erb*-A. *Nature* 320:134, 1986.

202. Leavitt WW, Chen TJ, Do YS, Carlton BD, Allen TC: Biology of progesterone receptors, in O'Malley BW, Birnbaumer L (eds): *Receptors and Hormone Action.* New York, Academic, 1978, vol 2, p 157.

203. Vedeckis WV, Schrader WT, O'Malley BW: The chick oviduct progesterone receptor, in Litwack G (ed): *Biochemical Actions of Hormones.* New York, Academic, 1978, vol 5, p 322.

204. Liao S: Receptors and the mechanism of action of androgens, in Pasqualini JR (ed): *Receptors and Mechanism of Action of Steroid Hormones.* New York, Marcel Dekker, 1976, pt 1, p 159.

205. Wilson JD, MacDonald PC: Male pseudohermaphroditism due to androgen resistance: Testicular feminization and related syndromes, in Stanbury JB et al (eds): *The Metabolic Basis of Inherited Disease.* New York, McGraw-Hill, 1978, p 894.

206. Higgins SJ, Baxter JD, Rousseau GC: Nuclear binding of glucocorticoid receptors, in Baxter JD, Rousseau GC (eds): *Glucocorticoid Hormone Action.* New York, Springer-Verlag, 1979, p 135.

207. Munck A, Foley R: Activation of steroid hormone-receptor complexes in intact target cells in physiological conditions. *Nature* 278:752, 1979.

208. Hollenberg SM, Weinberger C, Ong ES, Cerelli G, Oro A, Lebo R, Thompson EB, Rosenfeld MG, Evans RM: Primary structure and expression of a functional human glucocorticoid receptor cDNA. *Nature* 318:635, 1985.

209. Weinberger C, Hollenberg SM, Rosenfeld MG, Evans RM: Domain structure of human glucocorticoid receptor and its relationship to the v-erb-A oncogene product. *Nature* 318:670, 1985.

210. Anderson NS, Fanestil DW: Biology of mineralocorticoid receptors, in O'Malley BW, Birnbaumer L (eds): *Receptors and Hormone Action.* New York, Academic, 1978, vol 2, p 323.

211. Marver D, Goodman D, Edelman IS: Relationships between renal cytoplasmic and nuclear aldosterone-receptors. *Kidney Int* 1:210, 1972.

212. Dahmer MK, Housley PR, Pratt WB: Effects of molybdate and endogenous inhibitors on steroid-receptor inactivation, transformation, and translocation. *Annu Rev Physiol* 49:67, 1984.

213. Clark JH, Peck EJ, Hardin JW, Eriksson H: The biology and

pharmacology of estrogen receptor binding: Relationship to uterine growth, in O'Malley BW, Birnbaumer L (eds): *Receptors and Hormone Action.* New York, Academic, 1978, vol 2, p 1.

214. Glusker JP: Structural aspects of steroid hormones and carcinogenic polycyclic aromatic hydrocarbons, in Litwak G (ed): *Biochemical Actions of Hormones.* New York, Academic, 1979, vol 6, p 122.

215. Neri RO: Studies on the biology and mechanism of action of nonsteroidal androgens, in Martini L, Motta M (eds): *Androgens and Antiandrogens.* New York, Raven, 1977, p 179.

215a. Segal S, Baulieu E-E: *The Antiprogestin Steroid RU 486 and Human Fertility Control.* New York, Plenum (in press).

216. Naylor PH, Gilani SSH, Milholland RJ, Rosen F: Antiglucocorticoids: In vivo assay and evaluation of cortexolone, progesterone, and 6-β-bromoprogesterone. *Endocrinology* 107:117, 1980.

217. Marver D, Stewart J, Funder JW, Feldman D, Edelman IS: Renal aldosterone receptors: Studies with [^{3}H]aldosterone and the antimineralocorticoid [^{3}H]spironolactone (SC-26304). *Proc Natl Acad Sci USA* 71:1421, 1974.

218. Felsenfeld G: DNA. *Sci Am* 253:58, 1985.

219. Richmond TJ, Finch JT, Rushton B, Rhodes D, Klug A: Structure of the nucleosome core particle at 7Å resolution. *Nature* 311:532, 1984.

220. Felsenfeld G, McGee JD: Structure of the 30 nm chromatin fiber. *Cell* 44:375, 1986.

221. O'Malley BW, Schwartz RJ, Schrader WT: A review of regulation of gene expression by steroid hormone receptors. *J Steroid Biochem* 7:1151, 1976.

221a. Payvar F, DeFranco D, Firestone GL, Edgar B, Wrange Ö, Okret S, Gustafsson J.-A, Yamamoto KR: Sequence-specific binding of glucocorticoid receptor to MTV DNA at sites within and upstream of the transcribed region. *Cell* 35:381, 1983.

221b. Scheidereit C, Beato M: Contacts between hormone receptor and DNA double helix within a glucocorticoid regulatory element of mouse mammary tumor virus. *Proc Natl Acad Sci USA* 81:3029, 1984.

221c. Karin M, Haslinger A, Holtgreve H, Richards RI, Krauter P, Westphal HM, Beato M: Characterization of DNA sequences through which cadmium and glucocorticoid hormones induce human metallothionein-II$_A$ gene. *Nature* 308:513, 1984.

221d. von der Ahe D, Janich S, Scheidereit C, Renkawitz R, Schütz G, Beato M: Glucocorticoid and progesterone receptors bind to the same sites in two hormonally regulated promoters. *Nature* 313:706, 1985.

221e. von der Ahe D, Renoir J-M, Buchou T, Baulieu E-E, Beato M: Receptors for glucocorticosteroid and progesterone recognize distinct features of a DNA regulatory element. *Proc Nat Acad Sci* 83:2817, 1986.

221f. Bloom E, Matulich DT, Lan NC, Higgins SJ, Simons SJ, Baxter JD: Nuclear binding of glucocorticoid receptors. Relations between cytosol binding, activation, and the biological response. *J Steroid Biochem* 12:175, 1980.

221g. Johnson LK, Lan NC, Baxter JD: Stimulation and inhibition of cellular functions by glucocorticoids: Correlations with rapid influences on chromatin structure. *J Biol Chem* 254:7785, 1979.

222. Senior MB, Frankel FR: Evidence for two kinds of chromatin binding sites for the estradiol-receptor complex. *Cell* 14:857, 1978.

223. Barrack ER, Coffey DS: The specific binding of estrogens and androgens to the nuclear matrix of sex hormone responsive tissues. *J Biol Chem* 255:7265, 1980.

224. Goldberg GI, Collier I, Cassel A: Specific DNA sequences associated with the nuclear matrix in synchronized mouse 3T3 cells. *Proc Natl Acad Sci USA* 80:6887, 1983.

225. Barrack ER, Coffey DS: The role of nuclear structure in hormone action: The nuclear matrix, in Eriksson H, Gustafsson JA (eds): *Steroid Hormone Receptors: Structure and Function.* Amsterdam, Elsevier, 1983, p 221.

226. Ciejek EM, Tsai M-J, O'Malley BW: Actively transcribed genes are associated with the nuclear matrix. *Nature* 306:607, 1983.

227. Schimke RT, McKnight GS, Shapiro DJ, Sullivan D, Palacios R: Hormonal regulation of ovalbumin synthesis in the chick oviduct. *Recent Prog Horm Res* 31:175, 1975.

228. Katzenellenbogen B, Gorski J: Estrogen action in vitro: Induction of the synthesis of a specific uterine protein *J Biol Chem* 247:1299, 1972.

229. Birnberg NC, Lissitzky J-C, Hinman M, Herbert E: Glucocorticoids regulate *in vitro* at the levels of transcription and secretion. *Proc Natl Acad Sci USA* 80:6982, 1983.

230. Nakamura M, Nakanishi S, Sueoka S, Imura H, Numa S: Effects of steroid hormones on the levels of corticotropin messenger RNA activity in cultured mouse-pituitary-tumor cells. *Eur J Biochem* 86:61, 1977.

231. Yamamoto KR: On steroid regulation of gene expression and the evolution of hormone-controlled gene networks, in Eriksson H, Gustafsson JA (eds): *Steroid Hormone Receptors: Structure and Function.* Amsterdam, Elsevier, 1983, p 285.

232. Schrader WT, Compton JG, O'Malley BW: Progesterone receptor binding to the ovalbumin gene, in Eriksson H, Gustafsson JA (eds): *Steroid Hormone Receptors: Structure and Function.* Amsterdam, Elsevier, 1983, p 247.

233. Chambon P, Gaub MP, Lepennec J-P, Dierich A, Astinotti D: Steroid hormones relieve repression of the ovalbumin gene promoter in chick oviduct tubular cells, in Labrie F, Proulx L (eds): *Endocrinology.* Amsterdam, Elsevier, 1984, p 3.

234. Ashburner M: Chromosomal action of ecdysone. *Nature* 285:435, 1980.

235. Gronemeyer H, Pongs O: Localization of ecdysterone on polytene chromosomes of *Drosophila melanogaster. Proc Natl Acad Sci USA* 77:2108, 1980.

236. Palmiter RD, Moore PB, Mulvihill ER, Emtage S: A significant lag in the induction of ovalbumin messenger RNA by steroid hormones: A receptor translocation hypothesis. *Cell* 8:557, 1976.

237. Darnell JE, Jelinek W, Puckett L, Derman E, Bachenheimer S: Biochemical events in mRNA formation in mammalian cells, in Papaconstantinous J (ed): *The Molecular Biology of Hormone Action.* New York, Academic, 1976, p 53.

238. Abelson J: RNA processing and the intervening sequence problem. *Annu Rev Biochem* 48:1035, 1979.

239. Swaneck GE, Nordstrom JL, Kreuzaler F, Tsai M-J, O'Malley BW: Effects of estrogen on gene expression in chicken oviduct: Evidence for transcriptional control of ovalbumin gene. *Proc Natl Acad Sci USA* 76:1049, 1979.

240. Crick F: Split genes and RNA splicing. *Science* 204:264, 1979.

241. Lonberg N, Gilbert W: Intron/exon structure of the chicken pyruvate kinase gene. *Cell* 40:81, 1985.

242. Cochet M, Gannon F, Hen R, Maroteaux L, Perrin F, Chambon P: Organization and sequence studies of the 17-piece chicken conalbumin gene. *Nature* 282:567, 1979.

243. Royal A, Garapin A, Cami B, Perrin F, Mandell JL, LeMeur M, Bregegegre F, Gannon F, LePennec JP, Chambon P, Kourilsky P: The ovalbumin gene region: Common features in the organization of three genes expressed in the chicken oviduct under hormonal control. *Nature* 279:125, 1979.

244. Carey N: Unsuspected relatives of the ovalbumin gene. *Nature* 279:101, 1979.

245. Skoglund U, Anderson K, Strandberg B, Daneholt B: Three-dimensional structure of a specific pre-messenger RNP particle established by electron microscope tomography. *Nature* 319:560, 1986.

246. Edelman IS, Ismail-Beigi F: Thyroid thermogenesis and active sodium transport. *Recent Prog Horm Res* 30:235, 1974.

247. Larsen PR, Dick TE, Markovitz BP, Kaplan MM, Gard TG: Inhibition of intrapituitary thyroxine to triiodothyronine conversion prevents the acute suppression of thyrotropin release by thyroxine in hypothyroid rats. *J Clin Invest* 64:117, 1979.

248. Eberhardt NW, Apriletti JW, Baxter JB: The molecular biol-

ogy of thyroid hormone action, in Litwak G (ed): *Biochemical Actions of Hormones.* New York, Academic, 1980, vol 7, p 311.

249. Surks ML, Oppenheimer JH: Concentration of L-thyroxine and L-triiodothyronine specifically bound to nuclear receptors in rat liver and kidney: Quantitative evidence favoring a major role of T_3 in thyroid hormone action. *J Clin Invest* 60:555, 1978.

251. Cheng S-Y: Structural similarities in the plasma membrane 3,3′,5-triiodo-L-thyronine receptors from human, rat, and mouse cultured cells. Analysis by affinity labeling. *Endocrinology* 113:1155, 1983.

252. Cheng S-Y, Maxfield FR, Robbins J, Willingham MC, Pastan IH: Receptor-mediated uptake of 3,3′,5-triiodo-L-thyronine by cultured fibroblasts. *Proc Natl Acad Sci USA* 77:3425, 1980.

253. Alderson R, Pastan I, Cheng S-Y: Characterization of the 3,3′,5-triiodo-L-thyronine-binding sites on plasma membranes from human placenta. *Endocrinology* 116:2621, 1985.

254. Oppenheimer JH, Schwartz HL: Stereospecific transport of triiodothyronine from plasma to cytosol and from cytosol to nucleus in rat liver, kidney, brain, and heart. *J Clin Invest* 75:147, 1985.

255. Tata JR: Growth and developmental action of thyroid hormones at the cellular level, in: *Handbook of Physiology.* Washington, D.C., American Physiological Society, 1974, sec 7, vol 3, p 469.

255a. Cattini PA, Anderson TR, Baxter JD, Mellon P, Eberhardt NL: The human growth hormone gene is negatively regulated by triiodothyronine when transfected into rat pituitary tumor cells. *J Biol Chem,* in press.

255b. Beyer HS, Carr FE, Mariash CN, Oppenheimer JH: Hepatic messenger ribonucleic acid activity profile of rats subjected to alterations in thyroidal and adrenocortical states: Evidence for significant interaction. *Endocrinology* 116:2669, 1985.

256. Oppenheimer JH: Thyroid hormone action at the nuclear level. *Ann Intern Med* 102:374, 1985.

257. Shupnik ML, Ardisson LJ, Meskell MJ, Bornstein J, Ridgway EC: Triiodothyronine (T_3) regulation of thyrotropin subunit gene transcription is proportional to T_3 nuclear receptor occupancy. *Endocrinology* 118:367, 1986.

258. Samuels HH, Horowitz ZD, Stanley F, Casanova J, Shapiro LE: Thyroid hormone controls glucocorticoid action in cultured GH_1 cells. *Nature* 268:254, 1977.

259. Nyborg JK, Nguyen AP, Spindler SR: Relationship between thyroid and glucocorticoid hormone receptor occupancy, growth hormone gene transcription, and mRNA accumulation. *J Biol Chem* 259:12377, 1984.

259a. Casanova J, Copp RP, Janocko L, Samuels HH: 5′-Flanking DNA of the rat growth hormone gene mediates regulated expression by thyroid hormone. *J Biol Chem* 260:11744, 1985.

259b. Crew MD, Spindler SR: Thyroid hormone regulation of a transfected rat growth hormone promoter. *J Biol Chem* 261:5018, 1986.

260. Duesberg PH: Activated proto-onc genes: Sufficient or necessary for cancer? *Science* 228:669, 1985.

261. Land H, Parada LF, Weinberg RA: Cellular oncogenes and multistep carcinogenesis. *Science* 222:771, 1983.

262. Weinberg RA: The action of oncogenes in the cytoplasm and nucleus. *Science* 230:770, 1985.

263. Bishop JM: Cellular oncogenes and retroviruses. *Annu Rev Biochem* 52:301, 1983.

264. Marx JM: New oncogene targets? *Science* 224:272, 1984.

265. Marx JM: Oncogene linked to cell regulatory system. *Science* 226:527, 1984.

266. Der CJ, Finkel T, Cooper GM: Biological and biochemical properties of human ras^H genes mutated at codon 61. *Cell* 44:167, 1986.

267. Lacal JC, Srivastava SK, Anderson PS, Aaronson SA: Ras p21 proteins with high or low GTPase activity can efficiently transform NIH/3T3 cells. *Cell* 44:609, 1986.

268. Coussens L, Yang-Feng TL, Liao Y-C, Chen E, Gray A, McGrath J, Seeburg PH, Liberman TA, Schlessinger J, Francke U, Levinson A, Ullrich A: Tyrosine kinase receptor with extensive homology to EGF receptor shares chromosomal location with *neu* oncogene. *Science* 230:1132, 1985.

269. Newmark P: Another link in the chain. *Nature* 316:681, 1985.

270. Hunter T: Oncogenes and growth control. *Trends Biochem Sci* 10:275, 1985.

271. Waterfield MD, Scrace GT, Whittle N, Stoobant P, Johnson A, Wasteson A et al: Platelet-derived growth factor is structurally related to the putative transforming protein $p28^{sis}$ of simian sarcoma virus. *Nature* 304:35, 1983.

272. Johnson A, Betsholtz C, von der Helm K, Heldin CH, Westermark B: Platelet-derived growth factor agonist activity of a secreted form of the v-*sis* oncogene product. *Proc Natl Acad Sci USA* 82:1721, 1985.

273. Griffin JE, Wilson JD: The syndromes of androgen resistance. *N Engl J Med* 302:198, 1980.

274. Eil C, Liberman U, Rosen JF, Marx SJ: A cellular defect in hereditary vitamin D-dependent rickets type II: Defective nuclear uptake of 1,25-dihydroxyvitamin D in cultured skin fibroblasts. *N Engl J Med* 304:1586, 1981.

275. Liddle GW: The adrenals, in Williams RH (ed): *Textbook of Endocrinology.* Philadelphia, Saunders, 1981, p 249.

276. Chrousos GP, Vingerhoeds A, Brandon D, et al: Primary cortisol resistance in man: A glucocorticoid receptor-mediated disease. *J Clin Invest* 69:1262, 1982.

277. Chrousos GP, Renquist D, Brandon D, et al: Glucocorticoid hormone resistance during primate evolution: Receptor-mediated mechanisms. *Proc Natl Acad Sci USA* 79:2036, 1982.

278. Brown MS, Goldstein JL: Lowering plasma cholesterol by raising LDL receptors. *N Engl J Med* 305:515, 1981.

279. Aguilera G, Catt KJ: Regulation of vascular angiotensin receptors in the rat during altered sodium intake. *Circ Res* 49:751, 1981.

280. Wisgerhof M, Brown RD: Increased adrenal sensitivity to angiotensin II in low-renin hypertension. *J Clin Invest* 61:1456, 1978.

281. van Obberghen E, Kahn CR: Autoantibodies to insulin receptors. *Mol Cell Endocrinol* 22:277, 1981.

282. Fraser CM, Venter JC, Kaliner M: Autonomic abnormalities and autoantibodies to beta-adrenergic receptors. *N Engl J Med* 305:1165, 1981.

283. Drezner MK, Warner MB: Altered activity of the nucleotide regulatory site in the parathyroid hormone-sensitive adenylate cyclase from renal cortex of a patient with pseudohypoparathyroidism. *J Clin Invest* 62:1222, 1978.

284. Farfel Z, Brothers VM, Brickman AS, Conte F, Neer R, Bourne HR: Pseudohypoparathyroidism: Inheritance of deficient receptor-cyclase coupling activity. *Proc Natl Acad Sci USA* 78:3098, 1981.

285. Wolsdorf JI, Rosenfield RL, Fang VS, Kobayashi R, Razdan AK, Kim MH: Partial gonadotropin resistance in pseudohypoparathyroidism. *Acta Endocrinol* 88:321, 1978.

286. Spiegel AM, Levine MA, Marx SJ, Aurbach GD: Pseudohypoparathyroidism: The molecular basis for hormone resistance—a retrospective. *N Engl J Med* 307:679, 1982.

287. Hirata F, del Carmine R, Nelson CA, et al: Presence of autoantibody for phospholipase inhibitory protein, lipomodulin, in patients with rheumatic diseases. *Proc Natl Acad Sci USA* 78:3190, 1981.

288. Davies TF, Gomez-Pan A, Watson MJ, Mountjoy CQ, Hanker JP, Besser GM, Hall R: Reduced "gonadotropin response to releasing hormone" after chronic administration to important men. *Clin Endocrinol* 6:213, 1977.

289. Hanker JP, Bohnet HG, Muhlenstedt D, Nowack C, Schneider HPG: Gonadotropin release during chronic administration of D-Ser(TBU)[6] LH-RH-EA in functional amenorrhoea. *Acta Endocrinol* 89:625, 1978.

290. Sheehan KL, Casper RF, Yen SSC: Induction of luteolysis by luteinizing hormone-releasing factor (LRF) agonist: Sensitivity, reproducibility, and reversibility. *Fertil Steril* 37:209, 1982.

291. Belanger A, Labrie F, Lemay A, Caron S, Raynaud JP: Inhibitory effects of a single intranasal administration of $(TBU)^6$,des-[gly-NH_2^{10}]LHRH ethylamide, a potent LHRH agonist, on serum steroid levels in normal adult men. *J Steroid Biochem* 13:123, 1979.

292. Sundaram K, Connell KG, Bardin CW, Samojlik E, Schally AV: Inhibition of pituitary-testicular function with [d-Trp^6] luteinizing hormone-releasing hormone in rhesus monkeys. *Endocrinology* 110:1308, 1982.

293. Comite F, Cutler GB, Rivier J, Vale WW, Loriaux DL, Crowley WF: Short-term treatment of idiopathic precocious puberty with a long-acting analogue of luteinizing hormone-releasing hormone. *N Engl J Med* 305:1546, 1981.

294. Klijn JGM, DeJong FH: Treatment with a luteinizing-hormone-releasing-hormone analogue (Buserelin) in premenopausal patients with metastatic breast cancer. *Lancet* 1:1213, 1982.

295. Warner B, Worgul TJ, Diago L-D, et al: Effect of very high dose d-Leu^6-GnRH proethylamide on the hypothalamic-pituitary-testicular axis as treatment of prostatic cancer. *J Clin Invest* 71:1842, 1983.

296. Meldrum DR, Chang RJ, Lu J, Vale W, Rivier J, Judd HL: "Medical oophorectomy" using a long-acting GnRH agonist—a possible new approach to the treatment of endometriosis. *J Clin Endocrinol Metab* 54:1081, 1982.

297. Denef C, Andries M: Evidence for paracrine interaction between gonadotrophs and lactotrophs in pituitary cell aggregates. *Endocrinology* 112:813, 1983.

298. Wildt L, Hausler A, Marshall G, Hutchison JS, Plant TM, Belchetz PE, Knobil E: Frequency and amplitude of gonadotropin-releasing hormone stimulation and gonadotropin secretion in the rhesus monkey. *Endocrinology* 109:376, 1981.

299. Lyendecker G, Wildt L, Hansmann M: Pregnancies following chronic intermittent (pulsatile) administration of GnRH by means of a portable pump (Zyklomat)—a new approach to the treatment of infertility in hypothalamic amenorrhoea. *J Clin Endocrinol Metab* 51:1214, 1980.

300. Hoffman AR, Crowley WF: Induction of puberty in men by long-term pulsatile administration of low-dose gonadotropin-releasing hormone. *N Engl J Med* 307:1237, 1982.

6

Hormone Assays

Judith L. Vaitukaitis

Over the past several years, clinical endocrinology has moved from the form of an "art" toward applied biochemistry, physiology, and pharmacology with development of more sophisticated, sensitive, and specific measuring techniques. That advance was made possible by the isolation and subsequent biologic and biochemical characterization of a variety of highly purified polypeptide hormones, steroids, vitamins, and small polypeptide or amino acid derivatives classified as hormones, as well as methods of radiolabeling hormones to high specific activities. Many clinical endocrinologic states are recognized or at least suspected in settings in which too much or too little of a normally secreted hormone is present. Alternatively, either biologically inactive hormone or altered receptor function may be responsible for the clinical syndrome. The capacity to detect low levels of hormones in small volumes of biologic fluids has helped to simplify diagnostic evaluation.

Initially, relatively crude and cumbersome bioassays were developed to quantitate hormones present in biologic tissues and fluids. With the advent of more sensitive radioimmunoassay and radioreceptor techniques, more rapid and cost-effective methods became available, and they essentially have become the backbone of clinical endocrinology. In spite of their shortcomings, classic bioassays are essential for complete characterization of a hormone, especially when one suspects a dissociation between the hormone's biologic and immunologic activities. Fortunately, hormone concentrations determined by radioimmunoassay usually correlate well with those determined biologically. Consequently, hormone concentrations determined by radioimmunoassay provide an approximation of circulating biologically active hormone levels. The latter association is fortuitous, since the biologic and immunologic activities usually reflect different properties and even different segments of the hormone molecule.

In addition to simply permitting development of sensitive techniques for measuring hormone concentrations, highly purified hormone preparations have been invaluable probes for better understanding of their cellular action. With those advances, it has become apparent that clinical disorders may result not only from abnormal secretion but also from altered action of hormones resulting from qualitative or quantitative aberrations of specific hormone receptors, as well as altered intracellular biochemical mechanisms mediating hormone action. In this chapter, the general principles and requirements for valid bioassays, radioimmunoassays, and radioreceptor assays will be presented. It should become apparent that most tests are complex, requiring sophisticated instrumentation and expertise. Additionally, the time required for assay completion varies considerably with the hormone measured, so that "stat" results are rarely available. Nothing can be more frustrating to a laboratory director than a request for a serum parathormone level 10 min after the sample was delivered to the laboratory. The time required for assay completion ranges from a few hours to several days, depending on the assay technique and the nature of the hormone assayed.

BIOASSAYS

Results from hormone assays performed in different laboratories must be reported in terms of a common hormone standard. Bioassay results are usually reported in terms of units of an *international standard* distributed by the World Health Organization. Results may also be reported in terms of units of a *reference preparation* distributed by agencies to laboratories over a more restricted geographic area. Conversion factors for units of reference preparations and units of established international standards should be provided with assay results. Although polypeptide hormones are highly purified, small but significant contamination of these preparations exists and usually makes it impossible to report bioassay or other assay results in terms of mass of hormone. Most polypeptide hormone bioassay and radioimmunoassay determinations are reported in terms of previously established units set by the World Health Organization; but since steroid and thyroid hormones are available in chemically pure form, assay results for these are usually reported in terms of mass of hormone. Since the reagents and techniques differ slightly but significantly among laboratories, each laboratory must determine its own normal range of hormone concentrations for patient samples collected under standardized conditions and assayed with well-characterized reagents or bioassay models.

In Vivo Assays

Bioassays may be carried out in vivo or in vitro using graduated doses of an appropriate reference preparation or standard, against which one interpolates the physiologic effect induced by the hormone contained in an unknown sample. In general, a relatively specific end point is monitored in response to hormonal stimulation. For example, changes in target-organ weight in response to increasing doses of an unknown and a standard hormone preparation are compared for similarity of response. The dose-response lines of reference preparation and unknown must be parallel for valid assay results. The ventral prostate weight assay is a good example of an in vivo bioassay for luteinizing hormone (LH) or human chorionic gonadotropin (hCG) bioactivity. LH, a pituitary hormone, and hCG, a placental hormone, have indistinguishable biologic activities. In that assay, increasing amounts of urinary extracts are injected subcutaneously in divided doses into hypophysectomized, immature male rats for several consecutive days and the change in weight of the ventral prostate determined at the end of that time. Similarly, graduated doses of a reference preparation containing a known biologic specific activity for LH or hCG are injected and the resulting change in ventral prostate weight compared with that for the unknown. This bioassay is valid for measuring the biologic activity of LH or hCG because these hormones stimulate the rat's Leydig cells to synthesize and secrete testosterone, which in turn induces the animal's ventral prostate gland to increase in size through a series of biochemical steps. The increase in ventral prostate weight is proportional to the amount of testosterone secreted by the LH- or hCG-stimulated testis. Hypophysectomized animals are used to prevent testosterone synthesis and secretion in response to the animal's endogenous luteinizing hormone. This is one of the classic bioassays still used to characterize LH and hCG preparations. It was initially described by

Greep et al. more than 40 years ago and subsequently modified.[1,2]

Since the slopes of the dose-response line may vary considerably from bioassay to bioassay, even for the same hormone preparation, statistical analysis for parallelism between the slopes and the homogeneity of variance of the dose-response lines for the assay standard or reference preparation and the unknown is imperative for each assay. Ideally, at least three widely separated points along the dose-response range with three to five animals per point should be assayed for both standard and unknown. Only if parallelism and homogeneity of variance exist between standard and unknown can a valid estimate be made of the biologic potency of the unknown and its confidence limits. If parallelism does not exist, the potency of the unknown is invalid. It should be readily apparent that there is no place for single-point determinations in bioassays of any type.

The number of in vivo bioassays developed over the years is legion. Some have been crude, insensitive, and nonspecific—for example, insulin-induced convulsions in mice. Other bioassays are considerably more specific and sensitive and are currently used to characterize purified hormone preparations.

In Vitro Assays

Most in vivo bioassays require relatively large volumes of plasma, urine, or tissue extracts containing sufficient quantities of hormone to induce a significant biologic effect. Consequently, these techniques, although initially valuable in characterizing a variety of hormone preparations, are not practical for routine clinical application. Over the past several years, a variety of in vitro bioassays have been developed. The in vitro bioassays not only are specific but also require considerably smaller volumes of tissue extracts and biologic fluids, reflecting their greater sensitivity. Unfortunately, these assays require a level of expertise not available in most laboratories responsible for routine clinical tests.

In general, graduated doses of hormone serve as a reference preparation so that the response induced by an unknown sample can be interpolated relative to the assay standard. Graduated doses or volumes of unknown samples are studied in the same assay system, and response variables of both unknown and standard or reference preparation are analyzed for parallelism and homogeneity of variance to validate the appropriateness of the standard used for dose interpolation. This analysis is a requisite for validation of in vivo or in vitro hormone assays of any type.

The Leydig, or interstitial, cell assay is an example of an in vitro bioassay. As a result of LH or hCG stimulation, Leydig cells synthesize and secrete testosterone in a dose-dependent relationship. Leydig cells may be separated from the seminiferous tubules with established techniques.[3] The Leydig cells are divided equally among culture plates and stimulated with graduated concentrations of reference LH or hCG preparations and varying volumes of unknown sample. Testosterone is secreted into the culture medium and its concentration determined by specific radioimmunoassay.

A variety of end points for in vitro bioassays may be used, including changes in concentrations of steroids, enzymes, or cyclic nucleotides. In general, the in vitro bioassays are more sensitive than their in vivo counterparts, and consequently smaller volumes of serum, tissue, or urinary extracts are required. However, care must be taken in interpretation of in vitro bioassay results, since a hormone may be biologically active in that system yet exert little if any biologic effect in vivo. That disparity reflects the fact that not only must a hormone bind to its specific cell surface receptors and initiate biochemical changes, but it must also be transported to that cell's surface receptors in sufficiently high concentrations to ensure that sufficient numbers of receptors will be occupied to mediate its effects. In some cases, clearance of a hormone or related substance may be markedly altered because of seemingly minor modifications of that hormone's structure.

In order for a hormone to interact with a receptor it must be biologically active, as reflected by its assuming an appropriate conformation so that it can interact with its specific receptor with high affinity or binding strength. However, a hormone may be biologically active in vitro but not elicit significant biologic activity in vivo because of altered metabolic clearance secondary to its altered structure. When the biologic activity of desialylated hCG is studied in vivo and in vitro, a marked disparity between these activities is observed.[4–7] After the hCG molecule has had the sialic acid removed (desialylation), it exerts a biologic effect as great as, if not greater than, its native fully sialylated molecule in vitro.[6] On the other hand, when it is examined in vivo, little if any biologic activity is observed, reflecting the degree of desialylation of the hCG molecule. The disparity results because the plasma half-life of desialylated hCG is considerably shorter than that of its intact counterpart.[5] Consequently, sufficiently high concentrations of desialylated hCG do not perfuse its target cells to initiate a significant biologic effect.

In vitro bioassays are usually more sensitive than in vivo bioassays used to assay the same hormone. In fact, some in vitro bioassays have greater sensitivity than radioimmunoassays used to determine the concentration of hormone. Those in vitro bioassays which monitor biochemical end points other than specific receptor binding or adenyl cyclase activation usually have at least a 10- to 1000-fold greater sensitivity than that for sensitive radioimmunoassay techniques. In vitro bioassays currently do not constitute a routine tool for patient evaluation except in those unusual cases in which a dissociation between the biologic and immunologic activities of a hormone is suspected.

Recently, it has been recognized that circulating antibodies to some receptors may induce a biologic effect similar to that of the parent hormone when the circulating immunoglobulin binds to the plasma membrane receptor. For example, thyroid stimulating immunoglobulin may bind to the TSH (thyroid-stimulating hormone) receptor, with overstimulation of the thyroid resulting in Graves' disease.[7] Additionally, some patients with abnormal thyroid function may have circulating TSH receptor antibody which blocks endogenous TSH stimulation of its target cells.

Cytochemical Assays

A variant of the in vitro test is the cytochemical bioassay. This type of assay is usually more sensitive than radioimmunoassay but considerably more cumbersome and expensive. Cytochemical bioassay responses are quantitated from histologic sections with a special device, a microdensitometer. Histologic sections are prepared from specific hormone target tissues or cells previously exposed to graduated concentrations of standard hormone and unknowns. The densitometer is used to scan an area 250 to 300 nm in diameter to quantitate the chromogenic reaction resulting from changes in redox state induced by hormone stimulation. Histologic stains sensitive to those changes are used for quantitation.

The first cytochemical bioassay was developed for adrenocorticotropin (ACTH), using adrenal target tissue.[8] Other available bioassays for ACTH either are too insensitive or require large plasma volumes. Consequently, the redox cytochemical assay is a valuable tool for assessing normal and altered ACTH physiology of the hypothalamic-pituitary-adrenal axis. A cytochemical assay for luteinizing hormone has been developed, but considerable difficulty has arisen because of marked interassay variation and changing assay sensitivity, possibly reflecting the well-known biologic variation observed among animals.[9] Sensitive, specific cytochemical assays have been developed for parathormone, antidiuretic hormone, and thyrotropin.[10,11] With further sophistication of equipment to enhance the number of samples studied on a single assay, this technique may become more widely applicable. It is particularly attractive because no radiolabeled substances are required. Currently, cytochemical assays are not very practical for routine clinical purposes and serve primarily as sensitive research tools.

Table 6-1 lists a variety of in vivo or in vitro bioassays currently used to characterize polypeptide hormones. Unfortunately, no specific, sensitive bioassays have yet been developed for several hormones.

LIGAND ASSAYS

Radioimmunoassay

Radioimmunoassay is probably the most extensively applied technique currently used to quantitate hormones and a variety of other substances in biologic fluids. As the term suggests, radioimmunoassay is an immunologic technique using radiolabeled hormone or ligand and antibody. More than two decades ago, Berson and Yalow described the insulin radioimmunoassay.[26] The radioimmunoassay technique evolved from their observation that ^{131}I-labeled insulin bound to a circulating protein, subsequently shown to be a globulin, in the peripheral blood of insulin-treated diabetic patients. The importance of their observations and subsequent development of an insulin radioimmunoassay is underscored by the awarding of the Nobel Prize to Drs. Yalow and Berson for their contributions. Shortly after their initial observations, several other hormone assays were developed and reported from other laboratories. These assays used either antibody or serum proteins that bound specific hormones or ligand and radiolabeled hormone to compete with standard hormone or hormone in biologic fluids.

Thermodynamically, the interaction of antigen and antibody may be considered a pseudo-first-order reaction, presented schematically as follows:

$$\mathrm{Ag} + \mathrm{Ab} \underset{k_d}{\overset{k_a}{\rightleftharpoons}} \mathrm{AgAb}$$

$$^{*}\mathrm{Ag} + \mathrm{Ab} \underset{k_d}{\overset{k_a}{\rightleftharpoons}} {}^{*}\mathrm{AgAb}$$

where Ag = antigen or hormone
Ab = antibody to the antigen or hormone
*Ag = radiolabeled antigen or hormone
k_a = association rate constant
k_d = dissociation rate constant

The antigen-antibody reaction is reversible. The rate of dissociation of the antigen-antibody complex is considerably slower than its rate of association. The observed amount of hormone bound to antibody is

Table 6-1. In Vivo and in Vitro Bioassays

Hormone	Assay	End point	Reference
ACTH	In vivo—hypophysectomized rat	Adrenal ascorbic acid depletion in response to ACTH stimulation	12
ADH	In vivo—fasted and water-loaded rats	Decrease in urine flow rate or increase in urine specific gravity	13–16
Cholecystokinin	In vitro—rabbit gallbladder strips	CCK-induced contraction of strips	17
FSH	In vivo—immature female rats	FSH-induced ovarian weight increase	18
Growth hormone	In vivo—hypophysectomized rats	Increase in width of uncalcified epiphyseal cartilage of tibia	19
LH/hCG	In vivo—21-day-old hypophysectomized rats	LH-hCG–induced weight gain of ventral prostate	1,2
LH/hCG	In vitro—isolated Leydig cells	Hormone-induced increased synthesis and secretion of testosterone into culture medium	6
Parathormone	In vitro—rat renal cortex	cAMP generation in response to parathormone stimulation	20
Prolactin	In vitro—mouse mammary explants	Lactoseamine synthetase activity *or* phosphoprotein synthesis	21 22
Renin	In vitro—renin activity	Generation of angiotensin I from renin substrate	23
Somatomedin	In vitro—pelvic rudiments of 11-day-old chick embryo	$[^{35}S]$Sulfate incorporation	24
TSH	1. In vivo—intact mouse pretreated with ^{131}I and thyroxine	1. TSH-induced thyroidal release of ^{131}I into blood	25
	2. In vitro—cytochemical monitoring of guinea pig thyroid segments	2. Lysosomal naphthylamidase activity	11

the resultant of the rates of association and dissociation.

Since a fixed concentration of antibody and radiolabeled hormone is added to each assay tube, the number of counts bound to the antibody will be a function of the concentration of unlabeled hormone in a standard or an unknown sample; the higher the concentration of unlabeled hormone, the fewer the number of counts bound to the fixed concentration of antibody. Figure 6-1 depicts several methods commonly used for graphing data for radioimmunoassays. The top graph is a dose-response line plotted on a log-logit scale with number of counts bound to antibody normalized to maximum number of counts bound, B_0, when only antibody and labeled hormone (no unlabeled hormone) are incubated. Nonspecific counts, which reflect physically trapped hormone in the assay tube, are subtracted from both total and bound counts. The resulting log-logit plot is usually a straight line and facilitates visual dose interpolation of unknown samples. A variety of techniques have been used to transform data so that straight lines result, facilitating visual dose interpolation of unknowns. Most radioimmunoassay results are computerized, obviating the tedious, time-consuming effort to calculate assay results manually.

With availability of highly purified hormones, sensitive radioimmunoassays have been developed for accurately measuring low physiologic circulating levels of hormone, requiring relatively small volumes of biologic fluids. The requisites for sensitive radioimmunoassays include:

1. A highly purified hormone radioactively labeled to sufficiently high specific activity so that only trace amounts of the labeled hormone are added to each assay tube.
2. Immunoreactivity of the labeled hormone that is not markedly altered by reagents used in the radiolabeling reaction.
3. An antibody of sufficiently high sensitivity (affinity) and specificity to measure low physiologic levels of the desired hormone.
4. An appropriate reference preparation against which

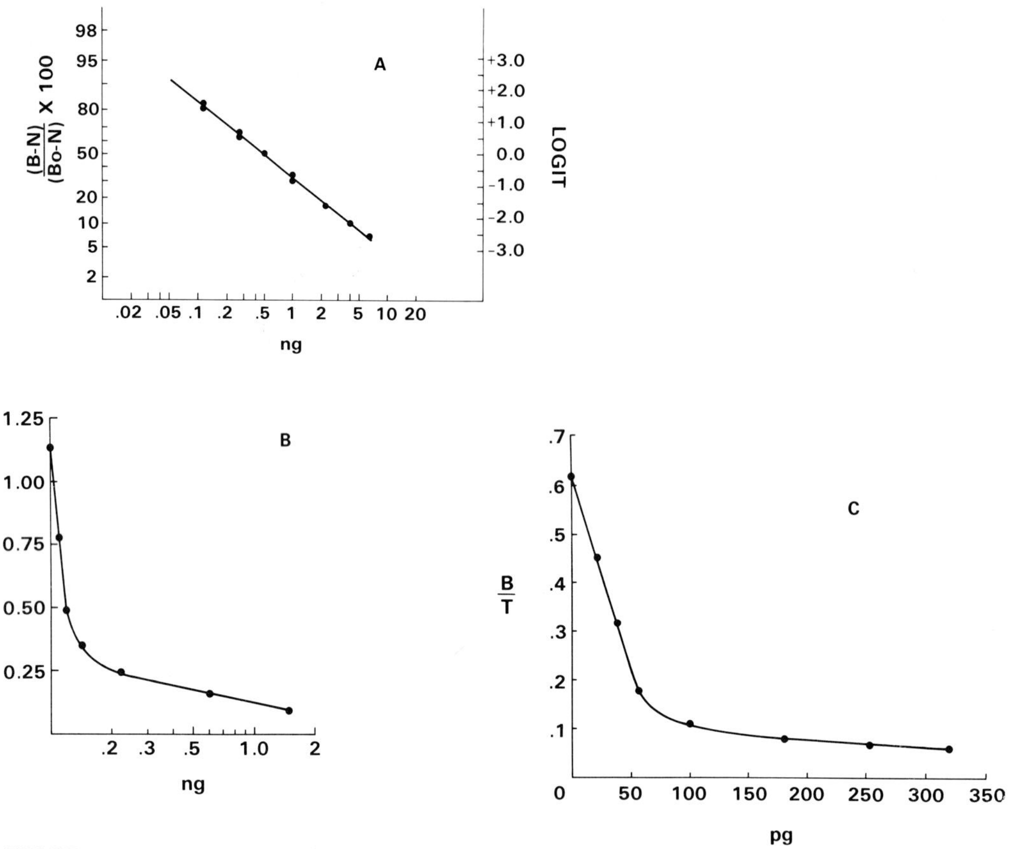

FIGURE 6-1 Dose-response lines for three different hormone assays depicted with three commonly used methods. Panel *A* depicts the log-logit transformation of data; panel *B* depicts bound/free versus log dose of hormone concentration; panel C depicts a dose-response line for a steroid hormone assay plotted as B/T versus dose of hormone. B, counts bound; F, free counts; T, total counts; N, nonspecific counts; B_0, maximum number of counts bound when only antibody and labeled hormone are incubated.

concentrations of unknown samples may be dose-interpolated. Both reference preparation and hormone must interact similarly with an antibody and exhibit parallel dose-response lines.

In a validated radioimmunoassay system, the concentration of labeled hormone and antibody is fixed. Consequently, as the concentration of unlabeled hormone increases, the probability of labeled hormone binding to antibody decreases, resulting in an inverse relationship between the number of labeled hormone molecules bound to antibody and the concentration of unlabeled hormone in the reaction mixture.

Several assumptions for interaction of antigen and antibody are made:

1. The hormone present is homogeneous and interacts with the antibody with similar affinity whether or not the antigen is radiolabeled.
2. The antibody is present in a homogeneous form, and one antibody molecule interacts with a single molecule of hormone.
3. The two molecular species, hormone and antibody, react until they reach equilibrium.
4. An effective means of separating hormone-bound antibody and free hormone is used, and that separation technique does not disturb the initial equilibrium attained between hormone and antibody.

The four points listed above are idealized, since both hormone and antibody are usually present in heterogeneous forms. Circulating hormone may be either partially metabolized or secreted in altered forms. Polyclonal antibody, reflecting a population of immunoglobulin molecules with varying specificities and sensitivities, may "recognize" many of these heterogeneous circulating hormone forms and bind with them in the assay. The radioimmunoassay technique measures concentrations of hormone which are usually unmeasurable by most in vivo bioassays. *Sensitivity*, or *least detectable dose*, is defined as that concentration of hormone which induces a significant change in percent of binding of radioactively labeled hormone to antibody when compared with a blank sample. The sensitivity of the assay is a function of the hormone's affinity for its specific antibody.

Iodination

Perhaps the most commonly used technique for iodinating proteins is a modification of the method initially reported by Greenwood, Hunter, and Glover.[27] Their chemical technique utilized the oxidizing agent chloramine T, which transforms $Na^{125}I$ to free iodide, which is then incorporated primarily by tyrosyl residues. Histidyl residues may also be iodinated by this technique. For maximum immunoreactivity, only one atom of ^{131}I or ^{125}I should be incorporated per molecule of hormone, since iodination to a greater extent usually results in decreased immunoreactivity and bioactivity, reflecting chemical damage to the hormone.[27]

Other iodination methods are currently used as well. Perhaps the second most popular technique is an enzymatic technique using lactoperoxidase.[28,29] Lactoperoxidase, catalyzed by hydrogen peroxide added directly to the reaction mixture, transforms $Na^{125}I$ to free iodide for selective incorporation of those atoms into tyrosyl residues. Since hydrogen peroxide is a strong oxidizing reagent, exposure of the hormone to high concentrations of that reagent may lead to chemical damage, and consequently, the hydrogen peroxide is usually added in two or three small aliquots and is quickly consumed within the reaction. Lactoperoxidase may also be catalyzed by activation of glucose oxidase. Another newer, but less popular, iodination method is that developed by Bolton and Hunter.[30] An intermediate derivative, 3-(*p*-hydroxyphenyl)propionic acid *N*-hydroxysuccinimide ester, is iodinated by the chloramine T reaction and then subsequently condensed with amino groups on the polypeptide hormone. This technique is somewhat cumbersome and has not yet gained widespread use.

Currently $Na^{125}I$ rather than $Na^{131}I$ is used because of its significantly longer half-life—59 vs. 6 days. However, care must be taken with assays using ^{125}I, since the specific gamma constant is considerably lower for ^{125}I than for ^{131}I. Differential quenching of ^{125}I may be observed with glass reaction tubes of variable thickness or lead content. Plastic reaction tubes are preferred. Steroid hormones and vitamin D are labeled with tritium, since higher specific activities are attained than by labeling with ^{14}C. Those small polypeptides or other molecules not containing tyrosyl or histidyl residues may be modified so that a tyrosyl residue is substituted within the polypeptide or steroid. A position within the molecule is selected so that the conformation of the native substance is not markedly altered. The modified molecule may then be iodinated.

Generation of Antisera

Antibodies selected for clinical assays belong to the class of immunoglobulins and are predominantly gamma globulins (IgG). The IgG molecule comprises four polypeptide chains—two heavy and two light chains symmetrically arranged and covalently bound by disulfide bonds. The molecule is schematically depicted in Fig. 6-2. The interaction of antigen or ligand with antibody may be considered a "lock and key" arrangement. The shape of the antibody combining site is complementary to that of the antigen. The antigen-antibody interaction is a combination of electrostatic, hydrogen-bonding, and van der Waals' interactions.[31,32] The amino acid sequence of the binding portion of the IgG molecule determines the "shape" of the binding site and, consequently, the affinity and specificity of the combining site for the desired antigen.[33]

For hormone assays, highly purified hormone is injected into laboratory animals to induce synthesis of immunoglobulin with sufficiently high specificity and sensitivity to be used in the radioimmunoassay. In general, immunogens having a molecular mass of less than 1000 daltons are not sufficiently immunogenic and consequently must be conjugated to a carrier molecule in order to be competent immunogens. An immunogen is a substance capable of inducing formation of antibody. Smaller molecules, or

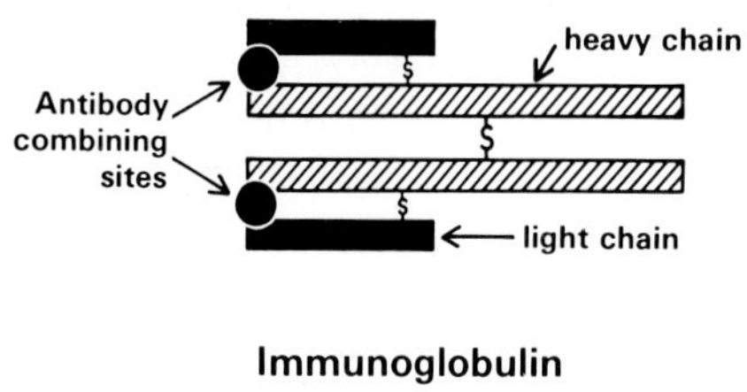

FIGURE 6-2 Schematic representation of a gamma globulin or antibody molecule. The hormone recognition sites contain the variable amino acid regions of the light and heavy immunoglobulin chains. The light chains are covalently linked to the heavy chains through a disulfide bond, schematically depicted as ∽ . A single disulfide bond exists between the two heavy chains. Recent data suggest that the immunoglobulin molecule assumes a Y conformation, with the antibody combining sites occupying the top portions of the Y.

haptens, must be conjugated to substances such as albumin, thyroglobulin, or hemocyanin to induce antibody formation. In general, the immunologic response is better for those carrier proteins which are intrinsically highly immunogenic. Consequently, substances such as albumin, thyroglobulin, and hemocyanin are good carrier proteins—in contrast to polylysine and other synthetic polyamino acids—for generating specific antibody to conjugated haptens. In general, steroids and the thyroid hormones triiodothyronine and thyroxine, as well as various forms of vitamin D, need to be conjugated to a carrier protein. Much care is taken to conjugate the steroid or other hapten through that part of the molecule which is least likely to alter its unique stereospecificity. For example, 17β-estradiol antibody is best generated by conjugating its 6-keto analogue covalently to albumin. Consequently, the 3- and 17-hydroxyl groups, as well as the A ring of that steroid, are undisturbed. The latter is especially important, since it is these structures that lend specificity to that particular estrogen.

A variety of immunization techniques have been developed over the years, and these techniques are essentially derivatives of the technique initially described by Freund.[34] The emulsion containing the hormone or immunogen, appropriate oils, and heat-killed tubercle bacilli is injected either intradermally or subcutaneously. With the advent of highly purified hormones and other derivatives, immunization techniques using small amounts of immunogen have been developed.[35] There is good experimental evidence supporting development of specific high-affinity antibodies with small doses of immunogen.[36] Antibody-forming cells with the highest affinity for the immunogen are more likely to be induced to form specific antibody when low doses of immunogen are used. Conversely, with higher doses of immunogen, there is a greater likelihood of developing lower-affinity antibody. With very high doses of immunogen, a phenomenon of tolerance may be induced in the immunized animal, resulting in no detectable circulating antibody or very low titers of that antibody.[37,38] With initial immunization, a minimum of 6 weeks is usually needed for significant antibody titers to appear. The affinity of the antibody continues to increase and usually peaks between 8 and 12 weeks after the initial immunization.[35,39] Empirically, rechallenge or boosting results in the best anamnestic responses when the animal is rechallenged at a time when its circulating antibody titer is falling. When the animal is rechallenged with one-half to one-quarter of the initial immunizing dose of hormone, a significant rise in circulating antibody titer is observed within a few days of reimmunization. The animal should be reimmunized over the same anatomic areas used for the initial immunization. Moreover, heat-killed tubercle bacillus is not needed for the anamnestic response and, in fact, may increase the likelihood of morbidity and mortality in the animal.

For generation of specific antibody, one selects an animal species that is readily available and not too expensive and in which there is significant structural difference between endogenous hormone and that with which it is to be immunized. For example, although growth hormones from different species have the same biologic activities, there are significant amino acid substitutions among growth hormones of different species. It is that primary structural difference and a variety of other poorly characterized factors that render a hormone immunogenic in another animal species. In some cases there may be relatively minor amino acid substitutions, consequently the animal species in which to generate hormone must be carefully selected. For example, insulin structure is quite similar in humans, rabbit, and sheep, but a larger structural difference exists between human and guinea pig insulin. Consequently, the guinea pig is the animal species most successfully used to generate specific insulin antibody.[40]

When an antiserum is generated with an in vivo immunization procedure, a population of immunoglobulin molecules with differing affinities and specificities is generated. In contrast, monoclonal antibody represents a single clone of immunoglobulin molecules with a single affinity and specificity for one antigenic site of a hormonal molecule. Typically, the monoclonal antibody is isolated in vitro after an animal, usually a mouse, has been immunized and antibody-producing cells from that animal's spleen or lymph nodes have been fused with a non-immunoglobulin-secreting myeloma cell line. Clones are selected from the hybridomas on the basis of their specificity and affinity for the desired antigen.[41] For routine clinical assays, a monoclonal antibody may not measure altered forms of circulating hormone if the antigenic site recognized by that monoclonal antibody has been altered during secretion or metabolism. However, that shortcoming can be theoretically overcome by mixing several monoclonal antibodies with different specificities, thus creating a "defined" polyclonal antibody.

Assay Sensitivity

After the antibody is harvested, studies are designed to assess the antiserum's sensitivity and specificity. The concentration of antibody within an antiserum is initially determined by checking, at serial dilutions, the binding of the antiserum to the radiolabeled hormone used for immunization. This technique is referred to as *titering*. Thus *titer* refers to the concentration of antibody molecules in serum. After the concentration of antibody which binds 30 to 40 percent of radiolabeled hormone at equilibrium is determined, the sensitivity and specificity of the antibody are ascertained. The development and characterization of a specific hCG or insulin assay for clinical use are extensively detailed elsewhere and may serve as guidelines to development of other specific radioimmunoassays.[40,42]

In reality, the "antibody" harvested for use in most clinical radioimmunoassays contains a population of antibodies with varying specificities and affinities. An antiserum is selected that has a population of antibodies with sufficiently high affinity and specificity for the hormone to be measured. One can operationally select out that population of high-affinity antibody within a polyclonal antibody by using the antiserum in sufficiently high dilution so that other lower-affinity, and possibly nonspecific, populations of antibody become relatively insignificant. If one chooses to use an antiserum at a significantly different dilution from that initially used to validate an assay, one must again determine the sensitivity and specificity of the antiserum at the new concentration, since other populations of antibody may now be present in relatively higher concentrations and may not be as sensitive and specific as when the antiserum was used at higher dilutions. This is graphically depicted in Fig. 6-3, in which the dose-response line for the highly purified ligand is shifted to the right, reflecting

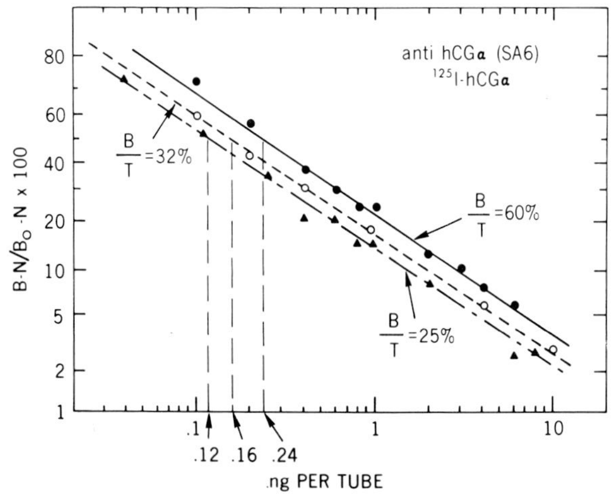

FIGURE 6-3 Dose-response lines for hCG-α assayed in a homologous hCG-α radioimmunoassay. The only variable among the three hCG-α dose-response lines is the concentration of hCG-α antibody. As the starting B/T increased from 25 to 60 percent, reflecting increased concentration of antibody, the 50 percent intercept increased from 0.12 to 0.24 ng per tube.

decreased sensitivity as the antibody concentration is increased. Since hormones circulate in relatively low concentrations ranging between 10^{-12} and 10^{-9} M, antibodies with both high affinity and high specificity must be selected. The affinity and specificity of each antibody must be empirically determined. Moreover, antisera harvested from the same animal at different times after immunization may have significantly varying affinities and specificities for the hormone to which it was immunized. In contrast, antibody secreted by selected clones has unvarying sensitivity and specificity, and theoretically can be maintained in perpetuity. Its specificity is unaltered by antibody concentration, but the assay sensitivity would decrease with higher antibody concentration.

Assay Specificity

Both the structure and the purity of a hormone used for immunization must be considered. The human glycoprotein hormones, luteinizing hormone, follicle stimulating hormone, thyroid stimulating hormone, and human chorionic gonadotropin, share a common quaternary structure of two dissimilar subunits, designated α and β.[42] The α subunits among these hormones are essentially identical in terms of their amino acid sequences. It is the β subunit that confers both immunologic and biologic specificity. Consequently, one must carefully select an antiserum generated to one of the glycoprotein hormones and carefully check whether it is sufficiently specific for measuring hormone concentrations in the presence of high levels of the other glycoprotein hormones in the same sample. In some cases, cross-reaction resulting from common antigenic determinants can be eliminated by adsorbing the antibody with the common antigen. For example, if a TSH antiserum cross-reacts with FSH and LH and that cross-reaction is due to common α subunit determinants, the antiserum can be adsorbed with free α or with hCG which contains α determinants. The adsorbed antiserum, ideally, is specific for TSH with little, if any, loss of sensitivity for that hormone.

To further complicate matters, the β subunits of hCG and LH share extensive structural homology, reflecting the indistinguishable biologic activities of these two molecules. Consequently, antibody generated to the entire LH or hCG molecule is most likely to lead to antibody which will detect either or both molecular species. Since some tumors ectopically secrete hCG and since high hCG concentrations are normally encountered during pregnancy, routine LH determination will result in spuriously high results, which should be interpreted with caution. Perhaps the best clinical clue to the predominance of hCG (not

LH) molecular species in peripheral blood is the marked disparity between circulating concentrations of LH and FSH determined on the same specimen.

Other technical problems may arise if a hormone preparation used to immunize an animal is cross contaminated with another hormone. Even with highly purified human pituitary hormone preparations, a small but significant amount of other pituitary hormones is present. Similar concerns are raised for hormones purified from the pancreas and gastrointestinal tract. Obviously, the immunized animal can then generate antibody to any of the molecular species injected, including the cross-contaminating hormone. Consequently, one must know the source of hormone, since other hormones may be copurified along with the desired hormone. Ideally, one should check structural similarity between hormones, since that may form the basis for cross reactivity between hormones for some antisera.

If only a relatively crude hormonal preparation is available for immunization, then a hybridoma approach is preferable, since one can select antibody-producing clones which are appropriately sensitive and specific for assay requirements.

Since there is extensive structural homology between the various steroids, between triiodothyronine and thyroxine as well as some of their metabolites, and between the various forms of vitamin D, it may not always be possible to generate a sufficiently specific antiserum to measure these hormones and their metabolites directly without initial extraction and separation techniques.

Effect of Serum Proteins

Several hormones circulate bound to specific carrier proteins or loosely bound to albumin. To prevent contamination of the radioimmunoassay reaction mixture with serum binding proteins, an initial solvent extraction usually must be carried out. If the antibody to the hormone is not sufficiently specific, an initial isolation step must be carried out as well. In some cases differential solvent extraction may suffice, but in others chromatographic separation is needed. Thin-layer chromatography, high-pressure liquid chromatography (HPLC), and LH-20 Sephadex column chromatography are among the processes more commonly used to separate structurally related steroids, biogenic amines, and small polypeptides. Since the larger polypeptide hormones do not circulate bound to carrier protein, an initial extraction step is not needed and an aliquot of the serum sample may be added directly to the test tube. However, circulating proteases may induce an artifactually low concentration of some polypeptide hormones. The degraded hormone may not react with antibody if its structure is significantly altered. One may need to add enzyme inhibitors to a sample to counteract the effect of proteases. Trasylol and benzamidine are among the protease inhibitors added to test tubes in which samples are collected for ACTH, glucagon, and other hormones likely to undergo rapid proteolytic degradation. In some cases, antioxidants or other inhibitors of proteolysis are added to biologic samples to prevent degradation of the substance to be measured.

Some polypeptide hormone assays are affected by nonspecific serum protein effects. These nonspecific protein effects can be overcome by adding blank serum to assay tubes not containing serum, so that all assay tubes contain comparable concentrations of interfering serum protein. Each antiserum must be empirically screened for nonspecific protein interference of the antigen-antibody reaction.

Separation of Bound and Free Hormone

Techniques for separating antibody-bound hormone and free hormone vary. Generally, polypeptide hormone assays use a *second antibody technique.* Since the initial hormone-antibody complex is soluble, simple centrifugation will not separate the two molecular species. A second antibody, generated to the IgG of the animal species in which the first antibody was generated, is added after equilibrium has been attained between the hormone and first antibody. Since the second antibody will now bind to the first antigen-antibody complex, an insoluble molecular species is created, and bound and free hormone can be separated by simple centrifugation, with bound hormone being precipitated. For example, if a gastrin antibody is generated in rabbits, a second antibody to rabbit IgG would be generated in another animal species such as horse, sheep, or goat. The horse antirabbit globulin would be added to the test tube after the reaction mixture containing ^{125}I-labeled gastrin and rabbit antigastrin serum has attained equilibrium. The time required for the second antibody reaction to attain equilibrium is a function of the concentration of carrier-rabbit serum in the reaction mixture. For example, if the first gastrin antibody is raised in rabbit, additional carrier-rabbit serum or globulin may be added to the test tube. If 2 percent of the volume in the tube is carrier-rabbit serum, a relatively large volume of second antibody (0.05 to 0.2 ml) will be required to precipitate the rabbit IgG present. Since the time required to attain equilibrium follows the first law of mass action, a relatively short time (a few hours) will be needed to attain equilibrium. That time is determined empirically initially, and the minimal optimal volume of second antibody needed is ascertained for each batch of second antibody harvested or purchased from a commercial source. Lower concentrations of carrier serum may be added to the assay tubes, and consequently a smaller volume of second antibody will be needed, but the time required for the second antibody reaction to attain equilibrium becomes greater. For separation of steroids, small polypeptides, and vitamin D, dextran-coated charcoal will adsorb free ligand. Consequently, antibody-bound hormone will be present in the supernatant of the reaction tube.

Other separation techniques may be used as well, including antibody coating on the inner surface of the test tubes so that bound and free hormone are separated by simple decanting of the supernatant which contains free hormone. Magnetic field separation of free and bound hormone with ferric oxide conjugated to the first antibody may also be used; no centrifugation step is required, since the antibody-bound hormone is pelleted in a magnetic field and free hormone in the supernatant can simply be decanted. The techniques presented here usually result in shorter incubation times and quicker assay results.

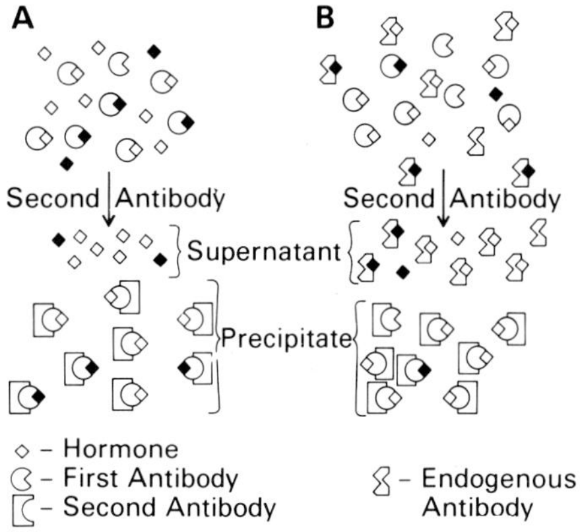

FIGURE 6-4 Schematic representation of a typical double-antibody radioimmunoassay reaction in panel *A*. In panel *B*, circulating endogenous antibody to the hormone is present, along with that added as a known reagent. The endogenous antibody will result in spurious hormone concentrations determined by the double-antibody technique, since some hormone-antibody complexes will not be precipitated by the second antibody directed to rabbit and not human gamma globulin. Shaded triangles represent labeled hormone or ligand.

Circulating Endogenous Antibody

If circulating endogenous antibodies are present in the patient's serum, spurious assay determinations may result. Theoretically, the radiolabeled hormone added to the test tube will bind either to the patient's antibody present within the serum sample or to the antibody added to the test tube. Since second antibody is generated to the IgG of the animal species used to generate the first antibody, the hormone bound to the human IgG will not be precipitated by that second antibody and will remain as a soluble complex in the supernatant. Consequently, fewer counts representing antibody-bound counts will appear in the pellet. Since the concentration of hormone in an assay tube is inversely proportional to the amount of radiolabeled hormone precipitated, a spuriously high hormone concentration will result. The foregoing is schematically depicted in Fig. 6-4. Other separation techniques will result in spurious hormone concentrations as well, simply because more antibody is present within the reaction mixture. Circulating antibodies are commonly encountered among diabetic patients receiving exogenous insulin. If one suspects circulating antibody in a patient, assay tubes containing labeled ligand and the patient's serum or plasma and buffer are incubated without exogenous antibody and ^{125}I-endogenous antibody complexes precipitated with appropriate concentrations of human immunoglobulin or ammonium sulfate.

Endogenous circulating antibody may be observed among insulin-dependent diabetic patients and those receiving hCG therapy as well as other hormone preparations which may differ structurally from endogenous native hormone.[43] Patients may develop antibodies to thyroglobulin which may render thyroglobulin assay results meaningless. Measurements of serial thyroglobulin levels can be useful in monitoring those patients who have well-differentiated thyroid cancer, since increase in those levels after the thyroid has been removed is evidence for functioning metastatic cancer. Other individuals may not have received hormonal therapy yet may have circulating antibody to thyroxine (T_4) or triiodothyronine (T_3), since circulating thyroglobulin contains bound thyroid hormone. The circulating complex is immunogenic, and antibodies to T_3 and T_4 may be generated. If one wishes to quantitate accurately the amount of antibody in a sample obtained from a patient with endogenous antibody to that hormone, additional sophisticated analysis must be carried out.

Steroid Assays

Steroid hormones usually circulate in serum bound to a variety of proteins. Since these serum proteins may have affinities similar to those for specific antibodies used for radioimmunoassay, the hormone usually must initially be extracted away from these serum proteins for valid assay analysis. Before the widespread development of radioimmunoassay, competitive protein-binding assays were developed using cortisol-binding globulin (CBG) to assay cortisol and other related steroids, e.g., progesterone, which bind to that carrier protein. These assays are no longer extensively used, since each batch of serum from which the CBG is harvested must be characterized, and more extensive thin-layer or other chromatographic separations of steroids are required. The added laboratory time needed for these initial steps, as well as the wider interassay variation, has relegated that assay approach to a secondary place.

The most common method of separating antibody-bound and free steroid hormones is with dextran-coated charcoal. With that technique, steroid not bound to antibody is adsorbed to the charcoal and consequently appears in the pellet. Conversely, the soluble hormone-antibody complex remains in the supernatant. For those steroid assays using tritiated hormone, the supernatant may be decanted into a vial containing an appropriate liquid scintillation-counting cocktail. A few steroid hormone assays are carried out with radiolabeled tyrosylated steroids. For those assays, a double-antibody or tube-coating method of separating bound and free hormone is commonly used.

Further Assay Validation

In addition to checking an antiserum's sensitivity, specificity, and susceptibility to nonspecific plasma or serum protein effects, one must ascertain whether the hormone standard used for dose interpolation of hormone concentration in patient samples is appropriate. Similarity of response between standard and clinical sample must be ascertained by constructing dose-response lines for each with either graduated doses of hormone or graduated volumes of sample to ascertain whether parallelism exists between the lines. As discussed above for hormone bioassays, parallelism must exist between hormone standard and unknown sample for valid dose interpolation. The slope and the 50 percent intercept of the dose-response line of the hormone standard should be monitored on each assay for quality control. In addition, pools of sera containing low, medium, and high concentrations of hormone should be assayed in replicate on each assay as an additional quality-control check. Considerably less interassay variation is observed than with bioassay, so most laboratories do not assay clinical samples at multiple volumes in routine radioimmunoassays unless hormone heterogeneity is suspected.

Finally, an independent check of the new assay's validity should be made with both physiologic and independent assay (preferably bioassay) correlates. Drugs and dietary intervention are perhaps the most common ways to perturb hormonal secretory patterns and are frequently used to assess whether the expected physiologic changes in hormone concentration are observed with the newly developed assay.

RADIORECEPTOR ASSAYS

The principle of radioreceptor assay is essentially the same as that for radioimmunoassay. Instead of binding to an antibody, a hormone binds to a specific hormone receptor in the plasma membrane or cytosol. The specific receptors for most polypeptide hormones are on the cell surface of plasma membrane, whereas biologically active steroids, as well as thyroxine and triiodothyronine, have specific intracellular receptors.[44] Radioreceptor-assay sensitivity is generally lower than that for radioimmunoassay and for most in vitro bioassays. The hormone must have the appropriate conformation to interact with its receptor and consequently must be biologically active. A hormone may fail to bind to its specific receptor but yet be detected by an antibody in a radioimmunoassay system. That disparity simply reflects the fact that radioimmunoassay and radioreceptor assays may detect different aspects of the hormone molecule.

A variety of radioreceptor assays have been developed. In general, tissue is harvested from hormone-specific target organs and receptor isolated by the use of standard techniques. Isolated particulate plasma membrane receptor is relatively stable on storage at temperatures lower than −20°C. However, solubilized polypeptide and steroid-hormone receptors derived from either plasma membranes or subcellular fractions without bound ligand are unstable, as reflected by their significantly decreased capacity to bind specific hormones even when they are stored frozen for a relatively short period of time.

Iodination of polypeptide hormones must be carried out with techniques which minimally alter the hormone's biologic activity. For preservation of biologic activity, one iodide atom is introduced per molecule of hormone. Excessive iodination usually markedly alters the hormone's biologic and immunologic activities. Moreover, some of the chemicals used in the iodination procedures are strong oxidizing or reducing agents, and consequently their concentration must be kept to a minimum. The variety of iodination techniques available is described above.

Immunoradiometric Assays

Immunoradiometric assays (IRMAs) differ from radioimmunoassays in that antibody is labeled instead of ligand or hormone. This technique provides a potential advantage in that iodinated immunoglobulin is usually stable for a longer time than iodinated hormones. However, a major disadvantage of IRMAs is that biologic samples must be assayed in at least two different volumes to be certain the concentration of hormone present is within the linear portion of the reference or standard dose-response range of the assay. Figure 6-5 depicts counts bound in the reaction tube versus the volume of sample added. When high concentrations of unknown are present in the reaction mixture, a "hook effect" is observed because there is a decrease in the counts bound with labeled antibody at higher hormone concentrations. For those biologic samples containing high hormone levels, a spuriously low hormone concentration may be reported if only a single aliquot of undiluted serum is assayed because of the hook effect. From a cost-effective laboratory standpoint, IRMA should be avoided for measurement of those hormones which may be present in high concentrations in pathologic states—for example, hCG, prolactin, or gastrin.

Enzyme-Linked Immunoassays

Enzyme-linked immunosorbent assays (ELISA) constitute another variety of immunoassay technique. In this case an enzyme may be covalently linked either to an antigen or to the specific antibody used to bind the

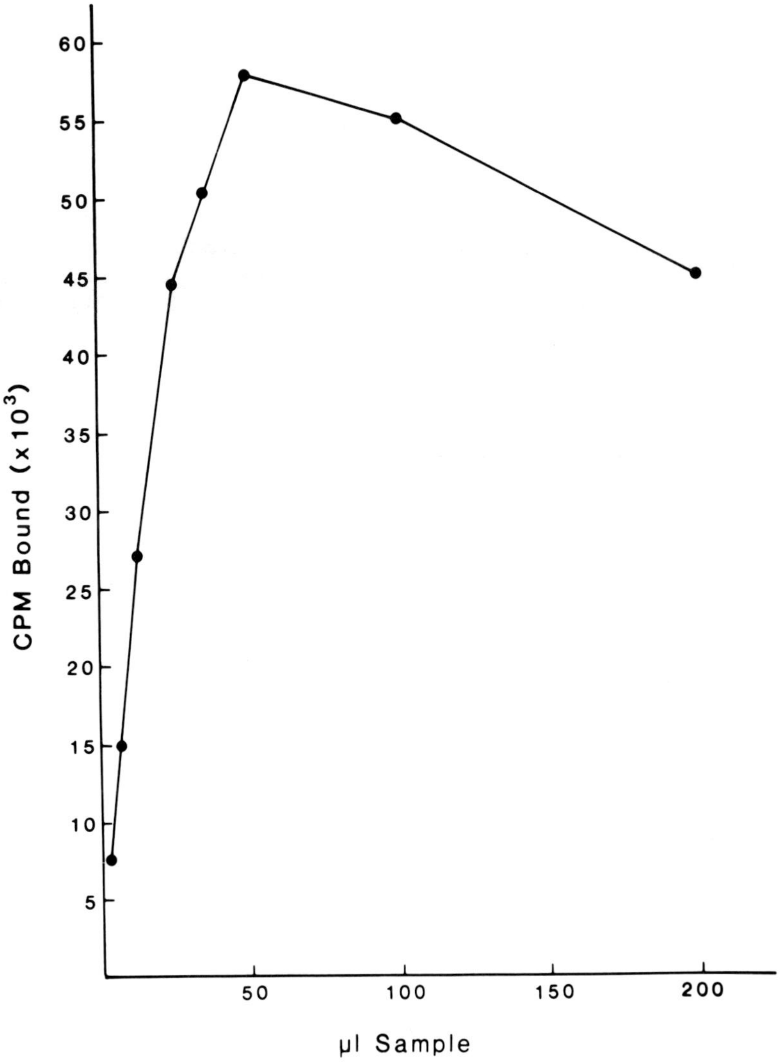

FIGURE 6-5 Dose-response line for graduated volume of a serum sample added to an immunoradiometric assay. A "hook effect" is observed beginning at 50 μl of sample added. If the concentration of hormone present in the sample were greater the hook effect would be greater, so that with increased volumes of serum added one would see the counts per minute bound approach the abscissa. In view of that relationship, it is imperative that all samples be assayed in at least two different volumes to be certain that the concentration of hormone is within the linear dose-response range of the IRMA.

desired substance. After the reaction has been allowed to proceed, the reaction product is measured spectrophotometrically. In general, the concentration of enzyme product is inversely related to hormone concentration. In some cases, second antibody is used in ELISA after having conjugated an enzyme to that second antibody. The enzymes most commonly used for these procedures include horseradish peroxidase, alkaline phosphatase, glucose oxidase, and beta-D-galactosidase. However, extreme care must be exercised to eliminate or at least minimize nonspecific interference with or modulation of the enzyme linked in the assay. Spurious assay results are more commonly observed with ELISA because nonspecific interfering substances appear in biologic samples. Currently, this problem has not been adequately addressed. Assay precision and sensitivity of ELISAs are comparable to those of most other radioimmunoassays.

Characterization of Hormone-Receptor Binding

A variety of mathematical analyses have been developed for characterizing hormone and receptor or antibody interaction. When a hormone $[H]$ interacts with its specific receptor $[R]$, a simple, bimolecular reversible reaction may be characterized at equilibrium by the following relationship:

$$[H] + [R] \underset{k_d}{\overset{k_a}{\rightleftharpoons}} [HR] \qquad (6\text{-}1)$$

where $[HR]$ represents the hormone-receptor complex. It is assumed that both hormone and receptor are homogeneous and univalent. The interaction of hormone and receptor may be further characterized by the following relationship:

$$K_a = \frac{k_a}{k_d} = \frac{[HR]}{[H]\,[R]} = \frac{1}{K_d} \qquad (6\text{-}2)$$

where K_a = equilibrium association constant, in liters per mole, or M^{-1}

k_a = association rate constant

k_d = dissociation rate constant

K_d = dissociation constant in moles per liter, or M

The relation between total receptor concentration and those sites occupied may be depicted as follows:

$$[R_0] = [HR] + [R] \qquad (6\text{-}3)$$

or

$$[R] = [R_0] - [HR]$$

where $[R_0]$ represents total receptor concentration, $[HR]$ represents bound receptor sites, and $[R]$ represents free receptor sites.

By rearranging the above equations, one can derive Eqs. (6-4a) and (6-4b), which, when plotted, usually will result in a straight-line relationship with a slope equal to $-1/K_d$ or $-K_a$.

$$\frac{[HR]}{[H]\,[R]} = \frac{1}{K_d} = K_a$$

$$\frac{[HR]}{[H]} = \frac{[R]}{K_d} = \frac{1}{K_d}([R_0] - [HR])$$

$$\frac{[HR]}{[H]} = -\frac{1}{K_d}[HR] + \frac{[R_0]}{K_d} \qquad (6\text{-}4a)$$

or

$$\frac{[HR]}{[H]} = -K_a[HR] + K_a[R_0] \qquad (6\text{-}4b)$$

Equations (6-4a) and (6-4b) are the mathematical representation of a Scatchard plot, perhaps the most frequently used transformation of receptor-hormone-binding data.[45,46] The above equations are also used to characterize hormone-antibody relationships. Figure 6-6 is a Scatchard plot. The intercept of the abscissa is $[R_0]$ and the ordinate intercept is $K_a[R_0]$ or $(1/K_d)[R_0]$. The slope of the line is $-K_a$ or $-1/K_d$. Consequently, when data are plotted, one can ascertain $[R_0]$ and $[HR]/[H]$ directly from the graph at the x- and y-axis intercepts, respectively. Since the term $-K_a[HR]$ of Eq. (6-4b) approaches zero as the amount of bound hormone $[HR]$ approaches zero, K_a can be calculated from the following:

$$\frac{[HR]}{[H]} = [R_0]K_a = \frac{B}{F}$$

where B = concentration of bound hormone

F = concentration of free hormone

or

$$K_a = \frac{[HR]}{[H]}\frac{1}{[R_0]} = \frac{B}{F}\frac{1}{[R_0]}$$

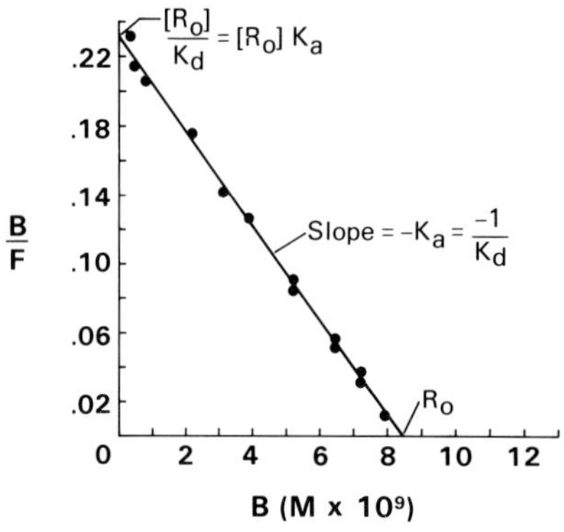

FIGURE 6-6 A Scatchard plot of data obtained from a radioreceptor assay.

Knowing the molar concentration of receptor, one can ascertain the number of binding sites per cell or per weight protein by multiplying the number of moles of receptor by 6.02×10^{23} (Avogadro's number, or the number of molecules per mole). The foregoing assumes that one hormone molecule may bind with one receptor site.

The association constants derived for a variety of hormone-receptor assays usually range between 1×10^{-11} and 1×10^{-9} M^{-1}. Not all Scatchard plots are linear, however. The nonlinearity reflects allosteric (receptor-receptor) interaction to enhance hormone binding after initial hormone binding (positive cooperativity) or to decrease hormone binding after initial hormone binding (negative cooperativity). One can further transform the data obtained from hormone-receptor-binding studies and determine whether significant allosterism is present by constructing a Hill plot.[47,48] If the slope of the line of the Hill plot is significantly different from 1, allostery exists. When one observes nonlinear Scatchard plots, factors other than allosterism must be considered, including artifacts introduced by carrying out the analyses under nonequilibrium conditions, inaccurate estimate of nonspecific binding, errors in separation of bound and free hormone, and significantly different affinities of labeled and unlabeled hormone for receptor.[49]

Hormone Receptors and Disease States

A variety of clinical states have been described in which the interaction between hormone and its specific receptor is altered. Those abnormalities have been ascribed to altered receptor number or affinity for hormone and to spontaneous formation of antibody to the hormone receptor. Patients with ataxia-telangiectasia may manifest extreme insulin resistance because of a marked decrease in the affinity of their receptors for insulin.[50] Some patients with myasthenia gravis have formed antibodies to their endogenous acetylcholine receptors, accounting for their clinical syndrome.[51] Similarly, patients with acanthosis nigricans exhibit marked insulin resistance clinically, and findings in those patients strongly suggest that an insulin receptor antibody contributed to their observed resistance.[52] The number of specific insulin receptors per cell may be reduced in obese patients, resulting in decreased insulin sensitivity; with weight reduction, the number of insulin receptors per cell increases, with restoration of normal insulin sensitivity.[53] Some patients with hyperthyroidism have circulating antibody to the TSH receptor. In contrast to patients with myasthenia gravis and diabetes, the circulating antibody of some patients with Graves' disease actually can stimulate the plasma membrane of thyroid tissue to induce increased production and release of thyroxine and triiodothyronine, resulting in a hyperthyroid state.[54]

In selected cases, the concentration of sex steroid hormone receptor can be helpful in selecting therapy.[55,56] Saturation analysis of breast cancer tissue to determine the concentrations of estrogen and progesterone receptors can be helpful in selecting patients for endocrine therapy. It is less cumbersome and more cost-effective than Scatchard analysis and many other forms of receptor kinetic analysis.

Saturation analysis provides a measure of the density of receptors available for estrogen or progestin binding but does not assess the affinity of these receptors. Excess labeled steroid is incubated with the cytosolic and/or nuclear fractions of tumor cells and allowed to attain equilibrium. Assuming there is no cooperativity between binding sites, the amount of ^3H-steroid or steroid analogue bound, corrected for nonspecific binding, is a direct measure of receptor concentration.

Premenopausal patients with breast cancer respond well to hormonal therapy if their breast cancers contain estrogen and/or progesterone receptors. Between 50 and 70 percent of women with significant tumor concentrations of estrogen receptor will respond to endocrine therapy, whereas less than 10 percent of those patients with receptor-negative tumors will respond to endocrine manipulation. The endocrine therapy commonly used is ablative surgery, including oophorectomy, adrenalectomy, and hypophysectomy. A variety of antiestrogenic drugs have been developed; these include nafoxidine, tamoxifen, and clomiphene. Premenopausal patients treated with a combination of endocrine therapy and adjunctive chemotherapy have significantly longer disease-free intervals than those women with tumors lacking significant concentrations of sex steroid receptor.[56]

PRACTICAL CONSIDERATIONS

Assay Variation

Quality control of radioimmunoassay, as well as both in vivo and in vitro bioassays, is imperative. The slope of the dose-response lines for the reference preparation and the unknown tested at several points must be parallel for valid results. In general, plasma or hormone pools are replicated on each radioimmunoassay or in vitro bioassay to provide an estimate of both within- and between-assay variations. The quality control system permits one to evaluate the long-term stability and reproducibility of the assay. In general, intraassay coefficients of variation are approximately half those for interassay variation. Consequently, when one expects relatively small but significant differences of hormone concentration among samples, it is best to determine hormone concentrations in one assay.

Hormone Stability

After secretion, several hormones are rapidly degraded and circulate as fragments. Probably the best example of this is parathormone (PTH), which, shortly after secretion into the peripheral blood, is broken down into amino-terminal and carboxy-terminal fragments. The carboxy-terminal fragment has a considerably longer blood half-life than the amino-terminal fragment has. However, it is the amino-terminal fragment which possesses the biologic activity of that hormone. When one generates antibody to native PTH, the immunized animal may generate antibody to predominantly amino-terminal, carboxy-terminal, or both portions of the molecule. The normal range of parathormone concentrations will differ according to the specificity of the antibody. Other hormones, such as β-endorphin, glucagon, and ACTH, may be rapidly degraded in plasma by circulating proteases. To avoid that problem, special sample handling is needed. In general, protease inhibitors, such as Trasylol or benzamidine, are added to the assay tubes upon collection.

Another technical problem is introduced when hormones are secreted in widely varying forms. For instance, there are several forms of gastrin—"minigastrin," "little gastrin," "big gastrin," "big big gastrin." Most gastrin assays will not differentiate among them when samples are assayed directly. Consequently, the samples must be subjected to gel filtration to ascertain the variety of physical forms present. Similar problems have been encountered with other hormones, such as prolactin, insulin, renin and ACTH. The larger forms usually represent precursor forms of the smaller biologically active native molecules.

Since serum hormone concentrations may vary with time of day, posture, metabolic state, and intrinsic rhythm over several minutes to weeks, sample collection must take place under uniform conditions. The normal range of values for a hormone is usually provided for samples collected under standardized conditions. It should be obvious, then, that hormone concentrations determined in well-controlled assays may be meaningless if they are obtained at inappropriate times or in inappropriate metabolic states. The metabolic state of the individual may be an important consideration, especially when one is measuring circulating concentrations of renin, aldosterone, growth hormone, insulin, or glucagon. Physical activity as well as stress may significantly affect baseline circulating levels of prolactin, ACTH, cortisol, renin, aldosterone, or growth hormone. Finally, a variety of drugs may affect hormone synthesis and secretion. Substances such as reserpine, methyldopa, and phenothiazines increase circulating levels of prolactin and, indeed, may induce clinically significant galactorrhea. Diuretics usually increase basal circulating renin levels. Consequently, both assay quality control and the setting in which a biologic sample is collected are important. Without optimization of both, assay results will be meaningless.

REFERENCES

1. Greep RO, Van Dyke HB, Chow BF: Use of anterior lobe of prostate gland in assay of metakentrin. *Proc Soc Exp Biol Med* 46:644, 1941.
2. McArthur JW: Identification of pituitary interstitial cell stimulation hormone in human urine. *Endocrinology* 50:304, 1952.
3. Dufau ML, Mendelson CR, Catt KJ: A highly sensitive in vitro bioassay for luteinizing hormone and chorionic gonadotropin: Testosterone production by dispersed Leydig cells. *J Clin Endocrinol Metab* 39:610, 1974.
4. VanHall EV, Vaitukaitis JL, Ross GT, Hickman JW, Ashwell G: Immunological and biological activity of hCG following progressive desialylation. *Endocrinology* 88:456, 1971.
5. VanHall EV, Vaitukaitis JL, Ross GT, Hickman JW, Ashwell G: Effect of progressive desialylation on the rate of disappearance of immunoreactive HCG from plasma in rats. *Endocrinology* 89:11, 1971.
6. Dufau ML, Catt KJ, Tsuruhara T: Retention of *in vitro* biological activities by desialylated human luteinizing hormone and chorionic gonadotropin. *Biochem Biophys Res Commun* 44:1022, 1971.
7. Bech K: Immunological aspects of Graves' disease and importance of thyroid stimulating immunoglobulins. *Acta Endocrinol* [suppl] Copenh 254:103, 1983.
8. Chayen J, Loveridge N, Daly JR: A sensitive bioassay for adrenocorticotrophic hormone in human plasma. *Clin Endocrinol* 1:219, 1972.
9. Kramer RM, Holdaway IM, Rees LH, McNeilly AS, Chard T: Technical aspects of the redox bioassay for luteinizing hormone. *Clin Endocrinol* 3:375, 1974.
10. Chayen J, Daly JR, Loveridge N, Bitensky L: The cytochemical bioassay of hormones. *Recent Prog Horm Res* 32:33, 1976.
11. Bitensky L, Alaghband-Zadek J, Chayen J: Studies of thyroid stimulating hormone and the long-acting thyroid stimulating hormone. *Clin Endocrinol* 3:363, 1974.
12. Sayers MA, Sayers G, Woodbury LA: The assay of adrenocorticotrophic hormone by the adrenal ascorbic acid–depletion method. *Endocrinology* 42:379, 1948.
13. Jeffers WA, Livezey MM, Austin JH: Method for demonstrating antidiuretic action of minute amounts of pitressin: Statistical analysis of results. *Proc Soc Exp Biol Med* 50:184, 1942.
14. Ames RG, Van Dyke HB: Antidiuretic hormone in serum or plasma of rats. *Endocrinology* 50:350,1952.
15. Thorn NA: A densimetric method for assay of small amounts of antidiuretic hormone. *J Exp Med* 105:585, 1957.
16. Baratz RA, Ingraham RC: Sensitive bioassay method for measuring antidiuretic hormone in mammalian plasma. *Proc Soc Exp Biol Med* 100:269, 1959.

17. Johnson AG, McDermott SJ: Sensitive bioassay of cholecystokinin in human serum. *Lancet* 2:589, 1973.
18. Steelman SL, Pohley FM: Assay of the follicle stimulating hormone based on the augmentation with human chorionic gonadotropin. *Endocrinology* 53:604, 1953.
19. Greenspan FS, Li CH, Simpson ME, Evans HM: Bioassay of hypophyseal growth hormone: The tibia test. *Endocrinology* 45:455, 1949.
20. Marcus R, Aurbach GD: Bioassay of parathyroid hormone in vitro with a stable preparation of adenyl cyclase from rat kidney. *Endocrinology* 85:801, 1969.
21. Loewenstein JE, Mariz IK, Peake GT, Daughaday WH: Prolactin by induction of *N*-acetyllactosamine synthetase in mouse mammary gland explants. *J Clin Endocrinol Metab* 33:217, 1971.
22. Turkington RW: Measurement of prolactin activity in human serum by the induction of specific milk proteins in mammary gland in vitro. *J Clin Endocrinol Metab* 33:210,1971.
23. Haber E, Koerner T, Page LB, Kliman B, Purnode A: Application of a radioimmunoassay for angiotensin I to the physiologic measurements of plasma renin activity in normal human subjects. *J Clin Endocrinol Metab* 29:1349, 1969.
24. Audhaya TK, Gibson KD: Serum inorganic sulfate and apparent somatomedin activity in an assay using chick embryo cartilage. *Endocrinology* 95:1614, 1974.
25. McKenzie JM: The bioassay of thyrotropin in serum. *Endocrinology* 63:372, 1958.
26. Berson SA, Yalow RS: Assay of plasma insulin in human subjects by immunological methods. *Nature* 184:1948, 1959.
27. Greenwood FC, Hunter WL, Glover JJ: The preparation of ^{131}I-labeled growth hormone of high specific activity. *Biochem J* 89:114, 1963.
28. Marchalonis JJ: An enzymatic method for the trace iodination of immunoglobulins and other proteins. *Biochem J* 113:299, 1969.
29. Miyachi Y, Vaitukaitis JL, Nieschlag E, Lipsett MB: Enzymatic iodination of gonadotropins. *J Clin Endocrinol Metab* 34:23, 1972.
30. Bolton AE, Hunter WM: The labeling of proteins to high specific radioactivities by conjugation to a ^{125}I-containing acylating agent. *Biochem J* 133:529, 1973.
31. Davies DR, Padlam EA, Segal DM: Three-dimensional structure of immunoglobulins. *Annu Rev Biochem* 44:639, 1975.
32. Poljak RJ, Amzel LM, Chen BL, Chiu YY, Phizackerley RP, Saul F, Yserm X: Three-dimensional structure and diversity of immunoglobulins. *Cold Spring Harbor Symp Quant Biol* 41:639, 1976.
33. Padlam EA, Davies DR, Pecht I, Givol D, Wright C: Model-building studies of antigen-binding sites: The hapten-binding site of MOPC-315. *Cold Spring Harbor Symp Quant Biol* 41:627, 1976.
34. Freund J: Some aspects of active immunization. *Annu Rev Microbiol* 1:291, 1947.
35. Vaitukaitis JL, Robbins JB, Nieschlag E, Ross GT: A method for producing specific antisera with small doses of immunogen. *J Clin Endocrinol Metab* 33:988, 1971.
36. Paul WE, Siskind GW, Benacerraf B: Specificity of cellular immune response: Antigen concentration dependence of stimulation of DNA synthesis in vitro by specifically sensitized cells as an expression of the binding characteristics of cellular antibody. *J Exp Med* 127:25, 1968.
37. Paul WE, Siskind GW, Benacerraf B: A study of the "termination" of tolerance to BSA with DNP-BSA in rabbits: Relative affinities of the antibodies for the immunizing and the paralyzing antigens. *Immunology* 13:147, 1967.
38. St. Rose JEM, Cinader B: The effect of tolerance on the specificity of the antibody response and on immunogenicity. *J Exp Med* 125:1031, 1967.
39. Eisen HN, Siskind GW: Variation in affinities of antibodies during the immune response. *Biochemistry* 3:996, 1964.
40. Starr JI, Horowitz DL, Rubenstein AH, Mako ME: Insulin, proinsulin, and C-peptide, in Jaffe BM, Behrman HR (eds): *Methods of Hormone Radioimmunoassay*. New York, Academic, 1978.
41. Kohler G, Milstein C: Continuous cultures of fused cells secreting antibody of predefined specificity. *Nature* 256:495, 1975.
42. Vaitukaitis JL, Ross GT, Braunstein GD, Rayford PL: Glycoprotein hormones and their subunits: Basic and clinical studies. *Recent Prog Horm Res* 32:289, 1976.
43. Johansen K: Human insulin—medical progress? *Metabolism* 32:528, 1983.
44. O'Malley BW: Steroid hormone action in eucaryotic cells. *J Clin Invest* 74:307, 1984.
45. Scatchard G: The attraction of proteins for small molecules and ions. *Ann NY Acad Sci* 51:660, 1949.
46. Scatchard G, Coleman JS, Shen AL: Physical chemistry of protein solutions: VII. The binding of some small anions to serum albumin. *J Am Chem Soc* 79:12, 1957.
47. Hill AV: A new mathematical treatment of changes of ionic concentration in muscle and nerve under the action of electric currents, with a theory as to their mode of excitation. *J Physiol (Lond)* 40:190, 1910.
48. Feldman HA: Statistics, in Rothfeld B (ed): *Nuclear Medicine in Vitro*. Philadelphia, Lippincott, 1983, pp. 10–34.
49. Rodbard D: Mathematics of hormone-receptor interaction: I. Basic principles, in O'Malley B, Means A (eds): *Receptors for Reproductive Hormones*. New York, Plenum, 1973.
50. Bar RS, Levis WR, Rechler MM, Harrison LC, Siebert C, Podskalny J, Roth J, Muggeo M: Extreme insulin resistance in ataxia telangiectasia: Defect in affinity of insulin receptors. *N Engl J Med* 298:1164, 1978.
51. Lindstrom JM, Seybold ME, Lennon VA, Whittingham S, Duane DD: Antiacetylcholine receptor antibody in myasthenia gravis: Incidences, clinical correlates and usefulness as a diagnostic test. *Neurology* 26:1054, 1976.
52. Kaplan SA: The insulin receptor. *J Pediatr* 104:327, 1984.
53. Bar RS, Gorden P, Roth J, Kahn CR, DeMeyts P: Fluctuations in the affinity and concentration of insulin receptors on circulating monocytes of obese patients: Effects of starvation, refeeding and diet. *J Clin Invest* 58:1123, 1976.
54. Mukhtar ED, Smith BR, Pyle GA, Hall R, Vice P: Relation of thyroid-stimulating immunoglobulins to thyroid function and effects of surgery, radioiodine and anti-thyroid drugs. *Lancet* 1:713, 1975.
55. Legha SS, Davis ML, Muggia FM: Hormonal therapy of breast cancer: New approaches and concepts. *Ann Intern Med* 88:69, 1978.
56. Lippman ME, Allegra JA: Current concepts in cancer: Receptors in breast cancer. *N Engl J Med* 299:930, 1978.

PART II

NEUROENDOCRINOLOGY AND THE PITUITARY

7

Neuroendocrine Physiology and Disease

Lawrence A. Frohman
Dorothy T. Krieger†

GENERAL CONCEPTS OF NEUROENDOCRINOLOGY

The neural and endocrine systems constitute the major integrative pathways in vertebrate species, effecting communication via synaptic neurotransmitter release and hormone secretion, respectively. The awareness that neurons can also secrete biologically active substances[1] and that neural tissue contains hormone receptors which modulate neurotransmitter and hypophysiotropic hormone release and/or activity has led to heightened awareness of the interrelations between these two systems, which together make up the substance of *neuroendocrinology*. This subject deals with (1) neural control of endocrine secretion, (2) hormonal effects on neural activity, and (3) broader problems of interactions between the central nervous system and the environment which affect and effect hormonal secretion. In the past the major emphasis has been on neural control of endocrine secretion, so much of the material presented in this chapter deals with this aspect, and more specifically with central nervous system control of anterior pituitary function. Neuroendocrine regulation of anterior pituitary function is conceptually and anatomically different from the classic mechanisms involved in neural regulation of posterior pituitary function (see Chap. 9). Central to this paradigm is the concept of the neurosecretory cell, whose secretion of hypophysiotropic factors (via the pituitary portal plexus) affects anterior pituitary function. The neurosecretory cell represents the final common pathway of neural control of the anterior pituitary, and as such is acted on (positively and negatively) by local tissue metabolites, target gland and pituitary hormones, neurotransmitters (i.e., monoamines, amino acids, acetylcholine), and neuropeptides, so that the final level of activity of the cell represents its response to the integrated effects of these agents. More recent studies have also delineated the presence in the vertebrate brain of peptides previously described as being localized to the pituitary and gastrointestinal tract, as well as peptides previously characterized in invertebrate organisms. Such peptides are thought to have neurotransmitter or neuromodulatory roles affecting major homeostatic systems as well as directly or indirectly influencing anterior pituitary function. It is believed, though yet unproved, that there is coordinate functional regulation of a given peptide in its central nervous system (CNS) and extra-CNS sites of production.

Feedback

One of the axioms of physiology has been Claude Bernard's concept of the constancy of the organism's internal environment. It has become apparent, however, that this is a relative matter, as manifested by changes occurring in response to changing environmental stimuli as well as by the presence of circadian

† Deceased.

variation. Despite such variation, it is still true that there is a relatively constant internal environment, which is achieved through the interaction of numerous bodily processes involving complex physiological control mechanisms for the accurate regulation and phasing of these interactions. The neuroendocrine system forms the major regulatory area in this regard. As can be seen in Fig. 7-1, it is essentially a closed-loop system, perturbed only by exteroceptive and interoceptive sensors, which may affect the function of neural pathways regulating basal endocrine function and of those pathways involved in rhythmic (circadian or ultradian) hormonal phenomena.

It can be seen from Fig. 7-1 that both long- and short-loop feedback systems are operative. The long-loop systems are those from the target gland to the anterior pituitary, hypothalamus, and other areas of the central nervous sytem; tissue metabolites may also function in such long-loop feedback systems. Most of these feedback processes are considered to be inhibitory; that is, the products of glandular secretion depress the release of the pituitary hormone that normally would act to stimulate the target gland. Such inhibition can occur directly at the pituitary level, or in the CNS, affecting the hypothalamic releasing hormone involved in stimulation of the given pituitary hormone or the neurotransmitters that regulate the releasing hormone. Occasionally feedback may be positive. For example, a low concentration of estrogen can stimulate the release of gonadotropin releasing

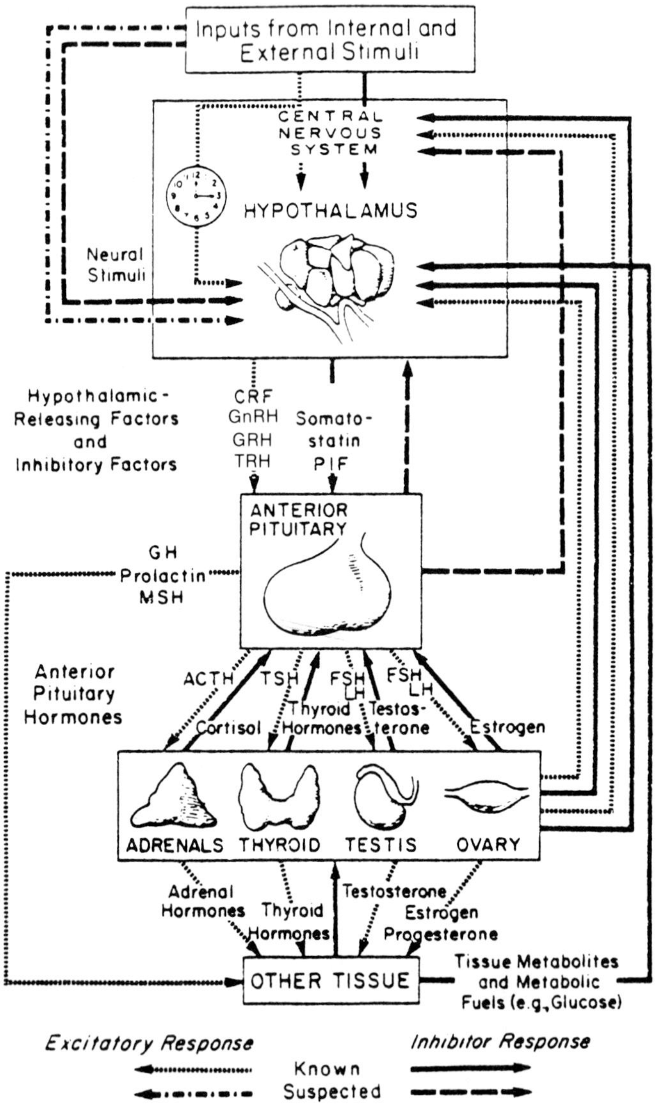

FIGURE 7-1 The basic feedback character of the neuroendocrine system is suggested in this schema, indicating the relationship among its components: the central nervous system, hypothalamus, anterior pituitary, and target glands and tissues. Hormone secretion is regulated by a balance of stimulatory and inhibitory effects. CRF, corticotropin releasing factor; GnRH, gonadotropin releasing hormone; TRH, thyrotropin releasing hormone; GRH, growth hormone releasing hormone; PIF, prolactin releasing inhibiting factor (dopamine ?).

hormone (GnRH). Such feedback processes also act within a certain "set point." This is similar to the concept involved in the setting of a thermostat. As an example, the cell regulating adrenocorticotropic hormone (ACTH) secretion is so programmed that it will normally stop secreting ACTH above a specific level of corticosteroid concentration and will initiate secretion when corticosteroid concentrations fall below a certain level. Under various conditions, e.g., stress or neuroendocrine disease, such set points may be changed, i.e., raised or lowered, allowing for deviation from normal feedback mechanisms. It has also been suggested that neurotransmitters acting on the neurosecretory cell responsible for releasing hormone release may modify hormonal feedback processes; this may give some insight into the mechanisms involved in resetting of set points. A change in the set point of gonadal steroid inhibition (raising of that point) has been invoked as an explanation for the onset of puberty, although the postulated change in neurotransmitter function that leads to set-point alteration has not yet been identified. Not indicated in the diagram are variations in the time course of the feedback pathways involved. For example, corticosteroid inhibition of ACTH release occurs rapidly, whereas the increase in ACTH following adrenalectomy appears to require several hours.

Short-loop feedback systems involving the effect of anterior pituitary hormones on releasing hormone concentrations have not been so thoroughly investigated. In the case of hypothalamic inhibitory hormones, the most information is available with regard to the effect of prolactin on dopamine, which is considered to be the main prolactin inhibiting factor. In this instance, elevated prolactin concentrations increase hypothalamic dopamine concentrations. It is believed that most such feedback systems are inhibitory in nature. Both short- and long-loop feedback systems are essentially closed loops, which allow self-regulation and avoid overshoot in the production of any secretory product. Such systems also respond to exteroceptive and interoceptive stimuli, though they are apparently not involved in the function of the hypothetical "clock(s)" which regulates the circadian periodicity of many pituitary and releasing hormone concentrations. Such periodicity persists in the absence of target organ gland secretions and exhibits phase characteristics similar to those seen in intact subjects, but at higher hormonal levels, which reflect the absence of target organ feedback processes.

In considering both long- and short-loop feedback processes, some mention should be made of the concept of the blood-brain barrier. This is based on the observation that many physiological substances can penetrate the central nervous system only poorly or not at all. Such penetration relates to molecular size, binding to plasma proteins, lipid solubility, presence of specific carrier-mediated mechanisms and active transport mechanisms, and presence of specific receptors within the nervous system. In certain areas of the nervous system no blood-brain barrier exists (the area postrema, the median eminence, the pineal body, and the interpeduncular tubercle); where it does exist, it is generally accepted that peptides do not penetrate the barrier whereas most steroid hormones and thyroid hormones do. Both the anterior and the posterior pituitary are outside of the blood-brain barrier. Whether peptide hormones arising from the pituitary will circumvent the blood-brain barrier via retrograde transport through pituitary portal veins into the median eminence and perhaps then via tanycytes into the cerebrospinal fluid (CSF) is currently under investigation (see below).

Hypophysiotropic Concept

It is generally accepted that central nervous system regulation of anterior pituitary function is mediated by hypophysiotropic hormones or factors. Although these hypothalamic hormones are called *releasing hormones* because of the rapidity with which they increase plasma levels of pituitary hormones, there is evidence that they also stimulate synthesis of the pituitary hormones. Electron-microscopic studies have indicated an increase in the number of pituitary secretory granules following administration of releasing hormones. Releasing hormones incubated with pituitary tissue in vitro cause an increase in the total pituitary content of the appropriate hormone and increased incorporation of radioactive precursors of the pituitary hormones. In vivo and in vitro studies have also demonstrated increase of the appropriate hormone in messenger ribonucleic acid (mRNA) in response to releasing factor administration. Lastly, in vivo administration of releasing hormones to animals with transplanted pituitaries leads to cellular differentiation of these previously inactive glands as well as hormone secretion.

Hypophysiotropic hormones are believed to be products of specialized neurosecretory cells which are concentrated within the hypothalamus but can also be found in extrahypothalamic areas. There is evidence, however, that the functions of such extrahypothalamic hypophysiotropic hormones and their regulatory controls are different from those affecting these same hormones within the hypothalamus.

The special role of the hypothalamus was emphasized in early studies in which fragments of anterior pituitary lobe tissue were transplanted into different parts of the hypothalamus of hypophysectomized and castrated rats.[2,3] Pituitary function was preserved only when the pituitary implants were placed in direct contact with a half-moon-shaped area in the hypothalamus extending from below the periventricular nuclei downward and backward on both sides of the inframammillary region (see Fig. 7-2). Such hypophysiotropic effects of these areas were believed to be independent of the median eminence capillary system (see below). This suggested that a substance essential for the maintenance of anterior pituitary function was present in the cell bodies within the hypophysiotropic region. Recent studies indicating that the blood supply of the hypophysiotropic area derives from vessels in the median eminence[4] may indicate the route by which hypophysiotropic factors reach such pituitary implants. Studies in which complete hypothalamic deafferentation has been performed—e.g., by severing all neural connections of the hypothalamus—also show fairly good preservation of adrenal and thyroid function, although in some species cyclic luteinizing hormone (LH) release is lacking.

It is obvious from these experiments, as well as from anatomic studies which demonstrated essential lack of innervation of the anterior pituitary, that pituitary function must be regulated by "humoral substances," i.e., the postulated hypothalamic regulatory factors, which normally would reach the pituitary gland via its portal vascular system supply. The possible role of the CSF in transporting the hypophysiotropic substances to the median eminence area and hence to the pituitary portal blood supply is now considered unlikely. Although the role of the hypophyseal portal vessel system in the neural regulation of anterior pituitary function by hypophysiotropic factors as originally postulated by Harris[5] is a critical one and such factors have been demonstrated in pituitary portal blood, it is now also recognized that (1) receptors for classic neurotransmitters such as acetylcholine, dopamine, and γ-aminobutyric acid (GABA) are present in the anterior pituitary,[6,7,8] (2) such neurotransmitters (dopamine, epinephrine, and possibly serotonin) are also present in pituitary portal blood,[9,10] and (3) uptake mechanisms for some neurotransmitters (such as serotonin) are also present in the anterior pituitary.[11] It has also been suggested that there is a regionalization of blood flow from a given

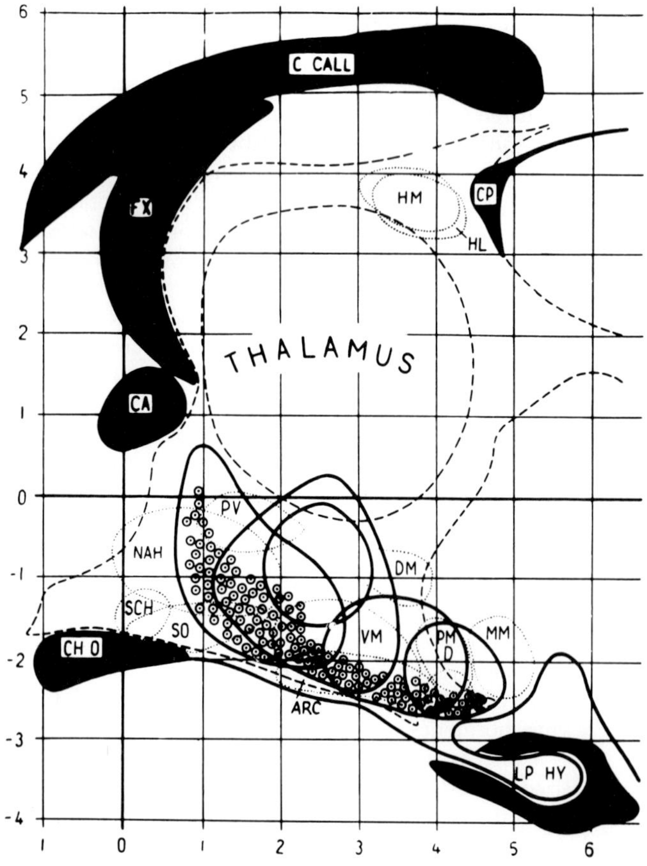

FIGURE 7-2 Localization of preserved PAS-positive basophil cells in hypothalamic anterior pituitary homografts. The thick outlines are the grafts and the small circles with dots in the center are the basophil cells, projected into the midsagittal plane. Irrespective of the location of the graft, basophils are found only in a well-defined region. (*From Szentagothai et al.*[2])

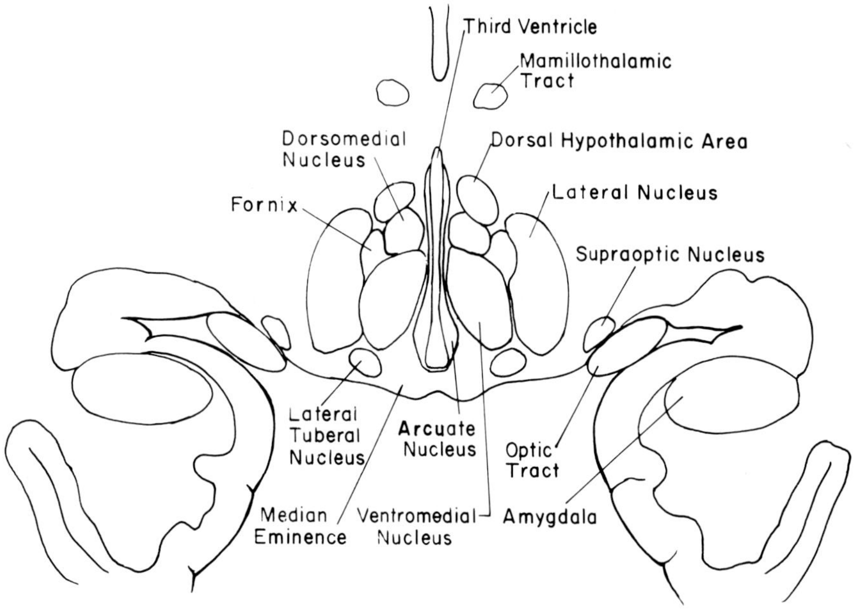

FIGURE 7-3 Frontal section of brain indicating major hypothalamic nuclear groups. (*From Krieger DT, Hosp Pract 6:87, 1971.*)

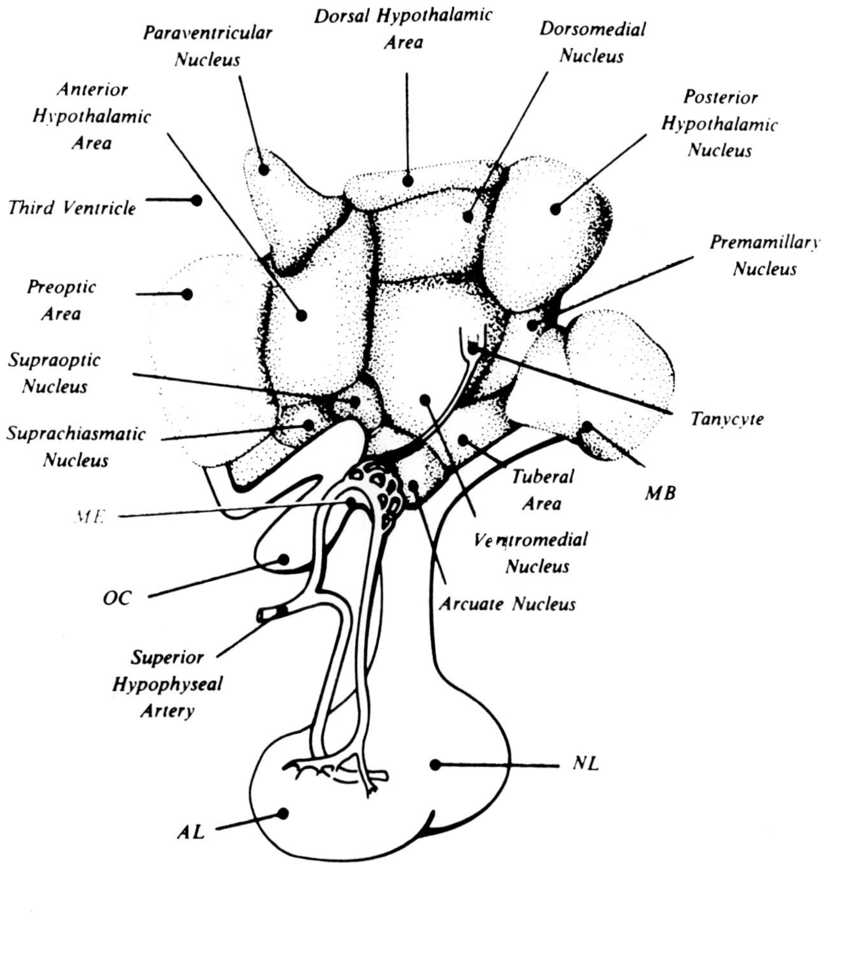

FIGURE 7-4 Nuclear organization in the hypothalamus shown diagrammatically in the sagittal plane, as it would appear from the third ventricle. Rostral is to the left and caudal to the right. The pituitary is shown ventrally. AL, anterior lobe; MB, mammillary body; ME, median eminence; NL, neural lobe; OC, optic chiasm. (*From Moore RY, in Reproductive Endocrinology, Philadelphia, Saunders, 1978, p 9.*)

hypothalamic area to a specific pituitary area,[12] though the various pituitary cell types are distributed throughout the gland.

ANATOMIC ASPECT

Hypothalamus

The anterior boundary of the hypothalamus is marked by the rostral edge of the optic chiasm, the posterior boundary by the mammillary bodies, the lateral boundaries by the optic tracts and the sulci formed with the temporal lobes, and the dorsal boundary by the overlying thalamus. The term *median eminence* refers to the specialized area of the hypothalamus located beneath the inferior portion of the third ventricle, whose external representation is grossly designated as the *tuber cinereum*. The hypothalamus can further be divided into medial and lateral subdivisions. The medial area is predominantly nuclear in composition (see Figs. 7-3 and 7-4); such nuclei are parvicellular, that is, composed of smaller cells than the classic neurosecretory cells in the magnocellular paraventricular and supraoptic nuclei. Its anterior portion contains the preoptic, suprachiasmatic, and magnocellular nuclei. Its tuberal portion contains the arcuate and ventromedial nuclei, which appear to give rise to neurons which enter the tuberoinfundibular tract and sweep around the lower part of the third ventricle to enter the median eminence of the hypothalamus. Other neural pathways which may give rise to fibers ending in the median eminence have been less well characterized but appear to originate within the suprachiasmatic nucleus, the preoptic area, and the dorsomedial hypothalamic nucleus. The posterior portion of the medial area contains the mammillary nuclei, only one of which (the tuberomammillary nucleus) may express endocrine functions. An additional cell group, the periventricular nuclei, lies beneath the ependymal floor of the third ventricle. The lateral hypothalamic area appears to be a major way station connecting the limbic forebrain with both hypothalamus and mesencephalon via the medial forebrain bundle (see Fig. 7-5).[13] Within this area, as well as in the medial hypothalamus, the bulk of axons are unmyelinated and exceedingly small; neurons of the lateral hypothalamic nucleus are mixed among the axons of the fiber bundles present.

It has become apparent that a given hypophysiotropic hormone is not specifically localized to a given

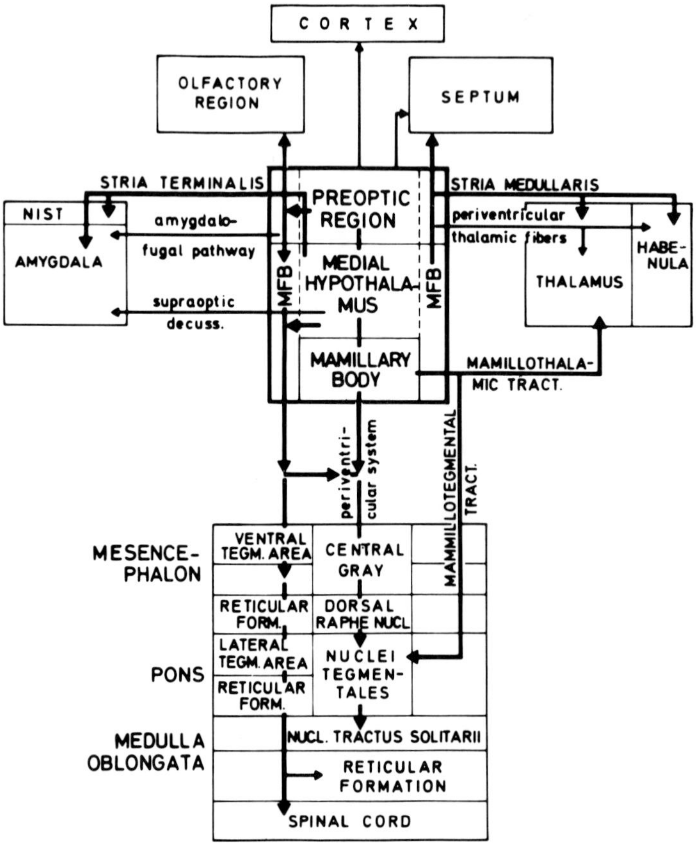

FIGURE 7-5 Summary of efferent connections of the hypothalamus (projections to the posterior pituitary not indicated). Afferent connections exist from the reticular formation, cortex, and limbic system (amygdala, septum, olfactory region, and hippocampus) to the lateral hypothalamic area. There are also afferent connections from the limbic system, the reticular formation, and the lateral hypothalamic area to the medial hypothalamic area. (*From Palkovits and Zaborszky.*[13])

Table 7-1. Gonadotropoin Releasing Hormone (GnRH), Thyrotropin Releasing Hormone (TRH), and Somatostatin in the Rat Hypothalamus

Region	GnRH, ng/mg protein	TRH, ng/mg protein	Somatostatin, ng/mg protein
Medial preoptic nucleus	<0.05	2.0 ± 0.1	14.0 ± 2.5
Periventricular nucleus	<0.05	4.2 ± 0.7	23.7 ± 9.0
Suprachiasmatic nucleus	Trace (<0.1)	1.8 ± 0.2	8.0 ± 0.6
Supraoptic nucleus	Trace (<0.1)	0.9 ± 0.2	3.2 ± 0.6
Anterior hypothalamic nucleus	<0.05	0.8 ± 0.3	8.6 ± 1.5
Lateral anterior nucleus	<0.05	0.7 ± 0.2	4.9 ± 1.1
Paraventricular nucleus	<0.05	2.6 ± 0.7	4.4 ± 1.8
Arcuate nucleus	2.9 ± 0.8	3.9 ± 0.9	44.6 ± 6.1
Ventromedial nucleus:			14.6 ± 2.1
Lateral part	0.6 ± 0.5	3.0 ± 0.6	
Medial part	Trace (<0.1)	9.0 ± 3.3	
Dorsomedial nucleus	<0.05	4.0 ± 0.8	5.4 ± 2.1
Perifornical nucleus	<0.05	2.0 ± 0.7	3.8 ± 0.7
Lateral posterior area	<0.05	1.2 ± 0.5	3.5 ± 0.7
Posterior hypothalamic nucleus	Trace (<0.1)	1.8 ± 0.2	3.8 ± 0.8
Dorsal premammillary nucleus	<0.05	1.5 ± 0.2	4.3 ± 0.7
Ventral premammillary nucleus	<0.05	1.3 ± 0.3	17.3 ± 4.4
Median eminence	22.4 ± 2.2	38.4 ± 8.3	309.1 ± 60.8

Source: Brownstein MJ et al, in *Frontiers in Neuroendocrinology*. New York, Raven, 1976, vol 4, p 1.

hypothalamic nuclear group. In general, it appears that while each type of hypophysiotropic factor thus far studied has a different pattern of distribution within the central nervous system, in every instance the highest concentrations are found in the median eminence. Most studies of such distribution have been performed in the rat. Table 7-1 and Fig. 7-6 indicate the patterns of distribution which have been observed.

Median Eminence–Portal System

The anatomic boundaries of the median eminence have already been described. Histologically this is the contact zone containing terminals of hypophysiotropic neurons and capillaries of the hypophyseal portal system. Figure 7-7 is a diagrammatic representation of the structual composition of the median eminence. It has already been noted that this region has a poorly developed blood-brain barrier. The portal-vein capillaries present in the median eminence are fenestrated, allowing the passage of high-molecular-weight substances from blood into the perivascular spaces of the median eminence. It is now generally accepted that most of the afferent blood supply of the pars distalis of the anterior pituitary has first been in contact with neural tissue. Branches of the hypophyseal arteries first break up into a capillary plexus situated in the median eminence, the pituitary stalk, and the posterior pituitary. These vessels constitute the primary plexus, which then recombines to form the portal veins. Long and short groups of portal vessels exist, and it has been postulated that each such vessel supplies a separate zone of the pars distalis, but this has not been proved. These long and short portal vessels break up into a secondary capillary plexus within the substance of the pituitary gland. Page, Munger, and Bergland have demonstrated in the rabbit pituitary stalk (1) the presence of vessels which connect the posterior pituitary gland to the hypothalamus, (2) the presence of connections between these vessels and the long portal vessels, (3) a common capillary bed between the posterior and anterior pituitary, and (4) the delivery of blood from the posterior pituitary to the ventricular surface of the median eminence.[14] These findings are of interest with regard to the reported presence of marked elevations in the concentration of immunoreactive LH, thyroid stimulating hormone (TSH), prolactin, ACTH, α-melanocyte stimulating hormone (α-MSH), and vasopressin in pituitary portal plasma in anesthetized male rats and differential effects of anterior and posterior pituitary lobectomy on the portal blood concentrations of these hormones.[15]

On the basis of these anatomic and biologic findings, it has been suggested that retrograde flow occurs

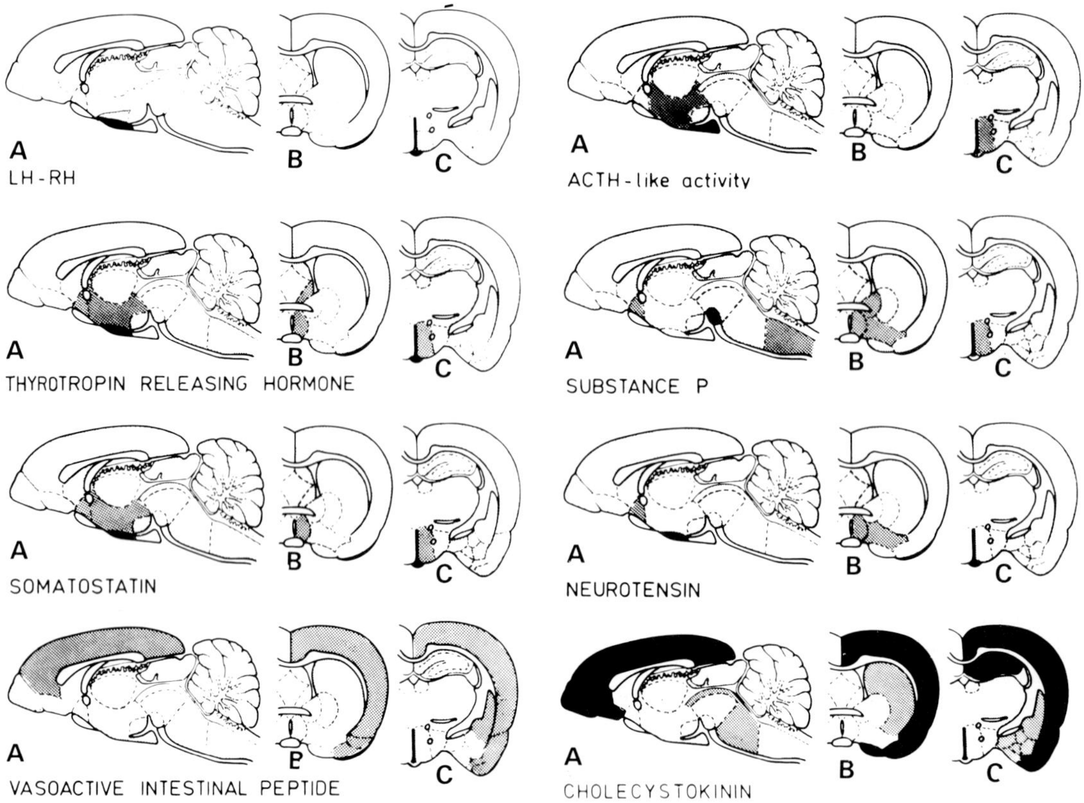

FIGURE 7-6 Diagrammatic representation of peptide distribution in central nervous system. Sagittal section (*A*) and coronal section (*B*) at anterior commissure level; coronal section at middle hypothalamic level (*C*). ■ = very high; ▩ = high; ▢ = moderate; □ = low density. (*From Palkovits M, Med Biol 58:188, 1980.*)

within the pituitary portal system and that this is of physiological significance.[16] More recent data, obtained in guinea pigs, indicate that at least in that species this is not the case,[17] although it is possible that retrograde transport could still occur along extracellular pathways from the pars distalis to the median eminence. It has been estimated that in the rat the blood flow in the combined median eminence-stalk is approximately 10 μl/min per milligram of tissue, which is among the highest of any tissue. The median eminence also contains in its inner palisade layer fibers of passage of the supraopticohypophyseal tract, and it has a high catecholamine content. Ultrastructural studies have demonstrated the occurrence of small and large granules which contain catecholamines, other granules which contain releasing factors, and neurons containing neurophysin, all of which end in close approximation to the capillary loops of the primary portal plexus. These granules are all found in the external palisade layer of the median eminence. An inner ependymal zone is also present, consisting of specialized cells termed *tanycytes* lining the third ventricle. These cells have ciliated apical processes that extend into the third ventricle lumen as well as elongated basal processes that extend to the primary portal capillary plexus. Although transport by these cells of material from the CSF to the median eminence as well as from the median eminence to the CSF has been demonstrated, the functional significance of such pathways is still not known.

Pituitary

A more detailed discussion of pituitary anatomy is given in Chap. 8. In all species the pituitary is a complex structure lying within a cavity, the sella turcica, whose anterior, posterior, and ventral boundaries are bone; whose superior boundary is formed by the diaphragma sellae (a reflection of the dura mater) through which the pituitary stalk and its accompanying blood vessels reach the main portion of the gland; and whose lateral boundaries are formed by the cavernous sinus on each side. In the adult human being there are only two lobes, an anterior and a posterior

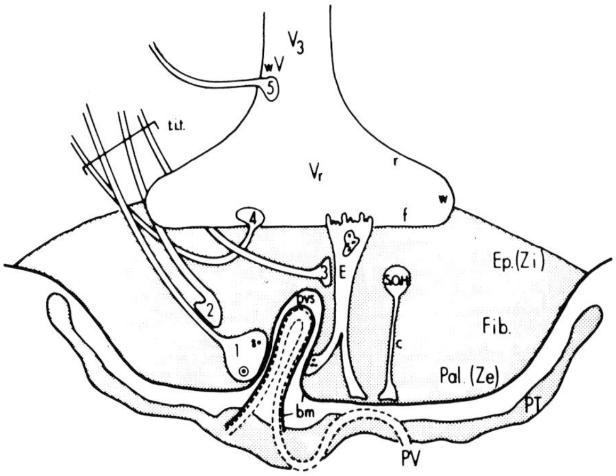

FIGURE 7-7 Schematic representation of basic structural arrangement and cellular composition of the median eminence. It is defined externally as that portion of the tuber cinereum in contact with the pars tuberalis (PT) of the anterior lobe and vascularized by the pituitary portal vessels (PV); internally it is demarcated by the wall (w) and floor (f) of the ventricular recess (V_r). The tissue between these two boundary planes constitutes the median eminence. No barrier exists between portal blood and the substance of the median eminence. It is generally organized into inner ependymal [Ep, zona interna (Zi)], middle fibrous (Fib), and outer palisade [Pal, zona externa (Ze)] layers. The tuberoinfundibular tract (t.i.t.) constitutes the major afferent system; its terminals (1) abut in the palisade zone upon the perivascular space (pvs), may form axoaxonic contacts (2), make "synaptoid" contacts with ependymal cells (3), and also have terminals that protrude into the third ventricle (4 and 5). Ependyma (E) line the floor of the third ventricle and, in addition, extend processes that traverse the width of the median eminence to terminate on the portal perivascular space. The middle fibrous layer contains axons of the supraopticohypophyseal tract (SOH) in transit to their termination in the neural lobe; some physiological evidence, but no substantive morphological data, suggest the possibility of collaterals (c) terminating in the palisade zone. wV, ependyma of wall of ventricle; V_3, third ventricle; r, ependyma of roof of ventricular abscess; bm, basement membrane. Not indicated are aminergic terminals (see Fig. 7-9), which may end either on capillary loops or on terminals of t.i.t. axons. *(From Knigge KM, Silverman AJ, in Handbook of Physiology. Washington, DC, American Physiological Society, 1974, vol 4, p 1.)*

lobe. A pars intermedia is present in the pituitary of most other vertebrates. In the human, this is present only in the fetal pituitary and possibly in the pituitary of pregnant women. The anterior lobe is made up of the pars distalis and the pars tuberalis, a layer of anterior pituitary cells capping the outer zone of the median eminence.

The characteristics of different cell types in the pars distalis vary between species. It appears that most of the major hormones are secreted by distinct cell types. Thus there are somatotrophs, lactotrophs, corticotrophs, thyrotrophs, and gonadotrophs, the latter secreting both follicle stimulating hormone (FSH) and LH. A substance resembling human chorionic gonadotropin (hCG) has also been described within human gonadotrophs,[18,19] as has renin- and angiotensin-like activity.[20,21] In addition to these secretory cells, there are stellate cells with long cytoplasmic processes adjacent to perivascular spaces, as well as other processes which connect with those from other stellate cells. It had been suggested that these cells play a nutritive role, since few if any secretory granules are present. More recently, such cells have been shown to contain S-100 protein,[22] previously believed to be unique to astrocyte-like cells. Media from clonal strains of rat anterior pituitary cells producing S-100 protein stimulate prolactin release,[23] providing an additional example of paracrine interactions between different pituitary cell types, as proposed by Denef and Andries.[24]

NEUROTRANSMITTERS, NEUROPEPTIDES, AND NEUROPHARMACOLOGICAL REGULATION

Neurotransmitter Regulation of Hypophysiotropic Neurosecretory Cells

It has already been noted that there are no unique anatomically or histologically demonstrable central nervous system areas that can be identified as being involved in the regulation of a specific hypophysiotropic hormone. Such regulation appears to reflect the integrated effects of various excitatory or inhibitory neurotransmitters and neuropeptides which impinge upon the neurosecretory cells, as modified by pH and the local concentrations of various ions and of target gland and pituitary hormones. Additionally, since neurally mediated pituitary hormone release occurs under different circumstances (periodic release, basal release, stress-mediated release), it may well be that different neurotransmitters are involved in each of these aspects of the regulation of a given pituitary hormone. The neurosecretory cell can therefore be pictured as having receptors for several neurotransmitters, each arriving via different anatomic pathways and activated by different stimuli. It has been shown for the hypothalamic-pituitary-adrenal system that a given neurotransmitter can activate ACTH release when implanted into one particular area but not other areas of the hypothalamus or limbic system, and a given hypothalamic area can be stimulated (resulting in ACTH release) by one neurotransmitter but not by others.

In attempting to delineate neurotransmitter control of hypophysiotropic hormones (see Fig. 7-8), it

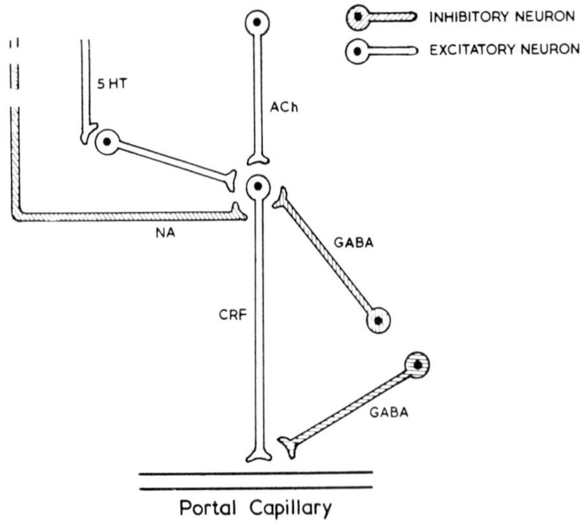

FIGURE 7-8 Suggested model for the control of corticotropin releasing factor (CRF) from the hypothalamus. Shown are (1) the CRF neuron with its axon terminating at a portal capillary, (2) a 5-hydroxytryptamine (5-HT) pathway that releases CRF after excitation of a cholinergic interneuron, and (3) the final common pathway to CRF release, which is cholinergic. Two cholinergic neurons are shown. One is the interneuron placed between the 5-HT pathway and the CRF cell (for control of the circadian rhythm?); the other cholinergic neuron does not have a 5-HT synapse and may control the stress-induced release of CRF. Also shown are (4) a noradrenergic (NA) pathway, which is inhibitory to CRF secretion, and (5) GABA inhibitory neurons which could provide either a pre- or postsynaptic input. (*From Jones MT, Hillhouse EW, Burden J, Ann NY Acad Sci 297:536, 1977.*)

should be realized that (1) such neurotransmitters may act either postsynaptically or by axoaxonal or axodendritic communication; (2) neurotransmitter regulation of hypophysiotropic hormones may be accomplished via multisynaptic pathways, so that a given neurotransmitter may be acting at a synapse proximal to that involved in the final regulation of the neurosecretory cell; and (3) as noted above, the effect of a given neurotransmitter may be modified by concentrations of other neurotransmitters, differential effects of low and high concentrations of the neurotransmitter, the point in time in the circadian cycle at which the neurotransmitter is acting, and the hormonal and physiological state of the subject. Neurotransmitter localization in discrete areas of the central nervous system has been greatly advanced by current immunocytochemical techniques. It is also necessary, however, to correlate changes in neurotransmitter content with those of neurotransmitter turnover and of hormone secretion to obtain an understanding of the role of a given neurotransmitter in the regulation of hormonal function. Virtually all the postulated neurotransmitters—catecholamines, indoleamines, acetylcholine, histamine, and GABA—have been identified in the hypothalamus and specifically within the median eminence area, as have the enzymes involved in their synthesis and metabolism.

Utilizing histochemical as well as chemical techniques, the distribution of monoaminergic neuronal networks has been plotted in great detail in the rat central nervous system (Fig. 7-9).[25-27] It appears that similar findings are present in humans. There is no direct procedure for visualizing acetylcholine; the knowledge of its distribution rests on the use of histochemical techniques and biochemical assay of choline acetyltransferase and acetylcholinesterase. There is also immunocytochemical evidence for the existence of GABA- and glutamate-containing networks of neurons,[28,29] which have been only partially mapped within the central nervous system.

To date, there is incomplete agreement as to the specific effects of a given neurotransmitter on a specific hypophysiotropic hormone. Table 7-2 summarizes the currently available evidence and indicates possible controversies, some of which stem from probable species differences, lack of drug specificity, and the use of different experimental paradigms.

The foregoing assumes that the effect of neurotransmitters on pituitary hormone release is the result of their effect on hypophysiotropic hormones. However, significant amounts of dopamine and serotonin are present in the anterior pituitary itself, and, as already noted, receptors or uptake mechanisms for these transmitters, as well as for acetylcholine, are also present. Especially in the case of prolactin, a direct action of dopamine on pituitary hormone secretion has been demonstrated, and it is now accepted that dopamine is the most physiologically important prolactin inhibiting factor (see below). It is also possible that biogenic amines may directly affect other pituitary hormones. α-Adrenergic stimulation of anterior pituitary ACTH release has been reported.[30]

Neurotransmitter Synthesis and Metabolism

There is currently considerable knowledge relating to the synthesis and metabolism of various neurotransmitters. This knowledge involves neuronal uptake of the specific amino acid precursor of the neurotransmitter, enzymatic synthesis, storage in specific granules in which the neurotransmitter is protected from degradation, release of such granules upon application of stimuli which cause neuronal depolarization, interaction of the released neurotransmitter with receptors on postsynaptic neurons, such as the neurosecretory cell containing the hypophysiotropic hormones, and metabolism of free neurotransmitter that has not

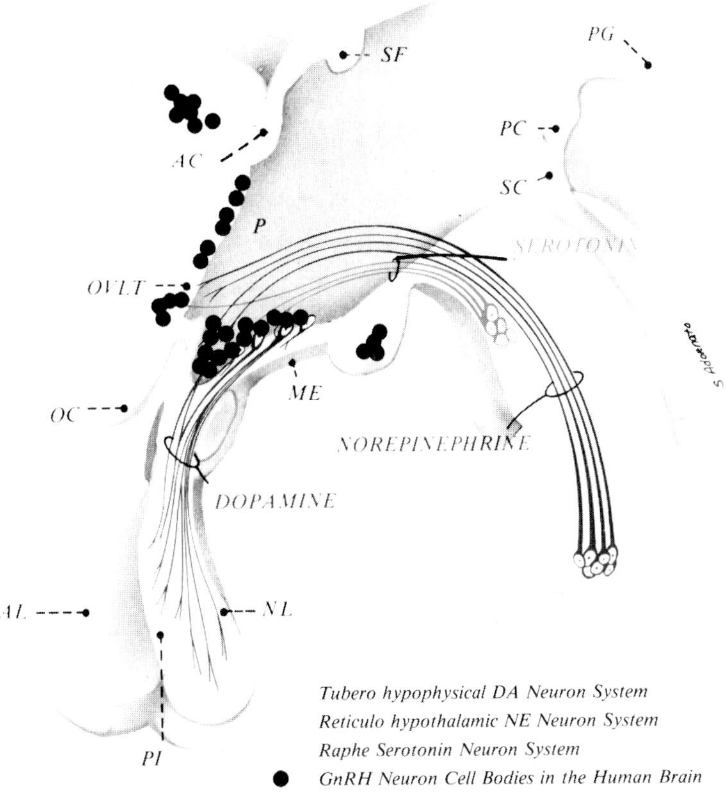

FIGURE 7-9 The monoamine neuron projections to the hypothalamus and pituitary are diagrammed in this drawing of the sagittal surface of the brain. Three major groups of monoamine neurons are shown: ascending brainstem norepinephrine neuron axons, arising mainly from cells in the neighborhood of the locus ceruleus, innervating most hypothalamic cell groups and the median eminence; ascending midbrain raphe serotonin neuron axons innervating the hypothalamus, median eminence, and organum vasculosum of the lamina terminalis (there is also evidence for an intrinsic serotonin pathway within the hypothalamus projecting to the pars intermedia); and dopamine neurons of the arcuate and paraventricular nuclei innervating the median eminence and neurointermediate lobe of the pituitary. The relation of the monoamine neuron innervation to the gonadotropin releasing hormone neurons (black circles) is evident. AC, anterior commissure; AL, anterior lobe; ME, median eminence; NL, neural lobe; OC, optic chiasm; OVLT, organum vasculosum of the lamina terminalis; PC, posterior commissure; PG, pineal gland; SC, superior colliculus; SF, subfornical organ; PI, pars intermedia. (*From Moore RH, in Reproductive Endocrinology. Philadelphia, Saunders, 1978, p 9.*)

reacted with receptors, either by reuptake into the presynaptic nerve ending (where it is subsequently metabolized or reincorporated into the storage granules) or by extracellular metabolism to biologically inactive compounds. Figure 7-10 depicts the major neurotransmitters in the central nervous system and the enzymes associated with their synthesis and degradation. Figure 7-11 depicts this process in a monoaminergic cell and its modification by various neuropharmacological agents (Table 7-3).

Neuropharmacological Effects

Pharmacological agents can affect neurotransmitter function and consequently hypophysiotropic hormone release at numerous sites. Some agents are used therapeutically for various conditions and it is important to know their endocrine side effects; others are used experimentally to delineate various aspects of neurotransmitter control. Table 7-4 summarizes some of the effects of pharmacological agents on hormone secre-

Table 7-2. Neurotransmitter Regulation of Pituitary Hormone Secretion

Neurotransmitter	Growth hormone	Prolactin	Gonadotropin	TSH	ACTH
Norepinephrine	↑	0	?↑	?↑	↓ or ↑
Dopamine	↑	↓	↓	↓	?↓
Serotonin	↑	↑	?↓	↑	↓ or ↑
GABA	↑	↓ or ↑	?↑	0	?↓
Histamine	0	↑	?↑	↑	?↑
Acetylcholine	↑	↓ or ↑	↑	0	↑

Key: ↑, increase; ↓, decrease; 0, no effect.

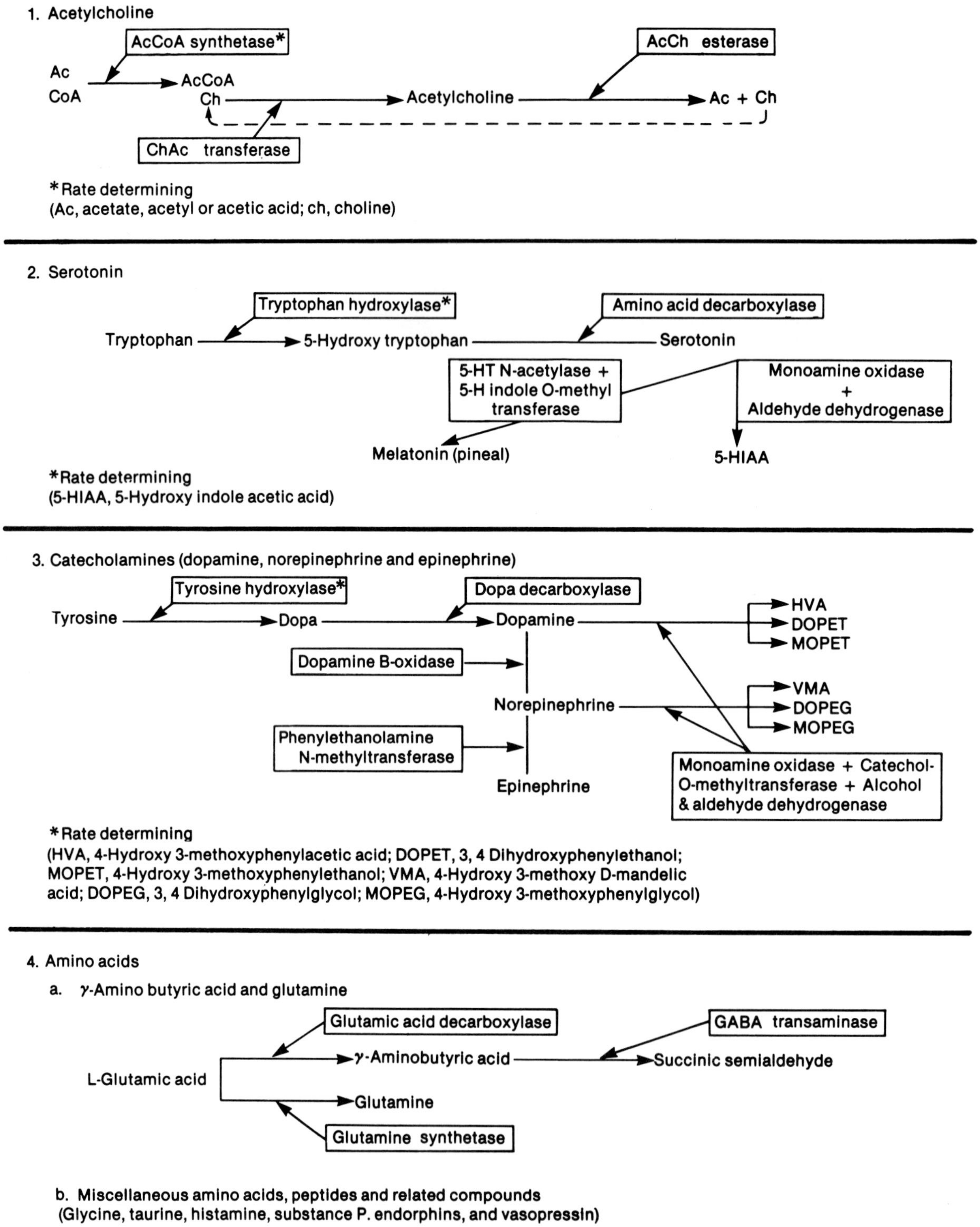

FIGURE 7-10 Neurotransmitters in the mammalian brain and their associated enzymes and major brain metabolites. (*From Samorajski T, J Am Geriatr Soc 25:337, 1977.*)

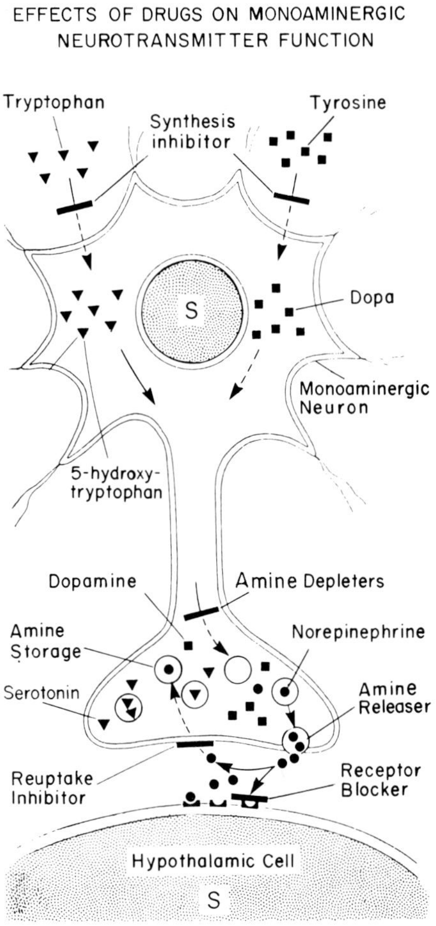

FIGURE 7-11 Schematic showing sites and modes of action of various categories of drugs (including many agents used therapeutically) that alter neurotransmitter function (see Table 7-3 for examples). Depending on a particular drug's mode of action, the result is a net increase or decrease in the secretion of a releasing or inhibitory factor by the hypothalamic cell. (*Modified from Frohman L, Hosp Pract 10:54, 1975.*)

tion. Comparison with Table 7-2 indicates the expected effects on anterior pituitary function; e.g., a drug that increases effective serotonin concentrations would be associated with evidence of increased growth hormone and prolactin secretion. Since some drugs have actions on several neurotransmitters, their hormonal effect would be a resultant of these actions.

Neuropeptides and Pituitary Hormone Release

A large number of peptides have been described and mapped within the central nervous system during the past decade.[31,32] These peptides are now believed to act as neurotransmitters or neuromodulators within the central nervous system. In this context, a *neurotransmitter* may be defined as a substance with an action highly localized to the synaptic region, which can produce physiological changes in the postsynaptic cell identical with those produced by stimulating the presynaptic cell. A *neuromodulator* has variously been defined as a substance which can modify the known actions of a classic neurotransmitter (monoamine, acetylcholine, amino acid), block the release of a given neurotransmitter, or alter the turnover of other neurotransmitters. Mention has already been made of the extrahypothalamic distribution of the hypophysiotropic hormones and the presumed functional differences in their actions in such sites. In this regard, the best evidence of a peptide acting as a conventional neurotransmitter has been obtained for GnRH, which is present in sympathetic ganglia.[33,34] It has been demonstrated that a GnRH-like peptide can be released from the ganglia by nerve stimulation via a calcium-dependent process, and that this peptide can act directly on sympathetic neurons to produce a depolarizing response lasting for minutes. This response can be blocked by the same GnRH analogues which inhibit GnRH-induced release of LH from pituitary gonadotrophs.

A number of differences exist between the mechanisms involved in the synthesis and activation of neuropeptides and those involved in the classic neurotransmitters described above, whether they are acting as neurotransmitters or as neuromodulators. Neuropeptides are synthesized (in many instances as parts of larger precursor molecules, as has been described for other polypeptide hormones) on ribosomes within the perikarya, at a considerable distance from the secretory site within the axon terminal. At the terminal, peptides are released via exocytotic mechanisms to act on postsynaptic membrane receptors. There is no evidence for presynaptic uptake–inactivating mechanisms for such peptides. The determination of the nature of the enzymes involved in termination of neuropeptide action is a field of great current interest.

In addition to their effects on a number of homeostatic systems,[35] neuropeptides have been shown to affect pituitary hormone secretion, in some instances via actions on hypophysiotropic or conventional neurotransmitter neurons and in others via direct pituitary action e.g., vasoactive intestinal polypeptide (VIP) has been demonstrated in pituitary portal blood;[36] its release is stimulated by serotonin; and its direct action is inhibited by glucocorticoids.[37] It has even been proposed to serve as a prolactin-stimulating hormone. Table 7-5 depicts some of the recently described endocrine effects of neuropeptides. It is believed that some of the central actions of VIP

Table 7-3. Drugs Affecting Monoaminergic Neurotransmitter Function

Drugs	Effects
Precursors	
Levodopa	Increases dopamine (DA) and norepinephrine (NE) levels
Tryptophan 5-Hydroxytryptophan	Increase serotonin levels
Receptor agonists	
Apomorphine Bromocriptine (Parlodel)	Stimulate DA receptors
Clonidine (Catapres)	Stimulates α-adrenergic receptors
Isoproterenol (Isuprel)	Stimulates β-adrenergic receptors
Quipazine Lysergide (LSD)	Stimulate serotonin receptors
Synthesis inhibitors and enzyme blockers	
α-Methyl-*p*-tyrosine (Demser)	Inhibits tyrosine hydroxylase, blocks synthesis of DA and NE
3-Iodotyrosine	
Disulfiram	Inhibits DA β-hydroxylase, blocks conversion of DA to NE
FLA 63	
Fusaric acid	
Methyldopa (Aldomet)	Converted to methylated monoamines, functions as false neurotransmitter
p-Chlorophenylalanine	Inhibits tryptophan hydroxylase, blocks synthesis of serotonin
Amine depleters	
Reserpine (Serpasil)	Interferes with storage of DA, NE, serotonin in nerve terminals
Reuptake inhibitors	
Tricyclic antidepressants	Block reuptake of neurotransmitters at nerve terminals
Amine releasers	
Amphetamines	Stimulate release of newly synthezized DA and NE by nerve terminals, also block uptake
Receptor blockers	
Phenoxybenzamine (Dibenzyline) Phentolamine (Regitine)	Block α-adrenergic receptors
Propranolol (Inderal)	Blocks β-adrenergic receptors
Metoclopramide (Reglan) Chlorpromazine (Thorazine) Haloperidol (Haldol)	Block dopaminergic receptors
Methysergide (Sansert) Cyproheptadine (Periactin)	Block serotonin receptors
Nerve ending poisons	Destroy terminals
6-Hydroxydopamine	Acts on dopaminergic and noradrenergic terminals
5,7-Hydroxytryptamine	Acts on serotonergic terminals

Source: Modified from Frohman L, *Hosp Pract* 10:54, 1975.

may be mediated via effects on cholinergic or opiate receptors and that the actions of opiates on prolactin secretion occur via changes in central dopamine and possibly serotonin turnover. Both transmitters have already been cited as affecting prolactin secretion. The evidence with respect to endocrine effects of opioids (see below) is of considerable interest, in view of previous reports of endocrine effects of morphine administration as well as the demonstration of opioid-containing terminals in the median eminence. Available data indicate that tolerance to the endocrine effects of opioids may develop. In addition to the central effects of opioids, there is suggestive evidence that opiate receptors are present on GnRH nerve endings and that β-endorphin administration can produce a marked reduction in rat pituitary plasma dopamine concentrations.[38] A possible direct action of opioids on anterior pituitary is suggested by reports of high concentrations of β-endorphin in pituitary portal blood[39] and the presence of high-affinity opiate-

Table 7-4. Effect of Drugs on Anterior Pituitary Hormone Secretion

Drugs	LH, FSH	Growth hormone	Prolactin	ACTH	TSH
Dopaminergic agonists					
Levodopa	0	↑	↓	0	Blocks response to TRH
Apomorphine	0	↑	↓	0	0
Bromocriptine					
Dopaminergic antagonists					
Haloperidol		↓ Response to stimuli	↑	0	0
Chlorpromazine		↓ Response to stimuli	↑	0	0
Metoclopramide	↑		↑	0	↑
Noradrenergic antagonists					
Phentolamine (α)	0	↓ Response to stimuli	0	?	0
Propranolol (β)	0	↑	0	?	0
Serotonin antagonists					
Cyproheptadine	0	↓	↓	↓	0
Catecholamine synthesis inhibitor					
Methyldopa			↑		
Catecholamine depleter					
Reserpine	? Blocks ovulation	↓	↑	↑Acutely	
Catecholamine reuptake inhibitor					
Imipramine	0	↓	↑	0	0
Catecholamine releaser					
Amphetamine		↑	↑	↑	
GABA agonist					
Muscimol	0	↑	↑		0

Key: ↑, increase; ↓, decrease; 0, no effect.

Table 7-5. Endocrine Effects of Peptides

Peptide	GH	AVP	Prolactin	LH
VIP	↑*		↑*	↑
Substance P	↑		↑*	↑↓
CCK	↑		↑	
Gastrin	↓			
Neurotensin	↑ ↓		↑*↓	↓
Opioid Peptides†	↑	↑↓	↑	↓

*Also direct pituitary effect.
†Refers to reported effects of either β-endorphin or met- or leu-enkephalin. Since these peptides are now known to be derived from different precursor molecules, have a different CNS distribution, and may act via different types of opiate receptors, more specific characterization of their effects is necessary.
GH, growth hormone; AVP, vasopressin; LH, luteinizing hormone; VIP, vasoactive intestinal polypeptide; CCK, cholecystokinin.

receptor-binding sites in the pituitary.[40] However, receptor densities are much higher in the posterior and intermediate lobes than in the anterior lobe.

THE HYPOPHYSIOTROPIC HORMONES: CHEMISTRY, DISTRIBUTION, EFFECTS

In the past 17 years, five factors have been isolated and definitively characterized: thyrotropin releasing hormone (TRH), GnRH, growth hormone release inhibiting hormone or somatotropin release inhibiting factor (somatostatin, SRIF), corticotropin releasing factor (CRF), and growth hormone releasing hormone (GRH). Their structures are shown in Fig. 7-12. Studies with each of these factors have underscored the complexities involved in characterizing the actions of hypophysiotropic hormones. For example, TRH

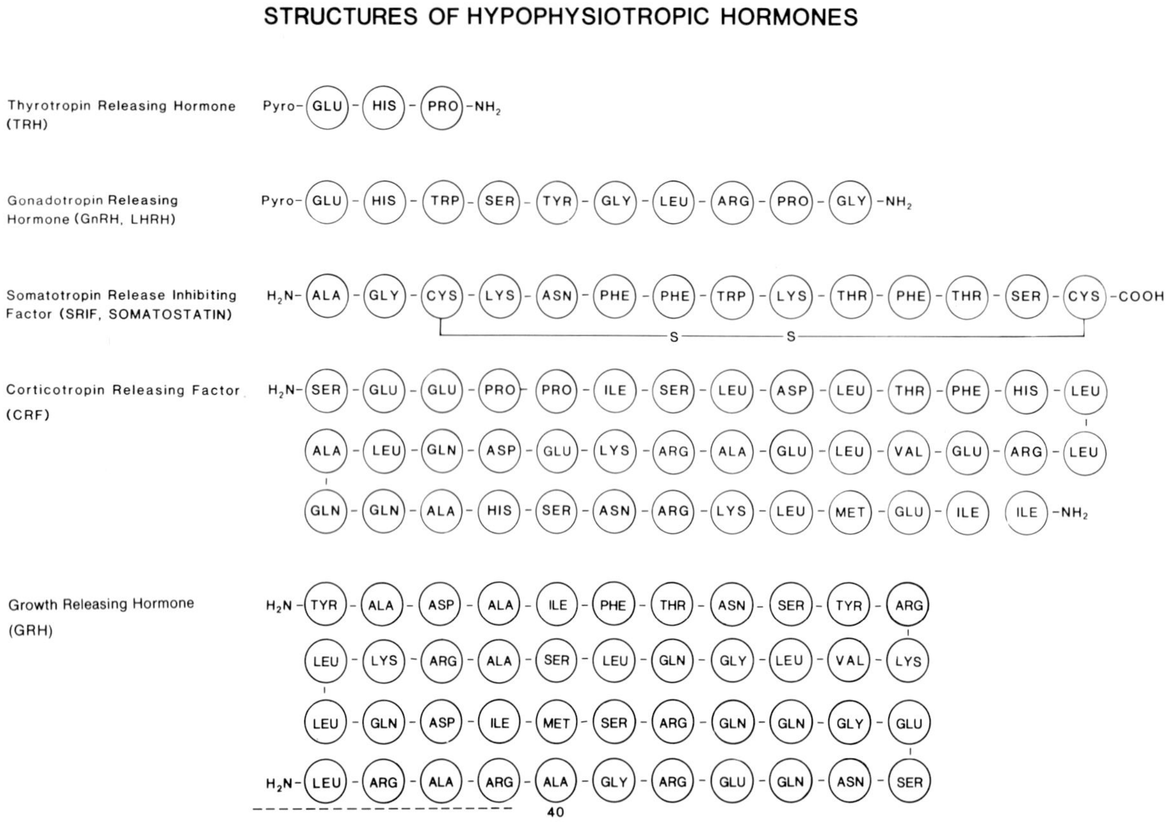

FIGURE 7-12 Structures of hypothalamic releasing and inhibiting hormones. The sequences of TRH, GnRH, and somatostatin are identical in all mammalian species studied. The sequence of human CRF, shown in the figure, has been deduced from that of its cDNA[41] and differs by seven amino acids from ovine CRF.[42] The sequence of GRH was originally derived from GRH ectopically produced by human pancreatic tumors. Two forms of GRH have been identified which differ only by the additional COOH-terminal tetrapeptide indicated by the broken line.[43,44] The identical 40- and 44-amino acid sequences are also present in human hypothalamus, while those of porcine and rat GRH differ by 3 and 14 residues, respectively.

affects more than one pituitary hormone; its administration causes the release of both TSH and prolactin. The question has therefore been raised as to whether TRH is the physiological prolactin releasing hormone (PRF) or whether other factors which stimulate prolactin release deserve this designation (see below). (It should be noted that the terms *factor* and *hormone* are interchangeably used for these substances, although *factor* was originally reserved for those substances whose chemical structure had not been characterized.)

TRH also exhibits behavioral as well as TSH-releasing effects, and these behavioral effects on the central nervous system can be demonstrated in the hypophysectomized animal. Additionally, with the development of new techniques for immunochemical identification of hypophysiotropic hormones, material with immunoreactivity similar to that of TRH has been detected throughout the central nervous system (see below), changing the terminology from that of *hypothalamic hormones* to *hypophysiotropic hormones.*

Similar findings exist with regard to GnRH. This factor is the physiological releaser of both LH and FSH (see below). In addition, extrahypothalamic localization of GnRH has been demonstrated, as have behavioral effects which also occur in the absence of the pituitary.

SRIF was the first of the hypophysiotropic factors identified which inhibits the release of a pituitary hormone. Its concentration in hypothalamic extracts has generally been sufficient to obscure the presence of growth hormone releasing hormone. The demonstration of SRIF in the peripheral nervous system, in the pancreas, and in cells in the gastrointestinal tract adds a still further dimension to the concept of hypophysiotropic factors. Additionally, somatostatin has been demonstrated to inhibit not only growth hormone and TSH release but also the release of insulin, glucagon, and gastrin.

With respect to CRF, preliminary findings indicate that its ACTH-stimulating potency is less than that occasioned by stress, indicating the involvement of cofactors (vasopressin, catecholamines) in mediating such responses. Unlike the previously described releasing factors, species differences in structure appear to exist, with seven amino acid differences between the human and ovine CRF. Synthetic human CRF has now become available and has been shown to exhibit comparable potency in humans. This occurs despite a more rapid clearance from circulation than that of ovine CRF.[44a] GRH, which exhibits greater species difference than CRF (13 amino acid differences between rat and human), was first characterized in pancreatic islet tumors associated with acromegaly.[43]

Thyrotropin Releasing Hormone

Thyrotropin releasing hormone, a tripeptide, was the first of the hypophysiotropic hormones to be identified. Table 7-1 indicates its distribution within hypothalamic nuclei, as determined by radioimmunoassay. Although TRH concentrations present in extrahypothalamic areas are small, they become significant when one considers that the weight of the hypothalamus is only 1 percent of the total weight of the brain in the rat. Extrahypothalamic TRH therefore accounts for as much as 70 percent of total brain TRH. There is evidence that almost all the TRH in the median eminence and much of that in the arcuate nucleus originates from neurons in the paraventricular nuclei,[45] although cell bodies are also present in other hypothalamic areas. Immunoreactive TRH has also been detected in the gastrointestinal tract, pancreatic islets, posterior pituitary, reproductive tract, and placenta in a number of species. These tissues might therefore be a source of the TRH detected in peripheral blood.

Some studies have suggested that TRH exists in higher-molecular-weight forms.[46,47] Such forms most likely reflect the presence of the biosynthetic precursor of TRH, whose structure has now been determined.[47a] There is also evidence that a metabolic product of TRH, histidyl-proline-diketopiperazine, may inhibit prolactin secretion,[48] although its other effects are similar to those of TRH. Formation of this metabolite is enhanced by TSH.

TRH has been widely used both experimentally and clinically. A number of analogues have been synthesized for determination of structure-activity requirements, as well as for attempts to produce antagonists of TRH action or longer-acting derivatives. TRH is usually administered as a bolus intravenous (IV) injection of 500 μg in normal subjects and is associated with increments in plasma TSH concentrations which peak approximately 20 min after injection. Clinical applications of TRH are covered in Chap. 8.

The estimated half-life of circulating TRH in the human being is approximately 4 min. TRH is rapidly inactivated in plasma by heat-labile enzymes.

TRH has been detected in rat peripheral plasma, with approximately 10-fold higher concentrations present in portal vein plasma.[49] No changes in peripheral plasma TRH concentrations have been found after cold exposure or the administration of thyroxine or propylthiouracil, although these procedures affect plasma TSH concentrations.[50] TRH content of rat brain and whole hypothalamus likewise appears unaffected by thyroidectomy or administration of T_4, α-methyl-*p*-tyrosine (α-MPT), or parachlorophenylalanine (PCPA)—drugs which affect central amine concentrations (see Fig. 7-11).[51]

Deafferentation decreases hypothalamic but not extrahypothalamic TRH concentrations, indicating that extrahypothalamic TRH is not produced by hypothalamic neurosecretory cells. The cause of the decrease of hypothalamic TRH following such deafferentation is open to conjecture. It has been postulated that this decrease is secondary to either removal of stimulatory (presumably α-adrenergic) neural inputs to hypothalamic TRH-producing cells, transsection of axons carrying TRH from areas outside the hypothalamus, or possible operative disruption of CSF flow interfering with transport of TRH from extrahypothalamic areas to the hypothalamus. Despite the decrease in hypothalamic TRH following deafferentation, normal TSH responsiveness to propylthiouracil or triiodothyronine and to cold exposure persists.

These responses, which are maintained in the deafferentated animal, are reduced by electrolytic destruction of the median eminence, which suggests that there is a pool of TRH within the arcuate nucleus–median eminence area which can maintain normal feedback and pituitary responsiveness, assuming that such lesions do not destroy pituitary cellular function.

The mechanism of TRH action on the pituitary involves activation of the adenylate cyclase–cyclic AMP system. This effect is inhibited by thyroid hormone through a mechanism involving synthesis of an inhibitory protein that inhibits the action of TRH. Corticosteroids also inhibit TRH stimulation of TSH release and probably also depress TRH secretion. Corticosteroids do not reduce the prolactin response to TRH, and thyroxine only partially reduces the prolactin response to TRH.

Somatostatin blocks TRH-induced secretion of TSH but not of prolactin. The similarity of the effects of thyroxine, cortisone, and somatostatin implies that the TRH receptors on the two types of cells (i.e., thyrotrophs, lactotrophs) are under different regulatory control or that the effects occur beyond the receptor.

Levodopa administration blocks both the TSH and the prolactin response to TRH. In patients with pituitary tumors or presumed pituitary tumors, i.e., in acromegaly, Cushing's disease, or tumors with FSH hypersecretion (but not in normal subjects), TRH stimulates the release of growth hormone, ACTH, and FSH, respectively. Abnormal growth hormone responses to TRH have also been reported in patients with anorexia nervosa, diabetes, cirrhosis, and depression. TRH has been shown to suppress the nocturnal elevation of plasma growth hormone levels. It has been postulated that when there are intact monoaminergic pathways, TRH acts on these to inhibit neurotransmitter-induced growth hormone release. Where there is abnormal function of such pathways (as postulated in acromegaly), TRH may act directly on the pituitary to induce an increase in growth hormone levels. There is also evidence for somatotroph TRH receptors in pituitary adenomas. TRH may similarly stimulate ACTH release only when CNS pathways are disrupted (anatomically or functionally). TRH can stimulate growth hormone release in the hypophysectomized rat bearing an ectopic pituitary[52] and in hypothyroidism.[52a]

TRH has been reported to have a wide variety of behavioral effects on motor activity, feeding and drinking behavior, and temperature regulation. Administration of TRH in pharmacological doses has been reported to dramatically ameliorate the consequences of spinal cord injury in cats.[53] This latter action may be mediated by known blocking effects of TRH on opioid actions other than analgesia.[54]

With regard to the noted behavioral effects of TRH, the demonstrated presence of TRH in the brain of primitive vertebrates that lack a pituitary or thyroid is consistent with the possibility that TRH may have a direct effect on CNS function. Although initial reports of the alleviation of depressive states by TRH administration have not been confirmed, TRH does lessen the duration of pentobarbital anesthesia, potentiates the behavioral effects of dopamine and serotonin, potentiates cholinergic excitatory effects, and raises the LD_{50} of pentobarbital while lowering the LD_{50} of strychnine. These observations are compatible with an excitatory effect of TRH on CNS function. Electrophysiological studies indicate that TRH may be involved in reduction of firing of a certain population of hypothalamic cells.

TRH may be effective behaviorally not only through an action on neural cells, as suggested by microiontophoresis studies, but also by altering the turnover of brain neurotransmitters (e.g., acetylcholine and norepinephrine. Accelerated norepinephrine turnover has been reported in the cerebral cortex of rats receiving intraperitoneal TRH.[55]

Gonadotropin Releasing Hormone

Immunoreactive GnRH (also known as luteinizing hormone releasing hormone), a decapeptide, has been demonstrated in the hypothalamus of several species. Avian, reptilian, and teleostean GnRHs are chemically distinct from the mammalian peptide but are in themselves indistinguishable, whereas amphibian GnRH appears to be identical to the mammalian peptide.[56] Although there are physicochemical differences in these vertebrate immunoreactive GnRHs, the biologically active regions of the molecule have been conserved, since GnRH from all species tested stimulates release of LH from ovine anterior pituitary cells in culture. By immunoassay, GnRH is present almost exclusively in the median eminence and organum vasculosum, with lesser concentrations in the arcuate and ventromedial nuclei. Table 7-6 indicates the immunocytochemical localization of GnRH-containing perikarya in several mammalian species.[57] There are major species differences related to the presence or absence of GnRH in perikarya in mediobasal hypothalamus, which have been shown for some rodent species (e.g., rat and mouse) but not in guinea pig or in rhesus monkey. Most studies indicate that the distribution of GnRH cell bodies forms a continuum from the septal nuclei through the anterior hypothalamic region, though projections from these areas differ. In the guinea pig and hamster, it appears that projections from septal GnRH neurons extend to the midbrain, whereas GnRH perikarya within the preoptic region send axons that terminate in the circumventricular organs, the median eminence, and the neural lobe. GnRH perikarya have also been observed in extrahypothalamic sites in the limbic system and cortex, as well as in the main and accessory olfactory bulbs. It is estimated that the total number of GnRH cells in the rodent brain varies between 500 and 2000. There is disagreement with regard to the effect of deafferentation on GnRH content within and outside the hypothalamus (differences perhaps based on the size of the hypothalamic island studied), in that different studies report either decreased or unchanged hypothalamic content, with no effect on extrahypothalamic content after deafferentation.

There is still also lingering controversy as to the existence of a distinct FSH-releasing factor and a report of a peptide with a greater molecular size than GnRH which stimulates FSH release.[58] Most available evidence, however, indicates that the differential effects of GnRH on FSH and LH release can be explained by variations in dose, time course, pulsatile frequency of administration, and steroid hormone interactions at the pituitary level in response to a sin-

Table 7-6. Immunocytochemical Localization of GnRH-Containing Perikarya in Several Mammalian Species

Species	C	OB	NT	H	A	S	POA/AHA	MBH	M
Human	–	–	–	–	–	++	++	++	0
Baboon	–	–	–	–	–	++	++	++	0
Macaque	–	–	+	–	+	++	++	+++	0
New world monkey	–	–	+	+	–	++	++	++	+
Prosimians	–	–	+	–	–	0	+++	0	0
Sheep	–	–	–	–	+	+	+++	+	–
Cow	–	–	–	–	–	0	0	++	–
Horse	–	–	–	–	–	–	+	++	–
Cat	–	–	–	–	–	–	++	0	0
Dog	–	–	–	–	–	+	++	++	+
Rabbit	–	–	+	–	–	+	++	++	+
Guinea pig	–	0	+	0	+	+	++	++	+
Rat	+	+	+	+	–	++	++	0	0
Mouse	–	–	–	–	–	++	++	0	0
Hamster	+	++	+	+	0	++	++	+	0

Abbreviations: C = cortex; OB = olfactory bulbs; NT = nervi terminales; H = hippocampal formation; A = amygdala; S = septum; POA/AHA = preoptic/anterior hypothalamic area; MBH = mediobasal hypothalamus; M = midbrain.
Key: –, region not studied; 0, region has been reported not to contain GnRH-positive structures; +, ++, +++, increasing numbers of GnRH cells in these regions.
Source: Modified from Krey and Silverman.[57]

gle releaser. Very recently, a GnRH-associated peptide (GAP) has been identified as part of the GnRH precursor and exhibits both gonadotropin-releasing as well as prolactin-inhibiting actions.[58a] Its physiological role, however, remains to be clarified.

There is evidence that GnRH release occurs episodically,[59] and this is reflected by detectable episodic elevations of the peptide in portal blood.[60] Knobil has reported that the frequency of episodic GnRH release determines the pattern of gonadotropin release.[59] Low-frequency pulsations (one pulse every 3 h) were associated with larger discharges of LH and FSH than frequencies of one pulse per hour. Higher LH/FSH ratios were seen with more frequent pulsing, in part dependent on the lower metabolic clearance rate of FSH as compared with that of LH and the greater magnitude of FSH release in response to the less frequent pulse. Variations in the amplitude of GnRH pulses were also associated with changes in LH/FSH ratios. When the magnitude of pulses was increased, there appeared to be a relative decrease in FSH response. In the primate, it appears that neurons in the arcuate nucleus are responsible for the frequency of episodic GnRH release. There is evidence that episodic release can be disrupted by the administration of neuropharmacological agonists and antagonists of a variety of neurotransmitters, indicating the role of numerous neuronal mechanisms in such regulation. Regulation of GnRH release by gonadal steroids also occurs. There are reports of increased amplitude of GnRH release in the portal blood of castrated rhesus monkeys.[60] If episodic LH release is believed to mirror that of GnRH, there are marked shifts in the frequency of episodic GnRH release during rodent and human reproductive cycles and following androgen administration to males. Gonadal hormones also modify gonadotropin response to GnRH. In humans, short courses of estradiol diminish gonadotropin response to GnRH, whereas prolonged estradiol treatment enhances responsiveness. Short-term progesterone treatment also diminishes GnRH-induced gonadotropin release. In male subjects, the administration of estrogen markedly reduces gonadotropin response to GnRH, whereas large doses of testosterone have only a slight suppressive effect. Corticosteroids have also been reported to diminish LH responsiveness to GnRH. GnRH, like TRH, has been reported to release growth hormone and ACTH in some patients with acromegaly and Cushing's disease.

GnRH is synthesized by mechanisms similar to those of other brain peptides,[61] and a larger precursor molecule has recently been identified.[62,62a] GnRH appears to be degraded by two primary peptidases.[63] Understanding of such cleavages has led to the development of GnRH analogues with amino substitutions at the positions of cleavage to prevent degradation. Such analogues have been of major clinical importance, acting both as superagonists and as antagonists.[64,65] As agonists, they have been used both in the treatment of hypogonadism and to induce fertility; as antagonists they are effective as contraceptive agents and in the treatment of precocious puberty, endometriosis, and cancer of the prostate, by producing a functional gonadectomy.

The central neurotransmitter regulation of GnRH release is still unclear. There is ample evidence that interactions occur between monoaminergic and GnRH neurons, in that there is a facilitatory action of the noradrenergic system in the production of the ovulatory surge of GnRH. The role of dopamine remains controversial, with most evidence suggesting inhibition of GnRH release. Norepinephrine reduces pulsatile LH release, while the circadian pattern of LH and presumably GnRH release is regulated by serotonergic neurons. Opioid inhibition of LH release has already been mentioned, and gonadal steroids have marked effects on the activity of both peptidergic and nonpeptidergic neurons, which may, in turn, affect the GnRH secretory cell.

In addition to its hypophysiotropic role, GnRH may also be involved in the species-specific behavior necessary for reproduction. Estrous behavior is induced by GnRH in estrogen-primed, oophorectomized, hypophysectomized animals.[66] GnRH is particularly effective in facilitating such responsiveness in the central gray area of the midbrain,[67] and GnRH antiserum infused into this area has a prolonged lordosis-inhibiting effect.[68] A role of GnRH in male sexual behavior has also been suggested, though not confirmed. The role of nonneural GnRH (the GnRH-like peptide(s) present in the male reproductive tract) in reproductive behavior is still unknown.

The electrophysiological basis of the behavioral effects of GnRH is not well defined. Electrophysiological studies show that variations in hypothalamic unit activity can be correlated with altered gonadotropin release and that GnRH administered microelectrophoretically appears to modify substantially the electrical activity of tuberoinfundibular, but not of preoptic, neurons.[69] Firing rates are altered by concomitant gonadal steroid administration.

Somatostatin

Somatostatin was first isolated from the hypothalamus and characterized as a tetradecapeptide (somatostatin-14). It exhibits profound inhibitory effects on growth hormone release. In human subjects, growth hormone responses to all stimuli thus far studied (i.e., hypoglycemia, stress, sleep, levodopa, and arginine infusion) are blocked by somatostatin. Somatostatin participates in the physiological regulation of growth hormone secretion, as evidenced by animal studies in which growth hormone release is enhanced following neutralization of endogenous somatostatin by antibodies to the peptide. Somatostatin secretion is regulated by a feedback system in which increased growth hormone concentrations as well as increased concentrations of somatomedin C stimulate somatostatin release.

It is now recognized that the originally described somatostatin-14 is contained within an amino-terminal-extended somatostatin (somatostatin-28) which, in turn, is contained within a larger molecular species. The structure of prosomatostatin has now been reported.[70] Somatostatin-28 is more potent than somatostatin-14 in certain systems and is secreted along with somatostatin-14; thus, somatostatin-28 appears to serve as a true hormone and not merely, as was originally suggested, as a prohormone for the smaller form.

Following the initial identification of somatostatin in the hypothalamus, the peptide was found to be widely distributed throughout the nervous system and in many extraneural tissues (secretory and neural elements of gastrointestinal tract, pancreas, parafollicular thyroid cells, salivary gland, and urinary excretory system). The structure of extraneural somatostatin in the GI tract and pancreas has been shown to be identical with that of hypothalamic somatostatin-14,[71,72] and somatostatin-28 has also been identified in these tissues. A structure similar or identical to somatostatin-14 has been detected in other vertebrate organisms in which somatostatin has been located, whereas the sequence of NH_2-terminal-extended somatostatin in these other species has not been so well conserved.

Somatostatin not only has a potent action on growth hormone release but inhibits the secretion of TSH, insulin, glucagon, virtually all exocrine gut hormones, and renin. It also impairs gastrointestinal motility and reduces intestinal absorption of all nutrient classes. Its effects on insulin and glucagon secretion, as well as on gastrointestinal motility, appear to be mediated via paracrine actions.

The mechanisms by which somatostatin inhibits pituitary growth hormone release are complex. Pituitary and pancreatic cAMP concentrations are reduced following exposure to somatostatin, as are the stimulatory effects of cAMP. It is known, however, that all the effects of somatostatin on hormone secretion involve changes in calcium flux, resulting in inhibition of cellular calcium uptake, and that the inhibitory effects of somatostatin may be reversed by the addition of calcium.[73] As seen in Table 7-1, the highest levels of somatostatin are found in the median eminence, and appreciable concentrations are found in other hypothalamic areas, as well as in the thalamus, cortex, preoptic area, midbrain, and spinal cord. Complete mediobasal hypothalamic deafferentation results in an increased growth rate and elevated plasma growth hormone levels associated with decreased somatostatin concentrations in the deafferentated area. It is possible than some neurotransmitter control of growth hormone release is mediated by effects on the release of somatostatin as well as on growth hormone releasing hormone though both mechanisms are probably involved. In vitro studies have demonstrated release of somatostatin from hypothalamic slices following exposure to acetylcholine, dopamine, and neurotensin, with decreases following exposure to GABA. A large number of other neurotransmitters and neuropeptides have also been reported to affect somatostatin release, sometimes with contrary results.[74] Growth hormone is capable of inhibiting its own secretion; this effect is in part mediated by changes in the release of somatostatin and growth hormone releasing hormone into portal vessels and also by direct effects on the pituitary. As with TRH and GnRH, direct application of somatostatin onto certain populations of single neurons in the hypothalamus and other areas, such as cerebral and cerebellar cortex and spinal cord, results in a significant depression of neuronal firing rates.[75] Recently excitatory effects of somatostatin on spontaneous neuronal activity have been reported.[76,77] The discrepancies may be secondary to dose-response characteristics of somatostatin. A number of behavioral changes believed to represent increased cortical excitability have been reported following intracerebroventricular injection of somatostatin.

Corticotropin Releasing Factor

Although CRF was the first hypophysiotropic factor whose activity was demonstrated in hypothalamic extracts, its chemical identity was not established until 1981.[42] Ovine CRF thus characterized was larger than the other previously reported hypophysiotropic factors, being a straight-chain peptide of 41 amino acids (see Fig. 7-12). Its reported concentration in rodent and human hypothalamus appears to be somewhat less than that of some of the other hypophysiotropic factors, although this may reflect decreased cross-reactivity of the ovine antiserum employed for human and rat CRF (which differ from ovine CRF by seven amino acids). In the one study performed on ovine brain, median eminence concentrations were in the range reported for somatostatin (see Table 7-1).[78] The majority of CRF-containing cell bodies have been identified in the paraventricular nucleus of several species.[79] This nucleus also contains subpopulations of cells in which either immunoreactive dynorphin 1–8 and CRF or immunoreactive CRF and vasopressin are colocalized.[80,81] Other CRF-containing cells are present in the basal telencephalon, hypothalamus, and brainstem, and scattered cells are found throughout most areas of the cerebral cortex. Projections from the paraventricular nuclear cells to the median eminence have been identified. CRF-containing fibers arising from cell bodies in other areas appear to be widely distributed, particularly in limbic areas and brainstem.[79] CRF-like material has been described in human and rat placental extracts,[82] and CRF-like immunoreactivity has also been reported in the vertebrate endocrine pancreas[83] and in the human gastrointestinal tract.[84] Whether extraneural CRF is the source of the tissue and circulating CRF-like material remains to be determined.[85] CRF has also been localized ultrastructurally within rat corticotrophs,[86] and it is possible that this represents internalized CRF bound to receptors.[87]

Elucidation of ovine CRF structure indicated a 50 percent amino acid homology with sauvagine, a 40-residue peptide isolated from the skin of the South American frog. Both peptides are closely related to a third peptide, urotensin I, isolated from fish neurohypophysis. There is also a four-amino acid homology of CRF with angiotensinogen, which is of interest in light of the ACTH-releasing activity of angiotensin. The size of CRF suggested it might be a prohormone for a smaller, more active ACTH-releasing fragment. This does not appear to be the case, since most shortened CRF analogues are much less active.[88] The cDNA for the ovine CRF precursor and the sequence of the human CRF precursor gene have been analyzed.[41,89] These analyses indicate the presence of a higher-molecular-weight precursor which may represent the high-molecular-weight material reported in earlier studies.[90] Comparison of the amino acid sequence of prepro-CRF with the sequences of the ACTH/β-lipotropic hormone (β-LPH) precursor and the arginine vasopressin/neurophysin II precursor suggests that these precursor proteins may be evolutionarily related.

CRF in vitro releases all the peptide components derived from the proopiomelanocortin (POMC) molecule.[91] There is some controversy as to whether CRF is effective in releasing intermediate lobe–derived POMC-like material. The anterior pituitary response to CRF is potentiated by both vasopressin[92] and catecholamines,[92,93] which is consistent with previous reports of such potentiation by native unpurified CRF-like preparations. These findings may explain the observations that in the human, the magnitude of the ACTH rise induced by CRF is less than that seen under stressful situations. Central administration of CRF has a number of systemic effects, such as increasing arterial blood pressure and heart rate and stimulating noradrenergic sympathetic nervous outflow.[94] CRF administration also increases locomotor activity.[95] It has been suggested that somatostatin or a related peptide may act within the CNS to inhibit hypothalamic release of CRF following stress.[96] Earlier reports, although contradictory, had indicated that hypothalamic bioactive CRF content increases after stress.[97] There are also discrepancies in the reported effects of adrenalectomy and hypophysectomy on bioactive CRF. However, more recent studies indicate that adrenalectomy and hypophysectomy are associated with increased staining intensity in CRF paraventricular median eminence pathways[79,98] and that decreases in immunoreactive content follow administration of dexamethasone.[99] These findings indicate that CRF concentrations are regulated by neuroendocrine feedback mechanisms.

Little is known about the mechanism of CRF action on the pituitary. Available studies indicate that it stimulates cAMP formation in a manner similar to that of the other releasing hormones.[100] Ovine CRF has been employed clinically as a test of pituitary ACTH reserve.[101] CRF increases plasma ACTH concentrations within 15 min following injection, although, as noted, the magnitude of this rise is less than is seen in other tests employed for detecting the integrity of the ACTH reserve. The widespread availability of synthetic CRF in the near future should help clarify the interrelations between vasopressin and CRF with regard to stress-induced ACTH release.

Growth Hormone Releasing Hormone

Extensive physiological studies have provided evidence for the existence of a growth hormone releasing hormone (GRH). Isolation of a peptide with growth hormone (GH) stimulatory effects has recently been reported.[43,44] Unlike the other hypophysiotropic peptides, this peptide, human pancreatic GRH (hpGRH), was first isolated and characterized not from the hypothalamus, but from pancreatic tumors associated with acromegaly in two patients, both of whom were successfully treated by removal of the pancreatic tumor. The delineation of GRH in these tumors confirmed previous reports in which GH-releasing activity was observed in partially purified extracts of pancreatic, carcinoid, and other neural crest tumors.[102,103] The sequence shown in Fig. 7-12 is the longest of three peptides found in one of the tumors;[44] a 40-amino acid nonamidated peptide, identical in sequence with the NH_2 terminus of the 44-amino acid peptide, was found in the other tumor.[43] Human hypothalamic GRH has now been fully characterized, and its sequence has been shown to be identical with that of hpGRH. The cloning of the human GRH cDNA and gene has also been reported.[104,104a] The cDNA sequence indicates the presence of a precursor containing a 25- or 26-amino acid carboxyl extension following the GRH sequence, the significance of which remains to be established. The structure of GRH from several other species has now been reported. In rat hypothalamic GRH, 30 percent of the residues differ from those described in human GRH,[105] though only one to three residues differ in bovine, ovine, caprine, and porcine GRH.[106] These sequence nonalignments thus reflect species rather than tissue site differences.

GRH 1–44 and GRH 1–40 appear to possess similar GH-releasing potency in vivo, though there is controversy concerning their relative effects in vitro.[105-109] The biologic activity is dependent on the presence of tyrosine or histidine at the amino terminus and fragments as short as GRH 1–29 exhibit full biologic activity. GRH is closely homologous with members of the glucagon/secretin family of peptides, including vasoactive intestinal polypeptide and peptide histidyl-isoleucine (PHI-27), though GRH is not present in the normal human pancreas and appears to be barely detectable in the intestinal tract.[103] Some of these peptides have previously been reported to stimulate GH secretion in various species, either in vivo or in vitro, though they are far less potent than GRH.

The tonic secretion of GH is inhibited by monoclonal antibodies to GRH, emphasizing its physiological importance in the regulation of GH secretion.[110] The effects of GRH are calcium-dependent and include the stimulation of cAMP efflux by pituitary cells in parallel to the release of GH. Its effects are blocked by somatostatin in a noncompetitive manner, while prostaglandin E_2 (PGE_2) in combination with GRH displays a true additive effect, implying that PGE_2 stimulates GH secretion by a mechanism different from that of GRH.[111] In addition to its effects on GH release, GRH also stimulates GH synthesis.[112,113] Treatment of pituitary cells with glucocorticoids enhances their response to GRH both in vitro and in vivo[114-116]—findings consistent with previous observations that glucocorticoids increase GH synthesis and content. The results imply disparate effects of glucocorticoids at hypothalamic and pituitary levels, in view of their known inhibitory effects in vivo on GH secretion.

Immunocytochemical studies indicate that antisera against GRH 1–40 specifically stain neuronal cell bodies in the arcuate nucleus of the human hypothalamus, with fibers projecting to the median eminence.[117] Cell bodies are also seen in the ventromedial nucleus, which had previously been proposed as a center for GRH secretion. Thus GRH, in contrast to somatostatin, exhibits a rather restricted localization in the hypophysiotropic area of the hypothalamus.

In normal subjects, peak GH responses to GRH-stimulated release occur at 15 to 30 min.[118] Responses are dose-related[107] and tend to decrease with age.[119,119a] Continuous infusions of GRH are associated with an attenuation of the GH secretory response due to mechanisms not entirely clear.[120] GRH, originally reported to have a relatively long half-life in circulation,[120a] is rapidly degraded to a biologically inactive metabolic lacking an NH_2-terminal dipeptide.[121]

Prolactin Inhibiting Factor

Available evidence suggests that much of the prolactin inhibitory factor–like activity of hypothalamic extracts may be accounted for by dopamine. Dopamine is present in high concentrations in the median eminence nerve terminals with cell bodies in the arcuate nucleus (tuberoinfundibular tract). Dopamine levels in portal blood are greater than those in peripheral blood, and high-affinity dopamine receptors are present on lactotrophs. Treatment of pituitary cells with dopamine and/or dopaminergic agents leads to rapid inhibition of prolactin secretion and of prolactin gene transcription.[122] Physiological experiments, however, indicate that dopamine does not appear to fully account for the hypothalamic inhibition of prolactin secretion; for example, the magnitude of the decrease in hypothalamic dopamine is insufficient to account for prolactin rises during suckling.[123] It has therefore been suggested that dopamine tonically stimulates the secretion of a separate prolactin inhibiting factor. Candidates for such an additional prolactin inhibiting factor are GABA, α-MSH, the previously noted TRH metabolite histidyl-proline-diketopiperazine, and the catechol estrogen 2-hydroxyestradiol. TRH and estradiol are recognized as stimulators of prolactin secretion, and the ability of their metabolites to limit such stimulation is an intriguing possibility. A recently discovered 56-amino acid peptide, located at the COOH-terminal end of the GnRH precursor, has been shown to exhibit potent prolactin-inhibiting activity[54a,124,125] (and also gonadotropin-releasing effects[124,126]).

Prolactin Releasing Factor

The stimulation of prolactin release by TRH has already been discussed. Recent studies have demonstrated that suckling increases TRH levels in hypophyseal stalk plasma[49] and prolactin responsiveness to TRH. There are also differential effects of TRH on prolactin and TSH secretion under specific conditions; certain stimuli that increase serum prolactin concentrations do not result in a rise in concentrations of serum TSH (e.g., stress, insulin hypoglycemia, or suckling). The observation that suckling is not associated with increases in TSH secretion may be explained by the finding that estradiol, which is present in high concentrations in this physiological state, markedly enhances prolactin responsiveness to TRH. A large number of substances have been reported to cause prolactin release via a direct action on the pituitary. These include VIP, serotonin, β-endorphin, met-enkephalin and leu-enkephalin, neurotensin, bombesin, PHI, angiotensin II, vasopressin, substance P, epidermal growth factor, fibroblast growth factor, cholecystokinin, and estradiol,[123] with VIP the most likely. This peptide is present in hypophyseal stalk plasma, its receptors are present in pituitary membranes, and its uptake in pituitary is localized to lactotrophs. Neutralization of endogenous VIP activity by treatment with anti-VIP serum inhibits the suckling-induced rise in prolactin in rats.[127] Epidermal growth factor has also been shown to rapidly stimulate prolactin gene transcription.[128]

Melanocyte Stimulating Hormone–Inhibiting Factor

Melanocyte stimulating hormone–inhibiting factor (MSH-IF; proline-leucine-glycine amide), obtained from an extract of bovine hypothalamus, has been demonstrated to be effective in causing skin lightening in the frog. This peptide is contained within the structure of oxytocin. A melanocyte stimulating hormone–releasing factor (MSH-RF), also described, is a pentapeptide consisting of the NH_2-terminal amino acids of oxytocin, and it has been suggested that oxytocin is a prohormone for both these peptides (MSH-RF and MSH-IF). There is evidence of species specificity among the related peptides with MSH-IF activity. There are no data in humans as to progressive increase in pigmentation after stalk section like that reported in frogs. MSH-IF does not appear to alter MSH levels in humans. This is consistent with the finding that MSH exists as a separate hormone only in animals with an intermediate lobe and is thus not present in humans. Indeed, in species with an intermediate lobe both dopaminergic and serotonergic innervation have been demonstrated, the former inhibitory to MSH release and the latter stimulatory.

NEUROPEPTIDES

In addition to the hypophysiotropic hormones, a large number of peptides have been demonstrated in vertebrate brain, some of which have been previously characterized in nonneural vertebrate tissues and other species.[32] These include gastrin, cholecystokinin (CCK), VIP, substance P, secretin, PHI, motilin, insulin, glucagon, angiotensin, bradykinin, calcitonin, α-MSH, growth hormone, prolactin, LH, TSH, renin, neurotensin, bombesin, and the endorphins and enkephalins. Except for substance P and neurotensin, for which sequence analysis is available, the similarity of the CNS form of these peptides to their form in other tissues has been determined only by immunochemical, biologic, chromatographic, and/or immunohistochemical means, which does not prove total identity. Only those peptides with demonstrated effects on pituitary hormone secretion are considered in the subsequent section.

Table 7-5 indicates the major reported endocrine effects of these peptides. In most instances, it is believed that the actions of these peptides on pituitary hormone secretion are mediated via neurotransmitters regulating hypophysiotropic secretion or the hypophysiotropic hormones themselves. A number of these peptides are present in high concentrations in the hypothalamus, in particular, the median eminence, raising the possibility of their portal blood transport, with a direct pituitary action; β-endorphin and VIP are among the peptides reported to be present in portal blood, and may serve as prolactin releasing factors. In addition to the data cited in Table 7-5, VIP has been shown to stimulate ACTH release from corticotropic tumors and ACTH-secreting pituitary cell lines but not from normal anterior pituitary tissue.

The contradictory effects noted for neurotensin on GH and prolactin release may be related to mode of administration. Intracerebroventricular administration of neurotensin is associated with inhibition of hormone release, while the stimulation seen following systemic administration may be secondary to the histamine-releasing effects of the peptide. CCK, as well as angiotensin, has been reported to directly stimulate ACTH secretion from anterior pituitary.

It can be seen from Table 7-5 that opioid peptides have a wide range of endocrine effects. Although considerable attention has been given to the central effects of opioid peptides, the pituitary concentrations of β-endorphin (derived from proopiomelanocortin) are significantly greater than those in the central nervous system (1000-fold greater in the intermediate lobe than in the hypothalamus, and 50- to 100-fold greater in the anterior lobe). The possibility of paracrine effects of opioids, therefore, must also be considered. Enkephalin and dynorphin are present in the pituitary, with highest concentrations in the neural lobe, and these concentrations also are greater than those in the hypothalamus. It has been suggested that the peptides in the hypothalamus may represent a storage pool for those in the posterior lobe.

The action of opioids on prolactin release is believed to be mediated via the turnover of dopamine and serotonin, both of which are known to affect prolactin secretion. In addition, opioids may block dopamine effects at the pituitary level. The inhibitory effects of opioids (both β-endorphin and met-enkephalin) on gonadotropin secretion appear to be physiologically significant. Opioid receptors are present on GnRH nerve endings, and this, as well as effects on monoamine turnover, may represent the mechanism(s) for inhibition of LH release. In addition, possible direct pituitary effects are suggested by the presence of opioid peptides in portal blood. Physiological studies indicate an increase in opioid inhibition in the latter half of the follicular phase of the human menstrual cycle. Additionally, opioids decrease pulsatile gonadotropin secretion. The reported effects and locus of action of opioids on ACTH secretion are controversial, with differences in responses between normal human subjects and patients with ACTH hypersecretion.

Assessment of opioid effects on vasopressin secretion is complex, in view of the presence of enkephalinergic and dynorphinergic fibers arising from the magnocellular nuclei in the posterior pituitary. Whether such fibers regulate vasopressin release or whether the opioids and vasopressin are cosecreted, with possible resultant effects on the posterior pituitary, remains to be elucidated. The presence of both stimulatory and inhibitory effects, as noted in Table 7-5, may reflect central versus peripheral actions similar to those of neurotensin.

Substance P

The demonstration of substance P in the brain resulted from studies in which attempts to purify CRF led to the identification of a sialagogic peptide, which was found to be identical with the substance P previously isolated from the gastrointestinal tract.[129] It is present in high concentrations in the hypothalamus, preoptic area, brainstem, and mesencephalon, with the highest levels noted in the reticular portion of the substantia nigra and differential concentrations found among various septal, preoptic, and hypothalamic nuclei.[130] Substance P appears to function as a neurotransmitter. Release from synaptosomes and perfused spinal cord has been demonstrated. Substance P inhibits CRF- or vasopressin-stimulated ACTH release but not basal ACTH release.[131]

Neurotensin

Neurotensin, a tetradecapeptide, was discovered during the isolation of substance P, because of its marked vasodilatory effects.[132] The hypothalamus contains 30 percent of its brain content, the greater part of the remainder being in the midbrain and brainstem. The total CNS content of neurotensin represents only one-tenth of that in small intestine. These brain and intestinal forms are chemically identical.

In addition to effects on circulation (causing vasodilatation and hypotension), neurotensin also causes marked hyperglycemia in hypophysectomized, adrenalectomized, or morphine-, phenoxybenzamine-, or propranolol-treated animals.[133] Its hyperglycemic effects are largely due to stimulation of glucagon secretion and inhibition of insulin secretion, which are mediated in part by the adrenal medulla and in part by histamine.[134] It also stimulates GH, prolactin, TSH, ACTH, and possibly gonadotropin secretion. Since these results are seen after intravenous injection, they do not rule out the possibility that the endocrine effects are secondary to the vasodilating effects. In contrast, cerebroventricular administration of neurotensin inhibits the release of GH, prolactin, and TSH[135] and also produces hypothermia.[136]

Angiotensin

Angiotensin I has been demonstrated within the CNS by both immunohistochemical and radioimmunoassay methods, with the highest concentrations in the subfornical organ, corpus callosum, hypothalamus, choroid plexus, and pars intermedia. Angiotensin II receptors have also been demonstrated within the CNS, with the highest specific binding in hypothalamic and midbrain thalamic regions. To date there has been no demonstration of intracellular synthesis or demonstration of release of neurally synthesized material. Intraventricular administration of angiotensin has been reported to cause water-replete animals to drink and also to stimulate vasopressin release. Since these effects have also been reported following systemic angiotensin administration, the role of the material presumably synthesized within the CNS is unclear.

Endorphins and Enkephalins

The discovery several years ago of the existence in the central nervous system of opioid peptide receptors (now known to include four subtypes—μ, δ, κ, and ϵ—with different affinities for the various types of opioids described below) and the subsequent identification of endogenous opioid peptides (endorphins, met-enkephalin and leu-enkephalin, and dynorphins) have generated considerable interest. Enkephalins are considered to be ligands for δ receptors, β-endorphin for both μ and δ receptors, and dynorphin and related peptides for κ receptors.

The demonstration that β-LPH, which contains within it the sequences of β-MSH, methionine-enkephalin, and β-endorphin 1–31, was present in brain as well as in its only previously described site of production, the pituitary, led to many studies characterizing the distribution of these diverse peptides, the possible precursor role of β-LPH in the formation of these fragments in the tissues in which they are present (other opioid peptides can be derived via posttranslational processing of β-endorphin: β-endorphin 1–27, β-endorphin 1–26, and their acetylated derivatives), and their physiological role. There is still considerable controversy as to the exact chemical nature and similarity of the various opioid peptides found in different regions of the central nervous system and in the pituitary gland and the exact anatomic sites of their distribution. Some of these difficulties lie in the absence of specific antisera with which to characterize the various fragments as well as the lack of sufficient material in some instances to allow for complete structural determination. β-LPH has been demonstrated in the anterior lobe of the pituitary in many species. Figure 7-13 shows the chemical structure of β-LPH and some of these other fragments. When initially detected in the brain, it was thought that β-LPH was the precursor of both brain endorphin and brain enkephalin. The 65 position in β-LPH is methionine, and this therefore could be the precursor only of met-enkephalin but not of leu-enkephalin, both of which have been demonstrated to occur in the brain of pigs, cows, and humans, though in varying proportions. It is now established that the enkephalins described in brain arise from a precursor, preproenkephalin A, which contains both met- and leu-enkephalin sequences.

There is some controversy as to the relative proportional localization of the opioid peptides (endorphins and enkephalins) in the pituitary lobes. An additional opioidlike peptide (dynorphin) has also been isolated from pituitary extracts.[137] This arises from still another precursor, preproenkephalin B, which, in addition to the dynorphin sequence, also contains leu-enkephalin sequences. These two precursors, in addition to proopiomelanocortin, appear to account for all known endogenous opioid peptides.

Although opioid receptors,[40] β-endorphin,[43] enkephalin,[45] dynorphin, and β-LPH[46] have been demonstrated within the central nervous system—the last three by either immunohistochemistry or specific radioimmunoassay—there is no precise correlation

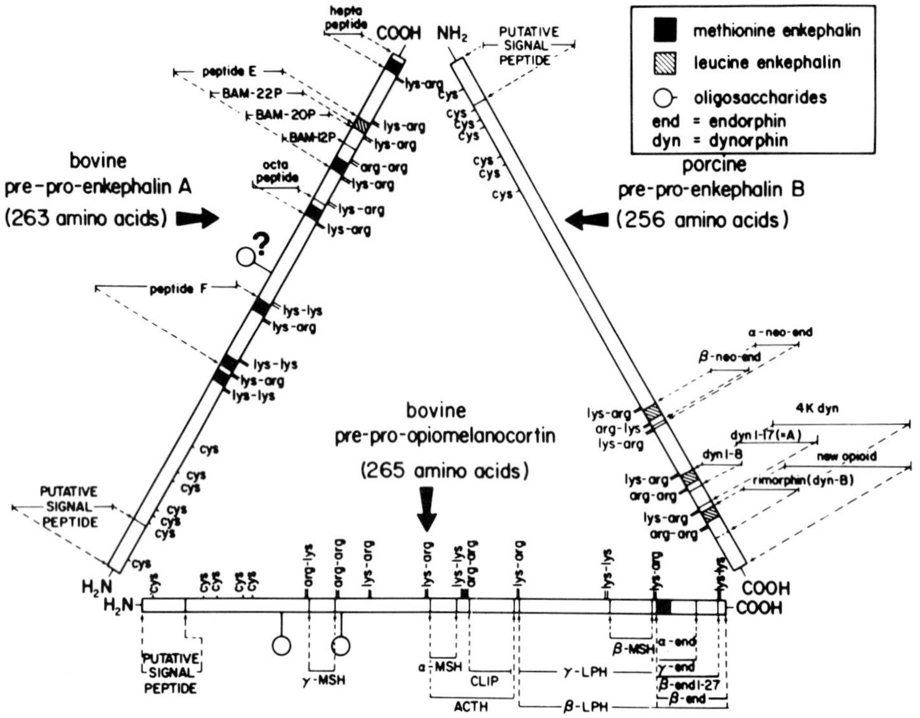

FIGURE 7-13 Schematic representation of bovine preproopiomelanocortin, bovine preproenkephalin A, and porcine preproenkephalin B. The heptapeptide is 6-arginyl-7-phenylalanyl-met-enkephalin; the octapeptide is 6-arginyl-7-glycyl-8-leucyl-met-enkephalin; BAM-P = bovine adrenal medulla peptides. γ-MSH occupies positions 61 to 77 in the NH_2-terminal fragment; γ_2-MSH occupies positions 51 to 62.

between concentrations of opioid receptors and those of either enkephalin or endorphin. There is likewise differential distribution of endorphin and enkephalin within the central nervous system. The cell bodies giving rise to enkephalinergic pathways are in the olfactory bulb, caudate, putamen, and paraventricular and supraoptic nuclei, whereas the arcuate nucleus is the source of β-endorphin-containing pathways. There is not always a strict correspondence between the density of a given opioid projection system in a given anatomic area and the number of opiate receptors present there. Incubation of β-LPH with extracts of rat brain or of posterior pituitary generates substances with opioid activity. The nature of the factors regulating central nervous system concentrations of opioidlike peptides is not clear; various agents seem to have different effects on concentration in brain, anterior pituitary lobe, and intermediate lobe. β-Endorphin concentrations appear to decrease in brain and intermediate lobe following estradiol administration, though the effects of stress or adrenalectomy do not appear to affect pituitary or brain concentrations of β-endorphin.

The relationship between the brain and the pituitary opioid systems is unclear, as is the normal mechanism of action of these opioid peptides. Whether the effects of endorphin and enkephalin and other opioid-like peptides are mediated solely by their effects on opioid receptors, whether they function as neurotransmitters or as neuromodulatory agents, and whether they affect the concentrations of other neurotransmitters are questions under active investigation. There are reports of increases in brain serotonin levels and inhibition of acetylcholine turnover following β-endorphin administration,[138] whereas enkephalin may decrease catecholamine turnover as well as that of acetylcholine.[139] Opioids acutely inhibit neuronal firing and hyperpolarize the membranes of most responsive cells. Among the second messenger mechanisms suggested as effecting opioid actions are their inhibition of Ca^{2+} uptake into nerve terminals and inhibition of basal and dopamine-stimulated adenylate cyclase activity (perhaps secondary to the inhibition of Ca^{2+} uptake), and as a result, impairment of protein phosphorylation. It has been suggested that electrical stimulation of centers in the central gray area of the brain inhibits the firing of nerves carrying pain signals into the spinal cord; similar effects have been produced by direct injection of morphine or endorphin into this area. Analgesia produced by electrical stimulation of these areas can be partially blocked by naloxone, a specific opioid antagonist, and it has recently been demonstrated that electrical stimulation of these areas results in endorphin release.

Analgesic doses of morphine injected into the periaqueductal region of the brain produce hyperactivity; injection of β-endorphin has been reported to induce both a catalepsy-like state[140] and a state of behavioral immobilization associated with rigidity or placidity and hyperactivity.[141] A possible relation of these peptides to mental disease has been suggested, but no convincing reports of effects of these peptides in mental illness are currently available. Other possible behavioral roles for the endorphins and enkephalins have been suggested. It has been reported that fragments of ACTH as well as lysine vasopressin derivatives have marked behavioral effects on animals (see below). β-Endorphin and the fragments β-LPH 66–69 and β-endorphin 51–76 are more active than ACTH fragments during psychological tests which are believed to reflect increased memory retention.

The role of endogenous opioids in addiction to or withdrawal from opioids is unclear. Neuroblastoma glioma cells have been shown to have opiate receptors. Acute exposure of clones of such cells to opioids results in inhibition of basal levels of adenylate cyclase. Chronic exposure of such cells to opioids leads to a compensatory increase in the amount of adenylate cyclase activity, and subsequent withdrawal of morphine from the tolerant cells leads to immediate large increases in cAMP levels above those normally found.[142]

There have been numerous reports of the stimulatory effect of morphine on release of ACTH, GH, and prolactin, and many of these effects are duplicated by opioidlike peptides. It has been suggested, on the basis of studies with opiate antagonists, that different types of opiate receptors mediate secretion of the various pituitary hormones: μ and ϵ receptors for prolactin, μ receptors for TSH and ACTH, δ or κ receptors for LH, and δ receptors for GH.[143] Some of these observations are complicated by the fact that in many instances modified enkephalins (with altered stereochemistry or receptor binding) or naloxone (assumed to act as a pure opioid antagonist, although it has agonist properties and may also interact with other neurotransmitter receptors) were used to investigate endocrine effects. Stimulatory effects of β-endorphin and met- and leu-enkephalin on prolactin and GH release have been reported following intraventricular injection.[144,145] The effect of leu-enkephalin on prolactin was not antagonized by naloxone,[146] but that on GH was;[147] the effects of β-endorphin and met-enkephalin were reported to be reversible by naloxone. No stimulatory effects were seen when endorphin was incubated with short-term cultured dispersed pituitary cells, suggesting a central nervous system site of action, perhaps through regulation of dopamine, despite the known presence of pituitary opiate receptors. γ-Endorphin and leu-enkephalin have been reported to release LH and FSH in vitro. The majority of observations, however, indicate that opioids suppress circulating LH and, to a lesser extent, FSH. Opioid antagonists increase the pulsatility of serum gonadotropin concentrations. There appears to be more "opioid tone" in the late follicular phase of the menstrual cycle. In vivo, morphine and met-enkephalin are reported to decrease serum LH and TSH concentrations; these effects are reduced by concurrent naloxone administration. Although acute morphine administration increases ACTH levels while chronic administration suppresses its release,[148] as yet no consistent effects of opioidlike peptides on the ACTH system have been reported.

EFFECT OF HORMONES ON BRAIN

The effects of hypophysiotropic hormones have been discussed in the preceding section. This section deals with the effects of pituitary and other peptides on brain function and those of target gland hormones administered exogenously, during physiological variations, and in disease.

Peptide Hormone–Nervous System Interactions

Evidence has been steadily accumulating that certain of the pituitary peptide hormones, namely, ACTH, β-endorphin, MSH, and vasopressin, have marked effects on learning and behavior in rats.[149] It has further been shown that even fragments of these peptides which are devoid of the endocrine effects of the parent hormones are effective. Additionally, these peptides and peptide fragments have marked effects in the absence of either the pituitary or the adrenals. Behavioral effects have been noted in hypophysectomized animals, and such defects are not corrected by corticosteroid administration. Administration of corticosteroids to hypophysectomized or intact animals has effects opposite to those of ACTH and its analogues. These studies imply, therefore, that these peptides and peptide fragments have direct effects on the central nervous system. In most instances the effects of these peptides are not marked in intact animals.

The parameters usually tested are the rate of acquisition of avoidance behavior (interpreted as facilitating learning), and inhibition of extinction of avoidance behavior (interpreted as facilitating short-term memory). The smallest effective fragment with regard to learning is the 4–7 amino acid sequence of the ACTH molecule; effects on memory can be elicited with the 4–10 fragment. It has been suggested that these compounds affect learning and memory by increasing the state of arousal of the animal.

β-Endorphin and smaller opioid fragments, as well as the enkephalins (see Fig. 7-13), exhibit behavioral effects. Facilitation of learning behavior has been reported for α- and β-endorphin and for minute doses of met-enkephalin and leu-enkephalin administered subcutaneously. γ-Endorphin usually produced opposite effects. Table 7-7 indicates the generally opposing behavioral effects of ACTH fragments and of β-endorphin.[150] This is consistent with reports that these two types of compounds have opposite effects on concentrations of brain neurotransmitters and of cAMP, as well as on neuronal firing rates. Also indicated in Table 7-7 are the behavioral effects of γ_2-MSH, a peptide present within the POMC sequence (see Fig. 7-13). γ_2-MSH and ACTH-related peptides appear to have opposite effects on certain brain functions while exhibiting similar effects on others. These findings, and the opposing behavioral effects of α- and γ-endorphin, raise the questions of whether there may be differential processing of POMC-derived peptides in different terminal areas as well as differential receptor distribution and whether the different peptides interact in a given area as a local feedback modulatory system.

There is also some evidence that ACTH and β-MSH antagonize morphine inhibition of spinal reflex activity. ACTH 4–10 has an affinity for opiate receptors, although the calculated dissociation constant is rather high. γ_2-MSH also has an affinity for opiate receptors. ACTH 1–39 and ACTH 1–24 antagonize the analgesic effect of morphine in the rat. This is not compatible, however, with the clinical observation that patients with adrenocortical insufficiency exhibit increased sensitivity to the effects of morphine. Such patients have markedly elevated levels of ACTH.

It has not yet been demonstrated that these fragments normally occur within the pituitary gland, nor is it clear whether the brain synthesizes such peptide fragments or whether they are either derived by retrograde portal blood flow or transport by the CSF or taken up from the bloodstream. In the latter instance one would postulate that the brain itself

Table 7-7. Various Effects of β-Endorphin, ACTH Neuropeptides, and γ_2-MSH in a Variety of Animal Experiments

	β-Endorphin	ACTH (1–24, 4–10)	γ_2-MSH
Avoidance and sexual behavior			
Extinction of pole-jumping avoidance behavior	−	−	+
Passive avoidance	+/−	+	−
Acquisition of shuttle box avoidance	N.D.	+	−
Motivation of sexual behavior	−	+	N.D.
Excessive grooming	+	+	−*
Opioid-related effects			
Opioid-induced antinociception	+	−	−
Opioid-induced hypothermia	+	−	−
Opioid-induced catatonia	+	−	N.D.
Tonic immobility	+	−	−
Pseudo abstinence syndrome (PAS)	N.D.	+	+
Acquisition of heroin self-administration	+	0	−
β-Endorphin-induced α-MSH release	+	N.D.	−
Naloxone binding	+	+	+
Electrical and neurochemical effects			
Single cell activity	−	+	N.D.
Hippocampal theta activity	+	+	N.D.
Catecholamine transmission	−	+	N.D.
Acetylcholine transmission	−	+	N.D.
cAMP activity in brain	−	+	N.D.

*ACTH induced excessive grooming.
Key: +, facilitation, induction; −, attenuation; N.D., not determined.
Source: De Wied D, *Prog Brain Res* 55:473, 1982.

might contain specific enzymes for production of the fragments from the intact ACTH molecule.

Animals lacking a posterior pituitary do not exhibit defects in memory retention. They do, however, exhibit defects in extinction of avoidance behavior. Although ACTH is also effective in correcting the defect in extinction of avoidance behavior, it does so only if administered during the extinction period, whereas vasopressin is effective irrespective of the time of treatment. Arginine vasopressin appears to be the most potent peptide of the vasopressin-like substances; oxytocin and arginine vasotocin have only 20 percent of the activity of arginine vasopressin. Analogues of vasopressin such as desglycinamide lysine vasopressin which have no endocrine effects produce behavioral effects similar to those of vasopressin. In some experimental paradigms, oxytocin has behavioral effects opposite to those of vasopressin. In addition to their effects on learning, vasopressin and vasopressin analogues facilitate the development of resistance to the analgesic action of morphine in mice and rats and also correct the reduction of the hippocampal θ frequency observed during paradoxical sleep in vasopressin-deficient Brattleboro animals.

The site of action of these peptides and peptide fragments has been explored in rats bearing lesions in various brain regions as well as by implantation of fragments in the brain. It appears that the parafascicular area of the thalamus is essential for ACTH fragment action. It is also likely that intact midbrain limbic connections are required for these neuropeptides to exert their behavioral effects. The parafascicular nuclei are sensitive to the administration of vasopressin, but they are not essential for its action. The midbrain limbic structures have an important role in mediating vasopressin effects on the persistence of learned responses.

The neurotransmitter basis for the effects of these peptides is a matter of question. ACTH 4–10 increases catecholamine turnover and synthesis in the brains of intact rats but does not do so in hypophysectomized or adrenalectomized animals, even though, as noted, it has behavioral effects in such animals. It has been suggested that the central effects of vasopressin are mediated by modulation of neurotransmission in catecholamine systems distributed throughout the dorsal adrenergic bundle. It has also been proposed that some behavioral effects of peripherally administered vasopressin are secondary to hemodynamic effects on central neurotransmitter concentrations; a pressor antagonist analogue of arginine vasopressin has been shown to abolish behavioral effects of peripheral vasopressin administration.[151,152] A number of peptides present in brain, including those derived from proopiomelanocortin, as discussed above, have marked effects on major body homeostatic systems such as blood pressure, feeding, and temperature (see Ref. 32 for review).

It is apparent that although a role for neuropeptides in cognitive function appears to have been shown, the specificity of the responses, their peripheral vs. central action, and their biochemical and physiological basis require extended investigation. Following initial reports in animals, studies were undertaken to assess their applicability to human learning and memory. There are both positive and negative reports that systemic administration of ACTH 4–10 can increase attention and visual discrimination; most such studies have been performed in young, healthy volunteers.[153,154] Administration of both lysine vasopressin and a synthetic analogue has been associated with improved performance in tests measuring long-term memory, while other reports have related improvement in patients suffering from retrograde amnesia.[155,156] Still unexplained is the long duration of the effect of administration of all the above-noted peptides on the behaviors tested.

Preliminary data show that CRF may produce central behavioral activation. The relation of such effects to alterations in brain concentrations of POMC-related peptides, as well as to vasopressin and to the reported stimulatory effects of CRF on adrenal medullary catecholamine secretion, remain to be investigated.

Effects of Target Gland Hormones on Central Nervous System Function

Disturbances in both cognitive and affective function have been described in many endocrine diseases, but most of these have not been systematically studied. Patients with Addison's disease are frequently described as manifesting confusion and depression. The EEG shows diffuse high-amplitude, slow-activity patterns, and thresholds for taste, smell, and hearing are decreased. No attempt has been made to separate these cases into primary and secondary adrenocortical insufficiency.

Patients with adrenocortical hyperfunction are also reported to exhibit anxiety, depression, and decreased cognitive function. In most instances, onset of psychiatric symptoms coincides with the onset of the physical stigmata of disease. There is an approximately 10 percent incidence of psychosis. In two reports[157,158] but not in another,[159] patients with adrenal adenomas (high cortisol, low ACTH levels) had a less severe neuropsychiatric disability than those with Cushing's disease. A higher prevalence of euphoria

(50 percent compared with 4 percent of patients with Cushing's disease) affords some insight into the effects of exogenous corticosteroid administration on central nervous system function. There was a similar prevalence of psychosis and a lesser prevalence of depression. The variability in symptoms appears to be dose-related with regard to exogenous steroids, although no correlation between the severity of depression and the level of circulating cortisol was seen in patients with Cushing's disease. The nature of the behavioral response does not appear to be correlated with the patient's pretreatment personality. Depression was rapidly relieved with effective therapy (either adrenalectomy or medical treatment) in cases of Cushing's disease and Cushing's syndrome. The relation of these behavioral disorders to the hypersecretion of cortisol in patients with endogenous depression remains to be clarified. The favorable therapeutic response of patients with Cushing's disease to lowering of plasma cortisol rather than ACTH concentrations indicates that the psychiatric disturbance in these patients is secondary to adrenal hyperactivity rather than the reverse.

Disturbances are also seen with parathyroid hyperfunction: 50 percent of patients show evidence of altered cognitive processes, whereas 10 percent manifest psychosis and another 30 percent exhibit unclassified psychiatric symptoms.[160] Limited data exist as to whether different causes of hyperparathyroidism are associated with different percentages of each of these defects. Some of the abnormalities are reversed with treatment of the disease. In hyperparathyroidism a linear relationship is present between impairment of cognition and increasing serum calcium level. Thirty percent of the patients manifest depression, and there is some evidence of reversal of this phenomenon with treatment of the hyperparathyroid state.

Patients with thyroid disease have classically been noted to manifest disturbances in nervous system function. Patients with hypothyroidism exhibit deterioration of recent memory and difficulty in concentration. In severe cases there is slowing of the dominant EEG frequency. The central nervous system is the first organ system to show improvement when thyroid medication is begun. Similar disturbances are reported in hyperthyroidism.

The nature of the affective disturbances, in contrast, appears to be related to an increase or decrease in thyroid hormone concentration. In hypothyroid patients the predominant disturbance is a marked depression of mood; some may manifest a peculiar facetiousness. In hyperthyroid patients the main complaints are anxiety, fatigue, and irritability; no severe depressive effect is present. Although motor activity is increased, these patients are not hypomanic in the generally accepted psychiatric sense. In both groups of patients there is usually a return to normal functioning with correction of the endocrine defect.

Mental changes seen in patients with pituitary disease can usually be related to those described above for target organ failure. Additionally a loss of libido is common. Corticosteroid replacement therapy corrects most of the abnormalities seen; libidinal changes are corrected by gonadal hormone therapy. There still may be some residual fatigue and apathy following such replacement—a role of growth hormone and perhaps other unknown pituitary hormones is possible.

The effects of hypoglycemia secondary to hyperinsulinism are not considered here, since these are not strictly manifestations of hormonal effects on the brain.

Behavioral changes have also been noted in relation to the menstrual cycle[161] and have become a matter of considerable legal interest.[162] The syndrome of premenstrual tension has been frequently described (with an incidence varying from 25 to almost 100 percent, depending on the criteria employed for definition), with manifestations varying among individuals (e.g., headache, depression, nausea, fluid retention, altered sexual desire, and irritability). There are also reports of exacerbation of psychiatric illness during the premenstrual period. It has been suggested that there are a variety of "premenstrual syndromes."[163]

No specific hormonal changes have been correlated with this syndrome to date, although there are claims that plasma progesterone levels are decreased. Double-blind studies have failed to confirm a therapeutic value of progesterone in treatment of premenstrual symptoms. The long list of other treatments (e.g., diuretics, aldosterone antagonists, tranquilizers, oral contraceptives, lithium) attests to their lack of efficacy and the lack of definition of the etiology of this syndrome. None of these treatments has survived rigorous controlled clinical testing. Recently, the efficacy of bromocriptine has been reported,[164] although there is no convincing evidence of hyperprolactinemia in these patients.

Plasma monoamine oxidase (MAO) levels have been reported to be elevated in premenstrual women. It has been suggested, but not proved, that this is inversely related to brain catecholamine rhythms. High MAO activity has also been associated with depression. There are still no data as to how steroids affect MAO levels or activity; observed interrelationships are conjectural at present. There is also no evidence that the peripheral changes in MAO activity during the cycle occur within the central nervous system.

Effects of Hormones on Sexual Dimorphism of the Brain

In both the rodent and the human, evidence suggests that exposure to prenatal (human) or neonatal (rat) androgen is associated with a sex-dependent difference in brain organization. In the rat exposure to neonatal androgen (endogenous in the male, exogenous in the female) is associated with acryclic (male-type) pituitary gonadotropin release and masculine sexual behavior responses. Female animals or males treated with neonatal estrogen exhibit female patterns of sexual behavior and of hormone release (the latter is especially true if estrogen is given to castrated neonatal males). Sexually dimorphic patterns of GH secretion are also altered by modifying the neonatal hormonal environment.[164a] There is a critical period for these effects; they are not seen if hormone treatment is withheld until after the neonatal period.[165] The critical period for mechanisms regulating cyclic secretion of gonadotropin and female sexual behavior differs from that for regulation of male sexual behavior.

Several questions arise with regard to the basis of these changes and the hormonal factors responsible. Sexual dimorphism has been demonstrated neuroanatomically in several areas in the rat (male rats have fewer nonamygdaloid synapses on dendrites in the preoptic area than do female animals; there is less axonal sprouting in the hippocampus of adult male rats following damage than in female rats; there are differences in the volume of the supraoptic and spinal bulbocavernosus nuclei in male and female animals). Electrophysiological studies show that more of the cells projecting to the mediobasal hypothalamus receive synaptic connections from the amygdala in male than in normal female animals or neonatally castrated males, while other neurons have a faster firing rate in normal female and neonatally castrated males than in normal males. Such dimorphism is also present in human brain. Asymmetry patterns of male and female brains differ: the splenium (the caudal or posterior portion of the corpus callosum) is larger in the female than in the male,[166] as is the planum temporale of the cortex. It is believed that such dimorphism can be correlated with known behavioral differences in male and female rodents, and perhaps in humans. Female rodents display more exploratory mobility than do males, and enhancement of sexual behavior in female rats has been reported following neonatal transplantation of brain tissue from males.[167] In humans, male dyslexic patients fail to show the hemispheric size discrepancy in the planum temporale seen in normal subjects.

Considerable effort has been spent on elucidating which gonadal hormones are involved in such sexual dimorphism.[168] The effects are not seen with dihydrotestosterone, which cannot be aromatized, but are seen with androgens which can be aromatized and also with 17β-estradiol. Rats treated with testosterone and an estrogen antagonist do not exhibit the syndrome of neonatal androgenization. Both estrogen and testosterone enhance neuritic proliferation in organotypic cultures of specific regions of the preoptic area; the nonaromatizable 5α-dihydrotestosterone has no such effect. There is a strong correlation between the presence of [^{3}H]-estradiol-concentrating neurons and the regional localization of the neuritic response.[169] Brain tissue is capable of aromatizing androgens, and it is believed that the effects of androgens are due to their intracellular conversion within brain, since the high levels of both circulating and CNS α-fetoprotein present in the neonate serve to bind maternal and fetal estrogen, making it unavailable for any interaction with brain steroid receptors. A major concern of this interpretation is that although there do appear to be periods during early development when circulating androgen levels are higher in males than in females, this difference is small and in many cases transient. The α-fetoprotein-protection hypothesis does not apply to all species, since in the human only approximately 0.1 percent of circulating α-fetoprotein binds estrogen. Other observations also are inconsistent with the idea that androgen acts entirely via conversion to estrogen.[170] 5α-Reductase is present in brain and is responsible for 5α reduction of both testosterone and progesterone, and it has been proposed that progesterone may attenuate testosterone action.[171,172] Cytosol estrogen-binding, progesterone-binding, and androgen-binding proteins have been demonstrated in the neonatal brain. Tissue concentrations of such receptors change rapidly during and after the critical period, as does their regional distribution. There is nuclear translocation of the estrogen receptor in neonatal male brains and in those of female animals treated with testosterone but not in brains from female and castrated male animals. It has also been noted that phenoxybenzamine can prevent the masculinizing action of testosterone. The possible interrelations of monoamines, hormone effects on monoamines, and receptor concentrations and/or affinity still remain to be explored.[173] It should also be stressed that there is species diversity in the neural organization that expresses sexual dimorphism and in the nature of the hormones that activate sexual responses and promote sexual differentiation.

Confirmation of such early hormonal effects in humans has been difficult. The most suitable subjects are those with congenital adrenal hyperplasia. Another group are patients whose mothers received oral progestins for treatment of high-risk pregnancy. It has been stated that girls in both categories exhibited a greater incidence of "masculine" behavior than matched controls and that patients in both groups have significantly higher IQ scores than the population norm. However, if one used unaffected siblings as the comparison group, it was noted that the entire families of patients with the adrenogenital syndrome showed higher IQs than expected. Such a consideration would not be applied to those subjects who were masculinized as a result of treatment with masculinizing synthetic progestogens.[174] A subsequent, more extensive study produced data at variance with the finding that an excess of androgenic steroids had a positive effect on IQ scores.[175]

Female patients with congenital adrenal hyperplasia (subsequent to treatment), as well as female primates exposed to perinatal androgen, can display cyclic gonadotropic release and female sexual behavior. There are also limited studies in primates and human beings suggestive of a sex-dependent difference in brain organization with regard to behavioral testing.[176–178] The evidence for a role of prenatal hormones in the development of sexual orientation is inconclusive.

THE PINEAL GLAND

The pineal gland originates as a neuroepithelial evagination protruding from the roof of the diencephalon. It is an extremely vascular organ. In the human two different types of cells are found, the pinealocytes of neuroepithelial origin, which no longer have the photoreceptor function seen in lower vertebrates, and modified glial cells. Cytoplasmic processes from the pinealocytes have been observed to terminate within the perivascular spaces. The pineal gland is in close contact with the cerebrospinal fluid of the aqueduct. It is not known whether there is direct pineal secretion into the CSF. Pineal secretion into the vascular system has been proposed to explain the finding (see below) of pineal hormones in plasma and urine, as well as in tissues which lack the enzyme activity required for their synthesis.

Synthesis of Pineal Principles

The innervation of the pineal is unique. It is derived almost completely from autonomic postganglionic fibers originating in the superior cervical ganglion. Such fibers form synapses on pineal parenchymal cells. The afferent projections to the superior cervical ganglia are believed to derive from either the inferior accessory optic tract or the retinohypothalamic fiber systems. Norepinephrine is found in the sympathetic nerve endings in the pineal gland, and in addition, serotonin is present in both the pinealocytes and the sympathetic nerve terminals. Serotonin serves as a precursor for one of the pineal "hormones," melatonin. Tryptophan is taken up by the pinealocytes and is converted to 5-hydroxytryptophan and then to serotonin. The conversion of serotonin to melatonin requires two enzymatic steps, the first a rate-limiting step involving serotonin *N*-acetyltransferase, which converts serotonin to *N*-acetylserotonin (*N*-acetyltransferase is stimulated by β-adrenergic input, which itself is potentiated by postsynaptic α-adrenergic receptors,[179] and the second, hydroxyindole-O-methyl transferase (HIOMT), which transfers a methyl group to *N*-acetylserotonin, leading to melatonin formation. HIOMT activity is highly concentrated within the pineal, although it has been detected in other organs such as the retina and the harderian gland, a small orbital structure in human beings.

Pineal serotonin, melatonin *N*-serotonin-acetyltransferase, and HIOMT concentrations exhibit a circadian variation. In the rat, maximum levels of serotonin and the two enzymes are attained during the daytime light period and fall markedly soon after the onset of darkness, at which time melatonin concentrations, which are low during the light period, begin to rise.[180]

The relationship of light, the sympathetic nervous system, and pineal indoles and hormones is illustrated in Fig. 7-14.[181] The effect of light is presumably mediated via a cholinergic input to the suprachiasmatic nucleus.[182] Lack of photo input (darkness) increases postganglionic sympathetic activity, thereby releasing norepinephrine from the terminals on the pineal cells. Resultant activation (via β-adrenergic receptor stimulation) of adenylate cyclase in the pinealocytes leads to increased activity of tryptophan hydroxylase (converting tryptophan to 5-hydroxytryptophan), serotonin *N*-acetyltransferase, and HIOMT, producing a decrease in serotonin concentrations and an increase in melatonin concentration. A reverse effect is seen following light exposure. As indicated in the figure, other manipulations which can activate the sympathetic system can overcome the inhibiting effect of light. Insulin-induced hypoglycemia or immobilization stress result in increased pineal enzyme levels.

The circadian variation in concentration of pineal melatonin (and of the constituent substances necessary for melatonin synthesis) is mirrored by a similar circadian variation in plasma and urine melatonin concentration. It is of interest that in both the rat, a nocturnal animal, and the human, a diurnal one, peak melatonin concentrations occur in the dark period. The circadian variation in plasma and urine melatonin

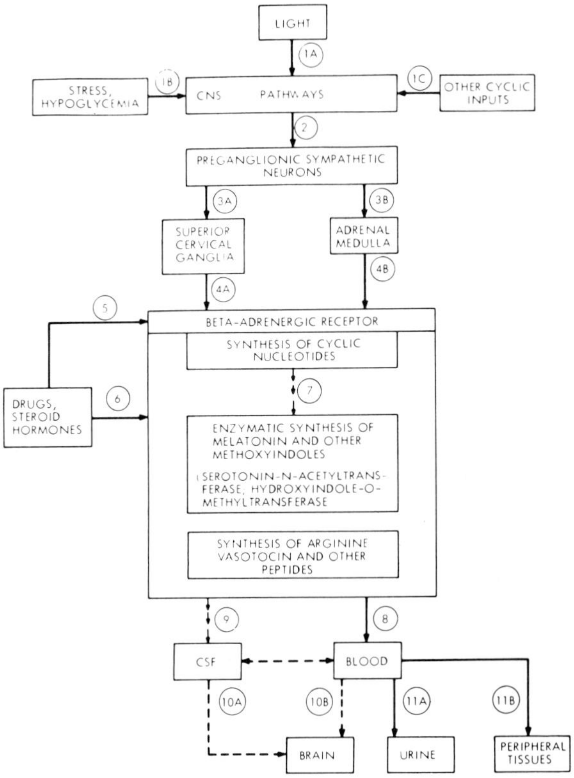

FIGURE 7-14 Schematic diagram showing the factors that control pineal hormone secretion and the delivery of pineal hormone (or hormones) to target organs. The major input controlling pineal melatonin synthesis is norepinephrine released from postganglionic sympathetic nerves (3A, 4A). The rate at which norepinephrine is released is decreased by environmental lighting (via a pathway involving the retinas and accessory optic tracts) and can be enhanced by stresses (1B) causing a generalized sympathetic activation; the latter also affect the pineal via epinephrine released into the circulation (3B, 4B). In the absence of cyclic changes in environmental lighting (e.g., when animals are housed under continuous darkness), melatonin synthesis and secretion continue to exhibit circadian rhythmicity, which requires the intactness of the pineal's sympathetic nerves (3A, 4A); hence another cyclic input (1C), perhaps of endogenous origin (i.e., within the brain), may also influence sympathetic nerves. Once released, the norepinephrine and epinephrine act via β-adrenergic receptors on the surface of the pineal cells (4A, 4B) to activate adenylate cyclase and thereby to raise pineal cyclic AMP levels; this compound may mediate the sympathetic nervous control of the enzymes that catalyze melatonin biosynthesis. Drugs that activate noradrenergic receptors directly or indirectly (e.g., levodopa) can also accelerate melatonin biosynthesis. Moreover, estrogens and related steroid hormones, acting by mechanisms that are not fully understood, can modulate the production of melatonin.

Besides melatonin, two other pineal products are thought to have hormonal activity: other methoxyindoles, such as 5-methoxytryptophol, and peptides, such as 8-arginine vasotocin. No information is available concerning control of pineal peptide synthesis.

Melatonin is found in human and calf cerebrospinal fluid in concentrations higher than those concurrently present in the blood; hence the hormone may be secreted directly into the cerebrospinal fluid and not the bloodstream. Its primary site of action is within the brain (10A, 10B), but it may also directly affect the pituitary and other peripheral organs (11B). The levels of melatonin in cerebrospinal fluid, blood, and urine (11A) all exhibit parallel daily variations, peaking during the hours of darkness in all species thus far examined. (*From Wurtman RJ, Moskowitz MA, N Engl J Med 296:1329, 1977.*)

disappears in the pinealectomized rat, in whom such concentrations are still measurable but at a lower level than in the intact animal. The existence of extrapineal sources of melatonin remains controversial; the low levels detected in pinealectomized animals may be related to methodological considerations. Patients with Shy-Drager syndrome or idiopathic orthostatic hypotension, diseases with central and peripheral sympathetic nervous system dysfunction, have reduced levels of plasma melatonin.[183] A possible menstrual-cycle variation in melatonin concentrations may also exist, with highest concentrations at the time of the menses and lowest concentrations at the time of the LH peak. Recent evidence also points to a role for melatonin in the timing of puberty. Nocturnal peaks of melatonin are greatest in childhood, diminish in the late prepubertal period, and are associated with the nocturnal secretory pulses of LH which herald the onset of puberty.

Hormones other than melatonin have also been described within the pineal gland. These include other methoxyindoles, arginine vasotocin, and possibly GnRH, TRH, and renin. It should be noted that the synthesis of such principles by the pineal has not yet been demonstrated. It may well be that there are additional pineal hormones which can explain some of the observed effects of pinealectomy and pineal extracts on endocrine function. In the experimental animal, pinealectomy results in evidence of stimulation of the pituitary-gonadal axis in both male and female animals. Prepubertal pinealectomy results in premature sexual development, and increased LH and FSH levels are found in the pituitaries of pinealectomized animals. Increased thyroid weight, ^{131}I uptake, and thyroid hormone secretion have been reported in such animals, as has evidence of adrenocortical activation manifested by both increased weight and increased hormonal secretion (aldosterone, corticosterone). Many but not all of these effects are reversed by melatonin administration. It has been suggested that such effects are mediated via serotonergic pathways. In animals, the nocturnal release of melatonin appears to relay the photoperiodic time cues through which seasonal species respond to the annual cycle in day length.

The locus of action of melatonin in producing its effects has been investigated mostly in the gonadal sphere. In some species, melatonin inhibits the pituitary LH response to injected GnRH both in vivo and in vitro. It has also been suggested that it suppresses gonadal function by an action on central nervous system GnRH. Intraperitoneal administration of melatonin has been shown to elevate brain serotonin concentrations, and uptake of melatonin by CNS has been demonstrated. Whether these are physiological or pharmacological effects remains to be determined. Other evidence for a CNS action of melatonin includes the observation that it causes EEG pattern changes consistent with sleep stages in cats and may cause sedation and sometimes sleep in cats and in human beings. Melatonin has been demonstrated in the cerebrospinal fluid, with steady-state levels in CSF being greater than those in peripheral blood. This has suggested, but not proved, that the pineal secretes melatonin into the CSF. There is some evidence for melatonin-binding sites in brain.

Under certain conditions a progonadal action of melatonin has been observed in certain species. The role of melatonin in human gonadal function has not been well characterized (see Diseases of the Pineal Gland, below). It should not be assumed that all the effects of pinealectomy are mediated by melatonin secretion, since it has already been noted that several other hormones exist within the pineal gland.

CNS RHYTHMS AND NEUROENDOCRINE FUNCTION

Rhythms in the levels of many bodily constituents are present throughout the evolutionary scale, though their origin, interrelationship, and biologic significance are matters of speculation.[185] The rhythms cover a large range of frequencies. The major classifications are daily, seasonal, and annual rhythms. Rhythms with approximately 24-h periodicity are called *circadian. Ultradian* rhythms are those with periods shorter than 24 h, and *infradian* rhythms are those with periods longer than 24 h. Rhythms are considered to be either endogenous (having an origin with the organism) or exogenous (existence depending upon a rhythmic input from the environment). Some endogenous rhythms may be synchronized by a periodic environmental influence (*zeitgeber*). These synchronizers may be tidal, day- and night-associated light changes, or the phases of the moon. In the presence of synchronizers having 24-h periodicity, a circadian rhythm is seen. If an organism is shielded from such a zeitgeber, its endogenous rhythms will tend to free run; that is, the period of the rhythm will deviate somewhat from that of the environment and may vary as much as 3 h from the environmentally determined 24-h rhythm.

In humans the bodily constituents most carefully studied with regard to periodicity have been those of the endocrine system. Studies of hormonal rhythms have led to important insights in clinical and experimental endocrinology and neuroendocrinology. The appreciation of rhythmicity has had major implications for delineating normal values of hormonal concentrations (dependent not only on time of day but on frequency of sampling), for determining treatment schedules of hormone medication, and for understanding the pathophysiology of disease states characterized by altered rhythmicity. An increased knowledge of the factors involved in such rhythmicity has led to new concepts of hormonal interrelationships, hierarchies of hormonal control, and neural regulation of hormonal function.

Although there is evidence of periodic function on a cellular as well as organic level, there is ample evidence of a hierarchy of rhythms, and it has been demonstrated that rhythms may be generated and entrained by the central nervous system, through thus far poorly understood anatomic and biochemical pathways. Circadian periodicity of CNS neurotransmitter and neuropeptide concentrations, of numbers of neurotransmitter receptors, and of effects of target gland feedback on CNS have been reported. A circadian periodicity of neural function has been demonstrated in isolated ganglion cells, as have circadian rhythms in the sensory responsiveness and activity of certain neurons in response to metabolic stimuli. Neuronal cells may be similar to other body cells in their inherent circadian periodicity. By virtue, however, of their inherent hierarchical role, they modulate an even more fundamental oscillatory function. It may well be that different areas of the nervous system are involved in rhythmic functions in different species. While pinealectomized sparrows become arrhythmic with regard to locomotor activity, this is not the case in pinealectomized rats. It has been suggested that the pineal may act as a neuroendocrine transducer responding to light input by secretion of a family of hormones which may then act on other centers, which in turn mediate or synchronize other biologic rhythms. Where these centers are is a matter of speculation. It has been suggested that the suprachiasmatic nucleus may serve as a "master clock" for many bodily rhythms. Its metabolic rate, as measured by 2-deoxyglucose uptake, has a circadian rhythm, and neurophysiological studies have shown a circadian rhythm of neural output in vitro as well as in vivo. Lesions of this area in the rat abolish circadian rhythms of running and drinking activity, estrous cyclicity, and plasma corticosteroid concentration.

The strongest evidence for central nervous system control of a circadian endocrine rhythm relates to the pituitary-adrenal system. Although a circadian periodicity of secretion is present in cultured adrenal cells, it is apparent in the intact organism that the level of plasma cortisol concentration follows the pattern of the ACTH rhythm and ultimately the rhythm of hypothalamic CRF secretion. It is also known that there is a rhythm of adrenal responsiveness to ACTH; this, however, does not explain circadian corticosteroid periodicity. The physiological development of rhythmicity in many hormonal parameters is dependent on a certain level of organismal maturity (see below). This is true with regard to the rhythmicity of plasma corticosteroid and plasma ACTH concentrations; such rhythmicity is not present in neonates but appears only during the prepubertal period. In the human, this circadian rhythmicity becomes evident between 2 and 5 years of age, concomitant with achievement of 24-h sleep patterns. In rodents, these rhythms appear by 3 weeks of age, although the time of appearance can be modified by neonatal handling, which accelerates the development of circadian periodicity. There is no decline in circadian periodicity in normal aged individuals.

Disruption of the circadian periodicity of both plasma ACTH and corticosteroid concentrations can be accomplished in the animal by hypothalamic deafferentation, suprachiasmatic nuclear lesions as noted above, or administration of agents which presumably alter central nervous system neurotransmitter content (i.e., anticholinergic or antiserotonergic drugs). Central nervous system neurotransmitters which have been implicated in the regulation of ACTH secretion themselves undergo circadian changes in concentration. Patients with disease involving the hypothalamic-limbic area manifest abnormal periodicity of plasma corticosteroid concentrations. This rhythm free-runs under constant conditions, e.g., blinding.

The pituitary-adrenal system exhibits endogenous periodicity. Evidence to date indicates that the circadian synchronization of its periodicity occurs via changes involved in the sleep-wake cycle rather than the light-dark cycle, and perhaps in the feeding cycle. The adrenal rhythm also does not shift phase immediately with a change in light-dark or sleep-wake cycles. The time needed to accomplish such a shift is variable, usually about 7 days. This is unlike other hormonal circadian rhythms such as those of GH, TSH, prolactin, and pubertal LH release, which have been found to be sleep-associated. The maximal levels noted for each of these hormones occur at specific intervals following sleep onset. Shifting the time of sleep onset immediately shifts the time when peak concentrations of these hormones are noted, the peak of each still maintaining a specific phase angle to the time of sleep onset.

The neurotransmitter basis for circadian periodicity of GH release appears to be cholinergic. The circadian rhythm of rodent LH secretion is obliterated following treatment with antiserotonergic drugs. As noted above, LH concentrations exhibit a circadian periodicity only in the pubertal period. There is no evidence of circadian rhythm in plasma LH concentrations either prior to this time or in the adult. However, despite the low range of oscillation, a circadian rhythm of plasma testosterone in the human male is well documented, though no such rhythms in female gonadal secretion have been demonstrated. Figure 7-15 depicts the periodicity of nine hormones. It remains to be seen whether endocrine rhythms are of two kinds, those which are circadian and those which are exclusively sleep-dependent, or whether a continuum exists between these two different types of rhythms.

The most evident human circadian rhythm is that of the menstrual cycle. A circadian periodicity in behavior, sensory detection, and sexual receptivity has also been reported in the human female, suggesting a relation between such periodicity and hormone fluctuation.

In addition to circadian rhythmicity of endocrine function, ultradian rhythms have also been noted. There seems to be an approximately 90-min cycle in the rapid-eye-movement EEG stage of sleep as well as in motor activity and oral activity. A similar variation may be seen in what has been described as episodic hormonal secretion. So far no rigorous proof has been provided that such episodic secretion is periodic, and the possibility of a mainly random distribution of such episodes still exists. In the case of LH there appears to be a rhythmic process underlying these patterns, with mean intervals between episodes of approximately 150 min. Episodic corticosteroid and ACTH secretion has also been reported, and there may be a correlation between the occurrence of some peaks of episodic secretion and times of daily meals. The physiological basis and significance of such episodic secretion is largely unknown. Whether the genesis of this periodicity is neural or pituitary is also an unresolved question. Episodic LH secretion can also be produced in oophorectomized, stalk-sectioned monkeys given a constant infusion of GnRH into the portal vein. In

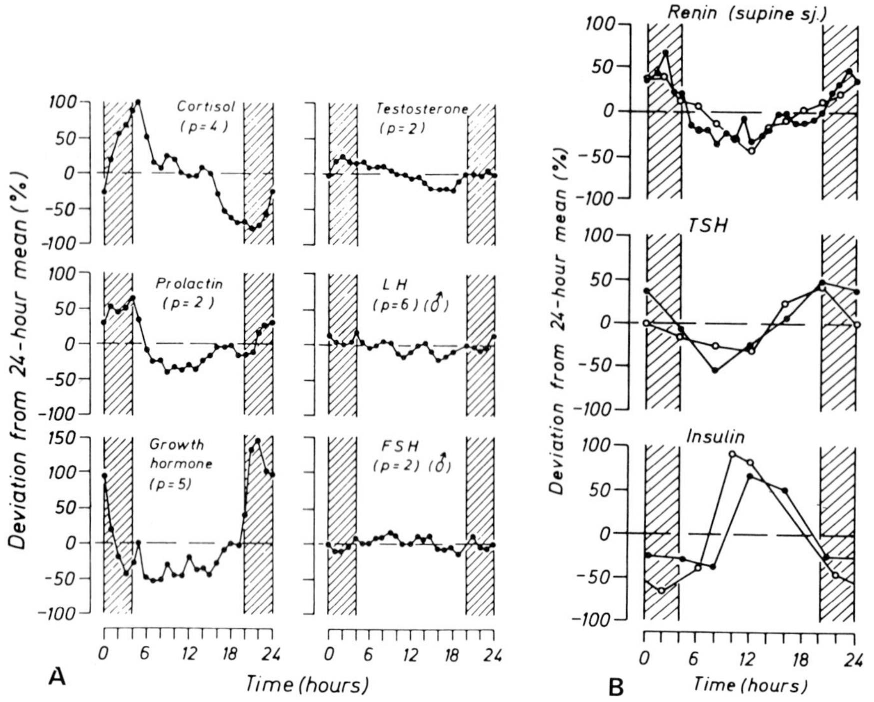

FIGURE 7-15 Circadian rhythms of several hormones in human plasma. Shaded area: approximate sleep time. (A) Mean values from a number of studies (p) with sampling at hourly intervals or more frequently. (B) Mean values from several subjects. (*From Krieger DT, Aschoff J, in Textbook of Endocrinology. New York, Grune & Stratton, 1979.*)

normal women, episodic secretion of progesterone is entrained to that of LH.[185a]

As noted above, there is in many species, including the human, an ontogenic development not only of endocrine rhythms but of a number of major physiological variables. The developmental pattern of GH in human studies shows no clear correlation between plasma levels and sleep-wake cycles in infants in the early neonatal period. In children over the age of 4 to 5 years and in adults, a major GH secretory peak following sleep onset, associated with the slow-wave stage of sleep, is consistently observed. This maturational change in the pattern of GH secretion is associated with maturational changes in the EEG characterization of sleep. It is of interest that the monophasic pattern of a single nocturnal sleep period and a single waking period is established beyond 5 years of age, i.e., at the time a major nocturnal GH secretory peak appears. LH concentration exhibits circadian periodicity only in the pubertal period. The ontogenic development of this rhythmicity is the subject of some controversy, since the detection of periodicity is, in part, dependent on the sensitivity of the assays employed. Although minor day-night differences in LH levels may be present prior to puberty, the association of increased LH secretion following sleep onset is consistently present only during adolescence. There are still questions as to when the ultradian variation in plasma LH concentration appears. Ultradian variation has been demonstrated in only about 50 percent of young children and may therefore be intermittent.

In certain endocrine diseases one of the hallmarks is the absence of normal periodicity. This is true of ACTH and cortisol in patients with Cushing's disease and syndrome and of GH in acromegaly. These observations, coupled with other evidence of altered central nervous system regulation of hormonal secretion in these diseases, have led to the suggestion that a functional abnormality in central nervous system activity, perhaps in neurotransmitter action or content, is responsible for these diseases, leading either to hyperplasia or to adenomas. Although time-zone displacement is not classically considered to be a disease state, the symptoms accompanying it are well known. Individuals vary in the rate of resynchronization of various rhythms when undergoing time-zone displacement. In the human, 6 to 9 days may be required for such resynchronization of plasma cortisol concentrations following a 12-h time-zone displacement. Since other body rhythms, such as that of temperature, resynchronize at different rates, it may be that some of the symptoms associated with phase shifting are secondary to the abnormal phase relationships of various body rhythms with one another and with regard to the external time period.

The significance of endocrine rhythms in normal body function can be considered only in general terms. Little is known concerning the adaptive significance of endocrine rhythms, especially in the human. In lower organisms, such rhythms may have evolved to synchronize behavior in relation to the external environment. Humans, however, are different from other species in that, with the ability to manipulate light-dark cycles, they are less dependent on adaptation to environmental changes. The presence of some rhythms in the human may therefore be a continuation of an evolutionary pattern or perhaps may represent acquired new functions. It is a role of biologic clocks to integrate the periodicity of the organism's internal milieu and functions with environmental periodicity. A full understanding of the underlying basis of hormonal rhythms may bring insights into normal behavior as well as lead to successful neuropharmacological treatment of disease states in which abnormal rhythmicity is present.

ENDOCRINE DISORDERS DUE TO CENTRAL NERVOUS SYSTEM DISEASE

Central nervous system disorders are frequently associated with altered hormone secretion. Careful observation of patients with CNS disorders has resulted in the recognition of new neuroendocrine disturbances, elucidation of the pathogenesis of previously unexplained diseases, demonstration of endocrine disturbances in neurological and behavioral disorders, and appreciation of the effects of altered hormone secretion on CNS function. Anatomically, attention was initially focused on the hypothalamus because of its unique role in neuroendocrine regulation. More recently, diseases of extrahypothalamic brain loci and nonlocalized disorders of the CNS have also been recognized as producing disturbances of endocrine function.

The clinical manifestations of endocrine disorders of extrahypothalamic CNS origin may be indistinguishable from those of hypothalamic disease, since they are frequently mediated via the hypothalamus. Similarly, hypothalamic dysfunction may simulate primary pituitary disease, though there are frequently distinguishing characteristics which can be recognized either clinically or by laboratory testing. Many disorders of CNS etiology described in this section are also discussed in association with the differential diagnosis of anterior and posterior pituitary (Chaps. 8 and 9), thyroid (Chap. 10), adrenal cortex (Chap. 12), and gonadal (Chaps. 16 and 17) diseases.

Diseases of the Hypothalamus

The anatomic structure of the hypothalamus exhibits a reticular organization. As in other brain regions arranged in a similar manner, some hypothalamic functions can be localized to a precise anatomic area (e.g., synthesis of vasopressin is limited to the magnocellular neurons of the supraoptic and paraventricular nuclei), while others are more widely distributed (e.g., temperature-sensitive neurons are scattered throughout a large region of the preoptic anterior hypothalamus, as are those involved with the regulation of anterior pituitary function). In addition, neurons in a single region may be involved in multiple hypothalamic functions (neurons in the ventromedial nucleus subserve both sympathetic pathways mediating hepatic glucose output and those involved in the control of growth hormone secretion). It is therefore the location rather than the size of a hypothalamic lesion which determines the extent of endocrine or metabolic disturbance.

Hypothalamic functions can generally be subdivided into two categories: those functions mediating anterior and posterior pituitary hormone secretion and those involved with nonpituitary function. The latter include sleep-wake behavior, cognition, emotional behavior, autonomic nervous system regulation, and neurometabolic control (eating and drinking behavior and caloric homeostasis). Extensive reviews of the nonpituitary aspects of hypothalamic function have recently appeared.[186–188]

Slowly growing lesions in the hypothalamus generally do not produce symptoms until they have reached considerable size (though exceptions to this rule occur), whereas rapidly enlarging lesions can cause dramatic clinical manifestations even when quite small, depending on their location. Acute damage to the hypothalamus is responsible for most disturbances of consciousness of hypothalamic origin, for sustained hyperthermia, and for severe disturbances of cardiovascular, gastrointestinal, or pulmonary function that are related to hypothalamic disease. Chronic damage to the hypothalamus, in contrast, is generally manifested by alterations in cognition and complex homeostatic functions involving neurometabolic regulation. Neuroendocrine control also tends to be altered primarily by chronic hypothalamic disturbances, though acute lesions (e.g., trauma) that destroy a final common pathway (e.g., the median eminence or pituitary stalk) are also seen. These complex functions require the integration of the hypothalamus with numerous other neural regions and result in effector mechanisms involving neuroendocrine or autonomic nervous system–mediated pathways. Although the component parts of the system can be shown to occur without the presence of an intact hypothalamus, the integrative functions of the hypothalamus are indispensable. The disturbances noted with chronic hypothalamic disease therefore tend to be alterations in normal regulatory tone rather than acute and severe fluctuations in consciousness, temperature, or autonomic discharge.

Hypothalamic neuronal projections in humans (with the exception of sympathetic efferent pathways) are not lateralized like those involving sensory and motor function. Unilateral hypothalamic damage consequently seldom causes significant or prolonged symptoms. Disturbances of hypothalamic function are therefore seen most commonly with infiltrative or inflammatory diseases which affect the region diffusely, with midline tumors which expand bilaterally and affect predominantly those structures adjacent to the third ventricle (paraventricular regions), and with diseases affecting the median eminence, the site of the final common effector pathway to the pituitary.

ETIOLOGY OF HYPOTHALAMIC DISEASE

Organic disease of the hypothalamus may result from many causes, which are summarized in Table 7-8. Within each age group the frequency of hypothalamic dysfunction attributable to the different diseases is listed in descending order. The nonpituitary and, to a limited extent, the anterior pituitary regulatory functions of the hypothalamus are not well developed at birth; therefore, certain types of damage to the hypothalamus may not be clinically recognized in the newborn.

In addition to the specific disorders listed, patients may exhibit disturbances of neuroendocrine or neurometabolic hypothalamic function unassociated with anatomic evidence of hypothalamic disease. Many of these disorders have been attributed to abnormalities of neurochemical function, though evidence that the primary disturbance involves the hypothalamus is still lacking, as is, in most instances, evidence of the nature of the specific biochemical abnormality.

Tumors

Tumors of the hypothalamus, particularly those derived from cell rests or developmental abnormalities, are most frequently located in the region of the third ventricle, and the disturbances produced depend upon their location. Tumors of the inferior portion of the third ventricle or the anterior mediobasal hypothalamus cause alterations in pituitary hormone secretion and in neurometabolic regulation and result in olfactory and/or visual disturbances. Tumors in the anterior and superior portion of the third ventricle may block the foramina of Monro, giving rise to internal hydrocephalus, may cause dementia by interfering with dorsomedial thalamic–frontal lobe pathways, and may result in symptoms of increased intracranial pressure (papilledema, headaches, nausea, and vomiting).

Table 7-8. Etiology of Hypothalamic Disease

Neonates:
- Intraventricular hemorrhage
- Meningitis: bacterial
- Tumors: glioma, hemangioma
- Trauma
- Hydrocephalus, hydranencephaly, kernicterus

1 month–2 years:
- Tumors: glioma, especially optic glioma, histiocytosis X, hemangiomas
- Hydrocephalus, meningitis
- "Familial" disorders: Laurence-Moon, Bardet-Biedl, Prader-Labhart-Willi, etc.

2–10 years:
- Tumors: craniopharyngioma, glioma, dysgerminoma, hamartoma, histiocytosis X, leukemia, ganglioneuroma, ependymoma, medulloblastoma
- Meningitis: bacterial, tuberculous
- Encephalitis: viral and demyelinating, various viral encephalitides and exanthematous demyelinating encephalitides, disseminated encephalomyelitis
- "Familial" disorders: diabetes insipidus, etc.
- Damage from nasopharyngeal radiation therapy

10–25 years:
- Tumors: craniopharyngioma, pituitary tumors, glioma, hamartoma, dysgerminoma, histiocytosis X, leukemia, dermoid, lipoma, neuroblastoma
- Trauma
- Subarachnoid hemorrhage, vascular aneurysm, arteriovenous malformation
- Inflammatory diseases: meningitis, encephalitis, sarcoid, tuberculosis
- Associated with midline brain defects: agenesis of corpus callosum
- Chronic hydrocephalus or increased intracranial pressure

25–50 years:
- Nutritional: Wernicke's disease
- Tumors: glioma, lymphoma, meningioma, craniopharyngioma, pituitary tumors, angioma, plasmacytoma, colloid cysts, ependymoma, sarcoma, histiocytosis X
- Inflammatory: sarcoid, tuberculosis, viral encephalitis
- Subarachnoid hemorrhage, vascular aneurysms, arteriovenous malformation
- Damage from pituitary radiation therapy

>50 years:
- Nutritional: Wernicke's disease
- Tumors: sarcoma, glioblastoma, lymphoma, meningioma, colloid cysts, ependymoma, pituitary tumors
- Vascular: infarct, subarachnoid hemorrhage, pituitary apoplexy
- Inflammatory: encephalitis, sarcoid, meningitis

Source: Adapted from Plum and Van Uitert.[186]

Tumors in the epithalamic or pineal region of the third ventricle cause disturbances of pupillary and extraocular muscle movements along with brainstem signs, while those located more posteriorly often produce hydrocephalus, ocular nerve palsies, and cerebellar and pyramidal tract signs. Gonadal dysfunction may also be seen, particularly if metastases occur along the floor of the third ventricle.

The most frequent tumors of the hypothalamus are craniopharyngiomas (see also Chap. 8), followed by astrocytomas and dysgerminomas. The majority of reported tumors, because of their developmental origin, are seen in patients under 25 years of age.

Endocrine disturbances associated with hypothalamic tumors generally result from a destruction of those neuronal elements required for normal pituitary function and are discussed later in this chapter. Hypothalamic neoplasms are occasionally associated with increased rather than decreased pituitary function. One category, the hamartoma, warrants special consideration (see below) in that its effects are due not to destruction of neural tissue but rather to the elaboration of a releasing factor.

Hypothalamic tumors are diagnosed by standard neuroradiological and neuroophthalmologic procedures. Computerized tomography and digital subtraction angiography have completely replaced pneumoencephalography and arteriography. The presence of atypical visual field defects (e.g., inferior field loss) and normal sellar structure in patients with hypopituitarism, particularly in the presence of diabetes insipidus and intact responses to releasing hormones, points to primary hypothalamic disease.[189]

The treatment of tumors originating in the substance of the hypothalamus is not very successful at present. The location of the tumor generally makes it difficult to remove without sacrificing intact hypothalamic tissue critical for maintenance of normal homeostatic mechanism. Developmental tumors, particularly the cystic varieties, tend to be slow-growing and may even undergo spontaneous growth arrest. Aspiration of the cystic fluid from such tumors, which is generally oily and cholesterol-rich, will frequently relieve pressure symptoms for long periods of time. Marsupialization of the cyst into the CSF has also been used successfully in some patients. Radiotherapy of craniopharyngiomas appears to be a useful technique both in adults and in children.[190-192] Treatment of other types of hypothalamic tumors is less successful, and lost endocrine function is virtually never restored, even with complete tumor removal.

HAMARTOMAS *Hypothalamic hamartomas* are collections of redundant, partially disoriented glial and ganglion cells located within the ventral hypothalamus. The term has also been applied (though technically incorrectly) to masses of neuronal elements lodged in an abnormal location such as the anterior pituitary. The latter tumors are more appropriately called *choristomas* or *gangliocytomas*. Hamartomas and related tumors have been associated with several hormonal hyperfunctional states: precocious puberty, acromegaly, and hyperprolactinemia. The pathogenic role of the hamartoma has been convincingly demonstrated for the first two syndromes by immunohistochemical demonstration of the appropriate releasing factor (GnRH or GRH) within the neurons of the tumor.

Hamartomas associated with precocious puberty consist of encapsulated nodules attached to the posterior hypothalamus at a point between the anterior portion of the mamillary body and the posterior region of the tuber cinereum. The neurons resemble those of the hypothalamus and contain membrane-bound granules similar in size and character to those in the hypothalamus and median eminence. The tumor's vascular supply usually originates from a fairly constant branch of the posterior communicating artery. The vessels in the hamartoma contain the characteristic fenestrations of those in the median eminence. These fenestrations allow transport of neurosecretory products directly into the bloodstream, with access to the pituitary portal system presumably provided by vessels of the tuber cinereum. The mechanism by which hamartomas induce early sexual maturation is not entirely clear. A report in which GnRH was detected in the spinal fluid of three patients with precocious puberty led to the suggestion that these tumors produce GnRH,[193] and this was subsequently confirmed by the demonstration of the releasing factor in tumor tissue by immunofluorescent techniques.[194] Clinical features and treatment of precocious puberty are discussed later in this section.

Hamartomas associated with acromegaly have been identified both in the ventral hypothalamus and within the anterior pituitary itself.[195,196] The tumors are morphologically similar to hamartomas associated with precocious puberty. Using antihuman GRH serum, the neurons within the tumors have recently been found to contain GRH. The mechanism of production of acromegaly (and, in addition, pituitary tumors) is presumably release of GRH into the pituitary portal system by the tumors located in the hypothalamus and a direct paracrine effect by the tumors within the anterior pituitary, whose neuronal processes can be shown by electron microscopy to exhibit contact with somatotroph tumor cells.[195]

An intrapituitary gangliocytoma has recently been observed in a patient with Cushing's disease and corticotroph hyperplasia.[197] Using a specific immunohistochemical stain, the tumor was found to contain

CRF. Although the tumor was intrapituitary, its morphological characteristics were those of a hypothalamic hamartoma. Thus, the effects of excessive CRF secretion are analogous to those of GRH and cause hyperfunction of the appropriate pituitary target cell.

Evidence for an etiologic role of hypothalamic hamartomas in the production of hyperprolactinemia is less convincing but must still be considered. A single case report has appeared of a neurohypophyseal neurosecretory body (hamartoma) identified in the pituitary stalk of a patient with an anterior pituitary prolactin-containing microadenoma.[198] Since the nature of the secretory product involved is unknown, the association of the two tumors must remain speculative.

In a series of 121 consecutive autopsies, 21 percent of brains exhibited nodular projections of the tuber cinereum in the posterior or lateral portion of the hypothalamus.[199] These nodules were labeled *hamartomatous* rather than true hamartomas, since they were clearly related to a lateral perforating vessel of the tuber cinereum and represented a displacement of tuberal tissue without obvious increase or disorientation of cells. Thus, they formed an integral part of the hypothalamus, in contrast to true hamartomas. However, an increased prevalence of multiple endocrine abnormalities and neoplasia was present in the affected subjects, suggesting that these hamartomatous nodules exhibit neuroendocrine function.

Immunologic Disorders

Numerous peripheral endocrine glands are affected by immunologic disorders (e.g., Graves' disease, autoimmune hypophysitis, type I diabetes mellitus), and recent data suggest that at least one neuroendocrine disease may have a similar pathogenesis. In a series of 30 patients with idiopathic diabetes insipidus, 11 were found to have circulating antibodies specific for the magnocellular vasopressin-secreting cells of the human hypothalamus.[200] The antibodies reacted with cellular components distinct from vasopressin, oxytocin, and the neurophysins. It thus appears that there is a subgroup of patients with diabetes insipidus who have an underlying immunologic disorder. No clinical or laboratory features have yet been identified which distinguish patients with autoantibodies from those without.

Inflammatory Disorders

SARCOIDOSIS Central nervous system involvement in sarcoidosis is relatively uncommon. It may appear early or late during the illness, and the course may be either self-limited or progressive. Manifestations of hypothalamic-pituitary dysfunction may range from polyuria and polydipsia, due to the presence of diabetes insipidus, and galactorrhea, due to hyperprolactinemia, to partial or total anterior pituitary insufficiency. A case of polyuria associated with elevated concentrations of plasma vasopressin has also been reported.[201] Infiltrative granulomatous nodules may be present in the stalk, the hypothalamus, or the pituitary. Other evidence of hypothalamic involvement may also be present, such as somnolence or hyperphagia. A case of panhypopituitarism has been reported in which on postmortem examination the anterior and posterior pituitary were intact but extensive hypothalamic involvement was present.[202] In occasional patients with granulomatous infiltrations of the hypothalamus and extrahypothalamic CNS, no peripheral evidence of sarcoidosis can be detected. Whether this condition represents a variant of the disorder or a separate entity is unknown. The diagnosis is facilitated by the presence of systemic manifestations of the disease and by CSF abnormalities, including elevated protein, pleocytosis, and, frequently, low glucose levels. Increasing experience with computed tomography has led to the recognition of characteristic changes consisting of localized regions of enhanced contrast medium uptake in the affected areas of both CNS and pituitary.[203] Although steroid therapy causes amelioration of many of the neurological manifestations of CNS sarcoidosis and, in occasional patients, of diabetes insipidus, it is generally ineffective in restoring deficient hormone production.

HISTIOCYTOSIS X This is a granulomatous disease of unknown etiology. When the central nervous system is involved, granulomas of the histiocytic type with eosinophilic elements occur in the tuber cinereum and the hypothalamus and may be associated with either diabetes insipidus or hypopituitarism similar to what has been described for sarcoid.[204] There are several clinical varieties of the disease: Hand-Schuller-Christian disease, the most common type, characterized by polyuria, exophthalmos, and skull defects; Letterer-Siwe disease, which is a much more rapidly progressive form; and eosinophilic granuloma, in which the same pathological findings are found in solitary bone lesions. Histiocytosis X should be considered as a possible diagnosis in any child presenting with diabetes insipidus. Although 90 percent of patients will eventually exhibit skeletal lesions, most commonly in the skull, diabetes insipidus may exist as a solitary abnormality for a long period. Diabetes insipidus occurs in almost 50 percent of patients with Hand-Schuller-Christian disease. Growth failure due to GH deficiency, hypogonadism, and panhypopituitarism may also be seen but is less common. The diagnosis is established by biopsy of a bone or an intracranial lesion. The course of the disease is generally favorable, with overall mortality of around 15 percent. Local forms of the disease are usually treated with curettage and radiotherapy of the bone lesions, while the disseminated forms may respond to high-dose glucocorticoid therapy or to chemotherapy utilizing alkylating agents. There are as yet no reports of reversal of the endocrine abnormalities with such treatment.[205,206]

Trauma

Head injury of any type may result in suprahypophyseal hypopituitarism. In patients with basilar skull fractures transsection of the pituitary stalk may lead to diabetes insipidus and panhypopituitarism. Comatose patients may exhibit TRH-responsive hypothyroidism and GnRH-responsive hypogonadism.[207] Plasma cortisol levels are elevated in patients with increased intracranial pressure through a mechanism that requires intact brainstem function.[208] After regaining consciousness, patients with severe head injuries exhibit paradoxical rises in GH secretion after oral glucose for up to 2 weeks.[209] The precise neurotransmitter or releasing factor disturbances which underly these changes are unclear.

Internal Hydrocephalus

Alterations in endocrine function have also been reported in cases of internal hydrocephalus, varying from primary amenorrhea, oligomenorrhea, decreased dexamethasone suppressibility, and absent insulin hypoglycemia responsiveness to panhypopituitarism.[210,211] Relief of the hydrocephalus has been associated with reversion of the abnormal tests or symptoms to normal in some patients.

Vascular Lesions

Vascular lesions of the hypothalamus generally occur as a result of rupture of aneurysms of the anterior or posterior communicating arteries. Both ischemic and hemorrhagic lesions have been observed.[212] Microhemorrhages have also been noted in the supraoptic and paraventricular nuclei. Though no studies of vasopressin secretion have been reported in such patients, evidence of impaired metyrapone responsiveness and a loss of the cortisol diurnal rhythm has been observed in a series of patients after subarachnoid hemorrhage.[213]

Radiation-Induced Damage

Radiation therapy for intracranial neoplasms (gliomas, ependymomas, medulloblastomas, and pituitary tumors) and for nasopharyngeal and maxillary sinus carcinomas has been associated with the subsequent development of signs and symptoms of hypopituitarism. The interval between radiation therapy and the appearance of hormone deficiencies may range from 1 to 10 years or possibly even longer. Growth failure associated with reduced GH responsiveness, hypogonadotropic hypogonadism, and hypothyroidism has been observed, and in some patients the preservation of pituitary hormone responsiveness to releasing factor stimulation has indicated the site of the abnormality to be the hypothalamus. This has now been documented for GH as well as other pituitary hormones.[213a] Children appear more susceptible than adults, and the critical dose is believed to be about 4000 rads.[214] Other manifestations of radiation necrosis include papilledema, dementia, and localized neurological signs. In occasional patients sarcoma formation has been observed. A commonly used practice of prophylactic head irradiation (2400 rads) in children with CNS leukemia has not to date appeared to produce any alterations in neurological function, though long-term follow-ups of neuroendocrine function are limited. No treatment is currently available other than replacement therapy of hormonal deficiencies. Growth deficiency can be treated with either GH or GRH.

DISTURBANCES OF PITUITARY FUNCTION DUE TO HYPOTHALAMIC DISEASE

Hypothalamic dysfunction can result in both quantitative and qualitative changes in pituitary hormone secretion. The early descriptions of endocrine abnormalities associated with hypothalamic tumors focused on diabetes insipidus and gonadal dysfunction (usually hypogonadism associated with anterior hypothalamic lesions or precocious puberty seen with lesions involving the posterior hypothalamus or pineal gland).[215] In many of these cases it was not ascertained whether pituitary histology and function were normal. Decreased secretion resulting from impaired hypophysiotropic effects can mimic hypopituitarism, though the extent of impairment is generally less than with primary pituitary disease. Panhypopituitarism has, however, been observed in patients with carcinoma metastatic to the brain. Impaired pituitary hormone secretion occurs primarily in relation to GH, prolactin, ACTH, LH, and vasopressin, and differentiation from primary pituitary disorders is not always possible. With increased understanding of hypothalamic control of anterior pituitary function has come an appreciation that abnormalities in endocrine function may be manifested by alterations in feedback, stress-induced release, or circadian periodicity (which are clinically less apparent) rather than by an effect on basal levels.

It therefore follows that abnormalities in CNS-endocrine regulation can be present without overt evidence of endocrine dysfunction. For example, alterations in plasma cortisol circadian rhythm are frequently seen in patients with lesions of the hypothalamus or involving the limbic system (from which pathways to the hypothalamus regulating ACTH secretion have been described) but are less common with CNS lesions outside these areas.[216] Patients with hypothalamic tumors also show a higher incidence of abnormal responses to metyrapone,[217,218] indicating a loss of the hypothalamic feedback mechanism, though the alterations in response do not correlate with change in circadian variation.

The following section illustrates those clinically recognized syndromes attributed to a hypothalamic disorder of releasing or inhibiting factor secretion, though it must be emphasized that in many of the examples, anatomic evidence for a specific hypothalamic disease is lacking.

TSH

Hypothalamic hypothyroidism or *tertiary hypothyroidism* is a disorder manifested by hypothyroidism, a low plasma TSH, and an exaggerated and delayed response to TRH. In most normal subjects the peak TSH value after TRH occurs at 15 to 30 min, while in these patients it may be as late as 90 or 120 min.[219] One series of children believed to have this disorder exhibited slightly elevated basal TSH levels but responded similarly to TRH.[220] TSH in these patients exhibits reduced biologic activity because of altered glycosylation, a process regulated by TRH.[220a] Hypothalamic hypothyroidism can be seen as an isolated defect or more commonly in children associated with deficiencies in gonadotropin, GH, and/or ACTH secretion. The frequency of this disease as a cause of hypothyroidism is unknown but is probably quite low. Most patients do not exhibit other evidence of CNS dysfunction. Thyroxine is used for treatment, as in primary hypothyroidism.

ACTH

Diminished secretion of ACTH secondary to hypothalamic or other CNS dysfunction is less common than that of the other anterior pituitary hormones for reasons which are not entirely clear. It may occur as an isolated hormone deficiency or in association with impaired secretion of other anterior pituitary hormones, usually in children. Preliminary information suggests that CRF testing may be useful in differentiating pituitary from hypothalamic deficiency. The presence of intact pituitary hormone responses to GnRH and TRH in children with idiopathic hypopituitarism implies a hypothalamic etiology for ACTH deficiency as well, and a recent report has demonstrated intact ACTH responses to CRF in these patients.[221]

Disturbances of the diurnal rhythm of ACTH secretion and of the normal suppressibility of ACTH are common in patients with a variety of intracranial diseases and reflect early deficiencies in neuroendocrine control mechanisms. These changes are not recognized to be of major clinical significance, but subtle effects on behavior cannot be excluded.

The etiology of Cushing's disease is still unsettled. Several of the manifestations of this syndrome (loss of circadian periodicity of adrenocorticosteroid levels, lack of responsiveness of plasma corticosteroid levels to stress, lack of normal suppressibility of corticosteroid levels following dexamethasone, abnormalities in GH responsiveness, and abnormalities in sleep EEG) may be explained by functional alterations in hypothalamic control mechanisms regulating periodicity, stress responsiveness, and the "set point" at which steroid suppression occurs.[222] There have been isolated case reports of the association of Cushing's syndrome with intracranial disease,[223] although today it may be questioned whether these might represent cases of ectopic ACTH production. A syndrome of periodic hypersecretion and unsuppressibility together with elevated plasma ACTH levels has been reported in which the only positive neurological findings were ventricular dilatation and cortical atrophy.[224] Similar findings have been reported in autopsied cases of classic Cushing's disease.[225] The response of some patients with Cushing's disease to cyproheptadine (a serotonin receptor antagonist)[226] and to sodium valproate (a GABA receptor antagonist)[227] may also be taken as evidence for a CNS etiology, since it is presumed that these drugs act primarily on receptors in the hypothalamus rather than in the pituitary gland, although direct pituitary effects on ACTH secretion have also been demonstrated in vitro.[228] It may well be that there are at least two types of Cushing's disease: one type secondary to excessive CRF production and one caused by a primary pituitary adenoma (see Chap. 8).[229] Two studies suggest that these subgroups of Cushing's disease may be distinguishable by their differential sensitivity to dexamethasone[230] or pulsatility of cortisol secretion.[230a]

LH and FSH

HYPOTHALAMIC HYPOGONADISM This is defined as an impairment in pituitary and gonadal function attributable to deficient or disordered secretion of GnRH. It can be seen in association with hypothalamic destruction or in the absence of pathological changes. The manifestations vary according to whether the disorder occurs before or after the onset of puberty.

Prepubertal The presence of hypothalamic hypogonadism prior to puberty results in failure of normal sexual maturation and, in girls, primary amenorrhea. In some children other pituitary hormone deficiencies are present, also on a hypothalamic basis. The nocturnal rise in plasma LH which normally occurs during puberty is absent, and clinically the disorder is similar to prepubertal primary hypopituitarism.

A key manifestation in some patients with prepubertal hypogonadotropic hypogonadism is anosmia or hyposmia. These findings constitute Kallmann's syndrome, or olfactory-genital dysplasia, which may be associated with other neurological defects such as color blindness and nerve deafness. It occurs primarily as a genetic disorder,[231] though sporadic cases have also been reported. Patients with this disorder usually exhibit absent or impaired gonadotropin responses to GnRH, although normal or, rarely, enhanced responses may also be seen. Clomiphene administration does not increase gonadotropin levels. One-fourth of patients demonstrate impaired cortisol responses to insulin hypoglycemia and impaired TSH responses to TRH, and nearly all exhibit impaired responses to dopaminergic receptor blockade. Although testicular response to gonadotropin administration is reduced in some male patients, an adequate response occurs in most. Occasional untreated patients may even be fertile. Some patients with Kallmann's syndrome exhibit defects in osmoreceptor function and abnormal thirst regulation, which indicate widespread hypothalamic dysfunction.[232] In some cases hypothalamic hypoplasia as well as hypoplasia of the region of the anterior commissure and the olfactory bulb, along with other midline defects, has been reported.[233] The importance of olfactory stimuli in lower mammals in the regulation of sexual behavior in both sexes and of gonadotropin cyclicity in females is well recognized, and there is some evidence that olfactory stimuli may play a role in gonadotropin regulation in primates[234] and even in humans.[235]

The gonadotropin responses to a single injection of GnRH are markedly impaired or absent in these patients, indicating a lack of prior (endogenous) GnRH function. If repeated administration of GnRH is provided to "prime" the gonadotrophs, a normal or even supranormal response will eventually be obtained, thereby providing a means to differentiate this disorder from primary hypopituitarism.[236] Therapy at present consists in the use of gonadal steroids for the development and maintenance of secondary sexual function and gonadotropins for promoting fertility. However, pulsatile administration of a GnRH analogue, using a portable infusion pump, has been found effective in promoting normal pubertal development and offers a more physiological approach to therapy.[237]

Postpubertal Postpubertal hypothalamic hypogonadism is a disorder predominantly of women. It is generally manifested by secondary amenorrhea or oligomenorrhea and occasionally by infertility associated with anovulatory cycles. The commonly used terms *functional* or *psychogenic* amenorrhea probably represent the same disorder(s). Patients may exhibit normal to decreased estradiol levels and inappropriately low LH and FSH levels.[238] Pulsatile fluctuations of serum LH levels typically seen in normal women are absent in most of these patients. Following a single injection of GnRH a rise in serum LH and FSH levels is observed, qualitatively similar to but often quantitatively greater than that seen in normal subjects, with relative enhancement of the FSH response. A normal response to clomiphene is usually also present. These data suggest the existence of a functional derangement in hypothalamic releasing mechanisms. Such secondary amenorrhea is usually a self-limited condition.

Similar physiological disturbances are seen in women with hyperprolactinemia irrespective of etiology (postpartum, idiopathic, pituitary tumor, or uremic). Extensive studies of women with nonphysiological hyperprolactinemia have indicated that gonadotropin responses to clomiphere are intact but that responses to estradiol are absent,[239] suggesting a selective effect of hyperprolactinemia on the positive feedback effect of estradiol on the CNS. Postmenopausal women with hyperprolactinemia exhibit increased FSH and LH levels, providing further evidence for preservation of the negative feedback mechanism. It is unclear at present whether the hypothalamic disturbance is specifically due to hyperprolactinemia or whether alterations in neurotransmitter mechanisms are responsible for altered secretion of both prolactin and gonadotropins. Some evidence exists for enhanced dopaminergic tone, which is inhibitory to LH secretion.[240] In men, hyperprolactinemia has been associated with varying degrees of hypogonadism, with the most frequent symptoms being diminished libido and potency.

Alterations in weight (both marked increases and decreases) and sustained exercise regimens are frequently accompanied by amenorrhea. Amenorrhea in ballet dancers and female athletes is quite common[241,242] and occurs in virtually all patients with anorexia nervosa.

Hypogonadism is also associated with other diseases with evidence of CNS dysfunction in which the nature of the CNS disorder and the cause of the hypogonadism still remain to be elucidated. These include the Laurence-Moon, Bardet-Biedl, and Prader-

Willi syndromes, all of which exhibit other similarities and are discussed later in this chapter.

Decisions concerning therapy depend on the nature of the primary disease and its reversibility, the extent of hypogonadism, and the patient's desire for fertility. Therapy of the underlying disease process should be attempted first, if possible. The severity of symptoms should determine the aggressiveness of the therapeutic approach. In most women no therapy is indicated unless restoration of menses and/or pregnancy is desired. In others, symptoms of hypoestrogenemia, primarily decreased libido and dyspareunia due to decreased vaginal secretions, and the increased risk of osteoporosis may warrant replacement therapy. Osteopenia has been noted in hyperprolactinemic women, though the risk of subsequent bone fractures remains to be determined. Replacement therapy with estrogen and progesterone is similar to that for primary or secondary hypogonadism. Fertility may be achieved either with the use of gonadotropins or by pulsatile administration of GnRH.[242a] In men, replacement therapy with testosterone is of value if endogenous hormone levels are subnormal, though suppression of hyperprolactinemia with bromocriptine may also be required.[243] For details of treatment, refer to Chaps. 8, 16, and 17.

HYPOTHALAMIC HYPERGONADISM In this condition, disordered pituitary-gonadal function occurs, in response to quantitatively increased or qualitatively disordered hypothalamic function, as two distinct clinical entities, one prepubertal and the other postpubertal.

Precocious Puberty The appearance of signs of sexual development in girls prior to 8 years or in boys prior to 9 years is defined as precocious puberty or sexual precocity. True precocious puberty (complete isosexual precocity) occurs in association with hypothalamic hamartomas which secrete GnRH (discussed above under Etiology of Hypothalamic Disease: Tumors), other CNS tumors (hypothalamic astrocytomas, neurofibromas, craniopharyngiomas), or inflammatory CNS disorders or may, in the absence of definable CNS disease, be idiopathic. In children with definable CNS disease there is no sex predilection, whereas the idiopathic form (which probably includes some patients with hamartomas), occurs predominantly in girls (> 90 percent). The age of onset of girls peaks at 6 to 8 years, suggesting the possibility of an extreme of the range of normal early onset, i.e., a normal variant. In this late-onset group the incidence of hamartomas is low compared with that of early onset, in which group hamartomas have been identified in more than one-third.[244]

The clinical features of precocious puberty are identical to those occurring during puberty at the normally expected age. They include not only physical but also behavioral manifestations. Patients with true precocious puberty must be differentiated from those with incomplete isosexual precocity. In boys the latter category includes hCG-secreting tumors of the CNS[245] or liver, increased testicular androgen secretion due to congenital adrenal hyperplasia, virilizing adrenal neoplasms, Leydig cell adenomas, and premature Leydig cell maturation. In girls, the differential diagnosis includes estrogen-secreting neoplasms, ovarian cysts, hypothyroidism, and exogenous sources of estrogen (e.g., meat from estrogen-fed cattle). The McCune-Albright syndrome, which occurs mostly in girls, consists of café au lait spots, intermittent signs of puberty (sporadic menstrual bleeding), polyostotic fibrous dysplasia, and eventually true precocious puberty due to activation of CNS mechanisms.[246,247]

Two problems warrant therapeutic consideration. First, the psychological impact of puberty, especially menstrual function during early childhood, is disconcerting to both the child and parents. Second, the premature secretion of estrogens or androgens results in an enhancement of bone growth disproportionate to the growth in height and leads to premature epiphyseal closure. As a consequence, most children with precocious puberty do not achieve a normal adult height, and many remain less than 5 ft.

Therapeutic alternatives until recently have been limited to the use of long-acting progesterone derivatives (e.g., medroxyprogesterone)[248] or weak androgenic anabolic steroids,[249] in an attempt to suppress cyclic gonadotropin function. While these drugs are fairly effective in preventing menstrual bleeding, the children exhibit, to varying degrees, androgenic side effects. More importantly, the effects of these steroids on bone maturation have been disappointing.

Recently, preliminary studies with a GnRH analogue have indicated promising results. Administration of a long-acting analogue of GnRH results in down regulation of pituitary GnRH receptors and desensitization of the pituitary gonadotropin response. Treatment with this agent has resulted in marked attenuation of the rate of bone maturation, which permits growth to considerably greater height.[250] Caution has been urged in the use of this agent because of uncertain long-term effects on the gonads. While long-term follow-up is essential to determine whether treatment affects the subsequent fertility of the patient, the use of GnRH analogues in the treatment of precocious puberty represents a major achievement.

Polycystic Ovary Syndrome The polycystic ovary (Stein-Leventhal) syndrome has been reported in association with a history of childhood CNS injury or "encephalitis."[251] In patients with this syndrome, LH levels have been consistently elevated, though below the level reached at the midcycle ovulatory peak in normal subjects. These findings are somewhat analogous to those seen in the neonatally androgenized rat, which also develops polycystic ovaries. However, polycystic rat ovaries transplanted into a normal host revert to normal, indicating that the ovarian alterations in the neonatally androgenized animal are secondary to nonovarian mechanisms. This had led to the suggestion that there may be a functional CNS disturbance in patients with Stein-Leventhal syndrome, which is supported by the demonstration of altered rhythmicity of LH secretion, particularly at night,[252] and by the clinical improvement noted in response to medroxyprogesterone therapy.[253] The association of the syndrome with either galactorrhea or hyperprolactinemia has also been observed,[254] and in these patients a stimulatory effect of prolactin on adrenal androgen synthesis has been suggested. For details of treatment, refer to Chap. 17.

Growth Hormone

GROWTH-HORMONE DEFICIENCY Idiopathic GH deficiency (IGHD) occurs as an isolated hormone deficiency or in association with other anterior pituitary hormone deficiencies as both a familial and a sporadic disorder. The causes appear to be heterogeneous. IGHD is a disease of childhood, with the diagnosis being made as early as 2 or 3 years of age. The GH deficiency may be complete (basal levels barely or not detectable) or partial (subnormal responses to provocative stimuli). In one form of complete GH deficiency, a deletion of the GH gene has been found.[255,256] The treatment of this disease with GH in some patients is limited because of GH-antibody development, confirming the "foreign" nature of GH in these children.

The lack of neuroradiographic abnormalities of the sella and the frequent coexistence of TRH- and GnRH-responsive deficiencies of TSH, LH, and FSH strongly suggest a hypothalamic cause in many of the patients. The limited histological studies of the pituitary and hypothalamus have not revealed any morphological abnormalities. Initial studies with GRH have demonstrated variable GH responses[257-259] and suggested that the response is inversely related to the duration of the disease. Repeated stimulation with GRH for as long as several weeks does not restore GH responsiveness to normal, in contrast to the LH response to repeated injections of GnRH.

It has been proposed that the disorder is secondary to a neurotransmitter abnormality rather than to a structural defect in the hypothalamus. There is one report of stimulation of GH release in children with IGHD by propranolol,[260] suggesting the existence of enhanced beta-adrenergic inhibitory tone. Increased growth in some children with IGHD has been achieved with bromocriptine, a dopaminergic agonist, raising the possibility of an impairment in dopaminergic neurotransmission.[260a]

Therapy for IGHD is limited to the prepubertal period and consists of human GH. Hypothyroidism, if present, must be treated concomitantly. A detailed description of the clinical presentation, diagnostic procedures, and therapeutic measures is provided in Chap. 26.

ACROMEGALY GH hypersecretion, acromegaly, and somatotroph tumors have on rare occasions been associated with hypothalamic hamartomas[196] and with intrapituitary gangliocytomas,[195] which have been demonstrated to contain GRH. In addition, GH hypersecretion, acromegaly, and pituitary somatotroph adenomas have been reported in the McCune-Albright syndrome in the absence of a demonstrable hypothalamic tumor,[261-263] presumably due to a functional overproduction of GRH. Peripheral plasma immunoreactive GRH levels are not elevated in such patients and plasma GH responses to GRH are intact.[263a] The differentiation of acromegaly due to excessive production of GRH from primary pituitary disease has to date not been possible with the exception of patients with extra-CNS GRH-secreting tumors in whom peripheral plasma immunoreactive GRH levels have been elevated.[103,264]

Prolactin

Idiopathic hyperprolactinemia (IH) has been defined as the presence of elevated prolactin levels in the absence of demonstrable pituitary or CNS disease or any other recognized cause of increased prolactin secretion (see Table 8-10). Prolactin levels may vary from slightly above normal (15 to 20 ng/ml) to values greater than 100 to 200 ng/ml. The diagnosis must at present remain inferential, since the coexistence of a nonvisualized pituitary microadenoma cannot be excluded. The dynamics of prolactin secretion have been extensively studied using a number of neuropharmacological agents (levodopa plus carbidopa, nomifensine, cimetidine, and metoclopramide) in an attempt to distinguish between normal individuals, patients with IH, and those with pituitary tumors, though no consistent differences have been found (Chap. 8). The possibility that IH represents an early stage of prolactin-secreting tumor formation cannot be excluded at present.

The development of IH was previously attributed to a CNS neurotransmitter defect related to dopamine metabolism, on the basis of observations that neuropharmacological agents which impair dopaminergic neurotransmission (most notably the neuroleptic dopamine receptor antagonists) increase prolactin secretion. Prolactin levels during chronic administration of neuroleptics, however, rarely exceed 100 ng/ml, and the site of action of these agents includes the pituitary as well as the CNS. Several studies have now demonstrated lactotroph dopamine resistance in patients with both IH and prolactin-secreting tumors,[265–267] in contrast to patients with known hypothalamic disease. The possibility that a hypothalamic prolactin-releasing factor (e.g., vasoactive intestinal polypeptide) may play a role in this disorder must be considered, though there is as yet no convincing evidence to support it.

The clinical manifestations of IH are similar to those of other forms of hyperprolactinemia: galactorrhea and amenorrhea. Therapy depends on the extent of inconvenience produced in individual patients. Bromocriptine (generally 2.5 mg bid) will suppress prolactin levels, eliminate galactorrhea, and restore cyclic menses and fertility.[268] Nearly 80 percent of patients will experience menses within 2 months of initiating therapy. The effect of the drug is of short duration, though, and hyperprolactinemia will usually recur within 48 h of its discontinuation. The most important site of bromocriptine action is at the pituitary, where it binds to dopamine receptors. In some patients, discontinuation of bromocriptine after prolonged therapy (6 to 24 months) is associated with restoration of normal prolactin secretory dynamics. In others, normal prolactin secretion may occur without specific therapy.

Galactorrhea can also occur in association with normal menses and the presence of normal prolactin levels and has been attributed to an increased sensitivity to endogenous prolactin, possibly because of an increase in breast prolactin receptor capacity or binding affinity. Suppression of prolactin secretion with bromocriptine has frequently proved effective in eliminating the galactorrhea. Similarly, occasional women with normoprolactinemic amenorrhea have had a restoration of cyclic menses with bromocriptine therapy, and it has been suggested that the etiology of the dysfunction is an increased CNS sensitivity to the effects of prolactin on the estrogen feedback mechanism.

Vasopressin (Antidiuretic Hormone)

Diabetes insipidus is considered elsewhere (see Chap. 9). The present section deals with the conditions of so-called cerebral hyponatremia and hypernatremia either secondary to organic central nervous system lesions or occurring as a result of drug therapy.

HYPONATREMIA The syndrome of inappropriate secretion of antidiuretic hormone (ADH), in addition to occurring with ectopic production of ADH by carcinomas, has been described in a variety of disease states involving the central and peripheral nervous system.[269] These include carcinoma metastatic to the brain, primary brain tumors, basal skull fracture, paroxysmal cerebral dysrhythmias, cerebral infarction, subarachnoid hemorrhage, meningitis, encephalitis, and acute intermittent porphyria. In all the case reports the criteria for the diagnosis of inappropriate ADH secretion have been fulfilled: hyponatremia, renal sodium loss, normal renal, pituitary, thyroid, and adrenal function, inability to excrete a dilute urine following water ingestion, resistance to correction by hypertonic saline, and reversibility following water restriction.

The increased excretion of sodium is a consequence of the expanded extracellular volume secondary to the inappropriate secretion of ADH, which then suppresses aldosterone secretion. Increased amounts of immunoreactive ADH have been found in the plasma of patients with this syndrome. It appears that a variety of mechanisms (osmoreceptor reset, ADH leak, peripheral resistance, random ADH secretion) may be responsible in individual cases.[270] Salt-retaining hormones can reverse the negative sodium balance but do not correct the dilutional effect, which is best treated by fluid restriction.

A number of hypoglycemic and antineoplastic drugs have been reported to induce hyponatremia. The former group includes chlorpropramide, tolbutamide, and less frequently the biguanides. The antineoplastic drugs include vincristine and cyclophosphamide. Additional implicated medications are carbamazepine (Tegretol), amitriptyline (Elavil), thioridazine (Mellaril), and clofibrate. Whereas the hypoglycemic agents act by augmenting the action of ADH on the renal tubule in addition to perhaps causing some stimulation of ADH release, vincristine has been shown to have direct neurotoxic effects on rat neurohypophyseal tissue with resultant ADH release. Clofibrate appears to act by release of endogenous ADH.[271]

In some instances, low serum sodium is accompanied by cerebral symptoms and an abnormal electroencephalogram which disappears with correction of the hyponatremia. In other patients, the underlying organic disease can explain most of the clinical manifestations.

HYPERNATREMIA There have been numerous reports of hypernatremia in patients with intracranial lesions, especially in the presence of serious disturbances of the sensorium or coma. The hypernatremia is a result of administration of large solute loads or impairment of normal fluid intake. Other cases, however, have been described in which hypernatremia and hyperosmolality occur in fully conscious patients.[272] In such instances there is evidence of normal renal function, an adequate fluid intake of 1 to 2 liters per day or more, absence of polydipsia or complaints of thirst, failure of forced fluid intake to correct the hyperosmolality and hypernatremia completely, defective release of ADH in response to osmotic stimuli, and occasionally anterior pituitary insufficiency and obesity. The constellation of findings seems to be best explained by impaired hypothalamic regulation of thirst as well as of ADH secretion. There is some evidence that the release of ADH in this disorder may be regulated primarily by changes in effective circulating volume rather than by plasma osmolality. It should be noted that the neural centers involved in the modulation of water ingestion and in the production and release of ADH lie in close proximity in the anterior hypothalamus. Experimentally a similar syndrome of adipsia, dehydration, hypernatremia, and obesity together with unstable temperature regulation has been produced by destruction of the ventromedial hypothalamus. Lesions involving these areas therefore might be expected to produce the described abnormalities. The syndrome has been described in cases of histiocytosis, craniopharyngiomas, optic nerve gliomas, inflammatory changes of undetermined origin, ruptured aneurysms, and pineal germinomas. The difficulty in correcting the hypernatremia with forced fluid intake points out the necessity for specific treatment, if possible, directed to the causative lesion. Qualitative disturbances in vasopressin secretion have also been reported in patients with anorexia nervosa.[273]

NONPITUITARY DISORDERS DUE TO HYPOTHALAMIC DISEASE

Hypothalamic disease can affect many non-pituitary-mediated functions including acute and chronic neurometabolic regulation, temperature control, behavior, sleep, and a large number of autonomic nervous system functions involving the cardiovascular, pulmonary, renal, hematopoietic, and gastrointestinal systems. This section deals primarily with metabolic and thermal regulation; the other topics are beyond the scope of this chapter and are reviewed elsewhere.[186,187]

Acute Disorders of Neurometabolic Regulation

The hypothalamus serves as an integrated locus of those components of the autonomic nervous system involved in the regulation of carbohydrate and lipid metabolism. These effects are mediated through direct neuronal connections with the pancreatic islets, liver, adipose tissue, and gastrointestinal tract and by the release of catecholamines from the adrenal medulla.[188] Acute disturbances of this regulatory system are most frequently seen in states of stress which result in activation of the sympathetic nervous system. Thus, in the presence of hypothermia, general anesthesia, trauma, sepsis, and burns, patients may exhibit hyperglycemia and hyperglucagonemia and/or impairment of insulin secretion.[274–277] In most instances these disturbances do not result in significant clinical problems, and reestablishment of metabolic homeostasis occurs with resolution of the stress. However, in patients with severe burns or sepsis where stress is prolonged, persistent and nonsuppressible hyperglucagonemia and gluconeogenesis have been implicated as etiologic factors in the accompanying catabolic state, which can be life-threatening.[274,278] Suppression of the enhanced sympathetic activity is difficult to achieve but may be the most important factor in reversing the catabolic state and improving the survival rate in these patients.

The "stress diabetes" which is seen in the same clinical disorders may represent a variety of phenomena. True diabetes mellitus may actually be first manifested under circumstances in which the enhanced secretion of cortisol, glucagon, catecholamines, and GH results in an impairment of insulin secretion and action. However, in many individuals the marked hyperglycemia may bear little relation to true diabetes mellitus. A syndrome which satisfies the generally accepted criteria of nonketotic hyperglycemia, with or without coma, may be seen after severe head injury, cerebrovascular thrombosis, encephalitis, and heatstroke; it represents the clinical counterpart of a phenomenon which can be produced in animals by stimulation of the ventromedial hypothalamus or intracerebroventricular administration of any of several neuropeptides (e.g., bombesin, CRF, TRH).[279] The severity of the hyperglycemia and its duration can be used to predict the probability of survival following head injury.[280] The possibility that peripheral adrenergic alpha-receptor blockade can reverse the hyperglycemia as it does in animal models remains to be adequately tested, although there is a preliminary suggestion that this can be effective.[281]

Hypoglycemia has only rarely been attributed to hypothalamic disease.[282] It has been seen in association with subdural hemorrhage, though the locus responsible for altered glucose regulation is unknown.

Chronic Disorders of Neurometabolic Regulation

The control of caloric homeostasis which is responsible for the maintenance of body weight is primarily a function of the ventromedial and ventrolateral hypothalamus, though there is considerable input from extrahypothalamic structures, in particular the limbic system and the telencephalon. A ventromedial satiety center and a ventrolateral feeding center have been well established through stimulation and lesion studies in animals, though controversy remains over the question of whether specific neuronal bodies within the nucleus or axonal fibers traversing the region are the critical elements. The signal for the activation of feeding or satiety behavior is also unknown. An early hypothesis of a glucose-mediated signal has had to be abandoned, and current belief is that the signal reflecting peripheral lipid stores is more likely, though its exact nature remains to be defined. The possibility of insulin involvement in the mediation of this control has been raised because of the presence of both insulin and insulin receptors within the CNS, though convincing evidence is still lacking. The mechanism of obesity development is complex and involves increased food intake, decreased activity, and autonomic nervous system–mediated effects on the pancreas, liver, adrenal medulla, and adipose tissue. A detailed discussion of the control of food intake and of the role of the hypothalamus in metabolic regulation is provided in Chap. 21 and in a recent review of the subject.[188,283]

Destruction of the ventromedial hypothalamus leads to a syndrome of obesity,[284] while damage to the ventrolateral hypothalamus results in anorexia and emaciation. The latter is less common, since bilateral lesions are required and the associated loss of other important homeostatic mechanisms is usually incompatible with prolonged survival.

In only a small percentage of patients with extensive obesity or inanition can the disorder be attributed to defined anatomic destruction of the hypothalamus. However, the inability to distinguish between clinical and biochemical features of obesity or inanition in patients with and without definable hypothalamic disease has supported the hypothesis that "functional" disorders of caloric balance (i.e., "essential" obesity and/or anorexia nervosa) represent biochemical disturbances of hypothalamic function that remain to be defined.

HYPOTHALAMIC OBESITY Ventromedial hypothalamic destruction as a result of tumor, trauma, vascular accident, pseudotumor cerebri, encephalitis, or infiltrative diseases (leukemia or histiocytosis X) has been associated with obesity.[285] Hyperphagia and weight gain continue until a new set point has been achieved, at which time food intake diminishes. Although some authors have commented on the tendency toward centripetal fat accumulation in hypothalamic obesity, the same can be seen in markedly obese patients without definable hypothalamic disease. It has been suggested that the hyperinsulinemia in hypothalamic obesity is greater than that in nonhypothalamic obesity,[286] but the number of patients studied is too small to permit firm conclusions. No differences in oxygen consumption, body composition, or adipose tissue metabolism have been found between patients with hypothalamic and "essential" obesity. The increase in adipose tissue mass in hypothalamic obesity is due primarily to adipocyte hypertrophy rather than hyperplasia. Insulin resistance is generally quite marked, and in some patients diabetes is present. GH secretion is invariably impaired, as in other types of obesity. Alterations in gonadal function and sexual behavior ranging from infertility or decreased libido to complete hypogonadism are common in severe obesity. In some patients this appears to be a secondary problem, since it is reversible upon successful weight reduction, whereas in others it is permanent and probably due to concomitant destruction of the hypothalamic loci controlling GnRH secretion.

A number of well-recognized syndromes associated with obesity have supported the idea of a primary hypothalamic etiology (Table 7-9). Many of these are familial disorders, though the mode of inheritance may vary. Evidence of other hypothalamic disturbances (hypogonadism, temperature intolerance, loss of diurnal rhythms) is present, but there are, in addition, extrahypothalamic disturbances (e.g., deafness, pigmentary retinopathy, mental retardation). In most of these syndromes the specific pathogenic mechanism is not known. However, a genetically altered sensitivity in a chemoreceptor cell within the hypothalamus could result in altered satiety or hunger signals and in changes in autonomic nervous system function which would enhance lipogenesis.

One subgroup, the Prader-Willi syndrome, has an estimated prevalence of about 1 in 25,000 births and has been extensively studied.[288,289] The features of the disorder are first noted during fetal life when decreased movement is often recognized. The classic features of hypotonia, small extremities, and cryptorchism are evident at birth and are accompanied by poor feeding. Mental retardation and obesity do not become prominent until several years later. Glucose tolerance is generally normal, though hyperinsulinemia is present. The TSH response to TRH is increased in relation to both obese and nonobese controls owing to unexplained causes, and GH responses are impaired, as is typical of all obese subjects. GnRH stimulation results in virtually no LH or FSH responses, but with clomiphene treatment, both basal and GnRH-stimulated gonadotropin levels return to normal (Fig. 7-16). In those patients studied at autopsy, no discernible CNS lesions have been found. In a few patients, a deletion or translocation of chromosome 15 has been noted.

Table 7-9. Syndromes of Hypothalamic Obesity

Syndrome	Clinical features	Etiology
Babinski-Froehlich	Obesity and hypogonadism	Craniopharyngioma or other tumor involving the ventromedial hypothalamus and median eminence
Kleine-Levin	Episodic hyperosmia, hyperphagia, hyperactivity when awake, hypersexuality	Preceding viral infection in some patients. Disorder seen primarily in teenage males. Usually disappears by mid-twenties. No histologic examinations performed. Possible paroxysmal limbic system or hypothalamic disease
Laurence-Moon	Pigmentary retinal degeneration, mental deficiency, spastic paraplegia, hypogonadism, obesity	Autosomal dominant inheritance. No gross or microscopic lesions of hypothalamus seen
Bardet-Biedl	Pigmentary retinopathy, mental deficiency, polydactylism, hypogonadism, obesity	No anatomic lesions seen
Allstrom-Hallgren	Pigmentary retinopathy, hypogonadism, deafness, obesity, diabetes	No anatomic lesions seen
Edwards	Pigmentary retinopathy, hypogonadism, gynecomastia, mental retardation, deafness, obesity, diabetes	Autosomal recessive inheritance. No histologic examinations performed
Prader-Willi	Hypogonadism, diabetes, short stature, obesity, temperature intolerance, loss of diurnal rhythms	No anatomic lesions seen

Sources: Adapted from McKusick,[286] Edwards et al,[287] Plum and Van Uitert,[186] and Bray et al.[288]

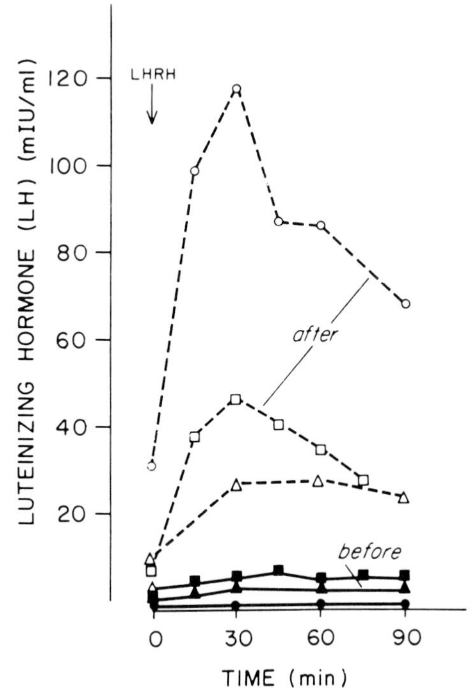

FIGURE 7-16 Effect of clomiphene on the LH response to gonadotropin releasing hormone (LHRH, GnRH) in patients with the Prader-Willi syndrome. Enhanced responses to 100 μg GnRH were observed after 28 to 70 days of clomiphene treatment. (*From Bray et al.*[288])

Therapy of hypothalamic obesity is for the most part unsuccessful. In children with CNS leukemia and hypothalamic infiltrates, chemotherapy-induced remission of the primary disease results in loss of hyperphagia and a reduction of weight to normal, implying that the critical hypothalamic structures have remained intact. However, once true hypothalamic destruction has occurred, the functional alterations are irreversible. Therapeutic measures aimed at treatment of the morbidly obese patient, described in Chap. 21, constitute the only alternative currently available.

DIENCEPHALIC SYNDROME OF INFANCY Approximately 70 infants have been described with a syndrome of emaciation and hyperkinesis, occasionally with large hands and feet, in association with invasive tumors (usually gliomas) which arise in the optic chiasm or anterior hypothalamus and remain confined to the anterior and tuberal regions at the time symptoms occur.[290] Most infants are alert and cheerful, though some may exhibit irritability, and they usually maintain a good appetite and exhibit normal linear growth. Very few patients have been adequately evaluated from an endocrine-metabolic standpoint, though some have been reported to exhibit absent circadian variation of plasma cortisol, lack of metyrapone responsiveness, and elevated GH levels associated with paradoxical responses to hyper- and hypoglycemia. Most children die within the first 2 years of life because of inanition and accompanying complications.

In the few infants who survive beyond 2 years of age the illness frequently undergoes a dramatic transformation. Appetite continues, emaciation ceases, and the child develops extreme obesity.[291] Increased irritability and even rage tend to replace the previous euphoric behavior and hyperactivity. The prognosis for survival improves greatly, but it is not known whether this is due to the altered metabolic activity or the growth characteristics of the tumor.[292]

It is unknown why destruction of the immature hypothalamus produces symptoms different from those in the older child and adult. However, experimental data indicate that the ventromedial nucleus function of controlling food intake does not play an important role until after weaning. Thus, a lesion in a nonfunctional ventromedial hypothalamus would produce relatively few symptoms, and the effects of ventrolateral hypofunction would predominate. With increasing maturity, the absence of the ventromedial hypothalamus would become clinically apparent and obesity would result.

ANOREXIA NERVOSA Anorexia nervosa is a disorder recognized for more than 300 years which is manifested predominantly by weight loss, amenorrhea, and behavioral disturbances occurring almost exclusively in young women of higher socioeconomic status. It has been attributed to a psychiatric disturbance, an endocrine-metabolic disorder, or a combination of the two.[293] The diagnosis in the past has been used loosely to describe many women with amenorrhea and weight loss, and this has led to considerable difficulty in assessing the true features of the disease and the responses to therapy. At present, most physicians agree that the diagnosis must be made on a psychiatric basis as well. The disease has several important features:

1. The age of onset is less than 25 years of age, and the peak period of onset is from 14 to 19 years. The disease occurs in males, but very infrequently (less than 5 percent).
2. There is weight loss of at least 25 percent of original body weight.
3. A distorted and implacable attitude toward eating and weight is present which overrides hunger, admonitions, threats, and reassurances. The patients deny their illness and fail to recognize their nutritional needs. They appear to enjoy losing weight and refusing to eat. They also exhibit a distorted body image of extreme thinness, which they cherish, and manifest unusual hoarding or handling of food. True anorexia does not appear until a late stage of the disease. Bulimia (excessive food intake) and vomiting represent the most severe disturbances of eating behavior and are seen in 50 percent of patients. Hypokalemia and arrhythmias are seen predominantly in this group.
4. Amenorrhea is present in virtually all female patients, and in 25 percent it may precede significant weight loss.
5. The absence of other medical and psychiatric illnesses is crucial in arriving at a diagnosis. Other features include bradycardia, hypotension, hypothermia, constipation, impairment in temperature regulation, lanugo hair growth, hypercarotenemia leading to yellow palms, occasional mild diabetes insipidus, and in severe cases, dependent edema.

Many studies have been performed on patients with anorexia nervosa to delineate the nature of the endocrine abnormalities. The amenorrhea is associated with reduced levels of estradiol, progesterone, and LH and FSH and a loss of the pulsatile secretion of LH seen in mature women (Fig. 7-17). This regression of the LH secretory pattern to the early prepubertal stage is characteristic of the disease. The gonadotropin responses to GnRH may be normal or reduced, and if reduced, the GnRH responsiveness and even ovulation can be restored by daily infusions of exogenous GnRH, implying a decreased secretion of endogenous GnRH.

GH levels are normal or at times elevated, particularly in the face of severe malnutrition, and a paradoxical increase in glucose is often seen. In some patients GH secretion is stimulated by TRH. TSH levels are normal, though there is frequently a delayed response to TRH.[294] T_4 levels are generally normal, though T_3 levels are often reduced and those of reverse T_3 increased. Plasma cortisol levels are in general elevated, and diurnal variation is lacking in 50 percent of patients. Responsiveness to insulin hypoglycemia is, however, maintained, as is dexamethasone suppressibility. Responses to CRF are reduced and have been attributed, in part, to the elevated cortisol levels.[294a] Adrenal androgen production, in contrast, is reduced. No abnormalities of prolactin secretion have been described.

Patients with anorexia nervosa are unable to shiver or to maintain basal body temperature in response to acute hypothermia or hyperthermia. One-third of patients also exhibit an impaired urine-concentrating ability during fluid deprivation which can be corrected by ADH administration, providing evidence for partial diabetes insipidus. There is also a dissociation between plasma vasopressin levels and osmolality, indicating disordered regulation of vasopressin secretion.[273]

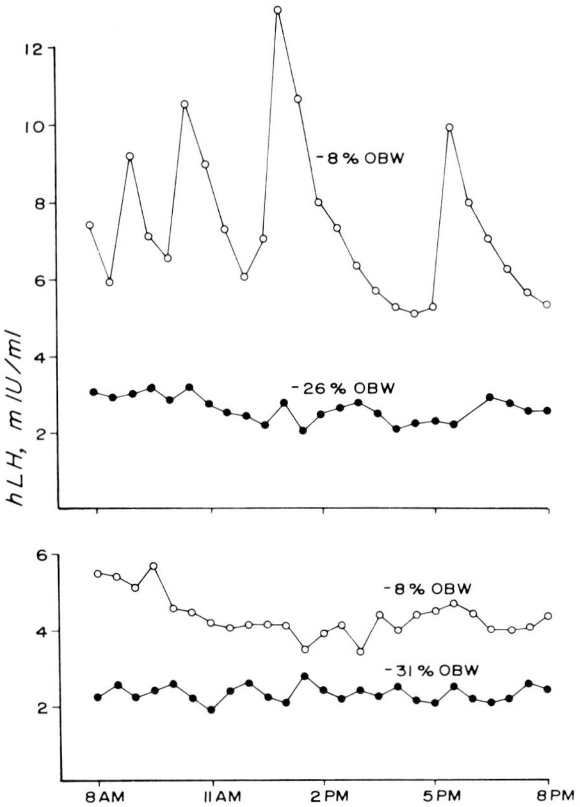

FIGURE 7-17 Loss of episodic LH secretion in anorexia nervosa. The patient in the upper panel exhibited no secretory bursts of LH when first studied at a time when she weighed 26 percent less than her original body weight (OBW). Following gain of weight to 8 percent below OBW, episodic LH secretion was reestablished. In one-third of patients, exemplified by the patient in the lower panel, lack of episodic LH secretion and amenorrhea persist despite comparable or even complete regaining of weight. (*Courtesy of Drs. L. A. Frohman and R. Casper.*)

The abnormalities in gonadotropin secretion, the delayed TSH response to TRH, and the alterations in GH and cortisol secretion suggest the presence of a hypothalamic defect. The return of normal pituitary hormone secretory patterns with successful therapy (with respect to weight gain) supports the hypothesis that the hypothalamic disturbances are secondary to weight loss. However, the persistence of amenorrhea in many patients even after restoration of weight to normal and an impaired response of plasma LH to clomiphene stimulation suggest that some factor in addition to malnutrition must be present.[295]

Therapeutic considerations in anorexia nervosa are to a large extent beyond the scope of this chapter and have recently been reviewed in detail elsewhere.[293] The basic approach relates to reinstitution of adequate dietary intake along with appropriate psychotherapeutic measures. A liquid diet beginning with 1200 to 1500 cal per day and increasing to 3000 cal per day within 1 week has been found useful in many patients. Introduction of solid foods should be accompanied by insistence on a balanced diet. Numerous psychopharmacological agents have been tried (cyproheptadine, neuroleptics, levodopa, antidepressants), but their limited efficacy and considerable side effects do not appear to justify their use.

The prognosis for reversal of the cachexia and for short-term weight gain is much better today than in the past. Mortality from the consequences of starvation (generally due to decreased resistance to infection) is about 5 percent or less.[295] The vast majority of patients will regain sufficient weight to return to within 10 percent of original body weight, but only about 40 percent of such patients will maintain this weight permanently and resume normal ovulatory menses. Another 25 percent will experience minor difficulties in weight maintenance, and in this group persistent amenorrhea is common. A similar percentage will have recurrent weight loss, exhibit severe depressive symptoms, and remain amenorrheic.

Disorders of Temperature Regulation

Maintenance of thermoregulation represents an integrated function of the hypothalamus involving thermoreceptors and pyrogen receptors in the preoptic and anterior hypothalamus, input from other CNS and peripheral thermoreceptors, and nonthermal stimuli including arousal level, diurnal rhythm, and menstrual cycle stage. The eventual set point reflects a combination of the multiple inputs rather than the local temperature at any given site. Heat dissipation and generation mechanisms activated by the hypothalamus consist of affective sensations of thermal discomfort leading to behavioral responses which attempt to modify the environment and physiological responses which include autonomic (vascular tone, sweating, panting) and endocrine (TSH) responses and activation of the sympathetic nervous system. The latter modifies the metabolic rate and the utilization of stored fuels, which provide the major source of thermogenesis during prolonged cold exposure. Serotonin has a stimulatory effect on thermoreceptors, norepinephrine exhibits an inhibitory effect, and cholinergic neurons appear to be involved in the pathways connecting thermosensing and thermoeffective neurons. The pharmacology and physiology of temperature regulation have been extensively reviewed elsewhere.[296,297]

Hypothalamic disorders in human beings can produce hypo- or hyperthermia by destroying heat-producing or -disseminating mechanisms or by causing an alteration in the set point.[186] The latter produces changes of body temperature irrespective of environmental temperature, while disturbances in heat production or dissemination require an ambient temperature either lower or higher, respectively, than body temperature. Sustained hypothermia is rare but may occur with anterior hypothalamic lesions and may be due to a chronically altered set point or to impairment of heat-generating mechanisms. Paroxysmal hypothermia, or attacks of lowered body temperature, have been reported in occasional patients, in some of whom diabetes insipidus has been present. Agenesis of the corpus callosum has been a common finding in these patients.

Sustained hyperthermia due to neuronal damage occurs only as a self-limited process—usually following craniotomy, trauma, or hemorrhage into the anterior hypothalamus or third ventricle. Cardiovascular changes are disproportionately small in such patients. Hypothalamic hyperthermia does not last for more than 2 weeks after the acute event. Paroxysmal hyperthermia is a rare disease consisting of episodes of shaking chills, spiking fever, and occasionally other autonomic phenomena. This condition must be considered as an exclusion diagnosis after other causes of intermittent fever have been eliminated. Anatomic evidence for the site of the abnormality is limited.

Relative poikilothermia (body temperature fluctuation of more than 2°C which coincides with charges in ambient temperature) is the most common neurogenic disorder of thermoregulation in human beings. Poikilothermia results from the loss of function of the final effector pathways in the posterior hypothalamus and mesencephalon and affects the thermal discomfort, behavioral regulation, and autonomic effector mechanisms. Patients with poikilothermia are unaware of their temperature imbalance and show no signs of discomfort with thermal stress. Because ambient temperature is generally below body temperature, most patients exhibit hypothermia. The lesions producing this disorder must be bilateral. Functionally, both newborns and the elderly exhibit moderate poikilothermia, as do patients with anorexia nervosa.

Other CNS Disorders

DISEASES OF THE PINEAL GLAND

Disorders of the pineal gland which produce endocrine disturbances include hypoplasia or aplasia, a rare disease often associated with precocious puberty, and tumors of the pineal region. Pineal tumors, which constitute less than 1 percent of all intracranial neoplasms, are of three types: pinealomas, tumors of pineal parenchymal tissue representing 20 percent of pineal neoplasms; glial tumors, which represent about 25 percent; and germinomas, which make up the remainder. Germinomas have also been called *ectopic pinealomas* (if their location is extrapineal) or *teratomas.*[298] They arise from embryonic germ cells which normally migrate from the yolk sac to the gonadal ridge but which may be found in aberrant locations, including the mediastinum and the midline paraventricular regions. They exhibit both histological and functional similarities to ovarian and testicular germ cell tumors. Tumors of this type infiltrate the third ventricle and floor of the hypothalamus and produce a characteristic triad of optic atrophy, diabetes insipidus, and hypogonadism. The enlarging tumor mass can also compress the aqueduct of Sylvius, giving rise to internal hydrocephalus with its characteristic headaches, vomiting, papilledema, and altered consciousness. Parinaud's syndrome (paralysis of conjugate upward gaze) due to pressure on the superior colliculi and disturbances of gait due to cerebellar or brainstem pressure may also be seen. Less common manifestations include disturbances of temperature regulation, hyperphagia, or anorexia secondary to compromising hypothalamic functional integrity. On rare occasions the tumors extend into the sella turcica and mimic a primary pituitary tumor. Some teratomas can develop into choriocarcinomas and secrete chorionic gonadotropin and free alpha subunit into the CSF and blood.

Since the first report of precocious puberty in a boy with a pineal tumor,[299] there has been considerable interest in this association, but when viewed in perspective, only a small percentage of such tumors cause sexual precocity.[300,301] In general, only those tumors which extend well beyond the pineal region have been associated with precocious puberty, and the basis for the endocrine disturbance is most likely a destruction of other brain regions which, during the prepubertal years, tonically inhibit GnRH and gonadotropin secretion. Nonparenchymatous pineal tumors are more commonly associated with precocious puberty than are parenchymatous tumors,[302] and on this basis, it has been suggested that destruction of the normal pineal by the tumor results in the loss of a pineal secretory product (perhaps melatonin, arginine vasotocin, or another factor) which normally inhibits the initiation of sexual maturation. There is also evidence that at least some pineal tumors exhibit endocrine function, and the production of an antigonadotropic factor by the tumor could provide an alternative explanation for the delayed puberty frequently encountered. Although there are no reports of elevated circulating melatonin levels in patients with pinealomas, a recent report has documented normal plasma melatonin levels prior to removal of a low-grade astrocytoma-pineoblastoma, with undetectable levels postoperatively.[303] While much additional investigation is required, it may well be that multiple mechanisms exist for the production of altered gonadal function in patients with pineal tumors. Because of their location, hypothalamic area pinealomas can generally not be resected without producing severe damage to surrounding structures. Although craniotomy has been routinely performed to establish a tissue diagnosis, in many instances the diagnosis can be made by measuring elevated hCG or alpha-fetoprotein levels in serum. In such instances radiotherapy is the treatment of choice, and long-term favorable results have been obtained.[304]

PSEUDOTUMOR CEREBRI

This syndrome, also known as *benign intracranial hypertension*, is characterized by headache, papilledema, and raised intracranial pressure in the absence of a focal CNS lesion or of obstructive hydrocephalus. The majority of cases are idiopathic, 90 percent occurring in obese females.[305] The clinical onset is usually abrupt, and severe headache or visual symptoms such as sudden loss or blurring of vision or diplopia occur in 35 percent of patients. Somnolence and hyperphagia may also be present. Twenty-five percent of patients experience spontaneous recovery. In others, recovery is coincident with repeated lumbar puncture alone or in combination with corticosteroid treatment.

In a small percentage of patients an association has been reported with venous sinus obstruction, vitamin A intoxication, iron deficiency anemia, steroid withdrawal, Addison's disease, pregnancy, or contraceptive medication, though an etiologic relationship has not been established. Sellar enlargement with evidence of an empty sella has also been noted in occasional patients, particularly when symptoms have been of prolonged duration. Endocrine studies, including basal prolactin, GH, and FSH and LH levels as well as cortisol and GH responses to insulin-induced hypoglycemia, circadian pattern of corticosteroid concentrations, and cortisol response to metyrapone, have usually been normal.

CEREBRAL GIGANTISM

This disease of children is characterized by a rapid growth rate (although final height is usually within the normal range), accelerated bone age, a normal sella turcica, and a nonprogressive cerebral disorder characterized by mental retardation.[306] Pneumoencephalography has demonstrated ventricular enlargement with no evidence of a focal CNS lesion. Studies of basal endocrine function have been normal; no elevation in plasma GH levels has been reported, although 24-h secretion studies have not been performed. A variant associated with lipodystrophy, pigmentation, hypertrichosis, hepatosplenomegaly, elevated 17-ketosteroids and 17-ketogenic steroids, abnormal glucose tolerance, hyperlipemia, and in one instance, increased plasma insulin-like activity has also been described.[307] Such cerebral gigantism is probably also different from that reported in cases of neurofibromatosis (with associated hypothalamic involvement),[308] in which paradoxical hypersecretion of GH has been reported and hypersecretion of GRH may be present.[309,310]

HUNTINGTON'S CHOREA

Pathological changes have been reported in the hypothalamus of patients with Huntington's chorea.[311,312] In some reports a disorder of dopaminergic metabolism has been suggested as an etiologic factor,[313] though this has not been confirmed by others.[314] Several neuroendocrine studies of basal and stimulated GH and prolactin concentrations have been reported, though the results have not been entirely consistent. Both elevated and depressed basal prolactin levels have been recorded along with normal or impaired responses to dopaminergic agonists and antagonists.[315–317] Similar conflicting results have been reported with respect to GH.[316,318–322] Attempts have been made to interpret these findings as indicative of a generalized dopaminergic neurotransmitter function in Huntington's chorea. However, the neural pathways involved in Huntington's disease are quite distinct from those which participate in neuroendocrine responses to the stimuli used for testing, and it is premature to draw any definitive conclusions from the studies reported to date.

Recently, increased concentrations of somatostatin and decreased concentrations of substance P have been noted in the basal ganglia of patients with Huntington's disease.[323] The relation of these changes to the underlying pathology of the disease and to the neuroendocrine disturbances is not known.

Behavioral Disorders

PSYCHIATRIC ILLNESS

It is readily apparent that behavioral changes accompany virtually every endocrine disease. In this section we will consider the endocrine correlates of psychiatric disease. There has been much recent interest in altered neurotransmitter metabolism in various categories of psychiatric disease. Neurotransmitters are known to be involved in the regulation of hypophysiotropic releasing factors, thereby acting directly or indirectly on pituitary hormone secretion. The interrelations between postulated neurotransmitter abnormalities, psychiatric disease, and endocrine disturbance are still unclear: are the last two independent variables responding to a change in neurotransmitter concentration, or does the altered behavior in itself directly produce endocrine changes? Many of the commonly used psychiatric drugs have endocrine effects, e.g., production of galactorrhea, alteration of corticosteroid metabolism by enzyme induction, or changes in gonadal and thyroid function. Morphine has long been known to have endocrine effects, and it is of interest that the endogenous opiates similarly affect pituitary hormone secretion, thus far being reported to elicit release of vasopressin, GH, and prolactin.

Depression

Of the various psychiatric conditions, those most thoroughly studied have been unipolar depression and the manic-depressive state. There appears to be general agreement that the circadian rhythm of plasma corticosteroids is normal in depression. Depressed patients, however, secrete more cortisol and have more secretory episodes and more minutes of active secretion throughout day and night, with a return to normal levels and episodic secretion on recovery.[324] Although these alterations in cortisol secretion were initially considered the result of stress, anxiety, or other nonspecific factors, careful studies have excluded these possibilities and have demonstrated a specific association with endogenous and generally unipolar depressive states. Depressed patients exhibit an enhancement both of cortisol production and metabolic clearance. They are more resistant than normal subjects to dexamethasone suppression,[325] an abnormality which also reverts to normal with successful treatment. While normal subjects given 1 mg of dexamethasone at 11 P.M. exhibit suppression of plasma cortisol levels to less than 5 μg/dl for at least 16 h, patients with depression escape from the effects of dexamethasone by this time.[326] The corticosteroid response to insulin-induced hypoglycemia is generally normal, though some instances of decreased responsiveness have also been noted.

It is apparent that depressed patients share many of the endocrine abnormalities seen in Cushing's disease. Since psychiatric manifestations may also be seen in Cushing's disease, the differential diagnosis may sometimes be difficult. However, depressed patients have none of the stigmata of hypercorticism (e.g., obesity, facial plethora, or striae), and as noted above, the finding of a normal circadian periodicity of plasma corticosteroid concentrations in depressed patients as well as normal corticosteroid responses to insulin-induced hypoglycemia and a diminished rather than enhanced ACTH response to CRF[327] should eliminate confusion with regard to differential diagnosis.

Circadian periodicity of plasma corticosteroids has been reported to be normal in mania. This, however, is based on infrequent sampling, and in view of the marked sleep disturbances in manic patients, a finding of altered periodicity might be expected under appropriate study conditions.

Growth hormone secretion is also altered in depression, with reduced responses to insulin hypoglycemia.[328,329] Since the GH response to insulin is related to urinary excretion of 3-methoxy-4-hydroxyphenylglycol, a metabolite of dopamine,[330] the impaired responses to insulin have been used in support of the hypothesis of a CNS catecholamine deficiency in some depressed patients. Studies of the secretion of other pituitary hormones in depression have been less consistent. The overall conclusion from these studies is that specific neuroendocrine abnormalities are present in affective disorders, which may be useful in assessing CNS biogenic amine function. However, for the most part, the results of such studies are of limited usefulness in establishing diagnoses or monitoring therapy.

Schizophrenia

Neuroendocrine studies in patients with schizophrenia have been carried out in an attempt to utilize the pituitary hormone responses as a "window to the brain," that is, as a means of probing for neurotransmitter abnormalities. The majority of studies have focused on dopaminergic agonists and antagonists because of interest in the hypothesis that dopamine overactivity has a pathogenic role in this disorder. GH responses to apomorphine, a dopamine agonist, are generally elevated in patients with acute schizophrenia,[331–333] whereas in chronic schizophrenia the responses tend to be blunted[332]—perhaps in part as a consequence of neuroleptic treatment. GH responses to apomorphine also exhibit an inverse correlation with platelet monoamine oxidase activity,[334] which is believed to reflect brain dopamine function and to have some predictive value in the antipsychotic response to lithium.[335] A degree of caution is required in interpreting these results, since the interrelation between the hypothalamic tuberoinfundibular dopaminergic tract, where apomorphine is believed to exhibit its GH-releasing action (through the release of GRH), and the mesolimbic dopaminergic tract, which is believed to be involved in the behavioral disturbances of schizophrenia, remains to be clarified.[336,337]

The neuroendocrine control of TSH secretion is believed to be impaired in schizophrenia. However, nearly half the acutely psychotic patients admitted to the hospital are found to have elevated serum thyroxine levels in association with clinical manifestations of thyrotoxicosis which return to normal within a few days without specific therapy.[338] The mechanism for the thyroid elevation and its resolution is unclear.

EMOTIONAL DEPRIVATION

The syndrome of emotional deprivation with growth failure (psychosocial dwarfism) is characterized by short stature, normal sellar size, and clinical findings suggestive of hypopituitarism (especially absent or diminished GH levels, both basally and in response to insulin-induced hypoglycemia, and diminished basal corticosteroid excretion and responsiveness to metyrapone).[339] Children with this disorder have a history of a disturbed home environment. The disorder is rapidly reversed on removal from this environment, concomitant with evidence of return of normal GH secretion. It has been suggested that excessive beta-adrenergic inhibitory effects may be one of the causative factors in the syndrome; there is one report of restoration of normal GH secretion by acute treatment with propranolol.[260]

REFERENCES

1. Scharrer E, Scharrer B: *Neurosecretion.* New York, Columbia University, 1961.
2. Szentagothai JP, Flerko B, Mess B, Halaz SZB: *Hypothalamic Control of the Anterior Pituitary,* 3d ed. Budapest, Akademia Kiado, 1968.
3. Halasz B: The endocrine effects of isolation of the hypothalamus from the rest of the brain, in Ganong WF, Martini L (eds): *Frontiers of Neuroendocrinology.* New York, Oxford University, 1969, p 307.
4. Ambach G, Palkovits M, Szentagothai J: Blood supply of the rat hypothalamus: IV. Retrochiasmatic area, median eminence, arcuate nucleus. *Acta Morphol Acad Sci Hung* 24:93, 1976.
5. Harris GW: Neural control of the pituitary gland. *Physiol Rev* 28:139, 1948.
6. Schaeffer MJ, Hsueh AJW: Acetylcholine receptors in the rat anterior pituitary gland. *Endocrinology* 106:1377, 1980.
7. Peters JR, Foord SM, Diequez C, Scanlon MF, Hall R: α_1-Adrenoreceptors on intact rat anterior pituitary cells: Correlation with adrenergic stimulation of thyrotropin secretion. *Endocrinology* 113:133, 1983.
8. Grandison L, Cavagnini F, Schmid R, Invitti C, Guidotti A: γ-Aminobutyric acid and benzodiazepine-binding sites in human anterior pituitary tissue. *J Clin Endocrinol Metab* 54:597, 1982.
9. Gudelsky GA, Porter JC: Sex-related difference in the release of dopamine into hypophysial portal blood. *Endocrinology* 109:1394, 1981.
10. Johnston CA, Gibbs DM, Negro-Vilar A: High concentrations of epinephrine derived from a central source and of 5-hydroxyindole-3-acetic acid in hypophyseal portal plasma. *Endocrinology* 113:819, 1983.
11. Johns MA, Azmitia EC, Krieger DT: Specific *in vitro* uptake of serotonin by cells in the anterior pituitary of the rat. *Endocrinology* 110:754, 1982.
12. Reymond MJ: Regionalization of dopamine secretion in the median eminence. *Proceedings of the 65th Meeting of the Endocrine Society,* 1983, p 175.
13. Palkovits M, Zaborszky L: Neural connections of the hypothalamus, in Morgane DJ, Panksepp J (eds): *Anatomy of the Hypothalamus.* Paris, Marcel Dekker, 1979, vol 1, p 397.
14. Page RB, Munger BL, Bergland RM: Scanning microscopy of pituitary vascular casts. *Am J Anat* 146:273, 1976.
15. Oliver C, Mical RS, Porter JC: Hypothalamic-pituitary vasculature: Evidence for retrograde blood flow in the pituitary. *Endocrinology* 101:598, 1970.
16. Bergland RM, Page RB: Pituitary-brain vascular relations: A new paradigm. *Science* 204:18, 1979.
17. Page RB: Directional pituitary flow: A microcinephotographic study. *Endocrinology* 112:157, 1983.
18. Matsuura S, Ohashi M, Chen HC, Shownkeen RC, Hartree AS, Reichert LE Jr, Stevens VC, Powell JE: Physicochemical and immunological characterization of an HCG-like substance from human pituitary glands. *Nature* 286:740, 1980.
19. Suginami H, Kawaoi A: Immunohistochemical localization of a human chorionic gonadotropin-like substance in the human pituitary gland. *J Clin Endocrinol Metab* 55:1161, 1982.
20. Maruse K, Celio MR, Takii Y, Inagami T: Immunohistochemical localization of renin in the luteinizing hormone containing cells in rat pituitary. *Proceedings of the 63rd Meeting of the Endocrine Society,* 1981, p 277.
21. Steele MK, Brownfield MS, Ganong WF: Immunocytochemical localization of angiotensin immunoreactivity in gonadotrops and lactotrops of the rat anterior pituitary gland. *Neuroendocrinology* 35:155, 1982.
22. Shirasawa N, Kihara H, Yamaguchi S, Yoshimura F: Pituitary folliculo-stellate cells immunostained with S-100 protein antiserum in postnatal, castrated and thyroidectomized rats. *Cell Tissue Res* 231:235, 1983.
23. Ishikawa H, Nogami H, Shirasawa N: Novel clonal strains from adult rat anterior pituitary producing S-100 protein. *Nature* 303:711, 1983.
24. Denef C, Andries M: Evidence for paracrine interaction between gonadotrophs and lactotrophs in pituitary cell aggregates. *Endocrinology* 112:813, 1983.
25. Ajika K: Relationship between catecholaminergic neurons and hypothalamic hormone-containing neurons in the hypothalamus, in Martini L, Ganong WF (eds): *Frontiers in Neuroendocrinology.* New York, Raven, 1980, vol 6, p 1.
26. Moore KE, Demarest KT: Tuberoinfundibular and tuberohypophyseal dopaminergic neurons, in Ganong WF, Martini L (eds): *Frontiers in Neuroendocrinology.* New York, Raven, 1982, vol 7, p 161.
27. Steinbusch HWM: Distribution of serotonin-immunoreactivity in the central nervous system of the rat—cell bodies and terminals. *Neuroscience* 6:557, 1981.
28. Storm-Mathisen J, Leknes AK, Boro AT, Vaaland JL, Edminson P, Haug F-MS, Ottersen OP: First visualization of glutamate and GABA in neurones by immunocytochemistry. *Nature* 301:517, 1983.
29. Perez de la Mora M, Fuxe K, Hokfelt T, Andersson K, Possani L, Tapia R: Gabaergic synapses: Distribution and interaction with other neurotransmitter systems in the brain, in Tapia R, Cotman CW (eds): *Regulatory Mechanisms of Synaptic Transmission.* New York, Plenum, 1981, p 71.
30. Beaulac-Baillargeon L, Di Paolo T, Raymond V, Giguere V, Labrie F: Alpha-adrenergic binding sites in bovine anterior pituitary gland and control of ACTH secretion in rat anterior pituitary cells in culture. *Proceedings, Meeting of the Society for Neuroscience,* 1980, vol 6, p 28.
31. Krieger DT, Martin JB: Brain peptides: I and II. *N Engl J Med* 304:876, 944, 1981.

32. Krieger DT: Brain peptides: What, where, and why? *Science* 222:975, 1983.

33. Jan YN, Jan LY, Kuffler SW: A peptide as a possible neurotransmitter in sympathetic ganglia of the frog. *Proc Natl Acad Sci USA* 76:1501, 1979.

34. Jan LY, Jan YN, Brownfield MS: Peptide neurotransmitters in synaptic boutons of sympathetic ganglia. *Nature* 288:360, 1980.

35. Krieger DT: Brain peptides, *Vitam Horm* 41:1, 1984.

36. Shimatsu A, Kato Y, Matsushita N, Katakami H, Yanaihara N, Imura H: Stimulation by serotonin of vasoactive intestinal polypeptide release into rat hypophysial portal blood. *Endocrinology* 111:338, 1982.

37. Rotsztejn WH, Dussaillant M, Nobou F, Rosselin G: Rapid glucocorticoid inhibition of vasoactive intestinal peptide–induced cyclic AMP accumulation and prolactin release in rat pituitary cells in culture. *Proc Natl Acad Sci USA* 78:7584, 1982.

38. Gudelsky GA, Porter JC: Morphine and opioid peptide–induced inhibition of the release of dopamine from tuberoinfundibular neurons. *Life Sci* 25:1697, 1979.

39. Wardlaw SL, Wehrenberg WB, Merin M, Carmel PW, Frantz AG: High levels of β-endorphin in hypophyseal portal blood. *Endocrinology* 106:1323, 1980.

40. Simantov R, Snyder SH: Opiate receptor binding in the pituitary gland. *Brain Res* 124:178, 1977.

41. Shibahara S, Morimoto Y, Furutani Y, Notake M, Takahashi H, Shimizu S, Horikawa S, Numa S: Isolation and sequence analysis of the human corticotropin-releasing factor precursor gene. *EMBO J* 2:775, 1983.

42. Vale W, Spiess J, Rivier C, Rivier J: Characterization of a 41-residue ovine hypothalamic peptide that stimulates secretion of cortocotropin and β-endorphin. *Science* 213:1394, 1981.

43. Rivier J, Spiess J, Thorner M, Vale W: Characterization of a growth hormone–releasing factor from a human pancreatic islet tumour. *Nature* 300:276, 1982.

44. Guillemin R, Brazeau P, Bohlen P, Esch F, Ling N, Wehrenberg WB: Growth hormone–releasing factor from a human pancreatic tumor that caused acromegaly. *Science* 218:585, 1982.

44a. Schurmeyer TH, Avgerinos PC, Gold PW, Gallucci WT, Tomai TP, Cutler GB Jr, Loriaux DL, Chrousos GP: Human corticotropin-releasing factor in man: Pharmacokinetic properties and dose response of plasma adrenocorticotropin and cortisol secretion. *J Clin Endocrinol Metab* 59:1103, 1984.

45. Brownstein MJ, Eskay RL, Palkovits M: Thyrotropin releasing hormone in the median eminence is in processes of paraventricular nucleus neurons. *Neuropeptides* 2:197, 1982.

46. Jackson IMD, Reichlin S: Distribution and biosynthesis of TRH in the nervous system, in Collu R, Barbeau A, Dacharme J, Rochefort J (eds): *Central Nervous System Effects of Hypothalamic Hormones and Other Peptides.* New York, Raven, 1979, p 3.

47. Rupnow JH, Hinkle PM, Dixon JE: A macromolecule which gives rise to thyrotropin-releasing hormone. *Biochem Biophys Res Commun* 89:721, 1979.

47a. Lechan RM, Wu P, Jackson IMD, Wolf H, Cooperman S, Mandel G, Goodman RH: Thyrotropin-releasing hormone precursor: Characterization in rat brain. *Science* 231:159, 1986.

48. Bauer K, Graf KJ, Faivre-Bauman A, Beier S, Tixier-Vidal A, Kleinkauf H: Inhibition of prolactin secretion by histidyl-proline-diketopiperazine. *Nature* 274:174, 1978.

49. Fink G, Koch Y, Ben Aroya N: Release of thyrotropin releasing hormone into hypophysial portal blood is high relative to other neuropeptides and may be related to prolactin secretion. *Brain Res* 243:186, 1982.

50. Reichlin S, Mitnick M: Biosynthesis of thyrotropin releasing hormone and its control by hormones, central monoamines and external environment, in Gual C, Rosemberg E (eds): *Hypothalamic Hypophysiotropic Hormones: Physiological and Clinical Studies.* Amsterdam, Excerpta Medica, 1973, p 124.

51. Kardon F, Marcus RJ, Winokur A, Utiger RD: TRH content of rat brain hypothalamus. *Endocrinology* 100:1604, 1977.

52. Udeschini G, Cocchi D, Panerai AE, Gil-Ad I, Rossi GL, Chiodini PG, Liuzzi A, Muller EE: Stimulation of growth hormone release by thyrotropin releasing hormone in the hypophysectomized rat bearing an ectopic pituitary. *Endocrinology* 98:807, 1976.

52a. Szabo M, Stachura ME, Paleologos N, Bybee DE, Frohman LA: Thyrotropin releasing hormone stimulates growth hormone release from the anterior pituitary of hypothyroid rats in vitro. *Endocrinology* 114:1344, 1984.

53. Faden AI, Jacobs TP, Holaday JW: Thyrotropin-releasing hormone improves neurologic recovery after spinal trauma in cats. *N Engl J Med* 305:1063, 1981.

54. Morley JE: Extrahypothalamic thyrotropin releasing hormone (TRH)—its distribution and its functions. *Life Sci* 25:1539, 1979.

55. Keller HH, Bartholini G, Pletcher A: Enhancement of cerebral noradrenaline turnover by thyrotropin-releasing hormone. *Nature* 248:528, 1974.

56. King JA, Millar RP: Heterogeneity of vertebrate luteinizing hormone–releasing hormone. *Science* 206:67, 1979.

57. Krey LC, Silverman A-J: Luteinizing hormone releasing hormone, in Krieger DT, Brownstein M, Martin JB (eds): *Brain Peptides.* New York, Wiley, 1983, p 687.

58. Fuchs S, Lundanes E, Leban J, Folkers K: On the existence and separation of the follicle stimulating hormone releasing hormone from the luteinizing hormone releasing hormone. *Biochem Biophys Res Commun* 88:92, 1979.

58a. Nikolics K, Mason AJ, Szonyi E, Ramachandran J, Seeburg PH: A prolactin-inhibiting factor within the precursor for human gonadotropin-releasing hormone. *Nature* 316:511, 1985.

59. Knobil E: The neuroendocrine control of the menstrual cycle. *Recent Prog Horm Res* 36:53, 1980.

60. Carmel PW, Araki S, Ferin M: Pituitary stalk portal blood collection in rhesus monkeys: Evidence for pulsatile release of gonadotropin-releasing hormone (GnRH). *Endocrinology* 99:243, 1976.

61. McKelvy JF, Lin C-J, Chan L, Joseph-Bravo P, Charli J-L, Pacheco M, Paulo M, Neale J, Barker J: Biosynthesis of brain peptides, in Gotto AM Jr, Peck EJ Jr, Boyd AE III (eds): *Brain Peptides: A New Endocrinology.* Amsterdam, Elsevier/North-Holland, 1979, p 183.

62. Curtis A, Fink G: A high molecular weight precursor of luteinizing hormone–releasing hormone from rat hypothalamus. *Endocrinology* 112:390, 1983.

62a. Seeburg PH, Adelman JP: Characterization of cDNA for precursor of human luteinizing hormone releasing hormone. *Nature* 311:666, 1985.

63. Griffiths EC, Kelly JA, Forbes R, Jeffcoate SL, White N, Milner RDG, Visser TJ: The role of enzymatic degradation of brain peptides in neuroendocrine control, in Gotto AM Jr, Peck EJ Jr, Boyd AE III (eds): *Brain Peptides: A New Endocrinology.* Amsterdam, Elsevier/North-Holland, 1979, p 197.

64. Crowley WF Jr, Beitins IZ, Vale W, Kliman B, Rivier J, Rivier C, McArthur JW: The biologic activity of a potent analogue of gonadotropin-releasing hormone in normal and hypogonadotropic men. *N Engl J Med* 302:1051, 1980.

65. Rivier C, Rivier J, Vale W: Chronic effects of [D-Trp^6,Pro^9-NEt]-luteinizing hormone–releasing factor in reproductive processes in the male rat. *Endocrinology* 105:1191, 1979.

66. Moss RL, McCann SM: Induction of mating behavior in rats by luteinizing hormone–releasing factor. *Science* 181:171, 1973.

67. Riskind P, Moss RL: Midbrain central gray: LHRH infusion enhances lordotic behavior in estrogen-primed ovariectomized rats. *Brain Res Bull* 4:203, 1979.

68. Sakuma Y, Pfaff DW: LH-RH in the mesencephalic central gray can potentiate lordosis reflex of female rats. *Nature* 283:566, 1980.

69. Moss RL: Actions of hypothalamic-hypophysiotropic hormones on the brain. *Annu Rev Physiol* 41:617, 1979.

70. Goodman RH, Jacobs JW, Dee PC, Habener JF: Somatostatin-28 encoded in a cloned cDNA obtained from a rat medullary thyroid carcinoma. *J Biol Chem* 257:1156, 1982.

71. Schally AV, DuPont A, Arimura A, Redding TW, Nishi N, Linthicum GL, Schlesinger DH: Isolation and structure of somatostatin from porcine hypothalami. *Biochemistry* 15:509, 1976.

72. Spiess J, Rivier JE, Rodkey JA, Bennett CD, Vale W: Isolation and characterization of somatostatin from pigeon pancreas. *Proc Natl Acad Sci USA* 76:2974, 1979.

73. Curry DL, Bennett LL: Does somatostatin inhibition of insulin secretion involve two mechanisms of action? *Proc Natl Acad Sci USA* 73:248, 1976.

74. Reichlin S: Somatostatin, in Krieger DT, Brownstein M, Martin JB (eds): *Brain Peptides.* New York, Wiley, 1983, p 711.

75. Renaud LP, Brazeau P, Martin JB: Depressant action of TRH, LH-RH and somatostatin on the activity of central neurons. *Nature* 255:233, 1970.

76. Ioffe S, Havlicek V, Friesen H, Chernick V: Effect of somatostatin (SRIF) and L-glutamate on neurons of the sensorimotor cortex in awake habituated rabbits. *Brain Res* 153:414, 1978.

77. Dichter MA, Delfs JR: Somatostatin and cortical neurons in cell culture. *Adv Biochem Psychopharmacol* 28:145, 1981.

78. Cote J, Lefevre G, Labrie F, Barden N: Distribution of corticotropin-releasing factor in ovine brain determined by radioimmunoassay. *Regul Pept* 5:189, 1983.

79. Swanson LW, Sawchenko PE, Rivier J, Vale WW: Organization of ovine corticotropin-releasing factor immunoreactive cells and fibers in the rat brain: An immunohistochemical study. *Neuroendocrinology* 36:165, 1983.

80. Roth KA, Weber E, Barchas JD, Chang D, Chang J-K: Immunoreactive dynorphin-(1-8) and corticotropin-releasing factor in subpopulation of hypothalamic neurons. *Science* 219:189, 1983.

81. Roth KA, Weber E, Barchas JD: Immunoreactive corticotropin releasing factor (CRF) and vasopressin are co-localized in a subpopulation of the immunoreactive vasopressin cells in the paraventricular nucleus of the hypothalamus. *Life Sci* 31:1857, 1982.

82. Shibasaki T, Odagiri E, Shizume K, Ling N: Corticotropin-releasing factor-like activity in human placental extracts. *J Clin Endocrinol Metab* 55:384, 1982.

83. Petrusz P, Merchenthaler I, Maderdrut JL, Vigh S, Schally AV: Corticotropin-releasing factor (CRF)-like immunoreactivity in the vertebrate endocrine pancreas. *Proc Natl Acad Sci USA* 80:1721, 1983.

84. Nieuwenhuijzen-Kruseman AC, Linton EA, Lowry PJ, Rees LH, Besser GM: Corticotropin-releasing factor immunoreactivity in human gastrointestinal tract. *Lancet* 2:1245, 1982.

85. Brodish A: Tissue corticotropin releasing factors. *Fed Proc* 36:2088, 1977.

86. Morel G, Hemming F, Tonon C-C, Vaudry H, Dubois MP, Coy D, Dubois PM: Ultrastructural evidence for corticotropin-releasing factor (CRF)-like immunoreactivity in the rat pituitary gland. *Biol Cell* 44:89, 1982.

87. Leroux P, Pelletier G: Radioautographic localization of corticotropin-releasing factor (CRF) receptors in the rat pituitary gland. *Proceedings of the 64th Meeting of the Endocrine Society*, 1982, p 277.

88. Vale WW, Rivier C, Spiess J, Rivier J: Corticotropin releasing factor, in Krieger DT, Brownstein M, Martin JB (eds): *Brain Peptides.* New York, Wiley, 1983, p 961.

89. Furutani Y, Morimoto Y, Shibahara S, Noda M, Takahashi H, Hirose T, Asai M, Inayama S, Hayashida H, Miyata T, Numa S: Cloning and sequence analysis of cDNA for ovine corticotropin-releasing factor precursor. *Nature* 301:537, 1983.

90. Yasuda N, Greer SE: Conversion of high molecular weight CRF (corticotropin-releasing factor) or PRF (prolactin-releasing factor) into lower molecular weight forms by boiling at low pH. *Biochem Biophys Res Commun* 85:1291, 1978.

91. Gibbs DM, Stewart RD, Liu JH, Vale W, Rivier J, Yen SSC: Effects of synthetic cortocotropin-releasing factor and dopamine on the release of immunoreactive β-endorphin/β-lipotropin and α-melanocyte-stimulating hormone from human fetal pituitaries *in vitro*. *J Clin Endocrinol Metab* 55:1149, 1982.

92. Gillies GE, Linton EA, Powry PJ: Corticotropin releasing activity of the new CRF is potentiated several times by vasopressin. *Nature* 299:355, 1982.

93. Giguere V, Labrie F: Additive effects of epinephrine and corticotropin-releasing factor (CRF) on adrenocorticotropin release in rat anterior pituitary cells. *Biochem Biophys Res Commun* 110:456, 1983.

94. Fisher LA, Jessen G, Brown MR: Corticotropin-releasing factor (CRF): Mechanism to elevate mean arterial pressure and heart rate. *Regul Pept* 5:153, 1983.

95. Sutten RE, Koob GF, Le Moal M, Rivier J, Vale W: Corticotropin releasing factor produces behavioural activation in rats. *Nature* 297:331, 1982.

96. Brown MR, Rivier C: Central nervous system (CNS) regulation of ACTH secretion: Role of somatostatins (SS). *Proc 65th Meeting Endocrine Soc*, 1983, p 321.

97. Yasuda N, Greer MA, Aizawa T: Corticotropin-releasing factor. *Endocr Rev* 3:123, 1982.

98. Merchenthaler I, Vigh S, Petrusz P, Schally AV: The paraventriculo-infundibular corticotropin releasing factor (CRF) pathway as revealed by immunocytochemistry in long-term hypophysectomized or adrenalectomized rats. *Regul Pept* 5:295, 1983.

99. Moldow RL, Fischman AJ: Physiological changes in rat hypothalamic CRF: Circadian, stress and steroid suppression. *Peptides* 3:837, 1982.

100. Giguere V, Labrie F, Cote J, Coy DH, Sueiras-Diaz J, Schally AV: Stimulation of cyclic AMP accumulation and corticotropin release by synthetic ovine corticotropin-releasing factor in rat anterior pituitary cells: Site of glucocorticoid action. *Proc Natl Acad Sci USA* 79:3466, 1982.

101. Grossman A, Nieuwenhuijzen-Kruseman AC, Perry L, Tomlin A, Schally AV, Coy DH, Rees LH, Comaru-Schally A-M, Besser GM: New hypothalamic hormone, corticotropin-releasing factor, specifically stimulates the release of adrenocorticotropic hormone and cortisol in man. *Lancet* 1:921, 1982.

102. Frohman LA, Szabo M, Berelowitz M, Stachura ME: Partial purification and characterization of a peptide with growth hormone–releasing activity from extrapituitary tumors in patients with acromegaly. *J Clin Invest* 65:43, 1980.

103. Frohman LA: Growth hormone releasing factor, a neuroendocrine perspective. *J Lab Clin Med* 103:819, 1984.

104. Gubler U, Monahan JJ, Lomedico PT, Bhatt RS, Collier KJ, Hoffman BJ, Bohlen P, Esch F, Ling N, Zeytin F, Brazeau P, Ponian MS, Gage LP: Cloning and sequence analysis of cDNA for the precursor of human growth hormone–releasing factor, somatocrinin. *Proc Natl Acad Sci USA* 80:4311, 1983.

104a. Mayo KE, Cerelli GM, Lebo RV, Bruce BD, Rosenfeld MG, Evans RM: Gene encoding human growth hormone-releasing factor precursor: Structure, sequence, and chromosomal assignment. *Proc Natl Acad Sci USA* 82:63, 1985.

105. Spiess J, Rivier J, Vale W: Characterization of rat hypothalamic growth hormone–releasing factor. *Nature* 303:532, 1983.

106. Frohman LA, Jansson J-O: Growth hormone-releasing hormone. *Endocr Rev* 7:223, 1986.

107. Vance ML, Borges JLC, Kaiser DL, Evans WS, Furlanetto R, Thominet JL, Frohman LA, Rogol AD, MacLeod RM, Bloom SR, Rivier J, Vale W, Thorner MO: Human pancreatic tumor growth hormone–releasing factor (hpGRF-40): Dose response relationships in normal man. *J Clin Endocrinol Metab* 58:838, 1984.

108. Rosenthal SM, Schriock EA, Kaplan SL, Grumbach MM: Synthetic human pancreas growth hormone–releasing factor ($hpGRF_{1-44}$-NH_2) stimulates growth hormone secretion in normal men. *J Clin Endocrinol Metab* 57:677, 1983.

109. Brazeau P, Ling N, Bohlen P, Esch F, Ying SY, Guillemin R: Growth hormone releasing factor, somatocrinin, releases pituitary growth hormone in vitro. *Proc Natl Acad Sci USA* 79:7909, 1982.

110. Wehrenberg WB, Brazeau P, Luben R, Bohlen P, Guillemin R: Inhibition of the pulsatile secretion of growth hormone by monoclonal antibodies to the hypothalamic growth hormone releasing factor (GRF). *Endocrinology* 111:2147, 1982.

111. Brazeau P, Ling N, Esch F, Bohlen P, Mougin C, Guillemin R: Somatocrinin (growth hormone releasing factor) in vitro bioactivity: Ca^{++} involvement, cAMP mediated action and additivity of effect with PGE_2. *Biochem Biophys Res Commun* 109:588, 1982.

112. Szabo M, Chu L, Frohman LA: Biological effects of an ectopic growth hormone–releasing peptide in cultured adenohypophyseal cells: Comparison with growth hormone-releasing activity from porcine hypothalamus. *Endocrinology* 111:1235, 1982.

113. Gick GG, Zeytinoglu FN, Esch FS, Bancroft FC: Effect of growth hormone–releasing factor on pituitary growth hormone release and GH-mRNA levels in vitro. *Proc 65th Meeting Endocrine Society*, 1983, abstr 13.

114. Webb CB, Szabo M, Frohman LA: Ectopic growth hormone–releasing factor and dibutyryl cyclic adenosine monophosphate–stimulated growth hormone release in vitro: Effects of corticosterone and estradiol. *Endocrinology* 113:1191, 1983.

115. Vale W, Vaughan J, Yamamoto G, Spiess J, Rivier J: Effects of synthetic human pancreatic (tumor) GH releasing factor and somatostatin, triiodothyronine and dexamethasone on GH secretion in vitro. *Endocrinology* 112:1553, 1983.

116. Wehrenberg WB, Baird A, Ling N: Potent interaction between glucocorticoids and growth hormone–releasing factor in vivo. *Science* 221:556, 1983.

117. Bloch B, Baillard RC, Brazeau P, Lin HD, Ling N: Topographical and ontogenetic study of the neurons producing growth hormone-releasing factor in human hypothalamus. *Regul Pept* 8:21, 1984.

118. Thorner MO, Spiess J, Vance ML, Rogol AD, Kaiser DL, Webster JD, Vale W, Rivier J, Borges JL, Bloom SR, Cronin MJ, Evans WS, MacLeod RM: Human pancreatic GHRF selectively stimulates GH secretion in man. *Lancet* 1:24, 1983.

119. Shibasaki T, Shizume K, Nakahara M, Masuda A, Jibiki K, Demura H, Wakabayashi I, Ling N: Age-related changes in plasma growth hormone response to growth hormone–releasing factor in man. *J Clin Endocrinol Metab* 58:212, 1984.

119a. Pavlov EP, Harman SM, Merriam GR, Gelato MC, Blackman MR: Responses of growth hormone (GH) and somatomedin-C to GH-releasing hormone in healthy aging men. *J Clin Endocrinol Metab* 62:595, 1986.

120. Frohman LA, Thominet JL, Webb CB, Vance ML, Uderman H, Rivier J, Vale W, Thorner MO: Metabolic clearance and plasma disappearance rates of human pancreatic tumor growth hormone releasing factor in man. *J Clin Invest* 73:1304, 1984.

121. Frohman LA, Downs TR, Williams TC, Heimer EP, Pan Y-CE, Felix A: Rapid enzymatic degradation of growth hormone releasing hormone by plasma in vitro and in vivo to a biologically inactive, N-terminally cleaved product. *J Clin Invest* 78:906, 1986.

121a. Webb CB, Vance ML, Thorner MO, Perisutti G, Thominet JL, Rivier J, Vale W, Frohman LA: Plasma growth hormone responses to constant infusions of human pancreatic growth hormone releasing factor: Intermittent secretion or response attenuation. *J Clin Invest* 74:96, 1984.

122. Maurer RA: Transcriptional regulation of the prolactin gene by ergocryptine and cyclic AMP. *Nature* 294:94, 1981.

123. Leong DA, Frawley LS, Neill JD: Neuroendocrine control of prolactin secretion. *Annu Rev Physiol* 45:109, 1983.

124. Phillips HS, Nikolics K, Branton D, Seeburg PH: Immunocytochemical localization in rat brain of a prolactin release-inhibiting sequence of gonadotropin-releasing hormone prohormone. *Nature* 316:542, 1985.

125. Adelman JP, Mason AJ, Hayflick JS, Seeburg PH: Isolation of the gene and hypothalamic cDNA for the common precursor of gonadotropin-releasing hormone and prolactin release-inhibiting factor in human and rat. *Proc Natl Acad Sci USA* 83:179, 1986.

126. Millar RP, Wormald PJ, Milton RC: Stimulation of gonadotropin release by a non-GnRH peptide sequence of the GnRH precursor. *Science* 232:68, 1986.

127. Abe H, Engler D, Molitch M, Reichlin S: Vasoactive intestinal peptide is a mediator of the suckling-induced prolactin release in the rat. *Proc 65th Meeting Endocrine Society*, 1983, p 223.

128. Murdoch GH, Potter E, Nicolaisen AK, Evans RM, Rosenfeld MG: Epidermal growth factor rapidly stimulates prolactin gene transcription. *Nature* 300:192, 1982.

129. Leeman SE, Hammerschlag R: Stimulation of salivary secretion by a factor extracted from hypothalamic tissues. *Endocrinology* 81:103, 1967.

130. Brownstein MJ, Mroz EA, Kizer JS, Palkovits M, Leeman SE: Regional distribution of substance P in the brain of the rat. *Brain Res* 116:299, 1976.

131. Jones MT, Gillham B, Holmes MC, Hodges JR, Buckingham JC: Influence of substance P on hypothalamo-pituitary-adrenocortical activity in the rat. *J Endocrinol* 76:183, 1978.

132. Carraway R, Leeman SE: The isolation of a new hypotensive peptide, neurotensin, from bovine hypothalami. *J Biol Chem* 218:6851, 1973.

133. Carraway RE, Demers LM, Leeman SE: Hyperglycemic effect of neurotensin, a hypothalamic peptide. *Endocrinology* 99:1452, 1976.

134. Nagai K, Frohman LA: Neurotensin hyperglycemia: Evidence for histamine mediation and the assessment of a possible physiologic role. *Diabetes* 27:577, 1978.

135. Maeda K, Frohman LA: Dissociation of systemic and central effects of neurotensin on the secretion of growth hormone, prolactin and thyrotropin. *Endocrinology* 103:1903, 1978.

136. Bissett G, Nemeroff CB, Loosen PT, Prange AJ Jr, Lipton MA: Hypothermia and intolerance to cold induced by intracisternal administration of the hypothalamic peptide, neurotensin. *Nature* 262:607, 1976.

137. Cox BM, Gentlemen D, Su T, Goldstein A: Further characterization of morphine-like peptides (endorphins) from pituitary. *Brain Res* 115:285, 1976.

138. Moroni F, Cheney DL, Costa E: β-Endorphin inhibits ACTH turnover in nuclei of rat brain. *Nature* 267:267, 1977.

139. Ferland L, Fuxe K, Eneroth P, Gustafsson J, Skett P: Effects of methionine enkephalin on prolactin release and catecholamine levels and turnover in the median eminence. *Eur J Pharmacol* 43:89, 1977.

140. Jacquet YF, Marks N: The C-fragment of β-lipotropin: An endogenous neuroleptic or antipsychotogen? *Science* 194:632, 1976.

141. Bloom F, Segal D, Ling N, Guillemin R: Endorphins: Profound behavioral effects in rats suggest new etiological factors in mental illness. *Science* 194:630, 1976.

142. Lampert A, Nirenberg M, Klee WA: Tolerance and dependence evoked by an endogenous opiate peptide. *Proc Natl Acad Sci USA* 73:3165, 1976.

143. Koenig JI, Mayfield MA, McCann SM, Krulich L: Differential role of the opioid μ and δ receptors in the activation of prolactin and growth hormone secretion by morphine in the male rat. *Life Sci* 34:1829, 1984.

144. Dupont A, Cusan L, Labrie F, Coy DH, Li CH: Stimulation of prolactin release in the rat by intraventricular injection of β-endorphin and methionine-enkephalin. *Biochem Biophys Res Commun* 75:76, 1977.

145. Dupont A, Cusan L, Garon M, Labrie F, Li CH: β-Endorphin: Stimulation of growth hormone release in vivo. *Proc Natl Acad Sci USA* 74:358, 1977.

146. Cocchi D, Santagostino A, Gil-Ad I, Ferri S, Muller EE: Leu-enkephalin-stimulated growth hormone and prolactin release in the rat: Comparison with the effect of morphine. *Life Sci* 20:2041, 1977.

147. Shaar CJ, Frederickson RCA, Dininger NB, Jackson L: Enkephalin analogues and naloxone modulate the release of growth hormone and prolactin—evidence for regulation by an endogenous opioid in brain. *Life Sci* 21:853, 1977.

148. Munson PL: Effect of morphine and related drugs on the corticotrophin (ACTH)-stress reaction. *Prog Brain Res* 39:361, 1973.

149. DeWied D: Behavioral effects of neuropeptides related to ACTH, MSH, and β-LPH. *Ann NY Acad Sci* 297:263, 1977.

150. Koob G, Bloom FE: Memory, learning, and adaptive behaviors, in Krieger DT, Brownstein MJ, Martin JB (eds): *Brain Peptides.* New York, Wiley, 1983, p 369.

151. Koob GF, LeMoal M, Bloom FE: Enkephaline and endorphin influences on appetite and aversive conditioning, in Martin JB et al (eds): *Endogenous Peptides and Learning and Memory Processes.* New York, Academic, 1981, p 249.

152. Bohus B: Effects of ACTH-like neuropeptides on animal behavior and man. *Pharmacology* 18:113, 1979.

153. Sandman CA, George J, Walker BB, Nolan JD, Kastin AJ: Neuropeptide MSH/ACTH 4-10 enhances attention in the mentally retarded. *Pharmacol Biochem Behav* 5(suppl 1):23, 1976.

154. Legros JJ, Gilot P, Seron X, Claessens J, Adam A, Moeglen JM, Audibert A, Berchiter B: Influence of vasopressin on learning and memory. *Lancet* 1:41, 1978.

155. Weingartner H, Gold P, Ballenger JC, Smallberg SA, Summers R, Robinow DR, Post RM, Goodwin FK: Effects of vasopressin on human memory functions. *Science* 211:601, 1981.

156. Oliveros JC, Jandali MK, Timsit-Berthier M, Remy R, Bengheazi A, Audibert A, Moeglen JM: Vasopressin in amnesia. *Lancet* 1:42, 1978.

157. Starkman MN, Schteingart DE: Neuropsychiatric manifestations of patients with Cushing's syndrome: Relationship to cortisol and adrenocorticotropic hormone levels. *Arch Intern Med* 141:215, 1981.

158. Cohen SI: Cushing's syndrome: A psychiatric study of 29 patients. *Br J Psychiatry* 136:120, 1980.

159. Jeffcoate WJ, Silverstone JT, Edwards CRW, Besser GM: Psychiatric manifestations of Cushing's syndrome: Response to lowering of plasma cortisol. *Q J Med* 191:465, 1979.

160. Petersen P: Psychiatric disorders in primary hyperparathyroidism. *J Clin Endocrinol Metab* 28:1491, 1968.

161. Steiner M, Carroll BJ: The psychobiology of premenstrual dysphoria: Review of theories and treatments. *Psychoneuroendocrinology* 2:321, 1977.

162. Brahams D: Premenstrual syndrome: A disease of the mind? *Lancet* 2:1238, 1981.

163. Moos RH: *Menstrual Distress Questionnaire: Preliminary Manual.* Stanford, CA, Stanford University Social Ecology Laboratory, 1969.

164. Benedek-Jaszmann LJ, Hearn-Sturtevant MD: Premenstrual tension and functional infertility. *Lancet* 1:1095, 1976.

164a. Jansson J-O, Eden S, Isaksson O: Sexual dimorphism in the control of growth hormone secretion. *Endocr Rev* 6:128, 1985.

165. Brown-Grant K: *Foetal and Neonatal Physiology.* Cambridge, MA, Harvard University, 1973, p 527.

166. de Lacoste-Utamsing C, Holloway RL: Sexual dimorphism in the human corpus callosum. *Science* 216:1431, 1982.

167. Arendash GW, Gorski RA: Enhancement of sexual behavior in female rats by neonatal transplantation of brain tissue from males. *Science* 217:1276, 1982.

168. McEwen BS: Neural gonadal steroid actions. *Science* 211:1303, 1981.

169. Toran-Allerand CD: Sex steroids and the development of the newborn mouse hypothalamus and preoptic area in vitro: II. Morphological correlates and hormonal specificity. *Brain Res* 189: 413, 1980.

170. MacLusky NJ, Naftolin F: Sexual differentiation of the central nervous system. *Science* 211:1294, 1981.

171. von Berswordt-Wallrabe R: Antiandrogenic action of progestins, in Bardin CW, Milgrom E, Mauvais-Jarvis P (eds): *Progesterone and Progestins.* New York, Raven, 1983, p 109.

172. Bardin CW: The androgenic, antiandrogenic, and synandrogenic actions of progestins, in Bardin CW, Milgrom E, Mauvais-Jarvis P (eds): *Progesterone and Progestins.* New York, Raven, 1983, p 135.

173. Raum WJ, Swerdloff RS: The role of hypothalamic adrenergic receptors in preventing testosterone-induced androgenization in the female rat brain. *Endocrinology* 109:273, 1981.

174. Money J, Ehrhardt AA: Gender dimorphic behavior and fetal sex hormones. *Recent Prog Horm Res* 28:735, 1972.

175. Reinisch JM: Effects of prenatal hormone exposure on physical and psychological development in humans and animals, in Sachar E (ed): *Hormones, Behavior, and Psychopathology.* New York, Raven, 1976, p 69.

176. Witelson SF: Sex and the single hemisphere: Specialization of the right hemisphere for spatial processing. *Science* 193:425, 1976.

177. Waber DP: Sex differences in cognition: A function of maturation rate? *Science* 192:572, 1976.

178. Hier DB, Crowley WF Jr: Spatial ability in androgen-deficient men. *N Engl J Med* 306:1202, 1982.

179. Klein DC, Sugden D, Weller JL: Postsynaptic α-adrenergic receptors potentiate the β-adrenergic stimulation of pineal serotonin *N*-acetyltransferase. *Proc Natl Acad Sci USA* 80:599, 1983.

180. Axelrod J: The pineal gland: A neurochemical transducer. *Science* 184:1341, 1974.

181. Wurtman RJ, Moskowitz MA: The pineal organ. *N Engl J Med* 296:1329, 1977.

182. Zatz M, Brownstein MJ: Intraventricular carbachol mimics the effects of light on the circadian rhythm in the rat pineal gland. *Science* 203:358, 1979.

183. Vaughan GM, McDonald SD, Bell R, Stevene EA: Melatonin, pituitary function and stress in humans. *Psychoneuroendocrinology* 4:351, 1979.

184. Cardinali DP: Melatonin: A mammalian pineal hormone. *Endocr Rev* 2:327, 1981.

185. Krieger DT (ed): *Endocrine Rhythms.* New York, Raven, 1979.

185a. Filicori M, Butler JP, Crowley WF Jr: Neuroendocrine regulation of the corpus luteum in the human. Evidence for pulsatile progesterone secretion. *J Clin Invest* 73:1638, 1984.

186. Plum F, Van Uitert R: Nonendocrine disease and disorders of the hypothalamus, in Reichlin S, Baldessarini RJ, Martin JB (eds): *The Hypothalamus.* New York, Raven, 1978, p 415.

187. Krieger HP: Sellar and juxtasellar disease: A neurologic viewpoint, in Krieger DT, Hughes J (eds): *Neuroendocrinology.* Sunderland, MA, Sinaur Associates, 1980, p 275.

188. Frohman LA: Hypothalamic control of energy metabolism, in Morgane PJ, Panksepp J (eds): *Handbook of the Hypothalamus.* New York, Marcel Dekker, 1980, p 519.

189. Sklar CA, Grumbach MM, Kaplan SL, Conte FA: Hormonal and metabolic abnormalities associated with central nervous system germinoma in children and adolescents and the effects of therapy: Report of 10 patients. *J Clin Endocrinol Metab* 52:9, 1981.

190. Kobayashi T, Kageyama N, Ohara K: Internal irradiation for cystic craniopharyngioma. *J Neurosurg* 55:935, 1981.

191. Carbezudo JM, Vaquero J, Areitio E, Martinez R, De Sola RG, Bravo G: Craniopharyngiomas: A critical approach to treatment. *J Neurosurg* 55:371, 1981.

192. Matson DD, Crigler JF Jr: Management of craniopharyngioma in childhood. *J Neurosurg* 30:377, 1969.

193. Bierich JR: Sexual precocity, in Bierich JR (ed): *Clinics in*

Endocrinology. Philadelphia, Saunders, 1975, vol 4, p 107.

194. Judge DM, Kulin HE, Page R, Santen R, Trapukdi S: Hypothalamic hamartoma. *N Engl J Med* 296:7, 1977.

195. Asa SL, Scheithauer BW, Bilbao JM, Horvath E, Ryan N, Kovacs K, Randall RV, Laws ER Jr, Singer W, Linfoot JA, Thorner MO, Vale W: A clinicopathologic study of six cases with hypothalamic gangliocytomas producing growth hormone-releasing factor. *J Clin Endocrinol Metab* 58:796, 1984.

196. Asa SL, Bilbao JM, Kovacs K, Linfoot JA: Hypothalamic neuronal hamartoma associated with pituitary growth hormone cell adenoma and acromegaly. *Acta Neuropathol (Berl)* 52:231, 1980.

197. Asa SL, Kovacs K, Tindall GT, Barrow DL, Horvath E, Taker Y: CRF-producing hypothalamic gangliocytoma associated with pituitary corticotroph cell hyperplasia: Evidence for a hypothalamic etiology of Cushing's syndrome. *Proc 65th Meeting Endocrine Society*, 1983, abstr 441.

198. Bergland RM: Neurosecretory bodies within the median eminence in association with pituitary tumors. *Lancet* 2:1270, 1979.

199. Sherwin RP, Grassi JE, Sommers SC: Hamartomatous malformation of the posterolateral hypothalamus. *Lab Invest* 2:89, 1962.

200. Scherbaum WA, Bottazzo GF: Autoantibodies to vasopressin cells in idiopathic diabetes insipidus: Evidence for an autoimmune variant. *Lancet* 1:897, 1983.

201. Kirkland JL, Person DJ, Goddard C, Davies I: Polyuria and inappropriate secretion of arginine vasopressin in hypothalamic sarcoidosis. *J Clin Endocrinol Metab* 56:269, 1983.

202. Selenkow HA, Tyler HR, Matson DD, Nelson DH: Hypopituitarism due to hypothalamic sarcoidosis. *Am J Med Sci* 238:456, 1959.

203. Brooks BS, Gammal TE, Hungerford GD, Acker J, Trevor RP, Russel W: Radiologic evaluation of neurosarcoidosis: Role of computed tomography. *Am J Neurol Radiol* 3:513, 1982.

204. Avery ME, McAfee JG, Guild HG: The course and prognosis of reticuloendotheliosis (eosinophilic granuloma, Schuller-Christian disease and Letterer-Siwe disease). *Am J Med* 22:636, 1957.

205. Kepes JJ, Kepes M: Predominantly cerebral forms of histiocytosis-X: A reappraisal of "Gagel's hypothalamic granuloma," "granuloma infiltrans of the hypothalamus" and "Ayala's disease" with a report of four cases. *Acta Neuropathol (Berl)* 14:77, 1969.

206. Vogel JM, Vogel P: Idiopathic histiocytosis: A discussion of eosinophilic granuloma, the Hand-Schuller-Christian syndrome and the Letterer-Siwe syndrome. *Semin Hematol* 9:349, 1972.

207. Rudman D, Fleischer AS, Kutner MH, Raggio JF: Suprahypophyseal hypogonadism and hypothyroidism during prolonged coma after head trauma. *J Clin Endocrinol Metab* 45:747, 1977.

208. Feibel J, Kelly M, Lee L, Woolf P: Loss of adrenocortical suppression after acute brain injury: Role of increased intracranial pressure and brain stem function. *J Clin Endocrinol Metab* 57:1245, 1983.

209. King LR, Knowles HC Jr, McLaurin RL, Brielmaier J, Perisutti G, Piziak VK: Pituitary hormone response to head injury. *Neurosurgery* 9:229, 1981.

210. Fiedler R, Krieger DT: Endocrine disturbances in patients with congenital aqueductal stenosis. *Acta Endocrinol* 80:1, 1975.

211. Kim CS, Bennett DR, Roberts TS: Primary amenorrhea secondary to noncommunicating hydrocephalus. *Neurology* 19:533, 1969.

212. Crompton MR: Hypothalamic lesions following the rupture of cerebral berry aneurysms. *Brain* 86:301, 1963.

213. Jenkins JS: Hypothalamic pituitary-adrenal function after subarachnoid hemorrhage. *Br Med J* 2:707, 1969.

213a. Lustig RH, Schriock EA, Kaplan SL, Grumbach MM: Effect of growth hormone-releasing factor on growth hormone release in children with radiation-induced growth hormone deficiency. *Pediatrics* 76:274, 1985.

214. Peck FC, McGovern ER: Radiation necrosis of the brain in acromegaly. *Neurosurgery* 25:536, 1966.

215. Bauer HG: Endocrine and metabolic conditions related to pathology in the hypothalamus: A review. *J Nerv Ment Dis* 128:323, 1959.

216. Krieger DT, Krieger HP: The circadian variation of the plasma 17-OHCS in central nervous system disease. *J Clin Endocrinol Metab* 26:929, 1966.

217. Hokfelt B, Luft R: The effect of suprasellar tumors on the regulation of adrenocortical function. *Acta Endocrinol* 32:177, 1959.

218. Krieger DT, Krieger HP: Effect of organic brain lesions on adrenal cortical activity, in Levine R (ed): *Endocrines and the Central Nervous System*. Baltimore, Williams & Wilkins, 1966, p 400.

219. Fleischer N, Lorente M, Kirkland J, Kirkland R, Clayton G, Calderon M: Synthetic thyrotropin releasing factor as a test of pituitary thyrotropin reserve. *J Clin Endocrinol Metab* 34:617, 1972.

220. Illig R, Krawczynska H, Torresani T, Prader A: Elevated plasma TSH and hypothyroidism in children with hypothalamic hypopituitarism. *J Clin Endocrinol Metab* 41:722, 1975.

220a. Beck-Peccoz P, Amr S, Menezes-Ferreira MM, Faglia G, Weintraub BD: Decreased receptor binding of biologically inactive thyrotropin in central hypothyroidism. Effect of treatment with thyrotropin-releasing hormone. *N Engl J Med* 312:1085, 1985.

221. Tsukada T, Nakai Y, Koh T, Tsuji S, Inada M, Nishikawa M, Shinoda H, Kawai I, Takezawa N, Imura H: Plasma adrenocorticotropin and cortisol responses to ovine corticotropin-releasing factor in patients with adrenocortical insufficiency due to hypothalamic and pituitary disorders. *J Clin Endocrinol Metab* 58:758, 1984.

222. Krieger DT: The central nervous system and Cushing's syndrome. *Mt Sinai J Med (NY)* 39:416, 1972.

223. Heinbecker P: Pathogenesis of Cushing's syndrome. *Medicine* 23:225, 1944.

224. Wolf SM, Adler BC, Buskirk ER, Thompson RH: A syndrome of periodic hypothalamic discharge. *Am J Med* 36:956, 1964.

225. Soffer LJ, Iannaccone A, Galbrilove JL: Cushing's syndrome. *Am J Med* 30:129, 1961.

226. Krieger DT, Amorosa L, Linick F: Cyproheptadine induced remission of Cushing's disease. *N Engl J Med* 293:893, 1975.

227. Dornhorst A, Jenkins JS, Lamberts SW, Abraham RR, Wynn V, Beckford U, Gillham B, Jones MT: The evaluation of sodium valproate in the treatment of Nelson's syndrome. *J Clin Endocrinol Metab* 56:985, 1983.

228. Lamberts SWJ, Klijn JG, de Quijada M, Timmermans HAT, Uitterlinden P, de Jong FH, Birkenhager JC: The mechanism of the suppressive action of bromocriptine on adrenocorticotropin secretion in patients with Cushing's disease and Nelson's syndrome. *J Clin Endocrinol Metab* 51:307, 1980.

229. Krieger DT: Pathophysiology of Cushing's disease. *Endocr Rev* 4:22, 1983.

230. Lamberts SWJ, Delange SA, Stefanko SZ: Adrenocorticotropin-secreting pituitary adenomas originate from the anterior or the intermediate lobe in Cushing's disease: Differences in the regulation of hormone secretion. *J Clin Endocrinol Metab* 54:286, 1982.

230a. Cauter EV, Refetoff S: Evidence for two subtypes of Cushing's disease based on the analysis of episodic cortisol secretion. *N Engl J Med* 312:1343, 1985.

231. Lieblich JM, Rogol AD, White BJ, Rosen SW: Syndrome of anosmia with hypogonadotropic hypogonadism (Kallmann's syndrome): Clinical and laboratory studies in 22 cases. *Am J Med* 73:506, 1982.

232. Hochberg Z, Moses AM, Miller M, Benderli A, Richman RA: Altered osmotic threshold for vasopressin release and impaired thirst sensation: Additional abnormalities in Kallmann's syndrome. *J Clin Endocrinol Metab* 55:799, 1982.

233. Gauthier G: La dyplasie olfacto-génitale (agénésie des lobes olfactifs avec absence de développement gonadique à la puberté). *Acta Neuroveg* 21:345, 1961.

234. Michael RP, Keverne EB: Pheromones in the communication of sexual status in primates. *Nature* 218:746, 1968.
235. McClintock MK: Menstrual synchrony and suppression. *Nature* 229:244, 1971.
236. Synder PJ, Rudenstein RS, Gardner DF, Rothman JG: Repetitive infusion of gonadotropin-releasing hormone distinguishes hypothalamic from pituitary hypogonadism. *J Clin Endocrinol Metab* 48:864, 1979.
237. Hoffman AR, Crowley WF Jr: Induction of puberty in men by long-term pulsatile administration of low-dose gonadotropin-releasing hormone. *N Engl J Med* 307:1237, 1982.
238. Yen SSC, Rebar R, Vandenberg G, Judd H: Hypothalamic amenorrhea and hypogonadotropism: Responses to synthetic LRH. *J Clin Endocrinol Metab* 36:811, 1973.
239. Aono T, Miyake A, Shioji T, Kinugasa T, Onishi T, Kurachi K: Impaired LH release following exogenous estrogen administration in patients with amenorrhea-galactorrhea syndrome. *J Clin Endocrinol Metab* 42:696, 1976.
240. Quigley ME, Judd SJ, Gilliland GB, Yen SSC: Effects of a dopamine agonist on the release of gonadotropin and prolactin in normal women and women with hyperprolactinemic anovulation. *J Clin Endocrinol Metab* 48:718, 1979.
241. Frisch RE, Wyshak G, Vincent L: Delayed menarche and amenorrhea in ballet dancers. *N Engl J Med* 303:17, 1980.
242. Feicht CB, Johnson TS, Martin BJ, Sparkes KE, Wagner WW Jr: Secondary amenorrhoea in athletes, *Lancet* 2:1145, 1978.
242a. Hurley DM, Brian R, Outch K, Stockdale J, Fry A, Hackman C, Clarke I, Burger HG: Induction of ovulation and fertility in amenorrheic women by pulsatile low-dose gonadotropin-releasing hormone. *N Engl J Med* 310:1069, 1984.
243. Carter JN, Tyson JE, Tolis G, Van Vliet S, Faiman C, Friesen HG: Prolactin-secreting tumors and hypogonadism in 22 men. *N Engl J Med* 299:847, 1978.
244. Cacciari E, Frejaville E, Cicognani A, Pirazzoli P, Frank G, Balsamo A, Tassinari D, Zappulla F, Bergamaschi R, Cristi GF: How many cases of true precocious puberty in girls are idiopathic? *J Pediatr* 102:357, 1983.
245. Sklar CA, Conte FA, Kaplan SL, Grumbach MM: Human chorionic gonadotropin–secreting tumor relation to pathogenesis and sex limitation of sexual precocity. *J Clin Endocrinol Metab* 55:656, 1981.
246. McCune DJ, Bruch H: Osteodystrophy fibrosa: Report of a case in which the condition was combined with precocious puberty, pathologic pigmentation of the skin and hyperthyroidism, with a review of the literature. *Am J Dis Child* 54:806, 1937.
247. Albright F, Butler AM, Hampton AO, Smith P: Syndrome characterized by osteitis fibrosa disseminata, areas of pigmentation and endocrine dysfunction with precocious puberty in females: Report of five cases. *N Engl J Med* 216:727, 1937.
248. Lee PA: Medroxyprogesterone therapy for sexual precocity in girls. *Am J Dis Child* 135:443, 1981.
249. Smith CS, Harris F: The role of danazol in the management of precocious puberty. *Postgrad Med J* 55 (suppl 5):81, 1979.
250. Mansfield MJ, Beardsworth DE, Loughlin JS, Crawford JD, Bode HH, Rivier J, Vale W, Kushner DC, Crigler JF Jr, Crowley WF Jr: Long term treatment of central precocious puberty with a long-acting analogue of luteinizing hormone–releasing hormone. *N Engl J Med* 309:1286, 1983.
251. Barturka DG, Eskin BA, Smith EM, Dacou C, Dratman MB: Brain damage, hypertrichosis and polycystic ovaries. *Am J Obstet Gynecol* 99:387, 1967.
252. Zumoff B, Freeman R, Coupey S, Saenger P, Markowitz M, Kream J: A chronobiologic abnormality in luteinizing hormone secretion in teenage girls with the polycystic-ovary syndrome. *N Engl J Med* 309:1206, 1983.
253. Wortsman J, Singh KB, Murphy J: Evidence for the hypothalamic origin of the polycystic ovary syndrome. *Obstet Gynecol* 58:137, 1981.
254. Thorner MO, NcNeilly AS, Hagan C, Besser GM: Long term treatment of galactorrhea and hypogonadism with bromocriptine. *Br Med J* 2:419, 1974.
255. Phillips JA III, Hjelle BL, Seeburg PH, Zachmann M: Molecular basis for familial isolated growth hormone deficiency. *Proc Natl Acad Sci USA* 78:6372, 1981.
256. Phillips JA III, Parks JS, Hjelle BL, Herd JE, Plotnick LP, Migeon CJ, Seeburg PH: Genetic analysis of familial isolated growth hormone deficiency type I. *J Clin Invest* 70:489, 1982.
257. Borges JL, Blizzard RM, Gelato MC, Furlanetto R, Rogol AD, Evans WS, Vance ML, Kaiser DL, MacLeod RM, Merriam GR, Loriaux DL, Spiess J, Rivier J, Vale W, Thorner MO: Effects of human pancreatic tumor growth hormone releasing factor on growth hormone and somatomedin C levels in patients with idiopathic growth hormone deficiency. *Lancet* 2:119, 1983.
258. Grossman A, Savage MO, Wass JAH, Lytras N, Sueiras-Diaz J, Coy DH, Besser GM: Growth hormone–releasing factor in growth hormone deficiency: Demonstration of a hypothalamic defect in growth hormone release. *Lancet* 2:137, 1983.
259. Takano K, Hijuka N, Shizume K, Asakawa K, Miyakawa M, Hirose N, Shibasaki T, Ling NC: Plasma growth hormone (GH) response to GH-releasing factor in normal children with short stature and patients with pituitary dwarfism. *J Clin Endocrinol Metab* 58:236, 1984.
260. Imura H, Nakai Y, Kato Y, Yoshimoto Y, Moridera K: Effect of adrenergic agents on growth hormone and ACTH secretion, in Scow RO (ed): *Endocrinology*. Amsterdam, Excerpta Medica, 1973, p 156.
260a. Huseman CA, Hassing JM, Sibilia MG: Endogenous dopaminergic dysfunction: A novel form of human growth hormone deficiency and short stature. *J Clin Endocrinol Metab* 62:484, 1986.
261. Lightner ES, Penny R, Frasier SD: Growth hormone excess and sexual precocity in polyostotic fibrous dysplasia (McCune-Albright syndrome): Evidence for abnormal hypothalamic function. *J Pediatr* 87:922, 1975.
262. Lightner ES, Penny R, Frasier SD: Pituitary adenoma in MuCune-Albright syndrome: Followup information. *J Pediatr* 89:159, 1976.
263. Chung KF, Alaghband-Zadeh J, Guz A: Acromegaly and hyperprolactinemia in McCune-Albright syndrome: Evidence of hypothalamic dysfunction. *Am J Dis Child* 137:134, 1983.
263a. Cuttler L, Levitsky LL, Zafar MS, Mellinger RC, Frohman LA: Hypersecretion of growth hormone and prolactin in McCune-Albright syndrome. Proceedings of the Annual Meeting of the Society for Pediatric Research, Washington, D.C., 1986.
264. Thorner MO, Frohman LA, Leong DA, Thominet J, Downs T, Hellmann P, Chitwood J, Vaughan JM, Vale W: Extrahypothalamic growth hormone releasing factor (GRF) secretion is a rare cause of acromegaly: Plasma GRF levels in 177 acromegalic patients. *J Clin Endocrinol Metab* 59:846, 1984.
265. Webb C, Thominet JL, Barowsky H, Berelowitz M, Frohman LA: Evidence for lactotroph dopamine resistance in idiopathic hyperprolactinemia. *J Clin Endocrinol Metab* 56:1089, 1983.
266. Serri O, Kuchel O, Buu NT, Somma M: Differential effects of a low dose dopamine infusion on prolactin secretion in normal and hyperprolactinemic patients. *J Clin Endocrinol Metab* 56:255, 1983.
267. Bansal S, Lee LA, Woolf PD: Abnormal prolactin responsivity to dopaminergic suppression in hyperprolactinemic patients. *Am J Med* 71:961, 1981.
268. Hokfelt B, Nillius SJ: The dopamine agonist bromocriptine: Theoretical and clinical aspects. *Acta Endocrinol [Suppl] (Kbh)* 88:1, 1978.
269. Joynt RJ, Afifi A, Harbison J: Hyponatremia in subarachnoid hemorrhage. *Arch Neurol* 13:633, 1965.
270. Robertson GL: The regulation of vasopressin function in health and disease. *Recent Prog Horm Res* 33:333, 1977.
271. Moses AM, Miller M: Drug-induced dilutional hyponatremia.

N Engl J Med 291:1234, 1974.

272. DeRubertis R, Michelis MF, Davis BB: Essential hypernatremia. *Arch Intern Med* 134:889, 1974.

273. Gold PW, Kaye W, Robertson GL, Ebert M: Abnormalities in plasma and cerebrospinal-fluid arginine vasopressin in patients with anorexia nervosa. *N Engl J Med* 308:1117, 1983.

274. Wilmore DW, Lindsey CA, Moylan JA, Faloona GR, Pruitt BA, Unger RH: Hyperglucagonaemia after burns. *Lancet* 1:73, 1974.

275. Baum D, Dillard DH, Porte D Jr: Inhibition of insulin release in infants undergoing deep hypothermic cardiovascular surgery. *N Engl J Med* 279:1309, 1968.

276. Rocha DM, Santeusanio F, Faloona GR, Unger RH: Abnormal pancreatic alpha cell function in bacterial infections. *N Engl J Med* 288:700, 1973.

277. Lindsey A, Santeusanio F, Braaten J, Faloona GR, Unger RH: Pancreatic alpha-cell function in trauma. *JAMA* 227:757, 1974.

278. Long CL, Kinney JM, Geiger JW: Nonsuppressibility of gluconeogenesis by glucose in septic patients. *Metabolism* 25:193, 1976.

279. Frohman LA: Effects of peptides on glucoregulation, in Krieger DT, Brownstein MJ, Martin JB (eds): *Brain Peptides.* New York, Wiley, 1983, p 281.

280. Wesemann W, Grote E: Diabetes insipidus: A syndrome of hypothalamic dysregulation. *Proc Ger Soc Neurosurg* 1974, p 208.

281. Robertson RP, Brunzell JD, Hazzard WR, Lerner RL, Porte D Jr: Paradoxical hyperinsulinaemia in alpha-adrenergic-mediated response to glucose. *Lancet* 2:787, 1972.

282. Hadfield MG, Vennart GP, Rosenblum WL: Hypoglycemia: Invasion of the hypothalamus by lymphosarcoma. *Arch Pathol* 94:317, 1972.

283. Schneider BS, Friedman JM, Hirsch J: Feeding behavior, in Krieger DT, Brownstein MJ, Martin JB (eds): *Brain Peptides.* New York, Wiley, 1983, p 251.

284. Celesia GG, Archer CR, Chung HD: Hyperphagia and obesity: Relationship to medial hypothalamic lesions. *JAMA* 246:151, 1981.

285. Bray GA, Gallagher TF Jr: Manifestations of hypothalamic obesity in man: A comprehensive investigation of eight patients and a review of the literature. *Medicine* 54:301, 1975.

286. McKusick VA: *Mendelian Inheritance in Man: Catalogs of Autosomal Dominant, Autosomal Recessive, and X-Linked Phenotypes.* Baltimore, Johns Hopkins University, 1975.

287. Edwards JA, Sethi PK, Scoma AJ, Bannerman RM, Frohman LA: A new familial syndrome characterized by pigmentary retinopathy, hypogonadism, mental retardation, nerve deafness and glucose intolerance. *Am J Med* 60:23, 1976.

288. Bray GA, Dahms WT, Swerdloff RS, Fiser RH, Atkinson RL, Carrel RE: The Prader-Willi syndrome: A study of 40 patients and a review of the literature. *Medicine* 62:59, 1983.

289. Jeffcoate WJ, Laurance BM, Edwards CRW, Besser GM: Endocrine function in the Prader-Willi syndrome. *Clin Endocrinol* 12:81, 1980.

290. Burr IM, Slonim AE, Danish RK, Gadoth N, Butler IJ: Diencephalic syndrome revisited. *J Pediatr* 88:439, 1976.

291. Gamstorp I, Kjellman B, Palmgren B: Diencephalic syndrome of infancy. *J Pediatr* 70:383, 1967.

292. Pelc S: The diencephalic syndrome in infants: A review in relation to optic nerve glioma. *Eur Neurol* 7:321, 1972.

293. Vigersky R (ed): *Anorexia Nervosa.* New York, Raven, 1977.

294. Casper RC, Frohman LA: Delayed TSH release in anorexia nervosa following injection of thyrotropin-releasing hormone (TRH). *Psychoneuroendocrinology* 7:59, 1982.

294a. Gold PW, Gwirtsman H, Avgerinos PC, Nieman LK, Gallucci WT, Kaye W, Jimerson D, Ebert M, Rittmaster R, Loriaux DL, Chrousos GP: Abnormal hypothalamic-pituitary-adrenal function in anorexia nervosa. *N Engl J Med* 314:1335, 1986.

295. Russell GFM: General management of anorexia nervosa and difficulties in assessing the efficacy of treatment, in Vigersky R (ed): *Anorexia Nervosa.* New York, Raven, 1977, p 277.

296. Gale CC: Neuroendocrine aspects of thermoregulation. *Annu Rev Physiol* 35:391, 1973.

297. Hensel H: Neural processes in thermoregulation. *Physiol Rev* 53:948, 1973.

298. DeGirolami U, Schmidek H: Clinicopathologic study of 53 tumors of the pineal region. *J Neurosurg* 39:455, 1973.

299. Huebner O: Tumor der Glandula pinealis. *Dtsch Med Wochenschr* 24:214, 1898.

300. Ringertz N, Nordenstam H, Flyger G: Tumors of the pineal region. *J Neuropathol Exp Neurol* 13:540, 1954.

301. Bing JF, Globus JH, Simon H: Pubertas praecox: A survey of the reported cases and verified anatomic findings. *J Mt Sinai Hosp* 4:935, 1938.

302. Kitay JI: Pineal lesions and precocious puberty: A review. *J Clin Endocrinol Metab* 14:622, 1954.

303. Lewy AJ: Biochemistry and regulation of mammalian melatonin production, in Relkin RM (ed): *The Pineal Gland.* Amsterdam, Elsevier/North-Holland, 1983, p 77.

304. Abay EO II, Laws ER Jr, Grado GL, Bruckman JE, Forbes GS, Gomez MR, Scott M: Pineal tumors in children and adolescents: Treatment by CSF shunting and radiotherapy. *J Neurosurg* 55:889, 1981.

305. Weisberg LA: Benign intracranial hypertension. *Medicine* 54:197, 1975.

306. Sotos JF, Dodge PR, Muirhead D, Crawford JD, Talbot NB: Cerebral gigantism in childhood. *N Engl J Med* 271:109, 1964.

307. Seip M: Lipodystrophy and gigantism with associated endocrine manifestations—a new diencephalic syndrome. *Acta Paediatr* 48:555, 1959.

308. Ford FR: *Diseases of the Nervous System.* Springfield, IL, CC Thomas, 1966, p 156.

309. Martin LG, Martul P, Connor TB, Wiswell JG: Hypothalamic origin of idiopathic hypopituitarism. *Metabolism* 21:143, 1972.

310. Woolf PD: Hypothyroidism and amenorrhea due to hypothalamic insufficiency. *Am J Med* 63:343, 1977.

311. Bruyn G: Huntington's chorea: Historical, clinical and laboratory synopsis, in Vinken PJ, Bruyn GW (eds): *Handbook of Clinical Neurology.* Amsterdam, North-Holland, 1968, vol 6, p 298.

312. Klintworth GK: Huntington's chorea—morphologic contributions of a century. *Adv Neurol* 1:353, 1973.

313. Barbeau A: Dopamine and basal ganglia disease. *Arch Neurol* 4:95, 1961.

314. Klawans HL: Cerebrospinal fluid homovanillic acid in Huntington's chorea. *J Neurol Sci* 13:277, 1971.

315. Caine E, Kartzinel R, Ebert M, Carter AC: Neuroendocrine function in Huntington's disease: Dopaminergic regulation of prolactin release. *Life Sci* 22:911, 1978.

316. Caraceni T, Panerai AE, Parati EA, Cocchi D, Muller EE: Altered growth hormone and prolactin responses to dopaminergic stimulation in Huntington's chorea. *J Clin Endocrinol Metab* 44:870, 1977.

317. Hayden MR, Paul M, Vinik AL, Beighton P: Impaired prolactin release in Huntington's chorea: Evidence for dopaminergic excess. *Lancet* 2:423, 1977.

318. Levy CL, Carlson HE, Sowers JR, Goodlett RE, Tourtelotte WW, Hershman JM: Growth hormone and prolactin secretion in Huntington's disease. *Life Sci* 24:743, 1978.

319. Phillipson OT, Bird ED: Plasma growth hormone concentrations in Huntington's chorea. *Clin Sci Mol Med* 50:551, 1976.

320. Keogh HJ, Johnson RH, Nanda RN, Sulaiman WR: Altered growth hormone release in Huntington's chorea. *J Neurol Neurosurg Psychiatry* 39:244, 1976.

321. Podolsky S, Leopold NA: Biogenic amines in the hypothalamus: Effect of L-dopa on human growth hormone levels in patients with Huntington's chorea. *Prog Brain Res* 39:225, 1973.

322. Podolsky S, Leopold NA: Growth hormone abnormalities in

Huntington's chorea: Effect of L-dopa administration. *J Clin Endocrinol Metab* 39:36, 1974.

323. Aronin A, Cooper PE, Lorenz LJ, Bird ED, Sagar SM, Leeman SE, Martin JB: Somatostatin is increased in the basal ganglia in Huntington's disease. *Ann Neurol* 13:519, 1983.

324. Sachar EJ, Hellman L, Roffwarg HP, Halpern FS, Fukushima DK, Gallagher TF: Disrupted 24-hour patterns of cortisol secretion in psychotic depression. *Arch Gen Psychiatry* 28:19, 1973.

325. Carroll BJ, Martin FIR, Davies B: Resistance to suppression by dexamethasone of plasma 11-OHCS levels in severe depressive illness. *Br Med J* 3:285, 1968.

326. Carroll BJ, Feinberg M, Greden JF, Tarika J, Albala AA, Haskett RF, James N McI, Kronfol A, Lohr N, Steiner N, de Vigne JP, Young E: A specific laboratory test for the diagnosis of melancholia: Standardization, validation, and clinical utility. *Arch Gen Psychiatry* 38:15, 1981.

327. Gold PW, Loriaux DL, Roy A, Kling MA, Calabrese JR, Kellner CH, Nieman LK, Post RM, Pickar D, Gallucci W, Avgerinos P, Paul S, Oldfield EH, Cutler GB Jr, Chrousos GP: Responses to corticotropin-releasing hormone in the hypercortisolism of depression and Cushing's disease. *N Engl J Med* 314:1329, 1986.

328. Greun PH, Sachar EJ, Altman N, Sassin J: Growth hormone responses to hypoglycemia in post-menopausal depressed women. *Arch Gen Psychiatry* 32:31, 1975.

329. Ettigi P, Brown GM, Seggie J: TSH and LH responses in subtypes of depression. *Psychosom Med* 41:203, 1979.

330. Garver DL, Pandey GN, Dekirmenjian H, Dehen-Jones F: Growth hormone and catecholamines in affective disease. *Am J Psychiatry* 132:1149, 1975.

331. Ettigi P, Nair NPV, Lal S, Cervantes P, Guyda H: Effects of apomorphine on growth hormone and prolactin secretion in schizophrenic patients, with or without oral dyskinesia, withdrawn from chronic neuroleptic therapy. *J Neurol Neurosurg Psychiatry* 39:870, 1976.

332. Tamminga CA, Smith RC, Pandey G, Frohman LA, Davis JM: A neuroendocrine study of supersensitivity in tardive dyskinesia. *Arch Gen Psychiatry* 34:1199, 1977.

333. Pandey GM, Garver DL, Tamminga C, Ericsen S, Ali SI, Davis JM: Postsynaptic supersensitivity in schizophrenia. *Am J Psychiatry* 134:518, 1977.

334. Malas LK, von Kammen DP, deFraites EA, Brown GM, Gold PW: Platelet monoamine oxidase and the growth hormone response to apomorphine in schizophrenia. *Biol Psychiatry* 18:255, 1983.

335. Hirschowitz J, Zemlan FP, Garver DL: Growth hormone levels and lithium ratios as predictors of success of Lithium Therapy in schizophrenia. *Am J Psychiatry* 139:646, 1982.

336. Frohman LA: Evaluation of neuropharmacologic strategies in schizophrenia, in Brown GM, Koslow SH, Reichlin S (eds): *Neuroendocrinology and Psychiatric Disorders.* New York, Raven, 1984, p 67.

337. Brown GM, Garfinkel PE, Grof E, Grof P, Cleghorn JM, Brown P: A critical appraisal of neuroendocrine approaches to psychiatric disorders, in Muller EE, MacLeod RM (eds): *Neuroendocrine Perspectives.* Amsterdam, Elsevier, 1983, vol 2, p 329.

338. Spratt DI, Pont A, Miller MB, McDougall IR, Bayer MF, McLaughlin WT: Hyperthyroxinemia in patients with acute psychiatric disorders. *Am J Med* 73:41, 1982.

339. Powell GE, Brasel JA, Raiti S, Blizzard RM: Emotional deprivation and growth retardation simulating idiopathic hypopituitarism: II. Endocrinologic evaluation of the syndrome. *N Engl J Med* 276:1279, 1967.

8

Diseases of the Anterior Pituitary

Lawrence A. Frohman

PITUITARY GLAND

Anatomy

The pituitary gland is located at the base of the skull in a saddle-shaped bone-lined cavity, the *sella turcica,* which forms a portion of the sphenoid bone. The anterior portion of the sella consists of the midline *tuberculum sellae* and the *anterior clinoid processes,* which are posterior projections from the sphenoid wings. Posteriorly, the sella is limited by the *dorsum sellae,* the lateral angles of which form the *posterior clinoid processes.* A thickened reflection of the dura mater, the *diaphragma sellae,* is attached to the clinoid processes and forms the roof of the sella. The external layer of the dura mater continues into the sella to form the periosteum of the pituitary fossa. As a consequence, the pituitary is considered to be extradural

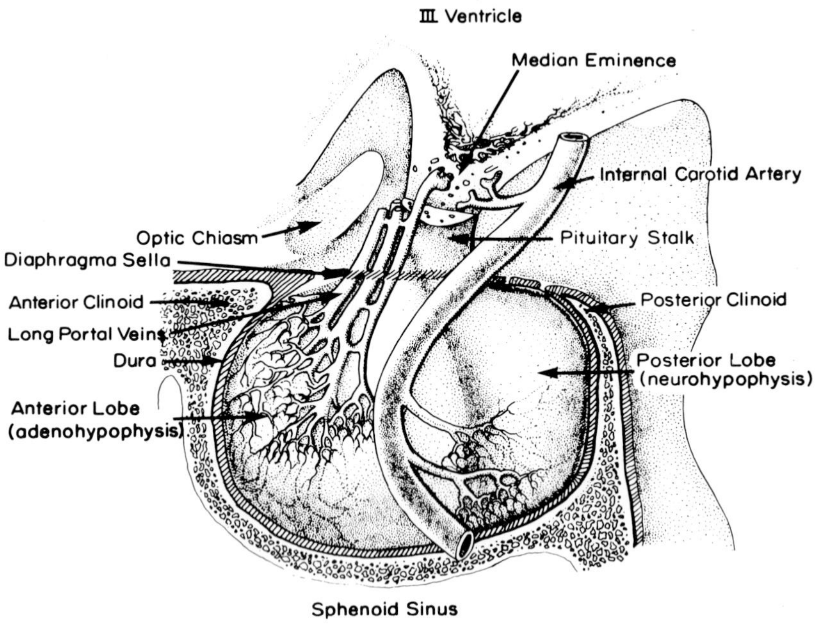

FIGURE 8-1 Schematic representation of the human pituitary gland in relation to its surrounding structures. Refer to text for detailed description.

and is normally not in contact with cerebrospinal fluid (CSF). The pituitary stalk and its associated blood vessels pass through a foramen in this membrane which may be incomplete or fenestrated (Fig. 8-1).

The shape of the pituitary gland varies from an ovoid to a true spheroid configuration. The shape of the sella turcica conforms to that of the pituitary, thus making the normal dimensions somewhat variable. Both age and sex influence the size of the sella. Thus, the frequently used dimensions of 10 by 13 by 6 mm must be regarded as only average figures.[1-4] Estimations of the volume of the pituitary from x-ray measurements have led to a suggested mean value of about 600 mm^3, though there is considerable variation. Measurements of size based on computed tomography (CT) tend to be smaller than those obtained at autopsy.[5] The pituitary weight varies from 0.4 to 0.9 g, being slightly greater in women than in men. During pregnancy the weight of the anterior lobe, which normally constitutes about 75 percent of the pituitary, increases up to twofold, primarily because of an increase in lactotrophs.

Blood and Nerve Supply

Scanning electron microscopy of digested vascular casts, together with direct observation of the direction of blood flow through portal vessels and measurement of pituitary hormone concentrations in these channels, has provided a greater understanding of the blood supply of the pituitary. The arterial blood supply of the pituitary originates from the internal carotid arteries via interconnecting branches of the circle of Willis and the superior, middle, and inferior hypophyseal arteries (Fig. 8-2). This network of vessels forms a unique portal circulation connecting the median eminence and the pituitary. Tiers from the first three vessels coalesce to form coiled capillary loops (*external plexus*) in the outer portion of the median eminence (*infundibulum*) and the upper portion of the pituitary stalk. These loops, along with capillaries from the inner median eminence (*internal plexus*), drain into a series of long portal vessels which traverse the pituitary stalk primarily on its anterior surface and terminate in a dense network of sinusoidal capillaries within the anterior lobe. The middle and inferior hypophyseal arteries, which provide the blood supply to the pituitary stalk and posterior pituitary, do not penetrate the substance of the anterior pituitary en route. Thus, it appears that the anterior pituitary receives no direct arterial blood supply and that all arterial blood flow first passes through the portal plexus.[6]

Venous drainage from the pituitary may follow one of several routes. There are sparse and probably insignificant lateral veins draining the anterior pituitary. Other veins join with the posterior pituitary veins and extend to the cavernous sinus. Whether these are of sufficient size to provide for drainage of all the blood entering the pituitary remains controversial. Venous blood from the anterior pituitary enters the posterior pituitary capillary bed, which is con-

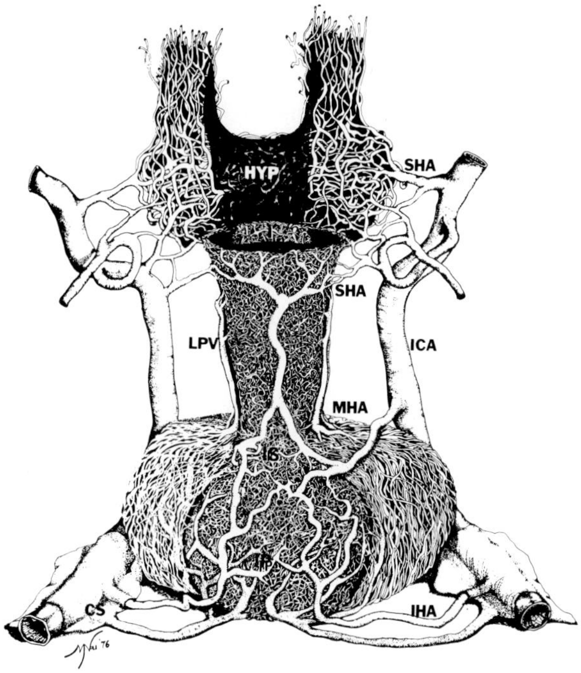

FIGURE 8-2 Vasculature of the rhesus monkey pituitary (posterior view), as constructed from photographs of digested vascular cast after intravenous injection of methyl methacrylate. I, infundibulum; IS, infundibular stem; IP, infundibular process; HYP, hypothalamus; SHA, superior hypophyseal arteries; MHA, middle hypophyseal artery; IHA, inferior hypophyseal artery; ICA, internal carotid artery; LPV, long portal vein; CS, cavernous sinus. The absence of a direct arterial supply to the anterior lobe and the paucity of venous drainage from the pituitary by a route other than via the stalk (infundibular stem) are evident. (*From Berglund and Page.*[6])

nected to both the long and short portal vessels on the posterior portion of the pituitary stalk. Retrograde blood flow from the posterior pituitary toward the median eminence has been observed in these vessels, and the concentrations of anterior pituitary hormones greatly exceed those in the systemic circulation.[7] Thus, a portion of the adenohypophyseal venous effluent appears to be carried toward the brain by vessels along the pituitary stalk.

The direction of the blood flow from the hypothalamus to the pituitary forms the basis for the portal vessel–chemotransmitter hypothesis of hypothalamic control of anterior pituitary function (see Chap. 7). Although the reverse blood flow provides a theoretical route for the direct feedback of pituitary hormones on the hypothalamus, the reverse flow is restricted to a distance of less than half the length of the stalk and thus does not reach the hypothalamus.[8,9] Blood flow to the anterior pituitary has been estimated to be 0.8 ml/g per min, which is the highest flow rate of any mammalian tissue.

The nerve supply of the anterior pituitary is quite sparse and represents almost exclusively postganglionic sympathetic fibers which accompany arteriolar branches and terminate on blood vessels. There is, however, little evidence to suggest that alterations in sympathetic nervous system activity affect the pituitary blood flow rate. Nerve fibers connecting the posterior and anterior lobes have also been described, though their function is unknown.

Embryology

An appreciation of the pattern by which the pituitary gland is formed is important in order to understand the anatomic distribution of pituitary cell types and the various types of congenital anomalies which occur, as well as the origin and potential directions in which pituitary tumors may grow. The glandular portion of the pituitary, or *adenohypophysis,* originates from Rathke's pouch, an ectodermal evagination of the oropharynx which eventually associates with an outpouching of the third ventricle region of the diencephalon of the developing embryo. This portion of the diencephalon subsequently differentiates into the *neurohypophysis,* or posterior lobe. The portion of Rathke's pouch which does not come into contact with the diencephalon enlarges to form the anterior lobe, or *pars anterior.* Early in development, two lateral outgrowths of tissue from the anterior lobes fuse across the midline and extend forward along the hypophyseal stalk. This structure, known as the *pars tuberalis,* forms a complete collar surrounding the stalk in some species; in humans it is limited to a group of cells along the anterior region of the stalk. That portion of Rathke's pouch which directly contacts the neurohypophysis develops less extensively than the opposite wall of the pouch and forms the intermediate lobe, or *pars intermedia.* In some animal species, such as the rat, this lobe remains a distinct anatomic region in adult life and can be easily recognized as such. In contrast, the cells of the pars intermedia in humans become intermingled with the anterior lobe, and the combined structure has been referred to as the *pars distalis.*

Cells of the pars intermedia develop the capacity to secrete corticotropin, or adrenocorticotropic hormone (ACTH), melanocyte stimulating hormone (MSH), lipotropin (LPH), and endorphins, whereas those in the pars anterior eventually secrete growth hormone (GH), prolactin, ACTH, LPH, thyroid-stimulating hormone (TSH), luteinizing hormone (LH), and follicle-stimulating hormone (FSH). Recent information gained from microsurgical removal of pituitary tumors indicates that the location of hormone-secreting tumors can, to some extent, be predicted on the basis of the embryogenesis of the cell type involved.

The lumen of Rathke's pouch in humans is obliterated by the developing pituitary gland. Remnants of the pouch may persist at the boundary of the neurohypophysis either as a cleft or as small colloid-filled cysts and are more prominent in children than in adults. The connection of the pouch to the oropharynx is disrupted quite early in development by a mesenchymal ingrowth which forms the sphenoid bone. A few cells of the lower portion of the pouch may persist into adult life within or beneath the sphenoid bone and are known as the *pharyngeal pituitary*. These cells contain secretory granules in which at least GH and prolactin are present, and it is possible that this structure could exhibit a significant endocrine function subsequent to removal or destruction of the pars distalis. These cells may also become neoplastic and develop into extrasellar, hormone-secreting pituitary tumors.[10]

The human fetal pituitary anlage is first recognizable at 4 or 5 weeks of gestation, and cytologic differentiation occurs rapidly, with basophilic cells apparent by the seventh week and acidophilic cells by the ninth to tenth week. Similar changes occur in the hypothalamus, with monoamine fluorescence noted in the median eminence by 13 weeks, followed shortly thereafter by development of the primary plexus of the portal vascular system. By the twentieth week the anatomic maturation of the hypothalamic-pituitary unit appears complete.

Secretory granules occur as early as the end of the first trimester and immunochemical measurements of hormones as early as the seventh week of gestation. There is considerable evidence for the importance of both the secretion of anterior pituitary hormones and their control by the central nervous system early in gestation, on the basis primarily of the decreased adrenal weight observed in anencephalic infants and the genital deformities associated with excessive ACTH and adrenal androgen secretion in the adrenogenital syndrome. True functional maturation, however, is a continuously developing phenomenon, and many aspects of feedback regulation are not developed until well into postnatal life.

Cell Types

The anterior pituitary is composed of numerous cell types, most of which have as their predominant function the synthesis, storage, and release of a specific hormone or hormones. Methods used to identify the cells in the anterior pituitary have changed dramatically in the past decade with the widespread use of histochemical staining techniques, electron microscopy, and, more importantly, immunocytochemistry. The classic staining methods used for many years revealed the presence of acidophil, basophil, and chromophobe cell types. The introduction of histochemical stains revealed the glycoprotein nature of the basophilic cells, and a combination of these techniques demonstrated that both basophils and acidophils consist of distinct classes of cells.[11] Detailed comparisons of the techniques used for distinguishing the morphologic characteristics of anterior pituitary cells are available.[12]

Among the problems with standard light microscopy is the frequent inability to discriminate between the various chromophobe cells, which represent more than half the cells in the anterior lobe. Thus, using light microscopy it is very difficult to distinguish between corticotropin-secreting cells, whose granules are too small and widely dispersed to be recognized, and other cell types in a state of active secretion which have become degranulated. Electron microscopy has made it possible to recognize that (1) secretory granules and the structure of certain cellular organelles, particularly the rough endoplasmic reticulum, vary greatly between cell types and (2) the size of secretion granules within a single cell type can vary considerably according to the functional state of the cell. Immunocytochemistry, using antisera specific for individual hormones or subunits, is currently the best available technique for the identification of individual cell types. For those hormones which share common subunits, e.g., the three glycoprotein hormones, which contain identical α subunits (see following section), antisera specific for the individual β subunits are required to distinguish between thyrotrophs and gonadotrophs. The use of these techniques has resulted in considerable uncertainty as to the validity of previous morphologic classifications because of the frequent lack of concordance between immunocytochemical and older histochemical procedures.[13] Characteristics of each of the recognized anterior pituitary cell types follow.

Somatrophs: Growth Hormone–Secreting Cells

The somatotroph cells can be recognized as acidophilic in standard hematoxylin and eosin preparations. Their association with GH secretion was originally proposed on the basis of their predominance in pituitary adenomas of patients with acromegaly. The presence of GH has been confirmed with immunofluorescence and immunocytochemical studies, and electron microscopy reveals the granule size to be approximately 300 to 400 nm in diameter. The somatotroph cells are located predominantly in the lateral portions of the anterior lobe.

Lactotrophs: Prolactin-Secreting Cells

The lactotrophs are a second class of acidophilic cell. They can be differentiated from somatotrophs by their irregular and coarse granulation on light microscopy. Immunologic techniques using antiprolactin serum have confirmed the presence of prolactin in the secretion granules, which electron microscopy shows to be smaller in size than those of GH (Fig. 8-3). Lactotrophs are also located in the lateral portion of the anterior lobe and generally develop peripherally to the somatotrophs. The percentage of lactotrophs in pregnancy and during fetal life is increased, reflecting the effects of elevated estrogen levels in pregnancy. Virtually all the increase in pituitary size during pregnancy is the consequence of lactotroph proliferation.

Thyrotrophs: TSH-Secreting Cells

The thyrotrophs, which are intensely basophilic-staining and polyhedral, tend to occur around the anterior edge of the pituitary near the midline, though they can also be found in deeper portions of the gland. The thyrotroph secretory granules, which are 50 to 100 nm in diameter, are smaller than the GH and prolactin granules and exhibit greater heterogeneity in density.[14] Under normal conditions thyrotrophs constitute about 6 percent of the anterior lobe cells. However, in primary hypothyroidism the cells undergo marked hypertrophy and exhibit the characteristic ultrastructural changes associated with increased secretory activity, including enlarged endoplasmic reticulum and hypertrophy of the Golgi apparatus. The number of secretory granules decreases markedly, indicating the depletion of intracellular hormone storage. These histologic characteristics of the cell are readily recognized and have led to its being named the "thyroidectomy cell." Following long periods of thyroid hormone deficiency, neoplastic transformation can also occur.[15]

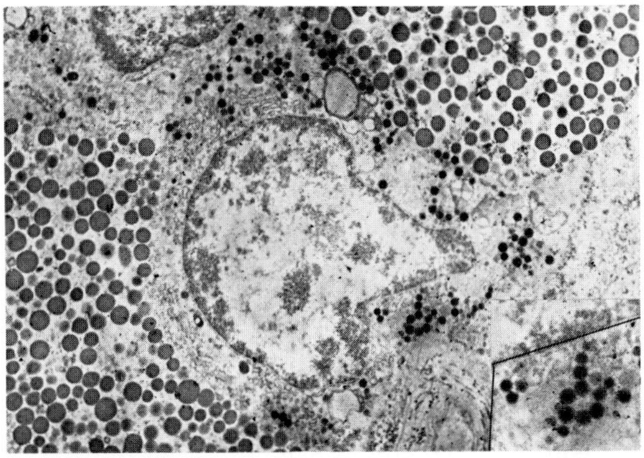

FIGURE 8-3 Immunohistochemical staining of a normal human lactotroph with anti-human-prolactin serum. The small size of the prolactin granules (mean diameter 185 nm), which appear black, contrasts with the nonstaining granules in the upper right and lower left of the field. The *inset* shows that only the small granules are covered with the immunochemical (peroxidase-antiperoxidase) stain; the others are stained by osmium tetroxide only. (*Courtesy of T. Duello, Colorado State University.*)

Gonadotrophs: LH- and FSH-Secreting Cells

LH and FSH were originally believed to be produced by separate basophilic cells. On the basis of immunocytochemical results using antiserum specific for the β subunits of the individual gonadotropins, however, it is clear that they originate from the same cells. These cells are located deep in the lateral portion of the lateral lobes in association with acidophilic, primarily lactotroph, cells. Hyperplasia of the gonadotrophs and, rarely, even tumor formation occur following surgical castration,[16] whereas a decrease is observed during pregnancy in association with chorionic gonadotropin production.

Corticotrophs: ACTH-Secreting Cells

A long-standing controversy as to whether ACTH and MSH are produced by the same or by separate cells has been resolved by the demonstration that ACTH and MSH (and β-endorphin) arise from the same precursor, proopiomelanocortin (POMC).[17] This cell type was originally considered chromophobic and later shown to be basophilic in its staining characteristics. Corticotrophs have been shown to be embryologically of intermediate lobe origin but residing most commonly in the medial mucoid region of the anterior lobe. A second group of corticotrophs appears to have migrated during development into regions of the posterior lobe which are in contact with the anterior lobe and also into the pars tuberalis. Ultrastructural studies have revealed the granules to be quite variable in size. Those cells in the anterior lobe exhibit sparse granulation and relatively poor staining, while those in the intermediate and posterior lobe region contain large electron-dense granules. Differences in the specific peptides found in the corticotrophs located in the anterior and intermediate lobes reflect differences in the processing enzymes present in individual corticotrophs that are responsible for converting the precursor to the mature hormone.[18]

The presence of increased glucocorticoids, whether endogenous or exogenous, produces a degranulation and microtubular hyalinization of corticotrophs known as *Crooke's hyaline degeneration*. The areas of hyaline deposits are associated with diminished immunostaining with anti-ACTH serum. In adrenal insufficiency, the sparsely granulated basophilic cells in the anterior lobe increase in number and the intensely staining basophilic cells of the intermediate and posterior lobe region decrease, suggesting that the former rather than the latter are of physiologic importance in the secretion of ACTH. Similar conclusions have been reached from laboratory studies in animals involving selective pituitary ablation.

Other Cell Types

Depending on the staining method used, some anterior pituitary cells, varying from 15 to 40 percent, appear to be chromophobic by light microscopy. Many of these cells resemble either basophils or acidophils, depending on the stain, and have been termed *amphophils*. Although a few secretory granules can be demonstrated by electron microscopy, no identifiable hormone secretory role has been established for these cells. It is possible that they represent actively secreting or even resting degranulated cells or that they are undifferentiated primitive secretory cells. Cells of this type have been associated with hypersecretory pituitary tumors.

Similarly, after immunohistochemical staining with antibodies to all the recognized pituitary hormones, a significant percentage of adenohypophyseal cells remain unstained. Some of these cells may be responsible for the secretion of other, yet to be characterized, pituitary hormones such as ovarian growth factor, fibroblast growth factor, and aldosterone stimulating factor.

Finally, a few cells exhibit a stellate shape, with cellular processes that often appear to extend into the perivascular spaces in an arrangement suggestive of primitive follicle formation. Secretory granules are uncommon in these cells, and their function also is unknown.

ANTERIOR PITUITARY HORMONES

There are six well-recognized hormones of the anterior pituitary whose structures have been identified, whose functions have been characterized, and for each of which precise measurements in tissues and biologic fluids are available. The hormones are polypeptide in nature and can be divided into three general categories, each of which exhibits unique characteristics: the corticotropin family of peptides (ACTH, MSH, LPH, β-endorphin, and related peptides), the glycoprotein hormones (LH, FSH, TSH, and the related chorionic gonadotropin), and the somatomammotropin hormones (GH, prolactin, and the related placental lactogen). A comparison of the chemical characteristics of these hormones is shown in Table 8-1.

Corticotropin-Related Peptides

Chemistry

Adrenocorticotropic hormone (corticotropin, ACTH) is a 39-amino acid, single-chain peptide. The NH_2-terminal (the end of the molecule containing the free amino group, conventionally designated as position 1) 24 amino acids are identical in all species studied to date, while there are variable but generally minor species differences in the COOH-terminal (the end of the molecule containing the free carboxyl group) region. The biologically active portion of the molecule is contained in the NH_2-terminal portion, with the first 18 amino acids being required for full biologic activity. Rapid degradation of synthetic $ACTH_{1-18}$ in vivo, however, has necessitated the use of a longer amino acid sequence, $ACTH_{1-24}$, to provide biologic activity in humans.

ACTH is only one of a number of peptides that are derived from a common precursor molecule, proopiomelanocortin (POMC), which has a molecular weight of approximately 29,000 and is glycosylated (Fig. 8-4).[19,20] Differential processing of this molecule occurs in various cell types, resulting in differing spectra of peptides in brain, posterior pituitary, and anterior pituitary. In addition, peptides once believed to be the final processing product, including ACTH itself, may be further cleaved to fragments that are secreted and bioactive. The POMC gene is located on chromosome 2.[21]

Two of these peptides share a portion of the ACTH molecule: α-melanocyte stimulating hormone (α-MSH), which is identical to $ACTH_{1-13}$ with an acetylated NH_2 terminus, and corticotropin-like intermediate lobe peptide (CLIP), which is identical to $ACTH_{18-39}$. α-MSH and CLIP are found primarily in species in which the intermediate lobe is more fully developed (e.g., rat and sheep). In the human they are normally found only during fetal life, when a distinct pars intermedia can be recognized. Neither appears to be secreted in humans.

A second hormone contained within POMC is β-lipotropin (β-LPH), which contains a heptapeptide sequence (β-LPH_{47-53}) that is identical to $ACTH_{4-10}$. This sequence is also present in several peptides

Table 8-1. Classification of Anterior Pituitary Hormones

Class	Members	Molecular weight	Amino acids	Carbohydrate	Other features
Corticotropin-lipotropin	ACTH	4500	39		All members of this class are derived from a single precursor
	α-MSH	1800	13		NH_2-terminal 13 amino acids of ACTH. In humans, found only in fetal life and in tumors
	β-Lipotropin	11,200	91		
	β-Endorphin	4000	31		COOH-terminal (amino acids 61–91) portion of β-LPH
Glycoprotein	LH	29,000	α subunit: 89 β subunit: 115	1% sialic acid	All have two subunits, with the α subunit being identical or nearly identical and the β subunit conferring biologic specificity
	FSH	29,000	α subunit: 89 β subunit: 115	5% sialic acid	
	TSH	29,000	α subunit: 89 β subunit: 112	1% sialic acid	
	Chorionic gonadotropin*	46,000	α subunit: 92 β subunit: 139	12% sialic acid	
Somatomammotropin	Growth hormone	21,800	191		All single-chain proteins with two to three disulfide bridges
	Prolactin	22,500	198	†	
	Placental lactogen*	21,800	191		

*Of placental origin and included for comparison purposes.
†Glycoprotein forms of prolactin have recently been identified.[116]

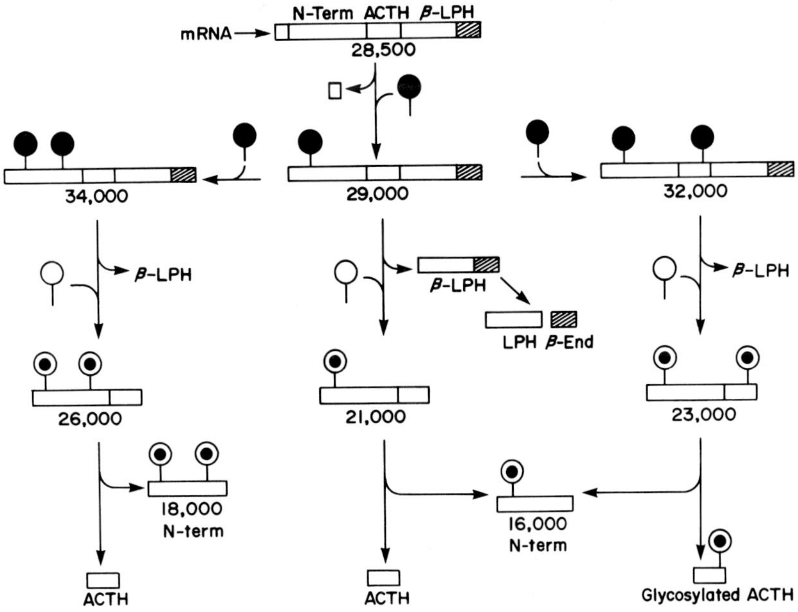

FIGURE 8-4 Biosynthetic pathway of ACTH- and β-LPH-related hormones. A single messenger RNA directs the translation of a precursor polypeptide which contains the amino acid sequences of an NH_2-terminal fragment (proposed to be a hormone but whose function has yet to be detected), ACTH, α-, β-, and γ-MSH, CLIP ($ACTH_{18-38}$), β-LPH, met-enkephalin, and β-endorphin. The earliest form of the molecule detected in the cell is one of molecular weight 29,000 containing carbohydrate in the positions indicated by the black circles. This molecule is further processed by additional glycosylation, yielding forms of 34,000 and 32,000 molecular weight. Subsequent modifications of the carbohydrate side chain are indicated by the white circles. The first proteolytic step involves cleavage of β-LPH from the COOH-terminal portion of the precursor. β-LPH can then be further processed to β-endorphin. Proteolysis of forms remaining after removal of the β-LPH fragment results in removal of the NH_2-terminal fragment, the molecular weight of which depends on its sugar content, and ACTH which is also present in glycosylated (13,000 mol wt) or nonglycosylated (4500 mol wt) forms. (*From Herbert E et al.*[18])

derived from cleavage of β-LPH: γ-LPH (β-LPH_{1-58}) and β-MSH (β-LPH_{41-58}). The structures of these peptides are shown in Fig. 7-13. β-MSH does not appear to be present in the human pituitary. Previous suggestions of a chemically distinct β-MSH (consisting of a 22-amino acid sequence) have been shown to be incorrect and caused by an artifact due to postmortem proteolysis during extraction procedures employed for its purification. Moreover, the immunologic reactivity ascribed to β-MSH in human plasma has been shown to be of a molecular size consistent with β-LPH and/or γ-LPH.[22] The presence of a true β-MSH thus appears to be restricted to those species possessing a distinct pars intermedia.

Two other β-LPH fragments, γ-LPH and β-endorphin, have been identified in postnatal human pituitary and are secreted. β-Endorphin itself can be further cleaved to yield the biologically active peptides α-endorphin and γ-endorphin. Although the structure of met-enkephalin is identical to that of the NH_2-terminal pentapeptide sequence of β-endorphin, a separate biosynthetic pathway exists for this peptide (see Chap. 7).

ACTH

Action

The primary effects of ACTH are on the adrenal cortex, where the hormone stimulates the secretion of glucocorticoids, mineralocorticoids, and androgenic steroids. ACTH binds to specific high-affinity receptors on adrenocortical cell membranes and stimulates steroidogenesis by enhancing the conversion of cholesterol to pregnenolone through an adenylate cyclase–mediated mechanism. ACTH also stimulates protein synthesis, leading to adrenocortical hypertrophy and hyperplasia.

Extraadrenal Effects

In addition to its effects on the adrenal, ACTH exhibits a lipolytic effect on adipose tissue and a hypoglycemic effect attributed to a direct insulin-releasing action on the pancreatic beta cell. Large doses of ACTH also stimulate GH secretion, enhance glucose and amino acid transport into muscle cells, and, in hypophysectomized animals, impair the hepatic degradation of cortisol, which prolongs its half-life in plasma. Except for patients with ACTH-secreting pituitary tumors, it is unlikely that plasma ACTH levels sufficient to achieve these effects ever occur.

The effects of ACTH on pigmentation have been well recognized for many years. Because ACTH is less effective as a melanin-dispersing agent than either α-MSH or β-MSH, it has been presumed that ACTH contributes relatively little to the hyperpigmentation seen in states of marked ACTH hypersecretion such as Addison's disease and ACTH-secreting pituitary tumors (Nelson's syndrome) (Table 8-2). However, with the recent data suggesting that neither α-MSH nor β-MSH exists in humans, the role of ACTH may well be greater than previously believed. In fact, even β-LPH may have significant pigmentation-enhancing effects in conditions where its blood level is markedly increased, e.g., chronic renal failure (see below).[23]

Measurement

Since the levels of plasma cortisol are directly related to those of ACTH under steady-state conditions, the measurement of cortisol serves as a functional bioassay of ACTH when adrenal function is normal. From a practical standpoint, plasma cortisol measurements are less expensive, more reliable, and generally more readily available for assessing ACTH function.

RADIOIMMUNOASSAY The radioimmunoassay for plasma ACTH has developed more slowly than for the other anterior pituitary hormones because of a variety of technical difficulties related to the low levels of ACTH in plasma, the relatively poor antigenicity of ACTH, and its susceptibility to destruction by plasma peptidases.[24] Furthermore, the existence of a family of peptides with partial structural homologies raises the question of the specificity of the assay unless the antiserum is carefully characterized and shown to react with structural determinants unique to ACTH. These limitations notwithstanding, the reliability of ACTH radioimmunoassays is improving, and they are becoming increasingly more useful in the diagnosis and management of selective disorders of ACTH secretion.

BIOASSAY The original techniques for measuring ACTH utilized changes in corticosterone levels in the adrenal gland, adrenal venous plasma, or peripheral plasma in hypophysectomized or neuropharmacologi-

Table 8-2. Pigmenting Effects of ACTH and Related Peptides

Hormone	Potency
α-MSH	100
β-MSH	50
ACTH	1
α-LPH	0.5
β-LPH	0.2

cally blocked rats. An improvement in sensitivity came with the development of in vitro techniques which at first utilized incubated rat adrenal quarters and more recently isolated adrenocortical cells in short-term culture. Although still primarily an investigative tool because of its difficulty, the latter system has sufficient sensitivity to measure levels of ACTH in normal human plasma.[25]

OTHER ASSAYS A radioligand, or receptor-binding, assay for ACTH utilizing partially purified adrenocortical membranes has been developed and exhibits a sensitivity almost equal to that of the radioimmunoassay.[26] The technical difficulty of this assay has precluded its application for the routine measurement of plasma ACTH levels. An elegant cytochemical assay for ACTH has also been reported[27] based on densitometric changes, enzymatically linked to ACTH-stimulated ascorbate depletion in slices of guinea pig adrenal. Its sensitivity far exceeds that of the other assays: it is capable of detecting 5 fg/ml (5×10^{-15} g/ml), and its specificity is excellent. The complexity of this technique, however, has limited its use to research.

Pituitary and Plasma Levels

The total pituitary content of ACTH is about 50 U, or 0.6 mg. Plasma levels of ACTH in healthy adults vary from less than 10 pg/ml (the lower limit of detection by RIA in most laboratories) to 80 pg/ml. ACTH is secreted episodically with a distinct diurnal rhythm. Peak ACTH levels occur in the early morning (5 to 8 A.M.), while the lowest levels occur at about midnight. Changes in plasma cortisol levels closely parallel those in plasma ACTH, with a short lag period. During stress, plasma ACTH levels can rise to 10 times normal values. Even with antibodies specific for ACTH, not all the ACTH immunoreactivity measured in plasma necessarily represents the ACTH monomer. Particularly in patients with malignant disease, larger-molecular-size forms of ACTH ("big" ACTH) have been observed and represent incompletely processed precursor molecules.[28]

Metabolism

Although ACTH is bound selectively by the adrenal cortex, most of the hormone disappears from circulation by other mechanisms, including intravascular enzymatic degradation. The disappearance rate (half-life) varies according to whether measurements are made by bioassay or radioimmunoassay, with bioactive ACTH disappearing more rapidly from circulation (half-life 3 to 9 min) than immunoreactive ACTH (half-life 7 to 12 min).[29] On the basis of the disappearance rate, a presumed tissue distribution equal to that of extracellular space, and a plasma level of 25 pg/ml, the daily secretory rate can be estimated to be 25 μg per day, which represents approximately 5 percent of the pituitary hormone content.

Control of Secretion

There are three major components of the control of ACTH secretion: an inherent diurnal rhythmicity (Fig. 8-5), a closed-loop feedback system which responds to changes in the levels of circulating cortisol, and an open-loop component relating to numerous neurally mediated stimuli commonly referred to as *stress*.

ACTH is secreted in a pulsatile manner which is a reflection of its neural control. A diurnal rhythmicity can be observed in both ACTH and cortisol secretion, which peaks in the morning about the time of normal awakening and then gradually decreases, reaching a trough around midnight. Reversal of the normal sleep-wake pattern, such as occurs with transoceanic plane travel, is followed by a corresponding change in the diurnal pattern of ACTH secretion.[30] The responsiveness of the hypothalamic-pituitary-adrenal axis to stimulation is therefore greatest in the late evening and lowest in the morning.

The closed-loop feedback control of ACTH secretion is mediated primarily by cortisol, which exhibits inhibitory effects on both the central nervous system (CNS) and the pituitary. The stimulation of the hypothalamic-pituitary-adrenal axis which occurs with a decrease in circulating cortisol levels is sensitive to both the absolute level and the rate of change. Elec-

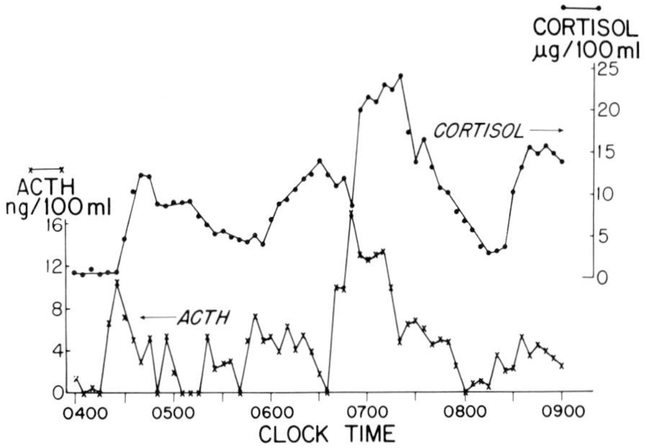

FIGURE 8-5 Concordance between ACTH and cortisol secretion during the early morning. The changes in plasma cortisol levels can be seen to follow those of ACTH with a relatively short lag period. (*From Gallagher TF et al: J Clin Endocrinol Metab 36:1058, 1973.*)

trophysiologic and binding studies indicate that there are probably both hypothalamic and extrahypothalamic sites of cortisol feedback which serve to suppress the release of corticotropin releasing factor (CRF). In addition, cortisol exhibits an inhibitory effect on the pituitary by suppressing the response of the corticotroph to CRF. The evidence currently available suggests that the inhibitory effects of cortisol at the level of the pituitary constitute the most important component of cortisol negative feedback in the physiologic regulation of ACTH secretion.

The open-loop component includes a variety of stimuli, all of which represent types of physical or emotional stress, e.g., pain, fever, anxiety, depression, and hypoglycemia. The trigger sites for these stimuli are undoubtedly different, though they all result in a release of CRF. Evidence for a peripheral β-adrenergic mechanism in the stimulation of ACTH secretion has been presented,[31] though the importance of this pathway in humans is unclear. While none of these stimuli is specific for ACTH (i.e., several lead to the release of GH and/or prolactin), the ACTH responses are mediated by separate neural pathways and are frequently dissociated from those of the other pituitary hormones. These responses are to a large extent unaffected by circulating cortisol levels, though with long-term high-dose glucocorticoid therapy they can be suppressed. Diurnal variation also frequently disappears during periods of stress. A full discussion of the neuroendocrine regulation of ACTH secretion is found in Chap. 7.

β-LPH, MSH, and Related Peptides

With the accumulating evidence that immunoreactive β-MSH in the human pituitary and plasma is not the 22-amino acid peptide, as previously believed, but a larger molecule representing β-LPH, γ-LPH, or a combination of the two, the reports of plasma β-MSH levels must now be reinterpreted. Furthermore, the use of antisera which recognize only γ-LPH and not β-LPH have also led to confusion concerning the secretory dynamics of these peptides. Current information indicates that the LPHs are present in normal human serum in the range of 10 to 40 pg/ml, that their secretory dynamics can be tested with the same stimuli used for evaluating ACTH secretion (insulin hypoglycemia, metyrapone, vasopressin), and that there is probably equimolar secretion of ACTH and the lipotropins in response to each of these stimuli.[32,33] The presence of both ACTH and LPH in the same parent molecule with enzymatic cleavage immediately prior to or concomitant with the secretory process provides an attractive explanation for these observations. In many aspects, the relationship between ACTH and LPH may be considered analogous to that between insulin and C peptide (see Chap. 19).

Dissociation of ACTH and LPH levels has been observed in two pathologic conditions. In patients on maintenance hemodialysis, elevated LPH-MSH levels have been reported[34] and correlate with both the extent of pigmentation and the length of time on dialysis.[23] This dissociation may well be explained by the facts that LPH, in contrast to ACTH, is stable in plasma (i.e., not subject to intravascular enzymatic degradation) and that its clearance in chronic renal failure is markedly prolonged. It also implies that LPH probably exerts relatively little feedback effect on its own secretion or that of ACTH. In patients with Addison's disease or Nelson's syndrome, the decrease in LPH levels in response to acute hydrocortisone administration is much slower than that in ACTH, again reflecting the differences in metabolic clearance rates.[35]

Endorphins and Enkephalins

Discovery of the existence of synaptosomal receptors in mammalian brain which bound opiates in a stereospecific manner led to a search for endogenous opiates and to the isolation of two pentapeptides, *leu-enkephalin* and *met-enkephalin*,[36] and the observation that the structure of the former was identical to residues 61 to 65 of β-LPH. Somewhat larger pituitary peptides with opiate activity were subsequently found,[37] and three endorphin peptides (α-, β-, and γ-endorphin) have been identified, each consisting of part or all of the COOH-terminal portion of β-LPH beginning with residue 61 (Fig. 7-8).[38,39] On the basis of studies demonstrating cleavage by pituitary enzymes, β-LPH is recognized as the precursor of the endorphins, though the absence of comparable enzymes in the brain as well as the difference in anatomic distribution of endorphins and enkephalins within discrete regions of brain and pituitary made it unlikely that the endorphins were the precursors of the enkephalins. A separate precursor for the enkephalins has now been identified (see Chap. 7). In the pituitary, β-endorphin has been localized primarily to the cells of the pars intermedia and to a small extent to the adenohypophisis and, using immunohistochemical techniques, has been demonstrated in the same cells as ACTH.

Radioimmunoassays (RIAs) for β-endorphin have been developed,[40,41] and the release of this peptide into the circulation, along with γ-MSH, another peptide with the MSH sequence contained in the NH_2-

terminal portion of POMC, parallels that of ACTH under nearly all conditions (following CRF,[42] metyrapone,[43] and insulin hypoglycemia[44] and in patients with Addison's disease and Nelson's syndrome).[45] The physiologic role of pituitary endorphin remains to be clarified. The peptide does not exhibit analgesic effects when infused systemically at concentrations leading to much higher blood levels than have been observed with endogenous endorphins, and altered states of pain perception (hypalgesia) have not been associated with clinical states of β-endorphin hypersecretion.

Extrapituitary ACTH and Related Peptides

ACTH, β-endorphin, and γ-MSH are located in numerous sites distant from the pituitary and CNS. These peptides have been identified in gastric mucosa,[46] pancreas,[47] semen,[48] and placenta.[49,50] No physiologic function has been evident to date for these peptides in any of the locations. However, a possible role for placental ACTH has been proposed to explain the increase in plasma cortisol levels during pregnancy, particularly with approaching parturition. This extrapituitary source of ACTH, unresponsive to normal feedback, could explain the rising cortisol level seen during pregnancy (presently attributed to an increase in cortisol-binding globulin), which is resistant to dexamethasone suppression.

Glycoprotein Hormones

Chemistry

The glycoprotein hormones of the pituitary include TSH (thyrotropin), LH, and FSH. In addition, a placental chorionic gonadotropin (CG) with both structural and biologic similarities to LH is included in this class of hormones.

The glycoprotein hormones are composed of two subunits, α and β, each consisting of a peptide core with branched carbohydrate side chains which contribute from 15 to 30 percent of the weight of the hormone. The sugars include fucose, galactose, galactosamine, glucosamine, mannose, and sialic acid, the presence of which is necessary for the hormones' biologic activity. In particular, deglycosylation of the α subunit impairs activation of the glycoprotein receptor once binding has occurred.[51] The sialic acid moiety serves to reduce the rate of metabolic degradation of the glycoprotein hormones but is probably not required for their recognition by target cell receptors.

Within a single species, including humans, the α subunits of the glycoprotein hormones are identical, or nearly identical, whereas the β subunits vary, providing the biologic specificity to each hormone. Even the β subunits exhibit considerable homology within a species: 50 percent of the amino acids of bovine TSH β and bovine LH β are either identical or consist of substitutions resulting from a single base pair change in the genetic code,[52] and human CG consists of human LH β plus an additional 30-amino acid residue at the COOH terminus.[53,54] Both α and β subunits also exhibit considerable cross-species homology: 70 percent identity exists between human and bovine TSH α subunits and 90 percent identity between the corresponding β subunits.[55] For these reasons, it is not surprising that the biologic activity of the glycoproteins is not species-specific and that hormones of bovine or ovine origin are active in humans. The isolated subunits are devoid of the biologic activity of the intact hormone, though there are suggestions that they may have some intrinsic activity of their own.[56] It is the β subunit which determines the biologic action of the hormone, since its combination with almost any homologous or heterologous α subunit will provide a biologically active hybrid molecule characteristic of the hormone.

Evidence for hormonal heterogeneity has been uncovered in preparations of LH from individual pituitaries and appears to be related to variations in the carbohydrate content (termed *microheterogeneity*). It has been proposed by some that the type of glycoprotein secreted (with different carbohydrate-containing forms possessing varying biologic activity) may be modified by changes in the endocrine milieu. Evidence for altered forms of glycoprotein hormone has recently been found for both LH and TSH (see below).

Biosynthesis

The gene for the α subunit is located on chromosome 6, and the genes for all the β subunits are on chromosome 19.[57] The linear peptides of the glycoprotein subunits are synthesized individually, and the addition of the carbohydrates appears to occur following completion of the peptide chain. Since the concentration of the free α subunit in the pituitary greatly exceeds that of the free β subunit, it is believed that glycoprotein hormone synthesis is regulated primarily at the level of β subunit synthesis. Recent evidence suggests that thyrotropin releasing hormone (TRH) specifically enhances glycosylation.[58]

TSH

Action

The effects of thyrotropin on the thyroid gland are to a large extent analogous to those of corticotropin on the adrenal cortex. Subsequent to the binding of thyrotropin to high-affinity receptors on the cell membrane, adenylate cyclase is stimulated, leading to increased intracellular cAMP, enhanced iodine transport and binding to protein, increased thyroglobulin and thyroid hormone synthesis, and increased proteolysis of thyroglobulin with the release of thyroid hormones. In addition, RNA and protein synthesis is stimulated, leading to an increase in thyroid size and vascularity of the gland. The effects of TSH are discussed in more detail in Chap. 10.

Measurement

RADIOIMMUNOASSAY The development of a specific RIA for TSH provided the opportunity to measure the hormone in plasma. The most specific TSH antibodies have been directed primarily toward antigenic sites on the β subunit and therefore exhibit little or no cross-reactivity with the other glycoprotein hormones. For routine clinical purposes, the RIA is the current method of choice. RIAs for the free α subunit and for TSH β, which exhibit only small degrees of cross-reactivity with the intact hormone, have also been developed.

BIOASSAY The McKenzie bioassay is based on the release of radiolabeled thyroid hormones from the mouse thyroid into the blood. Although a useful assay and one which provided the first documentation of the long-acting thyroid stimulator (LATS, or thyroid-stimulating immunoglobulins), the technique is relatively insensitive and incapable of quantitating levels of TSH in circulation of normal subjects. The radioligand assay and, in particular, the cytochemical assay for TSH possess the additional sensitivity necessary for measurement of plasma TSH levels, and values obtained by the latter correlate well with those determined by radioimmunoassay. Because of technical complexities, however, the cytochemical assay remains mainly a research procedure at this time.

Pituitary and Plasma Levels

PITUITARY The human pituitary content of TSH, determined by bioassay, is approximately 0.4 IU.[59] Although most of the TSH is stored as intact hormone, both the free α subunit and TSH β are present, with concentrations of the former exceeding that of the latter. The demonstration of free subunits in circulation of patients with hypothyroidism and in response to TRH reflects the presence of the free α subunit in the thyrotroph as well as in the gonadotrophs.[59,60]

PLASMA The reported levels of immunoreactive TSH in normal human plasma have been undergoing repeated downward revisions as higher affinity and more specific antisera have been developed. The precise limits for the normal range, therefore, vary from one laboratory to the next. The upper limit of normal in most laboratories is 6 μU/ml, though in some the upper limit is 3 μU/ml. The mean value of plasma TSH using the cytochemical assay is less than 1 μU/ml.[61] In most assays a few normal subjects have TSH levels beneath the lower limit of detectability, thus rendering basal levels useless for distinguishing between normal and subnormal values. TSH levels in primary hypothyroidism can rise to more than 100 μU/ml. Those in hyperthyroidism or hypopituitarism cannot generally be distinguished from normal levels by most RIAs, though they can by the cytochemical assay. However, a few assays, and in particular, those employing chemiluminescence, exhibit sufficient sensitivity to distinguish normal levels from the suppressed levels seen in patients with hyperthyroidism.[62] The free α subunit is detectable in plasma in about 80 percent of normal men and premenopausal women with levels of 0.5 to 2.0 ng/ml,[60] and the levels rise dramatically in response to TRH.[63] TSH β is undetectable in the plasma of normal subjects both under basal conditions and in response to TRH. In primary hypothyroidism the level of the α subunit is increased severalfold (~5 ng/ml), TSH β can be detected (~1.5 ng/ml), and the levels of both subunits rise in response to TRH stimulation.[64]

Immunologically detectable TSH in circulation is presumed to represent biologically active hormone. Where comparisons have been made (i.e., using the cytochemical bioassay), good correlations have been observed.[61] In some children with hypothyroidism believed due to primary hypothalamic disease slightly elevated plasma levels of immunoreactive TSH have been found.[65] Administration of TRH results in an exaggerated rise in plasma TSH but a subnormal increase in T_3, suggesting that the TSH secreted under basal conditions and in the absence of endogenous TRH may have reduced biologic activity.[66] This hypothesis has been confirmed by two separate bioassay methods.[67,68] A large-molecular-size form of TSH with reduced bioactivity has also been reported in a patient with hypothyroidism.[69]

Metabolism

The distribution space of TSH is just slightly greater than the plasma volume. The half-life of TSH in plasma is 75 to 80 min, and the secretion rate of the hormone is about 100 to 200 mU per day.[70] In hypothyroidism a small decrease in the metabolic clearance rate of the hormone is more than offset by the high plasma levels, leading to secretion rates of up to 10 to 15 times that in normal persons. Only small amounts of TSH are found in the urine, in contrast to the large quantities of gonadotropins that are excreted. The reason for this difference is not known. Attempts to demonstrate intravascular dissociation of TSH into its subunits have also been unsuccessful.

Control of Secretion

TSH secretion is controlled by two major factors: (1) the feedback effects of the thyroid hormones and (2) stimuli mediated by the central nervous system and the secretion of TRH and somatostatin. A fine-tuned feedback of thyroid hormones on the thyrotroph is responsive not only to the gross alterations in thyroxine (T_4) and triiodothyronine (T_3) observed in hypo- or hyperthyroidism but also to minor changes of these hormones within the normal range. The feedback affects both basal and TRH-stimulated TSH secretion through an inhibitory mechanism which involves protein synthesis within the thyrotroph. It has been shown that the administration of small amounts of thyroxine which do not increase plasma T_4 levels above the normal range can inhibit the TSH response to TRH and that the small decrease in thyroid hormones caused by short-term oral iodide administration is sufficient to increase both basal and TRH-stimulated TSH secretion. Both T_4 and T_3 are potent as feedback hormones on the thyrotroph. Thus, normal TSH levels are observed in patients with a variety of chronic illnesses in whom plasma T_4 levels are normal and plasma T_3 levels are decreased because of diminished peripheral deiodinase activity. Conversely, TSH secretion can be readily suppressed by the administration of T_3 in the presence of normal plasma T_4 levels.

Maintenance of the normal pituitary-thyroid axis is also CNS-dependent. Interruption of the normal hypothalamic-pituitary relationship, whether by hypothalamic destruction or by stalk section, impairs the ability of the thyrotroph to secrete TSH in response to decreasing thyroid hormone levels. In addition to this tonic role of the hypothalamus, there is a centrally mediated effect of temperature. In response to decreases in either environmental or core temperature, a neurally mediated rise in TSH occurs which leads to increased thyroid hormone secretion and enhanced calorigenesis. Cold-stimulated increases in TSH secretion are readily demonstrable in the rat but in humans are seen only in the newborn in response to the decrease in ambient temperature upon removal from the intrauterine environment and in infants subjected to hypothermia in association with cardiac surgery.[71] With increasing age and maturity of the sympathetic nervous system, the pituitary-thyroid axis appears to participate less in the acute metabolic adaptation to cold.

The participation of TRH in cold-induced TSH secretion has been shown by passive immunization studies in which the injection of anti-TRH serum blocks the rise in plasma TSH in the rat.[72] Studies in hypothyroid rats suggest that the acute removal of TRH only partially inhibits the secretion of TSH in response to acute decreases in thyroid hormone levels.[73] The role of TRH on the pituitary-thyroid axis can therefore be considered to be that of modulating the set point and the intensity of the TSH secretory response to decreasing thyroid hormone levels. Hypothalamic somatostatin secretion, in contrast, is enhanced by thyroid hormone and suppressed in hypothyroidism,[74] thereby serving to augment the direct effect of thyroid hormones on the pituitary. TSH is also secreted in a circadian manner, with peak levels occurring just prior to midnight.[75]

The secretion of TSH is also influenced by glucocorticoids, estrogens, and growth hormone.[76] Cortisol exhibits suppressive effects on basal and TRH-stimulated TSH, and a rebound in TSH secretion occurs following the withdrawal of glucocorticoid treatment. There is indirect evidence that a suppressive effect of glucocorticoids on TRH secretion may also occur.

Estrogen does not modify basal levels of TSH but does enhance the TSH response to TRH. This is reflected in the greater response seen (1) in women as compared with men, (2) during the late follicular phase of the menstrual cycle at the time of high estradiol levels, and (3) in men pretreated with estrogen. It is not known whether this effect of estrogen is responsible for the increased incidence of thyroid disease in women.

Somatostatin (SRIF, somatotroph release inhibiting factor) inhibits TSH secretion by an action on the thyrotroph. A physiologic role for this peptide has been provided by the demonstration of increased TSH levels after injection of anti-SRIF serum in animals.[77] Somatostatin has been shown to inhibit the nocturnal rise in TSH in normal humans and the elevated levels of TSH in patients with primary hypothyroidism. Treatment of GH-deficient children of presumed hypothalamic origin with GH has occasionally been complicated by the development of hypothyroidism associated with decreased TSH secretion in response to TRH. The inhibitory effect of GH is believed to be based on a stimulation of SRIF secretion, which in turn would inhibit the TSH response to TRH.[78]

Several neurotransmitters have also been shown to modulate TSH release.[76] Dopamine inhibits TSH secretion and has its major site of action on the thyrotroph; norepinephrine exhibits a stimulatory effect mediated through the α_1-adrenergic receptor; serotonin has a stimulatory effect mediated through TRH release. A physiologic role for the latter two monoamines in humans, however, still remains to be demonstrated.

Gonadotropins: LH and FSH

Action

The two pituitary hormones which regulate gonadal function are follicle stimulating hormone, which stimulates ovarian follicular growth and testicular growth and spermatogenesis, and luteinizing hormone, which promotes ovulation and luteinization of the ovarian follicle, stimulates testicular interstitial (Leydig) cell function, and enhances steroid production in both ovary and testis. On the basis of its function in the male, LH has in the past also been called interstitial cell stimulating hormone (ICSH). A third pituitary hormone which also exhibits effects on the ovary is prolactin (previously called luteotropic hormone, or LTH), which in rats assists in maintaining secretory activity and viability of the corpus luteum following ovulation.

FSH and LH bind to receptors in the ovary and testis, and their effects are mediated by mechanisms similar to those of the other pituitary tropic hormones. In the ovary, the target cell for FSH is the primordial follicle cell, whose growth and maturation are enhanced. LH stimulates progesterone production in the corpus luteum by increasing the conversion of cholesterol to pregnenolone and is required as well for the process of ovulation. Details of the actions of the gonadotropins on the ovary are discussed in Chap. 17. The primary target cell for FSH in the testis is the Sertoli cell, in which, together with testosterone, it stimulates the production of an androgen-binding protein which is secreted into the testicular lumen. The target cell of LH is the Leydig cell, where the production of androgens, particularly testosterone, is stimulated. The androgen-binding protein serves to bring a high concentration of testosterone into the tubular cells in the vicinity of the developing spermatogonia and thus promotes their development. Details of the effects of the gonadotropins and testosterone on the testis are provided in Chap. 16.

Measurement

RADIOIMMUNOASSAY Sensitive RIAs are available for measuring LH and FSH. The specificity of these assays is dependent on the particular antigenic determinants recognized by the antisera used. Although most assays discriminate between the two gonadotropins, cross-reactivity between the intact hormone and its individual subunits frequently occurs. From a practical consideration, this does not generally present a problem. Because of the great similarity between the structures of LH and chorionic gonadotropin, significant cross-reactivity is observed in assays for the intact hormones. In order to measure low levels of CG to aid in the early diagnosis of pregnancy, an assay for the β subunit of CG is used which exhibits only minimal cross-reactivity with LH.

Measurement of LH and FSH in urine by RIA, although less frequently performed because of the inherent advantages of plasma measurements in evaluating secretory dynamics, is still a useful procedure under certain circumstances, such as quantitating gonadotropin secretion during the early stages of puberty (see Chap. 26). The same RIAs used for plasma can be utilized for measurement of urinary gonadotropins, though there is evidence for some immunologic dissimilarity of urinary and plasma LH and FSH, presumably on the basis of chemical alteration of the hormones during excretion.

A minor problem in the plasma gonadotropin RIA relates to the choice of standards. The reference preparation used for bioassay originates from human urinary menopausal gonadotropin, is distributed by the Medical Research Council of Great Britain, and is known as the Second International Reference Preparation (Second IRP/HMG). Since plasma gonadotropin immunologic properties more closely resemble those of pituitary than of urinary gonadotropins, the reference standard currently provided by the National Hormone and Pituitary Program of the National Institutes of Health (LER 907) is a partially purified pituitary extract which has been calibrated against the Second IRP/HMG on the basis of its bioactivity: 20 IU FSH and 60 IU LH per milligram. Because urinary gonadotropin preparations have higher radioimmunoassay/bioassay potency ratios than pituitary preparations, comparison of values between laboratories is at times quite difficult. For purposes of comparison, it is recommended that values be expressed in terms of mIU equivalents of the Second IRP/HMG rather than as the actual weight of a partially purified reference preparation.

BIOASSAY Many bioassays for LH have been described, including the induction of ovulation, ovarian ascorbic acid depletion and progesterone secretion, and prostatic growth. FSH was measured initially by its enhancing effect on the size of female reproductive organs and its potentiating effect on LH. The limited sensitivity and precision of these assays restricted their usefulness to measurement of urinary (and pituitary) gonadotropins. Furthermore, alterations in the chemical structure of the gonadotropins, e.g., desialylation during excretion, could lead to underestimation of the actual quantities secreted. More sensitive bioassays have been developed and are important as investigative techniques. However, for routine clinical measurements RIA is the method of choice.

Radioligand assays have been developed for both LH and FSH in parallel with the other pituitary hormones. The receptor assays are highly specific[79,80] and possess sufficient sensitivity for the measurement of circulating levels of the gonadotropins. Together with the RIA, they have been valuable in investigating the secretion of biologically altered forms of gonadotropins. Increases in plasma LH bioassay/immunoassay ratios have been observed at the time of puberty[81] and in response to GnRH during the luteal phase of the menstrual cycle.[82] These differences have been attributed to variations in LH carbohydrate content.

Pituitary and Plasma Levels

PITUITARY The gonadotropin content of the pituitary in men and in premenopausal women is about 700 IU LH and 200 IU FSH. Postmenopausally, gonadotropin content increases more than twofold.

PLASMA Plasma levels of both LH and FSH rise shortly after birth to reach a peak at 1 to 4 months, with FSH levels in female infants exceeding those in males and the reverse being true for LH.[83] Values of both hormones subsequently decline to low levels until the time of puberty. A nocturnal rise in plasma LH and testosterone associated with non-REM sleep occurs in boys during puberty,[84] which results in a marked increase in urinary LH. In girls, cyclic secretion of FSH and to a lesser extent LH can be detected even prior to the menarche.

The pattern of LH and FSH secretion in the mature ovulating female is shown in Fig. 8-6. During the early follicular phase of the cycle, FSH levels rise slightly and then show a progressive decline. At the same time LH levels are generally stable or rise slightly. At midcycle an abrupt rise in LH, initiated by increasing estrogen secretion by the developing follicle, and to a lesser extent in FSH occurs which triggers ovulation. LH and FSH levels both decline during the luteal phase.

The levels of LH and FSH in males are similar to those in females during the follicular phase, with the exception of the ovulatory surge. There is a rise in FSH and LH associated with decreasing gonadal function in both sexes. In women the rise occurs at menopause, whereas in men there is a gradual increase during the sixth to eighth decades. Episodic secretion of LH is present in postpubertal men and women, with

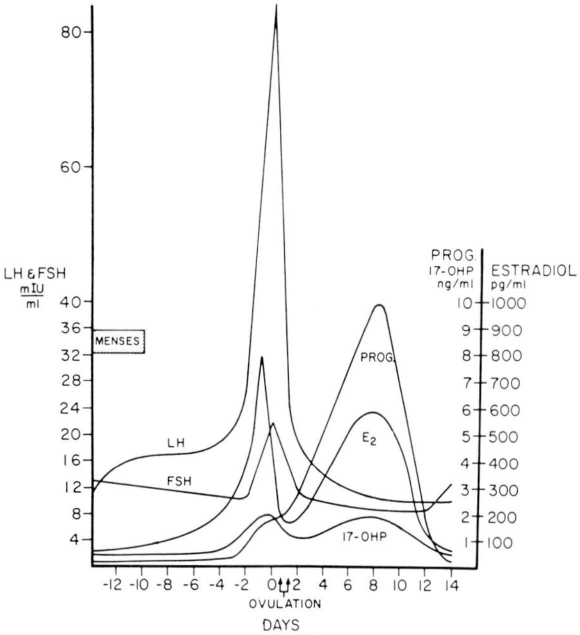

FIGURE 8-6 Changes in pituitary and ovarian hormones during a normal female menstrual cycle. The late follicular rise followed by a decline in estradiol levels can be seen to precede the midcycle surge of LH and FSH which triggers ovulation. (*From Speroff L et al, Am J Obstet Gynecol 109:234, 1971.*)

peaks occurring every 2 to 3 h. Secretory bursts of FSH are less marked and more difficult to detect, in part because of the more prolonged survival of FSH in circulation. They may or may not coincide with the pulses of LH.

The free glycoprotein α subunit has been identified in circulation by means of a specific RIA, and considerably greater levels are found in women after menopause. In response to GnRH, an increase occurs in both the α subunit and the LH β subunit.[85]

URINE Urinary gonadotropin measurements generally reflect those in plasma, with the notable exception of the prepubertal period, when urinary LH and FSH levels are disproportionately low in relation to their plasma values. The quantity of LH and FSH in a 3-h urine sample has been shown to correlate well with the integrated value of plasma gonadotropins during the same period[86] and can therefore provide a useful index of gonadotropin secretion.

Metabolism and Secretion Rate

Despite the similarities in structure, the metabolic clearance rates of the individual gonadotropins from plasma exhibit considerable variation.[87] The half-life of LH is approximately 50 min, while that of FSH is about 3 to 4 h and that of chorionic gonadotropin is even longer. The difference is attributed to the varying sialic acid content of the three hormones, since desialation markedly shortens the half-life in plasma. The secretion rate of LH has been estimated at 500 to 1000 IU per day and that of FSH at 50 to 100 IU per day in adults with normal gonadal function. Since the metabolic clearance rates are not altered in the postmenopausal period, the relative change in secretion rates is reflected by the plasma gonadotropin levels.

Control of Secretion

Gonadotropin secretion in the ovulating female is controlled by a complex and integrated circuitry involving the hypothalamus and the gonads. Gonadotropin levels and responses to gonadotropin releasing hormone (GnRH) in various clinical states are shown in Table 8-3. A progressive rise in estrogen secretion by the developing follicle, which is under the influence of both FSH and LH, exerts a stimulatory effect on the hypothalamus, leading to increased GnRH secretion. There is considerable evidence to suggest that the secretion of estrogen is to some extent under the influence of an intrinsic cyclicity of the ovary itself. Estrogen also sensitizes the gonadotrophs to the effect of GnRH, culminating in the ovulatory surge of LH and FSH. Progesterone secretion by the corpus luteum also enhances the gonadotropin response to GnRH in the presence of estrogen but appears to have a negative feedback effect on the hypothalamus. The estrogen feedback effects are actually considerably more complex, in that both stimulatory and inhibitory effects on the pituitary can be demonstrated, depending upon both dose and duration of exposure. Short-term effects of estrogen on basal LH release and the LH response to GnRH are suppressive.[88] With longer exposure to estrogen, particularly at lower doses, the gonadotropin response is enhanced.[89] More prolonged estrogen therapy will again inhibit the response. Gonadotropin secretion following GnRH is also enhanced by prior exposure to the releasing hormone itself, and this self-priming effect of GnRH is estrogen-dependent. Thus, the FSH and particularly the LH response to GnRH is increased with successive injections of the peptide, a process which is also enhanced by estrogen. In the absence of prior exposure to GnRH such as occurs following pituitary stalk section or in association with certain hypothalamic diseases, LH and FSH responses to an acute challenge with GnRH may be absent.

The sites of estrogen action on the hypothalamus are still open to controversy, but there appear to be two distinct loci, at least from a functional view. The positive feedback effect, that which enhances GnRH

Table 8-3. Gonadotropin Responses in Disorders of the Hypothalamic-Pituitary-Gonadal Axis

	Basal		Response to GnRH	
	LH	FSH	LH	FSH
Both sexes:				
Pituitary destruction	N or ↓	N or ↓	N → 0	N → 0
Primary hypothalamic disease	N or ↓	N or ↓	N or ↓*	N or ↓*
Isolated FSH deficiency	N	↓	N	↓ → 0
Precocious puberty	N	N	N	N
Males:				
Primary gonadal disease, complete	↑	↑	↑	↑
Azoospermia with normal testosterone	N	↑	N	↑
Testicular feminization	↑	↑	↑	↑
Kleinfelter's disease	↑	↑	↑	↑
Estrogen or GnRH agonist administration	↓	↓	↓	↓
Females:				
Postmenopausal state	↑	↑	↑	↑
Primary ovarian failure	↑	↑	↑	↑
Anorexia nervosa	N	N	N → ↓	N → ↑
Hyperprolactinemia	N	N	N	N → ↑
Polycystic ovary syndrome	N → ↑	N	N → ↑	N
Estrogen or GnRH agonist administration	N	N	↑ (early) ↓ (late)	↑ (early) ↓ (late)

0, absent; N, normal; *, normalized with repeated stimulation.

secretion, is seen only in the female and is believed to occur in that portion of the anterior hypothalamus which participates in the cyclicity of reproductive function. The negative feedback of estrogen occurs in the mediobasal hypothalamus and is most readily demonstrable after menopause or surgical castration, when estrogen therapy results in a reduction of LH and FSH to premenopausal levels.

In males, the regulation of gonadotropin secretion appears to be unaffected by cyclic function of either the hypothalamus or the testis. The feedback effects of testosterone appear to be primarily negative and can be shown to occur in both the hypothalamus and the pituitary. The elevated levels of LH and FSH often seen after the sixth decade as well as following castration are reduced by testosterone treatment. In contrast to the effects observed in women, estrogen exhibits only an inhibitory effect on gonadotropin secretion in men.

While it is well recognized that testosterone is the primary hormone involved in the feedback control of LH, its role in the control of FSH has been difficult to document. Although both androgens and estrogens undoubtedly play a role in modulating FSH secretion, there is substantial direct evidence that the testis and ovary produce another hormone, a polypeptide called *inhibin,* which exerts a major inhibitory feedback effect.[90,91] Inhibin has been identified in rete testis fluid of animals and in seminal plasma from normal men, as well as in ovarian follicular fluid, though it remains to be completely characterized. It has been shown to inhibit the secretion of FSH but not LH under basal conditions and in response to GnRH in several species,[91] and it therefore acts at the level of the pituitary. Inhibin also appears to inhibit FSH secretion after direct injection into the central nervous system, raising the possibility of multiple sites of action.

In addition to the feedback effects of gonadal hormones, the secretion of LH and FSH is influenced by prolactin. Inhibitory effects of prolactin may occur directly or through an intermediary compound such as dopamine at both pituitary and hypothalamic levels. Examples of prolactin effects include anovulation during physiologic postpartum lactation and in patients with prolactin-secreting pituitary tumors. The LH response to GnRH is diminished by glucocorticoid administration and in patients with Cushing's syndrome, indicating an inhibitory effect of glucocorticoids on LH secretion.

Other Glycoprotein Hormones

Several reports have suggested the existence of an aldosterone stimulating factor. One group has partially purified a glycoprotein of 26,000-dalton size from human urine and identified a similar material in human pituitary.[93,94] Evidence for biologic activity of peptides contained in the NH_2-terminal and COOH-terminal regions of proopiomelanocortin has also been reported.[95,96] Further studies will be required to confirm the existence of this putative hormone.

Somatomammotropic Hormones

Chemistry

The somatomammotropic hormones include two pituitary hormones, GH and prolactin, and one hormone of placental origin, placental lactogen or chorionic somatomammotropin, each consisting of a single peptide chain with interchain disulfide linkages. There is extensive interspecies similarity of both GH and prolactin (e.g., 73 percent of the amino acid residues in human and sheep prolactin are identical[97] as are 64 percent of the residues in human and sheep GH),[98] suggesting relatively limited changes in gene duplication during vertebrate evolution.[99] Despite this similarity, subprimate growth hormones are biologically inactive in humans. There is considerable homology between the primary structure of GH and placental lactogen; 159 (83 percent) of the 191 amino acid residues are identical. In contrast, there is only 16 percent residue identity between prolactin and GH and 13 percent identity between prolactin and placental lactogen. GH and placental lactogen each contain two disulfide bonds, whereas prolactin, which is seven amino acids longer than the other two, contains three. Despite the differences in their structures, each of the three hormones has intrinsic lactogenic and growth-promoting activity.

There are multiple copies of both the GH and placental lactogen genes.[100] The gene complex, consisting of five related genes, is located on chromosome 17,[101] while the prolactin gene, which has only a single copy, is on chromosome 6.[102] Only one of the GH genes (GH-N) is expressed in the pituitary and is responsible for directing GH synthesis. The other (GH-V), while present in GH-deficient patients who lack the GH-N gene,[103] is apparently incapable of substituting for the GH-N gene even though it can be expressed under certain experimental conditions,[104] and also in the placenta.[105] Two of the five placental lactogen genes appear to be expressed.

Extensive structure-function studies have been carried out with GH in an attempt to find the biologically active core of the molecule. Growth-promoting activity has been found to reside in fragments from several different areas of the molecule, most frequently in those containing part or all of residues 80 to 140. Activity has also been observed in synthetic fragments encompassing this region.

Biosynthesis

Studies derived from the translation of GH and prolactin messenger RNAs (mRNAs) in cell-free systems have indicated that both hormones are synthesized as species of higher molecular weight than the normally secreted form of the hormones. The precursor hormones, preprolactin and pre-GH, have a molecular weight of approximately 28,000, which is due primarily to an extra peptide of about 30 amino acids at the NH_2 terminus.[106] This precursor segment, which is highly hydrophobic, is common to other precursors and is believed to be important in the transportation of newly synthesized protein into the cisternae of the endoplasmic reticulum for subsequent packaging. Enzymes capable of removing the precursor segment from the hormone are present in the endoplasmic membranes.

In addition to the monomeric forms of these hormones, immunoreactive species of approximately twice the size of the monomer have been detected in pituitary extracts and in plasma ("big" GH, "big" prolactin, and "big" placental lactogen). Studies of all three hormones indicate that the big hormone may represent a dimer attached by interchain disulfide linkages rather than by peptide bonds.[107,108] Big GH has been shown to be secreted directly by the pituitary,[109] and there is a suggestion that its amino acid composition may differ from that of monomeric GH. Big GH binds to and displaces the GH monomer from hepatic membrane receptors,[110] though the biologic activity of the big moiety is less than that of the monomer and its physiologic significance remains to be determined.

One variant of GH, the 20,000-dalton fragment, has been extensively studied.[111] It differs from native GH by the absence of residues 32 to 46 and is a consequence of the exclusion of a corresponding RNA segment during the removal of one of the introns in the processing of premessenger RNA to mRNA.[112] This variant constitutes up to 10 to 20 percent of pituitary GH but is secreted only at low rates.[113] It does not appear to be selectively secreted in response to stimuli such as insulin hypoglycemia or GRH, and increased levels are not observed in acromegaly. It is claimed to lack the diabetogenic effects of native GH.[114]

Forms of GH and prolactin with higher molecular weights have also been observed in the pituitary gland and in circulation. Much of this material can be explained by aggregation of the hormone during the processes of extraction, purification, and analysis, though in one report, noncovalent aggregation of endogenous GH appeared to be responsible for impaired growth.[115] A small portion of GH within the pituitary also represents the nascent hormone, still bound to the ribosome.

A glycosylated form of prolactin has also been described recently in pituitary extracts.[116] It is presumed to originate from altered processing of prolactin mRNA, since only one copy of the prolactin gene is present in humans. It has a molecular size of 26,000 daltons and exhibits reduced biologic activity. A larger glycosylated form of prolactin has also been detected in the peripheral plasma of pregnant women[117] and may be related to a large and physiologically inactive form of prolactin in the circulation of women with idiopathic hyperprolactinemia but otherwise normal reproductive function.[118]

Growth Hormone

Action

Growth hormone was so named for its ability to produce an increase in linear growth which can be detected after a few days of treatment in hypophysectomized animals. The hormone also plays an important role in the regulation of metabolic processes. Interrelation between the metabolic effects of GH and the increase in body mass is only partially understood. The effects of GH can be categorized by tissue, by time of effect (acute vs. delayed), and by the type of metabolic effect produced (anabolic vs. diabetogenic).

Administration of GH to hypophysectomized animals and to GH-deficient humans is followed in a few days by a positive nitrogen balance, a decrease in urea production, a decrease in body fat, and a reduced rate of carbohydrate utilization, reflected by a decrease in the respiratory quotient. The effects observed after a single injection of GH are biphasic. Initially, decreases in concentrations of blood glucose, free fatty acids, and amino acids occur. Within a few hours, blood glucose and amino acid levels return to normal and free fatty acids rise above normal. Most of these effects can also be observed in normal persons, although to a lesser extent.

The mechanism responsible for these changes has been extensively studied by exposing isolated tissues and cultured cells to GH in vitro or by excising and examining tissues at various times after in vivo administration of the hormone.[119] Many of the acute effects of GH in isolated tissues resemble those of insulin. In muscle and liver, GH increases amino acid uptake and incorporation into protein. This process is independent of new RNA synthesis, although this is also stimulated. In muscle and adipose tissue, GH stimulates glucose uptake and enhances glucose utilization. In adipose tissue, GH antagonizes the lipolytic effect of catecholamines and stimulates RNA and mitochondrial protein synthesis.

With the exception of muscle protein synthesis, all these insulin-like effects of GH can be demonstrated at near-physiologic concentrations of the hormone, have a lag period of 10 to 30 min, and exhibit a characteristic refractory phenomenon. Within 3 to 4 h of their onset, the effects disappear and cannot be reinitiated by additional hormone. The refractoriness, which is specific for GH, requires both RNA and protein synthesis.

Concomitant with the disappearance of the acute effects of GH a series of delayed effects appear. They include (1) increased mobilization of free fatty acids from adipose tissue occurring as a consequence of increased triglyceride lipolysis, (2) increased sensitivity to the lipolytic effects of catecholamines, and (3) inhibition of both glucose uptake and glucose utilization, the latter on the basis of a decrease in pyruvate decarboxylation. All the late effects persist for many hours, are additive with additional exposure to GH, and form the basis of the diabetogenic effects of GH on carbohydrate and lipid metabolism.

The effects of GH administration on insulin secretion are complex and appear to be triphasic. There is initially an increase in insulin release which appears to be a direct effect of GH on the beta cell and can be observed within 5 min of injection in both normal and GH-deficient subjects.[120] During the subsequent 1 to 5 h, a slight inhibition of insulin secretion can be detected, the basis of which is not fully understood.[121] A more profound and persistent rise observed after longer periods of time is indirect and represents a secondary response to the impairment of carbohydrate utilization. With treatment of sufficient duration, and particularly in the presence of other factors such as glucocorticoids or an appropriate genetic background, overt diabetes may develop. The process is reversible upon removal of the GH influence, provided the secretory capacity of the beta cell has not been unduly compromised.

It has been recognized for some time that many of the effects of GH observed after its injection into intact animals could not be produced by exposure of tissues in vitro to the hormone. Furthermore, although GH binding to membrane receptors in a variety of tissues, including liver, breast, and circulating monocytes, can be readily demonstrated, correlation with its biologic effects is less evident than with other hormone receptor interactions. The demonstration that GH stimulates the incorporation of radiolabeled sulfate into cartilage proteoglycans by inducing a secondary "sulfation factor"[122] led to the recognition that normal plasma contains a number of GH-dependent growth factors which stimulate cellular processes involved with the growth of both skeletal and extraskeletal tissues. The term *somatomedin* was subsequently introduced to denote the more widespread spectrum of biologic activity involved. Investigators using differential experimental models found a close similarity between somatomedin C and non-(antibody-) suppressible insulin-like activity, soluble (in ethanol) (NSILA-s), a peptide that shares many properties with insulin, including binding to chick fibroblast insulin receptors, GH dependency, and sulfation activity in cartilage. Their identity has now been confirmed. The currently accepted name for these peptides, insulin-like growth factors (IGF), reflects their overall biologic effects.[123,124]

IGF-I (somatomedin C and NSILA-s) has a molecular size of 7500 daltons and a structure similar to that of proinsulin. It circulates in plasma primarily in association with a binding protein but also in a free form. It binds to specific receptors as well as (weakly) to insulin receptors and is believed to mediate many of the effects of GH. Injection of IGF-I stimulates growth in hypophysectomized rats.[125] After many years of attempts to identify a specific tissue of origin of IGF-I, i.e., a target organ for GH, it is now recognized that IGF-I is produced by many cell types, including liver, cartilage, kidney, and pituitary. Furthermore, there is evidence that IGF-I serves as a locally produced intracellular messenger of GH action rather than as a classic hormone.[126,127] For example, direct injection of GH into the tibial growth plate of a rat enhances cartilaginous growth to a greater extent than a subcutaneous injection, indicating that the effect of GH is local rather than systemic. In fact, there is now considerable question as to whether circulating IGF-I represents a source of tissue IGF activity, rather than a reflection of it.

IGF-II (identical to fibroblast multiplication factor) has also been sequenced and found to have a molecular size similar to that of IGF-I. It binds to a different receptor and exhibits tissue growth-promoting activity. However, its GH dependency has been less well established. Somatomedin A, a neutral protein, remains to be fully characterized but appears to be similar to somatomedin C. Somatomedin B is probably identical with epidermal growth factor.

GH has numerous effects on organ growth (e.g., cardiac and renal hypertrophy) and on specific hormone production and metabolism (e.g., aldosterone and renin production and thyroxine conversion to triiodothyronine,[128] the latter discussed in greater detail in subsequent chapters).

Measurement

RADIOIMMUNOASSAY The standard technique for measuring GH in circulating fluids is the radioimmunoassay. Antibodies to human GH are readily generated in rabbits, and the assay is reproducible from one laboratory to the next. The sensitivity of the assay, generally less than 10 pg, is more than adequate to measure basal circulating levels of the hormone. There is no significant cross-reactivity with any of the other pituitary hormones, though virtually all antibodies exhibit cross-reactivity with placental lactogen, which is structurally very similar. Because of the high levels of placental lactogen in pregnancy, measurement of GH levels by routine RIA is unreliable in pregnant women.

RADIORECEPTOR ASSAY Biologically active human GH can be measured by a radioreceptor assay using midpregnancy rabbit hepatic plasma membranes. This assay, though less sensitive than the radioimmunoassay, is capable of measuring plasma GH levels. It is also less specific, since prolactin exhibits considerable cross-reactivity. The radioreceptor assay has been of use in searching for biologically altered GH molecules, the presence of which has been suggested in acromegaly.[129]

BIOASSAY The original methods for assaying GH utilized its ability to increase linear growth in hypophysectomized rats. A more sensitive technique was subsequently developed which involved the measurement of tibial-epiphyseal cartilage width in hypophysectomized rats. This assay ("tibia test") remains useful for determining the biologic activity of GH extracted from pituitaries, but it has limited sensitivity (about 10 μg), making it impractical for the measurement of plasma levels. It is also affected by numerous other factors, making it relatively nonspecific for crude extracts of pituitary. To date, no cytochemical technique has been developed for GH.

Pituitary and Plasma Levels

PITUITARY The GH content of human pituitaries is approximately 2 percent of the wet weight, or 10 to 15 mg.[130] Males and females exhibit similar levels, and no significant changes in content occur with age. Less than 5 percent of the pituitary GH content is released each day, and it is believed that a considerable portion of the hormone in the pituitary undergoes destruction without ever being secreted.

PLASMA Plasma GH levels in the fasting, resting adult are generally less than 1 ng/ml, with levels occasionally at the lower limit of sensitivity. GH levels are slightly higher in women than in men, and the differences become more marked upon exercise, when levels increase in both sexes. GH levels are very high at the end of fetal life and during the first few days after birth (often more than 50 ng/ml). They rapidly decrease during the subsequent few weeks to levels just slightly higher than those in adults. GH is secreted episodically, with a periodicity of 3 to 4 h, and occasional values of 50 ng/ml or more may be observed, particularly in young adult males. Secretory bursts are less common after the fourth decade and rarely found after the sixth decade.

Only a small fraction of GH in plasma is excreted by the kidneys in an immunologically recognizable form. Urinary concentrations of GH reflect serum levels, being increased in states of GH hypersecretion and decreased in hypopituitarism; but this measurement is of little clinical value in the diagnosis of GH secretory disorders.

Metabolic Clearance and Secretion

GH is cleared from plasma primarily by the liver and to a lesser extent by the kidney. The half-life of GH in serum is 20 to 25 min,[131] and the metabolic clearance rate is approximately 110 ml/m^2 per minute, with little variation in states of GH over- or underproduction.[132] Decreased metabolic clearance rates have been reported in hypothyroidism and in diabetes. With these exceptions, therefore, the measurement of plasma GH provides an accurate reflection of the secretory rate of the hormone. GH secretion in normal men has been estimated at approximately 350 μg/m^2 per 24 h; in premenopausal women a value of about 500 μg/m^2 per 24 h is found.[133]

Control of Secretion

The regulation of GH secretion is mediated by both a releasing hormone (GRH) and an inhibiting hormone (somatostatin, SRIF) of hypothalamic origin. Alterations in the secretion of these two hormones represent the mechanism by which neural and extraneural factors regulate GH secretion under normal physiologic conditions. Since the secretion of these factors from the hypothalamus in vivo cannot presently be determined under physiologic conditions, it is their net effect on GH secretion which is measured. The recent availability of GRH has provided new insights into the regulation of GH secretion (see also Chap. 7). Its injection is followed by a rapid increase in GH release (Fig. 8-7), and its interaction with other factors affecting GH secretion is currently a subject of active investigation. Although several recently published reports suggest interactions of drugs affecting

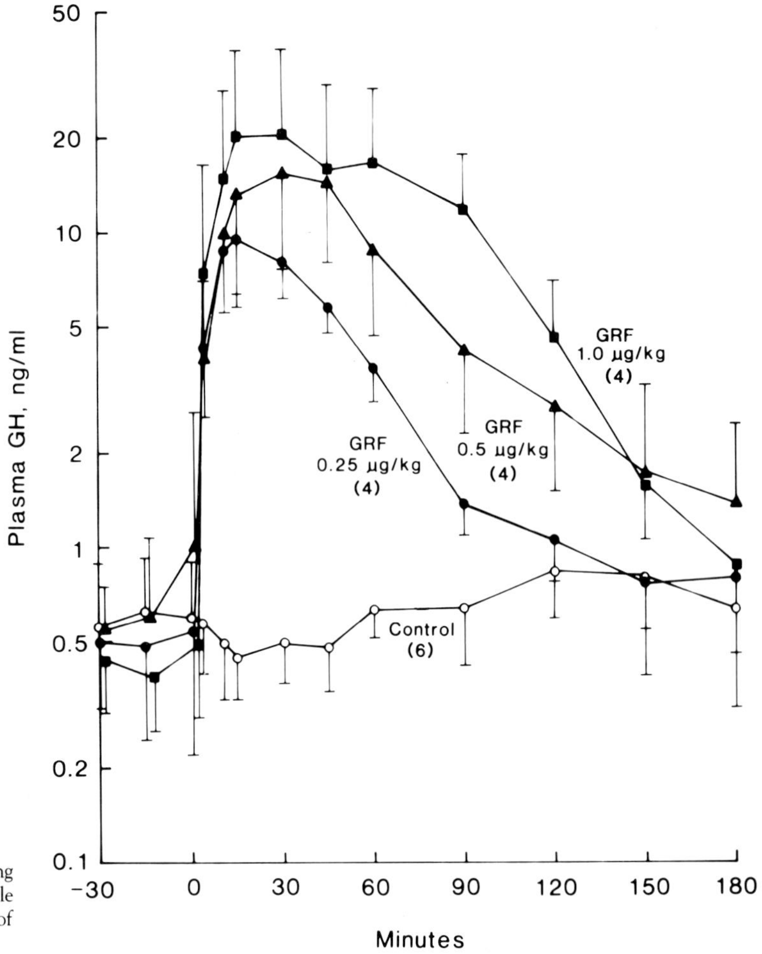

FIGURE 8-7 Plasma GH responses to increasing doses of GRH ($hGRH_{1-44}$-NH_2) given as a single intravenous injection in normal males. The dose of 1 µg/kg produces a maximal response.

neurotransmitter action with GRH at the pituitary,[134,135] possible effects on SRIF secretion have not been adequately examined.

Factors affecting the secretion of GH are summarized in Table 8-4. Because basal GH levels are so frequently near the lower limit of detectability, the demonstration of suppressive effects often requires the concomitant use of a stimulatory agent.

NEURAL Neural stimuli affecting GH release include both psychic and physical stress and episodic secretion unrelated to stress or recognizable metabolic events.[136] Sleep-associated bursts of GH secretion are most pronounced in infants, in whom they are seen during daytime naps as well as at night, and gradually decrease with age (Fig. 8-8). It has been estimated that 70 percent of the total GH secretion occurs during the night. These GH secretory episodes appear to be entrained by deep sleep, since they will not occur if sleep stage III or IV is prevented by awaking the subject. However, a close inspection of this relationship in individual normal subjects, in disease states associated with alterations in slow-wave sleep and GH secretion, and in the presence of pharmacologic agents (e.g., imipramine, flurazepam, methylscopolamine, and medroxyprogesterone) which can block the GH response has led to the conclusion that nocturnal GH secretion is frequently concomitant with sleep but is not closely linked to those neural processes required for slow-wave sleep.

METABOLIC Changes in the levels of circulating and, more importantly, intracellular fuels play an important role in regulating GH secretion.[136] Elevations of blood glucose by oral or intravenous glucose administration suppress GH secretion, a phenomenon which has been used extensively in confirming the diagnosis of acromegaly. In contrast, decreasing levels of blood glucose (and more specifically intracellular glucose metabolism), whether occurring as a result of insulin

Table 8-4. Factors Affecting Growth Hormone Secretion

Stimulative	Suppressive*
Physiologic	
Sleep	Postprandial hyperglycemia
Exercise	Elevated free fatty acids
Stress (physical or psychological)	
Postprandial hyperaminoacidemia	
Postprandial hypoglycemia (relative)	
Pharmacologic	
Hypoglycemia:	Hormones:
Absolute: insulin or 2-deoxyglucose	Somatostatin
Relative: postglucagon	Somatomedin C (IGF-I)
Hormones:	Growth hormone
Peptides (GRH, ACTH, α-MSH, vasopressin)	Progesterone
Estrogen	Glucocorticoids
Neurotransmitters, etc.:	Neurotransmitters, etc.:
α-Adrenergic agonists (clonidine)	α-Adrenergic antagonists (phentolamine)
β-Adrenergic antagonists (propranolol)	β-Adrenergic agonists (isoproterenol)
Serotonin precursors (5-hydroxytryptamine)	Serotonergic antagonists (methysergide)
Dopaminergic agonists (L-dopa, apomorphine, bromocriptine)	Dopaminergic antagonists (phenothiazines)
GABA agonists (muscimol)	Cholinergic (muscarinic) antagonists (pirenzepine)
Enkephalin analogues	
Pathologic	
Protein depletion and starvation	Obesity
Anorexia nervosa	Hypo- and hyperthyroidism
Chronic renal failure	Acromegaly: dopaminergic agonists
Acromegaly:	
TRH	
GnRH	

*Suppressive effects of some factors can be demonstrated only in the presence of a stimulus.

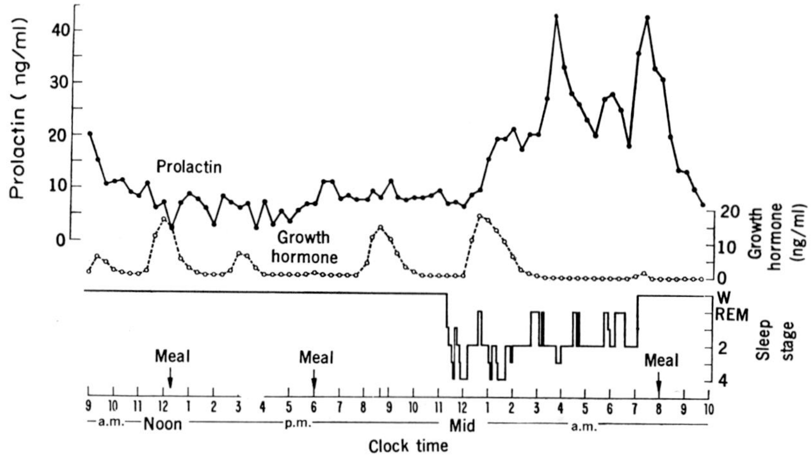

FIGURE 8-8 Sleep-associated changes in GH and prolactin secretion. The rise in GH accompanies the onset of slow-wave (EEG stages III and IV sleep, which usually occurs 90 to 120 min after sleep begins. The rise in prolactin secretion shows a sawtooth pattern, with peak values occurring at the end of the sleep period or shortly after awakening. (*From Sassin J et al: Science 177:1205, 1973.*)

hypoglycemia, during the descending portion of an oral glucose tolerance test, or several hours after a meal, stimulate GH release. The importance of intracellular metabolism is illustrated by the stimulatory effect of 2-deoxyglucose, which produces hyperglycemia with intracellular glucopenia by interfering with glucose phosphorylation. To date, insulin hypoglycemia has proved to be the most reliable stimulus for the evaluation of GH secretory capacity. Both the absolute glucose level and the rate of fall of glucose concentration are important determinants of the GH response, since a rapid decrease in glucose levels from hyperglycemic to normoglycemic levels can also cause GH release. Glucose-sensitive neurons in the ventral hypothalamus have been demonstrated, and these neurons are believed to trigger the release of GRH.

Oral administration or intravenous infusions of single amino acids (arginine, lysine, leucine, etc.), mixed amino acids, or proteins stimulate GH release. Elevations of plasma free fatty acids produced by infusions of a fat emulsion plus heparin (to activate lipoprotein lipase) acutely suppress GH secretion, while rapid decreases in plasma free fatty acids stimulate GH release. The mechanism of action as well as the specific central nervous system site involved in the effect of amino acids and free fatty acids remains to be determined.

HORMONAL GH secretion is affected by numerous hormones through a variety of processes. Estrogen enhances the growth hormone secretory response to many stimuli, as it does with prolactin, gonadotropins, and TSH. Progesterone is believed to suppress GH secretion, but the evidence is quite limited. GH responses to stimulation are suppressed by glucocorticoid therapy, endogenous hypercortisolism, hyperthyroidism, and hypothyroidism. Although steroids and thyroxine have both been shown to act directly on the somatotroph, their effects are clearly more complex and also involve actions on the hypothalamus and on generation of IGF-I (which is inhibited by both estrogens and glucocorticoids). GH exerts a negative feedback effect on its own secretion, in part mediated through IGF-I.[137] Both GH and IGF-I stimulate SRIF secretion,[138,139] and there are suggestions of effects on GRH as well. Clinical evidence of the role of IGF-I is provided by the Laron dwarf, in whom resistance to the actions of GH due to diminished binding to its receptor and possibly a postreceptor defect is associated with decreased IGF-I levels but elevated circulating GH levels.[140]

Several peptide hormones (vasopressin, ACTH and some of its fragments, and α-MSH) stimulate GH release acutely. Their effects, for the present, must be considered pharmacologic, perhaps due to an interaction with the GRH receptor on the somatotroph. Glucagon effects on GH secretion, on the other hand, are delayed and are most likely mediated by changes in carbohydrate metabolism.

NEUROTRANSMITTERS AND NEUROPHARMACOLOGIC AGENTS Studies on the neurochemical mediation of GH secretion and of the effects of neuropharmacologically active agents are extensive and have been reviewed in detail elsewhere.[136] The numerous reports which relate to GH secretion in normal humans can be summarized as follows: Irrespective of the nature of the extraneural stimuli, the mediation of the responses in the central nervous system and specifically within the hypothalamus involves one or more neurotransmitters and eventually results in alterations in the release of GRH or SRIF. The fact that these neurotransmitters are released locally and that two or more neurons involving more than a single neurotransmitter may be required for the response (see Chap. 7) can probably explain some of the apparent contradictions in the literature. It also follows that a neurotransmitter mediating a stimulatory response in one set of neurons can also mediate an inhibitory response in another.

There is, in general, evidence for the role of nearly all the classic monoamine neurotransmitters [norepinephrine, epinephrine, dopamine, serotonin, γ-aminobutyric acid (GABA), and acetylcholine] in the control of GH secretion. The beta-adrenergic receptor appears to be inhibitory and the alpha receptor stimulatory. Thus, beta receptor antagonists (e.g., propranolol) will enhance and alpha receptor antagonists (e.g., phentolamine) will suppress a variety of stimuli. Stimulation of the alpha receptor by clonidine also enhances GH release. Because of the lack of specificity of most of the receptor antagonists used clinically, however, caution is required in interpreting individual reports. The dopaminergic receptor is stimulatory, and agents such as L-dopa (the immediate precursor of dopamine), apomorphine, and bromocriptine (dopamine receptor agonists) all stimulate, while chlorpromazine and pimozide (dopamine receptor antagonists) impair GH responses to numerous stimuli. Serotonergic receptors are also stimulatory with respect to metabolic signals and possibly sleep-associated GH secretion, although the latter is still controversial. Cholinergic mechanisms appear to be involved as well in sleep-associated GH release. There is, in addition, evidence for a stimulatory effect of GABAergic neurons on GH secretion.[141]

Although several neuropeptides stimulate GH secretion in animal models, there is evidence only for enkephalins and α-MSH in humans. Enkephalin analogues capable of penetrating the blood-brain barrier stimulate GH secretion,[142] though the role of endogenous enkephalins in the regulation of GH is still unknown.

Prolactin

Action

The primary site of prolactin action is the breast, where, in conjunction with other hormones, it stimulates mammary tissue development and lactation. Prolactin is required for normal breast development in many species, although an essential role has yet to be demonstrated in humans. Pathologic elevations of prolactin may be but usually are not associated with an increase in breast size; in men, gynecomastia occurs in the presence of normal prolactin levels. During pregnancy, prolactin, in conjunction with estrogen, progesterone, and placental lactogen and in the presence of insulin and cortisol, results in additional breast development, leading eventually to milk formation. Prolactin specifically stimulates the synthesis of milk proteins, including lactalbumin, and of lipids and carbohydrates. Prolactin receptors have been demonstrated in normal mammary tissue and are located on the alveolar surfaces of cells. Prolactin receptors are also present in liver and kidney tissue, and prolactin appears capable of increasing the number of its own receptors.

Following parturition, the abrupt decrease in estrogen and progesterone of placental origin permits the initiation of lactation. Thus, estrogen, which plays a synergistic role in promoting breast development, antagonizes the effects of prolactin on lactation. This phenomenon forms the basis for the use of estrogens to inhibit lactation in the postpartum period and also explains the frequent appearance of galactorrhea in hyperprolactinemic women subsequent to discontinuation of oral contraceptives.

Continued secretion of prolactin is required to maintain lactation once it has begun. Inhibition of prolactin secretion by pharmacologic or surgical means is followed by a cessation of lactation. Prolactin secretion, which is stimulated by suckling, gradually diminishes to normal levels during the postpartum period. The actual milk "let-down" reflex, however, is not mediated by prolactin but by the release of oxytocin from the posterior pituitary. Oxytocin stimulates the contraction of myoepithelial cells around the terminal acinar lobules which expel their milk into the lobular ducts.

In the rat, prolactin is required for maintenance of the secretory activity of the corpus luteum and is therefore important in maintaining pregnancy during the early stages. This effect does not appear to be important in humans, although small amounts of prolactin are required for progesterone production by human granulosa cells.[143] Higher levels of prolactin are associated with progressive inhibition of progesterone secretion. Prolactin, along with FSH and LH, is present in follicular fluid, and there is evidence that prolactin may block the stimulating effect of FSH on estrogen secretion by the developing graafian follicle.

In addition to these effects on reproductive physiology, prolactin has effects on behavior and on fluid and electrolyte metabolism in several animal species, though evidence of these effects in humans is still unconvincing. In birds and in mice prolactin enhances maternal nurturing behavior, an action important in the life cycle of these species. Although prolactin levels increase in association with numerous psychic stimuli in humans (see below), the increased secretion of the hormone appears to be in response to rather than the cause of the stimuli. Prolactin also stimulates the retention of sodium, potassium, and water by the kidneys in several mammalian species and potentiates the effects of aldosterone and vasopressin. Attempts to demonstrate these actions in humans have to date been unsuccessful.

The metabolic effects of prolactin in hypophysectomized animals resemble those of GH and include stimulation of protein synthesis, calorigenesis, and chondroitin sulfate formation in cartilage. In humans, the administration of ovine prolactin to GH-deficient subjects produces nitrogen retention, hypercalciuria, lipid mobilization, carbohydrate intolerance, and limited skeletal growth. Hyperinsulinemia, reflecting insulin resistance, can also be demonstrated in patients with hyperprolactinemia and can be eliminated by suppressing prolactin secretion.[144]

Measurement

RADIOIMMUNOASSAY Prolactin is measured by a homologous radioimmunoassay. Antibodies are raised in rabbits, and the sensitivity of most assays is sufficient to measure basal levels of the hormone. The assay is quite specific and exhibits no significant cross-reactivity with either GH or placental lactogen.

RADIORECEPTOR ASSAY Radioligand assays for prolactin most commonly utilize pregnant rabbit mammary gland membranes.[145] Although this assay has sufficient sensitivity to measure prolactin levels in plasma, the binding of GH by the membrane and its displacement of radiolabeled prolactin has limited the usefulness of this technique. As with GH, comparison of radioimmunoassay and receptor assay potency may be important to distinguish between biologically active and inactive circulating prolactin in certain conditions. A large-molecular-size prolactin in serum has been reported to exhibit reduced biologic activity.[146]

BIOASSAY The stimulatory effect of prolactin on the crop sac of the pigeon provided the basis for a bioassay which was used for many years. Increased sensitivity was subsequently achieved by measuring lactose or casein synthesis in midpregnancy mouse mammary glands. Much of the early information on the plasma prolactin levels was obtained through the use of these assays, though they have been replaced by the RIA.

Pituitary and Plasma Levels

PITUITARY Measurement of prolactin content in the human pituitary by radioimmunoassay indicates levels of approximately 100 μg per pituitary. This concentration is considerably lower than that of GH (approximately 10 percent of the GH content) and also lower with respect to GH than in most mammalian pituitaries. There is some question as to the validity of this figure, possibly related to incomplete extraction techniques, since the estimated daily secretion rate of prolactin is several times that of the pituitary content (see below), which is unique among the anterior pituitary hormones.

PLASMA Reported levels of plasma prolactin from different laboratories have varied, with a downward trend observed as more specific antisera to prolactin have been used. Mean prolactin levels are approximately 5 ng/ml in men and 8 ng/ml in women, and most laboratories report an upper limit ranging from 15 to 20 ng/ml. Plasma prolactin values are detectable in all normal subjects.

Plasma prolactin levels are very high in the fetus and after the twentieth week of gestation may exceed 300 ng/ml. At term, umbilical vein levels are greater than those in maternal blood, indicating that the levels are due to fetal secretion. Similar levels are seen in anencephalic infants, indicating that the hypothalamus is not necessary for fetal prolactin secretion. Prolactin is also secreted by the chorion-decidua tissue of the placenta, and high concentrations of the hormone are present in amniotic fluid.[147]

Plasma prolactin levels in newborn infants decrease during the first few months of life to the values observed in adults. Levels in females begin to exceed those in males at puberty, primarily on the basis of estrogen effects. Prolactin levels in women decrease at menopause. Responses to almost all stimuli of prolactin secretion are greater in women than in men and are also increased in men by estrogen treatment. During pregnancy, prolactin levels rise continuously from early gestation to term. After parturition, levels begin to decline and, even with continued nursing, often return to the nonpregnant range after a few months.

Metabolic Clearance and Secretion

The limited availability of human prolactin has prevented extensive studies of the metabolic clearance rate of the hormone. Data obtained using radiolabeled prolactin indicate the metabolic clearance of prolactin to be about 40 ml/m^2 per minute, or about one-third that of GH.[148] A preliminary report using unlabeled prolactin gives similar findings.[149] The kidney is responsible for approximately 25 percent of prolactin clearance, and the remainder is believed to involve the liver. The half-life of prolactin in the circulation is approximately 50 min, or about three times that of GH. The prolactin secretion rate, based on metabolic clearance studies, is about 400 μg per day.

Control of Secretion

In contrast to the other anterior pituitary hormones, the neuroendocrine control of prolactin is predominantly inhibitory. Interruption of the integrity of the hypothalamic-pituitary axis, whether by pituitary stalk section or hypothalamic destruction or, in experimental animals, by transplantation of the pituitary to another region of the body, results in increased prolactin secretion. The major physiologic inhibitor (prolactin inhibiting factor, PIF) has appeared to this point to be dopamine. Dopamine has been identified in portal hypophyseal blood of rats at concentrations greater than in systemic blood and binds to specific receptors on the lactotroph, resulting in direct suppression of prolactin release. Recent studies have identified another prolactin-inhibiting peptide present as a COOH-terminal extension to GnRH in a common precursor.[150,151] This GnRH-associated peptide (GAP) is 56 amino acids in length, exhibits greater potency than dopamine in inhibiting prolactin secretion, and also stimulates LH and FSH secretion in vitro. Its significance in human physiology and disease must await appropriate clinical studies.

As with GH, there is a dual control of prolactin secretion consisting of a stimulatory as well as an inhibitory component. The stimulatory factor, which is influenced by serotonergic mechanisms, was at first believed to be TRH, which exhibits as great a stimulatory effect on prolactin as on TSH secretion. TRH binds to the lactotroph receptors, activates adenylate cyclase, and increases prolactin synthesis as well as secretion. However, neuroendocrine-mediated secretion of prolactin and TSH is more frequently discordant than concordant; that is, TSH, though not prolactin secretion, is increased by cold, and prolactin, though not TSH secretion, is increased by nursing and stress. These findings suggest that the prolactin stimulatory factor is not TRH. Several hypothalamic factors distinct from TRH have been described that stimulate prolactin release, including vasoactive intestinal peptide (VIP) and peptide histidyl-methionine (PHM), and VIP has been shown to play a physiologic role in relation to nursing.[152] These two peptides have also been shown to exist in the same precursor.[153]

Factors influencing prolactin secretion are listed in Table 8-5. Physiologic stimuli, in addition to those of pregnancy and nursing which are described above, include nipple stimulation, which can be demonstrated in both men and women, and sexual intercourse (in part also related to nipple stimulation). Sleep-associated rises in prolactin secretion can be readily demonstrated and begin about 60 to 90 min after the onset of sleep. Secretory bursts of prolactin continue throughout the sleep period, resulting in peak levels at 5 to 8 h after the onset of sleep. In contrast to GH secretion, sleep-associated prolactin secretion is not related to deep (stage III or IV) sleep (Fig. 8-8). Strenuous exercise also stimulates prolactin secretion, possibly by the same mechanisms as are involved in GH secretion, since like GH release, prolactin release is stimulated by hypoglycemia and frequently suppressed by hyperglycemia. Oral protein also stimulates prolactin secretion,[154] though the mediation of this response is not presently understood.

Prolactin secretion is influenced by many hormones. The effects of estrogen are exerted directly on the lactotroph, enhancing both basal and stimulated release, and can be seen within 2 to 3 days. Glucocorticoids diminish the prolactin response to TRH, by an effect that also occurs at the level of the pituitary. Thyroid hormone administration is not followed by changes in basal prolactin levels but suppresses the response to TRH. This response is increased in hypothyroidism and diminished in hyperthyroidism and reverts to normal with appropriate treatment. A minority of patients with primary hypothyroidism have hyperprolactinemia, and some exhibit galactorrhea.

A wide spectrum of agents with neuropharmacologic actions modify prolactin levels.[136] Agents which enhance dopaminergic activity, e.g., L-dopa (precursor), bromocriptine and apomorphine (dopaminergic agonists), and dopamine itself, all suppress prolactin secretion. The effects of dopamine and dopamine agonists are exerted directly on the pituitary, whereas those of dopamine precursors involve both pituitary and central mechanisms. Dopaminergic receptor antagonists, represented primarily by phenothiazine (chlorpromazine, prochlorperazine) and butyrophenone (haloperidol) neuroleptics, elevate prolactin levels and occasionally produce galactorrhea. The prolactin-elevating effects of these agents correlate well with their antipsychotic potency,[155] even though the maximal prolactin-stimulating effects are reached at doses below those required for psychotropic effects and despite evidence suggesting that the pituitary dopaminergic receptors are different from those in the

Table 8-5. Factors Affecting Prolactin Secretion

Stimulative	Suppressive
Physiologic	
Pregnancy	
Nursing	
Nipple stimulation	
Sexual intercourse (women only)	
Exercise	
Sleep	
Stress	
Pharmacologic	
Hypoglycemia	Hyperglycemia*
Hyperaminoacidemia	
Hormones:	Hormones:
Estrogen	Glucocorticoids*
TRH	Thyroxine
Neurotransmitters, etc.:	Neurotransmitters, etc.:
Dopaminergic antagonists (phenothiazines, butyrophenones, metoclopramide)	Dopaminergic agonists (L-dopa, apomorphine, dopamine, bromocriptine)
Catecholamine depletors and synthesis inhibitors (reserpine, α-methyldopa)	Serotonin antagonists (methysergide)
Serotonin precursors (5-HTP)	
GABA agonists (muscimol)	
Histamine H_2 antagonists (cimetidine)	
Opiates, etc. (morphine, enkephalin analogues)	
Pathologic	
Chronic renal failure	
Cirrhosis	
Hypothyroidism*	
Intercostal nerve stimulation (chest wall burns, herpes zoster, postmastectomy)	

*Occasionally observed.

CNS.[156] Reserpine, a central catecholamine depletor, has similar stimulatory effects. GABA does not affect prolactin secretion directly, but muscimol, a recently developed GABA analogue which crosses the blood-brain barrier after systemic administration, stimulates prolactin release.[141] The effects of histamine on prolactin secretion are incompletely understood. Histamine stimulates prolactin secretion by a central mechanism. The histamine H_2-receptor blockers cimetidine and ranitidine exhibit similar effects,[157,158] indicating a complex role for this neurotransmitter. Serotonergic mechanisms have been implicated in both stress and nursing-associated prolactin secretion on the basis of the suppression of these responses by serotonin receptor blockers. Prolactin secretion is also increased by opiates and endorphins.[142] The mechanism of this effect is related to the inhibitory action of opiates and endorphins on central dopamine release.

Prolactin secretion is increased with surgical stress, most dramatically during operations performed under general anesthesia, and some though not all of the response may be due to the anesthetic agent. The rise in prolactin secretion seen after chest wall trauma, burns, and thoracic operations may also be stress-mediated and is related to stimulation of afferent intercostal nerves from the area of the nipple.

Hyperprolactinemia is present in up to 65 percent of patients with chronic renal failure maintained on hemodialysis, and in women galactorrhea is frequently present.[159] Such patients exhibit impaired responses to short-term dopaminergic suppression and to TRH and chlorpromazine stimulation. Though the metabolic clearance of prolactin is decreased in uremia, the actual hormone secretion rate is increased, suggesting an impairment in feedback inhibition.[148] Renal transplantation is generally associated with a return of prolactin levels to the normal range.

HYPOPITUITARISM

Hypopituitarism does not become clinically evident until about 70 to 75 percent of the adenohypophysis is destroyed, though with currently available pituitary hormone function testing a diminished reserve is likely to be detected with less destruction. Total loss of pituitary secretion requires at least 90 percent destruction of the gland. In many patients with pituitary destruction, minimal clinical evidence of hypopituitarism may escape detection for long periods of time and may never be recognized.

Hypopituitarism is a disorder of diverse etiology, resulting in a partial or total loss of anterior and posterior pituitary hormone function. The clinical manifestations vary greatly according to the age of the subject, the rapidity of onset, the particular hormones involved, and the extent of their impaired secretion, as well as the nature of the primary pathologic process. Complete loss of hormonal secretion can rapidly become life-threatening and require immediate therapy.

Etiology

Hypopituitarism can be divided into two general categories: *primary* and *secondary*. Primary hypopituitarism is due to the absence or destruction of the hormone-secreting cells of the pituitary, secondary hypopituitarism to a lack of stimulation of pituitary hormone secretion caused by organic or functional disorders of the vascular and/or neural connections with the brain at the level of the pituitary stalk, hypothalamus, or extrahypothalamic central nervous system. Deficient anterior pituitary hormone secretion under such conditions is the result of lack of the appropriate releasing factors, while diminished posterior pituitary hormone secretion is due to lack of synthesis and axonal transport of the hormones from their site of origin in the anterior hypothalamus, discussed in detail in Chap. 9.

Table 8-6 lists the various diseases associated with hypopituitarism. Because of the many ways in which patients with hypopituitarism may present, the specific underlying pathologic process frequently cannot be reliably determined.

PRIMARY HYPOPITUITARISM

Simmonds, in his classic case of hypopituitarism following necrosis of the pituitary in a woman with severe puerperal sepsis,[160] was the first to associate the clinical disorder of hypopituitarism with ischemic necrosis of the pituitary, although the first report of acute pituitary necrosis appeared the previous year.[161] Simmonds emphasized the term *cachexia,* and for several decades this feature was erroneously considered an important feature of the disease. In fact, one emaciated patient whose picture appeared in several textbooks was subsequently shown at autopsy to have a normal pituitary gland and most probably had anorexia nervosa. The extensive work by Sheehan provided the first clear distinction between pituitary necrosis and hypopituitarism.[162] He demonstrated that fibrosis of the pituitary was a consequence of the ischemic necrosis and infarction that often occurred in association with postpartum hemorrhage and vascular collapse. He also provided convincing proof that cachexia is not an obligatory or even a common feature of the disease.

Table 8-6. Etiologic Factors in Hypopituitarism

- I. Primary
  - A. Pituitary tumors:
    - 1. Primary intrasellar (chromophobe adenoma, craniopharyngioma)
    - 2. Parasellar (meningioma, optic nerve glioma)
  - B. Ischemic necrosis of the pituitary:
    - 1. Postpartum (Sheehan's syndrome)
    - 2. Diabetes mellitus
    - 3. Other systemic diseases (temporal arteritis, sickle-cell disease and trait, arteriosclerosis, eclampsia)
  - C. Aneurysm of intracranial internal carotid artery
  - D. Pituitary apoplexy (almost always related to a primary pituitary tumor)
  - E. Cavernous sinus thrombosis
  - F. Infectious disease (tuberculosis, syphilis, malaria, meningitis, fungal disease)
  - G. Infiltrative disease (hemochromatosis)
  - H. Immunologic (granulomatous or lymphocytic hypophysitis)
  - I. Iatrogenic
    - 1. Irradiation of nasopharynx
    - 2. Irradiation of sella
    - 3. Surgical destruction
  - J. Primary empty sella syndrome
  - K. Metabolic disorders (chronic renal failure)
  - L. Idiopathic (frequently monohormonal and occasionally familial)
- II. Secondary
  - A. Destruction of pituitary stalk:
    - 1. Trauma
    - 2. Compression by tumor or aneurysm
    - 3. Iatrogenic (surgical)
  - B. Hypothalamic or other central nervous system disease:
    - 1. Inflammatory (sarcoid or other granulomatous disease)
    - 2. Infiltrative (lipid storage diseases)
    - 3. Trauma
    - 4. Toxic (vincristine)
    - 5. Hormone-induced (glucocorticoids, gonadal steroids)
    - 6. Tumors (primary, metastatic, lymphoma, leukemia)
    - 7. Idiopathic (frequently congenital or familial, often restricted to one or two hormones, and may be reversible)
    - 8. Nutritional (starvation, obesity)
    - 9. Anorexia nervosa
    - 10. Psychosocial dwarfism

The mechanism of acute ischemic necrosis is not entirely clear, but the condition is believed by most to be due to vasospasm of the hypophyseal vessels. Whether the changes in the pituitary during pregnancy associated with its marked increase in size under the influence of increased estrogen secretion result in enhanced sensitivity to vasoconstrictive stimuli or whether the gland becomes more sensitive to hypoxia is not known. However, the most frequent setting in which necrosis of the pituitary occurs is the immediate postpartum period in association with severe hemorrhage and hypotension. As many as 32 percent of women experiencing hemorrhage and vascular collapse during delivery will develop some degree of hypopituitarism.[163] The extent of pituitary necrosis and the subsequent hypopituitarism are related to the severity of the hemorrhage. A most important clue that pituitary necrosis has occurred is the inability to lactate in the postpartum period and the failure of cyclic menstruation to be reestablished. However, because of the slowly developing picture of hypopituitarism and its frequently incomplete clinical manifestations, the presence of postpartum lactation cannot be used to exclude the existence of at least partial pituitary insufficiency. The relatively large reserve capacity of the anterior pituitary is evident from the discrepancy between the incidence of ischemic pituitary necrosis and that of hypopituitarism.

With the improvement in obstetric care during the past half century, the syndrome of pituitary necrosis has become much less common. It must be emphasized, though, that significant hemorrhage and shock, while important predisposing factors, are not absolutely essential for its development. Ischemic necrosis of the pituitary can be seen in association with numerous other diseases, although the frequency is quite low. In diabetes mellitus a 2 percent incidence at autopsy has been reported,[164] though in most of the patients evidence of clinical hypopituitarism was lacking. When present, hypopituitarism can lead to a marked reduction in insulin requirement due primarily to the lack of glucocorticoids. Pituitary necrosis has been reported in epidemic hemorrhagic fever, but the rapid death of patients precluded assessment of their pituitary function. It has also been seen in association with a large variety of other diseases, including malaria, temporal arteritis, hemochromatosis, sickle cell disease, meningitis, eclampsia, and severe vitamin deficiency and occasionally without any predisposing illness.[165] In some patients there is sufficient destruction of the pituitary to result in signs and symptoms of hypopituitarism, whereas in others, detailed testing is required to document the impairment in hormone secretion.

Pituitary tumor is today the most common cause

of hypopituitarism involving multiple hormone deficiencies in the adult population. A full discussion of this subject is provided in the following section. Parasellar mass lesions can also invade the sella turcica and cause sufficient destruction of the pituitary to produce hypopituitarism. Similar destruction can be caused by aneurysms of the intracavernous portion of the internal carotid artery.

Hypopituitarism of varying degree may be secondary to an intrapituitary hemorrhage (*pituitary apoplexy*) associated with a functioning or nonfunctioning pituitary tumor.[166] The signs and symptoms may vary considerably. If bleeding occurs gradually, leading to compression of the pituitary, the symptoms of hypopituitarism will predominate, while if the hemorrhage is sudden, the presenting symptoms will be headache, ophthalmoplegia, and subarachnoid irritation. Patients typically present with features of sudden expansion of a preexisting pituitary adenoma. Most patients recover without acute surgical intervention, though in some it may be necessary to correct the visual abnormalities. In most patients some anterior pituitary function will be lost,[167] though posterior pituitary function is almost always preserved. During the acute period, glucocorticoid therapy should be provided.

With the changing spectrum of diseases and the advances in the treatment of infectious diseases over the past several decades, the classic examples of hypopituitarism found in diseases such as tuberculosis and syphilis have become exceedingly rare. However, more extensive investigations of patients with other diseases have revealed evidence of pituitary hypofunction. Nearly 50 percent of patients with hemochromatosis, in whom decreased gonadal function is a common and early manifestation, have evidence of impaired gonadotropin secretion.[168] In some patients adrenocortical insufficiency due to impaired ACTH secretion also occurs. The cause of the hypofunction relates to the iron deposition in the pituitary which commonly occurs in this disease. In some patients, however, hypopituitarism may be secondary to a disturbance of hypothalamic function.[169]

Hypopituitarism can also occur on an immunologic basis. There have been several recent reports of young women in the peripartum period who developed hypopituitarism associated with a presumed pituitary tumor.[170,171] At surgery, the pituitary tissue was mucoid, partially necrotic, and extensively infiltrated with lymphocytes. The pathogenesis of this disorder is at present unknown, as is its relation to giant cell granulomatous hypophysitis, a rare disorder seen primarily in middle-aged or older women.[172] The latter is distinct from pituitary sarcoidosis, which most commonly involves the posterior pituitary and is associated with diabetes insipidus. Isolated gonadotropin failure has also been reported in association with polyglandular failure, suggesting that autoimmune hypophysitis may also occur.[173]

The use of ionizing radiation for the treatment of malignant disease in the head and neck (nasopharyngeal carcinomas, brain tumors, leukemia treated with prophylactic cranial irradiation) is being recognized with increasing frequency as a cause of hypopituitarism on both a primary and secondary basis.[174,175] In children, the most common manifestation has been growth retardation or absence of onset of puberty, while in adults, symptoms of gonadotropin deficiency have been most prominent. Hypopituitarism can be detected within 6 to 12 months after a dose of about 3000 rads. The normal pituitary gland appears to be more susceptible to irradiation damage in children than in adults, in whom considerably greater doses (10,000 to 18,000 rads) are required to destroy the anterior pituitary in patients with breast cancer or diabetic retinopathy. The dose of irradiation used for the treatment of pituitary tumors is approximately 4500 to 5000 rads, and the short-term incidence of hypopituitarism is relatively low, as discussed in the following section. However, long-term evaluation of irradiated patients will be required to determine the true incidence of iatrogenic disease.

Surgical excision of the pituitary, which occasionally occurs during removal of a pituitary tumor or as intended therapy for breast cancer or diabetic retinopathy, produces panhypopituitarism requiring immediate therapy.

The primary empty sella syndrome, described below under Pituitary Tumors, is infrequently associated with hypopituitarism. Although most reported series of patients with this disorder include a small percentage in whom endocrine function testing reveals a defect in one or more pituitary hormones, the incidence of clinical (symptomatic) hypopituitarism is less than 10 percent.[176] An empty sella can occur secondary to Sheehan's syndrome,[177] sarcoidosis,[178] or other pituitary diseases in which varying degrees of hypopituitarism are present.

Hypopituitarism may occur without any detectable underlying disease and most frequently involves deficiencies in a single or a few rather than in all hormones. Although it is generally sporadic, there are reports of both autosomal and X-linked recessive varieties of hypopituitarism with small, normal, or even slightly enlarged sellae.[179–181] The manner of presentation and the specific characteristics of the various types of idiopathic hypopituitarism are discussed in relation to the specific hormone deficiencies encountered.

Impaired secretion of TSH and gonadotropins has been documented in chronic renal failure due to a combination of defects at both pituitary and hypothalamic levels.[182,183] Though the specific factor or factors responsible remain to be identified, the abnormalities appear reversible with renal transplantation.

Secondary Hypopituitarism

Secondary hypopituitarism can be caused by numerous central nervous system disorders, all of which have in common disruption of the normal delivery of releasing or inhibiting factors to the pituitary. Primary hypopituitarism can be differentiated from secondary hypopituitarism in the absence of anatomically defined disease of the pituitary or the central nervous system, in some but not all patients, by the use of hypothalamic releasing hormones. In addition, diabetes insipidus is more common in secondary than in primary hypopituitarism.

Pathologic processes involving the pituitary stalk are most frequently due to trauma. Basilar skull fractures occasionally lead to tearing of the stalk with rupture of both the neural and vascular connections. Parasellar tumors or aneurysms can also cause sufficient compression of the stalk to impair blood flow to the portal vessels, resulting in hypopituitarism. Pituitary stalk section has been performed to produce hypopituitarism as an alternative procedure to hypophysectomy. The results differ from those following hypophysectomy in that (1) prolactin levels frequently rise and remain elevated, owing to the loss of hypothalamic prolactin inhibiting factor, provided that sufficient blood flow remains to ensure lactotroph viability, and (2) neovascularization will occasionally lead to reestablishment of the hypophyseal portal vasculature and recovery of pituitary hormone function unless a barrier is inserted at the site of transsection.

Diseases of the central nervous system, primarily of the hypothalamus, which impair releasing factor secretion also produce hypopituitarism. Inflammatory diseases such as sarcoidosis and infiltrative processes, including the lipid storage diseases, hemochromatosis, and eosinophilic granuloma, often result in impaired TSH, gonadotropin, GH, and less commonly ACTH and vasopressin secretion. Prolactin levels are frequently elevated, confirming the suprasellar origin of the disease. The frequency of multiple hormone deficiencies in these as well as other hypothalamic diseases depends upon the size of the pathologic process and its location. The closer the location to the median eminence where the funneling effect of the hypothalamus occurs, the greater the possibility of multiple hormone deficiencies.

Trauma to the hypothalamus frequently occurs in serious head injuries. Evidence for hypopituitarism is often observed in patients with prolonged coma,[184-186] and recovery of pituitary function usually but not invariably parallels the improvement in neurologic status, though residual impairment is not uncommon.

Drugs used in the therapy of malignant disease (e.g., vincristine) may also have toxic effects on the hypothalamus resulting in impaired pituitary hormone secretion. Functional impairment of ACTH and the gonadotropins can also occur as the result of prolonged treatment with glucocorticoids, even with alternate-day therapy,[187] and with oral contraceptives as a result of continuous suppression of the specific releasing factors in an exaggeration of the normal negative feedback mechanism. Recovery of function usually occurs, though a moderately long period of time may be required. Recovery of the hypothalamic-pituitary-adrenal axis following the removal of an adrenocortical adenoma may require 12 to 24 months, and restoration of cyclic ovulation following discontinuation of oral contraceptives may take as long. Although impaired TSH reserve can be demonstrated transiently after prolonged treatment with exogenous thyroid hormone in euthyroid persons, clinical evidence of hypothyroidism is rare.

Tumors of the hypothalamus and third ventricle or hypothalamic involvement with lymphomatous or leukemic infiltrates can result in impaired pituitary function. With successful treatment of the underlying disease, some recovery may occur.

As with primary hypopituitarism, diminished pituitary hormone secretion may occur on the basis of central nervous system disorders which are unassociated with other subjective or objective findings. Single or multiple hormone deficiencies may be involved, and the disease may become evident at any age. A common cause of GH deficiency during childhood, either as an isolated hormonal defect or in association with TSH, gonadotropin, or ACTH deficiency, is a yet undefined abnormality in the secretion of or the response to the appropriate hypothalamic releasing hormones.[188] The most frequent disorder in adults is impaired gonadotropin secretion (hypothalamic hypogonadism or hypothalamic amenorrhea). In both children and adults hypothalamic hypopituitarism may be secondary to an emotional disturbance and thus reversible.

Hypothalamic dysfunction resulting in impaired gonadotropin secretion may occur as the result of marked changes in body weight. Both malnutrition and marked obesity are often associated with amenorrhea, which persists until a return to near-normal body weight. Amenorrhea also occurs with strenuous exercise, particularly in untrained women.[189,190] In patients with anorexia nervosa, secretion of gonadotropin and occasionally TSH may be diminished. Although weight loss contributes to the pathogenesis of the endocrine disorder, other still unknown factors are involved, since amenorrhea frequently precedes weight loss and can persist after weight is regained.[191] Stress, such as that associated with severe illness not affecting the CNS, also results in hypogonadism which is reversible upon recovery.[186]

Pinealomas are associated with both precocious puberty and hypogonadism. The secretion of a gonadotropin inhibitor by the tumor has been postulated, but the chemical nature of this substance is not yet known. These disorders are discussed in some detail in Chap. 7.

Clinical Features

The signs and symptoms of hypopituitarism vary according to the extent of diminished secretion of individual pituitary hormones and the rapidity of onset. Both factors are greatly influenced by the etiology of the disease. In the most extensive form of total absence of pituitary secretion, or *panhypopituitarism*, such as is seen after surgical hypophysectomy, severe pituitary apopolexy, or withdrawal of hormone therapy in hypophysectomized subjects, clinical features can develop within a few hours (diabetes insipidus) to a few days (adrenal insufficiency). In partial hypopituitarism, more commonly seen with tumors or infiltrative diseases, the signs and symptoms progress slowly and may be vague and nonspecific, with the diagnosis unsuspected for long periods of time. In general, the most common presenting manifestations are caused by gonadotropin deficiency in adults and GH deficiency in children. The spectrum of clinical features is best described by considering first the effects of deficiencies of the individual pituitary hormones and then their interrelationships.

ACTH

Deficiency of ACTH is manifested by diminished adrenocortical function, and many of the signs and symptoms of adrenal insufficiency are similar whether caused by pituitary or adrenal disease. Weakness, postural hypotension, and dehydration commonly occur during stress, although true addisonian crisis is infrequent because of the partial independence of the renin-angiotensin-aldosterone system from the secretion of ACTH. Thus, aldosterone secretion may be diminished in hypopituitarism but to a lesser extent than in primary adrenal insufficiency. Nausea, vomiting, and severe hypothermia may also occur. Hypoglycemia is occasionally seen, particularly after a prolonged fast and/or moderate alcohol ingestion, because of impaired gluconeogenesis. In patients with isolated ACTH deficiency this may be the only symptom of the disease. Unlike patients with primary adrenal insufficiency, in whom ACTH secretion is increased, those with ACTH deficiency show no hyperpigmentation; in fact, there may be depigmentation and diminished tanning after exposure to sunlight. Since impairment of ACTH secretion is frequently incomplete, patients may experience symptoms only during periods of stress (e.g., surgery, trauma, severe infections), and ACTH deficiency may thus remain undiagnosed for prolonged periods. The inability to excrete a water load, seen in Addison's disease, also occurs in ACTH deficiency but is less pronounced and often masked by a concomitant vasopressin deficiency (see below). The loss of adrenal androgens in males is of little consequence if testicular function is preserved. In females, however, it can contribute to decreased libido and is largely responsible for the loss of axillary and pubic hair. Calcification of auricular cartilage, once thought to be specific for Addison's disease, may also be seen with ACTH deficiency.[192]

TSH

Secondary or pituitary hypothyroidism is a term used to describe the thyroid deficiency state caused by diminished TSH secretion. Primary and secondary hypothyroidism are in general clinically indistinguishable from each other except in their severity. Patients with TSH deficiency exhibit cold intolerance, constipation, dry skin, pallor, mental slowing, bradycardia, and hoarseness. True myxedema occurs infrequently, and hypercholesterolemia and carotenemia are uncommon. Both increased and decreased menstrual flow may be observed. TSH deficiency occurring during childhood results in severe growth retardation unresponsive to treatment with GH. Isolated TSH deficiency has been observed on a familial basis[193] and in association with pseudohypoparathyroidism.[194]

LH and FSH

Gonadotropin deficiency in adult women is manifested by amenorrhea and clinical features of estrogen deficiency, including breast atrophy, dryness of skin, and a decrease in vaginal secretions often resulting in dyspareunia. A decrease in libido may also occur. In adult males, the loss of gonadotropins results in testes which are decreased in size, soft, and relatively nontender to pressure and in manifestations of decreased androgen production, consisting in diminished libido and potency, decreased rate of secondary sexual hair growth, and reduced muscular strength. Gonadotropin deficiency occurring prior to or during the period of sexual maturation results in total or partial impairment of secondary sexual development. In isolated gonadotropin deficiency or when GH secretion is unimpaired, the failure of sex steroid-induced epiphyseal closure in the long bones results in excessive growth of the limbs, leading to a eunuchoid appearance. Although both gonadotropins are usually deficient, an occasional patient has been reported to lack only FSH.[195]

Growth Hormone

Impaired secretion of GH in the adult does not result in significant clinical symptoms. Although the metabolic effects of GH deficiency can be readily demonstrated, other compensatory mechanisms presumably obscure clinical abnormalities. Impaired carbohydrate tolerance associated with hypoinsulinemia is present in GH-deficient subjects, but this disorder is distinguishable from diabetes mellitus, particularly by the absence of microangiopathy.[196] GH has been implicated in wound healing. It might be expected but has not been documented that repair of bone fractures would be delayed in GH deficiency. In children, GH deficiency is associated with growth retardation, as discussed in detail in Chap. 26. Fasting hypoglycemia occasionally occurs in GH-deficient children and is almost invariably present when there is associated ACTH deficiency.[197]

Prolactin

Prolactin deficiency is associated with only one clinical manifestation—the absence of lactation in the postpartum state.

Vasopressin

Decreased antidiuretic hormone secretion results in diabetes insipidus, described in detail in Chap. 9. The inability of the kidneys to reabsorb water leads to polyuria and polydipsia, and if fluid intake is not maintained, as frequently occurs in states of altered consciousness, severe dehydration can result. Patients exhibit extreme thirst, which is preferentially relieved by ice water. In the presence of ACTH deficiency, polyuria may not occur because of the requirement of glucocorticoids for the excretion of free water. The appearance of polyuria during the course of an ACTH test or following the institution of glucocorticoid therapy is highly suggestive of combined vasopressin and ACTH deficiency.

Oxytocin

The absence of oxytocin does not lead to any signs or symptoms in humans. Women with panhypopituitarism who become pregnant are able to initiate labor and to experience normal parturition despite the absence of this hormone.

General Features

In hypopituitary patients the skin frequently exhibits a loss of normal turgor and, in hypopituitarism of long duration, assumes a waxy character. Wrinkling, particularly around the mouth and eyes, leading to a prematurely aged appearance, is also common. Nutrition is in general well preserved; the cachexia which Simmonds originally attributed to this disease was probably due to anorexia nervosa. A moderate anemia is often present and is generally normocytic and normochromic but may also be hypochromic or macrocytic. Thyroid hormone deficiency is the most important contributory factor, though decreased testosterone secretion and impaired erythropoietin production also appear to be involved. Psychiatric disturbances are well recognized in hypopituitarism, with mental slowing or apathy being observed in nearly half the patients reported by Sheehan and Summers.[198] Other psychiatric symptoms include delusions and occasionally paranoid psychoses.

Carbohydrate metabolism is usually not markedly altered in nondiabetic hypopituitary patients. In contrast, hypopituitarism in insulin-requiring diabetic patients leads to a dramatic reduction in insulin dosage, frequently to 20 to 50 percent of the original level, and an increased tendency to hypoglycemic reactions. These changes persist even with full glucocorticoid replacement therapy, suggesting an important role of GH and also of epinephrine. The synthesis of epinephrine is decreased because of the absence of high levels of cortisol in the adrenal, required for normal levels of phenylethanolamine-N-methyl transferase, the enzyme that converts norepinephrine to epinephrine (see Chap. 13).

The relative frequency of the various features of hypopituitarism varies with the etiology of the disorder. Most recent series relate to patients with a pituitary tumor, which is today the most frequent cause of hypopituitarism. Although some disagreement exists among reports, loss of GH followed by loss of gonadotropins appears to be the earliest and thus the most frequent pattern encountered. ACTH and TSH deficiency occur less frequently and are also seen later in the natural history of the disease. The existence of single or selected hormonal deficiencies, however, precludes the evaluation of pituitary function on the basis of only one or two hormones.

Isolated Hormonal Deficiencies

Deficiencies of individual pituitary hormones frequently occur in the absence of detectable anatomic disease of the pituitary. The signs and symptoms associated with these disorders are described in the preceding section. TSH and gonadotropin deficiencies often cannot be distinguished clinically from decreased secretion of target organ hormones, whereas the absence of hyperpigmentation and salt craving serves to differentiate ACTH deficiency from primary adrenal insufficiency. The most common form of isolated pituitary hormone deficiency is GH deficiency, which is a disease of childhood and adolescence and is discussed in greater detail in Chap. 26. The site of the primary disorder in isolated pituitary hormone deficiencies, i.e., the CNS or the pituitary, can usually but not always be determined by detailed testing.

Differential Diagnosis

Hypopituitarism can be confused with two other disease categories. The first includes disorders of hormone hypofunction involving target glands or the region of the CNS (the hypothalamus) involved in neuroendocrine regulation. The second includes diseases that share some of the generalized signs and symptoms of hypopituitarism but are unassociated with endocrine hypofunction.

Target Organ and Hypothalamic Hypofunction

Primary failure of the thyroid, adrenals, or gonads must be differentiated from isolated pituitary hormone deficiencies. As indicated above, the signs and symptoms may be indistinguishable from those of hypopituitarism. In particular, the presence of multiple target gland (polyglandular) failure must be considered as a possibility. The diagnosis may be suggested by features of autoimmune disease, the presence of diabetes mellitus, moniliasis, or hypoparathyroidism, or a familial pattern, though none of these may be present. Although the severity of hormone deficiency in primary target organ disease is frequently greater than in hypopituitarism, this is not a distinguishing feature, since partial target organ failure can also occur.

Primary adrenal insufficiency is characteristically associated with hyperkalemia due to diminished aldosterone secretion. In hypopituitarism partial preservation of aldosterone secretion is sufficient to prevent elevations in serum potassium. The hyperpigmentation and salt craving of Addison's disease are also absent in hypopituitarism. In some patients with primary gonadal failure, there may be a discrepancy between the loss of gonadal steroid (androgen or estrogen) secretion and the loss of spermatogenesis or ovulation. In hypopituitarism, both aspects of gonadal function tend to be diminished to the same extent. The presence of hot flashes may be seen with primary ovarian failure, hypopituitarism, and GnRH deficiency.[199]

Hypopituitarism must also be distinguished from CNS disorders which affect releasing factor secretion. The presence of nonendocrine disturbances such as anosmia in Kallman's syndrome or progressive obesity may suggest the extrapituitary origin of these diseases. Laboratory studies are, however, crucial to distinguish this group of disorders, described in Chap. 7.

Nonendocrine Disorders

The possibility of hypopituitarism is frequently raised in patients with chronic malnutrition or liver disease who exhibit weakness, lethargy, cold intolerance, and decreased libido. As stressed above, cachexia is *not* a characteristic finding of hypopituitarism, and its presence should suggest another disease. Anorexia nervosa, a disorder primarily of young adult females, is often confused with hypopituitarism. The severe weight loss, characteristic psychiatric symptoms, and preservation of axillary and pubic hair are all useful in distinguishing anorexia nervosa from hypopituitarism. In chronic malnutrition and anorexia nervosa GH and ACTH secretion are intact and often increased. This disorder is discussed in Chap. 7.

Diagnostic Procedures

The diagnosis of hypopituitarism must be established by appropriate and carefully conducted studies of pituitary hormone secretion, since these provide the basis on which decisions are made concerning lifelong hormone replacement therapy. The studies must address two questions: (1) is pituitary hormone secretion diminished, and (2) is the disorder of pituitary or nonpituitary origin? In addition, nonendocrine (neuroanatomic) studies are required to determine the etiology of hypopituitarism. The latter procedures are discussed under Pituitary Tumors, below.

Diagnostic studies that evaluate the function of anterior pituitary hormones have undergone considerable change during recent years and are still being constantly revised, reflecting the change from indirect tests of pituitary function such as indexes of carbohydrate metabolism or assessment of target organ function by injection of pituitary hormones to direct measurement of circulating levels of pituitary hormones in response to releasing hormone stimulation. The availability of certain tests varies from one laboratory to the next, though most can be performed by regional reference laboratories if not in individual hospitals.

This section considers the evaluation of the six major anterior pituitary hormones and the differentiation of pituitary from extrapituitary sites of the primary disorder. The rationale for the various tests, their advantages, and their limitations are discussed here, while the specific details are provided at the end of the chapter under Details of Hypothalamic-Pituitary Testing.

ACTH

ACTH secretion is evaluated by measurement of both adrenocortical hormones and ACTH itself. The previously used urinary 17-OH corticoids have been replaced by cortisol, which is more specific. Although interpretation of cortisol levels requires knowledge of intrinsic adrenocortical function, cortisol measurement remains useful because it can be performed rapidly and is very reliable. Since the clinical significance of ACTH deficiency is adrenocortical insufficiency, measurement of plasma cortisol is a useful screening procedure. Morning values of < 10 μg/dl or values of < 20 μg/dl under conditions of stress are suggestive of hypopituitarism. In contrast to patients with primary adrenal insufficiency, patients with hypopituitarism may exhibit no appreciable clinical symptoms and yet have nearly undetectable circulating cortisol levels.

In order to attribute reduced cortisol levels to low (absolute deficiency) or normal (relative deficiency) ACTH secretion, it must be shown that the administration of ACTH (250 μg synthetic $ACTH_{1-24}$) is capable of eliciting a plasma cortisol response (measured at 30 min) while stimuli requiring the participation of the entire hypothalamic-pituitary-adrenal axis or of the pituitary-adrenal component are ineffective. Patients with prolonged ACTH deficiency usually develop adrenal atrophy and may not respond to an acute ACTH challenge. This lack of response has been used by some for an indirect assessment of ACTH secretion and has been reported to correlate with the response to insulin hypoglycemia (see below).[200] However, a response does not necessarily indicate an axis that will respond normally to surgical stress.[201] Treatment with long-acting corticotropin or continuous intravenous infusion of ACTH for 3 days almost always restores the response to an acute injection of ACTH to normal but does not correct the hypothalamic-pituitary suppression.

If cortisol levels are normal and an intact response to ACTH is present, the hypothalamic-pituitary axis can be evaluated by (1) stimulation with corticotropin releasing factor (CRF), (2) an insulin tolerance test, which measures the response to hypoglycemic stress, (3) metyrapone (Metopirone) administration, which measures the response to interruption of the negative feedback effects of cortisol, or (4) vasopressin, which exerts both hypothalamic and pituitary effects.

The most specific stimulus is CRF, which causes a rapid release of ACTH from the pituitary, followed by cortisol secretion by the adrenal. The plasma cortisol response to CRF is more reproducible than is the response of ACTH,[202,203] in part because of the short half-life of ACTH. The response to an intravenous injection of 100 μg CRF in normal subjects is a plasma cortisol increase of at least 10 μg/dl which peaks at 30 to 60 min. Side effects of CRF are minimal, consisting of facial flushing that may last for up to an hour. At the time of writing, CRF is still an investigational drug in the United States.

The stimulus of insulin hypoglycemia is based on the normal activation of the hypothalamic-pituitary-adrenal axis in response to central glucopenia (Fig. 8-9). An adequate stimulus requires that the blood glucose be reduced by 50 percent (or to 40 mg/dl). Normal subjects will experience adrenergic symptoms of hypoglycemia (diaphoresis, tachycardia, mild anxiety, headache), indicating that a sufficient decrease in blood glucose has occurred. The standard dose of 0.1 U/kg IV may need to be increased (to 0.15 or 0.2 U/kg) in patients with obesity, maturity-onset diabetes, acromegaly, or other states of insulin resistance, while in patients strongly suspected of hypopituitarism, a reduction of the dose to 0.05 U/kg is

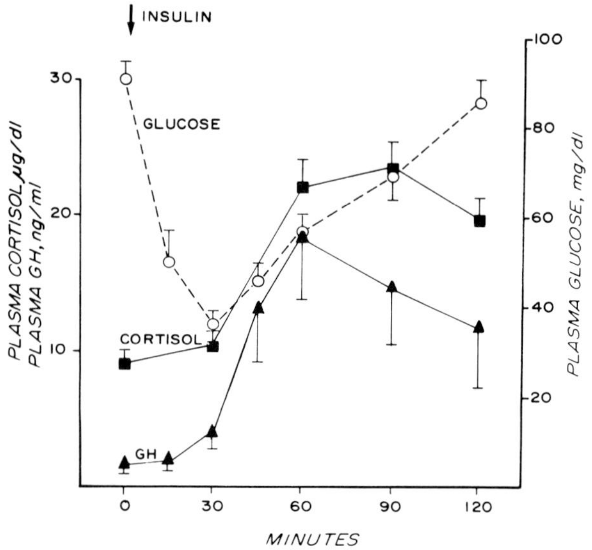

FIGURE 8-9 Plasma GH and cortisol responses to hypoglycemia produced by insulin 0.1 U/kg IV in normal subjects. Blood glucose should decrease by 50 percent or to 40 mg/dl to ensure an adequate stimulus.

recommended. The test should *not* be performed in patients with suspected Addison's disease, in those manifesting obvious clinical signs and symptoms of adrenal insufficiency, or in those with coronary artery or cerebrovascular disease.

Metyrapone impairs cortisol biosynthesis in the adrenal cortex by blocking the hydroxylation of 11-deoxycortisol and interrupts the negative feedback effect of cortisol on the CNS and pituitary. Administration of metyrapone therefore leads to an activation of the hypothalamic-pituitary axis and an accumulation of 11-deoxycortisol in the blood and tetrahydro-11-deoxycortisol in the urine. The latter is a 17-OH corticoid. Metyrapone (2.0 g for patients weighing < 70 kg, 2.5 g for patients 70 to 90 kg, 3.0 g for patients > 90 kg) is given orally at midnight, and plasma cortisol and 11-deoxycortisol are measured at 8 A.M.[204] In persons with a normal pituitary-adrenal axis, plasma 11-deoxycortisol should be < 7 μg/dl, whereas in patients with hypothalamic or pituitary disease, varying degrees of impairment are present. Variations in gastrointestinal absorption of the drug and increased degradation in patients on diphenylhydantoin (Dilantin) may interfere with the inhibition of 11-β-hydroxylase, and a plasma cortisol of < 10 μg/dl is required to confirm adequate enzyme inhibition. As with insulin hypoglycemia, the test is contraindicated in patients suspected of having primary adrenal insufficiency until this diagnosis has been excluded. It is important to emphasize that the patient must not be receiving any glucocorticoid therapy, since the basis of the test is the production of short-term adrenocortical insufficiency.

Vasopressin stimulates the release of ACTH by a direct action on the pituitary and probably also by enhancing hypothalamic CRF release. In some patients with CNS disease, an intact response to vasopressin can be seen in association with impaired responses to metyrapone or insulin. Side effects of vasopressin administration (primarily hypertension) make this procedure potentially hazardous to patients with coronary artery disease.

In determining which test(s) to use, it is important to consider the practical implications. The test is performed to identify patients with suspected relative adrenal insufficiency, i.e., those in whom a possible inadequate response to stress may occur. If the suspected disease is in the pituitary, then CRF or, as a second choice, insulin hypoglycemia should be used. The cortisol response to insulin hypoglycemia correlates well with the response to surgical stress. It also allows simultaneous evaluation of a second pituitary hormone,[205] as described below. The metyrapone response has a fairly high degree of concordance with that of insulin hypoglycemia, and therefore, until CRF is widely available, it remains a suitable alternative in patients in whom the risk of inducing hypoglycemia is not justified. Positive vasopressin responses have been reported in patients in whom no response to surgical stress was seen, and this procedure is consequently best used for characterizing the nature of ACTH deficiency due to disorders in the CNS.

The diagnosis of primary adrenal insufficiency is relatively easy to establish whether or not the patient is receiving replacement therapy when first seen, but prior glucocorticoid therapy, with its suppressive effects on the hypothalamus and pituitary, can complicate the workup of a patient with suspected hypopituitarism. The suppressive effects are most pronounced on metyrapone stimulation but can occur with other stimuli as well. A subnormal or absent response to any stimulus in a patient with a history of prolonged glucocorticoid therapy must therefore be interpreted with reservation. Glucocorticoids should be discontinued for at least 1 month, if possible, prior to definitive testing.

TSH

Basal plasma TSH levels in normal subjects are frequently at or near the lower limit of sensitivity of most assays and thus are not useful in distinguishing between normal and decreased TSH secretion. Consequently, plasma T_4 levels are used as an indirect measure of TSH function. If normal, they exclude a total though not necessarily a partial defect in TSH secretion. If T_4 and T_3 levels are decreased, an elevated TSH level is indicative of intact TSH function (primary hypothyroidism). Pituitary disease can sometimes be differentiated from hypothalamic disease by determining the TSH response to a maximal stimulatory dose of TRH (500 μg) (Fig. 8-10). In normal subjects peak TSH values occur at 15 to 30 min after TRH and generally reach a level of at least twice the upper limit of normal basal values. An impaired or absent response is indicative of decreased pituitary reserve. In patients in whom a hypothalamic disorder is responsible for the decreased TSH secretion, the response to TRH is often enhanced and the peak may be delayed, occurring at 60 to 120 min.[206] However, normal or impaired responses may also be seen, limiting the discriminating ability of this test. It is important that patients undergoing TRH testing be withdrawn from thyroid hormone therapy for at least 1 month prior to study to eliminate any suppressive effects of thyroid hormones on the TSH response to TRH.

LH and FSH

Basal levels of plasma LH and FSH in hypopituitary patients are often indistinguishable from those in the

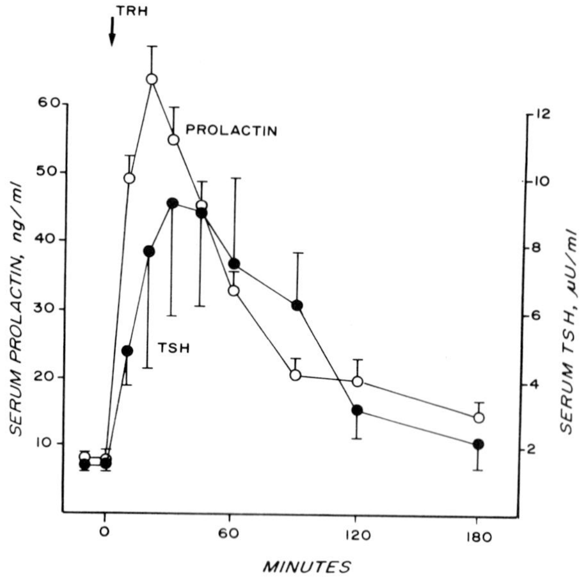

FIGURE 8-10 Plasma TSH and prolactin responses to TRH 500 μg IV in normal men and women. The dose used produces a maximal response. Delayed TSH responses are occasionally observed in patients with hypothalamic disease. (*Modified from Hershman JM, Pittman JA Jr: J Clin Endocrinol Metab 31:457, 1970; and from Jacobs L et al: J Clin Endocrinol Metab 36:1069, 1973.*)

lower part of the normal range for men and for women in the follicular phase. In a clinically hypogonadal female with low (< 30 pg/ml) or undetectable estradiol values or in a hypogonadal male with low plasma testosterone levels (< 3 ng/ml) associated with primary gonadal disease, plasma LH and FSH levels are elevated. The diagnosis of hypopituitarism can therefore be suspected in hypogonadal patients with levels of LH and FSH in the normal range. The differentiation between pituitary and suprapituitary (hypothalamic) causes of diminished gonadotropin secretion, however, is more difficult and cannot always be made with certainty. Three types of studies may be used: (1) direct stimulation of the pituitary with GnRH; (2) interference with the negative feedback of estrogen, using clomiphene; and (3) stimulation, in women, of the positive feedback effects of estrogen on GnRH secretion, using exogenous hormone.

Injection of GnRH at the most commonly used dose (100 μg IV) results in a rise of plasma LH to at least 3 times and often to 10 times basal levels, with peak values occurring within 15 to 30 min (Fig. 8-11). The FSH response, which is of lesser magnitude, exhibits a similar temporal pattern, though it is occasionally delayed.[207] In patients with hypopituitarism, a full range of gonadotropin responses may be seen despite clinical hypogonadism; i.e., there may be normal, diminished, or absent responses, depending on the extent of gonadotroph destruction. In contrast, patients with primary hypogonadism exhibit an enhanced LH and FSH response to GnRH as well as elevated basal gonadotropin levels. The loss of the LH response tends to occur more frequently than loss of the FSH response in patients with nonfunctioning pituitary tumors.[208] Repeated administration of GnRH to such patients does not enhance the LH or FSH response, indicating impaired functional residual capacity of the gonadotrophs. With isolated FSH deficiency, the LH response to GnRH is normal while the FSH response is impaired or absent.

In patients with gonadotropin deficiency of hypothalamic origin, the LH and FSH responses to GnRH may also be normal, diminished, absent, or even exaggerated. LH responses are usually absent in patients with congenital or prepubertal GnRH deficiency, whereas in those with adult-onset disorders, the response is intact. The LH response pattern in particular appears to be in part a reflection of endogenous GnRH secretion, and repeated injections of GnRH frequently restore a previously diminished or absent response to normal. Thus, while an impaired or absent LH and FSH response to GnRH cannot be used to distinguish hypothalamic from pituitary disease, the appearance of a response after repeated injections of GnRH indicates an intact pituitary functional reserve and points to the hypothalamus as the cause of the disorder.[209]

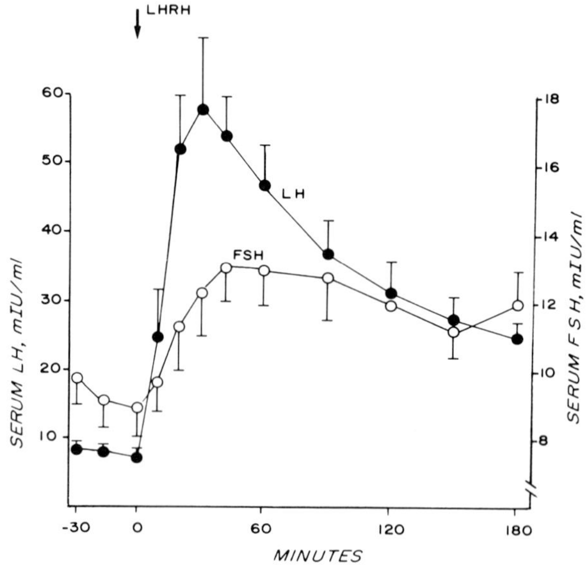

FIGURE 8-11 Plasma LH and FSH responses to GnRH 250 μg IV in normal men. The peak response of LH is greater and occurs earlier than that of FSH. LH (but not FSH) responses in normal women are affected by the stage of the menstrual cycle, with the greatest responses occurring at time of ovulation. (*Modified from Snyder P et al: J Clin Endocrinol Metab 41:938, 1975.*)

Evaluation of the hypothalamic component of the neuroendocrine regulation of gonadotropin secretion involves assessment of the negative and positive feedback effects of estrogen in women and the negative feedback effects of estrogen and testosterone in men. Clomiphene citrate, a weak estrogen, is capable of competing with estradiol for binding to receptors in the uterus, pituitary, and hypothalamus. When administered to adult women with near-normal estrogen levels, clomiphene acts as an estrogen antagonist and stimulates the release of endogenous GnRH, resulting in gonadotropin secretion. If gonadotropin secretion has been shown to be intact (by a normal response to GnRH) the absence of a gonadotropin response to clomiphene (100 mg per day for 5 days) indicates an impaired hypothalamic response to interruption of the negative feedback effect of estrogen.

The positive feedback effects of estrogen, demonstrated by elevating estradiol levels for at least 24 h (by injection of a long-acting estrogen preparation such as estradiol benzoate or estradiol valerate or by the continuous infusion of estradiol), are followed by a rise in LH but generally not in FSH, presumably mediated by a release of GnRH, which is maximal at 4 to 5 days. The inability of an anovulatory patient with intact gonadotropins to respond normally to exogenous estradiol administration indicates a hypothalamic defect related to the positive feedback effect of estrogen. This defect is characteristically seen in patients with hyperprolactinemia.

In men, estrogens have only inhibitory effects on LH secretion and are of no value as diagnostic agents. Clomiphene, however, is useful as a probe of the negative feedback effect of testosterone. After a dose of 100 or 200 mg per day for 6 to 7 days, LH increases to at least twice basal levels in normal men. Clomiphene is thus useful as a test of the hypothalamic-pituitary axis, provided that endogenous testosterone levels are at least 1 ng/ml.

Growth Hormone

Documentation of GH deficiency is important in children with short stature in whom therapy with exogenous hormone is under consideration. In adults, its importance relates to providing evidence for acquired hypopituitarism, such as that typically occurring with pituitary tumors. Nonresting levels of GH, particularly levels obtained 60 to 90 min after the onset of sleep in children, are often capable of distinguishing GH-deficient from normal subjects because of the frequent stimulatory bursts of the hormone. A plasma level of 6 ng/ml or more is evidence of normal GH secretion. In adults, in whom basal levels are lower and secretory bursts fewer, normal and GH-deficient subjects can generally not be distinguished without the aid of stimulation tests.

There are two types of stimuli for evaluating GH secretion: GH releasing hormone (GRH), which acts directly on the somatotroph, and a number of agents (insulin, arginine, L-Dopa, clonidine, ACTH, and propranolol plus glucagon) which evaluate the hypothalamic-pituitary axis and probably require the participation of endogenous GRH. The choice of the stimulus is determined by whether the physician wishes to assess pituitary GH reserves or the etiology of unexplained GH deficiency.

GRH is the most reliable stimulus for evaluating pituitary GH secretory capacity. The two forms of this hormone, GRH_{1-44}-NH_2 and GRH_{1-40}-OH, and also a GH fragment, GRH_{1-29}-NH_2, are equipotent in humans, and comparable response curves have been observed.[210,211] The intravenous injection of GRH produces a rapid increase in plasma GH level (Fig. 8-11), which peaks at 15 to 30 min and is dose-dependent. The most commonly employed dose is 1 μg/kg, which is a maximal stimulus and unaccompanied by any significant side effects. The response is variable, and peak GH values in normal subjects range from 10 to 100 ng/ml. In patients with hypopituitarism, the response is impaired or absent. In patients with hypothalamic disease, i.e., deficiency of endogenous GRH, GH responses to GRH appear to be intact, though reduced responses are seen in some patients with GH deficiency of unknown cause or long duration.[212] In general, about 30 to 50 percent of patients with idiopathic GH deficiency exhibit a normal GH response to GRH.[188,212] At the time of writing, GRH is still an investigational agent in the United States.

The most effective of the indirect stimuli for GH secretion is insulin hypoglycemia, described under ACTH, above (Fig. 8-9). GH levels peak at 60 to 90 min and should equal or exceed 10 ng/ml. Approximately 20 percent of normal subjects exhibit a subnormal response and a second stimulus must be used. Infusion of arginine (0.5 g/kg to a maximum of 30 g) is effective in raising GH to similar levels in 70 percent of normal persons, with a majority of the nonresponders usually being male. Although estrogen pretreatment will enhance the response, it is seldom used for practical reasons. L-Dopa (0.5 g PO) stimulates GH secretion in 60 to 70 percent of normal subjects to a level of at least 6 ng/ml, peaking at 60 to 150 min. Mild to moderate symptoms of nausea and vomiting occur in 15 to 20 percent of subjects because of concomitant stimulation of the emesis center. Clonidine (0.15 mg/m^2 or 25 μg PO), a centrally active α_2-adrenergic agonist, has been reported to stimulate GH secretion.[213,214] The mechanism of clonidine action is by stimulation of endogenous GRH release. Other stimuli, including propranolol plus glucagon and synthetic $ACTH_{1-24}$, do not offer any advantage over the previously described tests. Either L-dopa or arginine therefore serves as the most useful second choice stimulus if no response occurs with insulin. It should be noted that responses are generally absent in obesity, irrespective of whether the stimulus is direct (GRH)[215] or indirect[216] and even in obese children with normal linear growth. They are also impaired in hypothyroidism[217,218] and often restored to normal by thyroxine treatment.

Prolactin

The lower limit of plasma prolactin values in normal subjects extends to the lowest levels of detectability in many assays. Demonstration of prolactin responsiveness to TRH stimulation is the simplest and most useful method of documenting intact lactotroph function. Prolactin levels increase by at least twofold after TRH and peak at the same time as TSH levels (15 to 30 min), thus permitting both hormones to be assessed by use of the same stimulus. An alternative method of testing prolactin reserves is by injection of metoclopramide (10 mg IV), a D_2-dopaminergic receptor antagonist which is almost completely excluded from the CNS by the blood-brain barrier. Metoclopramide (and other dopaminergic blockers) bind to the lactotroph and stimulate prolactin release. Peak levels of 100 ng/ml or more are seen at 30 to 60 min in normal subjects. An impaired response is seen in pituitary disease with diminished lactotrophs, pituitary tumors, and disorders of neuroendocrine regulation (see Chap. 7), thus the test is not particularly helpful in the differential diagnosis. The prolactin response to insulin hypoglycemia also provides an index of the hypothalamic-pituitary axis.[219] The interpretation of an abnormal response (less than twofold rise) similarly requires information concerning the prolactin response to TRH.

Combined Pituitary Hormone Testing

Two protocols are available for testing pituitary hormone secretion on a combined basis. All four of the hypothalamic releasing hormones (TRH, GnRH, CRF, and GRH) can be injected simultaneously without altering the individual pituitary hormone responses.[220] This reduces substantially the time and effort required to assess pituitary function. Alternatively, insulin hypoglycemia may be combined with TRH and GnRH in a single injection to provide slightly different information, as indicated above.

Treatment

Replacement therapy in hypopituitarism must be considered for each individual hormone and the treatment goals specifically defined. The therapeutic use of anterior pituitary hormones is limited to GH for correcting problems of growth retardation and to gonadotropins for inducing ovulation or spermatogenesis, as described below. The use of hypothalamic releasing hormones and/or their synthetic analogues is currently restricted to GnRH for hypothalamic hypogonadism, though GnRH agonists have recently become available for precocious puberty and for non-pituitary-related use (prostatic carcinoma and endometriosis) and to the investigational use of GRH as therapy for certain types of GH deficiency. For the most part, however, therapy consists of replacing the target organ secretions by the use of natural hormones or synthetic analogues.

ACTH

ACTH deficiency is treated with adrenal glucocorticoids. Either cortisone (25 mg per day) or hydrocortisone (20 mg per day) given as a divided dose will provide adequate therapy for most patients under normal conditions. Because of the partial independence of aldosterone secretion from the pituitary, supplemental mineralocorticoid therapy is unnecessary. As a result, the physician can nearly always use prednisone (5 mg per day), which is considerably less expensive, in place of the natural glucocorticoids. Occasionally patients require full glucocorticoid replacement therapy (37.5 mg cortisone or 7.5 mg prednisone), though many will develop signs of steroid overdose (Cushing's syndrome) at these doses. Under conditions of stress (acute febrile illness, moderate to severe trauma, etc.) the dose should be increased two- to threefold and then gradually tapered as the stress subsides. If the patient is unable to retain oral medication, injectable hydrocortisone must be used (50 mg IM or IV q 6 h). The acute treatment of all severely ill hypopituitary patients requires the same dose of hydrocortisone (100 to 300 mg per day) as is used for primary adrenal insufficiency. Since some patients with hypopituitarism of long duration exhibit euphoric or even psychotic behavior with full replacement or larger doses of glucocorticoids, the minimal dose necessary should be used. Patients should take with them a supply of injectable steroids for emergency treatment if they plan to travel in areas where good medical care may not be immediately available. Preoperatively, patients should be treated as though primary adrenal insufficiency were present: hydrocortisone hemisuccinate 50 mg IM q 6 h prior to surgery and continuing through the immediate postoperative period, followed by a gradual tapering to maintenance by the second or third day.

The decision to treat a patient with glucocorticoids should be based on a low basal cortisol level or on signs or symptoms of adrenal insufficiency associated with normal cortisol levels but absent or impaired response to stimulation. A more difficult decision relates to the patient with partial ACTH deficiency without signs or symptoms in the nonstressed state. With adequate education, many patients in this category do not need maintenance glucocorticoid replacement and require therapy only in times of stress. Good medical practice dictates that these patients in particular, as well as all patients on maintenance glucocorticoid therapy, wear an appropriate medical identification tag.

The response to therapy is quite rapid and often dramatic, and many patients will recognize only in retrospect their malaise and weakness prior to therapy. The initiation of glucocorticoid therapy may also permit the clinical appearance of diabetes insipidus, manifested by polyuria and polydipsia. Treatment of diabetes insipidus is discussed in Chap. 9.

TSH

Treatment of patients with TSH deficiency is similar to that of patients with primary hypothyroidism. The indications for treatment are not based primarily on the TSH reserve, since patients with absent or impaired TSH responses to TRH may have normal serum thyroxine levels. Rather, they relate to the presence of a decreased serum thyroxine. The preferred treatment is with L-thyroxine, 0.15 to 0.2 mg per day, though in occasional patients an even lower dose may suffice. The clinical assessment of the patient, supplemented at appropriate intervals by measurement of serum thyroxine levels, is used to establish the appropriate dose. In this condition, unlike primary hypothyroidism, the measurement of plasma TSH is of no value.

It is most important to correct overt adrenal insufficiency prior to institution of thyroid hormone therapy, and patients with partial adrenal insufficiency may require glucocorticoid replacement therapy after thyroid hormone replacement is started. In severe or long-standing hypothyroidism, therapy should be initiated with a small dose of thyroxine (0.05 mg per day) and increased slowly until a maintenance dose is achieved. Long-term maintenance with triiodothyronine is not recommended, because its shorter biologic half-life results in the earlier appearance of symptoms of thyroid deficiency in the event therapy is omitted.

LH and FSH

Restoration of gonadal function requires consideration of two components: gonadal steroid replacement and treatment of infertility. These subjects are considered briefly here and discussed in greater detail in Chaps. 16 and 17.

WOMEN In premenopausal women, estrogen replacement therapy is indicated for many reasons, including the maintenance of secondary sex characteristics, i.e., breast size and vaginal and vulvar turgor and lubrication; prevention of osteoporosis and possibly of coronary artery disease; and preservation of a sense of well-being. A variety of estrogenic preparations can be used, including ethinyl estradiol 5 to 20 μg per day and conjugated estrogens (Premarin) 0.625 to 1.25 mg per day. The lowest possible dose which produces the desired clinical effects should be used. Because of the occasional development of cystic breast changes and, more importantly, the frequent breakthrough bleeding that occurs with continuous estrogen therapy, the hormone should be given for only 20 to 25 days each month and accompanied on the last 5 to 10 days by a progestational agent such as medroxyprogesterone acetate 5 to 10 mg per day, which will induce menstrual bleeding and prevent endometrial hyperplasia. Alternatively, one of the oral contraceptive preparations containing no more than the equivalent of 25 μg estradiol per day may be used. It is not known whether the increased risks of thromboembolism, hyperlipidemia, and carbohydrate intolerance associated with the use of oral contraceptives by normal women also occur in the hypopituitary patient. However, the benefits of restoring normal physiologic function in these women warrant the use of replacement estrogen therapy. It is still controversial whether the advantages of replacement therapy persist after the time of the expected menopause, i.e., mid- to late forties. The potential risks (endometrial carcinoma) and benefits (diminished rate of bone loss and clinically significant osteoporosis) should be frankly discussed with the patient in order to make an appropriate decision (see also Chap. 25).

Although dyspareunia and diminished satisfaction from sexual activity in hypopituitary women, attributable to local tissue changes, are usually corrected by estrogen therapy, the decreased libido due to the absence of adrenal androgens is often not. Libido can be restored by injection of a small dose of long-acting androgen such as testosterone enanthate, 50 mg every 1 to 2 months, or by orally active fluoxymesterone, 5 to 10 mg once or twice weekly. The lowest effective dose should be used to avoid the development of hirsutism. Inquiry regarding the patient's libido is important, since this information may not be volunteered and the patient may believe that no treatment is available.

Restoration of fertility is possible in a high percentage of gonadotropin-deficient women. In many patients with gonadotropin deficiency of hypothalamic etiology, clomiphene citrate therapy results in ovulation. If this is unsuccessful, GnRH administered every 3 h by an intermittent infusion pump will frequently be effective.[221] In the presence of primary pituitary disease, combined therapy with FSH-LH preparations is successful in up to 75 percent of patients. Treatment is initiated with daily injections of menotropins (Pergonal), an FSH-rich preparation of urine from postmenopausal women, to initiate follicular growth and maturation, which is monitored by measurement of plasma estradiol levels. When the estradiol value exceeds 1200 ng/ml (usually after 2 weeks), human chorionic gonadotropin is injected to induce ovulation. This form of therapy is expensive and in hyperstimulated ovaries (with multiple mature follicles) may result in superovulation leading to multiple births. It should be performed only under the direction of a physician with experience in this technique.

MEN Testosterone replacement therapy in adult males consists of either intramuscular injection of a long-acting testosterone preparation such as testosterone enanthate or cypionate, 200 mg every 3 weeks, or oral administration of fluoxymesterone, the only available oral preparation that is readily absorbable. The latter, however, is often less effective than injected testosterone because of variation in absorption. All oral preparations have been associated with the development of cholangiolitic hepatitis in a small percentage of patients, whereas the injectable forms of testosterone have not. These factors have made the parenteral preparations, which are also less expensive, the preferred agents. The end points of testosterone therapy are the restoration of full androgenization, which includes beard growth, generalized improvement in muscular strength, libido, and potency. Overdosage is associated with salt and fluid retention leading to edema, excessive sexual stimulation, priapism, nightmares, and occasionally gynecomastia, acne, and overaggressive behavior. The presence of testosterone is required for the development of baldness in a genetically predisposed person and this may occur in hypopituitary males as a result of therapy. Androgen therapy should be withheld as long as possible in the adolescent with growth retardation to avoid premature epiphyseal closure and limitation of potential for further linear growth (see Chap. 26).

Testosterone therapy may need to be given for many months before libido and performance are fully restored, depending on the duration of hypogonadism. In some patients in whom gonadotropin deficiency has developed before puberty, full androgenization may never occur. In other patients, the reverse problem may be seen. With long-standing hypogonadism, psychosocial behavioral changes develop which may pattern a patient's entire lifestyle including occupation and choice of a marital partner. The changes in libido and generalized behavior patterns which occur in response to replacement therapy can lead to major adjustment problems in both sexual and nonsexual relationships. This possibility must be carefully considered prior to initiation of replacement therapy.

The treatment of infertility follows the same principles in men as in women. If the disease is of hypothalamic origin, intermittent therapy with GnRH (2 μg q 2 h) using an infusion pump will frequently result in full androgenic stimulation and spermatogenesis.[222,223] Alternatively, or in patients with gonadotropin insufficiency of pituitary origin, human chorionic gonadotropin (hCG), alone or in combination with menotropins, will produce similar results. In patients with postpubertal onset of hypogonadism, an increase in sperm count occurs with hCG alone, while in those with prepubertal hypogonadism, menotropins must also be used.[224] The presence of prior cryptorchism, however, precludes normalization of the sperm count. Each form of therapy may be required for up to 3 months and possibly longer, and overall success (i.e., induction of fertility) occurs in only about 60 percent of patients in whom sperm counts become normal. It has also been suggested that fertile men about to undergo potentially destructive surgery to the hypothalamic-pituitary region consider the advisability of placing sperm in a sperm bank. Stored under the appropriate conditions, sperm can be kept viable for several years.

Growth Hormone

Treatment of GH deficiency is at present limited to children with significant growth retardation prior to the age of long-bone epiphyseal closure, which occurs at puberty. Two forms of therapy of GH deficiency are currently available: GH and GRH. Until mid-1985, the only GH preparation that could be used was derived from human pituitaries at autopsy, provided by the National Hormone and Pituitary Program and available commercially. The distribution of this preparation was stopped in the United States and throughout much of the world because of the discovery of several cases of Creutzfeldt-Jakob disease, a degenerative and invariably fatal CNS disease related to kuru and believed due to a slow virus, in patients who received human GH during the 1970s.[225] Although current purification methods are believed adequate to exclude the infectious agent, tests to validate this fact could require up to 3 to 5 years, are extremely costly, and have not yet been completed. GH of recombinant DNA origin has been extensively evaluated and is as effective as natural GH in promoting growth. It became available for clinical use in late 1985. The first preparation being distributed is methionyl-hGH, a single-amino-acid carboxy-terminal extension—the form that is synthesized by the bacteria containing the GH gene. Techniques for removal of the methionyl residue have been perfected, and GH structurally identical to the native hormone should be available shortly. The relatively unlimited supplies of GH will permit the efficacy of larger doses to be evaluated, and the currently recommended dose of approximately 2 units/kg three times a week may be modified.[226] It is thus unlikely that GH (or any other hormones) derived from human pituitaries will be used clinically in the future.

Since many children with GH deficiency are believed to have adequate stores of GH but lack an appropriate releasing mechanism, it is anticipated that as many as half may be responsive to therapy with GRH.[227,228] The route of administration (subcutaneous or intranasal), the dose required, and the possible use of GRH analogues are currently under active investigation.

Information is lacking concerning the potential value of GH therapy in the adult hypopituitary patient receiving thyroid, adrenal, and gonadal replacement therapy. With the forthcoming availability of biosynthetic GH, possible therapeutic benefits in this type of patient can be addressed. At the present time there are no indications for GH therapy in the adult. The use of GH as an anabolic agent in muscle-building programs has not been shown to be effective and, because of the potential side effects, represents a clear misuse of the hormone.

Prolactin

The extremely limited supply of human prolactin currently available has until recently precluded the use of this hormone in humans even for investigational purposes. Furthermore, concerns over the use of hormones extracted from human pituitaries (see above) has placed a moratorium on such studies until hormone of recombinant DNA origin is available. With the exception of an absence of postpartum lactation, disorders of prolactin deficiency, if they exist, are currently unrecognized. In women with impaired postpartum lactation, repeated administration of TRH has been reported to enhance milk production.[229]

PITUITARY TUMORS

Classification

Tumors of the pituitary gland can be classified by histologic characteristics and by functional activity. Both are important and reflect the spectrum of problems to be considered when evaluating a patient with a suspected pituitary tumor. There are two major histologic types of pituitary tumor: adenomas and craniopharyngiomas. In addition, tumors originating in the parasellar region, such as meningiomas, optic nerve gliomas, and sphenoid wing sarcomas, as well as metastatic tumors can be found within the sella turcica and must be differentiated from primary pituitary tumors. Although tumors originating within the pituitary can be locally invasive, truly malignant tumors are extremely rare, and concern over a possible malignant tumor need not influence decisions concerning diagnosis and treatment. Pituitary tumors can also be divided into those associated with hormone hypersecretion (*functioning*) and those without (*nonfunctioning*). The relative frequency of each type has changed considerably in the past decade as more functioning tumors have been recognized by measurement of circulating hormone levels rather than by clinical manifestations. Some tumors may synthesize hormones but, because of alterations in intracellular secretory mechanisms or degradative processes, may not release the hormones into the circulation.[230] Others may synthesize only portions of a hormone (e.g., the α subunit) which are biologically inactive.[231]

Pituitary Adenomas

Pituitary adenomas originate from one of the adenohypophyseal cell types and make up more than 90 percent of all pituitary neoplasms. They were for many years subdivided into chromophobic (originally synonymous with nonfunctioning) and chromophilic types, the latter being either eosinophilic (associated with acromegaly) or basophilic (associated with Cushing's syndrome). With the recognition that tumor histology frequently varied in different sections of individual tumors, that tumors from patients with acromegaly and Cushing's syndrome were frequently chromophobic, and that prolactin hypersecretion was often present in patients with chromophobic tumors, this cytochemical differentiation has ceased to be useful. At present the significance of a chromophobic appearance in an adenoma is merely that the tumor does not contain recognizable secretion (stored hormone) granules. Thus, the adenoma is either not producing a hormone, is storing a hormone in an altered chemical form which does not stain with the techniques used, or, most likely, is secreting the hormone immediately following synthesis without storage. Newer techniques involving electron microscopy and immunohistochemical stains have provided evidence to support the latter possibility.

In several large neurosurgical series, pituitary tumors accounted for 6 to 18 percent of all brain tumors,[232,233] and in an unselected autopsy series, microadenomas were found in one-third of patients, with 41 percent revealing immunohistochemical evidence of functional (prolactin) activity.[234]

There is no evidence to suggest that the growth pattern or biologic behavior of functioning tumors is any different from that of nonfunctioning tumors. Both may grow extremely slowly or may exhibit rapid growth. The slow-growing tumors which are nonfunctioning may never produce clinical manifestations and may be detected coincidentally at autopsy. In a series of 941 pituitary adenomas, over 50 percent were first discovered at autopsy.[235] Rapidly enlarging pituitary tumors are usually recognized because of the consequence of an enlarging intrasellar mass lesion, and the hormone hypersecretion is either incidental or else contributes in a minor way to the overall clinical problem. In contrast, the slow-growing functioning pituitary tumor allows for full development of the hormone hypersecretory disease. On the basis of the currently available radioimmunoassays for the anterior pituitary hormones, 70 to 80 percent of pituitary adenomas are believed to be functioning tumors, with the majority secreting prolactin.[236] The peak incidence of tumors in most series has been reported to be between 40 and 50 years,[235,237] though with earlier recognition now possible, the age at peak incidence will undoubtedly decrease. Most series report a similar incidence in males and females, though this also is changing with the increased awareness of prolactin-secreting tumors in women with amenorrhea.

Pituitary adenomas are generally solid tumors. They may, on occasion, be cystic, with evidence of hemorrhage within the tumor. At times the center of the cyst may communicate with the subarachnoid space and contain cerebrospinal fluid, giving rise to an empty sella. Calcification, if present, represents the end stage of organization of a previous hemorrhage.

Craniopharyngiomas

Craniopharyngiomas are benign tumors of congenital origin which may be partly or entirely cystic. Histologically they consist of bands of interwoven epithelium, often similar to tumors of the enamel organ of the teeth. The most superficial cells of the tumor often give rise to micro- or macrocysts, which frequently contain a brown fluid with a high cholesterol content and which develop calcifications in 50 percent of patients. The appearance of the tumor may vary, and it is often difficult to distinguish it from an ependymoma or epidermoid cyst. The tumor grows at a variable rate and may cease to grow entirely. Half the patients develop symptoms during childhood, one-fourth between ages 20 and 40, and the rest later in life.[238] The site of origin for most tumors appears to be in the midline at the upper end of the pituitary stalk, though some originate lower in the stalk and about 15 percent involve the upper part of the anterior lobe and are thus intrasellar. Large tumors push the chiasm upward and displace the hypothalamus and third ventricle. Downward pressure tends to compress the anterior lobe but more frequently results in atrophy of the posterior lobe because of damage to the stalk. Though it was previously believed that the tumor originated from remnants of Rathke's pouch, this has now been questioned because of the infrequency of a primary intrasellar site and the rarity of the tumor along the embryologic migration tract through bone.

Signs and Symptoms

The initial manifestations of pituitary tumors as well as their subsequent clinical features can be divided into three general categories: neuroanatomic, radiologic, and endocrinologic. The following sections are concerned primarily with those manifestations which relate to all pituitary tumors; the individual features of hormone-secreting tumors are considered separately.

The presenting symptoms of pituitary tumors have undergone a marked change in distribution frequency during the past two decades as refinements in neuroradiologic procedures and in pituitary hormone function testing have permitted their progressively earlier diagnosis and treatment. For example, whereas nearly 90 percent of patients in a large series of pituitary tumors diagnosed in the 1940s and 1950s exhibited visual disturbances,[237] more recent series indicate visual abnormalities to be present in only about 25 percent.[239,240] This percentage can be expected to decrease further. Visual field defects are particularly common in craniopharyngiomas and other tumors with suprasellar extension.[241] In contrast, abnormalities in endocrine function, most frequently amenorrhea, decreased libido, or infertility associated with prolactin-secreting pituitary tumors, now represent the most common presenting symptoms, whereas in earlier series only 25 to 35 percent of patients presented in this manner. The accidental discovery of a pituitary tumor in skull x-rays or CT scans continues to account for a small percentage of each reported series.

Endocrinologic Manifestations

Two types of endocrine symptoms are observed in patients with pituitary tumors: (1) hypofunction due to destruction of normal adenohypophyseal tissue by tumor compression or to interference with the delivery of portal blood, and (2) hyperfunction due to tumor and/or hyperplasia. The tumors involved in such hyperfunction, primarily growth hormone-, prolactin-, and ACTH-secreting tumors but also TSH- and FSH-secreting tumors, are described below. In addition, a combination of the two types of symptoms may be present, as in hypogonadism secondary to hyperprolactinemia.

The signs and symptoms of endocrine hypofunction have been described in the previous section. The most frequent symptoms relate to decreased gonadal function followed by symptoms of adrenal and thyroid insufficiency. The frequency of growth hormone deficiency is intermediate, but unless it occurs prior to the completion of the growth process it is of little clinical significance. Posterior pituitary dysfunction (diabetes insipidus) is quite uncommon with pituitary adenomas until the tumor is very large but occurs frequently with craniopharyngiomas or malignant disease metastatic to the pituitary.

Neuroanatomic Manifestations

The increase in size of an intrasellar tumor leads to compression of the surrounding pituitary tissue and pressure on the overlying dura which makes up the diaphragma sellae. This in turn results in headaches which are variable in nature and may be frontal, temporal, or retroorbital in location, generally dull in quality, unassociated with nausea or visual symptoms, unaltered by change in position, and inconsistently relieved by analgesics. With rupture of the dura the headaches often disappear. Many patients with pituitary tumors have headaches which are not attributable to the tumor and are not relieved by tumor removal. These are most readily differentiated in patients with microadenomas in whom the diaphragma sellae is normal.

Once the tumor has begun to expand in a suprasellar direction, the first structures encountered are the optic nerves, optic chiasm, or optic tracts. Most commonly it is the optic chiasm on which the tumor exerts its upward pressure, leading to the classic findings of bitemporal hemianopsia. If examined just after chiasmal pressure begins, the patient may exhibit only a superior temporal field defect, and asymmetric changes are frequently seen. With continued expansion of the tumor, visual loss may progress toward complete blindness, and optic atrophy will eventually develop. On occasion, tumor growth occurs primarily anterior to the chiasm, resulting in visual impairment limited to one eye. This is most common with a postfixed chiasm. When the chiasm is fixed anteriorly (prefixed), the pattern of visual field loss will reflect optic tract involvement. Papilledema is uncommon in pituitary adenomas but occurs in 27 percent of craniopharyngiomas.[238] With continued upward expansion of the tumor, symptoms of ventral hypothalamic compression may occur, including temperature fluctuations, hyperphagia, alterations in sleep pattern, and emotional disturbances. With pressure on the third ventricle, internal hydrocephalus may be seen. Rarely, there is compression of the temporal or frontal lobes causing behavioral changes and seizures, and midbrain compression may also be seen, resulting in long tract signs. Compression of extrahypothalamic structures occurs more frequently with craniopharyngiomas which may have an extrasellar origin than with pituitary adenomas. Expansion of the tumor in a lateral direction may lead to compression of cranial nerves III, IV, and VI as they pass through the cavernous sinus, resulting in ophthalmoplegia and diplopia. Tumor growth in an inferior direction results in rupture of the sellar floor and expansion into the clivus or into the sphenoid sinus, which may result in cerebrospinal fluid rhinorrhea. The reason for the direction of tumor growth is not known.

Although tumor growth is usually slow and the progression of symptoms gradual, sudden appearance of symptoms in a patient with a pituitary tumor may be caused by hemorrhage into the tumor, or *pituitary apoplexy*.[167] This complication of pituitary tumor was initially recognized only in its most dramatic form and often carried a very poor prognosis. However, it is now apparent that hemorrhage within the tumor mass occurs fairly frequently. In its mildest form it may cause no symptoms whatever or may be associated with sudden onset of headache of varying intensity which subsides after a few days. The bleeding often causes rapid expansion of the tumor, which can lead, if intrasellar, to the development of hypopituitarism and, if extrasellar, to sudden visual impairment or blindness. It may also result in the "spontaneous cure" of a hormone-secreting tumor.

The factors responsible for tumor growth are not entirely understood. Large doses of estrogen will cause pituitary tumors to develop in rats, but there is no evidence to date that this occurs in humans. It is important to recognize, however, that tumor growth may be accelerated during pregnancy. Women with evidence of a pituitary tumor who become pregnant have an increased risk of developing symptoms of chiasmal compression during the second or third trimester. Whether this represents growth of the tumor or only of the normal pituitary is unclear, since the symptoms generally regress spontaneously following parturition. Craniopharyngiomas have, on occasion, appeared to increase in size in children receiving GH therapy.

Neuroradiologic Presentation

A small percentage (5 to 15 percent) of pituitary tumors are initially discovered from skull x-rays obtained for unrelated purposes which reveal an enlarged or deformed sella. Because of the sensitivity of the current generation of computed tomography (CT) scanners, the differentiation of tumors from other nonneoplastic conditions must be carefully considered. The presence of endocrine symptoms and/or hormonal abnormalities becomes of great importance in the differential diagnosis (see below; also Table 8-7).

Diagnostic Procedures

The diagnostic procedures routinely employed are required (1) to differentiate between pituitary tumors and other parasellar disorders, (2) to determine the tumor size and extent of sellar and extrasellar destruction, (3) to define the hormone(s) hypersecreted, and (4) to determine the degree of hormone deficiency present. In addition, certain procedures are used to define precisely the anatomic boundaries of the tumor and the extent of distortion of surrounding normal structures to aid in decisions concerning therapy.

The endocrine evaluation of pituitary hypofunction is described elsewhere in this chapter and in Chap. 9, and that of hyperfunction follows in the next section. It is important that complete endocrine evaluation be carried out prior to definitive therapy if at all possible, since the degree of hypopituitarism may influence the type and extent of therapy. There are circumstances, however, in which this cannot be done, e.g., in a patient with rapidly deteriorating vision or with other progressive neurologic symptoms which necessitate immediate surgical intervention. Under such circumstances, the patient must be considered panhypopituitary and treated with steroids prior to invasive diagnostic procedures and surgery.

Radiographic Evaluation

INITIAL STUDIES The initial radiographic study to be obtained in a patient with a suspected tumor is determined by the degree of suspicion, based on the history and physical examination, and the type of tumor for which the physician is searching. The time-honored study is a lateral view of the skull—or possibly a "coned-down" view of the sella. This is the least expensive study and will detect evidence of nearly all large tumors such as overt enlargement or destruction of the sella (Fig. 8-12). There is considerable disagreement between experts as to what constitutes a normal sella on x-ray with respect to size, shape, and subtle variations in bony structure. Using a standard lateral view, the upper limit of the anteroposterior diameter, measured as the maximum distance from the anterior concavity of the sella to the anterior rim of the dorsum sellae, is 17 mm and the upper limit of the depth of the pituitary fossa, measured as the greatest distance between the floor to a perpendicular line between the top of the dorsum sellae and the tuberculum sellae, is 13 mm.[242] However, measurement of sellar dimensions provides limited help in the diagnosis of pituitary tumors,[243] since there is generally other evidence of sellar abnormality when the normal dimensions are ex-

Table 8-7. Presence of Clinical Symptoms in Patients with an Enlarged Sella

Clinical symptom	Primary intrasellar tumor [27], %	Extrasellar disease [13], %	Empty sella syndrome [25], %	Undiagnosed [10], %
Headache	85 (18)	100 (69)	48 (24)	80 (80)
CSF rhinorrhea	0	0	8 (8)	0
Endocrine	67 (67)	54 (31)	0	0
Visual	0	31 (0)	0	0
Asymptomatic	15 (15)	0	44 (44)	20 (20)

Note: The number of patients in each group is indicated in brackets in the column heads; the percentage of patients with each symptom at the time of diagnosis is indicated in each column followed, in parentheses, by the percentage of patients in whom it was a presenting symptom.
Source: Modified from Weisberg et al.[254] This series excluded 22 patients presenting with visual symptoms.

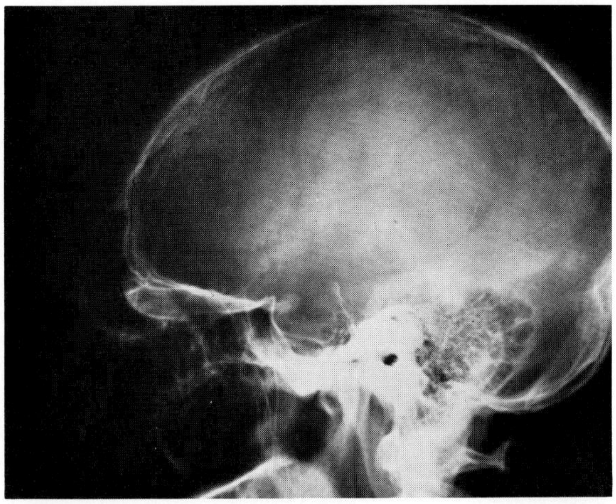

FIGURE 8-12 Neuroradiologic techniques for evaluation of pituitary disease, showing enlarged sella with destruction of floor and dorsum in a patient with a GH-secreting pituitary tumor. Note also the increased size of the sinuses.

ceeded, and sellae obviously abnormal by other criteria frequently have normal dimensions. Assessment of the shape of the sella involves a more subjective approach, and terms such as *bulging* or *ballooning* have been used to indicate the impression of minimal enlargement. None of these changes, however, is pathognomonic of a pituitary tumor. They can be seen with the empty sella syndrome, parasellar masses which have invaded the pituitary fossa, increased intracranial pressure, and, in their mildest forms, in patients with no endocrinologic or neurologic evidence of pituitary disease.

Intrasellar and extrasellar calcifications may also be seen on the lateral and anterior-posterior views of the sella. The presence of calcification, particularly in the suprasellar region, is highly suggestive of a craniopharyngioma, in which this change occurs in 50 percent of cases. No more than 5 percent of pituitary adenomas are associated with calcification. When seen, calcification is usually intrasellar, almost always curvilinear, and located in the tumor capsule or in the wall of cystic tumors.

Previously, numerous other diagnostic procedures were used for more detailed examination, including hypocycloidal tomography, pneumoencephalography, and carotid angiography. These have been completely replaced by CT scanning, which in many instances is the most appropriate initial procedure (see Fig. 8-13).

COMPUTED TOMOGRAPHY The availability of fourth-generation CT scanners has dramatically altered the radiologic evaluation of pituitary tumors. The resolution possible now permits recognition of tumors 3 to 4 mm in diameter, and the appropriate use of intravenous contrast material with dynamic scanning has further improved diagnostic accuracy. The technique of choice for evaluation of suspected pituitary tumors is coronal scanning of the pituitary region in conjunction with contrast injection. If a lesion is seen, dynamic scanning of a single cut after bolus injection of contrast will provide further information. The pituitary gland is outside of the blood-brain barrier and thus is enhanced by the contrast material. Shortly after injection the portal vessels and the tuft of vessels at the inferior end of the stalk are visualized, then the contrast material spreads to the entire pituitary. The maximal height of the normal pituitary gland, determined from coronal scanning of women of childbearing age, has been estimated to be between 9 and 10 mm (95 percent confidence limits),[244,245] though occasional values above 10 mm are encountered. In postpartum women, this value increases to 11.5 mm.[246] In men, the upper limit of normal is 6.0 to 6.5 mm. The upper contour of the pituitary is most commonly flat, but up to 44 percent of normal subjects exhibit convexity, resulting in an upward bulge previously believed to be indicative of a tumor.[245] The distribution of contrast material within the gland is usually homogeneous, but nonhomogeneity has been found in 40 to 75 percent of normal subjects. For the diagnosis of a pituitary microadenoma by CT, there should be a region of diminished uptake of contrast in conjunction with evidence of either bony erosion of the sellar floor on the ipsilateral side or lateral displacement of the pituitary vascular tuft or stalk to the contralateral side.[247,248] It is important to emphasize that the early changes of pituitary tumors on CT may be nonspecific, and differentiation from nonneoplastic changes is often impossible by radiographic techniques alone.[249]

The CT is also the best technique for demonstrating extrasellar extension of a pituitary macroadenoma. In the suprasellar region, macroadenomas will often appear enhanced in relation to the surrounding brain tissue. The position of the intracranial segments of the carotid artery can be determined, and their displacement, if any, is easily demonstrated. Differentiation of pituitary tumors from carotid aneurysms is generally no problem, though in occasional patients digital subtraction angiography may be necessary.

Diminished density within the sella (comparable to the density of CSF), seen in unenhanced scans, is suggestive of the empty sella syndrome. The diagnosis can be confirmed by repeat scanning after intrathecal injection of metrizamide, though this invasive technique is seldom required.

MAGNETIC RESONANCE IMAGING Magnetic resonance imaging (MRI) is a new technique that has the poten-

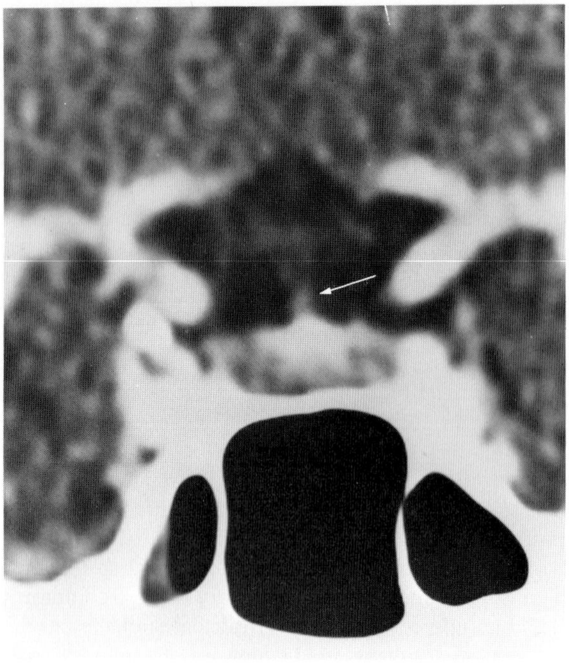
A

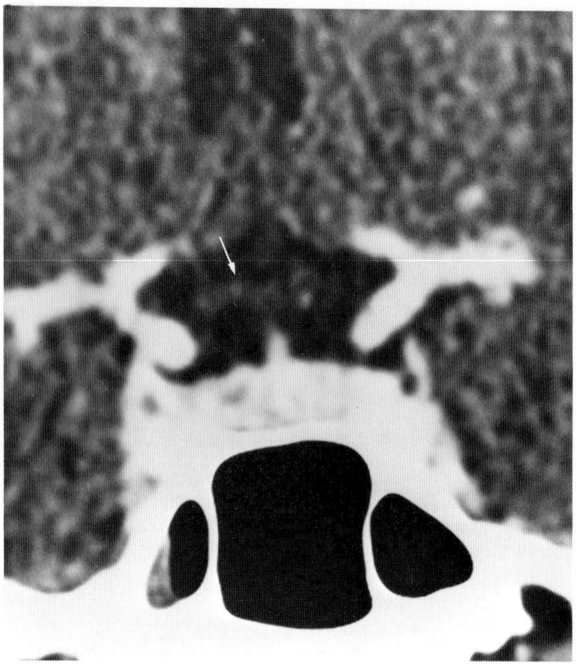
B

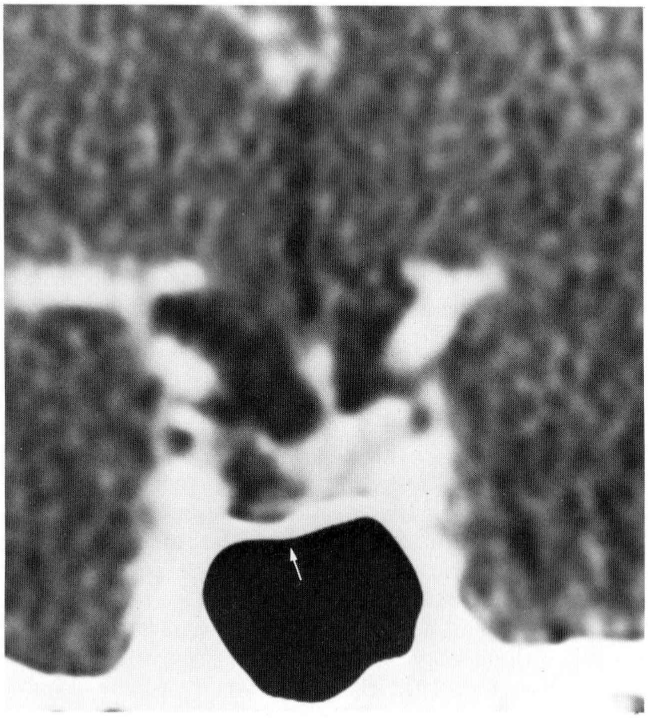
C

FIGURE 8-13 Computed tomography (coronal views) of the normal and abnormal pituitary. (*A*) Dynamic contrast scan of the normal pituitary. Shortly after the injection of contrast material, the pituitary stalk (arrow) and the vascular tuft at its base can be visualized. (*B*) Same, 3 s later. The stalk is still visible and the entire pituitary appears enhanced when compared with the brain. Some nonhomogeneity is commonly present. The horizontal structure above the stalk (arrow) is the optic chiasm. (C) Pituitary microadenoma. A hypodense area is present in the left side of the pituitary, associated with slight depression (arrow) of the sellar floor. The pituitary stalk is displaced to the contralateral side. (*D*) Pituitary macroadenoma. A large homogeneous mass extending in a suprasellar direction is evident without erosion of the sellar floor. (*E*) Empty sella. Contrast material outlines a rim of pituitary tissue in the inferior portion of the sella (arrow), the remainder of which exhibits low contrast comparable to that of cerebrospinal fluid. (*Courtesy of R. Lukin, University of Cincinnati Hospital.*)

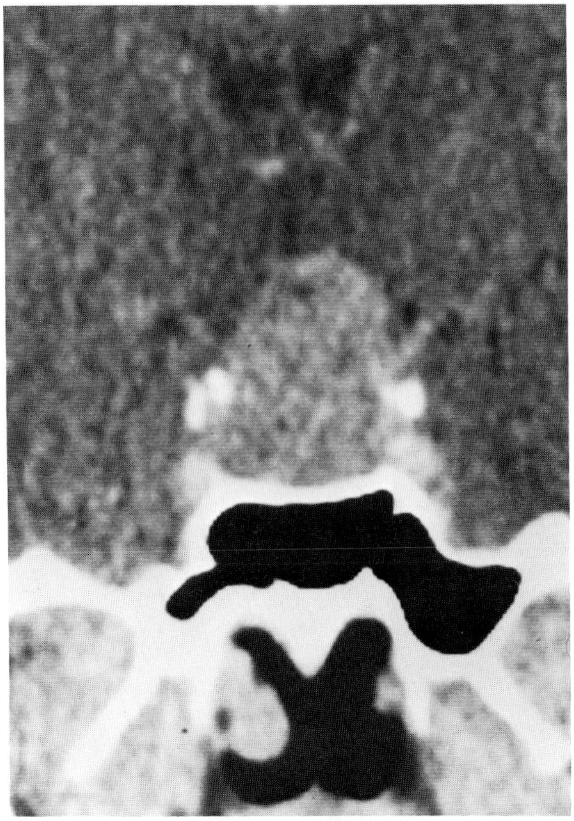

D

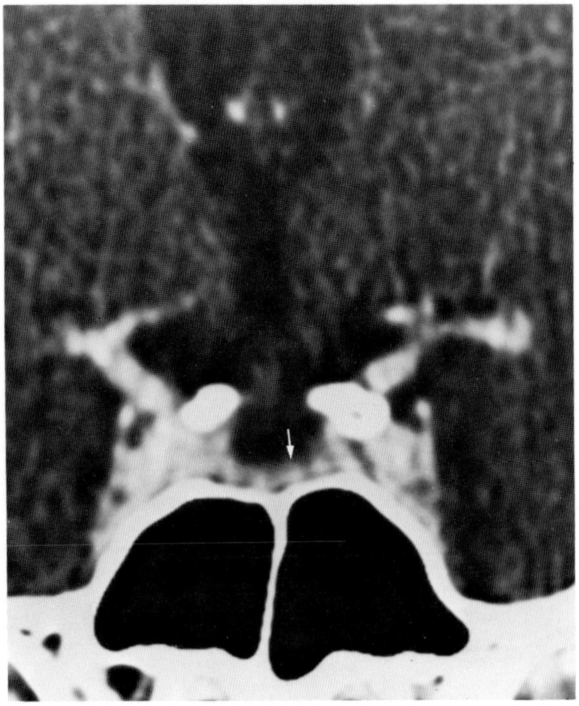

E

FIGURE 8-13 *(Continued)*

tial of adding a new dimension to the evaluation of the pituitary gland and surrounding structures (see Fig. 8-14). The ability to scan in many different planes, elimination of the requirement that the patient remain in awkward positions during the procedure, and noninterference by dental fillings result in satisfactory imaging in virtually all studies.[250] The absence of any radiation exposure provides a great advantage for repeated examinations, particularly in the frontal plane, where the risk of radiation injury to the eyes has been a limiting factor with CT. The only contraindication known to date is the presence of aneurysm clips, because of their potential movement, or of other metallic implants, including pacemakers.

The value of MRI in distinguishing between pituitary tumors and nontumorous dyshomogeneity of the pituitary requires further study, as has been necessary for CT evaluation. At present, specific changes in the "abnormal" pituitary gland which differentiate tumors have not been established. However, the potential for following the response of tumors to therapy and as a primary screening procedure in suspected tumors appears considerable.

Neuroophthalmologic Studies

VISUAL FIELDS A visual field examination performed at the bedside is a useful screening procedure. Because subtle defects are often missed by this technique, however, all patients with evidence of a suprasellar lesion should have formal visual field testing by perimetry. This procedure is currently performed by an automated method and provides an excellent assessment of both the central and peripheral visual fields. Its reproducibility and sensitivity make it extremely useful in following patients for serial changes (Fig. 8-15).

Though chiasmal compression with bitemporal field defects is the characteristic finding in pituitary tumors with suprasellar extension, it is neither specific for pituitary tumors nor the only change seen. In addition to pituitary tumors, bitemporal field defects may be seen with parasellar tumors, vascular abnormalities, demyelinating plaques in the chiasm, focal (sector) retinitis pigmentosa, adhesive arachnoiditis, and CNS sarcoidosis, as well as after irradiation of the chiasm and, rarely, with prolapse of the chiasm into the sella in association with the empty sella syndrome. Similarly, in a patient in whom the chiasm is fixed

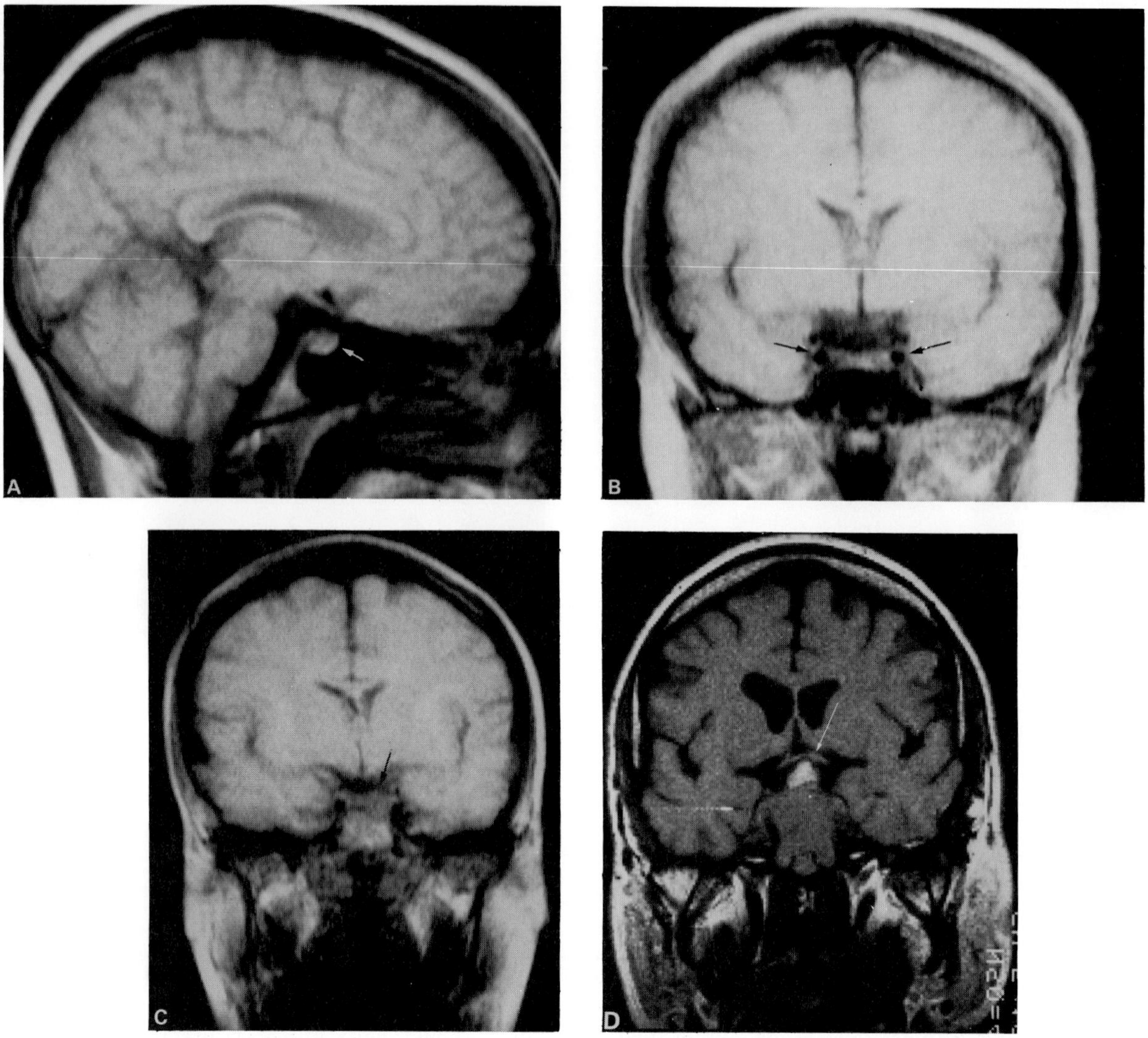

FIGURE 8-14 Magnetic resonance imaging of the pituitary. (*A*) Sagittal view of the normal adult female pituitary. The pituitary appears round (arrow) and isodense with the brainstem and the frontal lobes. The CSF appears black and demarcates the superior surface of the gland. (*B*) In the coronal view, the pituitary appears rectangular and contrasts superiorly with CSF and laterally with the circular low densities (arrows) of the intracavernous carotid arteries. (*C*) Macroadenoma of the pituitary. The right side of the gland reveals a slightly convex enlarged superior surface (arrow) and a pronounced downward enlargement. The higher (lighter) signal beneath the gland represents cancellous bone in the basisphenoid. (*D*) Microadenoma of the pituitary in frontal view. Superior displacement of the optic chiasm (arrow) is caused by suprasellar extension of the tumor. The high-intensity signal is caused by recent hemorrhage (apoplexy) within the tumor. (*From Kaufman.*[250])

anteriorly (prefixed) or posteriorly (postfixed), the predominant visual field defect may relate to one eye (optic nerve) or one field (optic tract). Finally, there are occasional patients with atypical field defects (asymmetric or even suggestive of superior pressure) associated with pituitary tumors in whom the defect disappears following removal of the tumor.

VISUAL EVOKED RESPONSE The visual evoked response procedure which has been used for studying abnormalities of the visual pathways, has been suggested as a more sensitive technique for detecting early chiasmal compression by pituitary tumors (Fig. 8-15). The procedure measures the pattern and latency of the electrical response from the occipital cortex produced by photic stimulation of the eyes. Portions of the individual fields can be evaluated selectively and effects on crossed and uncrossed pathways distinguished. With chiasmal pressure, a delayed response and/or reduction in the response can be seen in crossed as compared with uncrossed pathways. The advantages of the visual evoked response are its reliability and sensitivity along with

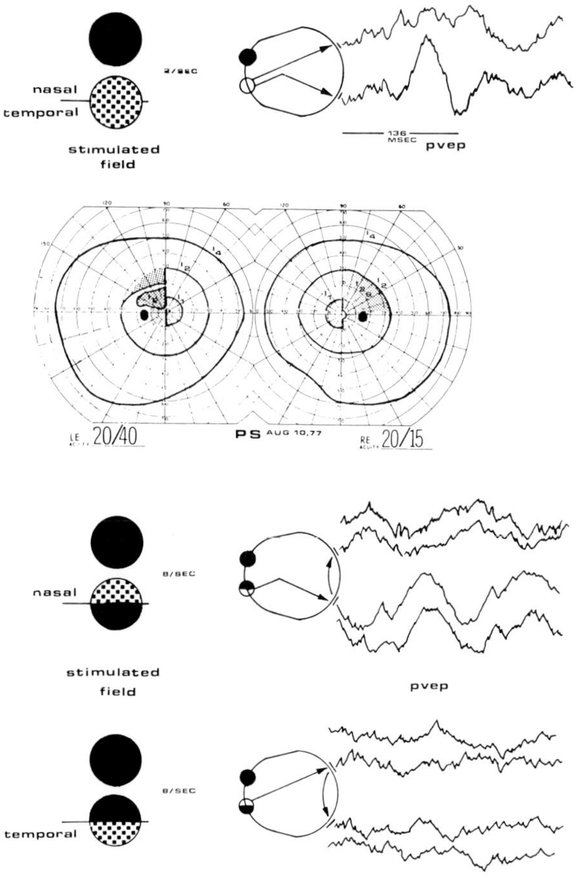

FIGURE 8-15 Visual fields and pattern visual evoked potential (PVEP) in a patient with suprasellar extension of a pituitary tumor. (*Top*) Stimulation of complete visual field (left eye) by a reversing checkerboard pattern. A large PVEP is elicited in the left occipital lobe, which receives input from the nasal field via uncrossed pathways in the chiasm. A low-amplitude distorted PVEP is produced in the right occipital lobe from the temporal field via crossed fibers in the chiasm. (*Middle*) Visual fields of the patient demonstrating low-grade upper temporal defects in both eyes. Fields were normal when all but the smallest targets were used. (*Bottom*) Separate stimulation of nasal and temporal fields of the left eye. A large sinusoidal PVEP occurs in the left hemisphere via uncrossed chiasmal pathways when the nasal field is stimulated. A low-amplitude response 180° out of phase is recorded over the right occipital lobe, which represents either volume conduction within the cranium or conducted activity across the corpus callosum (arrow). Stimulation of the temporal field fails to evoke a response at the right occiput. (*Courtesy of J. Goodwin, Michael Reese Hospital.*)

absence of influence by observer fatigue, which occasionally occurs during visual field testing.

Other Studies

Pituitary hormones have been demonstrated in the CSF, and it has been observed that the levels, normally lower than in peripheral blood, are increased in patients with pituitary tumors in the presence of suprasellar extension but not in patients whose tumors are entirely intrasellar in location, irrespective of whether the tumor is functional.[251,252] The single exception to this rule is with prolactin-secreting tumors, where increased prolactin levels in the CSF can be present even without suprasellar extension.[253] The elevated CSF hormone concentrations do not appear to be due to a loss of the normal blood-CSF barrier but most likely occur because of direct secretion by the pituitary.[252] Measurement of pituitary hormones in the CSF has not, however, proved to be of particular use in the evaluation of pituitary tumors.

Differential Diagnosis

The diagnosis of a pituitary tumor is made on two types of evidence: neuroanatomic confirmation of a tumor mass and, if present, demonstration of hormonal hypersecretion. If both exist, the diagnosis is established. The differential diagnosis of hormonal hypersecretion in the absence of neuroanatomic abnormalities is considered in the following section. If the tumor is hormonally inactive, the frequent lack of specificity of the neuroanatomic studies and clinical findings requires careful consideration of other diagnostic possibilities. It should be emphasized that hypopituitarism, whether partial or complete, in the presence of neuroradiologic evidence of sellar enlargement does not necessarily indicate the presence of a pituitary tumor.

The differential diagnosis of decreased pituitary function has already been presented. That of an enlarged sella is listed in Table 8-8 according to the frequency of occurrence. Among a series of patients with an enlarged sella without visual symptoms, the frequency of primary intrasellar tumors and the empty sella syndrome were similar (36 and 33 percent), extrasellar disease (including both tumors and granulomatous disease) was less common (17 percent), and no diagnosis could be established in the remaining 14 percent.[254] With newer neuroradiologic techniques, this percentage should decrease. The other disorders listed in Table 8-8 are relatively uncommon but necessitate markedly different diagnostic and therapeutic considerations.

Empty Sella Syndrome

Empty sella is a term applied to all sellae which exhibit low density on CT comparable to that of CSF. It results from an extension of the subarachnoid space into the intrasellar region and is often associated with flattening of the pituitary gland, usually along the posterior portion of the floor and dorsum. The sella turcica is generally, though not invariably, enlarged. The term *primary empty sella syndrome* has been used for those cases unassociated with prior surgical or radia-

Table 8-8. Differential Diagnosis of Nonfunctioning Pituitary Tumors

Diagnosis	Sella size	Sella deformity	Pituitary function	Other features
Empty sella syndrome	Generally increased	May be present Low-density contents	Almost always normal	Endocrine function testing may show mild abnormalities. Obesity and benign intracranial hypertension may occur.
Parasellar tumor	Normal or increased	Usually present	Normal or decreased	Headache pattern different. Extraocular nerve involvement frequent. Visual field defects atypical.
Intrasellar aneurysm	Normal or increased	Usually present	Normal or decreased	Throbbing headaches with vomiting may occur. Extraocular nerve involvement common. Symptoms begin suddenly and are often periodic.
Immunologic or granulomatous disease	Increased	May be present	Usually normal except for hyperprolactinemia	Decreased endocrine function, if present, is on hypothalamic basis. Diabetes insipidus present.
Primary hypothyroidism	Increased	May be present	Usually normal but may be decreased and prolactin may be increased	Elevated TSH and prolactin are suppressed by thyroxine.
Primary hypogonadism	Increased	May be present	Normal with increased gonadotropins	Gonadotropins suppressed by gonadal steroids.
Familial hypopituitarism	Increased	None	Decreased GH and TSH. Gonadotropins may also be decreased	Asymptomatic except for hormone deficiency.

tion therapy. A primary empty sella has been found in up to 24 percent of autopsy series, usually with no history of endocrine disease.[255]

The etiology of the primary empty sella syndrome is not known. It has been postulated that an incompletely formed diaphragma sellae permits CSF pressure to be transmitted to the contents of the sella, gradually leading to a herniation of the arachnoid with flattening of the adenohypophysis and remodeling of the sella. Other possibilities include the presence of a preexisting tumor or cyst with subsequent hemorrhage and resorption leading to a loss of tissue mass.

Nearly all patients with primary empty sella syndrome are asymptomatic. Although headache is frequently noted, it is probably unrelated and merely leads to the skull x-ray and the subsequent diagnostic evaluation. The syndrome is most frequently seen in obese women and is associated with an increased frequency of systemic hypertension, benign intracranial hypertension (pseudotumor cerebri), and CSF rhinorrhea, as indicated in Table 8-9.[175,176] Visual disturbances, more common in the secondary form of the syndrome (following surgery or radiotherapy), occur in the primary empty sella syndrome and include generalized peripheral field constriction, bitemporal hemianopsia, and papilledema.

The sella is usually symmetrically enlarged or ballooned (84 percent of patients) and may also be deformed (42 percent), most commonly showing a straightening of the dorsum with demineralization and less frequently asymmetry of the floor and erosion of the clinoids. The bony changes can be indistinguish-

Table 8-9. Features Commonly Associated with the Primary Empty Sella Syndrome

Feature	Frequency, %
Female sex	83.7
Obesity	78.4
Systemic hypertension	30.5
Benign intracranial hypertension (pseudotumor cerebri)	10.5
CSF rhinorrhea	9.7

Source: Modified from Jordan et al.[176]

able from those of pituitary tumors, though the diagnosis is readily confirmed by CT alone or after intrathecal metrizamide contrast.

Endocrine function testing of most patients with the primary empty sella syndrome is normal, though there are reports of occasional patients with diminished TSH and gonadotropin reserve, blunted growth hormone responses, hyperprolactinemia,[256] and, rarely, panhypopituitarism or diabetes insipidus.

The diagnosis of the primary empty sella syndrome is usually made during the course of a workup for a pituitary tumor. It should be suspected in a patient with an enlarged sella with no clinical symptoms or minimal symptoms and normal endocrine function. Under these conditions it is often unnecessary to perform invasive procedures, and the patient may simply be followed. It is important to remember, however, that the presence of an empty sella does not exclude the coexistence of a pituitary tumor. GH-, prolactin-, and ACTH-secreting tumors have all been reported in patients with the primary empty sella syndrome.[175,257,258] Fortunately, the diagnostic evaluation of the patients is guided by the hypersecretory features, and the presence of the empty sella syndrome, if discovered preoperatively, should not alter the planned therapy. To date there have been no reported cases of coexistence of a nonfunctioning pituitary tumor and the primary empty sella syndrome.

Parasellar Diseases

A number of diverse disorders arising in the parasellar area are associated with signs and symptoms which mimic those of pituitary tumors. They include inflammatory and granulomatous diseases (sarcoidosis, eosinophilic granuloma, arachnoiditis), degenerative disorders (aneurysms), and neoplasms (meningiomas, gliomas, sarcomas, hamartomas, and rarely metastatic tumors). By invading the sella, these disorders can cause enlargement and deformity of the bony structure and varying degrees of hypopituitarism in addition to their suprasellar manifestations. They must be distinguished from primary pituitary tumors if appropriate therapy is to be provided.

Suprasellar tumors usually present with predominantly neurologic manifestations: severe headache often associated with nausea and vomiting, asymmetric visual disturbances, papilledema, and extraocular nerve involvement. Tumors of the hypothalamus or third ventricle often produce symptoms of hypothalamic dysfunction and increased intracranial pressure.

In parasellar tumors, unlike pituitary tumors, endocrine manifestations tend to follow rather than precede the neurologic symptoms. Radiologic manifestations of suprasellar tumors frequently provide clues as to their origin, e.g., suprasellar calcification in craniopharyngiomas and meningiomas and erosion of the anterior clinoids with an otherwise intact sella. These are readily identified on CT scan.

Aneurysms of the internal carotid artery siphon or the anterior communicating artery can expand into the sella and, like suprasellar tumors, mimic a pituitary tumor.[259] Headaches, which are frequently throbbing and fluctuate in severity, are the predominant symptoms, and involvement of cranial nerves III, IV, and VI is also common. The diagnosis can be established preoperatively by CT and/or digital subtraction angiography.

Sarcoidosis and other granulomatous diseases affect primarily the hypothalamus, though pituitary involvement may also occur, leading to increased sellar size. The diagnosis is usually made on the basis of nonendocrine manifestations, and the assumption that the alterations in pituitary function are attributable to the granulomatous disease must be confirmed by the response to appropriate therapy and by long-term follow-up.

Pituitary Enlargement Associated with Other Endocrine Diseases

The presence of long-standing primary hypothyroidism or primary hypogonadism has been associated with the development of sellar enlargement, increased TSH or gonadotropin secretion, and in some patients, TSH-secreting pituitary tumors.[15–17,260] As can be shown in laboratory animals, long-standing target organ insufficiency results in hyperplasia of the tropic hormone-producing cells, leading eventually to tumor formation. Occasionally there is some overlap in hormone hypersecretion in that long-standing juvenile hypothyroidism has been associated with premature puberty. It is extremely important to recognize this syndrome, though it is quite uncommon, in its early stages, since the hypersecretion and hyperplastic changes can be reversed with appropriate therapy, i.e., thyroxine or gonadal steroids. Once adenoma formation has occurred this may no longer be possible, and surgical removal of the tumor may be required.

A syndrome of familial hypopituitarism involving growth hormone, TSH, and possibly gonadotropin secretion associated with an enlarged sella has also been described.[261] The basis for the enlarged but not deformed sella is not known, and the possibility of tumor formation has not been excluded, since surgical exploration has not been carried out in the patients described.

Therapy

Therapy of nonfunctional pituitary tumors is necessary to prevent or limit loss of pituitary function and the consequences of suprasellar extension on the optic chiasm and hypothalamus. The choice of therapy is between surgery and radiation, since pharmacotherapy is ineffective.[262]

Surgery

Pituitary surgery, which was established as a safe and effective procedure by Cushing, has been the conventional therapy for pituitary tumors. The transfrontal approach, which was standard until the past decade, remains the technique of choice for most parasellar tumors and craniopharyngiomas arising outside the sella and for primary intrasellar tumors with extensive suprasellar extension, particularly when separated from the intrasellar portion by a narrow neck. Tumors which have encircled the optic nerves can be removed only by the frontal approach. With the availability of high-dose glucocorticoid therapy, the postoperative mortality previously associated with operations in the region of the hypothalamus is no longer a problem. The operative mortality of transfrontal surgery has ranged from 1.2 percent to 10 percent in recent series, depending upon the type of cases included.[263,264]

The need to provide better exposure of the anterior and inferior portions of the pituitary, where the small functioning tumors are frequently located, led to the renaissance of transsphenoidal microsurgery by Guiot[265] and, subsequently, by Hardy.[266] This procedure, initially developed by Cushing, was abandoned because of the complications of CSF rhinorrhea and the invariably fatal meningitis in the preantibiotic era. Coupled with modern fluoroscopic aids and microsurgical techniques, the transsphenoidal approach is being used for the majority of pituitary tumors, with a mortality rate varying from a high of 3 percent to nearly zero.[266,267] Tumors with moderate suprasellar extension can be removed transsphenoidally, and even those tumors which require a frontal approach are often removed in a two-stage procedure, with the intrasellar portion of the tumor excised by the transsphenoidal route after removal of the suprasellar portion. This approach is specifically indicated where the intracranial route is associated with an unacceptably high risk as in the elderly, in patients nearly blind because of long-standing chiasmal compression, and in patients with inferior extension of the tumor into the sphenoid sinus. There are no absolute contraindications to the transsphenoidal approach, though an inadequately pneumatized sinus and anatomic variations in the position of the carotid siphon can make the procedure more difficult.

The preoperative endocrine evaluation of patients is of help in deciding on the extent of the surgical resection to be performed. If the patient has intact target organ function, a somewhat more conservative approach is indicated in order to preserve the remaining pituitary hormone-secreting tissue. If, however, hypopituitarism is documented preoperatively, there is little reason to be concerned with preservation of the contents of the sella. In practice, a small rim of adenohypophyseal tissue at the periphery of the sella is often sufficient to maintain pituitary function.

It is advisable to provide steroid coverage for the surgical period even in those patients with an intact pituitary-adrenal axis because of the possibility that more normal tissue will be removed than is anticipated preoperatively. Parenteral hydrocortisone, 50 mg q 6 h, beginning the morning of surgery or, if the patient is hypopituitary, at least 24 h before surgery, provides adequate coverage, and the dosage is rapidly tapered postoperatively. Pituitary function should be evaluated in the postoperative period to assess the need for replacement therapy.

Postoperatively, the patient must be carefully observed for the development of diabetes insipidus, particularly since an obtunded patient may not perceive thirst. Polyuria and increasing plasma osmolality commonly occur during the immediate postoperative period if there has been even mild trauma to the pituitary stalk. Persistence of these findings beyond the first 48 h usually indicates destruction of the stalk or posterior pituitary and some permanent impairment of function. However, most patients have clinical recovery. In some patients a recovery phase occurs which is followed by a permanent return of symptoms. The recovery period has been attributed to release of vasopressin from degenerating posterior pituicytes. Because the course of events during the first few postoperative days is unpredictable, fluid balance must be monitored carefully and the patient treated with desmopressin (DDAVP) 1 to 2 μg IM or aqueous vasopressin 5 U IM as necessary. A full discussion of the treatment of diabetes insipidus is provided in Chap. 9.

If rhinorrhea develops following transsphenoidal surgery, a glucose oxidase–impregnated strip (e.g., Dextrostix) should be used to determine whether the fluid is CSF. Postoperative CSF rhinorrhea frequently subsides spontaneously within 7 to 10 days. If it does not, surgical repair of the defect in the floor of the sella is required.

Radiation Therapy

As an alternative to surgical excision of pituitary adenomas a variety of radiotherapeutic procedures have been used. Patients considered to be candidates for radiotherapy are those without or with only limited suprasellar extension. In the presence of marked visual field defects, the use of external radiation carries an increased risk of further visual impairment because of the initial inflammatory response which occurs within the tumor. In addition, a larger field of radiation is required for tumors with marked suprasellar extension, leading to increased risk of damage to surrounding neural structures.

The dose of radiation currently used for most patients is 4500 to 5000 rads, which is an effective tumoricidal dose and is less than the 8000 to 9000 rads used to destroy normal pituitary tissue. The therapy is given in multiple divided doses with rotating ports and usually produces only minimal side effects with little or no hair loss. Long-term follow-up of patients receiving such therapy, however, reveals that a considerable percentage develop at least partial hypopituitarism.

Conventional irradiation employing high-energy sources (supervoltage) is the most commonly employed procedure. Stereotaxic implantation of ^{90}Y pellets was initially found to be an effective alternative, but the frequency of complications, including improper placement of pellets and CSF rhinorrhea, led to discontinuation of the procedure. Heavy particle (proton beam and alpha particle) irradiation is also an effective technique but is currently available in only the few locations with a cyclotron.[268–270] The dose can be administered within a few hours and produces results at least comparable with and possibly better than those of conventional irradiation. Neurologic complications, including oculomotor nerve palsies, visual field defects, and temporal lobe necrosis, are uncommon today because of the increased precision used in directing the therapeutic beam. Pituitary function, at least in the short term, is preserved in 80 to 85 percent of patients.

Craniopharyngiomas, unlike chromophobe adenomas, were initially considered to be radioresistant tumors. However, there are numerous reports of the efficacy of postoperative irradiation,[271,272] and most patients are now being treated in this manner.

Factors Relating to the Choice of Therapy

Many patients with pituitary tumors are candidates for either surgical or radiation therapy as primary treatment. The major advantages of surgery are (1) the immediate results, which are at times necessary in terms of visual symptoms and hormone hypersecretion (discussed below), and (2) the ability to obtain a tissue diagnosis and to treat effectively those tumors which are relatively radioresistant (e.g., cystic tumors and craniopharyngiomas). The disadvantages of surgery relate to the rare operative mortality and occasional morbidity, consisting primarily of damage to the frontal lobe, optic nerves, or pituitary stalk, pituitary hemorrhage, infection, and, particularly with the transsphenoidal procedure, CSF rhinorrhea.

Radiotherapy avoids the acute surgical complications and is a far simpler procedure for the patient. The disadvantages of radiotherapy include (1) unsuccessful outcome in the occasional patient with a radioresistant tumor (some radiotherapists insist on a histologic diagnosis prior to therapy), (2) slow response, coupled with the risk of acute swelling of the tumor, (3) occasional occurrence of pituitary apoplexy following therapy, (4) very infrequent episodes of damage to surrounding neural tissue, and (5) long-term development of hypopituitarism due to irradiation of normal adenohypophyseal tissue. Both surgery and radiotherapy share the problem of the occasional development of an empty sella syndrome with visual disturbances due to prolapse of the optic chiasm.

The major determining factors in the treatment of nonfunctioning pituitary tumors which meet the criteria for treatment by either modality relate to the long-term results with respect to preservation and/or restoration of vision, the maintenance of endocrine function, and the frequency of recurrence. Although most series do not distinguish between functioning and nonfunctioning pituitary tumors, the recurrence rates following surgery and radiotherapy appear to be similar.[267,273,274] It is encouraging to note that the recurrence rates reported in the past few years have been lower than those of one or two decades earlier for both procedures. It is also important to recognize, however, that the diagnostic criteria, therapeutic techniques, and posttherapy evaluation methods vary enormously among reports, thus the patient populations are in many respects not comparable. Nevertheless, the prognosis with respect to improvement of visual symptoms and recurrence appears excellent for most patients with other than extremely large pituitary tumors. Another important determinant in the choice of primary therapy is the availability of an experienced neurosurgeon and/or radiotherapist. Most neurosurgeons perform transsphenoidal pituitary surgery infrequently, and it is important to refer the patient to someone with extensive experience.

The relative frequency of hypopituitarism as a consequence of surgery or of irradiation is also roughly comparable (about 15 percent), although a difference exists with respect to time of onset: hypopituitarism following surgery is immediate, whereas that following irradiation tends to be delayed by up to several years. The use of irradiation as primary therapy for a nonfunctioning pituitary tumor does not interfere with subsequent surgical therapy in the event of recurrence, nor does initial surgery preclude subsequent irradiation. A most important use of radiation therapy is as an adjunct to surgery. Most, and in some series nearly all, tumors showing mass effects will recur within 5 years after surgical treatment alone.[275] Postoperative irradiation will prevent tumor regrowth in 90 to 95 percent of patients. It is therefore the author's practice to recommend surgery as primary therapy for nonfunctioning tumors except when medically inadvisable and to use radiation therapy postoperatively except in unusual circumstances.

PITUITARY TUMORS ASSOCIATED WITH HORMONE HYPERSECRETION

Most pituitary tumors (more than 70 percent) can be shown by RIA measurements of circulating hormone levels to be hyperfunctioning,[276] although in some patients the elevated hormone levels may not be associated with any clinical symptoms and thus serve only as biochemical tumor markers. The hormones secreted, in decreasing order of frequency, are prolactin, GH, ACTH, TSH, and FSH. Though the tumors are usually of a single-cell type and associated with overproduction of a single hormone, prolactin hypersecretion is not uncommonly seen in combination with GH, ACTH, and TSH hypersecretion. Pancreatic islet, carcinoid, and parathyroid tumors are frequently seen in association with hyperfunctioning pituitary tumors as part of the multiple endocrine neoplasia (type 1) syndrome (Chap. 28).

Therapeutic considerations of hormone-secreting pituitary tumors also differ from those of nonfunctioning tumors in that treatment sufficient to arrest the growth of the tumor may be inadequate to inhibit the hormone secretion. In addition, medical (neuropharmacologic) therapy directed at the hormone hypersecretion and reduction in tumor size is available as an alternative mode of treatment. This section describes those features unique to hormone-secreting tumors and stresses the differences in management of these tumors as compared with nonfunctioning tumors.

Growth Hormone–Secreting Pituitary Tumors: Acromegaly

GH hypersecretion is usually associated with a pituitary tumor which contains eosinophilic-staining granules in about 20 percent of patients and chromophobic granules in the remainder. By the use of electron microscopy together with special cytochemical and immunochemical staining techniques, however, almost all the chromophobe tumors associated with acromegaly can be demonstrated to have GH-containing secretory granules.[277] The presence or absence of abundant GH secretory granules in tumor cells does not correlate with plasma GH levels but is merely a reflection of the hormone storage capacity as compared with its synthesis and release. The absence of storage granules does, however, indicate a relatively less differentiated tumor, which in turn is reflected in its growth rate. Thus, eosinophilic adenomas tend to be smaller, grow more slowly, and permit signs and symptoms of GH hypersecretion to develop for a prolonged period, whereas chromophobe tumors frequently exhibit a more rapid growth rate and produce symptoms of an expanding tumor mass, with those of GH hypersecretion being less pronounced. Acromegaly can also be caused by somatotroph hyperplasia,[278,279] which is seen in association with GRH overproduction. Excessive GRH secretion, however, may also lead to somatotroph adenoma formation, suggesting that the hyperplasia is an intermediate stage.

Signs and Symptoms

The classic manifestations of GH-secreting tumors are produced by one or more of three factors: mass effects of the expanding tumor, pituitary hormone deficiencies, and GH hypersecretion. The clinical findings due to the first two have already been described, and their frequency in patients with GH-secreting tumors was once considerable. With earlier diagnosis, they are becoming relatively less common.

Signs and symptoms of GH hypersecretion are a result of the product of the GH concentration and the duration of hypersecretion. They may begin at any age, and the interval from onset to diagnosis may range from 1 or 2 years to several decades. The earliest recognizable findings are soft tissue swelling and hypertrophy involving the extremities and the face (Fig. 8-16). Photographs taken over a one- or two-decade span will frequently document the progressive changes in appearance. The acral changes are most prominent in the hands and feet, where spadelike changes develop in the fingers and increased soft tissue volume results in the need for progressively larger rings, gloves, and shoes. The skin becomes thickened and leathery and the prominence of skin folds increases. Generalized hirsutism may develop, as may increased pigmentation. Fibroma molluscum is seen in one-fourth of patients, and acanthosis nigricans is occasionally present. Sebaceous gland hypersecretion leading to oiliness of the skin and cyst formation is common, as is furrowing of the tongue. Most active acromegalic patients exhibit increased sweating,

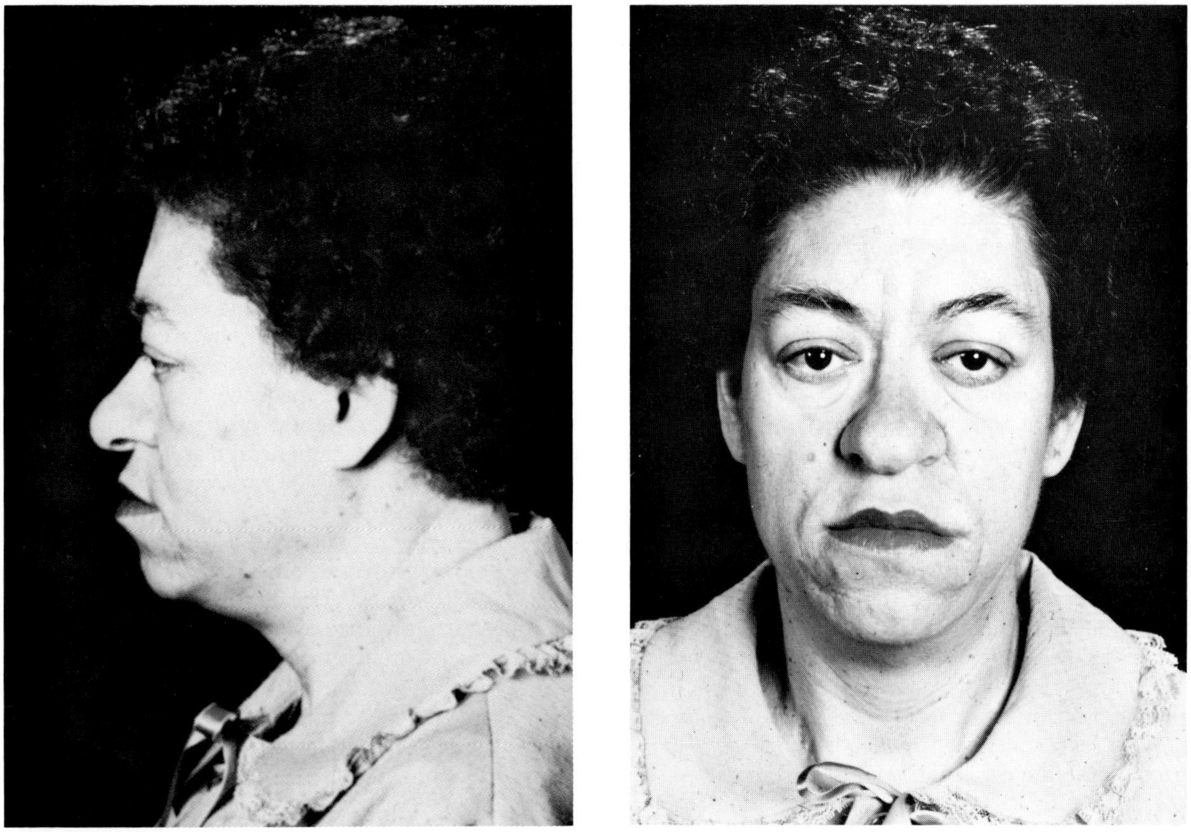

FIGURE 8-16 Facial appearance of a 43-year-old woman with acromegaly whose disease had been present for 15 years. Soft tissue overgrowth about the eyes, nose, and mouth has resulted in coarsening of the features. Lacrimal overgrowth is evident, as is thickening of the skin folds and the presence of fibroma molluscum (acrochordon).

which is a sensitive clinical indicator of the activity of the disease. The bony changes develop more slowly and include cortical thickening, osteophyte proliferation, and tufting of the terminal phalanges. Hypertrophic arthropathy associated with thickened and eventually degenerated articular cartilages and ligamentous hypertrophy cause symptoms ranging from mild arthralgias to deforming and crippling arthritis. The mandible undergoes marked enlargement, leading to prognathism and a significant overbite of the lower incisors. In addition, there is often increased spacing between the teeth. The bony ridges of the calvarium are thickened, and there is often overgrowth of the frontal, malar, and nasal bones. The sinuses are generally increased in size, which, along with hypertrophy of the vocal cords, leads to a deepening of the voice. Mucosal hypertrophy occasionally results in eustachian tube obstruction and serous otitis media.

When GH hypersecretion begins during childhood prior to fusion of the epiphyseal plates, the increase in skeletal growth tends to be proportional and leads to true gigantism. Because of the hypogonadism frequently present, epiphyseal closure is delayed and the period available for growth prolonged. The most celebrated pituitary giant (the Alton giant) reached a height of nearly 9 ft. It is more usual to see patients with an admixture of the features of gigantism and acromegaly, reflecting persistence of growth hormone hypersecretion in adult life. GH-secreting tumors currently constitute 20 percent of all pituitary adenomas diagnosed during childhood.[280]

Peripheral neuropathy is common and is due to a combination of (1) nerve entrapment due to overgrowth of the surrounding ligamentous and fibrous tissue—most commonly affecting the median nerve (e.g., carpal tunnel syndrome) and less frequently the spinal nerves and the cauda equina—and (2) axonal demyelination of peripheral nerves associated with a proliferation of the perineurial and subepineurial elements, resulting in palpable nerves.[281] Acromegalic patients exhibit paresthesias and sensory losses and characteristic proximal muscle weakness, which is usually not severe but may become debilitating. Muscle histology is relatively normal in most patients, although a few exhibit evidence of muscle degeneration.

Prolonged GH hypersecretion results in generalized visceromegaly that includes salivary glands, liver, spleen, and kidneys. The salivary gland enlargement is clinically apparent, while that of the other organs is generally not. Thus, significant hepatosplenomegaly usually implies the presence of a coexisting disease.[282] The renal hypertrophy is associated with an increase of both secretory and reabsorptive functions. Colonic polyps and carcinoma are also more frequent,[283,284] though the mechanism is unclear.

Enlargement and hyperfunction of other endocrine glands are common in acromegaly. Thyromegaly with adenomatous change is frequently seen, though true hyperfunction is infrequent. The presence of decreased thyroid-binding globulin and increased thyroid-binding prealbumin complicates the interpretation of thyroid function tests. Parathyroid hyperplasia and adenoma formation are common along with pancreatic islet tumors and carcinoid tumors as part of the multiple endocrine neoplasia (type 1) syndrome (though otherwise rare in acromegaly) and explain the frequent hypercalciuria and nephrolithiasis. A more specific role of carcinoid and islet tumors in the pathogenesis of acromegaly, as a result of their ectopic production of GRH, is discussed below. Galactorrhea, amenorrhea, and decreased libido, when they occur, are usually due to associated prolactin hypersecretion by the pituitary tumor, which may occur in up to one-third of patients.[285] The pathophysiology is discussed in the section on prolactin-secreting tumors. The decreased plasma testosterone levels occasionally seen may be secondary to hyperprolactinemia, but the reduced levels of testosterone-binding globulin are also a contributory factor.

The effect of GH on the cardiovascular system has been the subject of some controversy because of the limited numbers of patients evaluated, the method of their selection, and the investigative techniques used. Hypertension is frequently present beginning in the fourth to fifth decade but is generally mild and responsive to drug therapy. Cardiomegaly is routinely found at autopsy, but there appears to be no characteristic form of acromegalic heart disease.[286] Significant cardiac failure is present primarily in those patients with hypertension and does not correlate well with other parameters of GH hypersecretion. Yet there does appear to be an increased incidence of cardiovascular disease in acromegalic patients, which is associated with increased mortality.[287]

Weight gain is not a common feature of acromegaly. Less than one-third of patients are obese. However, alterations in carbohydrate metabolism have long been recognized and are due to the diabetogenic effects of GH. Glucose intolerance and hyperinsulinemia are common, and diabetes (defined as fasting hyperglycemia) is seen in about 25 percent of patients, primarily those with a positive family history of diabetes, suggesting that acromegaly may precipitate expression of an underlying genetic potential. Although diabetes is generally of the non-insulin-dependent type, large doses of insulin are frequently required because of insulin resistance, and occasional patients are ketosis-prone. Despite these alterations, the vascular complications of diabetes are extremely uncommon.[288] Although subtle evidence of retinopathy may be present, significant visual loss, renal failure due to diabetic nephropathy, peripheral diabetic neuropathy, and vascular insufficiency are extremely rare, even in long-standing disease.

In evaluating patients with acromegaly both prior to and following therapy, one occasionally encounters a patient with typical acral and facial features of long duration but with little evidence of recent metabolic activity. Such patients may either have truly inactive disease due to infarction of the tumor (with or without clinically evident pituitary apoplexy) or may be experiencing a plateau of the effects due to GH hypersecretion. Assessment of plasma hormone levels is necessary to distinguish between these alternatives.

Laboratory Studies

DIRECT The diagnosis of acromegaly is established by demonstration of an elevated plasma GH level which does not respond normally to stimulatory and suppressive agents. The upper limit of GH in normal adults is 5 ng/ml in males and 10 ng/ml in females. GH levels in patients with acromegaly may range from the upper normal range to more than 1000 ng/ml. The levels in general reflect the secretory activity of the tumor but not necessarily the duration of the disease or the severity of the clinical manifestations. Because normal children and younger adults may sporadically exhibit elevated GH levels of more than 50 ng/ml, dynamic studies of GH secretion are indicated unless the basal GH considerably exceeds this value. GH secretion in acromegaly is qualitatively distinct from that in normal subjects by many parameters. The suppressive effect of oral glucose administration in normal persons (to less than 2 ng/ml in males and less than 5 ng/ml in females) is absent in acromegaly, and assessment of this response is the most reliable method of confirming the diagnosis. It must be recognized, however, that plasma GH levels in acromegalic patients can decrease, remain unchanged, or even increase paradoxically in response to oral glucose. Changes in GH levels in response to glucose are seen in 70 to 80 percent of acromegalic patients.[289] When suppression occurs, however, GH levels do not decrease to the normal range.

Somatomedin C levels are uniformly elevated in acromegaly. There are conflicting data concerning the utility of plasma somatomedin C levels in providing a better correlation with the clinical manifestations of GH hypersecretion than with the GH level itself.[290–292] Since somatomedin C levels are influenced by many factors other than GH (see Chap. 26) and are one step removed from the hormone (GH) being hypersecreted, they can provide only ancillary help. In patients with only minimal elevations of plasma GH initially or after therapy, somatomedin C measurements may be useful in assessing the activity of the disease.

Plasma GH levels increase in response to TRH administration in 70 to 80 percent of acromegalic patients (but not in normal subjects), and this stimulus has been as reliable as glucose for establishing the diagnosis.[293] An increase in plasma GH is also seen after GnRH administration,[294] although both the magnitude of the response and the frequency are often less than after TRH. GRH stimulates GH release in most acromegalic patients (more than 90 percent), and in some the response is exaggerated.[295,296] The finding is, however, of little diagnostic help. Some patients with acromegaly also respond, occasionally in a paradoxical manner, to insulin hypoglycemia or arginine, but these stimuli are not useful in establishing the diagnosis. L-Dopa administration suppresses GH levels in most acromegalic subjects,[297] in contrast to normal persons. This effect can be duplicated by apomorphine and by systemic dopamine infusion and is due to a direct dopaminergic inhibitory effect on the tumor. Other differences in GH secretory patterns between acromegalic and normal subjects include a lack of deep sleep–associated GH secretion and a tendency to wide spontaneous fluctuations in GH levels, indicating intermittent secretory activity of the tumor.

INDIRECT Numerous indirect measurements of GH hypersecretion are no longer used or are obtained only as ancillary information because of the reliance on measurements of circulating GH levels. Serum inorganic phosphorus is often elevated, as is the tubular reabsorption of phosphate. Hyperinsulinemia with or without glucose intolerance is usually present, and somatomedin C levels, irrespective of the type of assay used, are also elevated. Radiographic changes include tufting of the terminal phalanges, enlargement of the sinuses, and an increased thickness of the heel pad. Hypercalcemia, if present, suggests the presence of hyperparathyroidism and the multiple endocrine neoplasia syndrome.

Differential Diagnosis

The clinical features of acromegaly are not readily confused with those of any other disease. Rather, one is more often confronted with the question of whether a patient's features (primarily facial and acral) are due to acromegaly or whether the disease may have been present at one time and is now inactive. Dynamic studies of GH secretion with more than one agent (glucose, TRH, GRH, or L-dopa) may be required to establish a diagnosis of "inactive" acromegaly. Gigantism during childhood has been reported to occur in the absence of GH hypersecretion (cerebral gigantism) and in some patients may be associated with increased somatomedin C production.

GH levels are elevated in patients with chronic renal failure, cirrhosis, starvation, anorexia nervosa, diabetes,[298] and protein-calorie malnutrition, and there is often a stimulatory response to TRH. Differential diagnosis presents no problem, however, because of the absence of the clinical features of acromegaly. Elevated levels of GH are also present in the Laron dwarf,[140] in whom there is a defect in somatomedin C production, though these children show clinical signs of GH deficiency rather than GH excess. GH responses to TRH are also seen in some tall adolescents,[299] but clinical features of acromegaly are not present and there is normal GH suppression with glucose.

Increased GH levels and features of acromegaly have been observed with central nervous system tumors (e.g., ependymomas of the third ventricle, hypothalamic hamartomas, intrapituitary gangliocytomas)[300,301] and in association with carcinoid and pancreatic islet tumors and small cell lung carcinomas.[278] Each of these tumors has been shown to secrete GRH ectopically, and tumor removal has often led to restoration of normal GH secretion. In those tumors secreting GRH into the systemic circulation, measurement of plasma GRH levels will confirm the diagnosis.[302] Although the frequency of ectopic GRH secretion as a cause for acromegaly is quite low ($<$ 1 percent),[303,304] the implications for therapy are sufficient to warrant a plasma GRH measurement in each newly diagnosed acromegalic patient. Plasma GRH levels are not elevated in patients with CNS or pituitary GRH-secreting tumors, as might be expected, since GRH is either secreted into the portal system or acts in a paracrine manner.

GH itself has been reported to be secreted ectopically, though rarely, by lung carcinomas,[305] carcinoid tumors,[306,307] and a pancreatic islet tumor,[308] alone or in combination with GRH. In only one report could acromegaly unequivocally be attributed to extrapituitary GH production.[308]

Pathogenesis of Acromegaly: Hypothalamic versus Pituitary Disease

Considerable uncertainty exists as to whether acromegaly is a primary pituitary disease due to de novo tumor formation or is of hypothalamic (or other CNS) origin, occurring as a consequence of excessive secretion of GRH or possibly decreased secretion of somatostatin (Fig. 8-17).

The evidence for a possible hypothalamic etiology is as follows:

1. GH secretion in most acromegalic patients is not autonomous but responds to stimuli mediated through the hypothalamus, such as glucose, insulin hypoglycemia, and arginine. This implies that the somatotrophs, even though neoplastic, are capable of responding to hypothalamic signals.
2. Nearly all GH-secreting pituitary tumors respond to GRH with normal to excessive GH secretion.
3. GH responses to glucose suppression and insulin stimulation, when examined following removal of a GH-secreting adenoma, generally remain abnormal, even when basal GH levels are normal.[309]
4. GH secretion in acromegaly is altered by neuropharmacologic agents (α-adrenergic antagonists and β-adrenergic agonists stimulate GH secretion)[310] believed to act within the CNS.
5. Some acromegalic subjects exhibit relative resistance to the inhibitory effects of somatostatin,[311] a phenomenon consistent with excessive stimulation by a releasing factor.
6. Most importantly, ectopic GRH secretion, whether from a pancreatic islet or carcinoid tumor with transport by the systemic circulation or from a pituitary tumor, results in not only GH overproduction but also somatotroph hyperplasia and eventually tumor formation. Thus, GRH acts not only as a releasing factor but also as a tropic factor.

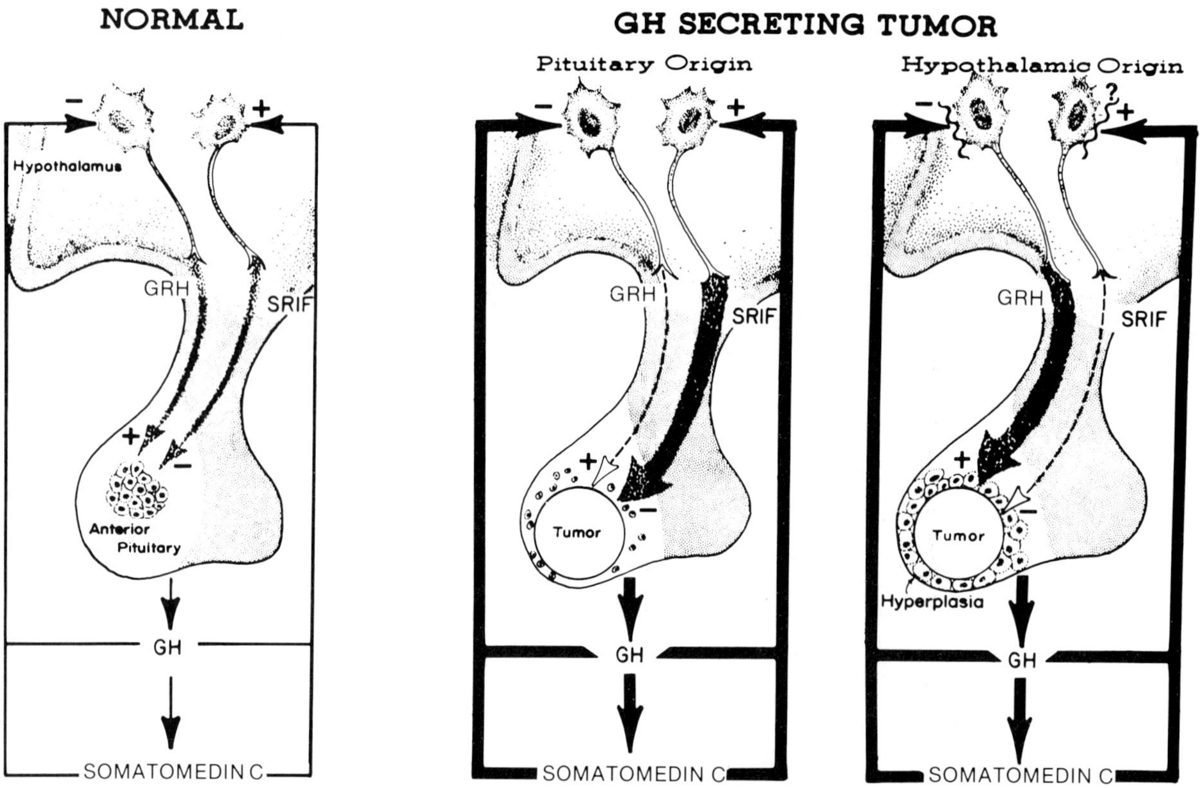

FIGURE 8-17 Possible neuroendocrine disturbances in the pathogenesis of GH-secreting pituitary tumors. (*Left*) Normal feedback regulation of GH secretion, which is mediated by GH alone or by some intermediate, possibly somatomedin C, and presumably involves both a stimulatory effect on somatostatin (SRIF) release and an inhibitory effect on GRH release. (*Middle*) Alterations which would occur if the pituitary tumor arose de novo. Enhanced GH secretion would lead to suppression of GRH and stimulation of SRIF release, resulting in hypofunction of the normal somatotrophs. It follows that the pituitary tumor must exhibit some resistance to the suppressive effects of SRIF for GH hypersecretion to occur. GH release in acromegaly is suppressed by exogenous SRIF, but the relative sensitivity as compared with normal subjects is not precisely known. (*Right*) Alterations which would occur with a hypothalamic etiology. The primary disturbance proposed is that of GRH hypersecretion leading to somatotroph hyperplasia and, eventually, tumor formation. Also implied are (1) an impairment of the negative feedback effect on GRH release and (2) a similar impairment of SRIF release or (3) a relative resistance to the effects of SRIF.

These arguments suggest a hypothalamic etiology for acromegaly and are consistent with the eventual development of an autonomous pituitary tumor.

The evidence that GH-secreting pituitary tumors may represent a primary pituitary disease is based on two observations: (1) in a few selected cases restoration not only of normal GH levels but of normal secretory responses to neurally mediated signals has been seen following complete excision of the tumor,[312] and (2) adenohypophyseal tissue surrounding the tumor, when examined histologically, does not appear to exhibit evidence of somatotroph hyperplasia.[313]

The conflicting nature of the available data does not permit a definitive conclusion at present. However, it is quite possible that two subgroups of acromegaly exist, with one being of hypothalamic and the other of pituitary origin. Detailed testing of patients before and for varying periods after tumor excision may permit distinction of these two groups, though specific and sensitive assays for circulating GRH and somatostatin of hypothalamic origin may be required for a definitive answer.

Therapy

Three forms of therapy can be used in patients with acromegaly: surgery, irradiation, and medical (pharmacologic) therapy. As in patients with nonfunctioning pituitary tumors, consideration must be given to the consequences of an expanding intracranial mass, to the need of preserving residual pituitary function, and to replacement therapy for hormone deficiencies. The presence of GH hypersecretion by the tumor does not alter the rationale for the therapy of pituitary tumors already presented. The present section is concerned primarily with the effectiveness of the various therapeutic modalities in reducing GH levels to normal and alleviating the clinical manifestations of hormone hypersecretion. The goals of therapy are to correct the metabolic disturbances, to reverse as much as possible the soft tissue changes, and to arrest the progression of the musculoskeletal complications. Slight regression of bony changes can occur, though this is relatively uncommon. The reduction of GH levels has been reported to improve existing cardiovascular disease in some but not all patients. Therapy of acromegaly does not at present depend on whether the disease is of pituitary or hypothalamic origin. However, prior to initiating therapy directed at the pituitary, consideration should be given to the possibility of an extrapituitary (carcinoid or pancreatic islet) GRH- or GH-secreting tumor, removal of which may reverse the GH hypersecretion.

SURGERY Surgical excision of GH-secreting tumors is a rapid and effective treatment for acromegaly. The surgical considerations, including the risks, are similar to those in nonfunctioning tumors, with the exception that once a diagnosis of acromegaly is established, surgical intervention is warranted even in the presence of only minimal radiographic findings. The success rate, which varies in different series, has been reported as high as 92 percent, using as criterion a reduction of plasma GH to normal levels.[313] Some variation in the definition of "normalization" of GH levels in the various reported series (10 ng/ml basal, 5 ng/ml basal, or 5 ng/ml after glucose) may explain some of the differences observed.[266,314,315] The success in restoring GH levels to normal is inversely related to the size of the tumor, with considerably less favorable results occurring with tumors greater than 2 cm or extending beyond the sella,[316] where complete removal of the tumor is not generally feasible. Although tumor size is not necessarily related to the level of circulating GH, the likelihood of normalization of plasma GH levels is substantially lower when the initial value is more than 40 ng/ml. Remission of clinical symptoms and metabolic alteration of acromegaly occur in nearly all patients in whom a moderate reduction of GH levels occurs. The rapidity with which these symptoms (e.g., diaphoresis and soft tissue swelling) remit is at times striking. However, these parameters do not always correlate with the degree of GH hypersecretion, and in some patients clinical features may disappear completely even with persistence of elevated GH levels. Thus, the levels of plasma GH are the most objective means of evaluating the effects of therapy. Tumor recurrence in patients whose GH levels have been normalized is infrequent (approximately 5 percent) and is almost always seen during the first year.[267,313,317] Postoperative testing with TRH may help define that subgroup of patients in whom the tumor is most likely to recur.[318] In the larger tumors where nearly the whole adenohypophysis may need to be removed for GH levels to revert to normal, it is preferable to leave sufficient residual tissue to retain anterior pituitary function and to treat the patient postoperatively with radiotherapy.

RADIATION THERAPY Two forms of external radiation are currently in use as primary therapy for acromegaly. Conventional (supervoltage) irradiation, available at most large medical centers, involves the use of 1 MeV or higher energy photon beams with radiation doses to the pituitary of 4000 to 5000 rads. Therapy is given in divided doses over a 4- to 6-week interval. Heavy-particle therapy (proton beam) provides a much higher energy particle (340 to 900 MeV), and a slightly greater dose of radiation (4500 to 6500 rads) can be delivered in a single treatment. Heavy-particle radiation is not indicated for tumors with more than minimal suprasellar extension because of the greater risk of damage to the optic nerves.

Improvement in clinical features and a reduction in GH levels is comparable with the two techniques, though GH is normalized in less than 20 percent of patients after 2 years. Additional improvement has been claimed with heavy-particle and conventional irradiation after 5 and 10 years,[319] with up to 70 percent of patients exhibiting GH levels < 5 ng/ml. However, the number of patients followed for this period of time is limited.

A direct comparison of irradiation with surgery for the treatment of GH-secreting tumors is difficult because of the differences in patient populations treated by each method, though the overall impression is that the two methods are comparable. The major difference is in the rapidity with which GH values are normalized and other anterior pituitary function lost. A comparison of the frequency of recurrence is also difficult because of the recent change in the size of the tumors being removed at surgery and the relatively shorter period of follow-up in most recent surgical series. The use of irradiation following surgical removal of GH-secreting tumors has been recommended as a means of decreasing the frequency of recurrence.[274] This suggestion should be followed whenever there is persistence of GH hypersecretion postoperatively. In those patients in whom GH levels return to normal following surgery, radiotherapy is probably unnecessary.

PHARMACOLOGIC THERAPY Pharmacologic therapy of acromegaly was initiated with the use of hormones which were presumed to act by antagonizing the peripheral effects of GH (estrogen) or by some incompletely defined action inhibiting the release of GH by the tumor (progesterone). Some regression of clinical features of the disease was occasionally seen, though most patients responded minimally if at all.

The observation that orally administered L-dopa acutely suppressed GH secretion in acromegaly[297] was followed by attempts to use the drug for chronic suppression. Partial suppression was achieved, though the drug's short duration of action and frequency of side effects at the doses required precluded its general acceptance. However, bromocriptine, an ergot derivative with strong dopamine agonist activity initially evaluated as a prolactin suppressant, was found to exhibit potent GH suppressive effects in acromegaly.[320] Although bromocriptine can cross the blood-brain barrier and exert central dopaminergic activity, its effects on GH secretion in acromegaly act directly on the tumor and are demonstrable in vitro.

The frequency with which acromegalic patients respond to bromocriptine or to a related drug, pergolide, with a reduction of GH to normal levels varies considerably in different series,[320–322] with the average range being 25 to 50 percent. The dose of bromocriptine varies from 2.5 to 15 mg per day given in two divided doses. Mild hypotensive symptoms and nausea (both due to central actions of the drug) are occasionally seen but generally disappear with time and can usually be prevented by initiating therapy with a small dose in the evening and gradually increasing the dose until the desired effect is achieved. Long-term experience with bromocriptine in a few patients indicates that it can be given for more than 10 years with continued effectiveness. Discontinuation of the drug is associated with return of GH hypersecretion, and therapy must therefore be continued indefinitely. Bromocriptine decreases the size of experimentally induced tumors in rats[323] and exhibits antitumor effects as well as hormone suppressive activity in acromegaly. However, at the present time there are no criteria for preselection of patients most likely to respond with the possible exception of concomitant prolactin hypersecretion. In mixed GH- and prolactin-secreting tumors, the suppression of prolactin secretion is not always accompanied by a reduction in GH levels. Overall, a reduction in tumor size can be expected in only about 25 percent of those patients whose GH levels have been normalized.[324]

Somatostatin has been shown to suppress GH secretion in acromegaly,[325] but the effects require continuous intravenous administration of the peptide. However, a recently synthesized octapeptide analogue of somatostatin, selective minisomatostatin (SMS 201-995), appears, in preliminary reports, to be effective in reducing GH levels to or near the normal range after subcutaneous administration three or four times a day and in improving the clinical manifestations of the disease.[326] Whether this agent has an effect on tumor size remains to be determined.

Thus, the current indications for pharmacologic therapy consist of those patients in whom surgery and/or radiation therapy has not restored GH levels to normal or in whom other forms of therapy are contraindicated.

Prolactin-Secreting Tumors: Amenorrhea-Galactorrhea Syndrome

The clinical manifestations of prolactin-secreting tumors were well recognized long before prolactin was identified as a separate hormone. Galactorrhea and amenorrhea were initially classified on the basis of whether they occurred during the postpartum period (Chiari-Frommel syndrome) or not (Ahumada-Del Castillo or Forbes-Albright syndrome). Long-term follow-up of both groups of patients, particularly the latter, revealed that a large percentage eventually developed signs of a pituitary tumor. With the development of the prolactin RIA, it was recognized not only that high levels of circulating prolactin were present in patients without demonstrable evidence of pituitary tumors but also that considerable numbers of patients with pituitary tumors and hyperprolactinemia did not exhibit galactorrhea. In fact, the incidence of elevated prolactin levels in pituitary adenomas ranges from 60 to 80 percent and is higher than that of any other pituitary hormone. The finding of unexplained hyperprolactinemia in a patient with amenorrhea, menstrual irregularity, or infertility in the absence of anatomic evidence of a pituitary tumor (idiopathic hyperprolactinemia) is increasingly common today.

Prolactin-secreting pituitary tumors often appear chromophobic with routine stains, which is why most pituitary tumors were originally believed to be nonfunctioning. With immunohistochemical staining techniques, prolactin can be demonstrated in almost all these tumors.[277]

Signs and Symptoms

Women with hyperprolactinemia present with galactorrhea, abnormalities of menstrual function, or infertility. The development of galactorrhea requires the presence of gonadal steroids as well as prolactin and therefore is not necessarily seen in all patients. It commonly occurs in association with oral contraceptives, either during their use or, more frequently, following their discontinuation. It is believed that the sudden decrease in estrogen and progesterone levels in a patient whose breasts have been prepared by the combination of gonadal steroids and hyperprolactinemia is responsible for the onset of galactorrhea, as occurs physiologically in the immediate postpartum period. The incidence of galactorrhea in patients with prolactin-secreting pituitary tumors varies from 50 to 90 percent[327–329] and reflects the changing spectrum of hyperprolactinemia caused by earlier recognition of the disorder.

Amenorrhea or oligomenorrhea with loss of normal cyclicity occurs in 60 to 90 percent of women with hyperprolactinemia and in nearly all with radiologic evidence of a pituitary tumor. The order of appearance of amenorrhea and galactorrhea can vary, with either symptom preceding the other by months to years. Hyperprolactinemia could interfere with the normal hypothalamic-pituitary-ovarian axis at three locations. First, prolactin suppresses progesterone production by ovarian granulosa cells.[330] However, the ovary of the hyperprolactinemic woman is capable of responding to exogenous gonadotropins, suggesting that ovarian function is intact. Second, prolactin could act within the pituitary to suppress the gonadotropin response to GnRH. This is unlikely, since numerous studies have demonstrated normal or increased gonadotropin responses to GnRH in hyperprolactinemic women.[331,332] Finally, hyperprolactinemia inhibits the ultradian secretion of LH, which requires a pulsatile release of endogenous GnRH.[333] It also inhibits the positive feedback response of exogenous estrogen on gonadotropin secretion[334,335] and possibly the negative feedback response as well. Thus, the most likely explanation for the hypogonadism of hyperprolactinemia is a derangement of hypothalamic GnRH secretion due either to an effect of prolactin itself or more likely to enhanced tuberoinfundibular dopaminergic tone secondary to the enhanced prolactin secretion (see below). In addition to anovulation, patients with hyperprolactinemia usually exhibit hypoestrogenemia accompanied by a decrease in vaginal secretion and dyspareunia, which may be responsible for a diminished libido. Many women with hyperprolactinemia have also noted mild hirsutism accompanied by an increase in dehydroepiandrosterone sulfate production by the adrenals.[336] Elevations of plasma free testosterone also occur and are attributed to decreased testosterone (estrogen)-binding globulin.[337] Decrease in bone density is present, though there is controversy as to whether it is caused by hypoestrogenemia or is an independent effect of hyperprolactinemia.[338,339]

The major clinical features of hyperprolactinemia in men are impotence and loss of libido and performance.[340] Prolactin-secreting tumors in men are usually quite large by the time medical attention is sought, unlike those in women, in whom the features of hyperprolactinemia often occur in the presence of microadenomas. Both gynecomastia and galactorrhea may be seen in men, though these findings are uncommon. Testosterone levels are uniformly depressed, and, as in women, the defect lies within the hypothalamus, since Leydig cell function, when tested by HCG administration, is normal, as are the pituitary LH and FSH responses to GnRH. The absence of a rise in LH in the presence of low testosterone levels under these conditions points to a defect in endogenous GnRH secretion analogous to the findings in women. Impotence is in part related to factors other than decreased testosterone production, since testosterone replacement therapy alone is often ineffective in restoring potency.[340] Oligospermia is also seen in some but not all hyperprolactinemic men.[336,341,342] Reduction of prolactin levels to the normal range usually restores both libido and sperm counts to normal.[342]

Laboratory Studies

Plasma prolactin levels in patients with prolactin-secreting tumors vary from just above the upper limit of normal (15 to 20 ng/ml) to values greater than 10,000 ng/ml. Prolactin levels greater than 200 ng/ml are almost always indicative of a pituitary tumor. Repeated sampling in individual patients reveals considerable variation in prolactin levels, suggesting, as in acromegaly, intermittent hormone secretion by the tumor. Since prolactin is a stress-responsive hormone, two or three separate plasma samples should be obtained for prolactin determination to confirm pathologic hyperprolactinemia.

Dynamic studies of prolactin secretion have revealed several differences between normal subjects and patients with tumors but are not generally useful in distinguishing between pituitary tumors and other causes of hyperprolactinemia. Prolactin responses to TRH in patients with prolactin-secreting tumors are decreased on a percentage basis when compared to normal persons. The absolute responses in tumor patients, however, may be absent or may be indistinguishable from normal responses. The explanation for the impaired response, when present, is that the tumor is secreting at maximal capacity and cannot be further stimulated or that TRH receptors are decreased in the neoplastic lactotrophs.

The prolactin response to dopamine receptor blockers is almost always reduced or absent in patients with tumors. This impaired response is not a consequence of hyperprolactinemia, since normal to enhanced responses are seen in postpartum hyperprolactinemic women.[343] Since agents excluded from the CNS (e.g., metoclopramide) and those with CNS activity (e.g., chlorpromazine and haloperidol) give similar results, the site of the abnormal response must be at or beyond the lactotroph dopamine receptor. The absence of an increase in prolactin therefore suggests that the tumor is not responding to the suppressive signal (dopamine) or that the signal itself is decreased or absent. The lack of prolactin response to dopamine antagonists, however, is also found in patients with hypothalamic disorders and is not of diagnostic help. L-Dopa and dopamine suppress prolactin secretion in most patients with pituitary tumors to an extent similar to that in normal subjects,[331,344] though in occasional patients no suppression is observed.[345] Unfortunately, the patients in whom the most clearly abnormal responses to all three agents are observed are those with markedly elevated prolactin values and with unmistakable radiologic evidence of a pituitary tumor, whereas in patients with only moderately elevated levels (less than 100 ng/ml) and normal radiologic findings, the responses are generally inconclusive.

Administration of L-dopa combined with the dopa-decarboxylase inhibitor carbidopa results in an inhibition of peripheral dopa decarboxylation and an enhanced uptake of L-dopa by the CNS. In normal subjects and in postpartum hyperprolactinemia, the persistence of prolactin suppression by the combination of these agents indicates a CNS-mediated suppressive action of L-dopa. In contrast, prolactin suppression is markedly attenuated in patients with prolactin-secreting tumors, suggesting a loss of the cental L-dopa effect.[344] However, patients with idiopathic hyperprolactinemia exhibit responses similar to those in patients with tumors.

The histamine H_2-receptor antagonist cimetidine increases prolactin secretion in normal subjects by an action involving the CNS[157] and linked to the histamine receptor.[158] Most patients with prolactinomas do not respond to cimetidine, but neither do patients with idiopathic hyperprolactinemia.[157] Nomifensine, an inhibitor of dopamine reuptake by synaptosomes, inhibits prolactin secretion in normal women and in postpartum hyperprolactinemia but in only a minority of patients with idiopathic hyperprolactinemia or prolactin-secreting tumors.[346,347]

Evidence for resistance to the prolactin-lowering effects of dopamine has now been reported by several groups in patients with hyperprolactinemia and prolactinomas but not in patients with hypothalamic disorders.[348,349]

Thus, several agents are capable of distinguishing between known hypothalamic disease and suspected prolactinomas, but none can reliably separate prolactinomas from idiopathic hyperprolactinemia. Since current therapeutic options do not require this distinction to be made, the use of stimulation/suppression tests has generally been discontinued.

Differential Diagnosis

It is likely that prolactin-secreting tumors are present in most patients with persistent elevation of prolactin levels without another explanation. An unequivocal diagnosis of a prolactin-secreting tumor requires neuroradiologic evidence of a tumor as well as hyperprolactinemia, and this is found with the greatest frequency in those patients with the most pronounced elevations of prolactin values. In patients with prolactin levels greater than 200 ng/ml, CT examination almost always provides evidence of a tumor. With levels of less than 200 ng/ml, radiologic findings may be nondiagnostic, though many patients previously considered to have idiopathic hyperprolactinemia on the basis of polytomography are today recognized by CT scan as having prolactinomas. The terms *microadenoma* and *macroadenoma* have frequently appeared in the literature in relation to prolactin-secreting tumors and in a general sense refer to estimates of pituitary tumor size based on neuroradiologic studies. These terms are unfortunately imprecise and are used differently by various authors; they are being redefined as newer and more sophisticated neuroradiologic procedures detect smaller areas of abnormality within the sella turcica. At present, the commonly accepted definition of a microadenoma is a tumor less than 1 cm in diameter and entirely intrasellar in location.

In the patient with hyperprolactinemia who does not exhibit radiographic evidence of a pituitary tumor, other causes must be considered (Table 8-10). Careful questioning may uncover a history of ingestion of drugs which can cause hyperprolactinemia. These drugs include primarily agents affecting central dopamine regulation or estrogen-containing medications. The most common drugs in use today include psychotropic dopamine receptor antagonists (phenothiazines, butyrophenones, thioxanthenes) and tricyclic antidepressants, antihypertensives (α-methyldopa, reserpine), phenothiazine antihistaminics (meclizine) and antiemetics (metoclopramide, prochlorperazine), and oral contraceptives. Galactorrhea has also been reported in heroin addicts and may be caused by stimulation of CNS enkephalin receptors.

Table 8-10. Differential Diagnosis of Hyperprolactinemia

Prolactin-secreting pituitary tumor
Pharmacologic agents:
Monoamine synthesis inhibitors (α-methyldopa)
Monoamine depletors (reserpine)
Dopamine receptor antagonists (phenothiazines, butyrophenones, thioxanthenes
Monoamine uptake inhibitors (tricyclic antidepressants)
Estrogens (oral contraceptives)
Narcotics (morphine, heroin)
Central nervous system disorders:
Inflammatory/infiltrative (sarcoidosis, histiocytosis)
Traumatic (stalk section)
Neoplastic (hypothalamic or parasellar tumors)
Other:
Hypothyroidism
Renal failure
Cirrhosis
Autoimmune or granulomatous hypophysitis
Chest wall diseases
Spinal cord lesions
Empty sella
Idiopathic hyperprolactinemia

Primary disorders of the CNS which interfere with the integrity of the hypothalamic-pituitary axis can also proclude hyperprolactinemia by decreasing the inhibitory CNS influence on prolactin secretion. Hyperprolactinemia and galactorrhea are occasionally seen in association with such granulomatous lesions of the hypothalamus as occur in sarcoidosis. The abnormalities generally respond to treatment with anti-inflammatory agents. Infiltrative disorders such as eosinophilic granuloma are often associated with hyperprolactinemia. Other evidence of hypothalamic dysfunction usually includes diabetes insipidus, which is rare in small pituitary tumors. Head injuries associated with basal skull fractures or penetrating wounds can cause trauma to the pituitary stalk leading to hyperprolactinemia. Similarly, parasellar tumors (meningiomas, optic gliomas, craniopharyngiomas) or tumors arising within the hypothalamus (ependymomas) can produce hyperprolactinemia along with evidence of hypopituitarism.

Patients with nonfunctioning pituitary macroadenomas may also exhibit hyperprolactinemia, usually less than 100 ng/ml. In some, suprasellar extension of the tumor with compression of the stalk or hypothalamus can explain the findings, while in others such an explanation is lacking. While it is always possible that a few prolactin-secreting cells may have escaped detection, an alternative explanation is that the tumor may have so altered intrapituitary blood flow as to eliminate the normal hypothalamic inhibitory tone. Clearly, such tumors should not be considered prolactinomas.

Patients with hypothyroidism frequently exhibit breast tenderness and, on occasion, galactorrhea. While prolactin levels are usually normal, they may be elevated, though rarely to more than 100 ng/ml. With long-standing hypothyroidism pituitary enlargement may occur and lead to the erroneous diagnosis of a pituitary tumor. In contrast to prolactin-secreting tumors, the prolactin response to TRH is increased in hypothyroidism.

Prolactin levels are increased in 60 to 70 percent of patients with chronic renal failure to values as high as 150 ng/ml. The prolactin response to TRH is impaired, but L-dopa and dopamine are ineffective in decreasing prolactin levels acutely, suggesting a receptor or postreceptor defect in the lactotroph.[159] These abnormalities, as well as the hyperprolactinemia, are unaltered by hemodialysis but are reversed by renal transplantation.

Hyperprolactinemia of two to three times normal levels has been observed in cirrhosis, particularly in patients with hepatic encephalopathy,[350] and has been attributed to the presence of false neurotransmitters, which have also been implicated in other CNS manifestations of the disease.

Galactorrhea and hyperprolactinemia can be seen following spinal cord lesions and injuries to the chest wall (burns, thoracic incisions, herpes zoster) involving the fourth to sixth intercostal nerves, stimulation of which produces nonpuerperal lactation.[351,352] Anesthesia of the intercostal nerves will suppress the prolactin levels and frequently the lactation.[352]

If none of the above disorders is present and there is no history of drug ingestion, the patient with elevated prolactin levels and a normal CT scan is considered to have idiopathic hyperprolactinemia. This disorder is often seen after discontinuation of oral contraceptives or for prolonged periods in the postpartum state. Galactorrhea may or may not be present. The differentiation between a "functional" disorder and an occult prolactin-secreting tumor is often difficult or impossible at this stage. Long-term follow-up of the patients has indicated that the vast majority remain unchanged or have a return of prolactin levels to normal, while only a small fraction (5 to 10 percent) exhibit increasing prolactin values or develop radiologic evidence of a tumor.[353–355] At the present time, there are no reliable means of distinguishing those patients who will show progression of their disease. Thus, continued observation for more than a decade may be required in some.

In those patients with galactorrhea who have normal prolactin levels, dynamic studies of prolactin secretion are usually normal, the likelihood of pituitary tumor is small, and continued ovulatory menstrual cycles and normal fertility can be predicted. This group of patients probably represents the most common type of nonpuerperal galactorrhea, termed *normoprolactinemic galactorrhea,* which is probably due to an enhanced sensitivity of the breast to normal circulating prolactin levels. This form of galactorrhea is commonly seen as a persistence of postpartum galactorrhea or following discontinuation of oral contraceptives.

Pathogenesis of Prolactin-Secreting Tumors: Hypothalamic vs. Pituitary Disease

There is general agreement that CNS (hypothalamic) dysfunction is probably responsible for the hyperprolactinemia seen following discontinuation of oral contraceptives and that persisting for excessive time periods in the postpartum state. Idiopathic hyperprolactinemia has also been attributed to an alteration of hypothalamic-pituitary dopaminergic mechanisms.[356] Whether the dopaminergic defect is in the hypothalamic tuberoinfundibular system or at the lactotroph receptors and whether a separate nondopaminergic abnormality exists are areas of disagreement (Fig. 8-18).

A hypothalamic etiology is supported by the following evidence:

1. The altered responses to dopamine receptor antagonists, to dopa decarboxylase inhibitors, and to dopamine reuptake inhibitors—all previously used to support the hypothesis of decreased central dopaminergic tone—could all be explained on the basis of lactotroph dopamine resistance with increased dopaminergic tone; evidence for the latter has now appeared on the basis of enhanced LH and TSH responses to dopamine receptor antagonists in hyperprolactinemic patients.[357,358] In addition, lactotroph dopamine insensitivity has been shown in vivo.[348,349] Since tumor tissue dopamine receptor and dopamine-binding capacity and affinity are unaltered when studied in vitro,[359,360] some type of extrapituitary factor that stimulates prolactin release, thereby antagonizing the effects of dopamine, must be postulated. Such a prolactin releasing factor has been proposed on the basis of animal studies, and two possible candidates are vasoactive intestinal peptide and PHM, both of which appear to play physiologic roles in prolactin secretion.[152,361]
2. Persistence of abnormalities related to dopaminergic regulation postoperatively in patients whose basal prolactin levels have returned to normal[362,363] argues for a continuation of the pathogenic mechanism even though the specific adenoma is no longer present.
3. Administration of bromocriptine to normal subjects produces a decrease in circulating dopamine, norepinephrine, and epinephrine levels through a CNS-mediated mechanism, whereas in patients with prolactin-secreting tumors, no decrease is observed either preoperatively or possibly postoperatively following reduction of prolactin levels to normal.[364] Thus, although hyperprolactinemia causes alteration of hypothalamic dopamine turnover,[365] abnormalities in central dopaminergic function appear to be in part independent of hyperprolactinemia.
4. Lactotroph hyperplasia has been found in up to one-third of patients with prolactin-secreting adenomas, supporting the hypothesis that a hyperfunctional disorder eventually leads to tumor formation.[366]
5. Prolactin-releasing activity has been described in the serum of patients with prolactin-secreting tumors.[367] The activity has been reported to be peptide in nature, but its identity is unknown.
6. Most importantly, there are several reports of recurrence of prolactinomas in 17 to 50 percent of patients previously considered cured.[368–370] Although recurrence is defined primarily as hyperprolactinemia

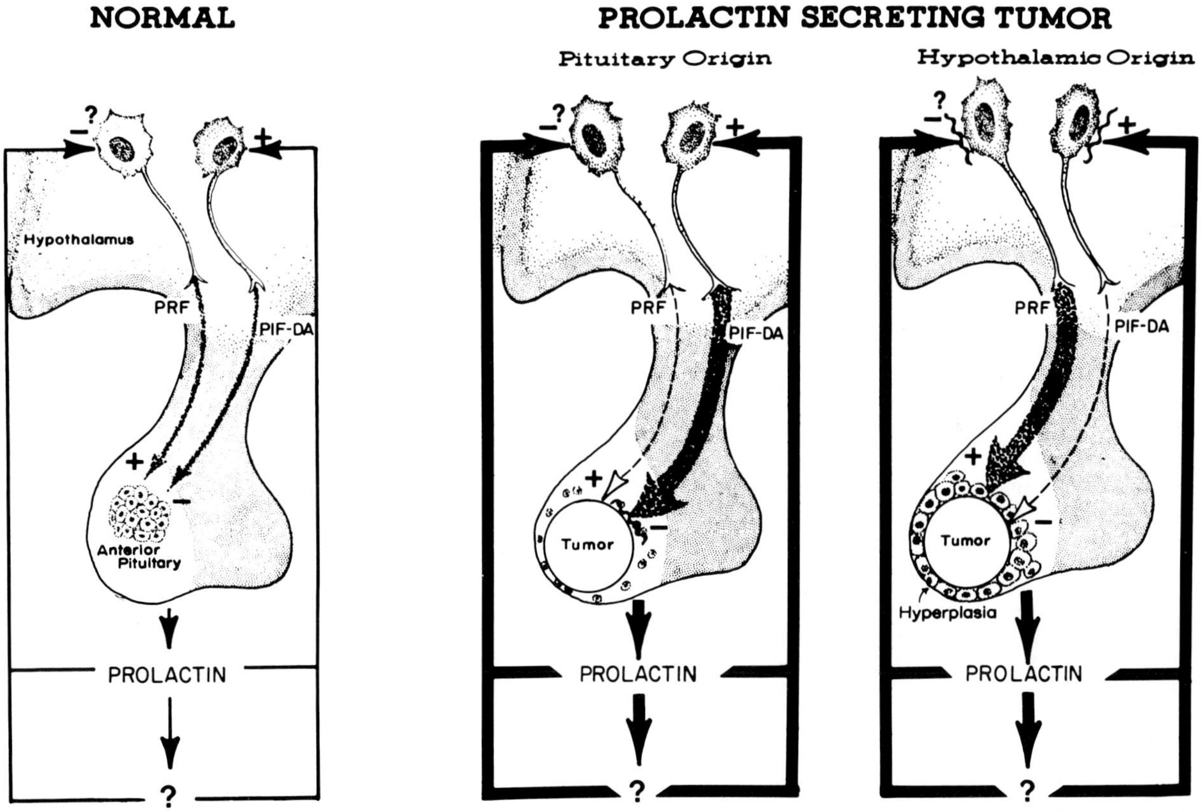

FIGURE 8-18 Possible neuroendocrine disturbances in the pathogenesis of prolactin-secreting pituitary tumors. (*Left*) Normal feedback regulation of prolactin secretion, which is mediated by prolactin itself or by some yet undefined intermediary and involves a stimulatory effect on dopamine (DA) and/or a separate prolactin inhibiting factor (PIF) and an inhibitory effect on a prolactin releasing factor (PRF). (*Middle*) Alterations which would occur if the pituitary tumor arose de novo. Increased prolactin secretion would lead to suppression of PRF and stimulation of DA-PIF, resulting in hypofunction of the normal lactotrophs. It follows that the pituitary tumor must exhibit some resistance to the suppressive effects of DA or PIF for prolactin hypersecretion to occur. Since prolactin-secreting tumors respond normally to exogenous dopaminergic suppression, this model would require that PIF be distinct from DA. (*Right*) Alterations which would occur with a hypothalamic etiology. The primary disturbance proposed is that of PRF hypersecretion or of DA-PIF hyposecretion leading to lactotroph hyperplasia and eventually tumor formation. Also implied are (1) an impairment of the negative feedback effect on PRF release and (2) a similar impairment of DA-PIF release or (3) a relative resistance to the effects of PIF.

rather than tumor mass reappearance, it again suggests a persistence of the pathogenic process.

The major evidence favoring a pituitary etiology is that following successful removal of microadenomas, prolactin secretion returns to normal, cyclic menses resume, and fertility is restored. It can thus be argued that reversal of the hyperprolactinemic state corrects the abnormalities related to gonadotropin secretion which were secondary changes. There are, however, only a few reports of detailed neuropharmacologic studies of prolactin secretion in postoperative patients with normal prolactin levels in which dopaminergic mechanisms appear to be restored to normal.[240,371,372] It has been argued that suppression of prolactin secretion by bromocriptine reverses the clinical syndrome, thereby proving that interruption of hyperprolactinemia at the pituitary level corrects the pathophysiologic process. However, this does not necessarily argue against a primary CNS process and, furthermore, bromocriptine also exerts significant effects within the CNS.

Thus, most of the evidence based on neuropharmacologic and epidemiologic studies favors a hypothalamic etiology for the disorder. However, the question cannot be completely answered at this time and will require detailed study and prolonged follow-up of patients after various types of therapy. It is possible that some prolactin-secreting tumors will be found to arise de novo while others will be shown to be secondary to altered hypothalamic influence. The latter possibility implies that a hyperplastic process may represent only an interim stage of autonomous tumor formation.

Therapy

The therapy of prolactin-secreting tumors remains an area of controversy. Because of the accumulating information available concerning the natural history of the disease, the recurrence rate following surgery, the risks to the patient of no treatment or of conservative management, and intercurrent pregnancy, separate therapeutic plans have been developed for macroadenomas, microadenomas, and idiopathic hyperprolactinemia, which consider the risk/benefit ratio for each entity.

Continued follow-up of untreated patients with idiopathic hyperprolactinemia indicates that only a small percentage will develop identifiable tumors over a 5- to 10-year period and that only a few patients with microadenomas will show an increase in tumor size over the same period of time.[353-355] In contrast, macroadenomas, once identified, can be expected to increase in size, sometimes quite rapidly; thus treatment of macroadenomas should not be delayed. The aggressive treatment of microadenomas to prevent macroadenoma formation is clearly not justified, even though at present it is not possible to identify those microadenomas which will enlarge.

A major concern to patients with prolactinomas is tumor enlargement during pregnancy. An extensive review of the risks of pregnancy in patients with prolactinomas indicates that the probability of symptomatic enlargement of microadenomas is only 3 to 5 percent and that the affected patients respond to pharmacologic treatment.[373] In contrast, patients with macroadenomas have a 22 percent chance of symptomatic tumor expansion during pregnancy, thus some form of antitumor therapy is indicated before pregnancy occurs.

The risk of sustained hyperprolactinemia to the nonpregnant patient has also been recently reevaluated. While initial considerations were limited to infertility or severe galactorrhea, it is now recognized that hyperprolactinemia may be associated with diminished libido in women as well as in men and, more importantly, that hypoestrogenemia, or possibly hyperprolactinemia itself, may represent a risk factor for subsequent development of osteoporosis.[338,339]

Therapeutic decisions are consequently based on the premises that (1) macroadenomas should be treated for the same indications as nonfunctioning tumors, i.e., the tumor mass should be excised or reduced before normal tissue is destroyed; (2) hyperprolactinemia should be corrected to restore normal gonadal function; and (3) an overall treatment plan involving pharmacotherapy, surgery, and/or irradiation should be established and carefully discussed with the patient.

MACROADENOMAS Therapy of macroadenomas was, until recently, approached in the same manner as that of nonfunctioning tumors. However, during the past decade it has become evident that pharmacotherapy with bromocriptine results not only in lowering of prolactin levels but, in many patients, decreases in tumor size. As a result, bromocriptine administration is gaining increasing acceptance as primary therapy. Its use in conjunction with surgery and irradiation is discussed below.

Pharmacologic Therapy For the past 12 years, pharmacologic therapy of prolactinomas has centered around one drug, bromocriptine (2α-bromoergocriptine), an ergot derivative with potent agonist activity on both pituitary and brain dopamine receptors.[374] Other ergot derivatives have been used in other countries and experimentally in the United States; pergolide and lisuride have also been shown to be effective.[322,375] Bromocriptine binds to the dopamine receptor with 5 to 10 times greater affinity than dopamine, has a long half-life in plasma, and is effective when administered every 8 to 12 h. The most marked effect of bromocriptine is in decreasing prolactin levels to subnormal values in normal subjects and into the normal range in patients with prolactinomas, at times representing a more than 99 percent decrease in prolactin secretion. The effects are rapid in onset (1 to 2 h) and the rate of fall is exponential, i.e., the greatest decrease in prolactin levels occurs at the start of therapy and normalization may take weeks or months. Virtually all patients with prolactinomas will respond to the prolactin-lowering effects, though the dose required varies from 5 to 20 mg per day. The biologic half-life of bromocriptine is similar to its plasma half-life. Discontinuation of the drug is followed in nearly all patients by a return of hyperprolactinemia, though in some, not to the initial values. Galactorrhea is eliminated or improved in many patients, even if prolactin levels remain slightly elevated. Similarly, cyclic menses and fertility may be restored without complete normalization of prolactin levels. The drug is also used for interruption of postpartum lactation.

Therapy is initiated with 1.25 mg given at bedtime, and the dose is increased at 3- to 4-day intervals to minimize the symptoms of nausea, vomiting, and postural hypotension which may otherwise occur. In most patients these side effects disappear within a few days, though in some they persist and in a few may preclude continued use of the drug.

The dose should be increased until the desired effect is achieved or side effects become the limiting factor. Patients should be advised concerning the restoration of fertility, and mechanical contraception should be used, if appropriate, to prevent pregnancy. On the basis of experience with more than 1000 patients, bromocriptine appears not to be teratogenic in humans. The frequency of fetal loss and of congenital malformation in infants of women receiving bromocriptine at the time of conception is not increased.[376] Nevertheless, women who become pregnant should be advised to discontinue the drug. Bromocriptine is equally effective in decreasing prolactin levels in men with prolactinomas and, as a result, in restoration of normal testosterone levels, libido, and potency. Treatment of such patients with testosterone alone, without reducing prolactin levels to normal, may be insufficient to restore sexual function.[340]

Of even greater importance is the antitumor effect of bromocriptine, which was initially not appreciated. Bromocriptine produces tumor shrinkage in 60 to 75 percent of prolactinomas, with size reduction averaging 50 to 70 percent.[375,377,378] The onset of action is extremely rapid, with effects apparent within 48 h, as manifested by improvement in visual fields. Size reduction may at times be dramatic. Large suprasellar tumor components may disappear, and a partial empty sella may even occur (Fig. 8-19). Histologic examination of bromocriptine-treated adenomas re-

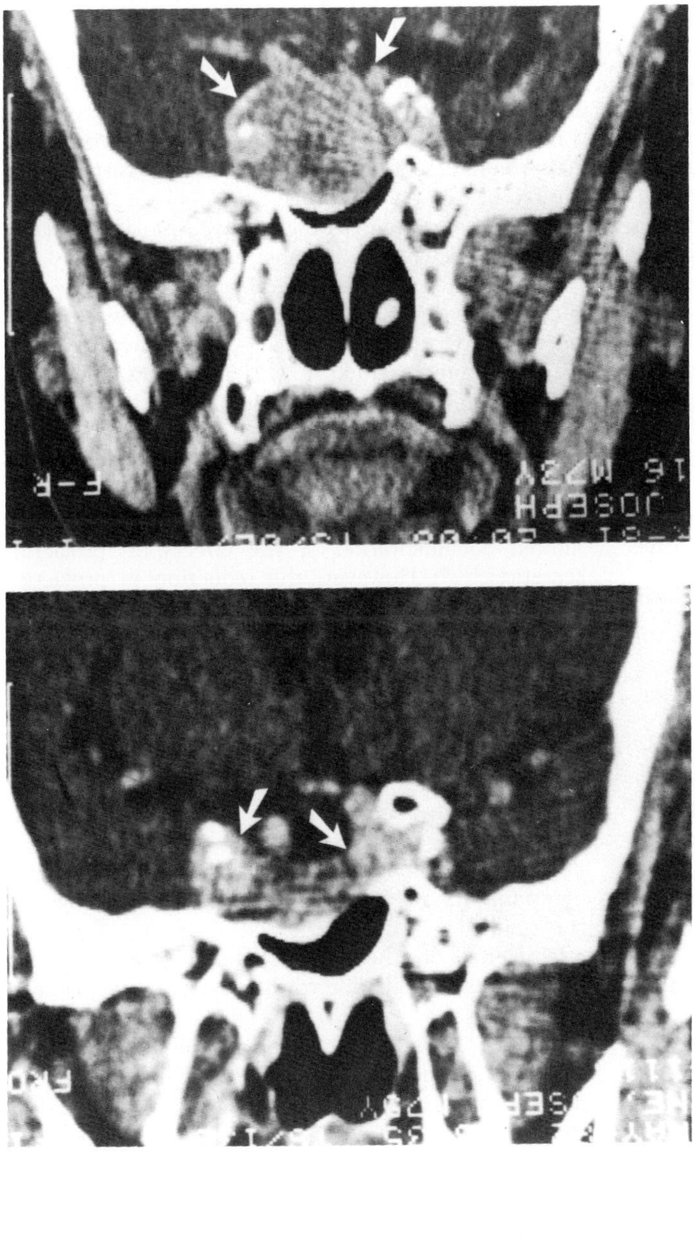

FIGURE 8-19 Effect of bromocriptine on reduction of prolactinoma size. (*Upper panel*) Pretreatment scan of a large macroadenoma with extensive suprasellar extension. (*Lower panel*) Effect of 1-year treatment. The upper border of the tumor is indicated by the arrows. (*From Molitch et al.*[378])

veals a decrease in both nuclear and cytoplasmic size, reduction in prolactin storage granules, and other changes indicative of a reduction of cell metabolic activity.[379] With long-term treatment, cytolysis has been noted in some tumors.[380] Although escape from the drug's effects does not occur even after many years, discontinuation of the drug may lead to rapid reexpansion of tumor size, particularly with short treatment periods. Therapy can be maintained for many years, often at doses lower than initially required.[375] After several years of therapy, most patients will not exhibit tumor reexpansion after discontinuation of therapy, though hyperprolactinemia often recurs.[381] Drug efficacy in reducing prolactin levels does not necessarily predict tumor size reduction: tumor shrinkage is seen even when prolactin levels are not normalized, and normalization of prolactin levels is not invariably accompanied by a decrease in size. Tumors most likely to respond are those which have the highest prolactin levels and which are not combined prolactin- and GH-secreting tumors. The macroadenoma with only modest hyperprolactinemia (less than 100 ng/ml) is less likely to exhibit size reduction. Histologic examination of such tumors often reveals moderate cystic or hemorrhagic changes and relatively few prolactin-secreting lactotrophs.

Surgical Therapy Prior to the availability of bromocriptine, surgical treatment of prolactinomas was the therapy of choice. Since bromocriptine is not curative, its use in the macroadenoma patient is still considered by some as only initial therapy, and surgical excision of the tumor is recommended, except when contraindicated for other reasons. It is currently believed that reduction in tumor size by preoperative use of bromocriptine will improve the surgical success rate,[382] though the hypothesis remains to be rigorously tested. The results of preoperative treatment of microadenomas with bromocriptine are still controversial, with some but not all reports suggesting that the drug causes the shrunken tumor to adhere to adjacent normal pituitary tissue,[382–385] making total removal more difficult. This has been noted primarily in the larger microadenomas and after 12 months of therapy. A prospective study is needed to resolve this issue.

The vast majority of macroadenomas can be resected by the transsphenoidal approach. Many adenomas can readily be dissected away from the surrounding tissue. After the tumor is excised, the application of alcohol to the tumor bed for a few seconds is believed by some to help destroy any residual tumor cells. There are, however, considerable numbers of tumors, particularly those greater than 10 mm in size, which cannot be clearly separated from the surrounding pituitary tissue, which contain necrotic or hemorrhagic centers, or which are cystic in nature. The cyst may even communicate with the subarachnoid space and give the appearance of a partially empty sella.

The frequency of surgical cure, defined as a return of prolactin levels to the normal range or the spontaneous resumption of menses, varies greatly between series, owing to a difference both in the selection of patients and in surgical technique. It is generally agreed that the smaller tumors (less than 10 mm in size or with preoperative prolactin levels of less than 200 ng/ml) yield the best results.[239,240,386] Cure rates as high as 94 percent have been described in this group,[240] although most series are somewhat lower. With the larger tumors, the outcome is less favorable, with only 20 to 30 percent of patients exhibiting a return of prolactin to normal levels, even though reductions of 70 to 80 percent are commonly seen. It is not uncommon for the entire tumor to appear to be removed, only to have the postoperative prolactin value remain elevated. Whether this represents residual or multicentric tumor, surrounding hyperplasia, or altered blood flow to normal lactotrophs is frequently difficult to determine. Residual hyperprolactinemia is readily corrected with bromocriptine.

The use of postoperative radiation is generally not recommended for small adenomas on the basis of postoperative hyperprolactinemia but is rather reserved for those tumors which show signs of invasiveness or which have been incompletely removed.

Radiotherapy Primary treatment of prolactin-secreting tumors with external radiation has received less attention than has surgery, and there is consequently limited documentation of the effects on prolactin secretion.[329,387] However, the reduction in prolactin levels occurs more slowly and less completely than after surgery. Radiotherapy has been suggested as an alternative to surgery in patients with hyperprolactinemia and minimal radiologic abnormalities of the sella who desire to become pregnant, prior to institution of pharmacotherapy.[388] The risk of tumor expansion during pregnancy in patients with clinically evident prolactin-secreting tumors who do not receive prior therapy provides a rationale for this procedure,[389] though long-term follow-up will be required to determine its ultimate value. Concern for damage to the residual normal anterior pituitary as well as the effectiveness of other forms of therapy has tended to limit the use of radiation to the postoperative patient.

MICROADENOMAS The basic principles in devising a therapeutic rationale for macroadenomas apply to microadenomas, except that the lesser concern for tumor expansion dictates a more conservative approach. Thus, while the immediate results of surgical treatment of this tumor type are generally excellent, it is now evident that almost all patients can be treated effectively with bromocriptine. Evidence for shrinkage of microprolactinomas has been shown by high-resolution CT scanning,[390] and the risk of tumor expansion during pregnancy is extremely low (3 to 5 percent).[373] Bromocriptine can be discontinued after several years in selected patients without resumption of hyperprolactinemia,[391] though the frequency with which this occurs is not yet known.

IDIOPATHIC HYPERPROLACTINEMIA The management of idiopathic hyperprolactinemia is pharmacologic. Bromocriptine should be used at the lowest possible dose that maintains normal prolactin levels and the drug withdrawn on a yearly basis to determine whether hyperprolactinemia recurs.

ACTH-Secreting Tumors: Cushing's Disease

The association of bilateral adrenocortical hyperplasia and the clinical features of hypercortisolism with pituitary adenomas was first described by Cushing.[392] The small size of the tumors and the infrequency with which they were detected at the time patients presented with signs and symptoms of adrenal hyperplasia resulted in attention being focused on the adrenal cortex as the site of the primary disease. On the basis of the results obtained with transsphenoidal surgery, it is now accepted that ACTH-secreting pituitary tumors coexist in nearly all patients with adrenal cortical hyperplasia (Cushing's disease). The appearance of pituitary tumors following bilateral adrenalectomy in patients with Cushing's disease was first described by Nelson et al., who demonstrated increased ACTH activity in plasma and postulated that an ACTH-secreting tumor could develop as a consequence of adrenalectomy.[393] At the same time, the demonstration of a variety of neuroendocrine disturbances in patients with Cushing's disease and the nature of the pituitary hormonal responses to neuropharmacologic agents have raised the possibility that the disease is of CNS origin.

Pituitary tumors in patients with Cushing's disease and Nelson's syndrome may exhibit basophilic staining (about 80 percent) or may be chromophobic. It is now known that the 31,000-dalton ACTH precursor is a glycoprotein and that the capacity of tumor cells to stain with basic dyes is dependent on the presence of this glycoprotein. With the use of immunohistochemical stains, both basophilic and chromophobic tumors can be shown to contain ACTH. In addition, β-LPH and β-endorphin may be present in tumor tissue and circulation of patients with ACTH-producing tumors.

Basophilic adenomas are found in about 5 percent of pituitaries at autopsy in patients without evidence of ACTH hypersecretion during life. Nonfunctioning tumors of this type may biosynthesize ACTH which is never released and undergoes intracellular (lysosomal) degradation, possibly owing to a defect in the secretory mechanism of the tumor cell.[230] ACTH-secreting tumors are usually benign. However, in contrast to other tumors of anterior pituitary origin, ACTH-secreting tumors can exhibit true malignant potential on rare occasions and metastasize both within and outside the CNS.[394,395] Mixed ACTH and prolactin-secreting tumors may also be seen.

Signs and Symptoms

The clinical features of ACTH-secreting tumors can be divided into two components: those related to adrenocortical hyperplasia and hypercortisolism and those involving extraadrenal effects of ACTH and associated peptides. Signs and symptoms of hypercortisolemia are similar irrespective of whether they are due to pituitary or extrapituitary ACTH hypersecretion, adrenocortical adenomas, or exogenous cortisol, as discussed in detail in Chap. 12. The major features include centripetal obesity, hypertension, diabetes, amenorrhea, hirsutism, acne, osteoporosis and compression fractures, muscular wasting, violaceous striae, capillary fragility, impaired would healing, decreased resistance to infection, and behavioral changes such as mania and psychosis.

The increased secretion of ACTH and probably β-LPH results in increased pigmentation similar to that seen in Addison's disease. Skin darkening occurs over the pressure points (knees, elbows, knuckles, belt and brassiere strap regions), in the areolae, genitalia, mucous membranes, and at the sites of new scar formation. Because ACTH secretion by pituitary tumors is not entirely autonomous but is partially suppressed by hypercortisolemia, hyperpigmentation is not pronounced in the early stages of the disease and is most prominent after adrenalectomy, when ACTH levels may increase markedly. It is a major feature of Nelson's syndrome and of extrapituitary ACTH-producing tumors. Although ACTH fragments and endorphins exert profound effects on the CNS, the behavioral changes seen in patients with Cushing's disease (euphoria, decreased sleep requirements, and occasionally true psychoses) can probably be explained by the elevated levels of plasma cortisol.

While once common, the frequency of symptoms due to the expanding pituitary tumor itself (headache, visual disturbances, hypopituitarism) is decreasing, owing to earlier diagnosis and therapy.

Laboratory Findings

A full discussion of the laboratory tests used in the differential diagnosis of adrenocortical hyperfunction is found in Chap. 12. This section relates primarily to the studies which are used to diagnose ACTH-secreting tumors. Patients with these tumors exhibit an increase in plasma ACTH and cortisol levels, elevated urinary excretion of cortisol and adrenocortical steroid metabolites, evidence of altered negative feedback of cortisol, and disturbances in neuroendocrine regulation (primarily periodicity) of GH and prolactin as well as ACTH.

Plasma ACTH values are elevated in about 50 percent of patients with Cushing's disease.[35,396] The upper limit of normal is in the range of 80 to 100 pg/ml but varies between laboratories. The reliability of the laboratory is of extreme importance for this determination. Diurnal variation is absent, and even the values in the normal range are relatively elevated in relation to circulating cortisol levels. Morning plasma cortisol values are elevated in most but not all patients with Cushing's disease. The upper limit of plasma cortisol is 25 μg/dl in the morning and 15 μg/dl in the evening. The diurnal variation observed in normal subjects is absent in patients with Cushing's disease, therefore elevation of plasma cortisol levels is more common in the late afternoon. The 24-h secretion of free cortisol is the most reliable urinary measurement for distinguishing between normal and increased adrenocortical function.[397] Normal values are less than 100 μg per 24 h. Urinary 17-OH corticoids, or corticosteroids (17-OHCS), are less discriminating and therefore not recommended. The upper level of normal is 10 to 12 mg per 24 h, depending upon technique. Though a 24-h urine collection has advantages over a single plasma sample in that it provides an integrated assessment of cortisol secretion, the completeness of collection when used as a screening procedure in ambulatory patients is at times questionable. In obese patients, however, it is a more discriminating screening procedure. Measurements of urine volume and creatinine are useful indicators of the reliability of the collection.

Assessment of the alteration in negative feedback control of the hypothalamic-pituitary-adrenal axis is the most reliable procedure available for distinguishing between normal subjects and those with Cushing's disease or adrenal tumors. The basis for this test is the characteristic decreased sensitivity of ACTH secretion by pituitary tumors to cortisol suppression. The screening procedure of choice is the overnight (rapid) dexamethasone suppression test. Dexamethasone, 1 mg, is given at 11 P.M. and the plasma cortisol level is measured at 8 A.M. the following day. Plasma cortisol levels < 5 μg/dl exclude the diagnosis, whereas values above this level warrant further study. The standard dexamethasone suppression test involves the measurement of serial morning cortisol levels and/or 24-h urine samples before and after 2 days of dexamethasone treatment at 2 mg per day and 8 mg per day, respectively.[398] In normal subjects the low dose of dexamethasone decreases urinary free cortisol to < 20 μg per 24 h and plasma cortisol to < 5 μg/dl at 4 P.M. of the second day.[399] In patients with ACTH-secreting tumors, urinary steroid secretion is impaired with the low dose but should be at least 50 percent with the high dose. Plasma cortisol should be ≤ 10 μg/dl at 4 P.M. of the second day.[399] Lack of suppression at the high dose is suggestive of an adrenal tumor. It must be emphasized, however, that exceptions to this pattern exist. Some patients with ACTH-secreting tumors show no suppression until 32 mg per day of dexamethasone is administered.

Stimulation of the hypothalamic-pituitary axis with metyrapone reveals an increased adrenocortical response in patients with Cushing's disease, reflecting the hyperresponsiveness of the entire axis to both CNS-mediated signals and the removal of the negative feedback. The cortisol response to exogenous ACTH administration is also increased. These procedures are particularly helpful when responses to dexamethasone suppression are atypical. The cortisol response to insulin hypoglycemia is decreased.

Patients with ACTH-secreting tumors exhibit a hyperresponsiveness to CRF, indicating a preservation of CRF receptors. Following successful tumor removal, the response returns to normal. The greatest utility of this procedure, however, is in its ability to distinguish between ACTH-secreting pituitary tumors and ectopic ACTH secretion, in which CRF does not stimulate ACTH release.[400]

CT scanning of the pituitary in patients with ACTH-secreting tumors identifies the tumor in about 50 percent. In patients in whom the diagnosis is in doubt, measurement of plasma ACTH levels in samples obtained by superior petrosal sinus sampling[401] will help differentiate pituitary from extrapituitary tumors and will frequently aid in localizing the pituitary tumor.

Differential Diagnosis

In approximately 80 percent of patients with Cushing's syndrome (excluding those secondary to exogenous hormone administration) the abnormality is due to an ACTH-secreting pituitary tumor or to corticotroph hyperplasia. In about 15 percent, an adrenal tumor is present, and in the remainder the abnormality is due to ACTH production by an ectopic source. The diagnosis is made on the basis of increased cortisol secretion, altered dexamethasone suppressibility, elevated plasma cortisol levels, and hyperresponsiveness of the hypothalamic-pituitary-adrenal axis in the absence of any evidence of another neoplasm and irrespective of findings on sellar tomography. There are two major steps in establishing the diagnosis. The first is to differentiate patients with hyperadrenocorticism from those with clinical features of the disease but with normal steroid secretion; the second is to differentiate mechanisms not dependent on the hypothalamic-pituitary axis for the hyperadrenocorticism. These topics are discussed further in Chap. 12. One entity deserving special emphasis is the ectopic ACTH syndrome (see also Chap. 29). ACTH is most commonly produced by small cell lung carcinomas, carcinoids, and pancreatic islet tumors. The disease can mimic pituitary-dependent Cushing's disease in its clinical and biologic features, though in patients with malignant tumors the weight gain is often absent and severe hypokalemia is a prominent feature. The results of dexamethasone suppression tests indicate a variable degree of suppressibility. Some of these tumors have been shown to secrete CRF rather than or in addition to ACTH,[402,403] which may explain the similarity in the dynamic responses. Removal of such tumors completely reverses the biochemical and clinical abnormalities.

Loss of periodicity of cortisol secretion and dexamethasone suppressibility and frequently mild elevations in plasma cortisol levels are seen in patients under stress, with alcoholism,[404] during periods of bereavement, and with emotional disorders, typically depressive illnesses.[405] Such patients, in contrast to those with Cushing's disease, may respond to insulin hypoglycemia with an increase in cortisol levels. While it may be impossible to distinguish these patients from those with ACTH-secreting tumors on a biochemical basis, the clinical features of the latter are generally absent.

Etiology of ACTH-Secreting Tumors: Hypothalamic vs. Pituitary Disease

Many of the arguments used in relation to GH- and prolactin-secreting tumors also apply to ACTH-secreting tumors. Cushing originally attributed the origin of the disease to the pituitary, but subsequent observations have suggested the possibility that the cause lies within the CNS (Fig. 8-20).[406]

The hypothesis of a hypothalamic etiology is based on the following:

1. Lesions have been noted at autopsy in the hypothalamic paraventricular and supraoptic nuclei of patients with Cushing's disease,[407] and there have been case reports of Cushing's disease associated with CNS tumors and increased intracranial pressure in which symptoms regressed following tumor removal. In particular, a CRF-producing gangliocytoma of the pituitary as well as other ectopic CRF-producing tumors can cause corticotroph hyperplasia and tumor formation.[205]
2. A 10 to 25 percent incidence of basophil hyperplasia has been found in pituitaries of patients with Cushing's disease at autopsy, and in one series, 87 percent of pituitaries removed transsphenoidally for treatment of Cushing's disease exhibited diffuse or nodular corticotroph hyperplasia, while tumors were found in 73 percent.[313] Similar changes were present in pituitaries from patients with Nelson's disease.
3. The similarity between the loss of ACTH and cortisol periodicity and glucocorticoid suppressibility in Cushing's disease and that occurring in primary CNS disorders suggests a common etiology mediated by increased CRF secretion, and the similar findings in CRF-producing lung tumors support this concept.
4. Studies of other periodic phenomena (GH and prolactin secretion and the percentage of time spent in slow-wave sleep) also suggest a primary CNS disturbance. Prolactin periodicity is lost in patients with Cushing's disease but not in Cushing's syndrome,[408] and the loss of GH and cortisol periodicity and the decrease in slow-wave sleep which occur in patients with active Cushing's disease disappear following normalization of cortisol levels after surgery in only some patients.[409]
5. Some patients with Cushing's disease respond to neuropharmacologic agents such as the serotonin receptor blocker cyproheptadine,[410] sodium valproate (a GABA agonist),[411] and bromocriptine,[412] which have been shown to affect CNS control of ACTH secretion in animals. The responses include restoration of normal glucocorticoid suppressibility of ACTH secretion[413] and amelioration of the clinical manifestations of the disease.[406]

The major argument for a pituitary etiology of Cushing's disease is based on the results of transsphenoidal surgery, with selective adenomectomy resulting initially in a deficiency of ACTH secretion followed by a recovery of the hypothalamic-pituitary axis.[396,414,415] The impairment in ACTH secretion is postulated to be secondary to a suppression of the normal corticotrophs by the ACTH-secreting tumors, analogous to that seen after removal of an adrenal cortical adenoma. The reestablishment not only of cortisol secretion but of normal diurnal periodicity

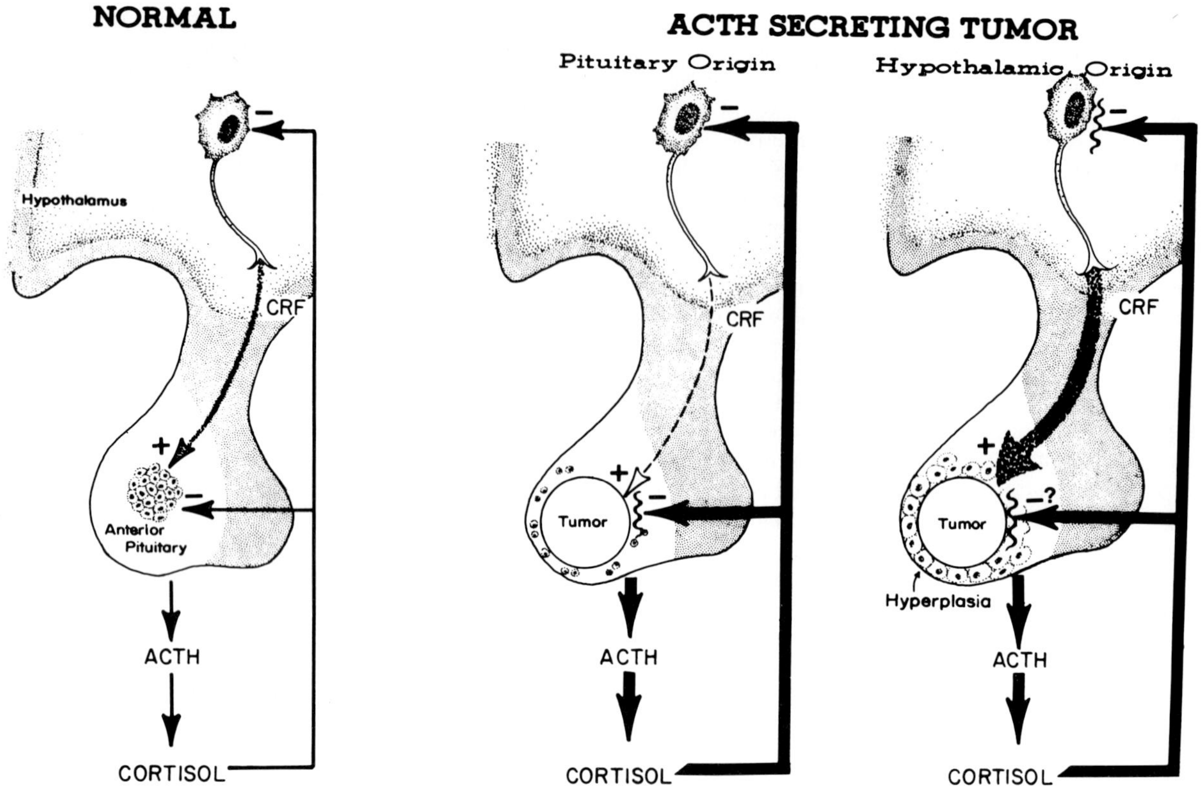

FIGURE 8-20 Possible neuroendocrine disturbances in the pathogenesis of ACTH-secreting tumors. (*Left*) Normal feedback regulation of ACTH secretion, which is mediated by cortisol and involves an inhibitory effect on both the pituitary and the hypothalamus (and possibly other CNS loci). The hypothalamic effects inhibit the release of corticotropin releasing factor (CRF), and the pituitary effects suppress the effects of CRF on ACTH release. (*Middle*) Alterations which would be expected if the pituitary tumor arose de novo. Increased ACTH and cortisol secretion would lead to suppression of CRF secretion and of its effects on the tumor. It follows that the pituitary tumor must exhibit some resistance to the suppressive effects of cortisol, for which there is abundant evidence. (*Right*) Alterations which would be expected with a primary hypothalamic disturbance. An increase in CRF secretion would lead to corticotroph hyperplasia and eventual tumor formation. Also implied are (1) an impairment of the negative feedback effects of cortisol on CRF release and (2) possibly a resistance to the suppressive effects of cortisol on the action of CRF.

and glucocorticoid suppressibility argues for a pituitary origin of the disease. Since glucocorticoids can suppress ACTH secretion at the level of the pituitary as well as by CNS-mediated mechanisms, the altered feedback sensitivity observed in ACTH-secreting tumors remains consistent with a pituitary etiology.

The major difficulties in reconciling the two arguments are the limited numbers of patients treated by the various methods and the relatively brief duration of follow-up in most patients. Thus, the frequency of long-term recurrence following pituitary adenomectomy remains unknown. It is also possible that there are two types of Cushing's disease, one of pituitary origin and the other secondary to excessive CRF secretion. The variation in results between different surgical series and the response to pharmacotherapy are compatible with a dual etiology, as are several other observations. An anatomic differentiation has been noted in the location of corticotroph adenomas. Most are in the anterior lobe, while others are in the midline, near the intermediate-posterior lobe boundary. It has been reported that the latter tumors are less sensitive to glucocorticoid suppression, are less likely to have normalization of ACTH levels postoperatively, and exhibit bromocriptine suppressibility.[412,416] A detailed analysis of circadian ACTH and cortisol secretion has suggested the existence of two subgroups, one with hyperpulsatility and the other with hypopulsatility.[417] Surgery is much more successful in the latter than in the former.

Therapy

Of all the hyperfunctioning pituitary tumors, those secreting ACTH provide the clearest indication for definitive therapy because of the problems associated with prolonged adrenocortical hypersecretion. Although the effectiveness of therapy directed at the pituitary was initially demonstrated by Cushing, subsequent attention was given to the adrenals, and the return to a pituitary focus occurred only after the reintroduction of transsphenoidal surgery. Simultaneously, improvement in pharmacologic therapy directed at both the adrenals and the CNS has provided the physician with several options. Before initiating therapy to the adrenals, pituitary, or CNS, a careful search must be made for an extrapituitary ACTH- or CRF-secreting tumor.

SURGERY Until recently, the most commonly employed technique was bilateral adrenalectomy. Earlier attempts to preserve a portion of one adrenal to permit residual adrenal cortical function were abandoned because of the frequent recurrence of disease due to hyperplasia of the remaining fragment under the influence of persistent and enhanced ACTH secretion. Similarly, attempts to transplant adrenal tissue to a readily accessible location (e.g., the forearm) were successful in only a few instances.[418,419] Following restoration of cortisol levels to normal by adrenalectomy, ACTH secretion increases markedly owing to a decrease of the inhibitory feedback effect of hypercortisolemia. With time, ACTH-secreting tumors characterized by generalized hyperpigmentation have appeared in approximately 10 percent of patients.[395] The latency of tumor appearance following adrenalectomy is highly variable (1 to 16 years), and a small percentage of tumors may show invasive and even metastatic behavior.[420] Although pituitary irradiation at the time of adrenalectomy has been advocated as a prophylaxis, the limited data available suggest that it is not completely effective.[395]

The current procedure of choice is a transsphenoidal approach with adenomectomy.[313,396,421] In ACTH-secreting tumors, unlike other hyperfunctioning pituitary tumors, operations are warranted on patients in whom the diagnosis has been established even in the presence of a normal CT scan. The tumors may be extremely small (2 to 3 mm) and may be located throughout the anterior lobe[396] as well as in the midline as originally described.[266] Although a total anterior hypophysectomy has been favored by one group because of the frequency of multicentric areas of hyperplasia,[313] most prefer simple adenomectomy as the initial procedure. Cure rates with this technique, based on the postoperative reduction in cortisol hypersecretion of 80 to 90 percent, have been reported for microadenomas,[396,421] though overall experience appears closer to 70 to 75 percent.[422] Following surgery, there is generally evidence of adrenocortical hypofunction, requiring glucocorticoid replacement therapy, which has been attributed to suppression of the hypothalamic-pituitary axis, as seen after removal of an adrenal adenoma. The duration of time required for recovery of the axis is usually 9 to 12 months but may extend to 2 years, and the frequency of recurrence remains to be determined. Patients may also experience steroid withdrawal syndrome (see Chap. 15). The surgical results in patients with Nelson's syndrome are not as encouraging, with reduction in hyperpigmentation and ACTH levels being seen in only 30 percent.[396]

RADIATION THERAPY Conventional radiotherapy is also effective as a primary therapeutic modality in the treatment of ACTH-secreting pituitary tumors. A cure rate of 80 percent has recently been reported in a large series of children with Cushing's disease.[423] Proton beam therapy is successful in reducing cortisol secretion in 90 percent of patients and in restoring levels to normal in approximately 60 percent.[270,273] The radiation dose used (6000 to 15,000 rads) is higher than that for other pituitary tumors. Dynamic studies of the hypothalamic-pituitary axis have not been extensively reported following irradiation, though the frequency of recurrence appears quite low.

PHARMACOLOGIC THERAPY Pharmacologic agents used in the treatment of Cushing's disease are directed at either cortisol biosynthesis by the adrenals (aminoglutethimide, metyrapone, *o′,p′*-DDD, or the experimental drug trilostane) or neurotransmitter metabolism within the CNS. Differences in the mechanism of action, doses, effectiveness, and side effects of the steroid synthesis inhibitors are described in Chap. 12. They were initially used as primary therapy directed to the adrenals and subsequently as an adjunct to radiation therapy to the pituitary. At present they are in use as alternative therapy when surgery is contraindicated or unsuccessful and in normalization of cortisol levels prior to surgery.

The combination of radiation and steroid biosynthesis inhibitors constitutes an improvement over radiation alone with respect to the rapidity with which cortisol secretion is restored to normal and is of particular benefit in patients with moderately severe clinical symptoms.

Metyrapone, given alone, has a rapid onset of action but occasionally causes hirsutism,[424] and some patients exhibit an escape phenomenon: with reduction of the negative feedback effect of cortisol, increased ACTH secretion overrides the block. Metyrapone given together with aminoglutethimide and dexamethasone is an effective means of both short- and long-term suppression of cortisol secretion.[425] This combination has been advocated for restoring cortisol secretion to normal prior to surgical removal of an ACTH-secreting adenoma. While probably unnecessary in most patients, some with florid disease may become better surgical risks with prior medical therapy. Because *o′,p′*-DDD has a much slower onset of action, it is used primarily for long-term therapy in doses smaller than those recommended for treatment of adrenal carcinoma.[426] A recent report suggests that ketoconazole, an imidazole broad-spectrum antimycotic, is effective in reducing the elevated cortisol secretion in patients with Cushing's disease.[427] Ketoconazole inhibits cortisol biosynthesis by blocking P450 enzymes associated with cholesterol side-chain cleavage[428] and inhibiting C_{17-20} lyase.[429] Additional experience with this agent is needed to evaluate its efficacy and safety.

A better understanding of the neurotransmitter control of ACTH secretion has led to the use of several neuropharmacologic agents in attempts to reduce ACTH secretion by central mechanisms. Experience with dopaminergic agents (L-dopa and bromocriptine) has been inconsistent, with most patients exhibiting little or no response.[430,431] On the basis of extensive evidence for a serotonin-mediated stimulatory control of ACTH secretion (see Chap. 7), cyproheptadine, a serotonin receptor blocker, has been used with encouraging results in the treatment of Cushing's disease.[410] Reductions of plasma ACTH, plasma cortisol, and the cortisol secretory rate to normal have been observed, as has a restoration of dexamethasone suppressibility and diurnal periodicity. Remission of clinical symptoms has occurred simultaneously with the biochemical changes. Doses of 24 to 32 mg per day are required, and the side effects include somnolence and hyperphagia. The latter may be difficult to control, particularly in children. The response rate is no more than 30 percent and probably less, and relapses occur in some patients while on therapy and in all patients upon discontinuation. There has not to the present time been any way to predict which patient will or will not respond to cyproheptadine. Responses have also been seen in patients with Nelson's syndrome. Cyproheptadine has also been used as an adjunct in patients treated with irradiation and may help produce a more rapid response.

TSH-Secreting Tumors

TSH-secreting pituitary tumors are quite uncommon and are recorded in the literature mainly as case reports rather than as a recognizable percentage of hyperfunctioning tumors. Histologic examination of the tumors usually reveals a chromophobe adenoma, though immunohistochemical staining has revealed the presence of TSH. These tumors are generally detected during the course of an investigation of a presumed nonfunctioning tumor or of patients with hyperthyroidism when an elevated rather than a normal or low plasma TSH level is present.[432] The clinical manifestations of TSH-secreting pituitary tumors consist of those related to the tumor mass (which may be absent if the tumor is small) and those of thyrotoxicosis. Tumors of mixed pituitary cell types have also been reported with concomitant GH or prolactin hypersecretion.

TSH secretion is not always autonomous in these tumors. Though the simultaneous presence of elevated TSH and thyroxine levels defines the loss of the inhibitory feedback effect of thyroxine on the pituitary, a reduction of thyroxine levels by methimazole often results in a further increase in TSH secretion, analogous to the pattern in ACTH-secreting pituitary tumors. The TSH response to TRH is variable, with only some patients responding,[433] and a lack of suppression by L-dopa has been reported, in contrast to the effect seen in patients with primary hypothyroidism. Elevated levels of the α-glycoprotein subunit have also been observed in patients with TSH-secreting and "non functioning" tumors.[434]

Patients with TSH-secreting tumors must be distinguished from those with an enlarged pituitary, thyrotroph hyperplasia, and elevated TSH levels secondary to long-standing hypothyroidism. The subnormal thyroxine levels and the suppressibility of the elevated TSH levels and reduction of pituitary size by exogenous thyroxine readily distinguish this group of patients. Patients with elevated TSH and thyroxine levels but no evidence of a pituitary tumor are more difficult to differentiate.[435,436] These patients have been considered to have a pituitary resistance to the feedback effects of thyroxine rather than a tumor. The absence of the clinical features of hyperthyroidism serves to differentiate these patients from those with tumors.

Therapy should be directed at the pituitary if a tumor can be identified. In the patient who is thyrotoxic, however, pharmacologic suppression of the thyroid to produce a euthyroid state prior to pituitary surgery is essential.

Gonadotropin-Secreting Pituitary Tumors

A few cases of FSH- or FSH- and LH-secreting pituitary adenomas have been reported.[437,438] In some patients, pituitary enlargement and tumor formation is believed to be secondary to long-standing hypogonadism, whereas in others the pituitary tumor is considered to be the primary disease. FSH levels may or may not respond to GnRH or clomiphene administration and are suppressed either subnormally or not at all by testosterone. The effects of elevated FSH secretion will generally preserve Sertoli cells, but testosterone levels are usually reduced, resulting in symptoms of hypogonadism and impairment of spermatogenesis. The tumors described have been relatively large, and restoration of normal pituitary and gonadal function following tumor removal has not been achieved. One patient with an FSH- and α-subunit-secreting tumor has responded to bromocriptine.[439]

α-Subunit-Secreting Pituitary Tumors

Measurement of the glycoprotein α subunit levels in plasma of patients with nonfunctioning tumors has revealed a subgroup with elevated levels.[440] The α subunit secreted by these tumors differs in degree of glycosylation from that produced by normal gonadotrophs and thyrotrophs. To date, no clinical consequences have been recognized, and the elevated α subunit serves merely as a tumor marker. There appear to be no particular diagnostic characteristics of this group of tumors, and their therapy is the same as for truly nonfunctioning tumors.

DETAILS OF HYPOTHALAMIC-PITUITARY TESTING

The testing procedures described below are not intended to constitute an exhaustive list but are those which have been found to have the greatest utility in diagnosing disorders of pituitary hormone secretion. The rationale for their use and a detailed interpretation of the results are provided in the preceding sections.

ACTH

Basal Measurements

The use of plasma ACTH determinations demands unquestioned reliability of the laboratory performing the procedure. Normal values range from 20 to 80 pg/ml, though their interpretation requires a simultaneous cortisol determination. Measurement of plasma cortisol still provides, for practical purposes, an excellent assessment of ACTH secretion when pituitary function is being evaluated, provided that adrenocortical function is intact. The normal range for most laboratories is 5 to 25 μg/dl. The normal diurnal variation is at least 5 μg/dl. The 24-h urinary excretion of 17-OH corticoids is 4 to 12 mg and of free cortisol is 20 to 100 μg in normal adults.

Stimulation Tests

CORTICOTROPIN RELEASING FACTOR At the time of writing, CRF is available only as an investigational agent in the United States.

Method CRF, 100 μg, is injected intravenously and blood samples are obtained at 0, 15, 30, 60, and 120 min. This test may be combined with GRH, TRH, and GnRH testing.

Normal Values The increase in cortisol should be at least 10 μg/dl. Peak values should occur by 30 to 60 min. Measurement of ACTH levels gives more variable results, and peak increments at 15 to 30 min may range from 20 to 50 pg/ml.

Interpretation In both hypothalamic and pituitary disease, the cortisol response is decreased. However, the ACTH response is intact if the cause of diminished function is in the hypothalamus. More extensive evaluation of this test in hypothalamic-pituitary disease is needed to define the reliability of the test in separating the two disease categories. Patients with ACTH-secreting pituitary tumors respond to CRF with a supranormal response, while those with ectopic ACTH secretion are unresponsive.

Risks There are no significant risks. Immediately following injection, patients experience facial flushing which may last for several minutes.

INSULIN HYPOGLYCEMIA *Method* This study should be performed in the morning after an overnight fast. An indwelling needle is inserted into a forearm vein and kept patent with heparinized saline. Regular insulin is injected intravenously at a dose sufficient to decrease the blood glucose by 50 percent or at least 40 mg/dl. The standard dose is 0.1 U/kg, though this is increased to 0.15 U/kg in states of presumed insulin resistance, e.g., obesity, acromegaly, and Cushing's syndrome, and reduced to 0.05 U/kg when hypopituitarism is strongly suspected. If signs and symptoms of adrenergic discharge occur, the hypoglycemic stimulus is adequate even if the extent of glucose reduction is not achieved. If none of these criteria is met, the test may need to be repeated with a larger dose of insulin. Dextrose (50%) should be immediately available in case of unexpectedly severe hypoglycemia. Blood glucose is measured at 0, 15, 30, 45, 60, 90, and 120 min. Plasma cortisol is measured at 0, 30, 60, 90, and 120 min. The insulin hypoglycemia test can be performed simultaneously with the TRH and GnRH tests if indicated.

Normal Values The minimal glucose value should occur at 30 to 45 min. A normal cortisol response consists of a rise of at least 10 μg/dl and a value of at least 20 μg/dl.

Interpretation A normal response indicates an intact hypothalamic-pituitary-adrenal axis. An impaired response does not identify the site of the abnormality. An ACTH stimulation test should be used to document intact adrenocortical function and a CRF test to evaluate the pituitary-adrenal axis. The response to insulin hypoglycemia may be blunted or absent if the initial cortisol level is high, as often occurs in patients under stress. It is also reduced in patients receiving exogenous glucocorticoids at the time of testing or in the recent past, in patients with Cushing's syndrome or Cushing's disease, and in patients with depressive illness.

Risks All subjects should be under the direct observation of a physician until the time of maximal hypoglycemia has passed. The test should not be performed in patients with clinical evidence of adrenocortical insufficiency and should be performed only with caution when a history of coronary or cerebrovascular insufficiency is present.

METYRAPONE Metyrapone stimulation was originally performed by administering the drug orally and collecting and measuring urine for four sequential 24-h periods. This time-consuming procedure has been shortened by substitution of plasma for urine steroid measurements.

Method Metyrapone, 0.75 g, is given PO at midnight (patient weight < 70 kg, 2.0 g; 70 to 90 kg, 2.5 g; > 90 kg, 3.0 g), and plasma cortisol and 11-deoxycortisol are measured at 8 the next morning.

Normal Values Plasma cortisol levels should be less than 10 μg/dl to ensure adequate suppression of hormone biosynthesis. Plasma 11-deoxycortisol value should equal or exceed 7 μg/dl.

Interpretation Adequate suppression of plasma cortisol confirms the reduction of the negative feedback effect. A normal 11-deoxycortisol rise indicates the ability of the hypothalamic-pituitary system to respond to interruption of the steroid feedback effect. An impaired response does not distinguish the site of the defect. Enhanced responses are seen in Cushing's disease, whereas the response is impaired in patients receiving exogenous steroids or with adrenocortical adenomas.

Risks The procedure is generally safe. However, in patients with only minimal residual cortisol secretion, irrespective of etiology, mild to moderate symptoms of adrenocortical insufficiency may occur during the course of the test and may require its interruption. The test cannot be performed if the patient is receiving glucocorticoid therapy and should not be performed in patients with primary adrenal insufficiency.

Suppression Tests

OVERNIGHT DEXAMETHASONE TEST *Method* The subject is given 1 mg dexamethasone PO at 11 P.M., and plasma cortisol is measured at 8 the following morning.

Normal Values The plasma cortisol level should be 5 μg/dl or less.

Interpretation This is the most commonly used screening test to exclude Cushing's syndrome. A lack of suppression requires that the standard dexamethasone suppression test be performed. Acutely ill or depressed patients and those who are under stress or are obese may also lack suppression.

STANDARD DEXAMETHASONE TEST *Method* This test requires the collection of six consecutive 24-h urine samples for free cortisol measurement or, alternatively, daily morning plasma samples for cortisol determinations. Dexamethasone, 0.5 mg every 6 h PO, is given on days 3 and 4 and 2.0 mg every 6 h on days 5 and 6.

Normal Values In normal subjects urinary free cortisol is decreased to less than 20 μg per 24 h on the low dose (2 mg per day) of dexamethasone. Plasma cortisol at 48 h should be < 5 μg/dl.

Interpretation A normal response excludes the diagnosis of Cushing's syndrome or Cushing's disease. In patients with Cushing's disease there is failure of adequate suppression on the low-dose dexamethasone, but a suppression of 50 percent is observed with the high dose. Patients with adrenocortical tumors characteristically do not show suppression even with the high dose. Lack of low-dose suppression can also be seen in patients with acute illness or stress. Occasionally, patients with Cushing's disease require larger doses of dexamethasone (up to 32 mg per day) for suppression. Urinary free cortisol measurement provides the best discrimination between normal and abnormal responses.

TSH

Basal Measurements

The plasma TSH determination is capable of distinguishing normal from elevated values and therefore is useful in differentiating primary from secondary hypothyroidism. Each laboratory must determine its own normal values for both basal and stimulated TSH levels. The normal range based on the TSH reference standard MRC 68/38 is up to 6 μU/ml. Elevated values have been occasionally seen in children with hypothalamic hypothyroidism. The possibility of spurious elevation due to cross-reacting antibodies to previously injected bovine TSH should be considered in patients with nonsuppressible elevation of TSH. Low values cannot be reliably distinguished from those in the normal range in most assays.

Stimulation Tests

THYROTROPIN RELEASING HORMONE (TRH) TEST *Method* TRH, 500 μg, is injected intravenously, and blood samples are obtained for TSH at 0, 15, 30, 60, and 120 min.

Normal Values The increase in TSH should be at least 6 μU/ml in females and in males under 40 years and at least 2 μU/ml in males over 40 years. Peak values should occur by 30 min.

Interpretation Occasionally, normal subjects may show a slightly decreased response, and differentiation from patients with a partial deficiency of TSH reserve may be difficult. In primary hypothyroidism the response to TRH is increased, whereas in hyperthyroidism or in patients receiving thyroxine, triiodothyronine, or pharmacologic doses of glucocorticoids and frequently in euthyroid Graves' disease it is absent. In hypothalamic hypothyroidism the TSH response to TRH is increased and the peak is often delayed to 60 min. The delayed response is, however, occasionally seen in patients with pituitary disease. Impaired responses are seen in patients with chronic renal failure.

Risks There are no significant risks. Immediately following injection subjects experience a sensation of warmth, nausea, a strange taste, and an urge to micturate, which persists for 30 to 60 s and then disappears.

LH and FSH

Basal Measurements

FSH and LH determinations vary with the methods and standards used by each laboratory. Most values are reported in relation to the Second IRP/HMG. FSH levels in postpubertal females are approximately 4 to 15 mIU/ml in the follicular and luteal phases, 10 to 50 mIU/ml at midcycle, and 30 to 200 mIU/ml postmenopausally. LH levels are 4 to 30 mIU/ml in the follicular phase, 30 to 150 mIU/ml at midcycle, 4 to 40 mIU/ml in the luteal phase, and more than 40 mIU/ml postmenopausally. Levels in males are similar to those in the follicular phase until the seventh or eighth decade, when increased values occur. Though it is usually not possible to distinguish low from normal values, the absence of elevated LH or FSH levels in patients with clinical and biochemical evidence of hypogonadism is indicative of hypothalamic or pituitary hypofunction.

Stimulation Tests

GONADOTROPIN RELEASING HORMONE (LHRH OR GNRH) TEST *Method* GnRH, 100 μg, is injected intravenously and blood samples are obtained for LH and FSH at 0, 15, 30, and 60 min.

Normal Values The normal response varies considerably between laboratories. In general, an LH response of more than 12 mIU/ml and an FSH response of more than 3 mIU/ml in females and an LH response of more than 8 mIU/ml and FSH response of more than 3 mIU/ml in males are considered normal. In females the LH responses vary with the phase of the menstrual cycle, with the greatest response being seen at midcycle. Peak values for LH occur within the first 30 min, though those of FSH may be delayed in some subjects.

Interpretation In patients with hypopituitarism the responses to GnRH may be normal, impaired, or absent, and the same is true of patients with hypothalamic disease. Thus, an intact response can exclude a pituitary etiology for hypogonadism, but an impaired or absent response cannot be used to define the anatomic site of the abnormality. The test does, however, reflect the functional capacity of the gonadotrophs, and if pituitary function is otherwise intact, an impaired response is suggestive of lack of exposure to endogenous GnRH. Repeat testing after 3 to 7 days of intermittent GnRH therapy permits the differentiation of hypothalamic from pituitary disease. Estrogen deficiency generally decreases the LH response more than the FSH response, resulting in a reversed FSH/LH response ratio. In women with secondary amenorrhea of hypothalamic origin (e.g., anorexia nervosa), the FSH response may be increased.

CLOMIPHENE TEST Clomiphene citrate, a synthetic steroid with weak estrogen activity, binds to estrogen receptors in the hypothalamus, where it exhibits antiestrogenic activity and in adults stimulates the secretion of GnRH and consequently LH and FSH. In prepubertal children, in whom no estrogen levels are present, clomiphene at low doses suppresses gonadotropin secretion. In early puberty a resistance to the effect is noted, and by mid- to late puberty the adult pattern of stimulation is seen.

Method for Women A dose of 100 mg is given PO each day for 5 days (beginning on day 5 of the cycle if the patient is menstruating). Blood samples for LH and FSH are obtained on days 0, 5, 7, 10, and 13.

Method for Men A dose of 100 mg per day is given for 1 to 4 weeks. Blood samples for LH and FSH are obtained twice weekly.

Normal Values In women, FSH and LH should rise and peak on the fifth day of treatment at a level usually above the normal range. After the last dose, the levels should decrease, with a secondary rise in LH between days 9 and 14. In men, a doubling of LH values is seen by 1 week, and the response increases with time. FSH levels rise similarly but to a lesser extent.

Interpretation A normal rise in gonadotropins indicates an intact hypothalamic response to interruption of the negative feedback effect of estrogen. An absent response coupled with a normal response to GnRH points to a hypothalamic origin for the gonadotropin deficiency. In the presence of an abnormal GnRH response, the clomiphene test is usually abnormal and does not distinguish between hypothalamic and pituitary disease. Responses are generally absent in anorexia nervosa and in hyperprolactinemic states.

Growth Hormone

Basal Measurements

A single GH value is occasionally sufficient to document adequacy of hormone secretion in patients with suspected GH deficiency or to exclude the presence of acromegaly. For the former, samples are obtained on one or several occasions. In children a GH measurement obtained 90 min after the onset of sleep is particularly helpful. A value of 6 ng/ml or more excludes GH deficiency. In patients with suspected acromegaly, a single sample can be obtained without any patient preparation or, preferably, 2 h after a meal. A value of < 5 ng/ml in females or < 2 ng/ml in males is sufficient to exclude active disease.

Stimulation Tests

GRH stimulation directly assesses the capacity of the pituitary to secrete GH. All other available stimulation tests require the presence of an intact hypothalamic-pituitary axis and therefore cannot be used to distinguish the anatomic site of an abnormality. With nearly all the stimuli, an elevated basal GH level usually results in an impaired or absent response. However, for diagnostic purposes, the elevated initial value is sufficient to exclude GH deficiency. An absent or decreased response to each of the tests is seen with sufficient frequency in normal subjects that a deficient response to at least two stimuli is needed to make a definitive diagnosis of GH deficiency.

GROWTH HORMONE RELEASING HORMONE At present GRH is available only as an investigational drug in the United States.

Method GRH (either GRH_{1-40} or GRH_{1-44}), 1 μg/kg IV, is injected and blood samples are obtained at 0, 15, 30, and 60 min. The test may be combined with CRF, TRH, and GnRH tests.

Normal Values GH responses in normal subjects are quite variable, with peak levels occurring at 15 to 30 min and ranging from 10 to > 50 ng/ml in normal young adults. Responses in women are slightly higher than in men, and initial reports suggest that responses decrease with age.

Interpretation Diminished responses are seen in hypothyroidism and obesity. Patients with GH deficiency secondary to hypothalamic disease should respond to initial GRH stimulation.

Risks Mild and transient facial flushing is seen occasionally at the recommended dose and more commonly at higher doses.

INSULIN TOLERANCE TEST Hypoglycemia stimulates the secretion of GH in normal subjects, and this test is the most frequently used method of evaluating GH reserve.

Method The details of testing, including dosage, criteria for adequate hypoglycemia, and times of blood sampling, are as described under ACTH testing. GH is measured at 0, 30, 60, 90, and 120 min.

Normal Values A peak value of 9 ng/ml or more, which usually occurs at 60 or 90 min, is considered a normal response. Responses in females are higher than in males, but this difference is of no diagnostic importance.

Interpretation A normal response excludes GH deficiency. However, up to 20 percent of normal subjects exhibit an impaired or absent response. Such responses are seen frequently but not exclusively when the initial value is elevated. Impaired or absent responses are also seen in obesity, depression, hypothyroidism, hyperthyroidism, Cushing's syndrome (including exogenous steroids), and chronic renal failure and frequently occur in acromegaly.

Risks The risks are as described under ACTH testing.

L-DOPA TEST L-Dopa stimulates GH secretion by enhancing CNS dopaminergic transmission, which, in turn, is believed to enhance GRH secretion. This test is often used as a secondary procedure for evaluating GH reserve.

Method L-Dopa, 0.5 g PO, is given to a fasting, resting subject, and blood samples for GH are obtained at 0, 60, 90, 120, 150, and 180 min.

Normal Values A normal response consists of a peak value of 6 ng/ml or more, usually between 90 and 150 min. Reduced or absent responses are more frequently observed when initial values are elevated.

Interpretation An intact response excludes GH deficiency but is seen in only 65 to 75 percent of normal subjects, particularly in older persons. Reduced or absent responses occur in obesity and hypothyroidism and in patients receiving α-methyldopa and neuroleptics. In most acromegalic patients, GH levels decrease after administration of L-dopa owing to a direct dopaminergic action on the neoplastic somatotroph.

Risks The major side effects of L-dopa are nausea and vomiting, which are due to stimulation of a dopamine-sensitive, CNS-mediated mechanism. They are seen in 20 to 25 percent of subjects, usually during the second hour, and while often mild can cause moderate discomfort. Symptoms are generally self-limited but can be controlled by administration of a dopamine receptor antagonist (e.g., perphenazine 5 mg) following completion of the study.

ARGININE INFUSION TEST L-Arginine stimulates GH secretion by an undefined CNS-mediated mechanism.

Method L-Arginine hydrochloride, 0.5 g/kg to a maximum dose of 30 g, is infused intravenously over a 30-min period to an overnight-fasted, resting subject. Blood samples for GH are obtained at 0, 30, 60, 90, and 120 min.

Normal Values A normal response consists of a peak value of at least 9 ng/ml, which usually occurs at 60 to 90 min. Responses are higher in females than in males.

Interpretation A normal response is seen in 65 to 75 percent of normal subjects. The response is decreased or absent in obesity and hypothyroidism, while in acromegaly it is variable and of no diagnostic significance.

Risks The test has virtually no risks or side effects except in patients with severe liver or renal failure, in whom it should not be used.

CLONIDINE Clonidine is a central adrenergic α_2-agonist that stimulates GH secretion by augmenting the release of endogenous GRH.

Method Clonidine is administered orally (25 μg) and plasma GH measured at 0 and 75 min.

Normal Values A GH rise of at least 7 ng/ml is seen in normal subjects.

Interpretation A normal response is indicative of an intact hypothalamic-pituitary GH axis. The test has been more extensively evaluated in children than in adults.

Risks Because of its central adrenergic actions, clonidine administration may be associated with postural hypotension and drowsiness, though at the dose recommended these effects are minimal.

TRH TEST *Method* The dosage and time of blood samples are as described under TSH testing.

Normal Values TRH does not stimulate GH secretion in normal persons.

Interpretation An acute rise, peaking at 15 to 30 min, is seen in 80 to 90 percent of patients with acromegaly, and the test is most useful along with glucose suppression in evaluating patients with minimal elevations of GH levels. Acute responses also occur in patients with chronic renal failure. Responses in starvation, protein-calorie malnutrition, anorexia nervosa, and cirrhosis are delayed, often peaking at 45 to 60 min.

Suppression Tests

GLUCOSE SUPPRESSION TEST This test is based on the suppression of GH secretion, which normally occurs in response to hyperglycemia.

Method A standard oral glucose tolerance test is performed (75 g of partially hydrolyzed carbohydrate or 100 g of glucose PO), and blood samples for GH are obtained at 0, ½, 1, 2, and 3 h. Additional samples at 4 and 5 h are often useful to demonstrate a GH rebound.

Normal Values Normal subjects will exhibit a decrease in GH levels to less than 2 ng/ml (males) or 5 ng/ml (females) within 2 h. At 4 and 5 h a rebound of GH to more than 7 ng/ml is common.

Interpretation This test is used to evaluate the patient suspected of having acromegaly. Absence of suppression, incomplete suppression, or even paradoxic stimulation is seen in acromegalic patients; normal suppression excludes the diagnosis. Patients with anorexia nervosa who exhibit increased GH levels may have only partial suppression of GH secretion. After a period of refeeding, however, normal suppression is regained.

Prolactin

Basal Measurements

Plasma prolactin values vary between laboratories according to the method and the reference standard utilized. With the most highly purified standards available (NIH VLS-2) the upper limit of normal is 15 ng/ml in men and 15 to 20 ng/ml in women. Levels in children are similar, though neonates exhibit levels as high as 150 ng/ml during the first few weeks of life. When a single determination is used as a screening tool to exclude hyperprolactinemia, more than one normal value may be required because of the intermittent elevations which are occasionally observed. Plasma prolactin values can be detected in all normal subjects, though in some, the values are near the lower limit of the assay sensitivity. Therefore, a distinction between normal and hypopituitary values is not always possible.

Stimulation Tests

Stimuli for prolactin secretion can be divided into those which act on the lactotroph dopamine or TRH receptors. Responses to the two types of stimuli are not generally helpful in distinguishing between pituitary and hypothalamic disease.

TRH TEST TRH stimulates prolactin secretion via direct action of the lactotroph through a mechanism associated with adenylate cyclase activation.

Methods The dosage and the times of blood sampling are as described under TSH testing.

Normal Values A prolactin rise of at least three times basal values and a peak level of more than 20 ng/ml at 15 or 30 min are seen in normal persons. The rise is greater in females than in males.

Interpretation A reduced or absent response in a patient with low basal levels indicates a deficient prolactin reserve and implies a primary pituitary disorder. A reduced or absent response in patients with hyperprolactinemia may be seen with prolactin-secreting tumors, drug-induced hyperprolactinemia, chronic renal failure, and idiopathic hyperprolactinemia. Furthermore, some patients with pituitary tumors exhibit a normal response to TRH. Thus, the test cannot be used to distinguish between prolactin-secreting tumors and other forms of hyperprolactinemia with any degree of certainty.

METOCLOPRAMIDE Prolactin secretion is increased following metoclopramide administration as the result of blockade of pituitary dopaminergic receptors.

Method Metoclopramide, 10 mg IV, is injected, and blood samples are obtained for prolactin at 0, 30, 60, and 120 min.

Normal Values An increase of prolactin to levels of at least 50 ng/ml should be observed, with the peak value at 60 min.

Interpretation This test is useful in evaluating the lactotroph responsiveness to alterations in dopaminergic tone. Nearly all patients with prolactin-secreting tumors as well as those with hypothalamic disorders have a reduced or absent response to metoclopramide, consequently the usefulness of the test is limited.

Risks Metoclopramide has no side effects and involves no risks.

INSULIN HYPOGLYCEMIA The mechanism by which insulin hypoglycemia stimulates prolactin secretion is not known. Prolactin is measured at the same time intervals as is GH. A normal response consists of a rise of 10 ng/ml or more and is seen in 70 percent of normal subjects. A decreased or absent response is seen in patients with pituitary tumors and hypopituitarism, but the test is not discriminatory.

Suppression Tests

Prolactin secretion can at present be suppressed only by stimulation of dopaminergic receptors. This can be done by administration of dopamine itself or of a dopamine agonist. The most commonly used agent is the dopamine precursor L-dopa.

L-DOPA TEST *Method* The dosage and the times of blood sampling are as described under GH testing.

Normal Values Prolactin levels are suppressed by at least 50 percent in normal subjects at 2 or 3 h.

Interpretation Prolactin suppression is seen in most patients with hyperprolactinemia. A few patients with prolactin-secreting tumors have impaired suppression, but prolongation of the observation period is usually associated with evidence of normal suppression. Thus, L-dopa, like other tests, does not distinguish those patients with prolactin-secreting tumors. Similar suppression is observed with a dopamine infusion (0.04 to 4 μg/kg per minute IV) or with bromocriptine (2.5 mg PO). Patients with chronic renal failure do not show acute suppression with L-dopa, dopamine, or bromocriptine.

Risks Risks are as described under GH testing.

REFERENCES

1. DiChiro G, Nelson KB: The volume of the sella turcica. *Am J Roentgenol* 87:989, 1962.
2. Swartz JD, Russell KB, Basile BA, O'Donnell PC, Popky GL: High-resolution computed tomographic appearance of the intrasellar contents in women of childbearing age. *Radiology* 147:115, 1983.
3. Brown SB, Murphy K, Enzmann DR: CT characteristics of the normal pituitary gland. *Neuroradiology* 24:259, 1983.
4. Syvertsen A, Haughton VM, Williams AL, Cusick JF: The computed tomographic appearance of the normal pituitary gland and pituitary microadenomas. *Radiology* 133:385, 1979.
5. Wolpert SM, Molitch ME, Goldman JA, Wood JB: Size, shape, and appearance of the normal female pituitary gland. *Am J Roentgenol* 143:377, 1984.
6. Berglund RM, Page RB: Can the pituitary secrete directly to the brain? (Affirmative anatomical evidence). *Endocrinology* 102:1325, 1978.
7. Oliver C, Mical RS, Porter JC: Hypothalamic-pituitary vasculature—evidence for retrograde blood flow in pituitary stalk. *Endocrinology* 101:598, 1977.
8. Mezey E, Palkovits M: Two-way transport in the hypothalamo-hypophyseal system, in Ganong WF, Martini L (eds): *Frontiers in Neuroendocrinology.* New York, Raven, 1982, vol 7, p 1.
9. Page RB: Directional pituitary blood flow: A microcinephotographic study. *Endocrinology* 112:157, 1983.
10. Warner BA, Santen RJ, Page RB: Growth of hormone and prolactin secretion by a tumor of the pharyngeal pituitary. *Ann Intern Med* 96:65, 1982.
11. Kovacs K, Horvath E, Ryan N: Immunocytochemistry of the human pituitary, in Delellis RA (ed): *Diagnostic Immunocytochemistry.* New York, Masson, 1981, p 17.
12. Baker BL: Functional cytology of adenohypophyseal pars distalis and pars intermedia, in Greep RO (ed): *Handbook of Physiology.* Washington, D.C., American Physiological Society, 1974, vol 4, p 45.
13. Duello TM, Halmi NS: Ultrastructural-immunocytochemical localization of growth hormone and prolactin in human pituitaries. *J Clin Endocrinol Metab* 49:189, 1979.
14. Moriarty GC, Tobin RB: Ultrastructural immunocytochemical characterization of the thyrotroph in rat and human pituitaries. *J Histochem Cytochem* 24:1131, 1976.
15. Samaan NA, Osborne BM, MacKay B, Leavens ME, Duello TM, Halmi NS: Endocrine and morphologic studies of pituitary adenomas secondary to primary hypothyroidism. *J Clin Endocrinol Metab* 45:903, 1977.
16. Bower BF: Pituitary enlargement secondary to untreated primary hypogonadism. *Ann Intern Med* 69:107, 1968.
17. Roberts JL, Herbert E: Characterization of a common precursor to corticotropin and beta-lipotropin: Cell-free synthesis of the precursor and the identification of corticotropin peptides in the molecule. *Proc Natl Acad Sci USA* 74:4826, 1977.
18. Herbert E, Roberts J, Phillips M, Allen R, Hinman M, Budarf M, Policastro P, Rosa P: Biosynthesis, processing and release of corticotropin, β endorphin, and melanocyte stimulating hormone in pituitary cell culture systems, in Martini L, Ganong WF (eds): *Frontiers in Neuroendocrinology.* New York, Raven, 1980, vol 6, p 67.
19. Mains RE, Eipper BA: Biosynthesis of adrenocorticotropic hormone in mouse pituitary tumor cells. *J Biol Chem* 251:4115, 1976.
20. Eipper BA, Mains RE, Guenzi D: High molecular weight forms of adrenocorticotropic hormone are glycoproteins. *J Biol Chem* 251:4121, 1976.
21. Owerbach D, Rutter WJ, Roberts JL, Whitfeld P, Shine J, Seeburg PH, Shows TB: The proopiocortin (adrenocorticotropin/beta-lipotropin) gene is located on chromosome 2 in humans. *Somatic Cell Genet* 7:359, 1981.
22. Tanaka K, Nicholson WE, Orth DN: The nature of the immunoreactive lipotropins in human plasma and tissue extracts. *J Clin Invest* 62:94, 1978.
23. Gilkes JJH, Eady RAJ, Rees LH, Munro DD, Moorhead JF: Plasma immunoreactive melanotrophic hormones in patients on maintenance hemodialysis. *Br Med J* 1:656, 1975.
24. Berson SA, Yalow RS: Radioimmunoassay of ACTH in plasma. *J Clin Invest* 47:2725, 1968.
25. Liotta A, Krieger DT: A sensitive bioassay for the determination of human plasma ACTH levels. *J Clin Endocrinol Metab* 40:268, 1975.
26. Lefkowiz RJ, Roth J, Pricer W, Pastan I: ACTH receptors in the adrenal: Specific binding of ACTH-^{125}I and its relation to adenylcyclase. *Proc Natl Acad Sci USA* 65:745, 1970.
27. Chayen J, Daly JR, Loveridge N, Bitensky L: The cytochemical bioassay of hormones. *Recent Prog Horm Res* 32:33, 1976.
28. Yalow RS: Heterogeneity of peptide hormone. *Recent Prog Horm Res* 30:597, 1974.
29. Krieger DT, Allen W: Relationship of bioassayable and immunoassayable plasma ACTH and cortisol concentrations in normal subjects and in patients with Cushing's disease. *J Clin Endocrinol Metab* 10:675, 1975.
30. Desir D, Van Cauter E, Fang V, Martino E, Jadot C, Spire J-P, Noel P, Refetoff S, Copinschi G, Goldstein J: Effects of "jet lag" on hormonal patterns: I. Procedures, variations in total plasma proteins and disruption of adrenocorticotropin-cortisol periodicity. *J Clin Endocrinol Metab* 52:628, 1981.
31. Mezey E, Reisne TD, Brownstein MJ, Palkovits M, Axelrod J: β-Adrenergic mechanism of insulin-induced adrenocorticotropin release from the anterior pituitary. *Science* 226:1085, 1984.
32. Gilkes JJH, Bloomfield GS, Scott AP, Lowry PJ, Ratcliffe JG, Landon J, Rees LH: Development and validation of a radioimmunoassay for peptides related to a melanocyte-stimulating hormone in human plasma: The lipotropins. *J Clin Endocrinol Metab* 40:450, 1975.

33. Krieger DT, Liotta AS, Suda T, Goodgold A, Condon E: Human plasma immunoreactive lipotropin in normal subjects and in patients with pituitary/adrenal disease. *J Clin Endocrinol Metab* 48:566, 1979.

34. Bertagna XY, Stone WJ, Nicholson WE, Mount CD, Orth DN: Simultaneous assay of immunoreactive β-lipotropin, γ-lipotropin, and β-endorphin in plasma of normal human subjects, patients with ACTH/lipotropin hypersecretory syndromes, and patients undergoing chronic hemodialysis. *J Clin Invest* 67:124, 1981.

35. Rees LH: ACTH, lipotrophin, and MSH in health and disease, in Besser GM (ed): *Clinics in Endocrinology and Metabolism: The Hypothalamus and Pituitary.* London, Saunders, 1977, vol 6, p 137.

36. Hughes J, Smith TW, Fothergill LA, Morgan BA, Morris HR: Identification of two related pentapeptides from the brain with potent opiate agonist activity. *Nature* 258:577, 1975.

37. Goldstein A: Opioid peptides (endorphins) in pituitary and brain. *Science* 193:1081, 1976.

38. Guillemin R, Ling N, Lazarus L, Burgus R, Minick S, Bloom F, Nicoll R, Siggins G, Segal D: The endorphins, novel peptides of brain and hypophyseal origin, with opiate-like activity: Biochemical and biologic studies, in Krieger DT et al (eds): *ACTH and Related Peptides: Structure, Regulation, and Action.* New York Academy of Science, 1977, p 131.

39. Li CH, Yamashiro D, Chung D, Doneen BA, Loh HH, Tseng L: Isolation, structure, synthesis and morphine-like activity of beta-endorphin from human pituitary glands, in Krieger DT et al (eds): *ACTH and Related Peptides: Structure, Regulation, and Action.* New York Academy of Science, 1977, p. 158.

40. Wilkes MM, Stewart RD, Bruni JF, Quigley ME, Yen SS, Ling N, Chretien M: A specific homologous radioimmunoassay for human beta-endorphin: Direct measurement in biologic fluids. *J Clin Endocrinol Metab* 50:309, 1980.

41. Nakao K, Oki S, Tanaka I, Nakai Y, Imura H: Concomitant secretion of σ-MSH with ACTH and beta-endorphin in humans. *J Clin Endocrinol Metab* 51:1205, 1980.

42. Jackson RV, DeCherney GS, DeBold CR, Sheldon WR, Alexander AN, Rivier J, Vale W, Orth DN: Synthetic ovine corticotropin-releasing hormone: Simultaneous release of proopiomelanocortin peptides in man. *J Clin Endocrinol Metab* 58:740, 1984.

43. Nakao K, Nakai Y, Oki S, Horii K, Imura H: Presence of immunoreactive β-endorphin in normal human plasma: A concomitant release of β-endorphin with adrenocorticotropin after metyrapone administration. *J Clin Invest* 63:1395, 1978.

44. Nakao K, Nakai Y, Jingami H, Oki S, Fukuta J, Imura H: Substantial rise of plasma beta-endorphin levels after insulin-induced hypoglycemia in human subjects. *J Clin Endocrinol Metab* 49:838, 1979.

45. Suda T, Liotta AS, Krieger DT: β-Endorphin is not detectable in plasma from normal human subjects. *Science* 202:221, 1978.

46. Tanaka I, Nakai Y, Nakao K, Oki S, Masaki N, Ohtsuki H, Imura H: Presence of immunoreactive gamma-melanocyte-stimulating hormone, adrenocorticotropin, and beta-endorphin in human gastric antral mucosa. *J Clin Endocrinol Metab* 54:1982, 1982.

47. Bruni JF, Watkins WB, Yen SS: Beta-endorphin in the human pancreas. *J Clin Endocrinol Metab* 49:649, 1979.

48. Sharp B, Pekary AE: Beta-endorphin 61–91 and other beta-endorphin-immunoreactive peptides in human semen. *J Clin Endocrinol Metab* 52:586, 1981.

49. Liotta AS, Krieger DT: In vitro biosynthesis and comparative posttranslational processing of immunoreactive precursor corticotropin/β-endorphin by human placental and pituitary cells. *Endocrinology* 106:1504, 1980.

50. Genazzani AR, Fraioli F, Hurlimann J, Fioretti P, Felber JP: Immunoreactive ACTH and cortisol plasma levels during pregnancy: Detection and partial purification of corticotrophin-like placental hormone: The human chorionic corticotrophin (HCC). *Clin Endocrinol* 4:1, 1975.

51. Sairam MR, Bhargavi GN: A role for glycosylation of the alpha subunit in transduction of biologic signal in glycoprotein hormones. *Science* 229:65, 1985.

52. Pierce JG, Liao TH, Carlsen RB: Structural relationships between the subunits of pituitary thyroid stimulating and luteinizing hormones. *Fed Proc* 30:1045, 1971.

53. Carlsen RB, Bahl OP, Swaminathan N: Human chorionic gonadotropin. *J Biol Chem* 248:6810, 1973.

54. Shome B, Parlow AF: Human follicle stimulating hormone: First proposal for the amino acid sequence of the hormone specific beta-subunit (hFSH-β). *J Clin Endocrinol Metab* 39:203, 1974.

55. Sairam MR, Li CH: Human pituitary thyrotropin: The primary structure of the α and β subunits. *Can J Biochem* 55:755, 1977.

56. Begeot M, Hemming FJ, Dubois PM, Combarnous Y, Dubois MP, Aubert ML: Induction of pituitary lactotrope differentiation by luteinizing hormone α subunit. *Science* 226:566, 1984.

57. Naylor SL, Chin WW, Goodman HM, Lalley PA, Grzeschik KH, Sakaguchi AY: Chromosome assignment of genes encoding the alpha and beta subunits of glycoprotein hormones in man and mouse. *Somatic Cell Genet* 9:757, 1983.

58. Taylor T, Weintraub BD: Thyrotropin-releasing hormone regulation of TSH subunit biosynthesis in normal and hypothyroid rat pituitaries. *Endocrinology* 116:1968, 1985.

59. Van Helaelst L, Bonnyns M, Golstein-Golaire J: Pituitary TSH in normal subjects and in patients with asymptomatic atrophic thyroiditis: Evidence for its immunological heterogeneity. *J Clin Endocrinol Metab* 41:115, 1975.

60. Kourides IA, Weintraub RD, Ridgway EC, Maloof F: Pituitary secretion of free alpha and beta subunits of human thyrotropin in patients with thyroid disorders. *J Clin Endocrinol Metab* 40:872, 1975.

61. Peterson V, Smith BR, Hall R: A study of thyroid stimulating activity in human serum with the highly sensitive cytochemical bioassay. *J Clin Endocrinol Metab* 41:199, 1975.

62. Mardell RJ, Gamlen TR, Winton MR: High sensitivity assay of thyroid stimulating hormone in patients receiving thyroxine for primary hypothyroidism and thyroid carcinoma. *Br Med J* 290:355, 1985.

63. Edmonds M, Molitch M, Pierce J, Odell WD: Secretion of alpha and beta subunits of TSH by the anterior pituitary. *Clin Endocrinol* 4:525, 1975.

64. Kourides IA, Weintraub BD, Ridgway EC, Maloof F: Pituitary secretion of free alpha and beta subunits of human thyrotropin in patients with thyroid disorders. *J Clin Endocrinol Metab* 40:872, 1975.

65. Illig R, Krawczynska H, Torresani T, Prader A: Elevated plasma TSH and hypothyroidism in children with hypothalamic hypopituitarism. *J Clin Endocrinol Metab* 41:722, 1975.

66. Faglia G, Ferrari C, Paracchi A, Spada A, Beck-Peccoz P: Triiodothyronine response to thyrotropin-releasing hormone in patients with hypothalamic-pituitary disorders. *Clin Endocrinol* 4:585, 1975.

67. Faglia G, Bitensky L, Pinchera A, Ferrari C, Paracchi A, Beck-Peccoz P, Ambrosi B, Spada A: Thyrotropin secretion in patients with central hypothyroidism: Evidence for reduced biological activity of immunoreactive thyrotropin. *J Clin Endocrinol Metab* 48:989, 1979.

68. Beck-Peccoz P, Amr S, Menezes-Ferreira M, Faglia G, Weintraub BD: Decreased receptor binding of biologically inactive thyrotropin in central hypothyroidism: Effect of treatment with thyrotropin-releasing hormone. *N Engl J Med* 312:1085, 1985.

69. Spitz IM, LeRoith D, Hirsch H, Carayon P, Pekonen F, Liel Y, Sobel R, Chorer Z, Weintraub B: Increased high-molecular weight thyrotropin with impaired biologic activity in a euthyroid man. *N Engl J Med* 304:278, 1981.

70. Kuku SF, Harsoulis P, Kjeld M, Fraser TR: Human thyrotrophic hormone kinetics and effects in euthyroid males. *Horm Metab Res* 7:54, 1975.

71. Fisher DA, Dussault JH, Sack J, Chopra IJ: Ontogenesis of hypothalamic-pituitary-thyroid function and metabolism in man, sheep and rat. *Recent Prog Horm Res* 33:59, 1977.

72. Szabo M, Frohman LA: Suppression of cold-stimulated thyrotropin secretion by antiserum to thyrotropin-releasing hormone. *Endocrinology* 101:1023, 1977.

73. Szabo M, Kovathana N, Gordon K, Frohman LA: Effect of passive immunization with an antiserum to TRH on plasma TSH levels in thyroidectomized rats. *Endocrinology* 102:799, 1978.

74. Berelowitz M, Maeda K, Harris S, Frohman LA: The effect of alterations in the pituitary-thyroid axis on hypothalamic content and *in vitro* release of somatostatin-like immunoreactivity. *Endocrinology* 107:24, 1980.

75. Weeke J: Circadian variation of serum thyrotropin level in normal subjects. *Scand J Clin Lab Invest* 31:337, 1973.

76. Peters JR, Foord SM, Dieguez C, Scanlon MF: TSH neuroregulation and alterations in disease states. *Clin Endocrinol Metab* 12:669, 1983.

77. Ferland L, Labrie F, Jobin M, Arimura A, Schally AV: Physiological role of somatostatin in the control of growth hormone and thyrotropin secretion. *Biochem Biophys Res Commun* 68:149, 1976.

78. Cobb WE, Reichlin S, Jackson IM: Growth hormone secretory status is a determinant of the thyrotropin response to thyrotropin-releasing hormone in euthyroid patients with hypothalamic pituitary disease. *J Clin Endocrinol Metab* 52:324, 1981.

79. Reichert LE Jr, Ramsey RB, Carter EB: Application of a tissue receptor assay to measurement of serum follitropin (FSH). *J Clin Endocrinol Metab* 41:634, 1975.

80. Catt KJ, Dufau ML, Tsuruhara T: Radioligand-receptor assay of luteinizing hormone and chorionic gonadotropin. *J Clin Endocrinol Metab* 34:123, 1972.

81. Lucky AW, Rich BH, Rosenfield RG, Fang VS, Roche-Bender N: LH bioactivity increases more than immunoreactivity during puberty. *J Pediatr* 97:205, 1980.

82. Dufau ML, Beitins IZ, McArthur JW, Catt KJ: Effects of luteinizing hormone releasing hormone (LHRH) upon bioactive and immunoreactive serum LH levels in normal subjects. *J Clin Endocrinol Metab* 43:658, 1976.

83. Winter JSD, Faiman C, Hobson WC, Prasad AV, Reyes FI: Pituitary-gonadal relations in infancy: I. Patterns of serum gonadotropin concentrations from birth to 4 years of age in man and chimpanzee. *J Clin Endocrinol Metab* 40:545, 1975.

84. Boyar RM, Finkelstein J, Roffwarg H, Kapen S, Weitzman E, Hellman L: Synchronization of augmented luteinizing hormone secretion with sleep during puberty. *N Engl J Med* 287:582, 1972.

85. Hagen C, McNeilly AS: Changes in circulating levels of LH, FSH, LH beta- and alpha-subunit after gonadotropin-releasing hormone, and of TSH, LH beta- and alpha-subunit after thyrotropin-releasing hormone. *J Clin Endocrinol Metab* 41:466, 1975.

86. Kulin HE, Bell PM, Santen RJ, Ferber AJ: Integration of pulsatile gonadotropin secretion by timed urinary measurements: An accurate and sensitive 3-hour test. *J Clin Endocrinol Metab* 40:783, 1975.

87. Cobel YD, Kohler PO, Cargille CM, Ross GT: Production rates and metabolic clearance rates of human follicle-stimulating hormone in premenopausal and postmenopausal women. *J Clin Invest* 48:359, 1969.

88. Keye WR Jr, Jaffe RV: Modulation of pituitary gonadotropin response to gonadotropin-releasing hormone by estradiol. *J Clin Endocrinol Metab* 38:805, 1974.

89. Lasley BL, Wang CF, Yen SSC: The effects of estrogen and progesterone on the functional capacity of the gonadotrophs. *J Clin Endocrinol Metab* 41:820, 1975.

90. Franchimont P, Verstraelen-Proyard J, Hazee-Huelskin MT, Renard C, Denoulin A, Bourguignon JP, Hustin J: Inhibin, from concept to reality. *Vitam Horm* 37:243, 1979.

91. Baker HWG, Bremmer WJ, Burger HG, de Kretser DM, Eddie LW, Hudson B, Keogh EJ, Lee WK, Rennie CG: Testicular control of follicle stimulating hormone secretion. *Recent Prog Horm Res* 32:429, 1976.

93. Sen S, Valenzuela R, Smeby R, Bravo EL, Bumpus FM: Localization, purification, and biological activity of a new aldosterone-stimulating factor. *Hypertension* 3 (suppl. 1):81, 1981.

94. Sen S, Bumpus FM, Oberfield S, New MI: Development and preliminary application of a new assay for aldosterone-stimulating factor. *Hypertension* 5 (suppl 1):27, 1983.

95. Lis M, Hamet P, Gutkowska J, Maurice G, Seidah NG, LaRiviere N, Chretien M, Genest J: Effect of N-terminal portion of proopiomelanocortin on aldosterone release by human adrenal adenoma in vitro. *J Clin Endocrinol Metab* 52:1053, 1981.

96. Matsuoka H, Mulrow PJ, Franco-Saenz R, Li CH: Effects of β-lipotropin-derived peptides on aldosterone production in the rat adrenal gland. *J Clin Invest* 68:752, 1981.

97. Shome B, Parlow AF: Human pituitary prolactin: The entire linear amino acid sequence. *J Clin Endocrinol Metab* 45:1112, 1977.

98. Li CH: The chemistry of human pituitary growth hormone: 1967–1973, in Li CH (ed): *Hormonal Proteins and Peptides*. New York, Academic, 1975, vol 3, p 1.

99. Niall HD, Hogan ML, Traeger GW, Segre GV, Hwang P, Friesen HG: The chemistry of growth hormone and the lactogenic hormones. *Recent Prog Horm Res* 29:387, 1973.

100. Miller WL, Eberhardt NL: Structure and evolution of the growth hormone gene family. *Endocr Rev* 4:97, 1983.

101. Owerbach D, Martial JA, Baxter JD, Rutter WJ, Shows TB: Genes for growth hormone, chorionic somatomammotropin and a growth hormone–like gene are located on chromosome 17 in humans. *Science* 209:289, 1980.

102. Owerbach D, Rutter WJ, Cooke NE, Martial JA, Shows TB: The prolactin gene is located on chromosome 6 in humans. *Science* 212:815, 1981.

103. Phillips JA III, Hjelle BL, Seeburg PH, Zachmann M: Molecular basis for familial isolated growth hormone deficiency. *Proc Natl Acad Sci USA* 78:6372, 1981.

104. Pavlakis GN, Hizuka N, Gorden PL, Seeburg P, Hamer DH: Expression of two human growth hormone genes in monkey cells infected by simian virus 40 recombinants. *Proc Natl Acad Sci USA* 78:7398, 1981.

105. Seeburg PH: Structural and functional features of the human growth hormone locus. Program, Endocrine Society 68th Annual Meeting, Baltimore, 1986, p 14.

106. Maurer RA, Gorski J, McKean DJ: Partial amino acid sequence of rat preprolactin. *Biochem J* 161:189, 1977.

107. Benveniste R, Stachura M, Szabo M, Frohman LA: Big growth hormone: Conversion to small growth hormone without peptide bond cleavage. *J Clin Endocrinol Metab* 41:422, 1975.

108. Lewis UJ, Peterson SM, Bonewald LF, Seavey BK, VanderLaan WP: An interchain disulfide dimer of human growth hormone. *J Biol Chem* 252:3697, 1977.

109. Stachura ME, Frohman LA: Growth hormone: Independent release of big and small forms from rat pituitary in vitro. *Science* 187:447, 1975.

110. Soman V, Goodman AD: Studies of the composition and radioreceptor activity of "big" and "little" human growth hormone. *J Clin Endocrinol Metab* 44:569, 1977.

111. Lewis UJ, Dunn JT, Bonewald LF, Seavey BNK, VanderLaan WP: A naturally occurring structural variant of human growth hormone. *J Biol Chem* 253:2679, 1978.

112. DeNoto FM, Moore DD, Goodman HM: Human growth hormone DNA sequence and mRNA structures: Possible alternative splicing. *Nucleic Acids Res* 9:3719, 1981.

113. Baumann G, MacCart JG, Amburn K: The molecular nature of circulating growth hormone in normal and acromegalic man: Evidence for a principal and minor monomeric form. *J Clin Endocrinol Metab* 456:946, 1983.

114. Lewis UJ, Singh RNP, Tutwiler GF: Hypoglycemic activity of the 20,000-dalton variant of human growth hormone. *Endocr Res Commun* 8:155, 1981.

115. Valenta LJ, Sigel MB, Lesniak MA, Elias AN, Lewis UJ, Friesen HG, Kershnar AK: Pituitary dwarfism in a patient with circulating abnormal growth hormone polymers. *N Engl J Med* 312:214, 1985.

116. Lewis UJ, Sinha YN, Markoff E, VanderLaan WP: Multiple forms of prolactin: Properties and measurement, in Muller EE, MacLeod RM, Frohman LA (eds): *Neuroendocrine Perspectives.* Elsevier, Amsterdam, 1985, vol 4, p 43.

117. Shoupe D, Montz FJ, Kletzky DA, Di Zerega GS: Prolactin molecular heterogeneity: Response to TRH stimulation of concanavalin-A bound and unbound immunoassayable prolactin during human pregnancy. *Am J Obstet Gynceol* 147:482, 1983.

118. Jackson RD, Wortsman J, Malarkey WB: Characterization of a large molecular weight prolactin in women with idiopathic hyperprolactinemia and normal menses. *J Clin Endocrinol Metab* 61:258, 1985.

119. Isaksson OGP, Eden S, Jansson J-O: Mode of action of pituitary growth hormone on target cells. *Annu Rev Physiol* 47:483, 1985.

120. Frohman LA, MacGillivray M, Aceto T Jr: Acute effects of human growth hormone on insulin secretion and glucose utilization in normal and growth hormone deficient subjects. *J Clin Endocrinol Metab* 27:561, 1967.

121. Adamson U, Cerasi E: Acute effects of exogenous growth hormone in man: Time- and dose-bound modification of glucose tolerance and glucose-induced insulin release. *Acta Endocrinol* 80:247, 1975.

122. Salmon WD Jr, Daughaday WH: A hormonally controlled serum factor which stimulates sulfate incorporation by cartilage in vitro. *J Lab Clin Med* 49:825, 1957.

123. Froesch ER, Schmid C, Schwander J, Zapf J: Actions of insulin-like growth factors. *Annu Rev Physiol* 47:443, 1985.

124. Zapf J, Froesch ER, Humbel RE: The insulin-like growth factors (IGF) of human serum: Chemical and biologic characterization and aspects of their possible physiological role. *Curr Top Cell Regul* 19:257, 1981.

125. Schoenle E, Zads J, Humbel RE, et al: Insulin-like growth factor I stimulates growth in hypophysectomized rats. *Nature* 296:252, 1982.

126. Isaksson OGP, Jansson J-O, Gause IAM: Growth hormone stimulates longitudinal bone growth directly. *Science* 216:1237, 1982.

127. Russell SM, Spencer EM: Local injections of human or rat growth hormone or of purified human somatomedin-C stimulate unilateral tibial epiphyseal growth in hypophysectomized rats. *Endocrinology* 116:2563, 1985.

128. Rezvani I, DiGeorge AM, Doroshen SA, Bourdony CJ: Action of human growth hormone on extrathyroidal conversion of thyroxine to triiodothyronine in children with hypopituitarism. *Pediatr Res* 15:6, 1981.

129. Gordon P, Lesniak MA, Eastman R, Hendricks CM, Roth J: Evidence for higher production of "little" growth hormone with increased radioreceptor activity in acromegalic plasma. *J Clin Endocrinol Metab* 43:364, 1976.

130. Raiti S: The National Hormone and Pituitary Program: Achievements and current goals, in Raiti S, Tolman RA (eds): *Human Growth Hormone.* New York, Plenum, 1986, p 1.

131. Parker ML, Utiger RD, Daughaday WH: Studies in human growth hormone: II. The physiologic disposition and metabolic fate of human growth hormone in man. *J Clin Invest* 41:262, 1962.

132. MacGillivray MH, Frohman LA, Doe J: Metabolic clearance and production rates of human growth hormone in subjects with normal and abnormal growth. *J Clin Endocrinol Metab* 30:632, 1970.

133. Thompson RG, Rodriquez A, Kowarski A, Blizzard RM: Growth hormone: Metabolic clearance rates, integrated concentrations and production rates in normal adults and the effect of prednisone. *J Clin Invest* 51:3193, 1972.

134. Imaki T, Shibisaki T, Shizume K, Masuda A, Hotta M, Kiyosawa Y, Jibiki K, Demura H, Tsushima T, Ling N: The effect of free fatty acids on growth hormone (GH)-releasing hormone mediated GH secretion in man. *J Clin Endocrinol Metab* 60:290, 1985.

135. Massara F, Ghigo E, Goffi S, Molinatti GM, Muller EE, Camanni F: Blockade of hpGRF-40-induced GH release in normal men by a cholinergic muscarinic antagonist. *J Clin Endocrinol Metab* 59:1025, 1984.

136. Frohman LA, Berelowitz M: Physiological and pharmacological control of anterior pituitary hormone secretion, in Dunn A, Nemeroff CB (eds): *Peptides, Hormones, and Behavior.* Holliswood, NY, Spectrum, 1984, p 119.

137. Berelowitz M, Szabo M, Frohman LA, Firestone S, Chu L, Hintz RL: Somatomedin-C mediates growth hormone negative feedback by effects on both the hypothalamus and the pituitary. *Science* 212:1279, 1981.

138. Berelowitz M, Firestone SL, Frohman LA: Effects of growth hormone excess and deficiency on hypothalamic somatostatin content and release and on tissue somatostatin distribution. *Endocrinology* 109:714, 1981.

139. Tannenbaum GS: Evidence for autoregulation of growth hormone secretion via the central nervous system. *Endocrinology* 107:2117, 1980.

140. Laron Z: Laron-type dwarfism (hereditary somatomedin deficiency): A review, in Frick P, Harnack G-A, Kochsiek K, Martini GA, Prader A (eds): *Advances in Internal Medicine and Pediatrics.* Berlin, Springer-Verlag, 1984, p 117.

141. Tamminga CA, Neophytides A, Chase TN, Frohman LA: Stimulation of prolactin and growth hormone secretion by muscimol, a gamma-amino-butyric acid agonist. *J Clin Endocrinol Metab* 47:1348, 1978.

142. Stubbs WA, Jones A, Edwards CRW, Delitala G, Jeffcoate WJ, Ratter SJ, Besser GM, Bloom SR, Alberti KGMM: Hormonal and metabolic responses to an enkephalin analogue in normal man. *Lancet* 2:1225, 1978.

143. McNatty KP, Sawers RS: Relationship between the endocrine environment within the graafian follicle and the subsequent rate of progesterone secretion by human granulosa cells in vitro. *J Endocrinol* 66:391, 1975.

144. Landgraf R, Landgraf-Leurs MMC, Weissmann A, Horl R, Von Werder K, Scriba PC: A diabetogenic hormone. *Diabetologia* 13:99, 1977.

145. Shiu RPC, Kelly PA, Friesen HG: Radioreceptor assay for prolactin and other lactogenic hormones. *Science* 180:968, 1973.

146. Soong YK, Ferguson KM, McGarrick G, Jeffcoate SL: Size heterogeneity of immunoreactive prolactin in hyperprolactinemic women. *Clin Endocrinol* 16:259, 1982.

147. Golander A, Hurley T, Barrett J, Hizi A, Handwerger S: Prolactin synthesis by human chorion-decidual tissue: A possible source of prolactin in the amniotic fluid. *Science* 202:311, 1978.

148. Sievertsen G, Lim VS, Nakawatase C, Frohman LA: Metabolic clearance and secretion of human prolactin in normal subjects and in patients with chronic renal failure. *J Clin Endocrinol Metab* 50:846, 1980.

149. Molitch ME, Raiti S, Baumann G, Reichlin S: Initial pharmacokinetic studies of IM and IV human prolactin administration to normal human subjects. Program, Endocrine Society 67th Annual Meeting, Baltimore, 1985, abstr 162.

150. Phillips HS, Nikolics K, Branton D, Seeburg PH: Immuno-

cytochemical localization in rat brain of a prolactin release-inhibiting sequence of gonadotropin-releasing hormone prohormone. *Nature* 316:542, 1985.
151. Nikolics K, Mason AJ, Szonyi E, Ramachandran J, Seeburg PH: A prolactin-inhibiting factor within the precursor for human gonadotropin-releasing hormone. *Nature* 316:511, 1985.
152. Abe H, Engler D, Molitch ME, Bollinger-Gruber J, Reichlin S: Vasoactive intestinal peptide is a physiological mediator of prolactin release in the rat. *Endocrinology* 116:1383, 1985.
153. Bloom SR, Christofides ND, Delemarter J, Buell G, Kawashima E, Polak JM: Diarrhea in vipoma patients associated with cosecretion of a second active peptide (peptide histidine isoleucine) explained by single coding gene. *Lancet* 2:1163, 1983.
154. Carlson HE, Wasser HL, Levin SR: Prolactin stimulation by meals is related to protein content. *J Clin Endocrinol Metab* 57:334, 1983.
155. Langer G, Sachar EJ, Gruen PH, Halpern FS: Human prolactin responses to neuroleptic drugs correlate with antischizophrenic potency. *Nature* 266:639, 1977.
156. Rick J, Szabo M, Payne P, Kovathana N, Cannon JG, Frohman LA: Prolactin-suppressive effects of two aminotetralin analogs of dopamine: Their use in the characterization of the pituitary dopamine receptor. *Endocrinology* 104:1234, 1979.
157. Gonzalez-Villalpado C, Szabo M, Frohman LA: Central nervous system–mediated stimulation of prolactin secretion by cimetidine, a histamine H_2-receptor antagonist: Impaired responsiveness in patients with prolactin-secreting tumors and idiopathic hyperprolactinemia. *J Clin Endocrinol Metab* 51:1417, 1980.
158. Knigge U, Wollesen F, Dejgarrd A, Theusen B: Comparison between dose-responses of prolactin, thyroid stimulating hormone and growth hormone to two different histamine H-2 receptor antagonists in normal men. *Clin Endocrinol* 15:585, 1981.
159. Lim VS, Kathpalia S, Frohman LA: Hyperprolactinemia and impaired pituitary responses to suppression and stimulation in chronic renal failure. Reversal following transplantation. *J Clin Endocrinol Metab* 48:101, 1979.
160. Simmonds M: Uber hypophysisschwund mit todlichem Ausgang. *Dtsch Med Wochenschr* 40:322, 1914.
161. Glinski LK: Anatomische Veranderungen der Hypophyse. *Dtsch Med Wochenschr* 39:473, 1913.
162. Sheehan HL: Postpartum necrosis of the anterior pituitary. *J Pathol Bacteriol* 45:189, 1937.
163. Sheehan HL, Murdoch R: Postpartum necrosis of the anterior pituitary: Pathological and clinical aspects. *J Obstet Gynaecol Br Empire* 45:456, 1938.
164. Brennan CF, Malone RGS, Weaver JA: Pituitary necrosis in diabetes mellitus. *Lancet* 2:12, 1956.
165. Kovacs K: Necrosis of anterior pituitary in humans. *Neuroendocrinology* 4:170, 1969.
166. Cardoso ER, Peterson EW: Pituitary apoplexy: A review. *Neurosurgery* 14:363, 1984.
167. Pelkonen R, Kuusisto A, Salmi J, Eistola P, Raitta C, Karonen S-L, Aro A: Pituitary function after apoplexy. *Am J Med* 65:773, 1978.
168. Stocks AE, Powell LW: Pituitary function in idiopathic hemochromatosis and cirrhosis of the liver. *Lancet* 2:298, 1972.
169. Williams T, Frohman LA: Hypothalamic dysfunction associated with hemochromatosis. *Ann Intern Med* 103:550, 1985.
170. Asa SL, Bilbao JM, Kovacs K, Josse RG, Kreines K: Lymphocytic hypophysitis of pregnancy resulting in hypopituitarism. *Ann Intern Med* 95:166, 1981.
171. Baskin DS, Townsend JJ, Wilson CB: Lymphocytic adenohypophysitis of pregnancy simulating a pituitary adenoma: A distinct pathological entity. *J Neurosurg* 56:148, 1982.
172. Rickards AG, Harvey PW: "Giant cell granuloma" and other pituitary granulomata. *Q J Med* 23:425, 1954.
173. Barkan AL, Kelch RP, Marshall JC: Isolated gonadotrope failure in the polyglandular autoimmune syndrome. *N Engl J Med* 312:1535, 1985.
174. Samaan NA, Bakdesh MM, Caderao JB, Cangir A, Jesse RH Jr, Ballantyne AJ: Hypopituitarism after external irradiation: Evidence for both hypothalamic and pituitary origin. *Ann Intern Med* 83:771, 1975.
175. Romshe CA, Zipf WB, Miser A, Miser J, Sotos JF, Newton WA: Evaluation of growth hormone release and human growth hormone treatment in children with cranial irradiation–associated short stature. *J Pediatr* 104:177, 1984.
176. Jordan RM, Kendall JW, Kerber CW: The primary empty sella syndrome. *Am J Med* 62:569, 1977.
177. Fleckman AM, Schubart UK, Danziger A, Fleischer N: Empty sella of normal size in Sheehan's syndrome. *Am J Med* 75:585, 1983.
178. Chiang R, Marshall MC Jr, Rosman PM, Hotson G, Mannheimer E, Wallace EZ: Empty sella turcica in intracranial sarcoidosis. *Arch Neurol* 41:662, 1984.
179. Schimke RN, Spaulding JJ, Hollowell JG: X-linked congenital panhypopituitarism. *Birth Defects* 7:21, 1971.
180. Ferrier PE, Stone EF Jr: Familial pituitary dwarfism associated with an abnormal sella turcica. *Pediatrics* 43:858, 1969.
181. Parks JS, Tenore A, Bongiovanni AM, Kirkland RT: Familial hypopituitarism with large sella turcica. *N Engl J Med* 298:698, 1978.
182. Lim VS, Fang VS, Katz AJ, Refetoff S: Thyroid dysfunction in renal failure: A study of the pituitary axis and peripheral turnover kinetics of thyroxine and triiodothyronine. *J Clin Invest* 60:522, 1977.
183. Lim VS, Henriquez C, Sievertsen G, Frohman LA: Ovarian function in chronic renal failure: Evidence suggesting hypothalamic anovulation. *Ann Intern Med* 93:21, 1980.
184. Rudman D, Fleischer AS, Kutner MH, Raggio JF: Suprahypophyseal hypogonadism and hypothyroidism during prolonged coma after head trauma. *J Clin Endocrinol Metab* 45:747, 1977.
185. King LR, Knowles HC Jr, McLaurin RL, Brielmaier J, Perisutti G, Piziak VK: Pituitary hormone response to head injury. *Neurosurgery* 9:229, 1983.
186. Woolf PD, Hamill RW, McDonald JV, Lee LA, Kelly M: Transient hypogonadotropic hyogonadism caused by critical illness. *J Clin Endocrinol Metab* 60:444, 1985.
187. Schurmeyer TH, Tsokos GC, Avgerinos PC, Balow JE, D'Agata R, Loriaux DL, Chrousos GP: Pituitary-adrenal responsiveness to corticotropin-releasing hormone in patients receiving chronic alternate day glucocorticoid therapy. *J Clin Endocrinol Metab* 61:22, 1985.
188. Chihara K, Kashio Y, Abe H, Minamitnai N, Kaji H, Kita T, Fujita T: Idiopathic growth hormone (GH) deficiency, and GH deficiency secondary to hypothalamic germinoma: Effect of single and repeated administration of human GH-releasing factor (hGRF) on plasma GH level and endogenous hGRF-like immunoreactivity level in cerebrospinal fluid. *J Clin Endocrinol Metab* 60:269, 1985.
189. Bullen BA, Skrinar GS, Beitens IZ, von Mering G, Turnbull BA, McArthur JW: Induction of menstrual disorders by strenuous exercise in untrained women. *N Engl J Med* 312:1349, 1985.
190. Carlberg KA, Buckman MT, Peake GT, Riedesel M: A survey of menstrual function in athletes. *Eur J Appl Physiol* 51:211, 1983.
191. Vigersky R (ed): *Anorexia Nervosa.* New York, Raven, 1977.
192. Barkan A, Glantz I: Calcification of auricular cartilages in patients with hypopituitarism. *J Clin Endocrinol Metab* 55:354, 1982.
193. Miyai K, Azukizawa M, Kumahara Y: Familial isolated thyrotropin deficiency with cretinism. *N Engl J Med* 285:1043, 1971.
194. Zisman E, Lotz M, Jenkins ME, Bartter FC: Studies in pseudohypoparathyroidism: Two new cases with a probable selective deficiency of thyrotropin. *Am J Med* 46:464, 1969.
195. Bell J, Benveniste R, Spitz I, Rabinowitz D: Isolated deficiency of follicle-stimulating hormone: Further studies. *J Clin Endocrinol Metab* 40:790, 1975.

196. Merimee TJ: A follow-up study of vascular disease in growth hormone–deficient dwarfs with diabetes. *N Engl J Med* 298:1217, 1978.
197. Goodman HG, Grumbach MM, Kaplan SL: Growth and growth hormone: II. A comparison of isolated growth hormone deficiency and multiple pituitary hormone deficiencies in 35 patients with idiopathic hypopituitary dwarfism. *N Engl J Med* 278:57, 1968.
198. Sheehan HL, Summers VK: The syndrome of hypopituitarism. *Q J Med* 18:319, 1949.
199. Gambone J, Meldrum DR, Laufer L, Chang RJ, Lu JKH, Judd HL: Further delineation of hypothalamic dysfunction responsible for menopausal hot flashes. *J Clin Endocrinol Metab* 59:1097, 1984.
200. Lindholm J, Kehlet H, Blichert-Toft M, Dinesen B, Riishede J: Reliability of the 30-min ACTH test in assessing hypothalamic-pituitary-adrenal function. *J Clin Endocrinol Metab* 47:272, 1978.
201. Borst GC, Michenfelder HJ, O'Brian JT: Discordant cortisol response to exogenous ACTH and insulin-induced hypoglycemia in patients with pituitary disease. *N Engl J Med* 306:1462, 1982.
202. Grossman A, Kruseman AC, Perry L, Tomlin S, Schally AV, Coy DH, Rees LH, Comaru-Schally AM, Besser GM: New hypothalamic hormone, corticotropin-releasing factor, specifically stimulates the release of adrenocorticotropic hormone and cortisol in man. *Lancet* 1:921, 1982.
203. Orth DN, Jackson RV, DeCherney GS, DeBold CR, Alexander AN, Island DP, Rivier J, Rivier C, Spiess J, Vale W: Effect of synthetic ovine corticotropin-releasing factor: Dose response of plasma adrenocorticotropin and cortisol. *J Clin Invest* 71:587, 1982.
204. Spiger M, Jubiz W, Meikle AW, West CD, Tyler FJ: Single-dose metyrapone test: Review of a four-year experience. *Arch Intern Med* 135:698, 1975.
205. Asa SL, Kovacs K, Tindall GT, Barrow DL, Horvath E, Vecsei P: Cushing's disease associated with an intrasellar gangliocytoma producing corticotrophin-releasing factor. *Ann Intern Med* 101:789, 1984.
206. Costom BH, Grumbach MM, Kaplan SL: Effect of thyrotropin-releasing factor on serum thyroid-stimulating hormone. *J Clin Invest* 50:2219, 1971.
207. Besser GM, McNeilly AS, Anderson DC, Marshall JC, Harsoulis P, Hall R, Ormston BJ, Alexander L, Collins WP: Hormonal responses to synthetic luteinizing hormone and follicle stimulating hormone releasing hormone in man. *Br Med J* 3:267, 1972.
208. Mortimer CH, Besser GM, McNeilly AS, Marshall JC, Harsoulis P, Tunbridge WNG, Gomez-Pan A, Hall R: Luteinizing hormone and follicle stimulating hormone releasing hormone test in patients with hypothalamic-pituitary-gonadal dysfunction. *Br Med J* 4:73, 1973.
209. Snyder PJ, Rudenstein RS, Gardner DF, Rothman JG: Repetitive infusion of gonadotropin-releasing hormone distinguishes hypothalamic from pituitary hypogonadism. *J Clin Endocrinol Metab* 48:864, 1979.
210. Vance ML, Borges JLC, Kaiser DL, Evans WS, Furlanetto R, Thominet JL, Frohman LA, Rogol AD, MacLeod RM, Bloom S, Rivier J, Vale W, Thorner MO: Human pancreatic tumor growth hormone releasing factor (hpGRF-40): Dose response relationships in normal man. *J Clin Endocrinol Metab* 58:838, 1984.
211. Gelato MC, Pescovitz OH, Cassorla F, Loriaux DL, Merriam GR: Dose-response relationships for effects of growth hormone releasing factor-(1–44)-NH_2 in young adult men and women. *J Clin Endocrinol Metab* 59:107, 1984.
212. Schriock EA, Lustig RH, Rosenthal SM, Kaplan SL, Grumbach MM: Effect of growth hormone (GH)-releasing hormone (GRH) on plasma GH in relation to magnitude and duration of GH deficiency in 26 children and adults with isolated deficiency or multiple pituitary hormone deficiencies: Evidence for hypothalamic GRH deficiency. *J Clin Endocrinol Metab* 58:1043, 1984.
213. Gil-Ad I, Topper E, Laron Z: Oral clonidine as a growth hormone stimulation test. *Lancet* 2:278, 1979.
214. Laron Z, Gil-Ad I, Topper E, Kaufman H, Josefsberg Z: Low oral dose of clonidine an effective screening test for growth hormone deficiency. *Acta Paediatr Scand* 71:847, 1982.
215. Williams T, Berelowitz M, Joffe SN, Thorner MO, Rivier J, Vale W, Frohman LA: Impaired growth hormone responses to growth hormone-releasing factor in obesity: A pituitary defect reversed with weight reduction. *N Engl J Med* 311:1403, 1984.
216. Sims EAH, Danforth E Jr, Horton ES, Bray GS, Glennon JA, Salans LB: Endocrine and metabolic effects of experimental obesity in man. *Recent Prog Horm Res* 29:457, 1973.
217. MacGillivray MH, Aceto T, Frohman LA: Plasma growth hormone response and growth retardation of hypothyroidism. *Am J Dis Child* 115:273, 1968.
218. Williams T, Maxon H, Thorner MO, Frohman LA: Blunted growth hormone response to growth hormone-releasing hormone in hypothyroidism resolves in the euthyroid state. *J Clin Endocrinol Metab* 61:454, 1985.
219. Woolf PH, Lee LA, Leebaw WF: Hypoglycemia as a provocative test of prolactin release. *Metabolism* 27:869, 1978.
220. Sheldon WR Jr, DeBold CR, Evans WS, DeCherney GS, Jackson RV, Island DP, Thorner MO, Orth DN: Rapid sequential intravenous administration of four hypothalamic releasing hormones as a combined anterior pituitary function test in normal subjects. *J Clin Endocrinol Metab* 60:623, 1985.
221. Hurley DM, Brian R, Outch K, Stockdale J, Fry A, Hackman C, Clarke I, Burger HG: Induction of ovulation and fertility in amenorrheic women by pulsatile low-dose gonadotropin-releasing hormone. *N Engl J Med* 310:1069, 1984.
222. Hoffman AR, Crowley WF Jr: Induction of puberty in men by long-term pulsatile administration of low-dose gonadotropin-releasing hormone. *N Engl J Med* 307:1237, 1982.
223. Skarin G, Nillius SJ, Wibell L, Wide L: Chronic pulsatile low dose GnRH for induction of testosterone production and spermatogenesis in a man with secondary hypogonadotropic hypogonadism. *J Clin Endocrinol Metab* 55:723, 1982.
224. Finkel DM, Phillips JL, Snyder PJ: Stimulation of spermatogenesis by gonadotropins in men with hypogonadotropic hypogonadism. *N Engl J Med* 313:651, 1985.
225. Brown P, Gajdusek DC, Gibbs CJ Jr, Asher DM: Potential epidemic of Creutzfeldt-Jakob disease from human growth hormone therapy. *N Engl J Med* 313:728, 1985.
226. Frasier SD: Human pituitary growth hormone (hGH) therapy in growth hormone deficiency. *Endocr Rev* 4:155, 1983.
227. Thorner MO, Reschke J, Chitwood J, Rogol AD, Furlanetto R, Rivier J, Vale W, Blizzard RM: Acceleration of growth in two children treated with human growth hormone-releasing factor. *N Engl J Med* 312:4, 1985.
228. Gelato MC, Ross JL, Malozowski S, Peskovitz OH, Skerda M, Cassorla F, Loriaux DL, Merriam GL: Effects of pulsatile administration of growth hormone (GH)-releasing hormone on short term linear growth in children with GH deficiency. *J Clin Endocrinol Metab* 61:444, 1985.
229. Tyson JE, Perez A, Zanartu J: Human lactational response to oral thyrotropin releasing hormone. *J Clin Endocrinol Metab* 43:760, 1976.
230. Kovacs K, Horvath E, Bayley TA, Hassaram ST, Ezrin C: Silent corticotroph cell adenoma lysosomal accumulation and crinophagy. *Am J Med* 64:492, 1978.
231. Kourides IA, Weintraub BD, Rosen SW, Ridgway EC, Kliman B, Maloof F: Secretion of alpha subunit of glycoprotein hormones by pituitary adenomas. *J Clin Endocrinol Metab* 43:97, 1976.
232. Younghusband OZ, Horrax G, Hurxthal LM, Hare HF, Poppen JL: Chromophobe pituitary tumors: I. Diagnosis. *J Clin Endocrinol Metab* 12:611, 1952.
233. Bakay L: The results of 300 pituitary adenoma operations. *J Neurosurg* 7:240, 1950.
234. Burrow GN, Wortzman G, Rewcastle NB, Holgate RC, Kovacs K: Microadenomas of the pituitary and abnormal sellar

tomograms in unselected autopsy series. *N Engl J Med* 304:156, 1981.
235. Earle JM, Dillard SH Jr: Pathology of adenomas of the pituitary gland, in Kohler PO et al (eds): *Diagnosis and Treatment of Pituitary Tumors.* Amsterdam, Excerpta Medica, 1973, p 3.
236. Wilson CB, Dempsey LC: Transsphenoidal microsurgical removal of 250 pituitary adenomas. *J Neurosurg* 48:13, 1978.
237. Furst E: On chromophobe pituitary adenoma. *Acta Med Scand* 180(suppl 452):1, 1966.
238. Bartlett JR: Craniopharyngiomas—a summary of 85 cases. *J Neurol Neurosurg Psychiatry* 34:37, 1971.
239. Wilson CB, Dempsey LC: Transsphenoidal microsurgical removal of 250 pituitary adenomas. *J Neurosurg* 48:13, 1978.
240. Tindall GT, McLanahan CS, Christy JC: Transsphenoidal microsurgery for pituitary tumors associated with hyperprolactinemia. *J Neurosurg* 48:849, 1981.
241. Crane TB, Yee RD, Hepler FS, Hallinan JM: Clinical manifestations and radiologic findings in craniopharyngiomas in adults. *Am J Ophthalmol* 94:220, 1982.
242. Taveras JM, Wood EH: *Diagnostic Neuroradiology.* Baltimore, Williams & Wilkins, 1964, p 1.101.
243. McLachlan MSF, Wright AD, Doyle FH: Plain film and tomographic assessment of the pituitary fossa in 140 acromegalic patients. *Br J Radiol* 43:360, 1970.
244. Brown SB, Irwin KM, Enzmann DR: CT characteristics of the normal pituitary gland. *Neuroradiology* 24:259, 1983.
245. Swartz MD, Russell KB, Basile BA, O'Donnell PC, Popky GL: High-resolution computed tomographic appearance of the intrasellar contents in women of childbearing age. *Radiology* 145:115, 1983.
246. Hinshaw DB Jr, Hasso AN, Thompson JR, Davidson BJ: High resolution computed tomography of the postpartum pituitary gland. *Neuroradiology* 26:299, 1984.
247. Hemminghytt S, Kalkhoff DK, Daniels DL, Williams AL, Grogan JP, Haughton VM: Computed tomographic study of hormone-secreting microadenomas. *Radiology* 146:65, 1983.
248. Chambers AL, Turski PA, LaMasters D, Newton TH: Regions of low density in the contrast-enhanced pituitary gland: Normal and pathologic processes. *Radiology* 144:109, 1982.
249. Taylor CR, Jaffe CC: Methodological problems in clinical radiology research: Pituitary microadenoma detection as a paradigm. *Radiology* 149:279, 1983.
250. Kaufman B: Magnetic resonance imaging of the pituitary gland. *Radiol Clin North Am* 22:795, 1984.
251. Linfoot JA, Garcia JF, Wei W, Fink R, Sarin R, Born JL, Lawrence JH: Human growth hormone levels in cerebrospinal fluid. *J Clin Endocrinol Metab* 31:230, 1970.
252. Jordan RM, Kendall JW, Seaich JL, Allen JP, Paulsen A, Kerber CW, VanderLaan WP: Cerebrospinal fluid hormone concentration in the evaluation of pituitary tumors. *Ann Intern Med* 85:49, 1976.
253. Schroeder LL, Johnson JC, Malarkey WB: Cerebrospinal fluid prolactin: A reflection of abnormal prolactin secretion in patients with pituitary tumors. *J Clin Endocrinol Metab* 43:1255, 1976.
254. Weisberg LA, Zimmerman EA, Frantz AG: Diagnosis and evaluation of patients with an enlarged sella turcica. *Am J Med* 61:590, 1976.
255. Bergland RM, Ray BS, Torack RM: Anatomical variations in the pituitary gland and adjacent structures in 225 human autopsy cases. *J Neurosurg* 28:93, 1968.
256. Gharib H, Frey HM, Laws ER Jr, Randall RV, Scheithauer BW: Coexistent primary empty sella syndrome and hyperprolactinemia. *Arch Intern Med* 143:1383, 1983.
257. Domingue JN, Wing SD, Wilson CB: Coexisting pituitary adenomas and partially empty sellas. *J Neurosurg* 48:23, 1978.
258. Ganguly A, Stanchfield JB, Roberts TS, West CD, Tyler FH: Cushing's syndrome in a patient with an empty sella turcica and a microadenoma of the adenohypophysis. *Am J Med* 60:306, 1976.
259. Arseni C, Chitescu M, Cristescu A, Mihaila G: Intrasellar aneurysms simulating hypophyseal tumors. *Eur Neurol* 3:321, 1970.
260. Valenta LJ, Tamkin J, Sostrin R, Elias AN, Eisenberg H: Regression of a pituitary adenoma following levothyroxine therapy of primary hypothyroidism. *Fertil Steril* 40:389, 1983.
261. MacCarty CS, Hanson EJ Jr, Randall RV, Scanlon PW: Indications for and results of surgical treatment of pituitary tumors by the transfrontal approach, in Kohler PO, Ross GT (eds): *Diagnosis and Treatment of Pituitary Tumors.* Amsterdam, Excerpta Medica, 1973, p 139.
262. Grossman A, Ross R, Charlesworth M, Adams CBT, Wass JAH, Doniach I, Besser GM: The effect of dopamine agonist therapy on large functionless pituitary tumors. *Clin Endocrinol* 22:679, 1985.
263. Ray BS, Patterson RH Jr: Surgical experience with chromophobe adenomas of the pituitary gland. *J Neurosurg* 34:726, 1971.
264. Wirth FP, Schwartz HG, Schwetschenau PR: Pituitary adenomas: Factors in treatment. *Clin Neurosurg* 21:8, 1974.
265. Guiot G, Thibaut B: L'Extirpation des adenomes hypophysiaire par voie transsphenoidale. *Neurochirurgie* 1:133, 1959.
266. Hardy JJ: Transsphenoidal surgery of hypersecreting pituitary tumors, in Kohler PO, Ross GT (eds): *Diagnosis and Treatment of Pituitary Tumors.* Amsterdam, Excerpta Medica, 1973, p 179.
267. Guiot G: Transsphenoidal approach and surgical treatment of pituitary adenomas: General principles and indications in nonfunctioning adenoma, in Kohler PO, Ross GT (eds): *Diagnosis and Treatment of Pituitary Tumors.* Amsterdam, Excerpta Medica, 1973, p 159.
268. Kjelberg RM, Kliman B: Bragg peak proton treatment for pituitary-related conditions. *Proc R Soc Med* 67:32, 1974.
269. Braunstein CG, Loriaux DL: Proton-beam therapy. *N Engl J Med* 284:332, 1971.
270. Lawrence JA, Chong CY, Lyman JT, Tobias CA, Born JL, Garcia JF, Manougian E, Linfoot JA, Connell GM: Treatment of pituitary tumors with heavy particles, in Kohler PO, Ross GT (eds): *Diagnosis and Treatment of Pituitary Tumors.* Amsterdam, Excerpta Medica, 1973, p 297.
271. Fischer EQ, Welch K, Belli JA, Wallman J, Shillito JJ: Treatment of craniopharyngiomas in children: 1972–1981. *J Neurosurg* 62:496, 1985.
272. Manaka S, Teramoto A, Takakura K: The efficacy of radiotherapy for craniopharyngioma. *J Neurosurg* 62:648, 1985.
273. Kjellberg RN, Kliman B: A system for therapy of pituitary tumors, in Kohler PO, Ross GT (eds): *Diagnosis and Treatment of Pituitary Tumors.* Amsterdam, Excerpta Medica, 1973, p 234.
274. Sheline GE: Treatment of chromophobe adenomas of the pituitary gland and acromegaly, in Kohler PO, Ross GT (eds): *Diagnosis and Treatment of Pituitary Tumors.* Amsterdam, Excerpta Medica, 1973, p 201.
275. Bakay L: The results of 300 pituitary adenoma operations. *J Neurosurg* 7:240, 1950.
276. Randall RV, Laws ER Jr, Trautmann JC: Results of transsphenoidal microsurgery for pituitary adenoma in 892 patients, in Camanni P, Muller EE (eds): *Pituitary Hyperfunction: Pathophysiology and Clinical Aspects.* New York, Raven, 1984, p 417.
277. Zimmerman EA, Defendini R, Frantz AG: Prolactin and growth hormone in patients with pituitary adenomas: A correlative study of hormone in tumor and plasma by immunoperoxidase technique and radioimmunoassay. *J Clin Endocrinol Metab* 38:577, 1974.
278. Frohman LA: Ectopic hormone production by tumors: Growth hormone releasing factor, in Muller EE, MacLeod RM (eds): *Neuroendocrine Perspectives.* Amsterdam, Elsevier, 1984, p 201.
279. Thorner MO, Perryman RL, Cronin ML, Rogol AD, Draznin M, Johanson A, Vale W, Horvath E, Kovacs K: Somatotroph hyperplasia: Successful treatment of acromegaly by removal of a pancreatic islet tumor secreting a growth hormone-releasing factor. *J Clin Invest* 70:965, 1982.

280. Richmond IL, Wilson CB: Pituitary adenomas in childhood and adolescence. *J Neurosurg* 49:163, 1978.
281. Low PA, McLeod JG, Turtle JR, Donnelly P, Wright RG: Peripheral neuropathy in acromegaly. *Brain* 97:139, 1974.
282. Sober AJ, Gorden P, Roth J, AvRuskin TW: Visceromegaly in acromegaly: Evidence that clinical hepatomegaly or splenomegaly (but not sialomegaly) are manifestations of a second disease. *Arch Intern Med* 134:415, 1974.
283. Klein I, Parveen G, Gavaler JS, Vanthiel DH: Colonic polyps in patients with acromegaly. *Ann Intern Med* 97:27, 1982.
284. Ituarte EA, Petrini J, Hershman JM: Acromegaly and colon cancer. *Ann Intern Med* 101:627, 1984.
285. Melmed S, Braunstein GD, Horvath E, Ezrin C, Kovacs K: Pathophysiology of acromegaly. *Endocr Rev* 4:271, 1983.
286. McGuffin WL, Sherman BM, Roth J, Gorden P, Kahn R, Roberts WC, Frommer PL: Acromegaly and cardiovascular disorders. *Ann Intern Med* 81:11, 1974.
287. Wright AD, Hill DM, Lowy C, Fraser TR: Mortality in acromegaly. *Q J Med* 39:1, 1970.
288. Ballantine EJ, Foxman S, Gorden P, Roth J: Rarity of diabetic retinopathy in patients with acromegaly. *Arch Intern Med* 141:1625, 1981.
289. Lawrence AM, Goldfine ID, Kirsteins L: Growth hormone dynamics in acromegaly. *J Clin Endocrinol Metab* 31:239, 1970.
290. Clemmons DR, Van Wyk JJ, Ridgway EC, Kliman B, Kjelberg RN, Underwood LE: Evaluation of acromegaly by radioimmunoassay of somatomedin-C. *N Engl J Med* 301:1138, 1979.
291. Stonesifer LD, Jordan RM, Kohler PO: Somatomedin C in treated acromegaly: Poor correlation with growth hormone and clinical response. *J Clin Endocrinol Metab* 53:931, 1981.
292. Rieu M, Girard F, Bricaire H, Binoux M: The importance of insulin-like growth factor (somatomedin) measurements in the diagnosis and surveillance of acromegaly. *J Clin Endocrinol Metab* 55:147, 1982.
293. Irie M, Tsushima P: Increase of serum growth hormone concentration following thyrotropin-releasing hormone injection in patients with acromegaly or gigantism. *J Clin Endocrinol Metab* 35:97, 1972.
294. Faglia G, Beck-Peccoz P, Travaglini P, Paracchi A, Spada A, Lewin A: Elevations in plasma growth hormone concentration after luteinizing hormone-releasing hormone (LRH) in patients with active acromegaly. *J Clin Endocrinol Metab* 37:338, 1973.
295. Gelato MC, Merriam GR, Vance ML, Goldman JA, Webb C, Evans WS, Rock J, Oldfield EH, Molitch ME, Rivier J, Vale W, Reichlin S, Frohman LA, Loriaux DL, Thorner MO: Effects of growth hormone–releasing factor upon growth hormone secretion in acromegaly. *J Clin Endocrinol Metab* 60:251, 1985.
296. Wood SM, Ch'ng JLC, Adams EF, Webster JD, Joplin GR, Mashiter K, Bloom SR: Abnormalities of growth hormone release in response to human pancreatic growth hormone releasing factor (GRF 1–44) in acromegaly and hypopituitarism. *Br Med J* 286:1687, 1983.
297. Liuzzi A, Chiodini PG, Botalla L, Cremascoli G, Silvestrini F: Inhibitory effects of L-dopa on GH release in acromegalic patients. *J Clin Endocrinol Metab* 35:941, 1971.
298. Kaneko K, Komine S, Maeda T, Ohta M, Tsushima T, Shizume K: Growth hormone responses to growth-hormone–releasing hormone and thyrotropin-releasing hormone in diabetic patients with and without retinopathy. *Diabetes* 34:710, 1985.
299. Evain-Brion D, Garnier P, Schimpff RM, Chaussain JL, Job JC: Growth hormone response to thyrotropin-releasing hormone and oral glucose-loading tests in tall children and adolescents. *J Clin Endocrinol Metab* 56:429, 1983.
300. Asa SL, Scheithauer BW, Bilbao JM, Horvath E, Ryan N, Kovacs K, Randall RV, Laws ER Jr, Singer W, Linfoot JA, Thorner MO, Vale W: A case for hypothalamic acromegaly: A clinicopathological study of six patients with hypothalamic gangliocytomas producing growth hormone–releasing factor. *J Clin Endocrinol Metab* 58:796, 1984.
301. Asa SL, Bilbao JM, Kovacs K, Linfoot JA: Hypothalamic neuronal hamartoma associated with pituitary growth hormone cell adenoma and acromegaly. *Acta Neuropathol* 52:231, 1980.
302. Frohman LA: Growth hormone releasing factor—a neuroendocrine perspective. *J Lab Clin Med* 103:819, 1984.
303. Thorner MO, Frohman LA, Leong DA, Thominet J, Downs T, Hellman P, Chitwood J, Vaughn JM, Vale W: Extra-hypothalamic growth hormone–releasing factor (GRF) secretion is a rare cause of acromegaly: Plasma GRF levels in 177 acromegalic patients. *J Clin Endocrinol Metab* 59:846, 1984.
304. Penny ES, Penman E, Price J, Rees LH, Sopwith AM, Wass JAH, Lytras N, Besser GM: Circulating growth hormone–releasing factor concentrations in normal subjects and patients with acromegaly. *Br Med J* 289:453, 1984.
305. Greenberg PB, Beck C, Martin PJ, Burger HG: Synthesis and release of human growth hormone from lung carcinoma in cell culture. *Lancet* 1:350, 1972.
306. Dabek JT: Bronchial carcinoid tumor with acromegaly in two patients. *J Clin Endocrinol Metab* 38:329, 1974.
307. Leveston SA, McKeel DW Jr, Buckley PJ, Deschryver K, Greider MH, Jaffe BM, Daughaday WH: Acromegaly and Cushing's syndrome associated with foregut carcinoid tumor. *J Clin Endocrinol Metab* 53:682, 1981.
308. Melmed S, Ezrin C, Kovacs K, Goodman RS, Frohman LA: Acromegaly due to secretion of growth hormone by an ectopic pancretic islet-cell tumor. *N Engl J Med* 312:9, 1985.
309. Decker RE, Epstein JA, Carras R, Rosenthal AD: Transsphenoidal microsurgery for pituitary tumors: Experience with 45 cases. *Mt Sinai J Med* 34:565, 1976.
310. Cryer PE, Daughaday WH: Adrenergic modulation of growth hormone secretion in acromegaly: Suppression during phentolamine and phentolamine-isoproterenol administration. *J Clin Endocrinol Metab* 39:658, 1974.
311. Pieters GFFM, Romeijn JE, Smals AGH, Kloppenborg PWC: Somatostatin sensitivity and growth hormone responses to releasing hormones and bromocriptine in acromegaly. *J Clin Endocrinol Metab* 54:942, 1982.
312. Hoyte KM, Martin JB: Recovery from paradoxical growth hormone response in acromegaly after transsphenoidal selective adenomectomy. *J Clin Endocrinol Metab* 41:656, 1975.
313. Ludecke D, Kautzky R, Saeger W, Schrader D: Selective removal of hypersecreting pituitary adenomas. *Acta Neurochir* 35:27, 1976.
314. Williams RA, Jacobs HS, Kurtz AB, Millar JGB, Oakley MW, Spathis GS, Sulway MJ, Nabarro JDN: The treatment of acromegaly with special reference to transsphenoidal hypophysectomy. *Q J Med* 44:79, 1975.
315. Laws ER Jr, Piepgras DG, Randall RV, Abboud CF: Neurosurgical management of acromegaly. Results in 82 patients treated between 1972 and 1977. *J Neurosurg* 50:454, 1979.
316. Baskin DS, Boggan JE, Wilson CB: Transsphenoidal microsurgical removal of growth hormone-secreting pituitary adenomas. *J Neurosurg* 56:634, 1982.
317. Schuster LD, Bantle JP, Oppenheimer JH, Seljeskog EL: Acromegaly: Reassessment of the long-term therapeutic effectiveness of transsphenoidal pituitary surgery. *Ann Intern Med* 95:172, 1981.
318. Arosio M, Giovanelli MA, Riva E, Nava C, Ambrosi B, Faglia G: Clinical uses of pre- and postsurgical evaluation of abnormal GH responses in acromegaly. *J Neurosurg* 59:402, 1983.
319. Eastman RC, Gorden P, Roth J: Conventional supervoltage irradiation is an important treatment for acromegaly. *J Clin Endocrinol Metab* 48:931, 1979.
320. Liuzzi A, Chiodini PG, Botalla L, Cremascoli G, Muller E, Silvestrini F: Decreased plasma growth hormone levels in acromegalics following CB 154 (2-Br-α-ergocryptine) administration. *J Clin Endocrinol Metab* 38:910, 1974.

321. Moses AS, Molitch ME, Sawin CT, Jackson IM, Biller BJ, Furlanetto R, Reichlin S: Bromocriptine therapy in acromegaly: Use in patients resistant to conventional therapy and effect on serum levels of somatomedin-C. *J Clin Endocrinol Metab* 53:772, 1981.
322. Kleinberg DL, Boyd AE III, Wardlaw S, Frantz AG, George A, Bryan N, Hilal S, Greising J, Hamilton D, Seltzer T, Sommers CJ: Pergolide for treatment of pituitary tumors secreting prolactin or growth hormone. *N Engl J Med* 309:704, 1983.
323. MacLeod RM, Lehmeyer JE: Suppression of pituitary tumor growth and function by ergot alkaloids. *Cancer Res* 33:849, 1973.
324. Oppizzi G, Liuzzi A, Chiodini P, Dallabonzana D, Spelta B, Silvestrini F, Borghi G, Tanon C: Dopaminergic treatment of acromegaly: Different effects on hormone secretion and tumor size. *J Clin Endocrinol Metab* 58:988, 1984.
325. Hall R, Besser GM, Schally AV, Coy DH, Evered D, Goldie DJ, Kastin AJ, McNielly BS, Mortimer CH, Phenekos C, Tunbridge WMG, Weightman D: Action of growth hormone–release inhibitory hormone in healthy men and in acromegaly. *Lancet* 2:581, 1973.
326. Gomez-Pan A, Rodriguez-Arnao MD, del Pozo E: Advances in somatostatin research, in del Pozo E, Fluckiger E (eds): *Dopamine and Neuroendocrine Active Substances.* London, Academic, 1985, p 223.
327. Jacobs HS, Frank S, Murray MAF, Hull MGR, Steele SJ, Nabarro JDN: Clinical and endocrine features of hyperprolactinaemic amenorrhoea. *Clin Endocrinol* 5:439, 1976.
328. Jaquet P, Grisli F, Guibout M, Lissitzky J-C, Carayon P: Prolactin secreting tumors: Endocrine studies before and after surgery in 33 women. *J Clin Endocrinol Metab* 64:459, 1978.
329. Antunes JL, Housepian EM, Frantz AG, Holub DA, Hui RM, Carmel PW, Quest DO: Prolactin-secreting pituitary tumors. *Ann Neurol* 2:148, 1977.
330. McNatty KP, Sawers RS, McNeilly AS: A possible role for prolactin in control of steroid secretion by the human graafian follicle. *Nature* 250:653, 1974.
331. Boyd AE III, Reichlin S, Turksoy RN: Galactorrhea-amenorrhea syndrome: Diagnosis and therapy. *Ann Intern Med* 87:165, 1977.
332. Spark RF, Pallota J, Naftolin F, Clemens R: Galactorrhea-amenorrhea syndromes: Etiology and treatment. *Ann Intern Med* 84:532, 1976.
333. Boyar RM, Capen S, Finkelstein JW, Perlow M, Sassin JF, Fukushima DK, Weitzman ED, Hellman L: Hypothalamic-pituitary function in diverse hyperprolactinemic states. *J Clin Invest* 53:1588, 1974.
334. Aono T, Miyaki A, Shioji T, Kinugasa T, Onishi T, Kurachi K: Impaired LH release following exogenous estrogen administration in patients with amenorrhea-galactorrhea syndrome. *J Clin Endocrinol Metab* 42:696, 1976.
335. L'Hermite M, Delogne-Desnoeck J, Michaux-Duchene A, Robyn C: Alteration of feedback mechanism of estrogen on gonadotropin by sulpiride-induced hyperprolactinemia. *J Clin Endocrinol Metab* 47:1132, 1978.
336. Carter JN, Tyson JE, Warne GL, McNeilly AS, Faiman C, Friesen HG: Adrenocortical function in hyperprolactinemic women. *J Clin Endocrinol Metab* 45:973, 1977.
337. Glickman SP, Rosenfield RL, Bergenstal RM, Helke J: Multiple androgenic abnormalities, including free testosterone, in hyperprolactinemic women. *J Clin Endocrinol Metab* 55:251, 1982.
338. Klibanski A, Neer RM, Beitens IZ, Ridgway EC, Zervas NT, McArthur JW: Decreased bone density in hyperprolactinemic women. *N Engl J Med* 303:1511, 1980.
339. Schlechte JM, Sherman B, Martin R: Bone density in amenorrheic women with and without hyperprolactinemia. *J Clin Endocrinol Metab* 56:1120, 1983.
340. Carter JN, Tyson JE, Tolis G, Van Vliet S, Faiman C, Friesen HG: Prolactin-secreting tumors and hypogonadism in 22 men. *N Engl J Med* 299:847, 1978.
341. Segal LS, Polishuk WZ, Ben-David M: Hyperprolactinemic male infertility. *Fertil Steril* 26:1425, 1976.
342. Said K, Wenn RV, Sharif F: Bromocriptine for male infertility. *Lancet* 1:250, 1977.
343. Rao R, Scommegna A, Frohman LA: Integrity of central dopaminergic system in women with postpartum hyperprolactinemia. *Am J Obstet Gynecol* 143:883, 1982.
344. Fine SA, Frohman LA: Loss of central nervous system component of dopaminergic inhibition of prolactin secretion in patients with prolactin-secreting pituitary tumors. *J Clin Invest* 61:973, 1978.
345. Kleinberg DL, Noel GL, Frantz AG: Galactorrhea: A study of 235 cases, including 48 with pituitary tumors. *N Engl J Med* 296:589, 1977.
346. Muller EE, Genazzani AR, Murru S: Nomifensine: Diagnostic test in hyperprolactinemic stages. *J Clin Endocrinol Metab* 47:1352, 1978.
347. Ferrari C, Crosignani PG, Caldara R, Picciotti MC, Malinverni A, Barattini B, Telloli P: Failure of nomifensine administration to discriminate between tumorous and nontumorous hyperprolactinemia. *J Clin Endocrinol Metab* 50:23, 1980.
348. Webb CB, Thominet JL, Barowsky H, Berelowitz M, Frohman LA: Evidence for lactotroph dopamine resistance in idiopathic hyperprolactinemia. *J Clin Endocrinol Metab* 56:1089, 1983.
349. Bansal S, Lee LA, Woolf PD: Abnormal prolactin responsiveness to dopaminergic suppression in hyperprolactinemic patients. *Am J Med* 71:961, 1981.
350. McLain CJ, Kromhout J, Van Thiel D: Prolactin levels in portal systemic encephalopathy. *Clin Res* 26:664A, 1978.
351. Boyd AE III, Spare S, Bower B, Reichlin S: Neurogenic galactorrhea-amenorrhea. *J Clin Endocrinol Metab* 47:1374, 1978.
352. Morley JE, Dawson M, Hodgkinson H, Kalk WJ: Galactorrhea and hyperprolactinemia associated with chest wall injury. *J Clin Endocrinol Metab* 45:931, 1977.
353. March CM, Kletzky OA, Davajan V, Teal J, Weiss M, Apuzzo MLJ, Marrs RP, Mishell DR Jr: Longitudinal evaluation of patients with untreated prolactin-secreting pituitary adenomas. *Am J Obstet Gynecol* 139:835, 1981.
354. von Werder K, Eversmann T, Fahlbusch R, Muller OA, Rjosk H-K: Endocrine-active pituitary adenomas: Long-term results of medical and surgical treatment, in Camanni P, Muller EE (eds): *Pituitary Hyperfunction: Pathophysiology and Clinical Aspects.* New York, Raven, 1984, p 385.
355. Martin TL, Kim M, Malarkey WB: The natural history of idiopathic hyperprolactinemia. *J Clin Endocrinol Metab* 60:855, 1985.
356. Lachelin GCL, Abu-Fadil S, Yen SSC: Functional delineation of hyperprolactinemia-amenorrhea. *J Clin Endocrinol Metab* 44:1163, 1977.
357. Quigley ME, Judd SJ, Guilliand GV, Yen SSC: Effects of a dopamine antagonist on the release of gonadotropin and prolactin in normal women and women with hyperprolactinemic anovulation. *J Clin Endocrinol Metab* 48:718, 1980.
358. Scanlon MF, Rodriguez-Arnao MD, McGregor AM, Weightman D, Lewis M, Cook DB, Gomez-Pan A, Hall R: Altered dopaminergic regulation of thyrotropin release in patients with prolactinomas: Comparison with other tests of hypothalamic-pituitary function. *Clin Endocrinol* 2:133, 1981.
359. Bression D, Brandi AM, Martres MP, Nousbaum A, Cesselin F, Radacot J, Peillion F: Dopaminergic receptors in human prolactin-secreting adenomas: A quantitative study. *J Clin Endocrinol Metab* 51:1037, 1980.
360. Cronin MJ, Cheung CY, Wilson CB, Jaffe RB, Weiner RI: ^{3}H-Spiperone binding to human anterior pituitaries secreting prolactin, growth hormone, and adrenocorticotropic hormone. *J Clin Endocrinol Metab* 50:387, 1980.
361. Kato Y, Shimatsu A, Matsushita N, Ohta H, Tojo K,

Kabayama Y, Inoue T, Imura H: Regulation of pituitary hormone secretion by VIP and related peptides, in Labrie F, Proulx L (eds): *Endocrinology*. Amsterdam, Elsevier, 1984, p 175.

362. Tucker HS, Grubb SR, Wigand JP, Taylor A, Lankford HV, Blackard WG, Becker SP: Galactorrhea-amenorrhea syndrome: Followup of forty-five patients after pituitary tumor removal. *Ann Intern Med* 94:303, 1981.

363. Frohman LA, Berelowitz M, Gonzalez C, Barowsky H, Rao R, Lim VS, Frohman MA, Thominet JL: Studies of dopaminergic mechanisms in hyperprolactinemic states, in Crosignani P, Rubin B (eds): *Serono Clinical Symposia on Reproduction*. London, Academic, 1981, vol 2, p 39.

364. VanLoon GR: A defect in catecholamine neurones in patients with prolactin-secreting pituitary adenoma. *Lancet* 2:868, 1978.

365. Hokfelt T, Fuxe K: Effects of prolactin and ergot alkaloids on the tuberoinfundibular dopamine neurones. *Neuroendocrinology* 9:100, 1972.

366. McKeel DW Jr, Fowler M, Jacobs LS: The high prevalence of prolactin cell hyperplasia in the human adenohypophysis. *Endocrinology* 102:353A, 1978.

367. Garthwaite TL, Hagen TC: Plasma prolactin-releasing factor-like activity in the amenorrhea-galactorrhea syndrome. *J Clin Endocrinol Metab* 47:885, 1978.

368. Rodman EF, Molitch ME, Post KD, Biller BJ, Reichlin S: Long-term follow-up of transsphenoidal selective adenomectomy for prolactinoma. *JAMA* 252:921, 1984.

369. Serri O, Rasio E, Beauregard H, Hardy J, Somma M: Recurrence of hyperprolactinemia after selective transsphenoidal adenomectomy of women with prolactinoma. *N Engl J Med* 309:280, 1983.

370. Schlechte J, Sherman B, VanGilder J, Chapler F: Recurrence of hyperprolactinemia after transsphenoidal surgery for prolactin-secreting pituitary tumors. *Clin Res* 33:828A, 1985.

371. Barbarino A, DeMarinis L, Maira G, Menini E, Anile C: Serum prolactin response to thyrotropin-releasing hormone and metoclopramide in patients with prolactin secreting tumors before and after transsphenoidal surgery. *J Clin Endocrinol Metab* 47:1148, 1978.

372. Molitch ME, Goodman RH, Post KD, Biller BJ, Moses AC, King LC, Feldman ZT, Reichlin S: Surgical cure of prolactinoma reverses abnormal prolactin response to carbidopa/L-dopa. *J Clin Endocrinol Metab* 55:1118, 1982.

373. Molitch ME: Pregnancy and the hyperprolactinemic woman. *N Engl J Med* 312:1364, 1985.

374. Hokfelt B, Nillius SJ: The dopamine agonist bromocriptine: Theoretical and clinical aspects. *Acta Endocrinol* (suppl) 88:1, 1978.

375. Liuzzi A, Dallabonzana D, Oppizzi G, Verde GG, Cozzi R, Chiodini P, Luccarelli G: Low dose dopamine agonists in the long-term treatment of macroprolactinomas. *N Engl J Med* 313:656, 1985.

376. Turkalj I, Braun P, Krupp P: Surveillance of bromocriptine in pregnancy. *JAMA* 247:1589, 1982.

377. Wollensen F, Anderson T, Karle A: Size reduction of extrasellar pituitary tumors during bromocriptine treatment. *Ann Intern Med* 96:281, 1982.

378. Molitch M, Elton RL, Blackwell RE, Caldwell B, Chang J, Jaffe R, Joplin G, Robbins RJ, Tyson J, Thorner MO, Bromocriptine Study Group: Bromocriptine as primary therapy for prolactin-secreting macroadenomas: Results of a prospective multicenter study. *J Clin Endocrinol Metab* 60:698, 1985.

379. Tindall GT, Kovacs K, Horvath E, Thorner MO: Human prolactin-producing adenomas and bromocriptine: A histological, immunocytochemical, ultrastructural and morphometric study. *J Clin Endocrinol Metab* 55:1178, 1982.

380. Gen M, Uozumi T, Ohta M, Ito A, Kajiwara H, Moro S: Necrotic changes in prolactinomas after long term administration of bromocriptine. *J Clin Endocrinol Metab* 59:463, 1984.

381. Johnston DG, Hall K, Kendall-Taylor P, Patrick D, Watson M, Cook DB: Effect of dopamine agonist withdrawal after long-term therapy in prolactinomas. *Lancet* 2:187, 1984.

382. Fahlbusch R, Buchfelder M: Transsphenoidal operations for prolactinomas, in Auer LM, Leb G, Tscherne G, Urdl W, Walter GF (eds): *Prolactinomas*. Berlin, de Gruyter, 1985, p 209.

383. Landolt AM, Osterwalder V: Perivascular fibrosis in prolactinomas: Is it increased by bromocriptine? *J Clin Endocrinol Metab* 58:1179, 1984.

384. Watanabe K, Fukushima T: Transsphenoidal microsurgical treatment of 77 prolactinomas. *J Clin Endocrinol Metab* 58:235, 1984.

385. Faglia G, Moriondo P, Travaglini P, Giovanelli MA: Influence of previous bromocriptine therapy on surgery for microprolactinomas. *Lancet* 1:133, 1983.

386. Sherman BM, Harris CE, Schlechte J, Duello TM, Halmi NS, VanGlider J, Chapler FK, Granner DK: Pathogenesis of prolactin-secreting adenomas. *Lancet* 2:1019, 1978.

387. Grossman A, Cohen BL, Charlesworth M, Plowman PN, Rees LH, Wass JAH, Jones AE, Besser GM: Treatment of prolactinomas with megavoltage radiotherapy. *Br Med J* 288:1105, 1984.

388. Thorner MO, Besser GM, Jones A, Dacie J, Jones AE: Bromocriptine treatment of female infertility: Report of 13 pregnancies. *Br Med J* 4:694, 1975.

389. Bergh T, Nillius SJ, Wide L: Pregnancies in 15 amenorrhoeic women with hyperprolactinemia and radiological signs of pituitary tumors—clinical course and outcome. *Br Med J* 1:875, 1978.

390. Bonneville JF, Poulignot D, Cattin F, Couturier N, Millet E, Dietemann JL: Computed tomographic demonstration of the effects of bromocriptine on pituitary microadenoma size. *Radiology* 143:451, 1982.

391. Eversmann T, Fahlbusch R, Rjosk HK, von Werder K: Persisting suppression of prolactin secretion after long-term treatment with bromocriptine in patients with prolactinomas. *Acta Endocrinol* 92:413, 1979.

392. Cushing H: The basophil adenomas of the pituitary body and their clinical manifestations (pituitary basophilism). *Bull Johns Hopkins Hosp* 50:137, 1932.

393. Nelson DH, Meakin JW, Dealy JB Jr, Matson DD, Emerson K Jr, Thorn GW: ACTH-producing tumor of the pituitary gland. *N Engl J Med* 259:161, 1958.

394. Scholz DA, Gastineau CF, Harrison EG Jr: Cushing's syndrome with malignant chromophobe tumor of the pituitary and extra-cranial metastasis: Report of a case. *Proc Staff Meet Mayo Clin* 37:31, 1962.

395. Moore TJ, Dluhy RG, Williams GH, Cain JP: Nelson's syndrome: Frequency, prognosis and effect of prior pituitary irradiation. *Ann Intern Med* 85:731, 1976.

396. Tyrrell JB, Brooks RM, Fitzgerald PA, Cofoid PB, Forsham PH, Wilson CB: Cushing's disease: Selective transsphenoidal resection of pituitary microadenomas. *N Engl J Med* 298:753, 1978.

397. Eddy RL, Jones AL, Gilliland PF, Ibarra JD Jr, Thompson JQ, McMurray JF Jr: Cushing's syndrome: A prospective study of diagnostic methods. *Am J Med* 55:621, 1973.

398. Liddle GW: Tests of pituitary-adrenal suppressibility in the diagnosis of Cushing's syndrome. *J Clin Endocrinol Metab* 20:1539, 1960.

399. Ashcraft MW, Van Herle AJ, Vener SL, Geffner DL: Serum cortisol levels in Cushing's syndrome after low- and high-dose dexamethasone suppression. *Ann Intern Med* 97:21, 1982.

400. Chrousos GP, Schulte HM, Oldfield EH, Gold PW, Cutler GB Jr, Loriaux DL: The corticotropin-releasing factor stimulation test. *N Engl J Med* 310:622, 1984.

401. Oldfield EH, Chrousos GP, Schulte HM, Schaaf M, McKeever PE, Krudy AG, Cutler GB Jr, Loriaux DL, Doppman JL: Preoperative lateralization of ACTH-secreting pituitary microadenomas

by bilateral and simultaneous inferior petrosal venous sinus sampling. *N Engl J Med* 312:100, 1985.
402. Upton GV, Amatruda TT Jr: Evidence for the presence of tumor peptides with corticotropin-releasing factor-like activity in the ectopic ACTH syndrome. *N Engl J Med* 285:419, 1971.
403. Carey RM, Varma SK, Drake CR Jr, Thorner MO, Kovacs K, Rivier J, Vale W: Ectopic secretion of corticotropin-releasing factor as a cause of Cushing's syndrome. *N Engl J Med* 311:13, 1984.
404. Lamberts SWJ, Klijn JGM, de Jong FH, Birkenhager JC: Hormone secretion in alcohol-induced pseudo-Cushing's syndrome: Differential diagnosis with Cushing's disease. *JAMA* 242:1640, 1979.
405. Carroll BJ, Curtis GC, Mendels J: Neuroendocrine regulation in depression: I. Limbic system-adrenocortical dysfunction. *Arch Gen Psychiatry* 33:1039, 1976.
406. Krieger DT: Pathophysiology of Cushing's disease. *Endocr Rev* 4:22, 1983.
407. Heinbecker P: Pathogenesis of Cushing's syndrome. *Medicine* 23:225, 1944.
408. Krieger DT, Howanitz PJ, Frantz AG: Absence of nocturnal elevation of plasma prolactin concentrations in Cushing's disease. *J Clin Endocrinol Metab* 42:260, 1976.
409. Krieger DT, Glick SM: Sleep EEG stages and plasma growth hormone concentration in states of endogenous and exogenous hypercortisolemia or ACTH elevation. *J Clin Endocrinol Metab* 39:986, 1974.
410. Krieger DT, Amorosa L, Linick F: Cyproheptadine-induced remission of Cushing's disease. *N Engl J Med* 293:893, 1975.
411. Jones MT, Gillham B, Beckford U, Dornhorst A, Abraham RR, Seed M, Wynn V: Effect of treatment with sodium valproate and diazepam on plasma corticotropin in Nelson's syndrome. *Lancet* 1:1179, 1981.
412. Lamberts SWJ, Klijn JGM, de Quijada M, Timmermans HAT, Uitterlinden P, de Jong FH, Birkenhager JC: The mechanism of the suppressive action of bromocriptine on adrenocorticotropin secretion in patients with Cushing's disease and Nelson's syndrome. *J Clin Endocrinol Metab* 51:307, 1980.
413. Lankford HV, Tucker HTS, Blackard WG: A cyproheptadine-reversible defect in ACTH control presenting after removal of the pituitary tumor in Cushing's disease. *N Engl J Med* 305:1244, 1981.
414. Lagerquist LW, Meikle AW, West CD, Tyler FH: Cushing's disease with cure by resection of a pituitary adenoma: Evidence against a primary hypothalamic defect. *Am J Med* 57:826, 1974.
415. Bigos ST, Robert F, Pelletier G, Hardy J: Cure of Cushing's disease by transsphenoidal removal of a microadenoma from a pituitary gland despite a radiographically normal sella turcica. *J Clin Endocrinol Metab* 45:1251, 1977.
416. Lamberts SWJ, de Lange SA, Stefanko SZ: Adrenocorticotropin-secreting pituitary adenomas originate from the anterior or the intermediate lobe in Cushing's disease: Differences in the regulation of hormone secretion. *J Clin Endocrinol Metab* 54:286, 1982.
417. van Cauter E, Refetoff S: Evidence for two subtypes of Cushing's disease based on the analysis of episodic cortisol secretion. *N Engl J Med* 312:1343, 1985.
418. Kaplan NM, Shires GT: Apparent cure of Cushing's disease by bilateral adrenalectomy and autotransplantation. *Am J Med* 53:377, 1972.
419. Hardy JD: Surgical management of Cushing's syndrome with emphasis on adrenal autotransplantation. *Ann Surg* 188:290, 1978.
420. Scholz DA, Gastineau CF, Harrison EG Jr: Cushing's syndrome with malignant chromophobe tumor of the pituitary and extracranial metastasis: Report of a case. *Mayo Clin Proc* 37:31, 1962.
421. Slassa RM, Laws ER Jr, Carpenter PC, Northcut RC: Transsphenoidal removal of pituitary microadenoma in Cushing's disease. *Mayo Clin Proc* 53:24, 1978.
422. Burch W: Survey of results with transsphenoidal surgery in Cushing's disease. *N Engl J Med* 308:103, 1983.
423. Jennings AS, Liddle GW, Orth D: Results of treating childhood Cushing's disease with pituitary irradiation. *N Engl J Med* 297:957, 1977.
424. Jeffcoate WJ, Rees LH, Tomlin S, Jones AE, Edwards CRW, Besser GM: Metyrapone in long-term management of Cushing's disease. *Br Med J* 2:215, 1977.
425. Child DF, Burke CW, Rees LH, Fraser TR: Drug control of Cushing's syndrome. *Acta Endocrinol* 82:330, 1976.
426. Orth DN, Liddle GW: Results of treatment in 108 patients with Cushing's syndrome. *N Engl J Med* 285:243, 1971.
427. Sonino N, Boscaro M, Merola G, Mantero F: Prolonged treatment of Cushing's disease by ketoconazole. *J Clin Endocrinol Metab* 61:718, 1985.
428. Loose DS, Kan PB, Hirst MA, Marcus RA, Feldman D: Ketoconazole blocks adrenal steroidogenesis by inhibiting cytochrome P450-dependent enzymes. *J Clin Invest* 71:1495, 1983.
429. Santen RJ, Van den Bossche H, Symoens J, Brugmans J, de Costar R: Site of action of low dose ketoconazole on androgen biosynthesis in men. *J Clin Endocrinol Metab* 57:732, 1983.
430. Lamberts SWJ, Timmermans HAT, DeJong FH, Birkenhager JC: The role of dopaminergic depletion in the pathogenesis of Cushing's disease and the possible consequences for medical therapy. *Clin Endocrinol* 7:185, 1977.
431. Besser GM, Jeffcoate WJ, Tomlin S: The use of metyrapone and bromocriptine in the control of Cushing's syndrome. Proceedings of the Fifth International Congress on Endocrinology, 1976, abstr 494, p 202.
432. Smallridge RC, Smith CE: Hyperthyroidism due to thyrotropin-secreting pituitary tumors: Diagnostic and therapeutic considerations. *Arch Intern Med* 143:503, 1983.
433. Reschini E, Giustina G, Cantalamessa L, Peracchi M: Hyperthyroidism with elevated plasma TSH levels and pituitary tumor: Study with somatostatin. *J Clin Endocrinol Metab* 45:924, 1976.
434. Kourides IA, Weintraub BD, Rosen SW, Ridgway EC, Kliman B, Maloof F: Secretion of alpha subunit of glycoprotein hormones by pituitary adenomas. *J Clin Endocrinol Metab* 43:97, 1976.
435. Emerson CH, Utiger RD: Hyperthyroidism and excessive thyrotropin secretion. *N Engl J Med* 287:328, 1972.
436. Gershengorn M, Weintraub BD: Thyrotropin-induced hyperthyroidism caused by selective pituitary resistance to thyroid hormone. *J Clin Invest* 56:633, 1975.
437. Beckers A, Stevenaert A, Mashiter K, Hennen G: Follicle-stimulating hormone-secreting pituitary adenomas. *J Clin Endocrinol Metab* 61:525, 1985.
438. Ridgway EC: Glycoprotein hormone production by pituitary tumors, in Black PM, Zervas NT, Ridgway EC, Martin JB (eds): *Secretory Tumors of the Pituitary Gland.* New York, Raven, 1984, p 343.
439. Vance ML, Ridgway EC, Thorner MO: Follicle-stimulating hormone and α-subunit-secreting pituitary tumor treated with bromocriptine. *J Clin Endocrinol Metab* 61:580, 1985.
440. Klibanski A, Ridgway EC, Zervas NT: Pure alpha subunit–secreting pituitary tumors. *J Neurosurg* 59:585, 1983.

9

Posterior Pituitary

Gary L. Robertson

POSTERIOR PITUITARY HORMONES

Anatomy

The *neurohypophysis* is an elongated extension of the ventral hypothalamus which attaches to the dorsal and caudal surface of the adenohypophysis (Fig. 9-1). In adult men and women it weighs approximately 100 mg and is divided into two parts by the diaphragm of the sella. The upper part is variously referred to as the *infundibulum* or *median eminence* and the lower part as the *infundibular process* or *pars nervosa.* The two parts are supplied with blood by branches from the superior and inferior hypophyseal arteries which arise from the posterior communicating and intracavernous portion of the internal carotid. In the pars nervosa, the arterioles break up into localized capillary networks which drain directly into the jugular vein via the sellar, cavernous, and lateral venous sinuses. In the infundibulum, the primary capillary networks coalesce into another system, the portal veins, which perfuse the adenohypophysis before discharging into the systemic circulation.

Microscopically, the neurohypophysis appears as a densely interwoven network of capillaries, pituicytes, and nonmyelinated nerve fibers containing many electron-dense neurosecretory granules.[1,2] These neurosecretory neurons terminate as bulbous enlargements on capillary networks scattered throughout all parts of the neurohypophysis, including the stalk and infundibulum. The neurosecretory neurons that form the pars nervosa originate primarily in the supraoptic nuclei and probably provide most if not all of the vasopressin and oxytocin in plasma. Those that terminate in the median eminence originate primarily in the paraventricular or other hypothalamic nuclei and release their hormones into the portal blood supply of the anterior pituitary.[1-3] Another and somewhat smaller division of vasopressin- or oxytocin-containing neurons projects caudally from the paraventricular nucleus to the medulla and spinal cord, where it appears to terminate on neurons in the nucleus tractus solitarii, substantia gelatinosa, and other areas thought to be involved in the regulation of autonomic function.[4-7] A third vasopressin-containing division of the paraventricular nucleus projects through the stria terminalis to the lateral amygdala,[4] and a fourth appears to terminate on the walls of the lateral and third ventricles, where the neurons probably secrete directly into the cerebrospinal fluid.[8] Multipolar cell bodies containing vasopressin or its associated neurophysin also have been identified in the suprachiasmatic nuclei of humans as well as other primates and most laboratory animals.[3-5] The neurons that arise in this nucleus are of relatively fine caliber and appear to project exclusively to other neurons in the amygdala, lateral septum, and mediodorsal thalamus.[3,4] The widespread distribution of vasopressin in the central nervous system has also been demonstrated by direct radioimmunoassay of tissue extracts.[9]

Oxytocinergic cell bodies appear less numerous than those containing vasopressin and are found primarily in discrete areas in or around the paraventricular and, to a lesser extent, supraoptic nuclei.[3] Most of these neurons project to the pars nervosa, but many also terminate in the lamina terminalis or the median eminence. In addition, a relatively large paraventricular division runs in parallel with vasopressinergic fibers to the medulla and spinal cord, where it terminates on or near the same neural elements.

Chemistry

The neurohypophysis contains several peptides which probably serve as neurohormones, but the only ones which have been extensively studied are vasopressin and oxytocin. Their structures were first established by du Vigneaud and coworkers more than 20 years ago.[10] Each is a nonapeptide composed of a six-member disulfide ring and a three-member tail on which the carboxy-terminal group is amidated (Fig. 9-2). Vasopressin differs from oxytocin only in the

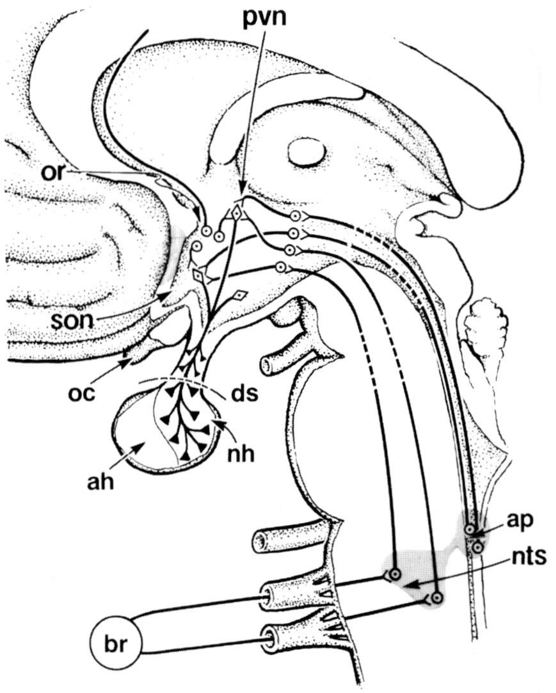

FIGURE 9-1 The neurohypophysis and its principal regulatory afferents. Key: nh, neurohypophysis; ah, adenohypophysis; ds, diaphragm of the sella; oc, optic chiasm; son, supraoptic nucleus; pvn, paraventricular nucleus; or, osmoreceptor; br, volume sensor and baroreceptor; nts, nucleus tractus solitarii; ap, area postrema (emetic center). Shading indicates areas which lack a blood-brain barrier and contain receptors for plasma insulin.

substitution of phenylalanine for isoleucine in the ring and of arginine for leucine in the tail. These two hormones have been found in all mammals except the suborder Suina, several species of which make a variant of vasopressin containing lysine instead of arginine in position 8.[11] Oxytocin also occurs in many birds, reptiles, amphibians, and bony fishes. Instead of vasopressin, however, the pituitaries of nonmammalian vertebrates contain arginine vasotocin. It differs structurally from vasopressin only by the presence of isoleucine at position 3 and has similar biologic effects. Because it is the only nonapeptide hormone found in some older vertebrate phyla, vasotocin is thought to be the precursor from which oxytocin and vasopressin evolved by genetic mutation and duplication.

The synthesis of a large number of structural analogues of vasopressin and oxytocin has made it possible to define more precisely the relationship between conformation and biologic activity.[12] Although changes in almost any part of the molecule may alter three-dimensional structure and biologic activity, it has been suggested that the side chains at positions 3, 4, 7, and 8 are most important for recognition and binding of the hormone to its receptor, while the side chain at position 5 influences intrinsic activity. The ratio of antidiuretic to pressor effects of vasopressin is increased markedly by substituting D-arginine for L-arginine at position 8. This modification, as well as removal of the terminal amino group from cystine, yields desamino-8-D-arginine vasopressin (DDAVP) (Fig. 9-2), a clinically useful analogue with prolonged and enhanced antidiuretic activity.[13] A number of analogues that antagonize selectively the antidiuretic or pressor action of vasopressin have also been synthesized.[14] They have been used effectively to help define the role of vasopressin in the regulation of water balance or blood pressure in health and disease and may also prove to be clinically useful in treating certain types of osmoregulatory or baroregulatory dysfunction.

Vasopressin and oxytocin are stored in the neurohypophysis as insoluble complexes with carrier proteins known as *neurophysins.* Separation of these neurophysins from the active hormones was first achieved by Acher and his colleagues over 20 years ago.[15] Only recently, however, has it been possible to isolate individual neurophysins in a form sufficiently pure to define their physicochemical characteristics.[16] In humans and most other mammals, two major types of neurophysin have been identified by both immunologic and chromatographic methods. One type is found exclusively in granules containing oxytocin, the other in granules containing vasopressin. Both appear to be single chain polypeptides which have a basic molecular weight of approximately 10,000 but readily form dimers and tetramers in concentrated solutions. Each type of neurophysin binds oxytocin and vasopressin equally well, indicating that the specific hormonal associations found in vivo are a function of anatomic compartmentalization. Binding of the hormones to neurophysin exhibits a pH optimum around 5.2 to 5.8 and a binding constant ($K°$) of approximately 2×10^4 M. These values favor complete dissociation of the neurophysin-hormone complex in plasma. The amino acid sequence of several neurophysins has been determined and found to have a considerable degree of internal homology in a part of the molecule thought to be the hormone binding site.

Biosynthesis and Release

Vasopressin and oxytocin are synthesized in the cell bodies of the supraoptic and paraventricular nuclei, packaged in granules with their respective neurophysins, and transported down the axons to be stored in terminal dilatations until their release.[2,17] Although each hormone is produced by a different population of neurons,[18] the biosynthetic mechanisms appear to be similar. The incorporation of amino acids into vasopressin requires the participation of ribosomes and

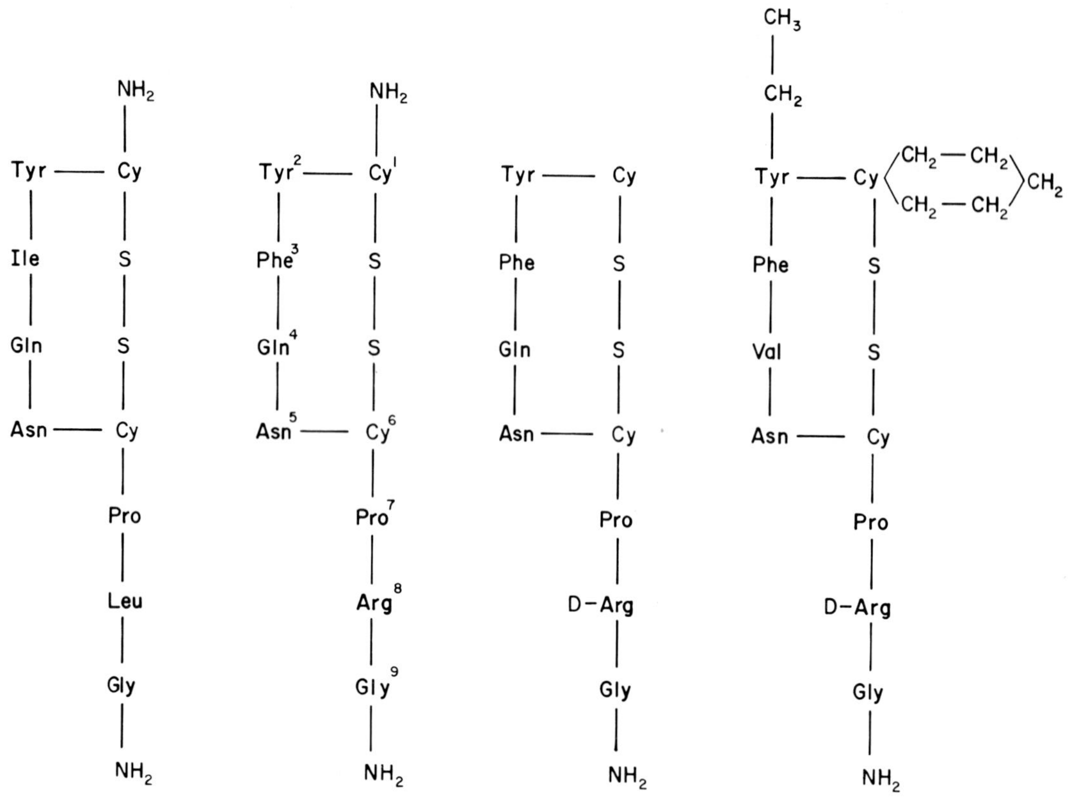

OXYTOCIN VASOPRESSIN dDAVP d(CH$_2$)$_5$ Tyr(Et) VDAVP

FIGURE 9-2 The amino acid sequence of oxytocin and vasopressin as well as a synthetic agonist, 1-desamino-8-D-arginine vasopressin (DDAVP), and an antagonist, d(CH$_2$)$_5$ Tyr(Et) (vDAVP), of vasopressin.

proceeds via formation of a macromolecular precursor or prohormone.[19] This precursor, which has been called *propressophysin,* has a molecular weight of approximately 20,000 and contains neurophysin as well as vasopressin and a relatively large glycosylated peptide. DNA cloning studies have shown that the vasopressin sequence is located at the amino terminus preceded by a signal peptide, the glycoprotein occupies the carboxyl terminus, and neurophysin is situated between them.[20] As in many other propeptides, the three parts are separated by lysine and/or arginine residues which mark the point of cleavage by proteolytic enzymes. Oxytocin and its neurophysin also are formed from a common precursor which is similar to propressophysin, except that the carboxy-terminal protein is not glycosylated.[19] Presumably, the prohormones are cleaved by proteolytic enzymes within the neurosecretory granules to yield the biologically active hormones and their respective neurophysins. The synthesis of vasopressin and oxytocin in humans probably proceeds by similar mechanisms, although the precursors have not been identified and may have different structures. Brattleboro rats, which synthesize oxytocin but have an inherited inability to make vasopressin, also lack its associated neurophysin.[18] The biosynthetic defect in the Brattleboro rat appears to be due to a single base deletion in the gene coding for the vasopressin precursor[21] and may result in the production of small amounts of an abnormal vasopressin precursor.

The synthesis of vasopressin and vasopressin mRNA is increased by stimuli, such as dehydration, which also increase secretion.[17,22] At least in rats, however, this compensatory response develops only gradually and may never completely match the increased rate of release. As a consequence, the neurohypophyseal stores of vasopressin tend to be severely depleted by a chronic stimulus such as prolonged water deprivation.[23]

The process by which the hormone and its neurophysin are packaged in granules and transported down the axon has not been completely defined. The granules are membrane-bound and appear in some species to arise from the Golgi apparatus in the perikaryon. Transport may be effected by the kind of axon flow phenomenon demonstrated for other nervous tissue or by some more rapid mechanism involving the microtubules.

The hormone and its associated neurophysin appear to be secreted by a calcium-dependent exocytotic process similar to that described for other neurosecretory systems.[24] According to this view, secretion is triggered by propagation along the neuron of an electrical impulse which causes depolarization of the cell membrane, an influx of calcium, fusion with the membranes of secretory granules, and extrusion of their contents.

Regulation of Secretion

VASOPRESSIN

Osmotic Factors

The secretion of vasopressin is known to be influenced by a number of variables.[25-29] Probably the most important under physiologic conditions is the effective osmotic pressure of plasma. Its influence on vasopressin is mediated by specialized neurons, known collectively as *osmoreceptors*, which appear to be concentrated in the anterolateral hypothalamus near but separate from the supraoptic nuclei (Fig. 9-1).[30-33] This part of the brain receives its blood supply from small perforating branches of the anterior cerebral and/or communicating arteries.[34] Interruption of these vessels disrupts the osmoregulation of thirst and vasopressin without affecting the neurohypophysis or its response to nonosmotic stimuli.[32,35]

The functional properties of the osmoregulatory mechanism resemble those of a discontinuous or "set point" receptor (Fig. 9-3A). Thus, at plasma osmolalities below a certain minimum or threshold level, plasma vasopressin is suppressed to low or undetectable concentrations. Above this point, plasma vasopressin rises steeply in direct proportion to plasma osmolality. The slope of this relationship indicates that a change in plasma osmolality of only 1 percent will change plasma vasopressin by an average of 1 pg/ml, an amount sufficient to significantly alter urinary concentration and flow (Fig. 9-3B). This extraordinary sensitivity confers upon the osmoreceptor the primary role in mediating the antidiuretic response to changes in water balance.

The sensitivity of the osmoregulatory system varies appreciably from person to person.[27] In a healthy adult population, as much as 10-fold differences in slope have been observed. In the most sensitive people, physiologically significant changes in vasopressin can be induced by changes in plasma osmolality as small as 0.5 mosmol/kg (0.17 percent), an amount far too small to be detected by even the best available laboratory osmometers. At the other extreme of normal, comparable changes in plasma vasopressin may require changes in plasma osmolality of up to 5 mosmol/kg (1.7 percent). These individual differences in osmoregulatory sensitivity are constant over prolonged periods of time and appear to be determined largely by genetic factors.[36] However, this property of the system is not totally immutable, since hypovolemia, angiotensin, glucopenia, hypercalcemia, insulinopenia, and lithium all increase the slope of the plasma vasopressin-osmolality relationship (see below). The sensitivity of the osmoregulatory system also appears to increase with age, at least in males.[37] The effect of sex and/or gonadal hormones on vasopressin secretion is controversial. One study found no differences in osmoregulatory function in adult males and females,[27] while others observed increased sensitivity in females and estrogen-treated males[38,39] and in estrogen-treated rats.[40]

The "set" of the osmoregulatory system also varies from person to person. In healthy adults, the osmotic threshold for vasopressin secretion ranges from 275 to 290 mosmol/kg, with an average of about 280 mosmol/kg.[27] Unlike sensitivity, however, these interindividual differences in the set of the osmoregulatory system are not constant over time but can rise or fall by as much as 5 mosmol/kg. The cause of this resetting is not known but may include changes in

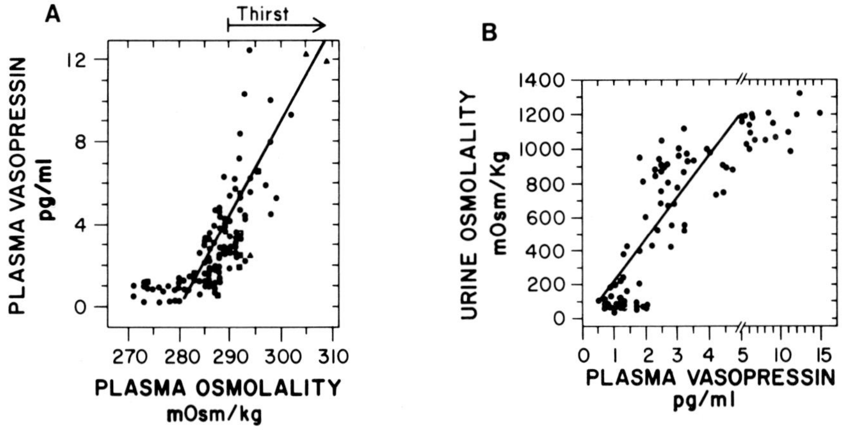

FIGURE 9-3 The relation of plasma vasopressin to plasma and urine osmolality in healthy adults in various states of hydration. (*Redrawn from Robertson et al.*[27])

blood pressure and/or effective blood volume (see below). The set of the osmoregulatory system is also reduced during pregnancy[41] and during the luteal phase of the menstrual cycle.[42,43] The mechanism is unknown but may involve hemodynamic stimuli.

It is uncertain whether the threshold concept accurately represents the operation of the osmoreceptor at its most fundamental level.[44-46] Some analyses of the relationship between plasma vasopressin and osmolality suggest that it may be described better by an exponential rather than a linear threshold model, while others find no significant difference in fit of the data. Indeed, it is uncertain whether current methods are sufficiently precise to distinguish between the two models or, if they could, whether the distinction would be important. Moreover, there is reason to think that vasopressin secretion reflects the balance of inhibitory as well as stimulatory input from a bimodal system of osmoreceptors.[29] If so, both types probably have a common set or null point that corresponds closely to the normal basal effective osmotic pressure of body water. For practical purposes, however, the concept of an osmotic threshold for vasopressin secretion remains for the present a useful if not valid way of describing many aspects of normal and abnormal osmoregulatory function in intact animals and in humans.

It is also uncertain whether vasopressin is secreted continuously or episodically in response to osmotic stimulation. When nonosmotic stimuli such as posture, activity, and blood pressure are controlled or constant, the infusion of hypertonic saline in humans usually produces a smooth progressive rise in systemic venous plasma vasopressin that correlates closely with the rise in plasma osmolality.[29,46,47] However, when samples are obtained from animals at a point nearer the source of the hormone, e.g., from the right atrium or internal jugular vein, large fluctuations in plasma vasopressin have been observed during osmotic stimulation.[48] Whether these fluctuations reflect an intrinsic property of the neurohypophysis or are artifacts of the experimental conditions is unknown. Irregular phasic firing of neurosecretory neurons has been observed by unit recording techniques,[49] but this activity is unlikely to be related to episodic fluctuations in plasma vasopressin, since the discharge cycles have a much shorter periodicity and are not synchronized from cell to cell.

The osmoregulatory mechanism is not equally sensitive to all plasma solutes (Fig. 9-4). Sodium and its anions, which normally contribute more than 95 percent of the osmotic pressure of plasma, are the most potent solutes known in terms of their capacity to stimulate vasopressin release.[50] However, certain sugars such as sucrose and mannitol are also very effective when infused intravenously.[25,51] In fact, particle for particle, mannitol appears to be nearly as potent as sodium chloride.[51] In this respect, therefore, the control mechanism behaves like a true osmoreceptor. However, a rise in plasma osmolality due to urea or glucose causes little or no increase in plasma vasopressin in healthy adults or animals.[27,51-53] These differences in response to various plasma solutes are independent of any recognized nonosmotic influence and are probably a property of the osmoregulatory mechanism per se. Precisely how and why the osmoreceptor discriminates so effectively between different kinds of plasma solutes is still unsettled. According to current concepts, the signal which stimulates the osmoreceptor is an osmotically induced decrease in the water content of the cell. If this hypothesis is correct, the ability of a given solute to stimulate vasopressin secretion ought to be inversely related to the rate at which it passes from plasma into the osmoreceptor neuron.[25] This concept agrees well with the observed inverse relationship between the effect of solutes such as sodium, mannitol, and glucose on vasopressin secretion and the rate at which they penetrate the blood-brain barrier. The latter observations are also consistent with the view that the osmoreceptors are actually sodium receptors located within the blood-brain barrier.[52-54] However, the sodium receptor theory is difficult to reconcile with the behavior of urea, which penetrates the blood-brain

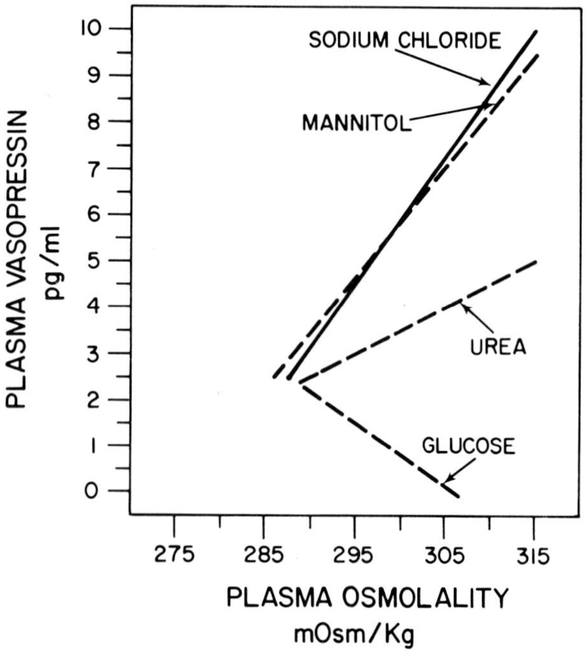

FIGURE 9-4 The relation of plasma vasopressin to elevations in plasma osmolality induced by various solutes in healthy adults. Each oblique line represents the mean regression function obtained during intravenous infusion of hypertonic solutions of the specified solutes. (*From Robertson.*[50])

barrier quite slowly yet is a relatively weak stimulus for thirst and vasopressin.[51,53] This singular disparity suggests that most if not all of the osmoreceptors are located outside the blood-brain barrier and that another factor, most likely the permeability of the osmoreceptor neuron per se, determines the specificity of the system.

The sensitivity of the osmoreceptors to stimulation by plasma glucose appears to be critically dependent on the level of plasma insulin. Thus, hyperglycemia stimulates thirst and vasopressin secretion in patients with insulin-deficient diabetes mellitus[55] but has no effect on either variable in healthy adults[51] or in patients with insulin-treated diabetes.[56] These observations probably explain the hyperdipsia and some of the hypervasopressinemia that occur in uncontrolled diabetic patients[57,58] and indicate that glucose uptake by osmoreceptor neurons is probably dependent on the action of insulin. This concept is supported by other evidence that high-affinity receptors for plasma insulin are present in an area of the anterior hypothalamus that is thought to contain the osmoreceptors.[59]

Hemodynamic Factors

The secretion of vasopressin is also affected by changes in blood volume and/or pressure.[25,26,28] These hemodynamic influences are mediated largely if not exclusively by neurogenic afferents that arise in pressure-sensitive receptors in the cardiac atria and large arteries, travel via the vagal and glossopharyngeal nerves, and synapse in the nucleus tractus solitarii in the brainstem (Fig. 9-1).[60–64] From there, postsynaptic pathways that are at least partly noradrenergic project to the region of the paraventricular and supraoptic nuclei.[65] The input from these pathways appears to be predominantly negative, or inhibitory, under basal normovolemic, normotensive conditions, since their elimination results in an acute rise in plasma vasopressin as well as arterial pressure.[66–68]

The functional properties of this baroregulatory system are exemplified in Fig. 9-5. In healthy adult humans, monkeys, and rats, acutely lowering blood pressure by any of several methods increases plasma vasopressin by an amount that is roughly proportional to the degree of hypotension achieved.[26,69–71] However, this stimulus-response relationship follows a distinctly exponential pattern. Thus, small decreases in blood pressure of the order of 5 to 10 percent usually have little effect on plasma vasopressin, while decreases in blood pressure of 20 to 30 percent result in hormone levels many times those required to produce maximum antidiuresis. The vasopressin response to changes in blood volume has not been so well defined but appears to be quantitatively and qualitatively similar

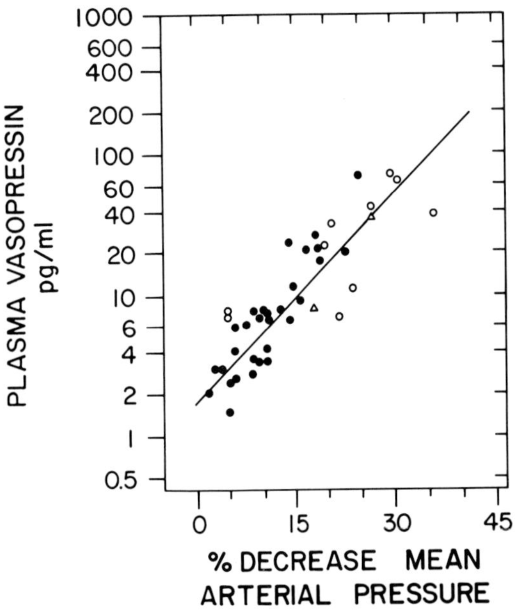

FIGURE 9-5 The relation of plasma vasopressin to percent fall in blood pressure in healthy adults and patients with idiopathic postural hypotension. In healthy adults, blood pressure was reduced by infusion of trimethaphan (Arfonad) (solid circle) or by orthostasis immediately after phlebotomy (open circle). In patients with orthostatic hypotension, blood pressure was reduced by tilting (triangle). (*From Robertson.*[50])

to the response to blood pressure (Fig. 9-6). In rats, plasma vasopressin increases as an exponential function of the degree of hypovolemia.[71] Thus, little or no rise in plasma vasopressin can be detected until blood volume falls by 6 to 8 percent. Beyond that point, plasma vasopressin begins to rise at a rapidly increasing rate in relation to the degree of hypovolemia and usually reaches levels 20 to 30 times normal when blood volume is reduced by 20 to 30 percent. The volume-vasopressin relationship in humans has not been so thoroughly characterized but appears to follow a similar pattern.[26,69,72,73] Thus, in healthy adults, plasma vasopressin is unchanged by a fall in blood volume of up to 7 percent, is doubled by a reduction of 10 to 15 percent, and increases markedly if the hypovolemia exceeds 20 percent. An acute rise in blood volume or pressure suppresses vasopressin secretion. This effect has been characterized even less well than that of hypotension or hypovolemia but seems to exhibit a similar quantitative relationship.

The minimal effect of small changes in blood volume and pressure on vasopressin secretion contrasts sharply with the extraordinary sensitivity of the osmoregulatory system (Fig. 9-6). Recognition of this difference is essential for understanding the relative contribution of each system to control of the hormone under

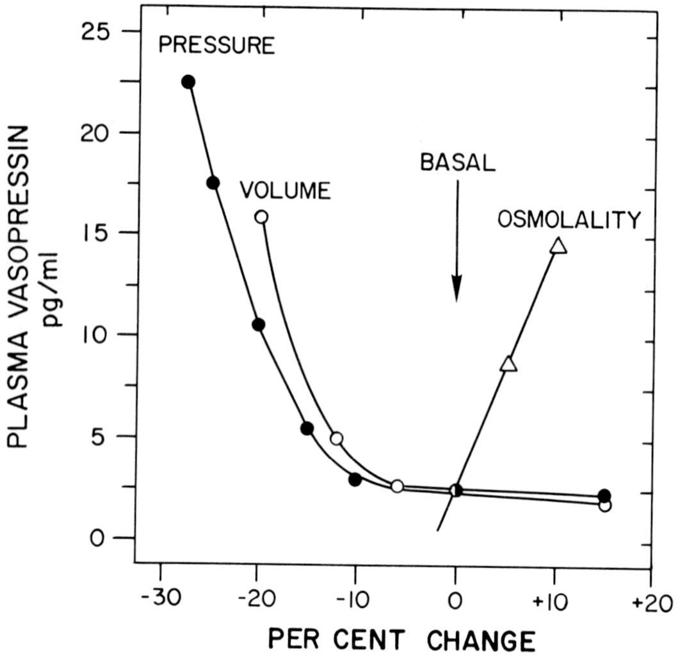

FIGURE 9-6 Schematic representation of the stimulus-response relationship between plasma vasopressin and percent change in plasma osmolality, total blood volume, and blood pressúre in healthy adults.

physiologic and pathologic conditions. Since day-to-day variations of total body water rarely exceed 2 to 3 percent, their effect on vasopressin secretion must be mediated largely, if not exclusively, by the osmoregulatory system.[71,74] This concept is consistent with the observation that patients with destruction of the osmoreceptor exhibit a markedly subnormal vasopressin response to changes in water balance, even though baroregulatory mechanisms are completely intact.[32] On the other hand, baroregulatory input may be responsible for the erratic and sometimes large fluctuations in plasma vasopressin that occur with normal activity,[75] since the latter is known to be associated with relatively large fluctuations in blood pressure and/or effective blood volume. Hence, hemodynamic and osmotic influences may be equally active under physiologic conditions, even though their determinants and effect on salt and water balance are quite different.

The baroreceptor also appears to mediate the effects of a large number of pharmacologic and pathologic influences (Table 9-1). Among the pharmacologic influences are diuretics, isoproterenol, nicotine, prostaglandins, nitroprusside, trimethaphan, histamine, morphine, and bradykinin, all of which stimulate vasopressin at least in part by lowering blood volume or pressure; and norepinephrine, which suppresses vasopressin by raising blood pressure.[60] In addition, upright posture, sodium depletion, congestive heart failure, cirrhosis, and nephrosis probably stimulate vasopressin by reducing total or effective blood vol-

Table 9-1. Variables that Influence Vasopressin Secretion

- Osmotic
  - Plasma osmolality
    - Changes in water balance
    - Infusion of hypertonic or hypotonic solutions
    - Deficiency of insulin and hyperglycemia
- Hemodynamic
  - Blood volume (total or effective)
    - Posture
    - Hemorrhage
    - Aldosterone deficiency or excess
    - Gastroenteritis
    - Congestive heart failure
    - Cirrhosis
    - Nephrosis
    - Positive pressure breathing
    - Diuretics
  - Blood pressure
    - Orthostatic hypotension
    - Vasovagal reaction
    - Drugs (isoproterenol, norepinephrine, nicotine, nitroprusside, trimethaphan, histamine, bradykinin, morphine)
- Emetic
  - Nausea
    - Drugs (apomorphine, morphine, nicotine)
    - Motion sickness
- Glucopenic
  - Drugs (insulin, 2-deoxyglucose)
- Other
  - Angiotensin
  - P_{CO_2}, P_{O_2}, pH
  - Stress(?)
  - Temperature (?)

ume,[76-78] while orthostatic hypotension, vasovagal reactions, and other forms of syncope markedly stimulate the hormone by reducing blood pressure.[69,79,80] This list probably could be extended to include almost every other hormone, drug, or condition known to affect blood volume or pressure. The only recognized exception is a form of orthostatic hypotension associated with loss of afferent baroregulatory function.[81]

Changes in blood volume or pressure large enough to affect vasopressin secretion do not necessarily interfere with osmoregulation of the hormone. Instead, they appear to act by shifting the set of the system in such a way as to increase or decrease the effect on vasopressin of a given osmotic stimulus (Fig. 9-7).[27,82-87] Thus, in the presence of a hemodynamic stimulus, plasma vasopressin can still be fully suppressed if plasma osmolality falls below the new, lower set point.[85] This aspect of the interaction is important because it ensures that the capacity to osmoregulate is not lost even in the presence of hemodynamic stimuli. It also indicates that the osmoregulatory and baroregulatory systems, though different in location and function, ultimately converge and act upon the same population of neurosecretory neurons.[27] How and where such integration occurs is unknown; but it most likely involves one or more interneurons that link the osmoreceptor to neurosecretory cells.[35]

Emetic Factors

Nausea is an extremely potent stimulus for vasopressin secretion in humans.[88,89] The pathway that mediates this effect has not been defined but probably involves the chemoreceptor trigger zone in the area postrema of the medulla (Fig. 9-1). It can be activated by a variety of drugs and conditions, including apomorphine, morphine, nicotine, alcohol, and motion sickness. Its effect on vasopressin is instantaneous and extremely potent (Fig. 9-8). Increases of 100 to 1000 times basal levels are not unusual, even when the nausea is transient and unaccompanied by vomiting or changes in blood pressure. Pretreatment with fluphenazine, haloperidol, or promethazine in doses sufficient to prevent nausea completely abolishes the vasopressin response. The inhibitory effect of these dopamine antagonists is specific for emetic stimuli, since they do not alter the vasopressin response to osmotic and hemodynamic stimuli. Water loading blunts, but does not abolish, the effect of nausea on vasopressin release, suggesting that osmotic and emetic influences interact in a manner similar to osmotic and hemodynamic pathways. Emesis is the only vasopressin stimulus known to exhibit significant species differences. In rats, apomorphine has little or no effect on vasopressin[88,90] but produces marked increases in oxytocin.[90]

Emetic stimuli probably mediate many pharmacologic and pathologic effects on vasopressin secretion. They may be responsible at least in part for the increase in vasopressin secretion that has been observed with intravenous cyclophosphamide,[91,92] vasovagal reactions,[79] ketoacidosis,[57,58] acute hypoxia,[93] and motion sickness.[94] Since nausea and vomiting are frequent side effects of many other drugs and diseases, additional examples of emetically mediated vasopressin secretion undoubtedly will be demonstrated. The potency and ubiquity of emetic stimuli create special problems for research studies of vasopressin secretion in animals and unconscious subjects, since the occur-

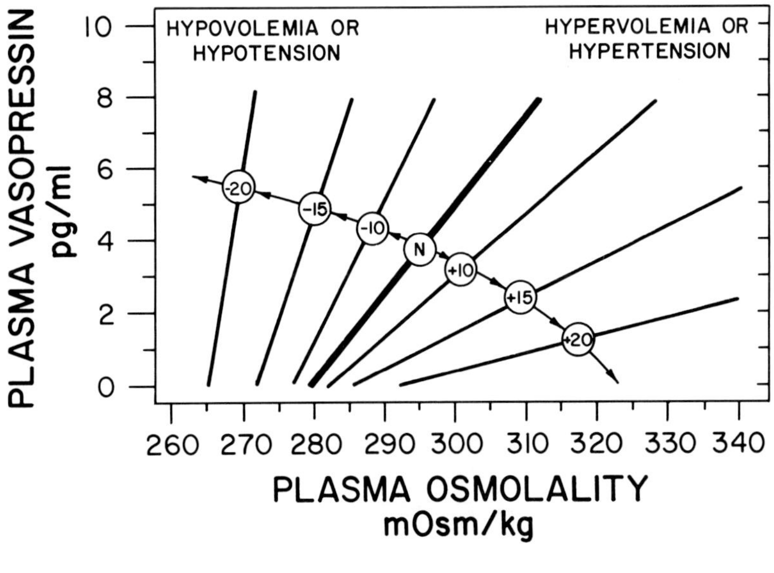

FIGURE 9-7 Schematic representation of the relationship between plasma vasopressin and plasma osmolality in the presence of differing states of blood volume and/or pressure. The line labeled N represents normovolemic, normotensive conditions. Minus numbers to the left indicate percent fall and positive numbers to the right percent rise in blood volume or pressure. (*From Robertson.*[50])

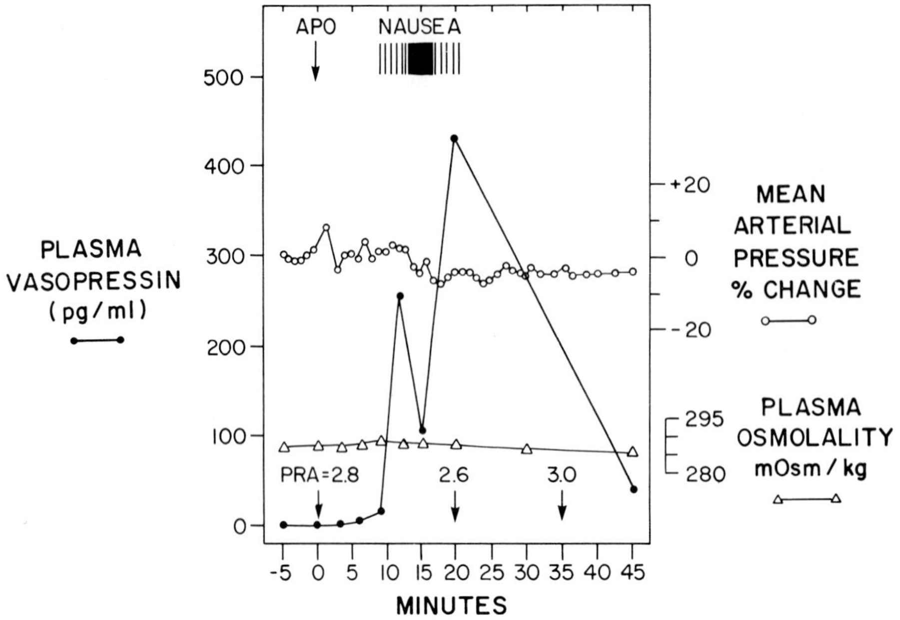

FIGURE 9-8 Relation of nausea to vasopressin secretion. Apomorphine (APO) was injected at the point indicated by the vertical arrow. Note that the rise in plasma vasopressin coincided with the occurrence of nausea and was not associated with detectable changes in plasma osmolality or blood pressure. (*From Robertson.*[50])

rence of nausea is difficult to ascertain except by verbal report.

Glucopenic Factors

Acute hypoglycemia is also a stimulus for vasopressin release,[95-98] but the effect is much less potent than that of nausea. The receptor and pathway that mediate this effect are unknown. However, they seem to be separate from those of other recognized stimuli, since hypoglycemia stimulates vasopressin secretion in patients who have lost selectively the capacity to respond to osmotic, hemodynamic, or emetic stimuli. The effect of hypoglycemia is not due to nonspecific stress, since it can occur in the absence of symptoms and is more pronounced in rats,[96] a species in which vasopressin secretion appears to be completely unresponsive to pain and other noxious stimuli (see below). The variable that actually triggers the release of vasopressin may be an intracellular deficiency of glucose or one of its metabolites, since 2-deoxyglucose is also an effective stimulus.[99,100]

The stimulus-response relationship to hypoglycemia appears to be exponential.[97] Thus, in healthy adults, a drop in plasma glucose of as much as 10 to 20 percent usually has little or no effect, whereas a decrease of 50 percent increases plasma vasopressin about threefold. The rate of fall in glucose is probably the critical determinant, however, since the rise in plasma vasopressin is not sustained even when the hypoglycemia persists.[96] In addition, the vasopressin response to hypoglycemia is accentuated by dehydration and abolished by water loading.[96] Thus, glucopenic stimuli probably act in concert with osmotic influences even though the osmoreceptors per se are unnecessary for the response.

Glucopenic stimuli are probably of little importance in clinical disorders of vasopressin secretion. Apart from acute hyperinsulinemia, there are few drugs or conditions that lower plasma glucose fast enough to stimulate release of the hormone. Moreover, even if secretion were increased, it would not be expected to influence perceptibly the regulation of water balance, since the effect tends to be transient and is prevented completely by a small decrease in plasma osmolality.

Renin-Angiotensin

The renin-angiotensin system has also been implicated in the control of vasopressin secretion.[101] The precise site and mechanism of action have not been defined, but central receptors seem likely, since angiotensin is most effective when injected directly into brain ventricles or cranial arteries.[102] Moreover, intraventricular administration of angiotensin antagonists inhibits the vasopressin response to osmotic and hemodynamic stimuli.[103] The level of plasma renin and/or angiotensin required to stimulate vasopressin release have not been determined but probably are quite high. When given intravenously, pressor doses of angiotensin increase plasma vasopressin only about two- to fourfold. The magnitude of the vasopressin response may depend upon the concurrent osmotic stimulus, since angiotensin has been observed to increase the sensitivity of the osmoregulatory system.[104] Hence, the effect of angiotensin on vasopressin may be imperceptible when plasma osmolality is depressed and exaggerated when plasma osmolality is high. This dependency on osmotic influences resembles that seen with glucopenic stimuli and may account for the failure of some investigators to demonstrate stimulation by exogenous angiotensin.[105]

Stress and Temperature

Nonspecific stress caused by factors such as pain, emotion, or physical exercise has long been thought to cause release of vasopressin.[106] However, it has never been determined whether this effect is mediated by a separate pathway or is secondary to another stimulus such as the hypotension and/or nausea that usually accompanies stress-induced vasovagal reactions. In rats at least, a variety of noxious stimuli capable of activating the pituitary adrenal axis and sympathetic nervous system do not stimulate vasopressin secretion unless they also lower blood pressure or alter blood volume.[26,107,108] The same stresses may stimulate the release of oxytocin,[109] but the role of other nonosmotic stimuli in the response has not been excluded. The marked rise in plasma vasopressin elicited by manipulation of the abdominal viscera in anesthetized dogs has been attributed to nociceptive influences,[110] but mediation by emetic pathways cannot be excluded in this setting. Environmental temperature can also influence vasopressin secretion.[76] In healthy adults, exposure to cold for a relatively short period of time depresses plasma vasopressin, while a hot environment has the opposite effect. These changes occur independent of changes in plasma osmolality but cannot as yet be disassociated from changes in effective blood volume or blood pressure. Hence, it is unclear whether there is a distinct thermoregulatory system for vasopressin secretion. Clarification of the possible role of nociceptive and thermal influences in vasopressin secretion is particularly important in view of the frequency with which painful or febrile illnesses are associated with osmotically inappropriate secretion of the hormone.

Hypoxia-Hypercapnia

Acute hypoxia and hypercapnia also stimulate vasopressin release.[93,111–114] In conscious humans, however, the stimulatory effect of moderate hypoxia (Pa_{O_2}>35 mmHg) is inconsistent[93,111] and seems to occur only in subjects who develop nausea or hypotension.[93] In conscious dogs, more severe hypoxia (Pa_{O_2}<35 mmHg) consistently increases vasopressin secretion without reducing arterial pressure.[113] Studies in anesthetized dogs suggest that the vasopressin response to acute hypoxia depends on the level of hypoxemia achieved. At Pa_{O_2} of 35 mmHg or below, plasma vasopressin is markedly elevated despite absence of change or even an increase in arterial pressure.[112,114] However, less severe hypoxemia (Pa_{O_2}>40 mmHg) has no effect on vasopressin.[112] These results indicate a hypoxemic threshold for vasopressin release and suggest that severe acute hypoxemia per se may also stimulate vasopressin secretion in humans. If so, it may be responsible, at least in part, for the osmotically inappropriate hormonal elevations noted in some patients with acute respiratory failure.[115] In conscious or anesthetized dogs, acute hypercapnia per se, independent of hypoxia or hypotension, also increases vasopressin secretion.[112,113] It has not been determined whether this response also exhibits threshold characteristics or otherwise depends on the degree of hypercapnia. It is also unknown whether hypercapnia has similar effects on vasopressin secretion in humans or other animals.

Pharmacologic Factors

A large number of drugs and hormones have also been shown to influence vasopressin secretion (Table 9-2).[116,117] Many stimulants, such as isoproterenol, nicotine, and high doses of morphine, undoubtedly act at least in part by lowering blood pressure or producing nausea.[60,118] Others, such as substance P, prostaglandin, endorphin, and other opioids, have not been studied sufficiently to define their mechanism of action[60,119–122] but probably work by one or both of the same mechanisms. As discussed elsewhere, insulin and 2-deoxyglucose seem to act by producing intracellular glucopenia, while angiotensin has an undefined but probably independent central effect. Vincristine may act by a direct effect on the neurohypophysis or peripheral neurons involved in the regulation of vasopressin secretion.[123] Lithium, which antagonizes the antidiuretic effect of vasopressin, also increases secretion of the hormone.[124–126] This effect is independent of changes in water balance and appears to result from an increase in sensitivity of the osmo-

Table 9-2. Drugs and Hormones that Affect Vasopressin Secretion or Action

Secretion	
Stimulate	Inhibit
Acetylcholine	Norepinphrine
Nicotine	Fluphenazine (emetic)
Apomorphine	Haloperidol (emetic)
Morphine (high doses)	Promethazine
Epinephrine	Oxilorphan
Isoproterenol	Butorphanol
Histamine	Morphine (low doses)
Bradykinin	Alcohol
Prostaglandins	Carbamazepine
β-Endorphin	Glucocorticoids
Cyclophosphamide (IV)	? Phenytoin
Vincristine	Clonidine
Insulin	Muscimol
2-Deoxyglucose	Diprenorphine (hypovolemic)*
Angiotensin	
Lithium	
? Chlorpropamide	
? Clofibrate	
Thiazides	
Action	
Potentiate	Inhibit
Chlorpropamide	Barbiturates
Indomethacin	Lithium
Thiazides	Tetracyclines
? Clofibrate	Methoxyflurane
? Carbamazepine	Glyburide
Acetaminophen	Isophosphamide
	Vinca alkaloids
	AVP antagonists
	Platinum
	? Glucocorticoids

*Experiment drug provided by National Institute of Drug Abuse.

regulatory system.[124] The stimulatory effects of chlorpropamide and clofibrate are still controversial.[127-130] Carbamazepine inhibits vasopressin secretion by diminishing the sensitivity of the osmoregulatory system.[131-133] This effect occurs independent of changes in blood volume, blood pressure, or blood glucose, suggesting that the ability of carbamazepine to produce antidiuresis in patients with neurogenic diabetes insipidus is due to an action on the kidney.

Vasopressor drugs such as norepinephrine inhibit vasopressin secretion indirectly by raising arterial pressure.[60] Dopaminergic antagonists such as fluphenazine, haloperidol, and promethazine probably act by suppressing the emetic center, since they inhibit the vasopressin response only to emetic and not to osmotic or hemodynamic stimuli. In low doses, a variety of opioids, including morphine, inhibit vasopressin secretion in rats[134-137] and in humans.[138-141] The inhibition by morphine, butorphanol, and oxilorphan is due to an increase in the osmotic threshold for vasopressin release[134,136] but is independent of changes in blood volume or pressure.[134] The inhibitory action of these opioids has not been completely defined but would appear to be an agonistic effect, since it is blocked completely by naloxone.[134-136] The inhibitory effect of alcohol[142-144] may be mediated at least in part by endogenous opiates, since it also is due to an elevation in the osmotic threshold for vasopressin release and can be blocked in part by treatment with naloxone.[145] Other drugs which have the capacity to inhibit vasopressin secretion include clonidine,[146,147] which appears to act via both central and peripheral adrenoreceptors,[146] and muscimol,[148] which is postulated to act as a gamma-aminobutyric acid (GABA) agonist.

Vasopressin and oxytocin may also feed back to inhibit or facilitate their own secretion.[149-151] In the case of vasopressin, at least, the feedback effect occurs following systemic as well as central administration and is not mediated by osmotic or hemodynamic influences.[149,150] The importance of local feedback effects on the physiology or pathophysiology of vasopressin secretion is uncertain because, so far, the phenomenon has been demonstrated only after exogenous administration of relatively large doses of the hormone.

OXYTOCIN

The regulation of oxytocin secretion has not yet been well defined, because simple and specific assays have been lacking. Bioassays, direct as well as indirect, have often been employed, but their specificity is suspect because vasopressin and possibly other peptides possess oxytocin activity. Radioimmunoassays have also been developed and used to characterize secretion of the hormone. However, even this information must now be viewed with caution, because some oxytocin and vasotocin assays have been found to cross-react with one or more plasma components other than oxytocin.[152] To further complicate matters, the ovary also synthesizes oxytocin or oxytocin-like peptides,[153] and this material may be the source of some of the immunoreactivity in plasma.

Studies employing specific assays have confirmed that nursing is a stimulus for oxytocin release in lactating postpartum women.[152] In rats, but not in other species, apomorphine also stimulates oxytocin release.[90] However, contrary to previous findings using less specific assays,[154] it now appears that pregnancy and/or high levels of estrogen do not result in increased secretion of oxytocin but do cause an increase in the plasma level of a novel peptide which may be structurally related to oxytocin.[152] The source and biologic action, if any, of this novel peptide are unknown.

However, it appears to be associated with estrogen-stimulated neurophysin and therefore is probably synthesized and secreted with it in a process similar to if not identical with vasopressin and oxytocin.

Distribution and Clearance

The concentration of vasopressin and oxytocin in plasma is determined by the difference between the rates of production and of removal from the vascular compartment. Unfortunately, studies of the volume of distribution, rate of clearance, and site of clearance of the hormone have given inconsistent results.[155] There seems to be agreement, for example, that in healthy adults, intravenously injected vasopressin distributes rapidly into a space roughly equivalent in size to the extracellular compartment.[26,156] In this initial, or "mixing," phase, the vasopressin has a half-life of 4 to 8 min, and the process is virtually complete in 10 to 15 min. The rapidity with which vasopressin diffuses across capillary membranes approximates that of many other small peptides and is consistent with its lack of binding to neurophysin or other macromolecular components of plasma. There is also agreement that the rapid mixing phase is followed by a second, slower decline that probably corresponds to the metabolic, or irreversible, phase of vasopressin clearance. However, there is considerable disagreement as to the half-life of the vasopressin in this second phase. Studies with one immunoassay yielded mean values of 10 to 20 min by both steady-state and non-steady-state techniques,[26,149,157] while non-steady-state measurements with another assay gave an average half-life of 82 min.[156] This discrepancy cannot be explained easily. Although the metabolic clearance rate can vary two- to threefold from person to person or from time to time in the same person,[26,157] these individual variations are not great enough to account for a fivefold difference in mean values. Some of the discrepancy may be explained by the ability of vasopressin to affect its own secretion (see above) and/or by differences in assay cross-reaction with metabolites. The rate of change in urine osmolality after water loading and injection of vasopressin supports the validity of the shorter half-life.[155] It should be noted that smaller animals such as the rat clear vasopressin much more rapidly than humans because their cardiac output is also much higher relative to their body weight and surface area.[155]

Although many tissues have the capacity to inactivate vasopressin in vitro, most metabolism in vivo appears to occur in liver and kidney.[155] This generalization seems to be true even in pregnant women, whose plasma contains an enzyme capable of rapidly degrading the hormones in vitro. The enzymatic processes by which the liver and kidney inactivate vasopressin have not been established with certainty but would appear to involve an initial reduction of the disulfide bridge followed by aminopeptidase cleavage of the bond between amino acid residues 1 and 2. The extent of further degradation and the peptide products, if any, that escape into plasma and urine are currently unknown.

Some vasopressin is excreted intact in the urine, but here too there is disagreement about the amounts and the factors that affect it. For example, in healthy, normally hydrated adults, the urinary clearance of vasopressin ranges from 0.1 to 0.6 ml per kilogram of body weight per minute under basal conditions and has never been found to exceed 2 ml per kilogram of body weight per minute even in the presence of a solute diuresis.[26] The mechanisms involved in the excretion of vasopressin have not been defined with certainty, but the hormone is probably filtered at the glomerulus and variably reabsorbed at one or more sites along the tubule. The latter process may be linked in some way to the handling of sodium in the proximal nephron, since the urinary clearance of vasopressin varies as much as 20-fold in direct relation to solute clearance.[26] Consequently, measurements of vasopressin excretion in humans do not provide a consistently reliable index of changes in plasma vasopressin and must be interpreted cautiously when glomerular filtration and/or solute clearance are inconstant or abnormal.

EXTRAHYPOPHYSEAL PATHWAYS

It is not altogether clear whether the factors which influence the release of vasopressin into plasma by the pars nervosa also affect secretion from the other divisions of the neurohypophyseal system. This uncertainty is particularly significant for the tuberoinfundibular tract, which, as noted previously, appears to secrete into the adenohypophysis by way of the portal veins. Plasma from these vessels has been shown to contain extremely high concentrations of vasopressin during the stress of major surgery and anesthesia,[158] but normal basal levels and the effect of other, more physiologic, stimuli are still unknown. Such information is of obvious importance for understanding the role of the vasopressin-containing neurons of the infundibulum in regulating anterior pituitary function.

The regulation of vasopressin and oxytocin secretion into spinal fluid is understood only slightly better. Most if not all of the vasopressin in CSF probably derives from direct secretion rather than diffusion from plasma.[8] In humans, the concentration of vasopressin in CSF appears to be slightly lower than in plasma,[8,159] although the opposite has also been reported in humans as well as animals.[160,161] Secretion into CSF seems to be influenced by some if not all of the same variables that stimulate release from the pars nervosa, since CSF concentrations correlate with those in plasma[8,159] and change appropriately during dehydration or rehydration in humans[8] or dogs,[161] during infusion of hypertonic saline,[161] and during hemorrhage.[161] However, the vasopressin concentration in CSF may also exhibit circadian variation, at least in cats.[162] The function of the vasopressin in CSF is unknown, but it may play some role in regulating brain hydration,[8] thirst,[163] or intellectual function.[164] CSF vasopressin is abnormal in the syndrome of inappropriate antidiuresis,[8] diabetes insipidus,[8] dementia,[165] affective disorders,[166] and benign intracranial hypertension,[167] but the role of the abnormalities in the pathophysiology of these disorders is unknown.

Biologic Action

The most important action of vasopressin is to conserve body water by reducing the rate of urine output. This antidiuretic effect is achieved by promoting the reabsorption of solute-free water in the distal and/or collecting tubules of the kidney (Fig. 9-9).[168] In the absence of vasopressin, the membranes lining this portion of the nephron are uniquely resistant to the diffusion of water as well as solutes. Hence, hypotonic filtrate formed in the more proximal part of the nephron passes unmodified through the distal tubule and collecting duct. In this condition, which is referred to as *water diuresis,* urine osmolality and flow in a healthy adult usually approximate 60 to 70 mosmol/kg and 15 to 20 ml/min, respectively. In the presence of vasopressin, the hydroosmotic permeability of the distal and collecting tubules increases, allowing water to diffuse back down the osmotic gradient that normally exists between tubular fluid and the isotonic or hypertonic milieu of the renal cortex and medulla (Fig. 9-9). Because water is reabsorbed without solute, the urine that remains has an increased osmotic pressure as well as decreased volume or flow rate. The amount of water reabsorbed in the distal nephron—hence also the degree of urinary concentration—varies as a function of the plasma vasopressin concentration (Fig. 9-3*B*). In healthy adults, this stimulus-response relationship is extremely sensitive, since the full range of urinary concentration and dilution is covered by a 10-fold or smaller change in plasma vasopressin. At maximally effective levels of vasopressin, urine osmolality and flow approximate 1200 to 1400 mosmol/kg and 0.3 to 0.6 ml/min, respectively. Certain other species, particularly rodents, can achieve much higher levels of urinary concentration, apparently because of longer renal papillae and correspondingly higher levels of hypertonicity in the medulla.

The effect of vasopressin on urinary concentration and/or flow can be markedly influenced by changes in the volume of filtrate presented to the distal tubule. In a normal adult, 85 to 90 percent of the approximately 200 liters of plasma filtered daily by the glomerulus is reabsorbed isoosmotically with salts and glucose in the proximal part of the nephron. The remaining 20 liters is made hypotonic by selective reabsorption of sodium and chloride in the ascending limb of Henle's loop, then presented to the distal nephron, where, depending on the level of vasopressin activity, additional water up to a maximum of 19 liters a day may be selectively reabsorbed. In situations in which the intake of salt is high or a poorly reabsorbed solute such as mannitol, urea, or glucose is present in increased amounts, considerably more than 10 to 15 percent of the filtrate may escape the proximal tubule. The resultant increase in the volume of fluid delivered to the distal nephron may overwhelm its limited capacity to reabsorb water and electrolytes. As a consequence, urine osmolality falls and the rate of flow rises even in the presence of supranormal levels of vasopressin. This type of polyuria is referred to as *solute diuresis* to distinguish it from that due to a deficiency of vasopressin action. Conversely, in clinical situations such as congestive failure, where the proximal nephron reabsorbs increased amounts of filtrate, the capacity to excrete solute-free water is greatly reduced even in the absence of vasopressin action.

The antidiuretic effect of vasopressin also may be inhibited by breakdown in the medullary concentration gradient. This may result from causes as diverse as chronic water diuresis, reduced medullary blood flow, or protein deficiency. However, probably because the bulk of the fluid issuing from Henle's loop can still be reabsorbed isotonically in the distal convoluted tubule and/or proximal collecting duct, loss of the medullary concentration gradient alone rarely results in marked degrees of polyuria.

The cellular mechanism by which vasopressin alters the hydroosmotic permeability of the distal nephron has not been fully determined. However, there is abundant evidence that it binds to receptors on the serosal surface of tubular epithelia, which, in turn, activate adenyl cyclase, thereby increasing the hydroosmotic permeability of the opposite or mucosal surface of the cell.[169] The exact nature and sequence of the biophysical events triggered by cyclic AMP are largely conjectural but would seem to involve the opening of highly specific channels or pores by a process requiring the participation of cellular microtubules.[170] There is also some evidence suggesting that

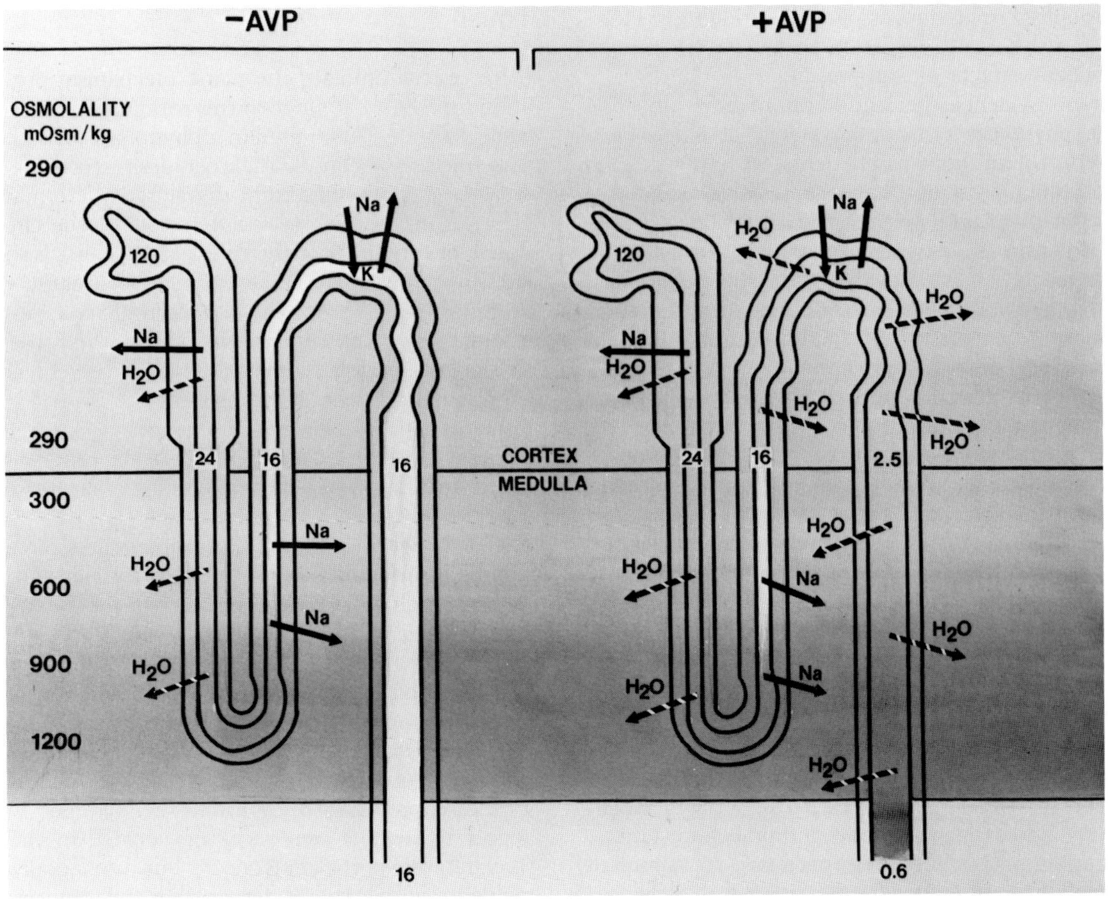

FIGURE 9-9 Schematic representation of the effect of vasopressin on the formation of urine by the nephron. The osmotic pressure of tissue and tubular fluid is indicated by the density of the shading. The numbers within the lumen of the nephron indicate typical rates of flow in milliliters per minute. Solid arrows indicate reabsorption of sodium (Na) or water (H_2O) by active mechanisms, broken arrows indicate reabsorption by passive mechanisms. Note that vasopressin acts only on the distal nephron, where it increases the hydroosmotic permeability of tubular membranes. The fluid which reaches this part of the nephron normally amounts to 10 to 15 percent of the total filtrate and is hypotonic because of selective reabsorption of sodium in the ascending limb of Henle's loop. In the absence of vasopressin the membranes of the distal nephron remain relatively impermeable to water as well as solute, and the fluid issuing from Henle's loop is excreted essentially unmodified as urine. With maximum vasopressin action, all but 5 to 10 percent of the water in this fluid is reabsorbed passively down the osmotic gradient which normally exists with the renal medulla.

the prostaglandins operate as a kind of local or short loop feedback system to modulate the actions of vasopressin on the kidney.[171] Thus, it has been shown that vasopressin stimulates the synthesis of prostaglandin E and that prostaglandin E, in turn, can inhibit the effect of the hormone on adenyl cyclase and hydroosmotic flow. Conversely, inhibitors of prostaglandin synthesis such as indomethacin or chlorpropamide potentiate the antidiuretic effect of the hormone. Renal prostaglandin synthesis can also be stimulated by angiotensin, bradykinin, and hypertonicity, suggesting that a variety of factors may be capable of influencing water balance by modifying the effects of vasopressin on the kidney.

As its name implies, vasopressin can also raise blood pressure by constricting vascular smooth muscle.[172] The pressor and antidiuretic effects of vasopressin are mediated by different parts of the molecule, since the two effects can be selectively altered by modifying the structure of the hormone[12,13] or treating with specific V_1 (vascular) or V_2 (antidiuretic) antagonists.[14] In dogs and some other quadrupeds, the pressor effect of vasopressin begins at plasma concentrations of around 50 pg/ml,[173,174] i.e., about 10 times that required to produce maximum antidiuresis. However, healthy adults appear to be more refractory to the pressor effects of vasopressin,[175,176] and there is as yet no evidence that the hormone plays any role in the physiology or pathophysiology of blood pressure control in humans. Patients with severe diabetes insipidus do not have appreciable defects in baroregulation, and neither the secretion nor the pressor action of vasopressin is increased in essential hypertension.[175,177,178] However, some patients with postural hypotension due to autonomic dysfunction appear to be supersensitive to the pressor effects of vasopressin,[179] and in some of these, failure to secrete the hormone normally in response to hypotension[81] may contribute to the baroregulatory defects.

The effects of vasopressin on the anterior pituitary are still unclear.[180] Although systemic administration of relatively large doses of vasopressin causes release of adrenocorticotropic and growth hormones, the weight of the evidence would seem to indicate that these effects are indirect. Endogenous secretion of vasopressin clearly is not necessary for activation of the pituitary adrenal system, since Brattleboro rats which lack the capacity to synthesize vasopressin exhibit little or no impairment in their corticosteroid response to various forms of stress.[181,182] Nevertheless, vasopressin has been shown to potentiate the effect of corticotropin releasing factor both in vitro[183] and in vivo,[184,185] indicating that under certain circumstances, the action of vasopressin is necessary to stimulate maximally the pituitary-adrenal axis.[186]

At physiologic concentrations, vasopressin also inhibits water loss from skin, lungs, and other extrarenal sites.[187,188] Other actions of vasopressin include inhibition of pancreatic flow,[189] stimulation of hepatic glycogenolysis,[190] and aggregation of platelets,[191] but the role of these effects in human physiology and pathology is unknown.

The major biologic action of oxytocin is to facilitate nursing by causing the ejection of milk. It is achieved by stimulating the contraction of myoepithelial cells in the lactating mammary gland. Oxytocin may also aid in parturition by stimulating contraction of the uterus. Whether the hormone has any significant effect in males is unknown. When given exogenously it may produce antidiuresis and/or natriuresis, but whether the kind of blood levels required to produce this effect ever occur as a result of endogenous secretion is unknown.

The neurophysins have no recognized biologic action apart from complexing oxytocin and vasopressin in neurosecretory granules of the neurohypophysis. Although present in plasma, they do not serve as binding or transport proteins, because the high pH and low concentration of the reactants favor complete dissociation.

Thirst

In terrestrial animals, the thirst mechanism provides an indispensable adjunct to the antidiuretic control of water balance. When used in a physiologic sense, *thirst* is defined as a conscious, inner desire to drink and must be distinguished from nondipsetic determinants of water intake such as social custom or the circumstance of eating. As might be expected, thirst is stimulated by many of the same variables that cause vasopressin release.[192,193] Of these, hypertonicity appears to be the most potent. In healthy adults, a rise in effective plasma osmolality of only 2 to 3 percent above basal levels produces a strong desire to drink.[194] This response is not dependent on changes in extracellular volume, since it occurs when plasma osmolality is raised by infusion of hypertonic saline[51,52] as well as by water deprivation.[194,195] The absolute level of plasma osmolality at which a desire for water is first perceived may be termed the *osmotic threshold* for thirst. It varies appreciably from one person to the next, but, among healthy adults, averages about 295 mosmol/kg.[26,51,194-196] This level is well above the osmotic threshold for vasopressin release and closely approximates that at which maximum concentration of the urine is normally achieved (Fig. 9-3).

The neuronal pathways that mediate osmotic dipsogenesis have not been totally defined but would appear to involve osmoreceptors located in the anterolateral hypothalamus near, but not totally coincident with, those responsible for vasopressin release.[27,31-33,197-201] The specificity of these two osmoreceptors appears to be similar, since plasma solutes such as urea and glucose, which have little or no effect on vasopressin secretion, are equally ineffective as dipsogens.[51,52] The sensitivities of the thirst and vasopressin osmoreceptors cannot be compared precisely but probably are equivalent. Thus, in healthy adults, intensity of thirst increases rapidly in direct proportion to plasma sodium or osmolality and generally becomes almost intolerable at levels only 3 to 5 percent above the threshold level.[196] Water consumption also appears to be proportional to the intensity of the thirst and under conditions of maximum osmotic stimulation may reach rates approximating 20 to 25 liters per day.

Hypovolemia and/or hypotension are also dipsogenic.[202] The degree of hypovolemia and/or hypotension required to produce thirst has not been defined for humans but appears to be greater even than that needed to effect vasopressin release. Thus, upright posture often induces a small but significant rise in plasma vasopressin but does not produce thirst. Hypovolemia may be a more potent dipsogen in rats, but even in that species reductions of less than 15 percent have little or no effect on water intake. The pathways by which hypovolemia and/or hypotension produce thirst are uncertain, but they are different from those that mediate osmotic dipsogenesis[203] and probably are close to if not identical with those that mediate the baroregulation of vasopressin. Hemodynamic stimuli also reset the osmotic threshold for thirst as they do for vasopressin.[204] The effects of hypovolemia on thirst and vasopressin may also be mediated partially via the renin-angiotensin system. The latter is a potent dipsogen in rats[205,206] but has not been shown to affect thirst in humans.

Thirst may also be affected by changes in plasma or CSF vasopressin.[207] Since osmotic and hemodynamic stimuli cause release of vasopressin into CSF as well as plasma (see above), the dipsogenic effect of dehydration may be mediated in part by increases in endogenous vasopressin secretion. However, the hormone probably does not play an essential or even a major role in the regulation of thirst, since dipsogenesis is normal in Brattleboro rats which lack the capacity to make vasopressin.

Maintenance of Salt and Water Balance

Water is by far the largest constituent of the human body.[208] In lean, healthy adults, it makes up 55 to 65 percent of body weight and is an even larger proportion in infants and young children. About two-thirds of body water is intracellular (Fig. 9-10). The rest is extracellular and is divided further into the intravascular (plasma) and extravascular (interstitial) compartments. Plasma is much the smaller of the two, being only about one-fourth of total extracellular volume. The solute compositions of intracellular and of extracellular fluid differ markedly, because most cell membranes possess an array of transport systems that actively accumulate or expel specific solutes. Thus, sodium and chloride are confined largely to extracellular fluid, whereas potassium, magnesium, and various organic acids or phosphates are predominantly intracellular. Glucose, which requires an insulin-activated transport system to enter most somatic cells and is rapidly converted therein to glycogen or other metabolites, is present in significant amounts only in extracellular fluid. Bicarbonate is present in both compartments but is about three times more concentrated in extracellular fluid. Urea is unique among the major naturally occurring solutes in that it diffuses freely across most cell membranes and is, therefore, present in similar concentrations in virtually all body fluids.

Despite marked differences in the concentration of particular solutes in the extracellular and the intracellular fluid, the total solute concentration is almost everywhere the same (Fig. 9-10). This osmotic equilibrium is due to the fact that most of the membranes that separate the various compartments are freely permeable to water.[210,211] Consequently, if the total solute concentration of one compartment becomes higher than the others, the difference in osmotic pressure induces a rapid influx of water from the neighboring compartments until equilibrium is restored. The osmolality determined by measurement of freezing point or vapor pressure of a fluid[212] must be distinguished from biologically effective osmolality. The former is a physicochemical property and is a function

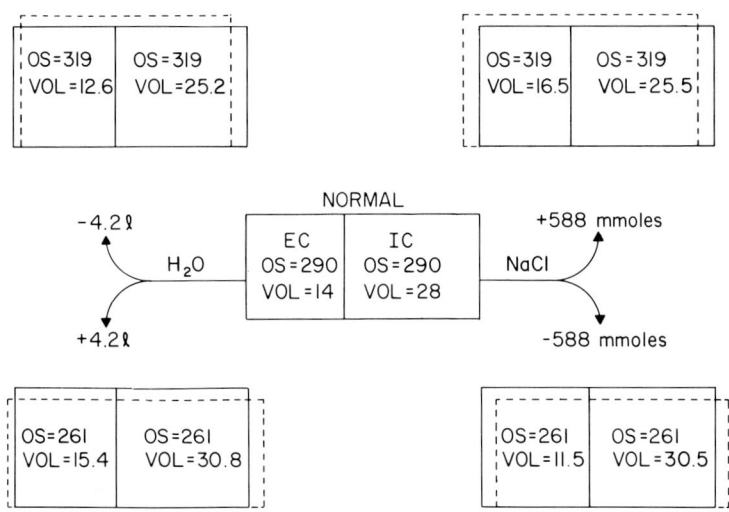

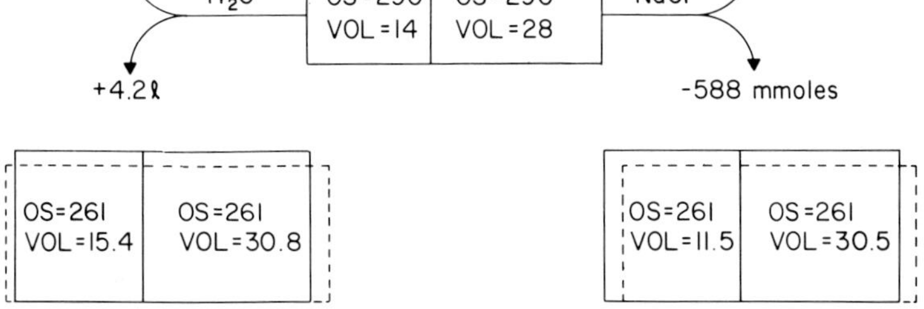

FIGURE 9-10 The osmolality and volume of intracellular and extracellular fluid under different conditions of salt and water balance. The vertical and horizontal dimensions of each box represent, respectively, the osmolality (OS) in milliosmols per kilogram and volume (VOL) in liters of the intracellular (IC) and extracellular (EC) compartments. The box in the center depicts the values in a typical 70-kg human. The values depicted with dotted lines to the left and right represent the changes that occur when total body water or sodium is altered by the amounts specified. Note that a 10 percent decrease in total body water and a 30 percent increase in total exchangeable sodium increase osmolality and decrease intracellular volume by about the same amount (10 percent) but have opposite and unequal effects on extracellular volume. The same is true for an increase in body water or decrease in sodium, except that all the changes in osmolality and volume are reversed. (*From Robertson and Berl.*[209])

of all the solutes present, regardless of their ability to penetrate biologic membranes. The effective osmolality of body fluid is a biologic property and is a function only of those solutes that can generate osmotic pressure—i.e., a concentration gradient for water—across the membranes of living cells. Thus, solutes such as sodium and chloride which are actively excluded from the intracellular compartment are osmotically effective. In contrast, urea is osmotically ineffective, because it diffuses rapidly across most cell membranes. Normally, the difference between the effective osmolality of body fluids and that determined by freezing point or vapor pressure osmometry is too small to be important, because most of the solute of plasma and extracellular fluid is composed of osmotically effective solutes such as sodium and its anions. However, in certain situations such as chronic renal failure, effective osmolality may be considerably less than that determined by conventional osmometry because the concentration of ineffective solutes such as urea is much higher than normal.

Because most cell membranes are freely permeable to water, any change in the effective osmolality of one compartment also changes its volume as well as the volume and osmolality of the other compartments (Fig. 9-10).[213] For example, a rise in extracellular osmolality induced by dehydration causes water to flow from the intracellular to the extracellular compartment. As a result, the water deficit distributes evenly throughout the body, causing a proportionally equal decrease in volume and increase in osmolality of each of the compartments. Conversely, a fall in extracellular osmolality induced by overhydration causes water to flow in the opposite direction thereby redistributing the excess to all compartments. However, if osmolality is changed by a gain or loss of solute, intracellular and extracellular volume change in opposite directions (Fig. 9-10). In each of these acute situations, the cells as a whole behave essentially like perfect osmometers—that is, the observed changes in the volume and osmolality of extracellular fluid conform closely to theoretical expectations. However, deviations from this kind of ideal behavior may occur when the disturbance in salt and water balance is particularly severe and/or prolonged. Under these conditions, many cells appear to be able to counteract osmotically induced changes in volume by reversibly activating or deactivating intracellular solute.[214] In addition, these acute disturbances in the osmolality and volume of body fluids bring into play a variety of other homeostatic mechanisms which, by altering total body content of salt and/or water, gradually restore the balance to normal (see below).

Both body water and solutes are in a state of continuous exchange with the environment. Ordinarily, the intake of water and solute is not determined by fluid and electrolyte requirements but is largely a byproduct of cultural influences and/or nutritional needs. In contrast, the excretion of water and solute is geared quite closely to the physiologic control of fluid and electrolyte balance. Normally, most water is excreted via the kidneys and is under the control of antidiuretic hormone. However, the rate of urine output is also influenced significantly by the rate of solute excretion and cannot be reduced below a certain minimum or obligatory level required to carry the solute load. The volume required for this purpose depends on the level of antidiuresis and the size of the load (Fig. 9-11). The amount of water lost by evaporation from skin and lungs also varies markedly, depending on several factors, including dress, humidity, temperature, and exercise,[215] as well as antidiuretic activity.[187,188] Under the conditions typical of modern urban life, insensible water loss in a healthy 70-kg man or woman approximates 1 liter per day (14 ml/kg). However, if antidiuretic hormone is absent or environmental temperature or activity increases, the rate of insensible water loss increases significantly and under extreme conditions may approximate the maximum rate of free water excretion by the kidney (Fig. 9-12). Thus, in quantitative terms, insensible loss and the factors that influence it are just as important to the economy of water balance as are the factors that regulate urine output.

In healthy adults, plasma osmolality and its principal determinant, plasma sodium concentration, are maintained within a remarkably narrow range. This stability is achieved largely by adjusting total body water to keep it in balance with sodium. The most important element in this homeostatic process is the threshold or set point of the osmoreceptors, which regulates thirst and vasopressin secretion. Through their ability to effect large increases in the rate of water intake or excretion, these two control functions provide almost insurmountable barriers to extreme over- or underhydration. The capacity of this osmoregulatory system to cope with disturbances in water balance is enormous. Because of the inverse exponential relationship between urinary osmolality and flow (Fig. 9-11), the suppression of plasma vasopressin to levels that permit maximum urinary dilution normally increases the rate of water excretion to more than 10 ml/min. Since outputs of this magnitude equal or surpass all but the most pathologically excessive rates of water intake, maximum suppression of vasopressin secretion normally provides an almost insurmountable barrier against water intoxication. Consequently, the osmotic threshold for vasopressin secretion effectively determines the lower limit for the osmotic pressure of body fluids. The upper limit is

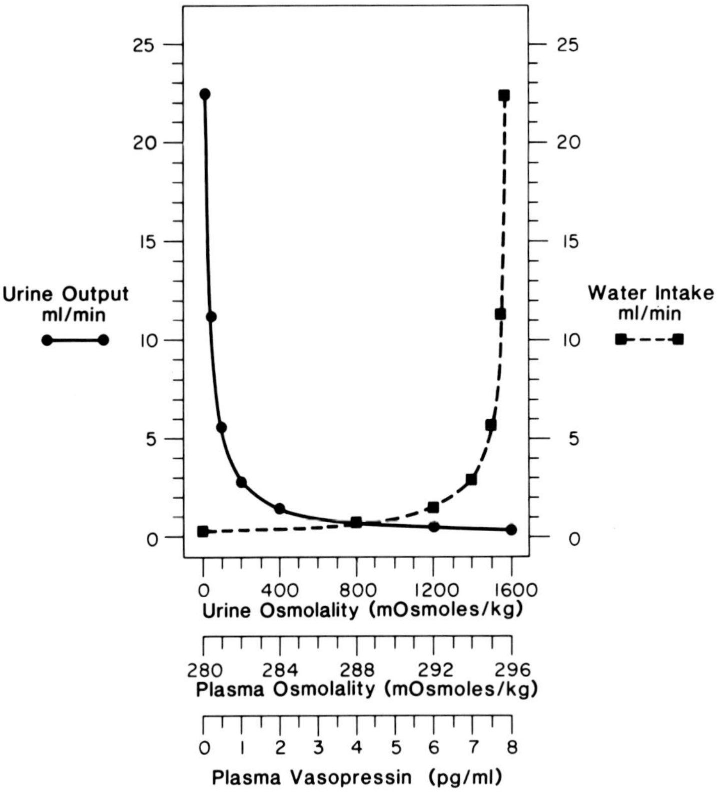

FIGURE 9-11 The relation of renal excretion or oral intake of water to urine osmolality, plasma osmolality, and plasma vasopressin in a typical 70-kg human. The line describing urine flow was calculated assuming a solute load of 800 mosmol/day. The line describing water intake was obtained by analyzing the relation of water intake to plasma osmolality in 12 healthy adults after infusion of hypertonic saline. The contributions of insensible loss and dietary water to total output and intake usually approximate 1.4 liters per day (1 ml/min). Neither is included in these calculations. (*From Robertson and Berl.*[209] *Water intake–plasma osmolality data courtesy of R. L. Zerbe and G. L. Robertson*).

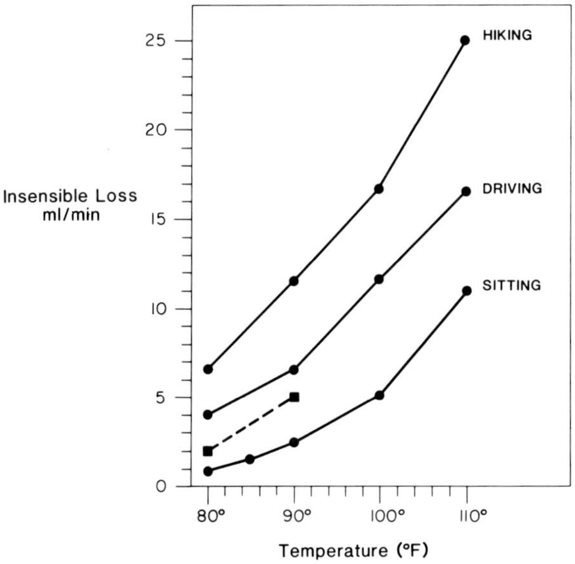

FIGURE 9-12 The effect of activity and temperature on insensible water loss in a typical 70-kg human. The solid lines indicate insensible loss for different activities in healthy adults. (*Redrawn from Adolph.*[215]) The broken line indicates insensible loss during minimal activity in a typical patient with neurogenic diabetes insipidus. (*Courtesy of G. L. Robertson.*)

established by the osmotic threshold for thirst. Provided access to fresh water is unrestricted, a rise in plasma osmolality above the threshold for thirst will increase the rate of water intake to levels sufficient to offset all but the most extraordinary rates of loss. To appreciate the effectiveness of this defense mechanism, it is necessary only to recall that many patients with severe neurogenic or nephrogenic diabetes insipidus excrete as much as 16 liters of urine per day for years, yet maintain their plasma osmolality at or only slightly above the upper limit of normal. Between the limits imposed by the osmotic threshold for thirst and vasopressin release, plasma osmolality may be regulated more precisely still by small, osmoreceptor-mediated adjustments in urine concentration and flow. The exact level at which stabilization occurs depends on individual differences in the rate of water loss from skin and lungs relative to the rate of gain from eating, nondipsetic drinking, and the metabolism of fat. On the average, however, overall intake and output come into balance at a plasma osmolality around 288 mosmol/kg, or about halfway between the thresholds for thirst and vasopressin release. From this position, minor deviations in free water balance can

Table 9-3. Causes of Diabetes Insipidus

- Vasopressin deficiency (neurogenic diabetes insipidus)
  - Acquired
    - Idiopathic
    - Trauma (accidental, surgical)
    - Tumor (craniopharyngioma, metastasis, lymphoma)
    - Granuloma (sarcoid, histiocytosis)
    - Infectious (meningitis, encephalitis)
    - Vascular (Sheehan's syndrome, aneurysm, aortocoronary bypass)
  - Familial (autosomal dominant)
- Excessive water intake (primary polydipsia)
  - Acquired
    - Idiopathic (resetting of the osmostat)
    - Psychogenic
  - Familial (?)
- Vasopressin insensitivity (nephrogenic diabetes insipidus)
  - Acquired
    - Infectious (pyelonephritis)
    - Postobstructive (prostatic, ureteral)
    - Vascular (sickle cell disease, trait)
    - Infiltrative (amyloid)
    - Cystic (polycystic disease)
    - Metabolic (hypokalemia, hypercalcemia)
    - Granuloma (sarcoid)
    - Toxic (lithium, demeclocycline, methoxyflurane)
    - Solute overload (glucosuria, postobstructive)
  - Familial (X-linked recessive)

be promptly counteracted by appropriate adjustments in vasopressin secretion and urine flow.

In humans and possibly other mammals, the operation of this osmoregulatory system is complicated somewhat by the superimposition of intermittent hemodynamic stimuli generated by standing and other activity. As noted previously, however, these influences do not interfere significantly with the control of vasopressin secretion by the osmoreceptor. Instead, they merely shift the set of the mechanism a few percent to the left or right, depending on whether blood pressure and/or effective blood volume are rising or falling. This constant resetting has the effect of widening slightly the allowable fluctuations in plasma osmolality but does not jeopardize the essential homeostatic function of the osmoregulatory system. It should be noted that the effects of vasopressin and thirst on the regulation of blood volume and pressure are normally trivial and occur largely as an indirect consequence of efforts to preserve osmolality. Indeed, in situations characterized by an abnormal increase in total body sodium, thirst and vasopressin act in such a way as to aggravate instead of ameliorate the underlying hypervolemia. The responsibility for coping with disturbances in volume per se rests primarily with those elements of the renal and endocrine systems which regulate sodium excretion. This distinction is useful to bear in mind when considering the role of the hypothalamic-neurohypophyseal system in the pathogenesis of clinical disorders of salt and water balance.

PATHOLOGIC HYPOFUNCTION

Etiology

Diabetes Insipidus

Deficient secretion of vasopressin is usually due to loss of the neurosecretory neurons that make up the neurohypophysis. This deficiency results in a clinical disorder commonly referred to as *neurogenic, central,* or *vasopressin-responsive* diabetes insipidus. It can be caused by a variety of pathologic processes (Table 9-3).[216] Probably the best-studied cause is hypophysectomy, or section of the pituitary stalk.[217–219] Autopsy studies after such procedures have revealed not only extensive destruction of the pars nervosa but also a loss of the large neurosecretory cells in the supraoptic and, to a lesser extent, paraventricular nuclei of the hypothalamus.[217] This hypocellularity requires 4 to 6 weeks to develop fully and presumably results from retrograde degeneration of axonal processes sectioned during the surgery. Because these axons normally terminate at all levels along the neurohypophyseal tract (Fig. 9-1), the extent of the degeneration depends on how high the damage extends. To destroy more than 80 percent of the supraoptic nucleus, the minimum required to produce significant polyuria, the stalk must be sectioned at the level of the infundibulum or above. This fact probably explains why tumors or other pathologic conditions confined to the sella turcica so rarely result in clinically apparent diabetes insipidus.

In many patients, the deficiency of vasopressin is idiopathic. The few neuropathologic studies performed on these patients also have revealed atrophy of the pars nervosa in association with a marked deficiency of neurosecretory cells in the supraoptic nuclei.[220–222] Not infrequently, idiopathic diabetes insipidus occurs on a familial basis.[221–225] It is inherited in an autosomal dominant fashion and is also associated with a marked loss of cells in the supraoptic nuclei.[221,222] This deficiency probably develops after birth, since affected family members often do not exhibit defects in antidiuretic function until 1 or 2 years of age and then progress gradually from partial to severe deficiencies of vasopressin during childhood and adolescence. The cause of the progressive loss of neurosecretory neurons is unknown, but it may be highly selective, since, in some patients at least, oxytocin production appears to be normal. Brattleboro rats also have a form of hereditary diabetes insipidus which follows an autosomal dominant or semirecessive mode of inheritance.[18] However, the defect in these animals is different, because it is present from birth and is due to a genetic failure in biosynthesis of vasopressin rather than a loss of neurosecretory neurons.[18,21] An X-linked form of familial vasopressin deficiency has been reported in humans,[223] but there is now reason to suspect that these patients may actually have had a recently discovered variant of partial familial nephrogenic diabetes insipidus.[226]

Other causes of acquired vasopressin deficiency include trauma,[227] tumors (particularly craniopharyngioma, lymphoma, large pituitary adenomas, and metastatic lung cancer),[216,228] granulomas (including sarcoid[229] and xanthoma disseminatum[230,231] as well as histiocytosis X[216]), infections,[216,232] autoimmunity,[233] and various vascular abnormalities.[234,235]

Osmoreceptor Ablation

Deficient secretion of vasopressin can also result from a lesion which destroys selectively the osmoreceptors without involving either the neurohypophysis or its other regulatory afferents.[32,35,236–240] This kind of lesion can be induced by a variety of hypothalamic disorders (Table 9-4), including tumors,[32,238–246] granulomas,[240,247] vascular occlusion,[32,240,248–250a] trauma,[236,240] hydrocephalus,[240] nonspecific inflammation,[240] degenerative disorders,[240] and developmental defects.[240,250b,251] In a few patients, no anatomic lesions were identified.[240,252,253] Autopsy studies delineating the precise location and histologic appearance of these lesions have not been reported. However, experiments in animals have shown that similar defects in vasopressin secretion can be produced by a lesion in an area of the anterolateral hypothalamus near the supraoptic nuclei.[33,198–201]

Table 9-4. Causes of Osmoreceptor Destruction

Tumors
Craniopharyngioma
Pinealoma
Meningioma
Metastatic
Granuloma
Histiocytosis
Sarcoidosis
Vascular
Occlusion of anterior communicating artery
Trauma
Penetrating
Closed
Other
Hydrocephalus
Developmental
Cysts
Inflammation
Degenerative
Idiopathic

Dipsogenic Diabetes Insipidus

Reduced secretion of vasopressin can also result from excessive water intake. This condition, which is often referred to as *primary polydipsia* or *dipsogenic diabetes insipidus,* can result either from a primary defect in the osmoregulation of thirst or, more commonly, as part of a general cognitive defect associated with schizophrenia or other mental disorders.[254–256] In humans, little is known about the precise location or nature of the lesions responsible for either type of polydipsia. However, organic lesions may be directly responsible in some cases, since dipsogenic diabetes insipidus has been associated with sarcoidosis of the central nervous system[257] and hyperdipsia can be produced experimentally in rats by making lesions in the midbrain,[258] septal nuclei,[259] and tegmentum.[260]

Nephrogenic Diabetes Insipidus

Polyuria and polydipsia can also result from insensitivity to the antidiuretic actions of vasopressin. This disorder, which is commonly referred to as *nephrogenic diabetes insipidus,*[261] was first recognized by Waring, Kadji, and Tappan,[262] who reported several patients with a familial form of the disorder. Subsequently, many additional examples have been recognized and studied.[263] These studies confirm that the disorder is carried by females and expressed most fully in their male offspring, indicating that it is transmitted by an X-linked semirecessive mode of inheritance. The pathogenesis of the defect has not been determined. Grossly, the kidneys, ureters, and bladder are sometimes enlarged, but this is probably a consequence rather than a cause of the disorder, since it also occurs in some patients with neurogenic diabetes insipidus. Microscopically, the kidney appears relatively normal unless complications, most commonly chronic infection, supervene. Biochemically, both decreases and increases in vasopressin-mediated cyclic AMP production by the kidney have been reported in these patients.[264,265] However, it is uncertain whether these defects relate in any way to the failure of vasopressin to cause urinary concentration, since most urinary cyclic AMP originates proximal to the distal tubule or collecting ducts. Nephrogenic diabetes insipidus can also be caused by various drugs[266] or other diseases (Table 9-2).[267]

Pathophysiology

Diabetes Insipidus

A deficiency of vasopressin secretion caused by destruction of the neurohypophysis results in a significant increase in the loss of water from renal and extrarenal sites.[217] As a consequence of the dehydration, there is a rise in plasma osmolality which stimulates the thirst mechanism and induces polydipsia. The resultant increase in body water restores balance between intake and output and stabilizes the tonicity of body fluids at a new, slightly higher level which closely approximates the osmotic threshold for thirst.

The development of diabetes insipidus in the period immediately following surgical or traumatic injury to the neurohypophysis can follow any of several different patterns.[218] In some patients, polyuria develops 1 to 4 days after injury and continues permanently. In others, the polyuria is transient and is followed in 4 to 7 days by a decline in urine volume to normal. In some of the latter, polyuria never recurs. In others, however, the interphase lasts only a few days and is followed by a second and permanent phase of polyuria. The functional and anatomic basis for the triphasic pattern of response is unknown. Presumably, however, the initial phase of polyuria reflects a kind of paralysis of vasopressin secretion secondary to neurohypophyseal damage. The interphase period during which urine output is normal may reflect degeneration and death of neurosecretory neurons, with release of stored vasopressin into the circulation. The final permanent phase of polyuria reflects degradation of released vasopressin and inability of surviving neurons to produce adequate amounts of the hormone.

It is important to note that the deficiency of vasopressin need not be complete for polyuria and polydipsia to occur.[217,268–277] *It is necessary only that the maximum plasma vasopressin concentration achievable at or below the osmotic threshold for thirst be inadequate to concentrate the urine.* The degree of neurohypophyseal destruction at which such failure occurs varies considerably from person to person, largely because of individual differences in solute load or the set and sensitivity of the osmoregulatory system.[36,272] However, an average value can be estimated from the known relationships between urine flow, urine osmolality, plasma vasopressin, plasma osmolality, and thirst in a typical healthy adult (Fig. 9-1). At an average rate of solute excretion, urine flow does not rise to symptomatic levels (>2.5 liters per day) until urine osmolality falls below 300 mosmol/kg. Thus, if renal sensitivity to vasopressin is normal, polyuria should not begin until the level of plasma vasopressin achievable at the osmotic threshold for thirst falls below 1.5 pg/ml, the amount required to maintain urinary concentration above 300 mosmol/kg (Fig. 9-3*B*). For this degree of deficiency to occur, secretory capacity must be reduced by at least 75 percent (Fig. 9-13). This estimate agrees relatively well with that obtained by neuroanatomic studies of cell loss in the supraoptic nuclei following pituitary surgery[217] and is also consistent with functional tests of secretory capacity in a large series of patients with diabetes insipidus of variable severity, duration, and etiology.[47,271]

Recognition of the fact that almost all patients with neurogenic diabetes insipidus retain a limited capacity to secrete vasopressin is the key to understanding many otherwise perplexing features of the disorder. For example, in many patients, restricting water intake long enough to raise plasma osmolality by only 1 to 2 percent will induce the release of enough vasopressin to concentrate the urine (Figs. 9-14 and 9-15). This response illustrates the relative nature of the vasopressin deficiency and underscores the importance of the thirst mechanism in preventing the use of residual secretory capacity under basal conditions of ad libitum water intake. Even in those patients who are unable to respond appreciably to hypertonicity, a more potent stimulus such as severe hypotension (Fig. 9-5) or nausea (Fig. 9-8) may evoke an increase in vasopressin secretion sufficient to concentrate the urine.[47] Consequently, when interpreting diagnostic or therapeutic procedures in these patients, it is necessary to be circumspect about the presence of drugs or associated diseases that can modify vasopressin secretion via nonosmotic mechanisms.

Neurogenic diabetes insipidus also is associated with changes in the renal response to vasopressin (Figs. 9-15 and 9-16). The most obvious change is a reduction in maximum concentrating capacity which is due to washout of the medullary concentration gradient caused by the chronic polyuria.[273–276] The severity of this defect is proportional to the magnitude of the polyuria and is independent of its cause.[271] Because of this defect, the levels of urinary concentration achieved at maximally effective levels of plasma vasopressin are reduced in all three types of diabetes insipidus (Fig. 9-16). In patients with neurogenic diabetes insipidus, this concentrating abnormality is offset to some extent by an increase in renal sensitivity to low levels of plasma vasopressin (Figs. 9-15 and 9-16). In this range, urine osmolality is usually supranormal for the amount of hormone present. The cause is unknown, but the supersensitivity may reflect upward regulation of vasopressin receptors secondary to a chronic deficiency of the hormone.[277]

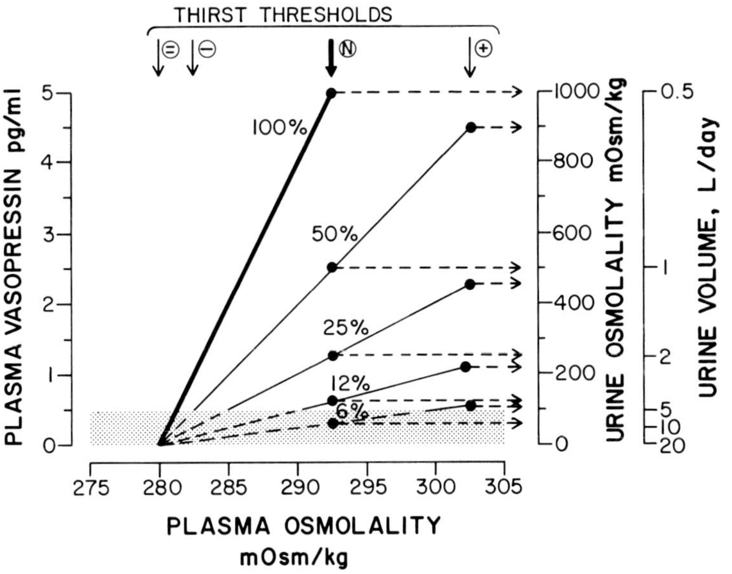

FIGURE 9-13 Plasma vasopressin and urine osmolality as a function of plasma osmolality in a typical healthy adult and in patients with various defects in thirst and/or hormone secretion. Each oblique line depicts schematically the relation between plasma vasopressin and plasma osmolality when secretory capacity is reduced to a specific percentage of normal. The vertical arrows indicate the osmotic threshold for thirst as it occurs in a typical healthy adult (N) and in patients in whom it is abnormally high (+), low (−), or very low (=). The solid circles on each oblique line indicate the highest level to which plasma osmolality and vasopressin are normally allowed to rise at each thirst setting. The broken horizontal arrows indicate the daily urine osmolalities that result when plasma vasopressin is limited to the specified levels. The shaded area indicates undetectable concentrations of plasma vasopressin. These figures assume a normal renal sensitivity to vasopressin. Note that the degree of impairment of vasopressin secretory capacity that results in urinary dilution depends on the "set" of the thirst mechanism. If the thirst threshold is normal, a significant water diuresis does not begin until secretory capacity falls to 15 to 25 percent of normal. However, if the thirst threshold is set 10 mosmol/kg higher, secretory capacity must be reduced to 12 percent of normal for the same concentrating defect to occur. Conversely, if the thirst threshold is set 10 mosmol/kg below normal, polyuria occurs even if vasopressin secretory capacity is normal. (*From Robertson and Berl.*[209])

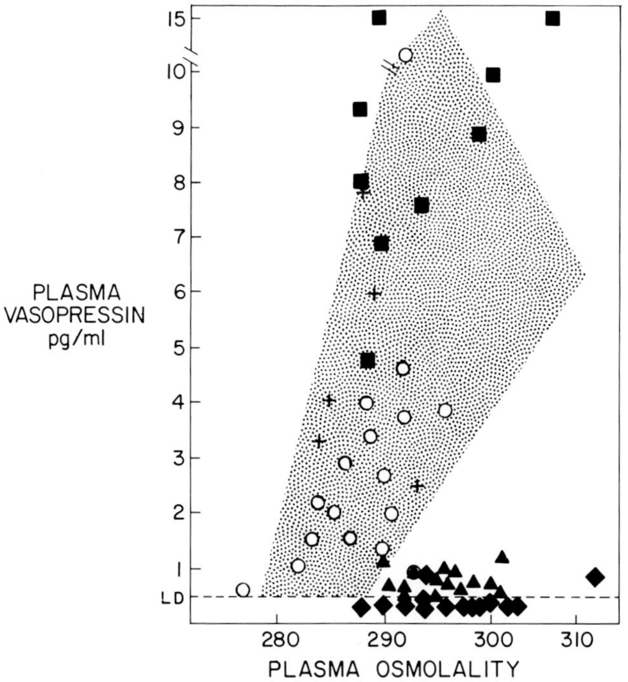

FIGURE 9-14 The relation of plasma vasopressin to concurrent plasma osmolality in patients with polyuria of diverse etiology. All measurements were made at the end of a standard dehydration test.[334] The shaded area represents the range of normal. In patients with severe (◆) or partial (▲) neurogenic diabetes insipidus, plasma vasopressin was almost always subnormal relative to plasma osmolality. In contrast, the values from patients with dipsogenic (○) or nephrogenic (■) diabetes insipidus were consistently within the above-normal range. Normal subjects are represented by the plus (+) symbol. (*From Robertson.*[256])

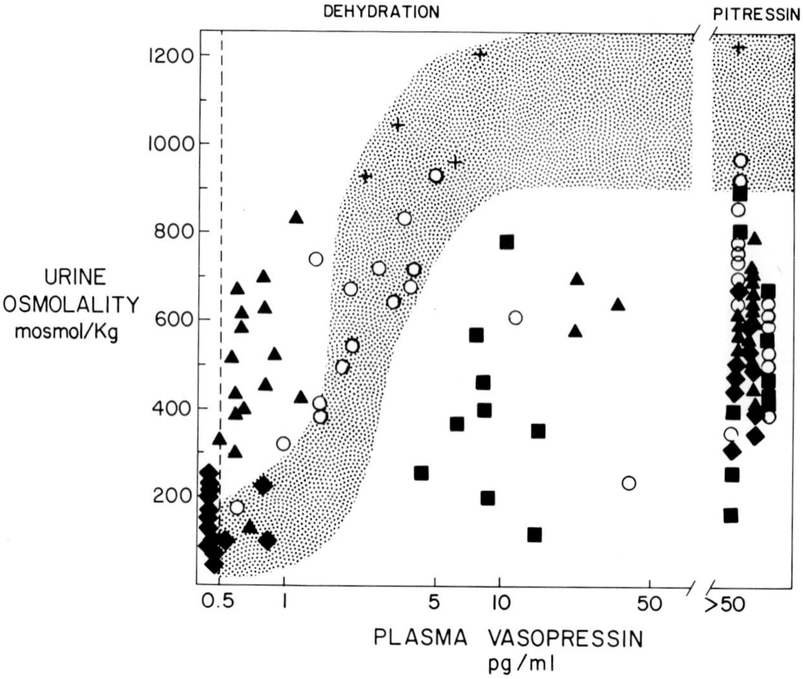

FIGURE 9-15 The relation of urine osmolality to concurrent plasma vasopressin in patients with polyuria of diverse etiology. All measurements were made at the end of a standard dehydration test.[270] The shaded area represents the range of normal. In patients with severe (◆) or partial (▲) neurogenic diabetes insipidus, urine osmolality is normal or supranormal relative to plasma vasopressin when the latter is submaximal. In patients with nephrogenic diabetes insipidus (■), urine osmolality is always subnormal relative to plasma vasopressin. In patients with dipsogenic diabetes insipidus (○), the relation is often normal, but urine osmolality may be subnormal when plasma vasopressin is supramaximal because of blunting of concentrating capacity. Normal subjects are represented by plus (+) symbol. (*From Robertson.*[256])

Osmoreceptor Dysfunction

The deficiency of vasopressin secretion that results from loss of osmoregulatory input usually produces a much different constellation of clinical abnormalities from that due to neurohypophyseal damage. Because the osmoreceptors for thirst and vasopressin secretion are located in overlapping if not identical areas of the hypothalamus (see above), destruction of one almost always results in equally serious damage to the other. Consequently, the predominant clinical manifestation of osmoreceptor destruction is chronic or recurrent

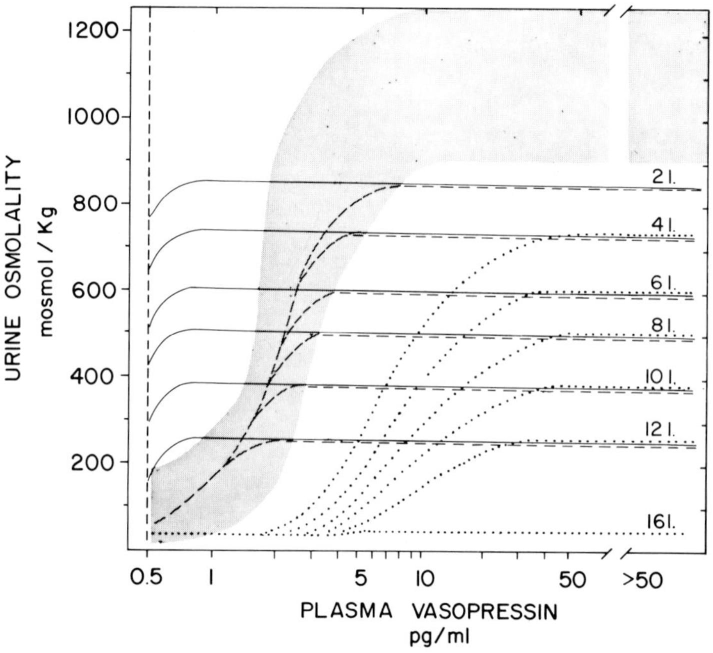

FIGURE 9-16 Schematic diagram of the relation between urine osmolality and plasma vasopressin in patients with diabetes insipidus of diverse etiology and severity. The shaded area represents the range of normal. The number at the common terminus of each family of lines indicates the magnitude of the basal polyuria. Note that, for any given level of urine output, maximum concentrating capacity is reduced to the same extent in all three kinds of diabetes insipidus. However, at submaximal or physiologic levels of plasma vasopressin, urine osmolality is above normal in neurogenic (—), normal in dipsogenic (---), and subnormal in nephrogenic (····) diabetes insipidus. (*From Robertson.*[256])

hypernatremia in association with hypodipsia and a *relative* deficiency of vasopressin. Except under certain conditions, polyuria is *not* a prominent feature of the syndrome and usually is not a major or even a contributing cause to the recurrent episodes of severe hypertonic dehydration. The primary, and in many cases only, cause is a failure of the thirst mechanism to maintain water intake at a level sufficient to replenish normal obligatory renal and extrarenal losses.[196,278] If sufficiently severe, the hypertonic dehydration may result in a variety of complications, including orthostatic hypotension, azotemia, hypokalemia, chorea, confusion, coma, convulsions, and paralysis, with or without rhabdomyolysis.[279-282]

Although polyuria is not a prominent feature of osmoreceptor ablation, defects in vasopressin secretion are a frequent if not constant feature of the syndrome. In most cases, however, these defects are not recognized clinically until efforts are made to correct the hypernatremia by water loading. At that time, one of two abnormalities appears. Most often, patients begin to form dilute urine and develop frank polyuria before dehydration succeeds in restoring plasma osmolality to normal. Originally, this abnormality was attributed to upward resetting of the osmostat, an entity sometimes referred to as *essential hypernatremia*.[283] However, regression analysis of the relation between plasma osmolality and urine osmolality or plasma vasopressin has shown that this abnormality in antidiuretic function can result from a marked reduction in the slope or sensitivity of the system (Fig. 9-17).[32,236,251] Since none of the patients reported to have essential hypernatremia was studied by the kind of regression methods needed to distinguish true from apparent resetting of the osmostat, it is possible that all of them actually had a normal threshold with reduced sensitivity of the system.

In some patients with hypodipsic hypernatremia, forced hydration results in hyponatremia in association with an inability to dilute maximally the urine.[32,236,240] This paradoxical defect resembles that seen in the syndrome of inappropriate antidiuresis and appears to result from two different mechanisms. One is a continuous or fixed secretion of vasopressin due to a total loss of osmoregulatory function (Fig. 9-17). In these patients, plasma vasopressin continues to circulate in small but biologically effective amounts irrespective of increases or decreases in hydration. In the other type of dilutional defect, urine osmolality remains high even when plasma vasopressin is suppressed to undetectable levels.[236] The cause of this abnormality is unknown but may involve supersensitivity of the kidney to low levels of vasopressin.

In many, if not most, patients with adipsic hypernatremia the deficient or absent vasopressin response to changes in hydration is due to selective loss of osmoreceptor function. The neurohypophysis and its other regulatory afferents appear to be totally intact, since vasopressin responds normally or even supranormally to hemodynamic, emetic, and glucopenic stimuli.[36,236-239,251]

Dipsogenic Diabetes Insipidus

Excessive intake of water causes expansion and dilution of body fluids. The resultant fall in plasma osmolality suppresses vasopressin secretion, thereby inducing dilution of the urine. As a consequence, the

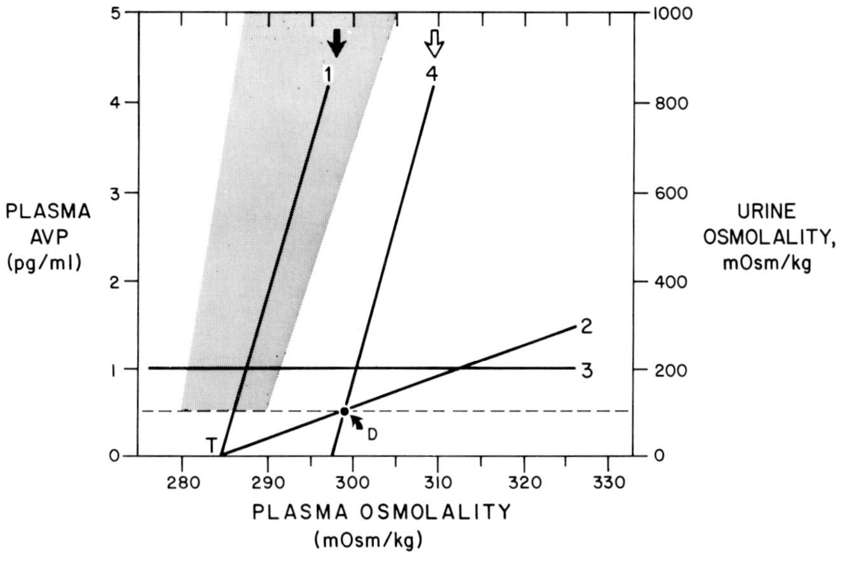

FIGURE 9-17 Schematic diagram of the relation of plasma osmolality to plasma vasopressin or urine osmolality in healthy adults and in patients with hypernatremia of diverse etiology. Line 1 represents a healthy adult. Lines 2 and 3 represent patients with partial and complete osmoreceptor destruction, respectively. Line 4 indicates the relation for a patient with the hypothetical entity of reset osmostat. The open and the solid arrows indicate the osmotic thirst threshold in the patient with resetting of the osmostat and in the healthy adult, respectively. The level of vasopressin at which urinary dilution occurs is indicated by D. Note that dilution of the urine at inappropriately high levels of plasma osmolality can result either from partial osmoreceptor destruction or resetting of the osmostat. (*From Robertson and Aycinena.*[278])

rate of water excretion rises to balance intake and the osmolality of body water stabilizes at a new, slightly lower level approximating the osmotic threshold for vasopressin secretion. The magnitude of the polyuria and polydipsia varies considerably, depending on the nature and/or intensity of the stimulus to drink. In a few patients, it is motivated by true thirst and appears to be due to an underlying abnormality in the osmoregulatory mechanism.[256] In such cases, the polyuria and polydipsia are usually moderate (4 to 10 liters per day) and relatively constant from day to day. In most patients, however, the polydipsia is not attributed to thirst but appears to be due to a more general cognitive defect associated with psychosis or other serious mental disorder.[254–256] Typically, these patients explain their water intake by other motives, such as an effort to cleanse their body of poison, relieve anxiety, or prevent kidney disease. In these patients, the amount of water ingested tends to fluctuate widely from day to day and, at times, may be incredibly large. Rarely, it rises to such extraordinary levels that it exceeds the excretory capacity of the kidney.[284] More often, however, the development of water intoxication in compulsive drinkers is due to an associated abnormality in the osmoregulation of vasopressin secretion.[285–287] Inappropriate secretion of the hormone can take any of several forms,[32] but most often it is due to resetting of the osmostat.[285] Patients with this condition often present with hyponatremia and maximum urinary dilution, suggesting that their water intoxication was caused by excessive drinking alone. However, if tested serially during water restriction, they begin to concentrate their urine before plasma osmolality and/or sodium return to normal. Since this diagnostic approach was not used in most previous studies, many patients in whom hyponatremia was attributed to polydipsia per se probably had resetting of the osmostat as an unrecognized contributory factor.[288]

Nephrogenic Diabetes Insipidus

Renal insensitivity to the antidiuretic effect of vasopressin also results in the excretion of increased volumes of dilute urine. The resultant decrease in body water causes a rise in plasma osmolality, which, by stimulating the thirst mechanism, induces a compensatory increase in water intake. As a consequence, the osmolality of body fluid stabilizes at a new and higher level which approximates the osmotic threshold for thirst. As in patients with neurogenic diabetes insipidus, the magnitude of the polyuria and polydipsia varies greatly, depending on a number of factors, including individual differences in solute load. It is important to note that the renal insensitivity to vasopressin need not be complete for polyuria to occur. It is necessary only that the defect be great enough to prevent concentration of the urine at plasma vasopressin levels achievable under ordinary conditions of ad libitum water intake, i.e., at plasma osmolalities near the osmotic threshold for thirst. Calculations analogous to those used for vasopressin deficiency indicate that this requirement will not be met until the renal sensitivity to vasopressin is reduced more than 10-fold. Studies of the relation between urine osmolality and plasma vasopressin in patients with familial and acquired forms of partial nephrogenic diabetes insipidus are consistent with these calculations.[226,289] When renal insensitivity to the hormone is incomplete, patients with nephrogenic diabetes insipidus are able to concentrate their urine when deprived of water[226,256,289,290] or given large doses of vasopressin.[226,289] In all likelihood, the X-linked form of familial vasopressin-responsive diabetes insipidus described by Forssman was really an example of partial nephrogenic rather than neurogenic diabetes insipidus.[223]

Diagnosis

Neurogenic Diabetes Insipidus

The diagnosis of neurogenic diabetes insipidus requires that it be differentiated from other causes of polyuria and polydipsia (Table 9-5). Confusion with diabetes mellitus is not a problem, since routine urinalysis usually reveals the glucosuria which is responsible for the solute diuresis. Differentiation from dipsogenic or nephrogenic diabetes is also relatively easy when the disorders are severe and present in the classic way. More often than not, however, this distinction cannot be made by conventional indirect tests,[270] because many patients with neurogenic or nephrogenic diabetes insipidus have a partial defect in vasopressin secretion or action and, as a consequence, are able to concentrate their urine to similar levels during a standard dehydration test.[268–271] To make matters worse, maximum concentrating capacity is reduced to variable degrees in all three forms of diabetes insipidus.[271,274,275] As a result, the absolute levels of urine osmolality achieved during water deprivation or vasopressin treatment can be similarly subnormal in all three types of polyuria (Fig. 9-16). This diagnostic dilemma usually cannot be resolved by other criteria such as measurements of basal plasma osmolality or sodium, because these values also overlap considerably in the various kinds of diabetes insipidus.[255]

To cope with this diagnostic problem, several auxiliary criteria have been proposed. One approach is to determine the ratio of urine to plasma osmolality at

Table 9-5. Diagnostic Evaluation of Nonglucosuric Polyuria

1. Measure plasma osmolality and/or sodium concentration under conditions of ad libitum fluid intake.
   A. If they are above 295 mosmol/kg and 143 meq/liter, respectively, primary polydipsia is excluded and the workup should proceed directly to a therapeutic trial of DDAVP (step 4) to distinguish between neurogenic and nephrogenic diabetes insipidus.
   B. If they are below 295 mosmol/kg and 143 meq/liter, the workup should proceed to step 2.
2. Perform a dehydration test.
   A. If urinary concentration does not occur before plasma osmolality and sodium reach 295 mosmol/kg and 143 meq/liter, primary polydipsia is excluded and the workup should proceed directly to step 4.
   B. If urinary concentration occurs during the dehydration test, measure plasma vasopressin and plasma osmolality and proceed to step 3.
3. Perform a hypertonic saline infusion and measure plasma vasopressin and osmolality (or sodium).
   A. If the plasma vasopressin value is subnormal relative to plasma osmolality and/or sodium, the diagnosis of neurogenic diabetes insipidus is established and therapy may be started.
   B. If the relation of plasma vasopressin to osmolality and/or sodium is normal, neurogenic diabetes insipidus is excluded. Differentiation between primary polydipsia and nephrogenic diabetes insipidus can be effected by examining the relation of urinary osmolality to plasma vasopressin during the dehydration test, or by proceeding to step 4.
4. Perform a therapeutic trial of DDAVP.
   A. If urinary volume and osmolality do not change, the diagnosis of nephrogenic diabetes insipidus is established and appropriate therapy may be initiated.
   B. If urinary output decreases and osmolality increases but polydipsia persists and/or dilutional hyponatremia and hypoosmolality develop, the diagnosis of primary polydipsia is likely and therapy should be discontinued until additional studies of vasopressin secretion and action can be performed.

the end of a brief period of fluid restriction.[291] Because most patients with diabetes insipidus can concentrate only in the face of supranormal dehydration, the ratio tends to be higher in normal subjects or patients with primary polydipsia. In a significant number of patients, however, the ratio falls between 1.8 and 2.2, a borderline zone which does not permit a clear distinction. The other indirect approach is a variation on that originally proposed by Barlow and de Wardener,[255] in which a comparison is made of the maximum urine osmolalities achieved after fluid restriction and vasopressin injection.[270] Although this test is sometimes helpful, it is tedious and cumbersome to perform and often gives ambiguous or erroneous results.[256,271]

A simpler and more definitive diagnostic approach is to measure plasma or urinary vasopressin following a suitable osmotic stimulus such as fluid restriction or hypertonic saline infusion.[271,292-294] For this method to be useful, the vasopressin values must be plotted as a function of the concurrent plasma osmolality (Fig. 9-14). With this approach, even patients with mild, partial defects in vasopressin secretion can be differentiated easily from those with other forms of diabetes insipidus. The diagnostic accuracy of this method also benefits from the fact that the functional properties of the osmoregulatory system do not seem to be appreciably altered by chronic dehydration or overhydration. Hence, the relation of plasma vasopressin to osmolality is usually within normal limits in both dipsogenic and nephrogenic diabetes insipidus. In most cases, the latter two disorders can be distinguished by measuring urine osmolality at the end of the dehydration test and relating it to the concurrent plasma vasopressin concentration (Fig. 9-15). However, this distinction is sometimes problematic, because maximum concentrating capacity is often severely blunted in patients with dipsogenic diabetes insipidus.[271] In such cases, the correct diagnosis usually can be made by examining the relationship at submaximal levels of plasma vasopressin (Fig. 9-16).[256,289] Under these conditions, patients with dipsogenic diabetes will almost always fall within the normal range, while those with nephrogenic diabetes insipidus will be clearly subnormal.

Occasionally, the measurement of vasopressin after fluid restriction does not provide a clear distinction between neurogenic and dipsogenic diabetes insipidus. This problem usually arises in patients who, because of excessive thirst and/or prompt antidiuretic response, fail to increase their plasma osmolality to 295 mosmol/kg, the lowest level at which a clear separation of normal and subnormal vasopressin values can be made. In this situation, it may be necessary to give a short intravenous infusion of hypertonic saline and obtain one or more additional measurements of plasma vasopressin. Patients with neurogenic diabetes insipidus may exhibit a further rise in plasma vasopressin, but it is always distinctly subnormal relative to the increment in plasma osmolality. In contrast, the slope of the response is normal in patients with dipsogenic or nephrogenic diabetes insipidus. Because of the solute diuresis, measurements of urine osmolality and/or vasopressin excretion during infusion of hypertonic saline are unreliable indicators of changes in hormone secretion and are of no diagnostic value.

As might be expected, most patients with diabetes insipidus also exhibit a subnormal rise in vasopressin secretion following hemodynamic, emetic, and glucopenic stimuli.[47,293] For diagnostic purposes, however, these nonosmotic tests of neurohypophyseal function do not appear to provide any particular advantage over dehydration and/or hypertonic saline infusion. Part of the problem is that orthostatic, emetic, and glucopenic stimuli are difficult to control and/or quantitate and normally result in a highly variable vasopressin response. Drug-induced hypotension permits more precise definition of the stimulus-response relation, but the procedure is cumbersome and potentially hazardous to perform. A more fundamental disadvantage with all nonosmotic stimuli is the real possibility of false-positive as well as false-negative results. A few patients have been found who exhibit little or no rise in vasopressin following hypotension or emesis, yet lack polyuria and have a normal response to osmotic stimuli.[81] Conversely, there are some patients with polyuria who exhibit little or no rise in plasma vasopressin during the infusion of hypertonic saline but have a relatively normal response to hypotensive, emetic, and glucopenic stimuli.[47,293] The latter observations suggest that diabetes insipidus may result rarely from a lesion which damages selectively the osmoreceptor that controls vasopressin release.

Osmoreceptor Dysfunction

Differentiating adipsic hypernatremia from other causes of vasopressin deficiency or hypernatremia is usually a simple clinical exercise (Table 9-6). In conscious adults, a lack of thirst when plasma osmolality and sodium concentration are greater than 310 mosmol/kg and 150 meq/liter, respectively, is almost always diagnostic of adipsic hypernatremia due to osmoreceptor dysfunction. In doubtful situations, thirst and plasma vasopressin can be monitored during dehydration or a standard infusion of hypertonic saline.[32,196]

Table 9-6. Differential Diagnosis of Hypernatremia

- I. Deficiency of body water
  - A. Inadequate intake
    - 1. Loss of thirst (adipsia)
      - *a.* Tumor (craniopharyngioma, pinealoma, germinoma, meningioma)
      - *b.* Granuloma (histiocytosis)
      - *c.* Vascular (ligation of anterior communicating artery or internal carotid artery)
      - *d.* Other (hydrocephalus, cysts, trauma)
    - 2. Physical limitation
      - *a.* Exogenous (desert, ocean)
      - *b.* Endogenous (coma, paresis)
  - B. Excessive loss
    - 1. Renal (neurogenic or nephrogenic diabetes insipidus)
    - 2. Extrarenal (lungs, perspiration)
- II. Excess of body sodium
  - A. Excessive intake (accidental substitution in infant formula)
  - B. Excessive retention (hyperaldosteronism)

Therapy

Neurogenic Diabetes Insipidus

Recovery of vasopressin secretion is extremely rare once the deficiency is established. Any spontaneous improvement in the polyuria almost always indicates progression of the underlying disease to involve the pituitary-adrenal axis[295,296] or the thirst mechanism. Rarely, it may indicate development of a malignant condition with ectopic production of vasopressin.[297] Although persistent polyuria and polydipsia do not pose a serious hazard for most patients, they are an annoying and embarrassing inconvenience and should be treated whenever possible. Fortunately, there are several safe, simple, and effective treatment methods.

For many years, the standard treatment for neurogenic diabetes insipidus was Pitressin tannate in oil, a partially purified extract of vasopressin prepared from animal pituitaries. Intramuscular injection of 5 to 10 USP units every 2 to 3 days gives satisfactory relief of the polyuria and polydipsia in most patients. Resistance due to the development of antibodies has been observed but is relatively rare.[298] A poor or erratic antidiuretic response is usually due to a failure to adequately emulsify the mixture by manually shaking and warming the vial immediately prior to use. Adverse reactions to the drug are uncommon and are usually allergic in nature. The major disadvantage of Pitressin therapy is the need for lifelong injections. Because its duration of action is only a few hours, aqueous Pitressin is not suitable for long-term treatment of diabetes insipidus, but it is useful for certain diagnostic tests.

Diapid is a preparation of synthetic lysine vasopressin which may be given by nasal spray. Since the antidiuretic effect of each spray lasts a maximum of only 4 to 6 h, it is generally used only as an adjunct to other forms of therapy.

A synthetic analogue of vasopressin, desamino-8-D-arginine vasopressin (DDAVP; Desmopressin) (Fig. 9-2) is now widely available for use in the United States.[299-301] Extensive experience indicates that it has many advantages in the treatment of diabetes insipidus. The modifications in positions 1 and 8 of the molecule double its antidiuretic therapy, eliminate its pressor actions, and increase significantly its resistance to metabolic degradation. Consequently, it has a much longer duration of action than the native molecule and can be given either parenterally or by nasal insufflation. In most patients, administration of 10 to 25 μg intranasally twice a day or 1 to 2 μg parenterally once a day affords prompt and complete relief of polyuria and polydipsia. Secondary failures are uncommon and usually are due to poor absorption of the nasal preparation caused by rhinitis or sinusitis. A poor initial response to DDAVP, particularly the parenteral form, almost always indicates that the patient has nephrogenic rather than neurogenic diabetes insipidus. Resistance due to antibody production has not been observed. Toxic side effects of DDAVP are also uncommon. Some patients with severe or long-standing neurogenic diabetes insipidus may develop water intoxication when first started on DDAVP therapy. However, the effect is usually transient and will subside with continued treatment. Severe or sustained hyponatremia is a reason to stop treatment and repeat diagnostic studies, since it usually indicates that the patient has dipsogenic diabetes insipidus or some associated defect in thirst regulation.

Largely by chance, several oral drugs have also been found to be efficacious in treating neurogenic diabetes insipidus. Chlorpropamide (Diabinese), a drug more commonly used to treat hyperglycemia, is the most potent. At conventional doses of 250 to 500 mg per day, it reduces polyuria by 25 to 75 percent in patients with neurogenic diabetes insipidus.[127,129,130,302,303] Contrary to long-held views,[303] this effect is independent of the severity of the disease.[127] It is associated with a proportionate rise in urine osmolality, correction of dehydration, and a reduction in drinking similar to that caused by small doses of vasopressin or DDAVP (Fig. 9-18). Chlorpropamide may also cause inappropriate antidiuresis in some patients with other diseases,[304–306] but for unknown reasons, this effect is much less pronounced than in patients with diabetes insipidus. Like vasopressin, chlorpropamide has no effect in patients with nephrogenic diabetes insipidus,[303] a fact suggesting that the drug and the hormone act via a similar mechanism. Potentiation of the renal tubular effects of small subthreshold amounts of vasopressin is probably the major mechanism of action,[127,129,130,307–311] although one study suggests that chlorpropamide may also stimulate release of the hormone.[129] A prolonged deficiency of vasopressin may be necessary for the antidiuretic effect of chlorpropamide to manifest itself, because its onset of action is slower in patients

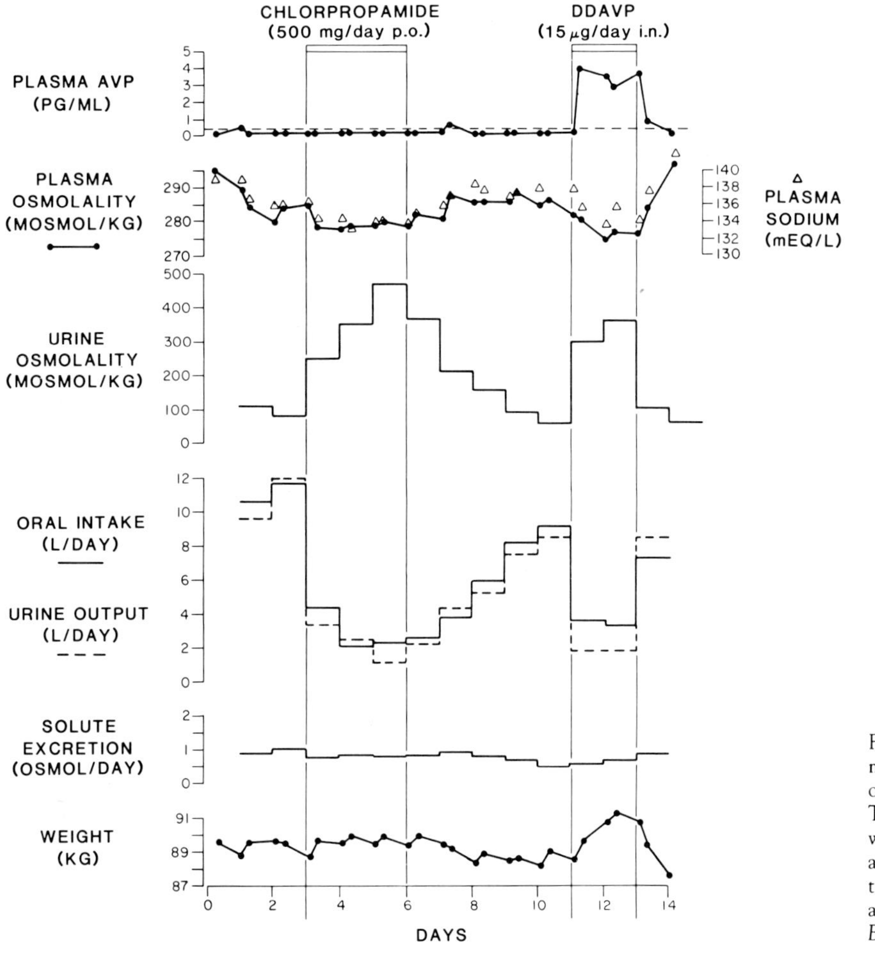

FIGURE 9-18 Effect of chlorpropamide and of DDAVP on water metabolism in neurogenic diabetes insipidus. The patient was a 32-year-old woman with severe familial diabetes insipidus and no detectable vasopressin secretion even during stimulation with apomorphine. (*From Robertson and Berl.*[209])

recently treated with vasopressin, and its antidiuretic effects can be reversed acutely by simultaneous administration of the hormone.[312]

Clofibrate (Atromid-S), a drug more commonly used to treat hyperlipidemia, also reduces polyuria and polydipsia in patients with diabetes insipidus.[128,313] At a maximum dose of 1 g tid, its antidiuretic effect is usually less than that of chlorpropamide,[314] although in a few patients it is more effective. Its mechanism of action is also uncertain. Like chlorpropamide, it is ineffective in patients with nephrogenic diabetes insipidus, and it has little if any antidiuretic action in normal subjects or patients with primary polydipsia. However, it has been difficult to show that clofibrate potentiates the renal actions of vasopressin, and there is evidence suggesting that the drug increases hormone secretion.[128]

The proper role of the oral drugs in the management of diabetes insipidus is currently uncertain. Used alone or in combination with thiazide diuretics, they can reduce polyuria to asymptomatic levels in virtually all patients with the disorder. However, they also have some undesirable side effects, such as hypoglycemia[303] or myalgia,[315] and the long-term safety, particularly of chlorpropamide, is open to question. When Pitressin tannate in oil was the only real alternative, many patients preferred those disadvantages to the discomfort and inconvenience of frequent injections. However, the advent of the long-acting analogue DDAVP probably will relegate the oral agents to a secondary therapeutic role.

Several other measures may be helpful in reducing polyuria in neurogenic diabetes insipidus. Restricting salt intake reduces urine output by reducing solute load. A similar effect may be achieved with thiazide diuretics, which deplete body sodium by inhibiting its reabsorption in the ascending limb of Henle's loop.[316] Because this step is necessary for maximum urinary dilution, the thiazides also raise urine osmolality and impair the ability to excrete a water load. Thus, if given to a patient with primary polydipsia, they may precipitate water intoxication.

The management of patients with diabetes insipidus also requires a careful search for its cause. At a minimum, this search should include x-rays of the chest and skull, visual field examination, and computed tomography of the pituitary-hypothalamic area. In some cases, a lumbar puncture or a nuclear magnetic resonance scan may also be needed to establish the presence or absence of treatable disease such as sarcoid or germinoma. Because of the possible coinvolvement of hypothalamic release factors, anterior pituitary function also should be evaluated even if there is no other evidence of intrasellar disease.

The management of diabetes insipidus in comatose and/or postoperative patients poses special problems, because medication cannot be given orally or intranasally and water intake is not regulated by the thirst mechanism. In this situation, the easiest and most effective approach is to maintain a relatively fixed level of antidiuresis by parenteral administration of DDVAP (1 μg IM or IV once or twice daily) and concentrate on adjusting fluid intake to match renal and extrarenal losses. Urine output and gastrointestinal losses, if any, should be measured during each nursing shift, and the total volume plus approximately 500 ml (to cover insensible losses) should be replaced with half-normal saline or dextrose and water during the succeeding 8-h shift. In addition, the effectiveness of the regimen should be monitored by measuring plasma osmolality or sodium at least twice a day. A rise in either variable indicates dehydration and should be treated by administering supplemental fluid. The amount will depend on the level of hypertonicity or hypernatremia and can be estimated by the formulas

$$H_2O = \frac{P_{os} - 295}{295} \times 0.6 \text{ BW}$$

or

$$H_2O = \frac{P_{Na} - 145}{145} \times 0.6 \text{ BW}$$

where

P_{os} = plasma osmolality in milliosmol per kilogram
P_{Na} = plasma sodium in milliequivalents per liter
BW = body weight in kilograms
H_2O = total water in liters

An excessive decrease in plasma osmolality or sodium indicates overhydration. It should be treated by reducing fluid intake by an amount estimated with the same formulas. Attempting to regulate water balance by altering the dose of antidiuretic hormone is not recommended, because the resultant changes in urine flow are impossible to control precisely and often lead to large and rapid fluctuations in salt and water balance.

Osmoreceptor Dysfunction

The treatment of adipsic hypernatremia is largely a matter of patient education. A regular schedule of water intake adjusted according to changes in hydration as determined by changes in body weight[196] will usually suffice to maintain plasma osmolality and sodium within 5 percent of normal. This regimen is particularly important in those patients with impaired urinary dilution, since they are prone to over- as well as underhydration. In patients in whom the development of polyuria interferes with the achievement or maintenance of normonatremia, the use of vasopressin or one of the oral agents to promote antidiuresis may be helpful.[239,248,250] The latter drugs may also slightly increase drinking, although this effect is mild at best and cannot be relied upon to replace other measures for maintaining water intake.

Dipsogenic Diabetes Insipidus

At present, there is no satisfactory treatment for dipsogenic diabetes insipidus. Administration of antidiuretic hormone or thiazides is hazardous because these agents diminish water excretion without reducing intake. The resultant water intoxication may develop rapidly and cause confusion, convulsions, coma, and even death. For this reason, any therapeutic trial in a patient in whom the cause of the polyuria is in doubt should always be conducted in the hospital with close monitoring of fluid balance. A few patients with dipsogenic diabetes insipidus due to resetting of the thirst osmostat can be managed effectively with antidiuretic therapy, because a fall in plasma osmolality inhibits thirst before significant water retention occurs.[256]

Nephrogenic Diabetes Insipidus

Some patients with nephrogenic diabetes insipidus can be treated by eliminating the drug or disease responsible for the disorder. In many others, however, the only practical form of treatment is to restrict sodium intake and/or administer thiazide diuretics.[316] The latter will generally reduce polyuria by about 50 percent and improve dehydration in all forms of nephrogenic diabetes insipidus. Thiazides work by a vasopressin-independent mechanism that involves inhibition of sodium reabsorption in the diluting segment of the nephron followed by increased reabsorption of glomerular filtrate in the proximal tubule.[316] Some patients with partial nephrogenic diabetes insipidus can be treated successfully with high doses of DDAVP. However, the great expense of this approach currently makes it an impractical form of treatment.

PATHOLOGIC HYPERFUNCTION

Increases in thirst and/or vasopressin secretion occur in many clinical conditions. Often they are an appropriate homeostatic response to some form of hyperosmolar dehydration. Not infrequently, however, they result from some other stimulus and are inappropriate for the osmolality of body fluids. These osmotically inappropriate increases in thirst and/or vasopressin secretion are customarily divided into three categories, based on the nature of the stimulus and the state of intravascular and extracellular fluid volume. Category 1 includes patients in whom total and/or effective blood volume is reduced but interstitial volume is increased as evidenced by the presence of generalized edema. Category 2 includes patients in whom interstitial as well as total and/or effective blood volume or blood pressure is reduced. Category 3, which is often referred to as the *syndrome of inappropriate secretion of antidiuretic hormone* (SIADH), includes patients in whom blood and extracellular volume as well as blood pressure are normal or slightly increased. The major clinical manifestation of all three categories is hyponatremia with impaired water excretion. However, the etiology, pathophysiology, and treatment of the underlying disturbance in salt and water balance is quite different in each category.

Etiology and Pathophysiology

Hypervolemic Hyponatremia

Severe low-output congestive failure is a common cause of abnormal retention of water and sodium.[317] This retention is thought to be secondary to low cardiac output or effective hypovolemia, which acts via several as yet incompletely defined mechanisms to stimulate proximal tubular reabsorption of filtered electrolytes and water. As a consequence, less filtrate is delivered to the distal tubular sites where free water is formed and the ability to excrete a water load is correspondingly diminished. In many cases, this deficiency is complicated by impaired urinary dilution, which is usually due to increased secretion of vasopressin.[77,78,318,319] Studies of osmotic stimulation and suppression indicate that this defect in vasopressin secretion is due to downward resetting of the osmostat,[320-322] probably as a consequence of the effective hypovolemia. If so, however, it probably is not mediated by the usual volume receptors, because left ventricular failure usually produces atrial distention, which suppresses vasopressin secretion.[323] For unknown reasons, some patients have impaired urinary dilution in the absence of detectable increases in vasopressin. In addition, thirst and/or water intake appear to be increased inappropriately in some patients. This combination of excessive intake and reduced excretion of water leads to the development of hyponatremia even though total body sodium is usually increased by more than 25 percent.

Patients with advanced cirrhosis and ascites also develop hyponatremia as a consequence of impaired water excretion.[324,325] The classic view suggests that the avid retention of salt and water characteristic of this disorder is also secondary to effective hypovolemia, although other explanations have been advanced.[326] In any event, osmotically inappropriate secretion of vasopressin also occurs in humans[327–329] as well as animals[330] with advanced cirrhosis. Earlier indirect studies anticipated this finding and suggested that the increase in vasopressin secretion may also be due to downward resetting of the osmostat secondary to effective hypovolemia.[331]

The nephrotic syndrome is also associated with hyponatremia and impaired water excretion[332] that is associated with increased secretion of vasopressin.[333] These abnormalities may also be due to a reduction in total or effective blood volume, since they are often associated with elevations in plasma renin and can be corrected at least in part by maneuvers which expand central blood volume.[334,335] However, in some patients total blood volume may be expanded,[336,337] suggesting some other cause for the antidiuretic defects.

The clinical hallmark of all patients with the defect of hypervolemic hyponatremia is generalized edema. It may be associated with various signs of volume depletion, including tachycardia, orthostatic hypotension, azotemia, hypokalemia, hyperaldosteronism, hyperreninemia, and low urinary sodium. In addition, if sufficiently severe, the hyponatremia may cause lethargy, anorexia, nausea, headache, confusion, seizures, and even coma.

Hypovolemic Hyponatremia

Use or abuse of diuretics is one of the most common causes of hyponatremia and impaired water excretion. The thiazides act primarily by interfering with sodium reabsorption in the diluting segment of the nephron.[316] As a consequence, maximum urinary dilution is impaired and urine flow decreases due to compensatory increases in the reabsorption of salt and water in the proximal tubule. Hypokalemia may also play a role,[338] possibly by increasing water intake,[339] since it inhibits both the secretion and the action of vasopressin.[340] The more potent loop diuretics and, in some cases, the thiazides may also produce significant volume depletion. The latter impairs water excretion by increasing reabsorption of filtrate in the proximal nephron[316] as well as by stimulating vasopressin secretion. In some patients, thirst may also be stimulated. As in other forms of hypovolemia, these abnormalities appear to be due to downward resetting of the osmostat.[85]

A deficiency of cortisol and/or aldosterone also causes hypovolemia, hyponatremia, and impaired water excretion.[278,341] In isolated mineralocorticoid deficiency, the abnormality in water balance is associated with hyperkalemia and appears to be secondary to a reduction in plasma and extracellular volume caused by sodium wasting. The hypovolemia interferes with water excretion both by reducing glomerular filtration and/or distal tubular delivery of filtrate[342] and by increasing vasopressin secretion.[343] As in other forms of hypovolemia, the increase in vasopressin secretion in the face of hypoosmolality is due to resetting of the osmostat,[278] and volume expansion alone is sufficient to correct the abnormalities in water metabolism.[344] Isolated deficiency of cortisol also causes hyponatremia and impaired water excretion,[345] but the mechanism of the defect is somewhat more complex and controversial. While it is clear that plasma vasopressin is usually elevated in this condition,[346–349] water excretion may also be impaired in the absence of detectable elevations in the hormone.[342,350,351] The cause of the increase in vasopressin secretion is also uncertain. It cannot be attributed to hypovolemia but may be due to reduced cardiac output[346,347] or a direct effect on the neurohypophysis.[349,352] The cause of the vasopressin-independent defect in water excretion is also unsettled and may be due to a change in renal hemodynamics. The abnormalities in water excretion that occur in Addison's disease reflect the combined effects of aldosterone and cortisol deficiency.

Diarrhea, bulimia, renal tubular acidosis, medullary cystic disease of the kidney, and many other disorders associated with sodium depletion also result in hypovolemia, hyponatremia, and impaired water excretion. Although not studied extensively, the pathophysiology of these two defects is probably similar to those seen with diuretic abuse, mineralocorticoid deficiency, and other forms of chronic hypovolemia and/or hypotension.

The symptoms and signs of hypovolemic hyponatremia are similar to those of hypervolemic hyponatremia except that edema is absent and urinary sodium excretion is not always low. In fact, in mineralocorticoid deficiency or renal sodium wasting, urinary sodium is usually elevated. In addition, plasma potassium may be elevated in the presence of mineralocorticoid deficiency.

Euvolemic Hyponatremia

The syndrome of inappropriate antidiuresis is also characterized by hyponatremia and impaired water excretion. However, it is distinguished by the fact that blood volume and pressure are normal or slightly increased and edema is absent. SIADH was first described in two patients with bronchogenic carcinoma.[353] Since then, it has been recognized with increasing frequency in association with a great many other diseases and drugs (Table 9-7). For reasons not altogether clear, these diseases usually involve the lungs or nervous system. Among the latter, patients

Table 9-7. Causes of the Syndrome of Inappropriate Antidiuretic Hormone

Neoplastic	
1. Bronchogenic carcinoma	6. Carcinoma of ureter
2. Carcinoma of duodenum	7. Lymphoma
3. Carcinoma of pancreas	8. Ewing's sarcoma
4. Thymoma	9. Carcinoma of the prostate
5. Mesothelioma	10. Carcinoma of the bladder
Nonneoplastic	
1. Trauma	
2. Pulmonary disease	
a. Pneumonia, bacterial or viral	*e*. Abscess
b. Cavitation (aspergillosis)	*f*. Asthma
c. Tuberculosis	*g*. Pneumothorax
d. Positive pressure breathing	*h*. Cystic fibrosis
3. Central nervous system disorders	
a. Meningitis, bacterial or viral	*i*. Psychosis
b. Head trauma	*j*. Delirium tremens
c. Brain abscess	*k*. Cerebral atrophy
d. Encephalitis, bacterial or viral	*l*. Cavernous sinus thrombosis
e. Guillain-Barré syndrome	*m*. Hydrocephalus
f. Subarachnoid hemorrhage	*n*. Rocky Mountain fever
g. Acute intermittent porphyria	*o*. Cerebrovascular accident
h. Peripheral neuropathy	*p*. Multiple sclerosis
4. Endocrine disease: Myxedema	
5. Idiopathic	
Pharmacologic	
1. Vasopressin and DDAVP	8. Nicotine
2. Oxytocin (Pitocin)	9. Phenothiazines
3. Vincristine	10. Cyclophosphamide
4. Chlorpropamide	11. Haloperidol
5. Thiazide diuretics	12. Tricyclic antidepressants
6. Clofibrate (Atromid-S)	13. Monoamine oxidase inhibitors
7. Carbamazepine	

with schizophrenia or other psychosis are noteworthy for the frequency and severity of the syndrome,[285–288] possibly because they also have a high incidence of psychogenic polydipsia.[288] Polydipsia alone is rarely capable of inducing water intoxication, because the excretory capacity of the kidneys is normally so great. However, by stressing the system, polydipsia probably brings out many subtle defects in vasopressin secretion that would otherwise go unrecognized. SIADH also occurs in some patients with myxedema.[354,355] However, water excretion is usually normal in uncomplicated hypothyroidism in humans, and those defects that can be demonstrated are usually mild and unrelated to inappropriate secretion of vasopressin.

A large number of drugs have also been implicated in the pathogenesis of SIADH. In most cases, however, it is difficult to distinguish an effect of the drug from that of the disease for which it was given. Moreover, certain drugs such as the phenothiazines or haloperidol may stimulate vasopressin release by producing orthostatic hypotension, while others, such as the thiazides, cyclophosphamide, or chlorpropamide, probably impair water excretion by vasopressin-independent mechanisms. Nevertheless, the clinical aspects of the hyponatremic disorders with which these drugs are associated are sufficiently similar to warrant inclusion in the category of SIADH.

In most patients with SIADH, secretion of the hormone is inappropriately high relative to the hypotonicity of body fluids (Fig. 9-19). Only rarely, however, is plasma vasopressin above the range found in normally hydrated recumbent adults. Consequently, hypersecretion can be identified with certainty only by measuring vasopressin under conditions of overhydration and relating it to plasma osmolality and/or sodium concentration.

Dynamic studies of vasopressin secretion in patients with SIADH have shown that it is a heterogeneous disorder which encompasses at least four distinct types of osmoregulatory defect (Fig. 9-20).[356] Each behaves in a characteristic way during water loading and/or hypertonic saline infusion and probably reflects a basically different pathogenetic mechanism. Type A is characterized by large and erratic fluctuations in plasma vasopressin which bear no relation whatever to changes in plasma osmolality. It is found in about 25 percent of all patients with SIADH and appears to be due to a total loss of

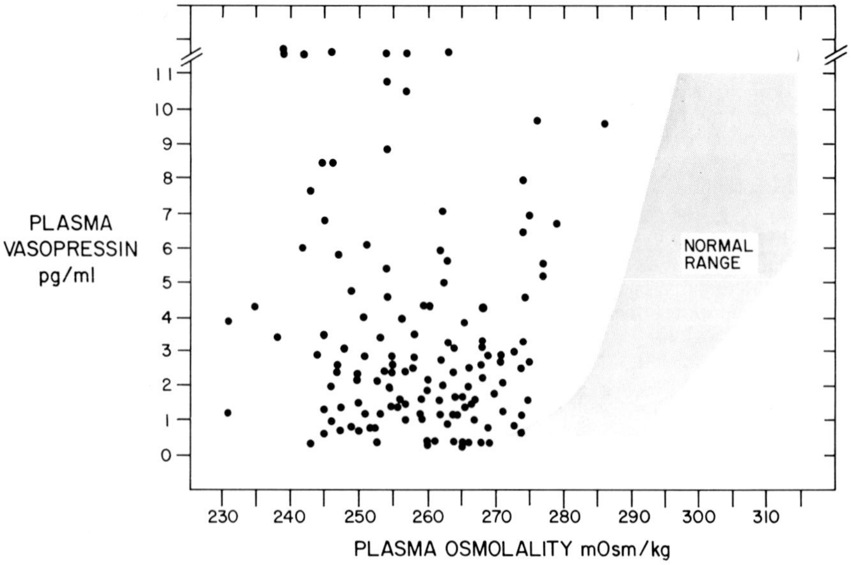

FIGURE 9-19 The relation of plasma vasopressin to plasma osmolality in the syndrome of inappropriate antidiuresis. Each value represents a single patient. (*From Robertson and Aycinena.*[278])

osmoreceptor control or intermittent stimulation by some unrecognized nonosmotic pathway. In the type B defect, plasma vasopressin remains fixed at an inappropriately high level until plasma osmolality rises into the normal range. At that point, plasma vasopressin begins to rise appropriately in close association with a further increase in plasma osmolality. This pattern also occurs in about 25 percent of all patients with SIADH. It appears to reflect a constant, nonsuppressible leak of vasopressin in the presence of otherwise normal osmoregulatory function. The type C defect is the most common, occurring in at least 35 percent of all patients. It is characterized by plasma vasopressin levels whose rise and fall are closely correlated with changes in plasma osmolality. Regression analysis of the relation between these two variables shows that the precision and sensitivity of the response are normal but the extrapolated threshold value is subnormal. Patients with this type of defect have resetting of the osmostat and exhibit clinical characteristics slightly different from those found in other forms of SIADH. Type D is much less common than the other three and probably represents a basically different defect in antidiuretic function. In these unusual patients, vasopressin secretion is stimulated and suppressed normally but urine osmolality remains fixed at a hypertonic level. The reason for this apparent dissociation between plasma vasopressin

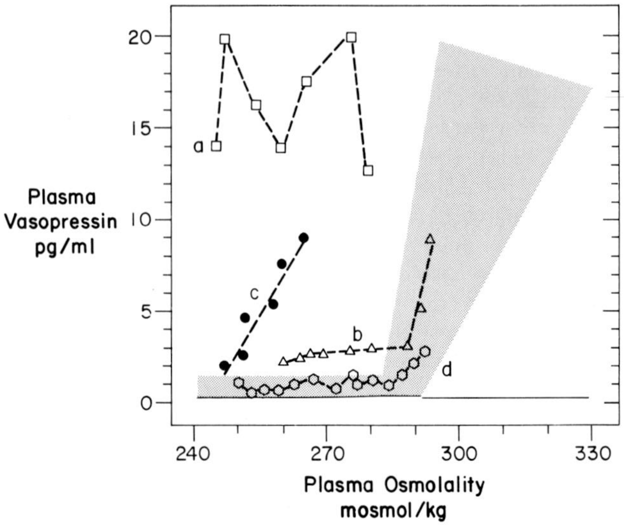

FIGURE 9-20 The relation of plasma vasopressin to osmolality during hypertonic saline infusion in four patients with the clinical syndrome of inappropriate antidiuresis. (*From Robertson.*[29])

and urinary concentration has not yet been determined. It could be due to hypersecretion of another antidiuretic hormone not detected by the radioimmunoassay or it could result from supersensitivity to the antidiuretic effect of normally low levels of vasopressin.

Except in those cases in which the hormone is produced ectopically by malignant disease or released from the neurohypophysis in response to emetic stimuli, the cause of the vasopressin secretion is unknown. There appears to be no relation between the type of osmoregulatory defect and the underlying disease.[356] Thus, it may be that the diseases most commonly associated with the syndrome can stimulate vasopressin secretion by any of several different mechanisms. It is particularly noteworthy in this regard that bronchogenic carcinoma has been associated with every type of osmoregulatory defect, including type C, the reset osmostat.[357] Since it is highly unlikely that anaplastic cells could acquire the normally separate capacities of osmoregulation and of vasopressin synthesis, many malignant diseases probably produce the syndrome by some mechanism other than ectopic production.

With the exception of the type C defect, the pathophysiology of the fluid and electrolyte disturbance in patients with SIADH is probably similar in most respects to that observed when healthy volunteers are treated with vasopressin.[358] If water intake is normal, i.e., between 1 and 2 liters a day, production of a fixed antidiuresis has little or no effect, because the combination of insensible loss and minimum urine output usually is sufficient to maintain water balance. However, if intake rises even slightly, a commensurate increase in output does not occur because plasma vasopressin and urine concentration are not suppressed normally by the fall in plasma osmolality. As a consequence, the excess water ingested each day accumulates, causing progressive dilution of solute concentration in all compartments of the body. When the expansion of body water reaches about 10 percent, the excretion of sodium begins to increase as a result both of decreased reabsorption in the proximal tubule and suppression of the renin-angiotensin-aldosterone system. This natriuresis has the effect of ameliorating the hypervolemia and increasing slightly urinary dilution and flow, but it also aggravates the hyponatremia and hypotonicity of body fluids. At this point, a new steady state may be achieved and plasma osmolality and sodium may stabilize unless some further change in intake occurs. If intake increases again, another cycle of water retention and natriuresis ensues, causing a further decline in plasma osmolality and sodium concentration. On the other hand, if water intake is sharply curtailed, the entire series of events reverses as water is lost, sodium is retained, and plasma osmolality and sodium gradually return to their original levels.

It should be noted that the clinical consequences of hypersecretion of vasopressin depend almost solely on the rate of water intake. If this is normal, inappropriate secretion will be clinically inapparent no matter how high plasma vasopressin may rise. If water intake is high, an increase in hormone secretion above the minimum level required to concentrate the urine will cause no appreciable worsening of the salt and water imbalance, because the rate of urine output falls only slightly when urine osmolality increases from 400 to 1200 mosmol/kg (Fig. 9-11). Once antidiuresis is established, only a change in water intake can appreciably alter the salt and water balance. In a real sense, therefore, hypersecretion of vasopressin plays only a permissive role in the series of events which leads to water intoxication. This role contrasts sharply with that of many other hormones such as insulin and parathormone, whose hypersecretion per se is sufficient to cause clinical abnormalities.

The pathophysiology of the fluid and electrolyte imbalance is much the same when vasopressin is produced endogenously. The only important difference occurs in patients with the type C defect, the reset osmostat. Because their threshold function is retained, increasing water intake leads eventually to maximum urinary dilution[359,360] and, consequently, a rate of water excretion sufficient to prevent further overhydration. As a consequence, plasma osmolality may stabilize, albeit at a markedly subnormal level. This variant constitutes an important exception to the rule that patients with SIADH are unable to excrete a maximally dilute urine. Most cases of reset osmostat probably go unrecognized, because the water loading and/or vasopressin studies necessary to demonstrate the condition are not employed routinely for diagnosis.

Patients with SIADH usually manifest few clinical symptoms and signs other than the neurologic abnormalities due to hyponatremia.[361] These include lethargy, confusion, muscle cramps, anorexia, pathologic reflexes, pseudobulbar palsy, coma, Cheyne-Stokes respiration, and seizures. These symptoms and signs are probably due to a swelling of brain cells that results from the decrease in extracellular osmolality (Fig. 9-10). Postmortem studies in patients who died with hyponatremia show cerebral edema, herniation of the brain, and, in a few cases, central myelinolysis.[362] The severity of the neurologic defects depends on several factors, including the degree of hyponatremia, the rate of decline, and the age of the patient.[361] Unless the patient has epilepsy or other preexisting brain disease, seizures and coma usually do not occur until plasma sodium falls below 120 meq/liter. If hyponatremia is chronic or slow to develop, cerebral swelling and symptoms appear to be less severe, probably because brain cells are able to inactivate or otherwise rid themselves of solute.[363] Although total body water is increased in SIADH, evidence of hypervolemia such as hypertension or edema does not occur unless there is also some abnormality in sodium excretion.

Diagnosis

In evaluating a patient with hyponatremia, the first step is to rule out factitious causes.[364] If plasma sodium is measured by flame photometer, its concentration will appear to be low in any disease in which plasma proteins or lipids are markedly elevated. This effect is an artifact caused by a relative decrease in the sodium-containing aqueous portion of the plasma. Since the *concentration* of sodium and its anions in plasma water are unaffected by the addition of lipid or protein, plasma osmolality or sodium as determined by ion-specific electrode are normal in the presence of hyperproteinemia or hyperlipidemia. A rise in the plasma concentration of glucose or mannitol will also produce hyponatremia. In this case, however, the fall in plasma sodium concentration is real, since it is due to an osmotically induced shift of water from the intracellular to the extracellular space. Therefore, plasma sodium will be low when measured by ion-specific electrode or flame photometer, but plasma osmolality will be normal or slightly increased. Thus, the *sine qua non* for true hyponatremia is a commensurate reduction in the osmolality and sodium concentration of heparinized plasma. Serum or ethylenediaminetetraacetic acid (EDTA) plasma should not be used for these measurements, since both are subject to significant artifacts in the osmolality measurements.

Differentiation between the three major categories of true hyponatremia is based largely on clinical assessment of the extracellular volume (Table 9-8). Generalized edema and/or association with a disease known to cause edema is pathognomonic of hypervolemic hyponatremia. In these patients, urinary sodium is usually low (< 20 meq per day), and plasma renin activity, aldosterone, and urea may be elevated because of a reduction in effective blood volume and glomerular filtration. The cardiac, hepatic, and nephrotic causes of this category of hyponatremia are differentiated by the usual clinical methods.

Hypovolemic hyponatremia is characterized by signs and symptoms of volume depletion *without* edema. Urinary sodium is usually low, but it may be increased if the condition is due to renal sodium wasting (e.g., adrenal insufficiency, diuretic abuse, or sponge kidney). Some degree of hypokalemia is the rule, except in patients with Addison's disease or isolated aldosterone deficiency, in whom serum potas-

Table 9-8. Diagnostic Evaluation of Hyponatremia

1. Measure plasma osmolality.
   - A. If it is decreased in proportion to plasma sodium (1 meq/liter = 2 mosmol/kg), true hyponatremia is present and the workup should proceed directly to step 2.
   - B. If it is not depressed, factitious hyponatremia should be suspected and evaluated by measuring plasma protein, lipids, and glucose. If they are normal, the presence of some abnormal osmogenic solute such as alcohol should be sought.
2. Examine the patient for evidence of edema, congestive failure, cirrhosis, nephrosis, hypotension, hypovolemia, adrenal insufficiency, or hypothyroidism.
   - A. If any of these abnormalities is present, the diagnosis of SIADH is excluded and therapy to correct the underlying disease should be started.
   - B. If these abnormalities are absent, proceed to step 3.
3. Measure urine osmolality.
   - A. If it is more than 100 mosmol/kg, the workup should proceed directly to step 4.
   - B. If it is less than 100 mosmol/kg, perform a dehydration test and repeat the measurement at hourly intervals. If urine concentration occurs before plasma osmolality and sodium reach 270 mosmol/kg and 130 meq/liter, respectively, the diagnosis of reset osmostat is likely and the workup should proceed to step 4. However, if urine concentration does not occur prematurely, a persistent defect in water excretion is excluded and the clinical history should be reviewed, looking for evidence of severe polydipsia (> 20 liters/day) and/or some transient antecedent stimulus to vasopressin release.
4. Measure urinary sodium.
   - A. If it is less than 20 meq/day, the diagnosis of SIADH is unlikely and further studies should be performed to determine whether there is evidence of diuretic abuse, chronic diarrhea, vomiting, or subclinical cardiac or hepatic failure.
   - B. If it is more than 20 meq/day, proceed to step 5.
5. Measure plasma vasopressin and renin activity while the patient is hyponatremic.
   - A. If plasma vasopressin is inappropriately high and renin is low, the diagnosis of SIADH is established and appropriate therapy should be started.
   - B. If both plasma vasopressin and renin are suppressed, a vasopressin-independent form of SIADH should be suspected.
   - C. If plasma vasopressin and renin activity are both elevated, diuretic abuse, adrenal insufficiency, or some other cause of sodium wasting should be sought.
6. A water load test may be performed if the hyponatremia remits before the other diagnostic studies are performed.
   - A. If the load is excreted normally, SIADH and all other forms of impaired water excretion are excluded.
   - B. If the load is not excreted normally, steps 1 through 4 should be performed to determine the cause of the defect.

sium is usually elevated. Normokalemia or hypokalemia does not exclude secondary adrenal insufficiency, so plasma cortisol should be measured in all cases in which hypotension or hyponatremia cannot be explained by other factors.

Euvolemic hyponatremia, or the syndrome of inappropriate antidiuresis, is distinguishable by the lack of any clinical signs of edema, hypovolemia, or hypotension. Thus, in contrast to the other two forms of hyponatremia, plasma urea and renin tend to be low while urinary sodium is high. The latter may be misleading, however, since the natriuresis can reverse quickly when the excess body water begins to decline.

Measurements of plasma vasopressin are of no help in distinguishing between the various types of hyponatremia, since it is usually elevated to the same extent in all three. However, plasma vasopressin levels may determine whether or not the hormone contributes to the impairment in urinary dilution and, if it does, which type of osmoregulatory defect is responsible. At present this information is of no clinical utility, since the therapy is essentially the same in any case. However, diagnostic studies of this type may prove more useful when and if more specific and effective methods for inhibiting the secretion or action of vasopressin come into general clinical use.

Therapy

Hypervolemic Hyponatremia

In patients with edema and hyponatremia, the ideal treatment would be to correct the cardiac, hepatic, or renal defect that is responsible for the impairment in water excretion. Indeed, some improvement in water excretion and/or hyponatremia may occur when cardiac output is increased[365] or ascitic fluid is shunted into the vascular space.[366] Usually, however, the basic hemodynamic defect cannot be completely rectified, and other methods must be used to correct the edema and hyponatremia. Since patients in this category have a greater increase in total body water than in sodium, the most rational and effective therapy is to combine fluid restriction with administration of an osmotic or loop diuretic.[367,368] Initially, infusion of mannitol will expand extracellular volume and increase hyponatremia by osmotically extracting cellular water. However, the fall in plasma sodium is inconsequential, because it is more than offset by the osmotic effect of the mannitol, and the hypervolemia and hyponatremia usually disappear in a few hours when the mannitol is excreted. Hypertonic saline should not be used in these patients, because they retain the sodium and develop more severe edema.

Hypovolemic Hyponatremia

These patients are usually the simplest to treat, since it is necessary only to expand blood and extracellular volume by oral or parenteral administration of salt and water. Since their sodium deficit is greater than their water deficit, the ideal combination is hypertonic—i.e., the ratio of sodium chloride to water should exceed 150 meq/liter. However, this approach is necessary only if the hyponatremia is severe and must be corrected quickly. In such a situation, an infusion of 3% saline at a rate of 0.1 ml/kg per minute for 2 h will raise plasma sodium by almost 10 meq/liter, an amount that is usually sufficient to eliminate the threat of serious neurologic complications. In most other situations, isotonic saline with or without supplementary potassium is sufficient to correct gradually the electrolyte imbalance. In addition, the cause of the sodium loss should be identified and, if possible, corrected. If the patient's pituitary-adrenal status is in question, parenteral cortisol should be administered pending completion of steroid measurements. If sodium wasting cannot be stopped (e.g., in a patient with chronic diarrhea due to bowel disease), intake of sodium and other electrolytes should be supplemented orally as needed to maintain balance. In no case should patients in this category be treated by water restriction or with vasopressin antagonists, since these measures only aggravate the underlying hypovolemia.

Euvolemic Hyponatremia

In patients with SIADH, the most rational therapy would be to correct the underlying abnormality in vasopressin secretion. However, it is rarely possible to do this except in those cases where the hormone is produced ectopically or secreted in response to emetic stimuli. Therefore, it is usually necessary to employ other methods to reduce the excess of body water which is responsible for the hyponatremia. The traditional method is to restrict water intake. To be effective, however, the *total* intake of water must be at least 500 ml a day less than the total of urinary and insensible output. Since the amount of water provided by food normally approximates insensible loss, discretionary intake of water must be kept at least 500 ml a day below urine output. In many patients, the requisite restriction is difficult to achieve because their urine is concentrated and/or their thirst is also inappropriately increased. And even if restriction is successful, the rate of decrease in body water and rise in plasma osmolality is only about 1 to 2 percent a day. Therefore, additional measures are almost always needed, particularly if the hyponatremia is symptomatic.

Infusion of hypertonic saline provides more rapid correction and is almost always indicated when the hyponatremia is sufficiently severe to cause neurologic abnormalities. When given IV as 3% saline at a rate of 0.1 ml/kg per minute, it will increase plasma sodium and osmolality at a rate of approximately 2 percent an hour. Since it acts both by producing a water-depleting solute diuresis and by correcting the sodium deficit, this approach is rational as well as rapid. In our experience and that of others, it is also safe.[369] However, there is some question whether in certain patients rapid correction of hyponatremia with hypertonic saline may be associated with central pontine myelinolysis,[370,371] a rare and often fatal neurologic disorder characterized by quadriparesis, dysphagia, and dysarthria. Therefore, hypertonic saline should be used cautiously in patients with SIADH and only to the extent necessary to raise plasma sodium to asymptomatic levels.

Body water can also be reduced by inhibiting the antidiuretic effects of vasopressin. Of the drugs that have been used for this purpose, demeclocycline (Declomycin) is probably the best.[372,373] At conventional doses of up to 1.2 g per day, it causes a reversible form of nephrogenic diabetes insipidus in almost all patients with SIADH. Its mechanism of action has not been defined precisely but appears to involve a step distal to the generation of cyclic AMP.[374] Because of other catabolic as well as nephrotoxic effects, it may cause a rise in plasma urea, which is reversible when the drug is stopped. However, demeclocycline can have serious or potentially lethal side effects in patients with edema and hyponatremia.[375,376] Hence, its use should be monitored closely and probably restricted to SIADH patients in whom the hyponatremia is chronic and symptomatic, strict fluid restriction is not feasible, and significant underlying cardiac, renal, or hepatic disease is not present. Lithium carbonate also causes a form of reversible nephrogenic diabetes insipidus. At conventional doses, however, it has a much less consistent inhibitory effect on urinary concentration and is even more prone to produce undesirable side effects.[377] For these reasons, its use to treat SIADH or other forms of hyponatremia is not recommended.

Other measures which can be useful in the treatment of chronic SIADH include the administration of oral sodium chloride with or without furosemide.[378] This regimen works much like an osmotic diuretic in that it increases free water excretion by increasing solute load. Much the same result can be obtained by giving salt or urea per os,[379] but the latter is unpalatable and may not be well accepted by patients.

Analogues capable of antagonizing the antidiuretic effect of vasopressin have also been developed and used to study the role of vasopressin in animal models of impaired urinary dilution.[14] These antagonists may eventually prove to be useful for treating some patients with SIADH or hypervolemic forms of hyponatremia.

TESTS USED IN DIAGNOSIS

Hypofunction

Fluid Restriction

This test is basic to the differential diagnosis of polyuria. It should not be used when basal osmolality and sodium concentration are above 295 mosmol/kg and 143 meq/liter, because in that situation it does not provide additional information of diagnostic value and may cause the patient unnecessary discomfort. If basal urine output is less than 6 liters per day, the test should be started at bedtime. Otherwise, it should be started early in the morning following an overnight fast. After obtaining initial samples of urine and plasma for the measurement of osmolality, the patient is weighed and instructed to stop all intake of fluids. The use of tobacco and unnecessary drugs is also prohibited, but lemon drops or other hard candy may be taken to assuage thirst or hunger. Every hour for the next 3 to 6 h, urine and plasma are collected for osmometry and the patient is reweighed. If urine osmolality does not rise above 300 mosmol/kg *before* plasma osmolality or sodium concentration reach 295 mosmol/kg or 143 meq/liter, the test is abnormal and a diagnosis of primary polydipsia is excluded. A measurement of vasopressin in the final plasma or urine sample or a therapeutic trial of DDAVP may then be used to differentiate neurogenic from nephrogenic diabetes insipidus.

If urine osmolality rises above 300 mosmol/kg before plasma osmolality or sodium reach the prescribed level, the dehydration test is inconclusive and should be supplemented with measurements of plasma vasopressin during hypertonic saline infusion to distinguish neurogenic diabetes insipidus from primary polydipsia.

If none of the urine samples is concentrated and the final plasma osmolality or sodium concentration does not exceed the prescribed level, surreptitious drinking should be suspected. If this is confirmed by finding that the changes in body weight or plasma osmolality are not commensurate with total urine output, the test is invalid and either should be repeated under closer observation or replaced by a hypertonic saline infusion.

Hypertonic Saline Infusion

This test is used to distinguish between primary polydipsia and neurogenic diabetes insipidus when the fluid restriction test is inconclusive or invalid. At the conclusion of the fluid restriction test, 3% saline is infused via intravenous catheter at a rate of 0.1 ml/min per kilogram of body weight for 1 to 2 h. Plasma samples for osmometry and vasopressin assay are collected from the opposite antecubital vein before and at 30-min intervals during the infusion. The results should be interpreted by plotting on a nomogram such as Fig. 9-14.

Therapeutic Trial of DDAVP

This test can be used to differentiate between primary polydipsia and neurogenic diabetes insipidus. The patient should be hospitalized in an environment where intake, output, body weight, and plasma electrolytes can be closely monitored. After at least 2 days of observation to determine basal values, DDAVP is given either by intramuscular injection (1 to 2 μg bid) or nasal insufflation (25 μg bid) for 1 to 3 days. Body weight and plasma sodium should be measured in the morning and late afternoon while daily intake and output continue to be monitored. If this treatment reduces polydipsia as well as polyuria and does not produce water intoxication, the patient probably has neurogenic diabetes insipidus. However, if DDAVP has no effect on water balance, the patient probably has nephrogenic diabetes insipidus and should be tried on a 10-fold higher dose of DDAVP to determine whether the renal resistance is partial or complete. On the other hand, if the standard dose of DDAVP reduces urine output without reducing intake or produces other signs of water intoxication (such as a gain in weight or fall in plasma sodium of more than 5 percent), the patient probably has some form of primary polydipsia, and all antidiuretic therapy should be discontinued until a definitive diagnosis is obtained.

Vasopressin Assay

Plasma or urinary vasopressin should be measured concurrently with plasma and urine osmolality during the dehydration test to verify the diagnosis of diabetes insipidus and differentiate the neurogenic and nephrogenic forms. The results should be interpreted by plotting on appropriate nomograms such as those in Figs. 9-14 and 9-15.

Hyperfunction

Vasopressin Assay

Measurements of plasma or urinary vasopressin can be used to verify the cause of impaired water excretion. However, they should be obtained only when plasma osmolality and sodium concentration are below 270 mosmol/kg and 130 meq/liter, respectively, and the results should be plotted on a nomogram like that in Fig. 9-19. Inadequate suppression of vasopressin is indicative of SIADH only if hypovolemia, hypotension, and certain other abnormalities are excluded (Table 9-8). Urinary sodium excretion or plasma renin activity may be measured concurrently as an indicator of blood volume status.

Water Load Test

This test is used primarily to verify suspected defects in water excretion at a time when plasma osmolality and sodium concentration are within normal limits. It may also be used in the presence of hypotonicity to test for resetting of the osmostat.

The test should be started in the morning 2 h after a light breakfast. After initial plasma and urine samples are obtained for osmometry, the patient is weighed and instructed to drink 20 ml of cool tap water per kilogram of body weight within 15 to 30 min. If necessary, lightly salted crackers may be eaten to overcome distate for the water. The patient is then placed in a semirecumbent position. Each hour for the next 4 h, a sample of plasma is obtained and the total urine output is collected for the measurement of osmolality and volume.

Normally this procedure should result in a fall in plasma osmolality of at least 5 mosmol/kg, a decrease in urine osmolality to less than 100 mosmol/kg, and a cumulative urine output of 90 percent of the water load or more within 5 h (Fig. 9-21). Failure to achieve either of the latter criteria in the presence of good absorption (i.e., a normal decline in plasma osmolality) is diagnostic of a defect in water and/or solute excretion. Some indication of the cause may be obtained by calculating solute excretion rate (urine flow in liters per minute times urine osmolality in milliosmols per kilogram) and plotting it along with urine osmolality on a suitable nomogram such as that in Fig. 9-21. A defect in distal delivery of filtrate is indicated by a subnormal rate of solute excretion. SIADH is characterized by a normal or supranormal rate of solute excretion in association with a less than maximum dilution of the urine. Measurements of plasma or urinary vasopressin on samples obtained 90 to 120 min after the load may be used to confirm the diagnosis.

General Considerations

The use of nicotine, caffeine, and all unnecessary drugs should be prohibited during any study of vaso-

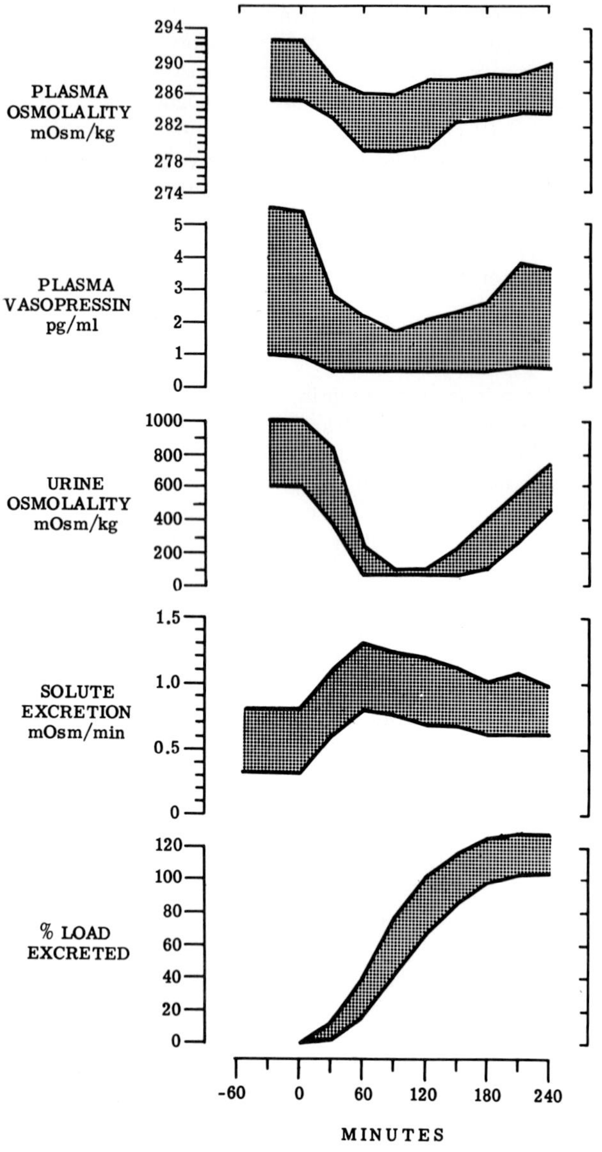

FIGURE 9-21 The effect of a standard water load on renal function. Shaded areas indicate the range of values obtained in 24 healthy adults. A water load of 20 ml per kilogram of body weight was given between 0 and 30 min. The bottom panel indicates cumulative excretion expressed as a percentage of the total load.

pressin function. The patient should also be monitored for symptoms of nausea or changes in blood pressure, which may confuse interpretation of the results.

Plasma for osmometry should always be collected in heparin with as little stasis as possible. Serum or EDTA produces relatively large artifactual increases in osmolality[380] which make interpretation of most vasopressin tests impossible. Osmometry should be performed only by freezing-point depression on equipment calibrated with a 290-mosmol/kg standard as well as 100- and 500-mosmol/kg standards. If the accuracy of the osmometry is poor or doubtful, measurements of plasma sodium should be substituted.

Samples of plasma and urine for vasopressin assay should always be collected, processed, and transported according to the specifications of the laboratory that is to carry out the test. The results should always be compared with normal values supplied by the same laboratory, since not all laboratories use the same reference standards.

REFERENCES

1. Haymaker W: Hypothalamo-pituitary neural pathways and the circulatory system of the pituitary, in Haymaker W et al (eds): *The Hypothalamus.* Springfield, Charles C Thomas, 1969, p 219.

2. Scharrer E, Scharrer B: Hormones produced by neurosecretory cells. *Recent Prog Horm Res* 10:183, 1954.

3. Zimmerman EA: The organization of oxytocin and vaso-

pressin pathways, in Martin JB, Reichlin S, Bick KL (eds): *Neurosecretion and Brain Peptides.* New York, Raven, 1981, pp 63–75.

4. Sofroniew MV, Weindl A, Schrell U, Wetzstein R: Immunohistochemistry of vasopressin, oxytocin and neurophysin in the hypothalamus and extrahypothalamic regions of the human and primate brain. *Acta Histochem [suppl]* 24:79, 1981.

5. Dierickx K, Vandesande F: Immunocytochemical localization of the vasopressinergic and the oxytocinergic neurons in the human hypothalamus. *Cell Tissue Res* 184:15, 1977.

6. Swanson LW: Immunohistochemical evidence for a neurophysin containing autonomic pathway arising in the paraventricular nucleus of the hypothalamus. *Brain Res* 128:346, 1977.

7. Nilaver G, Zimmerman EA, Wilkins J, Michaels J, Hoffman D, Silverman AJ: Magnocellular hypothalamic projections to the lower brain stem and spinal cord of the rat: Immunocytochemical evidence of predominance of the oxytocin-neurophysin system compared to the vasopressin-neurophysin system. *Neuroendocrinology* 30:150, 1980.

8. Luerssen TG, Robertson GL: Cerebrospinal fluid vasopressin and vasotocin in health and disease, in Wood JH (ed): *Neurobiology and Cerebrospinal Fluid.* New York, Plenum, 1980, vol 1, pp 613–623.

9. Glick SM, Brownstein MJ: Vasopressin content of rat brain. *Life Sci* 27:1103, 1980.

10. du Vigneaud V: Hormones of the posterior pituitary gland: Oxytocin and vasopressin, in *Harvey Lectures, 1954–1955.* New York, Academic, 1956.

11. Sawyer WW: Evolution of antidiuretic hormones and their functions. *Am J Med* 42:678, 1967.

12. Walter R, Smith CW, Mehta PK, Boonjarern S, Arruda JAL, Kurtzman N: Conformational considerations of vasopressin as a guide to development of biological probes and therapeutic agents, in Andreoli TE et al (eds): *Disturbances in Body Fluid Osmolality.* Bethesda, American Physiological Society, 1977, pp 1–36.

13. Vavra I, Machova A, Holecek V, Cort JH, Zaoral M, Sorm F: Effect of a synthetic analogue of vasopressin in animals and in patients with diabetes insipidus. *Lancet* 1:948, 1968.

14. Sawyer WH, Manning M: The development of vasopressin antagonists. *Fed Proc* 43:87, 1984.

15. Acher R, Chauvet J, Olivry G: Sur l'existence éventuelle d'une hormone unique hypophysaire: 1. Relations entre l'oxytocine, la vasopressine et la protein de Van Dyke extraites de la neurohypophyse du boeuf. *Biochim Biophys Acta* 22:421, 1956.

16. Breslow E: The neurophysins. *Adv Enzymol* 40:271, 1974.

17. Sachs H, Fawcett P, Takabatake Y, Portanova R: Biosynthesis and release of vasopressin and neurophysin. *Recent Prog Horm Res* 25:447, 1969.

18. Valtin H, Sokol HW, Sunde D: Genetic approaches to the study of the regulation and actions of vasopressin. *Recent Prog Horm Res* 31:447, 1975.

19. Russell JT, Brownstein MJ, Gainer H: Biosynthesis of vasopressin, oxytocin and neurophysins: Isolation and characterization of two common precursors (propressophysin and prooxyphysin). *Endocrinology* 107:1880, 1980.

20. Land H, Schutz G, Schmale H, Richter D: Nucleotide sequence of cloned cDNA encoding bovine arginine vasopressin-neurophysin II precursor. *Nature* 295:299, 1982.

21. Schmale H, Richter D: Single base deletion in the vasopressin gene is the cause of diabetes insipidus in Brattleboro rats. *Nature* 309:705, 1984.

22. Majzoub JA, Rich A, van Boom J, Habener JF: Vasopressin and oxytocin in mRNA regulation in the rat assessed by hybridization with synthetic oligonucleotides. *J Biol Chem* 258:14061, 1983.

23. Moses AM, Miller M: Accumulation and release of pituitary vasopressin in rats heterozygous for hypothalamic diabetes insipidus. *Endocrinology* 86:34, 1970.

24. Douglass WW: How do neurons secrete peptides? Exocytosis and its consequences including synaptic vesicle formation in the hypothalamo-neurohypophyseal system. *Prog Brain Res* 39:21, 1973.

25. Verney EB: Antidiuretic hormone and the factors which determine its release. *Proc R Soc Lond* [Biol] 135:25, 1947.

26. Robertson GL: The regulation of vasopressin function in health and disease. *Recent Prog Horm Res* 33:333, 1977.

27. Robertson GL, Athar S, Shelton RL: Osmotic control of vasopressin function, in Andreoli TE et al (eds): *Disturbances in Body Fluid Osmolality.* Bethesda, American Physiological Society, 1977, p 125.

28. Schrier RW, Berl T, Anderson RJ: Osmotic and nonosmotic control of vasopressin release. *Am J Physiol* 236(4):F321, 1979.

29. Robertson GL: Thirst and vasopressin function in normal and disordered states of water balance. *J Lab Clin Med* 101(3):351, 1983.

30. Jewell PA, Verney EB: An experimental attempt to determine the site of the neurohypophyseal osmoreceptors in the dog. *Philos Trans R Soc Lond* [*Biol*] 240:197, 1957.

31. Andersson B: Thirst and brain control of water balance. *Am Sci* 59:408, 1971.

32. Robertson GL: Physiopathology of ADH secretion, in Tolis G, Labrie F, Martin JB, Naftolin F, et al (eds): *Clinical Neuroendocrinology: A Pathophysiological Approach.* New York, Raven, 1979, pp 247–260.

33. Thrasher TN, Keil LC, Ramsey DJ: Lesions of the organum vasculosum of the lamina terminalis (OVLT) attenuate osmotically-induced drinking and vasopressin secretion in the dog. *Endocrinology* 110(5):1837, 1982.

34. Strong OS, Elwyn A: *Human Neuroanatomy.* Baltimore, Williams & Wilkins, 1948, p. 398.

35. Robertson GL: Control of the posterior pituitary and antidiuretic hormone secretion, in Brod J (ed): *Contributions of Nephrology.* Basel, Karger, 1980, vol 21, pp 33–40.

36. Zerbe RL: Genetic factors in normal and abnormal regulation of vasopressin secretion, in Schrier R (ed): *Vasopressin.* New York, Raven, 1985, pp 213–220.

37. Helderman JH, Vestal RE, Rowe JW, Tobin JD, Andres R, Robertson GL: The response of arginine vasopressin to intravenous ethanol and hypertonic saline in man: The impact of aging. *J Gerontol* 33:39, 1978.

38. Legros LL, Govaerts A, Demoulin A, Franchimont P: Interactions entre un dérive progestatif et l'ethinyl oestradiol sur l'élimination urinaire de neurophysine d'oxytocine et de vasopressine immunoactives et sur le taux de neurophysine sérique I et II chez l'homme normal. *C R Soc Biol (Paris)* 167(11):1668, 1973.

39. Vallotton MB, Merkelbach U, Gaillard RC: Studies of the factors modulating antidiuretic hormone excretion in man in response to the osmolar stimulus: Effects of oestrogen and angiotensin II. *Acta Endocrinol* 104:295, 1983.

40. Skowsky WR, Swan L, Smith P: Effects of sex steroid hormones on arginine vasopressin in intact and castrated male and female rats. *Endocrinology* 104:105, 1979.

41. Davison JM, Gilmore EA, Durr J, Robertson GL, Lindheimer MD: Altered osmotic threshold for vasopressin secretion and thirst in human pregnancy. *Am J Physiol* 246(15):F105, 1984.

42. Vokes T, Gaskill M, Robertson GL: Changes in the osmoregulation of thirst and vasopressin during the normal menstrual cycle, in *Excerpta Medica International Congress Series.* Amsterdam, Excerpta Medica, 1984, vol 652, p 1593.

43. Baylis PH, Spruce BA, Burd J: Osmoregulation of vasopressin secretion during the menstrual cycle, in Schrier RL (ed): *Vasopressin.* New York, Raven, 1985, pp 241–247.

44. Rodbard D, Munson PJ: Editorial comment. *Am J Physiol* 234:E340, 1978.

45. Wade CE, Bie P, Keil LC, Ramsay DJ: Osmotic control of plasma vasopressin in the dog. *Am J Physiol* 243:E287, 1982.

46. Hammer M, Ladefoged J, Olgaard K: Relationship between plasma osmolality and plasma vasopressin in human subjects. *Am J*

Physiol 238:E313, 1980.

47. Zerbe RL, Baylis PH, Robertson GL: Vasopressin function in clinical disorders in water balance, in Beardwell C, Robertson G (eds): *The Pituitary*. London, Butterworth, 1981.

48. Weitzman RE, Fisher DA, DiStefano JH III, Bennett CM: Episodic secretion of arginine vasopressin. *Am J Physiol* 233:E32, 1977.

49. Poulain DA: Electrophysiology of the afferent input to oxytocin- and vasopressin-secreting neurones: Facts and problems. *Prog Brain Res* 60:39, 1983.

50. Robertson GL: Regulation of vasopressin secretion, in Seldin DW, Giebisch G (eds): *The Kidney: Physiology and Pathophysiology*. New York, Raven, 1985, pp 869–884.

51. Zerbe RL, Robertson GL: Osmoregulation of thirst and vasopressin secretion in human subjects: Effect of various solutes. *Am J Physiol* 224:E607, 1983.

52. McKinley MJ, Denton DA, Weisinger RS: Sensors of antidiuresis and thirst: Osmoreceptors or CSF sodium detectors? *Brain Res* 141:89, 1978.

53. Thrasher TN, Brown CJ, Keil LC, Ramsay DJ: Thirst and vasopressin release in the dog: An osmoreceptor or sodium receptor mechanism? *Am J Physiol* 238:R333, 1980.

54. Olsson K, Kolmodin R: Dependence of basic secretion of antidiuretic hormone on cerebrospinal fluid [Na]. *Acta Physiol Scand* 91:286, 1974.

55. Vokes T, Robertson GL: Effect of insulin on the osmoregulation of thirst and vasopressin, in Schrier R (ed): *Vasopressin*. New York, Raven, 1985, pp 271–279.

56. Zerbe RL, Vinicor F, Robertson GL: The regulation of plasma vasopressin in insulin dependent diabetes mellitus. *Am J Physiol* 249(3):E317, 1985.

57. Zerbe RL, Vinicor F, Robertson GL: Plasma vasopressin in uncontrolled diabetes mellitus. *Diabetes* 28(5):503, 1979.

58. Walsh CH, Baylis PH, Malins JM: Plasma arginine vasopressin in diabetic ketoacidosis. *Diabetologia* 16:93, 1979.

59. van Houten M, Posner BI, Kopriwa BM, Brawer JR: Insulin binding sites in the rat brain: *In vivo* localization to the circumventricular organs by quantitative radioautography. *Endocrinology* 105(3):666, 1979.

60. Schrier RW, Berl T, Anderson RJ, McDonald KM: Nonosmolar control of renal water excretion, in Andreoli TE et al (eds): *Disturbances in Body Fluid Osmolality*. Bethesda, American Physiological Society, 1977, p 149.

61. Share L: Extracellular fluid volume and vasopressin secretion, in Ganong WF, Martini L (eds): *Frontiers in Neuroendocrinology*. New York, Oxford, 1969.

62. Brennan LA, Jr, Malvin RL, Jochim KE, Roberts DE: Influence of right and left atrial receptors on plasma concentrations of ADH and renin. *Am J Physiol* 221(1):273, 1971.

63. Wang BC, Sundet WD, Hakumaki OK, Goetz KL: Vasopressin and renin responses to hemorrhage in conscious, cardiac-denervated dogs. *Am J Physiol* 245(14):H399, 1983.

64. Kirchheim HR: Systemic arterial baroreceptor reflexes. *Physiol Rev* 56(1):100, 1976.

65. Sawchenko PE, Swanson LW: Central noradrenergic pathways for the integration of hypothalamic neuroendocrine and autonomic responses. *Science* 214:685, 1981.

66. Blessing WW, Sved AF, Reis DJ: Destruction of noradrenergic neurons in rabbit brainstem. *Science* 217:661, 1983.

67. Schrier RW, Berl T, Harbottle JA: Mechanism of the antidiuretic effect associated with interruption of parasympathetic pathways. *J Clin Invest* 51:2613, 1972.

68. Thames MD, Schmid PG: Cardiopulmonary receptors with vagal afferents tonically inhibit ADH release in the dog. *Am J Physiol* 237:H299, 1979.

69. Robertson GL: The role of osmotic and hemodynamic variables in regulating vasopressin secretion, in James VHT (ed): *Proceedings of the Fifth International Congress of Endocrinology, Hamburg, July, 1976*. Excerpta Medica International Congress Series No. 402. Amsterdam, Excerpta Medica, 1977, pp 126–130.

70. Fumoux F, Czernichow P, Arnauld E, Du Pont J, Vincent JD: Effect of hypotension induced by sodium nitrocyanoferrate (III) on the release of arginine-vasopressin in the unanaesthetized monkey. *J Endocrinol* 78:449, 1978.

71. Dunn FL, Brennan TJ, Nelson AE, Robertson GL: The role of blood osmolality and volume in regulating vasopressin secretion in the rat. *J Clin Invest* 52:3212, 1973.

72. Goldsmith SR, Francis GS, Crowley AW, Cohn JN: Response of vasopressin and norepinephrine to lower body negative pressure in humans. *Am J Physiol* 243:H970, 1982.

73. Davies R, Forsling M, Bulger G, Phillips T: Plasma vasopressin and blood pressure. *Br Heart J* 49:528, 1983.

74. Wade CE, Keil LC, Ramsay DJ: Role of volume and osmolality in the control of plasma vasopressin in dehydrated dogs. *Neuroendocrinology* 37:349, 1983.

75. Katz FH, Smith JA, Lock JP, Loeffel DE: Plasma vasopressin variation and renin activity in normal active hormones. *Hormone Res* 10:289, 1979.

76. Segar WE, Moore WW: The regulation of antidiuretic hormone release in man. *J Clin Invest* 47:2143, 1968.

77. Szatalowicz VL, Arnold PE, Chaimovitz C, Bichet D, Berl T, Schrier RW: Radioimmunoassay of plasma arginine vasopressin in hyponatremic patients with congestive heart failure. *N Engl J Med* 305:263, 1981.

78. Riegger GAJ, Liebau G, Kochsie K: Antidiuretic hormone in congestive heart failure. *Am J Med* 72:49, 1982.

79. Wiggins RC, Basar I, Slater JDH, Forsling M, Ramage CM: Vasovagal hypotension and vasopressin release. *Clin Endocrinol* 6:387, 1977.

80. Baylis PH, Heath DA: Influence of presyncope and postural change upon plasma vasopressin concentration in hydrated and dehydrated man. *Clin Endocrinol* 7:79, 1977.

81. Zerbe RL, Henry DP, Robertson GL: Vasopressin response to orthostatic hypotension: Etiological and clinical implications. *Am J Med* 74(2):265, 1983.

82. Quillen EW Jr, Crowley AW Jr: Influence of volume changes in osmolality-vasopressin relationships in conscious dogs. *Am J Physiol* 244:H73, 1983.

83. Robertson GL, Athar S: The interaction of blood osmolality and blood volume in regulating plasma vasopressin in man. *J Clin Endocrinol Metab* 42:613, 1976.

84. Wang BC, Sundet WD, Hakumaki MOK, Geer PG, Goetz KL: Cardiac receptor influences on the plasma osmolality–plasma vasopressin relationship. *Am J Physiol* 246(15):H360, 1984.

85. Weiss NM, Robertson G, Byun K: The effect of hypovolemia on the osmoregulation of thirst and AVP. *Clin Res* 32(4):786A, 1984.

86. Moses AM, Miller M, Streeten DHP: Quantitative influence of blood volume expansion on the osmotic threshold for vasopressin release. *J Clin Endocrinol Metab* 27:655, 1967.

87. Moses AM, Miller M: Osmotic threshold for vasopressin release as determined by saline infusion and by dehydration. *Neuroendocrinology* 7:219, 1971.

88. Rowe JW, Shelton RL, Helderman JH, Vestal RE, Robertson GL: Influence of the emetic reflex on vasopressin release in man. *Kidney Int* 16:729, 1979.

89. Coutinho EM: Oxytocic and antidiuretic effects of nausea in women. *Am J Obstet Gynecol* 105:127, 1969.

90. Verbalis J, Gardiner TW, McHale CM, Stricker EM: Neurohypophyseal secretion in response to nausea producing stimuli associated with learned taste aversions. *Soc Neurosci* 10:89A, 1984.

91. DeFronzo RA, Braine H, Colvin OM, Davis PJ: Water intoxication in man after cyclophosphamide therapy: Time course and relation to drug activation. *Ann Intern Med* 78:861, 1973.

92. Steele TH, Serpick AA, Block JB: Antidiuretic response to cyclophosphamide in man. *J Pharmacol Exp Ther* 185:245, 1973.

93. Heyes MP, Farber MO, Manfredi F, Robertshaw D, Weinberger M, Fineberg N, Robertson G: Acute effects of hypoxia on renal and endocrine function in normal man. *Am J Physiol* 243:R265, 1982.

94. Eversmann T, Guttsmann M, Uhlich E, Ulbrecht G, von Werder K, Scriba PC: Increased secretion of growth hormone, prolactin, antidiuretic hormone and cortisol induced by the stress of motion sickness. *Aviation Space Environ Med* 49:53, 1978.

95. Baylis PH, Heath DA: Plasma-arginine-vasopressin response to insulin-induced hypoglycemia. *Lancet* 2:428, 1977.

96. Baylis PH, Robertson GL: Rat vasopressin response to insulin-induced hypoglycemia. *Endocrinology* 107:1975, 1980.

97. Baylis PH, Zerbe RL, Robertson GL: Arginine vasopressin response to insulin-induced hypoglycemia in man. *J Clin Endocrinol Metab* 53:935, 1981.

98. Keller-Wood ME, Wade CE, Shinsako J, Keil LC, Van Loon GR, Dallman MF: Insulin-induced hypoglycemia in conscious dogs: Effects of maintaining carotid arterial glucose levels on the adrenocorticotropin, epinephrine and vasopressin responses. *Endocrinology* 112(2):624, 1982.

99. Baylis PH, Robertson GL: Vasopressin response to 2-deoxy-D-glucose in the rat. *Endocrinology* 107:1970, 1980.

100. Thompson DA, Cambell RG, Lilavivat U, Welle SL, Robertson GL: Increased thirst and plasma arginine vasopressin levels during 2-deoxy-D-glucose–induced glucoprivation in humans. *J Clin Invest* 67:1083, 1981.

101. Bonjour JP, Malvin RL: Stimulation of ADH release by the renin-angiotensin system. *Am J Physiol* 218:1555, 1970.

102. Mouw D, Bonjour JP, Malvin RL, Vander A: Central action of angiotensin in stimulating ADH release. *Am J Physiol* 220:239, 1971.

103. Yamaguchi K, Sakaguchi T, Kamoi K: Central role of angiotensin in the hyperosmolality- and hypovolaemia-induced vasopressin release in conscious rats. *Acta Endocrinol* 101·524, 1982.

104. Shimizu K, Share L, Claybaugh JR: Potentiation of angiotensin II of the vasopressin response to an increasing plasma osmolality. *Endocrinology* 93:42, 1973.

105. Cadnapaphornchai P, Boykin J, Harbottle JA, McDonald KM, Schrier RW: Effect of angiotensin II on renal water excretion. *Am J Physiol* 228:155, 1975.

106. Rydin H, Verney EB: The inhibition of water-diuresis by emotional stress and by muscular exercise. *Q J Exp Physiol* 27:343, 1938.

107. Husain MK, Manger WM, Rock TW, Weiss RJ, Frantz AG: Vasopressin release due to manual restraint in the rat: Role of body compression and comparison with other stressful stimuli. *Endocrinology* 104:641, 1979.

108. Keil LC, Severs WB: Reduction of plasma vasopressin levels of dehydrated rats following acute stress. *Endocrinology* 100:30, 1977.

109. Lang RE, Heil JWE, Ganten D, Hermann K, Unger T, Rascher W: Oxytocin unlike vasopressin is a stress hormone in the rat. *Neuroendocrinology* 37:314, 1983.

110. Ukai M, Moran WH, Zimmerman B: The role of visceral afferent pathways in vasopressin secretion and urinary excretory patterns during surgical stress. *Ann Surg* 168:16, 1968.

111. Baylis PH, Stockley RA, Heath DA: Effect of acute hypoxemia on plasma arginine vasopressin in conscious man. *Clin Sci Mol Med* 53:401, 1977.

112. Raff H, Shinsako J, Keil LC, Dallman MF: Vasopressin, ACTH, and corticosteroids during hypercapnia and graded hypoxia in dogs. *Am J Physiol* 244:E453, 1983.

113. Rose CE Jr, Anderson RJ, Carey RM: Antidiuresis and vasopressin release with hypoxemia and hypercapnia in conscious dogs. *Am J Physiol* 247:R127, 1984.

114. Raff H, Shinsako J, Keil LC, Dallman MF: Vasopressin, ACTH, and blood pressure during hypoxia induced at different rates. *Am J Physiol* 245:E489, 1983.

115. Farber MO, Weinberg MH, Robertson GL, Fineberg NS, Manfredi F: Hormonal abnormalities affecting sodium and water balance in acute respiratory failure due to chronic obstructive lung disease. *Chest* 85(1):49, 1984.

116. Miller M, Moses AM: Drug-induced states of impaired water excretion. *Kidney Int* 10:96, 1976.

117. Dyball REJ: The effects of drugs on the release of vasopressin. *J Pharmacol Chemother* 33:329, 1968.

118. Rockhold RW, Crofton JT, Wang BC, Share L: Effect of intracarotid administration of morphine and naloxone on plasma vasopressin levels and blood pressure in the dog. *J Pharmacol Exp Ther* 224(2):386, 1982.

119. Ukai M, Nagase T, Hirohashi M, Yanaihara N: Antidiuretic activities of substance P and its analogs. *Experientia* 37:521, 1981.

120. Bisset GW, Chowdrey HS, Feldberg W: Release of vasopressin by enkephalin. *Br J Pharmacol* 62:370, 1978.

121. Tseng LF, Loh HH, Li CH: β-Endorphin: Antidiuretic effects in rats. *Int J Pept Protein Res* 12:173, 1978.

122. Weitzman RE, Fisher DA, Minick S, Ling N, Guillemin R: β-Endorphin stimulates secretion of arginine vasopressin *in vivo*. *Endocrinology* 101:1643, 1977.

123. Robertson GL, Bhoopalam N, Zelkowitz LJ: Vincristine neurotoxicity and abnormal secretion of antidiuretic hormone. *Arch Intern Med* 132:717, 1973.

124. Gold PW, Robertson GL, Post RM, Kaye W, Ballenger J, Rubinow D, Goodwin FK: The effect of lithium on the osmoregulation of arginine vasopressin secretion. *J Clin Endocrinol Metab* 56(2):295, 1983.

125. Miller PD, Dubovsky SL, McDonald KM, Katz FH, Robertson GL, Schrier RW: Central, renal and adrenal effects of lithium in man. *Am J Med* 66:797, 1979.

126. Padfield PL, Park SJ, Morton JJ, Braidwood AE: Plasma levels of antidiuretic hormone in patients receiving prolonged lithium therapy. *Br J Psychiatry* 130:144, 1977.

127. Byun KY, Gaskill MB, Robertson GL: The mechanism of chlorpropamide antidiuresis in diabetes insipidus. *Clin Res* 32:483A, 1984.

128. Moses AM, Howanitz J, van Gemert M, Miller M: Clofibrate-induced antidiuresis. *J Clin Invest* 52:535, 1973.

129. Moses AM, Numann P, Miller M: Mechanism of chlorpropamide-induced antidiuresis in man: Evidence for release of ADH and enhancement of peripheral action. *Metabolism* 22:59, 1973.

130. Pockracki FJ, Robinson AG, Seif SM: Chlorpropamide effect: Measurement of neurophysin and vasopressin in humans and rats. *Metabolism* 30:72, 1978.

131. Gold PW, Robertson GL, Ballenger JC, Kaye W, Chen J, Rubinow DR, Goodwin FK, Post RM: Carbamazepine diminishes the sensitivity of the plasma arginine vasopressin response to osmotic stimulation. *J Clin Endocrinol Metab* 57(5):952, 1983.

132. Stephens WP, Coe JY, Baylis PH: Plasma arginine vasopressin concentrations and antidiuretic action of carbamazepine. *Br Med J* 1:1445, 1978.

133. Thomas TH, Ball SG, Wales JK, Lee MR: Effect of carbamazepine on plasma and urine arginine-vasopressin. *Clin Sci Mol Med* 54:419, 1978.

134. Kamoi K, White K, Robertson GL: Opiates elevate the osmotic threshold for vasopressin (VP) release in rats. *Clin Res* 27:254A, 1979.

135. Miller M: Inhibition of ADH release in the rat by narcotic antagonists. *Neuroendocrinology* 19:241, 1975.

136. van Wimersma Greidanus TB, Thody TJ, Verspaget H, deRotte GA, Goedemans HJH, Croiset G, van Ree JM: Effects of morphine and β-endorphin on basal and elevated plasma levels of

α-MSH and vasopressin. *Life Sci* 24:579, 1979.

137. Summy-Long JY, Keil LC, Deen K, Severs WB: Opiate regulation of angiotensin-induced drinking and vasopressin release. *J Pharmacol Exp Ther* 217:630, 1981.

138. Brownell J, del Pozo E, Donatsch P: Inhibition of vasopressin secretion by a met-enkephalin (FK 33-824) in humans. *Acta Endocrinol* 94(3):304, 1980.

139. Grossman A, Besser GM, Milles JJ, Baylis PH: Inhibition of vasopressin release in man by an opiate peptide. *Lancet* 2:1108, 1980.

140. Zerbe RL, Henry DP, Robertson GL: A new met-enkephalin analogue suppresses plasma vasopressin in man. *Peptides* 1:199, 1981.

141. Miller M: Role of endogenous opioids in neurohypophyseal function in man. *J Clin Endocrinol Metab* 50:1016, 1980.

142. Eggleton MG: The diuretic action of alcohol in man. *J Physiol* 101:172, 1942.

143. Kleeman CR, Rubini ME, Lamdin E, Epstein FH: Studies on alcohol diuresis: II. The evaluation of ethyl alcohol as an inhibitor of the neurohypophysis. *J Clin Invest* 34(3):448, 1955.

144. Helderman JH, Vestal RE, Rowe JW, Tobin JD, Andres R, Robertson GL: The response of arginine vasopressin in intravenous ethanol and hypertonic saline in man: The impact of aging. *J Gerontol* 33:339, 1978.

145. Oiso Y, Robertson GL: Effect of ethanol on vasopressin secretion and the role of endogenous opioids, in Schrier R (ed): *Vasopressin.* New York, Raven, 1985, p 265–269.

146. Reid IA, Ahn JN, Trinh T, Schackelford R, Weintraub M, Keil LC: Mechanism of suppression of vasopressin and adrenocorticotropic hormone secretion by clonidine in anesthetized dogs. *J Pharmacol Exp Ther* 229(1):18, 1984.

147. Roman RJ, Cowley AW Jr, Lechene C: Water diuretic and natriuretic effect of clonidine in the rat. *J Pharmacol Exp Ther* 211:385, 1979.

148. Iovino M, De Caro G, Massi M, Steardo L, Poenaru S: Muscimol inhibits ADH release induced by hypertonic sodium chloride in rats. *Pharmacol Biochem Behav* 19:335, 1983.

149. Engel P, Rowe J, Minaker K, Robertson GL: Effect of exogenous vasopressin on vasopressin release. *Am J Physiol* 246(9): E202, 1984.

150. Wang BC, Share L, Crofton JT: Central infusion of vasopressin decreased plasma vasopressin concentration in dogs. *Am J Physiol* 243(6):E365, 1982.

151. Moos F, Freund-Mercier MJ, Guerne Y, Guerne JM, Stoeckel ME, Richard P: Release of oxytocin and vasopressin by magnocellular nuclei in vitro: Specific facilitatory effect of oxytocin on its own release. *J Endocrinol* 102:63, 1984.

152. Amico JA, Ervin MG, Leake RD, Fisher DA, Finn FM, Robinson AG: A novel oxytocin-like and vasotocin-like peptide in human plasma after administration of estrogen. *J Clin Endocrinol Metab* 60(1):5, 1985.

153. Wathes DC, Swann RW, Birkett SD, Porter DG, Pickering BT: Characterization of oxytocin, vasopressin and neurophysin from the bovine corpus luteum. *Endocrinology* 113(2):693, 1983.

154. Amico JA, Seif SM, Robinson AG: Oxytocin in human plasma: Correlation with human plasma and stimulation with estrogen. *J Clin Endocrinol Metab* 52:988, 1981.

155. Lausen HD: Metabolism of the neurohypophyseal hormones, in Greep RO, Astwood EB, Knobil E, Sawyer WH, Geiger SR (eds): *Handbook of Physiology.* Washington, American Physiological Society, 1974, vol 4, pp 287–393.

156. Benmansour M, Rainfray M, Paillard F, Ardaillou R: Metabolic clearance rate of immunoreactive vasopressin in man. *Eur J Clin Invest* 12:475, 1982.

157. Robertson GL, Mahr EA, Athar S, Sinha T: Development and clinical application of a new method for the radioimmunoassay of arginine vasopressin in human plasma. *J Clin Invest* 52(9):2340, 1973.

158. Zimmerman EA, Robinson AG: Hypothalamic neurons secreting vasopressin and neurophysin. *Kidney Int* 10:12, 1976.

159. Jenkins JS, Mather HM, Ang V: Vasopressin in human cerebrospinal fluid. *J Clin Endocrinol Metab* 59(2):364, 1980.

160. Dogterom J, van Wimersma Greidanus TB, de Weid D: Vasopressin in cerebrospinal fluid and plasma of man, dog and rat. *Am J Physiol* 234(5):E463, 1978.

161. Szczepanska-Sadowska E, Gray D, Simon-Opperman C: Vasopressin in blood and third ventricle CSF during dehydration, thirst and hemorrhage. *Am J Physiol* 245:R549, 1983.

162. Reppert SM, Coleman RJ, Heath HW, Keutmann HT: Circadian properties of vasopressin and melatonin rhythms in cat cerebrospinal fluid. *Am J Physiol* 243:E489, 1982.

163. Szczepanska-Sadowska E, Sobocinska J, Sadowski B: Central dipsogenic effect of vasopressin. *Am J Physiol* 242:R372, 1982.

164. de Wied D: Behavioral effects of intraventricularly administered vasopressin and vasopressin fragments. *Life Sci* 19:685, 1976.

165. Sorensen PS, Hammer M, Vorstrup S, Gjerris F: CSF and plasma vasopressin concentration in dementia. *J Neurol Neurosurg Psychiatry* 46:911, 1983.

166. Gold PW, Goodwin FK, Ballenger JC, Post RM, Weingartner H, Robertson GL: Central vasopressin function in affective illness. *Int J Ment Health* 9(3–4):91, 1981.

167. Sorensen PS, Hammer M, Gjerris F: Cerebrospinal fluid vasopressin in benign intracranial hypertension. *Neurology* 32:1255, 1982.

168. Berliner BW, Levinsky NG, Davidson DG, Eden M: Dilution and concentration of the urine and the action of antidiuretic hormone. *Am J Med* 24:730, 1958.

169. Dousa TP, Valtin H: Cellular actions of vasopressin in the mammalian kidney. *Kidney Int* 10:46, 1976.

170. Andreoli TE, Schafer JA: Some considerations of the role of antidiuretic hormone in water homeostasis. *Recent Prog Horm Res* 33:387, 1977.

171. Dunn MJ, Hood VL: Prostaglandins and the kidney. *Am J Physiol* 233(2):F169, 1977.

172. Nakano J: Cardiovascular responses to neurohypophysial hormones, in Greep RO, Astwood EB, Knobil E, Sawyer WH, Geiger SR (eds): *Handbook of Physiology.* Washington, American Physiological Society, 1974, vol 4, pp 395–442.

173. Szczepanska-Sadowska E: Hemodynamic effects of a moderate increase of the plasma vasopressin level in conscious dogs. *Pfleugers Arch* 338:313, 1973.

174. Montani JP, Liard JF, Schoun J, Mohring J: Hemodynamic effects of exogenous and endogenous vasopressin at low plasma concentrations in dogs. *Circ Res* 47:346–355, 1980.

175. Graybiel A, Glendy RE: Circulatory effects following the intravenous administration of pitressin in normal persons and in patients with hypertension and angina pectoris. *Am Heart J* 21:481, 1941.

176. Padfield PL, Brown JJ, Lever AF, Morton JJ, Robertson JIS: Blood pressure in acute and chronic vasopressin excess. *N Engl J Med* 304:1067, 1981.

177. Ganguly A, Robertson GL: Elevated threshold for vasopressin release in primary hyperaldosteronism. *Clin Res* 28:330A, 1980.

178. Davies R, Forsling M, Bulger G, Phillips T: Plasma vasopressin and blood pressure studies in normal subjects and in benign essential hypertension at rest and after postural challenge. *Br Heart J* 49:528, 1983.

179. Mohring J, Glanger K, Maciel JA, Dusing R, Kramer HJ, Arbogast R, Koch-Weser J: Greatly enhanced pressor response to antidiuretic hormone in patients with impaired cardiovascular reflexes due to idiopathic orthostatic hypotension. *J Cardiovasc Pharmacol* 2:367, 1980.

180. Lymangrover BA Jr: The hypothalamic-pituitary-adrenocortical system, in McCann SM (ed): *International Review of Physiology.*

Baltimore, University Park, 1977, vol 2, pp 93–149.

181. McCann SM, Antunes-Rodrigues J, Nallar R, Valtin H: Pituitary adrenal function in the absence of vasopressin. *Endocrinology* 76:1058, 1966.

182. Arimura A, Saito T, Bowers CY, Schally AV: Pituitary adrenal activation in rats with hereditary hypothalamic diabetes insipidus. *Acta Endocrinol* 54:155, 1967.

183. Yates FE, Russell SM, Dallman MF, Hedge GA, McCann SM, Dhariwal APS: Potentiation by vasopressin of corticotropin release induced by corticotropin releasing factor. *Endocrinology* 88:3, 1971.

184. Liu JH, Muse K, Contreras P, Gibbs D, Vale W, Rivier J, Yeu SSC: Activation of ACTH-releasing activity of synthetic corticotropin releasing factor (CRF) by vasopressin in women. *J Clin Endocrinol Metab* 57:1087, 1983.

185. Rivier C, Vale W: Interaction of corticotropin releasing factor and arginine vasopressin on adrenocorticotropin secretion *in vivo*. *Endocrinology* 113:939, 1983.

186. Carlson DE, Gann DS: Effect of vasopressin antiserum on the response of adrenocorticotropin and cortisol to hemorrhage. *Endocrinology* 114:317, 1984.

187. Dicker SE, Nunn JE: The role of the antidiuretic hormone during water deprivation in rats. *J Physiol* 136:235, 1957.

188. Gaskill MB, Reilly M, Robertson GL: Vasopressin decreases insensible water loss. *Clin Res* 31:780A, 1983.

189. Schapiro H: Inhibiting action of antidiuretic hormone on canine pancreatic exocrine flow. *Am J Digest Dis* 20:853, 1975.

190. Heims DA, Whitton PD, Ma GY: Metabolic actions of vasopressin, glucagon and adrenalin in the intact rat. *Biochim Biophys Acta* 411:155, 1975.

191. Grant JA, Scrutton MC: Positive interaction between agonists in the aggregation response of human blood platelets: Interaction between ADP, adrenaline and vasopressin. *Br J Haematol* 44:109, 1980.

192. Fitzsimons JT: Thirst. *Physiol Rev* 52(2):468, 1972.

193. Andersson B: Regulation of water intake. *Physiol Rev* 58(3):582, 1978.

194. Wolf AV: Osmometric analysis of thirst in man and dog. *Am J Physiol* 161:75, 1950.

195. Rolls BJ, Wood RJ, Rolls ET, Lind H, Lind W, Ledingham JGG: Thirst following water deprivation in humans. *Am J Physiol* 239:R476, 1980.

196. Robertson GL: Abnormalities of thirst regulation (Nephrology Forum). *Kidney Int* 25:460, 1984.

197. Buggy J, Hoffman WE, Phillips MI, Fisher AE, Johnson AK: Osmosensitivity of rat third ventricle and interactions with angiotensin. *Am J Physiol* 5(1):R75, 1979.

198. Rundgren M, Fyhrquist F: A study of permanent adipsia induced by medial forebrain lesions. *Acta Physiol* 103:463, 1978.

199. Grossman SP, Dacey D, Halaris AE, Collier T, Routtenberg A: Aphagia and adipsia after preferential destruction of nerve cell bodies in hypothalamus. *Science* 202(3):537, 1978.

200. Buggy J, Johnson AK: Preoptic-hypothalamic periventricular lesions: Thirst deficits and hypernatremia. *Am J Physiol* 233(1):R44, 1977.

201. Coburn PC, Stricker EM: Osmoregulatory thirst in rats after lateral preoptic lesions. *J Comp Physiol Psychol* 92(2):350, 1978.

202. Fitzsimons JT: Drinking by rats depleted of body fluid without increase in osmotic pressure. *J Physiol* 159:297, 1961.

203. Kucharczyk J, Mogenson GJ: Separate lateral hypothalamic pathways for extracellular and intracellular thirst. *Am J Physiol* 228(1):295, 1975.

204. Kozlowski S, Szczepanska-Sadowska E: Antagonistic effects of vasopressin and hypervolemia on osmotic reactivity of the thirst mechanism in dogs. *Pflugers Arch* 353:59, 1975.

205. Epstein AN, Fitzsimons JT, Rolls BJ: Drinking induced by injection of angiotensin into the brain of the rat. *J Physiol* 210:457, 1970.

206. Simpson JB, Routtenberg A: Subfornical organ: Site of drinking elicitation by angiotensin II. *Science* 181:1170, 1973.

207. Szczepanska-Sadowska E, Kozlowski S, Sobocinska J: Blood antidiuretic hormone level and osmotic reactivity of thirst mechanism in dogs. *Am J Physiol* 227(4):766, 1974.

208. Altman PL, Dittmer DS (eds): *Blood and Other Body Fluids*. Washington, American Society of Experimental Biology, 1961.

209. Robertson GL, Berl T: Water metabolism, in Brenner BM, Rector FC (eds): *The Kidney*, 3d ed. Philadelphia, Saunders, 1985, pp 385–432.

210. Leaf A, Chatillon JY, Wrong O, Tuttle EP Jr: The mechanism of the osmotic adjustment of body cells as determined *in vivo* by the volume of distribution of a large water load. *J Clin Invest* 33:1261, 1954.

211. Wolf AV, McDowell ME: Apparent and osmotic volumes of distribution of sodium, chloride, sulfate and urea. *Am J Physiol* 176:207, 1954.

212. Hendry EB: Osmolarity of human serum and of chemical solutions of biologic importance. *Clin Chem* 7:156, 1961.

213. Darrow DC, Yanett H: Changes in distribution of body water accompanying increase and decrease in extracellular electrolytes. *J Clin Invest* 14:266, 1935.

214. Arieff AI, Guisado R, Lazarowitz VC: Pathophysiology of hyperosmolar states, in Andreoli TE et al. (eds): *Disturbances in Body Fluid Osmolality*. Bethesda, American Physiological Society, 1977.

215. Adolph EF: *Physiology of Man in the Desert*. New York, Hafner, 1969.

216. Coggins CH, Leaf A: Diabetes insipidus. *Am J Med* 42:807, 1967.

217. Maccubbin DA, Van Buren JM: A quantitative evaluation of hypothalamic degeneration and its relation to diabetes insipidus following interruption of the human hypophyseal stalk. *Brain* 86:443, 1963.

218. Randall RV, Clark EC, Dodge HW Jr, Love JG: Polyuria after operation for tumors in the region of the hypophysis and hypothalamus. *J Clin Endocrinol Metab* 20:1614, 1960.

219. Timmons RL, Dugger GS: Water and salt metabolism following pituitary stalk section. *Neurology* 19:790, 1969.

220. Blotner H: Primary or idiopathic diabetes insipidus: A system disease. *Metabolism* 7:191, 1958.

221. Braverman LE, Mancini JP, McGoldrick DM: Hereditary idiopathic diabetes insipidus: A case report with autopsy findings. *Ann Intern Med* 63(3):503, 1965.

222. Green JR, Buchan GC, Alvord EC Jr, Swanson AG: Hereditary and idiopathic types of diabetes insipidus. *Brain* 90(3):707, 1967.

223. Forssman H: Two different mutations of X-chromosome causing diabetes insipidus. *Am J Hum Genet* 7:21, 1955.

224. Cannon JF: Diabetes insipidus: Clinical and experimental studies with consideration of genetic relationships. *Arch Intern Med* 96:215, 1955.

225. Anderson KE, Arner B, Furst E, Hedner P: Antidiuretic responses to hypertonic saline infusion, water deprivation, and a synthetic analogue of vasopressin in patients with hereditary, hypothalamic diabetes insipidus. *Acta Med Scand* 195:17, 1974.

226. Robertson GL, Scheidler JA: A newly recognized variant of familial nephrogenic diabetes insipidus distinguished by partial resistance to vasopressin (type II). *Clin Res* 29:555A, 1981.

227. Notman DD, Mortek MA, Moses AM: Permanent diabetes insipidus following head trauma: Observations on ten patients and an approach to diagnosis. *J Trauma* 20(7):599, 1980.

228. Kimmel DW, O'Neill BP: Systemic cancer presenting as diabetes insipidus. *Cancer* 52:2355, 1983.

229. Winnacker JL, Becker KL, Katz S: Endocrine aspects of sarcoidosis. *N Engl J Med* 278(9):483, 1968.

230. Halprin KM, Lorincz AL: Disseminated xanthosiderohistiocytosis (xanthoma disseminatum). *Arch Dermatol* 82(2):171, 1960.

231. Kalz F, Hoffman MM, Lafrance A: Xanthoma disseminatum: Clinical and laboratory observations over a ten year period. *Dermatologica* 140:129, 1970.

232. Dorfman MSG, Ruark MGW, Agus ZS, Jacobs RL, Young RL: Transient diabetes insipidus with elevated serum osmolarity associated with "benign" febrile illness. *Arch Intern Med* 137:1479, 1977.

233. Scherbaum WA, Bottazzo GF: Autoantibodies to vasopressin cells in idiopathic diabetes insipidus: Evidence for an autoimmune variant. *Lancet,* 1:897, 1983.

234. Kuan P, Messenger JC, Ellestad MH: Transient central diabetes insipidus after aortocoronary bypass operations. *Am J Cardiol* 52:1181, 1983.

235. Verbalis JG, Nelson PB, Robinson AG: Reversible panhypopituitarism caused by a suprasellar aneurysm: The contribution of mass effect to pituitary dysfunction. *Neurosurgery* 10(5):604, 1982.

236. Halter JB, Goldberg AP, Robertson GL, Porte D Jr: Selective osmoreceptor dysfunction in the syndrome of chronic hypernatremia. *J Clin Endocrinol Metab* 44:609, 1977.

237. DeRubertis FR, Michelis MF, Beck N, Field JB, Davis BB: "Essential" hypernatremia due to ineffective osmotic and intact volume regulation of vasopressin secretion. *J Clin Invest* 50:97, 1971.

238. Rosansky SJ, Nidus BD: Volume receptor control of ADH release in essential hypernatremia. *NY State J Med* p 351, March 1981.

239. Kimura T, Matsui K, Ota K, Yoshinaga K: Hypothalamic hypernatremia due to volume-dependent ADH release and its treatment with carbamazepine and clofibrate. *Tohoku J Exp Med* 127:101, 1979.

240. DeRubertis FR, Michelis MF, Davis BB: "Essential" hypernatremia. *Arch Intern Med* 134:889, 1974.

241. Nichelli P, Baraldi A, Cappelli G: Hypernatremic thirst deficiency and memory disorders following hypothalamic lesions. *Arch Psychiatr Nervenkr* 231:459, 1982.

242. Nardi M, Harrington AR: Successful treatment of hypernatremic thirst deficiency with chlorpropamide. *Clin Nephrol* 10(3):90, 1978.

243. Zazgornik J, Jellinger K, Waldhausl W, Schmidt P: Excessive hypernatremia and hyperosmolality associated with germinoma in the hypothalamic and pituitary region. *Europ Neurol* 12:38, 1974.

244. Trust PM, Brown JJ, Chinn RH, Lever AF, Morton JJ, Padfield PL, Robertson JIS, Ireland JT, Melville ID, Thomson WST: A case of hypopituitarism with diabetes insipidus and loss of thirst: Role of antidiuretic hormone and angiotensin II in the control of urine flow and osmolality. *J Clin Endocrinol Metab* 41(2):346, 1975.

245. Khommami-Asadi F, Norman ME, Parks JS, Schwartz MW: Hypernatremia associated with pineal tumor. *J Pediatr* 90(4):605, 1977.

246. Sridhar CB, Calvert GD, Ibbertson HK: Syndrome of hypernatremia, hypodipsia and partial diabetes insipidus: A new interpretation. *J Clin Endocrinol Metab* 38:890, 1974.

247. Luciani JC, Conte-Devolx B, Fourcade JC, Barjon P: Chronic hypernatremia, hypovolemia and partial hypopituitarism in sarcoidosis: A case report. *Clin Nephrol* 13(5):242, 1980.

248. Takaku A, Shindo K, Tanaka S, Mori T, Suzuki J: Fluid and electrolyte disturbances in patients with intracranial aneurysms. *Surg Neurol* 11:349, 1979.

249. Cooper IS, MacCarty CS: Unusual electrolyte abnormalities associated with cerebral lesions. *Proc Staff Meetings Mayo Clin* 26:354, 1951.

250a. MacCarty CS, Cooper IS: Neurologic and metabolic effects of bilateral ligation of the anterior cerebral arteries in man. *Proc Staff Meetings Mayo Clin* 26:185, 1951.

250b. AvRuskin TW, Tang SC, Juan C: Essential hypernatremia, antidiuretic hormone and neurophysin secretion: Response to chlorpropamide. *Acta Endocrinol* 96:145, 1981.

251. Schaff-Blass E, Robertson GL, Rosenfield RL: Chronic hypernatremia resulting from a congenital defect in osmoregulation of thirst and vasopressin. *J Pediatr* 102(5):703, 1983.

252. Conley SB, Brocklebank JT, Taylor IT: Recurrent hypernatremia: A proposed mechanism in a patient with absence of thirst and abnormal excretion of water. *J Pediatr* 89(6):898, 1976.

253. Schaad U, Vassella F, Zuppinger K, Oetliker O: Hypodipsia-hypernatremia syndrome. *Helv Paediatr Acta* 34:63, 1979.

254. Sleeper FH, Jellinek EM: A comparative physiologic, psychologic and psychiatric study of polyuric and nonpolyuric schizophrenic patients. *J Nerv Ment Dis* 83:557, 1936.

255. Barlow ED, de Wardener HED: Compulsive water drinking. *Q J Med* 28:235, 1959.

256. Robertson GL: Diagnosis of diabetes insipidus, in Czernichow AP, Robinson A (eds): *Diabetes Insipidus in Man. Frontiers of Hormone Research.* Basel, Karger, 1985, vol 13, pp 127–155.

257. Stuart CA, Neelon FA, Lebovitz HE: Disordered control of thirst in hypothalamic-pituitary sarcoidosis. *N Engl J Med* 303:1078, 1980.

258. Coscina DV, Grant LD, Balagura S, Grossman SP: Hyperdipsia after serotonin-depleting midbrain lesions. *Nature [New Biol]* 235:53, 1972.

259. Blass EM, Nussbaum AI: Specific enhancement of drinking to angiotensin in rats. *J Comp Physiol Psychol* 87(3):422, 1974.

260. Grossman SP, Grossman L: Food and water intake in rats after transections of fibers en passage in the tegmentum. *Physiol Behav* 18:647, 1977.

261. Williams RH, Henry C: Nephrogenic diabetes insipidus: Transmitted by females and appearing during infancy in males. *Ann Intern Med* 27:84, 1947.

262. Waring AJ, Kadji L, Tappan V: A congenital defect in water metabolism. *Am J Dis Child* 69:323, 1945.

263. Bode HH, Crawford JD: Nephrogenic diabetes insipidus in North America—the Hopewell hypothesis. *N Engl J Med* 280(14): 750, 1969.

264. Bell NH, Clark CM Jr, Avery S, Sinha T, Trygstad CW, Allen DO: Demonstration of a defect in the formation of adenosine 3′,5′-monophosphate in vasopressin-resistant diabetes insipidus. *Pediatr Res* 8:223, 1974.

265. Ohzeki T, Igarashi T, Okamoto A: Familial cases of congenital nephrogenic diabetes insipidus type II: Remarkable increment of urinary adenosine 3′,5′-monophosphate in response to antidiuretic hormone. *J Pediatr* 104(4):593, 1984.

266. Singer I, Forrest JN Jr: Drug-induced states of nephrogenic diabetes insipidus. *Kidney Int* 10:82, 1976.

267. Bichet DG, Levi M, Schrier RW: Polyuria, dehydration and overhydration, in Seldin DW, Giebisch G (eds): *The Kidney: Physiology and Pathophysiology.* New York, Raven, 1985, p 957.

268. Lipsett MB, MacLean JP, West CD, et al: An analysis of the polyuria induced by hypophysectomy in man. *J Clin Endocrinol* 16:183, 1956.

269. Lipsett MB, Pearson OH: Further studies of diabetes insipidus following hypophysectomy in man. *J Lab Clin Med* 49:190, 1957.

270. Miller M, Dalakos T, Moses AM, Fellerman H: Recognition of partial defects in antidiuretic hormone secretion. *Ann Intern Med* 73:721, 1970.

271. Zerbe RL, Robertson GL: A comparison of plasma vasopressin measurements with a standard indirect test in the differential diagnosis of polyuria. *N Engl J Med* 305:1539, 1981.

272. Robertson GL: Osmoregulation of thirst and vasopressin secretion: Functional properties and their relationship to water balance, in Schrier R (ed): *Vasopressin.* New York, Raven, 1985, pp 202–212.

273. Epstein FH, Kleeman CR, Hendrikx A: The influence of bodily hydration on the renal concentrating process. *J Clin Invest* 36:629, 1957.

274. De Wardener HE, Herxheimer A: The effect of high water intake on the kidney's ability to concentrate the urine in man. *J Physiol (Lond)* 139:42, 1957.

275. Alexander CS, Filbin DM, Fruchtman SA: Failure of vasopressin to produce normal urine concentration in patients with diabetes insipidus. *J Lab Clin Med* 54:566, 1959.

276. Harrington AR, Valtin H: Impaired urinary concentration after vasopressin and its gradual correction in hypothalamic diabetes insipidus. *J Clin Invest* 47:502, 1968.

277. Block LH, Furrer J, Locher RA, Siegenthaler W, Vetter W: Changes in tissue sensitivity to vasopressin in hereditary hypothalamic diabetes insipidus. *Klin Wochenschr* 59:831, 1981.

278. Robertson GL, Aycinena P: Neurogenic disorders of osmoregulation. *Am J Med* 72:339, 1982.

279. Opas LM, Adler R, Robinson R, Lieberman E: Rhabdomyolysis with severe hypernatremia. *J Pediatr* 90(5):713, 1977.

280. Zierler KL: Hyperosmolarity in adults: A critical review. *J Chronic Dis* 7(1):1, 1958.

281. Simon RP, Freedman DD: Neurologic manifestations of osmolar disorders. *Geriatrics* p 71, June 1980.

282. Sparacio RR, Anziska B, Schutta HS: Hypernatremia and chorea: A report of two cases. *Neurology* 26:46, 1976.

283. Welt LG: Hypo- and hypernatremia. *Ann Intern Med* 56(1):161, 1962.

284. Smith WO, Clark ML: Self-induced water intoxication in schizophrenic patients. *Am J Psychiatry* 137(9):1055, 1980.

285. Hariprasad MK, Eisinger RP, Nadler IM, Padmanabhan CS, Nidus BD: Hyponatremia in psychogenic polydipsia. *Arch Intern Med* 140:1639, 1980.

286. Rosenbaum JF, Rothman JS, Murray GB: Psychosis and water intoxication. *J Clin Psychiatry* 40:287, 1979.

287. Raskind MA, Orenstein H, Christopher TG: Acute psychosis, increased water ingestion and inappropriate antidiuretic hormone secretion. *Am J Psychiatry* 132(9):907, 1975.

288. Robertson GL: Psychogenic polydipsia and inappropriate antidiuresis. *Arch Intern Med* 140:1574, 1980.

289. Weiss NM, Robertson GL: Effect of hypercalcemia and lithium therapy on the osmoregulation of thirst and vasopressin secretion, in Schrier R (ed): *Vasopressin.* New York, Raven, 1985, pp 281–289.

290. Cutler RE, Kleeman CR, Maxwell MH, Dowling JT: Physiologic studies in nephrogenic diabetes insipidus. *J Clin Endocrinol Metab* 22:827, 1962.

291. Dashe AM, Cramm RE, Crist CA, Habener JF, Solomon DH: A water deprivation test for the differential diagnosis of polyuria. *JAMA* 185(9):699, 1963.

292. Miller M, Moses AM: Urinary antidiuretic hormone in polyuric disorders and in inappropriate ADH syndrome. *Ann Intern Med* 77:715, 1972.

293. Baylis PH, Gaskill MB, Robertson GL: Vasopressin secretion in primary polydipsia and cranial diabetes insipidus. *Q J Med* 199:345, 1981.

294. Milles JJ, Spruce B, Baylis PH: A comparison of diagnostic methods to differentiate diabetes insipidus from primary polyuria: A review of 21 patients. *Acta Endocrinol* 104:410, 1983.

295. Skillern PG, Corcoran AC, Scherbel AL: Renal mechanisms in coincident Addison's disease and diabetes insipidus: Effects of vasopressin and hydrocortisone. *J Clin Endocrinol Metab* 16(2):171, 1956.

296. Martin MM: Combined anterior pituitary and neurohypophyseal insufficiency: Studies of body fluid spaces and renal function. *J Clin Invest* 38(6):882, 1958.

297. Takeda R, Hiraiwa Y, Hayashi T, Yasuhara S, Yanase E, Sakato T, Nakabayashi H, Takegoshi T, Nishino T, Tanino M, Yamaji T: Spontaneous remission of cranial diabetes insipidus due to concomitant development of ADH-producing lung cancer—an autopsied case. *Acta Endocrinol* 104:417, 1983.

298. Vokes T, Gaskill M, Robertson GL: Antivasopressin antibodies in neurogenic diabetes insipidus. *Clin Res* 32:275A, 1984.

299. Edwards CRW, Kitau MJ, Chard T, Besser GM: Vasopressin analogue DDAVP in diabetes insipidus: Clinical and laboratory studies. *Br Med J* 2:375, 1973.

300. Ziai F, Walter R, Rosenthal IM: Treatment of central diabetes insipidus in adults and children with desmopressin. *Arch Intern Med* 138:1382, 1978.

301. Cobb WE, Spare S, Reichlin S: Neurogenic diabetes insipidus: Management with dDAVP (1-desamino-8-D-arginine vasopressin). *Ann Intern Med* 88:183, 1978.

302. Arduino F, Ferraz FPJ, Rodriques J: Antidiuretic action of chlorpropamide in idiopathic diabetes insipidus. *J Clin Endocrinol Metab* 26:1325, 1966.

303. Webster B, Bain J: Antidiuretic effect and complications of chlorpropamide therapy in diabetes insipidus. *J Clin Endocrinol Metab* 30(2):215, 1970.

304. Weissman PN, Shenkman L, Gregerman RI: Chlorpropamide hyponatremia: Drug-induced inappropriate antidiuretic-hormone activity. *N Engl J Med* 284(2):65, 1971.

305. Hayes JS, Kaye M: Inappropriate secretion of antidiuretic hormone induced by chlorpropamide. *Am J Med* 263(3):137, 1972.

306. Garcia M, Miller M, Moses AM: Chlorpropamide-induced water retention in patients with diabetes mellitus. *Ann Intern Med* 75:549, 1971.

307. Mendoza SA, Brown CF Jr: Effect of chlorpropamide on osmotic water flow across toad bladder and the response to vasopressin, theophylline and cyclic AMP. *J Clin Endocrinol Metab* 388:883, 1974.

308. Berndt WO, Miller M, Kettyle M, Valtin H: Potentiation of the antidiuretic effect of vasopressin by chlorpropamide. *Endocrinology* 86(5):1028, 1970.

309. Miller M, Moses AM: Potentiation of vasopressin action by chlorpropamide in vivo. *Endocrinology* 86(5):1024, 1970.

310. Murase T, Yoshida S: Mechanism of chlorpropamide action in patients with diabetes insipidus. *J Clin Endocrinol Metab* 36:174, 1973.

311. Ingelfinger JR, Hays RM: Evidence that chlorpropamide and vasopressin share a common site of action. *J Clin Endocrinol Metab* 29:738, 1969.

312. Meinders AE, Van Leeuwen AM, Borst JGG, Cejka V: Paradoxical diuresis after vasopressin administration to patients with neurohypophyseal diabetes insipidus treated with chlorpropamide, carbamazepine or clofibrate. *Clin Sci Mol Med* 49:283, 1975.

313. de Gennes JL, Bertrand C, Bigorie B, Truffert J: Etudes preliminaires de l'action antidiuretique du clofibrate (ou atromid S) dans le diabète insipide pitressonsensible. *Ann Endocrinol* 31:300, 1970.

314. Thompson P Jr, Earll JM, Schaaf M: Comparison of clofibrate and chlorpropamide in vasopressin-responsive diabetes insipidus. *Metabolism* 26(7):749, 1977.

315. Sekowski I, Samuel P: Clofibrate-induced acute muscular syndrome. *Am J Cardiol* 30:572, 1972.

316. Earley LE, Orloff J: The mechanism of antidiuresis associated with administration of hydrochlorothiazide to patients with vasopressin resistant diabetes insipidus. *J Clin Invest* 41:1988, 1962.

317. Paller MS, Schrier RW: Pathogenesis of sodium and water retention in edematous disorders. *Am J Kidney Dis* 2:241, 1982.

318. Rondeau E, de Lima J, Caillens H, Ardaillou R, Vahanian A, Acar J: High plasma antidiuretic hormone in patients with cardiac failure: Influence of age. *Mineral Electrolyte Metab* 8:267, 1982.

319. Goldsmith SR, Francis GS, Cowley AW, Levine TB, Cohn JN: Increased plasma arginine vasopressin levels in patients with congestive heart failure. *J Am Coll Cardiol* 1:1385, 1983.

320. Takasic T, Lasker N, Shalhouh RJ: Mechanisms of hyponatremia in chronic congestive heart failure. *Ann Intern Med* 55:368, 1961.

321. Pruszczynski W, Vahanian A, Ardaillou R, Acar J: Role of antidiuretic hormone in impaired water excretion of patients with congestive heart failure. *J Clin Endocrinol Metab* 58:599, 1984.

322. Uretsky BF, Verbalis JG, Generalovich T, Valdes A, Reddy PS: Plasma vasopressin response to osmotic and hemodynamic stimuli in heart failure. *Am J Physiol* 248:H396, 1985.

323. deTorrente A, Robertson GL, McDonald KM, Schrier RW: Mechanism of diuretic response to increased left atrial pressure in the anesthetized dog. *Kidney Int* 8:355, 1975.

324. Klinger EJ Jr, Vaamonde CA, Vaamonde LE, Lancestremere RG, Morosi SJ, Frisch E, Papper S: Renal function changes in cirrhosis of the liver. *Arch Intern Med* 125:1010, 1970.

325. Arroyo V, Rodes J, Guitierrez-Lizarraga MA, Revert L: Prognostic value of spontaneous hyponatremia in cirrhosis with ascites. *Am J Digest Dis* 21:249, 1976.

326. Schrier RW: Mechanisms of disturbed renal water excretion in cirrhosis. *Gastroenterology* 84:870, 1983.

327. Bichet D, Szatalowicz V, Chaimovitz C, Schrier RW: Role of vasopressin in abnormal water excretion in cirrhotic patients. *Ann Intern Med* 96:413, 1982.

328. Bichet D, Van Putten VJ, Schrier RW: Potential role of increased sympathetic activity in impaired sodium and water excretion in cirrhosis. *N Engl J Med* 307:1552, 1982.

329. Reznick RK, Langer B, Taylor BR, Seif S, Blendis LM: Hyponatremia and arginine vasopressin secretion in patients with refractory hepatic ascites undergoing peritoneovenous shunting. *Gastroenterology* 84:713, 1983.

330. Linas SL, Anderson RJ, Guggenheim SJ, Robertson GL, Berl T: The role of vasopressin in the impaired water excretion in the conscious rat with experimental cirrhosis. *Kidney Int* 20:173, 1981.

331. Earley LE, Sanders CA: The effect of changing serum osmolality on antidiuretic hormone release in certain patients with decompensated cirrhosis of the liver and low serum osmolality. *J Clin Invest* 38:545, 1959.

332. Gur A, Adejuin PY, Siegel MJ, Hayslett JP: A study of the renal handling of water in lipoid nephrosis. *Pediatr Res* 10:197, 1976.

333. Usberti M, Federico S, Cianciaruso B, Becoraro C, Andreucci VE: Role of plasma vasopressin in the impairment of water excretion in nephrotic syndrome. *Kidney Int* 25(2):422, 1984.

334. Berlyne GM, Sutton J, Brown C, Feinroth MV, Feinroth M, Adler AJ, Friedman EA: Renal salt and water handling in water immersion in the nephrotic syndrome. *Clin Sci* 61:605, 1981.

335. Krishna GG, Danovitch GM: Effects of water immersion on renal function in the nephrotic syndrome. *Kidney Int* 21:395, 1982.

336. Dorhout Mees EJ, Roos JC, Boer P, Yoe OH, Simatupang TA: Observations on edema formation in the nephrotic syndrome in adults with minimal lesions. *Am J Med* 67:378, 1979.

337. Meltzer JI, Keim HJ, Laragh JH, Sealey JE, Jan K, Shien S: Nephrotic syndrome: Vasoconstriction and hypervolemic types indicated by renin-sodium profiling. *Ann Intern Med* 91:688, 1979.

338. Fichman MP, Vorherr H, Kleeman CR, Tefler N: Diuretic induced hyponatremia. *Ann Intern Med* 75:853, 1971.

339. Berl T, Linas SL, Aisenbrey GA, Anderson RJ: On the mechanism of polyuria in potassium depletion: The role of polydipsia. *J Clin Invest* 60:620, 1977.

340. Rutecki GW, Cox JW, Robertson GL, Francisco LL, Ferris TF: Urinary concentrating ability and antidiuretic hormone responsiveness in the potassium depleted dog. *J Lab Clin Med* 100:53, 1982.

341. Schrier RW, Linas SL: Mechanisms of the defect in water excretion in adrenal insufficiency. *Mineral Electrolyte Metab* 4:107, 1980.

342. Green HH, Harrington AR, Valtin H: On the role of antidiuretic hormone in the inhibition of acute water diuresis in adrenal insufficiency and the effects of gluco- and mineralocorticoids in reversing the inhibition. *J Clin Invest* 49:1724, 1970.

343. Boykin J, McCool A, Robertson G, McDonald K, Schrier R: Mechanisms of impaired water excretion in mineralocorticoid deficient dogs. *Mineral Electrolyte Metab* 2:310, 1979.

344. Ufferman RC, Schrier RW: Importance of sodium intake and mineralocorticoid hormone in the impaired water excretion in adrenal insufficiency. *J Clin Invest* 51:1639, 1972.

345. Agus ZS, Goldberg M: Role of antidiuretic hormone in the abnormal water diuresis of hypopituitarism in man. *J Clin Invest* 50:1478, 1971.

346. Boykin J, de Torrente A, Erickson A, Robertson GL, Schrier RW: Role of plasma vasopressin in impaired water excretion of glucocorticoid deficiency. *J Clin Invest* 62:738, 1978.

347. Linas SL, Berl T, Robertson GL, Aisenbrey GA, Schrier RW, Anderson RJ: Role of vasopressin in the impaired water excretion of glucocorticoid deficiency. *Kidney Int* 18:58, 1980.

348. Mandell IN, DeFronzo RA, Robertson GL, Forrest JN: The role of plasma arginine vasopressin in the impaired water diuresis of isolated glucocorticoid deficiency in the rat. *Kidney Int* 17:186, 1980.

349. Ahmed ABJ, George BC, Gonzalez-Auvert C, Dingman JF: Increased plasma arginine vasopressin in clinical adrenocortical insufficiency and its inhibition by glucosteroids. *J Clin Invest* 46:111, 1967.

350. Kleeman CR, Czaczkes JW, Cutler R: Mechanism of impaired water excretion in adrenal and pituitary insufficiency: IV. Antidiuretic hormone—primary and secondary adrenal insufficiency. *J Clin Invest* 43:1641, 1964.

351. Green HH, Harrington AR, Valtin H: On the role of antidiuretic hormone in the inhibition of acute water diuresis in adrenal insufficiency and the effects of gluco- and mineralocorticoids in reversing the inhibition. *J Clin Invest* 49:1724, 1970.

352. Silverman AJ, Hoffman D, Gadde CA, Krey LC, Zimmerman EA: Adrenal steroid inhibition of the vasopressin-neurophysin neurosecretory system to the median eminence of rat: Differential effects of corticosterone and desoxycorticosterone administration after adrenalectomy. *Neuroendocrinology* 32:129, 1981.

353. Bartter FC: The syndrome of inappropriate secretion of antidiuretic hormone (SIADH). *Disease-A-Month*, November 1973.

354. Skowsky WR, Kikuchi TA: The role of vasopressin in the impaired water excretion of myxedema. *Am J Med* 64:613, 1978.

355. De Rubertis FR, Michelis MF, Bloom ME, Mintz DU, Fidd JB, Davis BD: Impaired water excretion in myxedema. *Am J Med* 51:41, 1971.

356. Zerbe RL, Stropes L, Robertson GL: Vasopressin function in the syndrome of inappropriate antidiuresis. *Annu Rev Med* 31:315, 1980.

357. Robertson GL: Cancer and inappropriate antidiuresis, in Rudden RW (ed): *Biological Markers of Neoplasia: Basic and Applied Aspects.* New York, Elsevier North-Holland, 1978, pp 277–293.

358. Leaf A, Bartter FC, Santos RF, Wrong O: Evidence in man that urinary electrolyte loss induced by pitressin is a function of water retention. *J Clin Invest* 32:868, 1953.

359. Michelis MF, Fusco RD, Bragdon RW, Davis BB: Reset of osmoreceptors in association with normovolemic hyponatremia. *Am J Med Sci* 267:267, 1974.

360. DeFronzo RA, Goldberg M, Agus ZS: Normal diluting capacity in hyponatremic patients. *Ann Intern Med* 84:538, 1976.

361. Arieff AI, Llach F, Massry SG: Neurological manifestations and morbidity of hyponatremia: Correlation of brain water and electrolytes. *Medicine* 55:121, 1976.

362. Messert B, Ornson WW, Hawkins MJ: Central pontine myelinolysis. *Neurology* 29:147, 1979.

363. Covey CM, Arieff AI: Disorders of sodium and water metabolism and their effects on the central nervous system, in Brenner BM, Stein JH (eds): *Sodium and Water Homeostasis. Contemporary Issues in Nephrology*, vol. I. New York, Churchill Livingstone, 1978.

364. Smithline N, Gardner K: Gaps—anionic and osmolal. *JAMA* 236:1594, 1976.

365. Dzau VJ, Colucci WS, Williams GH, Curfman G, Meggs L,

Hollenberg NK: Sustained effectiveness of converting enzyme inhibition in patients with severe congestive heart failure. *N Engl J Med* 302:1373, 1980.

366. Yamahiro HW, Reynolds TB: Effects of ascitic fluid infusion on sodium excretion, blood volume and creatinine clearance in cirrhosis. *Gastroenterology* 40:497, 1961.

367. Schedl HP, Bartter FC: An explanation for an experimental correction of the abnormal water diuresis in cirrhosis. *J Clin Invest* 39:248, 1960.

368. Schrier RW, Lehman D, Zacherle B, Early LE: Effect of furosemide on free water excretion in edematous patients with hyponatremia. *Kidney Int* 3:30, 1973.

369. Ayus JC, Olivero JJ, Fromer JP: Rapid correction of severe hyponatremia with intravenous hypertonic saline solution. *Am J Med* 72:43, 1982.

370. Kleinschmidt-DeMasters BK, Norenberg MD: Rapid correction of hyponatremia causes demyelination: Relation to central pontine myelinolysis. *Science* 211:1068, 1981.

371. Norenberg MD, Leslie KO, Robertson AS: Association between rise in serum sodium and CPM. *Ann Neurol* 11:128, 1982.

372. Cherrill DA, Stote RM, Birge JR, Singer I: Demeclocycline treatment in the syndrome of inappropriate antidiuretic hormone secretion. *Ann Intern Med* 83:654, 1975.

373. deTroyer A: Demeclocycline: Treatment of syndrome of inappropriate antidiuretic hormone secretion. *JAMA* 237:2723, 1977.

374. Dousa TP, Wilson DM: Effect of demethylchlortetracycline on cellular action of antidiuretic hormone in vitro. *Kidney Int* 5:279, 1974.

375. Miller PD, Linas SL, Schrier RW: Plasma demeclocycline levels and nephrotoxicity: Correlation in hyponatremic cirrhotic patients. *JAMA* 243:2513, 1980.

376. Oster JR, Epstein M, Ulano HB: Deterioration of renal function with demeclocycline administration. *Curr Ther Res* 20:794, 1976.

377. Forrest JN, Cox M, Hong C, Morrisson G, Bia M, Singer I: Superiority of demeclocycline over lithium in the treatment of chronic syndrome of inappropriate secretion of antidiuretic hormone. *N Engl J Med* 298:173, 1978.

378. Decaux G, Waterlot Y, Genette F, Mockel J: Treatment of the syndrome of inappropriate secretion of antidiuretic hormone with furosemide. *N Engl J Med* 304:329, 1981.

379. Decaux G, Genette F: Urea for long term treatment of syndrome of inappropriate secretion of antidiuretic hormone. *Br Med J* 283:1081, 1981.

380. Redetzki HM, Hughes JR, Redetzki JE: Difference between serum and plasma osmolalities and their relationship to lactic acid values. *Proc Soc Exp Biol Med* 139:315, 1972.

PART III

THYROID DISEASE

10

The Thyroid: Physiology, Hyperthyroidism, Hypothyroidism, and the Painful Thyroid

Robert D. Utiger

Thyroid hormones are the only known iodine-containing compounds with biological activity. They have two important actions. In the maturing mammal, they are crucial determinants of normal development. In the adult, their major role is to maintain metabolic stability; in so acting they affect the function of virtually every organ system. To maintain thyroid hormone availability, there are substantial reservoirs of thyroid hormone in the blood and thyroid gland. The hypothalamic-pituitary system which regulates thyroidal hormone production is exquisitely sensitive to small changes in circulating hormone concentrations; it thus can maintain thyroid secretion within a narrow range.

Thyroid diseases are relatively common; they occur in the form of abnormalities in the size and shape of the thyroid gland (i.e., *goiter*) and abnormalities of thyroid secretion. Thyroid abnormalities may exist alone or in combination. Moreover, many nonthyroidal illnesses are accompanied by alterations in thyroid physiology, complicating the evaluation of thyroid status in many patients. Clinical observations provide the initial evidence or first suspicion that an individual patient has a thyroid disorder. However, because the symptoms and signs of thyroid diseases are frequently subtle or ambiguous, laboratory tests are important for establishing diagnoses. While many tests are available, the judicious use of only a few, selected and interpreted on the basis of an understanding of thyroid physiology, is usually sufficient to confirm or exclude suspected thyroid dysfunction.

PHYSIOLOGY AND ANATOMY

Clinical Anatomy

The normal adult thyroid gland weighs 15 to 20 g; it is composed of two encapsulated lobes, one on either side of the trachea (Fig. 10-1A), connected by a thin isthmus which crosses the trachea anteriorly just below the cricoid cartilage. The lobes may overlap the trachea to a considerable extent, but more often are beside it. Sometimes a pyramidal lobe is found extending superiorly from the isthmus in the midline, indicating the embryologic path along which the thyroid developed. Thyroid volume can be measured precisely by ultrasound. It ranged from 10 to 30 ml in one study of normal individuals.[1] Thyroid volume was slightly greater in men than women and increased slightly with age.

In the embryo, the thyroid develops as a pouch in the pharyngeal floor which elongates inferiorly as the thyroglossal duct and becomes bilobar as it descends through the neck. Rarely, one or both thyroid lobes fail to develop.[2] If migration is arrested, the thyroid may remain at the base of the tongue (lingual thyroid) or be found at other locations between the base of the tongue and the lower neck (thyroglossal duct remnants). Occasionally, the thyroid follows the developmental path of the thymus into the thorax where, decades later, it may become manifest as a substernal goiter, compressing the trachea or a recurrent laryngeal nerve or even causing superior vena cava obstruction.

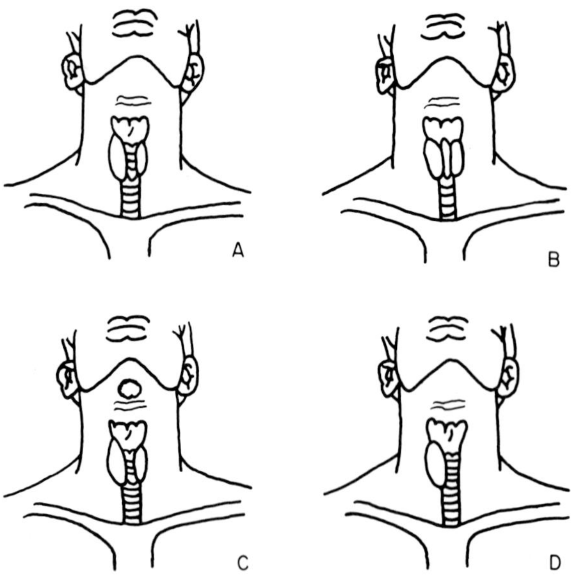

FIGURE 10-1 The normal thyroid gland and variations in thyroid anatomy. (*A*) Normal thyroid. (*B*) Pyramidal lobe between two normal thyroid lobes. (*C*) Thyroglossal remnant above larynx. (*D*) Agenesis of left thyroid lobe.

Some of these anomalies of development are shown in Fig. 10-1. The arterial supply of the thyroid is derived primarily from paired superior and inferior thyroid arteries. The former arise from the external carotid arteries and the latter from the thyrocervical trunks. The venous drainage is more complex and variable; usually there are paired superior, middle, and inferior thyroid veins. Normally, two pairs of parathyroid glands lie behind the upper and lower poles of the thyroid. The recurrent laryngeal nerves run along the trachea, medially and behind the lobes of the thyroid.

PHYSICAL EXAMINATION

First, the patient's neck should be inspected from the front before and during swallowing, with the patient's head slightly extended; the thyroid lobes may be seen and the presence of lobar enlargement or thyroid nodules noted. The examiner should then move behind the seated patient to palpate the neck. Both sides of the neck should be palpated while the patient swallows. First, the examiner's hands should be placed on the same side of the patient's neck; then each side of the neck should be palpated with the examiner's opposite hand. This maneuver allows lateral displacement of the sternomastoid muscle and thus often provides better delineation of the outline of each lobe. It is impossible to examine the thyroid adequately when the patient is supine. The thyroid is palpable in most normal individuals, the lobes being up to 3 cm long. The thyroid surface may be slightly irregular. Both size and consistency of the gland should be recorded, in addition to any local irregularities. For low-lying thyroids, it is helpful to have the patient extend the neck slightly.

In addition to the isthmus and the pyramidal lobe of the thyroid, several lesions may be found in the midline (Table 10-1). In addition to the thyroid lobes and thyroid lobe abnormalities, other masses may be palpable in the lateral neck regions (Table 10-1). Most such masses, however, can be distinguished from thyroid masses by their position and/or failure to move with swallowing.

The most practical way to determine the size of thyroid lobes and nodules is by measurement of their vertical and horizontal dimensions. The outline of the thyroid can be traced on thin, flexible paper. Estimates based on degree of enlargement or weight are so subjective as to be of little value at another time or to another examiner.

HISTOLOGY

Microscopically, thyroid tissue consists predominantly of spheroidal thyroid follicles. Each follicle consists of a single layer of cuboidal follicular cells surrounding a lumen filled with a viscid homogeneous material called *colloid.* When stimulated, the follicular cells become columnar and the follicles are depleted of colloid; when suppressed, the follicular cells become flat and colloid accumulates. The luminal surface of each follicular cell is covered with microvilli extending into the colloid. The cytoplasm is filled with membrane-bound microsomes on a rich endoplasmic reticulum. Near the apex of the cell are both exocytotic vesicles (secretory droplets) and endocytotic vesicles (colloid droplets), which are formed by the invagination of part of the luminal membrane. The formation of both

Table 10-1. Differential Diagnosis of Neck Masses

Midline mass
Thyroid isthmus, pyramidal lobe
Thyroglossal duct cyst
Pretracheal lymph nodes
Lateral neck mass
Thyroid lobes and intrathyroidal lesions
Anterior cervical lymphadenopathy
Branchial cleft cyst
Sternocleidomastoid fibrosis following trauma
Cystic hygroma
Arterial aneurysm
Carotid body tumor
Parathyroid masses

exocytotic and endocytotic vesicles is enhanced by hormonal stimulation.

Between the follicles and impinging on their surface are capillaries as well as adrenergic, cholinergic, and peptidergic nerve terminals. These abut both capillaries and follicles; their activation may alter not only thyroid blood flow but also thyroid hormone secretion.[3,4]

The thyroid also contains parafollicular or C cells in the interfollicular connective tissue and, in lesser numbers, within thyroid follicles. These cells produce calcitonin. Electron microscopy differentiates them from thyroid follicular cells because they have more numerous mitochondria and electron-dense granules surrounded by membranes which contain the storage form of calcitonin.

Chemistry of Thyroid Hormones

The structures of the thyroid hormones *thyroxine* (T_4) and *triiodothyronine* (T_3), their precursor iodotyrosines, thyronine, and several metabolites of T_4 and T_3 are shown in Fig. 10-2. The two thyroid hormones and many of their metabolites are iodinated thyronines; that is, they contain a phenyl ring attached via

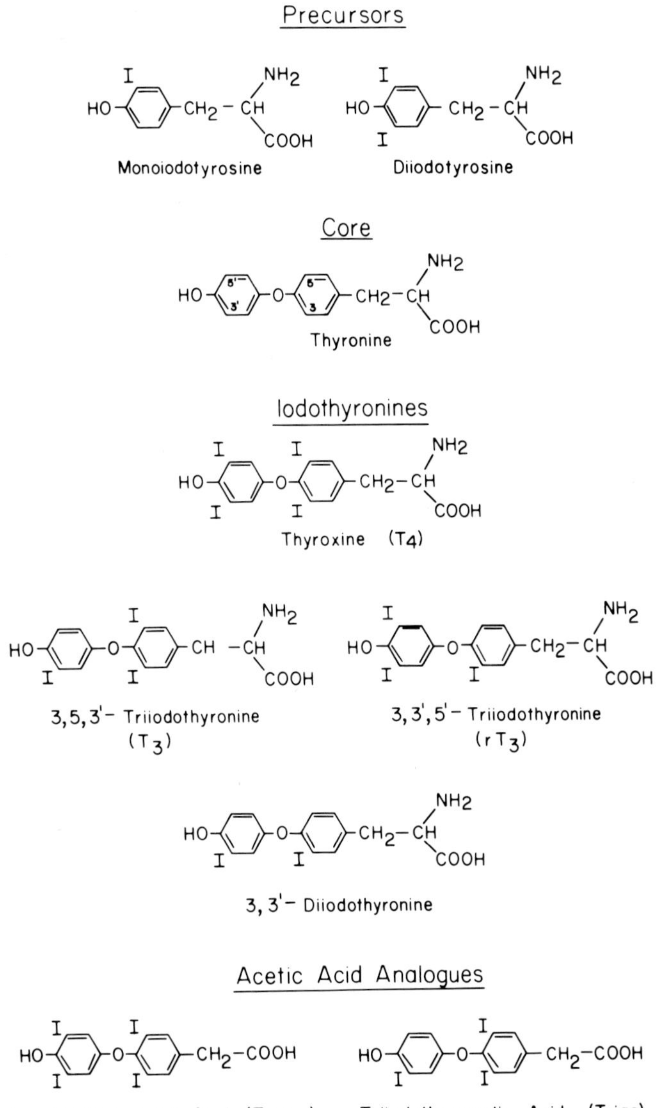

FIGURE 10-2 Structural formulas of various iodothyronines and analogues.

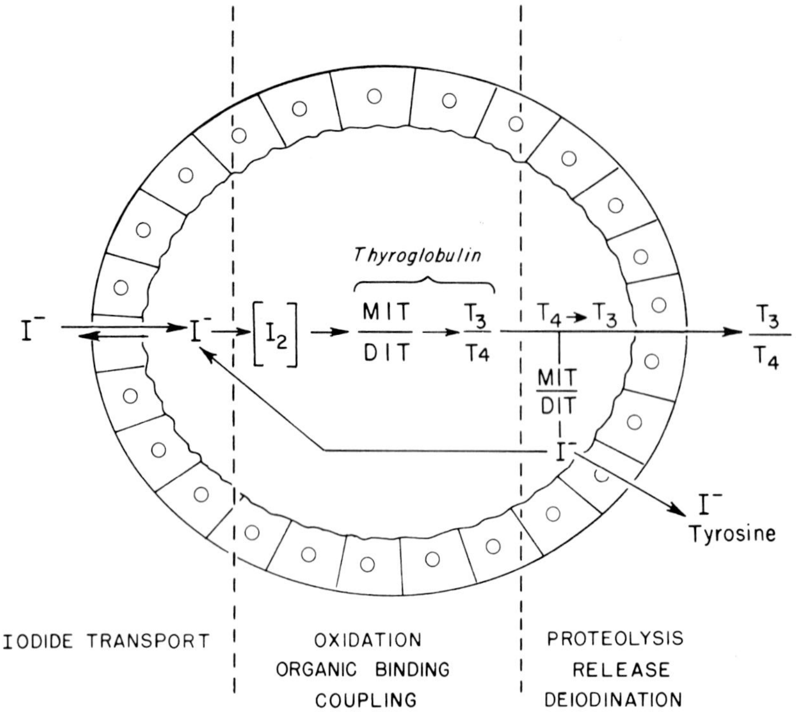

FIGURE 10-3 Outline of a thyroid follicle and the major steps of thyroid hormone biosynthesis and release.

ether linkage to tyrosine and from one to four iodine atoms. Thus, T_4 and T_3 are iodinated analogues of the amino acid tyrosine; they retain the α-amino carboxyl structure of amino acids. T_4 is 3,5,3′,5′-tetraiodothyronine, whereas T_3 is 3,5,3′-triiodothyronine, having one less iodine on the outer ring. If an iodine atom is removed from the *inner* ring of T_4 instead, the compound formed is 3,3′,5′-triiodothyronine, "reverse T_3" (rT_3). Diiodothyronine (T_2) can exist in three forms: two iodine atoms on the outer ring (3′,5′-T_2), two on the inner ring (3,5-T_2), or one on each (3,3′-T_2). When the amino group and a methylene group are removed from the alanine side chain of T_4, tetraiodothyroacetic acid (tetrac) is formed; T_3 similarly gives rise to triiodothyroacetic acid (triac).

Thyroid Hormone Biosynthesis

T_4 is solely a product of the thyroid gland, whereas T_3 is produced both by the thyroid and by deiodination of T_4 at extrathyroidal sites. The thyroid stores large amounts of T_4 and T_3 incorporated in thyroglobulin, the unique protein within which T_4 and T_3 formation occurs. Because of these stores, T_4 and T_3 can be secreted rapidly without the need for new hormone synthesis. The overall process of hormone production is shown in Fig. 10-3.

IODIDE ECONOMY

The major natural sources of iodine are food and water (see Chap. 11). Iodide intake varies greatly as a result both of varying iodide content of food and water and of dietary preferences; in many regions of the world iodide intake is inadequate or only barely adequate. In the United States, daily iodide intake averages about 500 μg because of the addition of iodide to salt and iodate to flour.[5] The recommended minimum intake is 150 μg daily, although the amount required to prevent goiter due to iodine deficiency in adults is about 50 to 75 μg daily. After its ingestion, iodide is absorbed rapidly and is distributed in the extracellular fluid, in which the iodide concentration is about 1 μg/dl. This pool receives not only dietary iodide but iodide that is released from the thyroid (normally about 50 μg per day) and iodide derived from peripheral iodothyronine deiodination. Iodide leaves this pool by two major routes, transport into the thyroid or excretion in the urine; small amounts also are lost via feces and sweat. Iodide is filtered by the glomeruli and partially reabsorbed passively, although it may be actively reabsorbed when chloride excretion is low. Normal renal iodide clearance is about

30 ml/min, while thyroid clearance ranges from 10 to 20 ml/min; as a result, the absolute thyroid iodide uptake rate is about 150 μg per day.

THYROIDAL HORMONOGENESIS

Thyroid Iodide Transport

Iodide is transported into thyroid follicular cells against both concentration and electrochemical gradients; it then rapidly diffuses toward the follicular lumen.[6] Iodide transport is a critical step in thyroid hormonogenesis, since sufficient iodide cannot be obtained by diffusion from the extracellular fluid to sustain T_4 and T_3 synthesis. Iodide transport occurs at the basal membrane of the follicular cell. It is an energy-dependent, saturable process, requiring oxidative metabolism and phosphorylation. Iodide transport is correlated with Na^+,K^+-ATPase activity and may involve a protein or phospholipid carrier. The transport mechanism is not specific for iodide; ions of similar size, shape, and charge, such as perchlorate, thiocyanate, and pertechnetate, are transported and thus are competitive inhibitors of iodide transport.

The ability of the thyroid to transport pertechnetate is used clinically; $^{99m}TcO_4^-$, a gamma-emitting radioisotopic ion with a short half-life, is used for thyroid scanning. Thyrotropin (thyroid-stimulating hormone, TSH) is an important stimulator of thyroid iodide transport. In addition, the thyroid autoregulates iodide uptake independently of TSH: iodide transport is depressed by excess iodide and increased by iodide deficiency.[7]

The gastric mucosa, salivary glands, mammary glands, choroid plexus, and placenta also transport iodide. The transport system in these tissues is very similar to that in the thyroid, except that it is not stimulated by TSH. Because iodide is not further utilized in these tissues, it rapidly diffuses back into the extracellular fluid.

Tyrosyl Iodination and Coupling

In the thyroid, iodide is very rapidly oxidized and then covalently bound ("organified") to tyrosyl residues of thyroglobulin[8] (Figs. 10-3, 10-4). These reactions occur in exocytotic vesicles fused with the apical cell membrane, in effect within the follicular lumen; activation of the reactions and exocytosis are closely linked. Both oxidation and organification are catalyzed by thyroid peroxidase, a heme-containing glycoprotein that is bound to the membrane wall of the exocytotic vesicle. The oxidized form of the iodine atom is not known, but hydrogen peroxide must be produced before iodide oxidation or organification can take

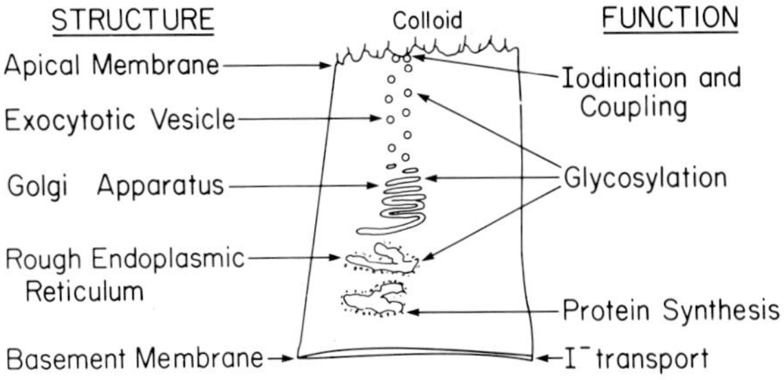

FIGURE 10-4 Schematic drawing of the path of thyroglobulin biosynthesis and iodination in the thyroid. The apical cell surface is at the top and the extracellular space at the bottom.

place. The hydrogen peroxide is probably generated by NADPH-cytochrome c reductase. This process results in mono- or diiodination of about 15 of the 120 tyrosyl residues of thyroglobulin.

Iodothyronines are formed by coupling of iodotyrosyl residues within the thyroglobulin molecule; thyronine per se is not found in thyroglobulin. The coupling reaction is an oxidative one; it, too, is catalyzed by thyroid peroxidase.[9] The most likely mechanism involves the removal of the iodinated ring from one iodotyrosyl residue, leaving a dehydroalanyl residue.[8] The iodinated ring is ether-linked to another iodotyrosyl residue of the same thyroglobulin molecule, thus forming T_4, T_3, or rT_3. Monoiodotyrosyl or diiodotyrosyl coupling to noniodinated tyrosyl residues occurs little if at all.

Thyroglobulin Synthesis

Thyroglobulin constitutes about 75 percent of the protein content of the thyroid, and is almost entirely found in the follicular lumen[10] (Fig. 10-4). Thyroglobulin is a 660,000-dalton glycoprotein composed of two identical noncovalently linked subunits; it contains about 10 percent carbohydrate. A 33-S (8600-nucleotide) mRNA coding for the subunit peptide has been isolated from human thyroid. Thyroglobulin mRNA is translated by large polyribosomes attached to the rough endoplasmic reticulum. Initial glycosylation occurs before release of the protein into the lumen of the endoplasmic reticulum. It continues during transfer of thyroglobulin to the Golgi apparatus and incorporation of thyroglobulin into the exocytotic vesicles that fuse with the apical cell membrane. Iodination and coupling only occur after these later steps; thyroglobulin which is not glycosylated cannot be readily iodinated.[11] Thus, fully glycosylated, iodinated, and iodothyronine-containing thyroglobulin is found only in the follicular lumen.

The unique feature of thyroglobulin which favors iodotyrosyl coupling is its primary structure. It is rather low, compared to other proteins, in tyrosine content; it contains 120 tyrosyl residues. Tyrosyl residues in all proteins can be iodinated, but only in thyroglobulin does coupling occur to any extent. Coupling does not occur randomly; rather, T_4 and T_3 are formed in one or more limited domains of the molecule which have unique amino acid sequences.[12]

The iodoamino acid content of thyroglobulin is dependent upon iodide availability. Normal thyroglobulin contains about six residues of monoiodotyrosine (MIT), four residues of diiodotyrosine (DIT), two residues of T_4, and 0.2 residue of T_3 per molecule. Only a minute amount of rT_3 is found. Poorly iodinated thyroglobulin has a lower total iodide content and higher MIT/DIT and T_3/T_4 ratios.[11]

Colloid Endocytosis and Hormone Release

Thyroglobulin is not only the site of formation, but also the storage form of T_4 and T_3. The process of hormone secretion requires that thyroglobulin be taken up by the thyroid follicular cells and T_4 and T_3 be liberated from it (Fig. 10-5). Thyroglobulin in the follicular lumen is taken up by pinocytotic extensions of microvilli from the apical membrane, forming endocytotic vesicles (colloid droplets). These vesicles fuse with lysosomes to form phagolysosomes. As these particles migrate toward the base of the cell, thyroglobulin is digested. Initially, digestion proceeds by reduction of sulfhydryl bonds; subsequently, proteolysis takes place and the particles regain their lysosomal appearance. The T_3 and T_4 resulting from thyroglobulin proteolysis diffuse into the extracellular fluid and enter the circulation. During this process, some of the T_4 is deiodinated to form T_3, so that thyroidal T_3 secretion is greater than expected on the basis of thyroglobulin T_3 content.[13] The iodotyrosines liberated by

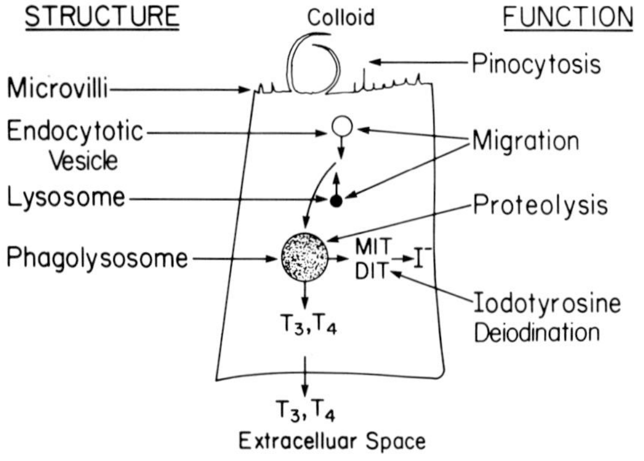

FIGURE 10-5 Schematic drawing of the path of thyroglobulin proteolysis and T_4 and T_3 release.

thyroglobulin hydrolysis are rapidly deiodinated by a separate microsomal deiodinase. Most of the iodide formed as a result of iodotyrosine deiodination is reused in the thyroid, but a small amount is released. Iodotyrosine deiodination provides two to three times more iodide for new hormone formation than does new iodide transport; it thus is of critical importance in maintaining iodothyronine synthesis. A small amount of thyroglobulin is not hydrolyzed and is released into the circulation.[10]

EXTRATHYROIDAL HORMONOGENESIS

Most of the T_3 produced each day results from extrathyroidal 5′-deiodination of T_4. This reaction is catalyzed by thyroxine 5′-deiodinase, a microsomal enzyme which requires reduced sulfhydryl groups as cofactors. The liver and kidneys have the highest T_4 5′-deiodinase activity per unit tissue;[14,15] these tissues may be the most abundant sources of circulating T_3. However, T_4 5′-deiodination has been identified in many tissues and is probably ubiquitous. There are two types of T_4 5′-deiodinase, distinguished by their sensitivity to inhibition by propylthiouracil (PTU). One form, called type 1 (PTU-sensitive), predominates in the liver, kidney, and thyroid, has a relatively high K_m (on the order of 1 μM) for T_4, and a considerably lower (nM) K_m for rT_3. The type 2 enzyme predominates in brain and pituitary, is not inhibited by PTU, and has K_m values for T_4 and rT_3 that are in the nM range and are similar to one another.[16–18]

Reverse-T_3 production is nearly all extrathyroidal. It is catalyzed by T_4 5-deiodinase. Little is known about the site(s) or regulation of rT_3 production. The placenta is a rich source of this enzyme; placental production of rT_3 probably accounts for the high rT_3 concentrations in fetal serum.[19] Both T_3 and rT_3 are metabolized in part by deiodination. While little is known about T_3 deiodination, that of rT_3 is catalyzed by a 5′-deiodinase which has many similarities to type 1 T_4 5′-deiodinase.[15]

THYROID HORMONE PRODUCTION AND METABOLISM

The total daily production of T_4 is 80 to 100 μg, all derived from thyroidal secretion (Fig. 10-6). The extrathyroidal pool contains 800 to 1000 μg of T_4, the majority of which is extracellular. The T_4 turnover rate is 10 percent per day. Thus, T_4 remains available for several weeks even in the absence of new secretion. Approximately 80 percent of the T_4 is metabolized by deiodination, about half to T_3 and the other half to rT_3. The other 20 percent is metabolized by conjugation with glucuronide and, perhaps, sulfate,

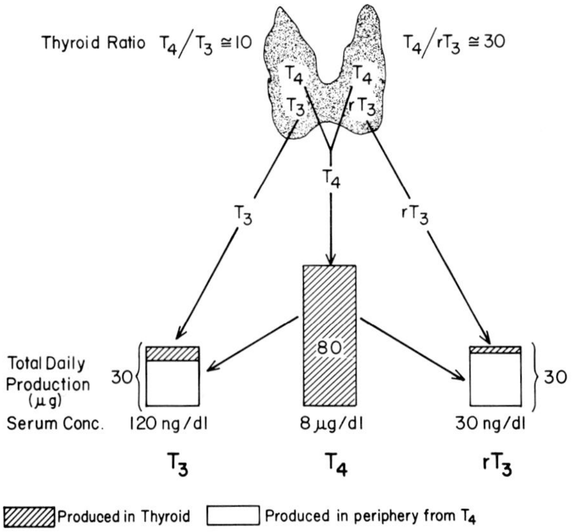

FIGURE 10-6 Sources and production rates of circulating T_4, T_3, and rT_3 in the normal adult. Shaded area of each bar represents production in thyroid; unshaded area represents production in periphery from T_4. Figures indicate total daily production of each compound (μg). Serum concentrations are: T_3, 120 ng/dl; T_4, 8 μg/dl; rT_3, 30 ng/dl. Thyroid ratios are: $T_4/T_3 \cong 10$; $T_4/rT_3 \cong 30$.

deamination to form tetrac, and cleavage of the ether link.[14] Deiodination of T_4 to form T_3 leads to enhanced biological activity, but all of the other metabolites of T_4 have little if any biological activity in the amounts produced in vivo. The extrathyroidal conversion of T_4 to T_3 is regulated by a variety of factors; production of T_3, the most active thyroid hormone, may therefore be altered independently of changes in pituitary-thyroid function.

T_3 is produced primarily (80 percent) by extrathyroidal deiodination of T_4; the remainder comes from the thyroid (Fig. 10-6). The total daily production is 30 to 40 μg. The extrathyroidal T_3 pool contains about 50 μg, most of which is intracellular. T_3 is much more rapidly degraded than is T_4; its turnover rate is about 75 percent per day. Hence, alterations in its production readily alter T_3 availability. Somewhat more than half of the T_3 produced each day is deiodinated to form 3,3′-diiodothyronine; sulfation probably precedes deiodination. A small amount is deiodinated to 3,5-diiodothyronine (Fig. 10-7), and the remainder is metabolized via deamination to form triac.[14]

Production of rT_3 also is largely extrathyroidal; over 90 percent of the 30 to 40 μg produced each day originates in this way (Fig. 10-6). Reverse T_3 is cleared rapidly from the circulation and degraded very rapidly in tissues. It is metabolized to both 3,3′-diiodothyronine and 3′,5′-diiodothyronine (Fig. 10-7); substantial amounts are also metabolized by other, as yet unidentified, pathways.[14] The various diiodothyronines also are very rapidly metabolized to monoiodothyronines and ultimately to thyronine, but little is known about the sites and regulation of these conversions. Table 10-2 shows the serum concentrations and production rates of some of these compounds. The serum concentrations of 3′- and 3-T_1 are less than 2 ng/dl.[20,21] Tetrac, triac, and the conjugates of T_4 and T_3 also are metabolized largely by deiodination.

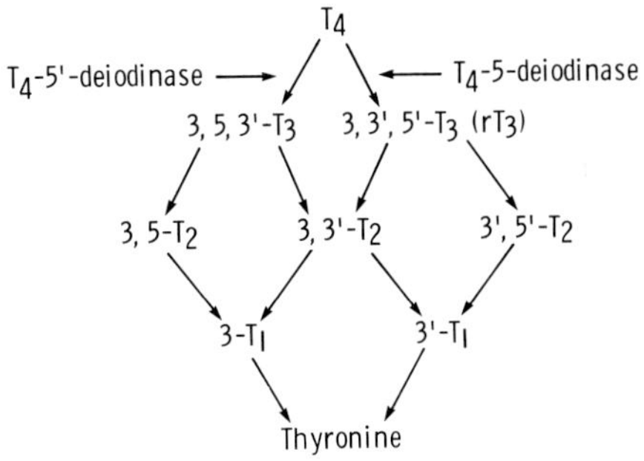

FIGURE 10-7 Pathways of deiodination of T_4 and its metabolites.

MIT and DIT are present in the circulation in low concentrations. They are derived both from dietary sources and from the thyroid gland. Both MIT and DIT are degraded rapidly by tyrosine deiodinase in peripheral tissues.

Transport and Cellular Binding of Thyroid Hormones

SERUM BINDING PROTEINS

Very little of the T_4 and T_3 in the circulation is free; more than 99.95 percent of T_4 and 99.5 percent of T_3

Table 10-2. Serum Concentrations and Production Rates of Various Iodothyronines

Compound	Serum concentration, ng/dl	Production rate, μg/day
T_4	5000–11,000	80–100
T_3	75–200	30–40
rT_3	20–50	25–35
3,3′-T_2	2–15	25–35
3,5-T_2	1–10	2–5
3′,5′-T_2	2–6	5–20
Tetrac	10–50	1–2
Triac	2–8	4–8

Abbreviations: tetrac, tetraiodothyroacetic acid, triac, triiodothyroacetic acid.
Source: Engler and Burger.[14]

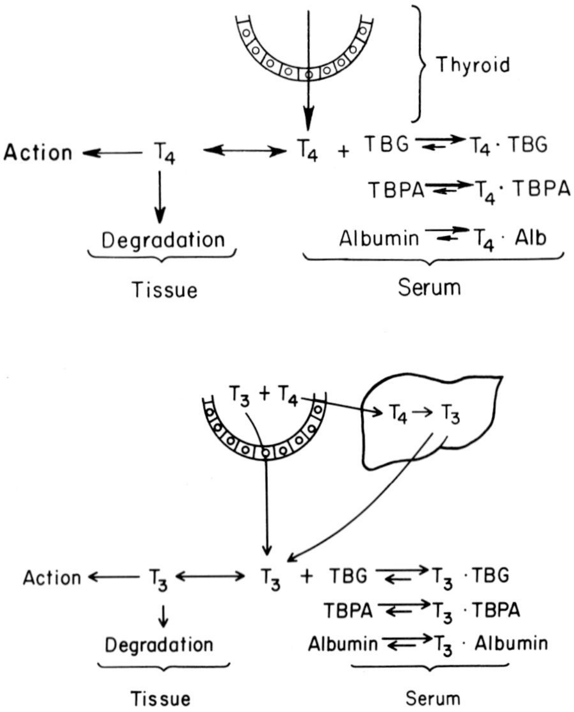

FIGURE 10-8 (*A*) Origin, circulation, and degradation of T_4; (*B*) origin, circulation, and degradation of T_3. Only the liver is shown as a site of T_4 conversion to T_3, but conversion occurs in many tissues.

are bound in reversible physicochemical equilibrium to serum proteins (Fig. 10-8*A* and *B*). These proteins are thyroxine-binding globulin (TBG), thyroxine-binding prealbumin (TBPA), and albumin. Under physiological conditions, approximately 80 percent of T_4 is bound to TBG, 15 percent to TBPA, and the remainder to serum albumin. In comparison, about 90 percent of T_3 is bound to TBG, 5 percent to TBPA, and 5 percent to albumin. Approximately 0.05 percent of the total serum T_4, or about 2 ng/dl, is free; the free T_3 concentration is about 0.4 ng/dl. Because so much of the T_4 and T_3 in serum is bound, changes in serum binding protein concentrations have a major effect on total serum T_4 and T_3 concentrations and fractional T_4 and T_3 metabolism; however, binding protein concentration changes do not alter free hormone concentrations or absolute rates of T_4 and T_3 metabolism.

These binding proteins serve to buffer the free thyroid hormone levels, act as reservoirs or storage sites from which free hormones can be made immediately available, and may serve to ensure uniform distribution of thyroid hormones within an individual tissue. If hormone production ceases, one day's normal utilization of T_4 in serum results in a 10 percent decline in its serum concentration, whereas if only free T_4 were available its supply would be exhausted within hours. While it is generally held that only the free hormone concentrations determine the amount of hormone available to tissues, some recent evidence suggests that albumin-bound T_4 and T_3 and perhaps TBG-bound T_3 are readily available to tissues such as the liver.[22] Moreover, other factors, such as vascular flow and permeability, tissue mechanisms for T_4 and T_3 uptake, and intracellular binding, also are important in determining T_4 and T_3 entry into cells.

Thyroxine-Binding Globulin (TBG)

Thyroxine-binding globulin (not to be confused with thyroglobulin) is an acid glycoprotein (molecular weight 54,000) which is synthesized in the liver. It has one binding site for T_4 or T_3. The affinity constant of TBG for T_4 is about 10^{10} M^{-1} (Table 10-3). T_4 binds to TBG considerably more avidly than does T_3. The serum TBG concentration in normal individuals is about 2 mg/dl; this amount of TBG is capable of binding about 20 μg of T_4. There is both intra- and interindividual genetic polymorphism of TBG.[24] Desialylation of TBG reduces its affinity for thyroxine 10-fold and results in accelerated TBG degradation.

Table 10-3. Properties of Serum Thyroid Hormone–binding Proteins

	Affinity constant, M^{-1}			Concentration, mg/dl	Mol wt	Half-life, days
	T_4	T_3	rT_3			
Thyroxine-binding globulin	2×10^{10}	2×10^{8}	2×10^{9}	2	54,000	5
Thyroxine-binding prealbumin	2×10^{8}	2×10^{7}		25	55,000	2
Albumin	2×10^{6}	1×10^{6}	2×10^{6}	4,000	69,000	15

Source: Robbins et al.[23]

Thyroxine-Binding Prealbumin (TBPA)

TBPA is a protein with a molecular weight of approximately 55,000. It has two T_4 binding sites per molecule. Occupation of one site by T_4 results in reduction of the affinity of the second site for T_4. The affinity constant of TBPA for T_4 is about 2×10^8 M^{-1}; its affinity for T_3 is only about one-tenth as great (Table 10-3). The serum concentration of TBPA is about 25 mg/dl, an amount capable of binding up to 200 μg of T_4. TBPA also binds another protein, retinol-binding protein (RBP) (molecular weight 21,000), which in turn binds one molecule of retinol (vitamin A). There are four such RBP binding sites on prealbumin. While adding T_4 has no effect on the affinity of TBPA for RBP, addition of retinol stabilizes the complex. Formation of the TBPA-RBP complex enhances affinity for retinol but not for T_4.

Albumin

Albumin has one binding site for T_4, with an affinity constant of 2×10^6 M^{-1}. There are four T_4-binding albumin isoforms; their affinity for T_4 varies.[25] Normally, less than 5 percent of the T_4 in serum is bound to albumin, so that changes in serum albumin levels have relatively little effect on serum T_4 levels.

CELLULAR HORMONE ENTRY AND BINDING

T_4 and T_3 enter cells primarily by diffusion (Fig. 10-9). Serum free T_4 and free T_3 are available for diffusion at any instant; so too may be T_4 and T_3 that are bound to low-affinity binding proteins such as albumin, from which they very rapidly dissociate. T_4 and T_3 uptake may also involve a transport process. Membrane binding sites for T_4 and T_3 and receptor-mediated internalization of T_4 and T_3 have been described in liver and some other tissues.[26] The contribution of this mechanism of cell hormone entry to overall intracellular hormone availability is unknown. Ultimately, virtually

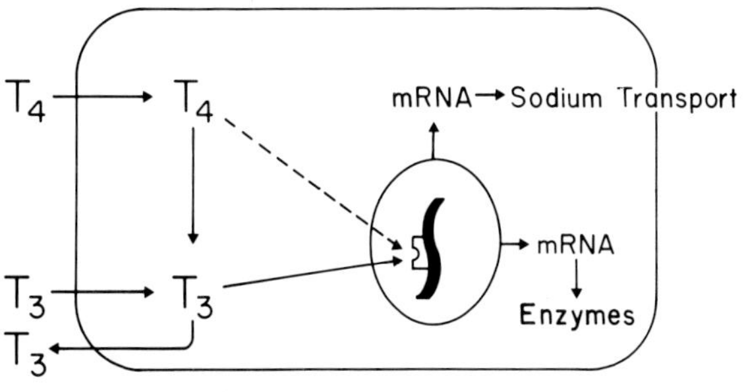

FIGURE 10-9 Schematic outline of extracellular and intracellular translocations of T_4 and T_3, and two cellular responses to binding of the hormones to nuclear receptors.

all serum protein–bound T_4 and T_3 molecules become available and may enter cells if the intracellular free hormone levels decline sufficiently.

T_3 is also available to cells because it is produced from T_4 in them (Fig. 10-9). Serum T_3 concentrations are near normal in athyreotic patients taking T_4, implying that free intracellular T_3 concentrations must be higher in some T_3-producing tissues, most likely including liver and kidney, than in the extracellular fluid; this would lead to outward diffusion of T_3. The T_3 is not all exported, however, since in many tissues some locally produced T_3 is bound to nuclear and, perhaps, other receptors linked to hormone action. Locally produced T_3 accounts for about 20 percent of nuclear T_3 in rat liver, about 50 percent in pituitary, and about 80 percent in cerebral cortex,[27] but virtually none in muscle.[28] Because of its production in peripheral tissue, its less intense serum binding, and its more intense intracellular binding, T_3 is the predominant intracellular hormone; about 90 percent of the total extrathyroidal T_3 pool of 50 μg is in the intracellular compartment.

T_4 and T_3 within cells exist both free and bound to cytosol, microsomes, mitochondria, and nuclei.[29] The cytosolic binding proteins probably have a passive role, similar to that of the iodothyronine-binding proteins in serum; thus, they probably have both buffering and storage functions within cells. The binding sites that best fit the criteria for receptors (specificity, saturability, limited capacity) are found in the nuclei of various tissues (Fig. 10-9).

T_3 enters the nucleus directly from the cytosol by diffusion or via a transport system in the nuclear membrane;[29] participation of a cytosol T_3-binding protein is not required. The receptor is an acidic nonhistone protein localized within chromatin; its location is not dependent on the presence of T_3.[30] The solubilized receptor has a molecular weight of about 50,000. It probably resides in chromatin because of its intrinsic DNA-binding properties. These receptors bind T_3 10 times more avidly than they do T_4 in vitro; in vivo about 85 percent of the specifically bound nuclear hormone is T_3 and 15 percent is T_4.[31] The affinity of the receptor for thyroid hormone analogues is generally proportional to the biological activity of the analogue. The hormone concentrations required for relative saturation of these nuclear sites by T_3 are linearly correlated to the relative hormone response in some tissues, such as the pituitary and heart. In other tissues, however, increases in receptor occupancy result in nonlinear, amplified responses. For example, in the liver an increase in receptor occupancy from 50 to 100 percent results in a 10-fold increase in the rate of production of some T_3-induced enzymes. Human tissues have nuclear receptors with specificities and affinities that are very similar to those in animal tissues.[32]

The cell content of nuclear receptors is generally high in those tissues most responsive to thyroid hormone, such as the pituitary and liver, whereas the concentrations are low in poorly responsive tissues, such as the spleen and testes. In rats, hepatic nuclear receptor content per cell is reduced by starvation, diabetes, uremia, and partial hepatectomy.[33-35] Such changes, if they occurred in humans, could represent an additional mechanism serving to limit the impact of thyroid hormone in patients with nonthyroidal illnesses (see Nonthyroidal Illness, below).

Much less is known about the nature and significance of thyroid hormone binding to other subcellular constituents. In most cases, the affinity and specificity of other intracellular receptors is much lower than that of nuclear receptors and their binding capacity is much higher. Nevertheless, some of them may mediate hormone action, since thyroid hormones may have actions that are not initiated by nuclear binding.

Actions of Thyroid Hormones

Thyroid hormones modulate a large number of metabolic processes. They do so by regulating the production and activity of many enzymes, the production and metabolism of most other hormones, and the utilization of substrates, vitamins, and minerals. As a result, thyroid hormones profoundly affect not only growth and development but also the function of virtually all tissues. They appear to do so, moreover, in several ways; no single biochemical site of action nor single reaction has yet been identified which satisfactorily explains all of their actions.

MOLECULAR MECHANISMS OF THYROID HORMONE ACTION

Some aspects of the molecular mechanisms by which thyroid hormones act deserve emphasis here. T_3 is the major physiological effector of thyroid hormone action, since it constitutes most of the nuclear-bound hormone; T_4 is predominantly a prohormone. T_3 activation of nuclear receptors results in stimulation of mRNA production. In some tissues there is an increase in total RNA synthesis; in others there is an increase in specific mRNAs, but no overall increase in mRNA synthesis. These changes in mRNA synthesis are due to altered rates of DNA transcription.[29]

The effects of thyroid hormone vary in different tissues. In some tissues, such as the pituitary, only a few cellular functions are affected; in others, such as the liver, there is stimulation of the synthesis of many proteins. Key functions or tissue components stimulated by thyroid hormone that mediate some of the hormone's physiological actions include production of growth hormone (GH) and nerve growth factor, beta-adrenergic receptors, Na^+, K^+-dependent ATPase and cardiac myosin ATPase, and enzymes that increase the rates of synthesis and degradation of other proteins, carbohydrates, and lipids.[36]

Several actions of thyroid hormones appear not to be due to effects on transcription. They include stimulation of myocardial adenyl cyclase activity, stimulation of amino acid and sugar transport in lymphoid cells, and reduction in cerebrocortical and pituitary type 2 T_4 5′-deiodinase activity.[37,38] Thus, either the T_3 nuclear receptor mediates extranuclear events or as yet undetected T_3 receptors with hormone-binding properties similar to those of the nuclear receptors exist at some other cellular location(s). (The molecular mechanisms of thyroid hormone action are discussed in more detail in Chap. 5.)

THERMOGENIC ACTIONS

Energy released by the oxidation of substrate and consumption of oxygen is either stored by the formation of ATP or liberated as heat. Use of ATP for ion transport, synthesis of cell constituents, and muscle contraction results in formation of ADP; rephosphorylation of ADP requires augmented mitochondrial oxidative metabolism. The single largest requirement for ATP in resting cells is for Na^+,K^+-ATPase-mediated sodium transport; thus, changes in the ATPase should have the greatest overall effect on oxidative metabolism.

Thyroid hormone stimulation of thermogenesis can be demonstrated both in vivo and in vitro in isolated tissues, such as muscle, liver, kidney, and intestine.[39] The degree of stimulation correlates with the number of nuclear T_3 receptors in most tissues except brain, which has a moderate number of receptors per cell but in which there is no thermogenic response.

There is a latent period of hours or days before thyroid hormone–induced increases in oxygen consumption occur. This increase correlates closely with increased sodium transport, as measured by increases in Na^+,K^+-ATPase activity. Inhibition of the enzyme by ouabain virtually completely inhibits the thyroid hormone–stimulated increase in oxygen consumption. Further studies of these processes indicate that increased sodium transport results from an increase in cell Na^+,K^+-ATPase production, i.e., in sodium pump units; the ATPase increase is due to new enzyme synthesis, since it is accompanied by increased incorporation of labeled amino acid into enzyme and is blocked by inhibitors of protein synthesis. Thus, thyroid hormone augmentation of thermogenesis can be explained by increased mitochondrial oxidative metabolism, driven by an increase in ATP hydrolysis which occurs as a result of increased Na^+,K^+-ATPase production. Despite the attractiveness of this scheme, there is evidence that thyroid hormone has direct mitochondrial actions which could mediate its thermogenic effect. Mitochondria contain T_3 binding sites. Thyroid hormones stimulate mitochondrial protein synthesis; inward transport of ADP, inorganic phosphate, and fuels; and ATP production and oxygen consumption.[40]

THYROID HORMONE-CATECHOLAMINE INTERACTIONS

Many of the signs and symptoms of thyroid disease appear to reflect increased sympathetic nervous system activity. However, plasma levels and production rates of norepinephrine are increased in hypothyroidism and normal in hyperthyroidism, while those of epinephrine are not altered by either.[41] Thyroid hormones do have several actions by which the apparent increase in sympathetic activity can be explained. First, they increase the number of beta-adrenergic receptors in myocardial tissue, skeletal muscle, adipose tissue, and lymphocytes and they decrease the number of myocardial alpha-adrenergic receptors.[42] Such changes might be expected to result in increased sensitivity to catecholamines. Second, thyroid hormones may alter catecholamine sensitivity at some postreceptor site. Third, thyroid hormones may have actions that mimic those of catecholamines. The available data, though often conflicting, indicate that thyroid hormone-catecholamine interactions vary considerably in different tissues. For example, in vivo myocardial contractile response and in vitro adenyl cyclase response to catecholamines are not altered by thyroid hormone excess or deficiency.[43,44] In contrast, adipose tissue lipolytic and adenyl cyclase responses to catecholamines are augmented by thyroid hormone.[42,45]

EFFECTS ON PROTEIN SYNTHESIS

Thyroid hormones stimulate the synthesis of many structural proteins, enzymes, and hormones. The consequences of this action are most obvious in the decreased neural and somatic growth that accompanies hypothyroidism in infants and children. The biochemical bases for increased protein synthesis are increased production of mRNA resulting from augmented gene transcription, proliferation of ribosomal constituents involved in protein synthesis, and increased translational efficiency.[29] Another potential mechanism for increased protein synthesis is increased amino acid availability, since thyroid hormones stimulate amino acid transport in several tissues by a rapid, cyclic AMP–mediated action independent of new protein synthesis.[37] As noted previously, in some tissues there is an increase in total cytoplasmic mRNA, including multiple poly(A)-containing RNAs, whereas in others only specific mRNAs are increased, without an increase in total mRNA. In some instances, the mRNA responses are coordinate, being influenced by T_3, GH, and dietary factors.

One of the best-studied protein responses is that of malic enzyme in liver. Increases in malic enzyme activity correlate with nuclear T_3 occupancy. After a lag period, T_3 receptor occupancy results in increases in the appropriate mRNA and, subsequently, proportional increases in enzyme protein concentration and catalytic activity.[29] However, not all thyroid hormone actions on synthetic processes are stimulatory. For example, thyroid hormones inhibit TSH secretion, at least in part by a process that is inhibited by protein synthesis inhibitors;[46] thyroid hormones also inhibit fibroblast glycosaminoglycan synthesis.[47] Moreover, the production of some hepatic poly(A)-containing RNA species is inhibited, although which proteins they code for is not known.[29]

EFFECTS ON CARBOHYDRATE AND LIPID METABOLISM

Thyroid hormones have major effects on carbohydrate and lipid metabolism. They increase hepatic glycolysis, decrease hepatic glycogen content, and increase gluconeogenesis and glycogenolysis, thus increasing hepatic glucose production.[48] All of these changes provide more glucose, the need for which would be expected in view of the calorigenic effects of thyroid hormone; in fact, glucose utilization does increase.[49] The biochemical mechanisms underlying these changes are not known.

Thyroid hormone effects on lipid metabolism are equally far-reaching; thyroid hormones affect fatty acid, triglyceride, and cholesterol production and metabolism. An important action is stimulation of hepatic fatty acid synthesis, which, at least in part, results from the increase in NADPH production due to increased malic enzyme activity. Mobilization of fatty acids and glycerol from adipose tissue stores also is increased by thyroid hormone; liberation of these compounds is a result of increased adipocyte lipogenesis and sensitivity to the lipolytic actions of catecholamines, as well as decreased sensitivity to the antilipolytic action of insulin. Thus, more fatty acids are available for ketogenesis and oxidation; the latter is an important component of the calorigenic action of thyroid hormone.[50,51] Hepatic triglyceride and cholesterol synthesis also are increased. However, triglyceride and cholesterol metabolism increases even more, due to increased lipoprotein lipase activity and increased numbers of cellular low-density lipoprotein (LDL) receptors.[52]

Regulation of Thyroid Hormone Production

Thyroid hormone production is regulated in two ways (Fig. 10-10). First, thyroidal secretion is regulated by pituitary thyrotropin (TSH). The secretion of TSH in turn is regulated by the circulating thyroid hormone concentrations and thyrotropin releasing hormone (TRH). Second, extrathyroidal production of T_3 from T_4 is regulated by a variety of nutritional, hormonal, and illness-related factors; the effect of these regulatory factors varies in different tissues. The first mechanism provides a sensitive defense to alterations in thyroid secretion. The second regulatory mechanism provides for the rapid alterations in tissue thyroid hormone availability in response to nonthyroidal illness which constitute an important adaptation to illness.

CONTROL OF THYROID SECRETION

Thyrotropin

Thyrotropin, a 28,000-dalton glycoprotein, is synthesized and secreted by thyrotrophs of the anterior pituitary (as described in greater detail in Chap. 8). TSH contains about 15 percent carbohydrate, and consists of two peptide subunits, an alpha subunit and a beta subunit, linked by noncovalent bonds. The alpha subunit of TSH is the same as that of luteinizing hormone (LH), follicle stimulating hormone (FSH), and chorionic gonadotropin (HCG). The beta subunit of TSH is unique; thus, it determines the biological specificity of TSH, although the beta subunits of all four hormones have considerable sequence homology. The two subunits are synthesized separately in the thyrotrophs; they then are glycosylated, rapidly linked together, and packaged into granules, which contain mostly intact TSH. Small amounts of the individual subunits are found in the thyrotrophs and in the circulation; their secretion is regulated in the same way as is that of intact TSH.[53]

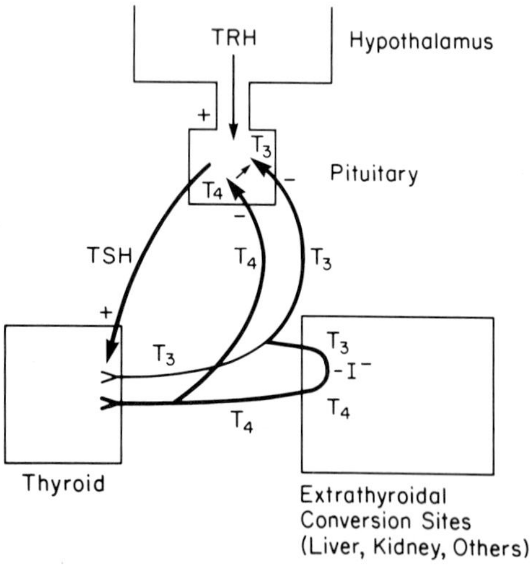

FIGURE 10-10 The hypothalamic-pituitary-thyroid-peripheral axis. TSH regulates thyroidal production of T_4 and T_3; T_3 is also produced in many other tissues. TSH secretion is regulated by serum T_4, serum T_3, T_3 produced from T_4 within the pituitary, and thyrotropin-releasing hormone (TRH). (−), inhibitory effect; (+), stimulatory effect.

Thyroid Hormone Regulation of TSH Secretion

T_3 and T_4 directly inhibit both TSH release and TSH synthesis (Fig. 10-11). Thyrotropin secretion in normal subjects is exquisitely sensitive to small changes in serum T_4 and T_3 concentrations when they are due to changes in thyroidal secretion; however, TSH release is not sensitive to T_3 changes when they are due to altered extrathyroidal T_3 production. Changes in thyroid secretion of as little as 15 to 20 percent result in reciprocal 50 to 100 percent changes in basal serum TSH concentrations and in TSH responses to exogenous TRH. Greater changes in serum T_4 and T_3 concentrations result in greater reciprocal changes in serum TSH concentrations. Such graded sensitivity to small changes in serum T_4 and T_3 concentrations prevents other stimuli (see below) from having more than a transient effect on TSH or thyroid secretion and thus serves to maintain thyroid secretion within narrow limits.

Circulating T_4 and T_3 both inhibit TSH secretion. Because the pituitary has considerable T_4 5′-deiodinase activity, circulating T_4 contributes more to the nuclear T_3 content in pituitary than in many other tissues.[18,27] The predominant role of T_4 from serum as a source of nuclear T_3 may explain the failure of serum TSH concentrations to increase in patients with nonthyroidal illnesses, in whom T_3 production by other peripheral tissues is impaired and serum T_3 concentrations are low (see Nonthyroidal Illness, below). In patients with abnormal thyroid glands or iodide deficiency, T_3 is produced and secreted by the thyroid in relatively more normal amounts than is T_4.[13,27] Since circulating T_3 contributes less to pituitary nuclear T_3 content than does serum T_4, TSH secretion remains elevated. Increased TSH secretion in such patients permits increased thyroid secretion.

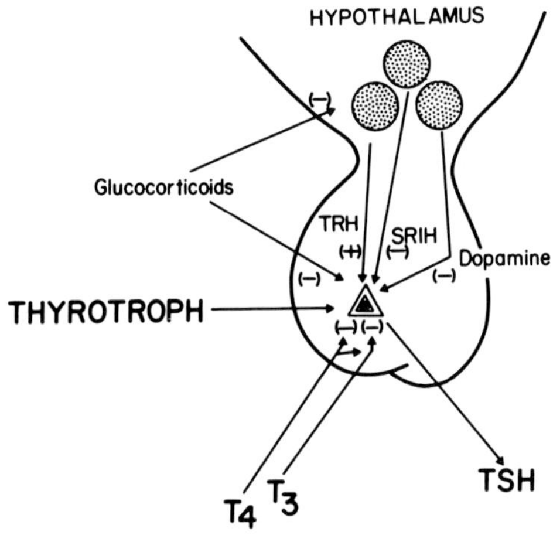

FIGURE 10-11 Factors regulating TSH secretion. (+), stimulatory effect; (−), inhibitory effect.

T_4 and T_3 inhibit TSH secretion by decreasing the number of TRH receptors and by decreasing TSH biosynthesis; these actions correlate with the extent of nuclear T_3 binding and are blocked by inhibitors of protein synthesis.[46,54] The rate and extent of thyroid hormone inhibition of TSH secretion is dependent on the initial serum TSH concentration, the hormone given, the dose, and time. Administration of a single large dose of 400 to 500 μg or more of T_3 or T_4 to a hypothyroid patient with increased TSH secretion results in a rapid decline in serum TSH concentrations within hours; TSH concentrations do not fall all the way to normal, however, and maximum inhibition of TSH secretion occurs long after peak serum T_4 or T_3 concentrations are achieved. Given in usual therapeutic doses, T_3 reduces serum TSH concentrations to normal in approximately a week, but the response to T_4 is considerably slower; full responses require several weeks or more. In normal subjects even smaller doses of T_4 or T_3 inhibit TSH secretion in a few days. When given continually, T_3 has about three times the potency of T_4 as an inhibitor of basal and TRH-stimulated TSH secretion.[55] Conversely, following treatment of hyperthyroidism or discontinuation of long-term thyroid therapy, recovery of basal TSH secretion and TSH responses to TRH takes several weeks or longer, depending on the duration and extent of the prior inhibition.

Thyrotropin Releasing Hormone

Thyrotropin releasing hormone is a tripeptide, pyroglutamyl-histidyl-prolineamide. The content of TRH is highest in the median eminence and arcuate nuclei of the hypothalamus, but some TRH is found in most hypothalamic nuclei.[56] The arcuate nuclei are considered the "thyrotropic" areas of the hypothalamus, since electrical destruction of them results in hypothyroidism.[57] Lesser amounts of TRH are found throughout the CNS and in the gastrointestinal tract, pancreatic islets, and reproductive tract.[58] Its physiological function (or functions) in these sites is unknown; it may serve as a local neuromodulator. TRH binds to receptors on thyrotroph cell membranes; the subsequent TSH release is mediated by altered calcium flux. TRH also stimulates TSH subunit biosynthesis and glycosylation.[59] The number of TRH receptors is depressed by TRH itself, as well as by thyroid hormones.[54]

Exogenously administered TRH causes a dose-dependent increase in serum TSH concentration in normal subjects (Fig. 10-11) (see Evaluation of Thyroid Function, below). When administered continuously for several days TRH stimulates the release of more TSH than does the same dose given intermittently, although in both situations serum TSH levels decline after about 1 day. TRH also stimulates prolactin release both in normal subjects and most hyperprolactinemic patients. In patients with various disorders, including acromegaly, chronic liver disease, hypothyroidism, and diabetes mellitus, exogenous TRH also stimulates GH secretion. However, endogenous TRH is not a physiological regulator of the secretion of either prolactin or GH.

TRH is required for maintenance of normal TSH secretion, and it determines the "set point" about which thyroid hormones regulate TSH secretion. Administration of anti-TRH serum as well as lesions of specific regions of the hypothalamus reduce serum TSH and thyroid hormone concentrations. Also, in some patients with hypothyroidism and low serum TSH levels, repeated TRH administration restores serum TSH, T_4, and T_3 concentrations to normal.[60] Moreover, thyroid deficiency results in smaller increases in TSH secretion and thyroid hormones more readily inhibit TSH secretion in patients or animals with TRH deficiency than in normal subjects. Alterations in TRH secretion may be responsible for the normal small diurnal increase in TSH concentration which occurs in the late evening hours in anticipation of sleep, the abrupt rise in serum TSH concentration that occurs in newborn infants, and the cold-induced rise in serum TSH concentration that occurs in children. Otherwise, there is little evidence that TRH levels are regulated.

TRH is very rapidly metabolized; the half-life of exogenously administered TRH in humans is 5 min.[61] Peripheral plasma TRH concentrations in normal subjects range from 25 to 100 pg/ml, and are not altered in either hypo- or hyperthyroidism.[62] However, the sources of TRH in peripheral plasma are unknown. In animals, peripheral and hypothalamic portal venous TRH concentrations and hypothalamic TRH content are not altered by either hypo- or hyperthyroidism. Administration of anti-TRH serum has relatively little effect on TSH secretion in hypothyroid animals. These results indicate that thyroid hormones do not alter TRH secretion, that the increased TSH secretion in animals with hypothyroidism is not due to excessive TRH secretion, and that the thyrotrophs are relatively protected from major alterations of TRH secretion, whether it originates from the hypothalamus or elsewhere; the protection is provided by rapid turnover of TRH as well as the direct actions of T_4 and T_3 on the thyrotrophs.

Other Factors Altering TSH Secretion

Several other factors, in addition to thyroid hormones and TRH, alter TSH secretion (Fig. 10-11). One is somatostatin.[57] Infusions of somatostatin reduce basal serum TSH concentrations and inhibit the serum TSH response to TRH. Conversely, infusions of somatostatin antiserum increase basal serum TSH concentrations and enhance TSH responses to several stimuli; hypothalamic lesions which reduce median eminence somatostatin content are accompanied by increased serum TSH concentrations. Thyroid hormones increase hypothalamic somatostatin content. Thus, somatostatin may be a physiologically important tonic inhibitor of TSH secretion whose production is in part regulated by T_4 and T_3.

Dopamine also may be a physiologically important inhibitor of TSH secretion.[57] Serum TSH concentrations decline during infusions of dopamine and after administration of the dopaminergic agonist bromocriptine; serum TSH levels are increased by dopaminergic antagonists, such as metoclopramide and domperidone, in both normal and hypothyroid subjects. Since domperidone does not traverse the blood-brain barrier, dopamine most likely has a direct action on the thyrotrophs.

Glucocorticoids inhibit basal TSH secretion, serum TSH responses to TRH, and the late-evening increase in serum TSH concentrations.[57] Conversely, metyrapone-induced decreases in glucocorticoid production are accompanied by increases in serum TSH concentrations. These changes probably reflect glucocorticoid effects on both the pituitary and the hypothalamus.

The overall importance of the effects of somatostatin, dopamine, and glucocorticoids in regulating TSH secretion in the long term is probably small. Most of the changes cited have been demonstrated in short-term studies; the changes in serum TSH responses to exogenous TRH are greater than are those in basal serum TSH concentrations. Transient increases in endogenous dopamine, somatostatin, or glucocorticoid production may temporarily decrease TSH secretion. However, sustained increases in the production of these factors do not lead to hypothyrotropic hypothyroidism, probably because the direct stimulatory effect of decreased thyroid hormone availability on TSH secretion largely overcomes any inhibition that might be induced by such agents. Occasional exceptions are the reversible hypothyrotropic hypothyroidism that can occur during GH therapy and in patients with prolactinomas.[63,64]

THYROTROPIN AND REGULATION OF THYROID SECRETION

TSH stimulates virtually every aspect of thyroid hormone biosynthesis and release by the thyroid. It also stimulates many steps in thyroid intermediary metabolism and protein and nucleic acid synthesis, and causes thyroid hyperplasia and hypertrophy. Most, but not all, of these responses are mediated by a receptor-adenyl cyclase system (see Chap. 5). TSH, through its beta subunit, binds to specific receptors in thyroid cell plasma membranes.[65] The receptors contain both high- and low-affinity TSH binding sites, which have molecular weights in the range of 60,000 to 80,000.[66] The binding sites may consist of both glycoprotein and ganglioside components. The TSH-receptor complex then activates a guanyl-nucleotide-binding protein component of the enzyme complex, which, in the presence of GTP, activates the catalytic component of adenyl cyclase. Stimulation of adenyl cyclase increases cyclic AMP formation, which then activates several protein kinases. How this process is linked to specific steps of iodide metabolism or other thyroid metabolic processes is not known. The cyclic AMP response to TSH is autoregulated, so that the response to subsequent TSH exposure is decreased.[67] This depression of the response seems to involve changes distal to the TSH receptor, since binding of labeled TSH is unaffected or may even increase after TSH administration.[67,68]

TSH stimulates most, if not all, aspects of intrathyroidal iodide metabolism, including iodide transport, oxidation, organification, and coupling; thyroglobulin proteolysis is also stimulated. The stimulation of iodide transport is slow, requiring 24 h of exposure to TSH; it is due to the production of additional transport units. The TSH-induced increase of iodothyronine formation is rapid, and occurs in the absence of measurable increases in H_2O_2 production or thyroid peroxidase activity. Stimulation of colloid endocytosis and thyroglobulin proteolysis is even more rapid; this occurs within minutes after TSH exposure. Finally, TSH stimulates thyroidal T_4 5′-deiodinase activity,[13] thus increasing the proportion of T_3 secreted. These TSH actions are mimicked by cyclic AMP.

TSH stimulates many other facets of thyroid cell function.[69] It increases thyroid oxygen consumption, glucose and fatty acid utilization, and phospholipid turnover. TSH leads to an increase in NADPH content, which is used for H_2O_2 generation; it also stimulates iodotyrosine deiodination and may stimulate iodothyronine deiodination. Besides its metabolic effects, TSH stimulates the synthesis and glycosylation of thyroglobulin, the synthesis of other proteins, and the synthesis of RNA and DNA. These TSH actions result in the morphological changes, namely hypertrophy and hyperplasia, that occur during protracted TSH stimulation. The thyroidal growth response to TSH, as measured by stimulation of thymidine incorporation, may reflect a non-cAMP-mediated response. It may be due either to linkage of the TSH receptor to some intracellular processes independent of adenyl cyclase or to TSH binding to a different receptor.

REGULATION OF THYROID SECRETION BY IODIDE

The thyroid gland uses iodide most efficiently when iodide is in scarce supply and limits its use when it is abundant. Much of this regulation is achieved by TSH, but iodide also participates in this process.[7] When little iodide is available, iodide organification and hormone synthesis are increased, even in the absence of TSH. With increasing iodide availability, the proportion of T_4 relative to that of T_3 in thyroglobulin increases; at higher iodide levels the attainment of sufficiently high intracellular iodide concentrations causes production of both hormones to decline. The dose of iodide at which production of T_3 and T_4 declines in vivo in humans is about 5 mg per day. The decline is blocked by drugs which inhibit organification, suggesting that inhibition of T_3 and T_4 production is due to an organic iodide compound. Thus, surges in iodide intake do not result in increases in thyroid hormone synthesis. When iodide intake is persistently increased, adaptation to this antithyroid effect of iodide occurs, so that hormone formation does not continue to be inhibited. The adaptation results from inhibition of iodide transport, so that intracellular iodide concentrations sufficient to maintain the block in hormone synthesis and thus cause thyroid deficiency do not develop.

Iodide also inhibits thyroglobulin proteolysis and, thus, release of T_4 and T_3 from the thyroid. This is the most rapidly developing effect of iodide, occurring within hours; it is the principal mechanism for the antithyroid effect of iodide in patients with hyperthyroidism. This action also appears to depend on the intracellular iodide concentration. The precise mechanisms of these regulatory actions are not known, but iodide deficiency augments and iodide excess inhibits the adenyl cyclase response to TSH.[69]

REGULATION OF EXTRATHYROIDAL TRIIODOTHYRONINE PRODUCTION

The activities of the extrathyroidal T_4 5′-deiodinases are altered by a number of factors (Table 10-4). The enzyme that predominates in liver and kidney (type 1) appears to produce most of the T_3 that returns to the circulation. The activity of this deiodinase is decreased in hepatic tissue from fetal animals and animals that are starved or hypothyroid or that have diabetes, uremia, or a variety of other nonthyroidal illnesses[14,15,18,27,70] (Fig. 10-12). Deiodinase activity is also decreased by PTU, glucocorticoids, oral cholecystographic agents, beta-adrenergic antagonists, and various iodothyronine analogues, most notably rT_3. Effects in renal tissue are similar, although fasting does not impair renal T_4 5′-deiodinase activity. Conversely, type 1 T_4 5′-deiodinase activity is increased by thyroid hormone administration and by high caloric intake.[71] There are several biochemical mechanisms which might cause alterations in tissue T_4 5′-deiodinase production. They include (1) altered substrate (T_4) production, (2) altered T_4 delivery to the enzyme, (3) altered enzyme activity and/or mass, and (4) altered cofactor availability. The drugs that reduce T_4 5′-deiodinase activity directly bind to and thus inhibit

Table 10-4. Conditions Altering Thyroxine 5′-Deiodinase Activity

Condition	Enzyme type affected* 1	2
Fetus	↓	↓
Hypothyroidism	↓	↑†
Hyperthyroidism	↑	↓†
Starvation	↓	n
Diabetes mellitus	↓	n
Uremia	↓	n
Administration of:		
Propylthiouracil	↓	n
Iopanoic acid	↓	↓
Propranolol	↓	?

*Type 1 enzyme predominates in liver and kidney, type 2 in brain and pituitary.
†Excluding pituitary thyrotrophs.
Symbols: ↓, activity decreased; ↑, activity increased; n, no change.
Source: Data from Refs. 14, 15, 18, 27, 34, 73, 133.

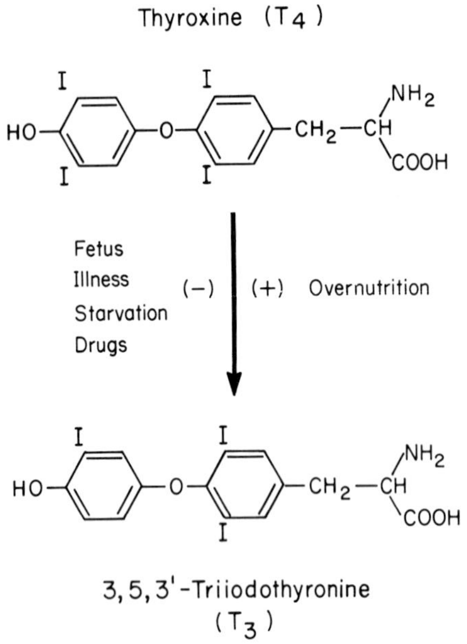

FIGURE 10-12 Effect of various diseases and drugs on T_4 conversion to T_3 in those organs (liver and kidney) which are the predominant sources of extrathyroidal T_3 production. Conversion is low in fetal tissues and is inhibited by illness, starvation, or certain drugs; overnutrition augments conversion.

the enzyme, whereas starvation may decrease hepatic T_3 production by reducing the amount of T_4 taken up into the liver;[72] in other situations, such as hypothyroidism, cancer, or diabetes mellitus, most available evidence suggests that alterations of enzyme mass or activity cause the decrease in T_3 production. The specific nutritional, hormonal, or toxic factors that cause the alteration of enzyme activity are not known.

The regulation of that T_4 5′-deiodinase which predominates in brain and pituitary (type 2) is different (Table 10-4). Its activity is increased by thyroid deficiency, little affected by nutritional deficiency and PTU, and decreased by thyroid hormone.[16–18,70,73] Such regulation serves to reduce the impact of systemic thyroid deficiency in these tissues by increasing the availability of T_3 for maintenance of neural and pituitary function and growth. The increase in pituitary T_4 5′-deiodinase activity that occurs in thyroid deficiency probably does not include the thyrotrophs; if it did, increased T_3 production in these cells would blunt increases in TSH secretion that are needed to defend against reductions in thyroidal T_4 and T_3 secretion.

Overall, these findings clearly indicate that T_3 production in various tissues is regulated in different ways. They also indicate that changes in thyroidal or even extrathyroidal thyroid hormone production, as manifested by circulating hormone concentrations, are not the only, and perhaps not the major, determinants of intracellular T_3 availability. Local regulation of T_3 production may be particularly important in limiting the effects of thyroid deficiency in tissues such as brain and pituitary,[73] and undoubtedly contributes to differences in T_3 availability in different tissues in patients with nonthyroidal illnesses.

Evaluation of Thyroid Function

Numerous tests are available for the evaluation of patients suspected of having abnormalities of the hypothalamic-pituitary-thyroid axis. Nevertheless, the single most important question to be answered in most such patients is how much thyroxine is being produced. The best initial tests for this purpose that currently are widely available are determinations of the total serum T_4 concentration and the number of unoccupied T_4 binding sites (T_3-resin uptake test) in serum. The combination of the two allows indirect estimation of the free T_4 concentration, which generally correlates well with clinical status. The routine use of additional tests as part of the initial evaluation should be avoided. Moreover, patients known not to have abnormalities of thyroid hormone–binding proteins on the basis of recent testing need not have repeated T_3-resin uptake tests every time their serum T_4 concentration is measured. If the results do not confirm the clinical impression, other tests may be needed. It is important to remember, however, that abnormalities in these tests occur in patients who have no disorder of thyroid function, especially those with nonthyroidal illnesses, and that treatment for thyroid disease should not be based on test results alone.

SERUM THYROXINE CONCENTRATION

The best method for measuring serum T_4 concentrations is radioimmunoassay (RIA). The assay uses specific T_4 antibody and requires the use of an agent such as 8-anilino-1-naphthalene sulfonic acid to render the T_4 bound to serum binding proteins available for reaction with the T_4 antibody. This is a reliable, specific, and inexpensive test. The normal range in adults in most laboratories is about 5 to 11 μg/dl. Two major factors alter serum T_4 concentrations, thyroid secretion of T_4 and the serum concentrations of thyroid hormone–binding proteins (Table 10-5). Therefore, serum T_4 concentrations are high in patients with hyperthyroidism and those with increased serum TBG concentrations, such as pregnant women (see Alterations in Serum Thyroid Hormone Binding, below). Rarer situations that result in raised T_4 concentrations are the presence of binding protein

Table 10-5. Conditions Altering Serum Thyroxine Concentrations, T_3-Resin Uptake, and Serum Free Thyroxine Index Values

	Serum T_4 concentration	T_3-resin uptake	Free T_4 index
Hyperthyroidism	↑	↑	↑
Increased serum TBG	↑	↓	normal
FDH	↑	normal	↑
Endogenous anti-T_4 Ab	↑	normal	↑
Generalized resistance to thyroid hormones	↑	↑	↑
Hypothyroidism	↓	↓	↓
Decreased serum TBG	↓	↑	normal
Inhibitors of TBG binding	↓	↑	normal
T_3 treatment	↓	↓	↓
Nonthyroidal illness	↓	normal or ↑	normal or ↓

Abbreviations: TBG, thyroxine-binding globulin; FDH, familial dysalbuminemic hyperthyroxinemia; Ab, antibody.

with increased affinity for T_4 (familial dysalbuminemic hyperthyroxinemia, FDH), autoantibodies that bind T_4, or decreased T_4 clearance. Thus, serum T_4 concentrations can be high in patients who are in fact euthyroid or hypothyroid. Conversely, serum T_4 concentrations are low in patients with hypothyroidism or decreased serum TBG concentrations, those who are receiving drugs that inhibit binding of T_4 to TBG, those receiving T_3 treatment, and those who are seriously ill as a result of nonthyroidal illness (Table 10-5). Misinterpretation usually can be avoided by simultaneous determination of serum T_4 binding capacity or direct measurement of the serum free T_4 concentration.

SERUM T_4 BINDING CAPACITY (T_3-RESIN UPTAKE) AND FREE THYROXINE INDEX

Since over 99.9 percent of the T_4 in serum is bound to TBG or other proteins, it is critical to determine the amount of protein binding to interpret properly the serum T_4 concentration. This is done most simply using the T_3-resin uptake test, which measures the number of unoccupied protein binding sites for T_4. The test is done by mixing radiolabeled T_3 with serum, adding a resin or other inert substance, and then determining the amount of radiolabeled T_3 bound to the resin. The test is outlined schematically in Fig. 10-13. In normal serum, the unoccupied protein binding sites, primarily TBG, take up about 45 to 65 percent of the radiolabeled T_3, and 35 to 55 percent of the label is bound to the resin, the "resin uptake"; these percentages depend upon the amount of serum and the particular type of inert substance used. Alternatively, the T_3-resin uptake may be expressed as the ratio of the amount of labeled T_3 bound to the resin in the presence of the test serum to that bound in the presence of normal serum (normal range 0.8 to 1.20). It should be emphasized that the T_3-resin uptake determination is not related to serum T_3 levels. Moreover, since the affinity of TBG for T_3 is low in comparison with that of TBG for T_4, the test is altered little by marked alterations in serum T_3 levels. Serum TBG concentrations can be measured directly, but such measurements have few advantages over the T_3-resin uptake test unless the specific cause of a binding abnormality is being sought.

There are three conditions in which the number of T_4 binding sites available in serum may be decreased, resulting in a high T_3-resin uptake: (1) when more binding sites are occupied with T_4, as in hyperthyroidism; (2) when binding sites are occupied by some ligand that competes with T_4 for binding to TBG, such as salicylate; or (3) when there is a decrease in the number of binding sites, as when TBG production is decreased (Table 10-5). The number of unoccupied T_4 binding sites in serum may be increased, resulting in a low T_3-resin uptake, when (1) fewer binding sites are occupied with T_4, as in hypothyroidism, or (2) there is an increase in the number of binding sites, as when TBG synthesis is increased (Table 10-5).

Thus, a serum T_4 value must be examined in conjunction with the T_3-resin uptake; if *both* T_3-resin uptake and serum T_4 concentration are high, or if both are low, thyroid secretion is altered. If the two results are discordant, a binding protein abnormality is likely (Fig. 10-13). The product of the serum T_4 con-

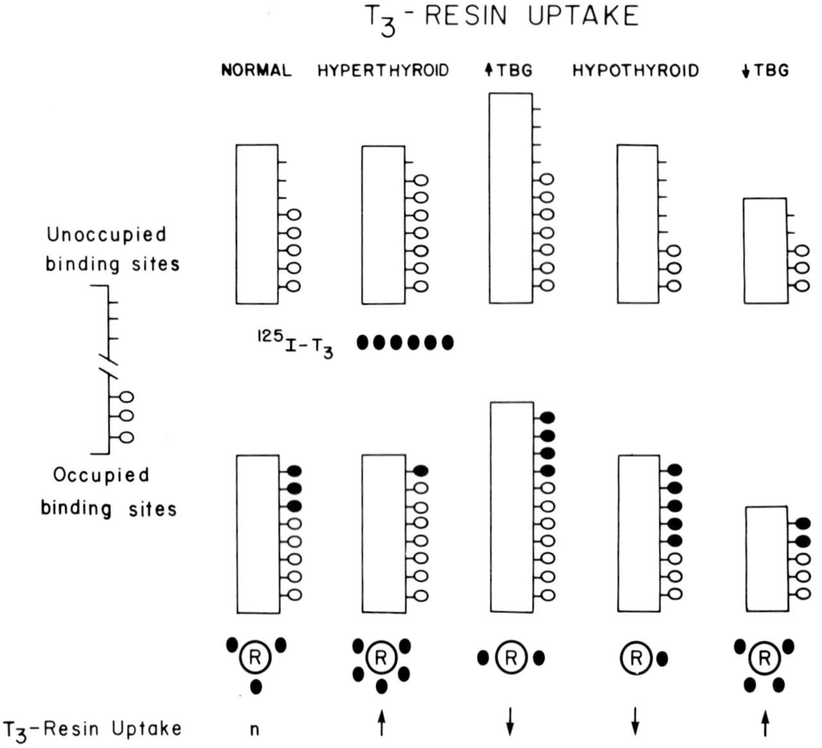

FIGURE 10-13 The T_3-resin uptake test. For clarity of representation the proportion of the total sites occupied by endogenous hormone is underrepresented in this figure.

centration and the T_3-resin uptake yields the free T_4 index. This value generally correlates well with direct measurement of the serum free T_4 concentration, although it may be inaccurate in patients with nonthyroidal illnesses, those with very large increases or decreases in serum TBG concentrations, and those with FDH.

SERUM FREE THYROXINE CONCENTRATION

If tracer quantities of radiolabeled T_4 are added to serum and the mixture dialyzed to equilibrium against protein-free buffer, the percentage of labeled T_4 that is dialyzable represents the proportion of the hormone in serum that is free (called percent free T_4 or dialyzable fraction of T_4). The product of this value and the serum T_4 concentration is the serum free T_4 concentration. This test is technically difficult, time-consuming, and expensive. Normal values range from 1 to 3 ng/dl. Serum free T_4 levels are high in hyperthyroidism and low in hypothyroidism, even in the presence of abnormal TBG concentrations. Free T_4 measurements are occasionally useful in determining whether a patient with an abnormality in thyroid hormone binding also has thyroid dysfunction.

Several assays that directly measure serum free T_4 concentration by nonequilibrium methods or with a radiolabeled thyroxine analogue that does not bind to TBG are available. Most such methods include a measurement of serum total T_4 concentration as well. In general, these methods provide reliable results in patients with thyroid disease or the common abnormalities in thyroid hormone transport. However, like serum free T_4 index values, the results of serum free T_4 determinations using these methods may be misleading in patients with nonthyroidal illnesses or those with abnormalities in serum thyroid hormone–binding proteins.

SERUM TRIIODOTHYRONINE CONCENTRATION

Serum T_3 concentrations are measured by RIA. The normal range in most laboratories is 75 to 200 ng/dl. Serum T_3 concentrations, like those of T_4, are altered by changes in thyroid secretion and changes in serum thyroid hormone–binding proteins. In patients with hyperthyroidism, serum T_3 concentrations characteristically are increased to a greater degree than are serum T_4 concentrations; in patients with hypothyroidism, they are more often within the normal range than are serum T_4 concentrations. Serum T_3 concentrations are low in patients with many nonthyroidal illnesses (see Nonthyroidal Illness, below). The major, if not only, indication for serum T_3 measurement is for the evaluation of patients with clinical manifestations of hyperthryoidism whose serum T_4 concentrations are within the normal range.

SERUM REVERSE TRIIODOTHYRONINE CONCENTRATION

Serum rT_3 concentrations in normal subjects range from 20 to 50 ng/dl. Serum rT_3 concentrations depend primarily on the level of T_4 secretion, since virtually all serum rT_3 is produced from T_4 at extrathyroidal sites. Serum rT_3 concentrations are only modestly altered by changes in serum iodothyronine-binding proteins, because the affinity of TBG for rT_3 is low. Elevations in serum rT_3 concentrations most characteristically occur in patients with nonthyroidal illnesses, in whom rT_3 degradation is decreased. Serum rT_3 measurements are not useful clinically because of both the wide variations that occur in patients with thyroid and nonthyroid disorders and alterations in thyroid hormone–binding proteins.

SERUM TSH AND TRH TESTING

Measurement of serum TSH concentrations provides a very precise indication of the availability of thyroid hormone to the pituitary in patients with hypothalamic, pituitary, and thyroid diseases (Fig. 10-14). Serum TSH concentrations in normal subjects range from 1 to 6 μU/ml. Serum TSH concentrations are increased in patients with even minor decreases in thyroid secretion, including those with few or no clinical manifestations of hypothyroidism. Therefore, a normal or undetectable serum TSH concentration in a hypothyroid patient is compelling evidence of hypothalamic or pituitary disease. Serum TSH concentrations are also within the normal range in patients with nonthyroidal illnesses in whom serum T_4 and/or T_3 concentrations are decreased; in fact, serum TSH concentrations may be depressed in some such patients (see Nonthyroidal Illness, below). Since most currently available TSH radioimmunoassays are not sufficiently sensitive to allow detection of TSH in all normal subjects, serum TSH determinations cannot now be used to distinguish normal from decreased TSH secretion, as occurs in hyperthyroid patients. Improved assays are becoming available which do allow this distinction to be made.[74]

Administration of TRH increases serum TSH concentrations in normal individuals. TRH testing is usually carried out by administering 400 or 500 μg of TRH as an intravenous (IV) bolus dose; serum TSH

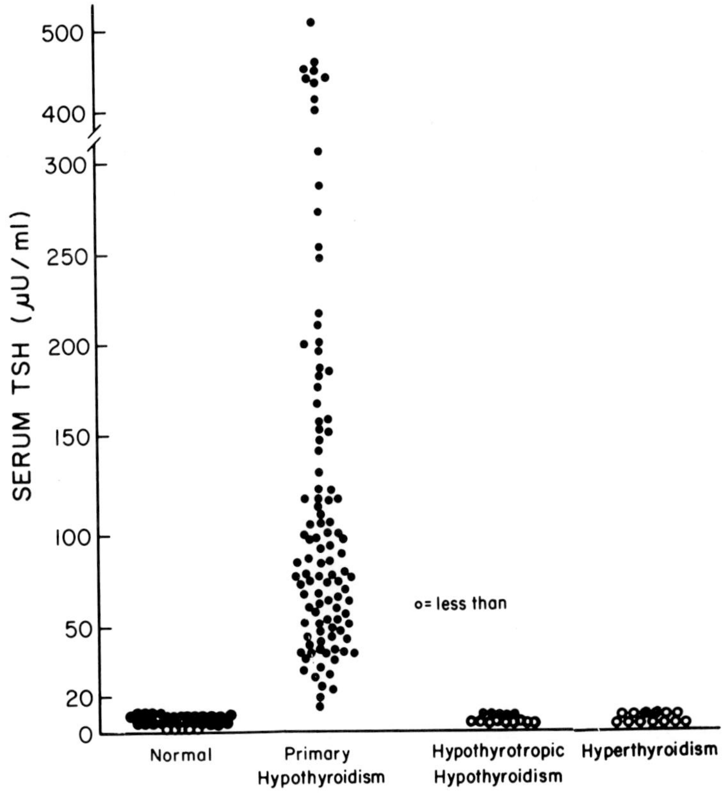

FIGURE 10-14 Serum TSH concentrations in patients with hypo- and hyperthyroidism.

concentrations increase two- to eightfold, to peak values of 5 to 25 μU/ml, 20 to 30 min after TRH administration. TRH administration usually is followed by transient nausea and an urge to micturate, and occasionally by transient hypertension; none of these side effects lasts more than 1 to 2 min. These doses of TRH produce maximal responses in normal subjects; smaller doses fail to increase serum TSH in some.

The response to TRH is characteristically increased in patients with primary hypothyroidism (see Hypothyroidism, below); the response is below normal and/or delayed in those with TSH or TRH deficiency. The response is inhibited by very small increases in serum T_4 and T_3 concentrations, so that TRH fails to increase serum TSH concentrations not only in patients with hyperthyroidism but also in euthyroid patients with autonomous thyroid secretion. Other factors, such as the actions of various drugs and nonthyroidal illnesses, also result in subnormal serum TSH responses to TRH. The only important clinical use of TRH is for the evaluation of patients suspected to have hyperthyroidism. In this setting, a normal serum TSH response to TRH conclusively rules out hyperthyroidism, but a subnormal response does not prove its presence (see Hyperthyroidism, below).

SERUM THYROGLOBULIN CONCENTRATION

Thyroglobulin is found in small amounts (5 to 25 ng/ml) in the circulation of virtually all normal subjects. Serum thyroglobulin is less iodinated than is thyroglobulin in the thyroid gland; this suggests that it is derived from the pool of most recently synthesized thyroglobulin. Serum thyroglobulin concentrations are increased in patients with hyperthyroidism, except when hyperthyroidism is due to exogenous thyroid administration. Thus, serum thyroglobulin concentrations can be used to differentiate spontaneous from iatrogenic or factitious hyperthyroidism. Serum thyroglobulin concentrations also are increased in some patients with endemic goiter, multinodular goiter, and benign and malignant thyroid tumors.[10] Serial serum thyroglobulin determinations may be useful in the follow-up of patients who have been treated for thyroid cancer, as an indicator of tumor recurrence. Thyroglobulin antibodies interfere with the measurement of thyroglobulin; therefore, serum thyroglobulin concentrations cannot be measured accurately in patients with such antibodies.

ANTITHYROGLOBULIN AND ANTITHYROID MICROSOMAL ANTIBODIES

Circulating antibodies to thyroglobulin are usually measured by the *tanned red cell agglutination* technique. High titers are commonly found in patients with autoimmune thyroid disease, especially autoimmune thyroiditis.[75] Since antithyroglobulin antibodies may be found in the serum of patients with Graves' disease, and less often in patients with subacute thyroiditis, nontoxic goiter, and carcinoma of the thyroid, tests for them have limited clinical usefulness.

Antibodies to thyroid microsomal antigen can be detected in serum by a variety of techniques. The most common tests presently used are a hemagglutination assay using a solubilized microsomal antigen and an immunofluorescent test using thyroid sections. If a very sensitive assay is used, such antibodies may be found in high titer in about 90 percent of patients with chronic autoimmune thyroiditis; antibodies are detected in lower titers in many patients with Graves' disease and in some patients with other thyroid diseases. Low titers of antithyroid microsomal (and, less often, antithyroglobulin) antibodies are also found in clinically and biochemically euthyroid subjects, particularly in elderly women, and in patients with other autoimmune diseases, such as pernicious anemia, idiopathic Addison's disease, and diabetes mellitus. Some of these patients have elevated serum TSH concentrations; they probably have chronic autoimmune thyroiditis.

RADIONUCLIDE AND OTHER TESTS

The characteristics of various isotopes useful for thyroid studies are shown in Table 10-6. Concern regard-

Table 10-6. Radiation Exposure from Isotopes Commonly Used for Thyroid Studies

			Average radiation exposure	
Isotope	Half-life	Usual scanning dose	Total body, mrad	Thyroid, rads*
^{123}I	13 h	200 μCi	6	2.6
^{131}I	8 days	50 μCi	36	65
$^{99m}TcO_4^-$	6 h	3 mCi	10–20	1

*Based on 25 percent 24-h uptake.
Isotopes given orally, except $^{99m}TcO_4^-$ given IV.

ing the radiation exposure from ^{131}I makes ^{123}I the iodine isotope of choice for clinical tests (as discussed in detail in Chap. 11). Pertechnetate 99m ($^{99m}TcO_4$) is used widely for thyroid imaging (scanning); it is transported into the thyroid, but since it is not organified it diffuses back into the circulation rapidly, and therefore does not accumulate in the thyroid. It is safe and easy to detect. Iodide isotopes are given orally, whereas pertechnetate is administered intravenously.

Measurement of thyroid radioiodine uptake, as the proportion of administered isotope concentrated in the thyroid per unit time, is still occasionally useful as an index of thyroid function. In patients in the United States, the percentage of radioiodine taken up by the thyroid is normally 5 to 15 percent in 2 to 4 h and 10 to 25 percent in the 24 h after administration of the isotope. In hyperthyroid patients, a low radioiodine uptake indicates thyroiditis or factitious hyperthyroidism. The test is necessary for choosing the dose of ^{131}I for therapy of hyperthyroidism. Because of the rather low values for radioiodine uptake in normal subjects, a low radioactive iodine uptake is not useful to distinguish hypothyroidism from euthyroidism, and some hypothyroid patients have high normal or increased radioiodine uptake. Radionuclides should not be administered to pregnant women.

Thyroid scanning is useful for detecting anatomic thyroid variations, locating ectopic thyroid tissue, and assessing regional function within the thyroid. In patients with nodular thyroid disease, scans indicate whether nodules can concentrate radioisotope and whether functioning nodules suppress extranodular tissue. Scanning may be done either with iodine radioisotopes or $^{99m}TcO_4$. The latter is preferable; it is less costly and more convenient for the patient, because the thyroid scan can be done 20 to 30 min after $^{99m}TcO_4$ administration, when thyroid pertechnetate uptake is at its peak. In contrast, peak radioiodine uptake occurs 24 h after it is administered so that a second visit is required. In either instance, proper interpretation of the scan requires examination of the patient's thyroid gland and of the scan at the same time. In most instances the results of scans using each isotope are similar; occasionally, a nodule concentrates pertechnetate but not iodide, because the nodule cannot organify iodide.

Ultrasonography and needle biopsy are discussed in Chap. 11.

TESTS OF THYROID HORMONE ACTION IN TISSUE

Thyroid hormones alter the function of many tissues. Measurements reflecting their impact on tissues would be expected to be useful adjuncts for the diagnosis of hyper- or hypothyroidism. However, the procedures now available for this purpose, such as measurements of myocardial contractility and serum cholesterol, sex hormone–binding globulin, and enzyme concentrations, are neither sensitive nor specific indicators of thyroid hormone availability. In the absence of hypothalamic or pituitary disease, the serum TSH concentration reflects thyroid hormone availability (its value for this purpose was discussed previously). There is a need for sensitive and specific tests reflecting thyroid hormone action in tissues other than the pituitary. Such tests would be particularly useful for evaluating the effects of the numerous changes that occur in patients with nonthyroidal illnesses.

Physiological Variables Affecting Pituitary-Thyroid Function and Tests

PREGNANCY

Serum T_4 and T_3 concentrations increase progressively throughout the first half of pregnancy, to values about 50 percent higher than those in men and nonpregnant women. Concentrations in serum remain constant during the latter half of pregnancy, returning to normal 4 to 6 weeks postpartum;[76] this increase is due to increased TBG production. There is a transient increase in serum free T_4 and T_3 concentrations in the first trimester, which coincides with the period of highest serum HCG concentration; it is probably due to the weak thyroid-stimulating action of HCG.[77] During this period serum TSH concentrations and serum TSH responses to TRH are slightly decreased. While pregnancy is a period of increased demand for iodide, there is no evidence that thyroid enlargement occurs during pregnancy in women whose iodide intake is adequate, as it is in the United States.[78]

FETAL THYROID FUNCTION

Thyroid function begins at about the tenth week of fetal life, and thyroxine secretion begins soon thereafter.[79] Serum T_4 concentrations are low until midgestation, and then increase progressively, reaching values similar to those in maternal serum at the time of delivery. Serum free T_4 concentrations are slightly higher, since TBG levels in fetal serum are lower than in maternal serum. Fetal serum T_3 concentrations, however, are very low and serum rT_3 concentrations are high. Fetal tissues have little T_4 5′-deiodinase activity. Placental tissue is rich in iodothyronine 5-deiodinase activity. T_3 is deiodinated to 3,3′-T_2 and T_4 to rT_3 very rapidly; thus, little maternal T_4 or T_3 reaches the fetus. The high level of placental conversion of T_4 to rT_3 also may explain the high fetal serum rT_3 concentrations.[80]

TSH becomes detectable in fetal serum at about the end of the first trimester, and thereafter rises gradually to levels of 5 to 15 μU/ml at term; maternal TSH does not reach the fetal circulation. TRH is detectable in the fetal hypothalamus by the end of the first trimester of gestation. However, the role of TRH in fetal pituitary-thyroid development is probably small, since anencephalic fetuses do not have hypothyroidism. Maternal TRH probably does not cross the placenta in important quantities, although large doses of TRH given to mothers shortly before delivery raise cord serum TSH concentrations.[80] The pituitary-thyroid system in the fetus responds appropriately to hypothyroidism, since maternal ingestion of antithyroid drugs or iodide causes fetal thyroid enlargement.

INFANTS AND CHILDREN

Serum TSH concentrations increase abruptly soon after birth, reaching levels from 50 to 100 μU/ml 1 to 2 h after delivery, and then gradually decline to adult values by the third or fourth day of life.[79] This surge in TSH concentration results in increased T_4 secretion. Serum T_4 concentrations increase 1.5 to 2 times in the first day of life, and then fall. However, they remain slightly higher than in adults throughout infancy and childhood, gradually declining to adult levels by puberty.[81] Serum T_3 concentrations increase four- to eightfold within the first day of life, due to increased thyroidal secretion, increased supply of T_4 for peripheral production of T_3, and rapidly increased extrathyroidal T_3 production. Serum T_3 concentrations also are slightly higher throughout childhood than in adults. The gradual decline in serum T_4 and T_3 concentrations throughout childhood is a result of gradually falling serum TBG concentrations; free hormone concentrations after the neonatal period are similar to those of adults. Serum rT_3 concentrations decline rapidly after birth, presumably due to rapid maturation of 5′-deiodinating pathways.

SEX

There are no significant differences in pituitary-thyroid function between women and men, either in regard to thyroid secretion, extrathyroidal thyroid hormone metabolism, or serum thyroid hormone–binding proteins. Thus, serum hormone concentrations do not differ. While TBG production is stimulated by estrogen and inhibited by androgen, serum TBG concentrations are similar in normal men and women, despite the disparities in gonadal steroid hormone concentrations (see Alterations in Serum Thyroid Hormone Binding, below).

AGING

The metabolic clearance rates of T_4 and T_3 gradually decrease with advancing age, as do T_4 and T_3 production rates. Serum T_4, T_3, and rT_3 concentrations in older adults are similar to those in younger adults, as are serum TSH concentrations; serum TSH responses to TRH, though, decrease slightly with age, more consistently in men than in women.[82] Reports that describe somewhat elevated serum TSH concentrations in the elderly, especially elderly women, reflect the inclusion of individuals with mild autoimmune thyroiditis: those individuals with elevated serum TSH concentrations usually have positive tests for antithyroid antibodies and histological thyroiditis.[83,84]

ENVIRONMENTAL FACTORS

Small variations in serum T_4 and/or T_3 concentrations occur as a result of seasonal variation; values are slightly lower in summer than in winter in temperate regions.[85] More convincing changes were found in T_4-treated hypothyroid patients in Japan; serum T_4 levels were lower and TSH concentrations higher in winter in patients receiving constant doses of T_4.[86] Cold exposure for several days raises serum T_4 and T_3 concentrations, although increases in serum TSH concentrations cannot be detected in adults exposed briefly to cold. Serum TSH concentrations do increase in cold-exposed infants, and the abrupt rise in serum TSH concentrations in the first hours after birth is due to cold exposure. Exposure to extreme high altitude (above 10,000 ft) also results in small increases in serum T_4, free T_4, and free T_3 concentrations, and variable increases in serum TSH concentrations. Other physical stresses such as intense or sustained physical exertion are not accompanied by significant changes in pituitary-thyroid function.

Alterations in Serum Thyroid Hormone Binding

Changes in serum thyroid hormone–binding proteins are important causes of altered serum T_4 concentrations, although they usually do not result in altered serum free T_4 concentrations or free T_4 index values. Most important in this regard are changes in serum TBG concentrations, because most of the T_4 and T_3 in serum is bound to TBG. If a binding protein is added to serum in vitro, the total T_4 or T_3 concentration does not change. Thus the changes in serum T_4 concentrations that occur in vivo require transient changes in pituitary-thyroid function and/or T_4 clearance to restore free hormone concentrations to normal. An increase in serum TBG concentration, for example, alters the equilibrium between free and bound T_4, raising the bound T_4 concentration and reducing the free T_4 concentration. This reduction in free T_4 concentration must result in transiently increased pituitary and thyroid secretion and/or decreased T_4 clearance until both the free T_4 concentration and the equilibrium between free and bound T_4 are restored. The converse occurs when TBG production decreases.

INCREASED SERUM BINDING

Increased serum TBG concentrations are most commonly caused by increased estrogen production, whether due to pregnancy, administration of estrogens or oral contraceptives, or estrogen-secreting tumors (Table 10-7). The increase is due to increased hepatic synthesis of TBG. The response to exogenous estrogens occurs over a period of 4 to 6 weeks and is dose-dependent.[87] The peak response is a twofold increase in serum TBG concentration, which results in a 50 percent increase in serum T_4 concentration. The serum TBG concentration returns to normal 4 to 6 weeks after termination of pregnancy or estrogen therapy. The amount of estrogen in most oral contraceptive agents now in wide use is too small to cause a major increase in serum TBG level.

Serum TBG concentrations may increase in patients with several liver diseases.[70] The greatest and most consistent increases occur in patients with acute hepatitis; chronic hepatitis and biliary cirrhosis raise serum TBG concentrations to a lesser extent. Some patients receiving methadone or heroin have increased TBG levels, although it is not certain whether the drugs or concomitant liver disease are the cause. Other drugs that increase serum TBG concentrations include clofibrate and 5-fluorouracil.[88] Other disorders that cause modest increases in serum TBG concentrations include acute intermittent porphyria and hypothyroidism. Increased TBG production also occurs as an X-linked inherited disorder.[89] Affected men have a twofold increase in serum TBG concentration; affected women have a lesser increase. The abnormality in transport protein production is limited to TBG; production of other hormone transport proteins such as corticosteroid-binding globulin and sex hormone–binding globulin is not increased.

Table 10-7. Important Conditions Altering Serum Thyroid Hormone Binding

TBG excess due to:	TBG deficiency due to:
Pregnancy	Heredity
Estrogen therapy	Nonthyroidal illness
Heredity	Androgen therapy
Acute hepatitis	
Familial	Competition for binding proteins:
Dysalbuminemic	Salicylates
Hyperthyroxinemia	Nonthyroidal illness

Increased serum T_4 concentrations also occur as a result of the production of abnormal binding proteins. One such syndrome is FDH.[90,91] Patients with this disorder are euthyroid. They produce increased quantities of those albumin isoforms which have higher affinities for T_4.[25] Binding of T_3 is not altered. As a result, serum T_4 concentrations are increased, but serum T_3 concentrations are not. Serum free T_4 concentrations are normal but serum free T_4 index values are increased, because T_3 does not bind to the albumin binding sites; the presence of the increased number of unoccupied binding sites is therefore not recognized by the T_3-resin uptake test. Serum TSH concentrations and TSH responses to TRH are normal, further confirming that the patients are euthyroid. This disorder is inherited as an autosomal dominant trait.

In a small number of patients, in whom hyperthyroxinemia is due to production of TBPA with increased affinity for or capacity to bind T_4, serum T_4, T_3, and TSH concentrations are very similar to those in patients with FDH.[92,93] The diagnosis of these disorders can be confirmed by the use of $[^{125}I]T_4$ instead of $[^{125}I]T_3$ in a resin uptake procedure; in such patients resin uptake of $[^{125}I]T_4$ is low because of the increased binding of $[^{125}I]T_4$ by albumin or TBPA.[94]

Hyperthyroxinemia, without hyperthyroidism, rarely is due to serum IgG or IgM autoantibodies which bind T_4.[95,96] The in vivo impact of such antibodies alone, in the absence of any thyroid dysfunction, is to raise the total serum T_4 and/or T_3 concentrations and slow the clearance of the hormones. When double-antibody RIA methods are used to measure T_4, as is done in most laboratories, such autoantibodies result in serum T_4 values that are falsely high, because the endogenous antibodies bind the labeled T_4 and effectively remove it from the assay system. When RIAs employing charcoal or other nonimmunologic methods to separate free from bound T_4 are used, falsely low serum T_4 concentrations are found. Endogenous thyroxine-binding autoantibodies also may bind thyroglobulin and/or T_3; in other patients autoantibodies binding only T_3 have been found. The antibodies may be mono- or polyclonal. Such iodothyronine-binding antibodies have been found most often in patients with autoimmune thyroid disease; most are euthyroid, but some are hypo- or hyperthyroid.

DECREASED SERUM BINDING

Decreased serum binding of thyroid hormones may occur as a result of decreased thyroid hormone–binding protein production or competitive interactions of drugs with the T_4 binding sites (Table 10-7). The greatest deficiency in serum TBG occurs in patients with an inherited defect in TBG production.[89] TBG deficiency is inherited as an X-linked recessive trait; affected men have virtually complete TBG deficiency whereas affected women have approximately half the normal serum TBG concentration. Disorders resulting in small reductions in serum TBG concentrations include acromegaly, Cushing's syndrome, and hyperthyroidism. TBG production also is decreased by administration of androgens and anabolic steroids; long-term, high-dose glucocorticoid therapy; and asparaginase therapy.[88,97]

Patients with many acute and chronic nonthyroidal illnesses have reduced serum T_4 and T_3 concentrations (see Nonthyroidal Illness, below). Among the causes of these changes are decreased serum TBG, TBPA, and/or albumin concentrations. Transient decreases in serum TBPA concentrations occur in patients with many acute illnesses. Serum TBPA concentrations also are low in those with chronic illnesses,[98] although the effect on serum T_4 concentrations is modest because of the relatively small contribution of TBPA to overall serum T_4 binding. The reduction in serum TBG concentrations that occurs in various nonthyroidal illnesses, such as chronic renal and hepatic disease, is usually modest.[99] Such patients also often have some degree of hypoalbuminemia. While albumin contributes even less than does TBPA to overall T_4 transport, hypoalbuminemia can contribute to decreased serum T_4 concentration in some patients. Whatever the specific causes or the degree of deficiency of the various thyroid hormone–binding proteins, there is little doubt that many patients with severe acute or chronic nonthyroidal illnesses have overall decreases in serum thyroid hormone binding, and thus high T_3-resin uptake values. In such patients the dialyzable fraction of T_4 is often relatively increased, so that serum free T_4 concentrations are more often normal than are serum free T_4 index values; sometimes serum free T_4 concentrations are increased.[70,99,100]

Substances which compete with T_4 for binding to TBG or other binding proteins, if present in sufficient concentration, alter the equilibrium between free and bound T_4. The result is an initial increase in serum free T_4 concentration; the free T_4 concentration then returns toward normal as a result of transiently decreased thyroid secretion and/or increased T_4 clearance. Thus, these patients have low serum T_4 concentrations and elevated T_3-resin uptake values, like patients with decreased serum levels of thyroid hormone–binding proteins. Seriously ill patients with nonthyroidal illnesses may have circulating lipid-soluble substances, perhaps fatty acids, which are derived from tissue, or serum IgM proteins, that inhibit serum T_4 binding.[101] Pharmacologic agents that competitively inhibit T_4 binding to TBG include salicylate, furosemide, and heparin; the last also displaces T_4 from intracellular binding sites.[88,102] Other drugs, such as phenytoin, phenylbutazone, and sulfonylureas, also inhibit T_4 binding, but not at concentrations achieved when used therapeutically.

Nonthyroidal Illness

A wide variety of abnormalities of pituitary-thyroid function, serum thyroid hormone binding, and extrathyroidal thyroid hormone metabolism occur in patients with nonthyroidal illnesses. These abnormalities frequently result in decreased serum T_3 concentrations; less often, they lead to decreased serum T_4 concentrations, and occasionally they produce decreased serum free T_4 concentrations. In general, the degree and extent of the abnormalities correlate with the severity of the nonthyroidal illness. The changes in serum hormone concentrations are accompanied by changes in T_4 conversion to T_3 which vary in different tissues; animal studies indicate that there are decreases in the number of nuclear T_3 receptors and postreceptor actions of thyroid hormones.

The conditions, considered together, mimic hypothyroidism. They are frequently referred to as the "euthyroid sick" syndrome,[70] but this term is inappropriate for several reasons. First, since the abnormalities vary in different patients, no single discrete set of abnormalities constitutes the syndrome. Second, while such patients have no overt clinical manifestations of hypothyroidism, there is evidence that thyroid hormone actions in some tissues are diminished. Therefore, it is more likely that these changes represent adaptive forms of hypothyroidism which serve to reduce the availability and action of thyroid hormones in order to lessen the physiological impact of the nonthyroidal illness; in other words, they are beneficial adaptations to illness. That no overt manifestations of thyroid deficiency occur may reflect the transient nature of the abnormalities, the variability of their impact in different tissues due to variations in local T_3 production, and the modifying effects of the nonthyroidal illness on tissue responses to thyroid deficiency. To further confuse matters, some patients with nonthyroidal illnesses have elevated serum T_4 concentrations. These various syndromes are shown schematically in Fig. 10-15; the derangements that contribute to them are listed in Table 10-8 (each is discussed in more detail below).

The frequency of these abnormalities in hospitalized patients is high. In one study of all patients

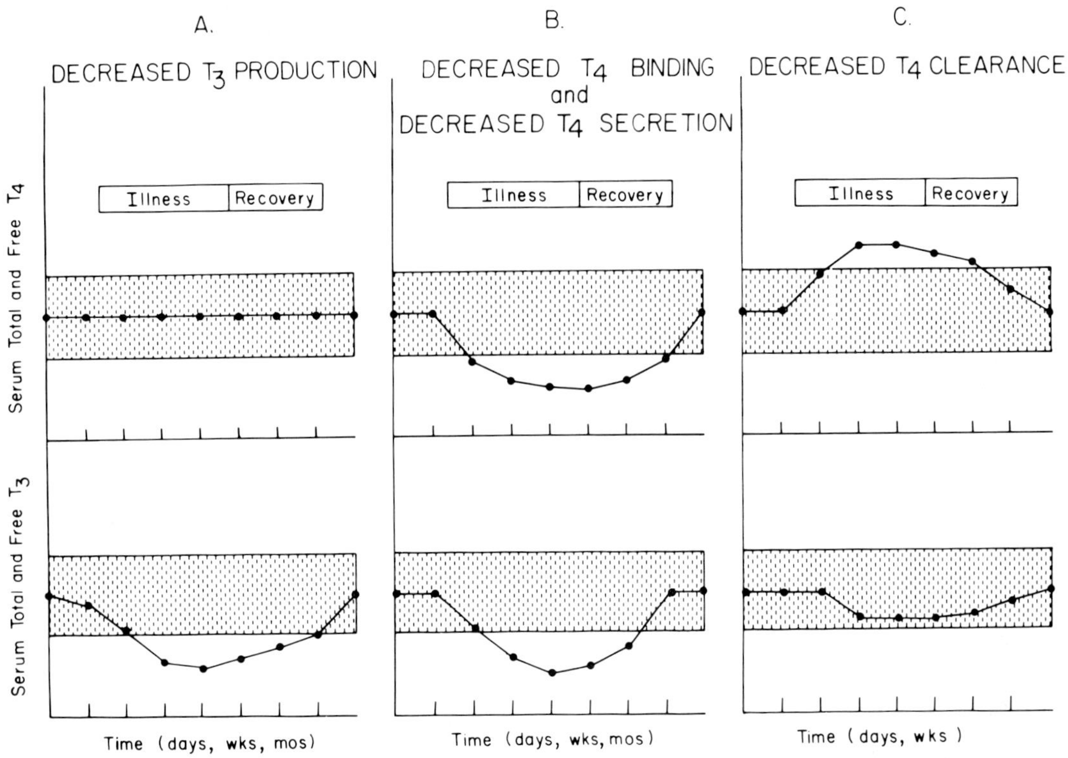

FIGURE 10-15 Patterns of the three major types of abnormalities in serum T_4 and T_3 concentrations that occur in patients with nonthyroidal illness; (A) Decreased extrathyroidal T_3 production. (B) Decreased T_4 binding and decreased T_4 secretion. (C) Decreased T_4 clearance.

admitted to a medical service on several days, 26 percent had decreased serum T_3 concentrations, 19.5 percent had decreased serum T_4 concentrations, 11.7 percent had decreased free T_4 index values, and 6.8 percent had decreased serum free T_4 concentrations.[103] Increased serum T_4 and free T_4 concentrations were found in 3.9 and 5.4 percent, respectively. Even higher frequencies of abnormal test results are found in patients admitted to emergency rooms or intensive care units.[104,105] It bears emphasis that these abnormalities do not occur in isolated forms and different degrees of abnormality may occur in individual patients. The occurrence of these abnormalities also means that care must be taken in diagnosing hypo- or

Table 10-8. Alterations in Pituitary-Thyroid Function in Nonthyroidal Illness

Alteration	Site	Cause
Decreased serum T_3 concentrations	Extrathyroidal tissue	Decreased T_4 5′-deiodinase activity
Decreased serum total T_4 concentrations	Extrathyroidal tissue	Decreased binding proteins Inhibitors of T_4 binding
Decreased serum free T_4 concentrations	Thyroid	Decreased TSH secretion
Decreased serum TSH concentrations	Pituitary	Decreased TRH secretion Increased dopamine secretion
Decreased T_3 action	Extrathyroidal tissue	Decreased T_3 receptors or postreceptor actions
Increased serum T_4 concentrations	Extrathyroidal tissue Thyroid	Decreased T_4 clearance Increased TSH secretion

hyperthyroidism, as those disorders are defined conventionally, in patients who have nonthyroidal illnesses.

DECREASED EXTRATHYROIDAL T_3 PRODUCTION

Decreased serum T_3 concentrations occur in patients with virtually all illnesses.[70] These include acute illnesses such as myocardial infarction, acute infection, reduced caloric intake, and the effects of trauma and surgery. Decreased serum T_3 concentrations also are found in patients with chronic illnesses such as diabetes mellitus; chronic liver, renal, cardiac, and pulmonary disease; and neoplastic disease. Administration of several drugs, such as glucocorticoids, propranolol, oral cholecystographic agents, amiodarone, and propylthiouracil, also results in decreased serum T_3 concentrations (see Effects of Various Drugs on Thyroid Function, below).

The fundamental cause of decreased serum T_3 concentrations in these situations is decreased extrathyroidal conversion of T_4 to T_3 (Fig. 10-15A). The identity of the particular organs in which T_3 production is impaired is not known. Presumably, they include the liver and kidneys; these organs are important sources of circulating T_3, and some patients have a circulating inhibitor of hepatic T_4 5′-deiodinase activity.[106] Serum total and free T_4 concentrations are usually normal. Serum rT_3 concentrations are characteristically high, due to decreased extrathyroidal 5′-deiodination of rT_3. Serum TSH concentrations are usually within the normal range, though they may be slightly increased or decreased; serum TSH responses to TRH are normal or diminished. The failure of serum TSH concentrations to increase may be due to continuing availability of T_4 for intrapituitary T_3 generation, altered thyrotroph sensitivity to decreased serum T_3 concentrations as a result of decreased TRH and/or increased somatostatin production, or intrinsic changes in thyrotroph function.[18,70]

The most widely studied model of this particular nonthyroidal illness syndrome is caloric deficiency. Normal subjects who ingest 600 kcal or less each day have an approximately 40 percent fall in serum T_3 concentrations and a 100 percent increase in serum rT_3 concentrations within 72 h. Both remain abnormal until refeeding, which may be accomplished with either carbohydrate or protein.[107] Serum T_4 and free T_4 concentrations do not change. Basal serum TSH concentrations and serum TSH responses to TRH may decline slightly,[70] but not sufficiently to decrease T_4 production.[108] The thyrotrophs remain exquisitely sensitive to increased amounts of T_3, since maintaining normal serum T_3 concentrations (i.e., a level characteristic of well-nourished individuals) during starvation by exogenous T_3 administration decreases serum TSH concentrations and virtually abolishes the serum TSH response to TRH.[109] The thyrotrophs also remain sensitive to the antithyroid effect of inorganic iodide, since iodide administration during fasting results in the same increase in TSH secretion as it does when food intake is normal.

When exogenous T_3 is given during fasting in doses which prevent decreases in serum T_3 concentrations, the acute metabolic responses to starvation are not altered, but urinary nitrogen and 3-methylhistidine excretion increase, suggesting that the decrease in T_3 production that occurs during fasting reduces protein catabolism.[109,110] Some manifestations of hypothyroidism occur when extrathyroidal T_3 production is reduced. These include reductions in cardiac contractility and rate; these reductions are reversed when small doses of T_3 are given.[111] Increased erythrocyte Na^+,K^+-ATPase activity also occurs.[112] In animals, reductions in extrathyroidal T_3 production and nuclear receptor T_3 content are accompanied by reductions in hepatic production of some enzymes, numbers of cardiac beta-adrenergic receptors, and cardiac myosin ATP isoenzymes. T_3 administration reverses these changes.[29,34,35,113–115]

Therefore, the reduction in extrathyroidal T_3 production is accompanied by some tissue responses indicative of decreased T_3 action. These responses should serve to conserve substrates and maintain tissue integrity. Thyrotroph function is altered in these situations so as to prevent increases in TSH secretion in response to decreased serum T_3 concentration. These findings suggest that reduced extrathyroidal T_3 production represents a beneficial adaptation to illness, and that raising serum thyroid hormone concentration in such patients is not warranted.

DECREASED SERUM THYROXINE CONCENTRATIONS

Both low serum T_4 and low serum T_3 concentrations are found in critically ill patients with various infectious, cardiac, pulmonary, renal, and other diseases; burns; and severe trauma[70,103,104] (Fig. 10-15B). Often only the serum total T_4 concentration is decreased, and the free T_4 concentration and free T_4 index value are normal. This change is due to diminished serum T_4 binding, resulting either from decreased serum concentrations of TBG, TBPA, and/or albumin or from inhibitors of T_4 binding in serum, which leads to increased T_4 clearance, as discussed previously (Table 10-4). However, in some patients serum free T_4 index values and, less often, serum free T_4 concentrations are decreased.[99,116,117] Such decreases are caused by increased T_4 clearance that is not compensated by increased TSH secretion. In fact, serum TSH concentrations in such patients are low normal or undetectable, serum TSH responses to TRH may be subnormal or even absent,[118,119] and T_4 production is decreased; these findings provide further evidence that TSH secretion is in fact decreased. The mechanisms responsible for decreased TSH secretion are unknown; they may include increased dopamine, somatostatin, or cortisol production or decreased TRH production. Further evidence that TSH secretion is decreased in such patients is that serum TSH concentrations may rise transiently above the normal range during recovery.[120]

These findings mimic those of hypothyroidism due to TSH or TRH deficiency; it is likely that they indicate more severe adaptive hypothyroidism, designed to produce greater reduction in thyroid hormone availability than occurs in patients who have only decreased extrathyroidal T_3 production, when more severe illness is present. (Nonthyroidal illnesses do not cause significant reductions in serum TSH concentrations in patients with primary hypothyroidism; therefore, the presence of coexisting primary hypothyroidism can be recognized in patients who have other illnesses.[121]) Clinical manifestations of hypothyroidism are not usually apparent in patients with nonthyroidal illnesses who have low serum T_4 concentrations. However, clinical assessment of thyroid function may be extremely difficult in seriously ill patients, who may, for example, be confused or obtunded, edematous, and hypothermic. There is evidence that low serum T_4 concentrations in such patients indicate a grave prognosis; in two studies, for example, more than 60 percent of patients with low serum free T_4 index values died.[104,122] One clue that such patients do not have preexisting chronic hypothyroidism is that their serum free T_4 values, whether measured directly or indirectly, are less depressed than are their serum T_4 values; in patients with hypothyroidism the converse is true. T_4 or T_3 treatment is of no benefit in this situation, and is potentially harmful.

INCREASED SERUM THYROXINE CONCENTRATIONS

Increased serum T_4 and free T_4 concentrations also may occur in patients with nonthyroidal illnesses.[14,123] Such findings have been reported most often in patients with psychiatric disorders, although their frequency in groups of such patients varies widely.[124,125] Serum total and free T_4 concentrations are also elevated in patients with various acute and chronic medical illnesses,[103,126,127] although increased levels are not characteristic of any one type of illness. T_4 levels are also elevated in some patients who have received certain drugs, such as amiodarone, oral cholecystographic agents, and propranolol (see Effects of Various Drugs on Thyroid Function, below). Serum T_3 concentrations are usually within the normal range. Basal and TRH-stimulated TSH concentrations also are usually normal, although the latter may be increased, normal, or decreased. These patients have few clinical manifestations of hyperthyroidism and their serum T_4 concentrations decline to normal within 1 or 2 weeks. There are several mechanisms by which such elevations in serum total and free T_4 concentrations may occur. One is transient increase in TSH secretion, which may be operative in patients with psychiatric disorders or those who received drugs which inhibit T_4 conversion to T_3 in the thyrotrophs. A second is decreased entry of T_4 into cells and/or decreased clearance of T_4. An additional abnormality that is probably invariably present is decreased extrathyroidal T_3 production.

In general, patients with elevated serum T_4 concentrations due to nonthyroidal illness are not severely ill. The diversity of illnesses and the transient nature of the abnormalities has made prospective study difficult; it is not now possible, except in the patients who received drugs, to identify the causes of the changes or to know their physiological significance. The practical significance is, however, clear: the diagnosis of hyperthyroidism in patients who are ill must be based on clinical evidence of hyperthyroidism, and not merely elevated serum T_4 and free T_4 values.

Effects of Various Drugs on Thyroid Function

GLUCOCORTICOIDS

Endogenous or exogenous glucocorticoid excess has multiple effects on pituitary-thyroid function;[70] increased endogenous cortisol production may account for some of the changes that occur in patients with nonthyroidal illness. Glucocorticoids inhibit TSH secretion, both at the hypothalamic and pituitary levels.[128,129] Large doses of glucocorticoids inhibit extrathyroidal T_3 production and can reduce serum T_3 concentrations within several days. They also decrease serum TBG concentrations and increase TBPA concentrations.[97] The net result of these various glucocorticoid actions in patients with spontaneous or iatrogenic Cushing's syndrome is low normal serum T_4, normal free T_4, and low serum T_3 concentrations; serum TSH concentrations are normal and serum TSH responses to TRH are somewhat decreased. Glucocorticoids also directly inhibit thyroidal T_4, T_3, and thyroglobulin release in patients with hyperthyroidism due to Graves' disease or thyroiditis.[130]

ADRENERGIC ANTAGONISTS

The beta-adrenergic antagonist propranolol, when given in large doses, is a weak inhibitor of extrathyroidal T_4 conversion to T_3; therefore, it reduces serum T_3 concentrations about 10 to 20 percent.[70] Serum T_4 concentrations modestly increase in occasional patients.[131] Other beta-adrenergic agents have a similar action.[132] In vitro, these drugs all inhibit T_3 production from T_4 in rat liver, but propranolol is the most potent.[133] The ability of beta-adrenergic antagonists to inhibit T_3 production is not related to their beta-adrenergic antagonist properties, since D-propranolol, which is not an adrenergic antagonist, is equally active.

PROPYLTHIOURACIL AND METHIMAZOLE

Propylthiouracil and methimazole (methylmercaptoimidazole, MMI) are commonly used antithyroid agents. Both of these drugs inhibit thyroid hormone biosynthesis (see Hyperthyroidism, below). In addition, PTU, but not MMI, rapidly inhibits the peripheral deiodination of T_4 to T_3, reducing serum T_3 concentrations within 24 h, while serum rT_3 concentrations increase.[134] PTU thus has a theoretical therapeutic advantage for the early treatment of hyperthyroidism. Monodeiodination of T_4 by the pituitary is not altered by PTU.[18]

IODIDE

Iodide administration, or iodide formed in vivo by deiodination of various iodide-containing drugs, alters thyroid hormone production in several ways (see Regulation of Thyroid Secretion by Iodide, below). Iodides have limited antithyroid actions in normal subjects,[135] but they may induce overt hypothyroidism in patients who previously received ^{131}I or surgical therapy for hyperthyroidism, or who have autoimmune thyroiditis.[136] Conversely, iodide may result in hyperthyroidism in patients with iodide deficiency or those with autonomously functioning thyroid tissue that concentrates iodide poorly[137] (see Hyperthyroidism, below).

IODINATED RADIOGRAPHIC CONTRAST AGENTS

Iodinated radiographic agents (iopanoic acid, sodium ipodate, and sodium tyropanoate) used for oral cholecystography transiently reduce serum T_3 and raise serum rT_3 levels for up to 2 weeks when given in single doses.[138] These agents are potent in vitro inhibitors of T_4 conversion to T_3 and rT_3 degradation in liver, kidney, and pituitary.[27] Serum T_4 concentrations increase slightly in some patients. Serum TSH concentrations and TSH responses to TRH also increase slightly, but usually not to above the normal range. The water-soluble iodinated contrast agents used for arteriography and pyelography do not alter pituitary-thyroid function. All of these agents contain large amounts of iodide, and are deiodinated in vivo, so that transient thyroidal effects of iodide may follow their use in appropriately susceptible patients (see above).

AMIODARONE

The antiarrhythmia and antiangina drug amiodarone is another iodine-containing agent that alters pituitary-thyroid function. In normal subjects, it inhibits extrathyroidal T_3 production and rT_3 deiodination, reducing serum T_3 and raising serum rT_3 concentrations.[139,140] T_4 clearance decreases, and serum T_4 concentrations increase, sometimes substantially, during the first several months of its administration. Serum TSH concentrations and TSH responses to TRH also increase slightly during this interval. After several months of therapy, serum TSH and T_4 levels return to normal. The changes in serum T_3 and rT_3 persist as long as amiodarone is given and for several months after it is discontinued, because it is stored in adipose tissue and very slowly metabolized or excreted. Because it also is in part metabolized by deiodination, it can cause either hyper- or hypothyroidism in appropriately susceptible individuals. Hypothyroidism develops more often in individuals whose iodine intake is high, as in the United States, whereas hyperthyroidism is more likely to occur in those whose iodine intake is limited.[141]

LITHIUM

Lithium is concentrated by the thyroid and inhibits the release of thyroid hormones.[142] It is thus goitrogenic, though only weakly so. Elevations in serum TSH concentrations occur in about 20 percent of patients receiving therapeutic doses of lithium carbonate, but overt clinical and biochemical hypothyroidism is rare.[143] Lithium also slows the rate of T_4 degradation, but does not decrease extrathyroidal T_3 production.

PHENYTOIN

Phenytoin (diphenylhydantoin) accelerates clearance of T_4 and perhaps T_3. As a result, serum T_4 and free T_4 concentrations decline by about 25 percent, while serum T_3 concentrations do not change. Serum TSH concentrations increase very slightly;[144] this increase may be due to direct inhibition of thyroid hormone action in the pituitary as well as the decrease in serum T_4 concentrations.

HYPERTHYROIDISM

Hyperthyroidism (thyrotoxicosis) is the clinical, physiological, and biochemical syndrome that results when tissues are exposed to excessive thyroid hormone concentrations. Thyroid hormones act in most tissues, and hyperthyroidism may result in abnormalities of virtually every organ system. The clinical manifestations of hyperthyroidism may be mild or severe; they may be modified by the patient's age, the presence of concomitant abnormalities in various organ systems, and the duration of the hyperthyroidism. Hyperthyroidism may be transient or persistent. The diagnosis may be obvious, confirmed readily by a few simple laboratory tests; or it may be difficult, requiring investigation of pituitary-thyroid regulation or prolonged observation. Hyperthyroidism is a rather common disorder. A community survey in Great Britain revealed a prevalence of 19/1000 women and 1.6/1000 men.[83] The annual incidence was estimated to be 2 to 3/1000 women (no comparable data are available for the United States). Thus, hyperthyroidism is much more common in women. This is true not only for Graves' disease, but also for hyperthyroidism due to most other causes as well.

Pathophysiology of Hyperthyroidism

Hyperthyroidism is due to the unregulated production of excessive amounts of T_4 and/or T_3, or ingestion of excessive amounts of T_4 and/or T_3. It may be due to intrinsic thyroid disease, excessive TSH secretion, excessive TRH secretion (theoretically), or production of abnormal thyroid stimulating hormones such as thyroid-stimulating autoantibodies (TSab) or HCG. Hyperthyroidism also may occur as a result of destruction of thyroid tissue with excessive release of T_4 and T_3. Any of these situations may exist without producing clinically significant hyperthyroidism, but hyperthyroidism cannot occur in their absence. Compensatory increases in thyroid hormone secretion may occur in patients who have accelerated hepatic T_4 and T_3 degradation or peripheral resistance to the actions of T_4 and T_3, but hyperthyroidism does not occur in such circumstances. Increased extrathyroidal T_4 conversion to T_3 should not cause hyperthyroidism, since any substantial increase in T_3 production via this pathway would result in decreased TSH and, therefore, decreased thyroidal T_4 and T_3 secretion.

In most patients with hyperthyroidism production of both T_4 and T_3 as well as serum T_4 and T_3 concentrations are increased. The increases in T_3 production rate and serum T_3 concentration characteristically are greater than are those in T_4 production rate or concentration.[145] Figure 10-16 shows a schematic summary of these findings. In one study of hyperthyroid patients, the mean T_4 production rate was increased 3.5 times, whereas the mean T_3 production rate was

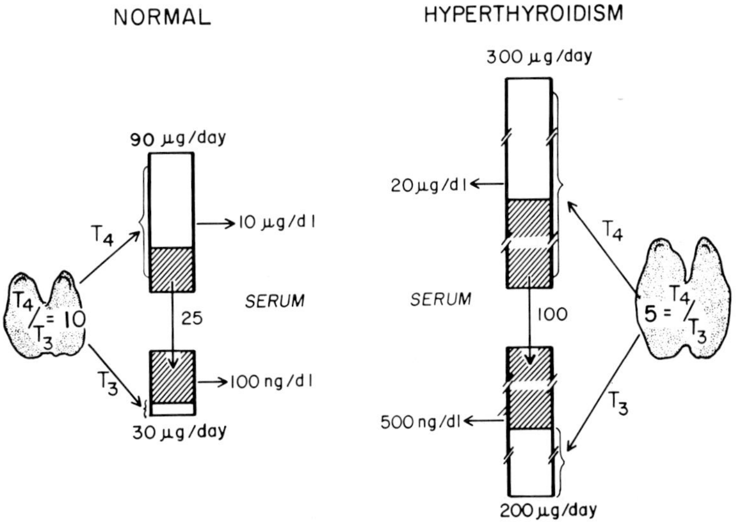

FIGURE 10-16 Diagram of thyroidal T_4/T_3 ratios, thyroidal and extrathyroidal production rates of T_4 and T_3, and serum T_4 and T_3 concentrations in normal subjects and patients with hyperthyroidism. The shaded areas indicate the amount of T_4 (upper bars) converted extrathyroidally to T_3 (lower bars). (*From Kaplan and Utiger.*[145])

increased over seven times.[146] The disproportionate increase in T_3 production has several sources. First, thyroid tissue from patients with hyperthyroidism has an increased T_3/T_4 ratio,[147] indicating that glandular synthesis of T_3 is increased to a greater extent than is that of T_4. Second, the rates of both thyroidal and extrathyroidal T_4 conversion to T_3 are increased.[13,148]

In some patients with hyperthyroidism, only serum T_3 concentrations, and presumably T_3 production, are above the normal range. This is referred to as *T_3 hyperthyroidism* (T_3 toxicosis), and is a result of marked discrepancy in the relative proportions of T_3 and T_4 that are produced. There are no characteristic clinical manifestations of T_3 hyperthyroidism. It is especially likely to occur in patients whose hyperthyroidism is due to a thyroid adenoma or recurrent Graves' disease, but may be due to hyperthyroidism of any cause. The frequency of T_3 hyperthyroidism varies widely; it is rare in the United States but more common in regions where iodide intake is limited. The abnormality resulting in T_3 hyperthyroidism is probably relative intrathyroidal iodine deficiency; greatly increased extrathyroidal T_4 conversion to T_3 in a patient who also had autonomous thyroid secretion also could cause the disorder.

A few patients with hyperthyroidism have elevated serum T_4 concentrations but normal serum T_3 concentrations (T_4 hyperthyroidism).[14,126,127] In addition to hyperthyroidism, most of these patients have another serious illness or have recently received oral cholecystographic contrast agents. Since extrathyroidal T_4 conversion to T_3 is decreased in patients with many nonthyroidal illnesses and by such radiographic contrast agents, the biochemical findings of T_4 hyperthyroidism are probably a result of excessive thyroidal T_4 and T_3 secretion and concomitantly impaired extrathyroidal T_3 production. In these patients, serum T_3 concentrations become elevated after recovery from the nonthyroidal illness.

Causes of Hyperthyroidism

An attempt should always be made to determine the cause of hyperthyroidism, since the various disorders which cause it differ in their natural history, and different forms of therapy may be required. (The causes of hyperthyroidism are listed in Table 10-9.) The cause of hyperthyroidism usually can be identified by history and physical examination. Important findings concern the duration of symptoms, and the presence of localized or diffuse thyroid enlargement, thyroid pain and tenderness, and extrathyroidal manifestations of Graves' disease. Laboratory procedures, such as determination of thyroid radioiodine uptake, thyroid scan, thyroid antibody tests, and TSH assay, occasionally may be helpful in identifying the cause but are usually unnecessary and need not be done routinely.

Table 10-9. Causes of Hyperthyroidism

Graves' disease
Thyroiditis
Subacute
Painless
Radiation-induced
Exogenous hyperthyroidism
Iatrogenic
Factitious
Iodine-induced
Toxic multinodular goiter
Toxic uninodular goiter (thyroid adenoma)
Ectopic hyperthyroidism (struma ovarii)
Thyroid carcinoma
TSH excess
Pituitary thyrotropin
Trophoblastic tumors

GRAVES' DISEASE

By far the most common cause of hyperthyroidism, Graves' disease most often occurs in young women but may occur in men or women at any age. It is not primarily a thyroid disease, but a multisystem disorder consisting of one or more of the following: hyperthyroidism, diffuse thyroid enlargement, infiltrative ophthalmopathy, infiltrative dermopathy (localized or pretibial myxedema), and thyroid acropachy. Most but not all patients with Graves' disease have both hyperthyroidism and goiter. As the two usually develop concurrently, Graves' disease is often referred to as *toxic diffuse goiter*. Extrathyroidal manifestations are less common; when present, they indicate that hyperthyroidism is due to Graves' disease. They may also occur in the absence of any evidence of thyroid disease.

A characteristic feature of hyperthyroidism due to Graves' disease is the presence of serum autoantibodies capable of reacting with and stimulating thyroid tissue. These thyroid-stimulating autoantibodies (TSab) can be detected in such patients by a variety of procedures, including in vitro and in vivo bioassays using thyroid tissue responses such as radioiodine release or thyroid hormone release, adenyl cyclase activation, cyclic AMP generation, and inhibition of TSH binding to thyroid tissue. Those assays that are based on measurement of a biological response in thyroid tissue are the most specific, albeit cumbersome; those that depend on inhibition of TSH binding are less specific because serum from patients with other thyroid diseases, notably chronic autoimmune thyroiditis, may contain immunoglobulins which inhibit TSH binding and TSH action. Using sensitive bioassays, TSab can be detected in the serum of nearly all patients with hyperthyroidism due to Graves' disease,[149-152] and at times in patients with nontoxic goiter;[153] whether the latter patients in fact have subclinical Graves' disease or the positive tests are due to nonspecific serum responses is not clear. TSab stimulate the thyroid when infused into normal subjects,[154] and the presence of TSab in the serum of newborn infants of mothers with Graves' disease correlates well with elevated thyroid function in the infants. Moreover, the presence of TSab correlates well with the presence of hyperthyroidism in untreated patients; in patients who have received antithyroid therapy TSab are associated with the presence of thyroid autonomy, as reflected by absent serum TSH responses to TRH.

TSab are components of the IgG fraction of serum. Their biological activity resides in the Fab fragment of IgG; it is inhibited by anti-IgG serum. Peripheral blood lymphocytes can produce TSab in vitro. Lymphocyte TSab production is stimulated by extracts of normal human thyroid tissue, and monoclonal TSab can be produced by immunization with lymphocytes from patients with Graves' disease.[155,156] Physicochemical studies indicate that TSab have limited heterogeneity but are not monoclonal. Thus, TSab are a family of IgG antibodies; the corresponding antigen is the TSH receptor or a region of the thyroid plasma membrane adjacent to it. When TSab bind to the thyroid cell, the TSH receptor is activated and hence thyroid function is stimulated. Therefore TSab are anti-thyrotropin-receptor autoantibodies, which cause hyperthyroidism by mimicking the action of TSH on thyroid tissue.

Serum from patients with hyperthyroid Graves' disease also may contain IgGs which stimulate thyroid growth, at least as measured in vitro by stimulation of thymidine incorporation; thyroid adenyl cyclase is not stimulated.[157,158] The presence or absence of such growth-stimulating immunoglobulins may account for the wide variations in the degree of thyroid enlargement seen in patients with hyperthyroid Graves' disease.

A third type of autoantibodies found are anti-idiotypic antibodies directed at the TSH combining site of TSab,[159] and presumably formed in response to production of TSab. Variations in production of such anti-idiotypic antibodies could modulate the severity of the disease.

If the hyperthyroidism of Graves' disease is caused by production of TSab, what factors initiate their production? One possibility is that TSab production is initiated by some thyroid injury which liberates a normal or abnormal thyroid component, which then provides the stimulus for TSab production by B lymphocytes. There is no evidence for such a mechanism; no known thyroid injury (e.g., thyroiditis, radiation damage) is followed by sustained TSab production, no structural thyroid tissue abnormality unique to Graves' disease has been found, and normal thyroid tissue stimulates TSab production in vitro. However, thyroid cells of patients with Graves' disease express class II (HLA-DR) histocompatibility antigens, unlike normal thyroid cells. Since T lymphocytes have HLA-DR receptors, the acquisition of class II antigens by thyroid cells could initiate abnormal lymphocyte function in such patients.

Another possibility is that some infectious or other agent stimulates production of antibodies which cross-react with thyroid tissue. A high frequency of antibodies to certain *Yersinia* serotypes has been reported in patients with Graves' disease, and some organisms, including those of *Yersinia* sp., have membrane TSH binding sites.[160,161] Thus, such infections could initiate production of antibodies that react with the thyroid TSH receptor.

A third explanation is that TSab production occurs because a normally suppressed population of B lymphocytes is activated to produce TSab. Such activation could occur as a result of increased B lymphocyte function per se or as a result of an abnormality in the function of the T lymphocytes which regulate B cell function. Either an increase in helper T lymphocyte function or a decrease in suppressor T lymphocyte function could cause increased B lymphocyte function.[162] Although the overall numbers of B and T lymphocytes in peripheral blood are normal in patients with Graves' disease, variable decreases in the proportion of T suppressor cells, as measured using monoclonal antibody techniques, have been reported, and thyroid tissue from patients with Graves' disease contains increased numbers of T lymphocytes.[159,162,163] When peripheral blood or thyroid T lymphocytes from patients with Graves' disease are exposed to particulate fractions of human thyroid tissue, they, in contrast to those from normal subjects, produce a lymphokine, *migration inhibition factor* (MIF).[164,165] This response is inhibited by T lymphocytes from normal subjects.[166] These results suggest that patients with Graves' disease have thyroid tissue–sensitized and –activated T lymphocytes and that their suppressor T lymphocyte function is deficient. By this formulation, TSab production, and thus hyperthyroidism, in Graves' disease reflect abnormal T lymphocyte regulation of B lymphocyte function; i.e., the underlying abnormality is one of T lymphocyte function. This hypothesis is outlined schematically in Fig. 10-17. The

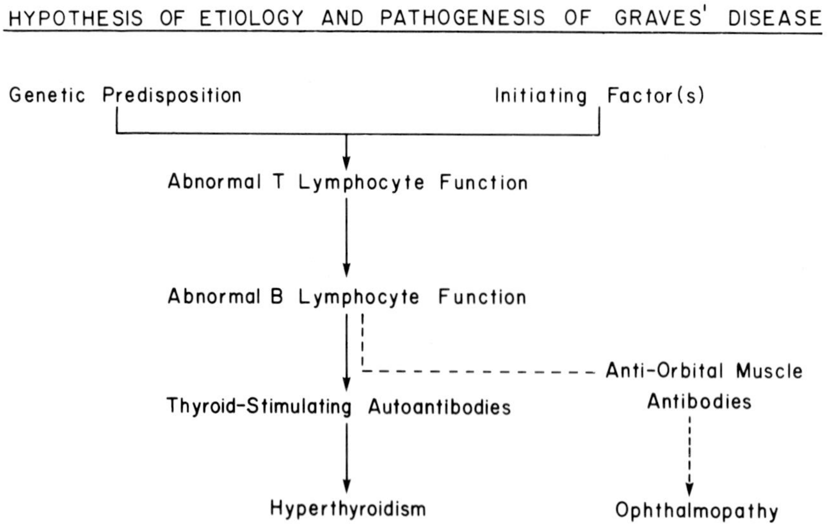

FIGURE 10-17 Hypothetical outline of the etiology and pathogenesis of hyperthyroidism and ophthalmopathy of Graves' disease.

genetic and initiating factors that might cause abnormal T lymphocyte function are obscure; one possibility is that the disease is initiated by some process whereby thyroid cells acquire class II histocompatibility antigens, as mentioned previously.

The causes of the extrathyroidal manifestations of Graves' disease, e.g., ophthalmopathy, localized myxedema, and acropachy, are not known. Clinically, they may not appear at the same time that hyperthyroidism develops. TSab do not seem to be involved in the pathogenesis of these manifestations of Graves' disease; many patients with ophthalmopathy without apparent thyroid disease (euthyroid Graves' disease) do not have serum TSab. Incubation of serum containing TSab with orbital tissue does not inhibit the thyroid-stimulating activity of TSab, whereas incubation with thyroid tissue does inhibit TSab activity.

If hyperthyroidism and goiter are due to autoantibodies, it is reasonable to suspect that the extrathyroidal manifestations of the disease are due to other autoantibodies which react with orbital and other affected tissues (Fig. 10-17). Several mechanisms have been proposed.[162,167] One is based on observations that immunoglobulins in the serum of patients with ophthalmopathy promote binding of TSH and its fragments to orbital tissue; such an interaction could presumably initiate an orbital inflammatory reaction.[168] However, TSH secretion is decreased in hyperthyroid patients and TSH fragments have not been identified in the circulation. A second hypothesis is that ophthalmopathy is due to binding of thyroglobulin to extraocular muscle, followed by reaction of thyroglobulin with free or lymphocyte-bound antithyroglobulin antibodies; or ophthalmopathy may result from binding of thyroglobulin-antithyroglobulin immune complexes to extraocular muscle.[169] Such events could initiate muscle injury and inflammation, which might be perpetuated by cellular immune reactions. Arguments against this hypothesis include: (1) many patients with Graves' disease have serum antithyroglobulin (and antithyroid microsomal) antibodies but relatively few have clinically severe ophthalmopathy, and (2) ophthalmopathy is rare in patients with chronic autoimmune thyroiditis who have high serum titers of antithyroid antibodies.

A third hypothesis is that ophthalmopathy results from an inflammatory reaction initiated by antibodies to extraocular muscle cytosolic or membrane antigens. Such antibodies can be detected in the serum of patients with ophthalmopathy,[170,171] but what initiates their production or how they cause ophthalmopathy is not known.

Even less is known about the pathogenesis of localized myxedema and acropachy, although they, too, likely have an autoimmune basis. Serum from patients with localized myxedema stimulates hyaluronic acid synthesis by fibroblasts in normal subjects, especially fibroblasts from the lower extremity; some monoclonal anti-TSH-receptor antibodies stimulate DNA synthesis and collagen biosynthesis in cultured fibroblasts.[172,173] These changes are in vitro correlates of localized myxedema.

There are several known risk factors for Graves' disease. One is female sex. A second is heredity. Evidence that hereditary factors predispose to the development of Graves' disease include an increased frequency of family history of hyperthyroidism in affected individuals; a high concordance rate in monozygotic twins; a high prevalence of antithyroid antibodies; abnormalities in thyroid regulation; and even TSab in other euthyroid family members of patients with Graves' disease.[162,174,175] The pattern of inheritance is probably polygenic. Compared to the general population, patients with Graves' disease have a predominance of certain HLA haplotypes at the B and D loci, especially HLA-B8/DR3, although the specific haplotype associations vary among different ethnic groups.[159,162] Previous suggestions that physical or emotional stresses are initiating factors remain unconfirmed.[176]

An important clinical feature of Graves' disease is the occurrence of spontaneous remissions. The abnormalities in cell-mediated immunity and TSab production decrease or disappear with time in many patients. For those patients whose hyperthyroidism is treated with antithyroid drugs, this means that prolonged therapy may not be required. The proportion of patients whose hyperthyroidism undergoes remission varies extremely widely, ranging from 20 to 80 percent in different series. The reasons for this variability are not known. One important factor is time, since higher rates of remission are usually achieved in patients treated with antithyroid drugs for several years.[177,178] Another factor may be dose-related immunosuppressive actions of antithyroid drugs; a third may relate to HLA haplotype.[179–181]

Remissions occur in patients who received no therapy, as well as those treated with antithyroid drugs and/or propranolol. Such remissions are usually accompanied by disappearance of TSab from serum.[149,151,159,162] TSab also gradually disappear from the serum of most patients late after treatment with radioactive iodine or subtotal thyroidectomy, although there are transient increases in TSab levels in the first several weeks after thyroidectomy; greater and more prolonged increases, lasting up to a year, occur after radioiodine therapy.[162]

Some patients who have a remission of hyperthyroidism have normal pituitary-thyroid regulation; this finding suggests that Graves' disease in such individuals has disappeared. In others, however, abnormalities of pituitary-thyroid regulation persist, suggesting that the Graves' disease continues, but at a subclinical level.[182,183] Presumably, in such patients TSab production persists, but in amounts too small to cause hyperthyroidism. Thus there is a pathophysiological, although not clinical, distinction between remission of hyperthyroidism alone and remission of Graves' disease. Remission of hyperthyroidism could also occur if thyroid failure takes place. Some patients studied many years after remission of their hyperthyroidism have evidence of hypothyroidism or, at least, thyroid damage, suggesting that thyroid failure can be the final stage in the natural history of Graves' disease.[182,184] If Graves' disease is considered a subset of thyroid autoimmune disease, with the other major subset being chronic autoimmune thyroiditis, then transition from the former to the latter could explain the later development of hypothyroidism. Conversely, hypothyroidism occasionally precedes the development of hyperthyroidism due to Graves' disease,[185] indicating that the reverse evolution can occur.

The gross thyroid pathologic finding of Graves' disease is diffuse enlargement. Microscopic examination reveals follicular hyperplasia. The thyroid follicles are small, contain decreased quantities of colloid, and are lined by columnar epithelium, which often projects into the follicular lumen (*papillary infolding*). The individual follicular cells have increased numbers of mitochondria, hypertrophic Golgi apparatus, and increased numbers of microvilli at the apical surface. The interfollicular spaces are richly vascular, often containing foci of lymphocytes and occasionally lymphoid germinal centers. Preoperative treatment in most patients causes reduction in follicular hyperplasia, vascularity, and lymphoid infiltration.

THYROIDITIS

Subacute Thyroiditis

Clinical manifestations of hyperthyroidism occur in approximately 50 percent of patients with subacute thyroiditis, although the frequency of biochemical hyperthyroidism approaches 100 percent.[186] Usually, however, hyperthyroidism is overshadowed by the nonspecific systemic inflammatory manifestations of the illness, as well as thyroid pain, tenderness, and enlargement. There is often a recent history of an acute upper respiratory infection. Hyperthyroidism lasts for a week to a month or so and then subsides, although it may recur transiently. Subacute thyroiditis rarely results in permanent thyroid disease[187] (this disorder is discussed more fully in The Painful Thyroid, below).

Painless Thyroiditis

Thyroiditis without pain or tenderness may be the second most common cause of hyperthyroidism. It occurs more nearly equally in men and women, compared to Graves' disease.[187,188] In women, it is particularly well recognized as a component of postpartum thyroid disease,[189] and may occur in the postpartum period in over 50 percent of women with a history of Graves' disease.[190] Characteristically, the hyperthyroidism is of recent onset and clinically mild; there is usually no history of preceding upper respiratory infection which is so common in patients with subacute thyroiditis. The thyroid is not painful or tender;

thyroid enlargement is slight or moderate. There are none of the extrathyroidal manifestations of Graves' disease. Thyroid radioiodine uptake is characteristically low. Sedimentation rate is usually normal and thyroid autoantibodies are present only in low titer.

Hyperthyroidism usually lasts for several weeks, but it may persist for several months. The hyperthyroid phase is followed by recovery, or by a transient period of hypothyroidism. Thyroid biopsies show evidence of lymphocytic thyroiditis.[191] Painless thyroiditis with hyperthyroidism thus is most likely a manifestation of chronic autoimmune thyroiditis, in which the thyroid inflammatory process is more intense than usual, but, since thyroid follicular cells are not destroyed, it is transient. Follow-up studies indicate that many patients have recurrent episodes of transient hyperthyroidism, including after subsequent pregnancies, persistent evidence of autoimmune thyroid disease, and/or later diminution of thyroid secretion.[187]

Radiation Thyroiditis

Radiation-induced thyroid follicular necrosis and inflammation following ^{131}I therapy can result in exacerbations of hyperthyroidism and/or thyroid pain and tenderness. These complications of ^{131}I therapy occur in the first 1 to 2 weeks after treatment, but fortunately are rare.

EXOGENOUS HYPERTHYROIDISM

Iatrogenic Hyperthyroidism

Hyperthyroidism is likely to occur in patients receiving L-thyroxine in doses of 0.3 mg per day or more, L-triiodothyronine in doses of 0.075 mg per day or more, or desiccated thyroid in doses of 180 mg per day or more (or the equivalent as combinations of synthetic T_4 and T_3). Somewhat smaller doses can cause biochemical and occasionally clinical hyperthyroidism. Iatrogenic hyperthyroidism is especially likely to develop when T_3 alone or T_4-T_3 combinations (whether synthetic or as desiccated thyroid) are used, because serum T_4 measurements underestimate the total dosage of thyroid hormone administered, particularly when T_3 alone is used. In euthyroid patients with autonomous (TSH-independent) thyroid function, whether due to Graves' disease, multinodular goiter, or an autonomously functioning thyroid adenoma, even the usual therapeutic doses of thyroid hormone, e.g., 0.1 to 0.15 mg of T_4 per day, may cause hyperthyroidism. Important clues to the presence of exogenous hyperthyroidism are absence of thyroid enlargement or failure of thyroid enlargement to regress significantly if the treatment was given for this purpose and normal or low serum T_4 concentrations. Such patients also have low thyroid radioiodine uptake values and low serum thyroglobulin concentrations.[192]

Factitious Hyperthyroidism

The biochemistry of factitious hyperthyroidism is similar to that of iatrogenic hyperthyroidism. Patients given thyroid therapy may increase the dosage themselves for a variety of reasons. Some patients perceive that larger doses of thyroid hormone provide more energy or allow greater food intake without weight gain. Other patients, particularly paramedical personnel, surreptitiously take larger doses of thyroid hormone because of psychologic disturbances. It is usually very difficult to obtain definite proof of the diagnosis, as most patients deny taking medication. They often have hysterical personality characteristics and usually decline psychiatric care.[193]

Iodide-Induced Hyperthyroidism

Iodide supplementation for inhabitants of endemic goiter regions results in a reduction in thyroid enlargement in most of the population, but it induces hyperthyroidism in some patients.[137] For this to occur, the patient must have some preexisting thyroid autonomy, but insufficient iodide intake to permit excessive thyroid hormone production. In iodide-deficient populations, iodide supplementation is followed by a transient two- to fivefold increase in the incidence of hyperthyroidism; most patients have evidence of Graves' disease, multinodular goiter, or an autonomously functioning thyroid adenoma.[194]

Iodide-induced hyperthyroidism also occurs in non-endemic-goiter regions.[137] Most patients have a multinodular goiter or a thyroid adenoma and develop hyperthyroidism several weeks or months after receiving pharmacologic doses of inorganic iodide, iodide-containing radiographic contrast agents, or iodide-containing drugs such as amiodarone. Induction of hyperthyroidism by iodide in such patients occurs because their autonomously functioning thyroid tissue has limited capacity for iodide transport; when large quantities of iodide are given, enough iodide may diffuse into the abnormal thyroid tissue to allow excessive thyroid hormone secretion.

TOXIC MULTINODULAR GOITER

Hyperthyroidism may be a late development in the natural history of multinodular goiter. Hyperthyroidism usually occurs in the sixth or seventh decade of life and mostly affects women. The usual multinodular goiter patient has a very long history of gradually increasing thyroid enlargement and develops hyperthyroidism insidiously. There is no ophthalmopathy or localized myxedema. Once present, hyperthyroidism persists unless it is treated or the autonomous thyroid tissue is destroyed by hemorrhage or infarction. The hyperfunctioning tissue is usually less efficient than normal; thus, the mass of autonomous thyroid tissue required to cause hyperthyroidism is large. Even so, hyperfunctioning regions account for only a portion of the total thyroid mass, as is evident on thyroid scan and pathologic examination.

The development of this type of goiter probably starts with the appearance of local areas of autonomous thyroid hyperplasia within individual follicles, followed by their continued replication and growth. The process is accompanied by extranodular involution so that functional and anatomic heterogeneity ("nodules") appears. As time progresses, some nodules may rupture, become hemorrhagic, or infarct, and considerable fibrosis occurs. If autonomous regions grow and function sufficiently, hyperthyroidism ensues. Such a formulation, based largely on autoradiographic and pathologic studies, explains the very gradual development of toxic nodular goiter, the fact that most patients with nodular goiter never become hyperthyroid, and the varied pathology of the disorder.

TOXIC UNINODULAR GOITER (THYROID ADENOMA)

Hyperthyroidism occurs in some patients with an autonomously functioning thyroid adenoma; its frequency in patients with this lesion is about 20 percent.[195,196] The female/male ratio is high, as in Graves' disease. Although thyroid adenomas occur in adults of all ages and occasionally in children, most patients with hyperthyroidism are in the older age groups. The adenomas in patients with hyperthyroidism are nearly always greater than 3 cm in diameter. For unknown reasons, hyperthyroidism rarely develops during follow-up of euthyroid patients with autonomously functioning thyroid adenomas who are not treated.[195]

The characteristic finding in a hyperthyroid patient with a thyroid adenoma is a solitary nodule. The thyroid scan shows intense isotope uptake in the location of the palpable nodule and almost no uptake in the remainder of the thyroid gland. T_3 hyperthyroidism is relatively more common in patients with a thyroid adenoma than in those whose hyperthyroidism is due to other causes.[195,197] Pathologically, these lesions are well-encapsulated masses of hyperplastic thyroid tissue, though they may be cystic. They are generally considered to be true tumors, in contrast to the nodules found in patients with multinodular goiter.

ECTOPIC HYPERTHYROIDISM (STRUMA OVARII)

The only recognized causes of hyperthyroidism due to excessive ectopic thyroid hormone secretion are dermoid tumors or teratomas of the ovary (*struma ovarii*). The ectopic thyroid tissue is the sole source of excessive thyroid hormone only when it contains a hyperfunctioning thyroid adenoma. This has been reported, but most patients with hyperthyroidism and struma ovarii have had a diffuse (Graves' disease) or multinodular goiter.[198] Thus, their hyperthyroidism was due to a more common cause, although the ectopic thyroid tissue contributed to it.

THYROID CARCINOMA

Thyroid hormone biosynthesis is virtually always very limited or nonexistent in thyroid carcinomas of all histologic types. However, hyperthyroidism occasionally occurs in patients with follicular carcinoma, usually many years after the initial appearance of the tumor and when the tumor burden is very large. Hyperthyroidism is rare in patients with thyroid carcinoma because few of these tumors transport iodide well, although many can synthesize thyroglobulin.[10]

THYROID-STIMULATING HORMONE EXCESS

Pituitary Thyrotropin

Excessive TSH secretion is a rare cause of hyperthyroidism. Patients with this abnormality have diffuse goiter but no ophthalmopathy. The majority of them have either a micro- or macroadenoma of the pituitary, but in some no tumor is evident, even after prolonged follow-up.[199,200] There may be concomitant hypersecretion of GH or prolactin as well. Characteristically, those patients with a TSH-secreting pituitary tumor have increased serum TSH and glycoprotein hormone alpha subunit concentrations that do not increase after TRH administration, although serum TSH concentrations increase during antithyroid therapy. In contrast, patients without a demonstrable tumor usually have normal basal alpha subunit concentrations; both alpha subunit and TSH concentrations increase after TRH and antithyroid therapy and decrease after exogenous thyroid hormone administration. Glucocorticoids regularly decrease TSH secretion and dopaminergic agonist drugs variably decrease TSH secretion in both groups.

Trophoblastic Tumors

Tumors of trophoblastic origin, i.e., hydatidiform mole, choriocarcinoma, or embryonal carcinoma of the testes, may cause hyperthyroidism. The evidence that the hyperthyroidism is due to a humoral product of the tumor is strong, since successful surgical treatment and/or chemotherapy of the trophoblastic disease results in cure of the hyperthyroidism. The thyroid stimulator is probably HCG, since (1) HCG has weak thyroid-stimulating activity and (2) there is a rough correlation between the HCG concentration and the thyroid-stimulating activity detected in bioassays of the serum of these patients.[201] While overt hyperthyroidism is uncommon in patients with trophoblastic disease, many have elevated serum T_4 and T_3 concentrations and impaired serum TSH responses to TRH.[202] The lack of overt hyperthyroidism in this group may be due to the limited duration of excess thyroid secretion and/or the severity of the manifestations of trophoblastic disease.

Clinical Manifestations of Hyperthyroidism

Hyperthyroidism is usually first suggested by evidence of increased thyroid hormone actions on one or more organ systems. However, hyperthyroidism may be discovered in patients who initially seek care for thyroid enlargement or ophthalmopathy. Since the actions of thyroid hormone are generally stimulatory, the manifestations of hyperthyroidism usually involve increased functions of various organ systems or inability of an organ system to meet the demands imposed by hyperthyroidism. The most common and specific symptoms and signs of hyperthyroidism are listed in Table 10-10. The diagnostic weights shown were developed on the basis of extensive clinical studies;[203] the scores presented may assist in the evaluation of patients with suspected hyperthyroidism.

The frequency and severity of the symptoms and signs of hyperthyroidism are influenced by many factors. These include the rate of onset, the age of the patient, and the vulnerability of different organ systems to excessive thyroid hormone action in individual patients. For example, the clinical manifestations of hyperthyroidism tend to be less severe when its onset is gradual, it is more debilitating in elderly patients and cardiovascular manifestations are more prominent in the elderly.[206]

Table 10-10. Frequency of Common Symptoms and Signs of Hyperthyroidism and Their Relative Discriminant Value

	Frequency in hyperthyroid patients, %	Diagnostic weight*	
		Present	Absent
Symptoms			
Nervousness	80–99	+2	
Increased sweating	50–91	+3	
Heat intolerance	41–89	+5	−5
Palpitations	63–89	+2	
Dyspnea	66–81	+1	
Fatigue and weakness	44–88	+2	
Weight loss	52–85	+3	−3
Increased appetite	11–65	+3	−3
Eye symptoms	55		
Hyperdefecation	12–33		
Signs			
Thyroid enlargement	37–100	+3	−3
Thyroid bruit	28–77	+2	−2
Ophthalmopathy	49–62	+2	
Lid retraction	38	+2	
Lid lag	48–62	+1	
Hyperkinesis	39–80	+4	−2
Tremor	40–97	+1	
Hands:			
Hot	72	+2	−2
Moist	76	+1	−1
Tachycardia (>90 bpm)	58–100	+3	−3
Atrial fibrillation	10–38	+4	

*A total score > +18 indicates hyperthyroidism, a score of +18 to +11 is equivocal, and a score of < +11 indicates the patient is euthyroid.
Source: Compiled from Refs. 203–206.

Hyperthyroidism is often tolerated well, particularly in younger patients, and some patients may feel better than when they were euthyroid, i.e., they may have more energy, can eat more without gaining weight, and are more comfortable in cool weather. Careful questioning usually reveals some less desirable changes, such as muscle weakness, emotional lability, or fatigue on exertion. However, hyperthyroidism is fundamentally a catabolic process; sooner or later more disabling manifestations are likely to develop if it persists.

Several clinical subtypes of hyperthyroidism with serious implications are recognized; they are *apathetic* or *masked hyperthyroidism* and *thyroid storm* or *crisis.* The term apathetic or masked hyperthyroidism is usually applied to elderly patients whose hyperthyroidism is manifested mainly by cardiac failure, atrial fibrillation, muscle weakness, or weight loss and who do not have the nervousness, heat intolerance, increased appetite, and general hyperactivity so common in younger patients. However, there is no evidence that apathetic hyperthyroidism is pathophysiologically different; more careful investigation will often elicit the presence of the latter type of symptoms and signs. (Thyroid storm is discussed later.)

GENERAL APPEARANCE

Figure 10-18 shows a woman with hyperthyroidism whose appearance alone should suggest the diagnosis. She appears to have lost weight and has a pained or apprehensive expression. Her skin is shiny and smooth, her eyelids are retracted, and she has an obvious goiter. Typically, she will be unable to sit quietly or talk calmly, but will speak rapidly and be restless and unable to concentrate.

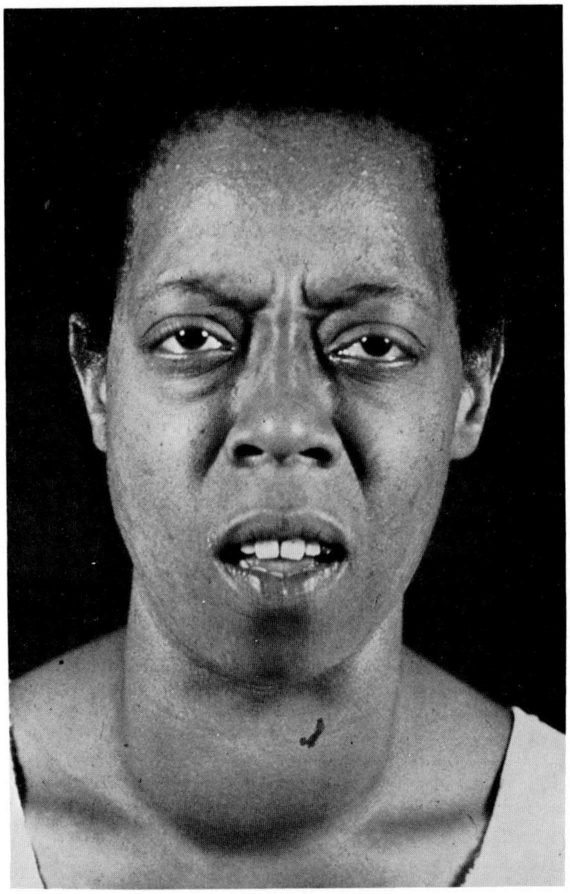

FIGURE 10-18 Photograph of a woman with hyperthyroidism and ophthalmopathy due to Graves' disease. Note the anxious expression, prominent eyes, periorbital edema, and diffuse thyroid enlargement.

SKIN AND APPENDAGES

The skin of patients with hyperthyroidism is warm and its texture smooth or velvety; erythema and pruritus may be present. Hyperhidrosis is a common complaint. Hair may become thin and fine in texture; alopecia can occur. The nails may be soft and separated from the nail bed (*onycholysis*). Other occasional findings are hyperpigmentation and vitiligo, the latter primarily in patients with Graves' disease. Localized myxedema, not a manifestation of hyperthyroidism per se, is described below (see Extrathyroidal Manifestations of Graves' Disease).

EYES

Two types of ocular abnormalities occur in hyperthyroid patients; noninfiltrative and infiltrative. The noninfiltrative signs, i.e., lid retraction and lid lag, occur in patients with hyperthyroidism of any cause. Usually, the upper lids are symmetrically retracted so that some sclera is visible, but lid retraction may be asymmetric and involve the lower lids as well. Lid retraction results in apparent proptosis, but not in forward protrusion of the eyes; it is often accompanied by subjective symptoms of conjunctival irritation. Lid lag is a common, but less reliable, finding. Infiltrative ophthalmopathy is discussed below (see Extrathyroidal Manifestations of Graves' Disease).

THYROID GLAND

Thyroid enlargement is a common finding and may be the initial or only clue to the presence of hyperthyroidism. In Graves' disease, both thyroid lobes are usually diffusely and symmetrically enlarged, but in about 25 percent of patients, the thyroid is not enlarged; absence of enlargement does not exclude the diagnosis of hyperthyroidism due to Graves' disease.[207] The goiter is usually moderate, i.e., the thyroid is two- to fourfold enlarged. The thyroid gland is sometimes slightly tender. Its consistency ranges from soft to firm; the surface is usually smooth, but it can be irregular or lobulated. A thyroid bruit or thrill, due to greatly increased thyroid blood flow, may be present. Thyroiditis results in slight or moderate diffuse thyroid enlargement; the thyroid is tender in subacute thyroiditis. Toxic multinodular goiters tend to be quite large, asymmetric, and uneven in consistency. A thyroid adenoma causing hyperthyroidism is usually at least 3 cm in diameter; no other thyroid tissue should be palpable.

CARDIOVASCULAR SYSTEM

Cardiovascular dysfunction is common in hyperthyroidism. In some patients cardiovascular symptoms dominate the illness. Heart rate, stroke volume, and cardiac output are increased and peripheral resistance is decreased. These changes are due both to direct inotropic and chronotropic effects of thyroid hormone and to increased peripheral oxygen requirements due to hypermetabolism. Either direct or oxygen-demand-mediated effects may predominate. Peripheral arteriovenous oxygen differences may be normal or decreased. Although cardiac output is increased, regional blood flow does not increase uniformly; skin, muscle, cerebral, and coronary flow are increased, whereas hepatic flow is not.[208,209] Other adaptive mechanisms augmenting peripheral oxygen delivery include increased red blood cell (RBC) mass and RBC 2,3-diphosphoglyceric acid concentrations.[210]

The changes in cardiovascular function may result in palpitations, tachycardia, atrial fibrillation or, less commonly, paroxysmal atrial tachycardia and heart failure. Atrial fibrillation may be the sole manifestation of hyperthyroidism.[211] The pulse pressure is increased, arterial pulsations are bounding, and systolic hypertension may be present. A jugular venous hum is often heard. Examination of the heart reveals a prominent apical impulse, accentuated heart sounds, systolic ejection or other murmurs, and, occasionally, cardiac enlargement. Other than disturbances in rhythm, electrocardiographic manifestations are limited to nonspecific ST and T wave abnormalities. Noninvasive studies show shortened systolic time intervals, rapid myocardial contraction, increased ventricular mass, and reduced left ventricular ejection fraction during exercise.[213,214]

The question of whether or not hyperthyroidism alone causes cardiac failure is controversial, particularly since heart failure with hyperthyroidism usually occurs in older patients presumed to have underlying cardiac disease. Heart failure, usually in association with atrial fibrillation, may occur in younger patients who have no evidence of cardiac disease when studied after treatment. Dynamic studies in patients with heart failure have shown both normal and increased resting cardiac output; in both groups, however, cardiac output is unchanged or decreased during exercise.[214] Symptomatic coronary artery disease, if present, is aggravated by hyperthyroidism.

RESPIRATORY FUNCTION

Abnormalities in respiratory function described in hyperthyroidism include decreased vital capacity, decreased pulmonary compliance, and increased minute ventilation.[215] Alveolar and arterial oxygen and CO_2 pressures (P_{O_2} and P_{CO_2}) are usually normal. Ventilatory responses to hypoxemia or hypercapnia are increased.[216] Dyspnea during exercise is a common symptom; it is best explained by respiratory muscle weakness.[217] Less often, dyspnea is due to cardiac dysfunction.

GASTROINTESTINAL SYSTEM

Appetite and food intake increase in hyperthyroid patients in response to increased calorie use. In most patients, however, compensation is inadequate and some weight loss occurs. Weight loss is usually modest, although in older patients weight losses of 20 lb (9 kg) or more are common.[206] The increased appetite and food intake are sometimes sufficient to cause modest weight gain; such patients probably eat to satisfy emotional needs.

The major abnormality in GI function is reduced bowel transit time. The most common symptom is increased frequency of bowel movements, though frank diarrhea may occur. Intestinal hypermotility and increased dietary fat intake cause steatorrhea in some patients.[218] Intestinal histology is normal, as is absorption of D-xylose and cyanocobalmin. Some abnormalities in hepatic function are found in the majority of patients. These include mild increases in concentrations of serum alanine and aspartate aminotransferase, alkaline phosphatase, and bilirubin; occasionally, jaundice is clinically evident. Serum angiotensin converting enzyme activity is often increased.[219] Serum albumin concentrations may be reduced. Liver histology is normal or shows mild hepatocellular necrosis.

HEMATOPOIETIC SYSTEM

Both red cell mass and plasma volume tend to be increased in hyperthyroidism; the volume increase predominates.[210] Thus, some patients have modest anemia; often, the RBCs are slightly microcytic.[220] Red cell survival is normal or slightly shortened. Serum vitamin B_{12}, folate, and iron levels and iron stores may be low. Iron clearance and serum erythropoietin concentrations tend to be increased. The bone marrow shows erythroid hyperplasia and, occasionally, megaloblastic changes. These findings, indicative of increased iron utilization and increased RBC production, are the expected responses to the need for increased peripheral oxygen delivery. The lack of an increase in red cell mass and consequent mild anemia in some patients is probably a reflection of deficiency of one or more hematopoietic nutrients. Pernicious anemia is found in 1 to 2 percent of patients with hyperthyroidism due to Graves' disease, though not necessarily close to it in time. Parietal cell antibodies are found in about 10 percent of such patients.[221]

Granulocytes and lymphocytes are usually normal in number, although mild lymphocytosis and granulocytopenia may be present.[220] Lymphadenopathy, thymic enlargement, and splenomegaly are occasionally found; it is not clear whether these are manifestations of hyperthyroidism per se or of Graves' disease. Some hyperthyroid patients bruise easily and are thrombocytopenic; their platelets contain increased amounts of IgG and aggregate abnormally.[222] Factor VIII–related antigen and coagulant activity tend to be increased.[223]

RENAL FUNCTION

Renal blood flow, glomerular filtration rate, and tubular reabsorptive and secretory capacities are increased, but electrolyte balance and serum electrolyte levels are normal. Plasma renin activity is often increased, although aldosterone production is normal. Renin and aldosterone levels and renal responses to sodium restriction and volume increase are normal.[224] Studies of water balance usually show impaired concentrating ability after both dehydration and vasopressin administration, probably due to increased renal medullary blood flow and, therefore, decreased intramedullary solute concentrations. Polydipsia and polyuria may be prominent symptoms; in such patients serum osmolality is lower than normal, indicating that primary thirst stimulation may be expected.[225] Given the heat sensitivity and physical and emotional lability common in hyperthyroidism, the occurrence of primary polydipsia is not surprising.

NERVOUS SYSTEM AND MUSCLE

Hyperthyroid patients often have symptoms of CNS dysfunction. Common complaints are nervousness, physical hyperactivity, emotional lability, anxiety, and distractibility. Patients become very restless and are unable to remain still for any length of time. Ability to concentrate on a task is decreased, and complaints of memory loss are common. Objective testing may show some impairment of cognitive function. Lability of mood is often striking: patients may become irritable and short-tempered, or may easily become depressed and prone to crying spells. Insomnia may be marked. These changes often result in significant impairment of work or school performance and disturbances in home and family life. Most patients are aware of these changes, but their extent often becomes clearer when a family member or friend is interviewed. At the other extreme, depression and withdrawal may occur in older patients. These striking clinical findings occur in the absence of gross abnormalities in cerebral oxygen consumption or substrate utilization.

Neuromuscular symptoms include tremor and muscle weakness. The tremor is usually limited to the hands and fingers and is most evident when the hands are extended. It may also involve the arms, legs, tongue, and head. The movements are rapid, uniform, and of low amplitude. Though not worsened by voluntary movement, performance of skills requiring fine coordination, such as threading a needle or writing, becomes difficult. The pathophysiology of the hyperthyroid tremor is unclear. It is not a manifestation of muscle weakness, although that may aggravate it, and it is decreased by propranolol.

Some evidence of myopathy is evident in most hyperthyroid patients.[226] Muscle weakness usually develops gradually. It varies from mild to severe, and may be accompanied by muscle wasting. The weakness and wasting affect proximal muscles primarily, thus causing difficulty in combing hair, reaching above the head, climbing stairs, or rising from a lying or sitting position. Deep tendon reflexes are hyperactive; both contraction and relaxation phases are accelerated, despite muscle weakness, and unsustained clonus may be present. Myopathy can also involve the respiratory and oropharyngeal musculature, causing hoarseness or difficulty in swallowing. Ophthalmoplegia, most commonly limitation of upward gaze, may occur; but ophthalmoplegia is a manifestation of infiltrative ophthalmopathy rather than extraocular muscle weakness due to hyperthyroidism per se. Serum concentrations of creatine phosphokinase and myoglobin are normal or low, although their release from muscle may be increased but overshadowed by increased catabolism. Electromyography shows reduced mean action potential duration and/or amplitude and, at times, polyphasic potentials; these are the findings of myopathy in general, and are not specific for hyperthyroidism.

Muscle biopsies show atrophy of both type 1 and type 2 muscle fibers, fibrosis, degeneration, and fatty infiltration.[227]

A syndrome of periodic muscle weakness that is clinically and pathophysiologically very similar to familial hypokalemic periodic paralysis occurs in patients with hyperthyroidism, particularly in Asians.[228] As in hypokalemic periodic paralysis, attacks may be induced by food or ethanol and infusions of glucose and insulin; patients may respond to potassium therapy and propranolol. These patients have no family history of periodic paralysis and no recurrences of paralysis after antithyroid treatment. Myasthenia gravis also can occur in patients with Graves' hyperthyroidism. Although there is no convincing evidence that its frequency is increased, the two diseases have some pathogenetic and demographic similarities, and antireceptor antibodies are a feature of each.

ENERGY AND INTERMEDIARY METABOLISM

A major consequence of hyperthyroidism is increased energy expenditure. Maintenance of basic physiological functions and mechanical work are both less efficient than normal. To counterbalance these changes, increased food intake, use of stored energy, and oxygen consumption occur, with attendant increased heat production. Major changes also occur in the metabolism of carbohydrate, lipid, and protein. Absorption of glucose is increased, as is the rate of glucose production from glycogen, lactate, glycerol, and amino acids.[49] Peripheral insulin sensitivity is normal or decreased, and hepatic insulin sensitivity may be decreased.[49,229] Muscle and adipose tissue glucose utilization is increased. Plasma glucose and insulin responses to an oral glucose load are usually normal. In about one-third of patients, however, oral glucose tolerance is impaired, insulin responses are inadequate, and glucagon secretion is not suppressed normally by glucose.[230] Thus, hyperthyroidism, like pregnancy and Cushing's syndrome, may uncover insulin secretory deficiency. In patients with preexisting diabetes mellitus, requirements for exogenous insulin increase due to accelerated insulin catabolism.[231]

Synthesis and clearance of cholesterol and triglycerides increase in hyperthyroidism; the clearance effect predominates. Thus, modest reductions in serum cholesterol, including both high-density lipoprotein (HDL) and LDL cholesterol, are the usual findings.[232] Serum triglyceride concentrations are usually normal. Hepatic lipase activity is decreased, but lipoprotein lipase activity is normal. Mobilization of adipose tissue lipid stores also is accelerated, resulting in increased plasma free fatty acid concentration. The latter falls normally after a glucose load, indicating normal in vivo adipocyte sensitivity to insulin.

Protein synthesis and catabolism are also increased, the latter to a greater extent. The net result is excessive protein catabolism and increased urinary amino acid excretion, resulting in negative nitrogen balance. Serum concentrations of albumin and other proteins, including TBG and TBPA, may be decreased.

ENDOCRINE SYSTEM

Pituitary Hormone Secretion

Modest increases in basal serum GH concentrations may be present, but serum GH may fail to increase normally after provocative stimuli. Serum somatomedin concentrations are normal. These findings do not suggest that augmented GH secretion causes the accelerated linear growth and skeletal maturation that is found in some prepubertal children with hyperthyroidism. Basal serum prolactin concentrations and prolactin responses to TRH are normal or slightly decreased.[233]

Adrenal Function

Hyperthyroidism results in significant acceleration in cortisol degradation, as manifested by a shortened cortisol half-life and increased urinary 17-hydroxycorticosteroid excretion. As a result, adrenocorticotropin (ACTH) secretion, the number of cortisol secretory episodes, and cortisol secretory rate are increased.[234] Serum cortisol concentrations and urinary cortisol excretion are normal, as are adrenal responses to ACTH and hypoglycemia.

Circulating levels and secretion rates of epinephrine and norepinephrine are normal.[41]

Gonadal Function

Menstrual cycles are normal in most women with hyperthyroidism, although some have hypomenorrhea or amenorrhea. The major biochemical abnormality is an increase in serum sex hormone–binding globulin (SHBG), due to the excess thyroid hormone. The increase in SHBG results in increased serum total estradiol and estrone concentrations, but low normal or low serum free estradiol and estrone concentrations. Serum LH and FSH concentrations are slightly increased during most of the cycle, as are LH and FSH responses to gonadotropin-releasing hormone, probably as a result of the reduced level of serum free estrogen. The midcycle serum LH and FSH peaks are subnormal in regularly cycling or hypomenorrheic hyperthyroid women, but these peaks are followed by increases in serum progesterone concentrations, indicating that ovulation occurred.[235] Thus, infertility should occur only in those women with amenorrhea. In postmenopausal women with hyperthyroidism, serum LH and FSH concentrations are appropriately elevated.

In men, hyperthyroidism results in loss of libido, decreased potency, and gynecomastia.[236] Semen volume and sperm density may be decreased. Serum SHBG concentrations are increased, resulting in increased serum total testosterone concentrations; serum free testosterone concentrations are normal. Extragonadal conversion of androgen to estrogen is increased, resulting in increased serum total and free estradiol concentrations. The increased estradiol concentrations cause gynecomastia and, perhaps, seminiferous tubule dysfunction. Serum LH and FSH concentrations may be slightly elevated, perhaps also due to increased estradiol levels or, possibly, impairment in the ability of testosterone to inhibit LH and FSH secretion.

Parathyroid-Vitamin D-Bone System

The major disturbance in calcium metabolism that occurs in hyperthyroidism is hypercalcemia, which is present in a modest proportion of patients.[237,238] Increased serum ionizable calcium concentrations occur more frequently. Serum phosphate concentrations are usually normal, and serum skeletal alkaline phosphatase activity may be increased. Hypercalcemia is usually neither severe nor symptomatic. It is due to stimulation of bone resorption by excess T_4 and T_3. Serum parathyroid hormone (PTH) and 1α,25-dihydroxycholecalciferol [$1\alpha,25\text{-}(OH)_2D_3$] levels and gastrointestinal calcium absorption are decreased as a consequence of the augmented skeletal calcium resorption. Although clinical osteopenia is rare, probably because hyperthyroidism is of short duration in most patients, evidence of osteopenia responsive to antithyroid therapy may be detected by bone densitometry, and histological studies show increased bone resorption and formation in most patients.[239,240]

Laboratory Diagnosis of Hyperthyroidism

SERUM THYROID HORMONE CONCENTRATIONS

Increased serum total and free T_4 and T_3 concentrations are the biochemical hallmarks of hyperthyroidism. There is some correlation between the clinical severity of hyperthyroidism and the magnitude of the serum T_4 and T_3 abnormalities, but there are numerous exceptions. Serum T_4 and T_3 concentrations in patients with thyroid storm (see Special Situations, below) are not different from those in patients with much less severe hyperthyroidism. Therefore, assessment of the severity of hyperthyroidism should be based on clinical and not laboratory findings. Since serum total T_4 concentrations are increased in many situations, such as pregnancy, confirmation of the diagnosis of hyperthyroidism requires demonstration that the serum free T_4 index or free T_4 concentration is increased as well. Even an elevated serum free T_4 value is not a totally specific indicator of hyperthyroidism, since elevated values also occur in patients with nonthyroidal illnesses or thyroid hormone resistance (see Hypothyroidism and Nonthyroidal Illness).

Serum total (and free) T_3 concentrations and free T_3 index values also are increased in nearly all patients with hyperthyroidism. Figure 10-19 shows that serum

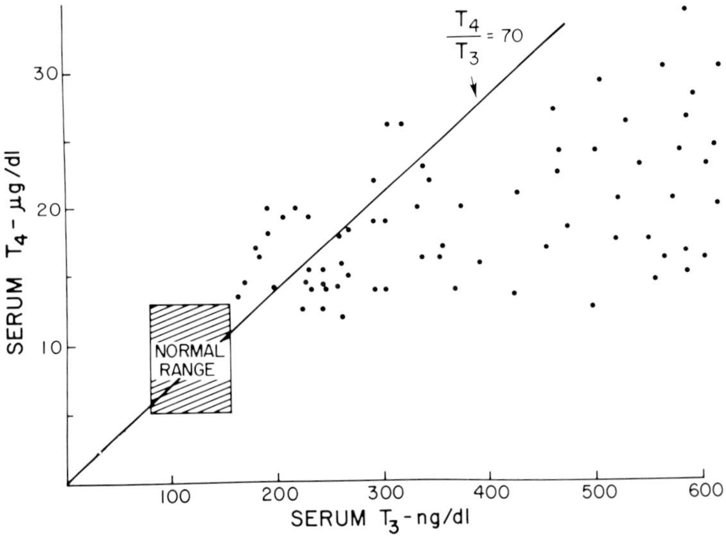

FIGURE 10-19 Serum T_4 and T_3 concentrations in patients with hyperthyroidism. Note that most of the points lie to the right of the line given by the normal T_4/T_3 ratio, indicating that most patients have a disproportionate increase in serum T_3 concentration.

T_3 concentrations are usually disproportionately elevated compared to serum T_4 concentrations. However, serum T_3 measurements are rarely needed and should not be done routinely. In addition, they are more expensive and less widely available than are T_4 measurements, and are subject to alteration by nonthyroidal illness. Serum T_3 determinations do help establish the diagnosis of hyperthyroidism in patients with borderline high or slightly elevated serum T_4 concentrations and free T_4 index values, and they are essential for the evaluation of patients with suspected T_3 hyperthyroidism whose serum T_4 and free T_4 index values are within the normal range.

Conversely, some patients with hyperthyroidism, especially those who are elderly, have increased serum T_4 but normal serum T_3 concentrations (T_4 hyperthyroidism).[14,126,127,241] The occurrence of this syndrome is evidence that nonthyroidal illness or pharmacologic agents can impair extrathyroidal conversion of T_4 to T_3, and thus lower T_3 production even in hyperthyroid patients. In other patients with various nonthyroidal illnesses, serum T_4 concentrations may be elevated and serum T_3 concentrations may be normal or low initially, but both return to normal during recovery. Serum TSH responses to TRH are subnormal or absent in patients with T_4 hyperthyroidism; those with transient, illness-related serum T_4 elevations initially may have subnormal responses as well. The two syndromes also may be distinguished by the lack of symptoms and signs of hyperthyroidism in patients with nonthyroidal illnesses, and by follow-up studies.

THYROID RADIOIODINE UPTAKE AND SCANNING

Thyroid radioiodine uptake is increased in most patients with hyperthyroidism. Important exceptions include patients with subacute thyroiditis, painless thyroiditis, and exogenous hyperthyroidism. Thyroid radioiodine uptake may be low or normal in patients with hyperthyroidism due to other causes, such as Graves' disease or toxic multinodular goiter, if they have recently received iodide-containing drugs or radiographic contrast agents. Even in the absence of such factors, thyroid radioiodine uptake measurement is an insensitive test of hyperthyroidism. Therefore, it is not indicated for routine evaluation of patients with possible hyperthyroidism and should be performed only to confirm a diagnosis of painless thyroiditis or exogenous hyperthyroidism.

Thyroid scans may be helpful in identifying a thyroid adenoma or multinodular goiter as a cause of hyperthyroidism. A scan should not be done in patients with diffuse thyroid enlargement, since it provides little information beyond that obtained by careful palpation of the thyroid gland.

SERUM TSH AND OTHER THYROID STIMULATORS

In most patients with hyperthyroidism serum TSH concentrations are undetectable. However, the diagnostic utility of serum TSH measurements is limited because serum TSH concentrations are undetectable in some normal subjects when measured by most currently available assays. For this reason, and because hyperthyroidism due to excessive TSH secretion is very rare, serum TSH concentrations should be measured only when specific indications of pituitary disease are present. Improved assays for TSH may make measurement of TSH useful in diagnosing hyperthyroidism in the near future.[74]

Patients with hyperthyroidism due to Graves' disease usually have TSab in their serum (see Causes of Hyperthyroidism, above). However, TSab may be found during or after treatment when the patient is euthyroid or hypothyroid. Thus, the presence of TSab is not necessarily indicative of the presence of hyperthyroidism. Moreover, tests for TSab are complex, are not widely available, and vary widely in their specificity and sensitivity.

TESTS OF PITUITARY-THYROID REGULATION

Serum TSH concentrations normally increase promptly following IV administration of TRH. In hyperthyroidism, the inhibition of TSH secretion resulting from T_4 and T_3 overproduction is accompanied by subnormal or absent serum TSH responses to TRH (Fig. 10-20). This is an extremely sensitive test of pituitary suppression; the responses are subnormal or absent not only in hyperthyroid patients but also in patients with euthyroid Graves' disease, thyroid adenoma, or multinodular goiter who are clinically euthyroid and whose serum T_4 and T_3 concentrations are within the normal range,[242] as well as in many patients with nonthyroidal illnesses. Thus, subnormal or absent TSH responses to TRH are indicative of thyroid autonomy or depressed pituitary function for other reasons, and do not prove the presence of clinically significant hyperthyroidism. However, a normal serum TSH response to TRH conclusively rules out the possibility of hyperthyroidism. This test of TSH response is easily performed, requiring only that serum TSH concentrations be measured before and 15 and 30 minutes following the IV administration of 400 or 500 μg of TRH.

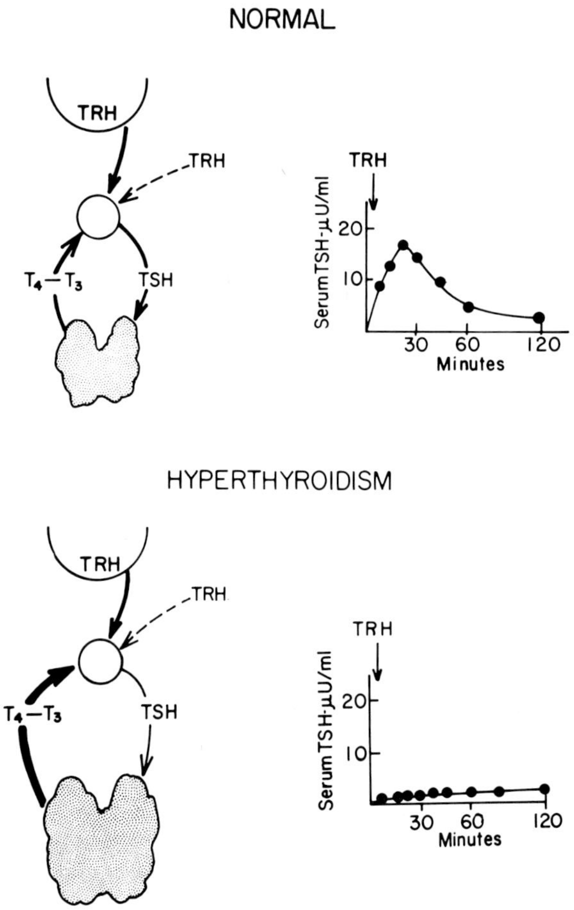

FIGURE 10-20 Hypothalamic-pituitary-thyroid interactions and the serum TSH response to TRH in normal subjects (*top*) and patients with hyperthyroidism (*bottom*). The thyroid outline at the bottom, showing diffuse thyroid enlargement, could just as well show a thyroid adenoma or multinodular goiter. (*Adapted from Kaplan and Utiger.*[145])

The thyroid suppression test provides the same information. When T_3 is given to normal subjects, TSH secretion is inhibited, and therefore thyroid function, as measured by radioiodine uptake or serum T_4 concentration, declines. In patients with thyroid autonomy, with or without clinical hyperthyroidism, thyroid function is not dependent on endogenous TSH secretion; therefore, the radioiodine uptake and serum T_4 concentration do not decline when exogenous T_3 is given. This test requires determinations of thyroid radioiodine uptake (or the serum T_4 concentration) before and after administration of T_3, 75 to 100 μg daily for 7 days. The test also can be done using a single 3-mg dose of T_4, in which case only thyroid radioiodine uptake can be measured. Either way, the thyroid suppression test is more hazardous, time-consuming, and expensive than the TRH test.

SUMMARY: DIAGNOSIS OF HYPERTHYROIDISM

A scheme for the evaluation of patients with suspected hyperthyroidism is shown in Fig. 10-21. The initial step should be measurement of the serum total T_4 concentration and T_3-resin uptake or serum free T_4 concentration. If these are elevated, the diagnosis of hyperthyroidism is confirmed and no further tests are required in most patients. If the results are normal or equivocal, and strong suspicion of hyperthyroidism persists, measurement of the serum T_3 concentration is indicated. When these analyses do not confirm the diagnosis and further evaluation is needed, a TRH stimulation test should be done. An abnormal response indicates the presence of thyroid autonomy, and is compatible with but not diagnostic for hyperthyroidism.

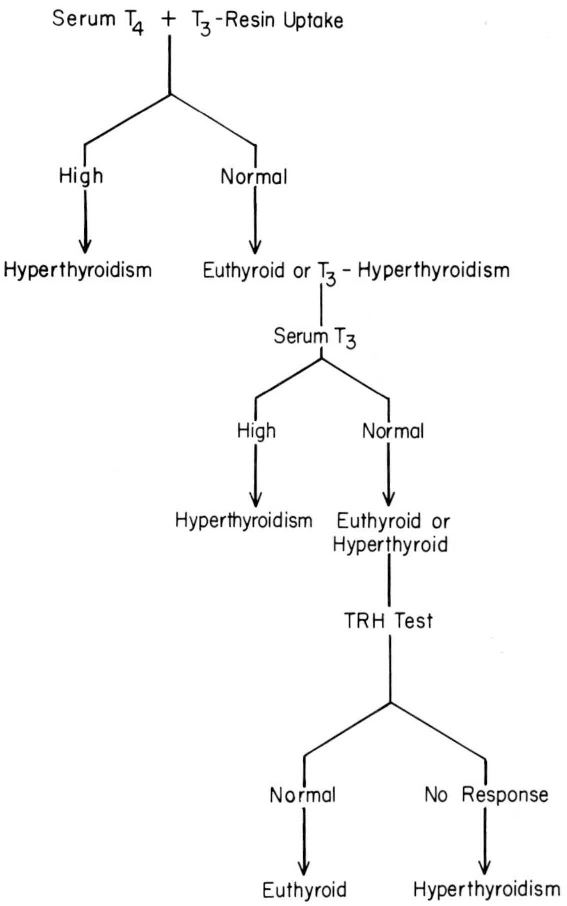

FIGURE 10-21 Diagnostic scheme for evaluation of patients with suspected hyperthyroidism. (*From Kaplan and Utiger.*[145])

OTHER LABORATORY MANIFESTATIONS OF HYPERTHYROIDISM OR DISEASES CAUSING IT

Many other physiological, biochemical, and serological abnormalities may be found in patients with hyperthyroidism. Some result from excessive thyroid hormone action on various tissues; others reflect the various diseases that cause hyperthyroidism. None are direct indicators of increased thyroid hormone production; therefore, they should not be used to confirm a diagnosis of hyperthyroidism. Tests indicative of thyroid disease include measurements of serum thyroglobulin concentration and antithyroid antibodies. (Tests of tissue thyroid hormone action were discussed previously.) Serum thyroglobulin concentrations are increased in most patients with hyperthyroidism, whether the hyperthyroidism is due to thyroid stimulation or thyroid inflammation, but not in those in whom hyperthyroidism is due to thyroid hormone administration.[10,192] Antibodies to thyroglobulin or thyroid microsomes are present in serum in most patients with Graves' disease, though not usually in the high titers found in patients with Hashimoto's disease.[75] However, these antibodies are in no way specific for thyroid autoimmune disease; they are found, though usually in low titer, in patients with many other thyroid diseases and some normal individuals as well.

Treatment of Hyperthyroidism

Ideal therapy for a patient with hyperthyroidism is elimination of its cause so that hyperthyroidism disappears and normal pituitary-thyroid function is restored. Various treatments for hyperthyroidism are listed in Table 10-11. However, for most patients, the fundamental cause of their hyperthyroidism is not known and no truly curative treatment is available.

The following sections deal with the treatment of hyperthyroidism due to Graves' disease, thyroiditis, multinodular goiter, and thyroid adenoma. The treatments of many of the rarer causes of hyperthyroidism listed in Table 10-9 are obvious. For patients with any of them, therapy with drugs which inhibit thyroidal production of thyroid hormones or relieve peripheral manifestations of hyperthyroidism may be needed before or during specific and permanent therapy. The considerations pertaining to the use of these drugs are the same as when they are given to patients with Graves' disease, as discussed below.

TREATMENT OF HYPERTHYROIDISM DUE TO GRAVES' DISEASE

Antithyroid drugs or radioactive iodine (^{131}I) are the two best treatments for the hyperthyroidism of Graves' disease. Both are effective, safe, and relatively inexpensive. Neither results in cure of Graves' disease and neither obviates the need for long-term observation of the patient. The major reason to choose antithyroid drug therapy is that a spontaneous remission of hyperthyroidism may occur, permitting drug therapy to be discontinued and leaving the patient with normal, and often normally regulated, thyroid function. Remissions of hyperthyroidism occur in about 30 to 50 percent of patients treated for a year and more often in those patients treated longer, but may occur even in the first months of therapy.[177–181] It is widely believed that a remission is more likely to occur in a patient whose hyperthyroidism is of recent onset and of mild or moderate severity, and whose thyroid enlargement is modest, although documentation of these impressions is sparse. The frequency of remission also may depend on HLA haplotype; some studies indicate that patients with the HLA-B8 or HLA-DR3 haplotype are less likely to have remissions.[179,181] The uncertainty concerning remission does not apply to ^{131}I therapy, since radiotherapy is destructive and its effects are ongoing. The hazards and expense of subtotal thyroidectomy are greater than are those of either antithyroid drugs or ^{131}I; surgery should be used rarely if at all in patients of any age.

The choice between antithyroid drug and ^{131}I therapy depends on several theoretical and practical considerations. A rough comparison of their features is shown in Table 10-12. The most important are the acceptability to the patient and the experience of the physician in the use of therapy. Antithyroid drugs are more rapidly effective, do not cause permanent thyroid damage, may not need to be given indefinitely, and are less expensive. For these reasons, they are the initial treatment of choice for most patients, both children and adults. If remission does not occur and the patient tires of taking medication, or if hyperthyroidism is difficult to control, ^{131}I can always be

Table 10-11. Therapy for Hyperthyroidism

Treatment of cause of hyperthyroidism
Antithyroid therapy
Drugs:
Propylthiouracil
Methimazole
Iodide
^{131}I
Subtotal thyroidectomy
Inhibition of peripheral T_3 production:
Propylthiouracil
Sodium ipodate and iopanoic acid
Propranolol
Glucocorticoids
Amelioration of thyroid hormone action
propranolol and similar drugs

Table 10-12. Comparison of Features of Antithyroid Drug and ^{131}I Therapy for Hyperthyroidism

	Drug therapy	^{131}I therapy
Dosage	Daily	Single dose
Initial response	4–6 weeks	8–12 weeks
Side effects*	Uncommon	Rare
Hypothyroidism	Uncommon	Common
Inadequate therapy	Uncommon	Rare
Cost of medication†	$25–50/year	$500–1000/treatment
Need for continuous or repeated therapy	Common	Rare
Long-term outcome	Euthyroidism or hyperthyroidism	Hypothyroidism
Outcome dependent on continued TSab‡ production	Yes	No
Use during pregnancy	Acceptable	Never

*Toxic drug effects and radiation thyroiditis.
†Excludes costs of follow-up examinations, serum hormone assays, and treatment of subsequent hypothyroidism in ^{131}I-treated patients.
‡TSab = thyroid-stimulating autoantibody.

given at some future time. ^{131}I treatment is simple, though not so rapidly effective, and hypothyroidism nearly always develops subsequently. With either form of treatment, no matter how effective in the early months after it is initiated, indefinite follow-up is necessary to ensure that hyperthyroidism has not recurred, that hypothyroidism has not developed, or, if it has, that replacement therapy is continuing.

Antithyroid Drugs

THIONAMIDES The thionamide drugs used in the United States are PTU and MMI. These drugs inhibit thyroid hormone biosynthesis by blocking iodine oxidation and organification and iodotyrosine coupling, reactions all catalyzed by thyroid peroxidase.[243] These drugs are concentrated and metabolized by the thyroid in reactions involving the peroxidase. Escape from the inhibitory effects of the drugs follows intrathyroidal drug metabolism. Thus, the drugs are less effective when iodide intake and intrathyroidal iodine stores are plentiful.[244] PTU also inhibits the extrathyroidal conversion of T_4 to T_3. Both thionamides are absorbed rapidly and nearly completely from the GI tract; peak serum concentrations are reached about 1 h after their ingestion.[245,246] PTU is metabolized more rapidly than is MMI; the plasma half-life of PTU is 1 to 2 h whereas that of MMI is 4 to 6 h. Because these drugs are concentrated in the thyroid, their intrathyroidal concentrations remain high for considerably longer than their serum levels.[247]

In addition to their antithyroid effects, both drugs have an immunosuppressive action and thus may ameliorate Graves' disease directly. For example, they may inhibit thyroid autoantibody production, and high-dose regimens may be accompanied by more frequent remissions.[180,248,249] Antithyroid drugs also inhibit lymphocyte function and viability in vitro,[250,251] although higher concentrations may be required than those achieved in vivo; they do not, however, alter antibody-dependent cell-mediated cytotoxicity.[252]

The initial goal of antithyroid drug therapy is to inhibit completely thyroid hormone synthesis. Even if achieved, release of intrathyroidal hormone stores, which may be substantial, continues until such stores are depleted. The usual initial doses are 300 to 600 mg of PTU per day, given in two or three divided doses, or 15 to 30 mg of MMI daily, given in one or two doses. The larger doses are usually given to patients who have more severe clinical hyperthyroidism and/or a large goiter. Single daily doses may be adequate, but, at least for PTU, divided doses result in more rapid responses.[253] The greater potency of MMI is due to its slower metabolism, its greater accumulation in thyroid tissue, and its greater potency as an inhibitor of thyroid peroxidase.

Failure of antithyroid drug therapy to effectively control hyperthyroidism may result from inadequate dosage or failure of the patient to comply with the regimen, usually the latter.[254] Noncompliance can be minimized by careful explanation of the need for therapy and its goals to the patient. In some patients, hyperthyroidism persists and the thyroid may enlarge further despite a fall in serum T_4 concentration; such patients have persistently high serum TSab and T_3 levels.[255,256] They do become euthyroid when the antithyroid drug dose is increased, but daily doses as high as 1000 mg of PTU or 100 mg of MMI may be required, and such patients are unlikely to have a remission.

The patient should be reevaluated 4 to 6 weeks after initiation of therapy. Some clinical and biochemical improvement is usually apparent after 1 or 2 weeks and is usually substantial after 4 to 6 weeks of treatment; serum T_4 and T_3 concentrations are normal in many patients by this time. If considerable improvement has occurred, the antithyroid drug dosage should be reduced by 25 to 50 percent. Further follow-up visits should occur at about 8-week intervals. Once the patient has become euthyroid, the goal of continued therapy is partial rather than complete inhibition of thyroid hormone biosynthesis, so that hypothyroidism does not occur. If antithyroid drug therapy rapidly reduces serum T_4 and T_3 concentrations to below normal, serum TSH concentrations may remain low for several weeks because of prior suppression of TSH secretion by hyperthyroidism. Prevention of hypothyroidism and further thyroid enlargement is best achieved by judicious reduction in antithyroid drug dosage; addition of thyroid hormone is not necessary or desirable.

Several programs for long-term therapy have been advocated. One is to administer gradually decreasing doses of an antithyroid drug with the goal of withdrawal of the drug as soon as possible. As improvement occurs, the dosage of antithyroid drug is reduced by 25 to 50 percent at approximately 8-week intervals; it may be given once daily. If the patient remains euthyroid while receiving 50 mg of PTU or 5 mg of MMI daily for 8 weeks, the drug is discontinued. It may be possible to discontinue therapy in as little as 4 to 6 months with such a regimen. If hyperthyroidism recurs after the dose is reduced or discontinued, remission obviously has not occurred and treatment is increased or resumed until the euthyroid state is achieved, at which time dosage reduction may be resumed. In such a pragmatic program, decisions are made largely on clinical grounds, supported when necessary by serum T_4 or occasional T_3 determinations.

A second treatment program is to simply continue therapy with the initial dose of antithyroid drug until the patient is clinically and biochemically euthyroid, at which time therapy is discontinued. In the study describing this regimen the mean duration of therapy was 4.8 months and the sustained remission rate was 29 percent.[257]

A third program involves prolonged treatment for 1 to 2 years. Such a program requires one or more reductions in dosage after the first several months of treatment. Prolonged antithyroid drug therapy results in higher remission rates, probably because remissions of hyperthyroidism continue to occur over time.[177,178,258] This program, with treatment for a fixed interval, is probably the most widely used, but it results in treatment of some patients for longer periods than are necessary. For this reason, the former programs are preferable.

TRH or thyroid suppression tests have been used to determine whether a remission of Graves' disease has occurred and whether therapy can therefore be discontinued. A normal result in either test indicates that pituitary-thyroid function is normal and therefore that Graves' disease is in remission; however, a patient may remain euthyroid despite abnormal pituitary-thyroid regulation when improvement, but not complete remission, of Graves' disease has occurred.[182,183] These tests require withdrawal of antithyroid drug therapy for several weeks; they are cumbersome and expensive, and their predictive value is limited. Measurements of serum TSab may prove useful for this purpose in the future, but current experience is limited and TSab assays are expensive and not readily available.

Thus, whatever therapeutic program is used, it is simpler merely to discontinue the drug at the end of the initial treatment period and reexamine the patient in 6 to 8 weeks; subsequently, examinations may take place less often if hyperthyroidism does not recur. Most recurrences develop in the first few months after drug withdrawal, and may be treated with an antithyroid drug. However, many patients choose ablative therapy if hyperthyroidism recurs after drug withdrawal. Those patients whose hyperthyroidism is easily controlled with small doses of drug may prefer to continue treatment for many years; there are no contraindications to such a program.

Toxic reactions to antithyroid drugs are uncommon; they occur in from 5 to 10 percent of patients.[259] There is little evidence that one drug is more toxic than the other. The most common reactions are dermatologic, consisting of pruritus, urticaria, or other rashes. They may subside with no treatment or symptomatic antihistamine therapy, and generally do not require discontinuation of antithyroid drug therapy. More serious side effects of both drugs include fever, arthralgias or arthritis, loss of taste, vasculitis, hepatitis or cholestatic jaundice, anemia, thrombocytopenia, and agranulocytosis; the last occurs in about 0.5 percent of patients.[259,260] All of these side effects disappear after the drug is discontinued. Agranulocytosis has been reported to be more common in older patients and when higher doses (30 mg per day or more) of MMI are used, but no dose relationship for PTU was found.[260] Agranulocytosis usually develops rapidly, so precautionary white blood cell counts are not useful.

To minimize the severity and consequences of the side effects of antithyroid drugs, patients should be carefully warned about the symptoms of these reactions and instructed to discontinue therapy and contact the physician immediately if any symptoms occur. Blood counts or liver function tests may then be indicated. Drug reactions are probably immunologic in nature, as antinuclear or antineutrophil antibodies or lymphocyte sensitization to PTU or MMI may be present; in vitro studies indicate patients who had agranulocytosis after receiving one drug may have lymphocyte sensitivity to the other, even though the structures of the two drugs differ considerably.[261] The more severe reactions usually occur during the first months of treatment and require discontinuation of antithyroid drug therapy. Treatment with ^{131}I, rather than trial of the other drug, is indicated when a serious antithyroid drug reaction has occurred.

The choice of antithyroid drug is largely a matter of individual preference. Both PTU and MMI are effective inhibitors of thyroidal hormone synthesis. Since PTU also inhibits extrathyroidal T_3 production, it causes a somewhat more rapid reduction in serum T_3 concentrations,[262] and thus may be theoretically preferable when a rapid response is desired. Methimazole is preferable, however, for the very practical reasons that its action is more prolonged, so that single daily doses are more likely to be effective, and equivalent dosage of MMI requires fewer tablets per day, since MMI is available in 5- and 10-mg tablets and PTU only in 50-mg tablets. However, PTU is preferable in pregnant women (see Hyperthyroidism during Pregnancy, below). The costs of equivalent doses of PTU and MMI are similar.

IODIDE Inorganic iodide inhibits thyroid hormone secretion primarily by inhibiting thyroglobulin proteolysis.[263] This action requires only 5 to 10 mg of iodide daily, though iodide is usually given in far greater doses, such as 5 to 10 drops of a saturated solution of potassium iodide (50 mg of iodide per drop) several times daily. Antithyroid effects of iodide are demonstrable in normal subjects, but they are much greater in those with hyperthyroidism. The major limitation of iodide as antithyroid therapy is that "escape" from its antithyroid effects occurs quickly. When iodide is given alone, serum T_4 and T_3 concentrations decrease by about 50 percent, reaching a nadir in 7 to 14 days; they then increase in most patients.[264] Therefore, iodide should not be used as the sole therapy for hyperthyroidism. Iodide given after ^{131}I therapy results in more rapid amelioration of hyperthyroidism, and escape does not occur in this setting.[265] Iodide is also used in preparation for thyroidectomy, for both its antithyroid action and because it reduces thyroid blood flow. Iodide produced by metabolism of organic iodine compounds has the same antithyroid actions.

The indications for iodide therapy are preparation for subtotal thyroidectomy, for which it is given for 7 to 10 days preceding surgery; thyroid storm (see below); and, occasionally, recent treatment with ^{131}I, when iodide is given for several months.

Drugs Inhibiting Extrathyroidal T_3 Production

Drug-induced inhibition of extrathyroidal T_3 production (see Effects of Various Drugs on Thyroid Function, above) results in decreased serum T_3 concentration, and thus might be expected to ameliorate hyperthyroidism. While a reasonable expectation, there is no evidence that such amelioration occurs, or that a drug which acts both on the thyroid and the periphery, such as PTU, is more effective clinically than a drug which acts only on the thyroid, such as MMI.

Propylthiouracil, oral cholecystographic agents, beta-adrenergic antagonists, and glucocorticoids inhibit extrathyroidal T_4 conversion to T_3. This action of PTU is manifest within 24 h; PTU treatment of hyperthyroid patients results in more rapid reduction in serum T_3 concentrations than does treatment with MMI.[139,262]

Ipodate and other oral cholecystographic agents, in doses of 1.5 to 3 g, rapidly inhibit extrathyroidal T_3 production; the iodide produced when these compounds are metabolized inhibits thyroid secretion. Ipodate administration therefore is accompanied by prompt reductions in both serum T_4 and T_3 concentrations, which are maintained for at least several weeks when daily doses are given.[266] Although experimental, these agents may be useful for short-term therapy for the occasional patient in whom antithyroid drug treatment or ^{131}I is contraindicated.

Propranolol and other beta-adrenergic antagonists cause a 10 to 20 percent reduction in serum T_3 concentrations, but not in serum T_4 concentrations after 1 to 2 weeks of therapy.[70,132] This modest and gradual fall in serum T_3 concentrations does not explain the clinical benefits of propranolol in hyperthyroidism (see below).

Glucocorticoids inhibit extrathyroidal T_3 production when given in large doses. They also inhibit thyroid hormone secretion in patients with hyperthyroidism due to Graves' disease,[130] but their toxicity precludes their use in all but emergency situations.

Drugs Ameliorating Peripheral Thyroid Hormone Action

A number of the manifestations of hyperthyroidism may be ameliorated by beta-adrenergic antagonist drugs. When propranolol is given in doses of 80 to 240 mg daily, it results in improvement in many of the common symptoms of hyperthyroidism, including palpitations, increased perspiration and heat intolerance, nervousness, tremor, and muscle weakness, in several days. However, such symptoms do not disappear completely, even during prolonged therapy.[267]

The pulse rate slows and myocardial contractility decreases. Little weight gain or changes in nitrogen balance, oxygen consumption, systolic time intervals, or other tissue responses occur.[268] Thus, propranolol alone is inadequate treatment for hyperthyroidism, and it has no beneficial effect when used in conjunction with antithyroid drugs.[269] Propranolol is contraindicated in patients with asthma and those with heart failure due to intrinsic cardiac disease. Other beta-adrenergic antagonists have similar actions in hyperthyroid patients, although they differ in their membrane-stabilizing properties, degree of selectivity as beta-adrenergic antagonists, potency as inhibitors of extrathyroidal T_3 production, and duration of action. These variables are not known to be important, but compliance may be better with use of the longer-acting analogues.

Beta-adrenergic antagonist drugs should not be used routinely in patients treated with antithyroid drugs or ^{131}I, and should never be used alone in patients with hyperthyroidism due to Graves' disease. They are useful for amelioration of hyperthyroid symptoms before and for several weeks after ^{131}I therapy, preceding subtotal thyroidectomy, during thyroiditis, and in thyroid storm.

Radioactive Iodine

The goal of ^{131}I therapy is to reduce the amount of functioning thyroid tissue. The effect of ^{131}I therapy is independent of whether or not a spontaneous remission of hyperthyroidism occurs. Although the occurrence of such a remission after ^{131}I therapy would contribute to the effectiveness of the therapy, in fact, TSab production often increases within the first year after ^{131}I therapy.[162]

The major advantages of ^{131}I therapy are that usually only a single dose is needed, it is safe, and its cost is relatively low. One disadvantage is that amelioration of hyperthyroidism usually requires several months. For markedly symptomatic patients, a period of antithyroid drug therapy before ^{131}I therapy is often advisable; the drug therapy must be discontinued 3 to 4 days before thyroid ^{131}I uptake is determined and the therapeutic ^{131}I dose given. Antithyroid drug therapy may then be resumed after several days, if indicated; its use then does not alter the efficacy of ^{131}I therapy.[270] Alternatively, propranolol can be given continuously for relief of symptoms before ^{131}I therapy is given and until its effects become apparent. Iodides should not be given before therapy and care should be taken to avoid iodide-containing drugs or contrast agents if ^{131}I therapy is planned. After ^{131}I therapy, iodide administration may be beneficial.[265]

Various methods for determining ^{131}I dosage have been employed; they are all subject to considerable error because thyroid gland size is difficult to estimate, isotope retention within the thyroid is variable, and radiation sensitivity is not predictable. Many now believe that a fixed dose of 8 to 12 mCi is appropriate for treatment of nearly all patients, with minor increments if thyroid radioiodine uptake is near normal or if thyroid enlargement is substantial. Such doses deliver approximately 100 to 200 μCi per gram of estimated thyroid weight, or 10,000 to 20,000 rads, to the thyroid. They result in significant clinical and biochemical improvement and reduction in thyroid size in 2 to 3 months; most patients are euthyroid, if not hypothyroid, in 3 to 6 months.

There are only two important untoward effects of ^{131}I therapy: persistent hyperthyroidism and hypothyroidism. Acute temporary exacerbation of hyperthyroidism and/or thyroid pain and tenderness, both due to radiation thyroiditis, are rare, though patients should be warned about the possibility of their occurrence. The risk of these effects is reduced by prior antithyroid drug therapy. Hypoparathyroidism is an even rarer consequence of ^{131}I therapy.[271] Persistent hyperthyroidism results from inadequate ^{131}I therapy, and not surprisingly is more common when lower doses of ^{131}I are given. For example, in a recent series in which the average dose was less than 5 mCi of ^{131}I, 34 percent of patients required re-treatment.[270] Even with large doses, a few patients require re-treatment.

Hypothyroidism is not so much a complication of treatment as an almost inevitable consequence of it. It may occur in the first few months after therapy or at any time thereafter; in the initial period after therapy it may be transient.[272] The frequency of early hypothyroidism (within a year after treatment) is about 80 percent in patients treated with 8 to 12 mCi of ^{131}I.[273] Such moderately aggressive treatment is the most appropriate therapeutic approach. Smaller doses result in early hypothyroidism less often, but the frequency of subsequent persistent hyperthyroidism is unacceptably high,[270] and the primary goal of therapy should be the permanent amelioration of hyperthyroidism as expeditiously as possible. Early hypothyroidism is the result of the acute destructive effects of ^{131}I. Hypothyroidism develops thereafter in additional patients (0.5 to 2 percent) each year for at least 10 years, whether the treatment dose was large or small. Thus, the occurrence of late hypothyroidism is independent of the ^{131}I dose given; it is due to damage to the replicative ability of thyroid follicular cells and, perhaps, autoimmune thyroid injury. It usually develops extremely slowly; many patients have elevated serum TSH concentrations but normal serum T_4 and T_3 concentrations (subclinical hypothyroidism) for several years before symptomatic hypothyroidism develops.[274]

Many physicians have been reluctant to use ^{131}I therapy in young adults, adolescents, and children. The reasons for this reluctance are that (1) post-^{131}I hypothyroidism is more likely to develop in patients whose life expectancy is longer, (2) ^{131}I might cause thyroidal or other neoplasms, (3) ^{131}I might cause gonadal damage, and (4) the patient may be pregnant. The possible induction of hypothyroidism is a less important consideration when large doses of ^{131}I are used because hypothyroidism so often occurs soon after therapy. Fears that ^{131}I therapy is a risk factor for thyroid or other neoplasms have proven unfounded.[275,276] The gonadal radiation dose after ^{131}I is no more than that which results from several diagnostic radiologic procedures. Follow-up of children and adolescents treated with ^{131}I has revealed neither impaired fertility nor increase in birth defects in their offspring.[277,279] Since ^{131}I crosses the placenta and can destroy the fetal thyroid, pregnancy is an absolute contraindication to its use.

Subtotal Thyroidectomy

The simplicity, safety, and economy of antithyroid drug and ^{131}I therapy have led to declining use of subtotal thyroidectomy for the treatment of hyperthyroidism. The goal of thyroidectomy, as of ^{131}I treatment, is reduction of the functioning mass of thyroid tissue. Subtotal thyroidectomy has little perioperative morbidity and mortality in properly prepared children and young adults. Preoperative treatment is generally accomplished by antithyroid drug treatment for 1 to 2 months and iodide treatment for 7 to 10 days. Short-term treatment with beta-adrenergic antagonists with or without concurrent iodide therapy for 10 to 14 days, also has proved to be safe and effective preoperative therapy.[280]

Postoperative problems after thyroidectomy include transient or permanent hypocalcemia, vocal cord paralysis, recurrent hyperthyroidism, and transient or permanent hypothyroidism. The frequency of nonthyroid complications is quite low. Transient hypocalcemia, lasting a few days to a few weeks, may be due to calcitonin release or temporary hypoparathyroidism. More chronic, but still transient, hypocalcemia may be due to healing thyroid osteopenia. Permanent hypoparathyroidism is rare, but it can be difficult to treat. Hyperthyroidism recurs now in less than 20 percent of patients;[270,281] it usually develops several years after thyroidectomy and is due to persistence of active Graves' disease. The long lag time reflects the time required for regrowth of sufficient thyroid tissue to sustain hyperthyroidism. Clinical and/or biochemical hypothyroidism may occur in the first 1 to 2 months after surgery in as many as 30 percent of patients, but in some patients thyroid hormone production returns to normal as a result of endogenous TSH secretion.[282] Therefore, a diagnosis of permanent hypothyroidism should not be made for at least 4 to 6 months after surgery. Currently, permanent hypothyroidism develops in the first year after surgery in from 25 to 75 percent of patients, because of more aggressive surgery intended to reduce the frequency of recurrent hyperthyroidism.[270,281,283] Subsequently, hypothyroidism occurs at a rate of about 0.5 percent/year. These data indicate that postoperative hypothyroidism is now nearly as common as is post-^{131}I hypothyroidism, and for the same reason, namely, the attempt to reduce the frequency of recurrent hyperthyroidism. Because subtotal thyroidectomy has nonthyroid hazards, both its overall risks relative to benefits and its expense render it unacceptable except for occasional hyperthyroid patients who have marked thyroid enlargement or who are pregnant and cannot tolerate antithyroid drugs.

THYROIDITIS

The diagnosis and treatment of subacute thyroiditis is discussed below (see The Painful Thyroid). Hyperthyroidism due to painless thyroiditis is more difficult to diagnose; clues to its presence are described above. Since it is transient and usually mild, most patients do not need any treatment. Propranolol can be given to the few patients who have many symptoms. Glucocorticoid therapy reduces serum T_4 and T_3 concentrations rapidly in patients with painless thyroiditis,[284] but its use is not warranted because of the mild nature and limited duration of hyperthyroidism in these patients.

TOXIC MULTINODULAR GOITER

Ablative treatment with ^{131}I is the treatment of choice for patients with hyperthyroidism due to multinodular goiter, since spontaneous remission of hyperthyroidism does not occur in this disease. Large doses of ^{131}I, e.g., 25 to 30 mCi, should be given, because thyroid ^{131}I uptake is usually only moderately increased, the pattern of uptake is heterogeneous, and persistent hyperthyroidism is especially to be avoided in these elderly patients. Doses of 30 mCi or more require hospitalization and special handling of excreta. Multiple doses may be required. Hypothyroidism rarely develops subsequently, because the thyroid gland contains some tissue whose function is suppressed; such tissue can regain function as needed. Since most patients with hyperthyroidism due to toxic multinodular goiter have serious cardiovascular manifestations of their disease, a period of treatment with an antithyroid drug before and after ^{131}I administration is often indicated. Such a regimen accelerates recovery, since antithyroid drugs are more rapidly effective than is ^{131}I, and minimizes the chances of radiation thyroiditis–induced exacerbation of hyperthyroidism after ^{131}I therapy.

THYROID ADENOMA

Thyroid adenomas are benign tumors which cause permanent hyperthyroidism, so that ablative therapy with ^{131}I is most appropriate. The dose used should be large (20 to 25 mCi), so that the nodule is effectively destroyed. Transient hypothyroidism then may occur until TSH secretion recovers. There is little risk of permanent hypothyroidism, as the suppressed extranodular tissue does not concentrate appreciable quantities of ^{131}I and recovers function as TSH secretion resumes.

Special Situations

THYROID STORM

Thyroid storm is severe, life-threatening hyperthyroidism. There are no fixed criteria for its diagnosis and no evidence that its pathophysiology differs from that of hyperthyroidism in general. Thyroid storm may occur after ^{131}I therapy,[285] but more often develops in a hyperthyroid patient who has another major stress or illness, such as an infection, injury, parturition, or a surgical procedure; it can also develop spontaneously.[286] Hyperthyroidism may or may not have been diagnosed previously, but the symptoms nearly always had been present for months. Clinical findings in patients with thyroid storm include fever, tachycardia, anorexia, nausea, vomiting, abdominal pain, and cardiac failure, as well as any of the manifestations of less severe hyperthyroidism. The patients usually have marked anxiety and agitation and, occasionally, acute psychosis; apathy, confusion, and coma may develop terminally. Manifestations of the precipitating illness may confuse the problem. Attributing findings such as fever or tachycardia either to thyroid storm or to the associated or precipitating illness may be impossible; a decision concerning therapy must often be made in the absence of any pathognomonic symptoms or signs.

There are no characteristic laboratory abnormalities in patients with thyroid storm, emphasizing that its diagnosis is a clinical one. Serum T_4 and T_3 concentrations are elevated, but no more so than in "ordinary" hyperthyroidism. Acute illness can decrease TBG and/or TBPA production, and thus decrease serum total T_4 and T_3 concentrations; it is thus possible that *free* hormone concentrations are increased more, in relation to *total* hormone concentrations, in these patients by comparison to most patients with hyperthyroidism.

The treatment of thyroid storm involves the use of agents which inhibit thyroidal production of T_4 and T_3, peripheral production of T_3, and peripheral actions of thyroid hormone, as well as general supportive measures and treatment needed to deal with any coexisting illness. PTU should be given in large doses, such as 250 mg every 6 h, by nasogastric tube if necessary. It is at least theoretically preferable to MMI because PTU inhibits extrathyroidal production of T_3, as well as inhibiting thyroidal synthesis of T_4 and T_3. Sodium iodide should be given orally or IV to inhibit release of T_4 and T_3 from the thyroid; the usual dose is 500 mg per day. Iodide should be given 1 to 2 h after PTU so that thyroid gland iodide content is not increased before T_4 and T_3 synthesis is blocked.

Propranolol, in a dose of 0.5 to 1 mg/min IV for 5 to 10 min, is the most effective treatment for the cardiac and neuromuscular manifestations of thyroid storm. Its effects last for several hours and it can be repeated as needed. If appreciable reductions in pulse rate are not achieved, larger doses may be given. Alternatively, propranolol can be given orally in doses of 20 to 40 mg every 4 to 6 h; higher doses may be used if necessary.

Parenteral glucocorticoids are usually given in large doses, such as 50 mg of cortisol or equivalent doses of a synthetic glucocorticoid every 8 h. The rationale for the use of corticosteroids is that ACTH and cortisol secretion may not increase sufficiently to meet cortisol requirements in a situation of increased need superimposed on accelerated cortisol degradation. Corticosteroids also inhibit thyroid secretion and extrathyroidal T_3 production.

These measures usually result in clinical improvement and reduction in serum T_4 and T_3 concentrations, especially the latter, in 24 to 48 h.[287] Supportive therapy should include measures to reduce hyperpyrexia and appropriate parenteral fluid and electrolyte therapy. Combined with aggressive treatment of coexisting illness, these measures collectively have resulted in substantially reduced mortality from thyroid storm.

HYPERTHYROIDISM DURING PREGNANCY

In most pregnant women with hyperthyroidism, the illness precedes the pregnancy. However, hyperthyroidism, nearly always due to Graves' disease, may first develop during pregnancy; it is usually recognized in the second trimester. Relapses of hyperthyroidism also occur during pregnancy in patients who were in remission and receiving no therapy prior to becoming pregnant;[190] such relapses are often transient and spontaneously subside by the third trimester. Since pregnancy is a hypermetabolic state, normally characterized by increased oxygen consumption, heat production, cardiovascular activity, and anxiety or nervousness, hyperthyroidism may be difficult to recognize. Findings that are particularly indicative of hyperthyroidism include marked tachycardia, muscle weakness, weight loss, and thyroid enlargement. Thyroid enlargement does not occur in normal pregnant women whose iodide intake is adequate.[78]

Hyperthyroidism is usually well tolerated in pregnant women, as it is in nonpregnant women of the same age. There is no increase in maternal mortality or morbidity in untreated patients, although postpartum thyroid storm has been reported.[288] In untreated hyperthyroid pregnant women, however, fetal loss is more common due to spontaneous abortion and premature delivery; some infants of hyperthyroid mothers are small for gestational age.[289]

The effects of maternal hyperthyroidism per se on the fetus are uncertain, but they are probably minimal. Normally, late in pregnancy, free T_4 concentrations are higher in fetal serum, and free T_4 concentrations are higher in maternal serum (see Physiological Variables Affecting Pituitary-Thyroid Function and Tests, above). Maternal hyperthyroidism could reverse the T_4 gradient and increase the T_3 gradient. However, active placental conversion of T_4 to rT_3 and deiodination of T_3 should minimize the transfer of increased maternal serum T_4 and T_3 to the fetus. Since hyperthyroidism in pregnant women is usually due to Graves' disease, transplacental passage of TSab may occur and cause fetal, as well as neonatal, hyperthyroidism. Fetal hyperthyroidism can be suspected by the presence of tachycardia. Treatment of the mother with an antithyroid drug reduces fetal tachycardia;[290] such therapy may be indicated even in mothers with previously treated hyperthyroid Graves' disease who are euthyroid.

The diagnosis of hyperthyroidism is confirmed by a serum total T_4 concentration that is above the normal range for pregnancy (which is about 50 percent higher than normal) and an elevated serum free T_4 concentration or free T_4 index. Similar abnormalities in serum total and free T_3 concentrations are present, but, as in nonpregnant individuals, T_3 measurement in a patient suspected of having hyperthyroidism is not warranted unless serum T_4 measurements are within the normal range. If the diagnosis is not established by these procedures, continued observation is the wisest course. TRH tests yield valid results in pregnant women,[291] but should be done only if an immediate conclusion regarding the presence of hyperthyroidism is required.

Antithyroid drug therapy is the most appropriate treatment for pregnant women with hyperthyroidism. Both PTU and MMI cross the placenta, but PTU is preferable because its fractional transplacental transfer is considerably less.[292] Only doses sufficient to ameliorate the clinical manifestations of hyperthyroidism and lower the total serum T_4 concentration to near or just within the normal range for pregnant women should be given. An appropriate initial dose is 300 mg daily. The patient should be evaluated at 3- to 4-week intervals and the dosage should be reduced as necessary to maintain this thyroid secretory level. Repeated attempts to discontinue therapy should be made. The rationale for this approach is that mild hyperthyroidism is tolerated well by pregnant women and the fetus is exposed to limited quantities of antithyroid drug. On the other hand, if severe hyperthyroidism is present, therapy initially should be aggressive since serious maternal illness threatens fetal development and survival.

PTU (and MMI) may cause fetal goiter and/or hypothyroidism, which subside soon after birth.[293] Transplacental passage of these drugs varies; for example, these abnormalities were found in only one twin of several sets of twins from mothers treated during pregnancy. The use of T_4 in addition to an antithyroid drug is not warranted, since (1) it increases the amount of antithyroid drug required to control hyperthyroidism in the mother and (2) it does not protect the fetus because transplacental transfer of T_4 and T_3 is so poor. Iodide and propranolol also are to be avoided. The fetal thyroid is very sensitive to the antithyroid effects of iodide; iodide thus may cause a large goiter. Propranolol is contraindicated except for brief use, as it may cause intrauterine growth retardation and neonatal CNS depression.

While subtotal thyroidectomy has been used for treatment of hyperthyroidism during pregnancy, it should be performed only when the previously mentioned side effects of antithyroid drugs preclude continuation of drug therapy. Surgery is safe only after some period of drug treatment. This may have been achieved with PTU or MMI before the side effects developed, or may require short-term treatment with iodide and/or propranolol. Additional hazards of subtotal thyroidectomy during pregnancy are abortion, premature labor, and fetal anoxia. ^{131}I therapy is absolutely contraindicated in pregnant women.

T_4 is present in breast milk in low concentrations.[294] Concentrations of MMI in milk are similar to those in serum;[246] milk concentrations of PTU are considerably lower.[295] While limited data indicate that not enough antithyroid drug is present in breast milk to cause difficulty in the newborn infant,[296] nursing probably should be avoided by women taking these drugs, or their infants should be followed closely for signs of thyroid deficiency, such as growth retardation.

NEONATAL HYPERTHYROIDISM

Infants of mothers who have Graves' disease may be hyperthyroid at birth or may develop hyperthyroidism several days after delivery. These infants may be born prematurely. They are hyperactive, tremulous, and irritable, and have tachycardia, feeding problems, diarrhea, and cardiac failure. Thyroid enlargement occurs variably; proptosis is common. Craniosynostosis may be present and skeletal development may be accelerated.[297] This syndrome of neonatal hyperthyroidism occurs in only a minority of infants born of mothers who have or have had hyperthyroidism due to Graves' disease.[298] In about half of the infants, the mother was hyperthyroid during the pregnancy. In the remainder the mother was euthyroid, having received antithyroid therapy prior to or during the pregnancy. The key variable is the maternal TSab level late in pregnancy. Neonatal hyperthyroidism is due to transplacental passage of TSab; it occurs primarily in those infants whose mothers have high serum TSab levels,[298,299] indicating that the degree of transplacental passage of TSab is limited. At birth TSab are detectable in the infant's serum but thereafter disappear within a period of weeks. The duration of the hyperthyroidism is a function of the initial TSab concentration and the rate of TSab metabolism, which is about 3 percent per day ($t_{1/2} = 14$ days).

Infants with neonatal hyperthyroidism have high serum T_4 and T_3 concentrations, although the hormone levels may not be elevated at birth in infants whose mothers received an antithyroid drug up to the time of delivery. Serum T_4 and T_3 concentrations in neonates must be interpreted in relation to norms that differ markedly from adult values and change rapidly following birth (see Physiological Variables Affecting Pituitary-Thyroid Function and Tests, above).

Neonatal hyperthyroidism should be treated with an antithyroid drug, for example 50 mg of PTU or 10 mg of MMI daily. If hyperthyroidism is clinically severe, iodide and propranolol should be given as well. The drugs subsequently should be gradually withdrawn as indicated by clinical evaluation and serum T_4 measurements. Withdrawal can usually be achieved within 6 to 8 weeks and is rarely followed by recurrence.

POSTPARTUM HYPERTHYROIDISM

Hyperthyroidism may occur in the first several months following delivery. Three forms of postpartum hyperthyroidism are recognized.[189,190] One is the new development of Graves' hyperthyroidism. A second is recurrence of Graves' hyperthyroidism, which may be persistent or transient. In all of these patients, thyroid radioiodine uptake is high. The third, and most common, is painless thyroiditis with hyperthyroidism. It can be recognized by low thyroid radioiodine uptake. The thyroiditis is often followed by transient hypothyroidism. Because postpartum hyperthyroidism is usually mild as well as transient, treatment is usually not necessary. However, propranolol may be useful in those patients with many symptoms.

Extrathyroidal Manifestations of Graves' Disease

INFILTRATIVE OPHTHALMOPATHY

Clinical evidence of ophthalmopathy is present in 20 to 40 percent of patients with hyperthyroidism due to Graves' disease, although measurements of orbital protrusion and orbital echographic studies indicate it is present to some degree in nearly all patients with Graves' hyperthyroidism.[300,301] Infiltrative ophthalmopathy usually develops concurrently with hyperthyroidism, but may precede or follow it.[167] There is little correlation between the severity of the hyperthyroidism and that of the ophthalmopathy. Occasionally, ophthalmopathy that is clinically indistinguishable occurs in patients who are euthyroid and did not have hyperthyroidism in the past (euthyroid Graves' disease).

The pathogenesis of infiltrative ophthalmopathy is poorly understood (see Graves' Disease, above). The major pathologic findings are edema, lymphocytic and plasma cell infiltration of the extraocular muscles and periorbital soft tissues, and, less commonly, optic neuropathy. Since there is little unoccupied space in the normal orbit, even a small increase in retroorbital tissue volume results in proptosis.

Clinical Manifestations

Patients with infiltrative ophthalmopathy may have symptoms referable to any of the orbital structures, as categorized in Table 10-13. These symptoms include pain the eyes, lacrimation, photophobia, diplopia, and blurring or loss of vision. The onset is usually gradual, but may be abrupt. Even when asymptomatic, ophthalmopathy may be very distressing to the patient for

Table 10-13. Clinical Classification of Eye Changes of Infiltrative Ophthalmopathy

Class	Finding
0	No symptoms or signs
1	Only hyperthyroid signs and mild proptosis (< 2 mm)
2	Soft-tissue involvement
3	Proptosis
4	Extraocular muscle involvement
5	Corneal involvement
6	Vision loss

Source: Werner.[302]

cosmetic reasons. The major signs are proptosis ("bulging eyes"), periorbital and conjunctival congestion and edema (chemosis), conjunctival injection, limitation of ocular mobility (Fig. 10-22), and increased intraocular pressure, especially on upward gaze.[303,304] Of these signs, proptosis is the most common. Since proptosis may be difficult to distinguish from lid retraction, it is best identified with an exophthalmometer, a device which measures the distance from the lateral orbital notch to the anterior surface of the cornea. In *true proptosis*, exophthalmometer readings are > 20 mm in white patients and > 24 mm in blacks; true proptosis is thus distinguished from "apparent" proptosis due to lid retraction alone. Proptosis is usually symmetric, although 1- to 2-mm differences in protrusion are common and more marked asymmetry is found occasionally. However, it is extremely unusual for one eye to be abnormal and the other normal in all respects; such a finding warrants special attention.

Extraocular muscle involvement most often results in limitation of upward gaze, but movement in any direction may be limited. Limitation of gaze is due to inflammatory restriction of muscle mobility rather than muscle weakness per se. Corneal ulceration and decreased visual acuity or visual field defects are,

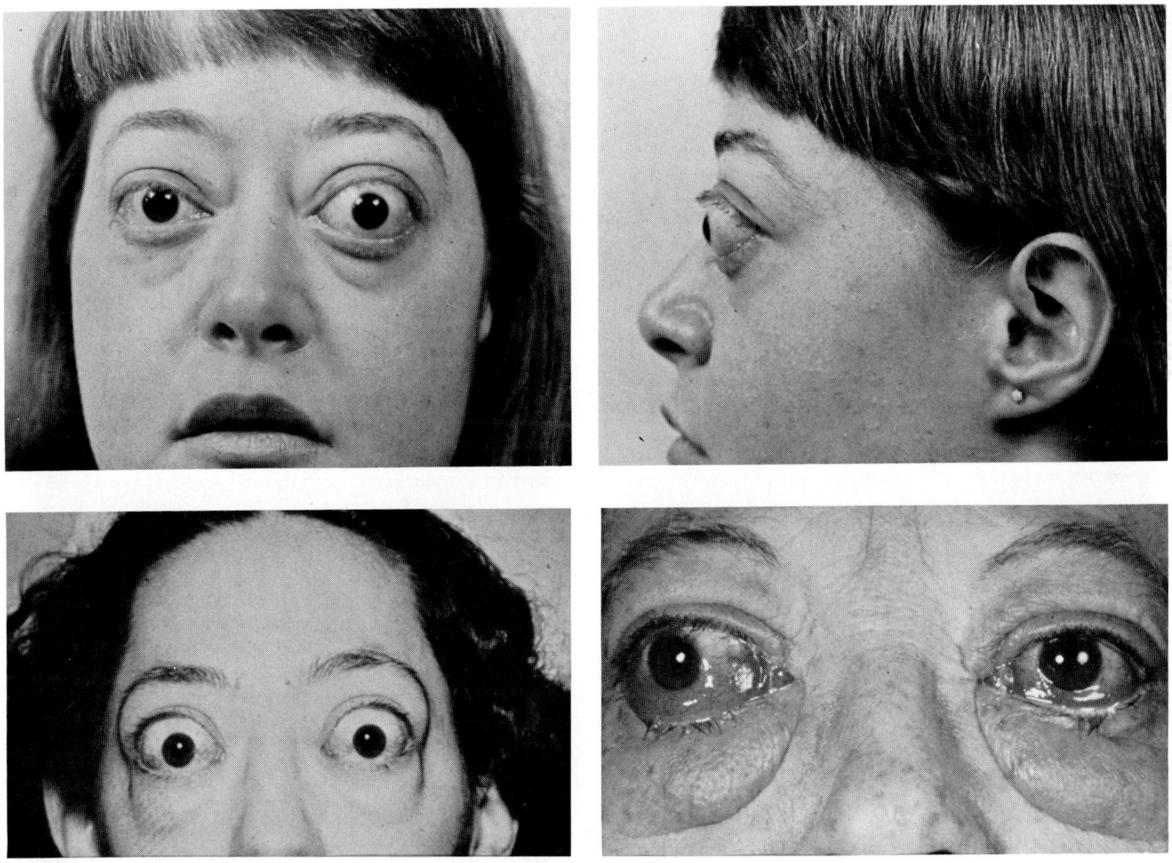

FIGURE 10-22 Photographs of three patients with ophthalmopathy due to Graves' disease. (*A*, *B*) A young woman with moderate asymmetric proptosis, with marked left eyelid retraction. This patient has few manifestations of ocular inflammatory disease. (*C*) A young woman with marked periorbital edema, bilateral lid retraction, and proptosis. (*D*) A middle-aged woman with marked infraorbital edema, conjunctival injection and chemosis, and muscle restriction of the right eye, but little proptosis.

fortunately, rare. The first defect is due to marked proptosis; the latter two may result from optic neuropathy or papilledema resulting from stretching or compression of the optic nerve or ophthalmic veins. The more severe signs, such as marked limitation of eye movement, marked proptosis, and visual impairment usually occur together, but there are exceptions. For example, an occasional patient may have visual impairment but only moderate proptosis; conversely, proptosis may be so great that the eye at times extends beyond the lid, but there is no visual loss.

The diagnosis of infiltrative ophthalmopathy when hyperthyroidism is or was present is usually not difficult, and no studies of orbital anatomy are needed. The diagnosis is inevitably less certain if the patient has euthyroid Graves' disease (see below). Other causes of bilateral ophthalmopathy include orbital pseudotumor, granulomatous diseases (sarcoidosis, Wegener's granulomatosis), arteriovenous malformations, and lymphoma and other tumors of the orbits. Tumors, vascular abnormalities, and pseudotumor are the usual causes of unilateral ophthalmopathy. If further study is deemed necessary, orbital ultrasonography or CT scan are the best procedures to confirm the presence of infiltrative ophthalmopathy and exclude most of the other disorders mentioned above.[301,305] Both of these procedures reliably show the characteristic finding of enlarged extraocular muscles (Fig. 10-23).

Euthyroid Graves' Disease

Euthyroid Graves' disease is a term applied to *euthyroid* patients who have infiltrative ophthalmopathy that is clinically and pathologically indistinguishable from the ophthalmopathy associated with hyperthyroidism due to Graves' disease. The disorder is uncommon, occurring with about 1 to 2 percent of the frequency of ophthalmopathy with hyperthyroidism. Patients with euthyroid Graves' disease have little or no thyroid enlargement. They may have serum antithyroid microsomal or antithyroglobulin antibodies and/or abnormal serum TSH responses to TRH; serum tests for TSab are weakly positive in

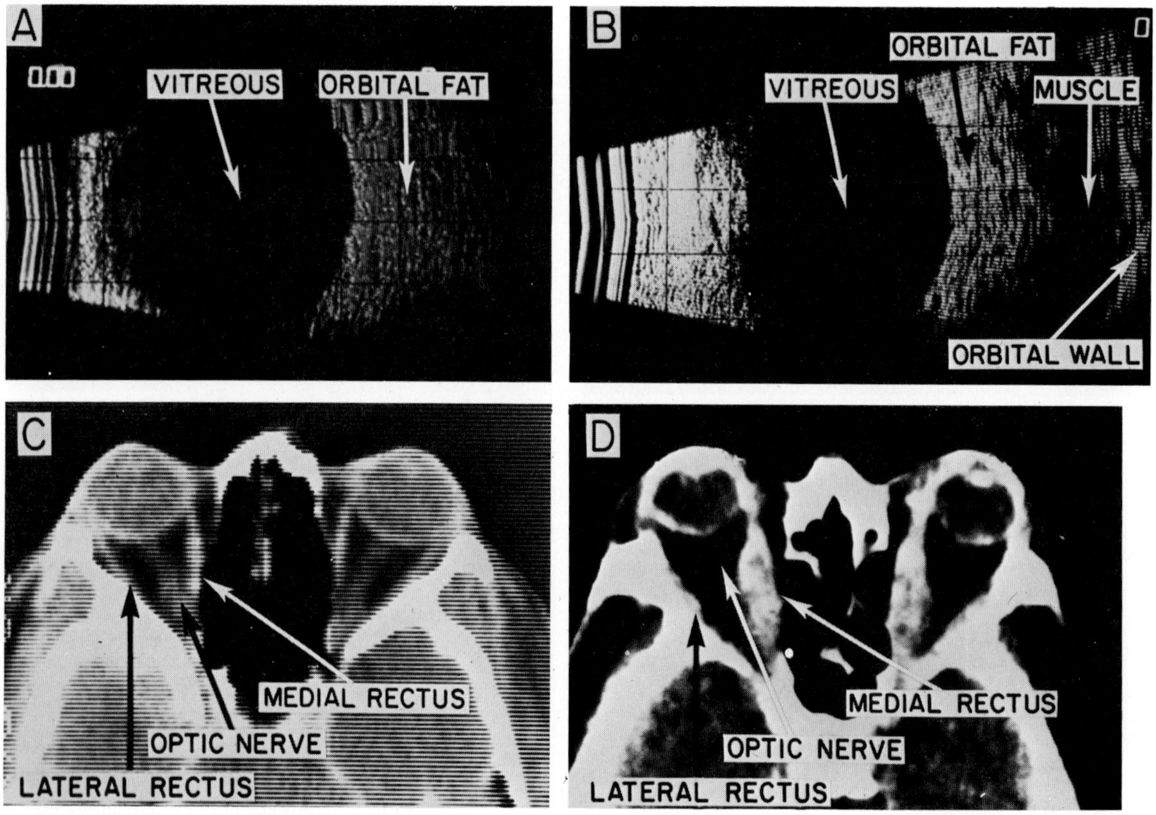

FIGURE 10-23 B-mode ultrasonograms and computed tomograms of the orbit. (*A, C*) Pictures from a normal subject. (*B, D*) Pictures from a patient with infiltrative ophthalmopathy due to Graves' disease. Note the sonolucent enlarged extraocular muscle in (*B*) and the enlarged medial rectus muscle in the tomogram (*D*).

about 50 percent.[306,307] The absence of hyperthyroidism in patients with abnormal thyroid regulation suggests that TSab are not present in sufficient quantity to cause hyperthyroidism, or else that the patient has autoimmune thyroiditis or some other thyroid disease that limits thyroid responsiveness to TSab. A few patients with ophthalmopathy have overt autoimmune thyroiditis; ophthalmopathy also may develop after external neck irradiation therapy for nonthyroid neoplastic disease.[308] The fact that some patients have no detectable TSab and a normal serum TSH response to TRH indicates that the ophthalmic process can occur entirely independently of any other manifestations of Graves' disease. When doubt exists concerning the cause of ophthalmopathy in a euthyroid patient, it is more appropriate to perform orbital echography or CT scan than a TRH stimulation test. The latter test provides only indirect evidence that the ophthalmopathy may be due to Graves' disease, whereas the other two tests provide detailed information about the orbital contents.

Course and Management

In most patients ophthalmopathy is at its worst before their hyperthyroidism is treated. During or after antithyroid treatment the patient's eyes feel and look better: noninfiltrative eye signs (lid retraction, apparent proptosis), local symptoms of irritation, and subjective diplopia often gradually improve. However, in the majority of patients, there is a modest 1- to 3-mm increase in proptosis in the first 1 to 2 years after treatment for hyperthyroidism. A longer-term study (up to 15 years) revealed that proptosis and ophthalmoplegia had changed little in most patients.[309,310] When ophthalmopathy progresses more, it usually does so within the first 1 to 2 years after antithyroid treatment; it is during this period that visual loss is most likely to develop. Although individual reports suggest that one or another form of antithyroid therapy is more likely to be followed by progression of ophthalmopathy, the differences are small and probably reflect the unpredictability of the process. Therefore, hyperthyroidism should be managed in the same way whether or not significant ophthalmopathy is present. The course of euthyroid Graves' disease is similar, although it may worsen somewhat more frequently; patients with euthyroid Graves' disease constitute a greater proportion of those patients requiring aggressive therapy.[311]

There is no satisfactory treatment for infiltrative ophthalmopathy.[167] For many patients, knowledge that their apparent proptosis will improve with treatment of their hyperthyroidism and that major progression is unlikely is very reassuring. When reassured in this way, most patients adapt to and tolerate significant degrees of ophthalmopathy and require no therapy. Hyperthyroidism, or hypothyroidism (if present), should be treated as otherwise indicated. Periorbital and eyelid edema may improve if the patient sleeps with the head raised; diuretics may also be helpful. Eye irritation and pain should be treated with 0.5% methylcellulose eye drops. For diplopia, prism lenses may be tried; occasionally, extraocular muscle surgery is needed, but this should not be undertaken until inflammatory signs have subsided spontaneously, or after corticosteroid treatment or decompression surgery.

Patients with severe inflammatory symptoms, severe periorbital congestion, edema and chemosis, marked proptosis, and, especially, optic neuropathy should be treated aggressively with corticosteroids, retroorbital radiotherapy, or orbital decompression.[167,312] All have been found reasonably effective and there are no established criteria for the selection of any one of them. Prednisone is given initially in doses of 60 to 80 mg per day. The dosage is reduced and the dose is given on alternate days as improvement occurs. As is often the case with corticosteroid therapy for inflammatory disorders, dose reduction may lead to exacerbations of the process, and therapy may be required for many months.

Transantral orbital decompression is the surgical treatment of choice, though it may be done transfrontally. Orbital decompression usually results in marked reduction in periorbital and conjunctival inflammation, a several-millimeter decrease in proptosis, and relief of optic neuropathy. Diplopia may persist or develop initially after the operation. Carefully directed retroorbital radiotherapy is safe and sometimes effective, particularly when combined with glucocorticoid therapy.[312]

When treatment is considered necessary, a reasonable approach is to start with corticosteroids in patients in whom periorbital and conjunctival edema and diplopia predominate, and with orbital decompression for those with marked proptosis and visual impairment; decompression should be used secondarily for those patients who do not respond to or tolerate corticosteroids. Experimental treatments for ophthalmopathy include plasmapheresis and administration of cyclosporin and other immunosuppressive drugs.

LOCALIZED MYXEDEMA AND THYROID ACROPACHY

Localized myxedema is a rare manifestation of Graves' disease. It usually occurs months or years after treatment for hyperthyroidism and in patients who also have significant ophthalmopathy. The lesions are usu-

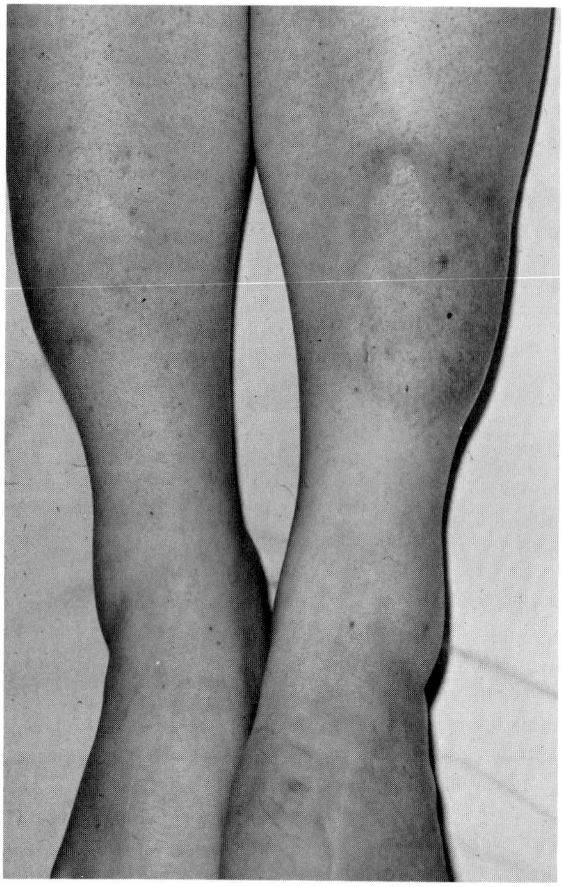

FIGURE 10-24 Localized myxedema. Note the raised, slightly hyperpigmented plaques on both anterolateral pretibial regions.

ally asymptomatic and rarely painful, but may be pruritic. They initially appear as shiny, erythematous, hyperpigmented, or slightly scaly plaques 10 to 20 mm in diameter, usually lying over the tibial or ankle regions anteriorly; they very rarely occur on the arms or trunk. The lesions are not tender, are indurated and nonpitting, and have an "orange peel" appearance (Fig. 10-24). Although the lesions may be unilateral when first detected, they usually become bilateral and symmetric. Some enlargement occurs after detection, but the lesions then usually slowly regress. In rare cases they extend to cover the entire pretibial region or encircle the leg, become bullous, ulcerate, or cause "foot drop" due to peroneal nerve entrapment. Biopsy reveals epidermal atrophy, fibrosis, and mucinous edema due to glycosaminoglycan deposition in the dermis. Most patients require no therapy. For those with extensive bullous or ulcerated lesions, 0.2% fluocinolone or other corticosteroid cream should be applied topically and covered by an occlusive dressing.[313] The cream should initially be used nightly or every other night, but when improvement occurs, treatment can be reduced to weekly or biweekly applications.

Thyroid acropachy is the rarest manifestation of Graves' disease. Nearly all reported patients have localized dermopathy, as well as hyperthyroidism (usually previously treated) and ophthalmopathy. Its manifestations are clubbing of the fingers and toes, subcutaneous edema and fibrosis of the hands and feet, and periosteal bone formation involving the phalanges and metacarpal and metatarsal bones. Thyroid acropachy usually causes no symptoms or deformity, but contractures may occur. The pathogenesis is not known. There is no known effective therapy.

HYPOTHYROIDISM

Hypothyroidism may be defined as the clinical and biochemical syndrome that results from decreased thyroid hormone production by the thyroid gland or, rarely, generalized resistance to thyroid hormones. The term *adaptive hypothyroidism* may be used (see Nonthyroidal Illness, above) to describe the reduction in extrathyroidal production of T_3 and the reduction in TSH secretion and thus thyroidal production of T_4 and T_3 that occur in patients with nonthyroidal illnesses. While such nonthyroidal illness–related reductions in serum T_3 and T_4 concentrations are the result of decreased thyroid hormone production, they are transient and not accompanied by clinical manifestations of hypothyroidism; thyroid hormone treatment is not indicated. This section is devoted primarily to a discussion of the causes, clinical manifestations, diagnosis, and management of hypothyroidism, as traditionally defined.

Hypothyroidism may result from thyroid disease (primary or thyroidal hypothyroidism), hypothalamic or pituitary disease (secondary or hypothyrotropic hypothyroidism), or generalized resistance to thyroid hormones. Primary hypothyroidism is by far the most common.

The severity of hypothyroidism varies widely. Some patients have no symptoms and normal serum T_4 and T_3 concentrations, but elevated serum TSH concentration; this is defined as *subclinical hypothyroidism.* In others, hypothyroidism is overt, causing symptoms and signs reflecting abnormal function of one or many organ systems. Rarely, it is so severe that it is a medical emergency (*myxedema coma*).

The frequency of hypothyroidism also varies considerably, depending on the population studied. Community surveys have revealed prevalences of overt hypothyroidism of 5/1000 to 13/1000 and annual incidence rates of 1/1000 to 2/1000 in women.[83] Hypothyroidism is considerably less common in men.

In patients seeking medical care, overt hypothyroidism may be found in 0.5 to 2 percent and subclinical hypothyroidism in 3 to 4 percent.[314]

Causes of Hypothyroidism

Hypothyroidism may result from thyroid, pituitary, or hypothalamic disease (Table 10-14). An attempt should always be made to determine how hypothyroidism arose, because it may be possible to treat it by removing the cause. Uncovering the cause of the disorder is important, moreover, because hypothyroidism may be the predominant or only manifestation of a potentially serious disease such as a pituitary adenoma. Often, the cause can be determined by history and physical examination. Particular attention should be paid to whether or not the patient has had thyroid disease or some antithyroid treatment in the past or is taking any drugs, and to palpation of the thyroid gland.

CHRONIC AUTOIMMUNE THYROIDITIS

Autoimmune thyroiditis is the most common cause of spontaneously occurring hypothyroidism in both children and adults. It most often occurs in women in their thirties or older, but can occur in men. It exists in two forms, *atrophic* (nongoitrous) and *goitrous* (*Hashimoto's disease*). The former type was previously called "idiopathic hypothyroidism," "primary myxedema," or "primary thyroid atrophy." The atrophic and goitrous forms of the disease differ clinically only in the presence or absence of goiter. Pathologically, the atrophic form is characterized by thyroid follicular atrophy, lymphocytic infiltration, and fibrosis; the goitrous form is characterized by thyroid follicular hyperplasia, lymphocytic and plasma cell infiltration, lymphoid germinal centers, and fibrosis.

Table 10-14. Causes of Hypothyroidism

Primary (thyroidal) hypothyroidism
Insufficient functional thyroid tissue due to:
Chronic autoimmune thyroiditis*
^{131}I therapy or thyroidectomy
Thyroid dysgenesis*
Infiltrations
Defective thyroid hormone biosynthesis due to:
Congenital defects*
Iodide deficiency*
Antithyroid agents*
Iodide excess*
Hypothyrotropic hypothyroidism
Pituitary hypothyroidism
Hypothalamic hypothyroidism
Generalized resistance to thyroid hormones*

*Hypothyroidism may be accompanied by goiter.

Patients with either form of autoimmune thyroiditis may be euthyroid or have subclinical or overt hypothyroidism. Some have rather specific defects in thyroid hormone biosynthesis, such as an iodide organification defect. Their thyroid glands may be very sensitive to the antithyroid action of inorganic iodide.[126] The disease also is characterized by the presence of antithyroid microsomal and antithyroglobulin antibodies in serum, often in very high titer.[75,162]

Both forms of autoimmune thyroiditis probably result from both cell- and antibody-mediated thyroid injury. Antithyroglobulin antibodies are not known to have biological activity. Antithyroid microsomal antibodies, however, may be cytotoxic.[315] The microsomal antigen is a vesicle-bound lipoprotein and may in fact be thyroid peroxidase. Its expression on the thyroid cell surface supports the possibility that antibodies reacting with it may be cytotoxic.[316] Serum from patients with autoimmune thyroiditis also may contain autoantibodies that inhibit TSH binding to thyroid cells, inhibit thyroid adenyl cyclase activity, or stimulate thyroid growth but not thyroid adenyl cyclase.[158,317-319] Thus, variations in the type(s) and amounts of autoantibodies produced may play an important role in determining the degree of thyroid dysfunction and determining whether the thyroid gland is atrophic or enlarged in individual patients with autoimmune thyroiditis.

Patients with autoimmune thyroiditis also have disordered mechanisms of cellular immunity. Their T lymphocytes are sensitized to thyroid tissue; the T cells produce migration inhibition factor (MIF) when exposed to thyroid tissue. Production of the lymphokine is inhibited by addition of normal T lymphocytes.[165,166] The ability of T lymphocytes from patients to inhibit antithyroglobulin antibody production by B lymphocytes is impaired.[320] These results suggest the presence of antigen-specific defects in suppressor T lymphocyte function. Some investigators have found reduced numbers of circulating suppressor T lymphocytes and/or increased numbers of "killer" T cells, using monoclonal antibody methods, but others have not.[162,163] Thyroid tissue may contain autoantibody-producing B lymphocytes and reduced numbers of suppressor T lymphocytes.[162,321] These data, although incomplete and at times conflicting, suggest that autoimmune thyroiditis results from both autoantibody and cell-mediated immunological disturbances. As in Graves' disease, however, the mechanisms that initiate these processes are not known.

The several known risk factors for autoimmune thyroiditis include female sex and heredity. Thyroid autoantibodies are found in up to 50 percent of siblings of patients, and with lesser but still substantial frequency in other relatives; the frequency of Graves' disease in siblings and relatives may be increased.[162] Predominance of certain HLA haplotypes, notably HLA-DR3 and -DR5, has been reported. Patients with autoimmune thyroiditis and their relatives may have autoantibodies to other endocrine tissues; occasionally they have other endocrine deficiency states, indicating the presence of the autoimmune polyglandular syndromes.[221]

The natural history of autoimmune thyroiditis is quite variable. In those patients with atrophic thyroiditis and subclinical hypothyroidism, overt hypothyroidism develops in from 5 to 25 percent per year;[322,323] disappearance of both antithyroid autoantibodies or normalization of serum TSH concentration is uncommon. Hypothyroidism also develops in time in the majority of patients with goitrous autoimmune thyroiditis who are not hypothyroid initially.[324] Treatment with T_4 results in decreased goiter size in about half of the patients. Repeated biopsies in patients show little change with time, and withdrawal of thyroid therapy usually results in recurrence of hypothyroidism. Thus, either form of autoimmune thyroiditis results in progressive and persistent thyroid failure, although remissions do occur.[324]

TRANSIENT AUTOIMMUNE THYROIDITIS

Autoimmune thyroiditis also causes transient hypothyroidism. This syndrome occurs most often in the postpartum period; transient hypothyroidism in other populations is rare. In two surveys of women followed closely after delivery, 3 and 5 percent had transient hypothyroidism within the first year.[189,325] It usually appears 3 to 6 months after delivery, and is characterized by the development of modest thyroid enlargement, hypothyroidism, and high titers of antithyroid microsomal antibodies; all such findings subside within several months.[325,326] Often, the hypothyroidism is subclinical, manifested only by transient elevations in serum TSH concentrations and antithyroid microsomal antibody titers. Recurrences are common following subsequent pregnancies.

Thyroid biopsies show lymphocytic thyroiditis, but the cellular infiltration is less intense than in chronic autoimmune thyroiditis and there are no germinal centers or fibrosis. Women with transient autoimmune thyroiditis probably have very mild chronic autoimmune thyroiditis, since they often have persistently positive tests for antithyroid microsomal antibodies, although the titers usually decline late in pregnancy and are lower after the postpartum illness.[325] It is likely, although not yet documented, that these women are destined to develop clinically significant, permanent chronic autoimmune thyroiditis.

HYPOTHYROIDISM FOLLOWING RADIOIODINE THERAPY

Hypothyroidism occurs within a year after therapy in a substantial number of patients treated with ^{131}I for hyperthyroidism; thereafter it occurs at a rate of 0.5 to 2 percent per year.[270,273] Hypothyroidism appearing within the first year after therapy is dependent on the dose of ^{131}I given. The rate at which hypothyroidism develops later is the same whether the initial dose of ^{131}I is large or small. Late hypothyroidism is preceded by a long period of subclinical hypothyroidism,[274] which attests to the ability of TSH hypersecretion to maintain nearly adequate thyroid secretion if the thyroid is not badly damaged. Late post-^{131}I hypothyroidism probably occurs because the thyroid follicular cells that survive acute irradiation with ^{131}I can maintain function but cannot replicate. However, autoimmune thyroid cellular injury may occur, just as it may occur long after antithyroid drug treatment of hyperthyroidism due to Graves' disease. Hypothyroidism is unusual following ^{131}I therapy for toxic uninodular goiter (thyroid adenoma) or multinodular goiter, since some of the thyroid tissue in these patients is atrophic at the time ^{131}I is given and thus does not concentrate the radioisotope.

External neck radiation therapy using doses of 2500 rads or more, as used for the treatment of patients with lymphoma, laryngeal carcinoma, and nasopharyngeal carcinoma, also causes hypothyroidism in children and adults.[327-329] Its effect is dose-dependent; hypothyroidism ultimately develops in over 50 percent of patients receiving more than 4000 rads. Like hypothyroidism occurring one or more years after ^{131}I therapy, overt hypothyroidism induced by external irradiation is usually preceded by months or years of subclinical hypothyroidism.

POSTOPERATIVE HYPOTHYROIDISM

Total thyroidectomy causes hypothyroidism within one month. The frequency of hypothyroidism following subtotal thyroidectomy for hyperthyroid Graves' disease is now high, ranging from 25 to 75 percent in the first year after surgery.[270,281,283] The current high rate of postoperative hypothyroidism is the result of more aggressive surgery, undertaken to reduce the frequency of recurrent postoperative *hyper*thyroidism. Hypothyroidism also may develop later than one year after surgery, at a rate of about 0.5 percent per year. Late postoperative hypothyroidism is probably due to destruction of the thyroid remnant by autoimmune mechanisms, since it is more likely to occur in patients whose excised thyroid tissue had histological evidence of autoimmune thyroiditis.

TRANSIENT HYPOTHYROIDISM

Hypothyroidism that is transient may occur within several weeks or months following ^{131}I therapy, subtotal thyroidectomy for Graves' disease, subacute thyroiditis, painless thyroiditis, or withdrawal of prolonged thyroid hormone therapy in patients who are euthyroid.[272,282,330,331] Following these events, serum T_4 and T_3 concentrations decline to subnormal levels and may remain low for several weeks or months. Initially, despite low serum T_4 and T_3 concentrations, serum TSH concentrations are low because of preceding thyroid hormone–induced inhibition of TSH secretion. Several weeks or months may be required for TSH secretion to recover, and symptoms of hypothyroidism may develop within this period. If the remaining thyroid tissue mass is small but otherwise normal, serum TSH concentrations rise to above normal until the thyroid grows large enough to maintain normal thyroid secretion. Thus, transient hypothyroidism in these settings may be associated with either decreased or increased TSH secretion.

THYROID DYSGENESIS (SPORADIC NONGOITROUS CRETINISM)

Developmental defects of the thyroid gland are the most common cause of hypothyroidism in the newborn. Some patients have virtually complete thyroid agenesis, but in about half, thyroid tissue is detectable by thyroid scan.[79] The thyroid tissue may be located in the midline anywhere from the base of the tongue to below the thyroid cartilage, or in the normal location on one or both sides of the neck. A midline neck mass, simulating a thyroglossal duct cyst, may be present, indicating that the dysgenetic tissue can enlarge in response to TSH. The cause of abnormal thyroid development is not known. One possibility is that it is due to transplacental passage of maternal thyroid autoantibodies that are cytotoxic. However, such antibodies are found with similar frequency in normal and hypothyroid neonates.[332] Transplacental passage of autoantibodies that inhibit TSH binding or action causes transient, but not permanent, neonatal hypothyroidism; such antibodies have been found only in infants whose mothers had clinically significant chronic autoimmune thyroiditis.[318,332]

HYPOTHYROIDISM DUE TO THYROID INJURY FROM OTHER CAUSES

A variety of other diseases may result in thyroid damage sufficient to cause hypothyroidism. *Cystinosis* is one such disease: hypothyroidism was found in 25 percent of patients in one study.[334] The thyroid tissue was atrophic and, in some patients, contained cystine crystals. Hypothyroidism also occurs occasionally in patients with hemochromatosis, amyloidosis, sarcoidosis, scleroderma, and frequently in those with fibrous invasive thyroiditis (Riedel's thyroiditis).

BIOSYNTHETIC DEFECTS IN THYROID HORMONOGENESIS

Thyroid hormone biosynthesis and secretion depend on the availability of iodide, and the ability of thyroid tissue to concentrate iodide, synthesize thyroglobulin, form iodotyrosines and iodothyronines, and hydrolyze thyroglobulin. The entire process is dependent on the TSH responsiveness of thyroid tissue. It is not surprising, therefore, that there are multiple genetic, nutritional, and pharmacologic causes of decreased thyroid hormone production.

Congenital Defects

Inherited defects of many of the steps of thyroid hormone biosynthesis occur. While rare, they have provided considerable insight into the normal mechanisms of thyroid hormone biosynthesis and release. Most of these disorders are inherited as autosomal recessive traits. In the homozygote, hypothyroidism is severe and becomes apparent early in life. The increase in TSH secretion in response to thyroid deficiency leads to thyroid enlargement, which may be minimal early in life but becomes marked later in childhood or in adult life. In presumed heterozygotes the abnormality is usually mild and only a variable degree of thyroid enlargement results.

IODIDE CONCENTRATION DEFECT This rare abnormality is characterized by partial or complete failure of thyroid tissue to transport iodide.[6] Thus, thyroid radioiodine uptake is very low despite the presence of goiter. The defect also is present in salivary tissue, gastric mucosa, and choroid plexus. Treatment with iodide in doses of 5 mg or more daily restores thyroid hormone secretion to normal, as a result of passive diffusion of iodide into the thyroid, but treatment with T_4 is more convenient.

IODIDE ORGANIFICATION DEFECTS The oxidation and organification of iodide are catalyzed by thyroid peroxidase. When peroxidase activity is subnormal, thyroidal iodide transport is normal but little further iodide is metabolized in the thyroid. Therefore, inorganic iodide accumulates in the thyroid; the iodide is "discharged" when perchlorate or thiocyanate is given. So-called discharge is in fact concentration-dependent outward diffusion made evident when inward iodide transport is inhibited by one of these agents. Perchlorate discharge tests are done by administering 500 mg of $KClO_4$ 1 h after a tracer dose of ^{131}I or ^{123}I is given. A fall in thyroid radioactivity of 10 percent or more 1 h after $KClO_4$ is given indicates defective iodide oxidation and organification.

Several different types of organification defect have been described.[8] They include quantitative deficiency of thyroid peroxidase, qualitative abnormalities, such as defective binding of the heme prosthetic group to the enzyme and abnormal intracellular enzyme localization, and deficient hydrogen peroxide generation. In some families, goiter, usually with only minimal hypothyroidism, occurs along with congenital sensorineural deafness (Pendred's syndrome). Such patients have a positive perchlorate discharge test, so they are considered to have an organification defect. Although thyroid tissue from most patients with Pendred's syndrome has normal peroxidase activity and forms iodotyrosines normally in vitro, little iodothyronine is formed; in some patients thyroglobulin formation is abnormal as well. Thus, the biochemical defect is uncertain, and may be heterogeneous. The deafness usually precedes the development of goiter. Deafness may occur in patients with no thyroid abnormality; on the other hand, patients with thyroid disease may have no deafness.

THYROGLOBULIN BIOSYNTHETIC DEFECTS Various abnormalities in thyroglobulin biosynthesis and secretion result in reduced T_4 and T_3 production.[8] Thyroglobulin production may be inadequate, although its structure is normal. It may be produced in adequate quantities but be structurally abnormal. Organification or iodotyrosyl coupling within it is then poor, or else it cannot be secreted into the thyroid follicular lumen. Abnormalities of either the amino acid or the carbohydrate composition may be responsible for the structural thyroglobulin abnormality. In these patients, serum and the abnormal thyroid tissue usually contain iodinated albumin or iodinated IgG immunoglobulins. Although these proteins may contain iodinated tyrosyl residues, their structure is such that little if any iodotyrosyl coupling occurs and therefore little T_4 and/or T_3 is formed. Thus, thyroglobulin biosynthetic abnormalities result in deficient coupling, but probably do not involve a coupling defect per se, considering the above findings and the lack of evidence of a separate thyroidal iodotyrosine coupling enzyme.

IODOTYROSINE DEIODINASE DEFECT Thyroid iodotyrosine deiodinase, which catalyzes the deiodination of iodotyrosines, plays an important role in the recirculation of iodine, and thus in iodide conservation. Deiodinase deficiency results in release of large quantities of mono- and diiodotyrosine from the thyroid gland.[8] Since extrathyroidal iodotyrosine deiodinase also is lacking in these patients, the iodotyrosines are excreted. Thus, iodide that normally is recycled and therefore available for reuse within the thyroid is lost, resulting in secondary iodide deficiency.

THYROID INSENSITIVITY TO TSH Several patients with congenital hypothyroidism without thyroid enlargement, in whom the defect is insensitivity to TSH, have been described.[8] Thyroid tissue is present, but is unresponsive in vivo either to high endogenous serum TSH concentrations or to exogenous TSH administration. In vitro studies demonstrate poor cyclic AMP or other responses to TSH in the thyroid tissue; whether these patients have a TSH receptor or postreceptor defect is not known. Thyroidal resistance to TSH also occurs in patients with pseudohypoparathyroidism; their thyroid tissue TSH receptors are normal but deficient activity of the guanine nucleotide regulatory protein results in reduced adenyl cyclase responses to TSH.[335]

In a patient with primary hypothyroidism in whom a congenital defect in thyroid hormone biosynthesis is suspected, thyroid radioiodine uptake should be determined. If iodine uptake is low and the patient has thyroid enlargement, the iodide concentrating defect is present. Low thyroid radioiodine uptake in a patient with no goiter indicates that the thyroid is insensitive to TSH. The other defects are associated with an increased thyroid radioiodine uptake. Iodide organification defects are associated with an abnormal perchlorate discharge test, as described previously. Recognition of the other abnormalities involves measurement of iodotyrosine deiodination or studies of thyroid tissue.

Iodide Deficiency

Dietary iodide deficiency results in inadequate production of thyroid hormone despite the presence of intrinsically normal thyroid tissue (see Chap. 11). The presence of infantile hypothyroidism (cretinism) in regions where iodide deficiency is endemic has long been recognized. Many more residents of such regions have thyroid enlargement, abnormalities in thyroid iodide metabolism and secretion, and elevated serum TSH concentrations, although their frequency varies greatly. The degree of iodide deficiency is the major determinant of the frequency of these findings, but other variables such as dietary goitrogens, genetic factors, and water pollution may be important contributory factors.

Antithyroid Agents

A variety of inorganic and organic compounds, both naturally occurring and synthetic, have antithyroid actions. Since these compounds inhibit thyroid hormone synthesis and secretion, usually by inhibiting iodide transport or iodide organification and coupling, they can cause hypothyroidism with goiter. PTU and MMI are the most potent antithyroid drugs; their use will usually be evident. Other agents that are commonly used which may cause hypothyroidism and goiter are iodide and lithium carbonate (see Effects of Various Drugs on Thyroid Function, above). Ethionamide and aminoglutethimide also have antithyroid actions.[336,337] Many other drugs, chemicals, and constituents of natural foodstuffs have antithyroid effects, and occasionally have been implicated as the cause of goiter and/or hypothyroidism in individual patients. These include thiocyanate, perchlorate, nitroprusside, sulfonamides, sulfonylureas, resorcinol, polybrominated biphenyl compounds, and *goitrin* (found in various plants).

Despite the multiplicity of drugs known to interfere with thyroid hormone biosynthesis, drugs are not important causes of hypothyroidism. First, other than PTU or MMI, most are very weak antithyroid agents. Second, other than lithium carbonate, none is widely used. Nevertheless, it is important to inquire about drug use in any patient with hypothyroidism.

Iodide Excess

Iodide excess, in addition to iodide deficiency, may result in subclinical or overt hypothyroidism. Patients who are susceptible to iodide-induced hypothyroidism are those who have abnormal thyroid tissue due to either chronic autoimmune thyroiditis or previous ^{131}I or surgical therapy for hyperthyroidism.[136] In such patients, escape from the antithyroid action of iodide does not occur, as it does in normal subjects and patients with hyperthyroidism; thus, iodides have sustained antithyroid action which persists as long as they continue to be administered.

HYPOTHYROTROPIC HYPOTHYROIDISM

Pituitary Hypothyroidism

TSH is required for normal thyroid secretion; decreased thyroid secretion and thyroid atrophy follow TSH deficiency. Deficiency of TSH is much less common than primary (thyroidal) hypothyroidism. It may be caused by destruction of the thyrotrophs by either functioning (GH- or prolactin-secreting) or nonfunctioning pituitary macroadenomas; most patients with microadenomas are euthyroid. If not present initially, TSH deficiency may result from surgical therapy of such tumors or, rarely, after external pituitary radiation therapy. TSH deficiency may also result from postpartum pituitary necrosis (Sheehan's syndrome), pituitary cysts, craniopharyngioma, carotid aneurysm, trauma, hemochromatosis, and infiltrative processes such as metastatic tumor, tuberculosis, and histiocytosis (Hand-Schüller-Christian disease). Sometimes the cause is not apparent; autoimmune mechanisms have been postulated but not established. In any of these situations, TSH deficiency may occur in association with other trophic hormone deficiencies or as an isolated abnormality. In infants and children, TSH deficiency may be caused by many of the same diseases. In addition, occasional patients with isolated familial TSH deficiency or pituitary aplasia or hypoplasia have been described.

In most hypothyroid patients with pituitary disease, serum TSH concentrations are undetectable or normal. In this setting, serum TSH concentrations within the normal range must be considered inappropriately low. Usually, there is little increase in serum TSH concentration after TRH administration.

Pituitary enlargement and hypothyroidism do not invariably indicate the presence of a primary pituitary tumor and pituitary hypothyroidism. Slight pituitary enlargement is present in many patients with severe primary hypothyroidism[338] due to compensatory hyperplasia and hypertrophy of the thyrotrophs. Occasionally, primary hypothyroidism causes radiologically and even clinically evident pituitary enlargement, for example, bitemporal vision defects.[339,340] Recognition that such abnormalities occur in patients with primary hypothyroidism is very important, however, so that these patients do not undergo unnecessary pituitary surgery. Serum TSH concentrations in these patients decline during thyroid hormone therapy, indicating that TSH secretion is not autonomous; the pituitary also diminishes in size.

Hypothalamic Hypothyroidism

TRH deficiency also causes hypothyroidism. As with TSH deficiency, TRH deficiency may be isolated or may coexist with other hypothalamic hormone deficiencies. Hypothalamic hypothyroidism occurs predominantly in children, in whom it is not accompanied by any anatomic abnormality. In both adults and children it may occur as a result of cranial irradiation, traumatic, infiltrative, and neoplastic diseases of the hypothalamus, or pituitary lesions which interrupt the hypothalamic-pituitary portal circulation (see Chap. 7). However, hypothalamic hypothyroidism is rare. Basal serum TSH concentrations are low or normal. The characteristic, but by no means specific, finding in hypothyrotropic hypothyroidism is a serum TSH response to TRH that is normal in magnitude but delayed in time.

Somatostatin inhibits TSH as well as GH secretion, and increased somatostatin secretion may account for the transient hypothyroidism that sometimes occurs in children treated with GH.[63] Patients with acromegaly also may have increased somatostatin production, which in turn could inhibit TSH secretion and cause hypothyroidism. Although removal of somatotroph adenomas has not been reported to ameliorate hypothyroidism in acromegaly, serum TSH responses to TRH do increase in such patients after successful surgery.[341] Similarly, patients with prolactinomas have increased dopamine secretion and reduced serum T_4 and T_3 concentrations, if not overt hypothyroidism, which may result from dopamine-induced depression of TSH secretion.[64]

In rare patients with hypothalamic hypothyroidism, elevated basal serum TSH concentrations are found.[342,343] The TSH in these patients is immunoreactive but biologically inactive, and its biological activity increases when the patients are given TRH. These patients may have either idiopathic hypothalamic disease or a hypothalamic tumor.

GENERALIZED RESISTANCE TO THYROID HORMONES

Generalized resistance to thyroid hormones is a rare disorder characterized by thyroid enlargement, variable clinical manifestations of hypothyroidism, and elevated serum total and free T_4 and T_3 concentrations. Some reported patients have physical abnormalities, such as deafness, stippled epiphyses, and short stature, indicative of hypothyroidism in infancy; others have only thyroid enlargement.[344] Their serum TSH concentrations and TSH responses are usually normal or slightly increased, unless they had been treated inappropriately for hyperthyroidism in the past.[345,346] The resistance to thyroid hormone is partial, since the high serum T_4 and T_3 concentrations result in normal or nearly normal peripheral tissue thyroid hormone actions. Additional thyroid hormone evokes little additional response unless very large doses are given.

Complete resistance to thyroid hormones would be expected to result in very severe infantile hypothyroidism no matter how much thyroid hormone could be produced, and it may not be compatible with life. Partial generalized resistance may occur sporadically or cluster in families. The cause of the abnormality in partially resistant patients is not known, but appears to be a postreceptor defect. Equilibrium T_3 binding to its nuclear receptor is normal, although the kinetics of T_3 nuclear uptake may be impaired.[347] Resistance to the biological action of T_4 and T_3 can be demonstrated in vitro as well as in vivo.[348,349]

Clinical Manifestations of Hypothyroidism

The clinical manifestations of hypothyroidism are highly variable; they depend on its cause, duration, and severity. Today, hypothyroidism is recognized in many patients with mild or vague clinical symptoms and signs previously attributed to other disorders or ignored. The improvement in diagnosis has come as a result of the availability of accurate methods for measuring serum T_4 and, more importantly, serum TSH concentrations.

The clinical manifestations of hypothyroidism indicate that some thyroid hormone is required for normal function of most organ systems. The term that best applies to organ system function in the presence of thyroid deficiency is *slowing:* there is slowing of physical and mental activity and of cardiovascular, gastrointestinal, and neuromuscular function. The more common symptoms and signs, their relative frequencies in several older studies, and their diagnostic importance are listed in Table 10-15. Hypothyroidism now can be diagnosed at a stage when fewer of these findings are present, and indeed when there are no symptoms or signs at all.

Many of the common symptoms and signs of hypothyroidism frequently occur in euthyroid patients. Certain symptoms, such as fatigue, lethargy, constipation, and dry skin, are so common that their diagnostic value is limited. The most *discriminating* (as opposed to *frequent*) symptoms and signs are slow movements, coarse skin, decreased sweating, hoarseness, paresthesias, cold intolerance, periorbital edema, and delayed reflexes[352] (Table 10-15). Also important in suggesting the diagnosis of hypothyroidism is a history of events that might cause it, such as ^{131}I therapy, thyroid surgery, or use of drugs such as iodide or lithium carbonate.

Spontaneously occurring hypothyroidism, as, for example, due to chronic autoimmune thyroiditis, usually develops gradually; as thyroid secretion declines, the resulting rise in TSH secretion limits the decline in thyroid secretion and may stabilize it. Thus, symptoms and signs of hypothyroidism often appear very slowly in such patients. When hypothyroidism develops more rapidly, for example, within the first year

Table 10-15. Frequency of Common Signs and Symptoms of Hypothyroidism and Their Relative Discriminant Value

	Frequency in hypothyroid patients, %	Diagnostic weight*	
		Present	Absent
Symptoms			
Dry skin	60–100	+3	−6
Cold intolerance	60–95	+4	−5
Hoarseness	50–75	+5	−6
Weight gain	50–75	+1	−1
Constipation	35–65	+2	−1
Decreased sweating	10–65	+3	−6
Paresthesias	50	+5	−4
Diminished hearing	5–30	+2	0
Weakness	90		
Signs			
Slow movements	70–90	+11	−3
Coarse skin and hair	70–100	+7	−7
Cold skin	70–90	+3	−2
Periorbital puffiness	40–90	+4	−6
Bradycardia	10–15	+4	−4
Slow reflex relaxation	50	+15	−6

*In patients without other illnesses and receiving no medication, a total score of > +19 usually indicates hypothyroidism, a score of +19 to −24 is equivocal, and a score of < −24 indicates euthyroidism.[352]
Source: From Refs. 203, 350–352.

after ^{131}I therapy or subtotal thyroidectomy, patients recognize the changes more readily; symptoms such as muscle cramps and weakness are more prominent. When hypothyroidism is due to hypothalamic or pituitary disease it is less likely to be associated with periorbital and peripheral edema, hoarseness, and weight gain.

The characteristic pathologic finding in patients with hypothyroidism is the accumulation of glycosaminoglycans, primarily hyaluronic acid, in interstitial tissue. Glycosaminoglycans are normal constituents of interstitial tissue, in which they exist in both free and protein-bound forms. Their accumulation is the result of increased synthesis.[47] Their hydrophilic properties lead to the mucinous edema characteristic of hypothyroidism; this is *myxedema*. Mucinous edema of the dermis produces some of the most obvious clinical manifestations of hypothyroidism (see below). In fatal cases, mucinous edema has been found in the interstitial tissue of many other organ systems;[353] it probably causes many of the functional abnormalities that accompany hypothyroidism.

GENERAL APPEARANCE

A patient with hypothyroidism may appear normal, have overt myxedema, or be comatose. Often the major presenting manifestations are subjective. The patient is chronically tired and weak, fatigues easily, and is unable to continue normal physical or mental activities. Cold intolerance may be marked, so that the patient uses extra clothing even in summer. It may not be possible to elicit a history of the other, more specific symptoms or signs of hypothyroidism; the patient has either not noted or cannot remember them. Too often such behavior is attributed to aging by the patient or the patient's relatives.

SKIN AND APPENDAGES

The characteristic appearance of the hypothyroid patient (Fig. 10-25) is primarily a reflection of subcutaneous mucinous edema, which results in facial, periorbital, and peripheral edema of both hands and feet. This edema is usually nonpitting. The facial features are coarse. Periorbital edema, often an early sign, causes the patient to look haggard. There is hyperkeratosis, which makes the skin rough, scaly, and thickened.

More often, the patient's appearance is much less altered. The patient may complain of dry, scaly skin, but the skin is not thickened or particularly rough. Periorbital and peripheral edema is mild. Good nursing care may render previously dry and scaly skin almost

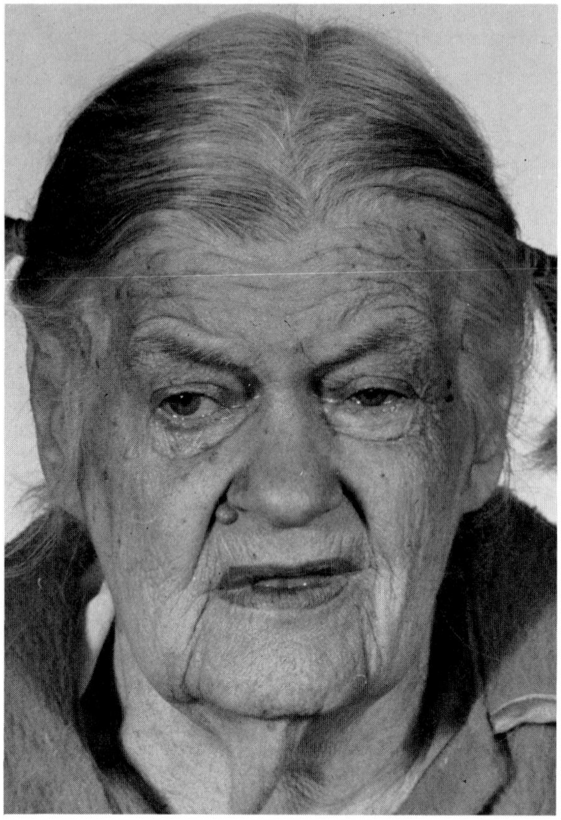

FIGURE 10-25 Photograph of a patient with hypothyroidism, showing facial puffiness and periorbital edema.

normal. At times, the edema is pitting, particularly in the legs; such a finding need not indicate the presence of cardiac or other disease. There is often pallor, due to the thickened dermis and epidermis, decreased cutaneous blood flow, and, sometimes, anemia. The yellowish hue of carotenemia may be evident. Skin thickening and decreased blood flow also result in coldness of the skin. Decreased sebaceous and sweat gland secretions add to the dryness of the skin. The hair may be coarse, dry, and brittle, and hair growth may slow or cease; hair may be lost on the scalp, the extremities, or the eyebrows. The nails also grow slowly, and may be thickened and brittle.

THYROID GLAND

The size of the thyroid may provide a valuable clue to the cause of hypothyroidism, and even to its presence, since thyroid enlargement may be the first objective sign of hypothyroidism. Goitrous autoimmune thyroiditis is characterized by diffuse thyroid enlargement, although the surface may be irregular or even nodular. The consistency of the thyroid gland is often described as firm or rubbery. The gland also is diffusely enlarged in patients with hypothyroidism that is due to iodide deficiency, congenital defects in thyroid hormone biosynthesis, or the action of any antithyroid agent. The thyroid is not palpable in atrophic autoimmune thyroiditis or hypothyrotropic hypothyroidism.

NERVOUS SYSTEM

Hypothyroid patients have many symptoms related to CNS dysfunction. Central nervous system glucose and oxygen consuption are normal in hypothyroid adults. Cerebral vascular resistance is increased and cerebral blood flow is reduced, in proportion to the decrease in cardiac output.[354] The reduced delivery of oxygen to tissue which uses it at a normal rate should result in some degree of cerebral hypoxia. Electroencephalography may show decreased amplitude and loss of alpha rhythm. Cerebrospinal fluid protein concentrations are often modestly elevated. Histological examination of CNS tissue from untreated patients reveals mucinous edema around neural tissue.

Clinical features reflect slowing of cerebral function. Complaints of tiredness, lethargy, and fatigue, or loss of ambition and energy, are common; anxiety and depression may result. The patient becomes complacent, less alert, mentally slow, and physically clumsy. Speech is slow and hesitant, as well as hoarse. Other than memory loss, intellectual capacity is usually preserved. Headache and hearing loss may be prominent complaints. The patient may sleep longer at night or may fall asleep frequently during the day. The patient may thus seem uncooperative and inattentive. Often the patient describes significant limitations of activity with inappropriate amusement and may accept such limitations with equanimity. Occasionally, dementia is marked; rarely, there is severe anxiety and agitation ("myxedema madness").

Hypothyroid patients often complain of paresthesias but usually have no objective neurological findings other than slow deep tendon reflexes. Several neurological syndromes that are reversible may occur, however. Perhaps most frequent is the carpal tunnel syndrome, due to mucinous edema of the flexor retinaculum of the wrist, resulting in median nerve compression. Occasional patients have either polyneuropathy, due directly to myxedema of peripheral nerves, or cerebellar dysfunction; signs of the latter include ataxia, intention tremor, and nystagmus.[355,356]

MUSCULOSKELETAL SYSTEM

Muscle dysfunction occurs in many hypothyroid patients.[357] Muscle cramps, myalgias, and stiffness are frequent symptoms. Movements may be slow and clumsy. Subjective weakness and fatigability are common. Objective muscle weakness also may be found, especially of the proximal muscles of the legs. Slow relaxation of tendon reflexes is common. Rarely, chronic hypothyroid myopathy results in increased muscle mass (pseudohypertrophy), muscle spasms, and pseudomyotonia.[358] Elevated serum creatine phosphokinase (CPK) levels are usually found in hypothyroidism, even in the absence of muscle symptoms.[359] Isoenzyme analysis indicates that the source is skeletal muscle, presumably caused by increased sarcolemmal permeability, but part of the increase may reflect slowed CPK clearance. Serum lactate dehydrogenase, alanine aminotransferase, and aldolase concentrations may be increased as well. Electromyographic abnormalities consist of decrease in size and duration of individual potentials and polyphasic potentials. Muscle biopsies show interstitial edema and muscle fiber enlargement, loss of striations, and sarcoplasmic degenerative changes.

Hypothyroid patients may complain of arthralgias and joint stiffness.[360] There may be synovial thickening and synovial effusions, usually of the knees. Synovial fluid may contain calcium pyrophosphate crystals, although the patients do not have pseudogout.

CARDIOVASCULAR-PULMONARY SYSTEM

Thyroid hormone deficiency results in decreases in the rate and force of cardiac muscle contractions.[361] It also reduces peripheral oxygen needs. Peripheral resistance is increased, and cerebral, cutaneous, and renal blood flow and blood volume are reduced. The physiological consequences are decreased cardiac output but no change in ventricular end-diastolic pressure, normal peripheral arteriovenous oxygen differences, and no pulmonary congestion. During exercise, cardiac output increases and peripheral resistance decreases appropriately, indicating that cardiac reserve is normal.[362] In fatal cases, swollen and vacuolated myocardial fibers and intercellular edema have been found.[353]

Symptoms and signs of cardiovascular dysfunction include bradycardia, evidence of poor peripheral circulation, such as pallor and cold skin, cold intolerance, decreased exercise tolerance, and fatigability. Hypertension that is reversible by thyroid therapy may be found.[363] Heart sounds may be distant. The lethargy, puffiness, edema, and diminished cardiac activity may suggest cardiac failure. In fact, this is rare, although occasionally it is caused by hypothyroid cardiomyopathy or massive pericardial effusion. Clinical and/or radiographic evidence of cardiac enlargement, whether due to pericardial effusion or cardiac dilatation, may be present. The pericardial effusion usually has a high protein concentration and may be rich in cholesterol as well. The electrocardiogram shows bradycardia and low-amplitude P waves and QRS complexes; atrioventricular or intraventricular conduction disturbances and nonspecific QRS and T wave abnormalities also may occur. Echocardiographic findings are those of pericardial effusion, septal cardiomyopathy, and slowed myocardial relaxation.[364-366]

The coexistence of angina pectoris and hypothyroidism in some patients warrants special mention. Although hypercholesterolemia and hypertriglyceridemia occur as a result of hypothyroidism, there is no compelling evidence that hypothyroidism is accompanied by accelerated atherogenesis. The development of hypothyroidism may ameliorate angina pectoris, either directly, because cardiac work and thus myocardial oxygen requirements are reduced, or simply because the patient becomes less active. The appropriate management of angina in a hypothyroid patient is controversial, since angina may worsen when T_4 therapy is given. Antiangina therapy combined with cautious T_4 therapy is the most appropriate treatment.[367] However, coronary revascularization, if otherwise indicated, can be safely carried out in untreated hypothyroid patients.[368]

Respiratory function abnormalities of several types occur in hypothyroidism. Chronic nasal congestion, due to mucinous edema of the nasal mucosa, may be present. Hoarseness due to vocal cord thickening is common, and may be an early or prominent complaint. Macroglossia and/or laryngeal myxedema may cause obstructive sleep apnea.[369] Lung volumes are normal, as is vital capacity and arterial P_{O_2}, P_{CO_2}, and pH. Maximum breathing capacity, compliance, and ventilatory drive may be reduced[370] due to respiratory muscle weakness and/or respiratory center depression. Pleural effusion(s) may be present without other evidence of lung disease.

FLUID AND ELECTROLYTE METABOLISM

Renal blood flow is reduced in proportion to the decrease in cardiac output, and the glomerular filtration rate is usually slightly reduced. Serum concentrations of urea, creatinine, and electrolytes are normal. There may be hyperuricemia due to decrased urate excretion. Modest proteinuria and defects in urine concentration and dilution may be present.[371] Impaired ability to excrete a water load and modest increases in plasma arginine vasopressin concentrations, in relation to plasma osmolality, are common; occasionally, significant hyponatremia is encountered.[372] Renin and aldosterone production are appropriate for volume status. These changes presumably reflect both renal and central effects of thyroid hormone deficiency.

Anatomic changes such as thickened glomerular and tubular basement membranes and tubular cell swelling and inclusions have been described.

Hypothyroid patients often appear puffy, even edematous, and their total body water and sodium contents are often increased. The causes are accumulation of hydrophilic glycosaminoglycans in extravascular tissue, increased vascular permeability, and decreased lymph flow.[373]

GASTROINTESTINAL SYSTEM

The tongue is often enlarged in hypothyroid patients. Decreased gastric emptying and intestinal motility may result in nausea, vomiting, abdominal distention, and constipation, especially the last. Hypomotility may be so severe as to produce ileus or megacolon, with the clinical picture of intestinal obstruction.[374] Liver size and function are usually normal; enzyme levels may be elevated, possibly in part be due to reduced hepatic enzyme clearance (as mentioned previously). The gallbladder may be dilated and empty poorly. Ascites is occasionally present, rarely as an early manifestation. Its presence is probably due to abnormal capillary permeability and reduced lymph flow.

Malabsorption of various nutrients may occur. Gastric atrophy and achlorhydria are common, and may be associated with vitamin B_{12} malabsorption. About 25 percent of patients with chronic autoimmune thyroiditis have antiparietal cell antibodies. Defects in acid secretion and vitamin B_{12} malabsorption are more frequent in patients with this type of hypothyroidism, some of whom have or develop pernicious anemia.

INTERMEDIARY METABOLISM

The decrease in energy expenditure and oxygen consumption in hypothyroidism is accompanied by decreased utilization of a variety of substrates. The result is decreased heat production, probably the major cause of cold intolerance so characteristic of hypothyroidism. Decreased metabolic activity and substrate utilization, as well as physical inactivity and mental depression, also result in decreased appetite and food intake. Body weight may increase modestly, but rarely increases markedly. When weight gain does occur, it is as much due to retention of salt and water in interstitial tissue as to fat deposition.

Patients with hypothyroidism have relatively normal carbohydrate tolerance, although glucose absorption may be delayed. Blood glucose concentrations do not fall excessively in the postabsorptive state and hepatic glycogen stores are normal. Overall glucose utilization is normal. Insulin responses to oral glucose are appropriate for the rise in glucose that occurs. Glucose administered intravenously is used more slowly than normal, because of decreased insulin secretion. In insulin-dependent diabetic patients, exogenous insulin degradation is slower than normal, so sensitivity to exogenous insulin may increase.

Synthesis of secreted, functional, and structural proteins in many tissues is impaired, most obviously in children (see Hypothyroidism in Newborn Infants and Children, below). Protein catabolism also is impaired. For several proteins, such as lipoproteins and albumin, degradation is impaired more than snythesis; thus increased quantities of the proteins are found. Since blood volume is reduced and plasma albumin concentrations are normal, the excess albumin is largely in the interstitial space.

Plasma fasting free fatty acid concentrations are low, while cholesterol and, less often, triglyceride concentrations are elevated.[375] Very low density lipoprotein production is decreased, but so is their conversion to LDL, since muscle, adipose tissue, and, probably, hepatic lipase activities are decreased. The increased concentrations of LDL cholesterol and its apoprotein B constituent primarily reflect decreased degradation. High-density lipoprotein cholesterol concentrations are unchanged or slightly decreased. Carotene also is transported by LDLs; thus, carotenemia may occur.

HEMATOPOIETIC SYSTEM

Mild anemia is found in about 25 percent of patients with hypothyroidism; reduced red cell mass occurs even more frequently.[210] The anemia may be normocytic, microcytic, or macrocytic. The hemoglobin concentration is rarely less than 10 g/dl. Serum erythropoietin level is normal or low. Serum iron concentration, iron-binding capacity, and vitamin B_{12} and folate concentrations usually are normal. The bone marrow is hypocellular. Kinetic studies indicate slowed iron clearance and incorporation. These findings are the anticipated adaptations to reduced peripheral oxygen needs; therefore, the reduced red cell mass may not reflect the presence of anemia. Occasionally, iron, folic acid, or vitamin B_{12} deficiency anemia with the appropriate peripheral blood and bone marrow findings may be present. Iron deficiency may result from excessive menstrual bleeding and/or poor iron absorption secondary to decreased gastric acid production. Megaloblastic anemia may be due to hypothyroidism-induced folic acid or vitamin B_{12} malabsorption, or to pernicious anemia in patients with chronic autoimmune thyroiditis.

Patients with hypothyroidism may bruise easily.[220] Bleeding time may be prolonged, platelet aggregation abnormal, and factor VIII antigen, factor VIII coagulant, and ristocetin cofactor activities may be decreased;[223,374] however, the coagulation factor abnormalities do not correlate well with bleeding time abnormalities.

ENDOCRINE SYSTEM

Hypothyroidism results in changes in the dynamics of several other endocrine systems. Rates of hormone degradation are decreased, resulting in compensatory reduction in the rate of hormone secretion; thus, plasma hormone concentrations usually are normal. In some patients, however, hypothyroidism causes clinically significant abnormalities in the function of other endocrine organs.

Pituitary Function

Growth hormone secretion is usually reduced in response to a variety of provocative stimuli, such as GH-releasing hormone, hypoglycemia, and arginine infusion. Curiously, GH secretion may increase in response to exogenous TRH. Little is known about physiological GH secretion. Serum somatomedin levels are low, and increase normally in response to exogenous GH.[376] These data suggest that hypothyroid patients have decreases in 24-h GH secretion sufficient to decrease somatomedin production. This would explain the short stature in hypothyroid children. Basal serum prolactin concentrations in most hypothyroid patients are within the normal range or slightly elevated,[377] although they may be as high as 200 ng/ml. Hyperprolactinemia is most likely to occur in patients with chronic hypothyroidism, and may result in amenorrhea-galactorrhea as it does in other hyperprolactinemic patients. Prolactin responses to TRH are augmented, but to a much smaller extent than are TSH responses to TRH.[233]

The various abnormalities of pituitary hormone secretion described above are functional abnormalities, and are reversed by treatment of hypothyroidism. Trophic hormone deficiencies may also occur as a result of hypothalamic or pituitary diseases that cause hypothyroidism.

Adrenal Function

Cortisol production is decreased,[378] because cortisol degradation is slowed as a result of decreased hepatic steroid catabolism. Therefore, excretion of urinary steroid metabolites falls. Plasma cortisol concentrations and urinary cortisol excretion are normal. Pituitary-adrenal responses to metyrapone, hypoglycemia, and ACTH are normal in most patients. Plasma cortisol levels increase normally in hypothyroid patients with other illnesses.[379,380]

Hypothyroidism due to chronic autoimmune thyroiditis and adrenal insufficiency due to autoimmune adrenalitis may occur in the same patient (autoimmune polyglandular syndromes).[381] Elevated serum TSH concentrations and, sometimes, overt hypothyroidism can occur in patients with adrenal insufficiency due to other causes.[382] Glucocorticoid replacement alone may result in restoration of normal thyroid function, indicating the sensitivity of autoimmune disease mechanisms to glucocorticoids.

Circulating levels and production rates of norepinephrine are increased, whereas those of epinephrine are normal.[41]

Gonadal Function

In hypothyroid women, production of sex hormone–binding globulin is decreased. Thus, serum estradiol concentrations are reduced, but free estradiol concentrations are normal. Estradiol and progesterone secretion and clearance are decreased, the former to a greater extent than the latter. Secretion of FSH and LH are usually in the normal nonovulatory range, though cyclic FSH and LH secretion may be interrupted. The clinical abnormalities that occur are anovulatory and irregular cycles, excessive menstrual bleeding, and occasionally amenorrhea. Infertility is common, but successful pregnancy can occur.[383] In postmenopausal women, serum FSH and LH concentrations may be somewhat lower than expected, and the response to GNRH reduced.[384]

In men, plasma testosterone concentrations may be lowered due to reduced sex hormone–binding globulin production, but serum free testosterone and gonadotropin concentrations are usually normal. Little is known about reproductive capacity, although hypogonadism in patients with long-standing primary hypothyroidism has been described.[385]

Parathyroid-Vitamin D-Bone System

Serum calcium and phosphate concentrations are normal, whereas those of PTH and $1\alpha,25\text{-}(OH)_2D$ may be increased.[239] Calcium absorption is decreased, as is bone resorption, suggesting the presence of some resistance to the actions of PTH and $1\alpha,25\text{-}(OH)_2D$. Further supporting the presence of resistance to the hypercalcemic effects of the calciotropic hormones are reports that recovery from induced hypocalcemia is delayed and primary hyperparathyroidism is ameliorated by hypothyroidism. Calcitonin deficiency also would be expected, because of destruction or removal of thyroid parafollicular cells; recovery from induced hypercalcemia is slowed in hypothyroid patients.

ILLNESS AND SURGERY IN HYPOTHYROID PATIENTS

Serum T_3 concentrations decline in hypothyroid patients as in normal individuals during nonthyroidal illnesses.[121] Serum TSH concentrations do not change during mild nonthyroidal illness, although they may fall during febrile illnesses or when corticosteroids or dopamine are given.[57] Such a change may make it more difficult to diagnose hypothyroidism.

Whether or not the course or outcome of nonthyroidal illness or surgery is altered in patients with hypothyroidism is not known. Some complications of surgery, such as hypotension, cardiac failure, and GI dysfunction, may be more common in hypothyroid patients, but overall morbidity and mortality do not appear to be increased.[386,387] Even so, hypothyroid patients should be given anesthetic, analgesic, and sedative drugs very cautiously, since metabolism of many drugs is prolonged in such patients.

Laboratory Diagnosis of Hypothyroidism

SERUM THYROID HORMONE AND TSH CONCENTRATIONS

Serum total and free T_4 concentrations in most patients with hypothyroidism are decreased. However, serum T_4 concentrations need not be below the normal range in patients with significant hypothyroidism;[338] on the other hand, low serum T_4 concentrations do not invariably indicate that hypothyroidism is present. Serum total T_4 concentrations may be reduced as a result of decreased production of TBG or by agents, such as salicylate, which competitively inhibit the T_4-TBG interaction. When T_4-TBG interaction is blocked, T_3-resin uptake tests indicate decreased numbers of unoccupied T_4 binding sites; therefore serum free T_4 concentrations and free T_4 index values are normal. Decreased serum total T_4, and sometimes free T_4, concentrations also occur in patients who are seriously ill as a result of nonthyroidal illnesses (see Nonthyroidal Illness).

Since most of the T_3 in serum is produced as a result of extrathyroidal deiodination of T_4, serum T_3 concentrations are usually low in patients with hypothyroidism. However, serum T_3 measurement is neither a specific nor a sensitive test for hypothyroidism. About 20 to 30 percent of patients with hypothyroidism and low serum T_4 concentrations have a normal serum T_3 concentration, due both to TSH-induced stimulation of thyroidal T_3 biosynthesis and thyroidal T_4 5′-deiodinase activity and an increased fractional conversion of T_4 to T_3 in the periphery.[13,338,388] Conversely, as discussed previously, serum T_3 concentrations are below normal in patients with a wide variety of nonthyroidal illnesses and those who are euthyroid and have normal serum T_4 and TSH concentrations but are receiving various drugs (see Nonthyroidal Illness).

Measurement of the serum TSH concentration is an indispensable test for the recognition of primary hypothyroidism and differentiation of primary from hypothyrotropic hypothyroidism, whether due to pituitary or hypothalamic disease. Serum TSH concentrations are elevated in all patients with overt primary hypothyroidism. They also are increased in many patients with chronic autoimmune thyroiditis or after subtotal thyroidectomy or ^{131}I therapy, even though such patients are clinically euthyroid and their serum T_4 and T_3 concentrations are not below the normal range.[274,322,338] Such a finding does not indicate imminent overt thyroid failure; such patients may remain clinically euthyroid for months or years. The elevated TSH concentrations in hypothyroid patients are due primarily to increased TSH secretion, although TSH clearance also is decreased.

In contrast, serum TSH concentrations are normal or undetectable in most patients whose hypothyroidism is due to pituitary or hypothalamic disease. Measurement of the serum TSH concentration, therefore, is not only an exquisitely sensitive test for the recognition of primary hypothyroidism, but also may be the first indication that hypothyroidism in an individual patient is due to pituitary or hypothalamic disease, thus indicating the need for neuroradiological studies and tests of pituitary function. Moreover, even if the patient has manifestations of pituitary disease or enlargement, such as hyperprolactinemia, sellar enlargement, or even visual impairment, the serum TSH concentration must be determined, since all of those findings may result from primary hypothyroidism and improve with T_4 therapy alone.[339,340] Serum TSH concentrations also are normal or undetectable in patients with severe nonthyroidal illnesses who have low serum total and free T_4 concentrations;[118,119] TSH measurements therefore cannot be used to differentiate between organic hypothalamic or pituitary disease and illness-related decreases in serum TSH concentrations.

The characteristic patterns of change in serum TSH level after administration of TRH in hypothyroid patients are shown in Fig. 10-26. Patients with primary hypothyroidism have augmented responses, but the test provides no additional information of value in a patient who has an elevated basal serum TSH level. The response also may be augmented in patients with very mild thyroid disease whose basal serum TSH concentrations are normal,[389] but such patients are clinically euthyroid. Characteristically, serum TSH concentrations fail to rise after TRH administration in

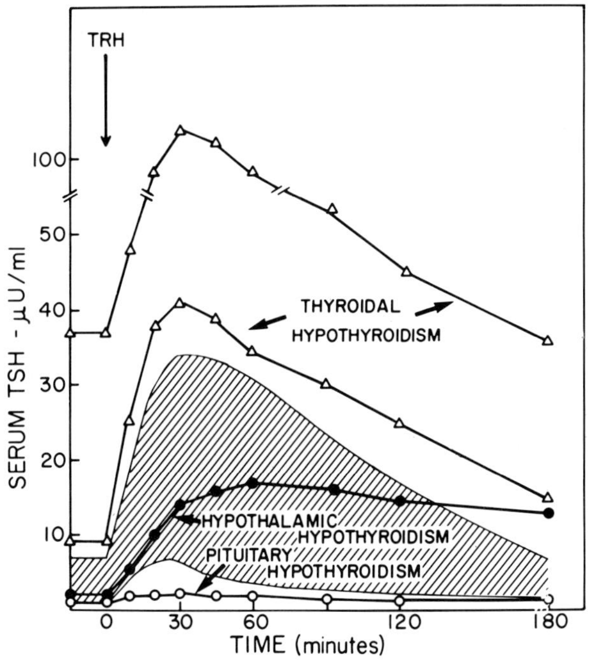

FIGURE 10-26 Serum TSH responses (in μU/ml) to TRH in various forms of hypothyroidism. Shaded area shows the range of responses in normal subjects.

patients with pituitary hypothyroidism. The significance of this finding is limited by the fact that TSH responses to TRH are below normal in many euthyroid patients with pituitary disease and many patients with nonthyroidal illnesses.[70,119] Responses that are normal in magnitude but are delayed are considered characteristic of hypothalamic hypothyroidism, but similar responses occur in patients with overt pituitary disease.[390] Thus, TRH stimulation tests do not reliably distinguish among patients with pituitary hypothyroidism, hypothalamic hypothyroidism, and severe nonthyroidal illness.

SUMMARY: DIAGNOSIS OF HYPOTHYROIDISM

A scheme for the evaluation of patients with clinically suspected hypothyroidism is shown in Fig. 10-27. The initial step should be measurements of the serum total T_4 concentration, T_3-resin uptake or serum free T_4 concentration, and serum TSH concentration. These procedures should confirm the diagnosis of hypothyroidism and establish its origin, though not its cause, in most patients who are otherwise reasonably healthy. Hypothyrotropic hypothyroidism and nonthyroidal illness (adaptive hypothyroidism) cannot be reliably differentiated as the cause of low serum total and free T_4 concentrations at a single point in time (see Nonthyroidal Illness, above). The distinction in such patients must be based on the presence or absence of symptoms and signs of hypothyroidism and hypothalamic or pituitary disease, results of T_3-resin uptake tests (uptake is low in patients with hypothyroidism and normal or high in those with nonthyroidal illnesses), and knowledge that hypothyrotropic hypothyroidism is rare.

OTHER LABORATORY PROCEDURES

Serum rT_3 concentrations are low in hypothyroid patients. Serum thyroglobulin concentrations are usually

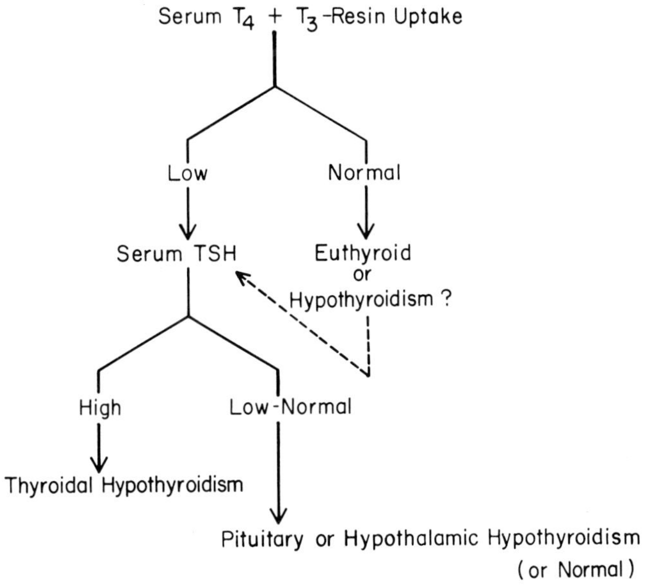

FIGURE 10-27 Diagnostic scheme for evaluation of patients with suspected hypothyroidism.

low, but may be elevated in patients with goitrous hypothyroidism; they may be artifactually high due to the presence of antithyroglobulin antibodies. The presence of antithyroglobulin or other thyroid autoantibodies indicates that autoimmune thyroiditis exists, but provides no information about thyroid secretion. Thyroidal radioiodine uptake is reduced in most patients with hypothyroidism, though normal or even high values may be found in patients with chronic autoimmune thyroiditis, iodide deficiency, and most inherited defects of thyroid hormone biosynthesis. Conversely, excess iodide intake, such as from drugs or radiographic contrast agents, reduces thyroidal radioiodine uptake to very low levels in normal subjects.

Measurements of radioiodine uptake or serum T_4 concentrations before and after the administration of exogenous TSH formerly were used to distinguish primary hypothyroidism (where there is no increase in ^{131}I uptake or serum T_4 concentration) from hypothyrotropic hypothyroidism (where there is an increase), but TSH assay has rendered the TSH stimulation test obsolete. More detailed information concerning intrathyroidal iodine metabolism can be obtained by measurements of thyroidal iodine turnover and retention or discharge of radioiodine after perchlorate administration.

Hypothyroidism is accompanied by a variety of biochemical and other changes which reflect decreased tissue actions of thyroid hormones. Basal metabolic rate is reduced. Achilles reflex half-relaxation time is prolonged. Serum concentrations of various enzymes, cholesterol, triglycerides, and carotene are frequently elevated, and serum angiotension-converting enzyme activity may be reduced. All of these findings, when encountered unexpectedly, may suggest the presence of hypothyroidism, but such measurements should not be used to confirm the diagnosis.

Treatment of Hypothyroidism

Treatment of hypothyroidism is simple and effective. Occasionally, all that is required is discontinuation of iodide, lithium, or some other medication. Consideration also should be given to the possibility that hypothyroidism is transient (see Causes of Hypothyroidism, above). For most patients, thyroxine administration is the appropriate treatment. Usually, lifelong treatment is required. The general principle is simple: to restore and maintain the euthyroid state. Besides prescription of medication, patients must be educated concerning the need for lifelong treatment and for periodic follow-up to evaluate the response to therapy, to confirm compliance, and to reinforce the need for therapy.

The initial dosage of thyroxine should be 0.1 to 0.15 mg per day orally in those patients who are young or otherwise healthy, or whose hypothyroidism is of short duration. For elderly patients or those with cardiac disease, the initial dosage should be less, 0.025 to 0.05 mg per day, because of the small risk of precipitation of angina, cardiac arrhythmia, or cardiac failure. Increases in pulse rate, serum enzyme concentrations, diuresis, and subjective feeling of well-being occur within 1 to 2 weeks, depending on the dosage. An appropriate time for the first follow-up visit is after 4 to 6 weeks. The dosage should not be increased sooner, because this amount of time is needed for complete expression of a given oral dose of T_4. Most symptoms and signs disappear within several months, although some abnormalities, such as anemia and abnormal GH and prolactin secretion, may persist for 4 to 6 months. There is a linear relationship between responses to T_4 and estimations of nuclear T_3 receptor occupancy.[391]

Adequate replacement in most patients requires 0.1 to 0.15 mg of T_4 daily; occasionally, larger doses are required (Fig. 10-28). Once-daily T_4 doses do not result in between-dose fluctuations in serum T_4, T_3, or TSH concentrations.[392] There is some evidence that elderly patients require less T_4, perhaps because their clearance of T_4 is decreased.[393] Some patients with hypothyroidism following ablative therapy for Graves' hyperthyroidism also may require less T_4 because their remaining thyroid tissue continues to secrete T_4, due to continued TSab production. T_4 also can be given in a single weekly dose of 1.5 to 2 mg.[394] From 40 to 70 percent of T_4 given orally is absorbed; absorption may be reduced in patients with various intestinal disorders,[395] so that larger doses may be required. Slightly larger doses may also be needed in patients receiving phenytoin[396] and in the winter in patients living in temperate zones.[86] There may be small variations in the potency or bioavailability of different T_4 preparations,[397] but the variations are so small that they are rarely of clinical importance. Very rarely, cutaneous allergy to T_4 associated with IgE anti-T_4 antibody occurs.[398]

Patients receiving prolonged therapy should be seen at 6-month intervals. Assessment of the adequacy of therapy should be based primarily on the clinical response, that is, the absence of symptoms and signs of hypothyroidism; small dosage adjustments may be made on this basis alone. In most patients who are clinically euthyroid while receiving T_4, serum T_4 and T_3 concentrations are within the normal range. However, since the range of serum T_4 concentrations in normal individuals is wide, restoration of serum T_4 concentrations merely to within the normal range may not be sufficient. An elevated serum TSH con-

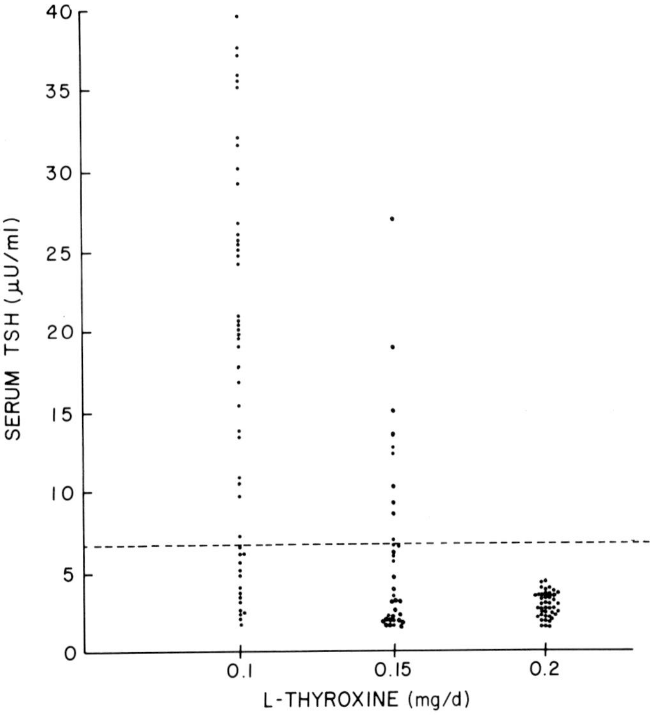

	0.1	0.15	0.2
Serum T_4 (μg/dl)	6.4	9.1	11.0
Serum T_3 (ng/dl)	79	111	123

FIGURE 10-28 Serum TSH concentrations in hypothyroid patients receiving prolonged treatment with 0.1, 0.15, and 0.2 mg of T_4 daily. Mean serum T_4 and T_3 concentrations shown at bottom.

centration is good evidence that therapy is inadequate. However, serum TSH measurements currently cannot be used to recognize excessive treatment, since some normal individuals have undetectable serum TSH concentrations. Some patients may feel best when their serum TSH concentrations are slightly increased, while others feel best when their serum T_4 concentrations are slightly high. From a practical point of view, therefore, dosage adjustments should not be made on the basis of test results alone.

A patient who cannot take T_4 orally, for example because of illness or surgery, need not be given parenteral T_4 for 5 to 7 days. If parenteral T_4 is given, the dose should be half of the usual oral dose, given intramuscularly or intravenously.

Controversy exists as to whether or not patients with subclinical hypothyroidism should be treated. By definition, such patients have no symptoms or signs of hypothyroidism and their serum T_4 concentrations are normal. Treatment may be warranted to reduce thyroid enlargement, if present,[399] or because of the presence of vague symptoms, although such symptoms also respond to placebo therapy. Treatment is not necessary merely to forestall the development of overt hypothyroidism, because progression to overt disease is often slow.[274,323]

Other thyroid hormone preparations are available for the treatment of hypothyroidism. They are T_3, combinations of T_4 and T_3, desiccated thyroid, and thyroglobulin. Serum T_3 concentrations fluctuate widely in patients treated with T_3, while serum T_4 concentrations remain low;[392] similar, but less marked, changes occur in patients receiving the other preparations. Serum T_4 measurements lead to underestimation of the efficacy of the dose that the patient is taking; hence patients taking T_3 or preparations containing it often are overtreated. These preparations therefore have important disadvantages, and no advantages, in comparison to T_4.

Special Clinical Situations

THYROID HORMONE WITHDRAWAL

Patients receiving thyroid hormone therapy may be encountered in whom the need for the treatment is questioned, either by the patient or the physician, and for whom either adequate documentation of hypothyroidism is unavailable or the hypothyroidism was transient. There is no simple way to establish the presence of hypothyroidism while thyroid therapy continues. The best course is to discontinue the therapy. The pituitary-thyroid axis, like any feedback-regulated endocrine system, will have been inhibited by the exogenous thyroid therapy. Normal individuals recover pituitary and thyroid function within 1 month after thyroid withdrawal, though they may have transient symptoms of hypothyroidism and subnormal serum T_4 concentrations for a few weeks after thyroid withdrawal.[330,331] In contrast, within 1 month virtually all hypothyroid patients develop symptoms and unequivocal laboratory evidence of hypothyroidism.

HYPOTHYROIDISM IN NEWBORN INFANTS AND CHILDREN

Hypothyroidism in the neonate may result in respiratory difficulty, cyanosis, persistent jaundice, umbilical hernia, lethargy, somnolence, poor feeding, hoarse crying, constipation, or the presence of large anterior or open posterior fontanels. However, severe biochemical hypothyroidism can be present in neonates who appear normal.[79,400] Because hypothyroidism during the first months of life results in irreversible mental and physical retardation, screening for it in newborns is now widespread. Screening usually employs measurements of the T_4 concentration in blood collected on filter paper in the first days of life. Permanent hypothyroidism is found in one of every 3500 to 4000 infants, and transient hypothyroidism, TBG deficiency, and illness-related abnormalities also can be identified.[400] Properly run screening programs miss few infants later found to have hypothyroidism in the first year or so of life, indicating that hypothyroidism rarely develops within this period. Infants identified by screening programs who are treated promptly develop and grow normally.

When hypothyroidism develops later in infancy or childhood, little permanent mental or physical retardation results. These older children have some form of acquired hypothyroidism, usually chronic autoimmune thyroiditis, and had normal thyroid secretion in the first year or so of life. They have symptoms of hypothyroidism similar to those in adults, as well as impaired skeletal growth and development, delayed epiphyseal maturation, and delayed dental development. The age of onset of hypothyroidism may be dated by determining, from school or other records, when growth slowed and by noting the appearance of the epiphyses; those formed before its onset are normal whereas those appearing after its onset are delayed or abnormal in appearance (epiphyseal stippling). Sexual maturation in some children is accelerated, serum gonadotropin concentrations being increased in relation to maturational, if not chronologic, age.[401] Overt sexual precocity has been described in both sexes; in some girls lactation occurs. In other children, however, sexual maturation is delayed, due to decreased gonadotropin secretion.

Hypothyroid infants and children also should be treated with T_4, but with the recognition that inadequate treatment is more hazardous in these patients since it may result in some impairment of mental and physical growth even in the absence of symptoms of hypothyroidism. The T_4 degradation rate is about 50 percent greater in children than in adults. Thus, on a weight basis, T_4 dosage should be relatively higher. Doses of 0.05 to 0.1 mg of T_4 daily are usually adequate in young infants; older children should receive 0.1 to 0.15 mg of T_4 daily. Despite the more rapid turnover of T_4 in children, these doses often result in some degree of hyperthyroidism, but are justifiable in view of the hazards of insufficient treatment. Thus, serum T_4 concentrations should be maintained in the upper normal range. Higher serum T_4 concentrations may be required to reduce serum TSH concentrations to within the normal range in children, probably because they have somewhat higher serum TBG levels than do adults.[81] Transient pseudotumor cerebri may occur following initiation of T_4 therapy in children.[402]

MYXEDEMA COMA

The development of coma in a patient with primary or hypothyrotropic hypothyroidism is a life-threatening emergency. Coma may develop spontaneously, as a result of severe prolonged hypothyroidism. The onset characteristically is gradual. It occurs more often in elderly patients, especially in the winter.[403] Progressive respiratory center depression and decreases in cardiac output and cerebral blood flow combine to result in cerebral hypoxia. Myxedema coma also may be precipitated by cold exposure, infection, respiratory disease, and inappropriate administration of narcotics and analgesics. Patients with myxedema coma usually have overt hypothyroidism. In addition to progressive stupor and coma, they may have seizures, hyponatremia, hypotension, hypoglycemia, and hypoventilation with hypercapnia and respiratory acidosis. Hypothermia is usually present; it is due to severely depressed metabolism and may precede the development of coma. Severity of hypothermia may be overlooked or underestimated because improperly prepared or calibrated thermometers do not register more than 1 to 2° below normal. Addition of any situation whereby heat loss is accelerated hastens the development of hypothermia in these patients. Hypoventilation may reflect the presence of respiratory muscle weakness, upper airway obstruction from the large tongue, or impairment in respiratory center function. Hyponatremia and water intoxication may be due to excessive vasopressin secretion and/or a direct renal effect of thyroid hormone deficiency. Hypoglycemia suggests that accompanying cortisol deficiency is present, but it may also result because gluconeogenesis is impaired by severe hypothyroidism per se.

Myxedema coma requires aggressive therapy both in terms of T_4 administration and ancillary measures. If myxedema coma is suspected, blood for T_4, TSH, and cortisol determinations should be obtained and therapy initiated immediately. While administration of large doses of thyroid hormone can be hazardous, the mortality risk of myxedema coma is such that aggressive therapy is justified. Thyroxine, in doses of 0.3 to 0.4 mg followed by 0.1 mg daily, should be given IV, as poor gastrointestinal function and peripheral circulation probably limit the availability of T_4 given orally or intramuscularly. Such a large dose should rapidly restore the serum T_4 concentration to normal; thus, substantial quantities of unbound T_4 should be available to the tissues.[404] With the use of large doses of T_4, improvements in pulse rate, blood pressure, temperature, and mental status occur within 24 h. Use of T_3 has been advocated, because (1) it acts more rapidly and (2) extrathyroidal T_3 production from T_4 is decreased in such seriously ill patients.[405] However, preparations of T_3 for parenteral use are not available, and there is some evidence that rapid increases in serum T_3 concentrations are more likely to lead to death.[406]

Cortisol should be given IV, since the patient may have concomitant ACTH or adrenal deficiency or impaired ACTH or adrenal responses to stress as a result of severe primary hypothyroidism. However, appropriate serum cortisol elevations occur in most hypothermic hypothyroid patients.[380] Supportive therapy is as important as hormonal treatment; indeed, it may be more important, as the patient may waken from coma without thyroid therapy. Ventilatory assistance may be required. Infection should be sought and appropriate therapy given. Fluid replacement may be needed, but should be given cautiously, as insensible fluid loss is decreased and water loads are excreted poorly. Water intoxication and hyponatremia, if present, should be treated by fluid restriction, but hypertonic saline is occasionally required. Further heat loss should be prevented by adequate covering; active rewarming is unwise since it may result in vasodilation and vascular collapse. A substantial proportion of patients thus treated recover.

THE PAINFUL THYROID

The thyroid is an encapsulated organ. Therefore, acute thyroid enlargement results in pain and tenderness. The pain may be confined to the thyroid region or referred to the ear, throat, jaws, or lateral neck regions. Thyroid diseases that cause these findings characteristically develop rapidly. They include subacute thyroiditis, hemorrhage into a thyroid nodule, radiation thyroiditis, and acute (suppurative) thyroiditis. Patients with many other thyroid diseases, such as Graves' disease, chronic autoimmune thyroiditis, and thyroid carcinoma, occasionally complain of discomfort in the thyroid region and have some thyroid tenderness. However, in such patients thyroid pain and tenderness are usually mild. Their illnesses (and thyroid enlargement) do not develop rapidly, and manifestations of thyroid dysfunction or a mass lesion, rather than inflammation, predominate. A variety of nonthyroid diseases, such as musculoskeletal disorders, pharyngeal and laryngeal inflammatory diseases, and globus hystericus, also cause neck pain and/or tenderness, but these disorders do not cause localized thyroid tenderness or thyroid enlargement.

Subacute Thyroiditis

Subacute thyroiditis (also known as granulomatous thyroiditis, de Quervain's thyroiditis, and nonsuppurative thyroiditis) is the most common cause of thyroid pain and tenderness. Its onset is usually abrupt, and is accompanied by malaise, myalgias, fatigue, and fever in most patients. A history of preceding upper respiratory infection is common.[186,407] The pain typically radiates to the upper neck, ears, throat, or jaws. The thyroid is nearly always moderately enlarged; although commonly diffuse, the enlargement, as well as pain and tenderness, may be confined to one thyroid lobe or shift from one lobe to another during the course of the illness. The thyroid is usually firm in consistency, and may even be quite hard. Cervical lymphadenopathy is rare. Clinical manifestations of hyperthyroidism occur in approximately 50 percent of patients with subacute thyroiditis although the frequency of biochemical hyperthyroidism approaches 100 percent.[186] The course of the illness is variable. In most patients it subsides within 2 to 6 weeks, but neck pain and tenderness and thyroid enlargement may persist or recur. Transient hypothyroidism may develop following extensive damage from the inflammatory process, but permanent hypothyroidism is rare.[187]

Considerable indirect evidence suggests that subacute thyroiditis is a viral illness, but conclusive proof is lacking. The disease has been associated with mumps, influenza, adenovirus, and other viral infections, and significant changes in titers of several antiviral antibodies have been found in many patients.[408] The seroconversions are probably anamnestic responses rather than responses to specific infection; no viruses have been isolated from thyroid tissue. An association with the HLA-B35 haplotype has been reported;[409] genetic predisposition may thus be a factor in the development of the disease.

Pathologically, the disease is characterized by disruption of thyroid follicles with polymorphonuclear or mononuclear cell infiltration, giant cell infiltration, microabscess formation, and fibrosis. This process results in unregulated and excessive thyroglobulin proteolysis and, therefore, increased serum T_4, T_3, thyroglobulin, and iodide concentrations and increased urinary iodide excretion. Thyroid radioiodine uptake is characteristically low early in the illness; this is due to the follicular damage, decreased TSH secretion, and increased serum iodide concentrations. Other common laboratory findings are mild anemia and an elevated erythrocyte sedimentation rate; leukocytosis is uncommon. Some patients have antithyroglobulin or other antithyroid antibodies transiently, but subacute thyroiditis does not result in persistent autoimmunization.

Both the inflammatory and hyperthyroid components of subacute thyroiditis may be so mild and transient that no therapy is necessary. More often, thyroid pain and tenderness result in sufficient discomfort to warrant anti-inflammatory therapy. Salicylates, in doses of 2.4 to 3.6 g per day, usually provide effective relief. Those patients with severe thyroid pain and tenderness, or those who do not improve rapidly with salicylates, may be treated effectively with prednisone in doses of 30 to 40 mg per day. Treatment should be continued for 2 to 3 weeks and then withdrawn gradually to minimize the likelihood of recurrence. Adequate anti-inflammatory therapy not only relieves the symptoms of subacute thyroiditis, but also probably reduces thyroid hormone release, thus accelerating recovery from hyperthyroidism. The latter usually requires no therapy, but propranolol, in doses of 20 to 40 mg given 3 or 4 times daily, may be used if clinically indicated. Hypothyroidism occurring during the recovery phase is usually mild and transient, and rarely requires therapy.

Hemorrhage in a Thyroid Nodule

The sudden development of pain, tenderness, and a localized thyroid mass is indicative of hemorrhage into a thyroid nodule. The nodule may or may not have been recognized previously. The distinction between this process and subacute thyroiditis may be difficult. The diagnosis of hemorrhage is supported by signs localized in the region of a nodule and by lack of systemic manifestations of inflammatory disease and hyperthyroidism. However, transient hyperthyroidism accompanying hemorrhagic infarction of a thyroid nodule has been reported.[410] A thyroid scan shows little isotope uptake in the region of the painful nodule, but normal uptake elsewhere. The pain and swelling may subside spontaneously, or require needle aspiration.

Radiation Thyroiditis

Clinically significant thyroiditis, with or without exacerbation of hyperthyroidism, is an occasional complication of ^{131}I therapy for hyperthyroidism. It develops 1 to 2 weeks after therapy and then subsides spontaneously.

Suppurative Thyroiditis

Bacterial or fungal infections of the thyroid are very rare. Routes of entry of organisms into the thyroid include blood vessels, a persistent thyroglossal duct, a fistula from the pyriform sinus, and direct trauma.[407,411] The thyroidal infection may develop abruptly or gradually, depending on the organism. Thyroidal involvement usually is asymmetric. Staphylococcal, streptococcal, or anaerobic organisms are usually the cause, but mycobacteria, other bacteria, or fungi may be found. In patients without evidence of systemic infection, a thyroglossal duct or pyriform sinus fistula should be sought.

REFERENCES

1. Hegedus L, Perrild H, Poulsen LR, Andersen JR, Holm J, Schnohr P, Jensen G, Hansen JM: The determination of thyroid volume by ultrasound and its relationship to body weight, age and sex in normal subjects. *J Clin Endocrinol Metab* 56:260, 1983.
2. Melnick JC, Stemkowski PE: Thyroid hemiagenesis (hockey stick sign): A review of the world literature and a report of four cases. *J Clin Endocrinol Metab* 52:247, 1981.
3. Melander A, Ljunggren J-C, Norberg K-A, Persson B, Rosengren E, Sundler S, Tibblin S, Westgren U: Sympathetic innervation and noradrenaline content of normal human thyroid tissue from fetal, young, and elderly subjects. *J Endocrinol Invest* 2:175, 1978.
4. Toccafondi RS, Brandi ML, Melander A: Vasoactive intestinal peptide stimulation of human thyroid cell function. *J Clin Endocrinol Metab* 58:157, 1984.
5. Oddie TH, Fisher DA, McConahey WM, Thompson CS: Iodine intake in the United States: A reassessment. *J Clin Endocrinol Metab* 30:659, 1970.
6. Wolff J: Congenital goiter with defective iodide transport. *Endocr Rev* 4:241, 1983.
7. Ingbar SH: Effects of iodine: Autoregulation of the thyroid, in

Werner SC, Ingbar SH (eds): *The Thyroid: A Fundamental and Clinical Text.* Hagerstown, Md., Harper & Row, 1978, p 206.

8. Lever EG, Medeiros-Neto GA, DeGroot LJ: Inherited disorders of thyroid metabolism. *Endocr Rev* 4:213, 1983.

9. Sugawara M: Coupling of iodotyrosine catalyzed by human thyroid peroxidase in vitro. *J Clin Endocrinol Metab* 60:1069, 1985.

10. Van Herle AJ, Vassart G, Dumont JE: Control of thyroglobulin synthesis and secretion. *N Engl J Med* 301:239, 1979.

11. Eggo MC, Burrow GN: Glycosylation of thyroglobulin: Its role in secretion, iodination, and stability. *Endocrinology* 113:1655, 1983.

12. Lissitzky S: Thyroglobulin entering into molecular biology. *J Endocrinol Invest* 7:65, 1984.

13. Laurberg P: Mechanisms governing the relative proportions of thyroxine and 3,5,3′-triiodothyronine in thyroid secretion. *Metabolism* 33:379, 1984.

14. Engler D, Burger AG: The deiodination of the iodothyronines and of their derivatives in man. *Endocr Rev* 5:151, 1984.

15. Kaplan MM, Utiger RD: Iodothyronine metabolism in rat liver homogenates. *J Clin Invest* 61:459, 1978.

16. Visser TJ, Leonard JL, Kaplan MM, Larsen PR: Kinetic evidence suggesting two mechanisms for iodothyronine 5′-deiodination in rat cerebral cortex. *Proc Natl Acad Sci USA* 79:5080, 1982.

17. Visser TJ, Kaplan MM, Leonard JL, Larsen PR: Evidence for two pathways of iodothyronine 5′-deiodination in rat pituitary that differ in kinetics, propylthiouracil sensitivity, and response to hypothyroidism. *J Clin Invest* 71:992, 1983.

18. Kaplan MM: The role of thyroid hormone deiodination in the regulation of hypothalamo-pituitary function. *Neuroendocrinology* 38:254, 1984.

19. Roti E, Fang SL, Green K, Emerson CH, Braverman LE: Human placenta is an active site of thyroxine and 3,3′,5-triiodothyronine tyrosyl ring deiodination. *J Clin Endocrinol Metab* 53:498, 1981.

20. Chopra IJ: A radioimmunoassay for measurement of 3′-monoiodothyronine. *J Clin Endocrinol Metab* 51:117, 1980.

21. Corcoran JM, Eastman CJ: Radioimmunoassay of 3-L-monoiodothyronine: Application in normal human physiology and thyroid disease. *J Clin Endocrinol Metab* 57:66, 1983.

22. Pardridge WM: Transport of protein-bound hormones into tissues in vivo. *Endocr Rev* 2:103, 1981.

23. Robbins J, Cheng S-Y, Gershengorn MC, Glinoer D, Cahnmann HJ, Edelhoch H: Thyroxine transport proteins of plasma: Molecular properties and biosynthesis. *Recent Prog Horm Res* 34:477, 1978.

24. Grimaldi S, Bartalena L, Ramacciotti C, Robbins J: Polymorphism of human thyroxine-binding globulin. *J Clin Endocrinol Metab* 57:1186, 1983.

25. Yabu Y, Amir SM, Ruiz M, Braverman LE, Ingbar SH: Heterogeneity of thyroxine binding by serum albumins in normal subjects and patients with familial dysalbuminemic hyperthyroxinemia. *J Clin Endocrinol Metab* 60:451, 1985.

26. Krenning EP, Docter R, Visser TJ, Hennemann G: Plasma membrane transport of thyroid hormone: Its possible pathophysiological significance. *J Endocrinol Invest* 6:59, 1983.

27. Larsen PR, Silva JE, Kaplan MM: Relationships between circulating and intracellular thyroid hormones: Physiological and clinical implications. *Endocr Rev* 2:87, 1981.

28. Van Doorn J, Van Der Heide D, Roelfsema F: Sources and quantity of 3,5,3′-triiodothyronine in several tissues of the rat. *J Clin Invest* 72:1778, 1983.

29. Oppenheimer JH: Thyroid hormone action at the nuclear level. *Ann Intern Med* 102:374, 1985.

30. Apriletti J, David-Inouye Y, Baxter JD, Eberhardt NL: Physicochemical characterization of the intranuclear thyroid hormone receptor, in Oppenheimer JH, Samuels HH (eds): *Molecular Basis of Thyroid Hormone Action.* New York, Academic Press, 1983, p 67.

31. Oppenheimer JH, Dillmann WH, Schwartz HL, Towle HC: Nuclear receptors and thyroid hormone action: A progress report. *Fed Proc* 38:2154, 1979.

32. Schuster LD, Schwartz HL, Oppenheimer JH: Nuclear receptors for 3,5,3′-triiodothyronine in human liver and kidney: Characterization, quantitation, and similarities to rat receptors. *J Clin Endocrinol Metab* 48:627, 1979.

33. Wiersinga WM, Frank HJL, Chopra IJ, Solomon DH: Alterations in hepatic nuclear binding of triiodothyronine in experimental diabetes mellitus in rats. *Acta Endocrinol* 99:79, 1982.

34. Lim VS, Passo C, Murata Y, Ferrari E, Nakamura H, Refetoff S: Reduced triiodothyronine content in liver but not pituitary of the uremic rat model: Demonstration of changes compatible with thyroid hormone deficiency in liver only. *Endocrinology* 114:280, 1984.

35. Grajower MM, Surks MI: Effect of decreased hepatic nuclear L-triiodothyronine receptors on the response of hepatic enzymes to L-triiodothyronine in tumor-bearing rats. *Endocrinology* 104:697, 1979.

36. Eberhardt NL, Apriletti JW, Baxter JD: The molecular biology of thyroid hormone action, in Litwack G (ed): *The Biochemical Actions of Hormones.* New York, Academic Press, 1980, vol 7, p 311.

37. Segal J, Ingbar SH: Plasma membrane-mediated effects of thyroid hormones, in Cumming IA, Funder JW, Mendelsohn FAO (eds): *Endocrinology 1980.* New York, Elsevier/North-Holland, 1980, p 405.

38. Leonard JL, Silva JE, Kaplan MM, Mellen SA, Visser TJ, Larsen PR: Acute posttranscriptional regulation of cerebrocortical and pituitary iodothyronine 5′-deiodinases by thyroid hormone. *Endocrinology* 114:998, 1984.

39. Guernsey DL, Edelman IS: Regulation of thyroid thermogenesis by thyroid hormones, in Oppenheimer JH, Samuels HH (eds): *Molecular Basis of Thyroid Hormone Action.* New York, Academic Press, 1983, p 293.

40. Sterling K: Thyroid hormone action at the cell level. *N Engl J Med* 300:117, 1979.

41. Coulombe P, Dussault JH, Walker P: Catecholamine metabolism in thyroid diseases. II. Norepinephrine secretion rate in hyperthyroidism and hypothyroidism. *J Clin Endocrinol Metab* 44:1185, 1977.

42. Bilezikian J, Loeb JN: The influence of hyperthyroidism and hypothyroidism on α- and β-adrenergic receptor systems and adrenergic responsiveness. *Endocr Rev* 4:378, 1983.

43. Forfar JC, Sawers JSA, Toft AD: Cardiovascular responses in hyperthyroidism before and during β-adrenoceptor blockade: Evidence against adrenergic hypersensitivity. *Clin Endocrinol* 16:441, 1982.

44. Williams RS, Lefkowitz RJ: The effects of thyroid hormone on adrenergic receptors, in Oppenheimer JH, Samuels HH (eds): *Molecular Basis of Thyroid Hormone Action.* New York, Academic Press, 1983, p 325.

45. Arner P, Wennlund A, Ostman J: Regulation of lipolysis by human adipose tissue in hyperthyroidism. *J Clin Endocrinol Metab* 48:415, 1979.

46. Gard TG, Bernstein B, Larsen PR: Studies on the mechanism of 3,5,3′-triiodothyronine-induced suppression of secretagogue-induced thyrotropin release in vitro. *Endocrinology* 108:2046, 1981.

47. Smith TJ, Murata Y, Horwitz AL, Philipson L, Refetoff S: Regulation of glycosaminoglycan synthesis by thyroid hormone in vitro. *J Clin Invest* 70:1066, 1982.

48. Sandler MP, Robinson RP, Rabin D, Lacy WW, Abumrad NN: The effect of thyroid hormones on gluconeogenesis and forearm metabolism in man. *J Clin Endocrinol Metab* 56:479, 1983.

49. Laville M, Riou JP, Bougneres PP, Canivet B, Beylot M, Cohen R, Serusclat P, Dumontet C, Berthezene F, Mornex R: Glucose metabolism in experimental hyperthyroidism: Intact in vivo

sensitivity to insulin with abnormal binding and increased glucose turnover. *J Clin Endocrinol Metab* 58:960, 1984.

50. Saunders J, Hall SEH, Sonksen PH: Glucose and free fatty acid turnover in thyrotoxicosis and hypothyroidism, before and after treatment. *Clin Endocrinol* 13:33, 1980.

51. Wennlund A, Arner P, Ostman J: Changes in the effects of insulin on human adipose tissue metabolism in hyperthyroidism. *J Clin Endocrinol Metab* 53:631, 1981.

52. Chait A, Bierman EL, Albers JJ: Regulatory role of triiodothyronine in the degradation of low density lipoprotein by cultured human skin fibroblasts. *J Clin Endocrinol Metab* 48:887, 1979.

53. Kourides IA, Weintraub BD, Ridgway EC, Maloof E: Pituitary secretion of free alpha and beta subunit of human thyrotropin in patients with thyroid disorders. *J Clin Endocrinol Metab* 40:872, 1975.

54. Gershengorn MC: Bihormonal regulation of the thyrotropin-releasing hormone receptor in mouse pituitary thyrotropic tumor cells in culture. *J Clin Invest* 62:937, 1978.

55. Sawin CT, Hershman JM, Chopra IJ: The comparative effect of T4 and T3 on the TSH response to TRH in young adult men. *J Clin Endocrinol Metab* 44:273, 1977.

56. Kubek M, Wilber JF, George JM: The distribution and concentration of thyrotropin-releasing hormone in discrete human hypothalamic nuclei. *Endocrinology* 105:537, 1979.

57. Morley JE: Neuroendocrine control of thyrotropin secretion. *Endocr Rev* 2:396, 1981.

58. Jackson IMD: Thyrotropin-releasing hormone. *N Engl J Med* 306:145, 1982.

59. Taylor T, Weintraub BD: Thyrotropin (TSH)-releasing hormone regulation of TSH subunit biosynthesis and glycosylation in normal and hypothyroid rat pituitaries. *Endocrinology* 116:1968, 1985.

60. Snyder PJ, Utiger RD: Repetitive administration of thyrotropin-releasing hormone results in small elevations of serum thyroid hormones and in marked inhibition of thyrotropin response. *J Clin Invest* 52:2305, 1973.

61. Bassiri RM, Utiger R: Metabolism and excretion of exogenous TRH in humans. *J Clin Invest* 52:1616, 1973.

62. Mallik TK, Wilber JF, Pegues J: Measurements of thyrotropin-releasing hormone-like material in human peripheral blood by affinity chromatography and radioimmunoassay. *J Clin Endocrinol Metab* 54:1194, 1982.

63. Frasier SD: Human pituitary growth hormone (hGH) therapy in growth hormone deficiency. *Endocr Rev* 4:155, 1983.

64. Holdaway IM, Evans MC, Sheehan A, Ibbertson HK: Low thyroxine levels in some hyperprolactinemic patients due to dopaminergic suppression of thyrotropin. *J Clin Endocrinol Metab* 59:608, 1984.

65. Buckland PR, Strickland TW, Pierce JG, Smith BR: TSH crosslinks to the TSH receptor through the beta subunit. *Endocrinology* 116:2122, 1985.

66. Nielsen TB, Totsuka Y, Kempner ES, Field JB: Structure of the thyrotropin receptor and thyroid adenylate cyclase system as determined by target analysis. *Biochemistry* 23:6009, 1984.

67. Field JB, Bloom G, Chou C-Y, Kerins ME: Inhibition of thyroid-stimulating hormone stimulation of protein kinase, glucose oxidation, and phospholipid synthesis in thyroid slices previously exposed to the hormone. *J Clin Invest* 59:659, 1977.

68. Davies TF: Positive regulation of the guinea pig thyrotropin receptor. *Endocrinology* 117:201, 1985.

69. Pisarev MA, Kleiman de Pisarev DL: Biochemistry of thyroid regulation under normal and abnormal conditions. *J Endocrinol Invest* 3:317, 1980.

70. Wartofsky L, Burman KD: Alterations in thyroid function in patients with systemic illness: The "euthyroid sick syndrome." *Endocr Rev* 3:164, 1982.

71. Danforth E, Horton ES, O'Connell M, Sims EAH, Burger AG, Ingbar SH, Braverman L, Vagenakis AG: Dietary-induced alterations in thyroid hormone metabolism during overnutrition. *J Clin Invest* 64:1336, 1979.

72. Jennings AS, Ferguson DC, Utiger RD: Regulation of the conversion of thyroxine to triiodothyronine in the perfused rat liver. *J Clin Invest* 64:1616, 1979.

73. Silva JE, Larsen PR: Comparison of iodothyronine 5′-deiodinase and other thyroid-hormone-dependent enzyme activities in the cerebral cortex of hypothyroid neonatal rat. *J Clin Invest* 70:1110, 1982.

74. Caldwell G, Gow SM, Sweeting VM, Kellett HA, Beckett GJ, Seth J, Toft AD: A new strategy for thyroid function testing. *Lancet* 1:1117, 1985.

75. Bigos ST, Hindson D, McCallum J: Serum thyroid-stimulating hormone and antimicrosomal antibodies as a screen for autoimmune thyroid disease. *J Lab Clin Med* 93:1035, 1979.

76. Weeke J, Dybkjaer L, Granlie K, Eskjaer Jensen S, Kjaerulff E, Laurberg P, Magnusson B: A longitudinal study of serum TSH, and total and free iodothyronines during normal pregnancy. *Acta Endocrinol* 101:531, 1982.

77. Guillaume J, Schussler GC, Goldman J: Components of the total serum thyroid hormone concentrations during pregnancy: High free thyroxine and blunted thyrotropin (TSH) response to TSH-releasing hormone in the first trimester. *J Clin Endocrinol Metab* 60:678, 1985.

78. Levy RP, Newman DM, Kejall LS, Barford DAG: The myth of goiter in pregnancy. *Am J Obstet Gynecol* 137:701, 1980.

79. Fisher DA, Klein AH: Thyroid development and disorders of thyroid function in the newborn. *N Engl J Med* 304:702, 1981.

80. Roti E, Gnudi A, Braverman LE: The placental transport, synthesis and metabolism of drugs which affect thyroid function. *Endocr Rev* 4:131, 1983.

81. Fisher DA, Sack J, Oddie TH, Pekary AE, Hershman JM, Lam RW, Parslow ME: Serum T4, TBG, T3 uptake, T3, reverse T3, and TSH concentrations in children 1 to 15 years of age. *J Clin Endocrinol Metab* 45:191, 1977.

82. Ingbar SH: The influence of aging on the human thyroid hormone economy, in Greenblatt RB (ed): *Geriatric Endocrinology*. New York, Raven, 1978, p 13.

83. Tunbridge WMG, Evered DC, Hall R, Appleton D, Brewis M, Clark F, Evans JG, Young E, Bird T, Smith PA: The spectrum of thyroid disease in a community: The Whickham survey. *Clin Endocrinol* 7:481, 1977.

84. Yoshida H, Amino N, Yagawa K, Uemura K, Satoh M, Miyai K, Kumahara Y: Associaton of serum antithyroid antibodies with lymphocytic infiltration of the thyroid gland: Studies of seventy autopsied cases. *J Clin Endocrinol Metab* 46:859, 1978.

85. Smals AGH, Ross HA, Kloppenberg PWC: Seasonal variation in serum T3 and T4 levels in men. *J Clin Endocrinol Metab* 44:998, 1977.

86. Konno N, Merikawa K: Seasonal variation of serum thyrotropin concentration and thyrotropin response to thyrotropin-releasing hormone in patients with primary hypothyroidism on constant replacement dosage of thyroxine. *J Clin Endocrinol Metab* 54:1118, 1982.

87. Geola FL, Frumar AM, Tataryn IV, Lu KH, Hershman JM, Eggena P, Sambhi MP, Judd HL: Biological effects of various doses of conjugated equine estrogens in postmenopausal women. *J Clin Endocrinol Metab* 51:620, 1980.

88. Wenzel KW: Pharmacological interference with in vitro tests of thyroid function. *Metabolism* 30:717, 1981.

89. Burr WA, Ramsden DB, Hoffenberg R: Hereditary abnormalities of thyroxine-binding globulin concentration. *Q J Med* 46:295, 1980.

90. Barlow JW, Csicsmann JM, White EL, Funder JW, Stockigt JR: Familial euthyroid thyroxine excess: Characterization of abnormal intermediate affinity thyroxine binding to albumin. *J Clin*

Endocrinol Metab 55:244, 1982.

91. Ruiz M, Rajatanavin R, Young RA, Taylor C, Brown R, Braverman LE, Ingbar SH: Familial dysalbuminemic hyperthyroxinemia. A syndrome that can be confused with thyrotoxicosis. *N Engl J Med* 306:635, 1982.

92. Moses AC, Lawlor J, Haddow J, Jackson IMD: Familial euthyroid hyperthyroxinemia resulting from increased thyroxine binding to thyroxine-binding prealbumin. *N Engl J Med* 306:966, 1982.

93. Rajatanavin R, Liberman C, Lawrence GD, D'Arcangues CM, Young RA, Emerson CH: Euthyroid hyperthyroxinemia and thyroxine-binding prealbumin excess in islet cell carcinoma. *J Clin Endocrinol Metab* 61:17, 1985.

94. Croxson MS, Palmer BN, Holdaway IM, Frengley PA, Evans MC: Detection of familial dysalbuminaemic hyperthyroxinaemia. *Br Med J* 290:1099, 1985.

95. Trimarchi F, Benvenga S, Costante G, Barbera C, Melluso R, Marcocci C, Cniovato L, De Luca F, Consolo F: Identification and characterization of circulating thyroid hormone autoantibodies in thyroid diseases, in autoimmune non-thyroid illnesses and in lymphoreticular system disorders. *J Endocrinol Invest* 6:203, 1983.

96. Rajatanavin R, Braverman LE: Euthyroid hyperthyroxinemia. *J Endocrinol Invest* 6:493, 1983.

97. Gamstedt A, Jarnerot G, Kagedal B: Dose related effects of betamethasone on iodothyronines and thyroid hormone-binding proteins in serum. *Acta Endocrinol* 96:484, 1981.

98. Helenius T, Liewendahl K: Abnormal thyroid function tests in severe non-thyroidal illness: Diagnostic and pathophysiologic aspects. *Scand J Clin Lab Invest* 39:389, 1979.

99. Kaptein EM, Macintyre SS, Weiner JM, Spencer CA, Nicoloff JT: Free thyroxine estimates in nonthyroidal illness: Comparison of eight methods. *J Clin Endocrinol Metab* 52:1073, 1981.

100. Chopra IJ, Hershman JM, Pardridge WM, Nicoloff JT: Thyroid function in nonthyroidal illnesses. *Ann Intern Med* 98:946, 1983.

101. Chopra IJ, Chua Teco GNC, Mead JF, Huang T-S, Beredo A, Solomon DH: Relationship between serum free fatty acids and thyroid hormone binding inhibitor in nonthyroid illnesses. *J Clin Endocrinol Metab* 60:980, 1985.

102. Stockigt JR, Lim C-F, Barlow JW, Wynee KN, Mohr VS, Topliss DJ, Hamblin PS, Sabto J: Interaction of furosemide with serum thyroxine-binding sites: In vivo and in vitro studies and comparison with other inhibitors. *J Clin Endocrinol Metab* 60:1025, 1985.

103. Gooch BR, Isley WL, Utiger RD: Abnormalities in thyroid function tests in patients admitted to a medical service. *Arch Intern Med* 142:1801, 1982.

104. Slag MP, Morley JE, Elson MK, Crowson TW, Nuttall FQ, Shafer RB: Hypothyroxinemia in critically ill patients as a predictor of high mortality. *JAMA* 245:43, 1981.

105. Kaplan MM, Larsen PR, Crantz FR, Dzau VJ, Rossing TH, Haddow JE: Prevalence of abnormal thyroid function test results in patients with acute medical illnesses. *Am J Med* 72:9, 1982.

106. Chopra IJ, Huang T-S, Beredo A, Solomon DH, Chua Teco GNC, Mead JF: Evidence for an inhibitor of extrathyroidal conversion of thyroxine to 3,5,3'-triiodothyronine in sera of patients with nonthyroidal illnesses. *J Clin Endocrinol Metab* 60:666, 1985.

107. O'Brian JT, Bybee DE, Burman KD, Osburne RC, Ksiazek MR, Wartofsky L, Georges LP: Thyroid hormone homeostasis in states of relative caloric deprivation. *Metabolism* 29:721, 1980.

108. Vagenakis AG, Portnay GI, O'Brian JT, Rudolph M, Arky RA, Ingbar SH, Braverman LE: Effects of starvation on the production and metabolism of thyroxine and triiodothyronine in euthyroid obese patients. *J Clin Endocrinol Metab* 45:1305, 1977.

109. Gardner DF, Kaplan MM, Stanley CA, Utiger RD: Effect of triiodothyronine replacement on the metabolic and pituitary responses to starvation. *N Engl J Med* 300:579, 1979.

110. Burman KD, Wartofsky L, Dinterman RE, Kesler P, Wannemacher RW: The effect of T3 and reverse T3 administration on muscle protein catabolism during fasting as measured by 3-methylhistidine excretion. *Metabolism* 28:805, 1979.

111. Osburne RC, Myers EA, Rodbard D, Burman KD, Georges LP, O'Brian JT: Adaptation to hypocaloric feeding: Physiologic significance of the fall in serum T3 as measured by the pulse wave arrival time (QKd). *Metabolism* 32:9, 1983.

112. Dasmahapatra A, Cohen MP, Grossman SD, Lasker N: Erythrocyte sodium/potassium adenosine triphosphatase in thyroid disease and nonthyroidal illness. *J Clin Endocrinol Metab* 61:110, 1985.

113. Lim VS, Henriquez C, Seo H, Refetoff S, Martino E: Thyroid function in a uremic rat model: Evidence suggesting tissue hypothyroidism. *J Clin Invest* 66:946, 1980.

114. Dillmann WH, Berry S, Alexander NM: A physiological dose of triiodothyronine normalizes cardiac myosin adenosine triphosphatase activity and changes myosin isoenzyme distribution in semistarved rats. *Endocrinology* 112:2081, 1983.

115. Sundaresan PR, Sharma VK, Gingold SI, Banerjee SP: Decreased β-adrenergic receptors in rat heart in streptozotocin-induced diabetes: Role of thyroid hormones. *Endocrinology* 114:1358, 1984.

116. Melmed S, Geola FL, Reed AW, Pekary AE, Park J, Hershman JM: A comparison of methods for assessing thyroid function in nonthyroidal illness. *J Clin Endocrinol Metab* 54:300, 1982.

117. Kaptein EM, Grieb DA, Spencer CA, Wheeler WS, Nicoloff JT: Thyroxine metabolism in the low thyroxine state of critical nonthyroidal illnesses. *J Clin Endocrinol Metab* 53:764, 1981.

118. Vierhapper H, Laggner A, Waldhausl W, Grubeck-Loebenstein B, Kleinberger G: Impaired secretion of TSH in critically ill patients with low T_4-syndrome. *Acta Endocrinol* 101:542, 1982.

119. Wehmann RE, Gregerman RI, Burns WH, Saral R, Santos GW: Suppression of thyrotropin in the low thyroxine state of severe nonthyroidal illness. *N Engl J Med* 312:546, 1985.

120. Bacci V, Schussler GC, Kaplan T: The relationship between serum triiodothyronine and thyrotropin during systemic illness. *J Clin Endocrinol Metab* 54:1229, 1982.

121. Shulkin BL, Utiger RD: Caloric restriction does not alter thyrotropin secretion in hypothyroidism. *J Clin Endocrinol Metab* 60:1076, 1985.

122. Kaptein EM, Weiner JM, Robinson WJ, Wheeler WS, Nicoloff JT: Relationship of altered thyroid hormone indices to survival in nonthyroidal illnesses. *Clin Endocrinol* 16:565, 1982.

123. Borst GC, Eil C, Burman KD: Euthyroid hyperthyroxinemia. *Ann Intern Med* 98:366, 1983.

124. Spratt DI, Pont A, Miller MB, McDougall IR, Bayer MF, McLaughlin WT: Hyperthyroxinemia in patients with acute psychiatric disorders. *Am J Med* 73:41, 1982.

125. Kramlinger KG, Gharib H, Swanson DW, Maruta T: Normal serum thyroxine values in patients with acute psychiatric illness. *Am J Med* 76:799, 1984.

126. Birkhauser M, Burer TH, Busset R, Burger A: Diagnosis of hyperthyroidism when serum-thyroxine alone is raised. *Lancet* 2:53, 1977.

127. Gavin LA, Rosenthal M, Cavalieri RR: The diagnostic dilemma of isolated hyperthyroxinemia in acute illness. *JAMA* 242:251, 1979.

128. Otsuki M, Dakoda M, Baba S: Influence of glucocorticoids on TRF-induced TSH response in man. *J Clin Endocrinol Metab* 36:95, 1973.

129. Re RN, Kourides IA, Ridgway EC, Weintraub BD, Maloof F: The effect of glucocorticoid administration on human pituitary secretion of thyrotropin and prolactin. *J Clin Endocrinol Metab* 43:338, 1976.

130. Williams DE, Chopra IJ, Orgiazzi J, Solomon DH: Acute effects of corticosteroids on thyroid activity in Graves' disease. *J*

Clin Endocrinol Metab 41:354, 1975.
131. Cooper DS, Daniels GH, Ladenson PW, Ridgway EC: Hyperthyroxinemia in patients treated with high-dose propranolol. *Am J Med* 73:867, 1982.
132. Perrild H, Hansen JM, Skovsted L, Christensen LK: Different effects of propranolol, alprenolol, sotalol, atenolol and metoprolol on serum T3 and serum rT3 in hyperthyroidism. *Clin Endocrinol* 18:139, 1983.
133. Shulkin BL, Peele ME, Utiger RD: β-adrenergic inhibition of hepatic 3′,3,5-triiodothyronine production. *Endocrinology* 115:858, 1984.
134. Saberi M, Sterling FH, Utiger RD: Reduction in extrathyroidal triiodothyronine production by propylthiouracil in man. *J Clin Invest* 55:218, 1975.
135. Vagenakis A, Rapoport B, Azizi F, Portnay GI, Braverman LE, Ingbar SH: Hyperresponse to thyrotropin-releasing hormone accompanying small decreases in serum thyroid hormone concentrations. *J Clin Invest* 54:913, 1974.
136. Vagenakis AG, Braverman LE: Adverse effects of iodine on thyroid function. *Med Clin North Am* 59:1075, 1975.
137. Pradkin JE, Wolff J: Iodide-induced thyrotoxicosis. *Medicine* 61:1, 1984.
138. Burgi H, Wimpfheimer C, Burger A, Zaunbauer W, Rosler H, Lemarchand-Beraud T: Changes of circulating thyroxine, triiodothyronine and reverse triiodothyronine after radiographic contrast agents. *J Clin Endocrinol Metab* 43:1203, 1976.
139. Melmed S, Nademanee K, Reed AW, Hendrickson JA, Singh BN, Hershman JM: Hyperthyroxinemia with bradycardia and normal thyrotropin secretion after chronic amiodarone administration. *J Clin Endocrinol Metab* 53:997, 1981.
140. Lambert MJ, Burger AG, Galeazzi RL, Engler D: Are selective increases in serum thyroxine (T4) due to iodinated inhibitors of T4 monodeiodination indicative of hyperthyroidism? *J Clin Endocrinol Metab* 55:1058, 1982.
141. Martino E, Safran M, Aghini-Lombardi F, Rajatanavin R, Lenziardi M, Fay M, Pacchiarotti A, Aronin N, Macchia E, Haffajee C, Odoguardi L, Love J, Bigalli A, Baschieri L, Pinchera A, Braverman L: Environmental iodine intake and thyroid dysfunction during chronic amiodarone therapy. *Ann Intern Med* 101:28, 1984.
142. Spaulding SW, Burrow GN, Bermudez P, Himmelhoch JM: The inhibitory effect of lithium on thyroid hormone release in both euthyroid and thyrotoxic patients. *J Clin Endocrinol Metab* 35:905, 1972.
143. Emerson CH, Dyson WL, Utiger RD: Serum TSH and T4 concentrations in patients receiving lithium carbonate. *J Clin Endocrinol Metab* 36:338, 1973.
144. Smith PJ, Surks MI: Multiple effects of 5,5′-diphenylhydantoin on the thyroid hormone system. *Endocr Rev* 5:515, 1984.
145. Kaplan MM, Utiger RD: Diagnosis of hyperthyroidism. *Clin Endocrinol Metab* 7:97, 1978.
146. Nicoloff JT, Low JC, Dussault JH, Fisher DA: Simultaneous measurement of thyroxine and triiodothyronine peripheral turnover kinetics in man. *J Clin Invest* 51:473, 1972.
147. Izumi M, Larsen PR: Triiodothyronine, thyroxine, and iodine in purified thyroglobulin from patients with Graves' disease. *J Clin Invest* 59:1105, 1977.
148. McGuire SB, Dennehey A, Cullen MJ: The effect of thyrotoxicosis and hypothyroidism on the extrathyroidal conversion of thyroxine to triiodothyronine in man, in Robbins J, Braverman L (eds): *Thyroid Research.* Excerpta Medica International Congress Series, no. 378, Amsterdam, 1976, p 259.
149. Zakarija M, McKenzie JM, Banovac K: Clinical significance of assay of thyroid-stimulating antibody in Graves' disease. *Ann Intern Med* 93:28, 1980.
150. Vitti P, Rotella CM, Valente WA, Cohen J, Aloj SM, Laccetti P, Ambesi-Impiombato FS, Grollman EF, Pinchera A, Toccafondi R, Kohn LD: Characterization of the optimal stimulatory effects of Graves' monoclonal and serum immunoglobulin G on adenosine 3′,5′-monophosphate production in FRIL-5 thyroid cells: A potential clinical assay. *J Clin Endocrinol Metab* 57:782, 1983.
151. Rapoport B, Greenspan FS, Filetti S, Pepitone M: Clinical experience with a human thyroid cell bioassay for thyroid-stimulating immunoglobulin. *J Clin Endocrinol Metab* 58:332, 1984.
152. Hensen J, Kotulla P, Finke R, Bogner U, Badenhoop K, Meinhold H, Schleusener H: Methodological aspects and clinical results of an assay for thyroid-stimulating antibodies: Correlation with thyrotropin binding-inhibiting antibodies. *J Clin Endocrinol Metab* 58:980, 1984.
153. Smyth PPA, Neylan D, O'Donovan DK: Association of thyroid-stimulating immunoglobulins and thyrotropin-releasing hormone responsiveness in women with euthyroid goiter. *J Clin Endocrinol Metab* 57:1001, 1983.
154. Arnaud CD, Kneubuhler HA, Seiling VL, Wightman BK, Engbring NH: Responses of the normal human to infusion of plasma from patients with Graves' disease. *J Clin Invest* 44:1287, 1965.
155. Sugenoya A, Trokoudes K, Row VV, Volpe R: The production of thyroid-stimulating immunoglobulin (TSI) by lymphocytes from patients with Graves' disease cultured with human thyroid subcellular fractions. *J Endocrinol Invest* 1:245, 1978.
156. Valente WA, Vitti P, Yavin Z, Yavin E, Rotella CM, Grollman EF, Toccafondi RS, Kohn LD: Graves' monoclonal antibodies to the thyrotropin receptor: Stimulating and blocking antibodies derived from the lymphocytes of patients. *Proc Natl Acad Sci USA* 79:6680, 1982.
157. Chiovato L, Hammond LJ, Hanafusa T, Pujol-Borrell R, Doniach D, Bottazzo GF: Detection of thyroid growth immunoglobulins (TGI) by [^{3}H]-thymidine incorporation in cultured rat thyroid follicles. *Clin Endocrinol* 19:581, 1983.
158. Valente WA, Vitti P, Rotella CM, Vaughan MM, Aloj SM, Grollman EF, Ambesi-Impiombato FS, Kohn LD: Antibodies that promote thyroid growth. *N Engl J Med* 309:1028, 1983.
159. Burman KD, Baker JR: Immune mechanisms in Graves' disease. *Endocr Rev* 6:183, 1985.
160. Bech K, Nerup J, Larsen JH: *Yersinia enterocolitica* infection and thyroid diseases. *Acta Endocrinol* 84:87, 1977.
161. Weiss M, Ingbar SH: Demonstration of a saturable binding site for thyrotropin in *Yersinia enterocolitica. Science* 219:1331, 1983.
162. Weetman AP, McGregor AM: Autoimmune thyroid disease: Developments in our understanding. *Endocr Rev* 5:309, 1984.
163. Wall JR, Baur R, Schleusener H, Bandy-Dafoe P: Peripheral blood and intrathyroidal mononuclear cell populations in patients with autoimmune thyroid disorders enumerated using monoclonal antibodies. *J Clin Endocrinol Metab* 56:164, 1983.
164. Totterman TH, Anderson LC, Hayry P: Evidence for thyroid antigen-reactive T lymphocytes infiltrating the thyroid gland in Graves' disease. *Clin Endocrinol* 11:59, 1979.
165. Okita N, Topliss D, Lewis M, Row VV, Volpe R: T-lymphocyte sensitization in Graves' and Hashimoto's diseases confirmed by an indirect migration inhibition factor test. *J Clin Endocrinol Metab* 52:523, 1981.
166. Okita N, Row VV, Volpe R: Suppressor T-lymphocyte deficiency in Graves' disease and Hashimoto's thyroiditis. *J Clin Endocrinol Metab* 52:528, 1981.
167. Jacobson DR, Gorman CA: Endocrine ophthalmopathy: Current ideas concerning etiology, pathogenesis, and treatment. *Endocr Rev* 5:200, 1984.
168. Kohn LD, Winand RJ: Experimental exophthalmos: Alterations of normal hormone-receptor interactions in the pathogenesis of a disease. *Isr J Med Sci* 10:1348, 1974.
169. Kriss JP, Konishi J, Herman M: Studies on the pathogenesis of Graves' ophthalmopathy, with some related observations regarding therapy. *Recent Prog Horm Res* 31:533, 1975.
170. Kendall-Taylor P, Atkinson S, Holcombe M: A specific IgG in Graves' ophthalmopathy and its relation to retro-orbital and

thyroid autoimmunity. *Br Med J* 288:1183, 1984.
171. Atkinson S, Holcombe M, Kendall-Taylor P: Ophthalmopathic immunoglobulin in patients with Graves' ophthalmopathy. *Lancet* 2:374, 1984.
172. Cheung HS, Nicoloff JT, Kamiel MB, Spolter P, Nimni ME: Stimulation of fibroblast biosynthetic activity by serum of patients with pretibial myxedema. *J Invest Dermatol* 71:12, 1978.
173. Rotella CM, Zonefrati R, Toccafondi R, Valente WA, Kohn LD: Ability of monoclonal antibodies to the thyrotropin receptor to increase collagen synthesis in human fibroblasts: An assay which appears to measure exophthalogenic immunoglobulins in Graves' sera. *J Clin Endocrinol Metab* 62:357, 1986.
174. Tamai H, Ohsako N, Takeno K, Fukino O, Takahashi H, Kuma K, Kumagai L, Nagataki S: Changes in thyroid function in euthyroid subjects with a family history of Graves' disease: A follow-up study of 69 patients. *J Clin Endocrinol Metab* 51:1123, 1980.
175. Banovac K, Zakarija M, McKenzie JM, Witte A, Sekso M: Absence of thyroid-stimulating antibody and long-acting thyroid stimulator in relatives of Graves' disease patients. *J Clin Endocrinol Metab* 53:651, 1981.
176. Gray J, Hoffenberg R: Thyrotoxicosis and stress. *Q J Med* 54:153, 1985.
177. Tamai HT, Fukino O, Ohsako N, Shinzato R, Suematsu H, Kuma K, Matsuzuka F, Nagataki S: Thionamide therapy in Graves' disease: Relation of relapse rate to duration of therapy. *Ann Intern Med* 92:488, 1980.
178. Sugrue D, McEvoy M, Feely J, Drury MI: Hyperthyroidism in the land of Graves: Results of treatment by surgery, radioiodine and carbimazole in 837 cases. *Q J Med* 49:51, 1980.
179. McGregor AM, Smith BR, Hall R, Petersen MM, Miller M, Dewar PJ: Prediction of relapse in hyperthyroid Graves' disease. *Lancet* 1:1101, 1980.
180. Romaldini JH, Bromberg N, Werner RS, Tanaka LM, Rodrigues HF, Werner MC, Farah CS, Reis LCF: Comparison of effects of high and low dosage regimens of antithyroid drugs in the management of Graves' hyperthyroidism. *J Clin Endocrinol Metab* 57:563, 1983.
181. Allannic H, Fauchet R, Lorcy Y, Gueguen M, Le Guerrier A-M, Genetet B: A prospective study of the relationship between relapse of hyperthyroid Graves' disease after antithyroid drugs and HAL haplotype. *J Clin Endocrinol Metab* 57:719, 1983.
182. Irvine WJ, Gray RS, Toft AD, Seth J, Lidgard GP, Cameron EHD: Spectrum of thyroid function in patients remaining in remission after antithyroid drug therapy for thyrotoxicosis. *Lancet* 2:181, 1977.
183. Gossage AAR, Crawley JCW, Copping S, Hinge D, Himsworth RL: Thyroid function and immunological activity during and after medical treatment of Graves' disease. *Clin Endocrinol* 19:87, 1983.
184. Wood LC, Ingbar SH: Hypothyroidism as a late sequela in patients with Graves' disease treated with antithyroid drugs. *J Clin Invest* 64:1429, 1979.
185. Skare S, Frey HMM, Konow-Thorsen R: Primary hypothyroidism followed by hyperthyroidism. Five case reports. *Acta Endocrinol* 105:179, 1984.
186. Christiansen NJB, Siersboek-Nielson K, Hansen JEM, Christensen LK: Serum thyroxine in the early phase of subacute thyroiditis. *Acta Endocrinol* 64:359, 1970.
187. Nikolai TF, Coombs GJ, McKenzie AK: Lymphocytic thyroiditis with spontaneously resolving hyperthyroidism and subacute thyroiditis. *Arch Intern Med* 141:1455, 1981.
188. Woolf PD: Transient painless thyroiditis with hyperthyroidism: A variant of lymphocytic thyroiditis. *Endocr Rev* 1:411, 1980.
189. Amino N, Mori H, Iwatani Y, Tanizawa O, Kawashima M, Tsuge I, Ibaragi K, Kumahara Y, Miyai K: High prevalence of transient postpartum thyrotoxicosis and hypothyroidism. *N Engl J Med* 306:849, 1982.
190. Amino N, Tanizawa O, Mori H, Iwatani Y, Yamada T, Kurachi K, Kumahara Y, Miyai K: Aggravation of thyrotoxicosis in early pregnancy and after delivery in Graves' disease. *J Clin Endocrinol Metab* 55:108, 1982.
191. Inada M, Nishikawa M, Naito K, Ishii H, Tanaka K, Imura H: Reversible changes of the histological abnormalities of the thyroid in patients with painless thyroiditis. *J Clin Endocrinol Metab* 52:431, 1981.
192. Mariotti S, Martino E, Cupini C, Lari R, Giani C, Baschieri L, Pinchera A: Low serum thyroglobulin as a clue to the diagnosis of thyrotoxicosis factitia. *N Engl J Med* 307:409, 1982.
193. Gorman CA, Wahner HW, Tauxe WH: Metabolic malingerers. *Am J Med* 48:708, 1970.
194. Adams DD, Kennedy TH, Stewart JC, Utiger RD, Vidor GI: Hyperthyroidism in Tasmania following iodide supplementation: Measurements of thyroid-stimulating autoantibodies and thyrotropin. *J Clin Endocrinol Metab* 41:221, 1975.
195. Hamburger JI: Evolution of toxicity in solitary nontoxic autonomously functioning thyroid nodules. *J Clin Endocrinol Metab* 50:1089, 1980.
196. Blum M, Shenkman L, Hollander CS: The autonomous nodule of the thyroid: Correlation of patient age, nodule size and functional status. *Am J Med Sci* 269:43, 1975.
197. Marsden P, Pacet P, Acosta M, McKerron CG: Serum triiodothyronine in solitary autonomous nodules of the thyroid. *Clin Endocrinol* 4:327, 1975.
198. Kempers RD, Dockerty MB, Hoffman DL, Bartholomew LG: Struma ovarii: Ascitic, hyperthyroid, and asymptomatic syndromes. *Ann Intern Med* 72:883, 1976.
199. Weintraub BD, Gershengorn MC, Kourides IA, Fein H: Inappropriate secretion of thyroid-stimulating hormone. *Ann Intern Med* 95:339, 1981.
200. Smallridge RC, Smith CE: Hyperthyroidism due to thyrotropin-secreting pituitary tumors. *Arch Intern Med* 143:503, 1983.
201. Kenimer JC, Hershman JM, Higgins HP: The thyrotropin in hydatidiform moles is human chorionic gonadotropin. *J Clin Endocrinol Metab* 40:482, 1975.
202. Nagataki S, Mizuno M, Sakamoto S, Irie M, Shizume K, Nakao K, Galton VA, Arky RA, Ingbar SH: Thyroid function in molar pregnancy. *J Clin Endocrinol Metab* 44:254, 1977.
203. Oddie TH, Boyd CM, Fisher DA, Hales IB: Incidence of signs and symptoms in thyroid disease. *Med J Aust* 2:981, 1972.
204. Vaidya VA, Bongiovanni AM, Parks JS, Tenore A, Kirkland RT: Twenty-two years' experience in the medical management of juvenile thyrotoxicosis. *Pediatrics* 54:565, 1974.
205. Crooks J, Murray IPC, Wayne EJ: Statistical methods applied to the clinical diagnosis of thyrotoxicosis. *Q J Med* 28:211, 1959.
206. Davis PJ, Davis FB: Hyperthyroidism in patients over the age of 60 years. *Medicine* 53:161, 1974.
207. Hegedus L, Hansen JM, Karstrup S: High incidence of normal thyroid gland volume in patients with Graves' disease. *Clin Endocrinol* 19:603, 1983.
208. Myers JD, Brannon ES, Holland BC: A correlative study on the cardiac output and the hepatic circulation in hyperthyroidism. *J Clin Invest* 29:1069, 1950.
209. Kontos HA, Shapiro W, Mauck HP, Richardson DW, Patterson JL, Sharpe AR Jr: Mechanism of certain abnormalities of the circulation to the limbs in thyrotoxicosis. *J Clin Invest* 44:947, 1965.
210. Das KC, Mukherjee M, Sarkar TK, Dash RJ, Rastogi GK: Erythropoiesis and erythropoietin in hypo- and hyperthyroidism. *J Clin Endocrinol Metab* 40:211, 1975.
211. Forfar JC, Miller HC, Toft AD: Occult thyrotoxicosis: A correctable cause of "idiopathic" atrial fibrillation. *Am J Cardiol* 44:9, 1979.
212. Nixon JV, Anderson RJ, Cohen ML: Alterations in left ventricular mass and performance in patients treated effectively for thyrotoxicosis: A comparative echocardiographic study. *Am J Med*

67:268, 1979.
213. Forfar JC, Muir AL, Sawers SA, Toft AD: Abnormal left ventricular function in hyperthyroidism: Evidence for a possible reversible cardiomyopathy. *N Engl J Med* 307:1165, 1982.
214. Graettinger JS, Muenster JJ, Selverstone LA, Campbell JA: A correlation of clinical and hemodynamic studies in patients with hyperthyroidism with and without congestive heart failure. *J Clin Invest* 38:1316, 1959.
215. Stein M, Kimbel P, Johnson RL Jr: Pulmonary function in hyperthyroidism. *J Clin Invest* 40:348, 1961.
216. Massey DG, Becklake MR, McKenzie JM, Bates DV: Circulatory and ventilatory response to exercise in thyrotoxicosis. *N Engl J Med* 276:1004, 1967.
217. Ayres J, Rees J, Clark TJH, Maisey MN: Thyrotoxicosis and dyspnoea. *Clin Endocrinol* 16:65, 1982.
218. Thomas FB, Caldwell JH, Greenberger NJ: Steatorrhea in thyrotoxicosis. *Ann Intern Med* 78:669, 1973.
219. Nakamura Y, Takeda T, Ishii M, Nishiyama K, Yamakada M, Hirata Y, Kimura K, Murao S: Elevation of serum angiotensin-converting enzyme activity in patients with hyperthyroidism. *J Clin Endocrinol Metab* 55:931, 1982.
220. Reddy J, Brownlie BEW, Heaton DC, Hamer JW, Turner JG: The peripheral blood picture in thyrotoxicosis. *NZ Med J* 93:143, 1981.
221. Eisenbarth GS, Jackson RA: Immunogenetics of polyglandular failure and related diseases, in Farid N (ed): *HLA in Endocrine and Metabolic Disorders*. New York, Academic Press, 1981, p 235.
222. Hymes K, Blum M, Lackner H, Karpatkin S: Easy bruising, thrombocytopenia, and elevated platelet immunoglobulin G in Graves' disease and Hashimoto's thyroiditis. *Ann Intern Med* 94:27, 1981.
223. Rogers JS, Shane SR, Jencks FS: Factor VIII activity and thyroid function. *Ann Intern Med* 97:713, 1982.
224. Cain JP, Dluhy RG, Williams GH, Selenkow HA, Milech A, Richmond S: Control of aldosterone secretion in hyperthyroidism. *J Clin Endocrinol Metab* 36:365, 1973.
225. Evered DC, Hayter CJ, Surveyor I: Primary polydipsia in thyrotoxicosis. *Metabolism* 21:393, 1972.
226. Ramsay ID: Muscle dysfunction in hyperthyroidism. *Lancet* 2:931, 1966.
227. Wiles CM, Young A, Jones DA, Edwards RHT: Muscle relaxation rate, fibre-type composition and energy turnover in hyper- and hypo-thyroid patients. *Clin Sci Mol Med* 57:375, 1979.
228. Conway MJ, Seibel JA, Eaton RP: Thyrotoxicosis and periodic paralysis: Improvement with beta blockade. *Ann Intern Med* 81:332, 1974.
229. Shen D-C, Davidson MB: Hyperthyroid Graves' disease causes insulin antagonism. *J Clin Endocrinol Metab* 60:1038, 1985.
230. Kabadi UM, Eisenstein AB: Glucose intolerance in hyperthyroidism: Role of glucagon. *J Clin Endocrinol Metab* 50:392, 1980.
231. Cooppan R, Kozak GP: Hyperthyroidism and diabetes mellitus: An analysis of 70 patients. *Arch Intern Med* 140:370, 1980.
232. Muls E, Blaton V, Rosseneu M, Lesaffre E, Lamberigts G, De Moor P: Serum lipids and apolipoproteins A-I, A-II, and B in hyperthyroidism before and after treatment. *J Clin Endocrinol Metab* 55:459, 1982.
233. Snyder PJ, Jacobs LS, Utiger RD, Daughaday WH: Thyroid hormone inhibition of the prolactin response to thyrotropin-releasing hormone. *J Clin Invest* 52:2324, 1973.
234. Gallagher TF, Hellman L, Finkelstein J, Yoshida K, Weitzman ED, Roffwarg HD, Fukushima DK: Hyperthyroidism and cortisol secretion in man. *J Clin Endocrinol Metab* 34:919, 1972.
235. Akande ED, Hockaday TDR: Plasma concentration of gonadotrophins, oestrogen and progesterone in thyrotoxic women. *Br J Obstet Gynaecol* 92:541, 1975.
236. Kidd GS, Glass AR, Vigersky RA: The hypothalamic-pituitary-testicular axis in thyrotoxicosis. *J Clin Endocrinol Metab* 48:798, 1979.
237. Burman KD, Monchik JM, Earll JM, Wartofsky L: Ionized and total serum calcium and parathyroid hormone in hyperthyroidism. *Ann Intern Med* 84:668, 1976.
238. Manicourt D, Demeester-Mirkine N, Brauman H, Corvilain J: Disturbed mineral metabolism in hyperthyroidism: Good correlation with triiodothyronine. *Clin Endocrinol* 10:407, 1979.
239. Bijlsma JW, Duursma GA, Roelofs JMM, derKinderen PJ: Thyroid function and bone turnover. *Acta Endocrinol* 104:42, 1983.
240. Toh SH, Claunch BC, Brown PH: Effect of hyperthyroidism and its treatment on bone mineral content. *Arch Intern Med* 145:883, 1985.
241. Caplan RH, Pagliara AS, Wickus G: Thyroxine toxicosis: A common variant of hyperthyroidism. *JAMA* 244:1934, 1980.
242. Utiger RD: Tests of thyroregulatory mechanisms, in Ingbar SH, Braverman LE (eds): *The Thyroid: A Fundamental and Clinical Text*. 5th ed. Hagerstown, MD, Harper & Row, 1986, p 511.
243. Engler H, Taurog A, Dorris ML: Preferential inhibition of thyroxine and 3,5,3′-triiodothyronine formation by propylthiouracil and methylmercaptoimidazole in thyroid peroxidase-catalyzed iodination of thyroglobulin. *Endocrinology* 110:190, 1982.
244. Azizi F: Environmental iodine intake affects the response to methimazole in patients with diffuse toxic goiter. *J Clin Endocrinol Metab* 61:374, 1985.
245. Cooper DS, Saxe VC, Maloof F, Ridgway EC: Studies of propylthiouracil using a newly developed radioimmunoassay. *J Clin Endocrinol Metab* 52:204, 1981.
246. Cooper DS, Bode HH, Nath B, Saxe V, Maloof F, Ridgway EC: Methimazole pharmacology in man: Studies using a newly developed radioimmunoassay for methimazole. *J Clin Endocrinol Metab* 58:473, 1984.
247. Jansson R, Dahlberg PA, Johnsson H, Lindstrom B: Intrathyroidal concentrations of methimazole in patients with Graves' disease. *J Clin Endocrinol Metab* 57:129, 1983.
248. McGregor AM, Petersen MM, McLachlan SM, Rooke P, Smith BR, Hall R: Carbimazole and the autoimmune response in Graves' disease. *N Engl J Med* 303:302, 1980.
249. Wenzel KW, Lente JR: Similar effects of thionamide drugs and perchlorate on thyroid-stimulating immunoglobulins in Graves' disease: Evidence against an immunosuppressive action of thionamide drugs. *J Clin Endocrinol Metab* 58:62, 1984.
250. Weiss I, Davies TF: Inhibition of immunoglobulin-secreting cells by antithyroid drugs. *J Clin Endocrinol Metab* 53:1223, 1981.
251. McLachlan SM, Pegg CAS, Atherton MC, Middleton S, Young ET, Clark F, Smith BR: The effect of carbimazole on thyroid autoantibody synthesis by thyroid lymphocytes. *J Clin Endocrinol Metab* 60:1237, 1985.
252. Weetman AP, Gunn C, Hall R, McGregor AM: The absence of any effect of methimazole on in vitro cell-mediated cytotoxicity. *Clin Endocrinol* 22:57, 1985.
253. Gwinup G: Prospective randomized comparison of propylthiouracil. *JAMA* 239:2457, 1978.
254. Cooper DS: Propylthiouracil levels in hyperthyroid patients unresponsive to large doses. Evidence of poor patient compliance. *Ann Intern Med* 102:328, 1985.
255. Wenzel KW, Lente JR: Syndrome of persisting thyroid stimulating immunoglobulins and growth promotion of goiter combined with low thyroxine and high triiodothyronine serum levels in drug treated Graves' disease. *J Endocrinol Invest* 6:389, 1983.
256. Takamatsu J, Sugawara M, Kuma K, Kobayashi A, Matsuzuka F, Mozai T, Hershman JM: Ratio of serum triiodothyronine to thyroxine and the prognosis of triiodothyronine-predominant Graves' disease. *Ann Intern Med* 100:372, 1984.
257. Bouma DJ, Kammer H, Greer MA: Follow-up comparison of short-term versus 1-year antithyroid drug therapy for the thyrotoxicosis of Graves' disease. *J Clin Endocrinol Metab* 55:1138, 1982.

258. Wilkin TJ, Beck JS, Crooks J, Isles TE, Gunn A: Time, carbimazole and the outcome of Graves' disease. *J Endocrinol Invest* 4:409, 1981.
259. Cooper DS: Antithyroid drugs. *N Engl J Med* 311:1353, 1984.
260. Cooper DS, Goldminz D, Levin AA, Ladenson PW, Daniels GH, Molitch ME, Ridgway EC: Agranulocytosis associated with antithyroid drugs: Effects of patient age and drug dose. *Ann Intern Med* 98:26, 1983.
261. Wall JR, Fang SL, Kuroki T, Ingbar SH, Braverman LE: In vitro immunoreactivity to propylthiouracil, methimazole, and carbimazole in patients with Graves' disease: A possible cause of antithyroid drug-induced agranulocytosis. *J Clin Endocrinol Metab* 58:868, 1984.
262. Laurberg P, Torring J, Weeke J: A comparison of the effects of propylthiouracil and methimazole on circulating thyroid hormones and various measures of peripheral thyroid hormone effects in thyrotoxic patients. *Acta Endocrinol* 108:51, 1985.
263. Wartofsky L, Ransil BJ, Ingbar SH: Inhibition by iodine of the release of thyroxine from the thyroid glands of patients with thyrotoxicosis. *J Clin Invest* 49:78, 1970.
264. Emerson CM, Anderson AJ, Howard WJ, Utiger RD: Serum thyroxine and triiodothyronine concentrations during iodide treatment of hyperthyroidism. *J Clin Endocrinol Metab* 40:33, 1975.
265. Ross DS, Daniels GH, De Stefano P, Maloof F, Ridgway EC: Use of adjunctive potassium iodide after radioactive iodine (^{131}I) treatment of Graves' hyperthyroidism. *J Clin Endocrinol Metab* 57:250, 1983.
266. Wu S-Y, Shyh T-P, Chopra IJ, Solomon DH, Huang H-W, Chu P-C: Comparison of sodium ipodate (Oragrafin) and propylthiouracil in early treatment of hyperthyroidism. *J Clin Endocrinol Metab* 54:630, 1982.
267. Mazzaferri EL, Reynolds JC, Young RL, Thomas CN, Parisi AF: Propranolol as primary therapy for thyrotoxicosis. *Arch Intern Med* 136:50, 1976.
268. O'Malley BP, Abbott RJ, Barnett DB, Northover BJ, Rosenthal FD: Propranolol versus carbimazole as the sole treatment for thyrotoxicosis. A consideration of circulating thyroid hormone levels and tissue thyroid function. *Clin Endocrinol* 16:545, 1982.
269. Kvetny J, Frederikesen PK, Jacobsen JG, Haas V, Feldt-Rasmussen U, Date J: Propranolol in the treatment of thyrotoxicosis: A randomized double-blind study. *Acta Med Scand* 209:389, 1981.
270. Sridama V, McCormick M, Kaplan EL, Fauchet R, DeGroot LJ: Long-term follow-up study of compensated low-dose ^{131}I therapy for Graves' disease. *N Engl J Med* 311:426, 1984.
271. Burch WM, Posillico JT: Hypoparathyroidism after I-131 therapy with subsequent return of parathyroid function. *J Clin Endocrinol Metab* 57:398, 1983.
272. Sawers JSA, Toft AD, Irvine WJ, Brown NS, Seth J: Transient hypothyroidism after iodine-131 treatment of thyrotoxicosis. *J Clin Endocrinol Metab* 50:226, 1980.
273. Cunnien AJ, Hay ID, Gorman CA, Offord KP, Scanlon PW: Radioiodine-induced hypothyroidism in Graves' disease: Factors associated with the increasing incidence. *J Nucl Med* 23:979, 1982.
274. Toft AD, Irvine WJ, Seth J, Hunter WM, Cameron EHD: Thyroid function in the long-term follow-up of patients treated with iodine-131 for thyrotoxicosis. *Lancet* 2:576, 1975.
275. Saenger EL, Thoma GE, Thompkins EA: Incidence of leukemia following treatment of hyperthyroidism. *JAMA* 205:855, 1968.
276. Holm L-E, Dahlqvist I, Israelsson A, Lundell G: Malignant thyroid tumors after iodine-131 therapy: A retrospective cohort study. *N Engl J Med* 303:188, 1980.
277. Robertson JS, Gorman CA: Gonadal radiation dose and its genetic significance in radioiodine therapy of hyperthyroidism. *J Nucl Med* 17:826, 1976.
278. Freitas JE, Swanson DP, Gross MD, Sisson JC: Iodine-131: Optimal therapy for hyperthyroidism in children and adolescents? *J Nucl Med* 20:847, 1979.
279. Hamburger JI: Management of hyperthyroidism in children and adolescents. *J Clin Endocrinol Metab* 60:1019, 1985.
280. Peek CM, Sawers JSA, Irvine WJ, Beckett GJ, Ratcliffe WA, Toft AD: Combinations of potassium iodide and propanolol in preparation of patients with Graves' disease for thyroid surgery. *N Engl J Med* 302:883, 1980.
281. Maier WP, Derrick BM, Marks AD, Channick BJ, Au FC, Caswell HT: Long-term follow-up of patients with Grave's disease treated by subtotal thyroidectomy. *Am J Surg* 147:266, 1984.
282. Toft AD, Irvine WJ, Sinclair I, McIntosh D, Seth J, Cameron EHD: Thyroid function after surgical treatment of thyrotoxicosis. *N Engl J Med* 298:643, 1978.
283. Farnell MB, van Heerden JA, McConahey WM, Carpenter HA, Wolff LH: Hypothyroidism after thyroidectomy for Graves' disease. *Am J Surg* 142:535, 1981.
284. Nikolai TF, Coombs GJ, McKenzie AK, Miller RW, Weir J Jr: Treatment of lymphocytic thyroiditis with spontaneously resolving hyperthyroidism (silent thyroiditis). *Arch Intern Med* 142:2281, 1982.
285. McDermott MT, Kidd GS, Dodson LE Jr, Hofeldt FD: Radioiodine-induced thyroid storm: Case report and literature review. *Am J Med* 75:353, 1983.
286. Mackin JF, Canary JJ, Pittman CS: Thyroid storm and its management. *N Engl J Med* 291:1396, 1974.
287. Croxson MS, Hall TD, Nicoloff JT: Combination drug therapy for treatment of hyperthyroid Graves' disease. *J Clin Endocrinol Metab* 45:623, 1977.
288. Kamm ML, Weaver JC, Page EP, Chappel CC: Acute thyroid storm precipitated by labor. *Obstet Gynecol* 21:460, 1963.
289. Mestman JH, Manning PR, Hodgman J: Hyperthyroidism and pregnancy. *Arch Intern Med* 134:434, 1974.
290. Volpe R, Ehrlich R, Steiner R, Row VV: Graves' disease in pregnancy years after hypothyroidism with recurrent passive-transfer neonatal Graves' disease: Therapeutic considerations. *Am J Med* 77:572, 1984.
291. Ylikorkala O, Kivinen S, Reinila M: Serial prolactin and thyrotropin responses to thyrotropin-releasing hormone throughout normal human pregnancy. *J Clin Endocrinol Metab* 48:288, 1979.
292. Marchant B, Brownlie BEW, Hart DM, Horton PW, Alexander WD: The placental transfer of propylthiouracil, methimazole and carbimazole. *J Clin Endocrinol Metab* 45:1187, 1977.
293. Cheron RG, Kaplan MM, Larsen PR, Selenkow HA, Crigler JF Jr: Neonatal thyroid function after propylthiouracil therapy for maternal Graves' disease. *N Engl J Med* 304:525, 1981.
294. Moller B, Bjorkhem I, Falk O, Lantto O, Larsson A: Identification of thyroxine in human breast milk by gas chromatography-mass spectrometry. *J Clin Endocrinol Metab* 56:30, 1983.
295. Kampmann JP, Johansen K, Hansen JM, Helweg J: Propylthiouracil in human milk: Revision of a dogma. *Lancet* 1:736, 1980.
296. Lamberg B-A, Ikonen E, Osterlund K, Teramo K, Pekonen F, Peltola J, Valimaki M: Antithyroid treatment of maternal hyperthyroidism during lactation. *Clin Endocrinol* 21:81, 1984.
297. McKenzie JM, Zakarija M: Pathogenesis of neonatal Graves' disease. *J Endocrinol Invest* 2:183, 1978.
298. Munro DS, Dirmikis SM, Humphries H, Smith T, Broadhead GD: The role of thyroid stimulating immunoglobulins of Graves's disease in neonatal thyrotoxicosis. *Br J Obstet Gynaecol* 85:837, 1978.
299. Zakarija M, McKenzie JM: Pregnancy-associated changes in the thyroid-stimulating antibody of Graves' disease and the relationship to neonatal hyperthyroidism. *J Clin Endocrinol Metab* 57:1036, 1983.
300. Amino N, Yuasa T, Yabu Y, Miyai K, Kumahara Y: Exophthalmos in autoimmune thyroid disease. *J Clin Endocrinol Metab* 51:1232, 1980.
301. Werner SC, Coleman DJ, Franzen LA: Ultrasonographic

evidence of a consistent orbital involvement in Graves's disease. *N Engl J Med* 290:1447, 1974.
302. Werner SC: Modification of the classification of the eye changes of Graves' disease: Recommendations of the ad hoc committee of the American Thyroid Association. *J Clin Endocrinol Metab* 44:203, 1977.
303. Gamblin GT, Harper DG, Galentine P, Buck DR, Chernow B, Eil C: Prevalence of increased intraocular pressure in Graves' disease: Evidence of frequent subclinical ophthalmopathy. *N Engl J Med* 308:420, 1983.
304. Allen C, Stetz D, Roman SH, Podos S, Som P, Davies TF: Prevalence and clinical associations of intraocular pressure changes in Graves' disease. *J Clin Endocrinol Metab* 61:183, 1985.
305. Enzmann D, Marshall WH, Rosenthal AR, Kriss JP: Computed tomography in Graves' ophthalmopathy. *Radiology* 118:615, 1976.
306. Solomon DH, Chopra IJ, Chopra U, Smith FJ: Identification of subgroups of euthyroid Graves's ophthalmopathy. *N Engl J Med* 296:181, 1977.
307. Tamai H, Nakagawa T, Ohsako N, Fukino I, Takahashi H, Matsuzuka F, Kuma K, Nagataki S: Changes in thyroid functions in patients with euthyroid Graves' disease. *J Clin Endocrinol Metab* 50:108, 1980.
308. Wasnich RD, Grumet FC, Payne RO, Kriss JP: Graves' ophthalmopathy following external neck irradiation for nonthyroidal neoplastic disease. *J Clin Endocrinol Metab* 37:703, 1973.
309. Gwinup G, Elias AN, Ascher MS: Effect on exophthalmos of various methods of treatment of Graves' disease. *JAMA* 247:2135, 1982.
310. Hales IB, Rundle FF: Ocular changes in Graves' disease. *Q J Med* 29:113, 1960.
311. Gorman CA: Temporal relationship between onset of Graves' ophthalmopathy and diagnosis of thyrotoxicosis. *Mayo Clin Proc* 58:515, 1983.
312. Bartalena L, Marcocci C, Chiovato L, Laddaga M, Lepri G, Andreani D, Cavallacci G, Baschieri L, Pinchera A: Orbital cobalt irradiation combined with systemic corticosteroids for Graves' ophthalmopathy: Comparison with systemic corticosteroids alone. *J Clin Endocrinol Metab* 56:1139, 1983.
313. Kriss JP, Pleshakov V, Rosenblum A, Sharp G: Therapy with occlusive dressings of pretibial myxedema with fluocinolone acetonide. *J Clin Endocrinol Metab* 27:595, 1967.
314. Riniker M, Tieche M, Lupi GA, Grob P, Studer H, Burgi H: Prevalence of various degrees of hypothyroidism among patients of a general medical department. *Clin Endocrinol* 14:69, 1981.
315. Bogner U, Schleusener H, Wall J: Antibody dependent cell mediated cytotoxicity against human thyroid cells in Hashimoto's thyroiditis but not Graves' disease. *J Clin Endocrinol Metab* 59:734, 1984.
316. Chiovato L, Vitti P, Lombardi A, Kohn LD, Pinchera A: Expression of the microsomal antigen on the surface of continuously cultured rat thyroid cells is modulated by thyrotropin. *J Clin Endocrinol Metab* 61:12, 1985.
317. Steel NR, Weightman DR, Taylor JJ, Kendall-Taylor P: Blocking activity to action of thyroid stimulating hormone in serum from patients with primary hypothyroidism. *Br Med J* 288:1559, 1984.
318. Konishi J, Iida Y, Kasagi K, Misaki T, Nakashima T, Endo K, Mori T, Shinpo S, Nohara Y, Matsuura N, Torizuka K: Primary myxedema with thyrotrophin-binding inhibitor immunoglobulins. *Ann Intern Med* 103:26, 1985.
319. Arikawa K, Ichikawa Y, Yoshida T, Shinozawa T, Homma M, Momotani N, Ito K: Blocking type antithyrotropin receptor antibody in patients with nongoitrous hypothyroidism: Its incidence and characteristics of action. *J Clin Endocrinol Metab* 60:953, 1985.
320. Mori H, Hamada N, DeGroot LJ: Studies on thyroglobulin-specific suppressor T cell function in autoimmune thyroid disease. *J Clin Endocrinol Metab* 61:306, 1985.
321. Jansson R, Totterman TH, Sallstrom J, Dahlberg PA: Thyroid-infiltrating T lymphocyte subsets in Hashimoto's thyroiditis. *J Clin Endocrinol Metab* 56:1164, 1983.
322. Tunbridge WMG, Brewis M, French JM, Appleton D, Bird T, Clark F, Evered DC, Evans JG, Hall R, Smith P, Stephenson J, Young E: Natural history of autoimmune thyroiditis. *Br Med J* 282:258, 1981.
323. Gordin A, Lamberg B-A: Spontaneous hypothyroidism in symptomless autoimmune thyroiditis. A long-term follow-up study. *Clin Endocrinol* 15:537, 1981.
324. Maagoe H, Reintoft I, Christensen HE, Simonsen J, Mogensen EF: Lymphocytic thyroiditis. II. The course of the disease in relation to morphologic, immunologic and clinical findings at the time of biopsy. *Acta Med Scand* 202:469, 1977.
325. Jansson R, Bernander S, Karlsson A, Levin K, Nilsson G: Autoimmune thyroid dysfunction in the postpartum period. *J Clin Endocrinol Metab* 58:681, 1984.
326. Amino N, Miyai K, Kuro R, Tanizawa O, Azukizawa M, Takai S, Tanaka F, Nishi K, Kawashima M, Kumahara Y: Transient postpartum hypothyroidism: Fourteen cases with autoimmune thyroiditis. *Ann Intern Med* 87:155, 1977.
327. Constine LS, Donaldson SS, McDougall IR, Cox RS, Link MP, Kaplan HS: Thyroid dysfunction after radiotherapy in children with Hodgkin's disease. *Cancer* 53:878, 1984.
328. Schimpff SC, Diggs CH, Wiswell JG, Salvetore PC, Wiernik PH: Radiation-related thyroid dysfunction. Implication for treatment of Hodgkin's disease. *Ann Intern Med* 92:91, 1980.
329. Shafer RB, Nuttall FQ, Pollak K, Kuisk H: Thyroid function after radiation and surgery for head and neck cancer. *Arch Intern Med* 135:843, 1975.
330. Vagenakis AG, Braverman LE, Azizi F, Portnay GI, Ingbar SH: Recovery of pituitary thyrotropic function after withdrawal of prolonged thyroid-suppression therapy. *N Engl J Med* 293:681, 1975.
331. Krugman LG, Hershman JM, Chopra IJ, Levine GA, Pekary AE, Geffner DL, Chua Teco GN: Patterns of recovery of the hypothalamic-pituitary-thyroid axis in patients taken off chronic thyroid therapy. *J Clin Endocrinol Metab* 41:70, 1975.
332. Dussault JH, Letarte J, Guyda H, Laberge C: Lack of influence of thyroid antibodies on thyroid function in the newborn infant and on a mass screening program for congenital hypothyroidism. *J Pediatr* 96:385, 1980.
333. Takasu N, Mori T, Koizumi Y, Takeuchi S, Yamada T: Transient neonatal hypothyroidism due to maternal immunoglobulins that inhibit thyrotropin-binding and post-receptor processes. *J Clin Endocrinol Metab* 59:142, 1984.
334. Chan AM, Lynch MJG, Bailey JD, Ezrin C, Frazer D: Hypothyroidism in cystinosis. *Am J Med* 48:678, 1970.
335. Levine MA, Downs RW Jr, Moses AM, Breslau NA, Marx SJ, Lasker RD, Rizzoli RE, Aurbach GD, Spiegel AM: Resistance to multiple hormones in patients with pseudohypoparathyroidism. *Am J Med* 74:545, 1983.
336. Drucker D, Eggo MC, Salit IE, Burrow GN: Ethionamide-induced goitrous hypothyroidism. *Ann Intern Med* 100:837, 1984.
337. Santen RJ, Wells SA, Cohn N, Demers LM, Misbin RI, Foltz EL: Compensatory increase in TSH secretion without effect on prolactin secretion in patients treated with aminoglutethimide. *J Clin Endocrinol Metab* 45:739, 1977.
338. Bigos ST, Ridgway EC, Kourides IA, Maloof F: Spectrum of pituitary alterations with mild and severe thyroid impairment. *J Clin Endocrinol Metab* 46:317, 1978.
339. Samaan NA, Osborne BM, MacKay B, Leavens ME, Duello TM, Halmi NS: Endocrine and morphologic studies of pituitary adenomas secondary to primary hypothyroidism. *J Clin Endocrinol Metab* 45:903, 1977.
340. Yamamoto K, Saito K, Takai T, Naito M, Yoshida S: Visual field defects and pituitary enlargement in primary hypothyroidism.

J Clin Endocrinol Metab 57:283, 1983.
341. Lamberg B-A, Pelkonen R, Aro A, Grahne B: Thyroid function in acromegaly before and after transphenoidal hypophysectomy. *Acta Endocrinol* 82:254, 1976.
342. Faglia G, Bitensky L, Pinchera A, Ferrari C, Paracchi A, Peccoz PB, Ambrosi B, Spada A: Thyrotropin secretion in patients with central hypothyroidism: Evidence for reduced biological activity of immunoreactive thyrotropin. *J Clin Endocrinol Metab* 48:989, 1979.
343. Beck-Peccoz P, Amr S, Menezes-Ferreira M, Faglia G, Weintraub BD: Decreased receptor binding of biologically inactive thyrotropin in central hypothyroidism. Effect of treatment with thyrotropin-releasing hormone. *N Engl J Med* 312:1085, 1985.
344. Refetoff S: Syndrome of thyroid hormone resistance. *Am J Physiol* 243:E88, 1982.
345. Refetoff S, DeGroot LJ, Barsano CP: Defective thyroid hormone feedback regulation in the syndrome of peripheral resistance to thyroid hormone. *J Clin Endocrinol Metab* 51:41, 1980.
346. Refetoff S, Salazar A, Smith TJ, Scherberg NH: The consequences of inappropriate treatment because of failure to recognize the syndrome of pituitary and peripheral tissue resistance to thyroid hormone. *Metabolism* 32:822, 1983.
347. Menezes-Ferreira M, Eil C, Wortsman J, Weintraub BD: Decreased nuclear uptake of [^{125}I]triiodo-L-thyronine in fibroblasts from patients with peripheral thyroid hormone resistance. *J Clin Endocrinol Metab* 59:1081, 1984.
348. Chait A, Kanter R, Green W, Kenny M: Defective thyroid hormone action in fibroblasts cultured from subjects with the syndrome of resistance to thyroid hormone. *J Clin Endocrinol Metab* 54:767, 1982.
349. Murata Y, Refetoff S, Horwitz AL, Smith TJ: Hormonal regulation of glycosaminoglycan accumulation in fibroblasts from patients with resistance to thyroid hormone. *J Clin Endocrinol Metab* 57:1233, 1983.
350. Wayne EJ: Clinical and metabolic studies in thyroid disease. *Br Med J* 1:1,78, 1960.
351. Watanakunakorn C, Hodges RH, Evans TC: Myxedema: A study of 400 cases. *Arch Intern Med* 116:183, 1965.
352. Billewicz WZ, Chapman RS, Crooks J, Day ME, Gossage J, Wayne E, Young JA: Statistical methods applied to the diagnosis of hypothyroidism. *Q J Med* 38:255, 1969.
353. Douglas RC, Jacobson SD: Pathologic changes in adult myxedema: Survey of 10 necropsies. *J Clin Endocrinol Metab* 17:1354, 1957.
354. Sensenbach W, Madison L, Eisenberg S, Ochs L: The cerebral circulation and metabolism in hyperthyroidism and myxedema. *J Clin Invest* 33:1434, 1954.
355. Sanders V: Neurologic manifestations of myxedema. *N Engl J Med* 266:547, 1962.
356. Swanson JW, Kelly JJ Jr, McConahey WM: Neurologic aspects of thyroid dysfunction. *Mayo Clin Proc* 56:504, 1981.
357. Khaleeli AA, Griffith DG, Edwards RHT: The clinical presentation of hypothyroid myopathy and its relationship to abnormalities in structure and function of skeletal muscle. *Clin Endocrinol* 19:365, 1983.
358. Klein I, Parker M, Shebert R, Ayyar DR, Levey GS: Hypothyroidism presenting as muscle stiffness and pseudohypertrophy: Hoffmann's syndrome. *Am J Med* 70:891, 1981.
359. Goldman J, Matz R, Mortimer R: High elevations of creatine phosphokinase in hypothyroidism. *JAMA* 238:325, 1977.
360. Dorwart BB, Schumacher HR: Joint effusion, chondrocalcinosis and other rheumatic manifestations in hypothyroidism. *Am J Med* 59:780, 1975.
361. Buccino RA, Spann JF, Pool PE, Sonnenblick EH, Braunwald E: Influence of thyroid state on the intrinsic contractile properties and energy stores of the myocardium. *J Clin Invest* 46:1669, 1967.
362. Graettinger JS, Muenster JJ, Checchia CS, Grisson RL, Campbell JA: A correlation of clinical and hemodynamic studies in patients with hypothyroidism. *J Clin Invest* 37:502, 1958.
363. Bing RF, Briggs RSJ, Burden AC, Russell GI, Swales JD, Thurston H: Reversible hypertension and hypothyroidism. *Clin Endocrinol* 13:339, 1980.
364. Khaleeli AA, Menon N: Factors affecting resolution of pericardial effusions in hypothyroidism: A clinical, biochemical and electrocardiographic study. *Postgrad Med* 53:473, 1982.
365. Santos AD, Miller RP, Mathew PK, Wallace WA, Cave WT Jr, Hinojosa L: Echocardiographic characterization of the reversible cardiomyopathy of hypothyroidism. *Am J Med* 68:675, 1980.
366. Vora J, O'Malley BP, Petersen S, McCullough A, Rosenthal FD, Barnett DB: Reversible abnormalities of myocardial relaxation in hypothyroidism. *J Clin Endocrinol Metab* 61:269, 1985.
367. Levine HD: Compromise therapy in the patient with angina pectoris and hypothyroidism. *Am J Med* 69:411, 1980.
368. Hay ID, Duick DS, Vlietstra RE, Maloney JD, Pluth JR: Thyroxine therapy in hypothyroid patients undergoing coronary revascularization: A retrospective analysis. *Ann Intern Med* 95:456, 1981.
369. Orr WC, Males JL, Imes NK: Myxedema and obstructive sleep apnea. *Am J Med* 70:1061, 1981.
370. Wilson WR, Bedell GN: The pulmonary abnormalities in myxedema. *J Clin Invest* 39:42, 1960.
371. Discala VA, Kinney JM: Effects of myxedema on the renal diluting and concentrating mechanism. *Am J Med* 50:325, 1971.
372. Skowsky WR, Kikuchi TA: The role of vasopressin in the impaired water excretion of myxedema. *Am J Med* 64:613, 1978.
373. Parving HH, Hansen JM, Nielsen SL, Rossing N, Munck O, Lassen NA: Mechanism of edema formation in myxedema: Increased protein extravasation and relatively slow lymphatic drainage. *N Engl J Med* 301:460, 1979.
374. Tachman MC, Guthrie GP Jr: Hypothyroidism: Diversity of presentation. *Endocr Rev* 5:456, 1984.
375. Valdemarsson S, Hansson P, Hedner P, Nilsson-Ehle P: Relations between thyroid function, hepatic and lipoprotein lipase activities, and plasma lipoprotein concentrations. *Acta Endocrinol* 104:50, 1983.
376. Chernausek SL, Underwood LE, Utiger RD, Van Wyk JJ: Growth hormone secretion and plasma somatomedin-C in primary hypothyroidism. *Clin Endocrinol* 19:337, 1983.
377. Contreras P, Generini G, Michelsen H, Pumarino H, Campino C: Hyperprolactinemia and galactorrhea: Spontaneous versus iatrogenic hypothyroidism. *J Clin Endocrinol Metab* 53:1036, 1981.
378. Peterson RE: The influence of the thyroid on adrenal cortical function. *J Clin Invest* 37:736, 1958.
379. Havard CWH, Saldanha VF, Bird R, Gardner R: Adrenal function in hypothyroidism. *Br Med J* 1:337, 1970.
380. Sprunt JG, Maclean D, Browning MCK: Plasma-corticosteroid levels in accidental hypothermia. *Lancet* 1:324, 1970.
381. Carpenter CCJ, Solomon N, Silverberg SG, Bledsoe T, Northcutt RC, Klinenberg JR, Bennett IL, Harvey AM: Schmidt's syndrome (thyroid and adrenal insufficiency). *Medicine* 43:153, 1964.
382. Topliss DJ, White EL, Stockigt JR: Significance of thyrotropin excess in untreated primary adrenal insufficiency. *J Clin Endocrinol Metab* 50:52, 1980.
383. Montoro M, Collea JV, Frasier SD, Mestman JH: Successful outcome of pregnancy in women with hypothyroidism. *Ann Intern Med* 94:31, 1981.
384. Distiller LA, Sagel J, Morley J: Assessment of pituitary gonadotropin reserve using LHRH in states of altered thyroid function. *J Clin Endocrinol Metab* 40:512, 1975.
385. de la Balze FA, Arrillaga F, Mancini RE, Janches M, Davidson OW, Gurtman AI: Male hypogonadism in hypothyroidism: A study of six cases. *J Clin Endocrinol Metab* 22:212, 1962.
386. Weinberg AD, Brennan MD, Gorman CA, March HM,

O'Fallon WM: Outcome of anesthesia and surgery in hypothyroid patients. *Arch Intern Med* 143:893, 1983.
387. Ladenson PW, Levin AA, Ridgway EC, Daniels GH: Complications of surgery in hypothyroid patients. *Am J Med* 77:261, 1984.
388. Bianchi R, Pilo A, Marian G, Molea N, Cazzoola F, Ferdeghin M, Bertelli P: Comparison of plasma and urinary methods for the direct measurement of the thyroxine to 3,5,3'-triiodothyronine conversion rate in man. *J Clin Endocrinol Metab* 58:993, 1984.
389. Bastenie PA, Bonnyns M, Vanhaelst L: Grades of subclinical hypothyroidism in asymptomatic autoimmune thyroiditis revealed by the thyrotropin-releasing hormone test. *J Clin Endocrinol Metab* 51:163, 1980.
390. Snyder PJ, Jacobs LS, Rabello MM, Sterling FH, Shore RN, Utiger RD, Daughaday WH: Diagnostic value of thyrotropin-releasing hormone in pituitary and hypothalamic diseases: Assessment of thyrotropin and prolactin secretion in 100 patients. *Ann Intern Med* 81:751, 1974.
391. Bantle JP, Dillmann WH, Oppenheimer JH, Bingham C, Runger GC: Common clinical indices of thyroid hormone action: Relationships to serum free 3,5,3'-triiodothyronine concentrations and estimated nuclear occupancy. *J Clin Endocrinol Metab* 50:286, 1980.
392. Saberi M, Utiger RD: Serum thyroid hormone and thyrotropin concentrations during thyroxine and triiodothyronine therapy. *J Clin Endocrinol Metab* 39:923, 1974.
393. Sawin CT, Herman T, Molitch ME, London MH, Kramer SM: Aging and the thyroid: Decreased requirement for thyroid hormone in older hypothyroid patients. *Am J Med* 75:206, 1983.
394. Sekadde CB, Slaunwhite WR Jr, Aceto T Jr, Murray K: Administration of thyroxine once a week. *J Clin Endocrinol Metab* 39:759, 1974.
395. Stone E, Leiter LA, Lambert JR, Silverberg JDH, Jeejeebhoy KN, Burrow GN: L-Thyroxine absorption in patients with short bowel. *J Clin Endocrinol Metab* 59:139, 1984.
396. Blackshear JL, Schultz AL, Napier JS, Stuart DD: Thyroxine replacement requirements in patients receiving phenytoin. *Ann Intern Med* 99:341, 1983.
397. Sawin CT, Surks MI, London M, Ranganathan C, Larsen PR: Oral thyroxine: Variation in biologic action and tablet content. *Ann Intern Med* 100:641, 1984.
398. Benvenga S, Trimarchi F, Barbera C, Costante G, Morabito S, Barberio G, Consolo F: Circulating immunoglobulin E (IgE) antibodies to L-thyroxine in a euthyroid patient with multinodular goiter and allergic rhinitis. *J Endocrinol Invest* 7:47, 1984.
399. Cooper DS, Halpern R, Wood LC, Levin AA, Ridgway EC: L-Thyroxine therapy in subclinical hypothyroidism: A double-blind, placebo-controlled trial. *Ann Intern Med* 101:18, 1984.
400. Fisher DA, Dussault JH, Foley TP Jr, Klein AH, LaFranchi S, Larsen PR, Mitchell ML, Murphey WH, Walfish PG: Screening for congenital hypothyroidism: Results of screening one million North American infants. *J Pediatr* 94:700, 1979.
401. Kugler JA, Huseman CA: Primary hypothyroidism of childhood: Evaluation of the hypothalamic-pituitary-gonadal axis before and during L-thyroxine replacement. *Clin Endocrinol* 19:213, 1983.
402. Van Dop C, Conte FA, Koch TK, Clark SJ, Wilson-Davis SL, Grumbach MM: Pseudotumor cerebri associated with initiation of levothyroxine therapy for juvenile hypothyroidism. *N Engl J Med* 308:1076, 1983.
403. Blum M: Myxedema coma. *Am J Med Sci* 264:432, 1972.
404. Ridgway EC, McCannon JA, Benotti J, Maloof F: Acute metabolic responses in myxedema to large doses of intravenous L-thyroxine. *Ann Intern Med* 77:549, 1972.
405. Pereira VG, Haron ES, Lima-Neto N, Medeiros-Neto GA: Management of myxedema coma: Report on three successfully treated cases with nasogastric or intravenous administration of triiodothyronine. *J Endocrinol Invest* 5:331, 1982.
406. Hylander B, Rosenqvist U: Treatment of myxoedema coma: Factors associated with fatal outcome. *Acta Endocrinol* 108:65, 1985.
407. Levine SN: Current concepts of thyroiditis. *Arch Intern Med* 143:1952, 1983.
408. Volpe R, Row VV, Ezrin C: Circulating viral and thyroid antibodies in subacute thyroiditis. *J Clin Endocrinol Metab* 27:1275, 1967.
409. Nyulassy S, Hnilica P, Buc M, Guman M, Hirschova V, Stefanovic J: Subacute (de Quervain's) thyroiditis: Association with HLA-Bw35 antigen and other abnormalities of the complement system, immunoglobulins and other serum proteins. *J Clin Endocrinol Metab* 45:270, 1977.
410. Hamburger JI, Taylor CI: Transient thyrotoxicosis associated with acute hemorrhagic infarction of autonomously functioning thyroid nodules. *Ann Intern Med* 91:406, 1979.
411. Berger SA, Zonszein J, Villamena P, Mittman N: Infectious diseases of the thyroid gland. *Rev Infect Dis* 5:108, 1983.

11

The Thyroid: Nodules and Neoplasia

Gerard N. Burrow

Public interest in the thyroid gland has centered on goiter and nodule formation. Goiter may be defined as a thyroid gland that is twice normal size, or about 40 g. Endemic goiter is the major thyroid disease throughout the world, affecting probably more than 200 million people. Many goitrous glands contain one or more nodules.[1] The introduction of iodized salt has eliminated goiter as a medical problem in developed countries, although it continues to be a major problem in developing countries whose geographic position makes them more susceptible to iodine deficiency. In North America and other developed areas sporadic nodular goiter and the thyroid carcinoma associated with it present problems in diagnosis and management. The concern about "lumps" and cancer seems particularly acute with respect to the thyroid, where a nodule is easily palpable and often observable by the patient.

GOITER

Classification of Goiter and Thyroid Neoplasia

To bring order out of chaos in the classification of goiter, the American Thyroid Association has suggested the terminology in Table 11-1. The classification is based on whether the nontoxic goiter is diffuse or nodular. The goiters are further subdivided according to whether they are endemic, sporadic, or compensatory and, if nodular, whether they are uninodular or multinodular and functional or nonfunctional.

Historical Overview

The thyroid gland was first described in detail by Vesalius in the sixteenth century. Thomas Wharton (1614–1673) named the gland from the Greek word *thureos* (shield). He noted:[2]

> It contributes much to the rotundity and beauty of the neck filling up the vacant spaces around the larynx and making its protuberant parts almost to subside, and become smooth, particularly in females to whom for this reason a larger gland has been assigned, which renders their necks more even and beautiful.

Goiter once was widely prevalent in Switzerland, Austria, and southern Germany as well as in northern Spain, southernmost France, and northern Italy. As a consequence, some of the earliest descriptions of goiter and cretinism came from these regions.

Endemic cretinism was described by the Swiss German physician Paracelsus (1493–1541) in the region around Salzburg.[3] Paracelsus pointed out that the cretinism occurred together with endemic goiter. Felix Platter (1536–1614), a Swiss physician who was professor of medicine in Basel, also described cretinism and associated mental deficiency and noted that affected individuals "frequently have a struma at the throat."

Swellings of the neck, particularly those due to the thyroid and glandular tuberculosis, had been treated for centuries with iodine-containing substances such as seaweed and burned sponge. In 1817, Bernard Courtois, a French manufacturer of saltpeter, discovered iodine. Subsequent research on iodine and its compounds led Jean François Coindet to introduce tincture of iodine for the treatment of goiter. In 1820, Coindet reported to the Swiss Scientific Society that he had administered iodine solution to 150 goiter patients without ill effects. Coindet's work strongly influenced other physicians, among them J.G.A. Lugol, who used an aqueous solution of iodine and potassium iodide (which was named for him). Awareness of potential problems associated with iodine eventually led to limitation of its use, especially after Kocher in 1910 described the production of toxic goiter (iod-Basedow) in goitrous patients treated with iodine. Marine popularized the use of iodized salt in North

Table 11-1. Classification of Nontoxic Goiter

Nontoxic diffuse goiter
Endemic, induced by:
Iodine deficiency
Iodine excess
Dietary goitrogens
Sporadic, due to:
Congenital defect in thyroid hormone biosynthesis
Chemical agents, e.g., lithium, thiocyanate, ρ-aminosalicylic acid
Iodine deficiency
Compensatory, following subtotal thyroidectomy
Nontoxic nodular goiter, due to causes listed above
Uninodular or multinodular
Functional and/or nonfunctional

Source: Modified from Werner SC: *J Clin Endocrinol* 29:860, 1969.

America for the prevention of simple endemic goiter beginning in 1917.[4]

Sporadic cretinism as distinct from the endemic form was described by Fagge, a physician at Guy's Hospital in London, before the Royal Medical and Surgical Society in 1871. Fagge expressed the view that sporadic cretinism was caused by absence of the thyroid gland.

Etiology of Goiter

Marine first developed the concept in 1924 that periods of iodide deficiency and repletion result in cyclic hyperplasia and involution of thyroid follicular cells with eventual development of nodular hyperplasia.[4] For want of a better explanation, this hypothesis is still used to explain goiter formation. Whatever the specific cause, the final common pathway appears to result from inadequate thyroid hormone secretion with compensatory thyroid stimulating hormone (TSH) secretion and eventual thyroid gland enlargement. The essential factor for the conversion of a hyperplastic, iodine-deficiency goiter into a colloid goiter appears to be an acute reduction of TSH stimulation.[5] Iodine deficiency is an extremely rare cause of goiter in North America. However, any situation that would result in periodic increases and decreases in TSH secretion might eventually result in the production of a nodular goiter.

The suggestion has also been made that thyroid nodules might be caused by the shunting of blood to a particular area of the thyroid with a subsequent increase in tissue growth. Thyroid follicles are bound together to form a lobule; a single artery supplies each lobule. In long-standing goiters, the blood supply may be greatly increased.

Recently, there has been increasing interest in the possibility that other growth factors in addition to TSH play a role in the etiology of goiter.[6–8] Immunoglobulin fractions capable of stimulating thyroid growth in a cytochemical bioassay based on DNA determinations have been obtained from patients with nontoxic goiter and with Graves' disease[7] (see Chap. 10). These thyroid growth immunoglobulins correlate with goiter size or lack of thyroid hormone suppressibility, rather than with thyroid hormone concentration. Epidermal growth factor has been found to stimulate thymidine incorporation in thyroid cells cultured in serum-free medium, again suggesting that factors other than TSH are capable of stimulating thyroid growth.[9–11]

TSH SECRETION

TSH secretion is controlled by the serum thyroid hormone concentration. As thyroid hormone concentration falls, TSH secretion increases; TSH secretion declines as the thyroid hormone concentration rises. Feedback control of TSH secretion by thyroid hormone occurs at the level of the pituitary. The hypothalamus modulates information from the rest of the central nervous system and provides the set point for TSH secretion in response to thyrotropin releasing hormone (TRH)[12] and other hormones, including estrogens, dopamine, and somatostatin (see Chap. 10).

There appear to be substantial variations between individuals in the relationships of serum thyroid hormone concentration to TSH concentration; these may reflect variations in cellular sensitivity of the pituitary to thyroid hormone, the degree of TRH release, or other factors (illustrated in Fig. 11-1). Two theoretical curves suggest that the same concentration of thyroid hormone may result in an elevated TSH concentration in one individual but a normal value in another. This difference in response could be reflected in goiters of varying sizes despite a similar degree of thyroid hormone deficiency.

As discussed in Chap. 10, the actions of thyroid hormone appear mostly to be due to T_3; T_4 serves predominantly as a prohormone. This function is particularly important in the case of the pituitary, where T_4 5′-deiodinase is most active.[13] This feature allows the gland to respond more readily to changes in T_4 release than do peripheral tissues (Fig. 11-2).

TSH STIMULATION OF THE THYROID GLAND

TSH is essential for the maintenance of normal thyroid hormone synthesis, although hypophysectomized

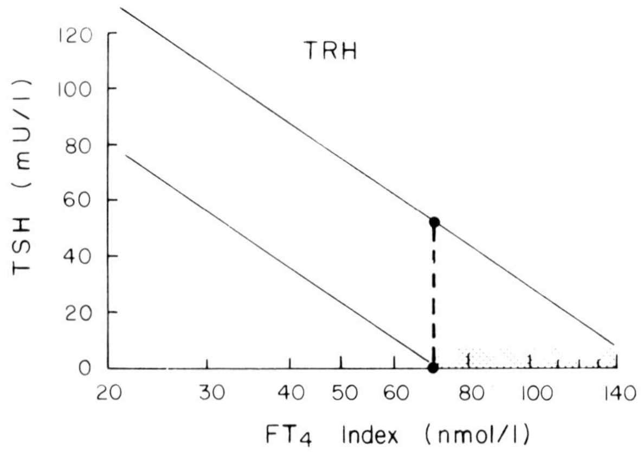

FIGURE 11-1 Speculative relationship among TRH, TSH, and thyroid hormone. A similar concentration of thyroid hormone as indicated here by the free T_4 index (see Chap. 10) results in widely disparate serum TSH concentrations. This may depend on the level of cellular sensitivity to TRH, which is governed by other factors. (*After Wilkin TJ, Storey BE, Isles TE, Crooks J, Beck JS: Br Med J 1:993, 1977.*)

animals secrete thyroid hormone to a very limited degree. The secretion of thyroid hormone is particularly sensitive to TSH and is proportional to the dose of administered TSH over a particular range. Under most physiologic conditions, TSH secretion maintains a stable serum concentration of thyroid hormone. However, the growth response of the thyroid to TSH has certain fixed limits; the thyroid is not capable of enlarging infinitely, and eventually a growth plateau is reached.

Evidence that goiter is due to increased TSH stimulation comes mainly from studies of endemic goiter. In a study of 285 patients from endemic goiter regions of New Guinea, mean serum TSH concentrations were found to be increased [16 μunits (μU)/ml] compared with normal values in North America (1.2 μU/ml).[14] However, within the group from the endemic goiter region, there was no difference in serum TSH concentration between goitrous and nongoitrous patients, suggesting that some factor in addition to TSH contributes to goitrogenesis. Perhaps the factor is differential sensitivity of the cells of the thyroid gland to TSH. In endemic goiter areas of Brazil, serum TSH concentrations were higher in goitrous patients from iodine-deficient areas compared with goitrous patients from iodine-replete areas.[15] Furthermore, there was a higher peak TSH response to TRH (see Chap. 10) in the iodine-deficient goitrous group. The authors suggested that there may have been an increase of the set point so that TSH secretion continued at a higher level. However, studies from Greece, another endemic goiter area, suggested that the iodine-deficient thyroid is more sensitive to the stimulatory effect of TSH.[16,17]

Studies of sporadic nontoxic goiter are even more complicated because the etiology is so diverse, ranging from thyroiditis to goitrogen ingestion. Serum TSH concentrations have been found to be increased slightly, and patients with sporadic nontoxic goiter often have an increased TSH response to TRH.[18] Patients with nodular goiter more often have an impaired or absent response to TRH compared with

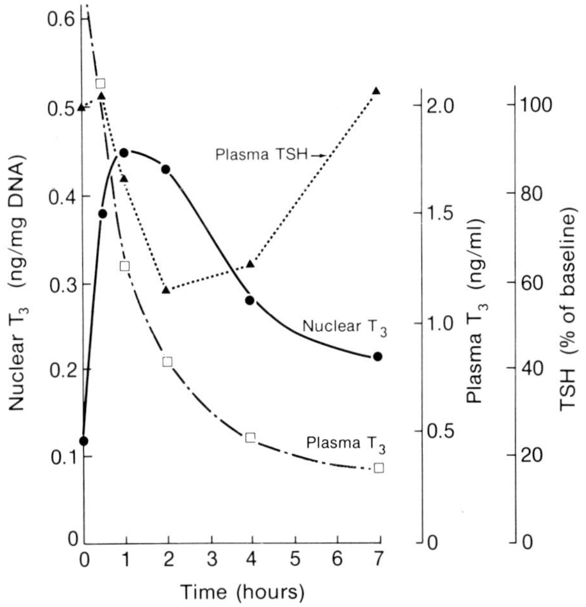

FIGURE 11-2 Time course of changes in pituitary nuclear T_3 and plasma T_3 and TSH levels. A single intravenous dose of T_3 was administered to thyroidectomized rats. The data suggest that the rapid inhibitory effect of T_3 on pituitary TSH release occurs through T_3 binding to receptors with kinetics similar to nuclear receptor binding. (*From Silva JE, Larson PR: Science 198:617, 1977.*)

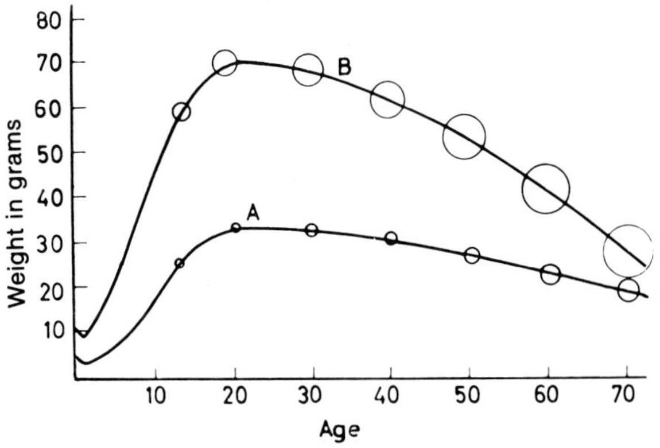

FIGURE 11-3 Goiter formation as a function of age. The size of the thyroid in grams is shown as a function of age for both nonendemic-goiter areas (*A*) and endemic goiter areas (*B*). The circles represent the relative size of thyroid nodules throughout life in both groups. (*From Farris in Deficiency Diseases. Springfield, IL, CC Thomas, 1958.*)

those with diffuse goiter. This impaired TSH response might indicate that there are areas of autonomy in the nodular gland, so that some thyroid hormone production is not under pituitary control; this would act to suppress the sensitivity of the pituitary to TRH. Serum TSH concentrations have been found to be higher in individuals who had goiters for less than a year.[19] Growth of the thyroid is more rapid early in life; the gland actually regresses later on (Fig. 11-3). TSH values also increase during the early decades; subsequently, TSH secretion and reserve progressively decrease.[20] The prevalence of thyroid nodules, however, may increase with age (Fig. 11-4).

The variability in TSH levels associated with goiter may be explained by the natural progression of the disease. Overall, in the early stages of the disease there is relative thyroid hormone deficiency; this results in increased TSH release, which then stimulates thyroid hypertrophy and hyperplasia. This increases the ability of the gland to produce thyroid hormone, which in turn results in a suppression of TSH levels toward normal. Further, in some cases, serum TSH stimulation might result in relatively autonomous foci of thyroid hormone–producing tissue within the gland, which could lead to depressed TSH levels. Thus, depending on the stage of the disease, TSH levels could be elevated, normal, or depressed.[14–20] However, it is also possible that individual variations in sensitivity of the gland to TSH and other growth factors are capable of stimulating thyroid gland growth[6–8] and may also participate in these variations.

Endemic Goiter

When the incidence of goiter in a population rises above 10 percent, the goiter becomes "endemic"; clearly, this is not a stringent criterion. However, it implies that an environmental factor is the causative agent. Worldwide, iodine deficiency is the major cause of goiter, but other goitrogens have been described which affect entire populations, usually in association with iodine deficiency.

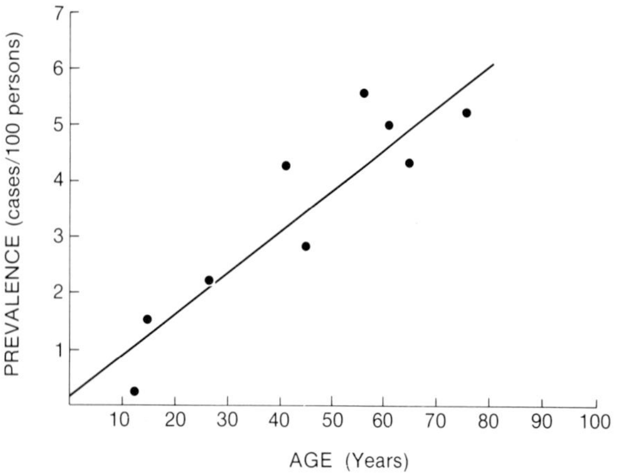

FIGURE 11-4 Prevalence of thyroid nodules with age. (*After Maxon et al.*[116])

GEOGRAPHY, DIET, AND IODINE ABUNDANCE

Although Noah may have saved the animals from extinction, the flood left their descendants susceptible to goiter. In areas subjected to flooding or intense glaciation in the last ice age, the iodine has been leached out of the soil. Newly formed soils are relatively iodine-deficient, although they are enriched by airborne iodine, the major source of which is seawater deposited in rain.

Although individual requirements vary, most people require more than 50 μg of iodine daily to replace iodine excreted in the urine (Table 11-2).[21] Diets inadequate to supply this amount of iodine are most often found in areas where the soil is poor in iodine. Individuals who live in villages in these areas and eat predominantly local food eat iodine-deficient diets. Iodine deficiency is less likely in larger cities because the food comes from a much wider geographic area. Similarly, members of upper socioeconomic classes are less apt to have goiter because they eat a more varied diet. In developed countries iodine added

Table 11-2. Urinary Iodide Content, Goiter, and Development

Severity of goiter	Urinary iodide excretion, μg/g creatinine	Percent with palpable goiter	Clinical spectrum
Mild	>50	10–20	Normal
Moderate	25–50	20–50	Occasional deafness and retardation; serum TSH elevated in 10–20%
Severe	<25	40–90	Cretinism in 1–10%; elevated serum TSH in 30–50%

Source: Modified from Ibbertson.[21]

to salt makes a major contribution to the iodine intake. With the exception of salt-water fish, there is relatively little iodine in natural food.

DEVELOPMENT OF ENDEMIC GOITER

Development of endemic goiter presumably follows the pattern of goiter in general. Decreased concentrations of circulating thyroid hormone resulting from iodine deficiency lead to increased TSH secretion and hyperplasia of the gland. As discussed above, factors other than TSH (such as the cellular sensitivity to TSH) also play a role in goiter formation;[22] it is necessary to invoke these factors to explain, for instance, why goiter is present in only certain individuals in areas of endemic goiter. There is no characteristic histological picture of endemic goiter. With the initial stimulation, hypertrophy of the follicular cells occurs, followed by hyperplasia of the follicles and a concomitant increase in the vascularity of the gland. All the follicles in the endemic goiter are not affected equally; radioautographic studies have shown an unequal distribution of radioiodine within the individual follicles.[23] This heterogeneity, combined with an overall increase in the size of the gland, might explain why some endemic goiters have been found to contain a higher than average total amount of iodine.[24] Also, some of this thyroidal iodine may be outside of the hormonally active pool. Nodular goiter might therefore be looked upon as an extreme variant of this heterogeneity. Part of the thyroid irregularity leading to nodule formation might be due to the accumulation of connective tissue, which, during periods of further stimulation, might serve as a focus of retraction and perhaps hinder the function of adjacent follicles.[5]

The human thyroid is limited in its ability to adapt to iodine deficiency, more so than to adapt to iodine excess. In severe deficiency, there is an inability of the thyroid to compensate completely for the low plasma inorganic iodide concentration by proportionally increasing the iodide clearance rate.[25] In the euthyroid patient with endemic goiter, total thyroid iodine stores may be normal, although the iodine concentration in the hormonally active pool is low. With less iodine, fewer iodothyronines are synthesized. Iodine deficiency also increases the monoiodotyrosine/diiodotyrosine ratio. These changes do not occur early in goiter formation, but they are often found in nodular glands. Iodine deficiency and perhaps the increased stimulation from TSH also result in a high T_3/T_4 ratio in these goiters. This adaptive effect results in production of the more potent T_3, despite deficiency of iodine.

CLINICAL FINDINGS IN ENDEMIC GOITER

In areas of severe iodine deficiency, virtually everyone is goitrous, regardless of sex or age. In less severely affected areas, surveys have shown that the thyroid gland may be moderately enlarged in early childhood but the incidence of goiter is usually at its height in pubertal children. The goiter of puberty is one of the more sensitive indicators of iodine lack in a particular region. A difference in gland size between the two sexes appears during puberty. Following puberty, the thyroid gland frequently diminishes in size in males, but not in females. Why females are more affected than males is not clear. In the endemic goiter area of New Guinea, thyroid enlargement was found to be related to breast development but not pregnancy, lactation, or parity.[26] The thyroid gland is more difficult to palpate in the male; this might account for some of the discrepancy. However, all thyroid disease is more common in females, and the difference is not solely due to estrogens. The diagnosis and treatment of goiter are discussed later in the chapter.

Relation to Thyroid Cancer

Despite continuing long-term interest in the problem, the relation between endemic goiter and thyroid cancer remains unclear. After the introduction of iodine prophylaxis, the incidence of both nodular goiter and certain adenocarcinomas and sarcomas of the thyroid decreased. Appreciation of this change was complicated by an increase in the incidence of papillary carcinoma of the thyroid. However, when geographic variation of goiter prevalence was compared with geographic patterns of mortality from thyroid cancer, there was no convincing evidence for the existence of an association between the two diseases.[27] In contrast, the comparison of the occurrence of goiter with that of hyperthyroidism showed the two to be highly significantly correlated.

Hyperfunction

Although data are not available, hyperthyroidism appears to be more common in areas of endemic goiter, especially after iodine therapy (iod-Basedow). Toxic nodular goiter (Plummer's disease) is common in association with endemic goiter; this may provide the explanation of the iod-Basedow phenomenon.[28] These hyperfunctioning nodules are avid for iodine and respond with a greatly increased production of thyroid hormone. An alternative has been suggested, that the iodine may damage the gland with release of stored hormone.[29]

CRETINISM

In areas of mild iodine deficiency the inhabitants are usually euthyroid; with more profound iodine depletion hypothyroidism may occur. A much more severe problem is the occurrence of *cretinism* in this population. Cretinism has been defined as permanent neurological and skeletal retardation resulting from an inadequate supply of thyroid hormone during fetal and neonatal life, in this case due to iodine deficiency.[21,24] Endemic cretins may present with neurological defects, particularly spastic diplegia and mental retardation, deafness, mutism, dwarfism, and hypothyroidism in varying combinations, depending upon the locale. Hypothyroidism can be diagnosed clinically by retarded linear growth and maturation of body proportions, myxedematous skin, and marked delay in sexual development (for further details see Chap. 10).

The various symptoms and signs of cretinism vary with the particular region, as illustrated in Fig. 11-5. The "myxedematous" type is characterized by hypothyroidism, dwarfism, and epiphyseal dysgenesis consistent with deficient hormone production. In contrast, the "nervous" type is characterized by mental retardation and deaf-mutism. Both groups may have goiter. The prevalence of cretinism observed in these regions also varies markedly and increases from 1 percent in Zaire to almost 6 percent in endemic goiter districts in Nepal. The clinical picture of endemic cretinism represents a spectrum of clinical and metabolic signs reflecting varying degrees of impairment of the nervous system and thyroid function[30,31] (Table 11-3).

Table 11-3. Types of Cretinism

Myxedematous	Neurological
Severe mental retardation	Severe mental retardation
Severe growth retardation	Mild growth retardation
Minimal neurological findings: delayed tendon reflexes	Severe neurological findings: Spastic diplegia, Neuromotor incoordination
Skeletal immaturity	Deaf-mutism (commonly)

Etiology of Cretinism and Iodine Deficiency

Endemic cretinism occurs only where long-standing severe endemic goiter is present. The prevalence of cretinism appears to be related to the severity of iodine deficiency. However, comparable states of iodine deficiency may be accompanied by cretinism in some areas but not in others.[33] Although the intrauterine period is important for the development of cretinism,[34] iodine administration can prevent it. In a severely iodine-deficient area in Africa, 40 percent of newborns had TSH concentrations greater than 2.5 standard deviations (SD) from controls whose mothers had received iodine.[32] In 6 of 34 iodine-deficient neonates, definite biochemical signs of hypothyroidism were encountered.

Endemic Goiter Due to Other Causes

Although iodine deficiency represents the major cause of endemic goiter, genetic factors and dietary goitrogens may also participate in endemic goiter formation. For example, a striking difference in the incidence of goiter was found between the inhabitants of two regions of an isolated island in Kivu Lake in Zaire, although the iodine intake in the two areas was the same and the two groups were ethnically similar.[32] Subsequent studies indicated that the goiter in this population was related to the consumption of cassava which, like several other chemical substances (dis-

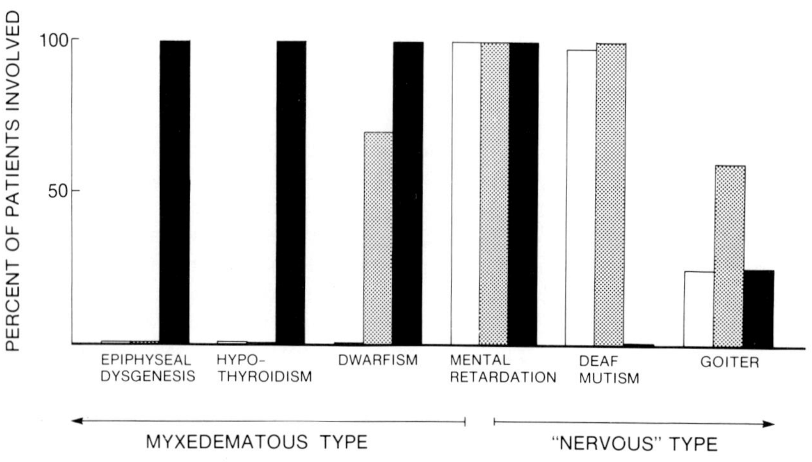

FIGURE 11-5 Regional variations of the clinical pattern of endemic cretinism. □, New Guinea; ▨, Ecuador; ■, Zaire. (*Modified from Delange et al.*[30])

cussed later), can impair the utilization of iodine by the thyroid gland. However, cassava appears to be active as a goitrogen only in the presence of severe iodine deficiency, since data from Vietnam indicate that the goitrogenic effect of this substance is easily overcome by supplementary iodine.[35]

Protein-calorie malnutrition (PCM) often is present in iodine-deficient areas and may contribute to the thyroid abnormalities. Malnutrition causes various alterations in thyroid gland structure and function; defective thyroid iodine concentration has been found despite adequate hormone secretion, which would further deplete iodine stores.[36] These abnormalities can be corrected by adequate protein and calorie intake. Studies from Senegal suggested that PCM might cause goiter by resulting in defective formation of the mannosyl retinene phosphate complex necessary for normal glycosylation of thyroglobulin.[37]

PROPHYLAXIS OF ENDEMIC GOITER

One of the strongest pieces of evidence supporting the contention that endemic cretinism is due to iodine deficiency is the disappearance of cretinism when iodine is added to the diet. Supplements of iodine to the daily diet have been widely employed since their efficacy was demonstrated by Marine and Kimball in 1917.[4,38] Similar favorable results have been duplicated throughout the world, but the total impact so far is small compared with the magnitude of the goiter problem. This apathetic approach may be partly due to the complexity of the etiologic aspects of endemic goiter; e.g., persistent endemic goiter which affects about 20 percent of schoolchildren in Colombia has been attributed to a goitrogenic agent in well water. However, despite these natural goitrogens or the possibility of genetically determined metabolic defects of thyroid hormone, studies have indicated that iodine is a highly effective agent for prevention of goiter.

Iodizing salt has been the most satisfactory method so far developed to provide populations with an adequate supply of iodine. Iodination of the water supply is effective but requires everyone to use a particular water supply. Iodized oil has been used successfully as an injectable form of goiter prophylaxis that lasts for three or more years. This form of goiter prophylaxis is particularly useful in less developed areas of endemic goiter, where distribution of iodized salt is difficult.

Iodine is more effective in preventing development of goiter than in suppressing an already enlarged thyroid gland. Early diffuse hyperplastic goiters may involute, but enlarged glands which have formed nodules and undergone cystic degeneration usually do not. After a diagnosis of cretinism is made, thyroid hormone therapy ensures an adequate hormone concentration, but the patient may not improve in growth or mentation and his or her behavior pattern may deteriorate.

Surgery may be indicated for goiter because of the large size (Fig. 11-6). The most important indication for surgery is pressure symptoms, which occur rarely in a goiter situated high up in the neck. Goiters that are low in the neck, intrathoracic goiters, or goiters that encircle the trachea are most likely to produce pressure symptoms.

Sporadic Goiter

Sporadic goiter can perhaps best be defined as goiter occurring in a non-endemic-goiter region. Although there are a number of known goitrogens and errors in thyroid hormone biosynthesis which may cause goiter, the majority of cases of sporadic goiter have no known etiology. The pathophysiology of sporadic goiter formation is presumably identical to that found in endemic goiter. Population studies have indicated that approximately 4 percent of individuals in a nonendemic area have thyroid nodules.[39] In autopsy studies

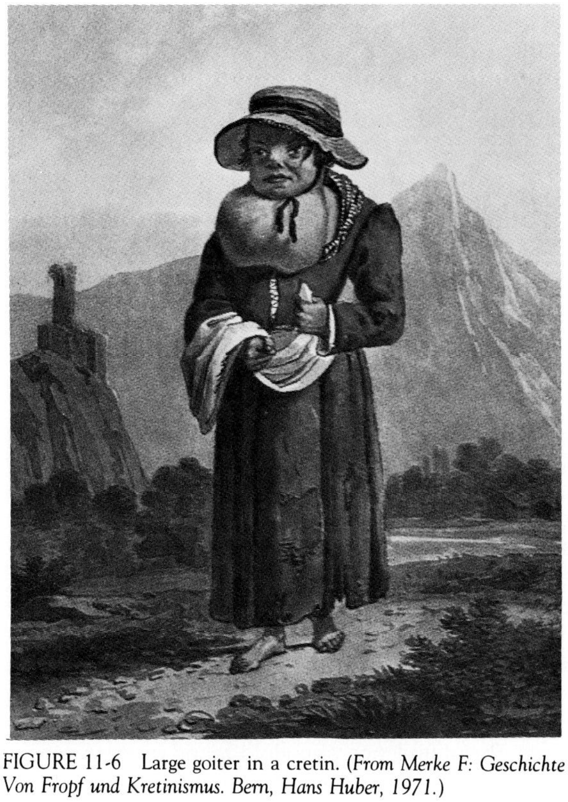

FIGURE 11-6 Large goiter in a cretin. (*From Merke F: Geschichte Von Fropf und Kretinismus. Bern, Hans Huber, 1971.*)

on unselected patients greater than 20 years of age, the incidence of nodules 1 cm or greater rose to 50 percent if the thyroid gland was sectioned serially.[40]

SEX AND AGE IN RELATION TO GOITER

Thyroid dysfunction of most kinds is approximately five times more common in females than in males, and goiter formation is no exception. Estrogens are an obvious source of this difference, but there is little evidence to support this possibility. In an effort to determine reasons for this sex difference, systematic comparisons of the development of the pituitary-thyroid axis in male and female rats were made.[41] Serum TSH concentration in adult male rats is 2.8 times higher than in females, but the serum T_4 concentration in males is 28 percent lower. Whether these findings are pertinent to the sex differences in human thyroid dysfunction remains to be determined.

Sporadic goiter does not usually occur before puberty. In endemic areas the highest incidence of goiter is found between ages 10 and 50; incidence decreases in later decades. In contrast, the incidence of sporadic goiter has no age peak. Frequently, the thyroid gland increases rapidly in size at the time of puberty, especially in girls. Whether this "physiologic" goiter represents relative thyroid hormone deficiency due to the stress of puberty is not clear, but the goiter tends to disappear subsequently without thyroid hormone therapy.

GENETIC INFLUENCES ON GOITER FORMATION

The suggestion has been made that, even in endemic goiter areas, those individuals who develop goiter are genetically distinct from nongoitrous individuals from the same area. In an endemic goiter region of Greece, a uniformly high thyroidal uptake of radioiodine occurred, but only certain individuals were goitrous.[42] Since these goiters were grouped within particular families, genetic factors might play a role in goiter formation. Goiter prevalence was compared in monozygotic and dizygotic twin pairs of like sex in order to obtain an index of the importance of inheritance in the etiology of goiter in healthy people.[43] The data suggested that a genetically determined tendency toward thyroid growth may exist. The suggestion that the goiter of puberty and pregnancy is a consequence of an increased requirement for thyroid hormone during a period of stress does not explain why only a minority of individuals develop the goiter. Nor does this hypothesis explain the results of radioiodine studies or the abundance of colloid found in most goiters of puberty.[44] The familial occurrence of thyroid disease in adolescents with the goiter of puberty again suggests a genetic predisposition.

A physiologic increase in thyroid size does appear to occur during some pregnancies. Histological examination of the typical thyroid gland during gestation reveals large follicles with abundant well-stained colloid and frequent vacuolation. Papillary infolding of thyroid follicles can be seen in 25 percent of cases, and the thyroid follicular cells are columnar rather than flat. All these findings reinforce the impression of thyroid hyperplasia. This histological picture is one of active formation and secretion of thyroid hormone.

In a study of pregnant women in Scotland, goiter was considered to be present if the thyroid gland was both palpable and visible.[45] By these criteria, 70 percent of pregnant women had goiter, compared with 38 percent of nonpregnant women. The prevalence of goiter did not appear to be affected by previous parity, since goiter occurred in 39 percent of nulliparous women and 35 percent of nongravid parous women. Thyroid enlargement occurred in each trimester with the same frequency, suggesting that goiter appears early and persists during pregnancy. When the same study was repeated in Iceland, no increase in goiter was found during pregnancy.[46] The difference in goiter incidence during pregnancy between the two countries was attributed to differences in dietary iodine content. Renal clearance of iodine is increased during pregnancy as a consequence of the increased glomerular filtration rate. Plasma inorganic iodine concentration decreases because more iodine is excreted in the urine and less is available for thyroid hormone biosynthesis. To compensate, the thyroid gland may enlarge and clear more plasma of iodine to ensure adequate thyroid hormone biosynthesis. Therefore, in areas of marginal iodine intake, pregnancy would be more likely to lead to goiter formation. A study done in the United States indicated that there was no significant difference in iodine balance between pregnant and nonpregnant women.[47] The high-iodine diet in North America may vitiate the increased iodine loss during pregnancy, and goiter is apparently not significantly more common during pregnancy.[48]

SPECIFIC INHERITED DEFECTS IN THYROID HORMONE BIOSYNTHESIS

The clearest examples of genetic influences on thyroid function and goiter formation are found in a small group of individuals with hypothyroidism and goiter. These persons have inherited specific autosomal recessive defects in hormone synthesis (Fig. 11-7). These defects lead to inadequate thyroid hormone production, which results in prolonged stimulation of TSH release, in some cases leading to an enlarged sella. The

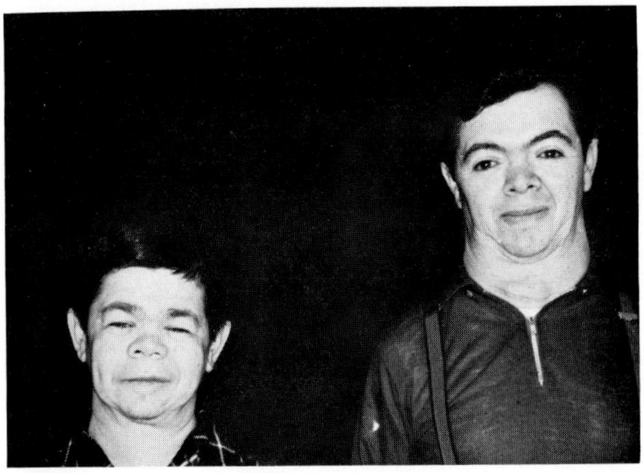

FIGURE 11-7 Two brothers with goitrous cretinism, due to a defect in thyroglobulin synthesis.

TSH hypersecretion leads to intense thyroid gland hyperplasia and goiter; the hyperplasia can be mistaken for malignancy. In fact, thyroid malignancy is uncommon in these patients.[49] These conditions apparently occur because of genetic defects of single enzymes or other proteins, presumably corresponding to each step in thyroid hormone biosynthesis (see Chap. 10). Recombinant DNA techniques should permit more intensive examination of the nature of these defects.[50]

As indicated in Fig. 11-8, there are five recognized defects in thyroid hormone biosynthesis, but it is almost certain that there are many more:

1. There may be a defect in the ability of the thyroid gland to trap iodine.
2. A defect may exist in the ability of the gland to convert inorganic iodide to an organic form, as an iodotyrosine. This defect is characterized by precipitate discharge of radioactive iodine from the thyroid after administration of thiocyanate or perchlorate; it may be associated with deafness. This is a heterogeneous group of defects related to the peroxidase system and associated with the various steps in organification.
3. Thyroid hormone is synthesized within the interstices of the very large thyroglobulin molecule. Defects in thyroglobulin synthesis lead to inadequate or absent thyroid hormone synthesis. This probably reflects a large, heterogeneous group of defects. Although no proof exists, a number of cases of sporadic goiter may in fact represent minor defects in thyroglobulin synthesis.
4. There may be coupling defects. These may be due to a variety of defects which impair iodothyronine formation.
5. The iodotyrosine deiodinase defect results in iodine loss from the gland. The enzyme usually deiodinates the iodotyrosines which have not coupled to form iodothyronines, which allows the iodine to be reused within the gland.

In addition to the defects listed above, there may be an impaired tissue response to TSH or to thyroid hormones (see Chap. 10). However, the former condition would not cause goiter. Whatever the specific defect, genetic influences lead to inadequate thyroid hormone production and goiter formation. Whether similar but less well defined genetic influences play a role in sporadic goiter remains to be determined.

SPECIFIC GOITROGENS

Any substance which interferes with the biosynthesis of thyroid hormone can be a goitrogen. This includes a number of chemical compounds which inhibit spe-

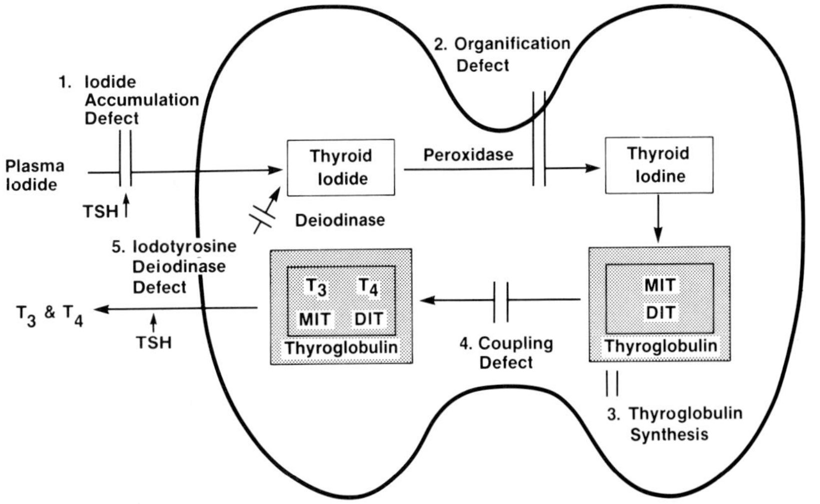

FIGURE 11-8 Defects in thyroid hormone biosynthesis.

cific steps of thyroid hormone biosynthesis, as well as dietary goitrogens in which the active compound is unknown.

Dietary Goitrogens

The development of antithyroid drug therapy began with the observation that rabbits fed cabbage developed goiters and, subsequently, that goiters developed in rats fed seeds of brassicas (cabbage, turnips, brussel sprouts, rutabagas, etc.).[51] This finding led to the appreciation of thiourea as a goitrogen and eventually to the introduction of thioamides as valuable therapeutic agents in hyperthyroidism. The quantity of the goitrogen, and perhaps the quality of the vegetables containing the goitrogen, are such that the chance of significant goiter formation in human beings is rare. Soybean milk has been observed to produce goiter in infants. The goitrogenic substance in soybean flour has not been identified, but supplementing the diet with iodide eliminates the problem. Certain foods like cassava contain compounds that on hydrolysis release free cyanide. After ingestion, the cyanide is converted to thiocyanate. Cassava has been suggested as a cause for endemic goiter in central Africa.[32] In Colombia, sulfur-containing compounds found in the water supply, which are derived from sedimentary rocks, are thought to be goitrogenic.[52]

Chemical Goitrogens

Various chemical goitrogens ranging from salts and minerals to complex nitrogen-containing heterocyclic compounds interfere with the synthesis of thyroid hormone (Table 11-4). Salts and minerals of interest include lithium, which has an inhibitory effect on the release of thyroid hormone, and cobalt, the action of which is unclear. The more complex chemical compounds which interfere with thyroid function by blocking iodination and the coupling reaction show some common structural features. None of the nitrogen heterocycles is as potent as the thioamides, e.g., propylthiouracil, but there is no apparent fundamental difference in their antithyroid action.

Table 11-4. Chemical Goitrogens

Effect within the Thyroid
Modifiers of iodine transport: complex anions: technetium perchlorate, thiocyanate (active principle of *Brassica* spp. and cassava)
Modifiers of iodination of thyroglobulin:
Thioamides: propylthiouracil, methimazole, carbimazole
Thiocyanate
Aniline derivatives: sulfonamides, *p*-aminosalicylic acid, amphenone B, aminoglutethimide, phenylbutazone
Effects on iodothyronine formation:
Thioamides
Sulfonamides
Influences on secretion of thyroid hormone:
Iodide
Lithium
Effect on Peripheral Disposal of Thyroid Hormone
Hormone deiodination: propylthiouracil, iopanoate, ipodate, amiodarone
Intestinal absorption of hormones: soy flour, resins (e.g., cholestyramine)
Hormone inactivation: inducers of hepatic drug-metabolizing enzymes (e.g., phenobarbital)

Environmental Goitrogens

Pollution of drinking water is known to precipitate goiter in low-iodine areas. McGarrison noted that goiter prevalence increased downstream from the water supply in a group of villages which make up Gilgit in the foothills of the Himalayans.[53] Goiter occurred in 12 percent of the inhabitants at the source; prevalence increased to 45 percent at the terminus of the river, which had served as a drinking channel and open sewer for the villages on its banks. McGarrison was able to produce goiter in himself and his colleagues by ingesting suspended matter from these goiter-producing waters.[53] The goiter did not occur if the water was boiled first. In subsequent studies, low urinary iodine excretion (4 to 6 μg/liter) was found in residents of this area, but equally low levels were found in both goitrous and nongoitrous individuals.

Nontoxic Goiter

Whatever the cause, both endemic and sporadic goiters present clinically as nontoxic goiters and, depending on duration, may be either diffuse or nodular. Some goiters which may be associated with hyperthyroidism were considered in Chap. 10. More frequently, some of the nodules may be autonomous, i.e., no longer responsive to normal pituitary-thyroid regulation.

INCIDENCE

The incidence of nontoxic goiter varies widely depending on whether goiter is endemic in the area. The discussion here centers on nonendemic areas like North America. The occurrence of goiter has been determined in both autopsy and clinical studies. In an unselected autopsy series of 1000 patients over 20 years old, the prevalence of goiter was 5 percent. Half the thyroids, when sectioned, contained nodules which were at least 1 cm across and would have been palpable if they had been anterior and superficial.[40] The study was carried out in Minnesota, which was an endemic goiter region before the introduction of iodine, and goiter may still be more common in these regions. However, similar results were found in Connecticut, a non-endemic-goiter area.[54]

PRESENTATION AND COMPLICATIONS

Nontoxic goiter is usually discovered during a routine examination. Occasionally, the patient will have noticed a lump in the throat. Rarely, the goiter may be symptomatic and cause pressure symptoms such as coughing, wheezing, dysphagia, or hoarseness. The last presentation is uncommon, so carcinoma of the thyroid or an unrelated condition could be ruled out. These symptoms are more likely to occur, with the exception of carcinoma, in a long-standing goiter low in the neck which is compressed by the sternum or which grows around behind the trachea. X-rays of the trachea may show deviation or even some compression. CT scanning of the thyroid may be helpful.[55] However, peak inspiratory and expiratory flow studies should be done to determine whether there is a decrease in airflow. Upper airway obstruction may actually be more common than realized.[56] Such obstruction is potentially dangerous because tracheitis with edema could result in severe compromise of the airway.[57] Occasionally, the thyroid may suddenly increase in size accompanied by pain and tenderness. This sudden change is often indicative of hemorrhage into a cystic area of the nodular goiter; it usually subsides within several weeks.

Complaints of a "lump in the throat" are most often due to globus hystericus, an anxiety reaction characterized by a constrictive feeling in the throat. This feeling is heightened by the presence of a nontoxic goiter, which presents a difficult problem for a physician. Patients frequently describe fluctuation in goiter size, often related to periods of emotional stress or to the menstrual cycle, but these changes are almost impossible to document. The position and irregular shape of the thyroid have made it difficult to estimate the size of the gland accurately over a period of time. The thyroid does have a rich blood supply, and changes in blood flow might change the volume of the gland. The ancient Romans are reputed to have believed that the thyroid gland swelled with sexual excitement; they used to measure the bride's neck as evidence that the marriage had been consummated.[58]

RISK OF CARCINOMA IN MULTINODULAR GOITER

One of the undesirable side effects of cancer education programs is that discovery of a "lump" frequently means cancer to the patient. Thus, the patient with a multinodular goiter is often very anxious, which may make the physician anxious enough to recommend surgery. If the patient demands that the physician guarantee that the thyroid nodule is not malignant, the demand can be met only if the nodule is excised and examined histologically. The decision to remove a thyroid nodule is thus a result of both the patient's and the physician's anxiety. Since as many as 50 percent of thyroid glands in adults may harbor a nodule 1 cm or greater, physicians must know exactly how suspicious they should be about the possibility of carcinoma occurring in a nontoxic multinodular goiter. (The solitary thyroid nodule is considered separately below.)

The questions to be answered are (1) what is the risk of thyroid carcinoma in the general population? and (2) does the presence of a nontoxic goiter increase this risk?

In two separate series of unselected autopsies, thyroid carcinoma was found in approximately 3 percent of the patients.[39,53] More recently, autopsy studies in Japan and Minnesota have indicated a prevalence of small histological malignancies in the thyroid as high as 17 percent when serial sections were carefully examined.[59] In contrast, the frequency of clinical thyroid cancer is about 39 cases diagnosed annually per 1 million population, or 0.0004 percent.[60] The reason for the marked discrepancy between histological and clinically apparent thyroid carcinoma is not clear. However, the histological diagnosis of small thyroid malignancies (minimal papillary thyroid carcinoma) does not appear to correlate with true invasiveness. Similar relationships have been found with prostatic carcinoma, where the incidence of the disease is much higher at autopsy than is clinically apparent during life.

The important question is whether the presence of a nontoxic goiter increases the incidence of clinically important thyroid cancer. The mortality rate for thyroid carcinoma was 10 times higher in Switzerland, where goiter is endemic, than in England.[61] Furthermore, as the use of iodized salt increased in Switzerland, deaths from thyroid carcinoma decreased. The difficulty with this type of study is that a higher rate of thyroid surgery with careful pathological examination may have resulted in the increased diagnosis of thyroid cancer. If the prevalence of goiter is based on medical examinations of draftees for World War I and II, and this difference is compared with the prevalence of thyroid carcinoma and hyperthyroidism, an estimate of the effect of goiter on thyroid carcinoma could be made.[27] The reduction in goiter prevalence between World War I and World War II was associated with the introduction of iodized salt. Despite the decrease in goiter frequency, the death rate for thyroid carcinoma changed very little during this time. Hyperthyroidism mortality rates increased immediately after the introduction of iodized salt, perhaps owing to the iod-Basedow phenomenon, and then decreased in parallel with the decrease in goiter. The comparison of goiter prevalence with hyperthyroidism strongly supports the hypothesis that endemic goiter is an important factor in the pathogenesis of hyperthyroidism. In contrast, comparison of thyroid cancer and goiter failed to provide convincing evidence for the existence of an association between these two diseases.

Thyroid malignancy can be induced experimentally in rats by prolonged TSH stimulation, but there is no convincing evidence that TSH stimulation is carcinogenic in normal individuals.[62,63] Although there are several reports of congenital goiters which have been intensely hyperplastic and have developed carcinomas, the intensely hyperplastic gland may also be mistaken for malignancy.[64,65] The balance of evidence seems to indicate that presence of goiter per se does not predispose to thyroid carcinoma.

LABORATORY EVALUATION

When a patient presents with a goiter, the questions to be asked are whether the goiter is toxic or nontoxic. If the goiter is nontoxic, is thyroiditis the cause? Is the goiter diffuse or nodular and is the nodule solitary or multiple? If the gland is nodular, are the nodules autonomous?

Evaluation of thyroid function is described in detail in Chap. 10. Patients with goiter should have a serum T_4 determination, resin T_3 uptake test, and assay for thyroid antibodies to determine the functional thyroid state and the presence of thyroiditis. A radioisotopic thyroid scan may be helpful in identifying nodularity and autonomy, but is not necessary.

THERAPY

Is the presence of goiter sufficient indication for thyroid hormone suppressive therapy? All goiters should be suppressed with thyroid hormone, with the exception of self-limited conditions like the goiters of puberty and of pregnancy. However, it is true that treatment of long-standing goiter may not result in a decrease in gland size because of the presence of fibrosis.

If the goiter is not large initially or is fibrotic and probably will not decrease in size, should the patient be subjected to long-term thyroid hormone therapy? Prolonged TSH stimulation results in dilated capillaries, which may rupture and result in a hemorrhagic cyst (Fig. 11-9). Furthermore, prolonged TSH stimulation may eventually lead to nodule formation. The presence of a thyroid nodule often makes both patient

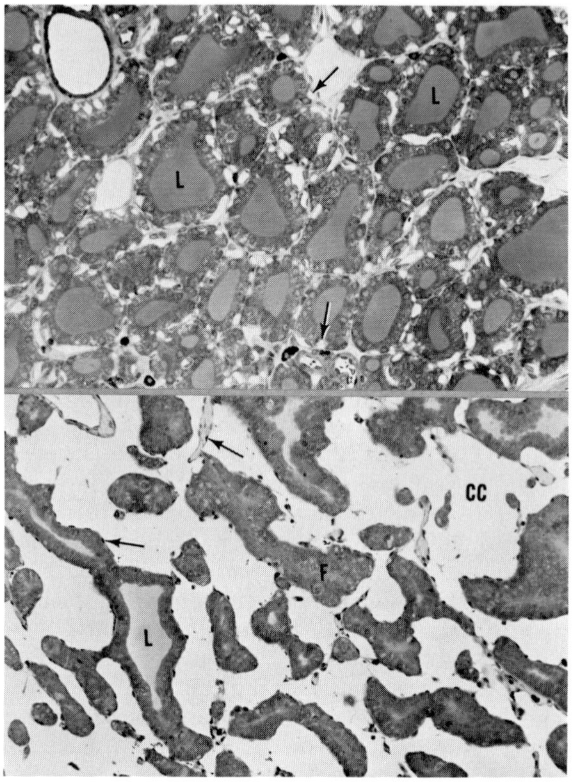

FIGURE 11-9 Histological sections of rat thyroid gland showing the gross increase in vascular space that occurs when animals are fed thiouracil, presumably reflecting TSH stimulation. Thyroid glands were fixed by perfusion; the white spaces are the interior of capillaries. *(Top)* Normal young adult rat. A large number of closely spaced follicles with lumens (L) are present. There are many small capillaries (arrows), most cut in cross section, around each follicle. The capillaries are approximately 5 μm in diameter. 220 ×. *(Bottom)* Young adult rat fed 0.25% thiouracil in low-iodine diet for 100 days. Follicles (F) are widely spaced and lumens (L) are generally narrowed. The space between follicles is the lumen of a cavernous capillary system (CC). Note the continuous line of flat, densely stained endothelial cell nuclei (arrows) on the basal surface of the follicle and on the other surface of connective tissue partitions, indicating that follicles and connective tissue partitions are covered with a continuous sheet of endothelium. The diameter of the cavernous capillary space is very variable; a single representative figure might be about 70 μm. 130 ×. *(Courtesy of SH Wollman.)*

and physician anxious and may lead ineluctably to the operating table.

The philosophy behind the tendency to treat all goiters with thyroid hormone is further predicated on the relatively low cost (only pennies per day) and relative lack of toxicity. A more toxic drug would have to be used much more carefully. Such long-term therapy is therefore recommended, with the caveat that autonomous areas of the goiter may be present which are not suppressible, resulting in too much circulating thyroid hormone. For this reason, thyroid function tests should be performed again 3 or 4 weeks after the initiation of therapy. A radioisotopic thyroid scan is not necessary.

Evaluation of Therapy

Despite the large number of patients receiving thyroid hormone suppression, there are relatively few large controlled studies which have examined carefully the efficacy of such treatment.[66–70] Two hundred and thirty patients with nontoxic goiter were each treated with 180 mg of desiccated thyroid and were observed at intervals of 1 to 3 months.[66] The goiter was regarded as diffuse if the entire gland was enlarged, even if the two lobes differed in size, or there was considerable irregularity in the shape of the gland. The goiter was called nodular only when conspicuous nodules were prominent or when a single nodule was found in an enlarged thyroid. A single nodule was diagnosed when there was an isolated nodule in an otherwise normal gland. Regression of the goiter with therapy was considered to be complete when the thyroid decreased to normal size. The response to therapy was called "moderate" for any unequivocal regression short of a complete response. The results, shown in Table 11-5, indicate that in one-fourth of patients with nodular goiter complete regression occurred and in one-half there was moderate regression.

Table 11-5. Response of Nontoxic Goiter to Thyroid Hormone Therapy. Usual Dose of 180 μg of Desiccated Thyroid Hormone Administered for Periods Ranging from 1 to More than 24 Months

Type of goiter	No. of patients	Percent with each level of response: Complete	Moderate	None
Diffuse	115	33	34	23
Nodular	78	24	52	24
Solitary nodule	37	27	27	46

Source: Astwood et al.[66]

Table 11-6. Response of Nontoxic Goiter to Therapy with Thyroxine and L-Triiodothyronine

Thyroid hormone	Decrease in goiter size, %: 12 weeks	28 weeks
T_3	55	73
T_4	39	49

Source: Shimaoka and Sokal.[68]

The effects of L-thyroxine and L-triiodothyronine were studied for their suppressive effect in 114 patients with goiter.[68] Five patients had diffuse goiters, 38 had multinodular goiters, and 71 had uninodular goiters on palpation. The patients were assigned randomly to T_3 (50 μg per day) or T_4 (200 μg per day) treatment groups. At the end of 12 weeks, patients with a significant reduction in goiter size (greater than 20 percent) continued to receive the same dose of the same thyroid hormone for 16 weeks. Patients who did not have a significant change in goiter size either were continued at the same dose or the suppressive dose of the drug was doubled, i.e., 100 μg per day of T_3 or 400 μg per day of T_4. The results are shown in Table 11-6. The duration of treatment rather than the dose of thyroid hormone was the major determinant of a decrease in goiter size. Responses among the patients who continued to receive thyroid hormone at the same dose were just as common as among those receiving the higher dose.

Thyroid Hormone Therapy

To decrease the size of the thyroid gland, sufficient thyroid hormone has to be given to suppress TSH secretion without inducing hyperthyroidism. Therapy with L-triiodothyronine results in markedly elevated serum levels of the hormone for several hours following ingestion. Although there is no evidence that the transient serum elevations of triiodothyronine in an otherwise healthy individual are harmful, it seems best to avoid these elevations if possible. Consequently, L-thyroxine should be used, since the hormone is slowly converted to triiodothyronine and elevated serum concentrations of T_3 do not occur. Triiodothyronine is less effective in maintaining TSH suppression.[13] Studies of TSH concentrations in hypothyroid women receiving L-thyroxine indicated that 90 percent of patients were optimally managed, as indicated by normal serum TSH concentration, by the daily administration of between 100 and 200 μg of L-thyroxine.[71] As mentioned previously, the presence of an autonomous nodule might result in excessive circulating thyroid hormone. The administration of 300 μg of T_4 daily has resulted in metabolic alterations suggestive of subclinical hyperthyroidism.[72] Older patients require less thyroid hormone, usually only 100 or 125 μg of T_4 daily.[73]

SOLITARY THYROID NODULES

Although the risk of thyroid carcinoma does not appear to be increased in patients with multinodular goiter, the risk is increased with the solitary thyroid nodule. In a series of 300 unselected autopsies of adults, 19 single thyroid nodules, or 6 percent, were found after sectioning of the gland.[54] The chance that a solitary thyroid nodule in this series would be a neoplasm, benign or malignant, was almost three times the number of neoplasms found in the entire group. The frequency of thyroid carcinoma in single nodules was almost four times the frequency in the entire series. Despite the difficulty in separating single from multiple thyroid nodules clinically, thyroid cancer has thus been found more frequently in the solitary thyroid nodule. Since thyroid carcinoma usually does not concentrate radioiodine as well as normal tissue, malignant thyroid nodules commonly appear as hypofunctioning or nonfunctioning ("cold") areas on a radioactive iodine scan of the thyroid gland.[74] However, it must be emphasized that thyroid carcinoma also occurs in functioning nodules, and the presence of a functioning thyroid nodule does not eliminate the possibility of malignancy. In one series of 202 patients with solitary thyroid nodules, there was an overall prevalence of thyroid carcinoma of 29 percent.[75] If cold solitary thyroid nodules had been the sole criterion for selection for surgery, 40 percent of the carcinomas would have been missed.

One of the major problems in estimating the risk of malignancies in thyroid nodules is to eliminate bias in case selection. This was attempted by studying patients with thyroid nodules who were referred for radioisotopic scan of the thyroid gland.[76] Presumably, most physicians in the community would obtain a radioisotopic scan before making any therapeutic decision. Solitary cold thyroid nodules were present in 130 patients; 68 of these patients came to thyroid surgery. Thyroid carcinoma was found in 18 percent of patients at surgery (Fig. 11-10). Factors that determined which patients were referred for surgery were impossible to ascertain, despite the study design. However, even if no further malignancies were found, the incidence of thyroid carcinoma in these presumably unselected patients with solitary cold thyroid nodules would have been about 9 percent.

Factors Predisposing to Thyroid Cancer

If there is an increased risk of malignancy in solitary cold thyroid nodules, are there criteria available to select those patients at higher risk?

GENDER

As mentioned earlier, most forms of thyroid disease are more common in females; this is true of thyroid

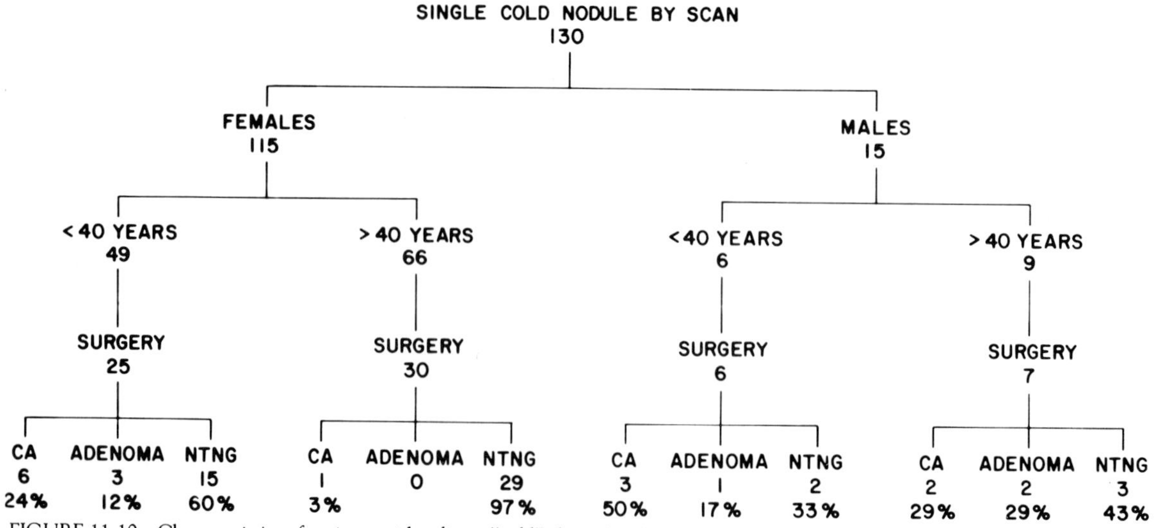

FIGURE 11-10 Characteristics of patients with solitary "cold" thyroid nodules on radioisotopic scan, number undergoing surgery, and frequencies of different end points. The number of individuals in each subgroup is shown. CA, carcinoma; NTNG, nontoxic nodular goiter. (*From Burrow et al.*[76])

malignancy as well. However, the male/female ratio is higher in nontoxic nodular goiter than in most other forms of thyroid disease. As a consequence, a solitary thyroid nodule occurring in a male is three times more likely to be malignant than a solitary nodule occurring in a female.

AGE

It has been estimated that one-half the thyroid nodules appearing in children may be malignant. The implication is not that thyroid cancer is more common in childhood but rather that thyroid nodules in general are uncommon in this age group. Eighty percent of the children with carcinoma of the thyroid who formed the basis of this estimate had a history of exposure to radiation.[77,78] The chance of malignancy in the thyroid nodule of children needs to be reappraised now that this type of irradiation has been practically discontinued.

In one study of 30 children with solitary thyroid nodules, only 4 children had a history of neck irradiation.[79] Nevertheless, there was a 40 percent incidence of carcinoma in the series, including the four irradiated children. These data suggest that thyroid carcinoma continues to be a significant risk in children with solitary thyroid nodules. However, in a study of 5179 schoolchildren in grades 6 through 12, nodularity of the thyroid was found in 93 (1.8 percent).[80] The nodularity represented adolescent goiter in 34 children and thyroiditis in 31. Only two thyroid cancers were found, which raised the question whether all thyroid nodules in children need to be removed surgically. However, 5 of 14 children with solitary thyroid nodules operated on in New York over a 10-year period had thyroid cancer without any history of external radiation.[81] Nodules that proved to be neoplasms were usually discrete, solitary, and of firm consistency and were unassociated with changes in the rest of the thyroid.

PREVIOUS IRRADIATION OF THE HEAD AND NECK

Previous irradiation of the head and neck markedly increases the chances of malignancy in a thyroid nodule. The observation in 1950 that 9 of 28 children with carcinoma of the thyroid had received radiotherapy to the thymus in infancy first highlighted this association, which was later confirmed in prospective studies.[82,83] Most instances of thyroid malignancy following neck irradiation were reported within 10 years after radiation therapy. Since this type of radiation therapy to the neck has been discontinued, a degree of complacency had developed among many physicians. However, recent reports indicating an increased incidence of thyroid carcinoma an average of 25 years after radiation exposure of the head and neck have dispelled this illusion.[84,85] Although radiation therapy for benign diseases of infancy and childhood was discontinued many years ago, the occurrence of radiation-associated thyroid carcinoma has apparently not declined.

Despite direct questioning, few patients with a thyroid nodule were able to give a history of irradiation during infancy. Public awareness increased dramatically after the relationship was featured in a television drama. This increased awareness was largely due to the fact that mothers are more knowledgeable than their children about medical history. (Perhaps all patients regardless of age should bring their mothers with them for the initial visit to the physician's office!)

The magnitude of the increase in thyroid carcinoma after irradiation to the neck is unknown, because appropriate age-matched control data are scanty. However, the increase in thyroid carcinoma is significant, and estimates have ranged from a twofold to a 100-fold increase in the frequency of thyroid cancer. In patients with a history of head and neck irradiation, only one-third had abnormal thyroid findings.[85] Carcinoma occurred in 37 percent of single nodules found on physical examination. Whether radioisotopic thyroid scans improve diagnostic capabilities is not clear.[86] Patients who had received head and neck radiation also had an increased incidence of other head and neck tumors, including parathyroid adenomas.[87] Probably any x-ray exposure has some carcinogenic potential. Previous irradiation to the thyroid is considered further under Thyroid Carcinoma, below.

PHYSICAL CHARACTERISTICS

Careful examination of the thyroid can be extremely helpful in determining how suspicious to be of underlying malignancy. A history of recent thyroid growth, dysphagia, or dyspnea should make the examiner suspicious of malignancy. Palpation of the thyroid should be done carefully, with particular attention to how regular and hard the nodule is, whether the gland is fixed to surrounding structures, and whether there are palpable regional lymph nodes. On the other hand, the presence of a multinodular goiter decreases the likelihood of malignancy.

A group of 53 patients with thyroid nodules were first classified clinically as to whether their nodules were benign or malignant, and these results were compared with the findings at surgery.[88] Thyroid cancer was found in 76 percent of cases thought to be malignant nodules clinically; 12 percent of cases thought to be benign clinically but symptomatic as indicated by pain, recent change in goiter size, or dysphagia; and 3 percent of patients whose nodules were thought to be benign and who were asymptomatic. In this particular study, only two patients with thyroid carcinoma were free of symptoms.

The most important physical sign of thyroid malignancy is the presence of a hard, irregular, thyroid nodule. Extreme hardness may be due to hemorrhage into a cyst with subsequent calcification. If the thyroid cancer has spread beyond the capsule and invaded surrounding structures, the clinical diagnosis becomes comparatively simple, although Riedel's struma (see Chap. 10) can also extend beyond the gland. Fixation to the strap muscles, trachea, or larynx is easily detected on physical examination. Recurrent laryngeal nerve paralysis is not a common presenting symptom in thyroid cancer but does occur.

Laboratory Diagnosis

The presence of a solitary thyroid nodule raises the question of thyroid malignancy, and the above predisposing factors may strengthen or allay suspicions about the individual patient. The next step in the evaluation of the solitary thyroid nodule is to use the laboratory to further discriminate which nodules may be malignant and which may be benign.

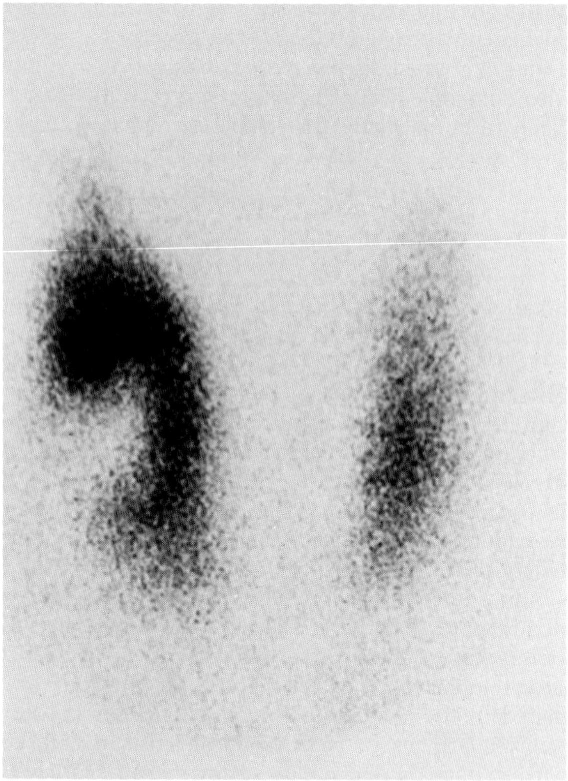

FIGURE 11-11 Radioisotopic scan of solitary nodules. A nonfunctioning solitary nodule is seen occupying lower pole of the right lobe of the thyroid.

RADIOISOTOPIC SCAN OF THE THYROID

Scanning of the thyroid after the administration of a tracer dose of radioactive iodine or technetium 99m permits the delineation of functioning and nonfunctioning areas of the thyroid (Fig. 11-11). Since even well-differentiated thyroid carcinomas do not concentrate iodine as efficiently as the normal thyroid, hypofunctioning, or cold, thyroid nodules have been considered to harbor a greater risk of malignancy. This classification is established by assessing the amount of radioactivity within the nodule relative to that in extranodular tissue. To be detectable under optimal conditions, the cold nodule must be at least approximately 1 cm in diameter. Large nodules may produce a well-defined focal defect, marginal indentation, or locally reduced parenchymal activity. Demonstration of a cold thyroid nodule is significant but unfortunately nonspecific. The majority of clinically significant thyroid nodules are less functional than the extranodular thyroid tissue.[89]

Iodine 131 has been the radionuclide most widely used for thyroid imaging, although the high radiation doses absorbed have been recognized with concern. This concern has heightened with the recurrence of interest in the delayed effects of neck irradiation.[90] The administration of 100 μCi of ^{131}I for a thyroid scan can result in a dose of 80 rads to the thyroid.[91] Since several scans would raise the dose of radiation delivered to the thyroid to a level which has been associated with subsequent thyroid cancer, alternative methods of thyroid imaging are highly desirable.

Iodine 123 is perhaps the ideal isotope for in vivo diagnostic studies of thyroid function and structure. The short half-life, 13.3 h, is suitable for routine uptake tests. Scans superior in resolution to those afforded by ^{99m}Tc or ^{131}I can be obtained with a radiation dose $^1/_{85}$ that for a comparable ^{131}I study. However, high-purity ^{123}I is not generally available, and, in its absence, technetium 99m is probably the most readily available isotope of choice for thyroid scanning at present. Technetium 99m delivers about 0.6 rads to the thyroid during a scanning procedure. The pertechnetate ion ($^{99m}TcO_4^-$) is rapidly trapped by the thyroid but is not organically bound and does not remain in the gland. The difference between the technetium and iodine radioisotopes has clinical significance because some thyroid malignancies trap pertechnetate but not ^{131}I, due to a defect in organification.[92]

The findings in most studies have been consistent with the physiologic considerations discussed above. Most of the thyroid cancers were found to be cold, but benign thyroid nodules are also predominantly cold. This lack of discrimination makes it difficult to use the thyroid scan to differentiate between benign and malignant thyroid nodules. Certainly, no patient with a solitary thyroid nodule should be either selected for surgery or screened from surgical consideration by a thyroid scan, although the scan would be helpful in eliminating the minority of solitary nodules with increased radioisotope uptake from serious consideration of malignancy.

ULTRASOUND

A cold nodule on thyroid imaging may represent either a solid nodule that does not trap the radionuclide or a cystic area in the gland. Diagnostic ultrasound employs acoustic properties to distinguish different soft tissues by passing ultrahigh sound frequencies into the nodule and analyzing the reflected echoes. The diagnostic principle is based on the partial reflection of ultrasound at boundaries or tissue interfaces. Analysis of ultrasound echoes may permit distinction of solid from cystic nodules. In solid thyroid nodules, multiple echoes are generated with high sensitivity levels, but this does not occur in a thyroid cyst.

The recording may involve analysis of a thin beam of sound as echo spikes, i.e., *A mode,* or a number of beams may be incorporated to form a two-dimensional image, i.e., *B mode.* The thyroid gland is not as acoustically dense as the surrounding tissue; tracheal cartilage represents the densest structure in the area (Fig. 11-12). Not only can solid and cystic thyroid nodules be distinguished, but enlargement of the thyroid due to tumor growth can also be differentiated from enlargement due to cystic or hemorrhagic degeneration.[93] The thyroid's volume can also be estimated by ultrasound.[69]

Cysts have been reported to occur in 20 percent of solitary thyroid nodules.[94] Although the possibility of malignancy is significant, particularly in a partially cystic lesion, malignancy is less common than in solid lesions. Thyroid hormone suppression has not been found to be helpful in preventing recurrence of benign cysts after initial aspiration.[95] Successful sclerosis of a recurrent thyroid cyst with injected tetracycline has been reported but is not indicated in the great majority of cases.[96] The use of ultrasound to evaluate solitary nodules over 4 cm is limited because

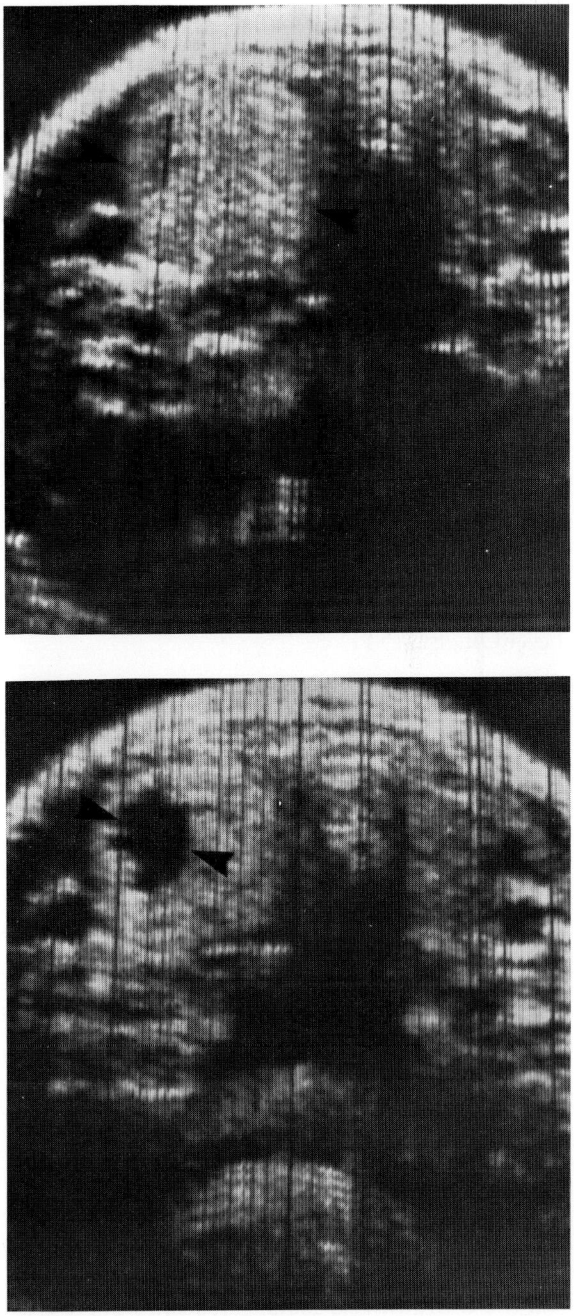

FIGURE 11-12 Ultrasound scan of solitary thyroid nodules. *Top:* Solid nodule. *Bottom:* Cystic nodule.

both solid and cystic lesions give rise to heterogeneous echoes. Small nodules are also difficult, and cystic lesions less than 1 cm in diameter may not be identified. Substernal goiters are difficult to study because the sternum reflects the sound. Despite the useful information that can be obtained, ultrasound does not differentiate between benign and malignant thyroid nodules.

OTHER IMAGING TECHNIQUES

Thyroid imaging techniques other than radioisotopic scan and ultrasound are available. The high Z number (i.e., radiographic density) of the thyroid has facilitated the use of the CT scan with or without prior loading with stable iodine.[55] However, the patient receives more radiation to the thyroid and the resolution of nodules is probably no better than with ultrasound. With growing interest in nuclear magnetic resonance (NMR) as an imaging technique, a study was conducted to show that NMR techniques are feasible in the detection of thyroid disease;[97] this technique may come into clincal use. Since the thyroid gland has a rich blood supply, angiography can be helpful in conjunction with other findings but is primarily of academic interest.[98]

THYROID BIOPSY

Although various diagnostic procedures may heighten suspicion that a particular solitary thyroid nodule is malignant, only a tissue diagnosis can ultimately diagnose or exclude thyroid cancer. Needle biopsy of the thyroid had been considered as an alternative to surgery, but fear that cancer might be disseminated along the track delayed acceptance of this procedure.[99,100] Spread of malignant cells has proved not to be a problem, and fine-needle aspiration biopsy of the thyroid has gained wide acceptance.[99,100] The most difficult thyroid lesions to diagnose are follicular carcinomas, because their identification often rests on the demonstration of vascular and capsular invasion. The small amount of tissue obtained means these areas may be missed. Lymphomas may be confused with thyroiditis.[101,102] Papillary carcinoma, on the other hand, usually is easily identified because of its unique histological characteristics.

Since the majority of patients who have had a biopsy of the thyroid do not have a subsequent thyroidectomy, comparison of the biopsy specimen with the entire thyroid gland is frequently impossible. In a series of 81 cases in which 93 percent of cutting needle biopsy diagnoses were confirmed by thyroid surgery, the errors were due to lymphoma complicating Hashimoto's disease, undifferentiated carcinoma diagnosed as nonspecific thyroiditis, and follicular carcinoma mistaken for follicular adenoma.[100] No serious complications occurred with the needle biopsy procedure, and in none of the primary cancers was there evidence of tumor implantation in the needle track. There was a single example of seeding in a renal cell carcinoma metastatic to the thyroid. If there is significant clinical suspicion of thyroid cancer, a negative needle biopsy should not deter immediate surgery. Thyroid biopsy with a cutting needle provides more tissue for examination but has the potential for more complications; this has made many physicians cautious about the procedure.

Fine-needle aspiration biopsy avoids the morbidity that may occur with cutting needles like the Vim-Silverman, and has become the determining factor in the management of the solitary thyroid nodule (Fig. 11-13).[103] In a review of 1330 patients, all of whom underwent surgery, 22 cases were diagnosed as negative by aspiration biopsy but were found to be malignant at surgery, an incidence of false negatives of 1.7 percent.[104] In the same study, the false-positive incidence was 0.5 percent. The diagnosis of malignancy by fine-needle aspiration biopsy had a specificity of 0.99 and a sensitivity of 0.73[100] (sensitivity measures the fraction of patients with thyroid cancer that is detected by the biopsy while specificity measures the fraction of patients correctly identified as having no thyroid malignancy). The results of the various diagnostic techniques for detecting thyroid cancer can be expressed according to Bayes' theorem, to give the predictive value of a positive test (Fig. 11-14).[105]

In the same study, three strategies were studied for diagnosis of thyroid nodules. Two began with a radioisotopic thyroid scan followed, if positive, by either aspirate biopsy or ultrasound; the third began with aspiration biopsy followed by scan.[103] The last was most cost-effective. Fine-needle aspiration biopsy was the most successful of the available tests when applied alone. Neither radioisotopic scan of the thyroid nor ultrasound has high specificity. Combination of the two procedures yields the highest sensitivity but does not improve specificity.

The use of needle biopsy in one large series of 455 patients with thyroid nodules decreased the number of patients sent to surgery by half and doubled the number of patients to be observed.[106] Operation for benign disease decreased 70 percent while thyroid carcinoma identified at operation increased 75 percent.[107] The accuracy depends both on sampling and ability to read the cytological determination.[108] A number of factors critical in assessing the value of thyroid biopsy are shown in Table 11-7.

Although most physicians agree that positive or undeterminable biopsies are indications for surgery, there is concern whether an apparently negative biopsy rules out the possibility of thyroid cancer. Only 100 to 1000 cells are examined out of perhaps a billion in the thyroid; sampling error may occur. A negative biopsy should not dissuade the physician from referring for thyroid surgery a patient who has significant risk

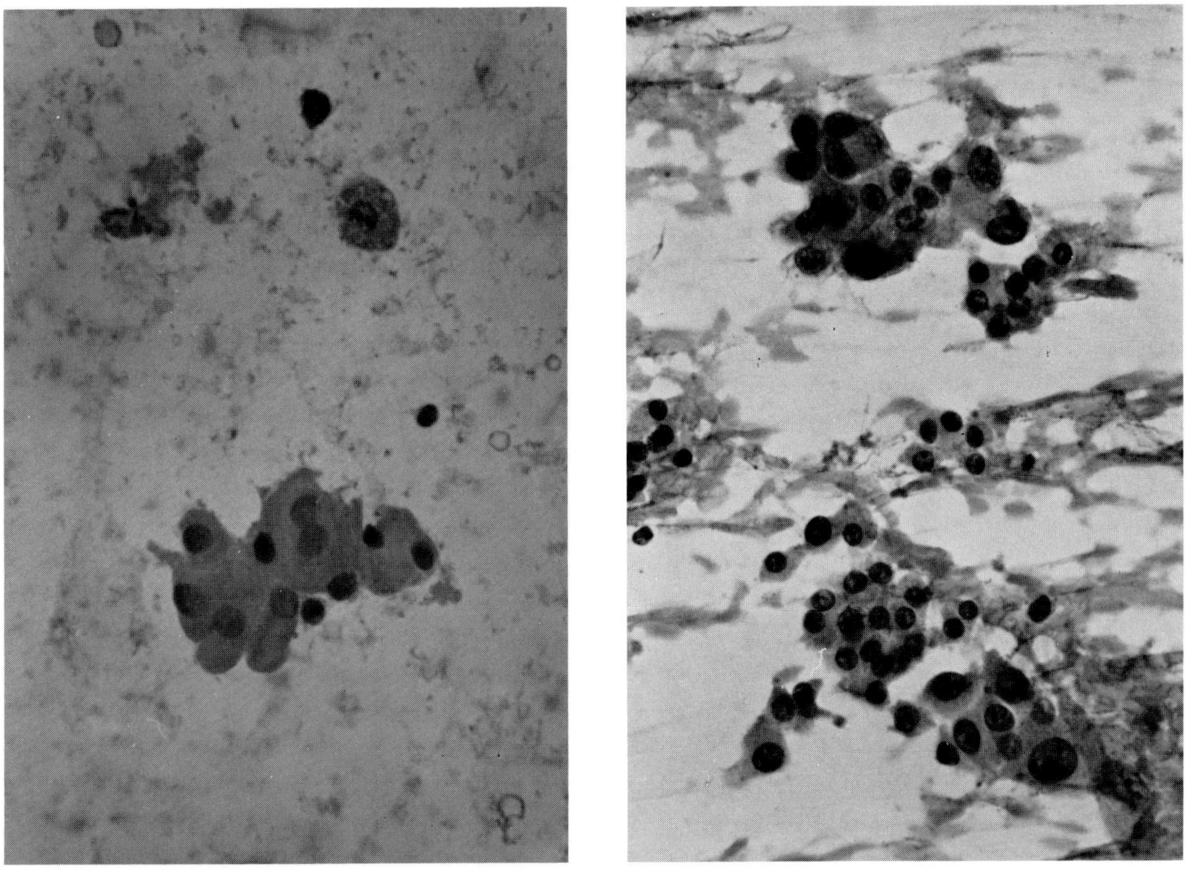

FIGURE 11-13 Fine-needle biopsy aspirate of thyroid. *Left:* Normal follicular cells. *Right:* Papillary carcinoma of the thyroid.

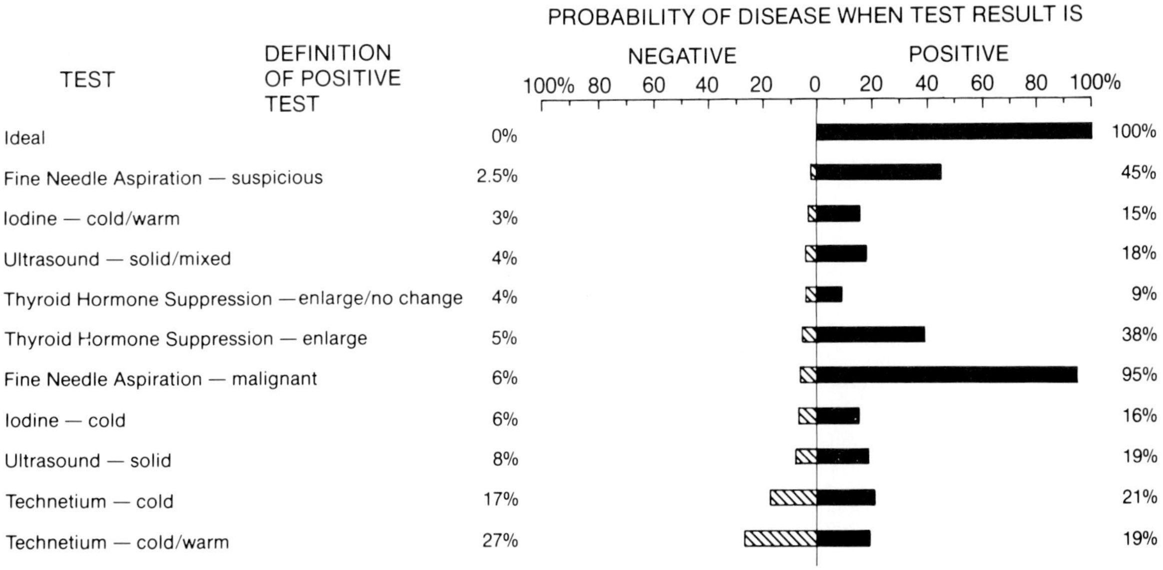

FIGURE 11-14 Probability of disease based on test results calculated according to Bayes' theorem. Hatched bars represent missed malignancies; solid bars represent percentage of surgeries in which malignancies were found. (*Modified from Van Herle et al.*[103])

Table 11-7. Factors in Assessing Fine-Needle Aspiration Biopsy of the Thyroid

	Percent of biopsies
Inadequate study	3–11
Undeterminable*	17–30
False negatives	2–4
False positives	0–3

*Frequency of carcinoma in undeterminable cases = 20 to 60 percent.
Source: Block MA: Surgery of thyroid nodules and malignancy, in Ravitch M (ed): *Current Problems in Surgery*. Chicago, Year Book Medical Publishers, 1983, vol 20, p 135.

factors, e.g., a young male with a firm, irregular thyroid nodule. However, this is a subjective decision.

Management of the Solitary Thyroid Nodule

A therapeutic decision must be made about the management of the solitary thyroid nodule. A decision tree for management is outlined in Fig. 11-15. A solitary thyroid nodule occurring in a child or individual with a history of neck irradiation should be operated upon immediately, as should the patient who has a clinically "malignant" thyroid on physical examination. Before surgery, it is important to be sure that a solitary nodule does not represent a single thyroid lobe with compensatory hypertrophy. If the other lobe cannot be palpated, a thyroid scan is indicated.

In the absence of immediate indications for surgery, the patient should have a thyroid scan. If the nodule is functioning, and if fine-needle aspiration biopsy is not diagnostic, the gland should be suppressed with thyroid hormone for 3 months; disappearance of the nodule is an indication for continued thyroid hormone suppression. An occasional patient may have an autonomous nodule and become hyperthyroid with thyroid hormone suppression; as mentioned previously, the presence of an autonomous nodule makes malignancy very unlikely. Therefore, thyroid function tests should be done several weeks after suppressive therapy has been started. If the response is incomplete and the patient is a young male, surgery is indicated. Otherwise, thyroid hormone suppression can be continued for another 3-month trial period.

If the solitary thyroid nodule is nonfunctioning,

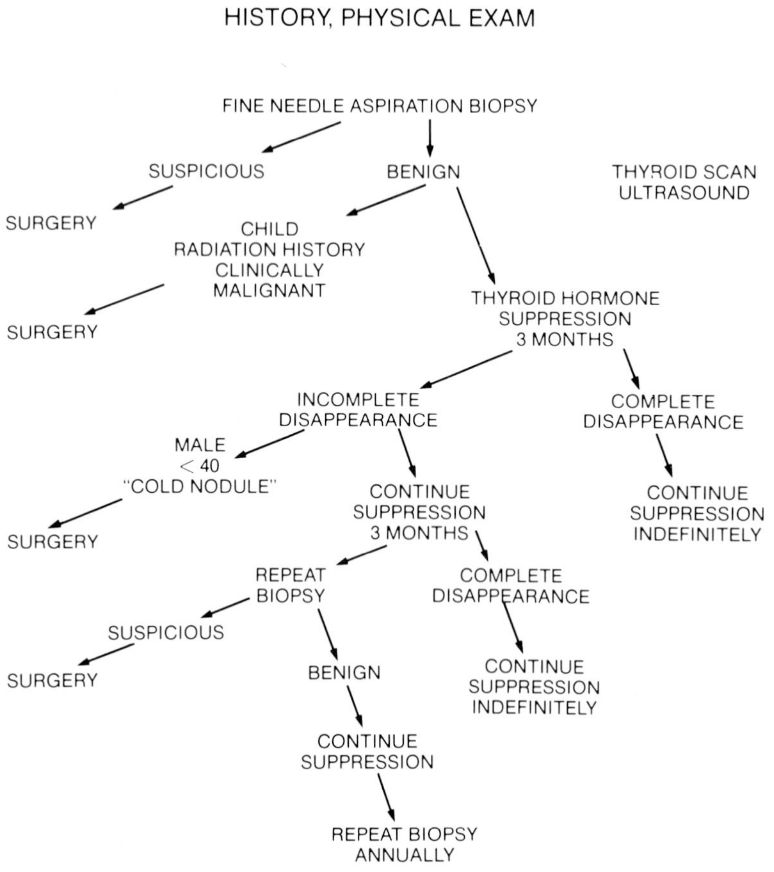

FIGURE 11-15 Management of the solitary thyroid nodule.

ultrasound may be used to determine whether it is solid or cystic, although the determination can also be made during aspiration. If it is cystic and aspiration does not reveal evidence of malignancy, thyroid hormone suppression can be attempted for 3 months. Complete disappearance of the nodule is an indication for continuation of thyroid hormone suppression therapy. All solitary thyroid nodules should be biopsied by fine-needle aspiration, including those in which the decision to operate has been made. Certain knowledge that the nodule is malignant is helpful to the surgeon. If malignancy is not found, the gland should be suppressed with thyroid hormone and managed like the functioning nodule; treatment depends on the response. Thus, although the degree of function in the thyroid nodule is used to separate patients into two branches, both groups are treated in similar manner. The presence of a cold nodule is a factor in the decision to continue suppression in patients with an incomplete response to thyroid hormone suppressive therapy.

Should management of the solitary thyroid nodule be altered in elderly patients? In a study of 100 patients who were more than 60 years old, two distinct groups could be identified.[109] Sixty-six patients were in the high-risk group, i.e., having a solitary cold nodule, hoarseness, etc; 11 of these patients had thyroid malignancies, 6 of which were poorly differentiated. There was no operative mortality. Surgery is indicated for elderly patients with thyroid nodules at risk for malignancy.

THYROID HORMONE SUPPRESSION

Once the decision not to operate has been made, the patient should be given a course of thyroid hormone suppression in an attempt to shut off TSH secretion and decrease the size of the nodule. The difference between thyroid hormone suppressive therapy for a diffuse or multinodular goiter and therapy of the solitary nodule is one of degree. The attempt should be made to treat the solitary nodule with the maximally tolerable dose of thyroid hormone so that TSH is suppressed as much as possible. Regardless of the dose of thyroid hormone administered, it is extremely difficult to suppress TSH secretion completely. Whether low circulating levels of TSH actually stimulate the thyroid is not clear. However, the circulating concentration of serum TSH should be lowered to the lowest level possible.

Questions have been raised about the practice of also using thyroid hormone suppression in solitary cold nodules, with the idea that cold means inactive. Actually, cold nodules have been shown to be more active biochemically than "warm" nodules.[110] They appear to have a defect in iodine trapping, but other parameters, such as glucose oxidation and cAMP level, are actually increased.[111] In one study, 50 percent of the cold nodules did decrease in size with thyroid hormone therapy.[68]

Dose of Thyroid Hormone

The usual suppressive dose of L-thyroxine is about 150 μg per day. The amount of thyroxine used for suppression of a solitary thyroid nodule can be adjusted to just below the dose that gives rise to hyperthyroid symptoms like palpitations, sleep disturbance, or excessive sweating. However, subclinical hyperthyroidism may result, which may be undesirable over the long term; the TRH test may be helpful in this situation.[112] TRH usually causes a temporary increase in serum TSH concentration, but effective thyroid hormone suppression should completely inhibit the TSH response to TRH.[113] Although complete suppression is desirable, in practice most patients are placed on 100 to 200 μg of L-thyroxine, unless there are extenuating circumstances such as heart disease.

Duration of Suppression

If the patient with a solitary thyroid nodule is to have a trial of thyroid hormone suppression, it is important to know how long thyroid hormone should be administered before deciding that the nodule is not going to regress with suppression of circulating TSH. Some goiters have not regressed until the treatment was continued for a year or longer.[66] In half the patients receiving thyroid hormone suppression therapy for nontoxic goiter in one series, thyroid nodules decreased in size after 3 months. When patients who had not responded were treated for another 4 months, one-third of the nodules decreased in size; it made no difference whether the dose of thyroid hormone was increased or not.[68] These data suggest a course of therapy for at least 3 months and preferably 6 months before the thyroid nodule is considered nonsuppressible. Other studies have indicated that no further suppression should be attempted after 3 months.[69] Reevaluation at 3-month intervals allows a management decision to be made based on factors such as sex and age in addition to thyroid hormone response.

If the thyroid nodule disappears completely, thyroid hormone suppression should be continued indefinitely. Regression of the solitary nodule does not eliminate the possibility of thyroid cancer but does indicate that the nodule is responsive to TSH. Thyroid hormone administration should be continued as long as there is no change in the size of the nodule; immediate surgery is advised if the nodule enlarges while on suppressive therapy. If the nodule does not regress completely, the decision whether or not to operate depends on the other factors discussed above.

Surgery

If the decision is made to operate, both thyroid lobes should be totally exposed even though the nodule is palpable in only one lobe before surgery. Multiple thyroid nodules are discovered at surgery in as many as 60 percent of cases diagnosed as a single nodule preoperatively by careful palpation and scan. If multinodular goiter is discovered at operation, the risk of carcinoma in the thyroid nodule is dramatically lower, but the surgeon should probably go on to remove the nodular tissue.

If only a single nodule is discovered at surgery on complete palpation and there are no suspicious signs of extrathyroid involvement, extracapsular lobectomy with removal of the isthmus is indicated. If the thyroid nodule appears benign on frozen section but turns out to be papillary carcinoma after review of the permanent sections, adequate surgery has probably been performed and reoperation is not indicated. The surgical approach to thyroid cancer is discussed later in the chapter.

THYROID CARCINOMA

The biologic behavior of thyroid cancer may vary markedly. Minimal papillary thyroid carcinoma is considered to have a negligible biologic risk, while anaplastic carcinoma of the thyroid is one of the most malignant of all human tumors.

Classification

Nearly all thyroid tumors arise from the follicular or parafollicular cells. These epithelial tumors of the thyroid are shown in the classification in Table 11-8. Thyroid carcinoma may be follicular, forming recognizable thyroid follicles, or these follicular cells may form papillary structures, either pure or mixed with follicles. Alternatively, the follicular cells may be largely undifferentiated and appear as giant spindle cells or small cells. Follicular cells may also grow as squamous cells. Carcinomas arising from parafollicular cells have different histological subtypes, but these have no definite clinical significance as yet; all are called *medullary*. Classification based on the histology of the tumor does have biologic significance. In a 5- to 30-year follow-up, 11 percent of patients with papillary carcinoma died of the disease, compared with 25 percent of patients with follicular carcinoma, 50 percent of patients with sporadic medullary carcinoma, and 90 percent of patients with undifferentiated carcinoma.

Table 11-8. World Health Organization Histological Classification of Epithelial Thyroid Tumors

Epithelial tumors
Benign:
Follicular adenoma
Others
Malignant:
Follicular carcinoma
Papillary carcinoma
Squamous cell carcinoma
Undifferentiated (anaplastic) carcinoma:
Spindle cell type
Giant cell type
Small cell type
Medullary carcinoma
Nonepithelial tumors
Benign
Malignant:
Fibrosarcoma
Others
Miscellaneous tumors
Carcinosarcoma
Malignant hemangioendothelioma
Malignant lymphoma
Teratoma
Secondary tumors

Source: World Health Organization: *International Histological Classification of Tumors*, no. 11: *Histological Typing of Thyroid Tumors*. Geneva, 1974.

Thyroid carcinoma may also be classified in regard to biologic behavior (Table 11-9). Papillary thyroid cancers occur in all age groups and tend to metastasize to lymph nodes; follicular carcinomas tended to have blood-borne metastases and occur in older age groups, while undifferentiated thyroid cancers occur predominantly in older patients and usually kill by local invasion. Although at present there is no completely satisfactory system for staging thyroid cancer, certain pathological characteristics relate to therapy and prognosis. The following prognostic factors for papillary and follicular thyroid carcinomas are thought to be of importance: (1) histological type, (2) age of patient, (3) extent of primary tumor, (4) distant metastases, (5) size of thyroid, (6) blood vessel invasion, (7) multiple foci, and (8) sex.[114]

Clinical staging of thyroid carcinoma has also been attempted (Table 11-10).

Table 11-9. Biologic Behavior of Thyroid Tumors According to Histological Classification

Tumor	Age group	Growth rate	Lymph node metastases	Distant metastases
Papillary	All	Slow	Common	Uncommon
Follicular	Middle-aged to old	Slow	Uncommon	Common
Medullary	All	Moderate	Common	Common
Undifferentiated	Older	Rapid	Extensive	Common (with local growth)

Source: Meissner.[114]

Incidence of Thyroid Carcinoma

Much of the confusion over the incidence of thyroid carcinoma is due to the presence of minimal papillary thyroid cancer, which can be defined as a tumor less than 1.5 cm in size. The prevalence of these small tumors has been reported to be as high as 28 percent in Japan and up to 13 percent in the United States.[115] Since the biologic risk of minimal papillary carcinoma is probably negligible, these tumors rarely are a cause of death. As a consequence, they are responsible for the disparity between thyroid cancer as a cause of death and thyroid cancer prevalence in some surgical series. The reported prevalence varies widely because diagnosis is exquisitely sensitive to the method of pathological examination of the thyroid gland. These thyroid tumors may be occult, and hence not grossly visible; as many as 300 to 900 slides per gland must be prepared to avoid missing the smallest tumor. If all thyroids were studied in this manner, as many as 10 to 30 million North Americans might be found to have minimal papillary thyroid carcinoma.[115] The magnitude of this problem is overwhelming, but from the patient's point of view probably biologically unimportant. However, the presence of such tumors does make it difficult to discuss incidence. Mortality from thyroid cancer approximates 0.8 deaths in females per 100,000 per year and 0.4 deaths per 100,000 per year in males; these data make deaths from tumors of the thyroid uncommon compared with deaths from other cancers.

Table 11-10. Clinical Stages of Thyroid Carcinoma

Stage I	Intrathyroidal lesions only
Stage II	Nonfixed cervical metastases
Stage III	Fixed lymph node metastases or invasion into the neck outside the thyroid
Stage IV	Thyroid tumors with metastatic disease outside the neck

Source: Modified from Smedal ML, Salzman FA, Meissner WA: *Am J Roentgenol* 99:352, 1967.

The Effects of Radiation on the Development of Thyroid Carcinoma

External irradiation of the thyroid, as mentioned earlier, is associated with an increased incidence of thyroid neoplasms, including carcinomas, after a delay of many years. There is no evidence at present that this radiation-associated increase in incidence of thyroid carcinoma disappears with time, so exposed individuals must be followed.

Fortunately, radiation-associated thyroid carcinomas are almost always well differentiated and have a good prognosis when detected in patients under 40. When data from several studies were combined, the absolute risk for thyroid cancers was found to be 1.5 cases per 1,000,000 per rad per year.[116,117] The estimated dose-response relationship between external radiation and thyroid cancer is shown in Fig. 11-16. Although not shown in the figure, there appears to be an upper limit to the radiation dose for inducing thyroid carcinoma; carcinogenesis is rare at doses above 2000 rads.[116] The protective effect of large doses of radiation has been thought to be due to complete destruction of thyroid cells, but there is no proof for this hypothesis. The failure of therapeutic doses of ^{131}I to result in an increased risk for thyroid carcinoma has also been explained by the destruction of thyroid cells. Therapeutic doses of ^{131}I given for hyperthyroidism result in delivery of 5000 to 8000 rads to the thyroid.[118] Doses of external radiation as low as 50 rads have been associated with an increased risk of thyroid carcinoma, and it is likely that any amount of radiation represents an increased risk. Since low doses of radiation may induce thyroid carcinoma, the use of ^{131}I for thyroid scans should be discouraged until better information is available.

The incidence of thyroid carcinoma peaks 20 to 25 years after radiation exposure and then appears to decline.[85] However, the decline is not statistically significant. If progression of the thyroid disease involves hyperplasia, adenoma formation, and, eventually, malignancy, there should be an age progression of radiation-induced malignancy through the group of

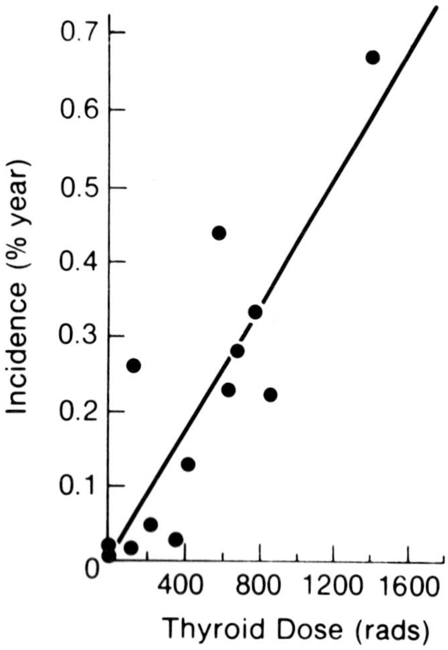

FIGURE 11-16 Incidence of thyroid cancer as a function of the dose of external radiation. (*After Maxon et al.*[116])

irradiated individuals. However, since progression did not continue, the data suggest that irradiation induced an immediate tendency to malignancy which then took several years to become clinically evident.

There is no clear relation between radiation dose and the interval between exposure and detection. Whether the size of the radiation dose or the length of the latency period can be related to the type of carcinoma is not clear.

The great majority of tumors have been papillary thyroid carcinoma. Malignancies found at the time of surgery do not just represent minimal papillary carcinoma. Approximately two-thirds of the carcinomas were greater than 1 cm in size and 59 percent were multi-focal, with lymph node metastases in 25 percent.[85] Although children are two to three times as susceptible as adults to radiation-induced thyroid nodules, they appear to be equally susceptible to the induction of thyroid carcinoma.[81] Although prophylaxis with thyroid hormone has not been shown to prevent new disease,[85] such suppression seems reasonable in patients exposed to external radiation to the head and neck until further information is available.[119]

Natural History of Thyroid Carcinoma

Carcinoma of the thyroid is three times more common in females than in males.[120] It has an incidence peak in the sixth decade, but ranges from infancy to old age. However, death from thyroid cancer has a very different age distribution. Mortality is low in the young, but the prognosis steadily worsens with age. This difference between mortality and incidence rates is related to the fact that most thyroid carcinomas in younger individuals are well differentiated while anaplastic thyroid carcinoma with its higher mortality is predominant in the elderly. The highly malignant anaplastic thyroid carcinoma seldom occurs before the age of 40; after 40, both mortality and the occurrence of metastases from thyroid carcinoma increase sharply.

PAPILLARY CARCINOMA

Papillary carcinoma is three times more common in females than in males and represents the great majority of thyroid cancers in childhood. Although more common, papillary carcinoma has a better prognosis in women and children compared with men. Nevertheless, the overall prognosis is generally good, and 80 percent or more of patients are alive after 10 years.

Histologically, the epithelial cells of the tumor have a definite papillary pattern (Fig. 11-17). Although follicular patterns with colloid-filled vesicles may be found frequently in the tumor, the follicular component apparently does not alter the behavior of the tumor; it is still classified as papillary. Approximately 40 percent of cases of papillary carcinoma contain laminated calcific spherules called *psammoma bodies.* These psammoma bodies can sometimes be identified as finely stippled calcifications on a properly exposed x-ray of the neck.[121] Xeroradiography may be particularly helpful but is not necessary. The tumor is slow-growing and usually of low-grade malignancy, which means that long follow-up periods are necessary. Spread occurs characteristically to the cervical lymph nodes; patients may actually present with enlarged cervical nodes rather than a mass in the thyroid.

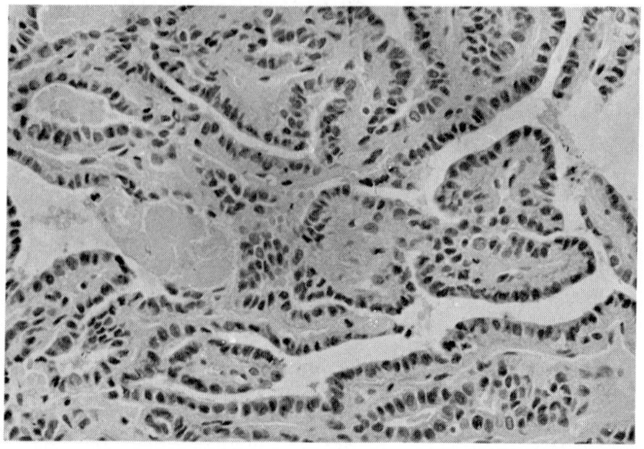

FIGURE 11-17 Papillary carcinoma of the thyroid. The papillae are lined by low columnar cells. Mitoses are absent.

Interestingly, the presence of metastases to the cervical nodes seems to have little deleterious effect on mortality.[122,123] Metastases to bones and lungs are much less common. Intraglandular metastases in both the same lobe as the primary tumor and the opposite lobe are not uncommon. Papillary carcinomas may remain indolent for long periods even with widespread metastases or may assume more aggressive properties. In the latter case the progression is often associated with a change to a more malignant type of thyroid cancer.

FOLLICULAR CARCINOMA

Follicular carcinoma accounts for about 15 percent of thyroid carcinomas and, like papillary carcinoma, is three times more common in women than in men. However, this tumor occurs less frequently in children; it is more a disease of middle and later years. Histologically, the tumor is characterized both by the formation of acinar structures with varying colloid content and by the absence of papillary elements (Fig. 11-18). Because of the relatively normal morphology the tumor may be very difficult to distinguish from follicular adenomas; usually, invasion of the capsule, adjacent thyroid, or blood vessels must be demonstrated. The initial appearance of follicular carcinoma may be as a distant metastasis with no thyroid lesion clinically evident. These tumors tend to metastasize by the bloodstream or invade adjacent structures rather than spread to local lymph nodes.

Prognosis depends on the extent of tumor invasion at the time of surgery. Follicular carcinomas that show minimal invasion and appear grossly similar to adenomas have a very high cure rate. With more extensive invasion, the prognosis becomes progressively poorer. In a study of 18 cases in which the patient died from follicular carcinoma of the thyroid, 56 percent had lung metastases, 89 percent had lymph node metastases, and 17 percent had skeleton, liver, or brain metastases.[124] The development of metastases may be delayed for as long as 10 to 20 years.

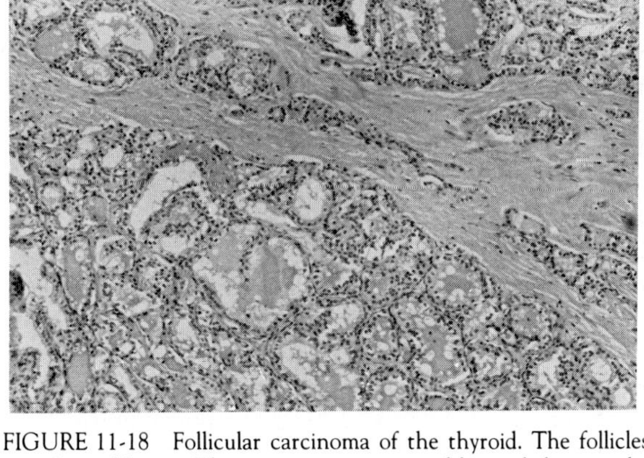

FIGURE 11-18 Follicular carcinoma of the thyroid. The follicles are of variable size. There is invasion into and beyond the capsule. Scalloping of colloid is present in some follicles.

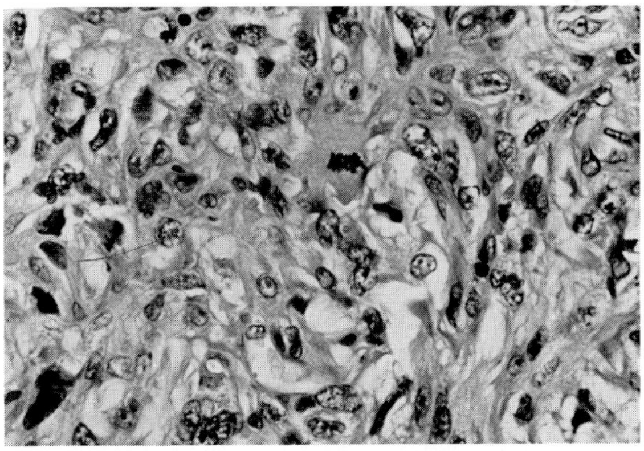

FIGURE 11-19 Anaplastic carcinoma of the thyroid, pleomorphic type. The cells are bizarre and pleomorphic, and many are elongated. The mitotic rate is high.

ANAPLASTIC CARCINOMA

The anaplastic carcinomas of the thyroid are those that form neither papillary nor follicular structures and do not have amyloid stroma. The cells tend to be strikingly pleomorphic and devoid of any special arrangement. Bizarre, multinucleated giant cells are encountered frequently (Fig. 11-19). A spindle cell growth pattern sometimes predominates; this may be suggestive of fibrosarcoma. Diffuse small-cell carcinoma of the thyroid forms a special group, which may be difficult to differentiate from lymphosarcoma; lymphosarcoma may be much more common in the thyroid.[125] The ratio of females to males is lower than in papillary or follicular carcinoma, and the mean age, 57 years, is older.

Anaplastic carcinomas grow rapidly, infiltrate neck structures, and may spread to regional lymph nodes, lungs, bones, and liver. Death may often occur as a result of rapid local spread before distant metastases appear. In one patient with anaplastic carcinoma of the thyroid it was necessary to readjust the cord around the neck which held the tracheotomy tube in place every 4 h because of tumor growth. Anaplastic thyroid tumors have a grim prognosis, with a 10-year survival rate of only about 1 percent.

Therapy of Thyroid Carcinoma

With such a wide variation in the behavior of differentiated tumors of the thyroid, how extensive the surgery should be remains controversial. Because of this wide range, methods of treatment can be compared only with difficulty even when cases are matched for age, sex, and histology. The risks of therapy must be weighed carefully against the prognosis for each individual. Radical procedures carry the risk of serious disability, e.g., recurrent laryngeal nerve paralysis and hypoparathyroidism, and should be used with restraint where the prognosis is good. Dangerous and disfiguring operations are virtually never indicated.

Radioactive iodine may be of real benefit in treating surgically inaccessible metastases without damaging surrounding tissue. Whether the isotope has a role in the routine ablation of the remaining thyroid gland after partial thyroidectomy for well-differentiated tumors remains a subject for debate. Hormone dependence of certain well-differentiated carcinomas of the thyroid is well established. There is good evidence that the induction of hypothyroidism with concomitant elevated serum TSH concentration has resulted in growth of thyroid metastases. Certainly, avoidance of hypopthyroidism and suppression of TSH levels are accepted parts of the therapy of thyroid carcinoma.

Table 11-11. Influence of Initial Treatment on Recurrence and Survival in Thyroid Papillary Carcinoma

	Recurrence, %	Deaths, %
Surgical therapy:		
Thyroidectomy:		
Subtotal	19.2	0.6
Total	10.9*	1.5
Lymphadenectomy:		
None	12.3	0.8
Simple	17.9	1.7
Excision	14.7	0.7
Medical therapy after surgery:		
None	40.0	10.0
Thyroid	13.1†	0.2
^{131}I and thyroid hormone	6.4	0.9

*Difference in recurrence frequency between patients with total vs. subtotal thyroidectomy statistically significant, $p < .01$
†Difference between patients with thyroid therapy vs. no therapy statistically significant, $p < .001$.
Source: Mazzaferri and Young.[123]

THERAPY OF PAPILLARY CARCINOMA

If the lesion is found at surgery to be minimal papillary carcinoma (< 1 cm), the procedure of choice is thyroid lobectomy on the affected side and removal of the isthmus.[122] Although there is still substantial controversy about the proper treatment of larger lesions, the evidence favors near-total thyroidectomy (leaving only enough of the gland to preserve the recurrent laryngeal nerve and the parathyroid glands). In one study, residual cancer would have persisted in remaining thyroid tissue in two-thirds of patients if only a lobectomy had been performed.[126] In a study of 576 patents with carcinoma of the thyroid, there was a significant inverse correlation between extent of surgery and recurrence of the tumor[122,123] (Table 11-11). The tumor recurred with twice the frequency after subtotal thyroidectomy as compared with near-total thyroidectomy, and the proportion of deaths from thyroid cancer was greater. Cervical lymph node metastases found at initial surgery were associated with higher recurrence rates but not higher mortality rates.

The major argument against total thyroidectomy is the increased risk of hypoparathyroidism and recurrent laryngeal nerve involvement.[125,126a] If the posterior capsule on the contralateral side is left intact, this risk can be reduced as low as 5 percent.[127] In one large series, hypoparathyroidism occurred in 13.5 percent of patients who had a total thyroidectomy and was clearly related to the extent of the surgery.[123] Recurrent laryngeal nerve paralysis occurred in 1.2 percent of the patients; it was also related to the extent of surgery. There was no evidence that extensive neck dissection in addition to total thyroidectomy improved survival or lessened recurrence, and major postoperative complications occurred in 44 percent of patients who were treated this way. In contrast, major complications occurred in only 13 percent of patients when total thyroidectomy was combined with selective regional lymph node excision.

As indicated in Fig. 11-20, medical therapy also significantly influenced survival and recurrence. The recurrence rate following thyroid hormone therapy was significantly less than with no therapy but was significantly greater than with ^{131}I plus thyroid hormone therapy. Differences in recurrence rates among these three subgroups were apparent within the first year after completion of previous therapy. The indication for therapy with ^{131}I was almost exclusively residual uptake in the neck, particularly in patients with larger tumors.[123] The average dose of radioactive iodine was 140 mCi; the dose was less than 200 mCi in 87 percent of the patients.

Although ^{131}I uptake occurs in as many as 80 percent of differentiated thyroid carcinomas, the benefits derived from therapy, particularly in patients with relatively small metastases in the neck, are not entirely certain. The data suggest that ablative doses of radioactive iodine should be given postoperatively to patients with papillary carcinoma whose lesions are multiple, metastatic, locally invasive, or larger than

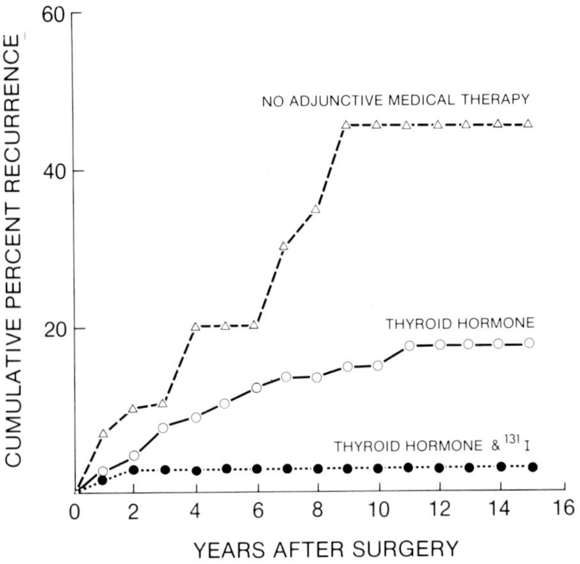

FIGURE 11-20 Cumulative recurrence rates for papillary carcinoma of the thyroid gland according to type of medical therapy used postoperatively. (*From Mazzaferri et al.*[122])

2.5 cm. For patients with papillary tumors less than 1.5 cm in diameter, less aggressive therapy, consisting of subtotal thyroidectomy and thyroid hormone suppression, may be adequate.[123] Treatment of these patients resulted in a lower recurrence and mortality rate.[122] Therapy should also be administered to patients with local or distant metastases, provided adequate ^{131}I uptake can be demonstrated.[128,129]

Numerous studies have indicated that thyroid carcinomas may be subject to endocrine control with depression of serum TSH concentration by thyroid hormone. Thyroid hormone was given to 19 patients with inoperable metastases of papillary carcinoma of the thyroid; this treatment resulted in regression of metastases in 12 of the patients for periods averaging 11 years.[130] The aim of thyroid hormone therapy in patients with thyroid carcinoma is not replacement but depression of serum TSH concentration. Total suppression of TSH secretion is difficult, regardless of the dose of thyroid hormone; however, TSH secretion should be inhibited as much as possible without inducing iatrogenic hyperthyroidism. Suppressive hormone therapy should be started as soon as possible, even before surgery if the diagnostic studies are completed. The TRH test (see Chap. 10) may prove helpful as an indicator of TSH suppression by thyroid hormone.[131] The patient is started on 0.15 mg of L-thyroxine daily; if there is any TSH response to the TRH bolus after 3 weeks of therapy, the dose of thyroid can be raised to 0.20 mg and the test repeated. This should be continued until the patient neither has an increase in serum TSH concentration with TRH stimulation nor is clinically hyperthyroid.

External irradiation at moderate dosage can eradicate microscopic papillary and follicular carcinoma; gross tumor also responds favorably, but the regression rate is slow.[132] External irradiation at present is indicated in patients who no longer respond to ^{131}I.

THERAPY OF FOLLICULAR CARCINOMA

The therapy of follicular carcinoma differs from the therapy of papillary carcinoma for several reasons. Follicular carcinoma is a more aggressive tumor and for that reason should be treated more aggressively. Blood-borne metastases are more common, often necessitating radionuclide therapy. Furthermore, patients in whom well-differentiated metastases outside the neck were ablated are three times more likely to survive than patients not freed of metastases.[133] For these reasons, total thyroidectomy is indicated even if the diagnosis must be made after reviewing the permanent sections, necessitating reoperation. The normal thyroid gland is so avid for iodine that radioactive iodine cannot be given for treatment of any metastases until the thyroid gland has been ablated. Therefore, total or near-total removal of the gland is indicated.[134] If follicular carcinoma was diagnosed in the distant past and a total thyroidectomy was not done, reoperation does not seem to be indicated. The patient in this situation should be followed expectantly. The thyroid remnant could also be ablated with radioactive iodine, but ablation of a normal-functioning remnant requires a large radioactive iodine dose, e.g., 60 mCi, which would contribute to the radiation dose imposed on the patient without significantly affecting the cancer. However, 30 mCi may be sufficient in most cases, providing a lower radiation burden.[135,136]

The immediate postoperative period is often difficult for patients with papillary carcinoma; making the patients hypothyroid accentuates the problems. Placing the patients on suppressive doses of L-thyroxine for 3 months and then switching them to 50 μg of T_3 per day for 4 weeks is preferred. The triiodothyronine is discontinued for 2 weeks and radioactive iodine given. This regimen appears to produce an optimal radioisotope uptake.[137,138] The patient is on suppressive therapy during this period and the risk of malignant growth is minimal. The patient could be kept on thyroid hormone suppressive therapy and 10 U of bovine TSH administered intramuscularly daily for 3 days. However, administration of bovine TSH may result in the development of antibodies and toxic reactions and should be avoided in most instances.[139,140]

Alternatively, the patient can be allowed to become hypothyroid immediately after surgery, e.g., 2 to 4 weeks after total thyroidectomy. When the serum TSH concentration is elevated in the range of 50 μU per ml, 2 mCi of ^{131}I can be given and a whole-body scan performed; the use of ^{123}I, if available, would lower the radiation dose for diagnostic purposes. If any uptake occurs in the thyroid or elsewhere, 100 mCi of ^{131}I should be given. The amount of ^{131}I taken up by the tumor should be maximized by decreasing the iodide pool.[141] This can be accomplished by placing the patient on a low-iodine diet for 3 weeks and administering hydrochlorothiazide, 50 mg daily, for the week before therapy. The administration of a cathartic and secretagogue on the day of ^{131}I therapy minimizes retention of radioactive iodine by the bowel and salivary glands.

There is some question whether the serum TSH concentration is as high with exogenous TSH stimulation as when endogenous TSH concentration is allowed to rise due to the induction of hypothyroidism.[140] In any case, the patient should not be allowed to remain hypothyroid any longer than absolutely necessary and thyroid hormone therapy should be restarted as quickly as possible.

THERAPY OF ANAPLASTIC CARCINOMA

For most patients, anaplastic carcinoma of the thyroid has progressed beyond the possibility of cure when they are first seen. Partial excision of the tumor as well as tracheostomy may be needed both to provide relief of tracheal compression and to decrease the amount of tumor to be irradiated. A tissue diagnosis can often be established by needle biopsy. Radical surgery has no role in the treatment of anaplastic carcinoma. Surgical procedures have failed to improve the prognosis; radiotherapy probably provides the best palliation. External radiotherapy may be given in a dose of 4000 to 5000 rads to the neck and upper mediastinum through a variety of ports. Shrinkage of the tumor may occur rapidly (hyperfractionation of the radiation dose, 100 rads qid at 3-h intervals, caused complete tumor regression in 6 of 14 patients[142]), but recurrence is the rule. The aim of radiotherapy in these cases is to prevent obstruction, ulceration, and hemorrhage. Although anaplastic carcinomas rarely pick up sufficient iodine to make treatment possible, a radioiodine uptake test and scan should be done before other therapy is attempted. Occasionally, an anaplastic carcinoma of the thyroid takes up sufficient ^{131}I to make therapy possible.[143]

Chemotherapy has not been very helpful in the treatment of these very aggressive tumors, but could be considered as an alternative to radiation therapy.[144] A partial remission associated with subjective improvement was achieved in 5 of 19 patients with anaplastic carcinoma treated with doxorubicin (Adriamycin).[145] All histological cell types responded, although spindle- and giant cell types appeared to be less responsive. The most significant toxicity encountered was Adriamycin-induced cardiomyopathy. Bleomycin is another antibiotic that has been suggested to be effective in thyroid cancer.[146]

Subsequent Follow-up

After surgery for differentiated thyroid carcinoma, residual thyroid tissue and metastases which concentrate radioiodine should be defined by a radioactive iodine scan as discussed previously. In addition, chest films should be taken on a yearly basis to rule out the possibility of metastases. Annual or biannual bone scans may also be helpful to check for possible bone metastases, particularly in follicular carcinoma.[147]

THYROGLOBULIN DETERMINATIONS

Recently, there has been interest in serum thyroglobulin concentration as an aid in the diagnosis and follow-up of thyroid carcinoma.[148–150] Although the assay is probably not specific in distinguishing benign from malignant thyroid tissue, it is valuable in assessing treatment of thyroid carcinoma and the course of the disease.[151] Circulating thyroglobulin concentrations tend to be high in patients with thyroid tumors but are also increased in a number of other thyroid diseases, including Graves' disease, subacute thyroiditis, and endemic goiter. Unfortunately, not all patients with thyroid neoplasms have elevated thyroglobulin concentration either. The major use of the thyroglobulin assay is probably in the follow-up of patients whose thyroid carcinoma has been removed and in whom postoperative thyroglobulin levels are very low or undetectable. Persistence of elevated thyroglobulin levels or an increase in previously low levels indicates that residual thyroid carcinoma should be searched for carefully.[152,153] Serum thyroglobulin concentration should be determined only if the assay is sufficiently sensitive (limit of detection less than 10 to 15 mg/ml) and no anti-thyroglobulin antibody has been demonstrated. Thyroid hormone withdrawal and concomitant TSH stimulation may significantly enhance serum thyroglobulin concentrations.[154] However, thyroglobulin concentrations < 10 ng/ml are rarely associated with significant disease, and thyroid hormone withdrawal and TSH are not routinely indicated.

In an effort to screen patients who had received irradiation to the head and neck for thyroid carcinoma, a battery of tests were done, including assays for serum thyroglobulin concentration, antithyroglobulin and antithyroid microsomal antibodies, and carcinoembryonic antigen.[155] Positive results were more frequent in the irradiated population than in the controls; however, with the exception of thyroglobulin, the tests did not clearly differentiate patients with benign or malignant lesions. Elevations of serum thyroglobulin concentration above 300 ng/ml were found only in patients with thyroid cancer, but the diagnosis was usually obvious in such patients.

IgG antibody to human thyroglobulin has been radiolabeled and successfully used to locate thyroid follicular and papillary tumors.[156] Results suggest that ^{131}I-antithyroglobulin scanning may be more sensitive than conventional [^{131}I]iodide scanning in locating metastases.

MEDULLARY CARCINOMA OF THE THYROID

Although medullary carcinoma comprises only 5 to 10 percent of all thyroid malignancies, there has been intense interest in this tumor because of a number of unique properties. Medullary carcinoma of the thyroid (MCT) differs from other thyroid carcinomas in that the cell of origin is the parafollicular C or light cell, which is of neural crest origin. As a result, the tumor has endocrine and biochemical properties that provide a distinctive means for early detection and follow-up and possibly prevention.

Natural History

MCT occurs over a wide age range from 5 to 80 years, without a particular predilection for age or sex. Most of these malignancies are apparently sporadic, in which case the tumors are usually unicentric and not associated with other endocrine lesions. However, in approximately 20 percent of patients, the disease is familial, transmitted as an autosomal dominant trait. The familial form usually occurs as Sipple's syndrome or multiple endocrine neoplasia (MEN) type 2 (see Chap. 28), characterized by the combination of MCT, bilateral adrenal pheochromocytomas, and parathyroid adenomas.[157] Cutaneous or mucosal neuromas involving the face, lips, and tongue may also occur in association with MCT and bilateral pheochromocytomas; they are thought to constitute a separate variant of the syndrome (MEN type 2b)[158] (Fig. 11-21).

The different characteristics of the hereditary and sporadic varieties of MCT may be explained by the two-hit theory proposed by Knudson.[159] In the hereditary form, the first event was postulated to be a germinal mutation resulting in many susceptible cells. This would be followed by a second somatic mutation which would transform the cell into a tumor cell. In the sporadic form, both mutational events were postulated to occur in somatic cells. Comparison of the ages of onset of hereditary and sporadic MCT have been consistent with this theory.[160] Further evidence was provided by studies with glucose-6-phosphate dehydrogenase in heterozygotes, indicating a clonal origin of medullary carcinoma.[161] The finding of C cell hyperplasia in patients with hereditary disease but not in those with sporadic forms is compatible with the theory and suggests that the hyperplasia was the expression of genetic mutation. The high degree of penetrance of the C cell hyperplasia suggests that the second somatic mutation must be ubiquitous.

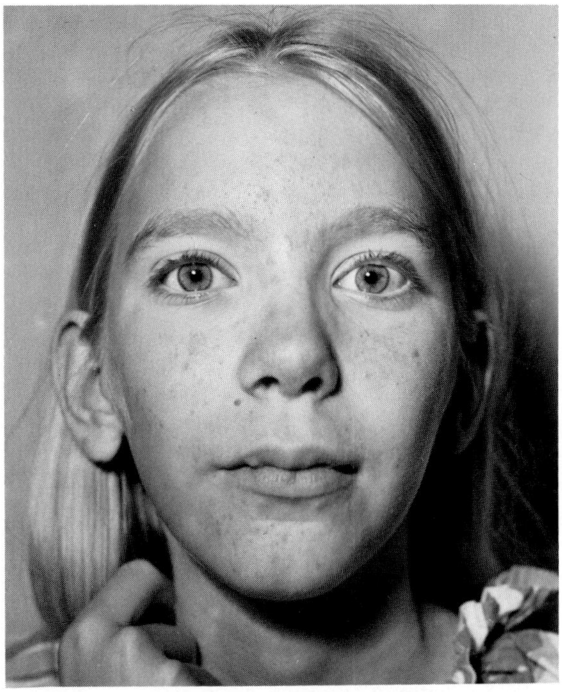

FIGURE 11-21 Typical facies of patient with MEN type 2b syndrome. (*From Khairi et al.*[158])

Clinical Course

MCT is intermediate in malignancy between follicular and anaplastic carcinoma; the 5-year survival rate is 70 to 80 percent.[162] Characteristically, the tumor runs a slow but progressive course; neck structures are invaded and metastases go both to cervical lymph nodes and distant sites. MCT may be sharply demarcated from surrounding normal thyroid or may infiltrate the adjacent thyroid. Smaller tumors are almost invariably located in the upper, posterior portion of the thyroid lobes. Microscopically, the tumor is distinguished by clusters of polyhedral, neoplastic cells (Fig. 11-22) arranged in compartments separated by hyaline amyloid-containing stroma, which is formed by the tumor cells. This organization, together with the absence of neoplastic follicles and papillary elements, is the diagnostic microscopic feature.

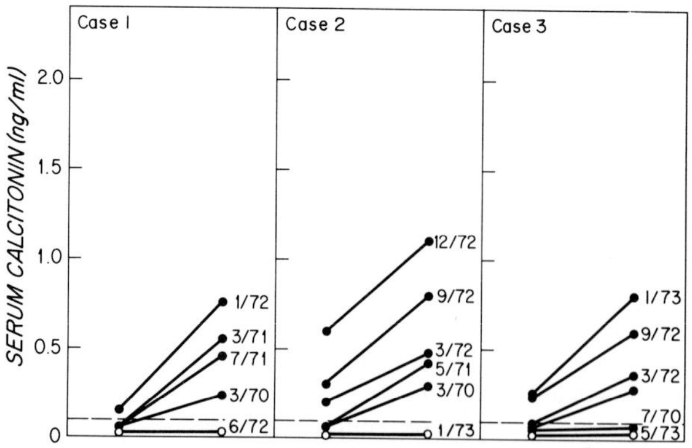

FIGURE 11-23 Serum calcitonin responses to calcium infusion in C cell hyperplasia: concentrations of calcitonin in serum before (*left*) and at the end (*right*) of calcium infusion tests in three patients with C cell hyperplasia. Broken line shows sensitivity of the assay; open circles show postoperative data. (*From Tashjian et al.*[163])

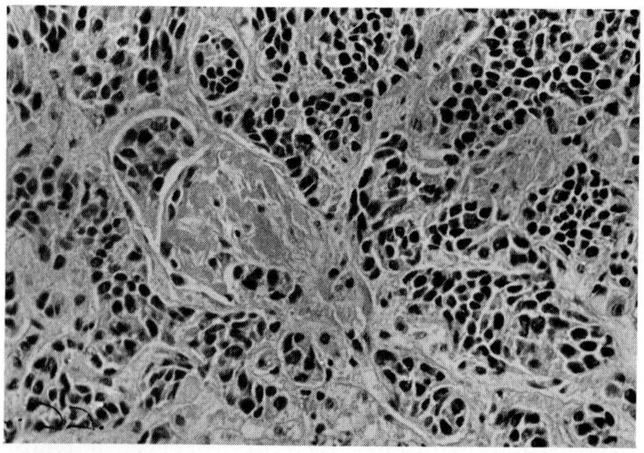

FIGURE 11-22 Medullary carcinoma of the thyroid. Anaplastic tumor cells are visible in clumps and cords. Some amyloid material is present in the stroma adjacent to tumor cells near the center of the micrograph.

Diagnosis

In contrast to the faint homogeneous calcification seen in other thyroid tumors, MCT has a tendency to calcify with a characteristic dense, irregular distribution of calcium throughout the tumor mass in both thyroid primary lesions as well as metastases.

The parafollicular cells of the thyroid which give rise to MCT secrete the calcium concentration–lowering peptide hormone calcitonin; virtually all patients with MCT have elevated calcitonin levels in their blood.[163] Some patients may have borderline elevated basal calcitonin values but respond with increased calcitonin secretion when calcium, glucagon, or pentagastrin is administered. The use of calcium and pentagastrin in combination appears to be superior to administration of either agent alone.[164] Normal individuals may have low circulating calcitonin levels, less than 250 pg/ml, because of a small number of calcitonin-producing C cells in the normal thyroid.

Since the tumor secretes large amounts of calcitonin, and this secretion can be stimulated, the calcitonin stimulation test has been used for the early diagnosis of MCT. However, in most cases of sporadic MCT, in contrast to the familial type, the disease is unsuspected either until surgery is performed or, occasionally, until fine-needle biopsy is done. There is a direct correlation between the basal level of calcitonin and the extent of the tumor. Calcitonin determinations are not indicated in the evaluation of all thyroid nodules. The long-range outcome for patients identified early in the course of the disease must await follow-up studies. When MCT was confined to the thyroid gland, serum calcitonin concentration was unmeasurable in 95 percent of cases for periods up to 3 years following surgery.[163] Other markers, like carcinoembryonic antigen, have also been studied, but their usefulness is questionable. High levels of histaminase activity have been found in MCT tissue and in serum of patients with the disease.[165] However, simultaneous measurements of serum histaminase and serum calcitonin levels in MCT patients have indicated that calcitonin assay is a more sensitive method of identifying the presence of MCT. In addition to calcitonin and histaminase, the tumors may secrete prostaglandins and serotonin as do other APUD (amine precursor uptake and decarboxylation) tumors, but measurement of these is not generally recommended.

Calcitonin stimulation tests have also been used to identify individuals who are at high risk by virtue of heredity[166] (Fig. 11-23). In kindreds with familial MCT, stimulation tests should be initiated by age 5 years and should continue annually until age 30;[167] after age 30 less frequent testing would be adequate [these recommendations are based on sequential testing of 445 members of 11 kindreds to determine the age-related probability for developing hereditary MCT (Fig. 11-24)]. With this screening procedure, individuals have been identified with early changes in C cell mass which could represent preinvasive hyperplasia of the cells. The thyroid glands in these cases were grossly normal. However, microscopic clusters of C

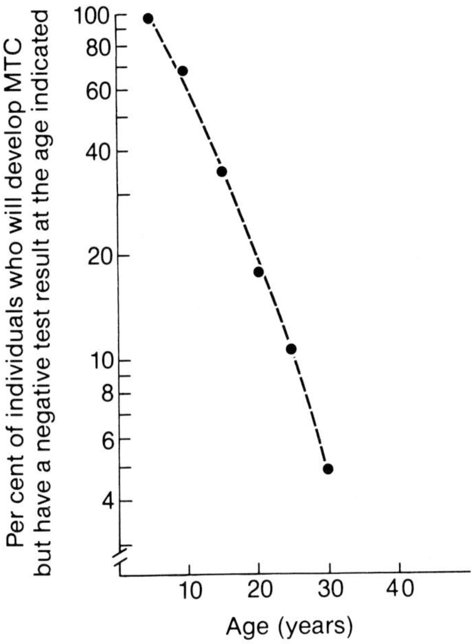

FIGURE 11-24 Semilogarithmic plot of the percentage of kindreds of patients with medullary thyroid carcinoma that convert from negative to positive on a calcitonin stimulation test as a function of age. (*Modified from Gagel et al.*[167])

cells occurred focally in the middle third or the junction of the middle and upper thirds of the lateral lobe (Fig. 11-25). No microscopic tumors or evidence of vascular or lymphatic invasion were found. If, in fact, parafollicular cell hyperplasia precedes invasive carcinoma in this disease, then the calcitonin stimulation test should lead to early recognition of the disease at a stage which is potentially curable. These screening procedures are of much more than academic interest in affected kindreds where half the group is potentially at risk to develop this aggressive neoplasm.

Therapy of Medullary Carcinoma

The treatment of MCT is surgical, but metastases have already occurred in more than half the patients with the sporadic form at the time of diagnosis; thus, complete excision of the tumor is difficult. If an affected kindred is followed with calcitonin screening, the presence of tumors will be detected at a much less advanced stage. Because of the frequent occurrence of multicentricity, near-total thyroidectomy is the procedure of choice. The initial surgical approach to MCT should include thorough central neck dissection of lymph nodes, extending as far substernally as possible.[162] The tumor often shows early aggressive behavior in terms of local metastases; this must be treated promptly. However, an extensive thyroidectomy should not be done at the expense of the recurrent laryngeal nerve and parathyroid glands, nor should disfiguring neck dissection be done. Since pheochromocytoma is a distinct possibility in these patients, this disease must be ruled out with appropriate tests, such as urinary catecholamine determinations, before thyroid surgery can be considered.

Medullary carcinomas rarely take up radioactive iodine; this modality should not be considered as a possible therapeutic measure. Although there have been reports of temporary responses to thyroid hormone, this form of therapy is not nearly as effective as in differentiated thyroid tumors.[168] No good therapy for MCT exists; therefore, a vigorous and effective

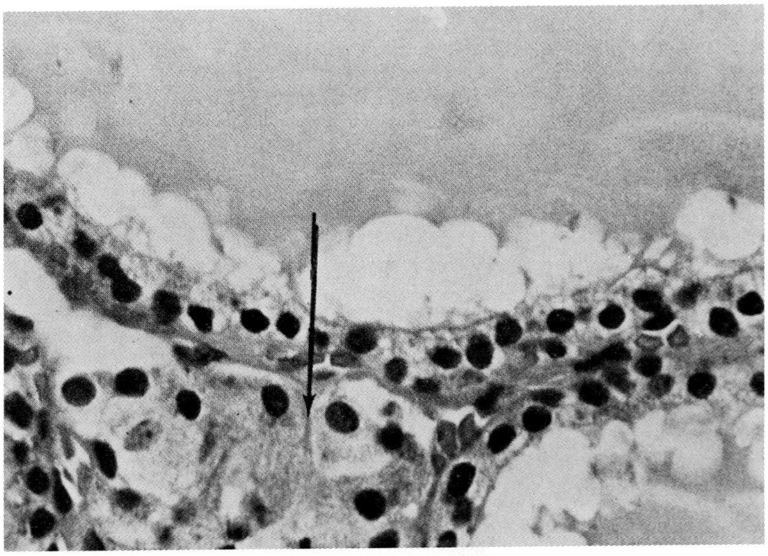

FIGURE 11-25 C cell hyperplasia. Clusters of polygonal to spindle-shaped C cells are seen in a parafollicular location. (*From Tashjian et al.*[163])

screening program offers the best chance for patient survival.

REFERENCES

1. Kelly FC, Snedden WW: Prevalence and geographical distribution of endemic goitre. *Bull WHO* 18:5, 1958.

2. Wharton T: *Adenographia: Sive, Glandularum Totius Corporis Descriptio*. London, 1656.

3. Rolleston HD: *The Endocrine Organs in Health and Disease*. London, Oxford University, 1936.

4. Marine D: Etiology and prevention of simple goiter. *Medicine* 3:453, 1924.

5. Studer H, Greer MA: *The Regulation of Thyroid Function in Iodine Deficiency*. Bern, Hans Huber, 1968.

6. Brown RS, Jackson IMD, Pohl SL, Reichlin S: Do thyroid-stimulating immunoglobulins cause non-toxic and toxic multinodular goitre? *Lancet* 1:904, 1978.

7. Drexhage HA, Bottazzo GF, Doniach D, Bitensky L, Chayen J: Evidence for thyroid-stimulating immunoglobulins in some goitrous thyroid diseases. *Lancet* 2:287, 1980.

8. Valente WA, Vitti P, Rotella CM, Vaughan MM, Aloj SM, Grollman EF, Ambesi-Impiombato FS, Kohn LD: Antibodies that promote thyroid growth: A distinct population of thyroid-stimulating autoantibodies. *N Engl J Med* 309:1028, 1983.

9. Roger PP, Servais P, Dumont JE: Stimulation by thyrotropin and cyclic AMP of the proliferation of quiescent canine thyroid cells cultured in a defined medium containing insulin. *FEBS Lett* 157:323, 1983.

10. Westermark K, Karlsson FA, Westermark B: Epidermal growth factor modulates thyroid growth and function in culture. *Endocrinology* 112:1680, 1983.

11. Eggo MC, Bachrach LK, Fayer G, Errick J, Kudlow JE, Cohen MF, Burrow GN: The effects of growth factors and serum on DNA synthesis and differentiation in thyroid cells in culture. *Mol Cell Endocrinol* 38:141, 1984.

12. Bowers CY, Lee KL, Schally AV: A study on the interaction of the thyrotropin-releasing factor and L-triiodothyronine: Effects of puromycin and cycloheximide. *Endocrinology* 82:75, 1968.

13. Larsen PR: Thyroid-pituitary interaction: Feedback regulation of thyrotropin secretion by thyroid hormones. *N Engl J Med* 306:23, 1982.

14. Chopra IJ, Hershman JM, Hornabrook RW: Serum thyroid hormone and thyrotropin levels in subjects from endemic goiter regions of New Guinea. *J Clin Endocrinol Metab* 40:326, 1975.

15. Medeiros-Neto GA, Penna M, Monteiro K, Kataoka K, Imai Y, Hollander C: The effect of iodized oil in the TSH response to TRH in endemic goiter patients. *J Clin Endocrinol Metab* 41:504, 1976.

16. Koutras DA, Alexander WD, Buchanan WW, Crooks J, Wayne EJ: Stable iodine metabolism in non-toxic goitre. *Lancet* 2:784, 1960.

17. Vegenakis AG, Koutras DA, Burger A, Malamos B, Ingbar SH, Braverman LE: Studies of serum triiodothyronine, thyroxine and thyrotropin concentrations in endemic goiter in Greece. *J Clin Endocrinol Metab* 37:485, 1973.

18. Dige-Petersen H, Hummer L: Serum thyrotropin concentrations under basal conditions and after stimulation with thyrotropin-releasing hormone in idiopathic non-toxic goiter. *J Clin Endocrinol Metab* 44:1115, 1977.

19. Young RL, Harvey WC, Mazzaferri EL, Reynolds JC, Hamilton CR Jr: Thyroid-stimulating hormone levels in idiopathic euthyroid goiter. *J Clin Endocrinol Metab* 41:21, 1975.

20. Bachtarzi H, Benmiloud M: TSH-regulation and goitrogenesis in severe iodine deficiency. *Acta Endocrinol* 103:21, 1983.

21. Ibbertson HK: Endemic goitre and cretinism. *Clin Endocrinol Metab* 8:97, 1979.

22. Van Herle AJ, Chopra IJ, Hershman JM, Hornabrook RW: Serum thyroglobulin in inhabitants of an endemic goiter region of New Guinea. *J Clin Endocrinol Metab* 43:512, 1976.

23. Pitt-Rivers R, Niven JSF, Young MR: Localization of protein-bound radioactive iodine in rat thyroid glands labeled with ^{125}I or ^{131}I. *Biochem J* 90:205, 1964.

24. Stanbury JB, Querido A: Genetic and environmental factors in cretinism: A classification. *J Clin Endocrinol Metab* 16:1522, 1956.

25. Dumont JE, Ermans AM, Bastenie PA: Thyroid function in a goiter endemic. V. Mechanism of thyroid failure in the Uele endemic cretins. *J Clin Endocrinol Metab* 23:847, 1963.

26. McCullagh SF: The Huon Peninsula endemic: III. The effect in the female of endemic goitre of reproductive function. *Med J Aust* 1:844, 1963.

27. Pendergrast WJ, Milmore BK, Marcus SC: Thyroid cancer and thyrotoxicosis in the United States: Their relation to endemic goiter. *J Chronic Dis* 13:22, 1961.

28. Studer H, Hunziker HR, Ruchti C: Morphologic and functional substrate of thyrotoxicosis caused by nodular goiters. *Am J Med* 65:227, 1978.

29. Boukis MA, Koutras DA, Souvatzoglou A, Evangelopoulou A, Vrontakis M, Moulopoulos SD: Thyroid hormone and immunological studies in endemic goiter. *J Clin Endocrinol Metab* 57:859, 1983.

30. Delange F, Costa A, Ermans AM, Ibbertson HK, Querido A, Stanbury JB: A survey of the clinical and metabolic patterns of endemic cretinism, in Stanbury JB, Kroc RL (eds): *Human Development and the Thyroid Gland, Relation to Endemic Cretinism*. New York, Plenum, 1972, p 175.

31. Editorial: Endemic goitre and cretinism. *Lancet* 2:1165, 1979.

32. Thilly CH, Delange F, Lagasse R, Bourdoux P, Ramioul L, Berquist H, Ermans AM: Fetal hypothyroidism and maternal thyroid status in severe endemic goiter. *J Clin Endocrinol Metab* 47:354, 1978.

33. Patel YC, Pharoah POD, Hornabrook RW, Hetzel BS: Serum triiodothyronine, thyroxine and thyroid-stimulating hormone in endemic goiter: A comparison of goitrous and nongoitrous subjects in New Guinea. *J Clin Endocrinol Metab* 37:783, 1973.

34. Pretell EA: Role of the placenta and of plasma hormone binding in the pathogenesis of cretinism, in Stanbury JB, Kroc RL (eds): *Human Development and the Thyroid Gland, Relation to Endemic Cretinism*. New York, Plenum, 1972, p 449.

35. Hershman JM, Due DT, Sharp B, My L, Kent JR, Binh LN, Reed AW, Phuc LD, Van Herle AJ, Thai NA, Troung TX, Van NV, Sugawara M, Pekary E: Endemic goiter in Vietnam. *J Clin Endocrinol Metab* 57:243, 1983.

36. Gaitan JE, Mayoral LG, Gaitan E: Defective thyroidal iodine concentration in protein-calorie malnutrition. *J Clin Endocrinol Metab* 57:327, 1983.

37. Ingenbleek Y, Luypaert B, De Nayer PH: Nutritional status and endemic goitre. *Lancet* 1:388, 1980.

38. Kimball OP: The prevention of simple goiter in man. *Am J Med Sci* 163:634, 1922.

39. Vander JB, Gaston EA, Dawber TR: The significance of nontoxic thyroid nodules. *Ann Intern Med* 69:537, 1968.

40. Mortensen JD, Bennett WA, Woolner LB: Incidence of carcinoma in thyroid glands removed at 1000 consecutive routine necropsies. *Surg Forum* 5:659, 1955.

41. Kieffer JD, Mover H, Federico P, Maloof F: Pituitary-thyroid axis in neonatal and adult rats: Comparison of the sexes. *Endocrinology* 98:295, 1976.

42. Malamos B, Miras K, Kostamis P, Mantzos J, Kralios AC, Rigopoulos G, Zerefos N, Koutras DA: Epidemiologic and metabolic studies in the endemic goiter areas of Greece, in Cassano C,

Andreoli M (eds): *Current Topics in Thyroid Research.* New York, Academic, 1965, p 851.

43. Greig WR, Boyle JA, Duncan A, Nicol J, Gray MJB, Buchanan WW, McGirr EM: Genetic and non-genetic factors in simple goitre formation: Evidence from a twin study. *Q J Med* 36:175, 1967.

44. Nilsson LR: Adolescent colloid goitre. *Acta Paediatr Scand* 55:49, 1966.

45. Crooks, J, Aboul-Khair SA, Turnbull AC, Hytten FE: The incidence of goitre during pregnancy. *Lancet* 2:334, 1964.

46. Crooks J, Tulloch MI, Turnbull AC, Davidsson D, Skulason T, Snaedal G: Comparative incidence of goitre in pregnancy in Iceland and Scotland. *Lancet* 2:625, 1967.

47. Dworkin HJ, Jacquez JA, Beierwaltes WH: Relationship of iodine ingestion to iodine excretion in pregnancy. *J Clin Endocrinol Metab* 26:1329, 1966.

48. Levy RP, Newman DM, Rejali LS, Barford DAG: The myth of goiter in pregnancy. *Am J Obstet Gynecol* 137:701, 1980.

49. Vickery AL: The diagnosis of malignancy in dyshormonogenetic goiter. *Clin Endocrinol Metab* 10:317, 1981.

50. Van Herle AJ, Vassart G, Dumont JE: Control of thyroglobulin synthesis and secretion. *N Engl J Med* 301:239,307, 1979.

51. Chesney AM, Clawson TA, Webster B: Endemic goitre in rabbits: I. Incidence and characteristics. *Bull Johns Hopkins Hosp* 43:261, 1928.

52. Gaitan E, Wahner HW, Correa P, Bernal R, Jubiz W, Gaitan JE, Llanos G: Endemic goiter in the Cauca Valley: I. Results and limitations of twelve years of iodine prophylaxis. *J Clin Endocrinol Metab* 28:1730, 1968.

53. McGarrison R: *The Thyroid Gland in Health and Disease.* London, Bailliere, Tindall and Cox, 1917.

54. Silverberg SG, Vidone RA: Carcinoma of the thyroid in surgical and postmortem material. *Ann Surg* 164:291, 1966.

55. Reede DL, Bergeron RT, McCauley DI: CT of the thyroid and of other thoracic inlet disorders. *J Otolaryngol* 11:349, 1982.

56. Jauregui R, Lilker ES, Bayley A: Upper airway obstruction in euthyroid goiter. *JAMA* 238:2163, 1977.

57. Cady B: Management of tracheal obstruction from thyroid diseases. *World J Surg* 6:696, 1982.

58. Medvei UC: *A History of Endocrinology.* Lancaster, U.K., MTP, 1982, p 57.

59. Sampson RJ, Key CR, Buncher CR, Iijima S: Thyroid carcinoma in Hiroshima and Nagasaki. I. Prevalence of thyroid carcinoma at autopsy. *JAMA* 209:65, 1969.

60. Cutler SJ, Young JL (eds): *Third National Cancer Survey: Incidence Data,* National Cancer Institute Monograph 41, U.S. DHEW publication (NIH) 75-787. Bethesda, 1975, pp 107, 111.

61. Taylor S, Goolden AWG: Thyroid and thymus, in Kunkler PB, Rains AJH (eds): *Treatment of Cancer in Clinical Practice.* Edinburgh, E & S Livingstone, 1959, p 410.

62. Money WL, Rawson RW: The experimental production of thyroid tumors in the rat exposed to prolonged treatment with thiouracil. *Cancer* 3:321, 1950.

63. Al-Saadi A: Precursor cytogenetic changes of transplantable thyroid carcinoma in iodine-deficient goiters. *Cancer Res* 28:739, 1968.

64. Elman DS: Familial association of nerve deafness with nodular goiter and thyroid carcinoma. *N Engl J Med* 259:219, 1958.

65. McGirr EM, Clement WE, Currie AR, Kennedy JS: Impaired dehalogenase activity as a cause of goitre with malignant changes. *Scott Med J* 4:232, 1959.

66. Astwood EB, Cassidy CE, Aurbach GD: Treatment of goiter and thyroid nodules with thyroid. *JAMA* 174:459, 1960.

67. Lamberg BA, Hernberg CA, Hakkila R: Treatment of nontoxic goitre with thyroid preparations. *Acta Endocrinol* 33:584, 1960.

68. Shimaoka K, Sokal JE: Suppressive therapy of nontoxic goiter. *Am J Med* 57:576, 1974.

69. Hansen JM, Kampmann J, Madsen SH, Skovsted L, Solgaard S Grytter C, Grontveldt T, Rasmussen SN: L-Thyroxine treatment of diffuse nontoxic goitre evaluated by ultrasonic determination of thyroid volume. *Clin Endocrinol* 10:1, 1979.

70. Clark OH: TSH suppression in the management of thyroid nodules and thyroid cancer. *World J Surg* 5:39, 1981.

71. Stock JM, Surks MI, Oppenheimer JH: Replacement dosage of L-thyroxine in hypothyroidism. *N Engl J Med* 290:529, 1974.

72. Braverman LE, Vagenakis A, Downs P, Foster AE, Sterling K, Ingbar SH: Effects of replacement doses of sodium-L-thyroxine on the peripheral metabolism of thyroxine and triiodothyronine in man. *J Clin Invest* 52:1010, 1973.

73. Rosenbaum RL, Barzel US: Levothyroxine replacement dose for primary hypothyroidism decreases with age. *Ann Intern Med* 96:53, 1982.

74. Shimaoka K, Sokal JE: Differentiation of benign and malignant thyroid nodules by scintiscan. *Arch Intern Med* 114:36, 1964.

75. Hoffmann GL, Thompson NW, Heffron C: The solitary thyroid nodule. *Arch Surg* 105:379, 1972.

76. Burrow GN, Mujtaba Q, Livolsi V, Cornog J: The incidence of carcinoma in solitary "cold" thyroid nodules. *Yale J Biol Med* 51:13, 1978.

77. Hempelmann LH: Thyroid neoplasms following irradiation in infancy, in DeGroot LJ (ed): *Radiation-Associated Thyroid Carcinoma.* New York, Grune & Stratton, 1977, p 221.

78. Winship T, Rosvoll RV: Childhood thyroid carcinoma. *Cancer* 14:734, 1961.

79. Rallison ML, Dobyns BM, Keating FR Jr, Rall JE, Tyler FH: Thyroid nodularity in children. *JAMA* 233:1069, 1975.

80. Kirkland RT, Kirkland JL, Rosenberg HS, Harberg FJ, Librik L, Clayton GW: Solitary thyroid nodules in 30 children and report of a child with a thyroid abscess. *Pediatrics* 51:85, 1973.

81. Silverman SH, Nussbaum M, Rausen AR: Thyroid nodules in children: A ten year experience at one institution. *Mt Sinai J Med* (NY) 46:460, 1979.

82. Duffy BJ Jr, Fitzgerald PJ: Cancer of the thyroid in children: A report of 28 cases. *J Clin Endocrinol Metab* 10:1296, 1950.

83. Pifer JW, Hempelmann LH: Radiation-induced thyroid carcinoma. *Ann NY Acad Sci* 114:838, 1964.

84. Refetoff S, Harrison J, Karanfilski BT, Kaplan EL, DeGroot LJ, Bekerman C: Continuing occurrence of thyroid carcinoma after irradiation to the neck in infancy and childhood. *N Engl J Med* 292:171, 1975.

85. DeGroot LJ, Reilly M, Pinnameneni K, Refetoff S: Retrospective and prospective study of radiation-induced thyroid disease. *Am J Med* 74:852, 1983.

86. Schneider AB, Pinsky S, Berkerman C, Ryo UY: Characteristics of 108 thyroid cancers detected by screening in a population with a history of head and neck irradiation. *Cancer* 46:1218, 1980.

87. Rao SD, Frame B, Miller MJ, Kleerekoper M, Block MA, Parfitt M: Hyperparathyroidism following head and neck irradiation. *Arch Intern Med* 140:205, 1980.

88. Bowens OM, Vander BJ: Thyroid nodules and thyroid malignancy. *Ann Intern Med* 57:245, 1962.

89. Miller JM, Hamburger JI, Mellinger RC: The thyroid scintigram: II. The cold nodule. *Radiology* 85:702, 1965.

90. DeGroot LJ (ed): *Radiation-Associated Thyroid Carcinoma.* New York, Grune & Stratton, 1977.

91. Esser PD: Absorbed radiation doses in adults, in Freeman LM, Johnson PM (eds): *Clinical Scintillation Imaging,* 2d ed. New York, Grune & Stratton, 1975, p 799.

92. Keyes JW, Thrall JH, Carey JE: Technical considerations in in vivo thyroid studies. *Semin Nucl Med* 8:43, 1978.

93. Blum M: Enhanced clinical diagnosis of thyroid disease using echography. *Am J Med* 59:301, 1975.

94. Miller JM, Zafar SU, Karo JJ: The cystic thyroid nodule. *Radiology* 110:257, 1974.

95. McCowen KD, Reed JW, Fariss BL: The role of thyroid therapy in patients with thyroid cysts. *Am J Med* 68:853, 1980.

96. Treece GL, Georgitis WJ, Hofeldt FD: Resolution of recurrent thyroid cysts with tetracycline instillation. *Arch Intern Med* 143:2285, 1983.

97. de Certaines J, Herry JY, Lancien G, Benoist L, Bernard AM, Le Clech G: Evaluation of human thyroid tumors by proton nuclear magnetic resonance. *J Nucl Med* 23:48, 1982.

98. Mojab K, Ghosh BC: Thyroid angiography. *Am J Surg* 132:620, 1976.

99. Maloof F, Wang CA, Vickery AL Jr: Nontoxic goiter—diffuse or nodular. *Med Clin North Am* 59:1221, 1975.

100. Vickery AL Jr: Needle biopsy and the thyroid nodule, in DeGroot LJ (ed): *Radiation-Associated Thyroid Carcinoma.* New York, Grune & Stratton, 1977, p 339.

101. Burke JS, Butler JJ, Fuller LM: Malignant lymphomas of the thyroid: A clinical pathologic study of 35 patients including ultrastructural observations. *Cancer* 39:1587, 1977.

102. Sirota DK, Segal RL: Primary lymphomas of the thyroid gland. *JAMA* 242:1743, 1979.

103. Van Herle AJ, Rich P, Ljung B-ME, Ashcraft MW, Solomon DH, Keeler EB: The thyroid nodule. *Ann Intern Med* 96:221, 1982.

104. Ashcraft MW, Van Herle AJ: Management of thyroid nodules. II: Scanning techniques, thyroid suppressive therapy, and fine needle aspiration. *Head Neck Surg* 3:297, 1981.

105. McNeil BJ, Keeler E, Adelstein SJ: Primer on certain elements of medical decision making. *N Engl J Med* 293:211, 1975.

106. Miller JM, Hamburger JI, Kini S: Diagnosis of thyroid nodules: Use of fine-needle aspiration and needle biopsy. *JAMA* 241:481, 1979.

107. Miller JM, Hamburger JI, Kini SR: The needle biopsy diagnosis of papillary thyroid carcinoma. *Cancer* 48:989, 1981.

108. Chu EW, Hanson TA, Goldman JM, Robbins J: Study of cells in fine needle aspirations of the thyroid gland. *Acta Ctyol* 23:309, 1979.

109. Clark OH, Demling R: Management of thyroid nodules in the elderly. *Am J Surg* 132:615, 1976.

110. Field JB, Larsen PR, Yamashita K, Mashiter K, Dekker A: Demonstration of iodine transport defect but normal iodide organification in nonfunctioning nodules of human thyroid glands. *J Clin Invest* 52:2404, 1973.

111. Shiroozu A, Inoue K, Nakashima T, Okamura K, Yoshinari M, Nishitani H, Omae T: Defective iodide transport and normal organification of iodide in cold nodules of the thyroid. *Clin Endocrinol* 15:411, 1981.

112. Hoffman DP, Surks MI, Oppenheimer JH, Weitzman ED: Response to thyrotropin releasing hormone: An objective criterion for the adequacy of thyrotropin suppression therapy. *J Clin Endocrinol Metab* 44:892, 1977.

113. Nilsson G, Pettersson U, Levin K, Hughes R: Studies on replacement and suppressive dosages of L-thyroxine. *Acta Med Scand* 202:257, 1977.

114. Meissner WA: The pathologic classification and staging of thyroid cancer, in DeGroot LJ (ed): *Radiation-Associated Thyroid Carcinoma.* New York, Grune & Stratton, 1977, p 45.

115. Sampson RJ: Prevalence and significance of occult thyroid cancer, in DeGroot LJ (ed): *Radiation-Associated Thyroid Carcinoma.* New York, Grune & Stratton, 1977, p 137.

116. Maxon HR, Thomas SR, Saenger EL, Buncher CR, Kereiakes JG: Ionizing irradiation and the induction of clinically significant disease in the human thyroid gland. *Am J Med* 63:967, 1977.

117. Maxon HR, Saenger EL, Thomas SR, Buncher CR, Kereiakes JG, Shafer ML, McLaughlin CA: Clinically important radiation-associated thyroid disease. A controlled study. *JAMA* 244:1802, 1980.

118. Holm L-E, Dahlqvist I, Israelsson A, Lundell G: Malignant thyroid tumors after iodine-131 therapy: A retrospective cohort study. *N Engl J Med* 303:188, 1980.

119. Getaz EP, Shimaoka K, Razack M, Friedman M: Suppressive therapy for postirradiation thyroid nodules. *Can J Surg* 23:558, 1980.

120. Schimpff SC: Specialty rounds. Well-differentiated thyroid carcinoma: Epidemiology, etiology and treatment. *Am J Med Sci* 278:100, 1979.

121. Margolin FR, Steinbach HL: Soft tissue roentgenography of thyroid nodules. *Am J Roentgenol* 102:844, 1968.

122. Mazzaferri EL, Young RL, Oertel JE, Kemmerer WT, Page CP: Papillary thyroid carcinoma: The impact of therapy in 576 patients. *Medicine* 56:171, 1977.

123. Mazzaferri EL, Young RL: Papillary thyroid carcinoma: A 10 year follow-up report of the impact of therapy in 576 patients. *Am J Med* 70:511, 1981.

124. Silliphant WM, Klinck GH, Levitin MS: Thyroid carcinoma and death: A clinicopathological study of 193 autopsies. *Cancer* 17:513, 1964.

125. Heimann R, Vannineuse A, De Sloover C, Dor P: Malignant lymphomas and undifferentiated small cell carcinoma of the thyroid: A clinicopathological review in the light of the Kiel classification for malignant lymphomas. *Histopathology* 2:201, 1978.

126. Clark OH: Total thyroidectomy: The treatment of choice for patients with differentiated thyroid cancer. *Ann Surg* 196:361, 1982.

126a. Foster RS Jr: Morbidity and mortality after thyroidectomy. *Surg Gynecol Obstet* 146:423, 1978.

127. Thompson NW, Harness JK: Complications of total thyroidectomy for carcinoma. *Surg Gynecol Obstet* 131:861, 1970.

128. Varma VM, Beierwaltes WH, Nofal MM, Nishiyama RH, Copp JE: Treatment of thyroid cancer. Death rates after surgery and after surgery followed by sodium iodide I 131. *JAMA* 214:1437, 1970.

129. Leeper RD: The effect of ^{131}I therapy on survival of patients with metastatic papillary or follicular thyroid carcinoma. *J Clin Endocrinol Metab* 36:1143, 1973.

130. Crile G: The endocrine dependency of papillary carcinoma of the thyroid, in Smithers D (ed): *Tumours of the Thyroid Gland.* Edinburgh, E & S Livingstone, 1970, p 269.

131. Lamberg B-A, Rantanen M, Saarinen P, Liewendahl K, Sivula A: Suppression of the TSH response to TRH by thyroxine therapy in differentiated thyroid carcinoma patients. *Acta Endocrinol* 91:248, 1979.

132. Simpson WJ, Carruthers JS: The role of external radiation in the management of papillary and follicular thyroid cancer. *Am J Surg* 136:457, 1978.

133. Beierwaltes WH, Nishiyama RH, Thompson NW, Copp JE, Kubo A: Survival time and "cure" in papillary and follicular thyroid carcinoma with distant metastases: Statistics following University of Michigan therapy. *J Nucl Med* 23:561, 1982.

134. Samaan NA, Maheshwari YK, Nader S, Hill CS Jr, Schultz PN, Haynie TP, Hickey RC, Clark RL, Geopfert H, Ibanez ML, Litton CE: Impact of therapy for differentiated carcinoma of the thyroid: An analysis of 706 cases. *J Clin Endocrinol Metab* 56:1131, 1983.

135. DeGroot LJ, Reilly M: Comparison of 30- and 50-mCi doses of iodine-131 for thyroid ablation. *Ann Intern Med* 96:51, 1982.

136. Beierwaltes WH: The treatment of thyroid carcinoma with radioactive iodine. *Semin Nucl Med* 8:79, 1978.

137. Hilts SV, Hellman D, Anderson J, Woolfenden J, Van Antwerp J, Patton D: Serial TSH determination after T_3 withdrawal or thyroidectomy in the therapy of thyroid carcinoma. *J Nucl Med* 20:928, 1979.

138. Goldman JM, Line BR, Aamodt RL, Robbins J: Influence of triiodothyronine withdrawal time on ^{131}I uptake postthyroidectomy for thyroid cancer. *J Clin Endocrinol Metab* 50:734, 1980.

139. Melmed S, Harada A, Hershman JM, Kirshnamurthy GT, Blahd WH: Neutralizing antibodies to bovine thyrotropin in immunized patients with thyroid cancer. *J Clin Endocrinol Metab* 51:358, 1980.
140. Hershman JM, Edwards CL: Serum thyrotropin (TSH) levels after thyroid ablation compared with TSH levels after exogenous bovine TSH: Implications for ^{131}I treatment of thyroid carcinoma. *J Clin Endocrinol Metab* 34:814, 1972.
141. Hamburger JI: Diuretic augmentation of ^{131}I uptake in inoperable thyroid cancer. *N Engl J Med* 280:1091, 1969.
142. Simpson WJ: Anaplastic thyroid carcinoma: A new approach. *Can J Surg* 23:25, 1980.
143. Smithers D (ed): *Tumours of the Thyroid Gland.* Edinburgh, E & S Livingston, 1970.
144. Shimaoka K: Adjunctive management of thyroid cancer. Chemotherapy. *J Surg Oncol* 15:283, 1980.
145. Gottlieb JA, Hill CS Jr: Chemotherapy of thyroid cancer with Adriamycin. *N Engl J Med* 290:193, 1974.
146. Harada T, Nishikawa Y, Suzuki T, Ito K, Baba S: Bleomycin treatment for cancer of the thyroid. *Am J Surg* 122:53, 1971.
147. Dewan SS: The bone scan in the thyroid cancer. *J Nucl Med* 20:271, 1979.
148. Charles MA: Comparison of serum thyroglobulin with iodine scans in thyroid cancer. *J Endocrinol Invest* 5:267, 1982.
149. Gebel F, Ramelli, F, Burgi U, Ingold U, Studer H, Winand R: The site of leakage of intrafollicular thyroglobulin into the blood stream in simple human goiter. *J Clin Endocrinol Metab* 57:915, 1983.
150. Van Herle AJ, Uller RP, Matthews NL, Brown J: Radioimmunoassay for measurement of thyroglobulin in human serum. *J Clin Invest* 52:1320, 1973.
151. Schneider AB, Favus MJ, Stachura ME, Arnold JE, Ryo UY, Pinsky S, Colman M, Arnold MJ, Frohman LA: Plasma thyroglobulin in detecting thyroid carcinoma after childhood head and neck irradiation. *Ann Intern Med* 86:29, 1977.
152. Charles MA, Dodson LE, Waldeck N, Hofeldt F, Ghaed N, Telepak R, Ownbey J, Burnstein P: Serum thyroglobulin levels predict total body iodine scan findings in patients with treated well-differentiated thyroid carcinoma. *Am J Med* 69:401, 1980.
153. Black EG, Cassoni A, Gimlette TMD, Harmer CL, Maisey MN, Oates GD: Serum thyroglobulin in thyroid cancer. *Lancet* 2:443, 1981.
154. Schneider AB, Line BR, Goldman JM, Robbins J: Sequential serum thyroglobulin determinations, ^{131}I scans, and ^{131}I uptakes after triiodothyronine withdrawal in patients with thyroid cancer. *J Clin Endocrinol Metab* 53:1199, 1981.
155. DeGroot LJ, Hoye K, Refetoff S, Van Herle AJ, Asteris GT, Rochman H: Serum antigens and antibodies in the diagnosis of thyroid cancer. *J Clin Endocrinol Metab* 45:1220, 1977.
156. Fairweather DS, Bradwell AR, Watson-James SF, Dykes PW, Chandler S, Hoffenberg R: Detection of thyroid tumours using radio-labelled anti-thyroglobulin. *Clin Endocrinol* 18:563, 1983.
157. Steiner AL, Goodman AD, Powers SR: Study of a kindred with pheochromocytoma, medullary thyroid carcinoma, hyperparathyroidism and Cushing's disease: Multiple endocrine neoplasia, type 2. *Medicine* 47:371, 1968.
158. Khairi MRA, Dexter RN, Burzynski NJ, Johnston CC Jr: Mucosal neuroma, pheochromocytoma and medullary thyroid carcinoma: Multiple endocrine neoplasia type 3. *Medicine* 54:89, 1975.
159. Knudson AG: Mutation and cancer: Statistical study of retinoblastoma. *Proc Natl Acad Sci USA* 68:820, 1971.
160. Jackson CE, Block MA, Greenawald KA, Tashjian AH: The two-mutational-event theory in medullary thyroid cancer. *Am J Hum Genet* 31:704, 1979.
161. Baylin SB, Hsu SH, Gann DS: Inherited medullary thyroid carcinoma: A final monoclonal mutation in one of multiple clones of susceptible cells. *Science* 199:429, 1978.
162. Hill CS Jr, Ibanez ML, Samaan NA, Ahearn MJ, Clark RL: Medullary (solid) carcinoma of the thyroid gland: An analysis of the M.D. Anderson Hospital experience with patients with the tumor, its special features, and its histogenesis. *Medicine* 52:141, 1973.
163. Tashjian AH Jr, Wolfe HJ, Voelkel EF: Human calcitonin. *Am J Med* 56:840, 1974.
164. Wells SA Jr, Baylin SB, Linehan WM, Farrell RE, Cox EB, Cooper CW: Provocative agents and the diagnosis of medullary carcinoma of the thyroid gland. *Ann Surg* 188:139, 1978.
165. Baylin SB, Beaven MA, Keiser HR, Tashjian AH Jr, Melvin KEW: Serum histaminase and calcitonin levels in medullary carcinoma of the thyroid. *Lancet* 1:455, 1972.
166. Wolfe HJ, Melvin KEW, Cervi-Skinner SJ, Al Saadi AA, Juliar JF, Jackson CE, Tashjian AH Jr: C-cell hyperplasia preceding medullary thyroid carcinoma. *N Engl J Med* 289:437, 1973.
167. Gagel RF, Jackson CE, Block MA, Feldman ZT, Reichlin S, Hamilton BP, Tashjian AH: Age-related probability of development of hereditary medullary thyroid carcinoma. *J Pediatr* 101:941, 1982.
168. Wahner HW, Cuello C, Aljure F: Hormone-induced regression of medullary (solid) thyroid carcinoma. *Am J Med* 45:789, 1968.

PART IV

ADRENAL DISEASE

12

The Adrenal Cortex

John D. Baxter
J. Blake Tyrrell

The adrenal cortex produces more than 50 different steroids. It is the sole source of glucocorticoids and mineralocorticoids and a major source of androgens in the female, but only a minor source of estrogens and progestins.

Glucocorticoids, named for their carbohydrate-regulating activities, are essential for maintenance of vital functions and are especially important for bodily responses to physical stress. They also regulate growth and developmental processes. Cortisol (hydrocortisone) is the major glucocorticoid in humans. A deficiency of this steroid, as occurs in Addison's syndrome, can be life-threatening. Cortisol excess results in Cushing's syndrome, with multiple deleterious manifestations.

The mineralocorticoids, of which aldosterone is preeminent in humans, were named for their salt-regulating activities and govern the balance of sodium and potassium ions. Mineralocorticoid excess can result in hypertension with sodium retention and hypokalemia; deficiency can cause sodium loss and hyperkalemia.

Although diseases of the adrenal cortex are relatively uncommon, many of the signs and symptoms of adrenal dysfunction mimic those commonly seen in office practice. Thus, diseases of the adrenal cortex must be considered in the differential diagnosis of common complaints. Further, because cortisol and its analogues (e.g., prednisone) are among the most commonly prescribed of all drugs and are used to treat a number of nonadrenal disorders, the physician is frequently confronted with the problems of iatrogenic glucocorticoid excess when these drugs are given and glucocorticoid deficiency following their withdrawal (Chap. 15).

In this chapter the physiology and diseases of the adrenal cortex are discussed. Chapter 15 deals more extensively with steroid therapy, and Chap. 14 addresses the mineralocorticoid excess syndromes and the relationships of the adrenocortical hormones to hypertension.

HISTORY OF STUDY OF THE ADRENAL CORTEX

The small suprarenal adrenal glands that surround the catecholamine-producing adrenal medulla may have been first described by Bartolomeo Eustacchio in 1563 (published by Lancisi in 1714 and cited in Ref. 1). However, scientific interest in them began with the description by Thomas Addison, in 1849 and 1855, of the classic features of adrenocortical deficiency, which included "general languor and debility, remarkable feebleness of the heart's action, irritability of the stomach and a peculiar change in the colour of the skin."[1] Addison's idea that the adrenal gland is essential for life received experimental support in 1856 from Brown-Sequard, who performed adrenalectomies on several species.[1]

By the turn of the century, the syndrome of glucocorticoid excess had been described in association with adrenal tumors and bilateral adrenocortical hyperplasia. In 1932, Harvey Cushing attributed the syndrome to basophilic pituitary adenomas.[2]

The roles of the adrenocortical hormones were generally elucidated with the increasing availability of more refined surgical techniques for removal of the pituitary and adrenal glands and of adrenocortical extracts to replace lost function. That the adrenal cortex is involved in regulating intermediary metabolism was established between 1908 and 1940.[1,3] The occurrence of hypoglycemia in adrenal-insufficient dogs and humans was appreciated by 1910 (see Ref. 3 for review). Maranon subsequently found that patients with coexisting diabetes and adrenal insufficiency were hypersensitive to insulin, and Cori and Cori noted a decrease in hepatic glycogen after adrenalectomy. Britten and Silvette subsequently proposed that loss of the carbohydrate-regulating properties of the adrenal gland was a factor in the debilitation and mortality in adrenal deficiency. Long, Katzin, and Fry reported in 1940 that the fall in blood glucose and liver glycogen levels in adrenalectomized animals deprived of food could be corrected by administration of adrenal extracts. These workers and Evans first noted that glucocorticoids have effects on nitrogen metabolism (cited in Refs. 1, 3, 4). Urinary nitrogen excretion increased in glucocorticoid-treated animals, but decreased in fasted adrenalectomized animals. These studies also suggested that glucocorticoids enhance gluconeogenesis. The same workers obtained evidence that glucocorticoids influence lipid metabolism with the finding that ketosis in diabetic animals could be abolished by adrenalectomy.

In 1927, Baumann and Kurland reported that adrenalectomy causes hyponatremia, hypothermia, and hyperkalemia (see Ref. 1 for review). Loeb and coworkers subsequently demonstrated that saline could extend the survival of adrenalectomized animals and patients with Addison's disease.

By 1937, it was perceived that although a high sodium intake enhanced survival in the adrenalectomized rat, it was not sufficient to prolong life indefinitely. With further study, it was found that these animals were susceptible to a host of stressful influences (e.g., toxins, trauma, drugs, strenuous exercise, infections, and emotional stimuli). These observations led to the realization that the glucocorticoid function of the adrenals was also necessary for survival. Hans Selye, who coined the terms *mineralocorticoid* and *glucocorticoid*, emphasized the relation of the adrenal glands to stress.

A pituitary role in regulation of adrenal function was suspected by about 1925 (see Refs. 1, 3). In 1930, Smith's landmark paper reported the effects of hypophysectomy, including atrophy of the adrenal glands, and the influences of replacement by administering fresh pituitary implants. In 1937, Ingle and Kendall demonstrated the existence of inhibitory feedback to the pituitary by adrenal hormones. They also noted the existence of additional regulatory mechanisms, since glucocorticoid feedback did not explain the adrenal secretory response to stress or the spontaneous circadian rhythm of adrenal and pituitary activity. Because survival after hypophysectomy was greater than after adrenalectomy, they correctly surmised that adrenal function is not completely pituitary-dependent.

ACTH (corticotropin or adrenocorticotropin), the pituitary factor that could restore adrenal function, was identified shortly thereafter and shown to stimulate steroid synthesis and release. It was purified by 1943 and its structure had been determined by 1956. It was subsequently established that ACTH is first synthesized as part of a larger precursor molecule that also contains the sequences of several other hormones, including β-lipotropin, β-endorphin, and the melanocyte stimulating hormones (MSH) (Chap. 8).

That the hypothalamus is important for ACTH release was perceived by 1950; shortly thereafter it was found that vasopressin could stimulate ACTH release.[5] Evidence for the presence of a factor other than vasopressin that could stimulate ACTH release was first reported in 1955.[6,7] However, it was not until 1981 that the structure of ovine corticotropin releasing factor (CRF), probably the major hypothalamic factor that regulates ACTH release, was obtained.[8]

The importance of the zona glomerulosa of the adrenal in the regulation of electrolyte balance, its control by dietary sodium and potassium, and the relative independence of this zone from the pituitary gland emerged from the studies of Deane and coworkers (cited in Ref. 4). In 1950, Deming and Luetscher detected a sodium-retaining factor in human urine (see Ref. 4). This factor, *aldosterone,* was isolated and characterized by Simpson et al., and its regulation by the renin-angiotensin system was subsequently described.[4,9] In 1955, Conn described the syndrome of aldosterone excess with hypertension and hypokalemia.[10]

The identification and synthesis of adrenal steroids and analogues of them led to detailed studies of their actions and use in therapy. In the 1930s, Steiger and Reichstein synthesized deoxycorticosterone (DOC), which had mineralocorticoid but not carbohydrate-regulating activity (see Refs. 1 and 3 for reviews). It was thought by some that this steroid might be the major sodium-regulating hormone. It was also found, however, that DOC did not prolong survival as well as did adrenal extracts containing steroid mixtures. The structure of corticosterone, the major rat glucocorticoid, was identified in 1937 by Reichstein, Kendall, and others, and by the late 1940s steroids with glucocorticoid activity were available. Results with 11-dehydrocorticosterone were disappointing, but cortisone was found to have the sought-after glucocorticoid activity. The synthesis of aldosterone proved to be much more difficult; it was finally achieved in the 1950s.[1,4]

The decision to try cortisone as an anti-inflammatory agent was made by Hench in 1941, who thought that the substance that ameliorated rheumatoid arthritis during pregnancy and jaundice might be an adrenal hormone.[11]

Sufficient material became available in 1949, when Hench, Kendall, Slocumb, and Polley found that cortisone and ACTH lessened articular, muscular, and other symptoms in patients with rheumatoid arthritis.[11] This finding was unexpected. Although anti-inflammatory effects of glucocorticoids had been reported as early as 1940 by Menkin, these were attributed to influences on fluid dynamics; most authorities did not anticipate an immunosuppressive and anti-inflammatory role for the steroids (see Ref. 1). The findings in rheumatoid arthritis led to wider use of these steroids in other diseases. However, it was also soon appreciated that the long-term use of glucocorticoids is accompanied by a number of adverse effects.

Over the past 30 years, more sophisticated experimental techniques have become available. These have led to a greater understanding of the responses elicited by the hormones, the mechanisms that regulate the plasma levels of the adrenal steroids, and the pathophysiology of the syndromes due to their excesses and deficiencies. Inquiry during the past two decades has also provided fundamental information about the molecular basis for adrenal steroid hormone action. The steroids bind to intracellular receptors, and the resulting complexes bind to the nuclear DNA and regulate the transcription of specific genes whose products mediate the hormonal effects. Such studies have provided not only information about the activities of secretions of the adrenal cortex, but also more fundamental information about the mechanisms by which the expression of genes in general is regulated. Finally, more recent experimental approaches have provided better means for diagnosing and treating conditions in which there is impaired or excess activity of the adrenal cortex.

STRUCTURE OF THE ADRENAL CORTEX

The adrenal glands are extraperitoneal at the upper poles of the kidneys (Fig. 12-1). They are located on the posterior parietal wall, on each side of the vertebral column, lateral to the eleventh thoracic to the first lumbar vertebrae.[12,13] The average gland weighs 4 g, irrespective of an individual's sex or size, and is 2 to 3 cm wide and 4 to 6 cm long.[12] It enlarges after stress (because of excessive ACTH secretion) and becomes smaller when ACTH production is inhibited. The gland is variably corrugated and nodular; it is surrounded by areolar tissue and a thick fibrous capsule. Unlike the kidneys, the adrenals are not displaced by changes in respiration or posture.[12,13] The right gland is pyramidal or triangular, whereas the left is more elongated, semilunar, and perhaps larger (Fig. 12-1).[12,13] The right gland tends to be higher and more lateral than the left, which frequently overlaps the abdominal aorta.

The adrenal arteries and veins do not run together (Fig. 12-1), as those of most other organs do. There are several short arteries that are terminal branches of the inferior phrenic artery, superior, middle, and infe-

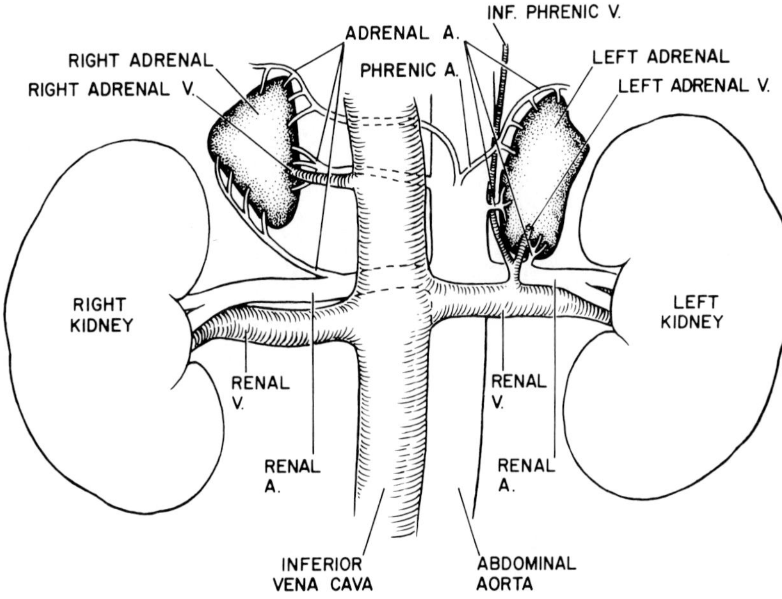

FIGURE 12-1 Schematic representation of the adrenal glands, their location, and their blood supply.

rior adrenal arteries, and, occasionally, the ovarian or the left spermatic artery.[13] Because there are several arteries, anemic infarction is unusual. Arterial blood enters a sinusoidal circulation in the cortex and usually drains into a single vein on each side. The adrenal vein empties directly into the vena cava on the right and into the renal vein on the left.[13] A few capillaries of the cortex extend into the medulla.

The innervation of the adrenal gland is autonomic.[13] Sympathetic preganglionic fibers are axons of cells in the lower thoracic and upper lumbar segments, whereas the parasympathetic fibers are from the celiac branch of the posterior vagal trunk; the latter may relay in ganglia in or near the gland. Most of the nerves are contained in an adrenal (suprarenal) plexus along the medial border of the gland, enter it as bundles near the hilus, and run through the cortex to the medulla. This innervation may participate in the control of adrenocortical growth and steroid secretion, and an afferent neural pathway from the adrenal to the hypothalamus mediates stress-induced feedback inhibition of ACTH secretion.[14]

In the adult the cortex makes up about 90 percent of the gland and surrounds the centrally located medulla.[12] The cortex comprises three zones: the zonae glomerulosa, fasciculata, and reticularis. The zona glomerulosa produces aldosterone but not cortisol and is present under the capsule in ill-defined foci that constitute about 15 percent of the cortex (Fig. 12-2).[12] The cells of this zone have a relatively small cytoplasmic volume, with small amounts of lipid. The cortisol-producing zona fasciculata (Fig. 12-2) comprises about 75 percent of the cortex. Its cells contain more cholesterol and cholesterol esters, giving them a vacuolated or clear appearance on stained sections.[12] Cells of the zona reticularis make up the inner zone and also produce cortisol, albeit at a much lower rate than the fasciculata cells.[15] They are relatively free of lipids and have a granular, compact appearance.[12] Adrenal androgens and estrogens are secreted

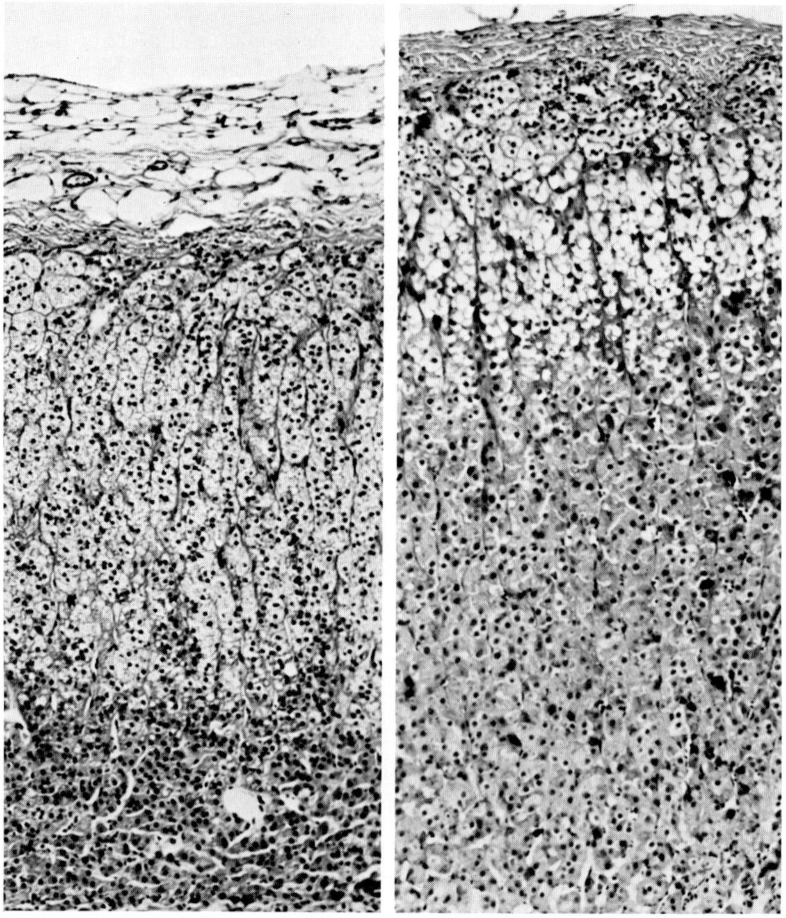

FIGURE 12-2 Normal adrenal cortex (*Left*) before and (*Right*) after ACTH stimulation. The focal zona glomerulosa under the capsule contains cells with a relatively small cytoplasmic volume. The clear cell zona fasciculata in the center and the compact cell zona reticularis at the bottom are clearly demarcated by an undulating border. After ACTH stimulation only a narrow rim of clear cells of the fasciculata remains on the outer aspect of the gland, the remainder of which consists of compact cells. Hematoxylin and eosin stain; 104X. (*From Neville and Mackay.*[12])

mostly by the fasciculata and reticularis;[13,15,15a,16] these zones are also the main producers of DOC and 18-hydroxydeoxycorticosterone (18-OH-DOC).[15]

ACTH has a dramatic effect on the adrenal.[12,16,17] Within 2 to 3 min after its administration, adrenal blood flow increases and there is cortisol release. Within hours, adrenal weight increases; ultimately, the adrenal can double in size. Also, the clear cells at the junction of the zonae fasciculata and reticularis (interface zone) lose their lipid content and are converted into compact cells. This conversion gradually extends outward, resulting in a broadening of the zona reticularis, which may reach the zona glomerulosa. This change is associated with an acquisition by the cells of the zona fasciculata of ultrastructural features of zona reticularis cells. Thus, the two inner zones function as a unit; whereas by light microscopy there appears to be an abrupt structural change between the two zones, electron microscopy reveals cells with intermediate ultrastructural features. Prolonged stimulation by ACTH causes both hypertrophy and hyperplasia.[17] By contrast, ACTH deficiency leads to atrophy of the zonae fasciculata and reticularis.[17]

The structure of the zona glomerulosa is affected by angiotensin II and potassium ion (see below). When concentrations of these substances are elevated, there is hyperplasia; when their levels are decreased there can be atrophy.[16]

Accessory adrenal glands composed of cortical tissue occasionally occur;[13,16] more rarely, such accessory glands contain both cortical and medullary tissue. This tissue may be present in the celiac plexus, kidney, spleen, or retroperitoneal area below the kidneys; along the aorta, pelvis, spermatic cord, or broad ligament of the uterus; or attached to the uterus. One adrenal gland may occasionally be absent but bilateral agenesis is rare.

The adrenal has the capacity to regenerate.[18] In animals this has been observed after enucleation of the adrenal,[18] and in humans it occurs after incomplete adrenalectomy for Cushing's disease.[16] In fact, in patients in whom adrenalectomy has been complete, hyperplasia of accessory adrenocortical tissue in response to ACTH excess can rarely give rise to hypercortisolism.[16]

Adrenocortical nodules, i.e., localized overgrowths of adrenocortical cells that are not true neoplasms, can occur.[12,16] They are usually bilateral, occur more commonly with increasing age, and contain mostly clear cells. They may contain hyalinized, myxomatous, or fibrous tissue, as well as hemorrhagic, myelolipomatous changes and osseous metaplasia. They can produce steroids, and may or may not respond to ACTH. They are not known to contribute to disease processes, although they are present in increased frequency in hypertension, Cushing's syndrome, and primary aldosteronism.

DEVELOPMENT OF THE ADRENAL CORTEX

The adrenal cortex is derived from mesodermal tissue, whereas the medulla originates from ectodermal tissue.[13] At the fifth to sixth week of development, cortical cells emerge from a proliferation of cells in the developing peritoneal epithelium at the base of the dorsal mesentery, near the cranial end of the mesonephros. These cells penetrate the retroperitoneal mesenchyme to form the primitive cortex, which soon becomes enveloped by a thick layer of more compactly arrayed cells to become the adrenal cortex. By the eighth week, the cortical tissue is closely associated with the cranial pole of the kidney, and becomes encapsulated with connective tissue. At this time the gland is much larger than the developing kidney.

The fetal cortex comprises a "fetal" zone that synthesizes predominantly estrogen and androgen precursors and a "definitive" zone that is more similar to the adult gland in its function. The fetal zone constitutes the chief bulk of the organ at birth. By the second week post partum, the adrenal weight decreases by one-third due to degeneration of the fetal zone (a process that begins in the last intrauterine month). This zone disappears by the end of the first year. Concurrently, the permanent cortex differentiates from cells of the outer portion of the gland, although the three adult zones are not completely developed until about 3 years of age. The adrenal cortex continues to grow (with accelerated growth just before and during puberty), reaching full size in the adult.

CHEMISTRY OF THE ADRENAL STEROIDS

The chemical structures of the major steroids synthesized by the adrenals[19] are shown in Fig. 12-3. These compounds contain four carbon-containing rings; the diversity of structure is due to the variable saturation of the carbon atoms and the presence of attached prosthetic groups. The numerical designation of the carbon atoms and the alphabetic designation of the rings are shown for pregnenolone in Fig. 12-3. The extent of angulation between the rings is also an important determinant of activity, and is affected by the saturation of the carbon atoms and the attached prosthetic groups. The latter can extend above or below the plane and are also of major importance in

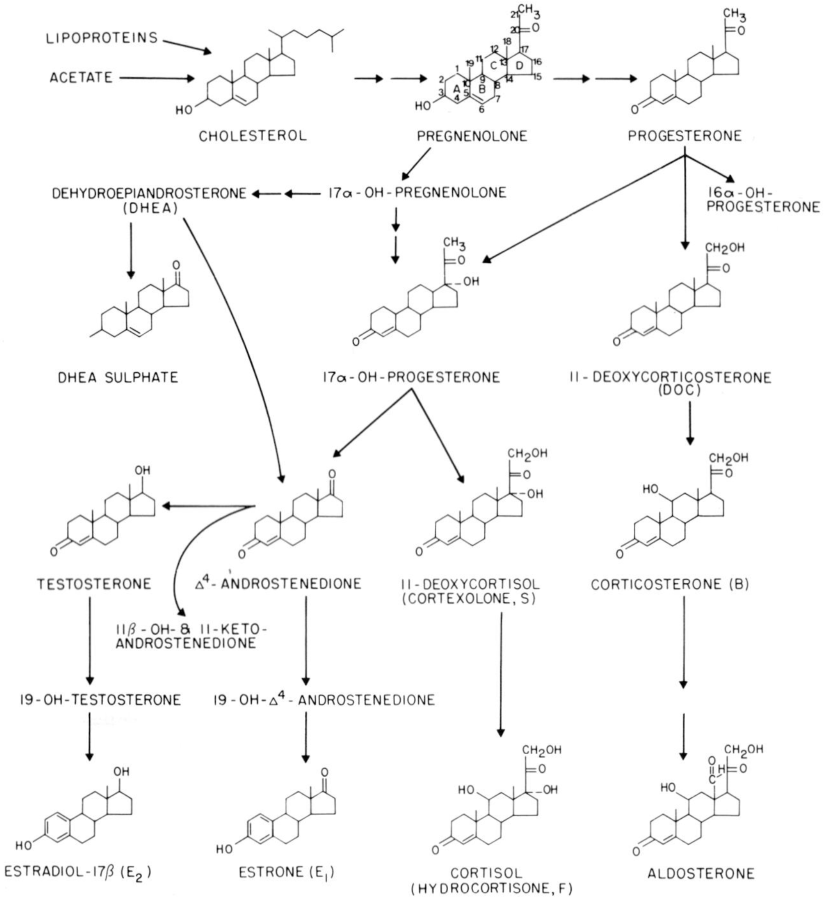

FIGURE 12-3 Steps in adrenal steroid biosynthesis. The numbers for the carbon atoms and the letters designating the rings of the steroid molecule are shown for pregnenolone. Arrows indicate the conversion pathways; the use of two arrows between intermediates indicates that more than one step is involved in the interconversion. The relative flow through each pathway varies in different cells of the adrenal (e.g., aldosterone production is favored in the glomerulosa and cortisol production is favored in the fasciculata), and some of the pathways are minor (e.g., very little testosterone, estrone, or estradiol is produced). The adrenal also catalyzes other steroid biosynthetic reactions that are not shown.

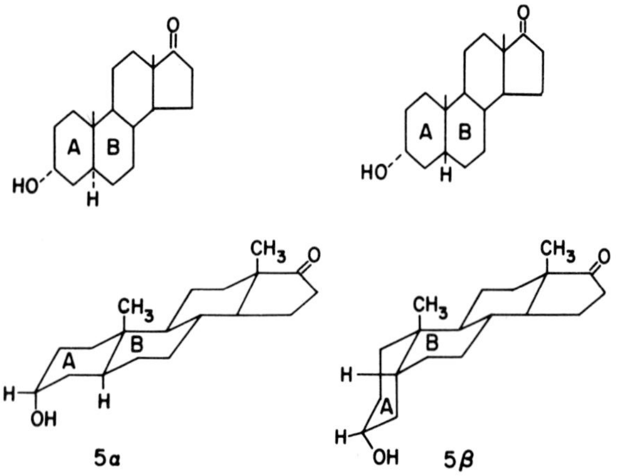

FIGURE 12-4 Effect of the hydrogen at position 6 on the conformation of the steroid molecule. The 5α-hydrogenated molecule is androsterone and the 5β-hydrogenated molecule is etiocholanolone. Shown at the top are the usual outline structural formulas and at the bottom the perspective views. (*From Bondy.*[19a])

determining activity (see below). Figure 12-4 shows the effect on the shape of the steroid molecule of the placement of a hydrogen atom in the 5α position (below the plane, dotted lines) and in the 5β position (above the plane, solid lines).

Steroids are identified by chemical (systematic) nomenclature; they are also given trivial names (Table 12-1).[15] The chemical system lists in order the hydroxyl groups, the aldehyde groups, the core ring structure (pregnane, pregnene, androstane, androstene), and the ketones, with the number of the carbon to which each is attached. In the case of carbon-carbon double bonds, the numbers of the two carbons, lower number first, are given; the presence of a double bond is alternatively indicated by the uppercase Greek delta (Δ) with a superscript indicating the lower-numbered carbon atom of the bond. A saturated ring structure is indicated by -ane (as in pregnane or androstane), whereas an unsaturated ring structure is indicated by -ene (as in pregnene or androstene). The core ring structure for the C_{21} steroids is termed *pregnane*, C_{19}

Table 12-1. Trivial and Systematic Names of Some Commonly Encountered Naturally Occurring and Synthetic Steroids

Trivial name	Systematic name
Aldosterone	11β,21-Dihydroxy-3,20-dioxopregn-4-en-18-al
Androsterone	3α-Hydroxy-5α-androstan-17-one
Corticosterone (compound B)	11β,21-Dihydroxypregn-4-ene-3,20-dione
Cortisol (hydrocortisone, compound F)	11β,17α,21-Trihydroxypregn-4-ene-3,20-dione
Cortisone (compound E)	17α,21-Dihydroxypregn-4-ene-3,11,20-trione
Cortol	5β-Pregnane-3α,11β,17α,20,21-pentol
Cortolone	3α,17α,20α,21-Tetrahydroxy-5β-pregnan-11-one
Dehydroepiandrosterone (prasterone, DHEA)	3β-Hydroxyandrost-5-en-17-one
11-Deoxycorticosterone (DOC)	21-Hydroxypregn-4-ene-3,20-dione
11-Desoxy-17-hydroxycorticosterone (11-deoxycortisol, cortexolone, compound S)	17α,21-Dihydroxypregn-4-ene-3,20-dione
Dexamethasone	9α-Fluoro-11β,17α,21-trihydroxy-16α-methylpregna-1,4-diene-3,20-dione
Estradiol	Estra-1,3,5(10)-triene-3,17β-diol
Etiocholanolone	3α-Hydroxy-5β-androstan-17-one
Fludrocortisone (9α-fluorocortisol)	9α-Fluoro-11β,17α,21-trihydroxypregn-4-ene-3,20-dione
17α-Hydroxypregnenolone	3β,17α-Dihydroxy-5β-pregnen-20-one
17α-Hydroxyprogesterone	17α-Hydroxypregn-4-ene-3,20-dione
Betamethasone	9α-Fluoro-11β,17α,21-trihydroxy-16β-methylpregna-1,4-diene-3,20-dione
Prednisone	17α,21-Dihydroxypregna-1,4-diene-3,11,20-trione
Prednisolone	11β,17α,21-Trihydroxypregna-1,4-diene-3,20-dione
Pregnanediol	5β-Pregnane-3α,20α-diol
Pregnanetriol	5β-Pregnane-3α,17α,20α-triol
Pregnenetriol	Pregn-5-ene-3β,17α,20α-triol
Pregnenolone	3β-Hydroxypregn-5-en-20-one
Progesterone	Pregn-4-ene-3,20-dione
Testosterone	17β-Hydroxyandrost-4-en-3-one
Tetrahydroaldosterone	3α,11β,21-Trihydroxy-20-oxo-5β-pregnan-18-al
Tetrahydrocortisol	3α,11β,17α,21-Tetrahydroxy-5β-pregnan-20-one
Tetrahydrocortisone	3α,17α,21-Trihydroxy-5β-pregnane-11,20-dione
Triamcinolone	9α-Fluoro-11β,16α,17α,21-tetrahydroxypregna-1,4-diene-3,20-dione

Source: *Biochem J* 113:5, 1969; modified from Brooks.[15]

steroids are *androstanes*, C_{18} steroids *estranes*, and C_{27} steroids *cholestanes*.

Although the chemical nomenclature is unambiguous, it is also cumbersome. Therefore, trivial names are ordinarily used. Several of the steroids have more than one trivial name. In general, the one listed first in Table 12-1 is preferred.

STEROID BIOSYNTHESIS

The steroid hormones are derived from cholesterol. Figure 12-3 shows the major pathways used by the adrenal gland in steroid biosynthesis (see also Chap. 4). The relative quantities of the numerous steroids that are produced vary considerably; this is due to differences in the activities of the enzymes responsible for the biosynthetic steps. These enzymes are located in the mitochondrial, microsomal, and soluble fractions of the adrenal cell; Chap. 4 provides a more in-depth analysis of the ultrastructural features of the adrenal relevant to steroid biosynthesis and of the subcellular localization of specific steps. Although the steps in steroid biosynthesis are described in terms of a series of individual reactions, as proposed recently, these might occur on biosynthetic units recently described as "hormonosomes," which can catalyze a series of steps.[20]

Cholesterol Uptake and Synthesis

The cholesterol for adrenal steroid synthesis is both synthesized by the adrenal gland and is taken up by the gland in low-density lipoprotein (LDL) or high-density lipoprotein (HDL) particles synthesized in the liver.[21-23] A lesser source of cholesterol is stored intracellular cholesterol esters.[23] Overall, about 80 percent of the adrenal steroids are derived from serum cholesterol under both basal and stimulated conditions[23] and blockade of cholesterol synthesis does not impair the cortisol response to ACTH.[24] Endogenous cholesterol synthesis is important only in the transient situation or with marked stimulation.[21] In contrast to other species that utilize predominantly HDL particles, humans rely predominantly on LDL particles[23,25] and HDL does not stimulate or sustain adrenal steroid biosynthesis.[23,25,26] In abetalipoproteinemia (absent LDL), there is a blunted cortisol response to ACTH; however, basal cortisol levels are normal and adrenal insufficiency has not been reported.[27] Thus, in this case de novo cholesterol biosynthesis and/or HDL may provide the alternative source of cholesterol. Steroids can also be synthesized from other precursors, such as desmosterol, but these play a minor role.[21]

LDL uptake involves association of the particles with specific binding sites (receptors) on the adrenal cell surface (B-E receptors).[21-23] The complexes congregate on small, specialized regions of the surface termed *coated pits* and are then internalized along with the receptors into vesicles that fuse with lysosomes.[21-23] These lysosomes contain degradative enzymes and release the cholesterol from the particles.[21-23] HDL cholesterol is delivered to the cell by a mechanism quite different from that for LDL.[28]

Acute stimulation with ACTH causes a rapid release of newly synthesized steroids derived from a small pool of free cholesterol in the gland that comes from increased hydrolysis of stored cholesterol esters.[17,21,23] Cholesterol synthesis is also activated.[21,23] With prolonged stimulation, there is accelerated uptake of cholesterol from plasma lipoproteins due to an increase in LDL receptors.[21] When the stimulation ceases, the cholesterol esters of the gland are replenished by continued LDL uptake, after which LDL receptors and uptake decrease and the gland returns to a basal state.[21]

Pregnenolone Formation

Cholesterol is converted to pregnenolone (Fig. 12-1), the precursor of all vertebrate steroid hormones. This conversion occurs in adrenal mitochondria and involves removal of a 6-carbon isocaproyl side chain from cholesterol and addition of a double-bonded oxygen at position 20 (Fig. 12-1).[29] Several steps are involved, and NADPH and oxygen are required.[15,29-31] The first step involves hydroxylation at the 22 position to yield (22*R*)-22-hydroxycholesterol, which is subsequently converted to the dihydroxy intermediate and then to pregnenolone.[29] The side chain cleavage system requires three proteins, a cytochrome P450-type hemoprotein ($p450_{scc}$), an FAD-containing flavoprotein called *NADPH-adrenodoxin reductase*, and an $Fe_2S_2^*$–type iron-sulfur protein dubbed *adrenodoxin.*[29] The conversion of cholesterol to pregnenolone is the rate-limiting step in adrenal steroid biosynthesis, which is determined by the amount of cholesterol bound to cytochrome $P450_{scc}$[29] and is controlled by the major regulatory factors (ACTH, angiotensin II, potassium ion).[15,17,29,31]

Modifications of Pregnenolone

Pregnenolone is modified mostly by one of two reactions in the endoplasmic reticulum.[15,29-31] Its 5,6 double bond (Δ^5) can first be converted to a 4,5 double bond by a 3β-hydroxysteroid dehydrogenase and a Δ^5-oxysteroid isomerase that are located in the smooth endoplasmic reticulum, resulting in progesterone. This is the preferred pathway in the glomerulosa,[15,31] and it accounts for DOC synthesis by the fasciculata. However, the major pathway in the fasciculata is probably hydroxylation of pregnenolone by 17α-hydroxylase, resulting in 17α-hydroxypregnenolone,[15,29,31,32] which is a precursor of cortisol, androgens, and estrogens. Pregnenolone can also be converted to 21-hydroxypregnenolone, which is a precursor to DOC.[15] These two hydroxylations require cytochrome P450s ($P450_{17\alpha}$ and $P450_{C21}$, respectively).[29]

Cortisol Synthesis

To synthesize cortisol,[15,29-31] the 5,6 double bond of 17α-hydroxypregnenolone is replaced by a 4,5 double bond by the 3β-hydroxysteroid dehydrogenase and isomerase enzymes in the endoplasmic reticulum (analogous to the conversion of pregnenolone to progesterone), resulting in 17α-hydroxyprogesterone. Two subsequent hydroxylations of 17α-hydroxyprogesterone then occur. The first is at position 21 by 21-hydroxylase in the endoplasmic reticulum, resulting in 11-desoxy-17-hydroxycorticosterone (DHC, also called 11-deoxycortisol, cortexolone, or compound S). The second, by 11β-hydroxylase (which also catalyzes 18-hydroxylation), occurs in the mitochondrion and results in cortisol (compound F). When cortisol is derived from progesterone, the pathway is progesterone → 17α-hydroxyprogesterone → DHC → cortisol (Fig. 12-3). Certain alternative pathways, although possible, apparently occur only to a minor extent. For instance, 17-hydroxylation does not occur after 21-hydroxylation, and there is very little 21-hydroxylation after 11β-hydroxylation.

The mitochondrial and microsomal hydroxylases require O_2, NADPH, a flavoprotein dehydrogenase, a nonheme iron-containing protein, and cytochrome P450. The cytochrome P450 that catalyzes 11β- and 18-hydroxylations is called cytochrome $P450_{11\beta}$. There is no evidence that hydroxyl groups are removed in the adrenal. Thus, once a steroid is hydroxylated, the products that can subsequently arise from it are more limited, in that they must contain the hydroxyl group.

Synthesis of Aldosterone, DOC, and Other Mineralocorticoids

Aldosterone is derived from progesterone via DOC, corticosterone, and 18-hydroxycorticosterone (Fig. 12-3).[15,29,31] Oxidation of the 18-hydroxy group to an aldehyde occurs as a result of the action of the mitochondrial enzyme 18-hydroxysteroid dehydrogenase.[15,29,31] This enzyme is apparently unique to the zona glomerulosa,[29,31] explaining why the zonae fasciculata and reticularis cannot make aldosterone. Conversely, the glomerulosa lacks the ability for 17α-hydroxylation and therefore does not synthesize cortisol.[15,29,31,32] Some aspects of the aldosterone biosynthetic pathway still need to be explained; for instance, in vitro corticosterone appears to be a better precursor for aldosterone biosynthesis than 18-hydroxycorticosterone.[33] Aldosterone may also be formed from 11-dehydrocorticosterone.[29,31,32]

As mentioned above, DOC can be synthesized in all three zones of the adrenal cortex. It can also be formed from extraadrenal conversion of progesterone, a pathway that can be major in certain circumstances, such as pregnancy and the luteal phase of the menstrual cycle.[34,35] However, because of the relative efficiencies of the various pathways, most of the DOC is produced by the fasciculata.[36] DOC can undergo further modification at the 18 position to form 18-OH-DOC[31] and at the 19 position to form 19-OH-DOC, 19-oxo-DOC, and 19-oic-DOC, which have some mineralocorticoid activity;[37,38] 19-oic-DOC can be converted in the kidney to 19-nor-DOC, a potent mineralocorticoid whose physiological importance is being investigated.[37]

The adrenal also synthesizes other steroids with mineralocorticoid activity; these include 19-hydroxyandrostenedione by hydroxylating androstenedione, in both the fasciculata-reticularis and glomerulosa zones;[39] 19-nor-corticocosterone;[40] 19-oxocortisol;[41] 18-hydroxycortisol;[42] and 18-hydroxycorticosterone.[33]

Synthesis of Adrenal Androgens

The adrenal also synthesizes steroids with 18 or 19 carbon atoms (C_{18} and C_{19} steroids) that have androgen activity and serve as androgen precursors. It secretes at least four 19-carbon compounds with androgenic activity; these are dehydroepiandrosterone, DHEA or prasterone, its sulfate (DHEA-S), androstenedione (and its 11β-analogue), and testosterone (Fig. 12-3 and Table 12-1). They are all derived from 17α-hydroxypregnenolone (Fig. 12-3). Most of the androstenedione and testosterone is probably derived from 17α-hydroxyprogesterone, although these compounds can also be synthesized via DHEA (Fig. 12-3).[19a]

DHEA and its sulfate conjugate DHEA-S are produced in the greatest quantities.[15,29–31,43,44] DHEA is synthesized by removal of the side chain at position 17, leaving a keto group. This reaction requires the presence of the 17α-OH group; the fact that 17-hydroxylation occurs in the fasciculata and reticularis but not the glomerulosa has been used as an argument that the former regions rather than the glomerulosa are responsible for adrenal androgen synthesis. The cleavage enzyme, C-17,20-lyase (which may be the same enzyme as 17α-hydroxylase[45]), that removes the side chain is located in the endoplasmic reticulum[15] and uses NADPH and O_2. A cytosolic 17β-hydroxysteroid dehydrogenase then reduces the hydroxyl to the keto moiety. DHEA is sulfated to DHEA-S by an adrenal sulfokinase,[15,31] by a reaction that occurs in the nonparticulate supernatant of adrenal homogenates. Most of the DHEA secreted by the adrenal is sulfated, but some of the plasma DHEA-S is also derived from the actions of peripheral sulfokinases.[43,44] Although the pathway is minor, the adrenal can synthesize DHEA from sulfated pregnenolone (and possibly sulfated cholesterol).[19a,32] The adrenal can also remove sulfate groups, so there is a constant interconversion of DHEA and DHEA-S in the gland.[19a]

Removal of the side chain at C-17 of 17α-hydroxyprogesterone or isomerization of DHEA (from Δ^5 to Δ^4) and conversion of the 3-hydroxyl to the 3-keto moiety can yield androstenedione (Fig. 12-3), which is secreted in appreciable quantities by the adrenal.[15,31,33] This compound has weak androgenic activity, but is converted to testosterone to a minimal extent in the adrenal and to a greater extent in peripheral tissues.

Synthesis of Estrogens

The adrenal synthesizes small quantities of estrone and estradiol (Fig. 12-3).[46] However, all four of the adrenal androgens discussed above can also serve as substrates for estrogen biosynthesis in peripheral tissues such as subcutaneous fat, hair follicles, and mammary tissue.[47]

THE FETAL ADRENAL

The adrenal cortex actively produces steroids during embryonic and fetal development. Fetal adrenal steroid production is coordinated with that of the placenta by complex interrelationships (see Chap. 17).[31,48–50] Most of the adrenocortical cells differentiating early in embryonic and fetal development constitute the fetal zone. These cells involute during the latter part of pregnancy, and this process is accelerated immediately after birth. The cells of the fetal zone are enveloped gradually by other cells of the definitive zone destined to become the adrenal cortex of the adult. Steroidogenesis appears in the fetal adrenal cortex around weeks 25 to 32 of pregnancy, and amnionic fluid steroid levels reflect, at least in part, fetal hormone secretion;[50] the measurement of maternal corticosterone sulfate concentration provides a good index of fetal cortisol production.[51]

The fetal zone has low 3β-hydroxysteroid dehydrogenase activity and synthesizes predominantly DHEA and DHEA-S.[48,52] There is little sulfatase activity, so the interconversion of DHEA-S and DHEA seen in the adult adrenal is minimal. These two steroids serve predominantly as precursors that are converted to estrogens by the placenta, accounting for about 90 percent of maternal estriol production and 50 percent of the estradiol and estrone production. Placental synthesis of estriol, however, occurs after DHEA and DHEA-S are converted to 16α-hydroxy-DHEA and 16α-hydroxy-DHEA-S in the peripheral tissues. DHEA and DHEA-S also serve as precursors for placental synthesis of testosterone and androstenedione.

The definitive zone synthesizes cortisol, corticosterone, DOC, progesterone, aldosterone, and androstenedione. The fetal adrenal accounts for about 65 percent of the fetal cortisol production; the remainder comes from placental transfer of cortisol and from conversion of cortisone to cortisol. About 85 percent of the cortisol crossing the placenta is converted to cortisone; the fetus has a very poor ability to convert cortisone to cortisol.[53] Cortisol in the amnionic fluid increases throughout pregnancy with a substantial increase between weeks 14 and 16 and a much greater increase after the 25th week.[50]

The factors controlling fetal adrenal growth and steroidogenesis in early pregnancy are poorly understood, but in anencephalic fetuses the adrenal gland develops normally for about 15 weeks.[48,49] Chorionic gonadotropin may be an important regulator during the first half of pregnancy. By midpregnancy in animals, both the fetal and the definitive zones are under ACTH control, and ACTH release can be suppressed by cortisol.[54] Although, in humans there is no evidence that the fetal hypothalamic-pituitary-adrenal axis can be suppressed by glucocorticoids at this time, this must occur subsequently.[55] In addition, the high levels of estrogens produced by the placenta can inhibit adrenal 3β-hydroxysteroid dehydrogenase activity.[52] Thus, these steroids may also serve a regulatory role by inhibiting cortisol production in this way with consequent shuttling of precursors into the alternate biosynthetic pathway, resulting in increased production of DHEA and DHEA-S required for placental estrogen synthesis.[52] Decreased cortisol production combined with a rapid clearance of cortisol by the placenta could result in low plasma cortisol levels and an enhanced ACTH release that would continue to drive the fetal adrenal to serve its dual role of producing both estrogen precursors and cortisol.[52] This model would also explain the fetal adrenal involution at birth; the placental source for estrogens (and thereby the block in 3β-hydroxysteroid dehydrogenase) would disappear, the production of cortisol relative to DHEA and DHEAS would increase and ACTH levels would be suppressed with consequent decreased stimulation of the adrenal.[52]

The estrogens produced by the placental-fetal unit enter the maternal circulation, and urinary excretion of these compounds and their metabolites during pregnancy is high. Estriol is the most abundant of these in human urine; measurement of its level can be useful in the detection of placental or fetal adrenocortical dysfunction.

QUANTITIES OF STEROIDS PRODUCED

Several techniques have been devised to estimate the secretion rates of the steroid hormones.[30,56] Although there are several methodological problems, reasonable estimates have been obtained;[43,44,56–60] some of these are shown in Table 12-2. Cortisol is the adrenal steroid secreted in the greatest quantity, and its production exceeds that of the only other major glucocorticoid, corticosterone, severalfold. The overall cortisol secretion rate shows some correlation with total body cellular mass.[61] The adrenal production of cortisone is only about 4 percent that of cortisol.[56] Adrenal production of DHEA-S is also high (accounting for about 90 percent of the steroid in females[62] and an even greater percentage in males). The gland also makes appreciable quantities of androstenedione (accounting for about 50 percent of the production in females and a higher percentage in males)[62] and its 11-oxygenated derivatives, 11-ketoandrostenedione and 11β-hydroxyandrostenedione.[19a,43] Androstenedione is converted to testosterone more readily than is DHEA or DHEA-S

Table 12-2. Secretion Rates and Plasma Concentrations of Various Steroids*

Steroid	Secretion rate, mg/24 h	Ref.	Plasma concentration, ng/ml	Ref.
Aldosterone	0.15	57	0.15–0.17	Chap. 14
Androstenedione	2.5 (F)	44	1.80 ± 0.21 (F)	43
	2.2 (M)	44	1.14 ± 0.21 (M)	43
Corticosterone	1–4	56–58	2.4 ± 1.5 (F)†	59
			4.2 ± 2.2 (M)†	59
Cortisol	8–25	56–58	85 (20–140) (F)	60
			116 (40–180) (M)	60
11-Deoxycorticosterone (DOC)	0.6	56–58	0.15–0.17	Chap. 14
11-Deoxycortisol	0.4	57	0.95–2.5	57
DHEA	0.7 (F)	57	5.34 ± 1.57 (F)	43
	3.0 (M)	43	5.53 ± 1.78 (M)	43
DHEA-S	6–8	43,44	1130 ± 280 (F)	43
			1260 ± 340 (M)	43
Etiocholanolone sulfate	—	—	17 ± 6 (F)	43
			15 ± 4 (M)	43
Etiocholanolone glucuronide			15 ± 5 (F)	43
			18 ± 7 (M)	43
Progesterone (M)			0.2 ± 0.09 (F)‡	59
			11.8 ± 7.00 (F)§	59
			0.18 ± 0.10 (M)	59
17α-Hydroxyprogesterone			0.58 ± 0.26 (F)‡	59
			1.96 ± 0.75 (F)	59
			0.18 ± 0.06 (M)	59
Testosterone	0.23 (F)	43	0.48 ± 0.14 (F)	43
			5.59 ± 1.51 (M)	43

*Values are for adults and are given as mean values alone, with ranges, or ± SD. F and M denote females and males, respectively. Data on 18-hydroxycorticosterone and 18-hydroxydeoxycorticosterone can be found in Chap. 14. For many of the steroids, plasma concentrations vary with the time of day and in females with the menstrual cycle. Levels also change with growth and development and with aging. Estradiol and estrone production in males is extremely low and is not listed. The selection of literature sources is somewhat arbitrary; values vary in different reports.

†Samples taken 8 to 9 A.M.

‡Follicular phase of the menstrual cycle.

§Luteal phase of the menstrual cycle.

(Fig. 12-3). Adrenal testosterone accounts for about 0 to 30 percent of the testosterone produced in the female,[62] but only a minor fraction in the male. The remainder of the testosterone produced in females (5 to 20 percent) comes from the ovaries[62] and peripheral production, mostly from androstenedione and, to a lesser extent, DHEA.[62] 17α-Hydroxypregnenolone and progesterone are produced in small quantities by the normal adrenal cortex and in much higher quantities in various pathological states.[43] Negligible quantities of testosterone or estradiol are produced by the adrenal. Aldosterone is produced in small quantities, but this steroid is active at low concentrations. Significant quantities of DOC are also produced.

INHIBITORS OF ADRENAL STEROID BIOSYNTHESIS

A number of compounds inhibit adrenal steroid biosynthesis; these can work at several different steps (Table 12-3).[19a,31,63,64] These compounds have been useful for research and the diagnosis and treatment of adrenal disorders. The use of metyrapone for evaluating the hypothalamic-pituitary axis is discussed below (see Laboratory Evaluation of Adrenocortical Function). This compound, as well as mitotane (*o,p'*-DDD) and aminoglutethimide, is used to treat spontaneous Cushing's syndrome. Aminoglutethimide also

Table 12-3. Inhibitors of Adrenal Steroid Biosynthesis*

Compound	Chemical and other names	Reactions inhibited
Amphenone B	3,3-Bis[4-aminophenyl]-2-butanone	11β-, 17α, and 21-hydroxylations Δ^5-3β-Hydroxyl to Δ^4-3-ketone oxidation
Metyrapone	SU-4885 2-Methyl-1,2-di-3-pyridyl-1-propanone	11β-Hydroxylation (in larger doses 21-hydroxylation and other reactions)
SU-9055	3-(1,2,3,4-Tetrahydro-1-oxo-2-naphthyl)pyridine	17α-Hydroxylation 18-Hydroxylation
SU-8000	3-(Chloro-3-methyl-2-indenyl)pyridine	18-Oxidation 17α-Hydroxylation
Cyanoketone	2α-Cyano-4,4,17α-trimethylandrost-5-en-17β-ol-3-one	3β-Hydroxysteroid dehydrogenation
Mitotane	2,2-Bis(2-chlorophenyl-4-chlorophenyl)-1,1-dichloralethane; *o,p′*-DDD	Mitochondrial, fairly specific for the adrenal
Aminoglutethimide	3-(4-Aminophenyl)-3-ethyl-2,6-piperidinedione 3-Ethyl-3-(*p*-aminophenyl)-2,6-dioxopiperidine	Cholesterol to 20α-hydroxycholesterol conversion 18-Hydroxylation
SKF 12185	*dl*-2-(*p*-Aminophenyl)-2-phenylethylamine	11β-Hydroxylation

*See Samuels and Nelson,[31] Bondy,[19a] Liddle,[63] and Aguilera and Catt[64] for documentation.

blocks the synthesis of adrenal estrogen precursors and the conversion of adrenal androgens to estrogens,[65] and is used for treatment of carcinoma of the breast.

The decreased cortisol production due to the inhibitors results in a compensatory increase in ACTH production (see Regulation of ACTH Release, below); this stimulation can override the enzymatic block. The override is not a problem in metyrapone testing since it does not occur soon enough to affect the test, which depends on an increase in ACTH production anyway. When decreased adrenal estrogen production is the aim, a glucocorticoid such as dexamethasone can be given simultaneously to block the compensatory increase in ACTH level.

A number of compounds other than those listed in Table 12-3 can also inhibit adrenal steroid biosynthesis. Macromolecular synthesis inhibitors block overall steroidogenesis; these have been useful for research.[31] Heparin can inhibit aldosterone biosynthesis in vivo but not in vitro.[31,63] This effect requires several weeks and sometimes occurs with heparin therapy.[66] Spironolactone can block aldosterone biosynthesis,[64,67] predominantly at the 11β-hydroxylation and 18-dehydrogenation steps.[65,67] This may contribute to the antimineralocorticoid actions of this compound (in addition to its antagonist actions, discussed below) and may explain why the plasma aldosterone concentration may not increase normally when renin levels rise following spironolactone therapy (Chap. 14).[67] Δ^9-Tetrahydrocannabinol is of interest since some effects of marijuana smoking resemble those of adrenal hypofunction. There is enhanced hypothalamic-pituitary axis activity in animals given Δ^9-tetrahydrocannabinol, possibly due to compensatory override of a drug-induced blockade of pregnenolone formation.[68] However, it is not clear whether this reaction is important in marijuana smokers. The antifungal drug ketoconazole has been shown to blunt the cortisol response to ACTH, although adrenal insufficiency has not been reported with usual doses.[69] This agent has been used to treat Cushing's disease.[69a,69b] Use of the anesthetic agent etomidate has been associated with unexpected mortality and low plasma cortisol levels; it inhibits adrenal mitochondrial cytochrome P450-dependent hydroxylation reactions.[70]

REGULATION OF ADRENAL STEROID BIOSYNTHESIS

Adrenal glucocorticoid and androgen production is controlled predominantly by the hypothalamic-pituitary axis, whereas aldosterone production is predominantly regulated by the renin-angiotension system and potassium ion. Interrelationships between the various tissues involved in steroid hormone synthesis and its regulation, peripheral uptake of steroids, and steroid metabolism and excretion are illustrated in Fig. 12-5. These systems allow modulation of the basal release of hormones by several factors; they also function so that steroid production can increase rapidly after more acute stimuli.

Regulation of Glucocorticoid Production

THE HYPOTHALAMIC-PITUITARY-ADRENAL AXIS

The hypothalamus, pituitary, and adrenal form a neuroendocrine axis whose primary function is to regulate

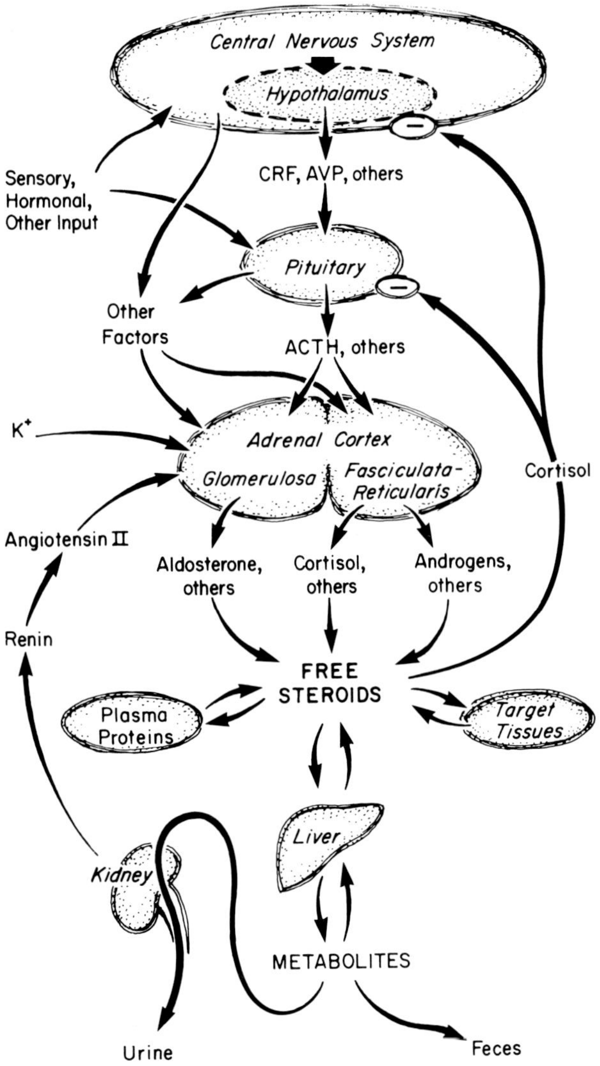

FIGURE 12-5 Interrelations between the various tissues and factors involved in the regulation of production of the adrenal steroids and their peripheral uptake, metabolism, and excretion.

the production of cortisol and some of the other adrenal steroids (Fig. 12-5). CRF, arginine vasopressin (AVP), and possibly other substances are released by the hypothalamus (Chap. 7) and pass through the portal vessels to the anterior pituitary gland, where they stimulate ACTH release (see Chap. 8). Other substances can also act at the level of the pituitary to influence ACTH release. ACTH in turn stimulates the release of cortisol and other steroids by the adrenal cortex. Steroid release is also influenced by the innervation of the adrenal and perhaps by other less well understood circulating factors.

Overall, three types of mechanism operate to control cortisol release (see also Chaps. 7–9). First, endogenous rhythms in the brain result in pulsatile releases of ACTH and cortisol that produce an episodic, circadian, and meal-stimulated pattern. Second, a number of other excitatory factors, both physical and emotional, can increase ACTH and cortisol release above the spontaneous pattern. Third, ACTH release is suppressed by cortisol. Hypothalamic and possibly other influences exert both trophic influences on the pituitary ACTH-producing cells in terms of their capacity to release ACTH and short-term influences on ACTH release. ACTH (Fig. 12-5) exerts short-term influences on adrenal steroid production, and it also has (directly or indirectly) a trophic influence on the gland that is important in determining the magnitude of steroid hormone responsiveness to an acute elevation of ACTH.

REGULATION OF ACTH RELEASE

The hypothalamus releases substances that stimulate ACTH release (discussed in Chap. 7). Two factors, CRF and AVP, are known to be important in regulating ACTH release. Other factors (discussed below), either released by the hypothalamus or acting directly on the pituitary, are probably also involved.

CRF and AVP are both produced predominantly in the paraventricular nucleus of the hypothalamus, and the peptides travel through neurons to the median eminence, from which they are released into the portal circulation (Chap. 7).[70a] As discussed in Chap. 7, several different neurotransmitter substances and pathways are apparently involved in regulating the secretion of these and other releasing substances.

CRF is a peptide of 41 amino acids[8,71] that arises from a much larger precursor protein. It is ordinarily not detectable in the peripheral circulation except in pregnancy,[72] implying that it acts mainly via the hypothalamic-pituitary portal system or through autocrine or paracrine mechanisms. By contrast, it has been found in the hypophyseal circulation in rats.[73] CRF acts at least in part by stimulating adenylate cyclase,[74] however, vasopressin (antidiuretic hormone, ADH) acts through other second messengers, probably Ca^{2+} (see Chap. 5.)[74] The ultimate effects are increased ACTH synthesis and release and these changes are also accompanied by an increase in corticotroph size.[75]

CRF also exerts actions outside of the pituitary (Chap. 7). The peptide and receptors for it are distributed extensively through the brain, gastrointestinal tract, and other regions.[76,77] It acts within the brain to stimulate sympathetic outflow, and in high doses can decrease blood pressure.[78,79] Overall, it may regulate stress responses and mentation, and abnormalities in CRF may be present in depression, in which the CRF level has been found to be elevated in the CSF.[80]

CRF is probably the most important overall stimulator of ACTH release. In vitro and in animals CRF is a more potent stimulator of ACTH release than any other known substance,[81,82] although at maximally effective doses in humans AVP can have an equivalent effect.[82,83] Nonetheless, given together, the two peptides act synergistically.[82–84] Antisera to CRF or antagonists of its actions can blunt ether-, restraint-, formalin-, CRF-, or AVP-induced increases in ACTH in rats.[82,85–87] That AVP is not essential for CRF action is suggested by the finding that Brattleboro rats that are deficient in AVP can respond to stress with increased levels of ACTH and cortisol.[88] CRF release may also be decreased by AVP[89] and increased by CRF[90] by short feedback loops. However, the pituitary release of ACTH is not totally CRF-dependent since stimulated but not basal release of ACTH can be blocked by antisera to CRF.[91]

AVP, although better characterized as a regulator of free water clearance and blood pressure (Chap. 9), is produced by the same neurons that synthesize CRF (see Chap. 7).[78] This peptide alone can stimulate ACTH release and acts synergistically with CRF.[82,83] It appears to play a physiologic role in stimulating ACTH, although, as discussed above, it is not essential for all responses.[82] Thus, in rats an antagonist to AVP blocked AVP-induced ACTH release, but failed to block stress-induced (i.e., by environmental change) increases in glucocorticoid production.[88] However, in the AVP-deficient Brattleboro rats there is a somewhat reduced activity of the hypothalamic-pituitary-adrenal axis;[88] in cats antiserum to AVP partially blocks the ACTH response to hemmorhage in the presence but not absence of glucocorticoids,[92] and in rats the AVP response to restraint- or formalin-induced stress is blunted by antisera to AVP and blocked by about 85 percent by the combination of antisera to both CRF and AVP.[82,87]

Although less is known about the role of other factors, these are operative and are of major importance in certain circumstances. The anterior pituitary contains receptors for a number of the classic neurotransmitters that could mediate the effects of such substances (Chap. 7). These include catecholamines,[74,82,93] angiotensin II,[74] opiates,[93,94] somatostatin,[93,94] and lymphocyte-derived factors.[95] In animals, oxytocin can affect ACTH release, but this appears not to be the case in humans.[96] The pituitary may respond to both α-adrenergic and β-adrenergic stimulation.[82] The role of lymphocyte-derived factors is a subject of active inquiry; for example, thymectomy in monkeys results in lower levels of ACTH-related peptides and cortisol.[95] ACTH release has been reported to be both stimulated[97] and inhibited[93] by opiates. Catecholamines of peripheral origin act on pituitary β-adrenergic receptors to regulate hypoglycemia-induced ACTH release,[94,98] although blockade of β- or α-adrenergic receptors does not prevent other stress responses.[82] ACTH release can be stimulated by serotonin.[99]

ACTH AND RELATED PEPTIDES

ACTH is predominantly of anterior pituitary origin, although it may be made in the intermediate lobe of the pituitary and in a number of extrapituitary tissues such as hypothalamus, amygdala, lymphoid cells, and placenta (see Chaps. 7 and 8).[100,101] There is no evidence that sources other than the anterior pituitary normally contribute significantly to circulating ACTH. However, as discussed below, ACTH can be produced by extrapituitary tumors. As discussed in Chap. 8, ACTH is produced by a discrete subset of anterior pituitary cells that constitute a minority of the cells of the gland.

The biosynthesis and methods for measurement of ACTH are discussed in Chap. 8. It arises from a larger protein of about 290 amino acids termed *proopiomelanocortin* (POMC) that also contains the sequences of several other proteins, including α-, β-, and γ-melanocyte stimulating hormone (MSH), β-lipotropin (β-LPH), β-endorphin, met-enkephalin, an NH_2-terminal fragment, and corticotropin-like intermediate-lobe peptide (CLIP).[102,103] ACTH contains 39 amino acids (Fig. 12-6), within which structure are the sequences of α-MSH and CLIP. ACTH can be phosphorylated and glycosylated, but glycosylation is negligible in humans.[104,105]

The structural features of ACTH required for its biological actions have been defined.[17] As Fig. 12-6 shows, the amino acids of the hormone are arranged in a single polypeptide chain. The amino-terminal 24 amino acids are constant in all species studied. Although $ACTH_{1-20}$, $ACTH_{1-23}$, and $ACTH_{1-24}$ are equipotent on a molar basis, the duration of adrenal stimulation is shorter than with $ACTH_{1-39}$. Thus, the presence of the carboxy-terminal portion of the molecule delays its breakdown. Biological activity requires amino acids 1 to 10. Further modifications in this region, for example replacement of the tryptophan at position 9 by phenylalanine, can result in a compound with antagonist activity.

ACTH is largely free in the circulation and it is rapidly cleared from it (Chap. 8) with a half-time of 10 min or less; the half-time is not known to be regulated by hormones or other stimuli.[17,108] Emphasized in Chap. 8 is that biological activity disappears from the circulation more rapidly than does radioimmunoassay-

```
     1               5                   10
H2N-Ser-Tyr-Met-Glu-His-Phe-Arg-Trp-Gly-Lys-

     11              15                  20
     Lys-Pro-Val-Gly-Lys-Lys-Arg-Arg-Pro-Val-

     21              25                  30
     Lys-Val-Tyr-Pro-Asn-Gly-Ala-Glu-Asp-Glu-

     31              35              39
     Ser-Ala-Glu-Ala-Phe-Pro-Leu-Glu-Phe-COOH
```

FIGURE 12-6 The amino acid sequence of human ACTH. The sequence for α-MSH comprises amino acids 1 to 13 and that for corticotropin-like intermediate lobe peptide (CLIP) comprises amino acids 18 to 39. (*Based upon data of Lerner and Buettner-Janusch*[106] *and Rinkler et al.*[107])

able activity, suggesting that there are inactive intermediates in ACTH breakdown that retain their ability to bind to antibodies to ACTH. Some of these are similar in size to ACTH, suggesting that minor modifications, possibly on the NH_2-terminal portion of the molecule, inactivate it. ACTH is catabolized by several tissues, although liver and kidney account for the greatest uptake.[108] Unlike certain other hormones (e.g., luteinizing hormone, LH), there is minimal excretion of ACTH into the urine.

ACTH can have actions other than on the adrenal and several of the other peptides arising from POMC have biological activities (Chap. 8). Thus ACTH can stimulate lipolysis in fat cells[109] and the peptide MSH and fragments of ACTH also have effects on learning and behavior in rats (Chap. 8). ACTH and MSH can also affect opiate action; the extensive actions of β-endorphin and other opiates are discussed in Chap. 8. MSH increases pigmentation, an important sign in states of ACTH excess (see below). This activity comes mostly from the α-MSH, β-MSH, and γ-MSH sequences contained within ACTH, β-LPH, and the NH_2-terminal fragments, respectively, since discrete MSH sequences have not been found in the circulation. The relative contributions of these sequences to pigment-stimulating activity is not known, although more activity comes from ACTH than β-LPH, since the activity of α-MSH within ACTH is about four times that of β-MSH within β-LPH and the plasma concentrations of ACTH and β-LPH are roughly equal. CLIP can stimulate pancreatic exocrine function,[110] and peptides of the NH_2-terminal fragment of POMC can stimulate adrenal steroidogenesis, the adrenal response to ACTH, adrenal growth, and natriuresis.[111–113] In general, the physiological importance of the actions of POMC-derived peptides other than ACTH is not known.

ACTIONS OF ACTH ON THE ADRENAL

ACTH stimulates an increased release of cortisol from the adrenal within 2 to 3 min, due largely to increased cortisol synthesis.[17,29,115] Although the concentrations of adrenal steroids are 100- to 1000-fold higher than the plasma levels, these levels do not provide an adequate reservoir.[116] Little is known about the factors that control this concentration gradient or whether there are active mechanisms that regulate release.[117,118] Adrenal androgens and smaller quantities of some of the intermediates in cortisol biosynthesis and other steroids are also released (Table 12-2). When ACTH concentrations fall, steroid biosynthesis rapidly declines. As mentioned above (see Structure of the Adrenal Cortex), ACTH also stimulates a very early increase in adrenal blood flow. With more prolonged stimulation, there are increases in total adrenal protein and RNA synthesis.[17,29,114,115] This leads to hypertrophy with increased adrenal cortical weight and protein and nucleic acid content. An increase in DNA content can be detected by 48 h and is progressive through 7 days of ACTH treatment. The size of the gland can double. There are also increases in the concentrations of most of the steroidogenic enzymes; these increases are greater than those of most of the other adrenal proteins and are due largely to increased enzyme synthesis.[29]

Conversely, when ACTH levels are low,[14] as in hypopituitarism or with glucocorticoid therapy or cortisol-producing adrenal adenomas, there is decreased adrenal protein and RNA synthesis and decreased activity of all of the steroidogenic enzymes.[17,29,114,115] The gland can be reduced to a fraction of its normal size. These changes are reversible upon readministration of ACTH or a return to normal pituitary function. However, in this case, steroidogenesis does not occur immediately as with the normal adrenal gland. There is some stimulation of steroidogenesis by 24 h, and a near-maximal effect can be achieved by 3 days (Fig. 12-7).

Receptors for ACTH have been found on adrenal cell membranes; these bind the hormone with an equilibrium dissociation constant (K_d) of about 1 nM.[119,120] Calcium is required for the binding.[119] However, others have argued that there are two sites with differing affinities for the hormone.[121,122] In isolated cells, the cellular concentration of ACTH receptors and other steps in the steroidogenic response are suppressed by the hormone.[119,120] However, the overall sensitivity of the adrenal gland to ACTH in vivo in states of ACTH excess is increased rather than decreased (see below).

The interaction of ACTH with adrenal cell membrane receptors activates adenylate cyclase.[17,29,114,115,121]

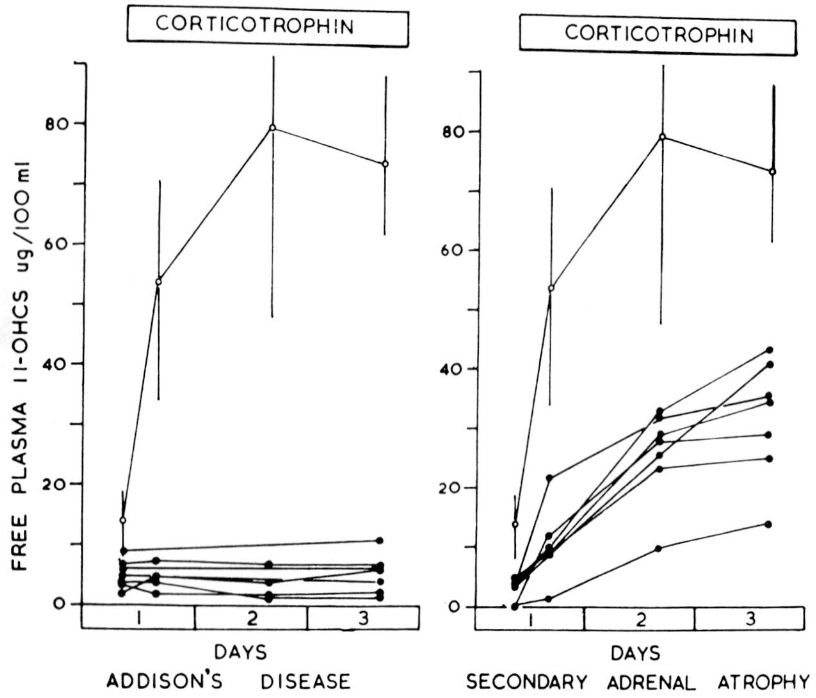

FIGURE 12-7 Response of total plasma cortisol (designated "free plasma 11-OHCS" on the ordinate) to ACTH in normal individuals and in individuals with Addison's disease and secondary hypoadrenalism. The lines indicate the responses in different individuals with primary adrenal insufficiency (Addison's disease, left) and secondary adrenal atrophy (right). The top curves show the ranges of normal responses. (*From Cope,*[118a] *based upon data of Mattingly.*)

The resulting increase in cyclic AMP (cAMP) concentration activates protein kinase (Chap. 5), which phosphorylates a number of proteins; it is not known which proteins involved in the process are actually phosphorylated.[123,124] During ACTH stimulation, changes in cAMP precede the stimulation of steroidogenesis and the extent of stimulation also correlates well with the occupancy by cAMP of the regulatory subunit of protein kinase (Chap. 5).[124]

Calcium ion is important for ACTH- or cAMP-stimulated steroidogenesis that is blocked by inhibitors of calmodulin;[29,115] therefore, this need may be due in part to Ca^{2+} binding of calmodulin.

The major effect of ACTH on steroidogenesis is to stimulate the rate-limiting step of the conversion of cholesterol to pregnenolone.[17,29,114,115] This may be due mostly to an ACTH-stimulated increase in the binding of cholesterol to the mitochondrial cytochrome $P450_{scc}$ involved in cholesterol-to-pregnenolone transformation.[29,115] This step involves enhanced transport of cholesterol to the cytochrome $P450_{scc}$ system present in the inner mitochondrial membrane.[29,115] It is blocked by inhibitors of protein synthesis and probably involves an ACTH-induced labile protein factor.[17,29,115] This factor may stimulate either the binding of cholesterol to the cytochrome $P450_{scc}$ by a mechanism involving calcium or the transfer of cholesterol to the inner mitochondrial membrane.[29] These actions could be mediated directly by the protein factor and/or through stimulating the synthesis of phospholipids that participate in the step.[29,115] The recently isolated adrenal steroid carrier protein that turns over rapidly and moves with cholesterol to the inner mitochondrial membrane in response to ACTH is a candidate to mediate these actions.[125] Other ACTH-stimulated proteins have also been found.[126,127] Intact cytoskeletal function is apparently required for the step.[115]

These actions on cholesterol side chain cleavage are likely mediated through increases in the de novo synthesis of phospholipids.[121,128] These include phosphatidic acid, phosphatidylinositides, polyphosphoinositides, phosphatidylcholine, and phosphatidylethanolamine.[121,128] These actions can be mimicked by cAMP, require intracellular Ca^{2+}, and are blocked by inhibitors of protein synthesis.[121,128] Further, phosphatidylinositide and polyphosphoinositides increase cholesterol side chain cleavage when added to isolated mitochondria.[129] The mechanisms for the ACTH-induced increase in phospholipid levels are not known, but might be due to cAMP-stimulated activity that initially yields phosphatidic acid; it is also likely that a labile protein is involved in the synthesis of phospholipids and therefore disappears rapidly when protein synthesis is blocked.

Other functions are also affected by ACTH. Most of the adrenal cholesterol is esterified. ACTH increases the activity of cholesterol esterase, possibly through ACTH-induced phosphorylation of the enzyme.[29] This increases the supply of free cholesterol that is required for the conversion of cholesterol to pregnenolone. It has also been suggested that pituitary factors other than ACTH, possibly a fragment of the NH_2-terminal portion of POMC, actually stimulate the hydrolase and participate in vivo with ACTH in the stimulation of steroidogenesis.[29,130] ACTH also decreases the activity of cholesterol ester synthetase, thereby decreasing the reverse reaction.[17] The stimulation of the esterase and inhibition of the synthetase by ACTH occur even when protein synthesis is blocked.[17] Lipoprotein uptake is also stimulated by ACTH, probably by increasing the LDL receptors.[21,115] Once the rate-limiting pregnenolone formation step is fully activated, however, the continuing supply of cholesterol through LDL uptake may become rate-limiting.[29]

It is unclear how ACTH exerts a trophic influence on the adrenal, and factors other than ACTH may participate in trophic influences traditionally attributed to ACTH. In animals, antiserum to ACTH impairs steroidogenesis, but does not decrease adrenal size.[131] Unilaterally adrenalectomized animals develop a compensatory hypertrophy that is dependent on both the pituitary and nervous stimulation, but is not associated with changes in plasma ACTH;[131] it is not prevented by antiserum to ACTH,[131] and, in fact, administration of ACTH at this time inhibits the usual increase in adrenal DNA content.[132] Finally, ACTH inhibits rather than stimulates growth in isolated adrenal cells.[133] Thus, ACTH itself may be growth-inhibitory but may in some way stimulate either the production of, availability of, or adrenal sensitivity to other growth factors that would act to override the effects of ACTH on both growth inhibitors and hormone responsiveness.

ACTIONS OF GLUCOCORTICOIDS ON THE ADRENAL

Glucocorticoids can inhibit steroidogenesis in isolated human adrenal cells.[133a] Thus, an additional short feedback loop may be present (Fig. 12-5). However, the role of glucocorticoids in humans may be minor, as ACTH excess states with hypercortisolism are associated with enhanced adrenal capacity for synthesis of steroids, and in vivo dexamethasone does not inhibit ACTH-stimulated cortisol production.[134]

ACTIONS OF OTHER FACTORS ON THE ADRENAL

The dominance of ACTH in regulating cortisol release is indicated by the fact that hypophysectomized individuals ultimately cannot produce cortisol. Nevertheless, other factors influence the adrenal release of cortisol and adrenal growth. (That the adrenal growth is influenced by innervation and perhaps other factors from the pituitary or from lymphoid cells is described above.) Innervation or other factors acting on the adrenal may participate in the circadian periodicity of cortisol release (see below). The adrenal cortex also contains β-adrenergic receptors that are coupled to adenylate cyclase stimulation.[135]

Some of these other factors probably regulate the responsiveness of the adrenal to ACTH. Opiate peptides can diminish the adrenal responsiveness to ACTH in hypophysectomized animals.[97] Hemorrhage can increase the adrenal sensitivity to ACTH.[136] Prostaglandins (PGs) and growth hormone have been reported to be capable of enhancing the effect of ACTH.[137,138]

SPONTANEOUS PATTERNS OF ACTH AND CORTISOL RELEASE

Most of the cortisol is released as a series of episodic bursts (Fig. 12-8).[139–145] Each episodic release of cortisol is characterized by a sharp rise in concentration, followed by a slower, generally smooth, decline. The intervals between these elevations range from around 40 min to hours. The basal plasma cortisol concentrations at which these secretory outbursts may occur vary greatly.

This adrenocortical activity results in rapidly fluctuating cortisol levels. However, the episodes of release are more frequent in the late evening and early morning hours than throughout the remainder of the day, such that overall there is a circadian rhythm in which plasma cortisol levels are higher at times when there are more releases and lower during the other times. During the period of minimal secretory activity, including the later afternoon and the early evening hours, the plasma cortisol can reach undetectable levels. In addition there are secretory episodes coincident with both lunch and dinner.[141,142] Several other episodes can occur during this period at irregular intervals. Nocturnal secretory episodes begin to increase during the third to fifth hours of sleep and are followed by the main secretory episodes during the sixth to eighth hours of sleep and the first 5 h of wakefulness, which account for most of the cortisol secreted. Aside from this general pattern, there is great variability in different individuals. Further, the secretory episodes in a given individual are not coincident on different days, as is evident in Fig. 12-8 for subject LC (cf. LC1 vs. LC2).

These bursts of cortisol secretion are triggered by intracranial events that are poorly understood. They result in episodic release of ACTH and are to some

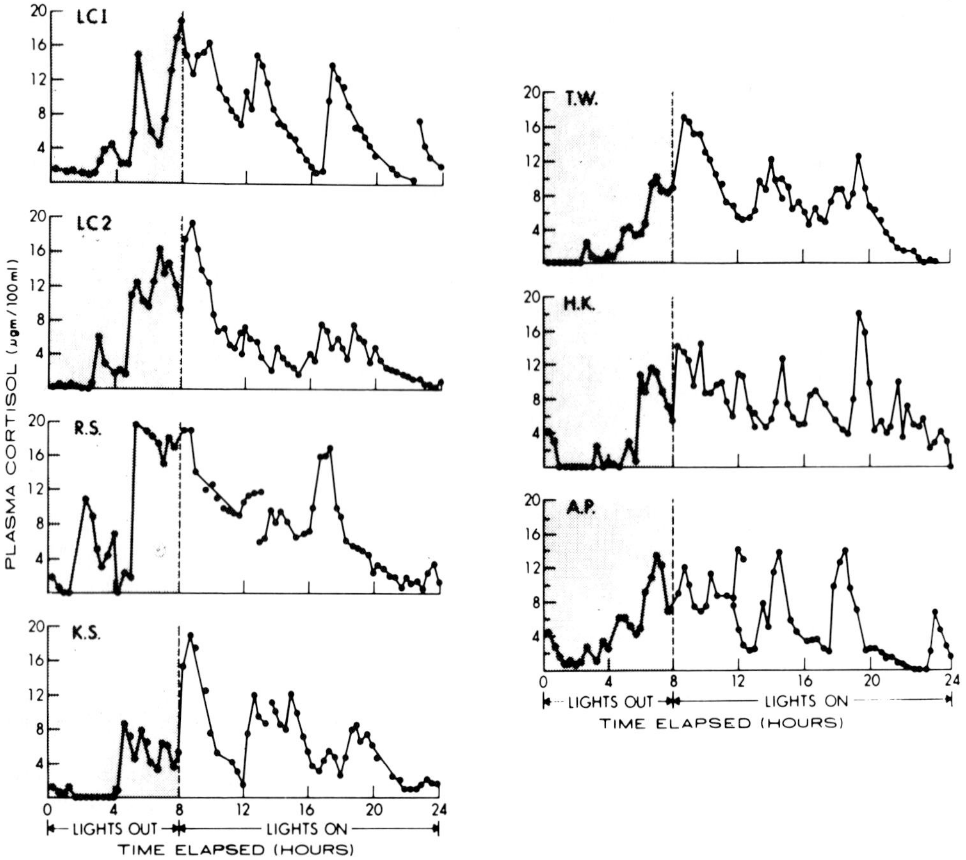

FIGURE 12-8 Plasma cortisol values of normal subjects for 24-h periods of study. Samples were obtained every 20 min. "Lights out" indicates the period available for sleep. LC1 and LC2 refer to studies done on the same subject in two different 24-h periods (*From Weitzman et al.*[139])

extent synchronized with peaks of plasma ACTH concentration (see Fig. 8-5).[140,143,144] There appears not to be circadian variation in the responsiveness of the pituitary to CRF.[140] There is a circadian periodicity in hypothalamic CRF content (that persists in hypophysectomized animals) with peak levels that precede by about 4 h the peak of plasma corticosteroid concentrations (see also Chap. 7);[140] however, the circadian rhythm is preserved when CRF is infused continuously.[145] Thus, to a significant extent, the rhythm is mediated by factors other than CRF.

In addition, aspects of the periodicity involve mechanisms independent of changes in pituitary ACTH release. There can be releases of cortisol that are not associated with ACTH release and vice versa.[140,144] In hypophysectomized animals given ACTH, cortisol rhythms can occur despite constant ACTH levels.[146] Further, in rats, spinal cord transection at T7 but not L1, or adrenal autotransplantation, abolishes the rhythm.[146] These data suggest that factors dependent on innervation may regulate the sensitivity of the adrenal to ACTH.[146]

In rats, the feeding schedule appears to be a major determinant of the circadian rhythm of glucocorticoid release, although there is some effect of light.[143,147] In rats, the peak plasma corticosteroid (corticosterone) level occurs after dark just prior to their nocturnal feeding. However, if the animals are fed only during the light period, the circadian period is altered and after about 10 days peak corticosterone concentrations occur coincident with the start of the feeding period. Thus, it appears that the endogenous rhythms of glucocorticoid release in the rat are primed to allow maximal release of corticosteroids during fasting and to decrease them at the time of feeding. Since glucocorticoids act to increase the blood glucose concentration (discussed below), the endogenous rhythms could conceivably serve in part as a relatively long-term regulatory mechanism to minimize the potential for developing hypoglycemia in times of fasting. Little is known about the mechanisms by which food affects the rhythm. The rhythm is present with pharmacological depletion of CNS serotonin or norepinephrine,[140] but changes in it in response to restricted food and water are abolished by lesions of the ventromedial nucleus of the hypothalamus (or fibers running through it).[148]

In humans, the mechanisms that regulate the circadian rhythm of cortisol release are less well understood. Although the influence of feeding on the overall rhythm has not been documented, episodes of cortisol release do occur before lunch and dinner, as mentioned above.[141,142] Further, these peaks do not occur in subjects accustomed to activity that does not include these meals.[142] The rhythm is not present until 3 to 8 years of age.[140] Once established, it is relatively resistant to change, and persists with prolonged bed rest, continuous feeding, and 2- to 3-day periods of sleep deprivation.[140] It remains normal in people who work night shifts but maintain a normal weekend life. When subjects totally change their sleep-waking-feeding patterns, as for instance when they move to a different part of the world, the circadian rhythm also changes, but only after 2 to 3 weeks.[149] In one study, the rhythm was affected by changing the period of light exposure independently of the feeding and sleeping schedule.[150] Thus, there may be several determinants of the rhythm in humans.

In addition, other factors, not as yet understood, acting on the adrenal in addition to ACTH, some of which may exhibit a circadian periodicity of their own, also modulate the adrenal secretory response.[140,144] This is evidenced by (1) the occasional increases of ACTH level without an increase in cortisol and (2) circumstances where there is a lack of proportionality between ACTH and cortisol peaks under different stimuli, such as spontaneous vs. provoked stimulations of ACTH release.[144,145a] Whereas in rats and monkeys there is evidence for an inherent circadian rhythm in adrenal sensitivity to ACTH, this has not been documented in humans.[140]

CHANGES IN THE SPONTANEOUS RHYTHM

The spontaneous rhythm of cortisol release can be interrupted by a variety of acute psychological and physical stresses and by a number of chronic conditions. These are generally mediated via the CNS (Chap. 7), although with insulin-induced hypoglycemia the effects are mediated via circulating catecholamines.[98] Although quantitative indexes of adrenal function, such as the mean 24-h cortisol concentration, do not change with age, the nadir and maximum periods of cortisol release tend to be earlier.[146]

Acute psychological stresses that result in increased cortisol release can be seemingly mild, such as the confrontation for venesection,[151] or more severe, such as the preparation for cardiac surgery.[152] The anticipation of and preparation for athletic competition or the stress of mental tasks such as university examinations can increase plasma cortisol levels.[145,153] However, with mild anxiety or in situations of prolonged stress, it is more difficult to predict whether there will be a stimulation of cortisol release.

Physical stresses that increase ACTH and cortisol release include severe trauma, major surgery, severe illness, hypoglycemia, fever, burns, cold exposure, irradiation, hypotension, severe dehydration, cigarette smoking, and moderate to intensive exercise.[14,19a,63,145,153] The response to surgery is illustrated in Fig. 12-9; such stresses can increase cortisol production sixfold.[63,154] Minor illnesses, such as upper respiratory infection, or

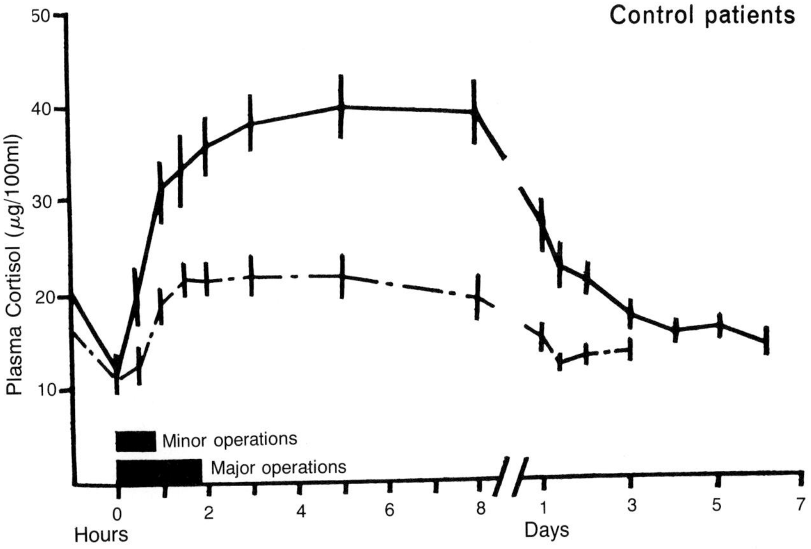

FIGURE 12-9 Plasma cortisol responses to major surgery (continuous line) and minor surgery (broken line) in normal subjects. Mean values and standard errors for 20 patients are shown in each case. (*From Plumpton et al.*[154])

minor surgery (Fig. 12-9)[154] may have little or no influence. The cortisol response to surgery can be blocked with the use of epidural anesthesia.[155] Changes in blood sugar level as little as from 81 to 64 mg/dl can result in some increase in cortisol;[156] the increases are much greater with more severe decreases in blood sugar level.

The circadian rhythm is also altered by chronic diseases.[157] It is abnormal in patients with liver disease or congestive heart failure (with hepatic congestion), in whom there is delayed cortisol removal.[149] The pattern is abnormal in patients with localized hypothalamic or limbic system disease and diffuse CNS disease with impaired consciousness.[149] In patients with marked depression, the number of secretory episodes is normal, but there is typically an increase in the magnitude and a reduced amplitude of the episodes associated with a decrease in the quiescent period and blunting of the circadian rhythm.[158,159] These changes result in an increase in the mean cortisol levels and are also probably associated with increased ACTH levels.[158,159] There is also an early nadir of cortisol secretion, and reduced latency between sleep onset and the nocturnal increase in cortisol secretion.[158,159] In depression, there is an elevation of CRF concentration in CSF, suggesting that the peptide contributes to the increased cortisol output,[80] and a decreased capacity of the axis to be suppressed by glucocorticoids (see also Central Nervous System under Actions of Glucocorticoids, below).[159] CRF hypersecretion may be present in anorexia nervosa, in which there is commonly cortisol hypersecretion, elevated cerebrospinal fluid CRF concentration, loss of the normal circadian rhythm, and blunted responses to dexamethasone suppression or CRF stimulation.[160] In Cushing's syndrome due to pituitary or ectopic ACTH hypersecretion or to an adrenal adenoma there occur continuous and irregular oscillatory patterns, with no increase in the proportion of peaks in the early morning hours.[148,149] Abnormal periodicity has been observed in over 50 percent of patients with intrasellar pituitary tumors without detectable abnormalities in basal adrenal function.[140] In hyperthyroidism, there is an increase in cortisol production with an exaggerated response to ACTH or metyrapone; the inverse occurs in hypothyroidism.[161] In blind subjects, the early morning increase in cortisol secretion usually occurs, but there are abnormal peaks throughout the day. However, ACTH release is decreased in women taking oral contraceptives,[162] and the serotonin antagonist cyproheptadine can inhibit both the circadian and hypoglycemia- or metyrapone-induced rises in ACTH level.[163,164] However, a number of drugs, including atropine, phenobarbital, reserpine, chlordiazepoxide, meprobamate, chlorpromazine, and phenytoin have been ineffective in blocking the circadian rise in cortisol production.[149]

FEEDBACK INHIBITION OF ACTH RELEASE

Glucocorticoids feedback inhibit the release of both CRF and ACTH.[14,156–167] Thus, in adrenal insufficiency plasma ACTH concentration may rise to levels as much as 10 to 20 times higher than normal, but can be reduced by physiological doses of cortisol. Stress-induced ACTH release is also greatly exaggerated in the adrenalectomized patient. Conversely, plasma ACTH concentrations and the ACTH response to stress are suppressed by high levels of glucocorticoids (Chap. 15). This feedback inhibition is elicited by all of the glucocorticoid agonists (defined below).[166,167a] The feedback inhibition is rapid and progressive with continued exposure to glucocorticoids.[14,165,166] It can be separated mechanistically into three components, a fast feedback occurring within seconds to minutes, an intermediate feedback occurring over 2 to 10 h, and a slow feedback occurring over hours to days.[165]

The fast feedback has been best studied in rats. Nevertheless, in humans a decrease in circulating ACTH concentration is detectable within 15 min (Fig. 12-10).[168] In rats the effect is apparent within

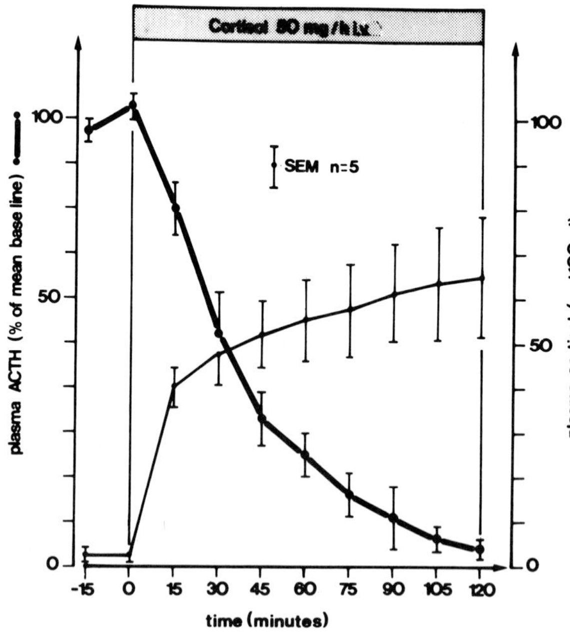

FIGURE 12-10 Time course of ACTH levels in response to a constant-rate infusion of cortisol at 50 mg/h in patients with Addison's disease. ACTH values are given as percent of the individual mean starting levels. The difference between ACTH values at 15 min and the starting value was significant ($p < 0.025$). (*From Fehm et al.*[168])

2 min and is not dose-dependent, but is proportional to the rate of increase of the level of a glucocorticoid.[165,166,168] It also blunts the ACTH responses to some stimuli (e.g., histamine), but the axis remains responsive to more major stimuli (e.g., major surgery).[14,63,166] The fast feedback is exerted at both the hypothalamus and the pituitary, although the effect on the hypothalamus may be more pronounced,[97,166,168a] since in rats the suppression can be overridden by CRF administration.[14,166] The fast feedback is too rapid to be accounted for by the classic glucocorticoid influences on mRNA (discussed below and in Chap. 5); glucocorticoids may affect more directly the release of CRF and ACTH by actions on the cell membrane. The fast feedback lasts less than 10 min in animals and is followed by a period of about 2 h in which there is little or no influence of certain stimuli on ACTH release; afterward, responses to these stimuli can again be suppressed and the intermediate feedback can be observed.[14,165,166]

The intermediate and delayed feedback mechanisms are progressive and proportional to the dose and duration of glucocorticoid administration. They are separable mechanistically in that the intermediate feedback lasts only a few hours, during which time there appears to be predominantly an inhibition of both CRF and ACTH release without major influences on the synthesis of the peptides. However, the intermediate feedback does require protein synthesis. These two mechanisms also differ in that during the intermediate feedback phase, the axis, although suppressed and unresponsive to certain stimuli (e.g., histamine), can respond to other stimuli, such as endotoxin. After several hours the delayed feedback sets in; it is associated with unresponsiveness to CRF with marked decreases in POMC mRNA and transcription of the POMC gene[167] and a decrease in the number of detectable pituitary ACTH-containing cells. However, there is no known loss of cells with the ultimate potential to produce ACTH. Glucocorticoid treatment has a much more modest effect, if any, on hypothalamic CRF mRNA,[169] although it does decrease hypothalamic CRF,[170] AVP,[78] and AVP mRNA[171] content. The feedback inhibition of CRF may also involve influences on other brain regions, such as the hippocampus, that influence releasing factor release.[172]

With time, the delayed feedback progresses to result in total unresponsiveness of the axis to even extreme stimuli, as is observed in patients with spontaneous Cushing's syndrome (see below) or on long-term high-dose glucocorticoid therapy (Chap. 15). The delayed feedback persists as long as steroid administration is continued.[165,166,168a,170] However, during the emergence of prolonged suppression (over a day to weeks of high-dose glucocorticoid therapy, for example), an intermediate capability to respond to various stimuli can be present. For instance, in some patients on glucocorticoids for 24 h or more there may be no cortisol response to surgery,[173] whereas other patients on more prolonged systemic corticosteroid therapy have impaired responses to insulin-induced hypoglycemia, but may maintain a normal or near-normal response to surgery.[154]

Following withdrawal of the glucocorticoid there is a return to normal function. The recovery period varies with the extent and duration of the suppression and can be from hours to many months; this is detailed in Chap. 15.[14,165,166]

There also exists a neural pathway not involving glucocorticoids by which feedback inhibition by the adrenal of the release of CRF and perhaps other hypothalamic factors occurs.[165] The overall importance of this mechanism is not known.[165]

The feedback inhibition can be altered in a number of disease states. These include spontaneous Cushing's syndrome, anorexia nervosa, alcoholism, depression, chronic illness, and renal disease. These states are described below (see Diagnosis and Differential Diagnosis under Cushing's Syndrome).

Regulation of Mineralocorticoid Production

The production of aldosterone by the adrenal zona glomerulosa is controlled by the renin-angiotensin system, K^+, Na^+, ACTH, serotonin, and possibly other factors. Although the renin-angiotensin system and potassium ion are the major regulators, there are complex interrelationships between all of these factors. Cortisol, corticosterone, DOC, and a number of the other steroids described above (under Synthesis of Aldosterone, DOC, and Other Mineralocorticoids) also have mineralocorticoid activity. Their potential importance is discussed below and in Chap. 14. DOC and its derivatives are synthesized in all three zones of the adrenal cortex, but production in the fasciculata in response to ACTH accounts for most of the plasma DOC.[36] The production of 19-nor-DOC (see also Chap. 14)[37,174–176] derived from 19-oic-DOC in peripheral tissues is regulated by the same stimuli as is DOC. Other steroids with C-18 substitutions, such as 18-OH-cortisol, 18-OH-corticosterone, and 18-oxo-cortisol, and possibly 19-OH-androstenedione, come predominantly from the adrenal glomerulosa and their release is controlled by the renin-angiotensin system.[33,39] In contrast to the case with reduced cortisol metabolites, some of the metabolites of aldosterone can have activity, although their importance is not known;[174] presumably, their production parallels that of aldosterone.

ANGIOTENSIN II

Angiotensin II is the major regulator of aldosterone release. This peptide has a number of other actions such as regulation of blood pressure and renin release; these and other aspects of the renin-angiotensin system are discussed in more detail in Chap. 14. Renin release is controlled by several factors, but the concentration of salt bathing the renal juxtaglomerular cells is a major factor (Figs. 12-11 and 12-12). A decrease in renal blood pressure (mediated via renal baroreceptors) and β-adrenergic action also stimulate renin release. Renin catalyzes the conversion of angiotensinogen (or renin substrate) to the decapeptide angiotensin I, which is then cleaved to form the octapeptide angiotensin II by converting enzyme in pulmonary and other tissues. In some species, angiotensin II is also converted to the desaspartyl$_1$ heptapeptide angiotensin III, which can also stimulate aldosterone production. Angiotensins II and III are rapidly degraded (with circulating half-lives of 1 or 2 min) to inactive forms by tissue angiotensinases.

Angiotensins II and III rapidly increase aldosterone production by the zona glomerulosa[177] but do not stimulate cortisol production. These two compounds have equipotent adrenal-stimulating activities, but the plasma concentrations of angiotensin III are perhaps only 20 percent of those of angiotensin II.[178] Thus, it appears that quantitatively angiotensin II is the more important.

Angiotensin II stimulates both early and late steps in aldosterone biosynthesis.[64,177,179] Thus, there is an increased conversion of cholesterol to pregnenolone and of corticosterone to 18-hydroxycorticosterone and aldosterone. Influences on the earlier step are more important in the initial actions of angiotensin II, although influences on the later steps are significant in long-term stimulation.

Angiotensin binds to glomerulosa cell surface receptors with an affinity of about 0.5 nM (Chap. 5).[180] The concentration of these receptors in glomerulosa cells is increased by angiotensin II and by potassium ion, and is decreased by low potassium concentration (Chaps. 5 and 14). The hormone does not stimulate adenylate cyclase.[181] The primary action of angiotensin II is probably to increase phosphatidylinositol hydrolysis via receptor activation; this in turn leads to Ca^{2+} mobilization from both intracellular and extracellular sources, with subsequent effects increasing phosphatidylinositol, phosphatidic acid, and polyphosphoinositide concentrations and activating C kinase; these mediators in turn stimulate cholesterol side chain cleavage and possibly the later steps in steroidogenesis, in a manner analogous to that described above for ACTH.[121,128,182] The major differences between angiotensin II and ACTH action are in the early steps and involve cAMP-dependent and -independent pathways, but the steps ultimately involve changes in Ca^{2+} and phospholipid levels. As with ACTH, angiotensin II actions require protein synthesis and the hormone does result in a stimulation of cholesterol binding to the putative cytochrome P450s that are involved in the biotransformation steps.[64,177] Unlike the case with ACTH, angiotensin II has not been reported to increase cholesterol ester hydrolysis or esterification.[177]

Angiotensin II actions may also be mediated in part by stimulation of prostaglandin biosynthesis.[183] PGE_1 and PGE_2 stimulate (in a manner additive with angiotensin II), whereas $PGF_{1\alpha}$ and $PGF_{2\alpha}$ inhibit aldosterone release, and angiotensin administration increases the plasma concentration of PGE_1.[183] Further, although there is controversy, the inhibitor of PG biosynthesis indomethacin can blunt both basal and angiotensin-stimulated release of aldosterone in vivo and in isolated adrenal cells.[183]

Angiotensin II also exerts a trophic influence on the glomerulosa. With prolonged stimulation, the sensitivity of the glomerulosa to the hormone increases; conversely, when renin and angiotensin II levels are suppressed, the sensitivity to angiotensin II is decreased (Chap. 14). However, in some low-renin states (i.e., low-renin essential hypertension), the sensitivity of the glomerulosa to angiotension II is increased (see Chap. 14).

POTASSIUM ION

Increases in plasma K^+ concentration stimulate aldosterone production.[128,179,182,184-186] Conversely, low potassium concentration decreases aldosterone producton and blunts the aldosterone response to sodium depletion. Changes in potassium concentration of as little as 0.1 meq/liter within the physiological range can influence the aldosterone secretion rate.[187] These effects are independent of sodium and angiotensin II levels.[179,182,184-186] In anephric humans, K^+ is probably the major regulator of aldosterone production, although plasma aldosterone levels are low. As is the case with angiotensin II, prolonged potassium loading produces a trophic influence with an increased sensitivity of the adrenal to K^+, an increase in the width of the zona glomerulosa, and structural changes similar to those seen with sodium depletion. Potassium ion does not affect the fasciculata or cortisol production. Potassium loading decreases and potassium deprivation increases renin release.[186,187] These influences could be mediated indirectly through effects on ion balance. Although the influences of potassium ion on renin tend to counterbalance those directly on aldosterone, the latter effect usually predominates.

In animals, potassium ion affects both the early (cholesterol to pregnenolone) and the late (corticosterone or DOC to aldosterone) steps in mineralocorticoid biosynthesis.[64,185] This may also be true in humans, since cells isolated from human subjects with a high potassium intake show an increase in the activity of the late pathway,[64] and hypokalemia increases the plasma ratio of 18-hydroxycorticosterone (the precursor to aldosterone) to aldosterone (Chap. 14).

Potassium probably acts by depolarizing the cell membrane, resulting in increased uptake of extracellular Ca^{2+}; this in turn results in increased phosphoinositide hydrolysis, with increased mobilization of intracellular Ca^{2+}, increased synthesis of phosphatidic acid, phosphatidylinositol, and polyphosphoinositides with a stimulation of steroidogenesis;[128,182] it can also have a weaker effect on cAMP.[121] Thus, the actions of K^+ and angiotensin II, although largely similar, differ in that the K^+ effect is primarily on Ca^{2+} uptake with secondary effects of decreasing phosphatidic acid and phosphoinositide formation, whereas angiotensin II initially affects phosphatidylinositol hydrolysis.

PITUITARY GLAND

The pituitary gland is not the major regulator of aldosterone production, but ACTH and perhaps other pituitary factors can have an influence. Hypophysectomy in humans or suppression of ACTH secretion by dexamethasone does not lower basal aldosterone secretion, nor prevent the increase following sodium deprivation.[187,188] However, when hypopituitarism has been present for months to years there may be little or no increase in aldosterone with sodium depletion.[187,188] This may be due to a deficiency of pituitary factors such as growth hormone.[187] However, decreased aldosterone production has also been observed with apparently isolated ACTH deficiency; this was corrected by glucocorticoid treatment.[189] Administration of ACTH to humans on a low or a normal sodium intake increases aldosterone secretion, but this effect is transient, lasting less than 24 h.[188] The transient response could be due to "down regulation" of ACTH receptors and responsiveness (discussed above); it may also be due to suppression of renin levels and angiotensin II production consequent to the mineralocorticoid actions of cortisol and/or aldosterone released in response to ACTH.[190] In the dog, prolonged ACTH treatment actually decreases both the size of the glomerulosa and its responsiveness to ACTH and angiotensin II.[187] Nevertheless, stresses that increase ACTH production increase aldosterone production; this effect is abolished by hypophysectomy or by hypothalamic lesions that abolish the ACTH responses to stress.[187] Hypophysectomy has a much greater effect on aldosterone production in the rat than in humans; it inhibits the rise of aldosterone concentration following sodium depletion. This effect is not completely overcome by ACTH, raising the possibility that other pituitary factors, such as other fragments of POMC, are also involved in regulating aldosterone biosynthesis.[113,187,188,191-193] In fact, β-endorphin has been reported to be as effective as ACTH in stimulating aldosterone release.[191] Further, aldosterone production can be stimulated by β-MSH (particularly in the presence of sodium deficiency)[192] and by the amino-terminal portion of POMC and γ_3-MSH.[195] The possible role of pituitary factors in regulating aldosterone release in primary aldosteronism is discussed in Chap. 14.

The mechanisms of ACTH action overall are similar to those used to stimulate cortisol synthesis. In the glomerulosa ACTH stimulates the conversion of cholesterol to pregnenolone and it stimulates the distal steps in aldosterone production in some species.[64,187] The actions of ACTH may involve both effects on cAMP and a stimulation of extracellular Ca^{2+} uptake.[121] Unlike the case with angiotensin II, the response to ACTH is only partially calmodulin-dependent.[182]

SODIUM ION

Sodium deficiency increases (Figs. 12-11 and 12-12) and sodium loading decreases aldosterone production. These effects are mostly due to the influences of sodium chloride on renin with consequent changes in angiotensin II levels (Fig. 12-12; Chap. 14). In addition, small changes in the sodium concentration can have a substantial effect on angiotensin II- and K^+-stimulated aldosterone production, independent of effects that may be due to osmotic influences of the ion and could account for blunted aldosterone responses during water deprivation.[194]

OTHER FACTORS

Several other factors affect aldosterone biosynthesis. Administration of ammonium chloride to normal subjects increases plasma aldosterone levels.[195] These influences might be direct or may be secondary to effects of the acidosis on renin and potassium concentration. Aldosterone output under stimulated conditions, but not in the basal state, appears to be under tonic dopaminergic inhibition.[187,196,197] This appears to be mostly a direct effect on the adrenal glomerulosa, exerted at the late steps in aldosterone biosynthesis,[196] although dopamine may also influence renin release under some circumstances.[187] The dopaminergic inhibition is demonstrable with the use of a dopamine antagonist (metoclopramide) and is probably maximal most of the time, since infusion of dopamine does not alter basal aldosterone levels or the aldosterone response to ACTH or angiotensin II.[187] Glucocorticoids may inhibit aldosterone production in isolated cells,[184] but whether this occurs in vivo has not been documented. The adrenal glomerulosa can also respond to vasopressin,[198] β-adrenergic stimulation,[199] serotonin,[187] and somatostatin.[200] Finally, the recently discovered atrial natriuretic factors (ANF) can block aldosterone release; these peptides can decrease basal aldosterone release and the sensitivity of the glomerulosa cells to ACTH and angiotensin II.[201] The peptides do not affect cortisol production. The physiological importance of these actions of vasopressin, β-adrenergic agonists, somatostatin, and ANF are not yet clarified.

SPONTANEOUS PATTERNS OF ALDOSTERONE RELEASE

The release of aldosterone (like cortisol) follows a circadian rhythm and is episodic (Fig. 12-11).[202] However, the variations tend to be much less than with cortisol.[202] In the supine individual on a normal salt intake, the plasma aldosterone levels usually vary synchronously with ACTH and cortisol (Fig. 12-11).[202] The mean plasma aldosterone concentration is highest from midnight to 8:30 A.M. and lowest from 4:30 to 11:30 P.M. Plasma renin activity is also lowest from 4:30 to 11:30 P.M., but it is highest between 9:00 A.M. and 4:00 P.M.[202] Thus, the peak aldosterone production under these conditions may be determined by factors other than renin. When dexamethasone is administered to block ACTH and cortisol production, the nocturnal rise in aldosterone persists, and correlates only partially with increased plasma renin activity (Fig. 12-11C).[202] This suggests that other factors, secreted synchronously with ACTH but not subject to glucocorticoid feedback inhibition, may determine the spontaneous rhythm.

When subjects' sodium intakes are restricted (10 meq/24 h), mean plasma aldosterone values are considerably higher (Fig. 12-11) and also show wide fluctuations.[202] In this case, the plasma aldosterone concentration shows a significant correlation with levels of both cortisol and renin (Fig. 12-11B);[202] presumably, it is the increased renin concentration in response to salt restriction (Chap. 14) that is responsible for the mean increase in aldosterone concentration.

INTERRUPTION OF THE SPONTANEOUS PATTERNS OF ALDOSTERONE RELEASE

A number of factors stimulate or inhibit aldosterone release and interrupt the spontaneous pattern described above. These mainly affect the renin-angio-

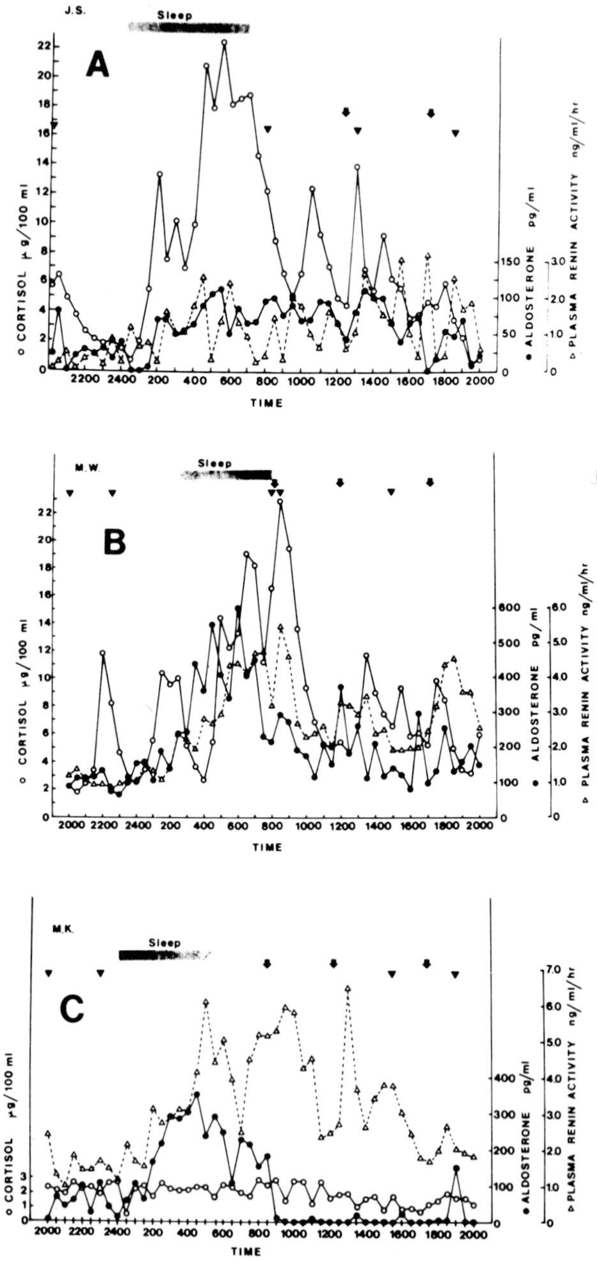

FIGURE 12-11 Patterns of aldosterone and cortisol release and plasma renin levels in normal individuals in supine position. (A) Normal sodium intake. (B) Sodium restriction (10 meq/24 h). (C) Dexamethasone treatment (1.5 mg per day). Arrows denote trips to the bathroom. (*From Katz et al.*[202])

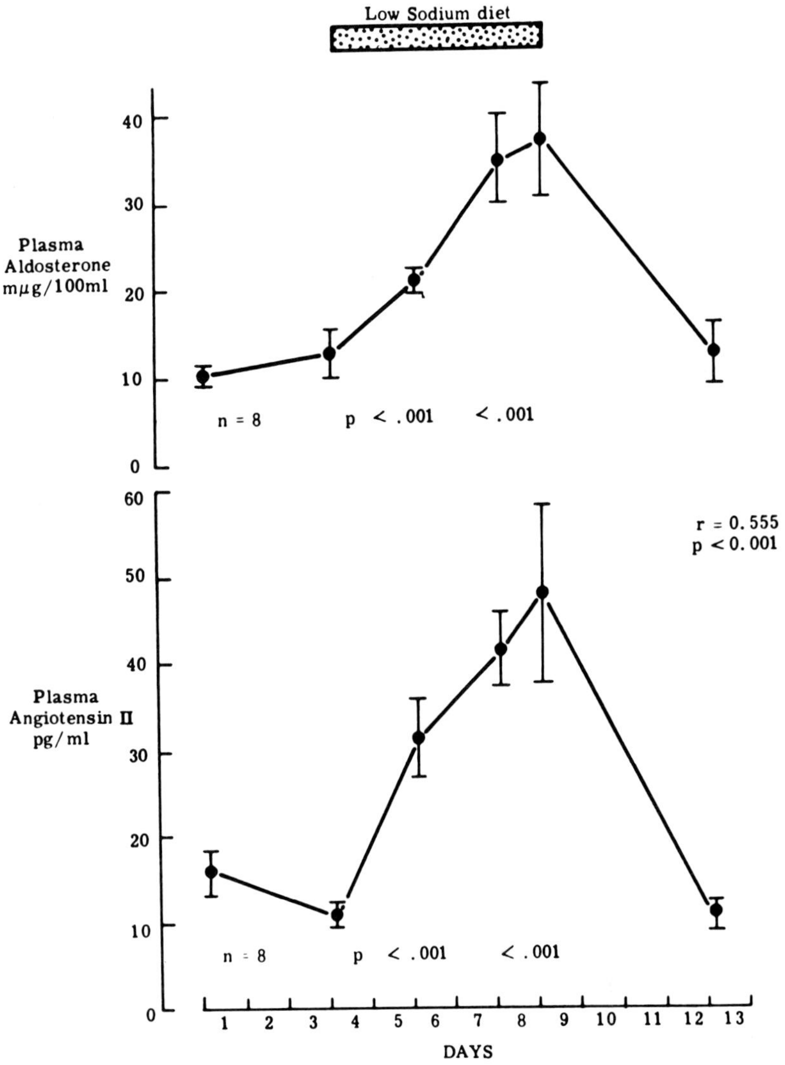

FIGURE 12-12 Effect of a low-sodium diet on plasma angiotensin II and aldosterone concentrations in normal subjects. (*From Brown et al.*[203])

tensin system and potassium and ACTH concentrations. Thus, salt restriction (Fig. 12-12),[203] dehydration, assumption of erect posture, physical exercise, carotid occlusion, and thoracic caval constriction all activate the renin-angiotensin system and increase aldosterone production. Hyperkalemia increases aldosterone production. Increases in ACTH levels transiently increase aldosterone production. Conversely, salt loading, hypokalemia, and prolonged ACTH deficiency decrease aldosterone production. Also, hyperreninemic hypoaldosteronism can occur in critical illness.[157] The regulation of aldosterone levels in hypertensive states is discussed in Chap. 14.

Regulation of Adrenal Androgen Production

ACTH regulates the production of adrenal androgens. Thus, plasma DHEA and androstenedione levels show both circadian and episodic variation, similar to cortisol.[43,204] This is not seen with DHEA-S, due to its slower metabolism and higher concentrations;[43] also, the plasma concentrations of DHEA-S, in contrast to the other steroids, are not elevated acutely by ACTH, although a later rise does occur.[43] Plasma androgen levels can also be suppressed when ACTH release is blocked by glucocorticoid treatment.[205] Plasma testosterone and 5α-dihydrotestosterone (DHT) concentrations also show circadian rhythms in spite of their multiple origins in women (ovaries, adrenal, and peripheral conversion from androstenedione) and testicular origin in men (see Chaps. 16 and 17).[206] Whereas these generally coincide with cortisol release, minor differences also occur.

The relation of adrenal secretion of androgens to that of cortisol varies in several circumstances.[137,207–212]

First, changes in DHEA and androstenedione levels in response to ACTH or dexamethasone suppression are less than those of cortisol.[212] Second, the ratios of adrenal androgen concentrations change at various times throughout life and in other circumstances.[137,209,211] They increase relative to cortisol at around ages 6 to 8 and again during puberty.[137,209] They are frequently increased in women with hirsutism.[212] They are decreased in fasting and anorexia nervosa and with aging.[137,202,209,210] They increase less than cortisol in response to stress,[137] and they recover more slowly than cortisol levels following long-term glucocorticoid suppression.[137,212]

These data imply that factors in addition to ACTH control adrenal androgen production. Among those considered are estrogens, prolactin, gonadotropins, growth hormone, lipotropins, PGs, other pituitary factors, and adrenal steroid content;[137] recently, a protein with such selective activity has been isolated from human pituitaries.[208] An additional proposal to explain the selective changes involves overall influences on adrenal mass and steroid concentrations that affect androgen production.[209] As described earlier (The Fetal Adrenal), increases in levels of several different steroids can partly inhibit 3β-hydroxysteroid dehydrogenase and result in increased relative shunting of steroids through the androgen pathway.[209] Measurements of intraadrenal steroid concentrations throughout life do correlate with the relative plasma concentrations of DHEA and cortisol.[116,209] Although it has been difficult to implicate growth hormone itself as a regulator of adrenal androgen secretion, recent correlations between altered adrenal androgen/cortisol ratios and somatomedin C levels in anorexia have suggested a specific role for somatomedin C.[137,207,210]

Although estrogens and prolactin can stimulate adrenal androgen production, it has been difficult to implicate them as physiologically important.[213] Gonadotropins do not affect the adrenal. Other products of POMC, although incompletely evaluated, have not been shown to be factors. Prostaglandins can stimulate cortisol production, but they have not been shown to specifically stimulate androgen production.[137] The fact that hypophysectomy in the chimpanzee alters the plasma DHEA/cortisol ratio has been taken as a possible indication of the existence of pituitary factors other than ACTH that selectively stimulate adrenal androgen production.[211]

Plasma androstenedione, testosterone, and DHT concentrations in women vary with the menstrual cycle; this is due to androstenedione production by the ovary and its peripheral conversion to testosterone and DHT.[43,206,214] Plasma androstenedione and testosterone concentrations average 125 ng/dl and 25 ng/dl, respectively, during the early follicular phase and 200 ng/dl and up to 50 ng/dl, respectively, during midcycle.[214] In the follicular phase, the adrenal accounts for about 67 percent of the testosterone, about 50 percent of the DHT (from peripheral conversion of testosterone, see Chap. 16), 55 percent of the androstenedione, 80 percent of the DHEA, and 96 percent of the DHEA-S.[214] The remainder comes from the ovaries. During midcycle the adrenal contribution to testosterone and androstenedione levels drops to 40 percent and 30 percent, respectively.[214]

In the male, the adrenal contribution to testosterone (and consequently DHT) is negligible, even though the peripheral tissues can convert androstenedione and DHEA to testosterone.[44]

Regulation of Adrenal Estrogen Production

Small amounts of estradiol and estriol are synthesized in the adrenal; however, the major adrenal contribution to estrogenic activity is due to conversion of androstenedione and, to a lesser extent, of DHEA and DHEA-S to estrogens in peripheral tissues.[19a] These steroids are under the control of ACTH and the other potential factors discussed above.

PHYSICAL STATE OF STEROIDS IN PLASMA

Cortisol and Other Glucocorticoids

The cortisol released by the adrenal gland is free. However, approximately 90 to 97 percent of the circulating cortisol is bound by plasma proteins.[215–220] About 90 percent of this binding is due to association of the steroid with corticosteroid-binding globulin (CBG, also termed transcortin) that binds cortisol specifically and with high affinity (i.e., it is saturable at moderately low concentrations of cortisol) (Fig. 12-13). A lesser quantity of cortisol is bound by albumin

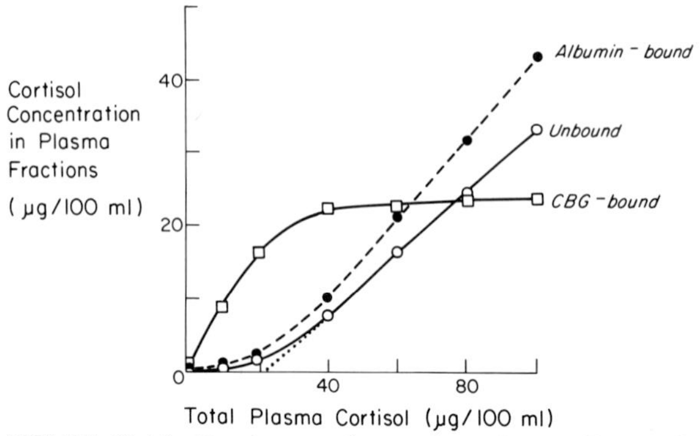

FIGURE 12-13 Distribution of cortisol in plasma. (*From Ballard.*[215])

and a negligible amount by other plasma proteins (Fig. 12-13).

CORTICOSTEROID-BINDING GLOBULIN

Some properties of CBG are listed in Table 12-4. The protein has been detected in all species examined, although the levels vary from about 1 μg/dl in the sheep to 100 μg/dl in the iguana and squirrel.[215] CBG is produced primarily in the liver;[215,220,221] however, it has also been found in a number of other tissues, including brain, pituitary, lung, kidney, muscle, and uterus, and in lymphocytes.[220,222] It has a molecular weight of around 50,000 and is glycosylated.[215,220] At usual concentrations in humans it can bind up to 25 μg/dl of cortisol[215] at physiological conditions (Fig. 12-13). Cortisol binds to and dissociates rapidly from the protein.[215-217,223] Its affinity for cortisol (K_d ~13 to 30 nM)[215,218] is such that at a total plasma cortisol of 10 μg/dl the protein is 50 percent saturated, and it is over 90 percent saturated at a total cortisol concentration of ~40 μg/dl. Since CBG is the major cortisol-binding protein, the free cortisol in plasma is almost linearly related to the total cortisol at normal concentrations. However, when total cortisol concentration rises above 25 μg/dl, CBG becomes more saturated with the steroid, and the proportion of the total cortisol that is free increases in a nonlinear fashion (Fig. 12-13). Thus, at a total plasma cortisol concentration of 40 μg/dl, the free cortisol (~10 μg/dl) would be tenfold higher than that at a total plasma cortisol concentration of 10 μg/dl (free cortisol concentration ≈1 μg/dl).

A number of other endogenous and synthetic steroids also bind to CBG (Table 12-5).[215,218,224] However, considering their affinity for CBG and/or their plasma concentrations, the extent of this binding in physiological circumstances is ordinarily minor and almost all of the CBG-bound steroid is cortisol. One exception is third-trimester pregnancy, where increased progesterone accounts for about 25 percent of the total CBG-bound steroid.[215,216] Also, in congenital adrenal hyperplasia (discussed below and in Chap. 18), several steroids can be elevated enough to occupy CBG to a major extent. These include corticosterone, 17α-hydroxyprogesterone, progesterone, 11-deoxycortisol, DOC, and 21-deoxycortisol. Most of the synthetic glucocorticoids used in therapy (prednisolone is an exception) have a low affinity for CBG (Table 12-5), and therefore bind negligibly to it (see also Chap. 15). Whereas prednisone and cortisone bind weakly, these compounds are converted to prednisolone and cortisol, which bind tightly.

The CBG concentrations in plasma vary between individuals and are also regulated by hormones and other factors. Estrogens increase CBG levels and therefore elevated concentrations are seen in pregnancy and with estrogen therapy and oral contraceptive use.[215-217] In pregnancy, CBG levels gradually rise and are twice normal in the third trimester.[216] With estrogen treatment, the effect is maximal in about 3 to 5 days and CBG levels return to normal 2 to 3 weeks following cessation of therapy.[216] Thyroid hormones increase CBG synthesis.[217] Thus, CBG levels are reduced in hypothyroidism and increased in hyperthyroidism.[217] Elevated CBG levels in some cases may have a genetic basis and can be associated with certain HLA types.[217,225] Elevated levels also occur in diabetes and certain hematological disorders.[225] CBG levels are subnormal in liver disease (decreased protein production), multiple myeloma, obesity, and the ne-

Table 12-4. General Properties of Corticosteroid-Binding Proteins in Human Serum

	CBG	Albumin	α_1 Acid glycoprotein
Molecular weight	52,000	69,000	39,000
Concentration, μM	0.71	550	18
Concentration, g/liter	0.037	38	0.18
Cortisol-binding capacity, μg/dl	25	>20,000	630
Equilibrium dissociation constant for cortisol at 37°C (K_d), M	3×10^{-8}	2×10^{-4}	8.5×10^{-6}
Cortisol-binding sites per molecule	1	1–20	1
Relative distribution of cortisol at 37°C, %	77.3	15.0	0

Source: Modified from Ballard;[215] data from Sandberg and Slaunwhite[216] and Westphal.[217]

Table 12-5. Relative Affinities of Steroids for CBG, Cytoplasmic Glucocorticoid Receptor, and Albumin in Humans

	CBG	Relative affinity for receptor*	Albumin
Cortisol	100	100	100
Fluocinolone acetonide	<1	1350	
Methylprednisolone	<1	1190	74
Dexamethasone	<1	710	>100
Betamethasone	<1	540	>100
Fluorometholone	<1	400	
9α-Fluorocortisol	<1	350	
Triamcinolone acetonide	<1	190	
Corticosterone	94	85	100
Prednisolone	58	220	61
Aldosterone	6	38	34
11-Deoxycorticosterone (DOC)	45	39	221
11-Deoxycortisol	77	19	
Progesterone	27	11	244
17α-Hydroxyprogesterone	70	>1	225
Prednisone	6	5	68
Cortisone	6	1	128
Testosterone	5	2	232
Pregnenolone	<1		
Estradiol	<1	5	1600
Estrone	<1		800
Androstenedione	<1	<1	223
Dehydroepiandrosterone (prasterone, DHEA)	<1		506

Note: Data for CBG and receptor obtained at 2°C; however, the relative binding at 37°C is similar overall.
*Human fetal lung.
Source: Ballard.[215]

phrotic syndrome (urinary loss of protein).[215,216,226] Glucocorticoids inhibit CBG synthesis in rats,[215] although this has not been convincingly demonstrated in humans. Complete absence of CBG has not been reported,[215] but there is a familial condition in which CBG levels are half normal with normal plasma-free cortisol concentrations and no clinical symptoms.[227]

ALBUMIN AND OTHER CORTISOL-BINDING PROTEINS

Cortisol binding to albumin has different characteristics. The kinetics of cortisol association with and dissociation from albumin are much more rapid than cortisol with CBG. The affinity of albumin for cortisol is much lower, but the capacity is over 1000-fold higher than that of CBG (Table 12-4).[215,217] At cortisol concentrations less than 20 μg/dl, about 7 percent of the plasma cortisol is albumin-bound.[218] With increasing cortisol level, CBG but not albumin becomes saturated with the steroid, and a larger proportion of the plasma-bound steroid is associated with albumin (Fig. 12-13).[215]

Synthetic glucocorticoids are bound by albumin with an affinity similar to or slightly exceeding that of cortisol.[215] For instance, 55 percent of the total prednisolone, 62 percent of the betamethasone, and 77 percent of the dexamethasone is bound by human plasma.[215]

Although the proportion of free steroid bound by albumin is relatively independent of the steroid concentration, it is affected by the plasma albumin concentration.[215] Thus, in premature infants and in hypoalbuminemia, the proportion of non-CBG-bound steroid that is free is increased.[215,218]

The α_1 acid glycoprotein that binds progesterone and other steroids also binds cortisol (Table 12-5), but this appears be of minor importance.[215]

PHYSIOLOGICAL ROLE OF PLASMA BINDING

The major function of CBG and other steroid-binding proteins is to serve as a reservoir to sequester steroids in an inactive form; this function ultimately influences the availability of steroids to tissues, and their receptors and steroid-metabolizing enzymes. These plasma-binding proteins are not necessary for transporting the steroids in the circulation, as the latter are sufficiently water-soluble at biologically active concentrations.[215] Further, humans with low CBG levels and animals such as sheep with extremely low CBG levels show no decrement in their responsiveness to glucocorticoids.[215,217,220]

The steroids are inactive when bound by plasma proteins.[215,220,223] For example, when tissue culture cells are incubated with cortisol and either CBG or albumin, the glucocorticoid dose response is reduced concomitantly to the extent of cortisol binding.[223] Further, the physiological mechanisms that control the plasma cortisol concentration respond to free rather than total cortisol levels, such that with variations in CBG levels the free cortisol concentrations do not change, even though total cortisol levels do.[215] The CBG-bound and, to a lesser extent, the albumin-bound cortisol is also protected from metabolic degradation, and when CBG levels are increased the rate of cortisol clearance is decreased.[215] Thus, the proteins can serve as a reservoir to sequester active steroids.

Whereas in any equilibrium situation the plasma-bound steroids are sequestered in an inactive state, they can become active through dissociation from the proteins. This can occur rapidly. Cortisol can dissociate from albumin with a $t_{1/2}$ of around 5 s at 37°C.[219]

Thus, as the free and protein-bound steroid circulates through the various tissues the free steroid binds specifically to receptors, steroid-metabolizing enzymes, and other proteins and nonspecifically to a number of cellular components. This reduces the free steroid concentration and shifts the equilibrium toward dissociation of plasma protein-steroid complexes. The dissociated steroid is then free for further tissue uptake. The net result is that the fraction of total cortisol available for tissue binding as the blood passes through a tissue exceeds the free cortisol concentration. This available fraction depends both on the extent of tissue uptake that shifts the equilibrium and the time of transport.[228] Since the rate of dissociation from albumin is more rapid than from CBG, steroid bound by albumin is a more readily available source. Since the capillary transit time through certain tissues such as liver is slower (around 5 s) than in other tissues such as brain (around 1 s), the former tissues can extract a larger proportion of the cortisol.[228] In fact, the brain uptake of corticosterone in the rat approximates the non-CBG-bound (free plus albumin-bound) steroid whereas in the liver it exceeds this fraction by three times and includes CBG-bound steroid.[219,220]

Plasma binding may also, by sequestering the relevant steroid and releasing it more gradually, serve to dampen the swings in plasma cortisol levels in plasma due to episodic pulsatile release of the steroid. This could protect the steroid from metabolic degradation and render changes in receptor occupancy more gradual.

Increasing evidence from rat studies suggests that CBG in the various tissues plays a role in regulating the occupancy by receptors of cortisol.[229–231] In the kidney, CBG or CBG-like proteins can sequester corticosterone and decrease its ability to bind to mineralocorticoid receptors, rendering them more available to be occupied by aldosterone. Conversely, in brain these proteins are either absent or low in concentration and the result is that corticosterone largely occupies the mineralocorticoid receptors. The net effect is to determine which type of steroid acts through these receptors. This issue is described further below (see Central Nervous System, Molecular Mechanisms of Glucocorticoid Action, and Molecular Mechanisms of Mineralocorticoid Action).

Except for the liver, where CBG is known to be synthesized,[215,221] in other tissues where there are substantial concentrations of CBG or CBG-like protein it has not yet been determined whether the presence of the protein is due to uptake or local synthesis.[219,222] In addition, there is active inquiry as to whether CBG with its associated steroid can function as a biologically active complex to facilitate steroid uptake,[219,220,230] although, as discussed above, the weight of the evidence suggests that the capacity of CBG to generate a free intermediate steroid through dissociation is the major mechanism.[228]

Aldosterone

There is no protein in plasma that is known to bind a substantial amount of aldosterone specifically and with high affinity, unlike the case with many other steroids. This steroid is mostly weakly associated with plasma proteins, including albumin and CBG.[216,218,228,232,233] It also associates with red cells.[234] At 37°C, about 60 percent of the total aldosterone in plasma is associated with proteins.[218,228] About 20 percent of the aldosterone is associated with CBG.[218] Although high concentrations of cortisol can decrease the total plasma binding of aldosterone slightly, the percent of free aldosterone in plasma is relatively invariant, even with wide fluctuations in the concentrations of this and other steroids.[235] The amount of aldosterone that is available for biological actions is decreased in proportion to the extent of plasma binding.[235] However, since aldosterone dissociates rapidly from the plasma proteins, it is likely that most of the aldosterone is available for biological actions as it passes through target tissues.

Although CBG binding of aldosterone is minor relative to the total plasma aldosterone, changes in aldosterone binding by this protein can affect the metabolic clearance rate of aldosterone.[232] This occurs, for instance, when cortisol concentrations are low. This greater influence of CBG compared to that of other proteins presumably results from the slower rate of dissociation of aldosterone from CBG than from other plasma binding proteins, resulting in more of the CBG-bound aldosterone surviving passage through the liver.

Deoxycorticosterone

About 97 percent of the circulating DOC is bound by plasma proteins.[218] About 60 percent and 36 percent are associated with albumin and CBG, respectively.[218] The extent of DOC binding by plasma varies little over a wide range of concentrations of this steroid (2 to 200 ng/dl).[235]

Adrenal Androgens and Estrogens

The adrenal androgens, i.e., DHEA and its sulfate conjugate and Δ^4-androstenedione and its 11β-hydroxylated derivatives, are bound extensively to plasma proteins, mostly to albumin.[44,215,218,220,228,236–238] About 98 percent of the testosterone circulating in plasma is bound both to albumin and to a specific testosterone-estradiol-binding globulin (TeBG) whose plasma concentration is increased by estrogens (as in pregnancy) and in hyperthyroidism and decreased by testosterone and in acromegaly (see Laboratory Evaluation of Adrenocortical Function, below, and Chaps. 16 and 17). The plasma binding of estrogens is discussed in Chap. 17.

METABOLISM OF ADRENOCORTICAL STEROIDS

The continuous dynamic control of the plasma concentrations of the adrenal steroids requires mechanisms for their removal from the body. The hydrophobic steroids are filtered by the kidney but actively reabsorbed (e.g., about 95 percent of cortisol and 86 percent of aldosterone)[239] and are mostly not excreted into the urine. Thus, the steroids undergo enzymatic modifications that transform them into inactive substances with increased water solubility that can be more readily removed.[15,239–241] The modifications result largely in the conversion of some of the less polar ketone groups to hydroxyl groups and the C-21 groups to acid forms. The hydroxyl groups can then be conjugated with glucuronide or sulfate groups, rendering them even more water-soluble. The liver is the major site of metabolic conversion, although most mammalian tissues, including the adrenal, metabolize steroids to some extent, and in pregnancy the placenta is quite active in metabolism of the steroids (see the section on The Fetal Adrenal).[239] These metabolized compounds are then excreted. Illustrative of their enhanced capacity to be excreted is the fact that the renal clearance of a major cortisol metabolite, tetrahydrocortisone glucuronide, is around 70 percent of the creatinine clearance.[239] In most cases, the kidney accounts for over 90 percent of the excretion of the metabolized steroids (DOC and corticosterone are exceptions; see below); the remainder is lost in the gut. Most of the metabolized steroids excreted into the gut are reabsorbed; in addition, and especially with aldosterone, there can be further metabolism by the intestinal flora prior to absorption.

Over 50 different metabolites of cortisol and aldosterone have been detected (Fig. 12-14).[15,239,240] These are generated by a limited number of types of metabolic conversions. Since many of the structural differences among the various steroid hormones are eliminated during metaboism, it is commonly difficult to identify the true precursor(s) of a given metabolite.

Cortisol

Cortisol is cleared with a half-time of 80 to 120 min in various studies (Chap. 15).[226,239] If radioactively labeled hormone is given, 70 percent of the radioactivity appears in the urine within 24 h and over 90 percent by 72 h (Table 12-6).[239] Approximately 3 percent is recovered in the feces.[239] Almost all of the radioactivity is present as cortisol metabolites; less than 1 percent appears as unchanged cortisol (Table 12-6).

Cortisol may be modified by several different enzymes. The most important initial reaction is the reduction of the 4,5 double bond by at least two Δ^4-reductases. This reaction is irreversible, inactivates the molecule, and results in dihydrocortisol, which may be in an α or β form depending on the orientation of the hydrogen in the 5 position; the $5\alpha/5\beta$ ratio is about 5:1.[239] Dihydrocortisol does not accumulate in appreciable quantities; instead, it is rapidly converted by a 3-hydroxysteroid dehydrogenase to tetrahydrocortisol (Table 12-6). Cortisol can be oxidized at the 11β-hydroxyl group to form the ketone (cortisone); this reaction does not occur after the A ring has been reduced.[239] The reaction is reversible,

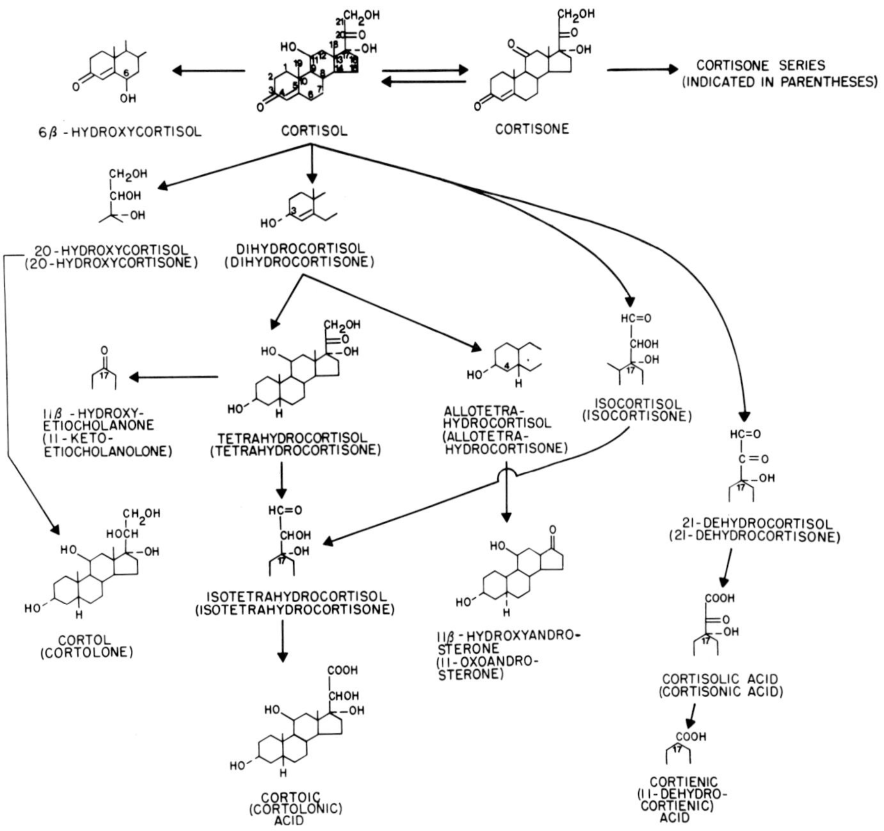

FIGURE 12-14 Pathways of cortisol and cortisone metabolism. Cortisol and cortisone are interconvertible. The steps shown are for cortisol metabolism; however, the metabolism of cortisone is similar. Thus, the name of the 11-keto metabolite resulting from cortisone metabolism is shown in parentheses for each cortisol metabolite. In many cases, only the portion of the steroid affected by the particular metabolic step is shown.

Table 12-6. Urinary Steroid Metabolites of Intravenously Administered Radioactive Cortisol*

Steroid	Percent in extract
Cortols (α and β)	7
Cortolones (α and β)	17
Allocortols and allocortolones	2
Tetrahydrocortisol	14
Tetrahydrocortisone	18
Allotetrahydrocortisol	6
Cortisol	1
6β-Hydroxycortisol	1
Cortisone	1
11β-Hydroxyetiocholanolone	4
11-Ketoetiocholanolone	2
11β-Hydroxyandrosterone	<1
Cortoic acids	10

*The data are taken from Peterson[239] and Monder and Bradlow.[240] The percentages of Peterson that did not include the cortoic acids were reduced by 25 percent (and rounded off) to include the contribution of the cortoic acids calculated from the data of Monder and Bradlow as based on the percentage of total cortoic acid relative to the sum of tetrahydrocortisol and tetrahydrocortisone. The numbers reported by different workers show considerable variation, and this table is intended to serve only as a rough estimate. It is also stressed that all of the known metabolites have not been included and that there are probably other, yet unidentified, metabolites.

but is probably mediated by two separate enzymes.[242,243] In general, the equilibrium is shifted to favor the 11-keto form.[242,243] Thus, there is substantial cortisol-to-cortisone conversion. This increases in hyperthyroidism and is marked in the fetus.[242,243] Cortisone is then, in general, metabolized similarly to cortisol and therefore it is also mainly converted via the dihydro derivative to the tetrahydro metabolite. The net result is that roughly similar quantities of unaltered cortisol and cortisone and their metabolites are excreted (Table 12-6).[239,240] Cortisol, cortisone, and their tetrahydro derivatives can be further reduced to the cortols and cortolones, respectively, via hydroxysteroid dehydrogenases (Fig. 12-14). There can also be oxidation at C-21 to form cortolic and cortolonic acids (Fig. 12-14), and conversion of the C-17 side chain to the C-20 acid.[240] The conversion to the acidic derivatives renders the steroid even more water-soluble.[240] Reduction of the C-20 keto group of cortisol or cortisone to 20-hydroxycortisol also occurs to a lesser extent. 6β-Hydroxylated or 16α-hydroxylated metabolites of cortisol and other steroids are formed ordinarily in small quantities;[239] however, the 6β-hydroxylation pathway can be of major importance in infants in whom the esterification mechanisms are not fully developed, in some disease states, and after treatment with certain drugs (discussed below),[239,244-246] and the 16α-hydroxylation pathway can be important for the conversion of estradiol to estriol. Finally, there can be some oxidative cleavage of the C-17 side chain to C_{19} 11-oxygenated 17-ketosteroids (5 to 10 percent).[239]

About 96 percent of the C_{19} and C_{21} metabolites of cortisol and cortisone is excreted as conjugates of cortisol and less than 1 percent as unchanged cortisol (Table 12-6);[239] 60 to 70 percent appears as conjugates at the 3α-hydroxyl position with glucuronic acid. A smaller amount of conjugates are formed with the sulfate through the C-21 hydroxyl.[247] The conjugation with glucuronide is due to the glucuronyl transferase and the glucuronide donor is uridine diphosphoglucuronic acid. Glucuronyl transferase is so active that reduced steroids are almost completely esterified when they leave the liver.[248] Further, this enzyme system differs from that responsible for conjugating bilirubin, because patients defective in the latter enzyme system have a much lesser defect in steroid conjugation.[244] Unlike their metabolites, the small quantities of cortisol and cortisone appearing in the urine (accounting for 1 percent or less of the cortisol removed in each case, Table 12-6)[239] are largely unconjugated.[239]

Corticosterone, 11-Deoxycortisol, and 11-Deoxycorticosterone

The metabolism of corticosterone, 11-deoxycortisol, and DOC is generally similar to that of cortisol except for minor quantitative differences.[239,240] For instance, more corticosterone than cortisol is excreted as the 21-conjugate,[239] its half-time of disappearance is shorter, C_{19} metabolites have not been found,[239] and more of the metabolites are excreted into the gut.[240] A much greater proportion of DOC (perhaps 50 percent) is excreted into the gut.[240]

Aldosterone

Aldosterone turns over rapidly,[239,249] with a half-time of 15 min or less; it is almost completely removed by one passage through the liver, and less than 0.5 percent appears in the urine in the free state.[15,239,249] About 35 percent of the aldosterone is excreted as tetrahydroaldosterone glucuronide (3 position; see the earlier discussion on cortisol metabolism); up to 20 percent appears as the glucuronide through the 18 position of aldosterone.[239] This metabolite is termed either the acid-labile conjugate (since free aldosterone can be released from it by hydrolysis at pH 1)[250] or the 3-oxo conjugate (since the 3-oxo group is intact). Determinations of urinary aldosterone usually measure the concentration of this metabolite. The remainder of the metabolized aldosterone is accounted for by a variety of other compounds, including a number of polar derivatives such as carboxylic acid and hydroxylated metabolites, and 21-deoxytetrahydroaldosterone.[249] This steroid is probably produced in the gut (after biliary excretion of tetrahydroaldosterone), reabsorbed, and secreted into the urine.[249] There is less metabolic modification of the 11β-hydroxy group of aldosterone than in cortisol, because this is protected by the steroid's cyclic 11,18-hemiacetyl form.[15] In the rat there are significant sex differences in aldosterone metabolism, with a greater proportion of various metabolites being present in male than in female tissues; also, aldosterone metabolism can be affected by both potassium ion and spironolactone.[249]

Androgens and Estrogens

The androgens are excreted predominantly as conjugates in the urine; a small fraction is excreted into the gut.[44] Over 80 percent of the androstenedione is removed from the circulation after one passage through the liver.[44] By contrast, only 44 percent of the testosterone is so removed.[44] DHEA-S of adrenal origin can be excreted unchanged; DHEA-S is also formed in liver and kidney. Both of these compounds can be further metabolized[44] by either hydroxylation at positions 7 and 16 or by transformation of the 17-keto group into a 17β-hydroxyl group (Fig. 12-15). DHEA is also irreversibly converted to androstenedione. As mentioned earlier, androstenedione is either converted to testosterone (mostly by extrahepatic tissues) or its 4,5 double bond is reduced, resulting in androsterone or etiocholanolone (Fig. 12-15). These steroids can be further reduced, respectively, to androstanediol and etiocholanediol (Fig. 12-15).[44] Testosterone is also converted in the androgen target tissues to DHT (Chaps. 16 and 18); the latter is reversibly inactivated, mainly by 3α-reduction to 3α-androstanediol;[251] a lesser amount is reversibly converted to 5α-androstanedione (Fig. 12-15). Both of these compounds can be converted to androsterone. All of these metabolites are further conjugated to glucuronides and, compared with cortisol metabolites, a larger proportion of them are converted to the sulfate derivatives (mostly through the 3 position). The sulfate conjugates are more slowly cleared and have a more prolonged half-life in plasma than the glucuronide conjugates. This is probably due to the fact that the sulfate conjugates bind more extensively to plasma proteins and are not filtered as well as are the glucuronides.

Testosterone and androstenedione are cleared two to three times more rapidly from plasma in men than in women.[44] Apparently, this is due to an effect of the

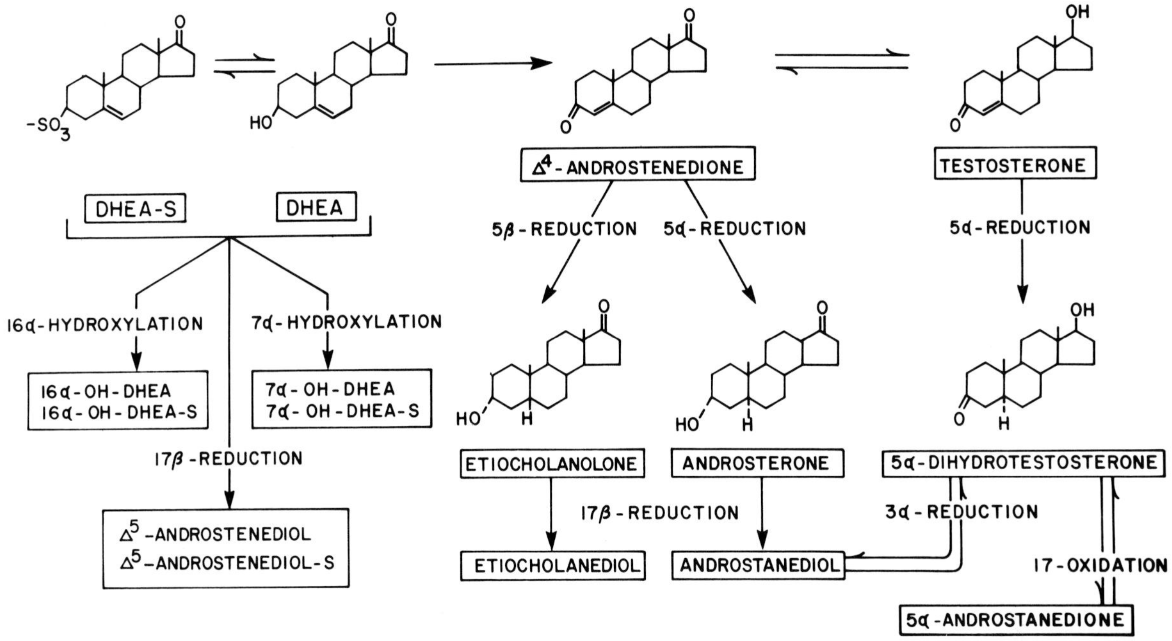

FIGURE 12-15 Major pathways in androgen metabolism. Most of the steps shown are involved in androgen degradation. However, the 5α reduction of testosterone occurs in androgen target tissues to yield the highly active 5α-dihydrotestosterone. See the text for details.

androgens on their own metabolism, as values more similar to the female are observed in the testicular feminization syndrome, in which plasma androgen concentrations tend to be elevated and there is peripheral insensitivity to androgens.[44]

VARIATIONS IN STEROID METABOLISM

The rate of metabolism of adrenal steroids is affected by a number of diseases, drugs, and other hormones. Plasma binding was discussed above; agents that increase plasma CBG levels also decrease the rate of cortisol clearance.[215,239] That plasma binding decreases aldosterone clearance was also discussed above.[232]

In chronic liver disease, the metabolism of cortisol and of estrogens is decreased.[239] These effects are relatively specific, since the metabolism of a number of other steroids (e.g., aldosterone, cortisone, and certain cortisol metabolites) is unaffected or minimally affected. This influence may be due to changes in specific metabolizing enzymes and does not result from alterations in hepatic circulation or CBG levels. The decreased metabolism of cortisol tends to decrease cortisol secretion, presumably by feedback inhibition of ACTH release. Thus, the urinary excretion of cortisol and other ACTH-dependent steroids (e.g., urinary 11-ketosteroids) are also low in chronic liver disease. However, plasma cortisol is normal unless CBG levels fall. By contrast, the decreased metabolism of estrogens in chronic liver disease results in elevated plasma concentrations of these steroids; such elevations may produce the feminizing features of cirrhosis.

The metabolism of cortisol, aldosterone, and several other adrenal steroids is increased in hyperthyroidism and decreased in hypothyroidism.[239] This apparently is a specific effect of the hormone mostly on biotransformation rather than conjugation and is not due to hypermetabolism per se, as the increase is not observed in other hypermetabolic states. There is also increased secretion of cortisol and aldosterone in hyperthyroidism and decreased secretion in hypothyroidism; these are felt to be compensatory effects on ACTH and renin release that in general normalize or nearly normalize the plasma steroid levels. They are also reflected by increased urinary 17-hydroxycorticosteroid (17-OHCS) levels in hyperthyroidism and decreased levels in hypothyroidism. The metabolism of progesterone and estrogens is much less affected by alterations in thyroid function, whereas the clearance of the androgens is, if anything, decreased.

The metabolism of corticosteroids is also altered in several other circumstances. Although renal disease affects the clearance of cortisol metabolites, it does not have a major effect on the metabolism of cortisol.[239] In congestive heart failure, there can be decreased clearance of aldosterone.[239] In general, there are no major differences in cortisol or aldosterone metabolism in chronic diseases, obesity, starvation, stress, anxiety, or depression.[239] In some of these cases, changes in steroid production can alter the amount of steroid excreted.[239] There can also be minor sex differences in the relative metabolic pathways.[249] The clearance of cortisol is decreased in the extremes of old age and infancy,[19a] but otherwise changes little throughout life.[239] Drugs such as mitotane (*o,p'*-DDD) (Table 12-3), phenytoin, rifampin, aminoglutethimide, and barbiturates result in differences in the patterns of urinary steroid secretion, including an increase in 6β-hydroxycortisol, but have only a minor influence on the total rate of disappearance of infused cortisol.[239,252] However, these drugs do increase the clearance of synthetic glucocorticoids such as dexamethasone and prednisolone, possibly by affecting the 6β-hydroxy modification and conjugation, which are more important in the metabolism of these steroids.[239,248] The 6β-hydroxycortisol pathway is also of increased importance in patients with liver disease,[245] in hyperestrogenic states,[245] and in cancer or prolonged terminal illness.[246] The antihypertensive agent minoxidil (unlike hydralazine) increases aldosterone clearance, possibly by hemodynamic influences.[253] In pregnancy, the cortisol clearance rate is lowered, probably as a result of the increased CBG levels.[239] Finally, there can be some impairment in cortisol clearance in anorexia nervosa and in protein-calorie malnutrition.[254]

ACTIONS OF GLUCOCORTICOIDS

The glucocorticoids are ubiquitous as physiological regulators and play a role in differentiation and development. They are essential for survival, at least to overcome certain stressful insults. Conversely, an excess of these hormones, particularly over a prolonged period of time, can lead to severe adverse influences (see Cushing's Syndrome, below). Nevertheless, glucocorticoids given in pharmacological dosages can also have useful therapeutic effects (see Chap. 15). Some effects of these steroids are observed only with glucocorticoid excess, as occurs with spontaneous Cushing's syndrome or glucocorticoid therapy. However, commonly, the manifestations of glucocorticoid excess are quantitatively greater influences that also occur in response to basal, unstimulated levels of cortisol. For these reasons it is not always possible to make distinctions between effects at physiological versus pharmacological concentrations in describing the biological actions of the glucocorticoids.

Intermediary Metabolism

Glucocorticoids were named for their glucose-regulating properties and have extensive influences on carbohydrate, lipid, protein, and nucleic acid metabolism. Although in humans these steroids are secondary to insulin in regulating glucose metabolism, they do influence blood sugar levels and serve a protective role against glucose deprivation (Chap. 1).[255] This latter role provides an excellent conceptual framework for considering many of the coordinated actions of the glucocorticoids on lipid, nucleic acid, protein, and carbohydrate metabolism (Fig. 12-16).

CARBOHYDRATE METABOLISM

Glucocorticoids in excess increase hepatic glycogen and glucose production, and decrease glucose uptake and utilization in peripheral tissues.[4,256-260] Although the relative quantitative importance of these various influences has not been clarified, they result in a tendency to hyperglycemia and decreased carbohydrate tolerance. Conversely, in glucocorticoid deficiency there is decreased glucose production and hepatic glycogen content and an increased sensitivity to insulin which may result in hypoglycemia. The extent of these effects depends on food intake and on insulin, which opposes many glucocorticoid actions and whose secretion increases in response to steroid-mediated increases in blood glucose concentration. Thus, in the nondiabetic individual exposed to an excess of glucocorticoids, increased insulin secretion counterbalances the glucocorticoid effect so that the fasting blood sugar level, although higher on average, is usually in the normal range, even though carbohydrate tolerance is impaired. In the diabetic patient with an inadequate insulin reserve, glucocorticoids in excess exacerbate the carbohydrate intolerance, resulting in an increased insulin requirement. Conversely, in the addisonian subject, feeding and a relative decrease in insulin secretion due to the lower blood sugar level blunt the tendency to hypoglycemia so that the fasting blood sugar level is commonly in the normal range.

Glucocorticoids increase glucose production by enhancing the liver's capacity for gluconeogenesis, the release of gluconeogenic substrate from peripheral tissues, and the ability of other hormones to stimulate gluconeogenesis.[258] In fed adrenalectomized animals basal gluconeogenesis is not impaired, but there is an impaired response to glucagon or catecholamines (Chap. 19). In fasted or diabetic animals, adrenalectomy results in a net reduction in hepatic gluconeogenesis which is reversible with cortisol administration.

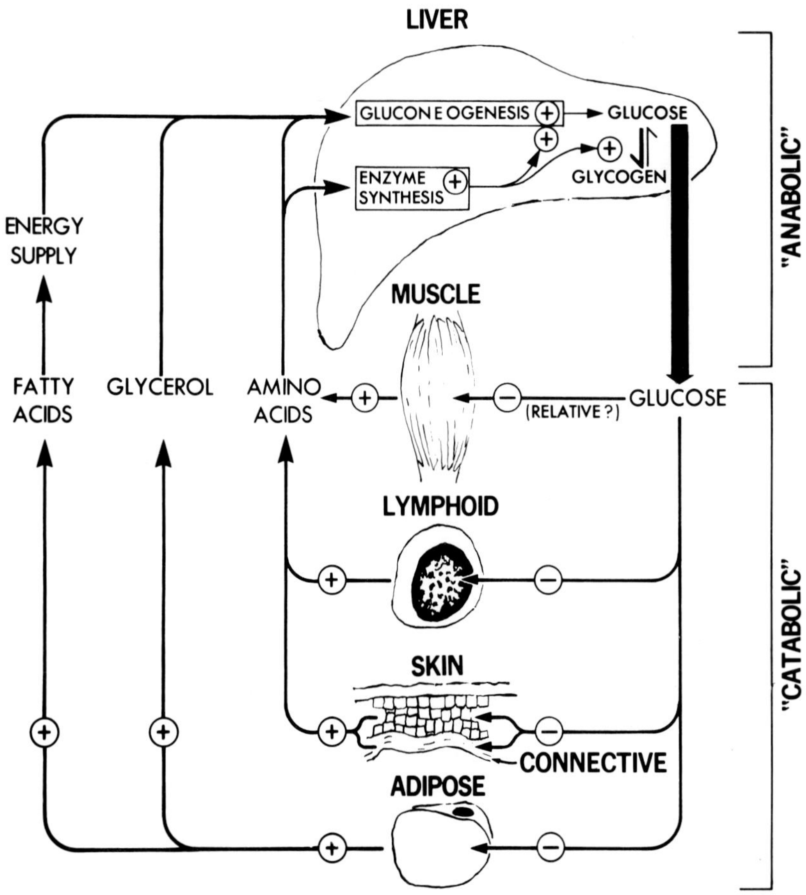

FIGURE 12-16 Glucocorticoid influences on peripheral tissues. Plus signs refer to stimulations and minus signs to inhibitions. (*From Baxter and Rousseau,*[3] *as modified from Baxter and Forsham.*[225a])

Thus, glucocorticoids are required for the responses of gluconeogenesis to fasting and insulin deficiency, but not for basal gluconeogenesis in the fed state.

It has been argued that essentially every step in the gluconeogenic pathway is increased by glucocorticoids.[256] Indeed, these steroids increase total hepatic protein synthesis and several of the transaminases are increased.[257] Of quantitative importance is alanine aminotransferase.[261] However, a probably greater influence on gluconeogenesis is on the steps distal to transamination. The steroid increases the activity of phospho*enol*pyruvate carboxykinase (PEPCK)[261] and possibly glucose 6-phosphatase. However, the changes in PEPCK may be offset by insulin, which depresses the activity of this enzyme.[258] There is little direct information about other gluconeogenic enzymes.

Glucocorticoids also play a permissive role (discussed below) by increasing the sensitivity of the liver to the gluconeogenic actions of glucagon and the catecholamines.[256-258,262] For instance, the effect of glucagon or α-adrenergic stimulation of hepatic gluconeogenesis is impaired by adrenalectomy.

Several types of glucocorticoid influences result in an increased release of gluconeogenic substrate from peripheral tissues.[256-258,263-266] Perfused muscle from adrenalectomized rats shows a net decrease in the release of amino acids which is reversed by glucocorticoids. The steroids decrease protein synthesis and can increase protein breakdown in several tissues, such as muscle, adipose, and lymphoid, resulting in an increased release of amino acids.[256-258,262,264-266] In rats, the inhibition of protein synthesis can be observed in the fed and fasted state and at the lower steroid doses, but an enhancement of protein breakdown is observed only in the fasted state and at higher doses.[262,264-266] Although the predominant glucocorticoid effect in muscle may be inhibition of protein synthesis,[258,262,264-266] increased proteolysis from other tissues in response to the steroid may be more prominent.[266] These influences are accompanied by increased urinary excretion of 3-methylhistidine, nitrogen, and plasma amino acids, primarily valine, leucine, isoleucine, tyrosine, phenylalanine, and histidine.[266,267] These amino acids serve as gluconeogenic precursors, and the conversion of leucine to alanine is increased, as are plasma pyruvate levels.[266] At early times, many of these influences can be observed in the absence of changes in plasma insulin and glycogen concentrations.[266] With time, the secondary hyperinsulinism can attenuate to some extent the increase in total protein breakdown.[264,265] In humans, the immediate net result of glucocorticoid excess is selective increases in the levels of several amino acids;[263,267] more persistently in the fed state only the alanine concentration is elevated,[263] mostly due to the conversion of other amino acids to alanine, which is the major gluconeogenic precursor and is used for the disposal of nitrogen from other amino acids. Glucocorticoids may also enhance the levels of amino acids available for gluconeogenesis by blocking the stimulatory effects of insulin in peripheral tissues on amino acid uptake and protein synthesis.[258]

Glucocorticoids also enhance the availability of gluconeogenic substrate by increasing glycerol release from fat cells (by stimulating lipolysis) and lactate release from muscle.[258] The latter influence appears to be due to a stimulation of the glycogenolytic actions of the catecholamines. The lipolysis also provides free fatty acids, which cannot themselves contribute to a net increase in gluconeogenesis, but can provide energy for gluconeogenesis and spare other substrate that can be converted into glucose.

A second major type of effect of glucocorticoids on carbohydrate metabolism results from their inhibition of glucose uptake and metabolism in peripheral tissues (Fig. 12-17).[257,266–268] There is a direct inhibition of glucose uptake in adipose tissue,[268,269] fibroblasts,[268] certain lymphoid cells,[268,270] and fat cells.[268] In the last case they decrease the number of glucose transporter molecules by mechanisms that require protein and RNA synthesis.[268] Even in muscle, which accounts for most of the glucose metabolism, the uptake of glucose (relative to blood glucose concentration) may be decreased, although a direct effect on glucose uptake has not been demonstrated.[256] The decrease in glucose uptake appears to be the major early influence on carbohydrate tolerance; following cortisol infusion the blood glucose concentration can rise with no change in glucose output (Fig. 12-17).[266,267]

Glucocorticoids have complex effects on insulin release and action.[260] Although the effects may require a day or more before they are manifest, glucocorticoid excess results in increased basal and glucose-stimulated insulin levels, and pancreatic beta cell hyperplasia occurs long-term.[260] These effects are due mostly to

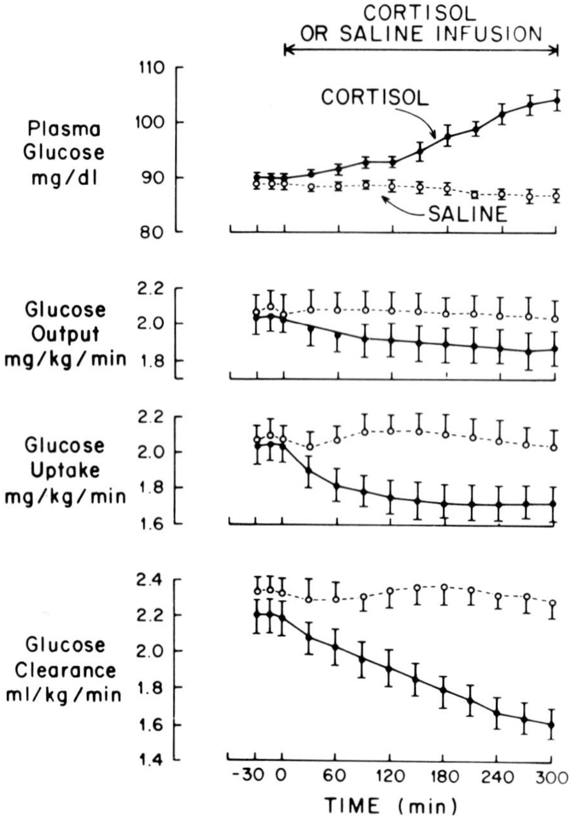

FIGURE 12-17 The effect of cortisol infusion on plasma glucose concentration and glucose kinetics in normal humans. (*From Shamoon et al.*[267])

the glucocorticoid-induced hyperglycemia; reports concerning direct effects of the steroids on the pancreatic islets are in conflict.[260] The elevated glucose and insulin levels imply that insulin resistance is present in the glucocorticoid excess states. This is due primarily to all of the anti-insulin actions described above, which are predominantly post-insulin-receptor events.[260,271] In addition, there may be more direct effects on insulin action. It has been reported that glucocorticoids can increase, decrease, or not affect insulin receptor levels, decrease the affinity of the insulin-receptor interaction, and stimulate insulin degradation, although the overall contribution of these influences to glucocorticoid action has not been clarified.[260,271]

GLYCOGEN METABOLISM

Glucocorticoids increase glycogen deposition in the livers of both fed and fasted animals.[259] After 12 to 24 h, glycogen content is slightly increased in muscle, but not kidney.[272] Conversely, adrenalectomy impairs hepatic glycogen synthesis; this effect is more prominent in fed than in fasted animals.[259] In this case, glucocorticoids and insulin have similar rather than opposing actions; however, the role of the steroid can be perceived as one to protect against long-term food deprivation by promoting glycogen storage, whereas that of insulin is more important for short-term lowering of the blood sugar level by shunting glucose into glycogen.

Glucocorticoids stimulate glycogen synthetase (UDPG-glycogen transglycosidase) activity by promoting its conversion from the inactive b form to the active a form[259] (Fig. 12-18). This may be a result of a stimulation of glycogen synthetase phosphatase (which activates glycogen synthetase) by blocking the actions of glycogen phosphorylase a which inhibits the phosphatase.[259] The steroid may induce a protein that inhibits the actions of phosphorylase a.[259]

A second effect of the steroid, of probably less importance, may be to inhibit glycogen breakdown by inactivation of phosphorylase a, which may occur by simulating, by unknown mechanisms, its conversion to (inactive) phosphorylase b (Fig. 12-18).[259] This may occur because the phosphatase (activated by glucocorticoids) that stimulates glycogen synthetase activity (Fig. 12-18) also inactivates the enzyme that converts phosphorylase b to phosphorylase a.[259] Such an effect would favor a decrease in amount of phosphorylase a.

Glucocorticoids also stimulate glycogen production in the fetal liver.[259] In this case, in addition to the mechanisms desribed above, the steroid may also increase the amount of glycogen synthetase itself.[259]

In vivo, glucocorticoid actions on glycogen accumulation appear to be predominantly, although not exclusively, insulin-dependent, since glycogen accumulation is markedly reduced in pancreatectomized animals.[259] Glucocorticoid-stimulated increases in insulin secretion promote further glycogen accumulation.[259]

LIPID METABOLISM

Obvious manifestations of glucocorticoids on lipid metabolism are observed in individuals with Cushing's syndrome who have excess fat in the neck, face, and trunk and loss of fat from the extremities. The steroid also increases the plasma-free fatty acid and lipoprotein concentrations.

Glucocorticoids increase lipolysis and increase plasma-free fatty acid levels.[264,269,272] Lipolysis and free fatty acid release are increased by the glucocorticoid-induced decrease in glucose uptake and metabolism that reduces glycerol production necessary for reesterification of fatty acids. The steroids also stimulate lipolysis by permissive actions (see below) that increase the efficiency of other lipolytic factors such as catecholamines.[269] The increase in free fatty acid release and possible augmentation of hepatic conversion of free fatty acids to ketones by glucocorticoids cause a tendency to ketosis.[267,269] These effects are ordinarily countered by increased insulin release and glucocorticoid-stimulated gluconeogenesis.

It is not known why in glucocorticoid excess states fat is lost in some areas and increased in others. However, fat deposition in certain areas may be due to lipogenic actions (see Chap. 19) of the increased plasma insulin concentrations. This is consistent with the finding that there can be overall fat loss in diabetic patients with Cushing's syndrome.[257] Increased fat deposition may also be due to stimulation of the appetite by glucocorticoids. Fat loss may be due to direct inhibitory actions of the hormones exerted on adipose tissue.[269] Thus, if different tissues vary in their relative sensitivity to glucocorticoids and insulin, there would be net fat deposition where sensitivity to insulin is dominant and fat loss where the glucocorticoid influence is dominant.

Glucocorticoids have been reported to affect the lipid content of membranes with influences on cholesterol and sphingomyelin.[273-274] The consequences of

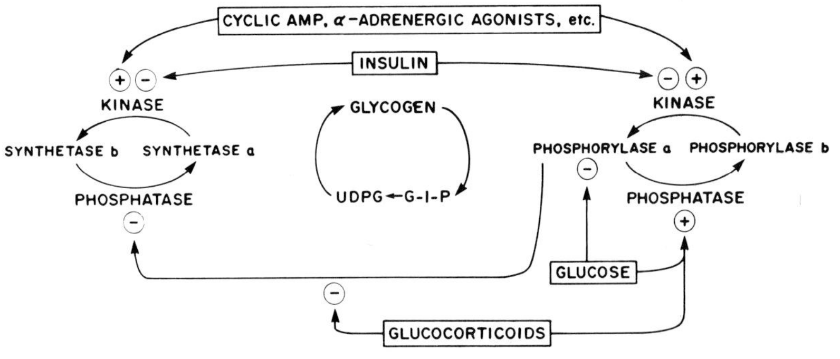

FIGURE 12-18 Actions of glucocorticoids on glycogen accumulation. The dominant effect of the steroid is to induce a factor or factors that block the inhibition by phosphorylase a of glycogen synthetase phosphatase. The steroid also decreases phosphorylase a, but this appears to be of secondary importance. Shown also are the actions of insulin, cAMP (as a mediator of glucagon action), α-adrenergic agonists (as mediators of epinephrine action), and glucose. Plus signs refer to stimulation; minus signs refer to inhibition. UDPG, uridine diphosphoglucose; G-1-P, glucose 1-phosphate.

these changes are not known, but they could influence the properties of cell membrane–localized receptors, enzymes, and other important molecules.

In glucocorticoid excess states there is an increase in very low density lipoproteins (VLDL), LDL, and HDL, with consequent elevations of total triglyceride and cholesterol levels.[275] The mechanisms for these changes are probably multifactorial, with influences on VLDL synthesis, free fatty acid production, hepatic endothelial lipase activity, and other components all possibly contributing.[275]

PROTEIN AND NUCLEIC ACID METABOLISM

The primary actions of glucocorticoid-receptor complexes are to regulate the transcription of specific genes with consequent changes in the levels of particular RNAs and their protein products (discussed below). The steroids also affect protein and RNA synthesis and breakdown and/or DNA synthesis and degradation more generally in a number of tissues.[257,276,277] The trend with protein and RNA is for the steroid to stimulate synthesis in the liver; to inhibit synthesis and stimulate breakdown in many peripheral tissues, such as muscle, skin, adipose, lymphoid, and fibroblastic (Fig. 12-16); and to have a lesser general influence on brain and cardiac tissue. The general effect on DNA synthesis is inhibitory, although there are some circumstances where DNA synthesis is stimulated, and rarely DNA breakdown can be stimulated (see below). This pattern may again be perceived as a general attempt by the body to provide substrate for hepatic gluconeogenesis from "less essential" tissues such as muscle and to decrease other types of substrate utilization while sparing certain critical tissues (e.g., brain and heart). However, in glucocorticoid excess states, other deleterious or beneficial effects (osteoporosis, immunosuppression, etc.) are more prominent. Many examples and more detail about these effects are provided in the following sections.

Liver

The liver is one of the few tissues in which there is an overall stimulatory influence of glucocorticoids on protein and RNA synthesis and the steroids cause a slight increase in the total hepatic protein and RNA content.[3,257] Nevertheless, the steroid effects are selective, since certain proteins (e.g., tyrosine aminotransferase and tryptophan oxygenase) are stimulated much more than others.[257,277a] Some of the other functions stimulated by the glucocorticoids (e.g., other gluconeogenic enzymes and glycogen accumulation) have been mentioned in preceding sections. However, there can be inhibitory glucocorticoid actions in liver, such as on hepatic DNA synthesis.[276,277]

Muscle

Glucocorticoid influences on muscle glucose and protein metabolism have already been discussed. The overall importance of these actions is underscored by the fact that muscle, because of its bulk, is a major source of gluconeogenic precursors and glucose utilization. Glucocorticoids also inhibit muscle DNA and probably RNA synthesis and promote RNA breakdown.[256,257,262–265,277] The extent to which these effects occur can be affected by other factors, such as insulin (which tends to oppose them) and diet, but they can lead to frank muscular wasting in glucocorticoid excess states. The effects on muscle are somewhat selective, with more pronounced influences on type 2 white glycolytic fibers than on type 1 fibers.[277b] The steroid both enhances proteolysis and decreases muscle synthesis; the proteolysis influence is probably the more important and it is associated with increases in certain proteolytic enzymes.[277b,277c]

Immunological and Inflammatory Responses

Glucocorticoids in excess suppress immunological and inflammatory responses[3,257,270,278–292] and are used extensively to treat diseases in which excessive inflammatory or immunological activity is damaging (see Chap. 15). These suppressive actions can also be deleterious, and infections are increased in frequency and severity in spontaneous Cushing's syndrome and with corticosteroid therapy (see Cushing's Syndrome, below, and Chap. 15).

In contrast to the well-documented immunosuppressive and anti-inflammatory actions of corticosteroids in excess, little is known about the role of basal levels of glucocorticoids in immunological and inflammatory responses. However, some role seems possible, since glucocorticoids can influence these responses at dosages that result in steroid levels equivalent to those that occur physiologically.

The role of increased cortisol secretion during stresses such as infection is also unknown. There is evidence for immunosuppression in postsurgical patients[282] and inflammatory reactions in these and other "stressed" patients may be blunted by the increased cortisol concentrations. It has been suggested that the increased cortisol in these circumstances may help prevent autoimmune responses to tissue antigens released by cellular injury.[282] The finding that corticosteroids can suppress autologous mixed leukocyte reactions without affecting allogenic reactions is consistent with such a role.[278,281] Nevertheless, the major role of the increased steroid levels in these circumstances may be to prevent a number of host responses recruited during the infection from becoming excessive;[284] this hypothesis is discussed below (see Glucocorticoids and Stress).

Much of the data on glucocorticoids and immunological responses have come from animal studies. Responses vary among species; for example, mouse, rat, and rabbit are relatively steroid-sensitive, whereas guinea pigs and humans are more steroid-resistant.[279] Nevertheless, these differences may be more quantitative than qualitative, and in various animal and human systems glucocorticoids have been shown to affect nearly every step in both the immunological and inflammatory responses.[257,270,278–291] They affect inflammatory reactions by inhibiting (1) the production and/or activity of vasoactive agents; (2) the movement of leukocytes to inflamed areas; and (3) the function of immunocompetent cells at the site of inflammation. The last includes actions on antigen processing by macrophages, specific B and T cell functions, antibody production and clearance, mobilization and functioning of polymorphonuclear and mononuclear cells, the liberation and actions of effector substances (prostaglandins, leukotrienes, interleukins, kinins, proteases such as plasminogen activator, etc.) at the site of cellular injury, and the fibroblastic proliferative response. Interestingly, glucocorticoids do not cause permanent damage to the immunological system. Thus, the precursor cells are steroid-resistant. This underscores the point that different stages in the response vary markedly in their sensitivity to glucocorticoids. The particular actions that are the most important in the observed responses are commonly unclear. In general, it appears that in humans the steroids affect cellular more than humoral processes, leukocyte distribution within body compartments more than function, and macrophages more than polymorphonuclear leukocytes and are more effective if given prior to or concurrent with a challenge than later.

EFFECTS ON VASOACTIVE AND OTHER INFLAMMATORY AGENTS

Early inflammatory changes at a site of injury result in enhanced vascular permeability and edema. These changes are mediated by a variety of inflammatory agents, including PGs, kinins, histamines, and the slow-reacting substance of anaphylaxsis (SRS-A).[284–292]

Arachidonic acid is the precursor of a number of molecules collectively called *eicosanoids*.[284–292] It is derived directly from the actions of phospholipase A_2 or indirectly from phospholipase C. Arachidonic acid can then be converted into prostaglandins, thromboxanes, hydroperoxyeicosatetraenoic acids (HPETEs), hydroxyeicosatetraenoic acids (HETEs), and leukotrienes.[287,289] A number of these compounds are relevant in inflammatory reactions, and their role is further suggested by the fact that certain nonsteroidal anti-inflammatory agents block the production of some of these substances.[285,287]

Glucocorticoids inhibit PG synthesis in a variety of cell types,[284–292] although this does not occur in all cases and in certain conditions total prostanoid levels or excretion may not be affected by the steroids.[283,292] These inhibitory actions on eicosanoid production may be due to the actions of a protein, termed *lipocortin* or *macrocortin*, that inhibits phospholipase A_2 and whose levels are increased by glucocorticoids.[283,287,289,291,293] These actions of glucocorticoids to inhibit phospholipase A_2 result in a more general inhibition of eicosanoid production than is the case with indomethacin and aspirin, and they may help to explain the greater anti-inflammatory actions of the steroids in comparison to these other molecules.

Glucocorticoids block the actions of bradykinin, which may also regulate PG synthesis.[285] They also block the release of histamine and SRS-A, which may be leukotrienes.[285]

LEUKOCYTE MOVEMENT

Glucocorticoid administration to human subjects causes a circulating lymphocytopenia, monocytopenia, and eosinopenia (Table 12-7).[278,294,295] Conversely, these cell types are increased in adrenal insufficiency.[257] The actions on lymphocytes and monocytes are maximal within 4 to 6 h and return to normal by 24 to 48 h, but persist with continued steroid administration.[278,285,294] These effects are mostly due to a redistribution of cells, with cells moving out of the circulation into other body compartments such as bone marrow, spleen, lymph nodes, and thoracic duct.[278,295] In other species, circulating lymphoid cells are also killed by the steroid, but this appears not to be the case with humans.[257,278,279] Although there are effects on both the T (thymus-derived) and B (bone marrow–derived) lymphocytes, the influence is much greater on the T lymphocytes, especially those with an Fc receptor for IgM (T_M) compared to those with a receptor for IgG (T_G).[278]

Glucocorticoid administration also increases (maximally after 4 to 6 h) the blood polymorphonuclear leukocyte concentration.[257,278,285,294] This is due to an accelerated release of neutrophils from the bone marrow, an increase in the half-life of circulating neutrophils, and reduced neutrophil egress from the blood.[278]

Glucocorticoids decrease markedly the number of

Table 12-7. Glucocorticoid Effects on Leukocyte Movements in Humans

1. Lymphocytes
   a. Circulating lymphocytopenia, due to redistribution of cells to other lymphoid compartments
   b. Depletion of recirculating lymphocytes
   c. Selective depletion of T lymphocytes (especially T_M subset) more than B lymphocytes
2. Monocyte-macrophages
   a. Circulating monocytopenia, probably due to redistribution
   b. Inhibition of accumulation of monocyte-macrophages at inflammatory sites
3. Neutrophils
   a. Circulating neutrophilia
   b. Accelerated release of neutrophils from the bone marrow
   c. Blocked accumulation of neutrophils at inflammatory sites, probably due to reduced adherence
4. Eosinophils
   a. Circulating eosinopenia, probably due to redistribution
   b. Decreased migration of eosinophils into immediate hypersensitivity skin test sites

Source: Modified from Parrillo and Fauci.[278]

polymorphonuclear leukocytes, monocyte-macrophages, and lymphocytes that accumulate at inflammatory sites; the effect is evident by 2 h.[257,279,282,285] Although the decreases are ordinarily similar for both monocytes and polymorphonuclear leukocytes, the effects on mononuclear cells appear to be longer-lived. These actions may be due in part to the fact that glucocorticoids can inhibit chemotactic and other factors such as plasminogen activator[285] that affect inflammatory cell accumulation at sites of injury, and may be a major mechanism of the anti-inflammatory actions of the glucocorticoids.[278]

The blood basophils are elevated in Addison's disease and depressed in Cushing's disease or with glucocorticoid therapy.[257] Presumably, the same mechanisms that regulate the levels of eosinophils are operative.

LEUKOCYTE FUNCTION

Glucocorticoids affect lymphocyte function and in some animals the steroids at high doses kill lymphocytes and cause involution of lymphoid tissues.[257,270] There are marked variations in the sensitivity of lymphoid cell subpopulations; for instance, in the mouse thymus, about 95 percent of the cells are killed by the steroid, whereas the remaining 5 percent are steroid-resistant.[257,270] This 5 percent must contain the precursor cells for immunological responses, since steroid treatment does not abolish certain thymic-dependent responses. Although most human lymphocytes are not killed by glucocorticoids, in some cases (e.g., cells of acute lymphocytic leukemia of childhood) there can by lymphoid cell killing (see also Chap. 15).[296] The actions of glucocorticoids on lymphocytes involve stimulation (or blockade) of specific functions; even the killing activity appears to involve specific programming and is associated with an early response in which a discrete set of proteins is induced.[297] One or a few of these ultimately result in cell killing, possibly through direct or indirect actions that induce or enhance the actions of a DNase that digests the cell's DNA.[298]

A number of specific lymphocyte functions are blocked by the steroids in instances where the cells are not killed (Table 12-8).[257,270,278,279,284,285] Again, there are variations in sensitivity. For instance, the lymphocyte-proliferative response to some but not other antigens can be suppressed.[278] The proliferative responses to antigens are more readily suppressed than are those to mitogens.[278] Nevertheless, blockage of some T cell mitogenic responses are observed; this may be due to steroid actions that block the release of T cell growth factor (interleukin 2).[284,285] This block is secondary to decreased leukotriene B_4 production resulting from the steroid-mediated inhibition of phospholipase A_2.[286] This action may help explain why the steroids are more effective when given early in an immunological response than later, because interleukin 2 is important for clonal expansion of cells early on but not later.[284,285] The steroids also suppress macrophage functions (see below) that affect T cell function. They suppress T lymphocyte production of γ interferon,[284] with subsequent effects on macrophages (see below), including on Fc receptors, activation of macrophages, and enhancement of natural killer cell activity and macrophage activating factor.[284,285] They

Table 12-8. Immunological Mediators Whose Production and/or Actions Can Be Blocked by Glucocorticoids

Bradykinin
Cachectin (tumor necrosis factor)
Collagenase
Colony stimulating factor
Eicosanoids (prostaglandins, leukotrienes, etc.)
Histamine
γ-Interferon
Interleukin 1 (lymphocyte activating factor)
Interleukin 2 (T cell growth factor)
Migration inhibition factor
Plasminogen activator

Note: The inhibitions are not always observed in all tissues. See text for References (see especially Ref. 284).

also block the production of colony stimulating factor, which stimulates granulocyte and macrophage production,[284] and of cachectin (tumor necrosis factor), which is involved in tumor rejection.[288] Whereas the steroids generally do not suppress antibody-dependent cell-mediated cytotoxicity of human cells, they can suppress spontaneous toxicity and cutaneous delayed hypersensitivity; the latter effect is probably due to an inhibition of lymphocyte-derived mediators (such as migration inhibition factor) that recruit cells (i.e., macrophages) necessary for the response.[278]

Overall, glucocorticoid effects on B cell functions are more modest. In humans, high-dose corticosteroid therapy causes a small decrease in immunoglobulin levels due both to decreased synthesis and increased catabolism,[299] and antibody responses to specific antigens are ordinarily not affected by glucocorticoids.[278] In vitro, the steroids can in some cases even stimulate immunoglobuin production by cultures of B and T lymphocytes.[300] However, immunoglobulin production by B cells is the result of a series of steps involving early activation, later B cell growth factor–mediated proliferation, and final differentiation to the immunoglobulin-producing state. These steps are affected by suppressor cell and helper cell functions and can be suppressed by glucocorticoids.[257,278,279,285] Studied in vitro, glucocorticoids affect substantially the early activation, have a lesser effect on the B cell growth factor response, and do not effect the final step.[301] Because of varying sensitivities and complex accessory cell effects on B and/or T cell function, it is possible to observe a variety of effects, either stimulatory or inhibitory. Inhibition of suppressor cell function may explain why, in sarcoidosis with anergy (that may be due in part to increased suppressor activity), glucocorticoids may increase immune responsiveness.[280]

Macrophage functions are relatively sensitive to glucocorticoid inhibitory actions.[278] The steroids induce a monocytopenia, suppress committed marrow-forming monocyte stem cells, and block the differentiation of monocytes into macrophages.[302] This may explain the effectiveness of glucocorticoids in treating many granulomatous diseases, since the monocyte is felt to be important in granuloma formation.[278] By blocking the production of γ interferon, glucocorticoids can also decrease the levels of Fc receptors (that bind the Fc portion of immunoglobulin) on monocytes and macrophages;[287] these receptors facilitate phagocytosis of particulate antigens and other functions of the cells in the inflammatory responses. Steroids can block the ability of the monocyte to bind to antibody-coated cells,[278] to elicit bactericidal activity and cytotoxicity,[278] and to release neutral proteases, including collagenase, elastase, and plasminogen activator,[285] that participate in the immunological and inflammatory responses. The steroids suppress the production by macrophages of lymphocyte activating factor, which is involved in T cell mitogenesis,[285] and of lymphocyte-derived macrophage factors that may block the exit of macrophages from inflammatory sites.[285] They block the production of macrophage activating factor by T cells and its actions on macrophages.[284] However, glucocorticoid actions are not always inhibitory: the steroids can increase the expression of mannose receptors in macrophages; this has an anti-inflammatory effect by enhancing the uptake and internalization of lysosomal enzymes.[290]

Actions of glucocorticoids on neutrophil functions other than regulating their trafficking are less definite. Suppression of functions such as phagocytosis, chemotaxis, and bactericidal activity has mostly been elicited at steroid concentrations that rarely if ever are achieved in vivo.[278]

Erythroid Cells and Thrombocytes

A mild polycythemia is observed occasionally in Cushing's syndrome, and there may be normochromic normocytic anemia in Addison's disease.[257] Thus, whereas the steroids do affect the hemoglobin concentration, glucocorticoids are not generally useful as stimulants for erythropoiesis except in several rare forms of congenital anemia of infancy and in certain forms of autoimmune hemolytic anemia.[257] In animals, glucocorticoids can inhibit erythroid colony formation.[303]

Glucocorticoids may acutely promote a rise in thrombocytes, but thrombocytopenia has also been reported after long-term administration.[257] The mechanisms for these influences are not known.

Fibroblastic and Epithelial Tissues

The actions of glucocorticoids on fibroblastic tissues are a major drawback to their long-term use in therapy.[3,257,304–306] These probably contribute to the thinning of the bone matrix and osteoporosis seen in glucocorticoid excess states (see Chap. 15). The steroids inhibit both specific matrix cell activities such as collagen and glycosaminoglycan formation and overall fibroblast function.[304–309] Inhibitory actions on fibroblasts also lead to easy bruising, poor wound healing, and a tendency to wound dehiscence following surgery in the glucocorticoid-excess state. The steroids do not appear to alter epithelialization of the wound, except indirectly through inhibition of the fibrous scar which serves as a scaffolding for the cells,[257] but they can inhibit epidermal epithelial cell proliferation in other circumstances; this action is useful in the treatment of psoriasis.[310]

Glucocorticoid effects on fibroblasts and epithelial cells are observed in isolated cells in culture. Both stimulation and inhibition of cellular functions have been reported.[304,311] Inhibitory effects lead to decreased uptake and metabolism of glucose, decreased protein and RNA synthesis, and inhibition of DNA synthesis.[312] The steroid can also affect collagen, fibronectin, and glycosaminoglycan formation.[307-309,311] These effects can also be specific and observed in the absence of major influences on most cellular functions. The effects on collagen involve a selective decrease in collagen mRNA, resulting in decreased collagen synthesis.[306] The steroids can also affect other enzymes involved in collagen metabolism, such as collagen galactosyltransferase and hydroxylase.[306] By contrast, stimulatory effects result in increased cell replication and incorporation of thymidine into DNA.[312] These seemingly paradoxical responses may be due to the fact that glucocorticoids can affect the actions or production of various growth factors either positively or negatively.[312a] In humans, the result is predominantly inhibitory.

Cardiovascular System and Fluid and Electrolyte Balance

Glucocorticoids affect the heart, vasculature, regulators of blood pressure, water excretion, and electrolyte balance. Some of these actions are direct; others involve mineralocorticoid-like actions.

In glucocorticoid-deficient states, there is hypotension with decreased responsiveness to pressor stimuli[313,314] and decreased cardiac output;[313] stresses such as surgery, infection, or trauma can precipitate an adrenal crisis with shock. This is partly due to a loss of the mineralocorticoid functions of the adrenal steroids. However, the importance of glucocorticoids in the maintenance of normal cardiovascular function is emphasized by the finding that the hypotension seen in patients with adrenal insufficiency crisis is not reversed by correction of volume or sodium losses or by administration of mineralocorticoids, such as DOC, that do not have glucocorticoid activity (Figs. 12-19 and 12-20).

Conversely, in glucocorticoid excess states there is hypertension, which occurs in almost all patients with spontaneous Cushing's syndrome[314] and in a lesser proportion of patients on glucocorticoid therapy (Chaps. 14 and 15), and enhanced responsiveness to pressors such as angiotensin II and norepinephrine.[313,314] Although mineralocorticoid actions may contribute to the hypertension in spontaneous Cushing's syndrome,

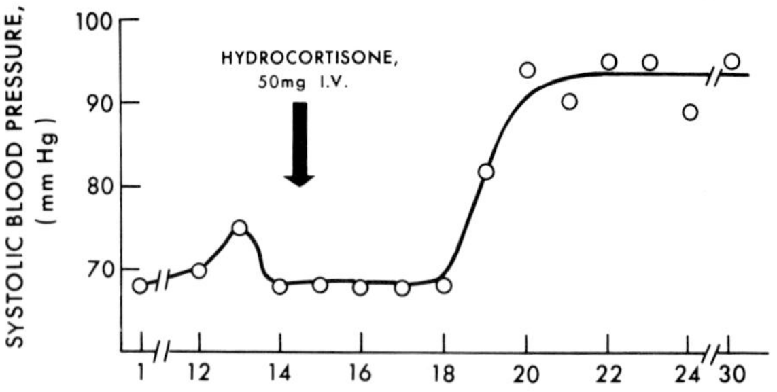

FIGURE 12-19 Effect of cortisol (hydrocortisone) on blood pressure in a patient with Addison's disease. The blood pressure had not responded to fluid replacement and other supportive measures. Cortisol was given when the diagnosis of adrenocortical insufficiency was suspected. (*From Baxter.*[257])

frank stigmata of mineralocorticoid excess such as depressed plasma renin level and hypokalemia are commonly not present, indicating that there are mineralocorticoid-independent effects of the glucocorticoids.[314] Further, in the rat glucocorticoid-induced hypertension is specifically blocked by glucocorticoid antagonists but not by low salt intake or mineralocorticoid antagonists.[315] Large doses of glucocorticoids may also be beneficial in shock due to gram-negative

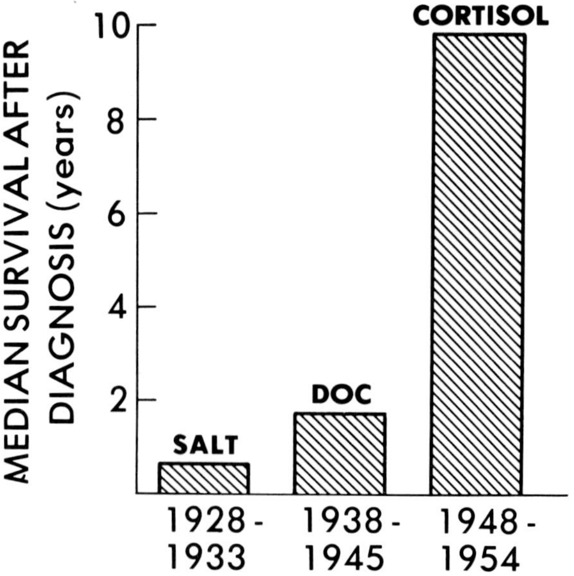

FIGURE 12-20 Median duration of survival of individuals with Addison's syndrome in years following the diagnosis, in relation to therapeutic advances. The specific time periods chosen were selected to avoid patients falling into overlapping therapy categories. However, the survival in the postcortisol era is actually greater than indicated since most of the individuals in this group were still alive at the time (1963) the data were collected,[398] and it is not clear that all the individuals who died actually received cortisol. (*From Baxter and Rousseau;*[3] *based upon data of Dunlop.*[398])

sepsis (see Chap. 15) and for treatment of refractory arrhythmias.[316,317]

The mechanisms of these vascular effects are complex and multifactorial. The steroids can have direct actions on the heart (discussed below). They can have permissive actions enhancing the activities of vasoactive substances (as described under Synergistic and Antagonistic Interrelationships, below). They may have direct actions on vascular smooth muscle[318,319] and endothelial cells.[320] The steroids can suppress the synthesis and actions of vasodilator and cardiac-suppressant substances that are produced in excess in adrenal insufficiency and/or in response to stress. (The role of PGs in this respect is discussed below, but this issue is addressed more comprehensively later, under Glucocorticoids and Stress.) Glucocorticoids can directly affect other components involved in blood pressure control, such as the renin-angiotensin system (see below).

The heart is a direct glucocorticoid target and in isolated preparations glucocorticoids can induce cardiac protein synthesis, increase the coupling between cardiac β-adrenergic receptors and adenylate cyclase, and have positive inotropic influences and effects on left ventricular work index.[320a] They have also been reported to induce cardiac ultrastructural damage.[321] Further, they probably do have mineralocorticoid-independent effects on cardiac output and stroke volume.[322]

The ability of glucocorticoids to decrease PG production probably contributes to these vascular responses,[283] and, although controversial[292] (see also Immunological and Inflammatory Responses, above), decreased urinary PGE_2 production has been reported in glucocorticoid excess.[314] In glucocorticoid-induced hypertension in the rat the renal medullary basal and angiotensin II–stimulated release of this PG is diminished even though plasma and urinary PGE_2 concentrations are increased.[322] PGI_2 is a potent vasodilator and is the principal product of arachidonic acid in arteries and veins. Its production is stimulated by angiotensin II and norepinephrine.[324] Thus, glucocorticoid inhibition of the production of this vasodilator could contribute significantly to the increased vascular reactivity and blood pressure in glucocorticoid excess states.[324] Conversely, overproduction of this mediator could result in decreased vascular reactivity and hypotension in the addisonian patient. PGI_2 also causes tachycardia, and excess PGI_2 could contribute to the presence of this sign in the addisonian individual.[324] It has been suggested that glucocorticoids stimulate the ability of mitochondria to retain calcium and thereby improve vascular responses by enhancing ATP generation.[325]

Glucocorticoids can increase the levels of prorenin[326] and renin substrate[314] and, in isolated cells,[327] the activity of angiotensin converting enzyme (see Chap. 14).[328] Whereas plasma renin levels are generally in the normal to high normal range in glucocorticoid excess states, this level of elevation is inappropriate in the face of hypertension.[314] A further indication that excess angiotensin II activity contributes to the hypertension in Cushing's syndrome is that it is decreased by the administration of inhibitors of converting enzymes (see also Chap. 14).[314,323] Conversely, angiotensin II generation is impaired in adrenal insufficiency in the face of elevated renin and converting enzyme levels, possibly as a result of decreased angiotensinogen, and this could contribute to the refractoriness of addisonian shock to therapy.[328,329]

Although glucocorticoids can affect salt and water excretion by binding to mineralocorticoid receptors (discussed below), they also have other actions that are not elicited through mineralocorticoid receptors. They increase the glomerular filtration rate (GFR).[330,331] Whether this is due to an increase in cardiac output or to direct influences on the kidney is not known. Glucocorticoids can increase the levels of cardiac ANF (see Chap. 14) and its mRNA,[332] which can increase GFR (Chap. 14). The increase in GFR can enhance the excretion of salt and water, and steroids such as dexamethasone, with much greater glucocorticoid than mineralocorticoid activity, sometimes produce a natriuresis rather than sodium retention.[330,331] Glucocorticoids increase Na^+,K^+-ATPase activity in the renal outer medullary tubules,[332a] erythrocytes,[333] and colon[334] and prekallikrein in the urine and on the basal membrane of distal tubular cells.[335] Although the physiological role of these actions has not been established, they imply that the steroid can have direct effects on renal hemodynamics and/or salt excretion.

Glucocorticoid deficiency results in a decreased ability to excrete water.[336] This effect is probably due both to the decreased GFR and to the fact that glucocorticoids can inhibit vasopressin release; in their absence, vasopressin levels are increased, leading to abnormal water retention.[336,337] In fact, water intoxication can occur rarely in panhypopituitarism with glucocorticoid but not mineralocorticoid deficiency.[336]

Glucocorticoids also affect potassium balance.[330,331,338,338a] Steroids such as cortisol can at higher concentrations produce hypokalemia through mineralocorticoid actions (see below and Chap. 14). However, their major effect is to produce a transient kaliuresis by increasing urine flow through increases in GRF and, possibly, protein catabolism with release of intracellular K^+. The net effect is that in glucocorticoid excess states and particularly in therapy using glucocorticoids with relatively weak mineralocorticoid potency, the plasma potassium concentration is usually normal or only slightly decreased (see Chap. 14). These effects on potassium ion also help to prevent hyperkalemia in response to a potassium load.

Glucocorticoids can increase renal acid output such that in glucocorticoid excess there is a tendency to alkalosis and in glucocorticoid deficiency a tendency to acidosis. These effects occur with minimal influences on urinary pH; they are due to stimulation of excretion of buffer as phosphate and ammonia by blocking tubular reabsorption of phosphate and increasing the production of ammonia.[339,340] The latter may occur due to a stimulation of Na^+–H^+ exchange in the proximal tubule brush border, which results in ammonia trapping.[340]

Bone and Calcium Metabolism

Glucocorticoids affect bone and calcium dynamics in a variety of ways. In Addison's disease, mild hypercalcemia can occur.[341–343] Conversely, glucocorticoids are used to treat certain hypercalcemias (see also Chap. 23);[344] these are largely granulomatous conditions such as sarcoidosis in which the steroid may block the formation of 1α,25-dihydroxycholecalciferol (1α,25-$(OH)_2D_3$) by the granulomatous tissues.[345] However, most hypercalcemias are not glucocorticoid-responsive and, in general, glucocorticoid excess does not result in lower serum Ca^{2+} levels.[346] Serum phosphate levels are lowered and urinary Ca^{2+} and phosphorus concentrations are elevated in glucocorticoid excess states.[346] Glucocorticoid excess ultimately leads to osteoporosis (see also Chaps. 15 and 24), the major limitation to their long-term use. Several independent actions contribute to these effects.

Glucocorticoids partly block intestinal calcium absorption (Chap. 23).[347,348] This is likely a direct effect on the gut that is more prominent in the duodenum and jejunum. However, there is either no effect or a stimulation of uptake by the ileum, and a stimulation of uptake in the colon.[349,350] Glucocorticoids apparently do not block vitamin D action in the intestine[349] and do not decrease vitamin D metabolite levels; renal vitamin D 1α-hydroxylase activity is increased by the steroid.[347,348,351] Earlier reports suggested that the steroid promotes a redistribution of calcium from extracellular into intracellular compartments,[325,352,353] but the significance of this is not known.

Glucocorticoids decrease renal reabsorption of calcium and phosphate and in excess cause hypercalciuria and renal calculi.[305,344,346] Hypercalciuria is the most consistent effect of glucocorticoids on calcium dynamics, and a major contributor to the negative calcium balance.[346,352]

The glucocorticoid-induced tendency to hypocalcemia induces a secondary rise in parathyroid hormone (PTH) level.[305,345,346,348] There may also be a direct increase of PTH release;[345,346] this action can explain why the steroid can increase both serum calcium and PTH levels in primary hyperparathyroidism.[345] However, glucocorticoids do cause hypocalcemia in parathyroidectomized animals maintained on a constant dose of PTH and are necessary for the induction of hypocalcemia in animals by thyroparathyroidectomy.[350]

Shortly after glucocorticoid administration there is enhanced bone accretion, but with continued administration inhibition is the predominant effect.[305] The inhibitory effects on accretion are probably due to decreased bone cell function and collagen formation; inhibition by glucocorticoids of bone cell proliferation and synthesis of protein, RNA, collagen, and hyaluronate have been demonstrated in vitro.[305,351,352,353a] Decreased bone synthesis in glucocorticoid excess states is probably also reflected by lower blood osteocalcin (bone Gla-protein) levels.[353b] This protein, whose function is unknown, is probably produced by osteoblasts; it comprises 20 percent of the noncollagenous protein of bone and binds tightly to hydroxyapatite.[353b]

Glucocorticoid excess also results in enhanced osteolysis with an increased number of osteoclasts and urinary secretion of hydroxyproline.[302] These steroids in vitro can stimulate the resorptive activity of macrophages, from which osteoclasts are derived, possibly by affecting cell surface glycoproteins involved in the association of these cells with bone.[302,353a] They can inhibit osteoclast function in vitro, but in vivo this function apparently is not predominant.[302,353a] Enhanced resorption may also be due to the increased PTH levels and by steroid augmentation of the actions of PTH, including its ability to stimulate cAMP accumulation in bone cells.[354,355] However, the increased osteolysis ordinarily is not profound enough to lead to bone changes typical of hyperparathyroidism (i.e., osteitis fibrosa cystica) in glucocorticoid excess states.[305] Glucocorticoids may also increase bone resorption by enhancing the sensitivity of bone cells to 1α,25-$(OH)_2D_3$, possibly by increasing the number of 1α,25-$(OH)_2D_3$ receptors, although in other instances they decrease osteoblast 1α,25-$(OH)_2D_3$ receptors.[356,357] Finally, glucocorticoids may block the inhibitory actions of calcitonin on bone resorption.[358]

These collective actions are summarized in Fig. 12-21. The decreased calcium absorption by the gut and increased urinary calcium and phosphate loss lead to a net negative calcium balance and a tendency to hypocalcemia and hypophosphatemia. This, plus direct steroid actions on the parathyroid gland, results in

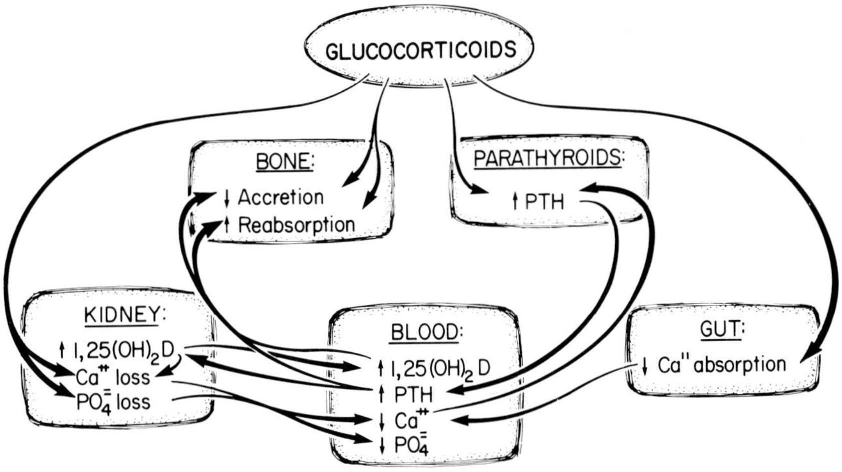

FIGURE 12-21 Effect of glucocorticoids on bone and calcium dynamics. See text.

increased PTH release that in turn results in increased 1α,25-$(OH)_2D_3$ formation. The increased PTH and 1α,25-$(OH)_2D_3$ blunt the hypocalcemic response and possibly the effect on intestinal calcium absorption, but they also, in combination with direct glucocorticoid effects, decrease bone accretion and increase bone resorption, resulting in an overall loss of bone mineral.

Central Nervous System

Glucocorticoids affect the brain in a number of ways. Thus, behavior, mood, neural activity, and a number of specific biochemical processes can be influenced by these hormones.[359,360] Glucocorticoids can penetrate the blood-brain barrier; their capability to do so is inversely proportional to their polarity, which is largely dependent on the number of hydroxyl groups.[361] They can also regulate the permeability of the blood-brain barrier to other substances and are used for therapy to reduce brain edema;[362] conversely, pseudotumor cerebri is rarely associated with glucocorticoid therapy.[338]

Mood changes (and, rarely, psychosis) are observed with both glucocorticoid excess and deficiency.[338,359] Patients receiving glucocorticoid therapy commonly have a feeling of well-being.[338,363,364] This may be due in part to a beneficial effect on the primary disease process, but there are additional independent influences. On the other hand, patients with spontaneous Cushing's syndrome are commonly depressed.[338] Patients with Addison's disease tend to be depressed, negativistic, irritable, seclusive, and apathetic.[364] Several types of psychoses have been reported (particularly in glucocorticoid excess states); neither the patient's psychiatric history nor personality traits prior to receiving glucocorticoids or developing Cushing's syndrome has been helpful in predicting whether a psychosis might occur;[363,364] interpretation of these effects is complicated by the fact that psychoses can occur due to the diseases for which glucocorticoid treatment is used. Patients with Addison's disease have anorexia,[363] whereas glucocorticoid excess stimulates the appetite.[338,363,364] In addition, high doses of glucocorticoids can affect sleep, with a trend toward increased wakefulness and a reduction in rapid eye movement (REM) sleep, an increase in stage II sleep, and an increase in the time to the first REM sleep.[365]

Conversely, in depressive syndromes there can be excessive glucocorticoid production with blunted circadian rhythm and decreased ability of glucocorticoids to suppress the hypothalamic-adrenal-pituitary axis (see above).[159,366] These abnormalities occur commonly in both unipolar and bipolar depression and are particularly frequent in delusional depression.[366] They also occur in schizoaffective disorders, catatonia, borderline character disorders, chronic pain syndromes, and bulimia, but they are uncommon in schizophrenia and in mania.[366] The abnormalities usually abate with clinical improvement; failure to do so is correlated with a high rate of relapse. The contribution of the glucocorticoid excess to these problems and the mechanisms of its development are not understood. The fact that dextroamphetamine, but not a number of other CNS active agents, can transiently decrease the cortisol hypersecretion in depression has been taken as suggesting that it may be due to cholinergic excess.[159]

Addisonian subjects can have increased sensitivity to a variety of sensory stimuli, including sound and taste, and impaired judgment and ability to discriminate sensory input.[359,364,367] In animals, bilateral adrenalectomy attenuates the circadian variations in paradoxical sleep.[359] Adrenal steroids can also facilitate extinction of previously acquired avoidance habits,[359] an effect opposite to that induced by ACTH and other POMC fragments.[359,368] However, this effect may not be glucocorticoid-specific,[359] since it can also be elicited by steroids, such as pregnenolone, that do not have glucocorticoid activity.

Glucocorticoids regulate a variety of developmental and other events in the brain.[360] In excess they can have detrimental effects on brain development in animals. They regulate the catecholamine biosynthetic pathway (discussed below), transsynaptic induction, the actions of nerve growth factor and epidermal growth factor on brain cells, the development of cholinergic ganglionic properties, glutamine synthetase, α-glycerophosphate dehydrogenase, myelination, γ-aminobutyric acid, and a neuron-specific phosphoprotein, protein 1.[360,368a] They can affect brain cell electrical activity and the EEG.[359,365] Most of these effects have been elicited at very high steroid concentrations, and therefore their importance is not understood.

Whereas most of these actions on the CNS are probably mediated by the glucocorticoid receptors (see below), some may be mediated through mineralocorticoid receptors. In the brain, unlike the case with the kidney, these receptors are present unassociated with high concentrations of the CBG-like protein that sequesters cortisol. Thus, in the absence of this protein, cortisol can have ready access to the receptor and in fact may keep it relatively saturated even under nonstimulated conditions.[229,230]

Adrenal Medulla

The adrenal cortex surrounds and is contiguous with the chromaffin tissue–containing medulla (Chap. 13), a gland that, like the cortex, is also involved in stress responses. The adrenal medulla receives adrenocortical venous effluent and thus is exposed to much higher cortisol concentrations than other tissues.[360] Glucocorticoids affect adrenal chromaffin cell phenotypic characteristics and the catecholamine biosynthetic pathway.[360] In the latter, they regulate phenylethanolamine *N*-methyltransferase (PNMT), tyrosine hydroxylase, and dopamine β-hydroxylase activities.[94,360] The effects are most prominent on PNMT, which catalyzes the formation of epinephrine, the principal catecholamine of the medulla, from norepinephrine.[94] Interestingly, in species in which the cortex and medulla are separated anatomically, norepinephrine is the principal catecholamine.[94] Consistent with these influences, resting and exercise-stimulated epinephrine levels are reduced in ACTH deficiency states; the physiological importance of this is not known.[369] Glucocorticoids can also increase adrenal medullary proenkephalin.[370]

Eye

Several types of ocular influences of glucocorticoids have been reported. Glucocorticoids in excess can increase the intraocular pressure in certain susceptible individuals, particularly in patients with primary open-angle glaucoma.[257,371] This appears to be due to a glucocorticoid effect on the aqueous outflow, perhaps through actions on the trabecular meshwork.[371] The role of the endogenous glucocorticoids in determining the intraocular pressure in normal individuals or patients with elevated intraocular pressure is not known, but the intraocular pressure tends to show a circadian variation that parallels, with about a 3-h lag, the overall fluctuations in plasma cortisol[371] and an increase in intraocular pressure can be observed in ocular hypertensive patients about 3 h after glucocorticoid administration.[371] Glucocorticoid therapy can stimulate cataract formation;[371] this is common in patients who have received high-dose glucocorticoid therapy for a long time.[371] Interestingly, more recent data suggest that this might be due to covalent linkage of the steroid molecules to the lens crystalline proteins.[372] Glucocorticoids decrease absorption of topical antibiotics, and therapy can result in nonspecific keratitis, refractive changes, papilledema due to intracranial hypertension, limitation of ocular movement, and changes in the aqueous and vitreous compositions.[372] Finally, glucocorticoids can influence certain enzymes in the developing chick retina.[257]

Gastrointestinal Tract

Several types of influences of glucocorticoids on the gastrointestinal tract have been reported. In animals, glucocorticoids at high doses inhibit DNA synthesis in gastric but not jejunal mucosa,[277] increase acid secretion in response to stimuli such as histamine,[257] and increase the incidence of gastric ulceration.[257] In humans, prolonged steroid treatment may increase acid output slightly.[373] Although the issue has been controversial,[374] it appears that glucocorticoids in high doses result in an increased incidence of peptic ulcers.[375] In an analysis of 71 controlled clinical trials in which a total of 3064 patients were randomly allocated to glucocorticoid therapy or nonsteroid therapy, 1.8 percent of the steroid-treated patients had ulcers, compared to 0.8 percent of the controls, and 2.5 percent of steroid-treated patients had hemorrhage, vs. 1.6 percent of controls.[375] Even in an earlier study in which it was concluded that ulcers are not more frequent in the steroid-treated group, the prevalences of proved peptic ulcer were 1.6 percent in patients on >20 mg of prednisone per day compared to 0.3 percent for the control population; 3.8 percent in steroid-treated patients with a prior ulcer compared to 2.3 percent in the control group; and 5.3 percent in patients who received a total dose of over 100 mg of prednisone per day compared to 2.3 percent for the control group.

In glucocorticoid-deficient states there can be nausea and vomiting. The mechanisms for this are not known, but, as discussed above, a deficiency of cortisol may lead to PGI_2 excess, which can produce such symptoms.[324]

Growth and Development

Glucocorticoids in excess inhibit linear growth; this limits their prolonged use in children.[276,277,376] These steroids also inhibit skeletal maturation; the result is that growth potential is maintained during and after therapy, and there can be further growth (sometimes with a growth spurt) after its withdrawal that compensates in part for the steroid inhibition of linear growth.

Glucocorticoids also inhibit growth (and cell division) in a number of individual tissues.[276,277] The effects on lymphoid, fibroblastic, epithelial, and bone cells have already been discussed. These actions are useful in steroid therapy, but they can also be detrimental. There are variations in sensitivity; in the growing rat, for instance, liver, heart, muscle, and kidney are more sensitive than gastric and jejunal mucosa, spleen, brain, and testis.[277] More information is needed with respect to humans.

In vitro, glucocorticoids can either stimulate or inhibit cell division of a larger number of cell types.[276–279,296,304,306,312,312a] Stimulation may occur by a steroid-induced augmentation of the actions of growth factors such as fibroblast growth factor[377] or somatomedin C,[378] and the steroid can also increase the levels of somatomedin C receptors.[379] Conversely, inhibition could be due to actions of the steroid in blocking growth factor (e.g., PG)[312a] production and/or action; it could also be due to other inhibitory actions of the glucocorticoids on the cell (discussed in Protein and Nucleic Acid Metabolism and Carbohydrate Metabolism, above).[257,276,278,279,296] The steroid-induced increase in fibronectin biosynthesis could also inhibit replication, since this extracellular glycoprotein may stimulate cell adhesion, which may inhibit cell replication.[311]

The mechanisms of inhibition of growth in the intact organism are not known.[276,277,376,380] They may in part be due to inhibitory influences on bone cells; for instance, chondrocyte proliferation can be inhibited by the steroids. Glucocorticoids also inhibit growth hormone production, but this action probably does not explain the growth-inhibiting effects of the steroid, since they are not overcome by administration of growth hormone. Although glucocorticoids do not decrease radioimmunoassayable levels of somatomedin in plasma, they do increase the levels of an inhibitor of somatomedin.

It is not known whether glucocorticoids at physiological concentrations play a role in regulating growth. In animals, physiologically equivalent concentrations of glucocorticoids do inhibit new cell accretion in several growing tissues.[276,376] It has also been reported that adrenalectomy increases the mitotic index in skin.[277]

Glucocorticoids accelerate developmental events in various species in several fetal and postnatal differentiating tissues, including liver (induce enzymes of intermediary metabolism), intestine (induce digestive enzymes), pancreas (regulate the production of insulin and induce digestive enzymes), stomach (induce pepsinogen), skin (induce epidermal proteins), retina (induce glutamine synthetase), brain (induce Na^+,K^+-ATPase), adrenal medulla (induce PNMT), placenta (induce enzymes for estrogen synthesis), mammary gland, and heart.[380a] The endogenous glucocorticoids may act similarly in the developing fetus, since plasma corticosteroid levels increase prior to term delivery, and this is associated with normal maturation of the tissues. In general, glucocorticoids tend to affect the timing and rate of differentiation, but not the sequence of development events. Thus, with adrenal insufficiency in utero there is continued development of the fetus and of certain specialized functions, but this differentiation is delayed.

The sensitivity to glucocorticoids varies during development, and various proteins may be regulated by the steroids only at certain stages.[380a] For instance, corticosteroids regulate surfactant synthesis in the fetal lung but not in the adult. In some instances (e.g., induction of intestinal sucrase activity), the steroid-induced changes are reversible, whereas in other instances (e.g., induction of glutamine synthetase in neural retina) the enzyme does not return to pretreatment levels following withdrawal of the steroid. There is also an increased sensitivity of certain responses to glucocorticoids just prior to the endogenous increase in glucocorticoid levels that precedes term delivery.

Little is known about the importance of these developmental influences in the child, but glucocorticoid effects on the fetus may prepare it for extrauterine existence. For instance, the actions on hepatic enzymes and the pancreatic islets are probably important for regulating glucose homeostasis, the effects on the adrenal medulla could aid in responsiveness to stress, and the surfactant-inducing actions permit the lung to carry out gas exchange.[380a] Some of these functions can be induced by glucocorticoids prior to the normal increase in steroid levels that precedes delivery. For example, treatment of the mother in spontaneous premature labor increases fetal surfactant levels and reduces the incidence and/or severity of the respiratory distress syndrome (hyaline membrane disease) associated with premature birth.

Production and Clearance of Other Hormones

Glucocorticoids can affect the production and/or clearance of other classes of hormones. In the liver, these steroids induce a specific cytochrome P450 that could participate in oxidative reactions involving a variety of drugs, steroids, bile acids, and other compounds.[381] The influences on ACTH, angiotensin II, vasopressin, somatomedin, growth hormone, insulin, glucagon, PTH, vitamin D, epinephrine, and PGs have been mentioned. Glucocorticoids in excess inhibit pancreatic polypeptide production,[382] basal and metoclopramide-stimulated prolactin release,[382] and basal and stimulated gastrin secretion.[382] They can stimulate the production of calcitonin and related peptides.[383]

Glucocorticoids affect thyroid stimulating hormone (TSH) release and thyroxine (T_4) metabolism. In glucocorticoid excess states there is a blunted TSH response to thyrotropin releasing hormone (TRH).[384] Plasma T_4 concentrations are generally in the low normal range in glucocorticoid excess states, but triiodothyronine (T_3) levels can be subnormal,[384] due to decreased conversion of T_4 to T_3 and increased conversion of T_4 to reverse T_3.[385] Glucocorticoids also increase thyroid hormone–binding prealbumin concentration.[385]

Reproductive Function

A variety of effects of glucocorticoids on reproductive function have been reported. These are predominantly inhibitory, are observed at high levels of the steroids, and may be part of an overall mechanism to delay reproductive function in times of stress. In men, glucocorticoid therapy and spontaneous Cushing's syndrome decrease plasma testosterone concentration.[386,387] This is likely due both to an inhibition of LH release and to direct actions on the testis.[386,388] In the short term there can be a decrease in testosterone concentration without a change in LH levels, whereas long-term testosterone levels are better correlated with depressed LH (but not follicle stimulating hormone, FSH) levels.[386,389] Glucocorticoids may also increase the ability of testosterone to block gonadotropin release by feedback inhibition.[387] They may also regulate factors that delay the onset of puberty.[390] In females, glucocorticoids in excess suppress basal and gonadotropin releasing hormone–stimulated LH (but not FSH) levels, plasma estrogen and progestin concentrations (variably), ovulation, and the onset of puberty. They result in a slight increase in testosterone clearance and have selective effects on FSH action.[390-392] In fat cells they increase the levels of aromatase, which converts androgens to estrogens.[392a]

Synergistic and Antagonistic Interrelationships between Glucocorticoids and Other Hormones

The complex interactions between the actions of glucocorticoids and other hormones have already been emphasized. Illustrative of these interrelationships are the synergism between glucocorticoids and glucagon or epinephrine and the antagonism between glucocorticoids and insulin. Glucocorticoids can modulate the cellular sensitivity to other hormones, regulate the same processes as other hormones, and have indirect influences that affect the overall response to other hormones. Conversely, other hormones can directly or indirectly affect glucocorticoid action.

Glucocorticoids can alter positively or negatively the cellular sensitivity to other hormones by shifting the dose-response curve or by influencing the maximal response obtained.[257,277a,393,394] In some cases, the cellular response to another hormone is amplified by the glucocorticoid and vice versa, effects termed by Ingle "permissive."[275a,393] Tissue synergistic and antagonistic actions can occur by influencing receptors for the other hormones or, more typically, by postreceptor mechanisms. Influences of the steroid on receptors mediating the actions of insulin and immunological mediators and on postreceptor steps in these processes are discussed above. Other permissive actions may explain glucocorticoid effects on blood pressure in addisonian individuals,[257] lipolysis,[269] and PTH action.[354,355] Many of the synergisms occur with hormones that activate adenylate cyclase (epinephrine, glucagon, PTH).[257,393] Occasionally, glucocorticoids increase cAMP levels by decreasing levels of the phosphodiesterase that degrades cAMP.[393] Conversely, cAMP can modulate glucocorticoid receptor action.[395] Glucocorticoids can affect β-adrenergic receptors: in adipocytes the steroid promotes a loss in β_1- and an increase in β_2-adrenergic receptors;[396] in human neutrophils glucocorticoids induce a tightened coupling of β-adrenergic receptors and adenylate cyclase and attenuate isoproterenol-induced uncoupling between receptors and cyclase activation.[397] Glucocorticoids increase β-adrenergic receptor density in several other cell types.[397] These actions may contribute to glucocorticoid effectiveness in treating asthma, in which the steroid can return desensitized bronchial tissue to normal.[397]

Glucocorticoids and Stress

Survival rate in patients with untreated adrenocortical insufficiency is decreased (Fig. 12-20).[398] Therapy with mineralocorticoids alone (e.g., with DOC, Fig. 12-20) increases life expectancy only slightly.[398] However, survival is increased markedly when cortisol is given.[398] Decompensation is usually precipitated by some stressful insult (surgery, infection, injury, etc.) and is associated with a variety of derangements, including an inability to maintain a normal blood pressure (Fig. 12-19). Thus, the view has emerged that these steroids are necessary to cope with stress.

It is generally thought that glucocorticoid levels higher than basal are required to combat stress. This would be consistent with the fact that glucocorticoid production is generally increased in stress and with the occasional finding of a patient in addisonian crisis who has a normal random plasma cortisol concentration. In fact, this point has not been rigorously documented and those addisonian individuals with normal random cortisol levels commonly have stigmata such as pigmentation and symptoms of adrenocortical insufficiency under nonstressed conditions that indicate decreased basal cortisol production.

The multiple actions of glucocorticoids on the cardiovascular system discussed earlier probably contribute to the steroidal stress-combating effect. Thus, these actions would improve vascular reactivity and cardiac performance.

The actions of glucocorticoids inhibiting production of mediators active on vascular and other systems may be especially critical in the response to stress.[284] The specific case with prostaglandins was discussed above (see Cardiovascular System and Fluid and Electrolyte Balance). In addition, many stressful stimuli such as serious infections recruit an increased production of numerous mediator substances, including kinins such as bradykinin; lymphokines such as γ-interferon, which stimulates the release of other inflammatory mediators; serotonin; histamine; collagenase, which causes tissue damage; plasminogen activator, which in excess can cause blood vessel leakage and hemorrhage; catecholamines; immunological mediators; fever-producing substances such as endogenous pyrogen (interleukin 1); PGs and related substances; vasopressin; myocardial depressant factor; cachectin, which has been implicated in endotoxin-induced shock;[288] and other vasoactive substances. It is possible that the actions of these substances are so profound that they can be harmful if left unchecked. Indeed, these could result in excessive vasodilatation, cardiac suppression, edema, fever, hemorrhage, and other deleterious effects. Glucocorticoids suppress the production and/or the actions of most of the mediators listed above.

Other specific influences may also contribute.[284] For example, the increase in GFR may facilitate the clearance of toxic products and combat against excessive fluid retention. The induction of glutamine synthetase in the brain may help to lower concentrations of the potentially toxic glutamate and ammonia, which are elevated in stress. The induction of hepatic cytochrome P450 may help to remove toxic foreign chemicals. The induction of metallothionein may help in the elimination of toxic metals such as zinc.

MOLECULAR MECHANISMS OF GLUCOCORTICOID HORMONE ACTION

The molecular events in glucocorticoid hormone action are similar to those of other classes of steroid hormones (Chap. 5).[257,399–401] The steroid probably enters the cell by passive diffusion. Whereas it traditionally has been thought that in the absence of the steroid the receptors are localized in the cytosol,[400] more recent data refute this and suggest a nuclear location.[402] However, confirmation of this is needed since in earlier studies using similar methodology a different conclusion was reached.[400] The receptors have a molecular weight of about 90,000 and may be phosphorylated.[403] There are from 5000 to 100,000 cytoplasmic receptors per cell.[257,399,400] They bind cortisol with an affinity constant (K_d) of around 20 to 40 nM; this value is close to the free cortisol concentration in plasma, suggesting that saturation of the receptors is probably ordinarily in the 10 to 70 percent range and that either increases or decreases in plasma cortisol will change the receptor occupancy and thereby the physiological responses. These receptors bind a variety of glucocorticoids in proportion to their biological activities.[257]

An analysis of cloned complementary DNAs to human receptor mRNA has provided details of receptor structure.[404,405] These cDNAs encode proteins of 777 (α) and 742 (β) amino acids and thus differ only in their codons for the carboxy-terminal amino acids (50 for α and 15 for β) and 3′-untranslated regions. Also, two α-cDNAs differ in the lengths of their 3′-untranslated regions. The α forms are more prevalent and bind steroid when expressed in vitro with the use of α-cDNA; since the in vitro-expressed β form does not bind steroid, it has been proposed that the steroid-binding site is contained on the carboxy-terminal portion of the molecule. The middle portion of the molecule in the region including amino acids 400 to 500 is enriched in the basic amino acids cysteine, lysine, and arginine. This region appears to contain the DNA-binding domain and also is homologous to the comparable region of the estrogen receptor (Chap. 5) and the *erbA* oncogene, suggesting that these domains were derived from a common evolutionary precursor. Presumably, the amino-terminal portion of the molecule encodes a function important for receptor function; this portion contains statistically significant homology with sequences of *Drosophila* homeotic genes that encode developmentally important regulatory proteins. The notion that this portion of the molecule is important is based on the fact that mutant glucocorticoid receptors from steroid-resistant lymphoma cells are truncated yet contain both steroid- and DNA-binding domains.[400]

As yet there is no clear answer as to how many forms of the glucocorticoid receptor there are. This is a critical issue. For example nuclear actions and non-nuclear events (e.g., rapid inhibition of ACTH release) might involve different receptors. Heterogeneity might result in receptors with subtle differences in their affinities for various steroids. Multiple receptor forms could arise from multiple genes, RNA processing events, or posttranslational modifications. To date, all these possibilities remain open. Probing of chromosomal DNA with receptor cDNA reveals sequences on several different chromosomes.[404,405] These could be pseudogenes or genes for related proteins or other classes of receptors. Nevertheless, in several cell types it appears that all of the expressed human receptor genes are on chromosome 5, which probably contains only one receptor gene copy,[404,405] and other data imply that the functional receptors in some cell types are expressed from a diploid complement of genes. That RNA processing heterogeneity can occur has already been discussed; in addition, RNA ("Northern") blotting experiments demonstrate receptor mRNA species as diffuse bands in the 5 to 7-kilobase range.[404,405] Thus, additional heterogeneity is possible.[405] Third, experiments with purified receptors demonstrate charge heterogeneity[406,407] that could be due to posttranslational processing differences.

Glucocorticoids are also known to be capable of binding to and acting through mineralocorticoid receptors.[229–231] As mentioned in the section on Physiological Role of Plasma Binding, the ability of the rat glucocorticoid corticosterone to bind to these receptors in the rat kidney is diminished by the presence of a CBG-like protein that sequesters corticosterone. These "mineralocorticoid" receptors are also present in certain regions of the brain where substantial quantities of the CBG-like proteins are not present. As a result, the receptors are occupied by corticosterone, which mediates certain effects of the steroid on brain cell metabolism, serotoninergic neurotransmission, and behavioral adaptation.[230] In fact, the affinity of corticosterone for these mineralocorticoid receptors is so high that in brain they are nearly fully occupied at basal levels of corticosterone;[230] this contrasts with the case with the glucocorticoid receptors. Nevertheless, most glucocorticoid effects in brain are probably mediated through the classic glucocorticoid receptors.

Hormone binding induces a conformational change in the receptors termed *activation* (or transformation), such that 50 to 70 percent of the hormone-receptor complexes then bind to sites in the chromatin of the nucleus termed *acceptors*.[400] Activation involves steroid-induced conformational changes in the receptors that affect their charge, tendency to aggregate at low ionic strength, and DNA-binding activity.[400] A variety of mechanisms have been proposed to account for these changes, including receptor dephosphorylation, disaggregation, and/or dissociation from heterologous molecules and association with other molecules.[400,408]

The receptor-glucocorticoid complexes bind to DNA sites in the nucleus termed *glucocorticoid regulatory elements* (GREs).[400,401] These DNA sites (Chap. 5) contain specific sequences that have a much higher affinity for binding the receptor-glucocorticoid complexes than does random DNA. It is possible that other proteins also participate in the binding in a stimulatory or inhibitory fashion.[400,408–410]

Binding of receptor-glucocorticoid complexes to GREs affects transcription of nearby genes. The effects can be to either stimulate or inhibit transcription. Thus, the GRE functions as a regulated enhancer element and it can function either upstream (with respect to transcription) or downstream (for instance, in an intron), in either orientation, and at a considerable distance away from the promoter for transcriptional initiation.[400,401,411,412] The mechanisms by which these effects occur are not understood, but the receptor-glucocorticoid complexes can induce rapid and local influences on chromatin structure that in turn could result in changes in polymerase access to or function at sites of transcriptional initiation.[400,401]

Changes in the production of RNA transcripts in response to the steroid are reflected by consequent influences on the respective mature mRNAs and their protein products. The steroid-regulated proteins are responsible for the steroid response. For example, these may be enzymes, such as those involved in gluconeogenesis, or hormones, such as POMC; the latter is an example where glucocorticoids inhibit transcription.[167] Inhibitory actions can also be mediated by inducing the synthesis of proteins (such as the phospholipase A_2 inhibitor) that block specific cellular functions.

These events probably explain most physiological and pharmacological actions of the glucocorticoids (possible exceptions are discussed below), and glucocorticoid receptors have been detected in most tissues.[400] This extensive tissue distribution of receptors contrasts with the much more restricted distribution of the receptors for other classes of steroids (Chap. 5) and is consistent with the notion that glucocorticoids affect most if not all mammalian tissues.

There is generally,[400] but not exclusively,[413] a close correlation between the relative saturation of the receptor by the hormone and the relative magnitude of the glucocorticoid hormone response, suggesting that the receptor concentration limits the magnitude of the steroid hormone response. This contrasts to a common case with polypeptide and catecholamine hormones in which "spare" receptors are present (Chap. 5).

A variety of factors can affect glucocorticoid responsiveness.[400,414,415] First, factors in the cell may modulate hormone-binding activity. Second, receptor levels can be regulated by glucocorticoids (ordinarily negatively), the cell cycle, or other factors. However, glucocorticoid receptors are not as extensively regulated as are those for polypeptide hormones. Finally, responsiveness is affected by many of the interrelationships with other hormones discussed above.

Glucocorticoid action is rapidly reversible. When steroid levels drop, the hormone dissociates from the receptor and the receptor dissociates from the DNA, resulting in a cessation of the effect on gene transcription. The hormone response, however, can be longer-lived, due to the persistence of the mRNAs and proteins whose levels were increased by the steroid.

The glucocorticoid hormone response is restricted to a small subset of the expressed genes in each cell type. For instance, in cultured pituitary cells, the steroid affects the rate of synthesis of only 1 percent or less of the detectable proteins.[400] In liver, the steroid affects 7 percent of 200 quantifiable proteins.[416] Further, the proteins induced are specific for each cell type; i.e., a given protein may be induced in only one or a few but not all glucocorticoid-responsive tissues. This also indicates that factors other than the presence of the glucocorticoid receptors determine whether expression of a given gene can be under glucocorticoid hormone control, since the receptors may be similar in the various glucocorticoid-responsive tissues.

Glucocorticoids may, in a minority of instances, act via nontranscriptional mechanisms.[400,417] For example, the rapid feedback inhibition of ACTH release after glucocorticoid administration (Fig. 12-10) occurs too rapidly to be due to changes in ACTH mRNA, although the delayed feedback is due at least in part to a decrease in POMC mRNA.[167] In addition, indirect evidence has implicated occasional glucocorticoid actions in regulating mRNA stability[418] or translation;[419] however, in some of these cases transcriptional steroid actions could affect the levels of proteins that influence such stability. Some of the effects of glucocorticoids given in very high doses, e.g., for gram-negative shock (Chap. 15),[316,317] might be due to nontranscriptional mechanisms. Glucocorticoids can influence membrane properties and enzymes at concentrations above those necessary to saturate the receptors; the biological relevance of these actions is unknown.[417,420,421]

GLUCOCORTICOID AGONISTS AND ANTAGONISTS

Cortisol, corticosterone, aldosterone, and the synthetic steroids used in steroid therapy (prednisolone, dexamethasone, triamcinolone, etc.) are glucocorticoid agonists and therefore elicit glucocorticoid responses.[257,422] The activity of these compounds depends on their affinity for the receptors and on their plasma concentrations. Cortisol and corticosterone have similar affinities for the glucocorticoid receptor (Table 12-5); however, cortisol is the more important glucocorticoid because it circulates at much higher concentrations (Table 12-2). In the 17α-hydroxylase deficiency syndrome (discussed below and in Chap. 14), corticosterone is the predominant glucocorticoid. Aldosterone is not an important glucocorticoid in humans, even in mineralocorticoid excess states, because it does not reach high enough concentrations.

A number of other steroids bind to the glucocorticoid receptor (Table 12-5)[257,422–424] but do not elicit glucocorticoid responses. These are antagonists (Chap. 5), because they can compete with agonists for binding to the receptors and can thereby block the agonist response. Some compounds have partial agonist (partial antagonist) activity such that full receptor occupancy by these steroids results in an intermediate response; when present at sufficient concentration they can also block agonist binding, in which case only the intermediate response of the partial agonist will be observed.

The differences in glucocorticoid agonists and antagonists are apparently due to the fact that antagonists, unlike agonists, do not promote the conformational changes in the receptors necessary for subsequent steps in the response.[400] In fact, in some cases, antagonist receptor complexes do not bind to the nucleus.[400] Relative to cortisol, the compounds that have antagonist or partial agonist activity tend to have ketone, hydrogen, or other substitutions of the 11-hydroxyl group; alterations or deletions of the side chain at C-17; C-21 substitutions; reduction of the 4,5 double bond; or bulky 9-position substitutions.[257,422,423,425] Although these substitutions have mostly been studied in animals, the compound RU-38486, containing several changes relative to cortisol, including a (*p*-dimethylamino)phenyl substitution at C-11, has been shown to be active in humans,[424] and may have utility in treating glucocorticoid excess states, although in patients with an intact hypothalamic-pituitary-adrenal axis compensatory increases in ACTH production may elevate endogenous glucocorticoid levels enough to overcome the effects of the antagonist.[424] Included among antagonists are cortisone and prednisone; however, these activities are ordinarily not significant in vivo, because their affinities for the glucocorticoid receptor are too low relative to their plasma concentratons in most natural or therapeutic situations.[257]

STRUCTURE-ACTIVITY RELATIONS OF GLUCOCORTICOIDS: BASIS FOR BIOLOGICAL ACTIVITY

The activities of a large number of synthetic and naturally occurring glucocorticoid agonists have been examined. Several factors, such as availability for receptor binding, intrinsic agonist activity, affinity, and clearance are important. For steroids that are useful for systemic glucocorticoid therapy, two major types of differences relative to cortisol have been found. First, some compounds are more potent than cortisol on a dose-administered basis (Chap. 15), due to increased affinity for the glucocorticoid receptors and/or a decrease in their metabolic clearance rate. Second, some compounds have less relative mineralocorticoid than glucocorticoid activity (see Chap. 15), due to enhanced glucocorticoid receptor affinity relative to mineralocorticoid receptor affinity. This property results in fewer mineralocorticoid side effects.

In the circulation, affinity is the major immediate determinant of steroid activity at a given time, and the rate of clearance determines the duration of exposure to the steroid. The overall steroid effect is a product of these two parameters. A study with dexamethasone illustrates the need to consider both parameters.[426] This steroid was found to be 17-fold more potent than cortisol when its effect on the suppression of cortisol secretion was extrapolated to zero time. By contrast, dexamethasone was 154 times more potent than cortisol when evaluated after 14 h. The early time estimate more nearly reflects the intrinsic activity differences between the two steroids, but underrates the long-term relative potency of dexamethasone because it does not fully consider the differences in cortisol and dexamethasone clearance. The later time values may overestimate the potency. This value exceeds the product of the measured differences in affinity (approximately sevenfold, Table 12-5) and clearance (about threefold),[426] and it may be an overestimate because by the 14-h time point, the cortisol effect is largely gone. Considerations such as these must be made in evaluating reports of relative potency. Prednisolone has about a twofold higher affinity for the receptor than does cortisol (Table 12-5) and is cleared more slowly;[426] its net activity is about five times that of cortisol (Chap. 15).

Other factors in evaluating steroid potency are discussed in Chap. 15. In brief, cortisol and the synthetic steroids used in glucocorticoid therapy are ordinarily readily absorbed by the gut and their potencies after oral or parental administration are similar. Uptake is a factor, however, when glucocorticoids are given topically or in "depo" injections (Chap. 15). The extent to which variations in the distribution of steroids within body compartments affect activity has not been determined. Conceivably, reservoirs such as CBG that sequester some steroids more than others (e.g., prednisolone more than dexamethasone) can affect their immediate availability for biological actions. With the exception of prednisone and cortisone, which need to be converted to prednisolone and cortisol, respectively, the endogenous or synthetic glucocorticoids do not need to be converted to other metabolites in vivo to be active.

Structural features that promote glucocorticoid activity confer on the steroid the ability to have agonist (rather than partial agonist or antagonist) activity, enhance the steroid's affinity for the glucocorticoid receptors, and decrease the rate of metabolic inactivation.[257,425] These structural features can be considered in terms of modifications of the progesterone skeleton (substitutions conferring antagonist or partial agonist activity are discussed in the preceding section). Features associated with higher affinity include: a reduced 4,5 or 1,2 double bond; a 9α-fluoro or 6α-methyl group; a C-17 side chain; hydroxyl groups at positions 11, 17, and 21; C-3 and C-20 keto groups; and the presence of certain 16- and 17-substitutions (16α- or 16β-methyl, 16,17-acetonide, etc.).

The ways that such changes affect activity are partly understood.[257,425] Receptor binding involves hydrophobic contact between the surface of the steroid molecule and the receptor protein; removal of hydrophilic water from the steroid via the hormone-receptor interaction is perhaps the major force driving the binding reaction. Thus, an increased surface area, such as with 9α-substitution (provided the substituent is not too large), can increase the strength of binding. Affinity is also enhanced by the presence of key hydroxyl and keto groups that form hydrogen bonds with particular amino acids in the receptor. There is a critical angle between the A and B rings; 9α-substitution and the addition of a 1,2 double bond alter the AB angle to a more optimal position and increase the affinity relative to cortisol. Other substitutions, for instance the Δ^1 substitution, render the molecule more resistant to metabolic degradation and decrease its clearance rate.

DEFINITION OF A GLUCOCORTICOID

The term *glucocorticoid* was coined to denote the glucose-regulating properties of these steroids.[1,4] However, these steroids have many actions that do not involve carbohydrate metabolism. As discussed in Structure-Activity Relations of Glucocorticoids, above, a class of proteins termed glucocorticoid receptors mediates these actions. Thus, similar to the way that drugs such as α- and β-adrenergic agonists are classified, it seems preferable to define adrenal steroid actions in terms of the receptors that mediate them.[4] Thus, a glucocorticoid effect is one mediated through a class of receptors termed glucocorticoid receptors. If, as discussed above, there is heterogeneity within the glucocorticoid receptor class that is functionally significant, then further subclassification may be necessary. In addition, as discussed earlier, certain glucocorticoids can also act by binding to other classes of receptors, for instance, through mineralocorticoid receptors, in which case the action would be termed mineralocorticoid even though it might have no relation to salt balance.

PHYSIOLOGICAL ACTIONS OF MINERALOCORTICOIDS

In humans, mineralocorticoid actions are predominantly due to aldosterone, cortisol, and occasionally DOC. In addition, a number of other steroids with mineralocorticoid activity, also produced by the gland (see below and Steroid Biosynthesis, above), are under investigation as potential mineralocorticoids under certain circumstances. Mineralocorticoids regulate ion balance and act on fewer tissues than the glucocorticoids; mineralocorticoid-responsive tissues include kidney, gut, salivary glands, sweat glands, vascular endothelium, brain, and possibly mammary gland and pituitary.[249,427–431] A major theme in these actions is a concerted effort to conserve sodium and to eliminate potassium and hydrogen ions.

Kidney

The kidney is the most important known site of mineralocorticoid action. Most if not all of the physiologically relevant effects occur in the connecting segment, cortical collecting tubules, and medullary collecting tubules.[249,427] Possible actions elsewhere in the kidney have been considered, but these appear either to be physiologically unimportant or to occur only at high aldosterone concentrations, in which case they are mediated through glucocorticoid receptors.[432]

Mineralocorticoids promote the reabsorption of sodium and the secretion of potassium in the cortical collecting tubules and possibly the connecting segment, and hydrogen ion secretion in the medullary collecting tubules.[249,427,433–437] Aldosterone also has a permissive effect on the osmotic water flux response to vasopressin in the cortical collecting tubule.[427] These effects can be observed after a lag of about 30 min to 2 h and require protein and RNA synthesis.[427] In mineralocorticoid deficiency states there is sodium loss, potassium retention, and decreased renal acid excretion, leading to dehydration, hyponatremia, hyperkalemia, and metabolic acidosis.[438] Conversely, in mineralocorticoid excess states there is an increase in total body sodium, hypokalemia, and a tendency to alkalosis (Chap. 14).[432]

Only a fraction of the filtered sodium is reabsorbed in response to aldosterone. Nevertheless, this fraction can have marked influences on electrolyte balance. The magnitude of the observed influence of aldosterone is dependent on the amount of solute delivered to the kidney.[432] Ordinarily, a decrease in urinary sodium excretion can be detected but this might not be observed with heavy salt loading, because the total reabsorption relative to the quantity of sodium passing through the cortical collecting tubules is minor.

The amount of sodium retention that can occur in response to an excess of mineralocorticoids in subjects with normal cardiac and renal function is limited.[432,439,440] Thus, in mineralocorticoid excess states, after an initial period of positive sodium balance, the body then adjusts to the excess sodium (the "escape" phenomenon, see Chap. 14) by reabsorbing less of the filtered sodium. This decrease occurs mostly in the proximal tubule, so that sodium intake ultimately equals excretion.[439] This may also explain why aldosterone excess does not ordinarily result in edema (Chap. 14).[439] Patients with edema from heart failure, cirrhosis of the liver, or nephrosis cannot respond normally and do not escape;[440] thus, secondary aldosteronism, when present in these conditions, contributes to the fluid retention and edema. The mineralocorticoid influence on potassium excretion does not show this escape phenomenon.[439,440]

The escape phenomenon may in part be mediated through secondary increases in ANF levels (Chap. 14), although other factors may contribute. ANF levels increase in response to volume expansion, as occurs after mineralocorticoid treatment, and they increase in dogs under conditions of escape.[441] This hormone produces natriuresis (Chap. 14). Cardiac output also increases under these conditions; this can increase GFR with secondary increases in sodium excretion.[441] This can be augmented, especially under conditions of volume excess. Volume increase caused by sodium retention also depresses proximal sodium reabsorption, although this is partly compensated by distal tubular reabsorption.[439] This effect can be independent of increases in GFR,[439] and may be due in part to an increase in renal interstitial pressure that lowers the tubular capacity for sodium reabsorption.[439] Urinary PGs and kallikrein increase in concentration after mineralocorticoid administration, have natriuretic actions, and also could conceivably participate in escape.[439] Finally, although escape can occur in the absence of afferent and efferent neural pathways, it is conceivable that the increased vascular volume stimulates volume receptors that decrease renal adrenergic activity, and that this decreases sodium transport directly and through renal vasodilatory mechanisms.[439]

The stimulation of potassium loss by mineralocorticoids depends largely on the sodium intake.[427,432,440,441] The sodium reabsorbed by the distal tubule increases the electronegativity of the lumen in relation to the peritubular fluid; this is important for passive diffusion of potassium ion into the tubule from which it is excreted. Thus, when there is sufficient delivery of sodium to the distal tubules, a kaliuretic effect of aldosterone is readily observed. By contrast, when sodium intake is restricted, there is minimal delivery of sodium to the distal tubule, since it is mostly reabsorbed in the proximal tubule. In this case, the necessary electronegativity is not generated and potassium excretion is not stimulated. This lack of a prominent kaliuretic effect can be apparent when aldosterone is present in excess in patients with cardiac failure, nephrosis, or cirrhosis who have a decreased GFR and increased proximal tubular reabsorption of sodium.

Changes in sodium and potassium concentrations do not always parallel each other. Further, there is not a stoichiometric relationship between sodium reabsorption and potassium excretion.[427,440] Potassium excretion may increase prior to an effect on sodium and vice versa.[427]

In addition to their role in the ordinary maintenance of potassium balance, mineralocorticoids also participate in the defense against chronic hyperkalemia.[427,440,442] Increased aldosterone secretion in response to hyperkalemia increases potassium excretion.

Several factors account for effects of mineralocorticoids on renal acid production. First, aldosterone produces a net decrease in urinary pH and therefore an increase in urinary acidification without much change in titratable acid.[339,443] This effect is due to an increase in the tubular fluid-to-blood pH gradients across the distal nephron and predominantly across the inner stripe of the outer medulla.[339,443] These effects on hydrogen ion can occur independently of those on sodium and potassium ions. Second, some of the sodium reabsorbed in response to aldosterone is exchanged for hydrogen ion, and this accelerates urinary loss of acid.[443,444] Thus, hydrogen ion loss due to mineralocorticoid excess can be decreased by reducing intake of sodium and thereby its delivery to the distal nephron.[443,444] Third, there is some movement of hydrogen ions into cells in exchange for the potassium lost in the urine.[443,444] Fourth, the potassium deficiency increases hydrogen ion excretion by increasing ammonia production and by decreasing the exchange of Na^+ for K^+ that enhances the exchange of Na^+ for H^+.[443,444] The production of alkalosis is blunted by the increased extracellular volume that suppresses bicarbonate reabsorption.[443,444] In adrenal insufficiency the opposite effect occurs and there are increases in bicarbonate removal and urinary pH and decreased excretion of titratable acid and ammonia.[444]

Mineralocorticoids also influence magnesium and calcium ion excretion.[440] Serum Mg^{2+} and Ca^{2+} concentrations are elevated in adrenal insufficiency. In primary aldosteronism magnesium concentrations are generally normal even though urinary magnesium excretion is increased. There is also increased urinary calcium excretion in primary aldosteronism. The mineralocorticoid actions increasing the excretion of magnesium and calcium are probably due to the sodium retention which decreases proximal tubular reabsorption of these ions.

Mineralocorticoids are not known to affect directly water excretion, GFR, renal plasma flow, or renin production. However, their effects on sodium and water retention with increased extracellular fluid volume indirectly increase GFR and renal plasma flow and suppress plasma renin concentration (Chap. 14).

In addition, these steroids (and also glucocorticoids) can enhance the vasopressin actions increasing water permeability.[427]

Mineralocorticoids increase the levels of urinary kallikrein, the enzyme that cleaves bradykinin from kininogen (Chap. 31). Urinary kallikrein level is increased in primary aldosteronism but not in most other forms of hypertension. Although the role of this influence is not known, bradykinin generated as a result of kallikrein action may block sodium reabsorption and serve to blunt aldosterone action.[445]

Extrarenal Tissues

Mineralocorticoid actions on extrarenal tissues, although probably of less importance in regulating ion balance, nonetheless contribute to concerted actions to retain sodium and excrete potassium. Mineralocorticoids decrease sodium excretion and enhance potassium loss in the ileum, colon, skin, and salivary glands.[440,446] Thus, patients with primary aldosteronism lose potassium in the stool, have a decreased level of stool sodium, have an increased potential difference across the colonic epithelium, and have a decreased salivary Na^+/K^+ ratio. In arterial smooth muscle the steroids stimulate passive and sodium pump–dependent transmembrane movements.[428] Direct actions on the heart and salt appetite have been proposed,[440] but the possibilities that the observed effects are indirect or that they are due to glucocorticoid actions of the steroids have not been excluded. Indirect influences of aldosterone outside the kidney (e.g., on blood pressure) are discussed in Chap. 14. Actions of glucocorticoids through mineralocorticoid receptors in brain are discussed under Molecular Mechanisms of Glucocorticoid Hormone Action, above).

MOLECULAR MECHANISMS OF MINERALOCORTICOID ACTION

The early molecular events in aldosterone action are similar to those of other classes of steroids (see above, Fig. 12-22, and Chap. 5). Thus, "cytosol" receptors for aldosterone are present in mineralocorticoid-responsive tissues; these have been best characterized in kidney and toad bladder.[427,431,432,437,447] They are similar to glucocorticoid receptors in their physical properties but can be distinguished from them by some differences, particularly in their binding characteristics. For example, they have a much higher affinity for certain mineralocorticoids such as aldosterone and DOC than do glucocorticoid receptors[427] and have a low affinity

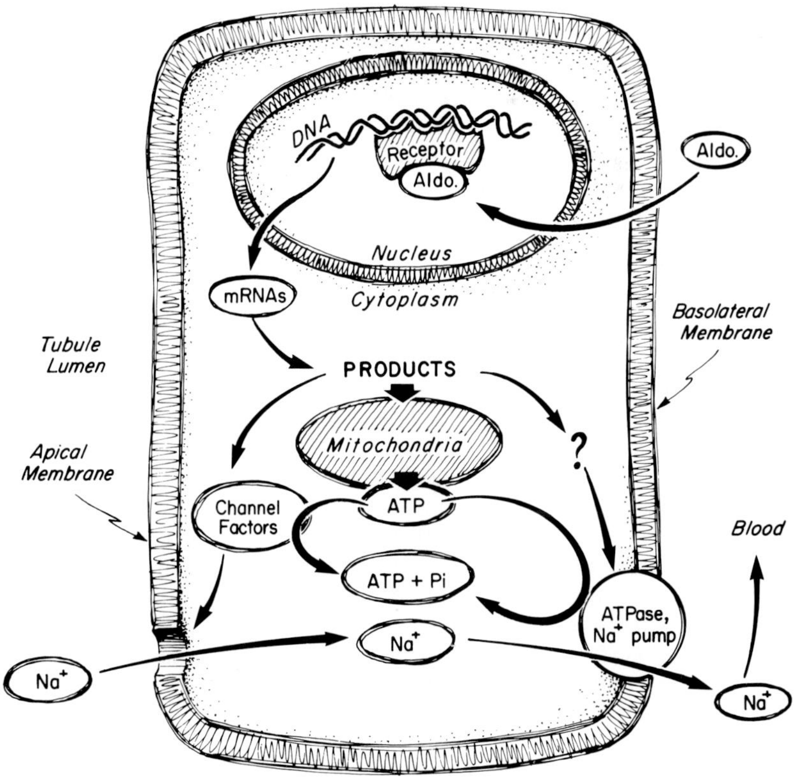

FIGURE 12-22 Steps in mineralocorticoid action. Illustrated are the early molecular events leading to the association of the aldosterone (Aldo.)-receptor complex with DNA with consequent induction of mRNAs that encode proteins that could affect the sodium channel, ATP generation, and Na^+ pumping activity.

for certain glucocorticoid receptor–specific compounds such as RU-26988.[429] Interestingly, they have a relatively high affinity (albeit lower than for aldosterone and DOC) for certain "classic" glucocorticoids such as cortisol, dexamethasone, and corticosterone.[447] In the kidney, these receptors are located in the branched collecting tubules, the cortical collecting tubules, and the outer medullary collecting tubules.[437] In intact cells, they bind aldosterone and DOC with a K_d of around 0.5 to 1 nM and cortisol with a K_d of around 50 nM,[447] although in isolated preparations the relative affinity for cortisol is higher.[229-231] The steroid enters the cell and binds to the specific receptor proteins; the receptor-mineralocorticoid complex then binds to the nuclear chromatin.[427] This probably results in an increase (or decrease) in the transcription of particular genes. Although this has not been clearly documented, actions of aldosterone do require RNA and protein synthesis.[432] Presumably, the protein products of these mineralocorticoid-regulated mRNAs then mediate the mineralocorticoid hormone responses.

As discussed earlier, the kidney is also a glucocorticoid target and contains glucocorticoid receptors. In addition, it contains a class of CBG-like sites (possibly with some differences) that occur at concentrations up to 100-fold those of the other receptors; these sites have a high affinity for cortisol and corticosterone but not aldosterone and other steroids.[229,448] Although these sites have been proposed to be receptors, there is no direct evidence that they are receptors; instead, they appear to modulate the accessibility to the mineralocorticoid receptors of steroids such as corticosterone (in the rat) and if extrapolated to the human, cortisol. Thus, when mineralocorticoid receptors are separated from this protein, their affinities for corticosterone and cortisol are, respectively, equal to and around one-tenth that of aldosterone.[229-231] The free cortisol concentrations in plasma are 100 times those of aldosterone in basal conditions. Thus, left unchecked, cortisol would be the major occupant of the mineralocorticoid receptor. The 50- to 100-fold lower apparent affinity for cortisol relative to aldosterone (reported in the preceding paragraph) appears to be due to the fact that these CBG-like proteins sequester cortisol and decrease its availability for receptor occupancy.[229-231,447] Since the proteins do not bind aldosterone appreciably, this steroid is more available for receptor occupancy and for mineralocorticoid actions. Nevertheless, even in the presence of such sequestration, cortisol may occupy the mineralocorticoid receptor to some extent.[447] However, when aldosterone levels are stimulated by postural or other stimuli, this steroid would be the major occupant of the receptor.

Sodium bathing the luminal surface passively enters the renal cell through channels in the apical membrane. The intracellular sodium ions are then pumped into the interstitial fluid on the serosal side of the cell by an Na^+,K^+-dependent ATPase. ATP is required to drive the pump and for maintenance of the Na^+ channels in the apical membrane. Aldosterone may act in three ways (Fig. 12-22):[249,427,432] (1) by increasing the cellular permeability to Na^+ by affecting channels in the apical membrane; (2) by affecting the energy-generating system and thus increasing cellular energy; and (3) by affecting the pump.

The hormone does increase the number of Na^+ specific apical membrane channels,[427,432] with an increase in the conductance of the apical membrane and an increased number of conducting sodium channels.[449] An aldosterone-regulated protein recruits these channels from a pool of nonconducting channels. This may be the earliest and primary effect. In toad bladder, aldosterone stimulates phospholipase activity, fatty acid synthesis, and acyltransferase activity.[427] These actions may affect membrane phospholipids and ion transport (Chap. 5) and may thereby mediate aldosterone action.

With respect to energy generation, aldosterone increases the renal $NADH/NAD^+$ ratio and the activities of mitochondrial enzymes involved in ATP generation, in particular citrate synthase,[427,451-453] and, in the toad bladder, cellular ATP levels.[450] These changes have been correlated kinetically with effects on Na^+ transport and may be due to increased enzyme synthesis. Thus, the effect of the hormone increasing the potential to generate ATP may drive both the Na^+ pump and affect the number of active Na^+ channels.

Aldosterone also increases the incorporation of riboflavin into renal flavin nucleotides and analogues of riboflavin that inhibit this incorporation also block the antinatriuretic effects of the steroid; more work is needed to determine the significance of these observations.[249]

Aldosterone also increases the Na^+,K^+-ATPase activity of the basolateral membranes of the cortical collecting tubule.[427,433-436,451,452] This may be due to an augmentation of the activity of pump sites, rather than an increase in Na^+,K^+-ATPase synthesis. Whether it involves the direct actions of an aldosterone-induced protein or is a secondary effect, occurring following initial effects on the apical membrane and possibly mediated by the increased sodium entry, is controversial. Nevertheless, this influence would further enhance sodium transport. These changes in the cortical collecting tubules are also associated with aldosterone-regulated increases in the basolateral cell membrane areas in which the Na^+,K^+-ATPase enzyme units are located.

Thus, several aldosterone-regulated proteins appear to act in a coordinated manner to stimulate sodium transport. Several other aldosterone-regulated proteins have also been identified,[427] and some of these could also affect energy generation, the apical channels, or other processes.

Much less is known about the way that aldosterone stimulates potassium or hydrogen ion secretion. The Na^+,K^+-ATPase action affects K^+ excretion by exchanging K^+ for Na^+. However, since effects on Na^+ can occur in the absence of influences on K^+, there might also be effects on a potassium pump or on the permeability of the luminal membrane to K^+.[427]

The effects on hydrogen ion appear to be exerted predominantly in the medullary collecting tubule and in this respect are independent of effects on Na^+, although the factors mentioned above are operative.[427] Suggested targets for aldosterone effects on hydrogen ion include effects on glutamine entry into or exit from mitochondria, on mitochondrial glutaminase, and on cytoplasmic PEPCK.[427]

MINERALOCORTICOID AGONISTS AND ANTAGONISTS

Naturally occurring and synthetic steroids can have mineralocorticoid agonist activity. Aldosterone, the predominant mineralocorticoid, contains an aldehyde at position 18 that is in equilibrium with the 11-hydroxyl function, forming a cyclic 11,18-hemiacetyl (Fig. 12-23). Cortisol, corticosterone, DOC, 19-nor-DOC, 19-OH-androstenedione, and other 18- and 19-substituted derivatives of these steroids have mineralocorticoid agonist activities (Chap. 14). Several synthetic steroids have mineralocorticoid activity. Of these, fludrocortisone (9α-fluorocortisol) is extremely potent and ordinarily is the steroid chosen for replacement mineralocorticoid therapy. Aldosterone and DOC are not suitable, since they are readily degraded by the liver after absorption (Chap. 14). Carbenoxolone, used to treat peptic ulcer, has mineralocorticoid activity which accounts for its principal side effects.[453]

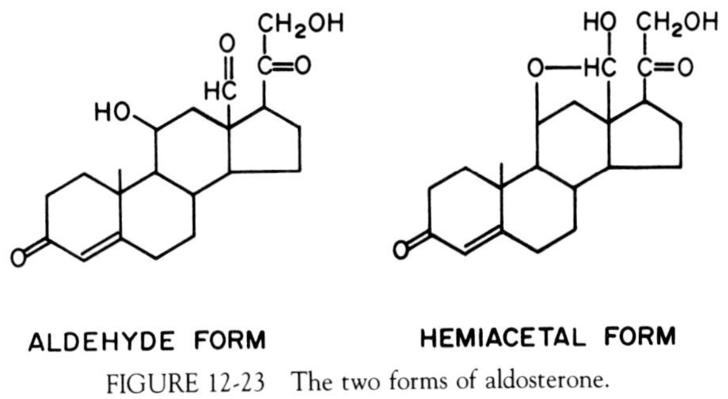

FIGURE 12-23 The two forms of aldosterone.

A number of compounds have mineralocorticoid antagonist activity. Progesterone is the most potent naturally occurring antagonist, but it probably has a minor physiological role in this respect, except possibly during the third trimester of pregnancy, in which progesterone concentrations rise to extremely high values (see Chap. 17).[454] Spironolactone is a steroid analogue and is the compound used clinically as a mineralocorticoid antagonist (Chap. 15). Mineralocorticoid antagonists competitively inhibit the binding of agonists by the receptors,[427] and as in the case of glucocorticoid receptors it appears that these receptor-antagonist complexes do not bind to the nuclear chromatin.[427]

The extent to which cortisol, DOC, 18- and 19-substituted derivatives of these steroids, and 19-OH-androstenedione contribute to mineralocorticoid activity has not been clarified. Radioreceptor assays suggest that, under ordinary conditions, almost all of the mineralocorticoid activity of human plasma can be accounted for by aldosterone and cortisol.[455,456] However, this may not be true in certain cases of hypertension (Chap. 14). Cortisol concentrations in plasma range from 100 to 5000 times higher than aldosterone concentrations, but the percentage of cortisol free in the plasma is much less than that of aldosterone (about 7 percent vs. 45 percent, see above). If the free fraction is assumed to be active, the effective free concentrations of cortisol are probably 15 to 750 times those of aldosterone. Considering the sequestration of cortisol by the CBG-like proteins discussed earlier, the effective relative binding of cortisol to the mineralocorticoid receptors may be about 1 percent that of aldosterone. In this case, the relative contribution of cortisol to mineralocorticoid receptor occupancy may vary from 15 to 750 percent that of aldosterone. It is therefore possible that, when aldosterone levels are higher, for instance standing or in the afternoon, cortisol would contribute little to mineralocorticoid receptor occupancy. By contrast, when aldosterone levels are low and cortisol is high, as occurs in the early morning in the supine subject, cortisol might account for more occupancy of the mineralocorticoid receptor. However, the net importance of aldosterone may be greater than these estimates, because glucocorticoids may have actions on sodium balance (discussed earlier) that mask their mineralocorticoid effects. Further, it has not been established that cortisol is a full rather than a partial agonist. DOC circulates at concentrations similar to those of aldosterone (see above and Chap. 14) and binds to mineralocorticoid receptors as tightly as does aldosterone.[456] However, because less than 5 percent of the circulating DOC is free compared to 45 percent of aldosterone,[218] it is likely that this steroid contributes negligibly to mineralocorticoid action under physiological circumstances. The physiological importance of 19-nor-DOC and 19-OH-androstenedione are currently under investigation and are potentially significant; since 19-nor-DOC is produced in the kidney, its plasma concentrations may not reflect its levels in the renal target tissue.[37,175,176] 19-OH-androstenedione is present in the circulation in concentrations about half those of aldosterone, although its plasma binding has not been reported.[37] The role of various steroids in mineralocorticoid-excess syndromes is discussed in Chap. 14.

DEFINITION OF A MINERALOCORTICOID

Because both glucocorticoids and mineralocorticoids affect salt balance, it is important to define the term mineralocorticoid. As already mentioned, there is a class of binding proteins that appears to mediate the actions of these steroids on ion movement, and these receptors can be distinguished from glucocorticoid receptors. Thus, analogous to the case with glucocorticoids, "mineralocorticoid" actions are referred to as those mediated through these receptors. This would also apply to actions of glucocorticoids on these receptors, for instance in brain (see above). Also, it is possible that other receptors mediating the actions of sodium-retaining steroids will be found. For example, some actions of steroids on sodium retention in rats[98a] or hypertension in sheep (Chap. 14) may not occur through classic mechanisms.

ACTIONS OF ADRENAL ANDROGENS AND ESTROGENS

The biological actions of the androgens are described in Chap. 16. The intrinsic androgenicity of androstenedione, DHEA, and DHEA-S is minimal, and their activity in physiological and pathological states is due to their peripheral conversion to testosterone (Chaps. 4 and 16) and DHT (Chaps. 4 and 16).[251] Whereas certain actions of the androgens can be mediated by testosterone, others, such as beard growth, receding of hairline, and full development of genitalia apparently require DHT.

Since most androgenic actions are due to testosterone and DHT, an estimate of the androgenic contribution of the adrenal is indicated by the relative contribution to the blood production rate of these two steroids by androstenedione (which, along with its precursors, is primarily of adrenal origin). As mentioned above, androstenedione can arise from DHEA-S and DHEA (Fig. 12-3), but it can also be formed from testosterone. In women, testosterone itself is made in low quantity, and therefore less than 5 percent of the blood production of androstenedione comes from testosterone.[44] In men, only about 5 percent of the testosterone is from extratesticular sources (see Chap. 16) and around 20 percent of the androstenedione can come from testosterone.[44] In women, a small amount of testosterone is produced (0.26 mg per day); about two-thirds of this comes from androstenedione.[44] Thus, it is thought that in normal circumstances the adrenal contributes greatly to the level of androgenic activity in women. The physiological role of androgens in women is poorly understood, but they may play some role in sexuality and libido.[44] In men, the contribution of the adrenals to the plasma testosterone content (production = 5.8 mg per day) is less than 5 percent.[44]

Other metabolites of the androgens are thought to have little androgenic activity; however, etiocholanolone injection can result in a transient fever and local inflammatory reaction and an increase in δ-aminolevulinate synthetase, an important enzyme in heme biosynthesis.[44] The importance of these effects is uncertain, as quantities (e.g., 25 mg) considerably in excess of those produced naturally are required.[44]

The biological actions of the estrogens are discussed in Chap. 17. The adrenal contribution to plasma estrogens results largely from the peripheral conversion of androstenedione.[46,457–459] In normal women, this accounts for less than 4 percent of the estrogen supply.[46] However, in postmenopausal women, the adrenal is the major source of estrogens.[47,457] The peripheral conversion occurs in subcutaneous fat, hair follicles, and mammary tissue.[46,458,459] In the male, about half of the estradiol comes from testosterone of testicular origin; most of the remainder comes from estrone that is derived mainly from androstenedione, although a small amount of estradiol is produced by the testis.[460] The adrenal production of estradiol is negligible.[460] In the fetus, a major role of the adrenal may be to provide a source for estrogens (discussed above and in Chap. 17).

LABORATORY EVALUATION OF ADRENOCORTICAL FUNCTION

Specific plasma assays allow precise determination of adrenal hormones, including the major glucocorticoids, mineralocorticoids, androgens, and estrogens. In many instances these assays have simplified the evaluation of adrenal dysfunction and have supplanted previously used determinations of urinary metabolites. In addition, plasma concentrations of the trophic hormones, i.e., ACTH and angiotensin, and of renin, which control adrenal secretion, can be determined with precision. However, urinary assays and in particular measurement of the 24-h urinary free cortisol can be useful in certain circumstances. The majority of the plasma steroid methods described measure the total hormone concentration; therefore, alterations in plasma binding proteins must be considered in their interpretation. The plasma concentrations of the adrenal hormones and their trophic factors ACTH, renin, and angiotensin II (Chap. 14) vary widely in normal individuals and in both endocrine and nonendocrine disorders. Thus, isolated plasma measurements are frequently not reliable in establishing definitive diagnoses and must be interpreted with regard to the time of the sample and the clinical situation. In general, more precise information is obtained by determining integrated assessments of hormone production and the responses of these hormones to appropriate stimulation and suppression tests (Fig. 12-24).

Plasma Cortisol and Related Steroids

Determination of the plasma cortisol concentration is essential in the evaluation of adrenal function. Current methods include competitive protein binding radioassay,[461,462] radioimmunoassay,[463,464] and measurement by high-pressure liquid chromatography (HPLC).[465,466] These methods have replaced the classic Porter-Silber method (adapted for plasma), which measures 17,21-dihydroxy-20-ketosteroids,[467,468] and are supplanting the fluorimetric determination of plasma 11-hydroxycorticosteroids.[469,470] Total plasma cortisol can also be measured by radioreceptor assay.[471] Other methods measure the biologically active fraction of plasma cortisol not bound to CBG ("plasma free cortisol"),[472,473] and this can also be estimated by measuring cortisol in saliva.[474] These latter assays may ultimately replace determinations of total plasma cortisol.

CORTISOL

Competitive Protein-Binding Radioassay

This assay permits rapid and precise determination of cortisol in small volumes of plasma. An extract of plasma is incubated with [^{3}H]cortisol and CBG. The plasma cortisol concentration is then determined by the extent of inhibition by the sample of [^{3}H]cortisol binding compared to a standard curve.[461] Thus, the procedure is similar to radioimmunoassay except that CBG is used instead of an antibody to cortisol.[461,462]

CBG also has a high affinity for other steroids, such as cortisone, corticosterone, 11-deoxycortisol, DOC, 21-deoxycortisol, progesterone, and 17α-hydroxyprogesterone (Table 12-5).[461,462] These are ordinarily present in negligible quantities and thus this assay usually is a valid estimate of plasma cortisol. However, in certain conditions levels of these cross-reacting steroids are elevated. These include pregnancy (progesterone), congenital adrenal hyperplasia (17α-hydroxyprogesterone, progesterone, corticosterone, DOC, 21-deoxycortisol, or 11-deoxycortisol), and adrenal carcinoma (11-deoxycortisol). The synthetic steroids prednisolone (also derived from prednisone) and methylprednisolone also have substantial affinity for CBG (Table 12-5) and thus cross-react in this assay system.

Although it is rarely necessary to do so, in cases where any of these potential competitors is present in significant quantity, greater specificity can be obtained by first separating them from cortisol prior to the assay. This can be achieved by solvent partition or by thin layer or column chromatography.[461,475] These modifications not only permit greater specificity of cortisol measurement, but they have also been used for simultaneous determination of the other steroids (see below).[475] A major advantage of this assay is the virtual absence of interference by other hormones and commonly used drugs and medications.[461]

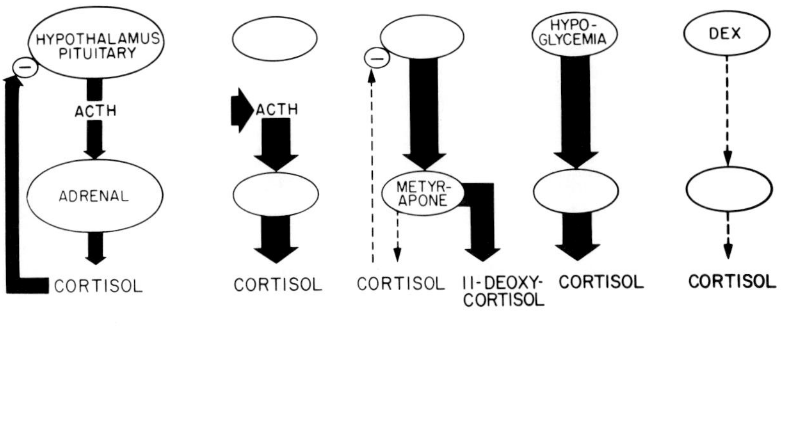

FIGURE 12-24 Tests used to evaluate the hypothalamic-pituitary-adrenal axis. The thickness of the arrow indicates the relative quantities of compounds present if the test is normal. Dotted lines show blocked pathway. See text for details.

Radioimmunoassay

Radioimmunoassay is also used extensively for the determination of plasma cortisol; its sensitivity allows the use of small plasma volumes. In early assays, the antisera varied greatly in specificity and exhibited cross-reactivity with 11-deoxycortisol, 21-deoxycortisol, 17α-hydroxyprogesterone, corticosterone, DOC, progesterone, cortisone, prednisone, and prednisolone.[436,476,477] However, antibodies are now available which have limited cross-reactivity with other steroids.[464,478,479] Because of variability of specificity, the characteristics of each antiserum must be determined. If a specific antibody is not available, steroids of interest can be separated as described above.[461,475,477] Commonly used drugs and medications also do not interfere with the radioimmunoassay.

Liquid Chromatography (HPLC)

In this assay cortisol is separated from other steroids by liquid chromatography and the concentration of the eluted cortisol is then measured by spectrophotometry or fluorometry.[465,466] The assay using fluorometry is not interfered with by drugs and medications nor does it detect prednisone, prednisolone, cortisone, dexamethasone, or other common natural and synthetic steroids.[466] This method is very accurate and reliable.

Fluorimetric Assay

Fluorimetric assay first allowed determination of plasma cortisol with ease and rapidity in relatively small volumes of plasma (1 to 2 ml);[469] it is being gradually supplanted by other methods. It depends on the fluorescence of Δ^4-steroids with 3-keto groups and steroids with 20-keto and 11β- and 21-hydroxy groups and is a measurement of plasma 11-hydroxycorticosteroid levels.[480] Thus, corticosterone and 21-deoxycortisol are also measured; however, except with congenital adrenal biosynthetic defects and certain adrenal carcinomas, these steroids do not circulate in significant amounts. Synthetic steroids such as prednisone, prednisolone, triamcinolone, dexamethasone, and betamethasone do not significantly interfere. Thus, the level of fluorimetric plasma 11-hydroxycorticosteroids usually reflects the plasma cortisol concentration.

The accuracy of this test is limited somewhat by nonspecific background fluorescence in plasma, which gives an average reading of 2 to 3 μg/dl of cortisol; thus, there is some overestimation of the cortisol concentration, particularly in the lower ranges.[469,470,480] This assay is also interfered with by several drugs and compounds which fluoresce, including spironolactone, mepacrine, fusidic acid, niacin, quinidine, and heparin preparations which contain benzyl alcohol. Nonspecific plasma fluorescence may also be present in uremic or jaundiced patients. Despite these limitations, the method is useful in the diagnosis of abnormal adrenal function.

Other Plasma Cortisol Methods

The radioreceptor assay depends on the ability of steroids in the sample to compete with a radiolabeled tracer steroid (e.g., [^{3}H]dexamethasone) for binding to glucocorticoid receptors.[471] The assay estimates the summed products of the affinities and concentrations of all glucocorticoid agonists and antagonists present. It usually reflects the total plasma cortisol concentration, since other steroids which bind appreciably are present in negligible amounts. The assay can also be used to measure the plasma concentrations of the exogenously administered steroids used for glucocorticoid therapy.[471]

Although measurements of the unbound fraction of circulating cortisol (plasma free cortisol) give a more accurate estimate of biologically active steroid levels, these methods have not come into general use because of their technical difficulty. The methods determine free cortisol after its separation from the bound steroid by equilibrium dialysis, gel filtration, or ultrafiltration.[471,472] Free cortisol can also be measured by a radioligand competition assay in which the ability of steroids in undiluted plasma to compete with [^{3}H]dexamethasone for binding to glucocorticoid receptors in intact cells is assessed.[473] Estimation of cortisol in saliva has also been shown to accurately reflect the plasma free fraction.[474]

Interpretation of Plasma Cortisol Determinations

Variations in plasma cortisol levels due to circadian changes, episodic release, and stimulation of the hypothalamic-pituitary-adrenal axis must be considered in evaluating the diagnostic significance of plasma cortisol determinations, and limit the usefulness of single measurements.[139,481–483] Subnormal or elevated levels should arouse suspicion of adrenal hypo- or hyperfunction, but in general more specific testing of the hypothalamic-pituitary-adrenal axis is required to establish diagnoses. Plasma cortisol levels are not altered with advanced age.[484]

The method used must be considered in interpreting the results of plasma cortisol determinations. Morning (8:00 A.M.) plasma cortisol levels measured by either competitive protein binding or radioimmunoassay average 10 to 12 μg/dl with a range of 3 to 20 μg/dl,[463,475,483] and values at 4 to 6 P.M. approximate 50 percent of morning levels. In one study using the competitive protein binding assay, values were 10.4 ± 4 (mean ± SD) at 8:00 A.M. compared to 4.0 ± 2.0 at 8:00 P.M., and less than 3 μg/dl between 10:00 P.M. and 2:00 A.M.[483] Mean plasma cortisol levels determined by the fluorimetric method at 7:00 to 8:00 A.M. average approximately 20 μg/dl (range 5 to 25 μg/dl),[470,481] at 9:00 A.M. are 13 to 14 μg/dl,[469,470] and at 9:00 P.M. are approximately 8 μg/dl.[483] Although the normal values reported for this assay are substantially higher than with competitive protein binding or radioimmunoassay, direct comparison of the fluorimetric and competitive protein binding assays in the same plasma specimens shows an excellent correlation except that values are approximately 2 to 3 μg/dl higher using the fluorimetric method (Fig. 12-25).[471,485]

Plasma cortisol is appropriately elevated with acute illness, trauma, or surgery[154,486] and levels tend to be elevated in patients with depression, alcoholism, severe anxiety, starvation, anorexia nervosa, and chronic renal failure.[487-490] Since the generally available assays measure total plasma steroid levels, the cortisol concentration is elevated in conditions with increased CBG levels, such as pregnancy and estrogen (including oral contraceptive) therapy.[162,215-217,487] In these instances plasma cortisol levels may be as high as 40 to 60 μg/dl and they may take several weeks to return to normal following delivery or cessation of estrogen therapy.[216,487] CBG levels may also be increased congenitally and in hyperthyroidism, diabetes, and certain hematological disorders;[217,225] decreased CBG levels also occur congenitally and in hypothyroidism, liver disease, nephrotic syndrome, multiple myeloma, and obesity.[215-217] CBG binding capacity may be measured in plasma, although this assay is not generally available.[215]

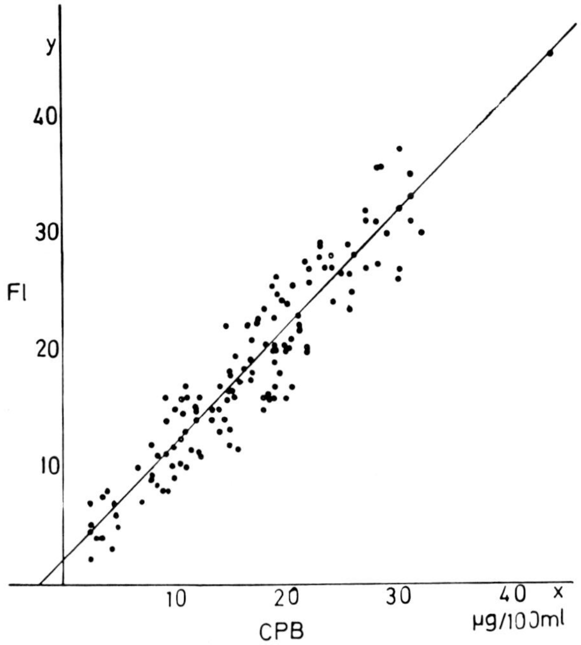

FIGURE 12-25 Correlation between plasma corticosteroid concentration in 131 samples measured by the competitive protein binding (CPB) and fluorimetric (FI) assays. Values are given in micrograms per deciliter. (*From Gore and Lester.*[485])

DETERMINATION OF OTHER PLASMA STEROIDS

Plasma androgen assays are discussed below and DOC and aldosterone assays are reviewed in Chap. 14. The precursors of both cortisol and aldosterone can be assayed in plasma, although these methods are not generally available. These steroids include pregnenolone, 17α-hydroxypregnenolone, progesterone, 17α-hydroxyprogesterone, DOC, corticosterone, and 11-deoxycortisol. The steroids are first separated by solvent extraction and/or chromatography and their concentrations are then measured by either competitive protein binding or radioimmunoassay;[461,475,491,492] their levels can also be measured by HPLC. The concentrations of these steroids may be elevated in the congenital adrenal biosynthetic defects (discussed below), in patients with adrenal carcinoma, and after administration of inhibitors of adrenal steroid biosynthesis (Table 12-3).

Plasma ACTH and Related Peptides

Specific and sensitive assays of plasma ACTH have been developed[493,494] and have simplified the diagnosis of pituitary-adrenal dysfunction. Sensitive bioassays have also been described, but they are technically difficult and have been largely restricted to research use. These bioassays measure plasma ACTH concentration by radioreceptor assay,[495] steroid response of dispersed adrenal cells,[496] or extremely sensitive cytochemical bioassay.[497] Thus, radioimmunoassay is the method in clinical use, but it is less available than methods for other polypeptide hormones. Many assays require extraction of plasma prior to assay, therefore 1 to 5 ml of plasma is needed. ACTH is unstable in plasma, is inactivated at room temperature, and adheres strongly to glass. Careful sample collection and preparation are essential; specimens must be collected with heparin or EDTA in plastic tubes on ice, centrifuged in the cold within an hour of collection and then frozen until assayed.

Antisera have been produced which react with

various sites on ACTH, i.e., antisera may react with the NH_2-terminal or COOH-terminal sequences or against the entire molecule.[498,499] In general, an antiserum should be chosen which reacts with the biologically active 1–24 sequence of human ACTH in order to reduce detection of biologically inactive fragments. With amino-terminal antisera the ratio of immunoreactive to bioassayable ACTH approximates 1.3 to 1.5 in normal subjects and in patients with untreated Cushing's disease.[500,501] Greater immunoreactivity than bioactivity is seen following hypoglycemia, metyrapone administration, and ACTH infusion and in patients with the ectopic ACTH syndrome.[501] The normal range of plasma ACTH concentration with specific assays is 20 to 120 pg/ml in the morning; the sensitivity of these assays is 5 to 20 pg/ml.[502] In addition to the same factors discussed above (in Plasma Cortisol and Related Steroids) (episodic secretion, circadian variation), the status of adrenal secretion must be considered in the evaluation of plasma ACTH levels.

Plasma ACTH levels are of greatest diagnostic utility in the differential diagnosis of spontaneous adrenal disorders. In the presence of subnormal adrenal responsiveness to exogenous ACTH, plasma ACTH levels greater than 250 pg/ml confirm primary adrenal insufficiency, whereas a level of less than 50 pg/ml is consistent with pituitary ACTH deficiency (secondary hypoadrenalism).[503]

In Cushing's syndrome, a suppressed plasma ACTH level (less than 20 pg/ml) is diagnostic of a primary glucocorticoid-producing adrenal tumor. In contrast, patients with pituitary ACTH hypersecretion have plasma ACTH levels in the normal to moderately elevated range (40 to 200 pg/ml) and, in general, patients with the ectopic ACTH syndrome have markedly elevated plasma ACTH concentrations (200 to $>$ 1,000 pg/ml).[502,504] However, the plasma ACTH level does not always correctly differentiate pituitary from ectopic sources of ACTH hypersecretion since a considerable overlap occurs in the range of 100 to 200 pg/ml.[504]

Radioimmunoassays have also been developed for human β-lipotropin; normal concentrations are 20 to 200 pg/ml.[505-507] β-LPH and ACTH are secreted simultaneously and thus the circadian variations of β-LPH follow those of ACTH.[507,508] β-LPH levels also respond to hypoglycemia, dexamethasone, and other factors that influence ACTH secretion.[507,508] β-LPH has a longer half-life and greater stability in plasma than ACTH; in addition, immunoassays are less difficult than for ACTH. However, this assay is not in general use and it is not yet clear that it has any specific advantage over the measurement of plasma ACTH concentration. Similarly, radioimmunoassays for plasma β-endorphin have been developed but their clinical utility is unknown, and β-LPH cross-reacts with all these assays.[509,510] Thus, precise measurement of β-endorphin concentration requires prior separation of the peptides by chromatography.

Urinary Corticosteroids

Several methods are available to measure levels of urinary cortisol and its metabolites. All of these involve 24-h urine collections, a feature that can be a disadvantage because of incomplete collections. However, these methods provide an integrated assessment of the amount of cortisol produced over a 24-h period and the problems of episodic release present with plasma assays can be bypassed. The 24-h urine sample is collected in a suitable preservative and is then stable when refrigerated.

FREE CORTISOL

In spite of the fact that less than 1 percent of the total cortisol secreted by the adrenal is excreted unchanged in the urine (see Variations in Steroid Metabolism, above),[511] a measurement of this fraction can give useful information. It is especially helpful when cortisol secretion is increased because the unbound plasma cortisol is elevated more than the total level since the capacity of CBG is exceeded.

Urinary free cortisol is measured by extraction of the steroid from the urine and assay of the extract by the competitive protein binding radioassay[512,513] or radioimmunoassay.[463] These assays are rapid and suitable for routine clinical use but have the same limitations of specificity described for the assay of plasma cortisol. The addition of a chromatographic purification step increases specificity by removing both steroidal and nonsteroidal interference,[514] but this modification is not required for routine use.[512,513] Normal values range from 0 to 100 μg/24 h,[502,513] although the sensitivity of the methods at values below 15 μg/24 h is unreliable unless the chromatographic step is used.[514] Elevated levels are nearly always found in spontaneous Cushing's syndrome. In contrast to urinary 17-OHCS, the urinary free cortisol excretion is not elevated in obesity.[512] This greatly enhances the diagnostic usefulness of this test in Cushing's syndrome. Levels are increased in acute illness and the other stresses discussed above, and may be slightly elevated in pregnancy.

17-HYDROXYCORTICOSTEROIDS (17-OHCS) AND 17-KETOGENIC STEROIDS

Measurements of urinary 17-OHCS and 17-ketogenic steroids (17-KGS) have been of major importance in the evaluation of adrenal function; these tests also provide an integrated assessment of adrenal function. Although it is argued that the 24-h urinary 17-OHCS excretion provides a better assessment of overall cortisol production than the determination of urinary free cortisol, this has not been true in our experience. The response of urinary 17-OHCS level to stimulation or suppression does have clinical utility; determination of urinary free cortisol and measurement of plasma cortisol with the rapid dynamic tests discussed below is preferred. Further, the urinary 17-KGS determinations are no longer used for the reasons outlined below.

Urinary 17-OHCS are assayed by the Porter-Silber reaction, which is specific for steroids with a 17,21-dihydroxy-20-keto configuration.[467,468] Steroids with this structure react with phenylhydrazine to form a compound which is measured colorimetrically. The urine is first treated with glucuronidase to cleave the conjugated steroids; the unconjugated steroids are then extracted with organic solvents before reaction with phenylhydrazine. The method ordinarily measures levels of the major urinary metabolites of cortisol and cortisone (discussed above), but, with inhibition of 11β-hydroxylase, as with metyrapone testing (see below), it determines the metabolites of 11-desoxy-17-cortisol.

The normal excretion rate of urinary 17-OHCS is 3 to 10 mg/24 h. Total urinary excretion is elevated in obesity, but this elevation can be compensated by comparing the result to urinary creatinine excretion.[502,515] Using this correction, the normal 24-h values range from 2.0 to 6.5 mg per gram of creatinine.[515] The urinary 17-OHCS may be decreased in starvation, renal failure, liver disease, pregnancy, and hypothyroidism, and increased in hyperthyroidism.[515–523] Drugs which are inducers of hepatic microsomal enzymes such as phenytoin, primidone, phenobarbital, and mitotane reduce urinary 17-OHCS excretion by increasing the steroid metabolism via the 6β-hydroxylation pathway, resulting in metabolites that are not measured by the Porter-Silber method.[487,523,524] Other drugs cause direct interference with urinary 17-OHCS determinations. These include spironolactone, chlordiazepoxide, hydroxyzine, meprobamate, phenothiazines, quinine, and troleandomycin.[525,526]

The 17-ketogenic steroids are those which are converted to 17-ketosteroids by oxidation and then measured colorimetrically by the Zimmerman reaction (discussed in Urinary Androgens, below).[527] Such steroids include the 17-OHCS (cortisol, cortisone, 11-deoxycortisol), the cortols and cortolones, steroids without a hydroxyl at position 21 (17α-hydroxyprogesterone and 21-deoxycortisol), pregnanetriol, and certain of their metabolites. In addition, the assay measures levels of the endogenous 17-ketosteroids. However, these can be determined separately, as described under Urinary Androgens, and the values can be subtracted from the total of ketogenic steroids to yield the actual level of 17-KGS. Normal values are 6 to 20 mg/24 h in most laboratories.

Although the assay of 17-KGS is still in widespread use, it does not have any advantages over the other tests and it does have several disadvantages.[19a,525,526] First, as with 17-OHCS, basal measurements are not particularly useful. Second, it is interfered with by a number of drugs. The result is spuriously elevated by large doses of penicillin G and is decreased by meprobamate, glucose, and radioopaque contrast reagents such as meglumine iodipamide and meglumine iothalamate. Third, the fact that pregnanetriol concentration is measured is a disadvantage in certain types of congenital adrenal hyperplasia in which the level of this steroid is elevated. Finally, the test is less reliable in the diagnosis of Cushing's syndrome than either determination of urinary free cortisol or response of urinary 17-OHCS to dexamethasone suppression (see below). Thus, this method is no longer used in a number of centers.

Cortisol Production Rate

Several methods are available for determination of the production or secretory rate of cortisol.[56] In principle, this is an excellent test to assess adrenal activity; however, technical complexity has largely limited its use to research situations.[43,56] Normal cortisol production is about 8 to 25 mg per day (Table 12-2). It is increased in Cushing's syndrome, obesity, pregnancy, hyperthyroidism, and other circumstances, discussed earlier, in which there is adrenal overactivity; it is decreased in adrenal insufficiency and hypothyroidism.[43] The method differentiates Cushing's syndrome from simple obesity if the cortisol production rate is expressed as mg per 24 h per gram of urinary creatinine.[515] Cortisol production in one study was less than 20 mg/24 h per gram of urinary creatinine in normal and obese controls and greater than 26 mg/24 h per gram creatinine in patients with Cushing's syndrome.[515]

Dexamethasone Suppression Tests

LOW-DOSE TESTS

Low-dose tests are used in the diagnosis of Cushing's syndrome and assess the integrity of negative feedback control by glucocorticoids of the hypothalamic-pituitary-adrenal axis (see above). Dexamethasone is used since it can be given in small amounts and thus is not measured in the plasma and urine corticosteroid assays employed. Thus, in normal individuals dexamethasone inhibits pituitary ACTH release and consequently adrenal cortisol secretion. In patients with Cushing's syndrome (in whom feedback control is abnormal) secretion is rarely normally suppressible with these tests.[487,502,528–530] Although these low-dose tests diagnose Cushing's syndrome they do not define the specific etiology.

Overnight Test

The overnight dexamethasone suppression test is a reliable screening test for Cushing's syndrome and requires only one plasma specimen. Dexamethasone (1.0 mg orally) is administered at 11:00 P.M. and plasma cortisol is measured at 8:00 A.M. the following morning. Although criteria vary (based on differing methods of cortisol assay), most studies agree that a plasma cortisol level below 5 μg/dl excludes Cushing's syndrome and that patients with Cushing's syndrome have plasma cortisol levels of above 10 μg/dl.[502] If the response is abnormal, Cushing's syndrome should be suspected and confirmed with other diagnostic tests.

Less than 2 percent of patients with Cushing's syndrome show normal suppressibility and only 1.1 percent of outpatient controls have false-positive results.[502] Thus, this test is valuable for outpatient screening. It is less useful in obese individuals, since 13 percent fail to show suppression, and it is of minimal usefulness in hospitalized or chronically ill patients, of whom approximately 25 percent have false-positive results.[502] False-positive responses may also occur in acutely ill patients, those with severe depression, anorexia nervosa, anxiety, alcoholism, or chronic renal failure, and in high-estrogen states (pregnancy, estrogen therapy, or oral contraceptive administration).[487] Lack of suppression can also occur in patients in whom accelerated metabolism of dexamethasone due to phenytoin, barbiturates, or other anticonvulsants results in failure to achieve plasma levels of the steroid sufficient to suppress ACTH secretion.[487] A cortisol suppression test for plasma corticosterone has been devised which circumvents this problem.[531]

Two-Day Test

This test was introduced by Liddle in 1960[532] and has been extensively used in the diagnosis of Cushing's syndrome. It provides the same information as the overnight 1-mg test, but is best standardized for urinary corticosteroids. The test is performed by first collecting a 24-h urine sample for baseline determination. Dexamethasone is then given in a dosage of 0.5 mg every 6 h for 2 days, with concurrent 24-h urine collections. Although the test can be performed on an outpatient basis, hospitalization may be required to ensure adequate urine collections. A normal urinary 17-OHCS response is suppression to less than 4 mg per day, from control values in the normal to elevated range, on the second day of dexamethasone administration.[502,532]

When these criteria are used, secretion in approximately 94 percent of patients with Cushing's disease is not suppressed and false-positive responses in controls are rare.[502] False-positive results occur rarely in obesity or high-estrogen states[487,515,533,534] but, as is the case with the overnight 1-mg test, false-positives occur with acute and chronic illness, depression, alcoholism, and phenytoin therapy.[487,535,536] Since some patients with Cushing's syndrome show normal suppression with this dose, a modification of the test was introduced in which dexamethasone is given in a dosage of 20 μg per kilogram of body weight per day. In this study, normal and obese controls had urinary 17-OHCS excretion of less than 1 mg per gram of creatinine whereas none of 15 patients with Cushing's syndrome displayed this degree of suppression.[515]

The response of the urinary free cortisol excretion to the 2-day low-dose dexamethasone test was assessed in two studies; the lower limit was 19 to 25 μg/24 h on the second day.[533,534] Using these criteria, function in 95.6 percent of patients with Cushing's syndrome failed to be suppressed normally and the frequency of false-positive responses in control subjects was 3 percent.[502] In one study plasma cortisol fell to less than 5 μg/dl in normal subjects in response to low-dose dexamethasone.[537]

HIGH-DOSE TESTS

High-dose dexamethasone tests are helpful in differentiating Cushing's disease from other types of hypercortisolism, once the low-dose dexamethasone suppression tests and the other steroid measurements described confirm the presence of Cushing's syndrome. These tests depend on the characteristic finding that the hypothalamic-pituitary axis in patients with Cushing's disease is suppressible with glucocorticoids, although higher than normal doses are required. Thus, ACTH and cortisol secretion decrease when large amounts of dexamethasone are administered.[502,532,538] In contrast, in patients with hypercortisolism secondary to autonomous adrenal tumors or the ectopic ACTH syndrome, high-dose dexamethasone characteristically fails to suppress cortisol hypersecretion, since it is not under the control of the hypothalamic-pituitary axis. Although extremely useful, a number of exceptions occur in the use of high-dose dexamethasone suppression tests. These are discussed below, under Diagnosis and Differential Diagnosis and Tumor Localization under Cushing's Syndrome, and include Cushing's syndrome with periodic hormonogenesis, nonsuppressible pituitary Cushing's disease, occasional ectopic ACTH-secreting tumors which are suppressible, and nodular adrenal hyperplasia.[487,502]

Overnight 8-mg Test

The overnight high-dose dexamethasone suppression test is more reliable and easier to perform than the standard 2-day test described below (Fig. 12-26).[539] A baseline morning cortisol specimen is obtained and a single dose of dexamethasone (8.0 mg) is administered orally at 11:00 P.M. Plasma cortisol is then measured at 8:00 A.M. the following morning.[539] Among 60 patients with Cushing's disease, plasma cortisol levels were suppressed below 50 percent of baseline in 55 (92 percent) whereas in no patient with either the ectopic ACTH syndrome or glucocorticoid-producing adrenal tumors ($N=16$) was this degree of suppression achieved. This single-dose test was found to be more reliable than the 2-day test when compared in the same patients, since in only 75 percent of patients with Cushing's disease was urinary 17-OHCS excretion suppressed with the 2-day test.[539] This overnight 8-mg high-dose dexamethasone suppression test is the procedure of choice because of its simplicity and reliability.

Two-Day High-Dose Test

This test first reliably differentiated Cushing's disease from other types of endogenous hypercortisolism.[502,532] A baseline 24-h urine sample is collected and then dexamethasone (2.0 mg every 6 h for 2 days) is administered with concurrent 24-h urine collection. Again, hospitalization may be required for accurate urine collection. The test is best standardized for urinary 17-OHCS; patients with Cushing's disease show suppression of urinary 17-OHCS level to below 50 percent of baseline levels.[532,539] In patients with adrenal tumors or the ectopic ACTH syndrome there is usually no decrease in urinary corticosteroid excretion.

The diagnostic accuracy of this procedure is limited in that in 15 to 30 percent of patients with pituitary-dependent Cushing's disease urinary

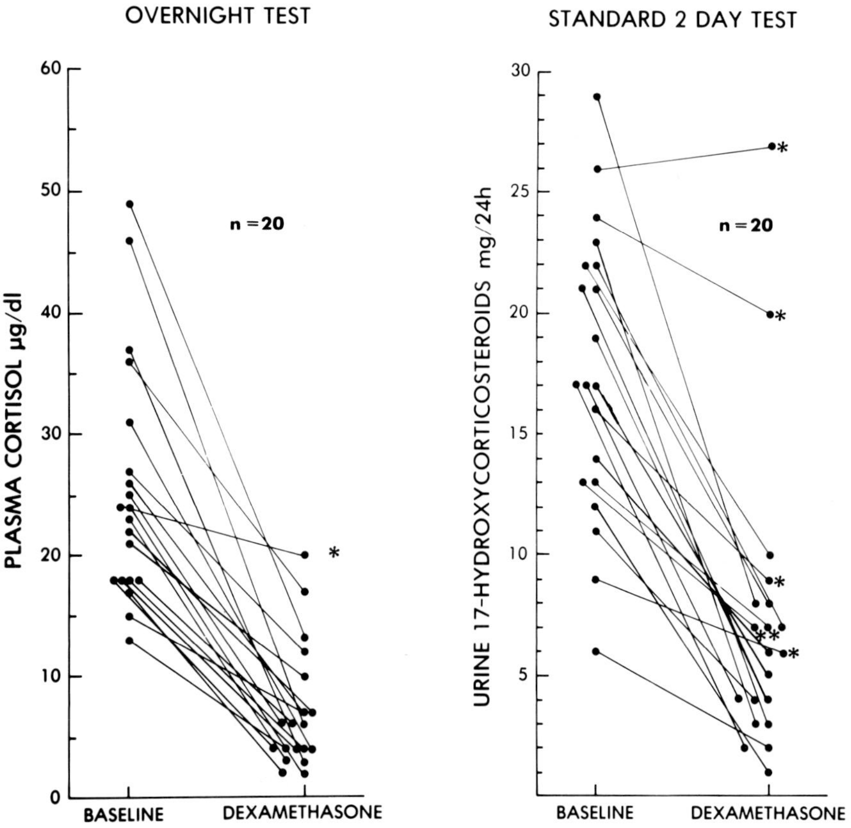

FIGURE 12-26 (*Left*) Plasma cortisol response to the overnight high-dose (8-mg) dexamethasone suppression test. (*Right*) Urinary 17-OHCS response to the standard 2-day, high-dose dexamethasone suppression test in 20 patients with Cushing's disease. Asterisks indicate tests in which response was not suppressed to < 50 percent of baseline level. (*Based upon data of Tyrrell et al.*[539])

17-OHCS excretion fails to be adequately suppressed.[487,502,539,540] The response of urinary free cortisol level has been less extensively studied, but in two series 16 percent of patients with Cushing's disease did not display 50 percent suppression.[533,534] Measurement of plasma cortisol does not increase diagnostic reliability[537,539] and measurement of urinary 17-KGS excretion is less reliable than that of urinary 17-OHCS.[502,534]

Tests of Pituitary-Adrenal Reserve

Tests of pituitary-adrenal reserve assess the functional capacity of the hypothalamic-pituitary-adrenal axis, its reserve capacity, and its ability to respond to stress. The four most reliable tests use: (1) ACTH, which directly stimulates adrenal glucocorticoid secretion; (2) metyrapone, which inhibits adrenal cortisol production and thereby indirectly stimulates pituitary ACTH secretion; (3) insulin-induced hypoglycemia, which acts via the pituitary to stimulate ACTH release;[98] and (4) human or ovine CRF to stimulate ACTH and cortisol release.[541-544] Measurement of the adrenal and pituitary responses to these tests is thus used to establish the diagnosis of primary or secondary adrenal insufficiency. Modifications of these tests that allow them to be performed more rapidly have, in general, supplanted traditional tests which require urine collections and several days to perform.

ACTH STIMULATION TESTS

The administration of ACTH results in direct stimulation of adrenal cortisol secretion. In primary adrenocortical insufficiency, the adrenal cortex is destroyed and, thus, cannot respond. In secondary adrenocortical insufficiency there is atrophy of the cortex; thus, there is an inadequate acute response to ACTH although cortisol secretion ultimately increases if ACTH stimulation is continued.

Rapid ACTH Stimulation Test

This test measures the acute response to ACTH; it is useful in the diagnosis of both primary and secondary adrenal insufficiency. The test can be performed on an outpatient basis at any time of the day, does not require fasting, and in emergencies requires only a 30-min delay in the institution of therapy. The potent synthetic ACTH derivative cosyntropin (or tetracosactrin) is used. It contains the first 24 amino acids of human ACTH and is preferred to previously used animal ACTH preparations, to which there is a greater incidence of allergic reactions.[545] Cosyntropin (250 μg) is administered intramuscularly (IM) or intravenously (IV) and samples for plasma cortisol determination are obtained prior to and at 30 to 60 min following the injection (Fig. 12-27). An additional basal plasma sample is collected prior to the injection; this is subsequently assayed for plasma ACTH if the response to cosyntropin is subnormal (see Adrenocortical Insufficiency, below).

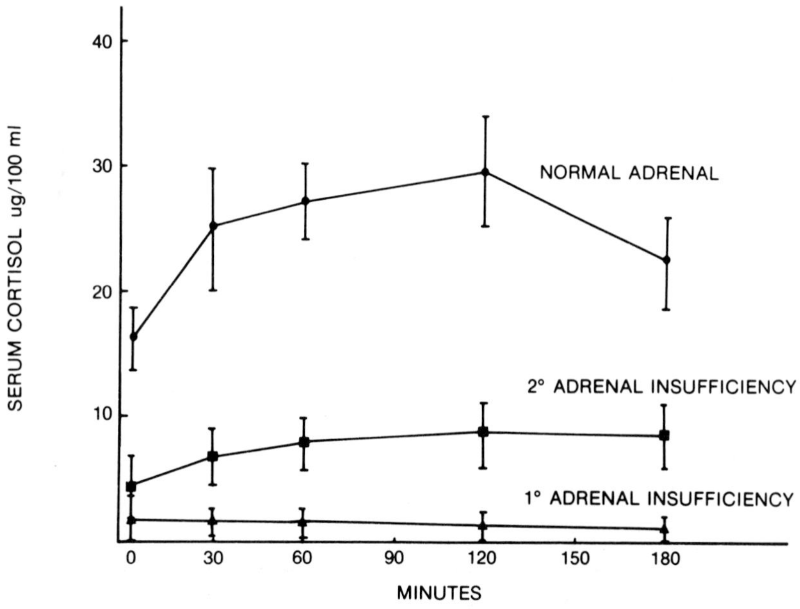

FIGURE 12-27 Serum cortisol response to 0.25 mg cosyntropin in nine normal individuals (normal adrenal), eight patients with hypopituitarism (secondary adrenal insufficiency), and seven patients with Addison's disease (primary adrenal insufficiency). (*From Speckart et al.*[546])

The following normal criteria were established using the fluorimetric cortisol assay.[545–547] The basal level of plasma cortisol should be greater than 5 μg/dl, with an ACTH-stimulated increment of >7 μg/dl and a maximal level of >18 μg/dl at 30 min. With the competitive protein binding cortisol assay performed at 60 min following ACTH injection, normal subjects and control patients all achieved peak cortisol levels of >15 μg/dl and 98.5 percent of 69 subjects had an increment of plasma cortisol >5 μg/dl.[548] In another study using cortisol immunoassay a normal response was defined as a peak cortisol of 20 μg/dl or greater regardless of the increment.[549] This study documented the frequently noted clinical finding that patients with high basal cortisol values may show no further increase in response to acute ACTH stimulation.

Subnormal responses to the rapid ACTH stimulation test establish the diagnosis of primary or secondary adrenal insufficiency. In primary adrenal insufficiency the cortex is damaged; cortisol secretion is reduced, endogenous ACTH secretion is increased, and any remaining cortical tissue is unable to increase cortisol secretion in response to maximal stimulation with exogenous ACTH (decreased adrenal reserve). In secondary adrenal insufficiency, inadequate ACTH secretion leads to atrophy of the zonae fasciculata and reticularis and therefore to adrenal unresponsiveness to brief (but not prolonged) stimulation with exogenous ACTH. In this setting a subnormal response to exogenous ACTH accurately predicts deficient responsiveness to insulin hypoglycemia, metyrapone, and surgical stress.[548–555] The cortisol determinations per se do not differentiate primary from secondary etiology; however, plasma ACTH concentration is elevated in the primary form but depressed in the secondary form (see Adrenocortical Insufficiency, below).

A normal response to the rapid ACTH stimulation test excludes the diagnosis of primary adrenal insufficiency, since it provides a direct assessment of adrenal reserve. However, the usefulness of this procedure in excluding secondary adrenocortical insufficiency or predicting normal pituitary responsiveness to stress is more controversial. The response is abnormal in almost all cases of secondary adrenocortical insufficiency; however, in partial ACTH deficiency, ACTH secretion may be sufficient to maintain adrenocortical function to the extent that atrophy does not occur, so adrenal responsiveness to exogenous ACTH stimulation remains normal or near normal. However, in these patients ACTH secretion is unable to increase further in response to stress because they have decreased pituitary reserve. In one study of glucocorticoid-treated patients, plasma cortisol responses to the rapid ACTH test or major surgery correlated well, although 4 of 17 patients with normal responses to ACTH had mildly subnormal cortisol responses to surgery; however, none of these had clinical evidence of adrenal insufficiency.[553] In another study seven glucocorticoid-treated patients were found with normal responses to the rapid ACTH stimulation test and subnormal responses to insulin hypoglycemia.[552] Of these, four had subnormal plasma cortisol responses to surgical stress, although, again, clinical adrenocortical insufficiency did not occur. Another study identified five patients with hypothalamic or pituitary disorders who had normal plasma cortisol responses to an ACTH infusion (10 U/h for 2 h) but deficient plasma cortisol responses to insulin hypoglycemia; one of these developed adrenocortical insufficiency during pneumoencephalography.[554] A more recent study confirmed the observation that normal responses to the rapid ACTH stimulation test do not necessarily predict normal hypothalamic-pituitary-adrenal axis responses to stress such as hypoglycemia.[555] Thus, a normal response to ACTH does not always predict a normal response to direct stimuli such as hypoglycemia or stress, and cannot be used to exclude partial secondary adrenal insufficiency with inadequate pituitary reserve.

The rapid ACTH stimulation test can also be used to measure plasma aldosterone responsiveness. This modification can be used to differentiate primary and secondary adrenocortical insufficiency.[556] In primary adrenal insufficiency destruction of all three zones of the cortex leads to deficient responses of both cortisol and aldosterone to exogenous ACTH. However, in most patients with secondary adrenal insufficiency aldosterone secretion is maintained by the renin-angiotensin system. Therefore, the aldosterone response to exogenous ACTH is normal even though cortisol does not respond. Patients with secondary adrenal insufficiency have an increment in plasma aldosterone of >4 ng/dl, whereas patients with primary Addison's disease have no response.[556]

Three-Day ACTH Stimulation Tests

Three-day ACTH stimulation tests have traditionally been used in the diagnosis of adrenal insufficiency and the differentiation of primary and secondary forms.[557] These tests are rarely performed at present.

The standard test is performed by first obtaining a baseline urine sample for 24-h 17-OHCS determination. ACTH (cosyntropin, 250 μg, or bovine ACTH, 40 U) is then given IV in 500 ml of saline over 8 h on three consecutive days with concurrent urine collections for 17-OHCS determination. In normal individuals, urinary 17-OHCS excretion increases two to three times greater than baseline on the first day of

ACTH stimulation. In patients with primary adrenal insufficiency, urinary 17-OHCS excretion fails to increase even with repetitive stimulation; however, in patients with secondary adrenal insufficiency, there is a minimal rise on the first day of ACTH infusion, but stepwise increments of urinary steroid levels occur with successive days of stimulation, to reach approximately three times basal levels on the third day.[557] A similar type of test in which plasma cortisol is measured is shown in Fig. 12-7. Patients with suspected primary adrenal insufficiency should be observed closely during 3-day ACTH stimulation tests, since prolonged adrenal stimulation may actually further decrease the adrenal secretory capacity and worsen the clinical state. Alternatively, these patients may be simultaneously treated with glucocorticoids and mineralocorticoids during the ACTH infusions.

The 3-day stimulation test has been simplified with the use of a long-acting cosyntropin (Synacthen) which is available in Europe and many other countries but not in the United States.[438] Basal plasma cortisol is first measured and the cosyntropin is then administered for 3 days in a dosage of 1.0 mg daily IM. Plasma cortisol is measured 6 h after the first and third injections. In normal individuals, plasma cortisol reaches a peak level of more than 25 μg/dl at 6 h following the first injection; such a response excludes adrenal insufficiency. In patients with primary adrenal insufficiency plasma cortisol fails to respond even with subsequent injections of syntropin depot. In patients with secondary adrenal insufficiency plasma cortisol does not increase normally with the first injection but rises to >25 μg/dl at 6 h following the third injection.[438]

INSULIN-INDUCED HYPOGLYCEMIA, PYROGEN, AND VASOPRESSIN STIMULATION TESTS

The response to insulin-induced hypoglycemia (insulin tolerance test) is the most sensitive and accurate test of the integrity of the hypothalamic-pituitary-adrenal axis[554,555,557,558] and its ability to respond to stress. The test is also used to simultaneously assess growth hormone responsiveness (see Chap. 7).[154,554,558,559] Hypoglycemia elicits a potent stress response via pituitary adrenergic receptors[98] and stimulates ACTH release. The test is performed after an overnight fast with measurement of plasma cortisol and glucose (and serum growth hormone, if desired) levels before and at 30, 45, 60, and 90 min after administration of IV regular insulin. Plasma glucose concentration is measured to assess the adequacy of the hypoglycemia; a value of less than 40 mg/dl is considered an adequate stimulus.[154] The usual dose of insulin is 0.15 U per kilogram of body weight but must be adjusted on the basis of the patient's clinical status and suspected pituitary function. In suspected hypopituitarism or adrenal insufficiency 0.1 U per kilogram of body weight is used and the usual dose of 0.15 U per kilogram of body weight is increased by 0.1 U/kg in patients with obesity, diabetes mellitus, endogenous Cushing's syndrome, or acromegaly, since these patients exhibit significant insulin resistance. An experienced physician must be in attendance, with careful monitoring of the patient and with IV glucose available. Most patients experience hypoglycemic symptoms, i.e., sweating, tachycardia, and hunger; the test should be terminated with IV glucose if significant symptoms of neuroglycopenia, such as confusion or disorientation, occur. The test is contraindicated in patients with seizure disorders, cardiovascular disease, and cerebrovascular disease and in those greater than 65 years of age. It should not be performed in acutely ill patients with suspected adrenocortical insufficiency since they may be extremely sensitive to insulin. When these precautions are observed there is little risk to the patient.

With adequate hypoglycemia, plasma cortisol levels peak 60 to 90 min following insulin injection. A normal response is an increment of plasma cortisol of >8 μg/dl and a maximum plasma cortisol level of >18 to 20 μg/dl when cortisol concentration is measured fluorimetrically.[154,550,554,558–561] Normal criteria using the competitive protein binding assay are an increment of plasma cortisol of >5 μg/dl and a maximal level >15 μg/dl.[548] Plasma ACTH concentration may also be measured during insulin hypoglycemia, but this is usually unnecessary since a normal increment of plasma cortisol demonstrates normal pituitary ACTH secretion. The normal response of plasma ACTH to hypoglycemia is not well standardized although various criteria have been reported.[507,561–563]

A normal plasma cortisol response to hypoglycemia excludes adrenal insufficiency and indicates an intact hypothalamic-pituitary-adrenal axis. The test is particularly useful in patients with prior glucocorticoid therapy (see Chap. 15) or suspected pituitary disorders as those with normal responses do not require glucocorticoid supplementation for stress or surgery.[154] A subnormal response proves primary or secondary adrenal insufficiency.

Pyrogen and vasopressin both stimulate pituitary ACTH release but are less frequently used than insulin-induced hypoglycemia in stimulation tests of pituitary-adrenal function. The procedures for and normal responses to these tests are discussed in Chap. 7.

METYRAPONE TESTING

Metyrapone stimulation assesses both pituitary and adrenal reserve and thus is used in the diagnosis of both primary and secondary adrenal insufficiency. Metyrapone inhibits adrenal 11β-hydroxylase (Table 12-3) and thereby blocks cortisol synthesis. The fall in circulating cortisol levels increases release of ACTH that in turn stimulates increased production of steroids proximal to the site of enzyme inhibition. As a result, plasma levels of 11-deoxycortisol increase, as does urinary 17-OHCS excretion (due to increased excretion of the tetrahydro metabolite of 11-deoxycortisol).[548,564,564a] The response to metyrapone correlates well with insulin-induced hypoglycemia,[548,564a] although occasional patients with either hypothalamic-pituitary disorders or prior glucocorticoid therapy have normal metyrapone responsiveness but subnormal plasma cortisol responses to insulin-induced hypoglycemia.[551,552] A normal metyrapone test predicts a normal response to surgical stress in virtually all patients.[552] Thus the metyrapone test and insulin-induced hypoglycemia are equally effective in predicting the integrity of the hypothalamic-pituitary axis. Because of its simplicity the metyrapone test is usually used in the assessment of glucocorticoid-treated patients whereas in patients with suspected hypothalamic-pituitary dysfunction from other causes, e.g., pituitary adenomas, the insulin-induced hypoglycemia test is usually employed since it allows simultaneous assessment of growth hormone reserve (see above).

Overnight Test

The overnight test is performed by administering a single dose of metyrapone at midnight, with a snack to minimize gastrointestinal upset. The dose of metyrapone is 2.0 g for patients weighing less than 70 kg, 2.5 g for patients weighing 70 to 90 kg, and 3.0 g for patients weighing more than 90 kg.[564] Blood for 11-deoxycortisol and cortisol is drawn at 8:00 A.M. Patients with a normal pituitary-adrenal axis have a post-metyrapone level of plasma 11-deoxycortisol >7 μg/dl, whereas patients with adrenal insufficiency do not respond.[564] Simultaneous plasma cortisol measurement is useful since 4 percent of normal subjects and patients on phenytoin have a rapid clearance or inactivation of metyrapone and thus adequate 11β-hydroxylase inhibition does not occur.[564] An 8:00 A.M. plasma cortisol level of <10 μg/dl indicates adequate 11β-hydroxylase inhibition.

A normal response to the overnight test indicates normal ACTH secretion and adrenal function since both are required to increase plasma 11-deoxycortisol concentration. A subnormal response indicates primary or secondary adrenal insufficiency, but does not differentiate between these.

Three-Day and Intravenous Test

The original 3-day protocol of the metyrapone test and an intravenous modification are less commonly used. The overnight test described above provides the same information and does not require either urine collections or IV administration of the drug. These procedures are described in Chap. 7.

CRF TESTING

Human and ovine CRF are available for experimental evaluation of the pituitary-adrenal axis.[541–544] These synthetic peptides are given IV in doses of 1 to 5 μg per kilogram of body weight. They directly stimulate pituitary secretion of the products of POMC, e.g., ACTH, β-LPH, and β-endorphin. Reported normal responses of ACTH and cortisol have varied and will need to be established for individual laboratories.

Patients with primary adrenal insufficiency have high basal ACTH levels and subnormal cortisol levels. In response to CRF, ACTH levels increase but cortisol levels do not, reflecting primary adrenal damage. In secondary adrenal insufficiency plasma cortisol also fails to respond to CRF, however, reported ACTH responses have been very variable and are probably not diagnostically reliable.

CRF has also been used to differentiate the various etiologies of Cushing's syndrome. In general, patients with Cushing's disease have normal or exaggerated plasma ACTH and cortisol responses to CRF, although an occasional patient fails to respond. Patients with the ectopic ACTH syndrome do not respond to CRF, although exceptions do occur.[543] Patients with adrenal tumors causing Cushing's syndrome do not respond to CRF.

Mineralocorticoids

The measurement of aldosterone, DOC, 18-OH-DOC, and other mineralocorticoid levels and the clinical evaluation of the renin-angiotensin-aldosterone axis are discussed in Chap. 14.

Androgens

Dynamic tests such as those described above for studying cortisol excess or cortisol deficiency states have not been developed for the evaluation of disorders of adrenal androgen production. Thus, greater reliance has been placed on measurement of basal plasma levels of the major adrenal androgens and the active metabolites derived from them (i.e., androstenedione, testosterone, and DHT). These steroids are assayed in small volumes of plasma after extraction and chromatographic separation. Additional techniques that measure the free fraction of testosterone (and other hormones) or the binding capacity of sex hormone–binding globulin (SHBG, TeBG) improve the diagnostic usefulness of the tests. Urinary assays of androgen metabolites have traditionally been used, but these are being replaced by the more sensitive plasma assays.

PLASMA ANDROGENS

Because of similarities in their structures, it has been difficult to assay the individual androgens in unfractionated plasma extracts.[491,492] However, DHEA-S concentration can be measured directly since it is present in plasma in relatively high concentrations.[491] The other androgens and their precursors require separation and purifications prior to assay. This is accomplished by solvent extraction, which fractionates steroids with differing polarity, and then chromatography.[491] After separation, the concentrations of steroids can be accurately measured by radioimmunoassay (even though the antibodies used are not completely specific)[491] or by competitive protein binding.[565] With these techniques total plasma levels of DHEA, DHEA-S, androstenedione, testosterone, and DHT can be measured simultaneously in approximately 5 ml of plasma.[491,492] The normal plasma levels of these steroids are listed in Table 12-2.

The plasma concentration of free testosterone may also be assayed by methods which include flow dialysis, charcoal adsorption, equilibrium dialysis, steady-state gel filtration, and ultrafiltration.[565–569b] Plasma free testosterone concentrations (mean $\pm$ SD) have been reported as follows: normal females, 5.39 $\pm$ 2.73 pg/ml (1 to 1.4 percent free); females on oral contraceptives, 6.59 $\pm$ 0.40 pg/ml (0.7 to 0.9 percent free); pregnancy, 4.64 $\pm$ 1.70 pg/ml (0.6 percent free); hirsute females, 16.1 $\pm$ 11.7 pg/ml (1.7 to 2.2 percent free); and normal males, 128 $\pm$ 57 pg/ml (1.7 to 2.5 percent free).[565,568] These free levels more clearly reflect biological activity of circulating testosterone than do total testosterone levels[565–573] (discussed further below). Recent studies have also confirmed the utility of measuring plasma androstanediol and androstanediol glucuronide concentrations in disorders of androgen excess. Levels of these metabolites of DHT are elevated in the majority of women with androgen excess and provide an assessment of tissue metabolism of androgens.[574]

The binding capacity of SHBG is estimated after its removal from plasma (by adsorption or precipitation) with the use of radiolabeled testosterone or DHT.[570,575] SHBG binding capacity is higher in normal women than in normal men. It is increased in pregnancy, cirrhosis, hyperthyroidism, and with estrogen (including oral contraceptive) therapy.[570,571,575] SHGB binding capacity is decreased in most females with hirsutism and in acromegaly.[570,571]

URINARY ANDROGENS

Measurement of urinary 17-ketosteroid excretion was the first method of quantification of adrenal hormone levels, but this method is a less useful index of androgenicity than the plasma methods described above.[576] This method measures the levels of urinary metabolites of plasma androgens; thus, the major contribution to urinary 17-ketosteroids is from DHEA and DHEA-S, the androgens secreted in greatest quantities (Table 12-2). Testosterone and DHT constitute less than 1 percent of the total urinary 17-ketosteroids.[576] The ketosteroids are first extracted from urine and then measured colorimetrically by the Zimmerman reaction, in which 17-ketosteroids react with *m*-dinitrobenzene in the presence of alkali to produce a reddish-purple pigment.[577] A number of modifications of the method have been reported;[577] normal excretion is generally in the range of 7 to 17 mg/24 h in males and 5 to 15 mg/24 h in females.[44] Drug interference is a disadvantage, i.e., chlorpromazine, ethinamate, meprobamate, nalidixic acid, penicillin, phenaglycodol, spironolactone, and troleandomycin falsely increase 17-ketosteroid levels and chlordiazepoxide, etryptamine acetate, progestins, propoxyphene, and reserpine artifactually decrease 17-ketosteroid levels.[525]

CLINICAL UTILITY

The assays described above are used in the evaluation of hyperandrogenic states. Idiopathic hirsutism and the polycystic ovary syndrome are the most frequent causes of elevated androgen secretion; however, androgen levels are also elevated in Cushing's syndrome, congenital adrenal hyperplasia, adrenal tumors, and ovarian tumors (see below and Chaps. 17 and 18). Hypoandrogenicity (hypogonadism) in the male is discussed in Chap. 16.

The utility of 17-ketosteroid determination is limited since this measurement is unreliable in the diagnosis of Cushing's syndrome[502,540] or androgen excess in hirsutism;[576] the diagnosis of congenital adrenal hyperplasia is best established by assay of more specific plasma steroids (see below). Plasma androgen assays are more useful; however, serial plasma samples and the assay of several plasma hormones may be required to document androgen excess.[569,573,576,578,579] In addition, assay of plasma free testosterone concentration is the best single indicator of androgen excess.[565-571,580] The use of these hormone assays is further discussed below (see Hirsutism and Virilism).

ADRENOCORTICAL INSUFFICIENCY

Impaired adrenal function results from deficient adrenal production of glucocorticoids and/or mineralocorticoids. Impairment of adrenal function is usually a consequence of destruction of the adrenal cortex (primary adrenocortical insufficiency, Addison's disease) or is secondary to deficient pituitary ACTH secretion (secondary adrenocortical insufficiency) (Fig. 12-28). Selective or general adrenal insufficiency may also be due to hyporeninemia (see Hyporeninemic Hypoaldosteronism, below), congenital aplasia of the adrenals, congenital enzyme deficiencies of the steroid biosynthetic pathways (see Congenital Defects in Adrenal Steroid Biosynthesis), adrenal unresponsiveness to ACTH, or isolated ACTH deficiency. Primary adrenocortical insufficiency is an uncommon disorder. However, it must be considered in the differential diagnosis of many common conditions that present with nonspecific complaints (weakness, lassitude, weight loss, anorexia, or vague gastrointestinal symptoms). Secondary adrenal insufficiency due to natural causes is also uncommon (see Chap. 7); however, iatrogenic secondary adrenocortical insufficiency is more frequent due to the large number of individuals who receive exogenous glucocorticoid therapy which suppresses pituitary ACTH production (see Chap. 15).

Primary Adrenocortical Insufficiency (Addison's Disease)

Adrenal destruction results from a variety of causes (Fig. 12-28; Table 12-9); however, at present, the

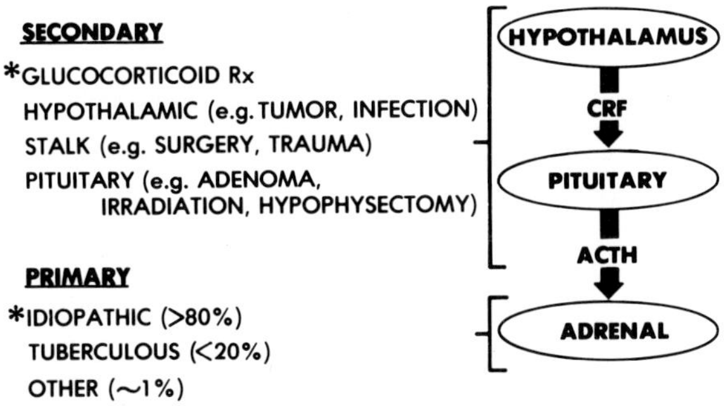

FIGURE 12-28 Causes of adrenocortical insufficiency. Secondary insufficiency can be due to lesions of either the hypothalamus or pituitary, although the most common cause (indicated by the asterisk) is iatrogenic and due to glucocorticoid therapy. The most common cause of primary adrenocortical insufficiency is idiopathic, also indicated by an asterisk.

Table 12-9. Etiology of Primary Adrenocortical Insufficiency

Idiopathic/autoimmune (~80%)
Tuberculosis (~20%)
Miscellaneous causes (~1%)
Vascular
Hemorrhage: sepsis, anticoagulants, coagulopathy, trauma, surgery, pregnancy, neonate
Infarction: thrombosis, embolism, arteritis
Fungal Infection: histoplasmosis, coccidioidomycosis, blastomycosis, candidiasis, torulosis
Acquired immune deficiency syndrome (AIDS)
Metastases
Lymphoma
Amyloidosis
Sarcoidosis
Hemochromatosis
Irradiation
Surgery: bilateral adrenalectomy
Enzyme inhibitors: metyrapone, aminoglutethimide, trilostane
Cytotoxic agents: mitotane
Heredity: adrenal hyperplasia, hypoplasia, familial glucocorticoid deficiency

Source: Irvine et al.[438] and Irvine and Barnes.[581]

autoimmune or "idiopathic" atrophic type of Addison's disease (autoimmune adrenal atrophy, autoimmune adrenalitis, lymphocytic adrenalitis) accounts for approximately 80 percent of cases.[438,581] Idiopathic Addison's disease is an autoimmune disease and there is evidence for disordered organ-specific immunity, a high incidence of associated immunologic and autoimmune endocrine dysfunction, and disorders of other tissues and organs.[582] In addition there are two (and perhaps three) distinct subtypes of these syndromes known as the polyglandular autoimmune syndromes (PGA types 1 and 2).[583-585]

Tuberculosis currently accounts for approximately 20 percent of cases of Addison's disease, with a higher prevalence in populations with poor control of this disease. This current distribution is a marked reversal of the relative frequency since the 1920s and 1930s when tuberculosis was responsible for 70 to 80 percent of reported cases (Table 12-10).[438,581,586] Adrenal insufficiency is relatively unusual in patients with tuberculosis, and even with adrenal involvement the extent of cortical destruction may not be sufficient to impair adrenal function.[587]

Other etiologies of primary adrenal insufficiency are distinctly unusual in larger published series (Table 12-9).[438,581,586] However, personal experience suggests that adrenal insufficiency due to invasive and hemorrhagic disorders may be becoming more commonly

Table 12-10. Changing Patterns in Primary Adrenocortical Insufficiency

	Percent*	
	1928–1938	1962–1972
Idiopathic	17	78
Tuberculous	79	21
Other	4	1

*Percent of cases with each of the three classes of adrenocortical insufficiency in each time period.
Source: Dunlop[398] and Irvine and Barnes.[581]

diagnosed. These etiologies include many systemic disorders (e.g., hemorrhagic disorders, neoplasia, infections, trauma, etc.) that involve a number of organ systems. The most common etiology of adrenal hemorrhage in adults is anticoagulant therapy[588] and in childhood is meningococcal and *Pseudomonas* septicemias.[589,590] Adrenal insufficiency may also occur in the acquired immune deficiency syndrome (AIDS), however, the exact cause and incidence are unknown.[591] Adrenal hypoplasia is a rare cause and may be familial.[592]

Primary adrenocortical insufficiency due to any cause is a rare disease; the exact incidence and prevalence are unknown. Current reports may underestimate the true incidence, since patients may die in acute crisis without an established diagnosis.[593] A prevalence of Addison's disease of 39 per million inhabitants in the 25 to 69 age groups in the United Kingdom was reported and there were 60 cases per million population in Denmark.[586,593] It is difficult to determine whether the dramatic alteration in the relative frequencies of idiopathic and tuberculous Addison's disease is due to an increase in the incidence of idiopathic cases or to a decrease in the number of cases secondary to tuberculosis. However, the series of Dunlop[398] suggests that the total incidence of Addison's disease is declining concomitant with control of tuberculosis, favoring the idea that the increase in the idiopathic variety is a relative one.

Tuberculous Addison's disease occurs predominantly in male patients, but idiopathic Addison's disease is more frequent in females. Thus, in recent series the female/male ratio approximates 1.25.[342] In idiopathic Addison's disease the female/male ratio is 2.6.[438]

Addison's disease is an unusual diagnosis at the extremes of life; approximately 60 to 70 percent of cases are diagnosed in the third to fifth decades.[438] The idiopathic variety occurs among all age groups but tuberculous Addison's disease is usually diagnosed in patients over the age of 40 years.[342,586,594] The mean ages of patients with idiopathic and tuberculous types were estimated to be 30 to 35 and 50 to 55 years, respectively; however, in a more recent report mean ages were 34 and 38 years.[342,438,586]

Only isolated information regarding death rates is available. Guttman estimated in 1930 that the death rate from Addison's disease was 4 per million population in the United States[587] and Stuart-Mason et al. reported an annual death rate of 1.4 per million population in the United Kingdom in the 1960s.[593]

IDIOPATHIC ADRENOCORTICAL INSUFFICIENCY

The etiology of the most common form of primary adrenocortical failure appears to be autoimmune in nature. Early in the course of the disease there is lymphocytic infiltration of the gland. There is a high incidence of associated endocrine disorders as well as of pernicious anemia, vitiligo, and other disorders. There is also a genetic predisposition. Antibodies to the adrenal gland and to other potentially affected organs are commonly present, and there is evidence for abnormal cell-mediated immunity.

Associated Disorders

In 1926, Schmidt described two patients with idiopathic Addison's disease who had chronic lymphocytic thyroiditis at autopsy.[595] In 1964, Carpenter et al. reviewed this association of hypoadrenalism and hypothyroidism and in addition noted the association of diabetes mellitus.[596] More recently, an association of idiopathic Addison's disease with gonadal failure, hyperthyroidism, hypothyroidism, Hashimoto's thyroiditis, vitiligo, hypoparathyroidism, and pernicious anemia has been established (Table 12-11).[342,438,581,586,594,597] One or more of these clinical disorders are present in

Table 12-11. Associated Clinical Disorders in Patients with Idiopathic Adrenocortical Insufficiency

Associated Disorder	Percent*
Primary ovarian failure	23
Thyroid	
Hyperthyroidism	7
Hypothyroidism/chronic thyroiditis	9
Diabetes mellitus	12
Vitiligo	9
Hypoparathyroidism	6
Pernicious anemia	4

Source: Irvine and Barnes[581,598] and Nerup.[586]

40 to 53 percent of patients with idiopathic Addison's disease and the presence of organ-specific antibodies is even more common. These disorders are not associated with Addison's disease due to tuberculosis or other invasive or infiltrative processes.

Although these associated disorders are common in patients with primary adrenal insufficiency, patients with more commonly occurring conditions such as diabetes mellitus or autoimmune thyroid disease rarely develop Addison's disease. Idiopathic hypoparathyroidism represents an exception since the two disorders commonly coincide and are frequently familial.[438,598,599]

The association of Addison's disease with one or more of these conditions has been referred to by a number of terms, including Schmidt's syndrome, autoimmune endocrine failure, and the polyglandular failure syndrome.

Gonadal Failure

Ovarian failure occurs in approximately one-quarter of female patients. These patients usually have secondary amenorrhea, although primary amenorrhea may also occur. The ovarian origin of the gonadal failure has been demonstrated by low estrogen levels and elevated gonadotropin levels.[598] These patients have either lymphocytic infiltration or total destruction of the ovary with only fibrous tissue remaining (streak gonad).[598] The ages of onset of amenorrhea and Addison's disease are closely correlated, suggesting a similar pathogenesis, i.e., autoimmunity directed at antigens which are identical in the steroid-secreting cells of both ovary and adrenal.[598] In addition, patients with both ovarian and adrenal failure have a very high incidence of hypoparathyroidism and thyroid disease.[581] Hypoparathyroidism is most frequent in those with primary amenorrhea.[598] Testicular failure is relatively unusual, occurring in only 3 of 79 patients in Irvine and Barnes's series.[598]

Thyroid Dysfunction

Clinical thyroid disorders are present in 16 percent of patients with Addison's disease; there is also a high prevalence of subclinical thyroiditis (as indicated by the presence of antithyroid antibodies; see below). Carpenter et al. documented lymphocytic thyroiditis in approximately 80 percent of patients with idiopathic Addison's disease[596] and a high frequency of elevated TSH levels has been reported.[600] Hyperthyroidism occurs in about 7 percent of patients with Addison's disease; virtually all of these patients are female and the thyrotoxicosis precedes the diagnosis of adrenal insufficiency in the majority.[598] Clinical hypothyroidism or Hashimoto's thyroiditis with goiter occurs in 9 percent of patients with idiopathic Addison's disease. Hypothyroidism has been reported to be reversible in a few addisonian patients following steroid replacement therapy; however, this appears to be an unusual occurrence.[601]

Diabetes Mellitus

Diabetes mellitus occurs in about 12 percent of patients with idiopathic Addison's disease, a prevalence which considerably exceeds that of the general population. More than 80 percent have insulin-requiring diabetes (type I) and the age at diagnosis of the two disorders is similar.[438] The mean age at diagnosis is approximately 30 years and the disorder occurs equally in both sexes. The similar age of onset and the increased prevalence of islet cell antibodies in these patients suggests a common pathogenesis.[438]

Vitiligo

Vitiligo is present in 9 percent of patients and may also have an autoimmune basis. Vitiligo may be the consequence of immunologic destruction of the melanocyte. It is rare in other causes of primary adrenal failure. In patients with vitiligo there is a high prevalence of circulating antibodies to the thyroid, parietal cells, and islet cells; however, to date, antimelanocyte antibodies have been described in only a few patients.[602] Since vitiligo occurs frequently in the normal population, its presence in patients with adrenal insufficiency does not establish the diagnosis of autoimmune adrenal dysfunction.

Hypoparathyroidism

The prevalence of hypoparathyroidism in idiopathic Addison's disease is 6 percent.[438] Both the hypoparathyroidism and the Addison's disease tend to occur at younger ages than the other disorders. The mean age at diagnosis of Addison's disease in patients with hypoparathyroidism is 12 years, compared to 32 years in those with diabetes mellitus and 41 years with thyroid disease or pernicious anemia.[583–585,598,599] There are also increased frequencies of ovarian failure and particularly of primary amenorrhea in this group. In Irvine and Barnes's series of five patients with Addison's disease and primary amenorrhea, four had associated hypoparathyroidism.[598] The histology of the parathyroids is characterized by atrophy, fibrosis, and lymphocytic infiltration and there is a high frequency of circulating parathyroid antibodies.

Pernicious Anemia

The association of pernicious anemia and Addison's disease is a remarkable coincidence, since Addison described each of these conditions. The prevalence of pernicious anemia is about 4 percent in idiopathic adrenal insufficiency; the majority of patients are female. In addition, subclinical atrophic gastritis, hypochlorhydria, and achlorhydria are frequent in patients who do not have overt pernicious anemia.[598]

Immunological Aspects

Anderson et al. demonstrated the presence of circulating antibodies to adrenal and thyroid tissue in a patient with Addison's disease in 1957,[603] and there is now extensive experience with antibody measurements in idiopathic Addison's disease.[438,582] The increased prevalence of antibodies to adrenal antigens and other tissues in idiopathic Addison's has not been found in adrenal failure due to tuberculous and other destructive etiologies. As might be anticipated, the occurrence of antibodies to other tissues is higher than the frequency of overt clinical evidence of glandular failure.

Circulating adrenal antibodies are present in approximately 60 percent of patients with idiopathic Addison's disease (Table 12-12).[438] Adrenal antibodies are rare in first-degree relatives of addisonian patients except in those who have primary adrenocortical insufficiency or hypoparathyroidism.[598] As already mentioned, the prevalence is also low in other organ-specific autoimmune diseases (hyperthyroidism, Hashimoto's thyroiditis, primary hypothyroidism, pernicious anemia, diabetes mellitus) in the absence of Addison's disease. However, in patients with idiopathic hypoparathyroidism there is an increased prevalence of antibodies to adrenal (11 percent), gastric (22 percent) and thyroid tissues (13 percent), even in the absence of adrenal insufficiency, pernicious anemia, or thyroid disease.[604,605]

Table 12-12. Circulating Antibodies in Idiopathic Adrenocortical Insufficiency

Antibodies to	Antibody prevalence (%)
Adrenal	64
Thyroid	
Cytoplasm	45
Thyroglobulin	22
Stomach	
Parietal cells	30
Intrinsic factor	9
Parathyroid	26
Gonad	17
Islet cell	8

Source: Adapted from Irvine et al.[438] and Blizzard et al.[604,605]

Antithyroid antibodies are present in 45 percent of patients with idiopathic Addison's disease. Antithyroid antibodies are present (two times) more frequently in female patients than is clinical thyroid dysfunction, especially hyperthyroidism. Since patients with elevated antibody levels may have impaired thyroid reserve, i.e., elevated TSH levels and decreased responsiveness to exogenous TSH administration,[600] these patients are probably at risk of developing subsequent hypothyroidism or Hashimoto's goiter. Thus, the incidence of clinical thyroid disease may increase as longer follow-up of addisonian patients is undertaken.

There are increased prevalences of gastric parietal cell (30 percent) and intrinsic factor (9 percent) antibodies in patients with idiopathic Addison's disease. Atrophic gastritis generally correlates with the presence of antiparietal cell antibodies, and intrinsic factor antibodies show a strong correlation with malabsorption of B_{12} and pernicious anemia.[438] Patients with intrinsic factor antibodies have severe atrophic gastritis, even in the absence of overt pernicious anemia.

Parathyroid antibodies are present in 26 percent of patients with idiopathic Addison's disease, as compared to 6 percent in normal controls.[604,605]

Antibodies reacting with steroid-producing cells of the ovary, testis, or placenta are present in 17 percent of patients, with a much higher prevalence in female patients (22 percent) than in males (5 percent). There is a strong correlation between the presence of circulating gonadal antibodies and premature ovarian failure, especially in patients with primary amenorrhea and idiopathic Addison's disease.[598] These antibodies react not only to gonadal tissue (both ovary and testis) but also to placental tissue and the adrenal cortex. It has also been demonstrated that sera from patients with Addison's disease contain antibodies which are cytotoxic to human granulosa cells grown in tissue culture.[606] The occurrence of antibodies to gonadal tissue is much less in male patients and correlates with the lower incidence of clinical testicular failure. These antibodies are not present in significant proportion in controls or in patients with amenorrhea who do not have Addison's disease.

Approximately 8 percent of patients with idiopathic Addison's disease have demonstrable circulating antibodies to islet cell tissue.[607,608]

With the exception, described above, of gonadal cells,[606] the circulating antibodies in Addison's disease are not considered cytotoxic; instead, it is thought that the adrenal destruction is the consequence of organ-specific cell-mediated immunological mechanisms. However, at present the evidence for abnormal cell-mediated autoimmunity in Addison's disease is less well documented than in thyroid diseases and diabetes mellitus, and the presence of immune complexes has not yet been reported.[438]

Genetic Aspects

Idiopathic Addison's disease is not infrequently familial and has been described in identical twins.[598] In families, Addison's disease may occur alone or may coexist with other autoimmune disorders. A strong familial association of Addison's disease and hypoparathyroidism occurs and an autosomal recessive pattern of inheritance has been suggested.[599] Irvine and Barnes found that 44 percent of patients with idiopathic Addison's disease had first- or second-degree relatives with one or more associated clinical disorders.[598] There is also an increased prevalence of the HLA types B8 and Dw3 in idiopathic Addison's disease, and one study also showed an increased frequency of the HLA-A1,B8 haplotype.[438,609] HLA-B8 also is present in high frequency in relatives of patients with Addison's disease, many of whom have one or more of the clinical disorders.[438,609]

Pathology

In idiopathic adrenal insufficiency there is early lymphocytic infiltration of the adrenal cortex, thus giving rise to the term *diffuse lymphocytic adrenalitis.* Subsequently, the adrenals are small, atrophic, and frequently difficult to locate at autopsy. The capsule is thickened and the normal cortical architecture is destroyed; however, the adrenal medulla is preserved. The cortical cells of all three zones are largely absent and those remaining are scattered, show degenerative change, and are surrounded by a fibrous stroma and lymphocytic infiltrates. The degree of lymphocytic infiltration is variable but its association with loss of cortical cells is the classic pathological feature.[438,587,610]

PRIMARY ADRENOCORTICAL INSUFFICIENCY DUE TO INVASIVE OR HEMORRHAGIC DISORDERS

Adrenal insufficiency secondary to invasive or hemorrhagic disorders is a consequence of total or near-total destruction of both glands and is often accompanied by advanced or disseminated systemic disease. Thus, destruction of the adrenal rarely occurs without involvement of other organs by the same disease process. In these conditions, the rate of development of adrenocortical insufficiency can vary markedly depending on the nature of the primary process. With septicemia or hemorrhage, the adrenal can be rapidly destroyed whereas with conditions such as tuberculosis a much longer period of time may be required.

Invasive Disorders

Adrenal tuberculosis is the consequence of bloodborne infection of the adrenal cortex. It is virtually always accompanied or preceded by tuberculosis infection elsewhere in the body, especially of the lung, gastrointestinal tract, or kidney.[587] In tuberculous Addison's disease, the adrenal glands are totally replaced by caseous necrosis with little or no remaining cortical or medullary tissue. CT scan shows adrenal enlargement in patients with tuberculous Addison's disease of less than 2 years' duration; in contrast, the adrenals are small or undetectable in patients with idiopathic Addison's disease.[611] Calcification of the adrenals is frequent and can be seen radiologically in approximately 50 percent of cases.[342,611]

When destruction is due to processes other than tuberculosis, the pathological findings in the adrenal are characteristic of the particular disorder, with loss of adrenal tissue and either scarring, inflammatory changes, or replacement of tissue with tumor, amyloid, etc.[611] Adrenal calcification is less common than with tuberculosis.

Adrenal Hemorrhage

Bilateral adrenal hemorrhage may cause rapid and total adrenal destruction, leading to acute loss of both glucocorticoid and mineralocorticoid secretion. In adults, adrenal hemorrhage usually occurs in patients over the age of 50 years, and anticoagulant therapy is the most common cause, contributing to one-third of the cases.[588,612] Adrenal hemorrhage can also occur in patients with either overwhelming infection with sepsis or with severe and frequently life-threatening major illnesses.[588–590,612,613] These include coagulation disorders, adrenal vein thrombosis, adrenal metastases, trauma, major surgery, severe cardiovascular disease, congestive heart failure, pulmonary emboli, acute renal failure, local infection, leukemias, lymphomas, malignancy, trauma, and severe burns.[588–590,612,613] In these cases the diagnosis is usually made at autopsy. In children, the most common cause of bilateral adrenal hemorrhage is fulminant meningococcemia or *Psuedomonas* septicemia.[589–590] Adrenal hemorrhage may also occur in the neonate following complicated delivery or in the presence of a coagulation disorder. Adrenal hemorrhage may also occur during complicated pregnancy or in the postpartum period.

The role of acute adrenal insufficiency in the mortality of these conditions is controversial.[588] It has been argued that adrenal hemorrhage does not significantly alter mortality in patients with sepsis or severe illness.[588,589,614] However, in a study of meningococcemia, six of seven patients with demonstrated adrenocortical insufficiency died (all had bilateral adrenal hemorrhage at autopsy), whereas 17 of 19 patients with appropriately elevated plasma cortisol concentrations survived.[589] Several cases of adrenal insufficiency secondary to anticoagulant-induced hemorrhage have been described with survival with corticosteroid therapy.[612] One patient with fulminant meningococcemia and adrenal insufficiency survived with steroid therapy and, when restudied after recovery, showed normal adrenal reserve.[614] Thus, it is possible that steroid therapy enhances survival in these patients and that adrenal damage is not always permanent.

The adrenal glands in this syndrome are enlarged, not infrequently to a massive degree, and the cortex may be totally destroyed.[611,612,615] The hemorrhage usually replaces the medulla and inner cortex; the outer cortex undergoes ischemic necrosis with only a thin rim of cortical cells remaining.[613] Venous thrombosis frequently accompanies the hemorrhage. In surviving patients the hematomas resolve and the adrenals may calcify.

FAMILIAL GLUCOCORTICOID DEFICIENCY

Familial glucocorticoid deficiency (hereditary adrenocortical unresponsiveness to ACTH) is a rare type of adrenal insufficiency characterized by glucocorticoid and adrenal androgen deficiency with elevated plasma ACTH levels.[616-618] Cortisol secretion does not respond to prolonged ACTH stimulation; however, aldosterone is normally responsive to posture and sodium deprivation, except in a few cases who have had partial mineralocorticoid deficiency.[616-618] The disorder usually presents in childhood, and may be accompanied by achalasia.[617,618] The features distinguishing this syndrome from idiopathic adrenocortical insufficiency are the maintenance of normal mineralocorticoid secretion with preservation of the zona glomerulosa histologically and the absence of lymphocytic infiltration in the degenerated zona fasciculata and reticularis. The etiology of this syndrome is unclear; it has been suggested that it is due to adrenal unresponsiveness to ACTH at the level of the ACTH receptor,[617] but others have proposed an inherited progressive degenerative process affecting the adrenal cortex.[618]

PATHOPHYSIOLOGY

The development of clinical manifestations of adrenocortical insufficiency requires loss of greater than 90 percent of both adrenal cortices. In the idiopathic and invasive types, destruction is usualy gradual, leading to the manifestations of chronic adrenocortical insufficiency; however, in one-third of cases there is a more rapid course, with a symptom duration of less than 3 months.[342] In addition, approximately 25 percent of patients are in crisis or impending crisis at the time of diagnosis.[342] Hemorrhagic destruction of the adrenals results in an abrupt state of adrenal insufficiency with sudden loss of both glucocorticoid and mineralocorticoid secretion.

With gradual destruction, normal regulatory mechanisms are able to compensate. Decreased cortisol production results in decreased feedback at the hypothalamus and pituitary with increased release of the POMC-derived peptides ACTH, β-LPH, and the NH_2-terminal fragment. The increased ACTH level results in increased stimulation of the remaining adrenal with normal cortisol production in the early stages, but inadequate production as the disease progresses. The MSH sequences within the POMC-derived peptides also lead to increased pigmentation, one of the cardinal signs of the disease (see below). In the minority of cases with more rapid adrenal destruction prominent hyperpigmentation may not be present. The decreased mineralocorticoid production leads to sodium loss and potassium retention. The sodium loss results in stimulation of renin release and angiotensin II production. The increased potassium and angiotensin II stimulate the remaining glomerulosa to produce more aldosterone, but with progressive adrenal destruction this mechanism also becomes inadequate.

When adrenal destruction is gradual there is a phase characterized by normal basal steroid secretion, but inability to respond to stress, i.e., decreased adrenal reserve. This may progress to a state where overall steroid production is diminished, but enough episodic releases of cortisol occur such that basal cortisol determinations can be in the normal range. In this state of partial adrenal insufficiency, the patient may have few complaints, but a history usually discloses symptoms and most of these patients show pigmentation because of increased POMC peptide production. In this state, a crisis can be precipitated by the stresses of surgery, trauma, or infection.

As destruction of the adrenal cortex progresses, mineralocorticoid and glucocorticoid secretion become inadequate and even basal cortisol levels are low. This leads to all of the metabolic derangements described above (see Actions of Glucocorticoids and Actions of Mineralocorticoids). These are reflected in manifestations of chronic adrenocortical insufficiency (see below).

CLINICAL FEATURES

The clinical presentation depends on the rate and degree of adrenocortical destruction and on extraadrenal factors which may precipitate a crisis. Thus, most cases with idiopathic or invasive etiologies are insidious in onset and gradually progressive, but a crisis may be precipitated by intercurrent stress.[342] Adrenal hemorrhage also presents with acute adrenal insufficiency. Because the presentations of these three subtypes of primary adrenocortical insufficiency differ, the clinical manifestations are discussed here separately.

Chronic Primary Adrenocortical Insufficiency

The gradual development of adrenal insufficiency may go unnoticed by the patient or physician until adrenocortical function is lost to a major degree. However, in retrospect, the symptoms are not infrequently present for months or even years before diagnosis or presentation.

Major clinical features and an estimate of their frequency are shown in Table 12-13.[342,581,598] These include weakness and fatigue, weight loss, anorexia, and gastrointestinal symptoms. The most distinctive physical finding is hyperpigmentation. Its presence in association with any of these other manifestations should elicit suspicion of Addison's disease. Weakness is always present and is accompanied by fatigue and malaise. It is generalized and usually manifested by an inability to complete routine tasks rather than being restricted to particular muscle groups. Weight loss is also very common, may vary from 2 to 15 kg, and becomes more severe as adrenal failure progresses.[398] It is largely due to tissue loss resulting from anorexia, but dehydration also contributes.

The majority of patients have gastrointestinal symptoms. Anorexia is extremely common and contributes to the weight loss. Nausea, vague abdominal discomfort, and vomiting occur more frequently with progressive adrenal failure. Diarrhea may be present but is less frequent. Gastrointestinal symptoms may be pronounced as adrenal crisis supervenes and may lead to the mistaken diagnosis of primary gastrointestinal disease. It is important for the physician to consider Addison's disease in patients with these symptoms, since radiologic studies that require enemas, cathartics, and fasting can precipitate shock and collapse.

Hypotension is common but in many patients may not be profound enough to suggest the diagnosis. Nevertheless, systolic blood pressure is <110 mmHg in over 90 percent of patients[398,581] and is frequently associated with complaints of orthostatic dizziness and, occasionally, syncope. In patients in crisis, recumbent hypotension or shock is an almost universal finding.

Hyperpigmentation of the skin and mucous membranes is the single most distinctive sign in chronic primary adrenocortical insufficiency and can be most useful, especially in an acutely ill patient with unexplained hypotension. It may precede other manifestations of adrenal insufficiency (Fig. 12-29). It is generalized, with accentuation in sun-exposed areas and pressure points such as the elbows, knees, knuckles, and toes and around the waist. Abnormal pigmentation should be suspected when it is present on palmar creases, nail beds, buccal mucosa, nipples, navel, areolae, and the perivaginal or perianal mucosa. Pigmentation of the buccal mucosa and gums is always accompanied by generalized hyperpigmentation.[438] Surgical scars acquired after the onset of Addison's disease are frequently hyperpigmented whereas previous scars remain unpigmented. The increased pigmentation is frequently accompanied by the appearance of numerous black or brown freckles. In people of dark-skinned races, pigmentation of the mouth, palmar creases, vulva, and anus may be normally present and the diagnosis of hyperpigmentation is frequently difficult. Pigmentation of the tongue is probably abnormal regardless of racial background. The hyperpigmentation is commonly misinterpreted as due to sun exposure, and the healthy appearance of the patient may lead to dismissal of other symptoms.

Vitiligo occurs in 4 to 17 percent of patients with idiopathic Addison's disease; however, it occurs rarely in those with tuberculosis.[342,581]

Salt craving is a significant feature in approximately 20 percent of cases;[619] some patients may actually eat salt by the spoonful despite anorexia.

Although both fasting and postprandial hypoglycemia were frequently reported in older series,[398,620] they appear to be less frequent in current patients.[341,581] The fasting blood sugar level is within the lower normal range in most patients; it is unusual for the patient with Addison's disease to present with or have symptomatic complaints of hypoglycemia, and severe hypoglycemia is rare, except in children. Hypo-

Table 12-13. Clinical Features of Chronic Primary Adrenocortical Insufficiency

Feature	Percent with condition
Weakness and fatigue	100
Weight loss	100
Anorexia	100
Hyperpigmentation	92
Hypotension	88
Gastrointestinal symptoms	56
Salt craving	19
Postural symptoms	12

Source: Adapted from Nerup[342] and Thorn.[619]

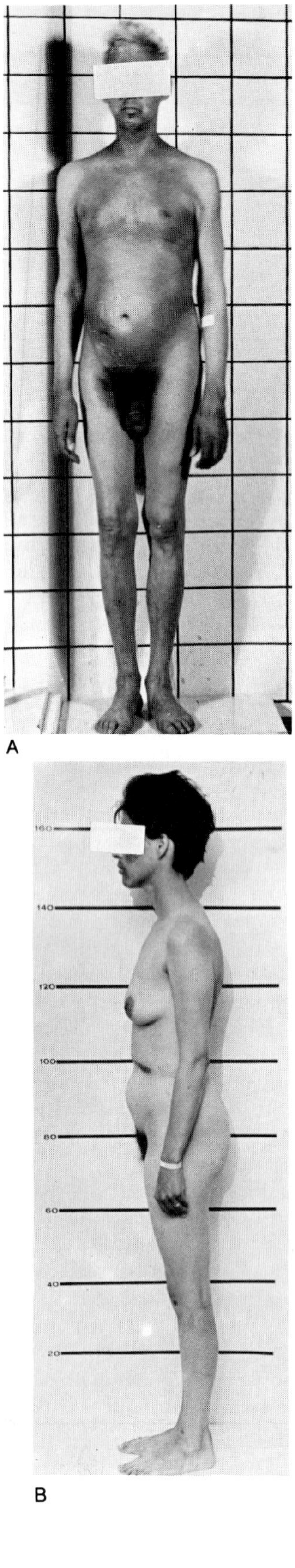

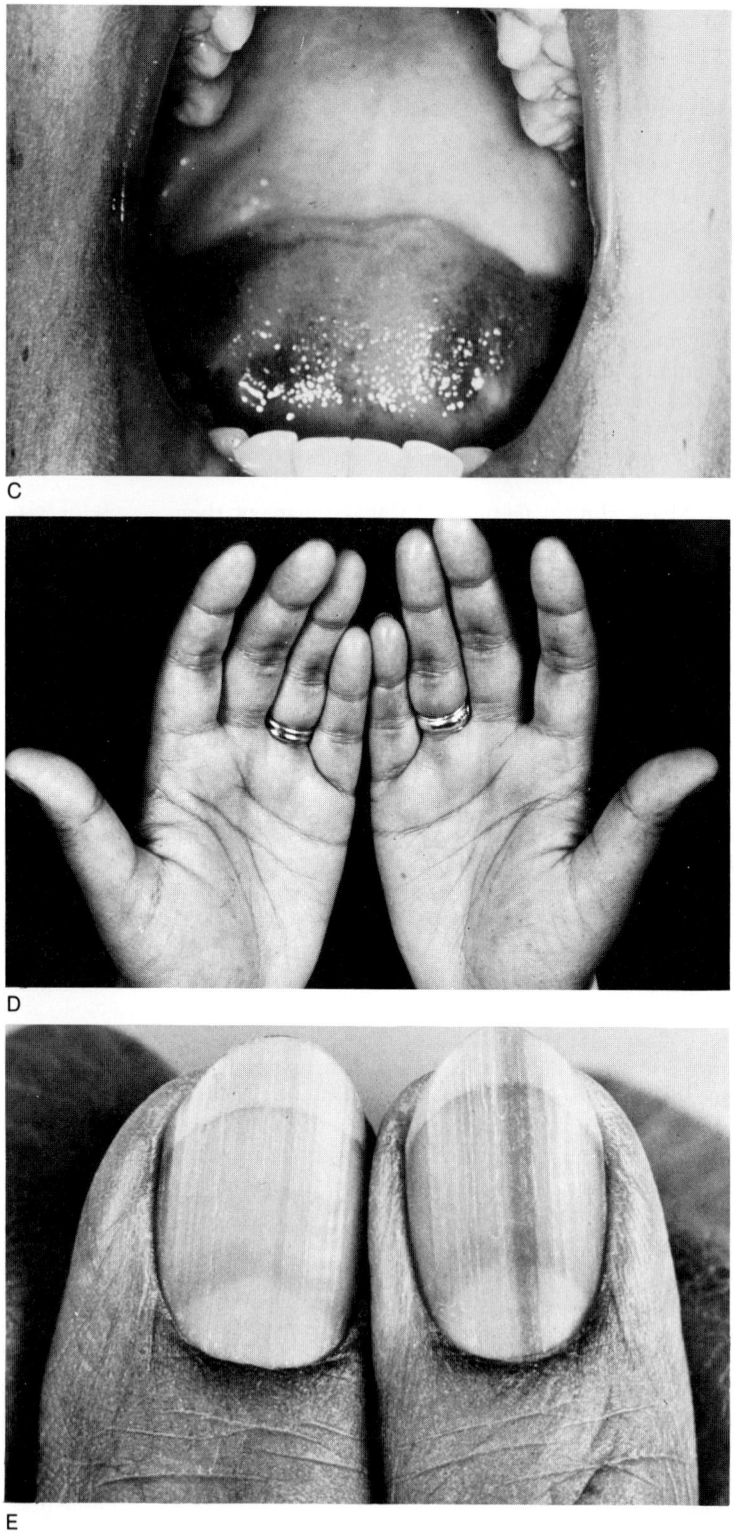

FIGURE 12-29 Abnormal pigmentation due to hypersecretion of ACTH and β-LPH. (*A*) Generalized hyperpigmentation with accentuation over exposed areas. (*B*) Pigmentation is noted mostly in exposed areas, although the abdominal surgical scar is markedly hyperpigmented. (*C*) Hyperpigmentation of the tongue. (*D*) Hyperpigmentation prominent in skin creases. (*E*) Hyperpigmentation of and around the nails.

glycemia may be provoked by fasting, fever, infection, or nausea and vomiting and may be present in acute adrenal crisis.[398,620] In the patient with preceding diabetes, improvement in blood sugar control and a decrease in insulin requirement tends to occur when Addison's disease emerges.

Amenorrhea is common in untreated Addison's disease patients and may be a manifestation of either weight loss and chronic illness or of primary ovarian failure from an associated immunological cause. Loss of axillary and pubic hair occurs in a minority of female patients, due to a loss of adrenal androgens.

Patients with idiopathic Addison's disease may also have symptoms of the associated disorders discussed earlier. Similarly, patients with tuberculosis or other invasive diseases causing adrenal insufficiency usually have involvement of other organ systems.

Acute Adrenocortical Insufficiency (Adrenal Crisis)

The most common emergency presentation of primary adrenal insufficiency is that of acute adrenal crisis in the patient with undiagnosed or treated Addison's disease who is exposed to stress such as infection, trauma, surgery, or dehydration due to salt deprivation, vomiting, or diarrhea. The requirement for increased glucocorticoid levels during stress has already been emphasized, although addisonian patients usually tolerate minor insults such as upper respiratory infections. Thus, the addisonian patient who does not receive therapy during these stresses may rapidly develop an acute adrenal crisis.

When acute adrenal insufficiency develops (Table 12-14), anorexia becomes profound and there is increased nausea and vomiting, which contributes to volume depletion and dehydration. Abdominal pain is frequent and may mimic an acute surgical abdomen. Specific localizing features are usually absent, although there may be tenderness and pain on deep palpation. The blood pressure falls further and hypovolemic shock develops with extreme weakness, apathy, and confusion. The patient may rapidly develop severe dehydration. Fever is frequent and hypoglycemia may be present. The fever may be due either to hypoadrenalism or to a precipitating infection. Hyperpigmentation is usually present in the patient with primary adrenocortical insufficiency and is an important clinical sign. Without appropriate therapy death may occur rapidly, with coma and shock. Hyponatremia, hyperkalemia, lymphocytosis, and eosinophilia should suggest the diagnosis of adrenal crisis and the possibility of adrenal insufficiency must be considered in any patient with unexplained shock. Since some other process commonly precipitates the adrenal crises, these manifestations may divert attention from the possibility of Addison's disease. For instance, in the patient with coexisting diabetes mellitus, ketoacidosis can precipitate or be caused by the crisis. In previously undiagnosed patients, it is frequently possible to obtain a history of preceding chronic adrenal insufficiency at the time of acute presentation; however, this is not always the case, because some patients may have enough basal glucocorticoid production to prevent chronic symptoms but adrenal reserve may be decreased in response to stress.

Table 12-14. Clinical Features of Acute Primary Adrenocortical Insufficiency (Adrenal Crisis)

Hypotension/shock (vascular collapse)
Weakness, apathy, confusion
Nausea, vomiting, anorexia
Dehydration, hypovolemia, hyponatremia, hypokalemia
Abdominal or flank pain
Hyperthermia
Hypoglycemia

Adrenal Hemorrhage Causing Acute Adrenal Insufficiency

The typical clinical picture in patients with bilateral adrenal hemorrhage and acute adrenal destruction is that of a progressively deteriorating course in an already complicated patient with major illness (Table 12-15).[588-590,612,613] The classic clinical features of Addison's disease, i.e., hyperpigmentation, weight loss, and preceding chronic gastrointestinal symptoms, are absent. The usual presenting symptoms are abdominal, flank, or chest pain with abdominal tenderness.[588,612] Abdominal distention, rigidity, or rebound tenderness occurs less frequently. Hypotension shock, fever, nausea, vomiting, confusion, and disorientation are common. Tachycardia and cyanosis are less frequent. With progression, severe hypotension, volume depletion, dehydration, hyperpyrexia, cyanosis, coma, and death ensue.[588,612] The diagnosis of acute adrenal hemorrhage should be considered in the deteriorating patient with unexplained abdominal or flank pain, vascular collapse, hyperpyrexia, or hypoglycemia.

LABORATORY FEATURES OF PRIMARY ADRENOCORTICAL INSUFFICIENCY

The specific laboratory diagnosis of Addison's disease depends on measurement of the plasma cortisol response to ACTH administration (see below). However, other laboratory abnormalities which are not diagnostic should suggest the diagnosis (Table 12-16).

Table 12-15. Clinical Features of Adrenal Hemorrhage

Features	Percent
General:	
Hypotension/shock	74
Fever	59
Nausea and vomiting	46
Confusion, disorientation	41
Tachycardia	28
Cyanosis/lividity	28
Local:	
Abdominal, flank, or back pain	77
Abdominal or flank tenderness	38
Abdominal distention	28
Abdominal rigidity	20
Chest pain	13
Rebound tenderness	5

Source: Adapted from Xarli et al.[588]

Hyponatremia and hyperkalemia secondary to mineralocorticoid deficiency are characteristic manifestations of primary adrenal insufficiency; in the absence of chronic renal failure their presence should suggest Addison's disease. Hyponatremia is present in 88 percent and hyperkalemia in 64 percent of patients at the time of diagnosis.[341]

A normocytic normochromic anemia is common, but may also be masked by dehydration and hemoconcentration. Pernicious anemia is present in 4 percent of patients with autoimmune Addison's disease.[581] The differential white count shows neutropenia, a relative lymphocytosis, and eosinophilia. Elevations of the blood urea nitrogen (BUN) and serum creatinine levels are ascribable to dehydration and hemoconcentration and are frequently accompanied by mild acidosis due to dehydration, hyperkalemia, and the loss of the acid-secreting properties of the mineralocorticoids.

Mild to moderate hypercalcemia occurs in approximately 6 percent of patients,[341] and may be mistaken for the hypercalcemia of dehydration. Hypocalcemia and hyperphosphatemia are present in patients with associated hypoparathyroidism.

Table 12-16. Laboratory Features of Primary Adrenocortical Insufficiency

Hyponatremia (88%)*	Eosinophilia
Hyperkalemia (64%)*	Lymphocytosis
Azotemia	Hypoglycemia
Anemia	Hypercalcemia

*Percent occurrence from Nerup.[342]

The heart can be small and vertical on x-ray. Routine radiographs of the abdomen are usually normal, but adrenal calcification is present in approximately 50 percent of cases due to tuberculosis[341,398] and can also be present with other invasive etiologies and after hemorrhagic destruction of the gland. With CT of the abdomen adrenal enlargement and/or calcification is demonstrated with tuberculosis, metastases, and adrenal hemorrhage, whereas, in the idiopathic form, the adrenals may be destroyed and thus are small or absent on abdominal scans.[611,615]

The electrocardiogram may reveal low voltage with a vertical QRS axis. There may be nonspecific abnormalities due to electrolyte imbalance (e.g., peaked T waves due to the hyperkalemia or a shortened QT segment).

With sudden adrenal destruction typical laboratory manifestations are usually absent. Hyponatremia and hyperkalemia occur in a minority; however, their presence should suggest the diagnosis.[588,612,613] Azotemia is common, whereas hypoglycemia is infrequent.[588,612,613] Increased circulating eosinophils or an increased total eosinophil count may be present and should also arouse suspicion of acute adrenal insufficiency.

Secondary Adrenocortical Insufficiency

ETIOLOGY

The causes of secondary adrenocortical insufficiency are reviewed in Chaps. 7 and 8. Therapy with pharmacologic doses of glucocorticoids is the most frequent cause (Chap. 15). If the steroid-treated population is excluded, tumors of the pituitary and/or hypothalamic region are the most common cause of pituitary ACTH deficiency, and surgical or radiation therapy for these tumors may also contribute to panhypopituitarism. In patients with hypothalamic or pituitary tumors, ACTH deficiency is virtually always accompanied by deficiencies of other anterior pituitary hormones, since the ACTH-producing cells are more resistant to pituitary damage. Growth hormone and gonadotropins are usually lost first, followed by loss of TSH and finally of ACTH (Chap. 8). Rarely, isolated ACTH deficiency can occur. Other less common causes of hypothalamic-pituitary dysfunction are discussed in Chaps. 7 and 8.

PATHOPHYSIOLOGY

The pathogenesis of secondary adrenal insufficiency differs from that of primary adrenocortical destruction since the predominant effect of ACTH deficiency is decreased cortisol and adrenal androgen secretion. In hypothalamic or pituitary tumors gradual growth of the lesion compresses the normal anterior pituitary, resulting in gradual destruction of corticotrophic cells with impairment of ACTH secretion. Initially, basal ACTH levels are maintained, however there may be impaired ACTH reserve; basal cortisol secretion is also normal but ACTH and cortisol levels cannot increase in response to stress. With progression, basal ACTH secretion becomes deficient, resulting in atrophy of the adrenal zonae fasciculata and reticularis and decreased cortisol secretion in the basal state. When this occurs, not only is there impaired ability to increase ACTH secretion in response to stress but the atrophic adrenal becomes unable to increase cortisol secretion in response to acute stimulation with ACTH.

In the rare syndrome of isolated ACTH deficiency, secondary adrenal insufficiency also develops, but, in contrast to pituitary tumors, there is no loss of other pituitary hormones,[621,622] except for other POMC-derived peptides.[622] It is not known whether deficient ACTH production in this case is due to a pituitary etiology or results from defective hypothalamic secretion of CRF.[621,622]

Glucocorticoid therapy also suppresses the pituitary-adrenal axis; the effect is both dose- and time-dependent (Chap. 15). Although growth hormone and gonadotropin secretion may be depressed, pituitary function is generally intact (see Actions of Glucocorticoids, above, Cushing's Syndrome, below, and Chap. 15).

The glucocorticoid deficiency present in these conditions results in manifestations similar to those seen in primary adrenocortical insufficiency except that derangements due to mineralocorticoid deficiency are usually absent. The functional status of the zona glomerulosa is initially preserved; in the early stages aldosterone secretion, controlled by the renin-angiotensin system, is normal. When ACTH deficiency is long-standing, mineralocorticoid deficiency may develop;[189,623] however, only a minority of patients with ACTH deficiency due to panhypopituitarism, prolonged steroid therapy, or other causes have clinical or electrolyte evidence of mineralocorticoid deficiency.[189] Of those with abnormalities, some maintain normal basal secretion with decreased responsiveness to sodium deprivation, whereas others have deficient basal and stimulated aldosterone secretion.[189,624] Thus, hyponatremia may be provoked in some of these patients by sodium deprivation.[189,624] The mechanism of this mineralocorticoid deficiency is unknown; it is possible that it is due to a loss of the effects of ACTH or other POMC-derived peptides on the glomerulosa (see Regulation of Mineralocorticoid Production, above). In addition, ACTH-deficient patients have been described in whom deficient aldosterone secretion was corrected by glucocorticoid administration; in one of these the hypoaldosteronism was associated with hyporeninemia.[189,623]

CLINICAL FEATURES

The clinical presentation of secondary adrenal insufficiency, like that of the primary type, is usually chronic. However, an acute presentation can occur in the undiagnosed patient during stress or in treated patients who do not receive increased steroid dosage during infection, surgery, or trauma. Pituitary apoplexy, i.e., hemorrhagic infarction of a pituitary tumor, may be accompanied by acute secondary adrenocortical insufficiency.

The usual presentation of secondary adrenal insufficiency is similar to that of primary adrenocortical insufficiency, with two important exceptions. First, since pituitary secretion of ACTH and β-LPH is deficient, the characteristic hyperpigmentation of Addison's disease is absent. In fact, patients with hypopituitarism frequently present with pallor of the skin. Secondly, as discussed above, the clinical features of mineralocorticoid deficiency are usually absent in the unstressed state, and therefore volume depletion, dehydration, and electrolyte abnormalities are usually absent. Hypotension is also less severe, except in acute presentations. Hyponatremia can be present, and is usually due to water retention and inability to excrete a water load rather than to sodium loss (see Cardiovascular System under Actions of Glucocorticoids, above). Thus, the clinical features of ACTH and glucocorticoid deficiency are nonspecific and consist predominantly of weakness, lethargy, easy fatigue, anorexia, nausea, and, occasionally, vomiting. Patients may also describe arthralgias, myalgias, and exacerbation of allergic responses. Hypoglycemia is occasionally the presenting feature and may be more prominent than in primary adrenal insufficiency due to the concomitant loss of growth hormone.[423] With acute decompensation, severe hypotension or shock may occur and be unresponsive to vasopressors unless glucocorticoids are administered.

Patients with secondary adrenal insufficiency (except those with isolated ACTH deficiency) commonly have associated historical or clinical features which suggest the diagnosis. There may be a history of glucocorticoid therapy or the presence of cushingoid features, suggestive of previous therapy (Chap. 15). Patients with hypothalamic or pituitary tumors and ACTH deficiency usually have loss of other pituitary function; i.e., hypogonadism and hypothyroidism are common and there may be hypersecretion of growth hormone or prolactin. Most patients also have local tumor manifestations such as visual field defects, headache, or enlargement of the sella turcica (see Chaps. 7 and 8).

LABORATORY FEATURES

Routine laboratory testing in secondary adrenal hypofunction may reveal a mild normochromic normocytic anemia, neutropenia, relative lymphocytosis, and eosinophilia. The serum sodium concentraton may be low, but potassium, BUN, creatinine, and bicarbonate concentrations are usually normal. Hypoglycemia may be present. Cardiac size on x-ray is normal, as is the ECG. CT scanning of the head may reveal the pituitary tumor and CT scan of the abdomen shows normal or atrophic adrenal glands.

Diagnosis

The typical clinical picture of Addison's disease is obvious in the majority of patients. Although the clinical suspicion must be confirmed by more definitive laboratory testing, therapy should not be delayed by prolonged diagnostic measures, nor should the patient be subjected to ancillary diagnostic tests which may lead to further volume loss, dehydration, and hypotension. In the acute situation, if rapid diagnostic tests are not available, therapy should be instituted and the diagnosis etablished later.

The diagnosis of adrenal insufficiency should not be established based on basal levels of either urinary or plasma steroids, since partial degrees of adrenal insufficiency occur. Thus, a normal plasma cortisol level (5 to 25 μg/dl) does not exclude the diagnosis of adrenocortical insufficiency in either chronic or acute situations, and it is not uncommon to find random cortisol determinations in the normal range with partial adrenal insufficiency. If the plasma cortisol is elevated (i.e., >25 μg/dl), the diagnosis is unlikely, but if the plasma cortisol is low or undetectable in a critically ill patient, adrenal insufficiency should be considered. However, tests which specifically measure adrenocortical reserve are necessary to establish the diagnosis (Fig. 12-30). These tests, discussed below in the context of their diagnostic utility in these conditions, are described in Laboratory Evaluation of Adrenocortical Function, above.

The rapid ACTH stimulation test using synthetic human $ACTH^{1-24}$ is a sensitive test of adrenal reserve and is the procedure of choice in the assessment of patients with possible adrenal insufficiency. This test is used as the initial diagnostic step in all suspected cases, either primary or secondary. Since the procedure requires only 30 min, it can usually be performed even in acute situations. In suspected primary adrenal insufficiency a normal response excludes the diagnosis and these patients do not require further evaluation. However, normal responses do not always exclude secondary adrenal insufficiency since some patients have decreased pituitary reserve or decreased responsiveness of the hypothalamic-pituitary-adrenal axis to stress but maintain the ability to respond to exogenous ACTH stimulation (discussed below and under Laboratory Evaluation of Adrenocortical Function).[551-555]

Subnormal responses to the rapid ACTH stimulation test establish the diagnosis of adrenocortical insufficiency, and correlate well with subnormal responsiveness of the pituitary-adrenal axis to metyrapone, insulin-induced hypoglycemia, and stress.[548-555] Three-day ACTH stimulation tests were traditionally used in the diagnosis of adrenocortical insufficiency, but are usually unnecessary and give little additional diagnostic information in the presence of a subnormal response to the rapid ACTH stimulation test.

If the rapid ACTH stimulation test indicates adrenal insufficiency, primary and secondary forms are readily differentiated by measurement of the plasma ACTH level. Plasma ACTH levels in patients with untreated primary adrenal insufficiency exceed 250 pg/ml and are usually between 400 and 2000 pg/ml (Fig. 12-31).[503] In secondary adrenal insufficiency due to pituitary ACTH deficiency, plasma ACTH levels are inappropriately low when compared to circulating cortisol levels and range from 0 to 50 pg/ml.[503]

If plasma ACTH assays are unavailable, the plasma aldosterone response to the rapid ACTH stimulation test or the three-day ACTH stimulation test can be used to differentiate primary and secondary adrenal insufficiency. However, experience with the aldosterone response is less extensive than with measurement of plasma ACTH levels (see Laboratory Evaluation of Adrenocortical Function, above).

Although a subnormal response to the rapid ACTH stimulation test establishes the diagnosis of adrenal insufficiency, a normal adrenal response to ACTH stimulation does not exclude partial ACTH deficiency. This problem usually arises in patients who have been treated with glucocorticoids (Chap. 15) and in patients with partial pituitary or hypothalamic dysfunction. When secondary adrenal insufficiency is still suspected in a patient with a normal response to the rapid ACTH stimulation test, more specific information regarding pituitary responsiveness can be obtained by testing with metyrapone or insulin-induced hypoglycemia. In these cases the overnight metyrapone test is ordinarily performed in patients with suspected hypothalamic or pituitary disorders in whom hypoglycemia is contraindicated and in those with prior glucocorticoid therapy. The overnight metyrapone

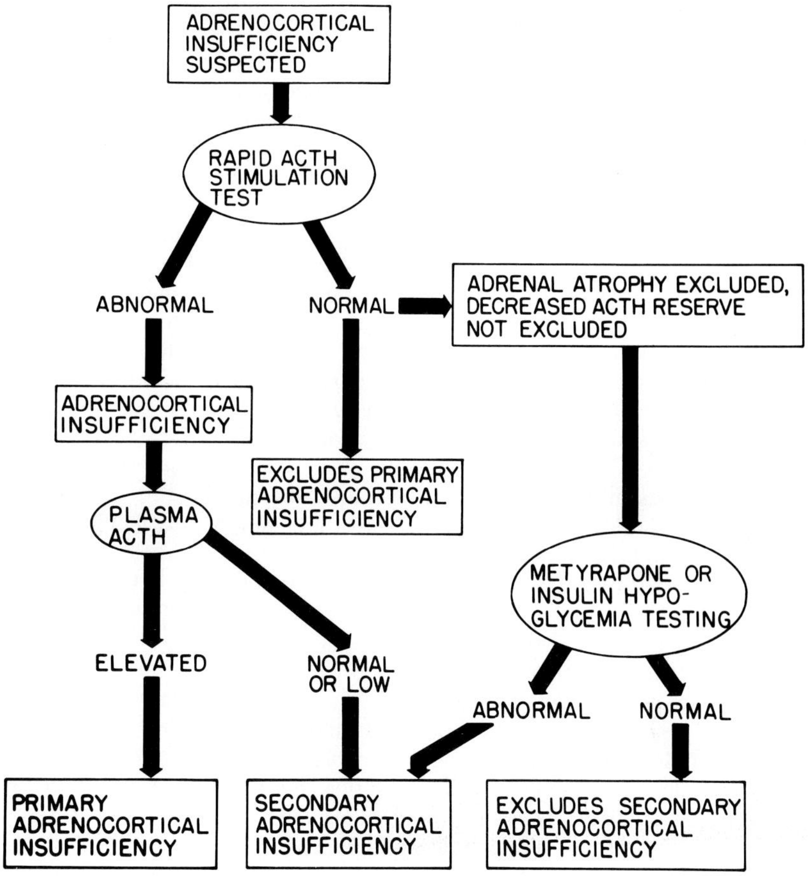

FIGURE 12-30 Evaluation of suspected primary or secondary adrenocortical insufficiency. Boxes enclose clinical decisions; circles enclose diagnostic tests.

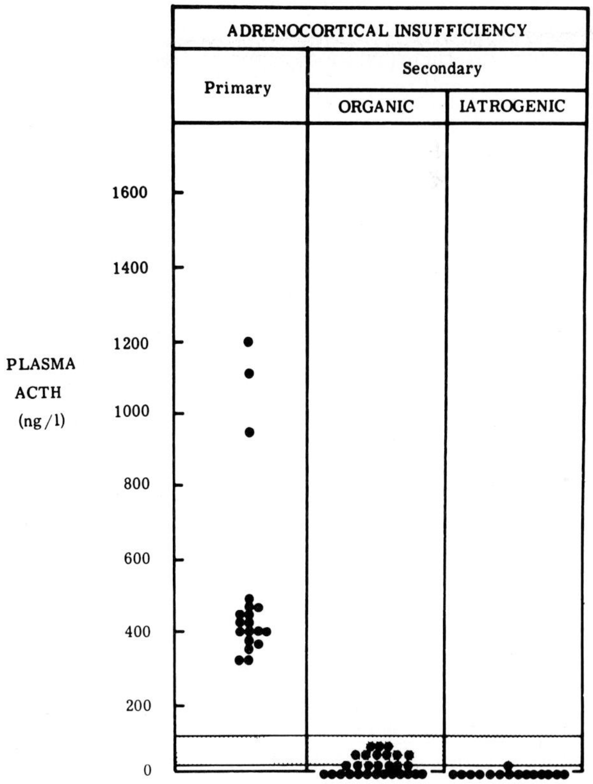

FIGURE 12-31 Basal plasma ACTH levels in primary and secondary adrenocortical insufficiency. (*From Irvine et al.*;[438] *based on data from Besser et al.*[503])

test is preferred because it is simpler, more rapid, and safer than the 3-day test. Insulin-induced hypoglycemia is usually used in patients with suspected hypothalamic or pituitary tumors, since both ACTH and growth hormone responsiveness are measured with this single procedure. A normal response to either metyrapone or hypoglycemia excludes secondary adrenocortical insufficiency (see Laboratory Evaluation of Adrenocortical Function, above). Subnormal responses to these tests establish the diagnosis of secondary adrenal insufficiency, since in these patients the primary form has been previously excluded by a normal rapid ACTH stimulation test and normal or subnormal plasma ACTH levels.

In primary adrenocortical insufficiency, tuberculosis must be ruled out by usual measures, including chest x-ray and skin tests. A urinalysis may show evidence of renal tuberculosis and adrenal CT scans may show adrenal enlargement and/or calcification. If tuberculosis is absent and if no other systemic disease is present, the adrenal insufficiency is probably idiopathic. The presence of adrenal antibodies confirms the diagnosis; however, assays for these antibodies are not generally available. The diagnosis of idiopathic Addison's disease is usually made by exclusion, but the presence of associated disorders provides confirmatory evidence. Since these associated disorders may not always be obvious by history and physical examination, screening tests are helpful. This evaluation should include a blood count; glucose, calcium, and phosphorus determinations; thyroid function tests; TSH assay; and test for thyroid antibodies. If there is oligomenorrhea or amenorrhea, FSH and LH levels should also be determined. Since there is a high frequency of disorders in first- and second-degree relatives, these individuals should also be screened by the same tests.

In secondary adrenocortical insufficiency the patient should be evaluated for other pituitary deficiencies and for the presence of a hypothalamic or pituitary tumor (see Chap. 7). The evaluation of patients with adrenal insufficiency resulting from steroid therapy is discussed in Chap. 15.

In the acutely ill patient with adrenal insufficiency, it is also imperative to determine the etiology of the condition that precipitates the crisis. For example, whereas fever can be due to glucocorticoid insufficiency, it may also be a manifestation of an underlying infection.

The patient who has been treated with glucocorticoids prior to establishment of a diagnosis presents a special problem, since the therapy may itself suppress the hypothalamic-pituitary-adrenal axis. This is especially true when high-dose glucocorticoids are given to an acutely ill patient. In general, such high-dose therapy is not needed for prolonged periods (for example, more than two weeks), so that when the steroid is tapered and the patient is placed on maintenance cortisol, normal hypothalamic-pituitary-adrenal responsiveness should be present and the rapid ACTH stimulation test can be used (see Chap. 15). In the exceptional circumstance in which longer high-dose therapy has been given, the 3-day ACTH stimulation test can be used; the overall management and diagnostic approaches in this case are discussed in Chap. 15.

Treatment

ACUTE ADDISONIAN CRISIS

Therapy in acute addisonian crisis should be instituted immediately if a strong clinical suspicion is present (Table 12-17). The rationale for high-dose glucocorticoids is based on the fact that the adrenal gland responds to serious illness with increased cortisol production. Therapy should include the administration of large doses of a soluble glucocorticoid preparation, the correction of hypovolemia and electrolyte abnormalities, general supportive measures, and treatment of coexisting or precipitating disorders. Since both mineralocorticoid and glucocorticoid deficiency are present in primary adrenocortical insufficiency, a preparation with sodium-retaining potency is recommended. The drug of choice is a soluble form of injectable cortisol (hydrocortisone hemisuccinate or hydrocortisone phosphate), which should be administered IV in doses of 100 mg every 6 h for the first 24 h. If the patient's progress is satisfactory and no additional complications are present, the dosage may be reduced to 50 mg every 6 h on the second day and then tapered gradually to oral maintenance doses by the fourth to fifth day. Mineralocorticoid therapy is usually required when the cortisol dose is decreased below 50 to 60 mg per day (see below). If a life-threatening condition is present at the same time, a dosage of 100 mg every 6 to 8 h should be continued until the patient improves.

Table 12-17. Treatment of Acute Adrenocortical Insufficiency (Adrenal Crisis)

1. Cortisol, 100 mg IV, every 6 h for 24 h. Reduce to 50 mg every 6 h if progress is satisfactory, and then taper to oral maintenance dose by day 4 or 5. Maintain or increase dosage to 200 to 400 mg/24 h if complications persist or occur.
2. IV saline and glucose.
3. Correction of precipitating factors.
4. General supportive measures.

Since patients in adrenal crisis may have profound dehydration, volume depletion, hypotension, and hypoglycemia, adequate replacement with IV glucose and saline must be given. Severe hyperkalemia and/or acidosis may occasionally require specific therapy. IM cortisone acetate should not be used in the treatment of acute adrenal insufficiency since there is poor absorption, failure to achieve adequate blood levels of cortisol and inadequate biological activity, as evidenced by failure to suppress ACTH levels.[625]

The patient with crisis due to secondary adrenocortical insufficiency usually does not have the severe electrolyte abnormalities seen with patients with primary adrenocortical insufficiency. Thus, the major requirement is for glucocorticoid replacement. Whereas the use of other glucocorticoids such as prednisolone or dexamethasone is probably acceptable, the regimen outlined above is standard, has been proved to be effective, and will provide adequate mineralocorticoid replacement in these patients with impaired aldosterone production.

CHRONIC ADRENAL INSUFFICIENCY

The treatment of chronic primary Addison's disease requires maintenance therapy with both glucocorticoids and mineralocorticoids (Table 12-18). The patient must be taught that a lifetime of therapy is required and that cessation of therapy may endanger life. In the majority of patients 20 to 30 mg of cortisol per day is sufficient, with two-thirds given in the morning and one-third in the late afternoon. This total dose approximates the daily production of cortisol. The higher morning than evening dose is given to approximate roughly the normal circadian rhythm of cortisol secretion. Cortisol is ordinarily used; it may have some theoretical advantage over some of the cortisol analogues (prednisone, prednisolone, dexamethasone, etc.), as it has greater mineralocorticoid potency and may therefore serve as partial replacement for the deficient mineralocorticoid function as well. However, superiority of cortisol has not been documented, as it appears that an equivalent dosage of a steroid such as prednisone, prednisolone, or dexamethasone is also acceptable.[626] Oral cortisone acetate (approximately 37.5 mg per day) is equally acceptable, since oral absorption is rapid and it is converted to cortisol.[625]

Table 12-18. Treatment of Chronic Primary Adrenocortical Insufficiency

1. Cortisol, 100 mg IV, every 6 h for 24 h. Reduce to 50 mg every 6 h if progress is satisfactory, and then taper to
2. 9α-Fluorocortisol: 0.05 to 0.1 mg in A.M.
3. Clinical follow-up: maintenance of normal weight, blood pressure, and electrolytes with regression of clinical features
4. Patient education plus identification card and/or bracelet
5. Increased cortisol dosage during stress

Mineralocorticoid replacement is given using 9α-fluorocortisol, 0.05 to 0.2 mg daily. Although the majority of patients require mineralocorticoid therapy, a minority do not and can be maintained on cortisol alone.[627] The major problem with omission of the mineralocorticoid is a tendency to develop hyperkalemia. The natural steroid aldosterone is not used; it is more expensive and is degraded rapidly after ingestion and adequate plasma concentrations are not achieved. DOC is also degraded rapidly after oral adminstration and is not recommended.

These doses are satisfactory in the majority of patients; they are accompanied by regression of the classic clinical features, including a return of a general feeling of well-being, weight gain, maintenance of normal blood pressure, improvement in pigmentation, and return to normal physical activity. Occasional patients who perform heavy manual labor may require up to 40 mg. Many of the subjective complaints of Addison's disease can be reversed within a few days; a somewhat longer period is required before strength returns to normal, and weeks may be required before the abnormal pigmentation subsides.

In evaluating the adequacy of glucocorticoid replacement, strong reliance is placed on the patient's subjective assessment. Excessive dosage is usually manifested by excessive weight gain; this is an indication to lower the dose. Since glucocorticoids given in excess can produce euphoria, occasional patients may increase the dosage on their own. Such excessive glucocorticoid replacement should be avoided. Inadequate dosage results in continuing manifestation of Addison's disease, especially weakness, fatigue, and excessive pigmentation. Caution should be exercised in the administration of other drugs since those, such as rifampin, which induce hepatic microsomal enzymes may result in accelerated glucocorticoid metabolism with induction of adrenal crisis.[628] This may also occur with phenytoin and phenobarbital. The timing of the doses can be varied to fit individual needs and activities; i.e., although most patients do well with twice-daily doses some feel better with three doses. The last dose is usually given at 4 to 5 P.M., since the cortisol may cause insomnia in some patients when given later in the evening. Plasma cortisol determinations are not usually necessary or helpful and there is currently no reliable biochemical method to assess the adequacy of glucocorticoid therapy. Thus, plasma ACTH levels have not proved useful because of episodic variation in secretion and the lack of sensitivity of the assay at low ACTH concentrations.

Adequate mineralocorticoid therapy is indicated by maintenance of normal blood pressure, sodium, potassium, and plasma renin levels.[627,629] Excessive therapy causes hypertension and hypokalemia[627] and inadequate therapy may result in persisting fatigue, orthostatic hypotension, hyponatremia, hyperkalemia, and hyperreninemia.[629] The dose may be altered using these parameters; the usual dose of 9α-fluorocortisol is 0.05 to 0.2 mg daily. Some patients may require variable doses at different times of the year, e.g., 0.1 mg and increased salt intake during the summer and 0.05 mg in the winter. Measurement of plasma renin concentration may be useful, since an increased level suggests inadequate replacement and a suppressed level may indicate excessive mineralocorticoid therapy.[627,629]

Every effort should be made to avoid adrenal crises. This can be achieved by patient education and an appropriate increase in steroid dosage during stress. It is therefore necessary to inform the patient fully of the nature of his or her disorder and of the necessity of obtaining prompt medical assistance in the event of illness or injury. Each patient should carry an identification card or bracelet to notify the treating physician of the diagnosis of Addison's disease and patients should be instructed to increase the dose of cortisol in the event of illness. Since it is difficult for the patient to assess the severity of illness it is best to err on the side of overreplacement rather than underreplacement during acute minor illnesses. Thus, patients are instructed to double or triple the cortisol dose at the onset of minor illnesses such as upper respiratory or viral infections. If the illness is minor the dose can be reduced to the usual maintenance level in 24 to 48 h; no adverse effects accompany this short-term increase. Should more severe or persisting symptoms develop, the patient is instructed to continue the increased cortisol dose and contact a physician. Increased dosage of 9α-fluorocortisol is not required during minor illnesses, provided that adequate cortisol is given. Patients with vomiting, and thus the inability to take oral cortisol, must seek immediate medical attention and receive parenteral cortisol, as must those with diarrhea, who may rapidly develop dehydration, volume depletion, and hypotension. Patients who may not have rapid access to medical attention should be provided with injectable cortisol and instructed in its use (available in preloaded syringes of hydrocortisone phosphate, 100 mg).

In patients with secondary adrenal insufficiency, mineralocorticoid therapy is usually not required and the cortisol doses listed above may be given without 9α-fluorocortisol except in the occasional patients with inadequate aldosterone production.

Patients with adrenal insufficiency due to previous high-dose glucocorticoid therapy are ordinarily maintained quite adequately on the same steroid they received for therapy (usually prednisone). The management of these patients is discussed in Chap. 15.

STEROID COVERAGE FOR ILLNESS, SURGERY, OR TRAUMA

Patients with primary or secondary adrenocortical insufficiency suffering trauma or acute illness should be treated according to the protocol described above for acute addisonian crisis. In patients undergoing elective surgery (Table 12-19), electrolyte status, blood pressure, and hydration should be assessed and, if necessary, corrected before induction of anesthesia. A regimen proven effective for increased steroid coverge is to administer 100 mg of soluble hydrocortisone IM on call to the operating room, 50 mg IM or IV in the recovery room, and then one dose subsequently every 6-h for three doses. On the second postoperative day, if the patient is progressing satisfactorily, the dosage may be reduced to 25 mg every 6 h. The dosage may then be tapered to normal maintenance levels over a period of 3 to 5 days. Should fever, hypotension, or other complications occur or persist, the dosage should be maintained at, or increased to, a total of 200 to 400 mg/24 h.

This protocol, a modification of that described by others,[629a] has been used successfully for the past 15 years in patients with either primary, secondary, or glucocorticod-induced adrenal insufficiency. It is also used routinely in patients undergoing adrenalectomy or pituitary surgery. No instance of acute adrenal insufficiency has been noted. IM cortisone acetate should not be used for coverage (see above), since adequate plasma cortisol concentrations are not achieved even if the cortisone acetate is administered 12 to 24 h prior to surgery.[625,629a] Intraoperative or postoperative shock has been reported in such patients

Table 12-19. Steroid Coverage for Surgery

1. Correct electrolyte levels, blood pressure, and hydration if necessary.
2. Give hydrocortisone phosphate or hemisuccinate, 100 mg IM, on call to operating room.
3. Give hydrocortisone phosphate or hemisuccinate, 50 mg IM or IV, in recovery room and every 6 h for the first 24 h.
4. If progress is satisfactory, reduce dosage to 25 mg every 6 h for 24 h; then taper to maintenance dosage over 3 to 5 days. Resume previous 9α-fluorocortisol dose when patient is taking oral medications.
5. Maintain or increase cortisol dosage to 200 to 400 mg/24 h if fever, hypotension, or other complications occur.

receiving injectable cortisone acetate in preparation for surgery.[630]

Prognosis and Survival

Prior to the availability of glucocorticoid therapy, primary adrenocortical insufficiency was a rapidly and uniformly fatal illness, and most patients died within 2 years of diagnosis (Fig. 12-19).[398] Life expectancy increased somewhat when mineralocorticoid therapy in the form of deoxycorticosterone acetate became available in the late 1930s (Fig. 12-19). However, despite correction of mineralocorticoid deficiency, hypotension, and electrolyte abnormalities, life expectancy was still usually less than 5 years and these patients were still susceptible to stress.[398] The introduction of glucocorticoid therapy in the late 1940s resulted in an immediate and marked increase in survival (Fig. 12-19).[398,593]

Survival in patients with either primary or secondary adrenocortical insufficiency now approximates that of the normal population when appropriate therapy, including patient education and increased coverage for stress, is carried out.[398,593] Deaths from adrenal insufficiency are rare in the diagnosed and appropriately treated patients and the majority of deaths occur in patients with a more rapid "acute" course, such as those with massive bilateral adrenal hemorrhage. These patients are frequently not receiving medical care; many die without diagnosis and the adrenocortical insufficiency is discovered only at autopsy.[593]

Hypoaldosteronism

Hypoaldosteronism may occur selectively or in association with an impairment in the production of cortisol. Hypoaldosteronism in association with hypocortisolism due to Addison's disease, hypopituitarism, and congenital adrenal biosynthetic defects are discussed in other sections. Selective hypoaldosteronism is commonly associated with a deficiency of renin secretion by the kidney (hyporeninemic hypoaldosteronism). It can also be due to defective adrenal release of aldosterone in association with normal or elevated plasma renin levels.[631,632] These occur with isolated adrenal biosynthetic defects (corticosterone methyloxidase deficiency, see below), with focal dysfunction of the adrenal glomerulosa with absent responsiveness to angiotensin II (hyperreninemic hypoaldosteronism), following resection of an aldosterone-producing adenoma (see Chap. 14), in pseudohypoaldosteronism (unresponsiveness to aldosterone), after heparin administration (discussed in Inhibitors of Adrenal Steroid Biosynthesis, above[31,63,66]), and with potassium deficiency.[632]

HYPORENINEMIC HYPOALDOSTERONISM

Hyporeninemic hypoaldosteronism occurs generally in older patients with renal disease who have hyperkalemia and hyperchloremic metabolic acidosis that is disproportionately more severe than expected based on the extent of renal impairment.[631–634] In a series of 22 patients, the mean creatinine clearance was 33 (range 11 to 56) ml/min per 1.73 square meter;[634] six patients had diabetes mellitus, one had multiple myeloma, and most of the remainder appeared to have interstitial nephritis.

The hypoaldosteronism is due to decreased renin release by the kidney.[631–634] Plasma renin levels are low and do not increase normally in response to postural changes or sodium restriction. Plasma aldosterone levels are also low and do not increase normally with postural changes and sodium restriction. However, they do increase appropriately relative to the small change in plasma renin levels, suggesting that the adrenal glomerulosa is normal.[632,633] In addition, angiotensin II infusion or ACTH administration results in prompt increases in aldosterone release.[631–634] In fact, the plasma aldosterone concentration is disproportionately high relative to the plasma renin concentration, possibly due to the associated hyperkalemia.[631–634] However, occasional patients with hyporeninemic hypoaldosteronism also have a defect in the late steps in adrenal aldosterone biosynthesis and plasma aldosterone levels do not respond normally to increased renin concentration (e.g., with diuretic treatment) or ACTH.[632–633] This may be due to the hyperreninemic syndrome discussed below.

The pathogenesis of the hyporeninemia is not clear.[631–636] It is likely that the renal disease in some way impairs the kidney's ability to release renin. This could be due to direct damage to the juxtaglomerular or macula densa cells or to some effector mechanism such as the efferent limb of the autonomic nervous supply, the functions that control exposure or responsiveness to ions, or the renal baroreceptor system (Chap. 14). It has also been speculated that there is either a defect in the conversion of prorenin to renin, or else an inhibitor of renin. Others have proposed that increased extracellular fluid volume causes a physiological suppression; indeed, an increase in extracellular fluid volume has been found in some patients, hypertension is present in about a third of cases, and renin and aldosterone concentrations have been shown to increase progressively as the extracellular fluid volume decreases with diuretic therapy, although it is not clear that renin level increases normally. Another postulated mediator of the hyporeninemia is ANF, which reduces renin levels and inhibits responsiveness to potassium (see above).[637a–639] In addition, deficiency of renal PG or prostacyclin production has been implicated in the renin deficiency.[637a,640]

The major consequence of the hypoaldosteronism in these patients is hyperkalemia; the serum potassium concentration is usually between 5.5 and 6.5 meq/liter.[632,633,635] Occasional patients have had third-degree heart block.[632–634] In fact, this condition appears to be the most common cause of chronic hyperkalemia in patients without severe renal disease (e.g., creatinine clearance less than 15 mg/min per 1.73 square meter).[632] Many patients do not lose sodium or develop dehydration, and a more common problem is the increased extracellular fluid volume and hypertension.[632] This lack of salt wasting may be due to the associated renal disease, to other primary factors, and to the fact that cortisol secretion is normal. However, hyponatremia is occasionally present.[635] The extent of hyperkalemia is related to dietary potassium intake and, in diabetics, to diabetic control.[632]

These patients also frequently develop hypochloremic acidosis,[632] which is accentuated by the renal insufficiency; the extent of acidosis is related to the degree of glomerular insufficiency. The acidosis is renal in origin and can be differentiated from renal tubular acidosis type 1 by the fact that the urine is acidotic and relatively bicarbonate-free during periods of acidosis; it can be distinguished from type 2 renal tubular acidosis by the fact that the extent of decreased reabsorption of bicarbonate at normal bicarbonate concentrations is not great enough to indicate defective proximal tubular dysfunction and by a lack of aminoaciduria, glucosuria, or increased renal phosphate clearance. Urinary excretion of ammonia is markedly reduced, even with an acidic urine. Thus, these changes, combined with evidence for low potassium clearance, have led to the classification of the dysfunction as *type 4* renal tubular acidosis. The acidosis itself appears to be due to both the hyperkalemia that reduces renal ammonia production and the reduced hydrogen secretory capacity.

The initial differential diagnosis includes all of the causes of hyperkalemia,[631–636] including the hypoaldosterone states mentioned above that have normal or elevated plasma renin levels. Pseudohypokalemia due to abnormal potassium release from clotting when elevated platelet or white blood cell counts are present can be excluded by obtaining heparinized blood with minimal turbulence and measuring the plasma K^+ concentration, which is normal in this condition. Use of drugs that elevate the serum potassium ion concentration (spironolactone, triamterene) can be excluded by history and also by the fact that the plasma aldosterone concentration is not abnormally low in these circumstances. Also, hyporeninemic hypoaldosteronism has been reported in association with chronic and massive intake of sodium bicarbonate.[637b] Addison's disease and adrenal biosynthetic deficiency states are usually associated with a high plasma renin concentration and may have other manifestations described above. However, as mentioned earlier, occasional patients with hyperkalemia and chronic renal disease have hypoaldosteronism with normal plasma renin levels. Oliguric renal failure and other causes of severe acidosis (e.g., diabetic ketoacidosis) can be excluded by the clinical setting. There are rare syndromes with hyperkalemia and lack of responsiveness to aldosterone (pseudohypoaldosteronism, see below); however, these patients have several distinguishing clinical characteristics, including high aldosterone and renin levels.

Patients with hyporeninemic hypoaldosteronism generally respond to mineralocorticoid replacement therapy using 9α-fluorocortisol with amelioration of the hyperkalemia and acidosis.[633–635] Dosages of around 0.2 mg per day are ordinarily required;[633–635] however, in some patients the kidneys appeared to be hyporesponsive to mineralocorticoids, and in these higher dosages of the steroid are required.[631] Mineralocorticoid replacement is not the therapy of choice in patients with hypertension and increased fluid volume. In many cases furosemide therapy can ameliorate both the hyperkalemia and the acidosis.[641] Further, in patients with severe hypoaldosteronism, the combination of furosemide and small doses of mineralocorticoids can be synergistic.[635,641] Thus, diuretics and mineralocorticoids should be used, alone or in combination, and the relative doses should be individualized, depending on the clinical setting and the response. Alternative measures depending on the individual patient can include the restriction of dietary potassium, the oral administration of sodium polystyrene sulfonate, a resin that binds potassium ion and releases sodium ion in the gastrointestinal tract, and the oral administration of sodium bicarbonate.[631]

NORMORENINEMIC OR HYPERRENINEMIC HYPOALDOSTERONISM

Normo- and hyperreninemic hypoaldosteronism appear to be the result of acquired dysfunction of the adrenal glomerulosa.[631,642–645] This occurs most commonly in critically ill patients with hypotension;[644,645] it has been reported in over 50 percent of such patients. These patients have hypoaldosteronism despite markedly increased plasma renin level; aldosterone secretion is subnormally responsive to stimulation with ACTH or angiotensin II.[644,645] The mechanism of impaired aldosterone production and the role of ischemia with potential anoxia and adrenal damage are not known, but the frequency of this condition should alert the physician to consider it in such patients. There is one report of a patient with hyperkalemia and moderate renal insufficiency who had hyperreninemia and subnormal plasma aldosterone responses to ACTH, upright posture, and sodium depletion.[642] This patient was shown to have antibodies against the zona glomerulosa, suggesting possible selective autoimmune destruction of the adrenal glomerulosa.[643]

PSEUDOHYPOALDOSTERONISM UNRESPONSIVE TO ALDOSTERONE

There exist rare cases in which patients do not exhibit a response to aldosterone.[631,632] This has been reported in infants without renal parenchymal disease and in children and adults with azotemia due to renal interstitial disease (salt-wasting nephropathy). These patients have hyperkalemia, metabolic acidosis, and renal sodium wasting with extracellular fluid depletion and hypotension, despite elevated plasma aldosterone and renin levels. These abnormalities do not respond to large doses of mineralocorticoids. These patients apparently have a renal defect whereby they cannot respond to mineralocorticoids, and treatment with sodium chloride and/or bicarbonate is ordinarily required to maintain them.

An additional rare syndrome has been termed *type 2 pseudohypoaldosteronism.*[631,646] It has been described in children and young adults and is characterized by hyperkalemia and hyperchloremia, metabolic acidosis with hypertension, hyporeninemia, and hypoaldosteronism. These patients differ from the hyporeninemic hypoaldosteronism patients in that they have normal GFRs. Like the case with pseudohypoaldosteronism, their renal potassium excretion fails to increase normally when large amounts of mineralocorticoids are administered, but unlike the case with pseudohypoaldosteronism, pseudohypoaldosteronism type 2 patients have a normal antinatriuretic and antichloriduric response to mineralocorticoids.[631] It has been suggested that the primary abnormality in the syndrome is a defect in the distal nephron for chloride reabsorption that increases distal NaCl reabsorption resulting in hyperchloremia, volume expansion, and hypertension that also limits the sodium- and mineralocorticoid-dependent voltage driving force for potassium and hydrogen secretion, resulting in hyperkalemia and hypertension;[631] the syndrome might also be explained by an isolated collecting tubule defect in potassium secretion.[631] Restriction of dietary NaCl or administration of a chloruretic diuretic ameliorates the hyperkalemia and acidosis in these patients.[631]

There can also be other circumstances where selective unresponsiveness to certain actions of mineralocorticoids occurs. Thus, after several days of mineralocorticoid excess, further sodium retention does not occur (the escape phenomenon), even though responses of potassium and hydrogen loss persist (see above). The lack of response of the kaliuretic actions of the mineralocorticoids occurs in the rare hypertensive syndrome with possibly increased chloride reabsorption (see above), and in pregnancy there is a relative resistance to the kaliuretic responses of the mineralocorticoids (discussed below).

ADRENOCORTICAL HYPERFUNCTION

Hyperfunction of the adrenal cortex can result from excessive activity of the zonae fasciculata and reticularis or the zona glomerulosa and from steroid-producing adenomas or carcinomas. Excessive stimulation of the zonae fasciculata and reticularis by ACTH is due to pituitary hypersecretion of ACTH (usually by a small adenoma), abnormal ACTH release by extrapituitary tumors (ectopic ACTH syndrome), or ACTH therapy. This results in increased secretion of cortisol, the adrenal androgens, and DOC. Excessive activity of the zona glomerulosa can be due to primary aldosteronism, with hyperplasia resulting from unknown causes (see Chap. 14), or it can be due to activation of the renin-angiotensin system by any of a number of causes. Adrenal adenomas usually produce either cortisol or aldosterone, and rarely androgens, whereas carcinomas frequently secrete a variety of steroids.

Cushing's Syndrome

Cushing's syndrome refers to the manifestations of glucocorticoid excess without regard to specific etiology; there may also be androgen excess. It is more commonly iatrogenic and due to glucocorticoid therapy (Chap. 15). Cushing's *disease* refers to the disorder resulting from pituitary ACTH hypersecretion. Spontaneous Cushing's syndrome is an uncommon disorder; however, it must be considered in the differential diagnosis of such diverse entities as obesity, hypertension, diabetes, weakness, osteoporosis, hirsutism, and menstrual disorders.

CLASSIFICATION, OCCURRENCE, AND AGE AND SEX DISTRIBUTIONS

Spontaneous Cushing's syndrome is either ACTH-dependent or ACTH-independent (Table 12-20). The ACTH-dependent types are Cushing's disease, the ectopic ACTH syndrome, and, more rarely, ectopic CRF production.[647–650] In these disorders chronic ACTH hypersecretion stimulates the zonae fasciculata and reticularis, resulting in bilateral adrenocortical hyperplasia with increased secretion of cortisol androgens, and DOC. ACTH-independent Cushing's syndrome is due to primary adrenocortical neoplasms, either adenomas or carcinomas; the resulting hypercortisolism suppresses the hypothalamic-pituitary axis.

Cushing's disease accounts for approximately 70 percent of adult patients in current series[16,647] and the majority of these patients have pituitary microadenomas (see below). There is a distinct female preponderance in Cushing's disease. In older series the female/male ratio was 3:1,[652] but it is 8:1 in current experience.[651] The age range in Cushing's disease is most frequently 20 to 40 years.[652]

Ectopic ACTH hypersecretion is responsible for approximately 15 percent of reported cases of Cushing's syndrome. This probably underestimates the true incidence since many patients lack the classic features of hypercortisolism. They are thus not brought to the attention of the endocrinologist; severe hypercortisolism and rapid death are common.[653] The tumors causing the ectopic ACTH syndrome are discussed below; oat cell carcinoma of the lung is the most common and ectopic ACTH secretion occurs in 0.5 to 2 percent of these patients.[654] In addition, immunoreactive and bioactive ACTH has been demonstrated in the majority of these tumors, even when clinical evidence of ectopic ACTH hypersecretion is not present.[635,655–657] The ectopic ACTH syndrome is more common in males (female/male = 1.3) and the peak incidence of 40 to 60 years reflects the greater incidence of malignancy in this age group.[16,658]

Table 12-20. Classification and Etiology of Cushing's Syndrome

	Percent
ACTH-dependent:	
Cushing's disease	68
Ectopic ACTH syndrome	15
ACTH-independent:	
Adrenal adenoma	9
Adrenal carcinoma	8
	100

Source: Huff.[647]

ACTH-independent primary adrenal tumors cause 17 to 19 percent of cases of Cushing's syndrome, with equal frequencies of adenoma and carcinoma in adults.[16,647] Adrenal adenomas causing Cushing's syndrome occur more frequently in females.[16] Adrenocortical carcinoma causing Cushing's syndrome also shows a female preponderance (approximately 66 percent of cases);[659] however, the prevalence of all types of adrenal carcinoma is higher in males.[659] The overall prevalence of adrenal carcinoma is approximately 2 per million population. Approximately 75 percent of cases occur after age 12, with the peak incidence in the fourth to sixth decades; the mean age at diagnosis is 38 years.[16,659,660]

Cushing's syndrome in childhood is distinctly unusual. Cushing's disease is responsible for only 35 percent of cases; the majority of these patients are 10 years old or older at the time of diagnosis[16,661–664] and the incidence by sex is approximately equal.[661–664] Adrenal tumors account for the majority (65 percent) of cases in childhood, with carcinoma responsible for 51 percent and adenoma 14 percent.[16] The majority of these tumors occur in girls and most occur between the ages of 1 and 8 years.[16]

PATHOLOGY

Anterior Pituitary

Pituitary adenomas are found either at surgery or autopsy in over 90 percent of patients with Cushing's disease[665–668] and confirm Cushing's original description of pituitary adenomas in six of his eight autopsied cases (Fig. 12-32). Approximately 80 to 90 percent of these are microadenomas (diameter less than 10 mm); 50 percent are 5 mm or less in diameter and microadenomas less than 2 mm in diameter have been reported.[666–668] Thus, these small adenomas do not result in sellar enlargement, although focal radiologic abnormalities may occur.[667] The remainder of the pituitary adenomas in Cushing's disease are larger than 10 mm; these cause sellar enlargement, frequently with extrasellar extension, and invasive tendencies are common.[669] Malignant tumors have occasionally been reported.[669]

The adenomas of Cushing's disease are characteristically basophilic, unencapsulated, and located within the anterior pituitary.[666,667] Chromophobe adenomas may also occur.[667] The tumors are composed of compact sheets of uniform, well-granulated cells with a sinusoidal arrangement and a high content of ACTH, β-LPH, and β-endorphin.[670,671] The cytoplasm usually contains abundant basophilic granules which, on immunocytochemical staining, are positive for ACTH and β-LPH. These cells frequently show a zone of

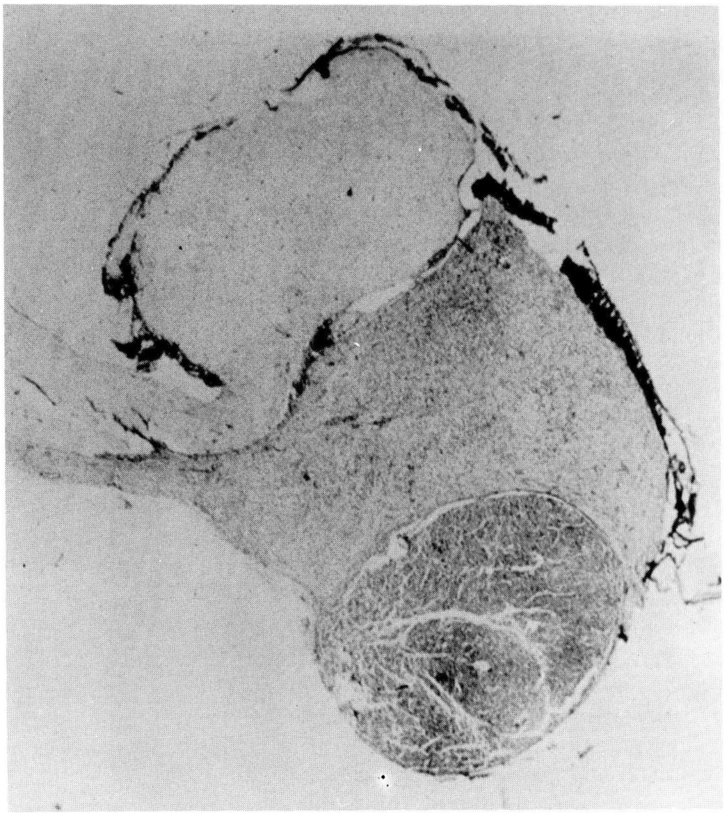

FIGURE 12-32 Basophilic anterior pituitary microadenoma from Cushing's original series. (*From Cushing.*[2])

perinuclear hyalinization known as *Crooke's changes* which is the result of exposure of the corticotrophs to hypercortisolism.[666] Electron microscopy demonstrates considerable heterogeneity of granule size (200 to 700 nm) and variability of the number of granules, which may be scattered throughout the cytoplasm or marginated along the cell membrane.[666] The hyaline changes seen on light microscopy appear as bundles of perinuclear microfilaments (average 7.0 nm in diameter) which encircle the nucleus.[666]

The portion of the anterior pituitary not involved by the adenoma has been less well studied. Hyperplasia of corticotrophs surrounding the tumor has been reported in some cases but not confirmed in others.[672,673] In addition, ACTH content in the paraadenomatous tissue is decreased, in contrast to the increased content in the adenoma cells themselves.[670,671] In an additional subgroup of cases tumors and adenomatous hyperplasia, postulated to arise from the intermediate lobe, occur.[674]

The subgroups of patients with Cushing's disease and no demonstrable pituitary adenoma usually have diffuse corticotroph hyperplasia,[675] although a few patients have no demonstrable pituitary abnormality.[676,677] Several patients with corticotroph hyperplasia have been found to have intrasellar gangliocytomas which secrete CRF,[648] and an additional two patients were found to have ectopic tumors that secreted CRF but not ACTH.[649,650]

In patients with adrenal tumors or the ectopic ACTH syndrome, and in those subjected to steroid therapy, the pituitary corticotrophs show prominent Crooke's hyaline changes with perinuclear microfilaments and reduced ACTH content.

Adrenal Cortex

ADRENOCORTICAL HYPERPLASIA Bilateral hyperplasia of the adrenal cortex occurs in patients with ACTH hypersecretion from either pituitary or ectopic sources.[16] Three types of hyperplasia have been described: simple, that associated with the ectopic ACTH syndrome, and bilateral nodular.[16]

With simple hyperplasia (usually secondary to Cushing's disease), the combined adrenal weight is between 12 and 24 g (normal weight is 8 to 10 g, see Structure of the Adrenal Cortex, above). The enlarged glands have a yellowish-brown color. On microscopic examination, the cortex is thickened because of approximately equal hyperplasia of the compact cells of the zona reticularis and the clear cells of the zona fasciculata, with normal ultrastructural features. The zona glomerulosa is normal.

The adrenals in the ectopic ACTH syndrome are usually much more enlarged, with combined weights of 24 to > 50 g.[16,658,660] The cut surface of the cortex is generally brownish. Microscopically there is, typically, marked hyperplasia of the zona reticularis with columns of hypertrophied compact cells extending to and into the zona glomerulosa. The clear cells of the zona fasciculata are markedly reduced; however, the zona glomerulosa is normal. These histologic features are consistent with the effects of the markedly elevated ACTH levels typically seen in the ectopic ACTH syndrome.[16]

Bilateral nodular hyperplasia is present in approximately 20 percent of cases.[16] The precise etiology of this pathological subtype is unclear, but most cases appear to result from pituitary ACTH excess[16,678] (see Cushing's Disease under Etiology and Pathogenesis, below). The adrenals are enlarged and adrenal weight is variable, depending on the number and size of the nodules present. The cut surface reveals at least one and usually multiple macroscopic yellow nodules which are usually bilateral. Rarely, this condition is associated with adrenal carcinoma.[679] The nodules consist mainly of clear cells which are similar to those of the normal zona fasciculata and the intervening cortex shows the typical features of simple hyperplasia described above.[16]

ADRENOCORTICAL TUMORS Benign hyperfunctioning adrenal adenomas causing Cushing's syndrome weigh from 10 to 70 g and range in size from 1 to 6 cm. They are encapsulated, with a well-delineated margin, and the cut surface is yellow with brown or red areas. Microscopically, clear cells of the zona fasciculata type predominate and make up the yellow areas, whereas the darker areas comprise cells resembling those of the compact zone of the reticularis. Rarely, these adenomas can be black due to the presence of lipofuscin.[660]

Adrenal carcinomas are generally quite large (over 100 g), may weigh in excess of several kilograms,[16] and are commonly palpable as abdominal masses. These tumors are encapsulated; the cut surface reveals a highly vascular tumor with necrosis, hemorrhage, and cystic degeneration. Calcification is not uncommon. Adrenal carcinomas may have a benign histological appearance with a predominance of compact cells, although variable degrees of pleomorphism occur, especially in larger tumors. The histologic features frequently do not predict the clinical behavior of the tumor.[16] Thus, in many cases, a definite diagnosis of malignancy can be established only if there is vascular invasion, local extension, or metastatic spread. These carcinomas spread by local invasion of the retroperitoneum, kidney, or liver or hematogenously to the liver and lungs.[659]

With both functioning adrenal adenomas and carcinomas there is atrophy of the cortex contiguous to the tumor and of the contralateral gland. The capsule of the uninvolved cortex is thickened, and the atrophic cortex is narrow and consists entirely of clear, lipid-containing cells. The zona reticularis is absent and the zona glomerulosa is normal.[658]

ETIOLOGY AND PATHOGENESIS

Cushing's Disease

Cushing's disease is caused by pituitary ACTH hypersecretion and pituitary adenomas are present in the great majority of patients (see Pathology, above, and Therapy of Cushing's Disease, below). A substantial body of evidence suggests that most cases of Cushing's disease are due to spontaneous ACTH-secreting pituitary adenomas and that hypothalamic abnormalities are secondary to hypercortisolism. However, others feel that this disorder is the result of a primary CNS abnormality with excessive stimulation of anterior pituitary corticotrophs by CRF or other factors with secondary adenoma formation (see below and Chaps. 7 and 8).[667,680,681]

Several endocrine abnormalities are characteristic of Cushing's disease. The primary endocrine abnormality (Table 12-21) is hypersecretion of ACTH with bilateral adrenocortical hyperplasia and hypersecretion of cortisol. The second major abnormality is absent circadian periodicity of ACTH and cortisol release; episodic secretion persists at a higher than normal frequency but is sporadic and without a diurnal pattern.[682,683] Third, there is absent responsiveness of

Table 12-21. Endocrine Abnormalities in Cushing's Disease

Hypersecretion of ACTH and cortisol
Absent circadian periodicity of ACTH and cortisol
Abnormal ACTH and cortisol responsiveness to stress (hypoglycemia, surgery)
Abnormal negative feedback regulation of ACTH secretion by glucocorticoids
Abnormal suppressibility with dexamethasone
Hyperresponsiveness to inhibition of cortisol synthesis with metyrapone
Subnormal responsiveness of growth hormone, thyrotropin, and gonadotropins to stimulation

ACTH and cortisol to stresses such as hypoglycemia or major surgery.[173,504] Fourth, although negative feedback regulation of ACTH secretion by glucocorticoids is present, higher than normal concentrations are required to suppress ACTH release and there is hyperresponsiveness of ACTH release when cortisol secretion is inhibited.[503,538] Fifth, abnormalities of other pituitary hormones are present in most patients; these include subnormal responsiveness of growth hormone, TSH, and the gonadotropins.[173,684,685] Finally, certain pharmacologic agents such as cyproheptadine and bromocriptine inhibit ACTH release in some patients with Cushing's disease.[680,681,686]

Evidence for a hypothalamic etiology of Cushing's disease is reviewed in Chaps. 7 and 8. It is postulated that there is a primary hypothalamic or CNS defect of neurotransmitter control with consequent hypersecretion of CRF and chronic stimulation of anterior pituitary corticotrophs,[680,681] which could lead to adenomatous changes. A primary CNS defect could explain the observed abnormalities of circadian periodicity, stress responsiveness, suppressibility by dexamethasone, and subnormal growth hormone responsiveness.[680–681] Also, inhibition of ACTH hypersecretion by cyproheptadine and bromocriptine could be due to inhibition of CRF release by the hypothalamus.[680] Abnormalities of sleep EEG stages in Cushing's disease have also led to the suggestion of a hypothalamic etiology, although they may be due to hypercortisolism per se.[681,687]

The theory that Cushing's disease is a primary pituitary disorder is based on the high frequency of pituitary adenomas, the response to their removal, and the interpretation of hypothalamic abnormalities as being secondary to hypercortisolism. This theory proposes that ACTH hypersecretion arises from a pituitary adenoma, that the resulting hypercortisolism suppresses the normal hypothalamic-pituitary axis and CRF release, and that this abolishes hypothalamic regulation of circadian variability and stress responsiveness.[667,688] This theory also postulates that the feedback control of ACTH secretion is mediated directly on the pituitary tumor and that other pharmacologic agents, such as vasopressin, cyproheptadine, and bromocriptine, directly inhibit the ACTH-secreting adenoma.[667,688] Finally, this theory presumes that abnormalities of growth hormone, TSH, and gonadotropin secretion are due to hypercortisolism and not to a primary hypothalamic disorder.[667,688]

An analysis of the response to therapeutic pituitary microsurgery or adrenalectomy sheds some light on these two possible etiologies. Selective removal of pituitary microadenomas by transsphenoidal microsurgery corrects ACTH hypersecretion and hypercortisolism in most patients.[667,688–693] This suggests that the adenoma and not generalized corticotroph hyperplasia is responsible for ACTH excess. Postoperatively, in 90 percent of these patients there is transient ACTH deficiency and secondary hypoadrenalism with preservation of other pituitary hormones.[667,689–693] This finding suggests that the normal hypothalamic-pituitary axis is suppressed by the hypercortisolism; this is supported by the in vitro demonstration of markedly decreased ACTH content in nonadenomatous pituitary tissue removed from patients with active Cushing's disease.[670,671] In cases studied following selective surgical removal of the adenoma there is a return to normal of (1) the circadian rhythm of ACTH and cortisol secretion, (2) the responsiveness of the hypothalamic-pituitary axis to hypoglycemic stress, (3) suppressibility of cortisol secretion by dexamethasone,[689–693] and (4) the formerly suppressed growth hormone, TSH, and gonadotropin responses.[690–694] Thus, in these patients, there is no evidence for a persisting hypothalamic abnormality. Recovery of ACTH and growth hormone responsiveness to hypoglycemia also occurs when patients with Cushing's disease are treated by bilateral adrenalectomy.[504,687] That these abnormalities are due to hypercortisolism rather than to a primary hypothalamic lesion is further supported by the fact that glucocorticoid administration can suppress ACTH responses to hypoglycemia as well as growth hormone, TSH, and gonadotropin responses.[173,384,693,694] Thus, the hypothalamic abnormalities of Cushing's disease are reversed simply by removing the source of hypercortisolism, suggesting again that the preoperative abnormalities were due solely to the pituitary adenoma with resulting hypersecretion of ACTH and cortisol.

The postulate that suppression of ACTH and cortisol secretion by high-dose dexamethasone in Cushing's disease occurs directly at the pituitary level is supported by evidence that the pituitary is an important site of glucocorticoid feedback (see above) and by the demonstration in vitro of a direct suppressive effect of glucocorticoids on ACTH secretion by adenomas removed from patients with Cushing's disease.[695–697]

A direct effect of other pharmacologic agents at the pituitary level in Cushing's disease is also supported by recent in vitro studies. Vasopressin, which stimulates ACTH release in patients with Cushing's disease and in normal individuals, also stimulates secretion in ACTH-secreting pituitary adenomas in vitro but does not release ACTH in the normal nonadenomatous anterior pituitary tissue from these patients.[695–697] Evidence that bromocriptine, cyproheptadine, and dopamine directly suppress pituitary ACTH secretion in patients with Cushing's disease is less direct; however, these agents suppressed ACTH secretion from an ACTH-secreting rat pituitary tumor.[686] In one pituitary adenoma from a patient with Cushing's disease, dopamine inhibited ACTH release[695] and in a tumor from a patient with Nelson's syndrome dopamine and cyproheptadine inhibited ACTH secretion.[698]

The Ectopic ACTH Syndrome

The ectopic ACTH syndrome is caused by ACTH hypersecretion from nonpituitary tumors. These tumors contain both immunoreactive and bioactive ACTH; they also secrete ACTH in vitro.[669,700] They also contain the mRNA of POMC and secrete β-LPH, β-endorphin, and both large and small ACTH fragments, suggesting that the ACTH is derived from a POMC similar to that of the anterior pituitary.[701–703] Ectopic tumors may also contain CRF-like activity;[701] the biological significance of this is unclear, since these tumors also contain and secrete ACTH. It is unlikely that the CRF in these cases is stimulating pituitary ACTH, since the histology of the gland in the ectopic ACTH syndrome shows Crooke's changes that are consistent with its suppression by hypercortisolism.[704] However, as mentioned above, several tumors have been described which secreted only CRF.[649,650]

The majority of cases of the ectopic ACTH syndrome are due to a small number of tumor types (Table 12-22).[702–705] Oat cell carcinoma of the lung is by far the most common type.[705] Other tumors in order of frequency are: epithelial thymoma; islet cell tumors of the pancreas; carcinoid tumors of the lung, gut, pancreas, and ovary; medullary carcinoma of the thyroid; and pheochromocytoma and its related neuroectodermal tumors.[705] Additional miscellaneous and rare cases include malignant melanoma, adenocarcinoma of the colon, ovarian arrhenoblastoma, parathyroid carcinoma, and nephroblastoma.[653,656,699,701,702,705] Undifferentiated or poorly differentiated carcinomas in the gall bladder, parotid, prostate, ovary, and cervix have been described with the ectopic ACTH syndrome, but the exact pathological classification and site of origin of these are difficult to ascertain.[705] The apparently diverse cell types from which these nonpituitary tumors arise also share a common neuroectodermal origin and the capability of amine precursor uptake and decarboxylation (see Chaps. 2 and 27).

Table 12-22. Tumors Most Frequently Causing the Ectopic ACTH Syndrome

Oat cell carcinoma of the lung
Thymoma
Pancreatic islet cell carcinoma
Carcinoid tumors (lung, gut, pancreas, ovary)
Thyroid medullary carcinoma
Pheochromocytoma and related tumors

Adrenal Tumors

Glucocorticoid-producing adrenal tumors, whether adenoma or carcinoma arise de novo and autonomously secrete adrenocortical steroids. Rarely, adrenal carcinomas occur in patients with nodular adrenal hyperplasia[679] or congenital adrenocortical hyperplasia, raising the possibility that in these special circumstances the development of carcinoma is promoted by prolonged ACTH stimulation of the adrenal. However, the majority of adrenal tumors develop spontaneously and are not associated with chronic ACTH excess.

PATHOPHYSIOLOGY

Cushing's Disease

In Cushing's disease, the pituitary adenomas release ACTH episodically without a circadian pattern,[682,683,692] and since the feedback inhibition of ACTH by glucocorticoids is defective,[538] the elevated cortisol secretion does not adequately decrease ACTH secretion (Fig. 12-33). Thus, a glucocorticoid excess state persists; it is the number and magnitude of ACTH and adrenal secretory episodes which accounts for the increase in total cortisol secretion. This episodic secretion results in variable plasma cortisol and ACTH levels, which may at times be moderately or markedly elevated and at other times be within the normal range.[538,682,683,692] However, measurement of cortisol production rate or urinary free cortisol excretion, or multiple cortisol sampling over 24 h, reveals cortisol hypersecretion (see Laboratory Features and Diagnosis, below, and Refs. 682, 683, and 692). Thus, the major differences in plasma ACTH and cortisol in Cushing's disease occur in the afternoon and at night when cortisol secretion is usually low in normal individuals. This overall increase in tissue exposure to glucocorticoids is sufficient to cause obvious Cushing's syndrome; however, the modest increase in ACTH secretion usually does not cause increased pigmentation. β-LPH is also hypersecreted.[505–507] Although this hormone may have actions on the adrenal, it is not known to contribute to the pathology of Cushing's disease, nor are the extraadrenal actions of ACTH (see Regulation of Glucorticoid Production and Regulation of Mineralocorticoid Production, above).

Although there is ACTH hypersecretion and resistance to suppression with glucocorticoids, the axis does not respond normally to stressful stimuli such as hypoglycemia or surgery.[173,504] This is probably due to

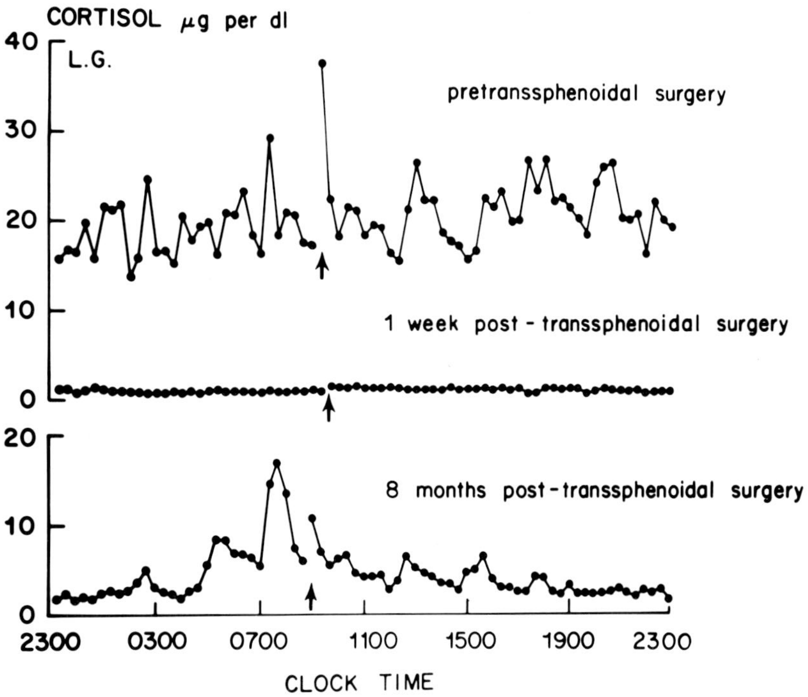

FIGURE 12-33 Twenty-four hour cortisol secretory patterns in a patient with Cushing's disease before treatment (*top*) and 1 week (*middle*) and 8 months (*bottom*) following transsphenoidal adenomectomy. Arrows denote the start of the sampling period. (*From Boyer et al.*[692])

the relative autonomy of the pituitary adenoma and suppression by glucocorticoids of the normal ability of the hypothalamic-pituitary axis to secrete CRF and ACTH.

The pathophysiologic basis for the clinical abnormalities due to the excess cortisol have already been described (see Actions of Glucocorticoids, above). Thus, the cortisol not only inhibits normal pituitary and hypothalamic function, affecting ACTH, TSH, growth hormone, and gonadotropin release, but also causes all of the peripheral effects described on most tissues of the body.

The secretion of adrenal androgens (also controlled by ACTH) is increased in patients with Cushing's disease; the extent of hypersecretion is roughly proportional to and parallels that of ACTH and cortisol. DHEA, DHEA-S, and androstenedione are all hypersecreted in Cushing's disease; these are converted peripherally to testosterone (also secreted from the adrenal in increased quantities) and DHT. Thus, plasma levels of these steroids are moderately increased in Cushing's disease and an androgen excess state develops. In the female, this causes the classic manifestations of hirsutism, acne, and amenorrhea. The latter is in part the consequence of androgen suppression of gonadotropin secretion.[685] In the male patient with Cushing's disease, testicular production of testosterone is decreased by the glucocorticoid excess state.[706] Thus, in spite of increased adrenal androgen production, the net result is the lowering of circulating testosterone levels, which is frequently accompaied by decreased libido and impotence. In male patients elevated cortisol secretion may also contribute to the suppression of pituitary gonadotropin release and testicular function (see Production and Clearance of Other Hormones under Actions of Glucocorticoids, above).

Because the influence of ACTH on glomerulosa cell function is transient, aldosterone production is usually not increased in Cushing's disease and the renin-angiotensin-aldosterone axis usually remains intact. Although there is some increase in DOC production, DOC and cortisol are not elevated enough to produce a frank mineralocorticoid excess state in most cases, in contrast to the case with the ectopic ACTH syndrome (Chap. 14).

Ectopic ACTH Syndrome

Patients with this syndrome usually have much more marked ACTH and cortisol hypersecretion than is seen in Cushing's disease. β-LPH and other peptides containing ACTH sequences are also secreted in excess (see Chap. 27).[701,702] ACTH and cortisol hypersecretion are also episodic, although at greatly elevated levels. With uncommon exception, the secretion of ACTH by the ectopic tumor is not suppressible even with high doses of glucocorticoids.

The marked ACTH hypersecretion results in a greater degree of hyperplasia of the zonae fasciculata and reticularis and of the secretion of cortisol, adrenal androgens, and DOC than with most cases of Cushing's disease.[16] Thus, plasma levels and urinary excretion of these steroids and their metabolites are usually markedly elevated.[707,708] However, in spite of the marked elevations of these steroids, the classic features of Cushing's syndrome are commonly absent.[708] This is presumably due to the rapid onset of hypercortisolism and the associated malignancy. Also, manifestations of androgen excess may not be prominent because most of these patients are male. However, the elevated DOC and cortisol concentrations (and possibly those of other steroids) frequently result in a frank mineralocorticoid excess syndrome with hypertension, hypokalemia, and suppressed plasma renin levels (Chap. 14). However, the suppression of plasma renin activity may be blunted by the effect of the elevated cortisol on the renin-angiotensin system (see above and Chap. 14).

Adrenal Tumors

Glucocorticoid-secreting primary adrenal tumors, whether adenomas or carcinomas, autonomously hypersecrete cortisol and suppress the hypothalamic-pituitary axis and circulating plasma ACTH levels.[504] This results in atrophy of the zonae fasciculata and reticularis not involved by the tumor.[16]

Adrenal adenomas causing Cushing's syndrome usually secrete only cortisol in significant excess; thus, the clinical picture is that of pure glucocorticoid excess. Cortisol secretion is again episodic, but feedback control of cortisol release is lost and thus these tumors typically show no response to either dexamethasone or metyrapone. The adrenal secretion of androgens may be subnormal, as manifested by low urinary 17-ketosteroid excretion or plasma DHEA-S levels.[709]

Adrenal carcinomas frequently secrete multiple steroids in an unpredictable pattern.[659] However, most commonly, cortisol and androgens are secreted in excess; less commonly, there is hypersecretion of aldosterone, DOC, or estrogens. Concentrations of plasma cortisol and its urinary metabolites are frequently markedly elevated in patients with adrenal carcinomas. In addition, androgen hypersecretion is frequently even more markedly elevated, with very high levels of urinary 17-ketosteroids or plasma DHEA and DHEA-S.[659] These patients usually have severe and rapidly progressive clinical manifestations of cortisol excess; in females androgen excess is prominent.[659] These patients also frequently have mineralocorticoid excess due to cortisol and DOC with resulting hypertension and hypokalemia.

CLINICAL AND LABORATORY FEATURES

Clinical Features

The clinical manifestations of Cushing's syndrome were well described by Cushing himself;[2] the frequencies of these features are listed in Table 12-23.[652,707] Although the frequency of presenting signs and symptoms has remained remarkably constant, the severity of the condition appears to be less in more recent series, presumably because of earlier clinical recognition and diagnosis.[652,707]

Obesity is the most common manifestation (Fig. 12-34) and weight gain is usually the initial symptom. Weight gain is classically central, affecting mainly the face, neck, trunk, and abdomen, with relative sparing of the extremities.[652] However, generalized obesity is equally frequent and was present in 60 percent of the cases described by Ross et al.[707] In children with Cushing's syndrome, obesity is invariably present and is usually generalized.[661–664] In addition to obesity, 85 percent of children with Cushing's syndrome have short stature and growth failure.[661] Whether central or generalized, the obesity of Cushing's syndrome has certain features which distinguish it from simple obesity. Accumulation of fat in the face leads to the typical "moon facies," which is present in 75 percent and which is accompanied by facial plethora in most

Table 12-23. Clinical Features of Cushing's Syndrome

Feature	Percent with feature
Obesity	94
Facial plethora	84
Hirsutism	82
Menstrual disorders	76
Hypertension	72
Muscular weakness	58
Back pain	58
Striae	52
Acne	40
Psychological symptoms	40
Bruising	36
Congestive heart failure	22
Edema	18
Renal calculi	16
Headache	14
Polyuria/polydipsia	10
Hyperpigmentation	6

Source: Modified from Plotz et al.[652] and Ross et al.[707]

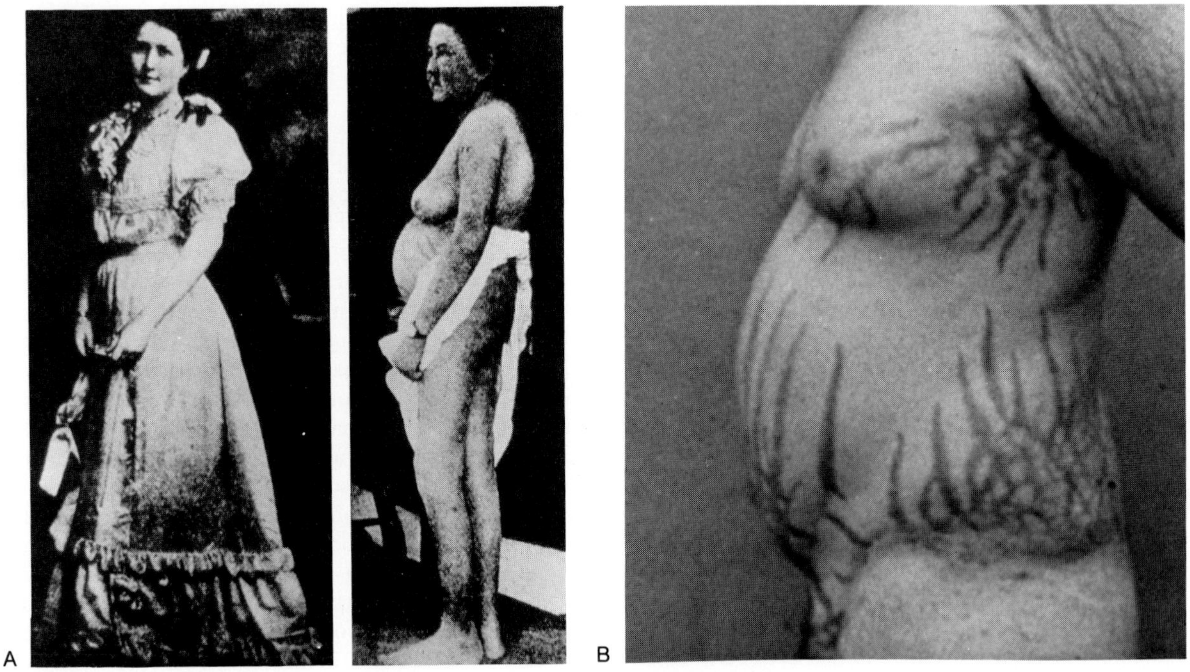

FIGURE 12-34 (A) Patient from Cushing's original series before and after development of clinical features. (B) Marked striae in a patient with Cushing's syndrome. (*Panel A from Cushing.*[2])

patients. Fat accumulation around the neck is prominent in the supraclavicular and dorsocervical fat pads; the fat deposition in the latter is responsible for the "buffalo hump." Adipose tissue accumulates over the thorax and frequently leads to protuberance of the abdomen. A minority of patients are not obese and do not gain weight; however, they usually have central redistribution of fat and a typical facial appearance.[652]

Although skin changes are less frequent, their presence should arouse suspicion of cortisol excess. Atrophy of the epidermis and its underlying connective tissue leads to thinning and a transparent appearance of the skin in advanced cases. This also accounts for the plethoric appearance. Easy bruisability with minimal trauma is present in 40 to 60 percent of patients. Such patients on occasion have been detected after referral for workup of a bleeding diathesis. Purple striae occur in 50 to 70 percent of patients; these are typically red to purple in color, depressed below the skin surface because of loss of underlying connective tissue, and wider (not infrequently 0.5 to 2.0 cm) than the pinkish-white striae seen with pregnancy or rapid weight gain. These striae are most commonly abdominal but may also occur over the breasts, hips, buttocks, thighs, and axillae. Minor wounds and abrasions frequently heal slowly and poorly, as do surgical incisions, which sometimes dehisce.[652] Mucotaneous fungal infections are frequent, including tinea versicolor, involvement of the nails, and oral candidiasis. Hyperpigmentation of the skin occurs rarely in patients with Cushing's disease or adrenal tumors but is more common in the ectopic ACTH syndrome.[707,708] Hirsutism is present in 65 to 70 percent of female patients due to hypersecretion of adrenal androgens; it is generally mild to moderate. Facial hirsutism is most common, but increased hair growth may also occur over the abdomen, breasts, chest, and upper thighs. Virilism is unusual except in adrenal carcinomas, in which it occurs in approximately 20 percent.[652,659] Acne (most frequently involving the face) and seborrhea usually accompany hirsutism.

Hypertension, a classic feature of spontaneous Cushing's syndrome, is present in 75 to 85 percent of patients. The diastolic blood pressure is >100 mmHg in over 50 percent of patients (Chap. 14).[707] In one series 23 of 24 patients over the age of 40 were hypertensive and of these 11 had congestive heart failure.[707] Hypertension and its complications contribute greatly to morbidity and mortality in spontaneous Cushing's syndrome; in the series of Plotz et al. 40 percent of those dying with the syndrome did so directly as a result of hypertension and/or atherosclerosis.[652] Peripheral edema was frequently described in early series,[652,709] but was present in only 18 percent of patients in the series of Ross et al.[707]

Gonadal dysfunction is extremely common due to elevated levels of androgens (in females) and cortisol (in males and to a lesser extent, females). Amenorrhea occurs in approximately 75 percent of premenopausal females and is usually accompanied by infertility.[652,707] Patients without amenorrhea have generally had a shorter duration of symptoms.[709] Male patients frequently have decreased libido and some have decreased body hair and soft testes.[707,709] Gynecomastia is unusual in male patients, but may be seen in patients with estrogen-producing adrenal carcinomas.

Psychological disturbances occur in approximately two-thirds of patients.[652] The presentation and severity of these features are extremely variable. Mild features include emotional lability and increased irritability. Increased anxiety, depression, decreased concentration, and poor memory may also be present. Some patients are euphoric and occasionally may manifest overtly manic behavior. The majority of patients also have disordered sleep with either insomnia or early morning awakening. A minority of patients exhibit more severe psychological disorders, which may include severe depression, psychosis with delusions or hallucinations, or paranoia, and some have committed suicide.[652] The patient's premorbid personality or psychiatric history has not been helpful in predicting the types of psychoses which occur.

Muscle weakness occurs in approximately 60 percent; it is most frequently proximal and is usually most prominent in the lower extremities.[707] Thus, patients typically first note difficulty in climbing stairs and in more severe cases may have difficulty arising from a chair.

Approximately 50 percent of patients have clinically obvious osteoporosis, although the incidence of this probably approaches 100 percent when refined measurements are made (Chap. 15). Back pain is an initial complaint in 40 percent.[707] Pathological fractures occur frequently in severe cases and most often involve the ribs and vertebral bodies.[707,709] Compression fractures of the spine are demonstrable radiographically in 16 to 22 percent and may be accompanied by loss of height and kyphosis.[707,709]

Renal calculi occur in approximately 15 percent of patients and renal colic may occasionally be a presenting complaint.[707] These calculi are the consequence of glucocorticoid-induced hypercalciuria, although a few patients have had associated primary hyperparathyroidism.[707] Thirst and polyuria may also occur in an occasional patient with hypercalciuria. Thirst and polyuria ascribable to overt hyperglycemia and diabetes mellitus occur in approximately 10 percent of patients, whereas glucose intolerance is much more frequent. Diabetic ketoacidosis is rare, as are diabetic microvascular complications.

Laboratory Features

Routine laboratory examinations are rarely of major diagnostic utility in the diagnosis of Cushing's syndrome, although certain abnormalities may suggest the diagnosis. The specific utility of ACTH and corticosteroid measurements and provocative testing is discussed below.

Patients with Cushing's syndrome frequently have high normal values of hemoglobin, hematocrit, and red cell count, but elevations into the range of polycythemia are rare.[707] The total white count is usually normal; however, the percentage of lymphocytes is below 25 in 50 percent of cases and the total lymphocyte count is subnormal in 35 percent.[707] The total eosinophil count is usually below 100/mm^3 and is less than 10/mm^3 in approximately 30 percent of patients. Serum sodium concentration is normal in most patients but is occasionally elevated. In patients with Cushing's disease, serum potassium and bicarbonate concentrations are usually normal but hypokalemia and alkalosis are frequent with the ectopic ACTH syndrome or adrenocortical carcinoma.[707,708] The degree of hypokalemia correlates well with adrenocortical hypersecretion; thus, it is not unexpected that hypokalemic alkalosis occurs most frequently in these latter two conditions, in which steroid levels are frequently markedly elevated.[708,710] Renal function is normal in uncomplicated Cushing's syndrome, but can be abnormal in those patients with long-standing hypertension, renal stones, nephrocalcinosis, or infection. Serum calcium and phosphorus concentrations are almost invariably normal; however, hypercalciuria occurs in 40 percent of patients and plasma phosphate concentrations are subnormal in almost half of the patients.[707] Fasting hyperglycemia occurs in 10 to 15 percent of cases and glucose intolerance with associated hyperinsulinemia occurs in the majority of patients.[652,707,709] Glycosuria is present in patients with fasting hyperglycemia and may also occur postprandially. Ketosis or ketoacidosis is rare; its presence suggests coexisting insulinopenic diabetes. Plasma lipoprotein (VLDL, LDL, and HDL) concentrations tend to be elevated, with consequent elevations of triglyceride and cholesterol levels,[275] especially in those patients with hyperglycemia.

Routine radiographs may reveal cardiomegaly due to hypertensive or atherosclerotic heart disease; rib or spinal compression features and renal calculi may be noted. The electrocardiogram may be abnormal in patients with long-standing disease in whom hypertensive or atherosclerotic myocardial injury has occurred.

FEATURES SUGGESTING A SPECIFIC ETIOLOGY

Although a definite diagnosis of the type of Cushing's syndrome present must be established biochemically, certain features suggest a specific etiology.

Patients with Cushing's disease present with the classic clinical picture. Women predominate, onset is generally between ages 20 and 40, and the clinical manifestations are usually slowly progressive over several years. Hyperpigmentation and hypokalemic alkalosis are rare. Cortisol and adrenal androgen secretion is increased moderately and androgenic manifestations are generally limited to acne and mild to moderate hirsutism.[707]

In contrast, the ectopic ACTH syndrome occurs predominantly in males, with highest incidence in the fifth to seventh decades.[708] The primary tumor is usually apparent but the clinical manifestations are frequently limited to weakness, hypertension, and glucose intolerance. Hyperpigmentation, hypokalemia, and alkalosis are common.[708] Weight loss and anemia due to malignancy are also common. The features of hypercortisolism are of rapid onset. Steroid hypersecretion is frequently severe, with equally elevated levels of glucocorticoids, androgens, and DOC.[708] Survival in these patients with both metastatic carcinoma and severe hypercortisolism is extremely limited.[708]

A minority of patients with the ectopic ACTH syndrome have more "benign" tumors, especially bronchial carcinoids, and present a more slowly progressive course with typical features of Cushing's syndrome. These patients may be clinically identical to those having pituitary-dependent Cushing's disease; the responsible tumor may not be apparent.[487,711a] Hyperpigmentation, hypokalemic alkalosis, and anemia are commonly absent. Further confusion may arise since a number of these patients with occult ectopic tumors may have ACTH and steroid dynamics typical of Cushing's disease (see below).[487,711a]

The clinical picture in patients with adrenal adenomas is usually that of glucocorticoid excess alone. Androgenic effects such as hirsutism are usually absent. The onset is gradual and the hypercortisolism is mild to moderate. Urinary 17-ketosteroid excretion and plasma androgen concentrations are usually in the low normal or subnormal range.[712]

With adrenal carcinomas in general the clinical features of excessive glucocorticoid, androgen, and mineralocorticoid hypersecretion have a rapid onset and are rapidly progressive.[659] Marked elevations of both 17-OHCS and 17-ketosteroid levels are usual. Hypokalemia is common. Abdominal pain, palpable masses, and hepatic and pulmonary metastases are also common at the time of diagnosis.[659]

DIAGNOSIS AND DIFFERENTIAL DIAGNOSIS

Diagnosis

The evaluation of Cushing's syndrome must first include a general assessment of the patient regarding the presence of other illnesses, drugs and medications,

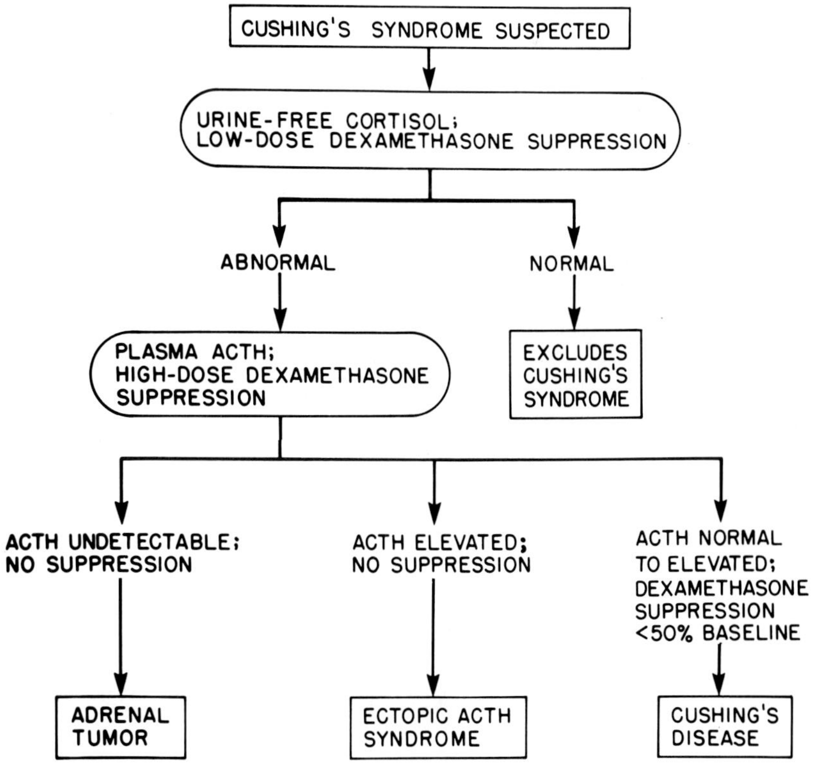

FIGURE 12-35 Evaluation of Cushing's syndrome. Boxes enclose clinical decisions and circles enclose diagnostic tests. See text for details and for the potential for false-positive and false-negative results.

alcoholism, and depression, since these may lead to misleading results. In suspected hypercortisolism, the overnight 1-mg dexamethasone suppression test is performed and a 24-h urine collection is obtained for assay of free cortisol on an outpatient basis (Fig. 12-35). If results of the overnight dexamethasone suppression test are normal (plasma cortisol concentration ≤ 5 g/dl), the diagnosis is very unlikely (Fig. 12-36); if the urinary free cortisol level is also normal (Fig. 12-37), Cushing's syndrome is excluded.[487,502] If these two tests are abnormal, hypercortisolism is present and the diagnosis of Cushing's syndrome is established, provided that conditions causing false-positive responses are excluded (see below).

In patients with equivocal or borderline results, the 2-day low-dose dexamethasone suppression test is performed, with measurement of urinary 17-OHCS or free cortisol excretion (normal responses: 17-OHCS $\leq$ 4 mg/24 h or $\leq$ 1.0 mg per gram of creatinine;[502,515,532] free cortisol $\leq$ 19 to 25 μg/24 h[502,533,534]). In this setting a normal response excludes Cushing's syndrome and abnormal suppressibility is consistent with the diagnosis, since the incidence of false-positive responses is negligible.[502]

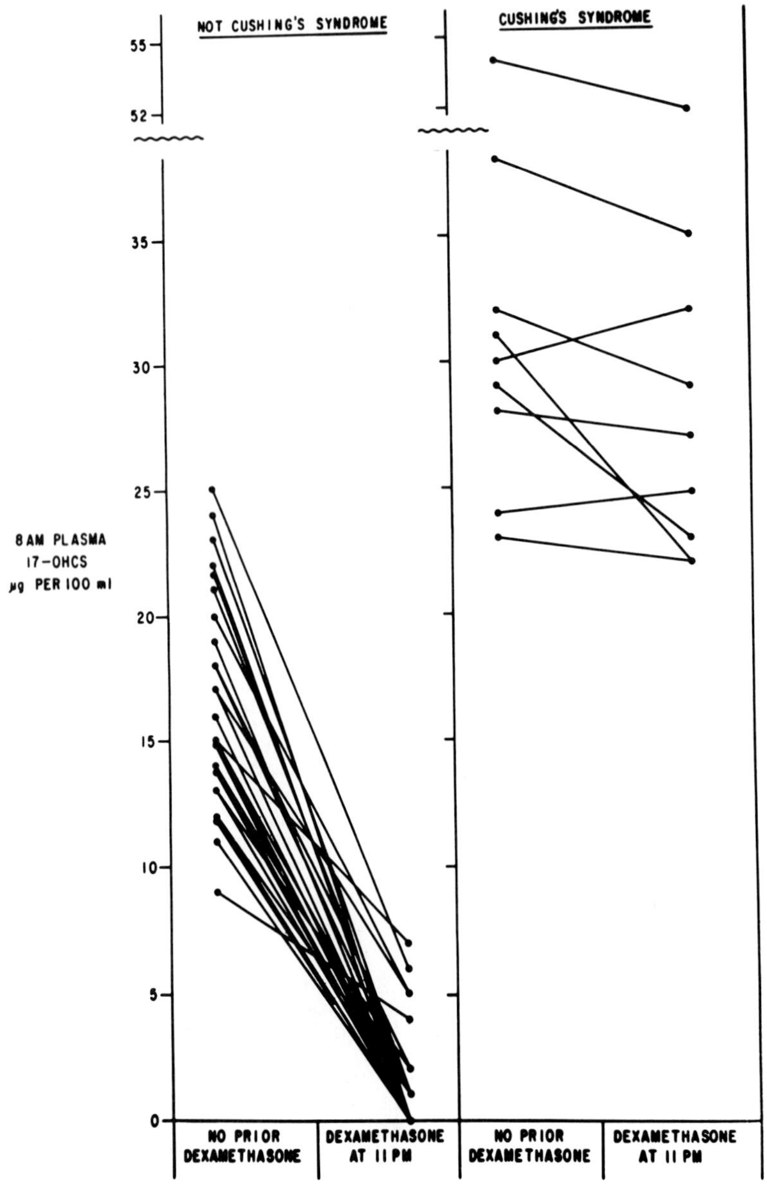

FIGURE 12-36 Plasma cortisol (8 A.M. plasma 17-OHCS) response to the low-dose dexamethasone suppression test (see text) in control subjects ("not Cushing's syndrome") and patients with Cushing's syndrome. (*From Nugent et al.*[711b])

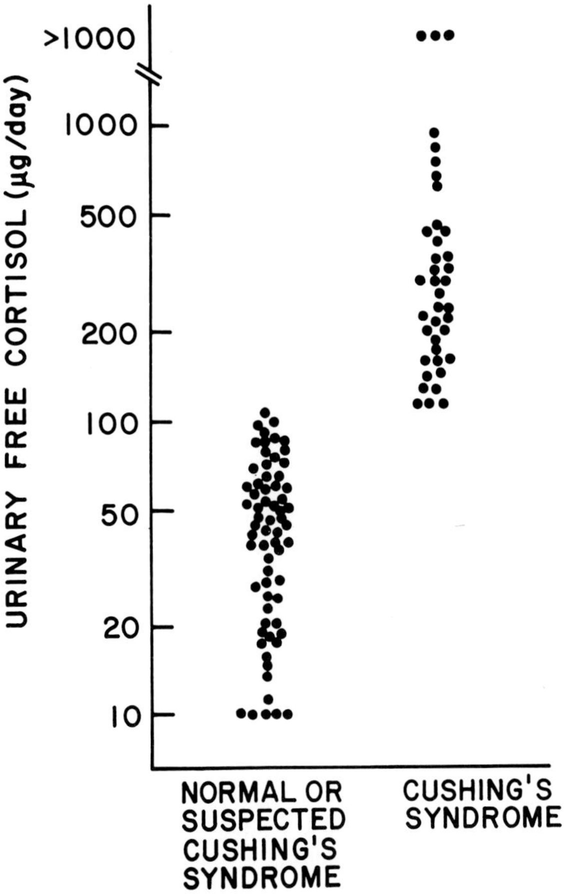

FIGURE 12-37 Urinary free cortisol excretion (measured by the competitive protein binding assay) in normal individuals, individuals with suspected but not substantiated hypercortisolism, and patients with Cushing's syndrome. (*Based upon data of Burke and Beardwell.*[534])

The measurement of late-evening (11:00 P.M. to 2:00 A.M.) plasma cortisol levels or cortisol production rate is also useful in the diagnosis of Cushing's syndrome,[502,525] but neither has come into general use, because of inconvenience.

Other tests and procedures are less reliable in the diagnosis and are no longer recommended since there is considerable overlap between patients with and without Cushing's syndrome.[502,540] These include basal morning cortisol levels; afternoon or early-evening diurnal cortisol level; basal 24-h urinary 17-OHCS, 17-KGS, or 17-ketosteroid excretion; and responsiveness to either ACTH or metyrapone stimulation tests (see Laboratory Evaluation of Adrenocortical Function, above).[502,540]

Problems in Diagnosis

Despite the generally clear separation of patients with and without Cushing's syndrome using a combination of the tests described above, several factors may complicate the diagnosis.[487,502] These include both rare false-negative results and, more commonly, false-positive results.

False-negative responses have been reported in several patients with Cushing's syndrome. First, there may be normal suppression of glucocorticoid secretion with low-dose dexamethasone because of delayed clearance of the steroid and higher than usual plasma levels of dexamethasone.[487,502,528,529] In this situation, urinary free cortisol level should be elevated and will assist in establishing the diagnosis.[487,529] The measurement of plasma dexamethasone concentrations, if available, will reveal the reason for normal suppressibility.[528,529] A second unusual cause of normal suppressibility is periodic or episodic hormonogenesis in Cushing's syndrome.[530,713,714] In these patients hypercortisolism is either cyclic, with a regular period of days to weeks, or episodic, without a regular pattern; cortisol secretion may be normal or near normal between cycles or episodes.[530,713] Thus, in these patients with spontaneously varying cortisol secretion, adrenal function may be normal at times and dexamethasone administration during phases of normal secretion may reveal normal suppressibility.[530] In these patients repeated evaluation is required to establish the diagnosis of hypercortisolism and additional difficulties may be encountered in the differential diagnosis (see below).

False-positive responses are more common. Patients with acute and/or chronic illnesses, especially those who are hospitalized, may have appropriately elevated glucocorticoid secretion. These patients may have elevated plasma cortisol and urinary free cortisol levels and their adrenal function is frequently nonsuppressible with the 1-mg overnight suppression test.[502] If Cushing's syndrome is suspected, diagnostic evaluation should be repeated when the acute stress has resolved.

Obesity is the most common differential diagnosis problem in Cushing's syndrome. The elevation of urinary 17-OHCS and 17-KGS excretion in obese patients is the major reason for the limited utility of these tests. The overnight 1-mg suppression test is also less useful, since approximately 13 percent of obese patients have abnormal responses.[502] However, the urinary free cortisol excretion is virtually always normal in simple obesity.[512,533,534] In addition, in those with an abnormal overnight test, the 2-day low-dose suppression test will resolve the problem, since in obese patients normal suppressibility of urinary 17-OHCS level is maintained.[487,515]

High-estrogen states (pregnancy, estrogen therapy, and oral contraceptive use) may also cause confusion since total plasma cortisol levels may be as high as

40 to 60 μg/dl because of increased CBG concentration and the result of an overnight 1-mg test may be abnormal; however, urinary free cortisol excretion is normal (except for late pregnancy). Further, if the overnight test is abnormal, the 2-day suppression test should be performed since suppressibility of urinary 17-OHCS level is normal.[487,515]

Patients on phenytoin and other anticonvulsants, including phenobarbital and primidone, can have false-positive results on low-dose dexamethasone tests; however, urinary free cortisol excretion is normal, as is the suppressibility of plasma corticosterone levels by oral hydrocortisone.[487]

A number of alcoholic patients have both clinical and biochemical features of Cushing's syndrome ("alcohol-induced pseudo-Cushing's syndrome").[487,715] The patients have elevated basal plasma cortisol levels with abnormal circadian variation, increased cortisol production rate, increased urinary corticosteroid excretion, and abnormal suppressibility by dexamethasone, i.e., steroid dynamics consistent with Cushing's syndrome.[487,715] The steroid dynamics revert to normal following cessation of alcohol intake; thus, if diagnostic test results are abnormal, testing should be repeated after abstention from alcohol for at least 4 weeks. In view of the frequency of excessive alcohol use, this possibility should be considered whenever hypercortisolism is suspected.

Similarly, patients with depression frequently have abnormal steroid dynamics which suggest Cushing's syndrome.[487] These patients also have increased cortisol secretion with elevated plasma levels, absence of diurnal variation, increased urinary free cortisol excretion, increased urinary 17-OHCS excretion, and impaired dexamethasone suppression.[487] The abnormal steroid dynamics revert to normal upon psychological recovery. These patients can be differentiated from those with true Cushing's syndrome since patients with depression alone maintain normal cortisol responsiveness to insulin-induced hypoglycemia, whereas in patients with Cushing's syndrome cortisol levels do not increase further during hypoglycemia.[487,504] CRF testing does not appear to adequately differentiate these etiologies.[716]

Patients with anorexia nervosa also have cortisol dynamics similar to those of Cushing's disease.[160] However, these patients can be distinguished from Cushing's disease patients by their clinical presentation and from those with the ectopic ACTH syndrome by high-dose dexamethasone suppression.

Determining the Etiology

When Cushing's syndrome is present the specific etiology must be defined. Thus, pituitary ACTH hypersecretion (Cushing's disease) must be differentiated from the ectopic ACTH syndrome and primary adrenal tumors (Fig. 12-35). The two most useful standard procedures are measurement of basal plasma ACTH levels (Fig. 12-38) and the performance of high-dose dexamethasone suppression testing (see Laboratory Evaluation of Adrenocortical Function, above and Refs. 487 and 717). The combined results of these two tests will establish the correct etiology in most instances.

Patients with Cushing's disease have normal to modestly elevated plasma ACTH levels, ranging from 40 to 200 pg/ml (normal = 20 to 100 pg/ml) and approximately 50 percent of patients have values consistently within the normal range.[504] The presence of detectable levels is consistent with the diagnosis. In patients with Cushing's disease, suppressibility of ACTH secretion characteristically is maintained with higher glucocorticoid doses, i.e., ACTH and cortisol secretion are suppressible to less than 50 percent of basal levels with the high-dose dexamethasone tests.

In the ectopic ACTH syndrome, plasma ACTH levels are frequently markedly elevated (500 to 10,000 pg/ml) and are above 200 pg/ml in 65 percent of patients.[504] However, since at lower levels these values overlap with the range seen in Cushing's disease, dexamethasone suppression testing must also be used. Since control of ACTH secretion is absent, cortisol secretion is classically not suppressible with high-dose dexamethasone. In addition, the primary tumor is clinically evident in the majority of patients.

Glucocorticoid-secreting adrenal tumors function autonomously and the resulting suppression of the normal hypothalamic-pituitary axis leads to undetectable plasma ACTH levels (≤ 20 pg/ml) and absent steroid suppression with high-dose dexamethasone.[502]

CRF testing has now been used quite extensively in Cushing's disease and Cushing's syndrome.[541–544,717] In Cushing's disease there is normal responsiveness or hyperresponsiveness of ACTH and cortisol to CRF administration; however, some patients do not respond.[544] In the ectopic ACTH syndrome, ACTH secretion does not increase further in response to CRF, although one exception has been reported.[543] In adrenal tumors basal ACTH levels are suppressed and do not respond to CRF. Current experience suggests that CRF responses will be useful in differential diagnosis of Cushing's syndrome, at the least to provide corroborative evidence. However, this procedure will probably not supersede the currently used procedures described above.[717]

Metyrapone testing has been used in the differential diagnosis of Cushing's syndrome.[502] However, it is usually unnecessary if reliable plasma ACTH levels are obtained. ACTH stimulation tests do not adequately

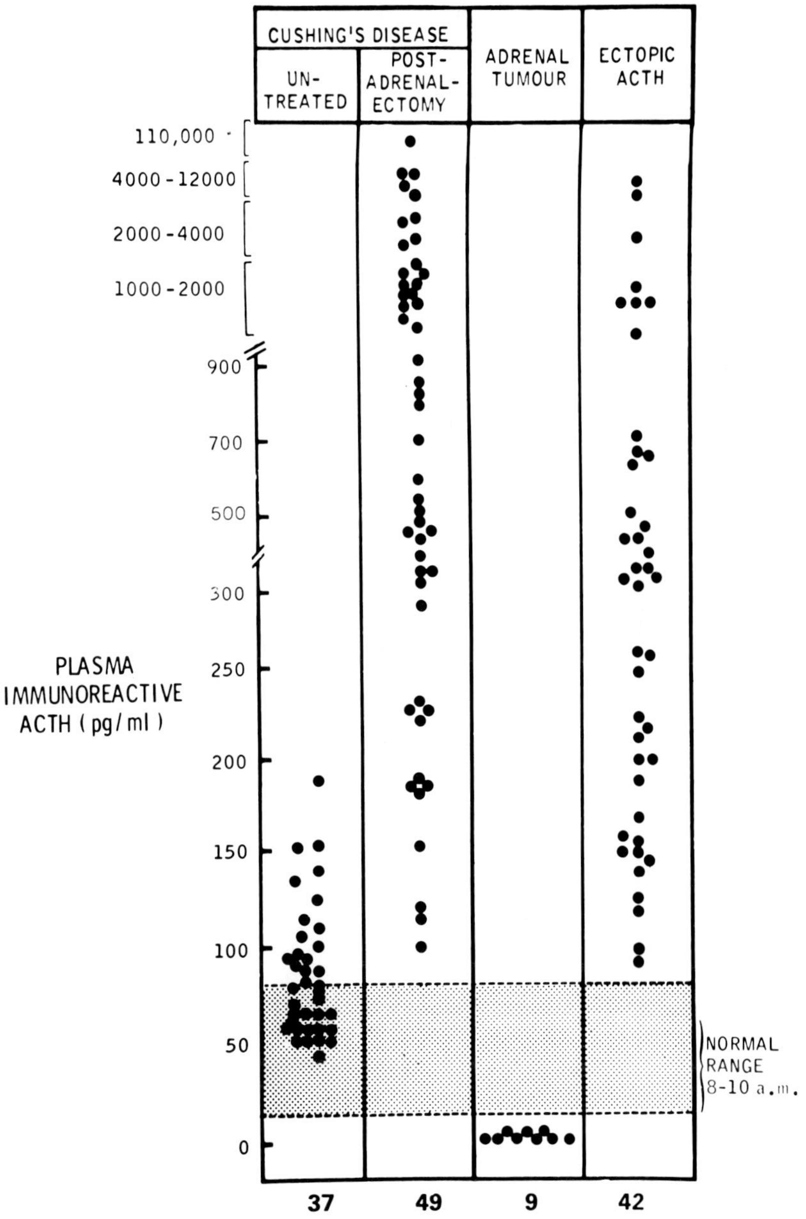

FIGURE 12-38 Basal plasma ACTH levels in patients with Cushing's disease before (untreated) and after bilateral adrenalectomy and with cortisol-producing adrenal adenomas and ectopic ACTH syndrome. (*From Besser and Edwards.*[504])

separate the various etiologies of Cushing's syndrome and are of little diagnostic utility.[502]

Problems in Determining the Etiology

Although the procedures described in the preceding section will establish a specific etiology in the majority of cases, sufficient exceptions occur to warrant discussion.

Problems are encountered in the rare patients with periodic or episodic hormonogenesis who may have either Cushing's disease, the ectopic ACTH syndrome, or adrenal tumors.[530,713,714] Thus, these patients may show normal suppression with the low-dose test if it is performed during certain periods; when studied at other times, secretion in these patients may be nonsuppressible or even show paradoxical increases during high-dose dexamethasone administration.[530,713] Repeated evaluations and use of the localizing procedures described below may be necessary to establish the correct etiology in such patients.

Urinary 17-OHCS excretion in approximately 10 to 30 percent of patients with Cushing's disease fails to be suppressed with the standard 2-day high-dose dexamethasone suppression test; in the presence of measurable ACTH levels this falsely suggests the ectopic ACTH syndrome.[487,502,539,540] This frequency of nonsuppressibility is decreased by the use of the overnight 8-mg high-dose dexamethasone suppression test.[539] Some of the patients with nonsuppressible function have nodular adrenal hyperplasia, which frequently causes diagnostic difficulties since approximately 75 percent of these patients have nonsuppressible function with the standard 2-day high-dose dexamethasone suppression test.[487,502,678] Plasma ACTH levels may be undetectable, normal, or elevated and may vary dramatically in the same patient.[502,678] In patients who do not show suppression with high-dose dexamethasone, in whom ACTH levels are not markedly elevated, and who do not have an obvious ectopic tumor, higher doses of dexamethasone (16 or 32 mg) should be administered and selective venous ACTH sampling performed (see below). If steroid suppression with higher doses of dexamethasone occurs and/or if selective venous sampling demonstrates a pituitary ACTH gradient, the diagnosis of Cushing's disease is established.[487,678] Also, the diagnosis may be established by the demonstration of nodular hyperplasia by CT scan of the adrenals.[487,678]

Although the ectopic ACTH syndrome is usually easily diagnosed by elevated ACTH levels and nonsuppressible steroid hypersecretion in the presence of an extrapituitary tumor, there are some cases in which the tumor is occult. In these, steroid secretion may be dexamethasone-suppressible and metyrapone-responsive.[487,711] In addition, the tumor may not reveal itself for a number of years following the onset of Cushing's syndrome.[487,711a] These occult tumors are usually bronchial carcinoids, and the plasma ACTH levels can be in the range of those seen with Cushing's disease.[487,711a] These findings may lead to the mistaken diagnosis of Cushing's disease and lead to inappropriate pituitary therapy. Although it is not possible to make this differentiation with certainty in all cases, certain features should increase suspicion of the presence of ectopic ACTH syndrome. These are male sex, rapid onset, severe hypercortisolism, hypokalemia, or weight loss. If the ectopic ACTH syndrome is suspected but no tumor is obvious, selective venous ACTH sampling is helpful. Thus, the demonstration of a pituitary venous ACTH gradient establishes the diagnosis of Cushing's disease.[718–722] In the absence of a pituitary gradient, the ectopic ACTH syndrome is likely, and selective venous sampling may localize the ACTH-secreting ectopic tumor.[702,720] If localization is not achieved by this method, additional diagnostic and radiologic procedures should be directed to the common sites of ACTH production, i.e., lungs, thymus, pancreas, thyroid, and adrenals.

Adrenal tumors rarely cause diagnostic difficulties since the typical features of undetectable ACTH levels and absent dexamethasone suppression are almost invariably present. Reproducible suppressibility by dexamethasone has not been documented[502] but might occur with episodic secretion.[714] Another rare exception is that of an ACTH-secreting adrenal carcinoma.[723]

Tumor Localization

These procedures, although useful in the localization of tumors in Cushing's syndrome, must be integrated carefully. They should be preceded when possible by a definite biochemical diagnosis since radiologic procedures can give misleading results.

In Cushing's disease neuroradiologic procedures are used to define sellar size, anatomy, and suprasellar tumor extension. In the 10 to 15 percent of patients with larger tumors (macroadenomas) plain radiography reveals sellar enlargement and may demonstrate erosion of the floor with sphenoid sinus extension of the tumor. Polytomography, angiography, and pneumoencephalography are rarely used at present.

The problem of tumor localization in patients with Cushing's disease who have microadenomas has not been solved and this remains a biochemical diagnosis.[667] Tomography and plain radiographs are normal in the majority and are not useful.[667,724] High-resolution CT of the sella turcica is the current radiologic procedure of choice.[725–727] This is performed with 1.5-mm collimation and can thus define normal pituitary anatomy.[725] The presence of a convex upper pituitary margin, increased height of the pituitary, deviation of the stalk, and focal "low-density" areas are the criteria on which a diagnosis of a pituitary adenoma are based. However, despite this precision, CT scans are abnormal in only approximately 50 percent of patients with Cushing's disease, presumably because adenomas less than 5 mm in diameter are too small to resolve with current techniques.[726,727] False-positive scans may also occur in patients with coincidental nonfunctional pituitary adenomas, interpituitary cysts, or the empty sella syndrome.[726] Magnetic resonance imaging (MRI) is currently being evaluated in the diagnosis of hypothalamic and pituitary lesions. Current techniques have resolution similar to that obtained with CT scans but MRI allows better definition of the pituitary stalk and optic chiasm. In a limited number of patients studied to date, an approximately 50 percent prevalence of abnormal scans has been found. Thus, the ultimate utility of MRI in localizing the pituitary adenomas of Cushing's disease remains to be determined.

Selective pituitary venous ACTH sampling is helpful in those patients in whom the source of ACTH hypersecretion is in doubt, e.g., non-dexamethasone-suppressible Cushing's disease, nodular adrenal hyperplasia, or an occult ACTH-secreting tumor (see above). It is also being used more extensively in patients with biochemical findings suggesting Cushing's disease in whom CT scans or MRI are normal. In these circumstances venous sampling may establish the pituitary as the source of ACTH and in some cases will localize an ectopic tumor.[702,718–720] The venous system is catheterized by the femoral route; ACTH samples are obtained from the inferior petrosal sinuses (a major site of venous drainage of the anterior pituitary), the jugular venous bulb, and other sites; these samples are compared to simultaneous peripheral vein samples. Simultaneous bilateral inferior petrosal sampling has also been described and may lateralize the pituitary adenoma.[721,722] This is probably beyond the current technical capacity of most centers. In patients with Cushing's disease, inferior petrosal sinus/peripheral ACTH ratios are usually greater than 2:1; samples from the jugular bulb and jugular vein are usually nondiagnostic because of venous admixture.[719] In patients with the ectopic ACTH syndrome, no inferior petrosal/peripheral ACTH gradient is demonstrable, but selective venous sampling may localize the ectopic tumor.[719]

CT scans are most commonly used to define adrenal pathology. However, ultrasonography and isotope scanning using radio-labeled cholesterol are useful.[728–730] In patients with ACTH hypersecretion these procedures exclude an adrenal tumor and confirm bilateral adrenal hyperplasia or nodular adrenal hyperplasia. These procedures also effectively localize adrenal tumors in most cases, since the tumors are usually greater than 2 cm in diameter (Fig. 12-39). However, nodular hyperplasia of the adrenals with a solitary or dominant nodule can be misinterpreted as an autonomous hyperfunctioning adenoma.[487,678] At present, invasive procedures such as arteriography and venography, which have significant morbidity, are usually used only to define blood supply, surgical anatomy, vena cava invasion by tumor, and hepatic metastases in patients with adrenal carcinoma.

TREATMENT OF CUSHING'S SYNDROME

The treatment of Cushing's syndrome, although not yet ideal, has been improved by advances in pituitary microsurgery and sophisticated radiotherapeutic techniques. Medical therapy is also becoming more effective in controlling ACTH and/or cortisol secretion in a minority of patients when other therapies are unsuccessful or are being contemplated. The aim of treatment in Cushing's syndrome is to remove or destroy the basic lesion, and thus correct hypersecretion of adrenal hormones without inducing pituitary and/or adrenal damage, which requires permanent replacement therapy for hormone deficiencies.[731]

Cushing's Disease

Treatment of Cushing's disease is currently directed at the pituitary to control ACTH hypersecretion; available methods include microsurgery, various forms of radiation therapy, and pharmacological inhibition of ACTH secretion. Treatment of hypercortisolism per se by surgical or medical adrenalectomy is less commonly used. Since pituitary adenomas in Cushing's disease are frequently not localized prior to treatment, a secure biochemical diagnosis of pituitary-dependent hypercortisolism must be established prior to therapy.

Transsphenoidal microsurgery is the current neurosurgical procedure of choice and is used at a number of centers as initial therapy for Cushing's disease in both adults and children.[664,667,668,689–692] Hypertension and hyperglycemia should be controlled prior to surgery and these patients should receive glucocorticoid coverage for surgery according to the protocol described above (see Adrenocortical Insufficiency). Since the pituitary tumors of Cushing's disease are small and are frequently within the anterior lobe tissue, an experienced surgeon and meticulous exploration of the intrasellar contents are required.[667,668] Once identified, the micro- or macroadenoma is selectively removed and the normal gland is left intact.

In patients with microadenomas (less than 1.0 cm in diameter), selective microsurgery is successful in correcting the biochemical abnormalities in approximately 85 percent.[664,667,668,689,690] Surgical damage to anterior pituitary function is rare, but the majority of successfully treated patients develop transient secondary adrenocortical insufficiency which is then followed by recovery of normal pituitary-adrenal function (see Etiology and Pathogenesis, above). In approximately 10 percent, the tumor is too small to locate at surgery and in adult patients past the reproductive age group total hypophysectomy may be performed.[667,668] In the remaining 5 percent of patients with microadenomas selective tumor removal fails to correct hypercortisolism. Patients with corticotroph hyperplasia or adenomatous hyperplasia will obviously not respond to selective pituitary microsurgery and must be treated with other modalities, as discussed below. Unfortunately, current diagnostic procedures cannot identify these patients preoperatively.

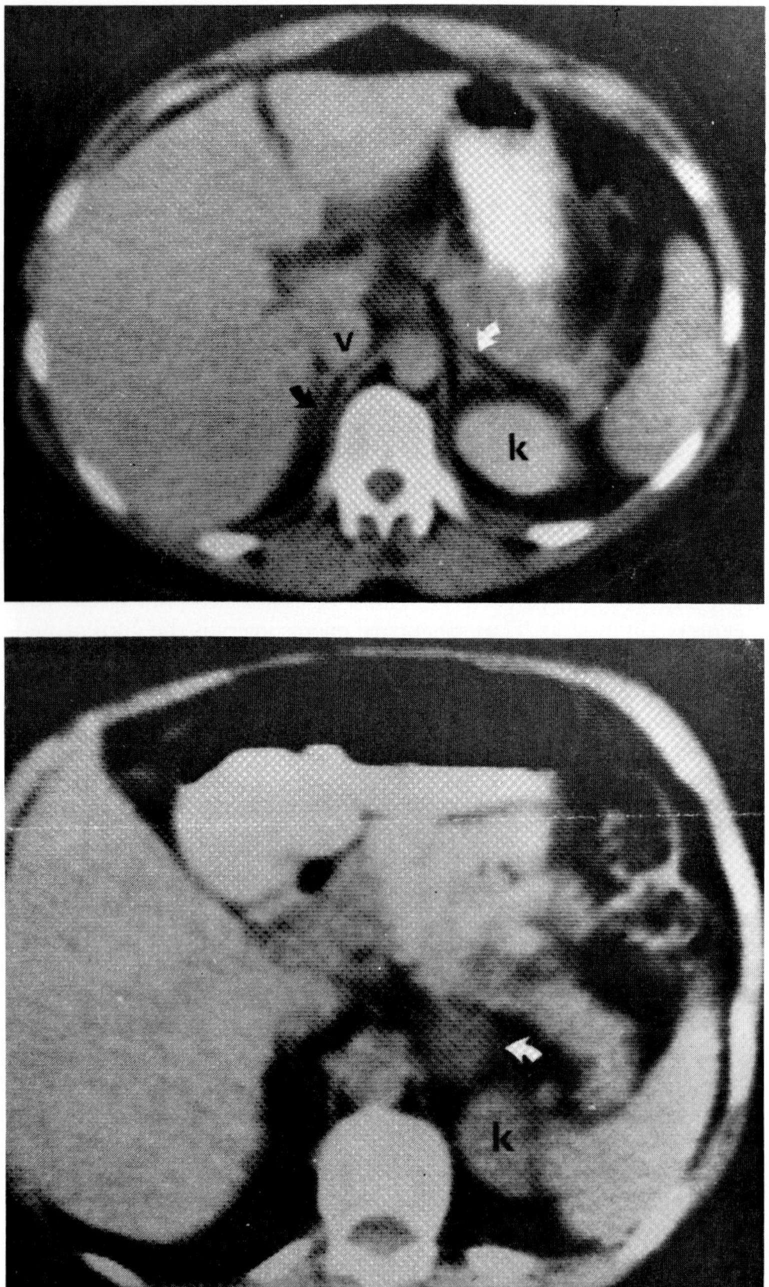

A

B

FIGURE 12-39 CT scans in Cushing's syndrome. (*A*) Patient with ACTH-dependent Cushing's syndrome. The adrenal glands are not detectably abnormal by this procedure. The curvilinear right adrenal (black arrow) is shown posterior to the inferior vena cava (v) between the right lobe of the liver and the right crus of the diaphragm. The left adrenal (white arrow) has an inverted Y appearance anteromedial to the left kidney (k). (*B*) A 3-cm left adrenal adenoma (white arrow) anteromedial to the left kidney (k). (*From Korobkin et al.*[729])

Transsphenoidal surgery is successful in only 25 percent of the approximately 10 to 15 percent of patients with Cushing's disease with pituitary macroadenomas or in those with extrasellar extension of the tumor.[668,690] These patients usually require multiple therapies (see below) and frequently present difficult problems in management. Rare patients with massive tumors and suprasellar extension may require craniotomy to achieve decompression of the optic chiasm and other vital structures.

Postoperatively, steroid coverage is reduced to maintenance doses of hydrocortisone (30 μg per day) by the seventh to tenth day. In these patients, who are accustomed to cortisol excess, the steroid withdrawal syndrome (see Chap. 15) may be prominent and this may necessitate increased cortisol dosage and slower tapering to maintenance levels. The pituitary-adrenal axis is reevaluated 4 to 6 weeks following surgery to ensure that hypercortisolism has been corrected; other pituitary hormones are also reevaluated at this time by measuring serum levels of prolactin, gonadotropins, TSH, and thyroid hormones. Since the majority of patients develop transient secondary adrenal insufficiency,[693] cortisol therapy is required until there is recovery of normal responsiveness of the pituitary adrenal axis (see Diagnosis under Adrenocortical Insufficiency, above, and Chap. 15). The complications of selective transsphenoidal microsurgery have been surprisingly few, considering the nature of the metabolic abnormalities in these patients. Transient diabetes insipidus occurs in approximately 20 percent and there is intra- or postoperative hemorrhage in an occasional patient.[667,668,688–690] Potential complications such as hypopituitarism, CSF rhinorrhea, infection, meningitis, visual impairment, or oculomotor dysfunction have not materialized in larger series.[668] Patients undergoing total hypophysectomy develop panhypopituitarism; in these diabetes insipidus may persist. The subsequent management of these patients is discussed in Chaps. 7 and 8 and above (see Treatment under Adrenocortical Insufficiency). Follow-up data in patients with successful surgical removal of microadenomas, although limited, are accumulating; the majority of patients achieve persisting control of Cushing's disease, although in a minority it recurs.[667,668,688–698] Thus, transsphenoidal microsurgery is an effective therapy for Cushing's disease and corrects hypercortisolism with minimal morbidity in the majority of patients with microadenomas.

Alpha particle or proton beam irradiation of the pituitary are also effective initial therapies for Cushing's disease, although these techniques are currently available in only one center in the United States.[732,733a] Since the size of the radiation field is limited, these methods are not applicable to patients with either suprasellar or sphenoid sinus extension of the tumor. Alpha particle radiation is effective in controlling hypercortisolism in 80 percent of patients with an incidence of hypopituitarism of approximately one-third.[732] Proton beam therapy is effective in 65 percent of patients and the incidence of hypopituitarism was reported to be 13 percent, although the follow-up period was not reported.[733] Neurological complications, including visual loss and oculomotor paralysis, rarely occur.[732,733a] With both of these techniques there is a lag period of 6 to 12 months before cortisol secretion returns to normal, and since the effects of radiation are prolonged, the incidence of hypopituitarism may increase with further follow-up.

Conventional pituitary irradiation has been used for many years; however, it is effective in only a minority of adults.[662,720,731] Additional disadvantages are the prolonged period of time (often 12 to 18 months) before it is effective and the occurrence of posttreatment hypopituitarism, which is increasingly being recognized.[733b] In children, conventional irradiation has been reported to be effective in 80 percent;[662] however, the potential for hypopituitarism and consequent growth failure must be considered. Because of the limitations of conventional radiotherapy in adults, various other maneuvers have been used to increase its efficiency. Pituitary irradiation combined with unilateral adrenalectomy increases the remission rate to 50 percent; however, this rate does not appear to justify use of both radiation and a major surgical procedure.[734] Radiation has also been combined with either metyrapone or mitotane.[720,735–737] These regimens have the advantage of reducing cortisol secretion more rapidly, although it appears that the ultimate response to radiation will still be unsatisfactory and prolonged drug therapy is required. Thus, conventional pituitary irradiation is not recommended as the primary therapy for adults with Cushing's disease. However, conventional radiation therapy should be used in those patients with larger tumors and in whom extrasellar extension precludes the use of heavy particle irradiation.

Implantation of radioactive seeds within the sella turcica has been used in Cushing's disease, although experience is limited.[663,738] In the largest reported series, remission occurred in 65 percent of those patients with no radiologic evidence of a pituitary tumor; however, in patients with possible tumors and those with definite tumors remission occurred in only 50 percent and 14 percent, respectively.[738,739] Replacement hormone therapy was required in 55 percent for total or partial hypopituitarism and 5 percent developed CSF rhinorrhea.[738] The same group reported successful treatment of juvenile Cushing's disease by pituitary implants; remission was attained in each of nine patients and partial or complete hypopituitarism developed in only two.[663] There were no complications in this group.

Pharmacologic inhibition of ACTH secretion in Cushing's disease has been attempted, with limited success. Cyproheptadine, a serotonin antagonist, and bromocriptine, a dopamine agonist, have been reported to control both ACTH hypersecretion and hypercortisolism in a few cases.[680,686,720] However, to date these agents are successful in only a minority of patients and cannot be considered definitive therapy since relapse occurs following their discontinuation. In addition, side effects frequently accompany their use (Chap. 7).

Treatment of Cushing's disease by adrenalectomy was the major form of therapy from the early 1950s until the 1970s. This method has now been largely replaced by therapy directed at the pituitary. Although bilateral adrenalectomy rapidly reverses hypercortisolism, it is accompanied by an operative mortality of 5 to 10 percent, a high incidence of postoperative complications (poor wound healing, infection, pancreatic injury, and thromboembolism), permanent glucocorticoid and mineralocorticoid deficiency, and a recurrence rate of approximately 10 percent.[720,740] Further, it may be followed by the development of large and progressive pituitary tumors (Nelson's syndrome; see below). Adrenalectomy should be used only in those few patients who cannot be treated successfully by other methods.

Pharmacologic agents which inhibit adrenal cortisol secretion are useful in Cushing's disease but mainly as adjunctive therapy.[628,720,737] Metyrapone and aminoglutethimide (Table 12-3) inhibit cortisol synthesis, although this is accompanied by increased ACTH levels which may overcome the enzyme inhibition. Adequate data are not available on the long-term use of these agents as the sole treatment of Cushing's disease; relapse occurs following discontinuation. Metyrapone is expensive and causes gastrointestinal side effects. Aminoglutethimide causes somnolence, skin rash, and goiter. Thus, these agents are ordinarily used while awaiting a response to therapy or in the preparation of patients for surgery.[720,737] More effective control of hypercortisolism with fewer side effects is obtained by combined use of these agents.[741] The adrenolytic drug mitotane not only inhibits cortisol synthesis, but also causes adrenal atrophy, predominantly of the zonae fasciculata and reticularis. It induces remissions in approximately 80 percent of patients with Cushing's disease, but 60 percent relapse following cessation of therapy.[742] Approximately 60 percent of patients experience gastrointestinal side effects; others include somnolence, depression, and skin rash. The high rate of relapse after treatment usually necessitates more definitive therapy.[742]

Ectopic ACTH Syndrome

Therapy of the ectopic ACTH syndrome is difficult in the setting of metastatic malignancy and accompanying severe hypercortisolism. Although therapy is directed at the primary tumor, this is usually unsuccessful and commonly other means must be used to correct the steroid excess state. Since severe hypokalemia may be present, it may be necessary to administer potassium replacement in large doses and spironolactone to block mineralocorticoid effects. Drugs which block steroid synthesis, including metyrapone and aminoglutethimide, are more useful in this situation than in Cushing's disease, since in the ectopic ACTH syndrome plasma ACTH levels usually do not increase in response to the lowered cortisol levels. Since these drugs may produce hypoadrenalism, steroid secretion must be monitored and replacement steroids given if necessary. In this setting mitotane is less useful because of its slow onset of action and because several weeks may be required to control cortisol secretion. Bilateral adrenalectomy rarely may be required if hypercortisolism cannot otherwise be controlled. Cure of the ectopic ACTH syndrome is usually possible only in tumors such as thymomas, bronchial carcinoids, or pheochromocytomas, which are frequently benign.[699,702,722] In patients with successful therapy plasma ACTH levels are useful to detect recurrence.[702]

Adrenal Tumors

Benign adrenal adenomas are successfully treated by unilateral adrenalectomy; the outlook is excellent. Since the hypothalamic-pituitary axis and the contralateral adrenal are suppressed by the prolonged autonomous cortisol secretion, these patients have postoperative adrenal insufficiency.[96] Thus, they require glucocorticoid but usually not mineralocorticoid therapy both during and following surgery, until the remaining adrenal recovers. This usually requires 6 to 12 months, but may be as long as 2 years (Chap. 15).[743]

Therapy of adrenocortical carcinoma is less satisfactory; the majority of patients have metastases at the time of diagnosis, usually to the retroperitoneum, liver, and lungs.[659,744] Surgery is the first step in therapy. Although surgical cure is rare, it serves to reduce the tumor mass and the degree of steroid hypersecretion. Curative surgery should be accompanied by essentially absent steroid secretion since the hypothalamic-pituitary axis and the contralateral adrenal are suppressed. Persisting nonsuppressible steroid secretion in the immediate postoperative period indicates residual or metastatic tumor. When metastatic or residual disease is present, mitotane is the drug of choice.[745] It is administered in doses of 6 to 12 g per day; however, the dose must be reduced due to side effects in 80 percent of patients (diarrhea, nausea, vomiting, depression, somnolence). Approximately 70 percent of patients display a reduction of steroid secretion, but only 35 percent show a reduction in tumor size.[744,745] Since mitotane reduces urinary 17-OHCS excretion by altering the hepatic metabolism of cortisol, these patients should be followed up by plasma cortisol or urinary free cortisol assays. Metyrapone and/or aminoglutethimide are useful in controlling steroid hypersecretion in patients who do not respond to mitotane. Radiotherapy and conventional chemotherapy have not been useful in this disease.

NELSON'S SYNDROME

Nelson's syndrome is due to the appearance or clinical progression of an ACTH-secreting pituitary adenoma following bilateral adrenalectomy for Cushing's disease.[746] Since pituitary adenomas are present in the majority of patients with untreated Cushing's disease, it is presumed that the tumors of Nelson's syndrome are due to progressive growth of preexisting pituitary adenomas. It is possible that the hypercortisolism in untreated cases restrains not only ACTH secretion but also growth of the adenoma. That ACTH secretion in Cushing's disease is restrained by the circulating cortisol levels is demonstrated by its stimulation with metyrapone. Further, the tumors in Nelson's syndrome are dexamethasone-suppressible, although larger doses may be required than with untreated Cushing's disease.[538] Thus, following adrenalectomy the suppressive effect of cortisol is no longer present, ACTH secretion increases, and the adenoma may progress. Conventional pituitary irradiation before or after adrenalectomy does not prevent the development of Nelson's syndrome and it may rarely occur following heavy particle irradiation.[732,747]

The incidence of Nelson's syndrome ranges from 5 to 78 percent in reported series.[747–749] It is higher in series studied with immunoreactive plasma ACTH levels and more sophisticated radiologic techniques such as sellar polytomography.[748,749] About 30 percent of patients adrenalectomized for Cushing's disease have been found to develop classic Nelson's syndrome. Another 50 percent develop evidence of a microadenoma without marked progression and about 20 percent never develop a progressive pituitary tumor. The reasons for these differences in clinical behavior are unknown and have not been predictable. Thus, patients who have undergone bilateral adrenalectomy for Cushing's disease require continuous observation by means of plasma ACTH assay, sellar radiology, and visual field examinations so that pituitary tumors may be diagnosed and treated early.

The pituitary tumors in patients with classic Nelson's syndrome are among the most aggressive and rapidly growing of all pituitary tumors.[669] These patients present with hyperpigmentation similar to but generally more severe than that seen in Addison's disease and the manifestations of an expanding intrasellar mass lesion usually within months to 2 years following adrenalectomy. Sellar enlargement, extrasellar extension, headache, visual field defects, and hypopituitarism are frequent.[669] Invasion of the cavernous sinus or cranial fossae may lead to extraocular muscle palsies and other neurological defects.[669] These tumors can occasionally be frankly malignant with local invasion and extracranial metastases,[669] and there is a high incidence of pituitary apoplexy (spontaneous hemorrhagic infarction of the tumor).[669] The diagnosis is usually obvious from the history of bilateral adrenalectomy followed by hyperpigmentation and the manifestations of an expanding pituitary tumor. Plasma ACTH levels are markedly elevated, usually to greater than 1000 pg/ml, and levels not infrequently are greater than 10,000 pg/ml.[504] Although an enlarged sella turcica is generally apparent on routine skull x-rays, additional neuroradiologic procedures such as polytomography, CT scanning, pneumoencephalography, and angiography are required to define the extent of tumor growth.

These tumors are treated by pituitary surgery and/or radiotherapy. Larger tumors, especially those with extrasellar extension, are frequently unresectable at surgery by either transsphenoidal or craniotomy approaches. Conventional radiation alone is satisfactory in only a minority of patients but should nonetheless be used postoperatively in those patients with extrasellar tumor extension.

Patients adrenalectomized for Cushing's disease who develop pituitary microadenomas generally present later and usually have a slower course accompanied by mild to moderate hyperpigmentation and plasma ACTH levels in the 500 to 4000 pg/ml range.[748,749] The sella turcica is usually normal in size; however, sellar polytomography reveals features of a pituitary microadenoma.[749] Extrasellar extension, visual defects, headache, and panhypopituitarism are unusual.[749] Spontaneous remission has occurred in such a patient ("silent pituitary apoplexy").[750] Transsphenoidal microsurgery or heavy particle irradiation is somewhat more successful in these patients with microadenomas. Although hyperpigmentation resolves, plasma ACTH levels frequently remain modestly elevated.

Patients who never manifest evidence of a progressive pituitary tumor after adrenalectomy for Cushing's syndrome do not develop hyperpigmentation, or abnormal pituitary function. However, plasma ACTH levels in these patients are mildly elevated in the range of 100 to 500 pg/ml and are not normally suppressible with low doses of dexamethasone.

PROGNOSIS

Untreated Cushing's syndrome is frequently a fatal illness. Mortality may be due to the underlying tumor itself, as in the ectopic ACTH syndrome and adrenal carcinoma. However, in many cases, death is the consequence of sustained hypercortisolism and its complications, including hypertension, cardiovascular disease, stroke, thromboembolism, and susceptibility to infection.[652,740] Thus, in one series reported in 1952,

50 percent of patients died within 5 years of onset of the disease.[652]

With current refinements in pituitary microsurgery and heavy particle irradiation, the great majority of patients with Cushing's disease can be treated successfully and the operative mortality and morbidity which attended bilateral adrenalectomy are no longer present. Although there is currently no statistical information regarding survival in these patients it appears that they live considerably longer. Patients with Cushing's disease who have large pituitary tumors at the time of diagnosis or those with Nelson's syndrome have a considerably less satisfactory prognosis and may die as the consequence of tumor invasion or persisting hypercortisolism.[669]

The prognosis in adrenal adenomas is excellent, although there is the mortality and morbidity of adrenalectomy in these patients.[744] In adrenal carcinoma the prognosis is almost universally poor and the median survival from the onset of symptoms is approximately 4 years.[659,744]

Prognosis is also poor in patients with the ectopic ACTH syndrome due to malignant tumors. In these patients with severe hypercortisolism survival is frequently only days to weeks.[653,708] However, a minority of patients respond to tumor resection or chemotherapy.[699,702] Prognosis is better in those with benign tumors producing the ectopic ACTH syndrome.[487,711]

Hyperaldosteronism

Hyperaldosteronism (aldosteronism) can occur as a "primary" adrenal problem or can be secondary to other metabolic derangements that stimulate its release.

PRIMARY HYPERALDOSTERONISM

Primary hyperaldosteronism (primary aldosteronism) results from adrenal tumors or from a hyperplastic adrenal glomerulosa and leads to hypertension and hypokalemia, as discussed in detail in Chap. 14.

SECONDARY HYPERALDOSTERONISM

Secondary hyperaldosteronism, due to stimulation of the adrenal glomerulosa by extraadrenal factors (usually the renin-angiotensin system) is classified in Table 12-24.[751] It can be physiological or can contribute to the pathology of disease states.

The factors that stimulate the renin-angiotensin system and the influences of aldosterone are discussed in preceding sections and in Chap. 14. The role of increased aldosterone in chronic hyperkalemia[440,442] has been discussed above (see Physiological Actions of Mineralocorticoids). Secondary hyperaldosteronism can occasionally occur on an iatrogenic basis due to oral contraceptive use (see Chap. 14).

Extrarenal Sodium Loss and Sodium Restriction

In these circumstances (Table 12-23 and Chap. 14), activation of the renin-angiotensin-aldosterone system serves to correct the deficiency by conserving sodium ion with minimal potassium wasting (see above).[751]

Changes in Aldosterone during the Menstrual Cycle and Pregnancy

Modest increases in plasma renin, angiotensin, and aldosterone concentrations of unknown cause occur during the luteal phase of the menstrual cycle and could be due to the marked increase (10- to 20-fold) in plasma progesterone level.[632] The mineralocorticoid antagonist properties of this steroid (discussed above) would block mineralocorticoid action, promoting sodium loss, and, in turn, stimulating renin release.[631] Levels of estrogens which induce renin substrate (Chap. 14) are also increased, but this has not been shown to be a significant factor.[631] The increased aldosterone concentration could contribute to the pathogenesis of premenstrual edema, but this is difficult to conceive of if the increased aldosterone concentration is secondary to natriuresis. Further, there is no correlation between the severity of edema and the levels of renin and aldosterone.[631]

Aldosterone secretion increases progressively during normal pregnancy, although its physiological significance is not known.[632,752] It is of maternal origin, is increased by the 15th week of gestation, and reaches levels in the third trimester 10 times those of nonpregnant women. The aldosterone contributes to sodium retention since blockade of aldosterone production by heparin results in natriuresis.[632] The increased renin levels may be due to the decrease in blood pressure that occurs in early pregnancy because of decreased systemic vascular resistance.[752] In addition, particularly in late pregnancy, progesterone levels are high and may further increase renin release by mechanisms discussed above.[632] However, renin levels are elevated more during the first trimester, whereas plasma aldosterone levels are highest during the third trimester.[632] This may be due to a progressive increase in the sensitivity of the glomerulosa to angiotensin II, due either to chronic exposure to angiotensin II (Chaps. 4 and 14) or to other unidentified factors. Whereas there is increased sodium retention in pregnancy, potassium loss does not occur.[632] This suggests that a functional mineralocorticoid excess state is not

Table 12-24. Classification of Secondary Hyperaldosteronism

Primary abnormality	Potassium loss	Edema	Hypertension	Effect of sodium load
Extrarenal sodium loss (e.g., from hemorrhage, thermal stress or gastrointestinal loss)	Absent	Absent	Absent	Repairs deficit
Sodium restriction	Absent	Absent	Absent	Repairs deficit
Abnormal distribution of sodium excess (e.g., from congestive heart failure, nephrotic syndrome, cirrhosis with ascites, or idiopathic edema)	Present	Present	Absent	Worsens edema
Abnormal renal electrolyte loss (e.g., from salt-losing renal disease*, Bartter's syndrome, diuretic abuse or renal tubular acidosis)	Present	Absent	Absent	Variable
Other renal lesions (e.g., renal artery stenosis, unilateral renal ischemia, accelerated hypertension, renin-secreting tumor or chronic renal failure*)	Present	Absent	Present	May worsen hypertension
Excessive potassium intake	Present	Absent	Absent	May facilitate kaliuresis
Luteal phase of menstrual cycle and pregnancy	Absent	May be present	Usually present	Supresses renin and aldosterone

Source: Modified from Stockigt.[75]
*Exception; no potassium loss.

present and that activation of the renin-angiotensin-aldosterone system is a compensatory response to other changes.

Since the renin-angiotensin-aldosterone axis is activated in pregnancy, there has been considerable interest in whether this contributes to the hypertension, edema, and other manifestations of toxemia.[632] If anything, levels of the components of the renin-angiotensin-aldosterone axis are decreased rather than increased in toxemia, although this condition is associated with an increased sensitivity to angiotensin II.[632,752] However, certain of the changes observed in toxemia (e.g., reduced uterine blood flow) are opposite to those elicited by angiotensin II (which leads to vasodilatation and increased blood flow in the uterine circulation, in contrast to its effects in other vascular beds; Chap. 14).[632]

Abnormal Distribution of Sodium Excess

The renin-angiotensin-aldosterone system is only one of several factors involved in the pathogenesis of edema.[632,751] In untreated patients with congestive heart failure, aldosterone excess is not consistently present, although it might be argued that normal aldosterone levels are inappropriate. In severe congestive failure, aldosterone excess may result from increased production as well as decreased clearance. Overall, aldosterone levels in congestive heart failure are the result of counterbalancing influences of decreased renal perfusion due to decreased cardiac output that increases renin and aldosterone release, and subsequent sodium retention that tends to suppress renin and aldosterone levels.

Secondary hyperaldosteronism ordinarily occurs when there is significant hypoalbuminemia and decreased plasma oncotic pressure associated with the nephrotic syndrome. Although aldosterone is only one factor, it does appear to play a role in the sodium retention that occurs.

In liver disease with ascites, renin and aldosterone concentrations are commonly elevated, but this is unusual in cirrhosis without ascites. There appears to be general agreement that mineralocorticoid excess plays little role in the initial development of ascites. The stimulus to renin release appears to be an effectively decreased arterial volume due to abnormal transudation of fluid from the vascular compartment. The increased renin level promotes aldosterone production; aldosterone levels rise and this is accentuated by the decreased clearance of aldosterone in this condition. The increased aldosterone concentration further promotes sodium retention and potassium loss; the sodium retention can be more marked than in other circumstances, because escape fails to occur in these patients, probably due to the lack of retention of the excess sodium in the intravascular space. Thus, in this condition administration of aldosterone antagonists can be particularly beneficial.

Aldosterone has been implicated in the pathogenesis of idiopathic edema, a form of dependent edema that occurs in women who do not have a history of heart, liver, kidney, or venous disease. These patients have an increased incidence of impaired carbohydrate tolerance and may be emotionally disturbed or may have an allergy history, subtle abnormalities in albumin metabolism with slightly low serum albumin concentrations, capillary permeability defects, and, occasionally, abnormalities in the sympathetic nervous system. The diagnosis is by exclusion of other causes of edema; these are commonly unveiled during the evaluation. Although aldosterone excretion is usually in the normal range, it has been argued that the values found are inappropriate relative to the increased extracellular fluid volume and that the patients do not adequately escape from the sodium-retaining actions of the mineralocorticoids. However, the syndrome has been described in addisonian patients with very low aldosterone levels and no specific mineralocorticoid replacement. Thus, this syndrome may not be a single entity and the various defects described above could contribute to the pathogenesis. In any event, it is unlikely that aldosterone is primarily responsible, since this syndrome differs significantly from primary aldosteronism, in which edema does not usually occur (Chap. 14). The edema ordinarily responds to conservative measures such as bed rest, use of elastic stockings, limitation of sodium intake, caloric restriction, intermittent diuretic use, and administration of aldosterone antagonists.

Abnormal Renal Electrolyte Loss

The renin-angiotensin-aldosterone system is stimulated by excessive salt loss by the kidney resulting from salt-losing nephropathy, Bartter's syndrome (discussed below), excessive diuretic use, or renal tubular acidosis. In these syndromes, the compensatory increase in aldosterone level does not correct the loss, but because there is increased sodium delivery to the distal nephron, aldosterone can accelerate potassium loss.[751]

Bartter's Syndrome

Bartter's syndrome is characterized by increased renin, angiotensin II, and aldosterone concentrations, hypokalemia and alkalosis, normal blood pressure, absence of edema, and hyperplasia of the renal juxtaglomerular cells.[631,753] In addition, there is decreased pressor responsiveness to angiotensin II, vasopressin-resistant impairment in urinary concentrating ability, variably decreased pressor responsiveness to IV norepinephrine, hypomagnesemia, hyperuricemia, and increased amounts of urinary PGE_2. The pathogenesis of this disorder is discussed in Chap. 29.

Other Renal Lesions

Hyperaldosteronism can occur with renal artery stenosis, unilateral renal ischemia, accelerated hypertension, and renin-secreting tumors. These disorders are associated with hypertension and are discussed in Chap. 14.

Hirsutism and Virilism

Hirsutism and virilism result from excessive adrenal or ovarian secretion of androgens. As discussed above, the secreted hormones are frequently only weakly androgenic in themselves, but their conversion in peripheral tissues to more biologically active hormones results in a hyperandrogenic state. Most cases of clinical androgen excess are associated with a measurable increase in circulating levels of androgens. However, a few patients have normal androgen production rates and plasma levels; these individuals may have increased androgen conversion in the target tissues or increased sensitivity of the peripheral tissues to normal androgen concentrations.[569]

Clinical consequences of excessive androgen production occur in children and women but not in men. In children, excessive androgens cause virilism; in women, mild to moderate androgen excess produces hirsutism and more severe excess leads to virilism. With hirsutism (excessive facial and body hair growth), facial hair growth is most frequent and in mild cases typically consists of increased coarse dark hair on the upper lip, chin, and sideburn areas; in more severe cases there may be extensive hair growth in the beard area which requires shaving or depilatories. Facial hair overgrowth is frequently accompanied by excessive body hair, particularly in the pubic area, lower abdomen (male pubic hair distribution), and also on the extremities, periareolar areas, and thorax. Hirsutism is usually accompanied by acne and oiliness of the skin and scalp, and amenorrhea is common in those with moderate to severe androgen excess (Chap. 17). Virilism is a more severe form of androgen excess and is usually accompanied by obvious androgen hypersecretion. Patients with virilism generally have severe hirsutism and, in addition, they have other systemic effects of androgen excess, which may include temporal recession of the hairline, male-type baldness, clitoral hypertrophy, deepening of the voice, increased muscle bulk, male habitus, and amenorrhea.

Androgen excess may be due to adrenal disorders such as congenital adrenal hyperplasia, Cushing's syndrome, adrenal carcinomas (see above and Chap. 18), and rare androgen-secreting adrenal adenomas.[754] Ovarian causes are the polycystic ovary syndrome, androgen-secreting tumors, and, rarely, stromal hyperthecosis (Chap. 17). Of these, the polycystic ovary syndrome is the most common; it appears to be responsible for most cases in adult females which are accompanied by moderate to severe hirsutism, anovulation, and amenorrhea (Chap. 17).[569] The other common etiology is that of idiopathic hirsutism, and some of these cases may be milder variants of the polycystic ovary syndrome without ovarian enlargement. Although the majority of patients with idiopathic hirsutism have measurable androgen excess, the source of androgen hypersecretion and the ovarian and/or adrenal contributions to this syndrome are unclear; studies using suppression testing with dexamethasone or estrogens, stimulation with ACTH or human chorionic gonadotropin, and the selective sampling of venous ovarian and adrenal androgen levels have failed to clarify this issue.[569] Thus the ovary, adrenal, or both glands may be responsible for androgen excess in hirsute females.

In evaluating these patients several clinical guidelines can be helpful. In children, manifestations of androgen excess are usually due to congenital adrenal hyperplasia or adrenal carcinoma. In adults, hirsutism accompanied by obesity, amenorrhea, infertility, and elevated plasma LH concentrations with or without bilateral ovarian enlargement is indicative of the polycystic ovary syndrome (Chap. 17) and the manifestations of glucocorticoid excess are present in Cushing's syndrome. Virilism in adults is commonly due to adrenocortical or ovarian tumors; virilization occurs in a minority of patients with the polycystic ovary syndrome and it is rare in Cushing's disease. In adult females, in the absence of these obvious syndromes, androgen excess (hirsutism with or without menstrual dysfunction) is commonly idiopathic or due to less severe cases of polycystic ovary syndrome.

In the patient with clinical evidence of androgen excess, an assessment of androgenic hormone levels should be undertaken. Plasma androgen assays are superior to urinary ketosteroid measurements, which are frequently normal in hirsute patients. Thus, in a study of patients with mild to moderate hirsutism, urinary 17-ketosteroid excretion was elevated in only 18 percent of determinations whereas plasma androgen concentrations were elevated in 85 percent.[576] However, since androgens are secreted episodically and vary both diurnally and with the menstrual cycle, single plasma levels may not predict overall secretion. Thus, several samples taken over a 24-h period or three samples obtained at hourly intervals more accurately represent mean plasma levels.[569,573] Alternatively, equal volumes of these individual samples may be pooled and assayed as one sample to save expense. Further, total plasma androgen concentrations may not accurately reflect the plasma concentration of the free androgens, because of the alterations in SHBG binding capacity. This is especially important since androgen excess reduces SHBG levels and binding capacity. Thus, in hirsutism, total plasma testosterone concentration is frequently normal, despite increased testosterone production and metabolic clearance rates, and elevated plasma free testosterone concentration.[565–571]

Measurement of the plasma free testosterone concentration, if available, is therefore recommended as the first step in evaluation, since these levels are elevated in 85 percent of patients with hirsutism, even when total testosterone levels are normal.[569,580] Levels are usually moderately increased in idiopathic hirsutism[565,568,569,580] and the presence of markedly elevated levels suggests an androgen-secreting tumor. In this setting, total plasma testosterone concentration should also be measured; in a female, a level above 2.0 μg/ml is indicative of an adrenal or ovarian tumor (Chap. 17). If the free testosterone level measurement is unavailable or within the normal range, total levels of plasma androgens should be measured. If multiple hormone concentrations are sampled, an elevation of at least one of them is present in virtually every patient with hirsutism and the majority have elevations of levels of several androgens; total plasma androgen levels are elevated as follows: DHT, 75 percent; DHEA-S, 66 percent; testosterone, 60 percent; androstenedione, 45 percent; and DHEA, 45 percent.[569,576,578,579] In the minority of patients with normal free testosterone and total plasma androgen concentrations, serial sampling may be required to document androgen excess. If androgen excess is present, the diagnosis of idiopathic hirsutism is basically one of exclusion of the other conditions mentioned above (and discussed in Chap. 17).

The treatment of idiopathic hirsutism involves local measures to remove hair growth and suppression of androgen secretion by hormones or antiandrogens. (The treatment of other disorders causing hirsutism and virilism is discussed in other sections and in Chap. 17.) Local measures include bleaching, use of depilatories, and electrolysis; these may be satisfactory in mild cases. Suppression of androgen secretion may be effected either with glucocorticoids (dexamethasone, 0.25 to 0.5 mg, given at bedtime)[569] or by the use of estrogen-progestin combination oral contraceptives (Chap. 17). Cyproterone acetate, a potent antiandrogen available in Europe but not in the United States, is effective in improving hirsutism in 60 to 80 percent of patients.[569] Spironolactone is also used to inhibit androgen action.[755]

CONGENITAL DEFECTS IN ADRENAL STEROID BIOSYNTHESIS

Defects in adrenal steroid biosynthesis, commonly known as congenital adrenal hyperplasia, are classic examples of inborn errors of metabolism in which an enzyme deficiency in a metabolic pathway leads to deficiency of the final products of the pathway and the accumulation of intermediates proximal to the site of the defective or deficient enzyme. Thus, the more common forms present with a mixed picture of steroid production abnormalities; the extent of the enzyme deficiency may be variable and thus the steroid secretory pattern and the clinical expression are also present in differing severity.[32,756,756a]

Each of these (except for corticosterone methyloxidase deficiency) is characterized by deficient cortisol secretion or decreased responsiveness to exogenous ACTH stimulation. The resulting ACTH hypersecretion leads to the classic manifestations of adrenal hyperplasia. If aldosterone secretion is also deficient, there are compensatory increases in renin and angiotensin II secretion. In addition, if the deficient enzyme is common to both adrenal and gonadal tissue, there is deficient production of ovarian or testicular steroids. Since the adrenal is persistently stimulated, steroids proximal to the deficient enzyme are hypersecreted and may lead to clinical manifestations of androgen or mineralocorticoid excess. Thus, the presentation of these syndromes is with variable degrees of glucocorticoid deficiency, mineralocorticoid excess or deficiency, androgen excess, sexual ambiguity, virilization, and sexual infantilism. Abnormalities of the external genitalia in these disorders are described in Chap. 18. The mineralocorticoid excess state with hypertension and hypokalemia that occurs in the 11β- and 17α-hydroxylase syndromes is described in Chap. 14. The normal pathways of steroid biosynthesis and the enzyme deficiencies which cause the syndromes are reviewed above (see Steroid Biosynthesis), in Refs. 32 and 756, and in Chap. 4.

21-Hydroxylase Deficiency

INCIDENCE, GENETICS, AND BIOCHEMICAL DEFECT

This type of congenital adrenal hyperplasia causes more than 90 percent of all reported cases and the incidence of the classical form of the disease has been reported to range from 1/5000 to 1/15,000 in Europe, the United States, and Japan.[757,757a] The 21-hydroxylase defect is inherited as an autosomal recessive trait; a similar pattern is likely in the other disorders although they are less well studied. The recessive gene locus responsible for the 21-hydroxylase deficiency is in close genetic linkage with the HLA region of chromosome 6.[756,758,759] Thus, HLA typing can be used to detect the heterozygous carriers in affected families and for prenatal diagnosis of the syndrome.[758,759] This locus contains two closely linked 21-hydroxylase genes, one of which is nonfunctional (a pseudogene) and the other of which encodes the cytochrome $P450_{c21}$ (see the section on Steroid Biosynthesis and Chap. 4) that is responsible for 21-hydroxylation.[759a,759b]

The clinical syndrome is the consequence of defective 21-hydroxylation of progesterone and 17α-hydroxyprogesterone, with resulting deficient production of DOC and 11-deoxycortisol, respectively (Fig. 12-40). This classically leads to subnormal production of cortisol and aldosterone, but milder forms occur (see below). Cortisol deficiency stimulates excessive ACTH secretion, causing adrenal hyperplasia and the shunting of adrenal biosynthesis toward the production of adrenal androgens, with elevated levels of adrenal precursors which are proximal to the 21-hydroxylase enzyme.

These disorders vary in the severity of the syndrome and of the steroid biosynthetic defect.[32,756] The most severe form (salt wasting form) is characterized by both aldosterone and cortisol deficiency and the presentation is with hypoadrenalism and salt wasting. Milder forms show predominantly virilization (simple virilizing form), and in these aldosterone secretion is normal, as is basal but not ACTH-stimulated cortisol secretion.

More recently, late-onset or attenuated forms (nonclassical forms) have been described in which there are either no symptoms (cryptic forms) or else the patients present with mild pubertal or postpubertal hirsutism, minimal evidence of virilism, and irregular menses or anovulation.[756a,758,760–765] All of these patients are homozygous for the defect and have the biochemical abnormalities in steroid secretion detectable by provocative testing. The asymptomatic patients have been detected by genetic screening studies[765] and they show the HLA locus linkage. Estimates

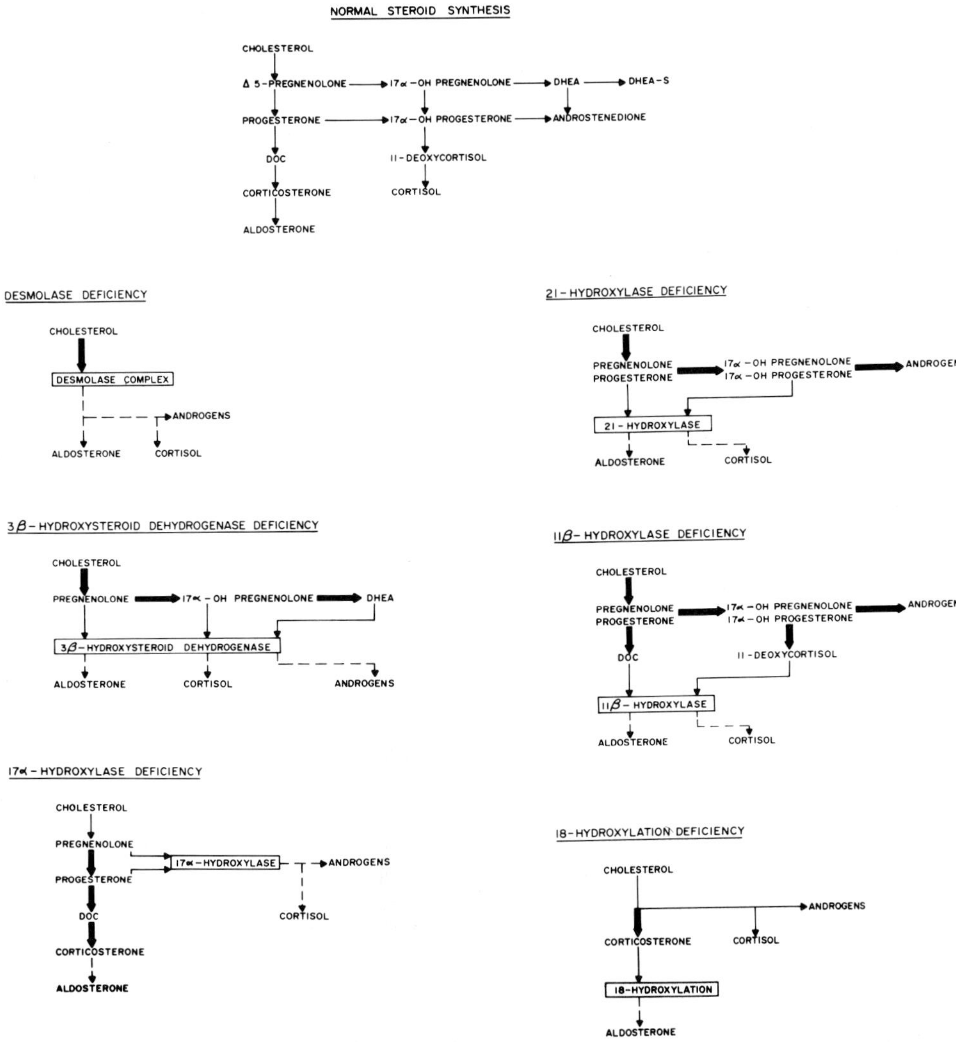

FIGURE 12-40 Schematic representation of the various inherited defects in adrenal steroid biosynthesis. Wide arrows denote pathways with increased synthesis proximal to the block. Dashed arrows denote pathways with decreased or absent steroid synthesis. The boxes show the deficient enzymes or steps. The overall effects are shown without regard to the particular functional zone of the adrenal cortex. In some cases, the decrease in steroid production results not from a deficient enzyme but from the consequences of other steroids secreted in excess. For instance, in the 17α-hydroxylation defect, DOC and corticosterone are secreted in excess and secondarily lead to suppression of the renin-angiotensin system and therefore of aldosterone secretion.

based on HLA associations combined with ACTH testing place the frequency of nonclassical 21-hydroxylase deficiency at 1 percent in Caucasians.[765a] This disorder is therefore one of the most frequently occurring known human autosomal recessive disorder.

Heterozygotes for either the classical or nonclassical forms of 21-hydroxylase deficiency have no symptoms but have demonstrable hypersecretion of 17α-hydroxyprogesterone in response to ACTH stimulation.[756a,766]

The defect in 21-hydroxylase deficiency appears to reside in the $P450_{c21}$ gene itself. In some patients with classical 21-hydroxylase deficiency, there may be deletions in the functional $P450_{c21}$ gene.[766a,766b] Gross defects in the gene have not been detected in the remaining patients with either the classical or nonclassical forms of the disorder, but based on their linkage to the HLA locus, it appears that defects in the $P450_{c21}$ gene will account for most cases.

The mechanisms for the variable clinical presentation are poorly understood. It is likely that to some extent the gene abnormalities in the milder forms of the disorder are overall less than those in the severe forms. It appears that a substantial reduction in 21-

hydroxylase activity is necessary for a clinically apparent defect, since heterozygotes do not have symptoms, and their hormonal responses to ACTH stimulation, although distinguishable from the general population on average, show considerable overlap with the latter group.[756a] Further, differences could not be detected in hormonal levels between individuals with cryptic or symptomatic nonclassical 21-hydroxylase deficiency.[766c] Whereas patients with the salt wasting classical form have a more severe defect in the glomerulosa than those with the simple virilizing form of the classical disorder, the two forms are indistinguishable in terms of the severity of the zona fasciculata defect.[766d] These findings, plus the probability that the same 21-hydroxylase gene functions in both zones of the adrenal, suggest that other factors participate in dictating the severity of the defect in the glomerulosa.

PATHOLOGY, PATHOPHYSIOLOGY, AND STEROID SECRETION

Irrespective of the nature of the enzymatic deficiency, there is defective 21-hydroxylation of progesterone and 17α-hydroxyprogesterone, and the pattern of steroid secretion reflects the site of defective steroid synthesis, the degree of enzyme deficiency, and the resulting ACTH excess. Thus, the steroid abnormalities are most marked in the salt-losing form with complete 21-hydroxylase deficiency, intermediate in the simple virilizing form, mild in the late-onset or attenuated and cryptic forms, and demonstrable in heterozygotes only by ACTH stimulation.

Plasma ACTH levels are increased as a result of cortisol deficiency.[764,767] Cortisol secretion rates, plasma cortisol concentration, and excretion of urinary 17-OHCS are low normal or subnormal and hyporesponsive to exogenous ACTH stimulation.[32] Plasma DOC, corticosterone, and 11-deoxycortisol levels and those of their urinary metabolites are also decreased. In mild cases cortisol secretion may be normal secondary to adrenal hyperplasia and ACTH excess, but unresponsive to stress and stimulation.

Plasma and urinary aldosterone levels are normal in milder cases and may respond to sodium restriction; however, aldosterone secretion is subnormal in cases with salt wasting, in spite of increased plasma renin levels, and is typically unresponsive to stimulation.[32] Levels of steroids proximal to the defective 21-hydroxylase enzyme are characteristically elevated.[32] Plasma 17α-hydroxyprogesterone concentration is increased 50 to 200 times; excretion rate of its urinary metabolite, pregnanetriol, is also markedly elevated, to 3 to 27 mg/24 h (normal = 0.1 to 1.5 mg/24 h). Plasma progesterone concentration is 6 to 10 times normal, as is that of its urinary excretion product, pregnanediol. Plasma 21-deoxycortisol concentration, which is normally less than 2 ng/ml, ranges from 20 to 100 ng/ml; its metabolite pregnanetriolone, which is normally undetectable in the urine, is excreted at a rate of 0.1 to 15 mg/24 h; the production rate of 21-deoxycortisol may be as high as 35 mg/24 h. Plasma pregnenolone and 17-hydroxypregnenolone concentrations are elevated two- to threefold, i.e., to a lesser extent than are levels of progesterone and 17-hydroxyprogesterone.

As a consequence of 21-hydroxylase deficiency and prolonged ACTH stimulation of the adrenals, excessive conversion of 17-hydroxypregnenolone and 17-hydroxyprogesterone to adrenal androgens occurs with elevated plasma levels of 11-hydroxyandrostenedione, androstenedione, DHEA, and DHEA-S.[32] The urinary excretion of metabolites of these steroids leads to a two- to threefold elevation of urinary 17-ketosteroid excretion. In addition, there is increased peripheral conversion of androstenedione to testosterone and DHT; these potent androgens lead to virilization.

CLINICAL FEATURES

The clinical features of 21-hydroxylase deficiency reflect the degree of enzyme deficiency and the abnormalities in steroid secretion.[768] Patients with the severe salt-losing form present with adrenal insufficiency and evidence of in utero androgen excess. These features are obvious within the first week following delivery and consist of anorexia, failure to gain weight, vomiting, dehydration, and shock. Death in adrenal crisis may occur unless appropriate therapy is instituted. These patients display salt wasting, hyponatremia, hyperkalemia, and acidosis. In females, adrenal insufficiency is accompanied by abnormal or ambiguous genitalia, which strongly suggests the diagnosis (Chap. 18). In male infants the presence of normal genitalia makes the diagnosis more difficult but it should be considered in any patient with evidence of adrenal insufficiency.[768]

The simple virilizing and the attenuated or cryptic forms usually do not present with manifestations of deficient glucocorticoid or mineralocorticoid secretion, but instead demonstrate variable manifestations of androgen excess.[32,756] In mild forms of the simple virilizing type children may be normal at birth and manifest no evidence of adrenal insufficiency; however, between the ages of 2 and 10 these children manifest rapid growth rates, premature development of pubic and axillary hair, penile growth in males, acne, and increased muscle development.[768,769] Although early growth is rapid, premature cessation of linear growth occurs owing to premature closures of the epiphyses, and these children ultimately have short stature.[769] Females at the time of expected puberty have absent breast development and absent menses and develop facial hirsutism and temporal balding. Males have absent testicular development and spermatogenesis does not occur. Thus, these patients fail to undergo normal puberty and the hypogonadotropic hypogonadism is a consequence of excess adrenal androgen secretion.[768,769]

In more severe enzyme deficiencies, virilization is present at birth. Females have clitoral hypertrophy and varying degrees of ambiguous genitalia, ranging from mild labioscrotal fusion to complete masculinization of the external genitalia, such that assignment of sex is difficult on clinical grounds (Chap. 18). Males are difficult to diagnose at birth since the external genitalia are normal. However, the penis may be enlarged and the scrotum hyperpigmented. In males the syndrome is recognized by rapid growth and early appearance of pubic and axillary hair.

In the attenuated or late-onset form, children are normal at birth and have normal childhood development and puberty; they subsequently develop hirsutism, infertility, and menstrual disorders, but virilization is minimal.[758–765]

DIAGNOSIS

The diagnosis of 21-hydroxylase deficiency should be suspected if ambiguity of the external genitalia or evidence of adrenal insufficiency is present. The classic diagnostic findings are elevated plasma ACTH concentration (250 to 2000 pg/ml), normal to decreased plasma cortisol and urinary 17-OHCS levels, and elevated urinary 17-ketosteroid levels. More specific documentation is obtained by measurement of urinary pregnanetriol or pregnanetriolone excretion, and the best available diagnostic test is the measurement of plasma 17α-hydroxyprogesterone concentration, which is elevated 50- to 200-fold in infants with 21-hydroxylase deficiency.[32,756] Further documentation of the disorder can be made by demonstrating deficient cortisol and excessive 17α-hydroxyprogesterone responsiveness to ACTH stimulation and suppression of excessive ACTH and adrenal secretion by dexamethasone.

It is also feasible to diagnose classical 21-hydroxylase deficiency with reasonable accuracy in the prenatal and neonatal periods. Prenatal diagnosis can be made in the second trimester by measuring 17α-hydroxyprogesterone in the amnionic fluid and by performing HLA genotyping on ammonia fluid cells.[769a] For neonatal diagnosis 17α-hydroxyprogesterone can be measured in blood specimens.[769b]

TREATMENT

Treatment of the patient with 21-hydroxylase deficiency is required to correct adrenal insufficiency, if present, and to suppress androgen hypersecretion in order to prevent further virilization and allow normal growth and gonadal maturation.[32,756,767,769,770] Infants or children with acute adrenal insufficiency should be treated with sodium and volume replacement and large doses of parenteral hydrocortisone (see Insufficiency, above, and Refs. 32, 756, 769, 770). In addition, since children with the virilizing and salt-wasting forms have decreased adrenal reserve, they should receive increased steroid doses during acute illness or in preparation for surgery.

Children with the simple virilizing form in general require only glucocorticoid therapy for chronic maintenance; the aim is the reduction of ACTH hypersecretion and the lowering of androgen levels to normal. Of major importance is the avoidance of excessive amounts of glucocorticoids; this may completely suppress ACTH and androgen secretion, but the glucocorticoid in excess will suppress linear growth.[769] Different steroids and dosage schedules have been used, but there appears to be no clear-cut advantage of any single one.[767,769] Average recommended doses (in mg per square meter of body surface per 24 h) optimal for reducing steroid hypersecretion and maintaining normal growth velocity are cortisol, 20 to 25 mg; cortisone acetate, 30 to 45 mg; and prednisone, 5 to 7 mg.[767,769] In infants parenteral therapy may be required, whereas oral administration is satisfactory in older children. An additional method has been the use of 0.125 to 0.175 mg of dexamethasone in the evening with a small dose of cortisol, 5 to 15 mg, in the morning.[767] Rigid dosage schedules should be avoided; the dose must be individualized in each patient and varied according to an assessment of the suppression of the plasma 17α-hydroxyprogesterone, urinary pregnanetriol or 17-ketosteroids, or ACTH levels and a careful follow-up of both linear growth and bone age progression.[767,769] Some have suggested that follow-up of the latter parameters is the best guide.[769] Excessive growth and progression of bone maturation indicate inadequate therapy, whereas delayed growth or bone maturation suggest steroid overdosage. Thus, continual reevaluation is required, especially during periods of rapid growth (e.g., during the first year of life and during puberty), and at these times frequent adjustment of the steroid dose may be required.[756,769]

Patients with the salt-losing form require maintenance mineralocorticoid replacement in addition to glucocorticoid therapy, as may those without salt-wasting but with increased plasma renin concentration, indicating partial aldosterone deficiency.[769,770]

This is given as 9α-fluorocortisol, 0.05 to 0.2 mg daily, as described above (see Treatment under Adrenocortical Insufficiency).[769,770] Ideally, these dosages should reduce plasma renin and potassium levels to normal.

With appropriate therapy further virilization is prevented and linear growth is normalized, although most children are ultimately somewhat shorter than their peers. In addition, the majority of children treated undergo spontaneous puberty and most have normal fertility if androgen excess is controlled.[769,771]

Early evaluation of children with ambiguous genitalia is essential for proper sexual assignment of the child and avoidance of the psychological consequences of virilization. Corrective surgery is indicated in female patients with moderate to severe degrees of masculinization of the external genitalia (Chap. 18).

The patient's siblings should be examined for the disorder and as described above, if pregnancy occurs, the syndrome can be diagnosed in utero by HLA typing and/or amniotic fluid steroid determination.[759,769a,772] Early diagnosis is desirable so that therapy can be instituted promptly; in fact, administration of dexamethasone to pregnant women carrying females afflicted with the syndrome may decrease the development of sexual ambiguity.[772a,772b]

11β-Hydroxylase Deficiency

11β-Hydroxylase deficiency is the second most common adrenal biosynthetic defect (see also Chap. 14) and is due to deficiency or defective function of the cytochrome $P450_{11\beta/18}$ hydroxylase enzyme.[32,756] This enzyme is now known to catalyze both 11β- and 18-hydroxylations in the fasciculata and glomerulosa and it has recently been shown to also perform the aldehyde synthetase function of the glomerulosa.[756,773,774] Deficient 11β-hydroxylation of 11-deoxycortisol and DOC interrupts the synthesis of cortisol, corticosterone, and aldosterone (Fig. 12-40), with resulting ACTH hypersecretion and overproduction of DOC, adrenal androgens, and other steroids.[32,768] The syndrome exhibits an autosomal recessive pattern of inheritance and variable degrees of clinical severity. As in the 21-hydroxylase syndrome, virilization may be present; however, this syndrome differs significantly, since hypertension presumably secondary to DOC excess is a common manifestation (Chap. 14).[32,768]

The exact mechanism of the defect is unknown (see also Chap. 14). It has been proposed that the 11β-hydroxylase systems in the zonae fasciculata and reticularis and the zona glomerulosa are regulated separately and that the defect is localized to the zonae fasciculata and reticularis.[32,773] Indeed, treated patients increase aldosterone production in response to a low-salt diet, although controversy exists as to whether this is normal; alternatively, it could be that a defect in 11β-hydroxylation is expressed more severely in the zonae fasciculata and reticularis than in the zona glomerulosa. Defective 18-hydroxylation has also been detected in the syndrome and may involve both the fasciculata/reticularis and the glomerulosa.[773,774]

Deficient cortisol secretion in the zonae fasciculata and reticularis is the primary abnormality; compensatory ACTH hypersecretion then leads to adrenocortical hyperplasia and accumulation of proximal steroids, including DOC and androgen precursors. Excess DOC causes a mineralocorticoid excess state with suppression of the renin-angiotensin system and of aldosterone synthesis in the zona glomerulosa (Chap. 14). Excess 17α-hydroxypregnenolone and 17α-hydroxyprogesterone lead to DHEA, DHEA-S, and androstenedione production and to virilization.

Pathologically, the adrenals are hyperplastic and similar to those of the 21-hydroxylase deficiency.

Plasma ACTH concentration is elevated; basal cortisol secretion varies from normal to unmeasurable and is subnormally responsive to ACTH stimulation. Plasma 11-deoxycortisol and DOC concentrations are elevated as are their urinary metabolites and the increased excretion of tetrahydro-11-deoxycortisol increases the urinary 17-OHCS excretion.[32] Plasma renin and aldosterone levels are characteristically suppressed (Chap. 14). Plasma DHEA, DHEA-S, androstenedione, and testosterone concentrations are elevated.[32]

The classic and more severe patients present in childhood, although milder adult-onset forms have been described.[756,775,776] In children the predominant feature is virilization, which is similar to but usually less severe than that seen with 21-hydroxylase deficiency (see above). Hypertension, sodium-retention, and hypokalemia are classic manifestations but are not always present or severe.[756,775,776] The milder late-onset forms present with hirsutism, menstrual irregularity, and pseudo precocious puberty in boys. These patients are usually normotensive and potassium and DOC levels may be normal.[775,776] The diagnosis is established by the demonstration of increased plasma concentrations of ACTH, 11-deoxycortisol, DOC, or their urinary metabolites. The elevations of levels of these steroids clearly separates this syndrome from 21-hydroxylase deficiency, in which they are subnormal. Therapy is with glucocorticoids to suppress ACTH and the adrenal hypersecretion of DOC and androgens (see Treatment under 21-Hydroxylase Deficiency, above, and Chap. 14).

17α-Hydroxylase Deficiency

17α-Hydroxylase deficiency syndrome is rare; approximately a dozen cases have been reported. The 17α-

hydroxylase enzyme is essential in both the adrenal fasciculata and the gonad for the synthesis of cortisol, estrogens, and androgens, however it is not normally present in the adrenal zona glomerulosa and is not required for DOC, corticosterone, and aldosterone synthesis (Chap. 14).

In the adrenal, decreased cortisol synthesis increases ACTH secretion, which in turn stimulates the accumulation of steroids proximal to the block. DOC and, possibly, corticosterone lead to the mineralocorticoid excess (Chap. 14). This suppresses renin and aldosterone secretion (Chap. 14). In the female the external genitalia are normal; however, deficient ovarian estrogen secretion results in primary amenorrhea and the failure to develop secondary sexual characteristics. In the male, androgen production by the fetal gonad is deficient and there is failure to develop masculine external genitalia fully (male pseudohermaphroditism; see Chap. 18).[777] FSH and LH secretion are elevated in both male and female patients, as a result of deficient gonadal steroid secretion. Milder forms occur in heterozygotes and family members.[778]

The diagnosis is established by the demonstration of increased ACTH, LH, and FSH concentrations; increased DOC level; and decreased or absent secretion of cortisol, estrogens, androgens, and aldosterone with suppressed plasma renin levels. Treatment is with glucocorticoids, as described in Chap. 14, and replacement therapy with gonadal steroids is also required.

Cholesterol Side Chain Cleavage Enzyme Deficiency

Approximately 40 cases of the rare enzyme defect, cholesterol side chain cleavage enzyme deficiency, also called congenital lipoid adrenal hyperplasia, have now been described.[23,756,779] The disorder is presumed to result from deficient conversion of cholesterol to pregnenolone. The single enzyme mediating this conversion is the cholesterol side chain cleavage enzyme ($P450_{scc}$), which binds cholesterol, performs both 20- and 22-hydroxylations, and cleaves the cholesterol side chain.[32,779] In vitro studies of adrenal tissue in one case showed markedly decreased activity of the entire complex,[780] whereas in another only deficient 20α-hydroxylation of cholesterol was detected.[781] Thus, it is possible that several types of defects may occur. The defect is also expressed in the ovary and testis, and the absence of testosterone in male fetuses with the disorder is suggested by the finding of incomplete masculinization of the external genitalia.

Plasma ACTH and gonadotropin concentrations have been elevated in the few cases in which they were reported.[779] The patients have hyperpigmentation and hyperplastic adrenal glands. The hyperplasia is marked and the gland is yellowish in color, with enlarged adrenal cells that stain strongly for lipid and contain cholesterol crystals.[32] Steroid studies are limited but show very low steroid secretion rates and absent responsiveness to ACTH stimulation.[32,782]

Males and females are equally affected and the majority of patients have died in infancy with salt wasting and adrenal insufficiency despite glucocorticoid and mineralocorticoid replacement.[32] The external genitalia are normal in females, whereas males have incompletely masculinized genitalia and may appear to be normal females. The testes are either intraabdominal or in the inguinal canals.

Because of the rarity of this disorder and the limited data available on steroid secretion patterns, firm diagnostic criteria have not been established.[779] Adrenal insufficiency should be suspected on clinical grounds and if electrolyte abnormalities are present. Deficiency of the $P450_{scc}$ can be established by demonstration of deficient secretion of all classes of adrenal steroids and their failure to respond to ACTH stimulation.[779,782] Chromosomal analysis is necessary to establish the correct genetic sex. In spite of the generally poor prognosis, several patients have survived with appropriate replacement therapy.[779,782]

3β-Hydroxysteroid Dehydrogenase Defect

The 3β-hydroxysteroid dehydrogenase defect[756] is caused by defective conversion of Δ^5-pregnenolone and 17-hydroxypregnenolone to progesterone and 17-hydroxyprogesterone, respectively.[32] The enzyme complex responsible for these conversions is the 3β-hydroxysteroid dehydrogenase–Δ^5-oxosteroid isomerase system. The defect affects both the adrenals and the gonads, resulting in decreased secretion of cortisol, aldosterone, androgens, and estrogens.[32] In severe cases, the only known biologically active adrenal steroid secreted is the weak androgen DHEA.

The cases described are of either a severe type with virtually complete enzyme deficiency or a milder type in which a partial enzyme deficiency is present.[527] The pathology of the adrenals in these patients is similar to that described for patients with severe forms of 21-hydroxylase deficiency. Steroid patterns in these cases are qualitatively similar in both forms. Urinary 17-OHCS excretion and plasma cortisol are decreased and urinary 17-ketosteroid excretion is increased because of increased DHEA and DHEA-S levels.[23] In severe cases, no cortisol metabolites have been found but in mild cases small amounts of cortisol, testosterone, and aldosterone metabolites are present.[527] Plasma levels of pregnenolone, 17-hydroxypregnenolone, and

DHEA are increased. Plasma cortisol fails to increase with ACTH stimulation but pregnenolone and 17-hydroxypregnenolone levels show excessive responses.[23]

Both sexes have ambiguous genitalia. Females have partial virilization (less severe than with 21-hydroxylase deficiency) with clitoral hypertrophy and mild labial fusion. The virilism is presumed to be due to the elevated levels of the weak androgen DHEA and to peripheral conversion of DHEA and DHEA-S to more potent androgens. Male patients have incomplete masculinization of the external genitalia with hypospadias, although in mild cases the external genitalia are normal.[527]

Presentation is in infancy with genital abnormalities, salt wasting, and adrenal insufficiency. Infants with the severe form have marked sodium wasting and usually die in the first several months of life, even with appropriate therapy. Patients with partial enzyme deficiency respond appropriately to steroid replacement therapy.

The diagnosis is suggested by ambiguous genitalia and adrenal insufficiency; the specific deficit is established by demonstrating elevated levels of Δ^5-3β-hydroxysteroids (pregnenolone, 17-hydroxypregnenolone, DHEA, and DHEA-S), which are responsive to ACTH stimulation, and decreased levels of cortisol, aldosterone, and testosterone, which are not.[32]

A late-onset form of this disorder has been described in women with postpubertal onset of hirsutism and menstrual abnormalities.[784a] The incidence of and diagnostic criteria for this late-onset disorder are not yet established.[784a]

Therapy consists of replacement of cortisol and mineralocorticoids. As stated above, the majority with the severe form die in infancy, despite treatment, whereas survival is usual in those with partial deficiencies. Children surviving may also require either androgen or estrogen replacement therapy at puberty.

Corticosterone Methyloxidase Deficiency Types 1 and 2 (18-Hydroxylation Defect)

This rare defect involves the mineralocorticoid pathway of the zona glomerulosa with defective conversion of corticosterone to aldosterone. The enzymes required are present almost exclusively in the zona glomerulosa.[784b–788] The exact sequence of enzyme steps and intermediates in the conversion of corticosterone to aldosterone has not been definitely established but is currently believed to involve two hydroxylations and two methyloxidase enzymes which convert corticosterone to aldosterone.[32] 18-Hydroxycorticosterone is not an obligatory intermediate; however, secretion rates of 18-hydroxycorticosterone and aldosterone are normally parallel, both in the basal state and during stimulation and suppression.[530] Discrepancies in their secretion rates in 18-hydroxylase deficiency have led to postulation of two types of congenital defects in corticosterone-aldosterone conversion: corticosterone methyloxidase defects types 1 and 2.[530] 18-Hydroxycorticosterone is also produced in the fasciculata; however, the second hydroxylation step, i.e., conversion of corticosterone to aldosterone, appears to occur only in the glomerulosa.[23]

In both types defective aldosterone synthesis leads to a mineralocorticoid deficiency state. Stimulation of the renin-angiotensin system increases production of aldosterone precursors, but these are inadequate to prevent the clinical manifestations of aldosterone deficiency. The patients have isolated aldosterone deficiency; ACTH, cortisol, and androgen secretion are normal.[23,528–530]

In type 1 there is absent aldosterone, subnormal levels of 18-hydroxycorticosterone metabolites, and elevated levels of corticosterone and its metabolites. DOC concentration is elevated to a lesser extent. These findings suggest that the initial hydroxylation of corticosterone is defective. Following deoxycorticosterone acetate therapy, the elevated levels of corticosterone and its metabolites fall toward normal.

The type 2 deficiency has a similar steroid pattern, except that 18-hydroxycorticosterone secretion is elevated, indicating a defect in the second hydroxylation step. Thus, in these patients there is low aldosterone secretion with increased secretion of 18-hydroxycorticosterone, corticosterone, and DOC.

The adrenals of one child who died were of normal weight and appeared grossly normal.[528] Microscopically the functional zones of the adrenal cortex were not well differentiated and the glomerulosa appeared poorly developed. There was a tubular aspect with inadequately developed columns of cells and adenomatous structures.

The clinical presentation of types 1 and 2 is isolated aldosterone deficiency; there is failure to gain weight, dehydration, vomiting, sodium wasting, hyponatremia, and hyperkalemia.[32,784b–787] Pigmentation is absent, and the genitalia are normal. An older sibling of one patient had typical biochemical features of type 1 and was maintained on an increased sodium intake without mineralocorticoid therapy.[784b] Two males with a partial form of type 2 presented with failure to gain weight, transient electrolyte abnormalities, and unresponsiveness to sodium deprivation.[32] Other family members have been described with biochemical evidence of type 2 who had no clinical manifestations.[785]

Methyloxidase deficiency is diagnosed by the demonstration of subnormal aldosterone, elevated corticosterone, and normal cortisol and androgen secretion.[32,786] 18-Hydroxycorticosterone is deficient in type 1 and its level is markedly elevated in type 2.[32,784b-787]

Children with this defect respond well to increased sodium intake and mineralocorticoid replacement. The prognosis appears to be good and sodium wasting tends to improve with increasing age.[784b,785,788]

REFERENCES

1. Gaunt R: History of the adrenal cortex, in Greep RO, Astwood EB (eds): *Handbook of Physiology: Endocrinology*, section 7. Washington, D.C., American Physiological Society, 1975, vol 6, p 1.
2. Cushing H: The basophil adenomas of the pituitary body and their clinical manifestations. *Bull Johns Hopkins Hosp* 50:137, 1932.
3. Baxter JD, Rousseau GG: Glucocorticoid hormone action: An overview, in Baxter JD, Rousseau GG (eds): *Glucocorticoid Hormone Action*. New York, Springer-Verlag, 1979, p 1.
4. Tan SY, Mulrow PJ: Aldosterone in hypertension and edema, in Bondy PK, Rosenberg LE (eds): *Metabolic Control and Disease*. Philadelphia, Saunders, 1979, p 1501.
5. McCann SM, Brobeck JR: Evidence for a role of the supraopticohypophyseal system in regulation of adrenocorticotropin secretion. *Proc Soc Exp Biol Med* 87:318, 1954.
6. Saffran M, Schally AU, Benfey BG: Stimulation of the release of corticotropin from the adenohypophysis by a neurohypophysial factor. *Endocrinology* 57:439, 1955.
7. Guillemin R, Rosenberg B: Humoral hypothalamic control of anterior pituitary: A study with combined tissue cultures. *Endocrinology* 57:599, 1955.
8. Spiess J, Rivier J, Rivier C, Vale W: Primary structure of corticotropin-releasing factor from ovine hypothalamus. *Proc Natl Acad Sci USA* 78:6517, 1981.
9. Fasciolo JC: Historical background of the renin angiotensin system, in Genest J, Koiw E, Kuchel E (eds): *Hypertension*. New York, McGraw-Hill, 1977, p 134.
10. Conn JH: Primary aldosteronism. *J Lab Clin Med* 45:661, 1955.
11. Hench PS, Kendall EC, Slocumb CH, Polley HF: The effect of a hormone of the adrenal cortex (17-hydroxy-11-dehydrocorticosterone compound E) and of pituitary adrenocorticotrophic hormone on rheumatoid arthritis. *Proc Staff Meeting Mayo Clin* 24:181, 1949.
12. Neville AM, Mackay AM: The structure of the human adrenal cortex in health and disease. *Clin Endocrinol Metab* 1:361, 1972.
13. Netter FH: Endocrine system and selected metabolic diseases, in *Ciba Collection of Medical Illustrations*. Summitt, NY, Ciba Pharmaceutical, 1965, vol 4, p 77.
14. Dallman MF: Adrenal feedback on stress-induced corticoliberin (CRF) and corticotropin (ACTH) secretion, in Jones MT, Gillham B, Dallman MF, Chattopadahyay S (eds): *Interaction within the Brain-Pituitary Adrenocortical System*. New York, Academic, 1979, p 149.
15. Brooks RV: Biosynthesis and metabolism of adrenocortical steroids, in James VHT (ed): *The Adrenal Gland*. New York, Raven, 1979, p 67.

15a. Eacho PI, Colby HD: Functional zonation of the guinea pig adrenal cortex: Differences in mitochondrial steroid metabolism between the inner and outer zones. *Endocrinology* 114:1463, 1984.

16. Neville AM, O'Hare MJ: Aspects of structure, function and pathology, in James VHT (ed): *The Adrenal Gland*. New York, Raven, 1979, p 1.
17. Gill GN: ACTH regulation of the adrenal cortex, in Gill GN (ed): *Pharmacology of Adrenal Cortical Hormones*. New York, Pergamon, 1979, p 35.
18. Skelton FR: Adrenal regeneration and adrenal regeneration hypertension. *Physiol Rev* 39:162, 1959.
19. Makin HLJ, Trafford DJH: The chemistry of the steroids. *J Clin Endocrinol Metab* 1:333, 1972.

19a. Bondy PK: The adrenal cortex, in Bondy PK, Rosenberg LE (eds): *Metabolic Control and Disease*. Philadelphia, Saunders, 1979, p 1427.

20. Lieberman S, Greenfield NJ, Wolfson A: A heuristic proposal for understanding steroidogenic processes. *Endocr Rev* 5:128, 1984.
21. Brown MS, Kovanen PT, Goldstein JL: Receptor-mediated uptake of lipoprotein-cholesterol and its utilization for steroid synthesis in the adrenal cortex. *Recent Prog Horm Res* 35:215, 1979.
22. Assman G: *Lipid Metabolism and Atherosclerosis*. Stuttgart, W. Germany, F.K. Schattauer Verlag, 1982, p 1.
23. Gwynne JT, Strauss JF III: The role of lipoproteins in steroidogenesis and cholesterol metabolism in steroidogenic glands. *Endocr Rev* 3:299, 1982.
24. Illingworth DR, Corbin D: The influence of mevinolin on the adrenal cortical response to corticotropin in heterozygous familial hypercholesterolemia. *Proc Natl Acad Sci USA* 82:6291, 1985.
25. Ohashi M, Carr BR, Simpson ER: Binding of high density lipoprotein to human fetal adrenal membrane fractions. *Endocrinology* 109:783, 1981.
26. Reaven E, Chen Y-DI, Spicher M, Azhar S: Morphological evidence that high density lipoproteins are not internalized by steroid-producing cells during in situ organ perfusion. *J Clin Invest* 74:1384, 1984.
27. Illingworth DR, Keny TA, Orwoll ES: Adrenal function in heterozygous and homozygous hypobetalipoproteinemia. *J Clin Endocrinol Metab* 54:27, 1982.
28. Kovanen PT, Schneider WJ, Hillman GM, Goldstein JL, Brown MS: Separate mechanisms for the uptake of high and low density lipoproteins. *J Biol Chem* 254:5498, 1979.
29. Simpson ER, Waterman MR: Regulation by ACTH of steroid hormone biosynthesis in the adrenal cortex. *Can J Biochem Cell Biol* 61:692, 1983.
30. Siiteri PK: Qualitative and quantitative aspects of adrenal secretion of steroids, in Cristy NP (ed): *The Human Adrenal Cortex*. New York, Harper & Row, 1971, p 1.
31. Samuels LT, Nelson DH: Biosynthesis of corticosteroids, in Greep RO, Astwood EB (eds): *Handbook of Physiology: Endocrinology*, sect 7. Washington, D.C., American Physiological Society, 1975, vol 6, p 55.
32. Finkelstein M, Shaefer JM: Inborn errors of steroid biosynthesis. *Physiol Rev* 59:353, 1979.
33. Fraser R, Lantos CP: 18-Hydroxycorticosterone: A review. *J Steroid Biochem* 9:273, 1978.
34. Casey ML, MacDonald PC: Extraadrenal formation of a mineralocorticosteroid: Deoxycorticosterone and deoxycorticosterone sulfate biosynthesis and metabolism. *Endocr Rev* 3:396, 1982.
35. Moghissi AE, Hawks D, Schneider T, Horton R: The origin of plasma deoxycorticosterone in men and in women during the menstrual cycle. *J Clin Endocrinol Metab* 56:93, 1983.
36. Tan SY, Mulrow PJ: The contribution of the zona fasciculata and glomerulosa to plasma 18-deoxycorticosterone levels in man. *J Clin Endocrinol Metab* 41:126, 1975.
37. Gomez-Sanchez CE, Gomez-Sanchez EP, Shackleton CHL, Milewick L: Identification of 19-hydroxy-deoxycorticosterone, 19-oxo-deoxycorticosterone, and 19-oic-deoxycorticosterone as products of deoxycorticosterone metabolism by rat adrenals. *Endocrinology* 110:384, 1982.
38. Kenyon KR, Saccoccio NA, Morris DJ: Further studies of the mineralocorticoid activity of 19-oxo-deoxycorticosterone. *Endocrinology* 115:535, 1984.

39. Sekihara H, Torii R, Osawa Y, Takaku F: Angiotensin II induces the release of 19-hydroxyandrostenedione in man. *J Clin Endocrinol Metab* 61:291, 1985.

40. Dale SL, Holbrook MM, Arison BH, Melby JC: 19-Nor-deoxycorticosterone metabolism by rat adrenal glands: Evidence for the formation of 19-nor-corticosterone and 19-nor-18-hydroxy-deoxycorticosterone. *Endocrinology* 116:118, 1985.

41. Gomez-Sanchez CE, Gomez-Sanchez EP, Smith JS, Ferris MW, Foecking MF: Receptor binding and biological activity of 18-oxocortisol. *Endocrinology* 116:6, 1985.

42. Gomez-Sanchez EP, Gomez-Sanchez CE, Smith JS, Ferris MW, Foecking M: Receptor binding and biological activity of 18-hydroxycortisol. *Endocrinology* 115:462, 1984.

43. Nelson DH: The adrenal cortex: Physiological function and disease, in Smith LH (ed): *Major Problems in Internal Medicine.* Philadelphia, Saunders, 1980, vol 18, p 1.

44. Migeon C: Adrenal androgens in man. *Am J Med* 53:606, 1972.

45. Nakajin S, Shively JE, Yuan PM, Hall PF: Microsomal cytochrome P-450 from neonatal pig testis. Two enzymatic activities (17α-hydroxylase and $C_{17,20}$-lyase) associated with one protein. *Biochemistry* 20:4037, 1981.

45. Yuen BH, Kilch RP, Jaffe RB: Adrenal contribution to plasma estrogens in adrenal disorders. *Biochemistry* 20:4037, 1981.

46. Yuen BH, Kilch RP, Jaffe RB: Adrenal contribution to plasma estrogens in adrenal disorders. *Acta Endocrinol* 76:117, 1974.

47. Vermeulen A: The hormonal activity of the postmenopausal ovary. *J Clin Endocrinol Metab* 42:247, 1976.

48. Seron-Ferre M, Jaffe RB: The primate fetal adrenal gland. *Annu Rev Physiol* 43:141, 1981.

49. Carr BR, Parker CR Jr, Porter IC, MacDonald PC, Simpson CR: Regulation of steroid secretion by adrenal tissue of anencephalic fetus. *J Clin Endocrinol Metab* 50:870, 1980.

50. Sippell WG, Muller-Holve W, Dorr HG, Bidlingmaier F, Knorr D: Concentrations of aldosterone, corticosterone, 11-deoxycorticosterone, progesterone, 17-hydroxyprogesterone, 11-deoxycortisol, cortisol, and cortisone determined simultaneously in human amniotic fluid throughout gestation. *J Clin Endocrinol Metab* 52:385, 1981.

51. deM Fencl M, Stillman RJ, Cohen J, Tulchinsky D: Direct evidence of sudden rise in fetal corticoids late in human gestation. *Nature* 287:225, 1980.

52. Fujieda K, Faiman C, Feyes FI, Winter JSD: The control of steroidogenesis by human fetal adrenal cells in tissue culture. IV. The effects of exposure to placental steroids. *J Clin Endocrinol Metab* 54:89, 1982.

53. Pasqualini JR, Nguyen BL, Uhrich F, Wiqvist N, Diczfalvay E: Cortisol and cortisone metabolism in the human fetoplacental unit at midgestation. *J Steroid Biochem* 1:209, 1970.

54. Wood CE, Rudolph AM: Negative feedback regulation of adrenocorticotropin secretion by cortisol in ovine fetuses. *Endocrinology* 112:1930, 1983.

55. Charnvises S, deM Fencl M, Osathanodh R, Zhu M-G, Underwood R, Tulchinsky D: Adrenal steroids in maternal and cord blood after dexamethasone administration at midterm. *J Clin Endocrinol Metab* 61:1220, 1985.

56. Zumoff B, Fukushima DK, Hellman L: Intercomparison of four methods for measuring cortisol production. *J Clin Endocrinol Metab* 38:169, 1974.

57. New MI, Seaman MP, Peterson RE: A method for the simultaneous determination of the secretion rates of cortisol, 11-deoxycortisol, corticosterone, 11-deoxycorticosterone and aldosterone. *J Clin Endocrinol Metab* 29:514, 1969.

58. Peterson RE: The miscible pool and turnover rate of adrenocortical steroids in man. *Recent Prog Horm Res* 15:231, 1959.

59. Schoneshofer M, Wagner GG: Sex differences in corticosteroids in man. *J Clin Endocrinol Metab* 45:814, 1977.

60. Zumoff B, Fukushima DK, Weitzman ED, Kream J, Hellman L: The sex difference in plasma cortisol concentration in man. *J Clin Endocrinol Metab* 39:805, 1974.

61. Streeten DHP, Anderson GH Jr, Dalakos TG, Seeley D, Mallov JS, Eusebio R, Sunderlin FS, Badawy SZA, King RB: Normal and abnormal function of the hypothalamic-pituitary-adrenocortical system in man. *Endocr Rev* 5:371, 1984.

62. Stearns HC, Sneeden VD, Fearl JD: A clinical and pathologic review of ovarian stromal hyperplasia and its possible relationship to common diseases of the female reproductive system. *Am J Obstet Gynecol* 119:375, 1974.

63. Liddle GW: Regulation of adrenocortical function in man, in Christy NP (ed): *The Human Adrenal Cortex.* New York, Harper & Row, 1968, p 41.

64. Aguilera G, Catt KJ: Loci of action of regulators of aldosterone biosynthesis in isolated glomerulosa cells. *Endocrinology* 104:1046, 1980.

65. Samojlik E, Veldhius JD, Wells SA, Santer RJ: Preservation of androgen secretion during estrogen suppression with aminoglutethimide in the treatment of metastatic breast cancer. *J Clin Invest* 65:602, 1980.

66. Wilson ID, Goetz FC: Selective hypoaldosteronism after prolonged heparin administration. *Am J Med* 36:635, 1964.

67. Tuck ML, Sowers JR, Fittingoff DB, Fisher JS, Berg GJ, Asp ND, Mayes DM: Plasma corticosteroid concentrations during spironolactone administration: Evidence for adrenal biosynthetic blockade in man. *J Clin Endocrinol Metab* 52:1057, 1981.

68. Warner W, Harris LS, Carchman RA: Inhibition of corticosteroidogenesis by delta-9-tetrahydrocannabinol. *Endocrinology* 101: 1815, 1977.

69. Wagner RL, White PF, Kan PB, Rosenthal MH, Feldman D: Inhibition of adrenal steroidogenesis by the anesthetic etomidate. *N Engl J Med* 310:1415, 1984.

69a. Pont A, Williams PL, Loose DS, Feldman D, Reitz RE, Bochra C, Steven DA: Ketoconazole blocks adrenal steroid synthesis. *Ann Intern Med* 97:370, 1982.

69b. Sonino N, Boscaro M, Merola G, Mantero F: Prolonged treatment of Cushing's disease by ketoconazole. *J Clin Endocrinol Metab* 61:718, 1985.

70. Kenyon CJ, Young J, Gray CE, Fraser R: Inhibition by etomidate of steroidogenesis in isolated bovine adrenal cells. *J Clin Endocrinol Metab* 58:947, 1984.

70a. Whitnall MH, Mezey E, Gainer H: Co-localization of corticotropin-releasing factor and vasopressin in median eminence neurosecretory vesicles. *Nature* 317:248, 1985.

71. Furutani Y, Morimoto Y, Shibahara S, Noda M, Takahashi H, Hirose T, Asai M, Inayama S, Hayashida H, Miyata T, Numa S: Cloning and sequence analysis of cDNA for ovine corticotropin-releasing factor precursor. *Nature* 301:537, 1983.

72. Sasaki A, Liotta AS, Luckey MM, Margioris AN, Suda T, Krieger DT: Immunoreactive corticotropin-releasing factor is present in human maternal plasma during the third trimester of pregnancy. *J Clin Endocrinol Metab* 59:812, 1984.

73. Gibbs DM: Measurement of hypothalamic corticotropin-releasing factors in hypophysial portal blood. *Fed Proc* 44:203, 1985.

74. Aguilera G, Harwood JP, Wilson JX, Morell J, Brown JH, Catt KJ: Mechanisms of action of corticotropin-releasing factor and other regulators of corticotropin release in rat pituitary cells. *J Biol Chem* 258:8039, 1983.

75. Westlund KN, Aguilera G, Childs GV: Quantification of morphological changes in pituitary corticotropes produced by in vivo corticotropin-releasing factor stimulation and adrenalectomy. *Endocrinology* 116:439, 1985.

76. Nieuwenhuijzen-Kruseman AC, Linton EA, Lowry PJ, Rees LH, Besser GM: Corticotropin-releasing factor immunoreactivity in human gastrointestinal tract. *Lancet* 2:1245, 1982.

77. De Souza EB, Perrin MH, Insel TR, Rivier J, Vale WW,

Kuhar MJ: Corticotropin-releasing factor receptors in rat forebrain: Autoradiographic identification. *Science* 224:1449, 1984.

78. Sawchenko PE, Swanson LW, Vale WW: Co-expression of corticotropin-releasing factor and vasopressin immunoreactivity in parvocellular neurosecretory neurons of the adrenalectomized rat. *Proc Natl Acad Sci USA* 81:1883, 1984.

79. Brown MR, Fisher LA, Spiess J, Rivier C, Rivier J, Vale W: Corticotropin-releasing factor: Actions on the sympathetic nervous system and metabolism. *Endocrinology* 111:928, 1982.

80. Nemeroff CB, Widerlov E, Bissette G, Walleus H, Karlsson I, Eklund K, Kilts CD, Loosen PT, Vale W: Elevated concentrations of CSF corticotropin-releasing factor-like immunoreactivity in depressed patients. *Science* 226:1342, 1984.

81. Gillies GE, Linton EA, Lowry PJ: Corticotropin releasing activity of the new CRF is potentiated several times by vasopressin. *Nature* 299:355, 1982.

82. Tilders FJH, Berkenbosh F, Vermes I, Linton EA, Smelik PG: Role of epinephrine and vasopressin in the control of the pituitary-adrenal response to stress. *Fed Proc* 44:155, 1985.

83. Lamberts SWJ, Verleun T, Oosterom R, de Jong F, Hackeng WHL: Corticotropin-releasing factor (ovine) and vasopressin exert a synergistic effect on adrenocorticotropin release in man. *J Clin Endocrinol Metab* 58:298, 1984.

84. Vale W, Vaughan J, Smith M, Yamamoto G, Rivier J, Rivier C: Effects of synthetic ovine corticotropin-releasing factor, glucocorticoids, catecholamines, neurohypophyseal peptides, and other substances on cultured corticotropic cells. *Endocrinology* 113:1121, 1983.

85. Rivier J, Rivier C, Vale W: Synthetic competitive antagonists of corticotropin-releasing factor: Effect on ACTH secretion in the rat. *Science* 224:870, 1984.

86. Rivier C, Vale W: Interaction of corticotropin-releasing factor and arginine vasopressin on adrenocorticotropin secretion in vivo. *Endocrinology* 113:939, 1983.

87. Linton EA, Tilders FJH, Hodgkinson S, Berkenbosch F, Vermes I, Lowry PJ: Stress-induced secretion of adrenocorticotropin in rats is inhibited by administration of antisera to ovine corticotropin-releasing factor and vasopressin. *Endocrinology* 116:966, 1985.

88. Mormede P: The vasopressin receptor antagonist dPTyr-(Me)AVP does not prevent stress-induced ACTH and corticosterone release. *Nature* 302:345, 1983.

89. Plotsky PM, Bruhn TO, Vale W: Central modulation of immunoreactive corticotropin-releasing factor secretion by arginine vasopressin. *Endocrinology* 115:1639, 1984.

90. Ono N, Bedran de Castro JC, McCann SM: Ultrashort-loop positive feedback of corticotropin (ACTH)-releasing factor to enhance ACTH release in stress. *Proc Natl Acad Sci USA* 82:3528, 1985.

91. Ono N, Samson WK, McDonald JK, Lumpkin MD, Bedran De Castro JC, McCann SM: Effects of intravenous and intraventricular injection of antisera directed against corticotropin-releasing factor on the secretion of anterior pituitary hormones. *Proc Natl Acad Sci USA* 82:7787, 1985.

92. Carlson DE, Gann DS: Effects of vasopressin antiserum on the response of adrenocorticotropin and cortisol to hemorrhage. *Endocrinology* 114:317, 1984.

93. Degli Uberti EC, Petraglia F, Trasforini G, Salvadori S, Margutti A, Bianconi M, Teodori V, Facchinetti F, Tomatis R, Genazzani AR, Pansini R: Dermorphin reduces the metyrapone-evoked release of adrenocorticotropin, β-endorphin, and β-lipotropin in man. *J Clin Endocrinol Metab* 61:1018, 1985.

94. Axelrod J, Reisine TD: Stress hormones: Their interaction and regulation. *Science* 224:452, 1984.

95. Healy DL, Hodgen GD, Schulte HM, Chrousos GP, Loriaux DL, Hall NR, Goldstein AL: The thymus-adrenal connection: Thymosin has corticotropin-releasing activity in primates. *Science* 222:1353, 1983.

96. Lewis DA, Sherman BM: Oxytocin does not influence adrenocorticotropin secretion in man. *J Clin Endocrinol Metab* 60:53, 1985.

97. De Souza EB, Van Loon GR: D-Ala^2-met-enkephalinamide, a potent opioid peptide, alters pituitary-adrenocortical secretion in rats. *Endocrinology* 111:1483, 1982.

98. Mezey E, Reisine TD, Brownstein MJ, Palkovits M, Axelrod J: β-Adrenergic mechanism of insulin-induced adrenocorticotropin release from the anterior pituitary. *Science* 226:1085, 1984.

99. Lewis DA, Sherman BM: Sterotonergic stimulation of adrenocorticotropin secretion in man. *J Clin Endocrinol Metab* 58:458, 1984.

100. Saito E, Odell WD: Corticotropin-lipotropin common precursor-like material in normal rat extrapituitary tissues. *Proc Natl Acad Sci USA* 80:3792, 1983.

101. Krieger DT: The multiple faces of pro-opiomelanocortin, a prototype precursor molecule. *Clin Res* 31:342, 1983.

102. Herbert E, Uhler M: Biosynthesis of polyprotein precursors to regulatory peptides. *Cell* 30:1, 1982.

103. Whitfeld PL, Seeburg PH, Shine J: The human pro-opiomelanocortin gene: Organization, sequence, and interspersion with repetitive DNA. *DNA* 1:133, 1982.

104. Miller WL, Johnson LK, Baxter JD, Roberts JL: Processing of the precursor to corticotropin and beta-lipotropin in man. *Proc Natl Acad Sci USA* 77:5211, 1980.

105. Mains RE, Eipper BA: Phosphorylation of rat and human adrenocorticotropin-related peptides: Physiological regulation and studies of secretion. *Endocrinology* 112:1986, 1983.

106. Lerner AB, Buettner-Janusch J: The structure of human corticotropin (adrenocorticotrophic hormone). *J Biol Chem* 236:2970, 1961.

107. Rinkler B, Sieber P, Rittel W, Zuler H: Revised amino-acid sequences for porcine and human adrenocorticotrophic hormone. *Nature (New Biol)* 235:114, 1972.

108. Nicholson WE, Liddle RA, Puett D, Liddle GW: Adrenocorticotrophic hormone biotransformation, clearance and catabolism. *Endocrinology* 103:1344, 1978.

109. Grunfeld C, Hagman J, Sakin EA, Buckley DI, Jones DS, Ramachandran J: Characterization of adrenocorticotropin receptors that appear when 3T3-L1 cells differentiate into adipocytes. *Endocrinology* 116:113, 1985.

110. Marshall JB, Kapcala LP, Manning LD, McCullough AJ: Effect of corticotropin-like intermediate lobe peptide on pancreatic exocrine function in isolated rat pancreatic lobules. *J Clin Invest* 74:1886, 1984.

111. Gaspar L, Chan JSD, Seidah NG, Chretien M: Urinary molecular forms of human N-terminal of pro-opiomelanocortin: Possible deglycosylation and degradation by the kidney. *J Clin Endocrinol Metab* 59:614, 1984.

112. Lowry PJ, Silas L, McLean C, Linton EA, Estivariz FE: Pro-γ-melanocyte-stimulating hormone cleavage in adrenal gland undergoing compensatory growth. *Nature* 306:70, 1983.

113. Lymangrover JR, Buckalew VM, Harris J, Klein MC, Gruber KA: Gamma-2-MSH is natriuretic in the rat. *Endocrinology* 116:1227, 1985.

114. Sayers G, Portanova R: Regulation of the secretory activity of the adrenal cortex: Cortisol and corticosterone, in Greep RO, Astwood EB (eds): *Handbook of Physiology: Endocrinology*, sect. 7. Washington, D.C., American Physiological Society, 1975, vol 6, p 41.

115. Hall PF: Trophic stimulation of steroidogenesis: In search of the elusive trigger. *Recent Prog Horm Res* 41:1, 1985.

116. Dickerman DR, Faiman GC, Winter JSD: Intraadrenal steroid concentrations in man: Zonal differences and developmental changes. *J Clin Endocrinol Metab* 59:1031, 1984.

117. Sibley CP, Whitehouse BJ, Vinson GP, Goddard C: Studies

on the mechanisms of secretion of rat adrenal steroids in vitro. *J Steroid Biochem* 13:1231, 1980.

118. Goddard C, Vinson GP, Whitehouse BJ, Sibley CP: Subcellular distribution of steroids in the rat adrenal cortex after incubation in vitro. *J Steroid Biochem* 13:1221, 1980.

118a. Cope CC: *Adrenal Steroids and Disease.* London, Pittman Medical, 1972, p 275.

119. Cheitlin R, Buckley DI, Ramachandran J: The role of extracellular calcium in corticotropin-stimulated steroidogenesis. *J Biol Chem* 260:5323, 1985.

120. Catalano RD, Stuve L, Ramachandran J: Characterization of corticotropin receptors in human adrenocortical cells. *J Clin Endocrinol Metab* 62:300, 1986.

121. Kojima I, Kojima K, Rasmussen H: Role of calcium and cAMP in the action of adrenocorticotropin on aldosterone secretion. *J Biol Chem* 260:4248, 1985.

122. Gallo-Payet N, Escher E: Adrenocorticotropin receptors in rat adrenal glomerulosa cells. *Endocrinology* 117:38, 1985.

123. Pedersen RC, Brownie AC: Failure of ACTH to mimic the stress-induced activation of rat adrenocortical cholesterol ester hydrolase in vivo. *J Steroid Biochem* 11:1393, 1979.

124. Hayashi K, Sala G, Catt KJ, Dufau ML: Regulation of steroidogenesis by adrenocorticotrophic hormone in isolated adrenal cells. *J Biol Chem* 254:6678, 1979.

125. Conneely OM, Headon DR, Olson CD, Ungar F, Dempsey ME: Intramitochondrial movement of adrenal sterol carrier protein with cholesterol in response to corticotropin. *Proc Natl Acad Sci USA* 81:2970, 1984.

126. Pederson RC, Brownie AC: Cholesterol side-chain cleavage in the rat adrenal cortex: Isolation of a cycloheximide-sensitive activator peptide. *Proc Natl Acad Sci USA* 80:1882, 1983.

127. Krueger RJ, Orme-Johnson NR: Acute adrenocorticotropic hormone stimulation of adrenal corticosteroidogenesis. *J Biol Chem* 258:10159, 1983.

128. Farese RV: Phospholipids as intermediates in hormone action. *Mol Cell Endocrinol* 35:1, 1984.

129. Farese RV, Sabir AM: Polyphosphoinositides: Stimulator of mitochondrial cholesterol side chain cleavage and possible identification as an adrenocorticotropin-induced, cycloheximide-sensitive, cytosolic steroidogenesis factor. *Endocrinology* 106:1869, 1980.

130. Pedersen RC, Brownie AC, Ling N: Pro-adrenocorticotropin/endorphin derived peptides: Coordinate action on adrenal steroidogenesis. *Science* 208:1044, 1980.

131. A Jagannadha Rao J, Long JA, Ramachandran J: Effects of antiserum to adrenocorticotropin on adrenal growth and function. *Endocrinology* 102:371, 1978.

132. Dallman MF, Engeland WC, Holzwarth MA, Scholz PM: ACTH inhibits adrenal growth after unilateral adrenalectomy. *Endocrinology* 107:1397, 1980.

133. Gill GN, Hornsby PJ, Simonian MH: Regulation of growth and differentiated function of cultured bovine adrenocortical cells, in Sato G, Ross R (eds): *Hormones and Cell Culture.* Cold Spring Harbor, NY, Cold Spring Harbor Laboratory, 1979, p 701.

133a. Saito E, Ichikawa Y, Homma M: Direct inhibitory effect of dexamethasone on steroidogenesis of human adrenal in vivo. *J Clin Endocrinol Metab* 48:861, 1979.

134. Rosenfield RL, Helke J, Lucky AW: Dexamethasone preparation does not alter corticoid and androgen responses to adrenocorticotropin. *J Clin Endocrinol Metab* 60:585, 1985.

135. Shima S, Komoriyama K, Hirai M, Kouyama H: Studies on cyclic nucleotides in the adrenal gland. XI. Adrenergic regulation of adenylate cyclase activity in the adrenal cortex. *Endocrinology* 114:325, 1984.

136. Dempsher DP, Gann DS: Increased cortisol secretion after small hemorrhage is not attributable to changes in adrenocorticotropin. *Endocrinology* 113:86, 1983.

137. Parker LN, Odell WD: Control of adrenal androgen secretion. *Endocr Rev* 1:392, 1980.

138. Castro-Magana M, Maddaiah VT, Collipp PJ, Angulo M: Synergistic effects of growth hormone therapy on plasma levels of 11-deoxycortisol and cortisol in growth hormone-deficient children. *J Clin Endocrinol Metab* 56:662, 1983.

139. Weitzman ED, Fukushima D, Nogeire C, Roffwarg H, Gallagher TF, Hellman L: Twenty-four hour pattern of the episodic secretion of cortisol in normal subjects. *J Clin Endocrinol Metab* 33:14, 1971.

140. Krieger DT: Rhythms in CRF, ACTH, and corticosteroids, in Krieger DT (ed): *Endocrine Rhythms.* New York, Raven, 1979, p 123.

141. Goldman J, Wajchenberg BL, Liberman B, Nery M, Achando S, Germek OA: Contrast analysis for the evaluation of the circadian rhythms of plasma cortisol, androstenedione, and testosterone in normal men and the possible influence of meals. *J Clin Endocrinol Metab* 60:164, 1985.

142. Follénius M, Brandenberger G, Hietter B, Siméoni M, Reinhardt B: Diurnal cortisol peaks and their relationships to meals. *J Clin Endocrinol Metab* 55:757, 1982.

143. Dallman MF: Viewing the ventromedial hypothalamus from the adrenal gland. *Am J Physiol* 246:R1, 1984.

144. Fehm HL, Klein E, Holl R, Voigt FH: Evidence for extrapituitary mechanisms mediating the morning peak of plasma cortisol in man. *J Clin Endocrinol Metab* 58:410, 1984.

145. Schulte HM, Chrousos GP, Gold PW, Booth JD, Oldfield ED, Cutler GB Jr, Loriaux DL: Continuous administration of synthetic ovine corticotropin-releasing factor in man. *J Clin Invest* 75:1781, 1985.

145a. Brandenberger G, Follénius M, Muzet A, Siméoni M, Reinhardt B: Interactions between spontaneous and provoked cortisol secretory episodes in man. *J Clin Endocrinol Metab* 59:406, 1984.

146. Sherman B, Wysham C, Pfohl B: Age-related changes in the circadian rhythm of plasma cortisol in man. *J Clin Endocrinol Metab* 61:439, 1985.

147. Kato H, Saito M, Suda M: Effect of starvation on the circadian adrenocortical rhythm in rats. *Endocrinology* 106:918, 1980.

148. Krieger DT: Ventromedial hypothalamic lesions abolish food-shifted circadian adrenal and temperature rhythmicity. *Endocrinology* 106:649, 1980.

149. Krieger DT: Rhythms of ACTH and corticosteroid secretion in health and disease and their experimental modification. *J Steroid Biochem* 6:785, 1975.

150. Orth DN, Island DP: Light synchronization of the circadian rhythm in plasma cortisol (17-OHS) concentration in man. *J Clin Endocrinol Metab* 29:479, 1969.

151. Davis J, Morrill F, Fawcett J, Upton V, Bondy PK, Spiro HM: Apprehension and serum cortisol levels. *J Psychosom Res* 6:83, 1962.

152. Czeister CA, Ede MCM, Regenstein QR, Kisch ES, Fang US, Ehrlich EN: Episodic 24-hour cortisol secretory patterns in patients awaiting elective cardiac surgery. *J Clin Endocrinol Metab* 42:273, 1976.

153. Sutton JR, Casey JH: The adrenocortical response to competitive athletics in veteran athletes. *J Clin Endocrinol Metab* 40:135, 1975.

154. Plumpton FS, Besser GM, Cole PV: Corticosteroid treatment and surgery: I. An investigation of the indications for steroid cover. *Anaesthesia* 24:3, 1969.

155. Brandt MR, Kehlet H, Skovsted K, Hansen JM: Rapid decrease in plasma triiodothyronine during surgery and epidural analgesia independent of afferent neurogenic stimuli and of cortisol. *Lancet* 2:1333, 1976.

156. Santeusanio F, Bolli G, Massi-Benedetti M, De Feo P, Angeletti G, Compagnucci P, Calabrese G, Brunetti P: Counterregulatory hormones during moderate, insulin-induced, blood glucose decrements in man. *J Clin Endocrinol Metab* 52:477, 1981.

157. Parker LN, Levin ER, Lifrak ER: Evidence of adrenocortical adaptation to severe illness. *J Clin Endocrinol Metab* 60:947, 1985.

158. Linkowski P, Mendlewicz J, Leclercq R, Brasseur M, Hubain

P, Goldstein J, Copinschi G, Van Cauter E: The 24-hour profile of adrenocorticotropin and cortisol in major depressive illness. *J Clin Endocrinol Metab* 61:429, 1985.

159. Sachar EJ, Asnis G, Halbreich U, Nathan RS, Halpern F: Recent studies in the neuroendocrinology of major depressive disorders. *Adv Psychoneuroendocrinology* 3:313, 1980.

160. Hotta M, Shibasaki T, Masuda A, Imaki T, Demura H, Ling N, Shizume K: The responses of plasma adrenocorticotropin and cortisol to corticotropin-releasing hormone (CRH) and cerebrospinal fluid immunoreactive CRH in anorexia nervosa patients. *J Clin Endocrinol Metab* 62:319, 1986.

161. Martin MM, Mintz DH: Effect of altered thyroid function upon adrenocortical ACTH and methopyrapone (SU-4885) responsiveness in man. *J Clin Endocrinol Metab* 25:20, 1965.

162. Carr BR, Parker CR Jr, Maddin JD, MacDonald PC, Porter JC: Plasma levels of adrenocorticotropin and cortisol in women receiving oral contraceptive steroid treatment. *J Clin Endocrinol Metab* 49:346, 1979.

163. Chimara K, Kato Y, Maeda K, Matsukura S, Imura H: Suppression by cyproheptadine of human growth hormone and cortisol during sleep. *J Clin Invest* 57:1393, 1976.

164. Plank J, Feldman JM: Modificaton of adrenal function by the antiserotonin agent cyproheptadine. *J Clin Endocrinol Metab* 42:291, 1976.

165. Keller-Wood ME, Dallman MF: Corticosteroid inhibition of ACTH secretion. *Endocr Rev* 5:1, 1984.

166. Jones MT: Control of adrenocortical hormone secretion, in James VHT (ed): *The Adrenal Gland.* New York, Raven, 1979, p 93.

167. Birnberg NC, Lissitzky J-C, Hinman M, Herbert E: Glucocorticoids regulate pro-opiomelanocortin gene expression in vivo at the levels of transcription and secretion. *Proc Natl Acad Sci USA* 80:6982, 1983.

167a. Byyny RL: Withdrawal from glucocorticoid therapy. *N Engl J Med* 295:30, 1976.

168. Fehm HL, Voigt KH, Kummer G, Lang R, Pfeiffer EF: Differential and integral corticosteroid feedback effects on ACTH secretion in hypoadrenocorticism. *J Clin Invest* 63:247, 1979.

168a. Widmaier EP, Dallman MF: The effects of corticotropin-releasing factor on adrenocorticotropin secretion from perfused pituitaries in vitro: Rapid inhibition by glucocorticoids. *Endocrinology* 115:2368, 1984.

169. Jingami H, Matsukura S, Numa S, Imura H: Effects of adrenalectomy and dexamethasone administration on the level of prepro-corticotropin-releasing factor messenger ribonucleic acid (mRNA) in the hypothalamus and adrenocorticotropin/β-lipotropin precursor mRNA in the pituitary in rats. *Endocrinology* 117:1314, 1985.

170. Suda T, Tomori N, Tozawa F, Mouri T, Demura H, Shizume K: Effect of dexamethasone on immunoreactive corticotropin-releasing factor in the rat median eminence and intermediate-posterior pituitary. *Endocrinology* 114:851, 1984.

171. Davis LG, Arentzen R, Reid JM, Manning RW, Wolfson B, Lawrence KL, Baldino F Jr: Glucocorticoid sensitivity of vasopressin mRNA levels in the paraventricular nucleus of the rat. *Proc Natl Acad Sci USA* 83:1145, 1986.

172. Sapolsky RM, Krey LC, McEwen BS: Glucocorticoid-sensitive hippocampal neurons are involved in terminating the adrenocortical stress response. *Proc Natl Acad Sci USA* 81:6174, 1984.

173. von Werder K, Smilo RP, Hane S, Forsham PH: Pituitary response to stress in Cushing's disease. *Acta Endocrinol* 67:127, 1971.

174. Gomez-Sanchez CE, Smith JS, Ferris MW, Gomez-Sanchez EP: Renal receptor-binding activity of reduced metabolites of aldosterone: Evidence for a mineralocorticoid effect outside of the classic aldosterone receptor system. *Endocrinology* 115:712, 1984.

175. Griffing GT, Wilson TE, Melby JC: Unconjugated and conjugated urinary 19-nor-deoxycorticosterone glucosiduronate. Elevated levels in essential hypertension. *Hypertension* 7(suppl 1):I12, 1985.

176. Griffing GT, Dale SL, Holbrook MM, Melby JC: Relationship of 19-nor-deoxycorticosterone to other mineralocorticoids in low-renin hypertension. *Hypertension* 5:385, 1983.

177. Kramer RE, Gallant S, Brownie AC: Actions of angiotensin II on aldosterone biosynthesis in the rat adrenal cortex. *J Biol Chem* 255:3442, 1980.

178. Goodfriend TL: Angiotensin receptors and specific functions of angiotensins I, II, and III, in Genest J, Kuchel O, Hamet P, Cantin M (eds): *Hypertension.* New York, McGraw-Hill, 1983, p 271.

179. Fraser R, Mason PA, Buckingham JC, Gordon RD, Morton JJ, Nicholls MG, Semple PF, Tree M: The interaction of sodium and potassium states, of ACTH and of angiotensin II in the control of corticosteroid secretion. *J Steroid Biochem* 11:1039, 1979.

180. Catt KJ, Harwood JP, Aguilera G, Dufau ML: Hormonal regulation of peptide receptors and target cell responses. *Nature* 280:109, 1979.

181. Fujita K, Aguilera G, Catt KJ: The role of cyclic AMP in aldosterone production by isolated zona glomerulosa cells. *J Biol Chem* 254:8567, 1979.

182. Farese RV, Larson RE, Sabir MA, Gomez-Sanchez CE: Effects of angiotensin II, K^+, adrenocorticotropin, serotonin, adenosine 3′,5′-monophosphate, guanosine 3′,5′-monophosphate, A23187, and EGTA on aldosterone synthesis and phospholipid metabolism in the rat adrenal zona glomerulosa. *Endocrinology* 113:1377, 1983.

183. Campbell WB, Gomez-Sanchez CE, Adams BV, Schmitz JM, Itskovitz HD: Attenuation of angiotensin II- and III-induced aldosterone release by prostaglandin synthesis inhibitors. *J Clin Invest* 64:1552, 1979.

184. Hornsby PJ, O'Hare MJ: The roles of potassium and corticosteroids in determining the pattern of metabolism of [^{3}H]deoxycorticosterone by monolayer cultures of rat adrenal zona glomerulosa cells. *Endocrinology* 101:997, 1977.

185. McKena TJ, Island DP, Nicholson WE, Liddle GW: The effects of potassium on early and late steps in aldosterone biosynthesis in cells of the zona glomerulosa. *Endocrinology* 103:1411, 1978.

186. Williams GH, Bailey LM: Effects of dietary sodium intake and potassium intake and acute stimulation on aldosterone output by isolated human cells. *J Clin Endocrinol Metab* 45:55, 1977.

187. Williams GH, Dluhy RG: Control of aldosterone secretion, in Genest J, Hamet P, Cantin M (eds): *Hypertension.* New York, McGraw-Hill, 1983, p 320.

188. Mulrow PJ, North R, Fernandez-Cruz A Jr: The diagnosis and management of disorders of aldosterone production, in Gill GG (ed): *Pharmacology of Adrenal Cortical Hormones.* New York, Pergamon, 1979, p 185.

189. Merriam GR, Baer L: Adrenocorticotropin deficiency: Correction of hyponatremia and hypoaldosteronism with chronic glucocorticoid therapy. *J Clin Endocrinol Metab* 50:10, 1980.

190. Aguilera G, Fujita K, Catt KJ: Mechanisms of inhibition of aldosterone secretion by adrenocorticotropin. *Endocrinology* 108:522, 1981.

191. Gullner H-G, Gill JR Jr: Beta-endorphin selectively stimulates aldosterone secretion in hyperphysectomized, nephrectomized dogs. *J Clin Invest* 71:124, 1983.

192. Yamakado M, Franco-Saenz R, Mulrow PJ: Effect of sodium deficiency on β-melanocyte-stimulating hormone stimulation of aldosterone in isolated rat adrenal cells. *Endocrinology* 113:2168, 1983.

193. Lis M, Hamet P, Gutkowska J, Maurice G, Seidah NG, Lariviere N, Chretien M, Genest J: Effect of N-terminal portion of pro-opiomelanocortin on aldosterone release by human adrenal adenoma in vitro. *J Clin Endocrinol Metab* 52:1053, 1981.

194. Scheider EG, Radke KJ, Ulderich DA, Taylor RE Jr: Effect of osmolality on aldosterone secretion. *Endocrinology* 116:1621, 1985.

195. Perez GO, Oster JR, Vaamondi CA, Katz FH: Effect of NH_4Cl on plasma aldosterone, cortisol and renin activity in supine man. *J Clin Endocrinol Metab* 45:762, 1977.

196. Sowers JR, Berg G, Martin VS, Mayes DM: Dopaminergic modulation of aldosterone secretion in the rhesus monkey: Evidence that dopamine affects the late pathway of aldosterone biosynthesis by inhibiting the conversion of corticosterone to 18-hydroxycorticosterone. *Endocrinology* 110:1173, 1982.

197. McKenna TJ, Island DP, Nicholson WE, Liddle GW: Dopamine inhibits angiotensin stimulated aldosterone biosynthesis in bovine adrenal cells. *J Clin Invest* 64:287, 1979.

198. Balla T, Enyedi P, Spat A, Antoni FA: Pressor-type vasopressin receptors in the adrenal cortex: Properties of binding, effects on phosphoinositide metabolism and aldosterone secretion. *Endocrinology* 117:421, 1985.

199. Pratt JH, Turner DA, McAteer JA, Henry DP: β-Adrenergic stimulation of aldosterone production by rat adrenal capsular explants. *Endocrinology* 117:1189, 1985.

200. Mazzocchi G, Robba C, Reubffat P, Gottardo G, Nussdorfer GG: Effect of somatostatin on the zona glomerulosa of rats treated with angiotensin II or captopril: Stereology and plasma hormone concentrations. *J Steroid Biochem* 23:353, 1985.

201. Atarashi K, Mulrow PJ, Franco-Saenz R: Effect of atrial peptides on aldosterone production. *J Clin Invest* 76:1807, 1985.

202. Katz FH, Romfh P, Smith JA: Diurnal variation of plasma aldosterone, cortisol and renin activity in supine man. *J Clin Endocrinol Metab* 40:125, 1975.

203. Brown JJ, Fraser R, Lever AF, Morten JJ, Oelkeis W, Robertson JIS, Young J: Further observations on the relationship between plasma angiotensin II and aldosterone during sodium deprivation. Exerpta Med Int Cong Ser: 302:148, 1973.

204. Hellman L, Kream J, Rosenfeld RS: The metabolism and 24-hour plasma concentrations of androsterone in man. *J Clin Endocrinol Metab* 45:35, 1977.

205. Grumbach MM: The neuroendocrinology of puberty. *Hosp Pract* 15:51, 1980.

206. Carter JN, Tysen JE, Warne GL, McNeilly AS, Faiman C, Friesen HG: Adrenocortical function in hyperprolactinemic women. *J Clin Endocrinol Metab* 45:973, 1977.

207. Winterer J, Gwirtsman HE, George DT, Kaye WH, Loriaux DL, Cutler GB Jr: Adrenocorticotropin-stimulated adrenal androgen secretion in anorexia nervosa: Impaired secretion at low weight with normalization after long-term weight recovery. *J Clin Endocrinol Metab* 61:693, 1985.

208. Parker LN, Lifrak ET, Odell WD: A 60,000 molecular weight human pituitary glycopeptide stimulates adrenal androgen secretion. *Endocrinology* 113:2092, 1983.

209. Byrne GC, Perry YS, Winter JSD: Kinetic analysis of adrenal 3β-hydroxysteroid dehydrogenase activity during human development. *J Clin Endocrinol Metab* 60:934, 1985.

210. Zumoff B, Walsh BT, Katz JL, Lerin J, Rosenfeld RS, Kream J, Weiner H: Subnormal plasma dehydroisoandrosterone to cortisol ratio in anorexia nervosa: A second hormonal parameter of ontogenic regression. *J Clin Endocrinol Metab* 56:668, 1983.

211. Albertson BD, Hobson WC, Burnett BS, Turner PT, Clark RV, Schiebinger RJ, Loriaux DL, Cutler GB Jr: Dissociation of cortisol and adrenal androgen secretion in the hypophysectomized, adrenocorticotropin-replaced cimpanzee. *J Clin Endocrinol Metab* 59:13, 1984.

212. Rittmaster RS, Loriaux DL, Cutler GB Jr: Sensitivity of cortisol and adrenal androgens to dexamethasone suppression in hirsute women. *J Clin Endocrinol Metab* 61:462, 1985.

213. Higuchi K, Nawata H, Maki T, Higashizima M, Kato K-I, Ibayashi H: Prolactin has a direct effect on adrenal androgen secretion. *J Clin Endocrinol Metab* 59:714, 1984.

214. Abraham GE: Ovarian and adrenal contribution to peripheral androgens during the menstrual cycle. *J Clin Endocrinol Metab* 39:340, 1974.

215. Ballard PL: Delivery and transport of glucocorticoids to target cells, in Baxter JD, Rousseau GG (eds): *Glucocorticoid Hormone Action*. New York, Springer-Verlag, 1979, p 25.

216. Sandberg AA, Slaunwhite WR Jr: Physical state of adrenal cortical hormones in plasma, in Christy NP (ed): *The Human Adrenal Cortex*. New York, Harper & Row, 1971, p 69.

217. Westphal U: *Steroid-Protein Interactions*. New York, Springer-Verlag, 1971.

218. Dunn JF, Nisula BC, Rodbard D: Transport of steroid hormones: Binding of 21 endogenous steroids to both testosterone-binding globulin and corticosteroid-binding globulin in human plasma. *J Clin Endocrinol Metab* 53:58, 1981.

219. Partridge WM, Sakiyama R, Judd HL: Protein-bound corticosterone in human serum is selectively transported into rat brain and liver in vivo. *J Clin Endocrinol Metab* 57:160, 1983.

220. Siiteri PK, Murai JT, Hammond GL, Nisker JA, Raymoure WJ, Kuhn RW: The serum transport of steroid hormones. *Recent Prog Horm Res* 38:457, 1982.

221. Wolf G, Armstrong EG, Rosner W: Synthesis in vitro of corticosteroid-binding globulin from rat liver messenger ribonucleic acid. *Endocrinology* 108:805, 1981.

222. Perrot-Applanat M, Racodot O, Milgrom E: Specific localization of plasma corticosteroid-binding globulin immunoreactivity in pituitary corticotrophs. *Endocrinology* 115:559, 1984.

223. Ogawa T, Sudea K, Matsui N: The effect of cortisol, progesterone, and transcortin on phytohemagglutinin-stimulated human blood mononuclear cells and their interplay. *J Clin Endocrinol Metab* 56:121, 1983.

224. Pugeat MM, Dunn JF, Nisula BC: Transport of steroid hormones: Interaction of 70 drugs with testosterone-binding globulin and corticosteroid-binding globulin in human plasma. *J Clin Endocrinol Metab* 53:69, 1981.

225. DeMoor P, Louwagie A, Van Baelen H, Van de Putte I: Unexplained high transcortin levels in patients with various hematological disorders and in their relatives: A connection between these high transcortin levels and HLA antigen B12. *J Clin Endocrinol Metab* 50:421, 1980.

225a. Baxter JD, Forsham PA: Tissue effects of glucocorticoids. *Am J Med* 53:573, 1972.

226. Kawai S, Ichikawa Y, Homma M: Differences in metabolic properties among cortisol, prednisolone and dexamethasone in liver and renal diseases: Accelerated metabolism of dexamethasone in renal failure. *J Clin Endocrinol Metab* 60:848, 1985.

227. Doe RP, Lohrenz FN, Seal US: Familial decrease in corticosteroid-binding globulin. *Metabolism* 14:940, 1965.

228. Pardridge WM: Transport of protein-bound hormones into tissues in vivo. *Endocr Rev* 2:103, 1981.

229. Krozowski ZS, Funder JW: Renal mineralocorticoid receptors and hippocampal corticosterone binding species have identical intrinsic steroid specificity. *Proc Natl Acad Sci USA* 80:6056, 1983.

230. Reul MJH, deKloet ER: Two receptor systems for corticosterone in rat brain: Microdistribution and differential occupation. *Endocrinology* 117:2505, 1985.

231. Beaumont K, Fanestil DD: Characterization of rat brain aldosterone receptors reveals high affinity for corticosterone. *Endocrinology* 113:2043, 1983.

232. Zager PG, Burtis WJ, Luetscher JA, Dowdy AJ, Sood S: Increased plasma protein binding and low metabolic clearance rate of aldosterone in plasma of low cortisol concentration. *J Clin Endocrinol Metab* 42:207, 1976.

233. Zipser RD, Meidor V, Horton R: Characteristics of aldosterone binding in human plasma. *J Clin Endocrinol Metab* 50:158, 1979.

234. Chanarri M, Luetscher JA, Dowdy AJ, Ganguly A: The effects of temperature and plasma cortisol on distribution of aldosterone between plasma and red blood cells: Influences on metabolic clearance rate and on hepatic and renal extraction of aldosterone. *J Clin Endocrinol Metab* 44:752, 1977.

235. Matulich DT, Morris JA, Bartter FC, Baxter JD: (Unpublished data).

236. Plager JE: The binding of androsterone sulfate, etiocholanolone sulfate and dehydroisoandrosterone sulfate by plasma protein. *J Clin Invest* 44:1234, 1965.

237. Forest MG, Rinarola MA, Migeon CJ: Percentage binding of testosterone, androstenedione and dehydroisoandrosterone in human plasma. *Steroids* 12:323, 1968.

238. Pearlman WH, Crepy O, Murphy M: Testosterone-binding levels in the serum of women during the normal menstrual cycle, pregnancy and the post-partum period. *J Clin Endocrinol Metab* 27:1012, 1967.

239. Peterson RE: Metabolism of adrenal cortical steroids, in Christy NP (ed): *The Human Adrenal Cortex.* New York, Harper & Row, 1971, p 87.

240. Monder C, Bradlow LH: Cortoic acids: Explorations at the frontier of corticosteroid metabolism. *Recent Prog Horm Res* 36:345, 1980.

241. Bradlow HL, Monder C, Zumoff B: Metabolism of cortoic acids in man. *J Clin Endocrinol Metab* 54:296, 1982.

242. Zumoff B, Bradlow HL, Levin J, Fukushima DK: Influence of thyroid function on the in vivo cortisol $\rightleftarrows$ cortisone equilibrium in man. *J Steroid Biochem* 18:437, 1983.

243. Abramovitz M, Branchaud CL, Pearson-Murphy BE: Cortisol-cortisone interconversion in human fetal lung: Contrasting results using explant and monolayer cultures suggest that 11β-hydroxysteroid dehydrogenase (EC 1.1.1.146) comprises two enzymes. *J Clin Endocrinol Metab* 54:563, 1982.

244. Ulstrom RA, Colle E, Burkey J, Gummelle R: Adrenocortical steroid metabolism in newborn infants. II. Urinary excretion of 6β-hydroxycortisol and other polar metabolites. *J Clin Endocrinol Metab* 20:1080, 1961.

245. Katz FH, Lipman MM, Frantz AG, Jailer JW: The physiologic significance of 6β-hydroxycortisol in human corticoid metabolism. *J Clin Endocrinol Metab* 22:71, 1962.

246. Werk EE, MacGee J, Sholiton LJ: Altered cortisol metabolism in advanced cancer and other terminal illnesses: Excretion of 6β-hydroxycortisol. *Metabolism* 13:1425, 1964.

247. Pasqualini JR, Jayle MR: Corticosteroid 21-sulphates in human urine. *Biochem J* 81:147, 1961.

248. Drucker WD, Sfikakis A, Borowski AJ, Christy NP: On the rate of formation of steroidal glucuronides in patients with familial and acquired jaundice. *J Clin Invest* 43:1952, 1964.

249. Morris DJ: The metabolism and mechanism of action of aldosterone. *Endocr Rev* 2:234, 1981.

250. Luetscher JA, Hancock EW, Camargo CA, Dowdy AJ, Nokes GW: Conjugation of 1,2-^{3}H-aldosterone in human liver and kidneys and renal extraction of aldosterone and labelled conjugates from blood plasma. *J Clin Endocrinol Metab* 25:628, 1965.

251. Wilson JD: The pathogenesis of benign prostatic hypertrophy. *Am J Med* 68:745, 1980.

252. Santen RJ, Lipton A, Kendall J: Successful medical adrenalectomy with aminoglutethimide: Role of altered drug metabolism. *JAMA* 230:1661, 1974.

253. Pratt JH, Grim CE, Parkinson CA: Minoxidil increases aldosterone metabolic clearance in hypertensive patients. *J Clin Endocrinol Metab* 49:834, 1979.

254. Doehr P, Fichter M, Pirke KM, Lund R: Relationship between weight gain and hypothalamic pituitary adrenal function in patients with anorexia nervosa. *J Steroid Biochem* 13:529, 1980.

255. Rousseau GG, Baxter JD: Glucocorticoids and the metabolic code, in Baxter JD, Rousseau GG (eds): *Glucocorticoid Hormone Action.* New York, Springer-Verlag, 1979, p 613.

255a. Baxter JD, Forsham PH: Tissue effects of glucocorticoids. *Am J Med* 53:573, 1972.

256. Cahill GF: Action of adrenal cortical steroids on carbohydrate metabolism, in Christy NP (ed): *The Human Adrenal Cortex.* New York, Harper & Row, 1971, p 205.

257. Baxter JD: Glucocorticoid hormone action, in Gill GN (ed): *Pharmacology of Adrenal Cortical Hormones.* Oxford, Pergamon, 1979, p 67.

258. Exton JH: Regulation of gluconeogeneis by glucocorticoids, in Baxter JD, Rousseau GG (eds): *Glucocorticoid Hormone Action.* New York, Springer-Verlag, 1979, p 535.

259. Stalmans W, Laloux M: Glucocorticoids and hepatic glycogen metabolism, in Baxter JD, Rousseau GG (eds): *Glucocorticoid Hormone Action.* New York, Springer-Verlag, 1979, p 517.

260. Lenzen S, Bailey CJ: Thyroid hormones, gonadal and adrenocortical steroids and the function of the islets of Langerhans. *Endocr Rev* 5:411, 1984.

261. Coufalik AH, Monder C: Stimulation of gluconeogenesis by cortisol in fetal rat liver in organ culture. *Endocrinology* 108:1132, 1981.

262. Goldberg AL, Tischler M, DeMortino G, Griffin G: Hormonal regulation of protein degradation and synthesis in skeletal muscle. *Fed Proc* 39:31, 1980.

263. Wise JK, Hendler R, Felig P: Influences of glucocorticoids on glucagon secretion and plasma amino acid concentrations in man. *J Clin Invest* 52:2774, 1973.

264. Tomas FM, Munro HN, Young VR: Effect of glucocorticoid administration on the rate of muscle protein breakdown in vivo in rats, as measured by urinary excretion of N-methylhistidine. *Biochem J* 178:139, 1979.

265. Odedra BR, Millward DJ: Effect of corticosterone treatment on muscle protein turnover in adrenalectomized rats and diabetic rats maintained on insulin. *Biochem J* 204:663, 1982.

266. Simmons PS, Miles JM, Gerich JE, Haymond MW: Increased proteolysis. An effect of increased plasma cortisol within the physiologic range. *J Clin Invest* 73:412, 1984.

267. Shamoon H, Soman V, Sherwin RS: The influence of acute physiological increments of cortisol on fuel metabolism and insulin binding to monocytes in normal humans. *J Clin Endocrinol Metab* 50:495, 1980.

268. Carter-Su C, Okamoto K: Effect of glucocorticoids on hexose transport in rat adipocytes. *J Biol Chem* 260:11091, 1985.

269. Fain JN: Inhibition of glucose transport in fat cells and activation of lipolysis by glucocorticoids, in Baxter JD, Rousseau GG (eds): *Glucocorticoid Hormone Action.* New York, Springer-Verlag, 1979, 547.

270. Munck A, Crabtree GR, Smith KA: Glucocorticoid receptors and actions in rat thymocytes and immunologically-stimulated human peripheral lymphocytes, in Baxter JD, Rousseau GG (eds): *Glucocorticoid Hormone Action.* New York, Springer-Verlag, 1979, p 341.

271. Rizza RA, Mandarino LJ, Gerich JE: Cortisol-induced insulin resistance in man: Impaired suppression of glucose production and stimulation of glucose utilization due to a postreceptor defect of insulin action. *J Clin Endocrinol Metab* 54:131, 1982.

272. Gaca G, Bernend K: Plasma glucose, insulin and free fatty acids during long term corticosteroid treatment in children. *Acta Endocrinol* 77:699, 1974.

273. Nelson DH: Corticosteroid induced changes in phospholipid membranes as mediators of their action. *Endocr Rev* 1:180, 1980.

274. Murray DK, Ruhmann-Wennhold A, Nelson DH: Adrenalectomy decreases the sphingomyelin and cholesterol content of fat cell ghosts. *Endocrinology* 111:452, 1982.

275. Taskinen M-R, Nikkila EA, Pelkonen R, Sane T: Plasma lipoproteins, lipolytic enzymes, and very low density lipoprotein triglyceride turnover in Cushing's syndrome. *J Clin Endocrinol Metab* 57:619, 1983.

276. Baxter JD: Mechanisms of glucocorticoid inhibition of growth. *Kidney Int* 14:330, 1978.

277. Loeb JN: Corticosteroids and growth. *N Engl J Med* 295:547, 1976.

277a. Ernest MJ, Feigelsen P: Multihormonal control of tyrosine aminotransferase in isolated liver cells, in Baxter JD, Rousseau GG (eds): *Glucocorticoid Hormone Action.* New York, Springer-Verlag, 1979, p 219.

277b. Clark AF, Vignos PJ: Experimental corticosteroid myopathy: Effect on myofibrillar ATPase activity and protein degradation. *Muscle Nerve* 2:265, 1979.

277c. Clark AF, Vignos PJ: The role of proteases in experimental glucocorticoid myopathy. *Muscle Nerve* 4:219, 1981.

278. Parrillo JE, Fauci AS: Mechanisms of glucocorticoid action on immune processes. *Annu Rev Pharmacol Toxicol* 19:179, 1979.

279. Glaman NH: How corticosteroids work. *J Allergy Clin Immunol* 55:145, 1975.

280. Saxon A, Stevens RH, Ramer SJ, Clements PJ, Yu DTY: Glucocorticoids administered in vivo inhibit suppressor T lymphocyte function and diminish B lymphocyte responsiveness in in vivo immunoglobulin synthesis. *J Clin Invest* 61:922, 1978.

281. Fauci AS, Dale DC, Balow JE: Glucocorticoid therapy: Mechanisms of action and clinical considerations. *Ann Intern Med* 84:304, 1976.

282. Craddock CG: Corticosteroid-induced lymphopenia, immunosuppression and body defense. *Ann Intern Med* 88:564, 1978.

283. Casey LM, MacDonald PC, Mitchell MD: Despite a massive increase in cortisol secretion in women during parturition, there is an equally massive increase in prostaglandin synthesis. *J Clin Invest* 75:1852, 1985.

284. Munck A, Guyre PM, Holbrook NJ: Physiological functions of glucocorticoids in stress and their relation to pharmacological actions. *Endocr Rev* 5:25, 1984.

285. Fahey JV, Guyre PM, Munck A: Mechanisms of anti-inflammatory actions of glucocorticoids, in Weissman G (ed): *Advances in Inflammatory Research.* New York, Raven, 1981, vol 2, p 21.

286. Goodwin JS, Atluru D, Sierakowski S, Lianos EA: Mechanism of action of glucocorticosteroids: Inhibition of T cell proliferation and interleukin 2 production by hydrocortisone is reversed by leukotriene B_4. *J Clin Invest* 77:1244, 1986.

287. Larsen GL, Henson PM: Mediators of inflammation. *Annu Rev Immunol* 1:335, 1983.

288. Beutler B, Cerami A: Cachectin and tumour necrosis factor as two sides of the same biological coin. *Nature* 320:584, 1986.

289. Goetzl EJ: Oxygenation products of arachidonic acid as mediators of hypersensitivity and inflammation. *Med Clin North Am* 65:809, 1981.

290. Johnson LK, Baxter JD: The mechanism of action of adrenocorticosteroids at the molecular level, in McCarty D (ed): *Landmark Advances in Rheumatology.* New York, Contact Associates, 1985, p 13.

291. Flower RJ: The mediators of steroid action. *Nature* 320:20, 1986.

292. Naray-Fejes-Toth A, Fejes-Toth G, Fischer C, Frolich JC: Effect of dexamethasone on in vivo prostanoid production in the rabbit. *J Clin Invest* 74:120, 1984.

293. Wallner BP, Mattalino RJ, Hession L, Cate RL, Tizard R, Sinclair LK, Foeller C, Chow EP, Browning JL, Ramachandran KL, Pepinsky RB: Cloning and expression of human lipocortin, a phospholipase A_2 inhibitor with potential anti-inflammatory activity. *Nature* 320:77, 1986.

294. Shoenfeld Y, Gurewich Y, Gallant LA, Pinkhas J: Prednisone-induced leukocytosis: Influence of dosage, method and duration of administration on the degree of leukocytosis. *Am J Med* 71:773, 1981.

295. Altman LC, Hill JS, Hairfield WM, Mullarkey MF: Effects of corticosteroids on eosinophil chemotaxis and adherence. *J Clin Invest* 67:28, 1981.

296. Lippman ME: Glucocorticoid receptors and effects in human lymphoid and leukemic cells, in Baxter JD, Rousseau GG (eds): *Glucocorticoid Hormone Action.* New York, Springer-Verlag, 1979, p 377.

297. Maytin EV, Young DA: Separate glucocorticoid, heavy metal, and heat shock domains in thymic lymphocytes. *J Biol Chem* 258:12718, 1983.

298. Compton MM, Cidlowski JA: Rapid in vivo effects of glucocorticoids on the integrity of rat lymphocyte genomic deoxyribonucleic acid. *Endocrinology* 118:38, 1986.

299. Butler WT, Rossen RD: Effects of corticosteroids on immunity in man. I. Decreased serum IgG concentration caused by 3 or 5 days of high doses of methylprednisolone. *J Clin Invest* 52:2629, 1973.

300. Grayson J, Dooley NJ, Koski IR, Blaese RM: Immunoglobulin production induced in vitro by glucocorticoid hormones. *J Clin Invest* 68:1539, 1981.

301. Cupps TR, Gerrard TL, Falkoff RFM, Whalen G, Fauci AS: Effects of in vitro corticosteroids on B cell activation, proliferation, and differentiation. *J Clin Invest* 75:754, 1985.

302. Bar-Shavit Z, Kahn AJ, Pegg LE, Stone KR, Teitelbaum SL: Glucocorticoids modulate macrophage surface oligosaccharides and their bone binding activity. *J Clin Invest* 73:1277, 1984.

303. Leung P, Gidari AS: Glucocorticoids inhibit erythroid colony formation by murine fetal liver erythroid progenitor cells in vitro. *Endocrinology* 108:1787, 1981.

304. Aronow L: Effects of glucocorticoids on fibroblasts, in Baxter JD, Rousseau GG (eds): *Glucocorticoid Hormone Action.* New York, Springer-Verlag, 1979, p 327.

305. Gordan GS: Drug treatment of the osteoporoses. *Annu Rev Pharmacol Toxicol* 18:253, 1978.

306. Cutroneo KR, Rokowski R, Counts DF: Glucocorticoids and collagen synthesis: Comparison of in vivo and cell culture studies. *Coll Relat Res* 1:557, 1981.

307. Furcht LT, Mosher DF, Wendelschafter-Crabb G, Woodbridge PA: Dexamethasone induced accumulation of a fibronectin and collagen extracellular matrix in transformed human cells. *Nature* 277:393, 1979.

308. Smith TJ: Dexamethasone regulation of glycosaminoglycan synthesis in cultured human skin fibroblasts. *J Clin Invest* 74:2157, 1984.

309. Sterling KM Jr, Harris MJ, Mitchell JJ, DiPetrillo TA, Delaney GL, Cutroneo KR: Dexamethasone decreases the amounts of type I procollagen mRNAs in vivo and in fibroblast cell cultures. *J Biol Chem* 258:7644, 1983.

310. Hammarstrom S, Hamberg M, Duell EA, Stawiski MA, Anderson TF, Voorhees JJ: Glucocorticoid in inflammatory proliferative skin disease reduces arachidonic and hydroxyeicosatetraenoic acids. *Science* 197:994, 1977.

311. Oliver N, Newby RF, Furcht LT, Bourgeois S: Regulation of fibronectin biosynthesis by glucocorticoids in human fibrosarcoma cells and normal fibroblasts. *Cell* 33:287, 1983.

312. de Asua LJ, Carr B, Clingan D, Rudland P: Specific glucocorticoid inhibition of growth promoting effects of prostaglandin F2α on 3T3 cells. *Nature* 265:450, 1977.

312a. Pratt WB, Aronow L: The effect of glucocorticoids on protein and nucleic acid synthesis in mouse fibroblasts growing in vitro. *J Biol Chem* 241:5244, 1966.

313. Christy NP: Adrenal cortical steroids in various types of hypertension, in Manger MW (ed): *Hormones and Hypertension.* Springfield, IL, CC Thomas, 1966, p 169.

314. Saruta T, Suzuki H, Handa M, Igarashi Y, Kondo K, Senba S: Multiple factors contribute to the pathogenesis of hypertension in Cushing's syndrome. *J Clin Endocrinol Metab* 62:275, 1986.

315. Grunfeld J-P, Eloy L, Moura A-M, Ganeval D, Ramos-Frendo B, Worcel M: Effects of antiglucocorticoids on glucocorticoid hypertension in the rat. *Hypertension* 7:292, 1985.

316. Sheagren JN: Anti-inflammatory steroid action: Infectious diseases, in Schleimer RP (ed): *Anti-inflammatory Steroid Action: Basic and Clinical Aspects.* New York, Academic, in press.

317. Sheagren JN: Glucocorticoid therapy in the management of

severe sepsis, in Root RK, Sande MA (eds): *Septic Shock*. New York, Churchill Livingston, 1985, p 201.

318. Nichols NR, McNally M, Campbell JH, Funder JW: Overlapping but not identical protein synthetic domains in cardiovascular cells in response to glucocorticoid hormones. *Hypertension* 2:663, 1984.

319. Nichols NR, Tracy KE, Funder JW: Glucocorticoid effects on newly synthesized proteins in muscle and non-muscle cells cultured from neonatal rat hearts. *J Steroid Biochem* 21:487, 1984.

320. Nichols NR, Lloyd CJ, Mendelsohn FAO, Funder JW: Glucocorticoid-induced proteins in bovine endothelial cells. *Mol Cell Endocrinol* 32:245, 1983.

320a. Davies AO, De Lean A, Lefkowitz RJ: Myocardial beta-adrenergic receptors from adrenalectomized rats: Impaired formation of high-affinity agonist-receptor complexes. *Endocrinology* 108:720, 1981.

321. Clark AF, Tandler B, Vignos PJ: Glucocorticoid-induced alterations in the rabbit heart. *Lab Invest* 47:603, 1982.

322. Sambhi MP, Weil MH, Udhoji VN: Acute pharmacologic effects of glucocorticoids: Cardiac output and related hemodynamic changes in normal subjects and patients with shock. *Circ Res* 31:523, 1965.

323. Nasjletti A, Erman A, Cagen LM, Baer PG, Matthews C, Killmar JT: Plasma concentrations, renal excretion, and tissue release of prostaglandins in the rat with dexamethasone-induced hypertension. *Endocrinology* 114:1033, 1984.

324. Axelrod L: Inhibition of prostacyclin production mediates permissive effect of glucocorticoids on vascular tone. *Lancet* 2:904, 1983.

325. White BC, Hoehner PJ, Wilson RF: Mitochondrial O_2 use and ATP synthesis: Kinetic effects of Ca^{+2} and HPO_4^{-2} modulated by glucocorticoids. *Ann Emerg Med* 9:396, 1980.

326. Krakoff LR, Elijovich F: Cushing's syndrome and exogenous glucocorticoid hypertension. *Clin Endocrinol Metab* 10:479, 1981.

327. Friedland J, Setton C, Silverstein E: Angiotensin converting enzyme induction by steroids in alveolar macrophages in culture. *Science* 197:64, 1977.

328. Stockigt JR, Hewett MJ, Topliss DJ, Higgs EJ, Taft P: Renin and renin substrate in primary adrenal insufficiency: Contrasting effects of glucocorticoid and mineralocorticoid deficiency. *Am J Med* 66:915, 1979.

329. Falezza G, Santonactaso CL, Parisi T, Muggeo M: High serum levels of angiotensin-converting enzyme in untreated Addison's disease. *J Clin Endocrinol Metab* 61:496, 1985.

330. Bengele HH, McNamara ER, Alexander ER: Natriuresis after adrenal enucleation: Effect of spironolactone and dexamethasone. *Am J Physiol* 233:F8, 1977.

331. Haack D, Mohring J, Mohring B, Petri M, Hackenthal E: Comparative study on development of corticosterone and DOCA hypertension in rats. *Am J Physiol* 233:F403, 1977.

332. Gardner DG, Hane S, Trachewsky D, Schenk D, Baxter JD: Atrial natriuretic peptide mRNA is regulated by glucocorticoids *in vivo*. *Biochem Biophys Res Commun* 139:1047, 1986.

332a. Klein LE, Hsiao P, Bartolomei M, Lo CS: Regulation of rat renal (Na^{+}+K^{+})-adenosine triphosphatase activity by triiodothyronine and corticosterone. *Endocrinology* 115:1038, 1984.

333. Kaji DM, Thakkar U, Kahn T, Torelli JA: Glucocorticoid induced alterations in the sodium potassium pump of the human erythrocyte. *J Clin Invest* 68:422, 1981.

334. Bastl CP, Barnett CA, Schmidt TJ, Litwack G: Glucocorticoid stimulation of sodium absorption in colon epithelia is mediated by corticosteroid IB receptor. *J Biol Chem* 259:1186, 1984.

335. Noda Y, Yamada K, Igic R, Erdos EG: Regulation of rat urinary and renal kallikrein and prekallikrein by corticosteroids. *Proc Natl Acad Sci USA* 80:3059, 1983.

336. Boykin J, deTorrente A, Erickson A, Robertson G, Shrier RW: Role of plasma vasopressin in impaired water excretion of glucocorticoid deficiency. *J Clin Invest* 62:738, 1978.

337. Schwartz J, Keil LC, Maselli J, Reid IA: Role of vasopressin in blood pressure regulation during adrenal insufficiency. *Endocrinology* 112:234, 1983.

338. Christy NP: Iatrogenic Cushing's syndrome, in Christy NP (ed): *The Human Adrenal Cortex*. New York, Harper & Row, 1971, p 395.

338a. Stanton B, Giebisch G, Klein-Robbenhaar G, Wade J, DeFronzo RA: Effects of adrenalectomy and chronic adrenal corticosteroid replacement on potassium transport in rat kidney. *J Clin Invest* 75:1317, 1985.

339. Wilcox CS, Cemerikic DA, Giebisch G: Differential effects of acute mineralo- and glucocorticosteroid administration on renal acid elimination. *Kidney Int* 21:546, 1982.

340. Freiberg JM, Kinsella J, Sacktor B: Glucocorticoids increase the Na^{+}-H^{+} exchange and decrease the Na^{+} gradient-dependent phosphate-uptake systems in renal brush border membrane vesicles. *Proc Natl Acad Sci USA* 79:4932, 1982.

341. Cope CL: *Adrenal Steroids and Disease*. London, Pitman, 1972, p 595.

342. Nerup J: Addison's disease—clinical studies. A report of 108 cases. *Acta Endocrinol* 76:127, 1974.

343. Downic WW, Gunn A, Paterson CR, Howie GF: Hypercalcaemic crisis as presentation of Addison's disease. *Br Med J* 1:145, 1977.

344. Ross EJ, Marshall-Jones P, Friedman M: Cushing's syndrome: Diagnostic criteria. *Q J Med* 35:149, 1966.

345. Breslau NA, Zerwekh JE, Nicar MJ, Pak CYC: Effects of short term glucocorticoid administration in primary hyperparathyroidism: Comparison to sarcoidosis. *J Clin Endocrinol Metab* 54:824, 1982.

346. Findling JW, Adams ND, Lemann J Jr, Gray RW, Thomas CJ, Tyrrell JB: Vitamin D metabolites and parathyroid hormone in Cushing's syndrome: Relationship to calcium and phosphorus homeostasis. *J Clin Endocrinol Metab* 54:1039, 1982.

347. Hahn TJ, Halstead LR, Baran DT: Effects of short term glucocorticoid administration on intestinal calcium absorption and circulating vitamin D metabolite concentrations in man. *J Clin Endocrinol Metab* 52:111, 1981.

348. Hahn TJ, Halstead LR, Teitelbaum SL: Altered mineral metabolism in glucocorticoid-induced osteopenia. *J Clin Invest* 64:655, 1979.

349. Lee DBN: Unanticipated stimulatory action of glucocorticoids on epithelial calcium absorption. *J Clin Invest* 71:322, 1983.

350. Williams GA, Peterson WC, Bowser EH, Henderson WJ, Hargis GK, Martinez NJ: Interrelationship of parathyroid and adrenocortical function in calcium homeostasis in the rat. *Endocrinology* 95:707, 1974.

351. Manolagas SC, Anderson DC, Lamb GA: Glucocorticoids regulate the concentration of 1,25-dihydroxycholecalciferol receptors in bone. *Nature* 277:314, 1979.

352. Hansen JW, Gordan GS, Purssin SG: Direct measurement of osteolysis in man. *J Clin Invest* 52:304, 1973.

353. Kimura S, Rasmussen H: Adrenal glucocorticoids, adenine nucleotide translocation, and mitochondrial calcium accumulation. *J Biol Chem* 252:1217, 1977.

353a. Chyun YS, Kream BE, Raisz LG: Cortisol decreases bone formation by inhibiting periosteal cell proliferation. *Endocrinology* 114:477, 1984.

353b. Reid IR, Chapman GE, Fraser TRC, Davies AD, Surus AS, Meyer J, Huq NL, Ibbertson HK: Low serum osteocalcin levels in glucocorticoid-treated asthmatics. *J Clin Endocrinol Metab* 62:379, 1986.

354. Chen TL, Feldman D: Glucocorticoid potentiation of the adenosine 3′,5′-monophosphate response to parathyroid hormone in cultured rat bone cells. *Endocrinology* 102:589, 1978.

355. Ng B, Hekkelman JW, Heersche JNM: The effect of cortisol on the adenosine 3′,5′-monophosphate response to parathyroid

hormone of bone in vitro. *Endocrinology* 104:1130, 1979.
356. Wong GL, Kukert BP, Adams JS: Glucocorticoids increase osteoblast-like bone cell response to 1,25(OH)$_2$D$_3$. *Nature* 285:254, 1980.
357. Chen TL, Cone CM, Morey-Holton E, Feldman D: Glucocorticoid regulation of 1,25(OH)$_2$-vitamin D$_3$ receptors in cultured mouse bone cells. *J Biol Chem* 257:13564, 1982.
358. Binstock ML, Mundy GR: Effect of calcitonin and glucocorticoids in combination in the hypercalcemia of malignancy. *Ann Intern Med* 93:269, 1980.
359. McEwen BS: Influences of adrenocortical hormones on pituitary and brain function, in Baxter JD, Rousseau GG (eds): *Glucocorticoid Hormone Action.* New York, Springer-Verlag, 1979, p 467.
360. Doupe AJ, Patterson PH: Glucocorticoids and the developing nervous system, in Ganten D, Pfaff D (eds): *Current Topics in Neuroendocrinology.* New York, Springer-Verlag, 1982, vol 2, p 23.
361. Pardridge WM, Mietus LJ: Transport of steroid hormones through the rat blood-brain barrier. *J Clin Invest* 64:145, 1979.
362. Long JB, Holaday JW: Blood-brain barrier: Endogenous modulation by adrenalcortical function. *Science* 27:1580, 1985.
363. Knowlton AI: Addison's disease: A review of its clinical course and management, in Christy NP (ed): *The Human Adrenal Cortex.* New York, Harper & Row, 1971, p 329.
364. Woodbury DM: Relation between the adrenal cortex and the central nervous system. *Pharmacol Rev* 10:275, 1958.
365. Gillin JC, Jacobs LS, Fram DH, Snyder F: Acute effect of a glucocorticoid on normal human sleep. *Nature* 237:398, 1972.
366. Sternberg DE: Biologic tests in psychiatry. *Psychiatr Clin North Am* 7:639, 1984.
367. Bohus B, de Kloet ER: Behavioral effects of neuropeptides (endorphins, enkephalins, ACTH fragments) and corticosteroids, in Jones MT, Gillham B, Dallman MF, Chattopadhyay S (eds): *Interaction within the Brain Pituitary-Adrenocortical System.* New York, Academic, 1979, p 7.
368. Sandman CA, George J, McCanne TR, Nolan JD, Kaswan J, Kastin AJ: MSH/ACTH 4–10 influences behavioral and physiological measures of attention. *J Clin Endocrinol Metab* 44:884, 1977.
368a. Nestler EJ, Rainbow TC, McEwen BS, Greengard P: Corticosterone increases the amount of protein 1, a neuron-specific phosphoprotein, in rat hippocampus. *Science* 212:1162, 1981.
369. Rudman D, Moffitt SD, Fernoff PM, Blackston RD, Faraj BA: Epinephrine deficiency in hypocorticotropic hypopituitary children. *J Clin Endocrinol Metab* 53:722, 1981.
370. Naranjo JR, Mocchetti I, Schwartz JP, Costa E: Permissive effect of dexamethasone on the increase of proenkephalin mRNA induced by depolarization of chromaffin cells. *Proc Natl Acad Sci USA* 83:1513, 1986.
371. Polansky JR, Weinreb RM: Anti-inflammatory agents: Steroids as anti-inflammatory agents, in Sears ML (ed): *Handbook of Experimental Pharmacology.* New York, Springer-Verlag, 1984, vol 69, p 459.
372. Manabe S, Bucala R, Cerami A: Nonenzymatic addition of glucocorticoids to lens proteins in steroid-induced cataracts. *J Clin Invest* 74:1803, 1984.
373. Fenster FL: The ulcerogenic potential of glucocorticoids and possible prophylactic measures. *Med Clin North Am* 57:1289, 1973.
374. Conn HO, Blitzer BL: Nonassociation of adrenocorticosteroid therapy and peptic ulcer. *N Engl J Med* 294:473, 1976.
375. Messer J, Reitman D, Sacks HS, Smith H, Chalmers TC: Association of adrenocorticosteroid therapy and peptic-ulcer disease. *N Engl J Med* 309:21, 1983.
376. Daughaday WJ, Herrington AC, Phillips LS: The regulation of growth by endocrines. *Annu Rev Physiol* 37:211, 1975.
377. Gospodarowicz D, Moran J: Stimulation of division of sparse and confluent 3T3 cell populations by a fibroblast growth factor, dexamethasone and insulin. *Proc Natl Acad Sci USA* 71:4584, 1974.
378. Conover CA, Rosenfeld RG, Hintz RL: Aging alters somatomedin-C-dexamethasone synergism in the stimulation of deoxyribonucleic acid synthesis and replication of cultured human fibroblasts. *J Clin Endocrinol Metab* 61:423, 1985.
379. Bennett A, Chen T, Feldman D, Hintz RL: Characterization of insulin-like growth factor I receptors on cultured rat bone cells: Regulation of receptor concentration by glucocorticoids. *Endocrinology* 116:1577, 1984.
380. Unterman TG, Phillips LS: Glucocorticoid effects on somatomedins and somatomedin inhibitors. *J Clin Endocrinol Metab* 61:618, 1985.
380a. Ballard PL: Glucocorticoids and differentiation, in Baxter JD, Rousseau GG (eds): *Glucocorticoid Hormone Action.* New York, Springer-Verlag, 1979, p 493.
381. Schuetz EG, Wrighton SA, Barwick JL, Guzelian PS: Induction of cytochrome P-450 by glucocorticoids in rat liver I. Evidence that glucocorticoids and pregnenolone 16α-carbonitrile regulate de novo synthesis of a common form of cytochrome P-450 in cultures of adult rat hepatocytes and in the liver in vivo. *J Biol Chem* 259:1999, 1984.
382. Lantiguce RL, Streck WF, Lockwood DH, Jacobs LS: Glucocorticoid suppression of pancreatic and pituitary hormones: Pancreatic polypeptide, growth hormone, and prolactin. *J Clin Endocrinol Metab* 50:298, 1980.
383. Muszynski M, Birnbaum Rs, Roos BA: Glucocorticoids stimulate the production of preprocalcitonin-derived secretory peptides by a rat medullary thyroid carcinoma cell line. *J Biol Chem* 19:11678, 1983.
384. Sowers JR, Carlson HE, Brautbar, Hershman JM: Effect of dexamethasone on prolactin and TSH responses to TRH and metoclopramide in man. *J Clin Endocrinol Metab* 44:237, 1977.
385. Burr WA, Griffiths RS, Ramsden DB, Black EG, Hoffenberg R, Meinhold H, Wenzel KW: Effect of a single dose of dexamethasone on serum concentrations of thyroid hormone. *Lancet* 2:58, 1976.
386. Karpas AE, Rodriguez-Rigau LJ, Smith KD, Steinberger E: Effect of acute and chronic androgen suppression by glucocorticoids on gonadotropin levels in hirsute women. *J Clin Endocrinol Metab* 59:780, 1984.
387. Vreeburg JTM, de Greef WJ, Ooms MP, van Wouw P, Wever RFA: Effects of adrenocorticotropin and corticosterone on the negative feedback action of testosterone in the adult male rat. *Endocrinology* 115:977, 1984.
388. Sapolsky RM: Stress-induced suppression of testicular function in the wild baboon: Role of glucocorticoids. *Endocrinology* 116:2273, 1985.
389. Cumming DC, Quigley ME, Yen SSC: Acute suppression of circulating testosterone levels by cortisol in men. *J Clin Endocrinol Metab* 57:671, 1983.
390. Novotny M, Jemiolo B, Harvey S, Wiesler D, Marchlewska-Koj A: Adrenal-mediated endogenous metabolites inhibit puberty in female mice. *Science* 231:722, 1986.
391. Schoonmaker JN, Erickson GF: Glucocorticoid modulation of follicle-stimulating hormone-mediated granulosa cell differentiation. *Endocrinology* 113:1356, 1983.
392. Suter DE, Schwartz NB: Effects of glucocorticoids on secretion of luteinizing hormone and follicle-stimulating hormone by female rat pituitary cells in vitro. *Endocrinology* 117:849, 1985.
392a. Simpson ER, Ackerman GE, Smith ME, Mendelson CR: Estrogen formation in stromal cells of adipose tissue of women: Induction by glucocorticosteroids. *Proc Natl Acad Sci USA* 78:5690, 1981.
393. Granner DK: The role of glucocorticoids as biological amplifiers, in Baxter JD, Rousseau GG (eds): *Glucocorticoid Hormone Action.* New York, Springer-Verlag, 1979, p 593.
394. Harris AW, Baxter JD: Variations in the cellular sensitivity to glucocorticoids: Observations and mechanisms, in Baxter JD,

Rousseau GG (eds): *Glucocorticoid Hormone Action.* New York, Springer-Verlag, 1979, p 423.

395. Gruol DJ, Campbell NF, Bourgeois S: Cyclic AMP-dependent protein kinase promotes glucocorticoid receptor function. *J Biol Chem* 261:4909, 1986.

396. Lai E, Rosen O, Rubin CS: Dexamethasone regulates the β-adrenergic receptor subtype expressed by 3T3-L1 preadipocytes and adipocytes. *J Biol Chem* 257:6691, 1982.

397. Davies AO, Lefkowitz RJ: In vitro desensitization of beta adrenergic receptors in human neutrophils. *J Clin Invest* 71:565, 1983.

398. Dunlop D: Eighty-six cases of Addison's disease. *Br Med J* 2:887, 1963.

399. Bloom E, Matulich DT, Higgins SJ, Simons SJ, Baxter JD: Nuclear binding of glucocorticoid receptors: Relations between cytosol binding, activation and the biological response. *J Steroid Biochem* 12:175, 1980.

400. Lan NC, Karin M, Nguyen T, Weisz A, Birnbaum MJ, Eberhardt NL, Baxter JD: Mechanisms of glucocorticoid hormone action. *J Steroid Biochem* 20:77, 1984.

401. Yamamoto KR: Steroid receptor regulated transcription of specific genes and gene networks. *Annu Rev Genet* 19:209, 1985.

402. Welshons WV, Krummel BM, Gorski J: Nuclear localization of unoccupied receptors for glucocorticoids, estrogens, and progesterone in GH_3 cells. *Endocrinology* 117:2140, 1985.

403. Singh VB, Moudgil VK: Phosphorylation of rat liver glucocorticoid receptor. *J Biol Chem* 260:3684, 1985.

404. Hollenberg SM, Weinberger C, Ong ES, Cerelli C, Oro A, Lebo R, Thompson EB, Rosenfeld MG Evans RM: Primary structure and expression of a functional human glucocorticoid receptor cDNA. *Nature* 318:635, 1985.

405. Weinberger C, Hollenberg SM, Rosenfeld MG, Evans RM: Domain structure of human glucocorticoid receptor and its relationship to the v-erb-A oncogene product. *Nature* 318:670, 1985.

406. Webb ML, Miller-Diener AS, Litwack G: Purification, characterization, and activation of the glucocorticoid-receptor complex from rat kidney cortex. *Biochemistry* 24:1946, 1985.

407. Smith AC, Harmon JM: Multiple forms of the glucocorticoid receptor steroid binding protein identified by affinity labeling and high-resolution two-dimensional electrophoresis. *Biochemistry* 24: 4946, 1985.

408. Schmidt TJ, Miller-Diener A, Webb ML, Litwack G: Thermal activation of the purified rat hepatic glucocorticoid receptor: Evidence for a two-step mechanism. *J Biol Chem* 260:16255, 1985.

409. Wrange O, Okret S, Radojeie M, Carlstedt-Duke J, Gustafsson J-Å: Characterization of the purified activated glucocorticoid receptor from rat liver cytosol. *J Biol Chem* 259:4534, 1984.

410. Dahmer MK, Tienrungroj W, Pratt WB: Purification and preliminary characterization of a macromolecular inhibitor of glucocorticoid receptor binding to DNA. *J Biol Chem* 260:7705, 1985.

411. Ponta H, Kennedy N, Skroch P, Hynes NE, Groner B: Hormonal response region in the mouse mammary tumor virus long terminal repeat can be dissociated from the proviral promoter and has enhancer properties. *Proc Natl Acad Sci USA* 82:1020, 1985.

412. Slater EP, Rabenau O, Karin M, Baxter JD, Beato M: Glucocorticoid receptor binding and activation of a heterologous promoter by dexamethasone by the first intron of the human growth hormone gene. *Mol Cell Biol* 5: 2984, 1985.

413. Svec F: The relationship between glucocorticoid biopotency and receptor binding in the AtT-20 cell. *Endocrinology* 114:1250, 1984.

414. Holbrook NJ, Bodwell JE, Munck A: Effects of ATP and pyrophosphate on properties of glucocorticoid-receptor complexes from rat thymus cells. *J Biol Chem* 258:14885, 1983.

415. Rousseau GG, van Bohemen GC, Lareau S, Degelaen J: Submicromolar free calcium modulates dexamethasone binding to the glucocorticoid receptor. *Biochem Biophys Res Commun* 106:16, 1982.

416. Beyer HS, Carr FE, Mariash CN, Oppenheimer JH: Hepatic messenger ribonucleic acid activity profile of rats subjected to alterations in thyroidal and adrenocortical states: Evidence for significant interaction. *Endocrinology* 116:2669, 1985.

417. Duval D, Durant S, Homo-Delarche F: Non-genomic effects of steroids: Interactions of steroid molecules with membrane structures and functions. *Biochim Biophys Acta* 737:409, 1983.

418. Raghow R, Gossage D, Kang AH: Pretranslational regulation of type I collagen, fibronectin, and a 50-kilodalton noncollagenous extracellular protein by dexamethasone in rat fibroblasts. *J Biol Chem* 261:4677, 1986.

419. Fulton R, Birnie DG, Knowler JT: Post-transcriptional regulation of rat liver gene expression by glucocorticoids. *Nucleic Acids Res* 13:6467, 1985.

420. Gelehrter TD: Glucocorticoids and the plasma membrane, in Baxter JD, Rousseau GG (eds): *Glucocorticoid Hormone Action.* New York, Springer-Verlag, 1979, p 97.

421. Thompson EB: Glucocorticoids and lysosmes, in Baxter JD, Rousseau GG (eds): *Glucocorticoid Hormone Action.* New York, Springer-Verlag, 1979, p 575.

422. Rousseau GG, Baxter JD: Glucocorticoid receptors, in Baxter JD, Rousseau GG (eds): *Glucocorticoid Hormone Action.* New York, Springer-Verlag, 1979, p 49.

423. Chrousos GP, Cutler GB, Sauer M, Simons SS Jr, Loriaux DL: Development of glucocorticoid antagonists. *Pharmacol Ther* 20:263, 1983.

424. Healy DL, Chrousos GP, Schulte HM, Gold PW, Hodgen GD: Increased adrenocorticotropin, cortisol, and arginine vasopressin secretion in primates after the antiglucocorticoid steroid RU 486: Dose response relationships. *J Clin Endocrinol Metab* 60:1, 1985.

425. Wolff ME: Structure-activity relationships in glucocorticoids, in Baxter JD, Rousseau GG (eds): *Glucocorticoid Hormone Action.* New York, Springer-Verlag, 1979, p 97.

426. Meikle AW, Tyler FH: Potency and duration of action of glucocorticoids: Effects of hydrocortisone, prednisone and dexamethasone on human pituitary adrenal function. *Am J Med* 63:200, 1977.

427. Marver D, Kokko JP: Renal target sites and the mechanism of action of aldosterone. *Min Elect Metab* 9:1, 1983.

428. Moura AM, Worcel M: Direct action of aldosterone on transmembrane ^{22}Na efflux from arterial smooth muscle: Rapid and delayed effects. *Hypertension* 6:425, 1984.

429. Quirk SJ, Gannell JE, Funder JW: Aldosterone-binding sites in pregnant and lactating rat mammary glands. *Endocrinology* 113:1812, 1983.

430. Nichols NR, Nguyen HH, Meyer WJ III: Physical separation of aortic corticoid receptors with type I and type II specificities. *J Steroid Biochem* 22:577, 1985.

431. Claire M, Oblin M-E, Steimer J-L, Nakane H, Misumi J, Michaud A, Corvol P: Effect of adrenalectomy and aldosterone on the modulation of mineralocorticoid receptors in rat kidney. *J Biol Chem* 256:142, 1981.

432. Ludens JH, Fanestil DD: The mechanism of aldosterone function, in Gill GN (ed): *Pharmacology of Adrenal Cortical Hormones.* New York, Pergamon, 1979, p 143.

433. Tomita K, Pisano JJ, Knepper MA: Control of sodium and potassium transport in the cortical collecting duct of the rat. *J Clin Invest* 76:132, 1985.

434. Petty KJ, Kokko JP, Marver D: Secondary effect of aldosterone on Na-K-ATPase activity in the rabbit cortical collecting tubule. *J Clin Invest* 68:1514, 1981.

435. Mujais SK, Chekal MA, Jones WJ, Hayslett JP, Katz AI: Modulation of renal sodium-potassium-adenosine triphosphatase by aldosterone. *J Clin Invest* 76:170, 1985.

436. Mujais SK, Chekal MA, Jones WJ, Hayslett JP, Katz AI: Regulation of renal Na-K-ATPase in the rat. *J Clin Invest* 73:13, 1984.
437. Kurt Lee S-M, Chekal MA, Katz AI: Corticosterone binding sites along the rat nephron. *Am J Physiol* (Renal Fluid Electrolyte Physiol 13) 244:F504, 1983.
438. Irvine WJ, Toft AD, Feek CM: Addison's disease, in James VHT (ed): *The Adrenal Gland.* New York, Raven, 1979, p 131.
439. Knox FG, Burnett JC Jr, Kohan DE, Spielman WS, Strand JC: Escape from the sodium-retaining effects of mineralocorticoids. *Kidney Int* 17:263, 1980.
440. Forman BH, Mulrow PJ: Effect of corticosteroids on water and electrolyte metabolism, in Greep RO, Astwood EB (eds): *Handbook of Physiology: Endocrinology.* Washington, D.C., American Physiological Society, 1975, vol 6, p 179.
441. Metzler CH, Gardner DG, Keil LC, Baxter JD, Ramsay DJ: Increased synthesis and release of atrial peptide during mineralocorticoid escape in conscious dogs. *Am J Physiol* (Renal Fluid Electrolyte Physiol), in press.
442. Cox M, Stevens RH, Singer I: The defense against hyperkalemia: The roles of insulin and aldosterone. *N Engl J Med* 299:525, 1978.
443. Seldin DW: Metabolic acidosis, in Brenner BM, Rector FC (eds): *The Kidney.* Philadelphia, Saunders, 1976, p 615.
444. Sebastian A, Sutton JM, Hulter HM, Schambelan M, Poler SM: Effect of mineralocorticoid replacement therapy on renal acid-base homeostasis in adrenalectomized patients. *Kidney Int* 18:762, 1980.
445. Lieberthal W, Oza NB, Arbeit L, Bernard DB, Levinsky NG: Effects of alterations in sodium and water metabolism on urinary excretion of active and inactive kallikrein in man. *J Clin Endocrinol Metab* 56:513, 1983.
446. Binder HJ: Efect of dexamethasone on electrolyte transport in the large intestine of the rat. *Gastroenterology* 75:212, 1978.
447. Lan NC, Graham B, Bartter FC, Baxter JD: Binding of steroids to mineralocorticoid receptors: Implications for in vivo occupancy by glucocorticoids. *J Clin Endocrinol Metab* 54:332, 1982.
448. Doucet A, Katz AI: Mineralocorticoid receptors along the nephron: [^{3}H]Aldosterone binding in rabbit tubules. *Am J Physiol* (Renal Fluid Electrolyte Physiol 10) 241:F605, 1981.
449. Park SC, Edelman IS: Dual action of aldosterone on toad bladder: Na^+ permeability and Na^+ pump modulation. *Am J Physiol* (Renal Fluid Electrolyte Physiol 15) 246:F517, 1984.
450. Cortas N, Abras E, Arnaout M, Mooradian A, Muakasah S: Energetics of sodium transport in the urinary bladder of the toad: Effect of aldosterone and sodium cyanide. *J Clin Invest* 73:46, 1984.
451. Park SC, Edelman IS: Effect of aldosterone on abundance and phosphorylation kinetics of Na-K-ATPase of toad urinary bladder. *Am J Physiol* (Renal Fluid Electrolyte Physiol 15) 246:F509, 1984.
452. El Mernissi G, Chabardes D, Doucet A, Hus-Citharel A, Imbert-Teboul M, Le Bouffant F, Montegut M, Siaume S, Morel F: Changes in tubular basolateral membrane markers after chronic DOCA treatment. *Am J Physiol* (Renal Fluid Electrolyte Physiol 14) 245:F100, 1983.
453. Karbowiak AI, Krozowski Z, Funder JW, Adam WR: The mechanism of mineralocorticoid action of carbenoxolone. *Endocrinology* 111:1683, 1982.
454. Wambach G, Higgins JR: Antimineralocorticoid action of progesterone in the rat: Correlation of the effect on electrolyte excretion and interaction with the renal mineralocorticoid receptors. *Endocrinology* 102:1686, 1978.
455. Speiser PW, Martin KO, Kao-Lo G, New MI: Excess mineralocorticoid receptor activity in patients with dexamethasone-suppressible hyperaldosteronism is under adrenocorticotropin control. *J Clin Endocrinol Metab* 61:297, 1985.
456. Lan NC, Matulich DT, Stockigt JR, Biglieri EG, New MI, Baxter JD: Radioreceptor assay of plasma mineralocorticoid activity. *Circ Res* 46(suppl):I94, 1980.
457. Yuen BH, Kelch RP, Jaffe RB: Adrenal contribution to plasma estrogens in adrenal disorders. *Acta Endocrinol* 76:117, 1974.
458. Nimrod A, Ryan KJ: Aromatization of androgens by human abdominal and breast fat tissue. *J Clin Endocrinol Metab* 40:367, 1975.
459. Schweikert HU, Milewich L, Wilson JD: Aromatization of androstenedione by isolated human hairs. *J Clin Endocrinol Metab* 40:413, 1975.
460. MacDonald PC, Madden JD, Brenner PF, Wilson JD, Siiteri PK: Origin of estrogen in normal men and women with testicular feminization. *J Clin Endocrinol Metab* 49:905, 1979.
461. Murphy BEP: Some studies of the protein-binding of steroids and their application to the routine micro and ultramicro measurement of various steroids in body fluids by competitive protein-binding radioassay. *J Clin Endocrinol Metab* 27:973, 1967.
462. Murphy BEP: Non-chromatographic radiotransinassay for cortisol: Application to human adult serum, umbilical cord serum and amniotic fluid. *J Clin Endocrinol Metab* 41:1050, 1975.
463. Ruder HJ, Guy RL, Lipsett MB: A radioimmunoassay for cortisol in plasma and urine. *J Clin Endocrinol Metab* 35:219, 1972.
464. Vecsi P: Glucocorticoids: Cortisol, corticosterone and compound S, in Jaffe BM, Behrman HR (eds): *Methods of Hormone Radioimmunoassay.* New York, Academic, 1974, p 393.
465. Kabra PM, Tsai L, Marton LJ: Improved liquid-chromatographic method for determination of serum cortisol. *Clin Chem* 25:1293, 1979.
466. Gotelli GR, Wall JH, Kabra PM, Marton LJ: Fluorometric liquid-chromatographic determination of serum cortisol. *Clin Chem* 27:442, 1981.
467. Porter CC, Silber RH: A quantitative color reaction for cortisone and related 17,21-dihydroxy-20-ketosteroids. *J Biol Chem* 185:201, 1950.
468. Nelson DH, Samuels LT: A method for the determination of 16-hydroxy-corticosteroids in blood: 17-Hydroxycorticosterone in the peripheral blood. *J Clin Endocrinol Metab* 12:519, 1952.
469. Mattingly D: A simple fluorimetric method for the estimation of free 11-hydroxycorticoids in human plasma. *J Clin Pathol* 15:374, 1962.
470. Nielsen E, Asfeldt VH: Studies on the specificity of fluorimetric determination of plasma corticosteroids ad Modum De Moor and Steeno. *Scand J Clin Lab Invest* 20:185, 1967.
471. Ballard PL, Carter JP, Graham BS, Baxter JD: A radioreceptor assay for evaluation of the plasma glucocorticoid activity of natural and synthetic steroids in man. *J Clin Endocrinol Metab* 41:290, 1975.
472. Robin P, Predine J, Milgrom E: Assay of unbound cortisol in plasma. *J Clin Endocrinol Metab* 46:277, 1977.
473. Lan NC, Baxter JD, unpublished observations.
474. Evans PJ, Peters JR, Dyas J, Walker RF, Riad-Fahmy D, Hall R: Salivary cortisol levels in true and apparent hypercortisolism. *Clin Endocrinol* 20:709, 1984.
475. Newsome HH, Clements AS, Borum EA: The simultaneous assay of cortisol, corticosterone, 11-deoxycortisol and cortisone in human plasma. *J Clin Endocrinol Metab* 34:473, 1972.
476. Willig RP, Blunck W: Quantitation of plasma cortisol and other C_{21}-steroids by radioimmunoassay, in Gupta D (ed): *Radioimmunoassay of Steroid Hormones.* Weinheim, Verlag Chemie, 1975, p 135.
477. West CD, Mahajan DK, Chavre VJ, Nabors CJ, Tyler FH: Simultaneous measurement of multiple plasma steroids by radioimmunoassay demonstrating episodic secretion. *J Clin Endocrinol Metab* 36:1230, 1973.
478. Dash RJ, England BG, Midgley AR, Niswender GD: A specific non-chromatographic radioimmunoassay for human plasma cortisol. *Steroids* 26:647, 1975.

479. Colburn WA: Radioimmunoassay for cortisol using antibodies against prednisolone conjugated at the 3-position. *J Clin Endocrinol Metab* 41:868, 1975.

480. De Moor P, Steeno O, Raskin M, Hendrikx A: Fluorimetric determination of free plasma 11-hydroxycorticosteroids in man. *Acta Endocrinol* 33:297, 1960.

481. Krieger DT, Allen W, Rizzo F, Krieger HP: Characterization of the normal temporal pattern of plasma corticosteroid levels. *J Clin Endocrinol Metab* 32:266, 1971.

482. Gallagher TF, Yoshida K, Roffwarg HD, Fukushima D, Weitzman ED, Hellman L: ACTH and cortisol secretory patterns in man. *J Clin Endocrinol Metab* 36:1058, 1973.

483. DeLacerda L, Kowarski A, Migeon CJ: Integrated concentration and diurnal variation of plasma cortisol. *J Clin Endocrinol Metab* 36:227, 1973.

484. Silverberg A, Rizzo F, Krieger DT: Nyctohemeral periodicity of plasma 17-OHCS levels in elderly subjects. *J Clin Endocrinol Metab* 28:1661, 1968.

485. Gore M, Lester E: Comparison of a fluorimetric and a competitive protein binding assay kit for the determination of plasma hydroxycorticosteroids. *Ann Clin Biochem* 12:160, 1975.

486. Jacobs HS, Nabarro JDN: Plasma 11-hydroxysteroid and growth hormone levels in acute medical illnesses. *Br Med J* 2:595, 1969.

487. Aron DC, Tyrrell JB, Fitzgerald PC, Findling JW, Forsham PH: Cushing's syndrome: Problems in diagnosis. *Medicine* 160:25, 1981.

488. Rao KSJ, Srikantia SG, Gopalan C: Plasma cortisol levels in protein calorie malnutrition. *Arch Dis Child* 43:356, 1968.

489. Walsh BT, Katz JL, Levin J, Kream J, Fukushima DK, Hellman LD, Weiner H, Zumoff B: Adrenal activity in anorexia nervosa. *Psychosom Med* 40:499, 1978.

490. Wallace EZ, Rosman P, Toshav N, Sacerdote A, Balthazar A: Pituitary adrenocortical function in chronic renal failure: Studies of episodic secretion of cortisol and dexamethasone suppressibility. *J Clin Endocrinol Metab* 50:46, 1980.

491. Abraham GE, Manlimos FS, Garza R: Radioimmunoassay of steroids, in Abraham GE (ed): *Handbook of Radioimmunoassay*. New York, Marcel Dekker, 1977, p 591.

492. Anderson DC, Hopper BR, lasley BL, Yen SSC: A simple method for the assay of eight steroids in small volumes of plasma. *Steroids* 28:179, 1976.

493. Berson SA, Yalow RS: Radioimmunoassay of ACTH in plasma. *J Clin Invest* 47:2725, 1968.

494. Landon J, Greenwood FC: Homologous radioimmunoassay for plasma levels of corticotrophin in man. *Lancet* 1:273, 1968.

495. Wolfsen AR, McIntyre HB, Odell WD: Adrenocorticotropin mesurement by competitive binding receptor assay. *J Clin Endocrinol Metab* 34:684, 1972.

496. Liotta A, Krieger DT: A sensitive bioassay for the determination of human plasma ACTH levels. *J Clin Endocrinol Metab* 40:268, 1975.

497. Daly JR, Fleisher MD, Chambers DJ, Bitensky L, Chayen J: Application of the cytochemical bioassay for corticotrophin to clinical and physiological studies in man. *Clin Endocrinol* 3:335, 1974.

498. Orth DN: Adrenocorticotropic hormone and melanocyte stimulating hormone (ACTH and MSH), in Jaffe BM, Behrman HR (eds): *Methods of Hormone Radioimmunoassay*. New York, Academic, 1974, p 125.

499. Ruhmann-Wennhold A, Nelson DH: Adrenocorticotropic hormone, in Antoniades HN (ed): *Hormones in Human Blood*. Cambridge, MA, Harvard University Press, 1976, p 325.

500. Krieger DT, Allen W: Relationship of bioassayable and immunoassayable plasma ACTH and cortisol concentrations in normal subjects and in patients with Cushing's disease. *J Clin Endocrinol Metab* 40:675, 1975.

501. Krieger DT: Plasma ACTH and corticosteroids, in DeGroot LJ et al (eds): *Endocrinology*. New York, Grune and Stratton, 1979, p 1139.

502. Crapo L: Cushing's syndrome: A review of diagnostic tests. *Metabolism* 28:955, 1979.

503. Besser GM, Cullen DR, Irvine WJ, Ratcliffe JG, Landon J: Immunoreactive corticotrophin levels in adrenocortical insufficiency. *Br Med J* 1:374, 1971.

504. Besser GM, Edwards CRW: Cushing's syndrome. *Clin Endocrinol Metab* 1:451, 1972.

505. Weidemann E, Saito T, Linfoot JA, Li CH: Radioimmunoassay of human β-lipotropin in unextracted plasma. *J Clin Endocrinol Metab* 45:1108, 1977.

506. Jeffcoate WJ, Rees LH, Lowry PJ, Beser GM: A specific radioimmunoassay for human β-lipotropin. *J Clin Endocrinol Metab* 47:160, 1978.

507. Krieger DT, Liotta AS, Suda T, Goodgold A, Condon E: Human plasma immunoreactive lipotropin and adrenocorticotropin in normal subjects and in patients with pituitary-adrenal disease. *J Clin Endocrinol Metab* 48:566, 1979.

508. Mullen PE, Jeffcoate WJ, Linsell C, Howard R, Rees LH: The circadian variation of immunoreactive lipotrophin and its relationship to ACTH and growth hormone in man. *Clin Endocrinol* 11:533, 1979.

509. Wardlow SL, Frantz AG: measurement of β-endorphin in human plasma. *J Clin Endocrinol Metab* 48:176, 1979.

510. Wiedemann E, Saito T, Linfoot JA, Li CH: Specific radioimmunoassay of human β-endorphin in unextracted plasma. *J Clin Endocrinol Metab* 49:478, 1979.

511. Beisel WR, Cos JJ, Horton R, Chao PY, Forsham PH: Physiology of urinary cortisol excretion. *J Clin Endocrinol Metab* 24:887, 1964.

512. Murphy BEP: Clinical evaluation of urinary cortisol determinations by competitive protein-binding radioassay. *J Clin Endocrinol Metab* 28:343, 1968.

513. Beardwell CG, Burke CW, Cope CL: Urinary free cortisol measured by competitive protein binding. *J Endocrinol* 42:79, 1968.

514. Meikle AW, Takiguchi H, Mizutani S, Tyler FH, West CD: Urinary cortisol excretion determined by competitive protein-binding radioassay: A test of adrenal cortical function. *J Lab Clin Med* 74:803, 1969.

515. Steeten DHP, Stevenson CT, Dalakos TG, Nicholas JJ, Dennick LG, Fellerman H: The diagnosis of hypercortisolism. Biochemical criteria differentiating patients from lean and obese normal subjects and from females on oral contraceptives. *J Clin Endocrinol Metab* 29:1191, 1969.

516. Smith SR, Bledsoe T, Chhetri MK: Cortisol metabolism and the pituitary adrenal axis in adults with protein-calorie malnutrition. *J Clin Endocrinol Metab* 40:43, 1975.

517. Bliss EJ, Migeon CJ: Endocrinology of anorexia nervosa. *J Clin Endocrinol Metab* 17:766, 1957.

518. Burke CW: Hormones in urine: Uses and misuses. *J R Coll Physicians Lond* 8:335, 1974.

519. McCann VJ, Fulton TJ: Cortisol metabolism in chronic liver disease. *J Clin Endocrinol Metab* 40:1038, 1975.

520. Peterson RE: The influence of the thyroid on adrenal cortical function. *J Clin Invest* 37:736, 1958.

521. Brown H, Englert E, Wallack S: Metabolism of free and conjugated 17-hydroxycorticosteroids in subjects with thyroid disease. *J Clin Endocrinol Metab* 18:167, 1958.

522. Hellman K, Bradlow HL, Zumoff B, Gallagher TF: The influence of thyroid hormone on hydrocortisone production and metabolism. *J Clin Endocrinol* 21:1231, 1961.

523. Garib H, Munoz JM: Endocrine manifestations of diphenylhydantoin therapy. *Metabolism* 23:515, 1974.

524. Bledsoe T, Island DP, Ney RK, Liddle GW: An effect of *o,p'*-DDD in the extraadrenal metabolism of cortisol in man. *J Clin*

Endocrinol Metab 24:1303, 1964.

525. Dillon RS: *Handbook of Endocrinology,* 2d ed. Philadelphia, Lea and Febiger, 1980, p 497.

526. Boruskek S, Gold JJ: Commonly used medications that interfere with routine endocrine laboratory procedures. *Clin Chem* 10:41, 1964.

527. Appleby JI, Gibson G, Normyberski JK, Stubbs RD: Indirect analysis of corticosteroids: 1. The determination of 17-hydroxycorticosteroids. *Biochem J* 60:453, 1955.

528. Caro JF, Meikle AW, Check JH, Cohen SN: "Normal suppression" to dexamethasone in Cushing's disease: An expression of decreased metabolic clearance for dexamethasone. *J Clin Endocrinol Metab* 47:667, 1978.

529. Meikle AW: Dexamethasone suppression tests: Usefulness of simultaneous measurement of plasma cortisol and dexamethasone. *Clin Endocrinol* 16:401, 1982.

530. Liberman B, Wajchenberg BL, Tambascia MA, Mesquita CH: Periodic remission in Cushing's disease with paradoxical dexamethasone response: An expression of periodic hormonogenesis. *J Clin Endocrinol Metab* 43:913, 1976.

531. Meikle AW, Stanchfield JB, West CD, Tyler FH: Hydrocortisone suppression test for Cushing's syndrome. *Arch Intern Med* 134:1068, 1974.

532. Liddle GW: Tests of pituitary adrenal suppressibility in the diagnosis of Cushing's syndrome. *J Clin Endocrinol Metab* 12:1539, 1960.

533. Eddy RL, Jones AL, Gilliland PF, Ibarra JD, Thompson JQ, McMurry JF: Cushing's syndrome: A prospective study of diagnostic methods. *Am J Med* 55:621, 1973.

534. Burke CW, Beardwell CG: Cushing's syndrome. An evaluation of the clinical usefulness of urinary free cortisol and other urinary steroid measurements in diagnosis. *Q J Med* 42:175, 1973.

535. Butler PWP, Besser GM: Pituitary-adrenal function in severe depressive illness. *Lancet* 1:1234, 1968.

536. Jubiz W, Meikle AW, Levinson RA, Mizutani S, West CD, Tyler FH: Effect of diphenylhydantoin on the metabolism of dexamethasone. Mechanism of the abnormal dexamethasone suppression in humans. *N Engl J Med* 283:11, 1970.

537. Ashcraft MW, Van Herle A, Vener SL, Geffner DL: Serum cortisol levels in Cushing's syndrome after low- and high-dose dexamethasone suppression. *Ann Intern Med* 97:21, 1982.

538. Cook DM, Kendall JW, Allen JP, Lagerquist LG: Nyctohemeral variation and suppressibility of plasma ACTH in various stages of Cushing's disease. *Clin Endocrinol* 5:303, 1976.

539. Tyrrell JB, Findling JW, Aron DC, Fitzgerald PA, Forsham PH: An overnight high-dose dexamethasone suppression test for rapid differential diagnosis of Cushing's syndrome. *Ann Intern Med* 104:180, 1986.

540. Nichols T, Nugent CA, Tyler FH: Steroid laboratory tests in the diagnosis of Cushing's syndrome. *Am J Med* 45:116, 1968.

541. Chrousos GP, Schuermeyer TH, Doppman J, Oldfield EH, Schulte HM, Gold PW, Loriaux DL: Clinical applications of corticotropin-releasing factor. *Ann Intern Med* 102:344, 1985.

542. Chrousos GP, Schulte HM, Oldfield EH, Gold PW, Cutler GB Jr, Loriaux DL: The corticotropin-releasing factor stimulation test: An aid in the evaluation of patients with Cushing's syndrome. *N Engl J Med* 310:622, 1984.

543. Lytras N, Grossman A, Perry L, Tomlin S, Wass JAH, Coy DH, Schally AV, Rees LH, Besser GM: Corticotrophin releasing factor: Responses in normal subjects and patients with disorders of the hypothalamus and pituitary. *Clin Endocrinol* 20:71, 1984.

544. Pieters GFFM, Hermus ARMM, Smals AGH, Bartelink AKM, Benraad TJ, Kloppenborg PWC: Responsiveness of the hypophyseal-adrenocortical axis to corticotropin-releasing factor in pituitary-dependent Cushing's disease. *J Clin Endocrinol Metab* 57:513, 1983.

545. Wood JB, Frankland AW, James VHT, Landon J: A rapid test of adrenocortical function. *Lancet* 1:243, 1965.

546. Speckart PF, Nicoloff JT, Bethune JE: Screening for adrenocortical insufficiency with cosyntropin (synthetic ACTH). *Arch Intern Med* 128:761, 1971.

547. Grieg WR, Jasani MK, Boyle JA, Maxwell JD: Corticotrophin stimulation tests. *Mem Soc Endocrinol* 17:175–192, 1968.

548. Nelson JC, Tindall DJ: A comparison of the adrenal responses to hypoglycemia, metyrapone and ACTH. *Am J Med Sci* 275:165, 1978.

549. May ME, Carey RM: Rapid adrenocorticotropic hormone test in practice. *Am J Med* 79:679, 1985.

550. Lindholm J, Kehlet H, Blickert-Toft M, Dinesen B, Rushede J: Reliability of the 30-minute ACTH test in assessing hypothalamic-pituitary-adrenal function. *J Clin Endocrinol Metab* 47:272, 1978.

551. Jasani MK, Boyle JA, Greig WR, Dalakos JG, Browning MCK, Thompson A, Buchanon WW: Corticosteroid-induced suppression of the hypothalamic-pituitary-adrenal axis: Observations on patients given oral corticosteroids for rheumatoid arthritis. *Q J Med* 36:261, 1967.

552. Jasani MK, Freeman PA, Boyle JA, Reid AM, Diver MJ, Buchanan WW: Studies of the rise in plasma 11-hydroxycorticosteroids (11-OHCS) in corticosteroid treated patients with rheumatoid arthritis during surgery: Correlations with the functional integrity of the hypothalamo-pituitary-adrenal axis. *Q J Med* 37:407, 1968.

553. Kehlet H, Binder C: Value of an ACTH test in assessing hypothalamic pituitary-adrenocortical function in glucocorticoid-treated patients. *Br Med J* 2:147, 1973.

554. Landon J, Greenwood FC, Stamp TCB, Wynn V: The plasma sugar, free fatty acid, cortisol and growth hormone response to insulin, and the comparison of this procedure with other tests of pituitary and adrenal function: II. In patients with hypothalamic or pituitary dysfunction or anorexia nervosa. *J Clin Invest* 45:437, 1966.

555. Borst GC, Michenfelder HJ, O'Brian JT: Discordant cortisol response to exogenous ACTH and insulin-induced hypoglycemia in patients with pituitary disease. *N Engl J Med* 306:1462, 1982.

556. Dluhy RG, Himathongkam T, Greenfield M: Rapid ACTH test with plasma aldosterone levels. Improved diagnostic discrimination. *Ann Intern Med* 80:693, 1974.

557. Thorn GW: Adrenal cortical insufficiency, in Conn HF, Clohecy R, Conn RB (eds): *Current Diagnosis.* Philadelphia, Saunders, 1966, p 445.

558. Jacobs HS, Nabarro JDN: Tests of hypothalamic-pituitary-adrenal function in man. *Q J Med* 38:475, 1969.

559. Greenwood FC, Landon J, Stamp TCB: The plasma sugar, free fatty acid, cortisol, and growth hormone response to insulin: I. In control subjects. *J Clin Invest* 45:429, 1966.

560. Krieger DT, Glick SM: Growth hormone and cortisol responsiveness in Cushing's syndrome. Relation to a possible central nervous system etiology. *Am J Med* 52:25, 1972.

561. Donald RA: Plasma immunoreactive corticotrophin and cortisol response to insulin hypoglycemia in normal subjects and patients with pituitary disease. *J Clin Endocrinol Metab* 32:225, 1975.

562. Fleischer MR, Glass D, Bitensky L, Chayen J, Daly JR: Plasma corticotrophin levels during insulin-hypoglycemia: Comparison of radioimmunoassay and cytochemical bioassay. *Clin Endocrinol* 3:203, 1974.

563. Staub JJ, Jenkins JS, Ratcliffe JG, Landon J: Comparison of corticotrophin and corticosteroid response to lysine vasopressin, insulin and pyrogen in man. *Br Med J* 1:267, 1973.

564. Spiger M, Jubiz W, Meikle AW, West CD, Tyler FH: Single-dose metyrapone test. Review of a four-year experience. *Arch Intern Med* 135:698, 1975.

564a. Staub JS, Noelpp B, Girard J, Baumann JB, Graf S, Ratcliffe JG: The short metyrapone test: Comparison of the plasma ACTH response to metyrapone and insulin-induced hypoglycemia. *Clin*

Endocrinol 10:595, 1979.

565. Moll GW, Rosenfield RL: Testosterone binding and free plasma androgen concentrations under physiological conditions: Characterization by flow dialysis technique. *J Clin Endocrinol Metab* 49:730, 1979.

566. Vermeulen A, Ando S: Metabolic clearance rate and interconversion of androgens and the influence of the free androgen fraction. *J Clin Endocrinol Metab* 48:320, 1979.

567. Vermeulen A, Stoïca T, Verdonck K: The apparent free testosterone concentrations: An index of androgenicity. *J Clin Endocrinol Metab* 33:759, 1971.

568. Fisher RA, Anderson DC, Burke CW: Simultaneous measurement of unbound testosterone and estradiol fractions in undiluted plasma at 37°C by steady-state gel filtration. *Steroids* 24:809, 1974.

569a. Vermeulen A, Rubens R: Adrenal virilism, in James VHT (ed): *The Adrenal Gland.* New York, Raven, 1979, p 259.

569b. Hammond GL, Nisker JA, Jones LA, Siiteri PK: Estimation of the percentage of free steroid in undiluted serum by centrifugal ultrafiltration-dialysis. *J Biol Chem* 255:5023, 1986.

570. Anderson DC: The role of sex hormone binding globulin in health and disease, in James VHT, Serio M, Giusti G (eds): *The Endocrine Function of the Human Ovary.* London, Academic, 1976, p 141.

571. Givens JR: Normal and abnormal androgen metabolism. *Clin Obstet Gynecol* 21:115, 1978.

572. Rosenfield RL: Studies of the relation of plasma androgen levels to androgen action in women. *J Steroid Biochem* 6:695, 1975.

573. Rosenfield RL: Plasma free androgen patterns in hirsute women and their diagnostic implications. *Am J Med* 66:417, 1979.

574. Horton R, Hawks D, Lobo R: $3\alpha,17\beta$-Androstanediol glucuronide in plasma: A marker of androgen action in idiopathic hirsutism. *J Clin Invest* 69:1203, 1982.

575. Nisula BC, Loriaux DL, Wilson YA: Solid phase method for measurement of the binding capacity of testosterone-estradiol binding globuin in human serum. *Steroids* 31:681, 1978.

576. Maroulis GB, Manlimos FS, Abraham GE: Comparison between urinary 17-ketosteroids and plasma androgens in hirsute patients. *Obstet Gynecol* 49:454, 1977.

577. Margraf HW, Weichselbaum TE: Laboratory procedures in diagnosis of adrenal cortical diseases, in Eisenstein AB (ed): *The Adrenal Cortex.* Boston, Little Brown, 1967, p 405.

578. Abraham GE, Maroulis GB, Buster JE, Chang RJ, Marshall JR: Effect of dexamethasone on serum cortisol and androgen levels in hirsute patients. *Obstet Gynecol* 47:395, 1976.

579. Abraham GE, Chakmakjian ZH: Plasma steroids in hirsutism. *Obstet Gynecol* 44:171, 1974.

580. Paulson JD, Keller DW, Wiest WG, Warren JC: Free testosterone concentrations in serum: Elevation is the hallmark of hirsutism. *Am J Obstet Gynecol* 128:851, 1977.

581. Irvine WJ, Barnes EW: Adrenocortical insufficiency. *Clin Endocrinol Metab* 1:549, 1972.

582. Doniach D, Cudworth AG, Khoury EL, Bottazzo GF: Autoimmunity and the HLA-system in endocrine disease, in O'Riordan JLH (ed): *Recent Advances in Endocrinology and Metabolism.* London, Churchill Livingston, 1982.

583. Neufeld M, Maclaren N, Blizzard R: Autoimmune polyglandular syndromes. *Pediatr Ann* 9:154, 1980.

584. Neufeld M, Maclaren NK, Blizzard RM: Two types of autoimmune Addison's disease associated with different polyglandular autoimmune (PGA) syndromes. *Medicine* 60:355, 1981.

585. Trence DL, Morley JE, Handwerger BS: Polyglandular autoimmune syndromes. *Am J Med* 77:107, 1984.

586. Nerup J: Addison's disease—a review of some clinical, pathological and immunological features. *Dan Med Bull* 21:201, 1974.

587. Guttman PH: Addison's disease: A statistical analysis of 566 cases and a study of the pathology. *Arch Pathol* 10:742, 895, 1930.

588. Xarli VP, Steele AA, Davis PJ, Buescher ES, Rios CN, Garcia-Bunuel R: Adrenal hemorrhage in the adult. *Medicine* 57:211, 1978.

589. Migeon CJ, Kenny FM, Hung W, Voorhess ML: Study of adrenal function in children with meningitis. *Pediatrics* 40:163, 1967.

590. Margaretten W, Nakai H, Landing BH: Septicemic adrenal hemorrhage. *Am J Dis Child* 105:346, 1963.

591. Guenthmer EE, Rabinowe SL, Van Niel A, Naftilian A, Dluhy R: Primary Addison's disease in a patient with the acquired immunodeficiency syndrome. *Ann Intern Med* 100:847, 1984.

592. Weiss L, Mellinger RC: Congenital adrenal hypoplasia—an X-linked disease. *J Med Genet* 7:27, 1970.

593. Stuart-Mason A, Mead TW, Lee JAH, Morris JN: Epidemiological and clinical picture of Addison's disease. *Lancet* 2:744, 1968.

594. Maisey MN, Lessof MH: Addison's disease: A clinical study. *Guy's Hosp Rep* 18:363, 1969.

595. Schmidt MB: Eine biglanduläre erkrankung (nebennieren und Schilddrüse) bei morbus Addisonii. *Verh Dtsch Ges Pathol* 21:212, 1926.

596. Carpenter CJ, Solomon N, Silverberg SG, Bledsoe T, Northcutt RC, Klinenberg JR, Bennett IL, McGehee HA: Schmidt's syndrome (thyroid and adrenal insufficiency): A review of the literature and a report of 15 new cases including 10 instances of co-existent diabetes mellitus. *Medicine* 43:153, 1964.

597. Turkington RW, Lebovitz HE: Extra-adrenal endocrine deficiencies in Addison's disease. *Am J Med* 43:499, 1967.

598. Irvine WJ, Barnes EW: Addison's disease, ovarian failure and hypoparathyroidism. *Clin Endocrinol Metab* 4:379, 1975.

599. Spinner MW, Blizzard RM, Childs B: Clinical and genetic heterogeneity in idiopathic Addison's disease and hypoparathyroidism. *J Clin Endocrinol Metab* 28:795, 1968.

600. McHardy-Young S, Lessof MH, Maisey MN: Serum TSH and thyroid antibody studies in Addison's disease. *Clin Endocrinol* 1:45, 1972.

601. Gharib H, Hodgson SF, Gastineau CF, Scholz DA, Smith LA: Reversible hypothyroidism in Addison's disease. *Lancet* 2:734, 1972.

602. McBurney EI: Vitiligo. Clinical picture and pathogenesis. *Arch Intern Med* 139:1295, 1979.

603. Anderson JR, Goudie RB, Gray KG, Timbury GC: Autoantibodies in Addison's disease. *Lancet* 1:1123, 1957.

604. Blizzard RM, Chee D, Davis W: The incidence of parathyroid and other antibodies in the sera of patients with idiopathic hypoparathyroidism. *Clin Exp Immunol* 1:119, 1966.

605. Blizzard RM, Chee D, Davis W: The incidence of adrenal and other antibodies in the sera of patients with idiopathic adrenal insufficiency (Addison's disease). *Clin Exp Immunol* 2:19, 1967.

606. McNatty KP, Short RV, Barnes EW, Irvine WJ: The cytotoxic effect of serum from patients with Addison's disease and autoimmune ovarian failure on human granulosa cells in culture. *Clin Exp Immunol* 22:378, 1975.

607. McCuish AC, Barnes EW, Irvine WJ, Duncan LJP: Antibodies to pancreatic islet-cells in insulin-dependent diabetes with co-existent autoimmune disease. *Lancet* 2:1529, 1974.

608. Bottazo GF, Florin-Christensen A, Doniach D: Islet-cell antibodies in diabetes mellitus with autoimmune polyendocrine deficiencies. *Lancet* 2:1279, 1974.

609. Eisenbarth GS, Wilson PW, Ward F, Buckley C, Lebovitz H: The polyglandular failure syndrome: Disease inheritance, HLA type and immune function. *Ann Intern Med* 91:528, 1979.

610. Symington T: *Functional Pathology of the Adrenal Gland.* Edinburgh, Livingstone, 1969.

611. Vita JA, Silverberg SJ, Goland RS, Austin JHM, Knowlton AI: Clinical clues to the cause of Addison's disease. *Am J Med* 78:461, 1985.

612. Amador E: Adrenal hemorrhage during anticoagulant ther-

apy. *Ann Intern Med* 63:559, 1965.
613. Greendyke RM: Adrenal hemorrhage. *Am J Clin Pathol* 43:210, 1965.
614. Bosworth DC: Reversible adrenocortical insufficiency in fulminant meningococcemia. *Arch Intern Med* 139:823 1979.
615. Lia L, Haskin ME, Rose LI, Bemis CE: Diagnosis of bilateral adrenocortical hemorrhage by computed tomography. *Ann Intern Med* 97:720, 1982.
616. Lanes R, Plotnick LP, Bynum TE, Lee PE, Casella JF, Fox CE, Kowarski AA, Migeon CJ: Glucocorticoid and partial mineralocorticoid deficiency associated with achalasia. *J Clin Endocrinol Metab* 50:268, 1980.
617. Spark RF, Etzkorn JR: Absent aldosterone response to ACTH in familial glucocorticoid deficiency. *N Engl J Med* 297:917, 1977.
618. Moshang T, Rosenfield RL, Bongiovanni AM, Parks JS, Amrhein JA: Familial glucocorticoid insufficiency. *J Pediatr* 82:821, 1973.
619. Thorn GW: *The Diagnosis and Treatment of Adrenal Insufficiency*. Springfield, IL, CC Thomas, 1951.
620. Thorn GW, Koepf GF, Lewis RA, Olsen EF: Carbohydrate metabolism in Addison's disease. *J Clin Invest* 19:813, 1940.
621. Nichols ML, Brown RD, Granville GE, Cunningham GR, Tanaka K, Orth DN: Isolated deficiency of adrenocorticotropin (ACTH) and lipotropins (LPHs). *J Clin Endocrinol Metab* 47:84, 1978.
622. Stacpoole PW, Interlandi JW, Nicholson WE, Rabin D: Isolated ACTH deficiency: A heterogeneous disorder. *Medicine* 61:13, 1982.
623. Major P, Kuchel O, Boucher R, Nowaczynski W, Genest J: Selective hypopituitarism with severe hyponatremia and secondary hyporeninism. *J Clin Endocrinol Metab* 46:15, 1978.
624. Lieberman AH, Luetscher JA: Some effects of abnormalities of pituitary, adrenal or thyroid function on excretion of aldosterone and the response to corticotropin or sodium deprivation. *J Clin Endocrinol Metab* 20:1004, 1960.
625. Fariss BL, Hane S, Shinsako J, Forsham PH: Comparison of absorption of cortisone acetate and hydrocortisone hemisuccinate. *J Clin Endocrinol Metab* 47:1137, 1978.
626. Khalid BAK, Burke CW, Hurley DM, Funder JW, Stockigt JR: Steroid replacement in Addison's disease and in subjects adrenalectomized for Cushing's disease: Comparison of various glucocorticoids. *J Clin Endocrinol Metab* 55:551, 1982.
627. Thompson DG, Stuart-Mason A, Goodwin FJ: Mineralocorticoid replacement in Addison's disease. *Clin Endocrinol* 10:499, 1979.
628. Kyriazopoulou V, Parparousi O, Vagenakis A: Rifampicin-induced adrenal crisis in addisonian patients receiving corticosteroid replacement therapy. *J Clin Endocrinol Metab* 59:1204, 1984.
629. Smith SJ, Markaandu ND, Banks RA, Dorrington-Ward P, MacGregor GA, Bayliss J, Prentice MG, Wise P: Evidence that patients with Addison's disease are undertreated with fludrocortisone. *Lancet* 1:11, 1984.
629a. Plumpton FS, Besser GM, Cole PV: Corticosteroid treatment and surgery: 2. The management of steroid cover. *Anaesthesia* 24:12, 1969.
630. Hayes MA: Surgical treatment as complicated by prior adrenocortical steroid therapy. *Surgery* 40:945, 1956.
631. Sebastian A, Hernandez RE, Schambelan M: Disorders of renal handling of potassium, in Brenner BM, Rector FC Jr (eds): *The Kidney*. Philadelphia, Saunders, 1986, p 519.
632. Mulrow PJ: Aldosterone in hypertension and edema, in Bondy PK, Rosenberg LE (eds): *Metabolic Control and Disease*. Philadelphia, Saunders, 1979, p 1501.
633. Schambelan M, Sebastian A: Hyporeninemic hypoaldosteronism. *Adv Intern Med* 24:385, 1979.
634. Schambelan M, Sebastian A, Biglieri EG, Brust NL, Chang BC, Hirai J, Slater KL: Prevalence, pathogenesis, and functional significance of aldosterone deficiency in hyperkalemic patients with chronic renal insufficiency. *Kidney Int* 17:89, 1980.
635. Phelps KR, Lieberman RL, Oh MS, Carroll HJ: Pathophysiology of the syndrome of hyporeninemic hypoaldosteronism. *Metabolism* 29:186, 1980.
636. Tuck ML, Mayes DM: Mineralocorticoid biosynthesis in patients with hyporeninemic hypoaldosteronism. *J Clin Endocrinol Metab* 50:341, 1980.
637a. Williams GH: Hyporeninemic hypoaldosteronism. *N Engl J Med* 314:1041, 1986.
637b. Oster JR, Perez GO, Rosen MS: Hyporeninemic hypoaldosteronism after chronic sodium bicarbonate abuse. *Arch Intern Med* 136:1179, 1976.
638. Atarashi K, Mulrow PJ, Franco-Saenz R: Effect of atrial peptide on aldosterone production. *J Clin Invest* 76:1807, 1985.
639. Obana K, Naruse M, Naruse K, et al: Synthetic rat atrial natriuretic factor inhibits in vitro and in vivo renin secretion in rats. *Endocrinology* 117:1282, 1985.
640. Nadler JL, Lee FO, Hsueh W, Horton R: Evidence of prostacyclin deficiency in the syndrome of hyporeninemic hypoaldosteronism. *N Engl J Med* 314:1015, 1986.
641. Sebastian A, Schambelan M: Amelioration of hyperchloremic acidosis with furosemide therapy in patients with chronic renal insufficiency and type 4 renal tubular acidosis. *Am J Nephrol* 4:287, 1984.
642. Williams JA Jr, Schambelan M, Biglieri EG, Carey RM: Acquired primary hypoaldosteronism due to an isolated zona glomerulosa defect. *N Engl J Med* 309:1623, 1983.
643. Carey RM, Schambelan M, Biglieri EG, Bright GM: Primary hypoaldosteronism due to zona glomerulosa defect. *N Engl J Med* 310:1395, 1984.
644. Zipser RD, Davenport MW, Mortin KL, Tuck ML, Warner NE, Swinney RR, Davis CL, Horton R: Hyperreninemic hypoaldosteronism in the critically ill: A new entity. *J Clin Endocrinol Metab* 53:867, 1981.
645. Stern N, Bech FWJ, Sowers JR, Tuck ML, Hsueh WA, Zipser R: Plasma corticosteroids in hyperreninemic hypoaldosteronism: Evidence for diffuse impairment of the zona glomerulosa. *J Clin Endocrinol Metab* 57:217, 1983.
646. Schambelan M, Sebastian A, Rector FC Jr: Mineralocorticoid-resistant renal hyperkalemia without salt wasting (type II pseudohypoaldosteronism): Role of increased renal chloride reabsorption. *Kidney Int* 19:716, 1981.
647. Huff TA: Clinical syndromes related to disorders of adrenocorticotrophic hormone, in Allen MB, Makesh VB (eds): *The Pituitary. A Current Review*. New York, Academic, 1977, p 153.
648. Asa SL, Kalman K, Tindall GT, Barrow DL, Horvath E, Vecsei P: Cushing's disease associated with an intrasellar gangliocytoma producing corticotrophin-releasing factor. *Ann Intern Med* 101:789, 1984.
649. Carey RM, Varma SK, Drake CR, Thorner MO, Kovacs K, Rivier J, Vale W: Ectopic secretion of corticotropin-releasing factor as a cause of Cushing's syndrome. *N Engl J Med* 311:13, 1984.
650. Belsky JL, Cuello B, Swanson LW, Simmons DM, Jarrett RM, Braza F: Cushing's syndrome due to ectopic production of corticotropin-releasing factor. *J Clin Endocrinol Metab* 60:496, 1985.
651. Findling JW, Aron DC, Tyrrell JB: Cushing's disease, in Imura H (ed): *The Pituitary Gland*. New York, Raven, 1985, p 441.
652. Plotz CM, Knowlton AI, Kagan C: The natural history of Cushing's syndrome. *Am J Med* 13:597, 1952.
653. Ratcliffe JG, Knight RA, Besser GM, Landon J, Stansfield AG: Tumor and plasma ACTH concentrations in patients with and without the ectopic ACTH syndrome. *Clin Endocrinol* 1:27, 1972.
654. Azzopardi JG, Freeman E, Pook G: Endocrine and metabolic disorders in bronchial carcinoma. *Br Med J* 4:528, 1970.
655. Gewirtz G, Yalow RS: Ectopic ACTH production in carcinoma of the lung. *J Clin Invest* 53:1022, 1974.
656. Knight RA, Ratcliffe JG, Besser GM: Tumor ACTH concen-

trations in ectopic ACTH syndrome and in control tissues. *Proc R Soc Med* 64:1266, 1971.

657. Bloomfield GA, Holdaway IM, Corrin B, Ratcliffe JG, Rees GM, Ellison M, Rees LH: Lung tumors and ACTH production. *Clin Endocrinol* 6:95, 1977.

658. Neville AM, Symington T: The pathology of the adrenal gland in Cushing's syndrome. *J Pathol Bacteriol* 93:19, 1967.

659. Hutter AM, Kayhoe DE: Adrenal cortical carcinoma. Clinical features of 138 patients. *Am J Med* 41:572, 1966.

660. Symington T: *Functional Pathology of the Human Adrenal Gland.* Edinburgh and London, E and S Livingston, 1969, p 121.

661. McArthur RG, Cloutier MD, Hayles AB, Sprague RG: Cushing's disease in children. *Mayo Clin Proc* 47:318, 1972.

662. Jennings AS, Liddle GW, Orth DN: Results of treating childhood Cushing's disease with pituitary irradiation. *N Engl J Med* 297:958, 1977.

663. Cassar J, Doyle FH, Mashiter K, Joplin GF: Treatment of Cushing's disease in juveniles with interstitial pituitary irradiation. *Clin Endocrinol* 11:313, 1979.

664. Styne DM, Grumbach MM, Kaplan SL, Wilson CB, Conte FA: Treatment of Cushing's disease in childhood and adolescence by transsphenoidal microadenomectomy. *N Engl J Med* 310:889, 1984.

665. Eisenhardt L, Thompson KW: A brief consideration of the present status of so-called pituitary basophilism. *Yale J Biol Med* 11:507, 1939.

666. Robert F, Pelletier G, Hardy J: Pituitary adenomas in Cushing's disease. *Arch Pathol Lab Med* 102:448, 1978.

667. Tyrrell JB, Brooks RM, Fitzgerald PA, Cofoid PB, Forsham PH, Wilson CW: Cushing's disease. Selective transsphenoidal resection of pituitary adenomas. *N Engl J Med* 298:753, 1978.

668. Boggan JE, Tyrrell JB, Wilson CB: Transsphenoidal microsurgical management of Cushing's disease. *J Neurosurg* 59:195, 1983.

669. Rovitt RL, Duane TD: Cushing's syndrome and pituitary tumors. Pathophysiology and ocular manifestations of ACTH-secreting pituitary adenomas. *Am J Med* 46:416, 1969.

670. Suda T, Abe Y, Demura H, Demura R, Shizume K, Tamahashi N, Sasano N: ACTH, β-LPH and β-endorphin in pituitary adenomas of the patients with Cushing's disease: Activation of β-LPH conversion to β-endorphin. *J Clin Endocrinol Metab* 49:475, 1979.

671. Suda T, Demura H, Demura R, Jibiki K, Tozawa F, Shizume K: Anterior pituitary hormones in plasma and pituitaries from patients with Cushing's disease. *J Clin Endocrinol Metab* 51:1048, 1980.

672. Lüdecke D, Kautzky R, Saeger W, Schrader D: Selective removal of hypersecreting pituitary adenomas. *Acta Neurochir* 35:27, 1976.

673. Peillon F, Racadot J, Oliver L, Vila-Porcile E: Microadenomas, structure and function, in Faglia G, Giovanelli MA, MacLeod RM (eds): *Microadenomas.* London, Academic, 1980, p 91.

674. Lamberts SWJ, DeLange SA, Stefanko SZ: Adrenocorticotropin-secreting pituitary adenomas originate from the anterior or the intermediate lobe in Cushing's disease: Differences in the regulation of hormone secretion. *J Clin Endocrinol Metab* 54:286, 1982.

675. McKeever PE, Koppelman MCS, Metcalf D, Quindlen E, Kornbluth PL, Strott CA, Howard R, Smith BH: Refractory Cushing's disease caused by multinodular ACTH-cell hyperplasia. *J Neuropathol Exp Neurol* 41:490, 1982.

676. Schnall AM, Kovacs K, Brodkey JS, Pearson OH: Pituitary Cushing's disease without adenoma. *Acta Endocrinol* 94:293, 1981.

677. Taylor HC, Velasco ME, Brodkey JS: Remission of pituitary-dependent Cushing's disease after removal of non-neoplastic pituitary gland. *Arch Intern Med* 140:1366, 1980.

678. Aron DC, Findling JW, Tyrrell JB, Fitzgerald PA, Brooks RM, Fisher FE, Forsham PH: Pituitary-ACTH dependency of nodular adrenal hyperplasia in Cushing's syndrome. *Am J Med* 71:302, 1981.

679. Anderson DC, Child DF, Sutcliffe CH, Buckley CH, Davies D, Longson D: Cushing's syndrome, nodular hyperplasia and virilizing carcinoma. *Clin Endocrinol* 9:1, 1978.

680. Krieger DT, Amorosa L, Linick F: Cyproheptadine-induced remission of Cushing's disease. *N Engl J Med* 293:893, 1975.

681. Krieger DT: Physiopathology of Cushing's disease. *Endocr Rev* 4:22, 1983.

682. Hellman L, Weitzman ED, Roffwarg H, Fukushima DK, Yoshida K, Gallagher TF: Cortisol is secreted episodically in Cushing's syndrome. *J Clin Endocrinol Metab* 30:686, 1970.

683. Sederberg-Olsen P, Binder C, Kehlet H, Neville AM, Nielsen LM: Episodic variation in plasma corticosteroids in subjects with Cushing's syndrome of differing etiology. *J Clin Endocrinol Metab* 36:906, 1973.

684. Duick DS, Wahner HW: Thyroid axis in patients with Cushing's syndrome. *Arch Intern Med* 139:767, 1979.

685. Smals AGH, Kloppenborg PWC, Benraad TJ: Plasma testosterone profiles in Cushing's syndrome. *J Clin Endocrinol Metab* 45:240, 1977.

686. Lamberts SWJ, Klijn JGM, De Quijada M, Timmermans HAT, Uitterlinden P, De Jong FH, Birkenhäger JC: The mechanism of the suppressive action of bromocryptine on adrenocorticotropin secretion in patients with Cushing's disease and Nelson's syndrome. *J Clin Endocrinol Metab* 51:307, 1980.

687. Krieger DT, Gewirtz GP: Recovery of hypothalamic-pituitary-adrenal function, growth hormone responsiveness, and sleep EEG pattern in a patient following removal of an adrenal cortical adenoma. *J Clin Endocrinol Metab* 38:1075, 1974.

688. Tyrrell JB: Cushing's disease. *Present Concepts in Internal Medicine* 13:5, 1980.

689. Salassa RM, Laws ER Jr, Carpenter PC, Northcutt RC: Transsphenoidal removal of pituitary microadenoma in Cushing's disease. *Mayo Clin Proc* 53:24, 1978.

690. Bigos ST, Somma M, Rasio E, Eastman RC, Lanthier A, Johnston NH, Hardy J: Cushing's disease: Management by transsphenoidal pituitary microsurgery. *J Clin Endocrinol Metab* 50:348, 1980.

691. Schnall AM, Brodkey JS, Kaufman B, Pearson OH: Pituitary function after removal of pituitary microadenomas in Cushing's disease. *J Clin Endocrinol Metab* 47:410, 1978.

692. Boyer RM, Witkin M, Carruth A, Ramsey J: Circadian cortisol rhythms in Cushing's disease. *J Clin Endocrinol Metab* 48:760, 1979.

693. Fitzgerald PA, Aron DC, Findling JW, Brooks RM, Wilson CB, Tyrrell JB: Cushing's disease: Transient secondary adrenal insufficiency after selective removal of pituitary tumors. Evidence for a pituitary origin. *J Clin Endocrinol Metab* 54:413, 1982.

694. Doerr P, Pirke KM: Cortisol-induced suppression of plasma testosterone in normal adult males. *J Clin Endocrinol Metab* 43:622, 1976.

695. Jaquet P, Lissitzky JC, Boudouresque F, Guibout M, Goldstein E, Grisoli F, Oliver C: Peptides lipocorticotropes dans la maladie de Cushing: Etudes in vitro, in vivo. Proceedings of the 23d International Symposium on Clinical Endocrinology, Paris, 1980, p 54.

696. Lüdecke DK, Westphal M, Schabet M, Höllt V: In vitro secretion of ACTH beta-endorphin and beta-lipotropin in Cushing's disease and Nelson's syndrome. *Horm Res* 13:259, 1980.

697. Gillies G, Ratter S, Grossman A, Gaillard R, Lowry PJ, Besser GM, Rees LH: ACTH, LPH and β-endorphin secretion from perfused isolated human pituitary tumor cells in vitro. *Horm Res* 13:280, 1980.

698. Ishibashi M, Yamaji T: TRH stimulation, and dopaminergic and antiserotonergic inhibition of ACTH release from cultured pituitary adenoma tissues of Nelson's syndrome. Program of the VIth International Congress of Endocrinology, Melbourne, 1980, p 407.

699. Liddle GW, Nicholson WE, Island DP, Orth DN, Abe K, Lowder SC: Clinical and laboratory studies of ectopic humoral syndromes. *Recent Prog Horm Res* 25:283, 1969.
700. Orth DN: Establishment of human malignant melanoma clonal cell lines that secrete ectopic adrenocorticotropin. *Nature (New Biol)* 242:26, 1973.
701. Hashimoto K, Takahara J, Ogawa N, Yunoki S, Ofuji T, Arata A, Kanda S, Terada K: Adrenocorticotropin, β-lipotropin, β-endorphin and corticotropin-releasing factor-like activity in an adrenocorticotropin-producing nephroblastoma. *J Clin Endocrinol Metab* 50:461, 1980.
702. Rees LH, Bloomfield GA, Gilkes JJH, Jeffcoate WJ, Besser GM: ACTH as a tumor marker. *Ann NY Acad Sci* 297:603, 1977.
703. Allen RG, Orwell E, Kendall JW, Herbert E, Paxton H: The distribution of forms of adrenocorticotropin and β-endorphin in normal, tumorous, and autopsy human anterior pituitary tissue: Virtual absence of 13K adrenocorticotropin. *J Clin Endocrinol Metab* 51:376, 1980.
704. Singer W, Kovacs K, Ryan N, Horvath E: Ectopic ACTH syndrome: Clinicopathological correlations. *J Clin Pathol* 31:591, 1978.
705. Azzopardi JG, Williams ED: Pathology of nonendocrine tumors associated with Cushing's syndrome. *Cancer* 22:274, 1968.
706. Luton J-P, Thieblot P, Valcke JC, Mahoudeau JA, Bicaire H: Reversible gonadotropin deficiency in male Cushing's disease. *J Clin Endocrinol Metab* 45:488, 1977.
707. Ross EJ, Marshall-Jones P, Friedman M: Cushing's syndrome: Diagnostic criteria. *Q J Med* 35:149, 1966.
708. Friedman M, Marshall-Jones P, Ross EJ: Cushing's syndrome: Adrenocortical hyperactivity secondary to neoplasms arising outside the pituitary-adrenal system. *Q J Med* 35:193, 1966.
709. Soffer LJ, Iannaccone A, Gabrilove JL: Cushing's syndrome: A study of fifty patients. *Am J Med* 30:129, 1961.
710. Prunty FTG, Brooks RV, Dupre J, Gilmette TMD, Hutchinson JSM, McSwiney RR, Mills IH: Adrenocortical hyperfunction and potassium metabolism in patients with "non-endocrine" tumors and Cushing's syndrome. *J Clin Endocrinol Metab* 23:737, 163.
711a. Finding JW, Tyrrell JB: Occult ectopic secretion of corticotropin. *Arch Intern Med* 146:929, 1986.
711b. Nugent CA, Nicols T, Tyler FH: Diagnosis of Cushing's syndrome: Single dose dexamethasone test. *Arch Intern Med* 116:172, 1965.
712. Yamaji T, Ishibashi M, Sekihara H, Itabashi A, Yanaihara T: Serum dehydroepiandrosterone sulfate in Cushing's syndrome. *J Clin Endocrinol Metab* 59:1164, 1984.
713. Bailey RE: Periodic hormonogenesis—a new phenomenon: Periodicity in function of a hormone-producing tumor in man. *J Clin Endocrinol Metab* 32:317, 1971.
714. Blau N, Miller WE, Miller ER, Cervi-Skinner J: Spontaneous remission of Cushing's syndrome in a patient with an adrenal adenoma. *J Clin Endocrinol Metab* 40:659, 1975.
715. Lamberts SWJ, Klijn JGM, DeJong FH, Birkenhäger JC: Hormone secretion in alcohol-induced pseudo-Cushing's syndrome: Differential diagnosis with Cushing's disease. *JAMA* 242:1640, 1979.
716. Gold PW, Loriaux DL, Roy A, Kling MA, Calabrese JR, Kellner CH, Nieman LK, Post RM, Pickar D, Gallucci W, Avgerinos P, Paul S, Oldfield EH, Cutler GB Jr, Chrousos GP: Responses to corticotropin-releasing hormone in the hypercortisolism of depression and Cushing's disease. *N Engl J Med* 314:1329, 1986.
717. Orth DN: The old and the new in Cushing's syndrome. *N Engl J Med* 310:649, 1984.
718. Corrigan DF, Schaaf M, Whaley RA, Czerwinski CL, Earll JM: Selective venous sampling to differentiate ectopic ACTH secretion from pituitary Cushing's syndrome. *N Engl J Med* 296:861, 1977.
719. Findling JW, Aron DC, Tyrrell JB, Shinsako JH, Fitzgerald PA, Norman D, Wilson CB, Forsham PH: Selective venous sampling for ACTH in Cushing's syndrome: Differentiation between Cushing's disease and the ectopic ACTH syndrome. *Ann Intern Med* 94:647, 1981.
720. Howlett TA, Rees HL, Besser GM: Cushing's syndrome. *Clin Endocrinol Metab* 14:911, 1985.
721. Manni A, Latshaw RF, Page R, Santen RJ: Simultaneous bilateral venous sampling for adrenocorticotropin in pituitary-dependent Cushing's disease: Evidence for lateralization of pituitary venous drainage. *J Clin Endocrinol Metab* 57:1070, 1983.
722. Doppman JL, Oldfield E, Krudy AG, Chrousos GP, Schulte HM, Schaaf M, Loriaux DL: Petrosal sinus sampling for Cushing's syndrome: Anatomical and technical considerations. *Radiology* 150:99, 1984.
723. Komanicky P, Spark RF, Melby JC: Treatment of Cushing's syndrome with trilostane (WIN 24,250), an inhibitor of adrenal steroid biosynthesis. *J Clin Endocrinol Metab* 47:1024, 1978.
724. MacErlean DP, Doyle DP: The pituitary fossa in Cushing's syndrome: A retrospective analysis of 93 patients. *Br J Radiol* 490:820, 1976.
725. Syvertsen A, Haughton VM, Williams AL, Cusick JF: The computed tomographic appearance of the normal pituitary gland and pituitary microadenomas. *Radiology* 133:385, 1979.
726. Findling JW, Tyrrell JB: The anterior pituitary, in Greenspan FS, Forsham PH (eds): *Basic and Clinical Endocrinology.* Los Altos, CA, Lange Medical Publications, 1983, p 38.
727. Turski PA, Damm M: Role of computed tomography in the evaluation of pituitary disease. *Semin Ultrasound CT MR* 6:276, 1985.
728. Sample WF, Sarti DA: Computed tomography and gray scale ultrasonography of the adrenal gland: A comparative study. *Radiology* 128:377, 1978.
729. Korobkin M, White EA, Kressel HY, Moss AA, Montagne J-P: Computed tomography in the diagnosis of adrenal disease. *Am J Roentgenol* 132:231, 1979.
730. Thrall JH, Freitas JE, Beirwaltes WH: Adrenal scintigraphy. *Semin Nucl Med* 8:23, 1978.
731. Orth DN, Liddle GW: Results of treatment in 108 patients with Cushing's syndrome. *N Engl J Med* 285:243, 1971.
732. Linfoot JA: Heavy ion therapy: Alpha particle therapy of pituitary tumors, in Linfoot JA (ed): *Recent Advances in the Diagnosis and Treatment of Pituitary Tumors.* New York, Raven, 1979, p 245.
733a. Kjellberg RN, Kliman B: Lifetime effectiveness—a system of therapy for pituitary adenomas, emphasizing Bragg peak proton hypophysectomy, in Linfoot JA (ed): *Recent Advances in the Diagnosis and Treatment of Pituitary Tumors.* New York, Raven, 1979, p 269.
733b. Sheline GE: Role of conventional radiation therapy in the treatment of functional pituitary tumors, in Linfoot JA (ed): *Recent Advances in the Diagnosis and Treatment of Pituitary Tumors.* New York, Raven, 1979, p 289.
734. Lamberts SWJ, DeJong FH, Birkenhäger JC: Treatment of Cushing's disease by unilateral adrenalectomy followed by external pituitary irradiation, in Fahlbush R, von Werder K (eds): *Treatment of Pituitary Adenomas.* Stuttgart, Georg Thieme, 1978, p 339.
735. Jeffcoate WJ, Rees LH, Tomlin S, Jones AE, Edwards CRW, Besser GM: Metyrapone in long-term management of Cushing's disease. *Br Med J* 2:215, 1977.
736. Schteingart DE, Tsao HS, Taylor CI, McKenzie A, Victoria R, Therrien BA: Sustained remission in Cushing's disease with mitotane and pituitary irradiation. *Ann Intern Med* 92:613, 1980.
737. Orth DN: Metyrapone is useful only as adjunctive therapy in Cushing's disease. *Ann Intern Med* 89:128, 1978.
738. Burke CW, Doyle FH, Joplin GF, Arnot RN, MacErlean DP, Russell Fraser T: Cushing's disease: Treatment by pituitary implantation of radioactive gold or yttrium seeds. *Q J Med* 42:693, 1973.

739. White MC, Doyle FH, Mashiter K, Joplin GF: Successful treatment of Cushing's disease using yttrium-90 rods. *Br Med J* 285:280, 1982.

740. Welbourn RB, Montgomery DAD, Kennedy TL: The natural history of treated Cushing's syndrome. *Br J Surg* 58:1, 1971.

741. Child DF, Burke CW, Burley DM, Rees LH, Russell Fraser T: Drug control of Cushing's syndrome: Combined aminoglutethimide and metyrapone therapy. *Acta Endocrinol* 82:330, 1976.

742. Luton JP, Mahoudeau JA, Bouchard PH, Thiebolt PH, Hautecouverture M, Simon D, Laudat MH, Touitou Y, Bricaire H: Treatment of Cushing's disease by *o,p'*-DDD: Survey of 62 cases. *N Engl J Med* 300:459, 1979.

743. Graber AL, New RL, Nicholson WE, Island DP, Liddle GW: Natural history of pituitary adrenal recovery following long-term suppression with corticosteroids. *J Clin Endocrinol Metab* 25:11, 1965.

744. Bertagna C, Orth DN: Clinical and laboratory findings and results of therapy in 58 patients with adrenocortical tumors admitted to a single medical center (1951 to 1978). *Am J Med* 71:855, 1981.

745. Hutter AM, Kayhoe DE: Adrenocortical carcinoma. Results of treatment with *o,p'*-DDD in 138 patients. *Am J Med* 41:581, 1966.

746. Nelson DH, Meakin JW, Dealy JB, Matson DD, Emerson K, Thorn GW: ACTH-producing tumor of the pituitary gland. *N Engl J Med* 259:161, 1958.

747. Moore TJ, Dluhy RG, Williams GH, Cain JP: Nelson's syndrome: Frequency, prognosis and effect of prior pituitary irradiation. *Ann Intern Med* 85:731, 1976.

748. Barwich D, Bahner F: Pituitary tumors in adrenalectomized patients with Cushing's disease, in Fahlbush R, von Werder K (eds): *Treatment of Pituitary Adenomas.* Stuttgart, Georg Thieme, 1978, p 326.

749. Weinstein M, Tyrrell JB, Newton TH: The sella turcica in Nelson's syndrome. *Radiology* 118:363, 1976.

750. Findling JW, Tyrrell JB, Aron DC, Fitzgerald PA, Wilson CW, Forsham PH: Silent pituitary apoplexy: Subclinical infarction of an ACTH-producing adenoma. *J Clin Endocrinol Metab* 52:95, 1981.

751. Stockigt JR: Mineralocorticoid excess, in James VHT (ed): *The Adrenal Gland.* New York, Raven, 1979, p 197.

752. Ferris TF: Toxemia of pregnancy: A model of human hypertension. *Cardiovasc Med* 2:877, 1977.

753. Gill JR: Bartter's syndrome. *Annu Rev Med* 31:405, 1980.

754. Spaulding SW, Masuda T, Osawa Y: Increased 17β-hydroxysteroid dehydrogenase activity in a masculinizing adrenal adenoma in a patient with isolated testosterone overproduction. *J Clin Endocrinol Metab* 50:537, 1980.

755. Cumming DC, Yang JC, Rebar RW, Yen SSC: Treatment of hirsutism with spironolactone. *JAMA* 247:1295, 1982.

756. Rosenfield RL, Miller WL: Congenital adrenal hyperplasia, in Mahesh VB, Greenblatt RB (eds): *Hirsutism and Virilism: Pathogenesis, Diagnosis and Management.* Boston, Litton, John Wright/PSG, 1983, p 87.

756a. New MI, Levine LS: Recent advances in 21-hydroxylase deficiency. *Ann Rev Med* 35:649, 1984.

757. Prader A, Anders GJPA, Habich H: Zur Genetik des kongenitalen adrenogenitalen Syndroms (virilisierende Nebennierenhyperplasie). *Helv Paediatr Acta* 17:271, 1962.

758. Migeon CJ, Rosenwaks Z, Lee PA, Urban MD, Bias WB: The attenuated form of congenital adrenal hyperplasia as an allelic form of 21-hydroxylase deficiency. *J Clin Endocrinol Metab* 51:647, 1980.

759. Pollack MS, Maurer D, Levine LS, New MI, Pang S, Duchon M, Owens RP, Merkatz IR, Nitowsky HM, Sachs G, DuPont B: Prenatal diagnosis of congenital adrenal hyperplasia (21-hydroxylase deficiency) by HLA typing. *Lancet* 1:1107, 1979.

759a. Higashi Y, Yoshioka H, Yamane M, Gotoh O, Fujii-Kuriyama Y: Complete nucleotide sequence of two steroid 21-hydroxylase genes tandemly arranged in human chromosome: A pseudogene and a genuine gene. *Proc Natl Acad Sci USA* 83:2841, 1986.

759b. White PC, New MI, Dupont B: Structure of human steroid 21-hydroxylase genes. *Proc Natl Acad Sci USA* 83:5111, 1986.

760. Blankstein J, Faiman C, Reyes FI, Schroeder ML, Winter JSD: Adult-onset familial adrenal 21-hydroxylase deficiency. *Am J Med* 68:441, 1980.

761. Kuttenn F, Couillin P, Girard F, Billaud L, Vincens M, Boucekkine C, Thalabard J-C, Maudelonde T, Spritzer P, Mowszowicz I, Boue A, Mauvais-Jarvis P: Late-onset adrenal hyperplasia in hirsutism. *N Engl J Med* 313:224, 1985.

762. Kohn B, Levine L, Pollack MS, Pang S, Lorenzen L, Levy D, Lerner AJ, Rondanini GF, Dupont B, New MI: Late-onset steroid 21-hydroxylase deficiency: A variant of classical congenital adrenal hyperplasia. *J Clin Endocrinol Metab* 55:817, 1982.

763. Lee PA, Rosenwaks Z, Urban MD, Migeon CJ, Bias WD: Attenuated forms of congenital adrenal hyperplasia due to 21-hydroxylase deficiency. *J Clin Endocrinol Metab* 55:866, 1982.

764. Chrousos GP, Loriaux DL, Mann DL, Cutler GB: Late-onset 21-hydroxylase deficiency mimicking idiopathic hirsutism or polycystic ovarian disease. *Ann Intern Med* 96:143, 1982.

765. Levine LS, Dupont B, Lorenzen F, Pang S, Pollack MS, Oberfield SE, Kohn B, Lerner A, Cacciari E, Mantero F, Cassio A, Scaroni C, Chiumello G, Rondanini GF, Gargantini L, Giovanelli G, Virdis R, Bartolotta E, Migliori C, Pintor C, Tato L, Barboni F, New MI: Cryptic 21-hydroxylase deficiency in families of patients with classical congenital adrenal hyperplasia. *J Clin Endocrinol Metab* 51:1316, 1983.

765a. Speiser PW, Dupont B, Rubinstein P, Piazza A, Kastelan A, New MI: High frequency of nonclassical steroid 21-hydroxylase deficiency. *Am J Hum Genet* 37:650, 1985.

766. Gutae JP, Kowarski AA, Migeon CJ: The detection of the heterozygous carrier for congenital virilizing adrenal hyperplasia. *J Pediatr* 90:924, 1977.

766a. Werkmeister JW, New MI, Dupont B, White PC: Frequent deletion and duplication of the steroid 21-hydroxylase gene. *Am J Hum Genet.*

766b. Rumsby G, Carroll MC, Porter RR, Grant DB, Hjelm M: Deletion of the steroid 21-hydroxylase and complement C4 genes in congenital adrenal hyperplasia. *J Med Gen* 23:204, 1986.

766c. New MI, Lorenzen F, Lerner AJ, Kohn B, Oberfield SE, Pollack MS, Dupont B, Stoner E, Levy DJ, Pang S, Levine LS: Genotyping steroid 21-hydroxylase deficiency: Hormonal reference data. *J Clin Endocrinol Metab* 57:320, 1983.

766d. Kuhnle U, Chow D, Rapaport R, Pang S, Levine LS, New MI: The 21-hydroxylase activity in the glomerulosa and fasciculata of the adrenal cortex in congenital adrenal hyperplasia. *J Clin Endocrinol Metab* 52:534, 1981.

767. Smith R, Donald RA, Espiner EA, Glatthaar C, Abbott G, Scandrett M: The effect of different treatment regimens on hormonal profiles in congenital adrenal hyperplasia. *J Clin Endocrinol Metab* 51:230, 1980.

768. Visser HKA: Inherited variation in the biosynthesis of adrenal corticosteroids in man. *Mem Soc Endocrinol* 15:145, 1967.

769. Brook CGD: Congenital adrenal hyperplasia: Pathology, diagnosis and treatment, in James VHT (ed): *The Adrenal Gland.* New York, Raven, 1979, p 243.

769a. Pang S, Pollack MS, Loo M, Green O, Nussbaum R, Clayton G, Dupont B, New MI: Pitfalls of prenatal diagnosis of 21-hydroxylase deficiency congenital adrenal hyperplasia. *J Clin Endocrinol Metab* 61:89, 1985.

769b. Pang S, Pollack MS, Loo M, Green O, Nussbaum R, Clayton G, Dupont B, New MI: Pitfalls of prenatal diagnosis of 21-hydroxylase deficiency congenital adrenal hyperplasia. *Ann NY Acad Sci* 458:111, 1985.

770. Horrocks PM, London DR: A comparison of three gluco-

corticoid suppressive regimes in adults with congenital adrenal hyperplasia. *Clin Endocrinol* 17:547, 1982.

771. Savage MD: Congenital adrenal hyperplasia. *Clin Endocrinol Metab* 14:893, 1985.

772. Pang S, Levine LS, Cederqvist LL, Fuentes M, Riccardi VM, Holcombe JH, Nitowsky HM, Sachs G, Anderson CE, Duchon MA, Owens R, Merkatz I, New MI: Amniotic fluid concentrations of Δ^5 and Δ^4 steroids in fetuses with congenital adrenal hyperplasia due to 21-hydroxylase deficiency and in anencephalic fetuses. *J Clin Endocrinol Metab* 51:223, 1980.

772a. David M, Forest MG: Prenatal treatment of congenital adrenal hyperplasia resulting from 21-hydroxylase deficiency. *J Pediatr* 105:799, 1984.

722b. Evans MI, Chrousos GP, Mann DW, Larsen JW, Green I, McCluskey J, Loriaux DL, Fletcher JC, Koons G, Overpeck J, Schulman JD: Pharmacologic suppression of the fetal adrenal gland in utero: Attempted prevention of abdominal external genital masculinization in suspected congenital adrenal hyperplasia. *J Am Med Assoc* 253:1015, 1985.

773. Levine LS, Rauh W, Gottesdiener K, Chow D, Gunczler P, Rapaport R, Pang S, Schneider B, New MI: New studies of the 11β-hydroxylase and 18-hydroxylase enzymes in the hypertensive form of congenital adrenal hyperplasia. *J Clin Endocrinol Metab* 50:258, 1980.

774. Yanagibashi K, Hanius M, Shively JE, Shen WH, Hall P: The synthesis of aldosterone by the adrenal cortex. *J Biol Chem* 261:3556, 1986.

775. Cathelineau G, Brerault J-L, Fiet J, Julien R, Dreux C, Canivet J: Adrenocortical 11β-hydroxylation defect in adult women with postmenarcheal onset of symptoms. *J Clin Endocrinol Metab* 51:287, 1980.

776. Zachmann M, Tassinari D, Prader A: Clinical and biochemical variability of congenital adrenal hyperplasia due to 11β-hydroxylase deficiency. *J Clin Endocrinol Metab* 56:222, 1983.

777. Bricaire H, Luton JP, Laudat P, Legrand JC, Turpin G, Corvol P, Lemmer M: A new male pseudohermaphroditism associated with hypertension due to a block in 17α-hydroxylation. *J Clin Endocrinol Metab* 35:67, 1972.

778. D'Armiento M, Reda G, Kater C, Shackleton CHL, Biglieri EG: 17α-Hydroxylase deficiency: Mineralocorticoid hormone profiles in an affected family. *J Clin Endocrinol Metab* 56:697, 1983.

779. Hauffa BP, Miller WL, Grumbach MM, Conte FA, Kaplan SL: Congenital adrenal hyperplasia due to deficient cholesterol side-chain cleavage activity (20,22-desmolase) in a patient treated for 18 years. *Clin Endocrinol* 23:481, 1985.

780. Koizumi S, Kyoya S, Miyawaki T, Kidani H, Funabashi T, Nakashima H, Nakanuma Y, Ohta G, Itagaki E, Katagiri M: Cholesterol side chain cleavage enzyme activity and cytochrome P-450 content in adrenal mitochondria of a patient with congenital lipoid adrenal hyperplasia (Prader disease). *Clin Chim Acta* 77:301, 1977.

781. Degenhart HJ, Visser HKA, Boon H, O'Doherty NJ: Evidence for deficient 20α-cholesterol-hydroxylase activity in adrenal tissue of a patient with lipoid adrenal hyperplasia. *Acta Endocrinol* 71:512, 1972.

782. Kirkland RT, Kirkland JT, Johnson CM, Horning MG, Librik L, Clayton GW: Congenital lipoid adrenal hyperplasia in an eight-year-old phenotypic female. *J Clin Endocrinol Metab* 36:488, 1973.

783. Martin F, Perheentupa J, Adlercreutz H: Plasma and urinary androgens and estrogens in a pubertal boy with 3β-hydroxysteroid dehydrogenase deficiency. *J Steroid Biochem* 13:197, 1980.

784a. Pang S, Lerner AJ, Stoner E, Levine LS, Oberfield SE, Engel I, New MI: Late-onset adrenal steroid 3β-hydroxysteroid dehydrogenase deficiency. I. A cause of hirsutism in pubertal and postpubertal women. *J Clin Endocrinol Metab* 60:428, 1985.

784b. Visser HKA, Cost WS: A new hereditary defect in the biosynthesis of aldosterone: Urinary C21-corticosteroid pattern in three related patients with a salt-losing syndrome, suggesting an 18-oxidation defect. *Acta Endocrinol* 47:589, 1964.

785. Velhuis JD, Kulin HE, Santen RJ, Wilson TE, Melby JC: Inborn error in the terminal step of aldosterone biosynthesis. Corticosterone methyl oxidase type II deficiency in a North American pedigree. *N Engl J Med* 303:118, 1980.

786. Ulick S: Diagnosis and nomenclature of the disorders of the terminal portion of the aldosterone biosynthetic pathway. *J Clin Endocrinol Metab* 43:92, 1976.

787. Lee PDK, Patterson BD, Hintz RL, Rosenfeld RG: Biochemical diagnosis and management of corticosterone methyl oxidase type II deficiency. *J Clin Endocrinol Metab* 62:225, 1986.

788. Rösler A: The natural history of salt-wasting disorders of adrenal and renal origin. *J Clin Endocrinol Metab* 59:689, 1984.

Diseases of the Sympathochromaffin System

Philip E. Cryer

The sympathochromaffin system is a prototype neuroendocrine system.[1] Its major biologically active products, the catecholamines, serve both as neurotransmitters and hormones.[2–6] The sympathochromaffin system includes two components: the sympathetic nervous system and the chromaffin tissues.[6] The major clusters of chromaffin cells that persist through postnatal life constitute the adrenal medullae. The catecholamines—epinephrine, norepinephrine, and dopamine—are neurotransmitters in the central nervous system. In the periphery, epinephrine serves as a hormone. Although regulated epinephrine secretion from extraadrenal chromaffin cells occurs, biologically effective plasma epinephrine levels are derived only from the adrenal medullae, at least in adults.[6] Outside of the central nervous system norepinephrine functions primarily as a neurotransmitter of sympathetic postganglionic neurons;[2] it may also serve a hormonal function under some conditions. The physiologic function(s) of extracentral nervous system dopamine is unclear, although it may also play a neurotransmitter role.[7,8]

The sympathochromaffin system is a component of the autonomic nervous system.[9] The autonomic nervous system consists of afferent, central nervous system, and efferent elements and is divided, on anatomic grounds, into parasympathetic and sympathetic divisions. Parasympathetic efferents include preganglionic and postganglionic neurons, the former, arising from the brainstem and sacral spinal cord and synapsing with the latter in ganglia which generally lie close to the innervated organs. Both preganglionic and postganglionic parasympathetic neurons release the neurotransmitter acetylcholine. Sympathetic efferents also include preganglionic and postganglionic neurons, the former arising from the thoracolumbar spinal cord. Some sympathetic preganglionic neurons innervate chromaffin cells including the adrenal medullae; the latter can be conceptualized as postganglionic neurons without axons. They release epinephrine, norepinephrine, or dopamine directly into the circulation. The remaining sympathetic preganglionic neurons synapse with postganglionic neurons in ganglia which are generally remote from the innervated organs (e.g., paravertebral ganglia). Like parasympathetic neurons, sympathetic preganglionic neurons release the neurotransmitter acetylcholine. A minority of sympathetic postganglionic neurons, such as those innervating sweat glands, also release acetylcholine. Some may release dopamine. But the vast majority of sympathetic postganglionic neurons release the neurotransmitter norepinephrine. In addition to catecholamines, components of the sympathochromaffin system contain a variety of peptides of potential, but as yet undefined, biologic importance.

The sympathochromaffin system is a rapid communication system. Its direct neural effects are virtually instantaneous and its hormonal effects are detectable within minutes. The rapidity of the latter is comparable to that of the actions of pancreatic hormones such as insulin and glucagon but contrasts with the more gradual onset of the actions of pituitary hormones such as growth hormone, the adrenocortical and gonadal steroids, and, particularly, the thyroid hormones.

It has long been appreciated that the sympathochromaffin system is critically involved in cardiovascular homeostasis and that the catecholamines have prominent metabolic effects. But the precise physiologic roles of the catecholamines in human metabolic regulation are only beginning to emerge. It can be anticipated that better understanding of their physiology will provide insight into the pathophysiologic roles of the catecholamines.

Abnormal sympathochromaffin function is known to cause three human disorders: hypertension due to a norepinephrine-secreting tumor (pheochromocytoma), postural (orthostatic) hypotension due to deficient release of norepinephrine from sympathetic postganglionic neurons, and hypoglycemia due to combined deficiencies of epinephrine and glucagon secretion. There is increasing evidence that these disorders are but the extremes of a spectrum of adrenergic pathophysiology and that several more common disorders lie between these extremes.

SYMPATHOCHROMAFFIN PHYSIOLOGY

Biochemistry of the Catecholamines

Amines containing a 3,4-dihydroxyphenyl (catechol) nucleus are termed *catecholamines.* These include epinephrine (adrenaline), norepinephrine (noradrenaline), and dopamine. The conventions of catecholamine nomenclature and the structures of these catecholamines are illustrated in Fig. 13-1.

CATECHOLAMINE BIOSYNTHESIS

Catecholamines are synthesized from the amino acid tyrosine through the sequence tyrosine → dihydroxyphenylalanine (dopa) → dopamine → norepinephrine (NE) → epinephrine (E).[10,11] As shown in Fig. 13-2, some systems (e.g., the adrenal medullae) contain all the necessary biosynthetic enzymes and produce epinephrine as the major product. Others, such as sympathetic postganglionic neurons, lack the final enzyme and release norepinephrine. Various central nervous system neurons release dopamine, norepinephrine, or epinephrine.

Tyrosine utilized in catecholamine biosynthesis is derived from the diet or formed from phenylalanine, in the presence of phenylalanine hydroxylase, in the liver (Fig. 13-2).[12]

The catecholamine biosynthetic sequence is illustrated in Fig. 13-3. The initial step, conversion of tyrosine to dopa, is catalyzed by tyrosine hydroxylase, the rate-limiting enzyme in catecholamine biosynthesis. Tyrosine hydroxylase (and phenylalanine and tryptophan hydroxylases) requires tetrahydrobiopterin as a

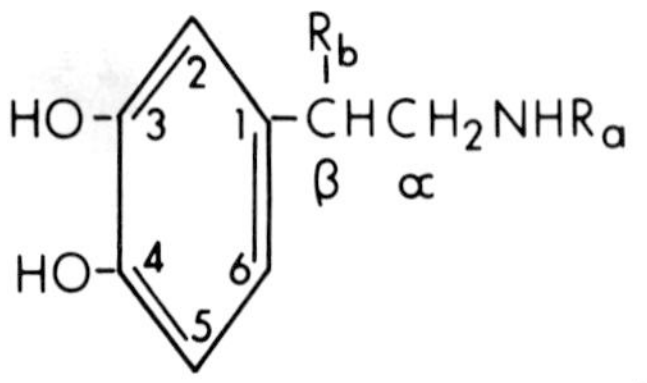

	R_a	R_b
DOPAMINE	H	H
NOREPINEPHRINE	H	OH
EPINEPHRINE	CH_3	OH

FIGURE 13-1 Conventions of catecholamine nomenclature.

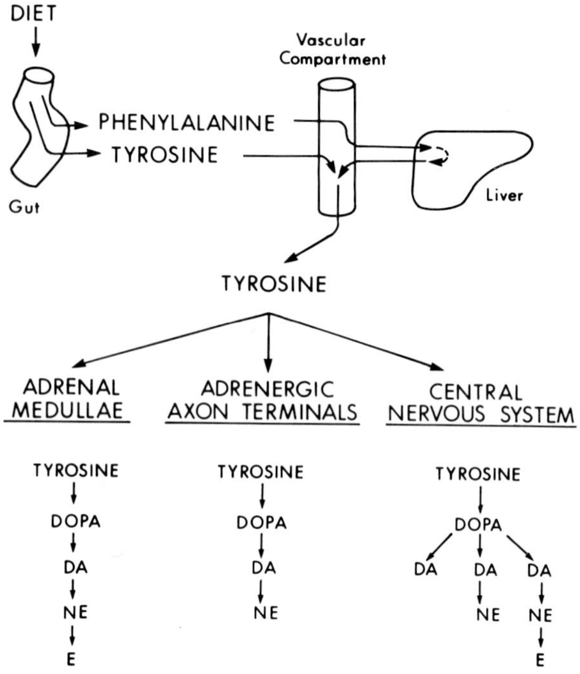

FIGURE 13-2 Sites of catecholamine biosynthesis from tyrosine and major end products in those sites.

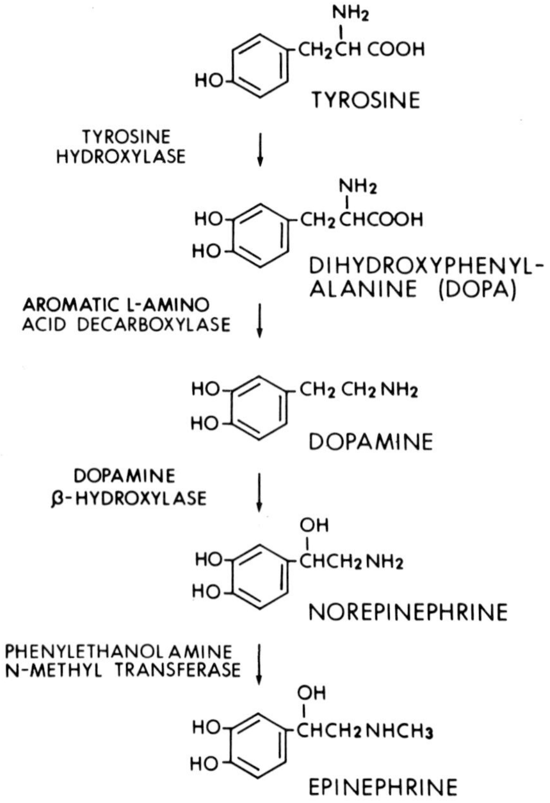

FIGURE 13-3 Catecholamine biosynthesis.

cofactor. Tetrahydrobiopterin deficiency results in deficient catecholamine biosynthesis.[13] Tyrosine hydroxylase activity is product-inhibited. Accordingly, intracellular catecholamine depletion results in a rapid increase in enzyme activity and catecholamine biosynthesis. Activation of tyrosine hydroxylation involves phosphorylation of the enzyme;[14,15] both phosphorylation and activation are stimulated by acetylcholine, the preganglionic neurotransmitter.[15] Further, prolonged sympathetic stimulation results in increased synthesis of tyrosine hydroxylase. Thus, tyrosine hydroxylase represents a major regulatory factor in catecholamine biosynthesis. Because of effective regulation of tyrosine hydroxylase, intracellular catecholamine stores are generally well maintained despite marked variation in catecholamine release.

In the presence of the relatively nonspecific enzyme aromatic L-amino acid decarboxylase, dopa is decarboxylated to form dopamine. As noted earlier, subsequent enzymes are missing from some catecholamine-forming neurons and dopamine is the final product.

In tissues containing dopamine β-hydroxylase, such as the adrenal medullae and sympathetic postganglionic neurons, dopamine is hydroxylated to form norepinephrine. Norepinephrine is the final product of most sympathetic postganglionic neurons.

In chromaffin tissues, such as the adrenal medullae, norepinephrine is methylated to form epinephrine in the presence of the enzyme phenylethanolamine *N*-methyl transferase (PNMT). The methyl donor is *S*-adenosyl-L-methionine. PNMT is a glucocorticoid-inducible enzyme, which may explain persistence of high activity of the enzyme in the adrenal medullae, which receive portal blood flow from the adrenal cortex. Indeed, histochemical studies suggest that norepinephrine-releasing adrenomedullary cells are located around medullary arteries, whereas epinephrine-releasing adrenomedullary cells appear to receive most of their blood supply from corticomedullary venous sinuses. Interestingly, patients with secondary adrenocortical insufficiency (ACTH deficiency) have been found to have reduced basal and postexercise plasma epinephrine concentrations.[16]

CATECHOLAMINE DEGRADATION

The catecholamines are degraded by two principal enzyme systems, catechol-*O*-methyl transferase (COMT) and monoamine oxidase (MAO).[10,11] The major pathways of norepinephrine and epinephrine degradation are illustrated in Fig. 13-4.

In the presence of COMT and the methyl donor *S*-adenosyl-L-methionine, norepinephrine and epinephrine are converted to their respective *O*-methyl metabolites, normetanephrine (NMN) and metanephrine (MN). These can be converted, in the presence of MAO, to an aldehyde (3-methoxy-4-hydroxymandelaldehyde), which, in the presence of an aldehyde oxidase, is converted to 3-methoxy-4-hydroxymandelic acid, better known as vanillylmandelic acid (VMA). Alternatively, norepinephrine and epinephrine can be converted, in the presence of MAO, to 3,4-dihydroxymandelaldehyde which, in the presence of an aldehyde oxidase, can be converted to 3,4-dihydroxymandelic acid. In the presence of COMT, the latter is also converted to VMA. Thus, VMA is a major end product of catecholamine degradation.

As indicated in Fig. 13-4, an alternative fate of the oxidative intermediate 3,4-dihydroxymandelaldehyde is *O*-methylation and conversion to 3-methoxy-4-hydroxyphenylglycol (MHPG). Although MHPG was formerly thought to be a marker for central nervous system norepinephrine metabolism, it is now known that MHPG is formed from catecholamines in the periphery as well as in the central nervous system and that nearly half of the MHPG formed is further converted to VMA.[17–19] It has been estimated that the brain accounts for only 30 percent of total body production of MHPG.[17] Thus, although MHPG is produced by the human brain,[20] and cerebrospinal fluid MHPG can be used as an index of central nervous system norepinephrine metabolism if corrected for plasma MHPG,[21] neither urinary nor plasma MHPG can be considered a measure of central nervous system catecholamine metabolism.

The degradation of dopamine (not shown in Fig. 13-4) is similar to that outlined for norepinephrine and epinephrine except that the dopamine metabolites lack the hydroxyl group present on the β-carbon of norepinephrine and epinephrine metabolites. For example, dopamine is converted to 3-methoxytyramine (via COMT) and to 3-methoxy-4-hydroxyphenylacetic acid (via MAO and COMT). Structurally, the latter compound, better known as homovanillic acid (HVA), corresponds to VMA save for the absence of the β-hydroxyl group.

Physiology of Adrenergic Axon Terminals and Chromaffin Cells

ORGANIZATION OF THE SYMPATHOCHROMAFFIN SYSTEM

Afferent signals for sympathetic reflexes, derived primarily from the viscera, reach the central nervous system via a variety of visceral afferent nerves.[9] Central sympathetic connections include those in the spinal cord and medulla oblongata, where many sympa-

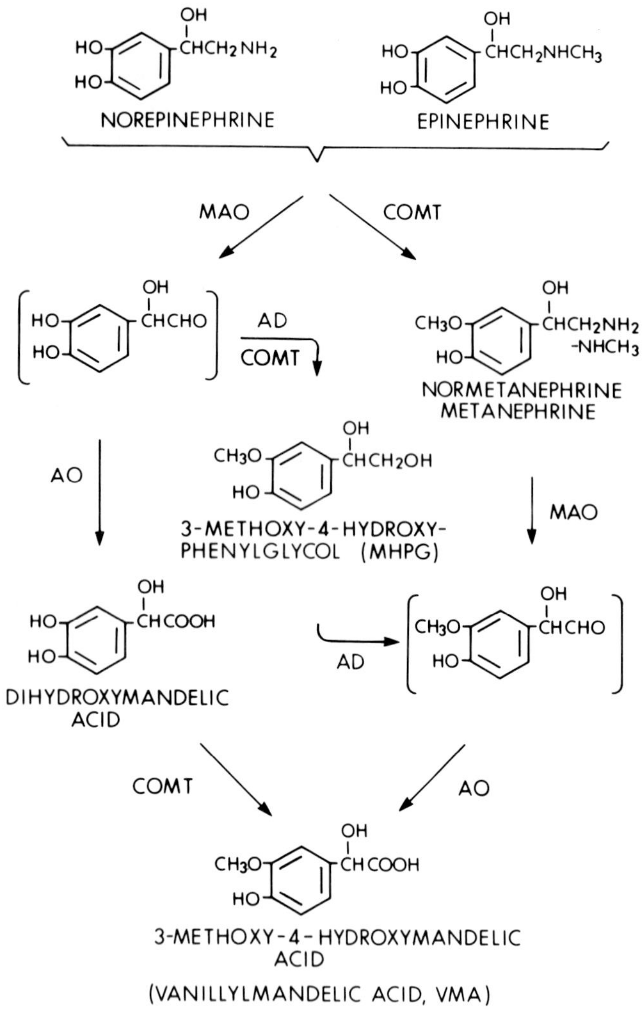

FIGURE 13-4 Catecholamine degradation. MAO, monoamine oxidase; COMT, catechol-O-methyl transferase; AD, alcohol dehydrogenase; AO, aldehyde oxidase.

thetic reflexes are mediated, and the hypothalamus, which is a principal site of autonomic integration. Efferent fibers from these and other central areas traverse the spinal cord and synapse, in the intermediolateral columns of the eighth cervical through the second or third lumbar cord segments, with cell bodies of sympathetic preganglionic neurons. The preganglionic axons leave the cord and synapse with sympathetic postganglionic neurons in the sympathetic ganglia. Preganglionic to postganglionic neurotransmission is cholinergic (mediated by acetylcholine). Neurotransmission from axon terminals of sympathetic postganglionic neurons to effector cells is, in the vast majority of instances, adrenergic (mediated by norepinephrine).

The sympathetic ganglia include the paravertebral, prevertebral, and terminal ganglia. Postganglionic axons extend from the paravertebral ganglia to sympathetically innervated structures of the trunk and extremities via somatic nerves, to those of the head and neck (from the superior cervical ganglion), to the heart (from the cervical ganglia, the stellate ganglia, and the upper thoracic ganglia), and to the lungs and pulmonary vasculature (from the stellate ganglia and the upper cervical ganglia). The major prevertebral sympathetic ganglia are the celiac (solar), aorticorenal, superior mesenteric, and inferior mesenteric ganglia. The greater splanchnic nerve carries preganglionic fibers to the adrenal medullae as well as to the celiac ganglion. Sympathetic postganglionic axons from the celiac ganglion project to the liver, spleen, pancreas, stomach, small intestine, proximal colon, and kidneys. The latter also receive postganglionic fibers from the aorticorenal ganglion. Postganglionic fibers from the superior mesenteric ganglion extend to the distal colon and those from the inferior mesenteric ganglion to the rectum, bladder, and external genitalia. Terminal sympathetic ganglia are found in the region of the bladder and rectum.

The anatomy of the sympathetic efferents leads to progressive spreading of signals. A given preganglionic axon may traverse several vertebral ganglia before synapsing and may synapse with several postganglionic neurons. The long axons of the postganglionic neurons are highly branched and studded with thousands of axon terminals which release their neurotransmitter directly at their effector cells. This anatomic arrangement does not, of course, preclude regional organization of sympathetic firing.

Chromaffin cells are widespread and intimately associated with the sympathetic nervous system during fetal life. Most degenerate after birth; the major residual clusters of chromaffin cells constitute the adrenal medullae. But extraadrenal chromaffin tissues adjacent to the aorta (paraganglia), in the carotid bodies, in the viscera, and within sympathetic ganglia persist in adult humans.[22] The physiologic functions, if any, of these extraadrenal chromaffin cells is unknown.

CATECHOLAMINE FORMATION, STORAGE, AND RELEASE

The catecholamine biosynthetic enzymes are themselves synthesized in cell bodies of chromaffin cells and postganglionic neurons. In the latter they are then transported by axoplasmic flow to the axon terminals where the catecholamines are formed. Tyrosine is taken up from the circulation and, in the presence of cytoplasmic enzymes tyrosine hydroxylase and aromatic L-amino acid decarboxylase, converted to dopa and then to dopamine. Dopamine is transported into cytoplasmic vesicles (storage or secretion or chromaffin granules) where, in the presence of dopamine β-hydroxylase, it is converted to norepinephrine. In chromaffin cells containing phenylethanolamine *N*-methyl transferase (mainly the adrenal medullae), which is located in the cytoplasm, norepinephrine must leave the granules to be converted to epinephrine, which must then be reincorporated into granules. Norepinephrine and epinephrine are taken up from the cytoplasm into granules by an energy-dependent process.

The chromaffin granules of adrenomedullary cells have been studied extensively.[23] They contain catecholamines bound to ATP in association with specific proteins called *chromogranins*, forming a nondiffusible complex. Interestingly, chromogranin A has been found recently to be present in a variety of peptide-producing tissues and tumors and may be a marker for peptide- as well as catecholamine-secreting cells.[24,25] Thus, chromogranins may be involved in storage mechanisms in a variety of granule-containing secretory cells. The adrenal medullae contain distinct epinephrine- and norepinephrine-containing cells distinguishable on the basis of differences in the electron microscopic appearance of the chromaffin granules as well as differences in biochemical composition.[26]

Catecholamine release into the extracellular fluid involves release of the entire soluble contents of chromaffin granules (including catecholamines, dopamine β-hydroxylase, and chromogranins) through fusion and rupture of adjacent granule and plasma membranes. This release process is termed *exocytosis.* It is normally the result of an acetylcholine-stimulated influx of calcium from the extracellular fluid into the cytoplasm.[27] Indeed, calcium-induced aggregation of chromaffin granules and displacement of membrane-associated particles has been visualized by electron microscopy.[28] Catecholamine release from isolated adrenomedullary cells is blocked by calcium-channel antagonists.[27] All-or-none calcium-dependent release of chromaffin granule contents during cell free interaction between adrenomedullary plasma membranes and chromaffin granules has been reported.[29]

Norepinephrine storage and exocytotic release from axon terminals of sympathetic postganglionic neurons is similar to that of chromaffin cells, just discussed. Despite wide variations in norepinephrine release, and some loss through intraneuronal oxidation (discussed below), the norepinephrine content of sympathetic axon terminals is normally well maintained. This is the result of regulated tyrosine hydroxylase activity and norepinephrine biosynthesis, discussed above, and reuptake and storage of released norepinephrine, discussed below. Because of release directly into the circulation rather than into a synaptic cleft, one might speculate that the adrenal medullae would less effectively recapture released catecholamines and, therefore, maintain their stores less effectively. Indeed, depletion of adrenomedullary catecholamines occurs in some experimental models of fasting hypoglycemia.[30]

BIOLOGIC INACTIVATION OF CATECHOLAMINES

A fundamental principle of neurotransmission is the existence of a mechanism or mechanisms capable of rapidly terminating the actions of released neurotransmitter. At cholinergic junctions, for example, the action of released acetylcholine is terminated rapidly by degradation of the neurotransmitter by acetylcholinesterase. Biologic inactivation of norepinephrine released from adrenergic axon terminals of sympathetic postganglionic neurons is accomplished by (1) axonal reuptake, (2) local metabolism, and (3) escape into the circulation.[31]

Axonal reuptake (uptake 1) is believed to be the major route of inactivation of released norepinephrine. Axonal reuptake is blocked by tricyclic antidepressants. Uptake 1 recognition sites have been measured with [^{3}H]desipramine and found to change in parallel with changes in norepinephrine content produced by MAO inhibition (increased norepinephrine) and by reserpine treatment (decreased norepinephrine).[32] Through the reuptake process, norepinephrine is returned from the synaptic cleft to the axon terminal, where it can be stored in granules or metabolized, largely via MAO. MAO is associated with mitochondria in axon terminals and is the major enzyme in the initial intraneuronal degradation of norepinephrine. In contrast, catechol-O-methyl transferase is an extraneuronal enzyme. COMT is present in cells adjacent to the synaptic cleft and mediates the initial degradation of released norepinephrine after its uptake (uptake 2) into those cells. COMT is widely distributed. Thus, both oxidized metabolites and released catecholamines, including those in the circulation, are rapidly O-methylated. As discussed earlier, the major products of norepinephrine metabolism are 3-methoxy-4-hydroxyphenylglycol and vanillylmandelic acid.

From the foregoing it is apparent that catecholamine metabolites in plasma and urine reflect not only local and systemic extraneuronal metabolism of released catecholamines but also metabolic degradation of catecholamines initiated within adrenergic axon terminals (or adrenomedullary cells). Indeed, it has been estimated that only 25 percent of urinary norepinephrine metabolites are derived from the extraneuronal degradation of released norepinephrine.[33]

Catecholamines are cleared rapidly from the circulation; plasma half-times are 1 to 2 min. Clearance is largely the result of cellular uptake and metabolism. Only 2 to 3 percent of the norepinephrine that enters the circulation is excreted unchanged in the urine.[33] Although the catecholamine clearance sites remain to be systematically defined and their quantitative importance determined, they are clearly widespread. Catecholamine removal by the liver, distal forearm, and lung has been demonstrated in humans.

In addition to cellular uptake and metabolism, catecholamines are conjugated, largely to the sulfate in humans, at least in part in the circulation.[8,34] The biologic importance of conjugation is unclear, but it is a potentially important route of inactivation, at least of circulating catecholamines. Plasma concentrations of conjugates are substantial. The concentrations of the corresponding sulfates exceed that of norepinephrine by about 50 percent and that of epinephrine about fourfold in the basal state. The ratio of the conjugated to the unconjugated form of dopamine is so high that some have suggested that dopamine per se does not circulate in the basal state in humans. Amounts of conjugates also exceed those of the catecholamines in the urine. At least during short-term physiologic adaptation, such as standing and exercise, changes in plasma catecholamine concentrations are not associated with corresponding changes in the plasma concentrations of the conjugates.

Axonal reuptake and storage or metabolism and extraneuronal uptake and metabolism are the major processes that inactivate norepinephrine released from axon terminals of sympathetic postganglionic neurons. Only a small fraction, estimated crudely to be less than 20 percent, of released norepinephrine escapes from the synaptic cleft into the circulation.[2]

Neurally stimulated norepinephrine release from adrenergic axon terminals may be modulated by several factors acting through receptors located on the axon terminals.[35,36] These prejunctional receptors include adrenergic receptors (discussed below): prejunctional α_2-adrenergic receptors mediate inhibition of norepinephrine release, whereas prejunctional β-adrenergic receptors mediate stimulation of norepinephrine release. Additional compounds that facilitate release through prejunctional receptors include angiotensin II. Those reported to diminish release include acetylcholine, prostaglandins of the E series, adenosine, histamine, serotonin, and opiates, as well as dopamine. The precise physiologic relevance of these factors remains to be determined.

Several pharmacologic agents are known to block norepinephrine uptake into axon terminals. These include cocaine, tricyclic antidepressants such as desmethylimipramine, and guanethidine. It should be emphasized that uptake across the plasma membrane from the synaptic cleft into the axonal cytoplasm and uptake from the cytoplasm into granules are separate processes. For example, the predominant effect of reserpine is to diminish uptake into granules.

MECHANISMS OF CATECHOLAMINE ACTION

In order to produce biologic actions, hormones and neurotransmitters made available to target cells must first interact with cellular receptors. Indeed, it is the presence of specific receptors linked to intracellular effector mechanisms that makes a given cell a target cell for a given hormone or neurotransmitter. Whereas steroid and thyroid hormones bind to intracellular receptors, the initial cellular interaction of the catecholamines (as well as acetylcholine and the peptide hormones) is at the external surface of the cell with receptors in the plasma membrane.[37,38] These concepts were discussed earlier in this book (Chap. 6).

Adrenergic (catecholamine) receptors are of two types, α- and β-adrenergic receptors (or adrenoceptors).[38–42] Each is divided into two subtypes, α_1- and α_2-adrenergic receptors and β_1- and β_2-adrenergic receptors. Originally classified on the basis of the potency sequence of various agonists,[43] they are now also classified by the potency sequence of various antagonists. Representative agonists and antagonists are listed in Table 13-1. Although the type (α vs. β) selectivity of antagonists is high, it is important to recognize that subtype selectivity is not absolute. For example, although metoprolol is a relatively selective β_1-adrenergic antagonist, it can produce β_2-adrenergic antagonism if used in a large enough dose.

It is fundamental to recognize that the endogenous catecholamines norepinephrine and epinephrine are mixed agonists. They interact with both α- and β-adrenergic receptors. Thus, the response of a given tissue is largely a function of the types (and subtypes) of adrenergic receptors that populate that tissue. As shown in Table 13-1, there are, however, some differences between the two agonists. In general, epinephrine has a higher affinity for adrenergic receptors and exhibits greater potency in vivo as well as in vitro than norepinephrine. Epinephrine has a particularly high affinity for β_2-adrenergic receptors relative to that of norepinephrine. Thus, β_2-mediated responses to epinephrine are more prominent than those to norepinephrine.

β-Adrenergic receptors are linked, through a guanine nucleotide regulatory protein, to adenylate cyclase on the inner aspect of the plasma membrane of target cells.[38,44–47] The biologic responses to interaction of agonists with β-adrenergic receptors (β_1 and β_2) are generally thought to be mediated by an increase in intracellular cyclic AMP and the biochemical cascade, including protein kinase activation, that results. Agonist interaction with α_2-adrenergic receptors causes inhibition of adenylate cyclase; receptor-cyclase coupling is mediated by an inhibitory guanine nucleotide regulatory protein.[45–47] The mechanism of α_1-adrenergic receptor coupling to intracellular events is unclear, but agonist interaction with α_1-adrenergic receptors results in calcium influx into the cell and acceleration of membrane phosphatidylinositol turnover.[46]

Adrenergic receptors are dynamic, not static, and are regulated by agonists.[41,42,46,48] This homologous regulation includes both down regulation (desensitization) in response to increased catecholamine levels and up regulation in response to decreased catecholamine levels. One mechanism of catecholamine-induced down regulation of β-adrenergic receptors is cellular internalization of the receptor; this appears to involve phosphorylation of the receptor.[49] More rapid regulation may involve changes in receptor affinity for agonist rather than changes in receptor density. There is also evidence that nonagonist hormones, including

Table 13-1. Adrenergic Receptors

Type	Subtype	Agonist potency sequence	Agonists: Selective	Agonists: Nonselective	Antagonists: Selective	Antagonists: Nonselective
Alpha	α_1	E>NE>ISP	Methoxamine		Prazosin	
				Phenylephrine Epinephrine Norepinephrine		Phenoxybenzamine Phentolamine
	α_2	E>NE>ISP	Clonidine		Yohimbine	
Beta	β_1	ISP>E≅NE	Prenalterol		Metoprolol Atenolol	
				Isoproterenol Epinephrine Norepinephrine		Propranolol Nadolol Timolol Oxprenolol Sotalol Alprenolol Pindolol
	β_2	ISP>E>NE	Terbutaline Salbutamol Soterenol		Butoxamine	

Key: E, epinephrine; NE, norepinephrine; ISP, isoproterenol.

thyroid hormones and steroids, regulate adrenergic receptors. The physiologic relevance of this heterologous regulation remains to be established.[50]

Dopamine interacts with specific dopaminergic receptors.[51] These are of at least two subtypes: D-1 receptors linked to stimulation of adenylate cyclase and D-2 receptors linked to inhibition of adenylate cyclase or not linked to adenylate cyclase. Dopamine is a full agonist at both D-1 and D-2 receptors. In contrast, apomorphine and the dopaminergic ergots such as bromocriptine are full agonists at D-2 receptors but only partial agonists at D-1 receptors. Phenothiazines and thioxanthenes are nonselective dopaminergic antagonists, whereas butyrophenones and related drugs (spiroperidol, haloperidol, domperidone) are relatively selective D-2 receptor antagonists; substituted benzamides such as sulpiride are also D-2 antagonists. A D-1 receptor antagonist has been described recently.[51a] A third subtype (D-3) of dopaminergic receptor has also been suggested from binding studies with brain tissue.[51]

Adrenergic receptors can be prejunctional (on axon terminals), postjunctional (on target cells adjacent to axon terminals) or extrajunctional (on noninnervated target cells). Prejunctional (presynaptic) α_2-adrenergic receptors on axon terminals of sympathetic postganglionic neurons mediate suppression of norepinephrine release; their blockade, as with phentolamine, results in increased norepinephrine release. Prejunctional β-adrenergic receptors may mediate facilitation of norepinephrine release. Postjunctional adrenergic receptors can be of the α_1 subtype (e.g., those that mediate arterial constriction), the α_2 subtype (e.g., those that mediate suppression of insulin secretion), or the β_1 subtype (e.g., those that mediate an increase in heart rate). Extrajunctional adrenergic receptors include those of the β_2 subtype (e.g., those that mediate lactate production and vasodilatation in skeletal muscle and those on lymphocytes) and those of the α_2 subtype (e.g., those that mediate platelet aggregation).

An interesting postulate, for which there is increasing evidence, is that there are physiologically distinct adrenergic receptors for neurally released norepinephrine and for circulating catecholamines such as epinephrine.[52–56] It was observed that tissues with little sympathetic innervation, such as skeletal, uterine, and tracheal muscle, are more sensitive to epinephrine than to norepinephrine and are populated predominantly by β_2-adrenergic receptors. In contrast, tissues with rich sympathetic innervation, such as heart and gut, tend to be more sensitive to

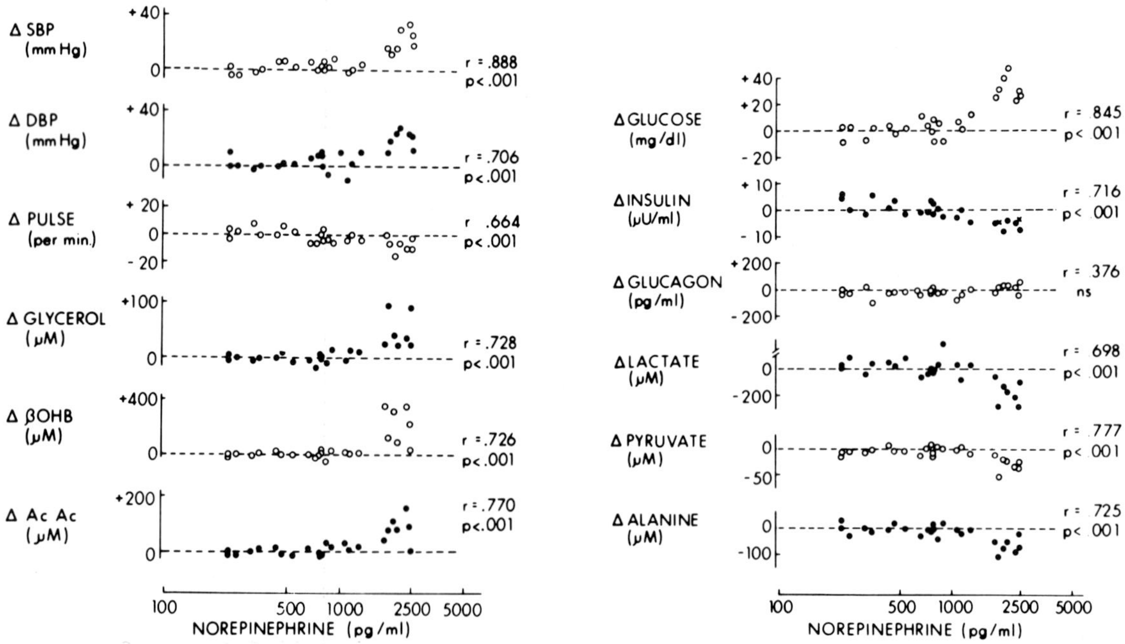

FIGURE 13-5 Relationship between steady-state venous plasma norepinephrine concentrations during 25 norepinephrine infusions in five normal humans and the change (Δ) in systolic blood pressure (SBP), diastolic blood pressure (DBP), and pulse rate; blood glycerol, β-hydroxybutyrate (βOHB), and acetoacetate (AcAc); plasma glucose, insulin, and glucagon; and blood lactate, pyruvate, and alanine. All values are after 60 min of norepinephrine infusion except those for plasma insulin, which are after 10 min of infusion. (*From Silverberg, Shah, Haymond, and Cryer.*[2])

norepinephrine and are populated predominantly by β_1-adrenergic receptors. Thus, it has been suggested that β_2-adrenergic receptors are extrajunctional and are the β-adrenergic receptors for the hormone epinephrine (β_H- or β_E-adrenergic receptors), whereas β_1-adrenergic receptors are postjunctional and are the β-adrenergic receptors for the neurotransmitter norepinephrine (β_T- or β_{NE}-adrenergic receptors). This notion is supported by the finding that neuronal catecholamine uptake inhibition potentiates β_1- but not β_2-adrenergic responses.[54] The findings that stimulated catecholamine release activates α_1- and β_1-adrenergic receptor processes at low doses of the releasing agent and α_2- and β_2-adrenergic receptor processes only at higher doses and that the latter is prevented by bilateral adrenalectomy[55] suggest a similar pattern for α-adrenergic receptors: α_2-adrenergic receptors are extrajunctional and are epinephrine receptors (α_H- or α_E-adrenergic receptors), and α_1-adrenergic receptors are postjunctional and norepinephrine receptors (α_T- or α_{NE}-adrenergic receptors). Nonetheless, it would seem too simplistic to consider all α_2- and β_2-adrenergic receptors to be hormone receptors, since prejunctional α_2- and β_2-adrenergic receptors are probably affected by released neurotransmitter.

Biologic Effects of the Catecholamines

Catecholamines produce a variety of effects in vivo. Many of these are illustrated in Figs. 13-5, 13-6, and 13-7.

Hemodynamic effects of the catecholamines—vasoconstriction (α), vasodilatation (β_2), and an increase in the rate and force of myocardial contraction

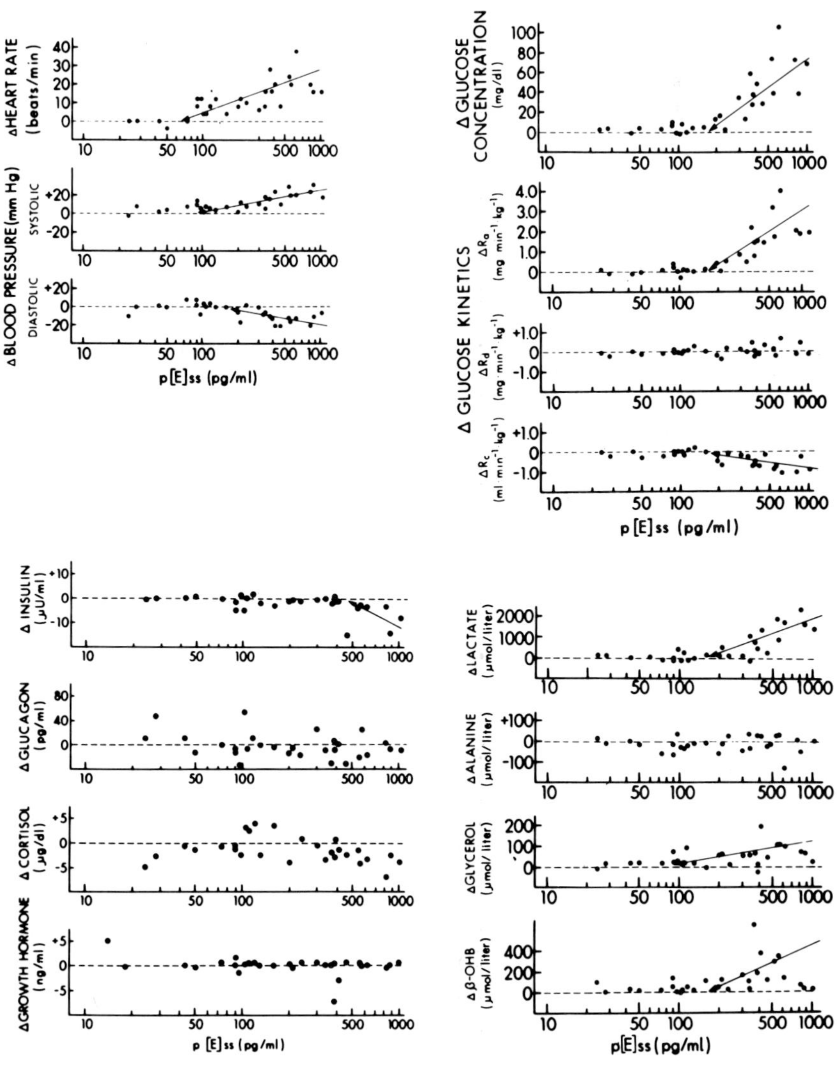

FIGURE 13-6 Relationship between steady-state venous plasma epinephrine concentrations (p[E]$_{ss}$) during 30 epinephrine infusions in six normal humans and the change (Δ) in heart rate and systolic and diastolic blood pressure; plasma insulin, glucagon, cortisol, and growth hormone; plasma glucose and the rates of glucose appearance (R_a), disappearance (R_d), and clearance (R_c); and blood lactate, alanine, glycerol and β-hydroxybutyrate (βOHB). All values are after 60 min of epinephrine infusion except those for blood glycerol (30-min values) and plasma insulin (average of 5- and 10-min values). The arrows indicate estimated plasma epinephrine thresholds for the epinephrine-responsive variables. (*From Clutter, Bier, Shah, and Cryer.*[3])

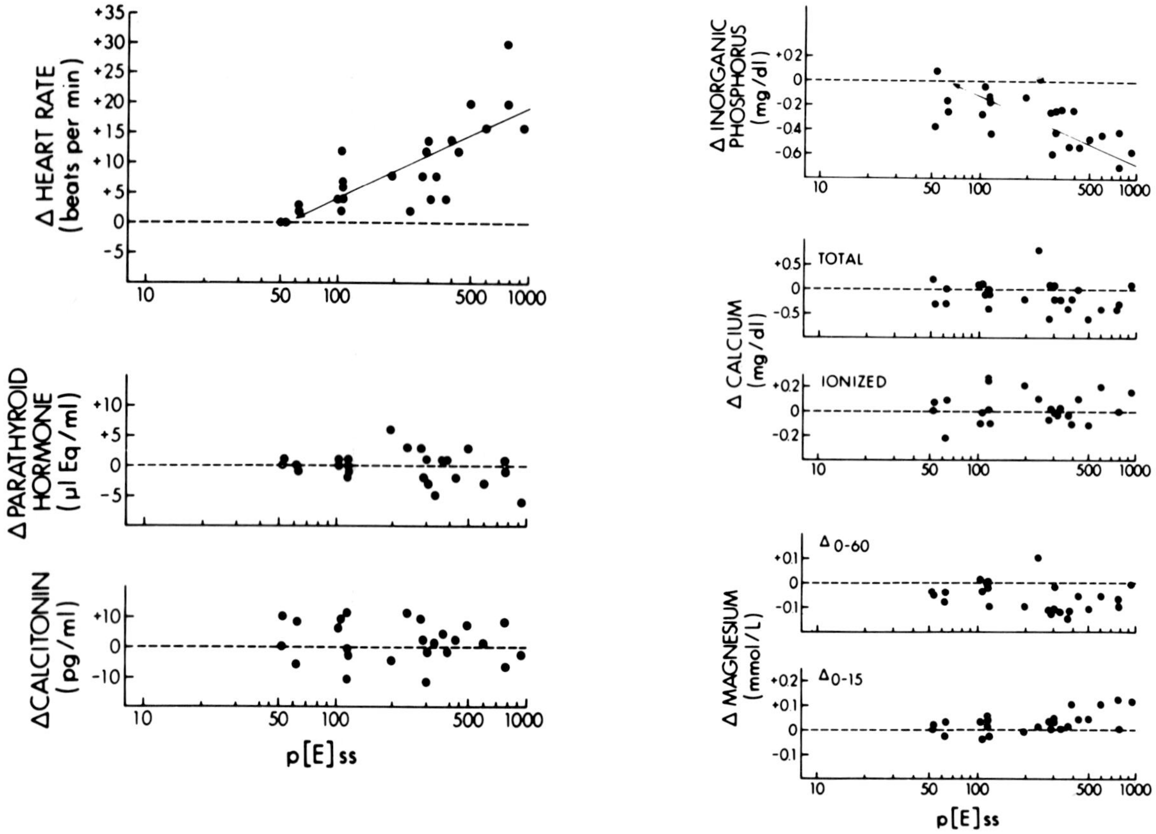

FIGURE 13-7 Relationship between steady-state venous plasma epinephrine concentrations ($p[E]_{ss}$, pg/ml) during 25 epinephrine infusions in six normal humans and the change (Δ) in heart rate; serum parathyroid hormone and calcitonin; and serum inorganic phosphorus, calcium (both total and ionized), and magnesium. All values are after 60 min of epinephrine infusion except as noted; magnesium values at 15 min are also shown. The arrows indicate estimated plasma epinephrine thresholds for the epinephrine-responsive variables. (*From Body, Cryer, Offord, and Heath.*[5])

(β_1)—are well known.[57] Norepinephrine causes generalized vasoconstriction and an increase in both systolic and diastolic blood pressure.[2] The latter causes reflex (parasympathetic) limitation of the increase in heart rate and cardiac output that would otherwise be expected. Epinephrine causes vasoconstriction in many vascular beds (e.g., skin, kidney, mucosae) but vasodilatation (β_2) in others (e.g., skeletal muscle). It also increases hepatic blood flow.[57] It causes substantial increments in heart rate and cardiac output. Systolic blood pressure increases. Diastolic blood pressure does not change at low doses but decreases with increasing plasma epinephrine concentrations that span the physiologic range.[3,4] Diastolic hypertension in patients with epinephrine-secreting tumors may reflect concomitant norepinephrine release; hypotension in such patients may reflect massive epinephrine release, although it is possible that other tumor products are responsible. Dopamine increases cardiac output, an effect mediated at least partially by β_1-adrenergic receptors; the increase may be the result of stimulation of norepinephrine release from adrenergic axon terminals.[57] Relatively small doses reduce mesenteric and renal vascular resistance but cause vasoconstriction in other vascular beds. Thus, systolic blood pressure rises more than diastolic blood pressure. The effect of dopamine on at least the renal vasculature is thought to be mediated by specific dopaminergic receptors.[57] In larger doses, dopamine can produce generalized vasoconstriction and substantial increments in blood pressure.

Other effects of catecholamines include bronchodilatation (β_2), mydriasis (α), decreased gastrointestinal motility (β_1), uterine contraction (α) and relaxation (β_2), and stimulation (α) and inhibition (β) of release of mast cell mediators.

Catecholamines produce multiple metabolic effects through both direct and indirect actions. Indirect actions are the result of catecholamine-induced changes in the secretion of hormones that regulate metabolic processes. For example, catecholamines both suppress (α_2) and stimulate (β_2) insulin secretion; the suppressive effect generally predominates. They also stimulate glucagon (β), growth hormone (α), and renin (β_1) secretion under some conditions. Indeed, there is evidence of adrenergic modulation of the secretion of most hormones, although the physiologic relevance of this remains to be determined in most instances. Thus, although limitation of insulin secretion plays an important role in epinephrine-induced hyperglycemia (discussed below), physiologic (as opposed to pharmacologic) elevations of plasma epinephrine do not alter parathyroid hormone secretion.[5]

Direct metabolic actions of catecholamines include (1) stimulation of hepatic glucose production—both glycogenolysis and gluconeogenesis—and glucose release ($\beta > \alpha$ in humans) and limitation of extracentral nervous system glucose utilization (β);[2-4,58-64] (2) stimulation of glycogenolysis and glycolysis with increased lactate and pyruvate release from tissues such as muscle (β_2);[2,3,64] (3) stimulation of release of some amino acids (e.g., alanine) from muscle (β);[65] (4) stimulation of lipolysis (β_1), with increased glycerol and fatty acid release, which predominates over inhibition of lipolysis (α_1) in fat;[66] (5) stimulation of hepatic ketogenesis, largely secondary to lipolysis and increased fatty acid delivery to the liver;[67] (6) stimulation of shifts of potassium (β) and phosphate into cells, causing hypokalemia and hypophosphatemia;[5,68] and (7) stimulation of thermogenesis (β_1).[69]

The mechanisms of the hyperglycemic effect of epinephrine are complex. They involve both indirect and direct actions of the hormone and both stimulation of glucose production and limitation of glucose utilization and are mediated through both β- and α-adrenergic receptors in humans.[3,4,58-64] These are shown schematically in Fig. 13-8.

Limitation of insulin secretion is an important indirect hyperglycemic action of epinephrine.[3,59,60] α-Adrenergic blockade prevents this effect of epinephrine and reduces the glycemic response;[59] in contrast, α-adrenergic blockade has little effect on the glycemic response to epinephrine when changes in insulin (and glucagon or glucose) are prevented, i.e., when only the direct hyperglycemic action is examined.[60] On the other hand, there is some insulin secretion, albeit limited, during sustained epinephrine elevations,[3,59] and this is physiologically important in that it normally limits the glycemic response to epinephrine.[63] Thus, patients with insulin-dependent diabetes mellitus, who are unable to release any insulin as the plasma glucose concentration rises, exhibit an enhanced glycemic response to epinephrine.[63] The role of epinephrine-stimulated glucagon secretion is less clear. Increments in plasma glucagon during epinephrine infusions have not been apparent in some studies[3,4,63] (see Fig. 13-6) but have been observed in several studies in humans and in dogs.[58,59,70] Although epinephrine-stimulated increments in glucose production clearly occur in the absence of glucagon release,[60,70] this does not exclude the possibility that glucagon may normally mediate part of the hyperglycemic effect. However, using a somatostatin dose that suppressed glucagon secretion but not insulin secretion (as judged by peripheral insulin levels) in dogs, Gray et al. found no effect on the glycemic response to epinephrine and concluded that the effect of epinephrine on glucose production is normally independent of glucagon.[70]

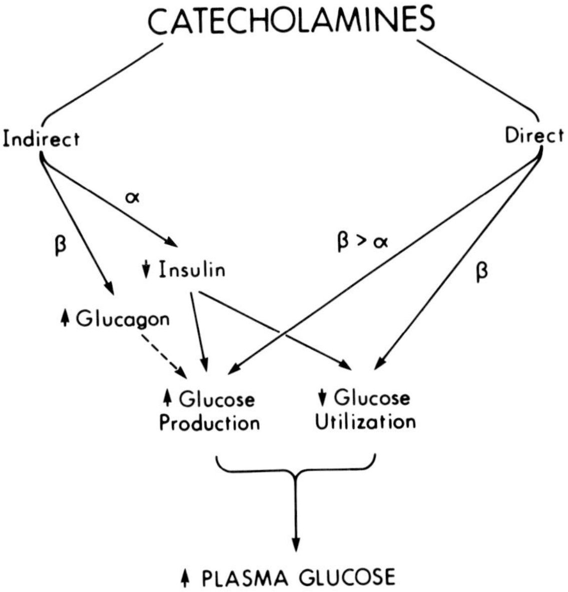

FIGURE 13-8 Model of the mechanisms of catecholamine-induced increments in plasma glucose concentration in humans. (*From Rosen et al.*[62])

The direct hyperglycemic actions of epinephrine involve both limitation of glucose utilization and stimulation of glucose production.[60,61] The first action is mediated through β-adrenergic mechanisms.[60,61] In humans, direct stimulation of hepatic glucose production is mediated predominantly through β-adrenergic (probably β_2-adrenergic) mechanisms,[60] although direct α-adrenergic stimulation of glucose production can be demonstrated under some conditions.[62] But there is also a large body of evidence indicating predominant (although not exclusive) α-adrenergic mediation in rats.[71]

The glucose concentration and kinetic responses to infused norepinephrine are similar to those during epinephrine infusion, although norepinephrine is less potent.[2,72] It is reasonable to assume that the mechanisms of the hyperglycemic effect of norepinephrine are the same fundamentally as those of the effect of epinephrine just discussed, although this has not been studied in detail.

Infusions of norepinephrine and of epinephrine, in doses that result in steady-state plasma norepinephrine and epinephrine concentrations that span the physiologic range, have been used to estimate the plasma concentration thresholds for hemodynamic and metabolic effects of these catecholamines in normal humans.[1-5] These studies are illustrated in Fig. 13-5 (norepinephrine) and Figs. 13-6 and 13-7 (epinephrine). It should be emphasized that these are estimates of *venous* plasma catecholamine threshold concentrations. Although relevant to comparisons with endogenous venous levels, they cannot be equated with biologic thresholds, because arterial epinephrine levels are commonly twice venous levels and venous norepinephrine concentrations tend to exceed arterial levels.[73]

It was estimated initially that plasma norepinephrine concentrations in excess of 1500 pg/ml were required to produce measurable hemodynamic and metabolic effects (Fig. 13-5). At least with respect to the pressor effect, this estimate may be somewhat high. Subsequent studies have demonstrated diastolic pressor responses at venous plasma norepinephrine levels of about 1000 pg/ml or perhaps somewhat lower.[74,75] For example, Grimm et al. found the mean extrapolated norepinephrine infusion rate that produced no change in mean arterial pressure in normal humans to correspond with plasma norepinephrine concentrations of about 800 pg/ml; that required to produce a 20-mmHg increase in mean pressure corresponded to plasma norepinephrine concentrations of approximately 3000 pg/ml.[74]

The estimated venous plasma concentration thresholds for epinephrine are as follows: cardiac chronotropic and hypophosphatemic effects, 50 to 100 pg/ml; systolic pressor and lipolytic effects, 75 to 125 pg/ml; hyperglycemic, glycolytic, and ketogenic effects, 100 to 200 pg/ml.[3-5] Thus, epinephrine is approximately 10 times more potent than norepinephrine.

Integrated Physiology of the Sympathochromaffin System

MEASUREMENT OF CATECHOLAMINES AND CATECHOLAMINE KINETICS

The development of sensitive and precise methods for measurement of catecholamines in plasma (as well as in urine and tissues) has stimulated renewed interest in the study of human adrenergic physiology and pathophysiology.[76] Single-isotope-derivative (radioenzymatic) assays have become the reference methods, but high-pressure liquid chromatography methods using various detection approaches including electrochemical detection (LCEC) are being used increasingly,[77] and a modification of the enzymatic method that employs radioimmunoassay of the derivative (metanephrine) has been developed.[78] Gas chromatography–mass spectroscopy (GC-MS) has also been used to measure catecholamines and their metabolites in plasma and urine.[79-81]

Venous plasma norepinephrine and epinephrine concentrations, determined with a single-isotope-derivative assay in normal humans sampled in the supine and standing positions and during insulin-induced hypoglycemia are summarized in Table 13-2.

Because the concentrations of catecholamines in urine are more than 100-fold higher than those in plasma, fluorometric methods are adequate for measurement of urinary catecholamines. They continue to be used for that purpose in many clinical laboratories. Similarly, spectrophotometric measurements of urinary catecholamine metabolites, such as metanephrines and vanillylmandelic acid, continue to be useful clinically. The clinically relevant analytical methods are discussed in more detail under Diagnostic Testing, below.

There is increasing interest in the application of newer analytical methods to estimations of catecholamine (particularly norepinephrine) kinetics. Since the plasma half-times of the catecholamines are short (1 to 2 min), steady-state plasma levels are achieved rather quickly during continuous catecholamine infusions. It is possible to estimate catecholamine clearance and plasma appearance rates from such infusions;[3,82] the metabolic clearance rate is the infusion rate divided by the difference between basal and steady-state plasma concentrations, whereas the plasma appearance rate is the product of the metabolic clearance rate and the basal plasma concentration. The calculated values are critically dependent upon the sampling site; because of arteriovenous differences,[73] epinephrine metabolic clearances so calculated from venous samples are about twice those calculated from arterial samples;[82] norepinephrine clearances calculated from venous samples would be expected to be somewhat lower than those calculated from arterial samples. Further, the calculations assume that endogenous catecholamine release does not change during infusions; this may not be a valid assumption.[82] Last, and perhaps most important, this method assumes that catecholamine flux into, or out of, the circulation is not altered by infusion of biologically active catecholamines, but there is evidence that this is not

Table 13-2. Venous Plasma Norepinephrine and Epinephrine Concentrations in Normal Humans (Single-Isotope-Derivative Assay)

	Supine	Standing, 10 min.	Hypoglycemia, peak values
Number of subjects	165	60	26
Norepinephrine (pg/ml):			
Mean	220	529	494
SD	83	199	291
Range	65–570	233–1040	179–1180
Epinephrine (pg/ml):			
Mean	30	50	1030
SD	17	29	1070
Range	<10–113	12–148	103–4570
Correlations (norepinephrine with epinephrine):			
r	0.115	0.080	0.829
p	n.s.	n.s.	<0.001

n.s., not significant.

a valid assumption.[3,82] For example, epinephrine infusions have been shown to increase the fractional extraction of epinephrine by the human distal forearm.[82] For these reasons, many investigators have abandoned the use of infusions of biologically active quantities of catecholamines to assess catecholamine kinetics.

An alternative approach is to calculate plasma appearance and plasma disappearance or clearance rates from infusions of tracer amounts of radioactive catecholamines, specifically norepinephrine.[83,84] At steady state the clearance of norepinephrine is the infusion rate divided by the plasma concentration of labeled norepinephrine and the plasma appearance rate is the infusion rate divided by the specific radioactivity of plasma norepinephrine. It should be emphasized that the plasma appearance rate is only some fraction (perhaps about 20 percent) of the rate of norepinephrine release, because released norepinephrine is largely dissipated locally, as discussed earlier;[2] Esler et al. have underscored this point by referring to the appearance rate as the "spillover" rate.[83] Nonetheless, the plasma norepinephrine appearance rate should reflect the biologically relevant synaptic cleft concentration, to the extent that norepinephrine is neurally derived. Again, the sampling site affects the absolute calculated values for reasons discussed earlier. Venous sampling has been used extensively,[83] but, since there is both removal and release of norepinephrine in an extremity, arterial sampling has been advised.[84] Indeed, since there is norepinephrine extraction across the lungs, truly mixed venous (pulmonary arterial) sampling might be ideal,[84] but this is debated.[83] This technique assumes, reasonably, that both labeled and unlabeled norepinephrine are handled identically in the body and, more problematically, that recycling of labeled norepinephrine from sympathetic axon terminals back into the circulation is negligible.

Despite these methodologic reservations, and others not discussed here, there is rather good agreement among the various methods used to calculate catecholamine kinetics. For example, from metabolic clearance rates determined from unlabeled norepinephrine infusions and venous sampling[2] and plasma norepinephrine concentrations in 60 subjects, one can calculate the plasma norepinephrine appearance rate to be 5.7 ± 2.0 (SD) ng/kg per min in basal normal humans. Mean values from tracer studies using arterial samples are zero to about 20 percent lower,[84,85] whereas those from tracer studies using venous samples are about 75 percent higher.[83] Similarly, the basal plasma norepinephrine metabolic clearance rate calculated from unlabeled norepinephrine infusions and venous sampling[2] is 25 ± 9 ml/kg per min. Mean values from tracer studies using arterial samples range from about 20 percent lower to about 25 percent higher,[84,85] whereas those from tracer studies using venous samples are about one-third higher.[83] The plasma epinephrine metabolic clearance rate determined from our unlabeled epinephrine infusions and venous sampling is 52 ± 9 ml/kg per min in basal normal humans,[3] a value very similar to that reported by others;[82] however, the value calculated from arterial samples is about 50 percent lower,[82] virtually identical to the plasma metabolic clearance rate of norepinephrine. But basal plasma epinephrine appearance rates calculated from arterial samples are less than one-third higher than the value of 1.8 ± 0.9 ng/kg per min derived from venous samples.[3,82]

In general, plasma norepinephrine concentrations

correlate with plasma norepinephrine appearance rates rather than norepinephrine metabolic clearance rates.[83,84,86] However, there are several examples in which altered clearance affects the plasma norepinephrine concentration.[83] For example, patients with a degenerative disorder of the sympathetic nervous system (see below) exhibit decreased norepinephrine clearance, because the axon terminals of sympathetic postganglionic neurons are major sites of catecholamine removal, as discussed earlier. Thus, plasma norepinephrine appearance rates are more clearly reduced than plasma norepinephrine concentrations in such patients. Tricyclic antidepressant drugs, such as desipramine, also decrease norepinephrine clearance into nerve terminals and tend to elevate plasma levels. β-Adrenergic antagonists such as propranolol also reduce the clearance of catecholamines (both norepinephrine and epinephrine) from the circulation.[83,87] This has little effect on basal plasma catecholamine concentrations but results in markedly elevated levels when catecholamine release is stimulated. The mechanism of this effect of β-adrenergic antagonists has not been established. Although we speculated that catecholamines might be cleared via β-adrenergic receptors per se,[87] it is quite conceivable that decreased catecholamine clearance during β-adrenergic blockade is the result of decreased cardiac output and the consequently decreased perfusion of catecholamine clearance sites. Indeed, reduced norepinephrine clearance in patients with cardiac failure has been reported.[88] Aging and reduced caloric intake have also been reported to decrease norepinephrine clearance.[83]

In a study of regional norepinephrine kinetics in humans, Esler and his colleagues surprisingly found 40 percent of the plasma norepinephrine appearance rate to be derived from the lungs, 17 percent from the kidneys, 8 percent from the splanchnic region including the liver, and 3 percent from the heart.[83] The origin of the remaining one-third of the plasma appearance rate is unknown, but muscle and its vasculature seem likely. With respect to norepinephrine clearance, Esler et al. found 45 percent of the plasma norepinephrine clearance rate to be into the lungs, 25 percent into the splanchnic region, 8 percent into the kidneys, and 1 percent into the heart.

A different approach to the estimation of norepinephrine production rates is measurement of the quantities of norepinephrine metabolites excreted in the urine.[19,89] This method assumes that extraurinary losses are negligible, requires corrections for epinephrine-derived metabolites and adrenomedullary catecholamine production, and, if used to estimate peripheral norepinephrine production, requires corrections for central nervous system–derived metabolites.[89] Further, it includes norepinephrine degraded intraneuronally, a major fraction of total norepinephrine degradation.[33] Thus, the norepinephrine production rate so calculated must be substantially greater than the norepinephrine release rate. Nonetheless, with this general approach it is possible to distinguish patients with degeneration of sympathetic postganglionic neurons, as well as those with decreased central sympathetic outflow, from normal subjects.[19]

PATTERNS DURING PHYSIOLOGIC ADAPTATION

Human plasma norepinephrine and epinephrine concentrations under a variety of physiologic and pathophysiologic conditions are illustrated in Figs. 13-9 and 13-10, respectively. Note that plasma catecholamine levels vary markedly. For example, plasma norepinephrine concentrations increase two- to threefold when a subject stands. Plasma epinephrine concentrations increase up to 100-fold during hypoglycemia. The plasma levels of both catecholamines increase severalfold during vigorous exercise. Note, also, that plasma epinephrine concentrations commonly exceed their thresholds for biologic actions discussed earlier. Plasma norepinephrine concentrations exceed their thresholds less commonly.

The sympathochromaffin system is well known to be intimately involved in the maintenance of cardiovascular homeostasis during daily activities. For example, maintenance of blood pressure in the standing position requires an intact sympathetic neural reflex arc. Defects in this arc result in postural hypotension and syncope, discussed later in this chapter. The roles of the sympathochromaffin system in metabolic regulation are only beginning to emerge. The importance of epinephrine, in concert with glucagon, in the prevention or correction of hypoglycemia is also discussed later in this chapter. It seems likely that epinephrine plays additional roles in the regulation of intermediary metabolism. Thus, the sympathochromaffin system can no longer be considered important only under conditions of "stress."

The Biologic Roles of Epinephrine and Norepinephrine: Hormones and Neurotransmitters

The biologic roles of epinephrine and norepinephrine outside of the central nervous system are shown schematically in Fig. 13-11. Epinephrine is a hormone of the adrenal medullae. Although regulated epinephrine secretion from extraadrenal chromaffin cells occurs, biologically effective plasma epinephrine levels are derived only from the adrenal medullae, at least in

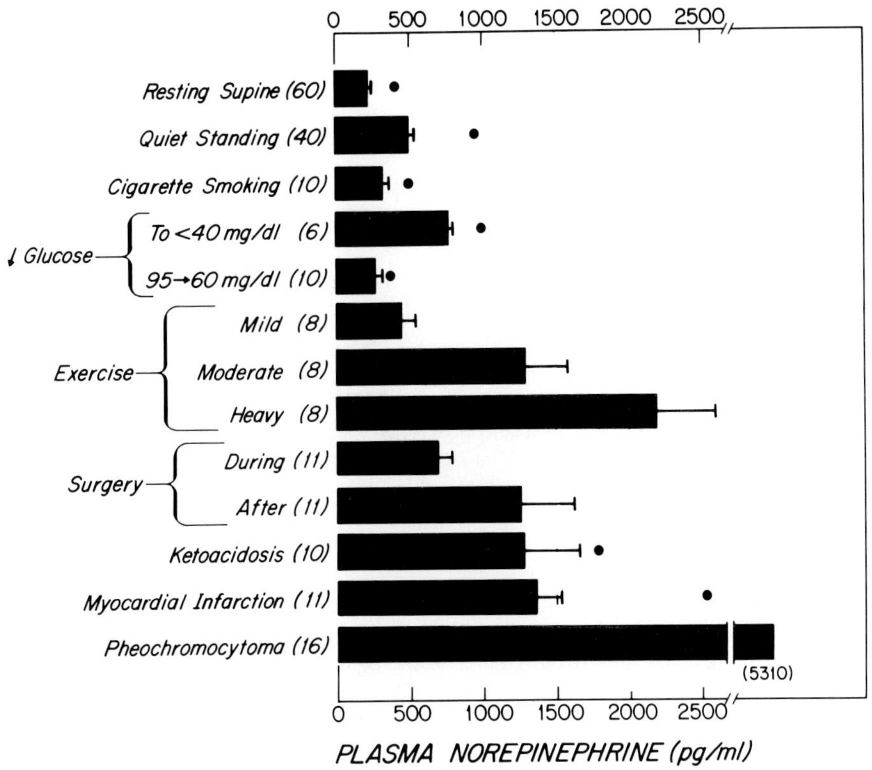

FIGURE 13-9 Mean (±SE) venous plasma norepinephrine concentrations in various physiologic and pathophysiologic states in humans. The numbers in parentheses indicate the number of subjects studied; solid circles represent the highest value observed. (*From Cryer.*[1])

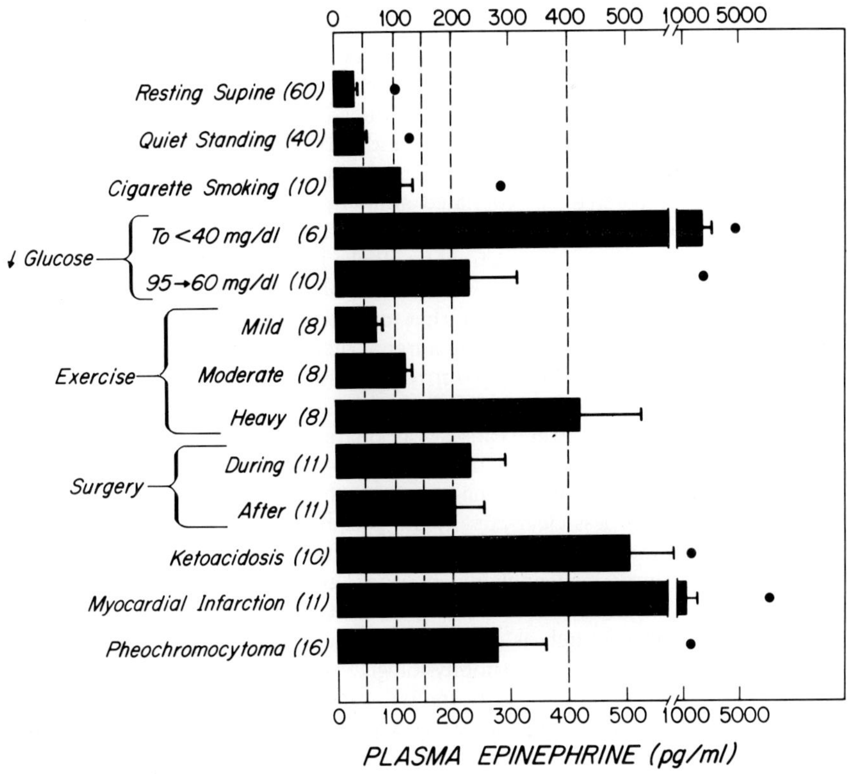

FIGURE 13-10 Mean (±SE) venous plasma epinephrine concentrations in various physiologic and pathophysiologic states in humans. The numbers in parentheses indicate the number of subjects studied; solid circles represent the highest value observed. (*From Cryer.*[1])

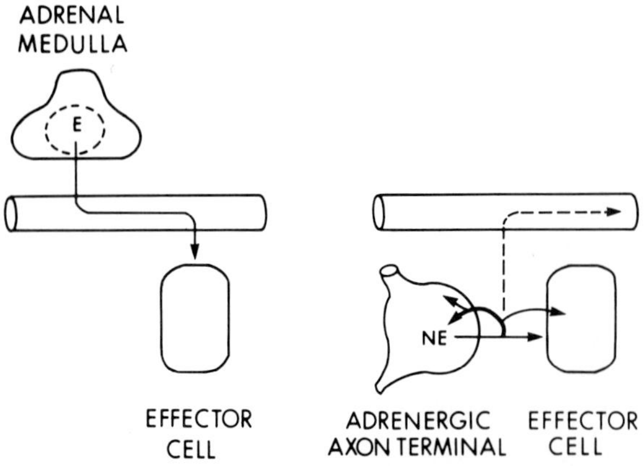

FIGURE 13-11 Schematic representation of the biologic roles of epinephrine (E) and norepinephrine (NE) outside of the central nervous system.

adults.[6] Thus, measurements of the plasma epinephrine concentrations can be interpreted like those of other hormones—as measurements of a biologically active substance en route to its target cells and to metabolic degradation and elimination. Although it seems most reasonable to view peripheral epinephrine strictly as a hormone at the present time, it is conceivable that it may also serve an autocrine, paracrine, or neurotransmitter function. For example, in an intriguing series of experiments in rats, Berecek and Brody observed that the hind limb vasodilator response to central (anteroventral region of the third ventricle) electrical stimulation was reduced by adrenalectomy or adrenal demedullation and further reduced by β-adrenergic blockade.[90] Further, in adrenalectomized or adrenal demedullated animals, the vasodilator response was restored by epinephrine infusions, an effect that was prevented by blockade of neuronal catecholamine uptake with desmethylimipramine. Thus, the authors suggested that circulating epinephrine, released largely from the adrenal medullae, is taken up into sympathetic axon terminals and then released in response to nerve stimulation and, acting as a neurotransmitter, causes vasodilatation in skeletal muscle.

The interpretation of plasma norepinephrine measurements is even less clear-cut. In the periphery, norepinephrine functions primarily as a neurotransmitter of sympathetic postganglionic neurons. Since its plasma concentrations exceed biologic thresholds under some conditions, such as during vigorous exercise and in a variety of pathophysiologic states (Fig. 13-9), it may also serve a hormonal function under those conditions. Nonetheless, to the extent that norepinephrine is derived from sympathetic neurons, its neurotransmitter function must be considered primary.

Norepinephrine is released from axon terminals of sympathetic postganglionic neurons in direct relation to postjunctional adrenergic receptors on effector cells. Transport via the circulation is not required to explain its biologic actions. As discussed earlier, only a fraction, perhaps about 20 percent, of neurally released norepinephrine escapes into the circulation,[2,89] but it should reflect the biologically relevant synaptic cleft norepinephrine concentration. Nonetheless, the plasma norepinephrine concentration is, at best, an *index* of sympathetic neural norepinephrine release.

There is considerable evidence (reviewed in Refs. 91 and 92) that the plasma norepinephrine concentration is a valid index of sympathetic neuronal activity under common physiologic conditions. Under basal conditions in humans the adrenal medullae have been estimated to produce only 2 to 8 percent of circulating norepinephrine;[89,93,94] bilaterally adrenalectomized humans have normal basal plasma norepinephrine concentrations and exhibit normal plasma norepinephrine increments in response to upright posture.[6] Further, plasma norepinephrine and epinephrine concentrations are not correlated in normal humans sampled in the supine, resting state or after 10 min of standing (Table 13-2), findings suggesting different sources (and regulation) of norepinephrine and epinephrine release. Thus, the plasma norepinephrine concentration is a reasonable index of sympathetic neuronal activity in the basal state and during ordinary upright activity. It is not, however, an optimally sensitive measure of sympathetic neuronal activity. It is conceivable that directionally different changes in sympathetic activity in different target tissues could occur with no change in the plasma norepinephrine concentration.[91] It is clear that increments in sympathetic activity sufficient to produce measurable biologic effects can be associated with small or even undetectable increments in plasma norepinephrine.[95,96] Last, as discussed earlier, altered norepinephrine clearance from the circulation can alter the impact of norepinephrine release on the plasma norepinephrine concentration.[83]

It cannot be assumed, however, that increments in plasma norepinephrine are derived from sympathetic neurons under all conditions. It has been estimated that the adrenal medullae contribute 30 to 45 percent of circulating norepinephrine in stressed animals.[92] Their contribution may be even greater during hypoglycemia. Studies in animals have consistently failed to demonstrate increased tissue (i.e., sympathetic neuronal) norepinephrine turnover during hypoglycemia despite increments in norepinephrine excretion;[30,97] the latter is prevented by adrenalectomy.[30] The capacity of the human adrenal medullae to release norepinephrine (along with large amounts of epinephrine) is well established.[93,94,98] Plasma norepinephrine and epinephrine concentrations are correlated highly during hypoglycemia in normal humans (Table 13-2), suggesting a predominant adrenomedullary source of the increments in norepinephrine. Further, in contrast to normal persons (Table 13-2), bilaterally adrenalectomized humans exhibit no increase in plasma norepinephrine during hypoglycemia.[6] Thus, the plasma norepinephrine response to hypoglycemia is derived predominantly from the adrenal medullae rather than from sympathetic neurons.[97] Clearly, the plasma norepinephrine concentration is not an index of sympathetic neuronal activity under this condition.

The origins of the increments in plasma norepinephrine (Fig. 13-9) that occur under other physiologic conditions such as exercise and in pathophysiologic states such as surgery, diabetic ketoacidosis, and acute myocardial infarction have not been established conclusively. However, since these are often associated with substantial increments in plasma epinephrine (Fig. 13-10), the adrenal medullae probably contribute to the circulating norepinephrine pool. Thus, the plasma norepinephrine concentration is best viewed as an index of net sympathochromaffin activity under these conditions.

SYMPATHOCHROMAFFIN PATHOPHYSIOLOGY

Pheochromocytoma

Pheochromocytomas are catecholamine-producing tumors that typically cause hypertension.[99,100] They are an uncommon cause of hypertension; approximately one in 1000 hypertensive patients harbors a pheochromocytoma.[101,102] Yet it is important to detect a pheochromocytoma when it is present, for several reasons. First, hypertension due to a pheochromocytoma is often curable by surgical removal of the tumor. Second, patients with a pheochromocytoma are at risk for a lethal hypertensive paroxysm. Third, there is an incidence, albeit probably less than 5 percent, of malignancy among pheochromocytomas,[99] and early detection and removal would be expected to reduce the frequency of metastatic disease. Extra-adrenal pheochromocytomas (paragangliomas) are more often malignant.[99] Fourth, the presence of pheochromocytomas can be a clue to the presence of associated endocrine and nonendocrine familial disorders.

Pheochromocytomas are components of the multiple endocrine neoplasia type 2 (MEN 2) and type 3 (MEN 3) syndromes.[103-106] These familial disorders are inherited as autosomal dominant traits. MEN 2 (Sipple's syndrome) includes medullary carcinoma of the thyroid, primary hyperparathyroidism, and pheochromocytoma. MEN 3 (sometimes called MEN 2b) includes medullary carcinoma of the thyroid, multiple mucosal neuromas, and pheochromocytoma. It is fundamental to exclude pheochromocytoma *before* neck surgery in a member of such a family, since an unrecognized pheochromocytoma can result in a fatal hypertensive paroxysm during surgery. Familial pheochromocytoma also occurs as an isolated disorder and in neurofibromatosis and in some kindreds with von Hippel-Lindau syndrome (including hemangioblastomas of the retinas, cerebellum, and other areas of the central nervous system). Pheochromocytomas occur in less than 1 percent of patients with neurofibromatosis but up to 25 percent in some kindreds with von Hippel-Lindau syndrome.[107]

Clinical manifestations of pheochromocytomas are generally the result of released catecholamines. They often contain a variety of peptides, including enkephalins,[108] somatostatin,[109] and calcitonin.[110] The clinical relevance of these, if any, is unknown. Pheochromocytomas can, however, be a source of clinically important ectopic hormone secretion.[111]

ORIGIN AND DISTRIBUTION

Pheochromocytomas arise from chromaffin cells. Chromaffin cells are widespread and generally associated with sympathetic ganglia during fetal life. Postnatally most chromaffin cells degenerate; the major residual clusters of chromaffin cells constitute the adrenal medullae. Thus, it is not surprising that approximately 90 percent of pheochromocytomas arise from the adrenal medullae. Extraadrenal pheochromocytomas have been found in sites ranging from the carotid body to the pelvic floor. However, the majority are associated with paravertebral sympathetic ganglia or the organ of Zuckerkandl near the aortic bifurcation in the abdomen, and most of the others with ganglia in the posterior mediastinum. Multiple pheochromocytomas, including bilateral adrenomedullary tumors, occur in up to 10 percent of apparently sporadic cases.

Bilateral adrenomedullary pheochromocytomas, with or without extraadrenal tumors, are the rule in familial pheochromocytoma associated with multiple endocrine neoplasia.[104] Bilateral adrenomedullary hyperplasia, thought to be a precursor to pheochromocytoma, has been found in members of such families.[105] Some have reasoned that bilateral tumors are inevitable in a member of an affected family who is found to have a pheochromocytoma and have advocated bilateral adrenalectomy at the initial operation.[104] However, at least in some patients, decades may pass between the removal of one pheochromocytoma and the emergence of a clinically apparent contralateral pheochromocytoma. Thus, a more conservative approach, coupled with careful, long-term follow-up, would seem reasonable.

CLINICAL MANIFESTATIONS

The majority of pheochromocytomas release norepinephrine, and most also release some epinephrine. Rarely, a pheochromocytoma releases epinephrine predominantly or even exclusively.[112,113] The clinical manifestations of pheochromocytomas are commonly due to the effects of released catecholamines, rarely to mass effects. There is marked variation in catecholamine release from a given pheochromocytoma and among different pheochromocytomas. Some pheochromocytomas are discovered at autopsy or incidentally at surgery.[99–102] Whether these synthesized catecholamines, which were degraded within the tumor and not released, released catecholamines at rates which did not produce plasma levels sufficient to cause biologic effects or caused clinical manifestations that the physician failed to recognize during the patient's life is conjectural. However, retrospective analysis of patients whose pheochromocytomas were missed often yields suggestive symptoms or signs. Melicow found that pheochromocytomas were not recognized in 30 of 100 affected patients.[99] From review of the medical records, he estimated that at least 13 of these 30 were clinically functional. In another series more than half the patients with unrecognized pheochromocytomas had hypertension.[102] Clearly, the physician must have a high index of suspicion if this generally curable disease is to be diagnosed appropriately.

Common symptoms of pheochromocytoma are headache, palpitations, diaphoresis, and anxiety.[100] Less common symptoms include abdominal or chest pain, gastrointestinal symptoms, weakness, or visual symptoms. Symptoms are typically paroxysmal and associated with increments in blood pressure. During a paroxysm patients are commonly pale, soaked with perspiration, and markedly hypertensive. Tachycardia is not striking with the common norepinephrine-releasing pheochromocytomas. Paroxysms often last only a few minutes but may persist for an hour or longer. Their frequency varies greatly.

Hypertension is sometimes truly intermittent; in many cases it is sustained but exhibits marked fluctuations, with peak values occurring during symptomatic episodes. In general, these paroxysmal clinical expressions can be explained by episodic catecholamine release; plasma catecholamine levels are higher during symptomatic hypertensive episodes than during asymptomatic, less hypertensive or even normotensive intervals. The event(s) that precipitates episodic catecholamine release is usually not identifiable. However, the relationship between plasma catecholamine concentrations and blood pressure is not close.[114] This may reflect contrasting effects of norepinephrine and epinephrine but raises the possibility that hypertension in a patient with a pheochromocytoma may not be exclusively the result of direct effects of circulating norepinephrine on the cardiovascular system. Indeed, it has been suggested that hypertension may be the result of catecholamine release from an expanded sympathetic neuronal pool.[114] This would explain the relatively weak relationship between blood pressure and the plasma norepinephrine concentration, the hypotensive response to clonidine without a decrease in plasma norepinephrine, and the occurrence of paroxysms that appear to be triggered by reflex mechanisms. However, it would require a coexistent abnormality of baroreflex regulation of sympathetic activity and conflicts with the concept of finely regulated norepinephrine stores in sympathetic neurons discussed earlier.

Metabolic features of pheochromocytoma include an increased metabolic rate (some patients complain of heat intolerance or weight loss, or both), limitation of insulin secretion, and an insulin-resistant state.[115] Glucose intolerance occurs, but overt diabetes is unusual and probably reflects a coexistent defect in insulin secretion, i.e., genetic diabetes mellitus.

The rare, predominantly epinephrine-releasing pheochromocytomas can produce different paroxysms. These may include systolic hypertension, tachycardia, hypotension, noncardiac pulmonary edema, and cardiac arrhythmias.[112,113] Even with these clinical features attributable to massive overproduction of epinephrine, substantial overproduction of norepinephrine may also be present.[113]

DIAGNOSIS

The diagnosis of pheochromocytoma is based upon clinical suspicion and biochemical confirmation. Pheochromocytoma should be suspected in patients with paroxysmal symptoms; hypertension that is intermittent, unusually labile, or resistant to conventional therapy; or conditions known to be associated with pheochromocytoma. Persons with a history of familial pheochromocytoma or other components of MEN 2 or 3 should be evaluated thoroughly, even if they are asymptomatic and normotensive. Radiographic studies should be used only to localize pheochromocytomas known, or suspected strongly, to be present on the basis of clinical and biochemical evidence.

Fluorometric measurement of catecholamines or spectrophotometric measurement of total metanephrines or vanillylmandelic acid (VMA) in 24-h urine collections are the three traditional approaches to the biochemical diagnosis of pheochromocytoma.[116,117] If predominant epinephrine release is suspected on clinical grounds, the urinary catecholamines may be fractionated into norepinephrine and epinephrine. Of the three, VMA determinations give a slightly higher frequency of false-negative findings. Nonetheless, the excretion of all three is substantially increased in the majority of patients with pheochromocytoma. For example, the urinary catecholamines were found to be more than twice the upper limit of normal in 90 percent of one large series.[116] These measurements provide somewhat different information. Catecholamine excretion (and perhaps that of metanephrines) provides an index of released catecholamines, whereas catecholamine degradation within the tumor also contributes to the excreted VMA.

With the development of sufficiently sensitive methods, specifically the single-isotope-derivative method discussed earlier, plasma catecholamine measurements have been effectively introduced into the diagnosis of pheochromocytoma.[118–122] From a direct comparison of plasma catecholamine measurements and 24-h urinary metanephrine and VMA measurements in the diagnosis of pheochromocytoma, Bravo and coworkers concluded that plasma catecholamine measurements were superior, because there was less overlap in the data between affected and unaffected hypertensive patients.[120] However, the two approaches yield somewhat different information. Urinary measurements provide an index of catecholamine release integrated over time. Thus, they might reflect intermittent plasma catecholamine elevations that could be missed by plasma measurements, which provide information relevant to a time frame of only a few minutes. Conceptually similar is the measurement of catecholamines in platelets. Platelets take up and store circulating catecholamines. The platelet catecholamine content has been shown to be elevated in some pheochromocytoma patients whose plasma catecholamine concentrations were within the normal range.[123,124]

Our experience with plasma norepinephrine and epinephrine measurements in patients with proven pheochromocytomas is summarized in Fig. 13-12. As can be seen, most patients have markedly elevated values. Three points, exemplified in Fig. 13-12, warrant emphasis, however. First, occasional patients with typical paroxysmal histories have normal plasma catecholamine concentrations when sampled during an asymptomatic, normotensive period. Second, some patients, commonly those investigated because of a family history of pheochromocytoma, have no symptoms or signs and have normal plasma catecholamine concentrations but are found to have pheochromocytomas. Measurement of epinephrine is particularly important in such patients.[105,106] These are not innocent tumors; lethal hypertensive paroxysms have occurred. Third, patients thought to have predominantly epinephrine-secreting pheochromocytomas on clinical grounds may also have substantial overproduction of norepinephrine.

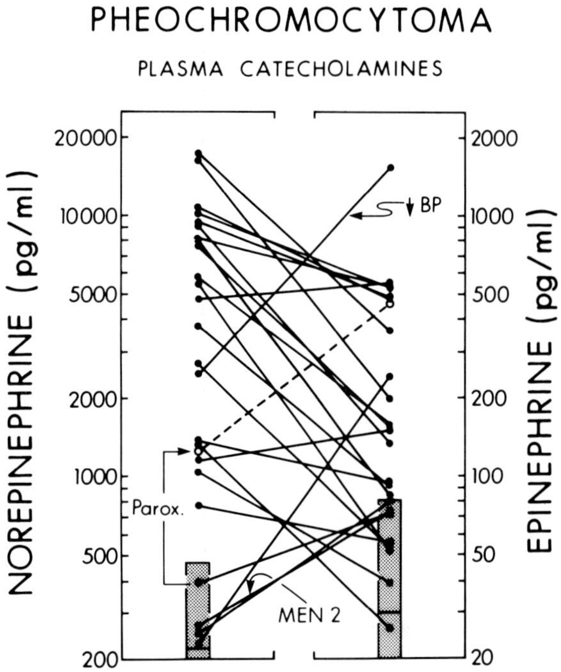

FIGURE 13-12 Venous plasma norepinephrine and epinephrine concentrations in 24 patients with pheochromocytomas. Note the log scales. The shaded areas show the mean plus 3 SD of values from 160 normal humans sampled in the supine position (see Table 13-2). Open symbols show values obtained during a symptomatic hypertensive paroxysm (parox.) in a patient with a pheochromocytoma but normal plasma norepinephrine and epinephrine concentrations during asymptomatic normotensive intervals. The patient with multiple endocrine neoplasia type 2 (MEN 2) was normotensive, had no history of paroxysmal hypertension, and had normal plasma catecholamine levels but had a pheochromocytoma. Because of episodes of hypotension, tachycardia, and noncardiac pulmonary edema, the patient whose values are marked BP was thought to have a pure epinephrine-secreting pheochromocytoma; however, her plasma norepinephrine concentrations (and tumor norepinephrine content) also were found to be increased.

Strict attention to the details of sample collection, handling, and storage, the sources of possible biologic variation, and the effects of drugs, as detailed later in this chapter under Diagnostic Testing, is critical if diagnostic error is to be avoided in the biochemical assessment of patients with suspected pheochromocytomas. Patients should be studied in the drug-free state if at all possible. Samples for plasma catecholamine determinations should be drawn after the patient has been supine for at least 15 min and preferably through an indwelling intravenous needle or catheter.

Samples for plasma norepinephrine and epinephrine should be obtained in the basal state, with the patient supine, when pheochromocytoma is suspected. Substantial elevations over reference values provide strong support for the diagnosis of pheochromocytoma and are commonly found in affected patients. Samples are also obtained during symptomatic paroxysms. However, the interpretation of such values is more open to judgment, since reference values cannot be defined precisely; patients without pheochromocytomas may be expected to have somewhat elevated plasma norepinephrine and epinephrine levels during such symptomatic episodes. Thus, the biochemical diagnosis of pheochromocytoma is more convincingly supported if plasma catecholamine levels are elevated in the basal state and rise further during symptomatic episodes.

It is useful to record the blood pressure and whether or not symptoms are present when plasma samples for catecholamine measurements are drawn from a patient suspected of having a pheochromocytoma. Normal plasma (or urinary) catecholamine values obtained when the patient is normotensive and free of symptoms do not exclude the presence of a pheochromocytoma. Theoretically, 24-h urinary catecholamine or metabolite measurements might detect intermittent catecholamine release missed by plasma sampling. Despite the absence of convincing examples of this phenomenon, measurement of 24-h urinary catecholamines and VMA as well as plasma norepinephrine and epinephrine is recommended unless the diagnosis is obvious.

Since substantial plasma norepinephrine elevations are required to produce hypertension in normal humans, as discussed earlier, and since plasma epinephrine elevations within the physiologic range do not raise the diastolic blood pressure, it is reasonable to consider normal or even minimally elevated plasma catecholamine levels measured when the patient is hypertensive to be evidence against the diagnosis of pheochromocytoma. It could be argued, however, that this reasoning is flawed if hypertension is the result of excessive norepinephrine release from an expanded neuronal pool, rather than the direct result of elevated circulating norepinephrine, as discussed earlier.

It should again be emphasized that most patients ultimately found to have pheochromocytomas have distinctly elevated plasma (and urinary) catecholamine levels. The considerations raised in the preceding paragraphs apply to the much less common patients in whom the diagnosis is less clear-cut and to the always difficult problem of the degree of certainty of a negative conclusion. Obviously, one can never be absolutely certain during life that a given patient does not have a pheochromocytoma. As in many other areas of medicine, a clinical judgment, based upon probability, must be made.

Blood pressure changes following administration of pharmacologic agents, e.g., a precipitous fall in blood pressure after phentolamine in a hypertensive patient or an exaggerated rise in blood pressure after histamine, tyramine, or glucagon in a normotensive patient, have been used in the past to test for pheochromocytoma. These tests are potentially dangerous, have unacceptably high false-positive and false-negative rates, and are not decisive. Consequently, they should not be used. Recently, oral clonidine (0.3 mg) has been reported to suppress plasma catecholamine levels in nonpheochromocytoma hypertensive patients but not in patients with a pheochromocytoma.[125] Thus, the clonidine suppression test has been suggested to separate essential hypertension patients with elevated basal plasma norepinephrine levels from those with hypertension due to a pheochromocytoma. The utility of this test awaits further experience. False negatives have already been reported.[126] Further, hypotension can follow administration of 0.3 mg of clonidine in persons who do not have a pheochromocytoma.

Given biochemical confirmation of pheochromocytoma, anatomic localization is desirable. Pheochromocytomas are rarely palpable, although those associated with the carotid body may be. The rare mediastinal pheochromocytomas are usually, but not invariably, seen on chest radiographs. A history of paroxysms precipitated by micturition suggests strongly that the pheochromocytoma is in, or adjacent to, the urinary bladder. In the absence of this history, a mass seen on chest radiographs, or a palpable neck mass, the pheochromocytoma is almost assuredly in the abdomen. In the past, insensitive methods such as intravenous urograms and suprarenal laminograms were used to attempt to localize adrenomedullary pheochromocytomas, and some physicians advised abdominal arteriography (after establishment of an α-adrenergic blockade) before recommending "blind" abdominal exploration of a patient with convincing clinical and biochemical evidence of pheochromocytoma. These approaches are seldom used today because of the development of more sensitive, noninvasive methods.

Normal adrenal glands can usually be imaged with modern computed tomographic (CT) scans,[127] and the majority of adrenomedullary pheochromocytomas can be seen with this technique.[128] CT scans are the recommended initial localizing procedure. It is conceivable that ultrasonography of the adrenals might be positive despite negative CT scans in an unusually thin patient. External scanning after the injection of radioactive agents that localize in pheochromocytomas has the conceptual advantage of measuring function rather than anatomy, the practical advantage of permitting scanning of the entire trunk of the body, and the likelihood of localizing extraadrenal pheochromocytomas better than CT scans. The initial experience with *m*-[^{131}I]iodobenzylguanidine (MIBG) scans has been encouraging in this regard.[129–132] This agent is concentrated in catecholamine-storing tissues. Such scans have been positive in uncommon patients with negative CT scans and have identified metastases and detected reasonably subtle abnormalities in members of MEN families.[131,132] The procedure requires administration of iodine to protect the normal thyroid gland and takes at least 2 days.

SCREENING

Since pheochromocytoma is a serious and generally treatable disease, it is tempting to suggest that all hypertensive patients should be screened for the presence of a pheochromocytoma, particularly since sensitive, noninvasive tests are available. However, given the high prevalence of hypertension in the population, the costs of screening would be appreciable. There are, of course, additional problems with screening. Screening tests require diagnostic sensitivity at the expense of specificity; false-negative tests are undesirable (since the diagnosis will be rejected), and some false-positive tests must, therefore, be accepted. The lower the prevalence of the disease sought in the population screened, the higher the number of false-positive tests. Clearly, the prevalence of pheochromocytoma is low (0.1 to 0.5 percent) in patients with hypertension.[99] Thus, screening results in a large number of false-positive tests. At the very least, these require repeat testing, expanding the cost. In some instances they could lead to more extensive diagnostic studies and perhaps unnecessary surgery, greatly expanding the dollar cost and making the human cost of screening inestimable. Some may view the dollar costs as justifiable and the human costs as avoidable and advocate screening of all hypertensive patients for pheochromocytoma. This is not my practice. Rather, a high index of clinical suspicion is used to select the patients in whom further testing is indicated for the diagnosis of pheochromocytoma.

TREATMENT

Most pheochromocytomas are benign and can be excised totally. Many believe that preoperative α-adrenergic blockade reduces surgical morbidity and mortality, although critical evidence to support this belief is lacking.[100] The premises are that preoperative α-adrenergic blockade will permit reexpansion of intravascular volume, for which there is evidence,[116] and that it will reduce the frequency and severity of intraoperative pressor episodes. The long-acting, orally effective α-adrenergic antagonist phenoxybenzamine (Dibenzyline) is often used. Starting with 10 mg twice daily, the dose is increased until the blood pressure is controlled and symptomatic paroxysms are prevented. Although total daily doses of 60 mg or more may be required, hypertension typically responds to phenoxybenzamine in patients with pheochromocytomas. Side effects include postural hypotension and, occasionally, the emergence of cardiac arrhythmias. The relatively selective α_1-adrenergic antagonist prazosin (Minipress) has also been used to prepare patients with pheochromocytomas for surgery.[100,133–135] Hypotensive responses to initial 1.0-mg oral doses of prazosin have been observed in patients with pheochromocytomas,[133–135] and an initial dose of 0.5 mg is recommended.[100] It has been suggested that prazosin might not be the preferred preoperative drug, because of its failure to prevent perioperative pressor episodes.[135] However, these can also occur in patients treated with phenoxybenzamine prior to surgery.

β-Adrenergic antagonists such as propranolol (Inderal) are generally not administered prior to surgery unless tachycardia or arrhythmias are, or become, a problem. It is generally recommended that a β-adrenergic antagonist be given only after effective α-adrenergic blockade is established, because β-adrenergic blockade alone might result in an increase in blood pressure as a result of unopposed α-adrenergic stimulation. However, this does not occur invariably.[136] Pulmonary edema has been reported to follow propranolol administration to patients with pheochromocytomas.[137]

Pheochromocytoma surgery is high-risk surgery that requires a surgeon and an anesthesiologist who have experience with this disorder. Careful monitoring of the blood pressure and electrocardiogram is fundamental. Plasma catecholamine levels vary widely;[138] severe hypertension, arrhythmias, or both can occur during induction of anesthesia, during manipulation of the tumor, or without obvious explanation. Pressor episodes can be treated with the rapid acting α-adrenergic antagonist phentolamine (Regitine) or nitroprusside intravenously. Arrhythmias can be treated with a β-adrenergic antagonist or another antiarrhythmic agent such as lidocaine. In view of the occurrence of multiple pheochromocytomas, including bilateral adrenomedullary ones, an anterior approach with thorough exploration after removal of a known intraabdominal tumor is most reasonable. Because of a high incidence of associated cholelithiasis, the gallbladder should also be examined.[100] Appropriate intraoperative fluid replacement is thought to reduce postoperative hypotension.[138]

Pheochromocytomas are occasionally first detected during pregnancy. Such patients have been treated to term with adrenergic antagonists and the baby delivered by cesarean section, with removal of the tumor at the same operation.[139]

Reported surgical cure rates in patients with benign pheochromocytomas vary.[117,140] In a recent series of 91 patients, 84 percent were normotensive following removal of tumors.[117] However, only 67 percent of those with sustained hypertension prior to surgery were normotensive after surgery. Persistent hypertension can be the result of missed pheochromocytoma, a surgical complication resulting in renal ischemia,[141,142] or underlying essential hypertension. The possibility that previous hypertension might have caused renal vascular changes that result in persistent hypertension is difficult to prove or disprove.[140] Relief of paroxysmal symptoms is the rule. Surgery cannot be curative of malignant pheochromocytomas, since this diagnosis is based upon the presence of metastases; histologic criteria are not reliable.

Although blood pressures are often normal prior to discharge in patients whose pheochromocytomas have been removed, some degree of hypertension in the first week after surgery does not preclude cure. Whether because of postoperative stress or an expanded catecholamine pool, plasma and urinary catecholamine values often remain elevated for about a week.[120,143] Thus, the patient should be assessed clinically and biochemically about 1 month after surgery.

The biochemical effects of unresectable pheochromocytomas can be treated medically with adrenergic antagonists. A tyrosine hydroxylase inhibitor, α-methyl-*p*-tyrosine (Demser) has also been used effectively, although it can cause side effects, including postural hypotension and central nervous system dysfunction.[144]

Malignant pheochromocytomas are generally resistant to radiotherapy and chemotherapy. Failures[145] and some success[146] with streptozotocin have been reported. Preliminary results with *m*-[^{131}I]iodobenzylguanidine have been reported.[147] The clinical course of patients with metastatic pheochromocytomas is quite variable: some die within months, others live for more than two decades. The 5-year survival rate is about 45 percent.[100]

OTHER SYMPATHOCHROMAFFIN TUMORS

Pheochromocytomas are tumors of differentiated neural crest cells, the chromaffin cells. Tumors of more primitive cells, and of cells differentiated toward neuronal elements, also occur. These include neuroblastoma,[148] a common malignant tumor of infancy and early childhood which is responsible for 15 percent of cancer deaths in children, as well as generally benign tumors such as ganglioneuromas.

Neuroblastomas arise commonly in the adrenal medullae (40 percent) or paravertebral sympathetic ganglia in the abdomen (25 percent); mediastinal, pelvic, or cervical ganglia are less common sites of origin.[148] These tumors synthesize catecholamines commonly but generally do not release sufficient quantities of biologically active catecholamines to produce clinical manifestations. Presumably, catecholamines are degraded within the tumors, since more than 90 percent of patients excrete excessive quantities of catecholamine metabolites such as homovanillic acid (HVA) and vanillylmandelic acid (VMA). Such measurements provide prognostic as well as diagnostic information: the duration of survival is correlated directly with the VMA/HVA ratio in patients with stage IV disease.[148] Measurements of catecholamine metabolites can also be used to follow the effects of therapy.

There have been notable advances in the treatment of neuroblastomas with surgery, radiation therapy, and chemotherapy.[148] A subset (about 10 percent) of patients with metastatic neuroblastomas, usually diagnosed at less than 1 year of age and with small primary tumors, is of particular interest because they exhibit a high spontaneous remission rate. More than 80 percent become long-term survivors with minimal therapy or none. Nonetheless, neuroblastoma is commonly a highly malignant tumor that requires aggressive therapy.

Autonomic Dysfunction

Assumption of the upright position causes a sharp reduction in venous return to the heart. In the absence of compensatory mechanisms, this would result in a corresponding decrease in cardiac output, arterial pressure, and central nervous system perfusion; cerebrovascular autoregulation notwithstanding, syncope would result from the simple act of standing. Obviously, there are effective compensatory mechanisms. The primary (if not the exclusive) compensatory mechanism is a baroreceptor-initiated, central nervous system–mediated sympathetic neural reflex that results in norepinephrine release from axon terminals within the tissues, which in turn results in a sharp increase in systemic vascular resistance (and limitation of the fall in venous return and cardiac output) and, thus, maintenance of the blood pressure in the standing position. Postural activation of this sympathetic reflex is reflected in a rapid, approximately twofold rise in plasma norepinephrine concentrations,[149] as shown in Table 13-2 and Fig. 13-13. Maximum levels are achieved within 5 min. Thus, measurement of the plasma norepinephrine response to standing provides a relatively simple means of assessing the integrity of this sympathetic reflex.

Defective postural adaptation results in a decrement in blood pressure upon standing—postural (orthostatic) hypotension. We have arbitrarily used a supine-to-standing decrement in mean blood pressure (diastolic pressure plus one-third of the pulse pressure) of 20 mmHg or more to define postural hypotension. Many use a supine-to-standing decrement in systolic pressure of 30 mmHg or more with a decrement in diastolic blood pressure of 15 mmHg or more.[150] These are conservative definitions. Lesser decrements may have diagnostic importance but seldom, if ever, cause symptoms. Postural hypotension is a common clinical finding,[150] especially in older persons.[151]

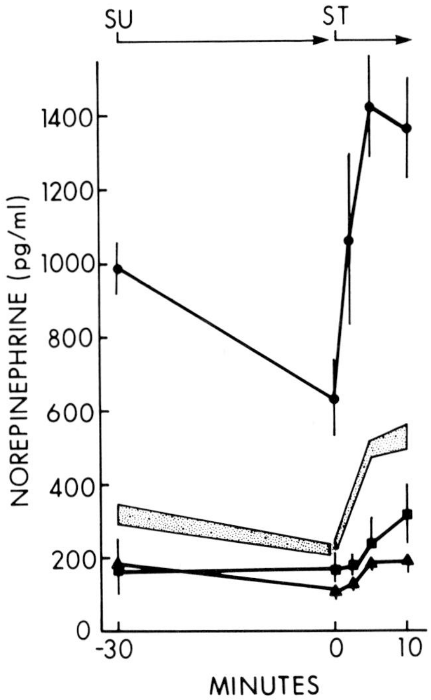

FIGURE 13-13 Mean (±SE) venous plasma norepinephrine concentrations, measured in the supine (SU) and standing (ST) positions, in posturally hypotensive patients with (1) severe sodium depletion (round symbols), (2) primary autonomic dysfunction (square symbols), or (3) diabetic adrenergic neuropathy (triangular symbols). The shaded areas encompasses 1 SE around the mean for normal subjects.

Upon standing, patients with postural hypotension note lightheadedness, blurring or even loss of vision, and a profound weakness that may culminate in syncope. Symptoms clear rapidly if patients lie down. Postural symptoms are commonly worse in the morning, after a meal, and after exercise. The clinical manifestations of postural hypotension syndromes can mimic other disorders, including angina pectoris.[150,152]

Conceptually, postural hypotension can be caused by one or more of three general mechanisms: (1) absolute or relative intravascular volume contraction; (2) resistance to the cardiovascular actions of norepinephrine; and (3) an afferent, central, or efferent defect in the sympathetic neural reflex arc. Patients with postural hypotension due to intravascular volume contraction or resistance to the action of norepinephrine exhibit an exaggerated plasma norepinephrine response to standing.[153,154] They have *hyper*adrenergic postural hypotension. In contrast, patients with postural hypotension due to a defect in the sympathetic reflex arc have a blunted plasma norepinephrine response to standing.[155–157] They have *hypo*adrenergic hypotension. These patterns are illustrated in Fig. 13-13.

In a posturally hypotensive patient a supine-to-standing plasma norepinephrine increment of less than 140 pg/ml—the smallest increment observed in a series of 40 normal subjects—is considered to be abnormally low and clearly indicative of hypoadrenergic postural hypotension. There is considerable scatter in the responses of normal subjects (Table 13-2). In a posturally hypotensive patient a maximum plasma norepinephrine concentration during standing of more than 1040 pg/ml—the highest value observed in normal subjects—is believed to be excessive and indicative of hyperadrenergic postural hypotension.

In practice, most patients with postural hypotension can be placed in the hyperadrenergic or hypoadrenergic categories on the basis of plasma norepinephrine measurements. Not infrequently, however, the plasma norepinephrine response overlaps the normal range. This may reflect the fact, discussed earlier, that plasma norepinephrine concentrations provide only an index of sympathetic activity, the scatter in the normal response, the presence of more than one mechanism of postural hypotension in a given patient, or a combination of these. One could reason that a normal norepinephrine response is inappropriately low, and thus indicative of a hypoadrenergic component, in a posturally hypotensive patient with intravascular volume contraction or resistance to norepinephrine. Obviously, this approach cannot be applied to all posturally hypotensive patients, since severely affected patients are unable to stand for any period of time.

The relative clinical utility of routine plasma

norepinephrine measurements in posturally hypotensive patients who are able to stand remains to be determined; I believe they are reasonable and have found them useful in individual patients. Typically, these are patients thought initially to have postural hypotension due to a defect in the sympathetic reflex arc, because of an associated disorder such as diabetes mellitus or because of the absence of any other clinically apparent mechanism, but found to have a hyperadrenergic pattern due to a potentially treatable abnormality.[154]

The heart rate and blood pressure should be recorded during supine and upright sampling for norepinephrine determinations. Although the heart rate response, which involves withdrawal of vagal tone as well as sympathetic stimulation, is not a sensitive measure for prediction of the hypotensive mechanism, a marked supine-to-standing increment in heart rate provides evidence against a defect in the sympathetic reflex arc. The forms of postural hypotension discussed here must, of course, be distinguished from bradycardic (vasovagal or vasodepressor) postural hypotension, which can occur in apparently normal persons and is generally not reproducible.

The causes of hyperadrenergic postural hypotension are listed in Table 13-3. These will not be discussed here. However, they should be considered in all patients with postural hypotension, including those with overt autonomic disease, because they are commonly treatable. A given patient can have multiple hypotensive mechanisms; correction of one can result in clinical improvement. For example, in a patient with relatively mild autonomic hypofunction, otherwise trivial sodium depletion can result in symptomatic postural hypotension that can be treated by sodium repletion.

Table 13-3. Postural Hypotension

Hyperadrenergic Postural Hypotension

A. Intravascular volume contraction
   1. Hemorrhage
   2. Severe chronic anemia
   3. Sodium (and water) depletion: aldosterone deficiency, diuretics, GI or renal diseases
   4. Relative volume contraction: pregnancy

B. Resistance to released norepinephrine
   1. Sodium depletion (see above)
   2. Glucocorticoid deficiency
   3. Bartter's syndrome
   4. Vasodilator drugs: nitroglycerin; hydralazine and minoxidil; prazosin, bromocriptine, and other α-adrenergic antagonists; guanethidine, bretylium, methyldopa

Hypoadrenergic Postural Hypotension

A. Secondary
   1. Brain lesions: vascular accidents involving the brainstem, toxic/nutritional encephalopathies, demyelinating and degenerative disorders, neoplasms, trauma, infections, tricyclic antidepressants, phenothiazines, and butyrophenones
   2. Spinal cord lesions: cervical transection, mass lesions (tumor, abscess), syringomyelia, combined systems disease, tabes dorsalis
   3. Peripheral nerve lesions: diabetic adrenergic neuropathy, alcoholism, amyloidosis, porphyria, vincristine

B. Primary
   1. Primary autonomic dysfunction
      a. Type 1: idiopathic orthostatic hypotension
      b. Type 2: idiopathic orthostatic hypotension with somatic neurologic deficit (Shy-Drager syndrome, multiple system atrophy)
   2. Familial dysautonomia (Riley-Day syndrome)

Hypoadrenergic postural hypotension can result from afferent, central, or efferent lesions in the sympathetic neural arc. Diseases recognized to cause secondary hypoadrenergic postural hypotension produce lesions in the brain, spinal cord, or peripheral nerves. These diseases are also listed in Table 13-3. In the absence of such diseases, autonomic hypofunction is considered to be idiopathic or primary. I prefer the less restrictive designation *primary autonomic dysfunction* for this syndrome over the more commonly used terms defined in the next paragraph.

Undoubtedly a heterogeneous group of disorders of unknown etiology, primary autonomic dysfunction can be divided into two clinical and pathophysiologic syndromes.[19,150,156,157] Primary autonomic dysfunction type 1, most commonly referred to as *idiopathic orthostatic hypotension,* is characterized by autonomic hypofunction in the absence of central nervous system disease. In addition to a blunted plasma norepinephrine response to standing,[155] common to both the type 1 and type 2 disorders, patients with the type 1 disorder as a group have low basal plasma norepinephrine concentrations.[156,157] They also have markedly reduced norepinephrine production rates as assessed by measurement of metabolite excretion and reduced plasma norepinephrine appearance and clearance rates.[19,83] They are thought to have lesions of sympathetic postganglionic neurons. Primary autonomic dysfunction type 2 is perhaps best known as the Shy-Drager syndrome; it has also been referred to as *multiple system atrophy* or *idiopathic orthostatic hypotension with somatic neurologic deficit.* In addition to autonomic hypofunction, patients with the type 2 disorder have degenerative central nervous system disease most commonly manifested as parkinsonism. Indeed, the disorder has been referred to as *parkinsonian multiple system atrophy.*[158] Its clinical manifestations are discussed in Refs. 158 and 159. Neurologic manifestations are outlined in Table 13-4. In general,

Table 13-4. Signs and Symptoms in 57 Selected Patients with Primary Autonomic Dysfunction

	Number of patients	Percent of patients
Symptoms		
Autonomic:		
Postural cerebral symptoms	54	95
Urinary dysfunction	37	65
Impaired libido/potency	29	51
Bowel dysfunction	17	30
Decreased sweating	6	11
Somatic neurologic:		
Gait disturbance	22	39
Speech disturbance	18	32
Generalized weakness	16	28
Tremor of limbs	15	26
Clumsiness of limbs	11	19
Impaired writing	10	18
Numbness of limbs	8	14
Swallowing disturbance	7	12
Signs		
Autonomic:		
Standing ↓DBP of 25 mmHg or greater*	57	100
Somatic neurologic:		
Corticobulbar/corticospinal:		
Hyperreflexia	48	84
Extensor toe signs	29	51
Dysarthria	17	30
Sucking reflex	13	23
Extrapyramidal:		
Masking of face	33	58
Rigidity	29	51
Monotony of voice	18	32
Resting tremor	16	28
Cerebellar:		
Intention tremor	23	40
Ataxic gait	22	39
Ataxic-dysarthric speech	2	4
Other		
Horner's syndrome	9	16
Anisocoria	8	14
Decreased ankle jerks	6	11
Intellectual impairment	4	7
Sensory impairment	1	<1

*A decrease in the supine-to-standing diastolic blood pressure (DBP) of 25 mmHg or more was a criterion for inclusion. Other autonomic signs were not reported.
Source: Schirger and Thomas.[159]

such patients have normal basal plasma norepinephrine concentrations (but reduced responses to standing),[19,156,157] although low basal norepinephrine concentrations occur. Their autonomic lesions are thought to be in the central nervous system.[19,156–159]

Impairment of parasympathetic as well as sympathetic neural functions is the rule in patients with primary autonomic dysfunction.[150,159,160] Thus, a variety of symptoms, such as diminished sweating and heat intolerance, difficulty in focusing, gastrointestinal symptoms, urinary and fecal incontinence, and impotence, in addition to postural symptoms, occur commonly (Table 13-4).

Patients with primary autonomic dysfunction have been found to have increased mononuclear leukocyte β_2-adrenergic receptor and platelet α_2-adrenergic receptor densities, probably representing receptor up regulation in response to decreased norepinephrine levels.[50] On the basis of increased cardiovascular sensitivity to agonists in vivo, receptor up regulation is thought to be a generalized phenomenon in such patients.

Although primary autonomic dysfunction type 1 is compatible with long survival, the prognosis is poor in patients with the type 2 disorder. In one large series, death followed the onset of neurologic manifestations by 4 to 5 years on average.[150]

Treatment of a patient with postural hypotension begins with a search for reversible pathogenic factors such as anemia, sodium depletion, or offending drugs.[150] This applies even if the patient has clear-cut autonomic failure, since treatment of such secondary factors can result in clinical improvement even though the basic neurologic disease cannot be corrected. In the absence of reversible factors, symptomatic therapy of postural hypotension is often required.

Mechanical measures are often recommended to patients with chronic postural hypotension.[150,161,162] These include sleeping with the head of the bed elevated and use of elasticized support garments that extend from the costal margin to the feet. The premise of the first is that it reduces fluid loss from the intravascular compartment during sleep and that of the second is that external pressure reduces venous pooling when the patient stands.

The objective of drug therapy of patients with postural hypotension is to raise the blood pressure in the upright position to a level that prevents symptoms. One does not attempt to normalize the standing blood pressure, since supine hypertension is a predictable result. Indeed, an increase in the supine blood pressure is a concomitant of most effective therapies.[150,161,162]

Administration of the mineralocorticoid hormone 9α-fluorohydrocortisone (Florinef), in doses of 0.1 to 0.3 mg or more daily, is the mainstay of symptomatic treatment of chronic postural hypotension.[150,161,162] This potent sodium-retaining agent often increases the standing blood pressure and relieves symptoms. If it is not in itself adequate, most physicians continue it and add additional drugs. It increases plasma volume only transiently; in the long term it increases vascular resistance, perhaps by increasing vascular sensitivity to norepinephrine.[163] To the extent that the efficacy of 9α-fluorohydrocortisone is the result of sodium retention, it would seem fundamental to ensure a liberal sodium intake, with sodium chloride tablets if necessary, and to document an initial positive sodium balance by serial measurements of body weight. Hypokalemia is a rather common complication and requires potassium supplementation. Cardiac failure is a potential, but relatively uncommon, complication. As with other therapies, supine hypertension occurs.[163] Administration of a β-adrenergic antagonist has been used to attempt to minimize this,[150,162] although it can precipitate cardiac failure.

Drugs of inconsistent efficacy in the treatment of chronic postural hypotension include monoamine oxidase inhibitors, indomethacin, and indirect sympathomimetics such as ephedrine, amphetamines, and dietary tyramine. β-Adrenergic antagonists have been used.[150] Interestingly, pindolol, a β-adrenergic antagonist with partial agonist activity, has been reported to be effective in patients with primary autonomic dysfunction type 1[164,165] but not in patients with the type 2 disorder, multiple system atrophy.[166] This is plausibly explained by very low receptor occupancy by endogenous norepinephrine in the former disorder, permitting expression of the agonist activity of pindolol. Similarly, severely affected patients with the type 2 disorder have been reported to have a pressor response to the α_2-adrenergic agonist clonidine.[167] Clonidine normally decreases blood pressure through a central action. Perhaps this did not occur in the patients because of their severe sympathetic disease; thus, the direct vasoconstrictor effect of the α_2-adrenergic agonist was expressed. Clearly, clonidine should not be given to patients with partial sympathetic failure.

Although α-adrenergic agonists such as phenylephrine have been disappointing in the treatment of chronic postural hypotension, agonists that constrict veins as well as arteries have shown promise. These include ergotamines[168] and midodrine.[172] Dihydroergotamine has been found effective during parenteral, but not oral, administration.[168–170] This is attributable to first-pass extraction, rather than malabsorption, of ingested dihydroergotamine.[169,170] Chobanian et al., however, found that long-term oral ergotamine tartrate administration produced increases in standing blood pressure and clinical improvement without recumbent hypertension in four patients.[171] Similarly, an initial trial of long-term treatment with the agonist midodrine led to improvement in postural symptoms and the standing blood pressure without symptomatic side effects and with supine systolic hypertension in only two of five patients.[172] The latter was responsive to a β-adrenergic antagonist. Clonidine, discussed above, also has a venoconstrictive effect.[167]

Among other treatments, atrial pacing has been helpful in some but not all patients.[173–175] Administration of DL-*threo*-3,4-dihydroxyphenylserine, an unphysiologic amino acid precursor of norepinephrine, was reported to increase plasma norepinephrine and blood pressure and to decrease postural symptoms in a patient with familial amyloid polyneuropathy.[176] Lastly, preliminary studies with a closed-loop computer-based system for blood pressure monitoring and controlled norepinephrine infusion have been reported.[177]

The preceding paragraphs have focused on supportive management of sympathetic hypofunction. Manifestations of parasympathetic hypofunction are common in patients with primary autonomic dysfunction. They are usually not treated. However, subcutaneous bethanechol chloride has been reported to improve tearing, salivation, sweating, and gastrointestinal and bladder functions.[178]

Hypoglycemia

The physiology of human glucose counterregulation—the mechanisms that prevent or correct hypoglycemia—has been clarified in the past decade (Fig. 13-14).[179–187] Glucose recovery from hypoglycemia is not due solely to dissipation of insulin; glucagon plays a primary counterregulatory role. Epinephrine, although not normally critical, compensates largely and becomes critical when glucagon secretion is deficient. Epinephrine may also serve in concert with glucagon to prevent hypoglycemia in glucose-lowering conditions under which the action of glucagon alone might be insufficient. Given adequate glucogenic reserves (hepatic glycogen and gluconeogenic precursors) and intact enzymatic systems, glucose counterregulation fails and hypoglycemia occurs only when both glucagon and epinephrine are deficient and insulin is present or when insulin action is excessive. Developed originally from studies of glucose recovery from insulin-induced hypoglycemia,[179–183] these principles also apply to the prevention of hypoglycemia in both the postprandial and postabsorptive states.[184–187]

Thus, prevention or correction of hypoglycemia is effectively accomplished by redundant glucose counterregulatory systems, primarily glucagon and secondarily epinephrine, coupled with dissipation of insulin. Other hormones, neural mechanisms, or autoregulation may be involved but need not be invoked and are not sufficiently potent to prevent or correct hypoglycemia when the key counterregulatory hormones, glucagon and epinephrine, are deficient or insulin action is excessive.

Developed initially from studies involving pharmacologic manipulations (somatostatin without and with hormone replacement, adrenergic antagonists, or both) and surgical epinephrine deficiency (bilateral adrenalectomy), as summarized in Fig. 13-14, these principles have been confirmed in that they predict the altered[188] and defective[189] glucose counterregulation that results from deficient glucagon and epinephrine secretory responses in patients with insulin-dependent diabetes mellitus (IDDM).[190–192] To the extent that they have deficient glucagon responses to plasma glucose decrements, as they commonly do, patients with IDDM are dependent upon epinephrine to promote recovery from hypoglycemia.[188] To the extent that they have deficient glucagon and epinephrine responses to glucose decrements, as they sometimes do, they are defenseless against hypoglycemia. Indeed, patients with combined deficiencies of their glucagon and epinephrine responses are at 25-fold higher risk for severe hypoglycemia during intensive treatment of the IDDM.[189] Thus, the presence of redundant defenses against hypoglycemia accounts for the rarity of hypoglycemia in nondiabetic persons and the ability of many intensively treated patients with

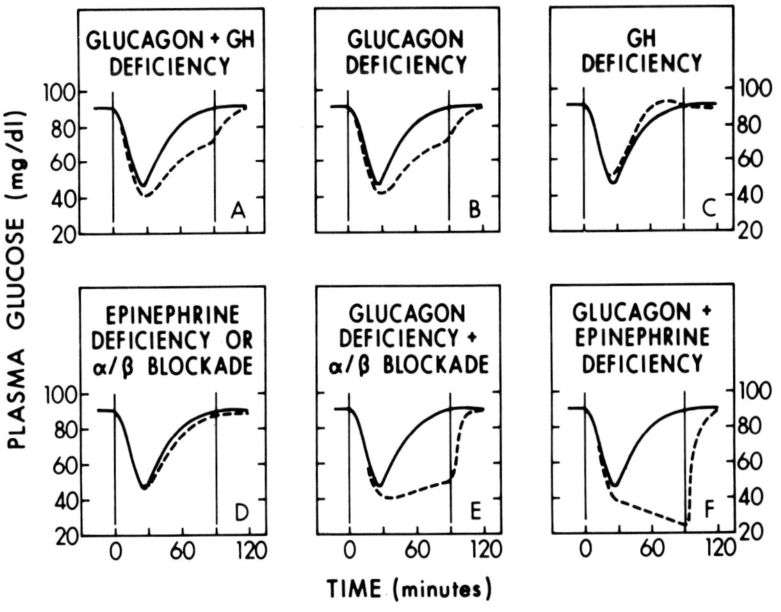

FIGURE 13-14 Plasma glucose curves following the intravenous injection of regular insulin at 0 min in human subjects during control studies (solid lines, same in all panels) and as modified (dashed lines) by (A) somatostatin infusion from 0 through 90 min (glucagon + GH deficiency); (B) somatostatin infusion with growth hormone replacement (glucagon deficiency); (C) somatostatin infusion with glucagon replacement (GH deficiency); (D) phentolamine plus propranolol infusion or studies in bilaterally adrenalectomized, glucocorticoid- and mineralocorticoid-replaced patients (α/β blockade or epinephrine deficiency); (E) somatostatin plus phentolamine and propranolol infusion (glucagon deficiency + α/β blockade); (F) somatostatin infusion in bilaterally adrenalectomized patients (glucagon + epinephrine deficiency). (*From Cryer.*[183])

IDDM to maintain their plasma glucose at levels sufficient for normal cerebral function despite hyperinsulinemia and deficient glucagon responses, as well as the susceptibility to hypoglycemia of those patients in whom epinephrine secretion is also deficient.

The role of the sympathochromaffin system, among other systems, in human glucose counterregulation and hypoglycemia is reviewed in Ref. 193.

Other Disorders

There is increasing evidence that the sympathochromaffin system is involved in the pathophysiology of a variety of human diseases, either as a factor in pathogenesis or as a result of the primary disorder. This evidence cannot be discussed in detail here; it is summarized briefly with reference to reviews or recent publications so that the interested reader can pursue selected topics.

ENDOCRINE-METABOLIC DISORDERS

DIABETES MELLITUS The role of deficient epinephrine secretion, probably a manifestation of diabetic autonomic neuropathy,[194] in the pathogenesis of hypoglycemia in intensively treated patients with IDDM[188–193] was discussed in the preceding paragraphs. Further, diabetic adrenergic neuropathy is a common, perhaps the most common, cause of deficient norepinephrine release from sympathetic neurons and the resultant hypoadrenergic postural hypotension,[153,157,195,196] as discussed earlier in this chapter. The possibility that autonomic, as well as peripheral, neuropathy may be a function of poor metabolic control remains a viable hypothesis.[197] If so, these may be treatable with better forms of therapy of diabetic patients.

The vast majority of patients with uncomplicated nonketotic diabetes mellitus have normal plasma catecholamine concentrations, although subtle elevations in integrated concentrations and increased responses to exercise have been demonstrated in poorly controlled patients, and markedly elevated plasma catecholamine levels occur in patients with diabetic ketoacidosis.[198] These revert to normal with effective therapy; it seems likely that they are secondary responses, perhaps to volume depletion. The catecholamines may well contribute to the perpetuation, if not the initiation, of diabetic ketoacidosis.[199,200] The finding that β-adrenergic blockade reduces late mortality after myocardial infarction, discussed later, appears to apply to patients with diabetes.[201]

Patients with IDDM exhibit increased glycemic responsiveness to epinephrine.[202] There is not a generalized alteration of adrenergic receptors in such patients.[50] The increased glycemic sensitivity to epinephrine is the result of their inability to secrete insulin as the plasma glucose concentration rises.[63] This does not, however, explain the observation of increased pressor sensitivity to norepinephrine.[203]

DISORDERS OF THYROID FUNCTION Although the data in humans are not compelling in my judgment, there is evidence that thyroid hormone excess increases sensitivity to catecholamines, at least in some tissues, in animal studies.[50,204] This appears to be the result of thyroid hormone–induced increments in β-adrenergic receptor densities; this may explain some of the clinical manifestations of thyrotoxicosis and their improvement during administration of a β-adrenergic antagonist, although this is a controversial point.[50,204] Decrements in β-adrenergic receptors in hypothyroidism have been found by some, but not all, investigators.[50,204]

ADRENOCORTICAL DISORDERS Although glucocorticoids and mineralocorticoids have been reported to modulate adrenergic receptors,[50] effects of human adrenocortical disorders on sensitivity to catecholamines have not been reported to my knowledge.

Diminished plasma epinephrine responses to exercise, presumably the result of decreased glucocorticoid induction of adrenomedullary phenylethanolamine-N-methyl transferase activity, in ACTH-deficient patients,[16] were discussed earlier.

GONADAL DISORDERS Despite substantial evidence that sex steroids modulate adrenergic receptors,[50] altered sensitivity to catecholamines in human gonadal disorders has not been reported. Effects of sex steroids and pregnancy on uterine sympathetic neurons are reviewed in Ref. 205. Maternal and neonatal plasma catecholamine levels are increased at the time of birth, especially with vaginal delivery.[206] We observed higher plasma epinephrine levels in luteal-phase women than in men or follicular-phase women, but the differences were small and of questionable biologic importance.[207]

PITUITARY DISORDERS Catecholamines modulate the secretion of pituitary hormones. Indeed, dopamine is thought to be the physiologic hypothalamic prolactin inhibiting factor that tonically restrains pituitary prolactin secretion. Although growth hormone secretory responses to L-dopa are qualitatively abnormal, there is little direct evidence that catecholamines are involved in the pathogenesis of chronic growth hormone hypersecretion and acromegaly.[50] The possibility that decreased dopaminergic action might underlie excessive prolactin secretion[50] is discussed elsewhere in this book (Chap. 8).

PARATHYROID DISORDERS Although β-adrenergic stimulation of parathyroid hormone secretion has been described in animal studies, plasma epinephrine concentrations that span the physiologic and pathophysiologic ranges in humans did not stimulate parathyroid hormone (or calcitonin) secretion.[5] Epinephrine is, however, a potent hypophosphatemic hormone.[5]

Patients with pseudohypoparathyroidism, including the subset with deficient guanine nucleotide regulatory protein activity in plasma membranes of cells of many tissues, have been shown to have blunted plasma cyclic AMP responses to isoproterenol,[208] but the plasma glucose and cardiovascular responses to isoproterenol were not demonstrably abnormal in those patients.

OBESITY Studies in rodents have established that underfeeding decreases and overfeeding increases norepinephrine turnover in a variety of tissues, including brown fat.[69,209] These changes in sympathetic neuronal activity are paralleled by changes in thermogenesis. A defective thermogenic response to overfeeding would be expected to contribute to obesity. There is, however, as yet no convincing evidence that defective thermogenesis commonly underlies the development of human obesity.[210] This is discussed in Chap. 21.

After studying lean women, obese women, and formerly obese women in the basal state, during standing, during passive vertical tilting, during norepinephrine infusion, in response to the Valsalva maneuver, and after caloric restriction, Jung et al. concluded that there appears to be no generalized abnormality in the sympathetic nervous system in obese women.[211] They did observe that during 2 weeks of caloric restriction (with constant sodium intake) there were reductions in plasma norepinephrine concentrations in both the supine and standing positions. Interestingly, the reductions in plasma norepinephrine were prevented by L-dopa administration during caloric restriction. They found no differences in plasma epinephrine concentrations, although they did not study exercise. Others have reported a reduced plasma epinephrine response to isometric exercise in obese women.[212]

An increase in platelet α_2-adrenergic receptor density and in platelet aggregation in association with weight loss was reported from a study of anorexiant drugs.[213]

IDIOPATHIC EDEMA Decreased urinary dopamine excretion by patients with idiopathic edema led Kuchel et al. to suggest that suppression of the renal dopaminergic system may contribute to excessive sodium retention in these patients.[214] This suggestion was supported by therapeutic responses to bromocriptine administration in such patients, although Sowers et al. suggested that decreased dopaminergic inhibition of aldosterone secretion might be an important pathogenic mechanism.[215]

BARTTER'S SYNDROME Patients with Bartter's syndrome exhibit decreased pressor responses to norepinephrine and increased endogenous plasma[216] and urinary[217] norepinephrine values. Further, the plasma norepinephrine response to standing is exaggerated in such patients. Some patients with Bartter's syndrome have postural hypotension, an example of hyperadrenergic postural hypotension due to resistance of the vasculature to norepinephrine, as discussed above. The enhanced sympathetic activity in Bartter's syndrome is, therefore, an appropriate compensatory response. Like many manifestations of the syndrome, it reverts toward or to normal during indomethacin administration.[216,217]

CARCINOID SYNDROME Excretion of dopamine, but not norepinephrine or epinephrine, was reported to be increased in some patients with carcinoid tumors, but platelet dopamine levels were found to be normal in patients with increased serotonin production.[218]

ACUTE INTERMITTENT PORPHYRIA The clinical picture of acute prophyria includes tachycardia and hypertension. These have been associated with increased catecholamine excretion and attributed to increased catecholamine levels. Beal et al. found that δ-aminolevulinic acid (ALA) and porphobilinogen (PBG) reduced uptake and accumulation of norepinephrine by platelets of patients with porphyria but not by platelets of controls.[219] The authors suggested that if platelet uptake serves as a model of adrenergic neuronal uptake, elevated catecholamines during acute attacks (when ALA and PBG levels are increased) could be the result of blockade of catecholamine uptake into sympathetic neurons.

LESCH-NYHAN SYNDROME Patients with the Lesch-Nyhan syndrome have been shown to lack a blood pressure response to the cold pressor test.[220] Since the heart rate response was normal, the defect would appear to be in the vascular response to released norepinephrine. Plasma dopamine β-hydroxylase activities were increased, suggesting increased catecholamine release.

NEUROFIBROMATOSIS The association of pheochromocytoma and neurofibromatosis was mentioned earlier in this chapter. The frequency of pheochromocytoma is probably less than 1 percent; the tumors are virtually unknown in children with neurofibromatosis.[221] Some patients with increased norepinephrine excretion but no demonstrable pheochromocytoma have been identified, and the possibility of catecholamine formation in, and release from, neurofibromas has been raised.[221]

CARDIOVASCULAR DISORDERS

ESSENTIAL HYPERTENSION It has long been suspected that increased sympathochromaffin activity is the cause of essential hypertension. Convincing evidence of this has not been forthcoming. In view of the antihypertensive efficacy of a variety of drugs that interfere with sympathetic outflow at the central (clonidine, methyldopa), ganglionic (trimethaphan camsylate), or peripheral (guanethidine, reserpine) levels or which block adrenergic receptors, it is clear that the sympathochromaffin system is involved in the maintenance of essential hypertension; but this does not establish a causal role for increased sympathetic activity in the pathogenesis of essential hypertension. It could represent interference with normal adrenergic maintenance of the blood pressure around an abnormal set point elevated by other mechanisms.

After reviewing a large, and conflicting, literature on plasma norepinephrine and epinephrine measurements in patients with essential hypertension, Goldstein concluded that the preponderance of evidence supports the hypothesis that increased plasma catecholamine concentrations occur in *some* patients with essential hypertension and suggested, again, a pathogenic role for increased sympathetic activity in a subset of patients—relatively young people with established hypertension.[222] Although the latter possibility is not excluded, tracer studies have shown that the plasma appearance rate of norepinephrine is normal in the majority of patients and in those with essential hypertension as a group.[86,223] Christensen,[224] while not rejecting the subset hypothesis, concluded that it is unlikely that sympathochromaffin activity is increased in the majority of patients with essential hypertension; rather, he favored the possibility of increased vascular sensitivity to norepinephrine in essential hypertension, for which there is considerable evidence. The mechanisms by which this might occur are reviewed in Ref. 225.

CORONARY HEART DISEASE β-Adrenergic antagonists are used widely to treat angina pectoris and cardiac arrhythmias. There is now a large body of evidence from controlled clinical trials that administration of a β-adrenergic antagonist following myocardial infarction reduces coronary heart disease mortality.[201,226–228] Although the mechanism of this effect is not established, the simplest explanation is that β-adrenergic blockade reduces myocardial oxygen demand. It is conceivable that this is due to a drug action other than β-adrenergic blockade, but the fact that reduced mortality has been observed with a variety of antagonists makes this unlikely. Thus, it appears that sympathochromaffin activity is involved in the pathogenesis of acute coronary heart disease events, presumably arrhythmias, and sudden death. This need not necessarily be increased sympathochromaffin activity, although it may well be.

Cigarette smoking is an established risk factor for coronary heart disease events. There is evidence that smoking accelerates atherosclerosis, and it is also possible that smoking may trigger such events acutely, since it stimulates the sympathochromaffin system.[95]

Plasma catecholamine concentrations increase promptly following acute myocardial infarction.[229,230] Although this may well be an appropriate compensatory response to a rapid decrease in cardiac output, its potentially deleterious effect on the heart is apparent. In experimental infarction the magnitude of the catecholamine response is directly related to infarct size.[229] Since the size can be reduced by adrenergic blockade,[226] it is reasonable to suggest that the magnitude of the catecholamine response is one of its determinants. However, a clear relationship between the catecholamine response and infarct size has not been established in humans.[230] Similarly, a clear relationship between abrupt increments in plasma catecholamine levels and cardiac arrhythmias has not been documented in humans. Obviously, these may be the result of infrequent sampling of these labile compounds, of the absence of true relationships, or of relationships with intramyocardial, rather than plasma, catecholamine levels.

Stable plasma norepinephrine elevations are the rule in patients with chronic cardiac failure. Decreased norepinephrine clearance may well be a factor.[83] However, increased norepinephrine release would be appropriate in view of the decreased sensitivity of the failing myocardium to norepinephrine. Indeed, decreased β-adrenergic receptor densities and adenylate cyclase and contractility sensitivities to isoproterenol have been demonstrated in myocardium from patients with heart failure.[231]

MITRAL VALVE PROLAPSE Elevated plasma catecholamine concentrations,[232] in both the supine and standing positions, and increased urinary catecholamine excretion[233] have been reported in patients with mitral valve prolapse. Further, plasma catecholamine levels were found to correlate with premature ventricular contractions during exercise in such patients.[233] The mechanisms and clinical relevance of these findings remain to be established. Increased sympathochromaffin responsiveness to upright posture during volume depletion has been reported;[234] postural hypotension occurs in some patients.[235]

RAYNAUD'S PHENOMENON It has been suggested that Raynaud's phenomenon is the result of increased sympathetic activity. Apparent plasma norepinephrine production rates, calculated from infusions of unlabeled norepinephrine, were found to be increased in patients with the secondary form of this disorder.[236] However, long-term treatment with α-adrenergic antagonists has not been proved effective.[237]

PULMONARY DISORDERS

BRONCHIAL ASTHMA There is evidence that some allergic persons exhibit α-adrenergic hyperresponsiveness, β-adrenergic hyporesponsiveness (correlated with circulating β-adrenergic receptor antibodies) and cholinergic hyporesponsiveness. Of these, only α-adrenergic hyperresponsiveness correlates with bronchial asthma.[238] It is of note that all three abnormalities have also been described in patients with cystic fibrosis.[239] The use of β-adrenergic agonists in the treatment of bronchospasm is associated with down regulation of β-adrenergic receptors.[50]

It has been suggested that nocturnal asthma may be the result of decreased plasma epinephrine levels in persons prone to release the mediators that trigger bronchoconstriction.[240]

CHRONIC OBSTRUCTIVE PULMONARY DISEASE Increased plasma norepinephrine concentrations, inversely related to the arterial oxygen saturation, occur in patients with chronic obstructive lung disease.[241]

CENTRAL NERVOUS SYSTEM DISORDERS

PARKINSON'S DISEASE Deficient dopamine release in the caudate and putamen, resulting from degeneration of neurons whose cell bodies reside in the substantia nigra, is the cause of parkinsonism.[242] This forms the basis of treatment with L-dopa and dopaminergic agonists.

MIGRAINE HEADACHES Catecholamines are among the various vasoactive substances that might mediate migraine headaches. The β-adrenergic antagonist propranolol is used to treat this disorder. Increased VMA excretion during attacks and, most interestingly, increased plasma norepinephrine concentrations prior to attacks[243] have been reported.

AUTONOMIC SEIZURES Metz et al. studied a patient with paroxysms of hypertension, tachycardia, and flushing attributed to diencephalic epilepsy.[244] Basal plasma catecholamine levels were normal, but these increased twofold during paroxysms. Administration of clonidine suppressed plasma catecholamine levels and flushing during spells. However, the blood pressure and heart rate increments were not abolished.

TREMORS Propranolol has been reported to be effective in the treatment of a variety of tremors.[245]

BEHAVIORAL DISORDERS

As central nervous system neurotransmitters, the catecholamines are reasonably thought to be critically involved in behavior.[246,247] Evidence of disordered catecholamine metabolism in patients with depression[248] and with schizophrenia[249] has been presented, and β-adrenergic antagonists have been used to treat anxiety. Tricyclic antidepressants decrease neuronal uptake of norepinephrine[83] and increase plasma norepinephrine concentrations.[250]

Persons with the type A behavioral pattern have been reported to exhibit enhanced plasma norepinephrine responses to mental work.[251]

GASTROINTESTINAL DISORDERS

CHRONIC LIVER DISEASE Portocaval shunting in dogs produces a model of chronic liver disease with hepatic encephalopathy. Shunting results in decreased metabolism of tyrosine through its major route (via hepatic tyrosine aminotransferase to 4-hydroxyphenylpyruvic acid, then to homogentisic acid) and increased decarboxylation of tyrosine to tyramine. Tyramine levels in plasma, cerebrospinal fluid, and brain are increased.[252] These changes correlate with the degree of encephalopathy. They are associated with increases in plasma and cerebrospinal fluid dopamine and norepinephrine, but in several brain areas dopamine and norepinephrine are depleted.[252] Thus, increased tyramine formation from tyrosine, with the subsequent increase in brain tyramine and depletion of brain catecholamines, may be the mechanism of hepatic encephalopathy. Increased plasma tyramine levels also occur in humans with hepatic encephalopathy.[253] Improvement in encephalopathy during administration of L-dopa and of bromocriptine to patients with cirrhosis has been reported.[254]

Plasma norepinephrine (and epinephrine) concentrations are elevated in patients with chronic liver disease and are even higher in patients with associated functional renal failure.[255–257] These elevations could be the result of decreased clearance (the liver is an important clearance site),[83] increased release, or both. Increased norepinephrine release could be an appropriate response to decreased vascular tone.[257] It has been suggested, however, that increased renal sympathetic activity may cause the sharply reduced renal blood flow that can lead to functional renal failure.[256,257] It has been further suggested that increased renal sympathetic activity may contribute to sodium and water retention in patients with chronic liver disease.[255,257]

DUODENAL ULCER Plasma norepinephrine concentrations have been reported to be elevated in patients with duodenal ulcers.[258]

RENAL DISORDERS

Plasma norepinephrine concentrations are elevated and found to be inversely related to blood volume in patients with end-stage renal disease requiring long-term dialysis.[259–263] Norepinephrine levels were found to be normal following renal transplantation in patients who had elevated values while receiving dialysis prior to transplantation.[260] The plasma norepinephrine production rate, calculated from the product of the plasma concentration and the metabolic clearance rate determined from infused unlabeled norepinephrine, was found to be elevated about threefold in patients with end-stage renal disease.[263] Thus, there is substantial evidence of increased sympathetic neural activity in patients with renal failure, at least those with end-stage renal disease treated with long-term hemodialysis. The cause of increased sympathetic activity is unknown; it could be a compensatory response.

Renal failure plasma contains a competitive inhibitor of catechol-O-methyl transferase.[263,264] Thus, the use of internal standards, or of external standards in renal failure plasma, is critical in the isotope-derivative measurement of catecholamines in renal failure plasma.[263,264]

MISCELLANEOUS DISORDERS

Defective catecholamine-stimulated lipolysis in lipomatous fat from patients with multiple symmetric lipomatosis has been reported[265] but not confirmed.[266] Essential hyperhidrosis is decreased by sympathectomy.[267] Decreased platelet α-adrenergic receptor density and responsiveness to epinephrine is found in samples from some patients with essential thrombocythemia.[268]

DIAGNOSTIC TESTING

Measurement of Catecholamines and Their Metabolites

Measurements of catecholamines and their metabolites in urine have been used clinically for decades. Although liquid chromatography with electrochemical detection is being used increasingly, urinary catecholamines continue to be measured fluorometrically in many clinical laboratories.[10] Catecholamines are extracted from urine and oxidized to their more intensely fluorescent trihydroxyindole derivatives. With use of two wavelengths or of oxidation at both pH 7.0 and 2.0, the proportion of norepinephrine and epinephrine can be estimated. Normal catecholamine excretion is generally less than 100 μg/24 h (approximately 80 percent norepinephrine), although some laboratories use 135 μg/24 h as the upper limit of normal. A few laboratories report upper limits of normal approximately twice the latter value; they may be including a hydrolysis step and measuring conjugates as well as catecholamines. This is not recommended, since the levels of conjugated catecholamines in urine (and plasma) are increased by foods such as bananas.[269] Alternatively, they may be including dopamine.

Urinary normetanephrine plus metanephrine (total metanephrines) and urinary VMA are commonly measured by selective extraction and conversion to vanillin, which is then measured spectrophotometrically.[10] Normal persons generally excrete less than 1 mg of total metanephrines and less than 7 mg of VMA per 24 h.

As discussed earlier, single-isotope-derivative (radioenzymatic) assays have become the reference method for measurement of catecholamines in plasma.[76] They have the sensitivity, specificity, and precision requisite to measurement of physiologic concentrations of epinephrine as well as norepinephrine in plasma.[264] They can, of course, be used to measure catecholamines in urine and tissues, but the high concentrations present do not require sensitive methods. Single-isotope-derivative methods are generally based upon the conversion of norepinephrine and epinephrine, in the presence of catechol-O-methyl transferase and S-adenosyl-L-methionine containing a tritiated methyl group, to their tritiated O-methyl derivatives, tritiated normetanephrine and tritiated metanephrine, respectively. These derivatives are then separated by thin-layer chromatography so that norepinephrine and epinephrine can be measured independently. A few laboratories omit the chromatography step and measure total catecholamines; others use phenylethanolamine-N-methyl transferase rather than catechol-

O-methyl transferase and isolate tritiated epinephrine, thus measuring only norepinephrine. Neither of the latter alternatives is advisable, since measurements of both norepinephrine and epinephrine are useful diagnostically.

Isotope-derivative methods are technically demanding, time-consuming, and relatively expensive, but they are now available in several commercial laboratories. An alternative approach to the measurement of catecholamines in plasma is high-performance liquid chromatography with electrochemical detection (LCEC).[77] Although not sensitive enough for measurement of physiologic fluctuations in plasma epinephrine in many laboratories, this method may well be sufficient to determine whether or not levels are distinctly elevated. It, too, is available commercially. A recent modification of the enzymatic approach employs conversion of the catecholamines to metanephrine and immunoassay of that derivative.[78] Assessment of the clinical utility of the latter assay must await further experience. As performed commercially, it measures biologically inactive conjugates as well as catecholamines.

Venous plasma norepinephrine and epinephrine concentrations, measured with a single-isotope-derivative method, in various physiologic and pathologic states in humans are shown in Figs. 13-9 and 13-10, respectively.

Catecholamine measurements are particularly susceptible to diagnostic misinterpretation. This can be the result of technical errors, biologic variation, or drug-induced alterations. These are discussed here in relation first to plasma catecholamine determinations and then to their relevance to measurements of urinary catecholamines and catecholamine metabolites.

Technical considerations include the selection of a clinically validated analytical method. The single-isotope-derivative method, with measurement of both norepinephrine and epinephrine, meets this criterion. When properly performed, the single-isotope-derivative method is sensitive to about 0.5 pg of norepinephrine and epinephrine, has a high degree of specificity, and is reasonably precise, with between-assay coefficients of variation of less than 10 percent.[264] Duplicate determinations require only 100 μl of plasma.

Catecholamines are readily oxidized. In general, they are most stable at low temperature and low pH and in the presence of an antioxidant. Erythrocytes contain catechol-O-methyl transferase. In whole blood catecholamines deteriorate at a rate of approximately 30 percent per hour at room temperature. Thus, blood samples for plasma catecholamine determinations should be drawn into iced tubes containing an anticoagulant and an antioxidant and the plasma promptly separated, preferably in a refrigerated centrifuge. Many laboratories, including our own, use the calcium-chelating agent EGTA and the antioxidant reduced glutathione. We add 20 μl of a solution containing 25 mmol EGTA and 20 mmol reduced glutathione per milliliter of blood to be drawn to standard heparinized tubes. Dithiothreitol, but not sodium metabisulfite or ascorbic acid, can be substituted for reduced glutathione. Once separated, plasma should be frozen quickly. Even in the presence of an antioxidant, catecholamines deteriorate at a rate of approximately 5 percent per month at −20°C. At −70°C catecholamines are stable for at least 1 year.[270]

With respect to biologic variation, the marked and rapid changes that occur in plasma catecholamine levels warrant emphasis. Plasma epinephrine levels can rise as much as 100-fold during hypoglycemia. Smaller, but substantial, changes in plasma norepinephrine and epinephrine occur rapidly during common activities (see Figs. 13-9 and 13-10). Thus, scrupulous attention to sampling conditions and reluctance to attach undue importance to single measurements are required if plasma catecholamine levels are to be interpreted correctly.

Physical and mental stress elevate plasma catecholamine levels. Indeed, even the stress of venipuncture increases mean values by about one-third and substantially increases the scatter in the data. Therefore, plasma catecholamine samples are best drawn through an indwelling intravenous needle or catheter inserted 30 min earlier. Because the upright posture roughly doubles plasma catecholamine concentrations (Table 13-2, Fig. 13-13), the patient should rest in the horizontal position between needle or catheter insertion and sampling. Additional physiologic factors should be kept in mind. Plasma norepinephrine concentrations increase slightly with increasing age; whether this is due to decreased clearance or increased release is controversial.[271] Sodium depletion due to disease, diuretics, or dietary sodium restriction ($<$3.0 g per day), elevates resting plasma norepinephrine concentrations and increases the norepinephrine response to standing.[98,272] Plasma glucose decrements from 95 to 60 mg/dl have been found to produce a 10-fold increase in mean plasma epinephrine,[273] a point potentially relevant to sampling from patients with insulin-treated diabetes.

Elevated plasma catecholamine concentrations are to be expected in any acute illness. Elevations, at times marked, have been well documented in patients with acute myocardial infarction, shock, burns, diabetic ketoacidosis, and cerebrovascular accidents, as well as during and immediately after surgery (see Figs. 13-9 and 13-10). Stable plasma catecholamine elevations also occur in patients with chronic disorders—hypothyroidism, congestive heart failure, chronic obstructive pulmonary disease, anemia, duodenal ulcer, etc.—as discussed earlier. Lastly, elevated plasma catecholamine concentrations have been found in some, but certainly not all, patients thought to have essential hypertension, as also discussed earlier.

Drug-induced alterations are perhaps the most common cause of erroneous interpretation of plasma catecholamine measurements. If at all possible, samples should be obtained when the patient is drug-free. Obviously, the catecholamines or drugs which are metabolized to catecholamines are expected to produce analytical artifacts. Methyldopa is a common offender. Although the parent compound does not interfere, its metabolites do. (In a commonly used chromatographic system the O-methyl derivative of α-methylnorepinephrine causes spuriously high epinephrine readings and that of α-methyldopamine, high dopamine readings.) Isoproterenol, metaproterenol, and terbutaline have been noted to increase measured catecholamine levels.

A variety of drugs alter sympathochromaffin physiology. Elevated plasma catecholamine concentrations can be the result of increased catecholamine release into the circulation or decreased catecholamine removal from the circulation.[83] Drugs that cause increased catecholamine release include (1) indirect-acting sympathomimetics, including amphetamines and ephedrine; (2) vasodilators, including nitrates and nitrites, hydralazine, minoxidil, methylxanthines, phenothiazines, and nifedipine among others; (3) α-adrenergic antagonists, including the α_1-adrenergic antagonists phenyoxybenzamine and prazosin and particularly those that also block prejunctional α_2-adrenergic receptors such as phentolamine;[95] (4) diuretics in doses sufficient to produce sodium depletion;[272] and (5) cigarette smoking,[95] marijuana smoking, and caffeine ingestion. Drugs known to decrease catecholamine removal from the circulation include the β-adrenergic antagonists.[87] Although propranolol and related drugs do not commonly produce striking plasma catecholamine elevations in the basal state, they cause disproportionate elevations when catecholamine release is stimulated physiologically. Tricyclic antidepressants increase plasma norepinephrine.[250] Drugs such as reserpine and guanethidine would also be expected to reduce catecholamine clearance; however, their long-term administration reduces catecholamine stores. Drugs that decrease plasma catecholamine levels by decreasing release include the α_2-adrenergic agonist clonidine[244] and the tyrosine hydroxylase inhibitor α-methyl-p-tyrosine. Bromocriptine, dexamethasone, and monoamine oxidase inhibitors have also been noted to lower plasma catecholamine concentrations.

Urine samples for catecholamine determinations are commonly collected in refrigerated containers to which 15 ml of 6*N* HCl has been added, since catecholamines are more stable at low temperature and low pH. Urine samples for metanephrines and VMA need not be acidified, but the analytical methods are compatible with this form of collection if catecholamines are also to be measured. The collection of a complete 24-h urine specimen requires careful instruction of the patient and, in the hospital, the nursing staff. The creatinine content should be measured in all specimens to detect major collection errors. Dietary restrictions are not necessary for specific measurements of urinary metanephrines and VMA and if conjugated catecholamines are not measured, as discussed earlier.

Catecholamine and catecholamine metabolite excretion is subject to the same sources of biologic variation as plasma catecholamine levels, discussed earlier. However, because these variations in catecholamine release are commonly brief, their effect on 24-h excretion is relatively small and sampling conditions need not be controlled rigorously. Nonetheless, major stress should be avoided during these collections, as conditions known to produce stable elevations in plasma catecholamine levels will produce corresponding elevations in urinary catecholamine and metabolite excretion.

Drug-induced alterations are also common. All the drugs that elevate plasma catecholamine levels, discussed earlier, would be expected to increase urinary catecholamine and metabolite values. In addition, some fluorescent drugs, tetracycline and erythromycin among others, cause artifactual elevation of fluorometric catecholamine determinations; L-dopa elevates urinary VMA. Methyldopa causes a characteristic pattern—elevated urinary catecholamines but not VMA. The methyldopa metabolite α-methylnorepinephrine is measured in most fluorometric assays. Because of the methyl group on the α carbon, however, the latter compound cannot serve as a substrate for monoamine oxidase and cannot be metabolized to VMA. Short-term administration of the mild analgesics acetylsalicylic acid, acetaminophen, and propoxyphene or of the sedative-tranquilizers diazepam, chlordiazepoxide, diphenhydramine, and phenobarbital does not alter catecholamine excretion.[274] Whether these drugs affect plasma catecholamine levels is not known.

In summary, physiologic plasma concentrations of norepinephrine and epinephrine can now be measured with a single-isotope-derivative method and used, along with measurements of urinary catecholamine and catecholamine metabolite excretion, to assess patients suspected to have disorders of sympathochromaffin function. However, particularly for the plasma measurements, the physician must pay strict attention to sample handling and storage, to the sampling conditions, and to the many sources of biologic variation. In view of the multitude of potential drug-induced alterations, patients should be sampled in the drug-free state if at all possible.

Indirect Tests of Autonomic Function

Selected indirect tests of the integrity of sympathetic neural function are outlined in Table 13-5. These have been reviewed in Refs. 195 to 197 and 257 to 281 and are not discussed here in detail. Measurement of the blood pressure in the supine and standing positions is the most widely used clinically and was discussed earlier in this chapter. Clearly, it is neither a sensitive nor a specific test of sympathetic function.

Table 13-5. Selected Indirect Tests of Sympathetic Neural Function

Maneuver	Mechanism	Normal responses	Usual interpretation of abnormal responses
Standing/tilting	Decreased cardiac output→sympathetic discharge	Maintenance of upright blood pressure	>20 mmHg decrease in standing mean blood pressure—sympathetic lesion (afferent, central, efferent)*
Valsalva maneuver	Decreased cardiac output→sympathetic discharge	<50% decrease in blood pressure (with tachycardia) during Valsalva and post-Valsalva blood pressure overshoot (with bradycardia)	>50% decrease in blood pressure and absence of post-Valsalva blood pressure overshoot—sympathetic lesion (afferent, central, efferent)*
Cold pressor test (extremity in ice water for 1–3 min) or mental stress	Centrally initiated sympathetic discharge	Increased blood pressure (with decreased limb blood flow)	No increase in blood pressure (or decrease in limb blood flow)—sympathetic lesion (central, efferent)*
Systemic infusions:			
Tyramine (1–3 mg)	Indirect (NE-releasing) adrenergic agonist	Increased blood pressure	No increase in blood pressure—sympathetic postganglionic lesion*†
Norepinephrine (0.07 μg/kg/min)	Direct adrenergic agonist	Increased blood pressure	Exaggerated increase in blood pressure—sympathetic postganglionic lesion (denervation hypersensitivity)†
Response to hyperthermia (1°C increase in core temperature)	Centrally initiated sympathetic stimulation including cholinergic postganglionic neurons	Sweating	No sweating—sympathetic lesion (central, efferent)*
Pupil responses to conjunctival sac instillations:			
Epinephrine (1:1000), phenylephrine (4%)	Adrenergic agonist	No effect (dilute solutions)	Mydriasis—sympathetic postganglionic lesion (denervation hypersensitivity)†
Hydroxyamphetamine (1%)	Indirect (NE-releasing) adrenergic agonist	Mydriasis	No response to either—sympathetic postganglionic lesion*†
Cocaine (4%)	Indirect (NE reuptake–inhibiting) adrenergic agonist		Response to hydroxyamphetamine but not to cocaine—sympathetic preganglionic or central lesion*
Homatropine (5%)	Cholinergic antagonist	Mydriasis	No mydriasis—sympathetic lesion*

*End-organ unresponsiveness is a possible alternative cause for these findings.
†It is conceivable that preganglionic or more central sympathetic lesions could also explain these findings.

Patients with other evidence of sympathochromaffin hypofunction may not have postural hypotension,[194,275] and postural hypotension can be the result of mechanisms other than sympathetic hypofunction, as discussed earlier. The utility of this maneuver is enhanced by simultaneous measurement of the plasma norepinephrine response.

Among tests of parasympathetic function, measurement of the variation in heart rate associated with deep breathing is commonly used.[195–197,275–281] The normal variation is determined largely by vagal inputs; variation is decreased by parasympathetic hypofunction. Although Pfeiffer et al. have emphasized that a potential β-adrenergic effect on heart rate variation should be prevented by propranolol administration during the test,[278] most do not give a β-adrenergic antagonist. A simple approach is to obtain an ECG recording during deep breathing at 5 to 6 cycles per minute in a resting subject.[281] RR intervals are measured and beat-to-beat variation calculated as the difference between maximal and minimal heart rate and expressed as the mean of differences in five successive respirations. Values less than 10 per minute are considered abnormal by Hilsted and Jensen.[281] Ewing et al. have assessed this approach, among other methods, found it to be independent of resting heart rate, and recommended it.[277]

These tests should be interpreted with caution for several reasons. First, normal responsiveness of the various end organs is assumed. Second, "abnormal" responses are sometimes found in overtly normal persons with no demonstrable autonomic defect. Third, certain assumptions concerning localization of the defect, although reasonable, have not been thoroughly established. For example, an exaggerated pressor response to infused norepinephrine (denervation hypersensitivity) is interpreted as evidence of a sympathetic postganglionic lesion, but it is conceivable that a more central primary lesion could produce a similar result.

ACKNOWLEDGMENTS The author is grateful for the efforts of his collaborators, whose names appear in the reference list, and for the support of U.S. Public Health Service grants AM 27085, RR 00036, and AM 20579. Particular thanks are due to Dr. William E. Clutter, for provocative and informative discussions as well as critical review of a draft of this manuscript, and to Ms. Theresa Lautner for tireless secretarial assistance.

REFERENCES

1. Cryer PE: Physiology and pathophysiology of the human sympathoadrenal neuroendocrine system. *N Engl J Med* 303:436, 1980.

2. Silverberg AB, Shah SD, Haymond MW, Cryer PE: Norepinephrine: Hormone and neurotransmitter in man. *Am J Physiol* 234:E252, 1978.

3. Clutter WE, Bier DM, Shah SD, Cryer PE: Epinephrine plasma metabolic clearance rates and physiologic thresholds for metabolic and hemodynamic actions in man. *J Clin Invest* 66:94, 1980.

4. Galster AD, Clutter WE, Cryer PE, Collins JA, Bier DM: Epinephrine plasma thresholds for lipolytic effects in man: Measurements of fatty acid transport with [1-^{13}C]palmitic acid. *J Clin Invest* 67:1729, 1981.

5. Body J-J, Cryer PE, Offord KP, Heath H III: Epinephrine is a hypophosphatemic hormone in man. *J Clin Invest* 71:572, 1983.

6. Shah SD, Tse TF, Clutter WE, Cryer PE: The human sympathochromaffin system. *Am J Physiol* 247:E380, 1984.

7. Lackovic Z, Relja M: Evidence for a widely distributed peripheral dopaminergic system. *Fed Proc* 42:3000, 1983.

8. Snider SR, Kuchel O: Dopamine: An important neurohormone of the sympathoadrenal system. *Endocr Rev* 4:291, 1983.

9. Mayer SE: Neurohumoral transmission and the autonomic nervous system, in Gilman AG, Goodman LS, Gilman A (eds): *The Pharmacological Basis of Therapeutics.* New York, Macmillan, 1980, pp. 56–90.

10. Nagatsu T: *Biochemistry of the Catecholamines.* Baltimore, University Park Press, 1973.

11. Mussachio JM: Enzymes involved in the biosynthesis and degradation of catecholamines, in Iversen LL, Iversen SD, Snyder SH (eds): *Handbook of Psychopharmacology.* New York, Plenum, 1975, vol 3, pp. 1–35.

12. Clarke JTR, Bier DM: The conversion of phenylalanine to tyrosine in man: Direct measurement by continuous intravenous tracer infusions of L-[ring-$^{2}H_5$]phenylalanine and L-[1-^{13}C]tyrosine in the postabsorptive state. *Metabolism* 31:999, 1982.

13. McInnes RR, Kaufman S, Warsh JJ, VanLoon GR, Milstien S, Kapatos G, Soldin S, Walsh P, MacGregor D, Hanley WB: Biopterin synthesis defect. *J Clin Invest* 73:458, 1984.

14. Ames MM, Lerner P, Lovenberg W: Tyrosine hydroxylase: Activation by protein phosphorylation and end product inhibition. *J Biol Chem* 253:27, 1978.

15. Haycock JW, Meligeni JA, Bennett WF, Waymire JC: Phosphorylation and activation of tyrosine hydroxylase mediate the acetylcholine-induced increase in catecholamine biosynthesis in adrenal chromaffin cells. *J Biol Chem* 257:12641, 1982.

16. Rudman D, Moffitt SD, Fernhoff PM, Blackston RD, Faraj BA: Epinephrine deficiency in hypocorticotropic hypopituitary children. *J Clin Endocrinol Metab* 53:722, 1981.

17. Blombery PA, Kopin IJ, Gordon EK, Markey SP, Ebert MH: Conversion of MHPG to vanillylmandelic acid. *Arch Gen Psychiatry* 37:1095, 1980.

18. Mardh G, Sjoquist B, Anggard E: Norepinephrine metabolism in man using deuterium labelling: The conversion of 4-hydroxy-3-methoxyphenylglycol to 4-hydroxy-3-methoxymandelic acid. *J Neurochem* 36:1181, 1981.

19. Kopin IJ, Polinsky RJ, Oliver JA, Oddershede IR, Ebert MH: Urinary catecholamine metabolites distinguish different types of sympathetic neuronal dysfunction in patients with orthostatic hypotension. *J Clin Endocrinol Metab* 57:632, 1983.

20. Maas JW, Hattox SE, Greene NM, Landis DH: 3-Methoxy-4-hydroxyphenethyleneglycol production by human brain in vivo. *Science* 205:1025, 1979.

21. Kopin IJ, Gordon EK, Jimerson DC, Polinsky RJ: Relation between plasma and cerebrospinal fluid levels of 3-methoxy-4-hydroxyphenylglycol. *Science* 219:73, 1983.

22. Coupland RE: *The Natural History of the Chromaffin Cell.* London, Longmans, 1965, p 77.

23. Winkler H, Westhead E: The molecular organization of adrenal chromaffin granules. *Neuroscience* 5:1803, 1980.

24. O'Connor DT, Burton D, Deftos LJ: Immunoreactive human chromogranin A in diverse polypeptide hormone producing tumors and normal endocrine tissues. *J Clin Endocrinol Metab* 57:1084, 1983.

25. Lloyd RV, Wilson BS: Specific endocrine tissue marker defined by a monoclonal antibody. *Science* 222:628, 1983.

26. Kryvi H: Comparison of the ultrastructure of adrenaline and noradrenaline storage granules of bovine adrenal medulla. *Eur J Cell Biol* 20:76, 1979.

27. Knight DE, Baker PF: Stimulus-secretion coupling in isolated bovine adrenal medullary cells. *Q J Exp Physiol* 68:123, 1983.

28. Schober R, Nitsch C, Rinne U, Morris SJ: Calcium-induced displacement of membrane-associated particles upon aggregation of chromaffin granules. *Science* 195:495, 1977.

29. Konings F, Majchrowicz B, DePotter W: Release of chromaffin granular content on interaction with plasma membranes. *Am J Physiol* C309, 1983.

30. Young JB, Landsberg L: Sympathoadrenal activity in fasting pregnant rats: Dissociation of adrenal medullary and sympathetic nervous system responses. *J Clin Invest* 64:109, 1979.

31. Axelrod J, Weinshilboum R: Catecholamines. *N Engl J Med* 287:237, 1972.

32. Lee C-M, Javitch JA, Snyder SH: Recognition sites for norepinephrine uptake: Regulation by neurotransmitter. *Science* 220: 626, 1983.

33. Maas JW, Benensohn H, Landis HD: A kinetic study of the disposition of circulating norepinephrine in normal male subjects. *J Pharmacol Exp Ther* 174:381, 1970.

34. Wang P-C, Buu NT, Kuchel O, Genest J: Conjugation patterns of endogenous plasma catecholamines in human and rat. *J Lab Clin Med* 101:141, 1983.

35. Starke K, Taube HD, Borowski E: Presynaptic receptor systems in catecholaminergic transmission. *Biochem Pharmacol* 26:259, 1977.

36. Shepherd JT, Vanhoutte PM: Local modulation of adrenergic neurotransmission. *Circulation* 64:655, 1981.

37. Baxter JD, Funder JW: Hormone receptors. *N Engl J Med* 301:1149, 1979.

38. Lefkowitz RJ, Michel T: Plasma membrane receptors. *J Clin Invest* 72:1185, 1983.

39. Motulsky HJ, Insel PA: Adrenergic receptors in man. *N Engl J Med* 307:18, 1982.

40. Minneman KP, Molinoff PB: Classification and quantitation of β-adrenergic receptor subtypes. *Biochem Pharmacol* 29:1317, 1980.

41. Hoffman BB, Lefkowitz RJ: Agonist interactions with α-adrenergic receptors. *J Cardiovasc Pharmacol* 4:S14, 1982.

42. Insel PA: *Adrenergic Receptors in Man.* New York, Marcel Dekker (in press).

43. Ahlquist RP: A study of adrenotropic receptors. *Am J Physiol* 153:586, 1948.

44. Spiegel AM, Downs RW Jr: Guanine nucleotides: Key regulators of hormone receptor–adenylate cyclase interaction. *Endocr Rev* 2:275, 1981.

45. Gilman AG: Guanine nucleotide binding regulatory proteins and dual control of adenylate cyclase. *J Clin Invest* 73:1, 1984.

46. Insel PA: Identification and regulation of adrenergic receptors in target cells. *Am J Physiol* 247:E53, 1984.

47. Limbird LE: GTP and Na^+ modulate receptor-adenyl cyclase coupling and receptor-mediated function. *Am J Physiol* 247:E59, 1984.

48. Harden TK: Agonist-induced desensitization of the β-adrenergic receptor linked adenylate cyclase. *Pharmacol Rev* 35:5, 1983.

49. Stadel JM, Nambi PN, Shorr RGL, Sawyer DF, Caron MG, Lefkowitz RJ: Catecholamine-induced desensitization of turkey erythrocyte adenylate cyclase is associated with phosphorylation of the β-adrenergic receptor. *Proc Natl Acad Sci USA* 80:3173, 1983.

50. Cryer PE: Adrenergic receptors in endocrine and metabolic diseases, in Insel PA (ed): *Adrenergic Receptors in Man.* New York, Marcel Dekker (in press).

51. Creese I, Silbey DR, Hamblin MW, Leff SE: The classification of dopamine receptors. *Annu Rev Neurosci* 6:43, 1983.

51a. Goldberg LI, Glock D, Kohli JD, Berger Y: Separation of dopamine receptors by a selective DA_1 antagonist (abstr). *Clin Res* 31:716A, 1983.

52. Ariens EJ, Simonis AM: Receptors and receptor mechanisms, in Saxena PR, Forsyth RP (eds): *Beta-adrenoceptor Blocking Agents.* Amsterdam, North-Holland, 1976, pp. 3–27.

53. Ariens EJ: The classification of beta-adrenoceptors. *Trends Pharmacol Sci* 2:170, 1981.

54. Hawthorn MH, Broadley KJ: Evidence from use of neuronal uptake inhibition that β_1-adrenoceptors, but not β_2-adrenoceptors, are innervated. *J Pharm Pharmacol* 34:664, 1982.

55. Wilffert B, Timmermans PBMWM, van Zwieten PA: Extrasynaptic location of alpha-2 and noninnervated beta-2 adrenoceptors in the vascular system of the pithed normotensive rat. *J Pharmacol Exp Ther* 221:762, 1982.

56. Zukowska-Grojec Z, Bayorh MA, Kopin IJ: Effect of desipramine on the effects of α-adrenoceptor inhibitors on pressor responses and release of norepinephrine into plasma of pithed rats. *J Cardiovasc Pharmacol* 5:297, 1983.

57. Weiner N: Norepinephrine, epinephrine and the sympathomimetic amines, in Gilman AG, Goodman LS, Gilman A (eds): *The Pharmacological Basis of Therapeutics.* New York, Macmillan, 1980, pp. 138–175.

58. Rizza RA, Haymond MW, Cryer PE, Gerich JE: Differential effects of physiologic concentrations of epinephrine on glucose production and disposal in man. *Am J Physiol* 237:E356, 1979.

59. Rizza RA, Haymond MW, Miles JM, Verdonk CH, Cryer PE, Gerich JE: Effect of alpha-adrenergic stimulation and its blockade on glucose turnover in man. *Am J Physiol* 238:E467, 1980.

60. Rizza RA, Cryer PE, Haymond MW, Gerich JE: Adrenergic mechanisms for the effect of epinephrine on glucose production and clearance in man. *J Clin Invest* 65:682, 1980.

61. Deibert DC, DeFronzo RA: Epinephrine-induced insulin resistance in man. *J Clin Invest* 65:717, 1980.

62. Rosen SG, Clutter WE, Shah SD, Miller JP, Bier DM, Cryer PE: Direct, α-adrenergic stimulation of hepatic glucose production in postabsorptive human subjects. *Am J Physiol* 245:E616, 1983.

63. Berk MA, Clutter WE, Skor DS, Shah S, Cryer P: Enhanced glycemic responsiveness to epinephrine in insulin-dependent diabetes mellitus is the result of the inability to secrete insulin. *J Clin Invest* 75:1842, 1985.

64. Chiasson J-L, Shikama H, Chu DTW, Exton JH: Inhibitory effect of epinephrine on insulin-stimulated glucose uptake by rat skeletal muscle. *J Clin Invest* 68:706, 1981.

65. Miles JM, Nissen S, Gerich JE, Haymond MW: Effects of epinephrine infusion on leucine and alanine kinetics in man. *Am J Physiol* 247:E166, 1984.

66. Fain JN, Garcia-Sainz JA: Adrenergic regulation of adipocyte metabolism. *J Lipid Res* 24:945, 1983.

67. Bahnsen M, Burrin JM, Johnston DG, Pernet A, Walker M, Alberti KGMM: Mechanisms of catecholamine effects on ketogenesis. *Am J Physiol* 247:E173, 1984.

68. Brown MJ, Brown DC, Murphy MB: Hypokalemia from beta_2-receptor stimulation by circulating epinephrine. *N Engl J Med* 309:1414, 1983.

69. Landsberg L, Saville ME, Young JB: Sympathoadrenal system and regulation of thermogenesis. *Am J Physiol* 247:E181, 1984.

70. Gray DE, Lickley HLA, Vranic M: Physiologic effects of epinephrine on glucose turnover and plasma free fatty acid concentrations mediated independently of glucagon. *Diabetes* 29:600, 1980.

71. Morgan NG, Blackmore PF, Exton JH: Age-related changes in the control of hepatic cyclic AMP levels by α_1- and β_2-adrenergic receptors in male rats. *J Biol Chem* 258:5103, 1983.

72. Sacca L, Morrone G, Cicala M, Corso G, Ungaro B: Influence of epinephrine, norepinephrine and isoproterenol on glucose homeostasis in normal man. *J Clin Endocrinol Metab* 50:680, 1980.

73. Halter JB, Pflug AE, Tolas AG: Arterial-venous differences of plasma catecholamines in man. *Metabolism* 29:9, 1980.

74. Grimm M, Weidmann P, Keusch G, Meier A, Glück Z: Norepinephrine clearance and pressor effect in normal and hypertensive man. *Klin Wochenschr* 58:1175, 1980.

75. Izzo J Jr: Cardiovascular hormonal effects of circulating norepinephrine. *Hypertension* 5:787, 1983.

76. Cryer PE: Catecholamines and metabolism. *Am J Physiol* 247:E1, 1984.

77. Hjemdahl P: Catecholamine measurements by high performance liquid chromatography. *Am J Physiol* 247:E13, 1984.

78. Raum WJ: Methods of plasma catecholamine measurement including radioimmunoassay. *Am J Physiol* 247:E4, 1984.

79. Wang M-T, Imai K, Yoshioka M, Tamura Z: Gas-liquid chromatographic and mass fragmentographic determination of catecholamines in human plasma. *Clin Chim Acta* 63:13, 1975.

80. Wang M-T, Yoshioka M, Imai K, Tamura Z: Gas-liquid chromatographic and mass fragmentographic determination of 3-O-methylated catecholamines in human plasma. *Clin Chim Acta* 63:21, 1975.

81. Elchisak MA, Polinsky RJ, Ebert MH, Kopin IJ: Kinetics of homovanillic acid and determination of its production rate in humans. *J Neurochem* 38:380, 1982.

82. Best JD, Halter JB: Release and clearance rates of epinephrine in man: Importance of arterial measurements. *J Clin Endocrinol Metab* 55:263, 1982.

83. Esler M, Jennings G, Korner P, Blombery P, Sacharias N, Leonard P: Measurement of total, and organ specific, noradrenaline kinetics in humans. *Am J Physiol* 247:E21, 1984.

84. Christensen NJ, Hilsted J, Hegedus L, Madsbad S: Effects of surgical stress and insulin on cardiovascular function and norepinephrine kinetics. *Am J Physiol* 247:E29, 1984.

85. Best JD, Halter JB: Effect of propranolol on norepinephrine release rate and clearance in man (abstr). *Clin Res* 30:86A, 1982.

86. Goldstein DS, Horwitz D, Keiser HR, Polinsky RJ, Kopin IJ: Plasma *l*-[^{3}H]norepinephrine, *d*-[^{14}C]norepinephrine and *d,l*-[^{3}H]-isoproterenol kinetics in essential hypertension. *J Clin Invest* 72:1748, 1983.

87. Cryer PE, Rizza RA, Haymond MW, Gerich JE: Epinephrine and norepinephrine are cleared through β-adrenergic, but not α-adrenergic, mechanisms in man. *Metabolism* 29:1114, 1980.

88. Ghione S, Palombo C, Pellegrini M, Fommei E, Pilo A, Donato L: The kinetics of plasma noradrenaline in normal and hypertensive subjects. *Clin Sci* 55:89S, 1978.

89. Hoeldtke RD, Cilmi KM, Reichard GA Jr, Boden G, Owen OE: Assessment of norepinephrine secretion and production. *J Lab Clin Med* 101:772, 1983.

90. Berecek KH, Brody MJ: Evidence for a neurotransmitter role for epinephrine derived from the adrenal medullae. *Am J Physiol* 242:H593, 1982.

91. Folkow B, DiBona GF, Hjemdahl P, Toren PH, Wallin BG: Measurements of plasma norepinephrine concentrations in human primary hypertension. *Hypertension* 5:399, 1983.

92. Goldstein DS, McCarty R, Polinsky RJ, Kopin IJ: Relationship between plasma norepinephrine and sympathetic neural activity. *Hypertension* 5:552, 1983.

93. Brown MJ, Jenner DA, Allison DJ, Dollery CT: Variations in individual organ release of noradrenaline measured by an improved radioenzymatic technique: Limitations of peripheral venous measurements in the assessment of sympathetic nervous activity. *Clin Sci* 61:585, 1981.

94. Planz G: Adrenaline and noradrenaline concentration in blood of suprarenal and renal vein of man with normal blood pressure and with essential hypertension. *Klin Wochenschr* 56:1109, 1978.

95. Cryer PE, Haymond MW, Santiago JV, Shah SD: Norepinephrine and epinephrine release and adrenergic mediation of smoking-associated hemodynamic and metabolic events. *N Engl J Med* 295:573, 1976.

96. Mancia G, Ferrari A, Gregorini L, Leonetti G, Parati G, Picotti GB, Ravazzani C, Zanchetti A: Plasma catecholamines do not invariably reflect sympathetically induced changes in blood pressure in man. *Clin Sci* 65:227, 1983.

97. Young JB, Rosa RM, Landsberg L: Dissociation of sympathetic nervous system and adrenal medullary responses. *Am J Physiol* 247:E35, 1984.

98. Cryer PE: Isotope derivative measurements of plasma norepinephrine and epinephrine in man. *Diabetes* 25:1071, 1976.

99. Melicow MM: One hundred cases of pheochromocytoma (107 tumors) at the Columbia-Presbyterian Medical Center. *Cancer* 40:1987, 1977.

100. Manger WM, Gifford RW Jr: Hypertension secondary to pheochromocytoma. *Bull NY Acad Med* 58:139, 1982.

101. Beard CM, Sheps SG, Kurland LT, Carney JA, Lie JT: Occurrence of pheochromocytoma in Rochester, Minnesota, 1950 through 1979. *Mayo Clin Proc* 58:802, 1983.

102. Sutton MGS, Sheps SG, Lie JT: Prevalence of clinically unsuspected pheochromocytoma: Review of a 50-year autopsy series. *Mayo Clin Proc* 56:354, 1981.

103. Steiner AL, Goodman AD, Powers SR: Study of a kindred with pheochromocytoma, medullary thyroid carcinoma, hyperparathyroidism and Cushing's disease: Multiple endocrine neoplasia, type 2. *Medicine* 47:371, 1968.

104. Lips KJM, Veer JVDS, Struyvenberg A, Alleman A, Leo JR, Wittebol P, Minder WH, Kooiker CJ, Geerdink RA, Van Waes PFGM, Hackeng WHL: Bilateral occurrence of pheochromocytoma in patients with the multiple endocrine neoplasia syndrome type 2a (Sipple's syndrome). *Am J Med* 70:1051, 1981.

105. DeLellis RA, Wolfe HJ, Gagel RF, Feldman ZT, Miller HH, Gang DL, Reichlin S: Adrenal medullary hyperplasia. *Am J Pathol* 83:177, 1976.

106. Hamilton BP, Landsberg L, Levine RJ: Measurement of urinary epinephrine in screening for pheochromocytoma in multiple endocrine neoplasia type II. *Am J Med* 65:1027, 1978.

107. Atuk NO, McDonald T, Wood T, Carpenter JT, Walzak MP, Donaldson M, Gillenwater JY: Familial pheochromocytoma, hypercalcemia and von Hippel-Lindau disease. *Medicine* 58:209, 1979.

108. Yoshimasa T, Nakao K, Li S, Ikeda Y, Suda M, Sakamoto M, Imura H: Plasma methionine-enkephalin and leucine-enkephalin in normal subjects and patients with pheochromocytoma. *J Clin Endocrinol Metab* 57:706, 1983.

109. Berelowitz M, Szabo M, Barowsky HW, Arbel ER, Frohman LA: Somatostatin-like immunoactivity and biological activity is present in a human pheochromocytoma. *J Clin Endocrinol Metab* 56:134, 1983.

110. Weinstein RS, Ide LF: Immunoreactive calcitonin in pheochromocytomas. *Proc Soc Exp Biol Med* 165:215, 1980.

111. Spark RF, Connolly PB, Gluckin DS, White R, Sacks B, Landsberg L: ACTH secretion from a functioning pheochromocytoma. *N Engl J Med* 301:416, 1979.

112. Page LB, Raker JW, Beberich FR: Pheochromocytoma with predominant epinephrine secretion. *Am J Med* 47:648, 1969.

113. Aronoff SL, Passamani E, Borowsky BA, Weiss AN, Roberts R, Cryer PE: Norepinephrine and epinephrine secretion from a clinically epinephrine-secreting pheochromocytoma. *Am J Med* 69:321, 1980.

114. Bravo EL, Tarazi RC, Fouad FM, Textor SC, Gifford RW Jr, Vidt DG: Blood pressure regulation in pheochromocytoma. *Hyper-*

tension 4(suppl 2):193, 1982.

115. Turnbull DM, Johnston DG, Alberti KGMM, Hall R: Hormonal and metabolic studies in a patient with a pheochromocytoma. *J Clin Endocrinol Metab* 51:930, 1980.

116. Sjoerdsma A, Engelman K, Waldmann TA, Cooperman LH, Hammond WG: Pheochromocytoma: Current concepts of diagnosis and treatment. *Ann Intern Med* 65:1302, 1966.

117. van Heerden JA, Sheps SG, Hamberger B, Sheedy PF, Poston JG, ReMine WH: Pheochromocytoma: Current status and changing trends. *Surgery* 91:367, 1982.

118. Engelman K, Portnoy B, Sjoerdsma A: Plasma catecholamine concentrations in patients with hypertension. *Circ Res* 26(suppl 1):141, 1970.

119. Geffen LB, Rush RA, Louis WJ, Doyle AE: Plasma catecholamine and dopamine β-hydroxylase amounts in phaeochromocytoma. *Clin Sci* 44:421, 1973.

120. Bravo EL, Tarazi RC, Gifford RW Jr, Stewart BH: Circulating and urinary catecholamines in pheochromocytoma. *N Engl J Med* 301:682, 1979.

121. Causon RC, Brown MJ: Catecholamine measurements in phaeochromocytoma: A review. *Ann Clin Biochem* 19:396, 1982.

122. Bravo EL: Pheochromocytoma. *Primary Care* 10:75, 1983.

123. Feldman JM, Klatt C: Elevated platelet norepinephrine concentration in patients with pheochromocytomas. *Clin Chim Acta* 117:279, 1981.

124. Zweifler AJ, Julius S: Increased platelet catecholamine content in pheochromocytoma. *N Engl J Med* 306:890, 1982.

125. Bravo EL, Tarazi RC, Fouad FM, Vidt DG, Gifford RW Jr: Clonidine suppression test: A useful aid in the diagnosis of pheochromocytoma. *N Engl J Med* 305:623, 1981.

126. Halter JB, Beard JC, Pfeifer MA, Metz SA: Clonidine suppression test for diagnosis of pheochromocytoma. *N Engl J Med* 306:49, 1982.

127. Wilms G, Baert A, Marchal G, Goddeeris P: Computed tomography of the normal adrenal glands: Correlative study with autopsy specimens. *J Comput Assist Tomogr* 3:467, 1979.

128. Welch TJ, Sheedy PF II, van Heerden JA, Sheps SG, Hattery RR, Stephens DH: Pheochromocytoma: Value of computed tomography. *Radiology* 148:501, 1983.

129. Sisson JC, Frager MS, Valk TW, Gross MD, Swanson DP, Wieland DM, Tobes MC, Beierwaltes WH, Thompson NW: Scintigraphic localization of pheochromocytoma. *N Engl J Med* 305:12, 1981.

130. Francis IR, Glazer GM, Shapiro B, Sisson JC, Gross BH: Complementary roles of CT and ^{131}I-MIBG scintigraphy in diagnosing pheochromocytoma. *Am J Roentgenol* 141:719, 1983.

131. Sutton H, Wyeth P, Allen AP, Thurtle OA, Hames TK, Cawley MID, Ackery D: Disseminated malignant phaeochromocytoma: Localisation with iodine-131-labelled metaiodobenzylguanidine. *Br Med J* 285:1153, 1982.

132. Valk TW, Frager MS, Gross MD, Sisson JC, Wieland DM, Swanson DP, Mangner TJ, Beierwaltes WH: Spectrum of pheochromocytoma in multiple endocrine neoplasia: A scintigraphic portrayal using ^{131}I-metaiodobenzylguanidine. *Ann Intern Med* 94:762, 1981.

133. Cubbeddu LX, Zarate NA, Rosales CB, Zschaeck DW: Prazosin and propranolol in preoperative management of pheochromocytoma. *Clin Pharmacol Ther* 32:156, 1982.

134. Glass AR, Ballou R: Pheochromocytoma, prazosin and hypotension. *Ann Intern Med* 97:455, 1982.

135. Nicholson JP Jr, Vaugh ED Jr, Pickering TG, Resnick LM, Artusio J, Kleinert HD, Lopez-Overjero JA, Laragh JH: Pheochromocytoma and prazosin. *Ann Intern Med* 99:477, 1983.

136. Plouin P-F, Menard J, Corvol P: Noradrenaline producing pheochromocytomas with absent pressor response to beta-blockade. *Br Heart J* 42:359, 1979.

137. Wark JD, Larkins RG: Pulmonary edema after propranolol therapy in two cases of phaeochromocytoma. *Br Med J* 1:1395, 1978.

138. Feldman JM, Blalock JA, Fagraeus L, Miller JN, Farrell RE, Wells SA Jr: Alterations in plasma norepinephrine concentration during surgical resection of pheochromocytoma. *Ann Surg* 188:758, 1978.

139. Leak D, Carroll JJ, Robinson DC, Ashworth EJ: Management of pheochromocytoma during pregnancy. *Can Med Assoc J* 116:371, 1977.

140. Farndon JR, Fagraeus L, Wells SA Jr: Recent developments in the management of phaeochromocytoma, in Johnston I, Thompson N (eds): *Endocrine Surgery*. London, Butterworth, 1983, pp. 189–201.

141. Hammerman M, Levitt R, Clutter WE, Meltzer V, Bobzein B: Persistent hypertension after resection of a pheochromocytoma. *Am J Med* 73:97, 1982.

142. Castle CH: Iatrogenic renal hypertension: Two unusual complications of surgery for familial pheochromocytoma. *JAMA* 225:1085, 1973.

143. Hengstmann JH, Dengler HJ: Evidence for extratumoral storage of catecholamines in pheochromocytoma patients. *Acta Endocrinol (Kbh)* 87:589, 1978.

144. Jones NF, Walker G, Ruthven CRJ, Sandler M: α-Methyl-*p*-tyrosine in the management of phaeochromocytoma. *Lancet* 2:1105, 1968.

145. Hamilton BPM, Cheikh IE, Rivera LE: Attempted treatment of inoperable pheochromocytoma with streptozotocin. *Arch Intern Med* 137:762, 1977.

146. Feldman JM: Treatment of metastatic pheochromocytoma with streptozotocin. *Arch Intern Med* 143:1799, 1983.

147. Sisson J, Shapiro B, Beierwaltes W, Satterlee W, Nakajo N, Glowniak J, Mangner T, Carey J, Swanson D, Copp J, Wieland D: Treatment of malignant pheochromocytomas with a new radiopharmaceutical (abstr). *Clin Res* 31:547A, 1983.

148. Seeger RC, Siegel SE, Sidell N: Neuroblastoma: Clinical perspectives, monoclonal antibodies and retinoic acid. *Ann Intern Med* 97:873, 1982.

149. Cryer PE, Santiago JV, Shah SD: Measurement of norepinephrine and epinephrine in small volumes of human plasma by a single isotope derivative method: Response to the upright posture. *J Clin Endocrinol Metab* 39:1025, 1974.

150. Thomas JE, Schirger A, Fealey RD, Sheps SG: Orthostatic hypotension. *Mayo Clin Proc* 56:117, 1981.

151. Caird FI, Andrews GR, Kennedy RD: Effect of posture on blood pressure in the elderly. *Br Heart J* 35:527, 1973.

152. Hines S, Houston M, Robertson D: The clinical spectrum of autonomic dysfunction. *Am J Med* 70:1091, 1981.

153. Cryer PE, SIlverberg AB, Santiago JV, Shah SD: Plasma catecholamines in diabetes: The syndromes of hypoadrenergic and hyperadrenergic postural hypotension. *Am J Med* 64:407, 1978.

154. Tohmeh JF, Shah SD, Cryer PE: The pathogenesis of hyperadrenergic postural hypotension in patients with diabetes. *Am J Med* 67:772, 1979.

155. Cryer PE, Weiss S: Reduced plasma norepinephrine response to standing in autonomic dysfunction. *Arch Neurol* 33:275, 1976.

156. Ziegler MG, Lake CR, Kopin IJ: The sympathetic nervous system defect in primary orthostatic hypotension. *N Engl J Med* 296:293, 1977.

157. Leveston SA, Shah SD, Cryer PE: Cholinergic stimulation of norepinephrine release in man: Evidence of a sympathetic postganglionic axonal lesion in diabetic adrenergic neuropathy. *J Clin Invest* 64:374, 1979.

158. Ropper AH, Davis KR, Parker SW, Hedley-Whyte ET: Clinicopathologic conference. *N Engl J Med* 308:1406, 1983.

159. Schirger A, Thomas JE: Idiopathic orthostatic hypotension: Clinical spectrum and prognosis. *Cardiology* 61(suppl 1):144, 1976.

160. McGrath BP, Stern AI, Esler M, Hansky J: Impaired pancre-

atic polypeptide release to insulin hypoglycaemia in chronic autonomic failure with postural hypotension: Evidence for parasympathetic dysfunction. *Clin Sci* 63:321, 1982.
161. Schatz IJ: Current management concepts in orthostatic hypotension. *Arch Intern Med* 140:1152, 1980.
162. Editorial: Management of orthostatic hypotension. *Lancet* 2:963, 1981.
163. Chobanian AV, Volicer L, Tifft CP, Gavras H, Liang C-S, Faxon D: Mineralocorticoid-induced hypertension in patients with orthostatic hypotension. *N Engl J Med* 301:68, 1979.
164. Frewin DB, Leonello PP, Penhall RK, Harding PE: Pindolol in orthostatic hypotension. *Med J Aust* 1:128, 1980.
165. Man in't Veld AJ, Boomsma F, Schalekamp MADH: Effects of β-adrenoceptor agonists and antagonists in patients with peripheral autonomic neuropathy. *Br J Clin Pharmacol* 13:367S, 1982.
166. Davies B, Bannister R, Mathias C, Sever P: Pindolol in postural hypotension: The case for caution. *Lancet* 2:982, 1981.
167. Robertson D, Goldberg MR, Hollister AS, Wade D, Robertson RM: Clonidine raises blood pressure in severe idiopathic orthostatic hypotension. *Am J Med* 74:193, 1983.
168. Fouad FM, Tarazi RC, Bravo EL: Dihydroergotamine in idiopathic orthostatic hypotension: Short-term intramuscular and long-term oral therapy. *Clin Pharmacol Ther* 30:782, 1981.
169. Bobik A, Jennings G, Skews H, Esler B, McLean A: Low oral bioavailability of dihydroergotamine and first-pass extraction in patients with orthostatic hypotension. *Clin Pharmacol Ther* 30:673, 1981.
170. Little PJ, Jennings GL, Skews H, Bobik A: Bioavailability of dihydroergotamine in man. *Br J Clin Pharmacol* 13:785, 1982.
171. Chobanian AV, Tifft CP, Faxon DP, Creager MA, Sackel H: Treatment of chronic orthostatic hypotension with ergotamine. *Circulation* 67:602, 1983.
172. Schirger A, Sheps SG, Thomas JE, Fealey RD: Midodrine: A new agent in the management of idiopathic orthostatic hypotension and Shy-Drager syndrome. *Mayo Clin Proc* 56:429, 1981.
173. Moss AJ, Glaser W, Topol E: Atrial tachypacing in the treatment of a patient with primary orthostatic hypotension. *N Engl J Med* 302:1456, 1980.
174. Kristinsson A: Programmed atrial pacing for orthostatic hypotension. *Acta Med Scand* 214:79, 1983.
175. Goldberg MR, Robertson RM, Robertson D: Atrial tachypacing for primary orthostatic hypotension. *N Engl J Med* 303:885, 1980.
176. Suzuki T, Higa S, Sakoda S, Hayashi A, Yamamura Y, Takaba Y, Nakajima A: Orthostatic hypotension in familial amyloid polyneuropathy: Treatment with DL-*threo*-3,4-dihydroxyphenylserine. *Neurology* 31:1323, 1981.
177. Polinsky RJ, Samaras GM, Kopin IJ: Sympathetic neural prosthesis for managing orthostatic hypotension. *Lancet* 1:901, 1983.
178. Khurama RK, Nelson E, Azzarelli B, Garcia JH: Shy-Drager syndrome: Diagnosis and treatment of cholinergic dysfunction. *Neurology* 30:805, 1980.
179. Garber AJ, Cryer PE, Santiago JV, Haymond MW, Pagliara AS, Kipnis DM: The role of adrenergic mechanisms in the substrate and hormonal response to insulin-induced hypoglycemia in man. *J Clin Invest* 58:7, 1976.
180. Clarke WL, Santiago JV, Thomas L, Haymond MW, Ben-Galim E, Cryer PE: Adrenergic mechanisms in recovery from hypoglycemia in man: Adrenergic blockade. *Am J Physiol* 236:E147, 1979.
181. Gerich J, Davis J, Lorenzi M, Rizza R, Bohannon N, Karam J, Lewis S, Kaplan S, Schultz T, Cryer PE: Hormonal mechanisms of recovery from insulin-induced hypoglycemia in man. *Am J Physiol* 236:E380, 1979.
182. Rizza RA, Cryer PE, Gerich JE: Role of glucagon, epinephrine and growth hormone in human glucose counterregulation: Effects of somatostatin and adrenergic blockade on plasma glucose recovery and glucose flux rates following insulin-induced hypoglycemia. *J Clin Invest* 64:62, 1979.
183. Cryer PE: Glucose counterregulation in man. *Diabetes* 30:261, 1981.
184. Tse TF, Clutter WE, Shah SD, Miller JP, Cryer PE: Neuroendocrine responses to glucose ingestion in man: Specificity, temporal relationships and quantitative aspects. *J Clin Invest* 72:270, 1983.
185. Tse TF, Clutter WE, Shah SD, Cryer PE: The mechanisms of postprandial glucose counterregulation in man: Physiologic roles of glucagon and epinephrine vis-a-vis insulin in the prevention of hypoglycemia late after glucose ingestion. *J Clin Invest* 72:278, 1983.
186. Rosen SG, Clutter WE, Berk MA, Shah SD, Cryer PE: Epinephrine supports the postabsorptive plasma glucose concentration, and prevents hypoglycemia, when glucagon secretion is deficient in man. *J Clin Invest* 73:405, 1984.
187. Cryer PE, Tse TF, Clutter WE, Shah SD: The roles of glucagon and epinephrine in hypoglycemic and nonhypoglycemic glucose counterregulation in man. *Am J Physiol* 247:E198, 1984.
188. Popp DA, Shah SD, Cryer PE: The role of epinephrine mediated β-adrenergic mechanisms in hypoglycemic glucose counterregulation and posthypoglycemic hyperglycemia in insulin dependent diabetes mellitus. *J Clin Invest* 69:315, 1982.
189. White NH, Skor D, Cryer PE, Bier DM, Levandoski L, Santiago JV: Identification of type 1 diabetic patients at increased risk for hypoglycemia during intensive therapy. *N Engl J Med* 308:485, 1983.
190. Cryer PE, Gerich JE: The relevance of glucose counterregulatory systems to patients with diabetes: Critical roles of glucagon and epinephrine. *Diabetes Care* 6:95, 1983.
191. Boden G, Hoeldtke RD: Making intensified insulin treatment safer. *Ann Intern Med* 99:268, 1983.
192. Santiago JV, White NH, Skor DA, Levandoski LA, Cryer PE: Defective glucose counterregulation limits the intensive therapy of insulin dependent diabetes mellitus. *Am J Physiol* 247:E215, 1984.
193. Cryer PE: Hypoglycemia, in Foster DW, Wilson JD (eds): *Williams' Textbook of Endocrinology*, 7th ed. Philadelphia, Saunders, 1985, p 989.
194. White N, Gingerich R, Levandoski L, Cryer P, Santiago J: Plasma pancreatic polypeptide response to insulin-induced hypoglycemia as a marker for defective glucose counterregulation in insulin-dependent diabetes mellitus. *Diabetes* 34:870, 1985.
195. Hilsted J: Pathophysiology in diabetic autonomic neuropathy: Cardiovascular, hormonal and metabolic studies. *Diabetes* 31:730, 1982.
196. Clarke BF, Ewing DJ: Cardiovascular reflex tests in the natural history of diabetic autonomic neuropathy. *NY State J Med* 82:903, 1982.
197. Young RJ, Ewing DJ, Clarke BF: Nerve function and metabolic control in teenage diabetics. *Diabetes* 32:142, 1983.
198. Cryer PE: Normal and abnormal sympathoadrenal function in patients with insulin dependent diabetes mellitus. *NY State J Med* 82:886, 1982.
199. Schade DS, Eaton RP: Pathogenesis of diabetic ketoacidosis: A reappraisal. *Diabetes Care* 2:296, 1979.
200. Alberti KGMM, Christensen NJ, Iversen J, Orskov H: Role of glucagon and other hormones in development of diabetic ketoacidosis. *Lancet* 1:1307, 1975.
201. Gundersen T, Kjekshus J: Timolol treatment after myocardial infarction in diabetic patients. *Diabetes Care* 6:285, 1983.
202. Shamoon H, Hendler R, Sherwin RS: Altered responsiveness to cortisol, epinephrine and glucagon in insulin infused juvenile onset diabetics. *Diabetes* 29:284, 1980.
203. Beretta-Piccoli C, Weidman P: Exaggerated pressor responsiveness to norepinephrine in nonazotemic diabetes mellitus. *Am J Med* 71:829, 1981.

204. Bilezikian JP, Loeb JN: The influence of hyperthyroidism and hypothyroidism on α- and β-adrenergic receptor systems and adrenergic responsiveness. *Endocr Rev* 4:378, 1983.
205. Marshall JM: Effects of ovarian steroids and pregnancy on adrenergic nerves of uterus and oviduct. *Am J Physiol* 240:C165, 1981.
206. Irestedt L, Lagercrantz H, Hjemdahl P, Hagnerik K, Belfrage P: Fetal and maternal plasma catecholamine levels at elective cesarean section under general or epidural anesthesia versus vaginal delivery. *Am J Obstet Gynecol* 142:1004, 1982.
207. Rosen SG, Berk MA, Popp DA, Serusclat P, Smith EB, Shah SD, Ginsberg AM, Clutter WE, Cryer PE: β_2- and α_2-adrenergic receptors and receptor coupling to adenylate cyclase in human mononuclear leukocytes and platelets in relation to physiologic variations of sex steroids. *J Clin Endocrinol Metab* 58:1068, 1984.
208. Carlson HE, Brickman AS: Blunted plasma cyclic adenosine monophosphate response to isoproterenol in pseudohypoparathyroidism. *J Clin Endocrinol Metab* 56:1323, 1983.
209. Young JB, Saville E, Rothwell NJ, Stock MJ, Landsberg L: Effect of diet and cold exposure on norepinephrine turnover in brown adipose tissue of the rat. *J Clin Invest* 69:1061, 1982.
210. Felig P, Cunningham J, Levitt M, Hendler R, Nadel E: Energy expenditure in obesity in fasting and postprandial state. *Am J Physiol* 244:E45, 1983.
211. Jung RT, Shetty PS, James WPT, Barrand MA, Callingham BA: Plasma catecholamines and autonomic responsiveness in obesity. *Int J Obesity* 6:131, 1982.
212. Gustafson AB, Kalkhoff RK: Influence of sex and obesity on plasma catecholamine response to isometric exercise. *J Clin Endocrinol Metab* 55:703, 1982.
213. Sundaresan PR, Weintraub M, Hershey LA, Kroening BH, Hasday JD, Banerjee SP: Platelet alpha-adrenergic receptors in obesity: Alteration with weight loss. *Clin Pharmacol Ther* 33:776, 1983.
214. Kuchel O, Cuche JL, Buu NT, Guthrie GP Jr, Unger T, Nowaczynski W, Boucher R, Genest J: Catecholamine excretion in "idiopathic" edema: Decreased dopamine excretion, a pathogenic factor? *J Clin Endocrinol Metab* 44:639, 1977.
215. Sowers J, Catania R, Paris J, Tuck M: Effects of bromocriptine on renin, aldosterone and prolactin responses to posture and metoclopramide in idiopathic edema: Possible therapeutic approach. *J Clin Endocrinol Metab* 54:510, 1982.
216. Silverberg AB, Mennes PA, Cryer PE: Resistance to endogenous norepinephrine in Bartter's syndrome: Reversion during indomethacin administration. *Am J Med* 64:231, 1978.
217. Gullner HG, Gill JR Jr, Bartter FC, Lake CR, Lakatua DJ: Correction of increased sympathoadrenal activity in Bartter's syndrome by inhibition of prostaglandin synthesis. *J Clin Endocrinol Metab* 50:857, 1980.
218. Feldman JM, Davis JA: Radioenzymatic assay of platelet serotonin, dopamine and norepinephrine in subjects with normal and increased serotonin production. *Clin Chim Acta* 109:275, 1981.
219. Beal MF, Atuk NO, Westfall TC, Turner SM: Catecholamine uptake, accumulation and release in acute prophyria. *J Clin Invest* 60:1141, 1977.
220. Rockson S, Stone R, van der Weyden M, Kelley WN: Lesch-Nyhan syndrome: Evidence for abnormal adrenergic function. *Science* 186:934, 1974.
221. Riccardi VM: von Recklinghausen neurofibromatosis. *N Engl J Med* 305:1617, 1981.
222. Goldstein DS: Plasma catecholamines and essential hypertension. *Hypertension* 5:86, 1983.
223. Esler M, Leonard P, Kelleher D, Jackman G, Bobik A, Skews H, Jennings G, Korner P: Assessment of neuronal uptake of noradrenaline in humans: Defective uptake in some patients with essential hypertension. *Clin Exp Pharmacol Physiol* 7:535, 1980.
224. Christensen NJ: Catecholamines and essential hypertension. *Scand J Clin Lab Invest* 42:211, 1982.
225. Abboud FM: The sympathetic system in hypertension. *Hypertension* 4(suppl 2):208, 1982.
226. Braunwald E, Muller JE, Kloner RA, Maroko PR: Role of β-adrenergic blockade in the therapy of patients with myocardial infarction. *Am J Med* 74:113, 1983.
227. Frishman WH, Furberg CD, Friedewald WT: β-Adrenergic blockade for survivors of acute myocardial infarction. *N Engl J Med* 310:830, 1984.
228. International Collaborative Study Group: Reduction of infarct size with the early use of timolol in acute myocardial infarction. *N Engl J Med* 310:9, 1984.
229. Karlsberg RP, Penkoske PA, Cryer PE, Corr PB, Roberts R: Rapid activation of the sympathetic nervous system following coronary artery occlusion: Relation to infarct size, site and haemodynamic impact. *Cardiovasc Res* 13:523, 1979.
230. Karlsberg RP, Cryer PE, Roberts R: Serial plasma catecholamine response early in the course of clinical acute myocardial infarction: Relationship to infarct extent and mortality. *Am Heart J* 102:24, 1981.
231. Bristow MR, Ginsburg R, Minobe W, Cubicciotti RS, Sageman WS, Lurie K, Billingham ME, Harrison DC, Stinson EB: Decreased catecholamine sensitivity and β-adrenergic receptor density in failing human hearts. *N Engl J Med* 307:205, 1982.
232. Pasternac A, Tubau JF, Puddu PE, Krol RB, DeChamplain J: Increased plasma catecholamine levels in patients with symptomatic mitral valve prolapse. *Am J Med* 73:783, 1982.
233. Boudoulas H, Reynolds JC, Mazzaferri E, Wooley CF: Metabolic studies in mitral valve prolapse syndrome. *Circulation* 61:1200, 1980.
234. Rogers JM, Boudoulas H, Malarkey WB: Mitral valve prolapse: Disordered catecholamine regulation with intravascular volume maneuvers (abstr). *Clin Res* 31:710A, 1983.
235. Santos AD, Matthew PK, Hilal A, Wallace WA: Orthostatic hypotension: A commonly unrecognized cause of symptoms in mitral valve prolapse. *Am J Med* 71:746, 1981.
236. Hooper M, Condemi JJ, Izzo JL Jr: Abnormal norepinephrine kinetics and increased sympathetic nervous system activity in Raynaud's syndrome (abstr). *Clin Res* 31:450A, 1983.
237. Nielsen SL, Vitting K, Rasmussen K: Prazosin treatment of primary Raynaud's phenomenon. *Eur J Clin Invest* 24:421, 1983.
238. Kaliner M, Shelhamer H, Davis PB, Smith LJ, Venter JC: Autonomic nervous system abnormalities and allergy. *Ann Intern Med* 96:349, 1982.
239. Davis PB, Shelhamer JR, Kaliner M: Abnormal adrenergic and cholinergic sensitivity in cystic fibrosis. *N Engl J Med* 302:1453, 1980.
240. Barnes P, Fitzgerald G, Brown M, Dollery C: Nocturnal asthma and changes in circulating epinephrine, histamine and cortisol. *N Engl J Med* 303:263, 1980.
241. Henriksen JH, Christensen NJ, Kok-Jensen A, Christiansen IB: Increased plasma noradrenaline concentration in patients with chronic obstructive lung disease: Relation to haemodynamics and blood gases. *Scand J Clin Lab Invest* 40:419, 1980.
242. Calne DB, Kebabian J, Silbergeld E, Evarts E: Advances in the neuropharmacology of parkinsonism. *Ann Intern Med* 90:219, 1979.
243. Hsu LKG, Crisp AH, Kalucy RS, Koval J, Chen CN, Carruthers M, Zilkha KJ: Early morning migraine: Nocturnal plasma levels of catecholamines, tryptophan, glucose and free fatty acids and sleep encephalographs. *Lancet* 1:447, 1977.
244. Metz SA, Halter JB, Porte D Jr, Robertson RP: Autonomic epilepsy: Clonidine blockade of paroxysmal catecholamine release and flushing. *Ann Intern Med* 88:189, 1978.
245. Winkler GF, Young RR: Efficacy of chronic propranolol therapy in action tremors of the familial, senile or essential varieties. *N Engl J Med* 290:984, 1974.
246. Antelman S, Caggiula AR: Norepinephrine-dopamine inter-

actions and behavior. *Science* 195:646, 1977.
247. Barchas JD, Akil H, Elliott GR, Holman RB, Watson SJ: Behavioral neurochemistry: Neuroregulators and behavioral states. *Science* 200:964, 1978.
248. Maas JW: Clinical and biochemical heterogeneity of depressive disorders. *Ann Intern Med* 88:556, 1979.
249. Lake CR, Sternberg DE, van Kammen DP, Ballenger JC, Ziegler MG, Post RM, Kopin IJ, Bunney WE: Schizophrenia: Elevated cerebrospinal fluid norepinephrine. *Science* 207:331, 1980.
250. Veith RC, Raskind MA, Barnes RF, Gumbrecht G, Ritchie JL, Halter JB: Tricyclic antidepressants and supine, standing and exercise plasma norepinephrine levels. *Clin Pharmacol Ther* 33:763, 1983.
251. Williams RB Jr, Lane JD, Kuhn CM, Melosh W, White AD, Schanberg SM: Type A behavior and elevated physiologic and neuroendocrine responses to cognitive tasks. *Science* 218:483, 1982.
252. Faraj BA, Camp VM, Ansley JD, Scott J, Ali FM, Malveaux EJ: Evidence for central hypertyraminemia in hepatic encephalopathy. *J Clin Invest* 67:395, 1981.
253. Faraj BA, Bowen PA, Isaacs JW, Rudman D: Hypertyraminemia in cirrhotic patients. *N Engl J Med* 294:1360, 1976.
254. Morgan MY, Jakobovits A, Elithorn A, James IM, Sherlock S: Successful use of bromocriptine in the treatment of a patient with chronic portasystemic encephalopathy. *N Engl J Med* 296:793, 1977.
255. Bichet DG, van Putten VJ, Schrier RW: Potential role of increased sympathetic activity in impaired sodium and water excretion in cirrhosis. *N Engl J Med* 307:1552, 1982.
256. Ring-Larsen H, Hesse B, Henriksen JH, Christensen NJ: Sympathetic nervous activity and renal and systemic hemodynamics in cirrhosis: Plasma norepinephrine concentration, hepatic extraction, and renal release. *Hepatology* 2:304, 1982.
257. Arroyo V, Planas R, Gaya J, Deulofeu R, Rimola A, Perez-Ayuso RM, Rivera F, Rodes J: Sympathetic nervous activity, renin-angiotensin system and renal excretion of prostaglandin E_2 excretion in cirrhosis: Relationship to functional renal failure and sodium and water excretion. *Eur J Clin Invest* 13:271, 1983.
258. Christensen NJ, Brandsborg O, Lvgreen NA, Brandsborg M: Elevated plasma noradrenaline concentrations in duodenal ulcer patients are not normalized by vagotomy. *J Clin Endocrinol Metab* 49:331, 1979.
259. Henrich WL, Katz FH, Molinoff PB, Schrier RW: Competitive effects of hypokalemia and volume depletion on plasma renin activity, aldosterone and catecholamine concentrations in hemodialysis patients. *Kidney Int* 12:279, 1977.
260. McGrath BP, Ledingham JGG, Benedict CR: Catecholamines in peripheral venous plasma in patients on chronic haemodialysis. *Clin Sci* 55:89, 1978.
261. Ban M, Matsumo T, Ogawa K, Satake T: Plasma norepinephrine and dopamine-beta-hydroxylase activity in chronic renal failure. *Jpn Circ J* 43:627, 1979.
262. Cannella G, Picotti GB, Movilli E, Cancarini G, DeMarinis S, Galva MD, Maiorca R: Plasma catecholamine response to postural stimulation in normotensive and dialysis hypotension prone uremic patients. *Nephron* 27:285, 1981.
263. Izzo JL Jr, Izzo MS, Sterns RH, Freeman RB: Sympathetic nervous system hyperactivity in maintenance hemodialysis patients. *Trans Am Soc Artif Intern Organs* 28:604, 1982.
264. Shah SD, Clutter WE, Cryer PE: External and internal standards in the single isotope derivative (radioenzymatic) measurement of plasma norepinephrine and epinephrine in normal humans and persons with diabetes mellitus or chronic renal failure. *J Lab Clin Med* 106:624, 1985.
265. Enzi G, Inelmen EM, Baritussio A, Dorigo P, Prosdocimi M, Mazzoleni F: Multiple symmetric lipomatosis: A defect in adrenergic stimulated lipolysis. *J Clin Invest* 60:1221, 1977.
266. Kather H, Schroder F: Adrenergic regulation of fat cell lipolysis in multiple symmetric lipomatosis. *Eur J Clin Invest* 12:471, 1982.
267. Burch GE, Jones RJ: Essential hyperhidrosis: Correlation of digital blood flow and capillary ultrastructure after unilateral sympathectomy. *Am J Med* 54:378, 1973.
268. Kaywin P, McDonough M, Insel PA, Shattil SJ: Platelet function in essential thrombocythemia: Decreased epinephrine responsiveness associated with a deficiency of platelet α-adrenergic receptors. *N Engl J Med* 299:505, 1978.
269. Davidson L, Vandongen R, Beilin LJ: Effect of eating bananas on plasma free and sulfate-conjugated catecholamines. *Life Sci* 29:1773, 1981.
270. Johnson GA, Kupiecki RM, Baker CA: Single isotope derivative (radioenzymatic) methods in the measurement of catecholamines. *Metabolism* 29(suppl 1):1106, 1980.
271. Christensen NJ: Sympathetic nervous activity and age. *Eur J Clin Invest* 12:91, 1982.
272. Romoff MS, Keusch G, Campese VM, Wang M-S Friedler RM, Weidman P, Massry SG: Effect of sodium intake on plasma catecholamines in normal subjects. *J Clin Endocrinol Metab* 48:26, 1978.
273. Santiago JV, Clarke WL, Shah SD, Cryer PE: Epinephrine, norepinephrine, glucagon and growth hormone release in association with physiologic decrements in the plasma glucose concentration in normal and diabetic man. *J Clin Endocrinol Metab* 51:877, 1980.
274. Cryer PE, Sode J: Drug interference with measurement of adrenal hormones in urine: Common analgesics and tranquilizer-sedatives. *Ann Intern Med* 75:697, 1971.
275. Hilsted J, Galbo H, Christensen NJ: Impaired responses of catecholamines, growth hormone and cortisol to graded exercise in diabetic autonomic neuropathy. *Diabetes* 29:257, 1980.
276. Bennett T, Farquahar IK, Hosking DJ, Hampton JR: Assessment of methods for estimating autonomic nervous control of the heart in patients with diabetes. *Diabetes* 27:1167, 1978.
277. Ewing DJ, Borsey DQ, Bellavere F, Clarke BF: Cardiac autonomic neuropathy in diabetes: Comparison of measures of R-R interval variation. *Diabetologia* 21:18, 1981.
278. Pfeiffer MA, Cook D, Brodsky J, Tice D, Reenan H, Swedine S, Halter JB, Porte D Jr: Quantitative evaluation of cardiac parasympathetic activity in normal and diabetic man. *Diabetes* 31:339, 1982.
279. Pfeiffer MA, Cook D, Brodsky J, Tice D, Parrish D, Reenan A, Halter JB, Porte D Jr: Quantitative evaluation of sympathetic and parasympathetic control of iris function. *Diabetes Care* 5:518, 1982.
280. Ewing DJ, Borsey DQ, Travis P, Bellavere F, Neilson JMM, Clarke BF: Abnormalities of ambulatory 24-hour heart rate in diabetes mellitus. *Diabetes* 32:101, 1983.
281. Hilsted J, Jensen SB: A simple test for autonomic neuropathy in juvenile diabetics. *Acta Med Scand* 205:385, 1979.

14

The Endocrinology of Hypertension

John D. Baxter
Dorothee Perloff
Willa Hsueh
Edward G. Biglieri

Hypertension, defined as persistent and inappropriate elevation of arterial pressure, is the most commonly treated disease in the United States. Approximately 20 percent of the adult population in the United States, or 60 million people, have blood pressures above 140/90 mmHg, the upper range of "normal" blood pressure (Table 14-1).[1-3] Hypertension accelerates the process of atherosclerosis and is one of the major risk factors for developing coronary artery disease and stroke.[4]

Regulation and maintenance of blood pressure levels sufficient for perfusion of vital organs is the result of complex interactions between multiple effectors and systems which are delicately balanced and counterbalanced with numerous feedback loops. This extensive network of effectors facilitates adjustments in pressure with physiological or pathologic perturbations, such as occur with gravity, when there are changes in posture, with exercise, or with fluid loss or overload, so that perfusion of vital organs is maintained.

Hormones play a key role in regulating the blood pressure. These hormones are produced in the kidney, adrenals, brain, peripheral nerves, heart, and a number of other organs. Most of them have multiple actions in influencing the blood pressure and also affect the release and actions of other hormones. For example, prostacyclin, a major product of the prostaglandin system, induces vasodilation and natriuresis and directly stimulates renin release. Angiotensin II, the active product of the renin system, stimulates prostacyclin production, induces vasoconstriction, and is antinatriuretic. These interactions are further modified by the state of sodium balance, the concentrations of major anions and cations, the hormonal milieu of other interacting systems, and a number of other interrelated factors.

In the majority of patients with hypertension, the mechanisms for the development of the elevated blood pressure are not understood. These cases are therefore ordinarily referred to as *essential* or *primary* hypertension. Based on what is now known, it is probable that essential hypertension is a heterogeneous disorder and that multiple genetic and environmental factors are operative in the etiology. Potential contributory influences under consideration include renal handling of sodium and water; release of pressor and depressor substances from the endocrine glands, the CNS, or organs such as the heart and kidney; and transmembrane transport of ions in various cells. Information concerning the mechanisms of essential hypertension is accumulating rapidly from a variety of sources. These include fundamental studies of the factors that control the blood pressure, lessons learned from patients with secondary forms of hypertension (see below) due to excessive levels of various hormones or renal disease, results from treatment of essential hypertension with specific pharmaceutical agents, and information from experimentally produced hypertension in animals such as Goldblatt dogs with one- and two-clip renal artery occlusion and deoxycorticosterone (DOC)-treated and salt-fed Dahl rats or inbred strains of rats that develop hypertension spontaneously.

In a small percentage of hypertensive individuals (see below), the blood pressure elevation is secondary to currently identifiable diseases of the kidney, endocrine glands, or other organs.[5-7] The common types of secondary hypertension in which a cause can be defined and which can potentially be cured by removal of these causes are listed in Table 14-2. Correction of the underlying defect can result in abolition of the hypertension in many of these patients. Selecting patients with secondary hypertension from among the

Table 14-1. Classification of Blood Pressure Levels

Pressure (mmHg)	Classification*
Diastolic	
< 85	Normal
85–89	High normal
90–104	Mild hypertension
105–114	Moderate hypertension
≥ 115	Severe hypertension
Systolic, when diastolic is < 90	
< 140	Normal
140–159	Borderline isolated systolic hypertension
≥ 160	Isolated systolic hypertension

*A classification of borderline isolated systolic hypertension (systolic blood pressure 140 to 159 mmHg) or isolated systolic hypertension (systolic blood pressure < 160 mmHg) takes precedence over a classification of high normal blood pressure (diastolic blood pressure 85 to 89 mmHg) when both occur in the same person. A classification of high normal blood pressure (diastolic blood pressure 85 to 89 mmHg) takes precedence over a classification of normal blood pressure (systolic blood pressure < 140 mmHg) when both occur in the same person.
Source: Ref. 2.

large population of hypertensive individuals and managing them appropriately, either surgically or medically, can potentially prevent the progressive complications of hypertension and the need for lifelong drug therapy in these patients.

In this chapter the role of hormones in hypertension is discussed. This is addressed first in terms of hormonal actions influencing the blood pressure. An understanding of these effects is useful in understanding hypertension in general and the syndromes in which hormones are known to contribute in a major way. Second, the approach to evaluating the patient with hypertension for the presence of a known secondary cause is discussed. Finally, the diagnosis and treatment of certain endocrine causes of hypertension is described, with focus on the mechanisms, diagnosis, and management of hypertension due to excessive levels of the mineralocorticoids, aldosterone or DOC, and of the hypertension due to activation of the renin-angiotensin-aldosterone (RAA) system in patients with renovascular hypertension. The lessons learned from these two forms of secondary hypertension can be applied to an understanding of blood pressure control in general.

The other forms of secondary hypertension, the endocrinology of thyroid disease, Cushing's syndrome, and pheochromocytoma are discussed in Chaps. 12, 13, and 15. The prostaglandins and the kallikrein-kinin system also have complex actions on the vasculature and on renal function and are discussed in detail in Chap. 31. Vasopressin is discussed in Chap. 9. Coarctation of the aorta is not discussed in this text; the mechanisms of hypertension in this condition are not well understood; both strictly mechanical mechanisms and activation of the RAA system have been postulated. The CNS plays a critical role in regulating the blood pressure and CNS dysfunction may explain much of essential hypertension. A discussion of such a role is outside the scope of this chapter. Similarly, CNS control of neuroendocrine secretions is intimately related to hormones that regulate the blood pressure; this is discussed in Chap. 7. The hypertension of renal parenchymal diseases caused by a failure of the kidney to act as an excretory organ and as a producer of depressor hormones is also not discussed.

GENERAL FEATURES OF HYPERTENSION

Some general information on the epidemiology, genetics, and pathophysiology of hypertension is relevant to an understanding of the role of hormones in hypertension and to the diagnosis and treatment of endocrine forms of hypertension. Many of the pathophysiological processes are common to all forms of hypertension. It is also important to consider epidemiologic and genetic factors as well as individual vascular and hemodynamic abnormalities to differentiate subgroups of patients with essential hypertension; such subgroups are defined by differences in levels of and responsiveness to particular hormones such as angiotensin II and in abnormalities of sodium transport and factors that influence it.

The Epidemiology of Hypertension

The importance of clinical hypertension as a risk factor for premature death and morbidity from cardiovascular disease was recognized long before modern treatment for hypertension was available.[8–10] These observations on hypertensive patients were amplified by prospective studies of large population groups (not patients) in the United States and Europe, as well as from life insurance company statistics.[11,12] They all showed a consistent increase in cardiovascular mortality and morbidity with increasing levels of blood pressure, both systolic and diastolic, even at levels not considered hypertensive. These studies were largely carried out before effective antihypertensive therapy was routinely used and thus are representative of the true natural history of hypertension.

Table 14-2. Types of Hypertension

- Systolic hypertension
  - Increased cardiac output
    - Aortic valvular insufficiency
    - Arteriovenous fistula, patent ductus arteriosus
    - Hyperthyroidism
    - Paget's disease of bone
    - Beriberi heart disease
    - Hyperkinetic circulation
    - Complete heart block
    - Rigidity of aorta and great vessels due to atherosclerosis
- Systolic and diastolic hypertension
  - Primary, essential, or idiopathic
  - Secondary
    - Renal
      - Renal parenchymal disease
        - Acute glomerulonephritis
        - Chronic nephritis: glomerulonephritis, pyelonephritis, interstitial, hereditary, irradiation
        - Polycystic disease
        - Connective tissue diseases
        - Renin-producing tumors
        - Hydronephrosis
      - Renovascular
        - Extrarenal arterial stenosis
        - Intrarenal arterial branch stenosis
        - Vasculitis
      - Renoprival
      - Primary sodium retention
        - (Liddle's syndrome, Gordon's syndrome)
    - Endocrine
      - Acromegaly
      - Hypothyroidism
      - Hyperthyroidism
      - Adrenal cortical
        - Cushing's syndrome
        - Primary aldosteronism
        - Congenital adrenal hyperplasia
      - Pheochromocytoma/neurofibroma/glioma
      - Hypercalcemia
      - Carcinoid syndrome
      - Exogenous
        - Estrogen/oral contraceptives
        - Glucocorticoids
        - Mineralocorticoids:
          - licorice, carbenoxolone
        - Sympathomimetics
        - Tyramine-containing foods and monoamine oxidase (MAO) inhibitors
        - Thyroid hormone
    - Coarctation of the aorta
    - Hypertensive diseases of pregnancy
    - Neurogenic
      - Psychogenic
      - Increased intracranial pressure
        - Respiratory acidosis (CO_2 retention): lung or CNS disease (polio)
        - Encephalitis
        - Brain tumor
      - Lead poisoning
      - Familial dysautonomia
      - Acute porphyria
      - Spinal cord damage
    - Miscellaneous
      - Polycythemia
      - Increased intravascular volume
      - Burns (extensive)

Source: Modified from Kaplan.[7]

The Build and Blood Pressure study of the Society of Actuaries reported in the 1950s[11] the mortality experience of 1 million middle-aged men; 45-year-old men with initial blood pressures of 152/95 and 162/85 mmHg had nearly twice and three times, respectively, the mortality rate within the first 10 years of follow-up as did men with a blood pressure less than 132/85 mmHg at entry. In the United States Pooling project studies begun in the 1950s,[12] men aged 40 to 59 with initial diastolic blood pressures between 90 and 104 mmHg had a 5 per 100 excess death rate, whereas those with entry diastolic blood pressures of 105 to 114 mmHg had an excess mortality of 12.5 per 100. Studies from Europe have yielded similar results.[13–16]

The Framingham study describes the course of 5127 men and women (a random sample of half the population of Framingham, Massachusetts), enrolled in 1944 and followed with biannual medical examinations for up to 36 years (Fig. 14-1).[17–21] The study focused especially on the incidence of clinical coronary artery disease.[20] At the 18-year follow-up, the age-adjusted average annual incidence of coronary

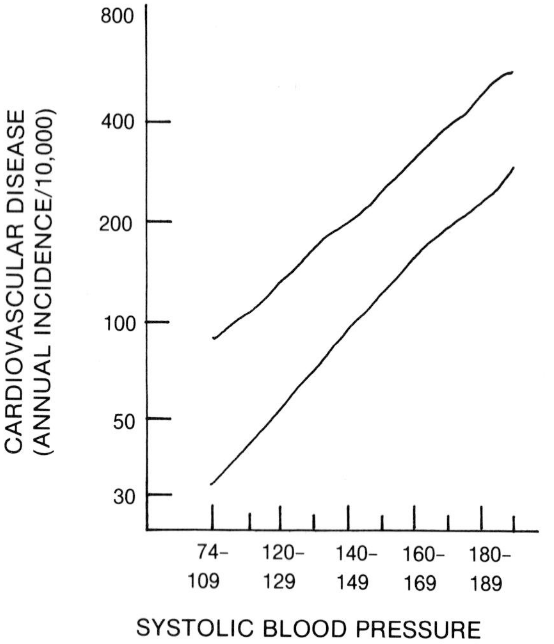

FIGURE 14-1 Annual incidence of cardiovascular disease among the Framingham group over an 18-year follow-up based on systolic blood pressure at the onset of the study. (*From Kaplan,*[7] *as drawn from data of Kannel and Sorlie.*[17])

artery disease events was three times as great in women with blood pressures > 160/95 mmHg than in those with pressures < 140/90 mmHg and nearly two and a half times as great in men.[21] The incidence of thrombotic strokes was seven to eight times as great in hypertensive as in normotensive persons, while that of heart failure was five to seven times as great. The Framingham study confirmed the importance of hypertension in conjunction with other predictors of cardiovascular disease: hyperlipidemia, cigarette smoking, glucose intolerance, and male sex and the additive or synergistic nature of these risk factors. Thus, when glucose intolerance, cigarette smoking, and left ventricular hypertrophy on the electrocardiogram are present in addition to the blood pressure and cholesterol elevation, a person with systolic blood pressure of 180 mmHg and a cholesterol level of 260 mg/dl has 12 times the risk of developing cardiovascular disease in 8 years as does a nonsmoker without glucose intolerance and a systolic blood pressure of 135 mmHg and a cholesterol level of 185 mg/dl.[20,21] However, even at a cholesterol level of 235 mg/dl, considered near average for the American population, the difference in morbidity between those with systolic blood pressures of 195 mmHg versus those with 135 mmHg was more than twofold.

Both systolic and diastolic blood pressure are determinants of cardiovascular risk, although different authors stress the relative greater importance of systolic vs. diastolic and vice versa.[19,22,23] Nevertheless, most recent drug intervention trials have used the diastolic blood pressure as the basic stratification for classification.

Of note is the fact that when hypertension is present without increased cholesterol level and in premenopausal women, the mortality is primarily from cerebrovascular disease; stroke is also common in Japan, where hypertension is very prevalent but cholesterol levels are low,[24] while in the United States and Europe, where average cholesterol levels are high and the diet is rich in fat, coronary artery disease, sudden death, myocardial infarction, and angina pectoris are more frequent than cerebrovascular accidents. The incidence of myocardial infarction and death from coronary heart disease was studied in samples of 45- to 68-year-old Japanese men living in Japan, Hawaii, and California.[25,26] The incidence rate was lowest in Japan where it was half that observed in Hawaii, while the incidence among Japanese men in California was nearly 50 percent greater than that of Japanese in Hawaii, suggesting that environmental or dietary factors play a major role in addition to that of hypertension. Presumably these men were genetically similar and the prevalence of hypertension was the same.[25,26]

Further data regarding the importance of hypertension as a risk factor come from studies on drug therapy of hypertension.[27] Before drug treatment was available, the mortality of patients with malignant or accelerated hypertension was 80 percent in one year.[28,29.] With intensive therapy available in the 1960s, this mortality was reduced to 15 percent in one year.[29] In the Veteran's Administration study 70 untreated control patients with prerandomization diastolic pressures of 115 to 129 mmHg developed 27 morbid cardiovascular events, including four deaths within 2 years, while of the 73 actively treated patients, whose blood pressures were lowered with triple drug therapy, only two developed such morbid events.[30] In patients with less severe degrees of hypertension, similar reduction in mortality and morbidity from hypertensive complications was achieved with drug therapy; however, the incidence of arteriosclerotic complications such as myocardial infarction was not as dramatically decreased in the drug-treated group.[31] In the Hypertension Detection and Follow-up Program, the 5-year mortality was 6.4 percent in the patients with diastolic blood pressure 90 to 104 mmHg (stratum 1) who were aggressively treated, versus 7.7 percent in the less intensively treated patients, a reduction of mortality of 20 percent.[32]

Genetic and Environmental Influences

The development of high blood pressure in a population depends on the interaction of both genetic and environmental influences. The incidence of hypertension is higher in men than women and in blacks than whites.[7,33] The distribution of blood pressures in families shows that the relatives of hypertensives have significantly higher mean blood pressure levels at all ages than the relatives of normotensives.[34a,34b] There is a correlation between maternal and infant blood pressure from birth.[34a–34c] A high proportion of the genetic component of blood pressure variability is attributed to dominance. Characteristics such as abnormal cation fluxes in red blood cells are indicators of the genetic influence on blood pressure. These abnormalities are inherited according to a dominant pattern in the families of hypertensive patients (see Sodium Transport and Blood Pressure, below). Genetic influences on the renin-angiotensin-aldosterone system may also play a part.

Among the environmental factors, the main influences that predict a rise in blood pressure are obesity, sodium intake (discussed below), and psychosocial stress.[7,33,34a] Alcohol has vasopressor actions and epidemiological surveys suggest that there is a higher incidence of hypertension in individuals who consume more than 60 to 80 g of ethanol per day.[35] Both obesity and lean body mass have been correlated with hypertension.[35,36] Blood pressure has been shown to be positively correlated with both blood glucose and insulin, and insulin resistance and/or hyperinsulinemia have been reported to be present in the majority of hypertensives.[35,36] The basic hypothesis is that the heritable component, a complex genetic predisposition, is expressed more when higher-risk genotypes are exposed to excessive environmental influences.

The Physiology of Blood Pressure Control

Mean arterial pressure is a function of systemic blood flow, cardiac output, and resistance to this flow in the regional circulation of the perfused organs.[37–39] These factors are interrelated. Systolic arterial hypertension results from increased cardiac output or increased total peripheral resistance, or both. Cardiac output is determined by cardiac filling pressure, which in turn is dependent on venous return, which depends on venous compliance, capacity of the venous bed, and total blood volume. The resistance to blood flow of a tissue determines the amount of blood perfusing it. The level of resistance is regulated by local factors, energy needs, metabolic or myogenic factors, and neural and humoral factors (remote regulation). Resistance to flow is determined largely by the radius of the lumen of the precapillary arteriole or "resistance" vessel. The cross-sectional area of this vascular bed depends on the number of resistance vessels and their reactivity to vasoactive stimuli. Resistance depends also on blood viscosity, which in turn depends on the hematocrit, the plasma viscosity, the deformability of erythrocytes by shear stresses during flow, and cell aggregation. A relationship between viscosity and plasma renin activity has also been described.[40]

Structural changes are seen in the arterioles of individuals with chronic hypertension. These probably represent an adaptive change in response to an increased local transmural pressure gradient and overperfusion.[37–39,41] The reasons for the elevation of this transmural pressure, i.e., the initiating events, are poorly understood. There is evidence that alteration in vascular smooth muscle function, including increased vasoconstrictor responsiveness, occurs early.[42,43] In experimental animals, the increased vascular reactivity occurs before blood pressure rises, while the structural changes occur later. Furthermore, functional changes may occur in vascular smooth muscles independent of wall stress and associated with similar changes in the systemic venous circulation.[42] The changes in reactivity have been attributed to changes in the cell membrane, including altered agonist responsiveness, calcium content, diffusion potential, and electrogenic ion transport. These could result in altered electrophysiological properties with a consequent increase in contractile activity of vascular smooth muscle.[43] The increased sensitivity to vasoactive drugs could be due to changes in binding of agonists to receptor sites on the cell membrane of the smooth muscle cell or to postreceptor influences (Chap. 5). Thus it appears that altered vascular cellular processes are the principal abnormalities causing changes in vascular smooth muscle function in hypertension.

The Autonomic Nervous System

The autonomic nervous system plays an important role in most types of hypertension, by its interaction with veins, arteries, and the heart, in controlling blood pressure (Chap. 13). These organs act not only as effector organs, but also as informers and modulators of nervous activity. The net effect of neural activity depends on the extent to which it modulates and integrates and either antagonizes or stimulates the other elements that control blood pressure, such as intra- and extravascular volume, cardiac activity, renal function, or humoral factors such as the RAA and vasodilator systems.[44-46b] Specific neural centers for blood pressure regulation have been identified in the brain and medulla. All elements of the renin-angiotensin system, in addition to other neuropeptides, have been identified in brain cells (see below). Angiotensin II also crosses the blood-brain barrier at the level of the area postrema, where it can stimulate the vasomotor center directly.

The baroreceptors which modulate blood pressure in response to short-term postural-gravitational changes can be reset to become activated at higher or deactivated at lower levels of pressure.[45] The nervous system probably plays a part in the mediation of cardiac hypertrophy and the vasoconstrictor changes in the resistance vessels. The autonomic nervous system also has an effect on extracellular fluid volume. Renin release can be modulated by sympathetic activity and angiotensin II can increase sympathetic activity both peripherally and centrally, as it enhances the effect of norepinephrine in the synaptic cleft.[46a,46b]

The Hemodynamics of Hypertension

The hemodynamic derangements in patients with hypertension have been studied in two groups of patients: those with mild, early, labile hypertension, now described as *borderline,* who are less than 35 years old, and in older patients with well-established, "fixed," moderate to severe hypertension of long duration.

BORDERLINE HYPERTENSION

In patients with borderline hypertension, cardiac output, stroke volume, and heart rate are generally high in relation to metabolic needs, while total peripheral resistance, though normal, is inappropriate for the elevated level of cardiac output.[47,48] These abnormalities are probably mediated via the sympathetic nervous system, since increased responsiveness to beta-adrenergic stimulation and increases in the levels of circulating catecholamines have been reported. Plasma volume is normal or is slightly decreased. Renal blood flow can also be decreased. Patients with borderline hypertension tend to have a relative polycythemia and increased hematocrit (Gaisböck's disease or stress polycythemia) possibly secondary to increased levels of atrial natriuretic factor (ANF, see below). This may contribute to the increased blood viscosity that has been reported.[40] The plasma renin activity can be normal, elevated, or suppressed (discussed in detail below). Myocardial contractility is also increased, but coronary reserve is decreased.[47,48] Anatomically these patients have normal cardiac and renal function. It is not clear whether the hemodynamic changes represent the earliest manifestations of hypertension or are somehow related to its etiology. Decreased arterial compliance, as measured by the ratio of pulse pressure to stroke volume and exponential analysis of diastolic blood pressure decay, and decreased pulse wave velocity have also been reported.[47] Additional studies in borderline patients have shown that, with exercise, cardiac output decreases, stroke volume does not increase sufficiently, and total peripheral resistance, instead of decreasing, actually increases. Safar has shown that total peripheral resistance is abnormal in patients with borderline hypertension, but only during upright tilt and exercise, while cardiac index and heart rate are elevated.[48] With upright tilt (a form of orthostatic stress) or exercise the total peripheral resistance increases more than in normal individuals without increases in cardiac index and stroke volume. These patients can also have a decreased plasma volume and attenuation of the microcirculation.[48,49]

ESTABLISHED HYPERTENSION

Patients with established or fixed hypertension, patients with long-standing hypertension, and older hypertensives characteristically have an increase in total peripheral resistance, attributable to structural changes in the resistance vessels.[42,47,49,50] In these patients cardiac output and cardiac index are normal or decreased and myocardial contractility is normal to increased, but early left ventricular filling is delayed, left ventricular compliance is decreased, and left ventricular mass is increased.[51a,51b] Circulating catecholamine levels are usually normal and renal blood flow is normal to decreased.

The Complications of Sustained Hypertension

Hypertension is a chronic disease which normally evolves over the course of 20 to 30 years. Most patients remain asymptomatic until target organ damage is well advanced. The primary complications resulting from sustained elevation of blood pressure include (1) effects on the heart, specifically the left ventricle, (2) acceleration of atherosclerosis, and (3) direct vascular structural changes which affect especially the brain, retina, and kidneys. Approximately 50 percent of hypertensive patients die of coronary artery disease, 30 percent die of stroke, and 10 to 15 percent die of renal failure.[7]

CARDIAC EFFECTS OF HYPERTENSION

Early in the course of hypertension, cardiac output, cardiac index, heart rate, and oxygen consumption are increased.[39] However, with exercise, the stroke volume does not increase as much as in normal individuals, and coronary reserve is reduced. With continued hypertension, in response to the increased wall stress, the left ventricle hypertrophies by increasing wall thickness. This is primarily due to an increase in cell size, not in cell number. According to Poiseuille's law, the increase in wall thickness maintains normal wall tension. This adaptive process keeps pace with the increased afterload, thus maintaining normal systolic cardiac performance. However, even with mild degrees of left ventricular enlargement, diastolic function of the heart becomes impaired. Delayed left ventricular filling is a sign of decreased left ventricular compliance or increased stiffness.[51a] Concurrent with the hypertrophy, structural changes occur in various vascular beds, including the coronary arteries. The acceleration of atherosclerosis produced by hypertension also affects the elastic and medium-sized muscular arteries, and the aorta and large conduit arteries, causing stiffening, decreasing elasticity, and tortuosity, resulting in altered aortic input impedance; this in turn affects the pressure and flow relationships, raising systolic pressure.[52a] Thus, the function of the left ventricle in hypertension depends on the level of the arterial pressure, the degree of left ventricular hypertrophy, and the structural changes in the coronary vascular bed. In the long run, the left ventricular systolic function becomes impaired, and hypertensive heart failure results.[51b] This complication has become rare in the absence of coronary artery disease, since the advent of antihypertensive medication, but in older epidemiologic studies hypertensive heart failure was a major cause of death.[10] In the Framingham study, cardiac decompensation developed six times more frequently among hypertensive than among normotensive individuals, and hypertension was the most common precursor of heart failure among the group aged 30 to 62 years.[17–21]

VASCULAR STRUCTURAL CHANGES IN HYPERTENSION

In established hypertension, structural alterations occur in the microvascular circulation.[43,49,50] These consist of increased thickness of the walls of the resistance arterioles due to hypertrophy of smooth muscle cells in the media. This increased bulk of tissue encroaches on the arterial lumen, resulting in resistance to flow even with maximal vasodilation. In addition, reduction in the number of arterioles occurs, reflecting a long-term autoregulatory reaction to overperfusion by the elevated arterial pressure, that probably is also mediated by neural and humoral factors.[43,49,50] The increased thickness of the media results from increased number and size of cells as well as osmotic trapping of water causing stiffness of these vessels. As discussed earlier, the arterioles are also more responsive to the vasoconstrictor effects of norepinephrine with a lower threshold for vasoconstriction; this change in sensitivity may actually precede the rise in blood pressure and increase in wall stress. In the precapillary arterioles the contractile mass and/or the number of smooth muscle cells in the media increase, and multinucleated or tetraploid cells can be present. Hypertension also accelerates the rate of endothelial cell turnover. These changes may play a part in the increased lipid transport and accumulation in the vessels of hypertensive patients.

ACCELERATION OF ATHEROSCLEROSIS IN HYPERTENSION

Hypertension accelerates the development of atherosclerosis in large elastic arteries and medium-sized muscular arteries such as the carotid, coronary, cerebral, mesenteric, aortoiliac, and renal arteries.[52a,52b] In experimental animals, hypertension results in an increase in fatty streaks, fibrous plaques, and severity of stenoses compared with normotensive animals.

The sequence of events in the development of an atherosclerotic plaque include: (1) Circulating blood cells (white cells and platelets) adhere to endothelial surfaces (possibly because of damage or denudation of the intima) and penetrate into the subendothelial space; intimal monocytes accumulate and endothelial cells proliferate. Macrophages derived from circulating monocytes, once inside the arterial wall, have receptors for low-density lipoproteins and accumulate lipids by phagocytosis, thus becoming "foam cells." These macrophages also secrete a fibroblast growth factor resulting in accumulation of connective tissue in the intima. (2) At the same time smooth muscle cells migrate from the media into the intima and proliferate. (3) Lysosomal enzyme activity is stimulated and enhanced arterial permeability to macromolecules results in accumulation of intimal lipid, especially when circulating lipid levels are elevated. (4) Monocytes are transformed to macrophages or foam cells which accumulate lipid and undergo necrosis, calcification, and fibrosis and form a fibrous cap. (5) Liberation of platelet-derived growth factor further stimulates smooth muscle cell proliferation and migration and DNA synthesis.[52b]

Hypertension accelerates these processes, leading to an increase in plaque formation, especially in the presence of increased levels of circulating lipids.[52a,52b] In the United States, where most of the population have cholesterol levels above the ideal, blood pressure elevation readily results in increased cardiovascular disease; in countries like Japan, where the population has a low level of lipoproteins, atherosclerotic coronary disease and its sequelae (but not cerebrovascular dissease) are rare despite a high prevalence of hypertension.[25,26]

The atherosclerotic process in turn leads to the development of thrombotic brain infarction, occlusive coronary artery disease, thromboembolic occlusive disease in the aortoiliac, mesenteric, and peripheral arteries as well as aneurysm formation. The incidence of these events is compounded by the association of additional risk factors for atherosclerosis such as advancing age, male sex, cigarette smoking, hyperlipemia, and glucose intolerance.[12,18,20]

THE EFFECT OF HYPERTENSION ON THE BRAIN

Hypertension affects the brain by accelerating atherosclerosis in the carotid and basilar arteries and in the main cerebral arteries connected by the circle of Willis. Occlusive lesions in these arteries result in thrombotic strokes, i.e., ischemic infarcts. Emboli composed of cholesterol and platelet clumps from ulcerating plaques at the carotid bifurcation and internal carotid arteries result in transient ischemic attacks, such as amaurosis fugax. Corticocerebral infarcts are the most common cause of stroke in hypertensive individuals. Seventy percent of these are due to extracranial carotid disease.[52a–52c]

A specific effect characteristic of hypertension is seen in the smaller cerebral arteries, in the lenticulostriate and the perforant thalamic arteries of the internal capsule and the pons, as well as the paramedian branches of the basilar artery. This process is known as *lipohyalinosis* and consists of deposition of hyalin material in the endothelium associated with hyperplasia and reduplication of the elastic lamina as well as intimal hyperplasia.[52d,53a,52b] Fatty macrophages and fibrinoid material are deposited in the wall of the arterioles, resulting in narrowing of the lumen and eventually obliteration of these vessels. Because the small cerebral arteries contain very little muscle tissue, hypertension promotes the development of small aneurysms, the Charcot-Bouchard aneurysms.[53a] These may thrombose, forming small infarcts, or rupture, leading to intracerebral hemorrhage. The small infarcts, known as "lacunar" infarcts,[53b] range in size from 0.2 to 15 mm^3.[53a,53b] Retinal changes reflect a similar process of medial and intimal thickening, formation of thrombi with microinfarcts, and eventual cerebral edema manifested as papilledema.[52a,53b]

In the condition known as *hypertensive encephalopathy*, the cerebral vessels lose their ability to autoregulate, that is, to vasoconstrict in response to a rise in blood pressure and to vasodilate in response to a fall in blood pressure.[54a] The extreme and rapid rise of blood pressure of this condition results in segmental overdistention of cerebral arterioles and ultrafiltration of red cells, plasma, and plasma protein into the stretched segments of the arterial wall. This results in cerebral edema, cerebral hemorrhage, herniation, and death unless the blood pressure is rapidly reduced.

Subarachnoid hemorrhage, mostly from ruptured aneurysms of the circle of Willis, occurs in hypertensive as in normotensive persons, but in the former the bleeding is often more extensive and devastating.[54b,54c]

RENAL EFFECTS OF HYPERTENSION

Although nephrosclerosis is common in the kidneys of hypertensives when examined at necropsy or by needle biopsy, death from renal failure is rare unless malignant hypertension develops.[28,29,55a] The pathologic changes include hyalinization of glomeruli; tubular atrophy; interstitial fibrosis; hyalinization of afferent arterioles, interlobular, and arcuate arteries; and medial hypertrophy and intimal fibrosis.[55a] Perera reported on 500 hypertensive subjects followed for 20 years in the era before effective drug therapy was available, and found that 212 developed proteinuria, but only 92 of these developed nitrogen retention.[8] However, in hypertensive blacks renal disease is more common.[55b]

One of the hemodynamic changes that occur in the kidneys of individuals with early hypertension is reduced renal blood flow with preservation of glomerular filtration rate, resulting in an increased filtration fraction. However, these changes have been observed in only about two-thirds of patients with essential hypertension.[55a,55c] Markers of early renal damage include microalbuminuria, perhaps reflecting permeability changes in the glomerulus secondary to hyperfiltration. Another possible marker of early renal damage is excretion of *N*-acetyl-β-D-glucosaminidase (NAG).[55a,55c] Messerli et al. showed that an increase in serum uric acid can be a reflection of increased intrarenal vascular resistance and decreased glomerular filtration rate.[55d]

In malignant hypertension, on the other hand, renal failure is a hallmark of the diagnosis and was the cause of death in up to 60 percent of patients before effective drug therapy was available.[28,29] The characteristic lesion is fibrinoid necrosis of the arterioles, perhaps due to physical disruption of the intima by the high perfusion pressure and consequent penetration of circulating plasma constituents into the arteriolar media, especially in the afferent arterioles.[28,29] The diagnosis is based on the presence of hematuria, granular casts, proteinuria occasionally in the nephrotic range, and progressive decrease in glomerular filtration rate with nitrogen retention.

HORMONAL MODIFIERS OF BLOOD PRESSURE

Many hormones affect the blood pressure. These include the steroid hormones (mineralocorticoids, glucocorticoids, estrogens), thyroid hormones, catecholamines (epinephrine and norepinephrine), the polypeptide hormones (angiotensin II, vasopressin, vasoactive intestinal peptide, ANF, and others), and as yet poorly characterized factors such as ouabainlike substances. Several of these are discussed below in relation to their effects on the blood pressure.

THE RENIN-ANGIOTENSIN SYSTEM

The renin-angiotensin system (Figs. 14-2 and 14-3) is important in the adaptive blood pressure responses and has been closely linked with both experimental and clinical hypertensive disorders. The effector substance of this system is angiotensin II, an octapeptide. An α-glycoprotein enzyme, renin, acts on an α_2-globulin substrate made in the liver to form the decapeptide angiotensin I, which is the precursor to angiotensin II. The two carboxy-terminal amino acids of angiotensin I are then cleaved in vascular beds, particularly in the pulmonary circulation, by converting enzyme to form angiotensin II. This octapeptide is inactivated by proteases in the circulation.

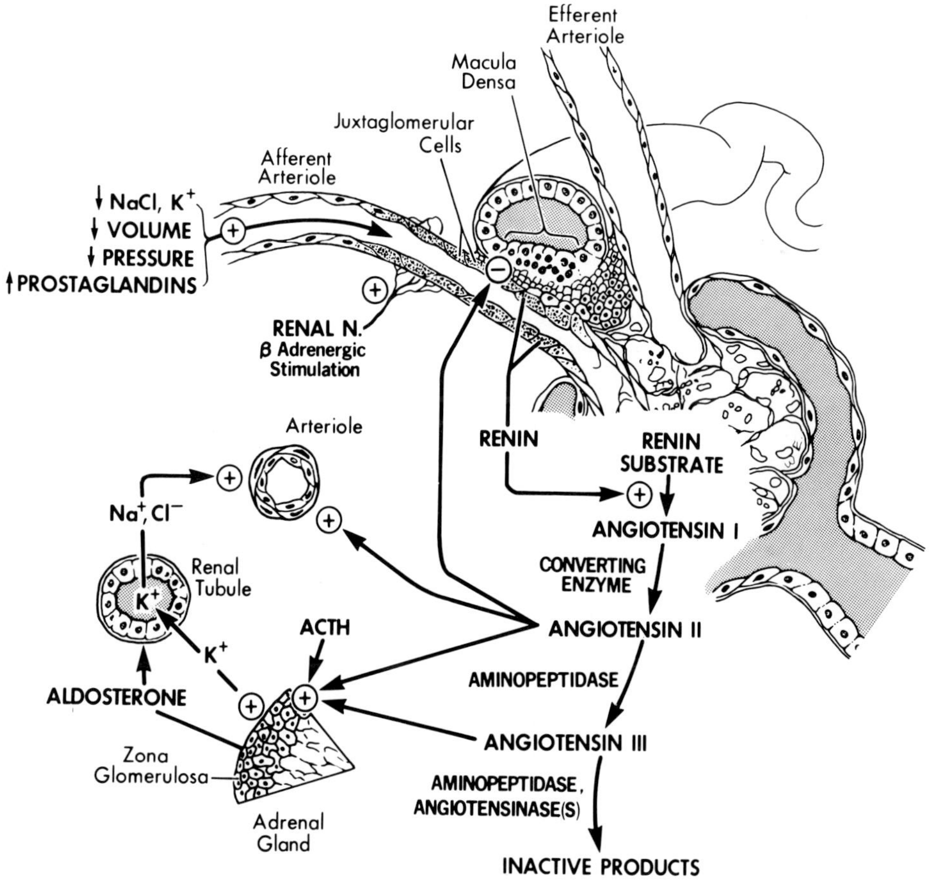

FIGURE 14-2 The renin-angiotensin system. Plus and minus signs indicate stimulation and inhibition, respectively.

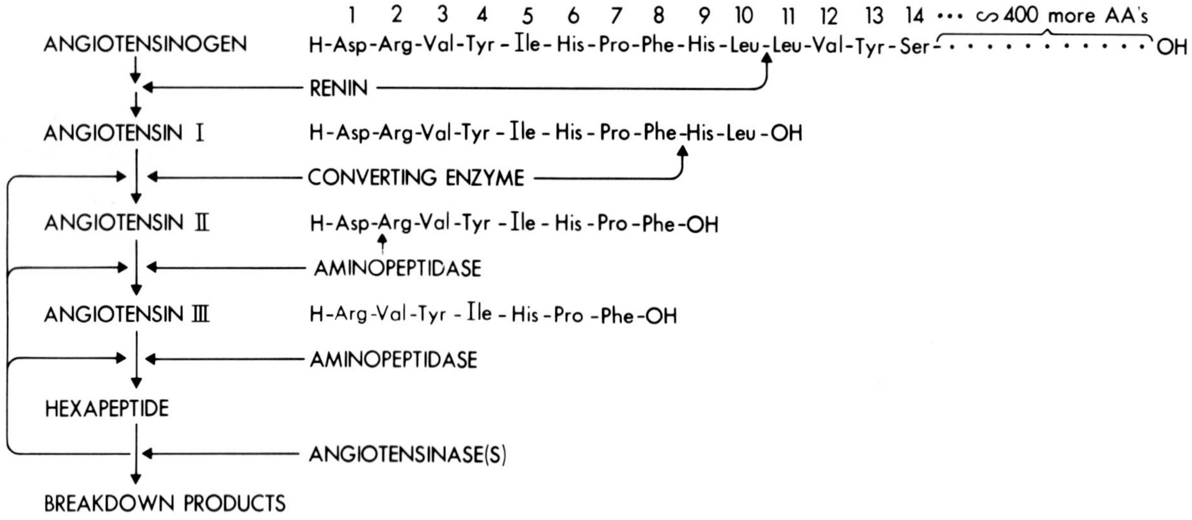

FIGURE 14-3 Formation and metabolism of angiotensins. (*Modified from Boucher et al.*[56a])

Components of the Renin-Angiotensin System

RENIN

Renin occurs in various forms at low concentrations in blood.[56a–61] The active form of this aspartyl protease has been purified from human kidney and from tissue of a renin-secreting tumor.[57–60] It has a molecular weight of about 40,000 and exists as four to five isoenzymes with differing isoelectric points. An inactive form of the enzyme (prorenin), which can be acid- or protease-activated, constitutes more than half of the renin proteins in the normal circulation. It has a molecular weight of 55,000 determined by gel filtration, or 47,000 by sodium dodecylsulfate (SDS)–polyacrylamide gel electrophoresis.[61,62] A direct radioimmunoassay for renin is on the horizon.[63] At present, renin is determined by the rate of generation of angiotensin II from renin substrate, angiotensin I. The concentration of the latter is then measured by radioimmunoassay.

Recently, the human renin gene[64–66] and cDNA to renin mRNA[67,68] have been cloned and sequenced, and from the DNA structure the amino acid sequence of preprorenin has been deduced. The human renin gene is located on chromosome 1.[69] A single gene appears to code for the enzyme.[64,65,69] Human preprorenin consists of 406 amino acids. A 20-amino-acid signal peptide is cleaved to form prorenin. Current studies strongly support the identity of prorenin and human inactive renin. The latter cross-reacts with antibodies generated against the "pro" segment of prorenin.[62,70–72] In addition, native human inactive renin and the prorenin product of the expressed gene share multiple biochemical similarities[73,73a] and activation characteristics.[71,72] Amino-terminal sequencing of pure human renal renin indicates that a 46-amino-acid amino-terminal pro segment is cleaved after the dibasic residues lysine-arginine.[60] The cleavage by a paired basic residue–specific protease is common to a number of systems, e.g., proopiomelanocortin, proinsulin, proglucagon, etc.[73b,74] Whether the prorenin processing enzyme is specific for prorenin remains to be determined.

The active form of renin in the circulation arises predominantly from the kidney. After nephrectomy, plasma renin activity (PRA) and angiotensin II concentration drop to undetectable levels.[75a,75b] This suggests that plasma angiotensin II concentrations are predominantly dependent on renin of renal origin. Several years after nephrectomy, the plasma prorenin level, but not that of active renin, increases in some patients to prenephrectomy values, suggesting extrarenal tissues can produce prorenin.[61] In the rat, prorenin release from extrarenal sources can be demonstrated within hours of nephrectomy.[61,71] Immunohistochemical studies in humans and animals have localized renin in the pituitary, several areas of the brain, vascular endothelial and smooth muscle tissue, cardiac myocytes, adrenal gland, chorion, pituitary, testes and ovary.[76,77] Renin mRNA has also been identified in some of these tissues, confirming their renin biosynthetic capability.[78a]

The finding that prorenin can be synthesized in extrarenal tissues and that these can contribute to material that circulates as prorenin suggests that these tissues and plasma have a very low capacity to convert prorenin to renin. This has led to speculation that prorenin may have actions other than those to generate angiotensin I. However, there is as yet no evidence for such actions. Alternatively, the pool of inactive renin in plasma could serve as a reservoir for local tissue production of active renin, or else small amounts of renin generated from local production of prorenin in these tissues might act there as part of a local renin-angiotensin system. This would be consistent with the finding that both converting enzyme and angiotensinogen are also produced in multiple tissues (see below). The possibility that these putative local renin-angiotensin systems play important roles in tissues such as the vasculature, brain, adrenal, and reproductive tissues is being studied intensively, although clear roles for them have not been established.[62,76,77,78a,78b]

There are other proteolytic enzymes that can generate angiotensin I or angiotensin II. Tonin, a serine protease, can act on angiotensinogen, on tetradecapeptide renin substrate, and on angiotensin I to form angiotensin II.[79] In the rat, tonin has been located in the submandibular gland and the kidney. It does not modify blood pressure when injected into intact rats, but it does produce a pressor effect in bilaterally nephrectomized animals. Tonin may also play a role in renovascular hypertension. Cathepsins can also generate angiotensins I and II. These are localized to the kidney, particularly in renin-containing granules, brain, white blood cells, and endothelial cells.[80,81] Their optimum pH of activity is 4 to 5; there is little generation of angiotensin I or II at physiological pH. The importance of these reninlike enzymes to overall blood pressure regulation is unknown.

Renal renin is synthesized in the juxtaglomerular cells of the afferent renal arteriole (Fig. 14-2) and stored as rhomboid-appearing granules.[82] It is released into both the bloodstream and the renal lymphatics in response to a number of stimuli (Fig. 14-2). These tend to act through three types of influences: (1) renal baroreceptors, (2) adrenergic receptors, and (3) circulating factors such as ions or hormones.[82] Renin release is stimulated[82] by a lowering of the blood pressure, changing from the supine to the erect posture, salt depletion, beta-adrenergic or central nervous system stimulation, and vasodilating prostaglandins and hormones, opiate peptides,[83] and kallikrein.[84] Renin release is inhibited by increases in the blood pressure (except with malignant hypertension), assumption of the supine posture, salt loading, angiotensin II, vasopressin, inhibitors of prostaglandin biosynthesis such as indomethacin, potassium (see Chap. 12), calcium,[82] and atrial natriuretic factor (ANF, discussed below). It is also inhibited by certain antihypertensive drugs, including beta-adrenergic blockers,[82] α-methyldopa,[85] and clonidine.[86] Renin is inactivated by proteolytic enzymes in the liver and plasma or is excreted by the kidney and in the bile. Its half-life in plasma is 10 to 20 min.[56a]

The macula densa is a specialized segment of the distal nephron where the distal tubule makes contact with the afferent arteriole just before it enters the glomerulus (Fig. 14-2).[82] It thus has an intimate anatomic relationship to the juxtaglomerular apparatus. In isolated preparations, the macula densa exerts an inhibitory influence on renin release that is increased when juxtaglomerular cells are separated from it.[87] This inhibitory influence may be due to the release of adenosine from the macula densa cells that act through α_1-adenosine receptors on the juxtaglomerular cells.[88]

Along with the juxtaglomerular cells, the macula densa appears to act as a sensor of renal tubular fluid composition and alters the rate of renin release. This occurs either through a direct sensor activity or through indirect influences as part of an intrarenal feedback mechanism that controls the state of glomerular filtration.[82] The macula densa detects the signal provided by renal tubular fluid sodium[82,89] or more likely the associated chloride concentration,[90] and translates this information to renin release. It may be that increases in the sodium chloride flux across the distal tubule increase adenosine release and decreases in sodium chloride flux decrease adenosine release. Whatever the precise mechanism, factors that reduce volume and/or lower the plasma sodium (and chloride) ion concentration such as dehydration or a loss of fluid or blood result in stimulation of renin release.

The renal baroreceptors stimulate the release of renin in response to decreases in renal perfusion pressure.[82] Apparently, changes are more important than the absolute perfusion pressure because they can effect renin release in the presence of either renal arteriolar constriction or dilation. These receptors can function independently of innervation and of influences of sodium chloride delivery to the macula densa. They are probably involved in stimulating renin release in response to fluid loss and decreases in blood pressure.

Renal sympathetic nerves that terminate in the juxtaglomerular cells and in the smooth muscle cells of the renal afferent arterioles secrete norepinephrine and stimulate renin release.[82] These nerves appear to be important in mediating central nervous system stimuli and the responses to posture, changes in the blood pressure, and even salt depletion. They can act independent of the baroreceptors and the salt influences on the macula densa. Activity of these nerves is stimulated primarily by the low-pressure cardiopulmonary venous receptors; an independent role for arterial baroreceptors has not been established, although effects through baroreceptors in concert with those through low-pressure receptors do appear to operate.[91]

A beta-adrenergic receptor mechanism can stimulate renin release.[82] These receptors probably mediate the effects of the norepinephrine released by the sympathetic nerves. Indeed, epinephrine, norepinephrine, and isoproterenol stimulate renin release, and this effect is abolished by the beta-adrenergic blocker propranolol, but not by alpha-adrenergic blockers in most studies. Although the question has not yet been resolved, it is possible that the efficacy of propranolol in the treatment of hypertension is in part due to the blocking of renin release. The actions of the catecholamines are in part due to their ability to induce vasoconstriction with the subsequent decrease in glomerular filtration rate and filtered load of sodium and chloride. However, the beta-adrenergic mechanism for stimulating renin release is independent of these vascular effects. Conversely, the effects of sodium and chloride (and possibly other influences) on renin release can occur independent of beta-adrenergic receptors.

Angiotensin II is a potent inhibitor of renin release.[92] This occurs under all conditions of sodium intake. Converting enzyme inhibition is a potent stimulus of renin release, even under conditions where it does not induce a hypotensive response.[93] This negative feedback inhibition appears to be calcium-dependent;[94] calcium channel blockers thus enhance renin release. However, calcium is also intimately involved in aldosterone production (see Chap. 12), so that calcium channel blockers inhibit aldosterone release and, thus, uncouple renin-aldosterone responses.

The effects of vasopressin are inhibitory and are observed at physiological concentrations of the hormone.[82] Although the precise role of vasopressin is not known, it has been proposed that the actions are direct and can be independent of influences of this hormone on hemodynamics or fluid volume.

There is a strong association between the renin-angiotensin system and the prostaglandin (PG) system (Chap. 31). Renal prostaglandins have been implicated as important mediators of the release of renin from the kidney, and may mediate baroreceptor and macula densa signals to release renin.[95] Administration of either the PG precursor arachidonic acid or various PGs themselves causes an increase in renin secretion. The vasodilator prostacyclin (PGI_2) has been shown to be the major prostaglandin produced in the renal cortex in humans.[96] PGI_2 consistently stimulates renin secretion when infused into the renal artery or when added to renal cortical slices.[97] Intravenous infusion of PGI_2 into humans induces a dose-dependent increase in PRA, which is independent of changes in renal hemodynamics or the sympathetic nervous system.[98] Inhibition of PG synthesis reduces renin production, further suggesting a role of PGs in renin release.[99] Treatment with indomethacin (a PG synthetase inhibitor) decreases supine renin levels, reduces levels that are normally stimulated by upright posture and furosemide,[100] reduces hyperreninemia associated with hemorrhage and Bartter's syndrome (see Chap. 12),[101] and induces the syndrome of hyporeninemic hypoaldosteronism in some patients with underlying renal disease (see Chap. 12).

The quantitative contributions of the nervous and vascular systems, the macula densa, and other influences to the regulation of renin release have not been fully delineated. It appears that each can act independently and that when one system is blocked (e.g., the kidney denervated and the vascular receptors blocked by papaverine), the other systems are capable of appreciable compensation.

Stimulation results in the release of both renin and prorenin, with a greater proportion of renin than prorenin. Further, during periods of relative suppression, there is more release of prorenin than renin. For example, with marked abrupt stimulation, such as occurs with removal of angiotensin II negative feedback (see below), active renin levels rise and plasma prorenin levels drop precipitously.[102] Thus, certain stimuli probably result in preferential processing of prorenin to renin. This could occur as a result of a preferential release, due to increased shuttling of newly synthesized protein to secretory granules that are more active in conversion of prorenin to renin. It is not known whether the processing itself is specifically regulated in some other way. PGs could play a role in regulating prorenin to renin conversion.[103a] In addition, studies in the rat show an increase in renin content and renin mRNA after prolonged stimulation, such as by salt deprivation, implying that the stimulation increases renin synthesis as well as release.[103b] In diabetic nephropathy there is an increase in prorenin but not renin levels, implying that tissue damage may impair the pathways that allow the conversion.[104]

Several compounds have been developed that can inhibit renin release.[105–107] These are analogues of renin substrate (angiotensinogen, see below). Although they are effective in blocking angiotensin production and can lower the blood pressure in certain circumstances (e.g., salt deprivation), they have not come into general clinical use, because, unlike converting enzyme inhibitors (see below), they must be injected, since after oral administration either they are inactive or extremely high doses are required.

ANGIOTENSINOGEN (RENIN SUBSTRATE)

Angiotensinogen is a glycoprotein synthesized predominantly in the liver, with a molecular weight of 50,000 to 100,000 (Fig. 14-3). The higher-molecular-weight forms are synthesized in greater quantities during pregnancy or oral contraceptive administration.[108] The protein is also synthesized at much lower levels in a variety of extrahepatic tissues, including kidney, brain, adrenal, aorta, heart, and testis.[109] The level of substrate is increased with estrogen excess[110] and by glucocorticoids and thyroid hormone.[111] A decrease in the concentration of this protein was demonstrated in certain patients with untreated Addison's disease.[112] However, this decrease may be due mostly to excessive angiotensinogen degradation resulting from the high levels of plasma renin in this state.[113] Under most circumstances, renin substrate appears to circulate at concentrations that do not greatly exceed the K_m for renin. The K_m for pure human renin and pure human renin substrate is 1.15 mM.[60] This means that at any given concentration of renin, variations in the concentration of substrate will have an influence on the amount of angiotensin that is generated. The angiotensin gene has been cloned[114] and angiotensinogen mRNA levels have been shown to increase with steroid and thyroid hormone treatment.[115]

ANGIOTENSIN-CONVERTING ENZYME

Angiotensin-converting enzyme is a zinc-containing glycoprotein that is found in the lung, plasma, the brush borders of the proximal renal tubule, the endothelium of vascular beds, the brain, and the testis.[116a,116b] The enzyme is mostly membrane bound, although a soluble form has also been found.[116b] This enzyme will remove two carboxy-terminal amino acids from a number of peptide substrates. Its two most important actions are the inactivation of bradykinin and the conversion of angiotensin I to angiotensin II (Figs. 14-2 and 14-3). It can also have actions on other proteins.[116b,117] The lung appears to be the most active tissue in converting angiotensin I to II.[118]

The converting enzymes have an enormous capacity for generating angiotensin II. Thus, even though in certain diseases (e.g., pulmonary disease) there can be a decrease in the measured concentration of converting enzyme in the plasma, this does not noticeably affect angiotensin II generation.[118a] However, whereas changes in converting enzyme have not been shown to markedly influence angiotensin II generation, more subtle changes might have more modest effects. Converting enzyme levels are increased in patients with essential and renovascular hypertension, by diuretic therapy, in some patients with diabetes mellitus,[118b] and in hyperthyroidism.[119,120] The activity of the enzyme is increased in isolated cells by glucocorticoid treatment (Chap. 12).

There are several compounds that can inhibit converting enzyme.[118a,121–130] These include chelating agents, certain metals, and sulfhydryl reagents; however, the class of inhibitors that hold perhaps the greatest clinical interest are peptide analogues of angiotensin I. The nonapeptides teprotide, captopril, and enalapril have been used extensively.[118a,122–130] They have been useful in defining the role of the renin-angiotensin system in regulating normal blood pressure, and they may be useful in the diagnosis and treatment of renin-dependent hypertension (see below).

The converting enzyme inhibitors have been shown to be efficacious in the treatment of essential hypertension as well as in the treatment of renin-dependent hypertension[123–125b] (see also Renovascular Hypertension, below). It is unclear whether they are less effective in the low-renin forms of hypertension (discussed below). However, they may be more effective in a subgroup of patients with essential hypertension and normal or high renin levels who are more salt-sensitive and in whom renal blood flow does not increase in response to a salt load.[125a] Since activation of the renin-angiotensin system has been shown to play a pathophysiological role in the development of congestive heart failure,[126] converting enzyme inhibitors have been demonstrated to improve hemodynamics in this condition. Another potentially exciting use of converting enzyme inhibitors may be in diabetic nephropathy, where captopril decreased proteinuria in hypertensive diabetics.[127,127a,127b] These agents may ultimately also have utility in preventing the progression of other forms of chronic renal disease.[124,128,129]

Interpretation of the actions of converting enzyme must be made in light of the fact that it also appears to play a role in the breakdown of the potent vasodilator substance bradykinin, and it can have other actions as well.[117,121-123b] The bradykinin-metabolizing activity has been termed kininase II or peptidyldipeptide hydroxylase. [Bradykinin is also inactivated by another enzyme, kininase I (carboxypeptidase N).[118a]] Inhibitors of converting enzyme decrease bradykinin breakdown; when these are given there is (briefly at least) a concomitant increase in the plasma bradykinin concentration along with a decrease in angiotensin II generation.[121,122] However, in the only long-term study reported to date, when captopril (which is active after oral administration) was administered for 8 months to patients with essential hypertension, plasma bradykinin concentrations were not increased.[123a] In dogs, converting enzyme inhibition reduces blood pressure more than does renin inhibition and decreases in blood pressure and angiotensin II levels in response to converting enzyme inhibition do not strictly parallel each other.[130]

ANGIOTENSINS I, II, AND III

Actions of Angiotensin

Angiotensin I is not known to have physiologically important actions, although it can (when given in very large doses) stimulate the adrenal medulla to produce catecholamines and the central nervous system to increase blood pressure and induce thirst.[76,131–134] A role for angiotensin I in the control of intrarenal blood flow has been proposed but has not been adequately documented.

Angiotensin II has potent vasoconstrictor activity and can cause an increase in blood pressure by direct vasoconstriction of the arteriole.[76] It acts within a few seconds and its duration of action is only a few minutes. It also directly inhibits the release of renin by the juxtaglomerular cells (Fig. 14-2).[81] It is one of the most potent stimulators of aldosterone production by the zona glomerulosa of the adrenal gland (see Chap. 12). It has unique effects on the kidney.[76,133] It decreases renal blood flow and glomerular filtration rate.[134] Administration of angiotensin II to the hypertensive patient results in natriuresis, whereas in the nonhypertensive normal subject sodium retention occurs. This effect on renal handling of sodium may be mediated through intrarenal changes in the kallikrein and prostaglandin systems initiated by the infused angiotensin II.[76,134]

In the brain, angiotensin II stimulates dipsogenic behavior, elevates blood pressure, and stimulates release of vasopressin, adrenocorticotropin (ACTH), prolactin, oxytocin, and luteinizing hormone (LH).[76] It can also stimulate the absorption of salt and water across extrarenal epithelial tissues such as jejunum and colon.[76] Other diverse effects include stimulation of uterine smooth muscle contraction, stimulation of erythropoietin, inhibition of glucagon effects on the liver, and stimulation of catecholamine production from nerve endings and adrenal medulla.[76] In addition, angiotensin II is an angiogenic factor, i.e., it induces formation of blood vessels.[76] Several other reported effects after infusion of moderate to high doses of angiotensin II include elevation of plasma lactate and blood glucose levels, increase in blood coagulation, and decrease in plasma fatty acid level; these may be secondary to vasoconstrictor effects.[55a]

The concentrations of angiotensin II in plasma vary between 5 and 100 pg/ml.[55a] Physiological stimuli may increase the plasma concentrations 10- to 25-fold. Angiotensin II may circulate partly bound by plasma proteins.[55a] It has a half-life of a very few minutes in plasma; 50 percent or more of the activity disappears in a single passage through the vascular beds.[55a]

There are several breakdown products of angiotensin II, but only the heptapeptide angiotensin III appears to have activity. Angiotensin III appears to be as active as angiotensin II on the adrenal gland and is perhaps one-half as active as a vasoconstrictor.[131] It has been proposed that angiotensin III contributes significantly to adrenal-stimulating activity in vivo, but this issue has not been clarified. Angiotensin III may also be formed through conversion of angiotensin I to des-1-aspartylangiotensin I, but the present data do not point to this pathway as being physiologically important.[135] The plasma concentrations of angiotensin III are perhaps only 20 percent of those of angiotensin II, and the former is even more susceptible to proteolytic degradation than the latter.

The molecular basis for angiotensin action involves its binding to specific receptors at the cell membrane (see Chaps. 5 and 12). Immediate postreceptor events involve effects on phospholipids and mobilization of intracellular calcium (Chaps. 5 and 12), which occur in all tissues which respond to angiotensin II. The mechanisms by which angiotensin II stimulates aldosterone release are described in Chap. 12. The initial events in the vasculature are mostly similar, and the actions of the peptide on Ca^{2+} mobilization can contribute to its pressor effects. In addition, effects on PG production may also contribute, although the precise role in this case has not been elucidated.[136]

There can be extensive regulation of the cellular sensitivity to angiotensin II, and this occurs, at least in part, through influences on the cellular content of the receptors (Chap. 5).[137] In the rat, the hormone appears to increase the concentration of adrenal receptors (an exception to the general case with polypeptide hormones) and to decrease the concentration of uterine (and possibly vascular) receptors.[137] In certain cases, prolonged infusions of angiotensin II have been shown to increase the sensitivity of the adrenal gland to the hormone. However, in some circumstances in which plasma angiotensin concentrations are chronically low (e.g., in low-renin essential hypertension), the sensitivity of the adrenal gland to angiotensin II is increased. Hyperkalemia can increase and hypokalemia can decrease the content of angiotensin receptors.[137] Their affinity for angiotensin can also be increased, albeit transiently, by sodium restriction.[137] As expected, decreased sodium intake increases and increased sodium intake decreases the adrenal content of angiotensin II receptors; this is due to the salt-induced changes in angiotensin II production.[137,138]

A number of substances have been synthesized that have angiotensin antagonist activity.[118] These bind to the angiotensin receptor and competitively inhibit the binding of agonists. In fact, the one mostly used clinically (Sar^1,Ala^8-angiotensin II, saralasin or P-113) is a partial agonist rather than a pure antagonist. Thus in states of low angiotensin II concentration its agonist activities are mostly seen, whereas in states of high angiotensin II concentration it shows its antagonist activities.[139] This partial agonist activity has limited its clinical usefulness.[140]

Maintenance of Blood Pressure

Information on the influence of angiotensin II on normal blood pressure has been provided by the development of angiotensin antagonists and converting enzyme and renin inhibitors. In sodium-replete normotensive individuals, blockade of the renin-angiotensin system by an angiotensin antagonist or converting enzyme inhibitor does not reduce blood pressure, even with changes in posture, but it does induce a significant fall in blood pressure in volume-depleted (salt-deprived, etc.) normotensive individuals.[141,142] However, the failure to reduce the blood pressure in the salt-replete state does not exclude a role of angiotensin II, since compensating mechanisms may be capable of normalizing the blood pressure under these conditions. However, the data on salt depletion indicate a limiting role for angiotensin II under these conditions.

Role of the Renin-Angiotensin System in Hypertension

EXPERIMENTAL HYPERTENSION

The hypothesis that excessive activity of the renin-angiotensin system can lead to hypertension has received support from studies with animal models with renal lesions.[143–145] The most extensively studied model systems are the one- and two-kidney Goldblatt preparations, in which a clamp is placed on the renal artery of one kidney and the other kidney is removed (one-kidney preparation) or is left intact (two-kidney preparation).

The two-kidney model resembles the acute stages of renovascular hypertension in humans. PRA and blood pressure increase immediately after the renal artery is clamped. Sodium balance tends to be positive in the early stages and to return to normal or become negative in the chronic phase. The sodium balance in this case tends to be inversely related to the degree of the hypertension. Inhibition of renin with anti-renin antibodies or inhibition of converting enzyme or angiotensin II action can cause a significant decrease in blood pressure in animals with two-kidney Goldblatt hypertension, at least in the early stages.[145] These data suggest that in the two-kidney model increased renin activity not only initiates the hypertension but is also a major factor in its maintenance. However, with longer periods of time (e.g., 2 to 4 months), the hypertension does become non-angiotensin-dependent and more volume-dependent.[145] This appears to be due to a hypertension-induced decrease in the ability of the contralateral kidney to excrete salt. At this stage the two-kidney preparation resembles the one-kidney preparation described below.

The sequence of events in the one-kidney Goldblatt model seems to be as follows.[144–146] There is a prompt increase in arterial blood pressure and an increase in PRA. During the chronic phase, hypertension persists, although the renin levels decrease to normal values. However, PRA is slightly elevated when compared with that in unilaterally nephrectomized rats. In the chronic phase, there is sodium retention; this may explain why PRA returns to normal levels. Use of an angiotensin antagonist or a converting enzyme inhibitor can prevent occurrence of hypertension early after the experimental lesion is produced, but neither is persistently effective. However, blood pressure can be reduced by inhibitors of angiotensin II action if the rats are first prepared by ingestion of a low-sodium diet. The hypertension can be reversed in the chronic phase by removal of the renal artery constriction, and this is accompanied by a negative sodium balance that correlates with the drop in blood pressure. Although the increase in renin activity is the primary initiating event, these observations suggest that other factors (most likely the sodium retention) participate more in the maintenance of the hypertension. The single (and compromised) kidney cannot excrete sodium adequately. This model may be useful for understanding chronic renovascular hypertension in humans. Rather than being renin-dependent, the hypertension becomes volume-dependent, possibly due to chronic hypertensive changes in the nonstenotic kidney. The hypertension during this phase in humans is not responsive to correction of the stenosis.

RENIN-SECRETING TUMORS

As described below there are rare occurrences of renin-secreting tumors (Fig. 14-4). These result in severe hypertension and hypokalemia. Removal of the tumor can result in amelioration of the hypertension and hypokalemia. This syndrome provides a clear example that renin in excess can lead to hypertension.

RENOVASCULAR HYPERTENSION

The animal models of experimental hypertension have aided greatly the understanding of renovascular hypertension (discussed in detail below). Thus, renal ischemia and hypoperfusion resulting from renal artery lesions lead to renin release with consequences similar to those in the animal. The overall result depends on the severity of the lesion and the functional capacity of both the contralateral and involved kidneys. Functional capacity depends both on the extent of preceding renal impairment as well as hypertension-induced changes. Because of these variables there are considerable differences in the clinical presentation, with plasma renin levels being high, normal, or low normal. These are in turn determined by the degree of stimulus induced by the ischemic kidney and the extent to which subsequent sodium retention suppresses the renin levels. The sodium retention is in turn affected greatly by the functional capacity of the kidneys. Thus, in general the hemodynamic and hormonal states of individual patients can be related to the various phases in the development of renovascular hypertension in animals. This heterogeneity of clinical presentation accounts in large measure for many of the problems in diagnosis and management of the renovascular hypertension. First, as mentioned above, there are significant variations in plasma renin levels, and normal renin levels can be present with clear angiotensin II–dependent hypertension. There are also substantial variations in patient responsiveness to both drug therapy and surgical intervention, and there are significant difficulties with the testing methods available to date in determining the functional importance of the lesions and in predicting the responses to drug therapy or surgical intervention. The approach to these problems is, however, addressed below.

OTHER FORMS OF SECONDARY HYPERTENSION

The issue of other types of secondary hypertension is complex because of the spectrum of causes of secondary hypertension. In cases in which the hypertension is more salt- or volume-dependent, primary aldosteronism for example, renin is suppressed. Unfortunately, many of the other syndromes are associated with hemodynamic abnormalities (e.g., excess catecholamine or glucocorticoid levels) that themselves have an effect on the renin-angiotensin system.

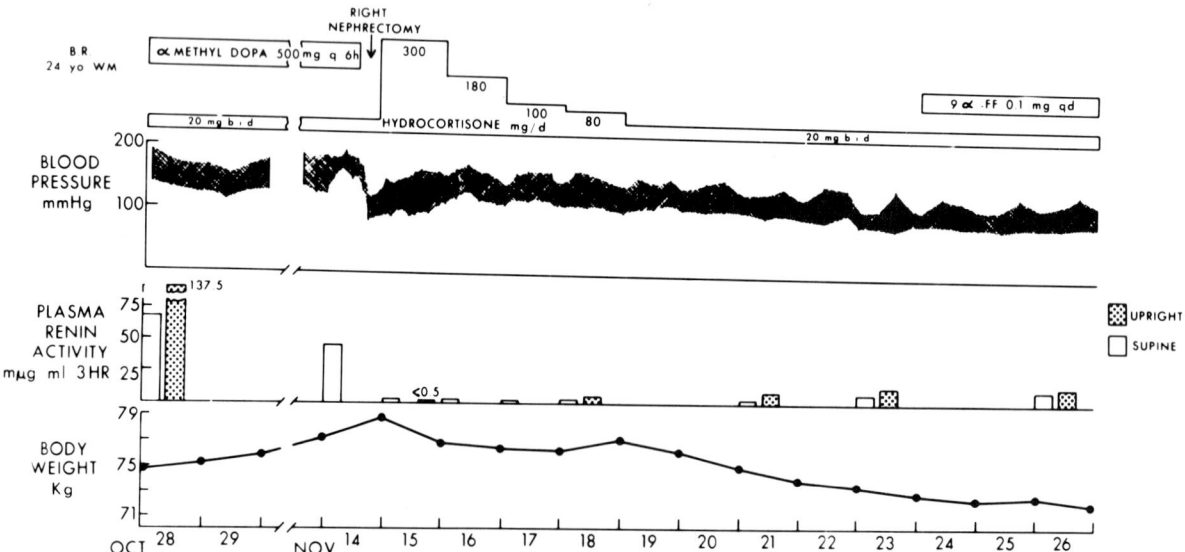

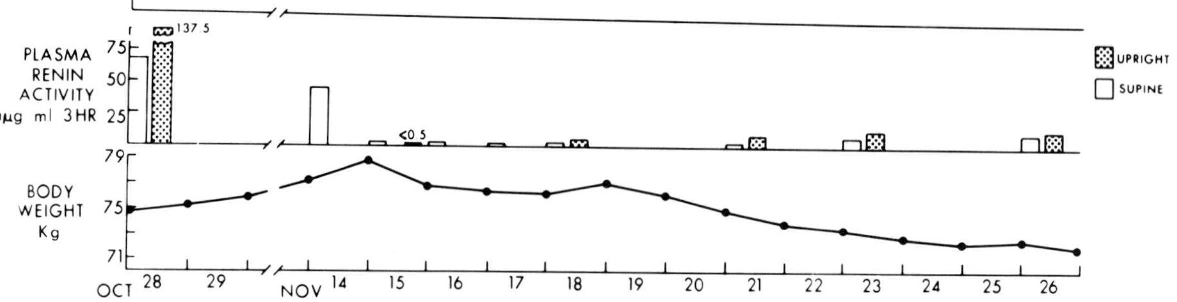

FIGURE 14-4 Preoperative and postoperative measurements of blood pressure, plasma renin activity (PRA), and body weight in a patient with a renin-secreting tumor (previous surgery was subtotal adrenalectomy). Note the prompt fall in blood pressure and PRA after right nephrectomy. Normal PRA was seen on the ninth postoperative day. Adrenal hormone replacement was required because of reduced adrenal mass from previous surgery. (*From Schambelan et al.*[379])

ACCELERATED HYPERTENSION

Accelerated hypertension is characterized by marked elevation of blood pressure, decreased renal function, and severe retinopathy. Renin levels are usually extremely high and result in secondary aldosteronism.[147,148] There are many reasons why the renin system should be activated in these patients, e.g., altered renal hemodynamics that result in ischemia, and these causes contribute to further vasoconstriction and arterial hypertension. Angiotensin antagonists can be effective in the acute vasospastic phase. Patients with chronic renal failure are particularly susceptible to this form of hypertension, and an increased blood volume usually aggravates the condition; in this case administration of diuretic agents or dialysis can be successful in normalizing the blood pressure. This renin-dependent form of accelerated hypertension occurs in a small subgroup of hypertensive patients and is an acute disorder that may require nephrectomy. The hypothesis that the hyperreninemia and aldosteronism are secondary rather than primary is suggested by the finding that renin and aldosterone levels usually return to the normal range after effective therapy.[148]

ESSENTIAL HYPERTENSION

The role of the renin-angiotensin system in essential hypertension is complex, due in large measure to the heterogeneity of the condition. Nevertheless, overall participation of the system is evidenced by the therapeutic effectiveness of blocking the system with converting enzyme inhibitors in clinical trials of patients with essential hypertension.[149,150] Overall, the converting enzyme inhibitors are probably as effective as diuretics or beta-adrenergic antagonists in treating mild to moderately severe hypertension and may be more effective overall in treating severe hypertension.

The participation of the system is more clearly understood, however, when individual patients with hypertension are studied. These vary markedly in their sensitivity to converting enzyme inhibition (see below). The physiological response to increased blood pressure is a suppression of plasma renin. This should occur in patients with volume excess, but volume is not increased in most patients with essential hypertension, irrespective of their plasma renin levels.[151–153] As shown in Figs. 14-5 and 14-6, the plasma renin levels as a function of urinary sodium excretion, a

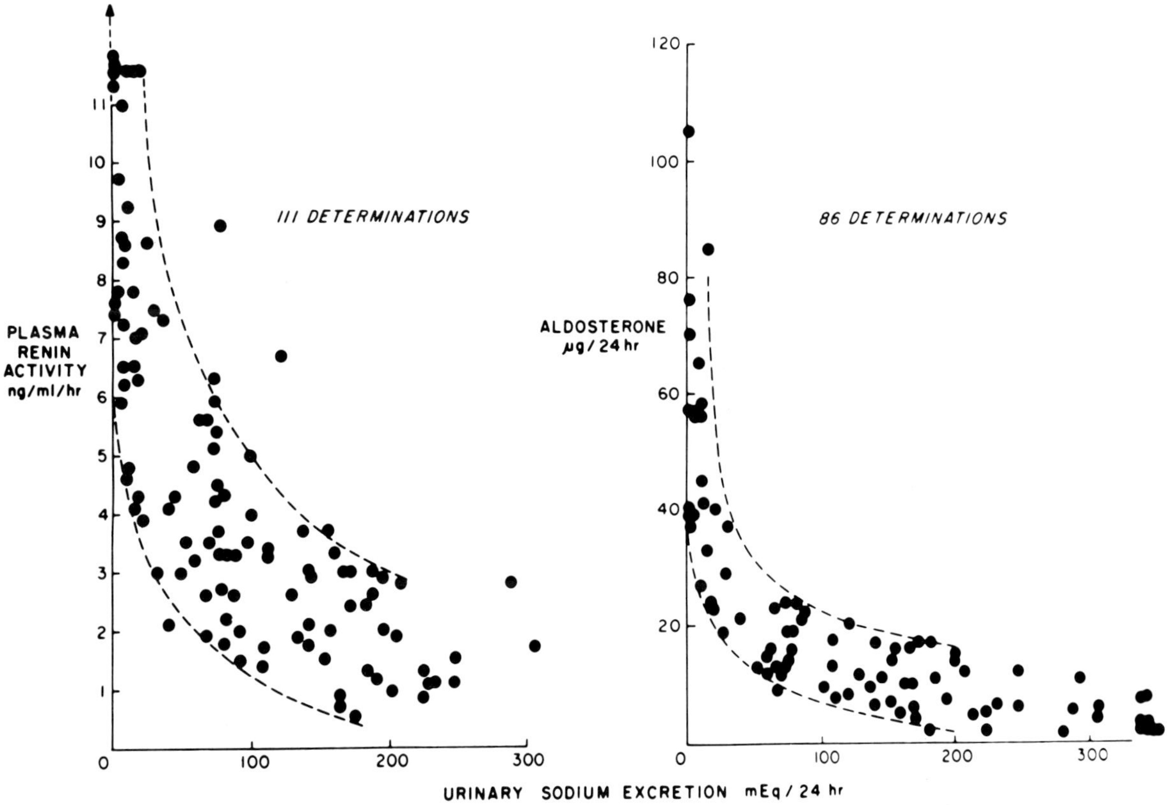

FIGURE 14-5 Relation of 4-h plasma renin activity (PRA, upright posture, *left*) or 24h urinary aldosterone levels (*right*) to the daily rate of sodium excretion in 52 normal subjects with 111 determinations. (*From Brunner et al.*[154])

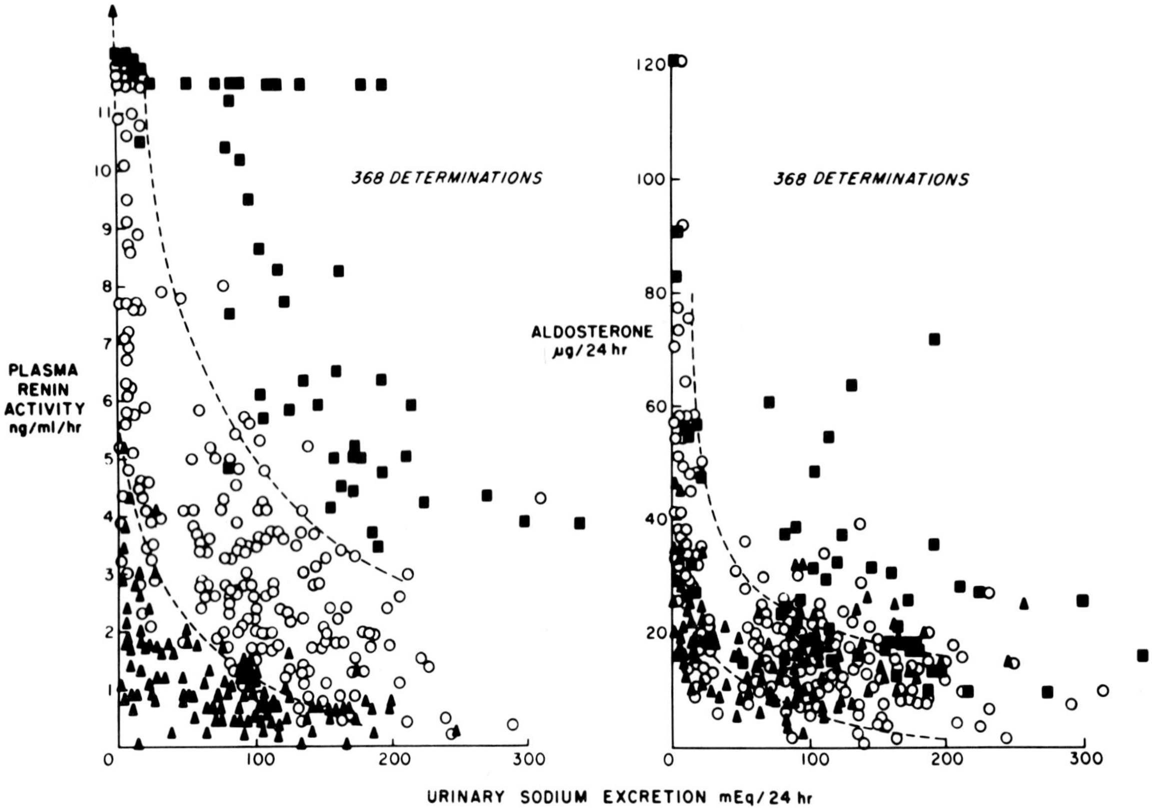

FIGURE 14-6 Plasma renin activity measured at noon after 4 h upright (*left*), and corresponding daily urinary aldosterone excretion (*right*) plotted against the concurrent daily rate of sodium excretion in 219 patients with essential hypertension. Plasma renin activity levels are indicated by triangles for low, open circles for normal, and squares for high activity. Values for 52 normal individuals are represented by the dotted line. In some cases, individual points fall outside the indicated classification. This is due to the fact that repeated samples in these patients mostly fall into another category. (*From Brunner et al.*[154])

reflection of sodium intake, show considerable variation in comparison to normal subjects.

The fact that there tends to be a spectrum of plasma renin concentrations in patients with essential hypertension without a clear separation of the low-renin subgroup raises the question of whether the low-renin state reflects an attempt by the body, which shows considerable variation among individuals and population groups, to adapt to the hypertensive state regardless of its cause. This could also explain the observation that on repeated study the renin values in certain patients shift into a different classification.[154] The idea that the renin values reflect adaptive responses to the hypertensive state is supported by the findings in several (although not all) studies of an inverse correlation between blood pressure and PRA in hypertensive and normotensive persons.[155] The possibility that plasma renin levels tend to decrease in response to hypertensive stimuli is further supported in studies of several animal systems[155] and by the finding that borderline hypertensive patients tend to have greater variations in their plasma renin levels than do age-matched normotensive control subjects.[156]

As discussed below, patients in the low-renin subgroup of essential hypertension, as might be expected, show lesser responses to converting enzyme inhibition.[143] This is consistent with their overall suppressed renin level, although the participation of angiotensin II in these patients can be somewhat greater than is reflected by their plasma renin levels, since these patients may be more sensitive to angiotensin II than normal-renin hypertensives.[157–159]

Within the normal-renin subgroup there is additional variability. As discussed below (see Sodium Chloride, below), patients with essential hypertension vary in the sensitivity of their blood pressures to a high salt intake. One group has examined salt sensitivity within the normal-renin groups and has separated patients into salt-sensitive ("nonmodulator") and salt-resistant ("modulator") types in terms of their blood pressure and other responses to an increased salt intake.[160,161] The modulators do not respond in terms of blood pressure lowering and other responses to converting enzyme inhibition, whereas the nonmodulators do. It is proposed that the nonmodulators have excessive intravascular angiotension II responses. The mechanisms of this are not known. It is equally unclear as to why the modulators do not respond to converting enzyme inhibition in the face of normal plasma renin levels. It is possible that members of this group resemble normal individuals, with the exception that their blood pressures are elevated and that the renin-angiotensin system is not contributing substantially to the elevated blood pressure. Although at present the classification of modulators vs. nonmodulators is cumbersome and restricted to research uses, ultimately drug therapy may be tailored to this type of evaluation.

IONS AND BLOOD PRESSURE

Actions of Individual Ions

SODIUM CHLORIDE

Sodium chloride is a major regulator of intravascular volume, and many of the hormones that regulate blood pressure also affect sodium dynamics. The role of sodium chloride in the pathogenesis of hypertension has been extensively studied. Epidemiologic evidence supports a role of sodium chloride in the genesis of hypertension.[162] In societies in which salt is added to food, blood pressure rises with age, but this is not seen in populations that have little access to salt. Some investigators have attributed this to the fact that sodium intake is inversely proportional to potassium intake, since societies which eat little salt tend to ingest more potassium-containing foods, e.g., fruits, vegetables, etc., and potassium may have blood pressure–lowering effects (see below). Nevertheless, when dietary sodium intake has been assessed by dietary history or by measuring 24-h urinary sodium excretion, several studies have demonstrated a significant relationship between both systolic and diastolic pressure and salt intake. The Framingham study in the United States and studies in several communities showed that the incidence of hypertension increases as sodium excretion increases.[163,164]

Blood pressure responses to altering dietary sodium intake and use of diuretics further suggest a role for sodium in the pathogenesis of hypertension. There is general agreement that a marked reduction of salt intake can lower the blood pressure in many patients with hypertension,[165] and overall there appears to be a correlation between the extent of the hypertension and the lowering effect of even moderate salt restriction (Fig. 14-7).[162] In Japan and Belgium, where there

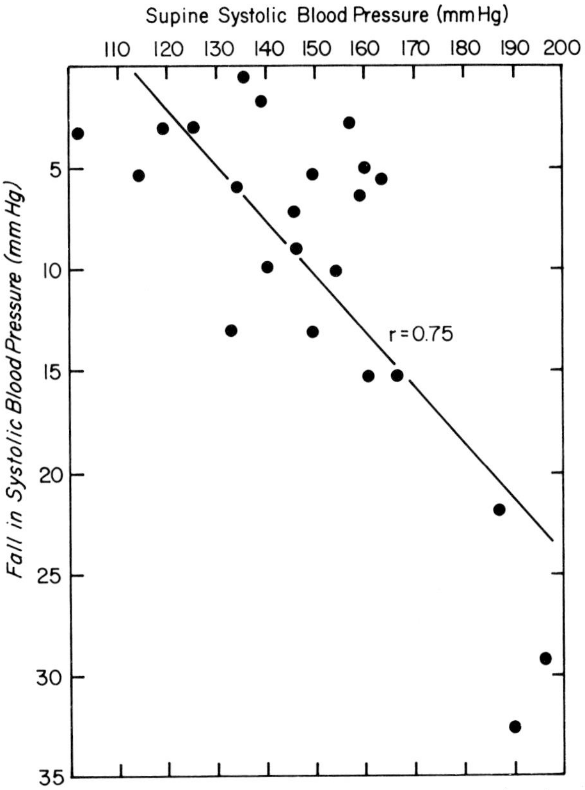

FIGURE 14-7 Fall in supine systolic blood pressure with sodium restriction plotted against pretreatment supine systolic blood pressure. The data were obtained from multiple studies. (*Reviewed in and redrawn from MacGregor.*[162])

are government campaigns to lower sodium consumption, a more modest reduction in salt intake was accompanied by a decreased prevalence of high blood pressure and a decrease in cerebrovascular mortality.[166,167] Increasing sodium intake in nearly all forms of experimental hypertension increases blood pressure.[168] The actions of diuretics to lower blood pressure in hypertensive patients are mainly sodium-dependent, since they can be nullified by ingesting a high-salt diet.[169] However, in other studies modest reductions in sodium intake have not been found to lower the blood pressure.[165]

The inconsistent overall reductions in blood pressure associated with modest reductions of salt intake in general populations of hypertensives may be explained in part by the existence of variations in sensitivity of individuals to the effects of salt on blood pressure. It has more recently been recognized that there exists a group of "salt-sensitive" patients with essential hypertension. The prevalence of salt sensitivity is around 25–50 percent, depending on the means of classification.[170,170a] These subjects are unable to excrete a sodium load. Several hypotheses, proven to varying degrees, exist to explain this defect in sodium handling. Defects in several components of the membrane handling of sodium and circulating inhibitors of the sodium pump have been found in hypertensive patients. The extent to which these changes are primary defects or are generated secondary to the hemodynamic and hormonal derangements of hypertension and the potential mechanisms by which abnormalities in sodium transport could lead to hypertension are discussed below (see Sodium Transport and Blood Pressure).

Williams and Hollenberg and coworkers have suggested that some sodium-sensitive hypertensive individuals have abnormal renal responses to angiotensin II resulting in sodium retention (nonmodulators).[125a,160,161] This group comprises about 50 percent of Caucasian patients with essential hypertension and normal or elevated renin levels (Fig. 14-8). In normal humans, low sodium intake enhances the aldosterone response to infused angiotensin II, while high sodium intake enhances the renal blood flow response. Unlike normotensive and hypertensive persons who are modulators, in nonmodulators a high dietary sodium intake does not alter aldosterone responses or renal blood flow responses to angiotensin II. Thus, on a high sodium intake, renal blood flow is not appropriately increased in the nonmodulators, and this leads to impaired sodium excretion. It has been suggested that this results from increased intrarenal levels of angiotensin II, since no differences in circulating levels of renin or angiotensin II could be demonstrated between modulators or nonmodulators. In addition the dose-response curve of renal blood flow following angiotensin II infusion shifts in modulators and normotensive subjects, while nonmodulators display an enhanced renovascular response after converting enzyme inhibition. Treatment with converting enzyme inhibitors is more effective in the nonmodulating salt-sensitive hypertensives than in the non-salt-sensitive modulators with hypertension. Whether nonmodulators also have defects in cellular sodium transport is currently under investigation.

Another mechanism of sodium sensitivity that has been suggested is abnormal sympathetic nervous system activity. In salt-sensitive hypertensive patients plasma norepinephrine levels do not decrease with high sodium intake, while in normal subjects and salt-resistant patients significant decreases in plasma norepinephrine concentration occur.[170] Salt-sensitive patients also display a greater increment in plasma norepinephrine concentration after 5 min of upright posture during a low or high sodium intake when compared to the non salt-sensitive patients. The mechanisms of the exaggerated activity of the sympathetic system are unknown. A central mechanism has been suggested in animal models.[168] For example, a high-salt diet in the spontaneously hypertensive rat increases norepinephrine content of the dorsomedial and anterior hypothalamic nuclei, areas of the brain which have been implicated in cardiovascular regulation. In the Dahl salt-sensitive rat strain, lesions in specific areas of the brain such as the paraventricular nucleus or the (AV3V) area could eliminate salt sensitivity.

The focus of studies of salt and hypertension has been on sodium; the role of the anion has received much less attention. Recent studies in salt-sensitive rats suggest that sodium with chloride is more effective in raising the blood pressure than it is with other anions.[171,172] Thus, it may be that chloride is necessary for the effects of sodium, although the importance of this in human hypertension is not known.

CALCIUM

Calcium is involved in mediating contractile responses (Chap. 5), including those of the vasculature, the actions of hormones and other extracellular and

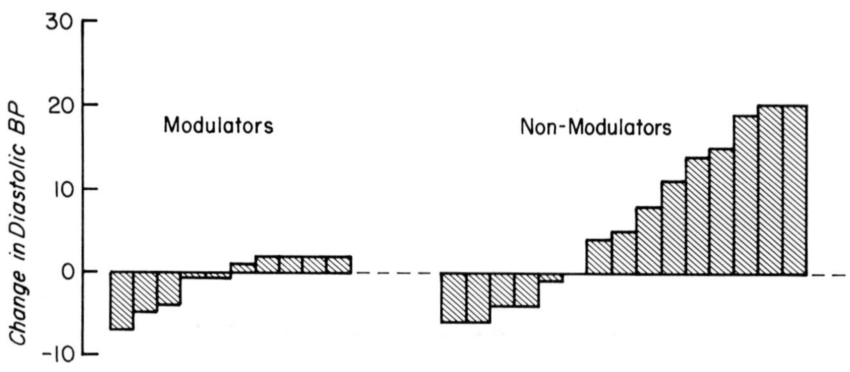

FIGURE 14-8 Frequency distribution of increment in diastolic blood pressure after 5 days of high sodium intake in 25 hypertensive subjects. The hypertensive subjects have been divided into modulators ($n=10$) and nonmodulators ($n=15$) according to their renal vascular response to angiotensin II. A significant pressor response (> 10 mmHg) with sodium loading occurred only in the nonmodulating group. The difference in the blood pressure response in the two groups was highly significant ($p < 0.004$). (*From Redgrave et al.*[125a])

intracellular effectors that regulate blood pressure (Chap. 5), secretion of hormones and other substances (Chap. 4), and neurological responses, and thus is centrally involved in blood pressure control. The participation of calcium in hypertension is illustrated by the success in using calcium channel blockers to treat essential and other forms of hypertension.[173] There has also been recent interest in the relationship between serum calcium levels, dietary calcium intake, and blood pressure.

Extracellular calcium is a major determinant of vascular reactivity. Contraction of cardiac muscle or vascular smooth muscle cannot occur in the absence of extracellular calcium. The relationship of extracellular calcium concentration and vascular smooth muscle contraction, however, is nonlinear.[174] In isolated strips of rat aorta, the relationship is parabolic because of the dual effects of calcium (Fig. 14-9). At lower concentrations, an increase in contraction occurs with increasing calcium concentrations up to a certain level of calcium. Then, relaxation of vascular smooth muscle occurs with increasing extracellular calcium levels. This dose-response curve shifts to the right in the hypertensive animal. It is likely that these dichotomous effects of calcium on vascular reactivity contribute to the controversial effects of calcium on blood pressure regulation.

Hypercalcemia has been shown to elevate the blood pressure in acute studies, and there is an increased incidence of hypertension in hyperparathyroidism.[174a]

In other studies, hypertensive individuals have been demonstrated to have lower levels of serum ionized calcium and higher calcium excretion for a given salt intake.[162] An inverse relation has been suggested from some studies between dietary calcium intake and blood pressure. Dietary calcium supplementation has lowered blood pressure in some but not all patients with essential hypertension.[175] However, the magnitude of the change was small (5 mmHg or less).[162] Thus, the possibility that some patients with hypertension have a relative or absolute deficiency of calcium has been suggested, but not proved. McCarron has postulated that adequate amounts of calcium are necessary to bind to calmodulin in order to promote Ca^{2+}-ATPase activity, lowering of intracellular free calcium levels, and vascular smooth muscle relaxation.[175]

Studies by Resnik and Laragh and associates have somewhat reconciled these seemingly incongruous observations.[176,177] They found that patients with the low-renin variety of essential hypertension appear to have a relative calcium deficiency, while patients with high-renin essential hypertension have a relative cal-

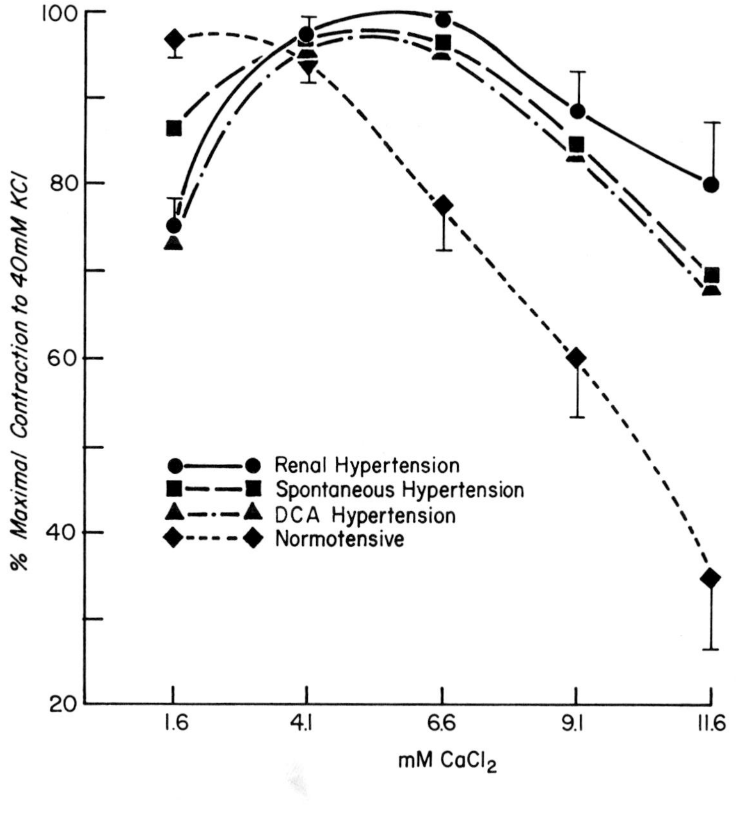

FIGURE 14-9 Normalized (see text) average of responses of aortic strips from normotensive, spontaneously hypertensive, renal hypertensive, and deoxycorticosterone hypertensive (DCA Hypt.) rats to 40 mM KCl at various calcium concentrations. The greatest response of strips (eight or nine from each group) from the normotensive rats was at 1.6 mM Ca^{2+}, from the spontaneously hypertensive rats was at 4.1 mM, and from the DCA and renal hypertensive rats was at 6.6 mM. Brackets indicate standard error and an asterisk indicates a significant difference from the normotensive value at $p < 0.05$. (*From Halloway and Bohr.*[174])

cium excess. Low-renin patients have lower serum ionized calcium levels, higher levels of parathyroid hormone, and a greater response to calcium channel blockade than the other renin subgroups of hypertension. High-renin patients or salt-insensitive patients have higher levels of ionized calcium, lower parathyroid hormone concentration, and less response to calcium channel blockade. These workers have proposed that due to aberrant transmembrane calcium transport, lower serum calcium levels in hypertensive patients may reflect increased levels of intracellular ionized calcium. In support of this idea, the free calcium concentration in platelets has been reported to be elevated in patients with essential hypertension.[177a]

The variations of calcium measurements and the heterogeneity of responses of patients with essential hypertension to calcium supplementation or calcium channel blockade is not surprising in view of the multifactorial etiology of this disease. Measurement of ionized calcium level in the hypertensive patient is currently only performed for research purposes. Administration of oral calcium as a treatment for hypertension is not recommended at this time. Although dietary calcium supplementation may reduce bone resorption, the side effects of calcium urolithiasis, milk-alkali syndrome, stimulation of gastrin secretion, etc., preclude the wide use of oral calcium as an antihypertensive modality.

MAGNESIUM

Magnesium was first suggested to play a role in hypertension because of observations that there is a high incidence of hypertension in geographic areas with soft drinking water or magnesium-poor soil.[178] Hypomagnesemia has been reported in a number of hypertensive populations.[176] The administration of magnesium salts has long been known to lower blood pressure, particularly in pregnancy-induced hypertension.[179] More recently, long-term administration of lower doses of magnesium salts has decreased requirements for antihypertensive drugs.[180]

The effect of magnesium on blood pressure is primarily through its ability to regulate vascular tone. Lowering the magnesium content of isolated vessels of animals or humans induces a rapid contractile response and potentiates the action of catecholamines, angiotensin II, and other vasoconstricting agents.[181] Acute hypermagnesemia decreases arteriolar and venous tone, resulting in decreased vascular resistance. Altura et al. recently demonstrated significant increases in blood pressure of rats made magnesium-deficient.[181] The lumen size of terminal arterioles and venules was also significantly smaller in magnesium-deficient animals. The severity of the blood pressure elevation and the decrease in lumen size correlated with the magnitude of the magnesium deficiency.

Current studies suggest that magnesium affects vascular smooth muscle by altering calcium flux and sodium content of the smooth muscle cells. Lowering extracellular magnesium concentration increases total exchangeable and intracellular free calcium levels in blood vessels.[182] Magnesium deficiency has been reported to enhance tissue uptake of sodium, increase sodium levels in blood vessels and blood cells, and impair sodium-calcium exchange.[181]

These effects of magnesium are important clinically because of the widespread use of diuretics in the treatment of hypertension, which enhance urinary magnesium loss. In addition, the hypomagnesemia resulting from diuretic treatment has been demonstrated to potentiate the risk of cardiac arrhythmias.[183] Specifically, a greater incidence of premature ventricular contractions, particularly during exercise, occurs with diuretic-induced hypomagnesemia. Oral magnesium supplementation in hypertensive patients on thiazide diuretics decreases both blood pressure and the incidence of exercise-induced premature ventricular contractions.[184]

POTASSIUM

Addison first suggested that "potassium salt regularly produced a decline in blood pressure . . . ."[185] Subsequently, Priddle reduced blood pressure in 45 consecutive hypertensive patients with potassium citrate therapy.[186] Since then, a number of studies under better-controlled conditions confirmed the blood pressure–lowering effect of oral potassium supplementation. In the United States, dietary potassium intake has been used to explain why in some geographic areas blacks have a higher prevalence of hypertension than whites. Blacks were demonstrated to have lower dietary potassium intake, since a large number were in a socioeconomic class which could not afford potassium-containing foods such as fresh fruits and vegetables. A relationship between potassium and blood pressure was also demonstrated in a study of 574 hypertensive and normotensive ambulatory subjects at Johns Hopkins Hospital.[187] Subjects with higher pressures had lower urinary excretion of potassium and lower potassium/creatinine ratios. No correlation with urinary sodium excretion was found. Ueshima et al. found a negative correlation between serum potassium concentration and the prevalence of hypertension in six populations.[188]

The effects of potassium on blood pressure appear to be mediated through its interaction with the autonomic nervous system and its natriuretic effects. A high-potassium diet has been demonstrated to decrease plasma norepinephrine levels in hypertensive persons on a normal diet.[189] Similarly, a high potassium intake decreased blood pressure and resting plasma norepinephrine levels in a group of students with a family history of hypertension and not in students without a familial predisposition to high blood pressure.[190] This study suggested a genetic predisposition to the effects of potassium on sympathetic activity. In a longer-term study (2 to 4 weeks) salt-sensitive hypertensive patients displayed a decreased pressor response to noradrenaline on a low-sodium and a low-sodium, high-potassium intake for the duration of the study. Potassium supplementation caused a fall in plasma norepinephrine levels and an increased sensitivity of baroreceptors. These changes occurred independently of a family history of hypertension. In humans and animals, potassium loading has been shown to decrease the pressor response to angiotensin II and noradrenaline, while sodium loading enhances vascular reactivity.[191] In some animal models, however, dietary potassium deficiency also impairs the vascular response to pressor agents.[192] In Dahl salt-sensitive rats, potassium feeding significantly diminishes activity of the CNS in response to intracerebroventricular injections of saline or angiotensin II, suggesting the CNS action may contribute to the protective effect of potassium against salt sensitivity in the animal.[193] Potassium has also been demonstrated to dilate the vascular bed of the dog gracilis muscle.[194] Ouabain blocked this effect, suggesting it is mediated by stimulation of membrane Na^+,K^+-ATPase.

In carefully controlled studies in dogs, an increase in potassium intake from 30 mmol per day to 200 mmol per day produced a 56 percent increase in sodium excretion despite an increase in aldosterone secretion.[195] Studies in the Goldblatt hypertensive rat also demonstrated natriuretic and hypotensive effects of potassium loading.[196] PRA also decreased in these animals. Micropuncture studies in the rat demonstrated that increased potassium concentration in the peritubular fluid directly inhibited proximal tubular sodium reabsorption.[197]

Whether or not diuretic-induced hypokalemia aggravates problems with blood pressure control in diuretic-treated hypertensive patients is unknown. Hypokalemia significantly increases the risk of cardiac arrhythmias,[184] so that potassium supplementation or use of a potassium-sparing agent is indicated if serum potassium concentration falls with diuretic administration.

Sodium Transport and Blood Pressure

The overall role of sodium in essential hypertension has already been discussed. The role of sodium chloride in mineralocorticoid hypertension and the effects of ANF on sodium dynamics are discussed below. The effects of sodium chloride on blood pressure are intimately linked to the transport of sodium and other ions between the intracellular and extracellular compartments. Sodium transport is a complex process involving several components, and it is affected by circulating factors that have not as yet been adequately characterized. It is also becoming clear that there are individual differences in sodium transport and that these may be important in the development of hypertension. These aspects of sodium transport are reviewed here.

CELLULAR ELEMENTS INVOLVED IN SODIUM TRANSPORT

The sodium content of a cell is determined by the rate of sodium entry into the cell and the capacity of the sodium pump to extrude it.[198,199] This is a complex process involving several cellular elements (Fig. 14-10). These have been best characterized in the erythrocyte because of its ease of study. However, leukocytes are a better model because their sodium-transporting activity is much greater and more similar to that in vascular, renal, and other cells that participate in blood pressure control and salt balance.[198,200]

Some of these elements are depicted in Fig. 14-10. These include the Na^+,K^+ pump with its associated ATPase activity, the Na^+-Na^+ countertransport (Na^+-Li^+ countertransport), the Na^+-K^+ cotransport, and passive mechanisms for Na^+ and K^+ permeability. Na^+ influx can also be linked to the uptake of glucose and amino acids, in the kidney with hydrogen exchange, and in several tissues with calcium exchange; however, these elements have not received adequate focus in terms of their role in hypertension.

Na^+,K^+-ATPase

The sodium pump, Na^+,K^+ ATPase, is an integral membrane protein that directly couples the hydrolysis of ATP to the vectorial transport of sodium and potassium ions across the plasma membrane. It contains an α subunit of mol wt 110,000 that is a transmembrane protein which contains all the known functional constituents, including the ATPase moiety and the binding site for ouabain.[201,202] There is also a β subunit of mol wt 55,000 whose function is not known. This protein complex is responsible for pumping sodium out of the cell and potassium into the cell and is the major element responsible for the intracellular-extracellular gradients of these ions and for the electrochemical gradients of Na^+ and K^+ that are the primary source of energy for the active transport of

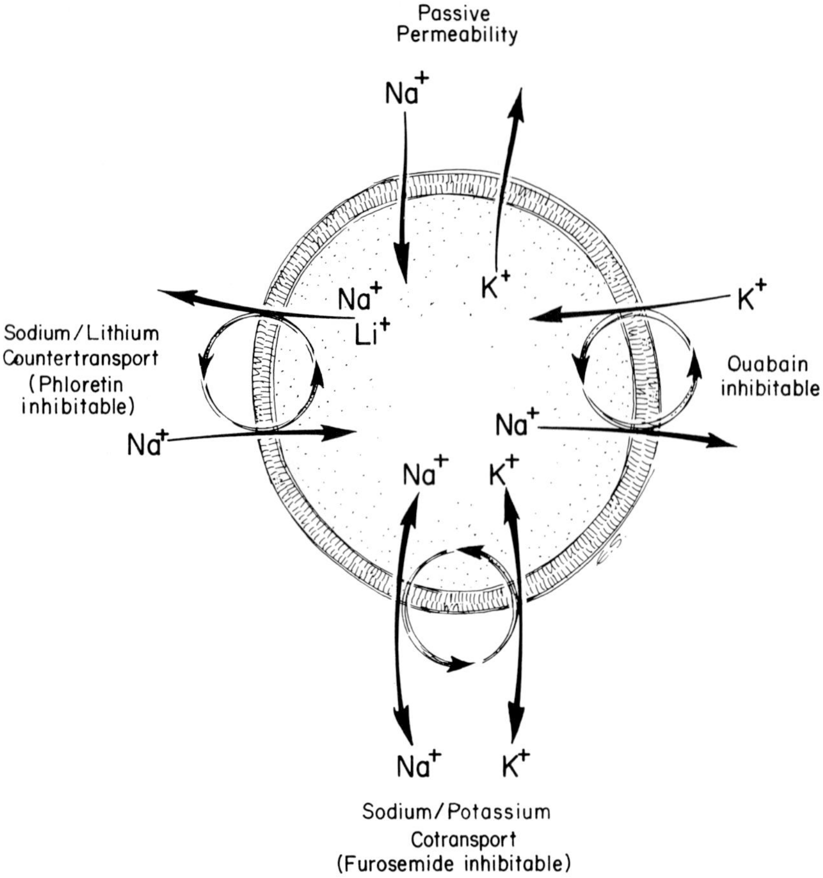

FIGURE 14-10 Cellular sodium transport systems.

nutrients across the cell membrane and for membrane polarization. Ordinarily, the activity of the ATPase is proportional to the intracellular sodium concentration; it is more active with higher intracellular sodium concentration and higher extracellular potassium concentration. Increased pumping hyperpolarizes the membrane and decreased pumping depolarizes it. More sodium ions than potassium ions are transported in each pump cycle.

The role of the ATPase in hypertension has mainly been studied in terms of circulatory factors that affect pump activity (discussed in detail below). However, erythrocyte pump activity has been found to be lower and cellular sodium concentration higher in normotensive blacks than in whites and in men than women; thus, it has been suggested that this could contribute to the higher prevalence of hypertension in blacks and men vs. whites and women.[203] It is also conceivable that additional individual differences in intrinsic pump activity could participate in the development of hypertension.

That potential abnormalities in sodium transport are present in hypertension has been suggested by a number of studies.[198] First, leukocytes from patients with essential hypertension have been reported to have an elevated intracellular sodium content and a reduced rate constant for sodium efflux by the sodium pump.[198] Further, increasing levels of diastolic blood pressure are associated with increasing levels of intracellular sodium concentration and diminishing values for the rate constant of sodium efflux.[198] Treatment with thiazide diuretics restores the normal pattern of sodium transport in these cells.[198] Although there has been controversy, it also appears that there is an increased intracellular erythrocyte sodium content in patients with essential hypertension, with differences from controls averaging around 13 percent.[198] These studies are in agreement with earlier ones showing an increased sodium content of renal arteries examined post mortem in patients with hypertension.[198] It has not been established that these abnormalities are inherited; studies of normotensive offspring of hypertensive patients have either failed to detect abnormalities or else found only marginal differences.[198]

Na^+-K^+ Cotransport

This is a facilitated diffusion mechanism in which sodium and potassium ions can enter or leave cells, depending on their concentrations. This process can be inhibited by furosemide. Its physiological role is still uncertain. A number of reports have suggested that Na^+-K^+ cotransport is reduced in patients with essential hypertension and also in normotensive offspring of these patients;[198,204] however, the extent of these abnormalities remains controversial.[198] Reduced cotransport could result in higher intracellular Na^+ concentrations, with consequent effects on blood pressure, as discussed below.

Na^+-Na^+ Countertransport (Na^+-Li^+ Countertransport)

This is a countertransport system in which sodium ions are exchanged for sodium ions by a passive facilitated diffusion process. Li^+ can substitute for Na^+. The activity of this element can be studied by loading cells with Li^+ and measuring Li^+ efflux; it is thus usually referred to as the Na^+-Li^+ countertransport system. This system can be inhibited by either furosemide plus phloretin or by phloretin alone.[198] The physiological importance of this system is also not known, although it has been speculated that in the kidney tubules this system can participate in the exchange of external sodium ions for internal hydrogen ions.[198]

A number of studies suggest that Na^+-Li^+ countertransport is abnormally high in erythrocytes from patients with essential hypertension,[198,199,205,206] and some studies suggest that normotensive offspring of the hypertensive patients have intermediate values. The studies of Na^+-Na^+ countertransport are, however, complicated by a number of factors that influence its activity, including hemodialysis, oral contraceptive use, hypokalemia, and physical training.[198]

Since the system does not affect net changes in sodium distribution some have regarded it as an epiphenomenon that might not contribute to the generation of hypertension. However, it has been speculated that this system is the same one responsible for Na^+-H^+ exchange in the proximal renal tubule.[198,205] If this were true, increased erythrocyte countertransport would be paralleled by increased proximal tubular Na^+-H^+ exchange with a resulting net increase in proximal tubular sodium reabsorption and relative decrease in the kidney's capacity to excrete sodium, which could be consistent with popular models for the pathogenesis of essential hypertension. In support of this notion, a recent study examined Li^+ clearance in hypertension as a potential reflection of the renal countertransport activity and found it to be decreased in subjects with essential hypertension.[205] Also, among the normotensive controls, Li^+ clearance was lower in individuals with at least one first-degree relative with hypertension. This hypothesis might explain the limitations in proximal tubular responses that have been reported in salt-sensitive human hypertension.

Although abnormalities of both cotransport and countertransport have been found in hypertension, these do not parallel each other and may reflect independent defects. The relative distribution of these defects varies among racial and geographic groups.[204] Low cotransport appears to be very frequent in European whites, elevated cotransport and countertransport are prevalent in North American whites, and low cotransport with normal countertransport is more prevalent in blacks.

CIRCULATING INHIBITORS OF SODIUM TRANSPORT

A large literature now documents the existence of inhibitors of sodium transport in human plasma and in extracts of hypothalamus and placenta. Whereas overall evidence for the existence of these factors is convincing, work in this area has been hindered because their structures have not been elucidated. Studies have also been hindered because numerous factors that are likely to be nonspecific, such as pH and ion effects, and high concentrations of certain lipids can affect the measurements.[207,208]

The results of the actions of these inhibitors are blockage of sodium reabsorption by the kidney and increases in blood pressure and contractility of the heart.[206] These actions are therefore ideal for eliminating fluid excess. They contrast with those of ANF (see below), which appear to be more related to immediate rescue from fluid excess; the ouabainlike substances might be thought of more as long-term correctors of fluid overload that can occur at the expense of higher blood pressure.

The presence of such inhibitors has been assessed by their capacity either to inhibit the sodium pump in vivo, to compete with ouabain for binding to the ATPase, or to react to antiserum to digoxin. In spite of extensive efforts at purification, the identity of these substances is not known. Most results suggest that they have a low molecular weight and in some studies they appear to be peptide in nature,[208] whereas in other cases they do not appear to be peptides.[207-209,210] The plasma levels of these inhibitor substances are increased with fluid loading.[206,209] They are also found in high concentrations in the plasma of patients with renal insufficiency[211] and in pregnancy;[212] the levels are higher in hypertensive pregnant women.[213]

It might be questioned why, if these substances

increase blood pressure, such actions are also not ordinarily observed for digitalis. These differences could be explained in several ways. First, it is not established that the ouabainlike binding activity and sodium pump inhibitory activity are due to the same material. Second, there may be several classes of binding sites for ouabain and related compounds, with the inhibitors overall acting preferentially at different sites than ouabain,[214] although to date analysis of the ATPase gene suggests there may be only one or a few copies.[201,202] Third, the substances may affect other parameters. For example, some fractions also inhibit Ca^+-ATPase.[213] Finally, ouabain has been reported to increase blood pressure in normal human subjects and dogs.[206]

Although the issue is still controversial, patients with hypertension have been shown to have increased sodium pump–inhibiting serum activity and increased sodium content of their leukocytes;[198,209] the magnitude of the effect has been found to be correlated with the degree of elevation of the diastolic blood pressure.[198] Comparable influences on erythrocytes have not been reported, although inhibition of isolated Na^+,K^+-ATPase preparations has been reported[198] and serum from hypertensive patients has also been shown to have an increased ability to compete with radiolabeled ouabain for binding to red cell ATPase; the latter was also found in normotensive offspring from these patients.[198] In some studies, the leukocyte inhibitory activity has been elevated predominantly in patients with low-renin essential hypertension.[206]

POSSIBLE ROLE OF SODIUM TRANSPORT ABNORMALITIES IN HYPERTENSION

Whereas the blood pressure–increasing effect of increased extracellular sodium concentration is clear, the influence of intracellular sodium is not as clear. Decreased activity of the sodium pump or Na^+-K^+ cotransport could result in increased intracellular sodium concentration, whereas increased Na^+ countertransport per se would not have an effect on intracellular sodium concentration. However, in the latter case the defect may reflect a decreased renal ability to eliminate sodium resulting in an increased extracellular sodium concentration.

One hypothesis to explain how increased intracellular sodium concentration could increase blood pressure is that it would result in a small reduction of the membrane potential that in turn would allow an increased calcium ion influx through voltage-dependent Ca^{2+} channels.[198] Alternatively, the increased intracellular Na^+ concentration might increase the intracellular Ca^{2+} level by increasing the Na^+-Ca^{2+} exchange mechanism known to exist in some tissues.[198] In either case, an increased intracellular calcium concentration in either vascular smooth muscle or its sympathetic nerve supply would increase vascular tone. Increased calcium uptake could also explain why the sympathetic nervous system appears to be more active in some forms of hypertension, particularly low-renin hypertension.[206]

As noted above, although there is some evidence linking abnormalities in the sodium pump and both the cotransport and countertransport systems to genetic factors, this has not been found with the circulating inhibitors. This has led to the suggestion that elevations of levels of these inhibitors in hypertension reflect secondary events. For example, it is possible that there is some tendency toward abnormal sodium retention in hypertensive subjects, through any of the mechanisms described above,[209] and that this recruits a secondary increase in concentrations of the sodium pump inhibitors. These inhibitors would then have the beneficial effect on the kidney of increasing sodium loss, but at the same time would have a deleterious effect on the vasculature, increasing blood pressure, which might be enhanced by the substances' positive inotropic effect on the heart, increasing cardiac output. The effects of the inhibitors could result in a normal or lower total extracellular sodium concentration than is ordinarily observed in essential hypertension. Elevations of levels of these inhibitors plus levels of other factors such as ANF would also explain why the ability of hypertensive patients to excrete a salt load is increased rather than decreased in essential hypertension.[173,209,215] These formulations would also be consistent with the finding that subjects with low-renin hypertension have an especially exaggerated natriuresis to a salt load. Low-renin hypertension is more common in blacks who more commonly have elevated levels of the inhibitors (see above) and who are more likely to have excessive volume as a critical factor.[215]

ATRIAL NATRIURETIC FACTOR

In opposition to mechanisms that elevate the blood pressure and conserve sodium, for instance in response to fluid loss, are counterbalancing effectors that serve to guard against excessive increases in blood pressure and fluid volume. Of these, the kallikrein-kinin system, which regulates bradykinin production, has been investigated in great detail (Chap. 31), as have the complex vasoconstrictor and vasorelaxant effects of the catecholamines (Chap. 13) and acetylcholine. The natriuretic actions of the Na^+,K^+-ATPase inhibitors are discussed above. In addition, other factors exist that participate in certain responses such as the "escape" from further fluid retention in response to continued mineralocorticoid administration or heart failure (Chap. 12).[216,217] It had been known that the cardiac atrium contains low-pressure baroreceptors and that stimulation of these receptors by distention causes diuresis, bradycardia, hypotension, and decreased vascular resistance.[217] It is now recognized that the heart is a major endocrine organ, and that atrial natriuretic peptides produced predominantly by the cardiac atria have many of these actions and may participate in these responses.

That the cardiac atria contain secretory granules was discovered in 1956 by Kisch, who speculated that this tissue secretes regulatory molecules.[216,217] Subsequent studies also demonstrated that the number of granules increases with sodium restriction and decreases with sodium loading.[216,217] Following this, studies by several groups, primarily deBold and coworkers,[217] found that atrial extracts possess vasodilatory and natriuretic activity. This work was accepted with guarded optimism until two groups isolated and sequenced a peptide that had the required activity.[217–221] Over the past few years the existence of such a hormone has been rigorously established and its role in physiology, pathology, and medical therapeutics is becoming understood. These peptides have variously been termed atrial natriuretic peptide, atrial natriuretic factor (ANF), cardionatrin, atriopeptin, atrin, auriculin, and other terms.

Synthesis and Release

Human ANF is the product of a single gene from which an mRNA is transcribed that encodes a 151-amino-acid protein (prepro-ANF).[221–223b] The precursor contains a signal peptide sequence that is cleaved from the precursor in association with its translation and insertion into the endoplasmic reticulum, yielding a 126-amino-acid protein (pro-ANF). This precursor appears to be the predominant form of the hormone that is stored in the heart.[217–219,224] Pro-ANF is cleaved, generating a carboxy-terminal peptide of 28 amino acids (ANF or $ANF_{1\text{-}28}$, Fig. 14-11) that appears to be the predominant biologically active form of the protein in humans[217,219,225,226] and rats.[221] Although several different terminologies have been proposed, a modified version of that proposed by Needelman and Greenwald is favored: ANF is used to refer to the 28-amino-acid form and pro-ANF to the 126-amino-acid precursor.[219] For other forms containing fewer of the 28 amino acids, numbers refer to the amino acids present.

A number of other active peptides containing various sequences of pro-ANF have been found, but the data overall suggest that these are not present in the heart or circulation at significant levels and are largely proteolytic degradative fragments generated during sample preparation. Although serum can degrade pro-ANF to ANF, this does not occur in plasma and infused pro-ANF is stable in the circulation.[227]

Sites of Synthesis

The major sites of ANF production are the cardiac atria. In fact, ANF mRNA is the most abundant mRNA in the atria, comprising around 2 percent of the total mRNA in the rat.[223b,224] Thus, the tissue probably devotes more of its synthetic efforts to produce ANF than any other protein. The levels of ANF and its mRNA are somewhat greater in the right than in the left atrium.[216,217] Further evidence that the atria are the major sources for circulating ANF comes from the fact that the levels of ANF in venous plasma from the coronary sinus that drains the atria are two to eight times those in the arteries or peripheral veins.[216]

ANF is also produced in much lower quantities in other tissues, as documented by the finding of ANF

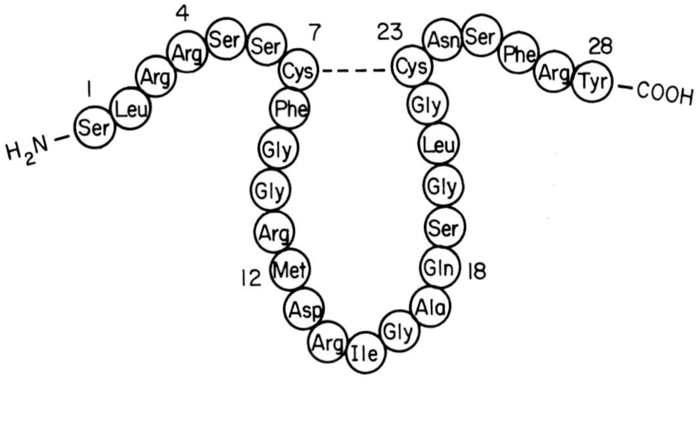

FIGURE 14-11 Structure of human atrial natriuretic factor residues 1 to 28 ($ANF_{1\text{-}28}$). (Data from Refs. 221 to 223b.)

and mRNA in these tissues. These include the subendothelial cells of the ventricles, selected cells of the lung, the aortic arch, selected regions of the central nervous system, and the pituitary.[228a,228b] Overall, the pattern suggested is that the peptide is present in areas of the body that respond to pressure stimuli. Because the quantities of ANF and ANF mRNA in these other tissues are only a fraction of a percent of those of the atria, it is unlikely that these sites contribute substantially to circulating ANF levels. Instead, these sites may produce ANF for local autocrine or paracrine actions.

Circulation

As stated, the major circulating ANF appears to be a 28-amino-acid protein. It has a half-life in the circulation of only a few minutes.[217] By contrast, infused pro-ANF is quite stable in rats, although it appears that little of this material is ever released.[227] It is not known to what extent it circulates free or bound to the plasma proteins. It is not yet clear how the peptide is degraded or what tissues are responsible, although the kidney may play an important role.

Both radioimmunoassays and radioceptor assays have been developed to measure ANF levels.[218,219,224] These assays yield normal values for ANF of 10 to 70 pg/ml or 7 to 21 pM.[219,224,226,229,230] ANF levels have been shown to be elevated in response to pressor agents such as angiotensin II or arginine vasopressin (AVP), saline infusion, and induced tachycardia.[216–219,224,231–234] They are elevated in congestive heart failure and renal failure.[216–219,224,231,232] ANF concentration has been reported to be normal to depressed in patients with cirrhosis and in renal failure patients following dialysis.[216–219,224,231]

Regulation of ANF Release and Synthesis

Consistent with a role for ANF in combating volume overload, ANF levels respond to stimuli that increase the atrial pressure.[216–219,224,229,232–235] Thus, these stimuli include pressor stimulants, atrial stretch volume increase due to fluid administration or postural changes, tachycardia, immersion in water, and immobilization. In vitro epinephrine, AVP, acetylcholine, and atrial distention all increase ANF release.[217,219] Release is not stimulated by ouabain, isoproterenol, and 40-mM potassium. The mechanisms for these effects are not clear, although it is possible that some of these actions are mediated through activation of sympathetic or parasympathetic cardiac efferent nerves,[236] and atrial stretch itself may be a direct stimulus.

As an index of synthetic activity, ANF mRNA levels are decreased by fluid deprivation and increased by fluid loading.[218,224] They are also increased by prolonged mineralocorticoid treatment[224,228c] and may be increased by glucocorticoids.[228d] Whereas ANF mRNA levels probably parallel synthesis, ANF content probably does so only on a long-term basis, but in the short term it fluctuates more in response to secretory stimuli.[224]

In humans, plasma ANF levels are elevated following ingestion of a high-salt diet, saline loading, atrial pacing, paroxysmal atrial arrhythmias, congestive heart failure, or chronic renal failure.[219,224] They have also been reported to be elevated in essential hypertension.[237] In the rat, levels are elevated following abrupt extracellular volume increase,[224] prolonged sodium loading,[224] or long-term DOC treatment.[224,228c] Little is known about the regulation of extraatrial ANF. Hypothalamic ANF levels have been reported to be increased with sodium loading and decreased with sodium deprivation, although it is not known whether this is secondary to changes in atria-derived plasma ANF levels.[219] Furthermore, in other studies water deprivation affected atrial but not brain ANF levels.[238]

Actions of ANF

The actions of ANF are complex, but overall they are natriuretic, diuretic, and vasorelaxant and they tend to oppose the effects of other sodium- and water-retaining and pressor stimuli (Fig. 14-12).

RENAL ACTIONS

ANF stimulates an increase in the glomerular filtration rate (GFR) and the renal excretion of water and sodium, chloride, magnesium, calcium, and phosphate ions.[224,230,239] The potency of the peptide as a diuretic is illustrated by the fact that 600 nmol of furosemide is required to elicit a diuresis equivalent to 0.4 nmol of ANF. It either has no effect or a minor effect on potassium and hydrogen ion excretion.

These renal actions are complex and are still being elucidated. The ANF increase in GFR is a relatively direct effect mediated at the glomerular level and occurs independently of changes in renal or glomerular plasma flows.[219,224,230,231,239] At lower doses, ANF increases total nephron GFR without changes in single-nephron GFR, but the latter also increases at higher ANF doses.[218] Ordinarily, increases in delivery to the distal tubule due to increases in GFR result in secondary decreases in GFR (tubular glomerular feed-

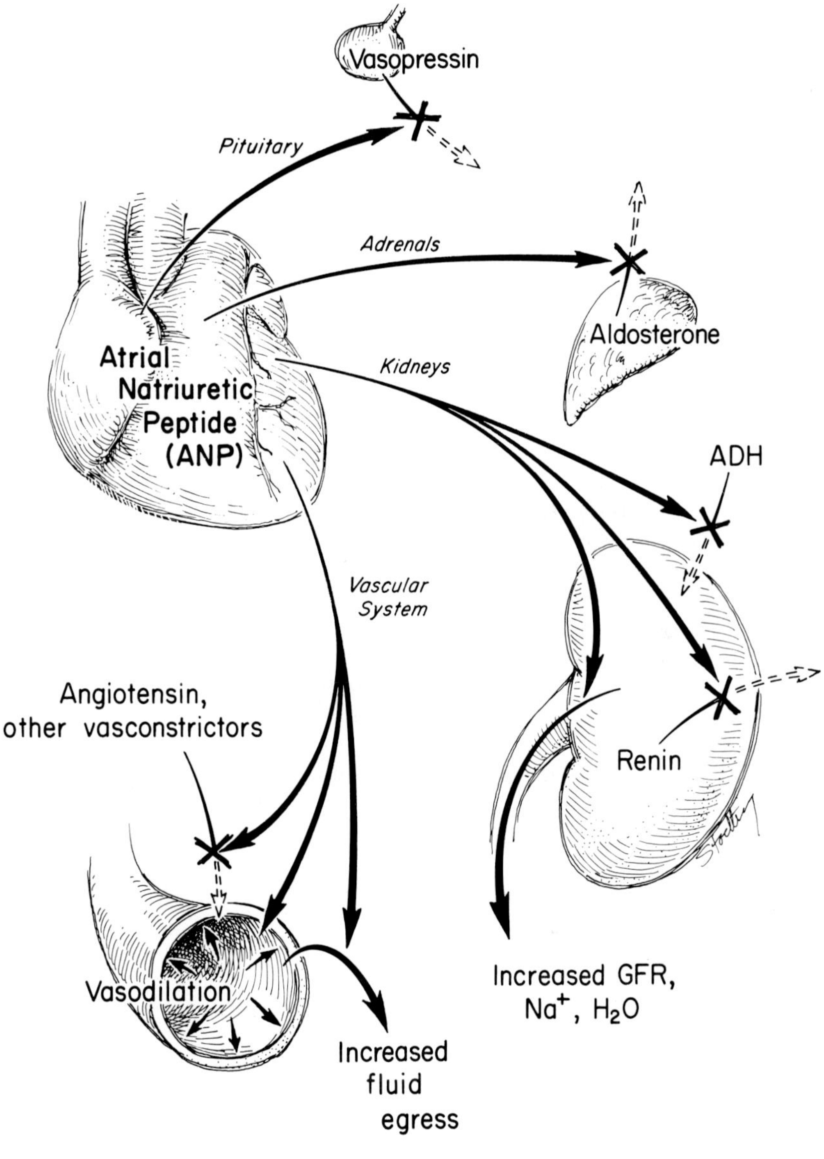

FIGURE 14-12 Actions of ANF.

back), but this does not occur when ANF is given.[219] These mechanisms are not completely understood, but may be due to increased efferent arteriolar resistance and/or dilation of the afferent glomerular arterioles entering the glomerulus with consequent hyperfiltration. It has also been suggested that the hormone modifies the glomerular cells to increase their surface area or permeability.[216] Effects on the GFR can be observed even in animals in whom renal failure has been reduced by five-sixths nephrectomy.[219] The hormone probably also modifies intrarenal hemodynamics by increasing the blood flow through the middle and outer cortices, the medulla, and the papilla.[219,224,239]

Effects on total renal blood flow are variable and do not account for the influences on GFR. In fact, in the isolated perfused kidney, ANF infusions can increase GFR with increased renal vascular resistance.[224] Nevertheless, the hormone does block renal artery vasoconstriction in response to other agents.[224,240] The effects on renal blood flow are more prominent at the higher doses, greater than are required for other renal influences,[224] although vasodilation does occur when renal vascular resistance is high due to treatment with agents such as angiotensin II, vasopressin, or norepinephrine.[224]

The GFR-increasing actions probably contribute substantially to the actions of the hormone increasing the excretion of salt, water, magnesium, calcium, and phosphate. However, it appears that the two- to threefold increased solute delivery to the distal tubule cannot account in full for the 10- to 50-fold increase in urinary solute excretion commonly found.[224] Further, the urinary sodium concentration commonly exceeds the plasma concentration following ANF administration.[224] This could be due in part to intrarenal hemodynamic influences resulting in hypernatric papillary interstitial fluid. It is also possible, although not established, that ANF may also block sodium resorption in the collecting tubules, possibly the medullary collecting duct.[216,218,238,241–243]

The effects on bicarbonate excretion are minimal in normal animals compared to humans,[219] but are significant in animals with chronic alkalosis; ordinarily, Cl^- is the predominant anion accompanying the Na^+ that is lost.[219,244] This further enhances sodium excretion and blunts potassium excretion.[224] The hormone does not block Na^+,K^+-ATPase activity.[224] Some have concluded that the hormone does not appear to block proximal tubular phosphate transport in the absence of changes in GFR; since ANF receptors in this segment have not been found, this could represent an indirect effect secondary to increased proximal tubular flow rates.[224]

The hormone also blocks the action of AVP increasing water reabsorption, which may participate in its action increasing water diuresis.[245a]

EFFECTS ON RENIN

ANF can blunt renin release in response to a variety of stimuli and can lower plasma renin levels in dogs.[219,224,230,231,233,239,245b] To date the reported responses do not yield totally consistent patterns, although overall the effects are more prominent in animals in which there is excessive renin production such as occurs with induced renovascular hypertension.[224] These effects could be due to increased delivery of NaCl to the macula densa, renal vasodilation, or direct effects on the juxtaglomerular cells.[224,230] ANF potentiated angiotensin II inhibition of renin release in renal cortical slices but did not affect the action of isoproterenol.[245b] However, an argument that at least some of the actions are secondary is derived from data in two-kidney, one-clip hypertensive rats in which blood pressure lowering in response to ANF was associated with increases in plasma renin levels.[231,233] Nevertheless, ANF has been reported to inhibit basal and stimulated renin release in the isolated rat renal cortex.[246]

EFFECTS ON ALDOSTERONE

ANF blocks the release of aldosterone under basal conditions and in response to angiotensin II, K^+, cAMP, PGE_1 or ACTH.[216,218,219,224,231] It does not affect basal or stimulated cortisol release. These actions involve the early steps in steroid biosynthesis, as the peptide decreases angiotensin II-induced pregnenolone accumulation. The data are conflicting as to whether ANF blocks the production of aldosterone from progesterone or 24-hydroxycholesterol. The peptide also does not block cAMP production in this case. The decrease in aldosterone release has been observed in normal human subjects on a normal sodium intake and in patients with hypertension.

AVP RELEASE

ANF can block AVP release.[240] This effect may combine with that blocking AVP action to enhance the excretion of water.

ACTIONS ON THE VASCULATURE

ANF has direct vasodilatory actions on isolated vascular preparations. In addition, it can oppose the actions of a number of vasoconstrictors, including catecholamines, angiotensin II, AVP, and carbachol.[216,224,247,248] A prominent effect is to inhibit smooth muscle contraction. These actions are relatively selective in their effects on specific vascular beds. Renal artery and isolated aortic strips are highly sensitive in vitro, whereas mesenteric, coronary, femoral, vertebral, and carotid arteries are less responsive. In vivo experiments have yielded conflicting results.[224] In rats ANF produced increases in renal, splanchnic, coronary, testicular, lung, and spleen blood flow without changes in cardiac output. In dogs there was an effect on renal blood flow but not on mesenteric, coronary, or iliac flows. When ANF was infused into rats, resulting in a decreased blood pressure due to decreased cardiac output, renal, mesenteric, and femoral vascular resistances increased. Thus, the effects are dependent on multiple factors.

INTRACELLULAR FLUID VOLUME

ANF appears to be capable of influencing the distribution of fluids in body compartments independent of its effect on fluid balance.[249] The peptide can increase the hematocrit to an extent that cannot be accounted for by its influences on fluid balance. This may be a major mechanism by which it increases the cardiac output in heart failure.[231,249,250] The mechanisms for these effects are not known.

CARDIAC ACTIONS

ANF has been shown to be capable of decreasing the cardiac output in patients or animals with hypertension and increasing cardiac output in heart failure.[231,249,250] Overall, it appears to have these influences by indirect mechanisms related to delivery of fluid to the heart and independent of direct cardiac influences. It may have some vasodilatory influence on the coronary arteries.

EFFECTS ON BLOOD PRESSURE

ANF causes a decrease in blood pressure in normal subjects[219,224,251,252] and in patients with hypertension.[253,254] These actions are complex and multifactorial and the predominant mechanisms may vary depending on the experimental circumstances. Although fluid loss due to renal influences may contribute, these probably do not explain the rapid blood pressure lowering actions.[250,252] In some circumstances decreased blood pressure may be predominantly due to decreases in cardiac output secondary to decreased venous return,[231,250] which may be due to the ANF-induced fluid shifts discussed above. The actions on the vasculature described above may also contribute. The peptide can also reduce the elevated blood pressure in rats that are genetically hypertensive or in whom two-kidney, one-clip (high-renin) or one-kidney, one-clip (low-renin) hypertension has been induced.[219,233,255] In spontaneously hyperreninemic rats, ANF levels are elevated, presumably in response to the elevated blood pressure.[233] A similar situation may exist in essential hypertension in humans[237,241] (also discussed above), although this has been disputed by others.[256] In the Dahl salt-sensitive rat, it has been proposed that increased renal resistance to ANF and a relative decrease in ANF level may contribute to the development of hypotension.[257]

EFFECTS ON WATER INTAKE

Intraventricular (third ventricle) or intravenous infusion of ANF promotes decreased water intake in rats.[258] Thus, central or peripherally derived ANF may decrease water intake as part of a mechanism to decrease overall volume.

INTEGRATED EFFECTS ON PHYSIOLOGY

The overall pattern of ANF action is to promote diuresis and natriuresis and lower blood pressure through a diverse combination of actions that blocks both production and actions of the renin-angiotensin system and vasopressin and the actions of vasoconstrictor substances. It has additional vasodilatory actions and effects on the kidney that contribute to its overall influence. What is less clear at present is which of these overall influences are most important under physiological and pathologic states.

Structure-Activity Considerations for ANF

A number of ANF analogues have been tested for activity.[216,219,230,231] It appears that the central ring structure (Fig. 14-11) containing the 17 amino acids with a disulfide bond is critical for ANF action; to date, analogues that lack the ring and the disulfide bond are relatively inactive. Whereas the 28-amino-acid structure is as, or nearly as, potent as any other structure reported to date, structures with more amino acids are also active at a reduced level. All of the amino-terminal peptides that contain the amino acids of the loop are active. Whereas deletion of the first seven amino acids does not decrease intrinsic activity, removal of carboxy-terminal amino acids does reduce activity.

Molecular Mechanisms of Action

ANF RECEPTORS

ANF receptors have been found in numerous tissues, including the blood vessels, adrenal glomerulosa, kidney, pituitary, and central nervous system.[218,219,224,259,260] The concentration of sites varies from 10,000 to 40,000 per cell. Whether there is a single class of ANP receptors has not yet been resolved,[260] although in many tissues only a single class of sites has been identified. Covalent labeling studies[224,251,261,262] have revealed several receptor peptides of molecular weight around 70,000 to 140,000. Binding constants have ranged from 0.15 to 5 nM.[218,260,263] The receptors are located on the cell surface, glycosylated,[224] and probably internalized and can be "down regulated" by a high salt intake.[224,263] This down regulation could be a significant factor in blunting the ability of ANF to lower the blood pressure in hypertension.[264a] In the kidney, the receptors are found in the visceral epithelial and mesangial cells of the glomerulus, in blood vessels, and to a somewhat lesser extent in the collecting ducts and the third part of Henle's loop, but not in the proximal tubules.[216]

POSTRECEPTOR ACTIONS

Several postreceptor actions of ANF have been described. The most consistent effect appears to be to increase cGMP levels.[219,224,264b] This has been observed in several tissues, including kidney slices, renal tubule cells, and cultured vascular smooth muscle cells.[219] In the kidney the effects are greatest in the glomeruli, less in the loop of Henle and the collecting ducts, and undetectable in the proximal tubules.[219] After ANF administration, both plasma and urinary cGMP levels increase; these may become useful markers for ANF action. Although the circulating cGMP level may be a marker for ANF action, circulating cGMP probably does not contribute to ANF action.[219]

In general, the concentrations of ANF required for stimulating responses are lower than those needed for increasing cGMP levels.[224] The hormone also increases guanylate cyclase activity in isolated cell fractions; this is probably the mechanism for increasing cGMP levels.

ANF also lowers cAMP levels in some tissues, such as aorta and kidney,[224] but not in all cells, and it can blunt the ability of other agents to elevate cAMP levels. It is unclear how these effects occur; there are reports that this is due to a decreased adenylate cyclase activity in some cases[219,224,259] and to an enhanced phosphodiesterase activity in other cases.[265] In the case of AVP action, the peptide blocks the effects of AVP but not of cAMP or forskolin.[245a] The effects on Ca^{2+} and phospholipid metabolism are less clear.

It has not been clarified to what extent these postreceptor effects are responsible for ANF actions. The currently prevalent view is that the effects on cGMP are largely responsible for the vasorelaxant and renal hemodynamic effects of ANF, as many of these can be elicited by dibutyl cGMP.[266,267] In addition, methylene blue, an inhibitor of guanylate cyclase, reduces the vasorelaxant activity of ANF.[224] These effects are analogous to those of the nitrosovasorelaxants,[219] although they may not be identical, since ouabain under certain circumstances can block ANF but not sodium nitroprusside action. cGMP presumably activates a specific protein kinase that in turn stimulates an increase in calcium ion sequestration in internal stores, with consequent vasorelaxant actions. The ANF-stimulated augmentation of angiotensin II action in renal slices is consistent with an influence on calcium ion.[245b] However, it has been reported that the inhibitory actions of ANF on aldosterone production in rat adrenal glomerulosa cells is independent of changes in cytosolic Ca^{2+} concentration, phospholipid turnover, or cGMP level, but may involve activation of phospholipase A_2.[268]

Role of ANF in Physiology and Disease

As stated above, ANF appears to have actions that protect against volume overload or pressure excess and its levels are increased when these perturbations occur. What is not clear as yet is how important the given elevations are in these settings. It is not known to what extent ANF is active under normal circumstances; in one preliminary report it was concluded, using antiserum to ANF, that under basal conditions in the rat the peptide does influence cardiac output, sodium excretion, and plasma volume, but not blood pressure and aldosterone level.[269] Although ANF concentration changes appropriately in disease states and has requisite natriuretic and other actions to defend against volume overload, it is not yet established how important the rises in ANF concentration are in these conditions.

ADRENAL STEROIDS AND HYPERTENSION

A number of the secretions of the adrenal gland have been implicated in hypertension. Commonly, an excess of more than one steroid is present in patients with disorders of the adrenal gland associated with hypertension; as a result, it has been difficult to unravel the relative roles of the glucocorticoids and mineralocorticoids in producing the blood pressure elevation (see Chap. 12 for definitions of "glucocorticoid" and "mineralocorticoid"). Nevertheless, it is now clear that an excess of mineralocorticoids can cause hypertension, and syndromes have been identified in which aldosterone, DOC, or cortisol appear predominantly to be responsible for the mineralocorticoid excess state. Two key investigations led to the identification of DOC and aldosterone as the mineralocorticoids causing elevations of blood pressure. In 1955 Conn described primary aldosteronism[270] and in 1956 Eberlein and Bongiovanni identified the tetrahydro metabolite of DOC in patients with the 11β hydroxylation deficiency type of congenital adrenal hyperplasia.[271] Further evidence that DOC excess can lead to hypertension was reported in 1966 with the discovery of the 17α-hydroxylase syndrome.[272] Hypertension is commonly present in patients with Cushing's syndrome with cortisol excess, although the question of the extent to which it is due to mineralocorticoid or glucocorticoid actions has not been clarified. There is also evidence that other adrenal steroids have potential actions raising blood pressure, although it is not known whether they contribute to human disease.

Mineralocorticoids

Mineralocorticoids in excess cause hypertension. This is documented by the clinical syndromes of mineralocorticoid excess with aldosterone[270] or DOC[271,272] excess. Administration of mineralocorticoids can also lead to iatrogenic hypertension (see below).[273]

The primary mechanisms of mineralocorticoid action are reviewed in Chap. 12. These steroids regulate ion transport in many secretory tissues, such as sweat glands, salivary glands, kidney, and the intestinal tract, and possibly in arterial walls (see Chap. 12). These actions lead to increased sodium retention, increase in the extracellular fluid volume, increase in total body sodium content, and potassium and hydrogen ion loss with consequent hypokalemia and a tendency to alkalosis. The result can be a cascade of events that ultimately leads to hypertension. The mechanisms and pathophysiology of these developments are detailed in the discussion of aldosterone excess.

ALDOSTERONE

Aldosterone is the major mineralocorticoid in humans (Chap. 12). Hypersecretion of this steroid in primary aldosteronism due to an aldosterone-producing adenoma results in hypertension, as discussed in the section on aldosterone excess. However, aldosterone may not be the only or even the major factor leading to hypertension in patients with primary aldosteronism and adrenal hyperplasia, since bilateral adrenalectomy in these patients does not usually normalize the blood pressure (see the discussion of aldosterone excess).

In contrast to cortisol, aldosterone is probably not important for maintenance of blood pressure under normal circumstances, and blockade of aldosterone action by mineralocorticoid antagonists in normotensive subjects who are not salt-depleted does not result in hypotension. The hormone instead is perceived as one that responds to posture or fluid loss to conserve sodium (Chap. 12).

As discussed in Chap. 12, a variety of conditions result in increases in aldosterone concentration, but in general the increase in level of the steroid in these states is secondary to conditions such as cirrhosis, fluid loss, and heart failure when other factors are the predominant regulators of the blood pressure. In these states the effects of aldosterone on sodium and potassium ions do contribute to the pathology that is present and may have some influence on blood pressure. Excess aldosterone in some cases with renin excess, such as renin-producing tumors or renovascular hypertension, may contribute to the elevated blood pressure although it is not the primary abnormality.

Aldosterone levels tend to be normal to low in patients with essential hypertension with normal or suppressed renin levels, and these patients do not have other stigmata of mineralocorticoid excess such as hypokalemia. Thus, this steroid appears to play a minor role in the pathogenesis of essential hypertension. This notion is also supported by the fact that administration of mineralocorticoid antagonists to patients with essential hypertension and normal to high plasma renin levels generally does not result in a lowering of the blood pressure. However, in the subgroup of patients with low-renin essential hypertension, the aldosterone levels may be contributing to some extent, since some reports, although not others, claim that there is a blood pressure–lowering effect with mineralocorticoid antagonist treatment (discussed below, under Low-Renin Essential Hypertension).

DEOXYCORTICOSTERONE

Although DOC is as potent as aldosterone in eliciting mineralocorticoid responses, its free concentration in plasma is ordinarily considered to be too low to contribute substantially to the plasma mineralocorticoid activity (Chap. 12). Exogenous DOC can lead to hypertension in certain animal models of hypertension and in humans.[274] As discussed in Chap. 12, the secretion of DOC is predominantly under ACTH control. Thus, in syndromes due to adrenal enzymatic defects (discussed below) and in some patients with Cushing's syndrome, particularly those with the ectopic ACTH syndrome, in which ACTH levels are extremely high (Chap. 12), DOC levels can be high enough to elicit significant activity and result in a mineralocorticoid hypertension syndrome. DOC excess also occurs with hypertension in rare patients with predominantly DOC-secreting tumors.

18-HYDROXYDEOXYCORTICOSTERONE

18-Hydroxy-DOC is a weak mineralocorticoid whose production is predominantly under ACTH control (Chap. 12). The level of this steroid tends to be elevated in states associated with ACTH excess and has been reported to be elevated in some patients with essential hypertension, but the levels observed are not high enough to be of clinical importance.[274]

18-HYDROXYCORTICOSTERONE

18-Hydroxycorticosterone (18-OHB) also has very weak mineralocorticoid activity but it has not been reported to occur at high enough levels to be of importance.[275] The steroid is useful, however, in the diagnosis and differential diagnosis of mineralocorticoid excess states (see below).

16α,18-DIHYDROXY-DOC, 19-HYDROXYANDROSTENEDIONE, AND 19-OXOANDROSTENEDIONE

These steroids, inactive by themselves, have been reported to potentiate the actions of aldosterone in rats, but there is no evidence for their participation in human disease.[274]

19-NOR-DOC

19-Nor-DOC is produced in the kidney and possibly other tissues from precursors synthesized in the adrenal (Chap. 12).[274] It has not been detected in plasma and therefore if it is important, it probably acts locally in the tissues in which it is produced.[274] The steroid has been shown to be highly active in producing hypertension in the rat, and it is a highly potent mineralocorticoid with activity equivalent to aldosterone.[274] Elevated levels of urinary 19-nor-DOC have been found in three animal models of hypertension, i.e., animals with adrenal regeneration hypertension, spontaneously hypertensive rats, and salt-sensitive Dahl rats.[274] Elevated levels have also been reported in some but not all patients with essential hypertension, including low-renin essential hypertension, and with primary aldosteronism. However, these levels are much lower than those of aldosterone.[276] Although production of the steroid is predominantly controlled by ACTH, which stimulates the production of its precursor (Chap. 12), converting enzyme inhibition results in a marked drop in urinary 19-nor-DOC levels, suggesting that renal actions of angiotensin II may affect its production.[277] Furthermore, the drop in 19-nor-DOC level correlates better than does the fall in aldosterone concentration with the decrease in urinary potassium excretion in respone to the inhibitor. Thus, the steroid is an interesting candidate for involvement in human hypertension, although whether it is of importance remains to be determined.

OTHER STEROIDS

A variety of other steroids can have mineralocorticoid activity or mineralocorticoid-like activity, but there is no information as to their importance in human hypertension. Some of the metabolites of aldosterone, dihydroaldosterone and tetrahydroaldosterone have been reported to have mineralocorticoid-like activity, to act through mechanisms other than mineralocorticoid receptors, and to be capable of inducing hypertension in adrenalectomized spontaneously hypertensive rats.[278,279] 18-Oxocortisol administration has hypertensive potency in rats susceptible to mineralocorticoid hypertension.[280]

Glucocorticoids

The diverse actions of glucocorticoids on blood pressure are discussed in detail in Chap. 12. The importance of these steroids in maintaining a normal blood pressure is amply demonstrated by the hypotension that occurs in the addisonian individual that is correctable with glucocorticoid but not mineralocorticoid replacement. By contrast, the importance of glucocorticoids in hypertension is less clear.

As discussed in Chap. 12 and later in this chapter, most patients with spontaneous Cushing's syndrome have hypertension. However, an analysis of the contributions of the glucocorticoid effects in this condition is complicated by the fact that the cortisol that is hypersecreted has both glucocorticoid and weaker mineralocorticoid activity and that sometimes other steroids such as DOC are produced in excess. Nevertheless, the fact that the hypertension is not predominantly due to mineralocorticoid excess is documented by the finding that two major stigmata of mineralocorticoid excess, suppression of plasma renin and hypokalemia are ordinarily not present (see below and Chap. 12).

A role for glucocorticoids in elevating blood pressure is more clearly seen with glucocorticoid therapy. Whereas many glucocorticoid-treated patients do not have hypertension, there does appear to be an increased prevalence of hypertension in patients treated with glucocorticoids. These prevalence estimates have ranged from 17 to 69 percent in more recent studies.[281-286] Thus, although glucocorticoids may not cause hypertension as reproducibly as other substances, such as epinephrine or angiotensin II, they are capable of elevating blood pressure in susceptible individuals.

Further evidence that glucocorticoids can cause hypertension has been obtained from studies of rats given high doses of dexamethasone (Chap. 12). In this case the steroid-induced increases in blood pressure are blocked by glucocorticoid but not mineralocorticoid antagonists (Chap. 12).[287]

It is not known which of the various actions of the glucocorticoids are predominantly responsible for their blood pressure–elevating activity. As detailed in Chap. 12, candidate actions include those that increase levels of the active constituents of the renin-angiotensin system. Thus, glucocorticoids can increase prorenin and angiotensinogen levels, and possibly those of converting enzyme. These actions may explain why plasma renin levels are not suppressed in Cushing's syndrome in the presence of hypertension and elevated mineralocorticoid activity. The hypertension in patients with high or normal PRA does respond to converting enzyme inhibition.[274] However, other actions on PG production, sensitivity to pressor substances such as epinephrine and angiotensin II, endothelial and smooth muscle cells, and the heart may also contribute. It is likely that a combination of these influences is operative (Chap. 12).[288]

LABORATORY TESTS FOR THE EVALUATION OF HYPERTENSION

Laboratory tests are used in patients with hypertension to determine whether there is a detectable underlying cause for the hypertension, localize the defect when relevant, determine the effects of therapy, and evaluate complications of the disease. These tests include blood measurements, radioligand procedures, and provocative measures. In this section are described some of the tests in general clinical use; tests that are used predominantly for research are either not described or are mentioned in the individual sections. Also, most of the tests that are used for particular diseases are described in the sections on those diseases.

Renin

Renin activity is measured by its ability to generate angiotensin I from the substrate angiotensinogen. In vivo this reaction occurs in the circulation, within blood vessel walls, and probably within some tissues. PRA is determined by incubation of plasma at 37°C followed by radioimmunoassay (RIA) of the generated angiotensin I.[289,290] The incubation pH is critical. A pH around 5.7 is used by some laboratories because this is the optimum pH for the reaction between human renin and human angiotensinogen; on the other hand, a pH around neutrality is used by others to mimic in vivo conditions and to eliminate the effect of any acid proteases in plasma which may have reninlike activity. Generation of angiotensin I at neutrality generally gives lower values of PRA than at pH 5.7. Another important factor is the presence of angiotensinase inhibitors which prevent destruction of the generated angiotensin I; the choice of inhibitors is dependent on the pH of incubation. The PRA is usually expressed as nanograms of angiotensin I generated per milliliter per hour and is dependent on the fact that angiotensin I generation is linear with time.

In human plasma, the reaction between renin and angiotensinogen occurs at substrate concentrations near the K_m for renin, so that the reaction rate is proportional to concentrations of both renin and substrate. Ordinarily, the plasma renin substrate concentration is quite constant. However, in some clinical conditions it may be altered, leading to a change in the measured rate of angiotensin I generation. During estrogen administration and pregnancy and in patients with syndromes of glucocorticoid excess, renin substrate concentration is increased, leading to elevated PRA. Renin substrate concentration is reduced in liver disease and in states of glucocorticoid deficiency.

Plasma renin concentration (PRC) is measured by generating angiotensin I in the presence of excess substrate so that the reaction between renin and angiotensinogen is not limited by the concentration of angiotensinogen (i.e., is zero order). Because of the difficulty in obtaining enough human substrate, animal substrate has been prepared from plasma of nephrectomized sheep, hogs, and other mammals. Except in situations where human substrate concentration is altered, PRA and PRC are directly proportional. The measurement of PRC is useful in situations where angiotensinogen concentration is altered or to better define a low-renin state, such as primary aldosteronism.

The plasma prorenin concentration is measured by acid or protease treatment of plasma.[61] Prolonged storage of plasma at temperatures just below freezing can result in slow activation of prorenin. Thus, plasma samples for renin determination must be processed quickly on collection (usually in tubes containing EDTA) and stored frozen at temperatures ≤ -20°C until assay. Some patients with diabetes mellitus, patients with renin-secreting tumors, and pregnant women have elevated plasma levels of inactive renin (5 to 10 times normal), resulting in cryoactivation of renin at 4°C. Thus, immediate processing of plasma samples from these patients for PRA measurements is critical.

PRA levels fluctuate spontaneously. They are influenced by many factors, including sex, race, age, sodium balance, position, activity, severity of hypertension, concurrent medication such as birth control pills and antihypertensive drugs, and illnesses such as diabetes mellitus, congestive heart failure, and cirrhosis (see above). Several protocols have been proposed to standardize the measurement of PRA. These include normal and low-sodium diet, pretreatment with a diuretic, and measurement of PRA after overnight recumbency before the patient arises; others measure PRA after the patient has been ambulatory and upright for 4 hours. Hence, "normal" values differ from laboratory to laboratory and under different circumstances.

PRA values (Table 14-3) should be interpreted relative to concurrent 24-h urinary sodium excretion rates after several days with a stable sodium intake and without diuretics. This relationship is referred to as the "renin-sodium index" (Fig. 14-5). If renal, endocrine, and cardiac functions are normal, the sodium excretion rate is a convenient marker for extracellular fluid volume. Sodium excretion and extracellular fluid volume normally are inversely related to PRA and plasma aldosterone level. The sodium/creatinine concentration ratio in a specimen of

Table 14-3. Normal Peripheral Plasma Renin Activity Values*

	Incubation pH	
	5.5	7.5
Supine 1 h	1–3	0–0.7
Standing 1 h	3–6	0.7–3.5
Sodium-restricted diet and standing	5–10	3.5–7.0

*Values in ng/ml per h for subjects on a normal sodium intake of ~110 meq/24 h. Low-salt diet or furosemide increase PRA two- to threefold; captopril increases PRA three- to fivefold. Data from Ref. 290.

urine collected at the same time as the blood for PRA can also be used as a marker of volume status. PRA falls with age and normal subjects above 55 years of age have PRA values that range up to 50 percent less than normal. Patients with diabetes mellitus with and without renal failure may have lower PRA levels. Illustrative values for normal peripheral PRA are shown in Table 14-3.

In hypertension, a PRA assay is useful when a secondary cause of hypertension is suspected such as primary aldosteronism, in which PRA is low, and renal vascular hypertension or a renin-secreting tumor, in which PRA may be increased. In tumor patients, plasma prorenin levels are also markedly elevated.[291] In patients with unexplained hyperkalemia, a PRA determination is necessary in the diagnosis of hyporeninemic hypoaldosteronism (Chap. 12).

To diagnose a low-renin state, PRA can be measured before and after stimulation of the renin system. Stimulatory maneuvers include provision of a low-sodium diet (10 to 20 meq of sodium per day for 4 to 5 days until the 24-h urinary sodium excretion is less than 20 meq) and standing (1 to 4 h), intravenous (IV) administration of furosemide (40 to 60 mg) and standing (1 to 4 h), or oral captopril (50 mg), and standing for 2 h.[92,290] In the presence of volume increase or with administration of drugs which suppress renin release, the renin response to these maneuvers may be difficult to interpret.

When an unprovoked PRA is elevated in the face of hypertension, the most common causes are high-renin essential hypertension and renovascular disease. Measurement of PRA following administration of inhibitors of the renin system such as saralasin or converting enzyme inhibitor has been reported to be helpful in differentiating patients with high-renin essential hypertension from those with renovascular hypertension (see also the sections on evaluation of renovascular hypertension).[292]

Measurement of PRA in both renal veins, if done under carefully standardized conditions, can be useful in establishing whether a lesion in the renal artery is causing hypertension and predicting the outcome of surgery in the patients with renovascular hypertension.[293] Blood for PRA is simultaneously collected from the vena cava and both renal veins. Because of the suppression of renin secretion from the unaffected side, the ratio between the PRA in the renal vein of the affected kidney and that of the contralateral one must be ≥ 1.5 for the test to be considered positive. In patients with a positive test surgery has an 80 to 90 percent cure rate, but a high frequency of false-negative tests has been reported (discussed in the section on renovascular hypertension). This incidence can be lowered by (1) stimulating the patient with a low-salt diet for several days prior to renal vein catheterization or (2) using a renin stimulator during catheterization; the latter may be administration of IV hydralazine (5 to 10 mg), slow tilt, head up, to 30 to 50° for 30 min, or (3) administration of a converting enzyme inhibitor (25 to 50 mg of captopril) before the test. It is essential that the catheters be in the appropriate places and their locations confirmed. This can be done either by dye injection under fluoroscopy or by oximetry, which should indicate that the oxygen content is higher (near 90 percent saturation) in renal venous blood compared with inferior vena caval blood (50 to 80 percent saturation). Patients with renin-secreting tumors will also display a high PRA in the renal vein of the affected kidney. In the event of a segmental or focal lesion of one kidney, it may be necessary to catheterize selectively the renal vein branch draining the abnormal segment in order to detect an elevated PRA.

Angiotensin II

Angiotensin II is the active component of the renin system. Its concentration can be measured by RIA or by reverse-phase high-pressure liquid chromatography.[294] Most antibodies directed against angiotensin II are highly cross-reactive with angiotensin I. The major problem with the angiotensin II assay is that angiotensin II is rapidly degraded in the plasma by proteases. Therefore, determination of angiotensin II is not used routinely for clinical purposes. However, careful measurements of plasma angiotensin II concentration indicate that the peptide's concentration varies in response to physiological maneuvers in the same direction as the PRA.

Aldosterone

Aldosterone production can best be assessed by measuring aldosterone excretion over a 24-h period.[295,296]

Ordinarily, the concentration of the urinary 18-glucuronide metabolite of aldosterone is measured. For this procedure, urine is collected at around pH 5 in the presence of a preservative to prevent bacterial growth. The urine is then treated with acid (at pH 1) to convert the 18-glucuronide metabolite of aldosterone to free aldosterone, which is then measured by RIA. The 18-glucuronidation occurs predominantly in the kidney and accounts for about 51 percent of the total aldosterone production. Less commonly, urinary tetrahydroaldosterone concentration is measured. Measurement of the plasma aldosterone concentration, although it provides information only for that moment in time, can provide an excellent assessment of mineralocorticoid production.[293] However, the conditions under which blood samples are obtained are critical in order to yield diagnostic information. Both plasma and urinary aldosterone measurements should be performed while the patient is on a high salt intake ($\geq$ 120 meq per day for at least 4 days), and after being recumbent overnight (at least 6 h). This is crucial, because in patients with essential hypertension any diminution of salt intake will normally increase the plasma aldosterone level and aldosterone production. In patients who have recently received diuretic therapy, both renin and aldosterone values may remain elevated until the extracellular fluid volume increases and sodium and potassium repletion has occurred.

Plasma aldosterone concentration can be measured in either heparinized or EDTA-treated blood. The steroid is extracted from the blood, separated by chromatography, and assayed by RIA.[297] For example, in normal subjects, plasma aldosterone concentrations at 8 A.M. after overnight recumbency range from 4 to 12 ng/dl.[298] In patients with an adenoma, they are always $>$ 20 ng/dl and may reach very high levels (Fig. 14-13). In patients with hyperplasia they are commonly $<$ 20 ng/dl but can be higher;[298a] in a group of 31 patients with hyperplasia the mean value was 13 $\pm$ 1.2 (standard error of the mean, SE) ng/dl (Fig. 14-14). Many of the values were in the normal range.

Typical normal urinary aldosterone excretion values range from 4 to 17 μg/24 h. In one series there were mean values of 37.6 $\pm$ 3.1 μg/24 h for adenoma and 22.5 $\pm$ 1.5 μg/24 h for hyperplasia.[298] Thus, the urinary measurements are superior to the plasma measurements for detecting abnormal production of aldosterone, but only the plasma measurements are useful in discriminating between adenoma and hyperplasia (compare Figs. 14-13 and 14-14).

The production of aldosterone is influenced by the potassium balance; it decreases with progressive hypokalemia (see Chap. 21). Such depletion may reduce both aldosterone production and plasma levels

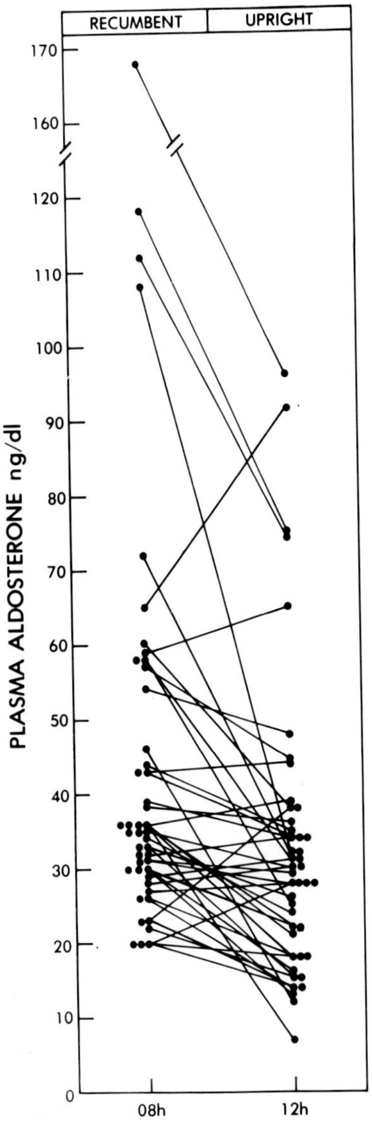

FIGURE 14-13 Effect of 4 h in the upright position after overnight recumbency in 47 patients with proven aldosterone-producing adenoma while on a sodium intake of 120 meq. Note: at 8 A.M. plasma aldosterone concentration is above 20 ng/dl.

into the normal or even below-normal range.[299] Thus, normal values in the presence of hypokalemia in these patients are really abnormal.

During normal sodium intake, a suppressed renin level accompanied by high urinary or plasma aldosterone levels in the presence of hypertension and hypokalemia confirm the diagnosis of primary aldosteronism. Suppression tests of aldosterone may be necessary for normal or borderline elevations of aldosterone concentration. These include (1) high-sodium diet (300 meq per day for 5 days), (2) fludrocortisone ace-

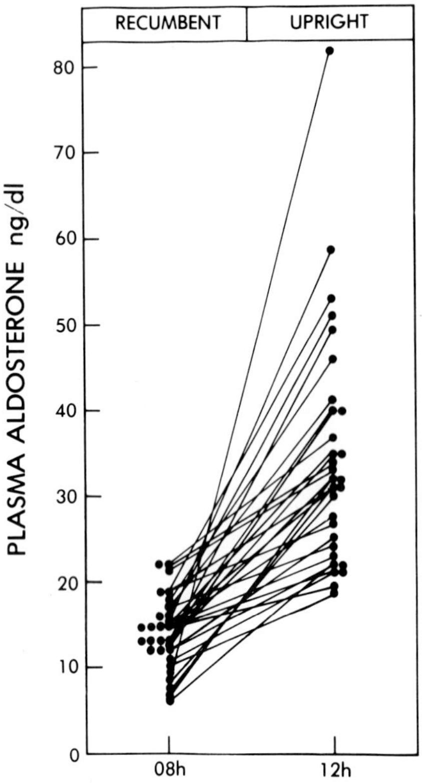

FIGURE 14-14 Effect of 4 h in the upright position after overnight recumbency in 31 patients on a sodium intake of 120 meq who have primary aldosteronism due to adrenal hyperplasia.

tate, 0.3 mg per day for 3 days, or (3) 2 liters of saline IV over 4 h.[300-302] In normal subjects, these maneuvers will decrease plasma aldosterone concentration to < 5 ng/dl, while in patients with hyperaldosteronism plasma aldosterone concentration is not reduced to less than 10 mg/dl (Fig. 14-15). In patients with primary aldosteronism, serum potassium level and blood pressure must be monitored carefully during these maneuvers, as the hypokalemia and hypertension are extremely sensitive to sodium loading.

Deoxycorticosterone

Deoxycorticosterone (DOC) is measured by RIA. In normal subjects circulating levels (4 to 12 ng/dl) probably contribute negligibly to the mineralocorticoid activity of plasma. In syndromes of DOC excess[302] where circulating levels are 10 times normal, hypertension and hypokalemia can ensue (discussed below).

18-Hydroxycorticosterone

18-Hydroxycorticosterone (18-OHB) concentration is measured by RIA. It is a key test to differentiate patients with primary aldosteronism due to adrenal adenoma from patients with adrenal hyperplasia or indeterminate hyperaldosteronism (see below). Plasma samples should be obtained in the supine position at 8 A.M. after overnight recumbency. Under these circumstances, normal values range from 10 to 30 ng/dl,[304] and the greatest differences in 18-OHB levels occur between patients with adenoma and those with hyperplasia (Fig. 14-16). Following this, values taken upright after several hours of ambulation in adenoma patients will have fallen while 18-OHB levels rise in hyperplasia patients. Administration of potassium or spironolactone decreases 18-OHB concentration and increases plasma aldosterone concentration in patients with adenoma, so that samples should probably not be obtained under these conditions. Unfortunately, at present this test is available in only a few centers, but it may become more generally available because of its utility.

Sodium and Potassium

Sodium and potassium concentrations are measured in blood and urine by flame photometry. Serum sodium concentration represents the amount of free water in the extracellular fluid. The normal range is around 135 to 148 meq/liter in most laboratories. This value is usually normal in hypertension, although diuretics can induce hyponatremia. It tends to be increased in primary aldosteronism, although diagnostic reliance cannot be placed on this. In the absence of diuretics, 24-h urinary sodium excretion is a good reflection of the body's volume state.

Potassium is the major intracellular cation. The normal range of concentration is 3.5 to 5.3 meq/liter in most laboratories in patients with a normal sodium intake. The most common cause of hypokalemia in the hypertensive patient is diuretic therapy. Unprovoked hypokalemia in the face of hypertension is indicative of a mineralocorticoid excess state. Primary or secondary hyperaldosteronism, excess DOC, glycyrrhizic acid ingestion, and, rarely, an excess of other mineralocorticoids should be considered. On a sodium intake of 120 meq per day or more, serum potassium concentration drops to ≤ 3.5 meq/liter in these conditions. Despite the hypokalemia, 24-h urinary potassium excretion is disproportionately elevated, > 20 meq/24 h, indicating excessive loss of potassium by the kidney.

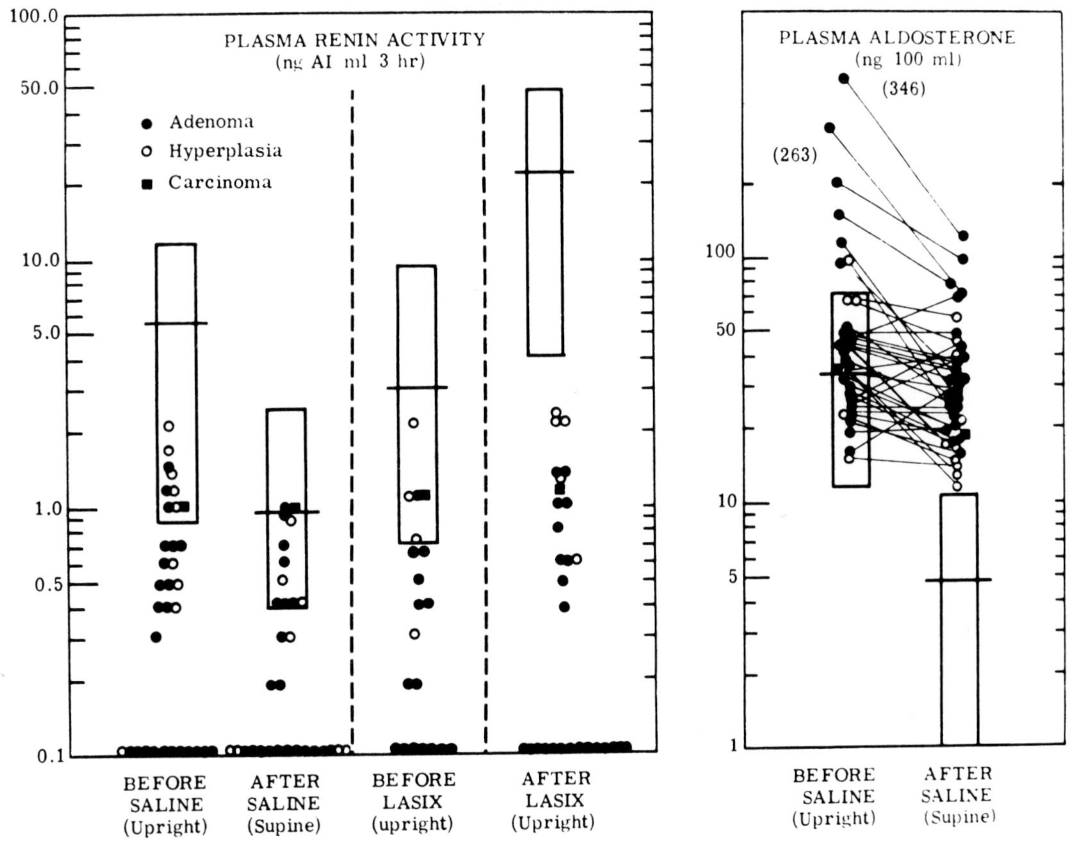

FIGURE 14-15 Responses of plasma renin activity (*left*) and plasma aldosterone concentration (*right*) to suppressive and stimulating maneuvers. Scales are logarithmic to accommodate the range of values. Normal values (114 subjects) are represented as mean (bars) ± 95 percent confidence limits (boxes). Values for patients with primary aldosteronism are indicated by symbols (see key); connecting lines for plasma aldosterone concentration represent values for a given patient. AI, angiotensin I. (*From Weinberger et al.*[295])

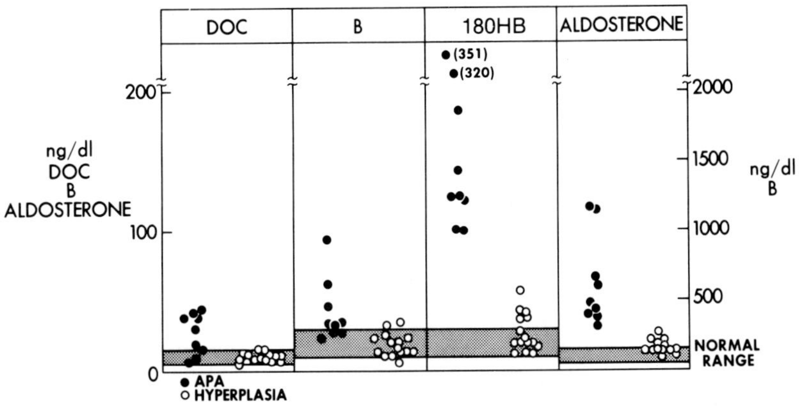

FIGURE 14-16 8 A.M. values (after overnight recumbency) of concentration of the steroids of the mineralocorticoid pathway [deoxycorticosterone (DOC), corticosterone (B), 18-hydroxycorticosterone (18-OHB), and aldosterone] in patients with primary aldosteronism due to an adenoma (APA) and hyperplasia.

EVALUATION OF THE HYPERTENSIVE PATIENT

Evaluation of the hypertensive patient is aimed at (1) confirming the presence and persistence of an inappropriately raised blood pressure; (2) determining the level of the blood pressure and the presence and degree of secondary end organ damage (in the heart, brain, kidneys, and arteries); (3) differentiating patients with curable or secondary hypertension from those with primary or essential hypertension (cause unknown); (4) establishing a baseline before initiating therapy; (5) providing indications for the selection of specific antihypertensive medications likely to be effective and for the urgency for initiating their administration; (6) assessing the coexistence and severity of other atherosclerosis risk factors, such as hypercholesterolemia, diabetes mellitus, or cigarette smoking, and of other illnesses, medications, or dietary factors contributing to the severity of the disease and complicating its management. This evaluation can be performed by a careful clinical history, physical examination, and certain screening laboratory tests.

The prevalence of secondary hypertension in the population is not known. Most published reports originate from large secondary and tertiary referral medical centers where the patient population is preselected, thereby biasing the data in favor of a higher prevalence of secondary hypertension than is present in the general population (Table 14-4).[305-307] Probably less than 5 percent of all unselected patients with hypertension have renovascular hypertension, the most common form of secondary hypertension. However, in certain groups of patients, such as those with accelerated or malignant hypertension, children under the age of 10, and those developing hypertension after the age of 50, the prevalence may approach 30 percent.[308,309] Nevertheless, since diagnosis of primary hypertension carries with it a life sentence of drug therapy, with accompanying costs, side effects, less than optimum blood pressure control, and potential for progressive renal failure, a careful search for a curable cause of hypertension is justified in all patients with significant hypertension.

The initial history should focus on the circumstances of the initial diagnosis of the hypertension; whether the patient had a blood pressure determination incidentally or seeks medical care because of symptoms; the known duration of hypertension; family history of hypertension and premature atherosclerosis; history of symptoms suggesting end organ damage or symptoms, illnesses, or operations providing clues to the presence of secondary hypertension; prior diagnostic evaluation; prior therapy, response to it, and reasons for discontinuation; the presence of other illnesses such as gout, diabetes, or peptic ulcer disease; medications, such as for asthma, nasal congestion, or arthritis, such as nonsteroidal anti-inflammatory agents, hormones, and oral contraceptives; dietary factors; and tobacco or alcohol use or drug abuse, which might relate to the hypertension or complicate its management.

Clinical features which are not usually found in patients with essential hypertension and which therefore suggest that a patient with hypertension should be further evaluated for the presence of renovascular or endocrine hypertension are listed in Table 14-5.

Physical Examination

Measuring Blood Pressure

On physical examination, careful attention should be paid to the accurate measurement of blood pressure on multiple occasions in both arms and in various positions. The classification of blood pressure recom-

Table 14-4. Frequencies of Various Diagnoses in Hypertensive Subjects

Diagnosis	Gifford[306a] (n = 4939), %	Ferguson[306b] (n = 246), %	Berglund[307] (n = 689*), %
Essential hypertension	89	90	94
Chronic renal disease	5	2	4
Renovascular disease	4	3	1
Coarctation	1		0.1
Primary aldosteronism	0.5	0.4	0.1
Cushing's syndrome	0.2		
Pheochromocytoma	0.2		
Oral contraceptive–induced		4	

*Men only.
Source: Modified from Kaplan.[7]

Table 14-5. Clinical Features Suggestive of Secondary Hypertension

No family history of hypertension
Abrupt onset of hypertension rather than gradual (over the course of months or years)
Onset of hypertension before the age of 20 or after the age of 50
Sudden acceleration of previously existing hypertension or development of malignant hypertension *de novo*
Rapid deterioration of renal function despite well-controlled hypertension or following treatment with converting enzyme inhibitors
Unresponsiveness to standard antihypertensive therapy
Rapid development of hypokalemia with standard doses of diuretics
History of renal trauma, flank pain, and hematuria, suggesting renal infarction
Sudden onset of hypertension in a patient with systemic emboli or vasculitis
Development of hypertension in association with lower-extremity ischemia, calf or buttock claudication, and erectile incompetence, abdominal angina, or aortic aneurysm
Nocturnal polyuria
Periodic paralysis or muscle weakness

mended by the Committee on Detection, Evaluation, and Treatment of High Blood Pressure is outlined in Table 14-1.[2]

Blood pressure variability is well recognized and complicates interpretations.[310,311] Blood pressure tends to be lower during rest and sleep, after several days of hospitalization, and with repeated measurements.[312] It tends to be higher during mental or physical arousal.[313] The "fight/flight reaction," preparing the body to deal with impending stress, results in increased blood pressure and heart rate. Thus, the anxiety in anticipation of the physical examination often results in pressure measurements in the physician's office which are not representative of most of the pressures during the day. These can lead to an erroneous diagnosis of hypertension, which has major implications in terms of prognosis, employability, and insurability. Erroneously high pressure readings can also set in motion an unwarranted, expensive workup for secondary hypertension and unnecessary or excessive drug therapy and life-style modification.

Several methods have been developed to determine "representative" blood pressures.[311] Multiple blood pressure determinations in a quiet, reassuring environment and after a period of rest are useful.[314] Blood pressure measured by paramedical personnel is often more representative than that measured by a physician. Home blood pressure measurements or repeated regular determinations of blood pressure by the patient or a family member at home or at the work site are often used.[315,316] Ambulatory blood pressures, using a portable automatic or semiautomatic device that measures and records blood pressure at 15- to 30-min intervals during a normal day's activities and at night have become available.[317,318] These are useful, especially in patients with borderline hypertension, difficult-to-control hypertension, or marked disparity between blood pressure level and end organ damage and for assessing the effect of drug therapy. Ambulatory blood pressures correlate better with the degree of end organ damage than do blood pressures measured in the physician's office.[319]

Another problem is the mechanics of measuring the blood pressure. Direct measurement via intraarterial needle is not feasible for general management of hypertensive patients. The indirect method of blood pressure determination, the technique of Korotkov, is therefore used.[320] The apparatus should be properly calibrated and the width of the cuff should be 40 percent of the upper arm circumference and its length 80 percent of the arm circumference.[321] Careful attention must also be paid to keep the antecubital fossa where the stethoscope is placed at the level of the heart (at the fourth intercostal space), the rate of deflation appropriate for the heart rate, and the stethoscope directly over the brachial artery pulsation. In addition, regular servicing and calibration of the equipment is recommended. It is now convention to use the fifth phase of the Korotkov sounds (the level of pressure at which the last sound is heard) as a measure of diastolic pressure. However, in children and patients with high cardiac output, such as in hyperthyroidism, aortic insufficiency, and pregnancy and after exercise, phase IV, or muffling of the Korotkov sounds, is a more accurate reflection of the diastolic pressure.[320]

It is advisable to obtain at least three separate elevated blood pressure determinations before labeling a patient hypertensive. Blood pressure should also be measured in supine, erect, and sitting positions. A marked postural fall in blood pressure (e.g., $>$ 10 mmHg systolic) suggests volume depletion, blunted baroreceptor reflexes or peripheral neuropathy.[320]

Other Aspects of Physical Examination

Several other aspects of the physical examination should receive special attention (Table 14-6). Examination of the skin should focus on the presence of striae, suggesting hypercortisolism, or café au lait spots, suggesting von Recklinghausen's disease. The optic fundi should be examined and the vascular changes classified according to the prognostic criteria of Keith, Wagener, and Barker:[322a]

Table 14-6. Findings on Physical Examination Suggestive of Secondary Hypertension

Presence of malignant hypertension, grade III or IV Keith Wagener retinopathy
Evidence of widespread occlusive vascular disease in the carotid, aortoiliac, or femoral arteries manifested by decreased pulses or bruits
Presence of an epigastric or flank bruit with both systolic and diastolic components
Presence of an abdominal aortic aneurysm
Positive Chvostek's or Trousseau's sign, suggesting alkalosis
Impaired autonomic reflexes; postural hypotension
Café au lait spots and neurofibromas
Central obesity with thinning of the extremities, hirsutism, etc., suggesting Cushing's syndrome
Tremor, weight loss, etc. suggesting thyrotoxicosis
Hypertension in the upper extremities only or radio-femoral pulse disparity (suggesting coarctation)

1. Arteriolar narrowing, i.e., ratio of venous to arterial caliber greater than 3:2
2. Arteriovenous compression and extensive focal or generalized arteriolar narrowing
3. Hemorrhages, exudates, cotton-wool spots (retinal microinfarcts)
4. Papilledema

The examination should include palpation of the peripheral pulses and auscultation for bruits over the carotid, radial, femoral, popliteal, dorsalis pedis, and posterial tibial arteries and careful palpation of the abdominal aorta for the presence of an aneurysm or bruits. Chest examination should include percussion and auscultation for detection of chronic obstructive pulmonary disease or asthma. The cardiac examination should include (1) palpation of the left ventricular impulse and (2) determination of rate and rhythm and presence of third or fourth heart sounds, accentuated aortic valve closing sound, and determination of the presence of murmurs suggesting aortic insufficiency, aortic sclerosis, left ventricular outflow obstruction, or mitral regurgitation. The presence of left ventricular hypertrophy can be recognized clinically by a palpable sustained left ventricular heave or evidence of left atrial enlargement reflected by the presence of a fourth heart sound. With progressive left ventricular hypertrophy, especially when it is asymmetric, there may also be associated left ventricular outflow tract murmurs. The late systolic murmur of coarctation of the aorta should be sought in the left second intercostal space and between the scapulae. Examination of the abdomen should include palpation for the presence of enlarged liver, spleen, and kidneys and an aortic aneurysm and determination of radiofemoral pulse delay, as is seen in coarctation of the aorta. The extremities should be examined for muscle wasting, deformities, and joint abnormalities.

Laboratory Tests

Laboratory tests should include a complete blood count and urinalysis and determinations of renal function, glucose, cholesterol, triglycerides, serum electrolytes, and uric acid. A measure of cardiac enlargement by electrocardiography or roentgenography of the chest (although the latter is less sensitive and specific) should also be made as a baseline reference. The electrocardiogram has traditionally been the most widely used test for determining the presence of left ventricular hypertrophy; however, the repolarization abnormalities seen with left ventricular hypertrophy are often difficult to differentiate from those of ischemia, and the voltage criteria for left ventricular hypertrophy have a low sensitivity and specificity, especially in young people.[322b] Echocardiography has, therefore, become the more widely used tool for determining the presence of early left ventricular hypertrophy. Left ventricular mass, wall thickness, and diastolic filling properties can all be determined by echocardiography.[322c]

There are a few specific clues from the routine laboratory evaluation that suggest hypertension due to renovascular or adrenal causes. These include proteinuria, impaired renal concentrating ability, impaired renal function, hypokalemic hypochloremic alkalosis, and glucose intolerance.

Although clues for the presence of secondary hypertension from the history, physical examination, and laboratory tests are useful when present, their absence should not preclude a thorough search for a cause for the hypertension in a young person with significant hypertension in whom successful cure of the hypertension would obviate the need for lifelong drug therapy. Even in older, more debilitated patients, a diagnosis of secondary hypertension should be sought if correction of this condition has potential for improving survival, renal function, or quality of life. Formerly, the pursuit of a diagnosis of secondary hypertension was discouraged in patients with chronic diseases and renal failure, since operative correction of a lesion, if found, carried a high morbidity and mortality. However, with the availability of digital subtraction angiography and transluminal angioplasty, even older patients with congestive heart failure or renal failure can be benefited by revascularization of a correctable lesion, with relatively low morbidity and mortality.

RENOVASCULAR HYPERTENSION

Historical Background

The first association of renal disease with hypertension is attributed to Bright, who noted in 1836 the association of cardiac enlargement with chronic renal disease.[323] Mahomed postulated in 1881 that high blood pressure was a cause of Bright's disease.[324] Tigerstedt and Bergmann later injected minced rabbit kidney into rabbits and produced a pressor response.[325] They named this pressor agent *renin*. Volhard and Fahr in 1914 described an association between necrotizing arteriolitis in the kidney and malignant hypertension.[326] There followed isolated case reports of hypertension in association with unilateral renal abnormalities.[327,328] Goldblatt and coworkers in 1934 produced chronic hypertension in the dog by renal artery constriction.[329] This experimental model became the stimulus and basis for subsequent work clarifying the relationship of renovascular disease to hypertension in humans (see above).[330] In 1936, Butler reported the correction of hypertension in a child with unilateral pyelonephritis following nephrectomy,[331] and Leadbetter and Burkland probably reported the first case of fibromuscular dysplasia.[332] However, it later became clear that in only a minority of patients with unilateral renal disease would nephrectomy cure the hypertension.[333,334]

Meanwhile, in 1939, Page in the United States and Braun-Menendez and coworkers in Argentina almost simultaneously described the renin-angiotensin system as the humoral mediator of hypertension in the ischemic dog.[335,336] Goormaghtigh later demonstrated that renin originates from cells in the juxtaglomerular apparatus of the afferent renal arteriole.[337] Angiotensin was subsequently identified, characterized, and synthesized.[338] Aldosterone was recognized and isolated in the 1950s and its relationship to potassium and extracellular fluid volume was clarified.[339] Subsequently, the link between aldosterone, renin, angiotensin II, the kidney, and hypertension was demonstrated, both experimentally and clinically.[340a] More recently, the development of antagonists of the renin-angiotensin system have furthered understanding of its role in the initiation, maintenance, and diagnosis of renovascular hypertension.[340b,340c]

Subsequent developments have improved markedly the capability to diagnose and treat renovascular hypertension. These include the use of renal arteriography, perfection of surgical techniques for revascularization, and development of methods for determining the physiological significance of identified arterial lesions. The medical treatment of renovascular hypertension with the beta-adrenergic blocking drugs and, subsequently, angiotensin antagonists and converting enzyme inhibitors followed. Percutaneous transluminal angioplasty has provided yet another alternative to surgical management.

The importance of renovascular disease as a remediable cause of hypertension in infancy and childhood is becoming ever more apparent. Likewise, the value of revascularization, surgically or by angioplasty, for the improvement of renal function is increasingly recognized and even older patients with extensive atherosclerotic disease are undergoing successful reconstruction with salvage of renal function.

The ideal, inexpensive, safe and simple, and 100 percent predictive outpatient screening test for renovascular hypertension is not yet available, although several are proposed. However, the need to search for a curable cause such as renovascular disease in persons with significant hypertension is generally recognized.

Pathologic Etiology of Renovascular Hypertension

The most common causes of renovascular hypertension are atherosclerosis (Fig. 14-17) and fibromuscular dysplasia (Fig. 14-18); other causes have been reported much less frequently. These causes are listed in Table 14-7.[340b,340c]

ATHEROSCLEROSIS

Atherosclerotic stenosis of the renal arteries resembles atherosclerotic lesions in other muscular arteries (Fig. 14-17). The atheromatous intimal plaque may be focal or extensive, eccentric or concentric; it consists of accumulations of lipid, collagen, and calcium in the intima and media. These atheromas may be complicated by adherent platelet clumps and hemorrhage into the plaque, resulting in dissection or occlusion of the lumen of the artery. Emboli from ulcerating plaques to distal vessels may also occur. Atherosclerotic lesions may be unilateral but are frequently bilateral and associated with plaques in the abdominal aorta. Atherosclerotic lesions are characteristically located at the orifice of or in the initial one-third of the renal arteries.

Atherosclerotic lesions occur predominantly in older patients, predominantly in men, and in patients with risk factors for atherosclerosis such as antecedent hypertension, adult-onset diabetes mellitus, hyperlipemia, and cigarette smoking.[340c,340d] In women, these lesions are seen in smokers and after the menopause.

Since hypertension is one of the most important risk factors for the development of atherosclerotic plaques in the renal arteries these plaques may occur in patients with preexisting hypertension, leading to an abrupt decrease in renal function or acceleration of

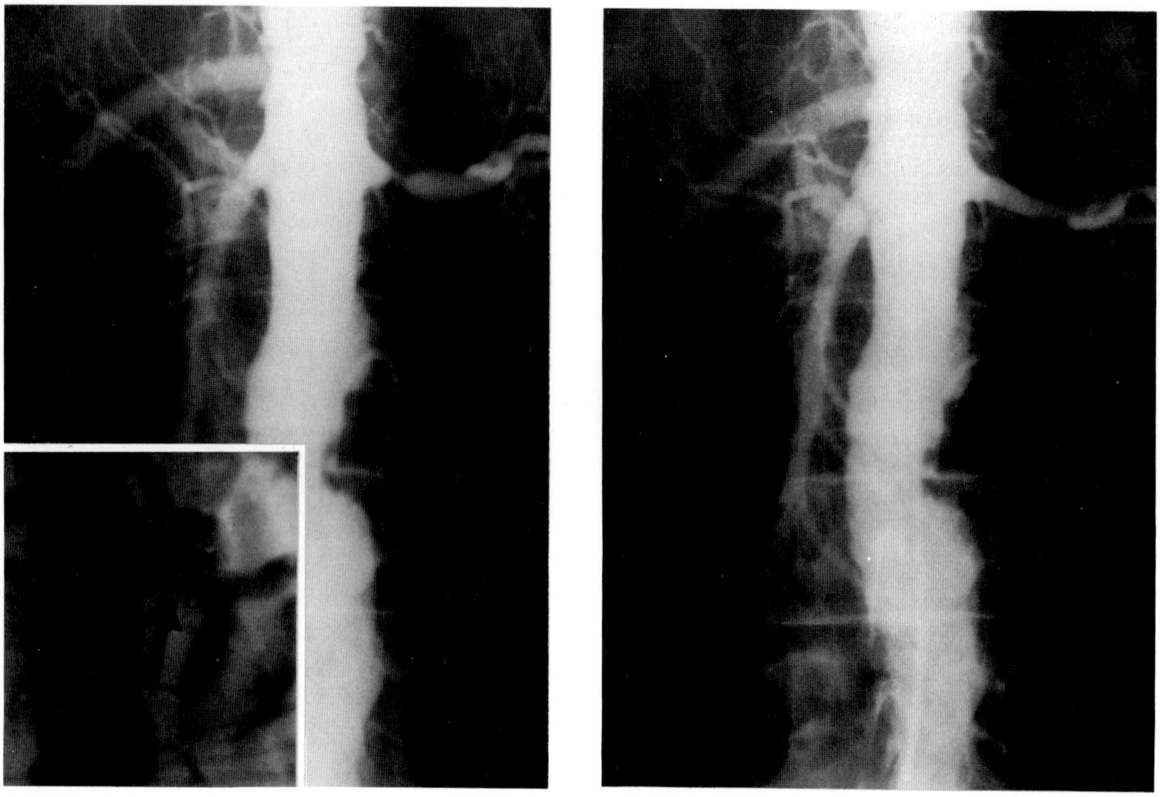

FIGURE 14-17 Renal arteriogram before (*left*) and after (*right*) balloon angioplasty. The insert in the left photograph shows the IV digital subtraction angiogram of the same lesion.

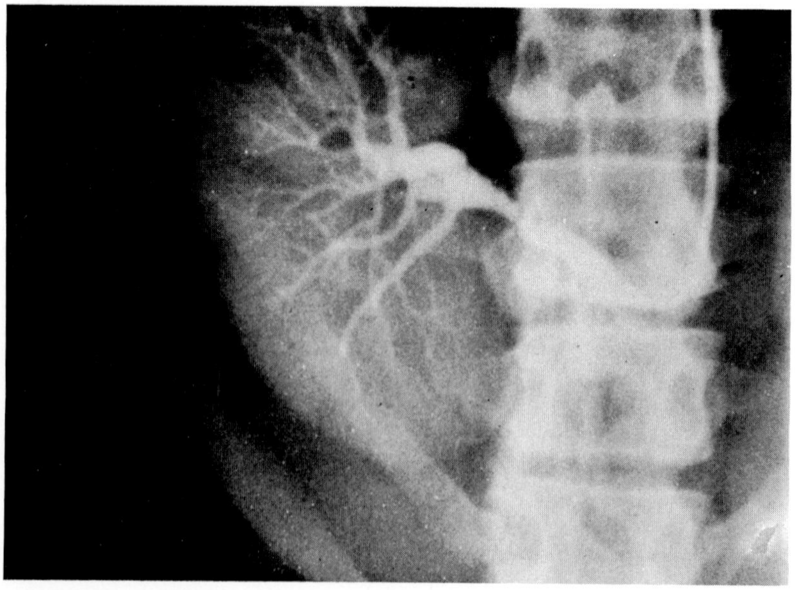

FIGURE 14-18 Renovascular hypertension due to fibromuscular disease. Note the "corkscrew" constriction with poststenotic dilatation.

Table 14-7. Anatomic Causes of Renal Artery Obstruction

Atherosclerosis
Fibromuscular dysplasia
Arterial emboli
Aortic dissection or isolated renal artery dissection
Extrarenal compression by tumor, neurofibroma, retroperitoneal fibrosis, perirenal or subcapsular hematoma, or scarring
Arteriovenous malformation, fistula, hemangioma,
Hypoplasia of suprarenal abdominal aorta
Renal artery aneurysm; intra- or extrarenal
Generalized arteritis, aortitis syndromes: Takayasu's disease
Stenosis in the artery supplying a transplanted kidney

the hypertension. On the other hand, incidental plaques have been observed at autopsy in the arteries of older patients without hypertension. In Perloff's series of 134 normotensive patients undergoing arteriography, 212 had minor atherosclerotic plaques, resulting in less than 50 percent stenosis of the renal arteries, and six had major arteriosclerotic stenoses (> 50 percent).[340e]

FIBROMUSCULAR DYSPLASIA

Lesions denoted as fibrous, fibrodysplastic, or nonatheromatous (Fig. 14-18) have been well described and classified by Harrison and McCormick.[340f] The subgrouping is based on (1) the location in the arterial wall of the predominant histopathology, whether intimal, medial, perimedial, or subadventitial, (2) the degree of destruction of the elastica interna and the elastica externa, and (3) the predominant cell type.[340g,341] These lesions occur predominantly in younger patients, infants and children, and women and have been described in arteries other than the renal arteries.[342–344] The cause of these lesions is not known.

Intimal Fibroplasia

Intimal fibroplasia is present in 5 to 10 percent of patients with fibrodysplastic lesions. This lesion is characterized by accumulation of irregularly arranged mesenchymal cells within a loose matrix of fibrous connective tissue in the subendothelium, resulting in long, irregular smooth focal tubular stenoses. This lesion is common in infants and children and occurs in both sexes.[340f–341,345–347] It may be associated with extensive arteritis of the aorta and with medial lesions. In some cases intimal lesions result from intimal trauma. Intimal fibroplasia is complicated by dissection and frequently progresses to involve other arteries. The lesion may be unilateral or bilateral. In pediatric cases, the elastica interna is reduplicated, and there is often some medial disorganization. In the adult, only intimal collagen accumulation is seen.

Medial Fibromuscular Dysplasia

Medial fibromuscular dysplasia is further subdivided into *medial fibroplasia, perimedial fibroplasia,* and *medial hyperplasia.*

MEDIAL FIBROPLASIA Also called *fibromuscular hyperplasia,* this is the most common of these dysplasias, occurring in perhaps 85 percent of patients with fibrodysplastic lesions, predominantly in women aged 25 to 50. The lesion is characterized by multifocal stenoses due to thick fibrous ridges and circumferential rings of thick collagen tissue replacing muscle, alternating with thinning of the arterial wall and aneurysm formation. This results in the typical "string of beads" appearance on the arteriogram.[348–350] The lesion is often bilateral, occurring in the middle and distal thirds of the renal artery, and may extend into the intrarenal branches. There is loss of normal media and internal elastica in the area of the aneurysm. These lesions rarely dissect or thrombose, and although progression has been reported, the lesion is often present in older patients.

MEDIAL HYPERPLASIA This is a much less common form of fibrodysplastic disease, occurring in 1 to 2 percent of patients. It is characterized by true hyperplasia of muscular and fibrous tissue cells in the media, resulting in smooth focal stenoses on the arteriogram. This process may involve either the main renal artery or its branches. The lesion occurs both in men and in women, is usually progressive, and is frequently complicated by dissection.[340f,341,351]

PERIMEDIAL FIBROPLASIA This type, also referred to as *subadventitial fibroplasia,* is intermediate in frequency between the above two varieties and is characterized by intense fibroplasia of the outer half of the media, forming a tight stenotic collar of collagen enveloping the artery to a variable extent. Replacement of the elastica externa by fibrous tissue is variable. The resulting appearance of the vessel is one of intermittent irregularities with small beads or "accordion pleating," but no true aneurysm formation.[340f,340g,342,352]

MEDIAL DISSECTION Medial dissection occurs in about 5 to 10 percent of fibrodysplastic lesions and may be bilateral, frequently involving the distal two-thirds of the artery and extending into the primary arterial branches. It can be isolated or associated with several of the above described lesions.[340f,340g]

Periarterial Hyperplasia

Periarterial hyperplasia is the least common of these dysplasias and is characterized by excessive collagen formation in the adventitia, surrounding the periarterial tissue. It is a rare condition and may be a variant of retroperitoneal fibrosis. Its natural history has not been well described.[340f,340g,352]

OTHER CAUSES OF RENOVASCULAR HYPERTENSION

Renal artery thrombosis may occur in situ or result from emboli composed of vegetations from endocarditis, mural thrombi (following myocardial infarction), cardiac tumors, paradoxical venous thromboemboli in a patient with a patent foramen ovale or atrial septal defect, and ulcerating atherosclerotic plaques in the aorta proximal to the orifice of the renal artery.[340e,346,352,353] Thrombosis in situ has been reported in a woman receiving oral contraceptives.[354]

Rarer causes of renovascular hypertension include aortic dissection,[355] renal artery aneurysm,[356,357] aortic arteritis syndromes such as Takayasu's disease[358–360] or generalized vasculitis[361–363] and retroperitoneal fibrosis, either idiopathic or due to tumor or infection, resulting in perirenal compression[364,365] as well as mechanical arterial compression due to neurofibromas or other mass lesions.[366–369] Many of these are particularly found in children.[346,370–372]

Stenosis in the artery supplying a transplanted kidney can result from superimposed atherosclerosis as well as from thrombosis or ischemic fibrosis and scarring at the anastomosis site because of intraoperative arterial trauma and fibrin deposits.[373–376]

RENIN-SECRETING TUMORS

Hypertension resulting from excessive renin secretion has on rare occasions been observed in patients with various types of renal and extrarenal tumors. Since Robertson and coworkers first described such a case,[377] numerous isolated case reports have appeared.[378,379] Most of these tumors are small benign encapsulated hemangiopericytomas or hamartomas composed of juxtaglomerular cells, but renin-secreting adenocarcinomas of the pancreas, lung, and ovaries as well as Wilms's tumors have been reported.[291,380,381] In addition, any expanding renal tumor or mass lesion that produces intrarenal ischemia by compression or distortion of arterial structures can result in hyperreninemia.

The diagnosis should be suspected in hypertensive patients with hyperreninemia, secondary hyperaldosteronism, and lateralization of renal vein renins, in whom no arterial lesion is seen on arteriography and who do not have evidence of malignant hypertension or diffuse arterial vasculitis.[379] Tomography or CT scanning of the hypersecreting kidney can be used to localize and identify the tumor.[378] Nephrectomy or segmental resection of this usually benign tumor results in a "cure" of the hypertension.[379]

Patients with renin-secreting renal adenomas often present with malignant or accelerated hypertension, severe headaches, and papilledema and symptoms of hyperaldosteronism, polyuria, thirst, muscle cramps, weakness, and hypokalemic alkalosis.[382,383] Patients with renin-secreting or extrarenal carcinomas may have lesser degrees of hypertension and symptoms due directly to the location of the tumor. Transient reduction of hypertension has been reported after surgical removal of a renin-secreting ovarian carcinoma, with recurrence of hypertension as metastases became widespread. If operative correction is not possible, however, converting enzyme inhibition can effectively control the hypertension.[384]

Laragh's group has found unusually high ratios of inactive to active renin in the plasma and tumor extracts in two patients with extrarenal carcinomas. His group suggested that such a high level of inactive or precursor renin is consistent with ineffective precursor processing by the neoplastic tissue.[61,385]

Natural History of Renal Artery Lesions

Information regarding the natural history of stenotic lesions in the renal arteries is derived from serial angiographic studies and autopsies.[340c,386–389] Both types of studies may overestimate the rate of progression since changes in the anatomic lesion may not result in worsening of renal function or hypertension, and patients without progressive renal failure or poor blood pressure control are less likely to be restudied. Arteriograms are often repeated in patients who have not undergone operations when their hypertension becomes difficult to control or their renal function deteriorates.[386] Operated patients are restudied to assess the development of new aortoiliac vascular disease or because hypertension has recurred postoperatively after an initial apparently successful reduction of blood pressure.[388] Normotensive patients are less likely to be restudied.

Arteriosclerosis is a generalized disease which progresses with advancing age and in response to other risk factors, and all investigators report progression of these lesions in an increasing percentage of patients the longer the interval between studies.[387] The degree of narrowing, the extent of narrowing, and the number of vessels involved increase. In addition, atherosclerotic lesions can thrombose, hemorrhage, embolize, or dissect.[389-391] Schreiber and coworkers reported that 37 of 85 patients with atherosclerotic lesions (44 percent) had progressive obstruction on repeat arteriography after a mean follow-up period of 52 months.[389] In some, the lesions progressed within a year and progression to occlusion occurred in 14; the higher the degree of stenosis on initial examination, the greater was the chance of progression to occlusion. Among the 37 with progressive stenoses, 70 percent had a decrease in renal size, serum creatinine concentration increased in 54 percent and 41 percent had poor blood pressure control. Blood pressure reduction with beta-adrenergic blocking agents and converting enzyme inhibitors can further reduce renal perfusion and raise serum creatinine concentration in patients with renal artery stenosis. This is sometimes a diagnostic clue to the presence of stenosis. Similar worsening of renal artery stenosis in patients with atherosclerotic lesions has been reported by other observers.[386,391,392]

Patients with fibromuscular dysplastic lesions have a variable rate of progression, especially since this group represents a variety of pathologic processes. Schreiber found progression in 22 of 66 patients (33 percent) with medial fibroplasia restudied after a mean interval of 45 months, but no progression to occlusion.[389] Only two patients had a rise in serum creatinine level, but kidney size decreased in six patients and blood pressure control became inadequate in nine. Progression to renal infarction has, however, been reported,[351] especially in patients with perimedial fibrosis or intimal fibroplasia. There are considerable differences in the rates of progression among the different subclassifications of fibromuscular dysplastic diseases. Thus, Stewart et al. found that in intimal fibroplasia, associated dissection is frequent and there is a tendency to progression in 60 to 100 percent of patients.[352] No dissection was found by Goncharenko et al. in medial fibroplasia and thrombosis occurred rarely.[351] Progression was seen in 13 of 40 patients over a 1- to 7-year follow-up by Meaney and coworkers.[386] However, progression was seen in none of the 28 patients over the age of 40. Sheps and coworkers did, however, see some progression in older patients.[388] Ekelund et al. found that medial hyperplasia usually progressed and often went on to dissection,[350] and Kincaid et al. described patients with perimedial fibroplasia progressing to severe stenosis.[342]

Patients with aneurysms may develop rupture, thrombosis, and enlargement with further compression of surrounding vasculature.[357,369] Patients with aortic dissection may have a second, more devastating dissection with further decrease in renal blood flow.[355] Arteritis such as Takayasu's often progresses but may arrest unpredictably.[358,393]

Clinical Characteristics of Patients with Renovascular Hypertension

Although there is considerable overlap in the clinical characteristics of patients with essential hypertension and those with renovascular hypertension, there are certain features that help to differentiate the two.[8,394-396] Patients with renovascular hypertension may develop hypertension abruptly rather than gradually, and before the age of 20 or after the age of 50. Hypertension beginning in infancy or childhood is especially likely to be secondary.[397,398] There is often no family history of hypertension and a short duration of hypertension. Although hypertension is more prevalent among blacks than whites in the United States, renovascular hypertension is rare among blacks.[399,400] In the Cooperative Study on Renovascular Hypertension, representing the combined experience with renal arteriography of 15 medical centers with 2442 patients, 30 percent of all patients studied were black but only 8 percent of those with renovascular hypertension were black.[394] Patients with renovascular hypertension may give a history of trauma to the flank, hematuria, or sudden pain in the kidneys and a source of systemic emboli; older patients with atherosclerotic lesions may have symptoms of occlusive vascular disease in other organ systems.[395,401] Patients with renovascular hypertension often give a history of poor response to medical therapy for hypertension. Also, renal function may deteriorate with converting enzyme inhibitor therapy.[402]

On physical examination patients with renovascular hypertension are more likely to have accelerated or malignant hypertension, with high blood pressure levels that have responded poorly to therapy, and they may have grade III and IV changes in the optic fundi.[309,403a,403b] An abdominal and/or flank bruit is commonly present;[395,401,404,405] in the Cooperative Study a bruit was heard six to nine times as often in patients with renovascular hypertension as in those with essential hypertension.[394] Evidence of occlusive aortoiliac disease or aortic aneurysm may also be a clue to renal artery involvement.[395]

The only routine laboratory clues to renovascular hypertension are hypokalemic alkalosis (due to secondary hyperaldosteronism), impaired renal function, and proteinuria.[309,403a,403b]

Specific Diagnostic Studies for Renovascular Hypertension

The definitive diagnosis of renovascular hypertension is made only in retrospect, when correction of a renal arterial lesion by revascularization or nephrectomy results in sustained reduction of blood pressure to normal levels. The only method for demonstrating the presence of an obstruction to renal arterial flow is renal arteriography. However, the presence of an anatomic lesion does not by itself prove a cause and effect relationship for the hypertension since major arterial stenoses occur in patients without hypertension.[406] Furthermore, renal arteriography is a relatively invasive procedure with a definite risk and considerable expense. Therefore, various screening tests are used to preselect patients in whom arteriography is most likely to reveal a functionally important lesion and therefore be worth performing, and to spare the large majority of patients with primary hypertension from unnecessary invasive procedures. These tests are also helpful in assessing the functional importance of the arterial lesion and for predicting the outcome of therapy. The individual tests are first described; following this the logic for choosing the tests is presented (see the subsequent section on Sequencing of Diagnostic Tests for Renovascular Hypertension).

Screening and predictive tests are based on either of two premises: (1) Unilateral renal arterial stenosis results in a unilaterally ischemic kidney whose function and structure can be shown to differ from the normal kidney. (2) If the renal arterial lesion is the cause of the hypertension, it operates by activation of the RAA mechanism; increased levels of renin or angiotensin II should be measurable in plasma, either directly or indirectly, and maneuvers that block the RAA system should result in an immediate fall in blood pressure. In the former category are tests such as the intravenous urogram, the isotope renogram, and the differential renal excretion or function tests (Howard-Stamey). These tests are relatively sensitive and specific in patients with unilateral disease, but may be equivocal in patients with bilateral disease. In the second category are tests such as the saralasin infusion test, converting enzyme inhibition (captopril) test, and measurement of renin levels, both in the peripheral venous blood and in the renal veins. These tests are relatively sensitive and specific when a careful protocol is followed, sodium intake is known, and renin determinations are done in an experienced laboratory, but they can be falsely positive or negative in patients receiving antihypertensive drugs or oral contraceptives or if the specimens are not handled according to strictly controlled methods.

A further confounding factor is that in patients with long-standing renovascular hypertension or hypertension of whatever cause, secondary mechanisms become activated, such as the development of nephrosclerosis and renal failure, which sustain the hypertension independently of the initiating mechanism and which result in renal sodium retention, volume increase, and secondary suppression of renin levels.[407] Progressive loss of functioning renal tissue can also result in loss of renal vasodepressor hormones, thus raising blood pressure by yet another mechanism. Under these circumstances, the measurement of renin levels can give misleading results.[147]

INTRAVENOUS UROGRAM

The rapid-sequence hypertensive intravenous urogram or pyelogram (IVP) is a useful test for determining the anatomic location, shape, and size of the kidneys in relation to other intraabdominal structures, and for providing information on renal excretory function, presence of ureteral obstruction, intra- and extrarenal masses, cysts, tumors, and vascular or other calcifications.[408] The technique involves rapid intravenous injection of a radiopaque contrast medium followed by serial radiography at 1, 3, 5, 10, 15, and 30 min after injection.

Specific features on the urogram which suggest unilateral renal ischemia, that is, decreased renal blood flow, decreased GFR, increased fractional sodium and water reabsorption, increased renal transit time, and renal atrophy or infarction, include the following:[395,408–411]

1. Disparity in size (decrease in pole-to-pole length of the ischemic kidney as compared to the "normal" kidney of 1.5 cm or more)[412]
2. Delayed appearance and diminished concentration of contrast medium in the calyces on 1- and 3-min post-injection films
3. Late hyperconcentration and delayed washout of contrast agent from the calyces

The likelihood that unilateral renal artery stenosis is present increases when several of these abnormalities are present.[395,408–411,413,414] Among 175 patients in the Cooperative Study on Renovascular Hypertension who were subsequently cured by revascularization or nephrectomy and thus had true renovascular hypertension, 83 percent had an abnormality on the IVP, but the remaining 17 percent had a falsely negative IVP.[409,410] Among patients with normal renal arteries, 11 percent had one or more abnormalities on the IVP. Delayed appearance was the single most common abnormality in patients with proven renovascular hypertension and was seen in 59 percent of patients with renovascular hypertension but in only 2 percent of patients with normal arteriograms, while disparity in size was seen in 38 percent of those with renovascular hypertension and 5.6 percent of those with normal arteries.[410] Since many patients in the Cooperative Study were referred for arteriography because of an abnormality on the intravenous urogram, these figures are misleading. A further analysis of the Cooperative Study results shows that among patients with 50 percent or more stenosis, 78 percent had an abnormal urogram, whereas among patients with 100 percent stenosis, 95.7 percent had an abnormal urogram. In patients with essential hypertension, less than 1 percent had two or more abnormalities on the urogram, as compared to 45 percent of patients with unilateral renovascular hypertension. In the 250 patients with bilateral renal artery stenosis, 60.7 percent had abnormal urograms.[415]

In patients with renal ischemia of short duration due to recently developed renal artery stenosis, the degree of secondary renal atrophy may be slight and therefore not detectable by urography. On the other hand, asymmetry of paired structures occurs not infrequently in normal people and thus disparity in renal length may be a false-positive finding.[340e,412] Furthermore, since the IVP is based on renal asymmetry due to unilateral ischemia, bilateral lesions can be missed, since the difference in degree of severity between the two kidneys may be negligible.

Atkinson and Kellet found that useful information that changed the course of management was found in only 1 percent of 952 hypertensive patients studied by IVP;[416] Thornbury et al., reviewing results from the University of Michigan, found a 41.6 percent false-negative rate in patients who had renal artery stenosis proven by arteriogram.[417] Thus, as a screening test, the intravenous urogram is not very reliable, and, in fact, in many centers it is no longer routinely performed as part of the evaluation of a patient for renovascular hypertension unless a parenchymal renal lesion is suspected.[418] As a predictor of surgical outcome the intravenous urogram also has its limitations.[419] In the Cooperative Study, 83 percent of those whose blood pressure fell after renovascular surgery had an abnormal urogram, compared with 81 percent of those who failed to respond to surgery.[415] Grim et al. found an abnormal urogram in 76 percent of surgical responders.[420]

However, the IVP remains a useful test for defining renal structure and function as well as perirenal and adrenal anatomy. It is easy to perform and does not require specialized equipment or training. Unless renal artery stenosis is strongly suspected, in which case an arteriogram should be performed directly, the IVP is a reasonable screening test in patients with impaired renal function of unknown etiology.

The water-soluble urographic contrast media used for both intravenous urography and renal arteriography include diatrizoate, iothalamate, and metrizoate,[421] are hypertonic in solution and have direct chemical toxicity.[422] Newly developed compounds include nonionic monomers, monoacidic dimers, and nonionic dimers such as metrizamide, iopamidol, and ioxaglate. These have a lower osmolality and less toxicity and provide equal or better opacification, but they are not yet generally available.

Rapid intravascular injection of hyperosmolar ionic compounds results in rapid fluid and ion shifts from extracellular space into the vascular compartment, resulting in as much as a 16 percent increase in blood volume and cardiac output.[422–424] This is a problem especially in children and in patients with impaired renal function. Other effects include an increase in pulmonary artery pressure, peripheral vasodilation with a fall in blood pressure, tachycardia, and an increase in cutaneous blood flow. Serum calcium concentration falls abruptly because of a chelating effect of disodium edetate and sodium citrate, which are present as stabilizing agents, and electrocardiographic changes are common. Direct chemical toxicity results in vascular endothelial damage, red cell aggregation, release of histamine, subclinical bronchospasm, pulmonary edema, and neurotoxicity.[423,424] In addition, allergic reactions to the iodide can occur.

Spataro estimated from a review of the literature that minor adverse reactions to contrast media occur in 5 percent of patients who undergo IVP.[421] These include nausea, vomiting, urticaria, rash, light-headedness, and dyspnea.[421] More serious reactions occur in 1 percent of patients, including extensive urticaria, facial edema, bronchospasm, laryngeal edema, dyspnea, chest pain, and hypotension. Severe reactions occur in 0.05 percent, including life-threatening laryngeal edema, pulmonary edema, refractory hypotension, circulatory collapse, severe angina, myocardial infarction, cardiac arrhythmias, convulsions, and coma; cardiac arrest occurs in 0.017 percent and 0.0025 percent die.[421]

Nephrotoxicity is seen particularly in children and patients with preexisting renal insufficiency, diabetes mellitus, and the extracellular volume depletion formerly prescribed as preparation for urography.[424] The nephrotoxicity is manifested as usually reversible oliguria, anuria, proteinuria, and azotemia. The prevalence of renal toxicity, although low in the general population of healthy individuals, may be as high as 0.6 percent after urography in hospitalized patients without renal disease and as high as 2 percent after arteriography. These complications can largely be prevented by avoiding unnecessary contrast procedures (urography and arteriography), using smaller doses, avoiding dehydration before the procedure, and ensuring adequate hydration afterward. Newer agents again appear to have less renal toxicity and fewer unpleasant side effects.

RADIONUCLIDE RENAL IMAGING (RENAL SCINTIGRAPHY)

The radioisotopic renogram is a noninvasive procedure which provides information on renal function and morphology, renal blood flow, effective renal plasma flow, and GFR for each kidney individually. The test is potentially useful both as a screening test for renovascular hypertension and for predicting outcome from a revascularization.[425,426] The test requires no patient preparation and takes 1 to 2 h to perform. An isotope-labeled substance which is cleared by the kidneys is injected intravenously, and, using a scintillation camera (the Anger camera), both static and sequential dynamic scintigraphic images can be obtained. The rate of accumulation of radioactivity (the upward slope of the curve) and the disappearance or clearance (downward slope of the curve) of the radiolabeled tracer represent renal blood flow and excretory function, respectively. Renal artery stenosis (reduced renal blood flow) prolongs the upslope, increases the time to peak amplitude, and delays the clearance of the radionuclide.[427] Confusing results are seen in patients with low urinary flow rates, renal parenchymal disease, and pelvoureteral obstruction. The radionuclides used give a low radiation dose to the kidney. The currently most commonly used compounds are sodium *o*-[^{123}I]iodohippurate and ^{99m}Tc-DTPA, technetium 99m diethylenetriamine pentaacetic (^{99m}Tc-pentetic) acid.[422,429] [^{123}I]Iodohippurate has replaced [^{131}I]iodohippurate because of the lower radiation delivered to the subject for an equivalent dose.[422]

The qualitative visual comparison of the curves of the two kidneys has been replaced by a high-resolution computerized system with a low-energy parallel-hole collimator and videotape recorder linked to a data processor, which provides absolute quantitative information on the function and flow characteristics of each kidney.[428] Analysis of tracer transit time, renal perfusion from initial renal/aortic slope ratio, whole kidney and parenchymal transit time by deconvolution analysis, and decomposition of renal transfer functions with capillary and tubular phases can all be determined with these new modifications.[428,430–435]

The sensitivity of this procedure for detecting functional renovascular lesions ranges from 79 to 85 percent and the specificity from 74 to 81 percent.[436] Because of the large number of false positives and the low incidence of renovascular hypertension, the predictive value of this test is low, although better than that of the IVP.[437–439] However, data obtained by renal isotope scanning correlated well with the Howard-Stamey divided renal function test, with the saralasin test, and with renal vein renin determinations.[439] The test is of value in assessing the functional hemodynamic significance of a lesion seen on arteriography and thus predicting response to revascularization. Isotopic renograms are also used in the postoperative evaluation of renal blood flow and function following revascularization and in patients with renal transplants.[440,441]

DYNAMIC COMPUTER TOMOGRAPHY OF THE KIDNEYS

This test is performed by rapid intravenous injection of a bolus of contrast material followed immediately by rapid serial scans of the kidney (up to six scans in 21 s).[442] Time-density curves for perfusion with contrast material of the right and left renal cortices are obtained and compared with the aortic time-density curve. Normally, renal cortical curves parallel the aortic curve. Flattening of the time-density curve is an indication of underperfusion of the renal cortex. Renal blood flow to each kidney can be determined by multiplying the area under the perfusion curve by the transit time. This test can be used both as a screening test for renovascular hypertension and following revascularization or renal transplantation to assess the adequacy of the repair and continued patency of the vessels.[442]

ULTRASONIC DUPLEX SCANNING

This is another newer noninvasive diagnostic technique which combines a high resolution B-mode ultrasound imager with a pulsed Doppler spectral analysis flow probe to obtain flow velocity information from specific locations along medium and large arteries.[443] This technique was originally used for classifying the degree of narrowing in the carotid arteries, but lower-frequency transducers and improved signal-processing methods have permitted the application of this technique to the renal arteries. The technique, which does not involve radionuclides or contrast medium, may become a valuable screening test for renovascular disease.[444,445]

RENAL ARTERIOGRAPHY

Renal arteriography is the definitive technique for visualizing the renal arteries in order to determine the presence, location, etiology, extent, and degree of obstruction (Figs. 14-17, 14-18). The original two-needle translumbar technique was associated with a high morbidity due in large part to mechanical damage such as hemorrhage, thrombosis, and spinal cord injury and to nephrotoxicity from the older hypertonic contrast media.[446,447] This technique has been supplanted by the retrograde percutaneous femoral catheter technique of Seldinger.[448] This technique makes it possible to make multiple injections of contrast material and obtain multiple views while changing the patient's position and respiratory phase in order to facilitate visualization of the renal artery orifices and "unfolding" of tortuous overlapping vessels.[449,450] With the Seldinger technique, it is also possible to obtain selective renal arteriograms for better visualization of the primary branches of the renal arteries as well as intrarenal vessels.[451,452]

Use of the Seldinger technique and new contrast agents has reduced the number of complications dramatically. In earlier studies with this technique there was a fatality rate of around 0.11 percent and a 0.4 to 1.2 percent incidence of major complications (hemorrhage, thrombosis, renal injury).[453,454] More recently, the rate of all kinds of complications has been reduced further.[455] Hessel found the fatality rate to be 0.03 percent and the total rate of complications, both major and minor, to be 1.7 percent in a recent survey of 83,068 arteriograms.[456] It appears that the reduction of complications correlates best with the increasing experience of the arteriographer, the number of procedures performed annually, and the use of newer, less toxic contrast agents.[422,456]

Renal arteriography, in addition to permitting visualization of the main renal arteries and determination of the presence, degree, and pathologic etiology of the obstruction, permits visualization of the branch renal arteries as well as the presence of collateral circulation, poststenotic dilatation, accessory renal arteries, arterial aneurysms, and vascular malformations.[452,457] Bookstein and coworkers have emphasized the value of demonstrating collateral blood flow around a stenotic renal artery, using a pharmacoangiographic manipulation as a method to predict the success of surgery.[458] The degree of renal artery stenosis, measured as percent reduction in luminal diameter, has been used as a predictor of response to revascularization.[459] However, several observers have found lesions that result in more than 50 percent narrowing of the renal arterial lumen in patients without hypertension, or at autopsy in patients without prior history of hypertension.[406,460,461] Furthermore, early reports of results of surgery based solely on the appearance of the artery indicated that not all patients with arterial lesions benefited from surgery. The physiological significance of the renal artery stenosis, i.e., its role in the genesis of the hypertension, must therefore be demonstrated by other techniques before corrective revascularization is undertaken.

DIGITAL SUBTRACTION ANGIOGRAPHY

Digital subtraction angiography (DSA) is a relatively new radiographic technique for visualizing arteries. It involves an image intensifier video system which digitizes, transmits, and stores the radiographic image in a computer which subtracts the precontrast from the postcontrast images, thus cancelling out overlying bone, gas, and soft tissue shadows.[462–464] The image is enhanced and magnified electronically and is displayed on an oscilloscope. The contrast medium can be injected as a bolus (equal to the volume used for the IVP) into a peripheral vein (called *IVDSA*) or through a centrally placed venous catheter into the superior vena cava. The same digital subtraction technique can be used for intraarterial injections of contrast agent; this route results in a sharper image and requires a much smaller volume of contrast medium.[465–467]

The advantage of the IV technique is that it can be easily performed in outpatients without prior enemas or other preparation and is less invasive than the intraarterial procedure. The disadvantage is that the image is not as sharp and detailed as that obtained with conventional arteriography, the visualized field is small, bowel gas motion and peristalsis may interfere, and selective views cannot be obtained. The problem of peristalsis can be partially relieved by abdominal compression and IV administration of glucagon.[467] In patients with a low cardiac output adequate contrast levels are not achieved. However, the procedure is widely used as a screening test for renovascular hypertension, both in adults and children, and as a quick and easy test to evaluate the results of angioplasty or surgical revascularization. Correlation with standard arteriography is reported to range from 71 to 100 percent.[465,466] False-negative and false-positive results are each reported in about 10 percent of studies. IVDSA is advocated by many investigators as a safe, simple, low-cost outpatient screening procedure for renovascular hypertension, with sensitivity and specificity better than that of the IVP.[468] Hillman suggested an algorithm for the use of IVDSA: a negative test is followed by medical therapy, a positive test leads to renal vein renin determination and angioplasty, and an indeterminate test is followed by conventional arteriography.[466] However, other investigators recommend that IVDSA not be used for widespread screening and that neither its sensitivity nor its specificity warrant such a use.[146,467–471] In patients with extensive arterial disease, surgeons often find the IVDSA insufficient for planning the surgical approach and require additionally the performance of a conventional arteriogram for accurate definition of the lesion.

Kerlan et al. prefer using the intraarterial DSA, which provides better detail of small vessels, requires less imaging time hence providing less chance for motion artifacts, and requires only a fraction of the usual contrast agent dose.[467] The facility for rapid display of the image, since there is no time required for film processing, is of particular use during angioplasty procedures where repeated injections are needed for assessing the adequacy of dilation. The low dose of contrast agent required is an advantage in patients with impaired renal function. With the use of smaller catheters the intraarterial technique can be safely performed in outpatients with little patient discomfort. The intraarterial DSA has the further advantage over IVDSA that selective arteriography can be performed after the initial midline aortography to evaluate branch vessels, thus often providing sufficient detail for planning extensive microsurgical procedures. However, despite the increased contrast resolution of DSA, the technique provides decreased spatial resolution compared with conventional arteriography.[467]

In centers where the equipment for DSA is available, both the IV and intraarterial techniques are likely to replace conventional arteriography in the majority of cases.

DIVIDED RENAL FUNCTION TESTS

Measurement of the function of each kidney separately was previously used as a screening test for unilateral renal ischemia and as a predictor of surgical outcome. The test was based on the observation that a reduction in renal blood flow produced by renal artery constriction is associated with a marked decrease in urinary flow and sodium excretion with consequent hyperconcentration of nonreabsorbable solutes such as inulin and creatinine by the ischemic kidney when compared to the contralateral normal kidney.[472–478] The technique involves the placement of catheters in each ureter. Following this, urine samples are collected from each kidney and are analyzed for volume, osmolality, sodium, potassium, creatinine, and chloride concentrations. *p*-Aminohippurate and inulin clearances can be assessed in each kidney as a measure of renal plasma flow and GFR, respectively.[477–480] A positive test is an excellent indicator of surgical curability; a negative test, however, does not exclude curability.[395,480,481]

Differential renal function studies are now rarely performed, because similar information can be obtained less invasively with newer modifications of the isotopic renogram.[455,482] In addition, the procedure is time-consuming, associated with significant morbidity, and is technically difficult.[473,478] Furthermore, the test is of little diagnostic value in patients with segmental arterial disease or with bilateral renal artery stenosis. However, information obtained with the differential renal function test may be of some use in patients in whom nephrectomy is proposed to determine whether the remaining kidney is capable of maintaining adequate renal function.[482]

BILATERAL RENAL BIOPSY

Bilateral renal biopsy was proposed previously in conjunction with arteriography to assess the presence of intrarenal vascular disease (nephrosclerosis) in the contralateral nonischemic kidney that might preclude success with revascularization procedure.[483–485] However, because of the complications of percutaneous renal biopsy, this test is not recommended and has been superseded by less invasive ones.

PLASMA RENIN DETERMINATION

Proof that an arteriographically demonstrated anatomic lesion is functionally related to the hypertension rests on demonstration that the renin-angiotensin system has been activated. PRA can be measured in the peripheral blood or in the venous blood draining the ischemic kidney, or indirectly by demonstrating a fall in blood pressure following treatment with converting enzyme blockers or competitive antagonists of angiotensin II (e.g., saralasin).[289,290,486–489] Human renovascular hypertension resembles the early phase of the two-kidney, one-clip Goldblatt animal model (discussed earlier) in that the kidney with decreased blood flow secretes increased amounts of renin and the opposite, nonischemic kidney is suppressed and secretes less renin.[486–489] However, in patients with longstanding renovascular hypertension, the pattern is more like the one-kidney, one-clip animal model and resistance to angiotension II blockade occurs unless the animal is sodium-depleted.[490,491] Although earlier studies showed that many patients with increased PRA benefited from surgery, there were patients with increased PRA who did not have renovascular hypertension and patients who benefited from operation whose PRA was not elevated.[491,492]

Basal Plasma Renin Level

PRA should be measured in association with quantification of 24-h urinary sodium excretion and antihypertensive medication must be withheld for at least 2 weeks before measurement. In a study by Marks and Maxwell only 109 (56 percent) of 196 patients with cured renovascular hypertension had an increased PRA.[491] But by standardizing the technique and determining PRA after 4 h of ambulation, Pickering et al. found an increased PRA in 80 percent of patients subsequently improved by angioplasty.[487] Since discontinuation of medication is not possible in patients with severe hypertension, 20 percent of patients with proven renovascular hypertension have normal to low PRA, and approximately 15 percent of patients with essential hypertension have elevated PRA, random determination of PRA per se has limited use in screening for renovascular hypertension.[491] Further, in chronic renovascular hypertension, especially if both renal arteries are stenotic, extracellular fluid volume can increase and PRA can be suppressed.[492]

Blockade of the Renin-Angiotensin System

The accuracy of peripheral PRA measurement can be enhanced by blocking the renin-angiotensin system. Administration of the angiotensin II competitive antagonist saralasin in individuals with high-renin hypertension usually results in a fall in blood pressure, especially after prior sodium depletion.[140,493,494] In patients with essential hypertension and low plasma renin levels, the partial agonist properties of saralasin usually result in a rise in blood pressure.[139] However, because of the pressor response seen in patients without renovascular hypertension, and because there is a high frequency of both false positive and false negative responses, the saralasin test is no longer used as a screening test for renovascular hypertension.[494]

More recently, converting enzyme inhibitors have been used with greater success.[140,293,495–498a] Oral administration of captopril usually reduces blood pressure in 10 to 15 min with a peak fall at 90 min, and the magnitude of blood pressure reduction is proportional to PRA.[495] In patients with correctable renovascular hypertension and high PRA, converting enzyme inhibition not only lowers blood pressure but produces a reactive hyperreninemia due to blockade of the negative feedback exerted by intrarenal angiotensin II. This reactive hyperreninemia is less pronounced in patients with essential hypertension.[140,293]

The protocol for the captopril test is as follows: antihypertensive medications are withheld for 2 weeks if possible, especially diuretics and nonsteroidal anti-inflammatory agents.[496–498a] The patient is maintained on a normal or high-sodium diet, and a baseline, 24-h urinary sodium excretion is measured. The patient is seated for at least 30 min and blood pressure measurements are taken at 20, 25, and 30 min and averaged for a baseline. A blood sample is drawn for PRA determination. A crushed 50-mg tablet of captopril dissolved in 10 ml of water is administered orally immediately prior to the test. Blood pressure is measured at 15, 30, 45, 50, 55, and 60 min after captopril; at 60 min another blood sample is taken for PRA determination (stimulated PRA). The test is positive and predictive of correctable renovascular hypertension if (1) the stimulated PRA is 12 ng/ml per hour or more, and (2) the absolute increase in PRA is 10 ng/ml per hour or more, and (3) the percent increase in PRA is 150 percent or more, or 400 percent or more if baseline PRA is less than 3 ng/ml per hour. Since the absolute values for PRA differ in various laboratories, these criteria, taken from Muller et al.,[498a] may need to be modified depending on the individual test used; conversion factors for the commonly used renin test kits have been proposed.[498a]

In the series of Muller et al.,[498a] these criteria identified retrospectively, among 200 hypertensive patients without evidence for renal dysfunction, all 56 patients with proved renovascular disease. False-positive responses occurred in only two of 112 patients with essential hypertension and in six with secondary hypertension. The test was not as specific or sensitive in patients with renal insufficiency. In this series the decreases in blood pressure in response to captopril were greater on average than in the patients with essential hypertension, but there was a significant overlap between the two groups in the blood pressure responses in individual subjects. Thus, this test is recommended as an excellent outpatient screening test for renovascular hypertension.

Differential Renal Vein Renin Determinations

These measurements are described in the section on laboratory testing and are used both as a screen before proceeding to arteriography and following arteriography if a stenotic lesion is demonstrated, to determine its functional importance. A ratio of ≥ 1.5 between the renin level of the ischemic kidney and that of the nonischemic kidney predicts a fall in blood pressure after revascularization in 90 percent of patients, but a lower ratio does not preclude a response to revascularization. As many as 51 percent of patients with a lower ratio were cured by revascularization in one series.[491] In this study of 412 patients, of the 286 patients with lateralizing ratios of 1.5 or greater and arteriographic evidence of unilateral stenosis, 93 percent improved or were cured by surgery.[491] Among the 126 with unilateral disease who did not have lateralizing renal vein renin ratios, 64 were improved by surgery.[491] This high frequency of false-negative tests is in part due to the fact that in chronic renovascular hypertension the renin secretion by the ischemic kidney can become suppressed and lateralization can no longer be seen, especially if the patient is on a high-sodium diet or has impaired renal function. In patients with bilateral stenosis, bilateral suppression is often seen due to volume increase and renal vein renin determinations are of little help. Other factors causing nonlateralization of renal vein renins include high sodium intake; sympatholytic drugs, especially beta-adrenergic blocking agents; volume increase; branch or segmental disease; sampling errors; and assay errors.[495,497] Nevertheless, the incidence of false-negative tests can be reduced by using one of the stimulatory measures described in the laboratory testing section, and these are recommended.

Techniques to improve the sensitivity and specificity of the renal vein renin ratio include, among others, the one suggested by Vaughn: comparing $(V - A)/A$, where V = venous renin activity and A = arterial activity.[495] An increment of $(V - A)/A$ of ≥ 0.50 in one kidney indicates hypersecretion, while if $(V - A)/A = 0$ in the contralateral kidney, contralateral suppression is suggested. Methods for increasing renin secretion with vasodilators, volume depletion, blood pressure reduction, and upright tilting tend to exaggerate the difference between the ischemic and nonischemic kidney.[140,487]

In summary, renal vein renin ratios of greater than 1.5 are highly suggestive of angiotensinogenic hypertension, but a negative test does not exclude a curable lesion.

Sequencing of Diagnostic Tests for Renovascular Hypertension

Various protocols have been suggested for pursuing a diagnosis of renovascular hypertension using the above diagnostic modalities as screening tests.[146,420,470] It is impossible to perform these tests in search of renovascular hypertension on all hypertensive patients since, given the low prevalence of this condition, this blanket approach would have a low yield and high overall cost.[499] Thus, those patients that are evaluated are ordinarily selected along the lines discussed in the section on evaluation of the hypertensive patient. Figure 14-19 shows possible algorithms.

Once the routine history, physical examination, and laboratory tests have been performed and the patient has been shown to have significant hypertension and no contraindications to surgery, if renovascular hypertension is strongly suspected, the next step can be visualization of the renal arteries by digital subtraction angiography or regular arteriography. If a lesion is found, its functional significance can be assessed using renal vein renin determinations.

In patients chosen for evaluation in whom renovascular hypertension is less strongly suspected, the captopril test or isotope renogram (or less preferably, the IVP) is recommended as the next test. If these are positive, then the arteriography should be performed followed by renal vein renins if indicated.

In general practice and in areas remote from major medical centers, many physicians instead initiate standard antihypertensive therapy and only reconsider the possibility of renovascular hypertension if standard treatment fails, hypertension accelerates, or renal function deteriorates. However, with the availability of beta-adrenergic blocking agents and converting enzyme inhibitors, many patients with renovascular hypertension can be effectively treated; blood pressure can be reduced to normal and renal function may not deteriorate for many years, especially in patients with unilateral disease. Hence, this approach can lead to overlooking patients with curable disease and sentencing them to a life of drug therapy instead of a "cure."

Medical Therapy for Renovascular Hypertension

Medical therapy for patients with renovascular hypertension is something of an anachronism, since many patients are originally investigated because medical therapy of their hypertension is unsuccessful or in the hope of finding a surgically curable cause. Patients who are not candidates for operation or transluminal angioplasty should not have been subjected to the diagnostic studies of arteriography or selective renal vein renin determinations in the first place.

However, before the general availability of transluminal angioplasty, a procedure with relatively low morbidity for revascularizing the renal arteries, but after the availability of potent antihypertensive drugs, there was considerable controversy regarding surgical vs. medical therapy.[500–502] Surgery offered the chance for a definitive cure of the hypertension and preservation of renal function, and obviation of continued medical therapy. Medical control offered a lower immediate mortality and morbidity, especially in older patients with widespread arteriosclerotic disease, in whom perioperative mortality was high. Furthermore, since both atherosclerotic and fibromuscular lesions are known to progress, patients operated on for renovascular hypertension do require continued medical supervision; the cure from surgery may not be permanent. In most centers with skilled surgeons, patients were generally referred for operation unless major medical problems produced unacceptable risks. High operative mortality rates among poorly selected

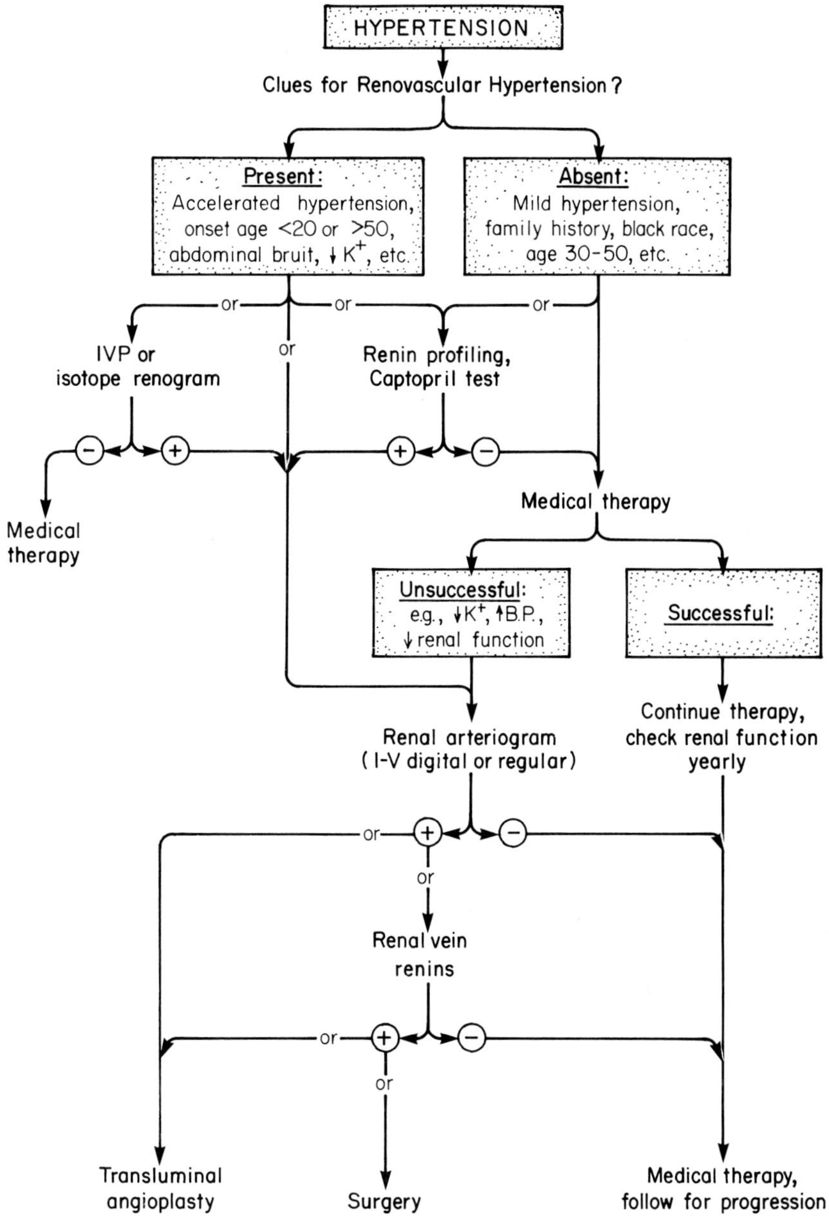

FIGURE 14-19 Algorithm for evaluating renovascular hypertension.

patients in centers with little experience favored a medical approach.

As radiologists and internists acquired skills in the use of balloon catheter angioplasty, this procedure has become more widely used, even in high-risk patients. Furthermore, the recognition that blood pressure reduction with converting enzyme inhibitors and beta-adrenergic blocking agents can cause renal failure in patients with bilateral renovascular disease or a stenotic artery to a solitary kidney has also helped to convince physicians that transluminal angioplasty or surgical revascularization is preferable to medical management in most patients, especially for preservation of renal function.[503-505]

Several investigators have compared the results of surgically vs. medically treated patients.[401,506-509] However, none of these series represents randomly selected patients and thus the results are difficult to interpret. Although atherosclerotic lesions are more likely to progress to renal failure if operation is not done, these patients are also likely to have a higher operative mortality and morbidity and a higher incidence of recurring hypertension as atherosclerosis progresses. On the other hand, patients with fibromuscular dysplasia tend to be younger and have a low operative mortality and morbidity, and surgery has a high success rate, but their lesions are less likely to progress if they are left unoperated and are treated medically. In an early report by Sheps and coworkers about 25 percent of medically treated patients with average follow-up of 20 months developed cardiovascular complications.[508] Most of these had atherosclerotic lesions. Similar results were reported by other investigators.[389,506,509] In these earlier studies it is possible that patients were selected for medical therapy because they were older and had more end organ damage, longer duration of hypertension, and greater risk for operative complications. Hunt and Strong reported in 1973 on 214 patients with renovascular hypertension and found that after 7 to 14 years the overall mortality was 16 percent among the surgically treated and 40 percent among the medically treated patients.[510] Many of these died despite relatively satisfactory blood pressure control. In another study of 41 patients with atherosclerotic lesions followed over 7 years, 42 percent (17) had a significant decline in renal function despite adequate blood pressure control.[504] Thus, it is important to obtain serial determinations of renal function in patients who are treated medically. Further, the adequacy of medical therapy varies widely in different centers. Hollenberg reviewed 11 reports between 1963 and 1982 on 269 patients with renovascular hypertension who were treated medically.[402] Controlled blood pressure was present in 29 to 92 percent of patients in various centers while failure of therapy was reported in 0 to 63 percent of patients.

In patients with renovascular hypertension, conventional therapy has been found to be moderately effective in the majority of patients. However, the oral converting enzyme inhibitors captopril and enalapril are particularly effective since they specifically block the effect of the hyperreninemia produced by the renal ischemia.[150] However, in patients with bilateral renal artery stenosis or stenosis in the artery to a solitary kidney, captopril and enalapril can lower intrarenal efferent arteriolar resistance to such a degree that GFR is reduced and acute oliguric renal failure results.[505,511] However, a similar decrease in renal function can occur following beta-adrenergic blocking agent therapy, which decreases cardiac output and hence renal blood flow.[512] Although the abolition of the autoregulation of glomerular filtration secondary to blockage of angiotensin II appears to be the primary cause, decreased arterial pressure, renal counterbalance, concurrent diuretic therapy, and other hemodynamic factors that maintain glomerular ultrafiltration pressure may also play a part. Nevertheless, these considerations emphasize the need for careful monitoring of renal function in these patients; if renal function deteriorates with medical therapy, revascularization therapy (discussed below) should be attempted.[513]

If a revascularization approach is planned, patients should be treated medically, with special attention to maintaining normal potassium levels, until the morning of the procedure. Intra- and postoperative hypertension can best be managed with continuous intravenous nitroprusside, which can be carefully titrated with a Harvard micropump or with intermittent boluses of 5 to 25 mg of hydralazine. Intravenous furosemide can be added on the third or fourth postoperative day when "third space" fluid mobilization occurs. Many patients, especially those with fibrodysplastic lesions, become normotensive immediately after surgery or angioplasty and require no further medical therapy. Patients with atherosclerotic lesions are slower to return to normal levels and may need to continue some of their preoperative medication for days to weeks after surgery.

Revascularization Approaches to Renovascular Hypertension

The only method for relieving an anatomic obstruction to renal blood flow is mechanical. Relief can be accomplished by transluminal balloon angioplasty or surgically, by resection, endarterectomy, bypass of the lesion, or replacement of the affected artery with endogenous or exogenous materials. Nephrectomy is indicated only if renal infarction or atrophy has occurred and revascularization is technically not feasible, since preserving functioning renal tissue is of prime importance.

The purpose of revascularization is to relieve the cause of the hypertension. In some patients, however, atherosclerotic renovascular hypertension is superimposed on preexisting long-standing essential hypertension, since hypertension accelerates the atherosclerotic process. In these patients, revascularization results in reversal of the superimposed accelerated hypertension, increases the ease with which blood pressure can be controlled medically, and preserves renal function, but does not "cure" the hypertension.

A successful outcome from revascularization is predicted by the tests described earlier and by certain clinical features including fibromuscular dysplastic lesions, young age, short duration of hypertension, unilateral focal lesions, evidence of collateral circulation, and normal renal function. A successful outcome from revascularization is less likely in older patients with atherosclerotic lesions, patients with impaired renal function, inadequate operative repair, residual intrarenal arterial disease such as nephrosclerosis, and coexistence of essential hypertension predating the development of renovascular hypertension.

Since none of the screening techniques for renal ischemia is 100 percent predictive, the considerations outlined above serve as guidelines for selecting the type of therapy. With the current availability of effective medications, as discussed above, nonoperative therapy can be selected in those patients who have poor prognostic indicators. Three factors have tilted the balance toward revascularization. One is the availability of percutaneous transluminal angioplasty, which can be safely performed even in elderly, seriously ill patients. As skill with this technique has become more widespread, more and more patients are undergoing angioplasty, since, even if stenosis recurs, repeat angioplasty is possible. The second factor is the recognition that in patients with bilateral renal artery stenosis or stenosis in the artery to a solitary kidney, especially if renal function is impaired, marked reduction of blood pressure can reduce renal perfusion to such a degree that renal failure can be precipitated. Revascularization, on the other hand, has the potential for improving both renal perfusion and function. Finally, the high perioperative mortality reported in older series, especially in debilitated patients with atherosclerotic lesions, bilateral lesions, and associated aortoiliac surgery, was largely due to associated coronary and cerebrovascular disease. Morbidity in these patients was due to postoperative myocardial infarction, congestive heart failure and cerebrovascular accidents, hemorrhage, hypotension, and acute renal tubular necrosis. It is the general policy now to perform carotid endarterectomy and coronary artery bypass grafting when indicated before undertaking renal and aortoiliac revascularization, thus decreasing the operative mortality and morbidity. Finally, operative techniques and experience have improved, and the perioperative management of patients in specially equipped intensive care units has reduced the perioperative morbidity and mortality considerably.[514a,514b]

SURGICAL TECHNIQUES

Endarterectomy

Endarterectomy, preferably transaortic, is an effective technique for removal of atherosclerotic plaques located in the aorta or at the orifices of the renal arteries. For more distal lesions, direct incision and endarterectomy is now rarely performed,[515] since bypass techniques are preferable.

Bypass Techniques

Various *bypass techniques* have been employed if resection of a lesion is not possible. Earlier experience using the splenic artery as a bypass to the left renal artery led to the use of other endogenous tissues such as the saphenous veins or hypogastric artery for bypass grafts.[516] Results using these techniques are detailed below in the section on results of revascularization procedures. Synthetic dacron grafts have also been employed, especially in patients in whom associated aortic aneurysm or extensive aortoiliac disease precludes the use of native vessels, and necessitates additional reconstructive grafting and bypassing. In patients with bilateral lesions, bypass grafting may be carried out as a one-stage or two-stage procedure.

Microsurgical Techniques

Revascularization by *microsurgical techniques* and autotransplantation is employed particularly for segmental disease, distal disease in the branches of the renal arteries, small intrarenal aneurysms, pediatric cases, and situations where "bench surgery" is necessary for repair of extensive lesions.[517]

Nephrectomy

Nephrectomy is now performed only if the kidney is atrophied and nonfunctioning or nearly totally infarcted, yet still produces renin. Although nephrectomy was formerly the procedure of choice, removal of potentially functioning renal tissue is now avoided if at all possible.[518] Even in patients with occlusion of a renal artery, if collateral circulation maintains some renal perfusion, revascularization is possible and should be attempted.[519] In patients with malignant hypertension, removal of a small ischemic kidney which is nevertheless "protected" from the impact of the markedly elevated blood pressure can actually result in progressive renal failure, since the remaining kidney which bears the brunt of the elevated pressure develops rapidly progressive nephrosclerosis.[520]

Segmental Resection

Segmental resection of a focal stenosis in a main renal artery with end-to-end reanastomosis of the artery is only applicable in arteries with focal stenotic segments due to intimal or medial fibroplasia. Not only is the lesion often too extensive to permit adequate excision and reapproximation of the cut ends of the vessel, but scarring and secondary stenosis may occur at the suture line. This technique is rarely used now.

TRANSLUMINAL ANGIOPLASTY

Transluminal angioplasty (PTLA) is a nonsurgical technique for relief of arterial stenoses applied first in peripheral vasculature, then in coronary arteries, and now widely used to dilate the renal arteries (Fig. 14-17). Dotter and Judkins in 1964 first performed PTLA in an elderly woman with femoral artery stenosis, using coaxial dilating catheters of successively greater diameters, passed over a guide wire.[521] In 1978 Grüntzig et al. reported the first successful use of the double-lumen balloon-tipped catheter for the treatment of renovascular hypertension.[522] The polyethylene double-lumen catheter is introduced percutaneously over a guide wire and is maneuvered so that the balloon is located at the site of the stenosis. It is then inflated to 4 to 6 atm for 10 s and deflated. This process can be repeated several times until a satisfactory result is demonstrated on angiography. Pressure gradients can be measured across the lesion before and after the procedure. The catheter is then withdrawn and prolonged pressure is applied at the femoral artery puncture site.[523] It is very important, however, to use a balloon size that will produce slight overdistention of the renal artery during dilation, otherwise stenosis is likely to recur. Sos and coworkers stressed the importance of a good initial cosmetic appearance following angioplasty as a predictor of long-term patency.[524]

Fibromuscular lesions can be "stretched" or dilated and atherosclerotic plaques can be fragmented, remodeled, and compressed or flattened against and into the vessel wall, thus enlarging the arterial lumen. Immediately after the procedure, the arteriogram shows roughening and fuzziness at the site of the lesion, suggesting that intimal abrasion and injury do occur, perhaps with rupture of the fibrous cap of the plaque in atherosclerotic lesions.[523] Hence, anticoagulation with heparin and antiplatelet drugs during and for a time following the procedure is generally recommended.

Angioplasty is a relatively low-risk procedure done under local anesthesia. The blood pressure usually falls promptly; the fall is maximal 6 h following the procedure. In experienced hands, complications with this technique occur in 5 to 10 percent of patients. The type of complications encountered include microcholesterol emboli in patients with atherosclerotic lesions, intimal dissection or raising of a subintimal flap, arterial thrombosis and acute renal infarction, arterial perforation, arterial spasm, hemorrhage at the percutaneous arterial puncture site, and balloon rupture.[523] In addition, in patients with impaired renal function, the load of contrast medium can lead to further deterioration of renal function.[467] Emergency surgery for arterial tear or balloon rupture or impaction is rarely necessary, but facilities should be available for such an eventuality.

Problems may also be encountered passing the catheter through tortuous femoral arteries. The axillary approach is associated with complications such as hematoma and brachial plexus injury. The most common reason for failure is inability to pass the guide wire across the stenosis in a lesion that is too tight, especially an arteriosclerotic lesion, or multiple lesions in a tortuous artery.[467]

Patients likely to respond well to angioplasty include especially those with fibromuscular dysplastic lesions which do not involve the primary branches and are not associated with aneurysms.[525] Atherosclerotic plaques can also be successfully fragmented and flattened, unless they are heavily calcified or contiguous with larger intraaortic periorifice plaques.[524] Transluminal angioplasty can be used in children and in stenoses occurring in the arteries to transplanted kidneys. Transluminal angioplasty is particularly useful for initial treatment of patients with renal insufficiency, especially high-risk patients with severe bilateral renal artery stenosis or critical stenosis in the artery to a solitary kidney, since revascularization can result not only in improved blood pressure control but also in improvement in renal function. In these patients, blood pressure reduction by medical means often results in further deterioration of renal function, and operative intervention carries a high morbidity and mortality.

Despite concerns voiced following the early experience, in many centers PTLA has become the first-line procedure for all patients with renal artery stenosis, unless they have indications mentioned above to exclude its use.[526] However, in centers where there is an active surgical revascularization program, surgery often continues to be the first-line approach.

RESULTS OF REVASCULARIZATION PROCEDURES

There is more information regarding the long-term results of surgery than of angioplasty. Stanley and Graham reviewed the operative results from six major medical centers spanning the period from 1958 to 1979.[527a] The combined results for 974 patients with atherosclerosis and 804 patients with fibromuscular dysplasia were: cure, 39 to 64 percent; improvement, 29 to 42 percent; failure, 11 to 35 percent; and operative mortality, 1.6 to 5.4 percent. The overall results from other studies were roughly comparable.[527b-531]

With better patient selection and preoperative establishment of the functional importance of arteriographically demonstrated lesions, improved surgical techniques, avoidance of nephrectomy, and careful perioperative management, the current surgical experience is much better. For example, recent reports from the Cleveland Clinic indicate nearly 90 percent improvement or cure with operative mortality of 0.5 percent.[530a] Overall, the more recent results from a number of medical centers are: among patients with fibrodysplastic lesions about 70 to 95 percent are cured or improved, with operative mortality approaching zero, while among patients with atherosclerotic lesions benefit was reported in 55 to 80 percent, with operative mortality ranging from 0 to 10 percent.[530b,531,532a–532c] Particularly dramatic results have been reported in children with renovascular hypertension;[532d] however, even in older (> 65 years of age) patients, marked benefit from revascularization is reported.[533a,533b] In addition, several authors have addressed the beneficial effect of revascularization on renal function, since this can continue to deteriorate despite or perhaps because of adequate blood pressure control in medically treated patients.[533c] Dean et al., using preoperative split renal function tests, were able to show improved function following surgical revascularization in 34 of 56 patients.[482]

Long-term results are excellent. In patients with an initial successful surgical result followed for a number of years, about one-third of patients with atherosclerotic disease and two-thirds with fibrodysplastic lesions have normal blood pressures.[534a,534b] Of the remainder, most have hypertension due to progression or recurrence of renovascular lesions, but some develop hypertension that does not appear to be renovascular in origin. Some patients with recurring or progressive disease can be re-treated.[534c] However, because of the progressive nature of both atherosclerotic disease and, to a lesser extent, fibrodysplastic lesions, continued regular follow-up of patients after surgery is important.

The earlier results of transluminal angioplasty of the renal arteries have been summarized in two reviews.[535,536] In five reported series of patients with fibromuscular dysplasia 47 to 83 percent were cured, 17 to 48 percent improved, and 5 to 18 percent were failures, with a total of 9 percent requiring nephrectomy for complications. In six reports on 173 patients with atherosclerotic lesions, from 4 to 44 percent were cured, 36 to 63 percent were improved, 8 to 60 percent were failures, and nephrectomy was subsequently required in up to 20 percent.[535,536] The earlier problems of intimal dissection and thrombosis with resulting renal infarction have largely been overcome by careful patient selection and antiplatelet therapy.

Martin and coworkers described subsequent results in successive groups of 100 angioplasties: the primary success rate increased from 93 to 97 percent, the total frequency of complications decreased from 20 to 13 percent, the rate of complications requiring surgical intervention decreased from 5 to 2 percent, and contrast-induced decreased renal function dropped in frequency from 10 to 5 percent.[537] These workers ascribe their success to new technical approaches for crossing the stenotic site, increased use of digital imaging during the procedure with less volume of contrast for each injection, better patient hydration and use of vascular sheaths at the femoral artery puncture site. Similar results are reported from other large centers where experience with angioplasty is accumulating rapidly.[538]

In a more recent summary of results from four centers with angioplasty in a total of 314 patients, the initial success rate was 85 to 94 percent and the patency rate, after 0.5 to 4.5 years, was 71 to 90 percent. Lack of a uniform method for follow-up makes these results somewhat difficult to compare, since only patients with recurring hypertension were restudied by some investigators while others performed repeat studies more routinely.[538]

It is apparent, therefore, that angioplasty as a first-line procedure is gaining popularity over surgical management in the majority of patients since it carries a lower cost, and morbidity and the initial results are comparable. The long-term role of angioplasty remains yet to be determined, and continued regular follow-up of all patients is necessary.

ALDOSTERONE EXCESS (PRIMARY ALDOSTERONISM)

Occurrence and Classification

Primary aldosteronism is the most frequent type of hypertension caused by the adrenal gland. Primary aldosteronism is defined as a condition in which there is increased and inappropriate production of aldosterone by the zona glomerulosa of the adrenal gland, leading to a mineralocorticoid excess state. Cortisol production is normal. This disorder should be considered in all hypertensive patients. The exact prevalence of this syndrome among hypertensive patients has yet to be defined precisely. Although it was originally predicted that up to 20 percent of patients with essential hypertension may have primary aldosteronism, it is more likely that less than 2 percent of unselected hypertensive patients have this disorder.[295,296] Primary aldosteronism occurs in all age groups but has its peak incidence during the third and fourth decades. This coincides with the peak decades of recognition of essential hypertension.

Three principal pathologic types occur (Table 14-8): unilateral benign adrenocortical adenoma, bilateral

Table 14-8. Syndrome of Primary Aldosteronism

Aldosterone-producing adenoma
Bilateral adrenocortical hyperplasia
Idiopathic aldosteronism
Glucocorticoid-suppressible aldosteronism
Surgically remediable aldosteronism
Unilateral adrenocortical hyperplasia
Adrenocortical carcinoma

adrenocortical micro- and macronodular hyperplasia, and adrenocortical carcinoma (rare). It is important to distinguish between adenoma and hyperplasia; patients with unilateral adenoma have excellent results from unilateral adrenalectomy, whereas most of those with hyperplasia do not respond to bilateral adrenalectomy. However, the hyperplastic syndromes show some heterogeneity in their presentation. The hypertension in a few patients does respond to bilateral adrenalectomy and more rarely responds to glucocorticoid treatment. There is also active inquiry as to whether hyperplasia represents an extreme variant of low-renin essential hypertension. All these subsets retain their characteristics with no progression from one hyperplastic syndrome to another. Thus, the possibility of a continuum or a progression from hyperplasia to adenoma seems unlikely. Most large series clearly indicate a greater incidence of adenoma in women (about 70 percent), but the prevalence of the hyperplastic disorders is equally divided between the sexes.[539]

Differences in pathophysiology and, hence, techniques to differentiate between these major forms of primary aldosteronism have been proposed because new mechanisms of aldosterone regulation have been recognized (see Chap. 12). In particular, pituitary factors have been implicated in the development of bilateral adrenocortical hyperplasia (discussed below).

ADENOMA

In the case of aldosterone-producing adenoma, increased production of aldosterone initiates a series of events that result in the clinical abnormality. However, it is not clear that excessive aldosterone production is the primary event in the case of hyperplasia, even though a number of the clinical features of hyperplasia and adenoma are similar. The following discussion focuses on the pathophysiology of primary aldosteronism due to aldosterone-producing adenoma.

The actions of aldosterone on ion transport (Chap. 12) lead to increased sodium retention, increased extracellular fluid volume, and an increase in total body sodium content, and they are further reflected by normal or elevated serum sodium concentrations and reduced hematocrit.[540] Although the effects on the kidney are the greatest quantitatively, the other secretory tissues also participate in this effect. Fecal excretion of sodium can be decreased so much that it is virtually absent.

Increases of the extracellular fluid and plasma volume are registered by stretch receptors at the juxtaglomerular apparatus and by sodium chloride flux at the macula densa with resultant suppression of renin secretion.[295] As a result, the usual parallel relationships between the renin system and aldosterone production are abolished or greatly suppressed. Thus, increased aldosterone production in the presence of a suppressed renin system identifies this disorder.

The increased distal tubular reabsorption of sodium and possibly other actions of the mineralocorticoids (see Chap. 12) lead to increased tubular electronegativity, which favors the movement of hydrogen and potassium ions into the lumen with resultant excretion in the urine.[541,542] Potassium depletion eventually develops, decreasing the total body concentration of the ion. Alkalosis and increased production of ammonia result from the progressive potassium depletion.[543] The hypokalemia also leads to decreased carbohydrate tolerance and resistance to vasopressin (nephrogenic diabetes insipidus).

There is compelling evidence that sodium and fluid overload is essential for the initiation of mineralocorticoid hypertension,[544] although it may not be the sole mechanism.[545,546] With the continued oversecretion of aldosterone and sodium retention, there is also a major redistribution of fluid with an increased intracellular sodium content in tissues.[547] This may explain the increased vascular reactivity that is present, which probably contributes further to the blood pressure elevation. It is also possible that direct actions of aldosterone on other organ systems such as the vasculature and the central nervous system contribute to the production of hypertension; however, there is no direct support for these ideas.

Potassium depletion and magnesium depletion may further contribute to the hypertension. With progressive depletion of potassium ion, abnormalities in baroreceptor functions have been demonstrated; postural falls in blood pressure without reflex tachycardia and a negative Valsalva maneuver without the hypertensive overshoot or bradycardia can be observed.[548] Thus, potassium depletion appears to diminish the activity of the adrenergic nervous system. The effect of this is to make the blood pressure even more dependent on the intravascular volume and less dependent on the nervous system than it ordinarily is. In this case, the mineralocorticoid-induced tendency to an increased intravascular volume has an even greater effect on the pressure than without hypokalemia. This also creates another problem with therapy. If a diuretic such as hydrochlorothiazide is administered to these patients (which should not be done), the combined loss of sodium and potassium can result in a precipitous lowering of the blood pressure and potassium concentrations to dangerously low levels. Hypomagnesemia increases vascular reactivity (see also the section on magnesium)[181] and further perpetuates the hypertension associated with primary aldosteronism.

With the development of sustained hypertension, as with all forms of hypertension, the body apparently attempts to compensate by decreasing the plasma volume. Thus, even though the increased level of exchangeable sodium and extracellular fluid volume persists, patients with long-established hypertension can have normal blood volumes.[547] Under these circumstances, the hypertension may be due, to a large extent, to the increased peripheral vascular resistance with normal cardiac output.[545-547] Nevertheless, even in this circumstance the continued actions of the excess mineralocorticoids contribute to the hypertensive state: removal of an adenoma or treatment of hyperplasia with mineralocorticoid antagonists can ameliorate the hypertension.

Some time (e.g., months to years) may in many cases be required for hypertension to develop. Indeed, short-term administration of large amounts of mineralocorticoids to normotensive subjects usually does not result in a sustained increase in blood pressure,[549] even though the mineralocorticoid does promote sodium retention. It is possible then that associated and more slowly developing events in the arteriole, such as intracellular changes in ionic concentrations or other long-term effects on vascular reactivity, must also take place in order to produce a sustained elevated blood pressure during the long-term administration of mineralocorticoid. Potentially, patients with primary aldosteronism who are not hypertensive may exist because those factors that determine the vascular response either are not present or have not yet emerged as a result of chronic oversecretion of the mineralocorticoid. Indeed, a history of transient hypertension during pregnancy is common in women who have this disorder. However, normotensive primary aldosteronism has only rarely been reported.[550]

The short-term effects of administration of large amounts of deoxycorticosterone acetate (DOCA) to normotensive subjects differ from those in patients with borderline or established hypertension. The borderline hypertensive patient becomes normotensive during hospitalization. Administration of DOCA to such patients results in sodium and water retention and a normal pattern of mineralocorticoid "escape" (see Chap. 12). At the moment of escape, hypertension recurs in these patients. It is inferred that either a structural or a biochemical abnormality not present in the normotensive subjects is triggered by the steroid at the point the escape mechanism comes into play in these patients, possibly by either volume increases or intracellular ionic changes.[551] The presence of such an abnormality may permit the more rapid development of hypertension in primary aldosteronism. When DOCA is administered to patients with sustained essential hypertension or primary aldosteronism, there is little or no acute sodium retention or change in the blood pressure, indicating that they are already in an escape state. This probably reflects the body's efforts to adapt to the hypertension from any of a number of causes by secreting salt maximally.[551]

Because aldosterone biosynthesis is intensified, it is not surprising that the entire biosynthetic pathway becomes activated. Steroids such as DOC, corticosterone, and 18-OHB, which are precursors to aldosterone, are present in increased amounts and released into the circulation.

HYPERPLASIA

In the case of primary aldosteronism due to bilateral hyperplasia of the adrenal glomerulosa, aldosterone excess and hypokalemia are present. In general, the aldosterone excess and the potassium depletion are not as severe in hyperplasia as in adenoma. Although suggestive, these parameters cannot be used as definitive markers to differentiate the two major forms of hyperaldosteronism.[295] However, as a consequence of the decreased aldosterone production, the production of other steroids in the aldosterone biosynthetic pathway (DOC, corticosterone, and 18-OHB) is not as increased, and measurement of plasma 18-OHB concentration has proved to be useful in differentiating adenoma from hyperplasia (see below). Although PRA is markedly suppressed, it responds slightly but significantly to postural or other stimuli and when this happens there is a substantial increase in aldosterone production.[552,553] The hyperplastic adrenal gland appears to be excessively sensitive to angiotensin II so that it is still stimulated by the low quantities of angiotensin II generated by the low renin levels. Also in contrast to the case with adenoma, aldosterone release can be suppressed in a few patients with hyperplasia by maneuvers such as sodium loading or mineralocorticoid treatment.[296] Thus, overall, aldosterone production with hyperplasia is not as autonomous as in adenoma.[296] The ability to suppress aldosterone levels with these maneuvers in some patients has sometimes led to their subclassification as "indeterminate hyperaldosteronism" (IHA).[296] In general these patients have less severe hypokalemia and less suppressed PRA. However, this classification has not been useful clinically, since these patients respond well to spironolactone therapy, and it is not clear whether the differences between these patients and others with hyperplasia are quantitative or qualitative.

In most cases of primary aldosteronism with hyperplasia the hypertension is not corrected by either adrenalectomy or blockade of aldosterone action by spironolactone, even though the latter does correct the hypokalemia. These observations suggest that factors other than aldosterone initiate and sustain the hypertension. Thus, the aldosterone excess may be an associated problem that could aggravate the hypertension and lead to hypokalemia, but is not itself the primary problem. However, it is not known what the primary initiating event is. Since there is increased adrenal sensitivity to angiotensin II, it might be speculated that the syndrome is due to an overall increased sensitivity to this peptide. Although this hypothesis needs further testing, consistent with it is the finding that the hypertension in many of these patients does respond to blockade of angiotensin II production with converting enzyme inhibitors.[554]

There is active inquiry as to whether other factors are involved in stimulating the adrenal in patients with hyperplasia. As reviewed in Chap. 12, several of the peptides of pro-opiomelanocortin (POMC) have been shown to either stimulate aldosterone production or augment the actions of the major stimuli to aldosterone release. For these reasons, analogous to Cushing's disease, pituitary factors are candidates as inducers of hyperplasia of the zona glomerulosa. A patient with bilateral adrenal hyperplasia with documented primary aldosteronism associated with basophilic hyperplasia of the anterior and intermediate lobes of the pituitary gland has recently been described.[555] Immunohistochemistry demonstrated the presence of ACTH-like peptides in the basophilic cells, which suggests that hyperplasia of the pituitary was related to adrenal hyperplasia in this patient. In other studies, circulating levels of pituitary factors have been found to be elevated in patients with hyperplasia but not those with adenoma. Plasma β-endorphin levels were elevated in 10 patients with hyperplasia and normal in four patients with adenoma.[556] The concentration of a putative plasma aldosterone stimulating factor (ASF) was elevated in seven patients with idiopathic hyperplasia, but was normal in four patients who had had adrenal adenomas surgically removed.[557] Urinary levels of ASF also were not suppressed by administration of dexamethasone. However, efforts to define this factor precisely have been unavailing. Griffing et al. reported that patients with idiopathic hyperaldosteronism have significantly higher levels of plasma immunoreactive α-melanocyte stimulating hormone (α-MSH) than patients with aldosterone-producing adenomas.[558] They suggested that this difference may be due to an abnormality of the pars intermedia, where POMC-derived products may be under positive serotonergic control and negative dopaminergic control and are unresponsive to glucocorticoid feedback inhibition. This was supported by the report that the serotonergic antagonist cyproheptadine acutely decreased aldosterone production in six patients with hyperaldosteronism due to hyperplasia, but not in eight patients with adenoma.[559]

A postulated mechanism for the development of hyperplasia is that hyperactivity of certain serotonergic neurons stimulates pituitary production of an ASF and some of the POMC derivatives. Increased levels of ACTH and Cushing's disease would not necessarily develop because of different processing of ASF and POMC by different areas of the pituitary.[560] Increased circulating levels of ASF would lead to hyperplasia of the zona glomerulosa and increased sensitivity of aldosterone production to angiotensin II.

The hypertension in a minority of patients with bilateral adrenal hyperplasia does respond to adrenalectomy or spironolactone therapy.[534] These patients could represent a fundamentally different subgroup. Alternatively, patients with hyperplasia may vary in the extent to which their blood pressures respond to aldosterone excess, and patients of this subgroup, whose hypertension responds to adrenalectomy, could be the ones whose blood pressures are more sensitive to the steroid. A patient with surgically correctable primary aldosteronism was recently described where aldosterone dynamics more nearly resembled those in patients with adenoma.[560a] This may represent a variant form of the disorder.

There is a glucocorticoid-remediable form of aldosteronism with hyperplasia that is rare, occurs primarily in young men, and can be familial.[561,562] In these patients all the biochemical abnormalities can be reversed after 2 to 3 weeks by moderately low doses of glucocorticoids (1 to 2 mg of dexamethasone daily). Although administration of dexamethasone in these doses can sometimes lower plasma aldosterone concentration into the normal range in the more common types of hyperplasia and even in patients with an adenoma, the plasma aldosterone concentration will return to elevated levels after 24 to 48 h.[563] However, in patients with glucocorticoid-remediable aldosteronism, normalization of the plasma aldosterone concentration and the other biochemical abnormalities including the hypertension will persist with continued therapy. The plasma aldosterone concentration is only mildly elevated in these patients; thus some as yet unidentified mineralocorticoid may also be operative in these persons. Observations with mineralocorticoid receptor studies support this hypothesis.[564] Recently, significantly increased urinary excretion of 18-oxocortisol, a relatively weak mineralocorticoid, has been described in this syndrome.[565] Gomez-Sanchez et al. postulated that patients with glucocorticoid-remediable aldosteronism may have a maturational abnormality of the adrenal cortex, resulting in increased capability of producing aldosterone, cortisol, and 18-oxocortisol, the last resulting from the metabolism of cortisol through the 18-methyloxidase enzyme system.[565] The mechanism whereby dexamethasone restores all the abnormalities to normal values is not clear, but the aldosterone (and other putative mineralocorticoids, if they exist) may be under ACTH control and their production may be blocked by the dexamethasone-mediated inhibition of ACTH production. Indeed, large doses of ACTH administered intravenously for 5 days to these patients produce sustained increases in both plasma and urinary aldosterone levels.[566] The normal mechanism whereby aldosterone production is only transiently stimulated by ACTH is not operative in these patients.[567]

A few cases of unilateral nodular adrenal hyperplasia have been described.[568] The dynamics of aldosterone release have shown variable patterns, such that they can resemble those with either adenoma or bilateral hyperplasia. The hypertension and hypokalemia in these patients responds to unilateral adrenalectomy, and of those patients so treated who have been followed for several years, recurrence of primary aldosteronism has not been reported.

History and Physical Findings

Patients usually present because elevated blood pressure was detected on a routine screening or because of symptoms of hypokalemia. Thus, the medical history may not reveal any characteristic symptoms. Mild potassium depletion may produce no symptoms at all or the nonspecific complaints of tiredness, loss of stamina, weakness, nocturia, and lassitude. If depletion is more severe with alkalosis, increased thirst, polyuria, paresthesias and cardiac palpitations due to arrhythmias may occur. This disease is now recognized earlier than in the past, and thus the incidence of flaccid paralysis resulting from extreme potassium depletion has decreased. Headache is a frequent incidental complaint.

Excessive production of mineralocorticoids produces no characteristic physical findings. The diagnosis is made after being aware of the possibility of the disorder in a hypertensive patient. Retinopathy is mild and hemorrhages are rarely, if ever, present. Postural falls in blood pressure without reflex tachycardia are observed in the severely potassium-depleted patient. Although the extracellular fluid volume is increased, clinical edema is practically never seen. A positive Trousseau's or Chvostek's sign may reflect the alkalosis accompanying severe potassium depletion. The heart is usually only mildly enlarged if at all, and electrocardiographic changes are usually those of modest left ventricular hypertrophy and potassium depletion, although arrhythmias may also be seen.

Hypertension

Blood pressure in patients with primary aldosteronism can range from borderline to severe hypertensive levels; the Hypertensive Research Unit in Glasgow has reported a value as high as 250/160 mmHg.[539] The mean blood pressure in the 136 patients reported by the unit was 205/123 ± 21/18 (SE) mmHg and the means for the adenoma and hyperplasia groups did not differ significantly. Accelerated (malignant) hypertension is extremely rare in patients with primary aldosteronism even though renal biopsies may occasionally show some fibrinoid necrosis typical of accelerated disease. Before primary aldosteronism was recognized and appropriately treated, long-standing hypertension resulted in the expected consequences, congestive heart failure, stroke, and repeated episodes of pyelonephritis and consequent renal failure. These complications occurred in all patients before the syndrome was defined and still occur in older patients. A history of transient hypertension during pregnancy is frequent in female patients who develop this disorder. Changes in the renin system during pregnancy may activate or intensify aldosterone production to levels that produce some clinical manifestations of an aldosterone-producing lesion in a subclinical state.

Initial Diagnosis

The hallmarks of this disease are hypertension with hypokalemia, suppression of the renin-angiotensin system, and increased aldosterone production in the presence of normal cortisol production. Determination of the presence or absence of hypokalemia is the initial most important screening procedure and should be carried out for all hypertensive persons. An outline of suggested steps in the workup is provided in Fig. 14-20.

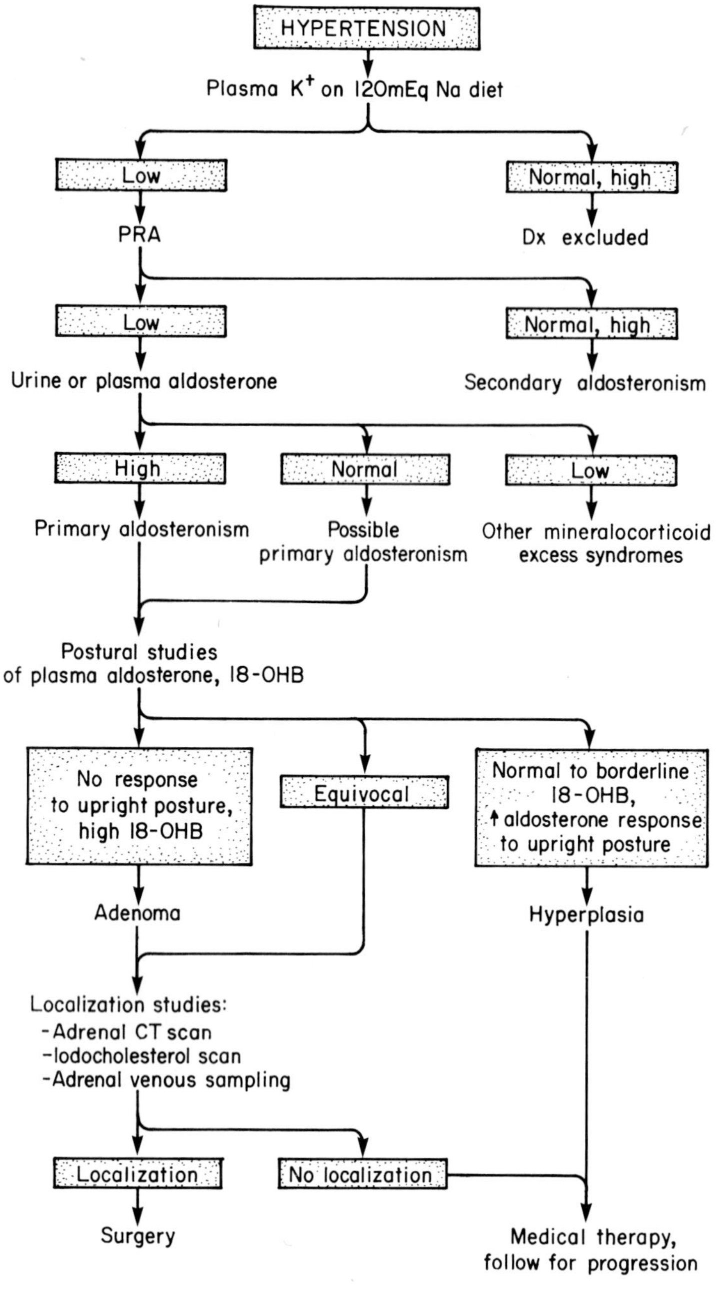

FIGURE 14-20 Flow diagram for diagnosis of primary aldosteronism and differentiation of adrenal adenoma from hyperplasia.

Care must be taken to control the sodium intake or balance in the patient before serum electrolyte levels are measured; serum potassium concentration and 24-h urinary excretion of potassium are closely related to and determined to a great extent by sodium chloride intake in these patients. A low-sodium diet can correct major potassium abnormalities by retarding potassium secretion in the distal tubule as the amount of sodium ion available for reabsorption and exchange is reduced. On sodium intakes greater than 120 meq per day, hypokalemia should be apparent in most patients with primary aldosteronism by the fourth day of this regimen (Fig. 14-21). Excessive renal potassium secretion should also be demonstrable under these conditions. Thus, a urinary potassium excretion of $>$ 50 meq/24 h is inappropriate in the presence of hypokalemia. However, up to 20 percent of patients with primary aldosteronism may have normal serum

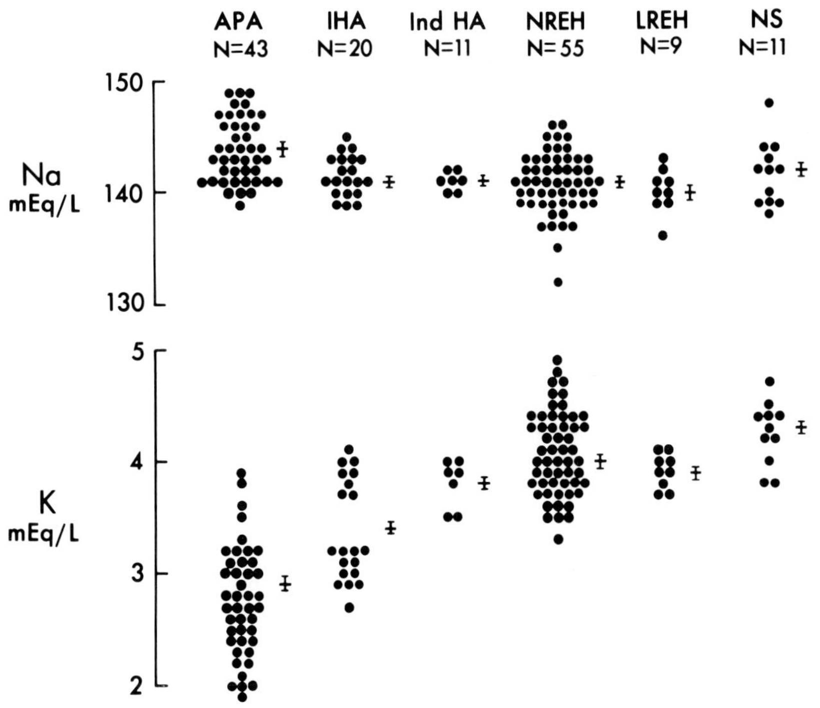

FIGURE 14-21 Serum sodium and potassium concentrations on a 120 meq sodium intake in patients with an aldosterone-producing adenoma (APA), idiopathic hyperplasia (IHA), indeterminate hyperaldosteronism (Ind HA), normal-renin essential hypertension (NREH), and low-renin essential hypertension (LREH) and in normal subjects (NS). High-salt challenge was not performed.

potassium concentrations, depending on the laboratory and its criteria for sodium intake;[295] many of these, however, are patients with hyperplasia (Fig. 14-21). Regardless, almost all patients with primary aldosteronism have a serum potassium concentration of < 4.0 meq/liter, whether or not this value is considered to be within the normal range for the laboratory (Fig. 14-21). In the presence of normal renal function and aldosterone excess, salt loading should be effective in unmasking hypokalemia as a manifestation of potassium depletion. Normokalemic aldosteronism under these conditions has been reported, and although its frequency is not established, it is probably rare.[539] Multiple measurements of serum potassium concentration during vigorous sodium loading would be necessary to determine the true prevalence of normokalemic aldosteronism.

In the United States, Japan, and Europe, among other areas, the average person consumes over 110 to 120 meq of sodium per day, enough to allow hypokalemia to be manifest. Thus, in practice, if such a dietary history is obtained and the serum potassium concentrations are normal on three occasions, further workup for primary aldosteronism is probably not indicated unless there are other reasons (e.g., inappropriate hypertension, Table 14-5) to pursue the diagnosis.

Previous diuretic therapy always poses a problem in interpreting serum potassium concentrations and is the most common cause of hypokalemia in patients with hypertension. The patient should be off diuretics for at least 3 weeks. Normal dietary intake of potassium will restore depleted potassium levels that are not related to primary aldosteronism. Potassium excretion may decrease immediately after cessation of diuretic treatment in the absence of primary aldosteronism. Sudden falls in serum potassium concentration when hypertensive patients are placed on diuretics are no indication that primary aldosteronism exists, but marked changes such as paralysis or profound weakness may reflect the disorder.

There are a number of other causes of hypokalemia in patients with hypertension. These include excessive gastrointestinal loss due to vomiting or diarrhea, other mineralocorticoid excess or "mineralocorticoid-excesslike" syndromes (discussed later), starvation, insulin and glucose therapy, metabolic alkalosis, renal disease, renovascular hypertension, and accelerated hypertension. These can be ruled out with the tests described below.

In the initial screening procedure, careful scrutiny of the serum or plasma concentrations of sodium (Fig. 14-21), potassium, and bicarbonate and the hematocrit also yields important clues to the presence or absence of a mineralocorticoid excess state. Carbohydrate intolerance and failure of urinary osmolality or specific gravity to increase are additional manifestations of the decrease in total body potassium. Careful attention should also be paid to the serum or plasma sodium concentration. In the absence of previous diuretic therapy, concentrations < 139 meq/liter are rare in primary aldosteronism, but they are common with diuretic therapy (Fig. 14-21). A high serum presence of a reduced hematocrit (due to increased extracellular fluid and plasma volume from sodium retention) is presumptive evidence of a mineralocorticoid excess state (Fig. 14-21).

If hypokalemia is documented, or if there are other indications that further evaluations are necessary, PRA and aldosterone should be measured (Fig. 14-20). A random measurement of unstimulated PRA is indicated, because in patients with primary aldosteronism the pathophysiology with increase in the extracellular fluid volume results in continuous suppression of PRA; therefore, factors such as posture, eating, exercise, salt intake, and to some extent even diuretic therapy tend to have a minimal influence on suppressed PRA in patients with this disorder. Thus, if PRA is normal or high in a patient who has been off diuretic therapy for 3 weeks, it is extremely unlikely that primary aldosteronism is present. If the random PRA is suppressed in this setting, no assessment is required in a stimulated state. If the random PRA is marginally suppressed and hypokalemia and aldosterone excess are present, further stimulating maneuvers of the renin system are indicated. These are discussed in the preceding section on renin laboratory testing. PRA that remains suppressed under these circumstances is strong corroborative evidence that a mineralocorticoid excess state exists, especially if hypokalemia is present. The risks must be carefully weighed, since these patients are extremely sensitive to volume depletion and show major changes in serum potassium concentration. Fainting and cardiac arrhythmias can occur.

If the random aldosterone concentration is ele-

Table 14-9. Common Biochemical Parameters and Blood Pressure Responses in Low-Renin Hypertension

	Syndrome of primary aldosteronism					
		Adrenal hyperplasia			Congenital adrenal hyperplasia	
	Aldosterone-producing adenoma	Idiopathic	Indeterminate	Glucocorticoid-remediable	11α-Hydroxylase deficiency	17α-Hydroxylase deficiency
PAC after overnight recumbency	> 20 ng/dl	< 20 ng/dl	< 20 ng/dl	V	↓	↓
PAC after 2–4 h upright	↓	↑	↑	V		
Cortisol	N	N	N	N	N to ↓	↓
Corticosterone	N	N	N	N	N to ↓	↑
DOC	occ ↑	N	N	N	↑	↑
18-OHB	↑	N to slight ↑	N	±	↓	↑
18-OHDOC	occ ↑	N	N	N	↓	↑
PRA	↓↓	↓	↓	↓	↓	↓↓
PAC after DOCA maneuver or fludrocortisone	0	0	↓	±	±	±
Blood pressure response to spironolactone	+	0	+	±	±	±
Blood pressure response to dexamethasone	0	0	0	+	+	+

Note: PAC, plasma aldosterone concentration; DOC, plasma deoxycorticosterone concentration; 18-OHB, plasma 18-hydroxycorticosterone concentration; 18-OHDOC, plasma 18-hydroxydeoxycorticosterone; PRA, plasma renin activity; N, normal; V, variable; ±, not established; ↑, increased; ↓, decreased; ↓↓, markedly suppressed; 0, no change; +, response; occ, occasionally.

vated in the face of suppressed PRA, the diagnosis of primary aldosteronism is confirmed. If the random plasma aldosterone determination is normal or only borderline elevated, a 24 h urinary aldosterone determination should be made. If this is also borderline, maneuvers to suppress aldosterone production should be performed. These include either the high-sodium diet, fludrocortisone acetate administration, or IV saline administration as described in the preceding section on renin laboratory testing. A clearly low aldosterone level suggests the presence of other mineralocorticoid excess syndromes.

Determination of the Etiology of Primary Aldosteronism

Several features are helpful in distinguishing an adenoma from hyperplasia (Table 14-9). First, an adenoma generally produces more aldosterone and secretes significantly larger amounts of the immediate biosynthetic precursor of aldosterone, 18-OHB.[304,554] Second, with the recent improvements in CT scanning, anatomic identification of the adrenal glands can be of major help in differentiating adenoma from hyperplasia.[554] If 18-OHB level and adrenal CT scanning do not confirm a diagnosis, other localization studies such as ^{131}I-cholesterol scanning[569,570] and adrenal vein catheterization and bilateral sampling[571,572] can be useful. In addition, the observation that the plasma aldosterone concentration in patients with hyperplastic glands is still under the control of the renin-angiotensin system, whereas that of patients with an adenoma is mostly under ACTH control, can be helpful. Finally, glucocorticoid treatment can be useful to identify rare patients with glucocorticoid-remediable aldosteronism. The diagnostic accuracy is listed in Table 14-10.[554]

Table 14-10. Diagnostic Tests Used to Differentiate Adenoma from Hyperplasia in Primary Aldosteronism

Test	Accuracy, %*
18-OHB determination	90
Postural testing	60–90
CT scan	~70
Iodocholesterol scan	80–90
Adrenal venous sampling	95

$$^{*}\%\ \text{Accuracy} = \frac{\text{Number of true positives plus number of true negatives}}{\text{Number of tests}} \times 100$$

Source: Taken from Ref. 554.

18-OHB

18-OHB concentration is invariably increased in patients with an adenoma to levels > 100 ng/dl, and there is no overlap of these levels with the normal or slightly elevated levels of this steroid in patients with hyperplasia when sampled at 8 A.M. after overnight recumbency (Fig. 14-16).[304] This clear-cut separation of 18-OHB levels without overlap is in part due to the fact that potassium depletion influences aldosterone production by retarding the final conversion of 18-OHB by dehydrogenation to aldosterone. The more normal the potassium concentration, the less likely that its influence on 18-OHB levels will be apparent.[304] Elevated levels of plasma 18-OHB concentration are less frequently observed in patients with adrenocortical hyperplasia because the plasma potassium concentration is generally not low enough to show the same influence.[296,304] Plasma DOC and corticosterone levels are frequently increased at 8 A.M. in patients with adenoma, whereas they are rarely elevated in patients with hyperplasia. Nevertheless, differences in 18-OHB levels between adenoma and hyperplasia patients are greater than for the other steroids, so that 18-OHB concentration is one of the best indicators of adenoma. In centers where this measurement cannot be made, reliance must be placed on the other means for differential diagnosis.

CT SCANNING

CT scanning is being used with reasonably good success in localizing adrenal tumors causing Cushing's syndrome or pheochromocytomas, which are rather large compared to aldosteronomas, many of which are 1 cm or less in diameter. It can nevertheless be used to identify the larger aldosteronomas.[554,573,574] In a study of 23 patients with adenoma causing primary aldosteronism, CT scan was 70 percent accurate in localizing the adenoma (Fig. 14-22). All nodules of ≥ 1.5 cm diameter were recognized and 50 percent of nodules 1.0 to 1.4 cm in diameter were identified.[573] High-resolution CT scanning improves the sensitivity of the technique, especially for smaller-size lesions. In comparison, bilateral adrenal venous sampling accurately located the tumor in 22 of the 23 patients; one patient had an adenoma diagnosed by CT scan, but venous sampling was insufficient. Problems with detection of small adenomas occur with CT scanning if the adenoma is totally surrounded by normal adrenal tissue, such that the tumor produces no defect in the center of the gland, or in patients who lack sufficient retroperitoneal fat, which is necessary to delineate adrenal anatomy. Nevertheless, continual efforts to improve the resolution capabilities of the CT scan

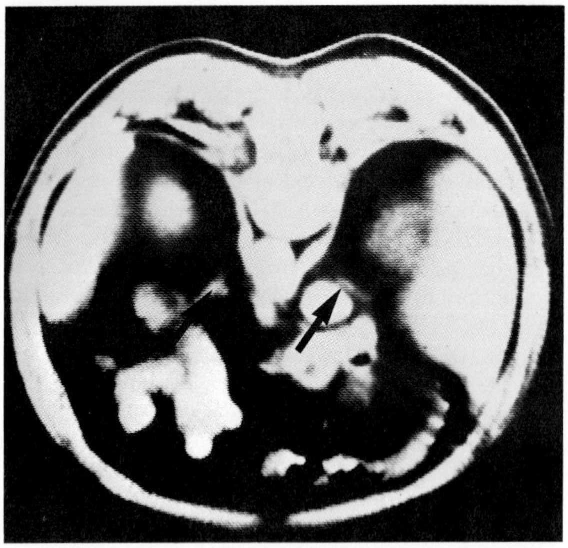

A

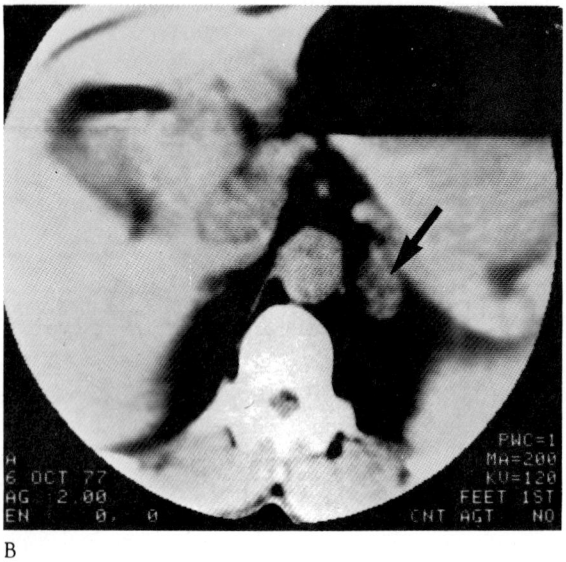

B

FIGURE 14-22 Coaxial computerized tomography of (*A*) hyperplasia and (*B*) an adrenal adenoma in patients with primary aldosteronism.

hold great promise to make this technique a standard diagnostic approach to differentiate adenoma from hyperplasia (Fig. 14-22).

BILATERAL ADRENAL VEIN CATHETERIZATION

Bilateral adrenal vein catheterization with sampling for plasma aldosterone and cortisol continues to be a useful procedure in determining the side the tumor is on.[554,571,572] This technique is currently used in the approximately 20 percent of patients with an adenoma that is not identifiable by CT scan and in the very small group in whom biochemical studies have not clearly differentiated an adenoma from hyperplasia. Samples from the caudal inferior vena cava are also obtained. A higher cortisol concentration in the adrenal vein sample than that in the caudal vena cava helps to document that the catheter is actually in or near the adrenal vein. Failure to catheterize the right adrenal vein is especially apt to happen because of visualization difficulties. A major increase in the concentration of aldosterone in one adrenal vein relative to that in the caudal vena cava or the contralateral adrenal vein is indicative of a unilateral source for the excess aldosterone. If the biochemical evidence strongly suggests a tumor, catheterization of only the left adrenal vein may yield sufficient information; i.e., if there is a considerable increase in the plasma aldosterone concentration between peripheral and left adrenal venous blood samples, the adenoma is most likely in the left adrenal gland. In contrast, if the plasma aldosterone concentration in the left adrenal vein is similar to that in the periphery, it can be inferred that aldosterone production by the left adrenal gland is markedly suppressed and therefore that the adenoma is in the right adrenal gland. One group of investigators has used simultaneous ACTH infusions to help block the possible episodic secretion of ACTH that can occur in patients with tumors,[295] although this has not been found to be necessary. The diagnostic accuracy of the results of bilateral adrenal vein catheterization has been adequately confirmed.[554,571] Thus, with technical proficiency and familiarity with adrenal vein sampling, which are essential, this is a valuable diagnostic tool.

Adrenal venography was one of the first techniques used to attempt to locate the tumor. This procedure was usually performed at the time of adrenal vein catheterization after the plasma samples for steroids had been taken. However, a number of difficulties have occurred, such as extravasation of dye, hemorrhage, and adrenal infarction,[575] making this a potentially traumatic procedure. Tumors < 1 cm in size are not located by this technique, and the success rate in identifying adrenal tumors has varied between 60 and 70 percent. Thus, this procedure is rarely performed.

IODOCHOLESTEROL SCANNING TECHNIQUE

For iodocholesterol scanning,[569,570,575,576] [^{131}I]6β-10-iodomethyl-19-nor-cholesterol (NP-59) is administered slowly (over 3 min) IV and the patient is scanned 1, 3, 5, and 7 days after the injection. Lugol's solution, three drops daily for 2 weeks, is given starting 1 to 2 days before iodocholesterol injection to avoid thyroid uptake of radioiodine. Dexamethasone, 1 mg every 6 h, is administered 7 days before the iodocholesterol injection and continued for the duration of the procedure to suppress zonae fasciculata and reticularis uptake of radioactivity. The patterns of uptake generally seen are: (1) unilateral uptake before 5 days after tracer injection, which usually indicates unilateral hyperfunction; (2) bilateral uptake before 5 days after tracer injection, consistent with bilateral hyperfunction; and (3) bilateral uptake 5 days or more after tracer injection, compatible with bilateral microscopic hyperplasia or normal function.[576] The diagnostic accuracy for localization of aldosteronomas by this technique has been reported to be $\geq$ 90 percent.[577]

CIRCADIAN AND POSTURAL CHANGES IN PLASMA ALDOSTERONE LEVEL

In addition to the information provided by the plasma aldosterone concentration at 8 A.M., the pathologic cause can be inferred by examining the circadian rhythm of aldosterone production. Under normal circumstances the rhythm has two peaks: an increase occurs with upright posture between 8 A.M. and 12 noon, followed by a decline throughout the day, and then a second peak occurs in the early morning hours[297,578] (see also Chap. 12). If the subject remains supine, only the early morning peak is seen; this is associated with increased ACTH release occurring at that time. Similarly, if a patient with primary aldosteronism remains recumbent for 24 h, the plasma aldosterone levels also follow the pattern of ACTH release. However, in patients with an adenoma, in contrast to normal subjects, the plasma aldosterone concentrations generally show no significant change or decrease in response to assumption of upright posture; after 2 to 4 h in the upright position the plasma aldosterone concentration falls in 90 percent of these patients (Fig. 14-13). Even in those (< 10 percent) who show a slight increase, the overnight recumbent value is > 20 ng/dl and the increases are less than in normal subjects, i.e., less than a doubling of the level. This general lack of a posture-induced increase in aldosterone levels in patients with adenoma is due to the renin system's profound suppression and consequent insensitivity to posture induced by the increased plasma volume attributable to excessive aldosterone production. The fall or downward drift of plasma aldosterone levels in these patients between 8 A.M. and noon may reflect the diminishing influence of ACTH due to its circadian rhythm. In contrast, the response to postural changes in patients with hyperplasia is quite different. The plasma aldosterone concentration almost always increases after 2 to 4 h in the erect posture (Fig. 14-14). In these patients with idiopathic aldosteronism, the observed increase in plasma aldosterone concentration is due in great part to the increased sensitivity of the hyperplastic gland to minute but definite changes in renin production that occur with assumption of upright posture (Fig. 14-14).[563]

The effectiveness of the postural studies is dependent on attention to the details of preparation. Thus, if clear-cut differences in the postural response in hypokalemic, hypertensive, renin-suppressed hyperaldosteronemic patients are present, the postural changes identify an adenoma over 90 percent of the time, although lower success rates were reported when different methods of patient preparation were employed.[295,554,579] Equivocal responses can be evaluated further by more frequent sampling during a 24-h period, which will yield a discriminating pattern, or by other studies described below. In interpreting the results, however, it must be kept in mind that episodic secretion of aldosterone, which may or may not be ACTH-dependent, occurs both in normal subjects and in patients with primary aldosteronism and that physiological stimuli such as posture or exercise can increase the plasma aldosterone concentration to quite high levels in normal subjects.

The adrenal sensitivity to angiotensin II in patients with hyperplasia led to the suggestion that there may be differential responses between hyperplasia and adenoma patients to inhibitors or agonists of the renin-angiotensin system. Although useful in differentiating primary aldosteronism from essential hypertension, converting enzyme inhibition does not differentiate adenoma from hyperplasia.[580] Saralasin, a partial angiotensin II agonist, does show promise in separating these two entities. Brown et al. demonstrated a significant increase in plasma aldosterone concentration following administration of saralasin to eight patients with hyperplasia, while no significant rises occurred in six patients with adenoma.[581]

SALINE INFUSION TEST

A saline infusion test has recently been developed that, based on a small number of patients, shows promise for the differentiation of patients with adenoma vs. hyperplasia.[581a] For the test, patients receiving a balanced diet containing 120 meq of sodium receive an IV infusion of 1250 ml of isotonic saline between 8 A.M. and 10 A.M. after overnight recumbency. Plasma samples are obtained immediately before and after the infusion, and the ratio of 18-OHB/cortisol is measured. This ratio increases in patients with aldosterone-producing adenoma but remains unchanged or decreases in patients with hyperplasia. The ratios increase in primary aldosteronism presumably due to the greater effect, over the time of study, of the diminishing circadian rhythm and ACTH on cortisol release from the normal adrenal compared to 18-OHB release from the adenoma. The saline infusion would have little influence on this ratio in adenoma, since the PRA is suppressed and the tumor is not under angiotensin II control. By contrast, the saline infusion decreases significantly the release of 18-OHB by the hyperplastic tissue that is in part under angiotensin II control, so that the 18-OHB/cortisol ratio will not increase. Similar results are obtained with measurements of the aldosterone/cortisol ratios, but these do not discriminate the two conditions as well.

GLUCOCORTICOID TREATMENT

Glucocorticoid treatment is useful to detect that subgroup of patients with bilateral hyperplasia who have the glucocorticoid-remediable form of the disorder, since it will normalize the blood pressure and hypokalemia in this subset of patients, but not in other forms of primary aldosteronism.[561-564] Patients identified as belonging to this subset can be treated long-term with a glucocorticoid such as dexamethasone.[561-564] Precise protocols for the diagnostic test have not been standardized, and, because of the rarity of the syndrome, most specialists do not perform the test in hyperplasia patients. However, it may be useful to perform the test in those patients with primary aldosteronism and hyperplasia who are younger, have a positive family history or have marked hypertension and hypokalemia inappropriate to their plasma and urinary aldosterone levels.

DIAGNOSIS OF SURGICALLY REMEDIABLE HYPERPLASIA (PRIMARY HYPERPLASIA)

The subset of patients with primary aldosteronism that has been designated as surgically remediable primary hyperplasia were identified in the past when adrenalectomy was performed for both adenoma and hyperplasia. The identification of responsive hyperplasia patients based on clinical features is difficult; the characteristics are mostly those of patients with idiopathic hyperplasia. These patients may have slight elevations in the plasma of precursor steroids, DOC, and 18-OHB, as well as plasma aldosterone concentration values that resemble 8 A.M. values associated with an adenoma, showing minimal changes with posture. Normalization of blood pressure and serum potassium concentration is achieved with spironolactone. At present, these slight differences do not appear to be sufficient indication to identify this group and therefore indicate surgery.

Treatment

Treatment depends for the most part on the precision of diagnosis. In patients with an aldosterone-producing adenoma without contraindication for surgical intervention, unilateral adrenalectomy is recommended. The blood pressure response to spironolactone before surgery provides a surprisingly close approximation of the actual response to surgery, although greater reductions often occur postoperatively, presumably because of a greater reduction of extracellular fluid volume. The surgical cure rate of hypertension associated with an adenoma is excellent (> 50 percent in several series, with reduction of hypertension in another 25 percent).[295,551,583-587] Normalization of blood pressure in 60 to 70 percent has been reported, and hypertension decreased in all other patients. However, it is disturbing that 10 years after surgery hypertension, but not primary aldosteronism, recurs in approximately 40 percent of patients[551] and usually requires antihypertensive drugs. Thus, the final evaluation of the effects on blood pressure of surgical removal of an adenoma may require a number of years.

Preoperative treatment with 200 to 400 mg of spironolactone daily is recommended. This should be continued until the blood pressure and serum potassium concentration are normalized. This drug is particularly beneficial owing to its unique mechanism of action, i.e., as an antagonist blocking steroid binding by the mineralocorticoid receptor. These high doses normalize blood pressure, reduce the expanded sodium spaces, restore normal serum potassium concentration, and promote potassium retention in 1 to 3 months. Once normalization of the blood pressure and the serum potassium level has occurred, the dosage can be reduced gradually to maintenance, approximately 100 to 150 mg of spironolactone per day. During the initial treatment period, further confirmation of the diagnosis can be obtained by demonstrating that PRA has not increased nor has aldosterone production been altered during the first few days. Spironolactone therapy also has the desirable effect of usually activating (after 1 or 2 months) the suppressed renin-angiotensin system.[588] This will stimulate the suppressed zona glomerulosa of the nonadenomatous adrenal gland so that postoperative aldosteronism with hyperkalemia is rare. Treatment will also permit reversal, to some extent, of some of the target organ changes that have been produced by the hypertensive and hypokalemic states.

The side effects of spironolactone stem largely from its antiandrogenic capabilities. Spironolactone has been demonstrated to both impair testosterone production and compete with testosterone for its cytosolic receptor on target organs.[589] Thus, loss of libido and gynecomastia have been reported in up to 80 and 40 percent, respectively, of male patients persistently ingesting spironolactone. Menstrual irregularities have been reported in women. Rash and epigastric discomfort occur rarely.

Interestingly, spironolactone bodies appear in the adrenal cortex during the first 4 to 5 weeks of therapy and then disappear. These intercellular whorls several microns in size are seen in the glomerulosa on histologic examination. Their function is unknown, but they often appear in relation to transient decreases in aldosterone production, which may result from interruption by the drug of the late steps of aldosterone synthesis[590] (also see Chap. 12).

Amiloride (a diuretic that retards potassium secretion and sodium entry), up to 20 to 40 mg per day, has been used instead of spironolactone and effected similar reductions in blood pressure and correction of hypokalemia.[554,586]

Since mobilization of intracellular calcium is a final common pathway for angiotensin II, potassium, and possibly even ACTH (see Chap. 12), calcium channel blockers may also be helpful in the medical management of primary aldosteronism.[298a,591] In addition, calcium antagonists inhibit smooth muscle contraction, thereby reducing vascular resistance. This is the major mechanism by which calcium channel blockers decrease blood pressure.[592,593] Nadler et al. demonstrated that nifedipine decreased blood pressure and plasma aldosterone levels in five patients with adenoma and five patients with hyperplasia.[298a] After 4 weeks of nifedipine administration (20 mg sublingually tid), four patients with hyperplasia and two with adenoma had decreases in plasma aldosterone levels and normalization of blood pressure and serum potassium levels. Addition of spironolactone with nifedipine led to supranormal elevations of serum potassium levels, which suggests that combinations of antialdosterone agents should be used with caution. In another study, nifedipine was found not to be as effective as spironolactone, so further evaluation of the effects of calcium channel blockers is necessary.[591]

The transperitoneal surgical approach has been employed for many years with good success.[585] However, with lateralization techniques the unilateral posterior approach has been employed with considerably less postoperative morbidity. Unilateral adrenalectomy is generally performed. If the tumor is identified at surgery, exploration of the contralateral adrenal gland is not indicated.

If there are contraindications for or if the patient refuses surgery, treatment with spironolactone can be effective. The initial dose of 200 to 400 mg of spironolactone per day must be continued for 4 to 6 weeks before the full effect on blood pressure is realized. With prolonged treatment aldosterone production increases, probably because of modest activation of the renin-angiotensin system by potassium replenishment and diminution of expanded sodium and fluid volume.

Medical therapy is recommended for patients with hyperplasia. Although surgery, such as with subtotal adrenalectomy, will correct the hypokalemia in these patients, it ordinarily does not normalize the blood pressure.[295,551,583-587] As mentioned earlier, even though there are occasional patients in whom removal of an adrenal mass has ameliorated hypertension,[295,585] identifying them prior to operation is difficult; because of the infrequent occurrence of this condition, subtotal adrenalectomy seems inadvisable at this time.

In patients with idiopathic hyperplasia, large doses of spironolactone alone are useful for treating the hypokalemia, but the drug alone is usually ineffective in controlling the hypertension. Thus, other antihypertensive measures must be added to normalize blood pressure. Calcium channel blockers may prove to be useful for treatment of hyperplasia,[298a] although they may not be effective in all patients.[591] Further understanding of the pathophysiology of hyperplasia may suggest new treatment modalities. For example, inhibitors of aldosterone stimulating factor, antagonists of the POMC derivatives whose concentrations are elevated in the plasma of patients with hyperplasia, or ANF may be useful. The antiserotonergic agent cyproheptadine has been reported to decrease aldosterone concentration in hyperplasia patients;[559] however, effects on blood pressure and potassium concentration and long-term effects on aldosterone production have not been reported. Whether other agents that alter neurotransmitter function will be helpful remains to be determined.

In patients with indeterminate aldosteronism, spironolactone alone is usually effective in controlling both the hypertension and the potassium-depleted state.[296] Often all other antihypertensive medications can be discontinued because of the effectiveness of spironolactone in these patients. In this respect, these patients resemble more those with aldosterone-producing adenoma than those with hyperplasia.[296]

In patients with glucocorticoid-remediable aldosteronism, a replacement dosage of 1 to 2 mg of dexamethasone per day normalizes blood pressure and hypokalemia in 3 to 4 weeks; prolonged treatment with 1 to 2 mg per day is necessary to maintain normal blood pressure and potassium concentration.

Pathologic Findings

A number of pathologic abnormalities are associated with primary aldosteronism. Adenomas are, with rare exception, unilateral.[295,539,585] In instances in which hyperplastic adrenal glands have been examined, micro- and macronodular forms of hyperplasia have been found. The characteristic adenoma (Figs. 14-22, 14-23) is readily identified by its golden yellow color. In addition, small satellite adenomas are often found, and distinction from micro- or macronodular hyperplasia can be difficult. In these patients the contiguous adrenal gland can show hyperplasia of the glomerulosa or micro- or macronodular hyperplasia throughout the gland.[539,585] Often this pathology is also present in the contralateral adrenal gland but is not associated with aldosterone abnormalities after removal of the primary adenoma.[585] The adenoma is composed of cell types resembling those of all three zones of the adrenal gland, including hybrid cells resembling zonae glomerulosa and fasciculata cells. These hybrid cells in monolayer cultures can produce aldosterone, corticosterone, and cortisol.[539]

The nodules of the hyperplastic adrenal gland are different and are composed of lipid-laden cells with the light and electron microscopic features of cells of the zona fasciculata. These nodules are reported to make cortisol but not aldosterone.[539]

Carcinoma

Adrenal carcinomas (see Chap. 12) exhibit a varied pattern of steroid production. Mineralocorticoids are secreted in excess in many cases, and when this occurs it is not unusual to find increased production of several different mineralocorticoid hormones; i.e., DOC, corticosterone, cortisol, and aldosterone.[594] In fact, it is rare to find a patient with a malignancy in whom aldosterone alone or its immediate precursors are the only steroids produced in excess. In the cases in which there is excessive production only by the mineralocorticoid pathway, the survival rate seems to be prolonged slightly; progression of the disease from local metastatic lesions usually takes years before more widespread metastasis occurs. Most patients with adrenal carcinomas are first seen because of symptoms related to excess androgens, glucocorticoid hormones, or mineralocorticoid hormones or a large tumor mass (see Chap. 12). The plasma concentrations of mineralocorticoid hormone can be extremely high. For instance, the finding of a plasma aldosterone concentration over 100 ng/dl should raise a strong suspicion of the possibility of malignancy. The disease is typified by the lack of any consistent pattern of the particular

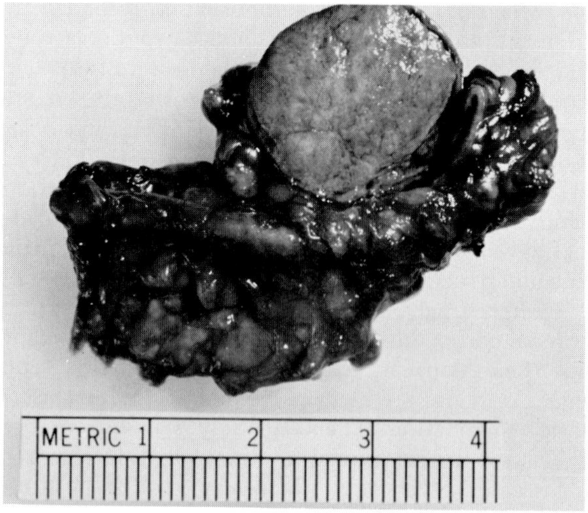

FIGURE 14-23 Aldosterone-producing adenoma. Note lack of suppression in the contiguous adrenal gland.

steroids whose concentrations are elevated. Furthermore, steroid production does not respond to stimuli such as postural changes, ACTH, and salt loading (Fig. 14-15). Changes in the clinical course are usually identifiable by sudden or gradual increases in aldosterone production and the appearance of increasing amounts of other adrenal steroids. Adrenal carcinomas associated with primary aldosteronism usually do not concentrate iodocholesterol. The reason for this is not clear, but it may well be related to the size of the tumor. Malignant lesions, when identified, are usually large, i.e., > 6 cm. Thus, the iodocholesterol may be too diffuse within the tumor itself to be adequately visualized by this technique. CT scan and intravenous pyelography may be adequate for locating the tumor.

DEOXYCORTICOSTERONE EXCESS HYPERTENSION

The best-defined circumstances in which DOC excess plays a role in hypertension are with the syndromes in which there is defective 11β or 17α hydroxylation of steroids. As discussed earlier, DOC excess may also occur and contribute to the hypertension in certain cases of Cushing's syndrome (particularly with ectopic ACTH production), adrenal adenoma and adrenal carcinoma. As discussed earlier, marked elevations of DOC level (e.g., > 70 to 100 ng/dl) are probably required for significant effects to occur, and these do occur in the following syndromes. Although the DOC excess in these states appears to be the major factor in inducing the hypertension, other steroids can be produced.

Hypertension and Congenital Adrenal Hyperplasia

Congenital adrenal hyperplasia is an autosomal recessive disorder (Fig. 14-24, Table 14-9; see also Chap. 12). Its most common type, 21-hydroxylase deficiency, is not associated with hypertension. The two forms associated with hypertension, 11β-hydroxylase and 17α-hydroxylase deficiencies, are rare but can usually be readily identified. The salient features of these disorders are listed in Table 14-9, and the site of the defect is depicted in Fig. 14-24.

11β-Hydroxylase deficiency syndrome is usually recognized in infants and children because of virilization and the frequent presence of both hypertension and hypokalemia. Although growth is accelerated, the ultimate height achieved by these patients tends to be abnormally low. Plasma levels of 17α-hydroxyprogesterone and its urinary metabolite pregnanetriol and urinary levels of 17-ketosteroids are increased, similar to the simple virilizing form, 21-hydroxylation deficiency. The defect is usually partial so that some cortisol is produced, but it does not increase with further stimulation by ACTH. The level of cortisol finally attained is in part due to the increased ACTH production in the presence of cortisol deficiency. Blood levels and production rates of cortisol are usually within normal limits or slightly decreased.[595] A partial defect of 11β hydroxylation with increased ACTH levels results in increased production and blood levels of DOC, 11-deoxycortisol (compound S), and androgens.[595-597] Hypertension results from excessive production of DOC by mechanisms previously described for aldosterone. The blood levels and production rates of aldosterone are normal or reduced.[596,598] Several mechanisms are proposed. First, there is partial inhibition of 11β hydroxylation in the zona glomerulosa, a required biosynthetic step for aldosterone synthesis. The constancy of this block is supported by the fact that after normalization of DOC production and correction of the hypertension, aldosterone production remains reduced[599] and is not increased by sodium restriction. In fact, a salt-losing state may be provoked by initial treatment with dexamethasone.[599] Second, suppression of renin release by increased production of DOC could suppress the normal production of aldosterone in the zona glomerulosa. This notion is supported by the increase in renin and aldosterone production after suppression of ACTH and reduction of DOC production.[598] Probably, both proposals are correct, depending on the degree of the retardation of aldosterone synthesis by the enzymatic block on one hand, and the increased DOC production suppressing renin on the other. The 11β-hydroxylating defect in the glomerulosa may not be manifest to the same degree in the fasciculata. This is suggested by the normal levels of 18-hydroxy-DOC (a zona fasciculata steroid) observed in this condition. Current evidence suggests that the 11β- and 18-hydroxylating enzymes are the same.[598,600]

The 17α-hydroxylase deficiency syndrome is usually recognized at the time of puberty in young adults by the presence of hypertension, hypokalemia, and primary amenorrhea in the female or pseudohermaphroditism in the male.[601,602] These features become more evident at this time because of the increased steroid production associated with puberty. In contrast to the 11β hydroxylation defect, there is no viril-

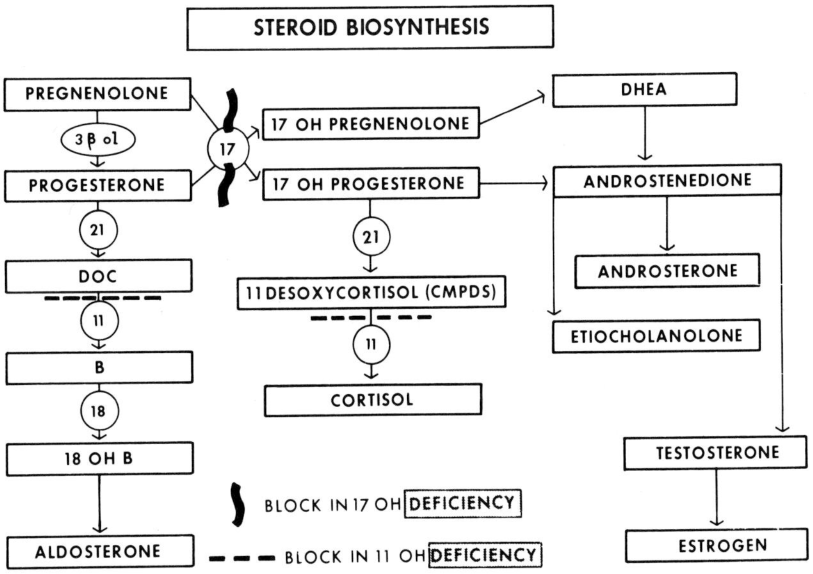

FIGURE 14-24 Enzymatic blocks in congenital adrenal hyperplasia associated with hypertension and 11β- and 17α-hydroxylase deficiencies.

ization or restricted growth. Patients often present with eunuchoid proportions and appearance. The usual measurement of 17α-hydroxyprogesterone, pregnanetriol, and ketosteroid concentrations is almost diagnostic by the virtual absence of these compounds.

The key location of the 17α-hydroxylating system in the steroid biosynthetic pathway prevents normal production of androgens and estrogens. There has been no instance in which the adrenal defect appears without a concomitant gonadal effect.[602] Thus, the defect seems to be one in a single gene that either codes for the enzyme or else affects the expression of the gene for the enzyme. The diminution of cortisol production with this deficiency syndrome precedes increased production of ACTH. Initially, the entire biosynthetic pathway of mineralocorticoids must presumably be increased, namely progesterone, corticosterone, 18-hydroxy-DOC, and aldosterone. Progressive overproduction of the mineralocorticoid pathway results in increases in the extracellular fluid and blood volumes, hypertension, and subsequent reduction and obliteration in most cases of PRA. Subsequent to this reduction, plasma aldosterone concentration virtually disappears in most patients studied. Thus, the principal mineralocorticoid hormones present in great quantities are DOC and corticosterone (renin-independent, ACTH-dependent steroids), although the levels of 18-hydroxy-DOC and 18-OHB are also increased. The mechanism by which 18-OHB concentration is increased in this condition in the absence of aldosterone has not been fully resolved.[603] Both 18-OHB and aldosterone seem to have a similar site of origin in the zona glomerulosa. The modestly elevated levels of 18-OHB could be due in part to the fact that it is also produced in other areas of the adrenal gland besides the zona glomerulosa or that in the hypokalemic state, which is present in all these patients, the final conversion of 18-OHB to aldosterone is impaired. This has been demonstrated in patients with primary aldosteronism in whom the 18-OHB/aldosterone ratio is increased by profound potassium depletion and is restored to normal by potassium repletion (see above).[304] Administration of ACTH to normal subjects on either normal or reduced sodium intakes results in patterns of steroids synthesized in the zona glomerulosa that are similar in certain respects to those seen in patients with the 17α-hydroxylase deficiency syndrome, namely, markedly increased production of corticosterone and DOC and normal or low aldosterone secretion.[604] This is also observed when ACTH is administered to patients with primary aldosteronism.[604] Thus, there is strong evidence that ACTH, through an intraadrenal event, can impede 11 hydroxylation and even 18 hydroxylation.[605]

The treatment of both these disorders, the 11β-hydroxylase deficiency syndrome and the 17α-hydroxylase deficiency syndrome, is similar to that of all non-salt-losing forms of congenital adrenal hyperplasia. Treatment with small doses of glucocorticoids such as dexamethasone restores blood pressure to normal levels, corrects potassium depletion, and reduces excessive DOC and corticosterone production in the 17α-hydroxylase deficiency syndrome, and reduces DOC and 11-deoxycortisol production in the 11β-hydroxylase deficiency syndrome. Prompt natriuresis usually occurs when treatment is started. In the 17α-hydroxylase deficiency syndrome, restoration of normal levels of DOC results in return of PRA and aldosterone concentration to normal values. In patients with extremely low cortisol production, care should be exercised during the early treatment period: a delay in the return of the suppressed reninaldosterone system toward normal can result in a hypovolemic crisis after the initial natriuresis and diuresis. It may take up to several years before the aldosterone and renin systems become normalized. The amount of glucocorticoid administered must be carefully determined because of apparently exquisite tissue sensitivity to glucocorticoid hormones. Cushingoid changes have been effected with as little as 0.125 mg of dexamethasone per day; often a very small dose must be given intermittently to suppress ACTH production to avoid complications of cushingoid features.

Deoxycorticosterone-Producing Adrenocortical Adenoma

A single case report has identified a patient with hypertension and hypokalemia associated with DOC excess, suppressed PRA, and low-normal plasma aldosterone and cortisol concentrations.[606] A large (240-g) adrenal tumor was removed; this resulted in correction of the abnormal biochemical findings and hypertension. Prolonged follow-up has not been provided, and the specter of malignancy must be considered in such a large adrenocortical tumor.

CUSHING'S SYNDROME AND ADRENAL MALIGNANCIES

Hypertension is a frequent finding in patients with spontaneous Cushing's syndrome. The prevalence varies in different reports but appears to be around 80 to 90 percent (Chap. 12).[284,607–609] Hypertension is almost always present whether the syndrome is due to Cushing's disease (excess ACTH production by the pituitary), ectopic ACTH production, or adrenal adenoma or carcinoma. In contrast, whereas the prevalence of hypertension is increased in patients with iatrogenic Cushing's syndrome due to glucocorticoid therapy (see the earlier section on adrenal steroids and hypertension), hypertension is not as consistently present in these patients as those with the spontaneous disease.

In patients with Cushing's disease, cortisol production is always increased, but aldosterone and corticosterone excretion and secretion are usually normal.[274,284,607–611] In some cases, urinary aldosterone excretion is low; rarely, it may be increased.[274,607,609,611] The lack of an increase in aldosterone level may not be surprising because stimulatory influences of ACTH on aldosterone production are only transient and, in fact, at high dosage or with prolonged use ACTH may actually inhibit aldosterone production. Plasma DOC concentrations are usually normal,[607,611] although modest increases in urinary DOC excretion have been reported.[609] Similarly, clear evidence for mineralocorticoid excess, i.e., hypokalemia and suppressed PRA, is commonly absent.[608,609] However, in one study the PRA values measured with the patient upright were low in 9 of 16 patients with Cushing's disease, even though the mean PRA for the group was normal and only three patients had plasma potassium concentration values of < 3.5 meq/liter.[607] However, PRA is high in some cases.[274] The lack of renin suppression is probably due in part to the actions of glucocorticoids on the renin-angiotensin system (see above and Chap. 12). Hypokalemia is observed more commonly in severe cases of Cushing's disease, with ectopic ACTH production, or with adenoma or carcinoma.[607–611] In the latter circumstances, the plasma cortisol concentrations may be higher than in most patients with Cushing's disease. In other cases, there can be excessive production of DOC, corticosterone, and possibly other steroids that have enhanced mineralocorticoid activity.[608,611,612]

In patients with adrenal malignancy, a variety of patterns of steroid production can be observed; elevated levels of DOC, corticosterone, and aldosterone concentration occur in some patients, whereas levels of cortisol and 11-deoxycortisol are elevated in others.[607,610–612] Of special interest are those patients with feminizing adrenocortical carcinoma (a rapidly fatal disease) and hypertension; longevity is greater in the hypertensive patients than in the normotensive patients with this malignancy. Two such patients exhibited mild 11-hydroxylation inhibition with increased production of DOC and 11-deoxycortisol.[613]

The mechanisms for the hypertension in spontaneous Cushing's syndrome are not clear; several factors may be operative. In cases in which there is hypokalemia and suppressed PRA, the pathogenesis of the hypertension is probably similar to that discussed earlier in the case of primary aldosteronism and DOC-excess hypertension. In cases in which DOC is found to be elevated to a major extent (i.e., > 75 ng/dl), this steroid may contribute substantially to the mineralocorticoid excess state. The actions of cortisol may also be contributory (Chap. 12). These combined actions could explain the occasional findings of hypokalemia and suppressed PRA in these patients.[274] However, the finding of normal to high renin levels and normal potassium concentration values in most patients with Cushing's syndrome indicates that other factors are involved. The first of these is the glucocorticoids, whose blood pressure–elevating properties independent of mineralocorticoid actions are reviewed in detail in Chap. 12 and above. These actions are likely to be the major ones responsible for inducing the hypertension. However, as discussed above (see Glucocorticoids under Adrenal Steroids and Hypertension), an excess of these steroids alone does not always result in hypertension. In spontaneous Cushing's syndrome the effects of glucocorticoids may be amplified by the presence of other effectors. These could be the modest increases in mineralocorticoid activity due to the contributions discussed above, or other factors such as other steroids or pituitary factors (see below).

Second, it is possible that adrenal steroids other than cortisol, aldosterone, or DOC contribute to the hypertension. As discussed in the earlier sections on adrenal steroids and hypertension and on glucocorticoid remediable primary aldosteronism, and in Chap. 12, a number of candidate steroids are being studied, but to date there is no evidence in humans that they are involved. Studies in sheep, however, are provocative in this respect. In this species, ACTH administration can induce hypertension without hypokalemia and suppressed PRA. The hypertension cannot be induced by administering cortisol, DOC, or other major glucocorticoids and mineralocorticoids in doses that mimic the ACTH-induced rises.[614] However, it can be induced when the steroids plus 17α-hydroxyprogesterone and $17\alpha,20\alpha$-dihydroxyprogesterone are given.[614]

Third, since in Cushing's disease and the ectopic ACTH syndrome cortisol hypersecretion is due to excess POMC production, it is possible that some of the other peptides of POMC (discussed in the preceding section on primary aldosteronism with hyperplasia) have a contributory role through direct actions or effects on other steroids. However, there is no direct evidence for this. Further, patients who underwent bilateral adrenalectomy for Cushing's disease and who developed Nelson's syndrome with marked ACTH hypersecretion on replacement of cortisol do not develop hypertension. Thus, these factors would require an intact adrenal to be effective. Overall, these studies indicate a need for continued investigation of the hypertension in Cushing's syndrome and search for as yet poorly characterized factors that may augment the effects of cortisol in inducing hypertension.

Cure or improvement of hypertension usually follows successful treatment of Cushing's syndrome and remission of other stigmata of the syndrome. However, this is not the case in about a third of the patients. This lack of consistent improvement is not unique to Cushing's syndrome but is seen with primary aldosteronism and other forms of secondary hypertension (see above).

OTHER LOW-RENIN HYPERTENSION SYNDROMES ASSOCIATED WITH HYPOKALEMIA

Using PRA and aldosterone measurements to classify types of hypertension, a small subgroup of patients with suppressed PRA and hypokalemia but normal or low concentrations of aldosterone was found.[615] It was within this group of patients that the syndrome of DOC-excess hypertension discussed in the preceding sections were first defined. However, in other patients similar characteristics are found but DOC concentrations are not elevated. The factors involved in producing the hypertension in these patients have not in all cases been as well delineated as those in primary aldosteronism or DOC-excess hypertension, and there appear to be several subtypes.

Iatrogenic Syndromes: Licorice, Carbenoxolone, or Steroid Ingestion

There are several circumstances in which iatrogenic mineralocorticoid-excess hypertension can occur. These include ingestion of large quantities of licorice,[616] use of chewing tobacco,[617] administration of carbenoxolone for gastric ulcer,[616] administration of moderate doses of fludrocortisone such as for postural hypotension,[618] and use of mineralocorticoid-containing nasal sprays.[619]

Licorice and tobacco contain glycyrrhizic acid, which appears to have mineralocorticoid activity. A number of cases have been reported of hypokalemic low-renin, low-aldosterone hypertension in persons ingesting large quantities (e.g., 1 lb per week) of licorice.

Carbenoxolone is a semisynthetic derivative of glycyrrhizic acid that has been used mostly in Europe for the treatment of gastric ulcers. The compound is available in the United States only for investigative use. It also apparently has mineralocorticoid activity and leads to a syndrome similar to that seen with licorice ingestion.

Mineralocorticoid hypertension with hypokalemia and suppressed PRA due to steroid ingestion is uncommon because compounds with predominant mineralocorticoid activity are not often used except for replacement therapy. However, fludrocortisone is sometimes used to treat postural hypotension, and this can lead to moderate hypertension (particularly in the supine state), hypokalemia, and a suppressed plasma renin level. Mantero and colleagues found mineralocorticoid-excess hypertension in several patients in Italy who were using a steroid-containing nasal spray (Biorinil) for allergic rhinitis.[619] The active component of the spray was found to be fluprednisolone, which was shown to have potent mineralocorticoid activity.

For all these syndromes the diagnosis depends on uncovering a history of ingestion of the offending substance in a patient with hypertension, hypokalemia, suppressed PRA, low aldosterone concentration, and no excess of other steroids. In all cases, the metabolic abnormalities become normal several weeks after discontinuance of the agent. Such a normalization also helps to confirm the diagnosis.

Low-Aldosterone Hypertension Unresponsive to Dexamethasone

Several other types of low-aldosterone, low-renin hypokalemic hypertension can be distinguished on the basis of the responsiveness of the clinical abnormalities to the aldosterone antagonist spironolactone and the resistance of the hypertension to dexamethasone therapy. However, it is possible that there are more than two subgroups within this type of hypertension.

SPIRONOLACTONE-RESPONSIVE SUBGROUP

New and coworkers,[620] Winter and coworkers,[621] and Shackleton et al.[622] reported several children with low-renin hypokalemic hypertension. The plasma concentrations of aldosterone were low and the plasma cortisol concentrations were low normal to low. The low renin levels, hypokalemia, and hypertension responded to spironolactone, suggesting that the abnormalities were due to the mineralocorticoids present. A further suggestion that this was the case was obtained from a finding by New et al.[620]: the hypertension was aggravated by administration of ACTH, even during salt restriction; thus steroids stimulated by ACTH may have been stimulating a redistribution of sodium in body compartments. The possibility that the hypertension was due to an as yet unidentified mineralocorticoid was also suggested. Abnormalities of steroid metabolism have been documented in the patient of New et al.[620] There is a persistently increased and abnormal ratio of tetrahydrocortisol to tetrahydrocortisone, suggesting a decreased level of 11β-hydroxyoxidoreductase.[623] In subsequent studies, Lan and coworkers with the use of a mineralocorticoid radioreceptor assay found a low total plasma mineralocorticoid activity.[624] They suggested that the syndrome was due to an enhanced cellular sensitivity to mineralocorticoids. Thus, the low concentrations of mineralocorticoids present may be sufficient to lead to a mineralocorticoid excess state. The consequent volume increase with suppression of PRA and the hypokalemia decrease aldosterone production; however, the normal (to low) concentrations of plasma cortisol persist because these are not subject to the same feedback inhibition. Thus, they suggested that the mineralocorticoid activity of cortisol, in the presence of excessive sensitivity to mineralocorticoids, could be sufficient to maintain a mineralocorticoid excess state. More recent studies support the idea that cortisol accounts for the mineralocorticoid excess state in these patients.[625]

SPIRONOLACTONE-UNRESPONSIVE SUBGROUP

Liddle and associates studied two siblings of a kindred with a probable familial renal disorder characterized by hypertension and hypokalemia with low aldosterone excretion and suppressed PRA.[625] Potassium depletion and low serum levels of potassium were not corrected by administration of spironolactone or a low-sodium diet. Triamterene, a diuretic that blocks sodium reabsorption in the distal collecting tubule and potassium excretion at a site distal to the mineralocorticoid site, reduces blood pressure and causes a rise in serum potassium concentration, but aldosterone levels remain low. A patient with this syndrome was found to have an increased intracellular sodium concentration and increased ouabain-insensitive sodium ion flux, suggesting that there is a primary abnormality in sodium transport that is manifest both in the kidney and in erythrocytes.

Dexamethasone-Responsive

As mentioned previously, patients with the 11β- and 17α-hydroxylase deficiency syndromes and a few patients with primary aldosteronism with hyperplasia respond to dexamethasone. There are also other patients who do not have an elevated plasma aldosterone or DOC concentration but whose hypertension, hypokalemia, and suppressed plasma renin concentration respond to treatment with dexamethasone.

SYNDROME OF PROBABLE INSENSITIVITY TO GLUCOCORTICOIDS

Vingerhoeldts and coworkers reported studies of a man who had hypertension, hypokalemia, suppressed plasma renin concentration, and low plasma concentrations of aldosterone and DOC.[627,628] This man was found to have a markedly elevated plasma cortisol concentration (50 μg/dl). The elevation could not be explained by an increased corticosteroid-binding globulin concentration, and the free plasma cortisol concentration was elevated. Despite this, he had no stigmata of Cushing's syndrome. Treatment with relatively large doses (5 mg per day) of dexamethasone normalized the blood pressure, serum potassium level, and plasma renin concentration. This dosage of dexamethasone did not effect signs or symptoms of glucocorticoid excess. Thus, it appears that the patient has a primary hyposensitivity to glucocorticoids without a major insensitivity to mineralocorticoids. Apparently, the hyposensitivity is generalized so that at normal cortisol concentrations cortisol does not inhibit ACTH production. With increased ACTH production, more cortisol is produced until the markedly high cortisol concentrations partly suppress the ACTH and also render the patient functionally euglucocorticoid. However, the elevated cortisol concentration still retains its mineralocorticoid activity. This in turn suppresses the plasma renin and consequently aldosterone concentration; it also causes hypertension and hypokalemia. There is also some evidence that other family members are similarly affected, but these have not been studied in detail. Although this is an isolated report, it probably does underscore the potential for cortisol to act as a mineralocorticoid.

POSSIBLE EXISTENCE OF AN AS YET UNIDENTIFIED MINERALOCORTICOID

Stockigt reported on a 17-year-old male who had hypertension, hypokalemia, suppressed PRA, and normal plasma concentrations of DOC, cortisol, and several other steroids.[564] This patient had, on several occasions, a mildly elevated plasma aldosterone concentration, but usually it was within normal limits. The clinical abnormalities responded to either dexamethasone or spironolactone. Using the mineralocorticoid radioreceptor assay, Lan and coworkers found that this patient's plasma mineralocorticoid activity was markedly elevated.[624] It decreased with dexamethasone therapy and returned to elevated levels after cessation of therapy. Only about half of the total plasma mineralocorticoid activity measured by the radioreceptor assay could be accounted for by the measured concentrations of aldosterone, cortisol, and DOC. In contrast, the plasma mineralocorticoid activity could be accounted for by the measured steroids in normal subjects and patients with primary aldosteronism. Thus, the possibility of production of a novel steroid in this patient is suggested. There are several earlier reports of patients with similar features;[629,630] they could also have an as yet unidentified mineralocorticoid hormone.

This syndrome is similar in many respects to the dexamethasone-suppressible form of primary aldosteronism discussed earlier. The distinction is based on whether or not there is excess aldosterone. However, plasma levels of this steroid can fall into the normal range in patients with primary aldosteronism with hyperplasia and were occasionally elevated in the patient of Stockigt.[564] Thus, it is possible that the two syndromes are identical and that mineralocorticoids other than aldosterone are also present in dexamethasone-suppressible primary aldosteronism.

PSEUDOHYPOALDOSTERONISM TYPE 2 LOW-RENIN HYPERTENSION WITH HYPERKALEMIA

An unusual familial form of low- to normal-renin hypertension is pseudohypoaldosteronism type 2.[631–633] It is inherited as an autosomal dominant trait. These patients present with hypertension and hyperkalemia, often as children, with low to normal renin and aldosterone production and normal renal sodium conservation and glomerular filtration. As a result of the apparent aldosterone resistance and hyperkalemia these patients also have a renal tubular acidosis with a defect in ammoniagenesis. It has been postulated that these patients have a generalized defect in potassium transport by cell membranes, an isolated defect in renal potassium excretion, or enhanced renal sodium reabsorption which leads to hypertension and suppressed plasma aldosterone production and hyperkalemia (also discussed in Chap. 12). Increased sodium reabsorption may be due to increased reabsorption of chloride by the distal nephron (resembling the reversal of the pathophysiology of Bartter's syndrome). The acidosis and hyperkalemia can be corrected by thiazide diuretics, which also improve blood pressure.

LOW-RENIN ESSENTIAL HYPERTENSION

Suppressed plasma renin levels are found in a substantial proportion of people with essential hypertension. Several methods have been devised to "diagnose" this condition. One is shown in Figs. 14-5 and 14-6. Comparison of PRA with urinary sodium excretion (an index of sodium intake) normally yields the pattern shown in Fig. 14-5. In contrast, in patients with essential hypertension, the pattern depicted in Fig. 14-6 is observed; it is of note that about 25 percent of the values fall below the normal range. These patients usually respond with only a slight increase in PRC in response to a low-salt diet or furosemide administration (Fig. 14-25). When aldosterone values are compared with the urinary sodium excretion, most of the patients with low-renin hypertension have normal

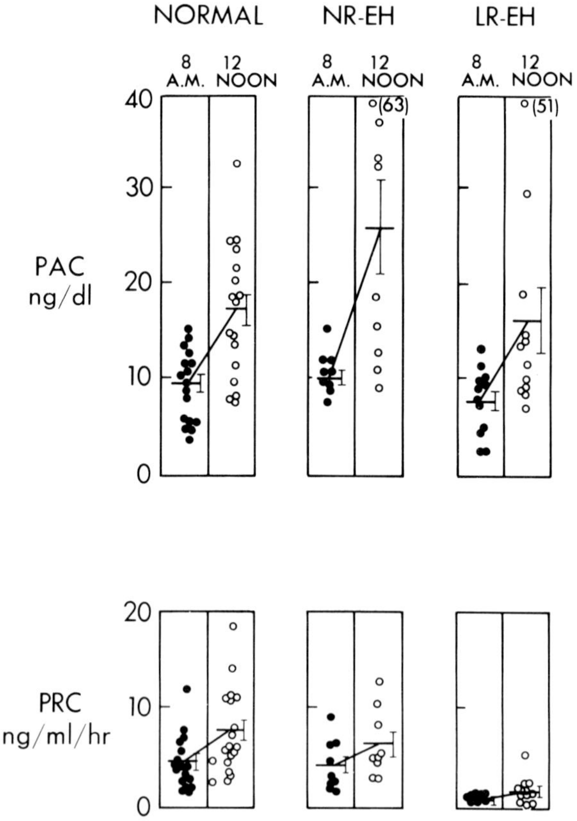

FIGURE 14-25 Response of plasma aldosterone concentration (PAC) and plasma renin concentration (PRC) to upright posture after overnight recumbency in patients with normal-renin (NR-EH) and low-renin essential hypertension (LR-EH) and in normal subjects. Note similar increases of PAC in normal subjects and LR-EH patients but no significant change in PRC in the latter.

urinary aldosterone excretion, although both low and high values are also seen (Fig. 14-6).

The finding of a suppressed renin level in these hypertensive patients naturally raised the question of whether or not the syndrome was similar to the other mineralocorticoid excess states. This notion was strengthened by the subsequent finding that the blood pressure of these patients responded more readily than that of other essential hypertension patients to spironolactone, other diuretics, or blockade of adrenal steroid synthesis.[152,634-636] Because plasma aldosterone concentrations are ordinarily not elevated, investigators began to search for other potential mineralocorticoids in these patients; indeed, there are reports of elevations of concentrations of several steroids,[152,155,634-637] including 16β-hydroxydehydroepiandrosterone and its 16-keto derivative, 18-hydroxydeoxycorticosterone, 18-OHB, and DOC. However, convincing evidence that these steroids are important has not been presented. Furthermore, in two studies the mineralocorticoid radioreceptor assay has failed to detect any major increase in plasma mineralocorticoid activity in patients with this disorder.[637]

Other features of low-renin essential hypertension are not suggestive of a mineralocorticoid excess state. First, hypokalemia is rare in these patients; in fact, the presence of hypokalemia should arouse suspicion of one of the previously described disorders. Second, whereas an increased total body sodium level in primary aldosteronism can be demonstrated, convincing evidence for this in low-renin essential hypertension has not been forthcoming.[638,639]

Although evidence for a new mineralocorticoid or even a major excess of mineralocorticoids in patients with low-renin essential hypertension is lacking, it can be argued that the amount of mineralocorticoid activity is excessive relative to the plasma renin concentration. Although the concentration of angiotensin II is, as expected, low because of the low plasma renin concentration, the amount of aldosterone produced in response to the small amount of angiotensin II present is excessive.[157-159] This suggests that there is an increased sensitivity of the adrenal gland to angiotensin II. However, the vascular system has not been shown to be more sensitive.

The suppression of renin in patients with low-renin essential hypertension is relative rather than absolute. Thus, there is a small rise in PRA after assumption of erect posture (Fig. 14-25), on a low-sodium diet, or with diuretic administration.[155] These changes in renin level result in a definite increase in aldosterone production due to the enhanced adrenal sensitivity to angiotensin II. These findings are similar to those of primary aldosteronism due to hyperplasia. In fact, they suggest that the latter is a more severe variant of low-renin essential hypertension.[640]

The role of angiotensin II in patients with low-renin essential hypertension has also been assessed with the use of converting enzyme inhibition. This resulted in a <3 percent lowering of the diastolic blood pressure, suggesting that the endogenous angiotensin II is contributing minimally to the hypertension.[641] In contrast, converting enzyme inhibition significantly lowered the blood pressure in patients with normal- or high-renin hypertension, suggesting that the hypertension in these patients is much more dependent on angiotensin II than in patients with low-renin hypertension.

Cognizance must be taken of the possibility that low-renin essential hypertension is a heterogeneous disease. The prevalence of this disorder tends to be higher in black persons and in the elderly.[615] In some, but not all, studies there is an increased prevalence of the low-renin type in women.[615]

As discussed in Essential Hypertension, under Role of the Renin-Angiotensin System in Hypertension, above, the presence of a low renin level could reflect an adaptive response to the hypertension. Alternatively, the suppressed renin could also reflect another process that is associated with or is responsible for the development of the hypertension. For instance, it has been suggested that there is a blunting of the peripheral beta-adrenergic receptor system in low-renin hypertension (see Chap. 13). This could result in lower plasma renin levels. Although it has been reported that there is a blunted rise in urinary norepinephrine excretion in response to upright posture in patients with low-renin essential hypertension, other studies suggest that these patients have a normally responsive sympathetic nervous system, implying that the low PRA may be due to a defective renin response to sympathetic nerve stimulation.[642]

Figure 14-26 summarizes some aspects of these thoughts. If endogenous factors of any type are stimulating the blood pressure to increase, then they or their influences on the renal baroreceptors may tend to suppress renin release. However, the extent to which this occurs could be variable and could even depend on the nature of the factors that cause the hypertension in the first place. Alternatively, the variations in plasma renin levels in patients with essential hypertension could be explained by the hypothesis that in some cases hypertensive stimuli (such as catecholamines, see Chap. 13) directly affect renin release (explaining why renin levels may be inappropriately normal or elevated), whereas in others

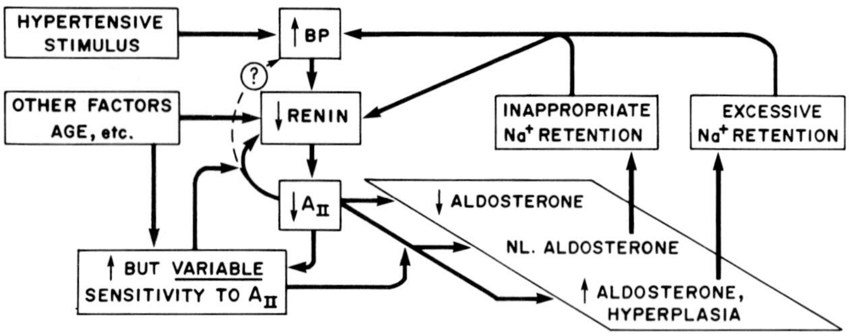

FIGURE 14-26 Possible explanation for abnormalities in low-renin essential hypertension.

they do not directly affect renin release, in which case renin levels might be suppressed by the resulting hypertension. Finally, as shown in the figure, it is possible that other factors (e.g., age- or race-related) could result in a variable tendency for renin release to be suppressed either in response to or independently of the hypertension. In any case, the low-renin state ultimately is associated with an increased sensitivity of the adrenal gland to angiotensin II, but the extent to which this occurs may be variable, such that in some cases aldosterone production would be markedly increased, in others it would be inappropriately normal, and in others it would be low (Fig. 14-26). In this context there is the possibility that as yet poorly characterized factors, such as pituitary factors (discussed above), are contributory. However, even when aldosterone production is normal, the steroid could be contributing to the increased blood pressure because the resulting mineralocorticoid activity could be excessive relative to the suppressed renin and hemodynamic state. In patients in whom aldosterone levels are markedly elevated, the consequent actions of the steroid in a similar setting could have an even greater effect on the hypertension and could be the major factor. This could be true in those patients with primary aldosteronism due to hyperplasia whose blood pressures respond to spironolactone; as discussed earlier, these cases may be part of a continuum of the large subgroup of patients with low-renin hypertension.

The mechanism(s) for the increased sensitivity to angiotensin II is not understood. In general, with polypeptide hormones, a lowering of the endogenous concentrations of the hormone results in an increased cellular sensitivity to it.[137] This appears to occur in the case of angiotensin II with respect to vascular and uterine receptors. However, in the rat, angiotensin II increases the cellular sensitivity of the adrenal gland to angiotensin II,[137] and in humans it appears to be needed for maintenance of the sensitivity of the glomerulosa to angiotensin (see Chap. 12). It is conceivable that in humans the increased adrenal sensitivity and elevated blood pressure might be induced initially by excessive angiotensin II activity. With increased angiotensin II action, renin and angiotensin II levels would gradually drop, but the progressively lower concentrations of angiotensin II might be sufficient to enhance or at least maintain the adrenal gland in a hypersensitive state. Such a hypothesis could explain the emergence of a partly volume-sensitive hypertension because this can occur in normal subjects given angiotensin II (but not norepinephrine) in progressively decreasing amounts.[152] However, there is no direct evidence to support this notion, and the available data raise the question of the possible existence of some as yet unidentified factor responsible for producing the enhanced adrenal sensitivity.

REFERENCES

1. U.S. Department of Health, Education, and Welfare: *Blood Pressure of Persons 18–74 Years, United States, 1971–72,* ser 11, no 150. DHEW publication 75-1632, National Center for Health Statistics, 1975.

2. Joint National Committee on Detection, Evaluation and Treatment of High Blood Pressure: The 1984 Report of the Joint National Committee on Detection, Evaluation and Treatment of High Blood Pressure. *Arch Intern Med* 144:1045, 1984.

3. Rowland M, Roberts J: Blood pressure levels and hypertension in persons 6–74 years: United States, 1976–80. *Advance Data, Vital and Health Statistics of the Center for Health Statistics,* no 84. Washington D.C., U.S. Department of Health and Human Service, 1982.

4. Kannel WB: Some lessons in cardiovascular epidemiology from Framingham. *Am J Cardiol* 37:269, 1976.

5. Berglund G, Andersson O, Wilhelmsen L: Prevalence of primary and secondary hypertension: Studies in a random population sample. *Br Med J* 2:554, 1976.

6. Bech K, Hilden T: The frequency of secondary hypertension. *Acta Med Scand* 197:65, 1975.

7. Kaplan NM: *Clinical Hypertension.* Baltimore, Williams and Wilkins, 1978.

8. Perera GA: Hypertensive vascular disease: Description and natural history. *J Chronic Dis* 1:33, 1955

9. Leishman AWD: Hypertension—treated and untreated. A study of 400 cases. *Br Med J* 1:5134:1361, 1959.

10. Sokolow M, Perloff D: The prognosis of essential hypertension treated conservatively. *Circulation* 23:697, 1961.

11. *Build and Blood Pressure Study*. Chicago, IL, Society of Actuaries, 1959, vol 1.

12. Pooling Project Research Group: Relationship of blood pressure, serum cholesterol, smoking habit, relative weight and ECG abnormalities to incidence of major coronary events: Final report of the Pooling Project. *J Chronic Dis* 31:201, 1978.

13. Tibblin G: High blood pressure in men aged 50: A population study of men born in 1913. *Acta Med Scand* suppl 470:1, 1967.

14. Bechgaard P: Arterial hypertension: A follow-up study of 1000 hypertonics. *Acta Med Scand* 172:3, 1946.

15. Keys A (ed): *Seven Countries—A Multivariate Analysis of Death and Coronary Heart Disease*. Cambridge, Harvard University, 1980.

16. Holme I, Waaler HT: Five-year mortality in the city of Bergen, Norway, according to age, sex and blood pressure. *Acta Med Scand* 200:229, 1976.

17. Kannel WB, Sorlie P: Hypertension in Framingham, in Paul O (ed): *Epidemiology and Control of Hypertension*. New York, Stratton, 1975, pp 553–590.

18. Dawber TR: *The Framingham Study. The Epidemiology of Atherosclerotic Disease*. Cambridge, Harvard University, 1980.

19. Kannel WB, Dawber TR, McGee DL, et al: Perspectives on systolic hypertension. The Framingham study. *Circulation* 61:1179, 1980.

20. Castelli WP, Anderson K: A population at risk: Prevalence of high cholesterol levels in hypertensive patients in the Framingham study. *Am J Med* 80:23, 1986.

21. Castelli WP: Epidemiology of coronary heart disease: The Framingham study. *Am J Med* 76:4, 1984.

22. Rabkin SW, Mathewson FAL, Tate RB: Predicting risk of ischemic heart disease and cerebrovascular disease from systolic and diastolic blood pressure. *Ann Int Med* 88:342, 1978.

23. Fisher CM: The ascendancy of diastolic blood pressure over systolic. *Lancet* 2:1349, 1985.

24. World Health Organization: *Epidemiological and Vital Statistics Report*. Geneva, 1967, vol 20, pp 535–710.

25. Robertson T, Kato H, Rhoads GG, et al: Epidemiological studies of coronary heart disease and stroke in Japanese men living in Japan, Hawaii and California. Incidence of myocardial infarction and death from coronary heart disease. *Am J Cardiol* 39:239, 1977.

26. Robertson T, Kato H, Gordon T, Kagan A, Rhoads GG, Land CE, Worth RM, Belsky JL, Dock DS, Miyanichi M, Kawamoto S, et al: Epidemiological studies of coronary heart disease and stroke in Japanese men living in Japan, Hawaii and California. Coronary heart disease risk factors in Japan and Hawaii. *Am J Cardiol* 39:244, 1977.

27. Perry HM Jr, Schroeder HA, Catanzaro FJ, et al: Studies on the control of hypertension. VIII. Mortality, morbidity and remissions during twelve years of intensive therapy. *Circulation* 33:958, 1966.

28. Schottstaedt MF, Sokolow M: The natural history and course of hypertension with papilledema (malignant hypertension). *Am Heart J* 45:331, 1953.

29. Harrington M, Kincaid-Smith P, McMichael J: Results of treatment in malignant hypertension: A seven-year experience in 94 cases. *Br Med J* 2:969, 1959.

30. Veteran's Administration Cooperative Study Group on Antihypertensive Agents: Effects of treatment on morbidity in hypertension. I. Results in patients with diastolic blood pressure averaging 115 through 129 mmHg. *JAMA* 202:1028, 1967.

31. Veteran's Administration Cooperative Study Group on Antihypertensive Agents: Effects of treatment on morbidity in hypertension. II. Results in patients with diastolic blood pressure averaging 90 through 114 mmHg. *JAMA* 213:1143, 1970.

32. Hypertension Detection and Follow-up Program Cooperative Group: Five-year findings of the hypertension detection and follow-up program. I. Reduction in mortality of persons with high blood pressure, including mild hypertension. *JAMA* 242:2562, 1979.

33. Kirkendall WM: Essential hypertension, in Genest J, Kuchel O, Hamet P, Cantin M (eds): *Hypertension*, 2d ed. New York, McGraw-Hill, 1983, pp 732–753.

34a. Page LB: Epidemiology of hypertension, in Genest J, Kuchel O, Hamet P, Cantin M (eds): *Hypertension*, 2d ed. New York, McGraw-Hill, 1983, pp 683–699.

34b. Cruz-Coke R: Etiology of essential hypertension. *Hypertension* 3(suppl II):191, 1981.

34c. Zinner SH, Lee YH, Rosner B, Oh W, Kass EH: Factors affecting blood pressure in newborn infants. *Hypertension* 2(suppl I): I-99, 1980.

35. Nonpharmacological approaches to the control of high blood pressure: Final report of the subcommittee on nonpharmacological therapy of the 1984 Joint National Committee on Detection, Evaluation, and Treatment of High Blood Pressure. *Hypertension* 8:444, 1986.

36. Weinsier RL, Norris DJ, Birch R, Bernstein RS, Wang J, Yang M-U, Pierson RN Jr, Van Itallie TB: The relative contribution of body fat and fat pattern to blood pressure level. *Hypertension* 7:578, 1985.

37. Dustan HP, Tarazi RC, Bravo EL: Physiological characteristics of hypertension. *Am J Med* 52:610, 1972.

38. Guyton AC: The relationship of cardiac output and arterial pressure control. *Circulation* 64:1079, 1981.

39. Lund-Johansen P: State of the art review. Hemodynamics in essential hypertension. *Clin Sci* 59:343, 1980.

40. Letcher RL, Chien S, Pickering TG, et al: Elevated blood viscosity in patients with borderline essential hypertension. *Hypertension* 5:757, 1983.

41. Schalekamp MADH, Man in't Veld AJ, Wenting GJ: The second Sir George Pickering Memorial Lecture: What regulates whole body autoregulation? Clinical observations. *J Hypertension* 3:97, 1985.

42. Folkow B: Physiological aspects of primary hypertension. *Physiol Rev* 62:347, 1982.

43. Webb RC, Bohr DF: Recent advances in the pathogenesis of hypertension: Consideration of structural, functional, and metabolic vascular abnormalities resulting in elevated arterial resistance. *Am Heart J* 102:251, 1981.

44. Gavras H, Hatzinikolaou P, North WG, et al: Interaction of the sympathetic nervous system with vasopressin and renin in the maintenance of blood pressure. *Hypertension* 4:400, 1982.

45. Krieger EM: Neurogenic mechanisms in hypertension: Resetting of the baroreceptors: State of the art lecture. *Hypertension* 8(suppl I):71, 1986.

46a. Abboud FM: The sympathetic system in hypertension. *State-of-the-art review. Hypertension* 4(suppl II):208, 1982.

46b. Tarazi RC: Pathophysiology of essential hypertension: Role of the autonomic nervous system. *Am J Med* 75:2, 1983.

47. Ventura H, Messerli FH, Oigman W, et al: Impaired systemic arterial compliance in borderline hypertension. *Am Heart J* 108:132, 1984.

48. Safar ME, Weiss YA, Levenson JA, et al: Hemodynamic study of 85 patients with borderline hypertension. *Am J Cardiol* 31:315, 1973.

49. Sullivan JM, Prewitt RL, Josephs JA: Attenuation of the microcirculation in young patients with high-output borderline hypertension. *Hypertension* 5:844, 1983.

50. Schwartz SM: Smooth muscle proliferation in hypertension. *Hypertension* 6(suppl I):56, 1984.

51a. Frohlich ED: Physiologic considerations in left ventricular hypertrophy. *Am J Med* 75:12, 1983.

51b. Massie BM: Myocardial hypertrophy and cardiac failure: A complex interrelationship. *Am J Med* 75:67, 1983.

52a. Chobanian AV, Brecher PI, Haudenschild CC: Effects of hypertension and antihypertensive therapy on atherosclerosis: State of the art lecture. *Hypertension* 8(suppl I):15, 1986.

52b. Ross R: The pathogenesis of atherosclerosis: An update. *N Engl J Med* 314:488, 1986.

52c. Weiner J, Spiro D, Lattes RG: The cellular pathology of experimental hypertension: II. Arteriolar hyalinosis and fibrinoid change. *Am J Pathol* 47:457, 1965.

53a. Ross RWR: Observations on intracerebral aneurysms. *Brain* 86:425, 1963.

53b. Mohr JP: Lacunar stroke. *Hypertension* 8:349, 1986.

54a. Strandgaard S, Olesen J, Skinhoj E, et al: Autoregulation of brain circulation in severe arterial hypertension. *Br Med J* 1:507, 1973.

54b. Phillips LH II, Whishnant JP, O'Fallon WM, Sundt TM Jr: The unchanging pattern of subarachnoid hemorrhage in a community. *Neurology* 30:1034, 1980.

54c. Sacco RL, Wolf PA, et al: Subarachnoid and intracerebral hemorrhage: Natural history, prognosis, and precursive factors in the Framingham study. *Neurology* 34:845, 1984.

55a. Lindeman RD, Tobin JD, Shock NW: Association between hypertension and the rate of decline of renal function. *Kidney Int* 26:861, 1984.

55b. Rostand SG, Kirk KA, Rutsky EA, Pate RA: Racial differences in the incidence of treatment for end-stage renal disease. *N Engl J Med* 306:1276, 1982.

55c. Ledingham JGC: Early assessment of organ involvement in hypertension: *J Hypertension* 3(suppl 2):s33, 1985.

55d. Messerli FH, Frohlich ED, Dreslinski GR, Suarez DH, Aristimuno GG: Serum uric acid in essential hypertension: an indication of renal vascular involvement. *Ann Intern Med* 93:817, 1980.

56a. Boucher R, Rojo-Ortega JM, Genest J: Description of renin-angiotensin system and methods of measurement, in Genest J, Koiw E, Kuchel O (eds): *Hypertension: Physiopathology and Treatment.* New York, McGraw-Hill, 1977, pp 140–155.

56b. Slater EE, Haber E: Inactive renin—"through a glass darkly." *N Engl J Med* 301:429, 1979.

57. Slater EE, Strout HV: Pure human renin: Identification and characterization of two molecular weight forms. *J Biol Chem* 256:8164, 1981.

58. Yokosawa H, Holladay LA, Inagami T, Haas E, Murakami K: Human renal renin: Complete purification and characterization. *J Biol Chem* 265:3498, 1980.

59. Galen FX, Devaux J, Guyenne TT, Menard RR, Corvol P: Multiple forms of human renin, purification and characterization. *J Biol Chem* 254:4848, 1981.

60. Do YS, Shinagawa T, Tam H, Inagami T, Hsueh WA: Characterization of pure human renal renin, evidence for its subunit structure. *J Biol Chem* 1986, in press.

61. Sealey JE, Atlas SA, Laragh JH: Prorenin and other large molecular weight forms of renin. *Endocr Rev* 1:365, 1980.

62. Hsueh WA, Do YS, Shinagawa T, Tam H, Baxter J, Shine J, Ponet P, Fritz L: Biochemical similarity of expressed human renin and native inactive prorenin. *Hypertension* 8(suppl II):78, 1985.

63. Galen FX, Guyenne TT, Devaux C, Auzan C, Corvol P, Menard J: Direct radioimmunoassay of human renin. *J Clin Endocrinol Metab* 48:1041, 1979.

64. Hobart PM, Fogliano M, O'Connor BA, Schaefer IM, Chirgwin JM: Human renin gene: Structure and sequence analysis. *Proc Natl Acad Sci USA* 81:5026, 1984.

65. Hardman JA, Hort YJ, Catanzaro DF, Tellam JT, Baxter JD, Morris BJ, Shine J: Primary structure of the human renin gene. *DNA* 3:457, 1984.

66. Miyazaki H, Fukamizu A, Hirose S, Hayashi T, Hori H, Ohkubo H, Nakanishi S, Murakami K: Structure of the human renin gene. *Proc Natl Acad Sci USA* 81:5999, 1984.

67. Imai T, Miyazaki H, Hirose S, Hori H, Hayashi T, Kageyama R, Ohkubo H, Nakamishi S, Murakami K: Cloning and sequence analysis of cDNA for human renin precursor. *Proc Natl Acad Sci USA* 80:7405, 1983.

68. Soubrier F, Panthier JT, Corvol P, Rougeon F: Molecular cloning and nucleotide sequence of a human renin cDNA fragment. *Nucleic Acids Res* 20:7181, 1983.

69. Chirgwin JM, Schaefer IM, Rotwein PS, Piccini N, Gross KW, Naylor SL: Human renin gene is on chromosome 1. *Somatic Cell Genet* 10:415, 1984.

70. Bohnik J, Fehrentz JA, Galen FX, Seyer R, Evin G, Castro B, Menard J, Corvol P: Immunologic identification of both plasma and human renal inactive renin as prorenin. *J Clin Endocrinol Metab* 60:399, 1985.

71. Atlas SA, Christofalo P, Hesson T, Sealy JE, Fritz LC: Immunological evidence that inactive renin is prorenin. *Biochem Biophys Res Commun* 132:1038, 1985.

72. Kim SJ, Hirose S, Miyazaki H, Ueno N, Higashimori K, Morinaga S, Kimura T, Sakakibara S, Murakami K: Identification of plasma inactive renin as prorenin with a site-directed antibody. *Biochem Biophys Res Commun* 126:641, 1985.

73. Hsueh WA, Do YS, Shinagawa T, Tam H, Ponte PA, Baxter JD, Shine J, Fritz LC: Biochemical similarity of expressed human prorenin and native inactive renin. *Hypertension* (suppl II)8: II-78, 1986.

73a. Fritz LC, Arfsten AA, Atlas SA, Baxter JD, Dzau VJ, Fiddes JC, Shine J, Cofer CL, Kushner P, Ponte PA: Characterization of human prorenin expressed in mammalian cells from cloned cDNA. *Proc Natl Acad Sci USA* 83:4114, 1986.

73b. Steiner DF, Docherty K, Carroll R: Golgi/granule processing of peptide hormone and neuropeptide precursors: A minireview. *J Cell Biochem* 24:121, 1984.

74. Loh YP, Parish DC, Tuteja R: Purification and characterization of a paired basic residue-specific pro-opiomelanocortin converting enzyme from bovine pituitary intermediate lobe secretory vesicles. *J Biol Chem* 260:7194, 1985.

75a. Schambelan M, Biglieri EG: Hypertension and the role of the renin-angiotensin-aldosterone system in renal failure, in Brenner BM, Rector FC Jr (eds): *The Kidney.* Philadelphia, Saunders, 1976, pp 1486–1521.

75b. Doi Y, Franco-Saenz R, Mulrow PJ: Evidence for an extrarenal source of inactive renin in rats. *Hypertension* 6:627, 1984.

76. Re RN: Cellular biology of the renin-angiotensin systems. *Arch Intern Med* 144:2037, 1984.

77. Naruse K, Murakoshi M, Osamura RY, Naruse M, Toma H, Watanabe K, Demura H, Inagami T, Shizume K: Immunohistological evidence for renin in human endocrine tissues. *J Clin Endocrinol Metab* 61:172, 1985.

78a. Deschepper CF, Mellon SH, Cumin S, Baxter JD, Ganong WF: Analysis by immunocytochemistry and in situ hybridization of renin and its mRNA in kidney, testes, adrenal and pituitary gland of the rat. *Proc Natl Acad Sci USA* 83:7552, 1986.

78b. Mikama H, Suzuki H, Smeby RR, Ferraro CM: Cerebrospinal fluid angiotensin II immunoreactivity is not derived from the plasma. *Hypertension* 7:65, 1985.

79. Schiffrin EL, Genest J: Tonin-angiotensin II system, in Genest J, Kuchel O, Hamet P, Cantin M (eds): *Hypertension,* 2d ed. New York, McGraw-Hill, 1983, pp 309–320.

80. Wintroub B, Klickstein LD, Watt KWK: A human neutrophil dependent pathway for generation of angiotensin II. *J Clin Invest* 68:484, 1981.

81. Taugner R, Yokota S, Buhrle CP, Hackenthal E: Cathepsin D coexists with renin in the secretory granules of juxtaglomerular epithelioid cells. *Histochemistry* 84:19, 1986.

82. Freeman RH, Davis JO: Factors controlling renin secretion and metabolism, in Genest J, Kuchel O (eds): *Hypertension,* 2d ed. New York, McGraw-Hill, 1983, pp 225–250.

83. Rabinowe SL, Taylor T, Dluhy RG, Williams GH: β-Endorphin stimulates plasma renin and aldosterone release in normal human subjects. *J Clin Endocrinol Metab* 60:485, 1985.

84. Beierwalters WH, Prada J, Carretero OA: Effect of glandular

kallikrein on renin release in isolated rat glomeruli. *Hypertension* 7:27, 1985.

85. Weidmann P, Hirsch D, Maxwell MH, Okun R, Schroth P: Plasma renin and blood pressure during treatment with methyldopa. *Am J Cardiol* 34:671, 1974.

86. Niarchos AP, Baer L, Radichevich I: Role of renin and aldosterone supression in the antihypertensve mechanism of clonidine. *Am J Med* 65:614, 1978.

87. Itoh S, Carretero OA: Role of the macula densa in renin release. *Hypertension* 7(suppl I):49, 1985.

88. Itoh S, Carretero OA, Murray RD: Possible role of adenosine in the macula densa mechanism of renin release in rabbits. *J Clin Invest* 76:1412, 1985.

89. Davis JO, Freeman RH: Mechanisms regulating renin release. *Physiol Rev* 56:1, 1976.

90. Kotchen TA, Galla JH, Luke RG: Contribution of chloride to the inhibition of plasma renin by sodium chloride in the rat. *Kidney Int* 13:201, 1978.

91. Egan BM, Julius S, Cottier C, Osterziel KJ, Ibsen H: Role of cardiovascular receptors on the neural regulation of renin release in normal men. *Hypertension* 5:779, 1983.

92. Williams GH, Hollenberg NK, Moore TJ, Dluhy RG, Barbi SZ, Solomon HS, Mersey JH: Failure of renin suppression by angiotensin in hypertension. *Circ Res* 42:46, 1978.

93. Mongeon R, Goldstone R, Carlson E, Hsueh W: Diagnosis of low renin states by converting enzyme inhibition. *7th International Congress on Endocrinology, Quebec,* 1984, p 1402 (abstr).

94. Antonipilla I, Horton R: Role of extra- and intracellular calcium and calmodulin in renin release from rat kidney. *Endocrinology* 117:601, 1985.

95. Oates J, Whorton AR, Gerkens JF, Branch RA, Hollifield JW, Frolich JC: The participation of prostaglandins in the control of renin release. *Fed Proc* 38:72, 1979.

96. Gerber JG, Olson RD, Nies AS: Interrelationship between prostaglandins and renin release. *Kidney Int* 19:816, 1981.

97. Whorton AR, Misono K, Hollifield J, Frolich JC, Inagami T, Oates JA: Prostaglandins and renin release. I. Stimulation of renin release from rabbit renal cortical slices by PGI_2. *Prostaglandins* 14:1095, 1977.

98. Patrono C, Pugliese F, Ciabattoni G, Patrignani PP, Maseri A, Chierchia S, Peskar BA, Cinotti GA, Simonetti BM, Peirucci A: Evidence for a direct stimulatory effect of prostacyclin on renin disease in man. *J Clin Invest* 69:231, 1982.

99. Tan SY, Shapiro R, Franco R, Stockard H, Mulrow PJ: Indomethacin induced prostaglandin inhibition with hyperkalemia: A reversible cause of hyporeninemic hypoaldosteronism. *Ann Intern Med* 90:783, 1979.

100. Patak RV, Mookerjee BK, Bentzel CJ, Hysert PE, Babej M, Lee JB: Antagonism of the effects of furosemide by indomethacin in normal and hypertensive man. *Prostaglandins* 10:649, 1975.

101. Bartter FC, Gill JR Jr, Frolich JC, Bowden RE, Hollifield JW, Radfar N, Keiser HR, Oates JA, Seyberth H, Taylor AA: Prostaglandins are overproduced by the kidneys and mediate hyperreninemia in Bartter's syndrome. *Trans Assoc Am Physicians* 89:77, 1976.

102. Goldstone R, Horton R, Carlson EJ, Hsueh WA: Reciprocal changes in active and inactive renin after converting enzyme inhibition in normal man. *J Clin Endocrinol Metab* 56:264, 1983.

103a. Hsueh WA, Goldstone R, Carlson EJ, Horton R: Evidence that the β-adrenergic system and prostaglandins stimulate renin release through different mechanisms. *J Clin Endocrinol Metab* 61:399, 1985.

103b. Nakamura N, Soubrier F, Menard J, Panthier J-J, Rougeon F, Corvol P: Nonproportional changes in plasma renin concentration, renal renin content, and rat renin messenger RNA. *Hypertension* 7:855, 1986.

104. Luetscher JA, Kraemer FB, Wilson DM, Schwartz HC, Bryer-Ash M: Increased plasma inactive renin in diabetes mellitus. *N Engl J Med* 312:1412, 1985.

105. Hofbauer KG, Wood JM, Gulati N, Heusser C, Menard J: Increased plasma renin during renin inhibition: Studies with a novel immunoassay. *Hypertension* 7(suppl I):61, 1985.

106. Wood JM, Gulati N, Forgiarini P, Fuhrer W, Hofbauer KG: Effects of a specific and long-acting renin inhibitor in the marmoset. *Hypertension* 7:797, 1985.

107. Kokubu T, Hiwada K, Murakami E, Imamura Y, Matsueda R, Yabe Y, Koike H, Iijima Y: Highly potent and specific inhibitors of human renin. *Hypertension* 7(suppl I):I-8, 1985.

108. Tewksbury DA, Dart RA: Molecular weight studies on high-molecular weight human angiotensin, in Sambhi (ed): *Heterogeneity of Renin and Renin-Substrate,* Amsterdam, Elsevier/North-Holland, 1981, pp 260–270.

109. Campbell DJ, Habener JF: Angiotensin gene is expressed and differentially regulated in multiple tissues of the rat. *J Clin Invest* 78:31, 1986.

110. Krakoff LR, Eisenfeld AJ: Hormonal control of plasma renin substrate (angiotensin). *Circ Res* 41(suppl 2):43, 1977.

111. Bouhnik J, Galen FX, Clauser E, Menard J, Corvol P: The renin-angiotensin system in thyroidectomized rats. *Endocrinology* 108:647, 1981.

112. Stockigt JR, Hewett MJ, Topliss DJ, Higgs EJ, Taft P: Renin and renin substrate in primary adrenal insufficiency: Contrasting effects of glucocorticoid and mineralocorticoid deficiency. *Am J Med* 66:915, 1979.

113. Clauser E, Bouhnik J, Jaramillo HN, Auzan C, Corvol P, Menard J: Angiotensin production and consumption in the adrenalectomized rat. *Endocrinology* 116:274, 1985.

114. Ohkubo H, Kageyama R, Ujihara M, Hirose T, Inayama S, Nakanishi S: Cloning and sequence analysis of cDNA for rat angiotensinogen. *Proc Natl Acad Sci USA* 80:2196, 1983.

115. Kalinyak JE, Chang E, Perlman AJ: Tissue specific regulaton of rat angiotensinogen gene. *Clin Res* 34:480A, 1986.

116a. Strittmatter SM, Thiele EA, DeSouza EB, Snyder SH: Angiotensin-converting enzyme in the testis and epididymis: Differential development and pituitary regulation of isozymes. *Endocrinology* 117:1374, 1985.

116b. Erdös EG, Skidgel RA: The unusual substrate specificity and the distribution of human angiotensin I converting enzyme. *Hypertension* 8(suppl I):I-34, 1986.

117. Skidgel RA, Erdös EG: Novel activity of human angiotensin I converting enzyme: Release of the NH_2- and COOH-terminal tripeptides from the luteinizing hormone-releasing hormone. *Proc Natl Acad Sci USA* 82:1025, 1985.

118a. Oparil S: Angiotensin I converting enzyme inhibitors and analogues of angiotensin II, in Genest J, Kuchel O, Hamet P, Cantin M (eds): *Hypertension,* 2d ed. New York, McGraw-Hill, 1983, pp 250–271.

118b. Liberman J, Sastri A: Serum angiotensin-converting enzyme: elevations in diabetes mellitus. *Ann Intern Med* 93:825, 1980.

119. Niarchos AP, Resnick LM, Weinstein DL, Laragh JH: Angiotensin I converting enzyme activity in hypertension: Relationship to blood pressure, renin-sodium profiles, and antihypertensive therapy. *Am J Med* 79:435, 1985.

120. Silverstein E, Schussler GC, Friedland J: Elevated serum angiotensin-converting enzyme in hyperthyroidism. *Am J Med* 75:233, 1983.

121. Mersey JH, Williams HG, Hollenberg NK, Dluhy RG: Relationship between aldosterone and bradykinin. *Circ Res* 40(suppl 1):84, 1977.

122. Williams GH, Hollenberg NK: Accentuated vascular and endocrine response to SQ 20881 in hypertension. *N Engl J Med* 297:184, 1977.

123a. Johnston CI, Millar JA, McGrath BP, Matthews PG: Long-term effects of captopril (SQ 14225) on blood pressure and hormone levels in essential hypertension. *Lancet* 2:493, 1979.

123b. Fantone JC, Schrier D, Weingarten B: Inhibition of vascular permeability changes in rats by captopril. *J Clin Invest* 69:1207, 1982.

124. Bauer JH, Reams GP: Hemodynamic and renal function in essential hypertension during treatment with enalapril. *Am J Med* 79(suppl 3C):10:13, 1985.

125a. Redgrave J, Rabinowe S, Hollenberg NK, Williams GH: Correction of abnormal renal blood flow response to angiotensin II by converting enzyme inhibition in essential hypertensives. *J Clin Invest* 75:1285, 1985.

125b. Helgeland A, Strφmmen R, Hagelund CH, Tretli S: Enalapril, atenolol and hydrochlorothiazide in mild to moderate hypertension: A comparative multicentre study in general practice in Norway. *Lancet* 1:872, 1986.

126. Editorial: Angiotensin-converting enzyme inhibitors in treatment of heart failure. *Lancet* 2:811, 1985.

127. Taguma Y, Kitamoto Y, Futaki G, Ueda H, Monma H, Ishizaki M, Takahashi H, Sekino H, Sasaki Y: Effect of captopril on heavy proteinuria in azotemic diabetics. *N Engl J Med* 313:1617, 1985.

127a. Björck S, Nyberg G, Mulec H, Granerus G, Herlitz H, Avrell M: Beneficial effects of angiotensin converting enzyme inhibition on renal function in patients with diabetic nephropathy. *Brit Med J* 293:471, 1986.

127b. Hommel E, Parring H-H, Mathiesen E, Edsberg E, Nielsen MO, Giese J: Effect of captopril on kidney function in insulin-dependent diabetic patients with nephropathy. *Brit Med J* 293:467, 1986.

128. Raij L, Chiou X-C, Owens R, Wrigley B: Therapeutic implications of hypertension-induced glomerular injury. *Am J Med* 79(suppl 3C):37, 1985.

129. Meyer TW, Anderson S, Rennke HG, Brenner BM: Converting enzyme inhibitor therapy limits progressive glomerular injury in rats with renal insufficiency. *Am J Med* 79(suppl 3C):31, 1985.

130. Blaine EH, Nelson BJ, Seymour AA, Schorn TW, Sweet CS, Slater EE, Nussberger J, Boger J: Comparison of renin and converting enzyme inhibition in sodium-deficient dogs. *Hypertension* 7:166, 1985.

131. Goodfriend TL: Angiotensin receptors and specific functions of angiotensins I, II and III, in Genest J, Kuchel O, Hamet P, Cantin M (eds): *Hypertension,* 2d ed. New York, McGraw-Hill, 1983, pp 271–280.

132. Bunag RD: Circulating effects of angiotensin, in Page I, Bumpus M (eds): *Angiotensin.* Berlin, Springer-Verlag, 1974, pp 441–454.

133. Navar LN, Langford HG: Effects of angiotensin in the renal circulation, in Page I, Bumpus M (eds): *Angiotensin.* Berlin, Springer-Verlag, 1974, pp 455–474.

134. Levens NR, Freedlender AE, Peach NJ, Carey RM: Control of renal function by intrarenal angiotensin II. *Endocrinology* 112:43, 1983.

135. Kano T, Fumitake I, Oseko F, Imura H, Endo J: Biological activity of des-Asp[1]-angiotensin I in man. *J Clin Endocrinol Metab* 50:40, 1980.

136. Diz DI, Baer PG, Nasjletti A: Angiotensin II-induced hypertension in the rat: Effects on the plasma concentration, renal excretion, and tissue release of prostaglandins. *J Clin Invest* 72:466, 1983.

137. Catt KJ, Harwood JP, Aguilera G, Dufau ML: Hormonal regulation of peptide hormone receptors and target cell responses. *Nature* 280:109, 1979.

138. Bellucci A, Wiles BM: Mechanism of sodium modulation of glomerular angiotensin receptors in the rat. *J Clin Invest* 74:1593, 1984.

139. Streeten DHP, Anderson GH, Freiberg JM, Dalakos TG: Use of an angiotensin II antagonist (saralasin) in the recognition of "angiotensinogenic" hypertension. *N Engl J Med* 292:657, 1975.

140. Case DB, Wallace JM, Keim HJ, Weber MA, Drayer JIM, White RP, Sealey JE, Laragh JH: Estimating renin participation in hypertension: Superiority of converting enzyme inhibitor over saralasin. *Am J Med* 61:790, 1976.

141. Haber E, Sancho J, Re R, Burton J, Barger AC: The role of the renin-angiotensin-aldosterone system in cardiovascular homeostasis in normal man. *Clin Sci Mol Med* 48(suppl 2):49s, 1975.

142. Noth RH, Tan SY, Mulrow PJ: Effects on angiotensin II blockade by saralasin in normal man. *J Clin Endocrinol Metab* 45:10, 1977.

143. Gavras H, Ribeiro AB, Gavras I, Brunner H: Reciprocal relation between renin dependency and sodium dependency in essential hypertension. *N Engl J Med* 295:1278, 1976.

144. Miller ED Jr, Samuels AI, Haber E, Barger AC: Inhibition of angiotensin conversion and prevention of renal hypertension. *Am J Physiol* 228:448, 1975.

145. Carretero OA, Romero JC: Production and characteristics of experimental hypertension in animals, in Genest J, Koiw E, Kuchel O (eds): *Hypertension: Physiopathology and Treatment.* New York, McGraw-Hill, 1977, pp 485–507.

146. Dzau VJ, Gibbons GH, Levine DC: Renovascular hypertension: An update on pathophysiology, diagnosis and treatment. *Am J Nephrol* 3:172, 1983.

147. Brown JJ, Davies DL, Lever AF, Robertson JIS: Variations in plasma renin concentration in several physiological and pathological states. *Can Med Assoc J* 90:201, 1964.

148. McAllister RG Jr, Van Way CW III, Dayani K, Anderson WJ, Temple E, Michelakis AM, Coppage WS Jr, Oates JA: Malignant hypertension: Effect of therapy on renin and aldosterone. *Circ Res* 28(suppl 2):160, 1971.

149. Waeber B, Gavras I, Brunner HR, et al: Safety and efficacy of chronic therapy with captopril in hypertensive patients: An update. *J Clin Pharmacol* 21:508, 1981.

150. Todd PA, Heel RC: Enalapril. A review of its pharmacodynamic and pharmacokinetic properties, and therapeutic use in hypertension and congestive heart failure. *Drugs* 3:198, 1986.

151. Bauer JH, Brooks CS: Volume studies in men with mild to moderate hypertension. *Am J Cardiol* 44:1163, 1979.

152. Laragh JH, Letcher RL, Pickering TG: Renin profiling for diagnosis and treatment of hypertension. *JAMA* 241:151, 1979.

153. Lebel M, Schalekamp MA, Beevers DG, Brown JJ, Davies DL, Fraser R, Kremer D, Lever SF, Morton JJ, Robertson JIS, Tree M, Wilson A: Sodium and the renin-angiotensin system in essential hypertension and mineralocorticoid excess. *Lancet* 2:308, 1974.

154. Brunner HR, Laragh JH, Baer L, Newton MA, Goodwin FT, Krakoff LF, Bard HR, Buhler FR: Essential hypertension: Renin and aldosterone, heart attack and stroke. *N Engl J Med* 286:441, 1972.

155. Dunn MJ, Tannen RL: Low renin essential hypertension, in Genest J, Koiw E, Kuchel O (eds): *Hypertension: Physiopathology and Treatment.* New York, McGraw-Hill, 1977, pp 349–364.

156. Kotchen TA, Guthrie GP Jr, Cottrill CM, McKean HE, Kotchen JM: Low renin-aldosterone in "prehypertensive" young adults. *J Clin Endocrinol Metab* 54:808, 1982.

157. Wisgerhof M, Carpenter PC, Brown RD: Increased adrenal sensitivity to angiotensin II in idiopathic hyperaldosteronism. *J Clin Endocrinol Metab* 48:266, 1979.

158. Wisgerhof M, Brown RD: Increased adrenal sensitivity to angiotensin II in low-renin essential hypertension. *J Clin Invest* 61:1456, 1978.

159. Marks AD, Marks DB, Kanefsky TM, Adlin VE, Channick BJ: Enhanced adrenal responsiveness to angiotensin II in patients with low-renin essential hypertension. *J Clin Endocrinol Metab* 48:266, 1979.

160. Williams GH, Hollenberg NK: Sodium-sensitive essential hypertension. Emerging insights into pathogenesis and therapeutic implications. *Contemp Nephrol* 3:303, 1985.

161. Williams GH, Hollenberg NK: Are non-modulating patients with essential hypertension a distinct subgroup? Implications for therapy. *Am J Med* 79:3, 1985.

162. MacGregor GA: Sodium is more important than calcium in essential hypertension. *Hypertension* 7:628, 1985.

163. Joossens JV: Dietary salt restrictions: The case in favour. *The Therapeutics of Hypertension. International Congress and Symposium Series, no 26.* London, Royal Society of Medicine, 1980, pp 243–250.

164. Dawber TK, Kannel WB, Kaga ANA, Donabedian RK, McNamara PM: Environmental factors in hypertension, in Stamler J et al (eds): *Epidemiology of Hypertension.* New York, Grune and Statton, 1967, pp 255–288.

165. Nicholls MG: Reduction of dietary sodium in western society. Benefit or risk? *Hypertension* 6:795, 1984.

166. Ministry of Health and Welfare: *National Survey on Circulatory Disorders.* Koseisho, Japan, 1980.

167. Joossens JV, Geboers J: Salt and hypertension. *Prev Med* 12:53, 1983.

168. Tobian L: Salt and hypertension. *Am J Nephrol* 3:80, 1983.

169. Winer BH: The antihypertensive actions of benzothiadiazines. *Circulation* 23:211, 1961.

170. Campese VM, Romoff MS, Levitan D, Saglikes Y, Friedler RM, Massry SG: Abnormal relationship between sodium intake and sympathetic nervous system activity in salt-sensitive patients with essential hypertension. *Kidney Int* 21:371, 1982.

170a. Bittle CC Jr, Molina DJ, Bartter FC: Salt sensitivity in essential hypertension as determined by the cosinor method. *Hypertension* 7:989, 1985.

171. Passmore JC, Whitescarver SA, Ott CE, Kotchen TA: Importance of chloride for deoxycorticosterone acetate-salt hypertension in the rat. *Hypertension* 7:I115, 1985.

172. Kurtz TW, Morris RC Jr: Dietary chloride as a determinant of "sodium-dependent" hypertension. *Science* 22:1139, 1983.

173. Laragh JH: Calcium metabolism and calcium channel blockers for understanding and treating hypertension. *Am J Med* 77:1, 1984.

174. Holloway ET, Bohr DF: Reactivity of vascular smooth muscle in hypertensive rats. *Circ Res* 33:678, 1973.

174a. Resnick LM: Calcium, parathyroid disease, and hypertension. *Cardiovascular Reviews and Reports* 3:1341, 1982.

175. McCarron DA, Morris CD: Blood pressure response to oral calcium in persons with mild to moderate hypertension. *Ann Intern Med* 103:825, 1985.

176. Resnick LM, Laragh JH, Sealey JE, Alderman MH: Divalent cations in essential hypertension: Relations between serum ionized calcium, magnesium, and plasma renin activity. *N Engl J Med* 309:888, 1983.

177. Resnick LM: Calcium and hypertension: The emerging connection. *Ann Intern Med* 103:944, 1985.

177a. Ernc P, Bürgisser E, Bolli P, Ji B, Bühler F: Free calcium concentration in platelets closely related to blood pressure in normal and essentially hypertensive subjects. *Hypertension* 6(suppl I): I-166, 1984.

178. Selig MS: *Magnesium Deficiency in the Pathogenesis of Disease.* New York, Plenum, 1980.

179. Pritchard JA: The use of magnesium ion in the management of eclamptogenic toxemias. *Surg Gynecol Obstet* 100:131, 1955.

180. Dyckner I, Wester PO: Effect of magnesium on blood pressure. *Br Med J* 286:1847, 1983.

181. Altura BM, Altura BT, Gebrewold A: Magnesium deficiency and hypertension: Correlation between magnesium-deficient diets and microcirculatory changes in situ. *Science* 223:1315, 1984.

182. Altura BM, Altura BT: Magnesium ions and contraction of vascular smooth muscles: Relationships to some vascular diseases. *Fed Proc* 40:2672, 1981.

183. Hollifield JW: Thiazide treatment of hypertension: Effects of thiazide diuretics on serum potassium, magnesium, and ventricular ectopy. *Am J Med* 80:8, 1986.

184. Helfant RH: Hypokalemia and arrhythmias. *Am J Med* 80(suppl 4A):13, 1986.

185. Addison W: The uses of sodium chloride, potassium chloride, sodium bromide and potassium bromide in cases of arterial hypertension which are amenable to potassium chloride. *Can Med Assoc J* 18:281, 1928.

186. Priddle WW: Observations on the management of hypertension. *Can Med Assoc J* 25:5, 1931.

187. Walker WG, Whelton PK, Saito H, Russell RP, Hermann J: Relation between blood pressure and renin, renin substrate, angiotensin II, aldosterone and urinary sodium and potassium in 574 ambulatory subjects. *Hypertension* 1:287, 1979.

188. Ueshima H, Tanigaki M, Jida M, Shimamoto M, Konishi M, Komacki Y: Hypertension, salt and potassium. *Lancet* 1:504, 1981.

189. Parfrey PS, Wright P, Goodwin FJ, Vandenburg MJ, Holly JMP, Evans SJW, Ledingham JM: Blood pressure and hormonal changes following alteration in dietary sodium and potassium in mild essential hypertension. *Lancet* 1:59, 1981.

190. Parfrey PS, Wright P, Holly JMP, Evans SJW, Condon K, Vandenburg MJ, Goodwin FJ, Ledingham JM: Blood pressure and hormonal changes following alteration in dietary sodium and potassium in young men with and without a familial predisposition to hypertension. *Lancet* 1:113, 1981.

191. Skrabsal F, Aubock J, Hortnagl H, Braunsteiner H: Effect of moderate salt restriction and high potassium intake on pressor hormones, response to noradrenaline and baroreceptor function in man. *Clin Sci* 59:157s, 1980.

192. Reid WD, Laragh JH: Sodium and potassium intake, blood pressure, and pressor response to angiotensin. *Proc Soc Exp Biol Med* 120:26, 1965.

193. Goto A, Tobian L, Iwai J: Potassium feeding reduces hyperactive central nervous system pressor responses in Dahl salt-sensitive rats. *Hypertension* 3(suppl I):128, 1981.

194. Chen WT, Brace RA, Scott JB, Henderson DK, Haddy FJ: The mechanism of the vasodilator action of potassium. *Proc Soc Exp Biol Med* 140:820, 1970.

195. Young DB, McCaa RE, Pan Y, Guyton AC: The natriuretic and hypotensive effects of potassium. *Circ Res* 38(suppl II):84, 1976.

196. Suzuki H, Kondo K, Saruta T: Effect of potassium chloride on the blood pressure in two-kidney, one clip Goldblatt hypertensive rats. *Hypertension* 3:566, 1981.

197. Brandis M, Keyes J, Windhager EE: Potassium-induced inhibition of proximal tubular fluid reabsorption in rats. *Am J Physiol* 222:421, 1972.

198. Hilton PJ: Cellular sodium transport in essential hypertension. *N Engl J Med* 314:222, 1986.

199. Golub MS, Eggena P, Sowers JR, Maxwell M: Hypertension symposium: Newer topics on normal and abnormal blood pressure regulatory mechanisms. *West J Med* 139:190, 1983.

200. Aalkjaer C, Parvin SD, Bing RF, Heagerty AM, Bell PRF, Swales JD: Cell membrane sodium transport: a correlation between human resistance vessels and leucocytes. *Lancet* 1:649, 1986.

201. Shull GE, Schwartz A, Lingrel JB: Amino-acid sequence of the catalytic subunit of the ($Na^+ + K^+$) ATPase deduced from a complementary DNA. *Nature* 316:691, 1985.

202. Schneider JW, Mercer RW, Caplan M, Emanuel JR, Sweadner KJ, Benz EJ Jr, Levenson R: Molecular cloning of rat brain Na,K-ATPase α-subunit cDNA. *Proc Natl Acad Sci USA* 82:6357, 1985.

203. Lasker N, Hopp L, Grossman S, Bamforth R, Aviv A: Race and sex differences in erythrocyte Na^+, K^+, and Na^+-K^+-adenosine triphosphatase. *J Clin Invest* 75:1813, 1985.

204. Montnari A, Sani E, Canali M, Simoni I, Schianchi P, Borghetti A, Novarini A: Low sodium cotransport in red cells with physiological internal sodium concentration in essential hypertension. *Hypertension* 6:826, 1984.

205. Weber AB: Red-cell lithium-sodium countertransport and renal lithium clearance in hypertension. *N Engl J Med* 314:198, 1986.

206. Haddy FJ: Abnormalities of membrane transport in hypertension. *Hypertension* 5:66, 1983.

207. Kelly RA, O'Hara DS, Canessa ML, Mitch WE, Smith TW: Characterization of digitalis-like factors in human plasma. *J Biol Chem* 260:11396, 1985.

208. Morgan K, Lewis MD, Spurlock G, Collins PA, Foord SM, Southgate K, Scanlon MF, Afzal Mir M: Characterization and partial purification of the sodium-potassium-ATPase inhibitor released from cultured rat hypothalamic cells. *J Biol Chem* 260:13595, 1985.

209. De Wardener HE, MacGregor GA: The natriuretic hormone and essential hypertension. *Lancet* 1:1450, 1982.

210. Carilli CT, Berne M, Cantley LC, Haupert GT Jr: Hypothalamic factor inhibits the (Na,K) ATPase from the extracellular surface. *J Biol Chem* 260:1027, 1985.

211. Graves SW, Brown B, Valdes R Jr: An endogenous digoxin-like substance in patients with renal impairment. *Ann Intern Med* 99:604, 1983.

212. Graves SW, Valdes R Jr, Brown BA, Knight AB, Craig HR: Endogenous digoxin-immunoreactive substance in human pregnancies. *J Clin Endocrinol Metab* 58:748, 1984.

213. Graves SW, Williams GH: An endogenous ouabain-like factor associated with hypertensive pregnant women. *J Clin Endocrinol Metab* 59:1070, 1984.

214. Kazazoglou T, Renaud J-F, Rossi B, Lazdunski M: Two classes of ouabain receptors in chick ventricular cardiac cells and their relation to (Na^+,K^+)-ATPase inhibition, intracellular Na^+ accumulation, Ca^{2+} influx, and cardiotonic effect. *J Biol Chem* 258:12163, 1983.

215. Rydstedt LL, Williams GH, Hollenberg NK: Renal and endocrine response to saline infusion in essential hypertension. *Hypertension* 8:217, 1986.

216. Cantin M, Genest J: The heart as an endocrine gland. *Sci Am* 254:76, 1986.

217. de Bold AJ: Atrial natriuretic factor: A hormone produced by the heart. *Science* 230:767, 1985.

218. Needleman P, Adams SP, Cole BR, Currie MG, Geller DM, Michener ML, Saper CB, Schwartz D, Standaert DC: Atriopeptins as cardiac hormones. *Hypertension* 7:469, 1985.

219. Needleman P, Greenwald JE: Atriopeptin: A cardiac hormone intimately involved in fluid, electrolyte, and blood-pressure homeostasis. *N Engl J Med* 314:828, 1986.

220. Currie MG, Geller DM, Cole BR, Siegel NR, Fok KF, Adams SP, Eubanks SR, Galluppi GR, Needleman P: Purification and sequence analysis of bioactive atrial peptides (atriopeptins). *Science* 223:67, 1984.

221. Schwartz D, Geller DM, Manning PT, Siegel NR, Fok KF, Smith CE, Needleman P: Ser-Leu-Arg-Arg-atriopeptin III: The major circulating form of atrial peptide. *Science* 229:397, 1985.

222. Seidman CE, Block KD, Zisfein J, Smith JA, Haber E, Homcy C, Duby AD, Choi E, Graham RM, Seidman JG: Molecular studies of the atrial natriuretic factor gene. *Hypertension* 7:31, 1985.

223a. Oikawa S, Imai M, Ueno A, Tanaka S, Noguchi T, Nakazato H, Kangawa K, Fokuda A, Matsuo H: Cloning and sequence analysis of cDNA encoding a precursor for human atrial natriuretic polypeptide. *Nature* 309:724, 1984.

223b. Greenberg BD, Bencen GH, Seilhamer JJ, Lewicki JA, Fiddes JC: Nucleotide sequence of the gene encoding human atrial natriuretic factor precursor. *Nature* 312:656, 1984.

224. Ballermann BJ, Brenner BM: Biologically active atrial peptides. *J Clin Invest* 76:2041, 1985.

225. Kangawa K, Fukuda A, Matsuo H: Structural identification of β- and γ- human atrial natriuretic polypeptides. *Nature* 313:397, 1985.

226. Yamaji T, Ishibashi M, Takaku F: Atrial natriuretic factor in human blood. *J Clin Invest* 76:1705, 1985.

227. Hilliker S, Vlasuk G, Borden L, Hancock N, Scarborough R, Schwartz K, Lewicki J: Fate of the atrial natriuretic peptide precursor in the circulation. *Proceedings of the 1st World Congress on Biologically Active Atrial Peptides,* New York, Raven, 1986, no 90A.

228a. Gardner DG, Deschepper CF, Ganong WF, Hane S, Fiddes J, Baxter JD, Lewicki J: Extra-atrial expression of the gene for atrial natriuretic factor. *Proc Natl Acad Sci USA* 83:6697, 1986.

228b. Gardner DG, Deschepper CF, Baxter JD: The gene for atrial natriuretic factor is expressed in the aortic arch. *Hypertension* 9:1986, in press.

228c. Metzler CH, Gardner DG, Keil LC, Baxter JD, Ramsay DJ: Increased synthesis and release of atrial peptide during DOCA escape in conscious dogs. *Am J Physiol,* 1986, in press.

228d. Gardner DG, Hane S, Trachewsky D, Schenk D, Baxter JD: Atrial natriuretic peptide in RNA is regulated by glucocorticoids in vivo. *Biochem Biophys Res Commun* 139:1047, 1986.

229. Burnett JC Jr, Kao PC, Hu DC, Heser DW, Heublein D, Granger JP, Opgenorth TJ, Reeder GS: Atrial natriuretic peptide elevation in congestive heart failure in the human. *Science* 231:1145, 1986.

230. Atlas SA: Atrial natriuretic factor: A new hormone of cardiac origin. *Rec Prog Hormone Res* 42:207, 1986.

231. Laragh JH: Atrial natriuretic hormone, the renin-aldosterone axis and blood pressure-electrolyte homeostasis. *N Engl J Med* 313:1330, 1985.

232. Tikkanen I, Metsarinne K, Fyhrquist F, Leidenius R: Plasma atrial natriuretic peptide in cardiac disease and during infusion in healthy volunteers. *Lancet* 1:66, 1985.

233. Lang RE, Tholken H, Ganten D, Luft FC, Ruskoaho H, Unger T: Atrial natriuretic factor—a circulating hormone stimulated by volume loading. *Nature* 314:264, 1986.

234. Sagnella GA, Shore AC, Markandu ND, MacGregor GA: Effects of changes in dietary sodium intake and saline infusion on immunoreactive atrial natriuretic peptide in human plasma. *Lancet* 2:1208, 1985.

235. Rascher W, Tulassay T, Lang RE: Atrial natriuretic peptide in plasma of volume-overloaded children with chronic renal failure. *Lancet* 2:303, 1985.

236. Sonnenberg H: Atrial natriuretic factor—a new hormone affecting kidney function. *Klin Wochenschr* 63:886, 1985.

237. Sagnella GA, Shore AC, Markandu ND, MacGregor GA: Raised circulating levels of atrial natriuretic peptides in essential hypertension. *Lancet* 1:179, 1986.

238. Morii N, Nakao K, Kihara M, Sakamoto M, Sugawara A, Shimokura M, Kiso Y, Yamori Y, Imura H: Effects of water deprivation and sodium load on atrial natriuretic polypeptide in rat brain. *Hypertension* 8:61, 1986.

239. Maack T, Camargo MJF, Kleinert HD, Laragh JH, Atlas SA: Atrial natriuretic factor: Structure and functional properties. *Kidney Int* 27:607, 1985.

240. Samson WK: Atrial natriuretic factor inhibits dehydration- and hemorrhage-induced vasopressin release. *Neuroendocrinology* 40:227, 1985.

241. Arendt RM, Gerbes AL, Ritter D, Zahringer J: Plasma-ANF in various disease states. *Proceedings of the 1st World Congress on Biologically Active Atrial Peptides,* New York, Raven, 1986, no 79A.

242. Gehr M, Clay S, Goldberg M: Mode of renal action of atrial natriuretic factor (ANF) in normal man. *Proceedings of the 1st World Congress on Biologically Active Atrial Peptides,* New York, Raven, 1986, no 82A.

243. Mimran A, Biollaz J, Nussberger J, Waeber B, Brunner HR: Effect of ANF on urinary kallikrein in normal man. *Proceedings of the 1st World Congress on Biologically Active Atrial Peptides.* New York, Raven, 1986, no 86A.

244. Cogan MG: Atrial natriuretic factor ameliorates chronic metabolic alkalosis by increasing glomerular filtration. *Science* 229:1405, 1985.

245a. Dillingham MA, Anderson RJ: Inhibition of vasopressin action by atrial natriuretic factor. *Science* 231:1572, 1986.

245b. Antonipillai I, Vogelsang J, Horten R: Role of atrial natriuretic factor in renin release. *Endocrinology* 119:318, 1986.

246. Obana K, Naruse M, Naruse K, Sakurai H, Demura H, Inagami T, Shizume K: Synthetic rat atrial natriuretic factor inhibits *in vitro* and *in vivo* renin secretion in rats. *Endocrinology* 117:1282, 1985.

247. Garcia R, Thibault G, Cantin M, Genest J: Effect of a purified atrial natriuretic factor on rat and rabbit vascular strips and vacular beds. *Am J Physiol* 16:R34, 1984.

248. Winquist RJ, Faison EP, Nutt RF: Vasodilator profile of synthetic atrial natriuretic factor. *Eur J Pharmacol* 102:168, 1984.

249. Cody RJ, Kubo SH, Atlas SA, Laragh JH, Ryman KS, Shaknovich A: Atrial natriuretic factor in heart failure: Endogenous activity and response to exogenous administration. *Proceedings of the 1st World Congress on Biologically Active Atrial Peptides,* New York, Raven, 1986, no 80A.

250. Kleinert HD, Volpe M, Odell G, Marion D, Atlas SA, Camargo MJ, Laragh JH, Maack T: Cardiovascular effects of atrial natriuretic factor in anesthetized and conscious dogs. *Hypertension* 8:312, 1986.

251. Richards AM, Ikram H, Yandle TG, Nicholls MG, Webster MWI, Espiner EA: Renal, haemodynamic, and hormonal effects of human alpha atrial natriuretic peptide in healthy volunteers. *Lancet* 1:545, 1985.

252. Weidmann P, Hasler L, Gnadinger MP, Lange RE, Uehlinger DE, Shaw S, Rascher W, Reubi FC: Blood levels and renal effects of atrial natriuretic peptide in normal man. *J Clin Invest* 77:734, 1986.

253. Richards AM, Nichols MG, Espiner EA, Ikram H, Yandle TG, Joyce SL, Cullens MM: Effects of α-human atrial natriuretic peptide in essential hypertension. *Hypertension* 7:812, 1985.

254. de Jong PE, Janssen WMT, van der Hem GK, de Zeeuw D: Blood pressure response to atrial natriuretic peptide (ANP) in essential hypertension (EH): Increased sensitivity after sodium depletion. *Proceedings of the 1st World Congress on Biologically Active Atrial Peptides.* New York, Raven, 1986, no 77A.

255. Seymour AA, Marsh EA, Mazack EK, Stabilito II, Blaine EH: Synthetic atrial natriuretic factor in conscious normotensive and hypertensive rats. *Hypertension* 7(suppl I):I-35, 1985.

256. Andersson OK, Persson B, Aurell M, Granerus G, Wysocky M, Hedner J, Hedner T: Basal and stimulated levels of immunoreactive atrial natriuretic peptide (α-hANP) in relation to central venous pressure, renal and central hemodynamics and sodium excretion in normotensive and hypertensive men. *Proceedings of the 1st World Congress on Biologically Active Atrial Peptides,* New York, Raven, 1986, no 79A.

257. Snajdar RM, Rapp JP: Atrial natriuretic factor in Dahl rats. *Hypertension* 7:775, 1985.

258. Antunes-Rodrigues J, McCann SM, Rogers LC, Samson WK: Atrial natriuretic factor inhibits dehydration- and angiotensin II-induced water intake in the conscious, unrestrained rat. *Proc Natl Acad Sci USA* 82:8720, 1985.

259. Quirion R, Dalpe M, Dam T-V: Characterization and distribution of receptors for the atrial natriuretic peptides in mammalian brain. *Proc Natl Acad Sci USA* 83:174, 1986.

260. Leitman DC, Murad F: Comparison of binding and cyclic GMP accumulation by atrial natriuretic peptides in endothelial cells. *Biochim Biophys Acta* 885:74, 1986.

261. Vandlen RL, Arcuri KE, Napier MA: Identification of a receptor for atrial natriuretic factor in rabbit aorta membranes by affinity cross-linking. *J Biol Chem* 260:10889, 1985.

262. Yip CC, Laing LP, Flynn TG: Photoaffinity labeling of atrial natriuretic factor receptors of rat kidney cortex plasma membranes. *J Biol Chem* 260:8229, 1985.

263. Ballerman BJ, Hoover RL, Karnovsky MJ, Brenner BM: Physiologic regulation of atrial natriuretic peptide receptors in rat renal glomeruli. *J Clin Invest* 76:2049, 1985.

264a. Schiffrin EL, St Louis J, Garcia R, Thibault G, Cantin M, Genest J: Vascular and adrenal binding sites for atrial natriuretic factor. *Hypertension* 8:141, 1986.

264b. Ishikawa S-E, Toshikazu S, Okada K, Kuzaya T, Kangawa K, Matsuo H: Atrial natriuretic factor increases cyclic GMP and inhibits cyclic AMP in rat renal papillary collecting tubule cells in culture. *Biochem Biophys Res Commun* 130:1147, 1985.

265. Lee MA, West RE, Moss J Jr: Atrial natriuretic factor suppresses cAMP content of human fibroblasts independent of the inhibitory guanyl nucleotide-binding regulatory component of adenylate cyclase. *Proceedings of the 1st World Congress on Biologically Active Atrial Peptides,* New York, Raven, 1986, no 90A.

266. Huang C-L, Ives HE, Cogan MG: Intrarenal arterial infusion of dibutyryl cyclic GMP (DBcGMP) can cause glomerular hyperfiltration: In vivo evidence that cGMP serves as the second messenger for ANF. *Proceedings of the 1st World Congress on Biologically Active Atrial Peptides.* New York, Raven, 1986, no 105A.

267. Rapoport RM, Draznin MB, Murad F: Endothelium-dependent vasodilator- and nitrovasodilator-induced relaxation may be mediated through cyclic GMP formation and cyclic GMP dependent protein phosphorylation. *Trans Assoc Am Physicians* 96:19, 1983.

268. Apfeldorf WJ, Barrett PQ, Rasmussen H: ANF inhibits the stimulation of aldosterone secretion by ANG II but not ANG II generation of $[Ca^{2+}]i$ transients. *Proceedings of the 1st World Congress on Biologically Active Atrial Peptides,* New York, Raven, 1986, no 100A.

269. Naruse M, Obana K, Inagami T: Antiserum to atrial natriuretic factor lowers urinary output, urinary sodium excretion and plasma renin activity. *Proceedings of the 1st World Congress on Biologically Active Atrial Peptides,* New York, Raven, 1986, no 109A.

270. Conn JW: Presidential address: Primary aldosteronism, a new clinical syndrome. *J Lab Clin Med* 45:3, 1955.

271. Eberlein WB, Bongiovanni AM: Plasma and urinary corticosteroids in the hypertensive form of congenital adrenal hyperplasia. *J Biol Chem* 223:85, 1956.

272. Biglieri EG, Herron MA, Brust H: 17-Hydroxylation deficiency in man. *J Clin Invest* 45:1946, 1966.

273. Funder JW, Adam WR, Mantero F, Kraft N, Ulick S: The etiology of a syndrome of factitious mineralocorticoid excess: A steroid-containing nasal spray. *J Clin Endocrinol Metab* 49:842, 1979.

274. Griffing GT, Melby JC: Adrenocortical factors in hypertension. *J Clin Pharmacol* 25:218, 1985.

275. Baxter JD, Schambelan M, Matulich D, Spindler BJ, Taylor AA, Bartter FC: Aldosterone receptors and the evaluation of plasma mineralocorticoid activity in normal and hypertensive states. *J Clin Invest* 58:579, 1976.

276. Griffing GT, Dale SL, Holbrook MM, Melby JC: 19-nor-Deoxycorticosterone excretion in primary aldosteronism and low renin hypertension. *J Clin Endocrinol Metab* 56:218, 1983.

277. Griffing GT, Wilson TE, Melby JC: Converting-enzyme inhibitor administration lowers urinary free 19-nor-deoxycorticosterone levels. *Hypertension* 7:178, 1985.

278. Gorsline J, Harnik M, Tresco PA, Morris DJ: Hypertensinogenic activities of ring A-reduced metabolites of aldosterone. *Hypertension* 8(suppl I):187, 1986.

279. Gomez-Sanchez CE, Smith JS, Ferris MW, Gomez-Sanchez EP: Renal receptor-binding activity of reduced metabolites of aldosterone: Evidence for a mineralocorticoid effect outside of the classic aldosterone receptor system. *Endocrinology* 115:712, 1984.

280. Hall CE, Gomez-Sanchez CE: Hypertensive potency of 18-oxocortisol in the rat. *Hypertension* 8:317, 1986.

281. Siegel RR, Luke RG, Hellebusch AA: Reduction of toxicity of corticosteroid therapy after renal transplantation. *Am J Med* 53:159, 1972.

282. Reed WP, Lucas ZJ, Cohn R: Alternate day prednisone therapy after renal transplantation. *Lancet* 1:747, 1970.

283. Soyka L: Treatment of the nephrotic syndrome in childhood. *Am J Dis Child* 113:693, 1967.

284. Gomez-Sanchez CE: Cushing's syndrome and hypertension. *Hypertension* 8:258, 1986.
285. Bulkley BH, Roberts WC: The heart in systemic lupus erythematosus and the changes induced in it by corticosteroid therapy. *Am J Med* 58:243, 1975.
286. Thomas TPL: The complications of systemic corticosteroid therapy in the elderly. *Gerontology* 30:60, 1984.
287. Grunfeld J-P, Eloy L, Moura A-M, Ganeval D, Ramos-Frendo B, Worcel M: Effects of antiglucocorticoids on glucocorticoid hypertension in the rat. *Hypertension* 7:292, 1985.
288. Saruta T, Suzuki H, Handa M, Igarashi Y, Kondo K, Senba S: Multiple factors contribute to the pathogenesis of hypertension in Cushing's syndrome. *J Clin Endocrinol Metab* 62:275, 1986.
289. Oparil S: Theoretical approaches to estimation of plasma renin activity: A review and some original observations. *Clin Chem* 22:583, 1976.
290. Bennett CM, Hsueh WA: Measurement of renin and interpretations of plasma renin activity, in Massry SG, Glassack RJ (eds): *Textbook of Nephrology*. Baltimore, Williams and Wilkins, 1983, pp 11.25–11.28.
291. Ruddy MC, Atlas SA, Salerno FG: Hypertension associated with a renin-secreting adenocarcinoma of the pancreas. *N Engl J Med* 307:993, 1982.
292. Case DB, Laragh JH: Reactive hyperreninemia in renovascular hypertension after angiotensin blockade with saralasin or converting enzyme inhibitor. *Ann Intern Med* 91:153, 1979.
293. Strong CG, Hunt JC, Sheps SG, Tucker RM, Bernatz PE: Renal-venous renin activity, enhancement of sensitivity of catheterization by sodium depletion. *Am J Cardiol* 27:602, 1971.
294. Wintroub BU, Klickstein LB, Kaempfer CE, Austen KF: A human neutrophil-dependent pathway for generation of angiotensin II: Purification and physicochemical characterization of the plasma protein substrate. *Proc Natl Acad Sci USA* 78:1204, 1981.
295. Weinberger MH, Grim CE, Hollifield JW, Ken DC, Ganguly A, Kramer NJ, Yune HY, Wellman H, Donohue JP: Primary aldosteronism: Diagnosis, localization, and treatment. *Ann Intern Med* 90:386, 1979.
296. Biglieri EG, Stockigt JR, Schambelan M: Adrenal mineralocorticoids causing hypertension. *Am J Med* 52:623, 1972.
297. Cain JP, Tuck ML, Williams GH, Dluhy RG, Rosenhoff SH: The regulation of aldosterone secretion in primary aldosteronism. *Am J Med* 53:627, 1972.
298. Biglieri EG: Effect of posture on plasma concentrations of aldosterone in hypertension and primary hyperaldosteronism. *Nephron* 23:112, 1979.
298a. Nadler JL, Hsueh W, Horton R: Therapeutic effect of calcium channel blockade in primary aldosteronism. *J Clin Endocrinol Metab* 60:1896, 1985.
299. Himathongkam T, Dluhy RG, Williams GH: Potassium-aldosterone-renin interrelationships. *J Clin Endocrinol Metab* 41:115, 1976.
300. Horton R: Stimulation and suppression of aldosterone in plasma of normal man and in primary aldosteronism. *J Clin Invest* 48:1230, 1969.
301. Kem DC, Weinberger MH, Mayes DM, Nugent CA: Saline suppression of plasma aldosterone in hypertension. *Arch Intern Med* 128:380, 1971.
302. Streeten DHP, Tomycz N, Anderson GH Jr: Reliability of screening methods for primary aldosteronism. *Am J Med* 67:412, 1979.
303. Biglieri EG: Rare causes of adrenocortical hypertension. *Cardiology* 72(suppl 1):70, 1985.
304. Biglieri EG, Schambelan M: Significance of elevated levels of plasma 18-hydroxycorticosterone in patients with primary aldosteronism. *J Clin Endocrinol Metab* 49:87, 1979.
305. Tucker RM, LaBarthe DR: Frequency of surgical treatment for hypertension in adults at the Mayo Clinic from 1973 through 1975. *Mayo Clin Proc* 52:549, 1977.
306a. Gifford RW: Evaluation of the hypertensive patient with emphasis on detecting curable causes. *Milbank Mem Fund Q* 47:170, 1969.
306b. Ferguson RK: Cost and yield of the hypertension evaluation: Experience of a community based referral clinic. *Ann Intern Med* 82:761, 1975.
307. Berglund G, Andersson O, Wilhelmson L: Prevalence of primary and secondary hypertension: Studies in a random population sample. *Br Med J* 2:554, 1976.
308. Loggie JMH: Hypertension in children and adolescents. I. Causes and diagnostic studies. *J Pediatr* 74:331, 1969.
309. Davis BA, Crook JE, Vestal RE, Oates JA: Prevalence of renovascular hypertension in patients with grade III or IV hypertensive retinopathy. *N Engl J Med* 301:1273, 1979.
310. Messerli FH, Glade LB, Ventura HO, Dreslinski GR, Suarez DH, MacPhee AA, Aristimuno GG, Cole FE, Frohlich ED: Diurnal variations of cardiac rhythm, arterial pressure, and urinary catecholamines in borderline and established essential hypertension. *Am Heart J* 104:109, 1982.
311. Perloff D, Sokolow M: The representative blood pressure: Usefulness of office, basal, home, and ambulatory readings. *Cardiovasc Med* 3:655, 1978.
312. Hossmann V, FitzGerald GA, Dollery CT: Influence of hospitalization and placebo therapy on blood pressure and sympathetic function in essential hypertension. *Hypertension* 3:113, 1981.
313. Pickering G: *High Blood Pressure,* 2d ed. New York, Grune and Stratton, 1968, p 35.
314. Carey RM, Reid RA, Ayers CR, et al: The Charlottesville blood pressure survey: Value of repeated blood pressure measurements to determine the prevalence of labile and sustained hypertension. *JAMA* 236:847, 1976.
315. Julius S, Ellis CN, Pascual AV, et al: Home blood pressure determination: Value in borderline ("labile") hypertension. *JAMA* 229:663, 1974.
316. Gould BA, Hornung RS, Kieso H, Cashman PMM, Raftery EB: An evaluation of self-recorded blood presure during drug trials. *Hypertension* 8:267, 1986.
317. Pickering TG, Harshfield GA, Devereux RB, Laragh JH: What is the role of ambulatory blood pressure monitoring in the management of hypertensive patients? *Hypertension* 7:171, 1985.
318. Littler WA, Honour AJ, Pugsley DJ, et al: Continuous recording of direct arterial pressure in unrestricted patients. Its role in the diagnosis and management of high blood pressure. *Circulation* 51:1101, 1975.
319. Sokolow M, Werdegar D, Kain HK, et al: Relationship between level of blood pressure measured casually and by portable recorders and severity of complications in essential hypertension. *Circulation* 34:279, 1966.
320. Kirkendall WM, Feinleib M, Freis ED, Mark AL: Recommendations for human blood pressure determination by sphygmomanometers. *Circulation* 62:1145A, 1980.
321. Maxwell MH, Schroth PC, Waks AU, Karam M, Dornfeld LP: Error in blood-pressure measurement due to incorrect cuff size in obese patients. *Lancet* 2:33, 1982.
322a. Keith NM Wagener HP, Barker NW: Some different types of essential hypertension: Their course and prognosis. *Am J Med Sci* 197:332, 1939.
322b. Romhilt DW, Bove KE, Norris RJ, et al: A critical appraisal of the electrocardiographic criteria for the diagnosis of left ventricular hypertrophy. *Circulation* 40:185, 1969.
322c. Liebson PR, Savage DD: Echocardiography in hypertension: A review. I. Left ventricular wall mass, standardization and ventricular function. *Echocardiography* 3:181, 1986.
323. Bright R: Cases and observations illustrative of renal disease accompanied with the secretion of albuminous urine. *Guy's Hosp Rep* 1:338, 1836.

324. Mahomed F: Chronic Bright's disease without albuminuria. *Guy's Hosp Rep* 25:295, 1881.
325. Tigerstedt R, Bergman G: Niere und Krieslauf. *Skand Arch Physiol* 8:223, 1898.
326. Volhard F, Fahr T: *Die Brightsche Nieren Krankheit Kinik Pathologie und Atlas.* Berlin, Springer, 1914.
327. Ask-Upmark E: Über junvenile maligne Nephrosklerose und ihr Verhältniss zu Störungen in der Nierenentwicklung. *Acta Pathol Microbiol Scand* 6:383, 1929.
328. Crabtree EG: Stricture formation in ureter following pyelonephritis of pregnancy. *J Urol* 18:575, 1927.
329. Goldblatt H, Lynch J, Hanzal RF, Summerville WW: Studies on experimental hypertension. 1. The production of persistent elevation of systolic blood pressure by means of renal ischemia. *J Exp Med* 59:347, 1934.
330. Goldblatt H: Studies on experimental hypertension. 5. The pathogenesis of experimental hypertension due to renal ischemia. *Ann Intern Med* 11:69, 1937.
331. Butler AM: Chronic pyelonephritis and arterial hypertension. *J Clin Invest* 16:889, 1937.
332. Leadbetter WF, Burkland CE: Hypertension in unilateral renal disease. *J Urol* 39:611, 1938.
333. Smith HW: Hypertension and urologic disease. *Am J Med* 4:724, 1948.
334. Smith HW: Unilateral nephrectomy in hypertensive disease. *J Urol* 76:685, 1956.
335. Page IH: On the nature of the pressor action of renin. *J Exp Med* 70:521, 1939.
336. Braun-Menendez E, Fasciolo JC, Leloir LF, Munoz JM: La substance hypertensive extraite du sang des reins ischemies. *C R Soc Biol* 133:731, 1940.
337. Goormaghtigh N: Facts in favor of an endocrine function of the renal arterioles. *J Pathol* 57:393, 1945.
338. Bumpus FM, Schwarz H, Page IH: Synthesis and pharmacology of the octapeptide angiotensin. *Science* 125:886, 1957.
339. Deming QB, Luetscher JA: Bioassay of desoxycorticosterone-like material in urine. *Proc Soc Exp Biol Med* 73:171, 1950.
340a. Laragh JH: The role of aldosterone in man: Evidence for regulation of electrolyte balance and arterial pressure by renal-adrenal system which may be involved in malignant hypertension. *JAMA* 174:293, 1960.
340b. Bumpus FM, Khosla MC: Pathogenetic factors involved in renovascular hypertension—state of the art. *Mayo Clin Proc* 52:417, 1977.
340c. Sheps SG, Wollenweber J, Davis GD: Clinical aspects of the natural history of atherosclerotic renovascular disease, in Brest AN, Moyer JH (eds): *Atherosclerotic Renovascular Disease: A Hahnemann Symposium.* New York, Appleton-Crofts, 1967, p 374.
340d. Poutasse EF, Dustan HP: Arteriosclerosis and renal hypertension: Indications for aortography in hypertensive patients and results of surgical treatment of obstructive lesions of renal artery. *JAMA* 165:1521, 1957.
340e. Perloff D, Sokolow M, Wylie EJ, Palubinskas AJ: Renal vascular hypertension: Further experiences. *Am Heart J* 74:614, 1967.
340f. Harrison EG Jr, McCormack LJ: Pathologic classification of renal arterial disease in renovascular hypertension. *Mayo Clin Proc* 46:161, 1971.
340g. Stanley JC, Gewartz BL, Boue EL, et al: Arterial fibrodysplasia: Histopathologic character and current etiologic concepts. *Arch Surg* 110:561, 1975.
341. McCormack LJ, Poutasse EF, Meaney TF, Noto TJ, Dustan HP: A pathologic-arteriographic correlation of renal arterial disease. *Am Heart J* 72:188, 1966.
342. Kincaid OW, Davis GD, Hallermann FJ, Hunt JC: Fibromuscular dysplasia of the renal arteries—arteriographic features, classification and observation on natural history of the disease. *Am J Roentgenol* 104:271, 1968.
343. Wylie EJ, Wellington JS: Hypertension caused by fibromuscular hyperplasia of the renal arteries. *Am J Surg* 100:183, 1960.
344. Wylie EJ, Binkley FM, Palubinskas AJ: Extrarenal fibromuscular hyperplasia. *Am J Surg* 112:149, 1966.
345. Schmidt DM, Rambo ON: Segmental intimal hyperplasia of the abdominal aorta and renal arteries producing hypertension in an infant. *Am J Clin Pathol* 44:546, 1965.
346. Sharma BK, Sagar S, Chugh KS, et al: Spectrum of renovascular hypertension in the young in north India: A hospital based study on occurrence and clinical features. *Angiology* 36:370, 1985.
347. Makker SP, Moorthy B: Fibromuscular dysplasia of renal arteries: An important cause of renovascular hypertension in children. *J Pediatr* 95:940, 1979.
348. Hunt JC, Harrison EG Jr, Kincaid OW, et al: Idiopathic fibrous and fibromuscular stenoses of the renal arteries associated with hypertension. *Mayo Clin Proc* 37:181, 1962.
349. Palubinskas AJ, Wylie EJ: Roentgen diagnosis of fibromuscular hyperplasia of the renal arteries. *Radiology* 76:634, 1961.
350. Ekelund L, Gerlock J, Molin J, Smith C: Roentgenologic appearance of fibromuscular dysplasia. *Acta Radiol [Diagn]* 19:433, 1978.
351. Goncharenko V, Gerlock AJ Jr, Shaff MI, Hollifield JW: Progression of renal artery fibromuscular dysplasia in 42 patients as seen on angiography. *Radiology* 139:45, 1981.
352. Stewart BH, Dustan HP, Kiser WS, et al: Correlation of angiography and natural history in evaluation of patients with renovascular hypertension. *J Urol* 104:231, 1970.
353. Poutasse EF: Occlusion of a renal artery as a cause of hypertension. *Circulation* 13:37, 1956.
354. Golbus SM, Swerdlin AR, Mitas JA, et al: Renal artery thrombosis in a young woman taking oral contraceptives. *Ann Intern Med* 90:939, 1979.
355. Slater EE, DeSanctis RW: Disease of the aorta, in Braunwald E (ed): *Heart Disease.* Philadelphia, Saunders, 1980, p 1548.
356. Poutasse EF: Renal artery aneurysm: Report of 12 cases, 2 treated by excision of the aneurysm and repair of renal artery. *J Urol* 77:697, 1957.
357. Smith JN, Hinman F Jr: Intrarenal arterial aneurysms. *J Urol* 97:990, 1967.
358. Ishikawa K: Natural history and classification of occlusive thromboaortopathy (Takayasu's disease). *Circulation* 57:27, 1978.
359. Shelhamer JH, Volkman DJ, Parrillo J, et al: Takayasu's arteritis and its therapy. *Ann Intern Med* 103:121, 1985.
360. Lagneau P, Michel JB: Renovascular hypertension and Takayasu's disease. *J Urol* 134:876, 1985.
361. White RH, Schambelan M: Hypertension, hyperreninemia, and secondary hyperaldosteronism in systemic necrotizing vasculitis. *Ann Intern Med* 92:199, 1980.
362. Scully RE, Mark EJ, McNeely BU: Weekly clinicopathological exercises: Case 36-1985. *N Engl J Med* 313:622, 1985.
363. Duffy J, Lidsky MD, Sharp JT, et al: Polyarthritis, polyarteritis and hepatitis B. *Medicine* 55:19, 1976.
364. Silver D, Clements JB: Renovascular hypertension from renal artery compression by congenital bands. *Ann Surg* 183:161, 1976.
365. Patel MR, Mooppan MM, Kim H: Subcapsular urinoma: Unusual form of "page kidney" in newborn. *Urology* 23:585, 1984.
366. Halpern M, Currarino G: Vascular lesions causing hypertension in neurofibromatosis. *N Engl J Med* 273:248, 1965.
367. Schurch W, Messerli FH, Genest J, et al: Arterial hypertension and neurofibromatosis: Renal artery stenosis and coarctation of abdominal aorta. *Can Med Assoc J* 113:879, 1975.
368. Flynn MP, Buchanan JB: Neurofibromatosis, hypertension, and renal artery aneurysms. *South Med J* 73:618, 1980.
369. Dodds WJ, Noyes WE, Hinman F Jr, Storey RJ: Renal artery aneurysm: A cause of segmental alteration in renal blood flow and hypertension. *Am J Roentgenol* 104:302, 1968.
370. Loggie JMH: Prevalence of hypertension and distribution of

causes, in New MI, Levine LS (eds): *Juvenile Hypertension.* New York, Raven, 1977, pp 1–12.

371. Stanley JC: Renal vascular disease and renovascular hypertension in children. *Urol Clin North Am* 11:451, 1984.

372. Watson AR, Balfe JW, Hardy BE: Renovascular hypertension in childhood: A changing perspective in management. *J Pediatr* 106:366, 1985.

373. Sagalowsky AI, Peters PC: Renovascular hypertension following renal transplantation. *Urol Clin North Am* 11:491, 1984.

374. Bennett WM, McDonald WJ, Lawson RK, et al: Post-transplant hypertension: Studies of cortical blood flow and the renal pressor system. *Kidney Int* 6:99, 1974.

375. Palleschi J, Novick AC, Braun WE, et al: Vascular complications of renal transplantation. *Urology* 16:61, 1980.

376. Klarskov P, Brendsrup L, Karup T, et al: Renovascular hypertension after kidney transplantation. *Scand J Urol Nephrol* 13:291, 1979.

377. Robertson PW, Klidjian A, Harding LK, Walters G: Hypertension due to a renin-secreting renal tumor. *Am J Med* 43:963, 1967.

378. Cohn JW, Cohen EL, Lucas CP, et al: Primary reninism. *Arch Intern Med* 130:682, 1972.

379. Schambelan M, Howes EL Jr, Stockigt JR, Noakes CA, Biglieri EG: Role of renin and aldosterone in hypertension due to a renin-secreting tumor. *Am J Med* 55:86, 1973.

380. Mitchell JD, Baxter TJ, Blair-West JR, et al: Renin levels in nephroblastoma (Wilms' tumour): Report of a renin-secreting tumour. *Arch Dis Child* 45:376, 1970.

381. Scully RE, Mark EJ, McNeely BN: Weekly clinicopathological exercises. Case 51-1985. *N Engl J Med* 313:1594, 1985.

382. Sheth KJ, Tang TT, Blaedel ME, et al: Polydipsia, polyuria and hypertension associated with renin-secreting Wilms' tumor. *J Pediatr* 92:921, 1978.

383. Genest J, Rojo-Ortega JM, Kuchel O, et al: Malignant hypertension with hypokalemia in a patient with renin-producing pulmonary carcinoma. *Trans Assoc Am Physicians* 88:192, 1975.

384. Aurell M, Rudin A, Tisell L-E, et al: Captopril effect on hypertension in patient with renin-producing tumour. *Lancet* 2:149, 1979.

385. Atlas SA, Hessen TE, Sealey JE, Dharmgrongartama B, Laragh JH: Characterization of inactive renin from renin-secreting tumors. *J Clin Invest* 73:437, 1984.

386. Meaney TF, Dustan HP, McCormack LJ: Natural history of renal arterial disease. *Radiology* 91:881, 1968.

387. Stanley JC: Morphologic, histopathologic and clinical characteristics of renovascular fibrodysplasia and arteriosclerosis, in Bergen JJ, Yao JST (eds): *Surgery of the Aorta and its Body Branches.* New York, Grune and Stratton, 1979, pp 255–376.

388. Sheps SG, Kincaid OW, Hunt JC: Serial renal function and angiographic observations in idiopathic fibrous and fibromuscular stenoses of the renal arteries. *Am J Cardiol* 30:55, 1972.

389. Schreiber MJ, Pohl MA, Novick AC: The natural history of atherosclerotic and fibrous renal artery disease. *Urol Clin North Am* 11:383, 1984.

390. Hunt JC, Strong CG: Renovascular hypertension: Mechanisms, natural history and treatment, in Laragh JH (ed): *Hypertension Manual.* New York, Yorke Medical, 1976, p 509.

391. Wollenweber J, Sheps SG, Davis GD: Clinical course of atherosclerotic renovascular disease. *Am J Cardiol* 21:60, 1968.

392. Black HR, Glickman MG, Schiff M Jr, et al: Renovascular hypertension: Pathophysiology, diagnosis and treatment. *Yale J Biol Med* 51:635, 1978.

393. Sreepada, Rao TK, Nicastri AD, Friedman EA: Natural history of heroin-associated nephropathy. *N Engl J Med* 290:19, 1974.

394. Simon N, Franklin SS, Bleifer KH, Maxwell MH: Cooperative study of renovascular hypertension: Clinical characteristics of renovascular hypertension. *JAMA* 220:1209, 1972:

395. Perloff D, Sokolow M, Wylie EJ, et al: Hypertension secondary to renal artery occlusive disease. *Circulation* 24:1286, 1961.

396. Perera GA, Haelig AW: Clinical characteristics of hypertension associated with unilateral renal disease. *Circulation* 6:549, 1952.

397. Londe S: Causes of hypertension in the young. *Pediatr Clin North Am* 25:55, 1978.

398. Malhotra KK, Sharma RK, Prabhakar S, Bhargava S, Bhuyan UN, Dhawan IK, Kumar R, Dash SC: Aortoarteritis as a major cause of renovascular hypertension in the young. *Indian J Med Res* 77:487, 1983.

399. Keith TA: Renovascular hypertension in black patients. *Hypertension* 4:438, 1982.

400. Gibson GS, Gibbons A: Hypertension among blacks. An annotated bibliography. *Hypertension* 4(suppl I):11, 1982.

401. Gifford RW Jr: Epidemiology and clinical manifestations of renovascular hypertension, in Stanley JC, Ernst CN, Fry WJ (eds): *Renovascular Hypertension.* Philadelphia, Saunders, 1984, pp 77–104.

402. Hollenberg NK: Medical therapy of renovascular hypertension: Efficacy and safety of captopril in 269 patients. *Cardiovasc Rev Rep* 4:852, 1983.

403a. Laidlaw JC, Yendt ER, Gornall AH: Hypertension caused by renal artery occlusion simulating primary aldosteronism. *Metabolism* 9:612, 1960.

403b. Foster JH, Pettinger WA, Oates JA, Rhamy RK, Klatte EC, Burke HC, Bolasny BL, Gordon R, Puyau FA, Younger RK: Malignant hypertension secondary to renal artery stenosis in children. *Ann Surg* 164:700, 1966.

404. Moser RJ Jr, Caldwell JR Jr: Abdominal murmurs: An aid in the diagnosis of renal artery disease in hypertension. *Ann Intern Med* 56:471, 1962.

405. McLoughlin MJ, Colapinto RF, Hobbs BB: Abdominal bruits: Clinical and angiographic correlation. *JAMA* 232:1238, 1975.

406. Blackman SS Jr: Arteriosclerosis and partial obstructon of the main renal arteries in association with "essential" hypertension in man. *Bull Johns Hopkins Hosp* 65:353, 1939.

407. Kashgarian M: Pathology of small blood vessel disease in hypertension. *Am J Kidney Dis* 5:A104, 1985.

408. Maxwell JM, Gonick HC, Wiita R, Kaufman JJ: Use of the rapid sequence pyelogram in the diagnosis of renovascular hypertension. *N Engl J Med* 270:213, 1964.

409. Bookstein JJ, Abrams HL, Buenger RE, Lecky J, Franklin SS, Reiss MD, Bleifer KH, Klatte EC, Maxwell MH: Radiologic aspects of renovascular hypertension. Part I. Aims and methods of the radiology study group. *JAMA* 220:1218, 1972.

410. Bookstein JJ, Abrams HL, Buenger RE, Lecky J, Franklin SS, Reiss MD, Bleifer KH, Klatte EC, Varady PD, Maxwell MH: Radiologic aspects of renovascular hypertension. Part 2. The role of urography in unilateral renovascular disease. *JAMA* 220:1225, 1972.

411. Don C: The changes on the intravenous pyelogram in renal artery disease. *Am J Roentgenol* 98:107, 1966.

412. Moëll H: Size of normal kidneys. *Acta Radiol* 46:640, 1956.

413. Correa RJ Jr, Stewart BH, Boblitt DE: Intravenous pyelography as a screening test in renal hypertension. *Am J Roentgenol* 88:1135, 1962.

414. Hunt JC, Sheps SG, Harrison EG Jr, Strong CG, Bernatz PE: Renal and renovascular hypertension: A reasoned approach to diagnosis and management. *Arch Intern Med* 133:988, 1974.

415. Bookstein JJ, Maxwell MH, Abram HL, et al: Cooperative study of radiologic aspects of renovascular hypertension—bilateral renovascular disease. *JAMA* 237:1706, 1977.

416. Atkinson AB, Kellet RJ: Value of intravenous urography in investigating hypertension. *J R Coll Physicians Lond* 8:175, 1974.

417. Thornbury JR, Stanley JC, Fryback DG: Hypertensive urogram: A non-discriminatory test for renovascular hypertension. *Am J Roentgenol* 138:43, 1982.

418. Lalli AF: Is the hypertensive urogram a necessary examination? *J Can Assoc Radiol* 32:11, 1981.
419. Webb JA, Talner LB: The role of intravenous urography in hypertension. *Radiol Clin North Am* 17:1, 1979.
420. Grim CE, Luft FC, Weinberger MH, et al: Sensitivity and specificity of screening tests for renal vascular hypertension. *Ann Intern Med* 91:617, 1979.
421. Spataro RF: Newer contrast agents for urography. *Radiol Clin North Am* 22:365, 1984.
422. Chervu LR, Blaufox MD: Renal radiopharmaceuticals—an update. *Semin Nucl Med* 12:224, 1982.
423. Stormorken H, Skalpe IO, Testart MC: Effect of various contrast media on coagulation, fibrinolysis and platelet function. An in vitro and in vivo study. *Invest Radiol* 21:348, 1986.
424. Misson RT, Cutler RE: Radiocontrast-induced renal failure (medical progress). *West J Med* 142:657, 1985.
425. Burbank MK, Hunt JC, Tauxe WN, Maher FT: Radioisotopic renography: Diagnosis of renal arterial disease in hypertensive patients. *Circulation* 27:328, 1963.
426. Maxwell MH, Lupu AN, Taplin GV: Radioisotope renogram in renal arterial hypertension. *J Urol* 100:376, 1968.
427. Rosenthal L: Radiotechnetium renography and serial radiohippurate imaging for screening renovascular hypertension. *Semin Nucl Med* 4:97, 1974.
428. Fommei E, Bellina CR, Carmellini M, Palla L, Palombo C, Ghione S: High sensitivity of a computerized radioisotopic method to evaluate unilateral renal blood flow reduction by firstpass analysis and static imaging with 99mTc-glucoheptonate. *J Nucl Med Allied Sci* 27:303, 1983.
429. Farmelant MH, Burrows BA: The renogram: Physiologic basis and current clinical use. *Semin Nucl Med* 4:61, 1974.
430. Tauxe WN, Maker FT, Taylor WF: Effective renal plasma flow: Estimation from theoretical volumes of distribution of intravenously injected 131-I orthoiodohippurate. *Mayo Clin Proc* 46:524, 1971.
431. Mackay A, Eadie AS, Cumming AMM, Graham AG, Adams FG, Horton PW: Assessment of total and divided renal plasma flow by 123-I-hippuran renography. *Kidney* 19:49, 1981.
432. Dubovsky EV, Russel CD: Quantitation of renal function with glomerular and tubular agents. *Semin Nucl Med* 7:308, 1982.
433. Szabo' Z, Vosberg H, Torsello G, Sandmann W, Feinendegen LE: Parameters of ^{99m}Tc-DTPA transfer in renal artery stenosis. *Cardiology* 72(suppl 1):46, 1985.
434. Giese J, Mogensen P, Munck O: Diagnostic value of renography for detection of unilateral renal or renovascular disease in hypertensive patients. *Scand J Clin Lab Invest* 35:307, 1975.
435. Keim HJ, Johnson PM, Vaughan ED, et al: Computer-assisted static/dynamic renal imaging: A screening test for renovascular hypertension? *J Nucl Med* 20:11, 1979.
436. Shovlin M: Radionuclide screening for renovascular hypertension. *J Nucl Med* 21:104, 1980.
437. DeGrazia JA, Scheibe PO, Jackson PE, et al: Clinical applications of a kinetic model of hippurate distribution and renal clearance. *J Nucl Med* 15:102, 1974.
438. McAfee JG, Thomas FD, Grossman Z, Streeten DHP, Dailey E, Gagne G: Diagnosis of angiotensinogenic hypertension: The complementary roles of renal scintigraphy and the saralasin infusion test. *J Nucl Med* 18:669, 1977.
439. Schaeffer AJ, Fair WR: Comparison of split function ratios with renal vein renin ratios in patients with curable hypertension caused by unilateral renal artery stenosis. *J Urol* 112:697, 1974.
440. Lamki L, Spence JD, MacDonald AC, Roulston M: Differential glomerular filtration rate in diagnosis of renovascular hypertension and follow-up of balloon angioplasty. *Clin Nucl Med* 11:188, 1986.
441. Gruenwald SM, Stewart JH, Simmons KC, Crocker EF: Predictive value of quantitative renography for successful treatment of atherosclcerotic renovascular hypertension. *Aust NZ J Med* 15:617, 1985.
442. Heinz ER, Dubois PJ, Drayer BP, Hill R: A preliminary investigation of the role of dynamic computed tomography in renovascular hypertension. *J Comput Assist Tomog* 4:63, 1980.
443. Kohler TR, Zierler RE, Martin RL, et al: Noninvasive diagnosis of renal artery stenosis by ultrasonic duplex scanning. *J Vasc Surg* 4:450, 1986.
444. Wood RFM, Nasmyth DG: Doppler ultrasound in the diagnosis of vascular occlusion in renal transplantation. *Transplantation* 33:547, 1982.
445. Rittgers SE, Norris CS, Barnes RW: Detection of renal artery stenosis: Experimental and clinical analysis of velocity wave forms. *Ultrasound Med Biol* 11:523, 1985.
446. Smith P, Rush TW, Evans AT: The technique of translumbar arteriography. *JAMA* 148:255, 1952.
447. Swartz RD, Rubin JE, Leeming BW, et al: Renal failure following major angiography. *Am J Med* 65:31, 1978.
448. Seldinger SI: Catheter replacement of the needle in percutaneous arteriography: A new technique. *Acta Radiol* 39:368, 1953.
449. Hodson CJ: Renal arteriography in hypertension. *Proc R Soc Med* 50:539, 1957.
450. Palubinskas AJ: "Stretching" of the arteries in renal arteriography. *Radiology* 82:40, 1964.
451. Kaufman JJ, Hanafee W, Maxwell MH: Upright renal arteriography in the study of renal hypertension. *JAMA* 187:977, 1964.
452. Staab EV, Smith CW, Burko H: The evaluation of routine selective arteriography: A new technique. *Cathet Cardiovasc Diagn* 2:143, 1976.
453. McAfee JG: Complications of abdominal aortography and arteriography, in Abrams HL (ed): *Angiography*. Boston, Little, Brown, 1971, vol 2, pp 717–728.
454. Reiss MD, Bookstein JJ, Bleifer KH: Radiologic aspects of renovascular hypertension. Part 4: Arteriographic complications. *JAMA* 221:374, 1972.
455. Foster JH, Dean RH, Pinkerton JA, Rhany RH: Ten-year experience with surgical management of renovascular hypertension. *Ann Surg* 177:755, 1973.
456. Hessel SJ: Complications of angiography and other catheter procedures, in Abrams HL (ed): *Angiography*. Boston, Little, Brown, 1983, pp 1041–1056.
457. Dean RH, Burko H, Wilson SP: Deceptive patterns of renal artery stenosis. *Surgery* 76:872, 1974.
458. Bookstein JJ, Walter JF, Stanley JC, et al: Pharmacoangiographic manipulation of renal collateral blood flow. *Circulation* 54:328, 1976.
459. May AG, Van de Berg L, De Weese JA, et al: Critical arterial stenosis. *Surgery* 54:250, 1963.
460. Holley KE, Hunt JC, Brown AL, Kincaid OW, Sheps GS: Renal artery stenosis: A clinico-pathologic study in normotensive and hypertensive patients. *Am J Med* 37:14, 1964.
461. Eyler WR, Clark MD, Garman JE, Rian RL, Meininger DE: Angiography of the renal areas including a comparative study of renal arterial stenoses in patients with and without hypertension. *Radiology* 78:879, 1962.
462. Osborne RW, Goldstone J, Hillman BJ, et al: Digital video subtraction angiography: Screening technique for renovascular hypertension. *Surgery* 90:932, 1981.
463. Hillman BJ, Ovitt TW, Nudelman S, et al: Digital video subtraction angiography of renal vascular abnormalities. *Radiology* 139:277, 1981.
464. Buonocore E, Meaney TF, Borkowski GP, et al: Digital subtraction angiography of the abdominal aorta and renal arteries. *Radiology* 139:281, 1981.
465. Smith CW, Winfield AC, Price RR, et al: Evaluation of digital venous angiography for the diagnosis of renovascular hypertension. *Radiology* 144:51, 1982.
466. Hillman BJ: Digital radiology of the kidney. *Radiol Clin North Am* 23:211, 1985.

467. Kerlan RK Jr, Pogany AC, Burke DR, Ring EJ: Recognition and management of renovascular hypertension (clinical conference). *Am J Roentgenol* 45:119, 1985.

468. Havey RJ, Krumlovsky F, delGreco F, Martin HG: Screening for renovascular hypertension: Is renal digital-subtraction angiography the preferred noninvasive test? *JAMA* 254:388, 1985.

469. Dunnick NR, Ford KK, Johnson GA, Gunnells JC: Digital intravenous subtraction angiography for investigating renovascular hypertension: Comparison with hypertensive urography. *South Med J* 78:690, 1985.

470. Thornbury JR, Stanley JC, Fryback DG: Optimizing work-up of adult hypertensive patients for renal artery stenosis. *Radiol Clin North Am* 22:333, 1984.

471. Sellars L, Siamopoulos K, Hacking PM, et al: Renovascular hypertension: Ten years' experience in a regional centre. *QJ Med* 56:403, 1985.

472. Connor TB, Berthrong M, Thomas WC, Howard JE: Hypertension due to unilateral renal disease with a report on a functional test helpful in diagnosis. *Bull Johns Hopkins Hosp* 100:241, 1957.

473. Howard JE, Berthrong M, Gould DM, et al: Hypertension resulting from unilateral renal vascular disease and its relief by nephrectomy. *Bull Johns Hopkins Hosp* 94:51, 1954.

474. Mueller C, Surshin A, Carlin M, White H: Glomerular and tubular influences on sodium and water excretion. *Am J Physiol* 165:411, 1951.

475. Blake WD, Negria R, Ward HP, et al: Effect of renal arterial constriction on excretion of sodium and water. *Am J Physiol* 163:422, 1950.

476. Selkurt EE: The effect of pulse pressure and mean arterial pressure modification on renal hemodynamics and electrolyte and water excretion. *Circulation* 4:541, 1951.

477. Stamey TA, Nudelman IJ, Good PH, Schwentker FN, Hendricks F: Functional characteristics of renovascular hypertension. *Medicine* 40:347, 1961.

478. Stamey TA: Functional characteristics of renovascular hypertension with emphasis on the relationship of renal blood flow to hypertension. *Circ Res* 11:209, 1962.

479. Rapaport A: Modification of the "Howard test" for the detection of renal artery obstruction. *N Engl J Med* 263:1159, 1960.

480. Birchall R, Batson HM Jr, Brannon W: Contribution of differential renal studies to the diagnosis of renal arterial hypertension with emphasis on the value of U sodium/U creatinine. *Am J Med* 32:164, 1962.

481. Hunt JC, Maher FT, Greene LF, Sheps SG: Functional characteristics of the separate kidneys in hypertensive man. *Am J Cardiol* 17:493, 1966.

482. Dean RH, Englund R, Dupont WD, et al: Retrieval of renal function by revascularization. Study of preoperative outcome predictors. *Ann Surg* 202:367, 1985.

483. Vertes V, Grauel JA, Goldblatt H: Renal arteriography, separate renal-function studies and renal biopsy in human hypertension. Selection of patients for surgical treatment. *N Engl J Med* 270:656, 1964.

484. Vertes V, Grauel JA, Goldblatt H: Studies of patients with renal hypertension undergoing vascular surgery. *N Engl J Med* 272:186, 1965.

485. Nochy D, Barres D, Camilleri JP, et al: Abnormalities of renin-containing cells in human glomerular and vascular renal diseases. *Kidney Int* 23:375, 1983.

486. Haber E, Koerner T, Page LB, et al: Application of a radioimmunoassay for angiotensin I to the physiologic measurement of plasma renin activity in normal human subjects. *J Clin Endocrinol* 29:1349, 1969.

487. Pickering TG, Sos TA, Vaughn ED Jr, et al: Predictive value and changes of renin secretion in patients undergoing successful renal angioplasty. *Am J Med* 76:398, 1984.

488. Gross F: The renin-angiotensin system in hypertension. *Ann Intern Med* 75:777, 1971.

489. Mohring J, Mohring B, Naumann JH, et al: Salt and water balance and renin activity in renal hypertension of rats. *Am J Physiol* 228:1847, 1975.

490. Sealey JE, Buhler FR, Laragh JH, et al: The physiology of renin secretion in essential hypertension: Estimation of renin secretion rate and renal plasma flow from peripheral and renal vein renin levels. *Am J Med* 55:391, 1973.

491. Marks LS, Maxwell MH: Renal vein renin: Value and limitations in the prediction of operative results. *Urol Clin North Am* 2:311, 1975.

492. Bean BL, Brown JJ, Casals-Stenzel J, et al: The relation of arterial pressure and plasma angiotensin II concentration: A change produced by prolonged infusion of angiotensin II in the conscious dog. *Circ Res* 44:452, 1979.

493. Brunner HR, Laragh JH: Saralasin in human hypertension: The early experience. *Kidney Int* 15:536, 1979.

494. Abramowicz M (ed): Saralasin for diagnosis of renovascular hypertension. *Med Lett* 24:3, 1982.

495. Vaughn ED Jr: Renovascular hypertension. *Kidney Int* 27:811, 1985.

496. Thibonnier M, Joseph A, Sassano P, Guyenne TT, Corvol P, Raynaud A, Seurot M, Gaux JC: Improved diagnosis of unilateral renal artery lesions after captopril administration. *JAMA* 251:56, 1984.

497. Sellars L, Shore AC, Wilkinson R: Renal vein studies in renovascular hypertension—do they really help? *J Hypertension* 3:177, 1985.

498. Delin K, Aurell M, Granerus G: Preoperative diagnosis of renovascular hypertension. The use of acute stimulation of renin secretion. *Acta Med Scand* 215:363, 1984.

498a. Muller FB, Sealey JE, Case DB, Atlas SA, Pickering TG, Pecker MS, Preikisz HJ, Laragh JH: The captopril test for identifying renovascular disease in hypertension patients. *Am J Med* 80:633, 1986.

499. McNeil BJ, Varady PD, Burrows BA, Adelstein SJ: Measures of clinical efficacy. Cost-effectiveness calculation in the diagnosis and treatment of hypertensive renovascular disease. *N Engl J Med* 293:216, 1975.

500. Vidt DG: Advances in the medical management of renovascular hypertension. *Urol Clin North Am* 11:417, 1984.

501. Breslin DJ, Swinton NW: Renovascular hypertension. Surgical versus medical therapeutic consideration. *Med Clin North Am* 63:397, 1979.

502. Schreiber MJ, Novick AC: Medical versus surgical management of renovascular hypertension. *Cardiovasc Clin* 2:93, 1982.

503. Bender W, LaFrance N, Walker WG: Mechanism of deterioration in renal function in patients with renovascular hypertension treated with enalapril. *Hypertension* 6:1193, 1984.

504. Dean RH, Kieffer RW, Smith BM, Oates JA, Nadeau JHJ, Hollifield JW, DuPont WD: Renovascular hypertension: Anatomic and renal functional changes during drug therapy. *Arch Surg* 116:1408, 1981.

505. Hricik DE, Browning PJ, Kopelman R, et al: Captopril-induced functional renal insufficiency in patients with bilateral renal-artery stenoses or renal artery stenosis in solitary kidney. *N Engl J Med* 308:373, 1983.

506. Owen K: Results of surgical treatment in comparison with medical treatment of renovascular hypertension. *Clin Sci Mol Med* 45(suppl):95, 1973.

507. Hunt JC, Bernatz PE, Harrison EG Jr: Factors determining diagnosis and choice of treatment of renovascular hypertension: Influence of location, severity, and type of stenosing lesions. *Circ Res* 21:211, 1967.

508. Sheps SG, Osmundson PJ, Hunt JC, et al: Hypertension and

renal artery stenosis: Serial observations on 54 patients treated medically. *Clin Pharmacol Ther* 6:700, 1965.

509. Whelton PK, Harris AP, Russell RP, et al: Renovascular hypertension: Results of medical and surgical therapy. *Johns Hopkins Med J* 149:213, 1981.

510. Hunt JC, Strong CG: Renovascular hypertension: Mechanisms, natural history and treatment. *Am J Cardiol* 32:563, 1973.

511. Crysant SG, Dunn M, Marples D, et al: Severe reversible azotemia from captopril therapy: Report of three cases and review of the literature. *Arch Intern Med* 143:437, 1983.

512. Epstein M, Oster JR: Beta blockers and renal function: A reappraisal. *J Clin Hypertens* 1:85, 1985.

513. Staessen J, Bulpitt CJ, Fagard R, Lijnen P, Amery A: Long-term converting enzyme inhibition versus surgical treatment in hypertensive patients with renovascular disease. *Neth J Med* 27:161, 1984.

514a. Horvath JS, Tiller DJ: Indications for renal artery surgery: A review. *J R Soc Med* 77:221, 1984.

514b. Novick AC, Straffon RA, Stewart BH, et al: Diminished operative morbidity and mortality in renal revascularization. *JAMA* 246:749, 1981.

515. Stoney RJ: Transaortic renal endarterectomy, in Rutherford RB (ed): *Vascular Surgery*. Philadelphia, Saunders, 1977, pp 1001–1066.

516. Wylie EJ, Perloff DL, Stoney RJ: Autogenous tissue revascularization technics in surgery for renovascular hypertension. *Ann Surg* 170:416, 1969.

517. Sinaiko A, Najarian J, Michael AF, Mirkin BL: Renal autotransplantation in the treatment of bilateral renal artery stenosis: Relief of hypertension in an 8-year-old boy. *J Pediatr* 83:409, 1973.

518. Poutasse EF: Surgical treatment of renal hypertension: Results in patients with occlusive lesions of renal arteries. *J Urol* 82:403, 1959.

519. Vogt PA, Pairolero PC, Hollier LH, Fowl RJ, Cherry KJ, Bernatz PE: The occluded renal artery: Durability of revascularization. *J Vasc Surg* 2:125, 1985.

520. Bauer H, Forbes GL: Unilateral renal artery obstruction associated with malignant nephrosclerosis confined to the opposite kidney. *Am Heart J* 44:634, 1952.

521. Dotter CT, Judkins MP: Transluminal treatment of atherosclerotic obstruction: Description of a new technique and a preliminary report of its application. *Circulation* 30:654, 1964.

522. Grüntzig A, Kuhlmann U, Vetter W, et al: Treatment of renovascular hypertension with percutaneous transluminal dilatation of a renal artery stenosis. *Lancet* 1:801, 1978.

523. Ring EJ, McLean GK: *Interventional Radiology: Principles and Techniques*. Boston, Little, Brown, 1981, pp 117–244.

524. Sos TA, Pickering TG, Sniderman K, et al: Percutaneous transluminal renal angioplasty in renovascular hypertension due to atheroma or fibromuscular dysplasia. *N Engl J Med* 309:274, 1983.

525. Tegtmeyer CJ, Elson J, Glass TA, et al: Percutaneous transluminal angioplasty: The treatment of choice for renovascular hypertension due to fibromuscular dysplasia. *Radiology* 143:631, 1982.

526. Slater EE: Renal artery angioplasty versus surgery: a hypertensionologist's dilemma. *Am J Roentgenol* 135:1085, 1980.

527a. Stanley JC, Graham LM: Renal artery fibrodysplasia and renovascular hypertension in Rutherford RB (ed): *Vascular Surgery*. Philadelphia, Saunders, 1984, pp 1145–1162.

527b. Fry WJ: Treatment of renovascular hypertension. *Adv Surg* 19:51, 1986.

528. Foster JH, Maxwell MD, Franklin SS, et al: Renovascular occlusive disease. Results of operative treatment. *JAMA* 231:1043, 1975.

529. Franklin SS, Young JD, Maxwell MH, et al: Operative morbidity and mortality in renovascular disease. *JAMA* 231:1148, 1975.

530a. Novick AC, Straffon RA: Surgical treatment of renovascular hypertension. *Urol Surv* 30:61, 1980.

530b. Sheps SG, Colville DS: Occlusive renovascular disease. *Cardiovasc Clin* 13:219, 1983.

531. Stanley JC, Whitehouse WM, Graham LM, et al: Operative treatment of renovascular hypertension. *Br J Surg* 69(suppl):63s, 1982.

532a. Morin JE, Hutchinson TA, Lisbona R: Long-term prognosis of surgical treatment of renovascular hypertension: A fifteen-year experience. *J Vasc Surg* 3:545, 1986.

532b. Jordan ML, Novick AC, Cunningham RL: The role of renal autotransplantation in pediatric and young adult patients with renal artery disease. *J Vasc Surg* 2:385, 1985.

532c. Fowl RJ, Hollier LH, Bernatz PE, Pairolero PC, Vogt PA, Cherry KJ: Repeat revascularization versus nephrectomy in the treatment of recurrent renovascular hypertension. *Surg Gynecol Obstet* 162:37, 1986.

532d. Stanley JC: Renal vascular disease and renovascular hypertension in children. *Urol Clin North Am* 11:451, 1981.

533a. Sellars L, Siamopoulos K, Hacking PM, Proud G, Taylor RM, Essenhigh DM, Wilkinson R: Renovascular hypertension: Ten years' experience in a regional centre. *Q J Med* 56:403, 1985.

533b. Dean RH, Krueger TC, Whiteneck JM, et al: Operative management of renovascular hypertension: Results after 15–23 years follow-up. *J Vasc Surg* 1:234, 1984.

533c. Luft FC, Grim CE, Weinberger MH: Intervention in patients with renovascular hypertension and renal insufficiency. *J Urol* 130: 654, 1983.

534a. Bardam L, Helgstrand U, Bentzen MH, Burchardt Hansen HJ, Engell HC: Late results after surgical treatment of renovascular hypertension. A follow-up study of 122 patients 2–18 years after surgery. *Ann Surg* 201:219, 1985.

534b. Starr DS, Lawrie GM, Morris GC Jr: Surgical treatment of renovascular hypertension. Long-term follow-up of 216 patients up to 20 years. *Arch Surg* 115:494, 1980.

534c. Stanley JC, Whitehouse WM Jr, Zelenock GB, Graham LM, Cronenwett JL, Lindenauer SM: Reoperation for complications of renal artery reconstructive surgery undertaken for treatment of renovascular hypertension. *J Vasc Surg* 2:133, 1985.

535. Treadway KK, Slater EE: Renovascular hypertension. *Annu Rev Med* 35:665, 1984.

536. Sos TA, Pickering TG, Saddekni S, Srur M, Case DB, Silane MF, Vaughan ED Jr, Laragh JH: The current role of renal angioplasty in the treatment of renovascular hypertension. *Urol Clin North Am* 11:503, 1984.

537. Martin LG, Casarella WJ, Alspaugh JP et al: Renal artery angioplasty: Increased technical success and decreased complications in the second 100 patients. *Radiology* 159:631, 1986.

538. Freiman DB: Transluminal angioplasty of the renal arteries. *Urol Clin North Am* 12:737, 1985.

539. Ferriss JB, Beevers DG, Brown JJ, Fraser R, Lever AF, Padfield PL, Robertson JIS: Low-renin ("primary") hyperaldosteronism. *Am Heart J* 95:641, 1978.

540. Biglieri EG, Forsham PH: Studies on expanded extracellular fluid and responses to various stimuli in primary aldosteronism. *Am J Med* 30:564, 1961.

541. Pelletier M, Ludens JH, Fanestil DD: The role of aldosterone in active sodium transport. *Arch Intern Med* 129:248, 1972.

542. O'Neil RG, Helman SI: Transport characteristics of renal collecting tubules: Influences of DOCA and diet. *Am J Physiol* 233:F544, 1977.

543. Tannen RL: Potassium handling by the kidney, in Tannen RL, Massry S, Glassock RJ (eds): *Textbook of Nephrology*. Baltimore, Williams and Wilkins, 1983, pp 3.31–3.48.

544. Slaton PE, Biglieri EG: Hypertension and hyperaldosteronism

of renal and adrenal origin. *Am J Med* 38:324, 1965.
545. Bravo EL, Dustan HP, Tarazi RC: Spironolactone as a nonspecific treatment for primary aldosteronism. *Circulation* 48:491, 1973.
546. Tarazi RC, Ibrahim MM, Brova EL, Dustan HP: Hemodynamic characteristics of primary aldosteronism. *N Engl J Med* 289:1330, 1973.
547. Went GJ, Man in't Veld AJ, Verhoeven RP, Derkx RP, Schalekamp MADH: Volume-pressure relationships during development of mineralocorticoid hypertension in man. *Circ Res* 40(suppl 1):163, 1977.
548. Biglieri EG, McIlroy MB: Abnormalities of renal function and circulatory reflexes in primary aldosteronism. *Circulation* 33:78, 1966.
549. August JT, Nelson DH, Thorn GW: Response of normal subjects to large amounts of aldosterone. *J Clin Invest* 37:1549, 1958.
550. Zipser RD, Speckart PF: "Normotensive" primary aldosteronism. *Ann Intern Med* 88:655, 1978.
551. Biglieri EG, Schambelan M, Slaton PE Jr, Stockigt JR: The intercurrent hypertension of primary aldosteronism. *Circ Res* 26/27 (suppl 1):195, 1970.
552. Stockigt JR, Collins RD, Biglieri EG: Determination of plasma renin concentration by angiotensin I immunoassay: Diagnostic import of precise measurement of subnormal renin in hyperaldosteronism. *Circ Res* 28/29(suppl 2):175, 1971.
553. Cain JP, Tuck ML, Williams GH, Dluhy RG, Rosenhoff SH: The regulation of aldosterone secretion in primary aldosteronism. *Am J Med* 53:627, 1972.
554. Melby JC: Primary aldosteronism. *Kidney Int* 26:769, 1984.
555. Franco-Saenz R, Mulrow PJ, Kin K: Idiopathic aldosteronism: A possible disease of the intermediate lobe of the pituitary. *JAMA* 251:2555, 1984.
556. Griffing GT, McIntosh T, Berelowitz B, Hudson M, Salzman R, Manson JE, Melby JC: Plasma β-endorphin levels in primary aldosteronism. *J Clin Endocrinol Metab* 60:315, 1985.
557. Carey RM, Sen S, Dolan LM, et al: Idiopathic hyperaldosteronism: A possible role for aldosterone-stimulating factor. *N Engl J Med* 311:94, 1984.
558. Griffing GT, Berelowitz B, Hudson M, et al: Plasma immunoreactive gamma melanotropin in patients with idiopathic hyperaldosteronism, aldosterone-producing adenomas, and essential hypertension. *J Clin Invest* 76:163, 1985.
559. Gross MD, Grekin R, Gniadek TC, Villareal JZ: Suppression of aldosterone by cyproheptadine in idiopathic aldosteronism. *N Engl J Med* 305:181, 1981.
560. Krieger DT: Physiopathology of Cushing's disease. *Endocr Rev* 4:22, 1983.
560a. Banks WA, Kastin AJ, Biglieri EG, Ruiz AE: Primary adrenal hyperplasia: A new subset of primary aldosteronism. *J Clin Endocrinol Metab* 58:783, 1984.
561. Sutherland DJA, Ruse JL, Laidlaw JC: Hypertension, increased aldosterone secretion, and low plasma renin actively relieved by dexamethasone. *Can Med Assoc J* 95:1109, 1966.
562. Giebink GS, Gotlin RW, Biglieri EG, Katz FH: A kindred with familial glucocorticoid-suppressible aldosteronism. *J Clin Endocrinol Metab* 36:715, 1973.
563. Schambelan M, Brust NL, Chang BCF, Slater KL, Biglieri EG: Circadian rhythm and effect of posture on plasma aldosterone concentration in primary aldosteronism. *J Clin Endocrinol Metab* 43:115, 1976.
564. Stockigt JR: Mineralocorticoid excess, in James VHT (ed): *The Adrenal Gland.* New York, Raven, 1979, pp 197–241.
565. Gomez-Sanchez CE, Montgomery M, Ganguly A, Holland OB, Gomez-Sanchez EP, Grim CE, Weinberger MH: Elevated urinary excretion of 18-oxocortisol in glucocorticoid-suppressible aldosteronism. *J Clin Endocrinol Metab* 59:1022, 1984.
566. Rauh W, Levine LS, Gottesdiener K, New MI: Mineralocorticoids, salt balance and blood pressure after prolonged ACTH administration in juvenile hypertension. *Klin Wochenschr* 56(suppl 1):161, 1978.
567. Biglieri EG, Schambelan M, Slaton PE Jr: Effect of adrenocorticotropin on deoxycorticosterone, corticosterone and aldosterone excretion. *J Clin Endocrinol Metab* 29:1090, 1969.
568. Ganguly A, Zager PG, Luetscher JA: Primary aldosteronism due to unilateral hyperplasia. *J Clin Endocrinol Metab* 51:1190, 1980.
569. Beierwaltes WH, Lieberman LM, Ansari AN, Nishiyama H: Visualization of human adrenal glands in vivo by scintillation scanning. *JAMA* 216:275, 1971.
570. Hogan MJ, McRae J, Schambelan M, Biglieri EG: Location of aldosterone-producing adenomas with ^{131}I-19-iodocholesterol. *N Engl J Med* 294:410, 1976.
571. Scoggins BA, Odie CJ, Hare WSC, Coghlan JP: Preoperative lateralization of aldosterone-producing tumors in primary aldosteronism. *Ann Intern Med* 76:891, 1972.
572. Horton R, Frinck E: Diagnosis and localization in primary aldosteronism. *Ann Intern Med* 76:885, 1972.
573. Geisinger MA, Zelch MG, Bravo EL, Risius BF, O'Donovan PB, Borkowski GP: Primary hyperaldosteronism: Comparison of CT, adrenal venography, and venous sampling. *Am J Roentgenol* 141:299, 1983.
574. Linde R, Coulam C, Battino R, Rhamy R, Gerlock J, Hollifield J: Localization of aldosterone-producing adenoma by computed tomography. *J Clin Endocrinol Metab* 49:642, 1979.
575. Bayliss RIS, Edwards OM, Starer F: Complications of adrenal venography. *Br J Radiol* 43:531, 1970.
576. Geisinger MA, Zelch MG, Bravo EL, et al: Primary hyperaldosteronism comparison of CT adrenal venographic and venous sampling. *AJR* 141:299, 1983.
577. Sarkar SD, Cohen EL, Beierwaltes WH: A new superior adrenal imaging agent, I-131-6-beta-10-iodomethyl-19-nor-cholesterol (NP-59): Evaluation in humans. *J Clin Endocrinol Metab* 45:353, 1977.
578. Ganguly A, Melada GA, Leutscher JA, Dowdy AJ: Control of plasma aldosterone in primary aldosteronism: Distinction between adenoma and hyperplasia. *J Clin Endocrinol Metab* 37:765, 1973.
579. Vetter H, Siebenschein R, Studer A, Witassek F, Furrer J, Glanzer K, Siegenthaler W, Vetter W: Primary aldosteronism: Inability to differentiate unilateral from bilateral adrenal lesions by various routine clinical and laboratory data and by peripheral plasma aldosterone. *Acta Endocrinol* 89:710, 1978.
580. Lyons DF, Kem DC, Brown RD, Hanson CS, Carollo ML: Single dose captopril as a diagnostic test for primary aldosteronism. *J Clin Endocrinol Metab* 57:892, 1983.
581. Brown RD, Kem DC, Hogan MJ, Hegstad RL: Evaluation of a test using saralasin to differentiate primary aldosteronism due to an aldosterone-producing adenoma from idiopathic hyperaldosteronism. *Metabolism* 33:734, 1984.
581a. Arteaga E, Klein R, Biglieri EG: Use of the saline infusion test to diagnose the cause of primary aldosteronism. *Am J Med* 79:722, 1985.
582. Gunnelles JC, McGuffin WL Jr, Robinson RR, Grim CE, Wells S, Silver D, Glenn JF: Hypertension, adrenal abnormalities, and alteration in plasma renin activity. *Ann Intern Med* 73:901, 1970.
583. George JM, Wright L, Bell NH, Bartter FC: The syndrome of primary aldosteronism. *Am J Med* 48:343, 1970.
584. Baer L, Sommers SC, Krakoff LR, Newton MA, Laragh JH: Pseudoprimary aldosteronism: An entity distinct from true aldosteronism. *Circ Res* 26/27(suppl 1):203, 1970.
585. Hunt TK, Schambelan M, Biglieri EG: Selection of patients and operative approach in primary aldosteronism. *Ann Surg* 182:353, 1975.

586. Ferriss JB, Beevers DG, Boddy K, Brown JJ, Davies DL, Fraser R, Kremer DL, Lever AF, Robertson JI: The treatment of low-renin ("primary") hyperaldosteronism. *Am Heart J* 96:97, 1978.

587. Grim CE, Weinberger MH, Kanand S: Familial dexamethasone-suppressible normokalemic hyperaldosteronism, in New MI, Levine LS (eds): *Juvenile Hypertension*. New York, Raven, 1977, pp 109–122.

588. Morimoto S, Takeda R, Murakami M: Does prolonged pretreatment with large doses of spironolactone hasten recovery of juxtaglomerular adrenal suppression in primary aldosteronism? *J Clin Endocrinol Metab* 31:659, 1970.

589. Horton R, Hsueh WA: Treatment of hyperaldosteronism, in Krieger D, Barden CW (eds): *Current Therapy in Endocrinology*, Philadelphia, CV Mosby, 1983, pp 127–131.

590. Conn JW, Hinerman DL: Spironolactone-induced inhibition of aldosterone biosynthesis in primary aldosteronism: Morphological and functional studies. *Metabolism* 26:1293, 1971.

591. Brano EL, Fouad FM, Tarazi RC: Calcium channel blockade with nifedipine in primary aldosteronism. *Hypertension* 8(suppl I): I-191, 1986.

592. Fleckenstein A, Frey M, Zorn J, Fleckstein-Grün G: Experimental basis of the long term therapy of arterial hypertension with calcium antagonists. *Am J Cardiol* 56:3H, 1986.

593. Calcium metabolism and calcium channel blockers for understanding and treating hypertension (panel discussion). *Am J Med* 771, 1984.

594. Biglieri EG, Slaton PE, Schambelan M, Kronfield SJ: Hypermineralocorticism. *Am J Med* 45:170, 1968.

595. New MI, Seaman MP: Secretion rates of cortisol and aldosterone precursors in various forms of congenital adrenal hyperplasia. *J Clin Endocrinol Metab* 30:361, 1970.

596. Finkelstein M, Shaefer JM: Inborn errors of steroid biosynthesis. *Physiol Rev* 59:353, 1979.

597. Bongiovanni AM, Root AW: The adrenogenital syndrome. *N Engl J Med* 268:1283; 268:1342; 268:1391, 1963.

598. Levine LS, Rauh W, Gottesdiener K, Chow D, Gunczler P, Rapaport R, Pang S, Schneider B, New MI: New studies of the 11β-hydroxylase and 18-hydroxylase enzymes in the hypertensive form of congenital adrenal hyperplasia. *J Clin Endocrinol Metab* 50:258, 1980.

599. Kowarski AA: Mechanism of salt loss in congenital virilizing adrenal hyperplasia, in Lee PA, Plotnick LP, Kowarski AA, Migeon DJ (eds): *Congenital Adrenal Hyperplasia*. Baltimore, University Park, 1977, pp 113–124.

600. Ulick S: Adrenocortical factors in hypertension: Significance of 18-hydroxy-11-deoxycorticosterone. *Am J Cardiol* 38:814, 1976.

601. New MI: Male pseudohermaphroditism due to 17α-hydroxylase deficiency. *J Clin Invest* 49:1930, 1970.

602. Biglieri EG, Mantero F: The characteristics, course and implications of the 17-hydroxylation deficiency in man, in Finkelstein Jungblut P, Klopper A, Conti C (eds): *Research on Steroids*, Rome, Societa Editrice Universo, 1973, vol 5, pp 385–399.

603. Biglieri EG: Mechanisms establishing the mineralocorticoid hormone patterns in the 17α-hydroxylase deficiency syndrome. *J Steroid Biochem* 11:653, 1979.

604. Biglieri EG, Schambelan M, Slaton PE Jr: Effect of adrenocorticotropin on deoxycorticosterone, corticosterone and aldosterone secretion. *J Clin Endocrinol Metab* 29:1090, 1969.

605. Biglieri EG, Schambelan M, Rost C: Adrenocorticotropin inhibition of mineralocorticoid hormone production. *Clin Sci* 57(suppl 5):307s, 1979.

606. Kondo K, Saruta T, Saito I, Yoshida R, Maruyama H, Matsuki S: Benign desoxycorticosterone-producing adrenal tumor. *JAMA* 236:1042, 1976.

607. Mantero F, Armanini D, Boscaro M: Plasma renin activity and urinary aldosterone in Cushing's syndrome. *Horm Metab Res* 10:65, 1978.

608. Krakoff L, Nicolis G, Amsel B: Pathogenesis of hypertension in Cushing's syndrome. *Am J Med* 58:216, 1975.

609. Cristy NP: Cushing's syndrome: The natural disease, in Christy NP (ed): *The Human Adrenal Cortex*. New York, Harper & Row, 1971, p 359.

610. Schambelan M, Slaton PE Jr, Biglieri EG: Mineralocorticoid production in hyperadrenocorticism: Role in pathogenesis of hypokalemic alkalosis. *Am J Med* 51:299, 1971.

611. Cassar J, Loizou S, Kely WF, Mashiter K, Joplin GF: Deoxycorticosterone and aldosterone excretion in Cushing's syndrome. *Metabolism* 29:115, 1980.

612. Hogan MJ, Schambelan M, Biglieri EG: Concurrent hypercortisolism and hypermineralocorticoidism. *Am J Med* 62:777, 1977.

613. Solomon SS, Swerise SP, Paulsen A, Biglieri EG: Feminizing adrenocortical carcinoma with hypertension. *J Clin Endocrinol Metab* 28:608, 1968.

614. Butkus A, Coghlan JP, Denton DA, Graham WF, Humphrey TJ, Scoggins BA, Whitworth JA: Adrenocortical steroid hormones in production of hypertension in sheep. *J Steroid Biochem* 11:1021, 1979.

615. Brunner HR, Laragh JH, Baer L, Newton MA, Goodwin FT, Krakoff LF, Bard RH, Buhler FR: Essential hypertension: Renin and aldosterone, heart attack and stroke. *N Engl J Med* 286:441, 1972.

616. Taylor AA, Bartter FC: Hypertension in licorice intoxication, acromegaly, and Cushing's syndrome, in Genest J, Koiw E, Kuchel O (eds): *Hypertension*. New York, McGraw-Hill, 1977, pp 755–767.

617. Blachley JD, Knochel JP: Tobacco chewer's hypokalemia: licorice revisited. *N Engl J Med* 302:784, 1980.

618. Chobanian AV, Volicer L, Tifft CP, Gavras H, Liang C-S, Faxon D: Mineralocorticoid-induced hypertension in patients with orthostatic hypotension. *N Engl J Med* 301:68, 1979.

619. Funder JW, Adam WR, Mantero F, Kraft N, Ulick S: The etiology of a syndrome of factitious mineralocorticoid excess: A steroid-containing nasal spray. *J Clin Endocrinol Metab* 49:842, 1979.

620. New MI, Levine LS, Biglieri EG, Pareira G, Ulick S: Evidence for an unidentified steroid in a child with apparent mineralocorticoid hypertension. *J Clin Endocrinol Metab* 44:924, 1977.

621. Winter JCD, McKenzie JK: A syndrome of low-renin hypertension in children, in New MI, Levine LS (eds): *Juvenile Hypertension*. New York, Raven, 1977, pp 123–131.

622. Shackleton CHL, Honour JW, Dillion MJ, Chantler C, Jones RWA: Hypertension in a four-year-old child: Gas chromatographic and mass spectrometric evidence for deficient hepatic metabolism of steroids. *J Clin Endocrinol Metab* 50:786, 1980.

623. Ulick S, Levine LS, Gunczler P, Zanconato G, Ramirez LC, Rauh W, Rosler A, Bradlow HL, New MI: A syndrome of apparent mineralocorticoid excess associated with defects in the peripheral metabolism of cortisol. *J Clin Endocrinol Metab* 49:757, 1979.

624. Lan NC, Matulich DT, Biglieri EG, Stockigt JR, New MI, Baxter JD: Radioreceptor assay of plasma mineralocorticoid activity: Role of aldosterone, cortisol, deoxycorticosterone in various mineralocorticoid excess states. *Circ Res* 46(pt II):194, 1980.

625. Oberfield SE, Levine LS, Carey RM, Greig F, Ulick S, New MI: Metabolic and blood pressure responses to hydrocortisone in the syndrome of apparent mineralocorticoid excess. *J Clin Endocrinol Metab* 56:332, 1983.

626. Liddle GW, Bledsoe T, Coppage WS Jr: A familial renal disorder simulating primary aldosteronism but with negligible aldosterone secretion. *Trans Assoc Am Physicians* 76:199, 1963.

627. Vingerhoeds ACM, Thijssen JHH, Schwartz F: Spontaneous hypercortisolism without Cushing's syndrome. *J Clin Endocrinol Metab* 43:1128, 1976.

628. Chrousos GP, Vingerhoeds A, Brandon D, Eil C, Pugeat M, DeVroede M, Loriaux DL, Lipsett MB: Primary cortisol resistance in

man: A glucocorticoid receptor-mediated disease. *J Clin Invest* 69:1261, 1982.
629. Sann L, Revol A, Zachmann M, Legrand JC, Bethenod M: Unusual low plasma renin hypertension in a child. *J Clin Endocrinol Metab* 43:265, 1976.
630. Werder E, Zachmann M, Vollmin JA, Veyrat R, Prader A: Unusual steroid excretion in a child with low renin hypertension, in Finkelstein M, Jungblut P, Klopper A, Conti C (eds): *Research on Steroids*, Rome, Societa Editrice Universo, 1975, vol 5, p 385.
631. Schambelan M, Sebastian A, Rector FC Jr: Mineralocorticoid-resistant renal hyperkalemia without salt wasting (type II pseudohypoaldosteronism): Role of increased renal chloride reabsorption. *Kidney Int* 19:716, 1981.
632. Licht JH, Amundson D, Hsueh WA, Lombardo JV: Familial hyperkalemic acidosis. *Q J Med* 213:161, 1985.
633. Gordon RD: Syndrome of hypertension and hyperkalemia with normal glomerular filtration rate. *Hypertension* 8:93, 1986.
634. Woods JW, Liddle GW, Stant EG Jr, Michelakis AM, Brill AB: Effect of an adrenal inhibitor in hypertensive patients with suppressed renin. *Arch Intern Med* 123:366, 1969.
635. Crane MG, Harris JJ: Effect of spironolactone in hypertensive patients. *Am J Med Sci* 260:311, 1970.
636. Adlin EV, Marks AD, Channick BJ: Spironolactone and hydrochlorothiazide in essential hypertension. *Arch Intern Med* 130:855, 1972.
637. Baxter JD, Schambelan M, Matulich D, Spindler BJ, taylor AA, Bartter FC: Aldosterone receptors and the evaluation of plasma mineralocorticoid activity in normal and hypertensive states. *J Clin Invest* 58:579, 1976.
638. Lebel M, Schalekamp MA, Beevers DG, Brown JJ, Daies DL, Fraser R, Kremer D, Lever SF, Morton JJ, Robertson JIS, Tree M, Wilson A: Sodium and the renin-angiotensin system in essential hypertension and mineralocorticoid excess. *Lancet* 2:308, 1974.
639. Bauer JH, Brooks CS: Volume studies in men with mild to moderate hypertension. *Am J Cardiol* 44:1163, 1979.
640. Davies DL, Beevers DG, Brown JJ, Cumming AM, Fraser R, Lever AF, Mason PA, Morton JJ, Robertson JIS, Titterington M, Tree M: Aldosterone and its stimuli in normal and hypertensive man: Are essential hypertension and primary aldosteronism without tumor the same condition? *J Endocrinol* 81:79P, 1979.
641. Case DB, Wallace JM, Keim HJ, Weber MA, Sealey JE, Laragh JH: Possible role of renin in hypertension suggested by renin-sodium profiling and inhibition of converting enzyme. *N Engl J Med* 296:641, 1977.
642. Campese VM, Myers MR, De Quattro V: Neurogenic factors in low renin essential hypertension. *Am J Med* 69:83, 1980.

15

Glucocorticoid Therapy

J. Blake Tyrrell
John D. Baxter

Glucocorticoids are among the most commonly used drugs; they are employed to treat a number of medical problems. These vary from self-limited processes such as poison ivy, poison oak, or other hypersensitivity reactions to life-threatening problems such as leukemia. A partial list of these is shown in Table 15-1.[1] Christy estimated in 1971[2] that some 5 million persons in the United States receive some form of steroids (Fig. 15-1) annually in therapy. The overall use has if anything increased with the expanding population. Because of such extensive use and the numerous conditions for which steroids are given, glucocorticoid-treated patients are encountered in all medical and surgical specialties.

Although glucocorticoids have many beneficial influences, their use is frequently accompanied by deleterious side effects. The physician must be aware of these and must also exercise judgment in the decision to use steroids in the first place. It is also important to be aware of methods to reduce the total dosage by manipulating the timing and route of administration while maximizing adjunctive measures.

Table 15-1. Selected Clinical Conditions for which Glucocorticoids Are Used

Addison's disease: replacement therapy

Adrenal hyperplasia due to enzymatic defects (e.g., 11β-, 17α-, and 21-hydroxylase syndromes)

Allergic diseases:
- Angioneurotic edema
- Bee stings
- Contact dermatitis
- Drug reactions
- Hay fever
- Serum sickness
- Urticaria

Arthritis, bursitis, and tenosynovitis; inflammatory complications of a variety of types of arthritis

Blood dyscrasias:
- Acquired hemolytic anemia
- Allergic purpura
- Autoimmune hemolytic anemia
- Idiopathic thrombocytopenic purpura
- Lymphoblastic leukemia
- Multiple myeloma

Collagen vascular disorders:
- Giant cell arteritis
- Lupus erythematosus
- Mixed connective tissue syndromes
- Polymyositis
- Polymyalgia rheumatica
- Rheumatoid arthritis
- Temporal arteritis

Eye diseases:
- Acute uveitis
- Allergic conjunctivitis
- Choroiditis
- Optic neuritis

Gastrointestinal diseases:
- Inflammatory bowel disease
- Nontropical sprue
- Regional enteritis
- Subacute hepatic necrosis
- Ulcerative colitis

Hypercalcemia (e.g., due to sarcoidosis; most hypercalcemias not responsive)

Infections (occasionally helpful to suppress excessive inflammation)

Malignant exophthalmos

Neurological diseases

Pulmonary diseases:
- Aspiration pneumonia
- Bronchial asthma
- Infant respiratory distress syndrome
- Sarcoidosis

Renal diseases: certain nephrotic syndromes

Skin conditions:
- Atopic dermatitis
- Dermatoses
- Lichen simplex chronicus (localized neurodermatitis)
- Mycosis fungoides
- Pemphigus
- Seborrheic dermatitis
- Xerosis

Transplantation: prevention of rejection

*This table is not meant to be comprehensive, nor are steroids always indicated for the conditions listed.
Source: Baxter and Rousseau.[1]

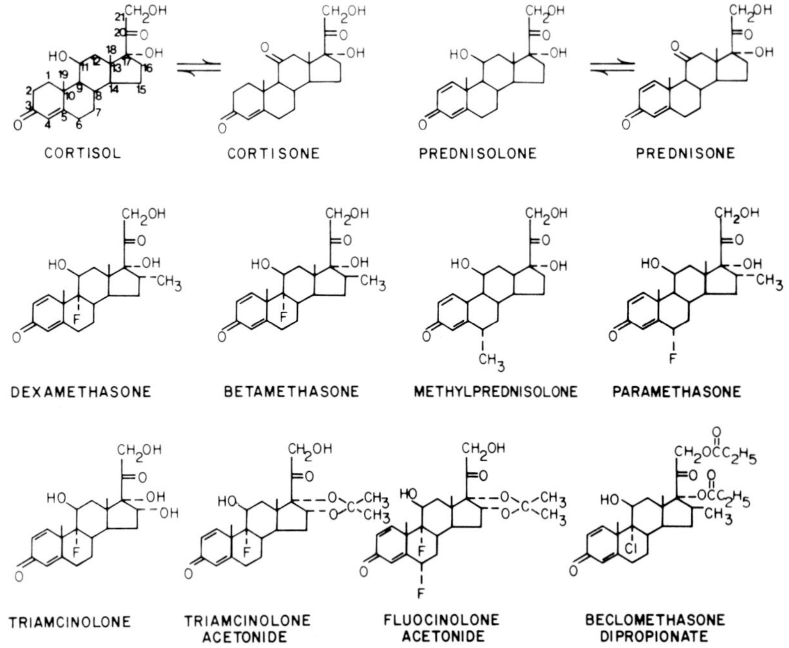

FIGURE 15-1 Structures of some steroids commonly used for glucocorticoid therapy. The numbers of the carbon atoms are shown for cortisol (upper left). Arrows indicate the interconvertibility of cortisol and cortisone, and prednisolone and prednisone. Dotted lines indicate side groups in the α position; solid lines indicate steroids in the β position (see also Chap. 12).

This allows maximum therapeutic benefit while minimizing adverse effects. Many of the sequelae of long-term glucocorticoid therapy are similar to those of the diseases for which steroids are given (weakness, bruising, etc.). Thus, the clinician must also know the features that can be helpful in differentiating the cause of such disturbances in glucocorticoid-treated patients.

Many endocrinologists encounter steroid-treated patients less commonly than do certain other specialists (e.g., nephrologists, rheumatologists, dermatologists), yet the endocrinologist commonly is asked to evaluate whether clinical stigmata are due to the steroid or some other process and to give advice on therapy or its withdrawal. The endocrinologist is also asked to evaluate the hypothalamic-pituitary-adrenal axis, which may be suppressed in glucocorticoid-treated patients, and to give advice on patient management in such situations.

Over the past 20 years, much has been learned about the pharmacokinetics of glucocorticoids and the mechanisms by which these steroids elicit their diverse effects (Chap. 12). This knowledge, although seriously incomplete, is helping to formulate more rational approaches to steroid therapy. This may increase the scope of steroid use in therapy and diminish the deleterious effects.

In this chapter, the pharmacology of the glucocorticoids is reviewed with the hope of providing a rational basis for the use of these steroids in therapy. For the most part, the specific clinical indications for glucocorticoid administration are avoided, as these require discussions of the particular diseases that are more appropriately found in the literature about them.

PHYSIOLOGICAL AND PHARMACOLOGICAL ACTIONS OF GLUCOCORTICOIDS IN RELATION TO STEROID THERAPY

Therapeutic Influences

The diverse actions of the glucocorticoids and the manifestations of excessive concentrations due to spontaneous or iatrogenic causes have been detailed in Chap. 12. Several different types of these actions are exploited in glucocorticoid therapy.

In most circumstances, the anti-inflammatory and/or immunosuppressive actions of the glucocorticoids are responsible for the therapeutic response. As detailed in Chap. 12, glucocorticoids can affect nearly every component involved in the inflammatory and immunological response, although in humans some components are more sensitive than others (e.g., cell-mediated more than humoral responses). What is less clear is which particular responses account for the beneficial therapeutic influences. For instance, the anti-inflammatory actions are clearly important when the steroids are given topically for inflammatory conditions. Thus, certain skin diseases benefit from glucocorticoid therapy, because the inflammatory response to the offending agent is excessive. In other cases (e.g., lupus erythematosus, other collagen vascular disorders, transplant rejection, and the nephrotic syndrome), it is not clear whether immunosuppressive or anti-inflammatory actions are more important. In general, glucocorticoid use for conditions of excessive inflammatory and/or immunological activity does not cure the primary condition, but instead ameliorates its manifestations. Sometimes this "buys time" for the body's natural defense to cure the problem or for more definitive therapy to work. Unfortunately, for many of the chronic problems for which glucocorticoids are used, the primary process is not curable by currently known measures and its manifestations return following withdrawal of steroid therapy. The result can be that, in spite of symptomatic improvement, steroid therapy either has no effect on the long-term prognosis or even worsens it.

When steroids are used to treat certain lymphoid cell malignancies, the direct actions to kill or inhibit the functions of the lymphoid cells mediate the response.[3] The different subpopulations of lymphoid cells vary markedly in their sensitivity to glucocorticoids (Chap. 12), and in humans under normal conditions (in contrast to certain animal species), glucocorticoids exhibit minimal lymphoid cell killing. Thus, many leukemias are steroid-resistant. Acute lymphoblastic leukemia of childhood is the most commonly occurring steroid-sensitive leukemia, and yet even this disease has the tendency to become steroid-resistant (see below).[3]

Whereas many malignancies are steroid-resistant, one occasionally observes patients with ordinarily steroid-resistant malignancies who do respond to glucocorticoids. For instance, in a study of patients with the preleukemic syndrome (hemopoietic dysplasia), 3 of 34 patients responded favorably to glucocorticoids.[4]

The actions of glucocorticoids on cell growth may also explain how these steroids inhibit solid tumors such as carcinoma of the breast and juvenile hemangiomas.[5]

In certain circumstances glucocorticoid therapy is used not to affect the primary process but to ameliorate some of the associated problems. This is true when these steroids are used to treat the hemolytic anemia that occurs sometimes in association with chronic granulocytic leukemia in the adult[5a] and to treat the hypercalcemias associated with malignancy or sarcoidosis (Chaps. 12 and 23).

Glucocorticoids are commonly used to treat severe or moderately severe asthma (Fig. 15-2)[6–14] and some patients with chronic obstructive pulmonary disease.[11,12] Pulmonary function in asthma can improve following steroid administration, although several hours are required for this to occur.[6,9] The improvement could be due to one or a combination of several types of influences. First, the steroid may directly promote bronchodilation by actions such as those that affect the sensitivity of the bronchioles to the effects of beta-adrenergic agonists (Chap. 12).[6,13] Second, glucocorticoids may also inhibit the action(s) or production of bronchoconstrictor substances, such as leukotrienes, other eicosanoids (Chap. 12), or histamine,[14] generated by immunological mechanisms. The actions of glucocorticoids to induce the phospholipase A_2 inhibitor may be of critical importance in this respect (Chap. 12). Third, the steroid might suppress inflammation in the lung and thereby improve pulmonary function.

There are several examples of steroid actions not primarily directed at inflammatory or immunological responses. For instance, in sarcoidosis the steroid may ameliorate the hypercalcemia by inhibiting the conversion of 25-hydroxycholecalciferol to 1α,25-dihydroxycholecalciferol (Chap. 23).[15] Glucocorticoids are used to decrease brain edema in certain patients with brain tumors, bacterial meningitis, or other conditions,[16–18] although they should not be used in certain circumstances.[18] In the cases where they are effective, it is not known to what extent the steroid effect is due to reduction of inflammation as opposed

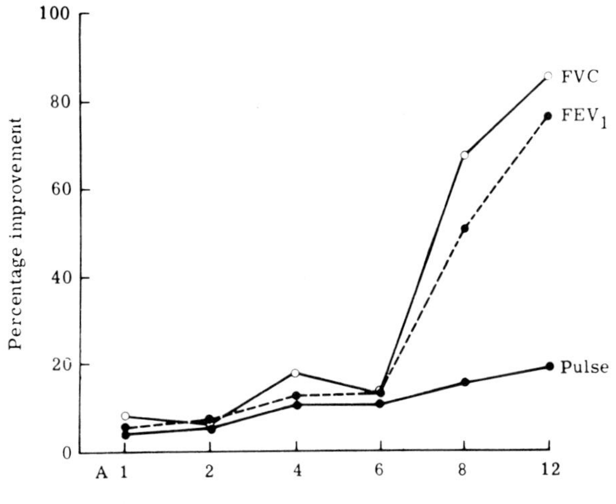

FIGURE 15-2 Effect of hydrocortisone hemisuccinate (4 mg per kilogram of body weight, followed in some cases by 3 mg per kilogram of body weight at 3-h intervals and in other cases by a continuous intravenous infusion at 3 mg per kilogram of body weight every 6 h) and of cosyntropin depot (1 mg IM) on pulmonary function (FEV_1 and FVC) in acute asthma. (*From Collins et al.*[6])

to other actions on brain fluid content, although the beneficial effects of steroids in conditions such as acute mountain sickness (believed to be due to cerebral edema unassociated with inflammation) argue for some role for the latter types of actions.[19] The antiemetic actions of the steroids are sometimes useful in cancer chemotherapy.[20]

Adverse Influences

Glucocorticoids have a number of adverse influences that lead to Cushing's syndrome and limit their usefulness in therapy. These problems are discussed in Chap. 12 and below. As with the beneficial influences, the actions on immunological and inflammatory responses play a dominant role in generating these adverse effects as these increase the incidence and severity of infections.[1,21–25] However, the actions on carbohydrate metabolism, fibroblasts, bone, and other tissues are much more prominent in the pathogenesis of iatrogenic Cushing's syndrome than with therapeutically beneficial responses.

MOLECULAR MECHANISMS FOR GLUCOCORTICOID-MEDIATED THERAPEUTIC INFLUENCES

As discussed in Chap. 12, it appears that most of the physiological and probably the pharmacological actions of the glucocorticoids are mediated through an intracellular receptor that binds the steroid, associates with the nucleus, and then affects the transcription of specific genes. Although a large body of evidence supports this model as a general mechanism for glucocorticoid action, in fact the molecular mechanisms for most therapeutic glucocorticoid responses have not been examined directly. The major reasons to presume that these mechanisms are generally involved are (1) the relative potency of steroids in eliciting therapeutic responses correlates with the receptor-binding activities of the steroids; (2) receptors are generally present in glucocorticoid-responsive tissues; and (3) glucocorticoid responses usually require hours to days to be observed, consistent with a requirement for influences on macromolecular synthesis.[26] Further, with lymphoblastic leukemic cells, discussed above and in Chap. 12, loss of the receptor is associated with unresponsiveness to glucocorticoids.[3] Nevertheless, in some cases glucocorticoids act by mechanisms that do not involve transcription [e.g., fast feedback of adrenocorticotropic hormone (ACTH) release; see Chap. 12]. Thus, a study of each therapeutic influence needs to be done before precise mechanisms can be assigned.

The receptor properties in most glucocorticoid target tissues are similar (Chap. 12), suggesting that an identical or near-identical receptor system is present in most cell types. This is true in spite of the fact that some actions of steroids with glucocorticoid activity in kidney, brain, and perhaps other tissues are mediated through mineralocorticoid receptors and despite the possibility that there is heterogeneity among the glucocorticoid receptors (as discussed in Chap. 12). The existence of similar receptors in many different tissues explains how glucocorticoids can influence all these tissues directly. The responses differ in the various tissues (e.g., killing in lymphoid cells or gluconeogenesis in liver) because of postreceptor cellular differentiation (Chap. 12). The fact that the receptors are similar in the different glucocorticoid-responsive tissues probably explains the failure of the pharmaceutical industry to find a steroid that, when administered systemically, has one type of beneficial therapeutic response (e.g., an immunosuppressive one) but not other deleterious ones (e.g., induction of osteoporosis); the compounds may bind to all the receptors and mediate all the responses. Thus, caution should be exercised in interpreting any differential effects of various glucocorticoids as being due to qualitatively different actions rather than to factors such as potency and duration of action.

However, when selecting the steroid to be used, cognizance should be taken of the fact that steroids such as cortisol (hydrocortisone) have sodium-retaining actions mediated through the mineralocorticoid receptor. The weaker mineralocorticoid/glucocorticoid activities of steroids such as prednisone, prednisolone, dexamethasone, or betamethasone (Chap. 12) constitute one reason these steroids are ordinarily used in preference to cortisol. The relative mineralocorticoid/glucocorticoid receptor-binding activities for several steroids are indicated in Table 15-2. This ratio is an approximation of the potential sodium-retaining activity, which is low for the steroids ordinarily used for glucocorticoid therapy.

Table 15-2. Affinities of Some Steroids for Human Glucocorticoid Receptors and Relative Mineralocorticoid-Glucocorticoid Receptor Affinities

Steroid	Affinity for the glucocorticoid receptor*	Mineralocorticoid/glucocorticoid receptor affinity ratio*
Cortisol	1.0	1.0
Fludrocortisone	3.5	11.6
Triamcinolone acetonide	1.9	
Prednisolone	2.1	0.9
Betamethasone	5.4	0.8
Dexamethasone	7.1	0.2
Fluocinolone acetonide	11.4	

*Relative to cortisol.
Source: Data for human receptor binding from Ballard et al.[27] Data for the ratio of affinities using rat mineralocorticoid receptors and human glucocorticoid receptors from unpublished data of Lan NC, Matulich DT, and Baxter JD.

KINETIC CONSIDERATIONS

Those actions of glucocorticoids which involve the interaction of the steroid with the receptors that have been studied, and the subsequent modulation of transcription of DNA into RNA, require some lag before a response is observed (Chap. 12). Similarly, in terminating the response, some time is required for the steroid to leave the circulation. When this occurs, dissociation of the steroid from the receptor occurs within a few minutes,[26] resulting in a termination of further steroid action. However, some time is required for the levels of the induced mRNAs and their protein products to return to baseline before the response is terminated.[28] Further, the response may be even more prolonged, because the steroid may have induced other factors that affect transcription; thus, a stimulation of transcription may occur for some time following removal of the steroid because of the period required for concentrations of these factors to decrease to basal levels. The time required for induced mRNAs and proteins to return to basal levels depends on their rates of turnover.[28] These rates vary for different mRNAs. The rates of protein and mRNA turnover also affect the kinetics of induction (for discussion see Ref. 28 and Chap. 12); for steroid-regulated mRNAs and proteins that turn over with a long half-life, a longer time is required for the response to reach a maximum (and to terminate) than with the more rapidly turning-over macromolecules. Thus, there may be considerable variation in the time required for the onset and disappearance of various glucocorticoid responses; these variations form the basis for alternate-day steroid therapy (discussed below), and they emphasize that the kinetics of each response must be determined independently in order to develop the most rational approach to glucocorticoid therapy.

MANIFESTATIONS OF IATROGENIC CUSHING'S SYNDROME

Comparisons with Spontaneous Cushing's Syndrome

Since iatrogenic Cushing's syndrome is due to chronic glucorticoid excess, the clinical features (with several exceptions) are similar to those of spontaneous Cushing's syndrome, described in Chap. 12. In fact, since many patients receive very high doses over prolonged time periods, the symptoms and signs are commonly more prominent than with spontaneous Cushing's syndrome, which is ordinarily diagnosed and treated before the sequelae become too severe. Thus, there can be weight gain with redistribution of fat to the truncal areas, "moon face," plethora, "buffalo hump," thin skin, easy bruising, osteoporosis, striae, poor wound healing, increased incidence of infections, psychiatric problems, myopathy and muscular weakness, decreased carbohydrate tolerance, negative nitrogen balance, renal calculi, and other stigmata. An extensive analysis of these and other factors and the pathophysiology is provided in Chap. 12.

The major differences between iatrogenic and spontaneous Cushing's syndrome (unless ACTH therapy is used) relate to the presence of androgens and mineralocorticoids. Since adrenal androgen excess is not present in the iatrogenic syndrome, the hirsutism and other virilizing features are not observed. However, glucocorticoid-treated individuals do develop an increase in fine lanugo hair on the face and elsewhere.[29] Steroids with less mineralocorticoid potency (relative to their glucocorticoid potency) than cortisol are ordinarily used for steroid therapy (Table 15-2). Further, steroids with mineralocorticoid potency, such as 11-deoxycorticosterone (DOC), are sometimes present in excess in spontaneous Cushing's syndrome (Chaps. 12 and 14). As a consequence, the sequelae of mineralocorticoid excess, i.e., hypokalemia (observed commonly with the ectopic ACTH syndrome), fluid retention with edema, and hypertension (Chap. 14), are much less common in the iatrogenic syndrome. However, in iatrogenic Cushing's syndrome there is an increased frequency of hypertension (Chaps. 12, 14), and fluid retention can be exaggerated in patients who have congestive heart failure and do not as readily "escape" from the sodium-retaining actions of the mineralocorticoids (Chap. 12).

Whereas steroid-treated patients can become euphoric or depressed, it appears that euphoria is more common in iatrogenic than spontaneous Cushing's syndrome. In some individuals this may be due to improvement in the disease for which steroids were given; however, others develop euphoria without any detectable beneficial effect on their primary disease.[2,17,30]

It has been reported that several other features are unique to iatrogenic Cushing's syndrome.[2,22] Some of these are uncommon; they include benign intracranial hypertension, pancreatitis, and vasculitis. Although it has been reported that an increased incidence of glaucoma and avascular necrosis of bone (discussed below) is unique to the iatrogenic syndrome,[2,31] glaucoma has been reported[32] and the authors have observed avascular necrosis of bone in the spontaneous syndrome. Whereas the deposition of fat in various body areas in Cushing's syndrome is well known, excessive deposition of fat around the spinal cord has been reported to date to occur rarely in iatrogenic Cushing's syndrome.[33] This can result in neurological symptoms and can be treated with diet, although surgical intervention has sometimes been required.[33]

Ocular Changes

Cataract occurs commonly in steroid-treated individuals (Chap. 12), especially with prolonged treatment.[34,35] It also occurs in the pediatric population, although it usually is not associated with detectable visual impairment.[36,37] As discussed in Chap. 12, there is some evidence that steroid-induced cataract may be a result of formation of covalent complexes between the steroids and lens proteins.[38]

Steroid-induced increases in the intraocular pressure with subsequent development of glaucoma occur in a subset of patients who are susceptible to this action.[34,35] There are a significant number of these individuals;[34] all glucocorticoid-treated patients should be monitored for changes in intraocular pressure.

Ischemic Necrosis of Bone

Avascular or ischemic necrosis of bone has been reported in up to 50 percent of patients in some series and is apparently related more to the dose than the duration of therapy.[38a] It is also more prevalent in patients with vasculitis and Raynaud's phenomenon, although it also occurs frequently with steroid therapy in other conditions such as in transplant recipients.[38a] It has been proposed that this complication is due to steroid-induced enlargement of intramedullary lipocytes with resulting pressure on the bone leading to ischemia.[38a]

Osteoporosis

Osteoporosis is one of the major limitations of long-term glucocorticoid therapy.[2,39-45] The precise prevalence is difficult to determine, since many studies have been performed in patients with diseases, such as rheumatoid arthritis, in which there is a high incidence of osteoporosis without glucocorticoid therapy.[2,40] However, in a retrospective study of 128 asthmatic patients who had received steroids for at least a year, there were 58 fractures in 14 patients (11 percent), compared with none in the control patients; in a prospective study, 8 of 19 patients and none of 11 control patients had fractures.[42] The long-term steroid-treated patients also had decreased trabecular but not cortical bone density, as measured by photon absorptiometry (Fig. 15-3), although within this group it was not possible to correlate bone density with dose or duration of therapy or to predict with the use of bone density measurements which patients would have a fracture.[42] Further, alternate-day steroid therapy (see below) was not found to protect against osteoporosis.[43] For bone density measurements, the ratio of cortical to trabecular mass appears to be the most sensitive index of glucocorticoid influence (Fig. 15-3).[42–44] This selectivity in influencing trabecular

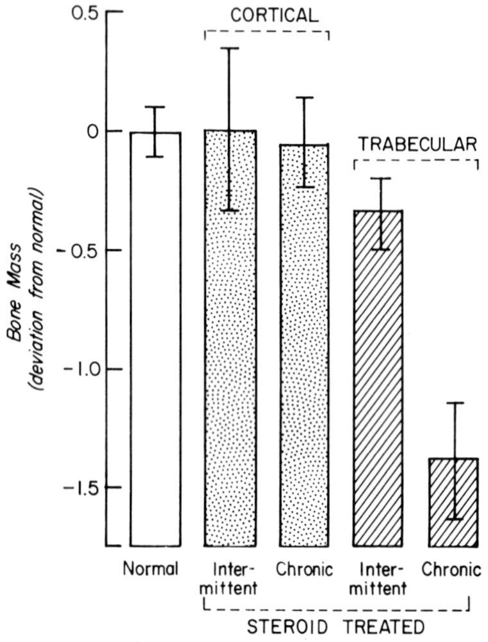

FIGURE 15-3 Trabecular and cortical bone mass in control and glucocorticoid-treated asthmatic patients. Bone mass was measured by single-photon absorption and was calculated by dividing the bone mineral content by bone width. Trabecular mass was taken from a metaphyseal site 2 cm proximal to the distal end of the ulnar styloid process, which contains a large proportion of trabecular bone. Cortical mass was taken from a diaphyseal site one-third the distance from the distal to the proximal end of the ulna, which is composed primarily of cortical bone. The bone mass is expressed as a fraction of the standard deviation of the mean of the normal value for the patient's sex and decade of age (z score). "Intermittent" refers to patients who had received intermittent courses of steroids but who did not require constant treatment for as long as a year. "Chronic" refers to patients who received daily or alternate-day corticosteroids for one year or more or at least eight short courses for 10 days or less of high-dose steroids for as long as a year. (*Data taken from Adinoff and Hollister.*[42])

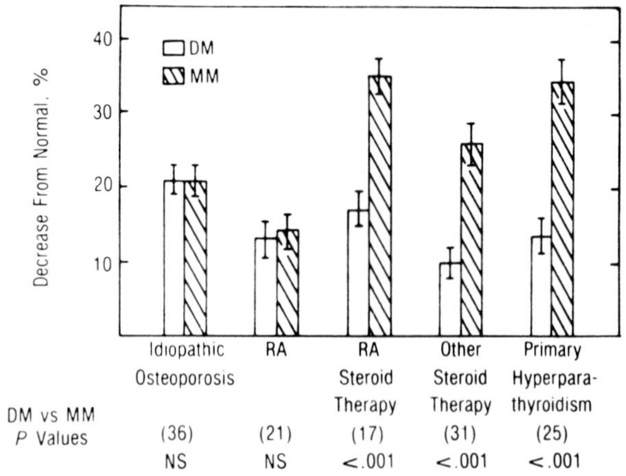

FIGURE 15-4 Decrease in bone mass (percent decrease from normal) estimated by photon absorption measurements of bone mass in the midshaft diaphyseal site (DM) and the distal metaphyseal site (MM) in patients with idiopathic osteoporosis, rheumatoid arthritis (RA) that was either not treated or was treated with glucocorticoids, and primary hyperparathyroidism. Vertical bars indicate mean percent decrease from normal for age and sex (± SEM). Number of patients studied is indicated in parentheses. (*From Hahn.*[40])

bone is also illustrated by the data of Fig. 15-4, which also compares patients with rheumatoid arthritis who were steroid-treated with those who did not receive glucocorticoids. This pattern of bone loss is similar to that seen with primary hyperparathyroidism, but differs from that observed in idiopathic osteoporosis (Fig. 15-4). The osteoporosis is most prominent in trabecular bone that has a high turnover rate with less dramatic changes in the more slowly turning-over cortical bone.[42–44] Thus, the most pronounced bone loss is in the axial skeleton, such as the ribs and vertebrae, more than in the long bones. Steroid-induced bone loss is more profound in patients with previously reduced bone mineral, e.g., postmenopausal or oophorectomized women, alcoholics in whom endogenous hypercortisolism may already be contributing to bone loss,[46] patients with bowel disease and decreased calcium absorption, or those with liver or renal disease and impaired vitamin D metabolism (Chap. 24). Children are also susceptible to steroid-induced osteopenia, presumably because of their lower bone mass and higher initial bone turnover.[40] The mechanisms of corticosteroid-induced bone loss are discussed in Chap. 12.

It is not yet clear whether specific measures should be taken to minimize glucocorticoid osteoporosis. Of course, major efforts should be made to decrease the steroid dose. Vitamin D (50,000 U three times weekly) or 25-hydroxyvitamin D (20 to 40 μg per day) and calcium (500 mg per day) have been shown to increase intestinal calcium absorption, decrease the elevated parathyroid hormone levels, and increase the trabecular bone mass of the distal radius in patients treated with glucocorticoids.[40,45] In addition, thiazide diuretic therapy will correct the hypercalciuria.[47] These measures will therefore partly correct the increased rate of bone resorption, but they probably will not prevent the glucocorticoid-induced depression of bone formation.[44] Sodium fluoride therapy can increase the trabecular bone mass, especially of the spine, but it apparently has little influence on the appendicular skeleton.[44] Thus, some have advocated the use of vitamin D, calcium, and sodium fluoride (66 to 88 mg per day) to treat selected patients,[43] and the use of a thiazide diuretic if hypercalciuria is present.[43,47] This approach seems reasonable, although no prospective study has as yet documented its usefulness.

It is also not clearly established which patients should receive this therapy.[39,44–46] Although osteoporosis may ultimately occur in 100 percent of patients treated for long enough, as stated above, it is not present in all patients. Thus, it has been argued that only selected patients should receive the regimen. However, it is far easier to prevent loss of bone than to replace it. At present, the best means to monitor bone loss is through photon absorptiometry.[40,42,44] One recommended approach is to measure bone mass in this way in the distal radius at the start of steroid therapy and every 3 to 6 months thereafter and to institute administration of the combination of fluoride, calcium, and vitamin D at the first sign that the loss exceeds that attributable to normal aging.[44] During therapy it is critical to monitor serum and urinary calcium levels at intervals of 1 to 2 months, to avoid inadvertent overdosage. Until more definitive data become available, this appears to be a reasonable approach.

Infections

Infections are a major problem with long-term glucocorticoid therapy (Chap. 12).[2,21–25,48,49] Several types of infections can occur (Chap. 12), including bacterial, viral, fungal, and parasitic; gram-negative and fungal infections appear to be particularly prevalent.[2,21–25,49] Except in specific situations (e.g., reactivation of quiescent tuberculosis, abscesses, osteomyelitis, etc.), it is not possible to predict the organism that will cause a complicating infection,[21] and opportunistic organisms can be responsible.[49] Hepatitis B virus poses a special concern because steroids are used to treat chronic active hepatitis[50] but can be harmful when this form of hepatitis is associated with hepatitis B surface antigen positivity.[51,52] Because glucocorticoids decrease the inflammatory response, it may be particularly difficult to detect and diagnose infections in glucocorticoid-treated individuals. The incidence, severity, and frequency of serious infections increase with both the dose and duration of steroid therapy.[53] Infectious complications may be decreased when alternate-day steroid therapy is used.[53] The mechanisms of glucocorticoid-mediated decreased host defense to infection are discussed in Chap. 12.

The probable increase in the incidence and severity of tuberculosis in steroid-treated patients with systemic disease has been of particular concern.[21,54] Diagnosis may be difficult in the presence of the systemic disease for which the steroid is being administered, and in addition the tuberculin response may be suppressed by glucocorticoids. However, reactivation of tuberculosis does not appear to occur with increased frequency in patients on long-term steroid therapy.[54] Thus, patients receiving glucocorticoids who are tuberculin-positive do not require antituberculosis therapy unless active disease is present.

Myopathy

Myopathy is a common manifestation of prolonged steroid therapy (Chap. 12).[2,22,55] Although the onset may be sudden, it usually occurs gradually and often requires weeks or months to develop. It first affects the proximal muscles, although distal muscles can also be involved. Muscle atrophy may be profound with prolonged high-dose therapy. Isolated muscular weakness has not been observed, but it must be considered in patients with connective tissue disease who complain of increasing weakness during therapy; in that setting weakness may be a consequence of treatment rather than an exacerbation of the primary disease. Myalgia is rather common when glucocorticoid-induced myopathy first appears, and it disappears shortly after discontinuing the dose; this symptom can therefore be useful in the differential diagnosis. Levels of serum enzymes [glutamic oxaloacetic transaminase (SGOT), creatine phosphokinase, and aldolase] are normal in glucocorticoid-induced myopathy, although they may be elevated in myopathy due to hypokalemia, polymyositis, or other causes.[55] However, creatine excretion is increased with glucocorticoid-induced and other myopathies and its measurement can be useful. Muscle biopsy has not been shown to be helpful. Changes in muscle may also be monitored with the use of CT and isokinetic dynamic testing.[55a] A recent study suggests that glucocorticoid-induced muscle wasting can be reversed by physical training;[55a] thus, steroid-treated patients should exercise when possible.

Atherosclerosis

Atherosclerosis has not traditionally been considered to be a complication of glucocorticoid therapy. However, there is a body of retrospectively obtained data that suggests that atherosclerosis is more prevalent in glucocortisol-treated individuals.[55b] Thus, although more data are needed, the potential for increasing the rate of progression of atherosclerosis should be considered in the overall decision to administer glucocorticoids on a long-term basis.

Dose and Time Dependency, and Reversibility

The manifestations of iatrogenic Cushing's syndrome are generally dose- and time-dependent, although the time required to develop particular features shows considerable variation. Further, some complications also occur less frequently with alternate-day therapy (see below). Increased appetite and euphoria can be observed within hours, whereas days to weeks are ordinarily required to develop a cushingoid appearance. Effects on carbohydrate metabolism can occur within hours, although these become more pronounced with time (Chap. 12). The time required to develop an increased susceptibility to infections is not known with certainty, although it is likely that this happens within hours, since influences on leukocytes and other factors involved in inflammatory and immunological responses occur by this time (Chap. 12). The development of frank osteoporosis[39–45] and muscular weakness[55,55a] usually occurs after weeks or months of therapy, although occasional patients have experienced onset of muscular weakness after a few days.[55] Psychiatric problems may develop soon after institution of therapy or may develop later.[2,17,56–58] Other, rarer stigmata due to glucocorticoid excess usually develop after weeks of therapy, although their appearance is unpredictable.

Most of the manifestations of glucocorticoid excess are reversible. Thus, within weeks to several months following the discontinuance of therapy, weight and fat distribution can return to normal, the skin changes and cushingoid appearance disappear, and muscular strength returns. The immunosuppressive and metabolic effects (e.g., on carbohydrate tolerance) return to normal within hours to days after discontinuing therapy. Unfortunately, the osteoporosis is not reversible with present therapy, even though further steroid-mediated bone destruction ceases.

DIAGNOSIS OF IATROGENIC CUSHING'S SYNDROME

The diagnosis of iatrogenic Cushing's syndrome is usually obvious from the clinical manifestations and the history of steroid therapy. Thus, further workup is ordinarily not required. However, occasional patients present with certain manifestations but deny a history of steroid use; the authors have seen one case evaluated in the hematology clinic for bruising in which even the patient's previous doctor denied prescribing a steroid.[27] The diagnosis in these circumstances can be made from the clinical features plus the finding of suppression of the hypothalamic-pituitary-adrenal axis (see below and Chap. 12). Thus, plasma cortisol and ACTH levels are low, and the rapid ACTH stimulation test result is abnormal. If clinical suspicion persists in the presence of a normal response to ACTH testing, metyrapone or insulin hypoglycemia testing (Chap. 12) can be used for a more definitive assessment of decreased ACTH reserve. If there is suspicion that steroid medication is being continued, the presence of a glucocorticoid can be identified with the use of the glucocorticoid radioreceptor assay,[27] by radioimmunoassay if the particular steroid in question is known, or by high-performance liquid chromatography (Chap. 12). Unfortunately, these assays are not generally available.

DETERMINANTS OF GLUCOCORTICOID POTENCY

The potency of a steroid depends on its absorption or "bioavailability," distribution, rate of metabolic clearance, concentration at sites of action, affinity for the glucocorticoid receptors, and ability to act as an agonist once bound (Chap. 12). It is important to consider each of these factors in using steroids for therapy.

Bioavailability

Most glucocorticoids are readily absorbed after oral administration. The estimates of fractional cortisol absorption expressed as bioavailability range from 0.45 to 0.8 (45 to 80 percent).[59] The absolute bioavailability of prednisolone from all forms of oral prednisone ranges from 77 to 99 percent.[59] Some preparations have groups attached to the C-21 position of the steroid that enhance their water solubility (e.g., hydrocortisone phosphate, hydrocortisone hemisuccinate). Ordinarily, these groups are not needed, since the steroids are soluble enough to be adequately absorbed. Although glucocorticoid uptake is not impaired in most patients with intrinsic intestinal disease,[59] this can occur rarely.[60] Food intake does not have an appreciable effect on uptake.[59] Uptake is generally not impaired in renal or pulmonary disease.[59]

In the case of intramuscular (IM) injections, the uptake of steroids can vary markedly depending on the preparation. For instance, triamcinolone acetonide is absorbed very slowly via the intramuscular route, so the effect of a single injection may last for several weeks (see also Intraarticular Preparations, below).[61] Intramuscular injections of cortisone acetate do not reproducibly yield adequate blood levels of cortisol in the first 4 to 6 h postinjections (Chap. 12),[62,63] although ultimately the steroid is absorbed. However, when more soluble derivatives of cortisol (e.g., hydrocortisone hemisuccinate) are injected IM, maximal cortisol levels are attained within an hour.[62,63] Thus, the physician must be especially aware of the properties of each preparation when the IM route is anticipated.

Compounds topically administered to the skin must penetrate the keratin layer of the stratum corneum in order to reach the squamous cell layer of the epidermis; high lipid solubility favors such penetration. For instance, the more lipophilic triamcinolone acetonide is 10 times as active topically as triamcinolone, but only equiactive systemically.[64–66] However, both these compounds are more active than cortisol, which penetrates very poorly. On the other hand, hydrocortisone butyrate appears to have an activity similar to triamcinolone acetonide.[65] Nevertheless, only a small fraction of the topically applied steroid is actually absorbed.[65,66] With cortisol only 1 percent is so taken up; the remainder rubs off, exfoliates with the stratum corneum, or washes off. Percutaneous penetration of glucocorticoids can vary in different anatomical regions. For instance, uptake by the scrotum and forehead is about 42 and 6 times, respectively, that of the forearm.[65] Absorption is enhanced when skin is damaged and when occlusive dressings are applied, particularly to open areas.[65] Uptake is affected by the vehicle; for example, ointment bases are better taken up than are creams or lotions.[65,66]

Uptake of steroids applied topically to the eyes presents a special problem in that they must penetrate both the corneal epithelium, which is hydrophobic, and the corneal stroma, which is hydrophilic.[34,35] For this, acetate steroid derivatives have been shown to be the most effective.[34,35] These are applied as aqueous suspensions and are most effective when applied frequently.[34,35]

Uptake in specific tissues after systemic administration can also vary. For example, in lung the uptake of cortisol and methylprednisolone is greater than that of prednisone.[67] Dexamethasone is sometimes given to mothers at risk for premature delivery to prevent respiratory distress syndrome in the newborn.[68] In this case, blood levels attained in the fetus are only a fraction of those reached in the mother.[68,68a] Whereas this may in part be due to decreased uptake, there is enhanced metabolism of the drug as well.[68a]

Distribution

The effect of distribution on steroid dynamics is discussed in Chap. 12; corticosteroid-binding globulin (CBG), other plasma proteins, and the peripheral tissues sequester administered steroids to a variable extent. For those steroids that bind to CBG, variations in the protein affect the rate of metabolic clearance. The presence of the protein also changes the rate of clearance of prednisolone following prednisone administration; this is more rapid shortly after the dose is given than later,[59] because at the early time the plasma prednisolone level exceeds the CBG binding capacity and more of the steroid is available for metabolic degradation or excretion. It has also been reported with prednisolone that individual patient differences in the volume of distribution may explain in part why certain patients are more prone to develop cushingoid side effects.[29] It has been reported that patients with low serum albumin concentrations are more likely to develop cushingoid side effects.[68b] This might affect the volume of distribution (although this was not measured), and other associated factors (e.g., the severity of the illness) might also contribute. Dexamethasone has only about sevenfold greater intrinsic activity than cortisol (Table 15-2), but was found in vivo to have 17 times the potency of cortisol when the data were extrapolated to zero time to eliminate any influence of clearance.[69] This greater activity may be due in part to enhanced availability of this steroid relative to cortisol because of less plasma binding.

Metabolism and Clearance

Metabolic pathways convert inactive compounds to active forms, and vice versa. Although most glucocorticoids are active without metabolic alteration, two commonly used compounds, prednisone and cortisone, are themselves antagonists, although their affinities for the glucocorticoid receptor (Chap. 12) are so low[27] that effectively these compounds are inactive. These

11-ketosteroids are, however, rapidly converted, mostly by the liver, to the 11-hydroxyl forms, prednisolone and cortisol, which have full agonist activity (Chap. 12). Ordinarily this conversion proceeds readily (Fig. 15-5); in the study shown, the concentration of prednisolone was 10 times that of prednisone even in the first 30 min following a 10-mg oral dose of prednisone.[70] However, it is possible that inadequate 11-hydroxylation could explain certain clinical findings such as the fact that cortisone, which can penetrate human skin, does not exhibit glucocorticoid activity when applied topically[65] or injected into joints[71] and that cortisone acetate injections are sometimes ineffective in the first few hours after injection[62,63] (see above and Chap. 12). In liver disease the conversion of cortisone to cortisol is rarely affected, although the conversion of prednisone to prednisolone can be impaired.[59] For this reason it is generally recommended that prednisolone rather than prednisone be used in patients with liver disease.[48,59] Other than with the 11-ketosteroids, there is very little role for metabolic conversion in the formation of more active steroids; instead, the rate of inactivation is an important determinant of biological potency. The plasma half-life is commonly used as an index of the rate of clearance of corticosteroids; this parameter has some utility. However, since both the distribution and the clearance can vary differentially for various steroids and in states where these parameters change, the use of half-life alone can sometimes be misleading and can underestimate true differences in clearance.[59]

The rates of clearance of the steroids used in therapy show considerable variation (Table 15-3), and the decreased clearance of many of the commonly used steroids (prednisone, dexamethasone, etc.) relative to cortisol is one of the most important factors explaining their enhanced potency.[59,69,72-76] To a large extent, it is the modification of the steroid molecule around the A ring and the AB ring angle that accounts for their delayed clearance, as these modifications decrease the ability of the liver to reduce the ring (Chap. 12). In these cases, the 6-methylation and 21-conjugation pathways become more important.

Although the issue has not received as much study as it deserves, there appear to be some variations in the rates of clearance of the steroids in different individuals.[77] For example, in one study, the half-life for prednisolone clearance in nine subjects ranged from 134 to 342 min.[60] Although it has been reported that the plasma clearance of prednisolone is less in steroid-treated patients who develop cushingoid side effects than in those who do not (Fig. 15-5),[29,78] this was not confirmed in a more recent study.[79] However, in the latter case, in the cushingoid steroid-treated patients the affinity of prednisolone for CBG was increased and plasma cortisol levels while on the steroid were higher.[79] The latter may imply that the hypothalamic-pituitary-adrenal axis is more resistant to suppression in the cushingoid patients, such that higher endogenous cortisol levels contribute to the development of side effects.

As outlined in Chap. 12, drugs and disease states can affect the clearance of administered glucocorticoids. There is impaired steroid clearance in liver disease.[59] In renal diseases, some have reported that the pharmacokinetics of steroids are unchanged;[59] however, a more recent report suggests that the clearance and half-life of prednisolone are decreased but those of dexamethasone are increased in renal disease.[80] Drugs such as phenytoin (diphenylhydantoin), phenobarbital, and rifampin can increase the rate of steroid clearance by inducing hepatic metabolizing enzymes.[59]

Table 15-3. Plasma Half-Life and Glucocorticoid and Mineralocorticoid Potencies of Some Commonly Used Glucocorticoid Preparations

Steroid	Half time, min	Ref.	Relative potency: Glucocorticoid	Relative potency: Mineralocorticoid	Ref.
Cortisol	80–120	59	1.0	1.0	73–76
Cortisone			0.8	0.8	73–76
Prednisone	200–210	72	3.5–4.0		73–75
			1.05–5.2		69
Prednisolone	120–300	59	4.0	0.8	74
Methylprednisolone	120–180	59	5.0	0.5	73,74
Triamcinolone			5.0	0	73,74
Dexamethasone	150–270	59	30.0	~0	73,74
			17–154		69
Betamethasone	130–330	59	25–30	~0	73,74

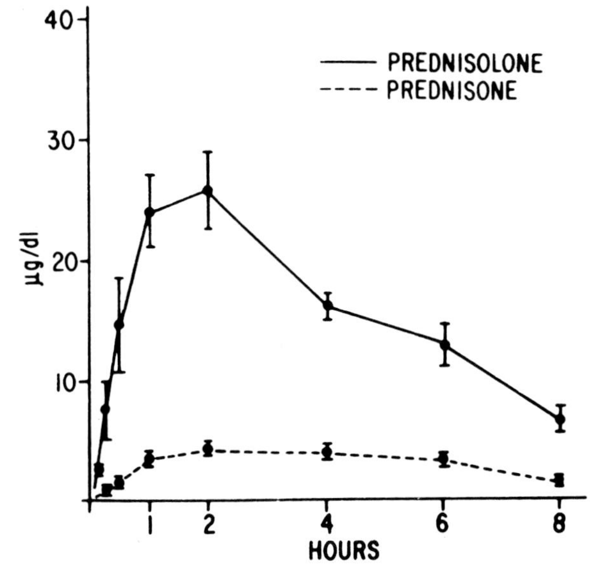

FIGURE 15-5 Plasma concentrations of prednisone and prednisolone following oral administration of 10 mg of prednisone. (*From Meikle et al.*[70])

The use of estrogen-containing oral contraceptives and estrogen therapy in general result in decreased clearance of administered steroid.[59,81] Nonsteroidal anti-inflammatory agents may increase steroid availability, although this has not been rigorously studied.[59] It appears that the use of antacids or cimetidine does not appreciably affect steroid pharmacokinetics.[59] In general, clearance is similar in children and adults, but may decrease slightly with advancing age.[59] As mentioned above, the metabolic clearance of dexamethasone in the fetus appears to be markedly enhanced relative to clearance in the mother.[69] Although the monitoring of steroid therapy with the use of plasma assays for free steroids is not performed today, this may be done in the future as such assays become more generally available and their interpretation better documented.

Concentration at Sites of Action

The potency of compounds with agonist activity, including all the major steroids used for glucocorticoid therapy (see the earlier discussions regarding the exceptions with cortisone and prednisone), is directly related to affinity for glucocorticoid receptors (Chap. 12, Table 15-2). Thus, once the steroid has been delivered to the target tissue, affinity is the overwhelming determinant of activity. For instance, dexamethasone and prednisolone have, respectively, about eight and two times the affinity of cortisol for the receptors;[27] initially, this is a major determinant of the relative differences in their potencies.

Agonist Activity

Most of the steroids that are used in glucocorticoid therapy are full agonists (Chap. 12). The major exceptions are those steroids with an 11-keto group, prednisone and cortisone (discussed above), which are rapidly converted in vivo to the agonists prednisolone and cortisol.

Overall Estimation of Glucocorticoid Potency

Because the relative potencies of steroids vary even with the time following administration, it is an oversimplification to consider only a single set of potency ratios. Thus, whereas dexamethasone and prednisone were found to be, respectively, 154 and 5.2 times as potent as cortisol when examined at 14 h, they were only 17 and 1.05 times as potent when the data were extrapolated to zero time.[69] Because other responses have different kinetics, it is likely that the changes in relative potency with time will also differ, depending on the particular response. For all these reasons, the safest way to develop clinical protocols would be to standardize each drug for each disease, adjust the dose for each patient (see below), and exercise caution when switching steroids.

Over the years, a number of estimates of relative potency have been made (Table 15-3). It is of interest that many writers now list the relative potencies without even documenting the source of the information. However, as the study by Meikle and Tyler shows,[69] it may be necessary to modify some of these values. In spite of the inherent problems, the relative potency values do serve as a rough index of relative activity; these relative activities are generally similar for various responses in a number of different tissues in animals and in humans (Chap. 4).[26] The data have been obtained from a variety of assays, including those that quantify glycogen deposition (Chap. 12), lymphocyte killing (Chap. 12), and clinical (e.g., antiarthritic[22]) responses.

Variations in Sensitivity to Glucocorticoids: Glucocorticoid Resistance

Variations in intrinsic sensitivity to glucocorticoids have been discussed in Chap. 12 and are reviewed in

Ref. 82. It is clear that marked and generalized hyposensitivity is rare; when this occurs, a mineralocorticoid excess syndrome occurs (Chap. 14). Similarly, there is no evidence for a syndrome of primary increased sensitivity to glucocorticoids. Nevertheless, there are known situations where steroid dosage must be altered because of either individual differences (discussed above, under Metabolism and Clearance) or therapy with other drugs (e.g., phenytoin or barbiturates) that increase the hepatic metabolism of glucocorticoids (Chap. 12). However, it is possible that there are also variations in intrinsic sensitivity between individuals and between various tissues in a given individual. Individual differences in the steroid's ability to suppress the hypothalamic-pituitary-adrenal axis could explain the higher cortisol levels in the cushingoid patients in the study of Benet et al.[79] If this were the case, it would be likely that the lowered sensitivity of the axis in certain individuals is also selective for the tissues involved in axis suppression, since the presence in these individuals of effects of the steroid sufficient to produce Cushing's syndrome indicates that other target tissues are sensitive to glucocorticoids. Individual differences could also explain why only subpopulations of patients with certain diseases respond to glucocorticoid therapy; the study quoted under Therapeutic Influences, above, in patients with the preleukemic syndrome[4] underscores this point.

The concentrations of glucocorticoid receptors, unlike receptors for other classes of hormones, such as the polypeptide and catecholamine hormones, are not extensively regulated; however, they can be regulated to some extent and other factors have a pronounced effect on the cellular sensitivity to glucocorticoids (Chap. 12). Although the clinical importance of these phenomena is not known at present, they could affect the sensitivity of selected target tissues to glucocorticoids and be of therapeutic relevance. It is possible that studies of these influences may in the future yield information that would facilitate the design of protocols to enhance specifically the effectiveness of glucocorticoids on certain tissues while minimizing those on other tissues.

In the treatment of lymphoid leukemias, patients who initially respond can become resistant to the steroid.[3] This appears to be due to a mutation in the gene for the receptor and the selection of a population of cells that have functionally defective receptors that cannot respond to the steroid (Fig. 15-6).

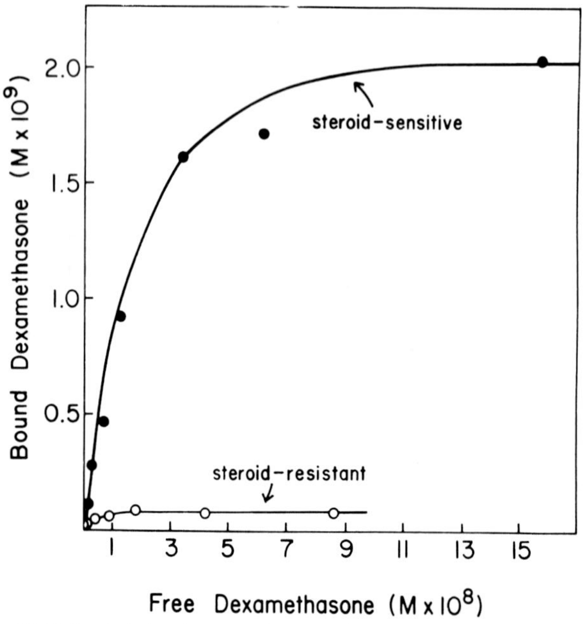

FIGURE 15-6 Binding of radioactive dexamethasone to receptors from glucocorticoid-sensitive lymphoma cells and to glucocorticoid-resistant cells selected by growing steroid-sensitive cells in the presence of dexamethasone (*From Rosenau et al.*[83])

GLUCOCORTICOID PREPARATIONS

Steroids with Glucocorticoid Activity Available for Therapy

A large number of steroids with glucocorticoid potency are available. Structures of some of the more commonly used synthetic glucocorticoid preparations are shown in Fig. 15-1. The modifications that enhance activity have been discussed above and in Chap. 12. The steroids may be given orally, parenterally, topically, intraarticularly, or as aerosols. The advantage of topical, intraarticular, or aerosol therapy is that certain areas (skin, joints, or the bronchial tree) can be exposed to high concentrations of glucocorticoids while minimizing systemic exposure and side effects.

Orally and Parenterally Active Preparations

In general, with oral administration, the unmodified steroid is given, since for the steroids commonly used (e.g., prednisone, prednisolone, dexamethasone, cortisol), substitutions (21-phosphate, etc.) are not needed for absorption (see Bioavailability, above).

Parenteral administration is indicated in the immediate treatment of the addisonian patient in crisis

(Chap. 12) and in patients who cannot take oral medications. There appears to be no acute danger in giving moderate does (1 g or less) intravenously (IV), although in general the oral route is effective. The preparations used intravenously are ordinarily compounds with C-21 substitutions to enhance solubility (Table 15-4). Intramuscular administration is described in the preceding section.

Four major considerations in selecting the particular steroid to be used are experience with it in the disease in question, duration of action, the possible need to avoid concomitant mineralocorticoid activity, and cost. Whereas in principle any of the various glucocorticoids should be effective given in equivalent doses, caution should be exercised in substituting because the relative potencies have not been established as clearly as has generally been assumed (see above and Chap. 12). Thus, in general, it is best to use preparations that have been shown to be effective for the particular condition. For instance, if a physician were treating an asthmatic crisis and wanted to administer the equivalent of 100 mg of cortisol, the prednisolone equivalent over the first few hours may be around 50 to 95 mg rather than the usually considered value of 20 to 25 mg (Table 15-2).[69] Whereas in the acute treatment of primary adrenocortical insufficiency cortisol is preferred because of its relatively greater mineralocorticoid activity, in other circumstances it is generally preferred to avoid sodium-retaining actions by giving a steroid with less mineralocorticoid activity. Duration of action is particularly relevant for alternate-day steroid therapy (discussed below). Finally, the physician should be aware that the various steroid preparations vary considerably in cost, and when possible less expensive preparations should be used.

Intraarticular Preparations

Glucocorticoids can be injected into joints for relief of inflammation.[22,71,84] Although these measures are usually for supplemental and temporary therapy, they can provide dramatic symptomatic relief. In general, the preparations are relatively insoluble and form microcrystals. Substitution with a *tert*-butylacetate or a hexacetonide group has proved to be particularly effective in this respect (Table 15-4).[22,71,84] These properties retard systemic absorption, promote retention within the joint space, and lead to a longer period of clinical effect; a single injection of such a preparation can last for weeks.[71] As stated earlier, preparations containing cortisone are not effective.[22,71,84]

When intraarticular preparations are used, generalized problems due to glucocorticoid excess, including suppression of the hypothalamic-pituitary-adrenal axis, are uncommon.[71] Intraarticular steroid administration is not, however, without risk. It is important to adhere to scrupulous aseptic technique and to avoid injection into potentially infected joints, as the steroids can worsen the course of such infections. Nevertheless, infections in the joint or needle tract occur infrequently in spite of strict aseptic techniques.[22] Other problems with intraarticular steroids include: the infrequent occurrence of synovitis, induced pre-

Table 15-4. Some Parenteral and Topical Glucocorticoid Preparations

Intravenous	Intraarticular
Hydrocortisone phosphate	Hydrocortisone acetate
Hydrocortisone hemisuccinate	Prednisolone tebutate
Prednisolone phosphate	Triamcinolone hexacetonide
Dexamethasone phosphate	Betamethasone acetate phosphate
Methylprednisolone hemisuccinate	Methylprednisolone acetate
Topical	
Lowest potency:	Low potency:
0.25–0.5% Cortisol	0.01% Fluocinolone acetonide
0.04–0.1% Dexamethasone	0.01% Betamethasone valerate
0.5% Prednisolone	0.025% Fluorometholone
0.2% Betamethasone	0.025% Triamcinolone acetonide
Intermediate potency:	High potency:
0.1% Betamethasone valerate	0.05% Betamethasone dipropionate
0.025% Halcinolone	0.5% Triamcinolone acetonide
0.1% Triamcinolone acetonide	0.2% Fluocinolone acetonide
0.025% Fluocinolone acetonide	0.1% Halcinonide

Source: Data on topical preparations from Robertson and Maibach.[65]

sumably by the steroid-containing crystals; occasional damage to the cartilage, supporting ligaments, and surrounding bone; partial absorption of bony margins; and cutaneous atrophy at the site of injection.[22,71,84] The last can be minimized by avoiding overdistention of the synovial cavity and leakage along the needle tract.[71]

Topical Preparations

The use of topical glucocorticoid preparations constitutes the major advance in the pharmacology of dermatology.[65,66] Some of the factors involved in topical uptake of glucocorticoids are discussed above under Determinants of Glucocorticoid Potency. Thus, many of the cortisol analogues are much more effective than cortisol itself. Some of the commonly used steroids are listed in Table 15-4. These come in ointment, cream, lotion, or aerosol vehicles and in varying strengths. The ointment bases tend to give better activity than do cream or lotion vehicles but tend to be less acceptable cosmetically to the patient, in spite of the fact that they are more soothing to dry skin.[65,66] However, hairy areas are best treated with lotions or aerosol vehicles.[65] The availability of several strengths helps the physician to provide the needed dosage while minimizing excess dosage. For most indications, high-potency steroid preparations are unnecessary; these carry a higher risk of local side effects (see below) and are used primarily on areas of skin that have been thickened by disease.[66] Although topical steroid preparations are commonly given without occlusion, they can be used (e.g., with plastic wrap, sometimes intermittently,[65] or with wet dressings[66]) to enhance penetration.[65,66] Single daily applications of an ointment are probably as effective as three daily applications.[65,66] In general, topical steroid use on ulcerated skin should be avoided. Except for circumstances under which there is markedly increased absorption, systemic toxicity, including suppression of the hypothalamic-pituitary-adrenal axis, is uncommon, although the possibility that this may develop must be kept in mind.[65] Other complications of topical therapy include exacerbation of an infection when the steroids are given inappropriately, localized striae (usually in areas of increased uptake such as the groin), rosacea-like eruptions, pustules (steroid acne), and, rarely, an allergic contact dermatitis from the steroids themselves.[65]

Corticosteroid Aerosols

Pressurized corticosterid aerosols are effective in the treatment of asthma.[36,85–88] Beclomethasone dipropionate and betamethasone valerate are the most commonly used preparations.[36,85–88] These preparations are advantageous over other steroids because they are not absorbed as well systemically as many other steroids such as cortisol.[36] More recently developed inhalers that deliver higher doses of up to 250 μg of beclomethasone dipropionate per puff have been shown to have significant efficacy.[88] In general, aerosols are used for maintenance therapy of asthma and are substituted for oral or parenteral steroids after these have induced a good response.[36] In some cases, delivery of the steroid to the lower bronchial tissue is enhanced by prior administration of a bronchodilator such as albuterol.[85] Delivery can be difficult during heavy sputum production. Although it is clear that steroids given in this way improve the ratio of therapeutic to toxic effects, this form of therapy is not without problems.[86] First, there is an increased incidence of fungal infections of the upper respiratory tract, including candidiasis of the pharynx.[86] Second, patients can experience dysphonia, which may be a steroid-induced myopathy of the phonatory muscle.[87] Suppression of the hypothalamic-pituitary-adrenal axis with corticosteroid aerosol therapy,[36] although it can occur, is overall much less severe than with the same dose given systemically; this can be minimized further in the asthmatic patient by holding the aerosol canister outside the mouth, using the inhaler before meals, rinsing the mouth and throat after inhalation, and using a spacer or holding chamber into which the medication is delivered.[36] The extent to which aerosols produce atrophy of the pharynx and airways has not yet been determined.[36]

ACTH

ACTH can be given instead of a glucocorticoid, and such preparations are occasionally used. Cosyntropin ($ACTH_{1\text{-}24}$, see Chap. 12) is commonly not used because of its short duration of action (unless continuous intravenous ACTH is given); instead, repository ACTH preparations are available for IM injection.[31] Given in this way, the peptide is released slowly and daily injections can be used to provide therapeutically effective steroid levels. These vary in composition and can include zinc or gelatin (the zinc preparations have a greater duration of action); 15 to 40 U of ACTH given in this way is roughly equivalent to 37.5 to 100 mg of cortisol.[31] However, a problem in comparing the efficacy of ACTH and glucocorticoids has been in determining the equivalency of dosages.[31]

ACTH stimulates the production of cortisol, adrenal androgens, and other steroids. Thus, the observed effects are due not only to cortisol but also to the other steroids, and they resemble spontaneous Cushing's syndrome, in which acne and hirsutism in females can be prominent.[73] Also, patients receiving ACTH appear to have a greater prevalence of hypertension than those receiving synthetic steroids.[31] This may be due to the greater mineralocorticoid activity of cortisol than that of the other more commonly used synthetic glucocorticoid preparations, and to the other reasons discussed in Chap. 14. Further, the ACTH itself can cause pigmentation.[31]

ACTH produces less suppression of the hypothalamic-pituitary-adrenal axis than do glucocorticoids. In almost all ACTH-treated patients, the responses to provocative testing with insulin-induced hypoglycemia are normal or only slightly impaired.[31] For instance, Daly et al. found a diminished plasma ACTH response but a normal cortisol response to insulin hypoglycemia testing.[89] These data suggest that ACTH therapy does suppress the axis to some extent, but that the adrenal, stimulated by the ACTH therapy, can respond to lower ACTH concentrations.[31] Further, some patients on prolonged ACTH therapy do show suppression of the pituitary-adrenal axis.[90] The decreased frequency of suppression of the axis by ACTH with respect to the frequency of suppression by glucocorticoids probably reflects differences in the maximal plasma glucocorticoid level attained and the duration of the effect. ACTH gel (20 to 40 U) given once daily results in only a moderate increase in plasma cortisol levels (maximum approximately 40 to 50 μg/dl), and these levels return to normal by approximately 16 h.[90] Thus, the effect of daily ACTH injections appears to be roughly comparable to that of a single morning dose of a short-acting glucocorticoid.[31] If ACTH were given twice daily, the degree of suppression of the axis might approximate that seen with glucocorticoids given in multiple doses. The fact that glucocorticoid concentrations are only moderately elevated and not sustained over 24 h by once-daily ACTH therapy[90] may also explain the observation that ACTH causes less suppression of linear growth in children than does daily glucocorticoid therapy.[31]

Further evidence that sustained, severe ACTH excess and the resulting hypercortisolism can suppress the hypothalamic-pituitary axis is seen in the ectopic ACTH syndrome, in which complete removal of the ectopic tumor is followed by hypocortisolism and the requirement for glucocorticoid therapy,[91] and Crooke's changes (the effect of hypercortisolism on anterior pituitary corticotropins) are the most prominent histological feature of the anterior pituitary (Chap. 12).

The disadvantages of ACTH therapy are the necessity for daily injection and the side effects of androgen excess and hypertension.[31] Since there is no clear advantage over oral glucocorticoids, ACTH, used in doses which achieve similar plasma glucocorticoid concentrations, is uncommonly used for prolonged therapy.

SOME GENERAL PRINCIPLES

Selection of Patients

The decision to use glucocorticoids implies that the benefits will outweigh the serious side effects. Thus, it should be clear that there is a reasonable chance that the patient will respond.

NEED FOR EMPIRICAL DATA

If there are no data to suggest that a given condition will respond to glucocorticoids, their use for that condition constitutes experimentation. Clearly, the decision to use corticosteroids should be based on some verification that the drugs are effective.

SHORT-TERM VERSUS LONG-TERM

The major complications of glucocorticoid therapy are ones that require a considerable time to develop (see above). Thus, in general, use of steroids over a short period of time is not associated with major risk. If steroids will significantly benefit a patient and need be given for only a few days, they should not be withheld. For instance, severe poison oak or poison ivy or an allergic skin reaction not responsive to topical steroids is an indication for a short course of systemic steroids.

The decision to initiate steroid therapy when it may involve treatment for a longer period of time is a more serious one. For instance, with asthma, once steroid therapy is started, it may be necessary to continue the drug for months to years. Clearly, the seriousness of the primary disease will commonly mandate this, but the physician must be aware of the consequences of such long-term therapy.

TESTING THE SENSITIVITY

With many conditions (e.g., acute lymphoblastic leukemia of childhood[3] and suppression of transplant rejection[23]), most patients will respond to glucocorticoids, whereas with other conditions only a subgroup of patients with the disease will respond. In the latter case it is sometimes possible to identify the patients who will respond. For instance, asthmatic patients with less fixed airway obstruction respond better than those with a greater complement of this.[86] Thus, documentation of such factors may assist in the selection of patients who will benefit from therapy. The identification of steroid-responsive patients may also be achieved by in vitro testing. This appears to be the case with the preleukemic syndrome mentioned under Therapeutic Influences, above. In this study, bone marrow cells of 34 patients were tested in vitro; the cells of five patients responded to the steroid, and three of these patients responded to glucocorticoid therapy.[4] In acute lymphoblastic leukemia and several other hematological malignancies, there is a good correlation between the concentration of glucocorticoid receptors measured in the malignant cells in vitro and responsiveness of the disease to glucocorticoid therapy.[3] In a recent study of T lymphocyte–mediated granulopoietic failure, prednisone-responsive patients could be identified by in vitro testing of the ability of the steroid to stimulate clonal growth of bone marrow cells.[92] It is to be hoped that approaches such as these will be applied to other conditions to increase the capability of detecting glucocorticoid-sensitive patients.

Dose-Response Considerations

The recommended doses of glucocorticoids used in therapy are based on empirical observations; this approach is reasonable and probably safest. As more is learned about glucocorticoid action, it will be possible to predict what doses will be required. This may facilitate the development of therapeutic trials and may help to optimize the dosage in order to minimize toxicity while maximizing therapeutic responses.

The application of current information about glucocorticoid receptors illustrates this point. For responses that are mediated by the receptors, doses resulting in steroid levels far in excess of those necessary to saturate the receptors will not provide a greater short-term benefit than those minimally required to do this. Such "excess' doses may, however, produce a greater effect, since higher levels of the steroid would be present longer.

As emphasized in Chap. 12, there is, in general, a close correlation between the relative saturation of the hormone by the receptor and the relative magnitude of the hormone response. In such cases, the effectiveness of a steroid can be calculated from its affinity for the receptor, and the free concentrations of the steroid with time. However, in vitro there appear to be circumstances[82] in which the steroid achieves a maximal response at concentrations lower than those required to fully saturate the receptors. Knowledge of whether this ever occurs in therapeutic situations would be particularly important, since lower than usual steroid concentrations might be used and these would have fewer undesirable side effects.

With human systems, precise data on the doses of steroids required to occupy the receptors have not been collected; however, from the known binding constants, free steroid levels, etc., it can be calculated that oral doses of 7.5 and 15 mg of prednisolone would result in blood levels 8 h after the dose that would bind the receptors to 42 and 63 percent, respectively, of saturation. Much higher doses (e.g., 100 mg or more) would be required to result in nearly complete receptor saturation for long periods of time. Thus, a dose this large given several times a day should stimulate near-maximal receptor-mediated responses.

There occur situations, such as acute renal transplant rejection,[23] gram-negative sepsis with shock,[16,93–97] tumors of the central nervous system,[17] and certain immune-mediated hematological dyscrasias,[98] in which the use of even larger doses of glucocorticoids has been recommended. Subsequent studies of renal transplant rejection indicate that such large doses actually decrease survival,[23] and for this indication the trend has been toward the use of progressively lower steroid doses.[99] Studies in baboons show clear beneficial effects of high-dose glucocorticoids given early in the course of bacteria-induced shock.[96] Dexamethasone at doses of 3 to 5 mg per kilogram of body weight per day has been shown to be beneficial in patients with suspected typhoid fever who are delerious, obtunded, stuporous, comatose, or in shock.[95] A single bolus of 30 mg per kilogram of body weight of methylprednisolone sodium succinate or of 6 mg per kilogram of body weight of dexamethasone sodium phosphate was associated with a reversal of shock during the first 24 h in 27 percent of patients with septic shock, vs. 0 percent of nonsteroid-treated patients and to reduce mortality early in the hospital course, although improvement in mortality was not evident on a long-term basis.[97] These workers suggested that this improved short-term survival and the reversal of shock may be beneficial in that they may allow the physician to buy time for institution of other measures.[97] Overall, it appears that glucocorticoids must be given early to be beneficial. It has not been demonstrated in these circumstances whether smaller doses of corticosteroids would have been equally effective. Based on the preceding considerations, these very large doses might not be expected to produce a greater effect than the large doses if the therapeutic influences are glucocorticoid receptor–mediated, and they might have other undesirable side effects. However, some argue that receptor-independent mechanisms, such as those due to membrane effects secondary to the lipid properties of the steroids, are operative in these conditions.[3,98]

The Use of Adjunctive Therapy

In the majority of conditions for which glucocorticoids are used, there are either alternative or adjunctive therapeutic modalities; these must be considered and if possible used prior to beginning steroid therapy, since their use may be associated with a lower incidence of complications. Further, if the patient's condition can be adequately controlled by such methods, glucocorticoid therapy may not be indicated. Conversely, the failure to respond to maximal utilization of conventional treatment may be an indication for the use of glucocorticoids in certain conditions.

If glucocorticoid therapy is used, adjunctive therapy should in most cases be continued, as it may be beneficial, improve the overall response to therapy, and allow the use of lower steroid dosages. For instance, in rheumatoid arthritis, the use of physical therapy, braces, salicylates, and other nonsteroidal anti-inflammatory agents may obviate the need for steroids or provide additional benefit. In asthma, other bronchodilators such as beta-adrenergic agents are used in conjunction with steroids. Immunosuppressants such as azathioprine, in addition to a glucocorticoid, may be helpful in the treatment of nephritis[100] or the prevention of renal transplant rejection.[23] Other chemotherapeutic agents can be helpful in malignancies or other conditions such as amyloidosis.[101]

Specific Measures to Reduce Side Effects

There is a growing awareness that certain specific measures may reduce side effects. The potential use of measures to reduce osteoporosis and myopathy, and of insulin to control diabetes, is discussed elsewhere in this chapter. An increased protein intake can reduce steroid-induced nitrogen wasting.[102] Vitamin A may decrease the steroid effect of impaired wound healing.[103]

Cognizance of Objective Criteria

In evaluating the response to steroid therapy, objective criteria should be used whenever possible since glucocorticoids themselves can induce a sense of well-being,[2,17,30,56–58] and this is not necessarily accompanied by improvement in the primary disease for which the steroids are being administered. Conversely, patients on long-term therapy frequently develop symptoms of steroid withdrawal when the dose is lowered (see below) and these symptoms may be misinterpreted as an exacerbation of the primary disease. For example, arthralgias and myalgias are common in steroid withdrawal and do not necessarily indicate increased activity of rheumatoid arthritis. Similarly, lowering the steroid dose in patients with inflammatory bowel disease may provoke anorexia and nausea which may not be due to an exacerbation of the gastrointestinal disorder. Thus, subjective changes may be misleading and may lead to inappropriate alterations in dosage. Although many of the disorders for which steroids are used have no clearly identifiable chemical criteria which can be used to quantify maximal benefit or improvement, objective criteria should be used when possible. Such criteria include pulmonary function studies or blood and sputum eosinophil determinations in patients with asthma,[104] gallium lung scanning or assay of serum angiotensin converting enzyme activity in sarcoidosis,[104a] evaluation of serum complement levels in patients with lupus erythematosus, determination of serum Ca^{2+} concentrations in patients with hypercalcemia, serial creatinine clearance measurements in patients treated for renal transplant rejection, and evidence for true joint inflammation in the case of arthritis.

The Circadian Rhythm

When moderate doses of glucocorticoids are given for a short time (e.g., a few days or less), the circadian rhythm of endogenous steroid production (Chap. 12) is ignored; the transient suppression of the hypothalamic-pituitary-adrenal axis in this setting is not a problem. When it is necessary to give moderate to large doses of steroids on a daily basis for a longer period, suppression of the axis is unavoidable and must be considered and dealt with as described below (see Withdrawal of Glucocorticoids and Suppression of the Hypothalamic-Pituitary-Adrenal Axis).

However, there are other circumstances in which it is important to tailor glucocorticoid therapy to the circadian rhythm; this is the case with alternate-day therapy (discussed below), replacement therapy in the patient whose hypothalamic-pituitary-adrenal axis is suppressed (discussed below), and sometimes when low doses of steroids are required. In the latter situation, a patient with lupus arthritis or asthma refractory to other therapy may sometimes respond to low dosages of glucocorticoids (e.g., 5 mg or less of prednisone per day). If these are given in the evening, there will be suppression of the rise in plasma ACTH concentration and therefore in cortisol level. In this case the total additional effect will be minor, since the suppression of endogenous cortisol production will offset the effect of the steroid administered. However, if the steroid is given in the morning, when

ACTH levels are spontaneously falling, the net effect can be additive, with a minimal influence on the body's normal rhythm of steroid secretion.

Adjusting the Dose

Once glucocorticoid therapy has been instituted, it is important to monitor the dose carefully. The major end point is clinical response; side effects can be minimized by decreasing the dose when the patient is responding. Alternatively, it may be necessary to increase the dose when the patient is not responding, and the literature regarding that condition suggests that higher doses might be more effective.

The factors that lead to variations in response were discussed earlier. Because variations exist in metabolism and distribution, absorption, and possibly even intrinsic sensitivity, it should be obvious that adherence to a fixed drug protocol is not ideal, although in certain situations this may be necessary because other information is not available.

It is hoped that plasma measurements of the glucocorticoids used in therapy will be used more in the future to minimize variations due to uptake, metabolism, and distribution. In this way patients in whom higher drug levels develop could have their doses lowered sooner, thereby minimizing cushingoid side effects. Conversely, patients in whom adequate blood levels are not attained could receive an increased dosage (and possible improvement) sooner.

ALTERNATE-DAY THERAPY

Alternate-day therapy emerged after it was found that, by giving a single dose of glucocorticoid once in the morning on alternate days, certain adverse effects of the steroid could be minimized while a therapeutically beneficial response could still be obtained.[31,36,105–107] Conditions in which alternate-day glucocorticoid therapy has been effective include certain nephrotic syndromes (particularly in children), renal transplantation rejection and other renal diseases, ulcerative colitis, rheumatoid arthritis and some other arthritic disorders, rheumatic fever, myasthenia gravis, muscular dystrophy, sarcoidosis, alopecia areata, chronic dermatoses, asthma, and pemphigus vulgaris.[31,36,54,108–110] However, alternate-day therapy has been shown not to be effective in giant cell arteritis.[111] Thus, before the use of alternate-day steroid therapy is contemplated, the specific literature about each condition should be examined.

Based on studies in which the same dose of steroid was given once in the morning on alternate days rather than over a 48-h period, it has been claimed that a number of cushingoid side effects are decreased.[31,36,107] These include suppression of the hypothalamic-pituitary-adrenal axis, growth inhibition in children, cushingoid facies, suprascapular fat deposition, obesity, excessive appetite, striae, easy bruisability, carbohydrate intolerance, infections, myopathy, and other features. The decrease in growth inhibition constitutes a major advantage of alternate-day glucocorticoid therapy in the pediatric group.[31,36,112]

The effect of alternate-day steroid therapy on the hypothalamic-pituitary-adrenal axis has been studied by ACTH stimulation, metyrapone testing, insulin hypoglycemia testing, and corticotropin releasing factor stimulation.[31,110,113–115] These studies do appear to show less suppression than with equivalent divided doses given on a daily basis. In one study, there was recovery of a suppressed axis when children were switched from daily to alternate-day therapy.[114] Some suppression of the hypothalamic-pituitary-adrenal axis does occur with alternate-day therapy.[31,110,113,115,116] For example, in a recent study of patients receiving from 5 to 60 mg of prednisone on alternate days,[115] the axis tended to be markedly suppressed on the day of treatment and mildly blunted on the day off treatment, as assessed by CRF testing. However, the cortisol response to ACTH was normal in all cases, indicating that enough ACTH was secreted to maintain normal basal adrenal function.[115] However, the extent of axis suppression in earlier reports was probably exaggerated, since some of the studies were performed when patients were taking either divided doses on the day of therapy or a long-acting glucocorticoid; in both cases, this would prolong the glucocorticoid effect (see below).

The precise mechanisms of the effectiveness of alternate-day therapy are not known. However, when various responses to glucocorticoids are examined, some of these persist on the "off steroid" day of alternate-day therapy, whereas other influences are present only during the "on" day. For instance, Fauci and Dale[109] found, in a study of patients with a variety of inflammatory diseases, that glucocorticoid-induced lymphocytopenia and monocytopenia returned to normal by 8 A.M. on the day off prednisone, yet at this time there was evidence that the steroid was suppressing disease activity. Considerations such as these underscore a general problem that must be faced with glucocorticoid therapy: the dose response and the kinetics of each particular beneficial and deleterious effect need to be known. It might then be possible to optimize even more precisely the dose and the interval between doses. However, other dosage intervals have been tried in some cases and were not found to be superior.[31,105,106]

If alternate-day therapy is used, one of the short-acting glucocorticoids should be administered (Table 15-5).[31,53,107,108] These are the steroids that are cleared more rapidly from the plasma (Table 15-3); they include prednisone, prednisolone, methylprednisolone, cortisol, and cortisone. As has already been stated, optimal alternate-day therapy requires that the steroid be administered in the morning (preferably before breakfast) as a single dose.[31,53,105,108] If the steroid is given in divided doses, the effect of the later doses may persist into the alternate day. Avoidance of late-afternoon and evening doses is especially important in terms of minimizing any suppression of the hypothalamic-pituitary-adrenal axis (discussed below), and with the short-acting steroid, morning-only administration will allow the steroid to be cleared from the circulation prior to the nocturnal increase in ACTH release. Steroids such as dexamethasone, betamethasone, triamcinolone, triamcinolone acetonide, and fluocinolone acetonide are cleared more slowly, are longer-acting, and should not be used for alternate-day therapy,[31,53,105,108] although in some cases certain of these have been successfully used on alternate days without uniformly causing suppression of the axis.[114]

Alternate-day therapy is best used for prolonged[114] therapy and is not in general indicated for initial treatment, especially when glucocorticoids are used for acute problems (Tables 15-1 and 15-5).[31,53,105,108,114] Thus, most people experienced in the use of steroids recommend that, even for chronic diseases, daily therapy should be used initially. In fact, if only short-term treatment is anticipated, alternate-day therapy may not be necessary. Thus, in instituting steroid therapy, the glucocorticoid first is given on a daily (or more frequent) basis and then, once there is amelioration or control, the patient is switched to alternate-day therapy. The change to alternate-day therapy should be made as soon as possible (within several weeks) after beginning steroid therapy and before there is major suppression of the hypothalamic-pituitary-adrenal axis, as the change is more difficult if the axis is suppressed.

Table 15-5. Recommendations Regarding Alternate-Day Glucocorticoid Therapy

1. Use a short-acting glucocorticoid.
2. Avoid in acute situations or if only short-term therapy (e.g., < 3 weeks) is anticipated.
3. Inform patient fully of the advantages; then be diligent.
4. Give special attention if there is already suppression of the hypothalamic-pituitary-adrenal axis.
5. Maximize adjunctive therapy, particularly on the "off" day.
6. Check the literature: may not be effective for certain diseases.

In patients in whom the axis is not suppressed, the change can be made abruptly. In changing to alternate-day therapy, it is generally best not to reduce the total dosage of steroid given.[31,53,105,107,108] In fact, sometimes it may be advantageous to increase the total dosage. Thus, the overall dosage for two days used with daily therapy can be administered as a single dose on the mornings of alternate days. Then, the overall dose can be reduced as indicated by the condition of the problem for which the steroid was given.

Patients on long-term daily multiple-dose therapy in whom the axis is suppressed frequently have manifestations of adrenal insufficiency and steroid withdrawal (discussed below) on the off day when switched abruptly to alternate-day therapy.[31,53,105,107,108] In these patients, the change can be made slowly; it may first require gradual reduction in the total dose, then a change to single daily doses, and finally a switch to alternate-day therapy. This can be done by gradually reducing (e.g., by 5 mg every 4 to 5 days) the steroid dose on alternate days and adding this dose to that given on the other days until the transition is achieved. In making this transition, the physician should be concerned not only with an exacerbation of the primary disease but also with the problem of a lack of well-being while off the steroid. This can be due to symptoms of adrenal insufficiency in cases where the hypothalamic-pituitary-adrenal axis is suppressed, to a lack of the general euphoric influences of the steroid independent of the primary disease, or to the primary disease. Thus, the patient is likely to complain on the off day. The physician and patient must be committed to alternate-day therapy once the decision to use it has been made, and special attention must be given, in the patient who has symptoms on the off day, to objective criteria and to the questions of whether the therapy is ineffective or is effective and whether the complaints are due to the other factors discussed above. However, during this time it may be necessary, if there is a documented flare-up of the primary disease, to switch to daily therapy for a short time, and several attempts at conversion to alternate-day therapy may be required. In switching to alternate-day therapy the physician should be especially aware of the use of adjunctive modalities (see above) that may minimize symptoms.

SPECIAL SITUATIONS

Pregnancy

There has been concern that the use of glucocorticoids in pregnancy might increase the incidence of fetal deaths or congenital abnormalities.[22,48,117,117a] Indeed, glucocorticoid-treated pregnant animals have an increased incidence of abortions, placental insufficiency, and congenital malformations, including cleft palate, in their offspring.[22,48,117,117a] Despite these valid concerns, there are circumstances in which pregnant patients with life-threatening conditions such as asthma or systemic lupus erythematosus may benefit from steroid therapy. Fortunately, the overall experience with glucocorticoids in pregnancy has not been so bad as expected.[22,48,117,117a] For instance, during 70 pregnancies in 55 asthmatic patients, there were 71 live births, only 1 spontaneous abortion, and possibly a slight increase in premature births.[117] Further, there were no fetal, maternal, or neonatal deaths, and the incidence of toxemia, uterine hemorrhage, or congenital malformations was not increased. In a series of 260 pregnancies (reviewed in Ref. 22), seven full-term infants had disorders. One had apparent adrenocortical failure for 3 days, and there were two cases of cleft palate. The latter has also been noted in a few instances in which steroids were used at the time of conception and continued for significant periods thereafter.[22] However, cleft palate was not observed in two other series of 46 mothers who were on steroids during and after conception.[22] Thus, glucocorticoids should not be used indiscriminately during pregnancy, and they should be avoided especially in the first trimester. However, they should not be withheld in conditions where the steroid may ameliorate life-threatening disease.

The use of steroid aerosols in pregnancy appears to be safe when recommended doses are used.[117a]

Diabetes

Glucocorticoids alter carbohydrate metabolism by increasing gluconeogenesis and antagonizing the peripheral uptake of glucose. However, in glucocorticoid-treated patients without subclinical or overt diabetes, significant clinical problems with hyperglycemia are unusual (Chap. 12). Thus, in most patients, fasting blood sugar levels are usually normal or only mildly elevated, although glucose tolerance may be impaired. However, in patients with subclinical or overt diabetes, steroid therapy may provoke or worsen hyperglycemia. Steroid therapy is not contraindicated in such patients although insulin therapy or an increase in insulin dose may be required. In the rare patient with insulin resistance ascribable to the development of anti-insulin antibodies, glucocorticoids may be beneficial and reduce the insulin requirement by suppressing the immune response.[22]

Surgery

It is generally recommended that patients on prolonged high-dose glucocorticoids must receive additional steroid coverage for the stress of surgery (discussed below and in Chap. 12). These patients also have an increased risk of serious postoperative complications. Local problems include poor healing, wound infections, and, occasionally, dehiscence of the incision; hematomas and abscesses may occur with abdominal or thoracic surgery. The courses of these patients may also be complicated by systemic infection. Thus, morbidity is increased and recovery is prolonged; if time allows, elective surgery should be deferred and the steroid dose decreased.

Psychiatry

Changes in mood and psychological state are frequent in glucocorticoid-treated patients, and although many patients initially note a feeling of mental well-being, depression and several types of psychosis may also occur.[2,17,30,56–58] The type of disorder that may occur is not predictable by the patient's pretherapy condition, but it is ordinarily reversible following discontinuation of therapy. Previous psychiatric disorders are in general not a contraindication to steroid therapy.

Peptic Ulcer

The relationship between glucocorticoid therapy and peptic ulcer disease is reviewed in Chap. 12. Although the issue is controversial, it appears that there is an increased incidence of peptic ulcer in glucocorticoid-treated individuals. Nevertheless, the prevalence is only in the range of 2 percent (Chap. 12). Thus, routine antacid treatment is not generally recommended for patients without ulcer disease, although glucocorticoid-treated patients should be monitored for ulcer stigmata and treated when appropriate. Also, whereas peptic ulcer disease does not constitute an absolute contraindication to steroid therapy, the possibility that this will be worsened by steroid therapy should be included in the overall decision to use steroids in these patients.

Pediatrics

In children, glucocorticoid therapy has the major additional disadvantage of causing growth failure (see Chap. 12). There tends to be a growth spurt following discontinuation of the steroid, since it also inhibits bone maturation (Chap. 12); fortunately, a more recent study suggests that long-term there may be no overall inhibition of height attainment.[112] Nevertheless, alternate-day therapy in children results in less inhibitory effect on growth (see above) and in decreased cushingoid effects in general.[36]

Kaposi's Sarcoma

Kaposi's sarcoma occurs with an increased prevalence in patients who are receiving immunosuppressive therapy, or who have the acquired immune deficiency syndrome (AIDS).[117b] There are several case reports of regression of their tumors in association with discontinuation of treatment with glucocorticoids.[117b] Thus, glucocorticoids should be used with caution in such patients, and their use should be avoided in patients who are at a greater risk for developing Kaposi's sarcoma.

WITHDRAWAL OF GLUCOCORTICOIDS AND SUPPRESSION OF THE HYPOTHALAMIC-PITUITARY-ADRENAL AXIS

As mentioned above, spontaneous Cushing's syndrome or glucocorticoid therapy can result in suppression of the hypothalamic-pituitary-adrenal axis. However, the suppression is most frequently encountered in glucocorticoid therapy because of the large number of patients receiving these steroids, and it must be considered in any patients who will discontinue or has discontinued glucocorticoid therapy.

Kinetics and Dosage Required for Suppression

Glucocorticoid suppression of the hypothalamic-pituitary-adrenal axis has been discussed in Chap. 12. Even a single dose of a glucocorticoid can for some hours prevent a response of the axis to a major insult such as surgery. However, with short exposure, i.e., one or two doses, the axis recovers rapidly and the suppression occurs for the most part while the glucocorticoid is present in the circulation.[118] Thus, after short-term glucocorticoid therapy, suppression of the hypothalamic-pituitary-adrenal axis is rarely pronounced for more than a few hours. With more prolonged therapy, suppression increases with both duration and total dose. When glucocorticoids are administered for a period of days, there may be both suppression of basal cortisol levels (Fig. 15-7), if doses are sufficiently high, and decreased responsiveness of both the hypothalamic-pituitary axis and the adrenal to stimulation.[118] Thus, in one study (Fig. 15-8), the administration of 50 mg of prednisone per day for 5 days resulted in decreased responsiveness to both insulin-induced hypoglycemia and exogenous ACTH 2 days after discontinuation of the steroid, but responses returned to normal at 5 days.[118] With lower doses, there may be suppression of basal secretion but normal responsiveness of the axis to stimulation, even when the steroid is given for a more prolonged period.[119] Finally, with long-term therapy, particularly in high doses, there is profound and prolonged suppression of the axis and absent responsiveness to major stimuli (Fig. 15-9).[119,120]

The degree of pituitary-adrenal suppression also depends on the timing of the dose and the steroid preparation used.[121] As discussed under Alternate-Day Therapy, above, longer-acting steroids such as dexa-

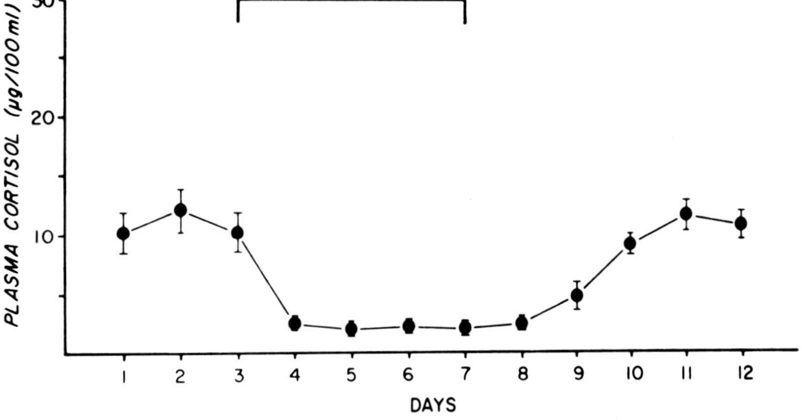

FIGURE 15-7 Fasting plasma cortisol levels (mean ± SEM) in 10 subjects before, during, and after the oral administration of prednisone, 25 mg twice daily on days 3 to 7. (*From Streck and Lockwood.*[118])

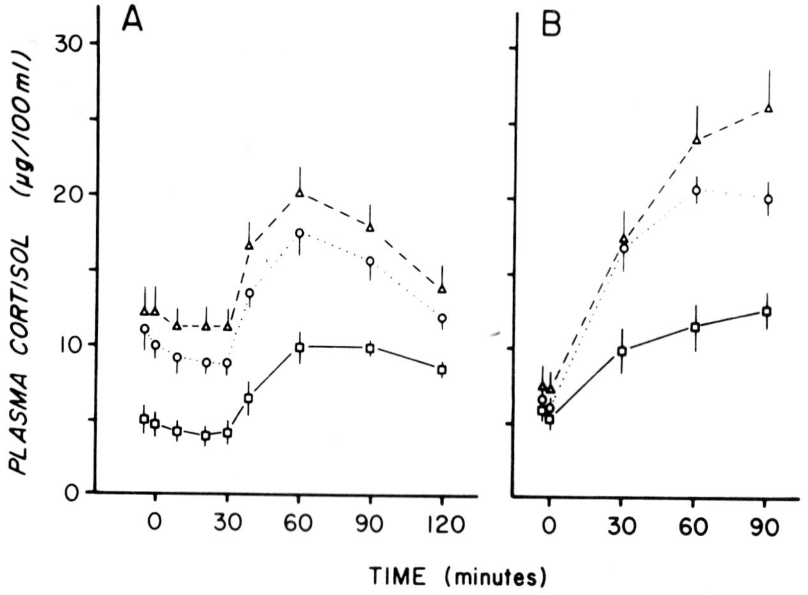

FIGURE 15-8 Plasma cortisol response (mean ± SEM) to insulin-induced hypoglycemia (*A*) and synthetic ACTH (*B*) in 10 subjects prior to (△), and at 2 days (○) and 5 days (□) after oral prednisone, 25 mg twice daily for 5 days. (*From Streck and Lockwood.*[118])

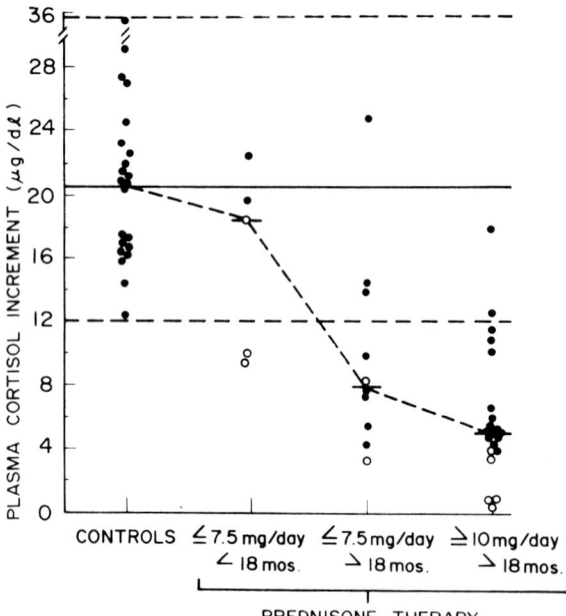

FIGURE 15-9 Plasma cortisol response (shown as the increment) after insulin hypoglycemia testing in control subjects and patients on various doses of glucocorticoids for various times. A dashed line connects median values, the solid line shows the median value for the control subjects, and the horizontal dashed lines show the upper and lower values for the control subjects. For the steroid-treated patients, open circles indicate that the test was performed while the patient was on steroids, and closed circles indicate that the test was performed 48 h after discontinuing therapy. (*Based on data from Livanou et al.*[119])

methasone result in greater suppression than do short-acting ones such as cortisol, prednisolone, or prednisone, since they are present in the circulation for a longer period of time.[77] Suppression is also greater if glucocorticoids are administered in the evening or at night, rather than in the morning, since this results in maximal suppression of the normal early-morning circadian rise in ACTH.[122] This timing of steroid administration is essential to the success of alternate-day therapy (see above).[113] Also discussed previously was the fact that therapy with ACTH, if given once daily, causes less suppression than does therapy with oral corticosteroids.[89,90]

Kinetics of Return to Normal Axis Function

The kinetics of the return of the hypothalamic-pituitary-adrenal axis are also time- and dose-dependent. Recovery of the axis may require hours to months.[118–120] Thus, as mentioned above, hypothalamic-pituitary-adrenal responsiveness remains normal following single doses and returns to normal within several days following short courses of glucocorticoids (Fig. 15-8).[118] When moderate doses of glucocorticoids have been continued for months to years, recovery is prolonged in general, although considerable individual variability is present (Fig. 15-10).[119] Recovery of both

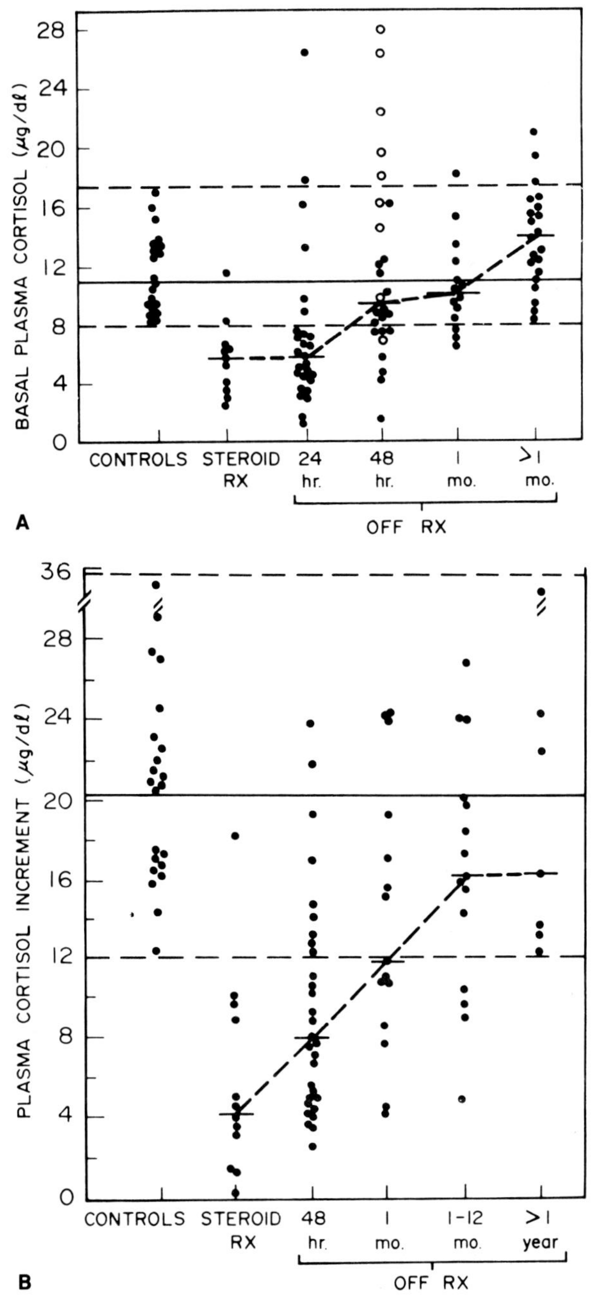

FIGURE 15-10 (*A*) Basal plasma cortisol levels in control subjects, patients on glucocorticoid therapy, and patients in whom glucocorticoid therapy had been withdrawn ("off Rx") for the indicated times. For the period 48 h after steroid withdrawal, open circles indicate the patients who had been on 7.5 mg of prednisone or less and closed circles indicate patients who had been on 10 mg of prednisone or more. (*B*) Plasma cortisol response to insulin-induced hypoglycemia testing in control subjects and patients on glucocorticoid therapy and after withdrawal of therapy for the indicated times. For both panels, heavy dashed lines connect median values. The solid line indicates the median value for the controls and the lighter dashed line shows the upper and lower values for the control subjects. (*Based on data from Livanou et al.*[119])

basal cortisol secretion and stress responsiveness is more rapid in patients receiving lower glucocorticoid doses (7.5 mg or less of prednisone per day) and in those in whom therapy was of shorter duration.[119] Basal plasma cortisol levels return to normal first, usually within 1 month of cessation of therapy, but months may be required before the response to insulin-induced hypoglycemia returns to normal (Fig. 15-10).[119]

The kinetics of return of the axis in patients exposed to higher glucocorticoid concentrations for more prolonged periods, i.e., 1 to 10 years, are shown in Fig. 15-11.[120] In the first month following withdrawal of glucocorticoid excess, both plasma cortisol and ACTH levels were subnormal. During the next several months, plasma ACTH levels increased to supranormal in most of the patients. Despite this, cortisol levels remained low and were subnormally responsive to stimulation with exogenous ACTH, indicating persisting adrenal atrophy.[120] However, at 5 to 9 months the plasma cortisol levels gradually increased into the normal range because of the trophic influence of ACTH, and in this study normal concentrations of plasma cortisol and ACTH were attained in all patients more than 9 months after glucocorticoid withdrawal.[120] Although suppression after more than a year is rare, the authors have followed one patient who had a successfully resected cortisol producing

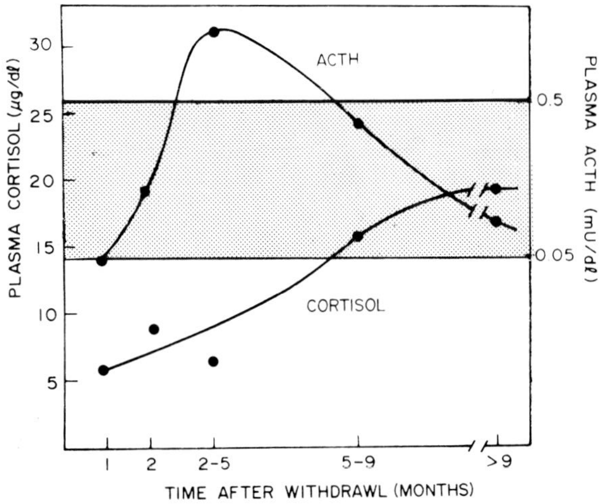

FIGURE 15-11 Median plasma cortisol and ACTH levels (at 6 A.M.) in patients following withdrawal of glucocorticoids. The shaded area indicates the range of values for control subjects. The data were obtained from eight patients with spontaneous Cushing's syndrome, following removal of an adrenal tumor, and from six patients on high-dose glucocorticoid therapy for 1 to 10 years. Glucocorticoids were not abruptly withdrawn in these patients but instead were tapered over periods of 1 to 4 weeks. The time after withdrawal indicates the period following complete cessation of therapy. (*Based on data from Graber et al.*[120])

adrenal adenoma whose axis has now remained suppressed for 2.5 years in spite of otherwise normal pituitary function. Thus, the return of normal axis function requires sequential recovery of the hypothalamus, pituitary, and adrenal. The recovery of pituitary ACTH secretion is the primary and limiting determinant for recovery; with recovery, ACTH levels gradually rise and stimulate the adrenal. However, they generally need to become elevated before adequate adrenal stimulation occurs with reversal of the adrenal atrophy. As plasma cortisol levels reach the normal range, the feedback inhibition by hydrocortisone begins to suppress ACTH production; as this happens, the axis returns to normal.

As mentioned in Chap. 12, administration of ACTH for 3 to 5 days can increase the responsiveness of the adrenal gland to normal or near normal.[119,123] It might, therefore, seem desirable to administer ACTH to restore such responsiveness to the adrenal. However, the limiting factor in the return of the axis is the ability of the pituitary to release ACTH. Thus, if ACTH is administered, the subsequent increase in steroid production may even impair the return of the pituitary to normal.[123] Further, once ACTH is withdrawn, it is still necessary to wait until the pituitary returns to normal function[123] before it can be predicted with confidence that the patient will respond to an insult requiring increased cortisol production. Thus, there is no evidence that ACTH administration hastens recovery of the axis[121,123,124] when given either as a single course or intermittently for months, and it is therefore not recommended.

Steroid Withdrawal Syndromes

The response to withdrawal of steroids can vary. First, the primary disease may remain in remission and the patient may be asymptomatic. Second, there may be a recurrence or worsening of the disease, and the patient may or may not experience other symptoms of withdrawal. Third, the patient may experience symptoms due to adrenal insufficiency. Fourth, the patient may experience symptoms similar to those of adrenal insufficiency and yet have no biochemical evidence of deficient adrenal secretion ("steroid withdrawal syndrome").[125,126] Perhaps a subclass within the last category is the case in which there is a general lack of well-being without other symptoms of adrenal insufficiency.

In the first case, in which there are no symptoms and the disease for which steroids were given is quiescent, has improved, or has resolved, it is necessary only to follow the disease and the potential of a suppressed axis. Many patients can have a suppressed hypothalamic-pituitary-adrenal axis without symptoms of adrenal insufficiency, and if these patients are exposed to stress (see Chap. 12), they can develop acute adrenal insufficiency. Thus, all the precautions outlined below in the withdrawal procedures should be taken.

In the second case, where there is an exacerbation of the primary disease, it may be necessary to reinstitute glucocorticoid therapy. Of course, there are times when it is not warranted. For instance, in acute lymphocytic leukemia of childhood, the development of glucocorticoid resistance precludes further glucocorticoid therapy. In other cases, serious complications of glucocorticoid therapy (e.g., compression fractures or severe osteoporosis) may be present to such an extent that further steroid administration might be more damaging than relief of the primary condition. In cases where therapy is not reinstituted, the precautions relative to hypothalamic-pituitary-adrenal axis suppression must be followed.

The symptoms of adrenal insufficiency that occur with a suppressed hypothalamic-pituitary-adrenal axis are similar to those of secondary adrenal insufficiency discussed in Chap. 12. Thus, the adrenal glomerulosa, with its electrolyte-regulating properties, is almost always intact, so that dehydration, hypotension, hyponatremia, and hyperkalemia are uncommon (see Chap. 12).

The steroid withdrawal syndrome is characterized by symptoms similar or identical to those of adrenocortical insufficiency in the patient who is either receiving physiological doses of glucocorticoids or has a normally responsive hypothalamic-pituitary-adrenal axis.[125,126] The syndrome occurs in patients in whom exogenous glucocorticoid doses are being either reduced or withdrawn. Thus, patients may develop the syndrome even though they continue to receive "physiologic" or even supraphysiological doses of glucocorticoids. The most prominent clinical features are anorexia, lethargy, malaise, nausea, weight loss, desquamation of the skin, headache, and fever.[126] Arthralgias, myalgias, and vomiting are less common; postural hypotension may occur occasionally.[126] These symptoms are variable and may be transient.[126] For example, the reduction of steroid dosage may be accompanied by mild to moderate symptoms that resolve within several days and permit continuation of the lower dose. However, in other patients, the symptoms may be severe and disabling. The persistence of severe symptoms for more than several days is an indication either to reinstitute glucocorticoids in small doses (e.g., 10 to 20 mg of cortisol) or to increase the steroid dosage to its former level and then to taper the dosage by smaller decrements over a more prolonged period of time.

The mechanisms of the steroid withdrawal syndrome are unknown; however, there are two potential explanations. First, it is possible that the transition from higher to lower doses of glucocorticoids, even when the lower dose is "normal," causes the same type of subjective findings as those observed in adrenal insufficiency. Second, it is possible that these patients have a relative state of glucocorticoid resistance that renders them effectively hypoadrenal. However, there is no evidence that this group is in danger of developing acute adrenal insufficiency, suggesting that any resistance, if present, is not severe or complete enough to prevent certain responses to stress.

Evaluation of Axis Function

The same considerations discussed in Chap. 12 for evaluation of adrenal insufficency apply in evaluating suppression of the hypothalamic-pituitary-adrenal axis. First, a normal random cortisol determination does not exclude significant suppression. Conversely, a subnormal random cortisol level does not prove suppression, as this may occur between periods of episodic cortisol secretion. If the plasma cortisol concentration is low or low normal during an obvious acute stress (e.g., during shock), significant suppression is likely. However, stimulation tests of the axis are usually required for verification.

The tests used to assess the integrity of the axis are discussed in Chap. 12. Of these, the rapid ACTH stimulation, metyrapone, and insulin-induced hypoglycemia tests are usually used. The rapid ACTH stimulation test is most commonly used because of its ease; it is a simple and safe outpatient procedure. If the cortisol response is subnormal, this test confirms suppression of the axis, since deficient cortisol responsiveness indicates adrenal atrophy secondary to ACTH deficiency. However, a normal response to this test does not necessarily predict normal pituitary responsiveness to stress (see Chap. 12), and in this circumstance more definitive information is obtained with metyrapone or insulin-induced hypoglycemia. Thus, in usual circumstances, a normal response to the rapid ACTH test is sufficient to exclude the necessity of daily maintenance therapy. However, if stress such as elective surgery is anticipated, further testing should be carried out or else the patient should receive glucocorticoid coverage (Chap. 12).

Withdrawal Protocols and Indications for Steroid Coverage

When the status of the disease being treated permits withdrawal of glucocorticoids, both the patient and the physician must be fully aware of the tedious nature and potential difficulty of the process. The patient should be informed of the symptoms of steroid withdrawal; this knowledge may allow differentiation of these symptoms from those due to worsening of the disease. The patient should also be aware of the potential time required for the return to normal of the axis.

Patients who have undergone only short courses of steroid usually do not have great difficulty during steroid withdrawal, but patients on high-dose long-term therapy may require close monitoring for as long as a year before pituitary-adrenal function returns to normal. In assessing these patients, the physician must assess the underlying disease and the potential symptoms of steroid withdrawal and in addition must serially assess the hypothalamic-pituitary-adrenal axis.[121]

In patients who have been on long-term glucocorticoid therapy, it is usually necessary to reduce the total dosage more gradually toward physiological levels, since abrupt changes may precipitate exacerbation of the underlying disease and steroid withdrawal symptoms. For instance, the glucocorticoid dosage might be reduced by 2.5 to 5.0 mg of prednisone (or its equivalent) per week. As the dosage is being reduced, an attempt should also be made to administer the dose either once daily in the morning or on alternate days to give the hypothalamic-pituitary-adrenal axis a beter chance to recover (see above). The dose may have to be increased if there is worsening of the underlying disease or if severe symptoms of steroid withdrawal develop. Acute flare-ups or unrelated acute illness should be managed by short-term administration of high-dose steroids with a return to the previous dosage as soon as the clinical situation permits. During this period, adjunctive therapy (see above) should also be continued or increased as this will assist in the control of the primary disorder.

When the total steroid dosage has been tapered to the equivalent of 20 to 30 mg of cortisol or 5 mg of prednisone given as a single morning dose, the function of the hypothalamic-pituitary-adrenal axis should be assessed. The simplest method is to measure basal morning cortisol levels prior to the daily glucocorticoid dose at 1- to 2-month intervals. When basal cortisol levels are normal, therapy may be withdrawn, since this indicates normal basal steroid secretion. Additionally, at this point serial assessment of the axis may be begun, also at 1- to 2-month intervals. Persisting subnormal responses to the rapid ACTH stimulation test indicate continuing suppression of the axis (Chap. 12). When normal responsiveness to ACTH occurs, the axis can be presumed to be normal in most patients; confirmation can be readily obtained by demonstrating a normal response to the overnight metyrapone test (Chap. 12). If the responses to both rapid ACTH stimulation and metyrapone tests are normal, the return of the normal function of the hypothalamic-pituitary-adrenal axis is demonstrated.

Supplementation with high doses of glucocorticoids may be required at any point in the withdrawal process for acute illness or elective surgery. In these circumstances increased steroid doses should be administered to those patients who have (1) a continuing requirement for glucocorticoid therapy, (2) subnormal basal cortisol levels, (3) subnormal responsiveness to the rapid ACTH stimulation test, or (4) a subnormal response to metyrapone testing. The patient who presents with an acute illness and for whom no previous data are available should empirically be covered with steroids, which may be withdrawn rapidly as the acute stress resolves. Similarly, patients undergoing surgery who have a history of prior glucocorticoid therapy may require additional steroid coverage. In these patients, a normal response to metyrapone indicates normal function of the axis, and glucocorticoid therapy is not required. If time does not allow assessment of hypothalamic-pituitary-adrenal axis function, steroid coverage should be given during surgery and the postoperative period. The dosages and ancillary procedures for treatment of acute illness and steroid coverage for surgery in these patients with secondary adrenocortical insufficiency due to glucocorticoid suppression are detailed in Chap. 12.

REFERENCES

1. Baxter JD, Rousseau GG: Glucocorticoid hormone action: An overview, in Baxter JD, Rousseau GG (eds): *Glucocorticoid Hormone Action.* New York, Springer-Verlag, 1979, p 1.

2. Christy NP: Iatrogenic Cushing's syndrome, in Christy NP (ed): *The Human Adrenal Cortex.* New York, Harper & Row, 1971, p 395.

3. Lippman ME: Steroids in malignant diseases: Progress in patient selection. *Hosp Pract* 19:93, 1984.

4. Bagby GC, Gabourel JD, Linman JW: Glucocorticoid therapy in the preleukemic syndrome (hemopoietic dysplasia). *Ann Intern Med* 92:55, 1980.

5. Brennan MJ: Corticosteroids in the treatment of solid tumors, in Azarnoff DL (ed): *Steroid Therapy.* Philadelphia, Saunders, 1975, p 134.

5a. Atkinson JP, Frank MN: Glucocorticoids in the treatment of hemolytic disorders, in Azarnoff DL (ed): *Steroid Therapy.* Philadelphia, Saunders, 1975, pp 49–61.

6. Collins JV, Clark TJH, Brown D, Townsend J: The use of corticosteroids in the treatment of acute asthma. *Q J Med* 44:259, 1975.

7. Littenberg B, Gluck EH: A controlled trial of methylprednisolone in the emergency treatment of acute asthma. *N Engl J Med* 314:150, 1986.

8. Fiel SB, Swartz MA, Glanz K, Francis ME: Efficacy of short-term corticosteroid therapy in outpatient treatment of acute bronchial asthma. *Am J Med* 75:259, 1983.

9. Fanta FH, Rossing TH, McFadden ER Jr: Glucocorticoids in acute asthma: A critical controlled trial. *Am J Med* 74:845, 1983.

10. Harrison BDW, Stokes TC, Hart GJ, Vaughan DA, Ali NG, Robinson AA: Need for intravenous hydrocortisone in addition to oral prednisolone in patients admitted to hospital with severe asthma without ventilatory failure. *Lancet* 1:181, 1986.

11. Mitchell DM, Gilfeh P, Rehahn M, Diamond AH, Collins JV: Effects of prednisolone in chronic airflow limitation. *Lancet* 2:193, 1984.

12. Mendella LA, Manfreda J, Warren CPW, Anthonisen NR: Steroid response in stable chronic obstructive pulmonary disease. *Ann Intern Med* 96:17, 1982.

13. Collins JV, Jones D: Corticosteroid mechanisms and therapeutic schedules, in Weiss EB (ed): *Status Asthmaticus.* Baltimore, University Park Press, 1978, p 235.

14. Bruce C, Weatherstone R, Seaton A, Taylor WH: Histamine levels in plasma, blood and urine in severe asthma and the effect of corticosteroid treatment. *Thorax* 31:724, 1976.

15. Frame B, Parfitt AM: Corticosteroid-responsive hypercalcemia with elevated serum 1-alpha,25-dihydroxyvitamin D. *Ann Intern Med* 93:449, 1980.

16. Tauber MG, Khayam-Bashi H, Sande MA: Effects of ampicillin and corticosteroids on brain water content, cerebral spinal fluid pressure and lactate in experimental pneumococcal meningitis. *J Infect Dis* 151:528, 1985.

17. Ellison GW: Corticosteroids in neurological disease. *Hosp Pract* 19:105, 1984.

18. Fishman RA: Steroids in the treatment of brain edema. *N Engl J Med* 306:359, 1982.

19. Johnson TS, Rock PB, Fulco CS, Trad LA, Spark RF, Maher JT: Prevention of acute mountain sickness by dexamethasone. *N Engl J Med* 310:683, 1984.

20. Markman M, Sheidler V, Ettinger DS, Quaskey SA, Mellits ED: Antiemetic efficacy of dexamethasone: Randomized, double-blind, crossover study with prochlorperazine in patients receiving cancer chemotherapy. *N Engl J Med* 9:549, 1984.

21. Dale DC, Petersdorf RG: Corticosteroids and infectious diseases, in Azarnoff DL (ed): *Steroid Therapy.* Philadelphia, Saunders, 1975, p 209.

22. Cope CL: *Adrenal Steroids and Disease.* London, Pittman Medical, 1977.

23. Vincenti F, Amend W, Feduska NJ, Duca RM, Salvatierra JRO: Improved outcome following renal transplantation with reduction in the immunosuppression therapy for rejection episodes. *Am J Med* 69:107, 1980.

24. Kass EH, Finland M: Corticosteroids and infections. *Adv Intern Med* 9:45, 1958.

25. Parrillo JE, Fauci AS: Mechanisms of glucocorticoid action on immune processes. *Annu Rev Pharmacol Toxicol* 19:179, 1979.

26. Rousseau GG, Baxter JD: Glucocorticoid receptors, in Baxter JD, Rousseau GG (eds): *Glucocorticoid Hormone Action.* New York, Springer-Verlag, 1979, p 49.

27. Ballard PL, Carter JP, Graham BS, Baxter JD: A radioreceptor assay for evaluation of the plasma glucocorticoid activity of natural and synthetic steroids in man. *J Clin Endocrinol Metab* 41:290, 1975.

28. Baxter JD, MacLeod KM: The molecular basis for hormone actin, in Bondy PK, Rosenberg LE (eds): *Metabolic Control and Disease.* Philadelphia, Saunders, 1979, p 104.

29. Gambertoglio JG, Vincenti F, Feduska NJ, Birnbaum J, Salvatierra O, Amend WJC Jr: Prednisolone disposition in cushingoid and noncushingoid kidney transplant patients. *J Clin Endocrinol Metab* 51:561, 1980.

30. Thorn GW, Jenkins D, Laidlow JC, Goetz FC, Dingman JF, Arons WL, Streeten DHP, McCraken BH: Medical progress: Pharmacological aspects of adrenocortical steroids and ACTH in

man. *N Engl J Med* 248:232, 284, 323, 369, 414, 588, 632, 1953.

31. Axelrod L: Glucocorticoid therapy. *Medicine* 55:39, 1976.

32. Bayer JM, Neuner H-P: Cushing-Syndrom und erhöhter Augeninnedruck. *Dtsch Med Wochenschr* 40:1791, 1967.

33. George WE Jr, Wilmot M, Greenhouse A, Hammeke M: Medical management of steroid-induced epidural lipomatosis. *N Engl J Med* 308:316, 1983.

34. Polansky JR, Weinreb RN: Anti-inflammatory agents: Steroids as anti-inflammatory agents, in Sears ML: *Handbook of Experimental Pharmacology*. Heidelberg, Springer-Verlag, 1984, vol 69, p 459.

35. Roberts AM, Leibowitz HM: Corticosteroid therapy of ophthalmologic diseases. *Hosp Pract* 19:181, 1984.

36. Ellis EF: Corticosteroid regimens in pediatric practice. *Hosp Pract* 19:143, 1984.

37. Brocklebank JT, Harcourt RB, Meadow SR: Corticosteroid-induced cataracts in idiopathic nephrotic syndrome. *Arch Dis Child* 53:30, 1982.

38. Manabe S, Bucala R, Cerami A: Nonenzymatic addition of glucocorticoids to lens proteins in steroid-induced cataracts. *J Clin Invest* 74:1803, 1984.

38a. Zizic TM, Marcoux C, Hungerford DS, Dansereau J-V, Stevens MB: Corticosteroid therapy associated with ischemic necrosis of bone in systemic lupus erythematosis. *Am J Med* 79:596, 1985.

39. Gordan GS: Drug treatment of the osteoporoses. *Annu Rev Pharmacol Toxicol* 18:253, 1978.

40. Hahn TJ: Corticosteroid-induced osteopenia. *Arch Intern Med* 138:882, 1978.

41. Chesney RW, Mayess RB, Rose P, Jax DK: Effect of prednisone on growth and bone mineral content in childhood glomerular disease. *Am J Dis Child* 132:768, 1978.

42. Adinoff AD, Hollister JR: Steroid-induced fractures and bone loss in patients with asthma. *N Engl J Med* 309:265, 1983.

43. Gluck OS, Murphy WA, Hahn TJ, Hahn B: Bone loss in adults receiving alternate day glucocorticoid therapy: A comparison with daily therapy. *Arthritis Rheum* 24:892, 1981.

44. Baylink DJ: Glucocorticoid-induced osteoporosis. *N Engl J Med* 309:306, 1983.

45. Hahn TJ, Halstead LR, Teitelbaum SL: Altered mineral metabolism in glucocorticoid-induced osteopenia. *J Clin Invest* 64:655, 1979.

46. Spencer H, Rubio N, Rubio E, Indreika M, Seitam A: Chronic alcoholism: Frequently overlooked cause of osteoporosis in men. *Am J Med* 80:393, 1986.

47. Suzuki Y, Ichikawa Y, Saito E, Homma M: Importance of increased urinary calcium excretion in the development of secondary hyperparathyroidism of patients under glucocorticoid therapy. *Metabolism* 32:151, 1983.

48. Claman HN: Glucocorticosteroids II: The clinical responses. *Hosp Pract* 18:143, 1983.

49. Graham BS, Tucker WS Jr: Opportunistic infections in endogenous Cushing's syndrome. *Ann Intern Med* 101:334, 1984.

50. Czaja AJ, Ludwig J, Baggenstoss AH, Wolff A: Corticosteroid-treated chronic active hepatitis in remission. Uncertain prognosis of chronic persistent hepatitis. *N Engl J Med* 304:5, 1981.

51. Lam KC, Lai CL, Ng RP, Trepo C, Wu PC: Deleterious effect of prednisolone in HBsAg-positive chronic active hepatitis. *N Engl J Med* 304:380, 1981.

52. Hoofnagle JH, Davis GL, Pappas C, Hanson RG, Peters M, Avigan MI, Waggoner JG, Jones EA, Seeff LB: A short course of prednisolone in chronic type B hepatitis: Report of a randomized, double-blind, placebo-controlled trial. *Ann Intern Med* 104:12, 1986.

53. Editorial: Tuberculosis in corticosteroid-treated asthmatics. *Br Med J* 2:266, 1976.

54. Fauci AS, Dale DC, Balow JE: Glucocorticosteroid therapy: Mechanisms of action and clinical considerations. *Ann Intern Med* 84:304–315, 1976.

55. Askari A, Vignos PJ, Moskowitz RW: Steroid myopathy in connective tissue disease. *Am J Med* 61:485, 1976.

55a. Horker FF, Scheidegger JR, Grünig BE, Frey FJ: Evidence that prednisone-induced myopathy is reversed by physical training. *J Clin Endocrinol Metab* 61:83, 1985.

55b. Nashel DJ: Is atherosclerosis a complication of long-term corticosteroid treatment? *Am J Med* 80:925, 1986.

56. Woodbury DM: Relation between the adrenal cortex and the central nervous system. *Pharmacol Rev* 10:275, 1958.

57. Gookler P, Schein J: Psychic effects of ACTH and cortisone. *Psychosom Med* 15:589, 1953.

58. Litz T, Carter JD, Lews BI, Suvratt C: Effects of ACTH and cortisone on mood and mentation. *Psychosom Med* 14:363, 1952.

59. Gustavson LE, Benet LZ: Pharmacokinetics of natural and synthetic glucocorticoids, in Anderson DC, Winter JSD (eds): *The Actual Cortex*. Cornwall, England, Butterworth, 1985, p 235.

60. Hsueh WA, Pay-Guevara A, Bledsoe T: Studies comparing the clearance rate of 11β,17,21-trihydroxypreg-1,4-diene-3,20-dione (prednisolone) after oral 17,21-dihydroxypreg-1,4-diene-3,11,20-trione and intravenous prednisolone. *J Clin Endocrinol Metab* 48:748, 1959.

61. Melby JC: Clinical pharmacology of adrenal steroids, in Thorn GW (ed): *Steroid Therapy*. Kalamazoo, MI, Medcom, 1974, p 16.

62. Fariss BL, Hane S, Shinsako J, Forsham PH: Comparison of absorption of cortisone acetate and hydrocortisone hemisuccinate. *J Clin Endocrinol Metab* 47:1137, 1978.

63. Plumpton FS, Besser GM, Cole PV: Corticosteroid treatment and surgery: 2. The management of steroid cover. *Anaesthesia* 24:12, 1969.

64. Wolff ME: Structure-activity relationships in glucocorticoids, in Baxter JD, Rousseau GG (eds): *Glucocorticoid Hormone Action*. New York, Springer-Verlag, 1979, p 98.

65. Robertson DB, Maibach HI: Topical corticosteroids. *Hosp Formulary* 16:1130, 1981.

66. Weston WL: Topical corticosteroids in dermatologic disorders. *Hosp Pract* 19:159, 1984.

67. Braude AC, Rebuck AS: Prednisone and methylprednisolone dispositin in the lung. *Lancet* 2:995, 1983.

68. Collaborative group on antenatal steroid therapy: Effect of antenatal dexamethasone administration on the prevention of respiratory distress syndrome. *Am J Obstet Gynecol* 141:276, 1981.

68a. Kream J Mulay S, Fukushima DK, Solomon S: Determination of plasma dexamethasone in the mother and the newborn after administration of the hormone in a clinical trial. *J Clin Endocrinol Metab* 56:127, 1983.

68b. Lewis GP, Jusko WJ, Burke CW, Graves L: Prednisone side effects and serum protein levels. *Lancet* 2:778, 1971.

69. Meikle AW, Tyler FH: Potency and duration of action of glucocorticoids: Effects of hydrocortisone, prednisone and dexamethasone on human pituitary-adrenal function. *Am J Med* 63:200, 1977.

70. Meikle AW, Weed JA, Tyler FH: Kinetics and interconversion of prednisolone and prednisone studied with new radioimmunoassays. *J Clin Endocrinol Metab* 41:717, 1975.

71. Gifford RH: Corticosteroid therapy for rheumatoid arthritis, in Azarnoff DL (ed): *Steroid Therapy*. Philadelphia, Saunders, 1975, p 78.

72. Rose JQ, Yurchak AM, Jusko WJ: Dose dependent pharmacokinetics of prednisone and prednisolone in man. *J Pharmacokinet Biopharm* 9:389, 1981.

73. Bondy PK: The adrenal cortex, in Bondy PK, Rosenberg LE (eds): *Metabolic Control and Disease*. Philadelphia, Saunders, 1979, p 1427.

74. Haynes RC Jr, Murad F: Adrenocorticotropic hormone;

adrenocortical steroids and their synthetic analogs; inhibitors of adrenocortical steroid biosynthesis, in: Gilman AG, Goodman LS, Rall TW, Murad F (eds): *The Pharmacological Basis of Therapeutics.* New York, Macmillan, 1985, p 1459.

75. Dluhy RG, Newmark SR, Lauler DP, Thorn GW: Pharmacology and chemistry of adrenal glucocorticoids, in Azarnoff DL (ed): *Steroid Therapy.* Philadelphia, Saunders, 1975, p 1.

76. Brooks RV: Biosynthesis of adrenocortical steroids, in James VHT (ed): *The Adrenal Gland.* New York, Raven, 1979, p 67.

77. Meikle AW, Clarke DH, Tyler FH: Cushing's syndrome from low doses of dexamethasone. *JAMA* 235:1592, 1976.

78. Kozower M, Veatch L, Kaplan MM: Decreased clearance of prednisone, a factor in the development of corticosteroid side effects. *J Clin Endocrinol Metab* 38:407, 1974.

79. Benet LZ, Frey FJ, Amend JC Jr, Lozada F, Frey BM: Endogenous and exogenous glucocorticoids in cushingoid patients. *Drug Intell Clin Pharm* 16:863, 1982.

80. Kawai S, Ichikawa Y, Homma M: Differences in metabolic properties among cortisol, prednisolone, and dexamethasone in liver and renal diseases: Accelerated metabolism of dexamethasone in renal failure. *J Clin Endocrinol Metab* 60:848, 1985.

81. Boekenoogen SJ, Szefler SJ, Jusko WJ: Prednisolone disposition and protein binding in oral contraceptive users. *J Clin Endocrinol Metab* 56:702, 1983.

82. Harris AW, Baxter JD: Variations in cellular sensitivity to glucocorticoids: Observations and mechanisms, in Baxter JD, Rousseau GG (eds): *Glucocorticoid Hormone Action.* New York, Springer-Verlag, 1979, p 423.

83. Rosenau W, Baxter JD, Rousseau GG, Tomkins GM: Mechanism of resistance to steroids: Glucocorticoid receptor defect in lymphoma cells. *Nature (New Biol)* 237:20, 1972.

84. Editorial: Intra-articular steroids. *Lancet* 1:38, 1984.

85. Clark RA, Anderson PB: Combined therapy with salbutamol and beclomethasone inhalers in chronic asthma. *Lancet* 2:70, 1978.

86. McAllen MK, Kochanowski SJ, Shaw KM: Steroid aerosols in asthma: An assessment of betamethasone valerate and a twelve month study of patients on maintenance treatment. *Br Med J* 1:171, 1974.

87. Editorial: Inhaled steroids and dysphonia. *Lancet* 1:375, 1984.

88. Editorial: High-dose corticosteroid inhalers for asthma. *Lancet* 2:23, 1984.

89. Daly JR, Fletcher MR, Glass D, Chambers DJ, Bitensky L, Chayen L: Comparison of effects of long term corticotrophin and corticosteroid treatment on responses of plasma growth hormone, ACTH and corticosteroid to hypoglycemia. *Br Med J* 2:521, 1974.

90. Bacon PA, Daly JR, Myles AB, Savage O: Hypothalamo-pituitary-adrenal function in patients on long-term adrenocorticotrophin therapy. *Ann Rheum Dis* 27:7, 1968.

91. Aron DC, Tyrrell JB, Fitzgerald PA, Findling JW, Forsham PH: Cushing's syndrome: Problems in diagnosis. *Medicine* 60:25, 1981.

92. Bagby GC Jr, Lawrence HJ, Neerhout RC: T-Lymphocyte-mediated granulopoietic failure: In vitro identification of prednisone-responsive patients. *N Engl J Med* 309:1073, 1983.

93. Schumer W: Steroids in the treatment of clinical septic shock. *Ann Surg* 184:333, 1976.

94. Sheagren JN: Septic shock and corticosteroids. *N Engl J Med* 305:456, 1981.

95. Hoffman SL, Punjabi NH, Kumala S, Moechtar A, Pulungsih SP, Rivai AR, Rockhill RC, Woodward TE, Loedin AA: Reduction of mortality in chloramphenicol-treated severe typhoid fever by high-dose dexamethasone. *N Engl J Med* 310:82, 1984.

96. Hinshaw LB, Archer LT, Beller-Todd BK, Coalson JJ, Flournoy DJ, Passey R, Benjamin B, White GL: Survival of primates in LD_{100} septic shock following steroid/antibiotic therapy. *J Surg Res* 28:151, 1980.

97. Sprung CL, Panagiota V, Caralis MD, Marcial RRT, Pierce M, Gelbard MA, Long WM, Duncan RC, Trendler MD, Karpf M: The effects of high-dose corticosteroids in patients with septic shock. *N Engl J Med* 311:1137, 1984.

98. Jacob HS: Pulse steroids in hematologic diseases. *Hosp Pract* 20:87, 1985.

99. Morris PJ, Chan L, French ME, Ting A: Low dose oral prednisolone in renal transplantation. *Lancet* 1:525, 1982.

100. Felson DT, Anderson J: Evidence for the superiority of immunosuppressive drugs and prednisone over prednisone alone in lupus nephritis. *N Engl J Med* 311:1528, 1984.

101. Kyle RA, Greipp PR, Garton JP, Gertz MA: Primary systemic amyloidosis: Comparison of melphalan/prednisone versus colchicine. *Am J Med* 79:708, 1985.

102. Cogan MG, Sargent JA, Yarbrough SG, Vincenti F, Amend WJ Jr: Prevention of prednisone-induced negative nitrogen balance: Effect of dietary modification on urea generation rate in hemodialyzed patients receiving high dose glucocorticoids. *Ann Intern Med* 95:158, 1981.

103. Hunt TK, Ehrlich HP, Garcia JA, Dunphy JE: Effect of vitamin A on reversing the inhibitory effect of cortisone on healing of open wounds in animals and man. *Ann Surg* 170:633, 1969.

104. Baigelman W, Chodosh S, Pizzuto D, Cupples LA: Sputum and blood eosinophils during corticosteroid treatment of acute exacerbations of asthma. *Am J Med* 75:929, 1983.

104a. Lawrence EC, Teague RB, Gottlieb MS, Jhingran SG, Lieberman J: Serial changes in markers of disease activity with corticosteroid treatment in sarcoidosis. *Am J Med* 74:747, 1983.

105. Harter JG, Reddy WJ, Thorn GW: Studies on an intermittent corticosteroid dosage regimen. *N Engl J Med* 269:591, 1963.

106. Harter JG: Alternate day therapy, in Thorn GW (ed): *Steroid Therapy.* Kalamazoo, MI, Medcom, 1974, p 42.

107. Fauci AS: Corticosteroids in autoimmune disease. *Hosp Pract* 18:99, 1983.

108. Fauci AS: Alternate-day corticosteroid therapy. *Am J Med* 64:729, 1978.

109. Fauci AS, Dale DC: Alternate day prednisone therapy and human lymphocyte subpopulations. *J Clin Invest* 55:22, 1975.

110. Fleisher DS, Pellecchier P: Pituitary-adrenal responsiveness after corticosteroid therapy in children with nephrosis. *J Pediatr* 70:54, 1967.

111. Hunder GG, Sheps SG, Allen GL, Joyce JW: Daily and alternate day corticosteroid regimens in treatment of giant cell arteritis: Comparison in a prospective study. *Ann Intern Med* 82:613, 1975.

112. Foote KD, Brocklebank JT, Meadow SR: Height attainment in children with steroid-responsive nephrotic syndrome. *Lancet* 2:917, 1985.

113. Ackerman GL, Nolan CM: Adrenocortical responsiveness after alternate-day corticosteroid therapy. *N Engl J Med* 278:405, 1968.

114. Fleisher DS: Pituitary-adrenal responsiveness after corticosteroid therapy in children with nephrosis. *J Pediatr* 70:54, 1967.

115. Schurmeyer TH, Tsokos GC, Avgerinos PC, Balow JE, D'Agata R, Loriaux DL, Chrousos GP: Pituitary-adrenal responsiveness to corticotropin-releasing hormone in patients receiving chronic, alternate day glucocorticoid therapy. *J Clin Endocrinol Metab* 61:22, 1985.

116. Wyatt R, Waschek J, Weinberger M, Sherman B: Effects of inhaled beclomethasone dipropionate and alternate-day prednisone on pituitary-adrenal function in children with chronic asthma. *N Engl J Med* 299:1387, 1978.

117. Schatz M, Patterson R, Zeit S, O'Rourke J, Melam H: Corticosteroid therapy for the pregnant asthmatic patient. *JAMA* 233:804, 1975.

117a. Greenberger PA, Patterson R: Beclomethasone dipropionate for severe asthma during pregnancy. *Ann Intern Med* 98:478, 1983.

117b. Real FX, Krown SE, Koziner B: Steroid-related development of Kaposi's sarcoma in a homosexual man with Burkitt's lymphoma. *Am J Med* 30:119, 1986.

118. Streck WF, Lockwood DH: Pituitary adrenal recovery following short-term suppression with corticosteroids. *Am J Med* 66:910, 1979.

119. Livanou T, Ferriman D, James VHT: Recovery of hypothalamo-pituitary-adrenal function after corticosteroid therapy. *Lancet* 2:856, 1967.

120. Graber AL, Ney RL, Nicholson WE, Island DP, Liddle GW: Natural history of pituitary-adrenal recovery following long-term suppression with corticosteroids. *J Clin Endocrinol Metab* 25:11, 1965.

121. Byyny RL: Withdrawal from glucocorticoid therapy. *N Engl J Med* 295:30, 1976.

122. Nichols T, Nugent CA, Tyler FH: Diurnal variation in suppression of adrenal function by glucocorticoids. *J Clin Endocrinol Metab* 25:343, 1965.

123. Donald RA, Espiner EA: The plasma cortisol and corticotropin response to hypoglycemia following adrenal steroid and ACTH administration. *J Clin Endocrinol Metab* 41:1, 1975.

124. Editorial: Steroid therapy and the adrenals. *Lancet* 2:537, 1975.

125. Dixon RB, Christy NP: On the various forms of corticosteroid withdrawal syndrome. *Am J Med* 68:224, 1980.

126. Amatruda TT, Hurst MM, D'Esopo ND: Certain endocrine and metabolic facets of the steroid withdrawal syndrome. *J Clin Endocrinol Metab* 25:1207, 1965.

PART V

GONADAL DISEASE

16

The Testis

Richard J. Santen

The human testis serves two separate functions, secretion of androgenic hormones and excretion of mature spermatozoa. Although the functional anatomy and physiologic control of these two processes are highly interrelated, this chapter approaches androgen secretion and germinal cell maturation separately from a conceptual viewpoint. This strategy minimizes the complexity of this system and reduces physiologic principles to their functional components. The important integrative interactions between the two testicular elements are addressed after full discussion of the discrete systems.

Recently, a large body of neuroanatomic, biochemical, physiologic, and clinical data regarding testicular function has accumulated. The breadth of this new information allows a more physiologic approach to the understanding of testicular function and provides a framework for presentation of pathophysiologic mechanisms.

ANATOMY

Central Nervous System and Hypothalamic-Pituitary Axis

Major regulatory centers for control of testicular function are highly concentrated within the hypothalamus.[1–3] Reference landmarks delineating the critical areas include the optic chiasma anteriorly, the mammillary body posteriorly, and the infundibulum (Latin for "funnel") inferiorly (Fig. 16-1A). Most important is a small triangular area within these boundaries called the *medial basal hypothalamus*. From this region, neural tissue extends down the pituitary stalk and into the *neural* or posterior lobe of the pituitary. The *glandular* or anterior pituitary lies in front of the neural lobe in the sella turcica but, superiorly, wraps around the pituitary stalk to form the *pars tuberalis*.

The medial basal hypothalamus contains a dense aggregation of structures involved in the integrated control of testicular function. The precise anatomic location of each of these neuronal regulatory components has been defined by immunohistochemical, fluorescence, or radioimmunoassay (RIA) studies. The major regulatory systems include the peptidergic neurons [i.e., gonadotropin releasing hormone (GnRH) and opiate systems], the aminergic systems (i.e., dopamine, norepinephrine, serotonin), and the steroid receptor–containing neurons.

PEPTIDERGIC SYSTEM

The greatest concentrations of neurons containing the peptide GnRH are found in two general regions: the anterior hypothalamic nuclear groups and the medial basal hypothalamus. The first include, specifically, the suprachiasmatic and preoptic nuclei, the retrochiasmatic areas, and the organum vasculosum of the lamina terminalis (OVLT); the medial basal hypothalamic region includes the arcuate nucleus and median eminence (Fig. 16-1*B*, Table 16-1).[2,4–8] While other parts of the brain also contain GnRH, concentrations are low; the functional significance of GnRH in other regions is unknown.[6] Axons from cell bodies in the anterior hypothalamus and medial basal hypothalamus terminate on the "neurohemal" contact

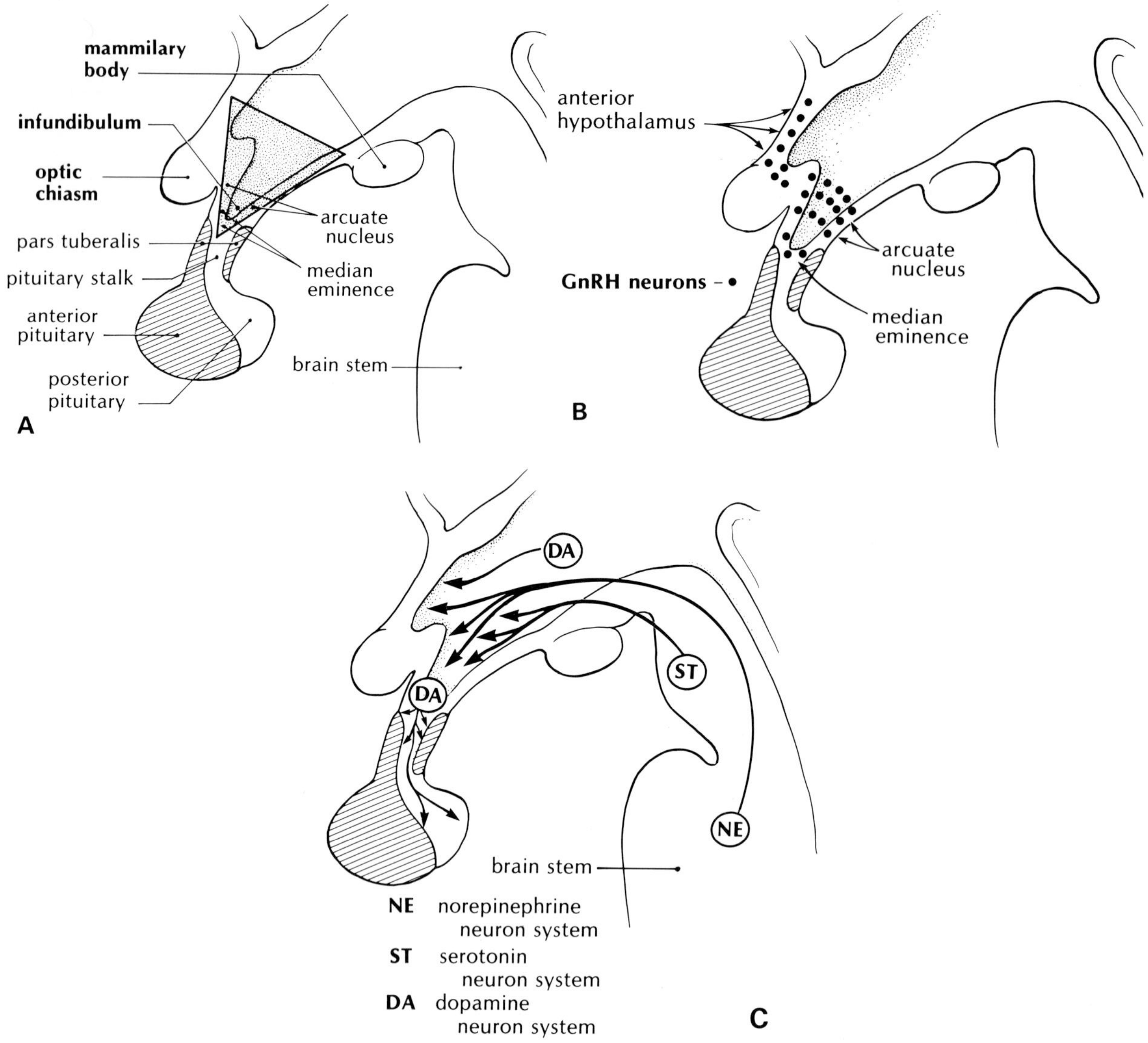

FIGURE 16-1 (*A*) Diagrammatic representation of the brainstem, hypothalamus, and pituitary with important anatomic landmarks labeled. The shaded triangular area indicates the region of the medial basal hypothalamus, a critical regulatory center. (*B*) Location of the major GnRH neuron cell bodies. (*C*) Diagrammatic representation of the aminergic neuronal systems. The superior dopamine system is called the *incertohypothalamic* and the inferior system is called the *tuberohypophyseal.* The serotonin pathway is called the *raphe* serotonin neuron system. The norepinephrine system arises from lateral tegmental cell groups in the caudal medulla, midpons, and rostral pons. (*Adapted from Moore.*[1])

zone (see below) which lies in the external as well as the internal portion of the median eminence. This region contains the highest concentration of GnRH found in the brain, 211 (±16) pg per microgram of protein (Table 16-1).[6] Here, GnRH is secreted into the pituitary portal capillaries for transport into the anterior pituitary.

The other peptidergic system of neurons contains the endogenous opiates.[9] The distribution of this system can be localized by measuring tissue levels of leu- or met-enkephalin or by detecting receptors for these

Table 16-1. GnRH Concentrations in the Hypothalamus

Structure	Concentration, pg/μg protein
Median eminence	211 ± 16
Organum vasculosum of lamina terminalis	46 ± 9
Arcuate nucleus	10 ± 1.5
Retrochiasmatic area	3.4 ± 0.5
Suprachiasmatic and preoptic nuclei	2.2 ± 0.2

Source: From data of Selmanoff et al.[6]

substances. The medial basal hypothalamus is rich in opiate receptors and contains measurable quantities of the enkephalins. High concentrations are present in the periventricular nucleus and in a dense band around the ventral floor of the hypothalamus. Lesser concentrations exist in the supraoptic nucleus, mammillary bodies, arcuate nucleus, median eminence, and suprachiasmatic nuclei.[9–14] The presence of endogenous opiates and their receptors in regions known to control gonadotropin secretion provides a neuroanatomic basis for recent physiologic observations that the opiates can modulate luteinizing hormone (LH) secretion.[14a]

AMINERGIC SYSTEM

Concentrated in the medial basal hypothalamus are aminergic neurons containing serotonin, norepinephrine, and dopamine (Fig. 16-1C). These axons represent the final termination of pathways carrying both stimulatory and inhibitory neural afferent systems into the hypothalamus.[1,2] The norepinephrine axons arise from cell groups in the medulla and pons. They enter the hypothalamus via the ventral tegmental area and course along the medial forebrain bundle in the lateral hypothalamus. They terminate on several anterior hypothalamic nuclei and are also densely aggregated in the area of the arcuate nucleus and median eminence.[1,15,16] The serotonin neurons originate in the midbrain raphe, project through the medial forebrain bundle, and also terminate on several medial hypothalamic nuclei, including the arcuate nucleus and median eminence.[1] The dopaminergic neurons (incertohypothalamic system) project from the posterior hypothalamus into the dorsal part of the dorsomedial nucleus and into the anterior hypothalamic areas. In addition, a local dopamine pathway (tuberohypophyseal) originates in the arcuate nucleus and periventricular nucleus and projects upon the median eminence, pituitary stalk, and posterior pituitary (Fig. 16-1C).[1,2,17–19] Axons from this system terminate directly on portal capillaries in the median eminence, which allows direct access of dopamine to the portal system.

STEROID RECEPTOR NEURONS

Autoradiographic techniques are used to localize steroid receptors. Special stains can demonstrate the neurons containing these receptors.[1,20] Steroid binding is most dense in the region along the third ventricle extending from the suprachiasmatic area to the caudal part of the arcuate nucleus. In the most intensely labeled areas, 4000 to 5000 molecules of estradiol are bound per neuron. Use of nonaromatizable androgens such as tritium-labeled dihydrotestosterone (DHT) has provided evidence for specific androgen receptors.[21] Concentrations of androgen receptors are much lower than concentrations of estrogen receptors in these areas. The receptors for both of these sex steroids are present in areas which largely overlap those of GnRH-containing neurons, a finding suggesting that a functional interaction takes place between peptidergic and sex steroid–binding neurons. It has been demonstrated that several groups of neurons in these areas contain receptors for both dopamine and estradiol ("estrodopaminergic neurons").[22] The close structural intimacy between catecholamine- and sex steroid–binding neurons implies that they are mutually involved in servomechanisms controlling gonadotropin secretion.[23]

TANACYTES

In addition to the various neuronal subgroups, the medial basal hypothalamus contains a structural matrix consisting of specialized cells called *tanacytes* (Fig. 16-2).[1,24] The cell bodies of the tanacytes border the

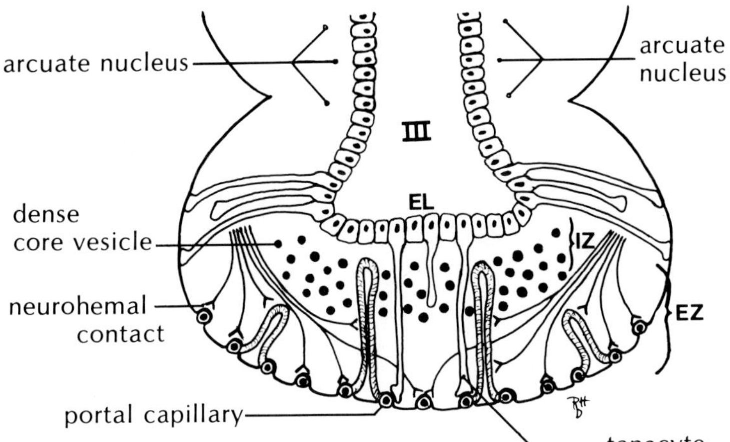

FIGURE 16-2 Diagrammatic representation of the median eminence and relationship of neurons to capillaries. III = third ventricle, EL = ependymal layer, IZ = internal zone, EZ = external zone. (*From Page RB, in Wilkins RH, Rengachary SS (eds): Neurosurgery. New York, McGraw-Hill, 1985, p 791.*)

third ventricle; their foot processes extend to the median eminence, where they terminate on pituitary portal capillaries. The function of these specialized ependymal cells is not currently known. Their anatomic features suggest the possibility that they have a transport function between CSF and the pituitary portal capillaries.

PORTAL VENOUS SYSTEM

The superior hypophyseal arteries deliver arterial blood at an extremely high rate of flow, 450 ml per 100 grams per minute, into the median eminence. Here, a capillary bed forms within a highly complex network of neurons. The unusual feature of this vascular bed is the termination of axons directly onto the walls of the capillaries.[25] This constitutes the "neurohemal" contact zone; it allows transport of GnRH and other substances from neurons into the vascular channels (Fig. 16-3). These capillaries form portal veins, which descend down the pituitary stalk to reform in a capillary bed in the anterior pituitary. Recent studies demonstrate that a continuous capillary network exists between the anterior and posterior pituitary.[26] An additional but contiguous capillary network extends up the pituitary stalk and into the median eminence. The venous drainage of the anterior and posterior pituitary consists of lateral pituitary veins which empty into the cavernous sinuses. It is apparent from the multiple interconnections of this vascular system that blood could flow in a circular fashion from the hypothalamus to the anterior and posterior pituitary and back to the hypothalamus. Alternatively, flow in the opposite direction from the anterior pituitary into the hypothalamus via the portal venous system is also possible. Dynamic flow reversal could deliver pituitary products back to the median eminence and provide a mechanism for impor-

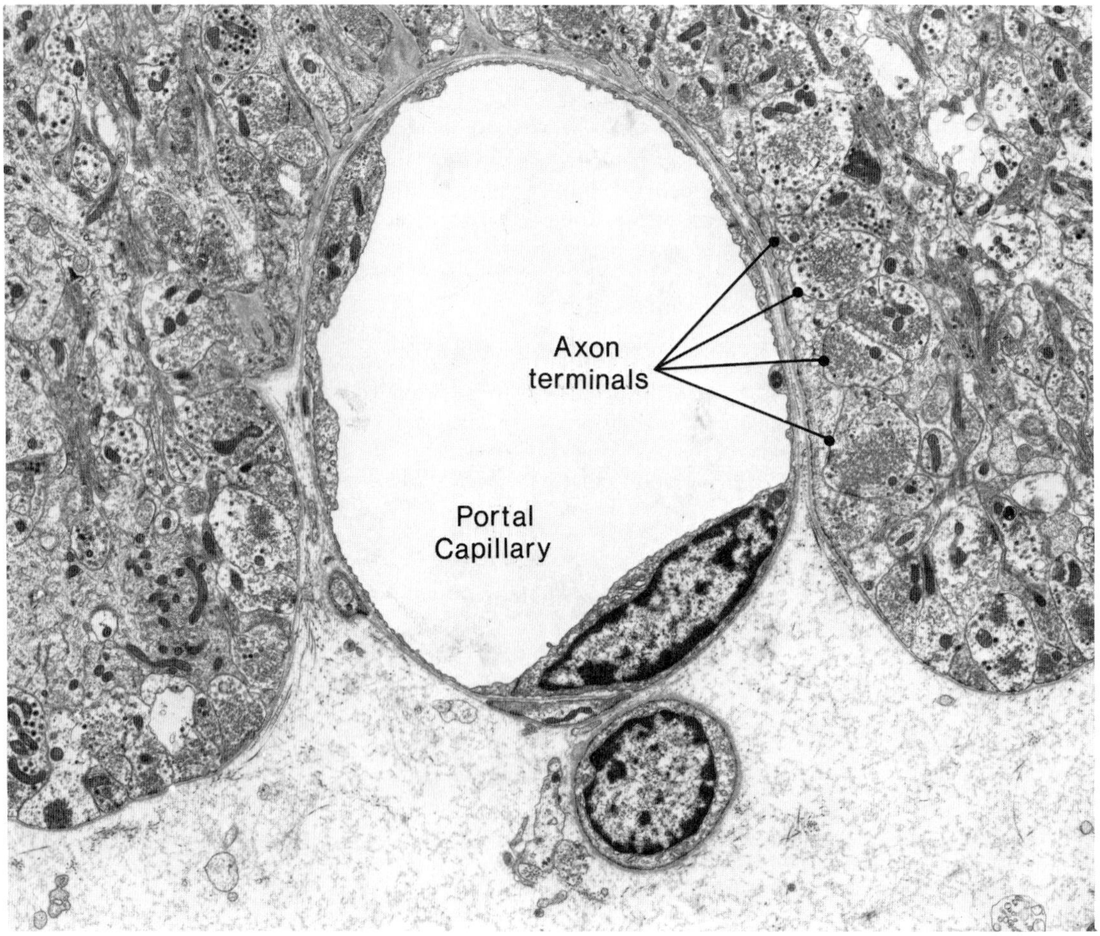

FIGURE 16-3 Electron micrograph of the neurohemal contact zone. A single portal capillary is surrounded by numerous axon terminals, only four of which are labeled. (*From Page and Dovey-Hartman.*[24])

tant regulatory control of this axis. Recent dynamic studies with rapid-sequence photography could not substantiate flow reversal, but this phenomenon may occur under certain pathologic conditions.[27]

ANTERIOR PITUITARY

The anterior pituitary is a glandular structure which lies below the diaphragma sella and is bordered by the cavernous sinuses laterally (Chap. 8). Bone comprises the floor as well as the anterior and posterior margins of the sella turcica. Interspersed among the multiple anterior pituitary cell types are the *gonadotrophs*, cells containing both LH and follicle stimulating hormone (FSH) and receptors for GnRH. Morphometric analyses indicate that most of these cells produce LH and FSH conjointly, and only a few contain LH or FSH exclusively.[28] The gonadotrophs can be identified on a highly specific basis by immunohistochemical studies; their propensity to concentrate acid dyes (acidophilia) and electron microscopic features are only relatively specific.

Testes

The testes are paired organs measuring approximately 5 × 3 cm and containing a volume of 20 to 30 ml. They hang in the scrotum in an environment with a temperature 2.2°C lower than in the abdomen. The *cremasteric* muscle allows retraction of the testes closer to the areas of core body temperature, a mechanism for maintaining testicular temperature relatively constant. Arterial blood to the testis is supplied by the internal spermatic, cremasteric, and vas deferential arteries. Venous blood drains into the pampiniform plexus and then into the internal spermatic veins. On the right, the internal spermatic vein enters the inferior vena cava; on the left, it drains into the renal vein. The close apposition of testicular arteries with the pampiniform plexus forms a functional countercurrent heat exchange mechanism and aids in the maintenance of testicular temperature at levels lower than in the body.[29] The anterior and lateral portions of the testes are covered by the *tunica vaginalis*. Beneath this, the entire testis is surrounded by the *tunica albuginea*, from which fibrous septa pass into the parenchyma and divide the testis into lobules.

The testis can be considered as two functional regions (Fig. 4*A* and *B*): the interstitial cell compartment with its androgen-secretory *Leydig* cells and the seminiferous tubular compartment containing *germinal* and *Sertoli* cells. Each serves a distinct function and, thus, is here considered separately.

INTERSTITIAL CELL COMPARTMENT

The Leydig or interstitial cells of the testis are highly specialized and have a typical appearance of highly active steroid-secretory tissue. In the adult male, the paired testes contain 432 (± 45) × 10^6 Leydig cells.[30] By light microscopy, these cells are polygonal and 10 to 25 μm in diameter; they make up approximately 5 percent of the total testicular volume (Fig. 4*A*). They contain lipid droplets and have prominent nucleoli; ratios of cytoplasm to nucleus are large.[31] These cells are contiguous to capillaries; they deliver the secreted steroids into the testicular veins and, less so, into the lymphatics draining the interstitial cell compartment. Clusters of Leydig cells are interspersed in the spaces adjacent to the seminiferous tubules. On electron microscopy (Fig. 16-5), Leydig cell cytoplasm contains large amounts of smooth endoplasmic reticulum, a morphologic structure characteristically abundant in steroid-producing cells, as well as numerous lipid droplets and mitochondria. Crystalloids of Reinke, a structure of unknown function unique to the Leydig cell, may also be seen.

SEMINIFEROUS TUBULAR COMPARTMENT

Individual seminiferous tubules are approximately 0.12 to 0.30 mm in diameter and up to 70 cm in length (Fig. 16-4*B*); they are tightly coiled. These structures provide a continuous pathway for delivery of sperm from the testes to the rete testis, caput epididymis, and vas deferens (Fig. 16-6). The seminiferous tubule is lined by a basal laminar layer and by myoid cells which impart the ability to propel fluids within the lumen (Fig. 16-7).[32] Immature stem cells, called *spermatogonia*, lie along the basal lamina, interspersed between Sertoli or supporting cells. Lateral projections of Sertoli cell cytoplasm envelop the spermatogonia, sealing these cells off from the remainder of the tubular contents and creating the basal or outer compartment (Fig. 16-7). Unimpeded diffusion across the basal lamina allows the spermatogonia free access to substances present in interstitial tissues. The Sertoli cells also project their cytoplasm upward toward the seminiferous tubular lumen. Specialized tight junctions between them form a blood-testis barrier and divide the tubule into the outer or basal compartment and the inner or adluminal compartment (Fig. 16-7). The inner segment contains the spermatocytes and spermatids, which rest within evaginations of Sertoli cell cytoplasm. Physiologic studies demonstrate that diffusion of dyes, steroids, proteins, and ions into the inner compartment is impeded and confirm the functional significance of the blood-testis barrier.[33]

SERTOLI CELLS

The Sertoli cells are basically columnar in form (Fig. 16-7). Their structural arrangement surrounding germinal cells, in conjunction with the anatomic distinction of the compartment formed by the blood-testis barrier, allows an intimate interaction between Sertoli cells and germ cells. By surrounding each cell type, Sertoli cell cytoplasm provides a controlled microenvironment and creates an immunologically protected space. Morphologically, the Sertoli cells have a basally placed trilobar nucleus with a prominent, centrally placed nucleolus. On electron microscopy the cytoplasm contains mitochondria, rough endoplasmic reticulum along the basal region, widely dispersed smooth endoplasmic reticulum, lysosomes, and numerous microtubular elements.

GERMINAL EPITHELIA

The human testis manufactures 123 ($\pm$ 18) $\times$ 10^6 sperm daily.[34] This requires a process of cellular replication with provision for a pool of undifferentiated cells held in reserve as well as a pool committed to full differentiation. The spermatogonia serve as the pool of undifferentiated cells (Figs. 16-8, 16-9). The majority undergo continuous mitotic division in a manner analogous to other somatic cells; in this way they provide a stem cell renewal pathway.[35,36] These cells remain in the outer or basal compartment. A minority become committed to further differentiation and undergo meiosis; meiosis involves a process unique to germinal cell tissue. These cells ultimately form mature spermatozoa; the series of maturing cells is detailed in Fig. 16-9. This process of differentiation of cells takes place in the inner, adluminal compartment.

In the process of meiosis a new complement of DNA is synthesized to replicate each of the 46 chromosomes.[37] In this way, chromosomes with twice the normal amount of DNA per chromosome are formed. Newly synthesized chromatin material progressively condenses. Each chromatid separates along its length, except at the common centromere (Fig. 16-10). During this process, crossing-over between contiguous chromosomes can take place. This mechanism allows formation of new combinations of maternal and paternal genetic material and explains the numerous translocations observed in banding studies during karyotype analysis.

The first meiotic division then takes place. Rather than splitting into daughter cells with 46 single chromosomes, the first meiotic division involves reduction into daughter cells with 23 chromosome pairs per cell. The *primary spermatocytes* formed by this meiotic division then quickly undergo a second meiotic division to produce daughter cells with 23 single chromosomes with a normal amount of DNA per chromosome. These *secondary spermatocytes* then mature further to spermatozoa, a process called *spermio-*

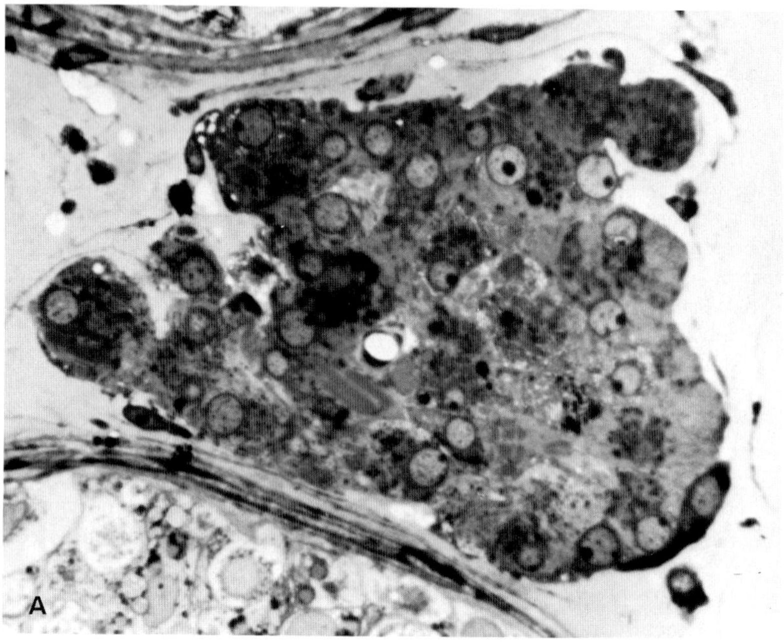

FIGURE 16-4 (A) Light microscopic appearance of Leydig cells from a human testis. (B) Light microscopic appearance of a seminiferous tubule from a human testis. (*Courtesy of Dr. Hugh F. English.*)

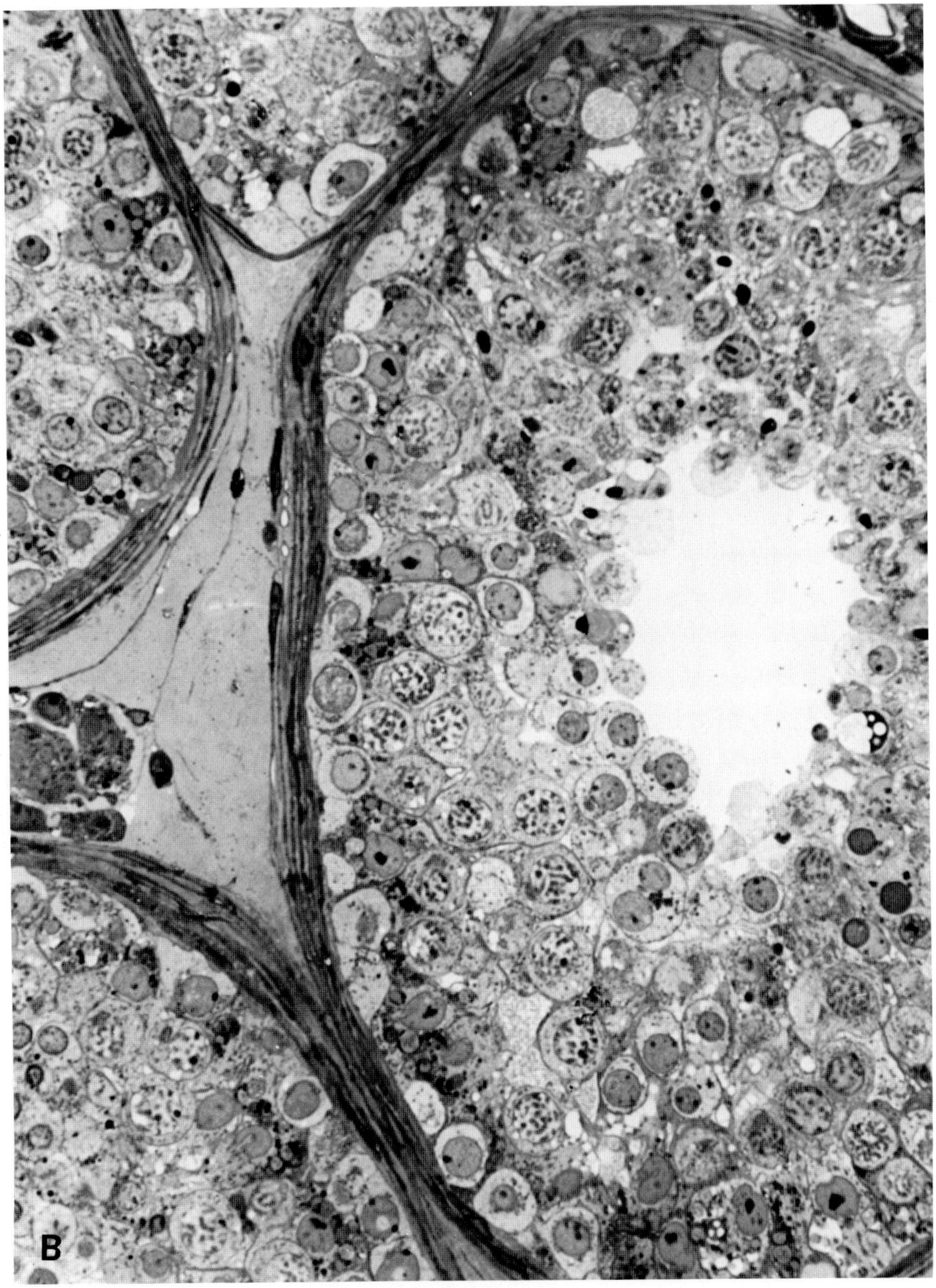

FIGURE 16-4 (*Continued*)

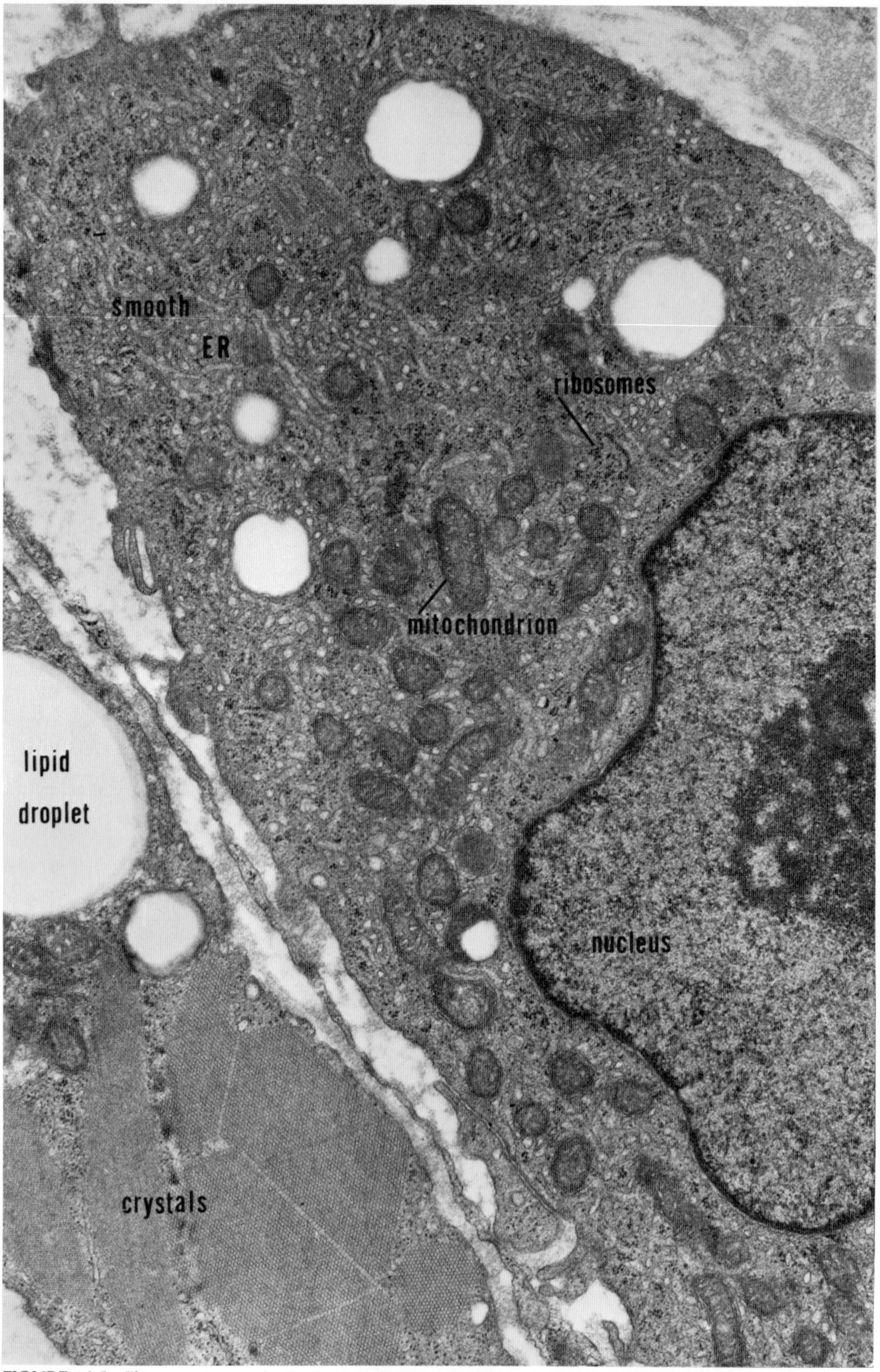

FIGURE 16-5 Electron micrograph of a Leydig cell from a human testis. Crystals refer to crystalloids of Reinke (see text). (*From Christensen.*[31])

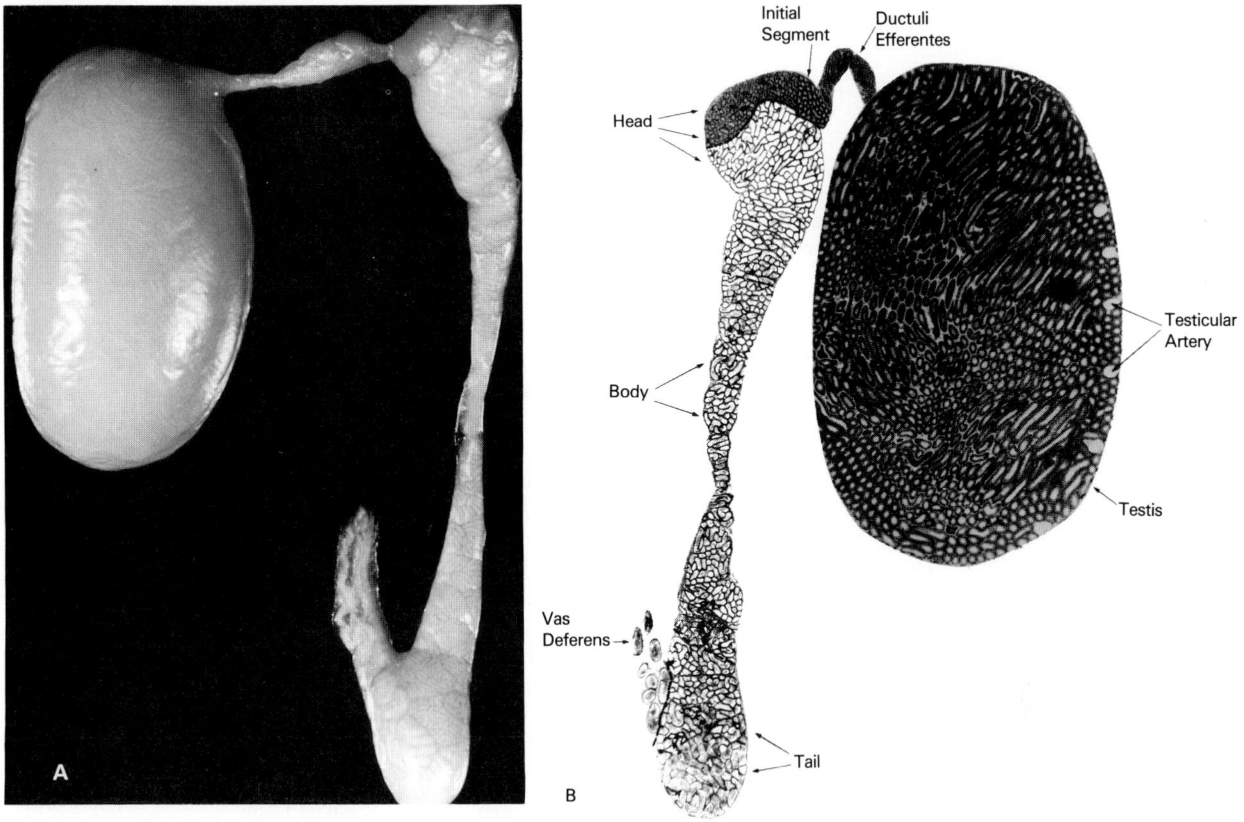

FIGURE 16-6 (A) Gross appearance of the testis, epididymis, and vas deferens in the rat. [*From Dym M, in Weiss L (ed): Histology, Cell and Tissue Biology, 5th ed. New York, Elsevier Biomedical, 1983, p 1041.*] (B) Contiguous excurrent ductal system illustrated from cut sections. (*From HF English, unpublished data.*)

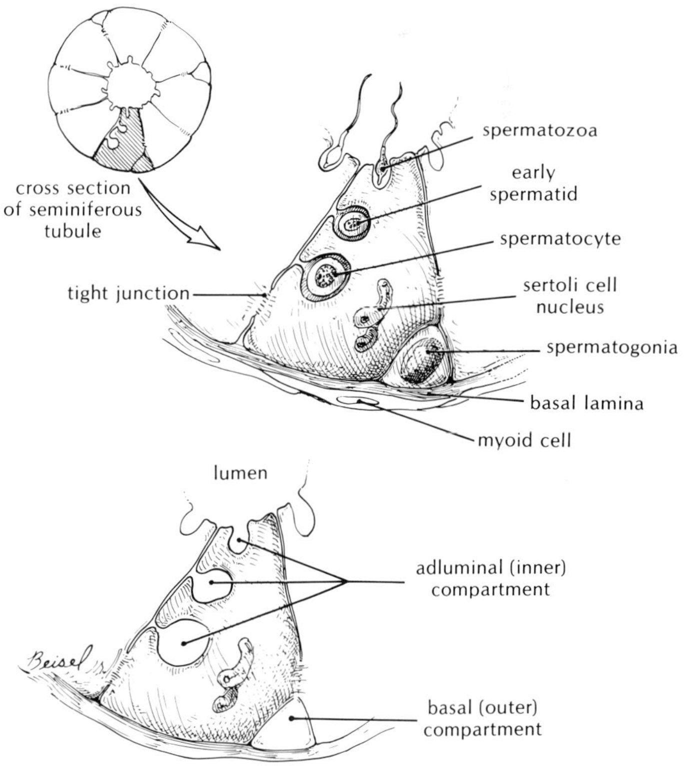

FIGURE 16-7 (*Top*) Diagrammatic representation of a seminiferous tubule to illustrate the relationship between the lining membrane structures (i.e., basal lamina and myoid cells), Sertoli cell cytoplasm, and germinal epithelial cells. (*Bottom*) As above with deletion of germinal cells. The basal or outer compartment lies outside of the tight-junction barrier formed by the Sertoli cells, whereas the adluminal compartment lies within it.

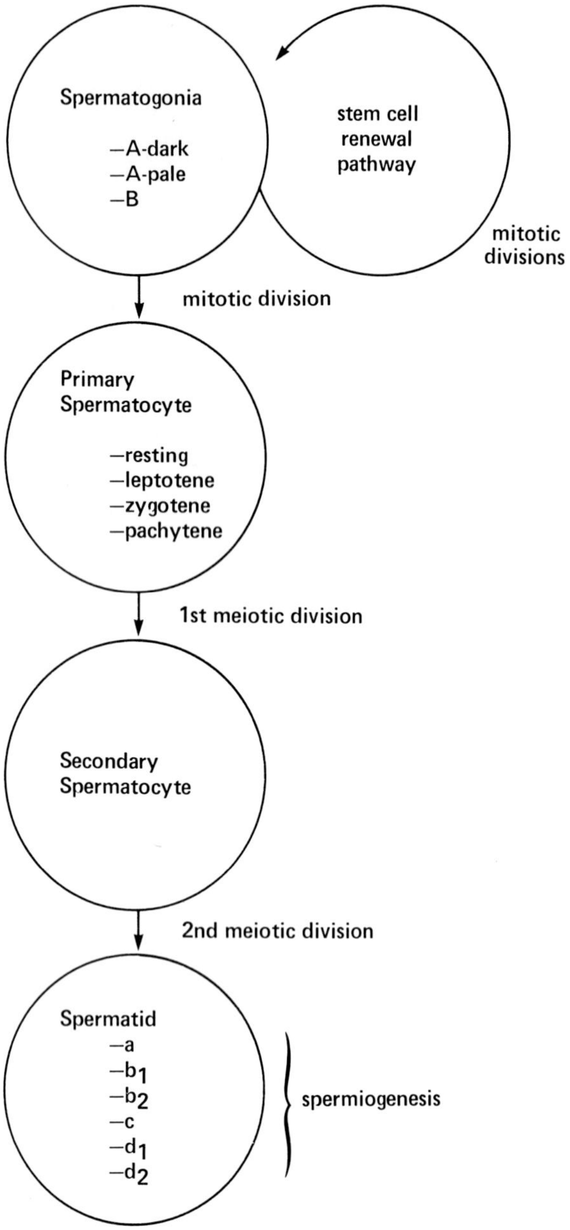

FIGURE 16-8 Diagrammatic representation of the stem cell renewal pathway and the differentiation pathway of the germinal cells. Specific cell types are listed for each major grouping.

genesis, and develop the cellular machinery necessary for motility. For cellular propulsion the sperm tail, a structure capable of generating linear, wavelike motion, is required (Figs. 16-11, 16-12). Called a *cilium,* this structure is highly conserved through phylogeny and appears monotonously similar from the lowest single-celled organism all the way to humans.[38] On electron microscopy the cilia contain 9 pairs of microtubules surrounding an additional central pair, the so-called 9 + 9 + 2 configuration (Fig. 16-12).[39] Pieces of electron-dense material, the *dynein* (outer and inner) arms, are connected to the outer pairs of tubules. Moderate variability in the presence of individual features occurs in a population of normal sperm.[39a] Reconstructed models (Fig. 16-12) reveal a series of linear tubules which can slide one against another to generate wave motion. Called the *sliding microtubule hypothesis,* this mechanism is invoked to explain the motility of all cilia or flagella.[40–42]

In many lower species, spermatogenesis is synchronous throughout the four quadrants of each seminiferous tubule.[35,36] Examination of teased tubules with a dissecting microscope reveals a progressive wave of maturation of each cell type along the length of the tubule. In the rat, this progression can be divided into 14 stages, each with a characteristic association of contiguous cells. On cross section, an identical pattern of cells is apparent in each quadrant of the seminiferous tubule; individual stages can be easily identified. This monotonous pattern throughout the four quadrants makes it quite easy to assess spermatogenesis in the rat quantitatively. In marked contrast, the process of spermatogenesis is asynchronous between various quadrants of each tubule in men. On superficial examination of cross sections, cell associations appear to be completely random. However, on closer inspection, precise patterns of spermatogenesis are seen in pie-shaped sections along the meridians of the tubule.[43] This asynchronous pattern renders quantitative assessment of spermatogenesis relatively difficult.

The elegant work of Heller and Clermont first ascribed order to the process of human spermatogenesis.[44] Cellular kinetic examination with [^{3}H]thymidine labeling techniques and careful morphometry revealed six separate stages of spermatogenic maturation. A complete cycle through six stages takes 16 days; 4.5 cycles (74 ± 5 days) are required for full spermatogenesis (Fig. 16-13). While these stages can be recognized by characteristic cell associations, several contiguous stages may be present at the same time in a given cross section of a tubule.

After the process of spermiogenesis is complete, the spermatozoa are released into the tubular lumen and carried by passive fluid flow to the rete testes, ductuli efferentes, and into the epididymis. The lining cells of this structure contain large amounts of carbonic anhydrase, carnitine, and glycerylphosphorylcholine, whose functions are not fully understood.[45] In the caput epididymis, the sperm first become actively motile, a process which requires exposure of the epididymal cells to androgen. Further spermatozoal maturation occurs during passage through the corpus and

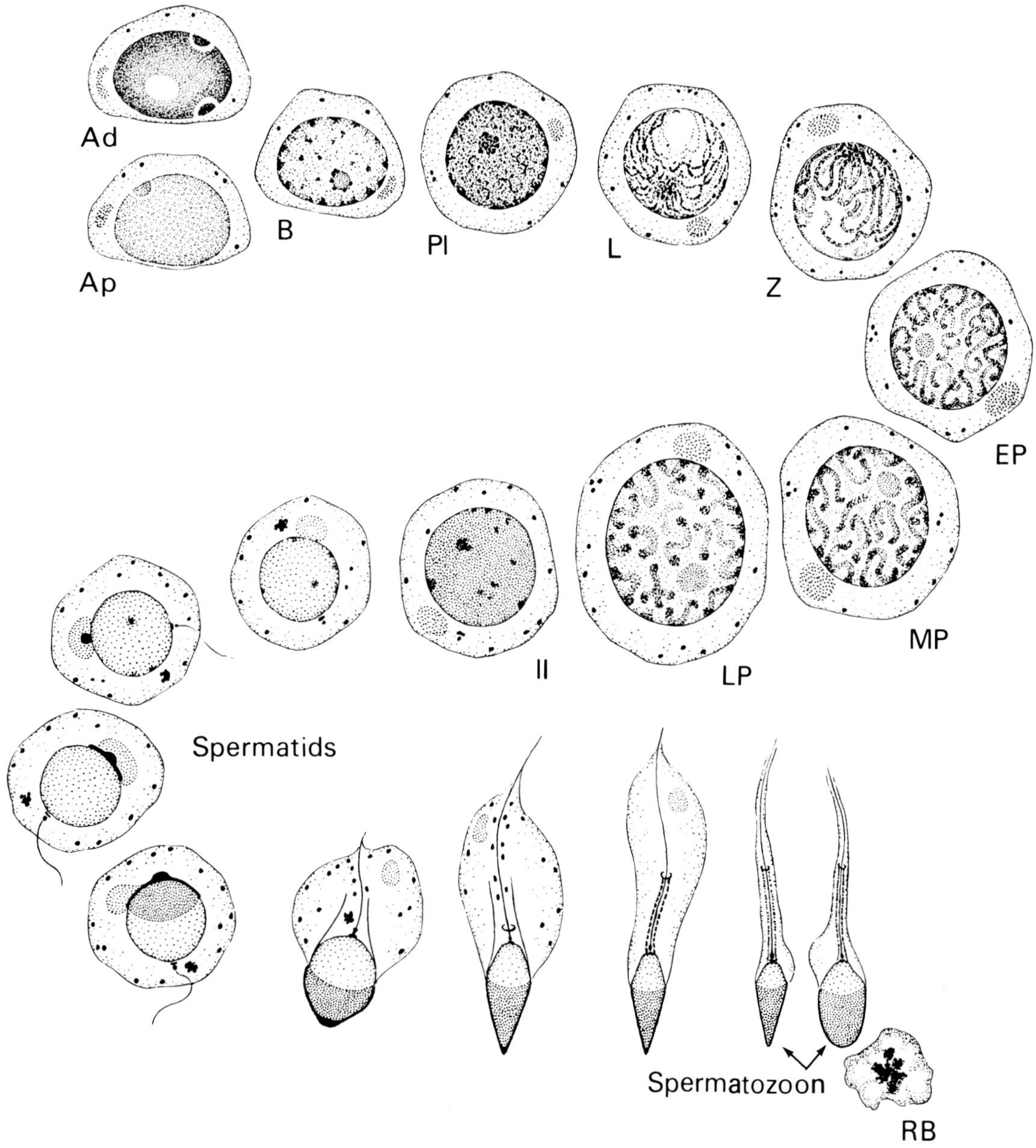

FIGURE 16-9 Appearance of the various germinal cell types in men. Ad, dark type A spermatogonium; Ap, pale type A spermatogonium; B, type B spermatogonium; R, resting spermatocyte; L, leptotene spermatocyte; Z, zygotene spermatocyte; P, pachytene spermatocyte; II, secondary spermatocyte; Sa, Sb_1, Sb_2, Sc, Sd_1, Sd_2, spermatids at different stages of spermatogenesis; RB, residual body. (*From Heller and Clermont.*[44])

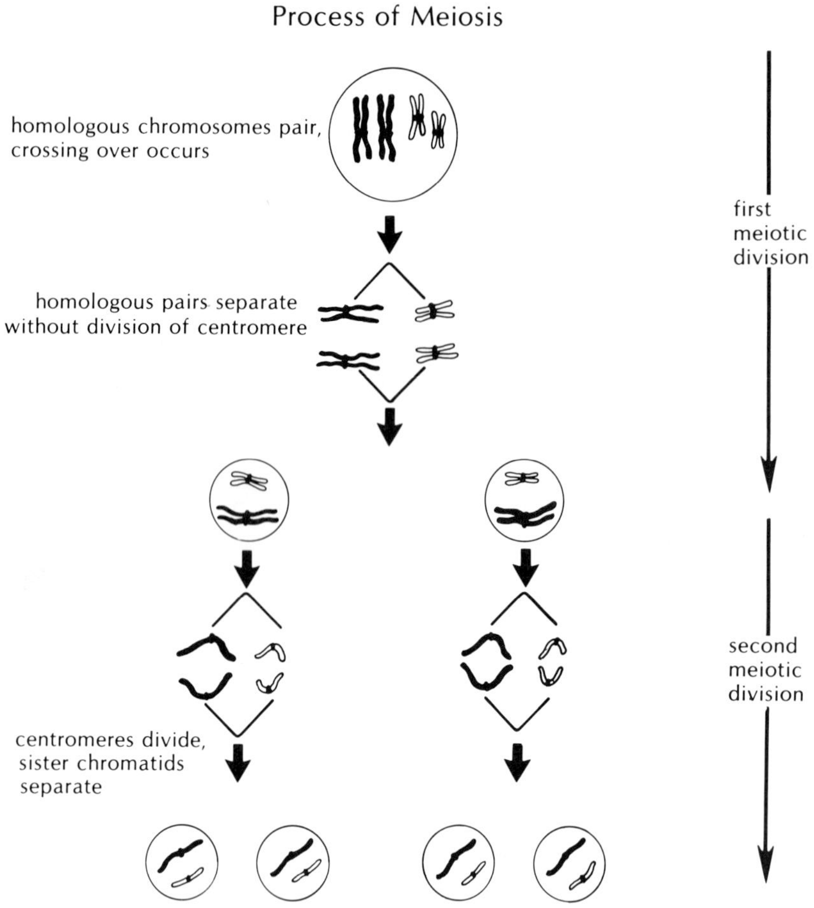

FIGURE 16-10 Diagrammatic representation of meiosis. (*Adapted from Flickinger et al.*[37])

cauda epididymides.[46] The average time for transit of sperm through the excurrent duct system is 12 days.[46,47] After ejaculation, these spermatozoa acquire fertilization potential through a process called *capacitation*, which takes place after entry into the female reproductive tract.[47,48] The fate of those not ejaculated is unclear; macrophage ingestion, local resorption, or passage into the urine are likely possibilities.[34]

PHYSIOLOGY

Hypothalamic-Pituitary-Leydig Cell Axis

OVERVIEW

An integrated, highly complex system regulates the level of circulating androgens within a relatively narrow range in humans. The hypothalamus plays a major regulatory role through release of GnRH, a decapeptide controlling both LH and FSH secretion. The pituitary secretes LH which, in turn, binds to Leydig cell receptors in the testes and stimulates androgen production. Superimposed upon this hypothalamic-pituitary-testicular regulatory axis are neuronal pathways imparting input from higher CNS centers.

HYPOTHALAMUS

Afferent Neural Input

The primary center for tonic control of gonadotropin regulation is located in the medial basal hypothalamus, primarily in the arcuate nucleus. Hormonal feedback exerted directly at this site and neural modulation from axons arising within or beyond the hypothalamus regulate GnRH secretion. The identities of the precise neuronal pathways involved and the specific neurotransmitters modulating these effects are controversial. The weight of current evidence suggests that catecholaminergic pathways using norepinephrine as a neurotransmitter (Fig. 16-1C) stimulate release of GnRH.[2,49,50] Dopaminergic pathways are inhibitory in

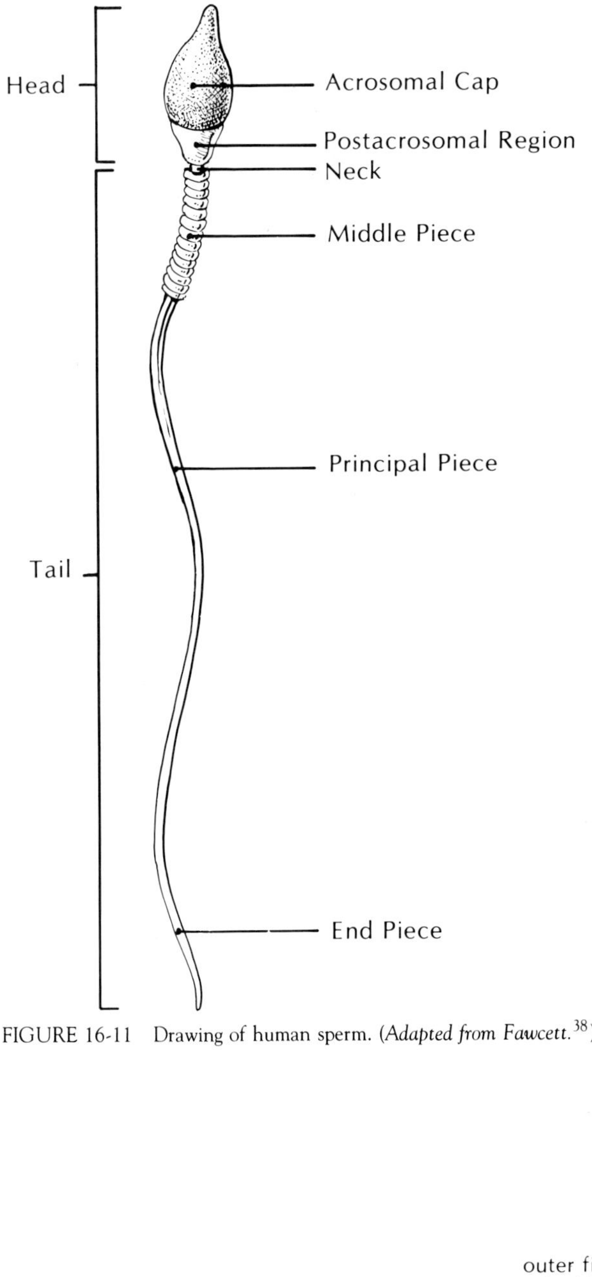

FIGURE 16-11 Drawing of human sperm. (*Adapted from Fawcett.*[38])

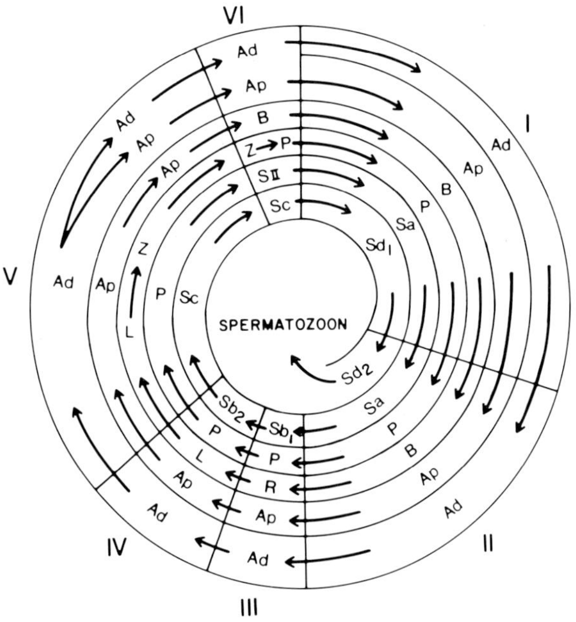

FIGURE 16-13 Germ-cell association (stage I to VI) comprising each cycle of spermatogenesis. (This illustration appeared originally in the first edition of "Endocrinology" in 1981. It is reproduced here by courtesy of Dr. Philip Troen.)

nature under certain experimental conditions and stimulatory under others.[2,51–55b]

Serotonergic neuronal systems are less well studied but generally appear inhibitory.[56,57] Several approaches are used to study the functional role of afferent neuronal pathways. These include electrical stimulation of specific brain nuclei or neuronal tracts; use of catecholamine agonists, antagonists, or depleting agents; and administration of agents such as 6-hydroxydopamine which destroy dopaminergic pathways.[2] Such experiments emphasize the precise anatomic localization of the afferent neural pathways and their potential

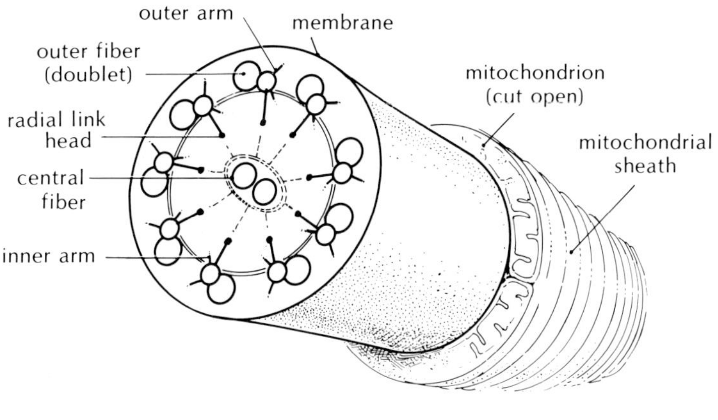

FIGURE 16-12 Drawing of cross section of midpiece of sperm and diagrammatic representation of its microtubules. Dynein represents outer and inner arms. Outer dense fibers not shown. (*Adapted from Fawcett.*[38])

importance in modulating reproductive processes. An integrated view of these regulatory pathways in humans, however, has not yet emerged.

Inhibitory neuronal pathways, particularly those modulated by endogenous opiates, have recently been a major topic of interest.[9,58-60] Whether the peptidergic neurons controlling the opiate system enter the hypothalamus from other CNS centers or arise exclusively within the hypothalamus is not currently known. Exogenous opiates suppress LH secretion under certain conditions, and opiate antagonists increase LH output.[61-64] Opiate antagonists added to human fetal hypothalamic preparations during in vitro perfusion experiments cause increased release of GnRH into the medium.[65] Opiate agonists block potassium-induced release of GnRH.[66] Based upon studies in animals, it has been postulated that a reduction in the tone of the opiate system may mediate the rises in gonadotropin concentrations which occur at puberty.[67]

Another potential inhibitory pathway involves the neural control of melatonin secretion by the pineal. This pathway appears important in the seasonal regression of reproductive activity in certain animal species, but is of uncertain import in primates.[68,68a]

Hypothalamic Pulse Generator

Release of GnRH is controlled by peptidergic neurons whose axons are highly concentrated in the arcuate

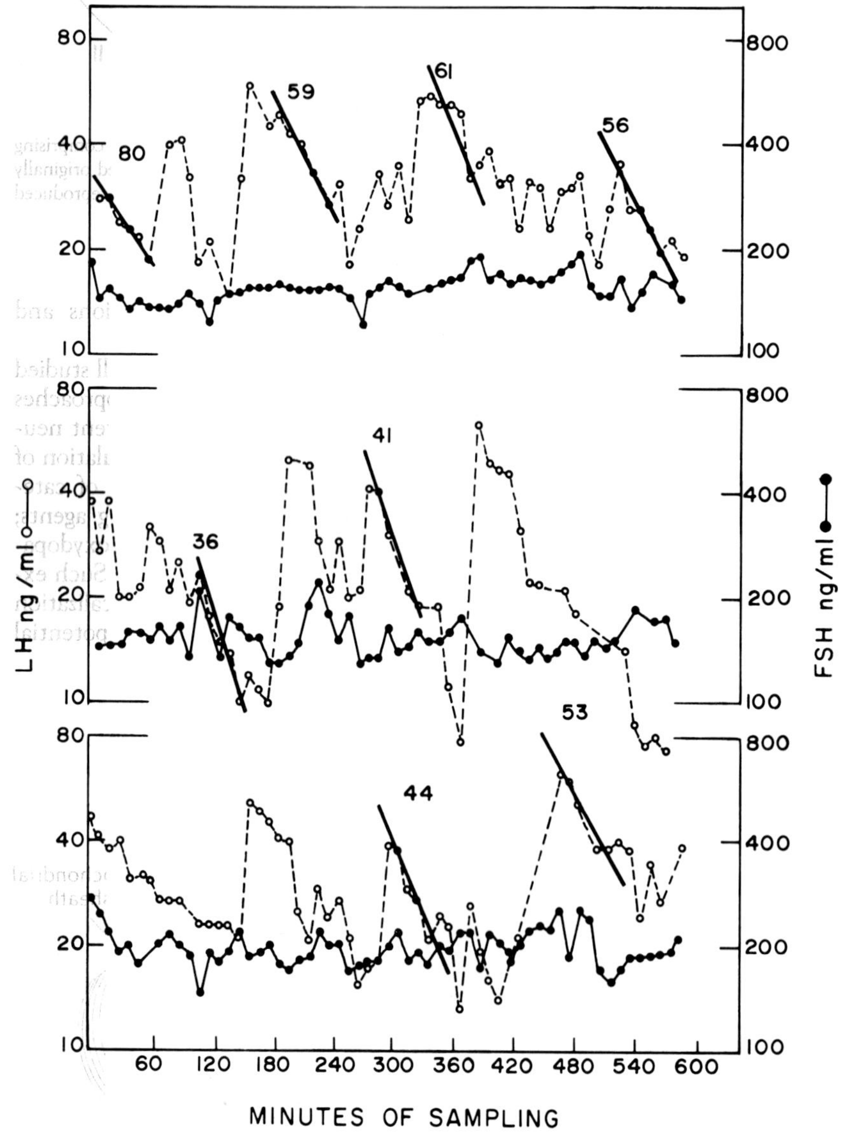

FIGURE 16-14 LH (open circles) and FSH (closed circles) levels in blood samples collected from three normal men at 10-min intervals over a 10-h period, demonstrating pulsatile LH (and FSH) release. Following pulses of LH, a linear decline (solid lines) in blood levels of this hormone is observed. The "apparent half-life" of LH following episodic release, determined then, is indicated by the numbers above the solid lines. (*From Santen and Bardin.*[70])

nucleus and median eminence. A characteristic property of neuronal function is an intrinsic periodicity of firing with variable amplitude and frequency modulation. The pattern of release of GnRH into the pituitary portal capillaries reflects the nature of its neuronal control. GnRH is secreted in a series of pulses with variable amplitude and frequency.[69] The pituitary responds to this releasing hormone with pulsatile secretion of LH and, to a lesser extent, FSH into the peripheral circulation (Fig. 16-14).[70] Simultaneous measurement of portal GnRH and peripheral plasma LH concentrations reveals an excellent concordance (Fig. 16-15).[69,71] Inference from a variety of observations regarding pulsatile LH secretion has led to the concept of a hypothalamic "pulse generator" (Fig. 16-16).[69-75] The neurons responsible for pulse generation reside primarily in the arcuate nucleus. Episodic neuronal firing in this area precedes each LH pulse by 2 to 5 min.[75-77] Highly selective radiowave lesions produced in the arcuate nucleus in the rhesus monkey completely abolish pulsatile LH release.[76,77] Sex steroid, catecholamine, and opiate agonists and antagonists can alter the amplitude and frequency of LH pulses, presumably through interactions with the neuronal pulse generator.[2,61,64,70,74,78] Afferent neuronal signals from other hypothalamic nuclei may also modulate pulse generation.[72]

The concentration of GnRH in the portal capillary system has not been directly measured in men, but is estimated indirectly to range from 30 to 300 pg/ml.[79] These levels are higher than the amounts found by direct measurements in sheep, 10 to 30 pg/ml.[69] Little GnRH accumulates in peripheral plasma because of the rapid rate of metabolism (802 ± 74 liters of plasma is cleared per day per square meter of body surface) of this releasing hormone.[79] Consequently, RIA methods for measurement of peripheral plasma levels of GnRH are insufficiently sensitive for routine clinical assessment. GnRH, as well as immunologically detectable cleavage products, is concentrated in the urine. Measurements in this biologic fluid correlate with LH and FSH secretion in adult men and increase appropriately during puberty in parallel with the plasma gonadotropins.[80]

Hypothalamic Behavioral Centers

Besides its integral role in GnRH regulation, the hypothalamus also exerts effects on behavioral patterning, at least in lower animals.[81] These actions can be divided into two types: those which exert organizational or permanent effects and those which are "activational" or transient. In the rat, reproductive behavior is at least partially controlled through sex steroid receptor–mediated organizational events. Morphologic correlates of established behavioral patterns can be observed in rodents and in several other species. The dimorphic nucleus in the rat hypothalamus undergoes recognizable structural change upon androgen administration.[82] Definable behavioral functions such as male-related singing behavior in the songbird or male lordosis patterns in the rat can be correlated

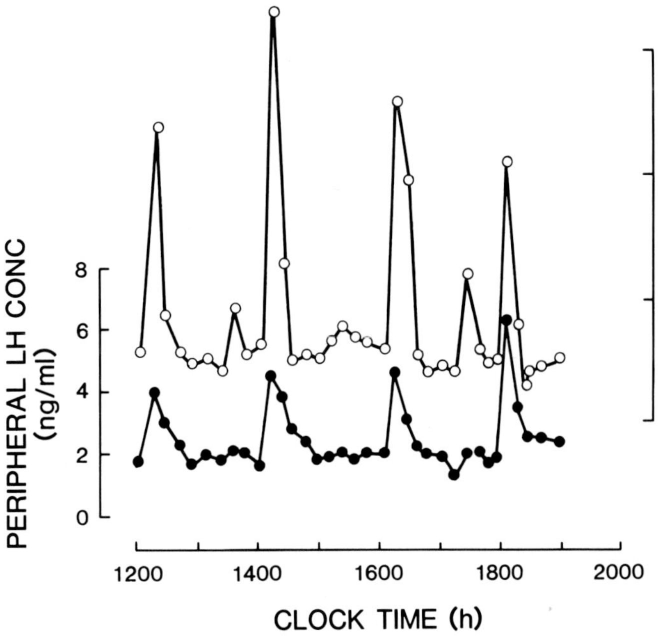

FIGURE 16-15 Simultaneous measurement of concentrations of GnRH in pituitary portal plasma and LH in peripheral plasma of the sheep. Open circles, GnRH; closed circles, LH. (*Adapted from Clarke and Cummins.*[69])

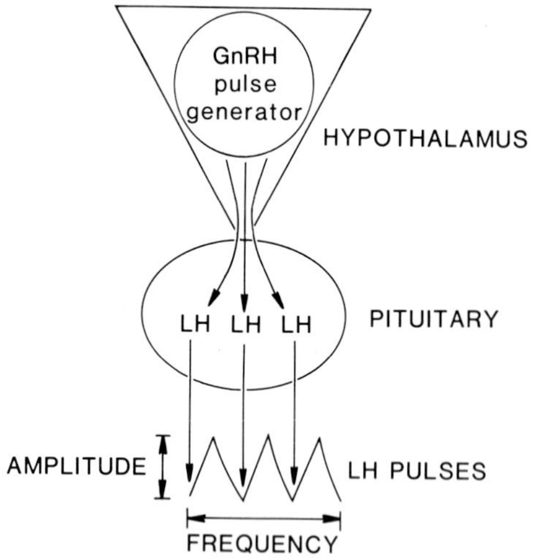

FIGURE 16-16 Diagrammatic representation of the GnRH pulse generator. Triangle = medial basal hypothalamus (see Fig. 16-1A); oval = pituitary. Pulsatile release of GnRH results in pulsatile LH release with measurable amplitude and frequency.

with characteristic hypothalamic histologic patterns.[81] Prenatal exposure to androgens imprints later patterns of gonadotropin regulatory control in the guinea pig, sheep, hamster, mouse, and rat.[81] In the rat, perinatal exposure to androgens influences aggressiveness and other definable behavioral parameters.[81]

The relevance of these structural studies in animals to understanding the behavioral effects of androgens in men has not yet been established. In a number of clinical disorders, exposure of the brain to androgen in the prenatal period had been altered. Males with androgen-resistant syndromes or 5α-reductase deficiency lacked appropriate prenatal androgen exposure; females with congenital adrenal hyperplasia or those who had been exposed to steroids prenatally were subjected to increased androgenic effects. These disorders may provide insight into the relative importance of prenatal androgen exposure vs. postnatal socialization on patterns of sexual behavior. However, no clear conclusions have emerged from observation of these disorders. It should be noted that little support has been provided for the concept of organizational imprinting of the brain by prenatal exposure to androgens in humans.[81] Further evidence against androgen imprinting comes from observations in men who had been castrated after prenatal androgen exposure.[83] Administration of estrogen in appropriate dosage causes a stimulatory release of LH in these subjects. In rodents and many other species, on the other hand, prenatal androgenic imprinting of the hypothalamus prevents such a stimulatory response.[81]

Specific behavioral effects of androgens in adult men are observable, but appear to be of the activational or transient type. The exact site which induces these actions is not known. Androgen deprivation reduces the frequency of nocturnal as well as spontaneous daytime erections; androgen replacement returns these functions to normal. Androgens also appear to influence libido, the behavioral activity which includes cognitive events leading to engagement in sexual activity.[84] While hypothalamic, cortical, or other CNS sites could mediate these actions, no data are available currently in men to localize these functions.

PITUITARY

The dominant factor controlling gonadotropin release by the pituitary is exposure to GnRH. This hormone binds to specific receptors on cells which synthesize and release both LH and FSH.[85] Binding of hormone to the GnRH receptor translocates uniformly distributed receptor units into patches, stimulates the mobilization of ionized calcium within the cell, and induces release of LH.[86-88] This coupling-activation sequence depends heavily upon calcium binding to the calcium-binding protein calmodulin for maximal function and also involves phosphokinase C activation and diacylglycerol.[85,89] Calcium channel blockers or calcium ionophores exert profound influences on this process. Some investigators have demonstrated an increase in cyclic AMP concentration following GnRH exposure,[90,91] but the requirement for this cyclic nucleotide remains a focus of controversy.[85]

In response to a discrete GnRH bolus, the pituitary promptly releases LH into the peripheral circulation.[92] With exposure to constantly infused GnRH for 2 to 4 h, a bimodal pattern of LH release becomes apparent.[93,94] After the initial burst of LH secretion over a 30-min period, the levels of this gonadotropin decline, only to increase slowly again over the next 4 h. This secretory pattern has been attributed to the presence of two functional pools of LH within the pituitary. Whether these pools represent molecular processing, compartmentalization of storage granules, or previously and newly synthesized hormone has not been established.

Exposure of the pituitary to two successive, discrete boluses of GnRH separated by 1 to 2 h enhances the response to the second dose.[95] Termed the *self-priming effect,* this phenomenon may reflect the same functional alterations observed during constant infusion, but could as well represent separate mechanistic changes.

LH is a glycoprotein with a molecular weight of 28,000 which is composed of two separate subunits. The α subunit contains 92 amino acids; it is identical to the α subunits of thyroid stimulating hormone

(TSH), FSH, and human chorionic gonadotropin (hCG); the β subunit contains 115 amino acids and is specific to LH. While the β subunit of hCG shares homology with the 115 amino acids of β-LH, β-hCG contains an additional 30 amino acids beyond the β-LH peptide sequence.[96] The gonadotrophs independently synthesize both the α and β subunits of LH from separate gene sequences and from separate mRNA.[97] After transcription and translation are completed, these subunits join to form the native LH molecule. During additional processing, a variable amount of carbohydrate is inserted into the molecule, resulting in a high degree of microheterogeneity. A family of LH molecules with various isoelectric points are demonstrable by isoelectric focusing techniques.[98] The amount of carbohydrate contained in the LH molecule after secretion is physiologically important, since this determines its rate of metabolic clearance in plasma and degree of inherent physiologic potency. A reduction in the carbohydrate content of LH enhances its rate of clearance and reduces its biologic potency when tested in vivo by bioassay.[99]

Recent studies suggest that qualitative differences exist in the molecular structure of circulating LH under various clinical circumstances. One sensitive marker for such qualitative changes is the ratio of biologic/immunologic activity of circulating LH. Recently available techniques allow both parameters to be determined in plasma samples.[100] In the most widely studied condition, pubertal maturation, the biologic/immunologic (B/I) ratio of LH progressively increases.[101–103] The B/I ratio of LH secreted during discrete LH pulses is higher than the ratio observed during intervals between pulses.[104] Exposure to exogenous GnRH analogues in high doses reduces the B/I ratio of LH.[105,106] In male rats, castration reduces the B/I ratio of LH in the pituitary.[98,99] The exact molecular modifications which mediate this change are currently unknown, but could relate to LH carbohydrate content.

The gonadotroph is ordinarily exposed to intermittent pulses of GnRH which occur at intervals of 90 to 120 min.[69,70] This periodicity of exposure appears necessary for preservation of normal secretory function. Paradoxically, exposure of the pituitary to constant amounts of GnRH for periods of 24 to 48 h suppresses LH production.[107] For this reason, potent synthetic analogues of GnRH which are resistant to metabolic cleavage and which bind to the GnRH receptor with higher than normal affinity produce a paradoxical inhibition of gonadotropin release upon long-term administration.[108]

Episodic exposure of the pituitary to GnRH results in LH pulses with quantifiable amplitude and frequency.[70] Several computer programs are currently available which allow precise estimation of pulse frequency and amplitude.[70,109,110] In men, pulse frequency averages 12 to 14 pulses/24 h. Pulse amplitude ranges from 20 to 400 percent between nadir and peak, with an average change of 70 percent. The levels of LH in plasma decline in a log-linear fashion following pulses. The "apparent half-lives" of this gonadotropin can be calculated from slopes of such decay curves.[70] The fact that apparent half-life approaches the known half-life of exogenously administered LH (i.e., 18 to 39 min for the first phase, 90 to 120 min for the second phase) suggests that pituitary LH secretion completely ceases during some intervals between pulses.[70,111,111a]

After release into the peripheral circulation, LH is cleared by the kidney, liver, and gonads and from other sites. The metabolic clearance rate of LH, determined by constant infusion of exogenous gonadotropin, is in the range of 34±3 ml/min for immunoactive LH[111a,112] and 26±3 ml/min for bioactive LH. Using the radiolabeled LH method, values are slightly higher, 44±8 ml/min.[112] The value determined for daily production rate depends on which assay is used for measurement of plasma LH concentration. Recent estimates include production rates of 600 IU/24 h for immunoactive LH and 1900 IU/24 h for bioactive LH.[111a] These generally correlate with the amounts of exogenous human LH necessary to maintain normal testosterone levels in patients with isolated gonadotropin deficiency.

Only a small fraction of LH is excreted intact into the urine; levels detected by immunoassay range from 12 to 60 IU/24 h.[112,113] Plasma LH concentration can be measured by RIA or by highly sensitive bioassay. The latter depends upon the stimulation of testosterone by Leydig cells isolated from rats or mice.[100] Bioassayable LH levels vary widely, depending upon the species of Leydig cell and standard utilized, but generally are 3.0 to 10 times higher than immunologic measurements. The degree of carbohydrate content, tertiary structure, and other minor molecular modifications appear to affect LH biologic activity to a greater extent than they do immunologic recognition.[99]

TESTIS

In the testes, the Leydig or interstitial cells contain membrane receptors which bind LH with high affinity. Studies of highly purified LH receptor preparations from ovary indicate that they have a molecular weight of 280,000 and an affinity constant of 7.6×10^{-11} M.[114] The molecular structure is dimeric; the monomers are of relatively equal molecular weights of 120,000 to 140,000. The monomers, in turn, contain 38,000- and 85,000-dalton subunits. These monomers appear specific for binding of the α and β subunits of LH, respectively. Ten percent of the receptor molecule consists of carbohydrate, including sialic acid, mannose, galactose, *N*-acetylglucosamine, and *N*-acetylgalactosamine.

The interaction of LH with its receptor initiates a cascade of events similar to those for other polypeptide hormones with their respective receptors. This sequence consists of receptor binding, aggregation of receptor proteins in the cell membrane, appearance of membrane pitting, activation of adenylate cyclase, interaction with a cyclic GMP–dependent protein, generation of cyclic AMP, binding to a regulatory protein, and release of the cyclic AMP–dependent catalytic subunits (see Chap. 4). These events induce an increase in Leydig cell steroidogenesis, and ultimately lead to an increase in testosterone production.[115] Only a small fraction of receptors must be occupied by hormone for testosterone stimulation to be maximal. The presence of "spare receptors" is not unique to the testes; spare receptors exist in many systems requiring binding of a peptide hormone to its receptor.

Exposure to high concentrations of LH over several hours reduces receptor content, a process of suppression generally termed "down regulation." The suppression process has been studied in the adult rat testis and ovary. It appears to result from inhibition of synthesis of new receptors via cyclic AMP–mediated processes.[116] However, it could also be due to increased receptor internalization and lysosomal degradation. The fetal testis, as opposed to the adult, is resistant to LH-induced suppression.[117] Reduced LH levels induce higher receptor concentrations ("up regulation"), a process which is prevented by addition of protein synthesis inhibitors.[116]

Extensive in vitro studies of rodent testis tissue demonstrated that the biologic consequences of receptor suppression involve inhibition of C_{17-20}-lyase and 17α-hydroxylase activities, both distal steps in the androgen biosynthetic pathway. These actions may be partially related to an associated increase in estradiol induced by the aromatase-stimulating effect of LH.[115,115a] Compatible with this hypothesis is the observation that antiestrogens or aromatase inhibitors can abolish the inhibitory effects of LH receptor "down" regulation." In addition, an estrogen-inducible protein is observed in the Leydig cell during the down regulation process.[115] When receptor levels are maximally reduced a further, more proximal block in steroidogenesis is observed with inhibition of pregnenolone production. The biologic relevance of the estrogen hypothesis is supported by the observation that estrogen-producing Leydig cell tumors are associated with precursor steroid patterns compatible with C_{17-20}-lyase inhibition.[115b]

Experiments in men given hCG also suggest the potential physiologic relevance of LH receptor suppression in patients. For example, increments in 17α-hydroxyprogesterone concentration greater than those of testosterone concentration, as a reflection of the C_{17-20}-lyase block, are observed for 1 to 2 days after exposure to high doses of hCG. The disproportionate rise in 17α-hydroxyprogesterone concentration correlates with increments in plasma estradiol concentration. Lower doses of hCG given more frequently caused exaggerated rises in neither 17α-hydroxyprogesterone nor estradiol concentrations.[118–120]

Receptor down regulation could explain why men with very high circulating levels of hCG due to choriocarcinoma secrete reduced and not increased amounts of testosterone. However, other studies call into question the general relevance of receptor down regulation in men. When physiologic amounts of hCG or LH are administered to men for long periods, Leydig cell responsiveness is not substantially altered.[121] Further correlation is thus necessary between in vitro studies using animal tissue and in vivo studies in humans to determine the precise significance of receptor down regulation in the regulation of intratesticular steroidogenic events.

Upon exposure to LH, the Leydig cells increase their rate of testosterone production by increasing pregnenolone synthesis. Substrate for this steroidogenic process can come from either de novo synthesis of cholesterol from acetate in the Leydig cells or tissue uptake of plasma cholesterol (Fig. 16-17).[122] Androgen biosynthesis in the human testis preferentially proceeds via the Δ^5 pathway from pregnenolone to dehydroepiandrosterone (DHEA) and androstenediol before entering the Δ^4 pathway as *androstenedione* (and testosterone). Cholesterol side chain cleavage occurs in mitochondria; conversion of pregnenolone to testosterone takes place in the microsomal fractions. Androgen precursors and products can be converted to steroid sulfates for storage in the testis. Enzymatic cleavage to the free steroids then precedes release into the circulation. The physiologic significance of this *sulfate storage shunt* remains a matter of controversy.[123]

The major androgen secreted by the testes is testosterone; approximately 7000 μg per day enters the peripheral circulation. By calculations from spermatic vein–peripheral vein gradients, the testes are also found to secrete microgram amounts (Fig. 16-18) of 17α-hydroxyprogesterone, androstenedione, and pregnenolone, as well as several other steroids.[124] It should be noted, however, that relatively little DHT is

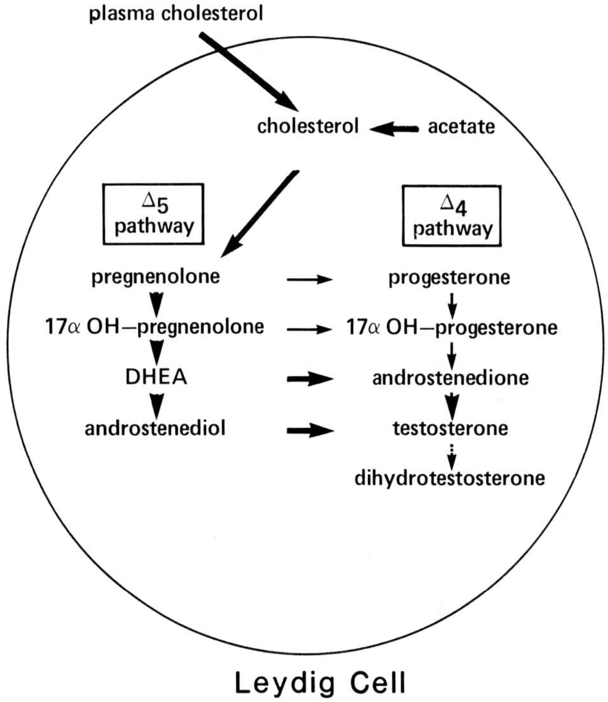

FIGURE 16-17 Diagrammatic representation of the androgen synthetic pathway in the Leydig cells of the testis. Preferred pathways are shown by heavy arrows. Only small amounts of dihydrotestosterone are synthesized from testosterone within the Leydig cell.

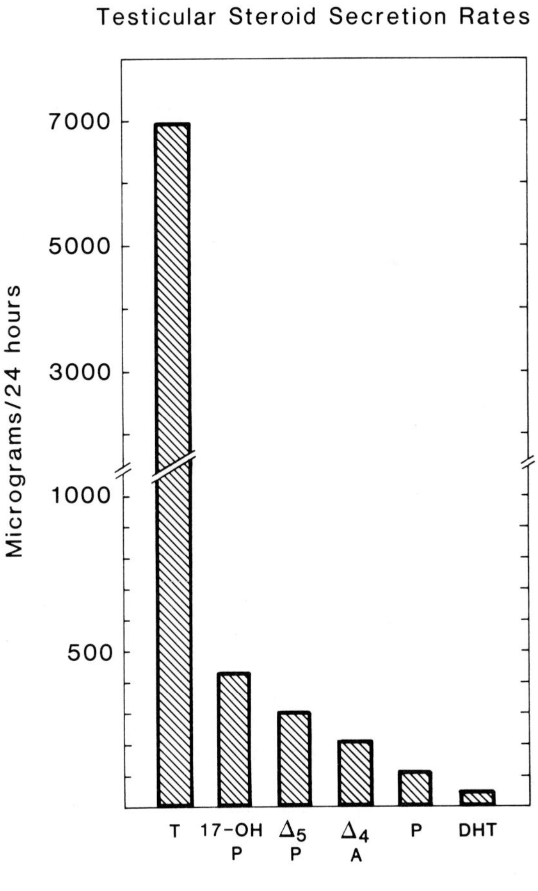

FIGURE 16-18 Testicular secretion rates of various androgens. T, testosterone; 17-OHP, 17α-hydroxyprogesterone; Δ^5P, pregnenolone; Δ^4A, androstenedione; P, progesterone; DHT, dihydrotestosterone. Secretion rates calculated from the arteriovenous (av) differences across the testis (as measured by Hammond et al.[124]). Calculations based upon assumptions used by Kirchner et al.[470] for adrenal secretion rates, represented by the formula

$$\text{Secretion rate (SR)} = \frac{\text{Assumed testosterone SR}}{\text{Testosterone av difference}} \times \text{av difference of steroid in question}$$

Testosterone SR assumed to be 7000 μg per day.

directly secreted by the testes (i.e., 69 μg/24 h) and even smaller amounts of estradiol are secreted (10 μg per day).[124,125]

Several clinical observations suggest that factors other than LH may modulate Leydig cell responsiveness. Growth hormone (GH) appears to enhance hCG-induced testosterone secretion in GH-deficient subjects.[126] When FSH is given to men with isolated gonadotropin deficiency during long-term hCG treatment, testosterone levels increase twofold.[127] Data accumulating from experimental animal studies also suggest that other peptide hormones play a role.[128] For example, GnRH, arginine vasopressin, oxytocin, and β-endorphin can inhibit testosterone biosynthesis in isolated Leydig cells in a dose-dependent fashion.[128] Convincing evidence exists from RNA hybridization experiments that at least some of these substances, such as β-endorphin, are synthesized directly in the testes.[129] On the other hand, much species variation exists. While receptors for GnRH can be demonstrated to exist in the testes of the rat, such is not the case in men, mice, or monkeys.[130,131] Therefore, a clear understanding of the importance of these substances (called gonadocrinins) will await further detailed studies in men.

Testosterone is secreted into the peripheral plasma via the spermatic veins in a pulsatile manner. While LH and testosterone pulses would be expected to be in concord, they appear to be poorly correlated in men.[132] Two factors probably explain this finding. First, testosterone is largely protein-bound in peripheral plasma.[133] The small fraction of newly secreted testosterone enters a large pool of bound testosterone; pulses are masked by this dilution factor. In support of this concept is the fact that excellent concordance between testosterone and LH pulses is observed in animal species lacking testosterone-binding proteins. Second, the response of the human testis to LH is relatively sluggish.[132] Although small rises in testosterone concentrations occur within 2 to 4 h after LH or hCG is administered, peak increases are not observed until 24 to 72 h later.[118] For these reasons, the variation in testosterone levels due to pulsatile secretion is only 25 percent; in comparison, LH pulses cause LH concentration to vary by 65 percent.[70,134]

A diurnal rhythm of testosterone level, with a peak at 4 to 8 A.M. and nadir concentration at 4 to 8 P.M., occurs in younger men and less so in elderly men.[132] The overall excursion from nadir to peak levels ranges from 20 to 30 percent. This rhythm is not associated with diurnal increments in LH. Its cause is unknown but may be related to nocturnal prolactin increments, changes in testosterone metabolic clearance rate, altered sensitivity of the testis to LH, or other factors.

The adrenal provides an additional source of testosterone. Direct measurements of testosterone concentration in adrenal venous plasma indicate that approximately 200 μg per day of testosterone arises from this source.[135] The peripheral conversion of androstenedione, secreted by the adrenal and converted into testosterone, accounts for another 200 to 300 μg. Therefore, adrenal sources provide approximately 5 percent of the total testosterone produced (i.e., 400 to 600 μg per day).[135]

A small percentage of testosterone (i.e., approximately 2 percent) circulates in a free state in plasma, whereas the remainder is bound either to testosterone-estrogen–binding globulin (TeBG), or to albumin (Fig. 16-19).[133] The affinity of TeBG for testosterone (1.6×10^{-9} M) is several orders of magnitude higher than that of albumin (4×10^{-4} M).[136] Several observations suggest that only TeBG binds testosterone with sufficiently high affinity to retard entry of this androgen into tissues. Vermeulen et al. initially demonstrated an excellent correlation between the levels of non-TeBG-bound testosterone and the rate of its metabolic clearance, a variable reflecting tissue entry.[137] Direct measurements of tissue entry using a highly sensitive bioassay technique demonstrate an excellent correlation between the non-TeBG-bound fraction of testosterone and entry into brain or liver.[133] Readily available clinical measures of non-TeBG-bound testosterone concentration, determined by ammonium sulfate precipitation, correlate with availability for tissue entry (Fig. 16-20).[138] Perturbation of the amount of TeBG present or drug saturation of its functional binding capacity alters the degree of tissue entry in a predictable fashion. Experimental studies and mathematical modeling have identified the major factors affecting the retardation of tissue entry by plasma protein binders. These include the affinity of the binder for the steroid, the half-time of release of the steroid from the binder, and the time taken for blood to traverse the organ in question.[133,136] Taking these factors into account, only TeBG-bound, but not albumin-bound, testosterone is retarded from tissue entry under most circumstances.

Several clinicopathologic events alter the absolute levels of TeBG in plasma (Fig. 16-19). Reduced TeBG levels occur in association with obesity, acromegaly, and hypothyroidism; increased levels accompany hyperthyroidism, use of birth control pills, cirrhosis, hypogonadism, and pregnancy. Estrogens stimulate and androgens inhibit its biosynthesis. Several drugs can alter the functional binding of TeBG. The most commonly observed effects occur with spironolactone and its metabolites; fluoxymesterone, danazol, methyltestosterone, megestrol, and a large group of natural and synthetic steroids also produce this effect.[136,139,140]

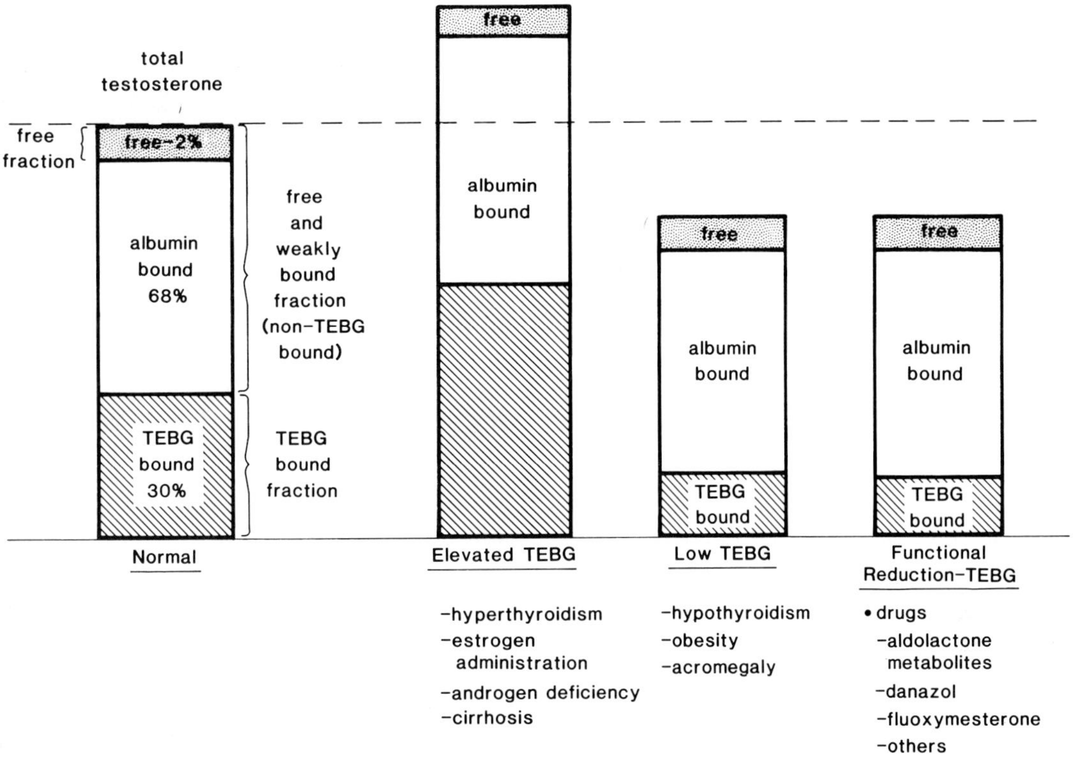

FIGURE 16-19 Fractions of bound, weakly bound, and free testosterone in normal men and in men with disorders producing high or low levels of testosterone-estrogen–binding globulin (TeBG).

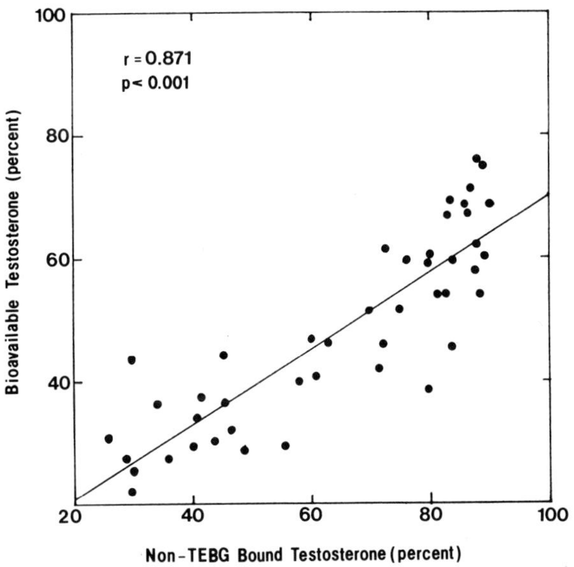

FIGURE 16-20 Correlation between non-TeBG-bound testosterone, as determined by the ammonium sulfate precipitation technique, and bioavailable testosterone measured by the Oldendorf method. (*From Manni et al.*[138])

Measurement of non-TeBG-bound testosterone provides a better indication of physiologically available testosterone than do total testosterone levels when conditions of altered TeBG concentrations or functional binding exist (see Fig. 16-20).

TeBG is a glycoprotein of molecular weight 84,000 composed of two subunits, form 1 and form 2, whose amino acid sequences are now known.[141–142a] Form 1 of TeBG is not a glycoprotein. Form 2, on the other hand, binds to concanavalin A, is eluted by α-methyl mannoside, and thus contains carbohydrate moieties. Form 1 of TeBG possesses major homology to sites in form 1 of the testicular androgen-binding protein (ABP), but the two species are distinct by peptide mapping. Form 2 of TeBG is virtually identical to form 2 of ABP by peptide mapping but differs in its carbohydrate composition. RIAs are now available for the specific measurement of the mass of TeBG in plasma.[143] Other methods for quantitating the level of this protein involve saturation analysis after purification on lectin or ion-exchange columns, quantitative polyacrylamide gel or agar gel electrophoresis, or precipitation with ammonium sulfate. For routine clinical purposes, the percentage of non-TeBG-bound androgen can be determined under equilibrium conditions using dialysis against an albumin buffer or precipitation with ammonium sulfate.[136,138,139]

Which clinical method is optimal for measuring the amount of testosterone free to enter tissue remains controversial. Because recent evidence indicates that non-TeBG-bound testosterone is the functionally free fraction (see above), measurement of this fraction is preferred for assessing testosterone levels. Such "free and weakly bound" testosterone measurements assess the albumin-bound as well as free fractions and correlate well with most clinical indexes of androgenicity. Measurement of the free fraction by methods not detecting albumin binding also correlate better with clinical findings than assay of total testosterone. However, the partition between albumin-bound and free testosterone is occasionally observed to be altered; this could confound interpretation of free testosterone measurements.[144] A potentially important approach, measurement of androgen concentrations in saliva, has been recently suggested.[145] This practical method assesses the mass of testosterone which has actually entered the tissue of the salivary glands before appearing in the saliva.

The peripheral metabolism of secreted testosterone involves a series of enzymatic steps which can either activate or degrade the hormone. Two activation pathways exist whereby testosterone serves as a prohormone and undergoes conversion to more potent metabolites. First, testosterone can be converted to estradiol, a compound with 200-fold greater gonadotropin-suppressive potency per unit mass than testosterone. The enzyme *aromatase,* which converts testosterone to estradiol, is present in fatty tissue, liver, muscle, hair follicles, Leydig and Sertoli cells, and specific sites in the brain. Approximately 0.4 percent of the 7000 μg of testosterone produced daily is converted to estradiol outside of the testes.[146] The 30 μg of estradiol produced in this manner and the 10 μg secreted directly by the testes[125] account for the majority of the 40 to 50 μg of estradiol made daily in males. The remainder arises from the peripheral aromatization of androstenedione to estrone and subsequent reduction to estradiol.

Testosterone can also be converted to DHT, an androgen with 2.5 times greater potency than testosterone itself. This reaction is catalyzed by the enzyme 5α-reductase, which is present in prostate, seminal vesicles, sebaceous glands, kidney, skin, brain, and other tissues.[147,148] Of the approximately 200 to 300 μg of DHT produced daily, the majority arises from peripherally converted testosterone; less than half is secreted by the testes.[124,147] From a study of men with congenital deficiency of 5α-reductase, DHT is inferred to be necessary for mediation of androgenic effects on beard growth, sebum production, and prostatic hypertrophy.[149] Stimulatory effects on muscle, germ cell epithelium of the testes, and sexual potency do not appear to require reduction at the 5α position. For potential exploration of these specific effects, inhibitors of 5α-reductase activity are currently being developed.

Degradative androgen metabolism takes place in liver (50 to 70 percent) as well as in peripheral tissues (30 to 50 percent). Nearly 50 percent of testosterone in the plasma is taken up by the liver during one pass through this organ (Figs. 16-21, 16-22). Testosterone is there converted to the inactive metabolites androsterone and etiocholanolone, both 17-ketosteroids, and to DHT and 3α-androstanediol. These compounds can then be converted to their glucuronide or sulfate derivatives for reentry into plasma and excretion into urine.

Biosynthetic activation of androgens can be hormonally regulated at specific target organ sites.[150–152] For example, in skin, 5α-reductase is under androgenic control. In conditions of androgen deficiency, such as hypogonadism in men, the levels of activity of this enzyme are reduced. Androgen administration increases the activity of 5α-reductase in these men.

Local degradative inactivation occurs in target organ sites as well but is not clearly androgen-regulated. DHT is reversibly converted to 3α-androstanediol and at some of these sites to 3α-androstanediol glucuronide as well. Each of these compounds can reenter plasma and ultimately be excreted in the urine.[153–155] Mauvais-Jarvis et al. first pointed out the significance of the local skin metabolic pathway for androgens.[155] They demonstrated that the quantity of urinary 3α-androstanediol glucuronide reflects not only the amount of androgen initially secreted into the plasma but also the rate of its metabolism in target tissues. Local metabolism of androgens in the skin increases in states of androgen excess; skin metabolism of androgens correlates with results of 3α-androstanediol glucuronide measurements in urine. Horton et al.[154] and others[156,157] later extended these observations by demonstrating a marked elevation of 3α-androstanediol glucuronide concentration in plasma in states of androgen excess. Taken together, these data suggest that 3α-androstanediol glucuronide measurements provide an excellent marker for peripheral androgen action in states of hormone excess or deficiency.

Testosterone induces its hormonal effects through a sequence of events which are analogous to those initiated by other steroid hormones. Either directly, in tissues such as the testis, or after metabolic activation to DHT, testosterone binds to a specific receptor.[158]

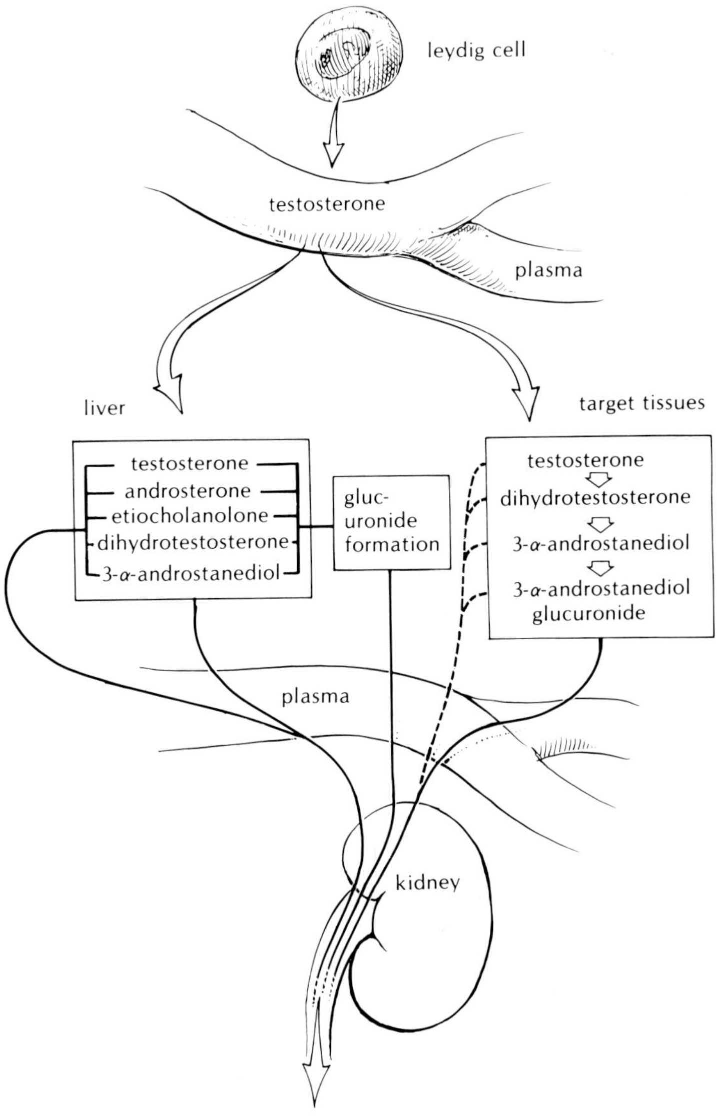

FIGURE 16-21 Diagrammatic representation of metabolism of testosterone. After secretion by the Leydig cell, testosterone travels through the plasma to liver or target tissues. After metabolism and conjugation, products are excreted into the urine.

The androgen receptor is an 86,000-dalton protein contained in androgen target organs which binds DHT with 1.2 times greater affinity than it binds testosterone.[159] The receptor-ligand complex binds to chromatin in the nucleus. The affinity of binding to specific nuclear structures varies. Certain nuclear receptor fractions elute under conditions of low salt concentration and others under high salt concentration, while others are highly resistant to extraction. Evidence is accumulating to suggest that only a small fraction of all nuclear androgen receptors mediate androgen effects.[160] This fraction binds preferentially to the nuclear matrix, the DNA cytoskeleton which forms a supporting infrastructure in the nucleus.[160]

Receptor binding to nuclear DNA initiates a sequence of events which involves activation of RNA polymerases I and II, initiation of protein synthesis, and induction of androgenic effects. Two general categories of androgenic actions on the body occur: those which are called anabolic effects and those which are more properly androgenic.[161] Assays more responsive to the anabolic effects of steroids (such as levator ani muscle mass assessment in the rat) or the androgenic effects (e.g., ventral prostate weight) have been developed in animals. Structural manipulations of the synthetic androgens can produce substances which are relatively more anabolic than androgenic and vice versa. However, the exact molecular basis for deter-

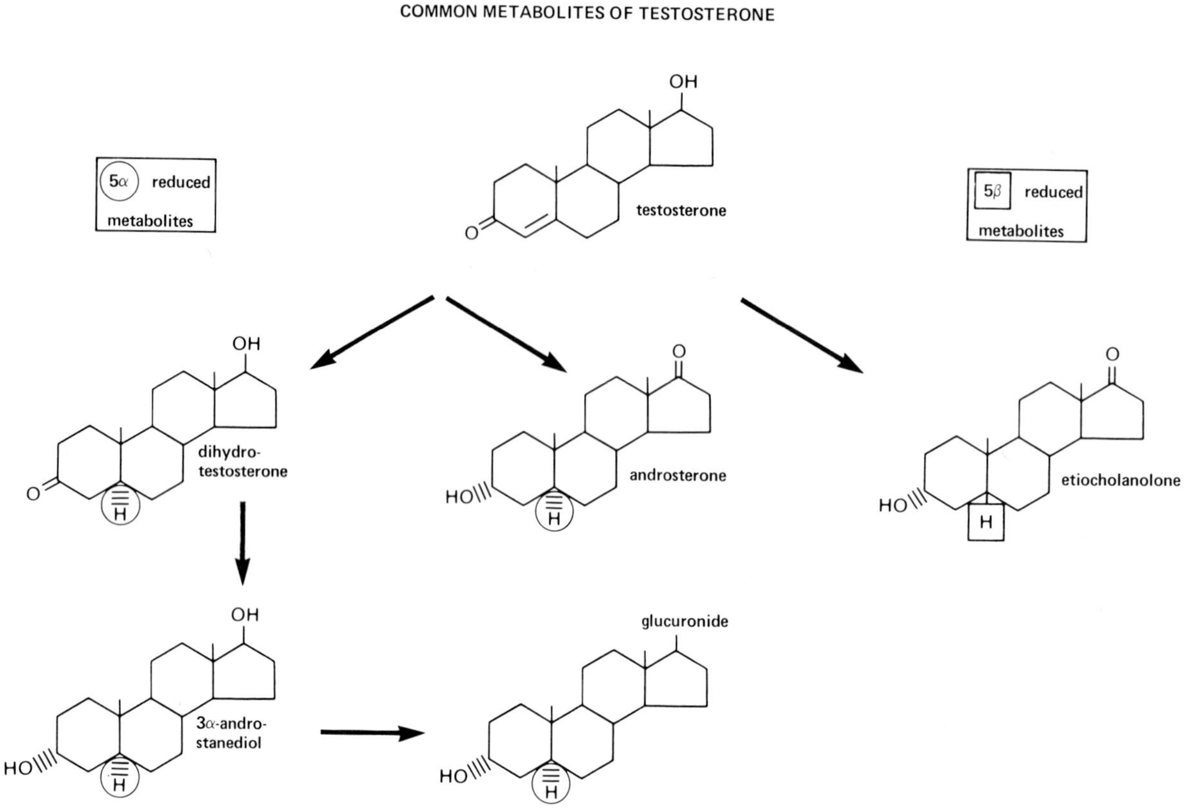

FIGURE 16-22 Structures of the testosterone metabolites.

mining whether actions will be androgenic or anabolic remains elusive at present.[161] The specific actions of androgens at various times in life are listed in Table 16-2. Anabolic and androgenic actions are not differentiated in the table because of the uncertainty in distinguishing these effects on a mechanistic basis.

FEEDBACK INTERACTION

Overview

As a reflection of the evolutionary necessity for propagation of each species, complementary and redundant servomechanisms have developed to control LH secretion precisely in men. Two steroids, testosterone and estradiol, independently control LH secretion at two separate anatomic sites, the hypothalamus and pituitary (Fig. 16-23).[74] Negative feedback, the primary mechanism of this control, consists of two phases: *suppressive* and *recovery* phases.[162] During the suppressive phase, an elevation of sex steroid concentrations causes a reduction in LH secretion (Fig. 16-24) and in pituitary mRNA levels for the LH subunits.[162a] Later, during the recovery phase, LH concentration returns to basal level upon lowering of the concentrations of sex steroids. Negative feedback effects can be mediated either by an alteration in LH pulse frequency or modulation of pulse amplitude. Another mechanism, positive feedback, allows estradiol but not testosterone to stimulate LH under precisely defined conditions.[83]

The degree of complexity of this system has gradually become apparent during ongoing studies over five decades. After initial identification of testosterone as a potent androgen in the 1930s, this steroid was considered to exert exclusive control over the release of LH through negative feedback inhibition. Later, the conversion of testosterone to estradiol through aromatization was demonstrated both in peripheral tissues and in specific hypothalamic nuclei. This observation led to the theory that all of the negative feedback effects of testosterone are mediated by aromatized estrogen products.[163] Several lines of evidence subsequently disproved this theory.[74,78,164–166] Nonaromatizable androgens such as DHT or fluoxymesterone inhibit LH. Testosterone, when administered with an aromatase inhibitor such as testolactone, suppresses LH release without a concomitant increase in estradiol concentration.[164] Androgens and estrogens produce differential effects on the frequency

Table 16-2. Clinical Actions of Androgen

In utero	
	External genitalia develop
	Wolffian ducts develop
Prepubertal	
	Possible male behavioral effects
Pubertal	
	External genitalia:
	Penis and scrotum increase in size and become pigmented
	Rugal folds appear in scrotal skin
	Hair growth:
	Mustache and beard develop; scalp line undergoes recession
	Pubic hair develops
	Axillary, body, extremity, and perianal hair appears
	Linear growth:
	Pubertal growth spurt
	Androgens interact with growth hormones to increase somatomedin C levels
	Accessory sex organs:
	Prostate and seminal vesicles enlarge and secretion begins
	Voice:
	Pitch is lowered because of enlargement of larynx and thickening of vocal cords
	Psyche:
	More aggressive attitudes are manifest
	Sexual potential develops
	Muscle mass:
	Muscle bulk increases
	Nitrogen balance is positive
Adult	
	Hair growth:
	Androgenic patterns are maintained
	Male pattern baldness may be initiated
	Psyche:
	Behavioral attitudes and sexual potency are maintained
	Bone:
	Bone loss and osteoporosis are prevented
	Spermatogenesis:
	Interaction with FSH modulates Sertoli cell function and stimulates spermatogenesis
	Hematopoiesis:
	Erythropoietin stimulated
	Direct marrow effect exerted on erythropoiesis

Source: Adapted from Bardin and Paulsen.[229]

of pulsatile LH secretion as well as on its amplitude. Finally, hypogonadal men are relatively resistant to the LH-suppressive effects of androgens but not estrogens.[166] Based upon these data, current opinion considers that two negative feedback systems, one mediated by androgens and the other by estrogens, operate independently (Fig. 16-23). Both of these systems exert rapid effects on LH secretion within a period of 3 to 6 h (Fig. 16-24).[78]

Testosterone Negative Feedback

Testosterone reduces the amount of GnRH released from hypothalamic tissue in vitro and the amount secreted into the pituitary portal circulation in vivo.[167,168] When given for a short period of time (i.e., 6 h to 4 days) testosterone inhibits LH exclusively through hypothalamic effects. This conclusion is inferred from the observation that the LH response to exogenous GnRH is not blunted during periods of androgen-induced LH suppression.[74,78,169] The mechanism of LH inhibition is through a specific effect on the frequency modulation of the pulse generator and involves the opiate pathway.[169a] Testosterone reduces GnRH pulse frequency from 1/100 min to 1/200 min on average.[74,78,169] This effect is observed both with testosterone and with androgens incapable of conversion to estrogens such as DHT or fluoxymesterone.[169,169a]

Whether androgens play an inhibitory role at the pituitary level in men is less certain. Androgen receptors are present in the pituitary of many species[21] and DHT lowers LH secretion and content when directly implanted into the rodent pituitary.[170] Cultured pituitary cells respond to DHT by decreasing the amount of LH released in response to GnRH.[171]

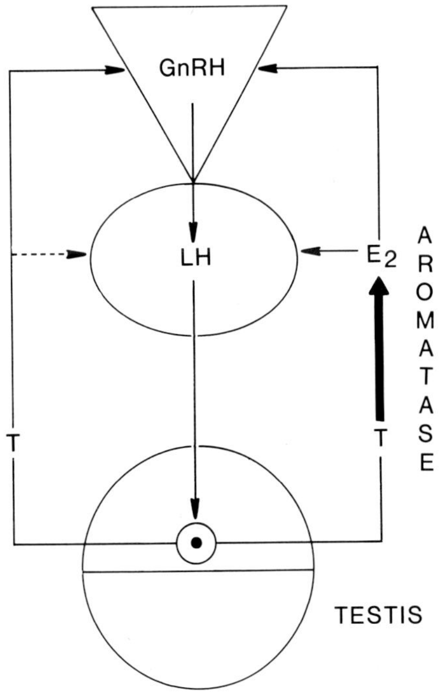

FIGURE 16-23 Diagrammatic representation of the hypothalamus (triangle), pituitary (oval), and testis (circle) with its Leydig cell depicted. T, testosterone; E_2, estradiol. Dotted line indicates questionable effect.

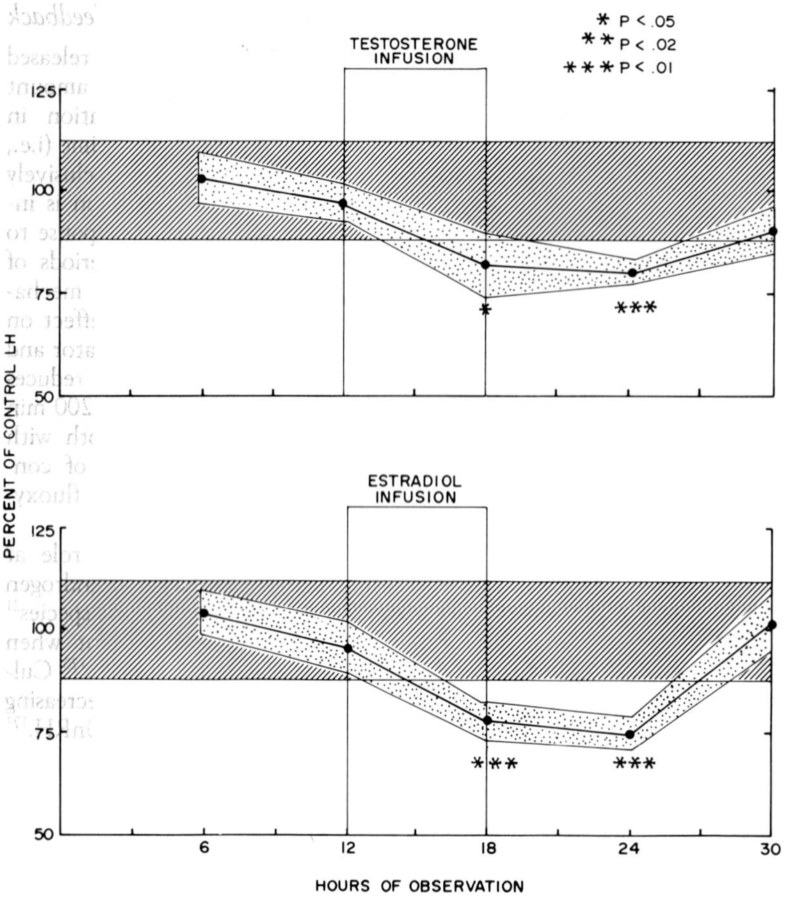

FIGURE 16-24 Effect of testosterone and estradiol infusions on mean LH concentration. Six-hour mean LH levels represented by solid circles; standard error of the mean represented by shaded area. With this method (6-h mean LH concentration), changes of > 12 percent (cross-hatched area) are significant. (*From Santen.*[78])

During prolonged testosterone administration in men (i.e., 3 to 4 weeks), responsiveness to exogenous GnRH is reduced.[172] In contrast to these suggestive studies, more direct observation in male monkeys suggests that the direct pituitary effects of androgens have only a minor role. Lesions made by radiofrequency waves are used to ablate the hypothalamic pulse generator in these animals; GnRH is then administered to reestablish these pulses artificially. Completely normal patterns of LH secretion persist in these animals in response to acute androgen depletion or repletion. Only during chronic androgen deprivation are minor effects on LH observed.[77] Taken together, these observations suggest that androgens play a major inhibitory role at the hypothalamic level and a minor role, perhaps only during persistent perturbation, at the pituitary.

Testosterone could act on the hypothalamus by binding to androgen receptors directly or by undergoing 5α reduction to DHT prior to receptor binding; no direct data are available to clearly establish which pathway predominates. 5α-Reductase exists in the hypothalami of several species.[148] Men with 5α-reductase deficiency exhibit slightly higher mean levels of LH and testosterone concentration than their unaffected siblings.[149] This observation suggests that there is a role for DHT, since levels of this steroid should be lower in the hypothalami of these patients. Definitive conclusions, however, await direct experimental evidence.

Estrogen Negative Feedback

In contrast to testosterone, the earliest effect of estradiol is mediated by a direct pituitary action. Within 3 to 6 h of estradiol administration, mean LH levels fall by 20 to 30 percent (Fig. 16-24), as do responses to exogenous GnRH.[74,78] This direct pituitary effect induces a 30 percent diminution in the amplitude of spontaneous LH pulses. Direct measurements of GnRH level in portal plasma in sheep further substantiate the direct pituitary effects of brief administrations of estradiol.[173] During more prolonged infusions (i.e., 4 days), GnRH responsiveness returns to normal levels, indicating that the direct pituitary effect is transient.[174] This is not surprising, since a variety of observations suggest that the pituitary responds to estrogen in a biphasic fashion.[175] When briefly exposed to estradiol, the pituitary initially responds to exogenous GnRH with blunted LH release; this is then followed by enhancement of LH release. While such an effect has not been tested directly in men, measurements of LH responses to GnRH during estradiol infusion suggest that a similar biphasic pattern occurs.[78,174]

Several studies imply that estrogens act on a hypothalamic site, in addition to directly affecting the pituitary. Receptors exist for estradiol in the hypothalamus as well as in the pituitary.[20] Estrogens inhibit the release of GnRH from neurons and increase hypothalamic tissue concentrations of this neuropeptide.[167,168] Neurons in the medial basal hypothalamus alter their firing rates upon exposure to estradiol.[176] Clinical observations also suggest that estradiol has a hypothalamic effect. In men, administration of an antiestrogen such as clomiphene stimulates LH secretion and pulse amplitude without enhancing the responsiveness to exogenous GnRH.[177,177a] By the fourth day of intravenous (IV) infusion of physiologic amounts of estradiol, mean LH levels are suppressed but responsiveness to exogenous GnRH is not.[174] The estradiol which acts at the hypothalamic level could be synthesized locally from androgen precursors or could be delivered to the hypothalamus from plasma. Aromatase, the enzyme which catalyzes the conversion of testosterone to estradiol, is present in the hypothalamus.[163] Aromatase is localized to certain hypothalamic nuclei; in the medial preoptic nucleus, for example, levels of aromatase are 10-fold higher than in the arcuate nucleus. This localization suggests that local estrogen production at these sites may play an important role (Fig. 16-25).[178,179] Experiments with aromatase inhibitors in dogs are most compatible with the hypothesis that local estradiol synthesis in the hypothalamus is required for LH feedback.[180] Taken together, these data imply that there are major negative feedback effects of the estrogens, both at the hypothalamic and pituitary levels.

Estrogen Positive Feedback

In women, administration of estrogens in an appropriate dosage and for an appropriate duration can transiently stimulate LH release after an initial inhibitory phase.[181] This positive feedback phenomenon is responsible for the abrupt midcycle rise in LH concentration which causes ovulation. An estrogen dosage equivalent to 50 to 100 μg of estradiol daily for 4 to 7 days is required to stimulate LH through positive feedback. Androgens blunt or abolish the positive

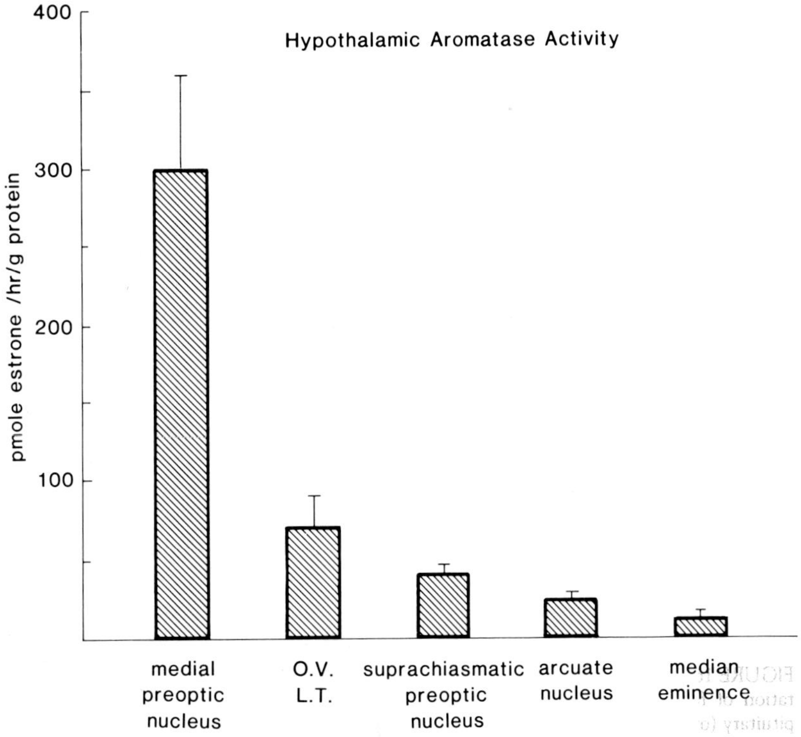

FIGURE 16-25 Aromatase activity in various areas of the rat hypothalamus. (*From data of Weisz J, reviewed in Goy and McEwen.*[179])

feedback response to estrogens. For this reason, castrated or hypogonadal men respond to estrogen with clearly defined positive feedback responses.[83] In contrast, men with normal circulating testosterone levels exhibit inconsistent and only modest LH concentration increases.[182]

Hypothalamic-Pituitary-Germ Cell Axis

OVERVIEW

In addition to their role in androgen secretion, the testes produce sperm and emit them via an excretory ductal system. Germinal cell function is controlled by FSH as well as by intratesticular androgens; the separate determinants of FSH secretion are emphasized in this section. The pituitary releases FSH, which stimulates the Sertoli cells of the testis to initiate secretion of a number of regulatory proteins. One of these, *inhibin*, enters plasma and exerts negative feedback effects on FSH secretion by the pituitary (Fig. 16-26).

HYPOTHALAMUS

GnRH stimulates FSH as well as LH release by the pituitary. The existence of a separate FSH-releasing factor has been suggested by electrostimulative and biochemical studies in rodents.[183] However, the discordance between FSH and LH levels observed in a variety of clinical conditions can be explained without postulating that a separate FSH-releasing factor exists. Based upon a variety of data, current opinion favors GnRH as the single physiologic releasing factor for FSH.

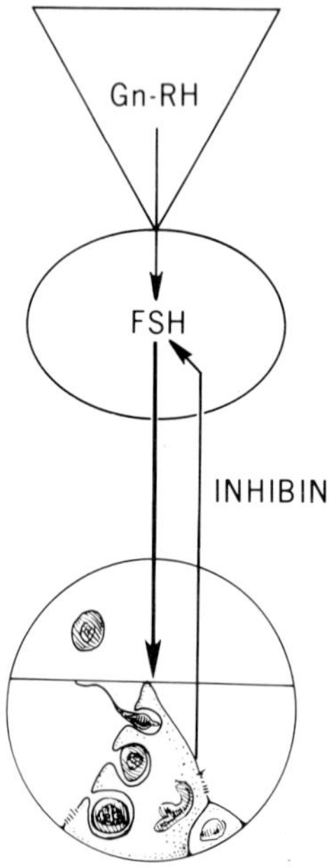

FIGURE 16-26 Control of FSH secretion. Diagrammatic representation of feedback relationship between hypothalamus (triangle), pituitary (oval), and testis (circle) with its Sertoli germ cell unit.

PITUITARY

One pituitary cell, the gonadotroph, releases FSH as well as LH upon exposure to GnRH. FSH is a glycoprotein with a unique β subunit and an α subunit identical to α-LH.[97] β-FSH contains 118 amino acids (or 108, according to some investigators). Posttranslational processing alters several properties of this molecule in an analogous fashion to processing of LH. The amount of carbohydrate introduced into its structure alters its intrinsic biologic activity, rapidity of clearance from the peripheral circulation, and ability to be recognized by RIA. The androgen depletion state associated with long-standing hypogonadism, the readministration of androgens, or therapy with estrogens can modulate the degree of posttranscriptional processing by the pituitary. Circulating FSH molecules are modified, as a result, so as to exert altered effects on gonadal stimulation. This process provides a potentially important regulatory step in controlling the male reproductive process.

Under a variety of circumstances, the amount of FSH released in proportion to that of LH increases. Mechanisms for controlling specific modulation of the amount of FSH released must, therefore, exist. As theorized by Franchimont et al., the gonadotroph releases FSH preferentially when exposed to minimal amounts of GnRH.[184] For example, fetal pituitary cultures secrete a predominance of FSH in the absence of GnRH in vitro.[185] FSH secretion predominates in a variety of clinical conditions characterized by reduced GnRH secretion, such as early puberty, hypothalamic amenorrhea, anorexia nervosa, and hyperprolactinemia.[186]

The frequency of GnRH pulses can also alter the amount of FSH secreted relative to that of LH.[187,187a] Administration of the same total dose of GnRH but in pulses every 3 h rather than every hour caused a twofold rise in FSH level without altering LH levels in men with isolated gonadotropin deficiency.[187] Generation of low-frequency GnRH pulses in monkeys also produces higher FSH than LH plasma levels.[188] High-frequency GnRH pulses, on the other hand, decrease the FSH/LH ratio.

The exposure of the pituitary to inhibin also alters the proportion of FSH/LH released in response to GnRH.[184] In culture, pituitary cells exhibit a dose-dependent decrease in FSH but not LH released in response to purified inhibin preparations.

After release into the circulation, FSH is cleared by the liver, kidneys, and other sites. Metabolic clearance rates (MCR) of 14 ml/min are found in premenopausal women, but have not yet been measured in men.[189,190] FSH production rates calculated from this MCR and mean plasma levels of 10 to 20 mIU/ml equal 140 to 280 IU per day. Approximately 5 percent of secreted FSH appears in the urine as immunologically detectable hormone (i.e., 5 to 20 IU per day).[113] The remainder is degraded in the liver and kidneys and at other sites. The half-life of FSH in plasma is markedly prolonged compared to that of LH. The first-phase half-life is 3.9 h and the second-phase half-life, 70.4 h.[111] Because the half-life of FSH is longer than that of LH in plasma, pulsatile FSH secretion is difficult to discern. With each secretory pulse, a small amount of newly released FSH enters a large, slowly turning-over pool of plasma FSH.[97] In contrast, newly secreted LH is added to a small, rapidly turning-over pool. Based upon these phenomena, LH pulses are readily apparent, whereas FSH pulses are less obvious. Under certain circumstances, pulsatile FSH secretion can be easily documented. With pulses of GnRH of high magnitude, discrete FSH secretory episodes can be observed.[70] As would be predicted, the concordance of FSH with LH pulses increases as LH pulse amplitude (and amount of GnRH released) increases.[70]

TESTIS

FSH binds to specific receptors located in the Sertoli cell.[191] The typical sequence of receptor binding, adenylate cyclase activation, stimulation of cyclic AMP, binding to the regulatory subunit, activation of the catalytic subunit, and protein phosphorylation occurs as for the other polypeptide hormones.[141] FSH induces increased synthesis and secretion of several Sertoli cell proteins. The best characterized is ABP, the intratesticular analogue of the plasma protein TeBG, with which it shares many amino acid homologies.[141,142,192] In the rodent, ABP is a dimeric glycoprotein of known amino acid sequence[192a] containing H and L monomers of molecular weights 45,000 and 41,000, respectively. Human ABP is similar, with monomers called *form 1,* which does not bind to concanavalin A, and *form 2,* a glycopeptide which does. Extensive physiologic studies in the rodent indicate that ABP synthesis is controlled by both FSH and testosterone.[141] ABP requires FSH for initial synthesis, but ABP levels can be maintained by high androgen concentrations after induction.

ABP is secreted into the seminiferous tubular lumen and travels by fluid flow to the epididymis; there, it is actively concentrated.[193] ABP has been suggested to play a physiologic role in maintaining high local testosterone concentrations in the seminiferous tubular compartment and epididymis, but this hypothesis has not been substantiated. In the rodent, ABP is also secreted into the peripheral plasma,[194] but this has not yet been demonstrated in men.[192]

Inhibin represents another well-studied Sertoli cell protein. Its activity is currently detected by its ability to inhibit FSH content or release in pituitary cell cultures.[184] Many other proteins, some of which are identical to serum proteins and others which are not,[141] are also secreted by the Sertoli cells. Two of these, somatomedin C and interleukin 1, serve as mitogens in other tissues and could exert similar effects on seminiferous tubule cells.[194a,194b] The responsiveness of most of these additional proteins to FSH is under study. Only aromatase, however, is known to be FSH-responsive.

The Sertoli cells serve a number of physiologic functions in the germinal cell compartment. These include the maintenance of potassium- and bicarbonate-rich tubular fluid in the seminiferous tubules, phagocytosis of damaged germ cells, regulation of germ cell maturation, and conversion of androgen precursors to estrogens by the action of aromatase.[141]

Control of the process of spermatogenesis is not completely understood at present. Data from studies in animals suggest that FSH is required to *initiate* spermatogenesis and that testosterone in high concentrations can *maintain* this process.[35,36] LH, by stimulating Leydig cells, produces high intratesticular testosterone levels. Testosterone or, alternatively, DHT then acts on the spermatogonia and primary spermatocytes to complete the meiotic divisions. FSH facilitates maturation of spermatids to spermatozoa during the process of spermiogenesis. After initiation of full spermatogenesis by this means, testosterone alone can maintain the process. After hypophysectomy in male monkeys and rats, prolonged administration of testosterone at high dosage can maintain spermatogenesis.[195,196]

How this proposed sequence relates to human physiology is problematic. The congenitally hypogonadotropic male serves as a model to study the initiation of spermatogenesis in patients. Administration of hCG, an LH-like material, stimulates germ cell maturation to the spermatid level but does not lead to production of mature spermatozoa. FSH is necessary to complete the process of spermiogenesis and allow exit of normal amounts of spermatozoa into the ejaculate.[127,197] These observations are consistent with the theories proposed to explain initiation of spermatogenesis in animals.

Another experimental paradigm is used to determine the requirement for *maintenance* of spermatogenesis in men.[198,199] Volunteers receive high doses of exogenous testosterone which inhibits the production of LH and FSH while it is being administered. Separate replacement of exogenous LH or FSH allows quantitative assessment of the effects of these individual gonadotropins on maintenance of spermatogenesis. With physiologic replacement amounts of pure LH, spermatogenesis is rapidly restored, presumably through induction of high intratesticular levels of testosterone. Of interest, FSH alone under these conditions also restores normal spermatogenesis.[198] Thus maintenance of spermatogenesis requires the presence of high intratesticular levels of testosterone and is facilitated by FSH. It should be noted that exogenous testosterone replacement in gonadotropin-deficient patients usually does not support spermatogenesis since high intratesticular concentrations are not maintained as with exogenous LH or hCG.

FEEDBACK CONTROL OF FSH RELEASE

A specific feedback interaction between the germ cell compartment of the testis and FSH was first suggested by isolated FSH elevations observed in syndromes of germ cell failure. Irradiation of the testis in animals or men[200,201] induces germ cell arrest and FSH increments without alterating LH and testosterone levels. Oligospermic males frequently exhibit monotrophic FSH increments.[202] These observations suggest that the germinal cell compartment, and specifically the Sertoli cells, secrete a substance into the peripheral plasma which specifically inhibits FSH. This factor, first called inhibin by McCullagh in 1932,[203] has been purified, sequenced by analysis of its complementary DNA, and tested in a variety of in vivo and in vitro systems.[184,204–204d] It consists of separate α and β subunits connected by a disulfide bridge and has a molecular weight of 32,000. Major homology exists between inhibin and a growth-regulatory peptide called transforming growth factor β (TGF_β). This observation and the fact that androgens stimulate inhibin production[204e] in the testis suggest that inhibin may exert local regulatory effects on spermatogenesis.[204d] Biologic studies, in conjunction with a variety of biochemical experiments, strongly suggest that inhibin functions as a separate regulator of FSH release. Most convincing in this regard are observations in male monkeys bearing arcuate nucleus lesions that ablate the LH pulse generator. Exogenous GnRH can be given by a computerized delivery system to maintain normal GnRH and LH secretion in these animals. Upon castration, these monkeys exhibit a dramatic monotrophic rise in FSH concentration with no demonstrable increase in LH concentration.[173] These and other data support the idea that inhibin exerts a direct inhibitory effect on the pituitary. Additional actions on GnRH synthesis at the hypothalamic level are suggested by other experiments, but the exact significance of these effects is unknown at present. TGF_β, on the other hand, stimulates FSH release by the pituitary but does not appear to be the separate FSH releasing factor postulated by several investigators.[183,204f]

Interactions between the LH-Leydig Cell and FSH-Germ Cell Axes

HYPOTHALAMUS AND PITUITARY

Since GnRH stimulates release of LH as well as FSH, regulation of GnRH affects both the Leydig cell and germ cell axes of the testis (Fig. 16-27). Through inhibition of GnRH release, testosterone and estradiol exert negative feedback effects on FSH as well as on LH at the hypothalamic level.[74] The differential effects of these sex steroids directly at the pituitary level have not yet been clearly delineated. Reports on the effect of testosterone are conflicting: in some studies LH secretion is suppressed to a greater extent than is that of FSH, whereas the converse is observed in other studies.[186] A similar lack of agreement exists regarding the differential effects of estradiol on LH

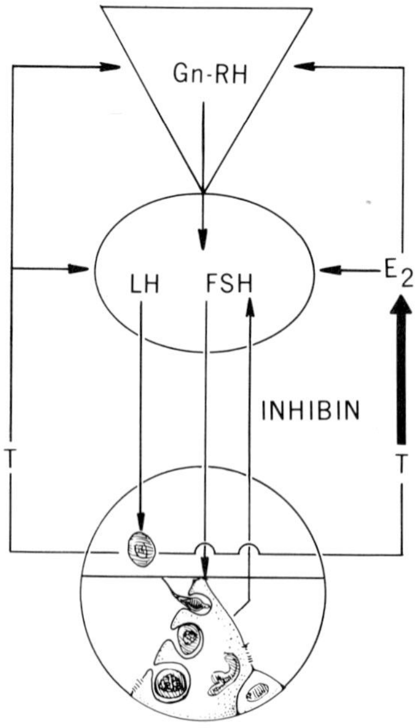

FIGURE 16-27 Integrated control of LH and FSH secretion involving both the Leydig cell and Sertoli cell compartments of the testis. T, testosterone; E_2, estradiol.

and FSH secretion at the pituitary level. Present data, then, indicate that there are multiple interactions between control of the LH-Leydig cell axis and the germ cell-FSH axis. Currently available models should allow further clarification of these interactions.

TESTIS

The germ cell and Leydig cell compartments are contiguous anatomically in order to facilitate local interactions between separate biologic functions, namely, testosterone production and manufacture and release of germ cells (Fig. 16-28). The Leydig cells maintain 100-fold higher testosterone concentrations locally in the testes than in peripheral plasma.[205] This facilitates concentration-dependent diffusion through the limiting blood-Sertoli cell barrier. As noted above, testosterone interacts with FSH to maintain ABP synthesis in the Sertoli cell.[141] While FSH is required to initiate ABP synthesis, large amounts of testosterone can maintain this process, at least in the rodent.[206] Androgen receptors are present in the germinal epithelium to mediate the effects of testosterone. Whether DHT or testosterone itself is the primary mediator of androgenic action on the germinal epithelium remains a matter of controversy.

The germinal cells can also influence Leydig cell function through local regulatory mechanisms. Within the Sertoli cell, sufficient aromatase is present to convert testosterone to estradiol. This enzyme and, thus, local estradiol synthesis are under the control of FSH.[141] Receptors are present in the Leydig cell for estradiol. A current hypothesis suggests that estradiol of Sertoli cell origin diffuses back into the Leydig cells, where it inhibits 17α-hydroxylase and C_{17-20}-lyase and modulates local testosterone production. Leydig cell aromatase may contribute to this process.[99] Support for this hypothesis derives from several observations. Antiestrogens facilitate testosterone synthesis by the Leydig cells and reduce the levels of 17α-hydroxyprogesterone and progesterone which accumulate as a result of estradiol-induced enzymatic blockade. Aromatase inhibitors effect similar alterations, both in vitro and in men receiving hCG for a long period.[99,208] When patients are given high doses of hCG, estradiol concentrations increase out of proportion to those of testosterone; this appears to induce an exaggerated rise in 17α-hydroxyprogesterone concentration.[118–120] In contrast, low-dose hCG administration causes no increase in estradiol concentrations and produces no differential increment of 17α-hydroxyprogesterone levels.[120] Based upon the estradiol inhibition hypothesis, aromatase inhibitors alone have been used to treat men with idiopathic oligospermia.[209] These drugs have also been given to men with isolated gonadotropin deficiency in conjunction with high doses of hCG.[208] Improved spermatogenesis has been observed in some but not all of these studies.

Not all investigators agree with the estradiol inhibition hypothesis. Hypogonadotropic patients given hCG for 4 to 6 months have persistent fourfold increases in estradiol concentration, but no alteration in testosterone biosynthesis.[121]

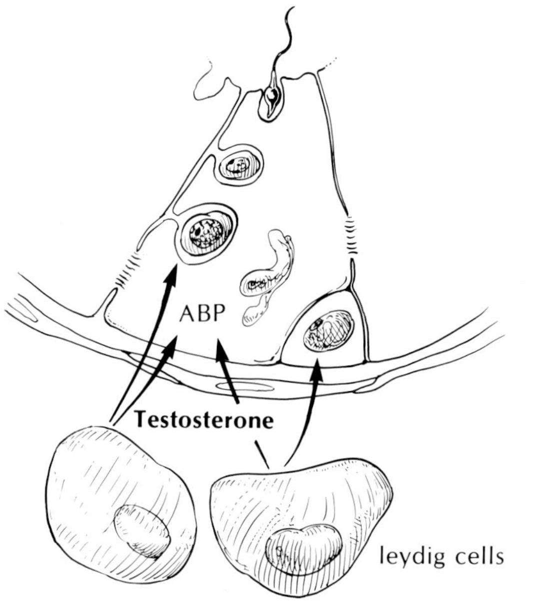

FIGURE 16-28 Diagrammatic representation of the relationship between the seminiferous tubular compartment of the testis and the Leydig cells. Testosterone crosses into the seminiferous tubular compartment where it stimulates spermatogenesis as well as synthesis of androgen-binding protein (ABP).

Prolactin Effects on Male Reproduction

Secretion of prolactin in physiologic amounts is required in animals for maintenance of testosterone biosynthesis. In the prolactin-deficient dwarf mouse, for example, testosterone production is impaired until prolactin is exogenously restored.[210] In men, such a role for prolactin is indicated by several indirect observations. At night, testosterone levels increase in association with prolactin rises whereas LH levels are unchanged. Testosterone but not LH concentration rises after administration of prolactin secretagogues such as haloperidol.[211] Prolactin may also influence the degree of tissue sensitivity to androgens by increasing androgen binding in reproductive tissues.[212]

Pharmacologic amounts of prolactin exert an opposite effect on testosterone synthesis both in men and animals. These actions are mediated primarily at the hypothalamic level. Prolactin inhibits GnRH release by influencing hypothalamic aminergic function.[57] Consequently, LH secretion is reduced and testosterone levels fall. In the clinic, men with prolactin-secreting adenomas and men given drugs such as chlorpromazine on a long-term basis are commonly found to experience these hormonal changes.[213] A direct testicular action of prolactin, while possible, is difficult to demonstrate in men. Prolactin receptors are present in the testes of several species, and perhaps also exist in men.[214,215] However, testosterone responses to hCG are completely normal in men with elevated prolactin levels. This is observed whether the prolactin increments are induced by pharmacologic means or by functioning tumors.[216,217]

Another important effect of prolactin is a reduction in 5α-reductase activity in peripheral tissues.[218] This results in a lower ratio of DHT to testosterone in plasma, both in the unstimulated state and during hCG stimulation.[217,219] Diminished androgenic effects at the tissue level would be expected but have not yet been clearly demonstrated. Hyperprolactinemic men do frequently complain of impotence. This symptom does not respond to testosterone administration until prolactin levels are normalized.[220] Whether this interesting observation can be explained by the 5α-reductase-inhibitory effects of prolactin or other mechanisms is currently unknown.

CLINICAL EVALUATION OF THE HYPOTHALAMIC-PITUITARY-TESTICULAR AXIS

Anatomic and Histologic Assessment

PITUITARY AND HYPOTHALAMUS

Plain skull x-rays or sella tomograms reveal the bony confines of the sella and demonstrate calcification within or above the sella turcica. Erosions of the bony structures produced by expanding tumors or vascular structures are apparent. CT scans with coronal views, particularly during contrast enhancement, provide evidence of lesions of low density or enhancing mass lesions. Nuclear magnetic resonance (NMR) scans can indicate the structural composition of mass lesions but do not yet have sufficient resolution to provide fine structural details. Digital subtraction angiography allows precise definition of vascular relationships between pituitary, hypothalamus, and surrounding structures.

TESTIS AND SURROUNDING STRUCTURES

The epididymis, vas deferens, and testes can be examined by palpation in the scrotal sac. Testis size is assessed by simple measurement of the longitudinal and horizontal axes (normal dimensions are: 4.0 to 5.5 cm long axis, 2.7 to 3.2 cm horizontal axis) or by comparison with a series of ellipsoids of increasing volume (normal volume = 20 to 30 ml) (Table 16-3) using an apparatus called a *Prader orchidometer*.[221] Special techniques of testicular examination must be used under certain circumstances. In boys with pseudocryptorchism or retractile testes, the gonads may only be palpated when the patient exits from a warm bath or assumes a squatting position. Dilatations of veins in the scrotum, a condition called *varicocele*, may only be detected when the patient is upright and performing a Valsalva maneuver.

Special diagnostic tools are available to provide further anatomic information.[222] Pelvic ultrasound can sometimes be of assistance in locating intraabdominal testicular structures in older boys or adults. This may be followed by spermatic venogram in selected cases to detect and delineate the location of cryptorchid testes.[223] Laparoscopy has also been used to detect the vas deferens and testicular structures. The presence of varicocele can be demonstrated by venogram with dye injected into the testicular vein. The vas deferens may be cannulated during surgery and injected with dye (called an *operative vasogram*) to establish patency of the epididymis and vas deferens.

Testis biopsy permits determination of the number of germ cells of each cell type and degree of hyalinization of the seminiferous tubules.[224,225] Determination of germ cell parameters is time-consuming and difficult. Special competence in processing (e.g., use of Cleland's or Buin's fixative rather than formalin) and in quantifying is required. The exact methodology is not standardized. A well-studied technique[224] expresses the number of germ cells as a function of the number of Sertoli cells present (Table 16-4). Biopsy data provide a precise definition of the total number of germ cells, degree of cellular maturation, and amounts of peritubular hyalinization and tubular sclerosis.

Before availability of plasma FSH assays, testis biopsy provided the only information regarding the degree of functional impairment of the spermatogenic

Table 16-3. Assessment of Testicular Size

Method	Prepubertal	Pubertal	Adult
Orchidometer*	1–6	8–15	20–30†
Ruler measurement‡			
Length	1.6–2.9	3.1–4.0	4.1–5.5
Width	1.0–1.8	2.0–2.5	2.7–3.2

*Measured in milliliters.
†24 ± 4 (SD) ml; n=44.
‡Measured in centimeters.
Source: Adapted from Sherins and Howards.[221]

Table 16-4. Abundances of Germinal Cell Components Quantified on Testicular Biopsy*

Cell type	Number/Sertoli cell	Range
Spermatogonia	1.77	1.05–2.83
Preleptotene	0.25	0.06–0.44
Leptotene	0.22	0.08–0.38
Zygotene + pachytene	1.96	1.03–2.86
Sa + Sb spermatids	3.05	1.59–4.87
Sc + Sd spermatids	2.14	1.44–3.63

*Cellular abundance is expressed as number of cells per Sertoli cell in cross sections of seminiferous tubules. Other methods are more practical but considered less precise.[463]
Source: Data adapted from Skakkebaek and Heller.[463]

process. Currently, plasma FSH measurements are also used to assess the amount of testicular damage, as FSH concentration rises with increasing testicular destruction.[202] For this reason, testis biopsy is now used less commonly. However, this procedure may be helpful in distinguishing obstructive azoospermia from idiopathic azoospermia with peritubular hyalinization. With obstruction, normal spermatogenesis is found on biopsy; with idiopathic azoospermia, severe tubular sclerosis and peritubular hyalinization are observed. FSH determination also distinguishes these two groups of patients since those with obstruction exhibit normal FSH levels while those with hyalinization have high titers.[226] Biopsies provide structural correlation with gonadotropin and sex steroid levels in patients with hyper- and hypogonadotropic states. However, this information usually does not influence the choice of specific therapy. Finally, serial biopsies allow assessment of various types of therapy for oligospermia, but their use in this situation is usually investigational. The clinician should be aware that testis biopsy causes a transient but reversible reduction in sperm count.[227]

SPERMATOZOA

Seminal fluid analysis provides information regarding the production of sperm by the testes and patency of the excurrent duct system. Standardized collection involves abstinence from ejaculation for three or more days, submission of the specimen by masturbation into a clean, dry, wide-mouthed container, and completion of sperm counting and other analyses within 2 h of collection. The presence of fructose indicates patency of the excurrent duct system beyond the seminal vesicles. Quantitative analysis of several sperm parameters provides information regarding the process of spermatogenesis. For several reasons, no absolute range exists to distinguish a fertile from an infertile specimen (Table 16-5). The sperm count in multiple specimens from the same subject can vary by an average of 75 percent but may vary more extremely.[228] For example, counts in samples from normal volunteers ranged from 5×10^6/ml to 200×10^6/ml in the same individuals over a 2- to 3-year period.[229] Several recent reports suggest that the mean sperm concentration for normal males has declined to a level below that found in classic studies in the 1940s and 1950s. This conclusion is controversial since in follow-up data from MacLeod and Wang in the 1960s and 1970s sperm counts were identical to those originally reported.[229a] Discordant findings may relate to the rigor with which the investigators insisted upon abstinence in the subjects for 3 days prior to submission of a specimen for analysis; frequent ejaculation significantly lowers total sperm count and can influence other variables as well.[228]

Independently assessed variables such as total sperm count, sperm concentration, percent motility, and percent normal forms covary in the same individual.[230] For example, specimens with decreased sperm counts commonly contain spermatozoa with decreased motility and percent normal forms. Under some circumstances, however, specimens with low counts (as

Table 16-5. Normal Values for Semen Analysis. Data from Five Studies

		Percent of fertile men with normal values				
Parameter	Normal value	MacLeod[464]	Rehan[465]	Nelson[466]	Smith[467] (Phila.)	Smith[467] (Houston)
Sperm concentration	$>20 \times 10^6$/ml	95	93	80	81	70
Total sperm in ejaculate	$>50 \times 10^6$	93	nr*	nr	76	67
Semen volume	>1 ml	97	92	95	nr	nr
Percent motile	>60	90	86	nr	nr	nr

*nr, not reported.

low as 5 × 10^6/ml) can be normal with respect to motility and morphology and, consequently, have high fertilization potential. For these reasons, only general ranges describing relative normality can be given (Table 16-5). It is recommended that a minimum of three samples collected over a 3-month period be obtained. The variability observed in single samples can be minimized by averaging the results from these separate collections.

The functional capability of sperm to fertilize can be examined in vitro with ova penetration tests. Ova from hamsters are stripped of the zona pellucida and incubated with human sperm. The number of sperm penetrating the ova under precisely defined conditions is counted. This measurement correlates with the in vivo fertilizing potential of the semen tested. The variability of methodology, difficulty in performing the test, and the sensitivity of the assessment to alterations in incubation medium have prevented wide application of this test at present.[231]

Assessment of Hormonal Status

BASAL LEVELS

GnRH circulates in plasma in concentrations too low for practical measurement. RIA of native GnRH or its degradative fragments in urine is feasible on an investigational basis but not practical clinically.[232] The pulsatile secretion of LH in plasma introduces an error in estimates from single samples of approximately ± 60 percent.[70] Measurement of LH concentration in a pool of samples taken over 1 h reduces the error by half. Sampling for 3 to 6 h decreases the variability further to 18 and 12 percent, respectively (Fig. 16-29). Because the longer half-life of FSH dampens the episodic fluctuations of the concentration of this gonadotropin compared to LH, fewer samples are required to accurately assess its mean level in plasma. Measuring LH or FSH concentration in timed 3-h (or longer) urine collections allows the kidney to integrate secretory pulses and provides a convenient method of accurately determining gonadotropin levels.[233] When coupled to a concentrating step, these urine techniques provide greater sensitivity in assaying the gonadotropins in states of markedly reduced secretion (Fig. 16-30).

Practical recommendations for gonadotropin assessment based upon cost and precision include either: (1) obtain single measurements of LH and FSH concentrations in plasma; confirm by repeat measurements in a pool of four samples taken at 20-min intervals if the initial level is borderline or clearly abnormal; or (2) measure LH and FSH concentrations in a precisely timed 3-h urine collection.

Research methodology is now available to measure

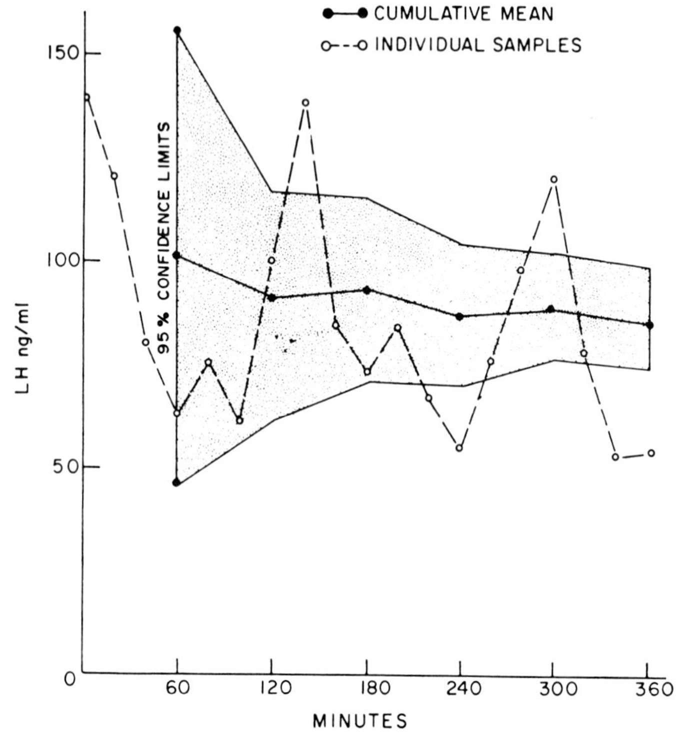

FIGURE 16-29 Solid line and shaded area are cumulative mean LH concentration and 95 percent confidence limits of the mean measured at hourly intervals for 6 h in a single patient. For comparison, dotted lines and open circles represent actual estimates of serum LH concentrations and samples obtained at 20-min intervals. (*From Santen and Bardin.*[70])

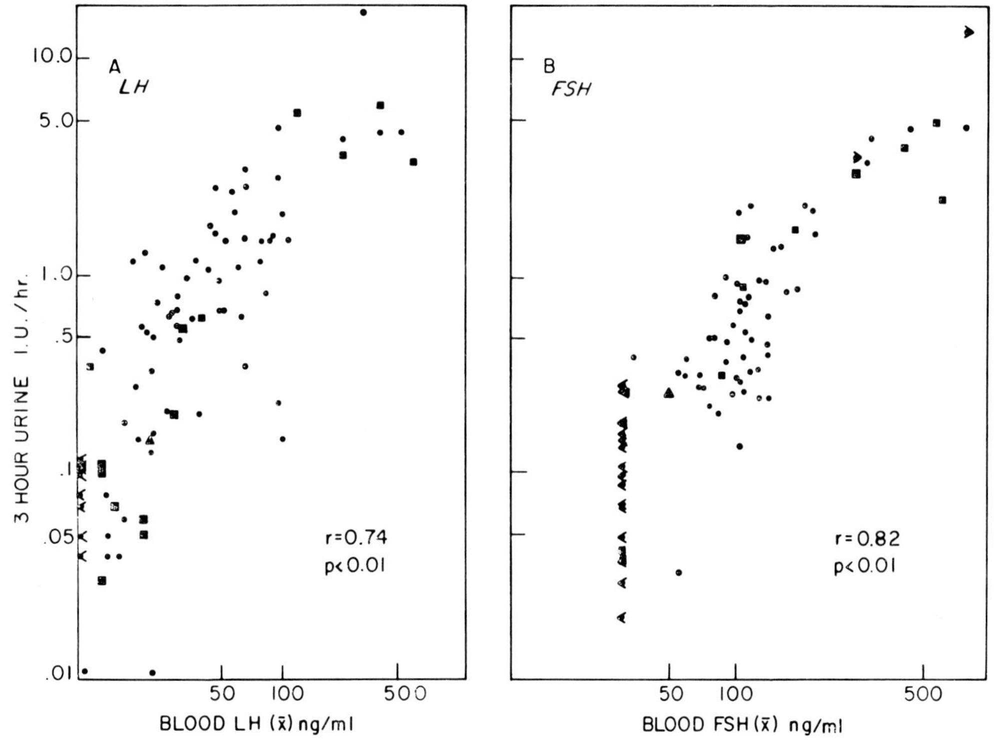

FIGURE 16-30 Correlation of LH levels (*left*) in matched samples of blood and urine; similar correlations of FSH levels (*right*). Arrows indicate samples that fall below (<) or above (>) assay sensitivity. Results indicate that either blood or timed 3-h urine samples may be used to assay basal gonadotropin levels. (*From Kulin et al.*[233] *and Santen and Kulin.*[468])

the biologic rather than immunologic activity of plasma LH. Testosterone production from isolated Leydig cells exposed to LH in vitro serves as the biologic end point. These techniques are highly sensitive and detect properties of the LH molecule other than the antigenic recognition sites which react with antibodies used in RIA systems. Most bioassays detect a greater amount of LH by bioassay than by immunoassay, which results in B/I ratios greater than unity. B/I ratios vary widely, depending on the assays used and upon the physiologic circumstances.[233a] Estimates of B/I ratios have been used to detect qualitative changes in the circulating LH molecule with aging, pubertal maturation, androgen deprivation, and estrogen administration.[100–104]

Measurement of gonadal steroid levels for clinical purposes presents fewer inherent problems than gonadotropin determinations. Assay sensitivity can be easily enhanced where necessary by extracting larger volumes of plasma prior to RIA. The lower amplitude of secretory pulses attenuates the error introduced by single-sample measurements to approximately half that for LH determinations.[132,134] Single samples are usually adequate for clinical assessment of testosterone and DHT levels. Testosterone levels, but not LH and FSH concentrations, vary diurnally; peak concentrations occur between 4 and 8 A.M. and nadir levels between 4 and 8 P.M.[234] Normal ranges should be established using early-morning samples and attempts should be made to collect patient samples at this same time of day. When abnormal values for total testosterone concentration are detected, attention should be directed toward the possibility of TeBG abnormalities (see Fig. 16-19) and free and weakly bound (i.e., non-TeBG-bound) testosterone levels should be specifically determined.

Certain clinical circumstances warrant measurement of concentrations of adrenal androgens. Determination of 17-ketosteroid level has been superseded by measurements of plasma DHEA sulfate concentration for this purpose.

DYNAMIC TESTS

Interruption of the estrogen negative feedback axis with clomiphene citrate (Fig. 16-31) stimulates release of LH and FSH and, secondarily, testosterone and estradiol.[235] Clomiphene is a potent estrogen antag-

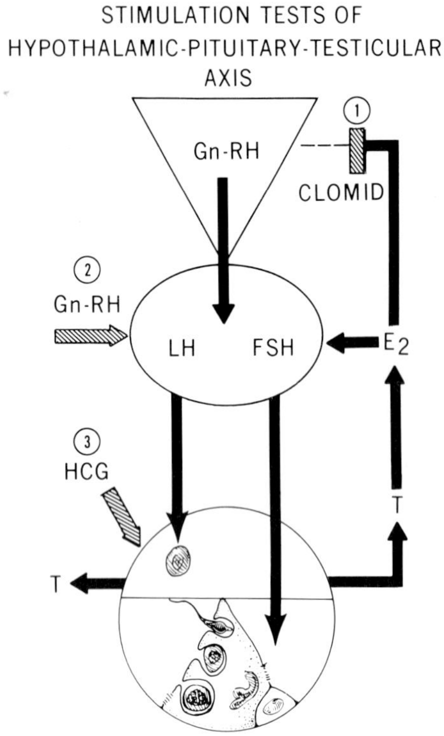

FIGURE 16-31 Diagrammatic representation of sites of action of stimulation tests of the testis: (1) clomiphene citrate, (2) GnRH, (3) hCG. Triangle = hypothalamus, oval = pituitary, circle = Leydig and germ cell compartments of the testis.

onist (and weak agonist) which exerts antiestrogenic effects predominantly at the hypothalamic level. In men, administration of 100 mg daily for 7 days can be used as a provocative test to evaluate the entire hypothalamic-pituitary axis (Fig. 16-32). A 100 percent rise in LH concentration and 50 percent rise in FSH concentration represent mean normal increments observed with this test (Table 16-6). When clomiphene is given over a 6-week period, LH concentration increases further by 200 to 700 percent and FSH by 70 to 360 percent, reaching a plateau at approximately 1 month.

The GnRH test evaluates the functional capacity of the gonadotrophs to release LH and FSH (Fig. 16-32). Two factors influence this response: the number of gonadotrophs present and the priming of these cells by prior exposure to endogenous GnRH. In states of reduced endogenous GnRH secretion, the gonadotrophs are not primed and the response to a single bolus of GnRH is limited. For this reason, use of the GnRH test to distinguish between hypothalamic and pituitary causes of reduced gonadotropin secretion is problematic. Operationally, the test consists of administration of 25 μg of GnRH as a single bolus with three measurements of plasma LH concentration before and three to six measurements after the injection over a 3-h period. Collection of timed 3-h urine samples before and after injection provides another well-defined method.[113] No general agreement exists whether results are best interpreted with respect to peak response, area under the response curve, absolute changes in gonadotropin level, or percent response. As a general guideline, a doubling of LH concentration and a 50 percent increase in FSH concentration would represent minimally normal results (Table 16-6).

A refinement of the GnRH test uses infusion of 0.25 μg of GnRH per min over a 4-h period. This method is based upon physiologic data indicating that polypeptide hormones are secreted in a bimodal fashion. Initially, presynthesized hormone is secreted in response to the initial stimulus; later, a secondary

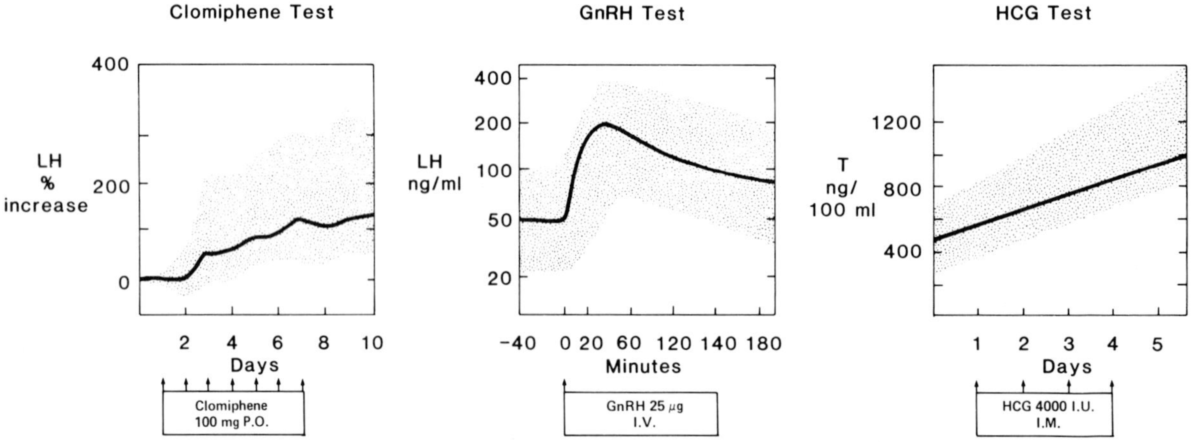

FIGURE 16-32 Mean (solid lines) and ranges (shaded areas) of LH and testosterone concentration increments during clomiphene, GnRH, and hCG stimulation tests. (*Data from Refs.* 78, 177, 235, 268, 468, 469.)

Table 16-6. Normal Basal and Stimulated Hormone Levels

	Basal	Stimulated, mean % increase*		
		Clomiphene	GnRH	hCG
Plasma concentration†				
LH	4–20 mIU/ml	100 (30–400)	450 (50–1200)	
FSH	4–20 mIU/ml	50 (20–200)	70 (9–176)	
Testosterone	300–1200 ng/100 ml	25 (0–65)	0	100 (50–200)
Urinary excretion rate				
LH	500–2500 mIU/h	100 (0–200)	100 (15–200)	
FSH	200–3300 mIU/h	100 (20–180)	63 (30–100)	

*Range of percent increase in parentheses.
†Normal ranges in laboratories that do not use external quality control standards vary.
Test protocols:
Clomiphene: 100 mg clomiphene citrate daily by mouth for 7 days; draw blood sample or collect timed 3-h urine samples before and on day 8.[177,235,468]
GnRH, plasma: 25 μg GnRH IV with collection of blood before and 30, 60, 90, 120 min later.[78,469]
GnRH, urine: 100 μg GnRH IV with collection of timed 3-h urine samples before and after injection.[113]
hCG: 5000 IU hCG IM daily for 4 days; draw blood sample before and on day 5.[268]

mode of release of newly synthesized or processed material occurs.[94]

Direct provocative testing of the testes requires administration of hCG and assessment of plasma testosterone concentration increments at various time intervals (Fig. 16-32). Traditional test procedures use multiple injections on a daily basis; however, recent data indicate that one injection of 1500 to 4000 IU intramuscularly (IM) is a sufficient stimulus.[236] Plasma testosterone concentration is then measured prior to and 5 days after hCG injections. Normal responses vary from a doubling of the initial testosterone level in adult patients to a rise greater than 150 ng/100 ml in prepubertal subjects (Table 16-6). Alternatively, a longer protocol can be used in prepubertal boys, with which testosterone reaches the adult male range after 16 days of stimulation.[237]

Biologic Effects of Sex Steroids on Target Organs

Structural changes of the epiphyseal growth centers in the wrists and hands occur in response to changes in testosterone levels during pubertal maturation. X-rays of these structures allow determination of bone age and provide functional information reflecting prior exposure of these structures to hormonal stimulation. In pubertal and prepubertal subjects, bone age correlates relatively well with the degree of pubertal maturation of the hypothalamus, provided that GH and thyroxine levels are normal.

Genetic Tests

Several disorders of testicular function are associated with abnormalities of chromosomes, particularly of the heterotopic sex chromatin. A number of methods are available to detect chromosomal abnormalities. When two X chromosomes are present, one of these condenses to form a Barr body, a dark-staining inclusion along the nuclear membrane of the cell. Examination of a buccal smear can therefore be used to detect an extra X chromosome in a man. Karyotype analysis of blood lymphocytes, skin fibroblasts, or gonadal tissues provides more definitive information. Special banding stains allow identification of individual chromosomes and portions of them. Special fluorescent stains are available which can identify the Y chromosomes in cells from buccal smears, from metaphase plates, or from meiotic spreads of gonadal tissue. Direct measurement of the H-Y–antigen, a 20,000-dalton protein controlled by the Y chromosome, is now possible.[238] Both RIA and bioassay techniques can quantify this material in plasma or in tissue extracts. These tests are discussed in Chap. 18.

AGE-DEPENDENT PHYSIOLOGIC CHANGES IN TESTICULAR FUNCTION

Prepuberty

During fetal life, hCG of placental origin stimulates testosterone secretion by the testes. Testosterone stimulates wolffian duct development directly; its metabolite DHT induces male differentiation of the external genitalia. Nearer to birth, pituitary LH probably supplants the effects of hCG, allowing achievement of normal penis size and, perhaps, testicular descent.[239] Consequently, congenital LH deficiency is associated with microphallus, a high incidence of cryptorchism, and subtle abnormalities in the morphologic appearance of Leydig cells.

During the first 2 months of life, LH and testosterone levels approach those which occur in adult life.[240] After this brief period, the hypothalamic-pituitary-testicular axis becomes quiescent during childhood, and LH and testosterone levels are low ($<$ 1 mIU/ml and $<$ 20 ng/100 ml, respectively). Testicular size is stable until age 6 and then gradually increases in proportion to somatic growth (Fig. 16-33).[241]

Puberty

The pubertal process begins on average at age 11.0 in boys (95 percent confidence limits, 9.0 to 13.0) with increases in LH, FSH, and testosterone secretion. The first physical evidence of puberty, testicular enlargement, appears approximately 6 months later, when the testes increase to greater than 2.9 cm on the long axis or 6 ml in volume. Once the process begins, pubertal testosterone increments occur relatively rapidly over a 10- to 12-month period and reach levels 20-fold greater than those observed in the prepubertal period.

During puberty, the major testosterone increase occurs during sleep, when simultaneous nocturnal LH and testosterone secretory pulses are observed (Fig. 16-34).[243] With progression into late puberty, the nocturnal LH increments cease but, inexplicably, the diurnal testosterone rhythm persists.

Two mechanisms are proposed to mediate these pubertal changes: (1) altered negative feedback sensitivity of the hypothalamus and pituitary (the *gonadostat* theory) and (2) an altered balance between the stimulatory and inhibitory neuronal pathways in the CNS which control gonadotropin secretion.[242] Various

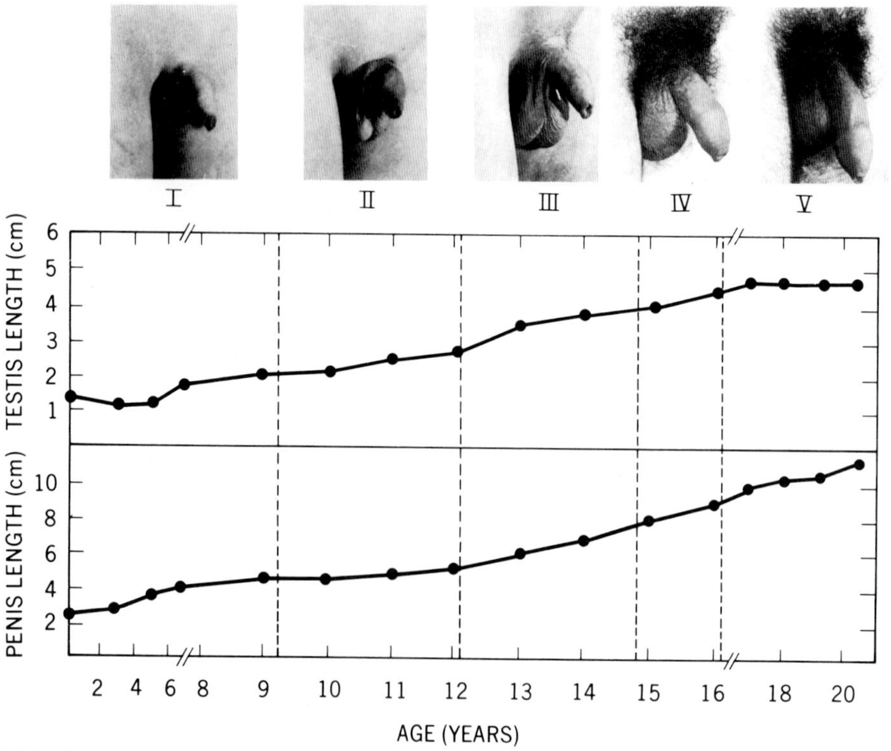

FIGURE 16-33 Hormonal and genital changes during puberty. I to V represent the pubertal stages of Marshall and Tanner.[471] (*From Faiman and Winter.*[241])

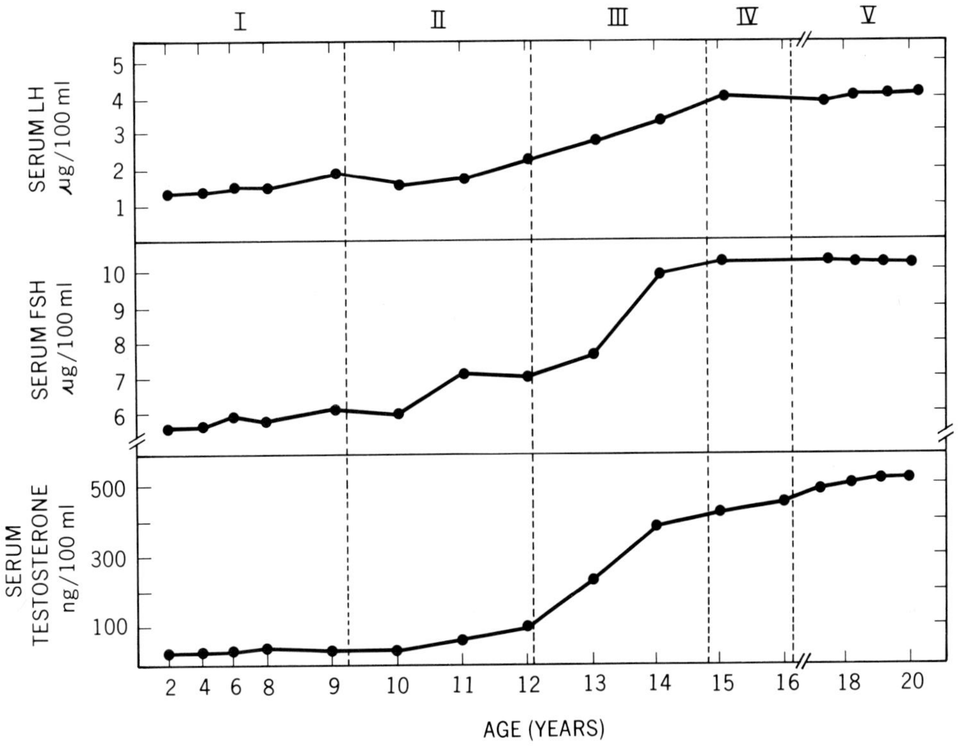

FIGURE 16-33 (*Continued*)

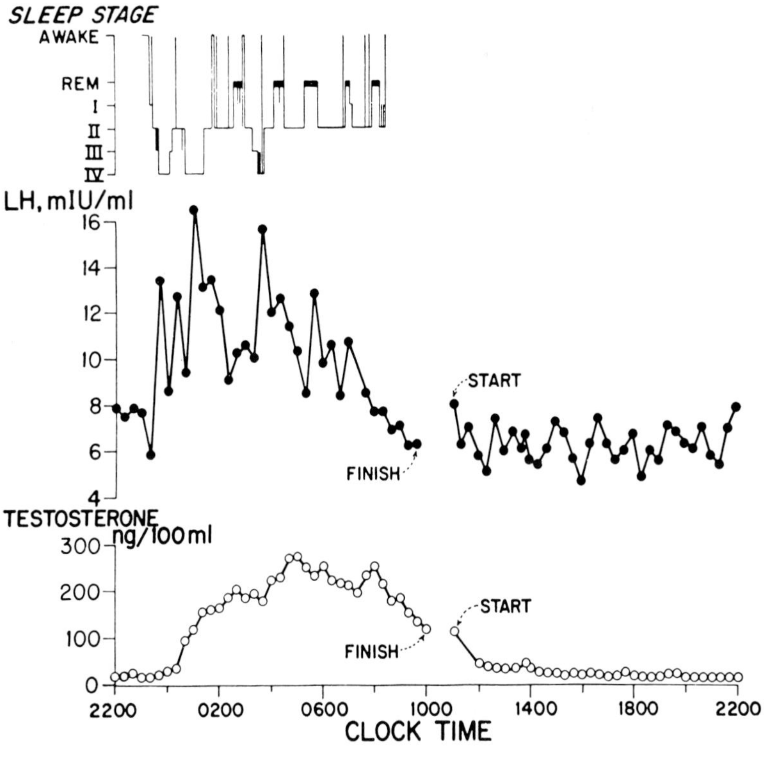

FIGURE 16-34 Levels of LH and testosterone concentration during sleep in a pubertal boy. (*From Boyar et al.*[243])

observations suggest that negative feedback sensitivity to sex steroids gradually decreases during the progression of puberty.[244] Larger amounts of sex steroids are required to inhibit LH and FSH in pubertal as opposed to prepubertal boys. This change in the set point of the negative feedback system (the "gonadostat") would explain gradually rising gonadotropin levels. This theory also explains why clomiphene citrate, a weak estrogen agonist or strong antagonist, inhibits gonadotropin secretion prior to puberty and stimulates it at midpuberty (Fig. 16-35).[245] Prior to puberty, the negative feedback centers are highly sensitive to the estrogenic properties of clomiphene; gonadotropin suppression occurs on clomiphene exposure. Later, these centers are not sufficiently sensitive to the estrogen-agonistic properties and, consequently, respond to the antagonistic actions of clomiphene. Interruption of estradiol negative feedback then stimulates further gonadotropin secretion.

Until recently, the gonadostat theory was considered an adequate explanation for the onset of puberty. However, increments in LH and FSH concentrations are now known to occur in castrated animals and in patients with gonadal dysgenesis at the time of puberty, even though sex steroid levels are negligible and invariant.[242,246] These data suggest that CNS events may be primary and that the pubertal process is mediated by activation of stimulatory neuronal pathways or diminution of inhibitory pathway messages. Brain lesion experiments designed to test this hypothesis are capable of inducing puberty; this supports the possibility that such CNS mechanisms are primary.[247] At present, the broadest perspective favors an interplay between both theories to explain the process of puberty. Thus, a change in the gonadostat probably occurs concomitant to accentuated hypothalamic neural stimulation. Both then interact to mediate pubertal gonadotropin changes.[248]

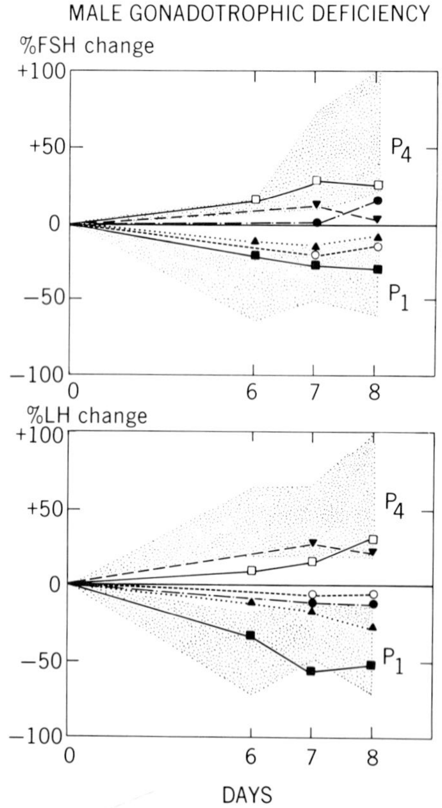

FIGURE 16-35 Percentage changes of plasma LH and FSH concentrations in male hypogonadotropic hypogonadism compared with normal responses to clomiphene (100 mg per day from day 1 to day 7) in prepubertal (P1) and pubertal boys (P4). Shaded area is the normal range. (*From Sizonenko.*[245])

Postpuberty

Following puberty, the hypothalamic-pituitary-testicular axis remains stable until approximately the fourth decade. Thereafter, the efficiency of Leydig cell steroidogenesis declines variably as a function of aging and of illness. The number of Leydig cells measured morphometrically falls from 432 (± 45) million per testis to 243 (± 27) million per testis in men older than 50. Each Leydig cell also decreases in size.[30,249] In general, LH levels gradually rise to compensate for reduced Leydig cell function (Fig. 16-36).[250] Responsiveness to exogenous hCG diminishes, as a reflection of this process.[251] Free testosterone levels are maintained in exceptionally healthy men; in studies of less highly selected subjects they later fall with aging.[250,252] Total testosterone concentration declines to a lesser extent than free testosterone level since TeBG concentration increases with age.[252] The diurnal rise in testosterone concentration which is easily observed in younger men becomes less pronounced.[253-255]

Studies to date have provided heterogeneous findings among different groups of men. Exceptionally healthy older men often compensate completely for testicular dysfunction and can maintain normal free testosterone levels even with far-advanced age.[252] Hospitalized patients and men with chronic illnesses, on the other hand, may exhibit a profound reduction in testosterone biosynthesis and mimic patients with primary testicular failure.[256,257] Although the data are not yet conclusive, the reduction in testosterone levels observed explains, to a degree, the decline in sexual activity of older men.[250,258]

Germ cell function in elderly men has been examined less rigorously.[259] However, in a group of very healthy grandfathers, age 60 to 88, spermatogenesis

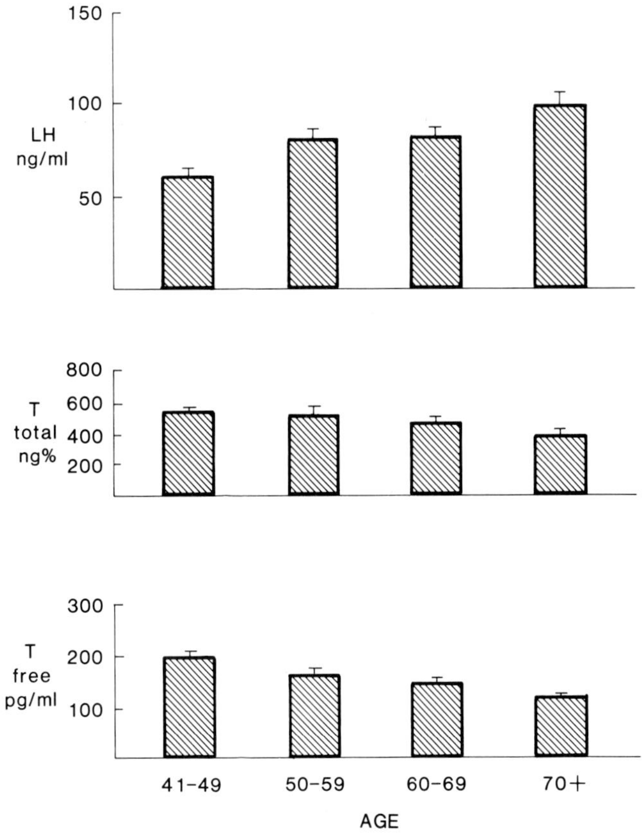

FIGURE 16-36 Age-related changes in LH and total and free testosterone concentrations in normal men. (*Adapted from data of Davidson et al.*[250])

appeared similar to that in young men.[260] Sperm concentration and total sperm output were not reduced in the older men, although percent motility was lower (50 ± 19 percent vs. 68 ± 14 percent). Functional testing in the ova penetration test revealed no abnormality in the grandfathers' sperm.[260] These observations are compatible with antecdotal reports of fertility in healthy men in their eighties; they indicate that infertility is not a corollary of senescence.

CLINICAL DISORDERS

Introduction

Physicians require a logical framework to direct their approach to patients with complaints that can be traced to reproductive dysfunction. A useful classification scheme, which provides a starting point upon which to initiate a rational evaluation, is based upon the functional status of gonadotropin secretion; it delineates hypogonadotropic, hypergonadotropic, and eugonadotropic syndromes. With this conceptual framework, Leydig cell and germinal cell dysfunction, considered separately, can be placed into one of these three categories.

Hypogonadotropic Syndromes

Hypogonadotropic syndromes are classified in Table 16-7 and depicted in Fig. 16-37.

ORGANIC CAUSES

Multiple

Prepubertal patients with multiple trophic hormone deficiencies (hypopituitarism) commonly present with severe growth retardation, whereas older boys present with delayed adolescence. Adults come to medical attention because of impotence, headaches, or visual disturbance. In children, examination of growth charts reveals a flattening of the growth curve as early as the second year of life in some instances or, more commonly, later in childhood. Height is usually retarded more than 3.5 standard deviations (SD) below the mean. A significant reduction in penis size for age

Table 16-7. Classification of Hypogonadotropic Hypogonadism

Organic causes
Multiple trophic hormone deficiencies (hypopituitarism)
Idiopathic
Secondary to tumor
Miscellaneous causes:
Histiocytosis X
Tuberculosis
Sarcoidosis
Collagen vascular diseases
Secondary to hyperprolactinemia
Isolated gonadotropin deficiency
Hypogonadotropic eunuchoidism (Kallmann's syndrome):
Complete
Partial: predominant LH deficiency ("fertile eunuch syndrome")
Variant form (isolated FSH deficiency)
Specific genetic syndromes:
Prader-Labhart-Willi
Laurence-Moon-Biedl
Other rarer disorders
Chronic illness
Malnutrition
Emotional disorders
Liver disease (one subgroup)
Renal disease (one component)
Hemochromatosis
Spinal cord damage
Miscellaneous
Functional cause: physiologic delayed puberty

may be present; this provides a diagnostic clue. In taking the patient's history, symptoms may be uncovered, such as lethargy or hypoglycemia, which suggest deficient secretion of TSH or ACTH. The patient may complain of progressive headache, visual disturbances, or symptoms of diabetes insipidus due to pituitary tumor. Idiopathic hypopituitarism is the most common cause of multiple pituitary hormone deficiencies in childhood or early adolescence. The onset of growth retardation at an early age may be the only feature in evidence of this etiology. Pituitary tumors are common in the adult patient. Specific etiologies include craniopharyngioma or other suprasellar lesions such as pinealoma, dysgerminoma, or glial tumors. A number of miscellaneous disorders which are recognizable by their extrapituitary manifestations may also cause hypogonadotropism (Table 16-7). These include histiocytosis X, tuberculosis, sarcoidosis, and certain collagen vascular diseases with CNS vasculitis.

LH, FSH, and testosterone concentrations are low in patients with each of these etiologies; release of these hormones in response to clomiphene is absent. GnRH produces release of LH and FSH variably, depending upon the degree of pituitary gonadotropin reserve and preexposure to endogenous GnRH from the hypothalamus.

Hyperprolactinemia

Recently, a functional defect in gonadotropin secretion due to elevated prolactin levels has been described as a cause of delayed puberty[261] or of adult-onset hypogonadotropism.[220] A variety of data suggest that prolactin acts upon the hypothalamus to alter aminergic function and thereby inhibit GnRH release.[262] With a small prolactinoma, the major clinical manifestations expected are delayed puberty in children or hypogonadism in adults as a result of gonadotropin deficiency.

Hyperprolactinemia reduces the concentration of 5α-reductase in androgen-dependent tissues.[218] A disproportionate reduction in DHT as opposed to testosterone level may then occur.[217,219] Impotence nearly always occurs. Most men with hyperprolactinemia and hypogonadotropism are found to have large prolactin-secreting pituitary tumors.[220] While this finding could reflect rapid tumor growth rates, it more likely indicates delayed clinical ascertainment: patients with this

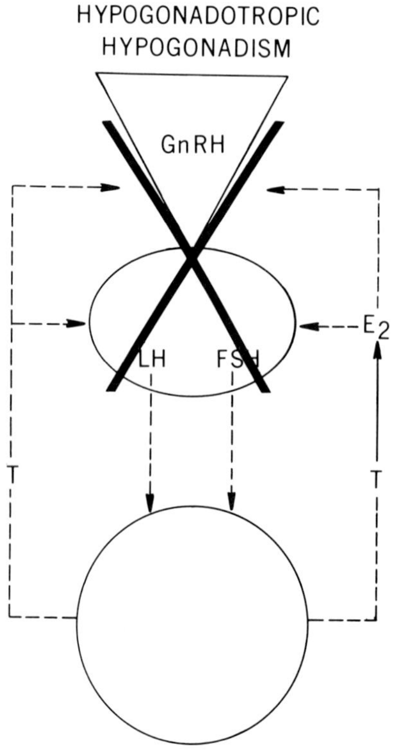

FIGURE 16-37 Diagrammatic representation of hypogonadotropic hypogonadism. Triangle, hypothalamus; oval, pituitary; circle, testis; T, testosterone; E_2, estradiol.

syndrome present late to the physician, often with headaches or visual problems rather than impotence.

Functional causes of hyperprolactinemia also produce hypogonadotropism, impotence, or gynecomastia. Drugs such as the phenothiazines commonly lower LH and testosterone levels in association with prolactin increments.[263] Antihypertensive medications with alpha- or beta-adrenergic or dopamine-blocking properties also produce this syndrome. The reduction of androgen secretion in association with hyperprolactinemia results predominantly from inhibition of GnRH and gonadotropin secretion. Pulsatile administration of GnRH in men with prolactinomas restores normal secretion of both LH and testosterone.[263a] A direct antagonistic effect of prolactin on the testis, a possibility suggested in early studies, is not supported by recent observations of normal hCG responsiveness in hyperprolactinemia of a variety of drug-induced or organic causes.[216,217] The impotence, on the other hand, is multifactorial. Correction of androgen deficiency alone is usually insufficient to relieve this symptom; reduction of prolactin concentration is also necessary. This observation, which suggests that prolactin has a direct role in the erectile process, remains to be explained by rigorous physiologic studies.

A small group of men with oligospermia and unexplained hyperprolactinemia have been reported.[264] A direct effect of prolactin on spermatogenesis in these patients, while possible, is unsupported by convincing evidence.

Evaluation of hypogonadotropism in men with hyperprolactinemia is directed toward identifying the cause or causes of prolactin excess. The associated gonadotropin deficiency may be related to one of three distinct mechanisms: (1) tumoral destruction of the gonadotrophs in the pituitary, (2) disconnection of the pituitary from the hypothalamus due to tumoral compression of the pituitary portal venous system, or (3) aminergic inhibition of GnRH release from the hypothalamus secondary to prolactin excess. Functional testing aids in distinguishing between these possibilities. A response to exogenous GnRH indicates that functional gonadotrophs are present and excludes the possibility of tumoral gonadotroph destruction in these patients. Increments in LH and FSH concentration during the clomiphene test indicate that anatomic integrity of the hypothalamus and pituitary has been preserved and suggest that there is aminergic inhibition of GnRH release.

Isolated Gonadotropin Deficiency

Gonadotropin deficiency without loss of other anterior pituitary hormones results from a number of different genetic disorders. All of the subjects with these conditions present with sexual infantilism or incomplete sexual development.[265] Osteopenia may be present as a result of androgen deficiency.[265a] The specific diagnosis may be made easily if a family history is elicited or if characteristic physical findings are demonstrated. The specific disorders and their associated anomalies are discussed below.

KALLMANN'S SYNDROME *Hypogonadotropic eunuchoidism* or *Kallmann's syndrome* is the most common cause of isolated gonadotropin deficiency; it is inherited either as an autosomal dominant syndrome with relative sex limitation to males[266] or by X-linked autosomal recessive inheritance in other kindreds.[267] This disorder results from a reduction in the secretion of GnRH by the hypothalamus. Abnormalities observed in subjects with this condition (shown in Fig. 16-38)

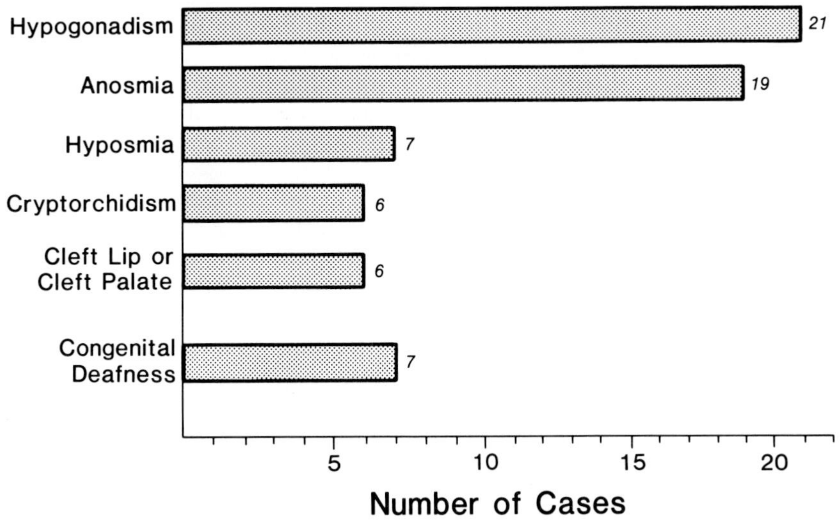

FIGURE 16-38 Frequency of anomalies in patients with Kallmann's syndrome. (*From Santen and Paulsen.*[266])

include hyposmia or anosmia, cryptorchism, cleft lip or cleft palate, and congenital deafness, in addition to the hypogonadism.[266,267] Most of these patients, when of late pubertal age, have eunuchoid proportions, with long arms and legs relative to total height; bone age is usually delayed. This somatic alteration results when the epiphyseal growth centers do not close under the influence of androgen at the appropriate age and long-bone growth continues.

No pathophysiologic distinction can be made at present between subjects with a familial pattern of gonadotropin deficiency and sporadic or nonfamilial forms. It is probably best to consider the familial and sporadic types of isolated gonadotropin deficiency together as a group, even though several discrete disorders may be represented. Clinically, approximately 80 percent of patients have anosmia or hyposmia, a marker specific for Kallmann's syndrome. Those lacking olfactory disorders or a positive family history cannot strictly be considered to have Kallmann's syndrome, but do not substantially differ, clinically, from the others.

The degree of gonadotropin deficiency in patients with Kallmann's syndrome may vary. In the complete form, both FSH and LH levels are low and no evidence of sexual maturation is apparent. With partial deficits, incomplete sexual development results. With partial GnRH deficiency, FSH secretion predominates and germinal cell maturation of the testis proceeds even to late spermatid or spermatozoa formation. These patients have been referred to as "fertile eunuchs," since spermatozoa may be present on testicular biopsy or in the ejaculate.[235] Few of these patients are actually fertile. On clinical examination, the presence of gynecomastia is more frequent in these subjects than in those with complete gonadotropin deficiency. The fertile eunuch syndrome is considered a variant of hypogonadotropic eunuchoidism, since anosmia and other anomalies of the genetic disorder may be present. Another variant, isolated FSH deficiency, has been described.[269] However, even in a well-documented recent case, the exact nature of the defect was unclear.

A large degree of heterogeneity of gonadotropin deficiency exists in patients with Kallmann's syndrome. For this reason, and because plasma gonadotropin assays are relatively insensitive, plasma LH and FSH levels in these patients may overlap the normal range. The degree of heterogeneity is best demonstrated with highly sensitive assays, such as those using concentrates of urine. In a group of 16 subjects with this disorder, basal urinary FSH excretion ranged from 10 to 500 mIU/h (a 50-fold variation), whereas LH excretion varied from 10 to 700 mIU/h (Fig. 16-39). Plasma testosterone concentration was as low as 5 ng/100 ml and as high as 60 ng/100 ml.[248] Heterogeneity in the amplitude and frequency of spontaneous LH pulses has also been observed.[270] Crowley demonstrated a spectrum of patterns of pulsatile LH secretion, ranging from absent LH pulses or only minimal pulses to pulses of normal amplitude but diminished frequency.[270] These latter subjects could be returned to normal testicular function by administration of GnRH episodically at a frequency comparable to that in normal individuals.

The severity of the gonadotropin secretory defect may have practical significance regarding therapy. Subjects with relative preservation of FSH may respond with normal spermatogenesis to treatment with hCG alone. Presumably, a sufficient amount of FSH is present to initiate and complete normal spermatogenesis after intratesticular testosterone levels are normalized by the effects of exogenous LH or hCG. Rowe et al. recently reported that two subjects developed normal spermatogenesis with testosterone treatment alone.[271]

The major problem in diagnosis of isolated gonadotropin deficiency is to differentiate patients with an organic defect from those with physiologic delayed puberty (see below); no definitive test is available to distinguish between these two groups of individuals. Serial measurements of LH and FSH concentrations over a period of several months strongly suggest physiologic delayed puberty if progressive increments in the levels of these hormones are observed (Fig. 16-40).

Demonstration of the nongonadal clinical abnormalities associated with hypogonadotropic eunuchoidism (e.g., anosmia, cleft lip) provides the best means of confirming the diagnosis of Kallmann's syndrome.[266,267] Approximately 80 percent of boys with hypogonadotropic hypogonadism exhibit either anosmia or hyposmia; therefore, this clinical finding is useful.[266] Precise determination of olfactory threshold may be accomplished using serial dilutions of thiophene, pyridine, and nitrobenzene.[272] Alternatively, a scratch, sniff, and smell test developed by Doty et al.[273] has been found to be clinically useful. If no associated congenital anomalies are present, the only definitive means of making the diagnosis of hypogonadotropic eunuchoidism may be to wait until the patient is older than 18 to 20 years of age, when most boys with physiologic delay will have undergone pubertal changes. It should be kept in mind, however, that some patients undergo spontaneous puberty even after age 20 (Fig. 16-41).

It was originally hoped that the gonadotropin response to GnRH might allow earlier differentiation between subjects with physiologic delay of puberty and those with isolated gonadotropin deficiency.

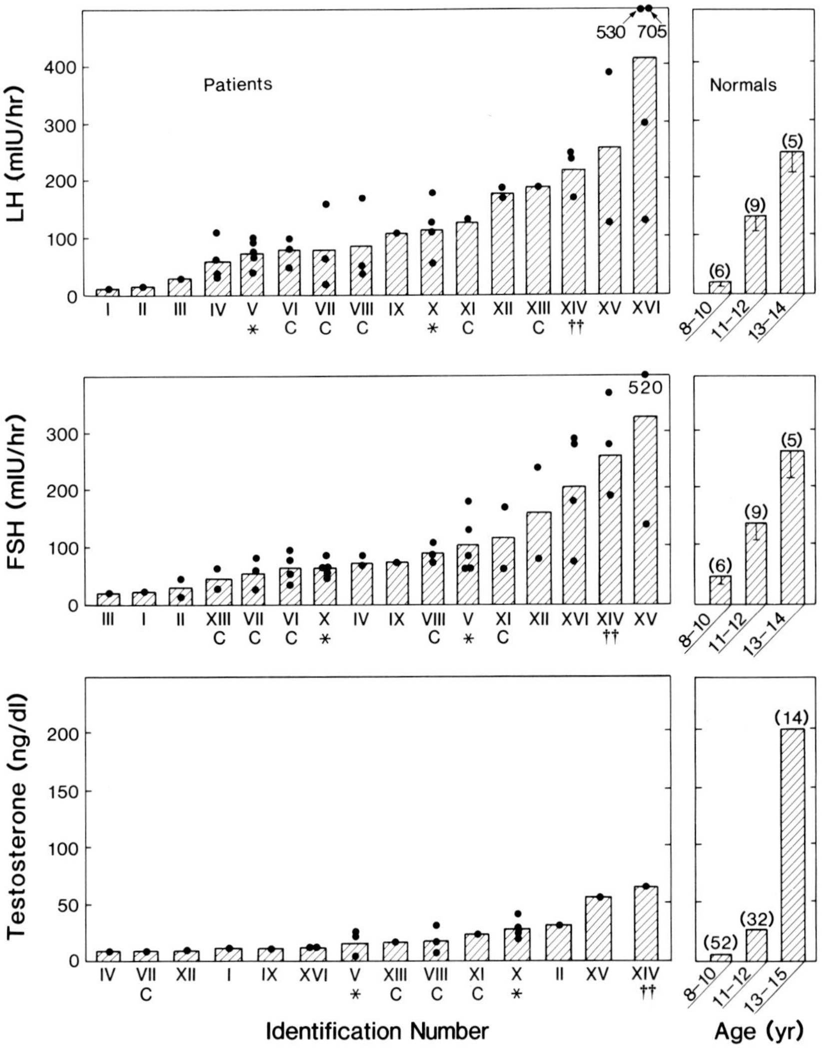

FIGURE 16-39 (*Top*) Levels of urinary LH were ranked according to increased concentration in subjects 1 to 16 with hypogonadotropic hypogonadism. Circles represent separate determinations; height of bar indicates mean level. For comparison (*middle, bottom*), levels of urinary FSH and plasma testosterone are shown. *, Testis size, 2.0 to 2.5 cm on the long axis, all others less than 2.0 cm; C, unilateral cryptorchism; ††, bilateral cryptorchism. Normal ranges and number of individuals in normal range (in parentheses) shown on right panels for comparison. (*From Santen and Kulin.*[248])

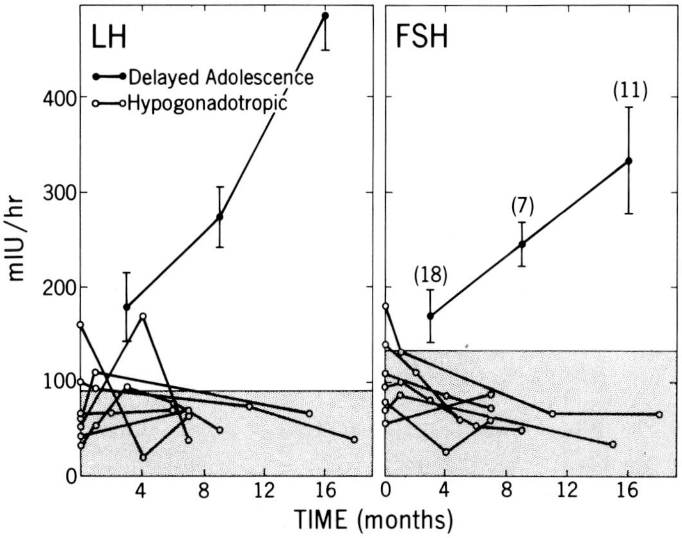

FIGURE 16-40 Sequential gonadotropin changes in 10 boys with constitutionally delayed adolescence and in seven patients with hypogonadotropic hypogonadism followed over a period of 6 to 28 months. Shaded areas indicate normal prepubertal male ranges. (*From Kulin and Santen.*[472])

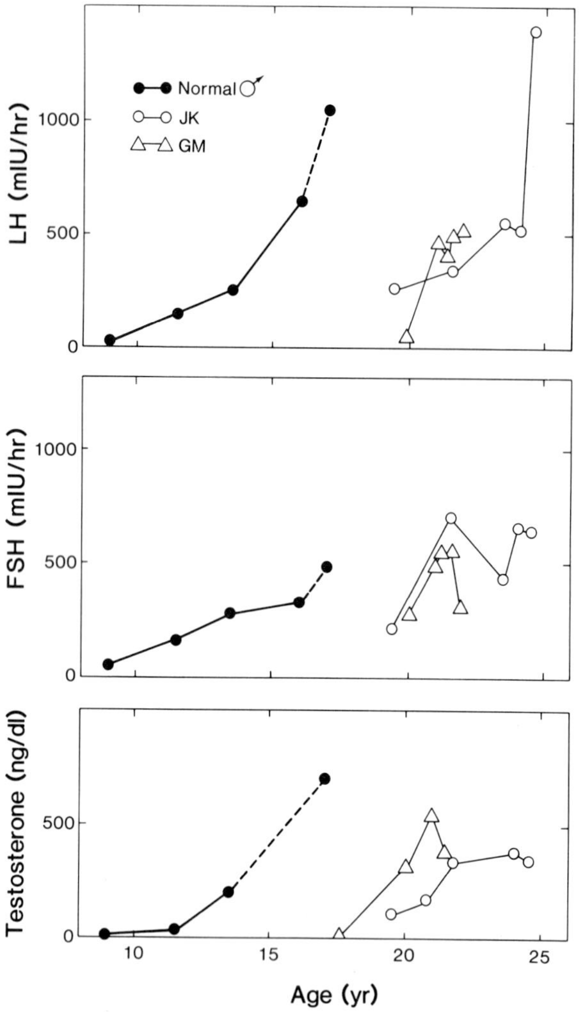

FIGURE 16-41 Urinary LH, urinary FSH, and plasma testosterone levels in two subjects with onset of puberty after age 20. Mean levels in normal males shown by solid line. (*From unpublished data of Santen and Kulin.*)

However, various increments in LH and FSH concentrations have been observed after single injections of GnRH in patients with hypogonadotropic eunuchoidism, particularly in those with the incomplete forms.[274-276] Patients with physiologic delayed puberty, on the other hand, may exhibit diminished responses to GnRH prior to the onset of testicular enlargement. When sexual maturation has progressed, as reflected by testicular enlargement, the LH concentration increments after GnRH stimulation then may become normal. Because of this variability, the overlap between normal boys and those with incomplete hypogonadotropic hypogonadism often makes the short GnRH test difficult to interpret (Fig. 16-42). Under these circumstances, correlation with other clinical parameters and serial clinical and laboratory observations may be necessary.

Other methods of administering GnRH, such as constant infusion over 4 h or intermittent pulses over 1 to 4 days, also produced variable responses in patients with hypogonadotropic eunuchoidism.[277-277c] Bremner et al.[277] observed definite increases in LH and FSH concentrations in some patients, but responses in others varied during GnRH infusion. The pattern of LH secretion was of interest in the boys with hypogonadotropic eunuchoidism. During the first 90 min, LH concentration increments in the responders were similar to those of normal adult men. However, between 90 and 240 min, the values in normal adult subjects and patients with hypogonadotropic eunuchoidism diverged. LH levels in the normal men increased progressively over this period, while stable or decreasing levels were observed in the patients with hypogonadotropic eunuchoidism. The lack of a late-phase rise in LH concentration may reflect lack of priming from prior exposure to endogenous GnRH. Barkan et al. found that responses to intermittent pulses of GnRH over 4 days also varied.[277c] The severity of the underlying GnRH secretory defect correlated with responses observed.

While a normal response to GnRH provides suggestive evidence of hypothalamic maturity, a negative or poor response may be difficult to interpret. Furthermore, the response parameters used have varied widely among different laboratories. Thus, gonadotropin measurements after brief GnRH administration have not allowed the reliable separation of boys with constitutionally delayed adolescence from those with hypogonadotropic eunuchoidism.

Stimulation of the hypothalamic-pituitary axis with clomiphene has also been suggested as a means to differentiate organic from physiologic disorders of sexual maturation. However, both boys with delayed puberty and those with hypogonadotropic eunuchoidism respond to clomiphene similarly, with a paradoxic suppression of LH and FSH concentrations (Fig. 16-35).[235,245] The fall in gonadotropin levels reflects their sensitivity to the minimally estrogenic properties of clomiphene. The combination of GnRH plus clomiphene may provide a provocative test with greater discriminatory ability, but this has not been widely accepted.[277b] Another proposed test involves stimulation of prolactin release with thyrotropin releasing hormone (TRH) or clorpromazine. Patients with physiologic delayed puberty exhibit normal prolactin concentration increments; those with isolated gonadotropin deficiency show blunted responses.[278] However, recent studies indicate that the observed differences are secondary to differences in endogenous androgen secretion: testosterone pretreatment of pa-

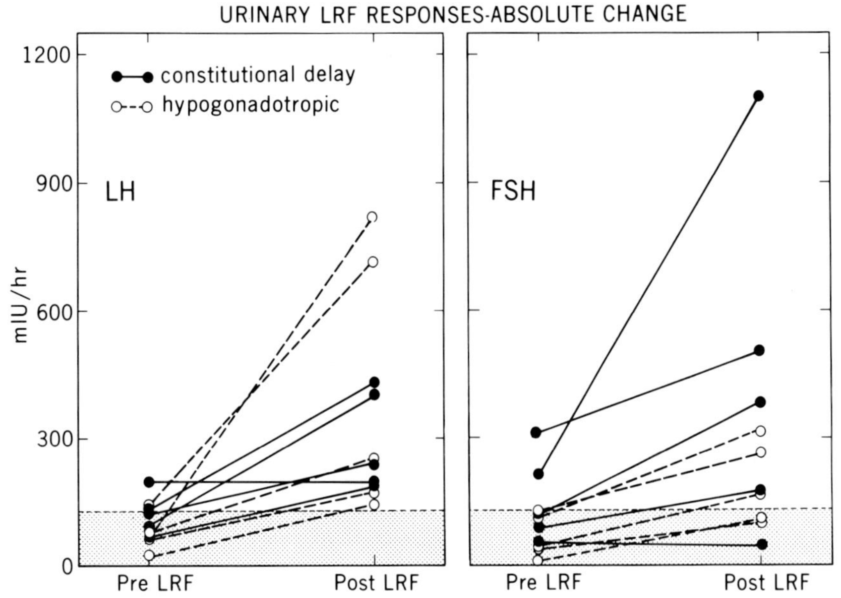

FIGURE 16-42 Response to GnRH in five males with constitutionally delayed adolescence and five with hypogonadotropic hypogonadism. LH and FSH concentrations were determined in urine specimens collected over a 3-h period before and after subcutaneous administration of 100 μg of GnRH. Shaded areas represent normal prepubertal male levels. (*From Kulin and Santen.*[472])

tients with isolated gonadotropin deficiency normalizes their prolactin responses to these stimuli. Because of the varying degrees of gonadotropin deficit in patients with isolated gonadotropin deficiency, these tests of prolactin level do not consistently separate patients with physiologic hypogonadotropism from those with organic hypogonadotropism.[278a]

Initial clinical observations suggested that certain patients with hypogonadotropic eunuchoidism may have Leydig cells that are relatively unresponsive to hCG.[279] This concept has been controversial, since the majority of patients in other series achieved normal testosterone levels if sufficient amounts of hCG were given for 6 to 8 weeks.[280] Recent data indicate that an associated Leydig cell defect is limited to patients with bilateral cryptorchism.[281]

Evaluation of patients with isolated gonadotropin deficiency requires a careful family history to identify other affected family members, many of whom may have hyposmia or anosmia without reproductive dysfunction. Quantitative estimation of olfactory threshold can identify 80 percent of subjects with this disorder. Measurements of LH, FSH, and testosterone concentrations define the degree of deficit. Additional evaluation includes demonstration of normal GH and thyroid function and exclusion of hyperprolactinemia and sellar or parasellar mass lesions. Assay of DHEA sulfate level, as an indicator of adrenal adrenarche, is useful in patients with Kallmann's syndrome. DHEA sulfate levels may be normal in these patients, whereas low levels are found with physiologic delayed puberty or organic lesions of the pituitary.

SPECIFIC GENETIC SYNDROMES WITH PREDOMINANT HYPOGONADOTROPISM *The Prader-Labhart-Willi Syndrome* Prader-Labhart-Willi syndrome[282,283] is an inherited disorder causing hypogonadism (Table 16-8). Boys with this disorder also have hypotonia (especially in infancy), obesity, mental retardation, short stature, and adult-onset diabetes mellitus. The mnemonic "HHHO syndrome" (hypomentia, hypotonia, hypogonadism, obesity) has been applied to this disorder. Other distinguishing features often present include acromicria, micrognathia, strabismus, fish-like or Cupid's-bow mouth, clinodactylism, and absence of auricular cartilage. The degree of hypogonadotropism in this disorder is variable but ranges from partial to severe. Some cases of hypergonadotropic hypogonadism or of diminished responsiveness to hCG have even been recognized.[283] The diagnosis is made by identifying the clinical stigmata of this syndrome and documenting the presence of reduced LH and FSH levels in blood or urine. Recently, a chromosomal defect has been described in a significant proportion of cases.[284] A few older subjects with this disorder have responded to clomiphene citrate with reversal of hypogonadotropism and onset of spontaneous puberty.[285] The pathogenetic mechanism for this response has never been fully explained.

The Laurence-Moon-Biedl Syndrome A rare form of hypogonadotropic hypogonadism called Laurence-Moon-Biedl syndrome is characterized by retinitis pigmentosa, obesity, mental retardation, and polydactylism (Table 16-8).[286] Early reports suggested that

Table 16-8. Clinical Features of Specific Genetic Hypogonadotropic Hypogonadal Syndromes

Prader-Labhart-Willi	Laurence-Moon-Biedl	Multiple lentigines	Rud	Hypogonadotropism/ataxia
Hypomentia	Retinitis pigmentosa	Multiple lentigines	Mental retardation	Cerebellar ataxia
Hypotonia	Obesity	Cardiac defects	Epilepsy	Pes cavus
Short stature	Polydactylism	Hypertelorism	Congenital ichthyosis	Spina bifida
Cupid's-bow mouth	Mental retardation	Short stature		
Diabetes mellitus		Deafness		
Hypogonadism*		Delayed or no puberty		
Obesity		Genital and urologic defects		

*A subset of these patients with hypergonadotropic hypogonadism has been reported.

hypogonadism occurs in about 85 percent of boys with the Laurence-Moon-Biedl syndrome. However, more than half of these patients were less than 15 years of age at diagnosis; examination of older boys revealed only a 50 percent prevalence of hypogonadism.[287] This finding suggests that delayed adolescence is a common feature of this syndrome. In the majority of patients, hypogonadotropic hypogonadism is found, although a minority exhibit primary testicular failure. In prepubertal boys, microphallus, hypospadias, and undescended testes are common. The major manifestations of this syndrome are apparent early in life. Retinal degeneration occurs between 4 and 10 years of age; obesity begins somewhat earlier.[287] Endocrine evaluation reveals low LH, FSH, and testosterone levels and no response to clomiphene. In the majority, the testes secrete testosterone normally in response to exogenous hCG.[288]

Other Syndromes Hypogonadotropic hypogonadism may also be associated with the multiple lentigines syndrome,[289] congenital ichthyosis,[290] Rud syndrome[290] and cerebellar ataxia.[291] Diagnosis of these disorders is made by recognizing the associated congenital anomalies (Table 16-8). A wide variety of other inherited disorders are associated with hypogonadotropic hypogonadism. The list is encyclopedic; the features cannot be systematically recalled by most clinicians. The approach suggested is to consult the compendium of genetic disorders written by Rimoin and Schimke[292] when unusual congenital malformations are noted in a patient with hypogonadism.[292]

Chronic Illnesses

SEVERE MALNUTRITION Any systemic illness of sufficient severity may cause hypogonadism in the adult.[292a] Severe malnutrition is a major unifying feature linking each of these disorders.[293,293a,293b] Studies in male primates suggest there is a defect in GnRH release at the level of the hypothalamic pulse generator during restricted food intake.[293c] Intestinal disease which produces weight loss or frank malabsorption may be associated with hypogonadotropic hypogonadism. Adolescents are particularly sensitive to the gonadotropin-suppressing effects of systemic illness and weight loss. Recurrent infections, repeated hospitalizations, severe burns, and neoplastic disease may also cause poor growth and delayed pubertal progression through the mechanism of malnutrition.[293b]

EMOTIONAL DISORDERS Adult men with anorexia nervosa present with gonadotropin deficiency and hypogonadism in association with weight loss. In adolescents, psychiatric illness or emotional stress may cause inhibition of gonadotropin secretion and delay the pubertal process. In children, severe psychiatric illness as a cause of delayed puberty is usually not difficult to diagnose. Milder forms of psychological problems, however, may be confirmed only by excluding the presence of organic disease. One variant of this condition appears to be a fear of becoming obese.[294] The mechanism underlying each of these forms of hypogonadotropism appears to be a reduction in GnRH secretion as a reflection of hypothalamic dysfunction.

LIVER DISEASE Hypogonadism, gynecomastia, and testicular atrophy are commonly observed in men with hepatic cirrhosis.[295] One of several different mechanisms may be responsible for these findings. Hypo- and hypergonadotropic subtypes are encountered. In the hypogonadotropic subgroup, LH and FSH levels may be suppressed because of associated malnutrition or because of enhanced aromatization of testosterone to estradiol and increased estrogen negative feedback.[295] The hypergonadotropic group has a form of primary gonadal disease characterized by high LH levels and diminished testosterone response to exogenous hCG. Direct steroidogenesis-inhibiting effects of alcohol on the testes[296] may partially explain this abnormality. Additional effects of alcohol on the liver which increase testosterone metabolic clearance rate may also lower circulating androgen concentrations.

RENAL DISEASE Chronic renal failure is associated with hypogonadism and hyperprolactinemia.[297] Impotence, partially related to the low androgen levels and partially to associated neuropathy and vascular disease, is a common complaint. The pathophysiology of the hypogonadism is complex. A reduced metabolic clearance rate of LH leads to an increased plasma LH concentration in patients with a marked reduction in renal function. A component of primary testicular failure leads to an increase in LH production rate in approximately 20 percent of men. However, the major defect involves hypothalamic dysfunction, which results in relative hypogonadotropism. Administration of the antiestrogen clomiphene citrate stimulates return of gonadotropin and testosterone secretion to normal in these patients, suggesting that an abnormality of negative feedback set point exists.[297]

HEMOCHROMATOSIS Hemochromatosis involves the pituitary; it produces gonadotropin deficiency and hypogonadism. Although testicular involvement is also present, the pituitary defect appears to predominate.[298] Marked iron deposition in the pituitary leads to functional impairment of the gonadotrophs.

SPINAL CORD DAMAGE Injury to the spinal cord induces a variable reduction in testosterone production, resulting in impotence and hypospermatogenesis in more than half of such patients.[299] No close correlation exists between the anatomic level of the injury and decreased testicular function. After the initial insult, malnutrition may be partially responsible for the inhibition of testosterone secretion. The levels of testosterone frequently return to normal after various intervals. Reflex neurogenic factors, disordered scrotal temperature-regulation mechanisms, and other factors may be responsible for the spermatogenic defect. Ejaculatory potential is lost, particularly with extensive lesions between the sixth thoracic and third lumbar vertebrae. In these subjects, retrograde ejaculation may be observed. In one study, only 7 percent of 84 patients could produce a semen specimen.[300]

Miscellaneous

In children, hypothyroidism or glucocorticoid excess may cause delayed growth and subsequent delayed adolescence. The latter may be iatrogenic; the administration of glucocorticoids for a variety of illnesses is a well-known cause of growth suppression in children. In adults, Cushing's syndrome and glucocorticoid administration are associated with reduced testosterone levels. Both central and direct gonadal effects of glucocorticoids are involved.[300a–300d] Autoimmune hypophysitis may also cause isolated gonadotropin deficiency.[300e]

PHYSIOLOGIC DELAYED PUBERTY (CONSTITUTIONAL DELAY)

Physiologic delayed puberty is a common disorder which often appears to be familial but may occur sporadically. From an early age, boys with this disorder lag 1 to 3 years behind their peers in growth and bone age; they may fall as low as the first percentile on growth charts. The diagnosis is suspected in a short, adolescent boy with no significant testicular enlargement whose father, brothers, or cousins initiated puberty between the ages of 14 and 18. In some instances, no family history can be elicited. The absence of hyposmia, anosmia, cryptorchism, or other congenital anomalies supports the diagnosis of physiologic delay. Retardation in bone age and/or height to more than 3.5 SD below the mean raises the possibility that there is an organic cause for delayed puberty. Additionally, clinical evidence of GH, thyroxine, or cortisol deficiency by history or physical examination points to organic rather than physiologic causes of delayed sexual maturation.

The major problem in diagnosis is the differentiation of boys with physiologic delayed puberty from those with complete or incomplete forms of hypogonadotropic eunuchoidism. There is no definitive means of establishing the diagnosis of delayed puberty other than prolonged observation. With physiologic delay, the pubertal process may occasionally be initiated as late as age 20 to 24 (Fig. 16-41).

Since it is inappropriate to withhold treatment until late in the teenage period, major efforts have been made to develop functional tests to identify the patients who will ultimately undergo sexual development. No definitive methods to make this distinction currently exist (see Kallmann's Syndrome, above). Progressive increments in gonadotropin titers over a period of months point to physiologic delayed adolescence rather than organic hypogonadotropic hypogonadism (Fig. 16-40). A clearly pubertal response to GnRH favors physiologic delay, although caution must be advised regarding definitive conclusions from this test.

Table 16-9. Classification of Hypergonadotropic Hypogonadism

Gonadal defects	
Genetic:	
	Klinefelter's syndrome
	Myotonic dystrophy
	Male Turner's syndrome
	XYY syndrome
	Down's syndrome
	Miscellaneous
Anatomic: functional prepubertal castrate	
Gonadal toxin-induced:	
	Drugs
	Ionizing radiation
Enzymatic:	
	17α-hydroxylase deficiency
	17-ketoreductase deficiency
Viral: Mumps orchitis	
Geronotologic	
Hormone resistance	
Androgen insensitivity	
LH resistance	

Hypergonadotropic Hypogonadism

OVERVIEW

Primary disorders of testicular function result in incomplete sexual maturation and hypogonadism (Table 16-9, Fig. 16-43). Demonstration of hypergonadotropism allows this group of patients to be differentiated from those with hypothalamic-pituitary disorders in whom gonadotropin secretion is diminished. The clinical presentation differs, depending on the patient's age. In boys, the defect in testosterone secretion is often partial; androgen-related somatic changes occur at puberty but are incomplete. Testicular growth is diminished because of the dysgenetic nature of the gonad. The gynecomastia which frequently develops during puberty is more severe than that observed in normal boys. In adults, testicular failure produces impotence as an early symptom; loss of secondary sex characteristics occurs later, often taking 5 to 10 years to develop.

GENETIC DISORDERS

Klinefelter's Syndrome

Klinefelter's syndrome, the most common disorder causing male hypogonadism, is defined as a type of testicular dysgenesis characterized by the presence of one or more supernumerary X chromosomes (Table 16-10). Classic and variant forms have been described. The classic (XXY) form occurs in approximately 1/500 males (0.21 percent of infants, 0.15 to 0.24 percent of adults).[229,301] This disorder is highly suspect in an adult with firm testes < 2.0 cm in length who has clinical signs of androgen deficiency of variable degree. Gynecomastia occurs in 85 percent of patients. The arm span is usually > 2 cm longer than the patient's height and the floor-to-pubis length is usually 2 cm greater than the distance from the pubis to the crown of the head. These disproportionate body measurements are called *eunuchoidal proportions.* It is a common misconception that short stature is associated with Klinefelter's syndrome; in general, these patients are of normal stature or tall. Large prospective surveys show that mean intelligence test scores and educational level achieved are lower in men with Klinefelter's syndrome compared to controls of similar age.[302] A slightly increased proportion of Klinefelter's subjects may have frankly subnormal intelligence;[303] however, case selection methods may bias these results toward identification of a greater number of patients of subnormal intelligence than occurs among the general population. Personality disorders are reported to occur more commonly in men with Klinefelter's syndrome than in the normal population. This finding could be ascribed to the problems encountered in adjusting to androgen deficiency and altered physical

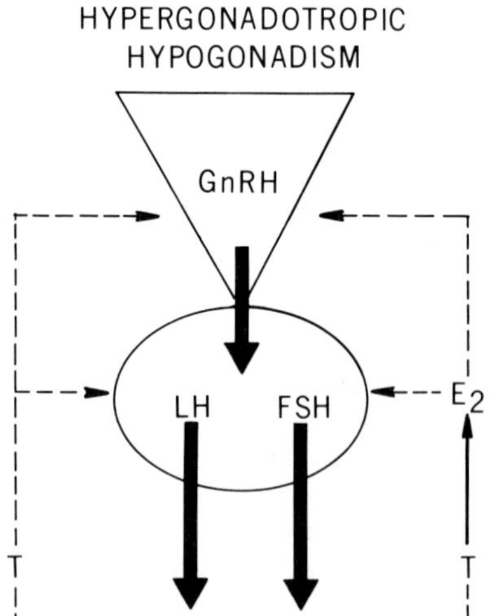

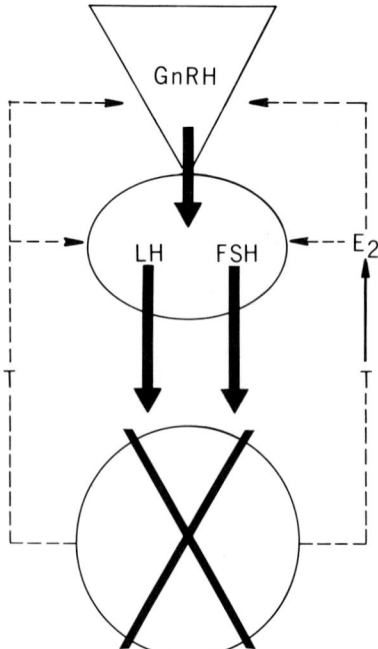

FIGURE 16-43 Diagrammatic representation of hypergonadotropic hypogonadism. Triangle, hypothalamus; oval, pituitary; circle, testis; T, testosterone; E_2, estradiol.

Table 16-10. Features of Klinefelter's Syndrome

Parameter	Classic form (XXY)	Variant forms* XX	Mosaic forms	Poly X + Y
Incidence	1/500	1/9000	Unknown	Unknown
Clinical features	Testes <2 cm and firm Eunuchoidal proportions Gynecomastia Personality disorder Androgen deficiency of variable degree	Shorter in stature Hypospadias	Testes may be normal-sized	Increased incidence of cryptorchism Radioulnar synostosis
Laboratory determinations	LH elevated FSH extremely elevated Testosterone lowered (in 50%) Barr body present			
Karyotype	47, XXY	46, XX	XXY/XY; XXY/XX	XXXY, XXXXY, XXXXXY
Spermatogenesis	Azoospermia		Impairment less severe	
Testis biopsy	Hyalinized tubules Relative Leydig cell hyperplasia		Less severe damage	

*Only divergent features are listed. (Adapted from Bardin and Paulsen.[229])

habitus or could occur as a primary manifestation of the genetic process.

Patients with this disorder most commonly are detected upon routine physical examination on the basis of small testes. Additional cases are discovered among patients with azoospermia (i.e., complete lack of spermatozoa) presenting to infertility clinics. Klinefelter's syndrome patients usually do not seek medical attention because of signs or symptoms of androgen deficiency, even though these features are commonly present. For this reason, the large majority of patients with this common syndrome escape diagnosis.

The exact mechanisms responsible for the testicular dysfunction are inferred from observations in animals. The presence of an extra X chromosome commits the germ cells to a shortened life span. In a variety of animal species as well as in humans, a normal complement of primordial germ cells is present in the fetal testis of XX males, but these die at an accelerated rate during childhood. Consequently, the testes of prepubertal boys with Klinefelter's syndrome are smaller than normal.[304] By adulthood, nearly all patients with classic Klinefelter's syndrome have lost their total complement of germinal cells in the testes. As a consequence, their semen contains no spermatozoa.

The exact mechanism causing the androgen deficiency in Klinefelter's is unknown and the degree of Leydig cell dysfunction is variable. Mean testosterone concentrations in patients with Klinefelter's syndrome as a group are approximately half those in normal men (i.e., 300 ng/100 ml compared to 600 ng/100 ml). However, 43 percent of men in one series had total testosterone levels in the normal (albeit low normal) range.[305] Plasma estradiol concentration, on the other hand, was twofold higher in patients than in control subjects (30 vs. 15 pg/ml).[305] This results from an increased fraction of testosterone converted into estradiol in peripheral tissues (0.60 percent in Klinefelter's syndrome vs. 0.38 percent in normal men).[305] In response to elevated estradiol concentration, plasma TeBG level increases and the fraction of non-TeBG-bound testosterone is reduced. Consequently, some patients with normal total testosterone levels exhibit low free and weakly bound testosterone concentrations.

Variant forms of Klinefelter's syndrome include individuals with a 46,XX karyotype, those with mosaic forms, and those with the poly X (XXX, XXXX, and XXXXX) + Y varieties (Table 16-10). The XX subtype (the "sex reversal syndrome") occurs in 1/9000 men; it mimics the XXY variety in most respects. The XX individuals, however, are shorter (168 ± 1.5 cm) than XXY males (177 ± 0.77 cm) and have a 9 percent incidence of hypospadias.[306] The H-Y–antigen, thought to be the testicular inducer substance, is uniformly present in these individuals. Presumably, the Y chromosomal material in this disorder has translocated to autosomal structures but is present to code for the testicular inducer substance.

The mosaic forms exhibit variable clinical features. Mosaicism may be present in cell lines from all tissues.[229] Supernumerary X cell lines may also exist exclusively in testicular tissue. Testicular biopsy with karyotyping of the testicular fibroblasts is required to diagnose such patients. Variable degrees of spermatogenesis and, occasionally, normal-sized testes may be present in some of these individuals; fertility is possible. Such individuals usually undergo a progressive loss of spermatogenesis, Leydig cell function, and testicular size if followed over time.

In the poly X + Y variant of Klinefelter's syndrome, the incidence of cryptorchism is increased, severe deficits in intellectual function occur, and radio-ulnar synostosis is found.[229]

The diagnosis of Klinefelter's syndrome of any type is presumed when buccal smear analysis reveals Barr bodies in a phenotypic male. Confirmation requires karyotype analysis of blood lymphocytes (commonly) or (rarely) of fibroblasts grown from testicular biopsy specimens. Elevation of plasma FSH concentration always occurs and LH elevation nearly always. Response to exogenous hCG is blunted, indicating that testicular reserve function is decreased.

Testis biopsy reveals peritubular hyalinization, tubular sclerosis, and adenomatous hyperplasia of Leydig cells. The hyperplastic appearance of the Leydig cells is deceiving; it reflects the marked reduction in seminiferous tubular mass with relative preservation of interstitial tissue. In actuality, quantitative morphometric studies reveal a reduced Leydig cell volume.

Treatment consists of counseling regarding the presence of infertility and provision of androgen replacement therapy where clinical circumstances warrant. Individuals with testosterone levels below the range of normal should nearly always be treated with androgen replacement. Individuals with testosterone levels in the low normal range in the face of high LH levels deserve a therapeutic trial of androgen replacement, even though they may not complain of androgen deficiency symptoms. Many of these individuals improve in state of well-being and sexual potency during such therapy. These patients may be considered analogous to subjects with high TSH levels but normal serum thyroxine concentrations (i.e., "compensated hypothyroidism").

Myotonic Dystrophy

Myotonic dystrophy is a familial disorder characterized by cataracts, baldness, muscle weakness, and hypogonadism in 80 percent of affected males. The testes are small and soft, resulting from partial to complete germinal cell destruction. Leydig cell morphology appears normal, but function is compromised and maintained only by secretion of high levels of LH. Testosterone concentration ranges from moderately reduced to low normal. Clinical signs of androgen deficiency vary; they correlate with level of plasma testosterone. FSH concentration was found to be increased in all of 32 patients by Harper et al.[307] Testicular biopsy revealed a range from complete tubular sclerosis and peritubular hyalinization to moderate derangement of spermatogenesis.[308] No treatment exists for the infertility; androgen replacement is available for patients with low testosterone levels.

Male Turner's Syndrome

The clinical association of diminished testicular function and phenotypic stigmata of Turner's syndrome has been called the *male Turner's syndrome.*[309] Clinical findings may include facies typical of Turner's syndrome in girls, webbed neck, short stature, low-set ears, ptosis, shield-like chest, cryptorchism, diminished spermatogenesis, decreased Leydig cell function, cubitus valgus, and cardiovascular anomalies. Also present may be mental retardation, low hairline, small penis, and lymphedema of the hands and feet, particularly at birth.

Diagnosis is made by observing the phenotypic features of Turner's syndrome and associated hypogonadism. Ninety-five percent of these patients have a normal XY karyotype, whereas 5 percent may have an XO cell line, usually as a mosaic form. Gonadotropin levels may be elevated, reflective of a reduction in germ cell or Leydig cell function. Sterility and cryptorchism are common. Testis biopsy reveals only Sertoli cells in the seminiferous tubules of some patients and a moderate reduction in germ cells in others. Treatment consists of androgen replacement when testosterone levels are low and orchiopexy for cryptorchism.

Some investigators divide these patients into two groups: the male Turner's category, who have an XO cell line, and the *Noonan syndrome* group, who have XY cells exclusively. The Noonan group may have severe pulmonic stenosis, mild mental retardation, and an autosomal dominant pattern of familial transmission. Small penis, cryptorchism, and sterility are also prominent in this group.[310] While separation into these two subgroups is open to question, the need for genetic counseling in families of patients with an XY karyotype and autosomal dominant transmission makes the division useful. Additional genetic and endocrine studies are needed for further characterization of these syndromes.

XYY Syndrome

A group of boys characterized by tall stature and severe nodular cystic acne in association with the XYY karyotype has been described. The frequency of the disorder is high; 0.1 to 0.2 percent of live male newborns are found to have this abnormality.[311,312] In adults, the disorder has been identified primarily in prisoners and in mental hospital patients. Early studies recorded aggressive tendencies in affected individuals and suggested that a behavioral effect is exerted by the extra Y chromosome. More recent observations suggest that the mean intelligence and educational level achieved in these patients is lower than in normal controls of the same age.[302] These individuals had a high incidence of convictions for criminal behavior, 45 percent, compared to 9.3 percent in a control group in one study.[302] However, the criminal behavior appears to relate more to the diminished intellectual function and its concomitant male adjustment patterns than to aggressive behavior imparted by the extra Y chromosome.

Endocrine studies reveal normal LH, FSH, and testosterone levels in the majority of these patients and elevated gonadotropin titers in a minority.[313,314] Early observations of increased testosterone excretion in the urine suggested that a higher than normal secretion rate of testosterone exists. However, data from more specific plasma testosterone assays document that testosterone secretion is normal. Numerous case reports of patients with an XYY karyotype with defective sperm production or Leydig cell function have appeared. The actual frequency of these abnormalities among all patients with this karyotype is unknown. The significance of an XYY karyotype in an otherwise normal boy is unclear; caution is advised with respect to alarming the patient or his parents if the diagnosis is made fortuitously on the basis of routine screening.

Down's Syndrome

LH levels are elevated in patients with Down's syndrome even though Leydig cells appear normal on testicular biopsy.[315] A moderate to severe reduction in patterns of all germ cell types, germ cell arrest, and Sertoli cells only can be seen. Peritubular hyalinization is not prominent. FSH level may be normal or elevated.

Miscellaneous Genetic Disorders

A variety of clinical syndromes involve testicular dysfunction as well as systemic manifestations. These entities are usually identified on the basis of their specific nontesticular features. One of these is sickle cell disease, which is associated with low testosterone levels in conjunction with high LH and FSH concentrations and a reduced response to exogenous GnRH.[316] Certain autoimmune disorders are associated with testicular failure and other endocrine deficiency states.[317] The reader is referred to the compendium of syndromes by Rimoin and Schimke[292] for identification of several additional disorders which occur rarely.

FUNCTIONAL PREPUBERTAL CASTRATE SYNDROME (ANORCHIA)

Individuals with functional prepubertal castrate syndrome[318,319] present with signs and symptoms of severe androgen deficiency and lack anatomically demonstrable or functioning testes. The appearance of the external genitalia is normal, with the exception of an empty scrotum. Since testosterone is required for development of the external genitalia during the critical fetal period of 8 to 14 weeks, it is assumed that testes were present at the time of fetal development; testicular degeneration must, then, have occurred at a later time. Bilateral testicular torsion likely explains the loss of testes in most patients with this disorder, but proof is usually lacking. Regardless of etiology, this disorder has been called a variety of names, including the syndrome of "vanishing testes," anorchia, and functional prepubertal castrate syndrome. This disorder may be partial, resulting from incomplete interference with the vascular supply to the testes. This occurs on occasion during bilateral hernia repair or performance of bilateral orchiopexy. Individuals may retain some degree of testicular tissue and ability to secrete testosterone.

Patients with complete anorchia present either with suspected bilateral cryptorchism prior to puberty or with sexual infantilism in the teenage or adult years. Palpation of the scrotum reveals the vas deferens or small masses of tissue consisting of wolffian duct remnants. With gonadtropin assays, elevated levels for age may be documented even in childhood.[320] In the pubertal years, the levels of LH and FSH increase and ultimately reach adult castrate levels in patients with anorchia. The finding of normal gonadotropin levels in a pubertal or adult patient suspected of having anorchia would serve to exclude this condition and prompt a search for cryptorchid testes.

The differential diagnosis between bilateral cryptorchism and anorchia can usually be made at any age by employing the hCG test.[321,322] After 2 to 3 weeks of administration of 1000 to 2000 IU of hCG 3 times per week, patients with functioning testes generally attain adult male testosterone levels whereas those without testes exhibit no increase in testosterone concentration. Exceptions to expected responses exist since patients with isolated gonadotropin deficiency and bilateral cryptorchism exhibit no rise in testosterone concentration for up to 6 weeks of hCG therapy. Cryptorchid testes often descend during this regimen.[322] Abdominal exploration may be avoided in anorchic patients if gonadotropin levels are high, provided that a prepubertal testosterone level is demonstrated and/or response to hCG is absent. Where intermediate responses are found, surgical exploration may still be indicated. Recent experience with laparoscopy indicates that this technique is useful.[222] When a blind-ending vas deferens and vascular structures are clearly seen, laparotomy may then be avoided.

GONADAL TOXINS

Cytotoxic drugs used as treatment of the nephrotic syndrome or of neoplastic diseases commonly produce testicular damage.[323] The alkylating agents are particularly common offenders. Radiation therapy that includes the gonads also results in testicular failure.[324] The degree of damage is more severe if exposure to the toxin occurs during or after puberty rather than before; damage is dependent upon both dose and duration of therapy.[323a] Spermatogenic elements are more sensitive than Leydig cells to radiation therapy or radiomimetic drugs. Consequently, each of these agents may compromise spermatogenesis to a greater extent than androgen production and monotrophic FSH rises may be observed. Radiation doses as low as 15 rads transiently compromise the pool of spermatogonial cells and 600 rads permanently destroys it.[201,325] Permanent Leydig cell dysfunction occurs with doses of 2000 to 3000 rads, as in treatment of lymphoblastic leukemia with testicular involvement.

When potential sterility is discussed with patients about to undergo cytotoxic therapy, the possibility of banking of sperm requires exploration. It should be recognized, however, that recent studies have revealed a high incidence of hypogonadism prior to initiation of therapy in groups of patients with malignant disorders.[326] Defects in both pituitary and gonadal function are encountered which explain their reduction in testosterone levels.

Environmental toxins or habitually abused agents which adversely affect Leydig cell function or spermatogenesis have been insufficiently investigated. Under experimental conditions, marijuana causes a reduction in sperm count and motility;[327] the frequency and severity of the abnormalities produced under uncontrolled conditions are currently unknown. Alcohol also exerts a direct effect on testicular steroidogenesis and may contribute to testicular dysfunction.[296] Industrial hydrocarbon exposure and, particularly, polychlorinated insecticides and dibromochloropropane have been associated with a reduction in sperm count.[328] At present, the clinician should be alert to and suspicious of other possible toxins which have not, as yet, been identified.

ENZYME DEFECTS

Genetic males with complete 17α-hydroxylase and 17-ketosteroid reductase deficiencies[329,330] present as phenotypic females with partial virilization at puberty. However, incomplete defects may result in androgenized males with lack of full pubertal development, hypospadias, and gynecomastia. In the 17α-hydroxylase defect, hypertension and hypokalemia are present because of increased adrenal mineralocorticoid production. Definitive diagnosis is made by demonstration of elevated levels of precursor steroids (i.e., progesterone in the 17α-hydroxylase defect and androstenedione in the 17-ketoreductase defect) during hCG testing. LH and FSH levels are high in these subjects.

VIRAL MUMPS ORCHITIS

In 15 to 25 percent of pubertal or postpubertal subjects, mumps involves the testes and produces a highly painful, inflammatory disorder. Cytoplasmic swelling of interstitial and germ cells progresses to complete germ cell sloughing. After the acute illness subsides, the germ cells gradually degenerate over a period of several years[331] and Leydig cell dysfunction develops. In later years, patients present with symptoms of androgen deficiency or infertility and relate a history of painful orchitis.[332] Gynecomastia and testicular atrophy may be present, as well as clinical evidence of androgen deficiency. Evaluation reveals low testosterone levels, low sperm counts, and high serum or urine LH and FSH concentrations. Testis biopsy specimens appear similar to those seen in Klinefelter's syndrome, with seminiferous tubular hyalinization and relative Leydig cell hyperplasia. The diagnosis is made in a patient with a clinical picture suggesting Klinefelter's syndrome but with a history of mumps and a normal blood cell karyotype. The disorder is treated with androgen replacement. This entity will probably be seen much less frequently in the future due to the advent of the mumps vaccine.

MALE CLIMACTERIC

The hormonal changes associated with aging include both gonadal and pituitary components.[250,258,333–336] In very healthy men, no decrease in the fraction of active testosterone (i.e., free testosterone, free and weakly bound testosterone) occurs and the male climacteric does not exist.[250–252] In other men, particularly those with systemic illnesses, free testosterone levels are lower than in younger men. Decreased sexual function may correlate with these changes.[250,258] Replacement of testosterone may be warranted as a therapeutic trial in highly selected patients after a clear demonstration of low androgen levels. Further study is required for development of clear guidelines in the evaluation and treatment of such patients.

HORMONE RESISTANCE

Androgen Insensitivity

The genetic male with complete insensitivity to androgens presents as a phenotypic female with primary amenorrhea and breast development, the so-called *testicular feminization* syndrome.[301,337] As a manifestation of androgen resistance, these individuals lack facial, axillary, and pubic hair and have female external genitalia. The distal two-thirds of the vagina is well developed but the proximal one-third, the uterus, and the fallopian tubes, are absent. Testosterone, estradiol, and LH levels are high, whereas FSH concentration is normal. Testis biopsy reveals immature germ cells because of the insensitivity to androgen. The Leydig cells are hyperplastic as a result of the elevated LH level and adenomatous clumps may be observed. The androgen resistance may be due to lack of androgen receptors, a defect in receptor function, or an abnormality in the biochemical steps which occur after binding of androgen to its receptor (i.e., postreceptor defect).

Incomplete insensitivity to androgens produces a clinical picture which confronts the physician differently. These patients experience pubertal onset at an appropriate age but usually fail to androgenize completely. Gynecomastia, hypospadias, bifid scrotum, and cryptorchism are common. The degree of androgen resistance ranges from severe to very mild. The disorder in these patients encompasses the entities previously called the syndromes of Rosewater, Dreyfus, Lubs, and Reifenstein.[338–341] Elevated LH levels in such patients reflect resistance to androgens at the hypothalamic-pituitary level.[342] FSH levels are usually normal because adequate amounts of estrogen and, presumably, inhibin are present to exert appropriate negative feedback effects. Testis biopsy reveals a variable picture; complete tubular sclerosis and peritubular hyalinization constitute one extreme and immature germ cells without sclerosis make up the other.

Recently, a group of men with azoospermia were reported to have partial androgen resistance and elevated LH/testosterone ratios.[343–343b] The incidence of this disorder in azoospermic men was found to be 40 percent in one study, but no definite cases were found in two others.[344,344a] The only manifestation of androgen resistance in these men was the reduction in sperm production. If the high prevalence of this disorder is confirmed in multiple studies, azoospermia with androgen resistance will represent the most common clinical syndrome caused by hormone resistance.

Another type of partial androgen resistance results from deficiency of 5α-reductase, which converts testosterone to DHT. These patients exhibit ambiguous genitalia at birth and are usually raised as girls. At puberty, partial virilization with penile growth and increase in muscle mass ensues. Facial hair, acne, and frontal balding are lacking but spermatogenesis is relatively preserved. In primitive cultures, these individuals take on a male role at puberty and adjust well psychologically to masculine behavioral patterns.[345,346]

LH Resistance

LH resistance was first described in the rodent. The predicted findings of elevated LH and low testosterone concentration and unstimulated testes were found.[301] Patients with this disorder exhibit similar features, in addition to sexual immaturity.[347] Secretion of an immunologically recognizable but biologically inactive LH molecule exactly mimics this syndrome. Measurement of LH concentration by bioassay as well as by RIA is required to identify the latter disorder.[348]

Treatment

Approaches to androgen treatment of hypogonadism differ, depending upon the clinical circumstances and desires of the patient (Table 16-11).

DELAYED ADOLESCENCE

Major psychological effects may result from a delay in adolescent sexual development. Precise differentiation of physiologic delayed adolescence from isolated gonadotropin deficiency may not always be possible in boys of pubertal age. These considerations favor empirical treatment in patients over 14 years of age when clinical circumstances warrant. The usual goal of therapy is to initiate androgenic effects with intermittent doses of less than replacement level testosterone (i.e., sufficient to maintain testosterone levels of 100 to 300 ng/100 ml) while observing for spontaneous maturational changes during periods off medication. Three therapeutic modalities are available: GnRH, analogues of LH, or direct androgen replacement.

GnRH treatment is still experimental and is limited to subjects with isolated GnRH deficiency; it requires administration in a pulsatile fashion by a pump

Table 16-11. Approaches to Treatment of Androgen Deficiency

		Treatment modality	
Disorder	Goal of treatment	Drug or hormone administered	Dosage
Delayed adolescence	Short-term maintenance of plasma testosterone concentration at 100–300 ng/100 ml	hCG	1000–4000 IU 1–3 times/wk, IM
		Testosterone enanthate or 17β-cypionate	50–100 mg q 3–4 wk, IM
Adult hypogonadotropic hypogonadism	Long-term maintenance of testosterone levels at 300–1200 ng/100 ml	GnRH*	2–20 μg q 2–3 h, SC
		hCG	1000–4000 IU 1–3 times/wk, IM
		Testosterone enanthate or 17β-cypionate	300 mg q 14–21 days, or 200 mg q 10–17 days, or 100 mg q 5–10 days
Adult hypergonadotropic hypogonadism	Long-term maintenance of testosterone levels at 300–1200 ng/100 ml	Testosterone enanthate or 17β-cypionate	300 mg q 14–21 days, or 200 mg q 10–17 days, or 100 mg q 5–10 days
	Provide subreplacement doses of androgen	Fluoxymesterone	5–10 mg qd, PO
		Methyltestosterone	25 mg qd, by linguet
		Testosterone undecanoate†	40–80 mg tid, PO

*Experimental; requires programmed pump.
†Not available in United States.
Abbreviations: IV, intravenous; IM, intramuscular; PO, peroral; SC, subcutaneous; q, every.

device.[349] Highly purified LH is available only in an investigational setting, whereas its analogue hCG is readily obtainable for routine use. hCG is efficacious in hypogonadotropic syndromes when Leydig cell responsiveness is adequate. Doses of 1000 to 4000 IU two to three times weekly stimulate testosterone secretion, raising testosterone levels into the normal range. This dosage of hCG can be used long-term if desired. Treatment for 3- to 4-month periods, interrupted by equal periods off therapy, is recommended until the diagnosis of organic hypogonadotropism is confirmed and physiologic delayed puberty excluded. Although one group reported better androgenic effects with hCG than with direct administration of androgen, this concept has not been widely accepted.[350] Antibodies to hCG develop but do not usually inhibit efficacy.[351] The major advantage of hCG treatment over direct androgen replacement is that testicular enlargement occurs during hCG treatment. The disadvantages are cost and frequency of administration.

An oral androgen which is fully effective in nontoxic doses is not yet available in the United States. Injectable esters such as testosterone enanthate or testosterone 17β-cypionate provide sustained endogenous androgen replacement. To initiate pubertal changes, 50 to 100 mg is administered IM every 3 to 4 weeks for 3 to 4 months, with cessation for an equal time. The goal is to promote development of secondary sex characteristics and normal linear growth. Evidence of spontaneous pubertal development such as testicular enlargement and increased gonadotropin and testosterone secretion should be sought during the 3 to 4 months off therapy. If no significant progression is noted, several intermittent courses of low-dose testosterone can be administered until spontaneous puberty is initiated or the need for long-term exogenous therapy is confirmed. Provided the doses are kept small, this regimen has no harmful effect on the potential for full somatic growth or subsequent testicular function.

ADULT HYPOGONADOTROPIC HYPOGONADISM

The treatment goal in adult hypogonadotropic hypogonadism is to maintain plasma testosterone levels in the normal adult range (i.e., 300 to 1200 ng/100 ml) over a prolonged period of time. Therapy with exogenous testosterone is usually chosen since this approach does not compromise later potential for fertility (Table 16-11).[351a] If hCG is chosen, 1000 to 4000 IU given IM two to three times per week is required; the exact dosage is established empirically in individual patients by monitoring testosterone concentration (Fig. 16-44). Testicular enlargement can be achieved, but the testes seldom exceed 3.5 cm in length on hCG alone. This approach is expensive, requires frequent injections, and has no advantage over direct androgen replacement therapy, unless fertility is an immediate goal. In that instance, FSH preparations such as Pergonal starting 6 to 12 months after hCG priming may be needed. hCG alone commonly suffices for patients with a postpubertal onset of hypogonadotropism, whereas Pergonal must usually be added in those with a prepubertal onset.[351b] A dose of 10 to 20 IU of Pergonal three times weekly (low-dose therapy) stimulates adequate spermatogenesis for fertility in 90 percent of these patients, whereas the others require 37.5 to 75 IU three times weekly.[351b,352]

HYPERGONADOTROPIC HYPOGONADISM

Direct replacement of androgen provides the only effective therapy in adults with hypergonadotropic hypogonadism and can be used as well in hypogonadotropic patients not immediately desiring to father children.[353] The goal of therapy is, again, to maintain plasma testosterone concentration in the range of 300 to 1200 ng/100 ml. After elapse of sufficient time, full secondary sex characteristics and sexual potency are attained. Testicular enlargement, an effect observed only with gonadotropin therapy, does not occur. Injectable testosterone esters are required for full androgen maintenance. Recent pharmacologic

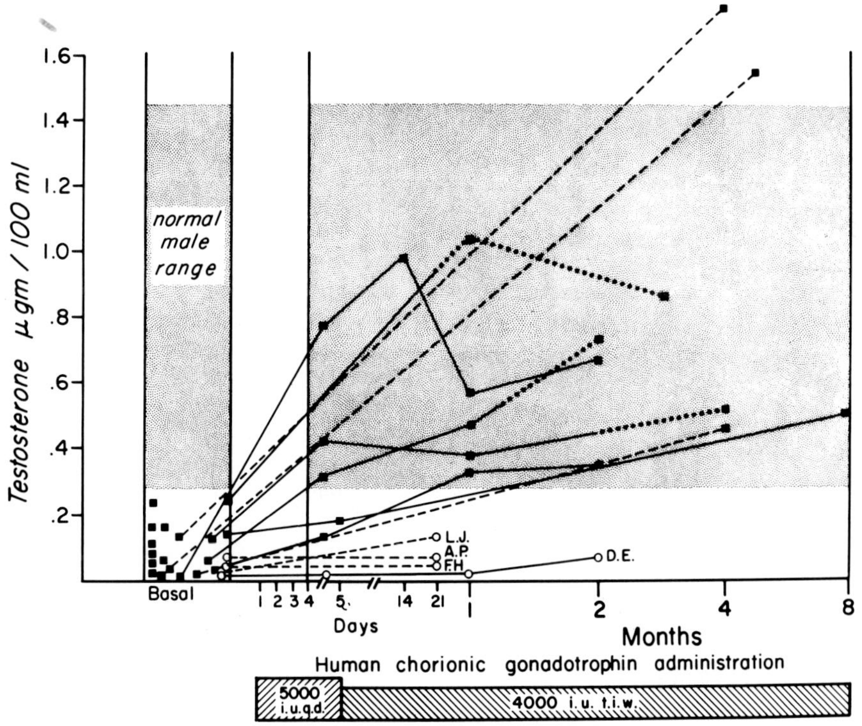

FIGURE 16-44 Basal and stimulated levels of serum testosterone concentration in men with hypogonadotropic hypogonadism. Open circles refer to men with bilateral cryptorchism. Broken lines refer to patients not studied with 4-day hCG stimulation. Dotted lines refer to nonconsecutive observations of serum testosterone concentration. (*From Santen and Paulsen.*[268])

studies fully characterized the profiles of dose response over time for the available agents (Fig. 16-45).[354] Higher doses produce more prolonged effects with the expense of higher peak levels.[353,354] As toxic effects of pharmacologic plasma concentrations of testosterone are quite rare, higher doses are usually chosen to prolong the effect. Suggested regimens include 300 mg of testosterone enanthate or testosterone 17β-cypionate every 14 to 21 days IM, 200 mg every 10 to 17 days, or 100 mg every 5 to 10 days. Measurement of plasma testosterone concentration at the nadir, just prior to the next injection, allows empirical adjustment of dosage. Levels of testosterone below 250 ng/100 ml during therapy can be perceived by certain patients as causing impaired sexual potency or reduced endurance during physical activity. Side effects or toxicity are uncommon. However, an increased hematocrit due to bone marrow stimulation,[355] acne, sleep apnea syndrome,[355a] gynecomastia as a result of aromatization of testosterone to estradiol, or prostatic hypertrophy in the elderly are physiologic consequences of this therapeutic approach. Rarely, hepatic tumors have occurred in patients receiving pharmacologic levels of androgen.[356] Cognizance of these problems and clinical monitoring allow prompt recognition and change of therapy when warranted.[356a]

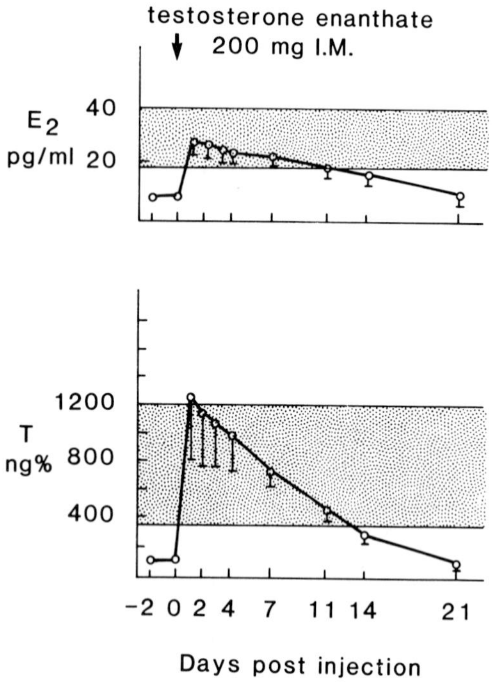

FIGURE 16-45 Testosterone and estradiol levels in hypogonadal subjects after a single dose of testosterone enanthate. (*Adapted from Sokol et al.*[354])

The available oral androgens are insufficiently potent for full androgen replacement at doses compatible with reasonable safety; they are useful, however, for achieving anabolic effects in selected patients. Either fluoxymesterone or methyltestosterone can be used. Testosterone undecanoate, another orally absorbable androgen ester, is not available for use in the United States,[353,353a] but is sufficiently potent for full androgen replacement. Patients should be monitored for development of cholestatic jaundice with liver function tests when receiving fluoxymesterone or methyltestosterone.

GERMINAL CELL FAILURE

Overview

Men with germinal cell failure usually come to medical attention during evaluation for the problem of infertility. If defined as a lack of conception for one year of adequate, unprotected intercourse, infertility occurs in 10 percent of marriages. In 30 to 50 percent of cases, the male partner in an infertile marriage is found to have oligospermia or azoospermia. Appropriate calculations indicate that the prevalence of germinal cell dysfunction in the general population approaches 3 to 5 percent. Thus, on a statistical basis, hypospermatogenesis constitutes one of the most common clinical disorders involving the endocrine glands.

Initial evaluation of the infertile male involves documentation of low sperm counts with at least three semen analyses at monthly intervals. If counts are consistently below 20×10^6 per ml or 50×10^6 total, germinal cell dysfunction should be highly suspected. A workup should then be initiated to identify possible causes. Disorders of germinal cell function can be classified as hypogonadotropic, hypergonadotropic, and eugonadotropic in type. The hypogonadotropic forms produce a clinical picture of Leydig cell dysfunction as well as germinal cell failure; they are best considered under the hypogonadotropic syndromes, discussed above. In contrast, germinal cell failure of the hypergonadotropic and eugonadotropic types produce only subclinical Leydig cell dysfunction and are generally recognized clinically because of infertility rather than testosterone deficiency. The germinal cell dysfunction accompanying cryptorchism is discussed below.

Hypergonadotropic Syndromes

When germinal cell mass or Sertoli cell function is sufficiently reduced, plasma or urinary FSH levels

(Fig. 16-46) increase, often without a compensatory rise in LH concentration. Current theory attributes this monotrophic FSH rise to a reduction in testicular inhibin production with partial interruption of FSH negative feedback.[184] Detailed clinical observations demonstrate an inverse correlation between the remaining germinal cell mass and the level of circulating FSH.[202] An exact relationship between FSH secretion and presence of a specific germinal cell type is not found. Several lines of evidence suggest that FSH secretion may directly correlate with Sertoli cell function and only indirectly with germinal cell maturation.[184,357] Regardless of the exact relationships, the degree of elevation of FSH concentration in plasma can be used as an index of the severity of germinal cell dysfunction.[202] An exaggerated release of FSH in response to GnRH appears to uncover lesser degrees of germinal cell failure.[358,359] Several specific disorders produce monotrophic FSH elevation or disproportionate FSH/LH ratios in association with germinal cell failure.[358-360]

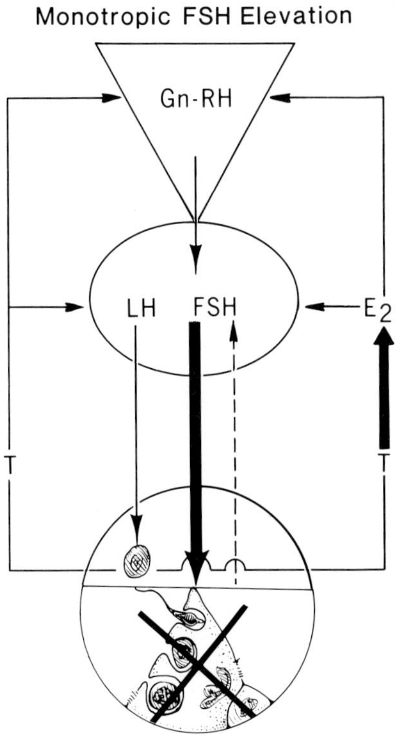

FIGURE 16-46 Diagrammatic representation of monotrophic FSH increments in patients with seminiferous tubular failure. Triangle, hypothalamus; oval, pituitary; circle, testis with Leydig cell and Sertoli cell compartments represented. T, testosterone; E_2, estradiol.

SERTOLI-CELL-ONLY SYNDROME

The Sertoli-cell-only syndrome probably results from multiple causes. It is characterized by a loss of germinal cell elements in the testis with relative preservation of Leydig cell function. Clinical examination reveals normal pubic and axillary hair but small, soft testes averaging 2 to 4 cm on their long axes (volume 10 to 20 ml). FSH levels are uniformly elevated; azoospermia is found on semen analysis. Half of the patients exhibit subclinical Leydig cell dysfunction, characterized by elevated LH concentration with normal or slightly reduced testosterone concentration and blunted response to hCG.[358,359] The seminiferous tubules are slightly reduced in diameter, contain only Sertoli cells, and are not sclerotic in appearance. No peritubular hyalinization is present. The Sertoli and Leydig cells appear normal by light microscopy but on electron microscopy contain minor abnormalities.[361] Occasional normal seminiferous tubules with full germinal cell maturation are seen, but the majority are completely depleted of germinal elements. A definitive diagnosis requires a testicular biopsy and demonstration of markedly depleted germinal cells. No treatment is available for the germinal cell failure. Testosterone replacement rarely is necessary for the subclinical Leydig cell defect.

IDIOPATHIC SEMINIFEROUS TUBULAR FAILURE WITH HYALINIZATION

In a major subgroup of men with oligospermia or azoospermia, no specific cause is found but FSH concentrations are elevated.[202] Testis biopsies reveal hyalinization of the peritubular elements in conjunction with variable degrees of germinal cell loss. Testis size may be reduced to below adult normal limits of 4.0 cm on the long axis or 20 ml. Because serum FSH level generally correlates with the degree of hyalinization and testicular damage, biopsy is usually not performed to establish this diagnosis. No treatment is currently available.

Eugonadotropic Germinal Cell Failure

IDIOPATHIC

Oligospermia or azoospermia of unknown cause may be less severe and associated with normal basal FSH level. Two subtypes have been described: arrest of germinal cell maturation at a specific step or generalized hypospermatogenesis affecting all germinal cell elements. Clinical examination reveals no abnormality; testis size is usually normal. On testis biopsy, only minimal peritubular hyalinization or normal peritubular elements are present. Subclinical hypergonadotropism can be uncovered in approximately 30 percent of these patients by the demonstration of exaggerated FSH (and often LH) increments after administration of exogenous GnRH.[358,359]

Numerous treatments for these patients have been proposed, including: (1) induction of rebound from testosterone or anabolic androgen-induced azoospermia; (2) administration of exogenous gonadotropins or gonadotropin releasing factors; (3) use of clomiphene citrate or tamoxifen to stimulate endogenous gonadotropin secretion; (4) administration of low doses of mesterolone, an oral synthetic androgen; and (5) use of an aromatase inhibitor such as testolactone.[362,363] A general review of available data reveals that sperm count increases in 20 to 40 percent of these patients in association with each of these treatments.[364] Few controlled, randomized trials using a placebo control have been conducted and no study has conclusively established the benefit of these treatments. One recently reported study suggests that a statistically significant effect is exerted only by clomiphene citrate but not by any of the other therapeutic modalities mentioned.[362] Strictly controlled studies of extensively characterized patients will be required to establish that any of the treatment modalities currently available has a role in reversing the deficiency.

VARICOCELE

Incompetence of the left testicular vein or, less commonly, the right results in the formation of dilated veins in the scrotum, a condition called *varicocele.* A series of observations suggests an etiologic association between varicocele and infertility.[221] Varicoceles can be palpated in approximately 40 percent of men with oligo- or azoospermia.[365] Sperm motility is often reduced and a stress pattern of sperm morphology, with increased numbers of immature or tapered forms, is commonly found.[221,366] Sperm from patients with varicocele penetrate into denuded ova from hamsters, as a test of sperm function, less well than normal sperm.[367] The majority of reports indicate that semen quality is improved in 60 to 70 percent of men and fertility is demonstrated in 30 to 40 percent after high venous ligation to correct the varicocele.[221] Because the mechanism of induction of oligospermia is unknown and prospective, controlled trials of treatment have not been done, some investigators question the etiologic association of varicocele and infertility.[368] Until further data are available, surgical treatment of varicocele remains a useful treatment option.

Detection of varicocele clinically requires examination of a standing patient during the Valsalva maneuver. Subclinical varicocele can be suggested by thermography and confirmed by retrograde testicular vein venography.[369] The significance of these subclinical varicoceles remains controversial. In the majority of patients, the levels of FSH, LH, and testosterone are normal, although subclinical gonadal dysfunction may occasionally be found.[370]

Treatment consists of ligation of the testicular veins high in the inguinal canal; the procedure is fully described in several recent reviews.[221,365,369] Venous occlusion can also be induced by injection of thrombogenic agents through a venous catheter.[369] Results of treatment depend upon the severity of the spermatogenesis defect. Azoospermic patients rarely respond to high venous ligation, whereas in 60 to 80 percent of those with sperm counts between 10 and 20×10^6/ml sperm quality improves after surgery. The clinician should be aware that 10 percent of varicoceles recur after surgery and can be detected upon careful repeat examination.[369]

Infections

In the majority of patients with eugonadotropic seminiferous tubular failure, no cause can be identified. A thorough search for infectious agents has identified a variety of organisms in the seminal fluid of men with oligospermia or with decreased sperm motility.[371] Mycoplasma infection, particularly by *Ureaplasma urealyticum*, has been suggested as a causative agent in infertility,[372] but this conclusion remains controversial.[373] *U. urealyticum* was found in 26 percent of 100 infertile men compared to 13 percent of 30 fertile men in one study. *Escherichia coli* has been implicated in other studies. No characteristic features are apparent by history or physical examination in these men.[371] The presence of an excess number of leukocytes in the seminal fluid suggests the possibility of infection. A cause-and-effect relationship between the documented infection and the associated infertility has not yet been established. However, most large infertility clinics routinely treat with antibiotics such as doxycycline when infection is suspected on the basis of the presence of pus cells on several seminal fluid examinations or positive cultures.[371,374]

Sinopulmonary-Infertility Syndrome

In a number of recently described disorders, a correlation between infertility and recurrent sinopulmonary infections is apparent (Table 16-12).[375] Although no one mechanism explains this association, consideration of these disorders as a group is useful for the clinician. In the *immotile cilia syndrome,* sperm motility and ciliary function in the respiratory tract are defective because of abnormal flagellar function.[376]

Table 16-12. Clinical Features of the Sinopulmonary-Infertility Syndrome

Syndrome	Sinopulmonary infection	Sperm and cilia ultrastructure	Vas and epididymis	Sperm analysis	Pancreatic function	Sweat test
Immotile cilia syndrome	Present	Abnormal*	Normal	Immotile sperm	Normal	Normal
Cystic fibrosis	Present	Normal	Malformation†	Azoospermia	Abnormal	Abnormal
Young's syndrome	Present	Normal	Obstruction by inspissated secretions	Azoospermia	Normal	Normal

*Biochemical variants with enzymatic defects may also exist.
†Rare cases with intact vas and epididymides and fertility have been reported.
Source: Adapted from Handelsman et al.[375]

One subtype of this syndrome is identified by electron microscopic study. It consists of absence of dynein arms on the sperm tail and respiratory cilia (Fig. 16-12). Partial deletions of the dynein arms may also exist but are difficult to detect because of considerable variability in the appearance of normal sperm tails on electron microscopy.[39a] Deficiency of protein carboxymethylase, an enzyme required for motility,[377] has been demonstrated in the sperm of patients with necrozoospermia.

Another disorder, *cystic fibrosis,* is characterized by congenital malformation of the vas deferens with azoospermia and tenacious bronchopulmonary secretions.[378] *Young's syndrome,* on the other hand, is associated with inspissated secretions in the vas deferens in association with azoospermia. Both disorders produce recurrent respiratory infections; the infections are severe in the case of cystic fibrosis and mild in those with Young's syndrome.[375]

Genetic Syndromes

Surveys of lymphocyte karyotype analyses or of meiotic chromosomes in men with infertility document the frequency of genetic disorders.[379,380] Fifteen percent of men with azoospermia are found to have various genetic abnormalities, including XXY and XYY karyotypes, reciprocal autosomal and robertsonian translocations, and a variety of other abnormalities.[379,380] The frequency of these disorders in oligospermic men with sperm counts of 1 to 20×10^6 per ml was 1.65 percent. In 2372 infertile men screened by Chandley, 24 had an XXY karyotype, 10 had reciprocal autosomal translocations, 5 were of XYY karyotype, 4 had robertsonian translocations, and 8 had miscellaneous abnormalities on somatic karyotype analysis.[379]

Autoimmunity

Infertility and oligospermia occur in association with certain autoimmune disorders such as Addison's disease and the familial autoimmune endocrine deficiency syndrome.[317] The presence of autoantibodies against the testis has been demonstrated in these subjects as well as in other patients with oligo- or azoospermia.[381] Indirect quantitative RIA detects antisperm antibodies on spermatozoa in seminal plasma and in the sera of men with oligospermia with greater frequency than in the normal population.[382,383] Anecdotal reports of successful immunosuppression with glucocorticoids in these patients have been published.[383] At present, the exact etiologic relationship between antibody formation and infertility is poorly understood.

Approach to the Infertile Male

After documentation of oligo- or azoospermia with three appropriate semen analyses, a carefully directed history (e.g., regarding previously undescended testes) and physical examination are required to rule out specific etiologies. A detailed history of drug and toxin exposure should be obtained, as well as information regarding respiratory illnesses. Since in utero exposure to diethylstilbestrol (DES) may be associated with infertility in males, information regarding this risk factor should be obtained.[383a] Examination of the scrotal veins during a Valsalva maneuver is required to exclude a minimal varicocele. Genital and rectal examination should exclude abnormalities of the vas deferens, epididymis, and prostate. Necessary laboratory data include measurement of LH, FSH, testosterone, and prolactin concentrations. Seminal fluid should be cultured if pus cells are detected on semen analysis or evidence of excurrent duct infection is apparent. Testicular biopsy may be requested in subjects with normal FSH levels to evaluate the degree of germ cell failure. Special techniques such as assessment of hamster egg penetration or anti-sperm antibodies are only available to certain investigative groups, but, under certain circumstances, may be useful. It should be emphasized that the female partner of the oligospermic male requires complete evaluation as well. Reproductive abnormalities commonly exist in both partners.

The clinician should keep in mind the relative prevalence of different etiologic disorders in infertile men. Five series which involved 3478 men[384–388] revealed the following frequencies of etiologies: idiopathic, 33 percent; varicocele, 25 percent; undescended testes, 7 percent; excurrent duct obstruction, 4.8 percent; mumps orchitis, 3.3 percent; hypogonadotropism, 2.3 percent; and Klinefelter's syndrome, 1.9 percent. A large category of miscellaneous etiologies remains. In another series of 280 men, testicular biopsy revealed hypospermatogenesis in 61 percent, maturation arrest in 15 percent, Sertoli-cell-only syndrome in 13 percent, normal appearance in 8 percent, hyalinized tubules in 2 percent, and immature testes in 1 percent.[384]

DISORDERS ASSOCIATED WITH NONPHYSIOLOGIC SECRETION OF GONADOTROPINS

Gonadotropin-Producing Tumors

Functioning tumors of the pituitary are usually recognized because of clinical signs of hormone excess, such as acromegaly or Cushing's syndrome. Gonadotropin-producing tumors result in no distinctive clinical features; they consequently remained unrecognized until recently. Routine preoperative screening in the last several years uncovered a group of men with large pituitary tumors and elevated FSH levels. Immunohistochemical staining of the tumor cells and demonstration of gonadotropin secretion in cell culture definitively established that these are functioning tumors.[388a] A recent series reported elevated FSH levels in 12 of 50 men with untreated pituitary adenomas, suggesting that this tumor is not rare.[389] Clinically, the majority of patients are men, tumors are large, and FSH concentrations correlate with tumor size. Even though LH levels are normal, these patients complain of impotence and have low testosterone levels. Physicochemical studies indicate that the majority of LH measurable by RIA consists of free α and β subunits, and not of intact LH.[390] FSH-producing tumors are variably autonomous and are incompletely suppressed during testosterone administration.[391] Clomiphene citrate, when given as a provocative test, results in a blunted stimulatory effect.[391] A major difficulty is to distinguish patients with FSH-secretory tumors from those with primary gonadal failure and FSH elevations.[389] In general, FSH but not LH concentration is increased in tumor patients, while both are increased in primary hypogonadism. Provocative testing with releasing factors allows further distinction. GnRH stimulates an increase in the concentration of the β subunit of FSH in all patients with gonadotropin-producing tumors and in none of the men with primary hypogonadism. Similarly, TRH stimulates LH α and β subunits in tumor patients but not in those with primary hypogonadism.[390]

Clinically, the majority of FSH-producing tumors arise de novo; the minority occur in the setting of long-standing testicular failure. Because there are no detrimental effects from the secretion of FSH in excess, treatment requires standard surgery and radiotherapy to control mass lesion effects.[392,393]

Precocious Puberty

"True" precocious puberty encompasses a group of disorders characterized by premature activation of the hypothalamic-pituitary-gonadotropic axis. Two forms occur, the cerebral and idiopathic types. Hamartomas, craniopharyngiomas, hydrocephalus, the McCune-Albright syndrome, congenital brain defects, tuberous sclerosis, neurofibromatosis, and postinfectious scarring are the specific pathologic causes of the cerebral type. Mental retardation, abnormal psychomotor development, and epilepsy are also associated with the cerebral type of true precocious puberty. Hamartomas are of special interest, since they contain a large amount of GnRH, have the electron microscopic characteristics of neurosecretory tissue, and may be considered GnRH-producing neoplasms.[394]

The idiopathic type includes cases of sexual precocity in which careful investigation reveals no CNS or gonadal lesion. Published series indicate an equal frequency of cerebral and idiopathic varieties of true precocious puberty in boys.[395] Availability of the CT and MRI scans, however, will probably increase the number of patients in whom specific CNS lesions are found. In patients with the Russell-Silver syndrome[395] and those with sexual precocity associated with hypothyroidism[396] elevated gonadotropin concentrations may be a cause of early maturation, but the pathogenesis is unknown. Rarely, primary gonadotropin excess from hCG-producing tumors, such as choriocarcinomas and hepatomas, may cause precocious puberty.

True sexual precocity begins at any time after birth and progresses in a normal, albeit premature, sequence. The clinical hallmark in boys is testicular enlargement, a sign which reflects increased circulating gonadotropin concentrations. Treatment with large amounts of the GnRH agonist analogues which paradoxically suppress LH secretion provides effective therapy for these patients.[397–397b] Medroxyprogesterone acetate lowers androgen secretion and reduces the clinical manifestations of androgen excess, but generally does not decelerate the rapid advance in bone age.[398]

Pseudo precocious puberty occurs as a result of a primary excess in androgen secretion, independent of gonadotropic control. Congenital adrenal hyperplasia is the most common cause,[399] followed by virilizing adrenal and testicular tumors. Recently, a type of testicular hyperplasia occurring independently of gonadotropin secretion, termed the *testis toxicosis* syndrome, has been described in several families.[400] Boys with this disorder have high testosterone but low gonadotropin levels. No etiology is apparent upon extensive study of these patients. Forms of the McCune-Albright syndrome with pseudo precocious puberty, in addition to those with true precocious puberty, have been described.[401]

Treatment of pseudo precocious puberty consists of adrenal suppression with cortisol for congenital adrenal hyperplasia and excision of virilizing tumors, if present. No satisfactory treatment for the testis toxicosis syndrome is currently available, although one report suggested the use of the androgen synthesis inhibitor ketoconazole.[401a]

CRYPTORCHISM

Pathophysiology

Cryptorchism is present when the testis does not occupy a scrotal position. In the clinical assessment of patients, two functional types of cryptorchism exist which should be considered separately. True cryptorchism requires that the testis reside outside the scrotum permanently. *Pseudocryptorchism* or *retractile testis* is present if the gonad at times occupies a scrotal position and at other times retracts into the inguinal canal. Compensatory hypertrophy of the contralateral scrotal testis is often observed in association with true cryptorchism.

The embryologic causes of true cryptorchism are incompletely understood. One view states that the primary defect is in the testis itself. Histologic studies demonstrate that severely atrophic or dysgenetic testes may be the cause of cryptorchism in some cases.[402,403] However, examination of a large number of cryptorchid testes biopsied during orchiopexy reveals that the majority of these gonads are not severely dysgenetic. The latter observations have led to the position that factors other than testicular atrophy are operative in most instances. Possible contributing causes include inadequate length of the spermatic vessels or vas deferens, insufficient size of the inguinal canal or superficial inguinal ring, and insufficient abdominal pressure to push the testes through the inguinal ring.

Another explanation, partial gonadotropin deficiency, has gained support from several recent observations. Basal LH level is low and response to GnRH is blunted in some boys with cryptorchism, but not all. Perhaps as a reflection of decreased testicular priming, testosterone concentration increments after hCG administration are diminished in some patients. While not all investigators can confirm these hormonal abnormalities, the possibility of gonadotropin deficiency has been raised.[404–407] LH, in addition to maternal hCG, may be involved in the process of testicular descent during fetal life. The *gubernaculum* (Latin for "helmsman") of the testis, which pulls the testis into the scrotum, is an androgen-dependent tissue.[408] Lack of LH late in gestation might lower testosterone concentration to a level supported only by residual hCG secretion. Consequently, gubernacular function might be insufficient to guide the testis into the scrotum. Two clinical observations support this hypothesis. First, patients with isolated gonadotropin deficiency or absent pituitaries (anencephalic patients) have a high incidence of cryptorchism.[409] Second, treatment of cryptorchid boys with endogenous GnRH to increase their LH levels induces testicular descent.[410]

Whatever the mechanism, the descent of the testis through its normal pathway may be arrested at an abdominal, inguinal, or high scrotal position (Fig. 16-47). A patent processus vaginalis often accompanies true cryptorchism. This evagination may extend considerably farther down the scrotum than the testis and predispose to inguinal hernia, which may be associated with cryptorchism in 50 to 80 percent of cases. In certain instances, the testis may migrate through an abnormal or ectopic pathway and occupy a pubic, femoral, peritoneal, or superficial inguinal position (Fig. 16-47). When this occurs, the testis is contained in the superficial inguinal pouch, a recessed line lateral to the superficial inguinal ring. Although it has been suggested that ectopic testes result from different etiologic factors from those leading to inguinal cryptorchid testes, the coexistence of both ectopic and inguinal testes in patients with bilateral cryptorchism

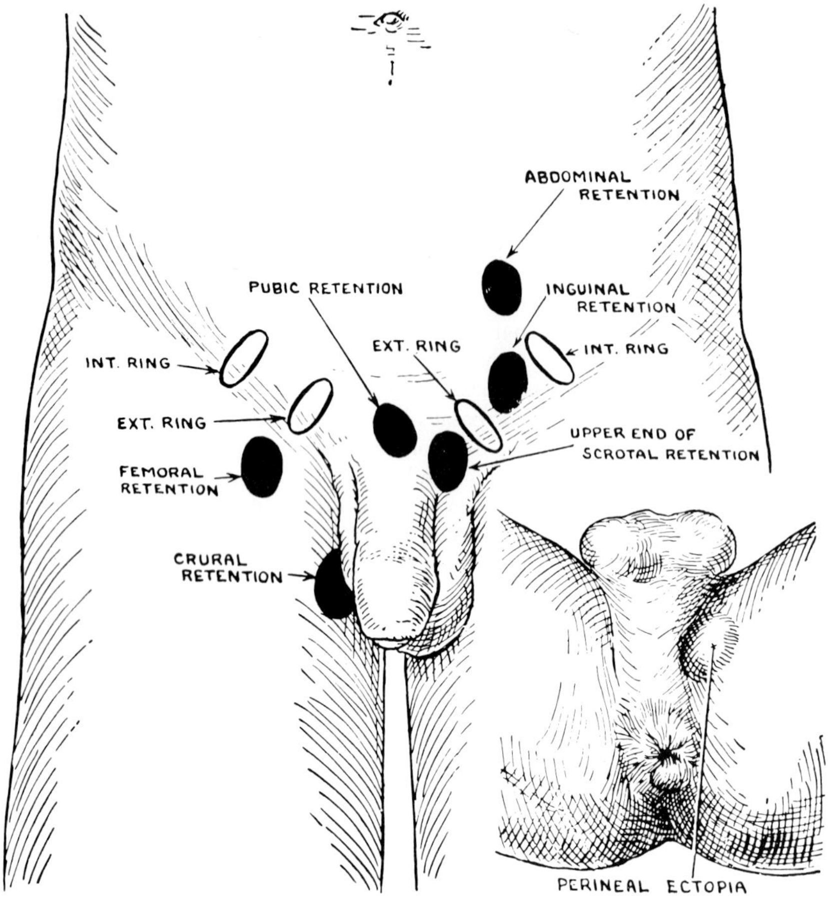

FIGURE 16-47 Sites of maldescent of the testes. (*From Santen RJ, Kulin HE, in Kelley VC (ed): Practice of Pediatrics. Philadelphia, Harper & Row, 1976.*)

suggests that similar causes are operative in both types.

Unilateral cryptorchism is a condition which occurs in 2 to 5 percent of newborn males. The incidence decreases to approximately 0.8 percent after the first 3 months of life.[395] Based on older studies, it was held that cryptorchid testes spontaneously enter the scrotum in late childhood or during early puberty. However, these studies failed to distinguish between retractile and truly cryptorchid testes. The natural history of pseudocryptorchid testes is that they occupy the scrotum for greater periods of time as the boy approaches puberty. Because of increasing gonadal size and a diminished cremasteric reflex, they eventually will permanently reside in the scrotum. No increased risk of infertility or testicular tumor is observed during long-term follow-up of patients with pseudocryptorchid testes.[411] On the other hand, truly cryptorchid testes never reach a normal scrotal position even though they may descend somewhat as the boy approaches puberty.

Bilateral cryptorchism occurs much less commonly than unilateral involvement. When present, this condition is more likely to be associated with a dysgenetic or defective testis than is unilateral cryptorchism. A primary cause of hypogonadism may be present; this should be suspected in patients with bilateral cryptorchism and androgen deficiency. Specific causes include isolated gonadotropin deficiency, idiopathic hypopituitarism, Prader-Labhart-Willi syndrome, Laurence-Moon-Biedl syndrome, poly X + Y Klinefelter's syndrome (but not classic XXY Klinefelter's), and various rarer syndromes.[292] Cryptorchism is also common in patients with cerebral palsy and occurs in 40 percent of patients with mental retardation.[412]

The evaluation of unilateral cryptorchism requires that the pseudocryptorchid or retractile testis be differentiated from the truly cryptorchid one. This involves repeated physical examinations and special techniques of examination. For example, the squatting position will often cause a retractile testis to descend spontaneously because of increased intraabdominal pressure. Examination after a warm bath may also reveal a scrotal testis when it had previously occupied an inguinal position. The parents can be instructed to examine the child at home after a bath to uncover this phenomenon.

Rationale for Treatment

Considerations regarding treatment are based on the known effects of cryptorchism on testicular function. It was initially recognized that the undescended testis is always smaller than the contralateral, descended one and that the undescended testis appears somewhat atrophic on histologic examination. In patients less than 8 years of age, the volume of the unilaterally cryptorchid testis is only 64 percent of normal.[413] These observations led to early speculations that cryptorchid testes are primarily dysgenetic and are not damaged further by occupying a cryptorchid position. However, more recent evidence from experimental studies in rats and clinical studies in men suggests that the cryptorchid position itself is detrimental and is the primary cause of the testicular damage. For example, surgically induced cryptorchism in rats produces a progressive diminution of germ cell maturation and ulimately leads to tubular atrophy. In response to the loss of germ cells, serum FSH concentration rises. In these animals, LH concentration also rises as a reflection of Leydig cell damage. It is likely that germ cell destruction results, at least in part, from an increase in testis temperature which is produced by the intraabdominal position. Similar disruption of germ cells can be produced in rats by warming the testis by immersion in warm water to the temperature occurring in the abdomen. In men, transient elevations of testicular temperature also may inhibit spermatogenesis.

Further evidence that the cryptorchid position is detrimental to germ cell maturation has been obtained by longitudinal studies. Mengel et al.[414] and Waaler[413] studied the histologic appearance of the cryptorchid testes in boys of increasing age and compared these with the subjects' contralateral normal testes. For precise characterization, they accurately counted the germ cells and measured the diameter of the seminiferous tubule. It was clear that the cryptorchid testis becomes progressively more atrophic when compared with the age-matched normal testis. From these observations, they concluded that the cryptorchid position itself produces progressive testicular damage. Additional studies have shown that the contralateral scrotal testis may also undergo progressive damage in boys with unilateral cryptorchism. Although this phenomenon can be produced experimentally in dogs, the mechanism is as yet unknown.[395]

An important practical question is whether cryptorchid testes brought into the scrotum recover function as a result of the altered testis position. Available data suggest that some improvement in the histologic appearance of cryptorchid testes may be expected if the operation is performed prior to the onset of puberty. The functional capacity for sperm production might be improved as well. Studies of patients with bilateral cryptorchism reveal that the fertility rate may be as high as 70 to 80 percent in subjects operated on before age 10. Without operation, such individuals are rarely fertile. Even though improvement in function occurs after orchiopexy, some degree of functional impairment persists after surgery. In one elegantly conceived study, unilateral vasectomy on the contralateral side allowed study of the function of the once-cryptorchid testis. Sperm were detected in only 4 of 12 men.[415] Follow-up studies have revealed elevations of FSH and, on occasion, LH concentrations in those boys operated on for bilateral cryptorchism. It is encouraging to note that serum gonadotropin levels remained normal in boys with unilateral cryptorchism who were treated by surgical intervention.

David et al.[416] extensively reviewed available literature regarding sperm counts in men who had previously undergone unilateral or bilateral orchiopexy. Fifty-two percent of 296 men with bilateral orchiopexy and 21 percent of 247 with unilateral orchiopexy exhibited azoospermia on later semen analysis. Similarly, spermatogenesis was adequate in only 13 percent and 30 percent, respectively. Unfortunately, the age at which these patients underwent surgery did not correlate with the degree of germ cell abnormalities found.

Another consideration regarding treatment is the malignant potential of a cryptorchid testis. It has been stated that the cryptorchid testis has a 20-fold greater chance of becoming malignant than a scrotal one if it resides in the inguinal canal and a 50-fold greater risk if it is intraabdominal. Testicular tumors are rare, however; they occur in approximately 1 to 2 per 100,000 males. Thus, the prevalence of malignancy in cryptorchid testes should only approximate 20 to 100 per 100,000. However, over a 60-year lifetime, the incidence may be as high as 6000/100,000 (6 percent). One recent study found a prevalence of malignancy of 8 percent,[417] predominantly carcinoma in situ, in prospectively biopsied cryptorchid testes.

Even when brought into the scrotum, the cryptorchid testis retains its malignant potential.[418,419] It has been argued that early detection of a testicular tumor is easier if the testis resides in the scrotum rather than in the inguinal canal. This rationale for treating by orchiopexy is not totally convincing; several investigators now recommend orchiectomy for unilaterally cryptorchid testes in older boys or when the testis is small or dysgenetic.

Treatment

A current recommendation is that orchiopexy be carried out between the ages of 6 months and 18 months if testicular descent is not observed after hCG therapy.[419] Medical treatment with hCG produces varying results, depending upon the group studied. When pseudocryptorchism was carefully excluded, 24 percent of patients with unilateral cryptorchism aged 2 to 5 responded with testicular descent in one study.[420] In a recent randomized trial, only 4 out of 33 boys experienced testicular descent with either hCG or with GnRH.[420a] As a matter of clinical practice, it is reasonable to administer a trial course of hCG, 1000 to 4000 IU three times weekly for 6 weeks, to avoid unnecessary surgery in those boys established to have true cryptorchism on repeated examination.[420b] GnRH therapy is still experimental in the United States. Subjects not responding to hCG (or GnRH) should undergo orchiopexy and correction of the associated hernia, if one is present.[420b]

GYNECOMASTIA

Overview

In prepubertal boys, as well as in girls, parenchymal and stromal cells with a potential for full breast development are present beneath the nipples. Experimental and clinical studies indicate that both stimulatory and inhibitory hormones control the growth and differentiation of these tissues (Fig. 16-48).[422,422a] Estradiol stimulates the cellular growth and proliferation of parenchymal epithelium to form ductal elements. Prolactin primarily acts upon differentiated breast acini to stimulate milk protein synthesis. In tissue culture, mammary cells require the presence of GH, insulin, and cortisol as permissive factors for growth, but specific effects on differentiated function are not clearly defined. Testosterone exerts a generalized inhibitory action on breast tissue growth and differentiation, perhaps through a specific antiestrogenic action.[422a] Also, certain regulatory hormones modulate systemic hormonal effects which, in turn, influence breast growth and differentiation. Thyroxine increases the levels of TeBG and serum estradiol concentration and thereby exerts indirect effects on the breast. Both cortisol and prolactin lower circulating testosterone levels through hypothalamic and testicular effects. Thus, they diminish inhibitory influences on the breast.

The application of these physiologic principles allows gynecomastia to be considered on a pathophysiologic basis. A disordered balance between secretion of stimulatory and inhibitory hormones underlies the development of the pathologic forms of gynecomastia in men. Gynecomastia may also occur as a normal physiologic process at various stages of life, as a reflection of hormonal changes. Major emphasis has

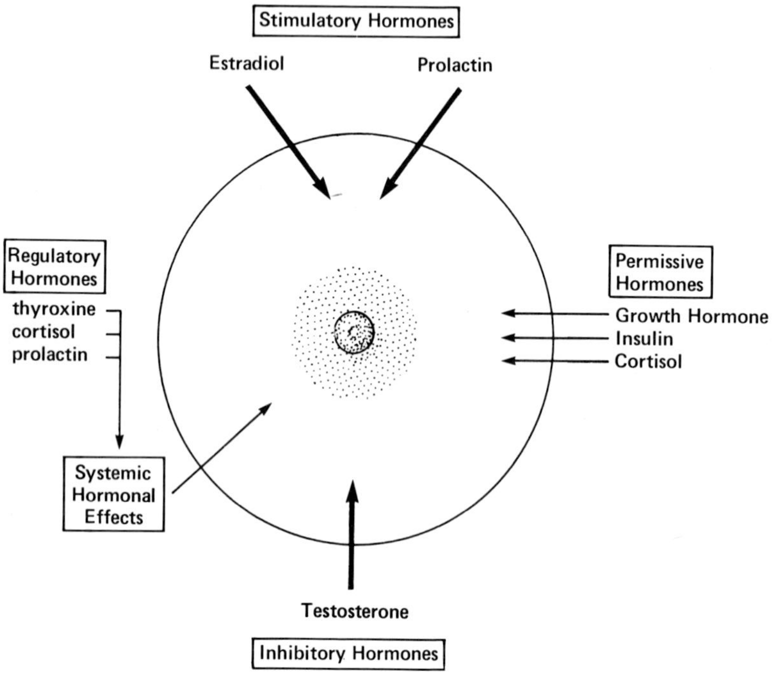

FIGURE 16-48 Diagrammatic representation of the hormones which affect breast tissue.

been placed on the balance between estradiol, the major facilitative hormone, and testosterone, as an inhibitor, in both the physiologic and pathologic types.

Physiologic Forms of Gynecomastia

During the early stages of puberty, the ratio of estradiol to androgens is increased, particularly during the daytime.[423,424] Beginning at age 11, approximately 30 percent of boys develop detectable gynecomastia (i.e., glandular tissue > 0.5 cm in diameter); by age 14, gynecomastia is detectable in 65 percent. The prevalence then decreases to 14 percent by age 16.[425] The reduced prevalence in early adulthood is associated with a diminution in estradiol/testosterone ratio. Three recent studies[426–428] found that gynecomastia later returns in adults with a surprising prevalence; patient and physician, however, were found to have minimal awareness of the existence of the condition. Thirty-three percent of men in their mid-twenties and 57 percent between ages 45 and 59 had palpable breast tissue which exceeded 2 cm in diameter. At autopsy, 40 percent of men have gynecomastia, 31 percent with stromal, and 9 percent with glandular predominance.[429] McFadyen et al.[430] reported that older men with gynecomastia as a group had higher estradiol/testosterone ratios than those without gynecomastia, providing further support for the androgen-estrogen imbalance theory of causation of gynecomastia.[430] Further studies are required to confirm this preliminary finding.

Pathologic Forms of Gynecomastia

In adolescence, a group of boys develop an exaggerated form of gynecomastia with breast development to Tanner stages III (i.e., > 4 cm of glandular breast tissue), IV (near-adult female), or V (normal adult female). This condition, called *persistent pubertal macromastia,* is not associated with specific endocrine disorders nor recognized hormonal or receptor abnormalities.[431]

As noted, gynecomastia may be a normal finding in adults. Consequently, the clinician must be concerned only when there is breast tenderness, a progressive increase in breast size, or enlargement beyond the physiologic range (i.e., 2 to 5 cm). A logical approach to the differential diagnosis can then be based upon known physiology (Table 16-13). An excess of breast-stimulatory hormones, a deficiency of inhibitory ones, a stimulatory-inhibitory or abnormalities of the regulatory hormones cause gynecomas-

Table 16-13. Causes of Gynecomastia

- Stimulatory hormone excess
  - Estradiol
    - Adrenal or testicular tumors
    - Drug therapy with:
      - Estrogens
      - Estrogen analogues: *digitoxin*
      - Estrogen precursors: aromatizable androgens
        - *Testosterone enanthate*
        - *Testosterone propionate*
    - Increased peripheral aromatase activity due to:
      - Heredity
      - Obesity
  - Prolactin
    - Pituitary tumor
    - Drug therapy with:
      - Catecholamine antagonists or depleters:
        - *Sulpiride* — *Phenothiazines*
        - *Metoclopramide* — *Reserpine*
        - *Domperidone* — *Tricyclic antidepressants*
        - *Methyldopa*
    - Hypothyroidism
- Inhibitory hormone deficiency
  - Androgen resistance
    - Complete testicular feminization
    - Partial: Reifenstein, Lubbs, Rosewater, and Dreyfus syndromes
  - Androgen antagonist drugs
    - *Spironolactone* — *Progestagens*
    - *Cimetidine* — *Flutamide*
    - *Marijuana*
- Stimulatory-inhibitory hormone imbalance
  - Hypergonadotropic syndromes
    - Primary gonadal diseases
    - Cytotoxic drug-induced hypogonadism from:
      - *Busulfan* — *Nitrosourea*
      - *Vincristine* — *Combination chemotherapy*
    - Tumor-related: hCG-producing tumors (testis, lung, GI tract, etc.)
    - hCG administration
  - Hypogonadotropic syndromes
    - Isolated gonadotropin deficiency, particularly "fertile eunuch syndrome"
    - Panhypopituitarism
  - Systemic illnesses
    - Severe liver disease
    - Renal disease
- Miscellaneous endocrine causes
  - Hyperthyroidism
  - Acromegaly
  - Cushing's syndrome
- Local trauma
  - Hip spica cast
  - Chest injury
- Primary breast tumor
- Uncertain causes
  - Refeeding
  - Other chronic illnesses
    - Pulmonary tuberculosis
    - Diabetes mellitus
  - Persistent pubertal macromastia
  - Idiopathic

Drugs are listed in italics.

tia in the majority of patients. The remainder of cases remain largely idiopathic or of uncertain cause.

The differential diagnosis of gynecomastia is extensive and difficult to remember because of the variety of causes. Two approaches are useful for the clinician: consideration of the various disorders on a pathophysiologic basis (Table 16-13) and practical attention to the most frequent causes of this condition (Fig. 16-49). With the first approach, the etiologies of gynecomastia are considered with respect to each specific hormone. Certain disorders, such as adrenal tumors, are associated with clear elevations of plasma estradiol secretion. Other conditions are characterized by increased conversion of androgens to estrogens in nonglandular tissues. The enzyme responsible for this conversion, aromatase, is present in fat, muscle, and liver as well as in breast tissue. Obesity, liver disease, and rare genetic disorders are associated with increased aromatase activity and gynecomastia. In addition, the gynecomastia associated with early puberty and administration of aromatizable androgens to hypogonadal men may be related to excess aromatase activity.[432]

Prolactin secretion is modulated by central aminergic neuronal pathways, particularly of the dopaminergic variety. A wide range of drugs with catecholamine-antagonizing or -depleting actions can stimulate prolactin release. Either by direct effects on the breast or by a regulatory alteration of gonadotropin and testosterone secretion, these drugs can cause gynecomastia.

Drugs which inhibit the biosynthesis or action of androgens may be associated with gynecomastia. Syndromes of androgen resistance represent experiments of nature in which a deficiency of androgen action causes gynecomastia. Among the most common examples of the androgen-antagonistic drugs are spironolactone, flutamide, and cimetidine.[427,433] Drugs with estrogenic effects such as digitoxin also cause gynecomastia.

The hypergonadotropic syndromes as a group are associated with relative deficiency of androgen secretion. The compensatory increase in LH and FSH secretion appears to induce a relative rise in estradiol concentration. The resulting imbalance between estrogen and androgen commonly produces gynecomastia. Klinefelter's syndrome, with an 85 percent prevalence of gynecomastia, is typical of this condition, but other genetic disorders and drugs can produce similar findings. Less well explained is the estrogen-androgen imbalance associated with hypopituitarism or systemic illness such as renal disease.

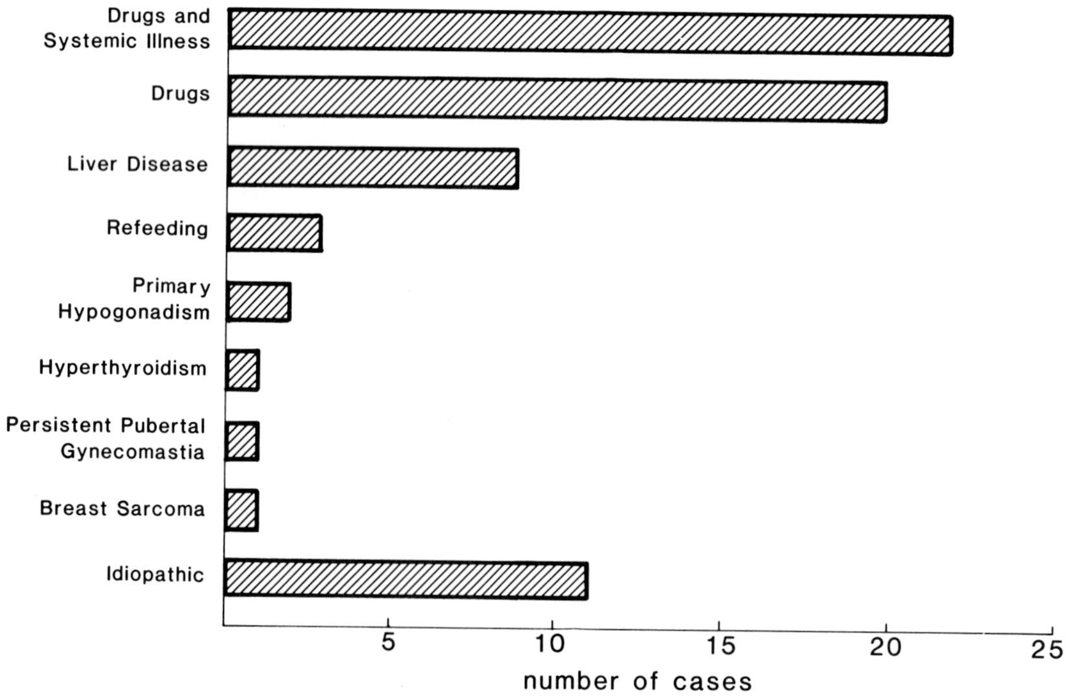

FIGURE 16-49 Frequency of etiologies of gynecomastia in men hospitalized at a Veterans Administration hospital. The "drugs and systemic illness" category included patients with male climacteric, cirrhosis, hepatitis, hyperthyroidism, refeeding syndrome, and primary hypogonadism. The "drug alone" category included α-methyldopa, phenothiazines, amitriptyline, imipramine, spironolactone, isoniazid, testosterone, narcotics, estradiol, amphetamines, and reserpine. (*From Carlson.*[427])

The rapid onset of gynecomastia in an adult patient should elicit suspicion of underlying neoplastic disease. Lung, GI, and testis tumors produce hCG, which stimulates estradiol out of proportion to testosterone and causes gynecomastia.[220]

Other endocrine disorders produce gynecomastia through secretion of hormones which indirectly influence breast growth. As examples, hyperthyroidism appears to increase estradiol levels[435] and cortisol excess inhibits testosterone production. Prolactin excess may cause gynecomastia by this mechanism as well, since it reduces testosterone secretion.[220]

Local chest trauma is associated with gynecomastia, probably related to local stimulation of breast tissue or afferent neurologic influences. Breast neoplasms characteristically are asymmetric. A hard nodule is palpable on examination. Breast carcinoma is rare in males and is not usually confused with gynecomastia.

The remaining causes of gynecomastia are uncertain. One form, associated with refeeding, was first recognized when prisoners of war in World War II were renourished after a period of starvation. A similar situation pertains when patients with chronic illnesses recover and regain weight. The gynecomastia associated with tuberculosis or diabetes mellitus may be similarly related to regain of weight.[427] An idiopathic category is also seen in which extensive evaluation reveals no definite cause.

For the clinician, knowledge of the frequency of these disorders provides information of practical use. To the general internist the most frequent causes of gynecomastia are (1) the combination of systemic illness and use of drugs known to cause gynecomastia, (2) use of drugs alone, (3) liver disease, and (4) regain of weight after a severe nutritional insult (refeeding gynecomastia) (Fig. 16-49). Patients with various disorders of hormone excess or gonadal insufficiency will be referred to the endocrinologist. Endocrinologists will also be asked to evaluate many patients in whom no etiology is diagnosed.

Evaluation

After deciding that the degree or rate of progression of gynecomastia is greater than normal, a directed evaluation should be initiated, including in all patients (1) a careful drug history; (2) identification of the presence of systemic renal, hepatic, cardiac, or pulmonary disease and, particularly, previous malnutrition due to these disorders; (3) detection of obvious signs and symptoms of underlying malignancy, especially testicular; (4) detection of clinically evident syndromes of estradiol, prolactin, GH, cortisol, or thyroxine excess or androgen deficiency.

If the initial evaluation is unrevealing, screening tests to exclude the presence of a neoplasm, including measurement of β-hCG as a tumor marker and a chest x-ray to rule out pulmonary carcinoma, should be performed on all patients. Clinical judgment then dictates whether additional studies such as thyroxine, prolactin, LH, FSH, estradiol, testosterone, and DHEA sulfate concentrations should be obtained. After this evaluation, many patients, particularly those referred to an endocrinologist, remain in the idiopathic category.

Treatment

Specific therapy for treatable diseases should be used where feasible and use of offending drugs should be discontinued. Reduction mammoplasty is required under certain clinical circumstances. Persistent pubertal macromastia is resistant to medical therapy; it requires surgical excision.[431] Reduction mammoplasty occasionally is necessary in men with painful or cosmetically disabling lesions. A highly experienced surgeon should be asked to perform this procedure because of the precise sculpturing necessary to produce an excellent cosmetic effect. Boys with pubertal gynecomastia can generally be reassured that regression occurs after 2 to 3 years in the majority of those with gynecomastia.[425] Use of antiestrogens to block estrogen action, stimulate testosterone secretion, and alter the estrogen-androgen balance has been evaluated in pubertal gynecomastia; improvement has been seen in some, but not all, patients.[436] In Europe, administration of nonaromatizable androgens, such as DHT, which lower estradiol concentration and increase androgen levels is associated with an improvement in gynecomastia.[437] The aromatase inhibitor testolactone has also been used to suppress estradiol but not androgen levels.[432] Each of these agents can be considered when pubertal gynecomastia is severe and psychologically debilitating. The pharmacologic agents mentioned can be used in adult patients with idiopathic gynecomastia, but experience with these drugs is limited and results have been disappointing.

IMPOTENCE

Impotence is defined as the inability to achieve or sustain an erection for a sufficient duration to have coitus and achieve an orgasm. In the largest available survey, difficulty in achieving an erection was reported to occur "frequently, regularly, or always" in 13 percent of men; it was reported "sometimes" in 17 percent and "infrequently" in 39 percent.[438] The causes of impotence can be divided into five general categories: psychogenic, vascular, neuropathic, endocrinologic, and drug-related. Psychogenic impotence is the most common etiology and the primary one in approximately 90 percent of individuals presenting with this complaint for the first time. Patients with psychogenic impotence often recount alternating periods of normal potency and impotence. Suggestive historical features include a history of premature ejaculation or stress-related premature detumescence, abrupt onset of impotence after heavy alcohol ingestion, and maintenance of normal libido but loss of potency. Characteristically, physiologic control of the erectile process remains intact; these individuals continue to experience morning and sleep-related erections and retain their ability to masturbate. The impotence of vascular insufficiency is often associated with symptoms of intermittent claudication, angina, or transient ischemic attacks of the anterior or posterior cerebral circulation. Historical features suggesting neuropathic impotence include stocking-glove paresthesias, symptoms of autonomic insufficiency, or a history of diabetes mellitus or renal disease. Endocrine-related impotence causes decreased libido as well as potency, loss of morning erections, inability to masturbate, and, after a prolonged period, loss of secondary sex characteristics. Drug-related impotence is obvious, provided that the physician considers the diagnosis.

Physical examination is directed toward careful assessment of secondary sex characteristics, testicular size, neurologic function, and peripheral pulses. Detection of normal prolactin and free testosterone concentrations in the morning (to eliminate diurnal variability) practically excludes an endocrinologic cause. The major clinical problem, then, is to distinguish between organic and psychogenic impotence. Quantitative assessment of nocturnal penile tumescence and correlation with EEG sleep stages is the best available method to exclude an organic cause. Qualitative methods to assess nocturnal erections (postage stamp test, strain gauge) are insufficiently sensitive and are discouraged.[439]

Detection of a low testosterone concentration favors the diagnosis of endocrine-related impotence. A specific etiology should then be sought and treated appropriately. Testosterone replacement, 200 mg of testosterone enanthate every 2 weeks, can then be given as a therapeutic trial. As confirmation of a physiologic rather than placebo response, the physician can substitute a sterile vehicle for 1-month periods, with androgen replacement therapy interspersed. The specific etiology of hyperprolactinemia, if present, should be evaluated. Prolactin levels should be lowered with bromocriptine before androgen therapy is initiated. As emphasized above, impotence often persists when prolactin levels are elevated even if the testosterone deficiency is corrected.

A different approach to diagnosis or therapy is needed if an organic cause of impotence is detected by nocturnal penile tumescence testing and endocrine causes are excluded. Diabetes or chronic renal failure most commonly produce sufficient degrees of peripheral neuropathy to cause impotence. Appropriate laboratory tests should be performed to rule these disorders in or out. Arteriosclerotic cardiovascular disease usually is the cause of large-vessel vascular disease with associated impotence. Treatment regimens for neuropathic or vascular impotence require implantation of prosthetic devices, either inflatable or noninflatable (the reader is directed to the review by Krane[440] which discusses the indications for, complications of, and use of these various devices).

The diagnosis of psychogenic impotence requires a treatment approach directed toward identifying precipitating features. The general internist or endocrinologist can identify major stress, alcohol ingestion, marital adjustment problems, excess fatigue, and other etiologic factors.[441] Frequently, attention to these conditions allows resumption of normal sexual function. If four or five visits to discuss these issues do not result in improvement, referral to a formal sexual dysfunction program is indicated. Success rates with the techniques used in these programs are approximately 50 to 75 percent, depending upon the duration of impotence and severity of underlying factors.

MALE CONTRACEPTION

Investigative groups worldwide are pursuing development of a practical male contraceptive.[442] Suppression of LH and FSH release with oral androgens and monthly or biweekly injections of testosterone enanthate do not produce azoospermia in all men. Pregnancies can occur in their partners even for men with oligospermia during these regimens; azoospermia is the only acceptable end point. Combinations of injectable testosterone with impeded androgens such as danazol, progestins such as medroxyprogesterone acetate, or antiandrogens such as cyproterone acetate are also incompletely effective. A more recent approach combines injectable testosterone with agonist analogues of GnRH, which paradoxically inhibit LH and FSH release. While azoospermia can be achieved in some men, uniform complete reduction of spermatogenesis may not be possible.[443] A direct inhibitor of spermatogenesis, *gossypol*, produces azoospermia without androgen deficiency.[444] Use of this contraceptive is efficacious in and has been acceptable to large groups of men undergoing therapeutic trial in China. However, hypokalemia is common and hypokalemic paralysis occurs in as many as 4.7 percent of Chinese men receiving this medication.

This brief summary of presently available data suggests that several years will be required for development of a safe, practical, acceptable pharmacologic contraceptive for men. In the meantime, vasectomy affords a generally applicable method. Immunologic abnormalities detected in the monkey as a complication of this procedure and accelerated coronary artery disease[445] have not been demonstrated in patients, although further surveillance in this regard will be required.

ANDROGEN-DEPENDENT NEOPLASIA

Sixty-thousand new cases of prostate cancer are diagnosed in the United States yearly. Eighty percent of these are androgen-dependent and regress after orchiectomy. Pharmacologic inhibition of testosterone production by the testis offers an alternative to surgical castration.[446,446a] This can be accomplished by administration of exogenous estrogen to suppress LH and, secondarily, testosterone secretion (Fig. 16-50). Doses of 5 mg of DES or its equivalent, given daily, inhibit testosterone adequately but accelerate the death rate from cardiovascular disease.[447] Use of a lower estrogen dose (e.g., 1 mg daily) reduces the risk of cardiovascular complications and continues to exert an antitumor effect. However, this dose may not suppress androgen production to castrate levels and may still exert cardiovascular toxicity. For these reasons, the potent analogues of GnRH ("superagonist analogues") have undergone extensive trial for the treatment of prostatic cancer. These compounds paradoxically inhibit LH and testosterone production, presumably by GnRH receptor suppression or postreceptor inhibitory effects. Testosterone concentration falls to levels similar to those observed after castration (i.e., 20 ng/100 ml). Controlled studies suggest that the superagonist analogues induce tumor regression as frequently as DES or orchiectomy with negligible long-term toxicity.[448,448a] Investigative work is currently directed toward addition of antiandrogens to the GnRH analogues in an attempt to produce a complete androgen blockade by antagonizing androgen action as well as inhibiting testicular secretion.[449] Direct inhibitors of androgen biosynthesis, such as ketoconazole, are also undergoing therapeutic trial.[450]

At present, symptomatic tumor metastasis is the major indication for androgen suppressive therapy or orchiectomy for prostate cancer. Prior studies by the Veterans Administration hospital cooperative groups demonstrated no survival benefit for earlier intervention. This concept is now being reexamined.

Only 10 to 40 percent of men respond to secondary hormonal therapy after initial orchiectomy or DES administration. The duration of response in these individuals is short (average 6 months) and the majority experience stabilization rather than objective

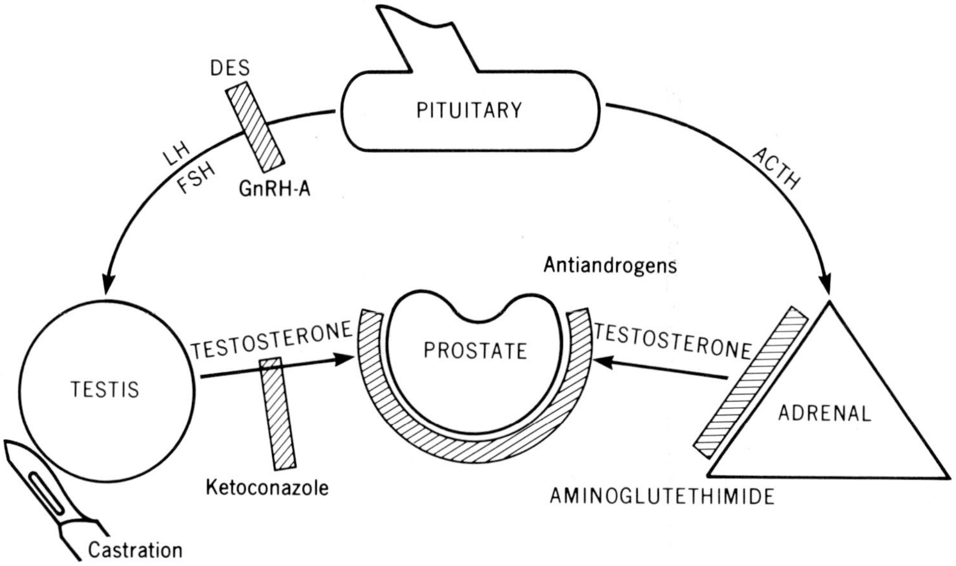

FIGURE 16-50 Diagrammatic representation of medical and surgical methods of ablating testosterone as treatments of men with prostatic carcinoma. GnRH-A, superagonist analogue of GnRH.

tumor regression. The reduced response rate compared to primary hormonal therapy probably represents the overgrowth of hormone-independent cell lines. Treatment strategies in these patients are directed toward a reduction in the 5 percent of remaining testosterone of adrenal origin. The adrenal inhibitor aminoglutethimide, in combination with replacement hydrocortisone as well as the antiandrogen flutamide, has been used with some success in these patients.[451,452]

TESTICULAR TUMORS

Testicular neoplasms represent 1 percent of all malignant tumors in men. They are 50-fold more common in cryptorchid or once-cryptorchid testes.[453] Four predominant types of germ cell malignancies affect the testis: seminomas, embryonal cell carcinomas, teratomas, and choriocarcinomas. Fourteen possible combinations of these basic types, called *compound tumors*, are observed. Two tumor markers, β-hCG and α-fetoprotein, provide useful information regarding prognosis at the time of initial evaluation and permit detection of early recurrence during follow-up observation. While seminoma has always been a highly curable tumor, major advances in chemotherapy of the other germinal cell tumors have markedly improved prognosis in these patients. The reader is referred to recent reviews for a full discussion of the diagnosis, surgery, and chemotherapeutic regimens for treatment of these neoplasms.[454–458]

Recent studies have identified an early form of testicular carcinoma in situ. This lesion was first recognized in 6 of 555 testes examined during studies of infertile men.[459,460] Within 1.3 to 4.5 years, four of these men developed invasive carcinoma. Skakkebaek and coworkers then recalled 180 men with corrected cryptorchism; 50 agreed to undergo biopsy of the testes. Eight percent were found to have carcinoma in situ on biopsy.[417] This preliminary observation suggests that testicular cancer may be identified early.

Nongerminal cell tumors of the testis are rare; they are diagnosed because of their steroid hormone–secreting nature. Sertoli or Leydig cell tumors may produce estrogens or androgens; they are generally benign.[115b,461,461a] Patients with these tumors develop gynecomastia or pseudo precocious puberty. Adrenal rest tumors occur in boys with incompletely treated congenital adrenal hyperplasia.[462] Tumor regression in them is observed after adequate suppression of ACTH with exogenous hydrocortisone. Gonadal, stromal, and compound tumors of nongerminal cell origin may also be encountered.

REFERENCES

1. Moore RY: Neuroendocrine regulation of reproduction, in Yen SSC, Jaffe RB (eds): *Reproductive Endocrinology*. Philadelphia, Saunders, 1978, p 3.

2. Barraclough CA, Wise PM: The role of catecholamines in the regulation of pituitary luteinizing hormone and follicle-stimulating hormone secretion. *Endocr Rev* 3:91, 1982.

3. Mess B: Functional anatomy of the hypothalamus and its afferent and efferent pathways, in Degroot LJ, Cahill GF, Odell WD, Martini L, Potts JT, Nelson DH, Steinberger E, Winegrad AI (eds): *Endocrinology*. New York, Grune and Stratton, 1979, vol 1, pp 3–14.

4. Palkovits M, Arimura A, Brownstein M, Schally AV, Saavedra JM: Luteinizing hormone releasing hormone (LH-RH) content of the hypothalamic nuclei in rat. *Endocrinology* 95:554, 1974.

5. Brownstein MJ, Palkovits M, Saavedra JM, Kizer JS: Distribution of hypothalamic hormones and neurotransmitters within the diencephalon, in Martini L, Ganong WF (eds): *Frontiers in Neuroendocrinology*. New York, Raven, 1976, vol 4, p 1.

6. Selmanoff MK, Wise PM, Barraclough CA: Regional distribution of luteinizing hormone-releasing hormone (LHRH) in rat brain determined by microdissection and radioimmunoassay. *Brain Res* 192:421, 1980.

7. Barry J: Immunohistochemistry of luteinizing hormone-releasing hormone-producing neurons of the vertebrates. *Int Rev Cytol* 60:179, 1979.

8. Merchenthaler I, Kovacs G, Lovasz G, Setalo G: The preoptico-infundibular LH-RH tract of the rat. *Brain Res* 198:63, 1980.

9. Morley JE: The endocrinology of the opiates and opioid peptides. *Metabolism* 30:195, 1981.

10. Bloom F, Battenburg E, Rossier J, Ling N, Guillemin R: Neurons containing β-endorphin in rat brain exist separately from those containing enkephalin: Immunocytochemical studies. *Proc Natl Acad Sci USA* 75:1591, 1978.

11. Sar M, Stumpf WE, Miller RJ, Chang KJ, Cuatrecasas P: Immunohistochemical localization of enkephalin in rat brain and spinal cord. *J Comp Neurol* 182:17, 1978.

12. Simantov R, Kuhar MJ, Uhl GR, Snyder SH: Opioid peptide enkephalin: Immunohistochemical mapping in rat central nervous system. *Proc Natl Acad Sci USA* 74:2167, 1977.

13. Adler MW: Opioid peptides. *Life Sci* 26:497, 1980.

14. Miller RJ, Meltzer HY, Fang VS: Distribution and pharmacology of the enkephalins, in Usdin E (ed): *Endorphins in Mental Health Research*. Oxford, Macmillan, 1979, p 3.

14a. Ferin M, van Vugt D, Wardlaw S: The hypothalamic control of the menstrual cycle and the role of endogenous opioid peptides. *Recent Prog Horm Res* 40:441, 1984.

15. Moore RY, Bloom FE: Central catecholamine neuron systems: Anatomy and physiology of the norepinephrine and epinephrine systems. *Annu Rev Neurosci* 2:113, 1979.

16. Dahlstrom A, Fuxe K: Evidence for the existence of monoamine-containing neurons in the central nervous system. I. Demonstration of monoamines in the cell bodies of brain stem neurons. *Acta Physiol Scand* 62(suppl 232):1, 1964.

17. Bjorklund A, Lindvall O, Nobin A: Evidence of an incertohypothalamic dopamine neurone system in the rat. *Brain Res* 89:29, 1975.

18. Bjorklund A, Falck B, Hromek F, Owman C, West KA: Identification and terminal distribution of the tubero-hypophyseal monoamine fibre systems in the rat by means of stereotaxic and microspectrofluorimetric techniques. *Brain Res* 17:1, 1970.

19. Bjorklund A, Moore RY, Nobin A, Stenevi U: The organization of tuberohypophyseal and reticulo-infundibular catecholamine neuron systems in the rat brain. *Brain Res* 51:171, 1973.

20. McEwen BS, Davis PG, Parsons B, Pfaff DW: The brain as a target for steroid hormone action. *Annu Rev Neurosci* 2:65, 1979.

21. Sheridan PJ: Androgen receptors in the brain: What are we measuring? *Endocr Rev* 4:171, 1983.

22. Grant LD, Stumpf WE: Localization of ^{3}H-estradiol and catecholamines in identical neurons in the hypothalamus. *J Histochem Cytochem* 21:404, 1973.

23. Sar M, Stumpf WE: Central noradrenergic neurones concentrate ^{3}H-oestradiol. *Nature* 289:500, 1981.

24. Page RB, Dovey-Hartman BJ: Neurohemal contact in the internal zone of the rabbit median eminence. *J Comp Neurol* 226:274, 1984.

25. Page RB: Pituitary blood flow: A review. *Am J Physiol* 243:E427, 1983.

26. Bergland RM, Page RB: Can the pituitary secrete directly to the brain? (Affirmative anatomical evidence.) *Endocrinology* 102:1325, 1978.

27. Page RB: Directional pituitary flow: A microcinephotographic study. *Endocrinology* 112:157, 1983.

28. Phifer RF, Midgley AR, Spicer SS: Immunohistologic and histologic evidence that follicle-stimulating hormone and luteinizing hormone are present in the same cell type in the human pars distalis. *J Clin Endocrinol Metab* 36:125, 1973.

29. Wiates GMH, Moule GR: Relation of vascular heat exchange to temperature regulation in the testis of the ram. *J Reprod Fertil* 2:213, 1961.

30. Neaves WB, Johnson L: Age-related change in numbers of other interstitial cells in the human testis: Evidence bearing on the fate of Leydig cells lost with increasing age. *17th Annual Meeting of the Society for the Study of Reproduction,* abstr 100, 1984.

31. Christensen AK: Leydig cells, in Hamilton DW, Greep RO (eds): *Handbook of Physiology: Endocrinology.* Baltimore, Williams and Wilkins, 1975, vol 5, p 57.

32. Fawcett DW: Ultrastructure and function of the Sertoli cell, in Hamilton DW, Greep RO (eds): *Handbook of Physiology: Endocrinology.* Baltimore, Williams and Wilkins, 1975, vol 5, p 21.

33. Waites GMH, Gladwell RT: Physiological significance of fluid secretion in the testis and blood-testis barrier. *Physiol Rev* 62:624, 1982.

34. Amann RP, Howards SS: Daily spermatozoal production and epididymal spermatozoal reserves of the human male. *J Urol* 124:211, 1980.

35. Steinberger E, Steinberger A: Spermatogenic function of the testis, in Hamilton DW, Greep RO (eds): *Handbook of Physiology: Endocrinology.* Baltimore, Williams and Wilkins, 1975, vol 5, p 1.

36. Parvinen M: Regulation of the seminiferous epithelium. *Endocr Rev* 3:404, 1982.

37. Flickinger CJ, Brown JC, Kutchai HC, Ogilvie JW: *Medical Cell Biology.* Philadelphia, Saunders, 1979.

38. Fawcett DW: The mammalian spermatozoon. *Dev Biol* 44:394, 1975.

39. Afzelius BA: Electron microscopy of the sperm tail. *J Biophys Biochem Cytol* 5:269, 1959.

39a. Wilton LJ, Teichtahl H, Temple-Smith PD, de Kretser DM: Structural heterogeneity of the axonemes of respiratory cilia and sperm flagella in normal men. *J Clin Invest* 75:825, 1985.

40. Satir P: Studies on cilia. III. Further studies on the cilium tip and a sliding filament model of ciliary motility. *J Cell Biol* 39:77, 1968.

41. Summers KE, Gibbons IR: Effects of trypsin digestion on flagellar structures and their relationship to motility. *J Cell Biol* 58:618, 1973.

42. Satir P: Introductory remarks: Cilia, eukaryotic flagella and an introduction to microtubules, in Goldman R, Pollard T, Rosenbaum J (eds): *Cell Motility.* New York, Cold Spring Harbor, 1976, vol C, p 841.

43. Clermont Y: The cycle of the seminiferous epithelium in man. *Am J Anat* 112:35, 1963.

44. Heller CG, Clermont Y: Kinetics of the germinal epithelium in man. *Recent Prog Horm Res* 20:545, 1964.

45. Flickinger CJ, Howard SS, English HF: Ultrastructural differences in efferent ducts and several regions of the epididymis of the hamster. *Am J Anat* 152:557, 1978.

46. Bedford JM: Maturation, transport, and fate of spermatozoa in the epididymis, in Hamilton DW, Greep RO (eds): *Handbook of Physiology: Endocrinology.* Baltimore, Williams and Wilkins, 1975, vol 5, p 303.

47. Rowley M, Teshima JF, Heller CG: Duration of transit of spermatozoa through the human male ductular system. *Fertil Steril* 21:390, 1970.

48. Chang MC: The meaning of sperm capacitation: A historical perspective. *J Androl* 5:45, 1984.

49. Drouva S, Gallo RV: Catecholamine involvement in episodic luteinizing hormone release in adult ovariectomized rats. *Endocrinology* 99:651, 1976.

50. Rubinstein L, Sawyer CH: Role of catecholamines in stimulating the release of pituitary ovulating hormones in rats. *Endocrinology* 86:988, 1970.

51. Huseman CA, Kugler JA, Schneider IG: Mechanism of dopaminergic suppression of gonadotropin secretion in men. *J Clin Endocrinol Metab* 51:209, 1980.

52. Leblanc H, Lachelin GCL, Abu-Fadil S, Yen SSC: Effects of dopamine infusion on pituitary hormone secretion in humans. *J Clin Endocrinol Metab* 43:668, 1976.

53. Lachelin GCL, Leblanc H, Yen SSC: The inhibitory effect of dopamine agonists on LH release in women. *J Clin Endocrinol Metab* 44:728, 1977.

54. Judd SJ, Rakoff JS, Yen SSC: Inhibition of gonadotropin and prolactin release by dopamine: Effect of endogenous estradiol levels. *J Clin Endocrinol Metab* 47:494, 1978.

55. Schneider HPG, McCann SM: Possible role of dopamine as transmitter to promote discharge of LH-releasing factor. *Endocrinology* 85:121, 1969.

55a. Kaufman J-M, Kesner JS, Wilson RC, Knobil E: Electrophysiological manifestation of luteinizing hormone-releasing hormone pulse generator activity in the rhesus monkey: Influence of α-adrenergic and dopaminergic blocking agents. *Endocrinology* 116:1327, 1985.

55b. Rasmussen DD, Liu JH, Wolf PL, Yen SSC: Gonadotropin-releasing hormone neurosecretion in the human hypothalamus: *In vitro* regulation by dopamine. *J Clin Endocrinol Metab* 62:479, 1986.

56. Fraschini J: Role of indoleamines in the control of the secretion of pituitary gonadotropins, in Martini L, Meites J (eds): *Neurochemical Aspects of Hypothalamic Function.* New York, Academic, 1971, p 141.

57. Pontiroli AE, Alberetto M, Pellicciotta G, de Castro e Silva E, De Pasqua A, Girardi AM, Pozza G: Interaction of dopaminergic and anti-serotoninergic drugs in the control of prolactin and LH release in normal women. *Acta Endocrinol* 93:271, 1980.

58. Delitala G, Giusti M, Mazzocchi G, Granziera L, Tarditi W, Giordano G: Participation of endogenous opiates in regulation of the hypothalamic-pituitary-testicular axis in normal men. *J Clin Endocrinol Metab* 57:1277, 1983.

59. Morley JE, Baranetsky NG, Wingert TD, Carlson HE, Hershman JM, Melmed S, Levin SR, Jamison KR, Weitzman R, Chang RJ, Varner AA: Endocrine effects of naloxone-induced opiate receptor blockade. *J Clin Endocrinol Metab* 50:251, 1980.

60. Grossman A, Moult PJA, Gaillard RC, Delitala G, Toff WD, Rees LH, Besser GM: The opioid control of LH and FSH release: Effects of a met-enkephalin analogue and naloxone. *Clin Endocrinol* 14:41, 1981.

61. Ellingboe J, Veldhuis JD, Mendelson JH, Kuehnle JC, Mello NK: Effect of endogenous opioid blockade on the amplitude and frequency of pulsatile luteinizing hormone secretion in normal men.

J Clin Endocrinol Metab 54:854, 1982.

62. Veldhuis JD, Kulin HE, Warner BA, Santner SJ: Responsiveness of gonadotropin secretion to infusion of an opiate-receptor antagonist in hypogonadotropic individuals. *J Clin Endocrinol Metab* 55:649, 1982.

63. Reid RL, Quigley ME, Yen SSC: The disappearance of opioidergic regulation of gonadotropin secretion in postmenopausal women. *J Clin Endocrinol Metab* 68:1107, 1983.

64. Veldhuis JD, Rogol AD, Williams FA, Johnson ML: Do α-adrenergic mechanisms regulate spontaneous or opiate-modulated pulsatile luteinizing hormone secretion in man? *J Clin Endocrinol Metab* 57:1292, 1983.

65. Rasmussen DD, Liu JH, Wolf PL, Yen SSC: Endogenous opioid regulation of gonadotropin-releasing hormone release from the human fetal hypothalamus in vitro. *J Clin Endocrinol Metab* 57:881, 1983.

66. Drouva SV, Epelbaum J, Tapia-Arancibia L, Laplante E, Kordon C: Opiate receptors modulate LHRH and SRIF release from mediobasal hypothalamic neurons. *Neuroendocrinology* 32:163, 1981.

67. Blank MS, Panerai AE, Firesen HG: Opioid peptides modulate luteinizing hormone during sexual maturation. *Science* 203:1129, 1979.

68. Ehrenkranz JRL, Tamarkin L, Comite F, Johnsonbaugh RE, Bybee DE, Loriaux DL, Cutler GB Jr: Daily rhythm of plasma melatonin in normal and precocious puberty. *J Clin Endocrinol Metab* 55:307, 1982.

68a. Plant TM, Zorub DS: Pinealectomy in agonadal infantile male rhesus monkeys (*Macaca mulatta*) does not interrupt initiation of the prepubertal hiatus in gonadotropin secretion. *Endocrinology* 118:227, 1986.

69. Clarke IJ, Cummins JT: The temporal relationship between gonadotropin releasing hormone (GnRH) and luteinizing hormone (LH) secretion in ovariectomized ewes. *Endocrinology* 111:1737, 1982.

70. Santen RJ, Bardin CW: Episodic luteinizing hormone secretion in man: Pulse analysis, clinical interpretation, physiologic mechanisms. *J Clin Invest* 52:2617, 1973.

71. Levine JE, Pau K-YF, Ramirez VD, Jackson GL: Simultaneous measurement of luteinizing hormone-releasing hormone and luteinizing hormone release in unanesthetized, ovariectomized sheep. *Endocrinology* 111:1449, 1982.

72. Carmel PW, Araki S, Ferin MP: Pituitary stalk portal blood collection in rhesus monkeys: Evidence for pulsatile release of gonadotropin releasing hormone (GnRH). *Endocrinology* 99:243, 1976.

73. Gallo RV: Neuroendocrine regulation of pulsatile luteinizing hormone secretion in the rat. *Neuroendocrinology* 30:122, 1980.

74. Santen RJ: Independent control of luteinizing hormone secretion by testosterone and estradiol in males, in Fotherby K, Pal SB (eds): *Hormones in Normal and Abnormal Human Tissues.* Berlin and New York, Walter de Gruyter, 1981, p 459.

75. Wilson RC, Knobil E: Central electrophysiologic correlates of pulsatile luteinizing hormone secretion in the rhesus monkey. *7th International Congress on Endocrinology*, Quebec, Canada, abstr S 204, 1984.

76. Plant TM, Krey LC, Moossy J, McCormack JT, Hess DL, Knobil E: The arcuate nucleus and the control of gonadotropin and prolactin secretion in the female rhesus monkey (*Macaca mulatta*). *Endocrinology* 102:52, 1978.

77. Plant TM, Dubey AK: Evidence from the rhesus monkey for the view that negative feedback control of LH by the testis is mediated by a deceleration of hypothalamic pulse frequency. *Endocrinology* 115:2145, 1984.

78. Santen RJ: Is aromatization of testosterone to estradiol required for inhibition of LH secretion in men? *J Clin Invest* 56:1555, 1975.

79. Huseman CA, Kelch RP: Gonadotropin response and metabolism of synthetic gonadotropin-releasing hormone (GnRH) during constant infusion of GnRH in men and boys with delayed adolescence. *J Clin Endocrinol Metab* 47:1325, 1978.

80. Bourguignon J-P, Hoyoux C, Reuter A, Franchimont P: Urinary excretion of immunoreactive luteinizing hormone-releasing hormone-like material and gonadotropins at different stages of life. *J Clin Endocrinol Metab* 48:78, 1979.

81. Pardridge WM, Gorski RA, Lippe BM, Green R: Androgens and sexual behavior. *Ann Intern Med* 96:488, 1982.

82. Gorski RA, Harlan RE, Jacobson CD, Shryne JE, Southam AM: Evidence for the existence of a sexually dimorphic nucleus in the preoptic area of the rat. *J Comp Neurol* 193:529, 1980.

83. Barbarino A, de Marinis L: Estrogen induction of luteinizing hormone release in castrated adult human males. *J Clin Endocrinol Metab* 51:280, 1980.

84. Kwan M, Greenleaf WJ, Mann J, Crapo L, Davidson JM: The nature of androgen action on male sexuality: A combined laboratory-self-report study on hypogonadal men. *J Clin Endocrinol Metab* 57:557, 1983.

85. Conn PM: The molecular basis of gonadotropin releasing hormone action. *Endocr Rev* 7:3, 1986.

86. Smith WA, Conn M: Microaggregation of the gonadotropin-releasing hormone-receptor: Relation to gonadotrope desensitization. *Endocrinology* 114:553, 1984.

87. Conn PM, Marian J, McMillian M, Stern J, Rogers D, Hamby M, Penna A, Grant E: Gonadotropin-releasing hormone action in the pituitary: A three-step mechanism. *Endocr Rev* 2:174, 1981.

88. Hazum E, Cuatrecasas P, Marian J, Conn PM: Receptor-mediated internalization of fluorescent gonadotropin-releasing hormone by pituitary gonadotropes. *Proc Natl Acad Sci USA* 77:6692, 1980.

89. Conn PM, Chafouleas JG, Rogers D, Means AR: Gonadotropin releasing hormone stimulates calmodulin redistribution in rat pituitary. *Nature* 292:264, 1981.

90. Borgeat P, Chavancy G, Dupont A, Labrie F, Arimura A, Schally AV: Stimulation of adenosine 3′,5′-cyclic monophosphate accumulation in anterior pituitary gland *in vitro* by synthetic luteinizing hormone-releasing hormone. *Proc Natl Acad Sci USA* 69:2677, 1972.

91. Naor Z, Koch Y, Chobsieng P, Zor U: Pituitary cyclic AMP production and mechanism of luteinizing hormone release. *FEBS Lett* 58:318, 1975.

92. Gual C, Rosemberg E (eds): *Hypothalamic Hypophysiotropic Hormones.* Amsterdam, Excerpta Medica, 1973.

93. Bremner WJ, Findlay JK, Cumming IA, Hudson B, de Kretser DM: Pituitary-testicular responses in rams to prolonged infusions of luteinizing hormone-releasing hormone (LHRH). *Biol Reprod* 15:141, 1976.

94. Bremner WJ, Paulsen CA: Two pools of luteinizing hormone in the human pituitary: Evidence from constant administration of luteinizing hormone-releasing hormone. *J Clin Endocrinol Metab* 39:811, 1974.

95. Evans WS, Uskavitch DR, Kaiser DL, Hellmann P, Borges JLC, Thorner MO: The self-priming effect of gonadotropin-releasing hormone on luteinizing hormone release: Observations using rat anterior pituitary fragments and dispersed cells continuously perifused in parallel. *Endocrinology* 114:861, 1984.

96. Odell WD: LH, in Degroot LJ, Cahill GF, Odell WD, Martini L, Potts JT, Nelson DH, Steinberger E, Winegrad AI (eds): *Endocrinology*, New York, Grune and Stratton, 1979, vol 1, p 151.

97. Chappel SC, Ulloa-Aguirre A, Coutifaris C: Biosynthesis and secretion of follicle-stimulating hormone. *Endocr Rev* 4:179, 1983.

98. Robertson DM, Foulds LM, Ellis S: Heterogeneity of rat pituitary gonadotropins on electrofocusing: Differences between sexes and after castration. *Endocrinology* 111:385, 1982.

99. Dufau ML, Nozu K, Dehejia A, Garcia Vela A, Solano AR, Fraioli F, Catt KJ: Biological activity and target cell actions of lu-

teinizing hormone, in Motta M, Zonisi M, Piva F (eds): *Serono Symposium, Pituitary Hormones and Related Peptides.* New York, Academic, 1982, pp 118–119.

100. Dufau M, Beitins I, McArthur J, Catt K: Bioassay of serum LH concentrations in normal and LHRH-stimulated human subjects, in Troen P, Nankin HR: *The Testis in Normal and Infertile Men.* New York, Raven, 1977, p 309.

101. Rich BH, Rosenfield RL, Moll GW Jr, Lucky AW, Roche-Bender N, Fang V: Bioactive luteinizing hormone pituitary reserves during normal and abnormal male puberty. *J Clin Endocrinol Metab* 55:140, 1982.

102. Reiter EW, Beitins IZ, Ostrea T, Gutai JP: Bioassayable luteinizing hormone during childhood and adolescence and in patients with delayed pubertal development. *J Clin Endocrinol Metab* 54:155, 1982.

103. Torresani T, Schuster E, Illig R: Bioactivity of plasma luteinizing hormone in infants and young children. *Acta Endocrinol* 103:326, 1983.

104. Dufau ML, Veldhuis JD, Fraioli F, Johnson ML, Beitins IZ: Mode of secretion of bioactive luteinizing hormone in man. *J Clin Endocrinol Metab* 57:993, 1983.

105. Evans RM, Doelle GC, Lindner J, Bradley V, Rabin D: A luteinizing hormone-releasing hormone agonist decreases biological activity and modifies chromatographic behavior of luteinizing hormone in man. *J Clin Invest* 73:262, 1984.

106. Santen R, Warner B, Dufau M: Decreased LH bio/immuno ratio during treatment with the superagonist analog of GnRH. *7th International Congress on Endocrinology,* Quebec, Canada, abstr 2254, 1984.

107. Nakai Y, Plant TM, Hess DL, Keogh EJ, Knobil E: On the sites of the negative and positive feedback actions of gonadotropin secretion in the rhesus monkey. *Endocrinology* 102:1008, 1978.

108. Corbin A, Bex FJ: Inhibition of male reproductive processes with an LH-RH agonist, in Cunningham GR, Schill W-B, Hafez ESE (eds): *Regulation of Male Fertility.* Hague, Boston, and London, Martinus Nijhoff, 1980, p 55.

109. Clifton DK, Steiner RA: Cyclic detection: A technique for estimating the frequency and amplitude of episodic fluctuations in blood hormone and substrate concentrations. *Endocrinology* 112: 1057, 1983.

110. Merriam GR, Wachter KW: Algorithms for the study of episodic hormone secretion. *Am J Physiol* 243:E310, 1982.

111. Yen SSC, Llerena LA, Pearson OH, Littell AS: Disappearance rates of endogenous follicle-stimulating hormone in serum following surgical hypophysectomy in man. *J Clin Endocrinol* 30:325, 1970.

111a. Veldhuis JD, Fraioli F, Rogol AD, Dufau ML: Metabolic clearance of biologically active luteinizing hormone in man. *J Clin Invest* 77:1122, 1986.

112. Pepperell RJ, de Kretser DM, Burger HG: Studies on the metabolic clearance rate and production rate of human luteinizing hormone and on the initial half-time of its subunits in man. *J Clin Invest* 56:118, 1975.

113. Kulin HE, Santner SJ, Santen RJ, Murray FT, Hammong JM: The use of urinary gonadotropin measurements to evaluate LRH responsiveness in hypogonadotropic states, in Berling CG, Wentz A (eds): *The LH-Releasing Hormone.* New York, Masson, 1980, p 75.

114. Dattatreyamurty B, Rathnam P, Saxena BB: Isolation of the luteinizing hormone-chorionic gonadotropin receptor in high yield from bovine corpora lutea. *J Biol Chem* 258:3140, 1983.

115. Nozu K, Dehejia A, Zawistowich L, Catt KJ, Dufau ML: Gonadotropin-induced receptor regulation and steroidogenic lesions in cultured Leydig cells: Induction of specific protein synthesis by chorionic gonadotropin and estradiol. *J Biol Chem* 256:12875, 1981.

115a. Tsai-Morris C-H, Aquilano DR, Dufau ML: Gonadotropic regulation of aromatase activity in the adult rat testis. *Endocrinology* 116:31, 1985.

115b. Bercovici JP, Nahoul K, Tater D, Charles JF, Scholler R: Hormonal profile of Leydig cell tumors with gynecomastia. *J Clin Endocrinol Metab* 59:625, 1984.

116. Schwall RH, Erickson GF: Inhibition of synthesis of luteinizing hormone (LH) receptors by a down-regulating dose of LH. *Endocrinology* 114:1114, 1984.

117. Warren DW, Dufau ML, Catt KJ: Hormonal regulation of gonadotropin receptors and steroidogenesis in cultured fetal rat testis. *Science* 218:375, 1982.

118. Forest MG, Lecoq A, Saez JM: Kinetics of human chorionic gonadotropin-induced steroidogenic response of the human testis. II. Plasma 17α-hydroxyprogesterone, Δ^4-androstenedione, estrone, and 17β-estradiol: Evidence for the action of human chorionic gonadotropin on intermediate enzymes implicated in steroid biosynthesis. *J Clin Endocrinol Metab* 49:284, 1979.

119. Padron RS, Wischusen J, Hudson B, Burger HG, de Kretser DM: Prolonged biphasic response of plasma testosterone to single intramuscular injections of human chorionic gonadotropin. *J Clin Endocrinol Metab* 50:1100, 1980.

120. Smalls AGH, Pieters GFFM, Boers GHJ, Raemakers JMM, Hermus ARMM, Benraad TJ, Kloppenborg PWC: Differential effect of single high dose and divided small dose administration of human chorionic gonadotropin on Leydig cell steroidogenic desensitization. *J Clin Endocrinol Metab* 58:327, 1984.

121. Matsumoto AM, Paulsen CA, Hopper BR, Rebar RW, Bremner WJ: Human chorionic gonadotropin and testicular function: Stimulation of testosterone, testosterone precursors and sperm production despite high estradiol levels. *J Clin Endocrinol Metab* 56:720, 1983.

122. Preslock JP: Steroidogenesis in the mammalian testis. *Endocr Rev* 1:132, 1980.

123. Ruokonen AO, Vihko RK: Quantitative changes of endogenous unconjugated and sulfated steroids in human testis in relation to synthesis of testosterone *in vitro. J Androl* 4:104, 1983.

124. Hammond GL, Ruokonen A, Kontturi M, Koskela E, Vihko R: The stimultaneous radioimmunoassay of seven steroids in human spermatic and peripheral venous blood. *J Clin Endocrinol Metab* 45:16, 1977.

125. Weinstein RL, Kelch RP, Jenner MR, Kaplan SL, Grumbach MM: Secretion of unconjugated androgens and estrogens by the normal and abnormal human testis before and after human chorionic gonadotropin. *J Clin Invest* 53:1, 1974.

126. Kulin HE, Samojlik E, Santen R, Santner S: The effect of growth hormone on the Leydig cell response to chorionic gonadotrophin in boys with hypopituitarism. *Clin Endocrinol* 15:463, 1981.

127. Sherins RJ, Winters SJ, Wachslicht H: Studies of the role of HCG and low dose FSH in initiating spermatogenesis in hypogonadotropic men. *Proceedings of the 59th Annual Meeting of the Endocrine Society,* abstr 312, 1977.

128. Sharpe RM: Intratesticular factors controlling testicular function. *Biol Reprod* 30:29, 1984.

129. Chen CLC, Mather JP, Morris PL, Bardin CW: Expression of proopiomelanocortin (POMC)-like gene in male reproductive tissues. *7th International Congress on Endocrinology,* Quebec, Canada, abstr 278, 1984.

130. Clayton RN, Huhtaniemi IT: Absence of gonadotropin-releasing hormone receptors in human gonadal tissue. *Nature* 299:56, 1982.

131. Clayton RN, Catt KJ: Gonadotropin-releasing hormone receptors: Characterization, physiological regulation, and relationship to reproductive function. *Endocr Rev* 2:186, 1981.

132. Baker HWG, Santen RJ, Burger HG, de Kretser D, Hudson B, Pepperell RJ, Bardin CW: Rhythms in the secretion of gonadotropins and gonadal steroids. *J Steroid Biochem* 6:793, 1975.

133. Pardridge WM: Transport of protein-bound hormones into tissues *in vivo. Endocr Rev* 2:103, 1981.

134. Goldzieher JW, Dozier TS, Smith KD, Steinberger E: Improv-

ing the diagnostic reliability of rapidly fluctuating plasma hormone levels by optimized multiple-sampling techniques. *J Clin Endocrinol Metab* 43:824, 1976.

135. Sanford EJ, Paulson DF, Rohner TJ Jr, Drago JR, Santen RJ, Bardin CW: The effects of castration on adrenal testosterone secretion in men with prostatic carcinoma. *J Urol* 118:1019, 1977.

136. Dunn JF, Nisula BC, Rodbard D: Transport of steroid hormones: Binding of 21 endogenous steroids to both testosterone-binding globulin and corticosteroid-binding globulin in human plasma. *J Clin Endocrinol Metab* 53:58, 1981.

137. Vermeulen A, Verdonck L, Van der Straeten M, Orie M: Capacity of the testosterone binding globulin in human plasma and influence of specific binding of testosterone on its metabolic clearance rate. *J Clin Endocrinol Metab* 29:1470, 1969.

138. Manni A, Pardridge WM, Cefalu W, Nisula BC, Bardin CW, Santner SJ, Santen RJ: Bioavailability of albumin-bound testosterone. *J Clin Endocrinol Metab* 61:705, 1985.

139. Pugeat MM, Dunn JF, Nisula BC: Transport of steroid hormones: Interaction of 70 drugs with testosterone-binding globulin and corticosteroid-binding globulin in human plasma. *J Clin Endocrinol Metab* 53:69, 1981.

140. Cunningham SK, Loughlin T, Culliton M, McKenna TJ: Plasma sex hormone-binding globulin levels decrease during the second decade of life irrespective of pubertal status. *J Clin Endocrinol Metab* 58:915, 1984.

141. Musto NA, Cheng CY, Gunsalus GL, Escobar N, Bardin CW: The use of androgen binding protein and other Sertoli cell products to monitor seminiferous tubular physiology and pathophysiology, in Santen RJ, Swerdloff RS (eds): *Male Sexual Dysfunction: Diagnosis and Management of Hypogonadism, Infertility and Impotence.* New York, Marcel Dekker, 1985.

142. Cheng CY, Musto NA, Gunsalus GL, Bardin CW: Purification of human testicular androgen binding protein (hABP): Comparison with serum testosterone-estradiol-binding globulin (hTeBG). *17th Annual Meeting of the Society for the Study of Reproduction,* Laramie, WY, abstr 34, 1984.

142a. Petra PH, Titani K, Walsh K: Purification and chemical characterization of SBP, the sex steroid binding protein of plasma. *First International Symposium on Binding Proteins: Steroid Hormones,* Lyons, France, 1986, p 1.

143. Cheng CY, Bardin CW, Musto NA, Gunsalus GL, Cheng SL, Ganguly M: Radioimmunoassay of testosterone-estradiol-binding globulin in humans: A reassessment of normal values. *J Clin Endocrinol Metab* 56:68, 1983.

144. Demisch K, Nickelsen T: Distribution of testosterone in plasma proteins during replacement therapy with testosterone enanthate in patients suffering from hypogonadism. *Andrologia* 15:536, 1983.

145. Walker RF: Assessment of endocrine function by salivary steroids, in Edwards RG (ed): *Research in Reproduction.* London, International Planned Parenthood Federation, 1983, vol 15, p 1.

146. Longcope C, Sato K, McKay C, Horton R: Aromatization by splanchnic tissue in men. *J Clin Endocrinol Metab* 58:1089, 1984.

147. Ito T, Horton R: The source of plasma dihydrotestosterone in man. *J Clin Invest* 50:1621, 1971.

148. Martini L: The 5α-reduction of testosterone in the neuroendocrine structures. Biochemical and physiological implications. *Endocr Rev* 3:1, 1982.

149. Peterson RE, Imperato-McGinley J, Gautier T, Sturla E: Male pseudohermaphroditism due to steroid 5α-reductase deficiency. *Am J Med* 62:170, 1977.

150. Mowszowicz I, Melanitou E, Kirchhoffer M-O, Mauvais-Jarvis P: Dihydrotestosterone stimulates 5α-reductase activity in pubic skin fibroblasts. *J Clin Endocrinol Metab* 56:320, 1983.

151. Deslypere J-P, Sayed A, Punjabi U, Verdonck L, Vermeulen A: Plasma 5α-androstane-$3\alpha,17\beta$-diol and urinary 5α-androstane-$3\alpha,17\beta$-diol glucuronide, parameters of peripheral androgen action: A comparative study. *J Clin Endocrinol Metab* 54:386, 1982.

152. Goos CMAA, Wirtz P, Vermorken AJM, Mauvais-Jarvis P: Androgenic effect of testosterone and some of its metabolites in relation to their biotransformation in the skin. *Br J Dermatol* 107:549, 1982.

153. Morimoto I, Edmiston A, Hawks D, Horton R: Studies on the origin of androstanediol and androstanediol glucuronide in young and elderly men. *J Clin Endocrinol Metab* 52:772, 1981.

154. Horton R, Hawks D, Lobo R: $3\alpha,17\beta$-androstanediol glucuronide in plasma: A marker of androgen action in idiopathic hirsutism. *J Clin Invest* 69:1203, 1982.

155. Mauvais-Jarvis P, Kuttenn F, Mowszowicz I (eds): *Hirsutism.* New York, Springer-Verlag, 1981.

156. Lookingbill DP, Horton R, Demers LM, Egan N, Marks JG Jr, Santen RJ: Tissue production of androgens in women with acne. *J Am Acad Dermatol* 12:481, 1985.

157. Samojlik E, Kirschner MA, Silber D, Schneider G, Ertel NH: Elevated production and metabolic clearance rates of androgens in morbidly obese women. *J Clin Endocrinol Metab* 59:949, 1984.

158. Chan L, O'Malley BW: Mechanism of action of the sex steroid hormones. *N Engl J Med* 294:1322, 1976.

159. Chang CH, Rowley DR, Tindall DJ: Purification and characterization of the androgen receptor from rat ventral prostate. *Biochemistry* 22:6170, 1983.

160. Barrack ER: The nuclear matrix of the prostate contains acceptor sites for androgen receptors. *Endocrinology* 113:430, 1983.

161. Saartok T, Dahlberg E, Gustafsson J-A: Relative binding affinity of anabolic-androgenic steroids: Comparison of the binding to the androgen receptors in skeletal muscle and in prostate, as well as to sex hormone-binding globulin. *Endocrinology* 114:2100, 1984.

162. Santen RJ, Friend JN, Trojanowski D, Davis B, Samojlik E, Bardin CW: Prolonged negative feedback suppression after estradiol administration: Proposed mechanism of eugonadal secondary amenorrhea. *J Clin Endocrinol Metab* 47:1220, 1978.

162a. Gharib SD, Bowers SM, Need LR, Chin WB: Regulation of rat luteinizing hormone subunit messenger ribonucleic acids by gonadal steroid hormones. *J Clin Invest* 77:582, 1986.

163. Naftolin F, Ryan KJ, Davies IJ, Reddy VV, Flores F, Petro Z, Kuhn M, White RJ, Takaoka Y, Wolin L: The formation of estrogens by central neuroendocrine tissues. *Recent Prog Horm Res* 31:295, 1975.

164. Marynick SP, Loriaux DL, Sherins RJ, Pita JC Jr, Lipsett MB: Evidence that testosterone can suppress pituitary gonadotropin secretion independently of peripheral aromatization. *J Clin Endocrinol Metab* 49:396, 1979.

165. Kuhn JM, Rieu M, Laudat MH, Forest MG, Pugeat M, Bricaire H, Luton JP: Effects of 10 days administration of percutaneous dihydrotestosterone on the pituitary-testicular axis in normal men. *J Clin Endocrinol Metab* 58:231, 1984.

166. Winters SJ, Sherins RJ, Loriaux DL: Studies on the role of sex steroids in the feedback control of gonadotropin concentrations in men. III. Androgen resistance in primary gonadal failure. *J Clin Endocrinol Metab* 48:553, 1979.

167. Gross DS: Effect of castration and steroid replacement on immunoreactive gonadotropin-releasing hormone in the hypothalamus and preoptic area. *Endocrinology* 106:1442, 1980.

168. Rudenstein RS, Bigdeli H, McDonald MH, Snyder PJ: Administration of gonadal steroids to the castrated male rat prevents a decrease in the release of gonadotropin-releasing hormone from the incubated hypothalamus. *J Clin Invest* 63:262, 1979.

169. Loriaux DL, Vigersky RA, Marynick SP, Janick JJ, Sherins RJ: Androgen and estrogen effects in the regulation of LH in man, in Troen P, Nankin HR (eds): *The Testis in Normal and Infertile Men.* New York, Raven, 1977, p 213.

169a. Veldhuis JD, Rogol AD, Samojlik E, Ertel NH: Role of endogenous opiates in the expression of negative feedback actions of androgen and estrogen on pulsatile properties of luteinizing hormone secretion in man. *J Clin Invest* 74:47, 1984.

170. Kingsley TR, Bogdanove EM: Direct feedback of androgens:

Localized effects of intrapituitary implants of androgens on gonadotrophic cells and hormone stores. *Endocrinology* 93:1398, 1973.

171. Leveque NW, Grotjan HE Jr: Testosterone inhibition of LRH-induced luteinizing hormone release by cultures of rat anterior pituitary cells: Effect of inhibitors of steroid 5α-reductase. *Acta Endocrinol* 100:196, 1982.

172. Caminos-Torres R, Ma L, Snyder PJ: Testosterone-induced inhibition of the LH and FSH responses to gonadotropin-releasing hormone occurs slowly. *J Clin Endocrinol Metab* 44:1142, 1977.

173. Clarke IJ: The relationships between GnRH and LH secretion. *7th International Congress on Endocrinology*, Quebec, Canada, abstr S 66, 1984.

174. Winters SJ, Janick JJ, Loriaux DL, Sherins RJ: Studies on the role of sex steroids in the feedback control of gonadotropin concentrations in men. II. Use of the estrogen antagonist, clomiphene citrate. *J Clin Endocrinol Metab* 48:222, 1979.

175. Frawley LS, Neill JD: Biphasic effects of estrogen on gonadotropin-releasing hormone-induced luteinizing hormone release in monolayer cultures of rat and monkey pituitary cells. *Endocrinology* 114:659, 1984.

176. Pfaff DW, McEwen BS: Actions of estrogens and progestins on nerve cells. *Science* 219:808, 1983.

177. Santen RJ, Ruby EB: Enhanced frequency and magnitude of episodic luteinizing hormone-releasing hormone discharge as a hypothalamic mechanism for increased luteinizing hormone secretion. *J Clin Endocrinol Metab* 48:315, 1979.

177a. Winters SJ, Troen P: Evidence for a role of endogenous estrogen in the hypothalamic control of gonadotropin secretion in men. *J Clin Endocrinol Metab* 61:842, 1985.

178. Roselli CE, Resko JA: Androgens regulate brain aromatase activity in adult male rats through a receptor mechanism. *Endocrinology* 114:1, 1984.

179. Goy RW, McEwen BS (eds): *Sexual Differentiation of the Brain.* Cambridge, MA, MIT, 1980, p 223.

180. Worgul TJ, Santen RJ, Samojlik E, Irwin G, Falvo RE: Evidence that brain aromatization regulates LH secretion in the male dog. *Am J Physiol* 241:E246, 1981.

181. Keye WR Jr, Jaffee RB: Strength-duration characteristics of estrogen effects on gonadotropin response to gonadotropin-releasing hormone in women. I. Effects of varying duration of estradiol administration. *J Clin Endocrinol Metab* 41:1003, 1975.

182. Kulin HE, Reiter EO: Gonadotropin and testosterone measurements after estrogen administration to adult men, prepubertal and pubertal boys, and men with hypogonadotropism: Evidence for maturation of positive feedback in the male. *Pediatr Res* 10:46, 1976.

183. Bowers CY, Currie BL, Johansson NG, Folkers K: Biological evidence that separate hypothalamic hormones release the follicle stimulating and luteinizing hormones. *Biochem Biophys Res Commun* 50:20, 1973.

184. Franchimont P, Demoulin A, Bourguignon JP, Santen R: Role of inhibin in the regulation of gonadotrophin secretion in the male, in *Pediatric and Adolescent Endocrinology: Cryptorchidism. Diagnosis and Treatment.* Basel, Karger, 1979, vol 6, p 47.

185. Pasteels JL, Sheridan R, Gaspar S, Franchimont P: Synthesis and release of gonadotrophins and their subunits by long term organ cultures of human foetal hypophyses. *Mol Cell Endocrinol* 9:1, 1977.

186. Franchimont P, Demoulin A, Bourguignon JP: Regulation of gonadotropin secretion, in Santen RJ, Swerdloff RS (eds): *Male Sexual Dysfunction: Diagnosis and Management of Hypogonadism, Infertility and Impotence.* New York, Marcel Dekker, 1986, pp 101–126.

187. Gross KM, Matsumoto AM, Southworth MB, Bremner WJ: The pattern of luteinizing hormone releasing hormone (LHRH) administration controls the relative secretion of follicle stimulating hormone (FSH) and luteinizing hormone (LH) in man. *Clin Res* 32:266A, 1984.

187a. Gross KM, Matsumoto AM, Berger RE, Bremner WJ: Increased frequency of pulsatile luteinizing hormone-releasing hormone administration selectively decreases follicle-stimulating hormone levels in men with idiopathic azoospermia. *Fertil Steril* 45:392, 1986.

188. Wildt L, Hausler A, Marshall G, Hutchison JS, Plant TM, Belchetz PE, Knobil E: Frequency and amplitude of gonadotropin-releasing hormone stimulation and gonadotropin secretion in the rhesus monkey. *Endocrinology* 109:376, 1981.

189. Coble YD Jr, Kohler PO, Cargille CM, Ross GT: Production rates and metabolic clearance rates of human follicle-stimulating hormone in premenopausal and postmenopausal women. *J Clin Invest* 48:359, 1969.

190. Amin HK, Hunter WM: Human pituitary follicle-stimulating hormone: Distribution, plasma clearance and urinary excretion as determined by radioimmunoassay. *J Endocrinol* 48:307, 1970.

191. Lipshultz LI, Murthy L, Tindall DJ: Characterization of human Sertoli cells *in vitro*. *J Clin Endocrinol Metab* 55:228, 1982.

192. Cheng CY, Frick J, Gunsalus GL, Musto NA, Bardin CW: Human testicular androgen-binding protein shares immunodeterminants with serum testosterone-estradiol-binding globulin. *Endocrinology* 114:1395, 1984.

192a. Joseph DR, Hall SH, French FS: Rat androgen binding protein: Structure of the gene, mRNA and protein. *First International Symposium on Binding Proteins: Steroid Hormones*, Lyons, France, 1986, p 1.

193. Becker RR, Gunsalus GL, Musto NA, Bardin CW: The epididymis contributes minimally to serum androgen-binding protein in the rat: A whole body kinetic study. *Endocrinology* 114:2354, 1984.

194. Gunsalus GL, Musto NA, Bardin CW: Immunoassay of androgen binding protein in blood: A new approach for study of the seminiferous tubule. *Science* 200:65, 1978.

194a. Khan SA, Soder O, Syed V, Ritzen M: Secretion of interkeulin-1 by the rat testis. *Fourth International Workshop on Molecular and Cellular Endocrinology of the Testis,* Capri, Italy, 1986, p 91.

194b. Benahmed M, Morera AM, Chauvin DC, Peretti E: Is somatomedin C a mediating factor between Sertoli and Leydig cells? *Fourth International Workshop on Molecular and Cellular Endocrinology of the Testis,* Capri, Italy, 1986, p 55.

195. Marshall GR, Wickings EJ, Ludecke DK, Nieschlag E: Stimulation of spermatogenesis in stalk-sectioned rhesus monkeys by testosterone alone. *J Clin Endocrinol Metab* 57:152, 1983.

196. Boccabella AV: Reinitiation and restoration of spermatogenesis with testosterone propionate and other hormones after a long-term post-hypophysectomy regression period. *Endocrinology* 72:787, 1963.

197. Paulsen CA, Espeland DH, Michals EL: Effects of hCG, hMG, hLH, and hGH administration on testicular function, in Rosemberg E, Paulsen CA (eds): *The Human Testis.* New York, Plenum, 1970, p 47.

198. Matsumoto AM, Karpas AE, Paulsen CA, Bremner WJ: Reinitiation of sperm production in gonadotropin-suppressed normal men by administration of follicle-stimulating hormone. *J Clin Invest* 72:1005, 1983.

199. Matsumoto AM, Paulsen CA, Bremner WJ: Stimulation of sperm production by human luteinizing hormone in gonadotropin-suppressed normal men. *J Clin Endocrinol Metab* 59:882, 1984.

200. Clifton DK, Bremner WJ: The effect of testicular-irradiation on spermatogenesis in man. *J Androl* 4:387, 1983.

201. Paulsen CA: The study of radiation effects of the human testis: Including histologic, chromosomal and hormonal aspects. *Final Progress Report AEC Contract AT(45-1)-2225,* Task agreement 6, RLO-2225-2, 1973.

202. de Kretser DM, Burger HG, Fortune D, Hudson B, Long AR, Paulsen CA, Taft HP: Hormonal, histological and chromosomal studies in adult males with testicular disorders. *J Clin Endocrinol Metab* 35:392, 1972.

203. McCullagh DR: Dual endocrine activity of the testes. *Science* 76:19, 1932.

204. de Jong FH, van Dijk S, van der Molen HJ: Purification of inhibin from bovine follicular fluid (BFF). *J Steroid Biochem* 20:1587, 1984.

204a. Godbout M, Labrie F: Isolation of "inhibin" from porcine follicular fluid following preparative polyacrylamide gradient gel electrophoresis. *J Steroid Biochem* 20:1587, 1984.

204b. Robertson DM, Foulds LM, Leversha L, Morgan FJ, Hearn MTW, Burger HG, Wettenhall REH, de Kretser DM: Isolation of inhibin from bovine follicular fluid. *Biochem Biophys Res Commun* 126:220, 1985.

204c. Miyamoto K, Hasegawa Y, Fukuda M, Nomura M, Igarashi M, Kanagawa K, Matsuo H: Isolation of porcine follicular fluid inhibin of 32K daltons. *Biochem Biophys Res Commun* 129:396, 1985.

204d. Mason AJ, Hayflick JS, Ling N, Esch F, Ueno N, Ying S-Y, Guillemin R, Nial H, Seeburg PH: Complementary DNA sequences of ovarian follicular fluid inhibin show precursor structure and homology with transforming growth factor-β. *Nature* 318:659, 1985.

204e. Verhoeven G, Franchimont P: Regulation of inhibin secretion by Sertoli cell-enriched cultures. *Acta Endocrinol* 102:136, 1983.

204f. Ying S-Y, Becker A, Baird A, Ling N, Ueno N, Esch F, Guillemin R: Type beta transforming growth factor (TGF-β) is a potent stimulator of the basal secretion of follicle stimulating hormone (FSH) in a pituitary monolayer system. *Biochem Biophys Res Commun* 135:950, 1986.

205. Takahashi J, Higashi Y, LaNasa JA, Winters SJ, Oshima H, Troen P: Studies of the human testis. XVII. Gonadotropin regulation of intratesticular testosterone and estradiol in infertile men. *J Clin Endocrinol Metab* 55:1073, 1982.

206. Hansson V, Ritzen EM, French FS, Nayfeh SN: Androgen transport and receptor mechanisms in testis and epididymis, in Hamilton DW, Greep RO (eds): *Handbook of Physiology: Endocrinology*, Baltimore, Williams and Wilkins, 1975, vol 5, p 173.

207. Setchell BP: Endocrinology of the testis, in Setchell BP (ed): *The Mammalian Testis*. Ithaca, NY, Cornell University, 1972, p 109.

208. Sherins RJ, Clark RV: Elevated estradiol prevents completion of spermatogenesis in hypogonadotropic men treated with HCG alone. *Annual Meeting of the Endocrine Society*, abstr no 941, 1983.

209. Vigersky RA, Glass AR: Effects of Δ^1-testolactone on the pituitary-testicular axis in oligospermic men. *J Clin Endocrinol Metab* 52:897, 1981.

210. Bartke A: Pituitary-testis relationship: Role of prolactin in the regulation of testicular function, in Hubinont PO (ed): *Progress in Reproductive Biology*, Basel, Karger, 1976, vol 1, p 136.

211. Rubin RT, Poland RE, Tower BB: Prolactin-related testosterone secretion in normal adult men. *J Clin Endocrinol Metab* 42:112, 1975.

212. Baranao JLS, Tesone M, Oliveira-Filho RM, Chiauzzi VA, Calvo JC, Charreau EH, Calandra RS: Effects of prolactin on prostate androgen receptors in male rats. *J Androl* 3:281, 1982.

213. Beumont PJV, Corker C, Friesen HG, Kolakowska T, Mandelbrote BM, Marshall J, Murray MA, Wiles DH: The effect of phenothiazines on endocrine function: II. Effects in men and postmenopausal women. *Br J Psychiatry* 124:420, 1974.

214. Klemcke HG, Bartke A, Borer KT: Regulation of testicular prolactin and luteinizing hormone receptors in golden hamsters. *Endocrinology* 114:594, 1984.

215. Wahlstrom T, Huhtaniemi I, Hovatta O, Seppala M: Localization of luteinizing hormone, follicle-stimulating hormone, prolactin, and their receptors in human and rat testis using immunohistochemistry and radioreceptor assay. *J Clin Endocrinol Metab* 57:825, 1983.

216. Martikainen H, Vihko R: hCG-stimulation of testicular steroidogenesis during induced hyper- and hypoprolactinaemia in man. *Clin Endocrinol* 16:227, 1982.

217. Bernini GP, Gasperi M, Franchi F, Luisi M: Effects of sulpiride induced hyperprolactinemia on testosterone secretion and metabolism before and after hCG in normal men. *J Endocrinol Invest* 6:287, 1983.

218. Magrini G, Pellaton M, Felber JP: Prolactin induced modifications of testosterone metabolism in man. *Acta Endocrinol* (suppl) 212:143, 1977.

219. Magrini G, Ebiner JR, Burckhardt P, Felber JP: Study on the relationship between plasma prolactin levels and androgen metabolism in man. *J Clin Endocrinol Metab* 43:944, 1976.

220. Carter JN, Tyson JE, Tolis G, Van Vliet S, Faiman C, Friesen HG: Prolactin-secreting tumors and hypogonadism in 22 men. *N Engl J Med* 299:847, 1978.

221. Sherins RJ, Howards SS: Male infertility, in Harrison JH, Gittes RF, Perlmutter AD, Stamey TA, Walsh PC (eds): *Campbell's Urology*, 4th ed. Philadelphia, Saunders, 1978, vol 1, p 715.

222. Lowe DH, Brock WA, Kaplan GW: Laparoscopy for localization of nonpalpable testes. *J Urol* 131:728, 1984.

223. Weiss RM, Glickman MG, Lytton B: Clinical implications of gonadal venography in the management of the non-palpable undescended testis. *J Urol* 121:745, 1979.

224. Skakkebaek NE, Hammen R, Philip J, Rebbe H: Quantification of human seminiferous epithelium. *Acta Pathol Microbiol Scand* (A) 81:97, 1973.

225. Müller J, Skakkebaek NE: Quantitative assessment of the seminiferous epithelium in male infertility, in Santen RJ, Swerdloff RS (eds): *Male Sexual Dysfunction: Diagnosis and Management of Hypogonadism, Infertility and Impotence*. New York, Marcel Dekker, 1986, pp 321–340.

226. Baker HWG, Burger HG, de Kretser DM, Hudson B: Relative incidence of etiologic disorders in male infertility, in Santen RJ, Swerdloff RS (eds): *Male Sexual Dysfunction: Diagnosis and Management of Hypogonadism, Infertility and Impotence*. New York, Marcel Dekker, 1986, pp 341–372.

227. Gordon DL, Barr AB, Heerigel JE, Paulsen CA: Testicular biopsy in man: Effect on sperm concentration. *Fertil Steril* 16:522, 1965.

228. Schwartz D, Laplanche A, Jouannet P, David G: Within-subject variability of human semen in regard to sperm count, volume, total number of spermatozoa and length of abstinence. *J Reprod Fertil* 57:391, 1979.

229. Bardin CW, Paulsen CA: The testes, in Williams RD (ed): *Textbook of Endocrinology*, 6th ed. Philadelphia, Saunders, 1981, p 293.

229a. MacLeod J, Wang Y: Male fertility in terms of semen quality: A review of the past, a study of the present. *Fertil Steril* 31:103, 1979.

230. Sherins RJ, Brightwell D, Sternthal PM: Longitudinal analysis of semen of fertile and infertile men, in Troen P, Nankin HR (eds): *The Testis in Normal and Infertile Men*. New York, Raven, 1977, p 473.

231. Aitken RJ, Warner P, Best FS, Templeton AA, Djahanbakhch O, Mortimer D, Lees MM: The predictability of subnormal penetrating capacity of sperm in cases of unexplained infertility. *Int J Androl* 6:212, 1983.

232. Bourguignon JP, Hoyoux C, Reuter A, Franchimont P: Urinary excretion of immunoreactive luteinizing hormone-releasing hormone-like material and gonadotropins at different stages of life. *J Clin Endocrinol Metab* 48:78, 1979.

233. Kulin HE, Bell PM, Santen RJ, Ferber AJ: Integration of pulsatile gonadotropin secretion by timed urinary measurements: An accurate and sensitive 3-hour test. *J Clin Endocrinol Metab* 48:783, 1979.

233a. Burstein S, Schaff-Blass E, Blass J, Rosenfield RL: The changing ratio of bioactive to immunoreactive luteinizing hormone (LH) through puberty principally reflects changing LH radioimmunoassay

dose-response characteristics. *Clin Endocrinol Metab* 61:508, 1985.
234. Nieschlag E: Circadian rhythm of plasma testosterone, in Aschoff J, Ceresa F, Halberg F (eds): *Chronobiological Aspects of Endocrinology.* Stuttgart, W. Germany and New York, Schattauer Verlag, 1977, p 117.
235. Santen RJ, Leonard JM, Sherins RJ, Gandy HM, Paulsen CA: Short- and long-term effects of clomiphene citrate on the pituitary-testicular axis. *J Clin Endocrinol Metab* 33:970, 1971.
236. Forest MG: How should we perform the human chorionic gonadotrophin (hCG) stimulation test? *Int J Androl* 6:1, 1983.
237. Saez JM, Bertrand J: Studies on testicular function in children: Plasma concentrations of testosterone, dehydroepiandrosterone and its sulfate before and after stimulation with human chorionic gonadotropins. *Steroids* 12:749, 1968.
238. Wachtel SS: HY antigen and the genetics of sex determination. *Science* 198:797, 1977.
239. George FW, Catt KJ, Wilson JD: Regulation of the onset of steroid hormone synthesis in fetal gonads, in Hamilton TH, Clark JH, Sadler WA (eds): *Ontogeny of Receptors and Reproductive Hormone Action.* New York, Raven, 1979, p 411.
240. Winter JSD, Hughes IA, Reyes FI, Faiman C: Pituitary-gonadal relations in infancy: 2: Patterns of serum gonadal steroid concentrations in man from birth to two years of age. *J Clin Endocrinol Metab* 42:679, 1976.
241. Faiman C, Winter JSD: Gonadotropins and sex hormone patterns in puberty, in Grumbach MM, Grave GD, Mayer EF (eds): *The Control of the Onset of Puberty.* New York, Wiley, 1974, p 32.
242. Ojeda SR, Andrews WW, Advis JP, White SS: Recent advances in the endocrinology of puberty. *Endocr Rev* 1:228, 1980.
243. Boyar RM, Rosenfeld RS, Kapen S, Finkelstein JW, Roffwarg HP, Weitzman ED, Hellman L: Human puberty. *J Clin Invest* 54:609, 1974.
244. Kulin HE, Maruca J: Sex steroid-gonadotropin feedback changes during childhood and adolescence, in Bhatnager AS (ed): *The Anterior Pituitary Gland.* New York, Raven, 1983, p 423.
245. Sizonenko PC: Endocrine laboratory findings in pubertal disturbances. *Clin Endocrinol Metab* 4:173, 1975.
246. Conte FA, Grumbach MM, Kaplan SL, Reiter EO: Correlation of luteinizing hormone-releasing factor-induced luteinizing hormone and follicle-stimulating hormone release from infancy to 19 years with the changing pattern of gonadotropin secretion in agonadal patients: Relation to the restraint of puberty. *J Clin Endocrinol Metab* 50:163, 1980.
247. Schultz NJ, Terasawa E: Further study on the causal relationship between developmental changes in LH release and the onset of puberty in female rhesus monkeys: Effects of posterior hypothalamic lesions. *7th International Congress on Endocrinology,* Quebec, Canada, abstr 2144, 1984.
248. Santen RJ, Kulin HE: Evaluation of delayed puberty and hypogonadotropism, in Santen RJ, Swerdloff RS (eds): *Male Sexual Dysfunction: Diagnosis and Management of Hypogonadism, Infertility and Impotence.* New York, Marcel Dekker, 1986, pp 145–190.
249. Kaler LW, Neaves WB: Attrition of the human Leydig cell population with advancing age. *Anat Rec* 192:513, 1978.
250. Davidson JM, Chen JJ, Crapo L, Gray GD, Greenleaf WJ, Catania JA: Hormonal changes and sexual function in aging men. *J Clin Endocrinol Metab* 57:71, 1983.
251. Longcope C: The effect of human chorionic gonadotropin on plasma steroid levels in young and old men. *Steroids* 21:583, 1973.
252. Harman SM, Tsitouras PD: Reproductive hormones in aging men. I. Measurement of sex steroids, basal luteinizing hormone, and Leydig cell response to human chorionic gonadotropin. *J Clin Endocrinol Metab* 51:35, 1980.
253. Bremner WJ, Vitiello MV, Prinz PN: Loss of circadian rhythmicity in blood testosterone levels with aging in normal men. *J Clin Endocrinol Metab* 56:1278, 1983.
254. Marrama P, Carani C, Baraghini GF, Volpe A, Zini D, Celani MF, Montanini V: Circadian rhythm of testosterone and prolactin in the aging. *Maturitas* 4:131, 1982.
255. Tsitouras PD, Hagen TC: Testosterone, LH, FSH, prolactin and sperm in aging healthy men. *7th International Congress on Endocrinology,* Quebec, Canada, abstr 1951, 1984.
256. Vermeulen A, Rubens R, Verdonck L: Testosterone secretion and metabolism in male senescence. *J Clin Endocrinol Metab* 34:730, 1972.
257. Baker HWG, Burger HG, de Kretser D, Hudson B, O'Conner S, Wang C, Mirovics A, Court J, Dunlop M, Rennie GC: Changes in the pituitary-testicular axis with age. *Clin Endocrinol* 5:349, 1976.
258. Tsitouras PD, Martin CE, Harman SM: Relationship of serum testosterone to sexual activity in healthy elderly men. *J Gerontol* 36:288, 1982.
259. McLeod J, Gold RZ: The male factor in fertility and infertility. VII. Semen quality in relation to age and sexual activity. *Fertil Steril* 4:194, 1953.
260. Nieschlag E, Lammers U, Freischem CW, Langer K, Wickings EJ: Reproductive functions in young fathers and grandfathers. *J Clin Endocrinol Metab* 55:676, 1982.
261. Patton ML, Woolf PD: Hyperprolactinemia and delayed puberty: A report of three cases and their response to therapy. *Pediatrics* 71:572, 1983.
262. Thorner MO, Evans WS, MacLeod RM, Nunley WC Jr, Rogol AD, Morris JL, Besser GM: Hyperprolactinemia: Current concepts of management including medical therapy with bromocriptine, in Goldstein M, Calne DB, Lieberman A, Thorner MO (eds): *Ergot Compounds and Brain Function: Neuroendocrine and Neuropsychiatric Aspects.* New York, Raven, 1980, p 165.
263. Bixler EO, Santen RJ, Kales A, Soldatos CR, Scharf MB: Inverse effects of thioridazine (Mellaril) on serum prolactin and testosterone concentrations in normal men, in Troen P, Nankin HR: *The Testis in Normal and Infertile Men.* New York, Raven, 1977, p 403.
263a. Bouchard P, Lagoguey M, Brailly S, Schaison G: Gonadotropin-releasing hormone pulsatile administration restores luteinizing hormone pulsatility and normal testosterone levels in males with hyperprolactinemia. *J Clin Endocrinol Metab* 60:258, 1985.
264. Rjosk HK, Schill WB: Serum prolactin in male infertility. *Andrologia* 11:297, 1979.
265. Spitz IM, Diamant Y, Rosen E, Bell J, David MB, Polishuk W, Rabinowitz D: Isolated gonadotropin deficiency. *N Engl J Med* 290:10, 1974.
265a. Finkelstein J, Klibanski A, Neer R, Greenspan S, Crowley W: Osteopenia in men with idiopathic hypogonadotropic hypogonadism (IHH). *Clin Res* 34:424A, 1986.
266. Santen RJ, Paulsen CA: Hypogonadotropic eunuchoidism: I. Clinical study of the mode of inheritance. *J Clin Endocrinol Metab* 36:47, 1973.
267. Lieblich JM, Rogol AD, White BJ, Rosen SW: Syndrome of anosmia with hypogonadotropic hypogonadism (Kallmann syndrome). *Am J Med* 73:506, 1982.
268. Santen RJ, Paulsen CA: Hypogonadotropic eunuchoidism. II. Gonadal responsiveness to exogenous gonadotropins. *J Clin Endocrinol Metab* 36:55, 1973.
269. Mozaffarian GA, Higley M, Paulsen CA: Clinical studies in an adult male patient with "isolated follicle stimulating hormone (FSH) deficiency." *J Androl* 4:393, 1983.
270. Spratt DI, Hoffman AR, Crowley WF Jr: Hypogonadotropic hypogonadism and its treatment, in Santen RJ, Swerdloff RS (eds): *Male Sexual Dysfunction: Diagnosis and Management of Hypogonadism, Infertility and Impotence.* New York, Marcel Dekker, 1986, p 227.
271. Rowe RC, Schroeder ML, Faiman C: Testosterone-induced fertility in a patient with previously untreated Kallmann's syndrome. *Fertil Steril* 40:400, 1983.
272. Henkin RI, Bartter FC: Studies on olfactory thresholds in normal man and in patients with adrenal cortical insufficiency: The

role of adrenal cortical steroids and of serum sodium concentration. *J Clin Invest* 45:1631, 1966.

273. Doty RL, Shaman P, Dann M: Development of the University of Pennsylvania smell identification test: A standardized microencapsulated test of olfactory function. *Physiol Behav* 32:489, 1984.

274. Bell J, Spitz I, Perlman A, Segal S, Palti Z, Rabinowitz D: Heterogeneity of gonadotropin response to LHRH in hypogonadotropic hypogonadism. *J Clin Endocrinol Metab* 36:791, 1973.

275. Ernould C, Bourguignon JP, Franchimont P: Usefulness and limits of GnRH test in boys with lack of sexual development. *Acta Paediatr* 32:105, 1975.

276. Job JC, Chaussain JL, Garner PE, Toublanc JE: Effect of synthetic luteinizing hormone-releasing hormone on the release of gonadotropins in hypophysogonadal disorders of children and adolescents. *J Pediatr* 88:494, 1976.

277. Bremner WJ, Fernando NN, Paulsen CA: The effect of luteinizing hormone-releasing hormone in hypogonadotropic eunuchoidism. *Acta Endocrinol* 54:1, 1977.

277a. Partsch C-J, Hermanussen M, Sippell WG: Differentiation of male hypogonadotropic hypogonadism and constitutional delay of puberty by pulsatile administration of gonadotropin releasing hormone. *J Clin Endocrinol Metab* 60:1196, 1985.

277b. de Lange WE, Sluiter WJ, Snoep MC, Doorenbos H: The assessment of hypothalamic pituitary maturation during puberty with combined clomiphene citrate/GnRH test in boys. *J Endocrinol Invest* 7:611, 1984.

277c. Barkan AL, Reame NE, Kelch RP, Marshal JC: Idiopathic hypogonadotropic hypogonadism in men: Dependence of the hormone responses to gonadotropin-releasing hormone (GnRH) on the magnitude of the endogenous GnRH secretory defect. *J Clin Endocrinol Metab* 61:1118, 1985.

278. Spitz IM, Hirsch HJ, Trestian S: The prolactin response to thyrotropin-releasing hormone differentiates isolated gonadotropin deficiency from delayed puberty. *N Engl J Med* 308:575, 1983.

278a. Moshang R Jr, Marx BS, Cara JF, Snyder PJ: The prolactin response to thyrotropin-releasing hormone does not distinguish teen-aged males with hypogonadotropic hypogonadism from those with constitutional delay of growth and development. *J Clin Endocrinol Metab* 61:1211, 1985.

279. Bardin CW, Ross GT, Rifkind AB, Cargille CM, Lipsett MB: Studies of the pituitary-Leydig cell axis in young men with hypogonadotropic hypogonadism and hyposmia: Comparison with normal men, prepubertal boys, and hypopituitary patients. *J Clin Invest* 48:2046, 1969.

280. Weinstein RL, Reitz RE: Pituitary-testicular responsiveness in male hypogonadotropic hypogonadism. *J Clin Invest* 53:408, 1974.

281. Santen RJ, Kulin HE: Hypogonadotropic hypogonadism and delayed puberty, in Burger H, de Kretser D (eds): *The Testis.* New York, Raven, 1981, p 329.

282. Tolis G, Lewis W, Verdy M, Friesen HG, Solomon S, Pagalis G, Pavlatos F, Fessas P, Rochefort JG: Anterior pituitary function in the Prader-Labhart-Willi (PLW) syndrome. *J Clin Endocrinol Metab* 39:1061, 1974.

283. Jeffcoate WJ, Laurence BM, Edwards CRW, Besser GM: Endocrine function in the Prader-Willi syndrome. *Clin Endocrinol* 12:81, 1980.

284. Pauli RM, Meisner LF, Szmanda RJ: Expanded Prader-Willi syndrome in a boy with an unusual 15q chromosome deletion. *Am J Dis Child* 137:1087, 1983.

285. Hamilton CR Jr, Scully RE, Kliman B: Hypogonadotropism in Prader-Willi syndrome. *Am J Med* 52:322, 1972.

286. Roth AA: Familial eunuchoidism: The Laurence-Moon-Biedl syndrome. *J Urol* 57:427, 1947.

287. Dekaban NS, Parks JS, Ross GT: Laurence-Moon syndrome: Evaluation of endocrinological function and phenotypic concordance and report of cases. *Med Ann DC* 41:687, 1972.

288. Perez-Palacios G, Uribe M, Scaglia H, Lisker R, Pasapera A, Maillard M, Medina M: Pituitary and gonadal function in patients with the Laurence-Moon-Biedl syndrome. *Acta Endocrinol* 84:191, 1977.

289. Gorlin RJ, Anderson RC, Blaw M: Multiple lentigenes syndrome. *Am J Dis Child* 117:652, 1969.

290. Bardin CW: Hypogonadotropic hypogonadism in patients with multiple congenital defects, in Bergsma D (ed): *Birth Defects, Original Article Services.* Baltimore, Williams and Wilkins, 1971, vol 7, p 175.

291. Volpe R, Metzler WS, Johnston MW: Familial hypogonadotropic eunuchoidism with cerebellar ataxia. *J Clin Endocrinol Metab* 23:107, 1963.

292. Rimoin DL, Schimke RN: The gonads, in Rimoin DL, Schimke RN (eds): *Genetic Disorders of the Endocrine Glands.* St. Louis, Mosby, 1971.

292a. Woolf PD, Hamill RW, McDonald JV, Lee LA, Kelly M: Transient hypogonadotropic hypogonadism caused by critical illness. *J Clin Endocrinol Metab* 60:444, 1985.

293. Kulin HE, Bwibo N, Mutie D, Santner SJ: The effect of chronic childhood malnutrition on pubertal growth and development. *Am J Clin Nutr* 36:527, 1982.

293a. Hoffer LJ, Beitins IZ, Kyung N-H, Bistrian BR: Effects of severe dietary restriction on male reproductive hormones. *J Clin Endocrinol Metab* 62:288, 1986.

293b. Vogel AV, Peake GT, Rada RT: Pituitary-testicular axis dysfunction in burned men. *J Clin Endocrinol Metab* 60:658, 1985.

293c. Dubey AK, Cameron JL, Steiner RA, Plant TM: Inhibition of gonadotropin secretion in castrated male rhesus monkeys (*Macaca mulatta*) induced by dietary restriction: Analogy with the prepubertal hiatus of gonadotropin release. *Endocrinology* 118:518, 1986.

294. Pugliese MT, Lifshitz F, Grad G, Fort P, Marks-Katz M: Fear of obesity. A cause of short stature and delayed puberty. *N Engl J Med* 309:513, 1983.

295. Baker HWG, Burger HG, de Kretser DM, Dulmanis A, Hudson B, O'Connor S, Paulsen CA, Purcell N, Rennie GC, Seah CS, Taft HP, Wang C: A study of the endocrine manifestations of hepatic cirrhosis. *Q J Med* 45:145, 1976.

296. Van Thiel DH, Lester R: Alcoholism: Its effect on hypothalamic pituitary gonadal function. *Gastroenterology* 71:318, 1976.

297. Emmanouel DS, Lindheimer MD, Katz AI: Pathogenesis of endocrine abnormalities in uremia. *Endocr Rev* 1:28, 1980.

298. Bezwoda WR, Bothwell TH, van der Walt LA, Kronheim S, Pimstone BL: An investigation into gonadal dysfunction in patients with idiopathic haemochromatosis. *Clin Endocrinol* 6:377, 1977.

299. Claus-Walker J, Scurry M, Carterre RE, Campos RJ: Steady state hormonal secretion in traumatic quadriplegia. *J Clin Endocrinol Metab* 44:530, 1977.

300. Munro D, Horne HW Jr, et al: The effect of injury to the spinal cord and cauda equina on the sexual potency of men. *N Engl J Med* 239:903, 1958.

300a. Luton JP, Thieblot P, Valcke JC, Mahoudeau JA, Bricaire H: Reversible gonadotropin deficiency in male Cushing's disease. *J Clin Endocrinol Metab* 45:488, 1977.

300b. Dubey AK, Plant TM: A suppression of gonadotropin secretion by cortisol in castrated male rhesus monkeys (*Macaca mulatta*) mediated by the interruption of hypothalamic gonadotropin-releasing hormone release. *Biol Reprod* 33:423, 1985.

300c. MacAdams MR, White RH, Chipps BE: Reduction of serum testosterone levels during chronic glucocorticoid therapy. *Ann Intern Med* 104:648, 1986.

300d. Evain D, Morera AM, Saez JM: Glucocorticoid receptors in interstitial cells of rat testis. *J Steroid Biochem* 7:1135, 1976.

300e. Barkan AL, Kelch RP, Marshall JC: Isolated gonadotrope failure in the polyglandular autoimmune syndrome. *N Engl J Med* 312:1535, 1985.

301. Bardin CW, Bullock LP, Sherins RJ, Mowszowicz I, Blackburn WR: Part II: Androgen metabolism and mechanism of action

in male pseudohermaphroditism: A study of testicular feminization. *Recent Prog Horm Res* 29:65, 1973.

302. Witkin HA, Mednick SA, Schulsinger F, Bakkestrom E, Christiansen KO, Goodenough DR, Hirschhorn K, Lundsteen C, Owen DR, Philip J, Rubin DB, Stocking M: Criminality in XYY and XXY men. *Science* 193:547, 1976.

303. Raboch J, Sipova I: The mental level in 47 cases of true Klinefelter's syndrome. *Acta Endocrinol* 36:401, 1961.

304. Ferguson-Smith MA: The prepubertal testicular lesion in chromatin-positive Klinefelter's syndrome (primary microorchidism) as seen in mentally handicapped children. *Lancet* 1:219, 1959.

305. Wang C, Baker HWG, Burger HG, de Kretser DM, Hudson B: Hormonal studies in Klinefelter's syndrome. *Clin Endocrinol* 4:399, 1975.

306. de la Chappelle A: Analytic review: Nature and origin of males with XX sex chromosomes. *Am J Hum Genet* 24:71, 1972.

307. Harper P, Penny R, Foley TP Jr, Migeon CJ, Blizzard RM: Gonadal function in males with myotonic dystrophy. *J Clin Endocrinol Metab* 35:852, 1972.

308. Drucker WD, Blanc WA, Rowland LP, Grumbach MM, Christy NP: The testis in myotonic muscular dystrophy: A clinical and pathologic study with a comparison with the Klinefelter syndrome. *J Clin Endocrinol Metab* 23:59, 1963.

309. Chaves-Carballo E, Hayles AB: Ullrich-Turner syndrome in the male: Review of the literature and report of a case with lymphocytic (Hashimoto's) thyroiditis. *Mayo Clin Proc* 41:843, 1966.

310. Collins E, Turner G: The Noonan syndrome: A review of the clinical and genetic features of 27 cases. *J Pediatr* 83:941, 1973.

311. Philip J, Lundsteen C, Owen D: The frequency of chromosome aberrations in tall men with special reference to 47,XYY and 47,XXY. *Am J Hum Genet* 28:404, 1976.

312. Friedrich V, Nielson J: Chromosome studies in 5,049 consecutive newborn children. *Clin Genet* 4:333, 1973.

313. Santen RJ, de Kretser DM, Paulsen CA, Vorhees J: Gonadotrophins and testosterone in the XYY syndrome. *Lancet* 2:371, 1970.

314. Schiavi RC, Owen D, Fogel M, White D, Szechter R: Pituitary-gonadal function in XYY and XXY men identified in a population survey. *Clin Endocrinol* 9:233, 1978.

315. Swersie S, Hueckel J, Hudson B, Paulsen CA: Endocrine, histologic and genetic features of the hypogonadism in patients with Down's syndrome. *53d Annual Meeting of the Endocrine Society*, San Francisco, abstr 440, 1971.

316. Abbasi AA, Prasad AS, Ortega J, Congco E, Oberleas D: Gonadal function abnormalities in sickle cell anemia. Studies in adult male patients. *Ann Intern Med* 85:601, 1976.

317. Elder M, Maclaren N, Riley W: Gonadal autoantibodies in patients with hypogonadism and/or Addison's disease. *J Clin Endocrinol Metab* 52:1137, 1981.

318. Abeyaratne MR, Aherne WA, Scott JE: The vanishing testis. *Lancet* 2:822, 1969.

319. Aynsley-Green A, Zachmann M, Illig R, Rampini S, Prader A: Congenital bilateral anorchia in childhood: A clinical, endocrine and therapeutic evaluation of twenty-one cases. *Clin Endocrinol* 5:381, 1976.

320. Winter JSD, Faiman C: Serum gonadotropin concentrations in agonadal children and adults. *J Clin Endocrinol Metab* 35:561, 1972.

321. Levine LS, New MI: Preoperative detection of hidden testes. *Am J Dis Child* 121:176, 1971.

322. Ehrlich RM, Dougherty LJ, Tomashefsky P, Lattimer JK: Effect of gonadotropin in cryptorchidism. *J Urol* 102:793, 1969.

323. Schilsky RL, Lewis BJ, Sherins RJ, Young RC: Gonadal dysfunction in patients receiving chemotherapy for cancer. *Ann Intern Med* 93:109, 1980.

323a. da Cunha MF, Meistrich ML, Fuller LM, Cundiff JH, Hagemeister FB, Velasquez WS, McLaughlin P, Riggs SA, Cabanillas FF, Salvador PG: Recovery of spermatogeneis after treatment for Hodgkin's disease: Limiting dose of MOPP chemotherapy. *J Clin Oncol* 2:571, 1984.

324. Bauner R, Czernichow P, Cramer P, Schaison G, Rappaport R: Leydig-cell function in children after direct testicular irradiation for acute lymphoblastic leukemia. *N Engl J Med* 309:25, 1983.

325. Ash P: The influence of radiation on fertility in man. *Br J Radiol* 53:271, 1980.

326. Chlebowski RT, Heber D: Hypogonadism in male patients with metastatic cancer prior to chemotherapy. *Cancer Res* 42:2495, 1982.

327. Hembree WC III, Nahas GG, Zeidenberg P, Huang HFS: Changes in human spermatozoa associated with high dose marihuana smoking, in Nahas GG, Paton WDM (eds): *Marihuana: Biological Effects.* New York, Pergamon, 1979, p 429.

328. Lantz GD, Cunningham GR, Huckins C, Lipshultz LI: Recovery of severe oligospermia after exposure to dibromochloropropane (DBCP). *Fertil Steril* 35:46, 1981.

329. Kershnar AK, Borut D, Kogut MD, Biglieri EG, Schambelan M: Studies in a phenotypic female with 17-alpha-hydroxylase deficiency. *J Pediatr* 89:395, 1976.

330. Imperato-McGinley J, Peterson RE, Stoller R, Goodwin WE: Male pseudohermaphroditism secondary to 17β-hydroxysteroid dehydrogenase deficiency: Gender role change with puberty. *J Clin Endocrinol Metab* 49:391, 1979.

331. Gall EA: The histopathology of acute mumps orchitis. *Am J Pathol* 23:637, 1947.

332. Ballew JW, Masters WH: Mumps, a cause of infertility. I. Present consideration. *Fertil Steril* 5:536, 1954.

333. Stearns EL, MacDonnell JA, Kaufman BJ, Padua R, Lucman TS, Winter JSD, Faiman C: Declining testicular function with age: Hormonal and clinical correlates. *Am J Med* 57:761, 1974.

334. Purifoy FE, Koopmans LH, Mayes DM: Age differences in serum androgen levels in normal adult males. *Hum Biol* 53:449, 1981.

335. Winters SJ, Troen P: Episodic luteinizing hormone (LH) secretion and the response of LH and follicle-stimulating hormone to LH-releasing hormone in aged men: Evidence for coexistent primary testicular insufficiency and an impairment in gonadotropin secretion. *J Clin Endocrinol Metab* 55:560, 1982.

336. Harman SM, Tsitouras PD, Costa PT, Blackman MR: Reproductive hormones in aging men. II. Basal pituitary gonadotropins and gonadotropin responses to luteinizing hormone-releasing hormone. *J Clin Endocrinol Metab* 54:547, 1982.

337. Migeon CJ, Brown TR, Fichman KR: Androgen insensitivity syndrome, in Josso N (ed): *Pediatric and Adolescent Endocrinology, the Intersex Child.* Basel, Karger, 1981, vol 8, p 171.

338. Rosewater S, Gwinup G, Hamwi GJ: Familial gynecomastia. *Ann Intern Med* 63:377, 1965.

339. Gilbert-Dreyfus S, Sebaoun CIA, Belaisch J: Case of familial androgenism with severe hypospadias, gynecomastia and excessive androgen production. *Ann Endocrinol* 18:93, 1957.

340. Lubs HA Jr, Vilar O, Bergenstal DM: Familial male pseudohermaphrodism with labial testes and partial feminization: Endocrine studies and genetic aspects. *J Clin Endocrinol Metab* 19:1110, 1959.

341. Reifenstein EC Jr: Hereditary familial hypogonadism. *Proc Am Fed Clin Res* 3:86, 1947.

342. Faiman C, Winter JSD: The control of gonadotropin secretion in complete testicular feminization. *J Clin Endocrinol Metab* 39:631, 1974.

343. Aiman J, Griffin JE: The frequency of androgen receptor deficiency in infertile men. *J Clin Endocrinol Metab* 54:725, 1982.

343a. Smallridge RC, Vigersky R, Glass AR, Griffin JE, White BJ, Eil C: Androgen receptor abnormalities in identical twins with oligospermia. *Am J Med* 77:1049, 1984.

343b. Migeon CJ, Brown TR, Lanes R, Palacios A, Amrhein JA, Schoen EJ: A clinical syndrome of mild androgen insensitivity. *J Clin Endocrinol Metab* 59:672, 1984.

344. Bouchard P, Wright F, Portois MC, Couzinet B, Schaison G, Mowszowicz I: Androgen insensitivity in oligospermic men: A reappraisal. *J Clin Endocrinol Metab,* 1986 (in press).

344a. Eil C, Gamblin GT, Hodge JW, Clark RV, Sherins RJ: Whole cell and nuclear androgen uptake in skin fibroblasts from infertile men. *J Androl* 6:365, 1985.

345. Wilson JD, Griffin JE, George FW, Leshin M: The role of gonadal steroids in sexual differentiation. *Recent Prog Horm Res* 37:1, 1981.

346. Imperato-McGinley J, Guerrero L, Gautier T, Peterson RE: Steroid 5α-reductase deficiency in man: An inherited form of male pseudohermaphroditism. *Science* 186:1213, 1974.

347. David R, Yoon DJ, Landin L, Lew L, Sklar C, Schinella R, Golimbu M: A syndrome of gonadotropin resistance possibly due to a luteinizing hormone receptor defect. *J Clin Endocrinol Metab* 59:156, 1984.

348. Beitins IZ, Axelrod L, Ostrea T, Little R, Badger TM: Hypogonadism in a male with an immunologically active, biologically inactive luteinizing hormone. *J Clin Endocrinol Metab* 52:1143, 1981.

349. Keogh EJ, Carati C, Meakin J, MacKellar A, Lawson-Smith C, Laing S, Barovic S, Curnow D, Mathews C: Clinical application of pulsatile gonadotropin releasing hormone (GnRH). *7th International Congress on Endocrinology,* Quebec, Canada, abstr 1166, 1984.

350. Clopper RR, Mazur T, MacGillivray MH, Peterson RE, Voorhees ML: Data on virilization and erotosexual behavior in male hypogonadotropic hypopituitarism during gonadotropin and androgen treatment. *J Androl* 4:303, 1983.

351. Claustrat B, David L, Faure A, Francois R: Development of anti-human chorionic gonadotropin antibodies in patients with hypogonadotropic hypogonadism. A study of four patients. *J Clin Endocrinol Metab* 57:1041, 1983.

351a. Ley SB, Leonard JM: Male hypogonadotropic hypogonadism: Factors influencing response to human chorionic gonadotropin and human menopausal gonadotropin, including prior exogenous androgens. *J Clin Endocrinol Metab* 61:746, 1985.

351b. Finkel DM, Phillips JL, Snyder PJ: Stimulation of spermatogenesis by gonadotropins in men with hypogonadotropic hypogonadism. *N Engl J Med* 313:651, 1985.

352. Sherins RJ, Winters S, Wachslicht H: Studies of the role of hCG and low-dose FSH in initiating spermatogenesis in hypogonadotropic men. *56th Annual Meeting of the Endocrine Society,* Chicago, abstr 312, 1977.

353. Snyder PJ: Clinical use of androgens. *Annu Rev Med* 35:207, 1984.

353a. Cantrill JA, Dewis P, Large DM, Newman M, Anderson DC: Which testosterone replacement therapy? *Clin Endocrinol* 21:97, 1985.

354. Sokol RZ, Palacios A, Campfield LA, Saul C, Swerdloff RS: Comparison of the kinetics of injectable testosterone in eugonadal and hypogonadal men. *Fertil Steril* 37:425, 1982.

355. Palacios A, Campfield LA, McClure RD, Steiner B, Swerdloff RS: Effect of testosterone enanthate on hematopoiesis in normal men. *Fertil Steril* 40:100, 1983.

355a. Sandblom RE, Matsumoto AM, Schoene RB, Lee KA, Giblin EC, Bremner WJ, Pierson DJ: Obstructive sleep apnea syndrome induced by testosterone administration. *N Engl J Med* 308:508, 1983.

356. Boyer JL, Preisig R, Zbinden G, de Kretser DM, Wang C, Paulsen CA: Guidelines for assessment of potential hepatotoxic effects of synthetic androgens, anabolic agents and progestagens in their use in males as antifertility agents. *Contraception* 13:461, 1976.

356a. Sokol RZ, Swerdloff RS: Practical considerations in the use of androgen therapy, in Santen RJ, Swerdloff RS (eds): *Male Reproductive Dysfunction: Diagnosis and Management of Hypogonadism, Infertility and Impotence,* New York, Marcel Dekker, 1986, p 211.

357. Leonard JM, Leach RB, Couture M, Paulsen CA: Plasma and urinary follicle-stimulating hormone levels in oligospermia. *J Clin Endocrinol Metab* 34:209, 1972.

358. Nankin HR, Troen P: Endocrine profiles in idiopathic oligospermic men, in Hafez ESE (ed): *Human Semen and Fertility Regulation in Men.* St. Louis, Mosby, 1976, p 370.

359. Bain J, Moskowitz JP, Clapp JJ: LH and FSH response to gonadotropin releasing hormone (GnRH) in normospermic, oligospermic and azoospermic men. *Arch Androl* 1:147, 1978.

360. Wu FCW, Edmond P, Raab G, Hunter WM: Endocrine assessment of the subfertile male. *Clin Endocrinol* 14:493, 1981.

361. Chemes HE, Dym DW, Fawcett DW, Jayadpour N, Sherins RJ: Patho-physiological observations of Sertoli cells in patients with germinal aplasia or severe germ cell depletion. Ultrastructural findings and hormone levels. *Biol Reprod* 17:108, 1977.

362. Wang C, Chan CW, Wong KK, Yeung KK: Comparison of the effectiveness of placebo, clomiphene citrate, mesterolone, pentoxifylline, and testosterone rebound therapy for the treatment of idiopathic oligospermia. *Fertil Steril* 40:358, 1983.

363. Vigersky RA, Glass AR: Effects of testolactone (Teslac) on pituitary-testicular axis in oligospermic men. *J Clin Endocrinol Metab* 52:897, 1981.

364. Schill WB: Recent progress in pharmacological therapy of male subfertility—a review. *Andrologia* 11:77, 1979.

365. Dubin L, Amelar RD: Varicocelectomy: 986 cases in a twelve-year study. *Urology* 10:446, 1977.

366. MacLeod J: Further observations on the role of varicocele in human male infertility. *Fertil Steril* 20:545, 1969.

367. Rogers BJ, McCarville C, Mygatt G, Soderdahk D, Hale R: The use of in vitro fertilization for monitoring changes in human spermatozoal fertilizing ability associated with repair of varicocele. *Fertil Steril* 34:311, 1980.

368. de Castro MPP, Mastrorocco DAM: Reproductive history and semen analysis in prevasectomy fertile men with and without varicocele. *J Androl* 5:17, 1984.

369. Comhaire FH: Evaluation and treatment of varicocele, in Santen RJ, Swerdloff RS (eds): *Male Sexual Dysfunction: Diagnosis and Management of Hypogonadism, Infertility and Impotence.* New York, Marcel Dekker, 1986, pp 387–406.

370. Ando S, Giacchetto C, Colpi G, Beraldi E, Panno ML, Lombardi A, Sposato G: Physiopathologic aspects of Leydig cell function in varicocele patients. *J Androl* 5:163, 1984.

371. Berger RE, Holmes KK: Infection and male infertility, in Santen RJ, Swerdloff RS (eds): *Male Sexual Dysfunction: Diagnosis and Management of Hypogonadism, Infertility and Impotence.* New York, Marcel Dekker, 1986, pp 407–438.

372. Swenson CE, Toth A, O'Leary WM: *Ureaplasma urealyticum* and human infertility: The effect of antibiotic therapy on semen quality. *Fertil Steril* 31:660, 1979.

373. Gump DW, Gibson M, Ashikaga T: Lack of association between genital mycoplasmas and infertility. *N Engl J Med* 310:937, 1984.

374. Toth A, Lesser ML, Brooks C, Labriola D: Subsequent pregnancies among 161 couples treated for T-mycoplasma genital-tract infection. *N Engl J Med* 308:505, 1983.

375. Handelsman DJ, Conway AJ, Boylan LM, Turtle JR: Young's syndrome: Obstructive azoospermia and chronic sinopulmonary infections. *N Engl J Med* 310:3, 1984.

376. Afzelius BA: "Immotile-cilia" syndrome and ciliary abnormalities induced by infection and injury. *Am Rev Respir Dis* 124:107, 1981.

377. Gagnon C, Sherins RJ, Phillips DM, Bardin CW: Deficiency of protein-carboxyl methylase in immotile spermatozoa of infertile men. *N Engl J Med* 306:821, 1982.

378. Kollberg H, Mossberg B, Afzelius BA, Philipson K, Camner P: Cystic fibrosis compared with the immotile-cilia syndrome: A study of mucociliary clearance, ciliary ultrastructure, clinical picture and ventilatory function. *Scand J Respir Dis* 59:297, 1978.

379. Chandley AC: Assessment of blood karyotypes and germinal cell meiosis in the evaluation of male inferility, in Santen RJ, Swerdloff RS (eds): *Male Sexual Dysfunction: Diagnosis and Management of Hypogonadism, Infertility and Impotence.* New York, Marcel Dekker, 1986, pp 457–477.

380. Chandley AC: The chromosomal basis of human infertility. *Br Med Bull* 35:181, 1979.

381. Rabin BS, Nankin HR, Troen P: Immunologic studies of patients with idiopathic oligospermia, in Troen P, Nankin HR (eds): *The Testis in Normal and Infertile Men*, New York, Raven, 1977, p 435.

382. Haas GG Jr, Cines DB, Schreiber AD: Immunologic infertility: Identification of patients with antisperm antibody. *N Engl J Med* 303:722, 1980.

383. Haas GG Jr: Evaluation of sperm antibodies and autoimmunity in the infertile male, in Santen RJ, Swerdloff RS (eds): *Male Sexual Dysfunction: Diagnosis and Management of Hypogonadism, Infertility and Impotence.* New York, Marcel Dekker, 1986, pp 439–456.

383a. Stenchever MA, Williamson RA, Leonard J, Karp LE, Ley B, Shy K, Smith D: Possible relationship between *in utero* diethylstilbestrol exposure and male fertility. *Am J Obstet Gynecol* 140:186, 1981.

384. Baker HWG, Burger HG, de Kretser DM, Hudson B: Relative incidence of etiologic disorders in male infertility, in Santen RJ, Swerdloff RS (eds): *Male Sexual Dysfunction: Diagnosis and Management of Hypogonadism, Infertility and Impotence.* New York, Marcel Dekker, 1986, pp 341–372.

385. Tyler ET, Singher HO: Male infertility—status of treatment, prevention and current research. *JAMA* 160:91, 1956.

386. Dubin L, Amelar RD: Etiologic factors in 1294 consecutive cases of male infertility. *Fertil Steril* 22:469, 1971.

387. Greenberg SH, Lipshultz LI, Wein AJ: Experience with 425 subfertile male patients. *J Urol* 119:507, 1978.

388. Abyholm T: Azoospermia and oligozoospermia. Etiology and clinical findings. *Arch Androl* 10:57, 1983.

388a. Snyder PJ, Bashey HM, Phillips JL, Gennarelli TA: Comparison of hormonal secretory behavior of gonadotroph cell adenomas *in vivo* and in culture. *J Clin Endocrinol Metab* 61:1061, 1985.

389. Snyder PJ, Bigdeli H, Gardner DF, Mihailovic V, Rudenstein RS, Sterling FH, Utiger RD: Gonadal function in fifty men with untreated pituitary adenomas. *J Clin Endocrinol Metab* 48:309, 1979.

390. Snyder PJ, Bashey HM: Secretion of free LH subunits by pituitary gonadotroph cell adenomas. *Clin Res* 32:487A, 1984.

391. Friend JN, Judge DM, Sherman BM, Santen RJ: FSH-secreting pituitary adenomas: Stimulation and suppression studies in two patients. *J Clin Endocrinol Metab* 43:650, 1976.

392. Borges JLC, Ridgway EC, Kovacs K, Rogol AD, Thorner MO: Follicle-stimulating hormone-secreting pituitary tumor with concomitant elevation of serum α-subunit levels. *J Clin Endocrinol Metab* 58:937, 1984.

393. Harris RI, Schatz NJ, Gennarelli T, Savino PJ, Cobbs WH, Snyder PJ: Follicle-stimulating hormone-secreting pituitary adenomas: Correlation of reduction of adenoma size with reduction of hormonal hypersecretion after transsphenoidal surgery. *J Clin Endocrinol Metab* 56:1288, 1983.

394. Judge DM, Kulin HE, Page R, Santen R, Trapukdi S: Hypothalamic hamartoma: A source of luteinizing-hormone-releasing factor in precocious puberty. *N Engl J Med* 296:7, 1977.

395. Santen RJ, Kulin HE: The male reproductive system, in Kelley VC (ed): *Practice of Pediatrics.* Hagerstown, MD, Harper & Row, 1976, vol 1, p 1.

396. Barnes ND, Hayles AB, Ryan RJ: Sexual maturation in juvenile hypothyroidism. *Mayo Clin Proc* 48:849, 1973.

397. Crowley WF Jr, Comite F, Vale W, Rivier J, Loriaux DL, Cutler GB: Therapeutic use of pituitary desensitization with a long-acting LH-RH agonist: A potential new treatment for idiopathic precocious puberty. *J Clin Endocrinol Metab* 52:370, 1981.

397a. Comite F, Pescovitz OH, Rieth KG, Dwyer AJ, Hench K, McNemar A, Loriaux DL, Cutler GB: Luteinizing hormone-releasing hormone analog treatment of boys with hypothalamic hamartoma and true precocious puberty. *J Clin Endocrinol Metab* 59:888, 1984.

397b. Styne DM, Harris DA, Egli CA, Conte FA, Kaplan SL, Rivier J, Vale W, Grumbach MM: Treatment of true precocious puberty with a potent luteinizing hormone-releasing factor agonist: Effect on growth, sexual maturation, pelvic sonography, and the hypothalamic-pituitary-gonadal axis. *J Clin Endocrinol Metab* 61:142, 1985.

398. Kaplan SA, Ling SM, Irani NG: Idiopathic sexual precocity: Therapy with medroxyprogesterone. *Am J Dis Child* 116:591, 1968.

399. Pescovitz OH, Comite F, Cassorla F, Dwyer AJ, Poth MA, Sperling MA, Hench K, McNemer A, Skerda M, Loriaux DL, Cutler GB Jr: True precocious puberty complicating congenital adrenal hyperplasia: Treatment with a luteinizing hormone-releasing hormone analog. *J Clin Endocrinol Metab* 58:857, 1984.

400. Wierman ME, Beardsworth DE, Mansfield MJ, Badger TM, Crawford JD, Crigler JF Jr, Bode HH, Loughlin JS, Kushner DC, Scully RE, Hoffman WH, Crowley WF Jr: Puberty without gonadotropins: A unique mechanism of sexual development. *N Engl J Med* 312:65, 1985.

401. Foster CM, Ross JL, Shawker T, Pescovitz OH, Loriaux DL, Cutler GB Jr, Comite F: Absence of pubertal gonadotropin secretion in girls with McCune-Albright syndrome. *J Clin Endocrinol Metab* 58:1161, 1984.

401a. Holland FJ, Fishman L, Bialey JD, Fazekas AT: Ketoconazole in the management of precocious puberty not responsive to LHRH-analogue therapy. *N Engl J Med* 312:1023, 1985.

402. Charney CW, Wolgen W (eds): *Cryptorchidism.* New York, Paul B. Hoeber, 1957.

403. Sohval AR: Histopathology of cryptorchism: Study based on comparative histology of retained and scrotal testes from birth to maturity. *Am J Med* 16:346, 1954.

404. Bergada C: Use of gonadotropins for the evaluation of testicular function and correlations to biopsy of cryptorchid testes, in Job JC: *Cryptorchidism*, Basel and New York, Karger, 1979, p 97.

405. Forest MG: Pattern of the response to hCG stimulation in prepubertal cryptorchid boys, in Job JC (ed): *Cryptorchism*, Basel and New York, Karger, 1979, p 108.

406. Gendrel D, Job JC, Chaussian JL, Roger M, Garnier P, Canlorbe P: Pituitary and gonadal responses to stimulation tests in cryptorchid children, in Job JC (ed): *Cryptorchidism.* Basel and New York, Karger, 1979, p 121.

407. Job JC, Gendrel D, Roger M: Gonadotrophins and testosterone secretion in infants with undescended testes, in Job JC (ed): *Cryptorchidism.* Basel and New York, Karger, 1979, p 130.

408. Elder JS, Isaacs JT, Walsh PC: Androgenic sensitivity of the gubernaculum testis: Evidence for hormonal/mechanical interactions in testicular descent. *J Urol* 127:170, 1982.

409. Ch'en KY: The endocrine glands of anencephalic foetuses. A quantitative and morphological study of 15 cases. *Chin Med J* (suppl) 2:63, 1938.

410. Illig R, Torresani T, Bucher H, Zachmann M, Prader A: Effect of intranasal LHRH therapy on plasma LH, FSH and testosterone and relation to clinical results in prepubertal boys with cryptorchidism. *Clin Endocrinol* 12:91, 1980.

411. Puri P, Nixon HH: Bilateral retractile testes—subsequent effects on fertility. *J Pediatr Surg* 12:563, 1977.

412. Cortada X, Kousseff BG: Cryptorchidism in mental retardation. *J Urol* 131:674, 1984.

413. Waaler PE: Morphometric studies in undescended testes, in Job JC (ed): *Cryptorchidism.* Basel and New York, Karger, 1979, p 27.

414. Mengel W, Heinz HA, Sippe WG, Hecker WC: Studies on cryptorchidism: A comparison of histologic findings in the germinative epithelium before and after the second year of life. *J Pediatr Surg* 9:445, 1974.

415. Alpert PF, Klein RS: Spermatogenesis in the unilateral cryptorchid testis after orchiopexy. *J Urol* 129:301, 1983.

416. David G, Bisson JP, Martin-Boyce A, Feneux D: Sperm characteristics and fertility in previously cryptorchid adults, in Job JC (ed): *Cryptorchidism.* Basel and New York, Karger, 1979, p 187.

417. Krabbe S, Skakkebaek NE, Berthelson JG, Eyben FV, Volsted P, Mauritzen K, Eldrup J, Nielsen AH: High incidence of undetected neoplasia in maldescended testes. *Lancet* 1:999, 1979.

418. Sumner WA: Malignant tumor of testis occurring 29 years after orchiopexy. *J Urol* 81:150, 1959.

419. King LR: Optimal treatment of children with undescended testes. *J Urol* 131:734, 1984.

420. Ehrlich RM, Dougherty LJ, Tomashefsky P, Lattimer JK: Effect of gonadotropin in cryptorchidism. *J Urol* 102:793, 1969.

420a. Rajfer J, Handelsman DJ, Swerdloff RS, Hurwitz R, Kaplan H, Vandergast T, Ehrlich RM: Hormonal therapy of cryptorchidism: A randomized, double-blind study comparing human chorionic gonadotropin and gonadotropin-releasing hormone. *N Engl J Med* 314:466, 1986.

420b. Colodny AH: Undescended testes—is surgery necessary? *N Engl J Med* 314:510, 1986.

421. Bernasconi S, Vanelli M, Rossi S, Ghinelli C, Ziveri M, Virdis R: Intranasal luteinizing hormone releasing hormone (LHRH) therapy in cryptorchid children. *J Androl* 5:116, 1984.

422. Casey RW, Wilson JD: Antiestrogenic action of dihydrotestosterone in mouse breast: Competition with estradiol for binding to the estrogen receptor. *J Clin Invest* 74:2272, 1984.

422a. Wilson JD, Aiman J, MacDonald PC: The pathogenesis of gynecomastia, in Stollerman GH (ed): *Advances in Internal Medicine.* Chicago, Yearbook Medical Publishers, 1980, vol 25.

423. Large DM, Anderson DC: Twenty-four hour profiles of circulating androgens and oestrogens in male puberty with and without gynaecomastia. *Clin Endocrinol* 11:505, 1979.

424. Moore DC, Schlaepfer LV, Paunier L, Sizonenko PC: Hormonal changes during puberty: V. Transient pubertal gynecomastia: Abnormal androgen-estrogen ratios. *J Clin Endocrinol Metab* 58:492, 1984.

425. Nydick M, Bustos J, Dale JH Jr, Rawson RW: Gynecomastia in adolescent boys. *JAMA* 178:449, 1961.

426. Nuttal FQ: Gynecomastia as a physical finding in normal men. *J Clin Endocrinol Metab* 48:338, 1979.

427. Carlson HE: Current concepts: Gynecomastia. *N Engl J Med* 303:795, 1980.

428. Ley SB, Mozaffarian GA, Leonard JM, Higley M, Paulsen CA: Palpable breast tissue versus gynecomastia as a normal physical finding. *Clin Res* 28:24A, 1980.

429. Williams MJ: Gynecomastia: Its incidence, recognition and host characterization in 447 autopsy cases. *Am J Med* 34:103, 1963.

430. McFadyen IJ, Bolton AE, Cameron EHD, Hunter WM, Raab G, Forrest APM: Gonadal pituitary hormone levels in gynaecomastia. *Clin Endocrinol* 13:77, 1980.

431. Eil C, Lippman ME, de Moss EV, Loriaux DL: Androgen receptor characteristics in skin fibroblasts from men with pubertal macromastia. *Clin Endocrinol* 19:223, 1983.

432. Siiteri PK, MacDonald PC: Role of extraglandular estrogen in human endocrinology, in Greep RO, Astwood EB (eds): *Handbook of Physiology.* Baltimore, Waverly, 1973, vol 2, p 615.

433. Jensen RT, Collen MJ, Pandol SJ, Allende HD, Raufman JP, Bissonnette BM, Duncan WC, Durgin PL, Gillin JC, Gardner JD: Cimetidine-induced impotence and breast changes in patients with gastric hypersecretory states. *N Engl J Med* 308:883, 1983.

434. Santen RJ, Van den Bossche H, Symoens J, Brugmans J, DeCoster R: Site of action of low dose ketoconazole on androgen biosynthesis in men. *J Clin Endocrinol Metab* 57:732, 1983.

435. Chopra IJ, Abraham GE, Chopra U, Solomon DH, Odell WD: Alterations in circulating estradiol-17β in male patients with Graves's disease. *N Engl J Med* 286:124, 1972.

436. Plourde PV, Kulin HE, Santner SJ: Clomiphene in the treatment of adolescent gynecomastia. *Am J Dis Child* 137:1080, 1983.

437. Kuhn JM, Laudat MH, Roca R, Dugue MA, Luton JP, Bricaire H: Gynécomasties: Effect du traitement prolongé par la dihydrotestosterone par voie per-cutanee. *La Presse Med* 12:21, 1983.

438. Hite S: *The Hite Report on Male Sexuality.* New York, Knopf, 1981.

439. Karacan I, Moore CA: Objective methods of differentiation between organic and psychogenic impotence, in Santen RJ, Swerdloff RS (eds): *Male Sexual Dysfunction: Diagnosis and Management of Hypogonadism, Infertility and Impotence.* New York, Marcel Dekker, 1986, pp 545–562.

440. Krane RJ: Surgical implants for impotence: Indications and procedures, in Santen RJ, Swerdloff RS (eds): *Male Sexual Dysfunction: Diagnosis and Management of Hypogonadism, Infertility and Impotence.* New York, Marcel Dekker, 1986, pp 563–576.

441. Spark RF, White RA, Connolly PB: Impotence is not always psychogenic. *JAMA* 243:750, 1980.

442. Steinberger E: Current status of research on hormonal contraception in the male, in Zatuchni GI (ed): *Research Frontiers in Fertility Regulation.* Hagerstown, MD, Harper & Row, 1980, vol 1, p 1.

443. Rabin D, Evans RM, Alexander AN, Doelle GC, Rivier J, Vale W, Liddle GW: Heterogeneity of sperm density profiles following 20-week therapy with high-dose LHRH analog plus testosterone. *J Androl* 5:176, 1984.

444. National Coordinating Group on Male Antifertility Agents: Gossypol—a new antifertility agent for males. *Chin Med J* 6:417, 1978.

445. Alexander NJ, Clarkson TB: Vasectomy increases the severity of diet-induced atherosclerosis in *Macaca fascicularis. Science* 201: 538, 1978.

446. Robinson MRG: Carcinoma of the prostate: Hormonal therapy. *Clin Oncol* 1:233, 1982.

446a. Catalona WJ (ed): *Prostate Cancer,* Orlando, Grune and Stratton, 1984.

447. Byar DP: The Veterans Administrative Co-operative Urological Research Groups: Studies of cancer of the prostate. *Cancer* 32:1126, 1973.

448. Leuprolide Study Group: Leuprolide versus diethylstilbestrol for metastatic prostate cancer. *N Engl J Med* 311:1281, 1984.

448a. Parmar H, Lightman SL, Allen L, Phillips RH, Edwards L, Schally AV: Randomized controlled study of orchidectomy vs. long-acting D-Trp-6-LHRH microcapsules in advanced prostatic carcinoma. *Lancet* 2:1201, 1985.

449. Labrie F, Dupont A, Belanger A, Lacoursiere Y, Raynaud JP, Husson JM, Gareau J, Fazekas ATA, Sandow J, Monfette G, Girard JG, Emond J, Houle JG: New approach in the treatment of prostate cancer: Complete instead of partial withdrawal of androgens. *Prostate* 4:579, 1983.

450. Trachtenberg J, Pont A: Ketoconazole therapy for advanced prostate cancer. *Lancet* 2:433, 1984.

451. Worgul TJ, Santen RJ, Samojlik E, Veldhuis JD, Lipton A, Harvey HA, Drago JR, Rohner TJ: Clinical and biochemical effect of aminoglutethimide in the treatment of advanced prostatic carcinoma. *J Urol* 129:51, 1983.

452. Stoliar B, Albert DJ: SCH 13521 in the treatment of advanced carcinoma of the prostate. *J Urol* 111:803, 1974.

453. Anderson T, Waldmann TA, Javadpour N, Glatstein E: Testicular germ-cell neoplasms: Recent advances in diagnosis and therapy. *Ann Intern Med* 90:373, 1979.

454. Webber BL: Germ cell tumors of the testis. *Cancer Treat Rep* 63:1629, 1979.

455. Einhorn LH: Testicular cancer as a model for a curable neoplasm: The Richard and Hinda Rosenthal Foundation Award Lecture. *Cancer Res* 41:3275, 1981.
456. DeWys WD, Muggia FM: Staging of testicular cancer. *Cancer Treat Rep* 63:1675, 1980.
457. Vugrin D, Herr HW, Whitmore WF Jr, Sogani PC, Golbey RB: VAB-6 combination chemotherapy in disseminated cancer of testis. *Ann Intern Med* 95:59, 1981.
458. Ball D, Barrett A, Peckham MJ: The management of metastatic seminoma testis. *Cancer* 50:2289, 1982.
459. Skakkebaek NE: Possible carcinoma-in-situ of the testis. *Lancet* 2:516, 1972.
460. Skakkebaek NE: Carcinoma-in-situ of the testis: Frequency and relationship to invasive germ cell tumors in infertile men. *Histopathology* 2:157, 1978.
461. Teilum G: Classification of testicular and ovarian androblastoma and Sertoli cell tumors. A survey of comparative studies with consideration of histogenesis, endocrinology and embryological theories. *Cancer* 11:769, 1958.
461a. Roth LM, Anderson MC, Govan ADT, Langley FA, Gowing NFC, Woodcock AS: Sertoli-Leydig cell tumors: A clinicopathologic study of 34 cases. *Cancer* 48:187, 1981.
462. Radfar N, Kolins J, Bartter FC: Evidence for cortisol secretion by testicular masses in congenital adrenal hyperplasia, in Lee PA, Plotnick LP, Kowarski AA, Migeon CJ (eds): *Congenital Adrenal Hyperplasia.* Baltimore, University Park, 1977, p 331.
463. Skakkebaek NE, Heller CG: Quantification of human seminiferous epithelium. I. Histological studies in twenty-one fertile men with normal chromosome complements. *J Reprod Fertil* 32:379, 1973.
464. MacLeod J, Gold RZ: The male factor in fertility and infertility. II. Spermatozoon counts in 1000 men of known fertility and in 1000 cases of infertile marriage. *J Urol* 66:436, 1951.
465. Naghma-E-Rehan, Sobrero AJ, Fertig JW: The semen of fertile men: Statistical analysis of 1300 men. *Fertil Steril* 26:492, 1975.
466. Nelson CMK, Bunge RG: Semen analysis: Evidence for changing parameters of male fertility potential. *Fertil Steril* 25:503, 1974.
467. Smith KD, Steinberger E: What is oligospermia?, in Troen P, Nankin HR (eds): *The Testis in Normal and Infertile Men.* New York, Raven, 1977, p 489.
468. Santen RJ, Kulin HE: Evaluation of gonadotropins in man, in Hafez ESE (ed): *Techniques of Human Andrology.* Amsterdam, Elsevier/North-Holland, 1977, p 251.
469. Santen RJ: Independent effects of testosterone and estradiol on the secretion of gonadotropins in man, in Troen P, Nankin HR (eds): *The Testis in Normal and Infertile Men,* New York, Raven, 1977, p 197.
470. Kirschner MA, Zucker R, Jespersen D: Idiopathic hirsutism—An ovarian abnormality. *N Engl J Med* 294:637, 1976.
471. Marshall WA, Tanner JM: Variations in the pattern of pubertal changes in boys. *Arch Dis Child* 45:13, 1970.
472. Kulin HE, Santen RJ: Normal and aberrant pubertal development in man, in Vaitukaitis JL (ed): *Current Endocrinology: Clinical Reproductive Neuroendocrinology.* New York, Elsevier, 1982, p 19.

17

The Ovary: Basic Principles and Concepts

A. PHYSIOLOGY*

Gregory F. Erickson

ANATOMY

Morphology

The mature human ovaries are oval-shaped bodies, each measuring 2.5 to 5.0 cm in length, 1.5 to 3 cm in width, and 0.6 to 1.5 cm in thickness. The medial edge of the ovary is attached by the mesovarium to the broad ligament, which extends from the uterus laterally to the wall of the pelvic cavity. The surface of the ovary is a layer of cuboidal cells resting on a basement membrane. This layer, termed the *germinal* or *serous* epithelium, is continuous with the peritoneum. Underlying the serous epithelium is a thin layer of dense connective tissue termed the *tunica albuginea.*

*This work was supported in part by National Institutes of Child Health and Human Development Research Center Grant HD-12303.

The ovary is organized into two principal parts: a central zone called the *medulla* surrounded by a particularly prominent peripheral zone called the *cortex* (Fig. 17A-1). One characteristic feature of the cortex is the presence of follicles containing the female gametes or *oocytes*. The number and size of the follicles vary greatly, depending on the age and reproductive state of the female. The existence of follicles of different sizes reflects internal changes associated with their growth and development. At the end of the follicular phase, one follicle reaches maturity and secretes its ovum into the peritoneal cavity (Fig. 17A-1). After ovulation, the wall of the follicle develops into a progestin-secreting organ called the *corpus luteum* (Fig. 17A-1). If implantation does not occur, the corpus luteum deteriorates and eventually becomes a nodule of dense connective tissue called the *corpus albicans*. Another class of cells in the cortex is that of the steroidogenic cells termed *interstitial* cells. These cells are found in nests or cords and are present throughout the life of the female. At the medial border of the cortex is a mass of loose connective tissue, the medulla. This tissue contains a network of convoluted blood vessels and associated nerves which pass through the connective tissue toward the cortex.

Blood Vessels

The arterial supply to the ovary originates from two principal sources: one, the ovarian artery, arises from the abdominal aorta; the other is derived from the uterine artery.[1] These two vessels, which enter the mesovarium from opposite directions, form an anastomotic trunk and become a common vessel called the *ramus ovaricus* artery. At frequent intervals, this artery gives rise to a series of primary branches which enter the hilum like teeth on a rake (Fig. 17A-2). Once in the hilum, numerous secondary and tertiary branches are given off to supply the medulla.

A characteristic feature of the secondary and tertiary arteries in the hilum and medulla is that they exhibit extensive spiralling.[1,2] The spiralling is in a counterclockwise direction with a gradually diminishing diameter (Fig. 17A-2). The degree of spiralling in the ovarian arteries undergoes dramatic changes during aging.[2] In the fetal ovary, there is little or no spiralling of the ovarian arteries; however, in the neonatal period, extensive spiralling and profuse branching of these arteries occur. The spiral ovarian arteries are most highly developed in the sexually mature woman and remain prominent throughout the reproductive

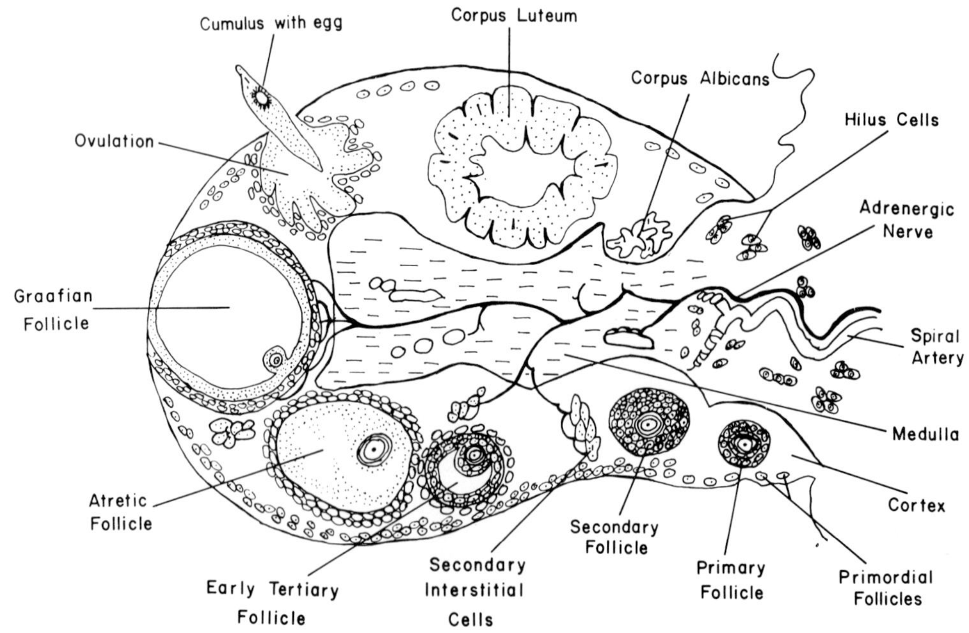

FIGURE 17A-1 Diagram summarizing the architecture of the human ovary during the reproductive years. The follicles, corpora lutea, and interstitial cells are located in the outer cortex, while the hilus cells, autonomic nerves, and spiral arteries are found in the medulla.

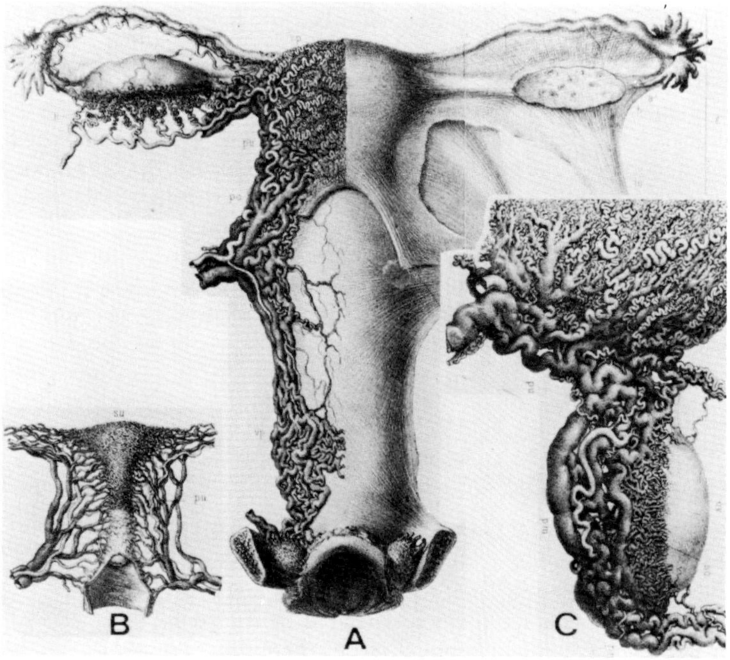

FIGURE 17A-2 Demonstration of extensive spiralling of arteries and veins in the genital tract of an adult woman. (*A*) Ovaries, fallopian tubes, uterus. (*B*) Details of uterus. (C) Details of ovary (note anastomoses of ovarian and uterine arteries). (*From Calza L: Arch Physiol Reils* 7:341, 1807.)

years. In the menopause, the spiral ovarian arteries diminish in number until finally only the main branches of the ovarian artery exist in the hilus.[2]

What is the importance of spiral arteries in the ovary? Evidence suggests that the number and distribution of ovarian spiral arteries are influenced by local changes in ovarian sex hormones,[1–3] in a manner not unlike that reported for spiral arteries in the uterus. During growth and development of the dominant follicle and the corpus luteum there occur tremendous increases in the vascular bed which supplies these two organs; such increases are associated with the induction of a high order of spiralling of the arteries that serve the organs. Thus, it seems that when the dominant follicle is selected, local control mechanisms are initiated whereby the arterial supply and degree of vessel spiralling increase. Although the nature of the inductive influences remains unknown, one such factor might be estrogen.[1,3] The physiological significance of this phenomenon would be the adaptation of the vasculature to accommodate differential ovarian growth, which occurs during the menstrual cycle. A physiological sequela of the increased spiralling could be to provide a mechanism for regulating the blood pressure within the ovary.[1]

Certainly the ovary contains within itself the ability of vascular adaptation. In this sense, it seems possible that disturbed vascular activities may be etiologic factors in pathological ovarian endocrine functions.

Innervation

Coursing through the human ovary is an extensive network of sympathetic and parasympathetic nerves reflecting both pre- and postganglionic fibers.[4] The preganglionic sympathetic fibers originate from cell bodies in the intermediolateral horn of the spinal cord at the 10th and 11th thoracic segments, and postganglionic sympathetic fibers originate from the ovarian and celiac plexuses. These nerves travel along the ovarian artery and enter the ovary at the hilus. The parasympathetic system consists of two main parts. One major part is derived from the vagus nerve and enters the hilum via the ovarian plexus. The other represents preganglionic parasympathetic fibers from the third and fourth sacral nerves, which are derived from the inferior hypogastric nerve. Thus, ovarian cells are capable of interacting with both adrenergic and cholinergic nerves.

The target tissues for adrenergic[5–8] and cholinergic[9] fibers are in the cortex and medulla, and include smooth muscle cells of large arteries and veins and the smooth muscle cells in the outermost layer of the follicle, the theca externa (Fig. 17A-1). In the past few years, considerable evidence has been generated showing that ovarian cells respond to specific neurochemical transmitters with changes in steroidogenesis. The best examples come from studies in which catecholamine stimulates corpus luteum function and granulosa cell activity.[11–13] However, the physiological significance of these studies remains unclear because neither corpora lutea nor the granulosa cells are innervated.[6,10,14]

Importantly, ultrastructural studies in laboratory animals have clearly demonstrated that naked sympathetic adrenergic axons end directly on steroidogenic interstitial cells.[7,15] The innervation between these cells is not a typical synapse but rather a "buton de passage" type often seen between adrenergic terminals and glandular cells.[15,16] The importance of nerves in regulating ovarian functions is an important issue, which is discussed below.

HISTOLOGY

Ovarian Follicles

In the mammalian ovary, all follicles are embedded in the loose connective tissue of the cortex, medial to the tunica albuginea. Each follicle exhibits a specialized cytologic character which is related to the steps in its development. In a broad sense, there are two major classes of follicles: nongrowing and growing. The nongrowing, referred to as *primordial*, follicles comprise 90 to 95 percent of the ovarian follicles throughout most of the life of the female. Once a primordial follicle has been recruited to initiate growth, its size, orientation, and relative position in the ovary change dramatically. Morphologically (Fig. 17A-3), the growing follicles can be divided into five classes: primary, secondary, tertiary, graafian, and atretic.[17] It is well established that an activated primordial follicle undergoes self-differentiation into the primary, secondary, and early tertiary stages in the absence of the pituitary.[18,19] Therefore, the mechanisms controlling differentiation along a pathway of preantral follicle development are under intraovarian regulation. By contrast, when a growing follicle reaches the early tertiary stage, its survival and continued development depend completely on the presence of follicle stimulating hormone (FSH) and luteinizing hormone (LH).[20,21]

PRIMORDIAL FOLLICLE

The primordial follicles represent a pool of nongrowing follicles from which all dominant preovulatory follicles are selected. In this sense primordial follicles are the fundamental reproductive units of the ovary. Morphologically, each primordial follicle is composed of an outer single layer of squamous epithelial cells, termed granulosa or follicle cells, and a small (approximately 15 μm in diameter) immature oocyte arrested in the dictyotene stage of meiosis; both the granulosa and oocyte are enveloped by a thin, delicate membrane termed the *basal lamina* (Figs. 17A-3, 17A-4). By virtue of the basal lamina, the granulosa and oocyte exist in a microenvironment in which direct contact with other cells does not occur. Although small capillaries are occasionally observed in proximity to primordial follicles, these follicles do not have an independent blood supply.[1-3]

Developmentally, the primordial follicles are formed in the cortical cords of the fetal ovaries between the sixth and ninth months of gestation (Fig. 17A-5).[22] During this period, the oocytes are stimulated to initiate meiosis in an asynchronous manner. Since the oocytes in the primordial follicles have entered meiotic prophase, all oocytes capable of participating in reproduction during a woman's life are formed at birth.[23] Soon after primordial follicle formation some are recruited or activated to initiate growth.[24] As successive recruitments proceed, the size of the pool of primordial follicles becomes smaller.[25] Between the times of birth and menarche[23] the number of primordial follicles (and thus oocytes) decreases from several million to several hundred thousand (Fig. 17A-6). As a woman ages, the number of primordial follicles continues to decline until at menopause they are difficult to find (Fig. 17A-7).

PRIMARY FOLLICLE

A primary follicle is defined as one which contains a growing oocyte surrounded by a single layer of granulosa cells which are becoming cuboidal or low-columnar in shape (Fig. 17A-4). During primary follicular growth, both the granulosa and the oocyte undergo striking changes. The first indication of primary follicle development (recruitment) is that individual granulosa cells begin to become round and appear cuboidal rather than squamous in shape; at about this time, the oocyte begins to change, primarily by increasing in size.[26] As oocyte growth progresses, small patches of glycoprotein material begin to form between the granulosa cells juxtaposed to the oolemma;[27-29] this material eventually covers the entire egg and is termed the *zona pellucida.* At the later primary stage, the oocyte is nearly full grown (100 μm in diameter) and is completely eveloped by a thin zona pellucida, a single layer of cuboidal granulosa cells, and a basal lamina (Fig. 17A-4).

SECONDARY FOLLICLE

During the stages of secondary follicle development, the granulosa cells proliferate and the oocyte completes its final growth. By the end of the secondary stage, the follicle is organized into a multilayered structure which is very strikingly symmetrical. In the

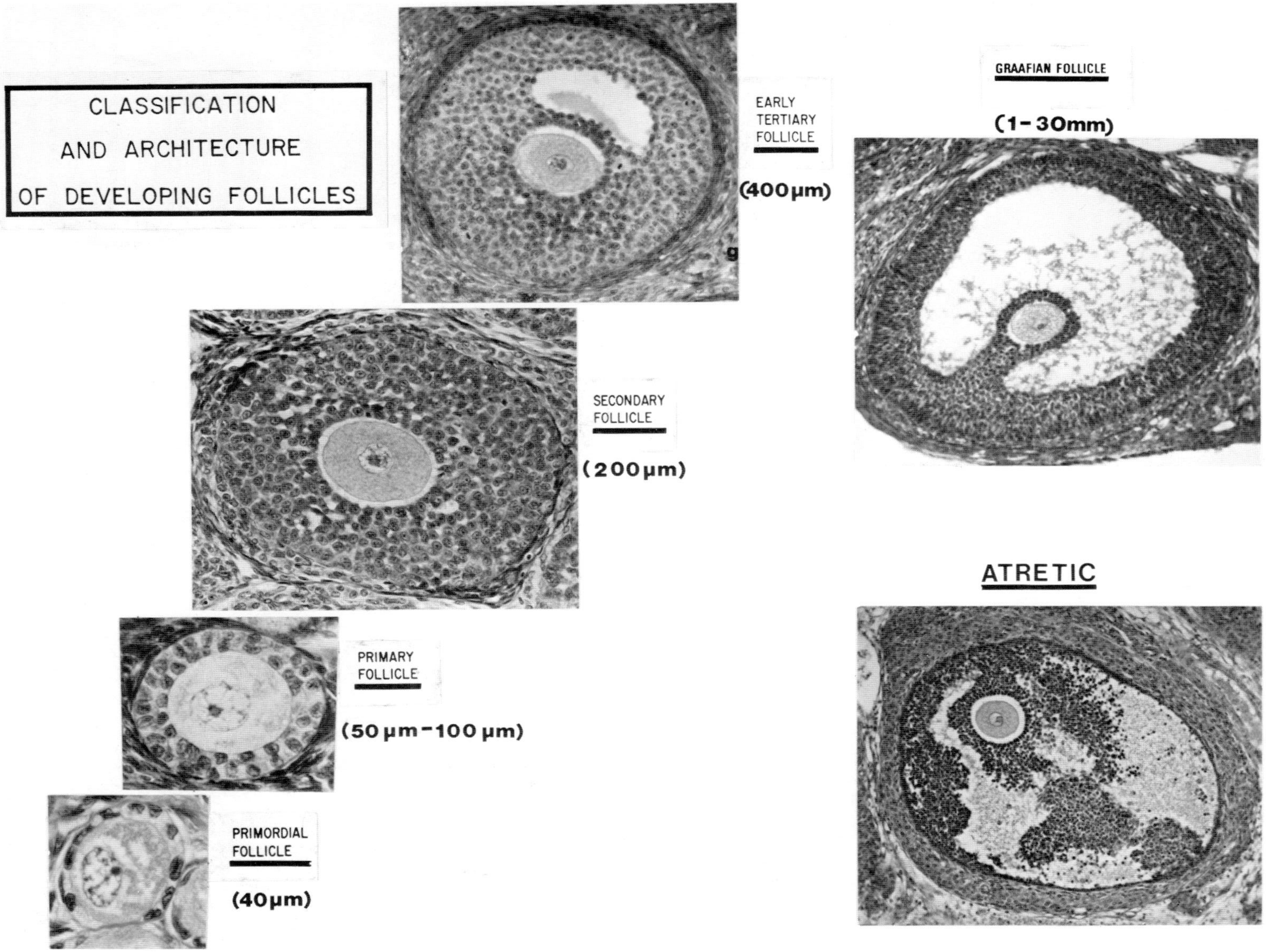

FIGURE 17A-3 Photomicrographs of stages of follicle growth and development. Recruitment occurs within the pool of primordial follicles; selection occurs between the early tertiary and graafian states. All unselected follicles die by atresia. (*From Erickson,*[99] *by permission of Elsevier Scientific.*)

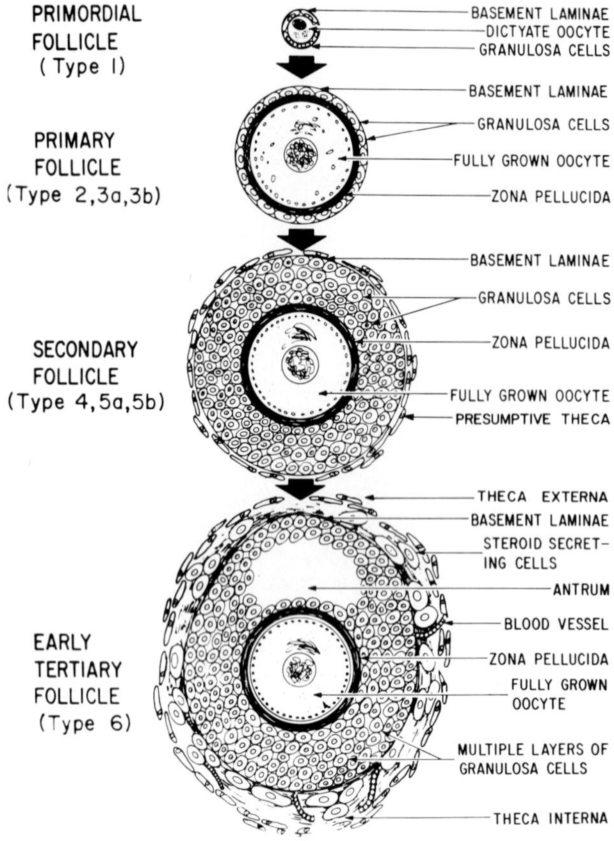

FIGURE 17A-4 Schematic drawing of the successive cellular events in preantral follicle development. (*Revised from Erickson,*[17] *by permission of JB Lippincott.*)

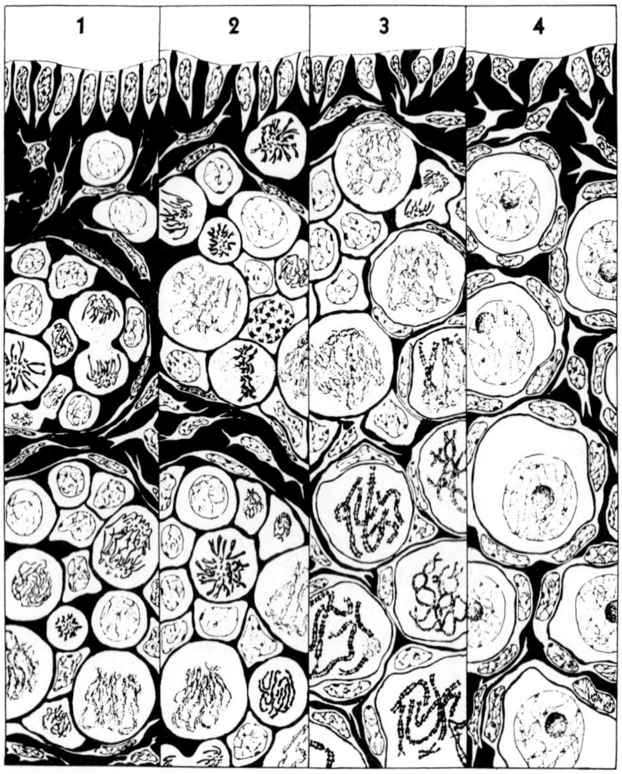

FIGURE 17A-5 Schematic drawing showing stages of meiosis in cortical cords of human fetal ovaries leading to the formation of primordial follicles. (*1*) At 3 months, oogonia engaged in mitosis; (*2*) at 4 months some oocytes deep within ovarian cords enter meiosis; (*3*) at 7 months the cords are no longer distinct and all germ cells are in meiotic prophase; (*4*) at 9 months the cortex is packed with primoridal follicles. (*From Ohno et al.,*[22] *by permission of S Karger.*)

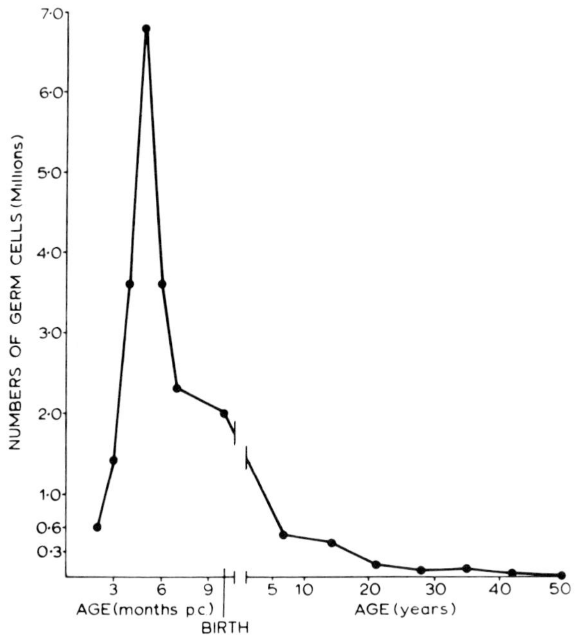

FIGURE 17A-6 Changes in the total number of germ cells in the human ovaries during aging. At early to midgestation the number of germ cells increases to almost 7×10^6. Shortly thereafter the number declines rapidly to about 2×10^6 at birth. The number continues to decline until no oocytes are detected at 50 years of age. (*From Baker and Sum,*[23] *by permission.*)

center is a full-grown oocyte (120 μm in diameter) covered by a thick zona pellucida, four to eight layers of stratified low-columnar granulosa cells, and a basal lamina (Figs. 17A-4, 17A-8).

During the course of secondary follicle development, several important morphologic events occur. One of the critical events involves the acquisition of cells of the prospective theca. When a secondary follicle acquires two to three layers of granulosa cells, a signal is generated which causes a stream of mesenchymal cells to migrate to the outer surface of the follicle.[18,19,30] The precise origin of these cells and the pathway that these cells take remain unknown, but there is evidence that they arise from stromal fibroblasts located outside the immediate vicinity of the secondary follicle.[31] After the mesenchymal cells reach the basal lamina, they align in parallel and form a radial arrangement of highly elongated, fibroblast-like cells around the entire follicle (Figs. 17A-4, 17A-8). This newly acquired connective tissue layer of the secondary follicle will ultimately give rise to both the theca interna and theca externa. It is apparent, therefore, that when a follicle reaches the secondary stage it has acquired a presumptive theca (Fig. 17A-8).

Another critical event which occurs during secondary follicle growth is the acquisition of an independent blood supply. At the secondary stage, a follicle becomes supplied by one or two arterioles which terminate in a wreathlike network of capillaries.[3] In a broad sense, the investing vessels form two sets of capillaries which are interconnected: an inner wreath

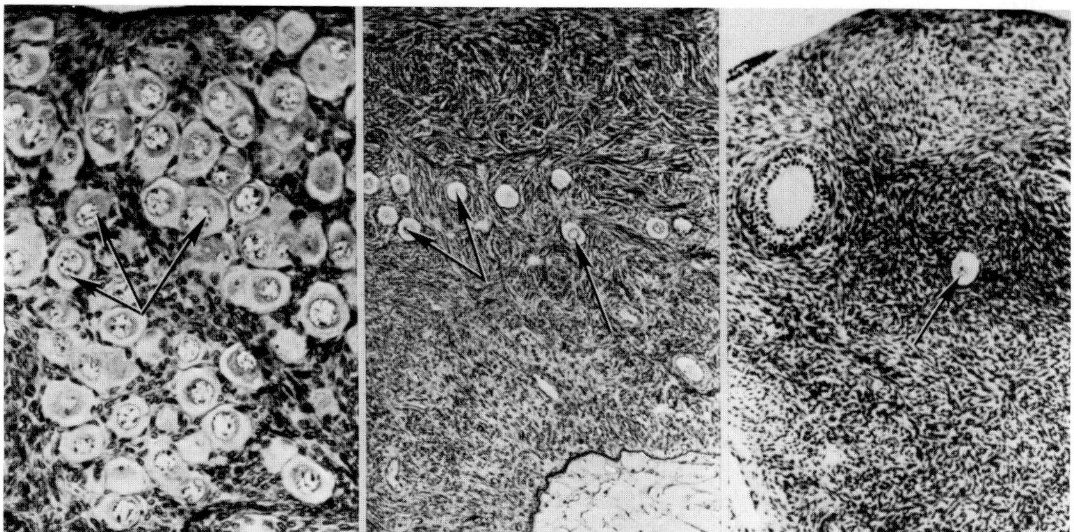

FIGURE 17A-7 Photomicrographs of sections through the cortex of human ovaries at different periods in life showing the progressive decrease in the number of primordial follicles (arrows).

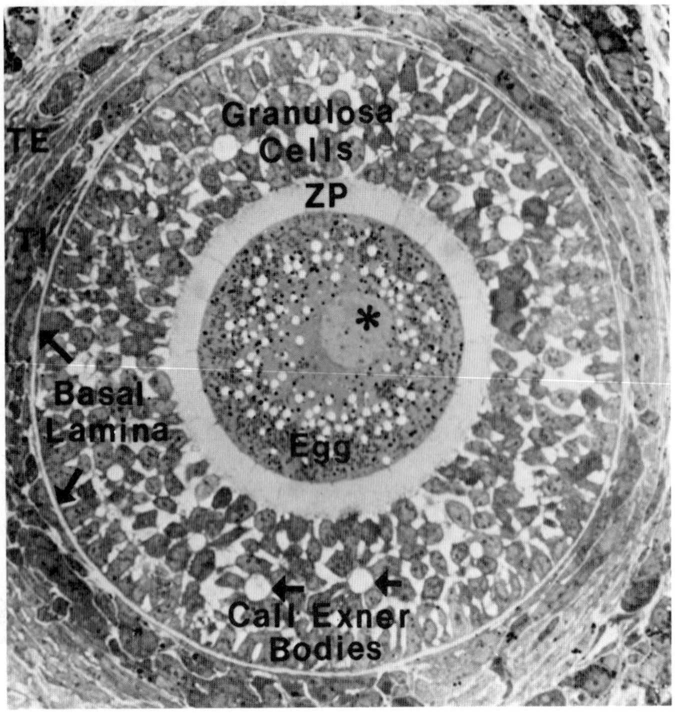

FIGURE 17A-8 Photomicrograph of a section through a secondary follicle. The dictyatene oocyte contains a large germinal vesicle (*) and a zona pellucida (ZP). The egg is surrounded by five layers of granulosa cells which in turn are enclosed by a basal lamina. The presumptive cells of the theca interna (TI) and theca externa (TE) have become associated with the follicle. (*Courtesy of Dr. Everett Anderson, by permission of WB Saunders.*)

of capillaries located in the theca interna, which is supplied by branches from an outer wreath of capillaries located in the theca externa. Characteristically, the capillaries of the inner wreath become closely associated with the basal lamina; however, they never penetrate beyond this membrane and thus the granulosa and egg are avascular. The inner capillary wreath is drained by small venules which connect in the theca externa into larger venules, which in turn enter the ovarian veins.[3]

One other interesting morphologic feature which appears in the secondary follicle is the formation of Call-Exner bodies among the granulosa cells (Fig. 17A-8). Although these bodies have been characterized ultrastructurally (Fig. 17A-9), nothing is known about the manner in which they form or their physiological importance. It is possible that they play a role in regulating granulosa differentiation by virtue of providing novel substrate-to-cell interactions.

TERTIARY FOLLICLE

The primary characteristic of a tertiary follicle is the presence of an antrum. Antrum formation occurs dramatically when a follicle reaches approximately 400 μm in diameter.[21] The process of antrum formation in its earliest phase is termed *cavitation* (Fig. 17A-4). This event is characterized by the uptake or accumulation of fluid between the granulosa cells and, there-

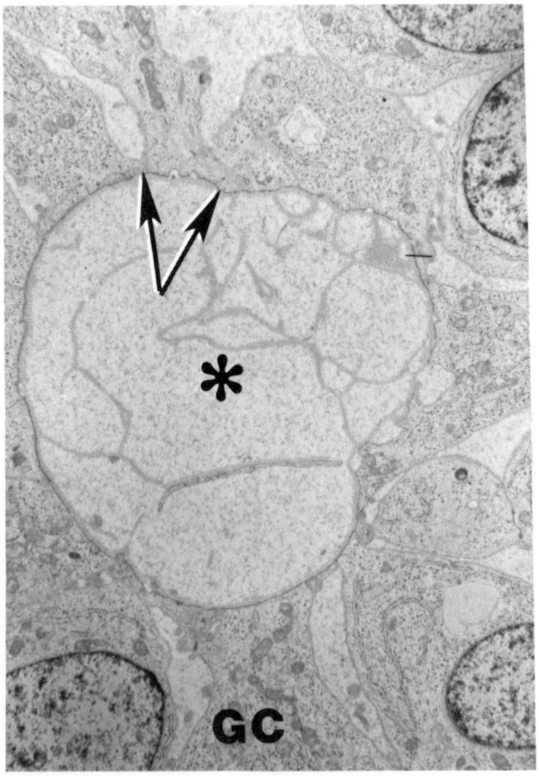

FIGURE 17A-9 Electron micrograph of a Call-Exner body. It consists of a distinct basal lamina (arrow) to which membrana granulosa cells (GC) are attached, and a cavity (*) with excess basal lamina material and a flocculant proteinlike material.

fore, the formation of a small internal cavity at one pole of the oocyte. Histologic evidence argues that the site of initiation of antrum formation is controlled in a highly specific manner (Fig. 17A-10). Although the underlying mechanism for cavitation is unknown, it occurs in the absence of the pituitary and thus seems to result from a developmental program constructed within the follicle itself.[21] As a result of cavitation, the follicle acquires an inherent polarity and internal organization which will remain throughout the rest of folliculogenesis (Figs. 17A-3, 17A-4).

Concurrent with the initiation of antrum formation, numerous histologic changes occur in both the theca interna and the granulosa cells. In the case of the theca interna,[18,19] subpopulations of stromal fibroblasts begin to transform into large epithelial cells termed *theca interstitial cells* (Fig. 17A-4). Eventually, the theca cells become highly differentiated steroidogenic cells which synthesize and secrete androgens in response to LH stimulation.[32]

At cavitation, there is a particularly dramatic cytologic event which occurs in the granulosa and the egg. Between the granulosa cells there develops a specialized contact termed a *gap junction* (Fig. 17A-11).[33,34] The gap junction, or nexus, is a membrane specialization composed of a protein called *connexin*.[35] Studies on the permeability of this cell-to-cell membrane channel indicate that molecules of up to 1800 daltons can pass from one cell to another.[36] Gap junctions also develop between the oocyte and presumptive corona radiata granulosa cells at cavitation.[37–39] It is apparent therefore that the granulosa and the oocyte become electrically and metabolically coupled when the follicle reaches early tertiary stage (400 μm diameter). Gap junctions have also been found between differentiating theca interstitial cells at cavitation.[40] The concept which emerges is that, by virtue of gap junctions, the entire follicle now has the potential to undergo a synchronized pattern of activities, either positive or negative, in response to hormone stimulation.

GRAAFIAN FOLLICLE

In response to gonadotropins brought to the follicle by the inner and outer capillary wreaths, the tertiary follicle increases tremendously in size.[20,21] If a developing human tertiary follicle is selected to ovulate it may grow 75-fold, increasing from 0.4 mm to 30 mm in diameter; the growth of the graafian follicle is accomplished by granulosa proliferation and follicular fluid accumulation in the antrum.[41] Contrary to preantral follicles, this change in size and differentiation is not under autonomous control but is dependent on FSH and LH.[20,21]

As seen in Fig. 17A-12, the graafian follicle is a highly structured mass of precisely positioned cells. Granulosa cells develop as pseudostratified epithelium and are limited peripherally by a basal lamina. By virtue of this architecture, the granulosa cells (and the egg) develop within the microenvironment of the follicular fluid. In the graafian follicle, both the number and size of the gap junctions between the granulosa cells increase, suggesting the levels of electrical and metabolic coupling in this tissue become amplified during folliculogenesis.[33,42]

During graafian follicle development the granulosa cells become different from one another with respect to polarity and relative position within the whole follicle (Fig. 17A-12). An important concept is

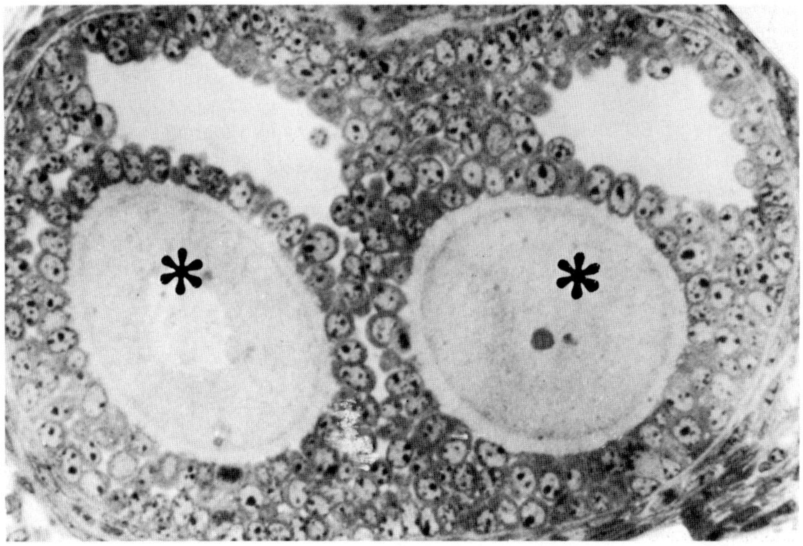

FIGURE 17A-10 Photomicrograph of a polyovular follicle at the early tertiary stage showing the sites of cavitation or early antrum formation (clear spaces) just above oocytes (*). This event, which is under intraovarian control, seems to arise in a specific synchronized manner and establishes the polarity of the follicle. (*From Zamboni,*[214a] *by permission of University Park.*)

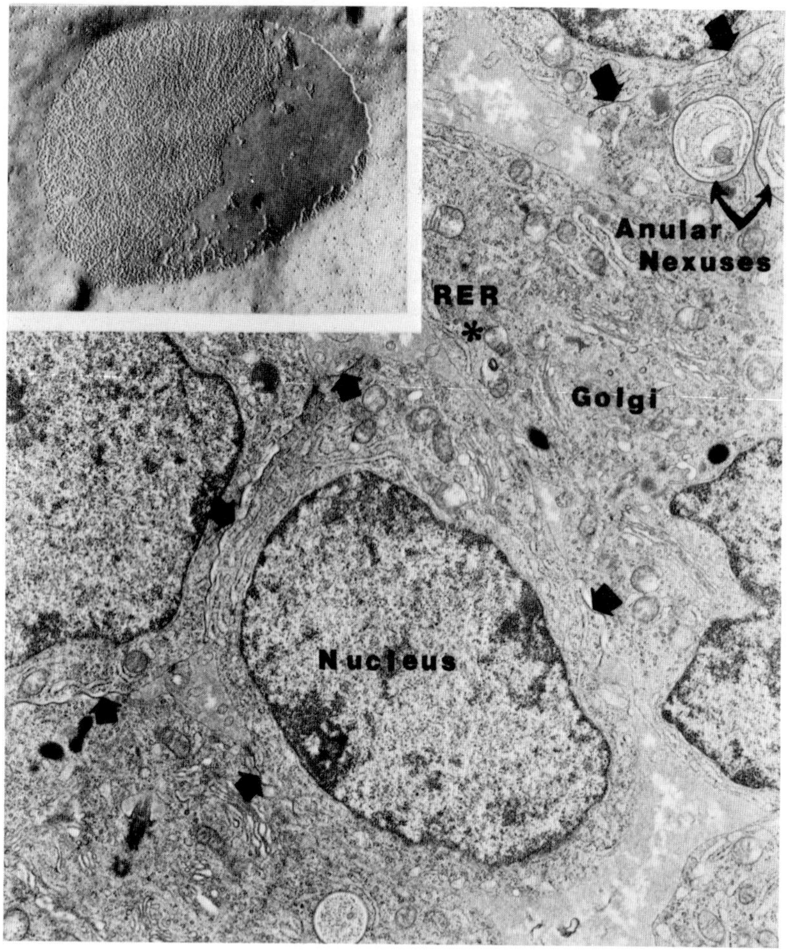

FIGURE 17A-11 Electron micrograph showing extensive gap junctional contacts (arrows) between granulosa cells of a healthy graafian follicle. (*Inset*) Replica of granulosa cell fracture showing the hexagonally ordered particles of the gap junction. (*Courtesy of Dr. David Albertini.*)

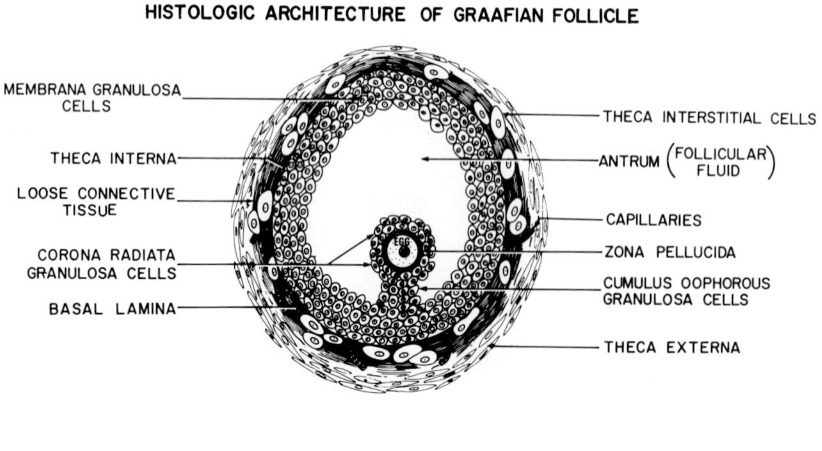

FIGURE 17A-12 Diagrammatic representation of the histology of a secretion through a dominant preovulatory graafian follicle. (*Revised from Erickson,*[99] *by permission of Elsevier Scientific.*)

that granulosa cells are a complex tissue containing several subgroups of different cell populations: the corona radiata cells, which make cell-to-cell contact with the egg and zona pellucida; the cumulus cells, which make cell-to-cell contact with both the corona and membrana granulosa cells; and the membrana cells, which make direct contact with the basal lamina and Call-Exner bodies (Fig. 17A-12). This has led to the concept of heterogeneity in granulosa cell organization and function. An interesting and basic question (considered below) is to what extent the relative position of a granulosa cell or a group of granulosa cells within the follicle can determine the direction in which that cell differentiates.

Throughout graafian follicle development, the morphologic characteristics of the theca established at cavitation remain. Highly differentiated theca interstitial cells progressively accumulate until there are eventually five to eight layers of these cells in a dominant preovulatory follicle (Fig. 17A-12). The production of theca interstitial cells results, through mitotic division of stem cells, in the theca interna.[43]

Electron microscopic studies of the theca externa of graafian follicles reveal the presence of smooth muscle cells[44–46] which contain actin and myosin.[8,47] The contractile cells in the theca externa (Figs. 17A-1, 17A-12) are innervated by both sympathetic and parasympathetic nerves,[4,9] and presumably the influence of the associated nerves directs to what extent the theca externa cells contract. Several lines of evidence point to a role of these cells in ovulation. This issue is addressed again below.

ATRETIC FOLLICLES

Once a primordial follicle is recruited to initiate growth, it either develops into a dominant preovulatory follicle or degenerates by a process termed *atresia*.[48] Atresia results in the selective death and clearance of the oocyte and granulosa, but the surrounding theca cells undergo extensive hypertrophy and eventually become interstitial gland cells, remaining permanently in the ovarian cortex.[49,50]

Differentiating between healthy and atretic follicles is difficult and not always clear-cut.[51] Most contend that a healthy follicle is completely free of degenerative necrotic changes; thus, any follicle which exhibits signs of cell death, regardless of how slight, would be atretic.[52]

In a broad sense, there are two types of atresia (Fig. 17A-13), *type* A atresia, in which primary changes occur in the oocyte, and *type B* atresia, in which there are primary changes in granulosa cells.[53] Type A atresia is most common in preantral follicles, whereas type B atresia is most common in graafian follicles. During the course of both types A and B atresia, three major successive changes have been identified morphologically: primary, secondary, and tertiary stages.

In the primary stage of type B atresia (in graafian follicles), necrotic changes first appear in some granulosa cells bordering the antrum.[54] In time, the margin of necrosis expands until all granulosa cells along the antrum are pyknotic. At the secondary stage, major zones of necrosis develop in the membrana granulosa

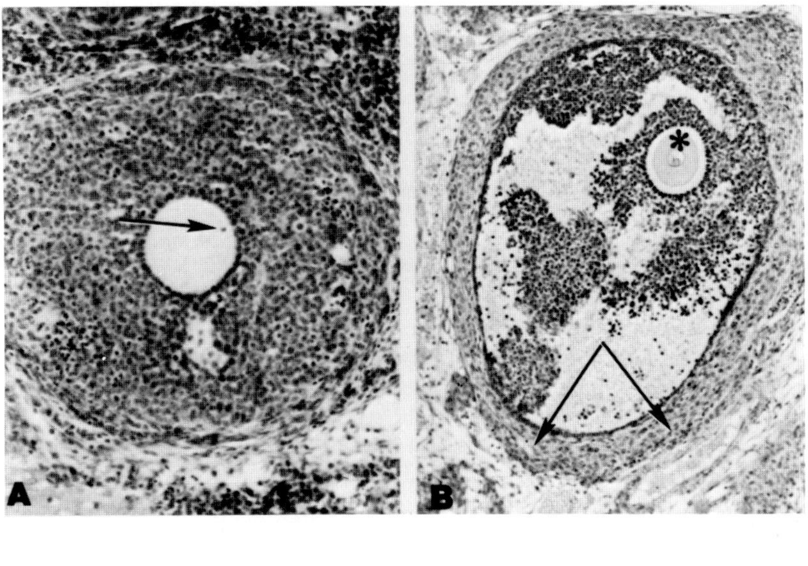

FIGURE 17A-13 Photomicrographs showing the two types of atresia. (A) Type A atresia takes place in preantral follicles; the primary changes occur in the oocyte with the initiation of meiotic maturation (arrow). (B) Type B atresia takes place in antral follicles, with primary degenerative changes occurring in the membrana granulosa cells while the oocyte-cumulus complex remains intact (*). Note striking hypertrophy of theca interna induced by atresia (arrows).

cells. As necrosis continues, large numbers of granulosa cells undergo autophagy and their nuclei begin to fuse, forming so-called atretic bodies.[54] Atretic bodies usually have a diameter of about 15 μm but occasionally reach 400 μm in size and may contain DNA equivalent to 500,000 pyknotic granulosa nuclei.[55] It seems that some membrana granulosa cells become phagocytic cells which engulf membrane, lipid bodies, mitochondria, chromatin, and gap junctions. It is interesting that located directly next to the granulosa cells that are extruding their cytoplasmic and nuclear contents are granulosa cells which appear healthy and show mitotic activity. In this light, cumulus cells show little or no sign of necrosis during secondary atresia, and thus seem to occupy a privileged position in comparison with membrana granulosa cells in the atretic process.[50,54] At the tertiary stage, the entire membrana granulosa is necrotic and large parts of it are often seen lying free in the antrum (Fig. 17A-13*B*).[53,55] During these late stages of atresia intense necrosis begins appearing in the cumulus cells and the first signs of oocyte degeneration are detected. In some cases, the cumulus breaks up and the oocyte, surrounded only by corona radiata, is set free within the antral cavity. Finally, there is the complete clearance of granulosa and oocyte; the follicle collapses. With the collapse of the follicle, the theca interstitial cells hypertrophy and become the secondary interstitial gland cells.[32,49]

The route taken in type A atresia (in preantral follicles) is completely different from that of the type B pattern. The first major morphologic event seen in type A atresia involves the oocyte rather than the granulosa cells.[53,55] In the early phases of type A atresia the oocyte initiates meiotic maturation and begins to exhibit maturation spindles and polar bodies (Fig. 17A-13A). In some instances, the activated oocytes in preantral follicles undergo pseudo cleavage or fragmentation into embryoid bodies.[56] It is possible that such activated eggs may be the source of ovarian teratomas. Subsequently, necrotic zones and atretic bodies develop in surrounding granulosa cells. This is followed by autophagy and removal of all granulosa and oocyte material from the preantral follicle. The basal lamina becomes hyalinized and the theca interna hypertrophies.[32,49]

Ovarian Interstitial Cells

A characteristic feature of the human ovary is the presence of several different types of interstitial cells which have the capacity to synthesize and secrete androgens. These cells are found in the stroma of both the cortex and medulla (Fig. 17A-1). Over the years, considerable attention has been paid to the development of these cells and, as a result, the life cycle of the ovarian interstitial cell type has been well worked out. In all cases, the cells which eventually give rise to interstitial cells are derived from mesenchymal cells in the ovarian stroma.[32] In the human, there are four major classes of ovarian interstitial cells: (1) primary, (2) theca interstitial, (3) secondary interstitial, and (4) hilus cells. Because ovarian interstitial cells produce androgens, they are central in regulating a number of fundamental reproductive processes, and therefore are of enormous physiological importance.[32]

PRIMARY INTERSTITIAL CELLS

The first interstitial cells to develop in the ovary are termed primary interstitial cells.[49,57] In the human, primary interstitial cells are first distinguished at 12 weeks of gestation in the fetal ovary; they remain visible there until about the 20th week.[58] During their presence in the fetal ovary, the primary interstitial cells are juxtaposed to the basal lamina of the ovarian cortical cords which contain the oogonia and oocytes (Fig. 17A-14).

The ultrastructural properties of primary interstitial cells are consistent with those of active, steroid-secreting cells. It is interesting that these cells bear a striking resemblance to the Leydig cells in the human fetal testis.[58] If their ultrastructure is considered, the hypothesis is suggested that primary interstitial cells are producing steroids, perhaps androgens, at high rates. This point is considered below.

THECA INTERSTITIAL CELLS

The most widely studied class of ovarian interstitial cells is that of the theca interstitial cells. Such cells are present in the theca interna of all tertiary follicles (Figs. 17A-4, 17A-12). In the human, theca interstitial cells are the site of follicular androgen, most notably androstenedione, synthesis.[59–64]

As pointed out earlier, presumptive theca interstitial cells first develop when a follicle reaches the secondary stage (Figs. 17A-4, 17A-8). At this point, some mesenchymal cells undergo significant change and become directed along a path of theca interstitial cell differentiation. This developmental shift involves acquisition of two constitutive molecules characteristic of a theca interstitial cell:[32,65] LH receptor and 3β-hydroxysteroid dehydrogenase (3β-HSD)–$\Delta^{4,5}$-isomerase enzyme. The stimulus which causes some mesenchymal cells to undergo this change is unknown, but it appears to be directed by local information emanating from the secondary follicle itself and is dependent of the pituitary.[18,19,21] In this sense, it appears the acquisition of LH receptors and 3β-HSD in theca cells is determined by a basic clock mechanism operating

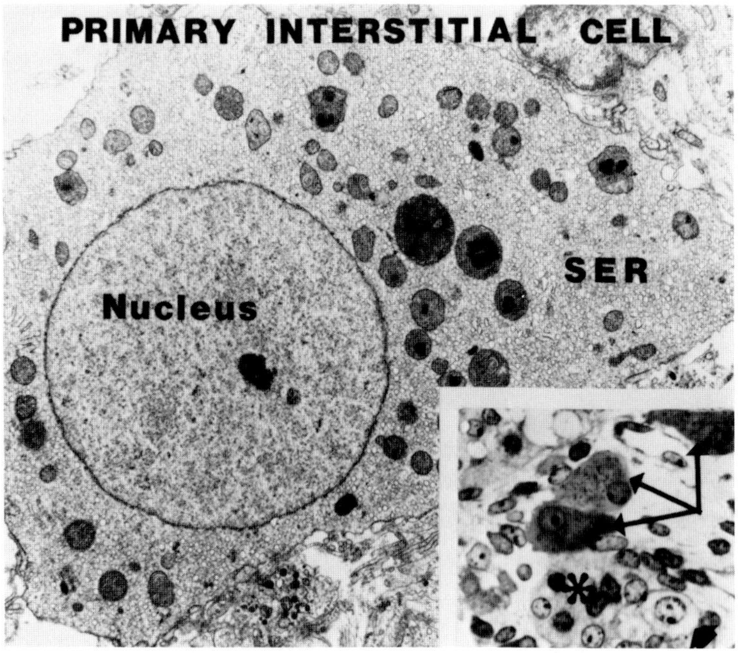

FIGURE 17A-14 Electron micrograph of primary interstitial cells in the human fetal ovary at 15 weeks of gestation. Such ovarian cells strongly resemble steroidogenically active Leydig cells. *Inset* shows the intimate relationship between primary interstitial cells (arrows) and oogonia (arrowhead) in the cortical cords (*). (*From Ref. 58, courtesy of Dr. B. Gondos, by permission of Williams & Wilkins.*)

within the secondary follicle. The remaining mesenchymal cells are thought to be pluripotent stem cells that can divide to produce other theca interstitial cells or differentiate into loose connective tissue as the follicle grows.[32]

The consequence of transforming from a mesenchymal to a theca interstitial cell is very evident. With the acquisition of LH receptors, theca interstitial cells are committed to respond to plasma LH, which is brought to the follicle by the inner capillary wreath. When a follicle reaches the early tertiary stage, the presumptive theca interstitial cells respond to LH by undergoing a major shape change from an elongated fibroblast to an epithelial cell.[18,19] Once the shape change is initiated (Fig. 17A-4), the cells begin to develop properties not found in the precursor stem cells. With increasing periods of time, theca interstitial cells increase markedly in size, to 15 to 20 μm in diameter, and acquire the fine structure typical of active steroid-synthesizing cells (Fig. 17A-15). This step is particularly striking and is characterized by the increased use of cytoplasmic organelles for androgen biosynthesis. As folliculogenesis proceeds, the number of terminally differentiated theca interstitial cells increases as a result of mitosis.[31,43] Within the theca interna of developing follicles are transitional cells whose ultrastructure reflects intermediate stages between the ultrastructure of unspecialized mesenchymal cells and that of fully differentiated steroidogenic cells, thus supporting the concept of a theca interstitial stem cell.[57]

A characteristic feature of the human theca interna is the presence of what seem to be subpopulations of differentiated theca interstitial cells (Fig. 17A-16). Electron micrographs show that the two main types (dark and light cells) both have the ultrastructure of active steroidogenic cells. Even though data are lacking, the demonstration of cytologic heterogeneity raises the possibility that within a follicle there may be theca interstitial cells with differing endocrine capabilities and responsiveness.[32] Whether these cells secrete different classes of steroids or are regulated independently is an intriguing and yet-unanswered question.

SECONDARY INTERSTITIAL CELLS

During the process of atresia, the granulosa and the egg degenerate; however, the theca interstitial cells[49] of atretic follicles undergo a striking hypertrophy (Figs. 17A-13, 17A-17) and survive as cords or clusters of large epithelial cells called *secondary interstitial cells.*[32,49,66,67] In this sense, secondary interstitial cells are direct descendants of theca interstitial cells of atretic follicles. Thus, theca interstitial cells never die, but are actually accumulated in the ovary. In humans, secondary interstitial cells maintain their specialized ultrastructure characteristic of active steroidogenic

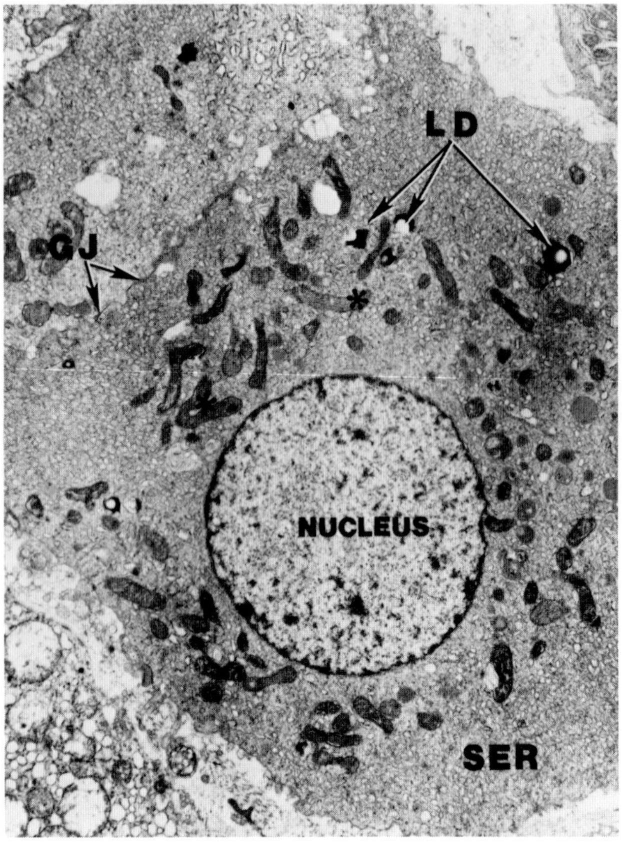

FIGURE 17A-15 Electron micrograph of two human theca interstitial cells in a 20-mm preovulatory follicle showing abundant smooth endoplasmic reticulum (SER), lipid droplets (LD) containing cholesterol esters, mitochondria with tubular cristae (*), and gap junctions (GJ).

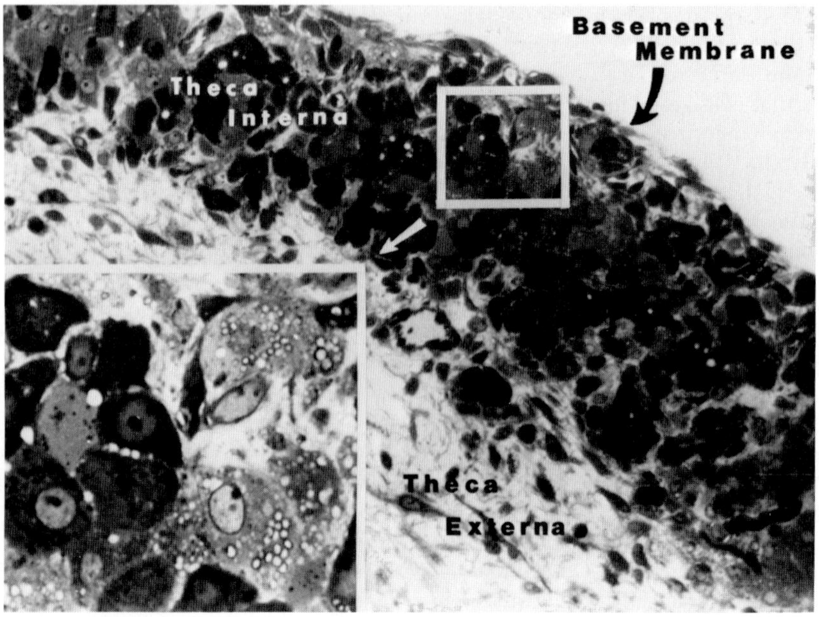

FIGURE 17A-16 Photomicrograph of theca interna of a 20-mm dominant preovulatory follicle in a human ovary at day 12 of the follicular phase. There are five to seven layers of highly differentiated theca interstitial cells between the basal lamina and the theca externa. Note the two distinct populations: the larger, paler theca cells and the smaller, darker ones. *Inset* shows higher magnification. Note granulosa cells have been removed from the basal lamina. (*From Erickson and Yen,*[231] *by permission of Thieme-Stratton.*)

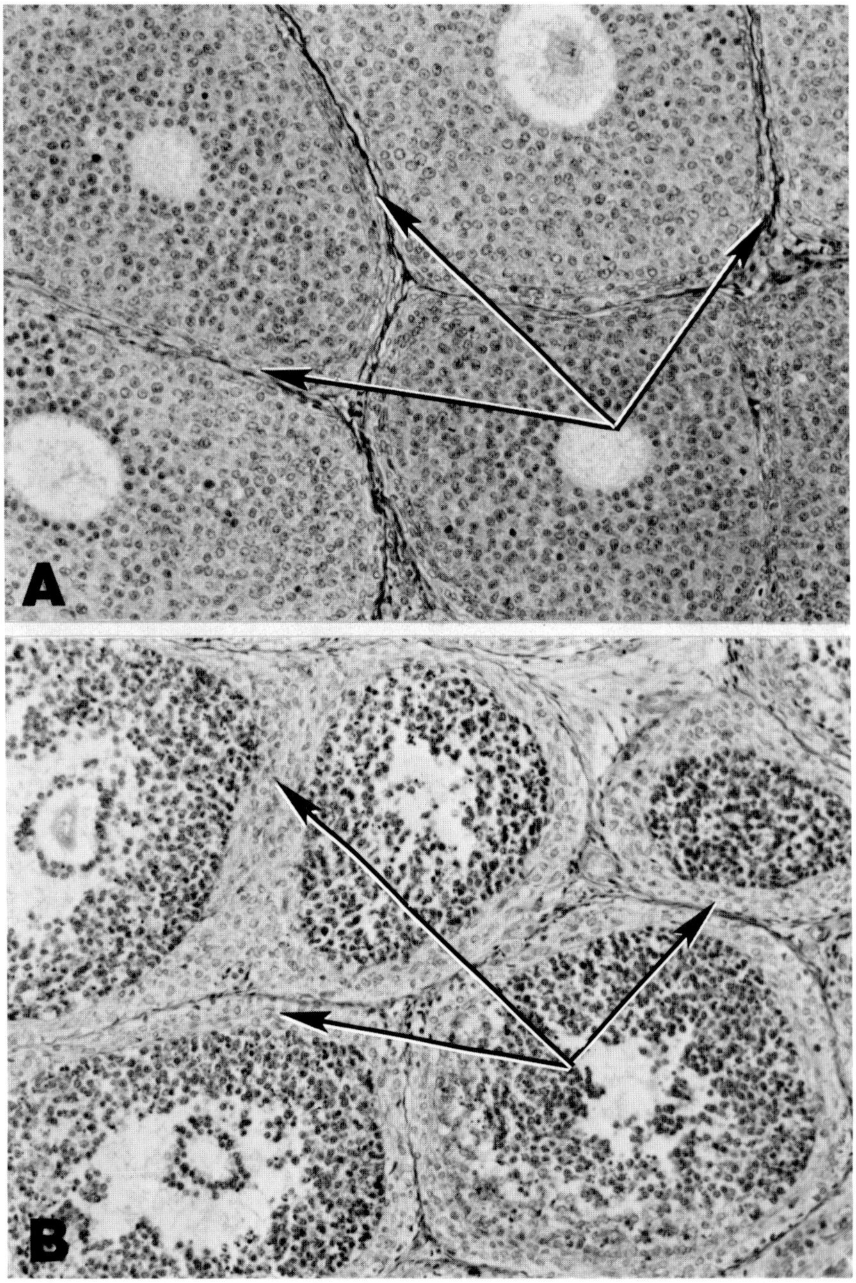

FIGURE 17A-17 Photomicrographs showing the hypertrophy of theca interstitial cells during atresia. (*A*) Concentric, thin layers of theca interna (arrows) in healthy, fully grown preantral follicles. (*B*) Hypertrophy of theca interna following experimental induction of atresia. When the atretic follicle collapses, the hypertrophied theca becomes secondary interstitial cells. (*Courtesy of Dr. Stephen Hillier.*)

cells (Fig. 17A-18) and continue responding to LH with increased androstenedione production.[62,68] This indicates that the secondary interstitial cells continue to exhibit properties of their precursors, the theca interstitial cells.

There is, however, one very important property that these two cell types do not have in common; the secondary, but not the theca, interstitial cell is innervated.[67] As mentioned earlier, secondary interstitial cells are unique in that they become innervated by sympathetic adrenergic nerves. Evidence in rodents strongly suggests the existence of point-to-point communication between neurons in the brain and the ovarian steroidogenic cells[69]: stimulation of selected hypothalamic nuclei in hypophysectomized and adrenalectomized rats stimulates or inhibits estrogen and

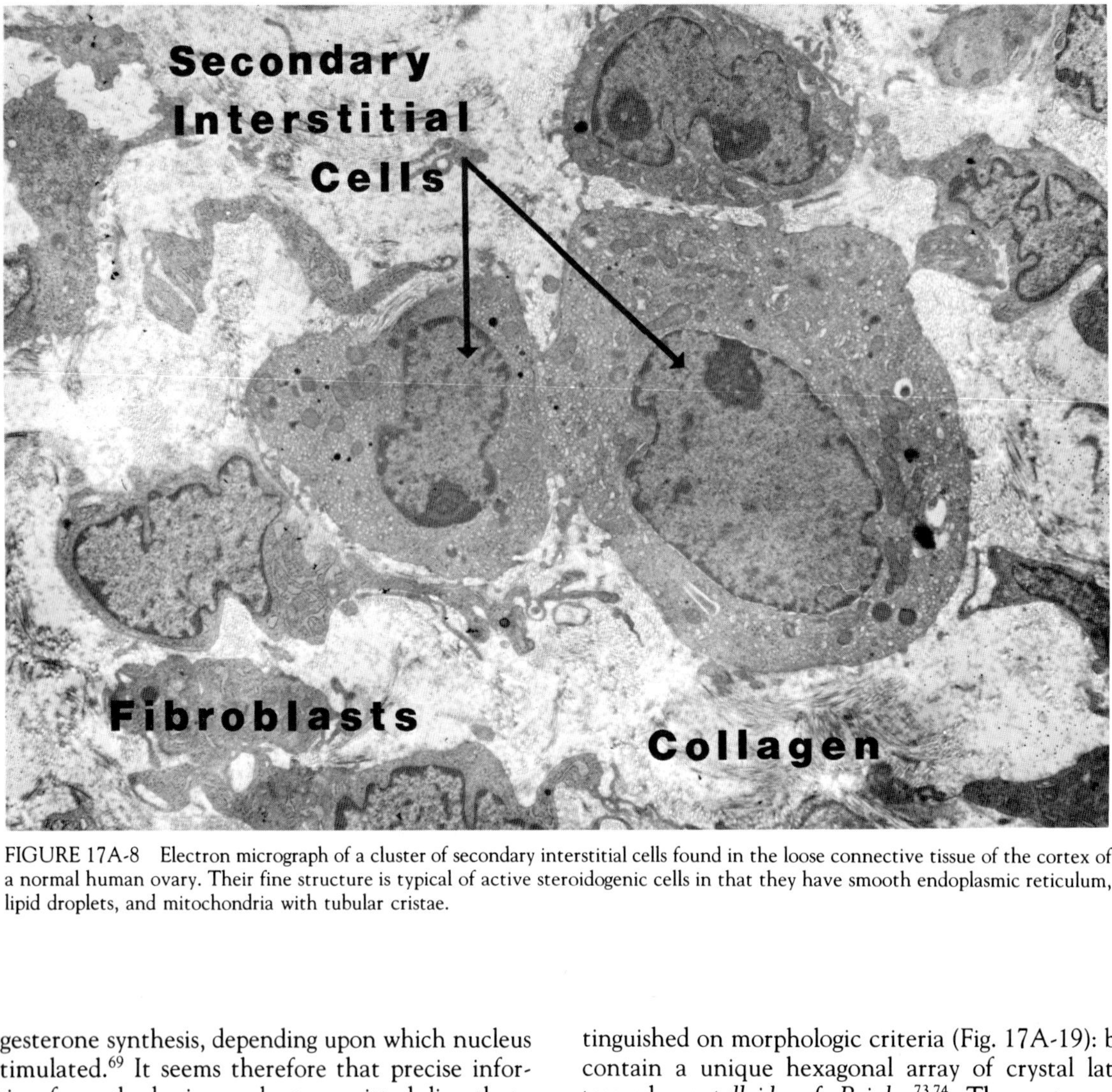

FIGURE 17A-8 Electron micrograph of a cluster of secondary interstitial cells found in the loose connective tissue of the cortex of a normal human ovary. Their fine structure is typical of active steroidogenic cells in that they have smooth endoplasmic reticulum, lipid droplets, and mitochondria with tubular cristae.

progesterone synthesis, depending upon which nucleus is stimulated.[69] It seems therefore that precise information from the brain can be transmitted directly to the ovaries via the secondary interstitial cells. In this regard, direct evidence that catecholamines can stimulate structure/function changes in secondary interstitial cells has been reported.[70] Thus, the concept which is emerging is that catecholamines passed across a synapse bind to catecholamine receptors and thereby regulate androgen activity in the secondary interstitial cell.

HILUS CELLS

Along the length of the ovarian hilus are clusters of large (15 to 25 μm in diameter) steroidogenic cells called *hilus cells* (Fig. 17A-1). These are highly unusual cells because all aspects of their structure and function are identical to those of differentiated testicular Leydig cells.[71,72] The hilus and Leydig cells can be distinguished on morphologic criteria (Fig. 17A-19): both contain a unique hexagonal array of crystal lattice termed *crystalloids of Reinke.*[73,74] The nature and importance of the crystalloids are unknown; however they might be albuminlike material which could provide a reservoir of binding sites for testosterone molecules. It has been established that hilus cells (like Leydig cells) synthesize and secrete testosterone in response to LH stimulation.[32,72,75-77] In this context, ovarian tumors of the hilus cell cause virilization.[72] For all intents and purposes, a hilus cell is an ovarian Leydig cell.

What are the endocrine controls and physical importance of ovarian hilus cells? One intriguing feature is the intimate association of hilus cells with nonmyelinated sympathetic nerve fibers (Fig. 17A-1)[72] and the ovarian spiral arteries.[1] Perhaps interactions occur between hilus cells and the nerves and blood vessels which could then directly or indirectly alter ovarian function. In this light, since testosterone

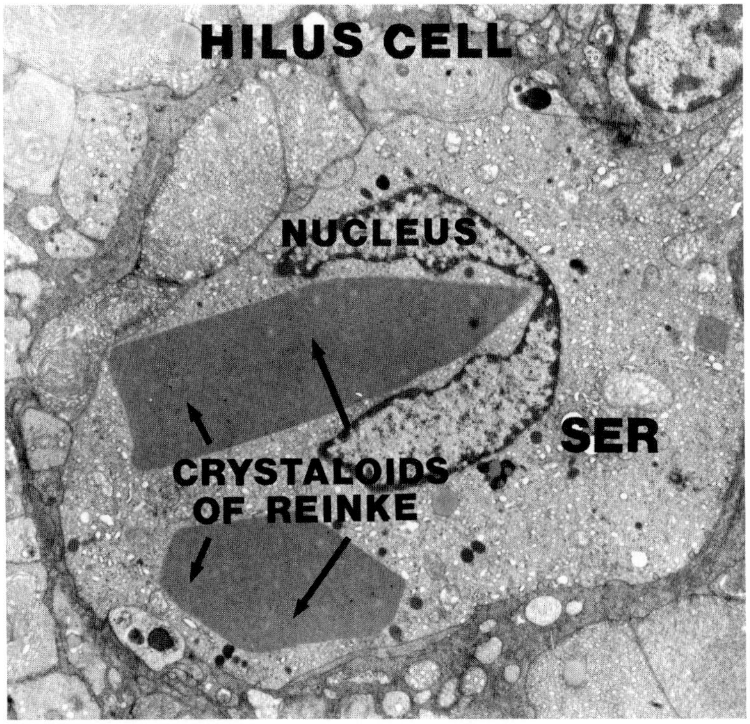

FIGURE 17A-19 Electron micrograph of a hilus cell showing both abundant smooth endoplasmic reticulum (SER) and numerous large crystalloids of Reinke. (*Courtesy of Dr. Norbert Schnoy, by permission of Springer-Verlag.*)

induces atresia, hilus cells may have an impact on the decision-making processes in follicular growth and development. Speculatively hilus cells may be a source of testosterone needed for increased striated muscle activities in women during exercise.[78]

Corpora Lutea

Following ovulation of the egg-cumulus complex, the follicle undergoes a series of histologic changes that result in the formation of a corpus luteum.[79] Cells that make up the corpus luteum are contributed by the membrana granulosa, theca interna, and theca externa. Morphologically, a corpus luteum is roughly equivalent to a graafian follicle (Fig. 17A-20; compare with Fig. 17A-12). In the center, where the antrum and liquor folliculi are located, is a fibrin clot in which there has been an invasion of loose connective tissue and blood cells. At ovulation the wall of the graafian follicle collapses resulting in a dramatic series of infolded tissue (Fig. 17A-20).

During luteinization the membrana granulosa cells undergo tremendous changes and attain a large size, 35 to 60 μm in diameter.[80] Such cells are termed *granulosa-lutein* cells. Perhaps the most dramatic event to occur in the newly forming granulosa-lutein cell is its transformation from a protein secretory-like cell[17] into a highly differentiated steroidogenic cell. In the cytoplasm prominent regions of smooth endoplasmic reticulum develop, the mitochondria develop tubular cristae, and large clusters of lipid droplets containing cholesterol esters accumulate (Fig. 17A-21). Importantly, granulosa-lutein cells contain substantial quantities of rough endoplasmic reticulum, indicating the granulosa lutein cells also have protein-synthesizing activity (Fig. 17A-21). These cells have a series of long microvilli which can measure 2 μm or more in length projecting from their apical surface.[80] In rodents these microvilli have been shown to contain the functional LH receptors, suggesting they may have important endocrine roles.[81]

During luteinization, the theca interstitial cells become incorporated into the corpus luteum, and are termed *theca lutein* cells. The theca lutein cells can be distinguished from granulosa-lutein cells (Fig. 17A-22) because they are typically smaller (15 μm in diameter) and stain more darkly.[80,82,83] Ultrastructurally they appear as active steroid-producing cells but also contain stacks of rough endoplasmic reticulum, suggesting they might also synthesize protein hormones.[80,83] Like theca interna (Fig. 17A-15), the theca lutein tissue contains cells with differing degrees of density (light, dark, intermediate) (Fig. 17A-22), suggesting there may be subpopulations of theca lutein cells.[80] Scattered throughout the corpus luteum are many macrophages,[82] the so-called K cells (Fig. 17A-22). Finally, as

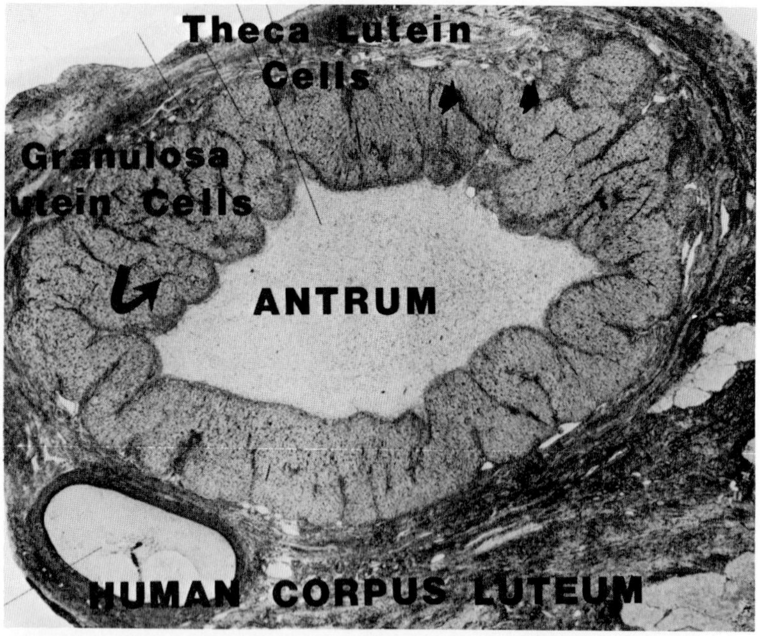

FIGURE 17A-20 Photomicrograph of a section of a human corpus luteum showing the fibrin clot in the antrum and the collapsed follicle wall composed of granulosa and theca lutein cells. (*Revised from Bloom and Fawcett,*[84] *by permission of WB Saunders.*)

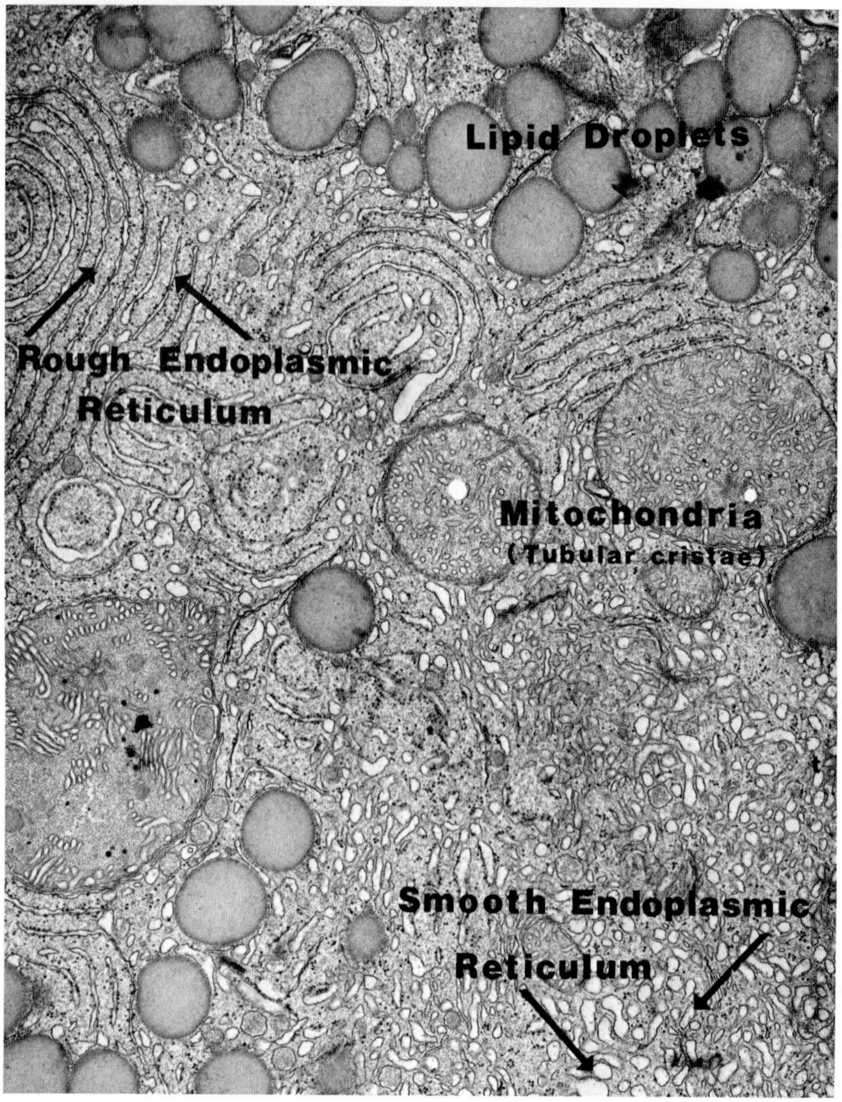

FIGURE 17A-21 Electron micrograph of a section through a human granulosa cell showing both protein-synthesizing (rough· ER) and steroid-synthesizing (smooth ER) potential. (*Courtesy of Dr. Tom Crisp, by permission of CV Mosby.*)

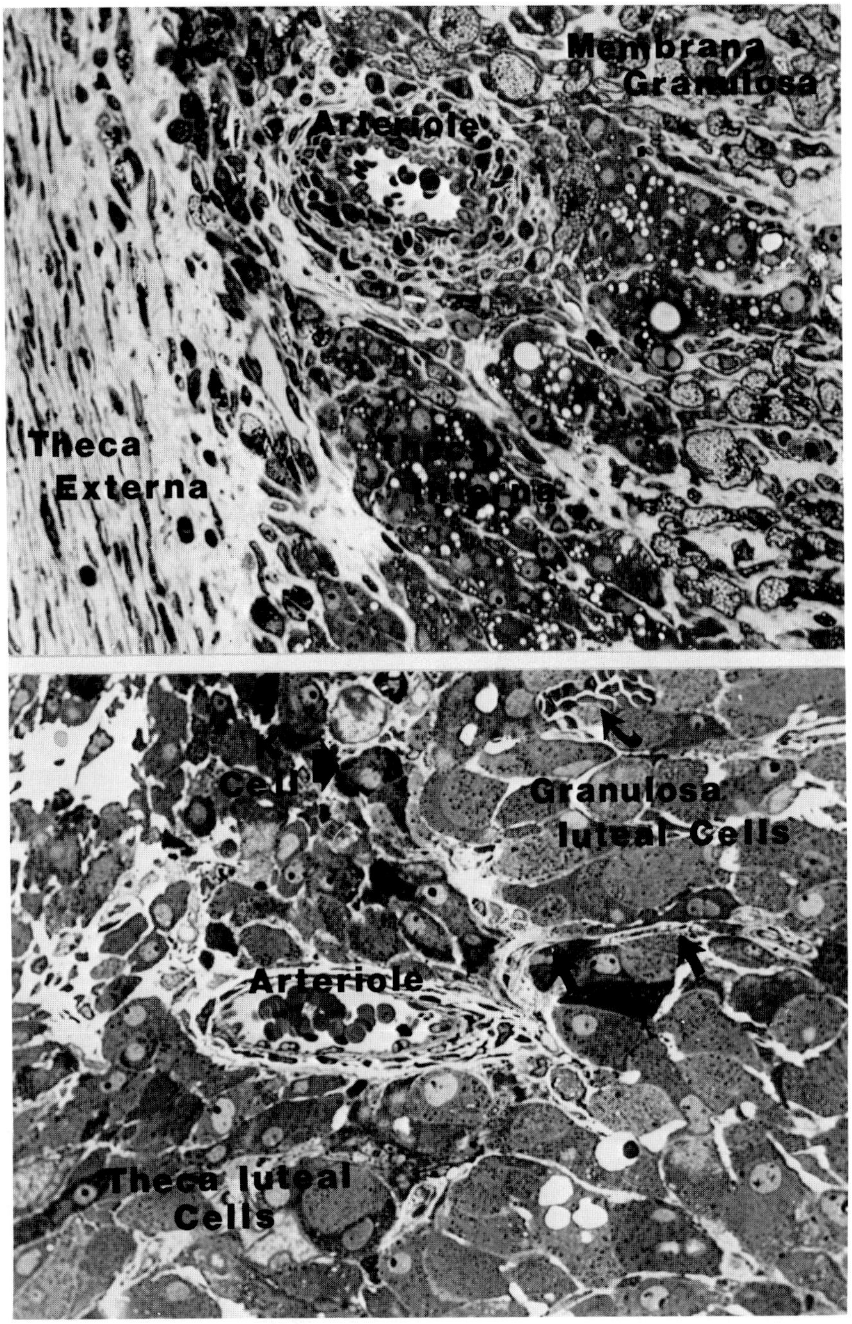

FIGURE 17A-22 Photomicrographs of a section through a human corpus luteum. (*Top*) The three main parts, theca externa, theca luteum, and granulosa luteum, are readily distinguished from one another. (*Bottom*) Larger pale granulosa-lutein cells readily distinguished from smaller (light and dark) theca lutein cells. Note intimate relationship between the K cell (macrophage) and luteal cells. (*Courtesy of Dr. Tom Crisp, by permission of CV Mosby.*)

with the follicle, the entire corpus luteum is surrounded by a theca externa.

If fertilization and implantation do not occur, the corpus luteum undergoes degeneration. This process, termed *luteolysis,* becomes apparent at 8 days after ovulation.[83] The first histologic indication of luteolysis is shrinkage of the granulosa-lutein cells. This is characterized by specific decreases in the amount of endoplasmic reticulum and general decreases in the amount of cytoplasmic matrix.[83] Initially the regression seems selective for granulosa-lutein cells as theca lutein cells actually become more prominent.[83] At this time, the theca layer is formed of tightly packed theca-lutein cells which contain profuse amounts of smooth endoplasmic reticulum and large mitochondria with tubular cristae. In this sense, luteolysis seems to be associated with hyperstimulation of the theca-lutein cells. This is followed by development of large zones of autophagy and necrosis. When the glandular corpus luteum disintegrates, all that is left is a nodule of dense connective tissue called the *corpus albicans.*

BIOGENESIS OF OVARIAN HORMONES

Steroids

In a broad sense, the adult human ovaries secrete three major types of biologically active steroid hormones: progesterone, androstenedione, and estradiol. The ability to produce these steroids depends on the presence of a special collection of enzymes termed *mixed function oxidases.* These enzymes are involved in a variety of oxidation-reduction reactions and require an NADPH-generating system and an oxygen transport system involving cytochrome P450.

An important concept in ovarian physiology is that steroidogenic enzymes are distributed throughout the endocrine compartments in a highly specialized manner.[85] The basis for this specification process is the selective transcription of genes which code for specific steroid-metabolizing enzymes. By virtue of differential gene activation, the various steroidogenic cells in the ovary respond to effectors with increases and/or decreases in selective classes of steroid hormones. Consequently, luteal cells secrete primarily C_{21} progestins and the interstitial cells preferentially produce C_{19} androgens. Importantly, the capacity to produce C_{18} estrogens de novo does not exist in any one cell type. Rather, ovarian aromatase enzymes are selectively expressed in the granulosa and granulosa-lutein cells.

CHOLESTEROL SUBSTRATE

All steroids are derived from cholesterol. Normally, three systems operate to provide a steroidogenic cell with cholesterol: (1) de novo synthesis from acetate, (2) mobilization from intracellular lipid droplets, (3) liberation from low-density lipoprotein (LDL). Under normal physiological conditions, the de novo synthesis of cholesterol provides little substrate for steroid hormone production by the ovary. Similarly, the storage pool of cholesterol esters in the lipid droplets is not a primary source of cholesterol under normal conditions.[86] The most important source of cholesterol used for steroid biosynthesis is the cholesterol liberated from LDL.[87] As seen in Fig. 17A-23, the process begins with the binding of LDL to a high-affinity receptor site and the subsequent internalization of the receptor-LDL particle in the form of a coated or endocytic vesicle.[88,89] This is followed by the delivery

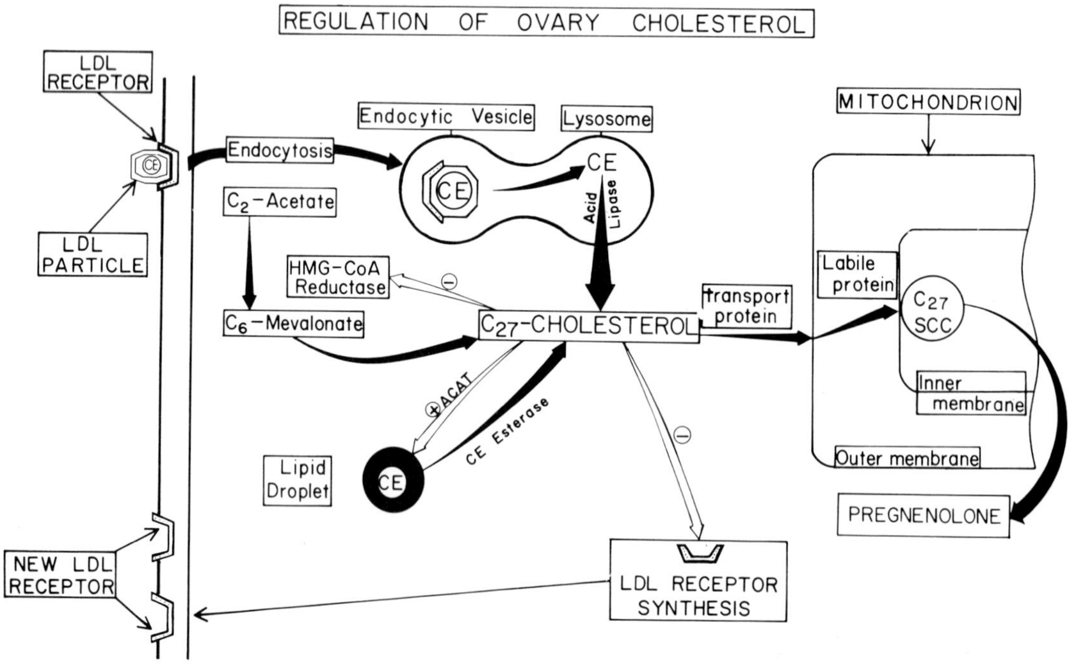

FIGURE 17A-23 Diagram showing the ovarian cellular responses to cholesterol with respect to steroidogenesis.

of the endocytic vesicle to a lysosome, where the LDL particle is hydrolyzed to amino acids by proteinases and the cholesterol esters are cleaved by an acid lipase to generate free cholesterol which leaves the lysosome for use in cell reactions.[90]

The cholesterol which is liberated from LDL initiates a set of feedback control mechanisms within the steroidogenic cell (Fig. 17A-23).[86,87,90] First, liberated cholesterol turns off de novo cholesterol synthesis from acetate by inhibiting 3-hydroxy-3-methyl-glutaryl coenzyme A reductase, which is the rate-controlling enzyme in cholesterol biosynthesis. Second, the LDL-derived cholesterol stimulates the enzyme acyl CoA:cholesterol acyltransferase, which reesterifies excess cholesterol and stores it as cholesterol ester lipid droplets. Third, the incoming cholesterol inhibits the synthesis of new LDL receptors, thereby preventing entry of LDL and overaccumulation of cholesterol.

INTRACELLULAR CHOLESTEROL TRANSPORT

The rate-limiting step in the conversion of cholesterol to steroid hormones is the transfer of the liberated cholesterol into the mitochondrion, where the side chain cleavage enzyme is located.[91] It is proposed that this process involves activation of the cytoskeletal systems (microfilaments and microtubules) by a cyclic AMP (cAMP)-protein kinase–dependent mechanism.[87] As a consequence of this putative transport system, free cholesterol accumulates in the outer membrane of the mitochondrion (Fig. 17A-23). Here, movement from the outer into the inner mitochondrial membrane, where the cholesterol side chain cleavage enzyme is located, depends on a labile protein.[91]

CHOLESTEROL SIDE CHAIN CLEAVAGE

The enzyme which is responsible for converting free cholesterol to pregnenolone (the initial step in steroidogenesis) is located at the inner mitochondrial membrane. In this enzyme complex, cytochrome P450 is a terminal oxidase of the mitochondrial electron transport system; the latter consists of a flavoprotein and an iron-sulfur protein which transports electrons from NADPH to O_2.[91] The consequence of the side chain cleavage is transformation of C_{27} cholesterol to C_{21} pregnenolone and a 6-carbon fragment called *isocaproic acid.*

METABOLISM OF STEROID HORMONES

Pregnenolone is the precursor to all steroid hormones. Once formed (Fig. 17A-24), pregnenolone is rapidly converted to the biologically active hormone progesterone through the action of Δ^5-3β-ol dehydrogenase–$\Delta^{4,5}$-isomerase. These enzymes are located within the outer mitochondrial membrane and in the smooth endoplasmic reticulum of steroid-secreting cells.[92] The main pathway of steroid synthesis in the human ovary is the Δ^4 pathway, which involves the conversion of progesterone to various C_{19} and C_{18} steroids. The enzymes in the Δ^4 pathway are involved principally with the stepwise removal of carbon atoms from the C_{21} skeleton of progesterone. The formation of C_{19} androgens involves two enzymes: 17α-hydroxylase and 17,20-lyase.[85] This dual enzymatic system is located in the smooth endoplasmic reticulum and is responsible for cleavage of the side chain of progesterone to yield Δ^4-androstenedione (Fig. 17A-24). In the ovary, these two enzymes are selectively found in the interstitial cells including the theca-lutein cells. Importantly, gran-

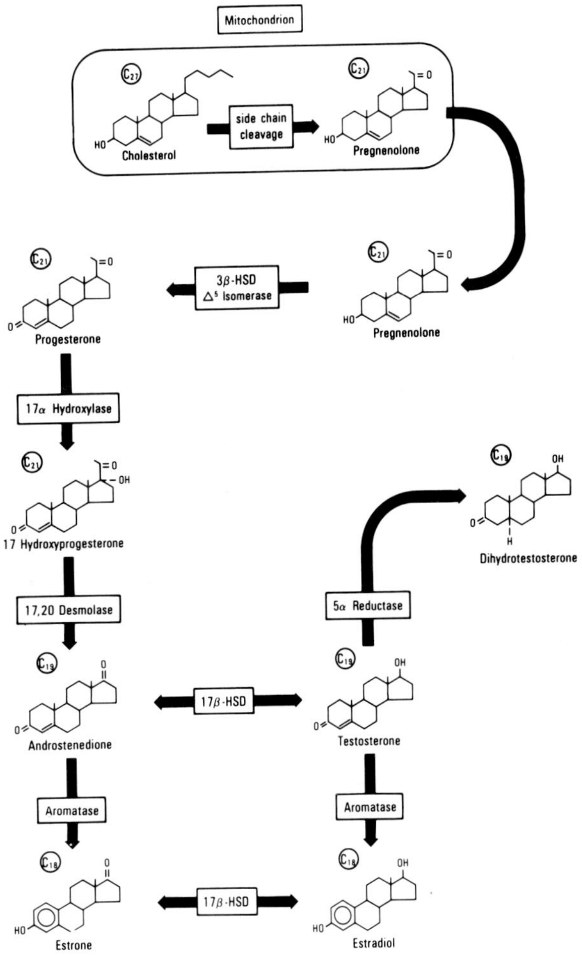

FIGURE 17A-24 Diagram showing how the ovary metabolizes steroid hormones beginning with the synthesis of pregnenolone. (*Revised from Erickson and Yen,*[231] *by permission of Thieme-Stratton.*)

ulosa cells do not contain these enzymes and therefore are unable to convert progesterone to androstenedione.[59–62]

The degree to which androstenedione is further metabolized depends on the ovarian cell type. The hilus cells, for example, contain the enzyme 17β-hydroxysteroid dehydrogenase, which converts androstenedione to testosterone.[75] This enzyme is also present in granulosa cells,[93] where it converts androstenedione to testosterone and estrone to estradiol (Fig. 17A-24). In the ovary one of the most important steps in androstenedione metabolism is its conversion to estrogen via a 19-hydroxylase-aromatase enzyme complex (Fig. 17A-24). This enzyme, which holds the key to so much that is characteristic of the female, is primarily found in the granulosa cells.[59,60,62] The presence of the aromatase leads to the removal of the angular carbon between rings A and B, followed by the aromatization of the A ring of the C_{18} steroid.[85] Finally, the interstitial cells contain a 5α-reductase (NADPH:Δ^4-3-ketosteroid-5α-reductase) which can convert ring A metabolites to 5α-reduced steroids.[94,95] The 5α-reductase is potentially an important enzyme because (1) the 5α-reduced steroids (like dihydrotestosterone, DHT) are extremely potent androgens and (2) they are competitive inhibitors of the aromatase.[96]

GONADOTROPIN CONTROL

The control mechanisms governing de novo steroid synthesis in the ovary are almost exclusively regulated by LH/LH and human chorionic gonadotropin (hCG). The ability of LH to stimulate de novo steroidogenesis involves both short- and long-acting mechanisms. The short term effects of LH occurs within minutes and involves cAMP-dependent activation of protein kinases and subsequent phosphorylation of regulatory proteins. The rate-determining step in ovarian steroid biosynthesis is the conversion of cholesterol to pregnenolone by the side chain cleavage.[91] LH, via cAMP, causes dramatic and rapid increases in the capacity of the side chain cleavage enzyme to convert cholesterol to pregnenolone.[97] The underlying control mechanism involves LH-induced increases in the amount of cholesterol which is specifically bound to the cytochrome P450 side chain cleavage enzyme.[98] The mechanism remains a mystery, but seems to involve LH-dependent increases in the amount or activity of the "labile protein" (Fig. 17A-24).[97,98] Thus, the basis of the immediate effect of LH on steroidogenesis seems to be a rapid delivery of cholesterol to the side chain cleavage enzyme.

The long-term effect of LH on steroidogenesis involves genetic expression of the steroid-metabolizing enzymes.[32,65,99] Specifically, LH stimulates the synthesis of cholesterol side chain cleavage enzyme, 3β-HSD, 17α-hydroxylase, 17,20-lyase, and 5α-reductase. Consequently, the long-term control of steroidogenesis by LH occurs at a rate which is governed by the rate of the expression of the genetic information. Although the relationship between FSH and de novo steroidogenesis is minimal, FSH plays a central role in regulating ovarian steroid formation by virtue of its control of the activities of the ovarian 17β-HSD[93] and aromatase enzymes.[61,100] In this sense, FSH is most important in controlling the immediate and long term estrogen responses in the ovary.

Protein

The ability of ovarian steroidogenic cells to produce protein hormones is a relatively new concept which has exciting physiological and pathological implications. The best-characterized protein produced by the human ovary is *relaxin.* This 6000-dalton peptide shows definite homologies with insulin-like growth factors and is preferentially produced by the corpus luteum of pregnancy.[101] Relaxin is released continuously by corpus luteum cells throughout gestation and its concentration is four times higher in the vein draining the ovary containing the corpus luteum of pregnancy than in either peripheral veins or the contralateral ovarian vein.[102] Histochemical studies at the ultrastructural level indicate that relaxin is present in both granulosa lutein and theca lutein cells and is localized to membrane-bound cytoplasmic vesicles.[103] It has been found that relaxin production by human luteal cells of pregnancy is under the control of hCG.[104] The search for a physiological role of relaxin has been unproductive. At present, there is no disease state which is causally linked to either hyper- or hyposecretion of relaxin. Relaxin has been proposed to have a paracrine function in the ovary during pregnancy. In this light, porcine theca interstitial cells are also a principal source of relaxin,[105] suggesting relaxin might play a role in regulating folliculogenesis during the menstrual cycle.

Other proteins which seem to be produced by the human corpus luteum are the neurohypophyseal nonapeptides oxytocin and arginine vasopressin.[106,107] The physiological role of the ovarian neurohypophyseal hormones is still unclear. In domestic species, oxytocin is secreted into the ovarian vein in response to prostaglandin ($PGF_{2\alpha}$).[108] In humans, oxytocin inhibits basal and hCG-stimulated progesterone synthesis by isolated corpus luteum cells.[109] Collectively, this evidence, together with other data,[110] has led to the proposal that ovarian neurohypophyseal hormones may be luteolytic factors and therefore play an important part in the control of the menstrual cycle.

Although less well documented, other studies suggest that the ovary may be the source of a number of other proteins, which include:

Inhibin, putatively a peptide produced by granulosa cells which, when delivered to the pituitary, inhibits preferentially FSH synthesis and secretion.[111]

Plasminogen activator, a peptide produced by granulosa cells of preovulatory follicles, which converts follicular fluid plasminogen to the active proteinase plasmin, which is capable of weakening the follicle wall.[112,113]

Oocyte maturation inhibitor, putatively a protein produced by membrana granulosa cells which interacts with the cumulus–corona radiata–egg complex to suppress the resumption of meiotic maturation.[114]

Follicular regulatory protein, putatively a peptide produced by granulosa cells which suppresses follicle responses to gonadotropin and thereby may be an inter- and/or intraovarian regulator of folliculogenesis.[115]

β-Endorphin, of which, with other pro-opiomelanocortin-derived peptides, granulosa[116] corpus luteum, and secondary interstitial cells[117] appear to be sources; there is no known function of these proteins, but a paracrine role has been proposed.

OVARIAN CYTODIFFERENTIATION: UNDERLYING CONTROL MECHANISMS

The changing morphologic pattern of the developing follicle and corpus luteum is accompanied by dramatic biochemical changes that reflect continuing processes of cellular differentiation. The underlying basis for the differentiation process is the acquisition of specific hormone receptors which provide cells with the competence to respond in a specific way to a set of hormonal signals. All such specializations occur in a highly predictable pattern and involve both intraovarian and extraovarian mechanisms. In essence, the continued transformation of cells from the undifferentiated to the fully differentiated state is the underlying principle of ovarian physiology.

THE GRANULOSA CELL

Cytodifferentiation

The differentiation of a granulosa cell begins in the primordial follicle when it is recruited to initiate growth. After becoming committed to the granulosa pathway, these morphologically unspecialized cells start to proliferate and produce new cells whose subsequent differentiation is under hormonal control. As such, granulosa cytodifferentiation can be divided into three levels (Fig. 17A-25) which parallel follicular morphology (Figs. 17A-3 and 17A-4).

FIRST LEVEL It is only when a primordial follicle is recruited that granulosa cytodifferentiation begins. After changing from a squamous to a cuboidal shape, the granulosa cells are shifted into mitosis. This transition is accompanied by the acquisition of FSH receptors in the plasma membrane.[118] Therefore, the first step in granulosa differentiation occurs in primary follicles and involves FSH receptor induction. The basis of FSH receptor induction is obscure, but seems to involve intraovarian control mechanisms. A role of FSH in the differentiation of the granulosa cell at this early time has been proposed,[119] but resolution of the question awaits more data. Kinetic binding studies indicate that when the follicle reaches the secondary stage, the granulosa cell has approximately 1500 specific high-affinity FSH receptors and that the number remains constant in the granulosa cells throughout the remainder of follicle development.[120] The conclusion therefore is that the first level of granulosa cytodifferentiation involves induction of a maximum number of FSH receptors (Fig. 17A-25).

SECOND LEVEL When a follicle reaches the secondary or early tertiary stage, granulosa cells reach the second level in their differentiation. The second transition (Fig. 17A-25) is accompanied by the "spontaneous" acquisition of intracellular receptors for estradiol,[121] progesterone,[122] testosterone,[123,124] and glucocorticoids[125] as well as the development of gap junctions in their membranes.[33] The factor responsible for inducing these important changes is unknown, but seems to be regulated by intraovarian processes. Clearly this differentiative change is fundamental because the granulosa cells (and thus the follicle) are now competent to react in a specific way to a set of very potent determinative stimuli which can modulate folliculogenesis for better or for worse.

THIRD LEVEL Up to this point, granulosa cytodifferentiation occurs independently from the pituitary. Such is not the case for its subsequent differentiation, which is completely dependent on pituitary FSH. FSH, which is brought to a tertiary follicle by capillaries in the theca interna, crosses the basal lamina where it binds to FSH receptor in the granulosa and stimulates cAMP synthesis. This causes an increase in the dissociation of a cAMP-dependent protein kinase, which then results in phosphorylation of regulatory proteins.[126] In this context, estrogen exerts a permis-

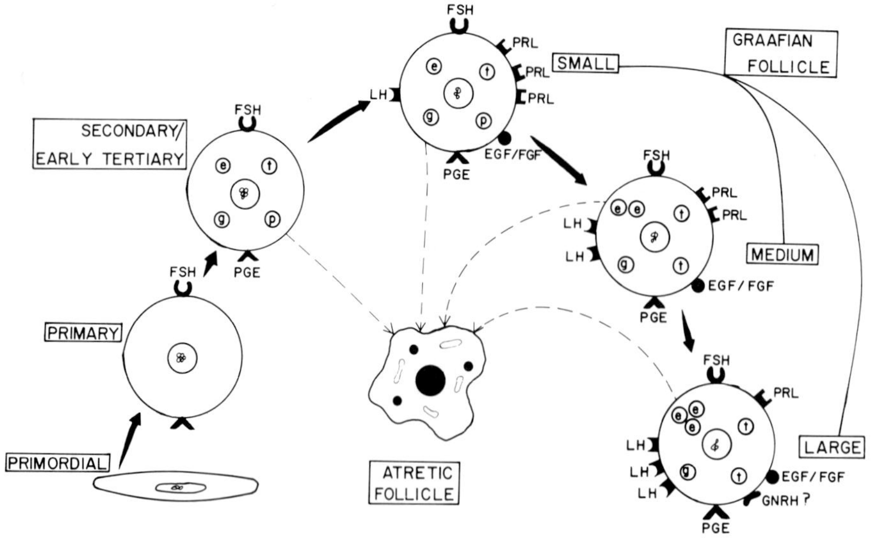

FIGURE 17A-25 Diagram showing qualitative and quantitative changes in hormone receptors in differentiating granulosa cells throughout follicle development.

sive role in FSH action by facilitating FSH-stimulated cAMP formation.[127] This action of estrogen is particularly important because it increases the sensitivity of the granulosa cell to FSH, which is known to be present in relatively low concentrations in follicular fluid.

The critical role of FSH in granulosa cytodifferentiation is illustrated by the number of specialized functions which are dependent on FSH stimulation. One of the primary consequences of FSH action is to activate proliferative cell cycles which lead to increased numbers of granulosa cells.[126,128] Obviously, this mitogenic effect of FSH on the granulosa cells is fundamental for follicle growth. In this light, the growth factors epidermal growth factor (EGF) and fibroblast growth factor stimulate human granulosa mitosis, presumably through receptor-mediated responses.[129] Another consequence of FSH interaction is to cause the granulosa cells to develop increasing amounts of aromatase enzymes.[61,100,231] This regulatory process is fundamentally important in the maintenance of the estrogen-synthetic activities of the follicle and thus the homeostatic activities of the female. Another important aspect of FSH action is to stimulate the induction of surface membrane receptors for prolactin[126,130] and LH,[126,131,132] the latter of which is central to the control of ovulation. These interactions clearly illustrate the fundamental role of FSH in controlling the differentiation processes that occur in granulosa cells during growth and development of the preovulatory follicle. Importantly, the FSH interactions involve the expression of new genes which code for characteristic proteins.[99,133]

A basic aspect of the third level of differentiation is that the prolactin and LH receptors, unlike FSH receptor, undergo characteristic changes during granulosa cell cytodifferentiation. During progress from the preantral to the small antral follicle (Fig. 17A-25), FSH induces a rapid increase in prolactin receptor number, after which the number declines steadily until granulosa cells in large follicles contain only a few prolactin receptors.[134] By contrast, the pattern of FSH induction of LH receptor is essentially the opposite.[126,135] Granulosa cells found in small and medium-sized antral follicles have few or no LH receptors;[135] it is not until the end of preovulatory follicle growth that FSH induces LH receptor in the granulosa cells; at this time the number of LH receptors increases rapidly (Fig. 17A-25), reaching a maximum of approximately 20,000 sites per cell in a dominant follicle just prior to the LH surge.[135]

An important sidelight is that once granulosa cytodifferentiation has been initiated by FSH, the cells become completely dependent on FSH for their survival. In this context, FSH withdrawal results in the loss of all available receptor and aromatase enzymes,[126,136] followed by cell death by atresia (Fig. 17A-25). Therefore, FSH is critical for the life of any granulosa cell that it has activated.

A prominent characteristic of the FSH control of granulosa differentiation is that it can be modulated.[99,137] At the level of endocrine action, this control is effected by a variety of hormones and factors, the sensitivity of which is determined by specific receptors. For example, the FSH stimulation of granulosa differentiation is blocked by prolactin,[138,180] glucocorticoids,[139] progesterone,[140,141] and growth factors,[142,143] but stimulated by estrogen[21,126] and insulin.[144] The conclusion is that granulosa differentiation is controlled by a balance of "plus" and "minus" factors. FSH provides the principal stimulatory signal to the granulosa cell; however, the intensity and duration of the FSH signal can be altered, either amplified or attenuated. The concept is that there is not a single hormone which is responsible for controlling granulosa differentiation, but rather the control is brought about by a complex push-pull type of interaction between a number of agonists and antagonists, any of which can alter the course of differentiation, for better or for worse.

Granulosa Heterogeneity

There is increasing evidence that groups of differentiating granulosa cells in the follicle respond to FSH differently.[99] Although each granulosa cell in a developing graafian follicle appears to possess FSH receptors,[131] when challenged by FSH in vivo or in vitro, the LH receptor[145,146] and aromatase enzymes[147] are selectively induced in the membrana granulosa cells, while prolactin receptor seems to be induced selectively in the corona radiata and cumulus granulosa.[148] These data argue strongly that the granulosa cells are not a simple equipotent cell type, even though they all presumably have FSH receptors. In this view it seems certain that the position of the granulosa cell within the follicle determines which way it will differentiate in response to FSH stimulation. How the relative position within the granulosa cell mass determines the direction of its differentiation is unknown, but probably involves the microenvironment of the follicular fluid as well as its contacts with the basal lamina, oocyte, and/or other granulosa cells.[99] The concept is that granulosa cells are really a complex tissue containing several subgroups of functionally different cells.

THE INTERSTITIAL CELLS

Androgens produced by interstitial cells are involved in both constructive and destructive processes in the ovary.[32] Follicular estradiol formation and the subsequent proliferation of granulosa cells are causally linked to androgens produced by interstitial cells. This contrasts with other evidence that androgens arising from interstitial cells can induce rapid necrosis and destruction of granulosa cells and ova through atresia. Therefore, androgens derived from interstitial cells are capable of controlling both cell proliferation and cell death in a follicle. Consequently, changes in interstitial androgen production will affect the direction of folliculogenesis and thereby could have important consequences for the reproductive state of the female.

The most important stimulating force in interstitial androgen production is LH.[32,65,149] All interstitial cells are competent to react to LH (or hCG) by way of specific high-affinity receptors in the plasma membrane.[32] LH binds to its receptor and activates adenylate cyclase, which converts ATP to the second messenger, cAMP; the cAMP activates specific protein kinases which subsequently add phosphate groups to cellular proteins.[65] As discussed earlier, LH-induced interstitial differentiation involves activation of genes which result in new RNA transcripts which code for specific rate-limiting enzymes in the pathway of androgen biosynthesis. The conclusion is that LH/hCG exerts its inductive and stimulatory effects on ovarian interstitial cells by genetic mechanism involving the process of differential gene expression.[32,99]

To what extent can the differentiation of interstitial cells be determined by interactions with other hormones? The concept which is emerging from animal studies is that the control of ovarian interstitial cytodifferentiation, as with the granulosa, is effected by a balance between activation and inhibition, rather than by simple stimulation.[32] There are two known activators or inducers which are capable of transforming presumptive interstitial cells into fully differentiated androgen-producing cells, namely, LH/hCG[60–65] and PGE_2;[32] however, the level of differentiation induced by these activators can be either amplified or attenuated by a variety of molecules. Two types of hormone have been found which are potent amplifiers of LH/hCG-stimulated androgen formation by ovarian interstitial cells: insulin[32,150] and the catecholamines (epinephrine and norepinephrine).[70] Conversely, the LH and PGE_2 stimulation can be severely inhibited by a number of physiological hormones including estrogen,[151,152] prolactin, gonadotropin releasing hormone (GnRH),[154] and EGF.[155] The current concept of how the ovarian interstitial cells is controlled is illustrated in Fig. 17A-26.

The conclusion is therefore reached that the differentiative function of ovarian interstitial cells, like those of the granulosa, is controlled by a balance of plus and minus factors. Once an ovarian fibroblast has been committed to become a presumptive interstitial cell, then LH and/or PGE_2 triggers the interstitial cell on the path of differentiation which leads to androgen biosynthesis. How far along that path the interstitial cell proceeds depends, however, upon interaction with a number of modulators, any one of which is capable of altering its interaction with the inducing substances. Given the importance of androgen in follicle development, it is clear that interaction with any one of the modulators could influence the reproductive state of the female.

THE CORPUS LUTEUM

Corpus luteum differentiation is typically divided into two periods. It begins in response to the preovulatory

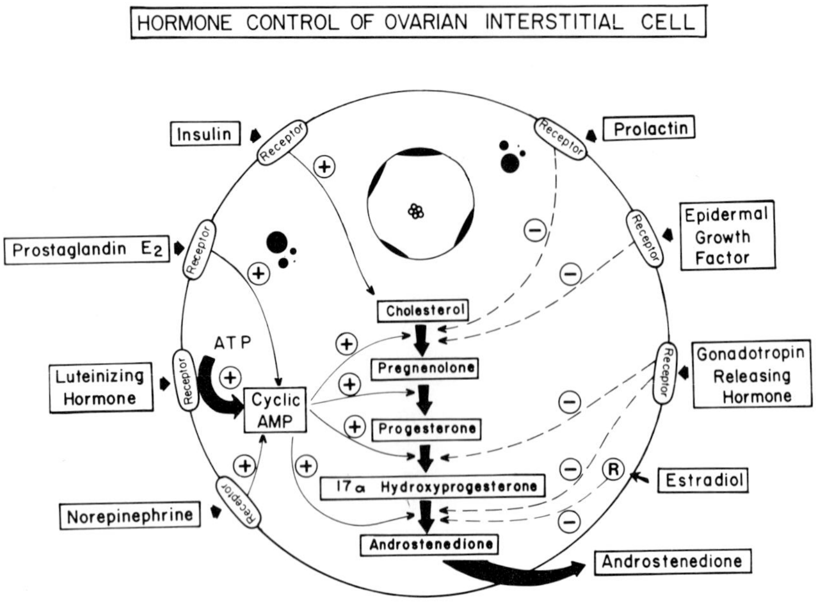

FIGURE 17A-26 Current concept of how hormones control the steroidogenic activity of the ovarian interstitial cells; (+) and (−) indicate sites of stimulation and inhibition, respectively.

surge of gonadotropins by the process termed luteinization. After maximal differentiated function is reached at the end of one week (day 21 to 22 of the cycle), the corpus luteum normally undergoes necrosis by the process of luteolysis. What are the primary events leading to luteinization and luteolysis?

Luteinization

Much of what is known about the control of the human corpus luteum has come from studies of hormone levels in peripheral and ovarian venous blood and follicular fluid.[156-161] Collectively, the evidence indicates that luteal differentiation is associated with a biphasic secretion of ovarian regulatory steroids, namely, progesterone, 17α-hydroxyprogesterone, androstenedione, and estradiol. This conclusion has been corroborated by in vitro experiments with isolated corpus luteum tissue.[162-164] The concept which emerges is that the biphasic production of a steroid in the corpus luteum is causally connected with biphasic changes of activities of steroidogenic enzymes in the Δ^4 pathway.

What agents are responsible for biphasic changes in corpus luteum steroidogenic enzymes? The fundamental regulator in promoting and maintaining the life of a corpus luteum is LH. LH is the inducer of luteinization and low levels of LH are critical for maintaining active luteal tissue during the early and midluteal phases.[165] Importantly, hCG produced by the blastocyst can prevent luteolysis and promote further increases in corpus luteum activity; however, the mechanism is totally obscure. The conclusion is therefore reached that induction and maintenance of the differentiated state of the corpus luteum is controlled directly by LH/hCG.

Considering the fact that LH/hCG action is mediated by receptors, the question of the factors involved in corpus luteum changes becomes intimately connected with how LH receptor is controlled by luteal cells. LH receptors in developing human corpora lutea undergo a predictable pattern of activity. As ovulation approaches, a striking decrease in LH receptor number occurs in granulosa cells, while during the early luteal phase LH receptor number increases sharply, reaching near-maximal level in the midluteal phase, where it remains until the end of the cycle.[166-169] It can be concluded therefore that the LH receptor is first "down regulated" and then reinduced during the process of luteinization.

Since reinduction of LH receptor is what renders the corpus luteum sensitive to hCG secreted by the implanting blastocyst, a most important question is how LH receptor is reinduced in the luteal cells. It has been found that FSH and prolactin are important in the induction and reinduction, respectively, of LH receptors in rodent granulosa cells.[126] In this light, functional FSH and prolactin receptors seem to be present in highest concentration in the early human corpus luteum,[168] during the time LH receptor number is being replenished. Although the question of the extent to which FSH and prolactin are involved in reinducing LH receptor during luteinization has not been answered, it is an important question clinically because foremost among the characteristics of luteal-phase defects in women is the inability of the corpus luteum to respond to LH/hCG.[170-172] Perhaps this defect is caused by inappropriate formation of new LH/hCG receptors.[170-172]

Luteolysis

At the time of luteolysis a program is initiated which leads to cell death approximately 5 to 7 days later. Once initiated, there is a striking decrease in progesterone production, an event which is unfavorable to pregnancy. What is the mechanism of luteolysis? Evidence suggests that aromatase activity may be particularly important. Aromatase activity in the corpus luteum increases prior to luteolysis and the concentration of estrogen in the corpus luteum reaches a peak then.[168,173,174] Can the two processes, decrease in progesterone production and increase in aromatase activity, be causally linked in luteolysis? In women, injection of estrogen directly into the ovary causes early onset of menstrual bleeding.[175] Furthermore, treatment with exogenous estrogen inhibits progesterone production by human corpus luteum cells in vitro.[176,177] The site of estrogen action seems to be directly at the level of the Δ^4-3β-HSD–$\Delta^{4,5}$-isomerase.[178] Consequently, the conclusion may be drawn that estradiol is an important luteolytic agent in the human.

With this concept in mind, a very important question in the differentiation of the corpus luteum is that concerning the underlying mechanisms for controlling estrogen biosynthesis. The mechanism controlling estrogen formation could act either directly at the aromatase and/or at the level of androgen substrate. LH/hCG can increase estrogen and progesterone secretion in human corpora lutea while FSH selectively stimulates estrogen but not progesterone production.[174] The picture emerging is that FSH and LH may be responsible for progressive increases in corpus luteum aromatase activity and progesterone levels, respectively, during the differentiation of the corpus luteum in the early to midluteal phases. If so, it can be concluded that progesterone and estradiol production by luteal cells are controlled independently.

In this context, clomiphene acts directly on human corpus luteum cells to decrease progesterone production while increasing 17-hyroxyprogesterone, androstenedione, and estradiol production.[179] How clomiphene exerts this action is unknown, but clomiphene can increase the aromatization of testosterone to estradiol. With respect to luteolysis, it may be that induction of aromatase activity by clomiphene results in increased concentrations of cellular estrogen, which then enters into the process of luteolysis. This scenario could have important implications for the way in which clomiphene induces luteal defects in women.

To what extent is luteal cytodifferentiation determined by interactions with modulators? It seems clear that LH, FSH, and hCG are the principal activators in corpus luteum differentiation. Several putative modulators of human corpus luteum function have been identified: prolactin, GnRH, $PGF_{2\alpha}$, estradiol, and oxytocin. These are discussed below.

In human granulosa cells which are undergoing luteinization in vitro, prolactin can inhibit LH/FSH-stimulated progesterone production[180] and prolactin inhibits basal and gonadotropin-stimulated progesterone and estrogen secretion by human ovaries in vitro. By contrast, experiments with human corpus luteum cells have failed to find consistent direct effects of prolactin on hCG-stimulated progesterone production, although prolactin was found to modulate hCG-stimulated estrogen formation.[181] Suffice it to say that, despite great clinical interest, the consequences of prolactin action on the human corpus luteum remain unsolved.

As with prolactin, a direct effect of GnRH on human ovarian cells is equivocal. Evidence suggests that human corpora lutea do not have high-affinity GnRH receptors[182] and GnRH does not influence steroidogenesis by human corpus luteum cells in vitro.[183] It has been reported that GnRH inhibits granulosa luteinization in culture,[184] but this was not subsequently confirmed.[185] Up to this point, the question of whether or not GnRH can modulate the differentiation of human corpus luteum cells is still controversial.

In some animals $PGF_{2\alpha}$ directly inhibits progesterone production by the corpus luteum and therefore has been termed a physiological luteolysin. In human corpora lutea, $PGF_{2\alpha}$ receptors have been reported[186] and luteal cells have the synthetic capability of producing PGs.[187,188] Again, despite considerable clinical interest, definitive evidence that $PGF_{2\alpha}$ is a physiological modulator in human luteal cytodifferentiation is lacking.[189]

As stated earlier, there is evidence that estradiol and oxytocin act directly on human corpus luteum cells to block LH/hCG activation of progesterone synthesis. Thus, the concept is emerging that the differentiation of the human corpus luteum (like the granulosa and interstitial cells) is controlled by multiple hormone responses, some of which are themselves the products of the corpus luteum. Importantly, in contrast to animal corpus luteum cells,[11,12] human corpus luteum cells do not seem responsive to catecholamines.[189]

THE OOCYTE

Primordial Germ Cells

The eggs within the ovary are derived from primordial germ cells (PGCs). These cells, which are set aside very early in embryonic development, arise in the yolk sac endoderm, far from the eventual site of gonad formation. In humans, PGCs can be selectively identified by virtue of an alkaline phosphatase which is located in the plasma membrane.[190] It is known that from their location in the hindgut they migrate through the dorsal mesentery and into the gonadal ridges; PGCs migrate to the gonad by ameboid movement, presumably by chemotaxis.[191]

When PGCs enter the female genital ridge, they migrate toward the germinal epithelium and become incorporated into cortical cords.[191] Coincident with the colonization of the gonad by the PGCs, epithelial cells from mesonephric tubules migrate into the genital area, where they probably become the granulosa and interstitial cells.[193] The conclusion, therefore, is that the presumptive follicle cells (oocyte, granulosa, theca) originate outside the gonadal blastoma.

Oogonia

In the PGCs, only one X chromosome in an XX female is expressed; however, once PGCs enter the presumptive ovary, both X chromosomes are expressed and the germ cells are now called *oogonia.*[194] Subsequently, oogonia initiate an active phase of proliferation and their number increases tremendously. As the oogonia proliferate, there are dramatic increases in the activity of X chromosome–encoded enzymes. The importance of expression of twice the gene product in developing female germ cells is emphasized by the fact that XO genetic females exhibit oocyte depletion and sterility.[195] The oogonium is a unique cell in that it is the only cell in which both X chromosomes are active.

As mitosis proceeds and the cortical cord growth continues, the dividing oogonia fail to complete cytokinesis. Consequently, subpopulations of oogonia remain joined together by intercellular bridges,[196] and their differentiation then proceeds synchronously, in a way resembling germ cell differentiation in the testis.

Oocytes

Beginning at 12 weeks of gestation[22] some of the connected oogonia (those in the deepest regions of the cortical cords nearest the medullary tissue) initiate meiosis (Fig. 17A-5). There is evidence that the mesonephric system is important in triggering the initiation of meiosis in the oocytes and their subsequent incorporation into primordial follicles.[197] In response to the putative meiosis-inducing substance, subgroups of oogonia initiate meiotic DNA synthesis and begin to proceed through leptotene, zygotene, pachytene, and diplotene of meiotic prophase (Fig. 17A-5). At diplotene, the paired homologous chromosomes become less condensed and the oocyte enters a protracted interphase-like stage called *dictyotene.* It is at this time that the oocytes become incorporated into primordial follicles (Fig. 17A-5).[22] At its shortest it can last 12 years (until puberty); at its longest it can last about 50 years (until the menopause).

OOCYTE GROWTH To understand oogenesis, two interrelated processes must be considered: oocyte growth and completion of meiosis. Oocyte growth is associated with the accumulation and storage of nutritional and informational materials, some of which are critical to the development of the preimplantation blastocyst. During growth the oocyte increases in diameter from 20 μm to 120 μm. The basis for growth resides in the active transcription of stable messenger RNA, ribosomal RNA, transfer RNA, and heterogeneous RNA by lampbrush chromosomes of the oocyte.[198–200] A fundamental concept is that the growth of the follicle relative to that of the oocyte can be divided into two distinct phases: initially, oocyte and follicle diameter are positively and linearly correlated until the follicle reaches the early tertiary stage (cavitation); after that the oocyte ceases to grow while follicular growth continues (Fig. 17A-27).

The presence of granulosa cells is an absolute requirement for oocyte growth.[201,202] As growth progresses, the oocyte is closely surrounded by corona radiata granulosa cells which interact directly with the oocyte via gap junctions and desmosomes.[37–39] By virtue of this metabolic coupling, the oocyte can capitalize on unique nutritional and/or regulatory capacities of granulosa cells. Results obtained with animal species indicate that 85 percent of the metabolites present in follicle-enclosed oocytes are originally taken up by the granulosa cell and then transferred into the oocyte through the gap junctions.[203,204] The concept which emerges is that the obligatory role of granulosa cells in oocyte growth involves special gap junctional contacts which are responsible for the transfer of fundamental nutrients into the oocyte.

During oocyte growth, the zona pellucida is formed. The zona pellucida is a relatively thick, translucent acellular coat which surrounds the oolemma of the fully grown oocyte. The zona pellucida plays an important role in a number of vital biological functions:[205] (1) it contains species-specific receptors for capacitated sperm, (2) it provides a block to polyspermy, and (3) it is critical in allowing the embryo to move freely through the fallopian tube into the uterus.

It is apparent that the proteins in the zona pellu-

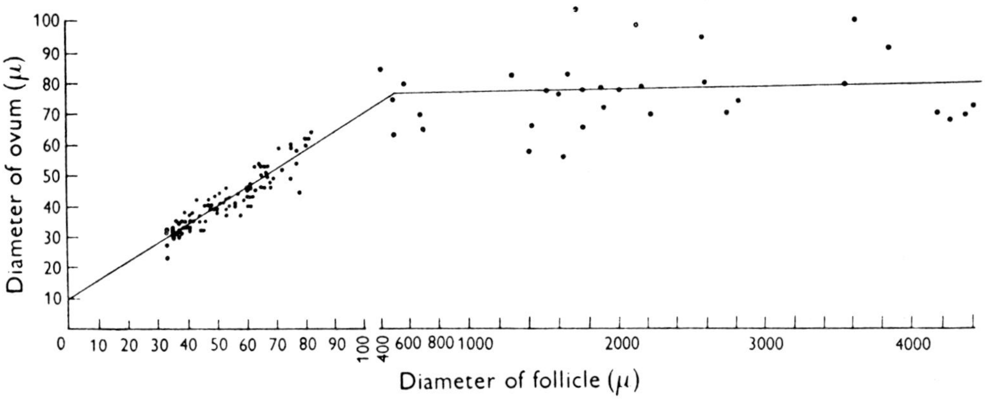

FIGURE 17A-27 Regression lines showing the relationship between the sizes of the oocyte and follicle in the human ovary. (*From Green and Zuckerman,*[264] *by permission of Cambridge University Press.*)

cida are synthesized and secreted by the growing oocyte.[29] The morphologic basis for this event involves multiple replications of the Golgi apparatus and their subsequent migration to the periphery of the oocyte, just beneath the oolemma.[28] The zona pellucida contains three glycoproteins, designated *ZP-1* (mol wt 200,000), *ZP-2* (mol wt 120,000), and *ZP-3* (mol wt 83,000).[206] The binding of species-specific sperm to the zona pellucida is believed to result from an interaction with the ZP-3 protein.[207] No function of the other zona-specific proteins is known.

MEIOTIC MATURATION The capacity to resume meiosis is acquired at a specific stage in oocyte growth and differentiation; the ability to complete meiotic maturation is acquired subsequently. Meiotic maturation or resumption of meiosis (Fig. 17A-28) is a process characterized by (1) the dissolution of the nuclear or germinal vesicle membrane, (2) the condensation of dictyotene chromatin into discrete bivalents, (3) the separation of homologous chromosomes, (4) the release of a first polar body, and (5) the arrest of the meiotic process at metaphase II. The completion of meiosis and release of the second polar body is triggered by fertilization or parthenogenetic activation.

During follicle development, the oocyte acquires the capacity to resume meiosis at the stage of cavitation or early antrum formation.[208] At this time the occyte has completed its growth and is surrounded by the zona pellucida and four to five layers of granulosa cells. The acquisition of the capacity for meiotic maturation seems to be a two-step process.[209] First, the oocyte acquires the capacity to undergo germinal vesicle breakdown and progress to metaphase I; second comes the acquisition of the capacity to complete the first reductional division and release the first polar body. The mechanisms responsible for the acquisition of meiotic potential are unknown, but again seem to be under intraovarian control.

Although the oocyte is capable of resuming meiosis early in follicle development, it is kept from doing so by an inhibitory influence. Under normal physiological conditions, the resumption of meiotic maturation is a highly selective process and occurs only in those oocytes which are in dominant preovulatory follicles. There is little doubt that the resumption of meiosis in these oocytes occurs as a result of the preovulatory surge of LH.[210] Based on a large body of data it is evident that fully grown oocytes from any tertiary or graafian follicle will undergo meiotic maturation spontaneously when the oocyte is placed in tissue culture. Collectively, these observations have led to the hypothesis that there is an inhibiting substance which blocks meiotic maturation in the follicle and that high levels of LH are capable of overriding the inhibitory influence.

Evidence suggests that granulosa cells supply to the ovum a substance which blocks meiotic maturation.[114] The substance, termed *oocyte meiotic inhibitor* (OMI), is putatively a protein (mol wt < 2000). What is the underlying mechanism by which LH and OMI regulate meiotic maturation? In this conception it is proposed that the membrana granulosa cells in response to gonadotropin stimulation secrete OMI into the follicular fluid. Evidence indicates that OMI does not act directly on the oocyte, but exerts its inhibitory influence indirectly, through interactions with the cumulus and corona radiata granulosa cells.[114] It has been proposed that OMI acts as a signal to these cells to stimulate cAMP, which subsequently diffuses through gap junctions into the oocyte where the cAMP suppresses meiotic maturation.[114] When the preovulatory surge of LH occurs, the membrana granulosa becomes desensitized and stops producing OMI.

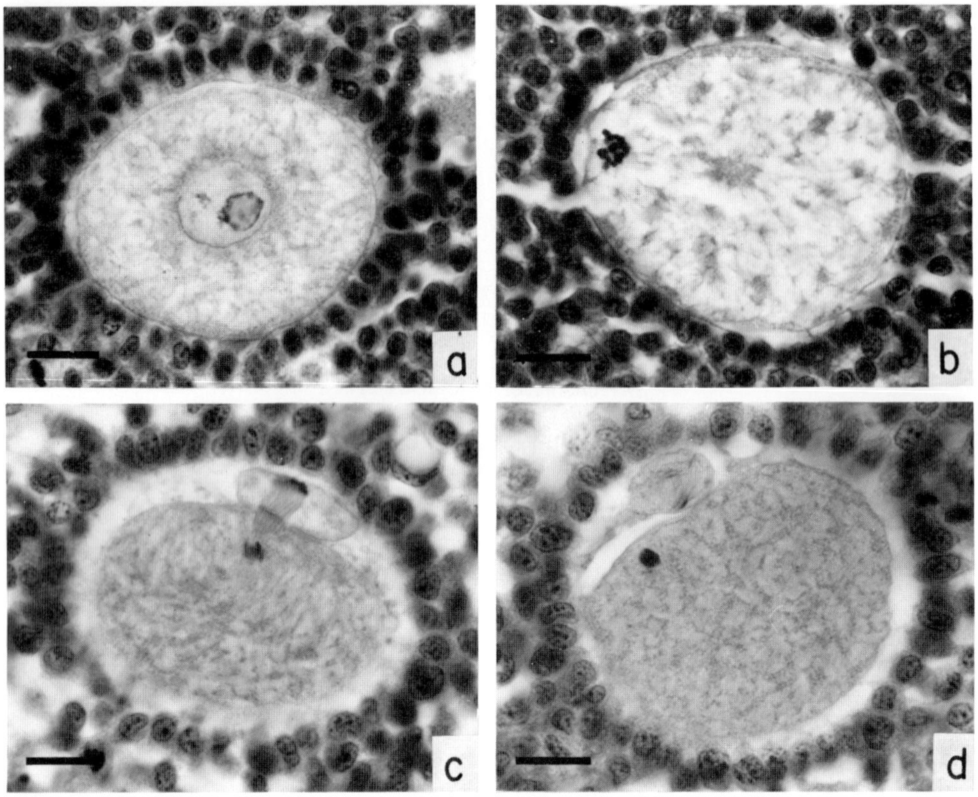

FIGURE 17A-28 Photomicrographs showing the process of meiotic maturation or resumption of meiosis. (*A*) Germinal vesicle stage; (*B*) germinal vesicle breakdown followed by condensation of chromosomes into bivalents; (*C, D*) release of first polar body and arrest of meiotic process at metaphase II. (*Courtesy of Dr. Carole Banka.*)

Ultimately this response leads to decreases in oocyte cAMP levels followed by a release of intracellular calcium stores and germinal vesicle breakdown.[211] This concept is illustrated in Fig. 17A-29.

An important aspect of this concept concerns the role of steroids in the initiation of meiosis. The best results to date have been obtained in animal species. High concentrations of estradiol are essential for normal cytoplasmic maturation of the oocyte. If there is inadequate estrogen support, meiotic maturation results in abnormalities in fertilization, delayed cleavage, and almost total failure of the embryo to undergo blastocyte formation.[212] The conclusion is that high levels of estradiol in the follicular fluid facilitate the complete differentiation of the egg in vivo and in vitro.

FOLLICLE DEVELOPMENT: CONTROL MECHANISMS

Recruitment

Recruitment is the process whereby a primordial follicle is stimulated to leave the pool of nongrowing follicles and initiate development. In the human, recruitment begins in the embryo when primordial follicles are first formed and ends at the menopause when the pool of primordial follicles is depleted.[22,23]

What mechanisms are responsible for recruitment? It is well established that the first transition to the recruited state is accompanied by the transformation of the granulosa cells from a squamous to a cuboidal shape.[213] Thus, the activation in the granulosa must be considered a major event in recruitment. As granulosa cells become round they acquire the capability to incorporate [^{3}H]thymidine and begin to divide, albeit very slowly.[213,214] When $\geq$ 90 percent of the granulosa cells are cuboidal, there occurs a dramatic activation in oocyte RNA synthesis which results in rapid growth of the cytoplasm and the germinal vesicle.[198–200] Since changes in synthetic activity of the oocyte arise after prior changes in the granulosa cells, it would seem that the granulosa either responds to or generates a signal that triggers the primordial follicle to follow the pathway of recruitment.

Although the whole process is very poorly understood, some information about the nature of the cues

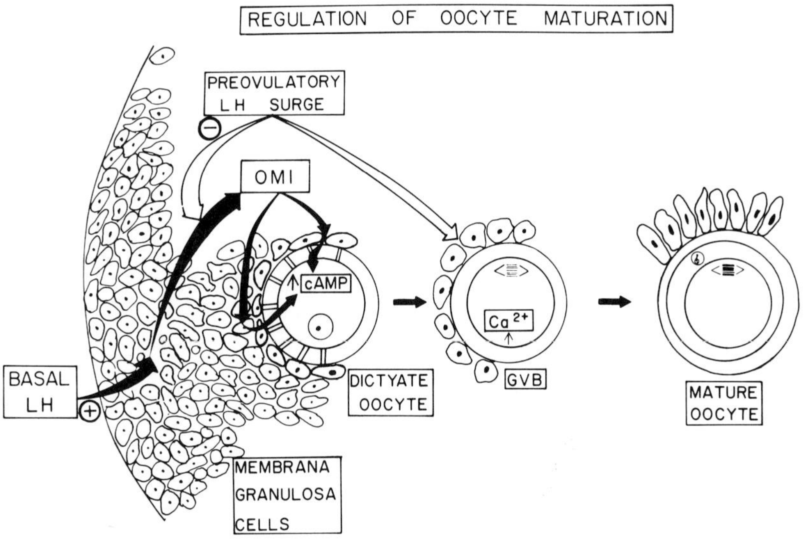

FIGURE 17A-29 Diagram of current concept of control of meiotic maturation.

for recruitment does exist. First, the ovaries are endowed with the message capable of initiating recruitment. It has long been recognized that recruitment (including oocyte growth and granulosa proliferation) does not depend on extragonadal hormones such as FSH and LH.[18,19] An exception to this may exist in the initiation of the first wave of recruitment in the embryo. It has been found that recruitment is markedly retarded in anencephalic fetuses[23] and hypophysectomized fetal monkeys.[215] Similarly, if ovaries are explanted in vitro prior to the initiation of recruitment, follicular growth does not occur, but recruitment can be initiated if the cultured ovaries are treated with exogenous gonadotropins.[216] It would appear, therefore, that FSH/LH may be responsible for initiating the program of recruitment in the fetus, but, once "blueprinted," the ovaries possess the power to autonomously produce recruitment molecules. The cellular source or chemical nature of recruitment inducers is unknown.

An important concept is that the process of recruitment can be modulated. Normally, the number of primordial follicles recruited is not constant but varies with age:[217] the greatest growth activity occurs early in life, after which the number of recruited follicles decreases progressively with advancing age.[218] This would argue that the normal inducers of recruitment are somehow regulated by the actual size of the pool of primordial follicles. In this context, there is a marked reduction (by 30 percent) in the number of follicles recruited during pregnancy, compared to the number during the cycle.[219] This suggests that the conditions leading to recruitment may be modulated by hormones. It is clear that the presence of testosterone severely reduces the number of primordial follicles and thereby influences the recruitment process.[220] On the basis of these experiments, it is proposed that recruitment is regulated by intraovarian androgens produced by the interstitial cells. Other experiments of a more complicated nature indicate that recruitment can also be modulated (i.e., attenuated) by the thymus gland,[221,222] food intake or starvation,[223] and opioid peptides.[224] Up to this point, no modulator has been found which can stimulate or amplify the process of recruitment.

Atresia

Of the estimated 2 million oocytes present in the female at birth (Fig. 17A-6), only about 400 are destined to leave the ovary through ovulation. Thus, 99.9 percent of the eggs are lost by the processes of atresia. There are two classes of atresia (see Ovarian Follicles, above): type A, which occurs in preantral follicles, and type B, which occurs in antral or graafian follicles (Fig. 17A-13). Evidence suggests that these two types of atresia are accomplished by different biochemical mechanisms.

The deleterious effect of testosterone on preantral follicles is clear. It has been found that if preantral follicles are exposed to testosterone then the oocyte and granulosa cells are destroyed. What mechanism must be operating to induce type A atresia? The fundamental role of estrogen in promoting the growth and development of preantral follicles is well established,[21] a permissive response which is mediated by the estrogen receptor.[126] It is clear that testosterone reduces or eliminates the sensitivity of the granulosa cell to estrogen, and that the mechanism by which testosterone antagonizes estrogen is to reduce the number of estrogen receptors in the granulosa cell.[225] The current concept of the physiological mechanisms which lead to type A atresia in preantral follicles is as follows: In some unexplained way, the theca and/or secondary interstitial cells surrounding a given preantral follicle respond to low levels of LH by secreting increased amounts of testosterone.[226–228] After diffusion into the granulosa cells, the testosterone binds to specific receptor molecules, acting to reduce the estrogen receptor levels. Consequently, the preantral granulosa cells become unresponsive to estrogen stimulation and subsequently die. The conclusion is therefore reached that the primary event in type A atresia involves LH-induced changes in testosterone production by local theca and/or secondary interstitial cells.

The basis for type B atresia in antral follicles seems also to involve causal relationships between LH and interstitial cells. In animals, treatment with antiserum to LH results in increased ovulation rates, the basis of which seems to involve the prevention of graafian follicle atresia.[229] The current concept for LH-induced type B atresia involves LH-induced switch in the hormone production by the theca interstitial cells from an androgen to a progesterone-secreting tissue.[230] Consequently, there occur dramatic decreases in available androgen for aromatization, resulting in decreased follicular estrogen levels. The effect is death in the granulosa, which needs the high levels of estrogen to survive. It seems, therefore, that the primary initiating event in graafian follicle atresia is an alteration in theca cell function, from an androgen- to a progesterone-secreting cell, and that LH is at the basis of the switch in steroid metabolism.

The concept emerging is that the most important generating forces in atresia involve LH-induced changes in steroid production processes of the ovarian interstitial cells that subsequently result in changes in either estrogen production or the sensitivity of the granulosa cells to estrogen hormones.

Selection

One of the most profound questions to concern ovarian physiologists has been how the dominant preovulatory follicle is selected from what appears to be a cohort of developing follicles. An important insight into the mechanism was obtained when it was found that this basic process requires both LH and FSH[20] as well as both granulosa and theca interstitial cells.[59] This has led to a fundamental principle in ovarian physiology, called the "two-cell–two-gonadotropin" principle of follicular estrogen biosynthesis. In response to LH stimulation, the theca interstitial cells synthesize and secrete androstenedione; the androstenedione diffuses across the basal lamina into the follicular fluid and then enters the granulosa cells, where it is metabolized to estradiol by aromatase enzymes induced by FSH (Fig. 17A-30). The newly synthesized estrogen is released into the follicular fluid and the peripheral circulation, where it leads to the formation of a permissive estrogenic environment. The presence and maintenance of this process is the basis of follicle selection.

What is the primary event leading to sustained follicle estrogen biosynthesis? Much of what is known has come from studies by McNatty and coworkers conducted on the microenvironment of developing follicles in normal women during the follicular phase of the menstrual cycle.[42,232,233] Some relevant data are illustrated in Table 17A-1. Focusing on the gonadotropins, it is evident that plasma FSH enters follicular fluid early on day 1 of the cycle, after which its concentration increases progressively with follicular growth. This finding is important because it strongly suggests that a selected follicle has the ability to sequester FSH against the declining FSH levels in the peripheral plasma. Interestingly, the situation is not the same for other gonadotropins. Table 17A-1 shows that the patterns of LH and prolactin concentrations in follicular fluid differ from each other and from that of FSH. This type of finding has implications for the way in which selection occurs, because it demonstrates that some mechanism is operating at the level of the follicle both to inhibit and stimulate the entry of potent regulatory molecules into the microenvironment of the follicular fluid.

Studies of human follicular fluid indicate that the major proteins are plasma proteins, and that both total protein and composition are basically the same in follicular fluid and serum. The relative proportions, however, of proteins in follicular fluid are strikingly different from those in plasma.[235] As a rule, the ability of a protein to enter follicular fluid is inversely proportional to its molecular weight. This has led to the concept that the follicle (most likely the basal lamina) filters thecal blood in a sievelike manner such that it blocks 50 percent of the proteins with mol wt 250,000 and is impermeable to proteins above 850,000 daltons. In this light, it could be argued that the gonadotropins, which are relatively small molecules, should have no difficulty in penetrating the blood-follicle barrier. It is apparent (Table 17A-1) that these molecules are not freely diffusible; thus, some mechanism must exist to account for their passage into and out of the follicles. The basis for this control is unknown but seems central to the selection process.[231]

To what extent is the estrogen potential of a follicle attributable to androgen substrate? It has been

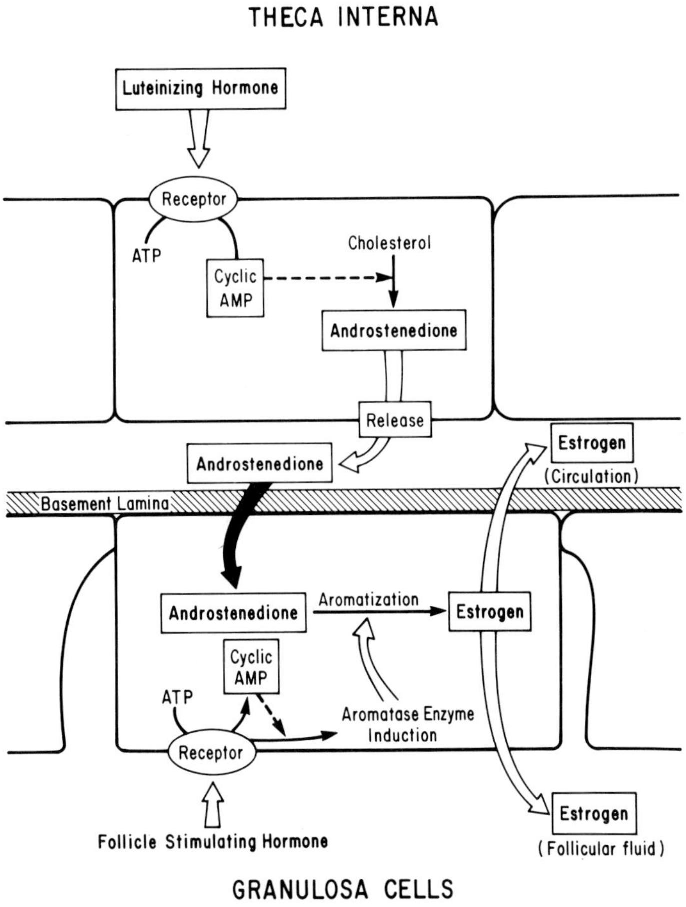

FIGURE 17A-30 Diagram of the two-cell–two-gonadotropin concept of follicular estrogen biosynthesis. (*From Erickson,[265] by permission of Harper and Row.*)

shown that aromatase substrate (androstenedione) in all follicles attains a maximum concentration of about 10^{-6} to 10^{-5} M at day 1 of the menstrual cycle (Table 17A-1). Despite these very high levels of aromatase substrate, the concentration of estradiol in the follicular fluid of all developing follicles is low during the first 7 days of the follicular phase. At the midfollicular phase, however, there occurs a rather sharp increase in estradiol concentration, reaching levels of about 1 to 2 μg/ml. Since androstenedione levels are so high, it can be concluded that the dramatic increases in follicle estradiol production that accompany selection are not causally related to the level of aromatase substrate. Rather, the underlying basis for the estrogen switch must depend on the induction or activation of follicular aromatase enzyme. An important sidelight is that the aromatase inhibitor DHT does not appear to be an important factor in regulating follicular estrogen

Table 17A-1. Microenvironment of Healthy Human Follicles

Day of cycle	Follicle size (mm)	Volume of follicular fluid (μl)	Hormone concentration (mIU or ng/ml)						
			FSH	LH	PRL	Δ4	E_2	P	DHT
1	4	30	2.5	ND	60	800	100	ND	100
4	7	150	2.5	ND	40	800	500	100	100
7	12	500	3.6	2.8	20	800	1000	300	100
12	20	650	3.6	6	5	800	2000	2000	100

Note: Data based on the work of McNatty et al.[41,62–64]
PRL=prolactin; Δ4=androstenedione; E_2=estradiol; P=progesterone; DHT=dihydrotestosterone; ND=nondetectable.

production because DHT (at a concentration found in follicular fluid; Table 17A-1) does not suppress aromatization of androstenedione by the human follicle.[236] This argues that the aromatase inhibitors do not play a role in the selection process.

The study of atretic follicles has been very valuable to understanding selection. One of the most characteristic features of the atretic or nondominant follicle is the absence of FSH in the follicular fluid (Fig. 17A-31). Given the evidence that FSH is the primary stimulus for the induction of aromatase enzymes in granulosa cells, the conclusion is drawn that the very essence of atresia in graafian follicles is the failure to sequester or concentrate FSH in the follicular fluid. Accordingly, there occur dramatic decreases in follicular fluid estradiol concentration and the follicle dies. It follows, therefore, that the mechanism controlling selection of a dominant preovulatory follicle most certainly involves the continued ability to selectively increase the concentration of FSH in the microenvironment. Physiologically, this would mean more aromatase enzyme and more estradiol, both of which would shift a follicle along the path of selection as opposed to atresia.

Inasmuch as the follicle contains two major populations of endocrine cells, the granulosa and theca interstitial, each with differing hormonal sensitivities and steroidogenic capacity, the question arises whether modulators are involved in the selection process. To become a dominant preovulatory follicle, the theca and the granulosa must complete all the steps in the selection process; interruption of the maturation sequence at any step in the process could potentially prevent selection and result in atresia. As pointed out earlier, many hormones and factors can alter follicular estrogen biosynthesis and thus hold potential for influencing the process of follicular maturation and selection. An interesting observation is that high concentrations of prolactin in human follicular fluid are associated with low estradiol levels.[237] This suggests that continued entry of prolactin into the follicle might lead to suppression of the physiological changes underlying estrogen biosynthesis (see Table 17A-1). Considering what is known about the control of gran-

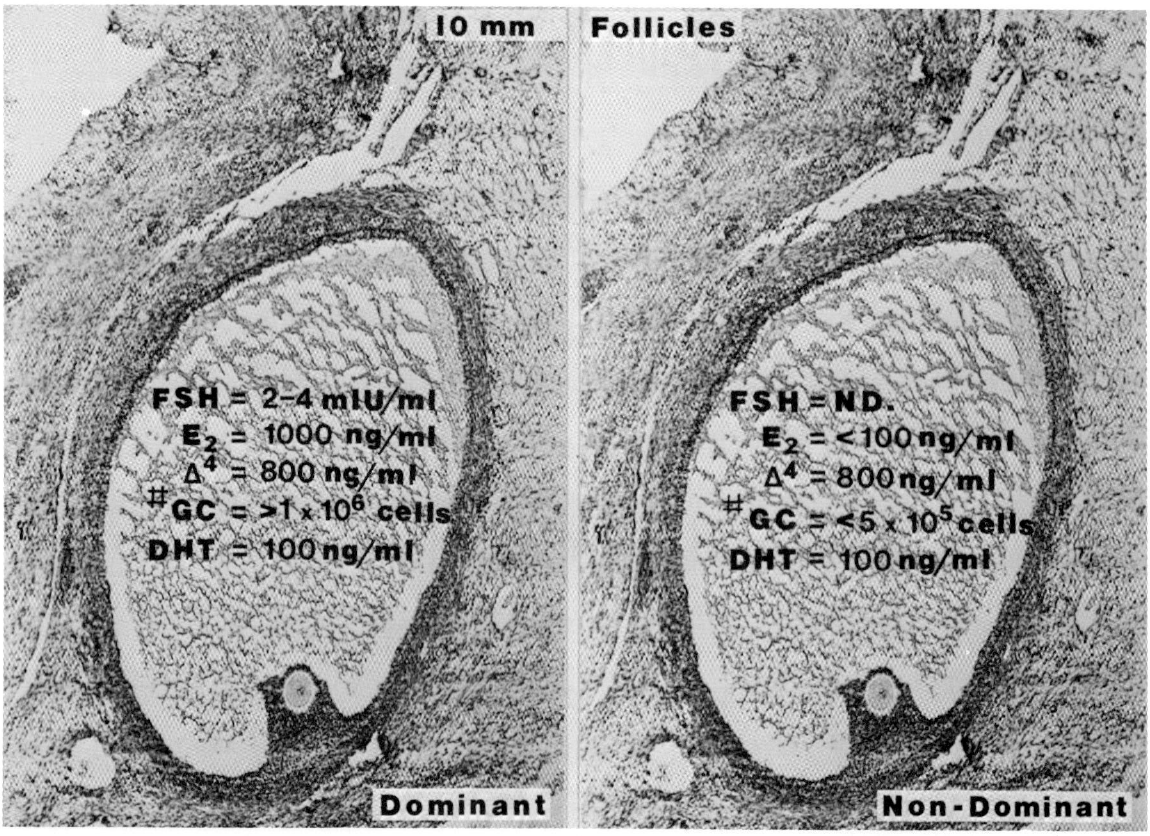

FIGURE 17A-31 Photomicrographs showing basic differences between the microenvironments of dominant and nondominant follicles at the midfollicular phase of the menstrual cycle. (*From Erickson and Yen,*[231] *by permission of Thieme-Stratton.*)

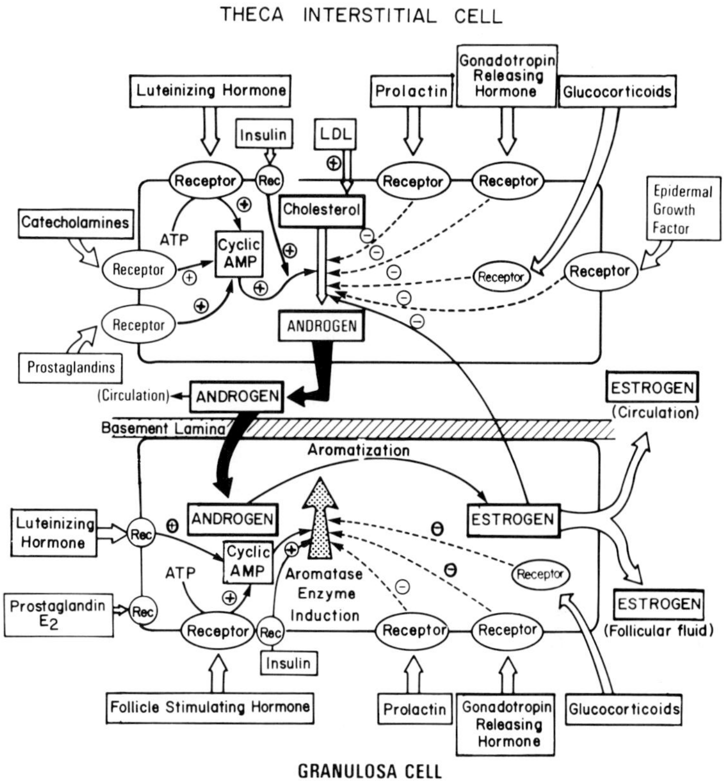

FIGURE 17A-32 Diagram of current concept of underlying controlling potentials of follicular estrogen biosynthesis in relation to the two-cell–two-gonadotropin principle. (*Revised from Erickson,*[99] *by permission of Elsevier Scientific.*)

ulosa and interstitial cell differentiation, then the implications for estrogen synthetic potential and therefore selection are obvious (Fig. 17A-32).

Ovulation

The expulsion of a mature oocyte from the ovary results from the release of hydrolytic enzymes in selected regions of the preovulatory follicle and a squeezing process in the basal region of the follicle wall (Fig. 17A-33). It follows, therefore, that questions concerning the phenomenon of ovulation center on the generation of proteolytic activity and contractile mechanisms in the theca externa.

There are seven cellular and extracellular components which together serve as a barrier to prevent the escape of the oocyte from the preovulatory follicle. Beginning at the surface of the ovary and moving inward, these components include: (1) the surface or germinal epithelium, (2) the basement membrane, (3) the dense connective tissue of the tunica albuginea, (4) the theca externa, (5) the theca interna, (6) the basal lamina of the follicle, (7) the membrana granulosa cells. It is evident that if an oocyte-cumulus complex is to exit from its follicle, then this organized

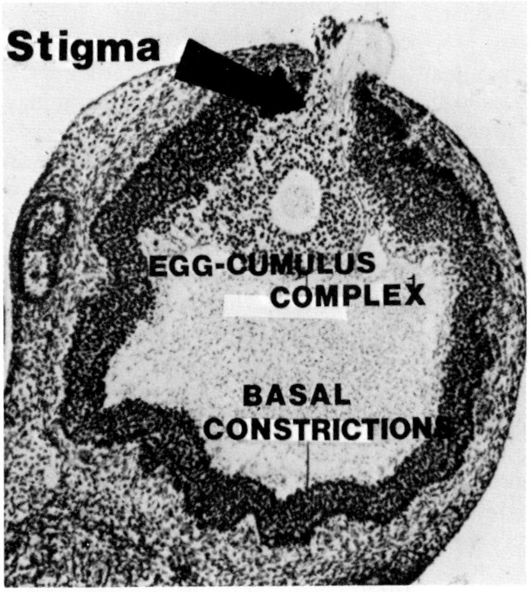

FIGURE 17A-33 Photomicrograph through a preovulatory follicle during ovulation. Note the selective destruction of tissue in the stigma and the constrictions of the basal follicular wall. (*From Hartman and Leathem,*[262] *by permission of Pergamon.*)

network of cells and extracellular material must be broken down.

One important aspect of the destructive mechanism is that it occurs in a highly localized area called the *stigma* (Fig. 17A-33). How do the cells in the presumptive stigma become activated to fulfill this fundamental degradative process? Morphologic and biochemical studies show that during the ovulatory period surface epithelial cells in the presumptive stigma become filled with large lysosomelike inclusions.[238] With increasing periods of time, the lysosomelike inclusions fuse with the plasma membrane and release their contents toward the tunica albuginea. This is accompanied by the progressive destruction of the basement membrane. This situation continues to progress medially, causing disruptive changes in the theca layers. It appears, therefore, that the steps leading to the formation of the stigma are initiated in a specialized population of surface epithelial cells and involve the formation and subsequent release of large amounts of hydrolytic enzymes. The question that must be analyzed is how this event occurs.

It is well established that the most important stimulating force in ovulation is LH. Although the basic mechanisms involved in LH-induced ovulation are unclear, some insights have been generated from studies carried out primarily in laboratory animals. First, the LH surge starts the preovulatory follicle on the path of progesterone production. An interesting observation in animals hypophysectomized during the preovulatory LH rise in that treatment with exogenous progesterone completely restores ovulation.[239] Consequently, it appears that progesterone plays a physiological role in the ovulation process and may be a mediator of LH action.

Results from an extensive variety of studies indicate that the mechanisms underlying ovulation involve the generation of PGs by the preovulatory follicle.[240,241] Following the preovulatory surge of LH and the stimulation of progesterone production, there occur marked increases in the synthesis of PGE and PGF. If an LH-stimulated preovulatory follicle is injected with indomethacin or antiprostaglandin serum, ovulation is completely blocked.[242] The conclusion emerging is that LH-stimulated PG production is an obligatory trigger eliciting ovulation. Interestingly, morphologic studies of indomethacin-treated ovaries suggest that the prostaglandins are involved in the steps by which the stigma is formed.[243] It appears, therefore, that the underlying mechanisms of LH-induced ovulation involve the following scenario: The elevated level of progesterone serves to activate PG production, which then promotes the release of hydrolytic enzymes by a subpopulation of surface epithelial cells, which then cause stigma formation (Fig. 17A-33).

Another highly active protease involved in ovulation is plasmin.[244] The follicular fluid of a preovulatory follicle contains the plasmin precursor *plasminogen* at the same levels as in serum. The granulosa cells in a preovulatory follicle are selectively stimulated by very low levels of FSH to release the protein plasminogen activator.[245] This substance then converts plasminogen to the active protease plasmin. Once the process is initiated, holes are formed in the basal lamina and there is a general weakening of the follicular wall, presumably due to the hydrolytic action of plasmin.[246] Questions concerning the physiological importance of the plasminogen activator in ovulation are unanswered, but the concept is intriguing and raises the possibility that FSH, like LH, plays a basic role in ovulation, perhaps by causing destructive changes in the follicular basal lamina.

To what extent are contractile mechanisms involved in ovulation? It has been established that cells with the ultrastructure of smooth muscle cells are found only in the basal hemisphere of the follicle and that these cells contract before follicle rupture.[247] A number of experiments have been done with human ovarian follicles with regard to the contractile effects of various hormones. The conclusion which emerges is that the smooth muscle cells in the theca externa have β-adrenergic receptors for norepinephrine and muscarinic receptors for acetylcholine, both of which, when activated by ligand, will stimulate follicle contraction.[248] Since smooth muscle cells in the theca externa are innervated by sympathetic and parasympathetic nerves, it seems certain that autonomic nerves are involved in the contractile mechanisms which occur prior to ovulation. Importantly, direct analysis of intrafollicular pressure during ovulation has ruled out a buildup of intrafollicular pressure in the ovulatory process.[249] These results suggest that contractile mechanisms do not play a direct role in follicular rupture. However, based on morphologic studies, there is little doubt that contractile mechanisms occur prior to ovulation and play an important role in the collapse of the follicle and the actual expulsion of the cumulus-egg complex onto the surface of the ovary.

PHYSIOLOGICAL CORRELATES OF OVARIAN ACTIVITY WITH AGING

The Fetal Period

To what extent is the human fetal ovary steroidogenically active? It was pointed out earlier that fetal ovaries at 12 to 20 weeks of gestation contain a population of differentiated primary interstitial cells (Fig. 17A-14). Analysis of steroid metabolism has led to the concept that the human fetal ovaries do not have the capability to synthesize steroids de novo, presumably because they are unable to metabolize cholesterol to pregnenolone.[250] Furthermore, if human fetal ovaries are incubated with either exogenous pregnenolone or progesterone, there is little or no metabolism to steroid hormones.[251,252]

By contrast, then fetal ovary cells at 12 weeks of gestation are incubated with pregnenolone sulfate, it is metabolized to pregnenolone, 17α-hydroxypregnenolone, dehydroepiandrosterone, and androstenedione, but not to estrogen or testosterone.[253] This finding indicates that the fetal ovaries at 12 weeks of gestation contain a very active sulfatase (three to seven times more active than in the fetal adrenal), as well as key steroidogenic enzymes in the Δ^5 pathway.[253] As development proceeds, there is a progressive decline in the steroidogenic enzymes such that, by 17 weeks, the ability of the fetal ovary to metabolize pregnenolone sulfate to C_{19} steroids is very low.[253] It follows from these types of experiments that cells in human fetal ovaries can effectively use pregnenolone sulfate to produce biologically active androgens. The physiological implications of this work lie in the fact that pregnenolone sulfate is present in very high concentrations in the fetal circulation.[254] Taken together, these various observations support the concept that, during their short existence (between 12 and 20 weeks of gestation), the primary interstitial cells are actively engaged in the production of biologically active androgens, using as substrate the steroid sulfates present in the fetal circulation. The physiological significance of the androgens produced by the fetal ovaries is unknown. Importantly, LH, FSH, and hCG do not stimulate steroid metabolism by fetal ovarian cells in vitro,[255] suggesting their activity is independent of gonadotropin control.

By 26 weeks of gestation, the fetal ovaries contain a population of graafian follicles that have well-developed thecae interna.[256] During the remainder of gestation, the frequency and size of graafian follicles increase; the largest diameter reached is about 5 mm at 28 weeks. No follicles progress beyond this size and all are destroyed by atresia. Nothing is known about the steroidogenic potential of the human fetal ovaries during this latter period, but the presence of well-developed theca interstitial cells implies they are active in androgen formation.

Premenarche

Typically, the normal ovary in childhood is a dynamic organ which is undergoing constant internal changes associated with recruitment, follicular growth, and atresia.[257–259] A characteristic feature of the human ovary from birth until menarche is the presence of large numbers of graafian follicles which measure between 1 and 6 mm in diameter (Fig. 17A-34). Generally, these follicles contain three to five layers of granulosa cells, a fully grown oocyte, and a thickened theca interna with apparently highly differentiated theca interstitial cells (Fig. 17A-34). In this sense, the infant and prepubertal ovary is morphologically indistinguishable from that of a woman with polycystic ovary syndrome (PCO). Although evidence is lacking, the premenarcheal ovaries (like those in PCO) may be actively engaged in androgen biosynthesis. Under normal circumstances, these follicles in the premenarcheal ovary grow to the graafian state, but all of them undergo atresia.[259] Thus, as in PCO, the regulatory mechanisms of selection are not operative in the prepubertal ovary.

Menarche

When a child reaches 6 years of age, some follicles begin to grow and develop beyond the 5- to 6-mm stage.[260] This situation is accompanied by progressive increases in the levels of estrogen in the plasma (Fig. 17A-35).[261] At the same time, there occur steady increases in FSH and LH concentrations in the peripheral plasma. Importantly, at about age 10, the concentration of FSH is greater than that of LH, similar to the situation in the early follicular phase of the menstrual cycle.[261] The underlying mechanism controlling the onset of follicular estrogen synthesis most certainly involves the stimulatory effect of LH and FSH, in particular the FSH induction of aromatase activity in the granulosa cells. As a result of this scenario, the prepubertal ovaries show a progressive increase in the capacity for estrogen production and follicular growth, a process which continues until the events responsible for the initiation of selection occur. After becoming committed to a dominant follicle, the ovulatory process is initiated and the follicle becomes a corpus luteum. At this time menarche occurs; the basis for the commitment toward menarche most certainly involves the steady increases in FSH level which, when high enough in the follicular fluid, drives granulosa cells in ovarian follicles to produce an appropriate estrogenic environment suitable for initiating the selection process.

Postmenarche: The Normal Menstrual Cycle

The menstrual cycle is accompanied by the sequence of recruitment, selection, ovulation, luteinization, and luteolysis. The underlying mechanisms responsible for these individual processes have already been described.

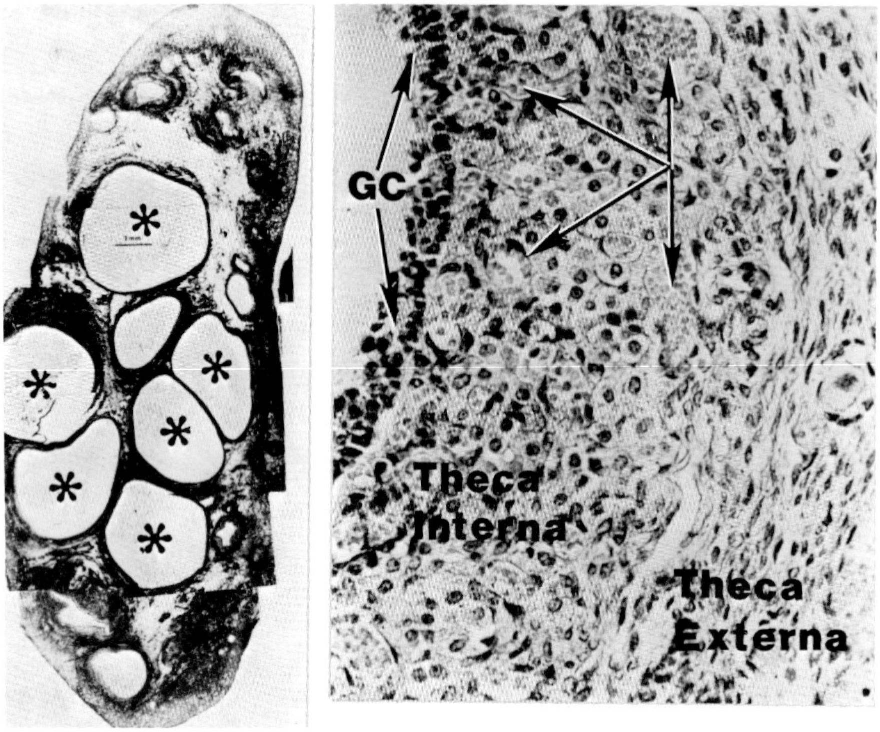

A B

FIGURE 17A-34 Photomicrographs of actively growing human ovary at 7½ years of age. (*A*) Ovaries are polycystic-like with large numbers of graafian follicles (*) measuring 2 to 6 mm in diameter. (*B*) Higher magnification of follicle shows paucity of granulosa cells (GC) and well-developed theca interna with five to seven layers of highly differentiated theca interstitial cells and numerous large capillaries (arrows). (*From Peters et al.*[258] *by permission of Periodical.*)

Typically, the menstrual cycle is divided into two major periods (Fig. 17A-36): the follicular phase (days 1 to 14) and the luteal phase (days 15 to 28); these major events are divided by ovulation, which occurs early on day 15. If the length of the normal menstrual cycle changes (becoming either shorter or longer), then the shift occurs in the length of the follicular phase; characteristically, the programming of the corpus luteum is highly constant at 14 days.

As the name implies, the follicular phase concerns

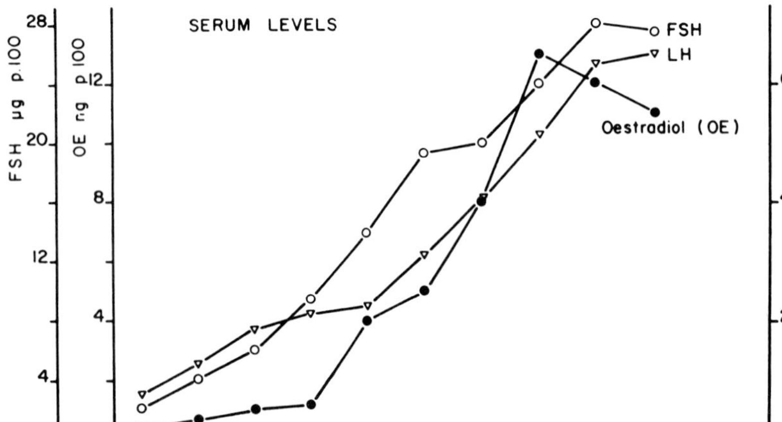

FIGURE 17A-35 Serum concentration of FSH, LH, and estradiol in girls of different ages. (*From Peters,*[263] *by permission of Gauthier Villars.*)

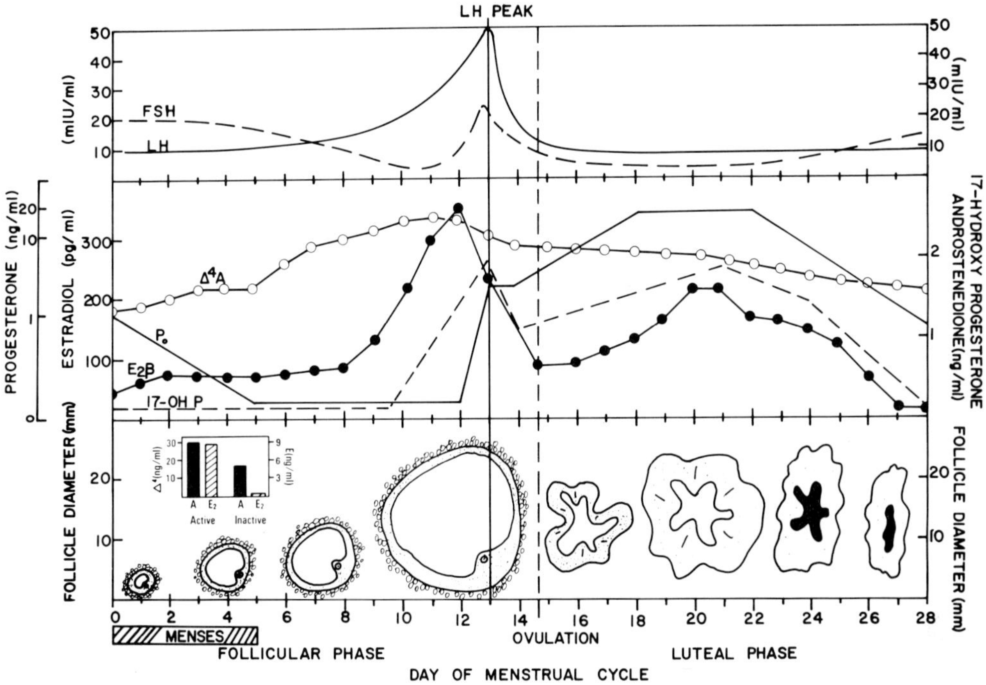

FIGURE 17A-36 Diagrammatic illustration of endocrine events in the human menstrual cycle. The *inset* (lower left) indicates differences in levels of steroids in ovarian venous effluent between ovaries with (active) and without (inactive) the selected follicle. Data are based on reports in Refs. 156–161. (*Revised from Erickson and Yen,*[231] *by permission of Thieme-Stratton.*)

the evolution and development of a preovulatory follicle. This important process is initiated during the preceding menstrual cycle. Results from studies in rodents indicate that at least 16 days are required for a primordial follicle to reach the early tertiary (Fig. 17A-4) or cavitation stage of 0.4 to 0.5 mm in diameter.[266] In sheep, it takes another 9 days for such a follicle to grow to a small graafian follicle, measuring about 4.5 mm in diameter.[267] If it is considered that the cohort of follicles ultimately responsible for producing a preovulatory follicle in women are 4 to 5 mm in diameter at the start of the follicular phase (Table 17A-1, Fig. 17A-36), then it would be argued that the presumptive preovulatory follicle is recruited approximately 25 days earlier, near the beginning of the previous menstrual cycle. Considering the fact that it takes 14 days for a selected follicle to ovulate, then the total time required for a primordial follicle to grow and develop to the preovulatory stage in the human would be 39 days ($16 + 9 + 14 = 39$ days).

The first question to consider is when and how a graafian follicle is selected in the follicular phase. Morphologic studies conducted on human ovaries strongly suggest that the follicle destined to ovulate is present in one ovary selected at the beginning of the follicular phase.[268] The chosen follicle is not necessarily the largest, but always shows the highest number of dividing granulosa cells.[268] Thus, at the beginning of the cycle, one follicle (about 5 to 6 mm in diameter) has received its signal and begun to differentiate in a specific manner toward ovulation. As discussed earlier, the nature of the selective influences involve FSH and estrogen. As illustrated in Fig. 17A-36, FSH is the predominant gonadotropin in the peripheral circulation when the dominant follicle is selected. The importance of elevated FSH concentration in selection is best revealed by studies employing estradiol implants.[269] When the FSH rise is blocked by estradiol, the selected follicle is rendered inactive and the follicular phase is substantially lengthened. In conjunction with the previous discussion, the basis for this process is that the chosen follicle sequesters plasma FSH which stimulates DNA synthesis and induction of aromatase activity in the granulosa cells, followed by dramatic increases in both granulosa cell number and follicular estrogen production (Table 17A-1). As a result of the selectivity of the FSH response, plasma estradiol levels begin to increase gradually between days 1 and 7, followed by a rapid and sharp increase of estrogen concentration, reaching peak values of about 300 pg/ml on day 12, when the dominant follicle reaches about 20 mm in diameter (Fig. 17A-36).

Unlike FSH, LH levels remain low and uniform during the early to midfollicular phase (Fig. 17A-36). Even though LH concentration is low, it is evident from the androstenedione levels that LH is stimulating theca interstitial cells to secrete large amounts of the aromatase substrate and that the amount formed is the same in both ovaries (Fig. 17A-36, *inset*). The concentration of androstenedione (1 to 2 ng/ml) in contrast to estradiol, in the peripheral plasma (and ovarian venous effluent) remains relatively constant throughout the menstrual cycle. This is supported by the fact that the concentration of follicular fluid androstenedione is maximal on day 1 of the cycle (Table 17A-1). Thus the conclusion is drawn that LH-stimulated androgen production in the follicular phase does not play an important role in the direction of estrogen synthesis by the selected follicle.

Once the estradiol levels rise, the gonadotropins (LH and FSH) undergo a predictable pattern of activity characteristic of negative and positive feedback, respectively (Fig. 17A-36). When LH reaches a concentration of about 30 to 40 mIU/ml (on day 12 of the cycle), a signal is triggered in the preovulatory follicle which results in the cessation of estradiol production. The mechanism underlying this change involves a selective inhibition of the 17,20-lyase enzyme in the theca interstitial cells.[270] Consequently, the selected follicle stops producing androstenedione (and therefore estradiol) and begins to secrete increased amounts of 17-hydroxyprogesterone. The physiological mechanism whereby the 17,20-lyase is suppressed seems to involve a local negative feedback action of estradiol directly on the theca interstitial cells.[271,272] Altogether, the increases in plasma 17-hydroxyprogesterone level during the late follicular phase seems to be a consequence of steroidogenic changes within the affected preovulatory follicle.

In response to the peak levels of LH and FSH which occur on day 13, the process of ovulation is initiated in the dominant follicle and an egg-cumulus complex is released 36 to 38 h later.[273] As a consequence of breaks in the basal lamina, LDL enters the granulosa cell microenvironment for the first time[274] and causes rapid increases in progesterone production. Considering the low levels of LH and FSH in the luteal phase (Fig. 17A-36), it is believed that LDL is the principal force stimulating corpus luteum progesterone production.[274] Normally, plasma progesterone concentration reaches maximum levels of 10 and 20 ng/ml on day 19 and remains elevated until day 22, when it declines sharply, reaching levels of about 0.8 ng/ml on the first day of menses.

It is evident that as the corpus luteum differentiates estrogen production is reinitiated and the corpus luteum begins progressively increasing estradiol secretion, reaching peak levels on days 21 to 22 of the luteal phase. Afterward a sharp decline in estradiol concentration occurs, reaching levels of about 40 pg/ml at the end of the luteal phase (Fig. 17A-36). Importantly, as estradiol levels decline in the late luteal phase, plasma FSH level begins to rise. Undoubtedly, this event is physiologically coupled with the selection of the dominant follicle which will generate the next menstrual cycle.

Menopause

The basis for the menopause is the depletion of the pool of primordial follicles (Fig. 17A-7). Consequently, the processes of recruitment and selection no longer occur, and the ovary loses its capability to synthesize and secrete estradiol and progesterone. Therefore the menstrual cycle ceases.

Although all the aspects of folliculogenesis cease, the postmenopausal ovaries are quite active steroidogenically. As discussed earlier, the theca interstitial cells of atretic follicles hypertrophy and subsequently accumulate in the ovarian stroma as the secondary interstitial cells. Thus, with increasing age, the number of secondary interstitial cells increases in human ovaries. It is obvious from the previous discussion that these cells, together with the hilar cells, respond to LH with increased synthesis of androstenedione and testosterone. During the menopause, plasma LH levels are elevated and therefore the interstitial cells in the postmenopausal ovaries are active secretors of potent androgens, but not of estradiol.[275,276] As might be expected, the androgenic capacity of the postmenopausal ovaries is greater than that found in ovaries of normal, nonhirsute women.

Altogether, it can be concluded that secondary interstitial and hilar cells in postmenopausal ovaries retain full capacity for androgen biosynthesis and are being constantly activated by the high levels of circulating LH in the peripheral plasma. The absence of estradiol production by the postmenopausal ovary most certainly is causally connected with the absence of follicular granulosa cells.

REFERENCES

1. Reynolds SRM: The vasculature of the ovary and ovarian function. *Recent Prog Horm Res* 5:65, 1950.

2. Delson B, Lubin S, Reynolds SRM: Vascular patterns in the human ovary. *Am J Obstet Gynecol* 57:842, 1949.

3. Bassett DL: The changes in the vascular pattern of the ovary of the albino rat during the estrous cycle. *Am J Anat* 73:291, 1943.

4. Neilson D, Jones GS, Woodruff JD, Goldberg B: The innervation of the ovary. *Obstet Gynecol Surv* 25:84, 1970.

5. Owman CH, Rosengren E, Sjöberg N-O: Adrenergic innervation of human female reproductive organs: A histochemical and chemical investigation. *Obstet Gynecol* 30:763, 1967.

6. Burden HW: Adrenergic innervation in ovaries of the rat and guinea pig. *Am J Anat* 133:455, 1972.

7. Lawrence IE, Burden HW: The autonomic innervation of the interstitial gland of the rat ovary during pregnancy. *Am J Anat* 147:81, 1976.

8. Walles B, Groschel-Stewart U, Owman CH, Sjöberg N-O, Unsicker K: Fluorescence histochemical demonstration of a relationship between adrenergic nerves and cells containing actin and myosin in the rat ovary with special reference to the follicle wall. *J Reprod Fertil* 52:175, 1978.

9. Burden HW, Lawrence IE: Experimental studies on the acetylcholinesterase-positive nerves in the ovary of the rat. *Anat Rec* 190:233, 1978.

10. Unsicker K: Qualitative and quantitative studies on the innervation of the corpus luteum of rat and pig. *Cell Tissue Res* 152:515, 1974.

11. Condon WA, Black DL: Catecholamine-induced stimulation of progesterone by the bovine corpus luteum *in vitro*. *Biol Reprod* 15:593, 1976.

12. Veldhuis JD, Harrison TS, Hammond JM: β_2-Adrenergic stimulation of ornithine decarboxylase activity in porcine granulosa cells *in vitro*. *Biochem Biophys Res Commun* 627:123, 1980.

13. Ratner A, Sanborn CR, Weiss GK: β-Adrenergic stimulation of cAMP and progesterone in rat ovarian tissue. *Am J Physiol* 239:E139, 1980.

14. Bahr J, Kao L, Nalbandov AV: The role of catecholamines and nerves in ovulation. *Biol Reprod* 10:273, 1974.

15. Capps ML, Lawrence IE, Burden HW: Ultrastructure of the cells of the ovarian interstitial gland in hypophysectomized rats: The effects of stimulation of the ovarian plexus and of denervation. *Cell Tissue Res* 193:433, 1978.

16. Ganong WF: Role of catecholamines and acetylcholine in regulation of endocrine function. *Life Sci* 15:1401, 1974.

17. Erickson GF: Follicular growth and development, in Sciarra JJ, Speroff L (eds): *Reproductive Endocrinology, Infertility and Genetics: Gynecology and Obstetris*. Hagerstown, MD, Harper & Row, 1981, vol 5, p 1.

18. Eshkol A, Lunenfeld B, Peters H: Ovarian development in infant mice: Dependence on gonadotropic hormones, in Butt WR, Crooke AC, Ryle M (eds): *Gonadotropins and Ovarian Development*. London, E and S Livingstone, 1970, p 249.

19. Eshkol A, Lunenfeld B: Gonadotropic regulation of ovarian development in mice during infancy, in Saxena BB, Gandy HM, Belling CG (eds): *Gonadotropins*. New York, Wylie, 1972, p 335.

20. Greep RO, Van Dyke HB, Chow BF: Gonadotropins of the swine pituitary. I. Various biological effects of purified thylakentrin (FSH) and pure metakentrin (ICHS). *Endocrinology* 30:635, 1952.

21. Hisaw FL: Development of the graafian follicle and ovulation. *Physiol Rev* 27:95, 1947.

22. Ohno S, Klinger HP, Atkin NB: Human oogenesis. *Cytogenetics* 1:42, 1962.

23. Baker TG, Sum OW: Development of the ovary and oogenesis. *Clin Obstet Gynecol* 3:3, 1976.

24. Pyrse-Davis J, Dewhurst CJ: The development of the ovary and uterus in the foetus, newborn and infant: A morphological and enzyme histochemical study. *J Pathol* 103:5, 1971.

25. Mandl A, Zuckerman A: The relation of age to the number of oocytes. *J Endocrinol* 7:190, 1951.

26. Arendsen de Wolff-Exalto E: Influence of gonadotropins on early follicle cell development and early oocyte growth in the immature rat. *J Reprod Fertil* 66:537, 1982.

27. Odor DL, Blandau RJ: Ultrastructural studies on fetal and early postnatal mouse ovaries. II. Cytodifferentiation. *Am J Anat* 125:177, 1969.

28. Kang Y-H: Development of the zona pellucida in the rat oocyte. *Am J Anat* 139:535, 1974.

29. Bleil JD, Wassarman PM: Synthesis of zona pellucida proteins by denuded and follicle-enclosed mouse oocytes during culture *in vitro*. *Proc Natl Acad Sci USA* 77:1029, 1980.

30. Peters H: The development of the mouse ovary from birth to maturity. *Acta Endocrinol* 62:98, 1969.

31. Hoage TR, Cameron IL: Folliculogenesis in the ovary of the mature mouse: A radioautographic study. *Anat Rec* 184:699, 1976.

32. Erickson GF, Magoffin D, Dyer CA, Hofeditz C: The ovarian androgen producing cells: A review of structure/function relationships. *Endocr Rev* 6:371, 1985.

33. Albertini DF, Anderson E: The appearance and structure of intercellular connections during the ontogeny of the rabbit ovarian follicle with particular reference to gap junctions. *J Cell Biol* 63:234, 1974.

34. Merk FB, Botticelli CR, Albright JT: An intercellular response to estrogen by granulosa cells in the rat ovary; an electron microscope study. *Endocrinology* 90:992, 1972.

35. Goodenough DA: The isolation of mouse hepatocyte gap junctions: Characterization of the principal protein, connexin: *J Cell Biol* 61:557, 1974.

36. Simpson I, Rose B, Lowenstein WR: Size limit of molecules permeating the junctional membrane channels. *Science* 195:294, 1977.

37. Anderson E, Albertini DF: Gap junctions between the oocyte and companion follicle cells in the mammalian ovary. *J Cell Biol* 71:680, 1976.

38. Gilula NB, Epstein ML, Beers WH: Cell-to-cell communication and ovulation: A study of the cumulus-oocyte complex. *J Cell Biol* 78:58, 1978.

39. Szöllösi D, Gérard M, Ménézo Y, Thibault C: Permeability of ovarian follicle corona cell-oocyte relationship in mammals. *Ann Biol Anim Biochem Biophys* 18:511, 1978.

40. Burghardt RC, Anderson E: Hormonal modulation of ovarian interstitial cells with particular reference to gap junctions. *J Cell Biol* 81:104, 1979.

41. McNatty KP, Moore-Smith D, Osathanondh R, Ryan KJ: The human antral follicle: Functional correlates of growth and atresia. *Ann Biol Anim Biochem Biophys* 19:1547, 1979.

42. Burghardt RC, Anderson E: Hormonal modulation of gap junctions in rat ovarian follicles. *Cell Tissue Res* 214:181, 1981.

43. Lane CE, Davis FR: The ovary of the adult rat. I. Changes in growth of the follicle and in volume and mitotic activity of the granulosa and theca during the estrous cycle. *Anat Rec* 73:429, 1939.

44. O'Shea JP: An ultrastructural study of smooth muscle-like cells in the theca externa of ovarian follicles in the rat. *Anat Rec* 167:127, 1970.

45. Okamura H, Virutamacen P, Wright KH, Wallach EE: Ovarian smooth muscle in the human being, rabbit, and cat. *Am J Obstet Gynecol* 112:183, 1972.

46. Bjersing L, Cajander S: Ovulation and the mechanism of follicle rupture. V. Ultrastructure of tunica albuginea and theca externa of rabbit graafian follicles prior to induced ovulation. *Cell Tissue Res* 153:15, 1974.

47. Amsterdam A, Lindner HR, Groschel-Stewart U: Localization of actin and myosin in the rat oocyte and follicular wall by immunofluorescence. *Anat Rec* 187:311, 1977.

48. Ingram DL: Atresia, in Zuckerman S, Mandl AM, Eckstein P (eds): *The Ovary*. New York, Academic, 1962, vol 1, p 247.

49. Dawson AB, McCabe M: The interstitial tissue of the ovary in infantile and juvenile rats. *J Morphol* 88:543, 1951.

50. Kingsbury BF: Atresia and the interstitial cells of the ovary. *Am J Anat* 65:309, 1939.

51. Oakberg EF: Follicular growth and atresia in the mouse. *In Vitro* 15:41, 1979.

52. Harman MT, Kirgis HD: The development and atresia of the graafian follicle and the division of intra-ovarian ova in the guinea pig. *Am J Anat* 63:79, 1938.

53. Spanel-Borowski K: Morphological investigations on follicular atresia in canine ovaries. *Cell Tissue Res* 214:155, 1981.

54. Hay MF, Cran DG: Differential response of components of sheep follicles to atresia. *Ann Biol Anim Biochem Biophys* 18:453, 1978.

55. Byskov AG: Atresia, in Midgley AR, Sadler WA (eds): *Ovarian Follicular Development and Function.* New York, Raven, 1979, p 41.

56. Krafka J: Parthenogenic cleavage in the human ovary. *Anat Rec* 75:19, 1934.

57. Quattropani SL: Morphogenesis of the ovarian interstitial tissue in the neonatal mouse. *Anat Rec* 177:569, 1973.

58. Gondos B, Hobel CG: Interstitial cells in the human fetal ovary. *Endocrinology* 93:736, 1976.

59. Ryan KJ, Petro Z, Kaiser J: Steroid formation by isolated and recombined ovarian granulosa and thecal cells. *J Clin Endocrinol Metab* 28:355, 1968.

60. Tsang BK, Moon YS, Simpson CW, Armstrong DT: Androgen biosynthesis in human ovarian follicles: Cellular source, gonadotropic control, and adenosine-3′,5′-monophosphate mediation. *J Clin Endocrinol Metab* 48:153, 1979.

61. Tsang BK, Armstrong DT, Witfield JF: Steroid biosynthesis by isolated human ovarian follicular cells *in vitro. J Clin Endocrinol Metab* 51:1407, 1980.

62. McNatty KP, Makris A, DeGrazia C, Osthanondh R, Ryan KJ: The production of progesterone, androgens and estrogens by granulosa cells, thecal tissue and stromal tissue from human ovaries *in vitro. J Clin Endocrinol Metab* 49:687, 1979.

63. McNatty KP, Makris A, Osthanondh R, Ryan KJ: Effects of luteinizing hormone on steroidogenesis by thecal tissue from human ovarian follicles *in vitro. Steroids* 36:53, 1980.

64. McNatty KP, Makris A, DeGrazia C, Osthanondh R, Ryan KJ: Steroidogenesis by recombined follicular cells from the human ovary *in vitro. J Clin Endocrinol Metab* 51:1286, 1980.

65. Magoffin DA, Erickson GF: Primary culture of differentiating ovarian androgen-producing cells in defined medium. *J Biol Chem* 257:4507, 1982.

66. Mossman HW, Koering MJ, Ferry D Jr: Cyclic changes of interstitial gland tissue of the human ovary. *Am J Anat* 115:235, 1964.

67. Guraya SS: Function of the human ovary during pregnancy as revealed by histochemical, biochemical and electron microscope techniques. *Acta Endocrinol* 69:107, 1972.

68. Rice BF, Savard K: Steroid hormone formation in the human ovary: IV. Ovarian stromal compartment; formation of radioactive steroids from acetate-1-^{14}C and action of gonadotropins. *J Clin Endocrinol* 26:593, 1966.

69. Kawakami M, Kubo K, Yemura T, Nagase M, Hagashi R: Involvement of ovarian innervation in steroid secretion. *Endocrinology* 109:136, 1981.

70. Dyer CA, ERickson GF: Norepinephrine amplifies hCG-stimulated androgen biosynthesis by ovarian theca-interstitial cells. *Endocrinology* 116:1645, 1985.

71. Berger L: Sur l'existence de glandes sympathicotropes dans l'ovaire et le testicule humains; leurs rapports avec la glande interstitielle du testicule. *C R Seances Acad Sci* 175:907, 1922.

72. Sternberg WH: The morphology, androgenic function, hyperplasia and tumors of the human ovarian hilus cells. *Am J Pathol* 25:493, 1949.

73. Merkow LP, Slifkin M, Acevedo HF, Greenberg WV: Ultr structure of an interstitial (hilar) cell tumor of the ovary. *Ob Gynecol* 37:845, 1971.

74. Schnoy N: Ultrastructure of a virilizing ovarian Leydig cell tumor. *Virchows Arch* (Pathol Anat) 397:17, 1982.

75. Corral-Gallardo J, Acevedo HA, Salazr JLP, Loria M, Goldzieher JW: The polycystic ovary VI. A hilus cell tumor of the ovary associated with PCO disease *in vivo* and *in vitro* studies. *Acta Endocrinol* 52:425, 1966.

76. Echt CR, Hadd HE: Androgen excretion patterns in a patient with a metastatic hilus cell tumor of the ovary. *Am J Obstet Gynecol* 100:1055, 1968.

77. Jeffcoate SL, Prunty FTG: Steroid synthesis *in vitro* by a hilar cell tumor. *Am J Obstet Gynecol* 101:684, 1968.

78. Jezova D, Vigas M: Testosterone response to exercise during blockade and stimulation to adrenergic receptors in man. *Horm Res* 15:141, 1981.

79. Corner GW Jr: The histological dating of the human corpus luteum of menstruation. *Am J Anat* 98:377, 1956.

80. Crisp TM, Dessouky DA, Denys FR: The fine structure of the human corpus luteum of early pregnancy and during the progestational phase of the menstrual cycle. *Am J Anat* 127:37, 1970.

81. Bramley TA, Ryan RJ: Interactions of gonadotropins with corpus luteum membranes. VII. Association of hCG-binding and adenylate cyclase activities with rabbit corpus luteum plasmamembranes. *Mol Cell Endocrinol* 12:319, 1978.

82. Gillim SW, Christensen AK, McLennan CE: Fine structure of the human menstrual corpus luteum at its stage of maximum secretory activity. *Am J Anat* 126:409, 1970.

83. Van Lennp EW, Madden LM: Electron microscopic observations on the involution of the human corpus luteum of menstruation. *Z Sellforsch* 66:365, 1965.

84. Bloom W, Fawcett DW: *A Textbook of Histology,* 10th ed. Philadelphia, Saunders, 1975.

85. Savard K: Comparative aspects of steroid-forming cells, in Whelan WS, Schultz J (eds): *Homologies in enzymes and metabolic pathways. Metabolic Alterations in Cancer.* New York, American Elsevier, p 176.

86. Strauss JF, Schuler LA, Rosenblum MF, Tanaka T: Cholesterol metabolism by ovarian tissue. *Adv Lipid Res* 18:99, 1981.

87. Gwynne JT, Strauss JF: The role of lipoproteins in steroidogenesis and cholesterol metabolism in steroidogenic glands. *Endocr Rev* 3:299, 1982.

88. Goldstein JL, Anderson RGW, Brown MS: Coated pits, coated vesicles, and receptor-mediated endocytosis. *Nature* 279:679, 1979.

89. Brown MS, Kovanen PT, Goldstein JL: Regulation of plasma cholesterol by lipoprotein receptors. *Science* 212:628, 1981.

90. Brown MS, Goldstein JL: Receptor-mediated endocytosis: Insights from lipoprotein receptor system. *Proc Natl Acad Sci USA* 76:3330, 1979.

91. Simpson ER: Cholesterol side-chaian cleavage, cytochrome P-450, and the control of steroidogenesis. *Mol Cell Endocrinol* 13:213, 1979.

92. Bara G, Anderson WA: Fine structural localization of 3β-hydroxysteroid dehydrogenase in rat corpus luteum. *Histochem J* 5:437, 1973.

93. Aono T, Kitamura U, Fukuda S, Matsumoto K: Localization of 4-ene-5α-reductase, 17β-ol-dehydrogenase and aromatase in immature rat ovary. *J Steroid Biochem* 14:1369, 1981.

94. Terakawa N, Kondo K, Aono T, Kurachi K, Matsumoto K: Hormonal regulation of 4-ene-5α-reductase in prepubertal rat ovaries. *J Steroid Biochem* 9:307, 1978.

95. Smith OW, Ofner P, Verra RL: In vitro conversion of testosterone-^{14}C to androgens of the 5α-androstane series by a normal human ovary. *Steroids* 24:311, 1974.

96. Hillier SG: Regulation of follicular oestrogen biosynthesis: A survey of current concepts. *J Endocrinol* 89:30, 1981.

97. Henderson KM, Gorban HMS, Boyd GS: Effect of LH factors regulating ovarian cholesterol metabolism and progesterone synthesis in PMSG primed immature rats. *J Reprod Fertil* 61:373, 1981.

98. Mori M, Marsh JM: The site of luteinizing hormone stimulation of steroidogenesis in mitochondria of the rat corpus luteum. *J Biol Chem* 257:6178, 1982.

99. Erickson GF: Primary cultures of ovarian cells in serum-free medium as models of hormone-dependent differentiation. *Mol Cell Endocrinol* 29:2, 1983.

100. Erickson GF, Hsueh AJW, Quigley ME, Reber RW, Yen SSC: Functional studies of aromatase activity in human granulosa cells from normal and polycystic ovaries. *J Clin Endocrinol Metab* 49:514, 1979.

101. Bryant-Greenwood GD: Relaxin as a new hormone. *Endocr Rev* 3:62, 1982.

102. Weiss G, O'Byrne EM, Steinetz BG: Relaxin: A product of the human corpus luteum of pregnancy. *Science* 194:948, 1976.

103. Mathieu PH, Rahier J, Thomas K: Localization of relaxin in the human gestational corpus luteum. *Cell Tissue Res* 219:213, 1981.

104. Goldsmith LT, Essig M, Sarosi P, Beck P, Weiss G: Hormone secretion by monolayer cultures of human luteal cells. *J Clin Endocrinol Metab* 53:890, 1981.

105. Evans G, Wathes DC, King GJ, Armstrong DT, Porter DG: Changes in relaxin production by the theca during the preovulatory period of the pig. *J Reprod Fertil* 69:697, 1983.

106. Wathes DC, Swann RW, Pickering BT, Porter DG, Hull MGR, Drife JD: Neurohypophysial hormones in the human ovary. *Lancet* 2:410, 1982.

107. Khan-Dawood FS, Dawood MY: Human ovaries contain immunoreactive oxytocin. *J Clin Endocrinol Metab* 57:1129, 1983.

108. Flint APF, Sheldrick EL: Ovarian secretion of oxytocin is stimulated by prostaglandin. *Nature* 297:587, 1982.

109. Tan GJS, Tweedale R, Biggs JSG: Oxytocin may play a role in the control of the human corpus luteum. *J Endocrinol* 95:65, 1982.

110. Flint APF, Sheldrick EL: Evidence for a systemic role for ovarian oxytocin in luteal regression in sheep. *J Reprod Fertil* 67:215, 1983.

111. Erickson GF, Hsueh AJW: Secretion of "inhibin" by rat granulosa cells *in vitro*. *Endocrinology* 103:1960, 1978.

112. Beers WH: Follicular plasminogen and plasminogen activator and the effect of plasmin on ovarian follicle wall. *Cell* 6:379, 1975.

113. Beers WH, Strickland S: A cell culture assay for follicle-stimulating hormone. *J Biol Chem* 253:3877, 1978.

114. Tsafriri A, Dekel N, Bar-Ami: The role of oocyte maturation inhibitor in follicular regulation of oocyte maturation. *J Reprod Fertil* 64:541, 1982.

115. DiZerega GS, Marrs RP, Campeau JD, Kling DR: Human granulosa cell secretion of protein(s) which suppress follicular response to gonadotropins. *J Clin Endocrinol Metab* 56:147, 1983.

116. Lim AT, Lolait S, Barlow JW, Sum OW, Zois I, Toh BH, Funder JW: Immunoreactive β-endorphin in sheep ovary. *Nature* 303:709, 1983.

117. Shaha C, Margioris A, Liotta AS, Krieger DT, Bardin CW: Demonstration of immunoreactive β-endorphin and melanocyte-stimulating hormone-related peptides in ovaries of neonatal, cyclic and pregnant mice. *Endocrinology* 115:378, 1984.

118. Presl J, Pospisil J, Figarova V, Krabec Z: Stage dependent changes in binding of iodinated FSH during ovarian follicle maturation in rats. *Endocrinol Exp* 8:291, 1974.

119. Hardy B, Danon D, Eshkol A, Lunenfeld B: Ultrastructural changes in the ovaries of infant mice deprived of endogenous gonadotropins and after substitution with FSH. *J Reprod Fertil* 36:345, 1974.

120. Nimrod A, Erickson GF, Ryan KJ: A specific FSH receptor in rat granulosa cells: Properties of binding *in vitro*. *Endocrinology* 98:56, 1976.

121. Richards JS; Estradiol receptor content in rat granulosa cells during follicular development: Modification by estradiol and gonadotropins. *Endocrinology* 97:1174, 1975.

122. Schreiber JR, Erickson GF: Progesterone receptor in the rat ovary: Further characterization and localization in the granulosa cell. *Steroids* 34:459, 1979.

123. Schreiber JR, Reid R, Ross GT: A receptor-like testosterone-binding protein in ovaries from estrogen-stimulated hypophysectomized rats. *Endocrinology* 98:1206, 1976.

124. Schreiber JR, Ross GT: Further characterization of a rat ovarian testosterone receptor with evidence for nuclear translocation. *Endocrinology* 99:590, 1976.

125. Schreiber JR, Nakamura K, Erickson GF: Rat ovary glucocorticoid receptor: Identification and characterization. *Steroids* 39:569, 1982.

126. Richards JS: Maturation of ovarian follicles: Actions and interactions of pituitary and ovarian hormones of follicular cell differentiation. *Physiol Rev* 60:51, 1980.

127. Richards JS, Jonassen JA, Rolfes AI, Kersey K, Reichert LE: Adenosine-3′,5′-monophosphate, luteinizing hormone receptor and progesterone during granulosa cell differentiation: Effects of estradiol and follicle-stimulating hormone. *Endocrinology* 104:765, 1979.

128. Rao MC, Midgley AR, Richards JS: Hormonal regulation of ovarian cellular proliferation. *Cell* 14:71, 1978.

129. Gospodarowicz D, Bialecki H: Fibroblast and epidermal growth factors are mitogenic agents for cultured granulosa cells of rodent, porcine, and human origin. *Endocrinology* 104:757, 1979.

130. Wang C, Hsueh AJW, Erickson GF: Induction of functional prolactin receptors by follicle-stimulating hormone in rat granulosa cells *in vivo* and *in vitro*. *J Biol Chem* 254:11330, 1979.

131. Zeleznik AJ, Midgley AR, Reichert LE: Granulosa cell maturation in the rat: Increased binding of human chorionic gonadotropin following treatment with follicle-stimulating hormone *in vivo*. *Endocrinology* 95:818, 1974.

132. Erickson GF, Wang C, Hsueh AJW: FSH induction of functional LH receptors in granulosa cells cultured in a chemically-defined medium. *Nature* 279:336, 1979.

133. Wang C, Hsueh AJW, Erickson GF: The role of cyclic AMP in the induction of estrogen and progestin synthesis in cultured granulosa cells. *Mol Cell Endocrinol* 25:73, 1982.

134. Rolland R, Hammond JM: Demonstration of a specific receptor for prolactin in porcine granulosa cells. *Endocr Res Commun* 2:231, 1975.

135. Channing CP, Kammerman S: Binding of gonadotropins to ovarian cells. *Biol Reprod* 10:179, 1974.

136. Uilenbroek JTJ, Woutersen PJA, Van der Schoot P: Atresia of preovulatory follicles: Gonadotropin binding and steroidogenic activity. *Biol Reprod* 23:219, 1980.

137. Hsueh AJW, Adashi EY, Jones PBC, Welsh TH: Hormonal regulation of the differentiation of cultured ovarian granulosa cells. *Endocr Rev* 5:76, 1984.

138. Wang C, Hsueh AJW, Erickson GF: Prolactin inhibition of estrogen production by cultured rat granulosa cells. *Mol Cell Endocrinol* 20:135, 1980.

139. Schoonmaker JN, Erickson GF: Glucocorticoid modulation of follicle-stimulating hormone-mediated granulosa cell differentiation. *Endocrinology* 113:1356, 1983.

140. Schreiber JR, Nakamura K, Erickson GF: Progestins inhibit FSH-stimulated steroidogenesis in cultured rat granulosa cells. *Mol Cell Endocrinol* 19:165, 1980.

141. Schreiber JR, Nakamura K, Truscello A, Erickson GF: Progestins inhibit FSH-induced functional LH receptors in cultured rat granulosa cells. *Mol Cell Endocrinol* 25:113, 1982.

142. Mondschein JS, Schomberg DW: Growth factors modulate gonadotropin receptor induction in granulosa cell cultures. *Science* 211:1179, 1981.

143. Knecht N, Catt KJ: Modulation of cAMP-mediated differentiation in ovarian granulosa cells by EGF and PDGF. *J Biol Chem* 258:2789, 1983.

144. Garzo VG, Dorrington JH: Aromatase activity in human

granulosa cells during follicular development and the modulation by follicle-stimulating hormone and insulin. *Am J Obstet Gynecol* 148:657, 1984.

145. Amsterdam A, Koch Y, Lieberman ME, Lindner HR: Distribution of binding sites for human chorionic gonadotropin in the preovulatory follicle of the rat. *J Cell Biol* 67:894, 1975.

146. Erickson GF, Wang C, Casper R, Mattson G, Hofeditz C: Studies on the mechanism of LH receptor control by FSH. *Mol Cell Endocrinol* 27:17, 1982.

147. Zoller LC, Weisz J: Identification of cytochrome P-450 and its distribution in the membrana granulosa of the preovulatory follicle using quantitative cytochemistry. *Endocrinology* 103:310, 1970.

148. Dunaif AE, Zimmerman EA, Friesen HG, Frantz AG: Intracellular localization of prolactin receptor and prolactin in the rat ovary by immunocytochemistry. *Endocrinology* 110:1465, 1982.

149. Parkes AS: Androgenic activity of the ovary. *Recent Prog Horm Res* 5:101, 1950.

150. Barbieri RL, Makris A, Ryan KJ: Effects of insulin on steroidogenesis in cultured porcine ovarian theca. *Fertil Steril* 40:237, 1983.

151. Magoffin DA, Erickson GF: Mechanism by which estradiol-17β inhibits androgen production in the rat. *Endocrinology* 108:962, 1982.

152. Magoffin DA, Erickson GF: Direct inhibitory effect of estrogen on LH-stimulated androgen synthesis by ovarian cells cultured in defined medium. *Mol Cell Endocrinol* 28:8, 1982.

153. Magoffin DA, Erickson GF: Prolactin inhibition of LH-stimulated androgen synthesis in ovarian interstitial cells cultured in defined medium: Mechanism of action. *Endocrinology* 111:2001, 1982.

154. Magoffin DA, Erickson GF: Mechanism by which GnRH inhibits androgen synthesis directly in ovarian interstitial cells. *Mol Cell Endocrinol* 27:191, 1982.

155. Erickson GF, Case E: Epidermal growth factor antagonizes ovarian theca-interstitial cytodifferentiation. *Mol Cell Endocrinol* 31:7, 1983.

156. Mikhail G, Zander J, Allen WM: Steroids in human ovarian vein blood. *J Clin Endocrinol Metab* 23:1267, 1963.

157. Baird DT, Guevara A: Concentration of unconjugated estrone and estradiol in peripheral plasma in non-pregnant women throughout the menstrual cycle, castrate, and postmenopausal women and men. *J Clin Endocrinol* 29:149, 1969.

158. Abraham GE, Odell WD, Swerdloff RS, Hopper K: Simultaneous radioimmunoassay of plasma FSH, LH, progesterone, 17-hydroxyprogesterone and estradiol-17β during the menstrual cycle. *J Clin Endocrinol* 34:312, 1972.

159. Thorneycroft IH, Sribyatta B, Tom WK, Nakamura RM, Mishell DR: Measurement of serum LH, FSH, progesterone, 17α-hydroxyprogesterone and estradiol-17β level at 4-hour intervals during the periovulatory phase of the menstrual cycle. *J Clin Endocrinol Metab* 39:754, 1974.

160. Baird DT, Burger PE, Heavon-Jones GD, Scaramuzzi RJ: The site of secretion of androstenedione in non-pregnant women. *J Endocrinol* 63:210, 1974.

161. Baird DT, Fraser IS: Blood production and ovarian secretion rates of estradiol-17β and estrone in women throughout the menstrual cycle. *J Clin Endocrinol Metab* 38:1009, 1974.

162. Huang WY, Pearlman WH: The corpus luteum and steroid hormone formation II. Studies on the human corpus luteum *in vitro*. *J Biol Chem* 238:1308, 1963.

163. Arceo RB, Ryan KJ: Conversion of androst-4-ene-3,17-dione-4-^{14}C to oestrogens by subcellular fractions of the human corpus luteum of the normal cycle. *Acta Endocrinol* 56:225, 1967.

164. Hammerstein J, Rice RB, Savard K: Steroid hormone formation in the human ovary: I. Identification of steroids formed *in vitro* from acetate-1-^{14}C in the corpus luteum. *J Clin Endocrinol* 24:597, 1964.

165. Vande Wiele RL, Bogumil J, Dyrenfurth I, Ferin M, Jewelewicz R, Warren M, Rizkallah T, Mikhail G: Mechanisms regulating the menstrual cycle in women. *Recent Prog Horm Res* 26:63, 1970.

166. Cole FE, Weed JC, Schneider GT, Holland JB, Geary WL, Rice BF: The gonadotropin receptor of the human corpus luteum. *Am J Obstet Gynecol* 117:87, 1973.

167. Lee CY, Coulam CB, Jiang NS, Ryan RJ: Receptors for luteinizing hormone in human corpora luteal tissue. *J Clin Endocrinol Metab* 36:148, 1973.

168. McNeilly AS, Kerin J, Swanston IA, Bramley TA, Baird DT: Changes in the binding of human chorionic gonadotropin/luteinizing hormone, follicle-stimulating hormone and prolactin to human corpora lutea during the menstrual cycle and pregnancy. *J Endocrinol* 87:315, 1980.

169. Rajaniemi HJ, Ronnberg L, Kauppila A, Ylostalo P, Jalkanen M, Saastamoinen J, Selander K, Paavo P, Vittko R: Luteinizing hormone receptors in human ovarian follicles and corpora lutea during menstrual cycle and pregnancy. *J Clin Endocrinol Metab* 108:307, 1981.

170. Jones GS: The luteal phase defect. *Fertil Steril* 27:351, 1976.

171. Wentz AC: Physiologic and clinical considerations in luteal phase defects. *Clin Obstet Gynecol* 22:169, 1979.

172. Soules MR, Hughes CL, Aksel S, Tyrey L, Hammond CB: The function of the corpus luteum of pregnancy in ovulatory dysfunction and luteal phase deficiency. *Fertil Steril* 36:31, 1981.

173. Fujita Y, Mori T, Suzuki A, Nihnobu K, Nishimura T: Functional and structural relationships in steroidogenesis *in vitro* by human corpora lutea during development and regression. *J Clin Endocrinol Metab* 53:744, 1981.

174. Hunter MG, Baker TG: Effect of hCG, cAMP and FSH on steroidogenesis by human corpora lutea *in vitro*. *J Reprod Fertil* 63:285, 1981.

175. Hoffman F: Unterschungen uber die hormonale Beeinflussung der Lebensdauer des corpus luteum in Zyklus der Frau. *Geburtshilfe Frauenheilkd* 20:1153, 1960.

176. Williams MT, Roght MS, Marsh JM, Lemaire WJ: Inhibition of human chorionic gonadotropin-induced progesterone synthesis by estradiol in human luteal cells. *J Clin Endocrinol Metab* 48:437, 1979.

177. Thibier M, El-Hassan N, Clark MR, Lemaire WJ, Marsh JM: Inhibition by estradiol of human chorionic gonadotropin-induced progesterone accumulation in isolated human luteal cells: Lack of mediation by prostaglandin F. *J Clin Endocrinol Metab* 50:590, 1980.

178. Depp R, Cox DW, Pion RJ, Conrad SH, Heinrichs WL: Inhibition of pregnenolone Δ^5-3β-hydroxysteroid dehydrogenase Δ^5-4-isomerase systems of human placenta and corpus luteum of pregnancy. *Gynecol Invest* 4:106, 1973.

179. Hagerman DD, Smith O, Day CF: Mechanism of the stimulatory effect of clomid on aromatization of steroids by human placenta *in vitro*. *Acta Endocrinol* 51:591, 1966.

180. McNatty KP, Sawers RS, McNeilly AS: A possible role for prolactin in control of steroid secretion by the human graafian follicle. *Nature* 250:5468, 1974.

181. Demura R, Ono M, Demura H, Shizume K, Oouchi H: Prolactin directly inhibits basal as well as gonadotropin-stimulated secretion of progesterone and 17β-estradiol in the human ovary. *J Clin Endocrinol Metab* 54:1246, 1982.

182. Clayton RN, Huhataniemi IT: Absence of gonadotropin-releasing hormone receptors in human gonadal tissue. *Nature* 299:56, 1982.

183. Casper RF, Erickson GF, Yen SSC: Studies on the effect of gonadotropin-releasing hormone and its agonist on human luteal steroidogenesis *in vitro*. *Fertil Steril* 42:39, 1984.

184. Tureck RW, Mastroianni L, Blasco L, Strauss JF: Inhibition of human granulosa cell progesterone secretion by gonadotropin-releasing hormone agonist. *J Clin Endocrinol Metab* 54:1078, 1982.

185. Casper RF, Erickson GF, Rebar RW, Yen SSC: The effect of

luteinizing hormone-releasing factor and its agonist on cultured human granulosa cells. *Fertil Steril* 37:406, 1982.

186. Rao CV, Griffin LP, Carman FR: Prostaglandin $F_{2\alpha}$ binding sites in human corpora lutea. *J Clin Endocrinol Metab* 44:1032, 1977.

187. Challis JRG, Calder AA, Dilley S, Foster CS, Hillier K, Hunter DJS, Mackenzie IZ, Thorburn GD: Production of prostaglandin E and F2α by corpora lutea, corpora albicantes and stroma from the human ovary. *J Endocrinol* 68:401, 1975.

188. Swanston IA, McNatty KP, Baird DR: Concentration of prostaglandin $F_{2\alpha}$ and steroids in the human corpus luteum. *J Endocrinol* 73:115, 1977.

189. Richardson MC, Masson GM: Progesterone production by dispersed cells from human corpus luteum: Stimulation by gonadotropins and $PGF_{2\alpha}$: Lack of response to adrenaline and isoprenaline. *J Endocrinol* 87:247, 1980.

190. McKay DG, Hertig AT, Adams EC, Danziger SL: Histochemical observation on the germ cells of human embryos. *Anat Rec* 117:201, 1953.

191. Eddy EM, Clark JM, Gong D, Fenderson BA: Origin and migration of primordial germ cells in mammals. *Gamete Res* 4:333, 1981.

192. Wartenberg H: Development of the early human ovary and the role of the mesonephros in the differentiation of the cortex. *Anat Embryol* 165:253, 1982.

193. Updahyay S, Luciani J, Zamboni L: The role of the mesonephros in the development of the indifferent gonads and ovaries of the mouse. *Ann Biol Anim Biochem Biophys* 19:1179, 1979.

194. Monk M, McLaren A: X-Chromosome activity in fetal germ cells of the mouse. *J Embryol Exp Morphol* 63:75, 1981.

195. Burgogne PS, Baker TG: Oocyte depletion in XO mice and their XX sibs from 12 to 200 days post partum. *J Reprod Fertil* 61:207, 1981.

196. Ruby JR, Dyer RF, Skalko RG: The occurrence of intercellular bridges during oogenesis. *J Morphol* 127:307, 1969.

197. Byskov AG: Regulation of meiosis in mammals. *Ann Biol Anim Biochem Biophys* 19:1251, 1979.

198. Moore GPM, Lintern-Moore S, Peters H, Faber M: RNA synthesis in the mouse oocyte. *J Cell Biol* 60:416, 1974.

199. Moore GPM, Lintern-Moore S: A correlation between growth and RNA synthesis in the mouse oocyte. *J Reprod Fertil* 39:163, 1974.

200. Moore GPM, Lintern-Moore S: Transcription of the mouse oocyte genome. *Biol Reprod* 17:865, 1978.

201. Bachvarova R, Baran MM, Tejblum A: Development of naked growing mouse oocytes *in vitro*. *J Exp Zool* 211:159, 1980.

202. Eppig JJ: A comparison between oocyte growth in coculture with granulosa cells and oocytes with granulosa cell-oocyte junctional contact maintained *in vitro*. *J Exp Zool* 209:345, 1979.

203. Heller DT, Cahill DM, Schultz RM: Biochemical studies of mammalian oogenesis: Metabolic cooperativity between granulosa cells and growing mouse oocytes. *Dev Biol* 84:455, 1981.

204. Brower PT, Schultz RM: Intercellular communication between granulosa cells and mouse oocytes: Existence and possible nutritional role during oocyte growth. *Dev Biol* 90:144, 1982.

205. Austin CR: *The Mammalian Egg.* Springfield, IL, CC Thomas, 1961.

206. Bleil JD, Wassarman PM: Structure and function of the zona pellucida: Identification and characterization of the proteins of the mouse oocyte's zone pellucida. *Dev Biol* 76:185, 1980.

207. Bleil JD, Wassarman PM: Mammalian sperm-egg interaction: Identification of a glycoprotein in mouse zonae pellucidae possessing receptor activity for sperm. *Cell* 20:873, 1980.

208. Erickson GF, Sorensen RA: *In vitro* maturation of mouse oocytes ioslated from late, middle and preantral graafian follicles. *J Exp Zool* 190:123, 1974.

209. Sorensen RA, Wassarman PM: Relationship between growth and meiotic maturation of the mouse oocyte. *Dev Biol* 50:531, 1976.

210. Dekel N, Hillensjo T, Kraicer PF: Maturational effects of gonadotropins on the cumulus-oocyte complex of the rat. *Biol Reprod* 20:191, 1979.

211. Whittingham DG, Siracuse G: The involvement of calcium in the activation of mammalian oocytes. *Exp Cell Res* 113:311, 1978.

212. Moor RM: Role of steroids in the maturation of ovine oocytes. *Ann Biol Anim Biochem Biophys* 18:477, 1978.

213. Lintern-Moore S, Moore GPM: The initiation of follicle and oocyte growth in the mouse ovary. *Biol Reprod* 20:773, 1979.

214a. Zamboni L: Comparative studies on the ultrastructure of mammalian eggs, in Biggers JD, Schuetz AW (eds): *Oogenesis.* Baltimore, MD, University Park, p 5.

214b. Peterson T: Determination of follicle growth in the ovary of the immature mouse. *J Reprod Fertil* 21:81, 1970.

215. Gulyas BJ, Hodgen GD, Tullner W, Ross GT: Effects of fetal or maternal hypophysectomy on endocrine organs and body weight in infant rhesus monkeys (*Macacca mulatta*) with particular emphasis on oogenesis. *Biol Reprod* 16:216, 1977.

216. Peters H, Byskov AG, Lintern-Moore S, Faber M, Anderson M: Effect of gonadotropin on follicle growth initiation in the neonatal mouse ovary. *J Reprod Fertil* 35:139, 1973.

217. Pedersen T: Follicular growth in the immature mouse ovary. *Acta Endocrinol* 62:117, 1969.

218. Krarup T, Pedersen T, Faber M: Regulation of oocyte growth in the mouse ovary. *Nature* 224:187, 1969.

219. Pederson T, Peters H: Follicle growth and cell dynamics in the mouse ovary during pregnancy. *Fertil Steril* 22:42, 1971.

220. Peters H, Byskov AGS, Sorensen IN, Krarup T, Pederson T, Faber M: The development of the mouse ovary after testosterone propionate injection on day 5, in Butt WR, Crooke AC, Ryle E (eds): *Gonadotropins and Ovarian Development.* London, Livingstone, 1970, p 351.

221. Lintern-Moore S: Effect of athymia on the initiation of follicular growth in the rat ovary. *Biol Reprod* 17:155, 1977.

222. Michael SD, Taguchi O, Nishizuka Y: Effect of neonatal thymectomy on ovarian development and plasma LH, FSH, GH and PRL in the mouse. *Biol Reprod* 22:343, 1980.

223. Lintern-Moore S, Everitt AV: The effect of restricted food intake on size and composition of the ovarian follicle population in the Wistar rat. *Biol Reprod* 19:688, 1978.

224. Lintern-Moore S, Supasri Y, Parasuthpaisit K, Sobhon P: Acute and chronic morphine sulfate treatment alters ovarian development in prepubertal rats. *Biol Reprod* 21:379, 1979.

225. Saiduddin S, Zassenhaus HP: Effect of testosterone and progesterone on the estradiol receptor in the immature rat ovary. *Endocrinology* 102:1069, 1978.

226. Harman SM, Louvet J-P, Ross GT: Interaction of estrogen and gonadotropins on follicular atresia. *Endocrinology* 96:1145, 1975.

227. Louvet J-P, Harman SM, Ross GT: Effects of human chorionic gonadotropin, human interstitial cell stimulating hormone and human follicle stimulating hormone on ovarian weights in estrogen-primed hypophysectomized immature female rats. *Endocrinology* 96:1179, 1975.

228. Louvet J-P, Harman SM, Schreiber JR, Ross GT: Evidence for a role of androgens in follicular maturation. *Endocrinology* 97:366, 1975.

229. Terranova PF, Greenwald GS: Increased ovulation rate in the cyclic guinea pig after a single injection of an antiserum to LH. *J Reprod Fertil* 61:37, 1981.

230. Terranova PF: Steroidogenesis in experimentally induced atretic follicles of the hamster: A shift from estradiol to progesterone synthesis. *Endocrinology* 108:1885, 1981.

231. Erickson GF, Yen SSC: New data on follicle cells in polycys-

tic ovaries: A proposed mechanism for the genesis of cystic follicles. *Sem Reprod Endocrinol* 2:231, 1984.

232. McNatty KP, Hunter WM, McNeilly AS, Sawers RS: Changes in the concentration of pituitary and steroid hormones in the follicular fluid of human graafian follicles throughout the menstrual cycle. *J Endocrinol* 64:555, 1975.

233. McNatty KP, Smith DM, Makris A, Osathanondh R, Ryan KJ: The microenvironment of the human antral follicle: Interrelationships among the steroid levels in antral fluid, the population of granulosa cells, and the status of the oocyte. *J Clin Endocrinol Metab* 49:851, 1979.

235. Shalgi R, Kraicer P, Rimon A, Pinto M, Soferman N: Proteins of human follicular fluid: The blood-follicle barrier. *Fertil Steril* 24:429, 1973.

236. Hillier SG, Van den Boogard AMJ, Reichert LE, Van Hall EV: Intraovarian sex steroid hormone interactions and the control of follicular maturation: Aromatization of androgens by human granulosa cells *in vitro*. *J Clin Endocrinol Metab* 50:640, 1980.

237. McNatty KP: Relationship between plasma prolactin and the endocrine microenvironment of the developing human antral follicle. *Fertil Steril* 32:433, 1979.

238. Cajander S, Bjersing L: Fine structural demonstration of acid phosphatase in rabbit germinal epithelium prior to induced ovulation. *Cell Tissue Res* 164:279, 1975.

239. Takahashi M, Ford JJ, Yoshinaga K, Greep RO: Induction of ovulation in hypophysectomized rats by progesterone. *Endocrinology* 95:1322, 1974.

240. Marsh JM, Yang NST, Lemaire WJ: Prostaglandin synthesis in rabbit graafian follicles *in vitro:* Effect of luteinizing hormone and cyclic AMP. *Prostaglandins* 7:269, 1974.

241. Armstrong DT: Role of prostaglandins in follicular responses to luteinizing hormone. *Ann Biol Anim Biochem Biophys* 15:181, 1975.

242. Armstrong DT, Grinwich DL, Moon YS, Zamecnik J: Inhibition of ovulation in rabbits by intrafollicular injection of indomethacin and PGF antiserum. *Life Sci* 14:129, 1974.

243. Downs SM, Long FJ: An ultrastructural study of preovulatory development in mouse ovarian follicles: Effects of indomethacin. *Anat Rec* 205:159, 1983.

244. Beers WH, Strickland S, Reich E: Ovarian plasminogen activator: Relationship to ovulation and hormonal regulation. *Cell* 6:387, 1975.

245. Beers WH, Strickland S: A cell culture assay for follicle stimulating hormone. *J Biol Chem* 253:3877, 1978.

246. Beers WH: Follicular plasminogen and plasminogen activator and the effect of plasmin on ovarian follicle wall. *Cell* 6:379, 1975.

247. Martin GG, Talbot P: The role of follicular smooth muscle cells in hamster ovulation. *J Exp Zool* 216:469, 1981.

248. Walles B, Falck B, Owman CH, Sjöberg N-O: Characterization of autonomic receptors in the smooth musculature of human graafian follicle. *Biol Reprod* 17:423, 1977.

249. Bronson RA, Bryant G, Balk MW, Emanuele N: Intrafollicular pressure within preovulatory follicles of the pig. *Fertil Steril* 31:205, 1979.

250. Jungman RA, Schweppe JS: Biosynthesis of sterols and steroids from acetate-^{14}C by human fetal ovaries. *J Clin Endocrinol Metab* 28:1599, 1968.

251. Bloch E: Metabolism of 4-^{14}C-progesterone by human fetal testis and ovaries. *Endocrinology* 74:833, 1964.

252. Taylor T, Coutts JRT, MacNaughton MC: Human foetal synthesis of testosterone from perfused progesterone. *J Endocrinol* 60:321, 1974.

253. Payne AH, Jaffe RB: Androgen formation from pregnenolone sulfate by the human fetal ovary. *J Clin Endocrinol Metab* 39:300, 1974.

254. Huhtaniemi I, Vinko R: Determination of unconjugated and sulfated neutral steroids in human fetal blood of early and mid-pregnancy. *Steroids* 16:197, 1970.

255. Wilson EA, Joe-Jowad M: The effect of trophic agents on fetal ovarian steroidogenesis in organ culture. *Fertil Steril* 32:73, 1979.

256. Pryse-Davies J, Dewhurst CJ: The development of the ovary and uterus in the foetus, newborn and infant: A morphological and enzyme histochemical study. *J Pathol* 103:5, 1971.

257. Valdes-Dapena MA: The normal ovary of childhood. *Ann NY Acad Sci* 142:597, 1967.

258. Peters H, Himelstein-Braw R, Faber M: The normal development of the ovary in childhood. *Acta Endocrinol* 82:617, 1976.

259. Himelstein-Braw R, Byskov AG, Peters H, Faber M: Follicular atresia in the infant human ovary. *J Reprod Fertil* 46:55, 1976.

260. Lintern-Moore S, Peters H, Moore GPM, Faber M: Follicular development in the infant human ovary. *J Reprod Fertil* 39:53, 1974.

261. Faiman C, Winter JSD: Gonadotropins and sex hormone pattern in puberty, in Grumbach MM, Grave GD, Mayer FE (eds): *The Control of the Onset of Puberty*. London, Wiley, 1974.

262. Hartman CG, Leathem JH: Oogenesis and ovulation, in: *Conference on Physiological Mechanisms Concerned with Conception*. New York, Pergamon, 1963, p 205.

263. Peters H: The development and maturation of the ovary. *Ann Biol Anim Biochem Biophys* 16:271, 1976.

264. Green SH, Zukerman S: Quantitative aspects of the growth of the human ovum and follicle. *J Anat* 85:373, 1951.

265. Erickson GF: Normal ovarian function. *Clin Obstet Gynecol* 21:31, 1978.

266. Pederson T: Determination of follicle growth rate in the ovary of the immature mouse. *J Reprod Fertil* 21:81, 1970.

267. Turnbull KE, Braden AWH, Mattner PE: The pattern of follicular growth and atresia in the ovine ovary. *Aust J Biol Sci* 30:229, 1977.

268. Gougeon A, Lefevre B: Evolution of the diameters of the largest healthy and atretic follicles during the human menstrual cycle. *J Reprod Fertil* 69:497, 1983.

269. Zeleznik AJ: Premature elevation of systemic estradiol reduces levels of FSH and lengthens the follicular phase of the menstrual cycle in rhesus monkeys. *Endocrinology* 109:352, 1981.

270. Suzuki K, Tamaoki B-I: Enzymological studies of rat luteinized ovaries in relation to acute reduction of aromatizable androgen formation and stimulated production of progestins. *Endocrinology* 104:1317, 1979.

271. Magoffin DA, Erickson GF: Mechanism by which 17β-estradiol inhibits ovarian androgen production in the rat. *Endocrinology* 108:962, 1982.

272. Magoffin DA, Erickson GF: Direct inhibitory effect of estrogen on LH-stimulated androgen synthesis by ovarian cells cultured in defined medium. *Mol Cell Endocrinol* 28:81, 1982.

273. Edwards RG: Studies on human conception. *Am J Obstet Gynecol* 117:587, 1973.

274. Carr BR, MacDonald PC, Simpson ER: The role of lipoproteins in the regulation of progesterone secretion by the human corpus luteum. *Fertil Steril* 38:303, 1982.

275. Mattingly RF, Huang W: Steroidogenesis of the menopausal and postmenopausal ovary. *Am J Obstet Gynecol* 103:679, 1969.

276. Asch RH, Greenblatt RB: Steroidogenesis in the postmenopausal ovary. *Clin Obstet Gynecol* 4:85, 1977.

B. CLINICAL

Robert I. McLachlan
David L. Healy
Henry G. Burger

In this section, an approach to the management of the clinical disorders of ovarian function is outlined, based on the particular setting in which patients present to the clinician, i.e., in teenagers, young adults, and individuals of middle age.

OVARIAN DISORDERS IN TEENAGERS

Primary Amenorrhea

The time of menarche varies widely among racial groups and families but is normally regarded as occurring between 9 and 16 years of age. It is preceded by an acceleration of growth and some development of secondary sexual characteristics, normally by the age of 14. These changes reflect the rise in estrogen secretion from the pubertal ovary and the consequent increase in circulating somatomedin concentrations. In addition, the development of pubic hair, reflecting a rise in androgen production (adrenarche), also precedes menarche by 1 to 3 years. Failure of menses to occur by the age of 16 years is termed *primary amenorrhea.* The clinical evaluation of a girl with primary amenorrhea commences with an assessment of her growth and development. The failure of normal growth and/or of any pubertal development to occur by the age of 14, or of menses to occur by 16, should lead to investigation.

A wide variety of disorders of the hypothalamic–pituitary–ovarian axis can result in primary amenorrhea. It is more helpful to classify these conditions clinically according to the girl's stature and the degree, timing, and nature of any pubertal change. The more common causes of primary amenorrhea are classified according to their clinical presentation in Table 17B-1.

SHORT STATURE AND NO PUBERTAL DEVELOPMENT

Gonadal Dysgenesis

TURNER'S SYNDROME Short stature, absence of a pubertal growth spurt, and absence of secondary sexual characteristics suggest the syndromes of gonadal dysgenesis which represent an important cause of primary amenorrhea. The most common is classic Turner's syndrome, a sporadic condition which affects approximately 1 in 3000 girls and results from a deficiency of one X chromosome, leading to a 45,XO karyotype. The mullerian duct derivatives and genitalia are female; however, the ovaries are represented by gonads devoid of primordial follicles. The characteristic phenotype includes short stature [$>$2.5 standard deviations (SD) below the mean for chronologic age, adult mean height $<$ 148 cm], infantile female genitalia, and absence of secondary sexual characteristics (Fig. 17B-1). Somatic abnormalities are usually but not invariably present and may include webbing of the neck, cubitus valgus, hypoplastic nails, shieldlike chest with wide-spaced nipples, micrognathia, and external ear abnormalities. Investigation shows low estrogen secretion and elevated gonadotropin concentrations; a 45,XO karyotype is diagnostic. Cardiovascular assessment is indicated in view of a 10 to 20 percent incidence of coarctation of the aorta. Thyroid function should also be measured because of an increased incidence of autoimmune thyroid disease. Routine diagnostic imaging of the kidneys is performed in the initial evaluation, in view of the increased incidence of renal tract abnormalities, especially horseshoe kidney.

Lifelong estrogen replacement is essential in Turner's syndrome. Significant acceleration of ulnar bone growth has been shown in short-term studies using low-dose estrogen replacement (5 μg ethinyl estradiol), while a dose of 10 μg ethinyl estradiol daily similarly accelerates bone growth but in addition induces breast budding.[1] Drug administration should be commenced at 10 to 12 years of age and the dosage gradually increased to 20 μg daily with cyclic progesterone (e.g., medroxyprogesterone acetate, 10 mg daily for 10 to 12 days every month) when the ethinyl estradiol dose exceeds 10 μg daily. Whether this therapy augments eventual adult height is controversial, but it has the clinical advantage of inducing pubertal change, menses, and a pubertal growth spurt in line with the patient's peers. The maintenance of bone

Table 17B-1. Clinical Classification of Primary Amenorrhea

- Short stature, no pubertal development
  - Gonadal Dysgenesis
    - Turner's syndrome (45,XO)*
    - Turner's mosaicism (e.g., 46,XX, 45,XO)
    - Abnormalities of X chromosome
    - Mosaicism 46,XX, 45,XO + Y variants
    - Pure gonadal dysgenesis
  - Hypopituitarism
    - Hypothalamopituitary dysfunction: idiopathic or associated with surgery, irradiation, trauma, tumor
- Normal stature, no or minimal pubertal development
  - Hypogonadotropic hypogonadism (Kallmann's syndrome)
    - Idiopathic*
    - Organic lesions
  - Idiopathic Delayed Puberty*
  - Malnutrition, systemic disease, intensive exercise*
- Normal stature and pubertal development
  - With adrenarche: mullerian (paramesonephric) duct derivative abnormalities
  - Without adrenarche: testicular feminization
- Virilization and/or anomalous genitalia
  - Miscellaneous rare disorders:
    - Partial testicular feminization
    - Inborn errors of testosterone biosynthesis or conversion to dihydrotestosterone
    - Untreated congenital adrenal hyperplasia

*Most common differential diagnoses

density and normal female lipid profiles (with a likely reduction in the risk of atherosclerotic vascular disease) are other important advantages of estrogen replacement.

Although these subjects have no oocytes and have been regarded as sterile, with the advent of donor oocyte in vitro fertilization (IVF) programs, fertility is now possible. Six ongoing pregnancies have been achieved at Monash University, Australia, with a schedule of steroid replacement, oocyte donation and embryo transfer in patients with no functioning ovaries.[2,3] Thus, a new optimism should permeate the paramedical and lay support groups for Turner's syndrome patients which are available in many centers for counseling of the patient, her parents, or her husband regarding the nature of this condition (see also Management of Premature Ovarian Failure, below).

MOSAICISM Compared to the XO karyotype, the XO/XX karyotype is associated with taller stature, fewer somatic abnormalities, and occasionally with menstruation and fertility. Pregnancies result in abortion 25 percent of the time and have 10 percent incidences of births with Down's and Turner's syndromes dictating the need for counseling and amniocentesis. Rare variants of gonadal dysgenesis include abnormalities of the short or long arms of the X chromosome, resulting in a phenotypic spectrum of amenorrhea, short stature, and somatic abnormalities.

Disorders incorporating XO/XY mosaicism lead to a range of phenotypes from male to female. Predominantly female phenotypes usually present with amenorrhea and a degree of genital virilization. The 30 to 70 percent frequency of gonadal tumors, especially dysgerminoma, warrants prophylactic removal of these gonads in teenagers with proven gonadal dysgenesis (see Chap. 18).

Hypopituitarism

Conditions that diminish pituitary function are often associated with inadequate growth hormone and

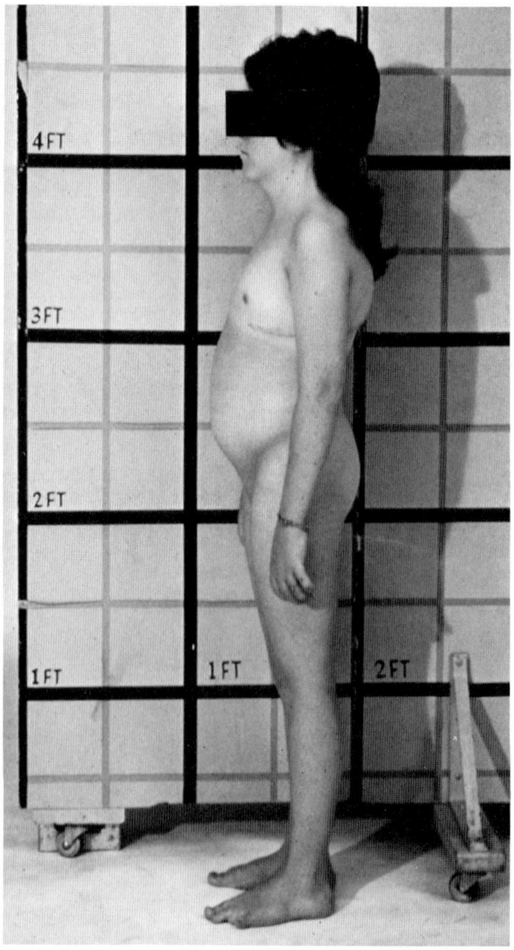

FIGURE 17B-1 Typical clinical stigmata of Turner's syndrome.

gonadotropin secretion, resulting in short stature and failure to enter puberty. Features of thyroid and adrenal deficiency may also be present. Often a history of head trauma, cranial tumor surgery, or irradiation will be elicited, although the patient may present with primary amenorrhea reflecting an underlying and often idiopathic hypothalamopituitary disorder. Depressed levels of gonadotropins and other pituitary hormones, which may be unresponsive to their normal trophic stimuli, will be found. Computerized tomography (CT) of the pituitary region is essential to exclude a neoplasm, especially craniopharyngioma. Therapy involves treatment of the underlying cause and replacement of sex steroids and other deficient hormones.

NORMAL STATURE AND NO OR MINIMAL PUBERTAL DEVELOPMENT

Hypogonadotropic Hypogonadism (Kallmann's Syndrome)

Delayed or absent pubertal change, particularly when associated with hyposmia or anosmia in a subject of normal height, suggests the possibility of idiopathic hypogonadotropic hypogonadism. This congenital, often familial, condition results from an isolated deficiency of hypothalamic gonadotropin releasing hormone (GnRH) and therefore of gonadotropins (Fig. 17B-2). Associated somatic abnormalities include cleft lip and palate and congenital deafness. Laboratory features include low ovarian steroid production and low to low normal gonadotropin levels. The pituitary, chronically deprived of GnRH stimulation, generally responds poorly to acute GnRH infusion, although normal or exaggerated responses have been described.[4,5] Basal levels of other pituitary hormones are normal although defects in TRH, prolactin, and cortisol responses have been described. CT scanning of the hypothalamopituitary region is also indicated in view of the occasional occurrence of tumor, hamartoma, empty sella syndrome, and disorders of the rhinencephalon. Induction of pubertal changes and menses is achieved with exogenous estrogen and progesterone. Women with this syndrome are characteristically unresponsive to clomiphene. Fertility can be achieved with exogenous gonadotropin ovulation induction (see below) or with pulsatile GnRH infusion therapy. The relative benefits of one or other of these therapies are not as yet clear.

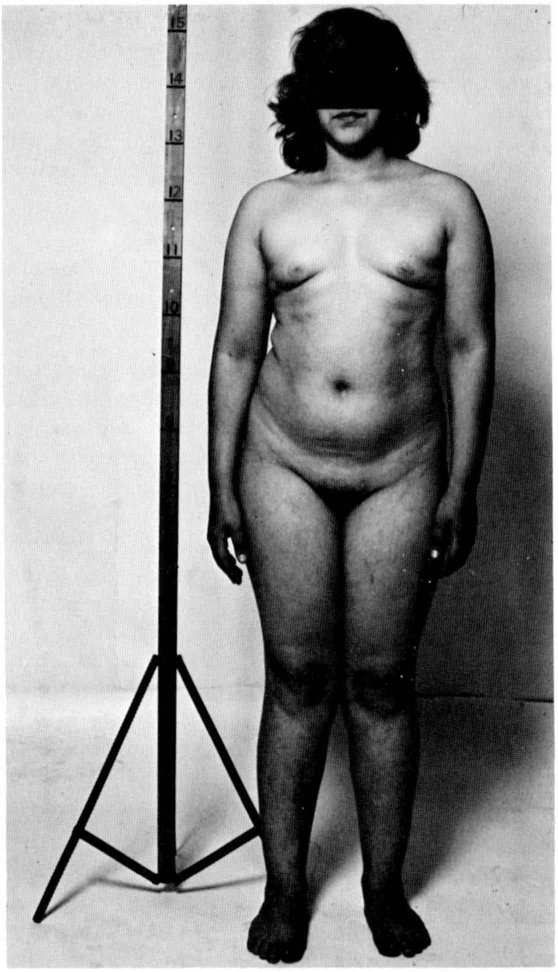

FIGURE 17B-2 Clinical appearance of a 19-year-old female with hypogonadotropic hypogonadism. Note the normal height (152 cm) and absence of a female body habitus. There was no breast development in this patient.

Idiopathic Delayed Puberty

The delay in menarche as a component of delayed puberty is a common cause of presentation with primary amenorrhea. Its differentiation from hypogonadotropic hypogonadism can be very difficult. Features supporting the diagnosis include a family history of delayed puberty, normal development in other respects, and usually some development and progression of pubertal changes by the time of consultation. These subjects are often short (3d to 10th percentile) with an appropriately delayed bone age. Serum gonadotropin and ovarian steroid secretion is either prepubertal or shows early pubertal changes corresponding with the degree of pubertal development. Neither GnRH infusion nor clomiphene testing leads to diagnostic discrimination between delayed puberty and hypogonadotropic hypogonadism. Therefore, having excluded other likely causes, reassurance and review of these patients should be rewarded by spontaneous menses between age 17 and 20 years. The pubertal growth spurt is also delayed but adult height is usually normal. Pubertal development can be hastened, if desired by the patient, by sex steroid replacement (as described above for Turner's syndrome) along with intermittent withdrawal to observe the underlying state of the pituitary ovarian axis.

Malnutrition, Systemic Disease, or Intensive Exercise

Normal puberty can be interrupted by intercurrent problems such as the severe weight loss seen in starvation, anorexia nervosa, or severe systemic diseases. Intensive athletic training, particularly ballet and running, can be associated with decreased body weight, particularly fat content, along with menstrual disturbances including amenorrhea. Although more commonly a cause of secondary amenorrhea, such activities undertaken and maintained from early puberty can produce primary amenorrhea. Restoration of good nutrition with weight gain or resolution of underlying illness should restore pubertal progression. In these settings serum gonadotropins show a prepubertal pattern of low levels (particularly of LH), lack of pulsatile secretion, and blunted response to GnRH.

NORMAL STATURE WITH NORMAL PUBERTAL DEVELOPMENT

MÜLLERIAN DUCT DERIVATIVE ABNORMALITIES Primary amenorrhea with normal growth and pubertal development to a stage where menses ought to be occurring suggests abnormalities of the mullerian duct–derived structures (uterine tubes, uterus, cervix, and upper vagina).[6] Ovarian function is normal but menses do not occur due to an absence of normal endometrial tissue or lack of a conduit for menstrual flow to the exterior. An imperforate vagina (often incorrectly diagnosed as an imperforate hymen) may lead to retention of menstrual fluid behind a membrane (hematocolpos) or cyclic abdominal pain from an accompanying hematosalpinx. The resultant mass may be sufficiently large to produce abdominal distention. Clinical examination, including examination under general anesthesia, will define these anatomical variations. Therapy will depend on the anatomy and may range from simple stellate incision of the vaginal membrane, drainage, and use of prophylactic antibiotics to laparotomy for excision of a noncommunicating uterine horn.

TESTICULAR FEMINIZATION A normal female phenotype, often with tall stature and breast development but absent or scanty pubic hair, suggests the possibility of testicular feminization. This is an X-linked dominant condition in which absent or defective cytosolic testosterone receptors result in androgen insensitivity in genetic males (46,XY). Testes are present but spermatogenesis does not occur and the testes lie in the inguinal canal or labia. This key examination feature underlines the importance of thorough examination of the inguinal and labial region. External genitalia are female; however, the vagina is a short pouch and no mullerian duct derivatives are present. The absence of a uterus can be confirmed by vaginal and/or rectal examination and ultrasound. Diagnostic features include a serum testosterone level in the normal male range while serum LH concentration is raised, underlining the insensitivity of the pituitary gonadotrophs to testosterone feedback. Testicular estrogen production and conversion of testosterone to estradiol, in the absence of testosterone effects, lead to pubertal breast development (Fig. 17B-3). Cytosolic androgen receptors are absent or defective. Therapy includes reinforcement of the female gender identity and orchidectomy at any time in the presence of a gonadal hernia or otherwise after puberty in view of an increased incidence of testicular neoplasia. Lifelong estrogen replacement is then required, with or without added progestogens (see Hormonal Replacement Therapy under Postmenopausal Problems, below).

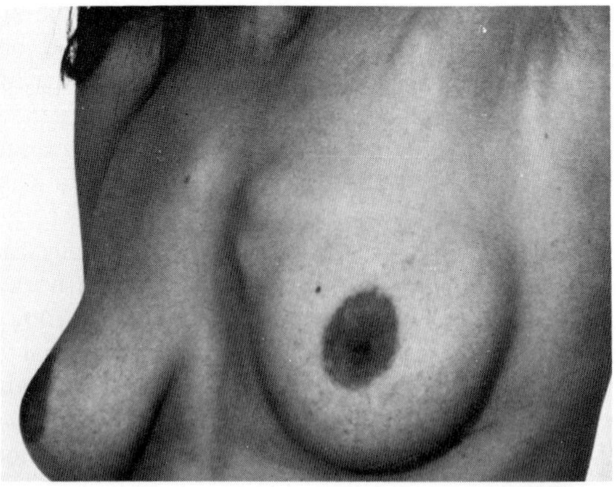

FIGURE 17B-3 Testicular feminization. Note the Tanner stage 5 breast development, resulting from testicular estrogen secretion, and the absence of axillary hair.

VIRILIZATION AND/OR ANOMALOUS GENITALIA

A range of rare disorders may present with amenorrhea and varying degrees of virilization and/or anomalous genitalia in a young girl. Partial testicular feminization occurs when the defect in the androgen receptor is incomplete. Some androgen effect therefore leads to labioscrotal fusion or clitoromegaly. Deficiency of the 5α-reductase enzyme is an autosomal recessive condition of genetic males wherein there are normal testosterone levels but inadequate conversion to the more potent androgen dihydrotestosterone (DHT). Ambiguous genitalia (varying degrees of labioscrotal fusion) with a blind-ending vaginal pouch occur. Virilization occurs at puberty while breast development fails. Finally, a range of inborn errors of the testosterone biosynthetic pathway are other rare causes of female or anomalous genitalia associated with amenorrhea in the genetic male. These conditions are outlined in Chap. 16. They require extensive investigation of steroid metabolism and androgen receptor activity, and anatomical delineation.

Menarcheal Menorrhagia

The mammalian uterus is a highly specialized fibromuscular and secretory organ in which the myometrium is elastic and whose contractile properties are responsive to a variety of hormonal regulators secreted both locally and distantly. In contrast, the inner lining of the uterus, the endometrium, is a distinctive tissue both in form and function. Throughout adult reproductive life in humans and other higher primates the endometrium grows and is shed cyclically as a bloody discharge (i.e., the menstrual cycle), typically recurring at about 28-day intervals. The temporal nature of this sequence (proliferation, differentiation, and sloughing of the endometrium) is the classic manifestation of an end organ response to the changing steroidal milieu imposed by the ovarian cycle. Until recently, little attention was given to the endometrium as the source of hormone secretion. Accordingly, traditional emphasis on clinical disorders of the ovary can now usefully be widened to include endometrial secretion of hormones that may act both locally and distantly. Increasing evidence suggests that endometrial tissue may have a central role in the complement of endocrine signals governing female fertility.[7]

Cyclic ovarian function normally commences in adolescent girls soon after menarche. Before the attainment of gonadotropin secretory capabilities sufficient to support follicular maturation leading to ovulation, a limited degree of intermittent estrogen secretion results in endometrial proliferation and irregular vaginal bleeding; that is, variable degrees and intervals of hypoestrogenism are interspersed with transient elevations of blood estrogen levels. The initial ovulatory cycles in these young women are often characterized by abbreviated intermenstrual intervals and serum progesterone levels below those of the normal adult in luteal phase. Clinically, these changes can be seen in the young teenager with heavy and irregular menses due to recurrent anovulation. In developed parts of the world, menarche normally occurs between 11.5 and 15.5 years (mean 13.5 years, SD 1.0 year). Menstruation occurs regularly; cycles between 21 and 35 days apart (28.0 ± 3.5 days) and persist for 3 to 7 days. Studies by Baird and associates have proven that dysfunctional uterine bleeding in this age group is often associated with a defect in the positive feedback response to estradiol.[8]

Heavy menarcheal bleeding is not rare. Assuming there is no possibility of pregnancy, the initial therapy should be medical, with progestogen treatment, such as 5 to 10 mg per day of norethindrone for 10 days (in the absence of cycles) or from day 5 to day 25 of the cycle, usually being effective since there has been sufficient estrogen secretion from the ovaries to induce progesterone receptors in the endometrium. If this has not occurred, it may be worth coadministering a conjugated estrogen preparation (e.g., Premarin) with a progestogen to induce this effect. In young teenagers curettage should be a last resort to attempt to control endometrial hemorrhage as well as to exclude rare diseases such as sarcoma botryoides. A hemorrhagic diathesis should always be excluded in a teenager who presents with catastrophic menarcheal bleeding. Fifty to eighty percent of patients with hemorrhagic diatheses have excessive menstrual blood loss.

OVARIAN DISORDERS IN YOUNG ADULTS

Secondary Amenorrhea

The cessation of menses for longer than 6 months in a patient who has previously menstruated is termed *secondary amenorrhea.* The commonest cause is pregnancy, although a pregnancy beyond 12 weeks gestation should not be missed clinically by any doctor. Early pregnancy findings are minimal and therefore a pregnancy test is essential in all patients with secondary amenorrhea. Serum gonadotropin assays in pregnancy will reveal a markedly elevated LH level, reflecting cross-reaction of human chorionic gonadotropin (hCG) in most LH radioimmunoassays, while follicle stimulating hormone concentration (FSH) is low normal. Another important physiological cause of amenorrhea is breast feeding. This is associated with a period of ovarian inactivity, the duration of which depends on the frequency and duration of suckling. It is associated with elevated prolactin levels, failure of positive feedback of estradiol on LH and FSH secretion, and disturbances of pulsatile LH release. With decreased breast feeding, ovarian function gradually returns, yielding periods of initially increased estradiol production without menses, menses without ovulation or with inadequate luteal function, and, finally, normal ovulatory cycles. Maternal undernutrition prolongs the period of lactational amenorrhea. Finally, the natural menopause generally occurs after age 40. The cessation of menses in the menopause can take the form of oligomenorrhea, menorrhagia, or abrupt cessation. Symptoms of estrogen deficiency (vaginal atrophy, hot flushes) are common and gonadotropin levels are in the postmenopausal range. A family history in cases of early menopause is common. The most important clinical disorders, after excluding the physiological causes of secondary amenorrhea, are outlined in Table 17B-2.

Table 17B-2. Clinical Classification of Secondary Amenorrhea

Physiological
Pregnancy
Lactation
Menopause
Premature ovarian failure
Congenital
Acquired:
Autoimmune
Idiopathic
Chemotherapy, irradiation
Surgery, trauma
Infection
Hyperprolactinemia and/or galactorrhea
Drug-associated
Prolactinoma:
Microadenoma
Macroadenoma
Systemic illness (e.g., hypothyroidism)
Nutrition/exercise-associated
Weight loss:
Simple
Anorexia nervosa
Systemic illness
Intensive exercise
Polycystic ovary syndrome
Rare conditions
Uterine synechiae: postcurettage endometritis
Pituitary deficiency:
Tumors, especially following surgery or irradiation
Sheehan's syndrome
Ovarian/adrenal neoplasia, empty sella syndrome

PREMATURE OVARIAN FAILURE

Premature ovarian failure (POF) can be defined as the syndrome of amenorrhea, hypoestrogenism, and elevated serum gonadotropin concentrations occurring before the age of 40 years. For practical purposes, 40 may reasonably be taken as the age after which cessation of menses is most likely due to spontaneous cessation of ovarian function. Cessation of ovarian function may occur in the teenage years as a rare cause of primary amenorrhea; most commonly it presents with secondary amenorrhea and accounts for about 5 percent of new cases.[9,10]

The clinical and hormonal features are similar to those of the normal menopause and commonly develop over a period of several years. Approximately half the subjects present with clinical features of hypoestrogenism (mainly vaginal dryness and hot flushes), while secondary sexual characteristics are usually normal. If the condition develops around the time of menarche then the secondary sexual characteristics may be underdeveloped. The combination of hot flushes and amenorrhea always warrants exclusion of premature ovarian failure. Serum gonadotropin concentrations are elevated and hyperresponsive to GnRH as after the normal menopause. As is also seen in the perimenopausal period, serum FSH level may fluctuate in and out of the normal range and serum estradiol levels may rise to the midfollicular range. These fluctuations may be seen over a period of several years with a gradual trend toward established hypoestrogenic hypergonadotropic amenorrhea. The variable natural history of this transition was underlined by a study of 67 women suspected of having premature ovarian failure on the basis of elevated FSH level.[11] Over one-quarter of these women resumed normal ovarian function in 1 to 5 years; six subjects conceived. Neither clinical features (e.g., age, mode of presentation) nor the degree of FSH concentration elevation predicted which subjects would resume ovarian function. Little is known of the natural history of premature ovarian failure, although clearly in some women spontaneous resumption of menses and fertility may occur.

Etiologies of Premature Ovarian Failure

GENETIC Chromosomal abnormalities, particularly variants of gonadal dysgenesis, may present with POF and secondary amenorrhea. The previous pattern of menses and physical findings may be normal and require that karyotyping be performed on nulliparous women under investigation for premature ovarian failure. Future management may be influenced by an abnormal karyotype, particularly one including a Y chromosome. The majority of subjects, however, have the normal 46,XX karyotype. A family history of premature ovarian failure is found in 10 percent of subjects. The pattern of inheritance is not clear but reports of vertical transmission of the trait are consistent with autosomal dominant or sex-linked inheritance.[12]

PHYSICAL AGENTS Pelvic surgery and viral (especially mumps) oophoritis are rare causes of POF. Gonadal irradiation and/or chemotherapy (especially with cyclophosphamide or busulfan) for malignant conditions are also well known to cause transient (especially with exposure before age 30) or permanent ovarian failure.[13] Finally, cigarette smoking, perhaps via an antiovarian action of polycyclic aromatic hydrocarbons, is associated with menopause 1 to 2 years earlier than in nonsmokers.

AUTOIMMUNE PREMATURE OVARIAN FAILURE Evidence for an autoimmune basis for some cases of POF is based on two observations. The association of POF with other autoimmune diseases, especially Hashimoto's thyroiditis and Addison's disease, has been reported. Recently, in a study of 33 women with POF, 39 percent had an associated autoimmune condition and 18 percent had a family history of such a condition.[14] Second, the presence of anti-ovarian antibodies, including anti-zona pellucida antibodies, in the serum of these patients has been reported. The methodology for assessing the presence of antibodies is not universally accepted and a direct pathogenic role for these antibodies has not been established. Overall, an autoimmune link with POF may be present in 20 to 50 percent of patients. Consideration of possible autoimmune thyroid or adrenal disease should be given in initial assessment and intermittently during a review of patients with POF.

Management of Premature Ovarian Failure

The diagnosis of POF is confirmed by the finding of sustained gonadotropin elevation associated with depressed estrogen secretion. Weekly serum gonadotropin determinations and tests of urinary estrogen and progesterone excretion over a 6-week period will establish a true baseline estimate of any ovarian follicular activity. Karyotyping is performed in nulliparous patients.

Therapy for POF involves first the replacement of cyclic estrogen and progesterone for the maintenance of normal secondary sex characteristics and libido and avoidance of the long-term sequelae of hypoestrogenism. Although achievement of fertility is unlikely, many spontaneous and therapy-associated pregnancies have been reported. Ovarian biopsy has been emphasized by some authors as necessary to differentiate oocyte depletion from the gonadotropin-resistant ovary syndrome, the latter allegedly being amenable to treatment. However, ovarian biopsy may not provide a representative tissue sample, and patients said to lack primordial follicles may subsequently ovulate. High-dose exogenous gonadotropin therapy has occasionally been associated with pregnancy, but results of this expensive therapy have generally been disappointing.[9,10] The majority of POF subjects who subsequently conceive have been exposed to estrogen. In theory, estrogen may be acting to induce FSH receptors in the remaining follicles, to prevent down regulation of ovarian gonadotropin receptors by suppressing circulating gonadotropin levels, or to increase the biological activity of the gonadotropins.

None of these therapies for POF has been subjected to proper prospective trial with due regard to the variable natural history of POF and the spontaneous pregnancy rate.[11,15] In view of these facts, POF patients requesting fertility are not routinely subjected to ovarian biopsy. Review of the underlying ovarian-pituitary axis during sex steroid replacement is undertaken every 3 to 6 months. The return of a normal serum FSH level may occur spontaneously even years after diagnosis, with the return of menses and fertility. Ovulation induction (see below) may be undertaken during the period of normal circulating FSH levels. Further studies of the natural history, autoimmunity, and ovarian histology of POF and prospective study of a range of therapies are needed to allow better categorization of POF and particularly to identify subgroups amenable to therapy.

At Monash University, an attempt has been made to manage infertile patients with POF by applying IVF techniques and oocyte donation.[16] This program has resulted in six pregnancies from 32 embryo transfers into patients with no functioning ovaries. These patients receive a schedule of cyclic steroid replacement.[17] A replacement schedule of oral estradiol valerate, up to 6 mg per day, and up to 100 mg per day of vaginal progesterone suppositories has been shown to produce plasma levels of estradiol and progesterone within the normal range of the spontaneous ovulatory cycle. The endometrium from patients on day 21 of these treatment cycles was consistent with the expected appearance according to the criteria of Noyes and associates.[18] In these treatments, the donor of the oocyte has either been anonymous or known to the recipient and the general phenotypic characteristics of the recipient and the donor have been matched, in a similar fashion to the matching of phenotypic characteristics which occurs in programs of artificial insemination using donor semen. The successes in this program suggest that patients with POF may be able to have healthy children despite an absence of oocytes.

HYPERPROLACTINEMIA AND GALACTORRHEA

Hyperprolactinemia is a common cause of female infertility, accounting for about 20 percent of cases, depending on the referral center. When sustained, hyperprolactinemia is usually associated with oligo- or amenorrhea and infertility. Impairment of reproductive capacity probably occurs at the hypothalamic level with disturbance of the dopaminergic control of pulsatile GnRH release. Defects in the positive feedback of sex steroids on the hypothalamus and a direct antiovarian action of prolactin have also been postulated. Galactorrhea is an important and frequent accompaniment of hyperprolactinemia. It is usually defined as any persistent milklike discharge from the nipple or overt lactation occurring in a nulliparous woman or a mother whose offspring has been weaned more than 6 months previously. It may be spontaneous or only apparent on manual expression. The majority of women with galactorrhea and secondary amenorrhea have hyperprolactinemia. Galactorrhea may, however, occur with normal prolactin concentrations and without menstrual disturbance. Such idiopathic galactorrhea was reported as the largest single category (32 percent) in 235 consecutive cases of galactorrhea.[19] The presence of galactorrhea always requires careful exclusion of the causes of hyperprolactinemia as detailed below. Serial sampling is routinely performed at 20-min intervals for 2 h when a single elevated prolactin value is detected, as the latter may be elevated by the stress of venipuncture or preceding breast examination.

Etiologies of Hyperprolactinemia

DRUG-RELATED Phenothiazines and other psychotropic agents that act to antagonize hypothalamic dopaminergic pathways are associated with mild to moderate elevations of prolactin concentration (up to four times normal).[20] Galactorrhea has been reported in one-quarter of female psychiatric patients on high doses of such medications. Amenorrhea in association is less common, occurring in 22 percent of patients with drug-induced galactorrhea. These symptoms generally resolve with cessation of medication.

Estrogens stimulate prolactin synthesis and mitotic activity in pituitary lactotrophs. Estrogen therapy, particularly the oral contraceptives, may lead to a mild elevation (approximately a doubling) of serum prolactin concentration. Estrogen has been implicated in the development of prolactinoma in cases of post-pill amenorrhea syndromes; however, most recent case-control studies have not supported this contention.[21]

HYPOTHALAMIC DISORDERS Pituitary prolactin secretion is under tonic inhibitory control by the hypothalamus via the postulated prolactin inhibitory factor(s) (PIF). Disruption of this system by hypothalamic tumor, infiltrative disease (e.g., sarcoidosis), or surgical or traumatic stalk section can lead to moderate prolactin concentration elevation four to six times normal. Galactorrhea and amenorrhea may result from the effect of elevated prolactin level combined with interference with GnRH production in some cases.

SYSTEMIC DISEASE Primary hypothyroidism is associated with elevated hypothalamic TRH secretion, which enhances pituitary TSH and prolactin secretion. It is therefore an uncommon but important cause of the amenorrheic galactorrhea syndrome and easily excluded by clinical assessment and thyroid function tests. Renal failure and hepatic cirrhosis are additional causes of hyperprolactinemia not usually presenting a diagnostic problem.

LOCAL FACTORS Repetitive nipple stimulation can be associated with hyperprolactinemia and galactorrhea; irritative chest wall diseases (thoracic scarring or herpes zoster) are rare causes.

POLYCYSTIC OVARY SYNDROME Inappropriately enhanced estrogen feedback leading to increased pituitary lactotroph secretion is likely to explain the modest (up to fivefold) elevation of prolactin concentration commonly seen in PCO. Disturbance in the normal dopaminergic control of GnRH release has also been described; this may further explain diminished PIF activity. Clinical features of hirsutism, obesity, and absence of galactorrhea assist in differentiation from prolactinoma, although occasionally further biochemical and radiological investigations are needed. The picture is somewhat confused by a purportedly increased risk of prolactinoma in PCO.

PROLACTINOMA Pituitary prolactinoma accounts for approximately 50 percent of cases of hyperprolactinemia. Its diagnosis depends upon the finding of the following:

1. Sustained hyperprolactinemia, often of marked degree.
2. Normal or suppressed serum gonadotropin levels and estrogen production, as is commonly seen in association with amenorrhea.

3. Radiological abnormalities of the pituitary. The high-resolution CT scanning procedure has now superseded plain x-ray and tomography, which are less sensitive and specific.[22] Conventionally, tumors are classified as microadenomas (less than 1 cm in diameter) or macroadenomas. The latter are less common in women; these larger tumors may extend beyond the pituitary fossa superiorly (suprasellar), laterally (parasellar), or anteroinferiorly into the sphenoid sinus.

Clinically, oligo- or amenorrhea may develop in association with prolactinoma at any reproductive age. With the widepsread use of oral contraceptives, the problem is frequently recognized when these are ceased. As previously mentioned, an etiologic role for this estrogen therapy in the genesis of prolactinoma has been suggested but not proved. Galactorrhea occurs in approximately 50 percent of cases. Occasionally, mild obesity and hirsutism are seen, again with the differential diagnostic problem of PCO. Estrogen deficiency resulting in frictional dyspareunia and loss of libido may occur. All these symptoms generally resolve upon restoration of normal prolactin levels. Symptoms of tumor enlargement (headache, visual field defects) are uncommon in females but can occur with macroadenomas and are an especially important consideration during pregnancy (see below).

IDIOPATHIC HYPERPROLACTINEMIA Idiopathic hyperprolactinemia is differentiated from prolactinoma by the inability to demonstrate a tumor on CT scanning. This distinction may be somewhat artificial in that the tumor may be simply too small to resolve even on the most sophisticated equipment. Therapeutically, the two conditions can be considered together. Various dynamic tests such as the prolactin response to TRH or levodopa have been suggested to differentiate tumorous from idiopathic hyperprolactinemia. None has been conclusively shown to be superior to CT scanning.

Management of Hyperprolactinemia

Therapeutic intervention may be indicated for the following reasons:

1. Tumor-related problems, particularly compressive features such as headache, visual field defects, or cranial nerve palsies.
2. Infertility.
3. Disabling galactorrhea.
4. Short-term symptoms and long-term side effects of chronic hypoestrogenemia, which may be avoided by restoration of normal menses and estrogen status.

Conservative therapy may be considered in selected cases.

BROMOCRIPTINE This dopamine agonist has now been established as the drug of choice in the management of hyperprolactinemia, including in some patients with PCO (see below). Control of hyperprolactinemia using bromocriptine is followed by restoration of ovulatory menses and fertility, and abolition of galactorrhea in 78 to 85 percent of patients.[23] A dramatic reduction in tumor volume is seen in up to three-quarters of subjects with a demonstrable prolactinoma.[22] Bromocriptine therapy is initiated with 1.25 mg at night with food and the dosage is gradually increased over 2 weeks until control of symptoms and hyperprolactinemia is achieved, usually at a dosage of 5.0 to 7.5 mg per day.[24] Side effects of nausea, vomiting, constipation, and postural hypotension are minimized with this gradual introduction of bromocriptine. Should side effects occur, a return to a lower dosage will usually be tolerated, although a few patients are unable to tolerate any dosage. Other dopamine agonists (e.g., lisuride, pergolide) are also effective but no advantage over bromocriptine has been shown.

Bromocriptine can maintain control of hyperprolactinemia, often in low dosage over long periods. The natural history of prolactinoma is poorly defined, but even so there is no evidence that long-term bromocriptine use adversely affects this. In a recent study of 15 subjects with micro- and macroadenomas, cessation of bromocriptine administration after 1.5 to 7 years of therapy was followed by a recurrence of symptoms and hyperprolactinemia but tumor or gland size did not increase in 13, decreased in 1, and increased minimally in the other.[25]

When fertility is desired in hyperprolactinemic women it can be achieved in 75 to 85 percent of patients using bromocriptine.[23] Therapy is ceased on confirmation of pregnancy. Enlargement of prolactinoma during pregnancy may occur; this probably relates to the trophic effect of high estrogen levels. A recent review of 16 studies indicates that tumor enlargement during pregnancy is uncommon in microadenomas or in macroadenoma previously treated with x-ray or surgical therapy.[26] However, untreated macroadenoma is associated with an approximately 5 to 10 percent risk of tumor enlargement. The authors seek symptoms of enlargement and perform visual field estimations every 2 months during pregnancy in all patients with a macroadenoma. CT scanning and reinstitution of bromocriptine is performed if deterioration occurs; control is usually achieved with bromocriptine. Adverse effects on the fetus have not been found when bromocriptine is ceased in the first few weeks of pregnancy nor in more limited studies in which it was continued throughout pregnancy.[27]

There appears to be no adverse long-term effect of pregnancy or breast feeding on the natural history of a prolactinoma. Serum prolactin concentration has been reported to fall by > 50 percent in one-third of patients 1 to 9 years post partum.[28]

Surgical management of prolactinoma has a limited role. Success of transsphenoidal surgery, as judged by short-term normalization of prolactin concentration and resolution of symptoms, has been claimed in 60 to 90 percent of microadenoma patients while the cure rate is much lower with larger tumors. Recent studies have indicated a late relapse rate of up to 20 percent at 5 years in those previously "cured" subjects.[29,30] In view of bromocriptine's efficacy the role of pituitary surgery is now seen as limited to those subjects who are intolerant of or resistant to bromocriptine and those with tumors causing compressive symptoms, where bromocriptine has had an inadequate effect.

NUTRITIONAL AMENORRHEA

Adequate nutrition is essential to the initiation and maintenance of reproductive capacity. Frisch and Revelle showed that mean weight of normal girls at the time of menarche was 48 kg, independent of their age at sexual maturation.[31] Subsequently, it was postulated that a critical percentage of body weight (17 percent) must be present as fat for menarche to occur and that during puberty this percentage increases, stabilizing at approximately 28 percent in adulthood.[32] The maintenance of normal ovulatory cycles requires about 22 percent body weight as fat. In practical terms weight loss below 10 to 15 percent of ideal body weight is sufficient to interfere with reproductive capacity. Improved nutrition over the past century may therefore be related to the trend toward an earlier menarche. Undernutrition of any cause can be associated with diminished reproductive capacity, the severity of which is proportional to the degree of weight loss.

The mechanism(s) by which body fat is related to reproductive state is obscure but probably is mediated through the hypothalamus and thereby pituitary gonadotropin release. There is a reversion toward a prepubertal pattern of diminished GnRH responsiveness and a decrease in levels of gonadotropins, particularly LH, which is proportional to the degree of fat loss (Fig. 17B-4).[33] Mediation of these effects by opiate peptide inhibition of GnRH secretion has been suggested; the opiate antagonist naloxone has been successful in restoring LH in weight loss–related amenorrhea.[34] Estrogen production by the ovary and from peripheral conversion of androgen in fat tissue is reduced even to prepubertal levels in these women. Overall, these can be considered appropriate adaptive responses to starvation. Other hormonal changes have been described in anorexia nervosa, including diminished serum triiodothyronine (T_3) and prolactin concentrations and increased hydrocortisone and growth hormone secretion.[35]

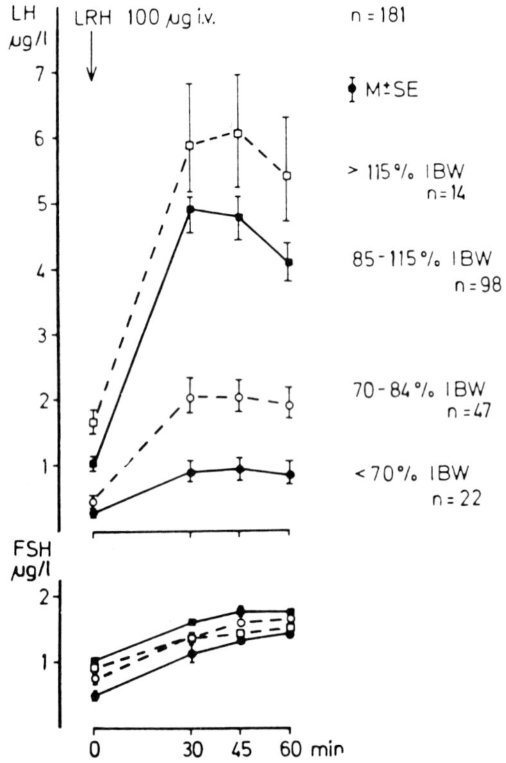

FIGURE 17B-4 As the proportion of body fat decreases, diminished gonadotropin responsiveness to GnRH occurs. (*Reproduced from Berg et al.,*[33] *by permission.*)

Etiologies of Nutritional Amenorrhea

The common etiologies of nutritional amenorrhea are summarized below. The endocrine changes outlined above are essentially common to all.

SIMPLE WEIGHT LOSS The most common presentation of secondary amenorrhea is that of a girl who complains of absence of menses without obvious cause, occurring either spontaneously or following discontinuation of the oral contraceptive pill. Careful questioning reveals a history of weight loss, often relatively rapid, of about 3 to 7 kg (7 to 15 pounds), usually because of a conviction that she is somewhat overweight. There may be an accompanying history of fairly intensive exercise. Such weight loss may occur while the contraceptive pill is being taken, in which case the postpill amenorrhea may be falsely ascribed to an effect of the pill rather than the incidental weight loss. There are usually accompanying drops in the levels of LH and estradiol. Regain of weight commonly leads to restoration of the hormone levels to normal and reinitiation of cyclic menses.

ANOREXIA NERVOSA This is a severe psychiatric condition featuring a distortion of body image and perceptions of feelings of hunger and satiety. Such patients are often adolescent girls with extremely manipulative personalities, making treatment attempts difficult. Avoidance of carbohydrate-rich foods in particular is typical; binging and self-induced vomiting (bulimia) may occur. Amenorrhea occurs with reduction of body weight and fat, the former being as low as 25 kg in severe cases. The causes of the psychological changes are unknown, but risk factors suggested are a high-achieving personality, upper socioeconomic class, and careers requiring avoidance of obesity (e.g., dancing). The condition is more subtle in the early stages and should always be considered in underweight amenorrheic subjects. Treatment occasionally involves hospitalization for severe cachexia but primarily involves intensive psychotherapy. Rates of successful treatment vary but are facilitated by early diagnosis. Mortality rates of 0 to 19 percent have been reported.[36]

EXERCISE-RELATED AMENORRHEA Intensive exercise programs require increased caloric intake for the maintenance of body weight. Weight loss and particularly a reduction in percent body weight as fat may occur if exercise programs are too severe and/or dietary intake is inadequate. In adolescent ballet dancers, a delay in the age of menarche compared to normal students matched for career stress has been reported.[37] An increased incidence of secondary amenorrhea in athletes has also been reported.[38] Of 23 runners, the incidence of amenorrhea was highest in those commencing running before age 30, those running more than 40 miles per week, and nulliparous compared to multiparous subjects.[39]

Management of Nutritional Amenorrhea

Resumption of menstruation and fertility usually accompany the regain of weight. Improved nutritional status requires treatment of any underlying psychiatric problem and modification of inappropriate diets or exercise programs. Attempts at ovulation induction in the presence of severe weight loss are usually unsuccessful[40] and inadvisable with respect to maternal and fetal health. If weight gain is not practicable, consideration should be given to estrogen replacement therapy in order to avoid long-term sequelae of hypoestrogenism, though such patients may be intolerant even of low-dose estrogen therapy. Exercise may not, as previously suspected, protect from the loss of bone density in amenorrheic runners.[41]

Polycystic Ovary Syndrome

The classic description of PCO is of a syndrome comprising oligo- or amenorrhea, infertility, hirsutism, obesity, and enlarged polycystic ovaries. It is now recognized that PCO is a heterogeneous group of disorders whose manifestations vary from the classic description to the isolated presence of one or more of the components. Assessment of its prevalence is difficult because of the lack of universally accepted diagnostic criteria. In the past, diagnosis has been based on the typical clinical features associated with an elevated plasma LH/FSH ratio and elevated plasma androgen levels. Histologic confirmation of polycystic ovaries has not been widely available. With the advent of high-resolution ovarian ultrasound, ovarian anatomy can be assessed noninvasively; this tool promises to reorganize present classifications. Polycystic ovaries defined ultrasonically have been described in nonhirsute, regularly ovulating women.[42] Therefore, this common condition has heterogeneous clinical, anatomical, and biochemical features. Surprisingly little is known about the primary nature of the problem.

CLINICAL FEATURES

Menstrual Disturbance

Menarche usually occurs normally in PCO, but there is menstrual irregularity with oligo- or amenorrhea persisting into adulthood. Menstrual bleeding may be heavy and painful in view of the continuous unopposed estrogen effect (see below). Cycles are often anovulatory or associated with a deficient luteal phase. Patients may seek help for irregular cycles per se, dysfunctional uterine bleeding, or infertility. The prevalence of PCO as a cause of infertility varies depending on the referral center but has been reported in up to 50 percent of cases.[42]

Hirsutism

A degree of hirsutism varying from mild to severe (i.e., masculine pattern) is common in PCO. It may be the primary reason for presentation or have frustrated cosmetic attempts at management.

Obesity

Weight gain at the time of puberty giving mild to moderate obesity is common in PCO, although many patients are of normal weight.

PATHOPHYSIOLOGY

The complex question of the primary defect in PCO remains unresolved, but the large body of knowledge available can be considered under the following headings. Figure 17B-5 depicts one schema for the pathogenesis of the PCO syndrome, which may be outlined as follows:

1. Defects in ovarian function
   a. Folliculogenesis
   b. Sex steroid secretion
2. Defects in hypothalamic-pituitary function
3. Abnormal androgen metabolism

These defects exist concurrently and interact to give a chronic anovulatory state with or without evidence of hyperandrogenemia. Whatever the primary defect, once these events are established they are usually self-maintaining.

Defects in Ovarian Function

FOLLICULOGENESIS Polycystic ovaries contain numerous small cysts (usually 2 to 4 mm in diameter) and characteristically increased stromal tissue, the latter being primarily responsible for increased ovarian volume. Granulosa cells from these cysts have a normal appearance and respond to FSH stimulation in vitro.[43] However, there is a failure of one follicle to become dominant and to develop to a preovulatory state with suppression of other follicles. The nature of this defect in intraovarian regulation is unknown.

SEX STEROID SECRETION Estrogen secretion in the absence of normal follicular development is acyclic with total estradiol levels in the early to midfollicular range. Increased ovarian and adrenal androgen secretion (see below) also bear directly on estrogen levels by acting as substrate for extraovarian estrogen production (especially of estrone), primarily in fat tissue. Androgens also act to lower sex hormone–binding globulin (SHBG) levels, thereby increasing the free androgen and estrogen levels. Abnormal sex steroid profiles are therefore present to feed back on the hypothalamic pituitary system.

Defects in Hypothalamic-Pituitary Function

Plasma LH levels are raised while plasma FSH levels are normal or depressed, leading to the characteristic, though not invariable, elevation in LH/FSH ratio.[44] Chronic acyclic elevation of free estrogen levels in PCO may explain this abnormal profile of gonadotropins. Unopposed estrogen feedback may enhance pituitary LH, but not FSH, release in response to GnRH exposure. Coordinated cyclic release of gonadotropins does not occur and failure of normal folliculogenesis results. A primary hypothalamic problem independent of abnormal sex steroid feedback has been suggested by the finding of abnormal LH secretory pulse fre-

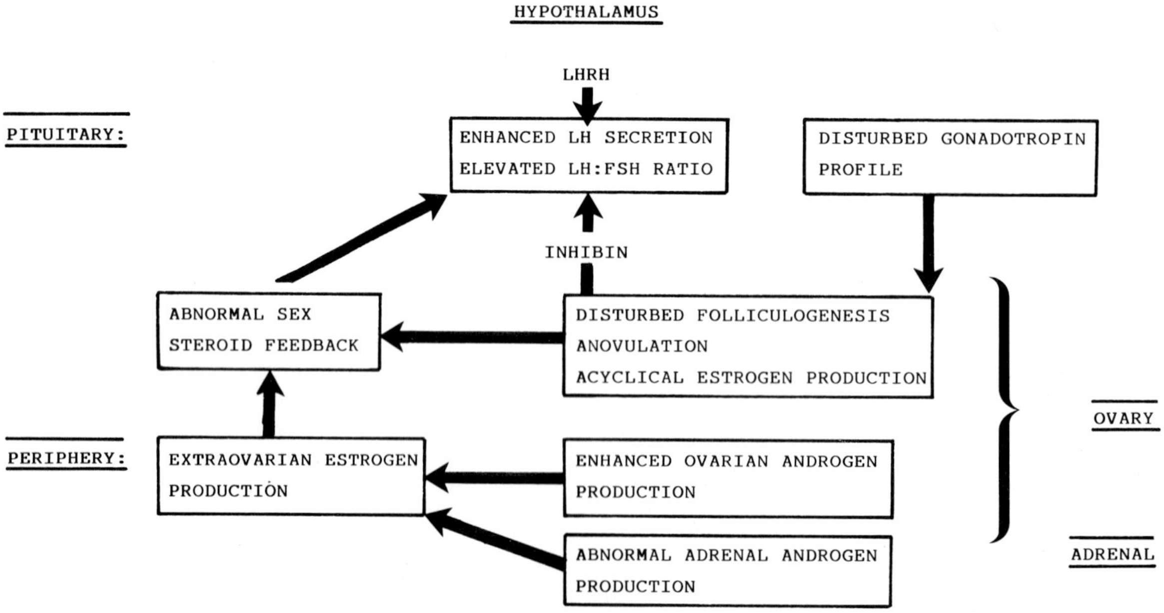

FIGURE 17B-5 Schema for the pathogenesis of the polycystic ovary syndrome.

quency in adolescent girls.[45] This may suggest alterations in hypothalamic GnRH pulsatility. However, other studies have shown normal LH pulse frequency in PCO.[46]

Abnormal dopamine metabolism has been reported in PCO syndrome, suggesting a hypothalamic problem. Moderate elevation of serum prolactin concentration (one to five times normal) was apparent in 27 percent of 394 PCO subjects in a review of several published series.[47] Increased LH sensitivity to dopamine inhibition in PCO syndrome compared to the sensitivity in the early follicular phase in normal women has been reported.[48] Finally, an increased risk of prolactinoma in PCO syndrome has been found, warranting careful exclusion of this tumor, particularly in patients with more marked elevations of prolactin concentration.[49]

The place of inhibin, a recently purified gonadal peptide which specifically acts to lower FSH secretion, in the abnormal gonadotropin profiles in PCO should be clarified now that a radioimmunoassay for human plasma inhibin has been reported.[50] Inappropriately high inhibin production by granulosa cells in polycystic ovaries is speculated to be a possible cause of PCO; some evidence for this has been reported.

Abnormal Androgen Secretion

Controversy has existed as to whether the ovary or the adrenal is the principal source of hyperandrogenemia in PCO. Approximately 50 percent of PCO subjects have elevated levels of total testosterone; with the suppression of SHBG seen in this condition, about 75 percent have elevated unbound levels.[51] The specific suppression of gonadotropins using GnRH analogues has been shown to suppress the elevated testosterone and androstenedione levels in PCO syndrome, suggesting that the ovary is the primary source of these androgens. Dehydroepiandrosterone sulfate (DHEA-S) is predominantly an adrenal androgen and its concentration is elevated in about 50 percent of PCO subjects.[52] The adrenal origin of this androgen is also suggested by an exaggerated DHEA-S response to ACTH and the well-known beneficial effect of dexamethasone suppression in PCO.

It is apparent, therefore, that in most subjects both the adrenal and ovary hypersecrete androgens, while in the remainder either or neither does so. It should be emphasized that hyperandrogenemia may be due to other causes, e.g., endocrine tumors or cryptic congenital adrenal hyperplasia, in which the elevation of 17-hydroxyprogesterone level, especially following ACTH infusion, is characteristic. These diagnoses should therefore be considered.

The interaction of these components is displayed in Fig. 17B-5. This self-perpetuating cycle of events can be followed commencing at the pituitary. In response to elevated and acyclic estrogen exposure and possibly abnormal inhibin levels, pituitary LH release is enhanced while the FSH/LH ratio is depressed and cyclic release of gonadotropins is abnormal. Orderly folliculogenesis fails to occur because of relative lack of FSH and therefore of aromatase activity, and ovulation does not occur. Enhanced ovarian and/or adrenal androgen secretion provides the substrate for peripheral estrogen production, lowers the SHBG level, and produces hirsutism in some patients. It must be emphasized that not all components of this schema need always be present.

MANAGEMENT OF POLYCYSTIC OVARY SYNDROME

Indications for therapeutic intervention in PCO syndrome can be summarized as

Control of menstrual cyclicity and/or bleeding
Management of infertility
Management of hirsutism

Menstrual Cyclicity

The use of a combined oral contraceptive can control irregular cycles in PCO syndrome. Heavy bleeding may occur in PCO in view of the anovulatory state, with continuous unopposed estrogen exposure leading to thickening of the endometrial lining. A course of progestogen (norethindrone, 5 to 10 mg daily for 10 days) will usually control this bleeding. A combined oral contraceptive or regular cyclic progestogen alone can then be used to maintain menstrual control. Induction of regular menses is advisable in anovulatory PCO syndrome in view of the reported increased incidence of endometrial hyperplasia and neoplasia.[53,54]

Infertility

Clomiphene citrate has conventionally been used for induction of ovulation. Its mechanism of action is presumed to be by the temporary relief of estrogen feedback on gonadotropins, especially FSH. Follicular development is permitted and estrogen level increases to stimulate an LH surge. Ovulation can be induced in the majority (80 percent) of PCO subjects, although the pregnancy rate is often reported as lower (39 percent).[55] In addition, there appears to be a high rate of spontaneous abortion in clomiphene-induced PCO pregnancy, 40 percent compared to 25 percent in non-PCO clomiphene-induced pregnancy. Nonetheless, clomiphene offers the most convenient form of ovulation induction for the majority of subjects. Doses of 50 to 150 mg daily for 5 days commencing on day 5 of the cycle are suggested. The response is monitored by charting basal body temperature and with ovarian ultrasound and luteal-phase progesterone concentration estimations.

For PCO subjects who fail to ovulate with clomiphene, a range of therapies has been applied, including the addition of hCG or glucocorticoids to clomiphene, although clear benefit over clomiphene alone has not been shown. Bromocriptine has also been shown to induce ovulation in some PCO women, especially when hyperprolactinemia is present.[56] Many such patients require ovulation induction with gonadotropins, while they are generally resistant to therapy with pulsatile GnRH. Newer approaches using preliminary treatment with GnRH agonists prior to gonadotropins are under evaluation, as is therapy with highly purified FSH.

Virilization and Hirsutism

CLINICAL ASSESSMENT AND INVESTIGATION

The number of advertisements offering the removal of superfluous hair suggests that hirsutism is indeed a fairly common disorder. It may be defined as the excessive growth of terminal hair in a male distribution and affects particularly the upper lip, chin, chest, sacral area, lower abdomen, and thighs. It is frequently perceived as being much more severe by the patient than by the doctor to whom she brings her complaint. In contrast, virilization is uncommon. It is manifested by male pattern baldness, clitoral hypertrophy, deepening of the voice, and increased muscularity in addition to hirsutism. The presence of virilization strongly suggests an underlying organic cause.

A variety of methods have been used to try to measure the degree of hirsutism and rate of hair growth. From a practical viewpoint, the scoring system of Ferriman and Gallwey has achieved widespread popularity.[57] The degree of hair growth is graded on a scale of 0 to 4 on the upper lip, chin, chest, upper back, lower back, upper abdomen, lower abdomen, upper arm, and thigh, giving a maximal possible score of 36 with an upper limit of normal of 7. Forty percent of normal Caucasian women have a score of 0. More cumbersome objective methods of assessing hair growth velocity have been described.[58]

There is considerable variation among different ethnic groups in the amount of hair growth which is perceived as normal. In Australian immigrants, those coming from the Mediterranean area have much more body hair than do women of Anglo-Saxon origin or those coming from southeast Asian countries.

Hirsutism may be classified as increased hair growth occurring in otherwise apparently normal subjects, for example, at puberty or in the late teens or early twenties, during pregnancy, or at the time of menopause. It may also occur in response to the administration of certain drugs including phenytoin, norgestrel, norethindrone, metronidazole, minoxidil, corticosteroids, anabolic steroids, androgens, and cyclosporin. Patients with hypothyroidism, acromegaly, and porphyria may develop increased hair growth, although the classic associations are with increased androgen production of either ovarian or adrenal source. Ovarian causes include the polycystic ovary syndrome, hyperthecosis, and ovarian tumor; the adrenal causes include tumors and congenital adrenal hyperplasia, particularly the late-onset adult type. Patients with Cushing's syndrome usually have some degree of hirsutism.

From a practical clinical viewpoint, by far the commonest clinical varieties of hirsutism are the idiopathic form and PCO syndrome. Terminology of the former is somewhat confused, as the majority of patients with idiopathic hirsutism actually have an increase at least in androgen production rate, though the cause of this remains undefined. An alternative term for this disorder is *functional androgen excess.* The concentration of a peripheral metabolite of DHT, androstanediol glucuronide, has been reported to be markedly elevated in hirsute patients and correlates with the degree of hirsutism.[59]

Idiopathic hirsutism is often associated with a family history of excess hair growth in either male or female relatives and tends to come on in the late teens or early twenties. The hirsutism is usually mild to moderate in extent and menstrual cycles usually remain regular and ovulatory. The PCO syndrome classically has its onset just before or at the time of puberty and is associated with obesity, menstrual irregularity (either oligomenorrhea or amenorrhea, which may be primary or secondary), and infertility. Both idiopathic hirsutism and PCO syndrome may be associated with acne and excessively oily skin. It has become increasingly recognized that a syndrome indistinguishable from PCO syndrome may occur in previously normal women who gain excess weight, often associated with one or more pregnancies, and who present in their late twenties or early thirties with obesity, hirsutism, and oligomenorrhea. In these patients, the obesity may be the primary disorder and restoration of menstrual periodicity and some decrease in hirsutism may accompany successful weight loss, though this is difficult to achieve. Other very rare associations of this disorder are insulin resistance and acanthosis nigricans (termed the HAIR-AN syndrome: *h*yper*a*ndrogenism, *i*nsulin *r*esistance, and *a*canthosis *n*igricans).[60]

The clinical assessment of patients presenting with hirsutism must include taking an appropriate history, including a family history with particular attention to the rapidity of onset of the hirsutism: an abrupt onset suggests the possibility of organic lesions such as an adrenal or ovarian tumor. A careful menstrual history with attention to symptoms suggesting the presence of ovulation should be recorded. It is important to determine whether the patient is also complaining of infertility and whether she requires contraception. Physical examination should include an assessment of the severity of the hirsutism. Using the Ferriman and Gallwey hormonal score with a maximum score of 36, mild hirsutism may be regarded as showing a score of 8 to 12, moderate hirsutism 13 to 18, and severe hirsutism > 19.[61] Careful assessment should be made for evidence of accompanying virilization (e.g., clitoral hypertrophy) and for stigmata of rare causes of hirsutism such as Cushing's syndrome or hypothyroidism.

An area of significant concern and controversy is the question of what degree of investigation should be undertaken in patients presenting with apparently uncomplicated hirsutism. Although it is of theoretical interest to establish whether excessive androgen secretion is arising from the ovary or the adrenal, in practice this may not significantly affect choice of management unless a specific adrenal lesion has been identified and suppressive therapy is contemplated.

Measurements which may be made include those of plasma testosterone concentration, either total or free; salivary testosterone determination is an alternative approach to assessing the unbound steroid level. DHT, DHEA-S, androstenedione, and androstanediol concentrations may be measured, together with that of 17-hydroxyprogesterone. A marked elevation in plasma testosterone level to more than twice the upper limit of normal is compatible with PCO syndrome, but if the testosterone level is substantially above that level, the possibility of an ovarian tumor in particular must be kept in mind and is best evaluated with pelvic examination and ultrasonography or CT scanning. A marked elevation in DHEA-S concentration to more than twice the upper limit of normal suggests the possibility of an adrenal tumor, which should again be excluded by CT scanning. Androstenedione and DHEA-S together with testosterone levels are frequently moderately elevated in PCO syndrome. An elevation in basal levels of 17-hydroxyprogesterone suggest late-onset congenital adrenal hyperplasia; in this disorder a stimulation test with ACTH may establish the diagnosis.[62] Measurements of FSH, LH, and prolactin levels may also be diagnostically helpful, with an elevation of LH concentration and a high LH/FSH ratio being typical of PCO syndrome. Prolactin-secreting pituitary adenomas may occasionally be associated with some excess of hair growth.

It is difficult to formulate entirely satisfactory general rules for the degree of investigation which should be undertaken in any individual patient. As a general guide, in mild to moderate hirsutism with normal menses investigations are of extremely doubtful value. An elevation of DHEA-S concentration may suggest an adrenal component from stress, but this is usually obvious from the history and patients can be counseled accordingly. In mild to moderate hirsutism with menstrual irregularity, investigations may be directed to establishing PCO syndrome as the cause with measurements of FSH, LH, and testosterone levels. It is well recognized that the free testosterone fraction is much more frequently elevated in hirsutism than is total plasma testosterone, but the observation is of little practical management value.

In severe hirsutism, levels of DHEA-S, testosterone, and 17-hydroxyprogesterone, with the latter's response to ACTH, should be assessed and, where indicated, abdominal CT scanning or ultrasound undertaken in order to clarify the diagnosis.

Where management with antiandrogens, particularly cyproterone acetate, is contemplated, it is also useful to measure baseline cholesterol and triglyceride levels, as cyproterone acetate may cause an increase in plasma lipid levels. In patients in whom spironolactone is to be used basal renal function should be assessed.

MANAGEMENT

The overall approach to the hirsute patient should be one of empathy and understanding with emphasis on the fact that it is a lifelong disorder for which cosmetic approaches provide the cornerstone of management. The available measures include simple plucking, waxing, shaving, and the use of depilatory creams, all of which require long-term use. Permanent cure may be achieved by properly performed electrolysis, which is however, tedious, uncomfortable, and expensive.

Medical measures include regimens of ovarian suppression (with a combination of estrogen and progestogen, e.g., the oral contraceptive) and adrenal suppression (with nocturnally administered corticosteroids such as prednisone, 7.5 mg daily, or dexamethasone, 0.5 mg daily). Results with such measures are slow to occur and often disappointing. More successful approaches have involved the use of antiandrogens, such as cyproterone acetate (given in reverse sequential form with cyclic estrogen[63]) or spironolactone in high doses (100 to 200 mg daily[64]). About two-thirds of hirsute patients will have satisfactory subjective and objective improvement in the rate and severity of excessive hair growth, commencing 2 to 3 months from the onset of treatment. Hirsutism almost always recurs when therapy is discontinued. It is mandatory that pregnancy be avoided during such therapy because of the risks of feminization of a male fetus.

Female Infertility: Management by Ovulation Induction

It has been estimated that one couple in 10 will experience difficulty with conception. Male and female factors are equally prevalent in causing infertility, although in many couples marginal subfertility exists in both partners. Thus, the recommendation for the clinical approach to the infertile couple emphasizes the importance of seeing both partners together and the recognition that anxiety and depression are common in one or both partners presenting with infertility. It is important to take time to speak with the couple at an initial interview rather than to hastily order many of the large number of investigations available for management, particularly in women with infertility and possible ovarian dysfunction. For example, care should be taken to determine the number and outcome of any previous pregnancies because, quite apart from the obstetric importance of this, the prognosis for secondary infertility is better than for primary infertility.

Previous medical treatments may cause permanent or temporary damage to folliculogenesis. These include not only use of cytotoxic agents and irradiation but also psychopharmacological agents such as tranquilizers or antidepressants. Surgical procedures obviously may affect fertility; these include not only gynecological procedures such as ovarian cystectomy and abdominal operations such as complicated appendectomy, but also tissue handling at laparotomy, which may cause adhesion formation in the pelvis which may affect tubal function. Environmental and occupational factors may be relevant to the chances of conception. For example, frequent night shift work may disturb ovarian function and make the possibility of intercourse in the fertile period less likely.

In a general physical examination use of a normal-weight chart is of great value; a weight index such as the Garrow index (weight in kilograms divided by squared height in meters) is recommended. Hair distribution should be scored according to the definitions of Ferriman and Gallwey.[57] Excessive hair growth may indicate excessive androgen secretion or action and this may be associated with anovulation. Hypoestrogenism may be indicated by incomplete breast development and should be recorded by the appropriate Tanner stage 2.[65] The presence of galactorrhea is detectable by gentle sustained pressure on the areolae. This secretion should not contain brown or blood-stained discharge, which would indicate that organic breast disease, including malignancy, should be excluded. In ideal circumstances, galactorrhea should be confirmed by testing for lactose and by microscopic examination for fat globules.

There are a number of possible tests of ovulation: charting of mucous symptoms and/or basal body temperature, determination of luteal-phase plasma progesterone concentrations, ultrasonic ovarian follicle assessment, and endometrial biopsy. The emphasis placed on each of these tests will depend on the clinical facilities at hand. The authors use plasma progesterone assay as a screening test of ovulation in either spontaneous or induced cycles. The blood sample is drawn either on day 21 of an expected 28-day cycle or approximately 7 days before the next anticipated menses in patients with oligomenorrhea.

In patients in whom chronic anovulation appears to be the major cause of infertility, a large number of ovulation induction agents are now available for therapy (Table 17B-3).

In amenorrheic women, low plasma estradiol concentrations ($<$ 100 pM) suggest that the response to antiestrogens, e.g., clomiphene citrate, will be inadequate. However, the progestogen withdrawal test does provide useful information and withdrawal uterine bleeding should be assessed by giving 10 mg per day of a progestogen such as medroxyprogesterone acetate or norethindrone orally for 5 days. If no vaginal bleeding occurs the test is negative; any bleeding up to one week following the test is positive and suggests that there is sufficient circulating estrogen present for antiestrogen therapy to be beneficial.

Table 17B-3. Ovulation-Inducing Agents

Category	Agents
Antiestrogens	Clomiphene, tamoxifen
Dopamine agonists	Bromocriptine, Lisuride
FSH, LH	hPG, hMG
Purified FSH	Metrodin
Surrogate LH	hCG
GnRH	
GnRH Agonists	Buserelin, Naferilin

Abbreviations: hPG = human pituitary gonadotropin; hMG = human menopausal gonadotropin; hCG = human chorionic gonadotropin

With the antiestrogen clomiphene citrate, treatment is commenced at 50 mg per day for 5 days beginning day 5 of the cycle and ovulation is assessed by charting basal body temperature as well as measuring serum progesterone concentration between days 21 and 24. Many patients find the prolonged recording of basal body temperature boring and these charts are not emphasized in reluctant patients. The serum progesterone level should be > 25 nM per liter in the midluteal phase to support the occurrence of ovulation. Clearly, the date of the next menses is of great significance in ensuring that the progesterone estimate was made on the appropriate day. The combination of these two tests for ovulation does allow for assessment of an adequate luteal phase. If the first progesterone estimate is made at a correct time but still suggests anovulation, the dose of clomiphene is increased in the next treatment cycle rather than continue with the previous dose. This stepwise increase in antiestrogen therapy is important to arrive at a dose which will consistently induce ovulation.

If a confident clinical diagnosis of hypoestrogenism can be made or a progestogen withdrawal test is negative, then the primary therapy should be gonadotropin or pulsatile GnRH treatment. A great number of different schedules have been reported for the administration of either human gonadotropin or GnRH to patients with persistent anovulation. Clearly, GnRH therapy is logical in patients who are demonstrably or clinically GnRH-deficient, such as individuals with Kallmann's syndrome (Fig. 17B-2). The introduction of pulsatile GnRH for ovulation induction appears to have some advantages over human gonadotropin treatment.[66,67] These advantages obviate the need for daily hormonal monitoring, twice-weekly monitoring being required mainly to confirm the timing of ovulation, and relative patient autonomy without the need to maintain daily physician contact for results of endocrine or ovarian ultrasound tests (Fig. 17B-6). In addition, there is a lower, although not negligible, risk of multiple pregnancy with pulsatile GnRH treatment (9 percent[68]) and a reduced risk of ovarian hyperstimulation. Nevertheless, there are disadvantages to GnRH therapy. These include cost, the need to wear a portable pump with a subcutaneous or intravenous needle, and the occurrence of local reactions. Other reported disadvantages are systemic infection or septicemia where an intravenous needle is employed, a low rate of success in patients with PCO syndrome, and patient stress in the initial weeks of treatment. Figure 17B-7 depicts changes in gonadotropin and GnRH concentrations during subcutaneous pulsatile administration of GnRH to a patient with hypothalamic amenorrhea.

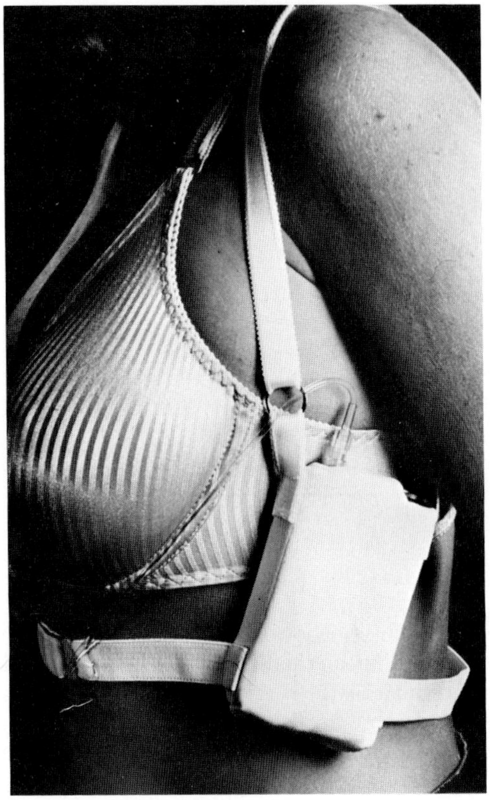

FIGURE 17B-6 Pulsatile GnRH infuser assembled to allow subcutaneous hormone administration in an ambulatory patient.

GONADOTROPIC OVULATION INDUCTION

Clinical use of human pituitary FSH resulting in pregnancy was first reported in 1960.[69] Human gonadotropins were prepared from cadaver pituitaries or crude preparations derived from the urine of postmenopausal women. More recently, highly purified FSH preparations from postmenopausal urine have been obtained.

From a clinical point of view, two schemes for the administration of gonadotropins for the induction of ovulation have been used. The first is a fixed dosage scheme, in which a predetermined dose of gonadotropin is administered in increasing concentrations in each cycle of treatment until a response occurs. In the second scheme, the dose of gonadotropin is determined by the patient's response during treatment, so that an effective dose is administered during each cycle. The advantage of the individual daily adjusted dosage regimen is the smaller number of cycles required per pregnancy, about half that of the predetermined schedule.[70,71]

The authors' clinic has used a daily adjusted sched-

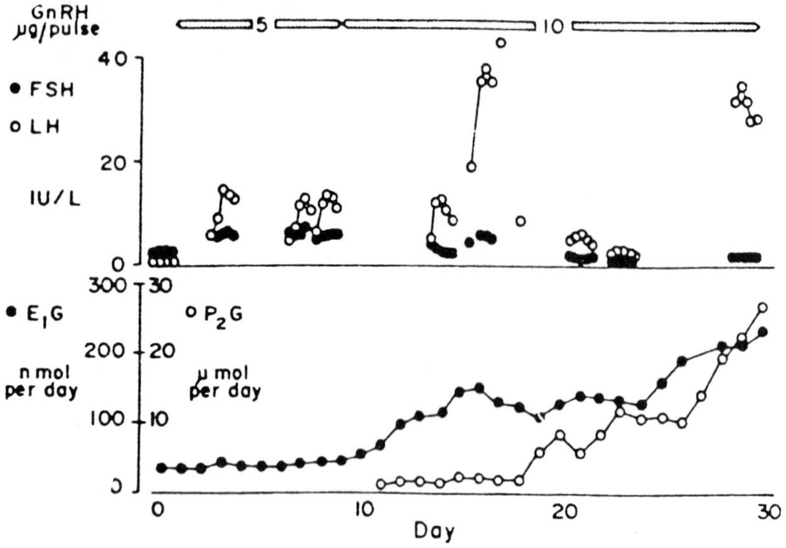

FIGURE 17B-7 Induction of ovulation in a hypogonadotropic patient using subcutaneous GnRH. The top of the figure indicates the amount of GnRH administered in each pulse. E_1G = estrone-1-glucuronide, P_2G = pregnanediol glucuronide. (*Reproduced from Hurley et al.,*[66] *by permission.*)

ule of human gonadotropin for ovulation induction since 1972. This method originally required monitoring by estimating 24-h total urinary estrogen excretion,[72] and more recently monitoring by the use of rapid radioimmunoassays of estrogen and pregnanediol glucuronides.[73] Other clinics have used daily plasma estradiol concentration estimates and/or ovarian ultrasound determinations for the same purpose, with equally good effect.[74] None of the various methods of monitoring folliculogenesis is believed to offer any particular advantage over another. The aim of human gonadotropin therapy in subjects with chronic anovulation should be to induce a pregnancy rate which is equivalent to the natural conception rate in the community, as assessed by life table analysis (Fig. 17B-8).[75]

With current human gonadotropin treatments, excessive stimulation of the ovaries is the major complication of therapy; this can be expressed in two forms. First, hyperstimulation may be clinically silent and detectable only by sex steroid excretion, or may present with a spectrum of clinical features varying from palpable ovarian cysts to its most severe form, which includes abdominal distention, nausea, hydrothorax, coagulopathy, and, occasionally, death.[76] Second, multiple ovulation and multiple pregnancy may be produced, with or without other signs of hyperstimulation; these occur in 20 to 30 percent of most gonadotropin series.[75]

Mean serum FSH and LH concentrations are markedly elevated during ovulation induction therapy with human gonadotropins.[77] Elevated FSH/LH ratios for more than 8 days provide unrelenting FSH exposure to the cohort of recruited follicles; this appears to be important in inducing disordered folliculogenesis in these patients. Two or more ovarian follicles develop in approximately 86 percent of gonadotropin-treated cycles, compared with only 23 percent of spontaneous

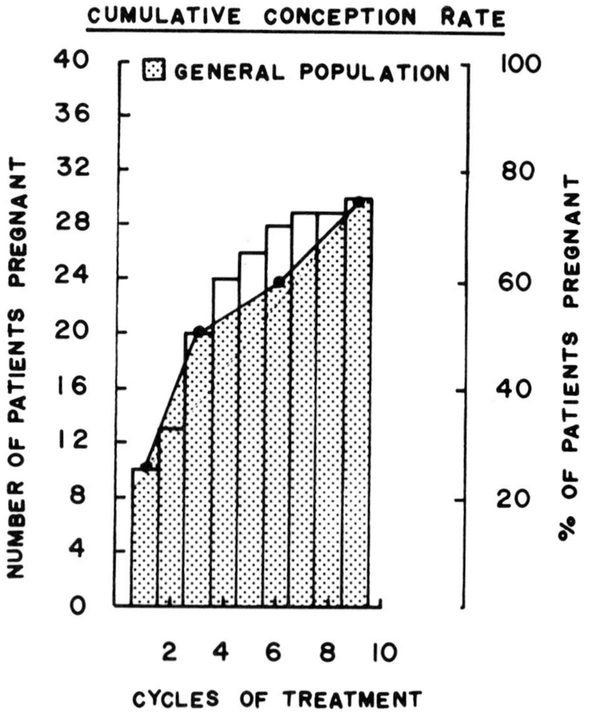

FIGURE 17B-8 Cumulative conception rate in a series of patients receiving human pituitary gonadotropin for ovulation induction. Stippled area shows the conception rate for the general population. (*Reproduced from Healy et al.*[75] *with permission.*)

Table 17B-4. Results of Ovulation Induction by Gonadotropin Therapy*

	Percent with follicles > 10 mm	
	2 Follicles	3 Follicles
Human gonadotropin–induced cycles ($n = 28$)	86	50
Spontaneous cycles ($n = 13$)	23	0

*Percent of cycles with 2 or 3 follicles developing to >10 mm diameter

cycles, and at least three follicles > 12 mm in diameter develop during 50 percent of gonadotropin-stimulated cycles (Table 17B-4).

Recently, small series of anovulatory patients treated by various permutations of human gonadotropin or GnRH therapy have been reported. These include the administration of human gonadotropin delivered in a pulsatile mode, pulsatile FSH therapy, and either of these treatments following a course of GnRH agonist suppression of endogenous pituitary function.[78] GnRH agonist administration has also been used in small groups of anovulatory patients in an attempt to induce pituitary down regulation and convert abnormal secretion of LH and FSH and aberrant LH/FSH ratios to more normal patterns (Fig. 17B-9). While the individual small series reported with each of these treatments are encouraging, larger groups of patients must be studied to be confident that these therapies offer a significant advantage over the current methods of ovarian stimulation. Indeed, there appears to have been no controlled studies comparing pulsatile LHRH with human gonadotropin therapy.

PULSATILE ADMINISTRATION OF GNRH

Leyendecker and colleagues were the first to report the use of pulsatile administration of GnRH in women

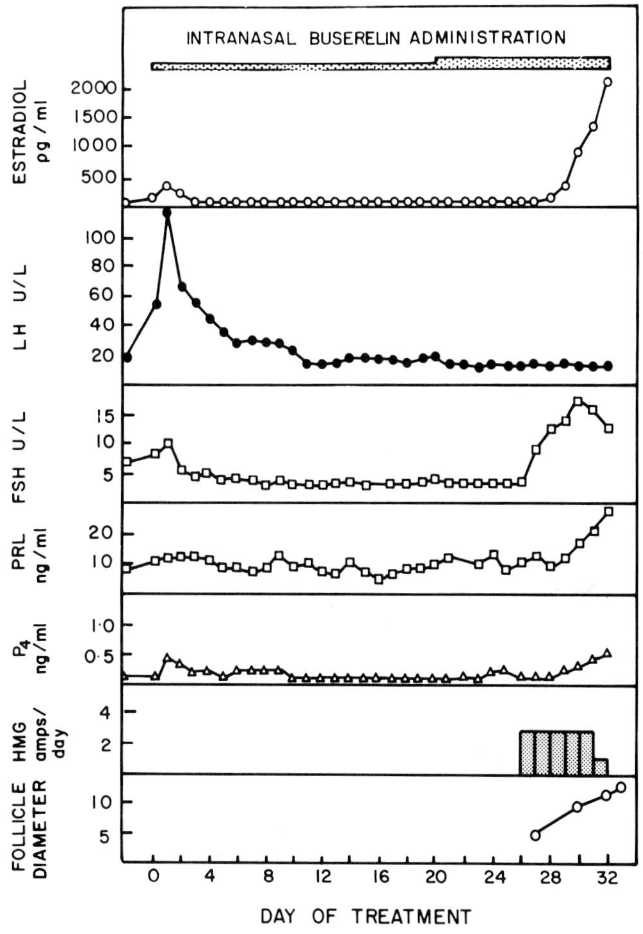

FIGURE 17B-9 Intranasal GnRH agonist (buserelin) administration to an anovulatory patient with polycystic ovary syndrome. Note the initial LH/FSH ratio, the suppression of plasma estradiol levels with buserelin therapy, the exponential increase in estradiol values when hMG treatment has begun, and the rapid increase in follicle growth.

with hypothalamic amenorrhea.[79] Since then many authors have reported the use of pulsatile administration of GnRH, by both intravenous and subcutaneous routes, to induce ovulation in patients with hypothalamic amenorrhea. In the authors' clinic, Hurley and associates[80] used 90-min subcutaneous pulses of GnRH, commencing at 5 μg per pulse and increasing by 5 μg every 7 to 14 days until a progressive rise in urinary estrone glucuronide level was observed. Twenty-three of the thirty ovulatory cycles with this therapy were induced with 10-μg pulses. There were 13 pregnancies in this group of 14 subjects. The largest series reported to date consisted of 28 patients treated with subcutaneous GnRH therapy.[81] Ovulation was induced in 100 percent of 80 treatment cycles, resulting in 25 pregnancies. Although there appeared to be no difficulties in this group of patients with subcutaneous GnRH administration, the anovulatory patients who did not respond to subcutaneous therapy did all subsequently ovulate and conceive when treated with intravenous GnRH. It therefore appears from the small numbers of patients so far reported, that if the more convenient and potentially less hazardous subcutaneous GnRH therapy is unsuccessful, then intravenous GnRH treatment should be attempted.

The incidence of multiple pregnancy is lower with GnRH therapy when compared with human gonadotropin treatment. Of reported series, a multiple pregnancy rate of 8 percent occurred, although it is noteworthy that several cases of triplet pregnancies and one quadruplet pregnancy have been reported, as have other instances of ovarian hyperstimulation.

Menorrhagia and Dysmenorrhea

The clinical problems of menorrhagia and dysmenorrhea are among the commonest which present to a gynecologist. In order to properly understand the basis of present clinical management of these disorders, a brief review of endometrial anatomy and physiology is relevant.

Endometrial Anatomy and Physiology

Normal endometrium consists of a simple columnar epithelium which contains estrogen-responsive and progesterone-dependent mucous glands on an underlying stroma. The endometrium is typically classified into a more superficial functional zone, which is supplied by coiled spiral arteries (Fig. 17B-10) and is shed at menstruation, and a deeper basal zone, which is supplied by straight arteries. This remains after menstruation and regenerates the endometrium. Moreover, the functional zone contains a superficial luminal zone (zone 1), an intermediate zone 2 where the glands are straight and widely separated by stroma, and a deeper layer, zone 3, where the glands are coiled and closely packed. These differences are clinically relevant, since the highest mitotic rates are observed in the upper third of human endometrium on days 8 to 10 of the cycle.

In 1950, Noyes, Hertig, and Rock established criteria for dating endometrial biopsies (Fig. 17B-11).[18] They found that the proliferative phase of the menstrual cycle was variable in length and the endometrial changes too indistinct to permit day-to-day recognition or "dating" of the endometrium. They recognized early proliferative, midproliferative, and late proliferative endometrium (Fig. 17B-11). Through these phases, the endometrium thickens due to an increase in the number and size of the glands, which become tortuous. Glandular diameter and volume are directly related to plasma estradiol concentrations.

In contrast to the proliferative phase, Noyes and colleagues found that secretory-phase endometrium developed in such a characteristic rate and fashion after ovulation that daily changes were recognizable; the endometrium could therefore be dated. Basal or subnuclear vacuolation of the glandular epithelium was found 36 to 48 h following ovulation and was the first endometrial sign of luteinization. This change was prominent from days 16 to 19 of a typical menstrual cycle. From day 19, basal vacuoles disappeared as the glycogen-enriched secretion passed by the gland nuclei and into the lumen. The nuclei were thus seen at the base of the epithelial cells. From days 21 to 23 the spiral arterioles acquired a cuff of stromal cells with enlarged nuclei and cytoplasm. This constituted the earliest predecidual or pseudodecidual change. Predecidua extended to beneath the epithelium by day 25 and at day 27 appeared as solid sheets of decidua-like cells infiltrated by leukocytes. These predecidual cells underwent mitosis as well as hypertrophy. If conception occurs, further enlargement forms polygonal decidual cells in a highly vascular stroma. After implantation, that portion of the decidua between the placenta and myometrium is called the *decidua basalis.* The part covering the blastocyst is the *decidua capsularis,* which fuses with the part lining the remainder of the uterus, the *decidua parietalis.*

In the young adult, menstrual blood loss can be measured by collecting tampons and/or sanitary pads and extracting the iron or hemoglobin. Hallberg and associates found in 476 women that the volume of menstrual blood loss was not normally distributed but rather was skewed in distribution:[82] median blood loss was 43 ml and 90 percent of randomly selected women had menstrual blood losses < 80 ml. Cole and colleagues examined 348 unselected women and con-

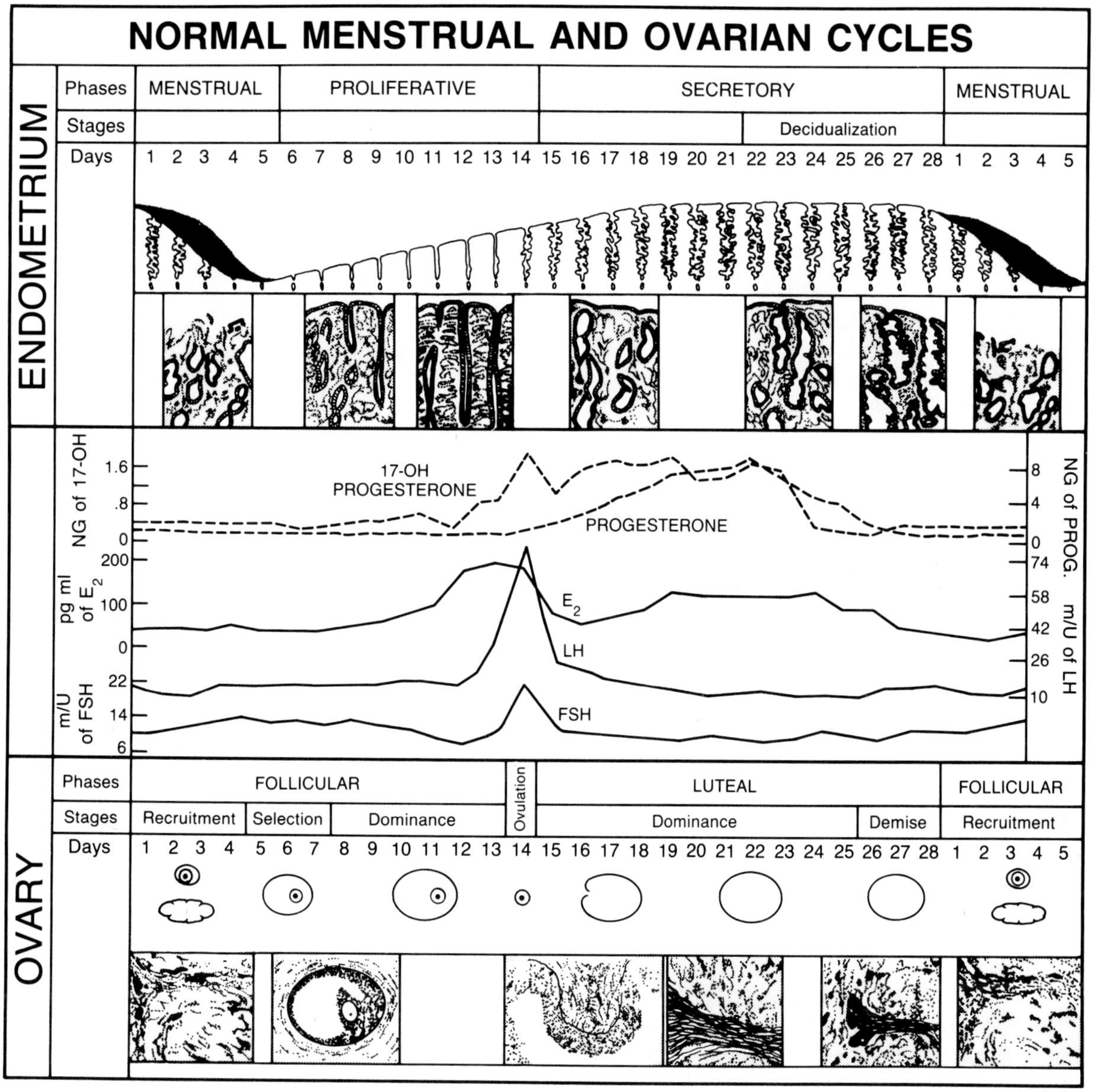

FIGURE 17B-10 Schematic representation of the interactions of the endometrium, pituitary, and ovaries during ovulatory menstrual cycles. (*Reproduced from Healy and Hodgen,*[7] *by permission.*)

firmed a skewed distribution of menstrual blood loss.[83] In their study, median blood loss was 28 ml; in only 20 percent of women was the difference in menstrual blood loss in consecutive periods $>$ 20 ml. Menstrual blood loss increased with parity, perhaps due to an increased endometrial area or vascularity or both, but did not increase with age. Above 80 ml menstrual blood loss, most women will probably develop iron-deficiency anemia.

Approximately 50 to 70 percent of the menstrual discharge is blood. The platelet count found in menstrual fluid is about 10 percent of that in blood. The remainder of the menses is fragments of endometrium and mucus. Normal menstrual blood does not readily clot. Although Buller reported that menstrual blood does not contain fibrin and that menstrual clots also contain no fibrin,[84] and thus are not true clots, more recent studies by Bonnar and colleagues[85] found fibrin in 85 percent of normal menstrual clots and in 88 percent of patients with dysfunctional uterine bleeding. They found no fibrinogen in menstrual blood, but did find large amounts of fibrin degradation products

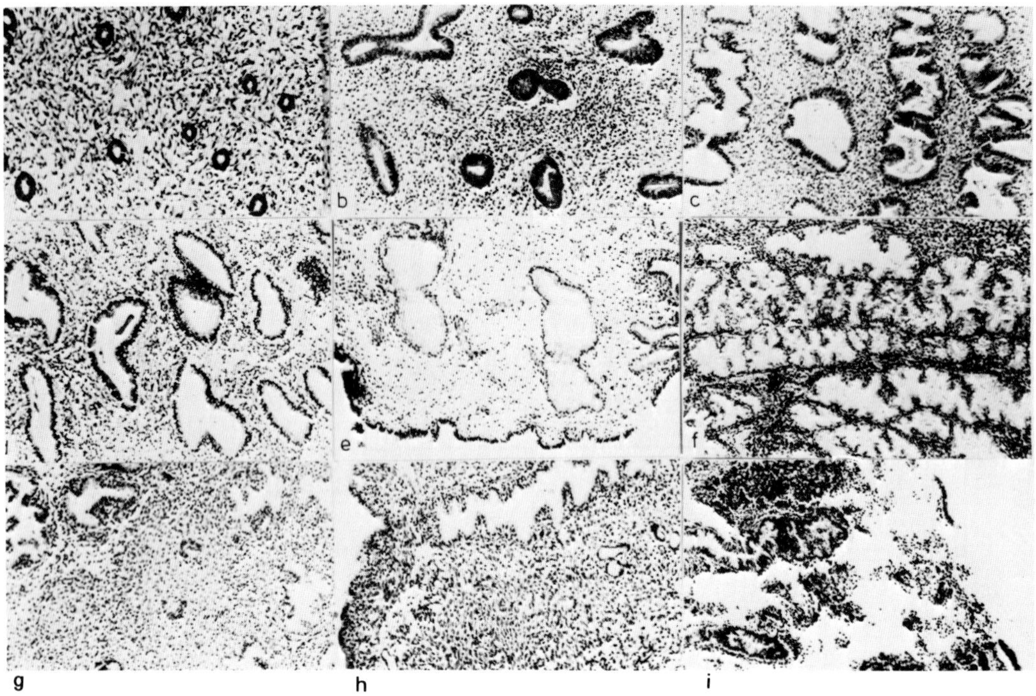

FIGURE 17B-11 Morphologic changes in human endometrium during a normal menstrual cycle. (*A*) Early proliferative. (*B*) Midproliferative. (*C*) Late proliferative. During the follicular phase, the endometrium thickens due to an increase in the number and size of the glands. Moderate tortuosity is seen as they become wider and longer. (*D*) Basal vacuolation of the gland epithelium is the earliest morphologic evidence of luteinization. Day 16 endometrium. (*E*) During the secretory stage, basal vacuoles disappear and nuclei are seen at the base of the epithelial cells. Note also stromal edema. Day 20 endometrium. (*F*) During the premenstrual stage, glands may present a pronounced sawtooth appearance. Day 25 endometrium (*G*) Stromal cells first show predecidual change around arterioles. Day 23 endometrium. (*H*) Just before menstruation, a compact layer of predecidual cells is formed. (*I*) During the menstrual phase, the endometrium typically crumbles away and is densely infiltrated with leukocytes.

and suggested that thrombin and plasmin generation are central to menstrual hemostasis. This active fibrinolytic system seems confined to the endometrial glandular epithelium. Not surprisingly, therefore, antifibrinolytic drugs such as ϵ-aminocaproic acid or tranexamic acid, 1 g every 8 h for 3 days, have proved effective in decreasing menstrual blood loss.

Endometrial Prostaglandins

Since the discovery of an acidic lipid with oxytocic properties in menstrual fluid,[86] later shown to be $PGF_{2\alpha}$ and PGE_2, these substances have been implicated in normal and abnormal menstruation. Figure 17B-12 presents a scheme of the interrelationships of the various PGs or prostanoids. Intrauterine PGs derive from arachidonic acid, originating predominantly from the essential fatty acid linoleic acid. Arachidonic acid is a polyunsaturated 20-carbon chain with four double bonds and no nitrogen and is liberated from cell membrane phospholipids by the enzyme phospholipase A_2 in response to many physical and hormonal stimuli. In the best-studied pathway, arachidonic acid is oxygenated rapidly by the enzyme PG synthetase or cyclooxygenase (COX) to form a family of prostaglandins; each contains only two double bonds. Later research discovered a second enzyme, lipoxygenase (LOX); its products, the *leukotrienes*, have a straight-chain conformation. *Eicosanoids* is the generic name for both COX and LOX products. In the COX path, the initial intermediates generated are two endoperoxides, PGG_2 and PGH_2. Both these substances are pivotal in liberating at least three groups of prostanoids. $PGF_{2\alpha}$ and PGE_2 are among the most studied, in part because of their potency in induction of myometrial contraction. $PGF_{2\alpha}$ and thromboxane A_2 (TXA_2) are potent vasoconstrictors; conversely, PGE_2 and especially prostacyclin (PGI_2) cause vasodilation. PGI_2 also dissociates platelets, while TXA_2 aggregates platelets. Both PGE_2 and TXA_2 are rapidly converted to more stable products, including 6-oxo-PGF_1 and TXB_2, respectively. Estrogen stimulates COX-mediated synthesis of endo-

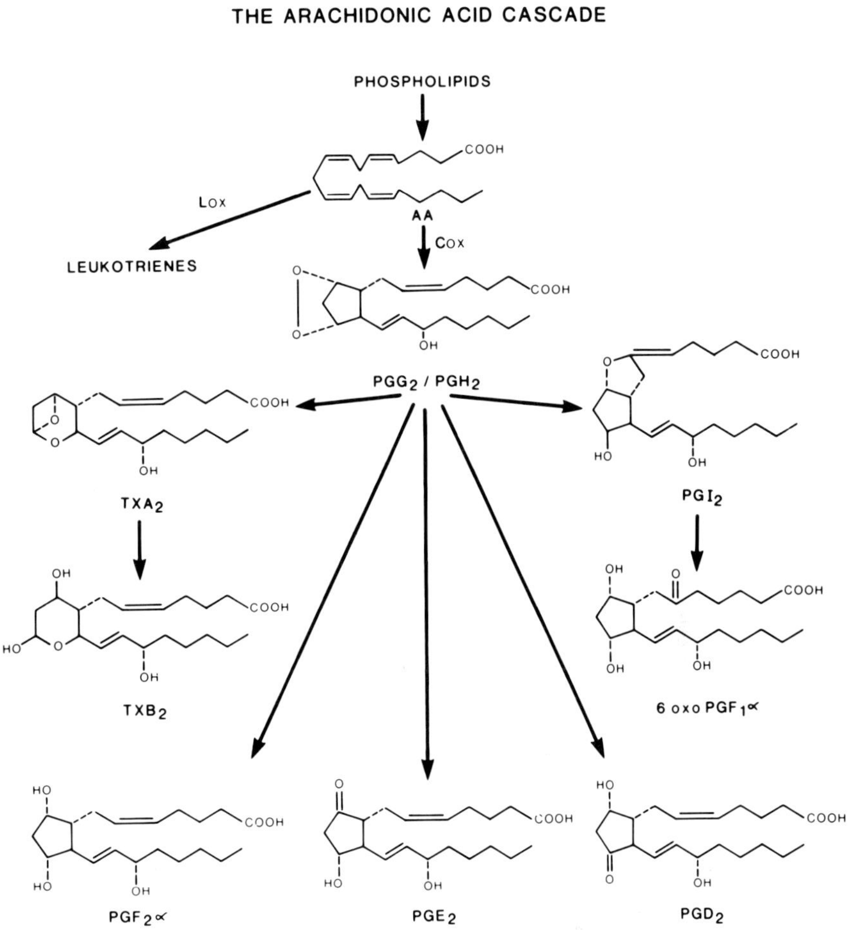

FIGURE 17B-12 The cyclooxygenase (COX) and lipoxygenase (LOX) cascade pathways of arachidonic acid (AA) metabolism. Note the pivotal position of the endoperoxide intermediates PGG_2 and PGH_2 in the production of the three classes of prostanoids, the thromboxanes (TXA_2 and TXB_2), prostacyclin (PGI_2), and the prostaglandins $PGF_{2\alpha}$, PGE_2, and PGD_2.

metrial $PGF_{2\alpha}$ and PGE_2 in women. In contrast, progesterone inhibits this production from proliferative and secretory phase endometrium. The precise intracellular mechanisms controlling steroid induction of PG synthesis are unknown.

$PGF_{2\alpha}$ is quantitatively the major endometrial prostanoid liberated during the human menstrual cycle. As estrogen does stimulate COX activity, it is not surprising that prostaglandin production rates are high in the proliferative phase of the menstrual cycle. In early human pregnancy, decidua contains less $PGF_{2\alpha}$ than is found in secretory endometrium. This chronic suppression appears due to an inhibitor of COX which is identifiable in amniotic fluid and maternal serum. The origin and nature of this endogenous inhibitor of prostaglandin synthesis by amniochorion is unknown, though suppression by decidual prolactin or a metabolite is possible.[87]

Excessive menstrual blood loss may affect up to 20 percent of women. In the majority of individuals, no organic cause for this menorrhagia is found and the diagnosis of dysfunctional uterine bleeding is made. Clinically, it is important to realize that only approximately one-third of the patients presenting with menorrhagia will indeed have excessive menstrual blood loss (> 80 ml).

It is now evident that excessive menstrual blood loss is associated with changes in PG production by the uterus. Endometrium from women with ovular dysfunctional uterine bleeding, which is common in young adults, synthesizes more PGE_2 than that of normal women, and the myometrial production of PGI_2 is markedly enhanced.[88] In women with anovular dysfunctional bleeding, excessive menstrual loss is associated with a relative deficiency of $PGF_{2\alpha}$ synthesis. There is, in fact, a direct relationship between the $PGE_2/PGF_{2\alpha}$ ratio and the amount of blood loss; it may be, therefore, that menstrual loss is determined by the relative synthesis of PGs with mainly vasoconstrictive properties on the one hand ($PGF_{2\alpha}$) as opposed to those with vasodilatory properties (PGE_2, and PGI_2) on the other.

Conventional gynecological management of menorrhagia in young adults, in whom pregnancy is excluded, is to prescribe a progestogen in an attempt to induce a secretory and regressed endometrium. Drugs such as norethindrone, 5 to 10 mg per day from days 5 to 25 of the cycle, are suitable for this purpose. Note that the first menses on this treatment may still be heavy; the patient should be forewarned about this. For the majority of patients, this long administration of an androgenic progestogen will usually lead to endometrial atrophy sufficient to reduce the amount of menstrual bleeding. An alternative drug is medroxyprogesterone acetate, 10 mg per day from days 5 to 25 of the cycle. Although it has been customary to state that oral progesterone is not clinically useful because of its erratic intestinal absorption, recent studies suggest that a dosage of 300 mg of progesterone (in micronized form) per day, if absorbed satisfactorily, leads to normal progesterone concentrations and to a normal secretory endometrium.[89] By not having the powerful androgenic side effects of many synthetic progestogens, micronized progesterone is expected to have a major place in the management of menorrhagia in the near future.

COX inhibitors reduce menstrual blood loss as well as reducing the pain of primary dysmenorrhea by reducing the formation of $PGF_{2\alpha}$ and PGE_2. Drugs such as mefenamic acid should be prescribed in relatively high dosage (1000 to 1500 mg per day), to prevent the generation of the prostaglandins contributing to these two gynecological disorders. The aim of treatment here is to prevent the synthesis of PGs; it is therefore important for the clinician to advise the patient to begin taking these tablets at the first sign of impending menstruation, rather than to try to avoid taking medication until the pain becomes unbearable.

In an important double-blind, crossover clinical trial, Shan and colleagues demonstrated that the PG synthetase inhibitor ibuprofen, at 1200 mg per day beginning 3 days before the expected onset of menses through 3 days after the onset of menses, decreased, by a factor of 3 to 4, both menstrual pain symptoms and $PGF_{2\alpha}$ concentrations measured in menstrual fluid.[90] In placebo cycles, there was a close correlation between the severity of menstrual pain, as assessed daily by the patient, and the level of $PGF_{2\alpha}$ released during the corresponding period.

Premenstrual Syndrome

There is no widely accepted definition of the common clinical entity of premenstrual syndrome (PMS) and the need exists for improved classification.[91] The incidence of PMS is not known, although 20 to 40 percent of menstruating women report some degree of recurrent mental or physical incapacitation prior to menses.[92] The range of symptoms commonly includes a disordered mood (irritability, depression), breast tenderness and abdominal bloating, headache, and altered appetite (especially carbohydrate craving) and libido. There have been many unsuccessful attempts to conclusively define clinical, menstrual, or hormonal parameters unique to PMS sufferers, including investigation of the sex steroid profile, the renin-angiotensin system, vitamin deficiency, glucose metabolism, and the opiate neuropeptides.[92,93] Recently, it has been suggested that ovulation occurs prematurely in PMS patients.[94] Although it may be a clinical disorder of the ovary, the PMS complex is still so imprecisely defined that other mechanisms are equally plausible. Social and psychological factors are important in the subjective assessment of PMS severity.[94,95] Not surprisingly, in view of the poorly defined pathophysiology, there are a large number of therapies available, commonly including relaxation therapy, pyridoxine, diuretics (including spironolactone), oral contraceptives, bromocriptine, and metronidazole, while recently "medical oophorectomy" using GnRH agonist therapy was reported to be of benefit.[96] All may be of some benefit in selected cases. It is suggested that a therapeutic trial be commenced using the most benign therapy and, if unsuccessful, other agents be tried in line with the severity of symptoms and the patient's desire for intervention.

OVARIAN DISORDERS IN MIDDLE AGE

Endocrinology of the Menopause

The menopause is the permanent cessation of menstruation which results from loss of ovarian follicular activity. The term *perimenopause*, or climacteric, signifies the period of months when the endocrine, biological, and clinical features of declining ovarian function commence until the first year after menses have ceased (Fig. 17B-13). The postmenopause dates from the menopause but, by convention, cannot be determined until spontaneous amenorrhoea has persisted for 12 months.[97] Uterine bleeding which recommences after 12 months of amenorrhoea in a woman over the age of 40 years requires investigation to exclude endometrial cancer.

The median age at menopause is about 50 years for women of European origin in developed countries, but there is no generally agreed range for this age, making the definition of premature menopause arbitrary. Cessation of ovarian function prior to the age of 40 years would be regarded widely as consistent with the concept of a premature menopause (see Prema-

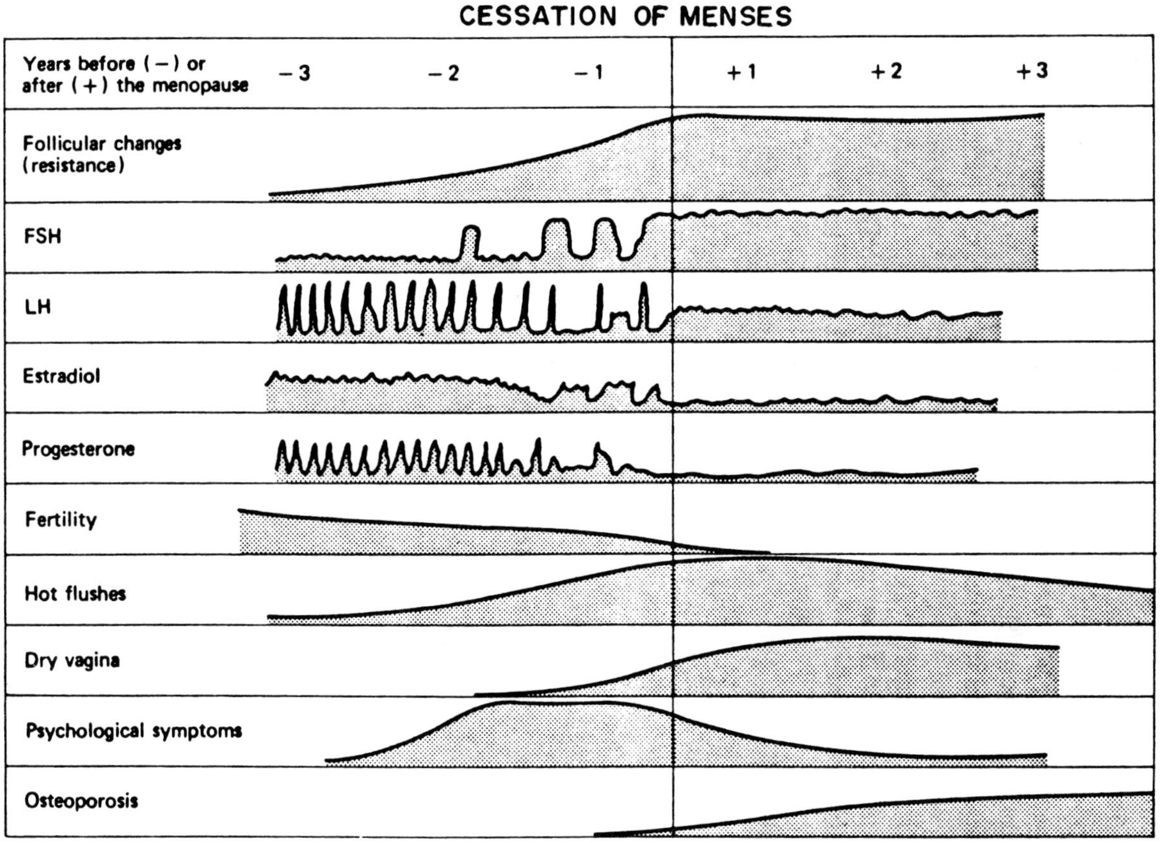

FIGURE 17B-13 Schematic representation of some clinical, biological, and endocrinological features of peri- and postmenopausal years.

ture Ovarian Failure, above). Cigarette smoking is associated with a slightly reduced age at menopause.[98]

Endocrinologically, the major features of the loss of ovarian function are a marked fall (by 90 to 95 percent) in circulating estradiol level (from normal follicular-phase levels of 200 to 500 pM to 30 to 50 pM) and marked elevations of FSH concentration (10- to 15-fold, from normal follicular-phase levels of 3 to 7 IU/liter to 40 to 50 IU/liter) and LH concentration (threefold, from 3 to 7 to 10 to 20 IU/liter) (Fig. 17B-14). Progesterone secretion virtually ceases. The increase in gonadotropin levels results from loss of steroidal feedback, and presumably also from loss of ovarian inhibin. During the transition between normal menstrual cyclicity and the postmenopausal period, a variety of hormonal patterns may be encountered. In women over the age of 45 who continue to have regular cycles, the follicular phase in particular may show moderate elevations in serum FSH levels and decreases in serum estradiol levels, with LH and progesterone secretion remaining unchanged.[99] The menopausal transition is marked by considerable variability in menstrual cycle length; during this phase, apparently bizarre hormonal changes are found,[100] including elevation of levels of FSH or LH alone, FSH with LH, and high or low levels of estrogens. In contrast to the decline in ovarian estrogen production, ovarian androgen production persists and there is little change in circulating testosterone concentration after the menopause. This may be an important consideration when decisions are made regarding removal of the ovaries in peri- and postmenopausal women. Because of the variability in FSH and estradiol levels, the diagnosis of the menopausal state may not be made reliably by means of hormonal measurements alone, especially in women who have experienced lack of menses for only a few months. From a practical viewpoint, the possibility of fertility cannot be excluded until 1 year after the menopause; estimates of the annual risk of pregnancy are 10 to 20 percent for women aged 40 to 44, and 2 to 3 percent for women aged 45 to 49.[101] The finding of a clearly elevated serum FSH concentration and a serum estradiol level < 50 pM in a woman with 6 months or more of

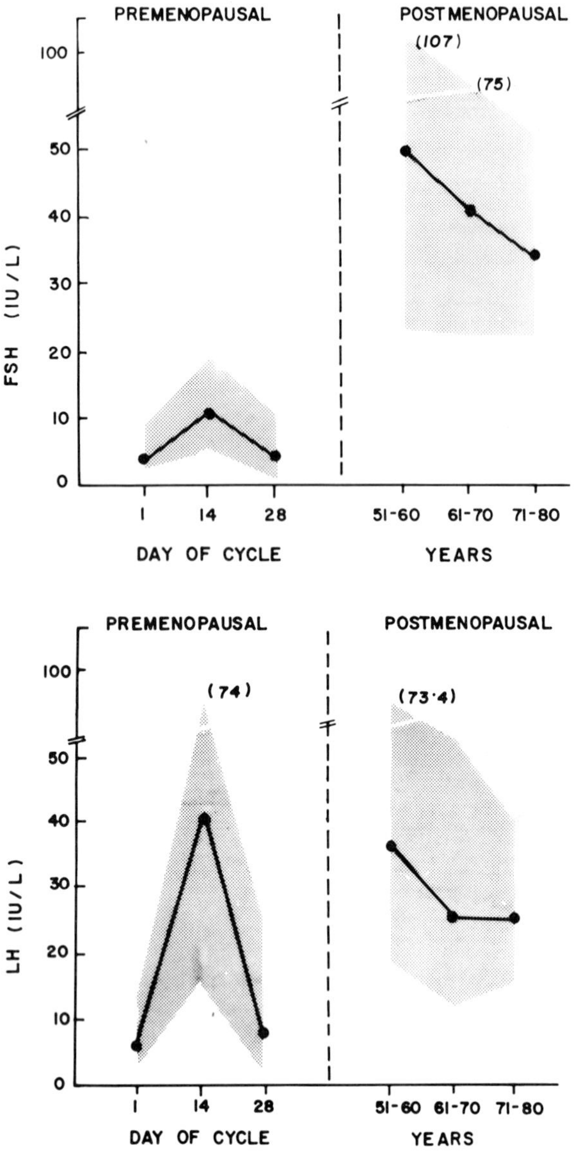

FIGURE 17B-14 Diagrammatic representation of serum FSH and LH concentrations during the follicular, periovulatory, and luteal phases of the normal menstrual cycle and during the postmenopausal period. Note that postmenopausal FSH levels greatly exceed those found during the menstrual cycle.

amenorrhea certainly makes the diagnosis of the postmenopausal state highly probable.

Climacteric Symptoms

Perimenopausal patients may seek medical advice regarding the desirability of hormone replacement therapy (HRT) when they are asymptomatic, because of widespread prominence given to such therapy in the media. Alternately, vasomotor symptoms, psychological complaints, and/or loss of sexuality, often in the context of menstrual irregularity, are frequent reasons for presentation.

The most characteristic perimenopausal symptom is the hot flush (or flash), found in one study in 17 percent of women in the age range 42 to 62 years still experiencing regular cycles, in 40 percent of those with irregular cycles, 65 percent of those in the 1 to 2 years after the menopause, and 35 percent of those 5 to 10 years post menopause.[102] The symptom is described as a brief sensation of heat usually involving the face and upper trunk; it is accompanied by a rise in skin temperature (up to 4°C or more), peripheral vasodilation, transient increase in heart rate, and lowering of skin resistance.[103] There may be sweating, chills, nervousness, irritability, and headache. Flushes are thought to be due to a sympathetic discharge[104] and occur more or less simultaneously with pulses of LH secretion, though they are not the result of such pulses.[105] Thus, it is likely that a hypothalamic event, in which there is a transient downward resetting of the central thermostat, occurs at the same time as the episodic discharge of GnRH.

Flush frequency is variable; occurrence during the night leads to sleep disturbance. Estrogen therapy specifically relieves the symptom, providing strong evidence for the role of estrogen withdrawal in its occurrence. Relief may also be afforded by the central α-adrenergic agonist drug clonidine and by progestogens, such as medroxyprogesterone. Techniques such as continual recording of such symptoms now allow objective monitoring of flush frequency, permitting proper study of the efficacy of various treatment regimens.[106]

Controversy has surrounded the specificity of psychological symptoms in relation to the menopause; the degree to which such symptoms as fatigue, irritability, depression, and a general sense of feeling unwell are a reflection of "general lack of well-being" or of more specific psychological states such as depression is unclear, but there is substantial evidence that estrogen replacement will also alleviate such symptoms, particularly in women who have no prior history of psychological disturbance.[107]

A decline in sexual interest of varying severity often occurs after the menopause.[108] There may be associated vaginal dryness and dyspareunia, but correction of the latter with local or systemic estrogens often fails to restore sexual interest and enjoyment.

Urinary symptoms, such as frequency and urgency of micturition, may be experienced for the first time by peri- and postmenopausal women, but their association with estrogen deficiency has not been established clearly. In the absence of another underlying cause, a trial of vaginal or systemic estrogen therapy may be rewarding.

Alterations in appearance due to declining skin quality are common complaints in perimenopausal women, and the skin has been shown to contain estradiol receptors.[109] Nevertheless, a clear relationship of skin texture to estrogen has not been established and thus the role of estrogen therapy in skin care for older women is unclear.

The symptoms of flushes, psychological disturbances, and loss of sexuality are self-limited, and respond very satisfactorily to HRT. The pressure of such symptoms constitutes a strong indication for at least short-term HRT, for a duration of 6 to 12 months. During such a limited period, the choice of estrogen is not a major issue, and oral therapy with a synthetic estrogen such as ethinyl estradiol (10 to 20 μg daily) or a natural estrogen [e.g., conjugated equine estrogens (Premarin), 0.625 to 1.25 mg daily, or estradiol valerate, 1 to 2 mg daily] is used conventionally. Although not mandatory with short-term therapy, it is prudent to add a cyclic progestogen (e.g., medroxyprogesterone, 10 mg daily for 12 days per month) in order to avoid unexpected vaginal bleeding. Topical vaginal estrogen cream is valuable for specific relief of vaginal dryness or dyspareunia. Contraindications to estrogen therapy include a history of breast cancer or endometrial cancer, recent undiagnosed genital bleeding, liver disease, or history of thromboembolism. For patients with loss of libido persisting despite adequate oral estrogen replacement, combined subcutaneous implants of estradiol (40 mg) and testosterone (50 mg) have proved very efficacious.[110]

Postmenopausal Problems

OSTEOPOROSIS

Osteoporosis is defined as a reduction in the mass of bony tissue relative to the volume of anatomical bone. Conventionally, the reference value for normal bones is taken as that derived from a normal young (premenopausal) adult population; a significant reduction is to less than 2 SD below that mean. A variety of techniques are available for measurement of bone mass; CT and densitometry of the forearm, spine, and neck of femur have been introduced relatively recently and are likely to enter widespread use. There is a growing tendency to make such measurements in women attending menopause clinics, in order to identify those at increased risk for the later development of osteoporotic fractures, which especially affect the radius, spine, and femoral neck. Loss of cortical bone in particular predisposes women to radial and femoral fractures while loss of trabecular bone leads to vertebral crush fractures.

The exact pathogenesis of postmenopausal osteoporosis is not understood; although there appears to be a clear association between cessation of ovarian function and loss of bone mass, there is no evidence for a direct effect of estradiol on the skeleton: no estrogen receptors have been found in bony tissue. It is hypothesized that estrogens somehow have a protective effect on bone, opposing bony resorption induced by parathormone, vitamin D, or both. Controversy exists regarding the role of calcitonin; there is some evidence that its levels fall after the menopause and are stimulated by estrogen. The mean daily calcium requirement to maintain calcium balance increases after the menopause from about 500 to about 1500 mg.[111] There is a slight rise in serum calcium and phosphate levels after the menopause, as well as in urinary calcium and hydroxyproline levels.[112] Measurement of the fasting urinary calcium/creatinine ratio provides a useful index of the rate of loss of calcium in the urine.

The prevention of postmenopausal osteoporosis is a major reason to consider long-term HRT (further discussed below); three separate case-control studies have shown a risk ratio for fractures of about 2 to 3 in favor of estrogen therapy.[113–115] Ensuring an adequate calcium intake (about 1500 mg daily) and encouragement of physical exercise are useful general measures.

The treatment of established osteoporosis is still controversial; increased calcium intake (e.g., effervescent calcium tablets containing 1 g calcium given at night), sodium fluoride (50 mg daily), calcitonin, and supplementary vitamin D are promoted, with or without added estrogen.[116] Recent reports have shown that calcium absorption can be normalized in women with postmenopausal osteoporosis using small doses (0.5 to 0.75 μg per day) of calcitriol.[117]

ATHEROSCLEROTIC CARDIOVASCULAR DISEASE

Because cardiovascular disease is a leading cause of death, its possible relationship to cessation of ovarian function and its possible prevention by HRT assume great importance.[118] It has been shown that the menopause is associated with increases in levels of serum cholesterol and triglycerides, accepted risk factors for atherosclerotic vascular disease.[119–121] Two population studies have examined the relationship between carefully defined cardiovascular disease and the menopause. In Goteborg, Sweden, systematic samples from birth cohorts of women were examined and classified on the basis of past history of myocardial infarction, angina pectoris, and electrocardiographic evidence of ischemic heart disease.[121] The observed cases were compared to unaffected members of their cohort in three age groups, and those in all three affected groups were found to have undergone earlier menopause. In the Framingham study, an increase in the incidence of coronary heart disease and in the severity of the presenting syndrome were found to occur after menopause among the 2873 women who had been followed up for up to 24 years after initial assessment.[125] No premenopausal women developed myocardial infarction or died of coronary heart disease, whereas such events were commonly seen among postmenopausal women. Within each of the age groups 40 to 44, 45 to 49, and 50 to 54 years, coronary heart disease was more than twice as common in postmenopausal as in premenopausal women, whether the menopause was spontaneous or surgical. In another study, of American nurses, those who had had bilateral oophorectomy before the age of 35 years had more than seven times the risk of having a nonfatal myocardial infarct as compared with premenopausal women of the same age and with the same risk factors.[127] Although there are other data not supportive of these associations, it can reasonably be concluded that the menopause is associated with an increase in the risks of morbidity and mortality from atherosclerotic cardiovascular disease.

Estrogen therapy alone, given to postmenopausal women, has beneficial effects on coronary risk factors, causing a fall in serum cholesterol and low-density lipoprotein levels, and an increase in concentration of high-density lipoprotein,[124,125] with variable effects on levels of plasma triglycerides. Synthetic progestogens tend to nullify these estrogen effects.[126] Effects of estrogen on blood coagulation factors are variable; dosage, route of administration and the nature of the estrogen preparation are important. Thus, oral estrogens cause increases in levels of factors VII, IX, X, and X complex[127,128] and lower concentrations of anticoagulation factors such as antithrombin III. Percutaneously administered estradiol is without effect on the last.[129]

Whether estrogen therapy leads to an alteration in the actual occurrence of cardiovascular disease remains controversial. At least one study of death from ischemic heart disease in a retirement community suggests a strong protective effect of oral estrogen (risk ratio with estrogen therapy 0.43).[130] A report from the Lipid Research Clinics Program follow-up study indicated a marked decrease in all-causes mortality in estrogen users compared with nonusers.[131] It is now clear that progestogen must be used routinely in patients on long-term HRT who have intact uteri; however, no epidemiological data are available which examine estrogen-progestogen combinations for their effect on heart disease. This remains a major unanswered question in the overall assessment of risk-benefit ratios for HRT.

Table 17B-5. Types of Estrogen Available for Therapeutic Use

Natural:
Estradiol
Estrone and estrone sulfate
Estriol
Conjugated (mixture of sodium estrone sulfate, sodium equilin sulfate, sodium equilenin sulfate, and sodium estradiol sulfate).
Synthetic
Ethinyl estradiol
Mestranol
Quinestrol
Diethylstilbestrol
Dienestrol

Long-Term Hormone Replacement Therapy

MODES OF ADMINISTRATION

From a therapeutic viewpoint, estrogens are arbitrarily classified into those which occur in nature and those which are synthetic (Table 17B-5). Natural estrogens include estradiol and its esters, estrone sulfate (including its piperazine salt), estriol, and conjugated equine estrogens (Premarin, a mixture of estrone sulfate, equilin, and equilenin). The major synthetic estrogen is ethinyl estradiol; mestranol and diethylstilbestrol are additional examples. Estrogens have most commonly been given orally, in daily doses listed in Table 17B-6. Although preparations differ in their relative potencies, depending on the assay end point, the doses listed are approximately equivalent in terms of FSH suppression (adapted from Ref. 132). The synthetic estrogens are relatively more potent than the natural estrogens in their hepatic effects.

Table 17B-6. Oral Estrogen Preparations and Approximately Equivalent Daily Doses

Preparation	Daily dose
Conjugated equine estrogens	0.625–1.25 mg
Piperazine estrone sulfate	1.25–2.5 mg
Estradiol valerate	1–2 mg
Micronized estradiol	1–2 mg
Ethinyl estradiol	10–20 μg

The estrogens may be given cyclically (3 weeks on, 1 week off) in the belief that this will minimize the likelihood of development of endometrial hyperplasia, but there is no evidence that continuous oral administration results in a greater risk,[133] and some patients suffer recurrence of hot flushes during the week off therapy on the cyclic regimen.

Oral estrogen administration results in "first-pass" effects on the liver, with maximal opportunity for effects on hepatic protein synthesis. Synthetic estrogens are particularly potent from this standpoint, and produce significant increases in the synthesis of renin substrate, SHBG, corticosteroid-binding globulin, thyroxine-binding globulin, and lipoproteins.[134] This has led to the development of various parenteral estrogen preparations, e.g., subcutaneous estradiol implants, estradiol gels for application to the skin, estrogen-containing vaginal creams, and, recently, transdermal therapeutic systems.[135] These preparations have little if any effect on hepatic protein synthesis, and may thus have at least theoretical advantages for long-term use. In addition, while all natural orally administered estrogens give rise to plasma levels of estrone markedly in excess of that of plasma estradiol, the parenteral preparations give plasma levels of estradiol greater than of estrone, mimicking the physiological situation of the normal follicular phase of the menstrual cycle.[135-137]

In women with an intact uterus, cyclic administration of a progestogen for a minimum of 10 and preferably 12 to 13 days each month is mandatory in order to avoid the risk of estrogen-induced endometrial hyperplasia, which may progress to endometrial carcinoma.[138] Other possible beneficial effects of the added progestogen (e.g., possible reduction in risk of occurrence of breast cancer, actual increase in bone mass), remain controversial and the potential adverse effects (neutralization of the possible beneficial effects of estrogens) have not been well defined. Because of some data indicating that 17-acetoxyprogestogens are metabolically more favorable than 19-norprogestogens,[126] it is common practice to recommend the use of medroxyprogesterone acetate at an oral dosage of 10 mg daily for 12 days per month, which may be given in the first 12 calendar days for simplicity. An alternative progestogen is norethindrone, 5 mg daily. There is evidence that much lower doses of 19-nortestosterone derivatives may be fully effective in preventing endometrial hyperplasia and regimens such as 0.7 mg daily of norethindrone or 60 μg of norgestrel (2 tablets of the relevant progestogen-only oral contraceptive preparation) given for 10 to 13 days per month may provide the necessary endometrial protection with few, if any, metabolic side effects. For patients who have had a hysterectomy, the use of progestogen is controversial, the major unanswered question being whether cyclic progestogens provide any protection against a possible small increased risk of breast cancer associated with estrogen therapy.[139]

Routine supervision of patients on long-term HRT should include blood pressure measurement, breast examination, and assessment of lipid levels, with endometrial sampling in any patient who develops unexpected uterine bleeding. Whether endometrial biopsy should be undertaken routinely before long-term HRT is instituted is controversial; in a patient previously untreated with estrogen, the procedure may be associated with significant discomfort, and if there is no history of abnormal uterine bleeding and a cyclic progestogen is used, endometrial biopsy is unlikely to yield clinically significant information. Especially in patients with a history of benign breast disease or a family history of breast cancer, routine mammography is desirable.

BENEFITS AND RISKS

The major potential benefits of long-term HRT are the established benefit of its prevention of osteoporosis and hence of lowering the risk of osteoporosis-associated fracture, particularly of the femoral neck, and the theoretical benefit of the prevention of atherosclerotic cardiovascular disease. If the latter is established on the basis of further epidemiological studies, it will be extremely important to consider using HRT more routinely in the community.

The major potential risks are of endometrial and breast cancer. Although it has been established that estrogen therapy without accompanying progestogen leads to a substantially increased risk of endometrial hyperplasia and carcinoma, this risk is abolished if regular cyclic progestogen is administered.[97,140] The question of whether HRT causes an increased risk of developing breast cancer is unresolved;[97,141] if a risk does exist, it is relatively small (risk ratio ~2). However, because breast cancer is an extremely frightening prospect for the individual patient, the risk must be taken into account in making a decision concerning long-term HRT. It has proved extremely difficult to arrive at an objective resolution of the benefit/risk ratio for HRT, and the situation has become ever more complex because there are few epidemiological data on the benefits (and risks) of long-term HRT using both estrogens and progestogens. Further, there are no comprehensive data on regimens of parenteral estrogen administration. The authors have adopted the approach of being ready to administer long-term HRT to any woman who seeks such therapy, provided that no contraindications are present, and provided that she is willing to tolerate the inconvenience of monthly withdrawal bleeding. A regimen commonly used is oral estradiol valerate, 1 to 2 mg, or conjugated equine estrogen, 0.625 to 1.25 mg daily, continuously with medroxyprogesterone acetate, 10 mg daily, for the first 12 calendar days each month. Patients are reviewed at 6- to 12-month intervals for assessment of blood pressure and breasts, and for measurement of serum lipids. Endometrial biopsy is undertaken only when abnormal uterine bleeding is reported.

It is likely that parenteral estrogen administration will become much more widely used in the future.

Postmenopausal Bleeding

Patients with or without HRT may develop bleeding more than 12 months after the cessation of their spontaneous menstrual cycles. Each patient with unanticipated postmenopausal bleeding must be thoroughly evaluated because of the increased incidence of endometrial adenocarcinoma, which in some series has reached 23 percent.[142] Outpatient curettage using a Novak or Randall cannula or suction devices such as the Vabra aspirator have all been reported to correlate with formal inpatient cervical dilatation and uterine curettage in approximately 90 percent of subjects.[143] In the 10 percent of outpatients in whom the endometrial cavity cannot be sounded or in whom repeated or persistent postmenopausal bleeding occurs, inpatient examination under anesthesia and curettage is mandatory. Gambrell and Greenblatt have emphasized the usefulness of progestogen and estrogen therapy to arrest heavy postmenopausal bleeding and the value of cyclic courses of progestogens to reverse hyperplasia of the endometrium.[144] Patients with any degree of endometrial hyperplasia must have repeat curettage after 3 months of progestogen treatment and hysterectomy if hyperplasia persists.

Acknowledgments

D.L.H. is a Wellcome Trust Senior Clinical Research Fellow. Jill Volfsbergs and Joan Williams have proved inexhaustible in typing this chapter and their superb efforts are greatly appreciated.

REFERENCES

1. Ross JL, Cassorla FG, Skerda NC, Valk IM, Loriaux DL, Cutler GB: A preliminary study of the effect of estrogen dose on growth in Turner's syndrome. *N Engl J Med* 309:1104, 1983.

2. Lutjen P, Trounson AO, Leeton JF, Findlay JK, Wood EC, Renou P: The establishment and maintenance of pregnancy using in vitro fertilization and embryo donation in a patient with primary ovarian failure. *Nature* 307:174, 1984.

3. Chan CLK, Findlay JK, Healy DL, Leeton JF, Lutjen PJ, Renou PM, Rodgers PA, Trounson AO, Wood EC: Oocyte donation and IVF for hypergonadotropic hypogonadism: Clinical state of the art. *Obstet Gynecol Surv* (in press).

4. Burger HG, Bremner WJ, de Kretser DM, Healy DL, Hudson B, Kovacs GT, Padron R, Wilson JD: Hypogonadotropic hypogonadism in male and female, in Crosignani PG, Reuben BL (eds): *Endocrinology of Human Infertility—New Aspects.* London, Toronto, Sydney, Academic, 1981, p 185.

5. Lieblich JM, Rogol AD, White BJ, Rosen SW: Syndrome of anosmia with hypogonadotropic hypogonadism (Kallmann's syndrome). *Am J Med* 73:506, 1982.

6. Dewhurst CJ (ed): *Integrated Obstetrics and Gynaecology for Postgraduates.* London, Blackwell, 1981.

7. Healy DL, Hodgen GD: The endocrinology of human endometrium. *Obstet Gynecol Surv* 38:509, 1983.

8. Fraser IS, Michie EA, Wide L, Baird DT: Pituitary gonadotropins and ovarian function in adolescent dysfunctional uterine bleeding. *J Clin Endocrinol Metab* 37:407, 1973.

9. Coulam CB: Premature ovarian failure. *Fertil Steril* 38:645, 1982.

10. Friedman CI, Barrows H, Kim MH: Hypergonadotropic hypogonadism. *Am J Obstet Gynecol* 145:360, 1983.

11. O'Herlihy C, Pepperell RJ, Evans JH: The significance of FSH elevation in young women with disorders of ovulation. *Br Med J* 281:1447, 1980.

12. Keelam CV, Stringfellow S, Frohoefnagel D: Evidence for a genetic factor in the etiology of premature ovarian failure. *Fertil Steril* 40:693, 1983.

13. Warne GL, Fairley KF, Hobbs JH, Martin FIR: Cyclophosphamide-induced ovarian failure. *N Engl J Med* 289:1159, 1973.

14. Alper MM, Garner PR: Premature ovarian failure: Its relationship to autoimmune disease. *Obstet Gynecol* 66:27, 1985.

15. Wright CSW, Jacobs HS: Spontaneous pregnancy in a patient with hypergonadotrophic ovarian failure. *Br J Obstet Gynaecol* 86:389, 1979.

16. Healy DL, Lutjen PJ, Chan CLK, Leeton JF, Trounson AO, Wood EC: Artificial menstrual cycles for IVF, in de Cherney A, Naftolin F (eds): *Serono Symposium: In Vitro Fertilization.* Paris, 1986.

17. Lutjen PJ, Findlay JK, Trounson AO, Leeton JF, Chan CLK: Effects on plasma gonadotropins of cyclic steroid replacement prior to embryo transfer in women with premature ovarian failure. *J Clin Endocrinol Metab* 62:419, 1986.

18. Noyes RW, Hertig AT, Rock AJ: Dating the endometrial biopsy. *Fertil Steril* 1:3, 1950.

19. Kleinberg BL, Noel GL, Francz AG: Galactorrhea: A study of 235 cases, including 48 with pituitary tumours. *N Engl J Med* 296:589, 197.

20. Hooper JH, Welch VC, Point P, Schackleford RT: Abnormal lactation associated with tranquilizing drug therapy. *JAMA* 178:506, 1961.

21. Shearman RP (ed): *Clinical Reproductive Physiology.* Sydney, Blackwell, 1985.

22. Bonneville JF, Poulignot D, Cattin F, Couturier M, Mollet E, Dietmann JL: Computed tomographic demonstration of the effects of bromocriptine on pituitary microadenoma size. *Neuroradiology* 143:451, 1982.

23. Pepperell RJ, Evans JH, Brown JB, Smith MA, Healy DL, Burger HG: Serum prolactin levels and the value of bromocriptine (CB154) in the treatment of anovulatory infertility. *Br J Obstet Gynaecol* 84:58, 1977.

24. Healy DL, Burger HG: Human prolactin. II. Recent advances in therapy. *Aust NZ J Obstet Gynaecol* 17:73, 1977.

25. Johnston BG, Hall K, Kendall-Taylor P, Patrick D, Watson M, Cook DV: The effect of dopamine agonist withdrawal after longterm therapy in prolactinomas. *Lancet* 2:187, 1984.

26. Molitch ME: Pregnancy and the hyperprolactinemic woman. *N Eng J Med* 312:1364, 1985.

27. Griffith RW, Turkal JI, Braun P: Pituitary tumours in pregnancy in mothers treated with bromocriptine. *Br J Clin Pharmacol* 7:393, 1979.

28. Rasmussen C, Berg HT, Nillius SJ, Wide L: The return of menstruation and normalization of prolactin in hyperprolactinemic women with bromocriptine-induced pregnancy. *Fertil Steril* 44:31, 1985.

29. Rodman EF, Molitch ME, Post KD, Boller BJ, Reichman S: Long-term followup of transsphenoidal selective adenomectomy for prolactinoma. *JAMA* 252:921, 1984.

30. Serri U, Rasio E, Beauregard H, Hardy J, Sommer AN: Recurrence of hyperprolactinemia after selective transsphenoidal adenomectomy in women with prolactinoma. *N Engl J Med* 309:280, 1983.

31. Frisch RE, Revelle ER: Height and weight at menarche and a hypothesis of critical body weight and adolescent events. *Science* 169:397, 1970.

32. Van der Spuy ZM: Nutrition and reproduction. *Clin Obstet Gynecol* 12:579, 1985.

33. Berg HT, Nillius SJ, Wide L: Serum prolactin and gonadotrophin levels before and after luteinising hormone releasing hormone in the investigation of amenorrhoea. *Br J Obstet Gynaecol* 85:945, 1978.

34. McArthur JW, Bullen BA, Beitins IZ, Pagano M, Badger TM, Klibanski A: Hypothalamic amenorrhea in runners of normal body composition. *Endocr Res Commun* 7:13, 1980.

35. Herd HP, Palumbo PJ, Gharib H: Hypothalamic-endocrine dysfunction in anorexia nervosa. *Mayo Clin Proc* 51:711, 1977.

36. Hsu LKG: Outcome of anorexia nervosa. *Arch Gen Psychiatry* 37:1041, 1980.

37. Warren MP: The effects of exercise on pubertal progression and reproductive function in girls. *J Clin Endocrinol Metab* 51:1150, 1980.

38. Feicht CB, Johnston TS, Martin BJ, Sparkes KE, Wagner WW Jr: Secondary amenorrhoea in athletes. *Lancet* 2:1145, 1978.

39. Baker ER, Mathur RS, Kirk RS, Williamson HO: Female runners and secondary amenorrhea: Correlation with age, parity, mileage, and plasma hormonal and sex-hormone-binding globulin concentrations. *Fertil Steril* 36:183, 1981.

40. Marshall JC, Fraser TR: Amenorrhoea and anorexia nervosa: Assessment and treatment with clomiphene citrate. *Br Med J* 4:590, 1971.

41. Drinkwater BL, Nilson K, Chestnut CH, Bremner WJ, Shainholtz S, Southworth MB: Bone mineral content of amenorrheic and eumenorrheic athletes. *N Engl J Med* 311:277, 1984.

42. Franks S, Adams J, Mason H, Poulson D: Ovulatory disorders in women with polycystic ovary syndrome. *Clin Obstet Gynecol* 12:605, 1985.

43. Erickson GS, Hsueh AJW, Quigley ME, Rebar RW, Yen SSC: Functional studies of aromatase activity in human granulosa cells from normal and polycystic ovaries. *J Clin Endocrinol Metab* 49:514, 1979.

44. Baird DT, Corker CS, Davidson DW, Hunter WN, Michie EA, Van Look PFA: Pituitary-ovarian relationships in polycystic ovary syndrome. *J Clin Endocrinol Metab* 45:798, 1977.

45. Zumoff B, Freeman R, Coupey S, Saenger P, Markowitz N, Krean J: A chronobiologic abnormality in luteinizing hormone secretion in teenage girls with the polycystic-ovary syndrome. *N Engl J Med* 309:1206, 1983.

46. Rebar J, Judd HL, Yen SSC: Characterization of the inappropriate gonadotropin secretion in polycystic ovary syndrome. *J Clin Invest* 57:1320, 1976.

47. Futterweit W: Pathologic anatomy of polycystic ovarian disease, in Futterweit W (ed): *Polycystic Ovarian Disease.* New York, Springer-Verlag, 1984, p 41.

48. Quigley ME, Rakoff JS, Yen SSC: Increased luteinizing hormone sensitivity to dopamine inhibition in polycystic ovary syndrome. *J Clin Endocrinol Metab* 52:231, 1981.

49. Futterweit W: Pituitary tumors and polycystic ovarian disease. *Obstet Gynecol* 62:74, 1983.

50. McLachlan RI, Robertson DM, Burger HG, de Kretser DM: The radioimmunoassay of bovine and human follicular fluid and serum inhibin. *Mol Cell Endocrinol* 46:175, 1986.

51. Lobo RA: Disturbances of androgen secretion and metabolism in polycystic ovary syndrome. *Clin Obstet Gynecol* 12:633, 1983.

52. Chang RJ, Loufer LR, Meldrum DR, De Fazio J, Lu JKH, Vale WW, Rivier JE, Hudd HL: Steroid suppression in polycystic ovarian disease after ovarian suppression by a long-acting gonadotropin-releasing hormone agonist. *J Clin Endocrinol Metab* 56:897, 1983.

53. Chamlian DL, Taylor HB: Endometrial hyperplasia in young women. *Obstet Gynecol* 36:659, 1970.

54. Jackson RL, Docherty NB: The Stein-Leventhal syndrome: Analysis of 43 cases with special reference to association with endometrial carcinoma. *Am J Obstet Gynecol* 73:161, 1950.

55. Garcia JE, Jones GS, Wentz AC: The use of clomiphene citrate. *Fertil Steril* 28:707, 1977.

56. Spruce BA, Kendall-Taylor P, Dunlop W, Anderson AJ, Watson MJ, Cook DB, Gray C: The effect of bromocriptine in the polycystic ovary syndrome. *Clin Endocrinol* 20:481, 1984.

57. Ferriman D, Gallwey JD: The clinical assessment of body hair growth in women. *J Clin Endocrinol Metab* 21:1440, 1961.

58. Burgess CA, Edwards CRE: Hirsutography. *Br J Photography* 8:770, 1978.

59. Lobo RA, Goebelsmann U, Horton R: Evidence for the importance of peripheral tissue events in the development of hirsutism in polycystic ovary syndrome. *J Clin Endocrinol Metab* 57:393, 1983.

60. Barbieri MD, Ryan KJ: Hyperandrogenism, insulin resistance, and acanthosis nigricans syndrome: A common endocrinopathy with distinct pathophysiologic features. *Am J Obstet Gynecol* 147:90, 1983.

61. Holdaway IM, Croxson MS, Frengley PA, Ibbertson HK, Sheehan A, Fraser A, Evans MC, Knox B, France JT, Graham F, Liggins GC: Clinical and biochemical evaluation of patients with hirsutism. *Aust NZ J Obstet Gynaecol* 24:23, 1984.

62. Chetkowski RJ, DeFazio J, Shamonki I, Judd HL, Chang RJ: The incidence of late-onset congenital adrenal hyperplasia due to 21-hydroxylase deficiency among hirsute women. *J Clin Endocrinol Metab* 58:595, 1984.

63. Hammerstein J, Cupceancu B: Behandlung des hirsutismus mit cyproteronacetat. *Dtsch Med Wochenschr* 94:829, 1969.

64. Shapiro G, Evron S: A novel use of spironolactone: Treatment of hirsutism. *J Clin Endocrinol Metab* 51:429, 1980.

65. Marshall WA, Tanner JM: Variations in pattern of pubertal changes in girls. *Arch Dis Child* 44:291, 1969.

66. Hurley DM, Brian R, Outch K, Stockdale J, Fry A, Hackman C, Clarke I, Burger HG: Induction of ovulation and fertility in amenorrheic women by pulsatile low-dose gonadotropin-releasing hormone. *N Engl J Med* 310:1069, 1984.

67. Lunenfeld B, Insler V: *Diagnosis and Treatment of Functional Infertility.* Berlin, Grosse Verlag, 1978.

68. Keogh EJ, personal communication.

69. Gemzell CA, Diczfalusy E, Tillinger KG: Clinical effect of human pituitary follicle stimulating hormone (FSH). *J Clin Endocrinol Metab* 18:1333, 1958.

70. Thompson CR, Hansen LM: Pergonal: A summary of clinical experience in the induction of ovulation and pregnancy. *Fertil Steril* 21:844, 1970.

71. Lunenfeld B, Insler V: Classification of amenorrheic states and their treatment by ovulation induction. *Clin Endocrinol* 3:223, 1974.

72. Brown JB, MacLeod S, MacNaughton C: A rapid method of measuring estrogens in human urine using a semi-automatic extractor. *J Endocrinol* 42:5, 1968.

73. McLean AR, Outch KH, Russel JM, Kovacs GT, Brian R, Burger HG, Dennis PM: The monitoring of induction of ovulation

by rapid radioimmunoassays of estrogen and pregnanediol glucuronides. *Ann Clin Biochem* 18:343, 1981.
74. O'Herlihy C, de Crespigny LJ, Robinson H: Monitoring ovarian follicular development with real time ultrasound. *Br J Obstet Gynaecol* 87:613, 1980.
75. Healy DL, Kovacs GT, Pepperell RJ, Burger HG: A normal cumulative conception rate with human pituitary gonadotropin. *Fertil Steril* 34:341, 1980.
76. Schenker JG, Polishuk WZ: Ovarian hyperstimulation syndrome. *Obstet Gynecol* 46:23, 1975.
76. Schenker JG, Polishuk WZ: Ovarian hyperstimulation syndrome. *Obstet Gynecol* 46:23, 1975.
77. Healy DL, Burger HG: Serum follicle-stimulating hormone, luteinizing hormone and prolactin during the induction of ovulation with exogenous gonadotropin. *J Clin Endocrinol Metab* 56:474, 1983.
78. Fleming R, Haxton MJ, Hamilton MPR, McGune GS, Black WP, MacNaughton MC, Coutts JRT: Successful treatment of infertile women with oligomenorrhea using a combination of an LHRH agonist and exogenous gonadotrophins. *Br J Obstet Gynaecol* 92:369, 1985.
79. Leyendecker G, Struve T, Potz EJ: Induction of ovulation with chronic intermittent (pulsatile) administration of LHRH in women with hypothalamic and hyperprolactinaemic amenorrhea. *Arch Gynecol* 229:177, 1980.
80. Hurley DM, Brian RJ, Burger HG: Ovulation induction with subcutaneous pulsatile gonadotropin-releasing hormone: Singleton pregnancies in patients with previous multiple pregnancies after gonadotropin therapy. *Fertil Steril* 40:575, 1983.
81. Mason P, Adams J, Morris DV, Tucker M, Price J, Voulgaris Z, Van der Spuy ZM, Sutherland I, Chambers GR, White S, Wheeler MJ, Jacobs HS: Induction of ovulation with pulsatile luteinising hormone releasing hormone. *Br Med J* 288:181, 1984.
82. Hallberg L, Hogdahl IEM, Nilsson L, Rybog T: Menstrual blood loss—a population study. *Acta Obstet Gynecol Scand* 45:320, 1966.
83. Cole SK, Billewicz WZ, Thomson AM: Sources of variation in menstrual blood loss. *J Obstet Gynaecol Br Cwlth* 78:933, 1971.
84. Buller FJ: Observations on the clotting of menstrual blood and clot formation. *Am J Obstet Gynecol* 111:535, 1971.
85. Bonnar J, Shepherd VL, Dockerey CJ: The haemostatic system and dysfunctional uterine bleeding. *Res Clin Forum* 5:277, 1983.
86. Pickles VR, Hall WS, Best FA, Smith GN: Prostaglandins in endometrium and menstrual fluid from normal and dysmenorrhoeic subjects. *J Obstet Gynaecol Br Cwlth* 72:185, 1965.
87. Healy DL: The clinical significance of endometrial prolactin. *Aust NZ J Obstet Gynaecol* 24:111, 1984.
88. Smith SK, Abel MH, Kelly RW, Baird DT: A role for prostacyclin (PGI_2) in excessive menstrual bleeding. *Lancet* 1:522, 1981.
89. Lane G, Sittle NC, Rider TA, Pryce-Davies J, Kine RJV, Whitehead MI: Dose-dependent effects of oral progesterone on the oestrogenised post-menopausal endometrium. *Br Med J* 287:1241, 1983.
90. Chan YW, Dawood MY, Fuchs F: Relief of dysmenorrhea with the prostaglandin synthetase inhibitor ibuprofen: The effect on prostaglandin levels in menstrual fluid. *Am J Obstet Gynecol* 135:102, 1979.
91. Freeman EW, Sondheimer S, Weinbaum PJ, Rickels K: Evaluating premenstrual symptoms in medical practice. *Obstet Gynecol* 65:500, 1985.
92. Reid RL, Yen SSC: Premenstrual syndrome. *Am J Obstet Gynecol* 139:85, 1981.
93. Bancroft J, Backstrom T: Premenstrual syndrome. *Clin Endocrinol* 22:247, 1985.
94. Wasp JSF, Butt WR, Edwards RL, Holder G: Hormonal studies in women with premenstrual tension. *Br J Obstet Gynaecol* 92:247, 1985.
95. Steege JF, Stout AL, Rupp SL: Relationships among premenstrual symptoms and menstrual cycle characteristics. *Obstet Gynecol* 65:398, 1985.
96. Muse KN, Cetel NS, Futterman LA, Yen SSC: The premenstrual syndrome: Effects of medical ovariectomy. *N Engl J Med* 311:1345, 1984.
97. Research on the menopause. Report of a WHO Scientific Group. World Health Organization technical report series 670, Geneva, 1981.
98. Kaufman DW, Slone D, Rosenberg L, Miettinen OS, Shapiro S: Cigarette smoking and age of natural menopause. *Am J Public Health* 70:420, 1980.
99. Sherman B, et al: The menopausal transition: Analysis of LH, FSH, estradiol, and progesterone concentrations during menstrual cycles of older women. *J Clin Endocrinol Metab* 42:629, 1976.
100. Metcalf MG, Donald RA, Livesey JH: Pituitary-ovarian function in normal women during the menopausal transition. *Clin Endocrinol* 14:245, 1981.
101. Gray RH: Biological and social interactions in the determination of late fertility. *J Biosoc Sci* (suppl) 6:97, 1979.
102. Jaszmann L, van Lith ND, Zaat JCA: The perimenopausal symptoms. *Med Gynaecol Sociol* 4:268, 1969.
103. Tataryn IV, Lomax P, Bajorek JG, Chesarek W, Meldrum DR, Judd HL: Postmenopausal hot flushes: A disorder of thermoregulation. *Maturitas* 2:101, 1980.
104. Sturdee DW, Wilson KA, Pipili E, Crocker AD: Physiological aspects of menopausal hot flush. *Br Med J* 2:79, 1979.
105. Casper RF, Yen SSC, Wilkes MM: Menopausal flushes: A neuroendocrine link with pulsatile luteinizing hormone secretion. *Science* 205:823, 1979.
106. Meldrum DR, Shamonki IM, Tataryn I, et al: Elevations in skin temperature of the finger as an objective index of postmenopausal hot flushes: Standardization of the technique. *Am J Obstet Gynecol* 135:713, 1979.
107. Dennerstein L, Burrows GD, Hyman GJ, Sharpe K: Hormone therapy and affect. *Maturitas* 1:247, 1979.
108. Hallstrom T: *Mental Disorder and Sexuality in the Climacteric.* Stockholm, Scandinavian University Books, Esselte Studium, 1973.
109. Hasselquist MB, Goldberg N, Schroeter A, Spelsberg TC: Isolation and characterization of the estrogen receptors in human skin. *J Clin Endocrinol Metab* 50:76, 1980.
110. Burger HG, Hailes J, Menelaus M, Nelson J, Hudson B, Balazs N: The management of persistent symptoms with oestradiol-testosterone implants: Clinical, lipid and hormonal results. *Maturitas* 6:351, 1984.
111. Heaney RP, et al: Calcium balance and calcium requirements in middle-aged women. *Am J Clin Nutr* 30:1603, 1977.
112. Crilly RG, et al: Steroid hormones, ageing and bone. *Clin Endocrinol Metab* 10:115, 1981.
113. Paganini-Hill A, et al: Menopausal estrogen therapy and hip fractures. *Ann Intern Med* 95:28, 1981.
114. Hutchinson TA, Polansky SM, Feinstein AR: Postmenopausal oestrogens protect against fractures of hip and distal radius. *Lancet* 2:705, 1979.
115. Weiss NS, et al: Decreased risk of fractures of the hip and lower forearm with postmenopausal use of estrogen. *N Engl J Med* 303:1195, 1980.
116. Riggs BL, Seeman E, Hodgson SE, Taves DR, O'Fallon WM: Effects of the fluoride/calcium regimen on vertebral fracture occurrence in post-menopausal osteoporosis. Comparison with conventional therapy. *N Engl J Med* 306:446, 1982.
117. Riggs BL, Nelson KI: Effect of long term treatment with calcitriol on calcium absorption and mineral metabolism in postmenopausal osteoporosis. *J Clin Endocrinol Metab* 61:457, 1985.
118. Bengtsson C, Lindquist O: Menopausal effects on risk factors for ischaemic heart disease. *Maturitas* 1:165, 1979.
119. Hjortland MC, McNamara PM, Kannel WB: Some athero-

genic concomitants of menopause: The Framingham study. *Am J Epidemiol* 103:304, 1976.
120. Shibata H, Matsuzaki T, Hapana S: Relationship of relevant factors of atherosclerosis to menopause in Japanese women. *Am J Epidemiol* 109:420, 1979.
121. Bengtsson C: Ischemic heart disease in women. *Acta Med Scand* (suppl) 549:75, 1973.
122. Gordon T, Kannell WB, Hjortland MC, McNamara PM: Menopause and coronary heart disease. The Framingham study. *Ann Intern Med* 89:157, 1978.
123. Rosenberg L, Hennekens CH, Rosner B, Belanger C, Rothman KJ, Speizer FE: Early menopause and the risk of myocardial infarction. *Am J Obstet Gynecol* 139:47, 1981.
124. Gustafson A, Svanborg A: Gonadal steroid effects on plasma lipoprotein and individual phospholipids. *J Clin Endocrinol Metab* 35:203, 1972.
125. Wallentin L, Larsson-Cohn V: Metabolic and hormonal effects of post-menopausal estrogen replacement. II. Plasma lipids. *Acta Endocrinol* 86:579, 1977.
126. Hirvonen E, Malkonen M, Manninen V: Effects of different progestogens on lipoproteins during postmenopausal replacement therapy. *N Engl J Med* 304:560, 1981.
127. Von Kaulla E, et al: Conjugated estrogens in hypercoagulability. *Am J Obstet Gynecol* 122:688, 1975.
128. Bonnar J, Haddon M, Hunter DH, Richards D, Thornton C: Coagulation system changes in postmenopausal women receiving oestrogen preparations. *Postgrad Med J* 52: (suppl 6) 30, 1976.
129. Elkik F: Potency and hepato-cellular effects of oestrogens after oral, percutaneous, and subcutaneous administration, in van Keep PA, Utian WH, Vermeulen A (eds): *The Controversial Climacteric,* workshop 12. Lancaster, England, MTP, 1982.
130. Ross RK, et al: Menopausal estrogen therapy and protection from ischaemic heart disease death. *Lancet* 1:858, 1981.
131. Bush TL, Cowan LD, Barrett-Connor E, Criqui MH, Karon JM, Wallace RB, Al Tyroler H, Rifkind BM: Estrogen use and all-cause mortality. *JAMA* 249:903, 1983.
132. Mashchak CA, Lobo RA, Dozono-Takano R, Eggena P, Nakamura RM, Brenner PF, Mishell DR: Comparison of pharmacodynamic properties of various estrogen formulations. *Am J Obstet Gynecol* 144:511, 1982.
133. Schiff I, Seta HK, Cramer D, Tulchinsky D, Ryan KJ: Endometrial hyperplasia in women on cyclic or continuous estrogen regimen. *Fertil Steril* 37:79, 1982.
134. Mandel FP, Geola FL, Lu JKH, Eggena P, Sambhi MP, Hershman JM, Judd HL: Biological effects of various doses of ethinyl estradiol in postmenopausal women. *Obstet Gynecol* 59:673, 1982.
135. Steingold KA, Laufer L, Chetkowski RJ, de Fazio JD, Watt DW, Meldrum DR, Judd HL: Treatment of hot flushes with transdermal estradiol administration. *J Clin Endocrinol Metab* 61:627, 1985.
136. Yen SSC, Martin PL, Burnier AM, et al: Circulating estradiol, estrone and gonadotropin levels following the administration of orally active 17-beta-estradiol in postmenopausal women. *J Clin Endocrinol Metab* 40:518, 1975.
137. Englund DE, Johansson EDB: Pharmacokinetic and pharmacodynamic studies on estradiol valerianate administered orally to postmenopausal women. *Acta Obstet Gynecol Scand* (suppl) 65:27, 1977.
138. Sturdee DW, Wade-Evans T, Paterson MEL, Thom M, Studd JWW: Relations between bleeding pattern, endometrial histology, and oestrogen treatment in menopausal women. *Br Med J* 1:1575, 1978.
139. Gambrell RD Jr, Maier RC, Sanders BI: Decreased incidence of breast cancer in postmenopausal estrogen-progestogen users. *Obstet Gynecol* 62:435, 1983.
140. Gambrell RD Jr: The prevention of endometrial cancer in postmenopausal women with progestogens. *Maturitas* 1:107, 1978.
141. Hulka BS: When is the evidence for "no association" sufficient? *JAMA* 252:81, 1984.
142. Keirse MJNC: Aetiology of postmenopausal bleeding. *Postgrad Med J* 49:344, 1973.
143. Kahler VL, Creasy RK, Morris JA: Value of the endometrial biopsy. *Obstet Gynecol* 34:91, 1969.
144. Gambrell RD, Greenblatt RV: Management of dysfunctional uterine bleeding with norgestrel-ethinyl estradiol. *Curr Med Dialogue* 42:80, 1975.

18

Sexual Differentiation

Jeremy S. D. Winter

Attempts to explain sexual dimorphism are as old as mankind itself, and countless theories have been promulgated to provide a rational basis for separate patterns of male and female development. Aristotle, with remarkable prescience, suggested that semen determined embryonic sex by its innate ability to impose maleness upon a process which otherwise tended to be female; the role of the female parent was seen to be essentially passive, providing the material and the environment for embryonic development. Two thousand years later, light microscopy led to the description of spermatozoa, ova, and the events of fertilization. It was probably Mendel who first perceived that sex might be a genetic character, obeying the laws of inheritance, but, like many of his ideas, the notion remained buried until this century. Painter in 1924 provided direct evidence for the role of the male parent in human sex determination when he showed that human primary spermatocytes contain an unequal pair of chromosomes, termed X and Y, which segregate into different gametes during the first meiotic division,[1] a finding which has since been confirmed by modern techniques of chromosome analysis.[2]

Sexual reproduction requires each parent to contribute equal (*haploid*) amounts of genetic material to the offspring, a mechanism which provides for rapid gene assortment, with increased opportunity for favorable combinations of genes to develop and be selected. In higher organisms the parents are of different sexes, maintained separate and distinct by the actions of unpaired sex chromosomes which contain the genetic information for sex determination. One sex (in mammals XX, or female) is homogametic while the other (XY, or male) is heterogametic. The Y chromosome contains important male-determining factors that direct the embryo away from an otherwise predetermined course of female differentiation. Fisher has pointed out that it is not necessary that all male characters be under the control of genes on the Y chromosome.[3] Rather, a single Y-linked gene need only cause male differentiation of the gonad; in turn, testicular hormones could activate or repress genes throughout the autosomal complement, a strategy which would allow any gene to become involved in producing sexual dimorphism.

The past quarter century has seen an increasing flood of new information and new insights into both the initial genetic process of sex determination and the endocrine mechanisms which subsequently direct sexual differentiation; indeed, it is probable that no aspect of prenatal development is better understood. Vital clues about these events have been provided by patients with various anatomical abnormalities of sexual differentiation. It is therefore fitting that these insights have led to the development of rapid and exact techniques for diagnosis and specific forms of therapy, which, if applied early and properly, can prevent much of the physical and psychological scarring which previously was the lot of these patients.

NORMAL SEX DETERMINATION AND SEXUAL DIFFERENTIATION

The appearance of a fertile adult with congruent secondary sexual characteristics and psychosexual orientation represents the denouement of a logical and ordered sequence which begins at conception with the establishment of *genetic sex.* In turn, the presence or absence of a male-determining Y chromosome defines *gonadal sex,* causing the indifferent embryonic gonad to become either a testis or an ovary. Subsequent differentiation of the internal genital ducts and the external genitalia follows a similar paradigm, in which indifferent common primordia show an innate tendency to feminize unless male patterns of development are imposed by secretions from the fetal testis. At birth the external genitalia provide the basis by which society assigns both gender role and legal sex. Later, during and after puberty, testicular or ovarian hormones induce secondary sexual characteristics which serve both to reinforce psychosexual identity and to signal adult reproductive capabilities. The six parameters of sexual dimorphism listed in Table 18-1 define the sum of what we mean by the terms *male* and *female.* In clinical situations of disordered sexual differentiation, the physician must be aware that complete diagnosis requires a definitive statement concerning each of these aspects of sexual development. In the absence of such information, the initiation of therapy, or even the assignment of sex of rearing, carries grave risk of a later psychosexual disaster.

Table 18-1. Parameters of Sexual Dimorphism

	Determining factors		
Aspect	Female development	Male development	Identified by
Genetic sex	Homogametic (XX)	Heterogametic (XY)	Karyotype
Gonadal sex	Oocytes	Possibly H-Y antigen	Histology
Genital ducts	Innate tendency	Antimüllerian hormone; testosterone	Examination
External genitalia	Innate tendency	Testosterone	Examination
Gender role	Psychosocial factors	Psychosocial factors	Observation
Puberty	Estradiol	Testosterone	Hormone assay

Genetic Sex

In some fish and amphibians complete sex reversal can be caused by environmental influences such as hormones, but in mammals sex is solely and decisively determined by chromosomal mechanisms. All physicians are now familiar with the systematized array of metaphase chromosomes known as a *karyotype* (Fig. 18-1). The 22 pairs of autosomes and the unpaired (X and Y) sex chromosomes can each be characterized according to size, centromeric position, and a distinctive pattern of banding. Various techniques are used to demonstrate these bands, including fluorescent staining with quinacrine (Q banding) or several methods of Giemsa staining (G, C, or R banding). The chemical basis for specific bands is not entirely clear, but the bands appear to reflect not only variations in DNA base composition but also the nature and quantity of associated histone and nonhistone proteins. *An International System for Human Cytogenetic Nomenclature,* first developed in 1960 and revised at intervals, provides a standard method for the description of the regions and bands of both normal and structurally altered chromosomes.[4]

CHROMOSOMAL ERRORS

Chromosomal abnormalities include both deviations from the normal number (*aneuploidy*) and various structural changes in individual chromosomes.

Aneuploidy

During cell division a chromosome may be lost; this circumstance, known as *anaphase lag,* is more likely if the chromosome is structurally abnormal. A more common mechanism to lose a chromosome (*monosomy*) or gain extra chromosomes (*trisomy* or *polysomy*) is primary nondisjunction; in this case a pair of sister chromatids (during mitosis) or homologous chromosomes (during meiosis) fails to separate at metaphase, so that one daughter cell receives both members of the pair while the complementary cell receives none.

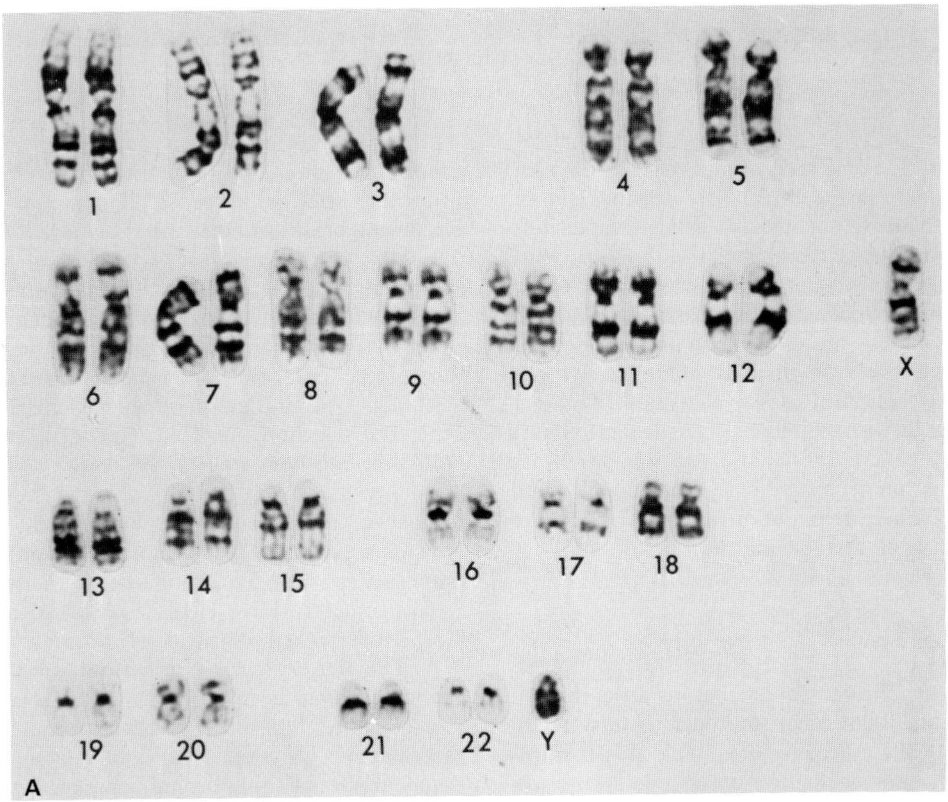

FIGURE 18-1 (A) Normal male karyotype (46,XY) pretreated with trypsin and Giemsa-stained to show characteristic banding patterns. (*B, next page*) Normal female karyotype (46,XX) stained with quinacrine dihydrochloride to show fluorescent bands of differing intensity.

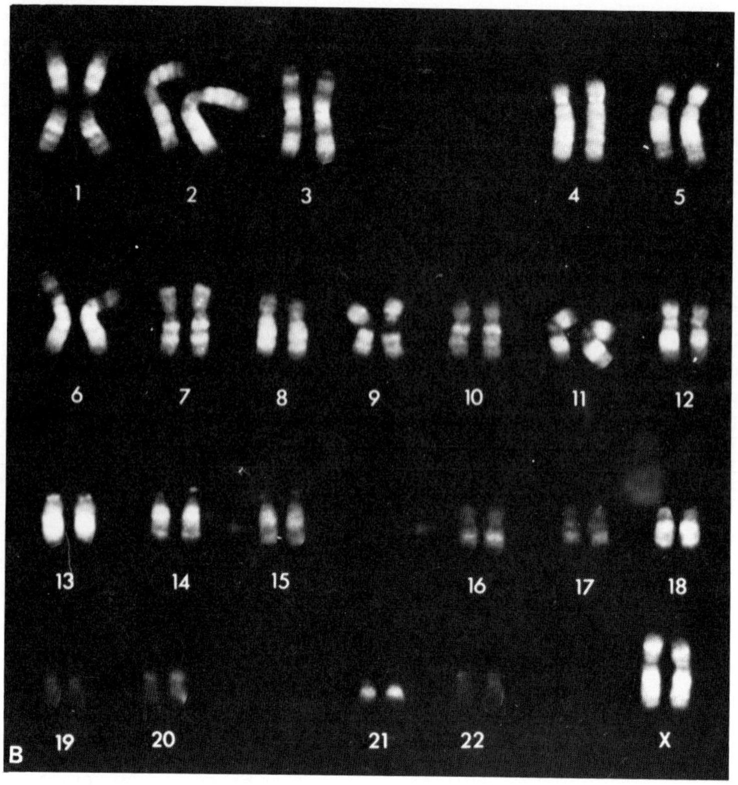

FIGURE 18-1 (B) (*continued*)

If nondisjunction occurs during meiotic division, aneuploid gametes will ensue and the resulting embryo will contain a single aneuploid cell line. Nondisjunction occurring after fertilization during an early mitotic division will produce an individual with two or more cell lines. Such mosaicism, particularly for the sex chromosomes, is not uncommon and can be ruled out only by karyotype analysis of relatively large numbers of cells from a variety of tissues. *Mosaicism*, in which the different cell lines have the same genetic origin, must be differentiated from the much less common situation of *chimerism*, in which double fertilization of a binucleate ovum or fusion of two zygotes leads to a single embryo having two cell lines of different genetic origin (e.g., 46, XY/46, XX).

Structural Anomalies

Aberrations of chromosome structure arise through breakage, often followed by improper reunion of the fragments; these can lead to phenotypic abnormalities through deficiency or duplication of genetic information or through a position effect. A simple *deletion* involves loss of either a portion of the short arm, designated *p* [e.g., 46,X,del(X)(p21), indicating deletion of the short arm of X distal to band Xp21], or of the long arm, designated *q*. *Ring chromosomes* occur following breaks in both the short and long arms, the ends of which then fuse, with loss of the acentric fragments [e.g., 46,X,r(X)]. *Duplications* may involve a portion of a single chromosome or *translocation*, in which genetic material is transferred from one chromosome to another. In the latter circumstance, although both chromosomes are structurally abnormal, the translocation may be balanced; however, an offspring receiving one of the translocation chromosomes without the other would be genetically unbalanced and presumably phenotypically abnormal. *Isochromosomes* result from loss of an entire arm with replication of the remaining one, so that the chromosome comes to have either two identical long arms [e.g., 46,X,iso(Xq)] or two short arms.

The frequency of chromosome abnormalities at conception has been estimated to be between 10 and 50 percent,[5] but most of these terminate in early spontaneous abortion. Studies of human spermatozoa show abnormal chromosome complements in about 9 percent (range, 0 to 28 percent in different donors), with aneuploidy and structural anomalies affecting every chromosome.[6] It is of interest that X-bearing sperm normally outnumber Y-bearing sperm by a ratio of 54:46, suggesting selective loss of the latter during gametogenesis. The incidence of significant abnormality involving the sex chromosomes is probably about 17 per 1000 conceptions;[7] most of these, particularly those with a 45,X karyotype, lead to early abortion. Surveys of unselected liveborn infants indicate that sex chromosome abnormalities (mainly 47,XYY, 47,XXY, and 47,XXX) occur in 0.3 percent of males and 0.15 percent of females. The low incidence of 45,X newborns (about 0.01 percent) is in sharp contrast to the high frequency of this karyotype in spontaneous abortions.

The frequency of chromosome abnormalities in adult patients is naturally biased by preselection for reproductive disorders. For example, approximately 25 percent of young women with primary amenorrhea and 4 percent with secondary amenorrhea show an abnormal karyotype, usually 45,X or one of its variants.[8] About 10 percent of males with azoospermia show an abnormality. Similarly, one may expect to find a chromosomal abnormality such as reciprocal autosomal translocation or mosaicism for X chromosome aneuploidy in about 10 percent of couples with a history of recurrent abortion.[9]

PROPERTIES AND FUNCTIONS OF THE SEX CHROMOSOMES

It is probable that the X and Y chromosomes evolved from an ancestral pair of autosomes by accumulation of sex-specific genes through translocation. Their common ancestry is demonstrated by the extensive regions of homology which still exist, particularly in the so-called pairing segment, which involves 95 percent of the short arm of Y and about 27 percent of the terminal short arm of the X chromosome. Such homologies might provide extensive opportunity for crossing-over and genetic interchange, but it seems that a mechanism exists to inhibit such X-Y interchange in order to preserve sex isolation.[10] Recent studies have shown, however, that this mechanism is imperfect and that X-Y genetic interchange does occur in, for example, situations of sex reversal such as the 46,XX male.[11]

The Y Chromosome

The normal Y chromosome, metacentric and slightly larger than the smallest chromosomes of the G group, has become highly specialized for sex determination. It is characterized by intense fluorescence of the distal two-thirds of its long arm, an area which shows up in quinacrine-stained interphase cells as the fluorescent Y body, usually adjacent to the nuclear membrane (Fig. 18-2A). The number of these Y bodies equals the number of Y chromosomes and thus can be a clue to Y chromosome aneuploidy. The length of this fluorescent segment, and thus of the Y chromosome itself, differs greatly between individuals; since it may be absent in apparently normal males, it seems probable that it is not involved in genetic transcription.

Patients with structural abnormalities of the Y chromosome are usually normal but may show genital ambiguity, with or without short stature. Karyotype-phenotype correlations to identify deleted Y-linked somatic determinants in these patients have been difficult, since the abnormal Y chromosome is frequently lost through anaphase lag, so that the patients also express a 45,X cell line. It seems likely that the Y

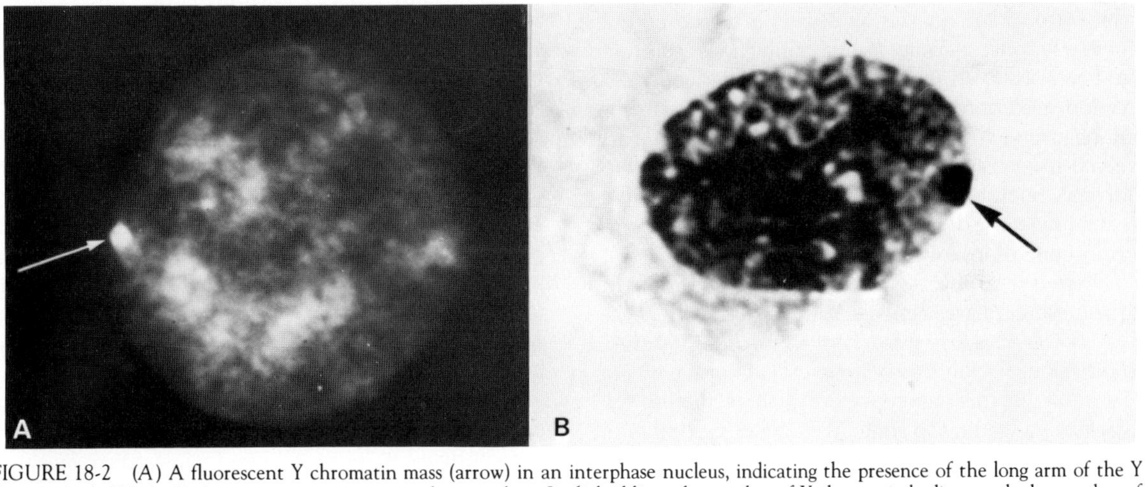

FIGURE 18-2 (A) A fluorescent Y chromatin mass (arrow) in an interphase nucleus, indicating the presence of the long arm of the Y chromosome. (B) An X chromatin mass in an interphase nucleus. In diploid lines the number of X chromatin bodies equals the number of X chromosomes minus one.

chromosome does contain some active genes related to stature and somatic development, since normal XY males do not show the short stature and anomalies characteristic of X monosomy. Conversely, the tall stature of some 47,XYY persons may reflect a dosage effect of these or related genes.

There is general agreement that the primary function of the Y chromosome is to direct male development by causing the indifferent embryonic gonad to differentiate into a testis. The critical male-determining genetic sequence appears to be located close to the centromere, most likely on the short arm (Yp), and may exist in multiple copies. This is the region which appears to be involved in the expression of H-Y antigen, the putative testis-organizing factor (see below); recent evidence suggests that it may represent a regulatory gene for H-Y synthesis rather than the structural gene locus.

The X Chromosome

The X chromosome is a large metacentric chromosome which contains about 5 percent of the total DNA in a haploid set (22 autosomes plus the X). In sharp contrast to the Y chromosome, the X chromosome is involved in the function of every system in the body and contains at least 200 mapped genetic loci.[12] These include genes that play important roles in the sexual differentiation of both males and females. There is evidence that X-linked genes are involved in both the regulation of H-Y antigen synthesis and the expression of the specific H-Y receptor necessary for its testis-inducing function. In addition, the gene for the dihydrotestosterone receptor, essential in the male for both genital differentiation and secondary sexual characteristics, is certainly X-linked.[13] Male carriers of X-autosome translocations, regardless of the position of the break point on the X, usually are azoospermic or severely oligospermic, while ambiguous genitalia have been observed in males carrying a pericentric X inversion. Deletion mapping has shown that genes on the long arm of X (between bands Xq11 and Xq22) are involved in expression of the stigmata of Klinefelter's syndrome. Such observations indicate the critical but still incompletely defined role that this chromosome plays in male reproductive function.[14]

There is a critical segment on the long arm of the X chromosome, lying between bands Xq13 and Xq26, which is essential for normal ovarian differentiation and function. Females with structural abnormalities or break points in this region present with premature follicular atresia leading to gonadal dysgenesis, primary or secondary amenorrhea, and infertility.[14] Although some deletions of the short arm (Xp) cause only short stature with normal sexual development, more severe abnormalities such as monosomy (45,X) or an isochromosome [46,X,iso(Xq)] give rise to the full Turner's syndrome, with gonadal dysgenesis, short stature, and somatic abnormalities.[15] It would appear, therefore, that determinants on both the short and the long arms of the X chromosome are necessary for normal female growth and development.

The X chromosome also contains a large number of unpaired genes not present on the Y chromosome, defects of which cause disease in hemizygous males or females with monosomy X. Examples of these X-linked traits include color blindness, hemophilia A (factor VIII), hemophilia B (factor IX), and glucose-6-phosphate dehydrogenase deficiency, the loci for which are located on the long arm. The steroid sulfatase (STS) locus, involved in X-linked ichthyosis and placental sulfatase deficiency, has been assigned to the distal part of the short arm.

Since normal 46,XX females obtain twice as many of these unpaired genes as normal males, a dosage difference with effects similar to those of aneuploidy might be expected were there not some mechanism for dosage compensation. This compensation is effected by inactivation of one X chromosome in the female early in development, so that the expressed dosage of X-linked genes is equivalent in males and females. This process is random but is fixed thereafter for each cell line; thus the female comes to be a mosaic of active paternal and maternal X chromosomes.[16] Regardless of the number of X chromosomes present in a cell, all but one are inactivated. Following inactivation, cell lines in which the active X is structurally abnormal may replicate less efficiently than their normal counterparts, so that selection against this line may occur.

The inactive X chromosome can be identified during cell division in the presence of [^{3}H]thymidine by its asynchronous delayed pattern of DNA synthesis. In interphase cells this late-replicating X can be stained and visualized as an X chromatin, or Barr body, of about 1 μm diameter applied to the inner surface of the nuclear membrane (Fig. 18-2*B*). In smears of female buccal mucosa X chromatin can be found in about 20 percent of cells. Sex chromatin also appears in the form of a drumstick-shaped accessory appendage on 1 to 15 percent of the nuclei of female polymorphonuclear leukocytes. The number of chromatin bodies in any diploid nucleus is one less than the total number of X chromosomes; thus the buccal smear of a 48,XXXY male will show two chromatin bodies, while a 45,X female will show none. Structural anomalies altering the size of the X chromosome may influence the size of the resulting mass of heterochromatin.

In recent years the concept of mammalian X inactivation and dosage compensation has been extended and modified to some degree.[17] In the embryo, even though X-linked genes become active in transcription as early as the two-cell stage, X inactivation does not occur until the early blastocyst stage. Thus very early female embryos show levels of X-linked enzyme activity twice as high as those of male embryos. The initiation of X inactivation seems to coincide with the beginning of cell differentiation and is seen first in the trophoderm, then in the primitive endoderm, and finally in the inner cell masses. Both somatic and germ cells appear to be derived from a common pool of X-inactivated cells. However, in females germ cells undergo genetic reactivation prior to entering meiosis so that both X chromosomes become active again in the primary oocytes of the fetal and postnatal ovary. This pattern is exactly the opposite of what occurs in the normal male during spermatogenesis, when the single active X chromosome undergoes apparent inactivation at the onset of meiosis.[18] These observations may underlie the accelerated oocyte degeneration seen in 45,X females and the azoospermia in 47,XXY males. In Turner's syndrome the lack of two active X chromosomes in the germ cell appears to accelerate follicular atresia; conversely, in Klinefelter's syndrome the extra, presumably active, X chromosome interferes with normal spermatogenesis.

In somatic cells and their descendants, X inactivation affects all but a single X chromosome and is irreversible. It has therefore been difficult to explain the somatic abnormalities of 45,X and 47,XXY subjects. Indeed, in polysomy X the severity of the somatic anomalies correlates with the number of X chromosomes, a finding which suggests that dosage compensation as achieved by X inactivation is incomplete. Recent evidence has partially resolved this paradox by the demonstration that several loci, including those for the Xg^a red blood cell antigen and for microsomal steroid sulfatase, both of which are located at the distal end of the short arm, escape complete inactivation and are expressed by both X chromosomes.[17] It therefore seems likely that X inactivation does not involve the entire chromosome and that females normally express some gene loci in double dosage.

The molecular basis of X chromosome inactivation is not entirely understood. It may involve methylation of DNA cytosine residues, since incorporation of 5-azacytidine to inhibit DNA methyltransferase can cause stable reactivation of loci on an inactive X chromosome.[19] Some authors have suggested that similar processes of DNA methylation and demethylation are involved in all specialized tissue differentiation, but this has not been confirmed.[20]

Gonadal Sex

Although a person's genetic sex is determined at conception, for the first few weeks of fetal life the gonadal anlagen maintain a similar appearance in both sexes. This indifferent gonad forms in the mesenchyme at the ventral edge of the cranial medial part of the mesonephros and is invaded in turn by primordial germ cells and cells originating from the mesonephros and the coelomic epithelium. The large spherical germ cells probably arise in or close to the yolk sac endoderm; from here they migrate through the hindgut region and the dorsal mesentery to reach the gonadal ridge around day 35 to 45, where they proliferate rapidly. The mesonephros itself contributes dense cell cords which in the male will form the rete testis and part of the epididymis and in the female remain as the rete ovarii. It has been suggested that mesonephric cells within the gonad may give rise to Sertoli and granulosa cells, while Leydig cells, theca, and ovarian stroma arise from mesenchyme.[21] These findings emphasize that although the testis and ovary differentiate into dissimilar organs, they continue throughout life to show numerous homologies in their gametogenic and steroidogenic functions.[22]

TESTICULAR DIFFERENTIATION

The earliest sign of male differentiation is the appearance at 6 to 7 weeks within the indifferent gonad of seminiferous cords containing germ cells and Sertoli cells. At 8 weeks typical Leydig cells equipped with cell membrane receptors for human chorionic gonadotropin (hCG) and luteinizing hormone (LH) begin to proliferate in the interstitium, and by 14 weeks they make up more than half the volume of the testis. The cytoplasm of these cells contains large amounts of tubular smooth endoplasmic reticulum and large round mitochondria with tubular cristae, features that are characteristic of active steroidogenesis. The histochemical appearance of 3β-hydroxysteroid dehydrogenase (3β-HSD) and other steroidogenic enzymes parallels these structural changes, with peak activities at 14 to 16 weeks gestation. After the end of the fourth month the number of fetal Leydig cells begins to decrease, but they do not disappear until several weeks after birth. As the seminiferous cords of the fetal testis grow they become coiled, thickened, and eventually canalized. Such tubules contain numerous spermatogonia, but further germ cell maturation and the onset of meiosis do not occur until puberty.

There is abundant evidence that differentiation of the somatic elements of the testis is independent of any germ cell influence.[32] Indeed, it appears that the Y chromosomal testis-determining factor first imposes testicular somatic development, and that this in turn is necessary for normal male germ cell differentiation.

The Role of H-Y Antigen

Awareness that male cells possess a sex-specific minor histocompatibility antigen, subsequently termed *H-Y antigen*, grew out of the observation that highly inbred female mice reject skin grafts from male donors, while female-to-male, female-to-female, and male-to-male grafts are readily accepted.[24] The demonstration that serum from these male-grafted female mice killed spermatozoa permitted the development of a specific complement-dependent sperm cytotoxicity assay for the serological detection of H-Y antigen in a variety of tissues.[25] A variety of assay systems have since been developed,[26] but all are difficult to perform and require experience for their proper interpretation.

The H-Y antigen shows a remarkable degree of phylogenetic conservation, having been found in the heterogametic sex of all vertebrates tested and possibly some prevertebrate species. It is found on XY (male) cells in XX/XY species such as humans; but H-Y or a closely related factor occurs also on ZW (female) cells in ZZ/ZW species such as the chicken. These observations led to the suggestion by Wachtel, Ohno, and associates that H-Y antigen is a primary determinant of gonadal sex, being the product of testis-determining genes in mammals but having an opposite, ovary-inducing function in species in which the heterogametic sex is female.[27]

There is considerable circumstantial support for the view that H-Y antigen is a testicular differentiation factor, influencing organogenesis through its effect on cell-cell recognition and interaction. Thus whenever even traces of testicular tissue are present in a mammal, H-Y serological tests are uniformly positive regardless of the actual karyotype (Table 18-2). It appears that the critical factor that correlates with testicular organogenesis is not just the presence of a Y chromosome but rather the expression of H-Y antigen (Fig. 18-3). It should be pointed out that occasional situations, notably in 45,X females, have been described in which gonadal differentiation and H-Y serological tests are discrepant. Such discrepancies may merely reflect the vagaries of difficult nonquantitative assay systems or may indicate that the testis-inducing function of H-Y antigen is dose-dependent. However, the alternative, more complex view that testis differentiation involves expression of several Y-linked and autosomal genes other than the H-Y locus[28] cannot be excluded. Indeed, some authorities maintain that the H-Y antigen detected by serological tests is different from the male-specific transplantation antigen and that neither may be necessary or sufficient alone for testicular differentiation.[29]

Direct evidence of a testis-organizing role for H-Y antigen has been provided by experiments in which cultured dissociated testicular cells were treated with an excess of H-Y antibody, sufficient to bind all H-Y antigen on the plasma membrane.[30] Instead of reaggregating to form testislike long tubular structures as

Table 18-2. Correlation of Testicular Development, Karyotype, and H-Y Antigen

Concordance
Testicular tissue present and H-Y antigen–positive:
XY normal male
XXY Klinefelter's syndrome and variants
XX or XO male
XX true hermaphroditism
XX/XY chimerism
XO/XY mixed gonadal dysgenesis
XY defects in testosterone synthesis
XY testicular feminization
Absence of testes and H-Y antigen–negative:
XX normal female
XY gonadal dysgenesis (testicular agenesis type)
XY campomelic dysplasia with sex reversal
Discordance
Testicular tissue absent but H-Y antigen–positive
XX normal female (possible carrier of autosomal recessive gene for sex reversal)
XO,XXp− and X,iso(Xq) forms of gonadal dysgenesis
XY gonadal dysgenesis (H-Y receptor defect)
Testes present but H-Y antigen–negative
No consistent examples

Source: Adapted from Wolf.[35]

with normal cells, anti-H-Y–treated cells formed spherical follicle-like structures, each containing a germ cell as in the ovary. Conversely, XX gonadal cells can be induced by "free" H-Y antigen in vitro to organize into testicular tubules containing oocytes and expressing hCG receptors;[31,32] this conversion can be blocked by specific H-Y antiserum. In vitro coculture of XY and XX gonadal cells similarly leads to coopting of ovarian cells to form testicular structures, providing direct evidence that H-Y antigen can be secreted by XY cells in order to influence the differentiation of indifferent gonadal tissue of either sex. An in vivo demonstration of the testis-inducing effect of H-Y antigen is provided by the bovine freemartin situation. When dizygotic twinning produces synchorionic twins of opposite sex in cattle, H-Y antigen can be detected in the blood of the female freemartin and may induce gonadal sex reversal. It is probable that this H-Y antigen is secreted by the male twin, but cells in the freemartin gonad may also be induced to secrete the material in some fashion.

H-Y antigen is composed of protein subunits of around 18,000 daltons polymerized by interchain disulfide bridges and resembles interferon in its hydrophobicity, amino acid composition, and lack of sugar residues. It is expressed by XY zygotes as early as the eight-cell stage and is subsequently produced by all male cells except immature premeiotic male germ cells, in which the X chromosome is presumably inac-

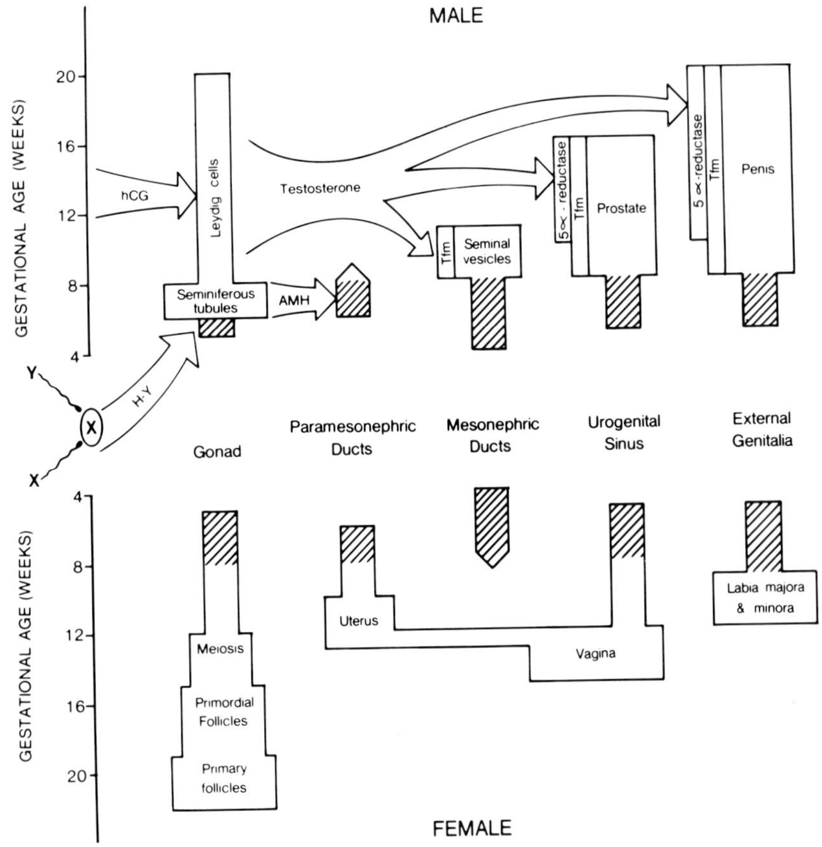

FIGURE 18-3 The major determinants of sexual differentiation: their impact on male (*top*) and female (*bottom*) development in relation to fetal age. The broad arrows show the effects of H-Y antigen, chorionic gonadotropin (hCG), antimüllerian hormone (AMH), and testosterone in directing male differentiation. Tfm indicates the cytosolic androgen receptor. The cross-hatched segment is a sexually undifferentiated structure.

tive. Primitive Sertoli cells in the embryonic testis appear to disseminate H-Y antigen, which is then bound to specific H-Y receptors on gonadal cells of either sex; such cells then become H-Y–positive on serological testing. In addition to these high-affinity gonad-specific H-Y receptors, there appear to be ubiquitous nonspecific membrane anchorage sites on male cells which involve α_2-microglobulin and cell surface components of the major histocompatibility complex. Thus the total system for testis differentiation may include the sex-specific H-Y antigen as a primary inducer, a gonad-specific receptor to guarantee selective action, and a general plasma membrane anchorage site involved in the action of a wide range of other organogenesis-directing proteins. Disorders of testicular differentiation may have their origin either in deficient synthesis of H-Y antigen or in some defect in gonad-specific receptor binding or function.

The Genetic Basis of H-Y Expression

The finding that the serological titer is increased in persons with two Y chromosomes[33] initially suggested that the structural gene locus was Y-linked and probably identical with the testis-determining locus. Subsequently, however, low titers of H-Y antigen have been detected in the absence of either a Y chromosome or testes, notably in patients with gonadal dysgenesis [45,X or 46,X,iso(Xq)]. Some authorities believe that testis-inducing H-Y antigen is expressed by the Y chromosome but that the material detected in gonadal dysgenesis is a cross-reacting protein expressed by a region of base sequence homology on the X chromosome;[34] such material might be involved in ovarian differentiation. An alternative theory suggests that the structural gene for H-Y antigen is located either on an autosome or the X chromosome and in turn is regulated both by a repressor locus on the distal end of the short arm of the X chromosome (absent in H-Y–positive Turner's syndrome) and by an activator locus on the short arm of the Y chromosome which can override the inhibitory influence of even several X chromosomes (as in 49,XXXXY males).[35] This latter hypothesis has been modified slightly by Adinolfi et al., who suggest that the autosomal locus may express an immunoreactive precursor peptide which is then either inactivated by the action of the X-linked gene or activated by the action of the

Y-linked testis-determining locus.[36] Finally, there is circumstantial evidence from studies of familial XY gonadal dysgenesis that the genetic locus for the specific gonadal H-Y receptor in both sexes is also X-linked.

OVARIAN DIFFERENTIATION

In contrast to testicular development, which appears to be independent of the presence of germ cells, differentiation of an ovary is to a great extent defined in terms of germ cell phenomena. The first definitive evidence of an embryonic ovary is the onset of meiotic prophase in primary oocytes at around 9 to 12 weeks gestational age. According to Byskov, this reflects the influence of a meiosis-inducing factor produced by the rete ovarii.[37] The first meiotic division is arrested at the diplotene stage and is not completed until ovulation occurs some 12 to 40 years later; the second meiotic division is not completed until after fertilization. By midpregnancy the ovaries contain 6 to 7 million germ cells, including oogonia, oocytes in various stages of meiotic prophase, and degenerating germ cells. After 20 weeks primitive granulosa cells organize around these oocytes to form single-layered primordial follicles and then multilayered primary follicles surrounded by thecal stroma. A few antral follicles may appear, but these degenerate without ovulation. Although it is probable that small amounts of steroid hormones are produced by either thecal or interstitial cells, both of which are homologous with Leydig cells, their nature and local significance remain undefined.

The most remarkable phenomenon of ovarian development during the latter half of pregnancy is a decline in the total germ cell population due to degeneration of oogonia and oocytes and atresia of many primordial and primary follicles. By term the ovaries contain about 2 million germ cells, and of these only about 400 will survive to ovulate during a woman's reproductive life.

Preservation of a viable follicle clearly requires an oocyte equipped with two active X chromosomes. Deletion mapping suggests that genes necessary for normal follicular development are found on both the long and the short arms of the X chromosome; the syndrome of autosomal recessive XX gonadal dysgenesis suggests that an autosomal gene may also be involved. It is not yet clear whether this process involves active secretion of an ovary-organizing factor analogous to the H-Y antigen of males. In 45,X fetuses, early fetal ovarian development appears to be normal but the primary follicles fail to acquire a complete layer of granulosa cells and soon degenerate.

Differentiation of the Genital Ducts

The mesonephric, or wolffian, ducts appear in the fetus at about 4 weeks gestation; they then grow caudally, become canalized, and open into the cloaca. The mesonephric nephrons, except for those contiguous with the rete system of the gonad, degenerate once the definitive kidney (metanephros) forms, but their ducts become incorporated into the genital system. The paramesonephric (müllerian) ducts originate at about 6 weeks gestation as solid cords of coelomic epithelial cells lateral to the mesonephric ducts which grow caudally and cross the latter ventrally to reach the urogenital sinus. These paired cords become canalized; caudally, where they meet in the midline, they fuse to form a single uterovaginal canal. Thus by 7 weeks gestation each fetus is equipped with the primordia of both male and female genital ducts (Fig. 18-4).

FEMALE INTERNAL GENITAL DEVELOPMENT

In female fetuses the mesonephric ducts degenerate relatively early, leaving only remnants of tubules that can be identified later as the epoophoron, paraoophoron, and Gartner's duct. The partially fused paramesonephric ducts provide the paired fallopian tubes, the midline uterine primordium, and, in collaboration with tissue contributed by the urogenital sinus, the vaginal primordium. Development of these structures does not depend upon any hormonal or other influences from the ovary. However, it is contingent upon prior appearance of the mesonephric ducts; thus renal aplasia is commonly associated with agenesis of the fallopian tube, uterus, and vagina. Although the female internal genitalia differentiate morphologically somewhat later than those of the male, there is evidence that they are functionally committed to become female by as early as 8 weeks gestation.[38]

MALE INTERNAL GENITAL DEVELOPMENT

The development of male internal genitalia involves two separate processes: regression of the paramesonephric ducts and stabilization of the mesonephric ducts. These processes are mediated by two secretions of the fetal testis: antimüllerian hormone (AMH) produced by the Sertoli cells and testosterone from the fetal Leydig cells (Fig. 18-3).

Antimüllerian Hormone

Regression of the paramesonephric ducts begins at about 8 weeks gestation, initially adjacent to the cau-

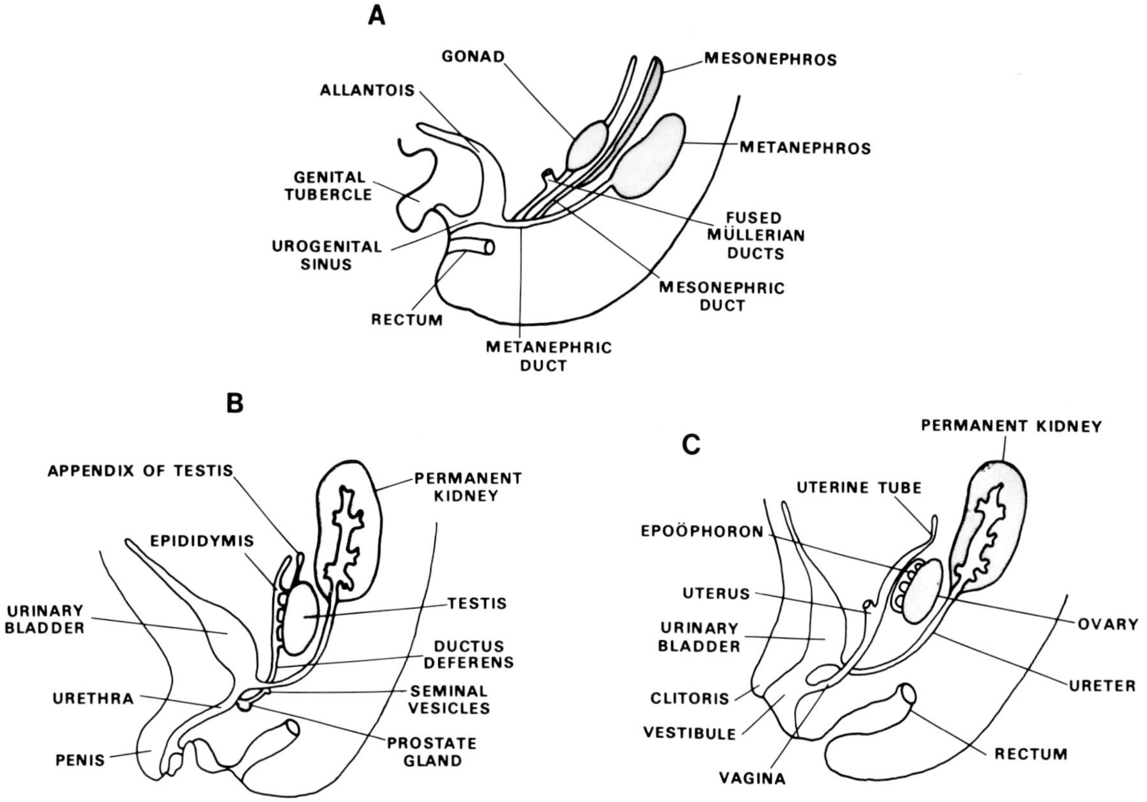

FIGURE 18-4 Diagrammatic sagittal sections of the internal genitalia of an 8-week fetus (*A*) and of a male (*B*) and female (*C*) fetus at 13 weeks gestation. [*From Smail P, Reyes FI, Winter JSD, Faiman C, in Kogan SJ, Hafez ESE (eds): Pediatric Andrology. The Hague, Martinus Nijhoff, 1981, p 11.*]

dal pole of the testis and then extending cranially and caudally. In the normal male only the cranial tip, which becomes the appendix testis, is spared. Close juxtaposition of the paramesonephric duct and the ipsilateral testis is necessary to initiate regression, but even large amounts of testosterone applied locally cannot duplicate the effect. Rather, paramesonephric regression is induced by the local paracrine action of AMH, secreted by Sertoli cells of the ipsilateral testis. Purified AMH appears to be a glycoprotein of approximately 140,000 daltons, composed of two or more identical subunits linked by disulfide bridges.[39,40] Although AMH is produced by Sertoli cells from the time seminiferous tubules appear until at least 2 years after birth, the paramesonephric ducts are responsive to its action only at a critical period, and the target cells can be rendered unresponsive by exposure to cyclic AMP.[41] Although steroids themselves cannot induce regression, reports of müllerian-derived squamous vaginal epithelium in females and persistent müllerian derivatives in males following prenatal exposure to diethylstilbestrol[42] raise questions about possible direct or indirect effects of estrogen upon this process.

With radioimmunoassay techniques it is possible to detect AMH in serum for some time after birth,[43] but as yet there is no evidence for any physiological effects on other tissues, nor is it clear what regulates secretion. It has been suggested that exogenous follicle stimulating hormone (FSH) may inhibit AMH secretion,[44] but pituitary regulation of its synthesis has not been confirmed. Recent studies have demonstrated that AMH is produced by granulosa cells of the mature ovary but not by the fetal ovary;[45] this observation provides further evidence of the homology between granulosa and Sertoli cells, but the role of AMH in the ovary remains unclear.

Testosterone

Stabilization and differentiation of the paired mesonephric ducts to form vasa efferentia, epididymis, vasa deferentia, ejaculatory ducts, and seminal vesicles is dependent upon local high concentrations of androgen from the ipsilateral testis. Androgen receptors in the ductal cells bind both testosterone and dihydrotestosterone; however, since only small amounts of the latter are synthesized by the testis and the ductal cells themselves appear to lack 5α-reductase until after differentiation, it is generally assumed that testosterone is the active intracellular mediator primarily responsible.[46]

In patients with asymmetric gonadal differentiation, duct development on each side correlates closely with the degree of testicular development on the same side. Patients with enzymatic defects in testosterone biosynthesis or defective androgen receptors show rudimentary mesonephric duct structures, but in genetic 5α-reductase deficiency male genital ducts are normal. That this effect of testosterone is a local paracrine effect rather than a blood-borne endocrine effect is underscored by the failure of adrenal androgens to prevent normal mesonephric duct regression in females with congenital adrenal hyperplasia.

Differentiation of the Urogenital Sinus and External Genitalia

For the first 2 months of prenatal development, the external genitalia are identical in both sexes. They consist of a midline genital tubercle (*phallus*) and lateral labioscrotal swellings. Behind these structures lies the urogenital sinus, into which open both the ureters and the internal genital ducts.

FEMINIZATION OF THE EXTERNAL GENITALIA

In females the phallus remains small and bends ventrally, the anogenital distance remains short, and the labioscrotal swellings and urethral groove do not fuse in the midline. The labioscrotal swellings become the labia majora, the separate genital folds the labia minora, and the phallic part of the urogenital sinus the vestibule (Fig. 18-5). The urogenital sinus is divided by downgrowth of a vaginal plate which approaches the perineum to provide separate urethral and uterovaginal access to the exterior. The contribution of paramesonephric duct tissue to the upper vagina is indicated by the abnormally shallow vagina of patients with complete testicular feminization, in whom the paramesonephric ducts regress. It appears that development of female external genitalia is independent of ovarian influence, although prenatal exposure to diethylstilbestrol can cause persistence of müllerian-derived vaginal epithelium, with vaginal adenosis and a predisposition to malignant transformation.

MASCULINIZATION OF THE EXTERNAL GENITALIA

During male differentiation the labioscrotal swellings and urethral folds fuse in the midline to form the scrotum and a penis enclosing the phallic urethra (Fig. 18-5). This process, imposed by testicular androgens, begins at 9 weeks and is complete by 14 weeks gestation. The urogenital sinus differentiates into the male urethra and the prostate. During the latter half of pregnancy the penis continues to enlarge, with a rate of growth three to four times that of the female clitoris.[47] During this same period the testes descend into the scrotum, a process that appears to be androgen-dependent, although other testicular factors may play a role.[48] In males with deficient testicular function the prostatic utricle, homologous to the female upper vagina, is commonly larger than normal.

Hormonal Sex: Differentiation of the Hypothalamic-Pituitary-Gonadal Axis

GONADAL STEROID PRODUCTION

By the time Leydig cells can be recognized at 6 to 7 weeks fetal age the fetal testis contains the necessary enzymes for synthesis of testosterone from various substrates, although the preferred substrate is probably circulating low-density lipoprotein cholesterol. Testicular concentrations of testosterone rise to a peak at 12 to 14 weeks gestation and then decline, a pattern which correlates closely with the growth and involution of fetal Leydig cells.[49] Although fetal ovaries of some mammalian species contain enzymes for both the synthesis of androgens and their aromatization to estrogen, there is as yet no evidence that the human fetal ovary secretes any significant amounts of sex steroids, at least during the first half of pregnancy when sexual differentiation is taking place.

SEX STEROIDS IN THE FETAL CIRCULATION

The initial local or paracrine action of fetal testosterone is to stabilize development of the ipsilateral mesonephric duct and possibly to stimulate growth of the testis itself. Soon, however, male fetal serum testosterone concentrations begin to rise, reaching peak concentrations of 200 to 600 ng/dl (7 to 21 nmol/l) at 16 to 18 weeks gestation, values which are in the adult male range.[49] After midpregnancy as Leydig cells involute male serum testosterone levels gradually decline, but they remain higher than female levels until term. At the same time the fetus is exposed to

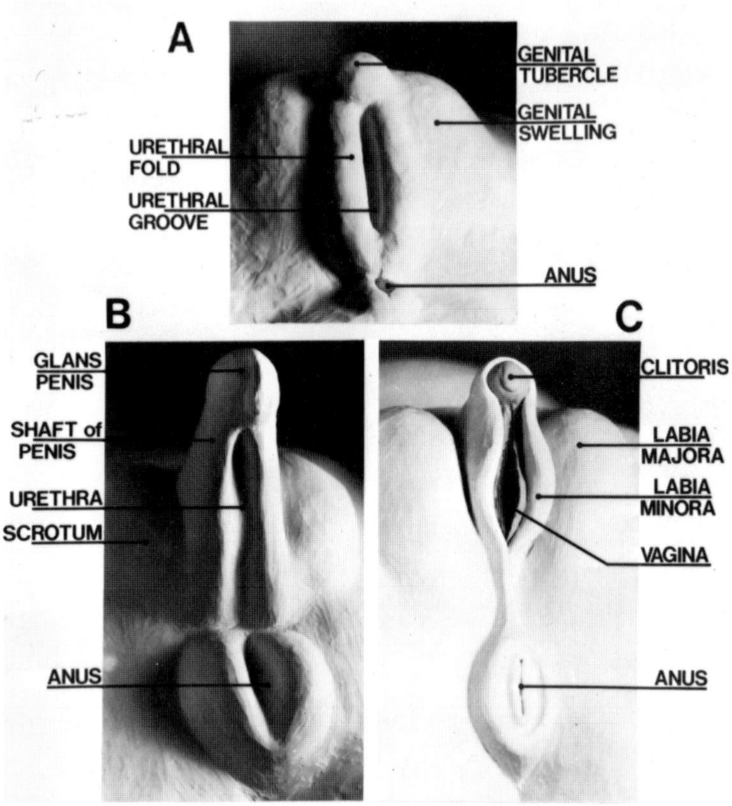

FIGURE 18-5 Models of the external genitalia in an 8-week undifferentiated fetus (*A*) and in a male (*B*) and female (*C*) fetus at 13 weeks gestation. [*From Smail P, Reyes FI, Winter JSD, Faiman C, in Kogan SJ, Hafez ESE (eds): Pediatric Andrology. The Hague, Martinus Nijhoff, 1981, p 12.*]

high concentrations of steroids from the placenta, notably estrogens and progesterone, and from the adrenal cortex, in particular dehydroepiandrosterone sulfate. There is no significant sex difference in serum concentrations of these steroids; presumably, therefore, they play no direct role in sexual differentiation, but they may influence the process through their effects on gonadal steroidogenesis, binding of steroids by serum proteins, and target cell receptor occupancy.

Serum levels of sex steroid–binding globulin (TeBG) are only about one-twentieth of those in maternal serum, and the human fetus does not appear to produce any other high-affinity androgen-binding protein. Although albumin serves as a low-affinity high-capacity carrier of many steroids, its concentration is also low in the fetal circulation. The effect of this low level of sex steroid binding is to increase the fraction of serum testosterone which is free and therefore presumably active.

ACTIONS OF SEX STEROIDS ON THE GENITALIA

The changing patterns of testosterone concentrations in the fetal testis and circulation, in relation to the major events of male genital development, are summarized in Fig. 18-6. Testosterone appears first in high concentrations in the testis itself, where, by a local paracrine effect, it induces masculinization of the ipsilateral mesonephric duct. Subsequently, circulating testosterone levels become sufficiently high to initiate masculinization of the urogenital sinus and external genitalia.

In all these target cells specific high-affinity androgen receptors can be found prior to differentiation (see Fig. 18-14). Androgens bind to this receptor protein, and the steroid-receptor complex is translocated to the nucleus, where it binds to specific chromatin acceptor sites to initiate transcription of new messenger RNA; in turn, this RNA is processed and transported to cytoplasmic ribosomes, where it is translated for synthesis of androgen-induced proteins. There is evidence that the actual target for these androgen effects is the mesenchyme of the genital anlagen, which in turn induces specific patterns of morphogenesis, cytodifferentiation, and functional activity in the overlying epithelium.[50]

The androgen receptor protein has a higher binding affinity for dihydrotestosterone than for testosterone itself. The enzyme necessary for this intra-

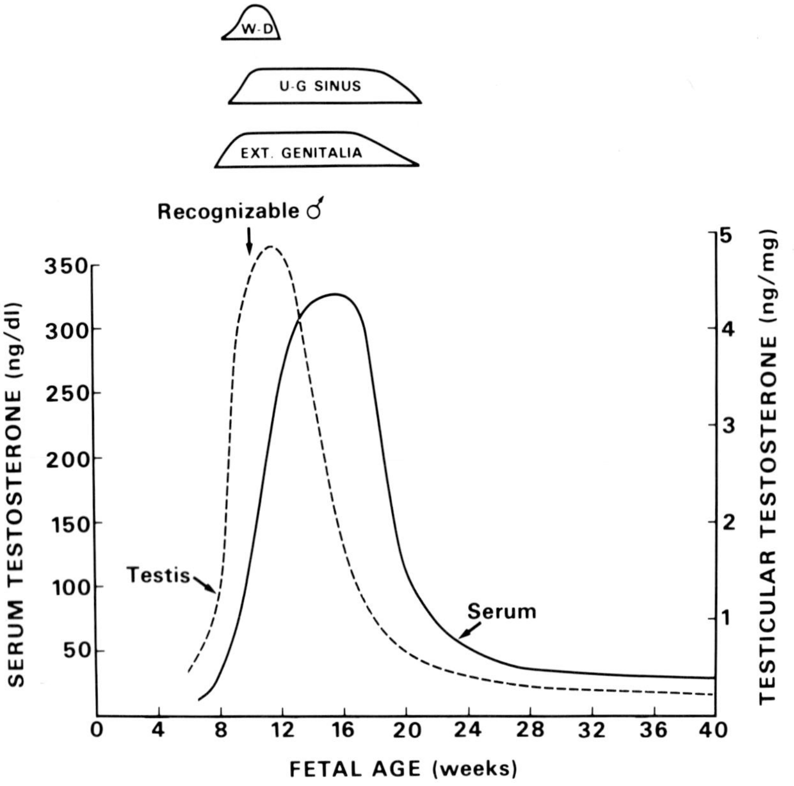

FIGURE 18-6 The relationship of changes in mean testicular and serum testosterone concentrations to the time of development of the mesonephric ducts (WD) and virilization of the urogenital (U-G) sinus and external genitalia in male fetuses. (*From Winter et al.*[49])

cellular conversion, 5α-reductase, does not appear in the mesonephric ducts until development is already well advanced, but high local concentrations of testosterone are sufficient to accomplish masculinization. The urogenital sinus and external genitalia contain active 5α-reductase as soon as testosterone appears in the circulation; it therefore seems likely that masculinization of these structures is accomplished by lower concentrations of the more potent androgen dihydrotestosterone.

The androgen receptor (Tfm) gene locus is on the X chromosome, while the 5α-reductase gene is autosomal. Thus in normal circumstances both sexes can respond to circulating androgen; the direction of genital differentiation is determined solely by testicular testosterone production. Defects in testosterone synthesis, deficient 5α-reductase activity, or an ineffective androgen receptor will each prevent normal genital masculinization of the genetic male, although in 5α-reductase deficiency mesonephric duct development is normal. Conversely, exposure of a female fetus to high levels of circulating androgen does not induce mesonephric duct development but does inhibit separation of the vagina from the urogenital sinus and promote labioscrotal fusion and clitoral hypertrophy.

CONTROL OF FETAL GONADAL FUNCTION

Chorionic Gonadotropin

There is considerable circumstantial evidence that Leydig cell testosterone synthesis during the period of genital differentiation is dependent upon hCG. Thus hypopituitary males do not demonstrate genital ambiguity, although micropenis and cryptorchism are often observed. Chorionic gonadotropin appears in the maternal circulation immediately after implantation of the blastocyst; levels rise to a peak at about 10 weeks fetal age and then decline, although significant placental production continues until term. The pattern in the fetal circulation of either sex is similar, but fetal hCG concentrations are only about one-thirtieth of those in the maternal compartment.[49]

Fetal Leydig cells, but not ovarian cells, have specific membrane receptors for LH and hCG; the number of these receptors increases to a maximum at 15 to 18 weeks gestation and then declines. Via a mechanism that appears to utilize cyclic AMP as the intracellular second messenger, hCG increases the number of low-density lipoprotein receptors, enhances de novo cholesterol synthesis, and stimulates mitochondrial cholesterol side-chain cleavage, all of which serve to increase the pool of available pregnenolone for androgen biosynthesis.[51]

Pituitary Gonadotropins

Although maternal pituitary gonadotropins do not cross the placental barrier, the fetal pituitary after about 9 weeks gestation produces significant amounts of FSH and LH. By 4 to 5 weeks fetal age the pituitary anlage has the ability to synthesize glycoprotein hormone α subunit, but gonadotropin releasing hormone (GnRH)–mediated hypothalamic stimulation is probably necessary for synthesis of hormone-specific β subunit and thus of intact FSH and LH.

Both gonadotropins appear in the fetal circulation at about 11 to 12 weeks and rise to peak concentrations at midpregnancy.[49] Serum FSH concentrations are much higher in female fetuses, in whom adult castrate values occur, than in male fetuses, in whom values are in the normal adult range. This sex difference demonstrates that a negative feedback mechanism mediated by testicular androgens is already operative by midgestation; in experimental animals, castration of the male fetus raises gonadotropin levels to the female range, while castration of the female has no effect. After 28 weeks gestation, serum gonadotropin levels decline in both sexes, a phenomenon that probably reflects maturation of placental estrogen–mediated feedback inhibitory mechanisms. The decline in Leydig cell testosterone production in the latter half of pregnancy would appear to result from the combined effects of a decline in circulating levels of hCG, FSH, and LH and direct inhibition of androgen biosynthesis by high levels of circulating placental estrogens.

The pattern of mean serum hCG and pituitary gonadotropin concentrations in the male fetus, in relation to changes in testicular morphology and function, is summarized in Fig. 18-7. While hCG is the major gonadotropin in the fetal circulation and clearly drives testosterone synthesis during genital differentiation, pituitary gonadotropins become relatively more significant in later gestation and influence such phenomena as phallic growth and testicular descent. It is of interest that the appearance of FSH in the fetal circulation coincides with the first transformation of primordial germ cells into spermatogonia. This, together with observations of reduced spermatogonial number in hypogonadotropic infants, suggests that seminiferous tubule maturation may also be dependent on the fetal pituitary.

The relationships between serum gonadotropins and ovarian development are summarized in Fig. 18-8. The timing of the appearance of primary follicles suggests that fetal pituitary FSH and LH may be necessary for normal follicular development. The ovaries of hypogonadotropic infants appear to contain only primordial and primary follicles and may show accelerated atresia with premature loss of germ cells.

There is considerable evidence that maturation of fetal pituitary function is regulated by the hypothalamus. Gonadotropin releasing hormone can be detected in fetal brain by 5 to 6 weeks of gestation. By 9 to 11 weeks, GnRH-secreting neurons can be demonstrated which have their perikarya in the pericommissural, preoptic, lamina terminalis, and perimamillary regions; their axons end in the median eminence apposed to capillaries which connect with the anterior pituitary, although a distinct hypothalamic-hypophyseal portal system forms later. Between 11 and 14 weeks gestation there is a 14-fold rise in hypothalamic GnRH content, which parallels the increase in pituitary gonadotropin secretion.[52]

Less is known about CNS regulation of fetal hypothalamic GnRH release. Certainly by midgestation hypothalamic nuclei are developed and can produce significant amounts of potential regulators such as dopamine, norepinephrine, and serotonin. Recent observations that neurons in the arcuate-median eminence unit of the fetal hypothalamus contain β-endorphin and that fetal hypothalamic GnRH secretion in vitro is responsive to naloxone suggest the possibility that endogenous opiates exert a tonic inhibitory influence on GnRH release at this time.[53] Both in vitro and in vivo, fetal pituitary cells respond to GnRH with increased gonadotropin secretion. In addition, material which immunologically resembles GnRH is produced by the placenta, but its relevance in the regulation of either fetal pituitary function or placental hCG synthesis has not been established.

Perinatal Adaptations of the Reproductive Endocrine System

By term, the pituitary-gonadal axis of the human infant is structurally complete and capable of relatively mature function.[54] Circulating levels of placental sex steroids such as estrone (900 to 4000 ng/dl), estradiol (200 to 1600 ng/dl), estriol (1200 to 15,000 ng/dl), 17-hydroxyprogesterone (1000 to 7000 ng/dl), and progesterone (12,000 to 50,000 ng/dl) are extremely high. Surprisingly, the only visible effects of these hormones on the neonate are occasional breast enlargement and some degree of endometrial hyperplasia. However, the feedback effect of these steroids suppresses serum FSH and LH secretion in both sexes. At term, cord serum hCG levels range from 20 to 9000 mIU/ml (median 50 mIU/ml). The only hormonal sex difference is in serum testosterone, which is still slightly higher in males than in females.

Immediately post partum, placental estrogens, progesterone, and 17-hydroxyprogesterone are cleared from the neonatal circulation. Concentrations of hCG fall more slowly, but by 4 days of age this go-

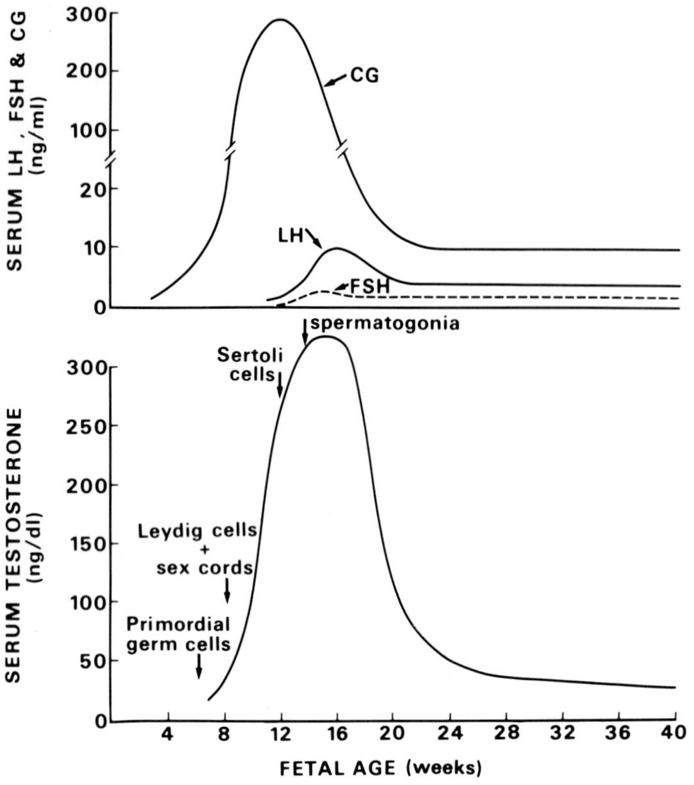

FIGURE 18-7 A schematic summary of the temporal relationship between mean serum concentrations of hCG, LH, and FSH, mean serum testosterone concentrations, and morphological development of the fetal testis. (*From Winter et al.*[49])

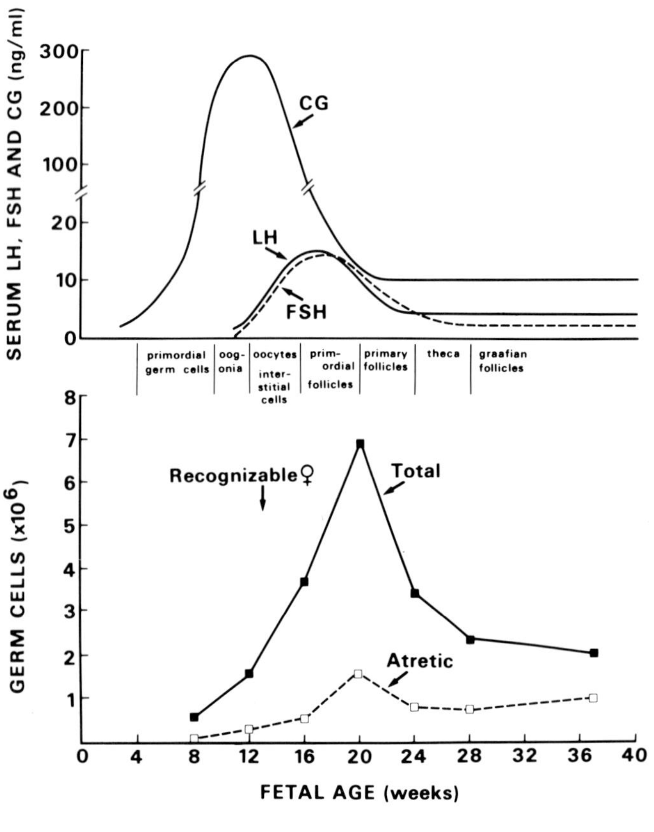

FIGURE 18-8 A schematic summary of the temporal relationships between mean serum concentrations of hCG, LH, and FSH, morphological development of the fetal ovary, and ovarian total content of germ cells. (*From Winter et al.*[49])

nadotropin is no longer detectable, while testosterone levels have become similar in both sexes. During the second week of life a remarkable phenomenon occurs in all normal infants, which can only be interpreted as an apparent onset of puberty. Released from the inhibitory influence of placental estrogens, there is brisk pulsatile secretion of pituitary gonadotropins, which is clearly driven by hypothalamic GnRH just as at adolescence.

In male infants serum gonadotropin levels rise until 1 month of age and then decline to prepubertal levels by 4 months. This rise is accompanied by a parallel rise and fall in serum testosterone concentration (see Table 18-6). In female or functionally hypogonadal infants, because of a relative lack of gonadal steroid feedback inhibition, serum FSH and LH levels continue to rise until 3 to 4 months of age and do not decline to their prepubertal nadir until 3 to 4 years. The steroidogenic response of the infant ovary to this postnatal gonadotropin surge is neither so immediate nor so dramatic as that of the testis. There is usually an increase in the number of large antral follicles, which can be observed by pelvic ultrasonography, but only a variable, unsustained rise in serum estradiol levels. The major clinical correlate of these events is the common appearance of transient breast enlargement in girls 1 to 2 years of age, referred to as *benign premature thelarche.*

The most interesting aspect of these neonatal phenomena is the decline in pituitary gonadotropin secretion which occurs in both sexes, even in the absence of gonads. This clearly reflects maturation of a central mechanism for inhibition of pulsatile hypothalamic GnRH secretion. This prepubertal suppression of pituitary gonadotropin secretion is the penultimate stage in sexual differentiation—the final phase is puberty, with the appearance of sexually dimorphic secondary sex characters and eventual acquisition of full adult reproductive function.

Gender Role and Psychosexual Differentiation

Gender role encompasses a person's psychosexual self-identity, legal and social gender designation, external manifestations such as dress and social comportment, and erotic responsiveness to one sex or the other. For years a nature-versus-nurture controversy has raged regarding the potential significance of prenatal androgen exposure as an organizer of these postnatal phenomena. At one extreme is the concept that each infant is psychosexually neuter at birth and gender identity is permanently imposed during the first few years of life by social and environmental influences. Numerous reports of persons raised in a sex discordant with their genetic or gonadal sex certainly testify to the importance of such influences, although it seems simplistic to assume that their effect is limited to infancy. More likely, gender role is continually reinforced through childhood and puberty by both external influences and awareness of one's genital and secondary sexual characteristics. The demonstration of spontaneous and successful gender role reversal in male pseudohermaphrodites following virilization at puberty[55] underscores the important influence of these sex hormone–mediated factors in later life.

The opposite viewpoint holds that postnatal behavior and intellectual function, to the extent that they are dimorphic, are programmed by sex steroids during a critical prenatal phase of neural differentiation. In its most extreme form this theory proposes that subtle deficiencies of androgen in genetic male fetuses can permit female organization of the brain and predispose to homosexuality.[56] Conversely, excess androgen in a genetic female might induce masculine postnatal behavior, homosexuality, and anovulatory infertility. It must be emphasized that this model invokes not just a direct and immediate activational effect of androgens, such as that upon energy expenditure and libido in adults, but rather an organizational effect on neuronal growth and synaptogenesis which is permanent and expressed for years after the actual hormone exposure. Such organizational effects can be readily demonstrated in female rodents, in whom brief exposure to sex steroids at a critical time can permanently impose male-type acyclic gonadotropin secretion and copulatory behavior in later adult life. Gorski et al. have described sexually dimorphic development of the preoptic area of rat brain which is dependent upon the level of circulating androgens during brain differentiation.[57] But it is not at all clear to what extent these phenomena have a counterpart in human brain development.

Prenatal exposure of female primates to testosterone in amounts sufficient to masculinize the genitalia may induce increased postnatal aggressiveness and lead to aberrant adult sexual behavior but does not block normal ovulatory cycles. The human parallel of this situation might be congenital adrenal hyperplasia, but here any permanent organizational effect has been difficult to prove. Early reports of higher IQ scores in androgen-exposed females have not been confirmed. No studies of the behavior of children with such endocrine disorders have been able to correct adequately for postnatal variations in sex steroid levels or for the impact that awareness of the disease, its treatment, and potential implications has upon both self-image and parental perceptions of behavior.

A reasonable viewpoint would suggest that prenatal androgen may play some role in the differentiation of human psychosexual behavior but is certainly not the decisive determinant.[58] Successful differentiation of gender role appears to depend primarily upon appropriate assignment of the sex of rearing plus continued unambiguous reinforcement by social interaction, concordant genital appearance, and appropriate secondary sexual characteristics. Even in adult life sex steroids continue to interact with psychological and sociocultural factors to maintain patterns of dimorphic behavior we identify as male and female.[59] The implications of this concept for the management of children with disorders of sexual differentiation should be obvious.

ABNORMAL SEXUAL DIFFERENTIATION

Under normal circumstances genetic sex is defined at conception. Subsequently unambiguous male or female differentiation is effected by the presence or absence of three key determinants: a testis-organizing factor, presumed to be H-Y antigen; antimullerian hormone; and testosterone. The synthesis of each is regulated by specific genetic loci, and each requires specific receptor mechanisms which are normally present in the target cells of either sex. Disordered differentiation may occur at any stage in this process and result in inadequate masculinization of a genetic male or inappropriate virilization of a genetic female. Some relatively common situations which should alert the clinician to the possible presence of such a disorder are listed in Table 18-3. In these situations the diagnostic process is not merely an attempt to assign a label but rather a logical stepwise evaluation of the operation of each of the three key determinants until the clinician can define or rationally infer the status of each of the parameters of sexual dimorphism listed in Table 18-1.

Such an approach can also be applied to the classification of disorders of sexual differentiation, as summarized in Table 18-4.

Table 18-3. Clinical Features Suggestive of a Possible Disorder of Sexual Differentiation

In the neonate or infant:
- Ambiguous external genitalia
- Cryptorchism and/or hypospadias
- Female with mass in the groin or labium majus
- Lymphedema or other stigmata of Turner's syndrome
- Family history of anomalous sexual development
- Maternal virilization or hormone ingestion

In the child or young adult:
- Female with short stature or other stigmata of Turner's syndrome
- Female with sexual infantilism or precocious ovarian failure
- Male with small testes, gynecomastia, or other stigmata of Klinefelter's syndrome
- Unexplained virilization

Errors of Primary Sex Determination

Disorders of sex determination involve sex chromosome abnormalities and/or defective gonad formation. For completeness the relatively common situations of trisomy X and the XYY syndrome are included in this category, even though neither produces any consistent abnormality of gonadal structure or function.

SEX CHROMOSOME ANOMALIES ASSOCIATED WITH FUNCTIONAL TESTES AND MALE PHENOTYPE

Klinefelter's Syndrome

In 1942 Klinefelter and his associates described in adult males a syndrome of seminiferous tubule dysgenesis characterized by small, firm testes, azoospermia, eunuchoid body habitus, and gynecomastia.[59a] Subsequent genetic studies disclosed that most of these patients had two X chromosomes; the term *Klinefelter's syndrome* is now usually restricted to persons with a 47,XXY karyotype, although variant forms with similar clinical features also occur.

The genetic abnormality arises from nondisjunction during the first or second meiotic division of gametogenesis. In 60 percent of cases the nondisjunctional error is maternal, therefore the frequency of this disorder is maternal age–dependent. Testis formation, paramesonephric duct regression, and mesonephric duct development are normal and the external genitalia are male, although micropenis may occur. There does not appear to be any excess prenatal wastage of 47,XXY embryos; the frequency in unselected newborns is approximately 1 per 1000 males. As a group, 47,XXY infants have a tendency to lower birth weights and minor somatic anomalies such as clinodactyly, but a clinical diagnosis at this time is unusual. There is some evidence that cord serum testosterone concentrations may be lower than those of controls, but as yet no data regarding the neonatal gonadotropin/testosterone surge are available.

During childhood many, but not all, patients with Klinefelter's syndrome show increased stature (above the 50th percentile), with relatively long legs, decreased head circumference, dull mentality, emotional immaturity, and poor neuromuscular coordination. Penile length and testis volume are usually in the low-

Table 18-4. A Classification of Abnormal Sexual Development

I. Errors of Primary Sex Determination
- A. Sex chromosome anomalies
  - 1. With testes and male phenotype
    - *a.* Klinefelter's syndrome (47,XXY and variants)
    - *b.* XYY syndrome
    - *c.* XX males (X-Y interchange)
  - 2. With ovaries and female phenotype
    - *a.* Trisomy X and variants
  - 3. With bisexual gonads
    - *a.* True hermaphroditism (X-Y interchange)
    - *b.* Chimeric (XX/XY) true hermaphroditism
    - *c.* Mosaic (XX/XXY) true hermaphroditism
  - 4. With dysgenetic gonads
    - *a.* Y chromosome anomalies (XYp−)
    - *b.* Mixed gonadal dysgenesis (45,X/46,XY)
    - *c.* Turner's syndrome (45,X and variants)
- B. Anomalies of gonadogenesis
  - 1. Defective ovary development
    - *a.* XX gonadal dysgenesis
  - 2. Defective testis development
    - *a.* XY gonadal dysgenesis
    - *b.* Dysgenetic male pseudohermaphroditism
    - *c.* Testicular regression syndromes (agonadism; rudimentary testis; anorchia)

II. Errors of Sexual Differentiation
- A. Inadequate masculinization of genetic male
  - 1. Defective paramesonephric duct regression
    - *a.* Persistent paramesonephric ducts
  - 2. Defective genital virilization
    - *a.* Leydig cell hypoplasia (LH/hCG receptor defect)
    - *b.* Inborn errors of corticosteroid and testosterone synthesis
      - (1) Cholesterol side-chain cleavage (20,22-desmolase) deficiency
      - (2) 3β-Hydroxysteroid dehydrogenase deficiency
      - (3) 17α-Hydroxylase deficiency
    - *c.* Inborn errors of testosterone synthesis
      - (1) 17,20-Desmolase deficiency
      - (2) 17β-Hydroxysteroid dehydrogenase deficiency
    - *d.* Inborn error of testosterone metabolism
      - (1) 5α-Reductase deficiency
    - *e.* Defective target cell response
      - (1) Complete testicular feminization
      - (2) Incomplete testicular feminization and variants
    - *f.* Environmental feminization
      - (1) Maternal ingestion of estrogen or progestin
    - *g.* Multigenic/multifactorial
      - (1) Isolated hypospadias and cryptorchism
      - (2) Multiple congenital anomaly syndromes
- B. Virilization of genetic female
  - 1. Adrenal androgens (congenital adrenal hyperplasia)
    - *a.* 21-Hydroxylase deficiency
    - *b.* 11β-Hydroxylase deficiency
    - *c.* 3β-Hydroxysteroid dehydrogenase deficiency
  - 2. Environmental hormones
    - *a.* Maternal virilizing disorders
    - *b.* Iatrogenic virilization
  - 3. Teratological malformation
    - *a.* Abnormal development of vagina or uterus
    - *b.* Multiple congenital anomaly syndromes

normal range. Before puberty the testes show reduced numbers of spermatogonia, but tubular hyalinization is not observed. Serum concentrations of FSH, LH, testosterone, and estradiol are in the normal prepubertal range, and responses to stimulation with GnRH and hCG are appropriate for age.[60]

Secondary sex characters usually appear at the normal age. Testis size often increases initially, but growth usually ceases before midpuberty at an average volume of 3.5 ± 1.5 ml.[61] Coincident with the onset of puberty, serum gonadotropin values increase abruptly to abnormal levels (Fig. 18-9). Presumably this hypergonadotropic state reflects diminished testosterone production; in turn it leads to progressive hyalinization and fibrosis of seminiferous tubules, clumping of Leydig cells, and enhanced testicular secretion of estrogen. Spermatogenesis is rarely present except in a few isolated tubules. Because of tubular shrinkage the Leydig cells appear hyperplastic, but in fact Leydig cell volume is not affected. Serum estradiol concentrations tend to be high-normal, while serum testosterone concentrations fail to rise above the low-normal adult range. In 50 to 75 percent of unselected patients, clinically apparent gynecomastia develops; in contrast to benign juvenile gynecomastia, this often persists into adult life.

Virtually all adult 47,XXY subjects are azoospermic; the occasional report of paternity may reflect hidden XY/XXY mosaicism or the appearance of a clone of XY spermatocytes through mitotic nondisjunction. Clinical problems possibly related to androgen deficiency include a eunuchoid body habitus, persistent gynecomastia, reduced lean body mass, decreased libido and seminal volume, and a lack of social drive and aggressiveness. It is not yet clear to what extent these physical and psychosexual handicaps can be prevented or ameliorated by supplementation with exogenous androgens from early puberty.

In addition to consistently elevated values of serum FSH and LH, adults with Klinefelter's syndrome show reduced circulating levels of testosterone (276 ± 156 ng/dl) and dihydrotestosterone (28 ± 9.4 ng/dl)

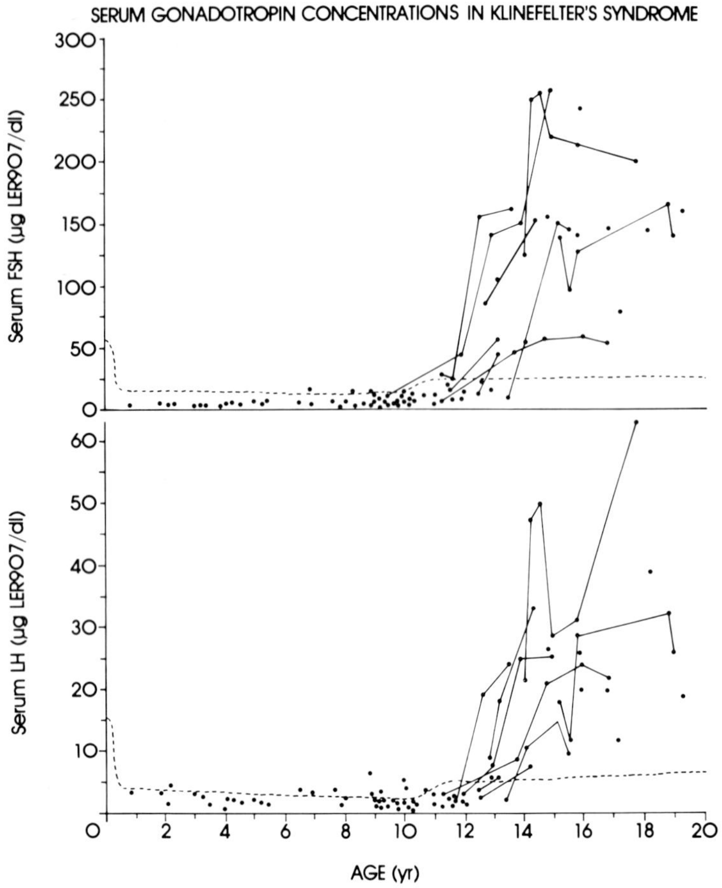

FIGURE 18-9 Basal serum FSH and LH concentrations in boys with Klinefelter's syndrome before and during puberty. The dotted lines show the upper limit of the normal male range. The gonadotropin values may be converted from micrograms of LER907 per deciliter to international units per liter by multiplying FSH by 0.5 and LH by 4.5. (*From Salbenblatt et al.*[60])

and increased levels of estradiol (2.8 ± 0.9 ng/dl); levels of adrenal androgens are not significantly different from normal.[62] With advancing age testicular function continues to decline, with a further decrease in serum testosterone levels and testosterone/estradiol ratios.

The prevalence of impaired glucose tolerance, chronic pulmonary disease, and varicose veins appears to be increased in adults with Klinefelter's syndrome. In addition there is a predisposition to various neoplasms, including germ cell tumors, bronchogenic carcinoma, acute lymphocytic leukemia, and carcinoma of the breast. The frequency of breast cancer in Klinefelter's syndrome patients is about 20 times that in normal men.[63]

The diagnosis of Klinefelter's syndrome may be suspected on the basis of the traditional phenotype but should be considered in any male with hypergonadotropic hypogonadism. The diagnosis is supported by the finding of a chromatin-positive buccal smear but should always be confirmed by karyotype analysis.

The most common variant form of Klinefelter's syndrome is 46,XY/47,XXY mosaicism; these patients show lesser degrees of hypogonadism, may be fertile, and may not complain of androgen deficiency until the fourth or fifth decades of life. Patients with more severe sex chromosome anomalies such as 48,XXYY, 48,XXXY, 49,XXXYY, or 49,XXXXY have the typical features of Klinefelter's syndrome but also are mentally retarded and show a wide range of somatic anomalies, particularly radioulnar synostosis, epiphyseal dysplasia, and patent ductus arteriosus. The presence of testes in these syndromes of X polysomy demonstrates the power of the Y chromosome to direct male gonadal differentiation.

The treatment of Klinefelter's syndrome is amelioration of hypergonadotropic hypogonadism and the resulting poor self-image. Most patients benefit psychologically and socially from surgery to reduce gynecomastia and administration of full replacement doses of oral testosterone undecanoate or intramuscular testosterone esters, coupled with long-term counseling by an informed and sympathetic physician.

XYY Males

Strictly speaking, the 47,XYY karyotype, which occurs in about 1 of every 1000 males, does not produce a disorder of sexual differentiation, since testicular, internal genital, and external genital development is male. There are no consistent physical anomalies, but hypotonia, delayed speech, and poor neuromuscular coordination appear to be relatively common. Tall stature is often described but is not a consistent finding. Testicular size is usually normal, but up to 10 percent may have small testes. Adolescent and adult testicular endocrine function is normal, with no evidence of hypergonadotropic hypogonadism. Although many XYY males are fertile and presumably have normal seminiferous epithelium, biopsy studies of institutionalized adult patients have described variable, but often severe, abnormalities of spermatogenesis. The XYY disorder initially gained notoriety when it was discovered that its incidence was increased in criminals with persistent violent or aggressive behavior. It is now generally recognized that various sex chromosome anomalies, including but not limited to XYY, may be associated with behavioral difficulties in children and adults, but the suggestion that criminality may be the inevitable result is both naive and simplistic.

XX Males

Although phenotypic males with a 46,XX karyotype occur only once in every 30,000 male infants, this situation provides a useful illustration of the central role played in male sexual differentiation by the testis-determining gene locus usually found on the Y chromosome. Even though these persons lack a Y chromosome, they are uniformly H-Y antigen–positive and have testes which resemble histologically those of XXY males. Recent studies have demonstrated that in XX males X-Y interchange has occurred during paternal gametogenesis, with the testis-determining segment and other DNA sequences normally located on the Y chromosome being translocated to the short arm of the X chromosome; in turn, the paternal X chromosome can be shown to have lost genetic material from its short arm.[64] Such X-Y translocation does not always lead to development of testes but may result in gonadal dysgenesis with a female phenotype if the testis-determining locus is not involved or is inoperative.[65] In the few XX males in whom Y-specific genetic material has not been detectable, the possibility has been raised that H-Y antigen synthesis and testis development could result from mutation or deletion of the putative X-linked repressor locus on both X chromosomes; such a genetic defect would explain the occasional autosomal recessive occurrence in the same pedigree of both XX males and true hermaphrodites.

Clinically, XX males resemble those with Klinefelter's syndrome, although they tend to be somewhat shorter (mean height 168 cm). Their internal and external genitalia are usually normal, but hypospadias, cryptorchism, or more severe genital ambiguity occurs in about 10 percent of cases. The testes are small and soft, with uneven hyalinization, peritubular fibrosis, and Leydig cell clumping after the onset of puberty. Spermatogonia are usually absent, possibly because of premature commitment of the XX germ cells to meiosis. It is of interest that while two functioning X chromosomes are essential to survival of germ cells in the ovary, they are detrimental to survival in a testicular environment. One-third of the patients develop significant gynecomastia. The hormonal profile of adult XX males confirms their hypergonadotropic hypogonadism, with increased serum concentrations of FSH and LH and reduced levels of testosterone. Basal and GnRH-stimulated androgen levels may be normal during childhood, as in Klinefelter's syndrome.

SEX CHROMOSOME ANOMALIES ASSOCIATED WITH OVARIES AND FEMALE PHENOTYPE

A 47,XXX karyotype occurs in about 1 per 1000 female infants, usually as a result of nondisjunction during maternal meiosis; thus, as in Klinefelter's syndrome, there is a maternal age effect. Sexual differentiation is female. No consistent pattern of somatic abnormalities is observed in this condition (*trisomy X*), but birth weight tends to be low and various minor anomalies have been reported.[66] Although one must be cautious regarding sampling bias due to investigation in institutions, triple-X females do seem to show a greater prevalence of mental retardation, cognitive dysfunction, and schizophreniform psychoses. There is a variable effect upon oogenesis: about one-quarter of patients experience some form of ovarian dysfunction, ranging from delayed menarche to premature ovarian failure, but fertility does occur. Naturally, the hormonal profile is dependent upon the degree of ovarian dysfunction. Similar abnormalities, but usually associated with more severe somatic anomalies, have been described in association with 48,XXXX and 49,XXXXX karyotypes.

SEX CHROMOSOME ANOMALIES ASSOCIATED WITH BISEXUAL GONADAL DEVELOPMENT

A person can be classified as a *true hermaphrodite* only if both testicular tissue with distinct tubules and ovarian tissue containing follicles or corpora albicantia are present. The more frequent finding of a dysgenetic gonad containing testicular elements plus fibrous stroma without follicles does not establish true hermaphroditism. About 30 percent of cases are classified as lateral, with a testis on one side and an ovary on the other; 50 percent have one ovotestis; and the rest have bilateral ovotestes containing distinct ovarian and testicular elements.[67]

All true hermaphrodites are H-Y antigen–positive, albeit in reduced titers. Approximately two-thirds show a 46,XX karyotype. In these the most common genetic mechanism is X-Y interchange during paternal gametogenesis, as in the XX male. Thus interchange between the X and Y chromosomes may result in an XX male (with or without hypospadias), true hermaphroditism, or gonadal dysgenesis, depending upon the efficacy of the translocated testis-determining DNA segment. Pedigrees containing both XX males and XX true hermaphrodites are thought to result from familial deletion of an X-linked repressor locus, permitting variable expression of an autosomal H-Y structural gene. The pathogenesis of the less common 46,XY form of true hermaphroditism is less clear but may involve undetected XX/XY chimerism. Such whole-body chimerism has been documented in several cases and presumably results from double fertilization (by an X and a Y sperm) of a binucleate ovum or fusion of XX and XY zygotes. Finally, a few cases of XX/XXY mosaicism have been described as a result of loss of a Y chromosome from a 47,XXY zygote at an early mitotic division. Thus a variety of genetic mechanisms may be operative, but all have the same end result: variable expression of H-Y antigen within the developing gonad.

The clinical presentation of true hermaphroditism depends upon the amount of functioning testicular tissue. In patients with a testis and an ovary, development of the mesonephric and paramesonephric ducts is consistent with the appearance of the ipsilateral gonad. With ovotestes, genital duct development is usually female. According to the level of circulating androgen, the external genitalia may appear female, may be ambiguous, or may be frankly masculine, although hypospadias and cryptorchism are common. Sometimes an inguinal hernia contains an ovotestis. At puberty virilization is variable. Breast development and menstruation are common, reflecting the low serum testosterone/estradiol ratio in most patients. If testicular function is minimal or if all testicular tissue has been removed, cyclical gonadotropin secretion, ovulation, and fertility may be observed. Spermatogenesis is rare, and male fertility has not been documented. Gonadal tumors, usually gonadoblastoma, dysgerminoma, or seminoma, occur in about 2 percent of true hermaphrodites.

The diagnosis of true hermaphroditism can be confirmed only by histological examination of the gonads. In an infant the sex of rearing should be assigned according to the degree of virilization of the internal and external genitalia. Any discordant or dysgenetic gonadal tissue together with inappropriate internal genital structures should be removed and plastic repair of the external genitalia undertaken. In children being raised as males it is probably wise to retain a testis only if it appears normal and is located in the scrotum, because of the risk of malignancy. Appropriate sex hormone replacement will usually be required at the age of puberty.

SEX CHROMOSOME ANOMALIES ASSOCIATED WITH DYSGENETIC GONADS

Structural Anomalies of the Y Chromosome

Abnormalities of the Y chromosome may include ring formation, deletions, dicentrics, inversions, and isochromosomes. Patients with extensive deletions of the short arm of Y may present with gonadal dysgenesis, female phenotype, and the somatic stigmata of Turner's syndrome. Conversely, if the short arm is intact, testes and male sexual differentiation may develop. However, the abnormal Y chromosome is frequently lost during an early mitotic division, producing a variable proportion of 45,X cells and some degree of gonadal dysgenesis. The clinical picture then becomes that of mixed gonadal dysgenesis.[68]

Mixed Gonadal Dysgenesis

It is not uncommon for a Y chromosome, particularly one that is structurally abnormal, to be lost from a 46,XY zygote by anaphase lag or mitotic nondisjunction. The karyotype will then show 45,X as well as 46,XY and/or 47,XYY cell lines in varying proportions, and the phenotype will depend upon the amount of testicular tissue present. If no testicular development occurs, the clinical presentation will be that of a female with bilateral streak gonads, although short stature and the somatic anomalies of Turner's syndrome (see below) may be less obvious than in the pure 45,X patient.

The term *mixed gonadal dysgenesis* is applied to those persons with 45,X/46,XY mosaicism in whom some prenatal virilization has occurred. These patients are H-Y antigen–positive and show either one dysgenetic testis (usually intraabdominal) and one streak gonad or bilateral testes, both usually dysgenetic to some degree. Internal genital differentiation depends upon the functional integrity of the ipsilateral gonad, but usually one or both paramesonephric ducts fail to regress and a rudimentary uterus is present. Depending upon the level of prenatal androgen secretion, the newborn patient may display isolated clitoral hypertrophy, ambiguous external genitalia, or even relatively normal male genitalia, with or without hypospadias.[69] Two-thirds of the reported patients have been raised as females.

The importance of identifying 45,X/46,XY mosaicism, regardless of the phenotype, lies in the potential for significant virilization at puberty and the propensity of the affected gonads to undergo malignant degeneration. In most cases there is fairly good correlation between the degree of genital masculinization and the secretion of testosterone at puberty; this can be assessed directly before puberty by observing the serum testosterone response to several days of hCG stimulation.

The risk of gonadal neoplasm, whether gonadoblastoma, dysgerminoma, or embryonal carcinoma, in patients with 45,X/46,XY mosaicism is approximately 20 percent overall and increases with age.[70] The risk of malignancy is probably greatest in dysgenetic testes and least in streak gonads. The occurrence of spontaneous breast development nearly always signals the presence of an estrogen-secreting gonadoblastoma. Often a gonadal neoplasm can be detected by pelvic ultrasonography or computerized tomography, but regardless of these findings or the clinical phenotype, it is a prudent policy to recommend prophylactic removal of streak gonads and undescended testes during the first decade in all children with 45,X/46,XY mosaicism. Occasionally in a phenotypic male, scrotal testes of normal consistency may be preserved under close and continuing observation.

Because of the continuum of genital differentiation seen in these patients, decisions regarding the sex of rearing should be based upon the potential for normal genital function. In females, clitoroplasty and vaginoplasty should be undertaken in infancy. In males all paramesonephric duct remnants should be removed, hypospadias repaired, and testicular prostheses placed in the scrotum. In either case prophylactic gonadectomy is desirable, and appropriate sex steroid replacement will be needed at puberty.

Turner's Syndrome

Classic Turner's syndrome consists of bilateral gonadal dysgenesis with streak gonads, female phenotype, and sexual infantilism plus short stature and a pattern of distinctive somatic stigmata (Fig. 18-10). The typical syndrome results from monosomy for the X chromosome (45,X), with or without mosaicism, but may also be seen in patients with two sex chromosomes in which one (X or Y) is structurally defective, producing effective monosomy.

Comparison of the frequency of the 45,X karyotype in spontaneous abortions (approximately 1 in 15) and in live births (1 in 20,000) demonstrates that monosomy X is nearly always lethal in utero; surviving patients often show some degree of mosaicism, indicative of a postfertilization mitotic error. It is of interest that Turner's syndrome is more frequently associated with young maternal age.[71] In 80 percent of 45,X survivors the single X chromosome is of maternal origin, suggesting preferential loss of the paternal sex chromosome either before or after fertilization. Mosaic forms are commonly the result of postzygotic loss of a sex chromosome that is structurally abnormal. Monozygotic twinning appears to be more frequent in such mosaicism situations; the twins may be discordant for the Turner's syndrome phenotype because of heterogeneous distribution of the 45,X and other (usually XX, XY, or XXX) cell lines.

The indifferent gonad of the 45,X fetus forms normally and is seeded by germ cells which become incorporated into primordial follicles. But the rate of follicular atresia and degeneration is greatly increased, so that by birth only a few primary follicles remain. Almost always these, too, disappear before puberty, leaving fibrous streak gonads, the consequence of which is sexual infantilism and primary amenorrhea. As one would expect, the internal and external genitalia are female. Any sign of prenatal or postnatal virilization indicates the presence of a Y-bearing cell line and some testicular tissue (mixed gonadal dysgenesis).

Generalized lymphedema with hygromatous neck masses is characteristic of the 45,X fetus. In newborn infants this same lymphatic hypoplasia can produce the Bonnevie-Ullrich syndrome, with distal lymphedema, loose skin folds at the nape, ascites, and pleural effusion. Birth weight and length are usually low for gestational age.

During childhood the dominant clinical feature is short stature. Height is invariably below the third percentile for age, while growth velocity is less strikingly reduced (between the 10th and 25th percentiles). Because of the sexual infantilism, untreated patients show no pubertal growth spurt, and radiological bone maturation becomes retarded after 11 years of age. The mean adult height is 147 cm, but height can range up to 155 cm, depending on parental stature.[72]

Accompanying this short stature is often a characteristic pattern of somatic abnormalities (Fig. 18-10). The skull is brachycephalic and the facies are distinctive, with a triangular shape, retruded mandible, epicanthal folds, ptosis, and a narrow high palate. The ears are low-set and often deformed. The nuchal hair line is low and the neck short in most cases, but frank webbing of the neck (pterygium colli) occurs in only 40 percent. The chest is usually square or shield-shaped, the nipples are relatively wide-spaced, and pectus excavatum may be present. There are com-

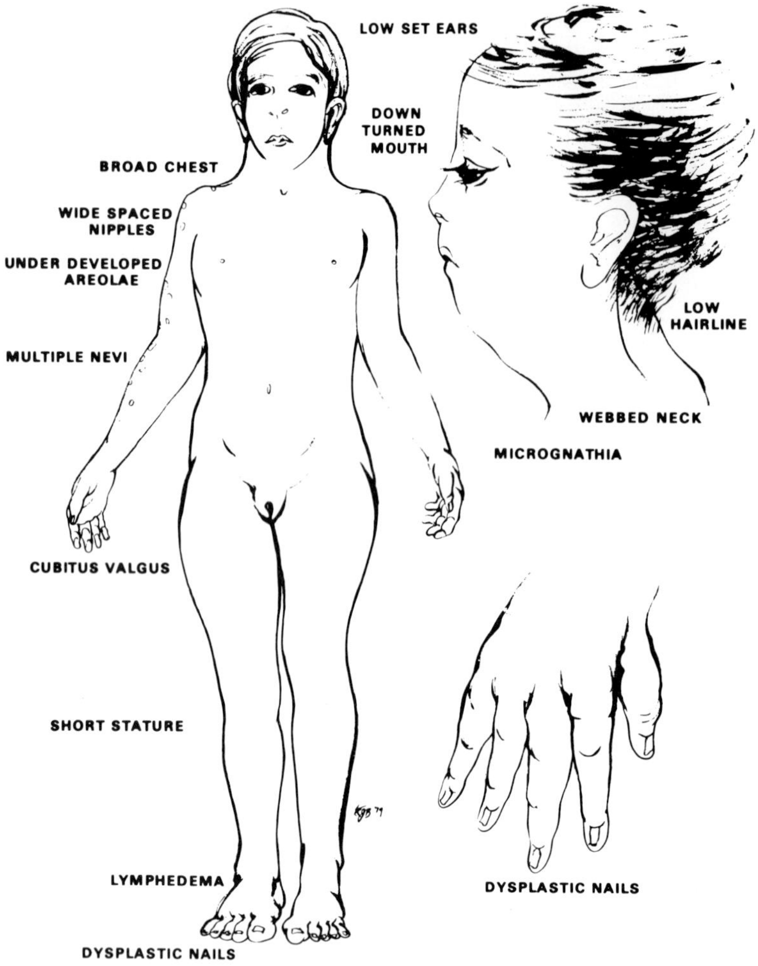

FIGURE 18-10 The major clinical features of a child with Turner's syndrome (45,X gonadal dysgenesis). [*From Dean HJ, Winter JSD, in Collu R, Ducharme JR, Guyda H (eds): Pediatric Endocrinology. New York: Raven, 1981, p 339.*]

monly many pigmented nevi over the face, arms, and chest. Anomalies of the extremities include cubitus valgus (in about 50 percent), lymphedema or puffiness of the hands and feet, shortening of the fourth metacarpal, and hypoplastic nails. Kyphoscoliosis is not uncommon. Renal anomalies, including unilateral aplasia, horseshoe kidney, and ureteral duplication, are found in 60 percent of cases. Coarctation of the aorta is the commonest cardiovascular anomaly (in 10 percent), but ventricular septal defect, aortic stenosis, and bicuspid aortic valve also occur. Occasionally gastrointestinal bleeding may result from congenital intestinal telangiectasia. Strabismus is not uncommon, and there may be hearing loss due to either sensorineural deficit or recurrent otitis media. Although most 45,X patients have normal intelligence and the incidence of severe psychopathology is not increased, they frequently demonstrate social immaturity and specific perceptual disability in areas of directional sense and space-form recognition.[72a]

Radiographic examination will often disclose characteristic bony anomalies, including shortening of the fourth metacarpal, the "carpal sign," or a reduced angle in the proximal row of carpals,[73] basilar impression of the skull, hypoplasia of cervical vertebrae, and occasional areas of aseptic necrosis, particularly around the knee. In adults who have not received sex steroids osteoporosis may become severe. Reactive enlargement of the pituitary fossa has also been described in adult patients with long-standing untreated hypergonadotropic hypogonadism. Excretory urography commonly discloses structural or positional abnormalities of the kidney, occasionally associated with significant ureteropelvic obstruction.

Several other disorders appear to be increased in patients with Turner's syndrome. Hypertension unrelated to aortic coarctation or renal disease occurs in about half of adult patients; although the initial rise in blood pressure occurs during the second decade, there does not seem to be an obvious relationship to estrogen therapy. The risk of autoimmune endocrine disease, particularly of the thyroid, is considerably increased. Antithyroid antibodies indicative of chronic lymphocytic thyroiditis can be detected in about a third of patients, and many of these in time develop goiter or become hypothyroid. Impaired carbohydrate tolerance can frequently be demonstrated, but frank diabetes mellitus is less common. Other autoimmune disorders, such as rheumatoid arthritis and inflammatory bowel disease, appear to be more frequent in Turner's syndrome. In addition to concern regarding possible gonadal neoplasms (see below), there is some evidence for an increased risk of nongonadal malignancy in these patients.

PHENOTYPE-KARYOTYPE CORRELATIONS The key genetic determinants which are absent in Turner's syndrome appear to be on the short arm of the X or Y chromosome, and the severity of the clinical presentation to some extent correlates with the amount of this loss. Patients with complete monosomy (45,X) or an isochromosome for the long arm [46,X,iso(Xq)] usually show the classic syndrome, with short stature, sexual infantilism, and multiple somatic stigmata. The latter patients are unlikely to show aortic coarctation or severe lymphedema but appear to be more at risk for autoimmune disorders such as Hashimoto's disease and diabetes mellitus. Patients with major deletions of the short arm [46,X(Xp−)] or a ring X chromosome [46,X,r(X)] tend to have fewer somatic stigmata, while those with deletions of the long arm [46,X(Xq−)] usually present with only sexual infantilism or primary amenorrhea, are of normal stature, and show none of the usual somatic stigmata. However, structurally abnormal sex chromosomes are frequently lost during an early mitotic division, leading to a variable proportion of 45,X cells, which will naturally confute phenotype-karyotype generalizations. For the same reason the buccal smear may be chromatin-negative or chromatin-positive, depending upon the relative proportion of 45,X and 46,XX cells in that tissue. Occasionally a clue to the presence of an isochromosome or major deletion may be provided by a sex chromatin body that is larger or smaller than normal.

There have been many reports of breast development, menses, and even fertility in patients with Turner's syndrome.[74] Most such patients show few physical stigmata and can be shown to have 45,X/46,XX or 45,X/47,XXX mosaicism. If mosaicism cannot be detected in peripheral leukocytes, it may be impossible to determine whether this spontaneous ovarian function represents hidden mosaicism or the rare survival of a 45,X oocyte. To date most reported patients with 45,X/46,XX mosaicism with secondary amenorrhea have also had short stature, but it is not clear to what extent this represents sampling bias.

Several interesting patients have demonstrated either pericentric inversion or balanced X-X or X-autosome translocation, that is, breakage and structural rearrangement of segments of the X chromosome without any detectable loss of genetic material. These studies demonstrate that there is a critical segment on the long arm of X (between bands Xq13 and Xq26) which is essential for normal gonadal development.[75] Females with break points or rearrangements affecting this segment often suffer from primary or secondary amenorrhea; males with the same defect may show disturbed spermatogenesis.

As described previously, patients with 45,X/46,XY or 45,X/47,XYY mosaicism may show varying degrees of virilization, depending upon the amount of functional testicular tissue. Not only may their genital development be female, ambiguous, or male, but the degree of short stature and the frequency of somatic anomalies are also highly variable. At puberty they may be virilized because of Leydig cell activity, may remain sexually infantile because of gonadal dysgenesis, or may be feminized because of an estrogen-secreting gonadal neoplasm. Because of their propensity to develop gonadoblastoma or malignant germinoma, the risk of which approaches 20 percent in the second decade, the streak gonads or dysgenetic testes of any patient with 45,X/46,XY mosaicism should be removed. However, in classic Turner's syndrome patients with no apparent prenatal or pubertal virilization and no cytogenetic evidence of a Y-bearing cell line, prophylactic gonadectomy does not appear to be necessary. Unfortunately, present-day assays for H-Y antigen are probably inadequate for the detection of small foci of dysgenetic testicular tissue, since all Turner's syndrome patients show low titers of H-Y antigen.[76]

DIAGNOSIS AND TREATMENT A definitive diagnosis of Turner's syndrome requires careful karyotype analysis, including banding and study of sufficient cells to confirm or exclude mosaicism. In equivocal situations, particularly when the presence of a Y-bearing or 45,X cell line is critical to patient management, consideration should be given to genetic analysis of additional tissues such as skin fibroblasts. Because of the relatively high proportion of patients with mosaicism, a buccal smear for sex chromatin is an inadequate diagnostic technique.

In the evaluation of females with short stature or late puberty, a clue to the presence of gonadal dysgenesis may be the finding of serum FSH concentrations which are above the age-specific normal range (Fig. 18-11). In contrast to the situation in Kline-

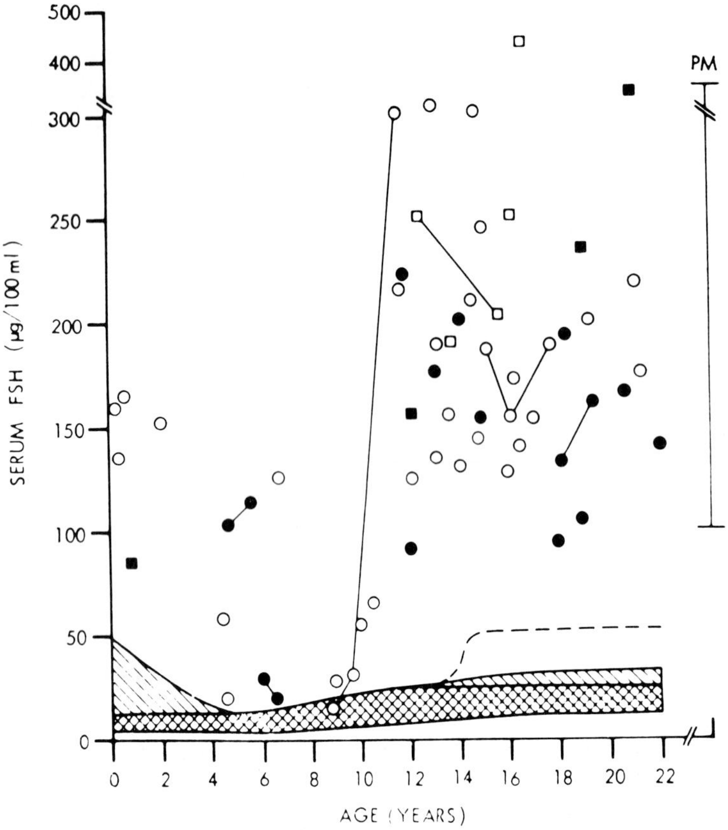

FIGURE 18-11 Serum FSH concentrations in agonadal subjects. The normal male and female ranges are shown by the hatched areas. The dotted line represents the adult female midcycle peak and the bar (PM) the postmenopausal range. Patients with gonadal dysgenesis are shown by open circles. (*From Winter and Faiman.*[77])

felter's syndrome, children with gonadal dysgenesis will usually show high serum FSH levels[77] and exaggerated responses to stimulation with exogenous GnRH. Even though the absence of gonadal negative feedback leads to increased gonadotropin secretion, the pattern of serum gonadotropin values in agonadal children parallels that in normal girls, with higher values in infancy, a decline in midchildhood, and a rise to the postmenopausal range again at the normal time of puberty.

The short stature of Turner's syndrome is present even before birth and is not the result of any endocrine deficiency. Growth hormone levels and responses to various stimuli are normal, and growth responses to the doses of exogenous human growth hormone used in hypopituitarism are insignificant. However, clinical acromegaly due to a growth hormone releasing hormone–secreting pancreatic neoplasm has been observed in a patient with Turner's syndrome, and there is therefore every reason to believe that, as in pituitary gigantism, a significant increase in final height might be obtained by treating affected children with large doses of growth hormone. The current availability of biosynthetic growth hormone will undoubtedly lead to studies which should serve to document both the growth impact and the metabolic side effects of such treatment.[78]

Patients with Turner's syndrome show normal serum levels of adrenal androgens and a normal adrenarchal rise in these values before the age of puberty; thereafter, because of deficient gonadal contribution, serum testosterone and androstenedione concentrations are slightly lower than in normal females.[79] Several studies have demonstrated improved growth velocity in patients treated with low doses of exogenous androgen (fluoxymesterone or oxandrolone, 0.1 to 0.3 mg per kilogram of body weight per day), but it has been difficult to ascertain whether such treatment has any significant effect upon eventual adult size.[80–82] A reasonable approach might be to restrict the use of androgen therapy to those situations in which short-term growth acceleration is desirable for psychological reasons.

While at the present time there does not appear to be any endocrine therapy which can consistently improve adult height in Turner's syndrome, there is no question that all patients with gonadal dysgenesis require replacement sex steroid therapy. Our approach has been to initiate estrogen replacement in low doses (ethinyl estradiol, 5 to 10 μg per day) at the age (usually 12 to 14 years) at which the patient's peers begin puberty. This will elicit gradual development of breasts and pubic hair and appears to induce at least a temporary acceleration of growth.[83,83a] Recently it has been suggested that even lower doses of ethinyl estradiol (100 ng per kilogram of body weight daily) might improve growth in younger children without producing secondary sex characteristics,[84] but in our experience even this amount eventually produces breast enlargement. Because of the significant risk of endometrial hyperplasia and carcinoma in patients treated only with estrogen, it is essential that patients after about 6 months be switched to a combination estrogen-progestin preparation administered in cyclic fashion. In our experience satisfactory secondary sexual maturation and regular menses can be maintained in young adults with daily doses of ethinyl estradiol or mestranol of 50 μg or less in combination with a progestin; there is reason to believe that such a regimen does not carry an increased risk of abnormal endometrial histology nor of breast cancer.[84a]

ANOMALIES OF GONADOGENESIS WITHOUT CHROMOSOMAL ABNORMALITY

Defective Ovary Formation

Defective ovary formation is exemplified by *XX gonadal dysgenesis,* in which patients have bilateral streak gonads but normal stature, a 46,XX karyotype, and none of the somatic stigmata of Turner's syndrome. Their internal and external genitalia are normal female, and the diagnosis is not suspected until sexual infantilism and hypergonadotropic hypogonadism become apparent at the normal age of puberty. Familial aggregation is common, and siblings may show hypoplastic ovaries and precocious menopause, suggesting variable expression of the basic genetic disorder. In several families gonadal dysgenesis and sensorineural deafness were observed together, but it is not clear whether this represented varied expression of a single mutant gene or coincident occurrence of two genetic disorders. An occasional patient has shown signs of postpubertal virilization, thought to reflect hilus cell hyperplasia within the streak gonads in response to high circulating gonadotropin levels. Gonadal neoplasia does not seem to be a feature of XX gonadal dysgenesis.

The common finding of consanguinity in affected families points to the presence of a rare X-linked or autosomal recessive gene which must be present in double dose to prevent normal ovarian development. Genetic heterogeneity seems likely, since occasional patients have shown short stature or various neurological deficits. The pathogenesis remains obscure, but presumably the mutant gene acts either to impair oogonial maturation and follicle formation or to accelerate the rate of germ cell attrition, as in Turner's syndrome. Because of the genetic implications of this disorder it is important to rule out 45,X/46,XX mosaicism with great care. Treatment of the hypergonadotropic hypogonadism is carried out with replacement estrogen and progestin as in other forms of gonadal dysgenesis.

Defective Testis Formation

XY GONADAL DYSGENESIS (SWYER SYNDROME) If in spite of normal male genetic sex (46,XY), testes fail to develop, the phenotypic result will be XY gonadal dysgenesis with streak gonads, female internal and external genitalia, and sexual infantilism at the time of puberty. The short stature and somatic stigmata of Turner's syndrome are not features of this syndrome and if present probably indicate undetected 45,X/46,XY mosaicism. However, different pedigrees have been described in which XY gonadal dysgenesis was associated with other somatic anomalies, notably camptomelic dwarfism, interstitial nephritis or renal failure, and ectodermal and cardiac anomalies.

This clinical variability underscores the genetic heterogeneity of this syndrome.[85] Some cases are sporadic; these tend to be H-Y antigen–negative and may represent a small deletion involving the H-Y antigen activator locus on the short arm of the Y chromosome. In addition there appears to be a male-limited autosomal recessive form which is also H-Y antigen–negative; this may represent a defect in an autosomal structural gene locus for H-Y antigen. Finally, about 70 percent of reported cases are in patients who are H-Y antigen–positive in spite of the absence of testes; the inheritance in these families appears to be X-linked recessive and may represent a defect in the gonadal receptor for H-Y antigen. In some of these families other members have shown bilateral dysgenetic testes and ambiguous genitalia, presumably reflecting variable expression of the same genetic defect. Thus XY gonadal dysgenesis may result from defects in the Y-linked activator locus (H-Y antigen–negative and sporadic because of sterility in the carrier); in the autosomal H-Y antigen structural gene locus (familial and H-Y–negative unless a serologically detectable but inactive molecule is synthesized); or in the X-linked H-Y antigen receptor locus (H-Y–positive and familial).

Regardless of the etiology, the usual clinical presentation is a phenotypic female with sexual infantilism and primary amenorrhea. Clitoromegaly can occur in untreated adults because of hyperstimulation of androgen-secreting hilus cells in the streak gonads. Spontaneous breast development does not occur unless an estrogen-secreting neoplasm appears.

As in other forms of defective testis development, there is a 20 to 30 percent risk of gonadal neoplasm, mainly gonadoblastoma or dysgerminoma. It is not yet clear whether the risk is higher in those patients who are H-Y antigen–positive and therefore more likely to have foci of testicular tissue. Until this issue is clearer it seems reasonable to suggest prophylactic gonadectomy for all patients with XY gonadal dysgenesis. Sex hormone replacement should be initiated in the same manner as in other forms of gonadal dysgenesis.

DYSGENETIC MALE PSEUDOHERMAPHRODITISM The term *dysgenetic male pseudohermaphroditism* does not define a distinct clinical entity but rather is a catchall phrase to describe patients with a 46,XY karyotype who present with bilateral dysgenetic testes (usually intraabdominal), incomplete masculinization with ambiguous external genitalia, and variable persistence of paramesonephric duct structures. In most such patients the disorder is not familial. It seems likely that many of these patients have a subtle structural anomaly of the Y chromosome [e.g., 46,X,(Yp−) or 46,X(Yp−)/46,XY mosaicism] or represent unrecognized cases of 45,X/46,XY mosaicism. The latter situation may prove impossible to detect if selective pressures mitigate against survival of the 45,X cell line in peripheral leukocytes or fibroblasts. Other patients may represent a less severe variant of XY gonadal dysgenesis with some testicular differentiation. A few pedigrees have been reported in which some members showed typical H-Y antigen–positive XY gonadal dysgenesis with bilateral streak gonads and female phenotype, while others appeared to demonstrate an incomplete variant with one or two dysgenetic testes, ambiguous genitalia, and rudimentary paramesonephric duct derivatives. It seems likely that this situation represents variable expression of a genetic defect involving the gonad-specific H-Y antigen receptor. Most of these patients will show some virilization at puberty if their testes remain, and they are at high risk to develop a gonadoblastoma or germinoma. As in any intersex situation in which sterility is inevitable, sex of rearing should be assigned so as to provide the greatest opportunity for normal genital function. Because of the high risk of neoplasia, early prophylactic gonadectomy should be performed; appropriate sex steroid replacement will be necessary at the time of puberty.

A subset of patients with dysgenetic male pseudohermaphroditism appear to have a teratological anomaly causing dysplasia of both the testes and the kidney.[86,87] In addition to ambiguous genitalia and persistent paramesonephric structures as a result of their dysgenetic testes, these infants have a constellation of renal abnormalities which may include hypertension, proteinuria and nephrotic syndrome, end-stage glomerulonephritis with renal failure, and Wilms's tumor. Several children have been described with bilateral aniridia (as well as cataracts or glaucoma), male pseudohermaphroditism (with hypospadias, cryptorchism, ambiguous genitalia, or gonadoblastoma), and early development of Wilms's tumor.[88]

TESTICULAR REGRESSION SYNDROMES The general term *testicular regression syndrome* applies to a heterogeneous group of conditions in which, for largely undetermined reasons, there is a cessation of testicular function during fetal life. Obviously the pathogenesis of these conditions is closely related to that of XY gonadal dysgenesis and dysgenetic male pseudohermaphroiditism. As shown in Table 18-5, the clinical phenotype depends on the degree of testicular function and its duration during sexual differentiation. Any of these disorders may be familial; the occasional reports of coexistence of, for example, XY gonadal dysgenesis and congenital anorchia in the same family suggest that all these syndromes of testicular regres-

Table 18-5. Clinical Features of Testicular Dysgenesis Syndromes

	XY gonadal dysgenesis	True agonadism	Rudimentary testes	Congenital anorchia
Genetic sex	46,XY	46,XY	46,XY	46,XY
Time of testis dysfunction (gestational)	Before 8 weeks	8–12 weeks	14–20 weeks	After 20 weeks
External genitalia	Female	Ambiguous	Micropenis	Male
Vagina	Complete	Blind pouch	Absent	Absent
Paramesonephric structures	Present	Rudimentary	Absent	Absent
Mesonephric structures	Absent	Absent	Present	Present
Gonads	Streak	Absent	Rudimentary testis	Absent

Source: Cleary, Caras, Rosenfield, and Young.[89]

sion may represent variable expressions of a common genetic defect.

So-called true agonadism probably is a variant form of dysgenetic male pseudohermaphroditism in which there is some testicular function during early development, after which the testes disappear.[89] The external genitalia are ambiguous, with a phallus the size of an enlarged clitoris, partial labioscrotal fusion, and a persistent urogenital sinus; both paramesonephric and mesonephric ductal structures are absent. Stimulation testing with chorionic gonadotropin in later life may sometimes induce a slight rise in plasma testosterone, even though testes cannot be found.[90] Associated craniofacial or vertebral anomalies have occasionally been observed, suggesting the action of some teratogen or an underlying connective tissue defect.

Bergada et al. have described a sibship in which the affected members were phenotypically male but had a micropenis and small testes (less than 1 cm in diameter) containing only a few tubules and occasional Leydig cells.[91] Suppression of paramesonephric structures was complete, suggesting that testicular function was relatively normal until around 14 weeks gestation.

Complete regression of the testes after 20 weeks gestation leads to congenital anorchia, in which male sexual differentiation is complete but testes absent. This situation can be distinguished from cryptorchism by the finding of high levels of serum FSH[77] and a failure of serum testosterone to rise following stimulation with hCG.[92] The mechanism underlying this late regression of the testes is unknown but is thought to involve torsion or occlusion of the testicular vascular supply.

Errors of Sexual Differentiation

Once structurally normal gonads have been formed, it is still possible for sexual differentiation to be aberrant if the testes are unable to accomplish normal masculinization of a genetic male (male pseudohermaphroditism) or if an abnormal source of androgen induces inappropriate prenatal virilization of a genetic female (female pseudohermaphroditism).

PERSISTENT PARAMESONEPHRIC DUCTS

A failure of paramesonephric (müllerian) duct regression, ranging from simple enlargement of the prostatic utricle to complete preservation of a uterus and tubes, is expected in disorders of testicular dysgenesis, in which case one also sees impaired testosterone-dependent differentiation.[93] However, more than 80 genetic males have been reported in whom normal male external genitalia were present but in whom at laparotomy or herniorrhaphy a cervix, uterus, and fallopian tubes were found in addition to normal male mesonephric duct structures.[94] This situation, referred to as *persistent müllerian duct syndrome* or *hernia uteri inguinalis,* is commonly associated with cryptorchism. Developmental anomalies of the vasa deferentia, epididymis, or tunica albuginea have been reported. Testicular endocrine function appears to be normal at puberty, spermatogenesis occurs, and fertility appears to be possible. There may, however, be an increased propensity to neoplastic degeneration of the testis. The disorder is often familial, most likely sex-limited autosomal recessive; it appears to involve defective or dissynchronous Sertoli cell synthesis of antimüllerian hormone, although a defective target cell receptor for this factor cannot be excluded. Therapy involves correction of undescended testes and hysterectomy, provided the latter can be accomplished without damage to the vasa deferentia contained within the broad ligaments.

DEFECTIVE GENITAL VIRILIZATION (MALE PSEUDOHERMAPHRODITISM)

Leydig Cell Hypoplasia

Leydig cell agenesis or hypoplasia is thought to represent a genetic defect in the LH-hCG receptor, resulting in Leydig cell unresponsiveness to gonadotropic stimulation and inadequate testosterone production before and after birth. These are 46,XY patients with female external genitalia, absent paramesonephric duct structures, and small intraabdominal testes lacking any Leydig cells.[95-97] There is no serum testosterone response to exogenous hCG, and testicular membrane preparations show defective receptor binding of hCG. However, some Leydig cell function may occur in fetal life, since occasional patients show minimal posterior labial fusion and some development of mesonephric duct structures (epididymis and vas deferens).

Inborn Errors of Testosterone Biosynthesis

Of the five known inborn errors of testosterone synthesis, three also impair adrenal secretion of cortisol and therefore cause variant forms of congenital adrenal hyperplasia (Fig. 18-12). In all cases prenatal androgen deficiency in affected genetic males results in either a female external genetic phenotype or ambiguous genitalia; at puberty there is sexual infantilism in both males and females because of inability to produce any sex steroids.

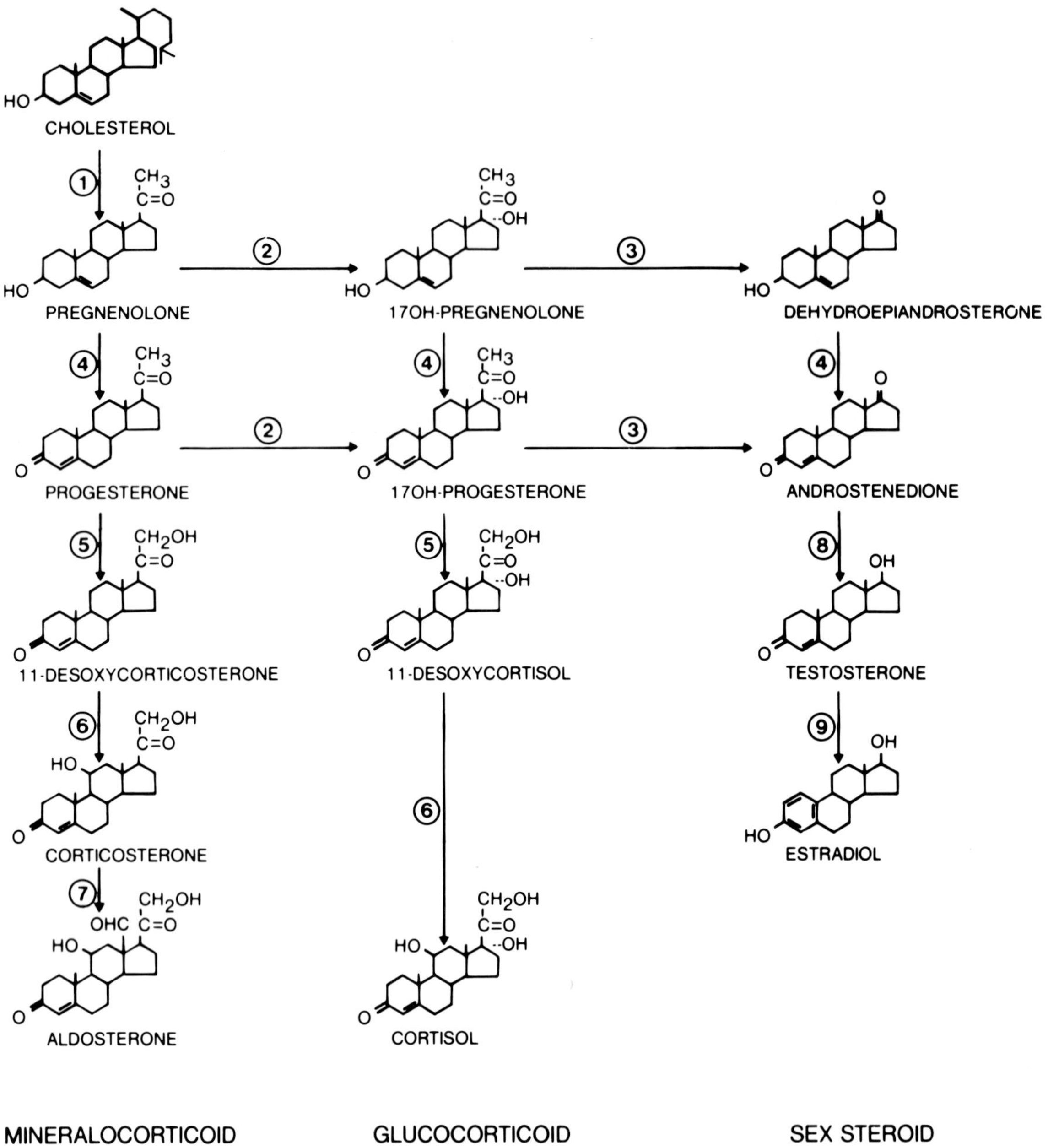

FIGURE 18-12 Pathways of steroidogenesis in the adrenal cortex and gonads. The steroidogenic enzyme systems shown include (1) cholesterol side-chain cleavage enzyme, (2) 17α-hydroxylase, (3) 17,20-desmolase, (4) 3β-hydroxysteroid dehydrogenase/isomerase, (5) 21-hydroxylase, (6) 11β-hydroxylase, (7) corticosterone methyl oxidase I and II, (8) 17β-hydroxysteroid dehydrogenase, and (9) aromatase.

CHOLESTEROL SIDE-CHAIN CLEAVAGE (20,22-DESMOLASE) DEFICIENCY Whether in the testis, ovary, or adrenal cortex, the initial and rate-limiting step in steroid hormone biosynthesis involves hydroxylation of cholesterol at the 20 and 22 positions followed by cleavage of the side chain at the C-20–C-22 bond to form pregnenolone. This step is catalyzed by a mitochondrial mixed-function oxidase, the side-chain cleavage (SCC) complex, which utilizes NADPH as an electron donor. The SCC complex is an electron transfer system composed of a flavoprotein (NADPH-adrenodoxin reductase), an iron sulfur protein (adrenodoxin), and a specific oxygenase (cytochrome $P450_{scc}$) which interacts with the substrate cholesterol. The role of trophic hormones such as LH/hCG or ACTH appears to be to enhance the availability and binding of free cholesterol to the $P450_{scc}$,[98] which is the substrate-specific component of the complex.

Cytochrome $P450_{scc}$ is a large (850,000-dalton) hemoprotein composed of 16 identical subunits. Although a clinical deficiency of SCC activity might result from abnormalities of adrenodoxin reductase or adrenodoxin or from abnormal binding of cholesterol to $P450_{scc}$, in at least one case the disorder was accompanied by a virtual absence of mitochondrial $P450_{scc}$ protein.[99] Patients with such a complete deficiency cannot synthesize any sex steroids, glucocorticoids, or mineralocorticoids; their adrenal glands are enlarged and laden with lipid, for which reason the disorder was formerly termed *congenital lipoid adrenal hyperplasia.*[100] Without replacement therapy, most affected infants die of severe mineralocorticoid and glucocorticoid insufficiency, although survival has been reported in at least one untreated infant thought to have a less severe variant.[101]

Affected males have either female or ambiguous external genitalia, hypoplastic mesonephric duct structures, and a blind vaginal pouch with no uterus or fallopian tubes. The testes appear normal and may be intraabdominal, inguinal, or in the labioscrotal area. Affected females have normal external and internal genitalia. Endocrine studies demonstrate low or negligible levels of glucocorticoids, mineralocorticoids, and sex steroids in the presence of high plasma levels of ACTH, renin activity, and gonadotropins. In the genetic female infant it may be necessary to differentiate this condition from congenital adrenal hypoplasia by radiographic demonstration of hyperplastic adrenals. Therapy of side-chain cleavage deficiency includes glucocorticoid and mineralocorticoid replacement and appropriate sex steroid replacement at puberty. To date all affected genetic males have been assigned a female sex of rearing but have required prophylactic orchiectomy to obviate any possible virilism at puberty. In the future, with early neonatal diagnosis of this form of male pseudohermaphroditism, testosterone therapy in infancy to render the penis normal in size, followed by genital plastic surgery, may be a more appropriate course of action.

3β-HYDROXYSTEROID DEHYDROGENASE DEFICIENCY All human biologically active steroid hormones, whether of adrenal or gonadal origin, have in common a Δ^4-3-keto configuration. The enzyme complex responsible for conversion of pregnenolone, 17-hydroxypregnenolone, and dehydroepiandrosterone to their respective Δ^4-3-keto forms (progesterone, 17-hydroxyprogesterone, and androstenedione) is 3β-hydroxysteroid dehydrogenase/isomerase, which utilizes NAD as cofactor and is located in the smooth endoplasmic reticulum, with lesser amounts in mitochondria. There is some evidence that the two steps of this process may involve separate enzymes, a 3β-hydroxysteroid dehydrogenase (3β-HSD) and a Δ^5-3-ketosteroid isomerase; indeed there may be several substrate-specific isomerases.[102] On the other hand, purified preparations of 3β-HSD retain both activities.[103] One remarkable characteristic of this enzyme is its susceptibility to inhibition by micromolar concentrations of circulating or intraadrenal steroids. Changes in ambient steroid concentrations appear to account for shifts in adrenal 3β-HSD activity during development;[104] thus in fetal and adult life, 3β-HSD normally becomes a rate-limiting step in cortisol biosynthesis, and large amounts of dehydroepiandrosterone are secreted by the adrenal cortex.

Infants affected with autosomal recessive 3β-HSD deficiency typically present with ambiguous genitalia plus severe adrenal insufficiency. The genitalia of affected females may be normal or show mild clitoromegaly, presumably a result of peripheral transformation of adrenal dehydroepiandrosterone to testosterone. At puberty there is no spontaneous breast development. Affected males typically show a small hypospadic phallus, partially fused labioscrotal folds, and a urogenital sinus with a blind vaginal pouch. Paramesonephric duct structures are absent, but surprisingly, mesonephric duct structures are normal, indicating that the prenatal testis was capable of some androgen production. At the time of puberty males show hypergonadotropic hypogonadism, with gynecomastia, inadequate masculinization, and spermatogenic arrest.

The diagnosis of 3β-HSD deficiency requires demonstration of increased concentrations of Δ^5-3β-hydroxysteroids such as dehydroepiandrosterone, Δ^5-androstenediol, and 17-hydroxypregnenolone in serum or increased urinary excretion of their metabolites. During the neonatal period attention must be paid to the normally high excretion of Δ^5-3β-hydroxysteroids at this time.[105] It is of interest that patients with 3β-HSD deficiency also characteristically show slightly increased serum levels of 17-hydroxyprogesterone and increased urinary pregnanetriol, presumably because of hepatic conversion of 17-hydroxypregnenolone. Therapy of this disorder requires glucocorticoid and mineralocorticoid replacement from birth and appropriate sex steroid replacement at puberty. Affected males should receive sufficient testosterone in infancy to correct the micropenis and permit satisfactory repair of hypospadias.

The clinical picture of severe adrenal insufficiency

in a male pseudohermaphrodite represents the most severe form of 3β-HSD deficiency, but many patients with milder variants have been described. Some of this biochemical and clinical heterogeneity may reflect synthesis of a functional 3β-HSD enzyme which is unduly susceptible to the type of steroidal inhibition described above. Thus some patients show apparent preservation of aldosterone secretion,[106] since intraadrenal steroid concentrations are normally lowest in the zona glomerulosa. In addition partial deficiencies of 3β-HSD have been documented in pubertal girls with clitoromegaly, hirsutism, and primary amenorrhea[107] and in males with hypospadias and pubertal gynecomastia.[108–110] Awareness of this genetic heterogeneity has not unreasonably led to the proposition that even more subtle defects, apparent only after ACTH stimulation, might cause postpubertal hirsutism or infertility resembling the polycystic ovary syndrome.[111]

As yet no data are available to establish whether placental 3β-HSD activity is also deficient when the fetus is homozygous for severe deficiency. If the syncytiotrophoblast (also of fetal origin) is not affected, as one might assume from the fact that pregnancies with such fetuses proceed to term, this would imply that 3β-HSD deficiency does not represent a primary lack of enzyme protein (as in cholesterol side-chain cleavage deficiency) but rather synthesis of an enzyme which can be effective in the placental but not in the adrenal or gonadal intracellular milieu.

17α-HYDROXYLASE DEFICIENCY Conversion of pregnenolone to 17-hydroxypregnenolone takes place in the adrenal cortex, testicular Leydig cells, and ovarian theca and granulosa cells. The enzyme complex, located in the smooth endoplasmic reticulum, is a typical mixed function oxidase; NADPH is the preferred electron donor, and the electron transport system involves a flavoprotein which interacts directly with the terminal cytochrome P450. Recently this cytochrome P450 (59,000 daltons) has been purified and shown to have not only 17α-hydroxylase but also 17,20-desmolase activity.[112,113] If a single enzyme catalyzes both these reactions, a new theoretical basis will have to be synthesized to explain the clinical situations in which one or other activity is apparently deficient. The gene for cytochrome $P450_{C17}$ has recently been assigned to chromosome 10.

In males, deficiency of 17α-hydroxylase results in variable genital ambiguity and mesonephric duct differentiation. The phenotype may vary from apparently female external genitalia with a blind vaginal pouch to hypospadic male with micropenis (Fig. 18-13). The testes are normally formed and may be intraabdominal, inguinal, or in the labioscrotal folds. Affected females have normal internal and external development. Hypertension, with or without hypokalemic alkalosis, due to excessive adrenal secretion of mineralocorticoids such as deoxycorticosterone, becomes evident by 2 years of age.[114] In both sexes there is failure of sexual maturation at puberty, although untreated males usually develop gynecomastia.

The diagnosis of 17α-hydroxylase deficiency can be confirmed by demonstration of increased serum concentrations of pregnenolone, progesterone, corticosterone, and deoxycorticosterone, with increased urinary excretion of their metabolites. Plasma renin activity and serum aldosterone levels are usually suppressed,[115] but plasma ACTH is increased. Affected males show low serum testosterone and cortisol values, with inadequate responses to hCG and ACTH. Serum FSH and LH levels are elevated into the age-specific agonadal range, because of the lack of sex steroid–mediated feedback inhibition.

Replacement glucocorticoid therapy (cortisol, 10 to 20 mg/m^2 daily) suppresses corticosterone and deoxycorticosterone secretion and corrects the hyper-

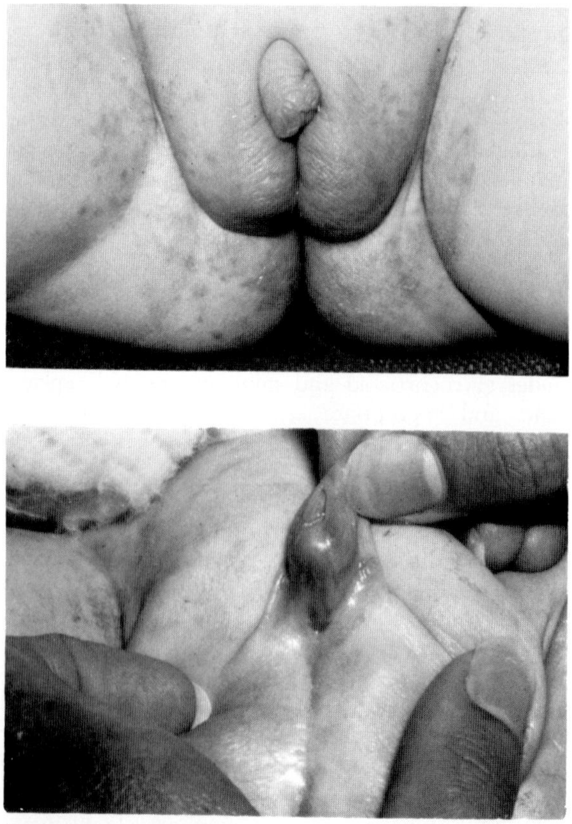

FIGURE 18-13 External genitalia of a male with 17-hydroxylase deficiency at 10 months of age. Testes were palpable in the labioscrotal folds. (*From Dean et al.*[114])

tension and hypokalemic alkalosis. Infant males should receive sufficient testosterone to produce a normal-sized penis, followed by surgical correction of the hypospadias.[114] In both sexes, appropriate sex steroid replacement is required at the time of puberty.

17,20-DESMOLASE DEFICIENCY Synthesis of testosterone involves two enzymes, 17,20-desmolase and 17β-HSD, which are not necessary for biosynthesis of cortisol or aldosterone (Fig. 18-12). Genetic deficiencies of these enzymes cause inadequate virilization of genetic males (male pseudohermaphroditism) without any associated adrenal insufficiency. They are autosomal recessive traits and should also present as sexual infantilism and primary amenorrhea in genetic females, since testosterone is a necessary precursor of estradiol biosynthesis. As yet few affected females have been described, presumably because of inadequate endocrine investigation of women presenting with hypergonadotropic hypogonadism.

If, as has been suggested, a single enzyme protein in both the gonad and adrenal gland catalyzes both 17-hydroxylation and side-chain cleavage of pregnenolone and/or progesterone, it is difficult to understand isolated 17,20-desmolase deficiency; in this syndrome 17-hydroxylation of C-21 steroids is maintained but subsequent cleavage to form C-19 steroids is severely impaired.[116] There are at least two genetic variants of this syndrome which differ in regard to the severity of the block in androgen biosynthesis.[117] Some affected genetic males present with female external genitalia and show little or no spontaneous pubertal development, owing to an almost complete inability to secrete testosterone. Others present as undervirilized males with micropenis, perineal hypospadias, and a bifid scrotum; the latter patients may show some Leydig cell response to hCG and will virilize to some extent at puberty. The testes in either case appear histologically normal, although tubular atrophy and hyalinization have been described after puberty. In most patients mesonephric duct structures are present, but a uterus is uniformly absent. Only one 46,XX female with 17,20-desmolase deficiency has as yet been recognized.[118] As would be expected, she presented with sexual infantilism and primary amenorrhea; her ovaries were enlarged but showed only primordial follicles and clusters of luteinized cells.

In vivo and in vitro studies confirm the inability of the gonad and adrenal cortex to convert pregnenolone or 17-hydroxypregnenolone to C-19 androgens, but secretion of cortisol and aldosterone is normal.[119] Serum concentrations of testosterone, androstenedione, and dehydroepiandrosterone are subnormal, while levels of C-21 precursors such as pregnenolone, 17-hydroxypregnenolone, and 17-hydroxyprogesterone are inappropriately high; this discrepancy is accentuated on stimulation with hCG or ACTH. Those patients with ambiguous genitalia excrete significant amounts of pregnanetriolone, a metabolite of 17-hydroxypregnenolone; conversely, the patients with female phenotype do not excrete pregnanetriolone, but some dehydroepiandrosterone is found in serum and urine.[116]

Patients who are identified at birth require plastic repair of the external genitalia and replacement therapy with testosterone. Those who have been raised as females and whose condition is not recognized until adolescence require castration and estrogen replacement therapy.

17β-HYDROXYSTEROID DEHYDROGENASE DEFICIENCY The final step in biosynthesis of testosterone is 17-keto reduction of androstenedione (Fig. 18-12). The enzyme which catalyzes this conversion, and also the conversion of estrone to estradiol, is 17β-HSD (also called *17-ketosteroid reductase*). Similar enzymes are found in various peripheral tissues which can catalyze this reaction in either direction.

Genetic males with 17β-HSD deficiency usually present with female external genitalia at birth (although a few show mild clitoromegaly or posterior labioscrotal fusion); thus the sex of rearing has almost always been female. The testes are usually inguinal or in the labioscrotal folds; in infancy such a condition may be misdiagnosed as testicular feminization. There is a blind vagina, and mesonephric duct structures are present.

The diagnosis is usually made at puberty, when, unless castration has already been performed, striking virilization occurs with marked enlargement of the phallus, hirsutism, acne, and deepening of the voice. Some breast enlargement may occur, but primary amenorrhea is constant. In some cases the degree of virilization has been such that successful transition to a male gender role has been possible.[120]

In vitro studies have confirmed reduced levels of 17β-HSD activity within the testis,[121] although there is some evidence that the activity in peripheral tissues is unimpaired, presumably owing to a different enzyme.[122] The diagnostic hallmark of this disorder is a markedly elevated serum concentration of androstenedione after puberty or hCG stimulation, with low-normal levels of testosterone. Serum estradiol values are normal, but estrone levels are increased. The reason for the discrepancy between the apparent lack of prenatal testosterone biosynthesis and the significant virilization which occurs at puberty is not clear. It may reflect postnatal peripheral conversion of androstenedione to testosterone, but in addition the abnormal testicular 17β-HSD may be affected by the high concentrations of placental steroids in the fetal circulation. As yet there have been no studies of placental 17β-HSD activity in this syndrome, and it is not known to what extent placental estradiol synthesis is affected.

Pedigree studies suggest that this disorder is autosomal recessive.[123] However, an X-linked recessive pattern cannot be ruled out, since as yet no affected homozygous females have been identified.

A deficiency of 17β-HSD should be considered in any male pseudohermaphrodite who has normal adrenal glucocorticoid and mineralocorticoid function and absent uterus, particularly if virilization occurs at puberty. Since these patients have generally already been assigned a female gender, the appropriate therapy is usually castration followed by estrogen replacement at puberty. When a male gender role is assigned or feasible, the patient requires plastic repair of the external genitalia and supplementary testosterone therapy. Spermatogenesis would not be expected, because of the lack of testicular testosterone.

Defects in Androgen Target Tissues

Current concepts regarding the cellular mechanisms by which androgens act are summarized in Fig. 18-14. The bulk of testosterone in the circulation is bound to either sex hormone–binding globulin or albumin, although levels of both proteins are markedly reduced in the fetus at the time of sexual differentiation. Unbound testosterone enters target cells by passive diffusion and is then converted to the more potent androgen dihydrotestosterone through the action of

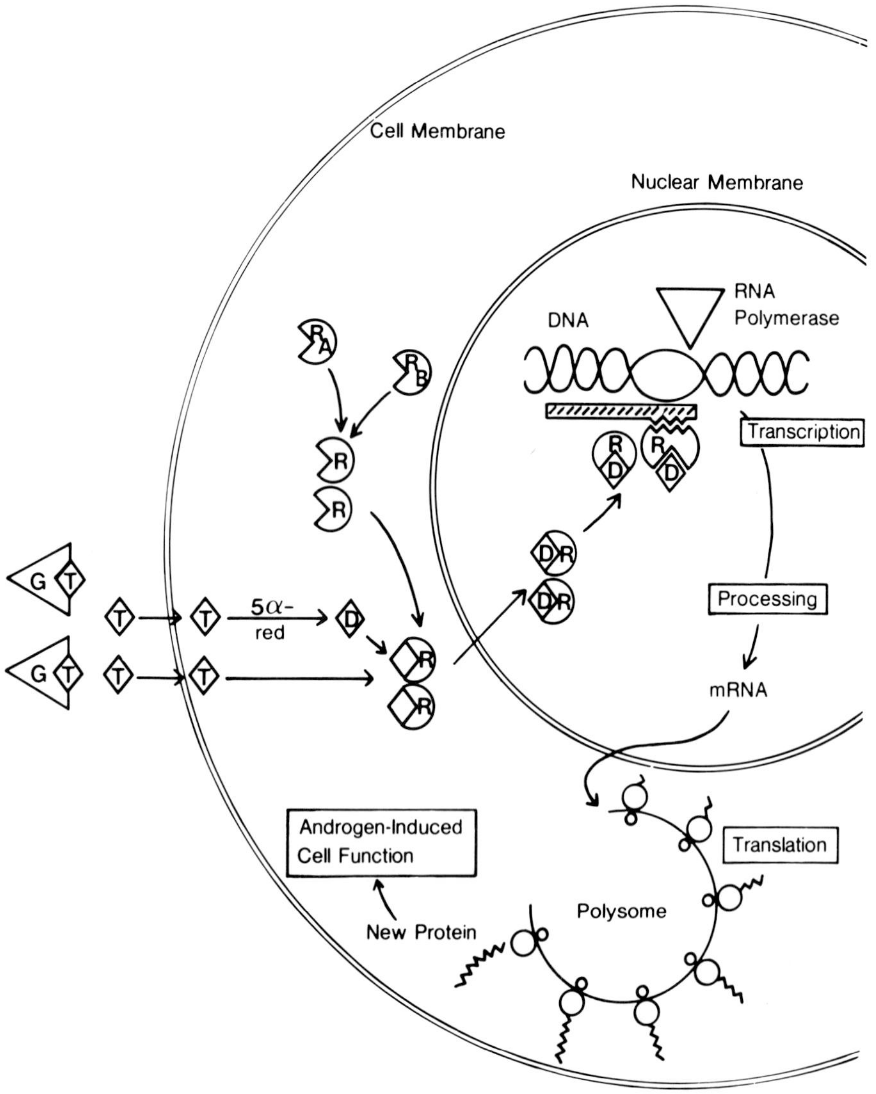

FIGURE 18-14 Mechanism of action of testosterone on target cell. In the circulation, testosterone (T) is largely bound to sex hormone–binding globulin (G). Free T diffuses through the plasma membrane and is metabolized by 5α-reductase (5α-red) to dihydrotestosterone (D). Both androgens can bind to cytosol receptor (R) to form a complex which is translocated to the nucleus and binds to an acceptor site on the target genome to activate gene transcription. New messenger RNA (mRNA) is processed and exported to cytoplasmic polysomes to direct the synthesis of androgen-induced proteins. Recent studies indicate that unoccupied estrogen receptors are entirely localized within the nucleus of target cells, rather than in the cytosol as formerly believed.[123a,123b] The precise subcellular location of the androgen receptor has not yet been resolved.

the enzyme 5α-reductase. Both androgens bind to a specific high-affinity protein receptor; the activated hormone-receptor complex is then translocated to the nucleus, where it binds to chromatin acceptor sites composed of DNA and nonhistone chromosomal protein. This interaction initiates transcription and processing of specific messenger RNAs which subsequently are translated to initiate ribosomal synthesis of new proteins. The androgen receptor is regulated by a gene on the X chromosome, while the gene for 5α-reductase is autosomal. Thus the cellular mechanisms for androgen action are present in target tissues of both sexes. There is evidence that dihydrotestosterone is the major androgen responsible for virilization of the external genitalia and later appearance of male secondary sexual characteristics at puberty; testosterone itself appears to mediate differentiation of the mesonephric duct and possibly also spermatogenesis and feedback control of gonadotropin secretion in adult life. In some forms of male pseudohermaphroditism, testosterone synthesis and paramesonephric duct regression are normal but prenatal masculinization of the external genitalia is inadequate because of target cell resistance to androgen. The molecular basis for such androgen resistance may include a defect in 5α-reductase, in the androgen receptor, or at one or more postreceptor loci.

DEFECTIVE ANDROGEN METABOLISM: 5α-REDUCTASE DEFICIENCY Genetic males with a deficiency of 5α-reductase present with a clinical picture formerly termed *pseudovaginal perineoscrotal hypospadias*. Typical features at birth include a clitoris-sized phallus with a hooded prepuce, ventral urethral groove, variable chordee, and a urogenital sinus opening on the perineum. Because paramesonephric duct regression is normal, there is a blind vaginal pouch opening into the urogenital sinus. The testes are normally formed and located in either the inguinal canal or the partially fused labioscrotal folds. Mesonephric duct structures (epididymis, vas deferens, seminal vesicle, and ejaculatory duct) are well differentiated and empty into the blind vagina. Most patients have been raised as females.

At puberty, if castration was not accomplished earlier, serum testosterone increases into the adult male range; variable virilization occurs, without gynecomastia. The phallus enlarges to as much as 8 cm in length, the testes enlarge and complete their descent, muscle mass increases, the voice deepens, and spermatogenesis may occur. However, prostatic enlargement, acne, facial and body hair growth, and temporal hair recession, features which are dihydrotestosterone-dependent, do not occur. Many such patients spontaneously and successfully change to a male gender identity and role, in spite of unambiguous assignment of female gender throughout childhood.[124] Such occurrences demonstrate the powerful influence that self-perception of genital and secondary sexual development have upon gender identity and cast serious doubts upon the previous notion that core psychosexual identity is always permanently imprinted during a critical period in infancy and early childhood.[125] Although most reported patients have chosen this postpubertal gender reassignment, some patients, particularly those with a relatively small phallus, have opted to retain their female psychosexual orientation.[126]

The absence of paramesonephric duct remnants differentiates 5α-reductase deficiency from disorders of gonadogenesis such as 45,X/46,XY mixed gonadal dysgenesis; however, detailed endocrine studies are necessary to rule out a disorder of testosterone biosynthesis or other forms of androgen resistance such as incomplete testicular feminization. Homozygous postpubertal males show normal or slightly increased levels of circulating FSH and LH. Serum testosterone concentrations are also normal or slightly elevated, but dihydrotestosterone concentrations remain relatively low; thus the testosterone/dihydrotestosterone ratio exceeds 35, in contrast to the normal adult male ratio of 8 to 16.[127] A similar pattern can be elicited in affected children following Leydig cell stimulation with hCG. Decreased conversion of ^{3}H-labeled testosterone to dihydrotestosterone has been confirmed in vivo. Study of urinary steroids shows diminished ratios of 5α-reduced to 5β-reduced C-19 and C-21 steroids (for example, a reduced androsterone/etiocholanolone ratio). Homozygous females show similar urinary steroid patterns but have no clinical manifestations; heterozygotes show intermediate 5α/5β steroid ratios. In vitro study of tissue slices or cultured genital skin fibroblasts may confirm the inability to convert [^{3}H]testosterone to 5α-reduced metabolites,[128] but the wide variation observed in normal control preparations can make interpretation of the results problematic. Mauvais-Jarvis et al. have suggested that the 5α-reductase activities of liver, nongenital skin, and genital skin may be due to separate enzymes;[129] the enzyme in nongenital skin appears to be induced by androgens, while that in genital tissues is independent of androgen exposure. It will be necessary to resolve these and other questions regarding the interpretation of in vitro 5α-reductase assays before issues such as genetic heterogeneity can be resolved.[130] In addition, it is necessary to differentiate primary genetic 5α-reductase deficiency from those disorders, such as complete androgen insensitivity, porphyria, hypothyroidism, or Cushing's syndrome, in which secondary defects in hepatic or peripheral 5α-reductase activity may occur. Although plasma concentrations of 3α-androstenediol glucuronide appear to reflect 5α-reductase activity, they are reduced in both primary and secondary deficiencies of the enzyme.

If the diagnosis of 5α-reductase deficiency is suspected and confirmed during the neonatal period, the sex of rearing should be male. Androgen (testosterone or dihydrotestosterone) therapy can be used to enhance penile growth and facilitate surgical repair of the genitalia. In such patients virilization can be expected at puberty, and fertility is theoretically possible. Those who are diagnosed later and who have an unambiguous female gender identity should undergo orchiectomy and receive estrogen therapy at the time of puberty.

ANDROGEN INSENSITIVITY: COMPLETE AND INCOMPLETE TESTICULAR FEMINIZATION The clinical phenotype in genetic males with various forms of androgen insensitivity may range from female through genital ambiguity to male with hypospadias or infertility, presumably a reflection of the severity of the receptor or postreceptor defect. In all these disorders, regardless of phenotype, the affected males have a 46,XY karyotype, are H-Y antigen–positive, and have testes capable of normal testosterone secretion.

The most common form of male pseudohermaphroditism is complete testicular feminization, an X-linked recessive disorder analogous to the Tfm mutation in the mouse.[131] Phenotypically the hemizygous male presents with normal female external genitalia, a blind vaginal pouch with absent cervix, uterus, and tubes, and absent or vestigial mesonephric duct structures. The testes may be intraabdominal, inguinal, or labial.

During infancy and childhood, complete testicular feminization should be considered in any girl with an inguinal hernia, particularly if it contains a palpable gonad; 1 in 50 girls with a hernia has this disorder. The diagnosis is almost certain if the karyotype is 46,XY and ultrasonography fails to demonstrate a uterus but should be confirmed by in vitro study of androgen receptors. After puberty the presenting complaint is primary amenorrhea, which in up to 10 percent of cases may be due to testicular feminization. At puberty these patients acquire a normal female body habitus and well-developed breasts, but the clitoris remains small and pubic and axillary hair is absent or sparse.

The testes are characterized by small seminiferous tubules devoid of spermatogenic elements other than spermatogonia. After puberty varying degrees of Leydig cell hyperplasia, frequently in adenomatous clumps, can be observed. These patients are predisposed to develop germ cell tumors of the testis, of which seminoma is the most common malignant variety. The incidence of malignant degeneration ranges from 5 to 20 percent and is clearly related to the age of the patient. Clinically apparent neoplasm rarely occurs before the third decade, but studies of even prepubertal testes frequently show carcinoma in situ.[132]

The hypothalamus and pituitary of these patients are resistant to the feedback effects of androgen, although gonadotropin suppression by estrogens is normal.[133] After puberty serum LH concentrations are higher than in normal men, and as a result, levels of testosterone, dihydrotestosterone, and estradiol are also elevated. In spite of defective spermatogenesis, serum FSH concentrations are usually normal or only slightly increased.

In most patients with complete testicular feminization, negligible or markedly reduced levels of cytosol androgen binding in vitro can be demonstrated in cultured genital skin fibroblasts.[134] This may reflect an absolute reduction in receptor protein, since these cells synthesize reduced amounts of two proteins which may be components of the oligomeric receptor.[135] However, several variant forms of androgen insensitivity have been identified in which intermediate or even normal levels of androgen binding can be demonstrated.[136] These receptor-positive patients show considerable clinical heterogeneity, even within the same pedigree, and some are more properly classified as incomplete testicular feminization. In some the androgen receptor appears to be defective, forming a steroid-receptor complex which is thermolabile, dissociates readily, is not stabilized by sodium molybdate, and cannot be normally translocated to the nucleus.[137–139] In others the receptor appears to be normal in amount and function even though the cells can be shown to be androgen-insensitive.[140,141] By exclusion such patients are considered to have a postreceptor defect, either at the level of the nuclear acceptor sites[142] or at some later step in gene expression.

Therapy of the androgen-insensitive patient requires positive reinforcement of the female gender identity, a process that will rarely be assisted by discussion of male chromosomes and gonads. The testes should probably be removed as soon as the diagnosis is made, particularly if herniorrhaphy is required. There seems to be little merit in retaining such testes in order to permit spontaneous puberty, since later prophylactic orchiectomy to prevent malignancy will be required as a second surgical procedure. Estrogen replacement therapy is required after castration to initiate and maintain secondary sex characters, but since no endometrium is present there is no need to provide this in cyclic fashion. The blind vagina will usually permit normal sexual intercourse, but occasionally dilatation is required. In adult life the female gender identity remains firm, and marital and maternal attitudes are clearly feminine.

About 10 percent of patients with androgen insensitivity show some evidence of prenatal and adolescent virilization and their condition is termed *incomplete testicular feminization.* Some of these patients show reduced levels of cytosol androgen binding, some have a defective androgen receptor, and some appear to have a postreceptor defect. In contrast to typical receptor-negative complete testicular feminization, there is considerable clinical heterogeneity even within the same pedigree. Furthermore, there is little if any correlation between the degree of virilization and the severity of the receptor abnormality demonstrable in vitro. In view of this clinical variability, there seems to be no value in retaining eponymic syndromes based upon phenotype, such as those of Reifenstein, Rosewater, Gilbert-Dreyfus, and Lubs.[130]

All these patients are 46,XY, have testes, and lack paramesonephric duct structures. In some the genitalia are female, as in complete testicular feminization, but distinct mesonephric duct structures can be identified. More commonly the genitalia are ambiguous, with varying degrees of clitoromegaly and labioscrotal fusion and a short blind vagina (pseudovaginal perineoscrotal hypospadias). At puberty such patients show, in addition to gynecomastia and primary amenorrhea, significant virilization with clitoral enlargement, masculine body habitus, and growth of pubic and axillary hair. In most the gender identity is female, and therapy involves immediate orchiectomy, genital reconstruction as necessary, and estrogen replacement.

The term *Reifenstein syndrome* was formerly applied to less severe variants of X-linked partial androgen insensitivity in which affected individuals presented as phenotypic males with hypospadias, inadequate pubertal virilization, gynecomastia, and infertility.[143] Cryptorchism is common; the testes are small, with normal Leydig cells but arrested spermatogenesis. Some patients show defective mesonephric duct development, such as severe hypoplasia of the vas deferens. More recently similar degrees of in vitro androgen insensitivity have been demonstrated in males presenting with only microphallus, simple penile hypospadias,[144] or idiopathic infertility.[145]

It is obvious that with this wide spectrum of clinical phenotypes, the diagnosis of partial androgen insensitivity is problematic unless there is an obvious family history. Serum concentrations of FSH, LH, testosterone, and estradiol are normal or moderately elevated after puberty. The diagnosis may be suspected because of a poor clinical response to administered androgen but must be confirmed by in vitro study of cytosol and nuclear androgen binding.

In patients with male sex of rearing, therapy is even more problematic in view of the limited response to testosterone. Any hypospadias or cryptorchism should be corrected surgically; mastectomy will often be required for gynecomastia. There is no evidence that the risk of gonadal neoplasm in this situation exceeds that in normal males with undescended testes.

Defective Virilization Due to Exogenous Sex Steroids

While normal exposure to placental estrogens and progesterone does not disturb fetal sexual differentiation, data derived from studies in experimental animals and some circumstantial epidemiological evidence have raised the possibility that maternal ingestion of synthetic sex steroids might lead to hypospadias or more severe genital ambiguity.[146] Variable degrees of incomplete masculinization can be induced in rats and rabbits by prenatal exposure to high doses of progestational compounds such as the 19-nor- and 17α-ethinyl derivatives of testosterone. In addition, there has been an apparent increase in the incidence of hypospadias in industrialized countries during the past decade, which might relate to the use of such drugs for threatened abortion or as a pregnancy test, or inadvertent ingestion of contraceptive steroids during early pregnancy. Several retrospective studies of hypospadiac boys demonstrate an increased rate of maternal sex steroid ingestion, with some correlation between the time of ingestion and the severity of the defect. However, prospective studies have failed to show an increased risk in the offspring of women exposed to synthetic progestogens in early pregnancy, perhaps because of the high incidence of spontaneous hypospadias.[147]

A case of male pseudohermaphroditism has been reported in which the mother received large doses of diethylstilbestrol during early pregnancy; in two surveys of boys similarly exposed, no increased incidence of hypospadias was found, although other genital anomalies such as meatal stenosis, epididymal cyst, and testicular hypoplasia were increased.[148,149] Estrogens are known to be potent inhibitors of the steroidogenic enzyme 3β-HSD, but as yet there is no proof that exogenous estrogens, even in combination with the high levels produced by the placenta, could cause significant inhibition of fetal testosterone biosynthesis. Progesterone itself and also the synthetic progestogen norethindrone have been shown to cause dose-dependent inhibition of 5α-reductase activity in genital skin fibroblasts,[150] but again the concentrations required make it seem unlikely that this mechanism could explain any teratogenic effect. A direct relationship between exogenous sex steroids and male pseudohermaphroditism cannot be said to have been confirmed, but the possibility remains that their influence may be significant in certain genetically predisposed persons.

Male Pseudohermaphroditism of Unknown Etiology

MULTIPLE MALFORMATION SYNDROMES The presence of ambiguous genitalia in a genetic male may alert the physician to the presence of associated somatic anomalies which require immediate therapy.[151] Such situations include the Smith-Lemli-Opitz syndrome, in which hypospadias is associated with mental retardation, short stature, and skeletal defects, and the Najjar syndrome of ambiguous genitalia, cardiomyopathy, and mental retardation.

ISOLATED HYPOSPADIAS Failure of fusion of the urethral folds is one of the commonest congenital malformations, with an incidence of about 5 per 1000 live male births. In most cases there is no obvious underlying endocrine defect; indeed, nonendocrine factors are suggested by the frequent coexistence of associated genitourinary and other anomalies. In about one-quarter of the cases another family member is affected. The overall risk factor for a subsequent male sibling has been estimated as 11 percent[152] but increases with more severe degrees of hypospadias, suggesting a multigenic form of inheritance. The concordance rate in identical twins is about 50 percent. Basal serum gonadotropin and testosterone concentrations are normal in unselected hypospadiac boys, but a slight diminution in mean testosterone levels has been reported in affected young adults.[153,154] More detailed testing even during childhood may reveal exaggerated FSH and LH responses to gonadotropin releasing hormone and reduced testosterone response to hCG stimulation, indicative of some degree of Leydig cell dysfunction.[155] Genital skin 5α-reductase activity appears to be normal in hypospadiac boys,[150,153] but cytosol androgen receptor levels may be reduced.[156] These findings only underscore the heterogeneous nature of simple hypospadias and its multigenic-multifactorial etiology.

CRYPTORCHISM The testes are frequently undescended in various forms of male pseudohermaphroditism and also in association with a number of multiple anomaly syndromes. In some of these latter situations, such as the Prader-Willi syndrome, the cryptorchism reflects hypogonadotropic hypogonadism. Because of the role of pituitary gonadotropins in the regulation of Leydig cell function during the latter half of pregnancy, the occurrence of microphallus and cryptorchism in an infant with otherwise normally formed genitalia should alert the clinician to a possible hypogonadotropic or hypopituitary condition. A high proportion of maldescended testes show abnormalities of germ cells, but it is not clear whether these represent a cause or effect of the maldescent.[157]

VIRILIZATION OF A GENETIC FEMALE (FEMALE PSEUDOHERMAPHRODITISM)

Exposure of a female fetus to inappropriate levels of circulating androgen does not affect ovarian or uterine development but results in some virilization of the external genitalia, or so-called female pseudohermaphroditism. The degree of genital ambiguity present at birth, which may be graded according to the classification of Prader,[158] depends mainly on the timing of the androgen exposure. Late exposure, after 12 weeks gestation, will cause only clitoral hypertrophy. However, exposure between 4 and 12 weeks gestation results in varying degrees of labioscrotal fusion; the urogenital sinus commonly opens on the perineum but occasionally may reach the tip of the phallus. The most common source of the offending androgens is the adrenal cortex, because of an inborn error of cortisol biosynthesis, but occasionally a maternal source of androgen can be identified. In addition, several nonendocrine malformation syndromes affecting the female external genitalia may produce a similar clinical picture.

Congenital Adrenal Hyperplasia

The virilizing syndromes of congenital adrenal hyperplasia (CAH) have in common reduced adrenal capacity to secrete cortisol (and in some forms also aldosterone). This cortisol deficiency, which during fetal life is exacerbated by rapid placental clearance of cortisol, leads to compensatory hypersecretion of ACTH, adrenocortical hyperplasia, and excessive synthesis of steroids proximal to the enzymatic block (Fig. 18-12). These steroids, such as 17-hydroxyprogesterone, may be converted to testosterone and cause virilization. The impact after birth upon salt and water handling depends on the specific enzymatic defect: thus in 11β-hydroxylase deficiency there is excessive secretion of steroids, such as 11-deoxycorticosterone, which have mineralocorticoid activity, but in 21-hydroxylase deficiency the predominant abnormal steroids, 17-hydroxyprogesterone and progesterone, have an antimineralocorticoid effect through their ability to compete for renal tubular aldosterone receptors.

These CAH syndromes are by far the most common cause of female pseudohermaphroditism and account for the majority of all neonates with ambiguous genitalia. Although it has been customary to consider each disorder, defined in vivo from its steroid secretion patterns, as a genetically distinct and homogeneous entity, recent evidence has demonstrated that there is remarkable phenotypic variation, which must reflect in part considerable genetic heterogeneity. It seems inevitable that future studies with cDNA probes will demonstrate many allelic variants at each steroidogenic gene locus, just as has been shown for the globin genes.

It may be useful to examine the variables which interact to determine the age of onset and severity of clinical abnormalities in any patient with CAH. These include both the factors which influence adrenal steroid secretion and those which regulate target cell responses. Obviously, the primary variable is the underlying genetic defect. This may be a major deletion which renders the gene incapable of transcription; such a defect is suggested in at least one patient with cholesterol side-chain cleavage deficiency in whom there was complete absence of the mitochondrial cytochrome $P450_{scc}$.[99] However, in most cases it is likely that varying amounts of gene product are formed which is defective in terms of substrate or cofactor affinity, maximal activity per cell, or susceptibility to intracellular inhibitors. In addition, genetic defects may occur in mitochondrial or microsomal proteins which serve to orientate enzymatic complexes; such factors may regulate the relative activities of those enzyme proteins (such as 17-hydroxylase/17,20-desmolase or 11β-hydroxylase/18-hydroxylase) which appear to catalyze two steps in steroidogenesis. The activities of steroidogenic enzymes are also regulated by hormones such as ACTH and angiotensin, electrolytes such as potassium, and the modulating effects of ambient intracellular steroids.[104]

Since steroids show a significant gradient across the adrenal cortex and these intraadrenal concentrations change with age and adrenal growth,[159] they may influence the relative secretion of mineralocorticoid, glucocorticoid, and androgen in both normal and CAH patients at different stages of development. ACTH and various unidentified mitogenic peptides interact to regulate the total mass of adrenal steroidogenic tissue. The interaction of all these variables determines the daily secretion of cortisol, aldosterone, and various other steroids, some of which are metabolically active while others are available for peripheral conversion to active steroids. Finally, the biological effect of secreted cortisol or aldosterone may be altered by the presence of steroids which bind competitively to plasma proteins or target cell receptors. These variables are probably sufficient to explain phenotypic variation in CAH without the need to postulate multiple age-, zone-, and substrate-specific steroidogenic enzymes, each under separate genetic control.

Prenatal virilization of a genetic female can result from defects of adrenal 21-hydroxylase, 11β-hydroxylase, or 3β-HSD. The more proximal defects of cortisol biosynthesis, such as cholesterol side-chain cleavage or 17-hydroxylase, also impair androgen synthesis; thus virilization of the female is not a clinical feature. All these CAH variants demonstrate an autosomal recessive pattern of inheritance.

21-HYDROXYLASE DEFICIENCY Over 90 percent of CAH patients have a deficiency of 21-hydroxylase. At least two clinical variants have been identified: the classic form, which causes prenatal and continuing postnatal virilization with varying degrees of apparent glucocorticoid and mineralocorticoid insufficiency, and a late-onset or attenuated form, which is expressed as hirsutism, virilism, or infertility during the second or third decades. The usual incidence of homozygous classic 21-hydroxylase deficiency is 1 per 10,000 live births; however, in one genetic isolate, the Yupik of Alaska, the incidence may reach 1 in 400 live births, or a gene frequency approaching 1 in 10.

The 21-hydroxylase complex, located in adrenal smooth endoplasmic reticulum, utilizes NADPH as cofactor, atmospheric oxygen, an intermediary flavoprotein, and a terminal substrate-specific cytochrome P450 of about 48,000 daltons.[160] This single enzyme complex catalyzes 21-hydroxylation of both 17-hydroxyprogesterone and progesterone (Fig. 18-12), but the former is the preferred substrate. Extraadrenal 21-hydroxylation does not appear to involve the same enzyme and is not impaired in CAH.

The gene locus (or loci, as there may be two) for 21-hydroxylase is on the short arm of chromosome 6, close to the HLA-B histocompatibility locus[161] and adjacent to the loci for complement factors C4a and C4b. This close linkage with histocompatibility and complement loci makes it possible to use extended HLA and complement haplotyping to trace inheritance of a particular 21-hydroxylase gene (Fig. 18-15). HLA testing combined with careful analysis of basal and ACTH-stimulated 17-hydroxyprogesterone levels can define accurately subjects who are homozygous for classic or late-onset 21-hydroxylase deficiency, genetic compounds carrying both genes, or heterozygous carriers.[162,163]

This close linkage of 21-hydroxylase with the major histocompatibility locus should not be confused with the phenomenon of genetic linkage disequilibrium, in which the frequency of certain HLA haplotypes differs in affected subjects from that observed in normal persons in the same population. Thus among northern European groups the haplotype Bw47DR7

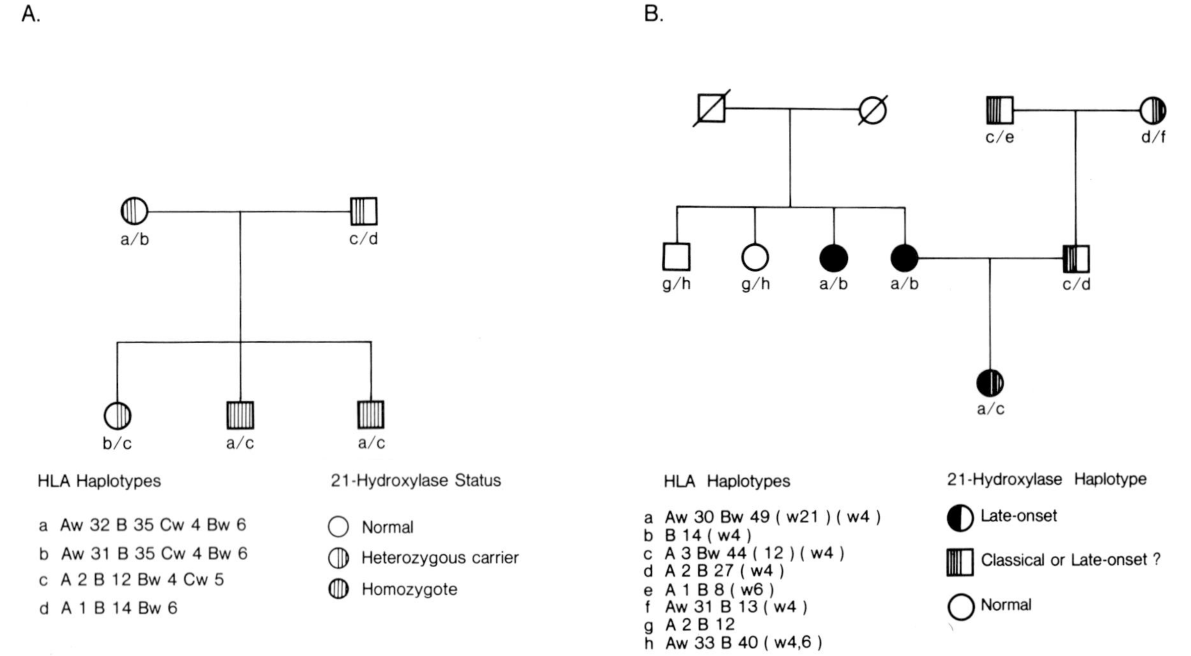

FIGURE 18-15 Application of HLA typing to genotyping of 21-hydroxylase deficiency. (*A*) Classic 21-hydroxylase deficiency in a family with two affected sons and one heterozygous daughter. (*B*) Pedigree in which the mother is homozygous for late-onset 21-hydroxylase deficiency, the father is heterozygous for 21-hydroxylase deficiency, and the daughter appears to be a genetic compound, showing elevated serum 17-hydroxyprogesterone levels but no virilization.

occurs with increased frequency in association with classic 21-hydroxylase deficiency, while the B8 haplotype frequency is reduced.[164] In the late-onset variant of 21-hydroxylase deficiency the frequency of the B14 haplotype appears to be increased.

The important clinical features of homozygous classic 21-hydroxylase deficiency are virilization and salt wasting. Their pathogenesis is summarized in Fig. 18-16. The primary impairment of cortisol synthesis causes increased pituitary secretion of ACTH, which in turn leads to excessive production of both 17-hydroxyprogesterone and progesterone. Side-chain cleavage of the former produces androstenedione, which is then available for adrenal and peripheral

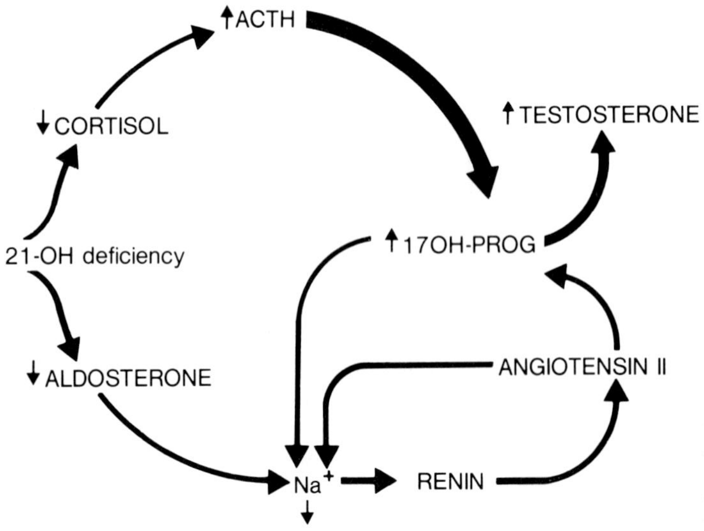

FIGURE 18-16 Pathogenesis of virilization and salt wasting in classic 21-hydroxylase deficiency, showing the close interrelation of these two aspects of the disease and the central importance of serum 17-hydroxyprogesterone (17OH-prog) and plasma renin activity for diagnosis and management. (*From Winter and Couch.*[179a])

conversion to the active androgen testosterone. In untreated patients plasma ACTH is moderately raised; levels of 17-hydroxyprogesterone, progesterone, androstenedione, testosterone, 21-deoxycortisol, and pregnenolone sulfate are markedly increased, with less striking increases in the levels of dehydroepiandrosterone and its sulfate conjugate. Even if basal serum cortisol levels are in the normal range, stress or ACTH testing may evoke only a blunted rise, in spite of a brisk increase in 17-hydroxyprogesterone. Metabolism of these abnormal steroids leads to increased urinary excretion of 17-ketosteroids and pregnanetriol.

Prenatal exposure to adrenal androgens has no effect on male sexual differentiation. The genitalia of affected males appear normal at birth, but continued androgen exposure becomes apparent by age 2 to 3 years, with rapid growth and skeletal maturation and precocious appearance of secondary sex characters in the absence of preceding testicular enlargement.

Genetic females who are homozygous for classic 21-hydroxylase deficiency have ambiguous external genitalia at birth (Fig. 18-17). Careful physical examination will demonstrate clitoromegaly, labioscrotal fusion without palpable testes, and a single urogenital sinus, opening usually on the perineum but occasionally on the phallus. By rectal examination one can usually palpate the cervix and thus confirm at once the presence of female paramesonephric structures. If appropriate therapy to suppress adrenal androgen production is not initiated, this virilism continues during childhood, causing further clitoromegaly, rapid growth,

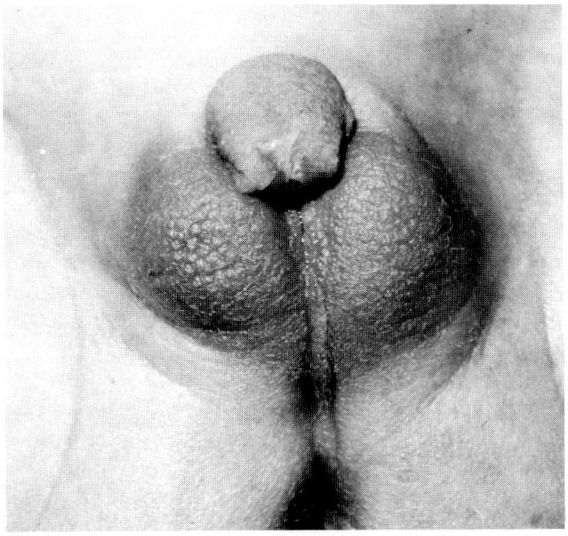

FIGURE 18-17 External genitalia of a newborn female with classic 21-hydroxylase deficiency. No gonads were palpable, and the cervix was felt on rectal examination.

and the appearance of pubic hair, acne, and a masculine body habitus. Even though growth is accelerated, precocious epiphyseal fusion leads to an arrest of growth by about 10 years of age, with marked reduction of adult height. Continued androgen exposure after puberty causes anovular infertility and amenorrhea.

The late-onset or attenuated variant of 21-hydroxylase deficiency is characterized by low-level androgen exposure which does not produce clinically apparent disease until late childhood or adolescence. Affected males are rarely detected unless they present with premature adrenarche. Homozygous females have normal genitalia at birth; the disorder may be suspected in a child with premature adrenarche or a young woman with mild clitoromegaly, hirsutism, or anovular infertility.[165] These patients show moderately increased basal serum concentrations of 17-hydroxyprogesterone and testosterone, with an exaggerated response of the former to ACTH stimulation.

A few persons who represent genetic compounds for the classic and late-onset variants of 21-hydroxylase deficiency have been identified (Fig. 18-15). They have normal genitalia, and postnatal signs of androgen excess or even infertility do not usually occur,[166] even though basal serum 17-hydroxyprogesterone levels are persistently increased. Heterozygous carriers for either variant are clinically normal and show normal basal serum concentrations of all adrenal steroids. Examination of basal and ACTH-stimulated 17-hydroxyprogesterone or 21-deoxycortisol values will usually permit appropriate categorization of individuals within an affected pedigree (Fig. 18-18).

Biochemical evidence of sodium depletion, as evidenced by increased levels of plasma renin activity or concentration, can be observed in virtually all untreated patients with homozygous classic 21-hydroxylase deficiency. However, clinically significant salt wasting develops in only about two-thirds of these patients,[167] usually during early infancy prior to diagnosis. In an affected neonate the first clues to an impending salt-losing crisis are hyperkalemia and rising levels of plasma renin activity, usually detectable by 1 week of age. If mineralocorticoid therapy is not initiated, progressive weight loss, vomiting, acidosis, hypoglycemia, and hyponatremic dehydration ensue, leading to peripheral vascular collapse by the third or fourth week. The clinical picture resembles that of hypertrophic pyloric stenosis except that in CAH, because of osmotic diuresis, urinary volume is often maintained in spite of obvious dehydration. The finding of hypernatremia and hyperkalemia in a dehydrated male (or virilized female) infant should lead immediately to investigation of adrenal function, including measurement of serum 17-hydroxyproges-

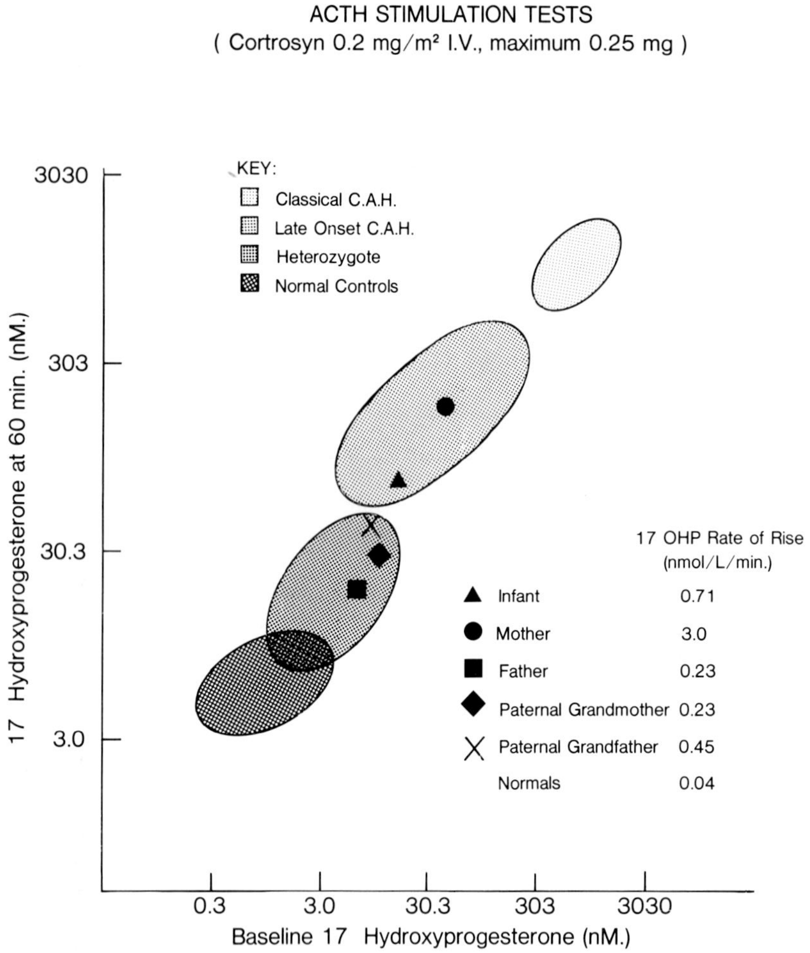

FIGURE 18-18 The relationship of baseline and 60-min ACTH-stimulated serum 17-hydroxyprogesterone concentrations in normal controls, heterozygous carriers, and patients with homozygous late-onset and homozygous classic forms of 21-hydroxylase deficiency. The application of the nomogram is illustrated, using data from individuals in pedigree *B* of Fig. 18-15. Data in nanomols per liter may be changed to nanograms per deciliter by multiplying by 33. (*Adapted from New et al.*[163])

terone levels. The differential diagnosis of a neonatal salt-losing crisis includes other forms of CAH, pyloric stenosis, congenital adrenal hypoplasia, and interstitial pyelonephritis.

Although 21-hydroxylase deficiency is certainly genetically heterogeneous, it is probably simplistic to assume that the presence or absence of a neonatal salt-losing crisis defines two genetically distinct disorders, a salt-losing variant and a simple virilizing variant. In later life most so-called salt losers show a persistent inability to tolerate sodium restriction, but some apparently gain the ability to conserve sodium relatively well. Similarly, one may observe apparent discordance between HLA-identical siblings as regards clinically significant salt wasting. It may be useful, therefore, to consider the variables which interact to determine whether and when a salt-losing crisis will occur.

One important determinant is the capacity to secrete aldosterone during sodium deprivation. Although all patients with 21-hydroxylase deficiency show evidence of an aldosterone biosynthetic defect[168] and hypovolemia, those with clinically apparent salt wasting have reduced plasma aldosterone levels and aldosterone secretion rates relative to their plasma renin activities, with little response to sodium restriction; aldosterone levels in those who are not salt losers are typically above normal and may rise further with sodium restriction.[169] However, this distinction is not absolute, as clinical salt wasting has been reported in infants with high aldosterone levels. This variability in aldosterone secretory capacity appears to reflect the severity of the defect in 21-hydroxylation, since persistent salt losers show more striking prenatal virilization and less capacity to secrete cortisol and 11-deoxycorticosterone during ACTH stimulation.[170] The observation that homozygous HLA Bw47 subjects are salt losers suggests that this haplotype is a marker for a more severe genetic defect, possibly a major deletion. The capacity to secrete aldosterone is also influenced by the total mass of the zona glomerulosa; although this aspect has not been carefully correlated with endocrine and genetic markers, it appears that salt-losing neonates show a deficient zona glomerulosa, while in older children with 21-hydroxylase deficiency this zone is usually hyperplastic.[171,172]

The second variable is the effect of high circulating levels of steroids such as 17-hydroxyprogesterone and progesterone, which bind to the renal tubular receptor for aldosterone and act as competitive inhibitors of mineralocorticoid action. This phenomenon greatly exacerbates salt wasting unless the patient can compensate by increased secretion of aldosterone. A salt-losing crisis tends to be self-accelerating (Fig. 18-16), since both ACTH and angiotensin levels rise, and both stimulate increased secretion of these antimineralocorticoid steroids.[173] Thus the glucocorticoid and mineralocorticoid abnormalities interact closely in this disorder: suppression of ACTH with glucocorticoid therapy serves to ameliorate the salt wasting, while suppression of the renin-angiotensin system by salt, fluids, and mineralocorticoid is essential for normalization of 17-hydroxyprogesterone secretion.

The third variable includes various nonendocrine aspects of fluid and electrolyte balance, such as body fluid compartment size, renal function, dietary intake of salt and water, and intercurrent infection, which may predispose the young infant to a salt-losing crisis under circumstances which would be less threatening in later life. In summary, therefore, the burden of current evidence suggests that severe and persistent salt wasting may be evidence of a more profound genetic defect in 21-hydroxylation, but one cannot differentiate genotypes solely by whether a neonatal salt-losing crisis has been recognized. A distinction between salt losing and simple virilizing forms of homozygous classic 21-hydroxylase deficiency has little impact on therapy, since it is now customary to provide sufficient mineralocorticoid to all patients to ensure normalization of plasma renin activity.

The diagnosis of classic 21-hydroxylase deficiency should be considered in three clinical situations: (1) the newborn with ambiguous genitalia (including apparent males with bilateral cryptorchism and hypospadias); (2) the young infant with dehydration, hyponatremia, and hyperkalemia; and (3) the child with precocious virilization. Investigation begins with the immediate determination of serum 17-hydroxyprogesterone levels,[174] at the same time as samples are being taken for karyotype analysis and assays of plasma renin activity. Umbilical-cord serum 17-hydroxyprogesterone values are high in normal infants (Table 18-6) but fall to below 200 ng/dl by 48 h (Fig. 18-19). Occasional values above 1000 ng/dl may be observed in sick or premature infants during the first week.[174a] In classic 21-hydroxylase deficiency, serum 17-hydroxyprogesterone levels greatly exceed normal, ranging from 3000 to 100,000 ng/dl,[175] and rise with age. Similar increases can be observed in levels of androstenedione, testosterone, progesterone, 21-deoxycortisol, and pregnenolone sulfate. Moderate increases in serum 17-hydroxyprogesterone are observed in 11β-hydroxylase deficiency, but in this disorder serum levels of 11-deoxycortisol are raised. Assays of urinary 17-ketosteroids and pregnanetriol were formerly used for the diagnosis of 21-hydroxylase deficiency, but the vagaries of neonatal steroid metabolism and urine collection can create serious errors of interpretation. Plasma renin activity is normal for the first few days of life, but by the fifth day all

Table 18-6. Normal Values of Hormones Commonly Used for the Diagnosis and Management of Congenital Adrenal Hyperplasia

	Serum					Plasma
	17-Hydroxyprogesterone (ng/dl)	Androstenedione (ng/dl)	Testosterone (ng/dl)		Aldosterone (ng/dl)	Renin activity (ng/ml per h)
			Male	Female		
Cord	1100–6500	50–200	5–50	5–50	95±10*	8±2*
1–2 days	65–400	20–100	60–400	20–70	7–850	25±8
3–6 days	60–250	10–100	15–25	10–25	35–210	12±2
1–3 weeks	20–220	10–150	50–350	3–25	15–105	6±2
1–12 months	5–150	5–50	5–350	3–20	5–95	6±1
1–3 years	5–90	3–40	3–15	3–15	10–80	5±2
3–6 years	5–90	3–40	3–15	3–15	10–70	3±1
6–15 years	10–160	5–150	10–770	10–60	10–70	2±0.3
Adult	10–285	50–200	260–1000	15–65	5–50	2±0.4

*Mean ± standard error of mean.

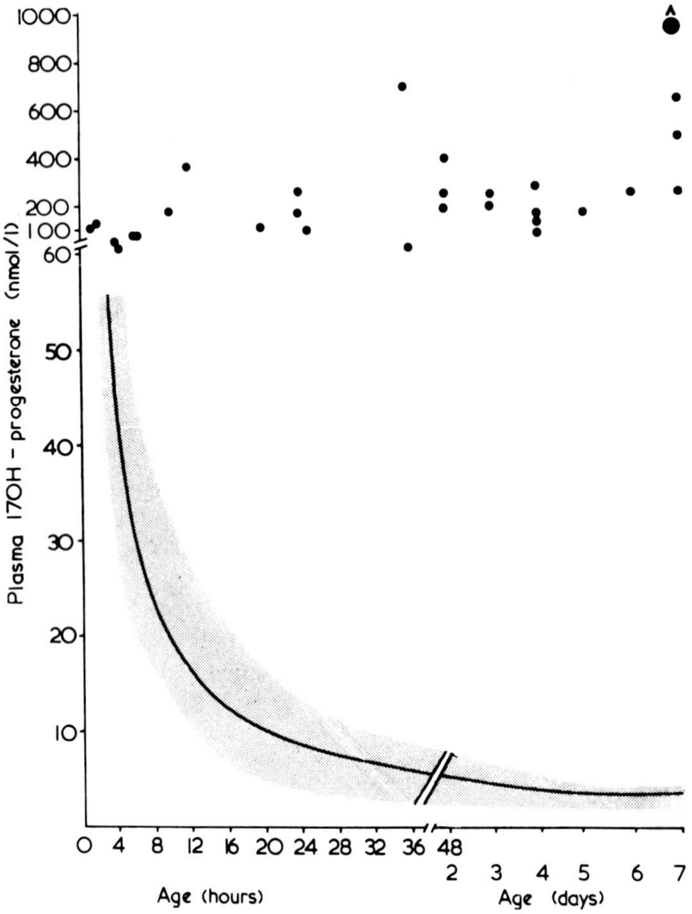

FIGURE 18-19 Plasma 17-hydroxyprogesterone concentrations in normal infants (shaded area indicates mean and range) and in untreated infants with classic 21-hydroxylase deficiency (individual dots) during the first 7 days of life. Values may be changed to nanograms per deciliter by multiplying by 33. (*From Hughes et al.*[175])

infants with classic 21-hydroxylase deficiency show elevated and rising values. There seems little merit in waiting to see if this signals a frank salt-losing crisis, and it is now customary to initiate mineralocorticoid therapy at this time.

Deficiency of 21-hydroxylase can be diagnosed prenatally after 14 weeks gestation by measurement of amniotic fluid concentrations of 17-hydroxyprogesterone, with confirmation by HLA typing of amniotic fluid cells.[176,177] Unfortunately this approach does not permit antenatal treatment in time to prevent virilization of affected females, and it remains to be seen whether the technique of chorionic villus biopsy will permit earlier diagnosis. Several investigators have demonstrated that the fetal adrenal cortex can be effectively suppressed during the period of sexual differentiation by administration of dexamethasone to the mother; such treatment at present must, however, be initiated without prior diagnosis and would prove to have been unnecessary in seven of eight pregnancies.

Neonatal screening for 21-hydroxylase deficiency by radioimmunoassay or enzyme immunoassay of 17-hydroxyprogesterone on filter paper blood spots is technically feasible.[178,179] Whether this technique should be added to existing screening programs for aminoacidopathies and congenital hypothyroidism should be decided for each jurisdiction after analysis of current mortality from unrecognized CAH. One way to estimate this is to compare the local incidence of recognized CAH in males and females, since males are at greatest risk for a salt-losing crisis before diagnosis.

The diagnosis of the late-onset or attenuated variant of 21-hydroxylase deficiency in patients with premature adrenarche, hirsutism, or infertility requires assessment of serum 17-hydroxyprogesterone concentrations before and after stimulation with ACTH.[163] In postmenarcheal females this test should be carried out in the early follicular phase, to avoid ovarian midcycle and luteal secretion of 17-hydroxyprogesterone. Some investigators feel that the test is more discriminating if preceded by overnight adrenal suppression with dexamethasone.

Successful treatment of congenital adrenal hyperplasia depends upon daily replacement of glucocorticoid and mineralocorticoid in the smallest doses sufficient to reduce pituitary ACTH secretion and the renin-angiotensin system to normal. If this is done correctly the affected patient can achieve normal growth, healthy psychosexual adjustment, and normal adult reproductive function. Other cornerstones of modern therapy include education of patient and family to ensure compliance and early perineal repair for affected females to provide normal genital appearance and function.

If the condition is diagnosed during a salt-losing crisis, treatment begins with intravenous fluids, initially with 5% glucose in saline (20 ml per kilogram of body weight in 1 h) to restore intravascular volume and then with a more gradual infusion of the same fluid or 3% saline to replace fluid and electrolyte losses. Hydrocortisone hemisuccinate (50 mg/m^2) is administered as an initial IV bolus, with a similar dose infused over the subsequent 24 h. If available, deoxycorticosterone acetate (1 to 3 mg IM every 12 h) or aldosterone (0.5 mg IV every 4 to 6 h) may be added, but mineralocorticoids tend to be relatively ineffective at first because of high levels of circulating 17-hydroxyprogesterone and other inhibitors. In small infants severe hyperkalemia may induce electrocardiographic changes and necessitate the use of rectal cation exchange resins.

Maintenance therapy seeks to provide sufficient glucocorticoid and mineralocorticoid to suppress adrenal 17-hydroxyprogesterone and androgen secretion without causing side effects such as growth failure or hypertension.[179a] Irrespective of the presence or absence of a previous frank salt-losing crisis, sufficient mineralocorticoid to reduce plasma renin levels to the age-specific normal range should always be provided.[180] In infancy 9α-fluorohydrocortisone (fludrocortisone) dosages of 0.15 to 0.2 mg per day are frequently necessary, but in older children and adults the same effect can be achieved with 0.05 to 0.1 mg per day. To avoid hypertension, the dose of 9α-fluorohydrocortisone should always be reduced if the plasma renin activity falls below normal. With such a regimen there appears to be no need for salt supplementation, but patients should not be denied access to salt, particularly during hot weather. Older forms of mineralocorticoid replacement such as IM injections or subcutaneous pellets of deoxycorticosterone are ineffective, cumbersome, and potentially dangerous.

Provided plasma renin activity is normal, adrenal androgen secretion can be suppressed by the use of oral hydrocortisone (cortisol), 10 to 20 mg/m^2 daily in three divided doses. Cortisone acetate appears to be less effective, with reduced bioavailability; more potent glucocorticoids such as prednisone or dexamethasone are useful in adults but carry too great a risk of growth inhibition for use during childhood.

Therapy should be monitored by measurements of plasma renin activity and serum 17-hydroxyprogesterone and testosterone at least every 3 to 6 months. The goal should be to maintain serum 17-hydroxyprogesterone values below 200 ng/dl and renin and testosterone values within the age- and sex-specific normal range (Table 18-6). The sensitivity of serum 17-hydroxyprogesterone to stress-induced fluctuations in ACTH release and its circadian rhythmicity demand careful attention to sampling details such as time of day, time since previous steroid administration, and successful initial venipuncture. Our approach for the past decade has been to measure plasma renin activity, serum 17-hydroxyprogesterone, and testosterone at 0900 h, just before ingestion of medication, and the serum steroid levels again 3 h later. Assays of salivary 17-hydroxyprogesterone and testosterone show excellent correlation with serum levels and provide a noninvasive technique for serial home monitoring.[181] Serum 17-hydroxyprogesterone and testosterone concentrations closely parallel each other in prepubertal children and females (Fig. 18-20), but naturally they deviate in adolescent boys.[182] Serum androstenedione, 17-hydroxypregnenolone, or 21-deoxycortisol determinations also correlate with 17-hydroxyprogesterone and can be used for monitoring therapy; however, levels of dehydroepiandrosterone (and its sulfate conjugate) remain markedly reduced after long-term glucocorticoid therapy and therefore do not provide a sufficiently sensitive index of day-to-day ACTH suppression. Assays of urinary 17-ketosteroids and pregnanetriol were formerly used to monitor therapy in CAH; however, they provide no advantage and are considerably less sensitive and more cumbersome.

In addition, patients should be monitored by careful attention to growth velocity and skeletal maturation, since there is no biochemical test for overtreatment. At all ages the smallest dose of cortisol which will normalize hormone levels should be used. During major infections the dose of cortisol should be doubled, and extra doses of oral or parenteral glucocorticoid should be provided prior to surgery requiring general anesthesia. It is our habit to instruct parents to repeat the previous medications any time the child vomits and to give IM cortisone acetate, 25 to 100 mg, and 1 to 3 mg deoxycorticosterone acetate (if available) if there is a second episode of vomiting; relatively large doses of cortisone acetate should be used, since this agent has been shown to have low bioavailability, due either to poor absorption or to incomplete conversion to cortisol.

Therapy of late-onset CAH requires only oral hydrocortisone in the same doses, without supple-

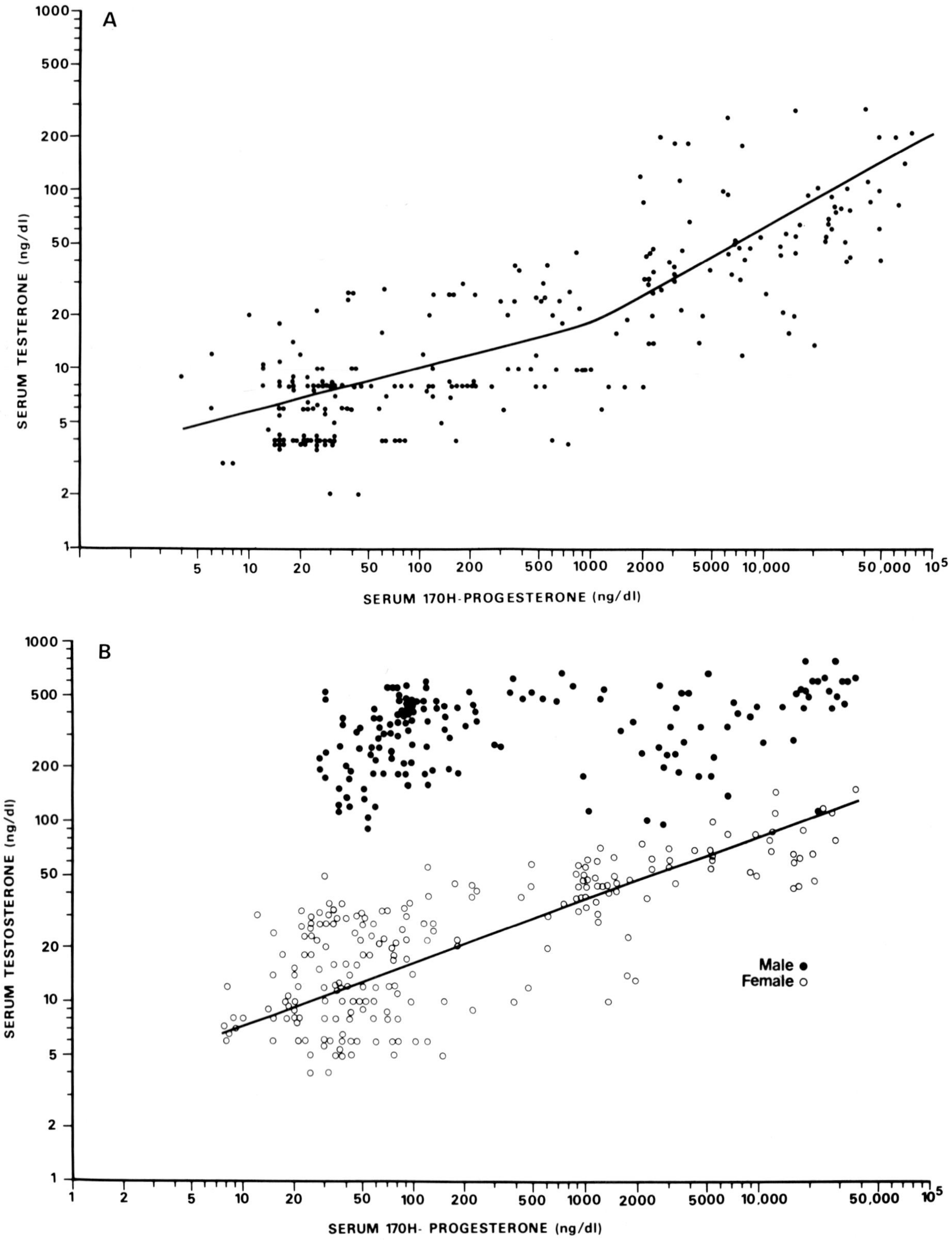

FIGURE 18-20 (*A*) Relation between log serum concentrations of 17-hydroxyprogesterone and testosterone in prepubertal patients with classic 21-hydroxylase deficiency. (*B*) Relation between log serum 17-hydroxyprogesterone and testosterone concentrations in adolescent male (closed circle) and female (open circle) patients with classic 21-hydroxylase deficiency. (*From Hughes and Winter.*[182])

mentary mineralocorticoid. Once growth is complete, satisfactory control and normal fertility can be achieved more easily with longer-acting agents such as dexamethasone.[183]

Occasionally, if the diagnosis of classic CAH has been delayed or therapy inadequate, significant advance of both skeletal maturation and hypothalamic-pituitary maturation may occur, with physical signs and hormonal evidence of true precocious puberty.[184] This complication may require adjunctive use of GnRH analogue therapy, as in other forms of true precocious puberty. From time to time other adjuncts, such as surgical or medical adrenalectomy (using aminoglutethimide) have been suggested to treat CAH. However, there is no evidence that such steps are necessary or even beneficial in patients who are compliant with standard glucocorticoid and mineralocorticoid replacement.

In all forms of female pseudohermaphroditism, including 21-hydroxylase deficiency, plastic repair of the external genitalia should be undertaken by 18 months of age, so that the child is never aware of the deformity. The appropriate procedure includes vaginoplasty, to provide labia majora and minora, and separate urethral and vaginal communication to the perineum, plus clitoroplasty, in which the separated crurae of the clitoris are placed under the symphysis pubis, leaving only the glans visible with its vascular and nervous supply intact. Occasionally the connection between the upper vagina and urogenital sinus is proximal to the external sphincter, so far from the perineum that it is necessary to delay creating the appropriate outlet to the perineum until after menarche. But in all cases the external appearance of the genitalia should be made normal in infancy, with no further surgical interference during childhood. Vaginal dilatation may be necessary in young women who underwent vaginoplasty in infancy, but thereafter sexual function is completely normal. It is our custom to recommend cesarean section in women who have undergone this repair, as we have no information regarding the effects of vaginal delivery.

If the diagnosis of 21-hydroxylase deficiency is made soon after birth and appropriate medical care is maintained through childhood, one can expect normal growth, intellectual and psychosexual development, adolescence, and adult reproductive function. In young women regular ovulatory menstrual cycles do not occur unless serum testosterone and 17-hydroxyprogesterone levels are reduced to normal.[183] Although apparent well-being and even normal spermatogenesis has been observed in occasional untreated adult males, it seems better to recommend lifelong therapy, since infertility due to suppression of gonadotropins is the more likely result of inadequate treatment.[185] Untreated adult males may also develop testicular tumors as a result of chronic ACTH stimulation of adrenal rest cells.

11β-HYDROXYLASE DEFICIENCY The enzyme complex which catalyzes conversion of 11-deoxycortisol to cortisol is a mitochondrial oxidase consisting of a flavoprotein, adrenodoxin, and a substrate-specific cytochrome P450. Immunochemical studies indicate that this single cytochrome P450 catalyzes both 11β- and 18-hydroxylation.[186] The gene for 11β-hydroxylase is not linked to the major histocompatibilty locus.

Deficiency of 11β-hydroxylase is the second most common form of CAH; it accounts, however, for only 5 percent of all CAH cases, although it is relatively more common among Jews of North African origin. It is an autosomal recessive disorder, in which the classic signs are virilization plus hypertension. Increased adrenal secretion of 11-deoxycorticosterone (DOC) and 11-deoxycortisol leads to ACTH-dependent hypertension of variable severity. Accumulation of steroids more proximal in the steroidogenic path (such as 17-hydroxyprogesterone) and their subsequent metabolism to androgens leads to prenatal masculinization of the external genitalia in genetic females, as in 21-hydroxylase deficiency.[187] Postnatally, untreated males and females show progressive virilization, with rapid skeletal maturation and eventual short stature. Prepubertal gynecomastia of uncertain pathogenesis has been reported in affected males. Severe virilization may occur without hypertension, but the reverse has not been observed. In addition to this classic form of 11β-hydroxylase deficiency, milder variants have been described, with onset of hirsutism, acne, amenorrhea, and variable hypertension in adolescence or even later.[188]

In untreated patients with the classic disorder, hypervolemia suppresses plasma renin activity and aldosterone secretion. Following glucocorticoid therapy and suppression of DOC production, plasma renin increases and there is a rise in aldosterone levels. However, the aldosterone response to sodium restriction is subnormal and salt wasting may occur, particularly in infants, after the initiation of therapy.[189] The ability of these patients to produce some aldosterone has been interpreted as evidence for separate 11β- and 18-hydroxylases in the fasciculata and glomerulosa but may only indicate that the defective gene product is relatively more effective within the microenvironment of the glomerulosa. In some cases the abnormal enzyme appears to be capable of 11β-hydroxylating 17-hydroxyprogesterone to form 21-deoxycortisol, the presence of which can mimic the hormonal pattern of 21-hydroxylase deficiency.[190]

The hallmark of 11β-hydroxylase deficiency is the

presence of elevated serum concentrations of 11-deoxycortisol and DOC and their suppression by exogenous glucocorticoid. Urinary excretion of metabolites such as tetrahydro-11-deoxycortisol (THS) is usually increased but may be normal during early infancy. Prenatal diagnosis is possible by determination of increased amniotic fluid concentrations of 11-deoxycortisol or increased maternal excretion of THS.[191] In obligate heterozygotes, however, basal and ACTH-stimulated 11-deoxysteroid levels cannot be distinguished from normal.[192]

Treatment of 11β-hydroxylase deficiency requires cortisol in doses similar to those used in other forms of CAH. With adequate treatment virilization ceases and hypertension usually disappears; serum concentrations of DOC and 11-deoxycortisol fall to normal, while plasma renin activity rises to the normal range. Early vaginoplasty and clitoroplasty are required for prenatally virilized females.

3β-HSD DEFICIENCY This disorder was discussed in detail earlier under Defective Genital Virilization (Male Pseudohermaphroditism), since it can cause genital ambiguity in both males and females. The originally described classic variant is an autosomal recessive disease which is not HLA-linked and which causes a major block in the biosynthesis of mineralocorticoid, glucocorticoid, androgens, and estrogens in both the adrenal cortex and the gonads (Fig. 18-12). Infant girls present with slight to moderate clitoral enlargement plus severe salt wasting; however, a few patients have been described who could maintain normal salt balance and apparently adequate aldosterone production by means of compensatory high renin-angiotensin stimulation. The virilization of affected females is presumably due to peripheral conversion of Δ^5-3β-hydroxysteroid precursors to androgen.

As in other forms of CAH, it is now recognized that 3β-HSD deficiency exists in several clinical variants, presumably reflecting underlying genetic heterogeneity. Genetic females with the milder late-onset variants have normal genitalia at birth and normal mineralocorticoid secretion; plasma renin activity may be normal or increased. They present during late childhood with premature adrenarche; during puberty with male-pattern hirsutism, acne, clitoromegaly, and primary amenorrhea; and in the older female with menstrual irregularity and infertility.[106,107,111] Obviously, this type of adrenal virilism can overlap with the presentation of polycystic ovary syndrome, particularly since adrenal androgens can produce the ovarian changes of the latter syndrome.

The diagnosis of 3β-HSD deficiency is indicated by the finding of high serum concentrations of dehydroepiandrosterone, pregnenolone, and 17-hydroxypregnenolone with their respective sulfate conjugates. Because of hepatic 3β-HSD activity, one may find increased serum levels of Δ^4-3-ketosteroids such as 17-hydroxyprogesterone and androstenedione, but these are never as markedly elevated as the Δ^5-3β-hydroxysteroids. There is a similar characteristic Δ^5/Δ^4 imbalance in the urinary excretion of Δ^5-pregnenetriol and pregnanetriol. In the classic variant, ACTH and hCG stimulation elicits little rise in circulating levels of cortisol and gonadal sex steroids. In the late-onset variants, basal hormone levels are frequently normal but a relative deficiency in 3β-HSD can be demonstrated by ACTH stimulation, which elicits a disproportionate increase in Δ^5-3β-hydroxysteroid levels.

Therapy of 3β-HSD deficiency requires replacement of cortisol, as in other forms of CAH, plus full mineralocorticoid replacement in any patient with elevated plasma renin activity or intolerance to sodium restriction. In addition, patients with the classic variant usually show defective pubertal development[193] and therefore require sex steroid (estrogen and progestin) replacement at the appropriate age. In the less severe variants, normal puberty and regular ovulatory menstrual cycles will usually follow suppression of adrenal androgen secretion.

Prenatal Virilization by Environmental Hormones

Masculinization of the external genitalia of female infants can also occur if the mother ingests androgens or has a virilizing disorder such as an ovarian tumor (usually arrhenoblastoma or hCG-dependent luteoma of pregnancy), adrenal neoplasm, or inadequately treated congenital adrenal hyperplasia. In addition, female pseudohermaphroditism of varying degrees has been observed in the offspring of women treated with synthetic progestins such as norethindrone, ethisterone, norethynodrel, or medroxyprogesterone.[194] Similar virilization may also occur following maternal ingestion of large doses of stilbestrol, perhaps because of inhibition of fetal adrenal 3β-HSD; such offspring would also be at risk for later development of adenocarcinoma of the cervix and vagina.

The only treatment necessary for this form of female pseudohermaphroditism is surgical repair of the external genitalia. There is no need for ongoing hormone replacement therapy, and subsequent physical and psychosexual development should be entirely normal.[58,195]

Teratological Malformations of the External Genitalia

Genital abnormalities, occasionally presenting as female pseudohermaphroditism, are frequently observed in association with renal agenesis, imperforate anus, and other malformations of the urinary and intestinal tracts.[196,197] Usually the internal genitalia are absent or abnormal. Similar apparently nonendocrine masculinization of a female fetus has been observed in association with multiple malformation syndromes, including cryptophthalmos, middle and outer ear maldevelopment, meningoencephalocele, and cardiac malformations; there may be familial recurrence of these anomalies, most of which have been lethal. A familial association of vaginal agenesis, middle ear malformations, and renal hypoplasia has been described.[198] Apparent clitoral enlargement giving the appearance of female pseudohermaphroditism can also occur in neurofibromatosis.[199]

CLINICAL APPROACH TO DISORDERS OF SEXUAL DIFFERENTIATION

The Newborn with Abnormal Genitalia

Genital ambiguity in a neonate presents a psychosocial crisis which demands rapid yet sophisticated investigation prior to therapy and sex assignment. Such infants should be transferred at once to a center capable of providing within days a definitive diagnosis in terms of genetic sex, gonadal and genital structure, and endocrine function. Although the resources and expertise of a team of physicians are often required, a single person, usually the pediatric endocrinologist, should be responsible for communication with the parents, to explain the problem and proposed investigations and to counsel regarding the prognosis for health, psychosexual adjustment, and reproductive function. Naming of the child should be delayed until gender assignment is decided; under no circumstances should parents be encouraged to select purposely a sexually ambiguous name. When reassignment of the sex of rearing is necessary because of a previous incorrect diagnosis or ignorance of the principles that govern gender assignment, it becomes doubly important that the reasons for this decision be explained to the parents in simple terms by a physician who is familiar with their cultural, religious, and educational background.

An abnormality of sexual differentiation should be suspected not only in the infant with obviously ambiguous genitalia but also in apparent males with hypospadias, cryptorchism, or micropenis and in apparent females with partial labial fusion, clitoromegaly, or an inguinal mass. An abbreviated flowchart for the logical application of genetic and endocrine investigations in these circumstances is presented in Fig. 18-21. Only rarely will the genitalia be sufficiently distinctive to diagnose a particular disorder. Rather, examination of the external genitalia serves to document specific points such as the size of the phallus, location of the urethral meatus, number and location of ventral frenula on the phallus, degree of labioscrotal fusion, and presence or absence of palpable gonads. It is usually possible by careful rectal examination of the newborn to determine whether a cervix is present. Finally, a careful assessment should be made of any associated congenital malformations, dehydration, or hyperpigmentation.

Initial laboratory investigation in the infant without palpable gonads includes karyotype analysis (supplemented by sex chromatin if the karyotyping will be delayed) and assays of serum 17-hydroxyprogesterone levels. The infant's intake, weight, and serum electrolytes should be monitored daily to assess any salt wasting, but assays of plasma renin activity are best delayed until after 4 days of age. During this period, ultrasonography or genitography may be performed in order to confirm the status of the paramesonephric duct structures.[200] The purpose of this approach is to identify the most common condition, 21-hydroxylase deficiency, before salt-losing complications appear. If, in a genetic female, the serum 17-hydroxyprogesterone concentrations are not significantly raised (over 3000 ng/dl) and rising by 5 days of age, one should consider other forms of female pseudohermaphroditism and assess serum levels of steroids such as 11-deoxycortisol, dehydroepiandrosterone, and 17-hydroxypregnenolone.

Any gonad felt in the labioscrotal or inguinal area almost certainly contains testicular tissue. If portions of it differ in consistency, one should consider a possible ovotestis or a gonad that has undergone neoplastic transformation. Absence of well-differentiated paramesonephric duct structures on one side is further evidence that the ipsilateral gonad contains testicular tissue. Complete absence of these structures shown by genitography in a 46,XY infant with ambiguous genitalia suggests one of the several forms of male pseudohermaphroditism; further investigation requires detailed analysis of hCG-stimulated androgen biosynthesis and of target cell receptors and metabolism.

With increasing frequency, a family history of abnormal sexual differentiation raises the question of possible prenatal diagnosis during a subsequent pregnancy. Ultrasonography may permit visualizaion of the external genitalia after the fifth month of gestation;[201] amniocentesis can often provide a biochemical diagnosis at 15 to 20 weeks; and chorionic villus biopsy offers the opportunity to assess at least genetic sex and HLA haplotype even earlier. Unfortunately, none of these techniques permits diagnosis in time to initiate therapy and prevent genital malformation. In the case of congenital adrenal hyperplasia the major

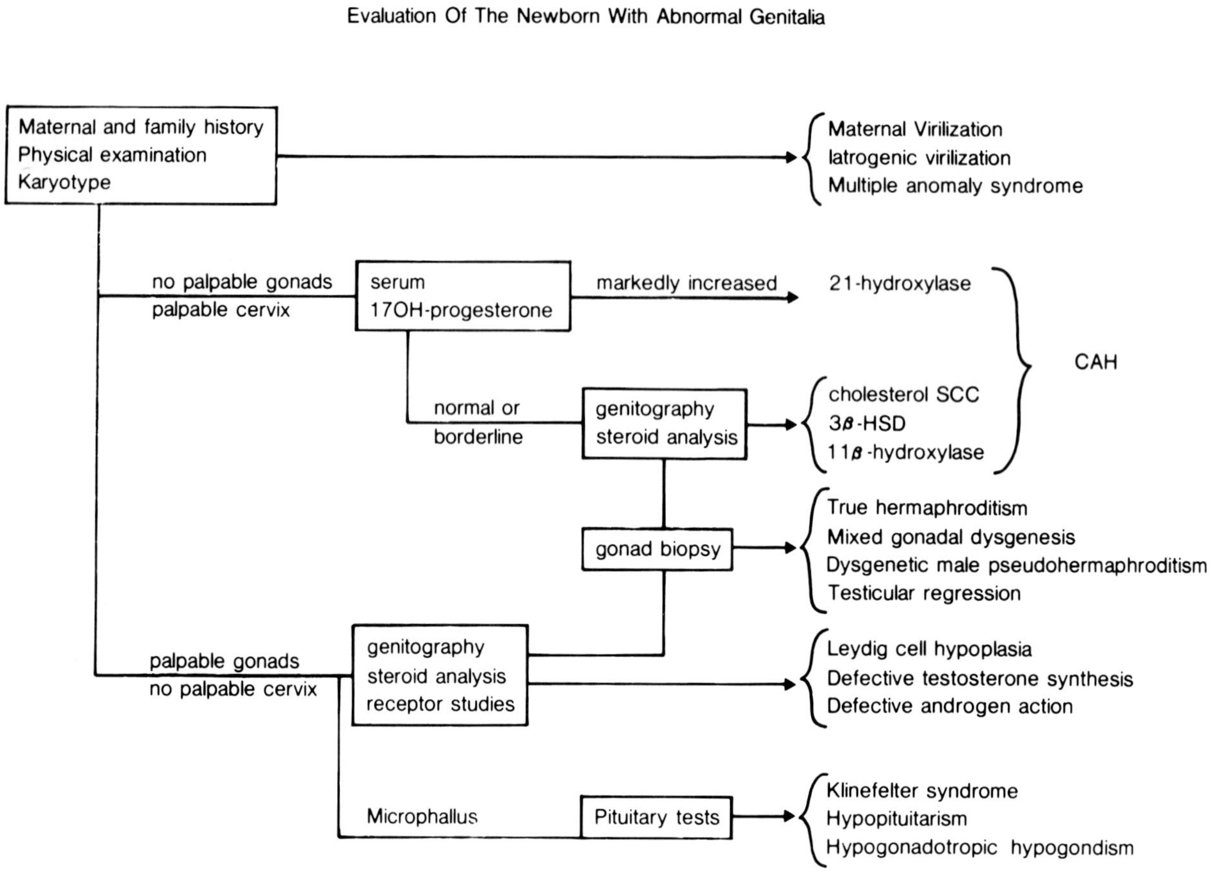

FIGURE 18-21 A simplified flowchart for the investigation and diagnosis of an infant with genital ambiguity.

purpose of prenatal diagnosis to date has been to justify therapeutic abortion for what is essentially a remediable disorder.

In a female pseudohermaphrodite capable of normal fertility, it is obvious that the sex of rearing should be female. Similarly, in the male with 5α-reductase deficiency the potential for dramatic virilization and adult male reproductive function requires that the infant be raised as male, regardless of genital appearance. However, in most intersex disorders there is no chance for fertility, and the prime consideration for gender assignment should be the potential to achieve functional and cosmetically acceptable external genitalia with endocrine and surgical therapy. Genetic males with microphallus often benefit from a course of androgen therapy (testosterone cyclopentylpropionate, 25 mg IM monthly for three doses) prior to any surgery. However, if a defect in androgen receptor activity has been demonstrated, such virilization is impossible and assignment of female gender is appropriate.

To ensure family acceptance and normal adjustment of the infant, reconstructive surgery to provide gender-compatible external genitalia should if possible be performed before 18 months of age. In females a type of vaginoplasty and clitoroplasty that preserves clitoral innervation and blood supply is most desirable. Thereafter, any further surgery should be delayed until late adolescence. In males the creation of a phallic urethra is more difficult and requires several procedures; if scrotal testes are not present, consideration should be given to the insertion of prostheses.

Where there is a significant risk of gonadal neoplasia, as in gonadal dysgenesis with a Y-bearing cell line, the gonads should be removed as early as is convenient. It has been customary in complete testicular feminization to leave the testes in place until after puberty, but when an infant is already undergoing repair of inguinal hernias it is probably more reasonable to remove the testes and then to provide estrogen replacement at the time of puberty. If the sex of rearing is female and there is any risk of even partial virilization at puberty (as in incomplete testicular feminization), the gonads should be removed during childhood.

Virilization during Childhood or Adolescence

The precocious appearance of pubic hair and acne or inappropriate hirsutism, clitoral enlargement, or other sign of virilization deserves careful investigation, as outlined in Fig. 18-22. A small but significant fraction of such patients will prove to have a late-onset variant of congenital adrenal hyperplasia (either 21-hydroxylase, 11β-hydroxylase, or 3β-HSD deficiency). Frequently ACTH stimulation as well as dexamethasone suppression testing are necessary to demonstrate the defect in steroidogenesis.

Delayed Puberty, Amenorrhea, and Infertility

The initial evaluation of the patient presenting with delayed or unsatisfactory pubertal development, primary or secondary amenorrhea, or unexplained infertility should include assessment of serum gonadotropin concentrations. Those with hypergonadotropic hypogonadism (Fig. 18-23) may turn out to have an unrecognized disorder of sexual differentiation. Females with gonadal dysgenesis may present early with pubertal failure or later with secondary amenorrhea and infertility. If an apparent female shows normal breast development, sparse sex hair, and primary amenorrhea, the likely diagnosis is testicular feminization.

REFERENCES

1. Painter TS: The sex chromosome of man. *Am Naturalist* 58:506, 1924.
2. Ford CE, Hamerton JL: The chromosomes of man. *Nature* 178:1020, 1956.
3. Fisher RA: *The Genetical Theory of Natural Selection.* Oxford, Clarendon, 1930.
4. National Foundation for Birth Defects: *An International System for Human Cytogenetic Nomenclature (1978). Birth Defects.* New York, 1978, vol 14, no 8; also *Cytogenet Cell Genet* 21:309, 1978.
5. Boué J, Boué A, Lazar P: Retrospective and prospective epidemiological studies of 1500 karyotyped spontaneous human abortions. *Teratology* 12:11, 1975.

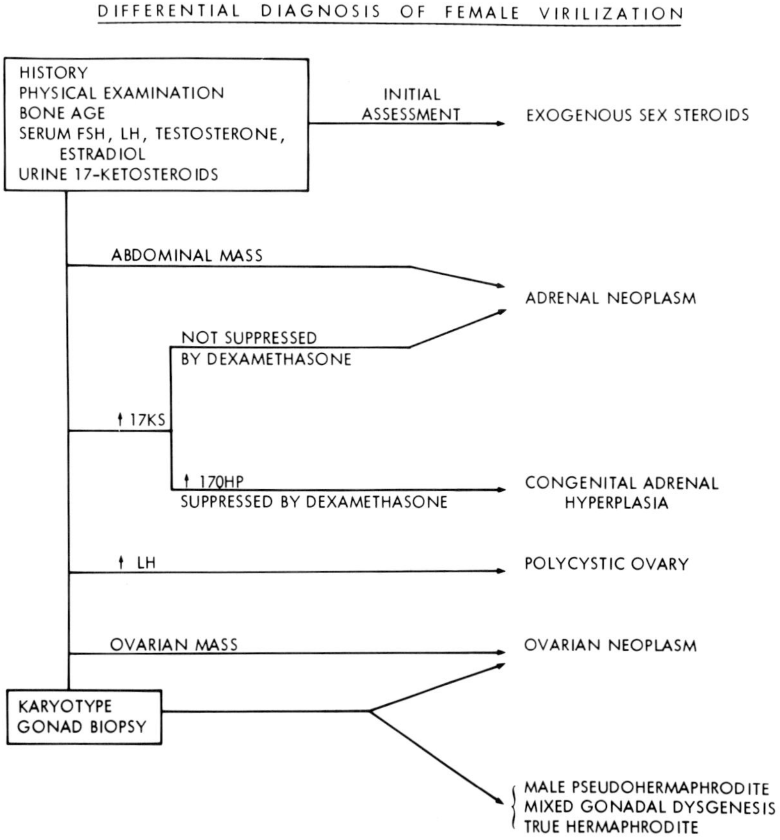

FIGURE 18-22 A flowchart illustrating a practical diagnostic approach to the child with inappropriate virilization. [*From Dean HJ, Winter JSD, in Collu R, Ducharme JR, Guyda H (eds): Pediatric Endocrinology. New York, Raven, 1981, p 350.*]

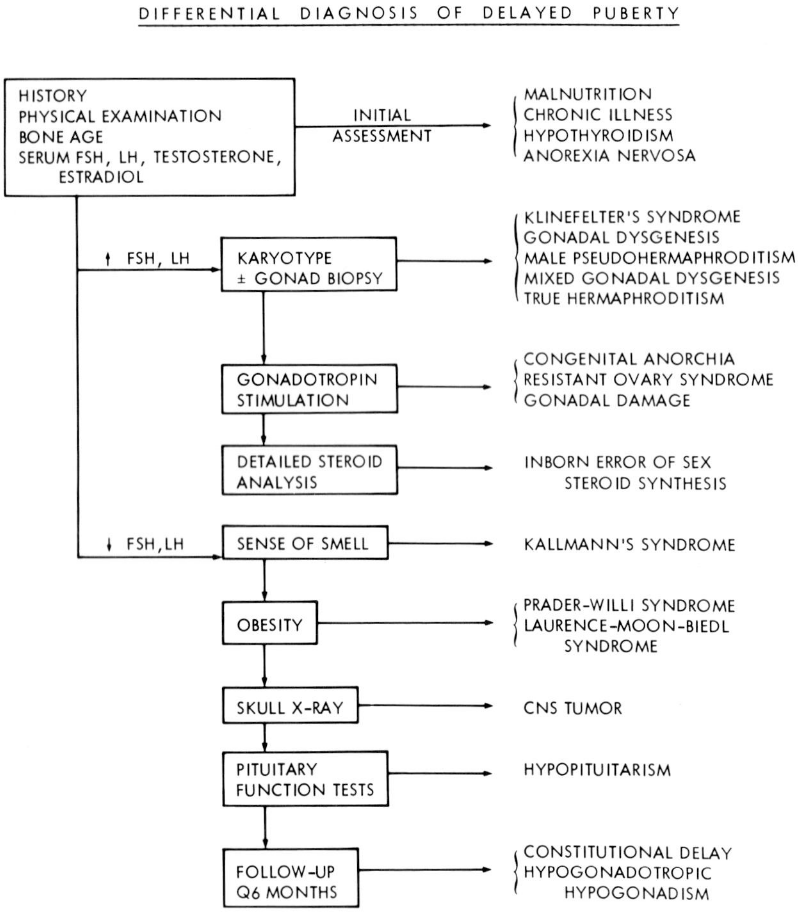

FIGURE 18-23 A flowchart illustrating a practical diagnostic approach to the patient with delayed puberty. [*From Dean HJ, Winter JSD, in Collu R, Ducharme JR, Guyda H (eds): Pediatric Endocrinology. New York, Raven, 1981, p 333.*]

6. Martin RH, Balkan W, Burns K, Rademaker AW, Lin CC, Rudd NL: The chromosome constitution of 1000 human spermatozoa. *Hum Genet* 63:305, 1983.

7. Jacobs PA: The incidence and etiology of sex chromosome abnormalities in man. The National Foundation, 1979.

8. Opitz O, Zoll B, Hansmann I, Hinney B: Cytogenetic investigation of 103 patients with primary or secondary amenorrhea. *Hum Genet* 65:46, 1983.

9. Diedrich U, Hansmann I, Janke D, Opitz O, Probeck H-D: Chromosome abnormalities in 136 couples with a history of recurrent abortions. *Hum Genet* 65:48, 1983.

10. Polani PE: Pairing of X and Y chromosomes, non-inactivation of X-linked genes and the maleness factor. *Hum Genet* 60:207, 1982.

11. Burgoyne P: The origins of men with two X chromosomes. *Nature* 307:109, 1984.

12. Miller OJ, Drayna D, Goodfellow P: Report of the committee on the genetic constitution of the X and Y chromosomes. *Cytogenet Cell Genet* 37:176, 1984.

13. Meyer WJ III, Migeon BR, Migeon CJ: Locus on human X chromosome for dihydrotestosterone receptor and androgen insensitivity. *Proc Natl Acad Sci USA* 72:1469, 1975.

14. Wolf U: X-linked genes and gonadal differentiation. *Differentiation* (suppl) 23:S104, 1983.

15. Therman E, Denniston C, Sarto GE, Uber M: X chromosome constitution and the human female phenotype. *Hum Genet* 54:133, 1980.

16. Lyon MF: Mechanisms and evolutionary origins of variable X-chromosome activity in mammals. *Proc R Soc Lond* [Biol] 187:243, 1974.

17. Gartler SM, Riggs AD: Mammalian X-chromosome inactivation. *Annu Rev Genet* 17:155, 1983.

18. Monesi V: Chromosome activities during meiosis and spermiogenesis. *J Reprod Fertil* 13:1, 1971.

19. Mohandas T, Sparkes RS, Shapiro LJ: Reactivation of an inactive human X chromosome: Evidence for X inactivation by DNA methylation. *Science* 211:393, 1981.

20. Cooper DN: Eukaryotic DNA methylation. *Hum Genet* 64:315, 1983.

21. Byskov AG: Gonadal sex and germ cell differentiation, in Austin CR, Edwards RG (eds): *Mechanisms of Sex Differentiation in Animals and Man.* London, Academic, 1981, p 145.

22. Ross GT, Lipsett MB: Homologies of structure and function in mammalian testes and ovaries. *Int J Androl* (suppl) 2:39, 1978.

23. McCoshen JA: Quantitation of sex chromosomal influence(s) on the somatic growth of fetal gonads in vivo. *Am J Obstet Gynecol* 145:469, 1983.

24. Eichwald EJ, Silmser CR: H-Y and serendipity. *Hum Genet* 58:6, 1981.

25. Goldberg EH, Boyse EA, Bennett D, Scheid M, Carswell EA: Serological demonstration of H-Y (male) antigen on mouse sperm. *Nature* 232:478, 1971.

26. Koo GC: Serology of H-Y antigen. *Hum Genet* 58:18, 1981.

27. Wachtel SS, Ohno S, Koo GC, Boyse EA: Possible role for H-Y antigen in the primary determination of sex. *Nature* 257:235, 1975.

28. Simpson E: Sex reversal and sex determination. *Nature* 300:404, 1982.

29. Silvers WK, Gasser DL, Eicher EM: H-Y antigen, serologically detectable male antigen and sex determination. *Cell* 28:439, 1982.

30. Ohno S, Nagai Y, Ciccarese S: Testicular cells lysostripped of H-Y antigen organize ovarian follicle-like aggregates. *Cytogenet Cell Genet* 20:351, 1978.

31. Zenzes MT, Wolf U, Engel W: Organization in vitro of ovarian cells into testicular structures. *Hum Genet* 44:333, 1978.

32. Muller U, Zenzes MT, Bauknecht T, Wolf U, Siebers JW, Engel W: Appearance of hCG-receptor after conversion of newborn ovarian cells into testicular structures by H-Y antigen in vitro. *Hum Genet* 45:203, 1978.

33. Wachtel SS, Koo GC, Breg WR, Elias S, Boyse EA, Miller OJ: Expression of H-Y antigen in human males with two Y chromosomes. *N Engl J Med* 293:1070, 1975.

34. Ohno S, Epplen JT, Cellini A: Evolutionary conserved sex-specific repeats, their transcripts and H-Y antigen, in Serio M, Motta M, Zanisi M, Martini L (eds): *Sexual Differentiation: Basic and Clinical Aspects.* New York, Raven, 1984, pp 17–31.

35. Wolf U: Genetic aspects of H-Y antigen. *Hum Genet* 58:25, 1981.

36. Adinolfi M, Polani P, Zenthon J: Genetic control of H-Y synthesis: A hypothesis. *Hum Genet* 61:1, 1982.

37. Byskov AG: Regulation of meiosis in mammals. *Ann Biol Anim Biochim Biophys* 19:1251, 1979.

38. Josso N, Picard JY, Tran D: The antimüllerian hormone. *Recent Prog Horm Res* 33:117, 1977.

39. Budzik GP, Powell SM, Kamagata S, Donahoe PK: Müllerian inhibiting substance fractionation by dye affinity chromatography. *Cell* 34:307, 1983.

40. Picard JY, Josso N: Purification of testicular anti-müllerian hormone allowing direct visualization of the pure glycoprotein and determination of yield and purification factor. *Mol Cell Endocrinol* 34:23, 1984.

41. Picon R: Testicular inhibition of fetal müllerian ducts in vitro: Effect of dibutyryl cyclic AMP. *Mol Cell Endocrinol* 4:35, 1976.

42. Gill WB, Schumacher GFB, Bibbo M: Pathological semen and anatomical abnormalities of genital tract in human male subjects exposed to diethylstilbestrol in utero. *J Urol* 117:477, 1977.

43. Vigier B, Tran D, du Buisson F du M, Heyman Y, Josso N: Use of monoclonal antibody techniques to study the ontogeny of bovine anti-müllerian hormone. *J Reprod Fertil* 69:207, 1983.

44. Bercu BB, Morikawa Y, Jackson IMD, Donahoe PK: Inhibition of müllerian inhibiting substance secretion by FSH. *Pediatr Res* 13:246, 1979.

45. Vigier B, Picard JY, Tran D, Legeai L, Josso N: Production of anti-müllerian hormone: Another homology between Sertoli and granulosa cells. *Endocrinology* 114:1315, 1984.

46. Siiteri PK, Wilson JD: Testosterone formation and metabolism during male sexual differentiation in the human embryo. *J Clin Endocrinol Metab* 38:113, 1974.

47. Feldman KW, Smith DW: Fetal phallic growth and penile standards for newborn male infants. *J Pediatr* 86:395, 1975.

48. Habenicht U-F, Newmann F: Hormonal regulation of testicular descent. *Adv Embryol Cell Biol* 81:1, 1983.

49. Winter JSD, Faiman C, Reyes FI: Sex steroid production by the human fetus: Its role in morphogenesis and control by gonadotropins, in Blandau RJ, Bergsma D (eds): *Morphogenesis and Malformation of the Genital System.* New York, Alan R. Liss, 1977, pp 41–58.

50. Cunha GR, Shannon JM, Neubauer BL, Sawyer LM, Fujii H, Taguchi O, Chung LWK: Mesenchymal-epithelial interactions in sex differentiation. *Hum Genet* 58:68, 1981.

51. Carr BR, Parker CR Jr, Ohashi M, MacDonald PC, Simpson ER: Regulation of human fetal testicular secretion of testosterone: Low density lipoprotein-cholesterol and cholesterol synthesized de novo as steroid precursor. *Am J Obstet Gynecol* 146:241, 1983.

52. Clements JA, Reyes FI, Winter JSD, Faiman C: Ontogenesis of gonadotropin-releasing hormone in the human fetal hypothalamus. *Proc Soc Exp Biol Med* 163:437, 1980.

53. Rasmussen DD, Liu JH, Wolf PL, Yen SSC: Endogenous opioid regulation of gonadotropin-releasing hormone release from the human fetal hypothalamus in vitro. *J Clin Endocrinol Metab* 57:881, 1983.

54. Winter JSD, Faiman C, Reyes FI: Sexual endocrinology of fetal and perinatal life, in Austin CR, Edwards RG (eds): *Mechanisms of Sex Differentiation in Animals and Man.* London, Academic, 1981, pp 205–253.

55. Imperato-McGinley J, Peterson RE, Gautier T, Sturla E: The impact of androgens on the evolution of male gender identity, in Kogan SJ, Hafez ESE (eds): *Pediatric Andrology.* The Hague, Martinus Nijhoff, 1981, pp 99–108.

56. Dorner G: Hormones, brain differentiation and the fundamental process of life. *J Steroid Biochem* 8:531, 1977.

57. Gorski RA, Gordon JH, Shryne JE, Southam AM: Evidence for a morphologic sex difference within the medial preoptic area of the rat brain. *Brain Res* 148:333, 1978.

58. Ehrhardt AA, Meyer-Bahlburg HFL: Effects of prenatal sex hormones on gender-related behavior. *Science* 211:1312, 1981.

59. Rubin RT, Reinisch JM, Hakett RF: Postnatal gonadal steroid effects on human behavior. *Science* 211:1318, 1981.

59a. Klinefelter HF Jr, Reifenstein EC Jr, Albright F: Syndrome characterized by gynecomastia, aspermatogenesis with A-leydigism, and increased excretion of follicle-stimulating hormone. *J Clin Endocrinol Metab* 2:615, 1942.

60. Salbenblatt JA, Bender BG, Puck MH, Robinson A, Faiman C, Winter JSD: Pituitary-gonadal function in Klinefelter syndrome before and during puberty. *Pediatr Res* (in press).

61. Topper E, Dickerman Z, Prager-Lewin R, Kaufman H, Maimon Z, Laron Z: Puberty in 24 patients with Klinefelter syndrome. *Eur J Pediatr* 139:8, 1982.

62. Forti G, Giusti G, Borghi A, Pazzagli M, Fiorelli G, Cabresi E, Mannelli M, Bassi F, Giannotti P, Fusi S, Serio M: Klinefelter's syndrome: A study of its hormonal pattern. *J Endocrinol Invest* 2:149, 1978.

63. Mies R, Fischer H, Pfeiff B, Winkelmann W, Würz H: Klinefelter's syndrome and breast cancer. *Andrologia* 14:317, 1982.

64. de la Chapelle A, Tippett PA, Wetterstrand G, Page D: Genetic evidence of X-Y interchange in a human XX male. *Nature* 307:170, 1984.

65. Hecht T, Cooke HJ, Cerrillo M, Mear B, Reck G, Hameister H: A new case of Y to X translocation in a female. *Hum Genet* 54:303, 1980.

66. Kohn G, Winter JSD, Mellman WJ: Trisomy X in three children. *J Pediatr* 72:248, 1968.

67. van Niekerk WA, Retief AE: The gonads of human true hermaphrodites. *Hum Genet* 58:117, 1981.

68. Yanagisawa S: Structural abnormalities of the Y chromosome and abnormal external genitals. *Hum Genet* 53:183, 1980.

69. Davidoff F, Federman DD: Mixed gonadal dysgenesis. *Pediatrics* 52:725, 1973.

70. Manuel M, Katayama KP, Jones HW Jr: The age of occurrence of gonadal tumors in intersex patients with a Y chromosome. *Am J Obstet Gynecol* 124:293, 1976.

71. Warburton D, Kline J, Stein Z, Susser M: Monosomy X: A chromosomal anomaly associated with young maternal age. *Lancet* 1:167, 1980.

72. Ranke MB, Pfluger H, Rosendahl W, Stubbe P, Enders H, Bierich JR, Majewski F: Turner syndrome: Spontaneous growth in 150 cases and review of the literature. *Eur J Pediatr* 141:81, 1983.

72a. Bender B, Puck M, Salbenblatt J, Robinson A: Cognitive development of unselected girls with complete and partial X monosomy. *Pediatrics* 73:175, 1984.

73. Kosowicz J: The roentgen appearance of the hand and wrist in gonadal dysgenesis. *Am J Roentgenol Radium Ther Nucl Med* 93:354, 1965.

74. Reyes FI, Koh KS, Faiman C: Fertility in women with gonadal dysgenesis. *Am J Obstet Gynecol* 126:668, 1976.

75. Madan K: Balanced structural changes involving the human X: Effect on sexual phenotype. *Hum Genet* 63:216, 1983.

76. Haseltine FP, De Ponte KK, Breg WR, Genel M: Presence of H-Y antigen in patients with Ullrich-Turner syndrome and X-chromosome rearrangements. *Am J Med Genet* 11:97, 1982.

77. Winter JSD, Faiman C: Serum gonadotropin levels in agonadal children and adults. *J Clin Endocrinol Metab* 35:561, 1972.

78. Rudman D, Goldsmith M, Kutner M, Blackston D: Effect of growth hormone and oxandrolone singly and together on growth rate in girls with X chromosome abnormalities. *J Pediatr* 96:132, 1980.

79. Apter D, Lenko HL, Perheentupa J, Söderholm A, Vihko R: Subnormal pubertal increases of serum androgens in Turner's syndrome. *Horm Res* 16:164, 1982.

80. Urban MD, Lee PA, Dorst JP, Plotnick LP, Migeon CJ: Oxandrolone therapy in patients with Turner syndrome. *J Pediatr* 94:823, 1979.

81. Lenko HL, Perheentupa J, Söderholm A: Growth in Turner's syndrome: Spontaneous and fluoxymesterone stimulated. *Acta Paediatr Scand (suppl)* 277:57, 1979.

82. Sybert VP: Adult height in Turner syndrome with and without androgen therapy. *J Pediatr* 104:365, 1984.

83. Lucky AW, Marynick SP, Rebar RW, Cutler GB, Glen M, Johnsonbaugh RE, Loriaux DL: Replacement oral ethinyloestradiol therapy for gonadal dysgenesis: Growth and adrenal androgen studies. *Acta Endocrinol* 91:519, 1979.

83a. Demetriou E, Emans SJ, Crigler JF Jr: Final height in estrogen-treated patients with Turner syndrome. *Obstet Gynecol* 64:459, 1984.

84. Ross JL, Cassorla FG, Skerda MC, Valk IM, Loriaux DL, Cutler GB Jr: A preliminary study of the effect of estrogen dose on growth in Turner's syndrome. *N Engl J Med* 309:1104, 1983.

84a. Pike MC, Henderson BE, Krailo MD, Duke A, Roy S: Breast cancer in young women and use of oral contraceptives: Possible modifying effect of formulation and age at use. *Lancet* 2:926, 1983.

85. Simpson JL, Blagowidow N, Martin AO: XY gonadal dysgenesis: Genetic heterogeneity based upon clinical observations, H-Y antigen status and segregation analysis. *Hum Genet* 58:91, 1981.

86. Barakat AY, Papadopoulou ZL, Chandra RS, Hollerman CE, Calcagno PL: Pseudohermaphroditism, nephron disorder and Wilms' tumor: A unifying concept. *Pediatrics* 54:366, 1974.

87. Drash A, Sherman E, Hartmann WH, Blizzard RM: A syndrome of pseudohermaphroditism, Wilms' tumor, hypertension, and degenerative renal disease. *J Pediatr* 76:585, 1970.

88. Di George AM, Harley RD: The association of aniridia, Wilms' tumor, and genital abnormalities. *Arch Ophthalmol* 75:796, 1966.

89. Cleary RE, Caras J, Rosenfield RL, Young PCM: Endocrine and metabolic studies in a patient with male pseudohermaphroditism and true agonadism. *Am J Obstet Gynecol* 128:862, 1977.

90. Parks GA, Dumars KW, Limbeck GA, Quinlivan WL, New MI: "True agonadism": A misnomer? *J Pediatr* 84:375, 1974.

91. Bergada C, Cleveland WW, Jones HW, Wilkins L: Variants of embryonic testicular dysgenesis: Bilateral anorchia and the syndrome of rudimentary testes. *Acta Endocrinol* 40:521, 1962.

92. Winter JSD, Taraska S, Faiman C: The hormonal response to hCG stimulation in male children and adolescents. *J Clin Endocrinol Metab* 34:348, 1972.

93. Josso N, Fekete C, Cachin O, Nezelof C, Rappaport R: Persistence of müllerian ducts in male pseudohermaphroditism, and its relationship to cryptorchidism. *Clin Endocrinol* 19:247, 1983.

94. Brook CGD, Wagner H, Zachmann M, Prader A, Armendares S, Frank S, Aleman P, Najjar SS, Slim MS, Genton N, Bozic C: Familial occurrence of persistent müllerian structures in otherwise normal males. *Br Med J* 1:771, 1973.

95. Berthezène F, Forest MG, Grimaud JA, Claustrat B, Mornex R: Leydig-cell agenesis: A cause of male pseudohermaphroditism. *N Engl J Med* 295:969, 1976.

96. Schwartz M, Imperato-McGinley J, Peterson RE, Cooper G, Morris PL, MacGillivray M, Hensle T: Male pseudohermaphroditism secondary to an abnormality in Leydig cell differentiation. *J Clin Endocrinol Metab* 53:123, 1981.

97. Eil C, Austin RM, Sesterhenn I, Dunn JF, Cutler GB Jr, Johnsonbaugh RE: Leydig cell hypoplasia causing male pseudohermaphroditism: Diagnosis 13 years after prepubertal castration. *J Clin Endocrinol Metab* 58:441, 1984.

98. Boyd GS, McNamara B, Suckling KE, Tocher DR: Cholesterol metabolism in the adrenal cortex. *J Steroid Biochem* 19:1017, 1983.

99. Koizumi S, Kyoya S, Mujawaki T, Kidani H, Funabashi T, Nakashima H, Nakamura Y, Ohta G, Itageki E, Katagiri M: Cholesterol side chain cleavage enzyme activity and cytochrome P_{450} content in adrenal mitochondria of a patient with congenital lipoid hyperplasia (Prader disease). *Clin Chim Acta* 77:301, 1977.

100. Kirkland RT, Kirkland JL, Johnson CM, Horning MG, Librik L, Clayton GW: Congenital lipoid adrenal hyperplasia in an eight-year-old phenotypic female. *J Clin Endocrinol Metab* 56:488, 1973.

101. Camacho AM, Kowarski A: Congenital adrenal hyperplasia due to a deficiency of one of the enzymes involved in biosynthesis of pregnenolone. *J Clin Endocrinol Metab* 28:153, 1968.

102. Cheatum SG, Douville AW, Warren JC: Site specificity of bovine adrenal 3β-hydroxysteroid dehydrogenase and Δ^5-3-ketosteroid isomerase. *Biochim Biophys Acta* 137:172, 1967.

103. Ford HC, Engel LL: Purification and properties of the Δ^5-3β-hydroxysteroid dehydrogenase-isomerase system of sheep adrenal cortical microsomes. *J Biol Chem* 249:1363, 1974.

104. Byrne GC, Perry YS, Winter JSD: Steroid inhibitory effects upon human adrenal 3β-hydroxysteroid dehydrogenase activity. *J Clin Endocrinol Metab* 62:413, 1986.

105. Bongiovanni AM: Urinary steroidal pattern of infants with congenital adrenal hyperplasia due to 3-beta-hydroxysteroid dehydrogenase deficiency. *J Steroid Biochem* 13:809, 1980.

106. Pang S, Levine LS, Stoner E, Opitz JM, Pollack MS, Dupont B, New MI: Nonsalt-losing congenital adrenal hyperplasia due to 3β-hydroxysteroid dehydrogenase deficiency with normal glomerulosa function. *J Clin Endocrinol Metab* 56:808, 1983.

107. Rosenfield RL, Rich BH, Wolfsdorf JI, Cassorla F, Parks JS, Bongiovanni AM, Wu CH, Shackleton CHL: Pubertal presentation of congenital Δ^5-3β-hydroxysteroid dehydrogenase deficiency. *J Clin Endocrinol Metab* 51:345, 1980.

108. Parks GA, Bermudez JA, Anast CS, Bongiovanni AM, New MI: Pubertal boy with the 3β-hydroxysteroid dehydrogenase defect. *J Clin Endocrinol Metab* 33:269, 1971.

109. Schneider G, Genel M, Bongiovanni AM, Goldman AS, Rosenfield RL: Persistent testicular Δ^5-isomerase-3β-hydroxysteroid dehydrogenase (Δ^5-3β-HSD) deficiency in the Δ^5-3β-HSD form of congenital adrenal hyperplasia. *J Clin Invest* 55:681, 1975.

110. Martin F, Perheentupa J, Adlercreutz H: Plasma and urinary androgens and oestrogens in a pubertal boy with 3β-hydroxysteroid dehydrogenase deficiency. *J Steroid Biochem* 13:197, 1980.

111. Bongiovanni AM: Acquired adrenal hyperplasia with special reference to 3β-hydroxysteroid dehydrogenase. *Fertil Steril* 35:599, 1981.

112. Nakajin S, Shively JE, Yuan PM, Hall PF: Microsomal cytochrome P-450 from neonatal pig testis: Two enzymatic activities (17α-hydroxylase and C17,20-lyase) associated with one protein. *Biochemistry* 20:4037, 1981.

113. Kominami S, Shinzawa K, Takemori S: Purification and some properties of cytochrome P-450 specific for steroid 17α-hydroxylation and C17—C20 bond cleavage from guinea pig adrenal microsomes. *Biochem Biophys Res Commun* 109:916, 1982.

114. Dean HJ, Shackleton CHL, Winter JSD: Diagnosis and natural history of 17-hydroxylase deficiency in a newborn male. *J Clin Endocrinol Metab* 59:513, 1984.

115. Kater CE, Biglieri EG, Brust N, Chang B, Hirai J: The unique patterns of plasma aldosterone and 18-hydroxycorticosterone concentrations in the 17β-hydroxylase deficiency syndrome. *J Clin Endocrinol Metab* 55:295, 1982.

116. Zachmann M, Vollmin JA, Hamilton W, Prader A: Steroid 17,20-desmolase deficiency: A new cause of male pseudohermaphroditism. *Clin Endocrinol* 1:369, 1972.

117. Zachmann M, Werder EA, Prader A: Two types of male pseudohermaphroditism due to 17,20-desmolase deficiency. *J Clin Endocrinol Metab* 55:487, 1982.

118. Larrea F, Lisker R, Banuelos R, Bermudez JA, Herrera J, Rasilla VN, Perez-Palacios G: Hypergonadotrophic hypogonadism in an XX female subject due to 17,20-desmolase deficiency. *Acta Endocrinol* 103:400, 1983.

119. Kaufman FR, Costin G, Goebelsmann U, Stanczyk FZ, Zachmann M: Male pseudohermaphroditism due to 17,20-desmolase deficiency. *J Clin Endocrinol Metab* 57:32, 1983.

120. Imperato-McGinley J, Peterson RE, Stoller R, Goodwin WE: Male pseudohermaphroditism secondary to 17β-hydroxysteroid dehydrogenase deficiency: Gender role change with puberty. *J Clin Endocrinol Metab* 49:391, 1979.

121. van Schakenburg K, Bidlingmaier F, Engelhardt D, Butenandt O, Unterburger P, Knorr D: 17-Ketosteroid reductase deficiency—plasma steroids and incubation studies with testicular tissue. *Acta Endocrinol* 94:397, 1980.

122. Akesode FA, Meyer WJ III, Migeon CJ: Male pseudohermaphroditism with gynecomastia due to testicular 17-ketoreductase deficiency. *Clin Endocrinol* 7:443, 1977.

123. Rosler A, Kohn G: Male pseudohermaphroditism due to 17β-hydroxysteroid dehydrogenase deficiency: Studies on the natural history of the defect and effect of androgens on gender role. *J Steroid Biochem* 19:663, 1983.

123a. King WJ, Greene GL: Monoclonal antibodies localize oestrogen receptor in the nuclei of target cells. *Nature* 307:745, 1984.

123b. Welshons WV, Lieberman ME, Gorski J: Nuclear localization of unoccupied oestrogen receptors. *Nature* 307:747, 1984.

124. Imperato-McGinley J, Peterson RE, Gautier T, Sturla E: Androgens and the evolution of male-gender identity among male pseudohermaphrodites with 5α-reductase deficiency. *N Engl J Med* 300:1233, 1979.

125. Money J, Hampson J, Hampson JL: An examination of some basic sexual concepts: The evidence of human hermaphroditism. *Bull Johns Hopkins Hosp* 97:301, 1955.

126. Cantu JM, Corona-Rivera E, Diaz M, Medina C, Esquinca E, Cortes-Gallegos V, Vaca G, Hernandez A: Post-pubertal female psychosexual orientation in incomplete male pseudohermaphroditism type 2 (5α-reductase deficiency). *Acta Endocrinol* 94:273, 1980.

127. Savage MO, Preece MA, Jeffcoate SL, Ransley PG, Rumsby G, Mansfield MD, Williams DI: Familial male pseudohermaphroditism due to deficiency of 5α-reductase. *Clin Endocrinol* 12:397, 1980.

128. Pinsky L, Kaufman M, Straisfield C, Zilahi B, Hall C St-G: 5α-Reductase activity of genital and nongenital skin fibroblasts from patients with 5α-reductase deficiency, androgen insensitivity, or unknown forms of male pseudohermaphroditism. *Am J Hum Genet* 1:407, 1978.

129. Mauvais-Jarvis P, Mowszowicz I, Kuttenn F: Significance of 5α-reductase activity in human sexual differentiation, in Serio M, Motta M, Zanisi M, Martini L (eds): *Sexual Differentiation: Basic and Clinical Aspects.* New York, Raven, 1984, pp 247–260.

130. Griffin JE, Wilson JD: The syndromes of androgen resistance. *N Engl J Med* 302:198, 1980.

131. Migeon BR, Brown TR, Axelman J, Migeon CJ: Studies of the locus for androgen receptor: Localization on the human X chromosome and evidence for homology with the Tfm locus in the mouse. *Proc Natl Acad Sci USA* 78:6339, 1981.

132. Müller J, Skakkebaek NE: Testicular carcinoma in situ testis in children with the androgen insensitivity (testicular feminization) syndrome. *Br Med J* 1:1419, 1984.

133. Faiman C, Winter JSD: The control of gonadotropin secretion in complete testicular feminization. *J Clin Endocrinol Metab* 39:631, 1974.

134. Keenan BS, Meyer WJ, Hadjian AJ, Jones HW, Migeon CJ: Syndrome of androgen insensitivity in man: Absence of 5α-dihydrotestosterone binding protein in skin fibroblasts. *J Clin Endocrinol Metab* 38:1143, 1974.

135. Risbridger GP, Khalid BAK, Warne GL, Funder JW: Differences in proteins synthesized by fibroblasts from normal individuals and patients with complete testicular feminization. *J Clin Invest* 69:99, 1982.

136. Amrhein JA, Meyer WJ III, Jones HW Jr, Migeon CJ: Androgen insensitivity in man: Evidence for genetic heterogeneity. *Proc Natl Acad Sci USA* 73:891, 1976.

137. Kaufman M, Pinsky L, Simard L, Wong SC: Defective activation of androgen-receptor complexes: A marker of androgen insensitivity. *Mol Cell Endocrinol* 25:151, 1982.

138. Griffin JE, Durrant JL: Qualitative receptor defects in families with androgen resistance: Failure of stabilization of the fibroblast cytosol androgen receptor. *J Clin Endocrinol Metab* 55:465, 1982.

139. Eil C: Familial incomplete male pseudohermaphroditism associated with impaired nuclear androgen retention. *J Clin Invest* 71:850, 1983.

140. Ozasa HT, Tominaga T, Nishimura T, Takeda T: Evidence for receptor dependent response to dihydrotestosterone in cultured human fibroblasts. *Endokrinologie* 77:129, 1981.

141. Kaufman M, Pinsky L, Feder-Hollander R: Defective upregulation of the androgen receptor in human androgen insensitivity. *Nature* 293:735, 1981.

142. Gyorki S, Warne GL, Khalid BAK, Funder JW: Defective nuclear accumulation of androgen receptors in disorders of sexual differentiation. *J Clin Invest* 72:819, 1983.

143. Amrhein JA, Klingensmith GJ, Walsh PC, McKusick VA, Migeon CJ: Partial androgen insensitivity: The Reifenstein syndrome revisited. *N Engl J Med* 297:350, 1977.

144. Warne GL, Gyorki S, Risbridger GP, Khalid BAK, Funder JW: Fibroblast studies on clinical androgen insensitivity. *J Steroid Biochem* 19:583, 1983.

145. Aiman J, Griffin JE: The frequency of androgen receptor deficiency in infertile men. *J Clin Endocrinol Metab* 54:725, 1982.

146. Aarskog D: Maternal progestins as a possible cause of hypospadias. *N Engl J Med* 300:75, 1979.

147. Mau G: Progestins during pregnancy and hypospadias. *Teratology* 24:285, 1981.

148. Gill WB, Schumacher GFB, Bibbo M: Structural and functional abnormalities in sex organs of male offspring of mothers treated with diethylstilbestrol (DES). *J Reprod Med* 16:147, 1976.

149. Henderson BE, Banton B, Cosgrove M, Baptista J, Aldrich J, Townsend D, Hart W, Mack TM: Urogenital tract abnormalities in

sons of women treated with diethylstilbestrol. *Pediatrics* 58:505, 1976.

150. Dean HJ, Winter JSD: The effect of five synthetic progestational compounds on 5α-reductase activity in genital skin fibroblast monolayers. *Steroids* 43:13, 1985.

151. Smith DW: *Recognizable Patterns of Human Malformation: Genetic, Embryologic and Clinical Aspects,* 3d ed. Philadelphia, Saunders, 1982, pp 98–111.

152. Bauer SB, Bull MJ, Retik AB: Hypospadias: A familial study. *J Urol* 121:474, 1979.

153. Svensson J, Eneroth P, Gustafsson J-A, Ritzen M, Stenberg A: Metabolism of androstenedione in skin and serum levels of gonadotrophins and androgens in prepubertal boys with hypospadias. *J Endocrinol* 76:399, 1978.

154. Raboch J, Pondelickova J, Starka L: Plasma testosterone values in hypospadias. *Andrologia* 8:255, 1976.

155. Nonomura K, Fujieda K, Sakakibara N, Terasawa K, Matsuno T, Matsuura N, Koyanagi T: Pituitary and gonadal function in prepubertal boys with hypospadias. *J Urol* 132:595, 1984.

156. Svensson J, Snochowski M: Androgen receptor levels in preputial skin from boys with hypospadias. *J Clin Endocrinol Metab* 49:340, 1979.

157. Müller J, Skakkebaek NE: Abnormal germ cells in maldescended testes: A study of cell density, nuclear size and deoxyribonucleic acid content in testicular biopsies from 50 boys. *J Urol* 131:730, 1984.

158. Prader A: Der Genitalbefund beim Pseudohermaphroditismus feminus des Kongenitalen Adenogenitalen Syndroms. *Helv Paediatr Acta* 9:231, 1954.

159. Dickerman Z, Grant DR, Faiman C, Winter JSD: Intra-adrenal steroid concentrations in man: Zonal differences and developmental changes. *J Clin Endocrinol Metab* 59:1031, 1984.

160. Hiwatashi A, Ichikawa Y: Purification and reconstitution of the steroid 21-hydroxylase system (cytochrome P_{450}-linked mixed function oxidase system) of bovine adrenocortical microsomes. *Biochim Biophys Acta* 664:33, 1981.

161. Levine LS, Zachmann M, New MI, Prader A, Pollack MS, O'Neill GJ, Yang SY, Oberfield SE, Dupont B: Genetic mapping of the 21-hydroxylase deficiency gene within the HLA linkage group. *N Engl J Med* 299:911, 1978.

162. Lejeune-Lenain C, Cantraine F, Dufrasnes M, Prevot F, Wolter R, Franckson JRM: An improved method for the detection of congenital virilizing adrenal hyperplasia. *Clin Endocrinol* 12:525, 1980.

163. New MI, Lorenzen F, Lerner AJ, Kohn B, Oberfield SE, Pollack MS, Dupont B, Stoner E, Levy DJ, Pang S, Levine LS: Genotyping steroid 21-hydroxylase deficiency: Hormonal reference data. *J Clin Endocrinol Metab* 57:320, 1980.

164. New MI, Dupont B, Grumbach K, Levine LS: Congenital adrenal hyperplasia and related conditions, in Stanbury JB, Wyngaarden JB, Frederickson DS, Goldstein JF, Brown MS (eds): *The Metabolic Basis of Inherited Disease,* 5th ed. New York, McGraw-Hill, 1982, pp 973–1000.

165. Blankstein J, Faiman C, Reyes FI, Schroeder M, Winter JSD: Adult-onset familial 21-hydroxylase deficiency. *Am J Med* 68:441, 1980.

166. Levine LS, Dupont B, Lorenzen F, Pang S, Pollack MS, Oberfield SE, Kohn K, Lerner A, Cacciari E, Mantero F, Cassio A, Scaroni C, Chiumello G, Rondanini GF, Gargantini L, Giovanelli G, Virdis R, Bartolotta E, Migliori C, Pintor C, Tato L, Barboni F, New MI: Genetic and hormonal characterization of cryptic 21-hydroxylase deficiency. *J Clin Endocrinol Metab* 53:1193, 1981.

167. Fife D, Rappaport EB: Prevalence of salt-losing among congenital adrenal hyperplasia patients. *Clin Endocrinol* 18:259, 1983.

168. Ulick S, Eberlein WR, Bliffeld AR, Chu MD, Bongiovanni AM: Evidence for an aldosterone biosynthetic defect in congenital adrenal hyperplasia. *J Clin Endocrinol Metab* 51:1346, 1980.

169. Pham-Huu-Trung MT, Raux MC, Gourmelen M, Baron MC, Girard F: Plasma aldosterone concentrations related to 17α-hydroxyprogesterone in congenital adrenal hyperplasia. *Acta Endocrinol* 82:572, 1976.

170. Kuhnle U, Chow D, Rappaport R, Pang S, Levine LS, New MI: The 21-hydroxylase activity in the glomerulosa and fasciculata of the adrenal cortex in congenital adrenal hyperplasia. *J Clin Endocrinol Metab* 52:534, 1981.

171. Osterwalder H: Die juxtaglomerulaeren Zellen beim virilisierenden kongenitalen adrenogenitalen syndrom mit und ohne Salzverlustsyndrom. *Schweiz Med Wochenschr* 101:1298, 1971.

172. Neville AM, O'Hare MJ: *The Human Adrenal Cortex.* Berlin, Springer-Verlag, 1982, p 162.

173. Schaison G, Couzinet B, Gourmelen M, Elkik F, Bougneres P: Angiotensin and adrenal steroidogenesis: Study of 21-hydroxylase-deficient congenital adrenal hyperplasia. *J Clin Endocrinol Metab* 51:1390, 1980.

174. Hughes IA, Winter JSD: The application of a serum 17OH-progesterone radioimmunoassay to the diagnosis and management of congenital adrenal hyperplasia. *J Pediatr* 88:766, 1976.

174a. Murphy JF, Joyce BG, Dyas J, Hughes IA: Plasma 17-hydroxyprogesterone concentrations in ill newborn infants. *Arch Dis Child* 58:532, 1983.

175. Hughes IA, Riad-Fahmy D, Griffiths K: Plasma 17OH-progesterone concentrations in newborn infants. *Arch Dis Child* 54:347, 1979.

176. Forest MG, Betuel H, Couillin P, Boué A, David M, Floret D, Francois R, Guibaud P, Plauchu H, Rappaport R: Prenatal diagnosis of congenital adrenal hyperplasia (CAH) due to 21-hydroxylase deficiency by steroid analysis in the amniotic fluid of mid-pregnancy: Comparison with HLA typing in 17 pregnancies at risk for CAH. *Prenatal Diagn* 1:197, 1981.

177. Hughes IA, Laurence KM: Prenatal diagnosis of congenital adrenal hyperplasia due to 21-hydroxylase deficiency by amniotic fluid steroid analysis. *Prenatal Diagn* 2:97, 1982.

178. Pang S, Murphey W, Levine LS, Spence DA, Leon A, LaFranchi S, Surve AS, New MI: A pilot newborn screening for congenital adrenal hyperplasia in Alaska. *J Clin Endocrinol Metab* 55:413, 1982.

179. Cacciari E, Balsamo A, Cassio A, Piazzi S, Bernardi F, Salardi S, Cicognani A, Pirazzoli P, Zappulla F, Capelli M, Paolini M: Neonatal screening for congenital adrenal hyperplasia. *Arch Dis Child* 58:803, 1983.

179a. Winter JSD, Couch RM: Modern medical therapy of congenital adrenal hyperplasia. A decade of experience. *Ann NY Acad Sci* 458:165, 1985.

180. Griffiths KD, Anderson JM, Rudd RT, Virdi NK, Holder G, Rayner PWH: Plasma renin activity in the management of congenital adrenal hyperplasia. *Arch Dis Child* 59:360, 1984.

181. Hughes IA, Read GF: Simultaneous plasma and saliva steroid measurements as an index of control in congenital adrenal hyperplasia: A longitudinal study. *Horm Res* 16:142, 1982.

182. Hughes IA, Winter JSD: The relationship between serum concentrations of 17OH-progesterone and other serum and urinary steroids in patients with congenital adrenal hyperplasia. *J Clin Endocrinol Metab* 46:98, 1978.

183. Hughes IA, Read GF: Menarche and subsequent ovarian function in girls with CAH. *Horm Res* 16:100, 1982.

184. Penny R, Olambiwonnu NO, Frasier SD: Precocious puberty following treatment in a six-year-old male with congenital adrenal hyperplasia: Studies of serum luteinizing hormone (LH), serum follicle-stimulating hormone (FSH) and plasma testosterone. *J Clin Endocrinol Metab* 36:920, 1973.

185. Wischusen J, Baker HWG, Hudson B: Reversible male infertility due to congenital adrenal hyperplasia. *Clin Endocrinol* 14:571, 1981.

186. Watanuki M, Tilley BE, Hall PF: Cytochrome P_{450} for 11β-

and 18-hydroxylase activities of bovine adrenocortical mitochondria: One enzyme or two? *Biochemistry* 17:127, 1978.

187. Rosler A, Leiberman E, Sack J, Landau H, Benderly A, Moses SW, Cohen T: Clinical variability of congenital adrenal hyperplasia due to 11β-hydroxylase deficiency. *Horm Res* 16:133, 1982.

188. Cathelineau G, Brerault J-L, Fiet J, Julien R, Dreux C, Canivet J: Adrenocortical 11β-hydroxylation defect in adult women with postmenarchial onset of symptoms. *J Clin Endocrinol Metab* 51:287, 1980.

189. Zadik Z, Kahana L, Kaufman H, Benderli A, Hochberg Z: Salt loss in hypertensive form of congenital adrenal hyperplasia (11β-hydroxylase deficiency). *J Clin Endocrinol Metab* 58:384, 1984.

190. Finkelstein M, Litvin Y, Mizrachi Y, Neiman G, Rosler A: Apparent double defect in C11β and C21-steroid hydroxylation in congenital adrenal hyperplasia. *J Steroid Biochem* 19:675, 1983.

191. Schumert Z, Rosenmann A, Landau H, Rosler A: 11-Deoxycortisol in amniotic fluid: Prenatal diagnosis of congenital adrenal hyperplasia due to 11β-hydroxylase deficiency. *Clin Endocrinol* 12:257, 1980.

192. Pang S, Levine LS, Lorenzen F, Chow D, Pollack M, Dupont B, Genel M, New MI: Hormonal studies in obligate heterozygotes and siblings of patients with 11β-hydroxylase deficiency congenital adrenal hyperplasia. *J Clin Endocrinol Metab* 50:586, 1980.

193. Zachmann M, Forest MG, De Peretti E: 3β-Hydroxysteroid dehydrogenase deficiency: Followup study in a girl with pubertal bone age. *Horm Res* 11:292, 1979.

194. Ishizuka N, Kawashima Y, Nakanishi T, Sugawa T, Nishikawa Y: Statistical observations on genital anomalies of newborns following the administration of progestin to their mothers. *Obstet Gynecol Surv* 19:496, 1964.

195. Lynch A, Mychalkiw W, Hutt SJ: Parental progesterone: I. Its effect on development and on intellectual and academic achievement. *Early Hum Dev* 2:305, 1978.

196. Carpentier PJ, Potter EL: Nuclear sex and genital malformations in 48 cases of renal agenesis, with special reference to nonspecific female pseudohermaphroditism. *Am J Obstet Gynecol* 78:235, 1959.

197. Franks RC, Northcutt R: Female pseudohermaphroditism and renal anomalies. *Am J Dis Child* 105:490, 1963.

198. Winter JSD, Kohn G, Mellman WJ, Wagner S: A familial syndrome of renal, genital, and middle ear anomalies. *J Pediatr* 72:88, 1968.

199. Kenny FM, Fetterman GH, Preeyasombat C: Neurofibromata simulating a penis and labioscrotal gonads in a girl with von Recklinghausen's disease. *Pediatrics* 37:456, 1966.

200. Josso N, Fortier-Beaulieu M, Faure C: Genitography in intersexual states: A review of 86 cases, with new criteria for the study of the uro-genital sinus. *Acta Endocrinol* 62:165, 1969.

201. Birnholz JC: Determination of fetal sex. *N Engl J Med* 309:942, 1983.

PART VI

FUEL METABOLISM

19

The Endocrine Pancreas: Diabetes Mellitus

Eleazar Shafrir
Michael Bergman
Philip Felig

The histologic identification by Paul Langerhans in 1869 of the islet cells which constitute the endocrine portion of the pancreas preceded by 20 years the classic studies of Minkowski and Von Mering, which demonstrated that pancreatectomy results in diabetes. Fifty-two years later the discovery of insulin as the internal secretion of the pancreas by Banting and Best heralded a new era in the treatment of diabetes. The significance of insulin secretion and action with respect to human disease is underscored by the ranking of diabetes mellitus as the third leading cause of death and the leading cause of blindness in the United States, and its elevation of the risk of coronary artery disease fourfold or more.[1] The role of diabetes in early mortality varies with the level of development in different parts of the world; in most countries it ranks between fourth and eighth as a cause of death.[2]

The islets of Langerhans consist of ~2 million clusters of pale-appearing cells dispersed among the pancreatic acinar cells which comprise <2 percent of the total pancreatic volume. On the basis of histochemical, ultrastructural, and immunofluorescent techniques, as well as identification of their hormonal secretory products, the islets cells are recognized as consisting of three distinct cell types (Table 19-1): *alpha* cells, which produce glucagon; *beta* cells, which produce insulin; and *delta* (or $alpha_2$) cells, which are the cells of origin of gastrin and somatostatin. All three cell types contain cytoplasmic granules within membrane-bound vesicles. The beta cells may be identified by their positive staining with aldehyde fuchsin and lack of staining with silver nitrate by the Hillman-Hellerstrom procedure. Both the alpha and delta cells fail to stain with aldehyde fuchsin, but the latter are argyrophilic with the silver nitrate method.[3] The granules in the alpha cells display an electron-dense core with a paler periphery; the beta cells show crystalloid pleomorphic granules, while the delta cells contain less-dense, uniform-appearing granules which extend to the limiting membrane of the vesicle (Fig. 19-1). The various islet cells are believed to arise from the neural crest; along with other secretory cells (e.g., anterior pituitary cells, adrenal medullary cells, thyroid parafollicular cells), they belong to a family of cells designated the APUD (amine precursor uptake and decarboxylation) series.[4]

Of the various disease states associated with abnormalities of the endocrine pancreas, diabetes mellitus, a disorder characterized by an absolute or relative lack of insulin, is by far the most common; it is the basis of this chapter. Abnormalities in the secretion of glucagon are frequently observed as a secondary phenomenon in diabetes and in very rare instances (e.g., the glucagonoma syndrome) may be the primary factor responsible for disturbances in metabolism. They, too, are discussed below. The consequences of excess gastrin secretion are covered in Chap. 26. The clinical syndromes associated with insulin-producing beta cell tumors are discussed in Chap. 20.

PHYSIOLOGY OF FUEL METABOLISM

Diabetes mellitus is characterized by changes in the metabolism of each of the major body fuels (carbohydrate, fat, and protein) and is associated with primary or secondary disturbances in the secretion of and/or sensitivity to a variety of hormones (insulin, glucagon, catecholamines, growth hormone (GH), and cortisol). The normal physiology of these substrates and hormones is therefore considered here.

Table 19-1. Characteristics of Pancreatic Islet Cell Types

Cell type and percentage of total	Hormone secreted	Staining characteristics	EM* appearance of secretory granules
Alpha (15%)	Glucagon		Dense core, pale periphery
Beta (65%)	Insulin	Aldehyde function	Crystalloid, pleomorphic
Delta (20%)	Gastrin, somatostatin	Silver nitrate	Homogeneous, low density, fill membrane

*EM, electron microscopic

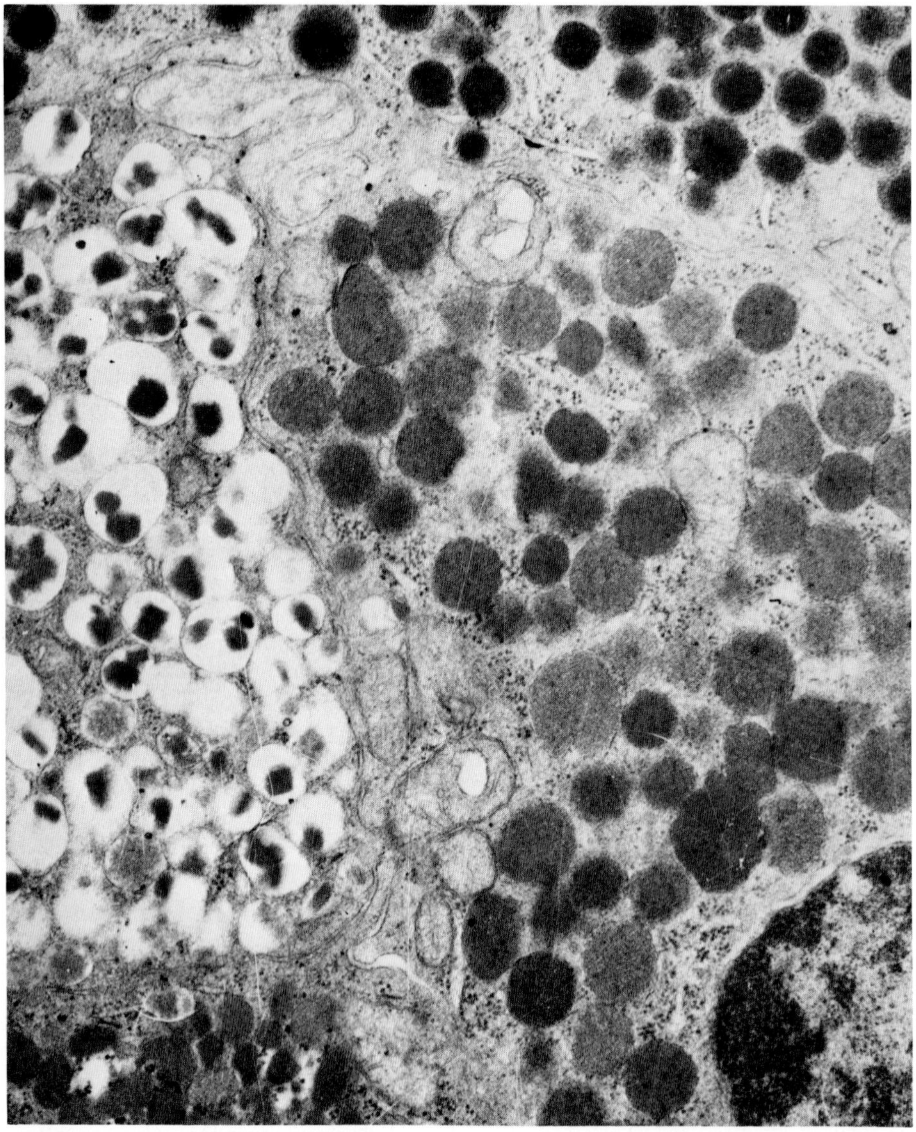

FIGURE 19-1 Electron micrograph of portion of normal human islet showing alpha, beta, and delta cells. In the alpha cell (upper right), the secretory granules show a dense core and pale periphery. In the beta cells (left), there are pleomorphic granules with a crystalloid matrix. In the delta cell (center), the secretory granules are homogeneous and fill the vesicles. Also shown is a delta cell with granules, believed to be gastrin, which are comparable to those observed in patients with ulcerogenic islet cell tumors.

Carbohydrate Metabolism

Carbohydrates are molecules of three or more carbon atoms combined with hydrogen and oxygen in a proportion of two hydrogen atoms per oxygen atom, or simple derivatives of these basic molecules. Most Americans and Europeans obtain 40 to 45 percent of their dietary calories in the form of carbohydrate. Despite the diversity of forms and sources of dietary carbohydrate, the end products of digestion which are absorbed in the intestine are the hexoses glucose, fructose, and galactose. Of these simple sugars, glucose is by far the largest constituent.

Little if any free glucose is present as such inside cells, since glucose taken up by tissues undergoes rapid metabolic transformation (Fig. 19-2). The major fates of glucose after it enters the cells are (1) intermediate storage as glycogen; (2) anaerobic metabolism via the glycolytic pathway to pyruvate and lactate; (3) continued aerobic oxidation in the main energy-yielding pathway, the tricarboxylic acid (TCA, or Krebs) cycle; (4) conversion to fatty acids (*lipogenesis*) and storage as triglyceride; and (5) to a small extent, oxidation via the pentose pathway.

Regardless of its ultimate metabolic fate, the first intracellular reaction involving glucose is phosphorylation to glucose-6-phosphate (G6P) (Fig. 19-2). In the liver this reaction is controlled by two different enzymes, *hexokinase* and *glucokinase*. The former, which is not specific, in that it can accept other hexoses as well as glucose, has a K_m of 10^{-5} M, indicating that the enzyme is half-saturated at a glucose concentration of only 0.18 mg/dl. In contrast, glucokinase, which is about four times as active in catalyzing phosphorylation of glucose as fructose, has a K_m of 10^{-2} M, so that it is half-saturated only when the ambient glucose concentration has risen to 180 mg/dl (10 mM). The difference in K_m between the two enzymes is critical, since hexokinase always functions at saturation, whereas the degree of saturation of glucokinase increases with postprandial increments of plasma glucose concentration. Hexokinase is a constitutive enzyme; its activity is quite stable under varying physiologic conditions and is little affected by endocrine influences. In contrast, glucokinase is an inducible enzyme under the control of insulin; its activity declines with fasting or in insulin-deficient diabetes and rises on refeeding or insulin administration. In muscle and adipose tissue, into which glucose entry is insulin-dependent, only low-K_m hexokinases are present. In these tissues, the rate-limiting step in the metabolism of glucose (regardless of its ultimate fate) is the transport of glucose into the cell.

GLYCOGENESIS AND GLYCOGENOLYSIS

Carbohydrate is stored inside cells in the form of *glycogen*, a branched, treelike, high-molecular-weight polysaccharide composed of glucose units linked in 1,4 bonds, with branch points of 1,6 glucosidic linkage (Fig. 19-3). The addition of glucosyl residues in 1,4 linkage constitutes the rate-limiting step in glycogen synthesis; it requires, as a primer, a polysaccharide chain of at least four glucose residues. The reaction

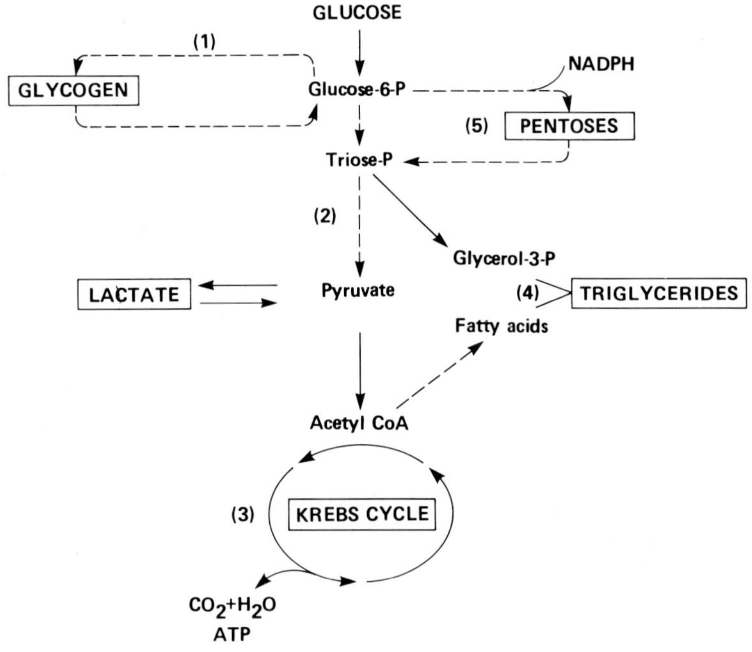

FIGURE 19-2 The major metabolic fates of glucose in humans. For delineation of the pathways, see text above.

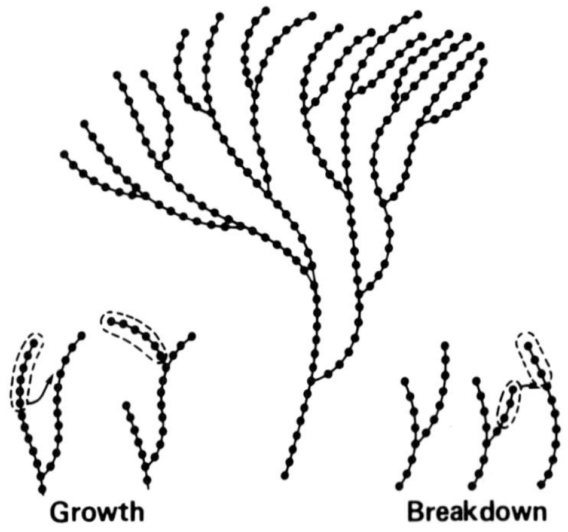

FIGURE 19-3 Part of an idealized glycogen particle represented as a continually branching tree without a main stem. Glucose residues (-●-) are linked in 1:4 glycosidic bonds; branches are attached by 1:6 bonds. The ratio of 1:4 to 1:6 bonds varies from 12 to 18 *Growth*: *Glycogen synthase* successively transfers glucose residues from uridine diphosphate glucose (UDPG) to the outer branches of glycogen; a preexisting small glycogen particle is obligatory to prime the reaction. When the chain length reaches 10 to 12 residues a group of 6 residues is transferred to a neighboring shorter chain to allow further elongation to take place. This is carried out by a "branching" enzyme, *amylo-1,4→1,6-transglucosidase* forming a 1:6 bond (*left*). Glycogen may attain a mass of 10^7 daltons in muscle and as much as 10^9 daltons in the liver. *Breakdown*: Phosphorylase degrades the 1:4 bonds on the outer branches of the glycogen particle, yielding glucose 1-phosphate, down to four glucose residues proximate to the 1:6 bonds. At this stage *α-1,4-α-1,4-glucan transferase* translocates the three-glucose segment to a neighboring chain, exposing the 1:6 bond to the "debranching" enzyme *amylo-1,6-glucosidase* (*right*). This is a specific hydrolytic cleavage yielding glucose, so that altogether up to 8 percent of the glycogen particle may be released as free glucose. The phosphorolysis of the branch may proceed after the removal of the 1:6 glucose stub.

depends on the activity of the enzyme *glycogen synthase*, which exists in two rapidly interconvertible forms, an active and an inactive one (Fig. 19-4). Phosphorylation of glycogen synthase inactivates this enzyme; activation is associated with loss of phosphate groups, which is effected enzymatically by *phosphoprotein phosphatase 1*. This enzyme appears to be controlled by insulin by a not yet completely understood mechanism. By virtue of the influence of phosphorylation, the activity of glycogen synthase is inversely related to the intracellular level of cyclic adenosine 3′,5′-monophosphate (cAMP), which promotes phosphorylation of proteins by activating protein kinases. The tissue levels of cAMP may be influenced by glucose-regulatory hormones: cAMP concentration is increased by glucagon and epinephrine; such hormonally induced increases are reversed by insulin. The activity of glycogen synthase therefore constitutes an important regulatory step in the hepatic disposal of glucose.

In addition to changes in glycogen synthase activity which are primarily hormonally mediated (via insulin or counterregulatory hormones), direct substrate control may also be possible. Hers[5] has advanced the thesis that an increase in cellular glucose concentration can of itself increase glycogen synthase activity. Support for such an action of glucose (in the presence of permissive concentrations of insulin) derives from studies involving the perfused liver in which increments in glucose concentration of ~50 mg/dl (2.8 mM) result in net uptake of glucose by the liver in the absence of changes in insulin concentration. In addition, in vivo studies in humans demonstrate that marked hyperinsulinemia in the absence of hyper-

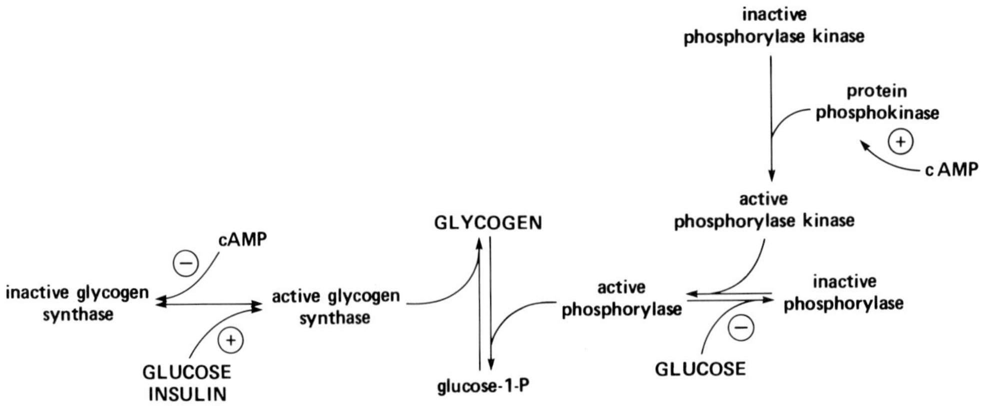

FIGURE 19-4 Regulation of glycogen synthesis and breakdown. Glycogen formation requires the activation of *glycogen synthase* and inactivation of *glycogen phosphorylase*. These processes are stimulated by glucose and/or insulin. Glycogen breakdown requires activition of phosphorylase and inactivation of synthase. These processes are regulated in a reciprocal fashion by a fall in insulin concentration and by increased concentrations of glucagon and epinephrine which act via a cAMP–protein kinase mechanism.

glycemia results in an inhibition of glucose production, but causes only minimal net hepatic glucose consumption. However, concurrent hyperglycemia augments net hepatic uptake of glucose.[6] As discussed below, the levels of both glucose and glucoregulatory hormones determine net glucose balance across the liver.

The initial step in the breakdown of glycogen involves the removal of glucose residues from the terminal 1,4 linkages by the action of *phosphorylase,* which splits off the glucose bond, inserting a phosphate at C-1 and releasing glucose 1-phosphate. Phosphorylase likewise exists in an inactive form which must be activated. However, in this case, phosphorylation of the enzyme by *phosphorylase kinase (ATP)* (Fig. 19-4) activates rather than inhibits the enzyme. Phosphorylase kinase is activated by cAMP, which in turn is formed from ATP by the action of the membrane-associated enzyme *adenyl cyclase.* Stimulation of *adenyl cyclase* is a primary factor in expressing the effect of many hormones. In this instance the classic phosphorylation cascade leading to the activation of phosphorylase is triggered by epinephrine or glucagon through β-adrenergic receptors. It should be noted, however, that epinephrine-mediated stimulation of glycogenolysis may also occur via α-adrenergic mechanisms, independent of changes in concentration of cAMP.[7,7a] In addition, the activities of phosphorylase and glycogen synthase can be influenced by alterations of the circulating glucose concentration independent of changes in the levels of hormones or cAMP.[5] Furthermore, in humans, so long as basal insulin concentrations are present a rise in plasma glucose concentration of itself inhibits glycogenolysis, presumably via a decrease in the activity of phosphorylase.[8]

The glucose-1-phosphate released from glycogen is converted by the action of the freely reversible, bidirectional enzyme *phosphoglucomutase* to G6P, which may then enter the glycolytic pathway (see below) or be converted to free glucose. The latter reaction is catalyzed by the regulatory unidirectional enzyme G6Pase, which is present in liver but not in muscle. As a result, stimulation of glycogenolysis in muscle tissue results in the release of lactate and pyruvate as the end products of glycolysis, since the G6P formed in glycogenolysis cannot be converted to free glucose but enters the glycolytic pathway.

GLYCOLYSIS

The anaerobic catabolism of glucose to pyruvate and lactate is termed *glycolysis.* This catabolic pathway, with its enzymes and intermediate metabolites, was the first to be elucidated; it has been referred to as the *Embden-Meyerhof* pathway. By this pathway, the energy of glucose is made available for cellular processes in the form of high-energy phosphate bonds in ATP; the mechanism involves oxidation-reduction reactions which may occur in the absence of oxygen. Under such anaerobic circumstances the end product of glycolysis is lactate. In aerobic conditions pyruvate, following conversion to acetyl CoA, enters the TCA cycle and is oxidized to CO_2 (Fig. 19-5). The enzymes involved in glycolysis are located within the cytoplasm and are present in virtually all cells throughout the body. However, glycolysis is quantitatively a major route of glucose utilization in only specific cell types: (1) brain, which has limited access to substrates which do not cross the blood-brain barrier; (2) red blood cells, which lack the aerobic oxidative pathway; (3) skeletal muscle, particularly during vigorous exercise; and (4) heart muscle during circumstances of impaired perfusion (e.g., coronary artery disease). The overall glycolytic catabolism of glucose involves three simultaneously coordinated processes: (1) breakdown via a series of enzymatic steps of the six-carbon skeleton of glucose, an aldehyde, to two molecules of a three-carbon acid, pyruvic acid (or pyruvate), in equilibrium with lactic acid (or lactate); (2) transfer of energy by the net resynthesis of two molecules of ATP; and (3) transfer of electrons via a sequence of oxidation-reduction reactions, resulting in a major ATP gain.

Of the 11 enzymatic steps involved in the conversion of glucose to lactate, only three are thermodynamically irreversible, nonequilibrium reactions and constitute regulatory points: the reactions catalyzed by (1) hexokinase or glucokinase, (2) phosphofructokinase, and (3) pyruvate kinase, which catalyzes the formation of pyruvate from phospho*enol*pyruvate (Fig. 19-5). The hexokinase/glucokinase reaction and its regulation was discussed above. A key position in glycolysis is the step at which 6-phosphofructo-1-kinase (PFK-1) catalyzes conversion of fructose-6-phosphate (F6P) to fructose-1,6-bis(dihydrogen phosphate) (fructose-1,6-diphosphate, $F1,6P_2$).[5a,9,10] A recently discovered enzyme, 6-phosphofructo-2-kinase (PFK-2), tightly associated with this step, converts F6P to fructose-2,6-diphosphate ($F2,6P_2$), which is not a metabolic intermediate but a prominent intracellular regulator. In circumstances of glucose abundance (e.g., during carbohydrate alimentation), F6P acts both as a substrate and activator of PFK-2; the product of its action, $F2,6P_2$, acts in turn as a potent allosteric effector of PFK-1 activity (Fig. 19-5).

The case of PFK-1 illustrates an important regulatory principle: a nonequilibrium, unidirectional reaction, conditioned to magnify the flow of metabolites in one direction, is coincidently reinforced by a reciprocal effect curtailing the flow in the opposite direction. This is accomplished by the same PFK-1 effector,

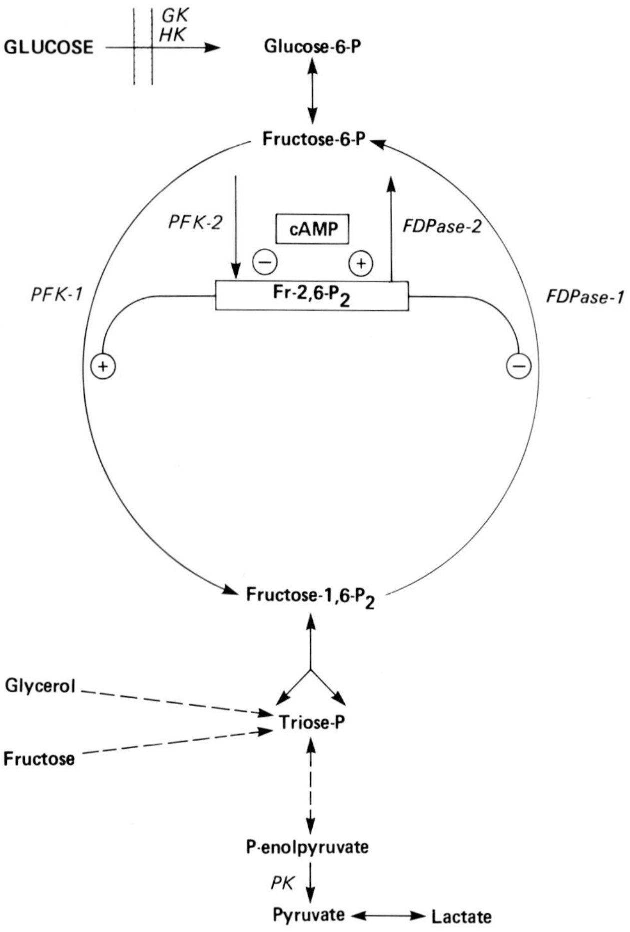

FIGURE 19-5 Regulatory steps in glycolysis stressing the nonequilibrium sites of *glucokinase* + *hexokinase* (GK+HK), *6-phosphofructo-1-kinase* (PFK-1) and *fructose 1,6-diphosphatase* (FDPase-1), and *pyruvate kinase* (PK). For the mechanisms of inhibition and activation of *PFK-1* and FDPase-1 by the regulatory activities of *PFK-2*, *FDPase-2* and fructose 2,6-diphosphate (F-2,6-P_2) see text.

F2,6P_2, which inhibits the activity of fructose 1,6-diphosphatase (FDPase-1) by allosterically raising its K_m for the substrate F1,6P_2. In this way, not only is efficient glycolysis secured, but the waste of ATP by cycling between F1,6P_2 and F6P is kept to a minimum. The potential for such "futile" cycling is not fortuitous; its existence provides a mechanism for rapidly switching, influenced by proximate cellular effectors, into a reverse direction whenever a physiologic need for glucose production arises.

PFK-2 is a unique bifunctional enzyme acting also as FDPase-2, which catalyzes the conversion of F2,6P_2 to F6P. Both activities are located on the same protein molecule and their expression is regulated by cAMP-dependent protein phosphorylation (and modulated by F6P concentration). The phosphorylated enzyme performs as FDPase-2; the dephosphorylated enzyme performs as PFK-2. Thus, the expression and the direction of orientation of this regulatory enzyme is under control of hormones affecting the cellular cAMP content (insulin, epinephrine, and glucagon).

PFK-1 activity is also susceptible to modulation by other intracellular substances such as citrate, ATP, and AMP. Citrate is a potent inhibitor, but this inhibition is not always relevant. It does not occur in the liver, where citrate concentration rises during glycolysis on the route to fatty acid synthesis. It may be pertinent in muscle, where the concentration of citrate rises in diabetes and starvation. In the latter condition, PFK-1 inhibition contributes to glucose sparing by muscles. ATP inhibits PFK-1 and AMP activates it; the converse is true of FDPase-1. Activation of PFK-1 by AMP is aimed to augment glycolysis whenever needed. Since ATP is in equilibrium with AMP (ATP + AMP $\rightleftharpoons$ 2ADP) and the cellular concentration of ATP greatly exceeds that of AMP (by about 50:1), a decrease even in a small fraction of ATP results in a large relative increase in AMP content. This represents an amplification of the signal for enhancement of glycolysis and consequent ATP replenishment through nonhormonal PFK-1 activation. This is of special importance in anoxia and exercise, where a sudden decrease in ATP concentration triggers a corrective, AMP-mediated burst in glycolysis.

Pyruvate kinase is an enzyme with two mechanisms of regulatory adjustment. One form of control is rapid: alterations in activity are effected by protein phosphorylation/dephosphorylation or conformational changes;[10,11] the latter include both feed-forward activation by F1,6P_2, which accumulates during brisk glycolysis as a result of enhanced PFK-1 activity, and inhibition by alanine released from muscles on fasting. The second aspect effects long-term regulation; it involves the acceleration of enzyme protein transcription. Insulin and diets rich in carbohydrate have distinct effects on this adaptive rise in enzyme level; in contrast, diabetes and starvation cause its decline. Pyruvate kinase is an enzyme with high activity, one of the highest among the 11 enzymes of glycolysis; it might thus appear to be unsuitable for control of glycolytic flow. While its activation may be superfluous for the accommodation of the maximal rate of glycolysis dictated by glucokinase and PFK-1, it seems of value for the control of the glycolytic metabolism of other substrates, such as fructose, a hexose which enters the pathway below the PFK-1 step. The enzyme responsible for phosphorylation of fructose to fructose-1-phosphate, *fructokinase,* has a capacity several times higher than that of glucokinase and hexokinase combined.[12]

Control of pyruvate kinase is particularly important when a reversal of the metabolite flow toward glucose production is required (see Gluconeogenesis, below). To limit the wasteful breakdown of newly synthesized phospho*enol*pyruvate on its way to glucose, pyruvate kinase activity has to be severely restrained. cAMP-dependent phosphorylation, promoted by lack of insulin, and/or glucagon excess greatly reduces the enzyme's activity, as does allosteric inhibition by alanine and other amino acids when they become abundant during the need for gluconeogenesis.

The final step in glycolysis is the conversion of pyruvate to lactate by the enzyme *lactate dehydrogenase.* In this reductive reaction, NADH formed earlier in glycolysis (by the oxidation of glyceraldehyde 3-phosphate to 3-phosphoglycerate) is reconverted to NAD^+. The equilibrium of this reaction favors the formation of lactate, particularly in muscles and brain. The importance of this reaction is that it permits the continued breakdown of glucose by providing NAD^+ at this critical site, at the expense of lactate formation. The lactate formed in glycolysis diffuses freely from cells and enters the bloodstream, from which it is removed mainly by the liver.

GLUCONEOGENESIS

Gluconeogenesis refers to the formation of glucose from noncarbohydrate sources. The principal precursor substrates from which glucose may be derived are pyruvate, lactate, glycerol, and amino acids. Most of the constituent amino acids in tissue proteins (except the "ketogenic" amino acids, leucine, isoleucine, and valine) can ultimately be converted to glucose. However, the pattern of amino acid uptake by the liver is such that alanine is the major gluconeogenic substrate released from peripheral protein reservoirs. Conversion of even-chain fatty acids (accounting for >95 percent of total fatty acid content) to glucose is not possible in mammalian liver, because there is no mechanism for net glucose synthesis from their final two-carbon oxidation product, acetyl CoA. A precursor for glucose must contain at least a three-carbon chain. When odd-chain fatty acids are oxidized, the final product, propionyl CoA, may serve as a glucogenic substrate by conversion to methylmalonyl CoA and succinyl CoA. Recently, a metabolic pathway has been uncovered which can use another three-carbon product of incomplete fatty acid oxidation, acetone, and convert it to lactate and glucose (see below).

With the exception of glycerol, each of the gluconeogenic precursors must be converted to pyruvate and/or oxaloacetate prior to the formation of glucose. The enzymatic steps involved in the formation of glucose from pyruvate differ from those involved in glycolysis, since they must bypass in the opposite direction the three irreversible steps of glycolysis, outlined in Fig. 19-5. They involve (1) the synthesis of phospho*enol*pyruvate from pyruvate by the enzymes *pyruvate carboxylase* (PC) and *phospho*enol*pyruvate carboxykinase* (PEPCK), (2) dephosphorylation of F1,6P_2 to F6P by FDPase-1, and (3) dephosphorylation of glucose 6-phosphate to glucose by *glucose-6-phosphatase* (G6Pase) (Fig. 19-6). These enzymes are unique to gluconeogenesis and are present in liver, kidney, and intestinal epithelium but not in muscle or heart. Quantitatively, the liver is the most important site of gluconeogenesis in physiologic circumstances such as fasting and exercise, and in pathologic conditions such as diabetes. The kidney becomes an important gluconeogenic organ during prolonged starvation.[13]

The moment-to-moment regulation of gluconeogenesis depends on substrate availability, enzyme activity, and the hormonal milieu. In the postabsorptive state (e.g., overnight fast) and during short-term starvation, a reduction in serum insulin concentration enhances protein breakdown and amino acid mobilization, providing a supply of glucose precursors. However, as starvation continues for prolonged periods,

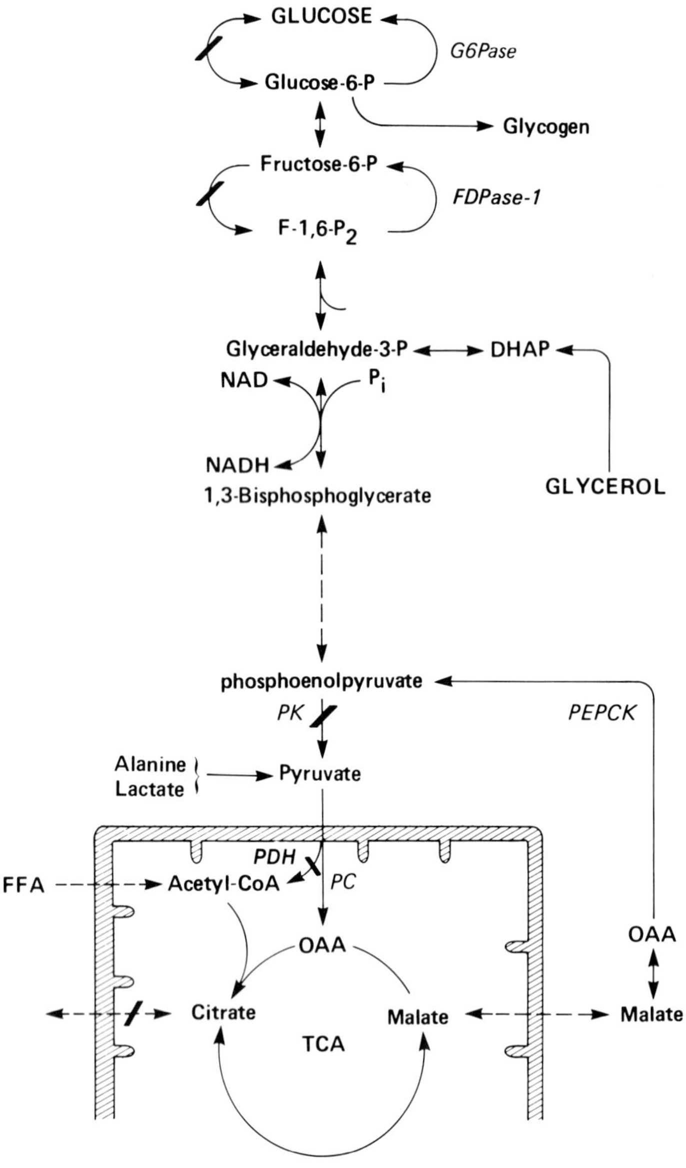

FIGURE 19-6 Regulatory steps in hepatic gluconeogenesis under the conditions of fasting and insulin deficiency. Pyruvate, mainly derived from extrahepatic lactate and alanine, enters the mitochondria to be carboxylated to oxaloacetate (OAA) by *pyruvate carboxylase* (PC) rather than converted to acetyl CoA by *pyruvate dehydrogenase* (PDH). The increased hepatic concentration of acetyl CoA, arising from large FFA inflow, is instrumental in this change (see text). Citrate is formed from the OAA in the tricarboxylic acid cycle (TCA); however, its transport into the cytosol is reduced in this condition. On the other hand, most of the OAA is exported, via malate, into the cytosol and converted to phospho*enol*pyruvate by *phosphoenolpyruvate carboxykinase* (PEPCK) bypassing the *pyruvate kinase* (PK) reaction, which is strongly inhibited in this situation by alanine and cAMP-dependent protein phosphorylation. A further step on the route to glucose involves *phosphoglycerate kinase*. The direction of action of this enzyme is determined by the NADH/NAD^+ ratio, which in this situation favors glyceraldehyde 3-phosphate production due to ample supply of NADH from increased fatty acid oxidation. Glycerol, derived from the enhanced lipolysis of adipose tissue triglycerides, joins the pathway of gluconeogenesis at this point, following phosphorylation by *glycerokinase* and oxidation to dihydroxyacetone phosphate (DHAP) by *glycerophosphate dehydrogenase*. The next regulatory points include the cleavage of $F1,6P_2$ by *FDPase-1* (see Fig. 19-5) and the final phosphorolysis of glucose 6-phosphate to free glucose by the microsomal *glucose 6-phosphatase* (G6Pase).

availability of precursor substrates becomes the rate-limiting process, as peripheral release of alanine is markedly reduced.[14]

Starvation as well as diabetes is characterized by massive mobilization of free fatty acids (FFA) from adipose tissue; these serve as a major oxidative substrate in the liver. As a consequence, the hepatic acetyl CoA concentration is markedly elevated while that of free coenzyme A is commensurately reduced. This change profoundly affects the activity of the two enzymes for which pyruvate is the substrate: *pyruvate dehydrogenase* (PDH) and PC. PDH is prevented from converting pyruvate to acetyl CoA by scarcity of CoA and is inhibited by acetyl CoA. Conversely, PC is allosterically activated by acetyl CoA. Thus, pyruvate is preferentially channeled to oxaloacetate (Fig. 19-6).

These initial reactions related to gluconeogenesis occur in the mitochondria. The next step, entailing the combined decarboxylation and phosphorylation of oxaloacetate to phospho*enol*pyruvate, is carried out by PEPCK in the cytosol. Oxaloacetate does not readily cross the mitochondrial membrane; it is transported out via malate. Regulation of PEPCK activity is effected mainly by transcriptional changes in the synthesis of this enzyme, which has a rapid turnover rate.[15,16] Insulin deficiency in starvation or diabetes results in marked enzyme induction, whereas ingestion of a diet plentiful in carbohydrate or administration of insulin reduces the synthesis of PEPCK. Insulin swiftly suppresses the synthesis of the enzyme protein, probably at the point of transcription initiation. The concentration of cAMP, which rises under glucagon stimulation or when glucose is in short supply, also has a strong promoting effect on PEPCK activity, not by protein kinase–mediated phosphorylation of the enzyme but by interfering with its synthesis at the mRNA level. PEPCK is also induced by glucocorticoid and thyroid hormones. These hormones also promote gluconeogenesis through their catabolic effects on tissue proteins, thereby increasing the availability of gluconeogenic amino acid precursors. The PEPCK is the rate-limiting reaction of gluconeogenesis; the subsequent regulatory point on the pathway toward glucose, at FDPase-1, was discussed above.

G6Pase controls the last step before glucose is released into the circulation. This enzyme is insoluble; it is linked to the endoplasmic reticulum. Its activity is determined by membrane translocation, giving it increased access to substrate within the cytosol, as well as by protein synthesis induction, abetted by insulin deficiency or glucocorticoid excess.

INTEGRATION OF GLYCOLYSIS AND GLUCONEOGENESIS: THE LACTATE (CORI) AND ALANINE CYCLES

While within a given tissue, such as the liver, the net movement of carbon atoms is in the direction of either glycolysis or gluconeogenesis, in the organism as a whole both glycolysis and gluconeogenesis generally proceed simultaneously, albeit in different tissues. Net glucogenic activity begins in the liver approximately 3 h after ingestion of a carbohydrate-containing meal and continues as long as food is withheld. On the other hand, lactate is continuously produced by the formed elements of the blood, resting muscle, and, to a much larger extent, exercising muscle. The combined activity of gluconeogenesis and glycolysis results in a cycling of carbon skeletons as glucose and lactate between liver and muscle known as the *Cori cycle* (Fig. 19-7). Glucose is released by the liver into the bloodstream and is taken up by muscle tissue. Within muscle the glucose undergoes glycolysis, and its carbon skeleton is released to the bloodstream as lactate and pyruvate.

Lactate is a means for the release of unused pyruvate, the end point of glycolysis, in tissues in which the oxidative capacity of the TCA cycle is lower than that of glycolysis. Alanine, produced by amination of pyruvate by *alanine aminotransferase,* is another end product of glycolysis released from muscles (the

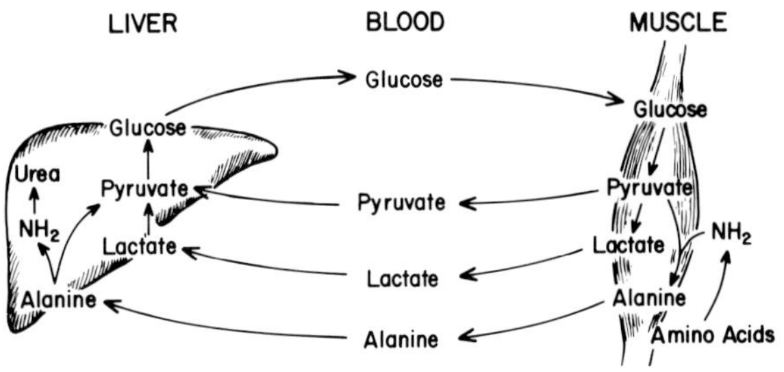

FIGURE 19-7 The lactate-glucose (Cori) and alanine-glucose cycles. In both cycles glucose is taken up by muscle and converted to pyruvate and lactate. Some of the pyruvate undergoes transamination in muscle to form alanine. The glucose-derived lactate and alanine are released into the bloodstream and taken up by the liver, where they are reconverted to glucose.

glucose-alanine cycle[14] is further discussed under Amino Acid Metabolism, below). The liver extracts lactate, pyruvate, and alanine from the blood and, by the process of gluconeogenesis, reconverts these substrates to glucose and glycogen. The recycling of carbon skeletons between lactate and glucose has been estimated to account for 20 percent of the total turnover of each of these substrates.[14]

The Cori cycle does not appear to result in the net production of new glucose, although lactate may substantially contribute to hepatic glycogen repletion even in the early postprandial state, when glucose becomes available. It does, however, provide a means whereby the end products of glycolysis may reenter the anabolic pathway rather than accumulate within the bloodstream or undergo further oxidation. Furthermore, the Cori cycle permits redistribution of glycogen stores from resting to exercised muscle in the recovery period after prolonged exercise.[17]

Despite the rapid turnover of glucose via the Cori and alanine cycles, the circulating levels of lactate are normally <1 mM. However, lactate accumulation occurs in circumstances of increased anaerobic glycolysis whether due to physiologic (e.g., exercise) or pathologic stimuli (e.g., cardiovascular collapse due to hypovolemia, sepsis, or cardiogenic shock). Lactate also accumulates when the Cori cycle is interfered with by substances which suppress gluconeogenesis from pyruvate, such as ethanol. The antigluconeogenic effect of ethanol derives from a marked increase in the $NADH/NAD^+$ ratio incident to the metabolism of ethanol by the enzyme alcohol dehydrogenase. As a result of excessive accumulation of NADH, conversion of lactate to pyruvate is inhibited. Furthermore, the pyruvate formed from alanine is also rapidly sequestered as lactate and becomes unavailable for gluconeogenesis. In contrast, gluconeogenesis from glycerol or fructose, both of which enter the gluconeogenic pathway at the triose phosphate level (Fig. 19-4), is not inhibited by ethanol.

Gluconeogenesis is not the sole metabolic fate of lactate released into the bloodstream. Within the liver and, to a much larger extent, heart and kidneys, lactate undergoes oxidation to CO_2; it is also a good substrate for fatty acid synthesis in the liver.

TRICARBOXYLIC ACID CYCLE

The enzymatic process whereby aerobic tissues utilize oxygen and produce CO_2 (i.e., undergo cellular respiration) is the TCA or Krebs cycle (Fig. 19-8). This sequence of metabolic conversions represents the final common pathway of aerobic oxidation and CO_2 formation for all substrates, carbohydrates, fatty acids, and amino acids. The enzymes catalyzing the TCA cycle are located within the mitochondria. Within those organelles they are in close association with the respiratory chain, a sequence of proteins which permits the energy liberated in the oxidation reactions of the TCA cycle products to be coupled with the formation of ATP, e.g., the process of oxidative phosphorylation. The TCA cycle thus is quantitatively the most important pathway for generation of the energy inherent in various metabolic fuels.

The reaction linking the glycolytic pathway with the TCA cycle is the oxidative decarboxylation of pyruvate to acetate and condensation of the latter with CoA to form acetyl CoA. This process is catalyzed by PDH. PDH is inhibited in the presence of high concentrations of ATP; in contrast, when the ATP level is reduced, the oxidation of pyruvate is accelerated. PDH activity is also regulated by phos-

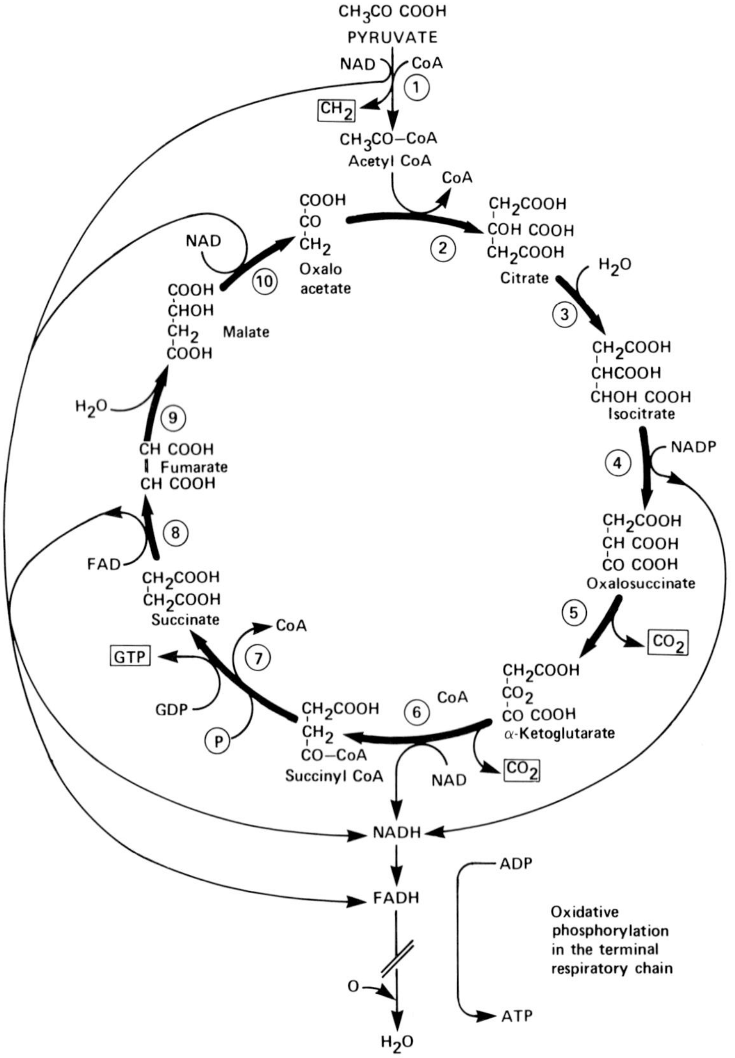

FIGURE 19-8 Enzymatic steps within the tricarboxylic acid cycle leading to NADH and FADH formation, which are oxidized along the tightly linked respiratory chain, coupled to phosphorylation of ADP. For each atom of oxygen consumed in oxidation of NADH 3 mol of ATP are obtained. Oxidation of FADH results in 2 mol of ATP, since it starts at a second phosphorylation site. Overall, one turn of the cycle oxidizing a pyruvate molecule produces 15 high-energy phosphate bonds, whereas glycolysis to pyruvate results in net production of 2 mol ATP altogether.

$$CH_3COCOOH + \tfrac{1}{2}O_2 + 15P_i + 14ADP + GDP \rightarrow 3CO_2 + 2H_2O + 14ATP + GTP$$

Enzymes involved are: (1) pyruvate dehydrogenase, (2) citrate synthase, (3) aconitase, (4,5) isocitrate dehydrogenase, (6) α-ketoglutarate dehydrogenase, (7) succinate thiokinase, (8) succinate dehydrogenase, (9) fumarase, (10) malate dehydrogenase.

phorylation/dephosphorylation of the enzyme protein, albeit not mediated by cAMP. Hormones affect this process, especially insulin; when insulin is abundant the enzyme exists in dephosphorylated, fully activated form.[18,19]

PDH activity is strongly influenced by the rate of FFA oxidation. Intramitochondrial elevation of acetyl CoA concentration deactivates the enzyme both by direct inhibition and trapping of free CoA necessary for enzyme function. In the liver this situation results in redirection of pyruvate flow back to glucose via PEPCK (Fig. 19-6), whereas in muscles it interferes with glucose oxidation (see The Glucose–Fatty Acid Cycle, below). An inhibitory effect of leucine (an amino acid catabolized to acetyl CoA) on glucose oxidation in muscle tissue has also been attributed to inhibition of PDH.[20]

Acetyl CoA is the final carbon product of all metabolic fuels entering terminal oxidation in the TCA cycle. The cyclic nature of this pathway derives from the fact that the substrate combining with acetyl CoA in the first reaction of the cycle, oxaloacetate, is reconstituted in the final reaction. The product of this initial reaction is citrate, a tricarboxylic acid (hence the terms TCA or citric acid cycle).

The overall activity of the TCA cycle is determined by the availability of ATP and substrate, enzyme activities, and hormonal milieu. These controlling influences are largely interdependent. For example, when insulin levels are low and the gluconeogenic pathway is markedly activated, oxaloacetate may be increasingly siphoned to PEP so as to limit activity of the TCA cycle.

The major determinant of TCA cycle enzyme activity is the relative concentrations of ATP, ADP, and AMP, which change according to general energy requirements and determine the respiratory chain activity; this in turn, dictates the rate of TCA cycling. Fine regulation of the enzymes is dependent on relationships among the intramitochondrial intermediates and various nucleotides. In circumstances of decreased ATP availability and increased levels of ADP, the activities of both *citrate synthase,* which catalyzes the condensation of acetyl CoA and oxaloacetate, and *isocitrate dehydrogenase* are increased. In contrast, these enzymes are inhibited when ATP levels are high and those of ADP are low. In this manner, the consumption of ATP by muscular contraction accelerates glucose oxidation, whereas in the resting state glucose oxidation by muscle is virtually nil.

OTHER PATHWAYS OF GLUCOSE METABOLISM

A number of alternate pathways of glucose metabolism exist; the activity of some is largely determined by the concentration of circulating glucose. These pathways comprise enzymes with a high K_m for glucose which are not insulin-dependent; their share in glucose metabolism may rise from < 3 percent at normal glucose concentration to > 15 percent in the presence of marked hyperglycemia and insulin deficiency (as occurs in uncontrolled diabetes).

Pentose Shunt

G6P, in addition to undergoing glycolysis and aerobic oxidation via the TCA cycle, may be metabolized via the *pentose shunt* pathway, in which it is oxidized by the $NADP^+$-dependent enzyme *glucose-6-phosphate dehydrogenase,* resulting in the formation of 6-phosphogluconate. The latter may then be converted via a sequence of intermediate reactions to the pentoses ribulose, ribose, and xylulose. The major purposes of this pathway are the formation of pentoses required for nucleic acid synthesis and generation of reducing equivalents in the form of NADPH, which are necessary in the reductive synthesis of fatty acids and sterols. Consequently, the pentose pathway is of some importance in the metabolism of glucose both in liver, the major site of fatty acid biosynthesis in humans, especially in circumstances of glucose abundance when active lipogenesis proceeds, and adrenal tissue and testis (sites of sterol biosynthesis). In contrast, virtually no pentose pathway activity is demonstrable in muscle.

Polyol Pathway

Glucose may be converted to the polyhydroxy alcohol *sorbitol* by the enzyme *aldose reductase* (Fig. 19-9). Aldose reductase is present in most mammalian tissues, including some highly specialized ones that are prone to lesions in diabetes, such as nerves, lens, retina, and vascular endothelium.[21] Aldose reductase is relatively nonspecific, capable of converting several aldohexoses to their respective alcohols; hence the general term "polyol pathway." Sorbitol generally traverses cellular membranes poorly and tends to accumulate within the cells unless it is converted by *sorbitol dehydrogenase* to more readily passable fructose. The cellular retention of sorbitol is, therefore, dependent to a large extent on the relative activities of aldose reductase and sorbitol dehydrogenase. The suggested mechanism of damage in cells accumulating sorbitol is inhibition of Na^+,K^+-ATPase activity probably linked to reduced uptake of *myoinositol,* a cyclic hexanol and precursor of phosphorylated cellular metabolism effectors[21a] and of membrane phospholipids, of importance in Schwann cells.[22,23] This suggestion led to current attempts to prevent these complications, which are associated with protracted diabetic

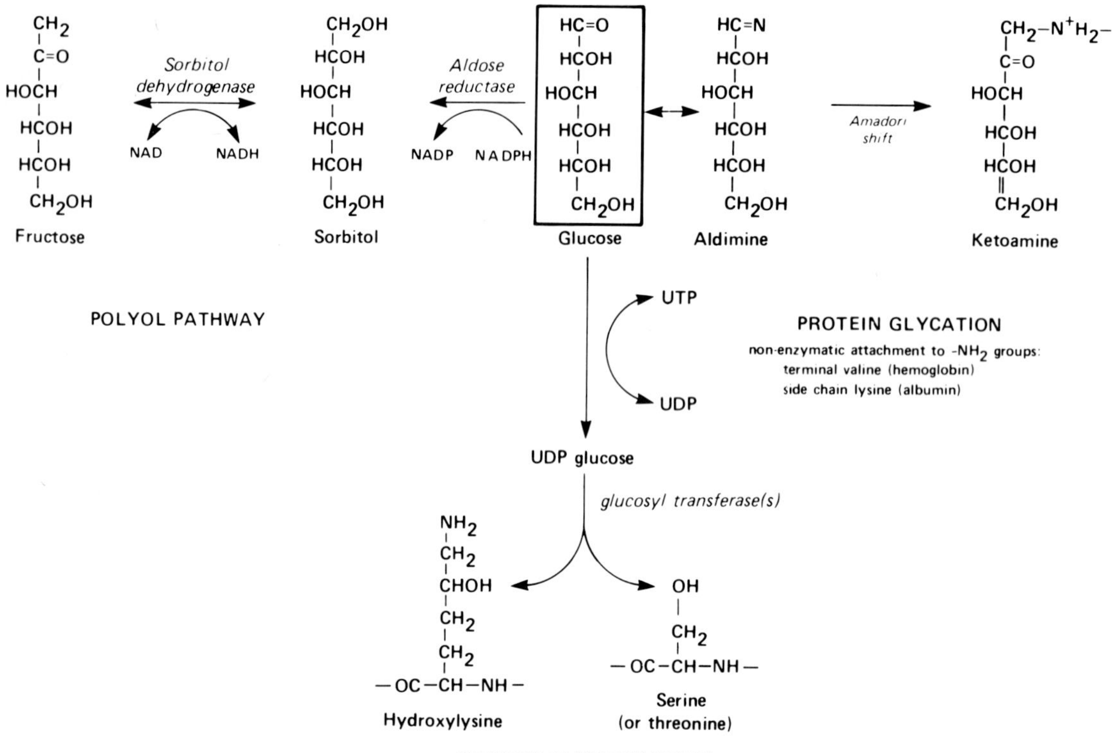

FIGURE 19-9 Glucose, especially at higher than normal concentrations, may enter several pathways apparently associated with deterioration of the function of the affected cell types or proteins.

Polyol pathway: $NADP^+$-dependent *aldose reductase* reduces aldohexoses to the corresponding polyhydroxy alcohols. The alcohols are trapped within the cells unless converted to freely diffusible fructose by a *polyol dehydrogenase*.

Protein glycation: In a two-stage mechanism, glucose reacts with exposed amino groups on proteins, resulting in conversion into ketohexoses, covalently attached for the life span of the protein molecule.

Protein glycosylation: Glucose alone or together with other hexoses may be increasingly linked to the hydroxyl groups within a defined amino acid sequence on cellular proteins. The acceptor groups are mainly serine and threonine as well as 5-hydroxylysine, present mainly in collagen; the last arises as a result of posttranslational hydroxylation. Glycosylation involves prior formation of UDP-glucose from UTP and glucose-1-phosphate by a pyrophosphorylase reaction followed by the transfer of the glucose residue to the hydroxyl acceptor by a transferase.

hyperglycemia, by the use of aldose reductase inhibitors[24-26] (see Diabetic Neuropathy, below).

Protein Glycation

The term *glycation* implies a nonenzymatic covalent bonding of glucose to the exposed amino groups in proteins, in distinction to *glycosylation*, which represents an enzymatic linkage of hexose molecules to hydroxyl groups on proteins; previously, the term glycosylation was widely and inaccurately used. At high concentrations, glucose forms first a reversible and unstable ketimine (Schiff base) in association with the amino group of terminal valine (in hemoglobin) or the ε-amino group of lysine (in albumin). The ketimine then undergoes a slow, spontaneous internal (Amadori) rearrangement, forming a stable covalent bond, involving a change from an aldo- into a ketohexose (Fig. 19-9).

The excessive glycation in the presence of hyperglycemia has generally a detrimental influence on the function of proteins due both to alterations in configuration and surface charge and to susceptibility to degradation. Hemoglobin (Hb) was one of the first proteins reported to undergo glycation to glycohemoglobin (HbA_{Ic}).[27,28] Both the terminal valine on the β chain and the intrapeptide lysines are glycated, but loss of the terminal amino group increases the electrophoretic and chromatographic mobility of Hb. The concentration of HbA_{Ic} is roughly proportional to blood glucose concentration and may be used as an indicator of therapeutic control of diabetic hyperglycemia[29,30] (see below). Albumin,[31,32] lipoproteins,[33,34] other plasma proteins, and cellular membranes are also targets of glycation.

Protein Glycosylation

Glycoproteins comprise a variety of proteins including circulating plasma constituents (fibrinogen, immunoglobulins), hormones (gonadotropins), enzymes (ribonuclease B), mucous secretions, collagen, and basement membrane. The addition of hexoses or other carbohydrate components in covalent linkage with amino acids in the course of protein synthesis imparts a diversified structure and expands the capacity of the protein to perform specific functions. The attachment of various carbohydrate moieties to serine or threonine hydroxyl groups on the polypeptide chains involves initial reaction of the hexose with uridine triphosphate (UTP) to form the UDP derivative. Specific transferases then catalyze the transfer of carbohydrate to the polypeptide.

In the hyperglycemia of diabetes, excessive posttranscriptional glycosylation of proteins does occur, with presumed deleterious consequences for cell function; the glomerular basement membrane, collagen, and other cellular proteins are affected.[35–38]

The various pathways of glucose metabolism involving polyol formation, glycation, and glycosylation have been implicated in the microvascular complications, i.e., neuropathy, retinopathy, and nephropathy, which occur with long-standing diabetes (see Pathogenesis of Diabetic Complications, below).

Fat Metabolism

Fatty acids are stored in adipose tissue and, to a lesser extent, in other cells as esters of the trihydroxy alcohol *glycerol;* hence the name triacylglycerols or, trivially, *triglycerides.* The triglycerides constitute the most important fuel depot in mammalian organisms, accounting for > 80 percent of total energy stores.

SYNTHESIS OF FATTY ACIDS AND TRIGLYCERIDES

The precursor of fatty acids is acetyl CoA, which is mainly derived from glucose via pyruvate by the pyruvate dehydrogenase reaction (see above). Actually, the acetyl CoA formed by this reaction in the mitochondria is not directly available for fatty acid synthesis, which occurs in the cytosol; it has to be transferred out via citrate. Citrate is synthesized by condensation of acetyl CoA with oxaloacetate and transported into the cytosol where it is cleaved to acetyl CoA by the enzyme *ATP-citrate lyase* (Fig. 19-10). Citrate, which becomes abundant in liver cells during the period of carbohydrate alimentation, is not only the initial substrate but also an important effector of lipogenesis.

The first committed step in the pathway of fatty acid synthesis in the cytosol is the carboxylation of acetyl CoA to form *malonyl CoA.* The catalysis of this reaction, by *acetyl CoA carboxylase,* is the rate-limiting step in fat biosynthesis.[39] The enzyme requires biotin as a cofactor. The short-term regulation of its activity is effected by citrate (which promotes conversion of inactive monomers to the active tetrameric enzyme), by cAMP-dependent phosphorylation (which reduces activity), and by the end products of fatty acid synthesis, the long-chain fatty acyl derivatives (which may inactivate the enzyme). Long-term regulation of acetyl CoA carboxylase is dependent on insulin-modulated

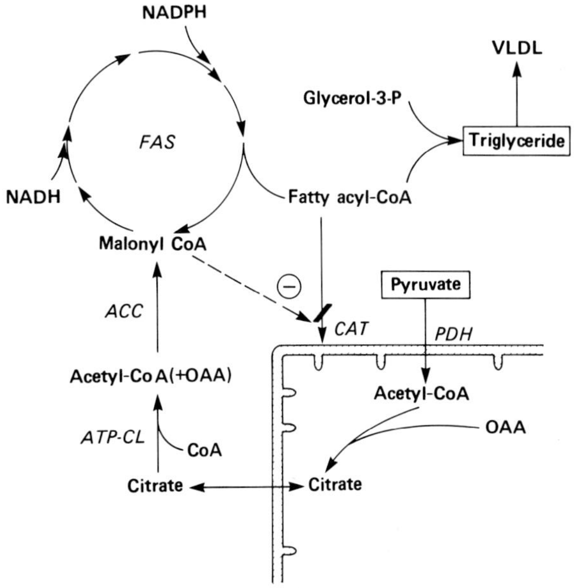

FIGURE 19-10 Hepatic fatty acid synthesis. The starting substrate for fatty acid synthesis is citrate, which is copiously produced in mitochondria from acetyl CoA and oxaloacetate whenever the rate of glycolysis, following a carbohydrate-rich meal, exceeds the energy requirements met by the TCA cycle. Citrate is actively transported out into the cytosol by a membrane transporter and cleaved by an insulin-induced enzyme, *ATP-citrate lyase* (CL). *Acetyl CoA carboxylase* (ACC) converts acetyl CoA to malonyl CoA by a rate-limiting process involving "fixation" of aqueous CO_2. The fatty acid chain is synthesized by a repetitive cyclic process catalyzed by several enzymes aggregated on an acyl-binding protein; termed *"fatty acid synthase"* (FAS). This "enzyme" is also insulin-dependent. Each cycle results in elongation by two carbon atoms. Reducing equivalents, particularly NADPH, are provided by the $NADP^+$–malate dehydrogenase and pentose shunt pathways. Fatty acid synthesis usually stops at 16 (14 to 18) carbon atoms; the fatty acyl CoA moieties are linked with glycerol 3-phosphate by an esterification system located on the endoplasmic reticulum, converted to triglycerides (or phospholipids) and transferred into the Golgi apparatus for secretion in plasma lipoproteins. Malonyl CoA exerts a feed-forward effect by preventing the entry of long-chain fatty acyl CoA into the mitochondria by inhibiting *carnitine acyltransferase* (CAT). Accumulation of long-chain fatty acyl CoA may have a feedback effect by inactivating ACC.

synthesis of the enzyme protein. Thus, the levels of the enzyme are decreased in starvation and diabetes and are increased during refeeding. Malonyl CoA, the product of acetyl CoA carboxylation, is, in turn, a potent inhibitor of fatty acid oxidation and ketogenesis.[40,41] In this manner a futile cycle, whereby fatty acid synthesis and oxidation are simultaneously stimulated, is avoided.

For storage as fat droplets in cells and transport out of liver cells in lipoproteins, fatty acids must be esterified with *glycerol 3-phosphate* to form triglycerides. Glycerol 3-phosphate may be generated by the glycolytic breakdown of glucose to *dihydroxyacetone phosphate,* which can then undergo reduction in the presence of NADH. Alternatively, glycerol 3-phosphate may be formed from free glycerol (liberated in the breakdown of triglycerides) by the enzyme *glycerol kinase* (ATP). The latter enzyme is present in liver but is virtually absent in adipose tissue. Consequently, triglyceride formation and storage in adipose tissue requires not only the availability of fatty acyl CoA esters (present in situ or derived from circulating lipoproteins), but also the uptake of glucose and its metabolism via the glycolytic pathway so as to generate glycerol 3-phosphate.

The enzymes required for fat synthesis are present in a variety of tissues, notably liver. In contrast to many other mammals, in humans adipose tissue exhibits low rates of glucose incorporation into fatty acids.[42] De novo lipogenesis in humans occurs largely in the liver, from which lipids are secreted as triglycerides in very low density lipoproteins (VLDL). VLDL transport triglycerides to adipose tissue; there, the insulin-dependent enzyme *lipoprotein lipase,* which is localized to the endothelium, catalyzes hydrolysis of triglycerides to glycerol and FFA, which then enter the cell. The reesterification reaction within the adipose cells occurs between glucose-derived glycerol 3-phosphate and lipoprotein-derived fatty acids. The synthetic function of human adipose tissue is thus mainly confined to the formation of glycerol 3-phosphate (Fig. 19-11).

MOBILIZATION OF FATTY ACIDS

Although fat is transported for storage as VLDL-borne triglycerides, its uptake and combustion by tissues (heart, muscle, liver) require its release from depot stores as FFA, which are transported in the blood bound to plasma albumin (Fig. 19-11). The breakdown of triglycerides in adipose tissue is regulated by an intracellular tissue lipase which catalyzes the reaction

$$\text{Triglyceride} + 3H_2O \longrightarrow 3\text{FFA} + \text{glycerol}$$

This process, which is termed *lipolysis,* is under the regulation of a variety of hormones. Lipolysis is increased by epinephrine, glucagon, GH, adrenocorticotropic hormone (ACTH), or thyroid hormone and is reduced by insulin. The relevant lipase is consequently often referred to as *hormone-sensitive lipase* (although other lipases are hormone-regulated too). In general, an increase in cAMP concentration accom-

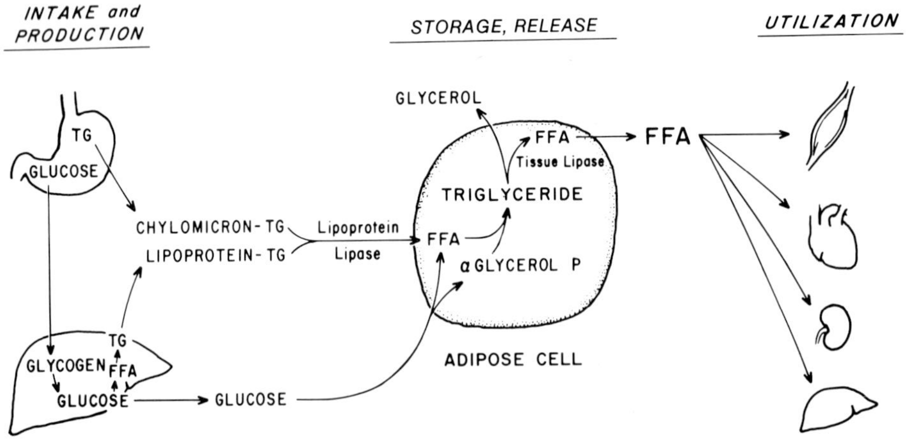

FIGURE 19-11 Fat homeostasis in humans. Fatty acids either enter the body as dietary triglyceride (TG) or are synthesized in the liver from glucose. Transport from the gut and liver is in the form of chylomicrons and very low density lipoproteins, respectively. Uptake by the fat cell requires initially the action of endothelial lipoprotein lipase, which liberates free fatty acids (FFA). FFA enter the cell and are reesterified to triglycerides with endogenously elaborated glycerol 3-phosphate. Release from the fat cell is regulated by an intracellular hormone-sensitive tissue lipase. FFA may then be taken up by muscle, heart, kidney, liver, and other tissues.

panies the protein kinase–mediated activation of the lipase, while a decrease in cAMP concentration is associated with inactivation. From a physiologic viewpoint, epinephrine and, to a lesser extent, thyroid hormone are the most important activators of the hormone-sensitive lipase, while insulin is the most important inhibitor. It is unlikely that ACTH or glucagon contributes to the physiologic modulation of lipolysis; inordinately high concentrations of these hormones are required to increase lipase activity.

The net rate of FFA outflow is also influenced by glucose utilization in adipose tissue. As indicated in Fig. 19-11, triglycerides are retained by reesterification so long as an adequate supply of glycerol 3-phosphate is maintained. Since adipose tissue lacks glycerol kinase, the availability of glycerol 3-phosphate is determined by the rate of glycolysis. Consequently, in circumstances of increased glucose utilization, the outflow of FFA is reduced because of both increased substrate availability for esterification and reduction in activity of the hormone-sensitive lipase.

OXIDATION OF FATTY ACIDS

The process whereby fatty acids are oxidized to provide high-energy phosphate in the form of ATP has been termed *β oxidation*, since it involves a series of consecutive oxidations of the β carbon to yield a β-ketoacid, which undergoes cleavage to produce acetyl CoA. In this process the fatty acid is shortened by two carbon atoms. The steps are repeated until the entire fatty acid has been oxidized to acetyl CoA, which enters the TCA cycle for oxidation to CO_2 (Fig. 19-12).

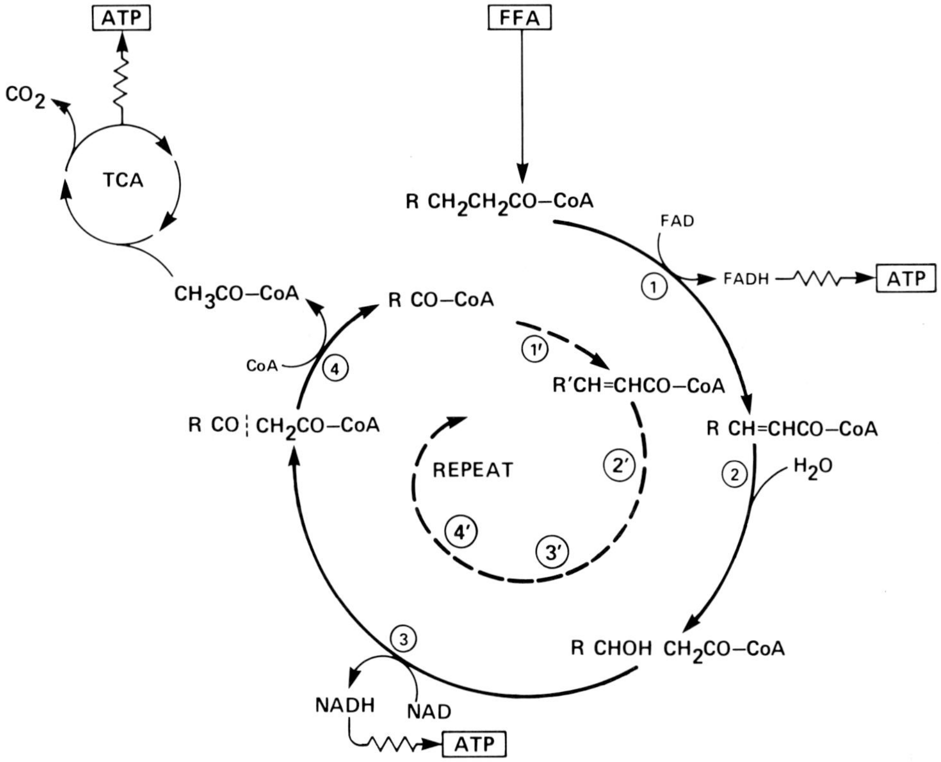

FIGURE 19-12 Fatty acid oxidation pathway. Long-chain FFA, flowing into the liver or muscles, are first acylated outside the mitochondria to form fatty acyl CoA esters by the enzyme *acyl CoA synthase* (thiokinase):

$$RCH_2CH_2COOH + ATP + CoA \rightarrow RCH_2CH_2COCoA + AMP + PP_i$$

Short-chain FFA (≤10 carbons) are acylated within the mitochondria. The fatty acid chain is rapidly shortened by two carbons in a four-step cycle by an enzyme complex collectively termed "*fatty acid oxidase*": (1) desaturation by FAD^+-dependent acyl CoA dehydrogenase, (2) hydration by Δ^2-enoyl CoA hydratase, (3) dehydration by NADH-dependent β-hydroxyacyl CoA dehydrogenase, (4) cleavage by β-ketothiolase. The acetyl CoA produced is oxidized in the TCA cycle, whereas the shortened FFA goes through repeated deacylation cycle. Each turn of the cycle, tightly associated with the terminal respiratory chain, generates 5 ATP (2 from FADH and 3 from NADH); the oxidation of acetyl CoA in the TCA cycle yields 12 more ATP bonds.

The initial step in the mitochondrial oxidation of fatty acids is their activation in the cytosol by the formation of the acyl CoA derivative. However, the long-chain fatty acyl CoA derivatives (12 or more carbons) cannot penetrate the mitochondrial membrane. Consequently, a carrier molecule, *carnitine* (γ-amino-β-hydroxybutyric acid trimethylbetaine), is required. The enzyme *carnitine acyltransferase 1* (CAT 1) catalyzes the formation of the fatty acyl-carnitine derivative, which crosses the inner mitochondrial membrane. The fatty acyl group is transferred to intramitochondrial CoA by the action of the enzyme CAT 2. Free carnitine is regenerated and is thus available for shuttling of additional fatty acyl residues into the mitochondria (Fig. 19-13). Recent data strongly indicate that CAT 1 is inhibited by malonyl CoA,[40,41] the first committed intermediate in the pathway of fatty acid biosynthesis (Fig. 19-10). Thus, mitochondrial β oxidation is controlled by three factors: (1) the rate of FFA supplied by fat-storing tissues (lipolysis), (2) the cytosolic concentration of malonyl CoA, and (3) the availability of carnitine. These factors are regulated, in turn, by insulin. An increase in insulin concentration prevents adipose tissue lipolysis, decreases carnitine availability, and promotes lipogenesis from glycolysis-derived acetyl CoA, thereby increasing malonyl CoA levels and inhibiting CAT 1. Absence of insulin causes increased FFA mobilization, increased carnitine availability, and depression in lipogenesis, together with decline in malonyl CoA concentration, effecting a rise in CAT 1 activity (Fig. 19-13). The latter two prerequisites for facilitation of mitochondrial entry of fatty acyl CoA are enhanced by the concomitant rise in glucagon concentration.[41] The regulatory relationship between the intermediate of fatty acid biosynthesis (malonyl CoA) and fatty acid

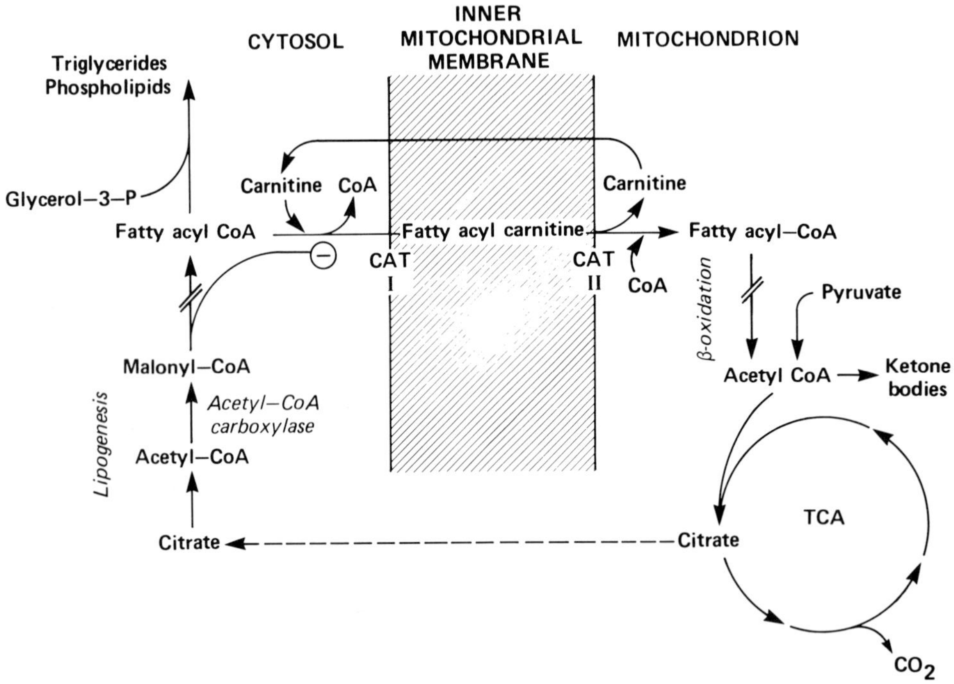

FIGURE 19-13 Fatty acid transport into mitochondria. The controlling step is the rate of transfer of fatty acyl CoA derivatives across the mitochondrial membrane, as determined by the activity of the transporter system composed of carnitine and carnitine acyltransferases (CAT) I and II. Carnitine, β-hydroxy-α-timethyl-ammonium butyrate, is synthesized in the liver but widely distributed among tissues, particularly muscles. Transfer of long-chain fatty acyl CoA is activated by an increased availability of free carnitine and a fall in the level of malonyl CoA, the latter reflecting reduced lipogenesis. CAT I, on the outer side of the membrane, allows penetration by cleaving the CoA bond and forming an acylcarnitine complex. The activity of CAT I is thought to be modulated by competitive binding of fatty acyl CoA and malonyl CoA to the regulatory site of the enzyme. CAT II, on the inner side, catalyzes the interaction of acylcarnitine with mitochondrial CoA. Fatty acyl CoA is re-formed and the liberated free carnitine is transported in the opposite direction in synchrony with acylcarnitine. Activation of short-chain FFA ($\leq$10 carbon atoms) occurs within the mitochondria independently of carnitine.

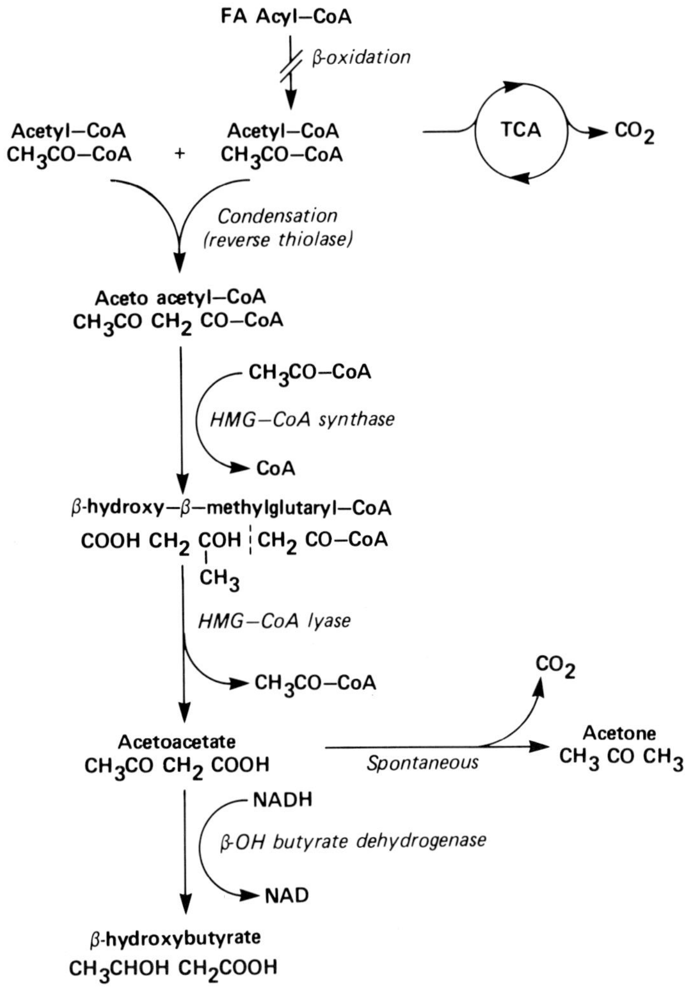

FIGURE 19-14 Ketogenesis pathway. In the presence of large amounts of acetyl CoA, derived from excessive FFA oxidation, condensation into acetoacetyl CoA takes place in liver mitochondria. Earlier it was thought that, during enhanced ketogenesis, acetoacetate may be directly formed by deacylation of acetoacetyl CoA, an intermediate in the last stage of β-oxidation. It is known today that the main pathway requires an additional condensation with acetyl CoA to form β-hydroxy-β-methylglutaryl CoA (HMG-CoA) catalyzed by *HMG-CoA synthase.* Acetoacetate is formed and released from the mitochondria after cleavage of HMG-CoA by *HMG-CoA lyase,* which also results in the recovery of acetyl CoA. Acetoacetate may be converted to β-hydroxybutyrate, which is quantitatively the predominant ketone body in the circulation, or decarboxylated to acetone. Neither of the above reactions is rate-limiting; FFA supply is the major determinant of ketogenesis.

oxidation thus assures that, in circumstances of anabolism (i.e., fat synthesis), there is a concomitant inhibition of catabolism (fat oxidation).

KETOGENESIS AND KETONE UTILIZATION

When there is an unrestrained increase in FFA mobilization, the rate at which acetyl CoA is produced in the course of β oxidation may exceed the capacity of the TCA cycle. In such circumstances, the surplus of acetyl CoA is shifted into the production of acetoacetate, β-hydroxybutyrate, and acetone. These substances are collectively termed *ketone bodies.* It should be emphasized that ketone bodies are products of incomplete fat oxidation. Only a fraction of the total ketone bodies can be used; excretion of the remainder constitutes a loss of energy. When produced in marked excess, as occurs in uncontrolled diabetes, acetoacetate and β-hydroxybutyrate cause metabolic acidosis (i.e., diabetic ketoacidosis, DKA). The large quantities of acetone present in various forms of ketosis do not contribute to the metabolic acidosis but impart a characteristic fruity odor to the patient's breath.

The initial step in formation of ketone bodies from acetyl CoA (Fig. 19-14) involves condensation of two molecules of acetyl CoA to form acetoacetyl CoA. The conversion of acetoacetyl CoA to acetoacetate requires conversion to β-hydroxy-β-methylglutaryl CoA, which is then cleaved to acetoacetate and acetyl CoA. Formation of β-hydroxybutyrate from acetoacetate involves a reversible oxidation-reduction employing NADH as the cofactor. Acetone is produced from acetoacetate by a nonenzymatic spontaneous decarboxylation.

Neither the esterification of FFA (for triglyceride formation) nor the rate of acetyl CoA oxidation via the TCA cycle is necessarily inhibited in the ketogenic liver. In fact, the hepatic triglyceride formation may be enhanced together with ketone production if

FFA delivery is massive. As a consequence, a fatty, triglyceride-laden liver and an elevation of circulating VLDL concentrations are common findings in patients with poorly regulated diabetes. On the other hand, synthesis of fatty acids from acetyl CoA is strongly inhibited in the ketogenic liver.

The acetoacetate and β-hydroxybutyrate produced in the liver enter the bloodstream and circulate in a ratio of approximately 1:3. The circulating ketones are oxidized by extrahepatic tissues and, in circumstances of prolonged starvation, taken up and oxidized by the brain.[42] The first step in the pathway of ketone utilization involves oxidation of β-hydroxybutyrate to acetoacetate. Acetoacetyl CoA is then formed by a transferase-catalyzed reaction with succinyl CoA (Fig. 19-15). The enzymes required for these reactions are present in muscle, brain, and fetal liver but not in adult liver.[43] In starvation the utilization of ketone bodies by extrahepatic tissues appears to be proportional to the ketone body concentration in the blood; their utilization, in addition to glucose or FFA, contributes to fuel economy. Saturation occurs at ~70 mg/dl, at which level the ketones are mostly excreted in urine or exhaled.

Recently, pathways for the metabolism of acetone have been outlined. Acetone may be converted to acetate and acetyl CoA[43a] and may also serve as a substrate for the synthesis of nonnegligible amounts of glucose in nondiabetic starving animals[44,45] or humans.[46] This pathway operates by conversion of acetone to pyruvaldehyde (methylglyoxal) in the liver or 1,2-propanediol in extrahepatic tissues (Fig. 19-15).

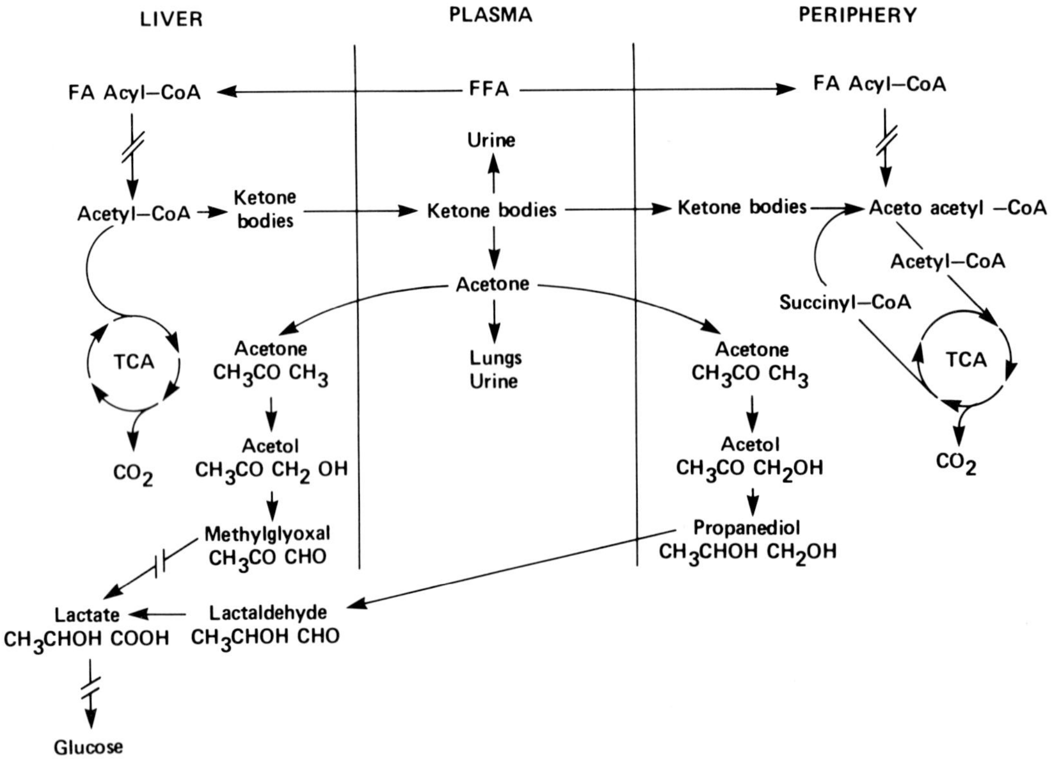

FIGURE 19-15 Distribution and utilization of ketone bodies. Ketone bodies are released from the liver into plasma. In uncontrolled diabetes large amounts may be excreted in urine. The volatile acetone may also be exhaled. In prolonged fasting, when ketone production is not excessive and glucose is scarce, there is an adaptation for ketone utilization in extrahepatic tissues. Acetoacetate is converted to acetoacetyl CoA in the mitochondria by a CoA transferase reaction using TCA cycle–derived succinyl CoA as a CoA donor. Direct acylation of acetoacetate by a thiokinase reaction is thought to be minimal. Acetoacetyl CoA is then cleaved into two acetyl CoA molecules by the action of *thiolase* and is catabolized in TCA cycle. A fraction of acetone may be used for gluconeogenesis after conversion to 1-hydroxy-2-propanone (acetol) by the mitochondrial *NADPH-acetone monoxygenase*, an enzyme probably related to the respiratory chain. The activity of this enzyme was found to be elevated in fasting rats. Acetol is converted to pyruraldehyde (methylglyoxal) in the liver by NADPH-alcohol dehydrogenase and to lactate by a mechanism not yet well-defined. In peripheral tissues 1-hydroxy-2-propanone is converted to 1,2-propanediol, then to lactaldehyde in the liver by NAD^+-aldehyde dehydrogenase.

Interactions of Fat and Carbohydrate Metabolism

The convergence of pathways of fat and carbohydrate metabolism via a shared intermediate (acetyl CoA) and the effects of intermediates derived from one process on enzymatic reactions in other pathways result in a variety of regulatory relationships between fat and carbohydrate metabolism. These relationships are best illustrated by the effects of augmented carbohydrate utilization on fat metabolism and the effects of augmented fat utilization on carbohydrate metabolism. These interactions are summarized in Table 19-2.

When the supply of carbohydrate is increased (e.g., after a carbohydrate-containing meal) and glucose utilization is stimulated, changes are observed in fat metabolism with respect to lipolysis, ketogenesis, and lipogenesis. The increase in glucose uptake decreases FFA release from adipose tissue by enhancing the availability of glycerol 3-phosphate for FFA reesterification. In addition, the rise in circulating glucose concentration stimulates the secretion of insulin, which in turn suppresses the hormone-sensitive lipase in adipose tissue. Thus, the antilipolytic action of carbohydrate is both substrate- and hormone-mediated.

The utilization of carbohydrate also promotes the net synthesis of long-chain fatty acids. The rate-limiting enzyme in fat biosynthesis, acetyl CoA carboxylase, is induced by carbohydrate feeding. This effect is mediated by hormonal changes (increased insulin concentration) as well as substrate-induced changes; the latter include augmented availability of citrate, which is an activator of the enzyme, and reduction in fatty acyl CoA esters, which inactivate the enzyme. The utilization of glucose along the pentose pathway also supplements the NADPH necessary for brisk fat biosynthesis.

Ketogenesis is also markedly inhibited by carbohydrate utilization. This effect is mediated via the

Table 19-2. Interrelationships between Fat and Carbohydrate Metabolism

Carbohydrate utilization		Metabolic effects and changes in enzyme activity and concentrations of intermediates		Fat utilization (starvation, diabetes)
↑		Glycolysis		↓
	↑	Phosphofructokinase-1	↓	
	↓	Fructose diphosphatase-1	↑	
	↑	$F2,6P_2$	↓	
	↑	Pyruvate kinase	↓	
	↑	Pyruvate dehydrogenase	↓	
↑		Lipogenesis and fat storage		↓
	↑	Acetyl CoA carboxylase	↓	
	↑	Hepatic citrate	↓	
	↑	VLDL production	↓	
	↑	TG esterification	↓	
	↑	Lipoprotein lipase	↓	
↓		Fat oxidation and ketogenesis		↑
	↓	Lipolysis and FFA release	↑	
	↓	Adipose tissue intracellular lipase	↑	
	↓	Carnitine acyltransferase	↑	
	↑	Malonyl CoA	↓	
	↑	Muscle glucose oxidation	↓	
↓		Gluconeogenesis		↑
	↓	Pyruvate carboxylase	↑	
	↓	Phospho*enol*pyruvate carboxykinase	↑	
	↓	Acetyl CoA and fatty acyl CoA	↑	
	↑	Free CoA	↓	

inhibition of lipolysis, which decreases the supply of FFA for oxidation by the liver. As noted above, fatty acid oxidation is influenced not only by the rate of lipolysis but also by the activity of the enzyme CAT 1, which in turn is influenced by the availability of carnitine and malonyl CoA. Thus, augmented rates of ketogenesis in diabetes or starvation are a consequence of substrate delivery (lipolysis) as well as augmented intrahepatic fatty acid oxidation. Hormonal changes accompanying carbohydrate utilization (increased insulin and reduced glucagon concentrations) also reduce the availability of free carnitine necessary for the transport of fatty acid derivatives across the mitochondrial membrane.

When fat utilization is increased, as occurs with restriction of dietary carbohydrate intake, total starvation, and diabetes, changes in glucose production as well as utilization are observed. An increase in gluconeogenesis generally accompanies augmented fat utilization and ketogenesis. The mechanism whereby fat oxidation stimulates gluconeogenesis is based in large measure on inverse modulation of enzymes: activation of PC and inhibition of PDH. This causes the oxaloacetate to flow to phospho*enol*pyruvate (as the gluconeogenic intermediate) in the cytosol (Fig. 19-6). Thus, while fatty acids cannot generally provide carbon skeletons for glucose synthesis, their oxidation enhances gluconeogenesis by regulation of enzyme activity.

Increases in fat oxidation are accompanied by inhibition of lipogenesis from acetyl CoA. Acetyl CoA carboxylase synthesis is reduced in the insulin-deficient hormonal milieu; this enzyme may be further inactivated by high intrahepatic levels of long-chain fatty acyl CoA.

In studies with muscles in vitro an inhibitory effect of FFA on glucose utilization via glycolytic and aerobic pathways has been observed.[47,48] The points of inhibition of glucose utilization are the steps catalyzed by PFK and PDH. Citrate, a potential PFK inhibitor, accumulates in fat-utilizing heart muscle to levels which may affect the activity of PFK; the coincident increase in the acetyl CoA/free CoA ratio is detrimental to PDH activity. This relationship has been termed by Randle et al. the *glucose–fatty acid cycle*;[49] they proposed that an elevation in circulating FFA interferes with glucose oxidation. Whether this relationship applies to all muscles is unclear. For example, during exercise an *increase* in glucose utilization is observed together with a rise in FFA oxidation by the contracting muscles. Nevertheless, a reciprocal relationship between fat and glucose oxidation serves to prevent superfluous glucose utilization in starvation or exercise, for the benefit of glucose-obligatory tissues (e.g., brain).

Amino Acid Metabolism

Maintenance of steady-state concentrations of circulating amino acids is dependent upon the net balance between release from endogenous protein stores and utilization by various tissues. Since muscle accounts for > 50 percent of the total body pool of free amino acids and the liver is the repository of the urea cycle enzymes necessary for nitrogen disposal, these two organs may be expected to play a major role in determining the circulating levels and turnover of amino acids.

In the postabsorptive state (e.g., following a 12- to 14-h overnight fast), there is a net release of amino acids from muscle tissue (Fig. 19-16A). The pattern of this release is quite distinctive: the output of alanine and glutamine exceeds that of all other amino acids and accounts for > 50 percent of total α-amino nitrogen release. Complementing the amino acid deficit in muscle tissue is the consistent uptake of amino acids across the splanchnic bed. As in the case of peripheral output, alanine and glutamine predominate in the uptake of amino acids by splanchnic tissues. In fact, there is a fairly close correspondence between the relative outputs of most amino acids from the periphery and their uptake by splanchnic tissues. Within the splanchnic bed, the liver is the site of uptake of alanine, while the gut is the site of utilization of glutamine. Most of the amino groups of the glutamine extracted by the gut are released as alanine or free ammonia. The major site of glutamine disposal is the kidney, where it provides nitrogen for ammoniagenesis.

THE GLUCOSE-ALANINE CYCLE

The primacy of alanine in the overall availability and uptake of amino acids by the liver and the rapidity with which the liver converts alanine to glucose indicate the importance of alanine as the key protein-derived glucose precursor. The predominance of alanine in the outflow of amino acids from muscle cannot be explained on the basis of its availability in constituent cellular proteins, since no more than 7 to 10 percent of the amino acid residues in muscle proteins is alanine. This discrepancy led to the recognition that alanine is synthesized de novo in muscle tissue by transamination of pyruvate and formulation of the *glucose-alanine cycle.*[14,50,51] By this formulation alanine is synthesized in muscle by transamination of glucose-derived pyruvate and is transported to the liver, where its carbon skeleton is reconverted to glucose (Fig. 19-7). The branched-chain amino acids (valine, leucine, isoleucine) have been suggested as the

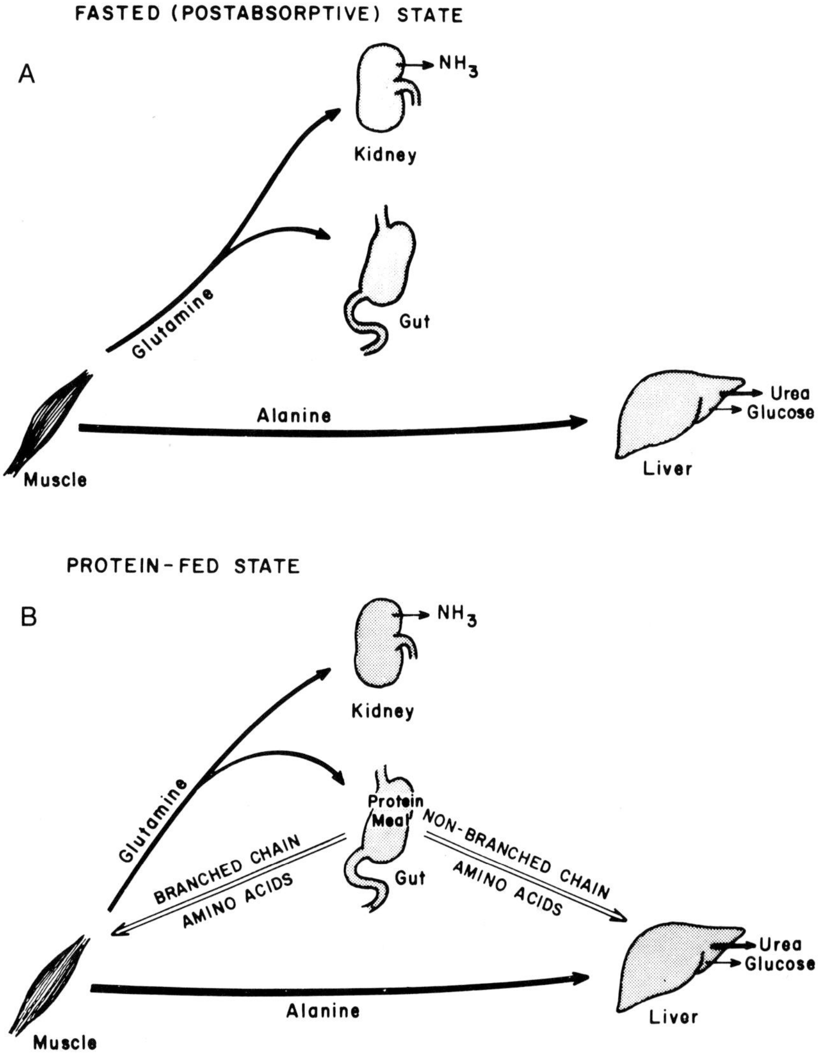

FIGURE 19-16 The effect of protein feeding on the exchange of amino acids between organs. In the fasted (postabsorptive) state there is net outflow of amino acids from muscle involving primarily alanine and glutamine (*A*). After a protein meal is eaten (*B*) the branched-chain amino acids (valine, leucine, and isoleucine) in the ingested protein are delivered to muscle tissue where they are used for protein synthesis and as an oxidative fuel. In contrast, only a small proportion of all other amino acids are taken up by muscle; they are largely extracted by the liver, where they are converted to glucose, oxidized, or used for protein synthesis.

origin of the amino groups for muscle alanine synthesis, inasmuch as extrahepatic tissues, particularly muscle, have been demonstrated to be the sites of oxidation of these amino acids.

Studies using [^{14}C]glucose indicate that 60 percent of the carbon skeletons of alanine residues released by muscle is derived from endogenous glucose, while virtually none of the carbon skeletons are derived from the in situ catabolism of other amino acids.[51] Quantitatively, as end products of peripheral glucose utilization as well as precursors of hepatic glucose production, carbon skeletons are recycled along the glucose-alanine cycle at a rate approximately 50 percent of that observed for the Cori (lactate) cycle.[14,51]

Although the glucose-alanine cycle does not yield new carbon skeletons for de novo glucose synthesis, it is of importance in glucose homeostasis as well as nitrogen and energy metabolism. A deficiency of alanine has been implicated in the accelerated starvation observed in pregnancy,[52] ketotic hypoglycemia of infancy,[53] and hypoglycemia of maple syrup urine disease.[54] Alanine also provides a nontoxic alternative to ammonia in the transfer of amino groups, derived from the catabolism of branched-chain amino acids in muscle, to the liver. Hyperalaninemia is observed in a variety of disorders of urea cycle enzymes, where it may moderate the hyperammonemia.[14]

The glucose-alanine cycle may also be useful with respect to ATP production. Conversion of glucose to alanine provides 8 mol of ATP compared with 2 mol provided by conversion to lactate. Furthermore, to the extent that alanine formation facilitates the oxidation of the branched-chain amino acids, an additional 30 to 40 mol ATP is generated per mol of amino acid oxidized.

PROTEIN REPLETION AND FEEDING

Since muscle tissue nitrogen balance in the fasting state is negative, repletion of muscle nitrogen depends on net uptake of amino acids in response to protein feeding. Ingestion of a protein meal (e.g., lean beef) is followed by a large output of amino acids, predominantly the branched-chain amino acids, from the splanchnic bed.[55] Valine, isoleucine, and leucine together account for 60 percent of the total of amino acids entering the systemic circulation, despite the fact that they contribute only 20 percent of the total amino acids in the protein meal. Simultaneous with the release of amino acids from the splanchnic bed, peripheral muscle exchange of most amino acids reverts from the net output observed in the basal state to net uptake. As in the case of splanchnic exchange, the uptake of amino acids across peripheral muscle tissue is most marked for the branched-chain amino acids.[55] Since the branched-chain amino acids constitute only 20 percent of the amino acid residues in muscle proteins, it is likely that these amino acids are not solely used for protein synthesis but are also metabolized within muscle.

These effects of protein feeding on interorgan amino acid exchange and the key role of the branched-chain amino acids are summarized in Fig. 19-16*B*. A nitrogen "shuttle" is observed, in which branched-chain amino acids provide for nitrogen repletion in muscle tissue in the fed state. The nitrogen thus delivered is released as alanine and glutamine in the fed as well as the fasted condition. The elevation of circulating and intracellular levels of branched-chain amino acids induced by protein feeding may have importance beyond delivery of nitrogen. The branched-chain amino acids, particularly leucine, may have a regulatory role in stimulating protein synthesis.[56] Furthermore, the overall uptake of branched-chain amino acids by muscle is regulated by insulin and is impaired in diabetic individuals.[55]

Insulin

HISTORY

Von Mering and Minkowski, in 1889, showed that removal of the pancreas of dogs caused serious disturbances of glucose metabolism, with elevation of the blood glucose concentration and the clinical picture of diabetes mellitus. The assumption that this effect was due to removal of a necessary hormone was confirmed in 1921 when Banting and Best prepared a pancreatic extract capable of lowering the blood glucose concentration. This substance, named *insulin*, was crystallized by Abel in 1926. Sanger determined the amino acid composition of insulin. However, synthesis of insulin was difficult because of inability to direct its two component chains into proper alignment (Fig. 19-17). Nevertheless, in 1965, Katsoyannis succeeded in chemically synthesizing small amounts of insulin.

The three-dimensional structure of insulin was determined by x-ray diffraction techniques in 1969. *Proinsulin*, the larger biosynthetic precursor of insulin, was discovered by Steiner in 1967,[57] clearing the way to large-scale insulin production. In 1979, biosynthesis of insulin by bacteria was accomplished using the techniques of recombinant DNA.[58] This procedure is now employed in the commercial production of human insulin which is increasingly used in clinical practice. Thus, insulin is the first protein hormone to be isolated, crystallized, sequenced, and synthesized, to have its precursor defined, and to be cloned.

CHEMISTRY

The human insulin molecule consists of two polypeptide chains, designated *A* and *B*, connected by two disulfide bridges. There is, in addition, a disulfide bridge between the sixth and eleventh amino acid residues of the A chain (Fig. 19-17). The complete unit contains 51 amino acids and has a molecular weight of 5800 and an isoelectric pH of 5.35. By definition, 1 mg of the pure substance contains 24.0 international units (IU). The amino acid composition is constant among the various species except for residues number 4, 8, 9, and 10 of the A chain and 1, 2, 3, 27, 29, and 30 of the B chain. Porcine insulin differs from human insulin only in the presence of a terminal alanine rather than threonine in the B chain; there are two additional differences between bovine and human insulin, at positions 8 (alanine replaces threonine) and 10 (valine replaces isoleucine) (Fig. 19-17). According to x-ray crystallographic studies, the unit cell of crystalline porcine insulin consists of an insulin hexamer made up of three dimers arranged around an axis on which lie two atoms of zinc; the zinc content of most crystalline preparations of insulin is 0.4 to 0.5 percent. In dilute solution insulin is adsorbed to glass or plastic [e.g., intravenous (IV) infusion sets]; adsorption can be minimized by the addition of albumin. Insulins derived from porcine and bovine pancreases were the most commonly used until biosynthetic human insulin became available.

Splitting of insulin into its constituent A and B chains by oxidation or reduction of the disulfide bridges results in complete loss of biological activity. In contrast, the activity of the insulin molecule is not

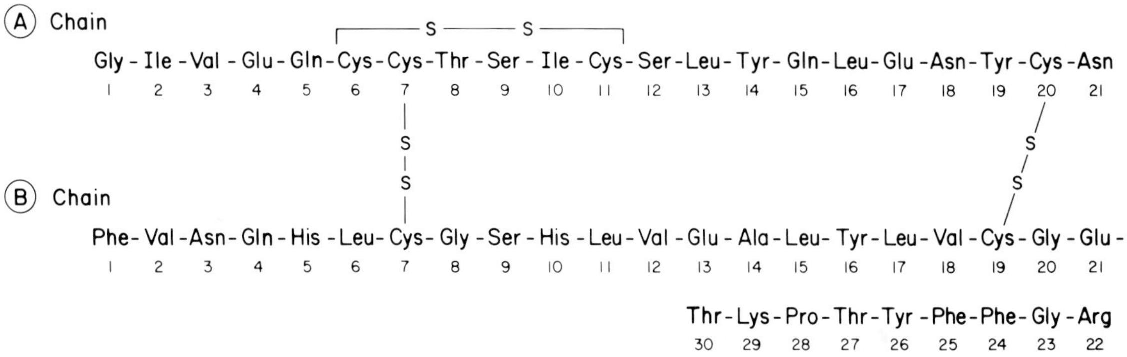

FIGURE 19-17 Amino acid sequence in human insulin. In porcine insulin alanine rather than threonine is the terminal amino acid in the B chain. Bovine insulin differs from human insulin in having an alanine at position 30 in the B chain, alanine (rather than a threonine) at position 8 in the A chain, and valine (rather than isoleucine) at position 10 in the A chain.

appreciably affected by removal of the amide group from the asparagine on the carboxyl end of the A chain or removal of the carboxy-terminal alanine from the B chain. When the entire asparagine (or aspartate) residue is removed from the carboxyl terminal of the A chain and the alanine is removed from the analogous position on the B chain, ~95 percent of the activity is lost. Removal by trypsin digestion of eight amino acids (residues 23 through 30) from the carboxyl terminal of the B chain (deoctapeptide insulin) eliminates all detectable activity. The region between residues 22 and 26 of the B chain is considered of crucial importance in the binding of insulin to its receptor, as well as in the overall action of insulin.[59]

BIOSYNTHESIS

Insulin is synthesized in the beta cells of the islets of Langerhans as a single-chain precursor, proinsulin, which has a molecular weight of ~9000.[57] Studies using cell-free systems indicate that the immediate translation product of proinsulin messenger RNA is a larger peptide of 11,500 daltons containing 23 additional amino acid residues at the amino terminal (Fig. 19-18). This precursor has been designated *preproinsulin;* it is converted to proinsulin by microsomal proteases within minutes of its synthesis. The peptide extension in preproinsulin is similar in size, partial amino acid composition, and amino-terminal location to the additional sequences found on the in vitro translation products of the mRNAs for a variety of hormones such as proparathyroid hormone and GH, as well as nonhormonal proteins such as immunoglobulin light chains.[60]

The intracellular sites where preproinsulin is synthesized and rapidly cleaved to proinsulin are the polysomes of the rough endoplasmic reticulum (Fig. 19-18). Proinsulin is then transferred, by an energy-dependent process, to the Golgi apparatus. At the Golgi, packaging into smooth-surfaced microvesicles takes place so as to form storage or secretory granules (Fig. 19-18). Beginning within the Golgi complex and continuing in the secretory granules, membrane-bound specific proteases cleave proinsulin into equimolar amounts of insulin and C *peptide,* the latter composed of 26 to 31 amino acid residues, according to species. The insulin, along with zinc, accumulates within the central core of the maturing secretory granule, which becomes progressively more electron-dense; the C peptide is localized in the peripheral clear space of the secretory granule.

In contrast to the minor differences in the amino acid sequences of A and B chains in various species, considerably greater variability is observed in the structure of the corresponding C peptides. Thus, human and porcine insulin differ by a single amino acid, whereas human C peptide, a 23-amino-acid chain of 3021 daltons, differs from porcine C peptide by 10 residues and contains two fewer amino acids.[61] This lack of interspecies homology is in keeping with the lack of a specific hormonal function of C peptide. Although proinsulin cross-reacts to a small degree with antibodies to insulin, it has only 3 to 7 percent of the biological effectiveness of native insulin. It is unsettled as to whether this small degree of biological activity is a genuine effect of proinsulin or a consequence of its conversion to insulin by target tissues. As compared with insulin, human proinsulin has been shown to have a relatively greater effect on hepatic than peripheral glucose metabolism.

Release of the contents of the mature secretory granules involves progressive migration of the granules to the plasma membrane of the cell followed by extrusion of insulin and C peptide. Within the cytosol of the beta cells, microtubules, 24-nm-diameter dimeric structures composed of 120,000-dalton subunits known as *tubulin*, act to guide granule movement to the plasma membrane. A series of microfilaments, 4- to 8-nm structures which are thought to be composed of the contractile protein *actin*, form a network near the plasma membrane and surround the secretory granules. The "final common path" of secretion is believed to involve the intracellular entry of calcium resulting in contraction of the microfilaments.[62] As a result, the secretory granules are moved to the cell surface, where their membranes fuse with the plasma membrane and their contents are discharged into the extracellular space. This process of membrane fusion has been termed emiocytosis, a form of exocytosis.

The development of methods of chemical DNA synthesis combined with recombinant DNA technology has permitted the synthesis of human insulin by bacterial cells (*Escherichia coli*).[57,63] The synthetic plan involves either the reverse transcription of messenger RNA coding for proinsulin so as to obtain the complementary DNA (cDNA) for proinsulin, or the chemical synthesis of smaller DNA fragments coding for

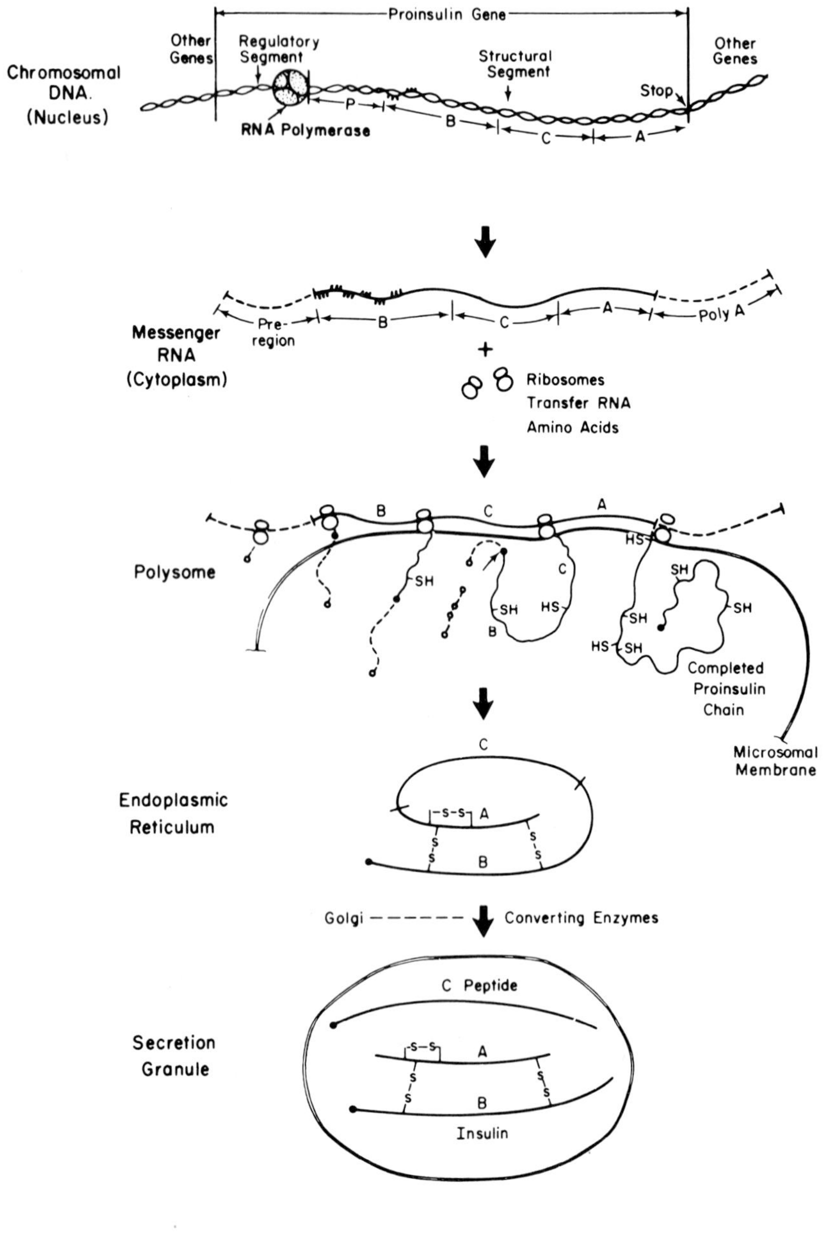

FIGURE 19-18 Schematic representatory of the biosynthesis of proinsulin and its conversion to insulin and C peptide. The proinsulin gene is represented in the upper panel. These genes contain introns that are processed out in forming mature messenger RNA. The mRNA serves to guide the formation of preproinsulin chains on the polysomes. Preproinsulin, indicated as "completed proinsulin chain" on the right-hand side of the polysome band in the middle panel, is cleaved and folded into the proinsulin molecule. The single-chain proinsulin, kept in configuration with the aid to two disulfide bonds, is then transferred to the Golgi apparatus and inserted into secretory granules. During secretion, proinsulin is cleaved into two-chain, biologically active insulin, by a protease specific to arginine and lysine bonds at positions 1 and 30 (Fig. 19-17). Together with insulin, equimolar amounts of a biologically inactive connecting peptide (C peptide) of 26 to 31 amino acids (lower panel). (*Adapted from Steiner.*[57])

the A and B chains of human insulin. The synthetic genes are then fused with a gene normally expressed in the *E. coli* host (e.g., the genes for penicillinase or β-galactosidase) so as to provide efficient transcription and translation to yield a stable precursor protein and (in the case of a periplasmic protein such as penicillinase) to facilitate transport outside the cell. The vectors used for the transfer of the foreign and bacterial DNA into the bacterial cell are either bacteriophages or plasmids. The bacterium containing the plasmid transcribes its own gene as well as the inserted sequences, thereby producing the desired polypeptide (Fig. 19-19). The fact that eukaryotic DNA sequences can be cloned and expressed in prokaryotic (bacterial) cells was successfully used for the production of human insulin, which may ultimately replace the current extraction procedures of porcine or bovine pancreas (see below).

INSULIN SECRETION

Basal Concentrations

The concentration of insulin in peripheral venous or arterial plasma or serum in healthy subjects after an overnight fast is generally 10 to 20 μU/ml (0.4 to 0.8 ng/ml). As noted above, equimolar amounts of C peptide are released with insulin during the secretory process and are present in concentrations of 0.9 to 3.5 ng/ml in the fasting state. The relatively higher level of C peptide, as compared to insulin, reflects the slower metabolic clearance of this substance.[61] Since the pancreatic islets drain into the portal vein and the liver removes 50 to 60 percent of the insulin presented to it, the portal/peripheral ratio of insulin in the basal state is 3:1. Following bursts of secretion (e.g., in response to administration of glucose or amino acids) the portal/peripheral ratio of insulin may reach a value of 9:1. The higher concentration of insulin in the portal vein may, in part, account for the fact that small increments in insulin secretion alter hepatic glucose metabolism in the absence of changes in peripheral glucose utilization.[64]

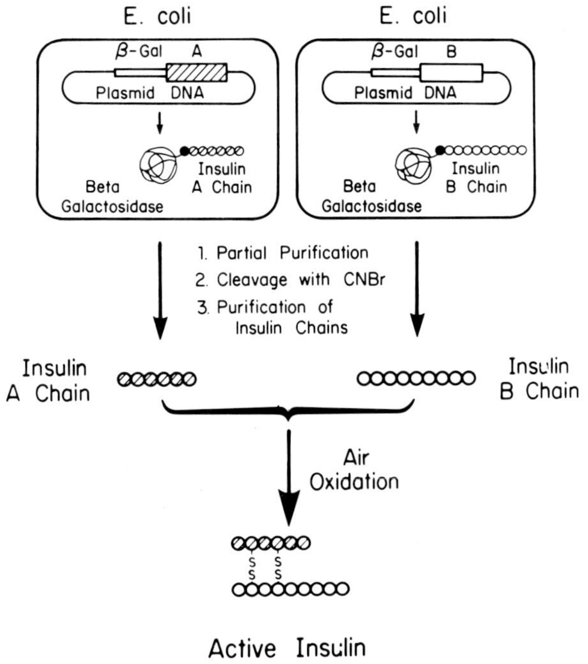

FIGURE 19-19 Schematic summary of the synthesis of the A and B chains of insulin by bacteria (*E. coli*) using recombinant DNA techniques. (*From Riggs A, Itakura K: Am J Hum Genet* 31:531, *1979*.)

Although proinsulin may be found in peripheral plasma, it generally accounts for < 15 percent of total circulating insulin immunoreactivity. In familial hyperproinsulinemia, an asymptomatic genetic defect with autosomal dominant inheritance, 65 to 90 percent of total plasma insulin immunoreactivity is accounted for by proinsulin.[65] This defect probably represents an abnormality in an intermediate formed on cleavage of proinsulin. A mutation affecting the dibasic amino acids arginine and lysine, which link the C peptide to the A chain of insulin, impairs the conversion of proinsulin to insulin.[66] Increased plasma levels of proinsulin are also observed in patients with insulinoma (see Chap. 20), chronic renal failure, and hyperthyroidism,[67] and in association with hypokalemia. Absolute elevations in proinsulin concentration are only rarely observed in diabetics and fail to account for the glucose intolerance observed in a variety of hyperinsulinemic states (e.g., obesity, pregnancy, hyperadrenalism). Elevations in proinsulin concentration in these conditions are generally proportional to those in insulin concentration.[66]

In insulin-treated diabetic patients the presence of antibodies precludes the measurement of circulating insulin concentration by conventional radioimmunoassay (RIA) techniques. In such circumstances the determination of C peptide provides a means of evaluating residual insulin secretory reserve.[61,61a] In patients with hypoglycemia and hyperinsulinemia, the measurement of C peptide concentration can indicate whether circulating insulin is of endogenous origin (high C peptide levels) or due to surreptitious insulin administration (low C peptide levels). Plasma C peptide determinations may also be helpful in assessing the pancreatic insulin secretion capacity in young individuals suspected, on the basis of islet antibody findings, of developing type I diabetes (see below).

The insulin secretory rate necessary to maintain normal basal concentrations of insulin is in the range of 0.25 to 1.5 U/h. These basal rates of secretion are normally present in the intervals between meal ingestion; their significance is underscored by studies showing that programmed insulin infusion systems, which provide insulin in basal as well as premeal doses, are more effective in normalizing blood glucose concentrations in type I diabetes than are premeal insulin doses alone.[68]

Carbohydrate

Of the various factors capable of stimulating insulin secretion, glucose is physiologically the most important. This is reflected by the moment-to-moment fluctuations in plasma insulin concentration which accompany fluctuations in plasma glucose concentration (Fig. 19-20). The precise mechanism whereby glucose acts on the beta cells to cause insulin release has not been entirely clarified. The preponderance of data indicates that glucose metabolism within the cell, rather than a signal from a membranal "glucose receptor" produces the stimulus for insulin release. Supporting this contention are the observations that (1) metabolizable sugars (hexoses or trioses) are more potent stimulators of insulin secretion than are nonmetabolizable carbohydrates (e.g., mannose), (2) glucose increases the concentration of glycolytic intermediates within islet cells, (3) compounds which inhibit glucose metabolism (mannoheptulose and 2-deoxyglucose) interfere with insulin secretion, and (4) the alpha anomer of glucose, a better substrate for glycolysis than the beta anomer, is more effective in stimulating the insulin secretion. The stereospecificity resides at the level of the phosphoglucose isomerase or phosphoglucomutase reaction.[69] Glycolysis may promote insulin secretion via increases in cellular NADH and NADPH concentrations as well as H^+ concentration.[70]

In the context of a glucose metabolism initiation of insulin release, two aspects have been advocated: (1) glucokinase might function as the glucose sensor, being an enzyme rate-limiting for overall glycolysis at the point of entry, rate-potentiated by glucose concentration, insulin-inducible and glucose-protected;[71,72] (2) beta cell PFK-1 is highly activated by $F2,6P_2$ (see Fig. 19-5). A burst of the glycolytic cascade, in association with increased insulin outflow, occurs rapidly after the formation of $F2,6P_2$, subsequent to the extracellular availability of glucose.[73] Another hexose diphosphate, glucose, 1,6-diphosphate, formed by the action of phosphoglucomutase, also activates PFK-1 markedly, acting in concert with $F2,6P_2$.[73] These findings indicate that the activation of PFK-1 may represent another critical event in the regulation of the glycolytic rate in the beta cell which mediates the acceleration of insulin secretion.

As in the case of a large number of intracellular processes, cAMP participates in the insulin secretory process. cAMP is believed to act as a positive synergistic modulator of a glucose-sensitive secretory step. An increase in cAMP concentration is not of itself sufficient to stimulate insulin secretion, as indicated by the fact that theophylline (an inhibitor of phosphodiesterase) elevates cAMP concentration but has a weak stimulatory action on insulin secretion unless glucose is present.

As noted above, an increase in intracellular calcium concentration is believed to be the final trigger-

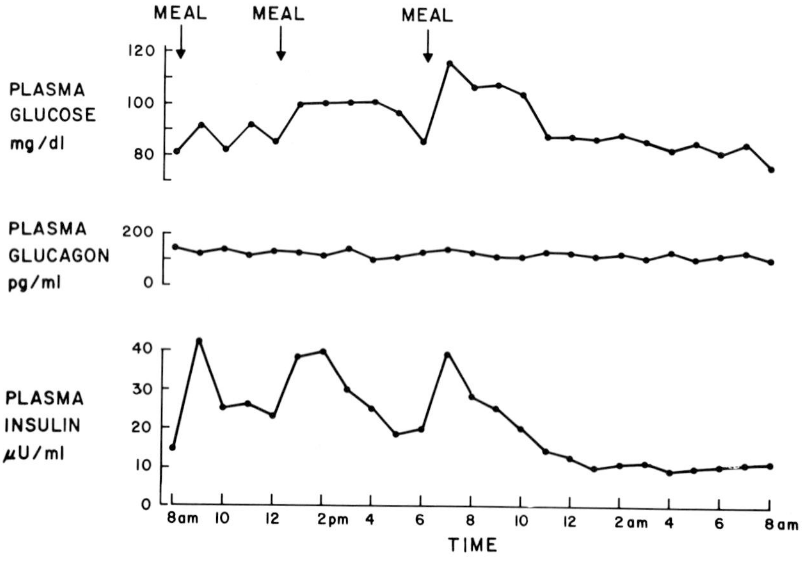

FIGURE 19-20 Fluctuations in plasma glucose, glucagon, and insulin concentrations over a 24-h period in normal healthy subjects ingesting mixed meals. The maximal excursion in plasma glucose concentration over 24 h is generally less than 30 mg/dl. The minimal degree of fluctuation of plasma glucose level is a consequence of the feedback relationship to insulin secretion and the enhancement of insulin secretion by gastrointestinal hormones in response to meal ingestion. In contrast to the changes in plasma insulin concentration, there is virtually no change in plasma glucagon level when mixed meals are fed. (*Modified from Tasaka et al.*[389])

ing mechanism whereby glucose or other stimuli result in the release of insulin from beta cells. Glyceraldehyde, a weak stimulator of calcium release in vitro, was shown to increase free calcium concentrations in beta cells.[74] The increased calcium uptake appeared to be due to a decrease in potassium permeability, resulting in depolarization. These alterations in calcium concentration are a consequence of inhibition of calcium efflux by glucose and enhanced mobilization of stored intracellular calcium by cAMP. The importance of changes in intracellular calcium concentration is strongly supported by studies using ionophores, molecules that act as membrane carriers for ion transport. In the presence of A23187, a specific divalent cation ionophore which transports calcium across biological membranes, addition of calcium to beta cells results in a burst of insulin secretion in the absence of rises in glucose availability or intracellular cAMP concentration.[75]

It should also be noted that glucose, in addition to stimulating calcium entry, may, under certain conditions, lead to intracellular sequestration and extrusion of calcium.[76] Therefore, high levels of glucose may paradoxically cause an inhibition of insulin release, which may be a factor in the low beta cell function noted in persons with poorly controlled type II diabetes.

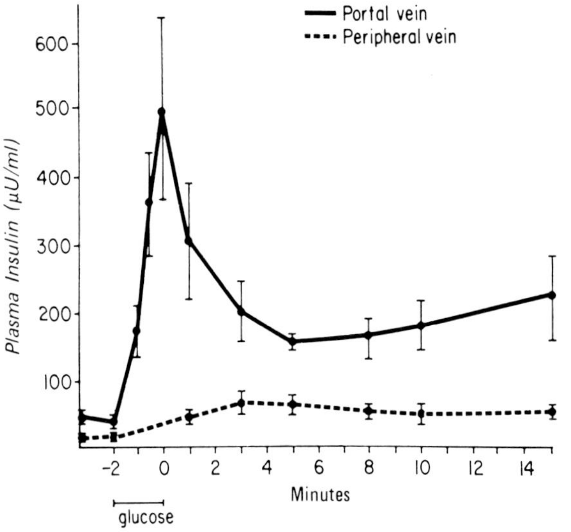

FIGURE 19-22 Plasma insulin concentrations in portal and peripheral venous blood before and after IV administration of glucose. The portal concentration of insulin is three times the peripheral level in the fasting state and may increase to 10 times the peripheral level immediately after glucose is infused. The changes in portal insulin concentration indicate the presence of a biphasic secretory response by the beta cell in which an acute rise in insulin release is followed by a slower, more sustained increment. (*From Blackard WG, Nelson NC: Diabetes 19:302, 1970.*)

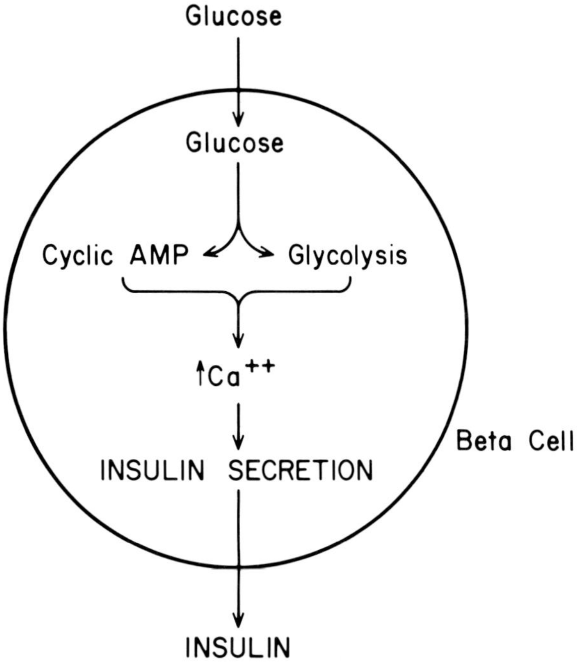

FIGURE 19-21 A simplified scheme of intracellular events underlying the stimulatory effect of glucose on insulin secretion by the beta cell. The entry of glucose into the beta cell is followed by an increase in glycolysis and a rise in cAMP concentration. These metabolic changes result in the accumulation of cytosolic calcium, rises in NADH and NADPH levels, and membrane depolarization, which are all involved in propelling the extrusion of insulin secretory granules.

The overall sequence of events leading to glucose-stimulated insulin secretion is summarized in Fig. 19-21. A characteristic kinetic feature of the insulin response to glucose is its biphasic nature (Fig. 19-22). An initial rapid secretory burst begins within 1 min of presentation of a glycemic stimulus, reaches a peak within 2 min, and declines over the ensuing 3 to 5 min. A second phase, characterized by a more gradual increase in insulin levels, commences 5 to 10 min after the initiation of glucose infusion and continues over the next hour. In the perfused pancreas, puromycin, an inhibitor of protein synthesis, attenuates the second phase but has no effect on the early phase of insulin release. These observations have led to the concept that insulin exists within the beta cell in a two-pool system.[77] An immediately releasable pool consisting of preformed insulin is rapidly discharged during the early secretory phase. A continuing release pool, composed of newly synthesized insulin and small amounts of proinsulin in addition to stored insulin, is gradually discharged during the second phase. The mechanism whereby glucose stimulates the synthesis of insulin is posttranscriptional; it is independent of new mRNA synthesis.[78]

Gastrointestinal Hormones

As early as 1906, Moore et al.[79] suggested that the duodenum provides "a chemical excitant for the internal secretion of the pancreas." Subsequently, La Barre demonstrated a hypoglycemic response to crude preparations of secretin and in 1926 postulated the existence of an "incretin," a factor produced by the gastrointestinal tract which stimulates the internal secretion of the pancreas. Interest in incretins was renewed with the demonstration that the plasma insulin response to an oral glucose load is two or more times greater than after an IV load, despite lower or equal plasma glucose levels (Fig. 19-23).

The GI tract may influence insulin secretion via three mechanisms: (1) provision of high local nutrient concentrations upon absorption and entry into the systemic circulation, (2) release of GI hormones, and (3) emission of neurogenic signals induced by food ingestion (Fig. 19-24). The precise nature of the GI hormones which enhance glucose-stimulated insulin secretion has been the subject of extensive study.[80] To qualify as a physiologic regulator of insulin secretion, a polypeptide should meet two criteria: its concentration must increase after nutrient ingestion, and it must stimulate glucose-mediated insulin release at physiologic concentrations (e.g., at plasma levels comparable to those observed after nutrient ingestion). Of the various gut hormones postulated to influence insulin secretion only gastric inhibitory peptide (GIP) fulfills the necessary criteria. Neither secretin, cholecystokinin (CCK), nor vasoactive inhibitory polypeptide (VIP) show an increment in plasma levels after oral glucose administration. CCK may, however, contribute to the incretin effect observed with oral glucose.

After an oral glucose load, serum levels of GIP increase before or simultaneously with the rise in serum insulin concentration.[81] IV infusion of purified GIP, in amounts resulting in plasma concentrations comparable to those observed after oral glucose administration (1 ng/ml), causes an enhancement of glucose-induced insulin secretion. Furthermore, an insulinotropic effect of endogenous GIP is suggested by the observation that ingestion of corn oil, a potent stimulus for GIP secretion, increases the insulin response to IV glucose. It is likely, however, that gut hormones other than GIP are insulinotropic. The augmented insulin response to oral glucose persists in patients following recovery from resection of the gastric antrum, duodenum, proximal jejunum, and head of the pancreas (Whipple procedure). Furthermore, injection of a potent GIP antiserum reduces but does not abolish the exaggerated insulin response to intraduodenal glucose.[82] These findings suggest that several incretins may exist and may be produced in areas distal to the jejunum.

Amino Acids and Fat-Derived Substrates

Ingestion of protein or infusion of single or multiple amino acids stimulates insulin secretion. As in the case of glucose, stimulation of insulin secretion by orally ingested amino acids exceeds that of IV-administered amino acids, suggesting that enhancement of GI hormones takes place. Protein-stimulated secretion of GIP may mediate this effect.[83] Nonmetabolizable analogues of leucine and arginine have been shown to stimulate insulin secretion, suggesting that membrane recognition (receptor interaction) rather than intracellular metabolism may trigger insulin secretion in this case.[84]

"Redundant regulation" by fat-derived substances is an attractive concept. Accordingly, FFA, or their oxidation products the ketones, whose concentrations are initially elevated by insulin deficiency, subsequently sustain basal insulin secretion at low glucose

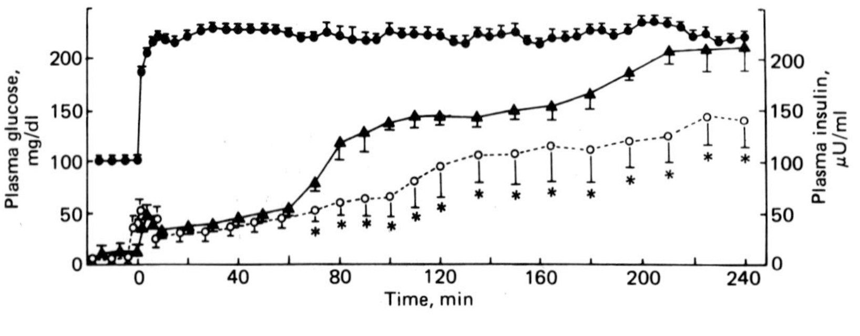

FIGURE 19-23 Enhancing effect of the oral route of glucose administration on plasma insulin response to hyperglycemia. Hyperglycemia was induced and maintained constant (●) by a variable IV infusion of glucose. After 60 min additional glucose was ingested by mouth while the plasma glucose level was maintained at the same hyperglycemic plateau. Despite the constancy of the plasma glucose level, there was a significantly greater rise in plasma insulin concentration after oral glucose (▲) than when hyperglycemia was maintained solely via the IV administration of glucose (○). (*From DeFronzo et al.*[6])

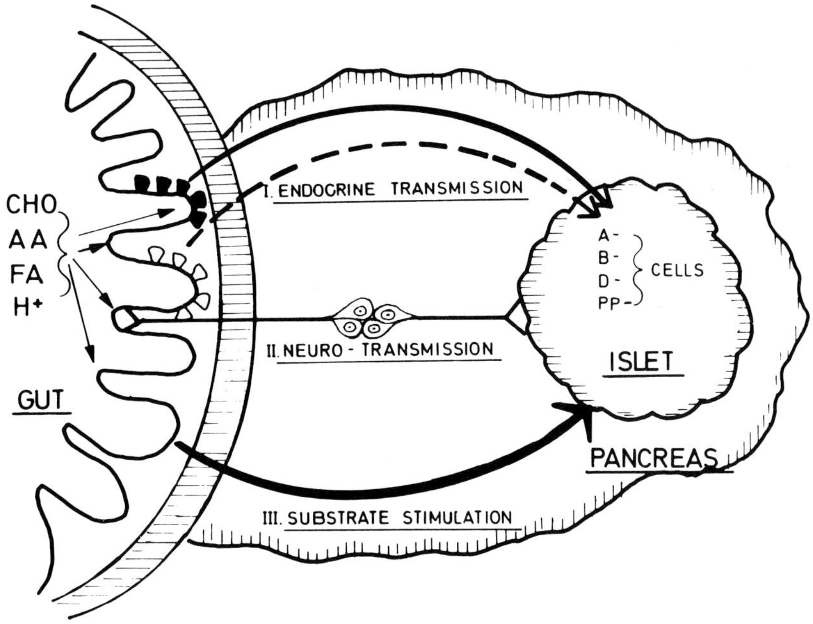

FIGURE 19-24 The enteroinsular axis. Entry of nutrients into the gut influences the secretion of islet cell hormones via three mechanisms: (1) endocrine transmission (e.g., release of gastric inhibitory polypeptide); (2) neurotransmission (e.g., vagal stimulation); and (3) substrate stimulation (e.g., glucose absorption resulting in hyperglycemia). CHO, carbohydrate; AA, amino acids; FA, fatty acids. (*From Creutzfeldt.*[80])

concentration, to prevent unrestrained fat loss from adipose tissue. Evidence supporting this concept is available primarily from animal studies.[47,84a] In obese human subjects bolus injections of acetoacetate cause a small rise in plasma insulin concentration, but this is not observed in nonobese subjects.[85] A small increment in insulin levels has been observed in normal humans following ingestion of medium-chain triglycerides. However, more evidence is needed to establish the validity of an insulin-secretory role of ketones or FFA in humans.

Neural and Neurohumoral Regulation

The catecholamines epinephrine and norepinephrine inhibit glucose-stimulated insulin release via actions mediated by α-adrenergic receptors in the islet cells. That β-adrenergic receptors are present as well is indicated by the stimulatory effect of isoproterenol, which in turn is inhibited by the β-adrenergic blocking agent propranolol. Despite this dual receptor system in the beta cells, the α-adrenergic action of epinephrine predominates; the net effect of epinephrine is therefore inhibition of glucose-stimulated insulin secretion, particularly the rapidly releasable pool. The adrenergic receptors in the islet cells appear to influence insulin secretion via alterations in intracellular cAMP concentration.[86]

The regulatory role of the autonomic nervous system and circulating catecholamines in the control of insulin secretion is manifested both in the physiologic hypoinsulinemia which accompanies exercise and pathologic circumstances such as stress hyperglycemia. During moderate or severe exercise, plasma insulin levels decline in association with a rise in plasma catecholamine concentrations. In stress hyperglycemia (e.g., with severe body burns or compound fractures), the failure of basal insulin levels to rise in association with increases in blood glucose concentration is probably a consequence of catecholamine action. Catecholamines also contribute to the blunted insulin response observed in patients with pheochromocytoma. On the other hand, very modest (two- to threefold) increments in plasma epinephrine concentration, as occur, e.g., with a mild viral illness, result in glucose intolerance by interfering with insulin action rather than inhibiting secretion[87] (see below).

In contrast to the action of epinephrine, the result of stimulation of the parasympathetic nervous system (e.g., the vagus nerves) is increased insulin secretion. However, the effect of atropine administration on insulin secretion in humans is only modest.

Participation of the central nervous system in the regulation of insulin secretion is indicated by the response to stimulation or destruction of hypothalamic nuclei. Stimulation of the ventromedial nuclei suppresses insulin release. This effect is reversed by adrenalectomy, suggesting that mediation occurs via adrenomedullary catecholamines. In contrast, destruction of the ventromedial nuclei leads to hyperinsulinism and hyperphagia.[88]

Other neurohumoral agents which have been

identified within islet tissue and have also been shown to influence insulin secretion are serotonin and dopamine.[89] The response to serotonin is species-specific: serotonin stimulates or has no effect on insulin secretion in the dog and human; it inhibits insulin release in the golden hamster and rabbit. Dopamine has been shown to diminish insulin release in vitro.

An inhibitory effect of prostaglandin A on insulin secretion has been observed in dogs and humans. Diminished insulin secretion in type II diabetes may in part be mediated by prostaglandin synthesis.[90] The cyclooxygenase pathway has been found to exert an inhibitory effect on glucose-induced insulin secretion, whereas the lipooxygenase pathway stimulates insulin release.[91] Naturally occurring opioids (enkephalins, endorphins) may not in themselves stimulate insulin secretion but may potentiate the effect of glucose or glyceraldehyde.[92] This may occur by a mechanism involving an increase in cAMP level and calcium uptake. The endocrine pancreas appears to have several types of opioid peptide receptors.[92]

Somatostatin

Somatostatin is a tetradecapeptide originally isolated from the hypothalamus as a GH release inhibitory factor and subsequently identified by immunofluorescent techniques in pancreatic islet cells, stomach antrum, jejunal cells of the GI tract, and a variety of areas of the brain.[93] In addition to interfering with release of GH, somatostatin is a potent inhibitor of both insulin and glucagon secretion. This effect of somatostatin on islet hormones represents a direct action which is demonstrable with in vitro techniques. Within the islets of Langerhans, somatostatin is localized to the delta cells located at the periphery of the islets. An increase in somatostatin-containing cells has been observed in rats rendered diabetic by streptozotocin and in some forms of genetic diabetes in experimental animals.

In addition to altering islet cell and GH secretion, somatostatin has been demonstrated to inhibit a variety of GI hormones, including gastrin, CCK, and secretin.[93] Diminished absorption of glucose and protein, decreased splanchnic blood flow,[94] and decreased gastrointestinal motility have also been noted. In addition, in patients with islet cell tumors composed of somatostatin-containing cells (somatostatinomas), steatorrhea is a prominent symptom.[95]

A major unresolved question concerns the physiologic role of somatostatin in the regulation of insulin and glucagon secretion as well as nutrient absorption. A rise in somatostatin concentration has been reported after glucose or fat ingestion and has been proposed to be a modulator of nutrient absorption.[96] Somatostatin has also been proposed to regulate insulin and glucagon secretion by release into the interstitial environment of the beta and alpha cells, a phenomenon which has been designated a paracrine effect. Undoubtedly, the myriad inhibitory effects of somatostatin on endocrine secretion and GI function (secretion, absorption, and motility) are at least in part pharmacologic in nature (Fig. 19-25).

Other Hormones

In GH-deficient dwarfs, diminutions in basal, glucose-stimulated, and arginine-induced insulin levels are observed. In contrast, hyperinsulinemia is a characteristic finding in acromegaly. A stimulatory action of glucagon on beta cell secretion has been demonstrated with the perfused pancreas. However, the small increments in plasma insulin concentration observed during in vivo infusions of glucagon in physiologic doses are probably a result of the accompanying rise in plasma glucose concentration.

Hyperinsulinemia has been observed with exogenous administration or endogenous increments of adrenocorticosteroids, estrogens, progestins, and parathyroid hormone. Since glucose levels are not reduced and sometimes are even raised in these situations, it may be inferred that resistance to the effectiveness of insulin accompanies these hormonal changes. There is no convincing evidence that these hormones have a direct effect on insulin secretion. Alternatively, some feedback signal from the insulin-resistant tissues or hyperglycemia may provide the necessary insulinotropic stimulus to the beta cells.

Obesity

The most common hyperinsulinemic condition encountered in humans is obesity. High plasma insulin levels are observed in obese individuals in the basal state as well as after meal ingestion. That hyperinsulinemia is a consequence rather than a cause of obesity is indicated by the fact that loss of weight results in a fall in insulin level while gain in weight in previously lean individuals is followed by a rise in plasma insulin concentration. The various factors determining the magnitude of hyperinsulinemia in obesity include (1) the extent of adiposity, (2) the caloric and carbohydrate content of the meals ingested, and (3) the extent of physical activity. The correlation between plasma insulin levels and body weight is due to adiposity rather than augmented muscle mass (as in weight lifters). On the other hand, a decrease in carbohydrate content of the diet or an overall reduction in caloric intake results in normalization of insulin

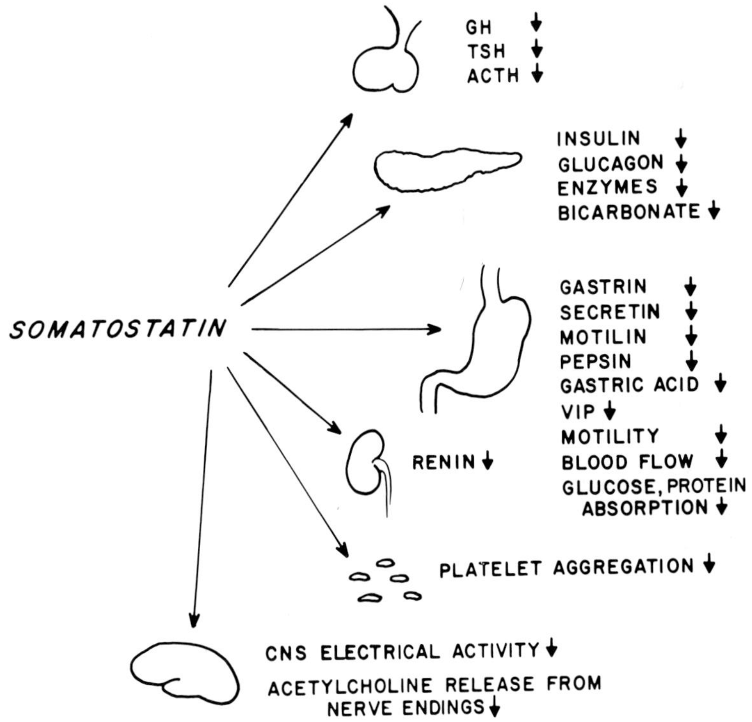

FIGURE 19-25 The multisystem inhibitory effects of somatostatin. In addition to inhibiting GH, insulin, and glucagon secretion, somatostatin has been shown to inhibit a variety of GI functions: secretion of GI hormones and splanchnic blood flow are decreased, motility is inhibited, and absorption of glucose and amino acids is reduced.

levels well before ideal body weight has been attained. In addition, physical training may result in a fall in insulin level independent of weight loss.[97]

The precise signal responsible for basal and postmeal hyperinsulinemia in the obese has not been established; hyperaminoacidemia has been suggested as a possible mechanism.[57] Inasmuch as obesity is not accompanied by hypoglycemia and in fact is associated with a tendency to develop type 2 diabetes (see below), the obese condition is clearly an insulin-resistant state.

INSULIN ACTION

Insulin is the primary factor which controls the storage and metabolism of ingested metabolic fuels. After a meal, secretion of insulin facilitates the uptake, utilization, and storage of glucose, fat, and amino acids. Conversely, a reduction in circulating insulin concentration leads to mobilization of endogenous fuels and reduced uptake of ingested nutrients. The action of insulin involves all three major metabolic fuels, carbohydrate, protein, and fat, and occurs in three principal tissues, liver, muscle, and adipose tissue. In each of these tissues there are anticatabolic as well as anabolic effects of insulin which act to reinforce each other (Table 19-3).

Carbohydrate Metabolism

The liver is a major site of insulin action in the disposal of an oral glucose load.[99-101] Since glucose is absorbed via the portal system, the extent to which an oral glucose load is available for uptake by peripheral tissues depends upon its escape from the splanchnic bed. During the 3-h period following the ingestion of 100 g of glucose, 30 to 60 g is taken up by the liver and used for glycogen synthesis and triglyceride formation. Of the total ingested glucose, it appears that only ~10 percent is taken up on the first pass. Since the major portion of glucose in the portal vein is recirculating, the hepatic glucose uptake exceeds 50 percent of the total. In addition, ~15 percent of the hepatic glycogen is promptly synthesized from three-carbon glucose precursors formed from peripheral and hepatic glucose degradation.[101a]

The relative amount of glucose directly deposited as glycogen in the liver vs. the amount requiring resynthesis from the three-carbon compounds can be inferred from randomization of labeled glucose carbons upon incorporation into glycogen. These estimates may vary with species. The role of the liver as the primary site of glucose uptake was questioned when the proportion of directly vs. indirectly formed glycogen in fasting rats was found as low as ~1:2.[102] Similar proportion was obtained in another study in

Table 19-3. Insulin Action on Liver, Adipose Tissue, and Muscle

	Liver	Adipose tissue	Muscle
Anticatabolic effects	Glycogenolysis Gluconeogenesis Ketogenesis	Lipolysis	Proteolysis Amino acid output
Anabolic effects	Glycogen synthesis Fatty acid synthesis	Fatty acid uptake, synthesis, and esterification	Amino acid uptake Protein synthesis Glycogen synthesis

rats,[102a] in which ^{13}C-glucose labeling pattern was traced by NMR spectroscopy.

Recently the randomization was assessed by trapping of carbons from UDP-glucose (the direct precursor of glycogen). Administration of diflunisal, a drug requiring hepatic glucuronidization for its excretion, and isolation of the UDP-glucose–derived glucuronide from urine of humans receiving the labeled hexose permitted the estimate that 70 to 75 percent of hepatic glycogen is formed directly from glucose.[102b]

In circumstances of mixed-meal intake, the blood glucose concentration in normal humans generally rises only by 30 to 40 mg/dl (1.7 to 3.4 mM) over 24 h (Fig. 19-20). This fine tuning of blood glucose regulation is determined by the exquisite sensitivity of the liver to small changes in insulin secretion. When blood glucose concentration rises by only 10 to 15 mg/dl (0.6 to 0.8 mM), there is a 60 to 100 percent increase in peripheral insulin levels and virtually complete inhibition of hepatic glucose output (i.e., sparing of hepatic glycogen and cessation of gluconeogenesis) with no stimulation of peripheral glucose utilization.[64] Thus, as compared with the liver, muscle and adipose tissue are less sensitive with respect to responses to small increases in plasma insulin concentration. In fact, the plasma concentration of insulin necessary for half-maximal stimulation of peripheral glucose uptake is several times higher than that required for half-maximal inhibition of hepatic glucose output.[101] Nevertheless, with significant peripheral hyperinsulinemia, glucose uptake by fat and muscle tissue helps minimize the fluctuations in systemic blood glucose level.

In view of the permeability of the hepatocyte to glucose, uptake of glucose by the liver is not rate-limiting. The first potential control point is initiation of glucose metabolism by phosphorylation to G6P. As mentioned above, phosphorylation in the liver takes place under the influence of hexokinase and glucokinase. While hexokinase is saturated at physiologic glucose concentrations, glucokinase is only half-saturated at the glucose concentration of 180 mg/dl (10 mM). Consequently, hepatic glucose uptake, by fully using glucokinase capacity, adjusts to the changing blood glucose concentration.

As noted above (see Glycolysis), a second crucial step in the glycolytic pathway involves the phosphorylation of F6P by PFK-1 activated by $F2,6P_2$ (Fig. 19-5). When insulin is plentiful this is efficiently accomplished and has significance not only with regard to stimulation of glycolysis but also with respect to inhibition of gluconeogenesis. In contrast, insulin deficiency results in reduced levels of $F2,6P_2$, decreased activity of PFK-1, and activation of FDPase. The net effect is a reversal of substrate flow from pyruvate (and alanine) to glucose, a catabolic process.

The glycogen content of the liver in patients with diabetic acidosis is significantly reduced but is promptly restored following insulin administration. This effect of insulin is due to its ability to activate glycogen synthase and reduce the activity of phosphorylase (Fig. 19-4) within a few minutes after it is administered.

The salient effect of insulin on the output of glucose from the liver is not only promotion of glycogen synthesis, but mainly, inhibition of gluconeogenesis. The rate-limiting step in the gluconeogenic pathway lies between pyruvate and phospho*enol*pyruvate, which depends on the relative activities of PC and PEPCK on the one hand and pyruvate kinase on the other hand (Fig. 19-6). The activities of these enzymes are adjusted inversely either through rapid inhibition by specific metabolites or by slower, insulin-dependent induction/deinduction, as discussed above (see Fig. 19-6 and corresponding text).

In addition to influencing hepatic gluconeogenesis by altering FFA availability, it has been suggested that insulin diminishes gluconeogenesis by decreasing the supply of precursor amino acids. A number of studies, however, do not support this hypothesis. For example, exogenous insulin fails to inhibit release of alanine, the key glucogenic amino acid, from peripheral muscle tissues. In like manner, plasma alanine levels show no consistent diminution after stimulation of endogenous insulin secretion. In contrast, glucose-stimulated insulin secretion results in a fall of hepatic alanine uptake, despite unchanged arterial alanine levels. The bulk of the evidence thus indicates that insulin regulates gluconeogenesis, primarily by altering intrahepatic processes rather than by influencing the rate of precursor supply.[99–101]

Inhibition of gluconeogenesis requires greater amounts of insulin than are necessary for inhibition of glycogenolysis. Thus, a 60 to 100 percent increase in plasma insulin concentration results in virtually complete inhibition of glycogenolysis, yet hepatic uptake and conversion of alanine, lactate, and pyruvate to glucose persists in the face of such minor increments of insulin concentration.[64,103] It should be noted that net liver glycogen storage has been suggested to occur in the face of active conversion of three-carbon precursors to G6P.[102] Thus, gluconeogenesis need not always be accompanied by net output of glucose from the liver.

A major question in the overall control of hepatic glucose metabolism concerns the relative importance of hyperinsulinemia and hyperglycemia as regulatory signals. Soskin and Levine in the 1940s proposed that blood glucose concentration is the primary stimulus that determines glucose uptake or glucose output by the liver. Support of this hypothesis derives from studies demonstrating that (1) glycogen synthase and phosphorylase are exquisitely sensitive to the ambient glucose concentration,[5] (2) hyperglycemia at constant insulin concentration inhibits hepatic glucose output from human[8] and rat liver[104] and (3) in the absence of hyperglycemia, hyperinsulinemia fails to induce net uptake of glucose by the liver.[6] When insulin concentration is raised between 400 to 600 μU/ml in euglycemic men, splanchnic uptake accounts for only < 8 percent of total glucose metabolism.[101] In contrast, other data emphasize the importance of insulin in regulating hepatic glucose output: (1) in insulin-deficient diabetic subjects, hyperglycemia induced by glucose infusion fails to inhibit hepatic glucose output;[105] (2) in perfused liver insulin activates glycogen synthase in the absence of added glucose;[105] and (3) much smaller increments in blood glucose concentration (10 to 15 mg/dl) effectively inhibit hepatic glucose output when accompanied by a rise in insulin concentration as compared with the increments in arterial glucose concentration (60 mg/dl) required to inhibit hepatic glucose output when insulin concentrations are kept at basal levels. There is also evidence that, even in the face of hyperglycemia and hyperinsulinemia, net uptake of glucose by the liver is relatively small (<15 percent of total glucose utilization) unless the glucose is administered orally[6] or via the portal vein.[106,107] It has also been suggested that in the postprandial phase dietary carbohydrate is converted into liver glycogen indirectly, mostly via lactate and alanine flowing in from the periphery. In this situation the G6P elaborated from pyruvate would be preferentially directed to glycogen rather than to glucose.[100]

The overall data thus indicate that hyperinsulinemia, hyperglycemia, and possibly signals from the GI tract, portal vein,[106,107] and glucogenic substrate flow contribute to the regulation of hepatic glucose balance. A rise in insulin concentration markedly increases the sensitivity of the liver to the inhibitory effects of glucose on hepatic glucose release. In like manner, a rise in glucose concentration facilitates and is probably essential for insulin-induced uptake of glucose by the liver. The net uptake of glucose by the liver is further stimulated when glucose is administered orally rather than IV.[6] A "portal factor" rather than a "gut factor" has been postulated to promote hepatic glucose uptake, since intraportal rather than peripheral delivery of glucose may cause greater hepatic uptake.[106,107]

Unlike the situation in the hepatocyte, the rate of entry of glucose into the muscle cell, at physiologic concentrations of plasma glucose, is the slowest (and therefore the rate-limiting) step. A major effect of insulin in this tissue is to control the transport of glucose across the cell membrane; the major end product of glucose uptake in nonexercising muscle is glycogen. The PFK system in muscle is also influenced by insulin, via a mechanism similar to that in the liver, except that the reverse reaction, in the direction of glucose production, is of little significance in this tissue. It should be emphasized that glucose uptake by exercising muscle is not dependent on an increase in insulin secretion (see Exercise, below).

In the fat cell, too, insulin acts primarily to stimulate transport of glucose across the cell membrane. An effect is also observed on glycogen synthase and on PFK. The major end products of glucose metabolism in the adipose cell are fatty acids and glycerol 3-phosphate. The latter is important for fat storage because it provides the glycerol moiety necessary for triglyceride synthesis. As noted above, most synthesis of carbohydrate-derived fatty acids in humans occurs in the liver rather than adipose tissue (Fig. 19-11).

Amino Acid and Protein Metabolism

Insulin increases the transport of most amino acids into muscles, stimulates protein synthesis, and inhibits protein catabolism.[108] In intact humans, intrabrachial arterial infusion of insulin in physiologic amounts results in diminished output of amino acids from deep forearm tissues. This effect is particularly prominent with respect to the branched-chain amino acids leucine and isoleucine, as well as tyrosine and phenylalanine. The action of insulin on muscle amino acid exchange probably accounts for its ability to lower systemic amino acid levels. In the absence of adequate insulin, e.g., in the diabetic patient in ketoacidosis, elevations are observed in plasma levels of valine, leucine, and isoleucine. In addition, the uptake of these amino acids by muscle tissue after the ingestion of a protein meal is reduced in the absence of adequate amounts of insulin.[55,108] Thus the stimulatory effect of ingested protein on insulin secretion (see above) serves to promote the uptake and anabolic utilization of the constituent amino acids.

In addition to its effect on protein synthesis, the overall anabolic action of insulin derives from its ability to inhibit protein catabolism. Insulin was shown to inhibit the diabetes-induced rise in the activity of a protease bound to the myofibrils of skeletal muscle.[109,110] The oxidation of branched-chain amino acids by muscle tissue is also inhibited by insulin and is accelerated in the diabetic state. Insulin thus increases body protein stores via at least four mechanisms: (1) increased tissue uptake of amino acids, (2) increased protein synthesis, (3) decreased protein catabolism, and (4) decreased oxidation of amino acids.

Fat Metabolism

In the liver the synthesis of fatty acids is stimulated at high insulin concentration. This effect reflects several actions: (1) the increased flow of substrate down the glycolytic pathway into the TCA cycle increases the availability of citrate, which stimulates the liposynthetic pathways, particularly the activity of acetyl CoA carboxylase (Fig. 19-10); (2) the reduction of FFA inflow removes the inhibitory influences which may be exerted on acetyl CoA carboxylase; (3) the availability of NADPH, which is a necessary hydrogen donor for synthesis of fatty acids, is increased by insulin through the induction of pentose shunt and $NADP^+$-malate dehydrogenase enzymes; (4) insulin directly stimulates aetyl CoA carboxylase both by promoting its synthesis and preventing its phosphorylation. In the human, stimulation of hepatic lipogenesis is tantamount to stimulation of total body fat production, since the triglycerides are mostly liver-derived and VLDL-transported for deposition in adipose tissue; all these processes are insulin-dependent.

Insulin accelerates the removal of circulating triglycerides derived from exogenous or endogenous sources by inducing the synthesis of the adipose tissue "entry" enzyme, lipoprotein lipase. In addition, insulin is extremely effective in inhibiting the intracellular (hormone-sensitive) lipase which catalyzes the hydrolysis of stored triglycerides and liberation of FFA. The antilipolytic effect occurs at concentrations of insulin below those necessary to promote glucose transport; this is considered the most sensitive action of insulin. Furthermore, a large proportion of the glucose from insulin-promoted uptake in the fat cell is used for the formation of glycerol 3-phosphate for FFA esterification. The net effect of these antilipolytic, glycerogenic, lipogenic, and lipid-assimilating actions of insulin is to increase total fat.

In addition to affecting fatty acid metabolism, insulin has a profound suppressive effect on circulating blood ketone concentrations. The formation and accumulation of β-hydroxybutyrate and acetoacetate are consequences of three distinct metabolic events: (1) unrestrained mobilization of FFA from adipose tissue; (2) surplus of hepatic acetyl CoA due to excessive FFA oxidation; the acetyl CoA has to be converted to ketones because of TCA cycle saturation; and (3) a reduction in ketone utilization by peripheral tissues. As already noted, insulin is a powerful antilipolytic hormone. In addition, insulin decreases the liver's capacity to oxidize fatty acids irrespective of substrate availability. This antiketogenic action of insulin is intimately related to both its regulation of hepatic carnitine levels and its stimulation of fatty acid synthesis, which increases malonyl CoA availability. These two factors are instrumental in rerouting fatty acyl CoA; they prevent it from entering the oxidative spiral in the mitochondria and redirect it into microsomal esterification to triglycerides (Figs. 19-10 and 19-13). The net result is a reduction in the ketogenic capacity of the liver. In addition, in the presence of insulin, the uptake and oxidation of ketone acids by muscle tissue is accelerated.[111]

The diverse effects of insulin on body fuel metabolism tend to reinforce each other (Table 19-3). Thus, the inhibition of gluconeogenesis spares amino acids for protein synthesis. Similarly, the inhibition of lipolysis decreases the availability of acetyl CoA needed for stimulation of gluconeogenic enzymes. Enhancement of fat synthesis increases the availability of malonyl CoA, which antagonizes the oxidation of fatty acids; fatty acid concentration is also reduced by insulin's antilipolytic effects.

Potassium and Sodium Metabolism

Insulin deficiency in diabetes is known to be associated with plasma cation losses due to increased use of cations for neutralizing organic acids, particularly ketoacids, thus enabling excretion of the acids. The drain affects particularly the total pools of body sodium and potassium (the latter is also released from tissues to meet the neutralization requirements).

Administration of exogenous insulin or stimulation of endogenous insulin secretion reverses the potassium outflow and results in a fall in serum potassium concentration. This hypokalemic action of insulin is due to stimulation of potassium uptake by muscle and liver tissue, which may occur independently of changes in glucose metabolism. The regulatory role of insulin in potassium metabolism is underscored by the changes in serum potassium concentration which accompany a reduction in basal insulin level. In association with a 50 percent decline in fasting insulin level induced by somatostatin, serum potassium concentration increases by 0.5 to 1.0 meq/l.[112] This hyperkalemic effect of modest insulinopenia is not due to altered renal handling of potassium. The sensitivity of body potassium homeostasis to minor changes in insulin secretion may in part explain the tendency of diabetic patients to develop hyperkalemia in the absence of uremia or acidosis.

Insulin has also been shown to influence sodium metabolism, although this action (in contrast to the effects on potassium) is a consequence of altered renal secretion of this cation.[112a] Following a physiologic increase in plasma insulin concentration, urinary sodium excretion falls in the absence of changes in glomerular filtration rate (GFR) or aldosterone excretion. In contrast, inhibition of basal insulin secretion by somatostatin is accompanied by a 50 percent increase in urinary sodium excretion. The antinatriuretic effect of insulin may account for the edema which occasionally appears in hyperglycemic diabetic patients following blood glucose regulation by insulin treatment. Similarly, the refeeding edema observed after starved or malnourished subjects are refed and the diuresis which accompanies starvation may be mediated in part by altered secretion of insulin.

INSULIN RECEPTORS

Receptor Interaction and Structure

As in the case of other polypeptide hormones, insulin initially binds to a specific receptor on the plasma membrane of the cell. A model of the insulin receptor is depicted in Fig. 19-26. The receptor is a symmetrical tetrameric protein composed of two α and two β subunits linked by disulfide bonds forming a $\beta\alpha\alpha\beta$ structure. The receptor is designed to carry out three functions:[113] (1) recognition of insulin by binding the hormone with high specificity, (2) transmission of a signal which results in activation of intracellular metabolic pathways and, (3) endocytosis of the complex leading to lysosomal proteolysis of insulin with recycling of the subunits to the membrane.

The α subunit, of 135,000 daltons, is the binding unit; the 95,000-dalton β subunit is the effector unit. The latter possesses an insulin-sensitive protein kinase activity, specifically phosphorylating tyrosine residues in proteins, and is responsible for signal transduction across the plasma membrane. Both subunits have been found to be glycoproteins, containing carbohydrate side chains which are involved in insulin binding.[114]

The physiologic essence of a hormone receptor is its specificity of binding and the close relation of this binding to the expression of hormone action. In studies involving over 40 insulin analogues, a direct relation has been demonstrated between the affinity of different insulins and insulin analogues for the recep-

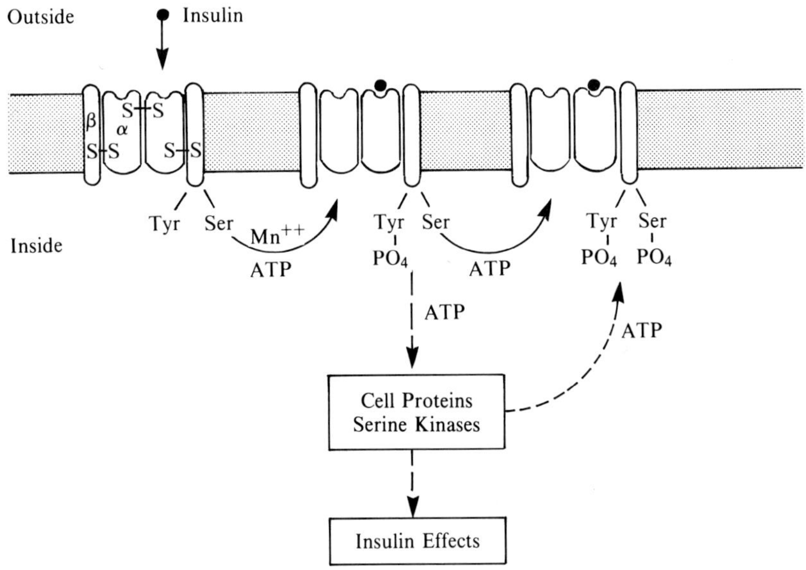

FIGURE 19-26 Model of the membranal insulin receptor and the intracellular transmission of the signal generated by insulin binding. Insulin binds to the external α subunit of the receptor. As a result, the tyrosine kinase activity on the internal segment of the β-subunit becomes activated (left) and the insulin receptor undergoes autophosphorylation (middle). Three factors affect the activity of tyrosine kinase: (1) receptor-bound insulin, which increases V_{max}; (2) M_n^{2+}, which decreases the K_m toward ATP; (3) the state of receptor phosphorylation, which sustains the activity after removal of insulin. The activated receptor kinase is cytosol-oriented and most probably continues to phosphorylate other intracellular proteins and enzymes with regulatory function, thereby propagating the insulin message. In addition, serine residues on the receptor are also phosphorylated (right) in the basal state; their phosphorylation increases in the course of signal transmission. (*From Kahn and Crettaz.*[113])

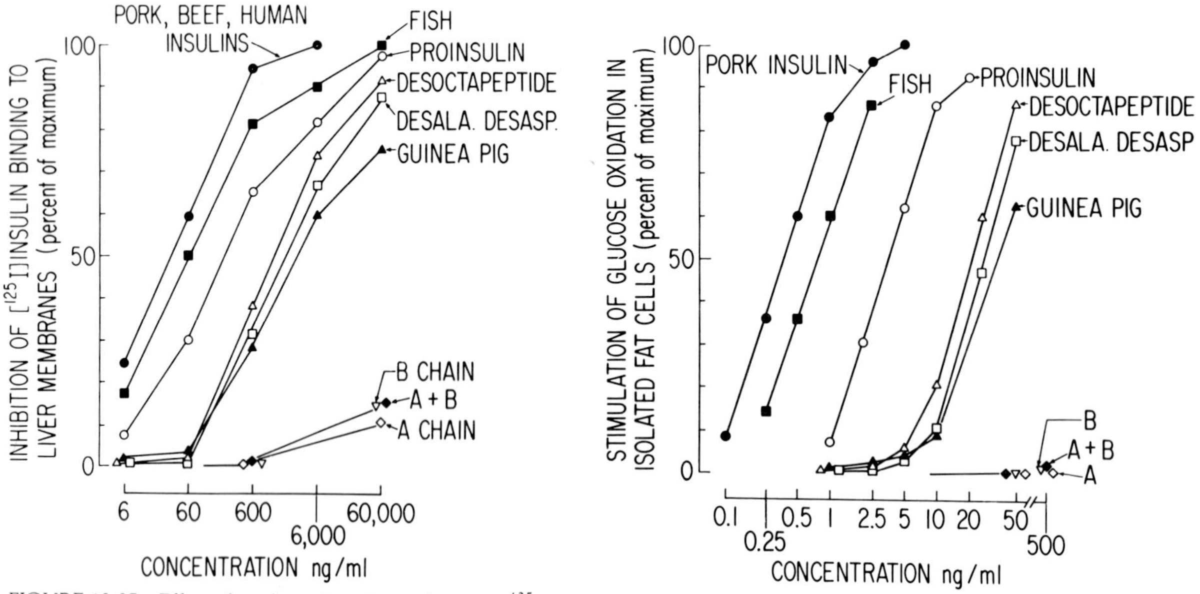

FIGURE 19-27 Effect of insulin and insulin analogues on ^{125}I-labeled insulin binding to liver membranes (*left*) and glucose oxidation in fat cells (*right*). Note the close correlation between affinity for the receptor (*left*) and biological effect (*right*). (*From Freychet P et al: Proc Natl Acad Sci USA 68:1833, 1971.*)

tor and the biological activity resulting from this interaction (Fig. 19-27).

The interaction between insulin and its receptor is not a simple, reversible bimolecular reaction with a single affinity or equilibrium constant; it is more complex, demonstrating heterogeneity of ligand affinity. This complexity is revealed by the curvilinear nature and upward concave shape of the plots obtained when insulin binding data are subjected to Scatchard analysis.[115] These findings have been interpreted as indicating the presence of "negative cooperativity," a phenomenon in which increasing occupancy of receptors results in decreased affinity for additional insulin molecules due to site-site interactions.[116] Negative cooperativity can occur either by allosteric transformation of the second subunit after insulin has interacted with the first subunit, or alteration of receptor affinity, resulting from the formation of receptor oligomers. The varous steric forms of the receptor are postulated to be in equilibrium in the plasma membrane of the cell, changing with insulin concentration. Although strong evidence was submitted for the negative cooperativity model, other explanations for the Scatchard plot pattern exist. They are based on the presence of two distinct classes of receptors, one with high affinity and low capacity, the other with low affinity and high capacity.[117,118] The existence of different classes of binding sites is suggested by the evidence that there are high-molecular-weight oligomeric forms of the receptor,[119,120] which seem to involve complexes of α, β, or α and β subunits exhibiting decreased affinity for insulin. Formation of receptor oligomers could account for receptor aggregation, which may be important in modifying insulin action. Such a model of the insulin receptor has been compared to the association of adenyl cyclase with its receptor,[113] effecting the formation of cAMP from ATP. In both systems, linkage of the biologically active form of the receptor to an effector system results in increased molecular weight and decreased receptor affinity. Whereas in the insulin receptor the β (effector) subunit is linked to the α subunit by disulfide bridges, the G protein effector in the adenyl cyclase system is noncovalently bonded.[121]

Insulin receptors have been found to be ubiquitous in mammals. They have been demonstrated in insulin-responsive tissues as well as those tissues and cells not directly responsive to insulin, such as the brain,[122] erythrocytes,[123] vascular endothelial cells,[124] gonadal cells,[125] and placenta.[125a] Presence of receptors may signify a dependence on slow, long-term effects of insulin, e.g., growth. Insulin receptors may vary in structure, depending on the tissue in which they are found. Small differences have been found in molecular weight, nature of disulfide bonding of subunits, and state of receptor aggregation.

Insulin Receptor Turnover

Insulin receptors constantly turn over, as do other membrane proteins. The receptor is probably synthesized from a partially glycosylated proreceptor of

190,000 daltons.[114] After further glycosylation and cleavage, the α and β subunits are inserted into the plasma membrane.[126] This takes from 1.5 to 3 h.

Electron microscopic studies have provided direct evidence that, following the binding of insulin to its receptor, the hormone-receptor complex enters the cell by endocytosis, where the hormone and the subunits may be degraded in lysosomes[127] (Fig. 19-28). However, most of the internalized receptors are recycled back to the membrane.[128] Degradation is enhanced by exposure to insulin: the half-life of the receptor is 7 to 12 h, but this can be shortened to 2 to 3 h in the presence of insulin.[114] A single receptor makes several cycles before being degraded.[129] Recent studies have suggested that the hormone-receptor complex is concentrated in Golgi-enriched endosomes to a greater degree than in lysosomes.[130] The endosomes may function as a clearinghouse wherein the hormone-receptor complex is dissociated; the hormone may then be directed to lysosomes and the receptor recycled back to the cell surface.[130] Alternatively, the receptor can be degraded by lysosomal proteolysis or remain sequestered. The proportion of receptors recycled, degraded, or sequestered determines the final receptor concentration and the amount found on the cell surface at any particular time, which varies with the type of tissue.[130,131]

A salient regulatory feature of the insulin receptor is its susceptibility to the ambient insulin concentration. In circumstances of hyperinsulinemia (e.g., obesity), the number of insulin receptors is reduced ("*down regulation*") while the reverse ("*up regulation*") occurs with hypoinsulinemia (e.g., starvation). These changes apply to the membrane concentration of the receptors, which are shifted to intracellular storage, sequestration, and/or degradation.[130,131] In addition, they may also involve formation or dissociation of oligomeric forms.

Insulin Receptor Phosphorylation

Phosphorylation, the process whereby phosphate groups are transferred from high-energy donors (e.g., ATP) to hydroxyl acceptors on amino acid residues on proteins, is mediated by protein kinases. Binding of insulin to the receptor activates the tyrosine-specific protein kinase which effects receptor autophosphorylation.[132,132a] Although the precise physiologic role of the receptor tyrosine kinase activity is not fully established, it is likely that this activity is a transmembrane signal leading to the biological effects of insulin. The receptor kinase activity is probably reflected in continuing phosphorylation of intracellular proteins, some of them possibly with protein kinase activity. These kinases may, in turn, continue the phosphorylation cascade with resultant activity modulations of the phosphorylation-sensitive cellular metabolic systems.

The insulin receptor is also phosphorylated on serine residues[132,132a] (Fig. 19-26), both in the basal state

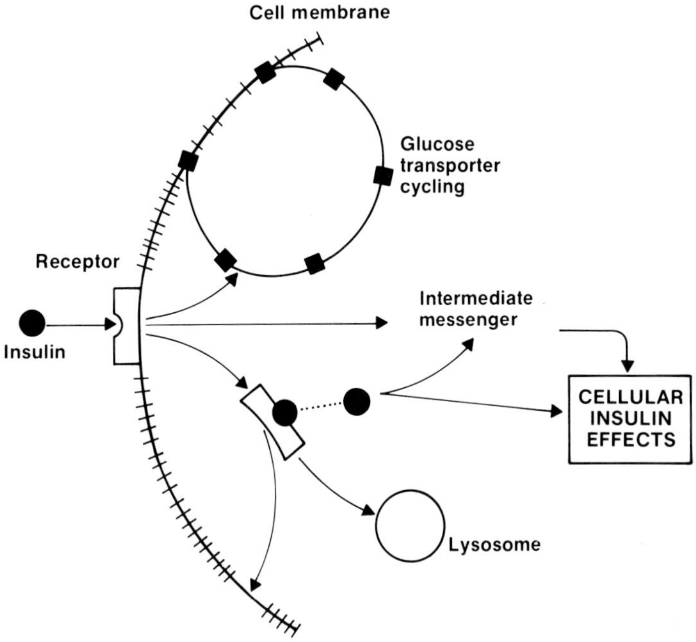

FIGURE 19-28 Events following the interaction of insulin with its receptor. Binding of insulin results in autophosphorylation and increased receptor kinase activity (as outlined in Fig. 19-26), which may transduce the insulin message by phosphorylating intracellular proteins. In addition, generation of an intermediate "second messenger" was postulated to transmit the insulin signal to intracellular proteins regulating various metabolic and protein-synthetic pathways and to initiate nuclear synthetic events. Following insulin binding there is increased internalization of the receptor translocating to the lysosomes and Golgi apparatus for degradation or recycling to the membrane. Intracellular actions of the activated receptor and of bound or dissociated insulin are possible. Furthermore, binding of insulin triggers a brisk cycling of glucose transporters, facilitating glucose entry into insulin-dependent cells.

and in the course of insulin binding. Phorbol esters, known for their insulin-like action, have been recently found to promote the phosphorylation of serine residues on the receptor,[133,134] which probably extends to other proteins as well. Thus, one of the intracellular phosphorylation substrates of the receptor kinase could be protein kinase C, a Ca^{2+}- and phospholipid-dependent serine-phosphorylating enzyme involved in the regulation of metabolic processes and cell growth and proliferation. The interaction of the tyrosine- and serine-specific kinases is not known; it has been suggested that they may mediate insulin action on metabolism and growth in dual or sequential modes.[132a] It is pertinent that some receptors for insulin-like growth factors also undergo autophosphorylation upon emergence of tyrosine kinase activity; they include epidermal growth factor,[135] platelet-derived growth factor,[136] and insulin-like growth factor 1 (IGF 1, or somatomedin C)[137] (see below).

Insulin is known to stimulate the synthesis of certain phospholipids, especially diacylglycerol and 1,4,5-triphosphoinositol as well as the activity of phospholipase C.[138] Insulin receptor itself has a phosphoinositol kinase activity.[139] These phospholipids are postulated to act as intracellular "second messengers" of insulin.[140,141] Diacylglycerol stimulates protein kinase C activity; diacylglycerol and insulin synergistically stimulate DNA synthesis and cell growth.[141] In addition, protein kinase C, in stimulating serine phosphorylation of the receptor (as it does elsewhere), may exert desensitizing feedback action, since excessive serine phosphorylation weakens the activity of tyrosine-phosphorylated receptors.[113]

POSTRECEPTOR EVENTS

While the kinetic phenomena related to insulin-receptor interaction are reasonably characterized, the molecular mechanisms leading to the modification of cellular processes such as glucose transport, glycogen synthesis and breakdown, lipolysis proteolysis, enzyme transcription, and translation remain to be elucidated. Studies reviewed recently[142–146] support the following concepts (Fig. 19-28):

1. The intracellular transport of glucose, early identified as a prominent effect of insulin, has now been shown to be carried out by membrane vesicles, termed *glucose transporters*.[147,148] Within seconds of insulin binding to the receptor translocation of the glucose transporters from an intracellular pool to the plasma membrane occurs, with acceleration of the cycling of transporters. These are probably the most immediate events in the receptor-mediated stimulation of glucose transport (see also Chap. 21).
2. Alterations in intracellular enzyme activities may be mediated via a cAMP-independent phosphorylation cascade subsequent to autophosphorylation at the membrane site, by contact of receptor kinase with subcellular sites before or during internalization. It may be assumed that among the many affected proteins there are also certain protein phosphatases which become activated by phosphorylation. Thus, dephosphorylation, which is usually characteristic of the insulin-mediated switch from catabolic to anabolic processes (e.g., the inhibition of glycogen phosphorylase), would be actually accomplished by phosphorylation of regulatory proteins. Such effects would offset cAMP-dependent phosphorylations. Other cAMP-mitigating effects of insulin could be stimulation of phosphodiesterase[149] or direct inhibition of protein kinase activities.[150]
3. Generation of a family of cytoplasmic mediators of insulin action. These mediators could be low molecular weight peptides[143] or phospholipids.[144,150a] They may interact with various enzyme systems directly[144] or may become phosphorylated independently of cAMP and/or carry out phosphorylations and dephosphorylations.[151,152]
4. The intracellular effects of insulin may be facilitated by internalization of the receptor-insulin complex. Contact with the microsomal and nuclear systems involved in protein synthesis could be made possible by dissociation of insulin from the internalized receptor. Which cellular actions (e.g., membrane function, enzyme dephosphorylation) are dependent on such internalization remains to be established.

The proposed mechanisms are not mutually exclusive. They could function in concert or amplify each other.

INSULIN RESISTANCE

Insulin resistance is generally recognized by diminished response to either endogenous insulin (e.g., hyperinsulinemia in association with normal or elevated blood glucose concentration) or exogenous insulin (e.g., diabetes requiring very large doses of insulin). Such resistance may be due to changes in insulin receptors, postreceptor events, or both. Although the number of insulin receptors per cell is estimated to vary between 50,000 (in adipocytes) and 250,000 (in hepatocytes), maximal biological effects depend on occupation of a certain *number* of receptors, which may represent a small fraction ($<$ 10 percent) of those present. The functional correlate of the existence of "spare receptors" is that in circumstances of reduced numbers of receptors (e.g., obesity), if the insulin concentration is sufficiently elevated, the number of receptor-hormone complexes will ultimately reach the critical concentration necessary to trigger a biological event (i.e., the dose-response curve for insulin is shifted to the right). This type of receptor-mediated insulin resistance occurs without a change in the maximal response (i.e., maximal rates of glucose utilization do not change); it is termed decreased *insulin sensitivity*. In contrast, a decrease in the maximal tissue response (i.e., a reduction in the maximal rate of glucose utilization) may be observed when insulin resistance is due to a postreceptor defect. Such a downward shift in the insulin dose-response curve is termed decreased *insulin responsiveness* (Fig. 19-29). Whether the insulin dose-response curve shifts rightward or downward has thus been used to identify receptor-mediated or postreceptor-mediated mechanisms of insulin resistance; a mixed mechanism produces both right- and downward shifts. In fact, in most cases of type II diabetes or obesity a mixed type of resistance is seen, due to both reduced insulin sensitivity and responsiveness.

Studies of insulin receptors in humans have been extensive.[153] Many of them assessed the binding of insulin to monocytes removed from the circulation, which were demonstrated to mirror insulin binding in target tissues of insulin action (liver, muscle, and fat tissue). How the conditions of tissue response vary with the availability of insulin in vivo is exemplified by Fig. 19-30.

Changes in insulin receptors in insulin-resistant states as well as in circumstances of hypersensitivity to insulin[154] are outlined in Table 19-4. Some patients with lipoatrophic diabetes; and patients with the syndrome of *acanthosis nigricans*, exhibit extreme insulin resistance. In the last syndrome, receptor function is decreased in some patients due to the presence of a circulating antireceptor antibody, which interferes with insulin binding.[154] In other patients there appears to be a decrease in receptor synthesis as well as an increase in receptor degradation.[155] The most common insulin-resistant state is obesity, in which a decrease in insulin binding has been observed in monocytes, adipocytes, hepatocytes, and muscle cells. Altered receptor function has also been observed in hyperinsulinemic, nonobese type II diabetics. Receptor phosphorylation decreases concomitantly with the decrease in insulin binding but several insulin-resistant individuals with virtually normal insulin binding but defective receptor kinase activity have also been identified.[156] Newer evidence suggests that a basal impairment in receptor-kinase activity exists in most of the common insulin-resistant states.[132a] Conversely, in trained athletes, anorexia nervosa patients,[157] and individuals

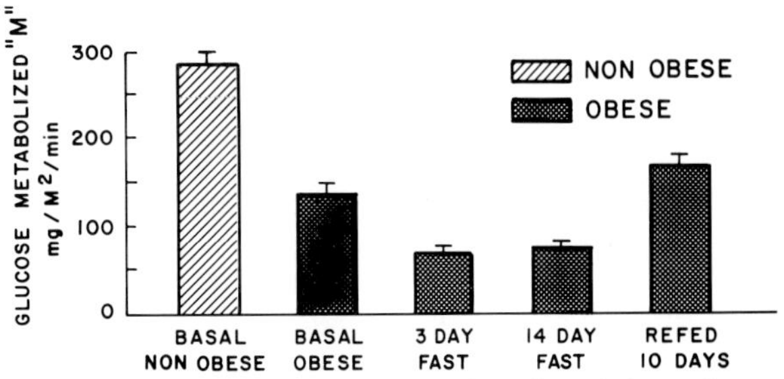

FIGURE 19-30 Insulin action in normal-weight and obese subjects in the basal (overnight-fasted) state and after 3- and 10-day fasts. Insulin action is indicated as the rate of glucose metabolized (M) during physiologic hyperinsulinemia achieved with the insulin clamp technique. In the basal state decreased insulin action in obesity is associated with a reduction in insulin binding, demonstrating that the receptor binding is a rate-limiting step in insulin action. In contrast, after fasting, insulin action is further reduced despite a rise in insulin binding, indicating that postreceptor events are rate-limiting. (*Based on data of DeFronzo R et al.*[159])

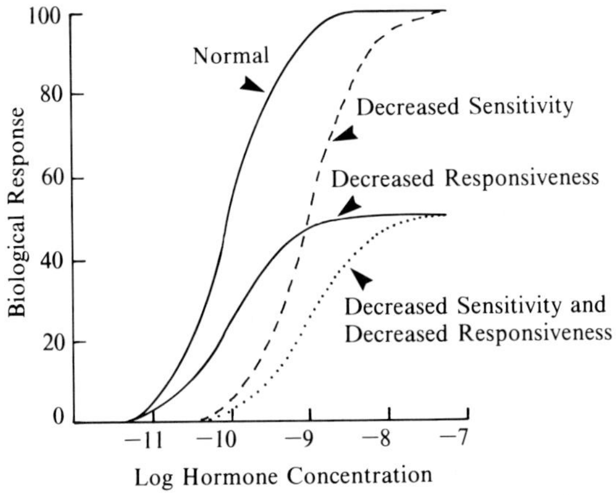

FIGURE 19-29 Types of resistance to insulin. Partial loss of high-affinity receptors or defective receptor function results in reduced binding due to decreased *sensitivity*. This is characterized by a shift of the dose response curve to the right without a change in maximal response. In a postreceptor defect or in the absence of sufficient receptor-binding capacity, the maximal insulin effect is lower, causing decreased *responsiveness*. Often, both receptor sensitivity and postreceptor responsiveness are reduced. (*From Kahn and Crettaz.*[113])

Table 19-4. Relationship between Insulin Binding and Insulin Action and Causes of Changes in Insulin Response

Insulin resistance: decreased insulin binding	
	Obesity
	Maturity-onset diabetes
	Severe insulin resistance and acanthosis nigricans
	Growth hormone excess
	Glucocorticoid excess
	Lipoatrophic diabetes
Insulin hypersensitivity: increased insulin binding	
	Athletic training
	Anorexia nervosa
	Glucocorticoid deficiency

with GH or glucocorticoid deficiency, augmented insulin sensitivity is accompanied by an increase in insulin binding.

A decrease in insulin binding may not, however, be the sole of even major mechanism of insulin resistance for a given target cell. For example, in obesity, a defect in intracellular glucose oxidation is demonstrable at maximal concentrations of insulin and cannot be accounted for by a diminution in insulin binding.[158] Decreases in the intracellular and plasma membrane pools of glucose transporters may account at least in part for insulin resistance in type 2 diabetes.[158a] Furthermore, during starvation, insulin binding to monocytes and adipocytes increases, yet intracellular utilization of glucose declines.[159] These findings indicate that insulin resistance may be a consequence of a variety of mechanisms at the receptor and/or postreceptor intracellular sites. As noted above, most patients with type 2 diabetes and/or obesity have a mixed defect.

INSULIN DEGRADATION

The biological half-life of insulin is in the range of 6 to 10 min. The major site of insulin degradation is the liver, where 40 to 60 percent of the hormone is removed in a single passage. As noted above, insulin is internalized by liver cells after it binds to the receptor and is translocated to lysosomes, the intracellular site of a variety of degradative enzymes. At least two insulin-degrading enzymes have been identified. *Glutathione-insulin transhydrogenase* cleaves the disulfide bonds of insulin, releasing intact A and B chains. Proteases inactivate insulin by peptide bond cleavage.[160]

The kidney accounts for 15 to 20 percent of insulin degradation. The renal clearance of insulin is larger than the GFR, indicating that the hormone is removed from the blood by the tubules as well as by filtration. In patients with renal insufficiency, insulin uptake by the kidney may fall to ~9 percent.[161] This accounts in part for the diminished insulin requirements sometimes seen in patients with diabetic glomerulosclerosis. The kidney assumes increased importance in the degradation of exogenous insulin since subcutaneously injected insulin is absorbed via the systemic circulation while endogenous insulin is released into the portal vein.

Glucagon

CHEMISTRY AND BIOSYNTHESIS

Glucagon is a polypeptide consisting of a single chain of 29 amino acids, with a molecular mass of 3485 daltons. Recent studies of structure-activity relationships indicate that the terminal amino group is active in both binding and cellular action of the hormone. However, the terminal carboxyl group confers the high affinity of the hormone for its receptor, which permits hormone binding and action at physiologic concentrations. Unlike insulin, the amino acid sequence of glucagon is identical in all mammalian species examined.

The alpha cells of the islets of Langerhans are the site of glucagon biosynthesis. Immunofluorescent studies indicate that these cells are situated on the outer rim of the islets and constitute ~25 percent of the islet cell population.[162] Within the islet cells, synthesis of glucagon involves the initial formation of a larger precursor: preproglucagon (a 180-amino-acid protein), which is converted to proglucagon. The latter is made up of 69 amino acid residues (9000 daltons) and is also referred to as *glicentin* or glucagon-like immunoreactivity (GLI)-1;[163] the secretory granules of alpha cells contain glucagon as the central core with glicentin in the outer band.[164] Following cleavage of this molecule to glucagon, the contents of the secretory granules are discharged by the process of exocytosis (emiocytosis), which is analogous to that described for insulin.

GLI (enteroglucagon) resides in the carboxy-terminal section of glicentin. It has 10 to 20 percent of the potency of glucagon and binds to the glucagon receptor. GLI stimulates adenyl cyclase of the oxyntic mucosa of the stomach and inhibits gastric acid secretion.[165,166]

CIRCULATING GLUCAGON

Advanced and specific immunoassay and gel filtration techniques have demonstrated that only 40 to 50 percent of human plasma glucagon represents biologically active hormone (i.e., of 3485 daltons). Most of the remaining glucagon immunoreactivity (of 160,000 daltons) elutes together with plasma proteins in the void volume. This fraction has been termed "*big plasma glucagon*" (BPG); it probably is devoid of biological activity. Two small additional fractions of ~9000 and ~2000 daltons have been identified in normal plasma. The biological significance of these fractions remains to be determined, although the 9000-dalton material is thought to represent proglucagon. The concentration of this fraction is increased in patients with chronic renal failure, presumably because of impaired renal removal.[167]

In pancreatectomized humans, glucagon has been reported to be absent from the circulation.[168] However, GLI polypeptides (of gut origin) may be capable of being converted to glucagon once they have entered the circulation.[169] This may account for the measurable glucagon levels following total pancreatectomy in humans. Extrapancreatic glucagon-containing cells may also be present in the digestive tract.[170,171] Although basal levels of immunoreactive glucagon (75 to 150 pg/ml) represent the biologically active and inactive components described above, alterations in circulating immunoreactivity in response to physiologic stimulation (e.g., by amino acids) or suppression (e.g., by glucose) generally reflect changes in the biologically active true pancreatic (3485-dalton) component of the immunoreactivity. Familial hyperglucagonemia is a rare asymptomatic autosomal dominant trait in which total plasma glucagon reactivity is increased two to ten times, but 85 percent of this immunoreactivity consists of biologically inactive, high-molecular-weight components[172] (see below).

SECRETION

Glucagon secretion does not markedly fluctuate throughout the day in normal subjects receiving mixed meals (Fig. 19-20). The relative constancy of glucagon concentration thus contrasts with the fluctuation of insulin concentration which accompanies mixed-meal ingestion or even minor changes (10 to 20 mg/dl) in blood glucose concentration (Fig. 19-20). The major physiologic stimuli of glucagon secretion in normal humans are protein ingestion, infusion of amino acids, and exercise, particularly if strenuous or prolonged.[173] Increases in glucagon secretion are also observed with acute hypoglycemia, after the infusion of large doses of epinephrine, and in association with hypercorticism.[173,174] The hyperglucagonemia observed with starvation is largely due to decreased catabolism rather than augmented secretion (see below). Hypoglycemia may provoke glucagon secretion by an α-adrenergic mechanism independent of insulin.[174] In type 1 diabetes, the stimulating effect of hypoglycemia on glucagon secretion is markedly reduced.

Suppression of glucagon secretion occurs after the ingestion or infusion of glucose. The hypoglucagonemic effects of glucose may depend on insulin-mediated uptake of glucose by the alpha cells and/or the absence of marked hyperglycemia.[174] In diabetic patients glucose fails to inhibit glucagon secretion, but this effect is restored following insulin treatment.[175] As noted above, somatostatin is a potent inhibitor of glucagon as well as insulin and GH secretion. In fact, the inhibitory action of somatostatin on alpha cell function has been the basis, in part, of its use as an adjunct in the management of insulin-dependent diabetes.[93]

ACTION

Although glucagon was discovered in the 1930s in crude insulin preparations as a "hyperglycemic-glycogenolytic factor," its physiologic role and mechanism of action have only recently been elucidated. Early studies were hampered by the inability to produce a pure glucagon-deficient state without concomitant insulin deficiency and the lack of data on circulating levels and secretory rates of glucagon.

It is now apparent that physiologic increments in glucagon concentration produce a rise in blood glucose concentration by stimulating hepatic glycogenolysis and gluconeogenesis (Fig. 19-31). In contrast, a fall in glucagon concentration to below basal level results in a decrease in hepatic glucose production.[176] However, when an increment in glucagon concentration is accompanied by a small (50 to 150 percent) rise in circulating insulin concentration, hepatic glucose production remains unchanged. The latter phenomenon accounts for the importance of the bihormonal response (i.e., rise in glucagon concentration as well as insulin concentration) to ingestion of a protein meal (Fig. 19-32). The insulin response, engendered by the protein meal, ensures the cellular uptake and utilization of amino acids contained in the meal. However, the rise in insulin concentration alone would inhibit hepatic glucose output, resulting in hypoglycemia. The simultaneous increase in glucagon concentration mitigates such an effect by ensuring that glucose production is maintained (Fig. 19-32). A speculation is that, since mixed meals fail to alter glucagon levels (Fig. 19-20), glucagon's role in evolution may relate primarily to carnivorous populations, feeding on infrequent but large protein meals.

In contrast to insulin, whose effects on various target tissues are ongoing so long as hypoglycemia does not occur, glucagon's stimulatory action on hepatic glucose production lasts only 30 to 60 min (Fig. 19-31).[173] However, once a given level of plasma glucagon concentration has been established, a further increase or decrease is followed, respectively, by a rise or fall in glucose production. Thus, hepatic glucose metabolism is influenced by *changes* in glucagon levels rather than by absolute glucagon concentration. The liver thus shows ongoing responsiveness to pulsatile alterations in circulating glucagon concentration, but the effect of any alteration is evanescent, both in vivo[177] and in vitro.[177a]

Because of the opposing actions of insulin and glucagon on the liver, and inasmuch as glucose suppresses glucagon secretion while stimulating insulin secretion, Unger has suggested that the insulin/glucagon molar ratio (I/G) rather than the concentration of either hormone alone governs overall carbohydrate homeostasis.[174] The applicability of this bihormonal hypothesis to the intact organism has been seriously challenged in studies involving infusions of glucagon in physiologic doses.[178,179] Those studies demonstrated

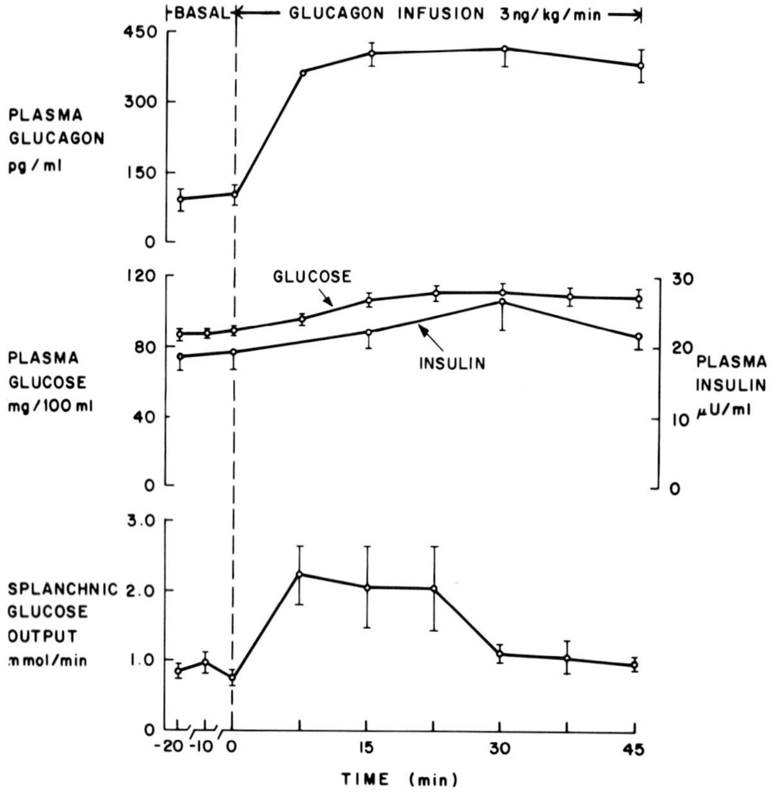

FIGURE 19-31 Stimulation by glucagon of hepatic (splanchnic) glucose production in normal humans. Physiologic hyperglucagonemia causes a prompt rise in hepatic glucose production. The effect is transient, however, lasting less than 45 min. The stimulatory action of glucagon on glucose production results thus from changes in concentrations of glucagon rather than absolute concentrations themselves. (*From Felig P et al.*[178])

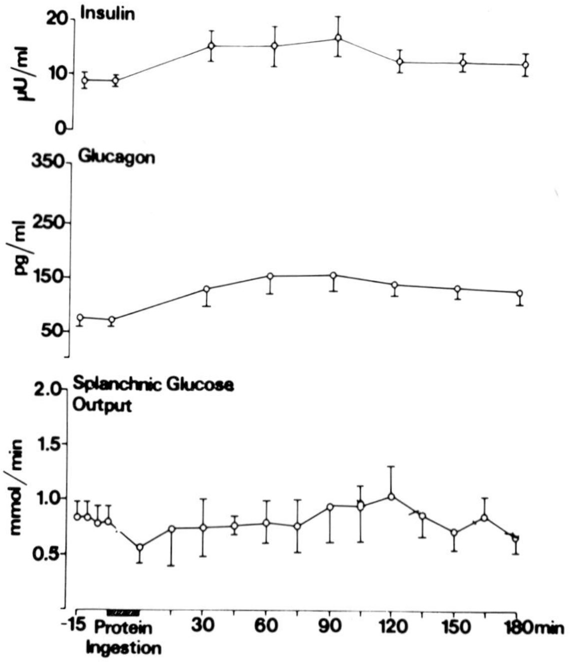

FIGURE 19-32 Influence of protein feeding on plasma insulin and glucagon concentrations and on splanchnic (hepatic) glucose production normal humans. The rise in glucagon concentration, induced by protein feeding, is necessary for the uptake and anabolic utilization of the amino acids contained in the protein meal. (*Based on the data of Wahren J, Felig P, Hagenfeldt, LJ: J Clin Invest 58:761, 1976.*)

that high plasma glucagon levels of 300 to 400 pg/ml (comparable with those observed in a variety of hyperglucagonemic states) fail to alter glucose tolerance in normal subjects. This conclusion is supported by the finding that, despite a marked fall in I/G (from 34:1 to 6:1) induced by glucagon infusion, no change in glucose tolerance occurs.[173] Glucagon-induced changes in glucose tolerance thus require either an absolute deficiency of insulin, pharmacologic doses of glucagon, or (in some circumstances) the presence of a glucagon-producing tumor (see below). Furthermore, while glucose administration normally suppresses glucagon secretion, hypoglucagonemia is not necessary for normal glucose disposal so long as insulin secretion is normal.[178,179]

In addition to its action on carbohydrate metabolism, glucagon is involved in the regulation of ketogenesis. Livers obtained from rats given physiologic doses of glucagon display augmented ketone production from FFA.[40] In vivo, ketonemia may occur in the absence of glucagon, as in pancreatectomized patients.[168] However, in the insulin-deficient diabetic, hyperglucagonemia increases the ketogenic capacity. It should be emphasized that glucagon's effects in raising blood glucose concentration and in enhancing ketosis are entirely a consequence of its actions on the liver.

Increases in FFA oxidation and ketogenesis result from glucagon's inhibitory effect on hepatic lipogenesis decreasing malonyl CoA availability rather than from stimulation of peripheral lipolysis.

The first step in the action of glucagon on the liver is interaction with a specific receptor on the cell membrane; this appears to be different and somewhat simpler than signal transmission with insulin. Binding to the receptor activates a coupled catalytic effector unit (E) containing the enzyme adenyl cyclase, which converts ATP to cAMP, the intracellular glucagon messenger. A GTP-dependent regulatory protein (G) mediates the cyclase activation.[180] Rodbell[180a] suggested that the G protein may dissociate into smaller molecules upon the GTP and hormone activation; these molecules may serve as messengers of the hormone, in addition to cAMP. At the same time the change in G protein may also transiently decrease the binding affinity of the receptor. The rise in cAMP concentration triggers several phosphorylation reactions resulting in activation of glycogen phosphorylase and simultaneous inhibition of glycogen synthase (Fig. 19-4). Insulin antagonizes this action by reducing the activity of cAMP-dependent protein kinase[150,150a] and/or augmenting the activity of phosphodiesterase responsible for cAMP degradation.[149] The glucagon-sensitive, cAMP-mediated steps in control of substrate flow toward gluconeogenesis are at the level of conversion of pyruvate to phospho*enol*pyruvate by induction of PEPCK synthesis and phosphorylation of pyruvate kinase as well as FDPase-2 (Figs. 19-5 and 19-6).

Administration of glucagon has been observed to lower serum potassium and calcium concentrations, decrease gastric acid and pancreatic enzyme secretion, raise serum GH secretion, and increase myocardial contractility. However, each of these effects requires pharmacologic doses of the hormone.

DEGRADATION

In contrast to insulin, glucagon degradation is carried out primarily in the kidney rather than the liver. As a result, plasma glucagon concentration is elevated in uremia despite the absence of hypersecretion.[173] Glucagon removal by the kidney normally exceeds the filtered load, suggesting that peritubular uptake contributes to renal clearance. A reduction in glucagon catabolism is also the major factor responsible for the hyperglucagonemia observed in short-term (3-day) starvation.[173] Although hyperglucagonemia is observed in cirrhosis patients, particularly when accompanied by portal hypertension, augmented secretion rather than diminished degradation is the major mechanism of the elevated plasma glucagon concentration in such patients.[181]

Catecholamines

Epinephrine and norepinephrine inhibit glucose-stimulated insulin secretion via an α-adrenergic effect. Studies in patients with cervical cord transections, however, indicate that increased rather than basal levels of plasma catecholamine concentrations and sympathetic nervous system activity are important in the regulation of basal or glucose-stimulated insulin secretion in the resting state.

Apart from altering insulin secretion, catecholamines raise the blood glucose concentration by at least five additional mechanisms: (1) activation of glycogenolysis, (2) stimulation of gluconeogenesis, (3) inhibition of insulin-mediated glucose uptake, (4) increased lipolysis, and (5) stimulation of glucagon secretion.

The glycogenolytic effect of epinephrine is considerably greater than that of norepinephrine and occurs in liver as well as muscle tissue. Since muscle lacks G6Pase, glycogen breakdown in muscle brings about a rise in blood glucose concentration via indirect mechanisms. Enhanced glycogenolysis in muscle is followed by an increase in glycolysis resulting in the release of lactate. The latter is transported to the liver, where it serves as a gluconeogenic substrate. The glycogenolytic effect of epinephrine in muscle tissue is mediated via β-adrenergic receptors and a rise in cAMP concentration (Fig. 19-4). However, in liver tissue glycogenolysis is not necessarily dependent on β-adrenergic receptors; it may be triggered by α-adrenergic receptors.[7,7a]

In addition to stimulating glycogen breakdown, epinephrine interferes with insulin-mediated glucose uptake. A physiologic rise in plasma epinephrine concentration (500 pg/ml) results in a 60 to 90 percent fall in the rate of glucose disposal, induced by postprandial increments in plasma insulin concentration (100 μU/ml).[182] This effect is mediated via β-adrenergic receptors. The insulin-antagonistic action of epinephrine is also observed with minimal plasma elevations of epinephrine concentration (25 to 50 pg/ml), which are comparable with those accompanying a mild viral illness and which are insufficient to interfere with insulin secretion.[87] The fall in glucose clearance (the rate of glucose uptake relative to the plasma glucose level) induced by epinephrine accounts for its having a substantially greater hyperglycemic effect than comparable doses of glucagon despite the fact that glucagon causes a greater rise in glucose production.[183]

Epinephrine is a potent lipolytic agent by virtue of its stimulation of the cAMP-dependent lipase in adipose tissue. Decreased glucose uptake induced by epinephrine also limits the availability of glycerol 3-phosphate for reesterification.

In contrast to its inhibitory effects on insulin

secretion, epinephrine stimulates the secretion of glucagon. The hyperglycemia after epinephrine administration represents thus a composite effect of two hormones; it is blunted when hyperglucagonemia is prevented by concurrent administration of somatostatin. This effect of somatostatin persists when glucagon is given in replacement doses, suggesting that somatostatin may blunt the hepatic response to epinephrine independent of glucagon availability.[184]

The major stimuli of catecholamine secretion and augmented sympathetic nervous system activity are exercise, trauma, fever, surgery, and hypoglycemia. The homeostatic responses to hypoglycemia are dependent on an intact sympathetic nervous system and are blunted but not entirely eliminated in adrenalectomized patients.[185] In type 1 diabetes glucagon secretion in response to hypoglycemia is attenuated. This leads to a greater dependence on catecholamines to counteract insulin-induced hypoglycemia.

Glucocorticoids

It has been recognized since the classic experiments of Long and Lukens and Houssay in the 1930s that the secretions of the adrenal cortex have a diabetogenic effect. Subsequent work has established that adrenal corticosteroids stimulate proteolysis while increasing gluconeogenesis and glycogen formation, hence the name *glucocorticoids.*

Glucocorticoids also raise blood glucose levels by decreasing the responsiveness of muscle and adipose tissue to insulin-stimulated glucose uptake. This effect of glucocorticoids is mediated, at least in part, by a decrease in binding of insulin to its receptor.[186] The insulin-antagonistic effect of cortisol is generally accompanied by hyperglycemia and a rise in serum insulin concentration. Thus, in Cushing's syndrome of spontaneous or iatrogenic origin, hyperinsulinemia and insulin resistance are characteristic findings. Whether such patients develop diabetes depends in part on the insulin-secretory capacity of their beta cells, determining whether enough insulin can be released to withstand the long-lasting hyperglycemic stimulus and meet the demands of their insulin-resistant tissues.

In contrast to the insulin antagonism induced by epinephrine, which is demonstrable within minutes, the effects of glucocorticoids require hours to days to become fully manifest. This time course of action is due to selective modulations in the rates of synthesis of several enzymes and other proteins involved in the transport and metabolism of glucose.

Growth Hormone

GH decreases glucose utilization while promoting the formation of tissue proteins and stimulating lipolysis. The antagonistic effects of GH on insulin-stimulated glucose uptake may be mediated by a change in insulin receptors.[154] In general, this action of GH results in a compensatory increase in insulin secretion so that glucose tolerance remains normal. However, if large enough quantities of GH are involved, either from the pituitary or by injection, or if insulin secretion is impaired (e.g., a genetic tendency to diabetes), the blood glucose concentration may rise to abnormal levels, or previously established diabetes may be aggravated.

During fasting, blood glucose level falls to strikingly lower concentrations in GH-deficient dwarfs than are observed in normal controls.[187] Growth hormone thus has an important role in setting the basal blood glucose concentration ("glucostat" effect).

In contrast to the insulin-antagonizing effects of prolonged or repeated administration of GH, the early response to this hormone is characterized by a fall in blood glucose concentration and other insulin-like effects. This action of GH may derive from its induction of secondary substances in serum, initially termed "sulfation factor," due to stimulation of bone matrix sulfation and Ca^{2+} deposition on the sulfated cartilage. More recently, these proteins were termed *somatomedins,* mediating the action of GH in stimulating protein synthesis and growth (see Chap. 7). There is now good evidence that the somatomedins are closely related to or identical with IGFs (see below). It has also been demonstrated that serum somatomedin activity is reduced in rats with streptozotocin-induced diabetes and that this reduction is prevented or reversed by insulin therapy. Growth failure in diabetes may thus be related to decreased somatomedin activity.[188]

Insulin-like Growth Factors

Prior to the advent of RIA procedures, plasma insulin was bioassayed by measuring in vitro glucose uptake by rat epididymal adipose tissue or diaphragm. Subsequent determinations revaled that only ~10 percent of the total insulin-like activity measured by bioassay corresponds to true pancreatic insulin as determined by RIA. The remainder of the circulating insulin-like activity persists even after pancreatectomy or the precipitation of insulin by specific antibodies and was consequently termed nonsuppressible insulin-like activity (NSILA). NSILA has been shown to consist of two polypeptides (mol wt ~7500) which promote growth of chick embryo fibroblasts (increase cell multiplication and DNA synthesis) and have consequently been termed IGF 1 and 2.[189] An unexpected finding was the extensive homology between the primary structures of IGF 1 and 2 on the one hand and the A and B chains of insulin on the other.[190] Structural homology also exists with respect to tertiary structure, accounting for cross-reactivity of IGFs with the insulin receptor.

In contrast to insulin, the C peptide region in circulating IGF 1 and 2 is conserved and there is no resemblance in amino acid sequence in the C peptide region.[190]

The IGFs mimic many actions of insulin; insulin is more potent in producing metabolic effects while the IGFs have greater growth-promoting effects (Table 19-5). Two IGF plasma membrane receptors have been identified. The type 1 receptor has a structure homologous to the insulin receptor with α and β subunits, one responsible for hormone binding and the other undergoing tyrosine phosphorylation.[113] The type 2 receptor contains a single polypeptide chain and does not appear to have tyrosine kinase activity.[191] Insulin, IGF 1, and IGF 2 have differing affinities for the three receptors. Insulin binds strongly to its own receptor, has a low affinity for the IGF 1 receptor, and has virtually no affinity for the IGF 2 receptor. The IGF 1 receptor has considerably greater affinity for IGF 1 than for IGF 2 in most mammalian cells nd the same affinity for both IGFs in chick cells.[190] The IGF 2 receptors preferably bind IGF 2 and multiplication-stimulating activity (the rat homologue of IGF 2 secreted by liver cells).

Another difference between IGFs and insulin is that the former are bound to specific proteins in the circulation whereas insulin is not. IGFs are bound to two proteins of ~50,000 and ~200,000 daltons; this binding provides a half-life of 4 h in the rat and 16 h in humans, in contrast to <10 min for insulin. Small amounts reach target organs in the dissociated form. Diurnal variations in IGF plasma concentrations were not demonstrated.

Under ordinary circumstances, IGF 1 levels are regulated by GH. However, in disease states such as malnutrition, IGF 1 deficiency occurs despite increased GH levels. Poorly regulated diabetes is also associated with relative or absolute IGF 1 deficiency, correctable with insulin therapy. Pygmies and dwarfs have normal pituitary function but are deficient in IGF 1.[191]

Pancreatic Polypeptide

This 36-amino-acid polypeptide originates in islet cells which are distinct from alpha, beta, and delta cells. Protein ingestion, fasting, exercise, and hyperglycemia raise the plasma levels of this polypeptide. Elevations have also been observed in diabetic patients and those with insulinomas.[192] The physiologic action of pancreatic polypeptide on nutrient metabolism has not yet been established.

Regulatory and Counterregulatory Hormones

The large number of hormones which influence body fuel metabolism may be categorized as favoring either the storage or dissipation of energy. In this regard, insulin is unique because it favors the storage of each of the major body fuels (glucose, fat, and protein). In contrast, five hormones (epinephrine, glucagon, cortisol, GH, and thyroid hormone) promote the dissipation of body fat, glycogen, and/or protein. These hormones may also be classified with respect to the feedback effect of plasma glucose concentration on their secretion and in terms of their action on blood glucose concentration. Insulin is the only hormone whose secretion is influenced on a moment-to-moment basis by physiologic fluctuations in blood glucose concentration (Fig. 19-20) and which brings about a fall in blood glucose concentration. In contrast, each of the energy-dissipating hormones (except for thyroid) causes a rise in blood glucose concentration. Furthermore, an increase in their secretion requires either the

Table 19-5. Properties of Insulin and Insulin-like Growth Factors

	Source	No. of amino acids	Mode of secretion	Regulator(s)	Plasma concentration, ng/ml	Plasma carrier protein	Half-life	Physiologic role
Insulin	Beta cells	51	Pulsatile	Glucose, amino acids	0.3–2.0	No	< 10 min	Control of metabolism
IGF 1*	Liver	70	Constant	GH, nutrition	~1	Yes	16 h	Skeletal and cartilage growth
IGF 2†	Diverse	67	Unknown	Unknown	~1	Yes	Unknown	Unknown

*Also called somatomedin C.
†Also called multiplication-stimulating activity.

development of frank hypoglycemia or the interposition of signals other than a change in blood glucose concentration (e.g., protein feeding, exercise, stress). Consequently, with respect to blood glucose control, insulin is generally considered the major regulatory hormone, while glucagon, catecholamines, cortisol, and GH are collectively referred to as *counterregulatory* hormones[193] (Table 19-5). The actions of the counterregulatory hormones in raising blood glucose concentration may result from coordinate effects on glycogen metabolism and/or gluconeogenesis or antagonism of insulin-mediated glucose uptake (Table 19-6).

Fuel-Hormone Interactions

The homeostasis of body fuels is dependent not only on the availability of enzymatically regulated pathways and a variety of hormonal signals but on finely coordinated substrate-hormone interactions. These are best understood by considering the changes which occur in conditions of fuel availability (the fed state), fuel need (starvation, exercise), or fuel imbalance ("stress" hyperglycemia). These perturbations, however, require an understanding of normal body composition (e.g., fuel stores) and the conditions which exist in the basal state.

BODY COMPOSITION

The caloric composition of a typical American or western European diet consists of 40 to 45 percent carbohydrate, 40 percent fat, and 15 to 20 percent protein. The composition of the fuels stored in the human body is far different from that of fuels ingested in the diet (Table 19-7). Carbohydrate represents a calorically insignificant fuel store. The combined caloric value of liver glycogen (70 g), muscle glycogen (200 g), and circulating blood glucose (20 g) amounts to ~1200 kcal, well below the average caloric expenditure of a single day. Nevertheless, liver glycogen represents an important source of carbohydrate for the ongoing supply to the brain and the needs of muscle during exercise (see below). The teleologic basis of the limitation for storing carbohydrate derives not only from its low caloric density (4 kcal/g, as compared with 9 kcal/g in fat) but also from the large amount of tissue water obligatory for the storage of glycogen (4 ml/g).

By far the largest reservoir of body fuel is fat, stored as triglyceride. In a nonobese subject, body fat amounts to ~20 percent of total body weight, representing 130,000 to 140,000 kcal and *accounting for 80 percent* of total body fuel depots. The compact nature of this large fuel depot is due to its caloric density and its anhydrous nature. To store an equivalent number of energy as carbohydrates would require more than eight times the weight of fat. The fat depot is sufficient to meet the caloric requirements for ~2 months. In obese subjects, fat tissue may provide for the storage of over 500,000 kcal. Regardless of the degree of adiposity, fat clearly represents the most expendable as well as the most plentiful fuel available to humans.

Table 19-6. Regulatory and Counterregulatory Hormones in the Control of Blood Glucose Concentration

	Secretion stimuli	Actions
Insulin	Moment-to-moment fluctuations in blood glucose concentration	↓ Blood glucose
		↑ Glucose uptake ↑ Glycogen synthesis ↓ Glycogenolysis ↓ Gluconeogenesis
Counterregulatory hormones:	Frank hypoglycemia (blood glucose concentration < 50 mg/dl), exercise, stress, protein feeding	↑ Blood glucose
Glucagon		↑ Glycogenolysis ↑ Gluconeogenesis
Catecholamines		↑ Glycogenolysis ↓ Glucose uptake
Cortisol		↑ Gluconeogenesis ↓ Glucose uptake
Growth hormone		↓ Glucose uptake

Table 19-7. Body Composition and Fuel Reserves in a Normal 70-kg Human

Fuel	Tissue	Weight, kg	% Body weight	Energy value, kcal
Fat	Adipose tissue	11–17	15–25	100,000–150,000
Protein	Muscle (primarily)	8–12	12–17	32,000–48,000
Carbohydrate	Liver (glycogen)	0.070	<1	280
	Muscle (glycogen)	0.200	<1	800
	Blood (glucose)	0.020	<1	80

The major reservoir of body protein is in muscle tissue, amounting to 10 kg (exclusive of tissue water) or 40,000 kcal. Because of protein's indispensability in body structure, muscle function and as a catalytic agent (e.g., enzymes), loss of >50 percent of body protein is incompatible with survival, despite residual mobilizable fat tissue. Death in starvation results not from hypoglycemia but from dissolution of protein stores: loss of respiratory muscle function leads to terminal pneumonia.

Of particular importance in considering the homeostatic response to fuel need is the interchangeability of body fuels. Body protein (by virtue of its constituent amino acids other than leucine or valine) is readily converted to glucose (gluconeogenesis). Carbohydrate availability for glucose-dependent tissues (e.g., brain) thus does not cease with depletion of liver glycogen. On the other hand, fatty acids can not generally be converted to glucose, since mammalian tissue lacks the enzymatic capacity for net gluconeogenesis from substrates with less than three carbons, e.g., acetyl CoA. Thus to the extent that glucose is terminally oxidized (by brain) and must be replenished by gluconeogenesis, there is an obligate dissolution of body protein stores in total starvation.

THE BASAL STATE

The basal or postabsorptive state, the condition which exists 6 to 12 h after food ingestion, represents the change from feeding to fasting. While this interval represents a nonsteady state, it is nevertheless a readily identifiable reference point with which various perturbations may be compared. In the postabsorptive condition, adipose tissue releases FFA to meet the fuel requirements of muscle and heart as well as parenchymal tissues (liver, kidney). The respiratory quotient of most muscles is close to 0.7, reflecting virtual dependence on fat oxidation. Carbohydrate utilization occurs primarily in the brain, which terminally oxidizes glucose at a rate of 100 to 125 g per day. Smaller amounts of glucose are utilized by resting muscle and by obligate anaerobic tissues such as the formed elements of the blood and the renal medulla (Fig. 19-33).

While several tissues contribute to glucose utilization, production of glucose is virtually limited to the liver. Maintenance of euglycemia depends on release of glucose from the liver at a rate equal to the combined utilization in brain and peripheral tissues (150 to 250 g per day, 2 to 3 mg/min per kilogram of body weight; ~75 percent of the glucose produced during an overnight fast is derived from glycogen; the remainder is formed by gluconeogenesis from lactate, alanine, and, to a lesser extent, pyruvate and glycerol.[12] In the complete absence of hepatic glucose production, the blood glucose level would be halved in 40 to 60 min. The increased delivery of FFA to the liver results in the formation of ketone bodies. However, the rate of ketogenesis in the basal state is such as to maintain the concentration of circulating ketone acids at <0.5 mM only.

The hormonal signal which permits the initiation of glycogenolysis, gluconeogenesis, and ketogenesis in the basal state is the fall in plasma insulin concentration from the level observed in the fed state (30 to 100 μU/ml) to values of 10 to 20 μU/ml. Glucose utilization in the basal state is thus largely (~70 percent) non-insulin-dependent, occurring primarily in the brain. On the other hand, the presence of basal insulin levels (and basal secretory rates of 0.25 to 1.5 U/h) ensures maximal efficiency in fuel economy by preventing excessive gluconeogenesis and unrestrained FFA mobilization and ketogenesis. There is an apparent "redundant regulation" of insulin secretion at low glucose levels, probably by FFA or products of their oxidation. Thus, the rates of glucose and ketone production do not exceed the rates of glucose and ketone utilization, thereby precluding the development of hyperglycemia and hyperketonemia. When there is no basal insulin secretion (as in type I diabetes) or if hormonal perturbations occur which interfere with basal insulin action (see Stress Hyperglycemia, below), the blood glucose and ketone concentrations rise.

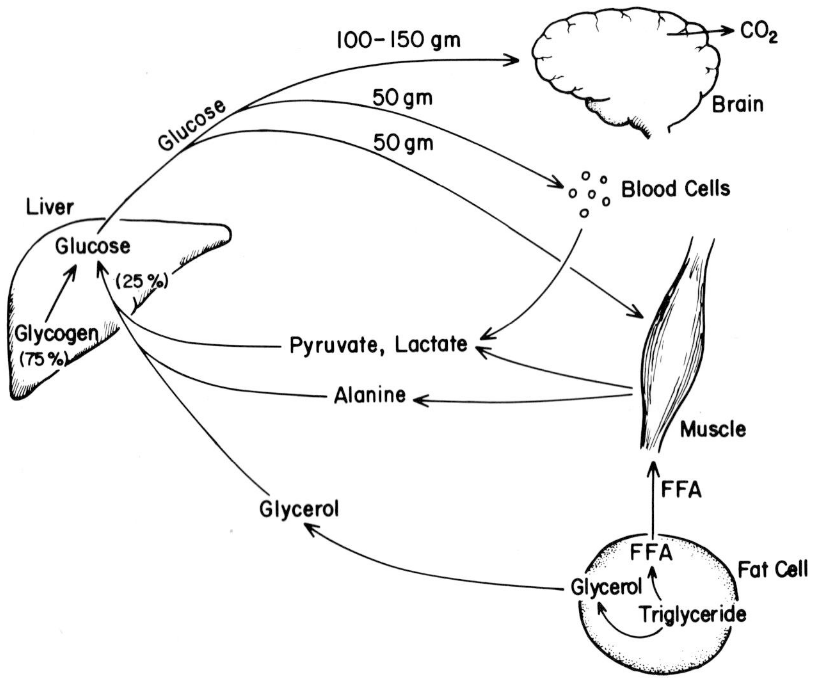

FIGURE 19-33 Glucose turnover in the basal (overnight-fasted) resting state in normal humans. The liver is the sole site of the production of glucose, by glycogenolysis (75 percent) and gluconeogenesis (25 percent). The brain is the major site of glucose utilization, consuming glucose at a rate of 100 to 150 g per day. Smaller amounts of glucose are taken up by the formed elements of the blood and by resting muscle. The latter is a source of glucose precursors in the form of alanine and the glycolytic intermediates lactate and pyruvate. The adipocyte contributes small amounts of glycerol for gluconeogenesis.

FUEL AVAILABILITY: THE FED STATE

The hormonal response to the fed state is determined in part by the nature of the ingested substrate (Table 19-8). If pure glucose is ingested, a multihormonal response ensues, involving a rise in insulin concentration and decreases in glucagon and GH concentrations. If pure protein is ingested, the multihormonal response consists of a rise in insulin as well as glucagon and GH concentrations. In contrast, when mixed meals are fed (the usual dietary intake), only a rise in insulin level is observed. Regardless of the substrate ingested, the rise in insulin concentration is the key signal which shifts metabolism to the fed state by stimulating cellular uptake of glucose, amino acids, or both and inhibiting lipolysis. When the rise in insulin concentration is not accompanied by a rise in glucagon concentration (e.g., with glucose or mixed-meal ingestion), glucose output from the liver is inhibited and net hepatic uptake of glucose occurs. The accompanying fall in GH concentration may enhance insulin's antilipolytic effects. When both insulin and glucagon levels rise (e.g., with protein feeding), glucose output from the liver is maintained at basal rates (Fig. 19-32). The importance of the latter derives from the fact that ingested protein cannot of itself provide for the fuel requirements of the brain. Note that feeding

Table 19-8. Hormonal Response to Altered Fuel Availability or Need

Condition	Insulin	Glucagon	Growth hormone	Epinephrine	Cortisol
Fuel availability:					
Glucose ingestion	↑	↓	↓	±	±
Protein ingestion	↑	↑	↑	±	±
Mixed-meal ingestion	↑	±	±	±	±
Fuel need:					
Starvation	↓	↑	↑ or ±	↑ or ±	↓
Acute hypoglycemia	↓	↑	↑	↑	↑
Exercise	↓	↑	↑	↑	↑

Abbreviations: ↑, increased secretion; ↓, decreased secretion; ±, unchanged.

fails to alter abruptly the secretion of catecholamines or cortisol (Table 19-8).

FUEL NEED

Starvation

If the basal state is not perturbed by the ingestion of food, the metabolic response progresses to that which characterizes starvation (starvation is considered in detail in Chap. 20). The major hormonal signals governing the fasting state are a fall in insulin concentration and, to a lesser extent, a rise in glucagon concentration. The progressive decline in insulin concentration is triggered by a small decline in blood glucose concentration but may be initiated by caloric lack per se.[194] The hypoinsulinemia leads to an increase in lipolysis and hepatic fatty acid oxidation, resulting in a gradual increase in ketogenesis. The outflow of amino acids (particularly alanine) from muscle as well as hepatic gluconeogenesis is also stimulated. In this manner hepatic glucose production is sustained despite the fact that liver glycogen stores are depleted within 24 h.

When starvation is prolonged for > 3 weeks, the rate of gluconeogenesis as well as glucose utilization is markedly reduced. In this circumstance ketones become an important substrate for the brain (replacing some glucose) and may provide the signal to muscle whereby protein catabolism and alanine outflow are diminished.[195] Even some acetone may be converted to glucose, as discussed earlier. Although growth hormone levels rise with starvation, the increment is transient and not essential for the lipolytic or ketogenic response.

Exercise

A marked increase in fuel requirements occurs in either fed or fasted humans during muscular exercise. The major fuel consumed (carbohydrate or fat) depends on the duration as well as the intensity of the exercise performed[196] (Fig. 19-34). With very brief exercise (a run lasting only a few minutes) the major fuel consumed is muscle glycogen. With longer periods of exercise, extending to 1 to 2 h, blood-borne glucose accounts for ~40 percent of the increased fuel consumption the rest being provided by FFA. The rate of glucose uptake by muscle is stimulated up to 40 times the resting level, while total body glucose turnover may increase three- to fourfold. With very prolonged exercise, there is progressively less dependence on glucose and increased utilization of fat.

The stimulatory effect of exercise on glucose utilization occurs in the face of a declining insulin concentration. The multihormonal response to exercise (Table 19-8) is thus largely directed at providing a milieu which favors hepatic glycogenolysis and gluconeogenesis as well as lipolysis. The response to exercise is further discussed below (see Treatment of Diabetes).

Hypoglycemia

When the blood glucose level is suddenly lowered by the administration of insulin, there is an immediate need to restore circulating glucose levels lest brain function be irreversibly disturbed (see Chap. 20). The homeostatic response consists of a marked increase in the secretion of each of the counterregulatory hormones and inhibition of endogenous insulin secretion (Table 19-8). As a result, within 15 to 30 min of the bolus administration of insulin, a reversal of its inhibitory effects on hepatic glucose production is observed. The lowered blood glucose level may of itself contribute to the reversal of insulin's action on the liver, independent of the rises in concentrations of counterregulatory hormones.[197]

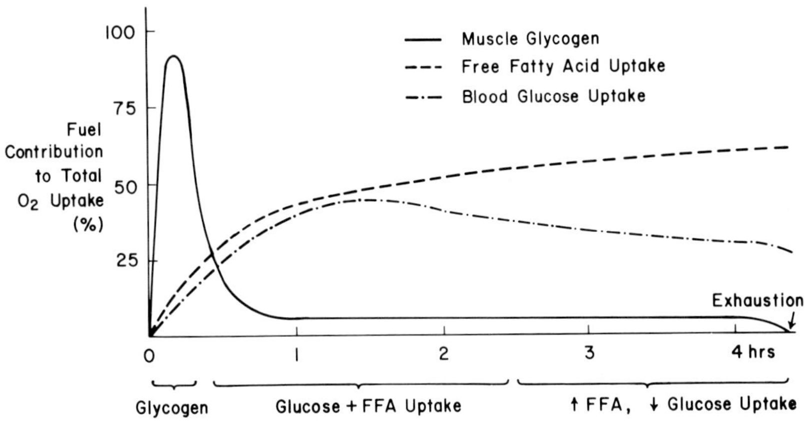

FIGURE 19-34 Pattern of fuel utilization by muscle during exercise of varying duration. During the initial few minutes of exercise, muscle glycogen is a major fuel for the production of ATP. Between 10 and 40 min of exercise blood-borne glucose and FFA each account for 40 percent of the total fuel oxidation. Thereafter (i.e., with very prolonged exercise), there is a progressive rise in the utilization of FFA and lessened uptake of blood glucose. Although muscle glycogen makes only a small contribution to fuel utilization in prolonged exercise, its total depletion is associated with the development of fatigue.

FUEL-HORMONE IMBALANCE

Stress Hyperglycemia

The hormonal response characteristic of acute fuel need (low insulin concentration and increased glucagon, catecholamine, cortisol, and GH concentrations) is occasionally observed in the absence of starvation, exercise, or hypoglycemia. In patients with various types of stress (extensive body burns, compound fractures, sepsis, etc.), high levels of counterregulatory hormones and a low plasma insulin concentration are often noted. In the absence of a stimulus for glucose utilization (e.g., exercise), such a hormonal pattern results in a rise in blood glucose concentration (*stress hyperglycemia*). This phenomenon involves overproduction as well as underutilization of glucose. It is due to synergistic interaction among the various counterregulatory hormones.[183,193] Thus, while glucagon, epinephrine, or cortisol causes only minor rises in blood glucose concentration when elevated individually, the effect of a multihormonal response is far more than additive (Fig. 19-35). The synergism derives from the fact that while cortisol itself has little effect on glucose production, it converts the transient hepatic effect of glucagon or epinephrine to one of sustained glucose overproduction. In addition, epinephrine, by virtue of its suppressive effects on insulin secretion as well as its antagonism of insulin action, exaggerates the hyperglycemic response by decreasing glucose utilization. If insulin levels are already reduced, as in the diabetic, the effect of such a multihormonal response is to intensify the diabetic state.

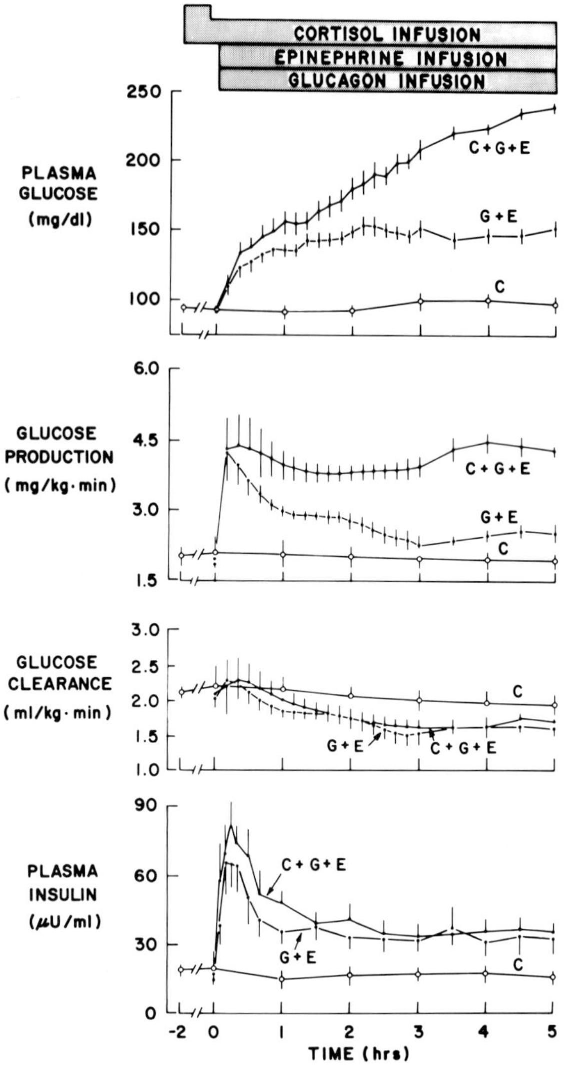

FIGURE 19-35 The synergistic effects of cortisol (C), glucagon (G), and epinephrine (E) in raising plasma glucose concentration, stimulating glucose production, and reducing glucose clearance. The hyperglycemic response to the triple hormone infusion (C + G + E) is far greater than the additive response to all three hormones given singly or the response to any combination of two hormones given together plus one hormone given singly. The development of "stress" hyperglycemia is a consequence of this hormonal synergism, which also includes GH. (*From Eigler et al.*[183])

DIABETES MELLITUS

History

The historical background to diabetes was reviewed by Mann.[198] The writings ascribed to the ancient Hindu Susruta (600 B.C.) contain what is probably the earliest recorded reference to diabetes mellitus: "When the doctor states that a man suffers from honey urine, he has declared him incurable." A more detailed clinical description, which included mention of the "melting down of the flesh into urine," excessive thirst, and increased urination, is provided in the works of Aretaeus of Cappadocia (A.D. 81–138).

With respect to the pathogenesis of diabetes, as early as 1682, Brunner noted that partial removal of a dog's pancreas made the animal drink and urinate copiously. A causal relationship between human diabetes and lesions in the pancreas was suggested by Lancereaux in 1877 on the basis of studies in two patients. It remained, however, for Minkowski to demonstrate definitively in 1889 that pancreatic extirpation produced diabetes. The histologic studies of Opie in 1901 suggested that the pancreatic lesion responsible for human diabetes was located in the islets of Langerhans. In 1920, Moses Barron hypothesized that the islets secrete a hormone which regulates carbohydrate metabolism. Finally, in December 1921, Banting and Best presented their findings that injection of an extract of pancreatic tissue, obtained 6 to 8 weeks after ligation of the pancreatic duct, resulted in reversal of the hyperglycemia and glucosuria of diabetic animals.

Definition and Classification

Diabetes mellitus is a chronic disorder of metabolism due to an absolute or relative lack of insulin. It is characterized by hyperglycemia in the postprandial and/or fasting state and in its most florid forms is accompanied by ketosis and protein wasting. When present for prolonged periods the disease is complicated by the development of small-vessel disease (*microangiopathy*) involving particularly the retina and renal glomerulus, neuropathy, and accelerated atherosclerosis. Clinically, diabetes mellitus may vary from an asymptomatic disorder detected on the basis of an abnormal blood glucose level determined during a routine examination to a fulminant, potentially catastrophic condition in which there is shock and/or coma (e.g., DKA).

Diabetes has long been classified on the basis of specific clinical features (age of onset, insulin dependence) into two major types: juvenile-onset and maturity-onset diabetes. The large overlap of age of onset among insulin-dependent and non-insulin-dependent diabetics indicates that these descriptive terms, though time-honored, are often inaccurate. Studies on the role of genetic and acquired factors in the etiology of diabetes indicate that primary diabetes is not a single disorder but a syndrome which is heterogeneous with respect to etiology as well as pathogenesis.[199] These findings suggest that potential etiologic factors such as the presence of islet cell antibodies and specific HLA (histocompatibility) haplotypes (see below) should be considered in the classification process. According to a new classification recommended by the National Institutes of Health (NIH), five major diagnostic groups are recognized: spontaneous diabetes which is insulin-dependent or non-insulin-dependent, secondary diabetes, impaired glucose tolerance, and gestational diabetes (Table 19-9).

Table 19-9. Classification of Diabetes Mellitus

- Spontaneous diabetes mellitus
  - Type I (insulin-dependent) diabetes (formerly called juvenile-onset diabetes)
  - Type II (non-insulin-dependent) diabetes (formerly called maturity-onset diabetes)
- Secondary diabetes
  - Pancreatic disease (pancreoprival diabetes, e.g., due to pancreatectomy, pancreatic insufficiency, hemochromatosis)
  - Hormonal: excess secretion of counterregulatory hormones (e.g., acromegaly, Cushing's syndrome, pheochromocytoma)
  - Drug-induced (e.g., potassium-losing diuretics, contra-insulin hormones, psychoactive agents, phenytoin)
  - Associated with complex genetic syndromes (e.g., ataxia telangiectasia, Laurence-Moon-Biedl syndrome, myotonic dystrophy, Friedrich's ataxia)
- Impaired glucose tolerance (formerly called chemical diabetes, asymptomatic diabetes, latent diabetes, and subclinical diabetes): fasting plasma glucose concentration normal; 2-h value on glucose tolerance test $>$ 140 mg/dl but $<$ 200 mg/dl
- Gestational diabetes: transient glucose intolerance which has its onset in pregnancy

Source: National Diabetes Data Group: *Diabetes* 28:1039, 1979.

In over 90 percent of cases diabetes is a spontaneous disorder which cannot be ascribed to some other more primary disease process. Two major types of spontaneous diabetes are recognized: type I or insulin-dependent diabetes (formerly called juvenile-onset diabetes) and type II or non-insulin-dependent diabetes (formerly called maturity-onset diabetes). The contrasting clinical, genetic, and immunologic characteristics of these two types of diabetes are summarized in Table 19-10. Insulin-dependent diabetes is characterized by absolute requirement for insulin treatment, a marked tendency to ketosis, onset generally but not exclusively below age 40, absence, in most patients, of obesity, and presence, in 80 percent or more of patients, of circulating islet cell antibodies at time of diagnosis. Non-insulin-dependent diabetes generally appears beyond age 40, does not lead to ketosis, and often (but not always) does not require treatment with insulin; in 80 percent of cases the patients are obese and circulating islet cell antibodies are not present. Fajans and colleagues have called attention to a form of insulin-independent diabetes which they have designated maturity-onset diabetes of young people (MODY).[199] In this form of diabetes there is neither ketosis nor insulin dependence, but asymptomatic hyperglycemia is observed in children, adolescents, and young adults and is associated with autosomal dominant transmission.[199] Regardless of the type of spontaneous diabetes, there is a progressive increase in vascular and neuropathic complications as the disease continues.

Secondary diabetes (accounting for <5 percent of all cases) is that form of the disease which occurs in patients with primary pancreatic disease or hypersecretion of hormones antagonistic to insulin, following administration of drugs which interfere with carbohydrate metabolism, or in association with complex genetic syndromes in which hyperglycemia is a characteristic feature (Table 19-9). The clinical spectrum of

Table 19-10. Clinical, Genetic, and Immunologic Characteristics of Insulin-Dependent and Non-Insulin-Dependent Diabetes

	Insulin-dependent diabetes (type I)*	Non-insulin-dependent diabetes (type II)†
Age of onset	Usually < 30	Usually > 40
Ketosis	Common	Rare
Body weight	Nonobese	Obese (80% of patients)
Prevalence	0.5%	4–5%
Genetics	HLA-associated; 40–50% concordance rate in twins	Non-HLA-associated; 95–100% concordance rate in twins
Circulating islet cell antibodies	50–85%	<10%
Treatment with insulin	Necessary	Usually not required
Complications	Frequent	Frequent

*Formerly "juvenile-onset" diabetes.
†Formerly "maturity-onset" diabetes.

these secondary forms of diabetes is quite variable, and an association with long-term complications is often difficult to establish.

Those patients in whom an abnormality in carbohydrate homeostasis is demonstrable only on the basis of the findings on a glucose tolerance test (i.e., the fasting plasma glucose concentration is normal) and in whom the elevation in plasma glucose concentration at the 2-h point in the test is <200 but >140 mg/dl (<11.1 but >7.8 mM are classified as having *impaired glucose tolerance* rather than overt diabetes. The basis for this separate classification (rather than inclusion in type II diabetes) is the observation that overt diabetes develops in such patients at a rate of only 1 to 5 percent per year and that such impairment in glucose tolerance may not be associated with an increased risk of long-term microangiopathic and neuropathic complications. The criteria for the diagnosis of overt diabetes and impaired glucose tolerance are further discussed below (see Diagnosis). When impaired glucose tolerance first appears in pregnancy, it is referred to as *gestational diabetes* (see Pregnancy and Diabetes, below).

Etiology

No single causative factor has been identified as the basis of the etiology of spontaneous diabetes. Increasing evidence has accumulated which indicates that diabetes is a heterogeneous group of disorders with varying etiologies. The major factors which have been identified are inheritance, autoimmunity, viral infections, and nutrition.[200,201]

GENETICS

A familial clustering of diabetes has long been recognized. In large population surveys the prevalence of the disease among relatives of diabetic patients has been reported as four to ten times greater than in control subjects. In addition, diabetes may occur with unusually high frequency in certain ethnic groups (e.g., type II diabetes in the Pima group of American Indians). Such aggregation may, however, reflect common environmental factors (e.g., diet) rather than inheritance. More compelling evidence for genetic transmission is provided by twin studies. Among monozygotic twins the concordance rate for diabetes (whether type I or type II) is substantially greater than in dizygotic twins.[202] While inheritance is an important etiologic factor in both types of diabetes, the genetic basis of type I diabetes is clearly different from that of type II diabetes. When monozygotic twin pairs are segregated on the basis of age of onset of diabetes, a concordance rate of 92 percent is found among those in whom diabetes began at age 40 or more in the index twin, while the concordance rate is < 50 percent when diabetes was diagnosed in the index twin before the age of 40. The different concordance rate not only indicates a distinction between type I and type II diabetes with regard to genetic input but also suggests a relatively greater role for environmental (i.e., acquired) factors in the development of type I diabetes. That the two major types of diabetes have different genetic inputs is also indicated by the fact that the prevalence of type II diabetes in the ancestors of type I diabetics is no greater than in the families of nondiabetics.

A second line of evidence indicating genetic differences between type I and type II diabetes patients and even among type I patients derives from studies of HLA antigens.[203–208] The HLA complex in humans consists of a cluster of four gene loci (designated A, B, C, and D) on the short arm of the sixth chromosome which determine the major histocompatibility antigens. Among type I diabetics a significantly increased frequency of HLA antigens B8 and B15 was initially recognized. Subsequent studies demonstrated that the association with the B locus is secondary, the primary association being with the DR (D-related) locus, specifically the *DR3* and *DR4* alleles. The presence of one of the haplotypes increases the relative risk for type I diabetes five- to sixfold and 14-fold when both alleles (*DR3* and *DR4*) are present (Table 19-11). In fact, 90 percent or more of patients with newly detected type I diabetes carry either or both *alleles.*[203] Interestingly, the presence of the *DR2* or *DR7 allele* appears to confer some protection against the development of type I diabetes. In marked contrast, no association between specific HLA types and type II diabetes has been observed.

With respect to their role in the pathogenesis of diabetes, the various HLA alleles may not of themselves be responsible for the predisposition to diabetes; they appear to exist in linkage disequilibrium with other genes that are more directly related to diabetes susceptibility. The linkage of the HLA system to the specific immune response genes has raised the possibility that the diabetic genotype operates by permitting the interaction of a virus (see below) with specific antigens on the beta cell membrane. It has also been postulated that viral infection or other environmental agents may trigger the expression of HLA-DR alleles on endocrine epithelial cells, which may allow presentation of autoantigens to T cells followed (in genetically predisposed individuals) by activation of autoreactive immunocytes.[209]

The discovery of the HLA population associations with type I diabetes has thus far failed to provide a clear-cut understanding regarding the mode of inheritance of this disorder. Simple modes of inheritance (e.g., autosomal recessive with two alleles, one normal and one diabetogenic) and more complex modes (e.g., two or more diabetogenic alleles in linkage disequilibrium with *DR3* and *DR4* respectively, or multiple loci) have been suggested.[205] The preponderant evidence does not support simple autosomal inheritance via a single gene linked to HLA, but favors two or more genes. First, the susceptibility to diabetes is substantially greater in *DR3DR4* heterozygotes than *DR3DR3* and *DR4DR4* homozygotes or when either allele is present alone.[203,205] Also, *DR3DR4* heterozygotes are twice as common in identical twin pairs concordant for type I diabetes as an identical twin pairs discordant for type I; in contrast, *DR3* or *DR4* homozygotes are not more common in concordant than in discordant pairs.[204] The number of *DR3DR4* heterozygotes in various diabetic population groups significantly exceeds the number of *DR3DR3* and *DR4DR4* homozygotes. There is also evidence that an additional non-HLA-linked gene or genes on loci other than those on chromosome 6 may influence susceptibility to type I diabetes (e.g., near the Kidd blood group and Km immunoglobulin loci on chromosome 2 and/or near the Gm immunoglobulin locus on chromosome 14).[205]

Table 19-11. Risk of Type I Diabetes for Various HLA Phenotypes Relative to the General Population

DR3	DR4	DR3 + DR4	DR2	DR7
5.0	6.8	14.3	0.1	0.1

Source: Wolf et al.[203]

In addition to genetic heterogeneity of type I diabetes as reflected by two or more susceptibility genes, phenotypic heterogeneity with respect to clinical, epidemiologic, and immunologic factors has also been suggested to exist. At present there is evidence that type I diabetes in patients with the *DR4* haplotype may be clinically more severe at the time of onset and that *DR4* patients more often have a history of viral infection and are more apt to have raised antibody titers against Coxsackie B viruses.[206]

The mode of inheritance in type II diabetes is also complex. Simple recessive inheritance is unlikely since only 30 to 50 percent of the offspring of two diabetic parents develop the disease. Incomplete penetrance cannot be invoked as the explanation of the latter phenomenon, inasmuch as virtually 100 percent concordance rates are observed among homozygotic twin pairs with type II diabetes (see above). Thus, it is most likely that transmission of type II diabetes is polygenic.

Studies examining the inheritance pattern of MODY[199] provide evidence of genetic transmission which differs from that observed in type I diabetes or the more typical, adult-onset type II diabetes. In the families of MODY patients several features point to autosomal dominant inheritance: (1) there is vertical transmission of diabetes through three generations in almost half the families; (2) 85 percent of affected patients have an affected parent; and (3) one-half of the siblings are diabetic.

In summary, genetic factors contribute to the development of all clinical forms of spontaneous diabetes, but the mode of inheritance is distinct for each type. In MODY patients an autosomal dominant pattern has been identified. In type I and type II patients complex patterns of inheritance have been determined, but it is clear that environmental factors are of great importance in type I diabetes. Furthermore, the inherited susceptibility for type I but not type II diabetes is linked to the HLA system; it is likely to involve at least two diabetogenic alleles and possibly more than one locus. Because of the complexity of the modes of inheritance, accurate counseling and prospective identification of the "prediabetic" subject on a genetic basis are not feasible at present.

VIRAL INFECTIONS AND OTHER ENVIRONMENTAL FACTORS IN TYPE I DIABETES

The high frequency (50 percent) with which type I diabetes occurs in one member of a monozygotic twin pair but not in the other indicates a strong role for nongenetic, acquired factors in the etiology of type I diabetes. Among potential environmental causes, viral infections have elicited interest.[201,210–214] The evidence for a viral etiology of diabetes derives from histologic and epidemiologic studies, case reports of viral isolation from diabetic patients, viral diabetes production in animals, and instances of transmission of diabetes from a human patient to an experimental animal by inoculation.

The histologic appearance of the islets in patients dying with type I diabetes is characterized by infiltration with mononuclear cells, particularly lymphocytes, and degeneration of islet cells (Fig. 19-36). The presence of this inflammatory response, termed *insulitis*, is compatible with a viral and/or autoimmune process. Further circumstantial evidence for a viral etiology is provided by the seasonal variation in the onset of type I diabetes; the peak incidence occurs in late summer or winter, and few cases appear in spring or early summer.

Mumps, rubella, Coxsackie B, mengo- and encephalomyocarditis (EMC) viruses have been impli-

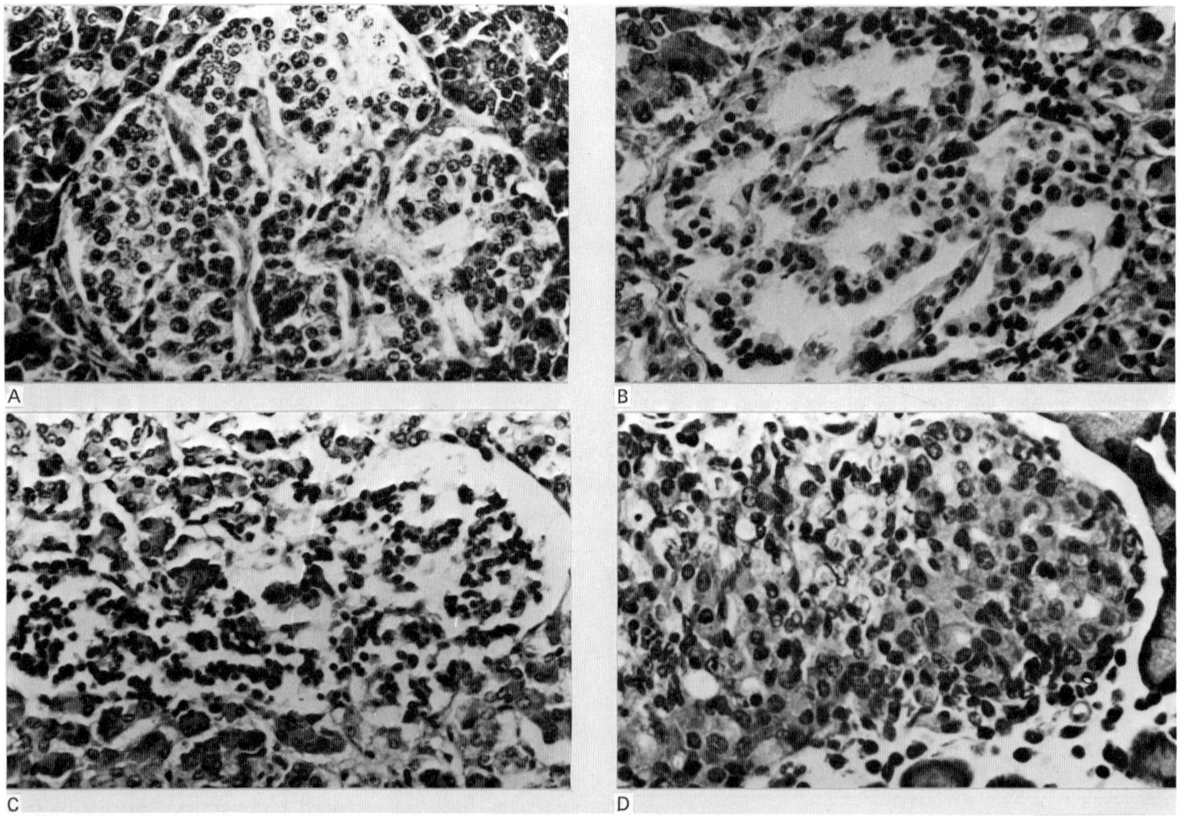

FIGURE 19-36 Insulitis in islet cells of a fatal case of virus-induced human diabetes. (*A*) Normal human pancreas with a single islet of Langerhans. Sections of pancreas from the patient (*B*) show moderate accumulation of inflammatory cells at the periphery of the islet and (*C*) an extensive inflammatory infiltrate with loss of normal islet architecture and islet cell degeneration. (*D*) Section of pancreas from a mouse 7 days after infection with the human isolate, showing inflammatory cells and marked islet cell degeneration. (*From Yoon et al.*[215])

cated as possible etiologic agents. A temporal association of diabetes onset with prior mumps infection has been noted. Diabetes has also been observed in the congenital rubella syndrome with a frequency as high as 20 percent. However, it is noteworthy that, in the decade following the institution of immunization against measles, mumps, rubella, and poliovirus, neither the incidence nor the age of onset of type I diabetes changed significantly in the United States. Coxsackie virus B4 was initially implicated on the basis of high titers of neutralizing antibodies in the sera of patients at the onset of diabetes. Subsequent studies demonstrated that mumps virus as well as Coxsackie viruses B3 and B4 were capable of replicating in human pancreatic beta cells maintained in cell culture. Furthermore, repeated passage of Coxsackie virus B4 in mouse beta cell cultures led to isolation of a diabetogenic strain which produced hyperglycemia when injected into intact mice. On the other hand, case-control studies of antibodies to Coxsackie B virus antibodies fail to show consistent evidence of an association with type I diabetes.[213] The most convincing evidence for a viral etiology in some cases of type I diabetes is provided by reports of isolation of Coxsackie virus from islet tissue of infants or children with fatal diabetes; the virus isolated caused diabetes upon inoculation of mice[213]

If infection with Coxsackie virus plays a role in the etiology of type I diabetes the question remains as to why type I diabetes develops in <0.5 percent of the population, yet evidence of infection with Coxsackie virus B4 is present in about half the population. The possibility exists that variants of the virus tropic for beta cells only rarely produce clinical disease. An alternative explanation derives from studies with the murine EMC virus. Inoculation of mice with EMC virus produces insulitis and hyperglycemia, provided that the mice have the appropriate genetic susceptibility as determined by one or more recessive genes.[201] The weight of evidence thus supports the conclusion that common viruses such as Coxsackie B viruses may bring about islet cell injury and/or destruction in some patients, but genetic and autoimmune factors are probably of greater importance in the causation of type I diabetes.

An additional environmental agent which has been implicated as a causative factor in the development of diabetes is the rodenticide pyriminil (Vacor), a nitrophenylurea derivative. Over 20 cases of insulin-dependent diabetes have been reported after the accidental ingestion of this poison.[201] These observations are significant in that they raise the possibility that some chemical in the environment may act as diabetogenic agents.

AUTOIMMUNITY IN TYPE I DIABETES

The possibility that an autoimmune process is involved in the development of type I diabetes has been suspected on the basis of several lines of evidence from human and animal studies:[214–220] (1) the presence of mononuclear cell infiltrates in the islets of newly discovered type I diabetes (insulitis); (2) the long-recognized clinical association of diabetes with autoimmune endocrinopathies (Addison's disease, Schmidt's syndrome, Graves' disease) and nonendocrine autoimmune disorders (myasthenia gravis, pernicious anemia); and (3) the relationship between diabetes and the HLA complex (see above). More direct evidence of an autoimmune process has emerged from studies of circulating islet cell antibodies (ICA) and, more recently, from the demonstration that intervention with cyclosporin A, a potent nonmyelotoxic immunosuppressant may induce a remission in patients with newly discovered type I diabetes.[221,222] Using immunofluorescent and/or complement-fixing techniques, ICA directed against cytoplasmic antigens have been detected in 60 to 98 percent of type I diabetics at the time of diagnosis; the percentage of patients with antibodies declines thereafter to only 20 percent after 3 years. By contrast, ICA were found in <10 percent of type II diabetic subjects and in only ~ 1 percent of the normal population. These antibodies are of the IgG class and are organ-specific, reacting with all types of islet cells. The antibodies are not directed at the islet hormones (insulin or glucagon) but at cytoplasmic organelles. ICA directed at beta cell surface antigens (islet cell surface antibodies, ICSA) have also been observed in patients with newly detected type I diabetes. A cytotoxic effect on beta cells is generally demonstrable with ICSA but not with cytoplasmic ICA.[220] Whereas the presence of these antibodies is usually a transient phenomenon closely related to the time of onset of diabetes, in patients with associated autoimmune polyendocrinopathy (Schmidt's syndrome), the antibody titer may remain persistently elevated.

Antipancreatic cell-mediated autoimmunity has also been described in type I diabetes on the basis of the leukocyte migration inhibition test. In 50 to 65 percent of patients, migration of leukocytes was inhibited when they were incubated with porcine or human pancreatic homogenates. Lymphocytes from diabetics have also been observed to lyse cultured human insulinoma cells.[223]

The precise pathogenic role of ICA and cell-mediated immunity in the development of type I diabetes has not been established. Whether these autoimmune phenomena are primary events, secondary effects of beta cell damage due to some other cause, or mediators of the histopathologic interactions between a genetically predisposed beta cell and some environmental agent (e.g., a virus) remains to be determined. Evidence for a pathogenic role in inducing diabetes derives from the observation that the appearance of ICA precedes rather than follows the appearance of type I diabetes by as much as 5 years.[207,219] A linear correlation between loss of beta cell function and elevated ICA titer was found.[224] On the other hand, first-degree relatives of individuals with type I diabetes may show transient increases in ICA titer and yet retain normal glucose tolerance.[209]

Autoimmune phenomena may be mediators in response to environmentally induced beta cell injury, as suggested by studies with the diabetogenic antibiotic streptozotocin in experimental animals. When administered in repeated small doses, streptozotocin produced diabetes associated with insulitis and evidence of activation of murine virus (type C) in genetically susceptible rats. Prior administration of antilymphocyte serum exerted a protective effect, suggesting an immune mechanism is involved in the development of diabetes in the susceptible animals.[225] In human subjects, acute diabetes induced by the accidental ingestion of the rodenticide Vacor has also been accompanied by the presence of ICA.[226] This observation indicates that ICA either mediate the effects of beta cell toxins or are merely a reflection of islet cell destruction.

Advances have been made in the understanding of the autoimmune factor in the etiology of diabetes by a fortunate discovery of an experimental model, the BB rat.[227–229] This animal becomes spontaneously insulin-dependent after about 2 months of life; severe insulitis is associated. The onset of clinical diabetes is preceded by the appearance of circulating ICSA and lymphocyte antibodies for several weeks. A marked correlation was found between the decrease in beta cell function and antibody titers in the latent period of lesion development. The study of the nature, formation process, and suppression of these antibodies is expected to aid in the evolution of national and testable strategies for the treatment and prevention of human type I diabetes.

Perhaps the most compelling evidence for the autoimmune etiology of human type I diabetes derives from studies with cytosporin A. Stiller et al.[221] and Feutren et al.[222] have shown that, when initiated within a few weeks of clinical onset of type I diabetes, treatment with cyclosporin A induces a significantly higher rate of remission than treatment with placebo (24.1 vs. 5.8 percent after 9 months of cyclosporin administration).[222] These findings raise hopes for even greater success of immunosuppressive intervention during the "silent" prediabetic period when the beta cell mass is not yet extensively destroyed (see Future Treatment).

OBESITY AND NUTRITION IN TYPE II DIABETES

In contrast to viral and autoimmune agents implicated as potential etiologic factors in type I diabetes, obesity is the most important acquired factor that contributes to the development of the type II disorder. The prevalence of obesity among type II diabetics is >80 percent. Conversely, in the obese population the prevalence of diabetes is increased; diabetes in this group depends on the duration rather than the degree of obesity. Ingestion of carbohydrate has not been shown to increase the likelihood of diabetes except by virtue of contributing to excessive weight gain. The mechanism whereby obesity predisposes to the development of diabetes is intimately related to the insulin resistance accompanying excessive weight gain (see below). Thus, in the genetically predisposed individual with a limited capacity for insulin secretion, the development of obesity engenders a demand for insulin that exceeds the beta cells' secretory capacity. The initial impairment of glucose tolerance may still be reversed by weight reduction. Gradually, fasting hyperglycemia and overt diabetes develop. These changes in insulin secretion and action in type II diabetes are discussed more fully below (see Pathogenesis). While obesity invariably precedes the development of diabetes, the possibility that the genetic input in the type II diabetic includes a disordered mechanism of appetite regulation or energy expenditure has not been excluded. It has been suggested, for example, that the insulin resistance of type II diabetes may accelerate the development of obesity by interfering with the thermogenic response that normally accompanies overeating.[230]

SUMMARY OF ETIOLOGIC FACTORS

Etiologically as well as clinically, diabetes is not a single disease entity. In type I diabetes a genetic predisposition linked to the HLA system is of importance but is not sufficient to bring about the disease. Acquired factors such as viral infection and/or autoimmunity are of greater significance, since they are capable of causing diabetes in the genetically susceptible host only. Genetic predisposition involves a complex mode of inheritance mediated by at least two alleles (linked to loci DR3 and DR4, respectively) which have a synergistic effect. A sequence of events which may be postulated is that in a genetically predisposed individual a viral infection triggers an autoimmune process, leading to islet cell damage (Fig. 19-37). In type II diabetes the mode of inheritance is also complex but, in contrast to type I diabetes, genetic predisposition rather than acquired beta cell injury is

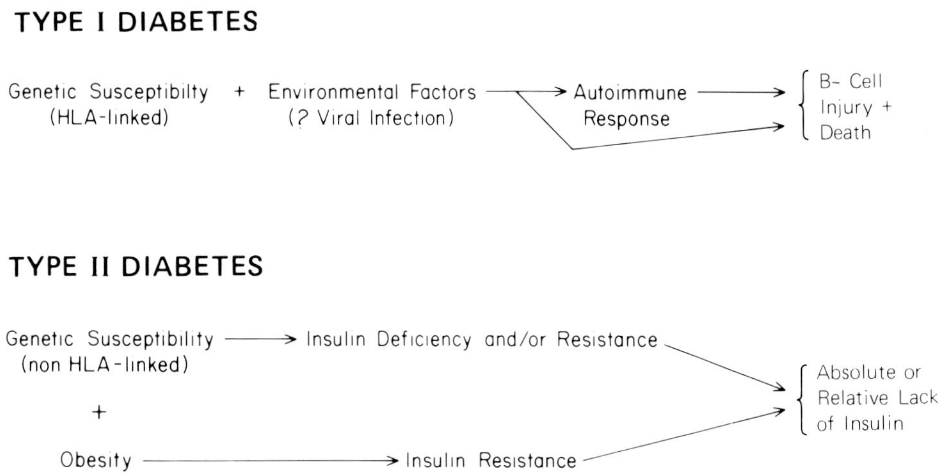

FIGURE 19-37 Etiologic factors in type I (insulin-dependent) and type II (non-insulin-dependent) diabetes. In type I diabetes genetic susceptibility (often HLA-linked) plus acquired environmental factors are necessary. The latter may take the form of a viral infection which either directly or via an autoimmune response leads to beta cell defects. In type II diabetes genetic factors are of even greater importance than in type I diabetes. The genetic susceptibility entails a secretory disorder and/or resistance to insulin. The latter is intensified by obesity (present in 80 percent of cases), resulting in an absolute or relative deficiency of insulin.

of the utmost importance. In this circumstance, most commonly, obesity leads to the clinical expression of insulin deficiency by increasing the demand for insulin secretion from genetically impaired beta cells (Fig. 19-37).

Pathogenesis

The available data clearly indicate that failure of insulin secretion is the primary pathogenic factor in type I diabetes. Glucagon excess may exaggerate the effects of insulin lack in such patients. In type II diabetes changes in tissue sensitivity to insulin (i.e., insulin resistance) have been implicated. The pattern of insulin secretion is heterogeneous; most commonly there is a relative deficiency in insulin secretion. However, resistance to insulin is more prominent and earlier apparent than the low beta cell capacity.

INSULIN SECRETION

The defect in insulin secretion in type I diabetes involves both the early and the late phases of insulin release; it rapidly progresses to nearly total secretory deficiency. In children with newly discovered type I diabetes a transient remission often occurs, the so-called honeymoon phase, and is associated with a recovery of insulin secretory ability (Fig. 19-38). Ultimately, an irreversible loss of insulin secretion occurs,

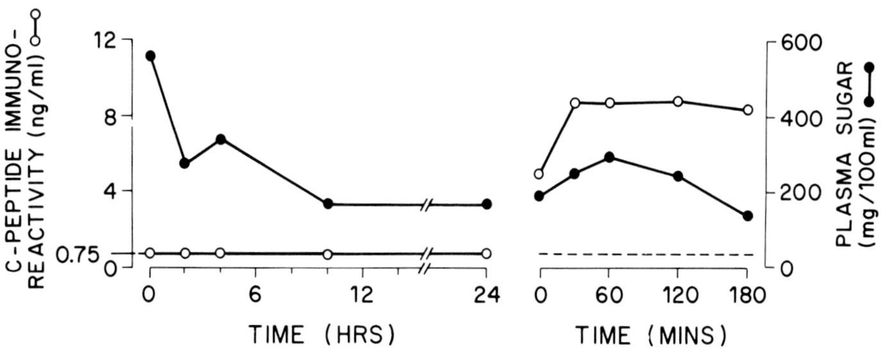

FIGURE 19-38 Changes in C peptide immunoreactivity during therapy for marked hyperglycemia in type I (insulin-dependent) diabetes (*left*) and in response to oral glucose and during a remission phase (*right*). The dotted line represents the lower limit of sensitivity of the C peptide assay. The data indicate the total absence of endogenous insulin secretion in patients with type I diabetes and moderate to severe hyperglycemia (*left*). A return of insulin secretion is seen in the transient remission phase (*right*). (*From Rubenstein AH et al: Arch Intern Med 137:625, 1977.*)

and hyperglycemia returns. Nevertheless, the defect in insulin secretion in the type I diabetic is generally not a complete failure of beta cell function. C peptide measurements have shown evidence of residual insulin secretion in patients with long-standing insulin-treated diabetes. In fact, the persistence of endogenous insulin secretion may be a major determinant of the ease with which the blood glucose concentration can be regulated using exogenous insulin.[230]

The absence of insulin secretion is evident with nonglucose stimuli as well. This lack of insulin responsiveness to all stimuli in type I diabetes represents a difference from type II diabetes, where partial responsiveness to nonglucose stimuli is preserved.[231] With the onset of fasting hyperglycemia, the response to nonglucose stimuli deteriorates.[232]

Insulin resistance also occurs to a certain extent in type I diabetes. Decreased disposal of glucose in the presence of normal and high insulin levels has been demonstrated in patients with poorly controlled type I diabetes.[233,234] The defect appears to be due to postreceptor unresponsiveness. It seems to be reversible upon insulin therapy, as suggested by experiments in dogs with alloxan-induced diabetes.[235,236] Hepatic glucose overproduction in type I diabetes is most probably not due to insulin resistance but to insulin deficiency, abetted by glucagon excess.

In type II diabetes the situation with regard to insulin secretion is less clear-cut; it never involves the severe degree of hyposecretion observed in type I patients. Early reports that insulin concentrations in type II diabetics were comparable with those in healthy individuals suggested that an impairment in insulin action exists, rather than in secretion. Such studies, however, failed to take into account the importance of obesity and the ambient glucose concentration.[237] When type II diabetics (most of whom are obese) are compared with weight-matched nondiabetic subjects, a decrease in insulin secretion, particularly in the early phase, is evident (Fig. 19-39). Furthermore, when the hyperglycemic glucose tolerance curve of such diabetics is simulated in normal individuals, the insulin response of the normal subjects clearly exceeds that of the diabetics.[238] Thus, the seeming hyperinsulinemia in most type II diabetics is a consequence of either obesity or a delay in early insulin release, which leads to hyperglycemia and secondary hyperinsulinemia late in the course of the glucose tolerance test. The insulin-secretory pattern in nonobese type II diabetics is not uniform, however; in some patients a markedly hyperinsulinemic response is observed in the absence of obesity and in the face of hyperglycemia[199,239] (Fig. 19-40). In such patients insulin resistance is the more important pathogenic factor (see below).

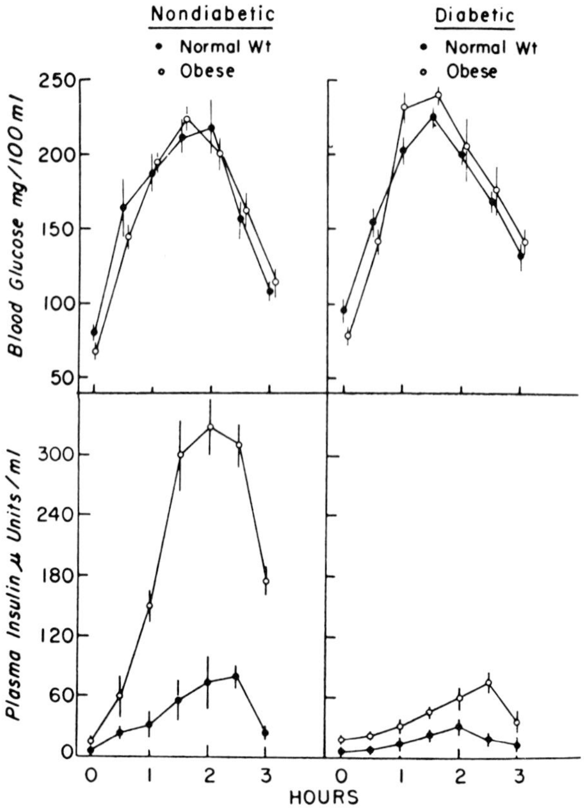

FIGURE 19-39 Plasma insulin response to a diabetic blood glucose profile (induced by intravenous glucose) in normal nonobese subjects, obese nondiabetics, nonobese diabetics, and obese diabetics. (*From Perley M, Kipnis DM: J Clin Invest 46:1954, 1967.*)

A failure of glucose recognition and/or metabolism despite the presence of an otherwise normal insulin-secretory process has been suggested to account for the hyposecretion of insulin in relation to ambient glucose concentration in most type II diabetics. Evidence for such beta cell abnormality has come from studies demonstrating a loss of early (i.e., acute-phase) insulin secretion in response to glucose stimulation even though secretory response to isoproterenol, secretin, and arginine remains normal.[231] That the decrease in glucose-stimulated insulin secretion may be mediated by the adrenergic nervous system is suggested by the improvement in secretion seen with α-adrenergic blockade and treatment with indomethacin, an inhibitor of prostaglandin synthesis.[90] Type II diabetics with severe fasting hyperglycemia ($>$250 mg/dl, or $>$14 mM) are generally severely insulinopenic and display abnormalities not only in first-phase insulin release but in the second-phase response to glucose as well.[231] The hyperglycemia of type II diabetes may actually serve to enhance the insulin response to non-

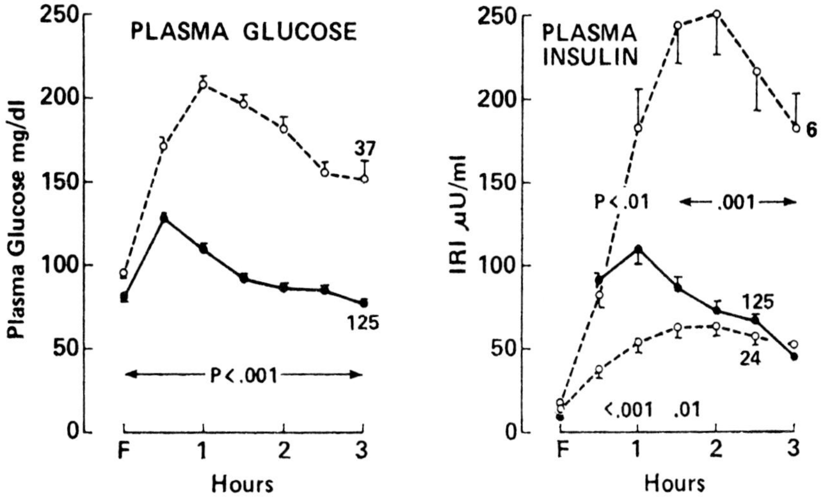

FIGURE 19-40 Heterogeneity of the insulin response to oral glucose challenge in patients with insulin-independent (type II) diabetes: ○, diabetic patients, age 18 to 25 (mean 22.0) years; ●, healthy subjects, age 18 to 25 (mean 22.3) years. The diabetic population shows two types of response, either a hyperinsulinemic or a hypoinsulinemic response to the glucose level. (*From Fajans.*[199])

glucose stimuli, since reduction of plasma glucose concentration to normal levels results in a lowering of the acute-phase insulin response to a nonglucose stimulus.[240]

INSULIN RESISTANCE

The coexistence of hyperglycemia or normoglycemia with hyperinsulinemia suggests that insulin resistance is present. More direct evidence of insulin resistance is provided by demonstrating that the in vivo effectiveness of exogenous insulin in stimulating glucose uptake by various target tissues is reduced.[158] On the basis of these criteria, obesity is clearly the most commonly encountered insulin-resistant state in humans. Its association with type II diabetes in > 80 percent of cases underscores its importance in unmasking the metabolic consequences of an inherited deficiency of beta cell function in such patients (Fig. 19-37).

Insulin resistance comprises a wide spectrum of reduced tissue sensitivity and/or reduced responsiveness to insulin. In its initial stages the enhanced insulin secretion may compensate for the reduced glucose utilization or increased gluconeogenesis. Gradually, hyperglycemia may develop and prevail in the face of insufficient insulin secretion. Even in the absence of obesity, some type II diabetic patients are hyperinsulinemic in the face of hyperglycemia.[241] Further evidence of insulin resistance in such patients was provided by studies of Reaven et al.,[239] in which the response to exogenous insulin was measured. Endogenous insulin secretion was suppressed by a combined infusion of epinephrine and propranolol at a steady rate of insulin and glucose infusion. Since similar steady plasma insulin concentrations were achieved, the steady-state plasma glucose level (SSPG) could be taken as a measure of insulin resistance; the higher the SSPG the greater the insulin resistance. In normal subjects these investigators found SSPGs of ~125 mg/dl as compared with SSPG values of 200 to 350 mg/dl in patients with type II diabetes. An alternative approach, which avoids the infusion of epinephrine and propranolol (which may of themselves alter insulin sensitivity), is the "insulin clamp" technique. In this procedure insulin is infused in physiologic doses and euglycemia is maintained by means of a variable glucose infusion. Since all the glucose infused must be metabolized, the rate of glucose infusion serves as an index of insulin-mediated glucose uptake. Using this procedure DeFronzo et al.[242] have shown a 30 to 40 percent decrease in insulin response in type II diabetes. Examination of the individual responses, however, indicates the heterogeneity of insulin resistance in this disorder. In about one-half of the subjects tissue responsiveness to insulin is reduced, while in the remainder it is normal (Fig. 19-41).

Insulin Receptors in Diabetes

The more severe the postprandial hyperglycemia in type II diabetes the greater the magnitude of insulin resistance.[243] Muscle appears to be a major site of reduced glucose uptake due to insulin resistance in type II diabetes.[244] In patients with mild fasting hyperglycemia (< 115 mg/dl or 6.4 mM) a rightward shift in the glucose dose–insulin response curve has been demonstrated while the maximal response remains unaffected. This is consistent with a decrease in number of high-affinity insulin receptors (i.e., lowered

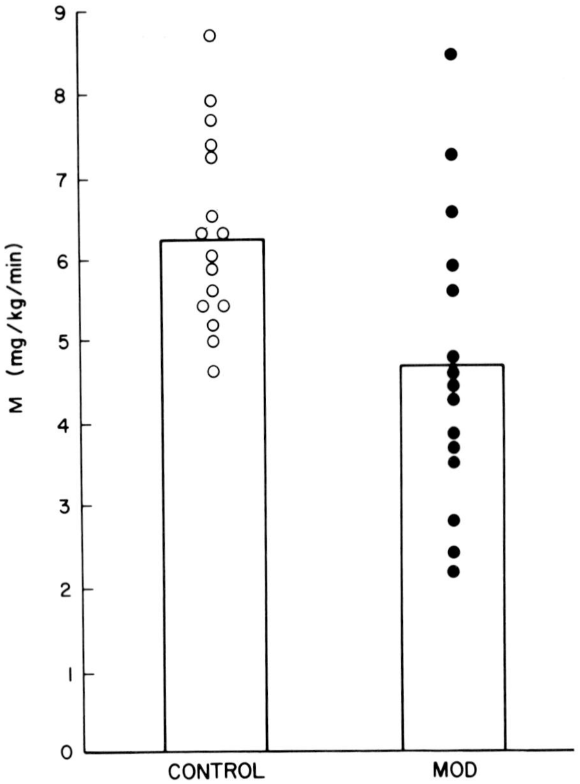

FIGURE 19-41 The heterogeneity of tissue sensitivity to insulin in insulin-independent (type II maturity-onset) diabetes (MOD). Insulin sensitivity is indicated as the rate of insulin-mediated glucose metabolism (M) during physiologic hyperinsulinemia induced by the insulin clamp technique. In the diabetic group, insulin sensistivity decreased in approximately half of the subjects compared with healthy controls. (*From DeFronzo et al.*[242])

insulin sensitivity, Fig. 19-29). With more severe diabetes, both a greater rightward shift in the insulin response curve as well as a decrease in the maximal rate of glucose disposal (impaired sensitivity and responsiveness) is seen. In the liver, the dose-response relationship for insulin-mediated suppression of glucose output shifts to the right without a decrease in the maximal response, suggesting a decline in the biological effect of insulin due solely to decreased insulin binding. This is manifested by rising fasting hyperglycemia. These observations suggest the presence of a postreceptor defect in peripheral tissues in overt type II diabetes, although a coincident decrease in the number of high-affinity receptors in both hepatic and peripheral tissues is evident.[245]

In obesity, resistance to insulin is closely related to diminished insulin binding, as assessed by measurements on adipocytes as well as circulating monocytes.[158] In nonobese, hyperinsulinemic type II diabetics, a decrease in insulin binding has also been observed. This decrease is due to a fall in the number of insulin receptors per cell rather than a change in binding affinity. Interestingly, the decrease in insulin binding is observed only in hyperinsulinemic type II diabetes and correlates closely with the insulin insensitivity.[158] As noted previously, the ambient insulin concentration has been demonstrated to regulate the number of insulin receptors.[153] Thus, decreased insulin binding and the accompanying reduction in insulin response observed in type II diabetic patients may be a consequence of down regulation by the hyperinsulinemia rather than an initiating event. This concept received strong support shown by progressive decrease in both insulin sensitivity and responses in adipocytes cultured in the presence of insulin.[246]

Postreceptor Defects

Although type II diabetic patients may have normal or raised insulin levels in the basal state, they mount a hypoinsulinemic response to a glucose challenge. It has, therefore, been postulated that the insulin deficiency may lead to a postreceptor defect which is manifested as insulin resistance. When the insulin-deficient state is corrected by intensive insulin therapy, the response to insulin improves. In this setting, the maximal rates of insulin-stimulated glucose disposal and glucose transport into adipocytes are restored. However, inhibition of hepatic glucose output during the euglycemic clamp may not be altered after intensive insulin therapy, suggesting the persistence of a receptor-mediated defect. This may be due to a further reduction in insulin receptor number resulting from intensified insulin therapy.[247,248]

Acanthosis Nigricans

Decreased insulin binding has also been shown to be of importance in some rare cases of extreme insulin resistance associated with acanthosis nigricans. In patients with this disorder insulin binding is reduced by 50 to 100 percent. Analysis of the clinical findings and receptor function permits classification of these patients into two groups.[154] In type A, the patients are younger and show evidence of virilization. In type B, the patients are older and manifest immunologic abnormalities, including a circulating anti-receptor antibody which is responsible for the decrease in insulin binding. The decrease in receptor number observed in the type A syndrome was initially theorized to have been due to down regulation as a result of the prevailing hyperinsulinemia. Evidence for the decrease in receptor number as the primary defect comes from studies involving fasting and tissue culture models. When type A patients fast, plasma insulin levels return to normal although insulin binding remains abnormal. In contrast, obese subjects who fast show an increase in insulin binding. Furthermore, in vitro tissue culture studies have demonstrated the persistence of insulin binding abnormalities in cells from patients with the type A syndrome.[249–251]

GLUCAGON SECRETION

Unger has suggested that the metabolic defects in diabetes are not solely due to insulin lack but that diabetes is a bihormonal disorder to which relative or absolute hyperglucagonemia is an essential contribution.[175] Evidence that altered secretion of glucagon is important in the pathogenesis of diabetes is presented by a variety of observations. In diabetics glucose fails to suppress glucagon secretion and administration of protein or amino acids causes hypersecretion of glucagon[55] (Fig. 19-42). In contrast, the glucagon response to hypoglycemia is blunted in type I diabetics, suggesting a defect in a glucose receptor on the alpha cell.[252] In addition, in experimental animals, diabetes induced by pancreatectomy is accompanied by excessive extrapancreatic production of glucagon.[175] Furthermore, a

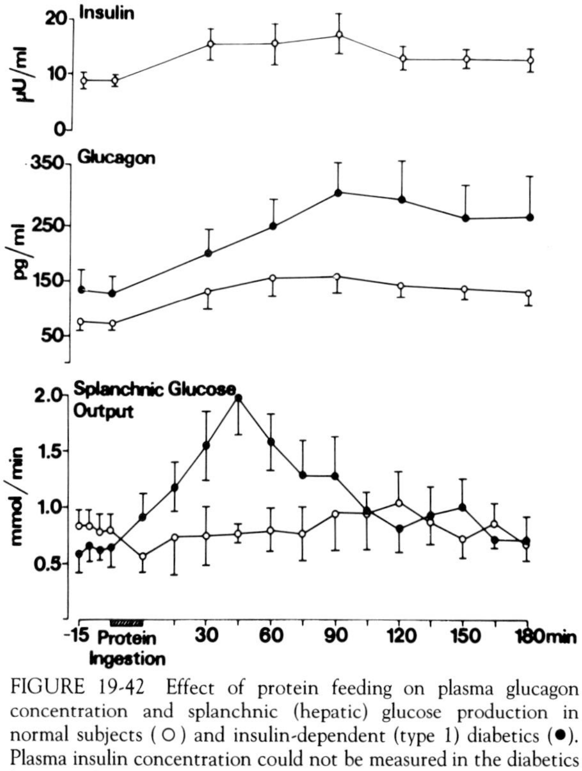

FIGURE 19-42 Effect of protein feeding on plasma glucagon concentration and splanchnic (hepatic) glucose production in normal subjects (○) and insulin-dependent (type 1) diabetics (●). Plasma insulin concentration could not be measured in the diabetics because of prior treatment with insulin. The protein meal results in a marked increase in glucose production in the diabetics but not in normal individuals. This difference is due to the exaggerated rise in plasma glucagon level in a setting of absolute insulin deficiency. (*Based on the data of Wahren et al.*[55])

reduction in plasma glucagon concentration induced by somatostatin results in amelioration of diabetic hyperglycemia.[93]

Despite the attractiveness of the bihormonal concept other findings have cast serious doubt on the essentiality of glucagon or the presence of a primary defect in alpha cell function in spontaneous human diabetes.[174,178] So long as insulin is available, an elevation in plasma glucagon concentration (produced by infusion), which simulates the hyperglucagonemia of diabetes or other hyperglucagonemic states, fails to cause glucose intolerance in normal humans or to precipitate deterioration of glucose control in known diabetics.[253] In pancreatectomized humans, extrapancreatic glucagon is not produced, yet hyperglycemia and ketosis develop.[168] In like manner, prolonged suppression of glucagon and insulin secretion by somatostatin results in transient hypoglycemia that is followed by fasting hyperglycemia and glucose overproduction (i.e., a diabetic state), despite ongoing suppression of glucagon.[178] In insulin-dependent diabetics, in whom somatostatin substantially reduces postprandial hyperglycemia, the effect is largely a consequence of diminished carbohydrate and protein absorption rather than enhanced carbohydrate use.[94] Finally, treatment with insulin results in suppression of hyperglucagonemia in human diabetes and in restoration of normal alpha cell function in experimentally induced animal diabetes.[176]

The major role of glucagon in diabetes is thus to intensify the consequences of insulin deficiency. Accordingly, meal-induced glucagon secretion in poorly controlled diabetes exaggerates the degree of postprandial hyperglycemia. In addition, the hyperglucagonemia enhances hepatic ketogenesis and gluconeogenesis.[41] A primary role for glucagon in the development of hyperglycemia has been observed in patients with the glucagonoma syndrome (see Endocrine Associated Diabetes, below).

OTHER HORMONES

Persistent hypersecretion of glucocorticoids (Cushing's syndrome) or GH (acromegaly) often results in secondary diabetes (see below). In both conditions hyperglycemia is a consequence of hormone-induced insulin resistance, mediated, at least in part, by a diminution in insulin binding.[154] In contrast, in primary spontaneous diabetes (either type I or type II), circulating levels of GH, cortisol, and catecholamines are usually normal. However, in DKA and in response to exercise in poorly controlled diabetes, marked increments of concentrations of each of the counterregulatory hormones are observed. The secondary nature of these abnormalities is suggested by the fact that normalization of plasma glucose concentration by insulin treatment restores normal testing and postexercise levels of the counterregulatory hormones.[254] Nevertheless, during surgery or other forms of stress, hypersecretion of counterregulatory hormones may cause a worsening of an already-manifest diabetic state or the transient development of hyperglycemia in a previously normal patient (see Stress Hyperglycemia, above).

Pathophysiology

The metabolic alterations observed in diabetes primarily reflect the degree to which there is an absolute or a relative deficiency of insulin. Since insulin is the major storage hormone, minimal insulin deficiency results in diminished ability to increase the reservoir of body fuels because of inadequate disposal of ingested foodstuffs. With a major deficiency of insulin, not only is fuel accumulation hampered in the fed state, but excessive mobilization of endogenous metabolic fuels (e.g., hyperglycemia, hyperaminoacidemia, and elevated FFA concentration) occurs in the fasting condition and even in the face of hyperphagia. In the most severe form of diabetes (DKA) there is overproduction of glucose and marked acceleration of catabolic processes (e.g., lipolysis, proteolysis).

CARBOHYDRATE METABOLISM

The mildest type of abnormality in carbohydrate metabolism related to diabetes is a decrease in glucose tolerance in association with a normal fasting blood glucose concentration. In this circumstance ingested glucose fails to elicit an adequate insulin response (because of either a secretory defect or tissue resistance to insulin); glucose consequently escapes uptake by the liver and is more slowly metabolized by peripheral tissues.[255]

When absolute or relative insulin deficiency occurs in the basal state, an elevation in fasting blood glucose concentration ensues. In this situation, normal basal levels of insulin may be maintained, but only with the cost of developing fasting hyperglycemia. In such patients, glucose production (determined by either radioactive tracer techniques or splanchnic balance studies) is generally normal or only slightly increased,[104] while fractional glucose turnover (glucose utilization relative to plasma glucose concentration) is reduced. In a normal individual even mild hyperglycemia is sufficient to inhibit hepatic glucose output (because of an accompanying rise in insulin concentration[64]), however, the diabetic patient with fasting hyperglycemia is always in a state of relative or absolute glucose overproduction. Furthermore, the relative contribution of gluconeogenesis to total hepatic glucose output is increased twofold.[104] This enhancement of gluconeogenesis with moderate deficiency of insulin is in keeping with the relatively greater amounts of insulin necessary to inhibit gluconeogenesis as compared with glycogenolysis.[64,102] In addition, the failure of hepatic glucose uptake after feeding results in glycogen depletion.

With the progress to total beta cell failure, an ever-increasing fasting blood glucose level fails to elicit a beta cell secretory response. In the absence of the restraining influence exerted by insulin, glucose production by the liver increases to three or more times normal, largely as a consequence of accelerated gluconeogenesis. The clinical correlate of this sequence of events is severe hyperglycemia, as is observed in DKA or nonketotic hyperosmolar coma.

Although the kidney also possesses the enzymes necessary for gluconeogenesis, a significant addition of glucose to the bloodstream by the kidney has not been observed in compensated human diabetes;[256] renal production of glucose may, however, become substantial on prolonged fasting.[257] Renal gluconeogenesis plays an important physiologic role by regulating the ammonia ion supply in response to shifts in acid-base status.[258,259] In the acidotic stage of diabetes cations are extensively required in order to permit excretion of keto- and other acids. The kidney responds by deaminating glutamine and glutamic acid, thereby producing NH_4^+. This is achieved by direct activation of a phosphate-dependent glutaminase and adaptive induction of PEPCK. The enhanced gluconeogenesis actually serves as a removal pathway for carbon skeletons of glutamine. Thus, alleviation of the acidemia involving oral and urinary cation loss in DKA carries the expense of aggravating the hyperglycemia.

PROTEIN AND AMINO ACID METABOLISM

Severe insulin deficiency is accompanied by negative nitrogen balance and marked protein wasting. In insulin-dependent diabetics, growth retardation is a frequent complication of poor diabetes control. Such changes are not surprising, since insulin, when present in normal amounts, stimulates protein synthesis and muscle amino acid uptake and inhibits protein catabolism and the output of amino acids from muscle. The changes in protein metabolism also involve gluconeogenesis, inasmuch as glucose overproduction in ketotic diabetic patients depends in part on augmented utilization of protein-derived precursors. The alterations in amino acid metabolism which characterize the diabetic state are, however, demonstrable even in the absence of severe insulin deficiency; they occur in the fasted (postabsorptive) as well as the protein-fed state.

In the insulin-dependent diabetic with mild to moderate hyperglycemia, changes in circulating amino acid levels, hepatic amino acid uptake, and muscle output of amino acids are demonstrable. A reduction in the plasma concentration of alanine and elevations in branched-chain amino acid concentrations (valine, leucine, and isoleucine) have been repeatedly shown in spontaneous diabetes in humans[108] as well as in experimental diabetes in animals. Despite the reduction in plasma alanine concentration, uptake of glucogenic amino acids and other glucose precursors by the liver is increased twofold or more.[104] As a consequence of this increase in substrate uptake, gluconeogenesis can account for > 30 percent of hepatic glucose production, as compared with 15 to 20 percent in normal humans. Since circulating alanine levels are reduced in diabetic patients, augmented fractional alanine extraction by the liver is responsible for the increase in alanine uptake. In the absence of the normal restraining effect of insulin on gluconeogenesis, the liver acts as a sink, depleting arterial alanine.

In contrast to the decrease in circulating alanine level, elevations in plasma concentrations of branched-chain amino acids are demonstrable in the fasting state in diabetes. Studies in experimental animals indicate that oxidation of leucine, isoleucine, and valine, once they enter muscle tissue, is accelerated in the diabetic state.[260] Repletion of muscle nitrogen after protein feeding is also reduced in diabetics. In contrast to the large, persistent uptake of branched-chain amino acids by muscle tissue which follows the ingestion of a protein meal by normal subjects, in diabetics amino acid uptake is only transient. As a consequence, total amino acid uptake by muscle is decreased and the plasma levels of the branched-chain amino acids are abnormally elevated after protein feeding.[55,108] These observations are in keeping with the known stimulatory effect of insulin on muscle amino acid uptake, which is most marked for the branched-chain amino acids. The arterial accumulation and reduced uptake of amino acids after protein feeding indicate that diabetes is characterized by protein as well as glucose intolerance. The defect in protein metabolism in diabetic individuals is further accentuated by the fact that those amino acids which are taken up by muscle tissue are preferentially catabolized rather than incorporated into protein.

PROTEIN-CARBOHYDRATE INTERACTIONS

In addition to the abnormalities in amino acid metabolism, protein feeding exacerbates the changes in carbohydrate homeostasis characteristic of diabetes. In normal, healthy subjects after protein feeding, blood glucose levels and splanchnic glucose output remain unchanged, despite an elevation in plasma insulin concentration (Figs. 19-32 and 19-42). This constancy of hepatic glucose production and blood glucose concentration is a consequence of protein-stimulated glucagon secretion which counteracts the effects of the concomitant rise in plasma insulin concentration. In marked contrast, in diabetic patients protein feeding results in a 150 percent increase in splanchnic glucose output (Fig. 19-42), as well as an exaggerated rise in plasma glucose concentration.[55] The stimulatory effect of protein feeding on hepatic glucose production is probably a consequence of the rise in plasma glucagon concentration; in the diabetic the glucagon concentration increase is exaggerated and occurs in a setting of absolute insulin deficiency. However, despite ongoing hyperglucagonemia, the increase in hepatic glucose production in the diabetic does not persist (Fig. 19-42). This transient hepatic response is in keeping with the only evanescent stimulatory effect of physiologic increments in glucagon concentration on hepatic glucose output.[174,178] Thus, the progressive increase in blood glucose concentration which accompanies a protein meal in the insulin-deficient diabetic does not reflect ongoing glucagon-mediated stimulation of hepatic glucose production. Rather, the hyperglycemia reflects the persistent failure (engendered by insulin lack) to metabolize the increased amount of glucose which is delivered to the periphery as a consequence of a transient elevation in hepatic glucose output.

FAT METABOLISM AND DIABETIC HYPERLIPIDEMIA

Elevation of plasma lipid concentration in diabetes is well documented. Mean levels of plasma triglycerides and cholesterol in individuals with various types of diabetes are higher than levels in nondiabetic subjects, reflecting an elevation in at least 50 percent of patients.[261] However, the individual values vary widely, depending on the severity of diabetes, its therapeutic control, and the composition of the diet.

In decompensated type I diabetic patients, the plasma FFA concentration is elevated as a result of increased FFA outflow from fat depots, where the balance of the FFA esterification–triglyceride lipolysis cycle is displaced in favor of lipolysis. The hepatic FFA inflow exceeds the energy requirement. One obvious outcome is increased ketone formation; the other entails reesterification of the FFA and reassembly of the triglycerides into VLDL, with return to the circulation.[262,263] Thus, the increased uptake of preformed FFA by the liver and their reexport as VLDL-borne triglycerides is one of the mechanisms leading to hyperlipidemia. This is not a strictly proportional relationship; in severe insulin deficiency VLDL secretion may be retarded due to a disturbance in apolipoprotein synthesis, and the liver triglyceride content may considerably increase (diabetic "fatty liver").

Another mechanism leading to the retention in plasma of either VLDL elaborated in the liver or chylomicrons produced from exogenous fat in the gut is decreased uptake by peripheral tissues.[264] The low capacity for triglyceride storage can be attributed in large measure to the reduction in lipoprotein lipase, an enzyme specifically oriented to cleave VLDL- and chylomicron-borne triglycerides, located on the capillary endothelial walls. The low activity of this rapidly turning-over enzyme in adipose tissue in experimental and human diabetes results from insulin deficiency, since its synthesis is induced by insulin.[265] However, despite the importance of adipose tissue lipoprotein lipase in triglyceride removal, its overall contribution to diabetic hyperlipidemia must be viewed in the context that adipose tissue constitutes $<$ 15 percent of body weight and that substantial lipoprotein lipase activity resides in other tissues, notably heart and skeletal muscle. Generally, a reciprocal relationship exists between adipose tissue and muscle lipoprotein lipase activity; the latter increases in conditions of insulin deficiency,[266,267] exercise,[268] and glucocorticoid-induced insulin antagonism.[269] Thus, even if the total body capacity to remove triglycerides is somewhat lowered, a redistribution in sites of triglyceride uptake occurs in diabetes, in keeping with the shift from triglyceride storage in adipose tissue to triglyceride utilization in muscles and other tissues.

Therefore, factors additional to the suppression of adipose tissue lipoprotein lipase activity may be instrumental in eliciting the diabetic hyperlipidemia, e.g. alterations in apolipoprotein composition of VLDL and chylomicrons, notably a decrease in the apoprotein E component. This change is associated with delayed removal of these particles from the circulation presumably due to an altered recognition pattern by tissue receptors.[270,271]

Plasma triglyceride (e.g., VLDL) concentration is elevated more frequently in diabetes than is cholesterol level. When total plasma cholesterol concentration is elevated, this often represents an increase in VLDL cholesterol concentration. However, the presumption that a high-carbohydrate diet, advocated for maintenance of diabetic patients, may result in hypertriglyceridemia and deterioration of diabetes control has not been supported.[272,273]

Hypertriglyceridemia is present in type II diabetes as well. However, in contrast to the increased FFA recirculation associated with insulinopenia, the hypertriglyceridemia in type II diabetes may be attributed to hyperinsulinemia (Fig 19-43). This enhances de novo fatty acid and VLDL synthesis in the liver as well as transport and storage of triglycerides in the periphery. The combined impact of hyperglycemia plus hyperinsulinemia promotes lipogenesis from carbohydrate, as insulin resistance at the hepatic level does not appear to affect the lipogenic pathway.[269] Thus, hypertriglyceridemia in most patients with type II diabetes is

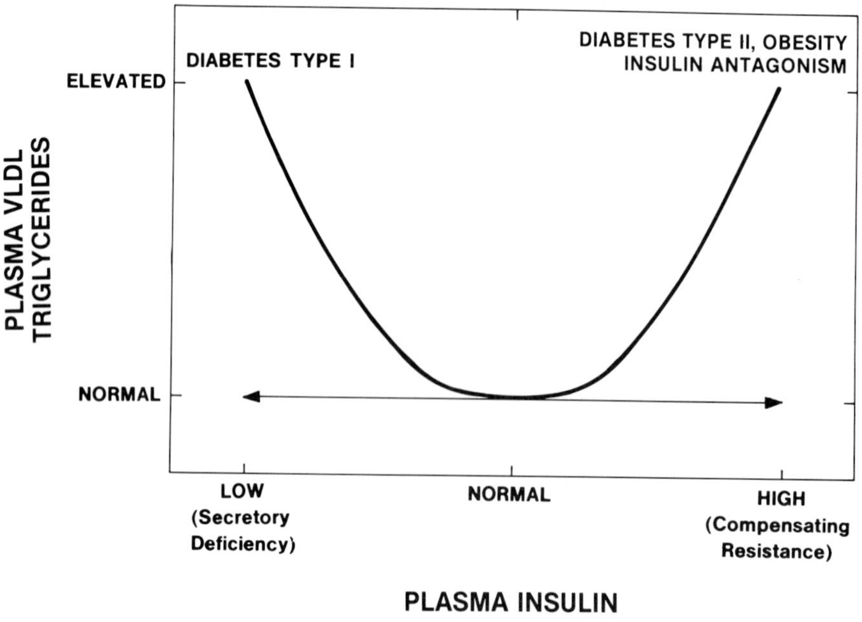

FIGURE 19-43 Summary representation showing that hypertriglyceridemia in diabetes may be elicited by both insulin deficiency and excess. In type I diabetes low insulin availability causes an increased transfer of FFA from adipose tissue to the liver. The liver responds with esterification and return of a part of the preformed FFA surplus into the circulation as VLDL-borne triglycerides. In type II diabetes the liver responds to the elevated insulin and glucose concentrations in the circulation with stimulation of the lipogenic pathway, resulting in de novo lipogenesis, reduced FFA oxidation, and enhanced VLDL production.

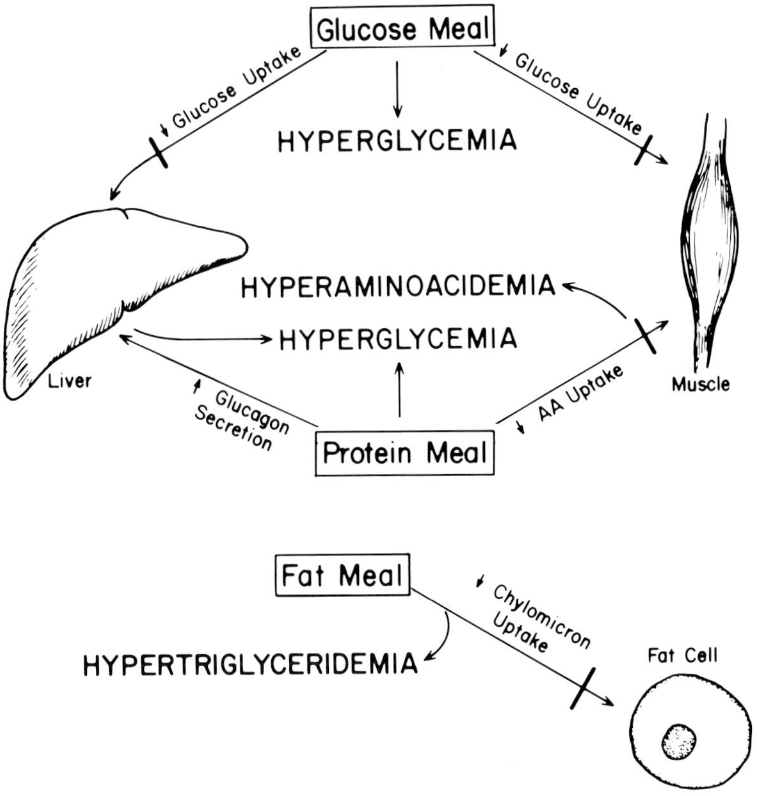

FIGURE 19-44 Pathophysiology of the metabolic abnormalities in the insulin-deficient diabetic in the fed state. Failure of glucose uptake by liver and muscle results in hyperglycemia after a carbohydrate meal. Following a protein meal hyperaminoacidemia occurs because of failure of amino acid (AA) uptake in muscle; hyperglycemia occurs because of the unopposed action of excessive increments in plasm glucagon concentration. After a fatty meal diminished activity of lipoprotein lipase results in decreased clearance of chylomicrons by adipose tissue, leading to hypertriglyceridemia. Increased production of triglycerides by the liver may also occur as a consequence of increased FFA delivery to the liver and recirculation of FFA in VLDL.

associated with increased adipose tissue mass leading to increased plasma FFA concentration;[274] the hepatic triglyceride synthesis is further aided by increased availability of preformed FFA, which is characteristic of obesity.[275,276] Studies of triglyceride turnover confirm the existence of VLDL overproduction in type 2 diabetes.[277] The defect in FFA turnover is potentially reversible with improved metabolic control.[260,278]

Both the frequency and the mechanism of plasma cholesterol concentration elevation in diabetes remain unsettled.[279,280] A consistent relationship between plasma glucose and serum cholesterol concentrations has not been observed. Furthermore, total sterol synthesis is not necessarily elevated in the patient with poorly regulated diabetes. The complexity of cholesterol metabolism is illustrated by the stimulation of intestinal cholesterologenesis in diabetes[281] while the hepatic cholesterol synthesis is uninfluenced or suppressed. Increased glycosylation of tissue collagen[282] and glycation of cholesterol-carrying low-density lipoproteins (LDL),[33] occurring under the conditions of hyperglycemia, lead to the retention of LDL cholesterol in the circulation due to delayed entry into the cells. In any event, hypercholesterolemia, together with hypertriglyceridemia, should be regarded as a factor contributing to accelerated atherosclerosis and the high incidence of coronary heart disease in the diabetic population.[280] The enhanced atherosclerotic process may also be related to a decrease in plasma HDL and apoprotein A-1 concentrations,[283–285a] particularly in patients with suboptimal treatment and/or high VLDL levels.

SUMMARY

Mild or moderate insulin lack is characterized by a failure to replete or augment body fuel stores in response to feeding (Fig. 19-44). Consequently, when a glucose-containing meal is eaten, failure of hepatic and muscle uptake of glucose results in hyperglycemia which is augmented by inadequate suppression of hepatic gluconeogenesis. When protein is ingested, insulin deficiency results in decreased amino acid uptake by muscle accompanied by hyperaminoacidemia. Hypersecretion of glucagon in response to the protein meal causes hyperglycemia. When a fat-containing meal is eaten, postprandial hypertriglyceridemia occurs because of inadequate removal of the circulating chylomicrons, mainly as a result of diminished activity of lipoprotein lipase. The hypertriglyceridemia is caused mainly by hepatic recirculation of the high levels of plasma FFA in the form of VLDL-borne triglycerides (in type I diabetes) or de novo lipogenesis in the liver (in type II diabetes).

With severe insulin lack, plasma elevations of concentrations of each of these fuels (glucose, amino acids, FFA) are observed in the fasted as well as the fed state (Fig. 19-44). The increased levels of circulating substrates are due to accelerated breakdown of body fuel reserves through increased proteolysis and lipolysis, as well as to overproduction of glucose and ketones from the respective precursors (amino acids and FFA).

Diagnosis

There is extensive evidence of altered secretion of insulin and/or sensitivity to insulin and changes in plasma concentrations of FFA and other metabolic fuels in diabetes. Nevertheless, for the clinician diagnosis of diabetes rests on the demonstration of the presence of hyperglycemia. In the patient who is clearly symptomatic, with polydipsia, polyuria, polyphagia, and weight loss, hyperglycemia is likely to be present in the fasting as well as the postprandial state. However, in the asymptomatic patient with a normal or nearly normal fasting plasma glucose level, the criteria for diagnosis and the indications for glucose tolerance testing have been the subject of debate.[286] Regardless of the criteria employed, proper understanding of the technical and physiologic factors which influence the glucose concentration is necessary for correct interpretation of laboratory data.

Since the introduction of automated laboratory methods, plasma or serum rather than whole blood has generally been employed for glucose measurement. The lower glucose concentration within red cells as compared with extracellular fluid accounts for the fact that glucose concentrations when measured in whole blood are ~85 percent of those observed in plasma. The analytical procedures currently employed to measure plasma glucose concentration are based on specific enzymatic methods (glucose oxidase or hexokinase). Formerly used methods, based on the reducing properties of the aldehyde group of glucose, are being phased out because of their low specificity; in situations such as uremia or in patients taking large doses of ascorbic acid, falsely elevated glucose concentration values were obtained with the former methods. In the laboratory, glucose concentration should be promptly determined or the blood samples should be centrifuged and the plasma (or serum) frozen until analyzed.

FASTING PLASMA GLUCOSE CONCENTRATION

In normal subjects the fasting plasma glucose concentration generally is < 110 mg/dl (< 6 mM) after an overnight (10- to 14-h) fast. A fasting plasma glucose level of > 140 mg/dl (> 8 mM) is definitely abnormal; if documented on more than one occasion (to exclude the possibilities that the patient has failed to recall having eaten breakfast or an error has been made, such a plasma glucose level establishes the diagnosis of diabetes. Many of the factors discussed below which influence glucose tolerance (e.g., age, diet, activity) have little effect on fasting plasma glucose level. On the other hand, intercurrent disease, by virtue of its "stress" effects (see Stress Hyperglycemia, above), may cause fasting hyperglycemia which reverts to normal following resolution of the underlying disease process. Individuals with this type of hyperglycemia, however, may be prone to the subsequent development of permanent diabetes.

ORAL GLUCOSE TOLERANCE TESTING

If the fasting plasma glucose concentration is normal (between 110 and 140 mg/dl or 6 to 8 mM), carbohydrate metabolism may nevertheless be abnormal as reflected by the plasma glucose response to an oral or IV glucose load. The procedure most commonly employed to evaluate carbohydrate metabolism is the oral glucose tolerance test. For proper interpretation of data, the testing conditions must be standardized. The test should be performed in the morning after an overnight, 10- to 14-h fast. The patient is seated or supine during the test and is not permitted to smoke. After a fasting blood sample is obtained, a glucose solution (generally a commercial cola-flavored preparation) is ingested over 5 min in a dose of 1.75 g glucose per kilogram of body weight up to a maximum dose of 100 g (the results do not differ if a maximum dose of 75 g is used). Thereafter, venous blood samples are obtained at 60, 90, and 120 min. In patients in whom the diagnosis of hypoglycemia is suspected, additional blood samples are obtained at 3, 4, and 5 h and at any time that the patient notes the development of symptoms.

The ingestion of a diet rich in carbohydrate (300 g per day) for at least 3 days prior to glucose tolerance testing was recommended in the past as a necessary preparation to avoid the glucose intolerance associated with starvation-like conditions. However, a reduction in dietary carbohydrate intake to as little as 100 g per day fails to diminish glucose tolerance.[287] Consequently, only if the patient has been following a severely restricted dietary regimen is any increase in carbohydrate intake necessary prior to testing.

Factors Affecting Glucose Tolerance

The ability to metabolize a glucose load is influenced by the patient's age, activity, and diet; drugs; and intercurrent disease (Table 19-12). Aging is recognized

Table 19-12. Factors Diminishing Performance in Glucose Tolerance Testing

Age: blood glucose concentration increases 10 mg/dl per decade beyond the fifth decade
Inactivity
Diet (if < 100 g carbohydrate per day)
Drugs
Potassium-wasting diuretics
Phenytoin
Alcohol (large amounts)
Corticosteroids
Oral contraceptives
Psychoactive drugs
Intercurrent disease
Endocrine abnormalities
Renal failure
Cirrhosis
Nonspecific severe stress
Myocardial infarction
Sepsis

as one of the most important factors influencing performance on glucose tolerance tests.[288] As compared with younger individuals, a progressive rise in 1- and 2-h glucose concentration values is observed beyond age 50. A decrease in tissue sensitivity is the major factor responsible for the diminution in glucose tolerance.[289] Although physical inactivity and reduction in lean body mass may be contributory factors, the aging process per se contributes to the development of insulin resistance. In general, the 1- and 2-h values on the glucose tolerance test rise by 10 mg/dl for each decade beyond the fifth. Consequently, unless the diagnostic criteria (see below) are age-adjusted, as many as 70 percent of patients above age 70 would be labeled "diabetic."

Inactivity associated with prolonged bed rest (i.e., several weeks or more) also results in a rise in postprandial plasma glucose level. As in the case of aging, the effect of inactivity is to diminish tissue response to insulin rather than insulin secretion. In contrast, a marked increase in physical activity (as in the trained athlete) enhances sensitivity to insulin. Very active individuals nevertheless show normal glucose concentration increments during glucose tolerance testing, but only minimal elevations in plasma insulin concentration.[290] Circadian factors also influence carbohydrate metabolism; a mild decrease in glucose disposal is observed in the late afternoon and evening. As noted above, severe restriction in dietary carbohydrate (<100 g per day) diminishes glucose tolerance.

A variety of drugs also may influence glucose tolerance. Consequently, where possible, their intake should be discontinued 3 days prior to testing. Large amounts of alcohol, thiazides, and other potassium-wasting diuretics (e.g., furosemide and chlorthalidone) and high doses of phenytoin (which interferes with insulin release) are associated with a lessening of glucose tolerance. The oral contraceptive agents (estrogen-progestins) cause a deterioration in glucose tolerance; this is due primarily to the estrogen component. Psychoactive agents such as phenothiazines and tricyclic antidepressants (amitriptyline, imipramine, nortriptyline) reduce glucose disposal. However, depression per se is associated with a fall in glucose tolerance, which is restored to normal with improvement in mood. A variety of endocrine disorders such as acromegaly and spontaneous and iatrogenic Cushing's syndrome as well as renal failure and hepatic cirrhosis are associated with an increased frequency of glucose intolerance. In renal failure, resistance to insulin, hyperglucagonemia, and augmented sensitivity to glucagon have been implicated as pathogenic factors.[174] In cirrhosis, portal-systemic shunting, resulting in failure of hepatic glucose uptake, resistance to insulin, decreased insulin secretion, and hyperglucagonemia, may be a contributory factor.[181] Glucose tolerance may also be diminished as a result of the nonspecific stress effects of any serious acute illness, e.g., myocardial infarction or sepsis (see Stress Hyperglycemia, above).

Diagnostic Criteria

The criteria for the diagnosis of diabetes on the basis of glucose tolerance testing have varied widely. The criteria widely employed in the past were those established by Fajans and Conn (Table 19-13). However, it may be argued that these criteria, even when age-adjusted, fail to provide a meaningful diagnosis of diabetes. First, large surveys in most population groups fail to reveal a bimodal distribution (a clear grouping of values around a normal as well as an abnormal peak). Consequently, any criteria employed (e.g., two standard deviations above the mean) are somewhat arbitrary. Second, many subjects may exceed the normal limits on the first test and then revert to a normal response on repeated glucose tolerance testing. Third, no more than 10 to 50 percent of patients diagnosed as abnormal on the basis of the Fajans-Conn or similar criteria develop overt diabetes (fasting hyperglycemia) over the ensuing 10 years (1 to 5 percent per year);[291] a similar proportion revert to normal on repeat testing. Fourth, while patients with a mildly abnormal glucose tolerance response are at increased risk of large-vessel cardiovascular disease (atherosclerosis),

Table 19-13. Criteria for Diagnosis of Diabetes by Oral Glucose Tolerance Testing
Two different standards for evaluation of plasma glucose concentrations at various time points after glucose ingestion

		NIH international workgroup*	
Time, min	Fajans-Conn	Overt diabetes	Impaired glucose tolerance
30		1 value > 200 (30, 60, 90)	1 value > 200
60	195		
90	165		
120	140†	> 200	> 140† but < 200

Note: all plasma glucose concentrations in mg/dl.
*National Diabetes Data Group: *Diabetes* 28:1039, 1979.
†In patients above age 50 add 10 mg/dl for each decade beyond the fifth.

they fail to develop the microangiopathy (retinopathy, nephropathy) observed in patients with overt diabetes.[292] Finally, studies in the Pima have shown a bimodal distribution on glucose tolerance testing; a 2-h value > 200 mg/dl separates the diabetic from the nondiabetic group.[293] The individuals with 2-h plasma glucose concentration values > 200 mg/dl also experience the long-term complications of diabetes such as retinopathy and neuropathy.

On the basis of the above considerations, an international study group sponsored by the NIH recommended new criteria for the establishment of a diagnosis of diabetes in patients without fasting hyperglycemia (Table 19-13). In the absence of fasting hyperglycemia, overt diabetes is present if the 2-h glucose concentration is > 200 mg/dl (11.1 mM) and one other value (at 30, 60, or 90 min) is also > 200 mg/dl. Plasma glucose concentrations which are intermediate between normal and overt diabetes (2-h value 140 to 200 mg/dl plus one value at 30 to 90 min > 200 mg/dl) are defined as *impaired glucose tolerance*. Such patients were previously described as having "chemical," "latent," or "subclinical" diabetes, terms which should be abandoned in view of the questions raised above as to whether such patients are in fact diabetic. Nevertheless, they are more prone than the general population to develop cardiovascular disease and to progress to overt diabetes.

The "Flat" Glucose Tolerance Curve

Frequently, patients are referred for consultation to the diabetologist for evaluation of a "flat" glucose tolerance curve, i.e., one in which a minimal elevation in blood glucose concentration is observed during the early part of the glucose tolerance test. Such patients occasionally are misdiagnosed as having hypoglycemia, "mild" diabetes, or malabsorption. It should be noted that, following the administration of a 100-g glucose load, the 1-h glucose concentration value remains below 100 mg/dl (5.6 mM) in as many as 35 percent of normal subjects and does not exceed 90 mg/dl (5.0 mM) in 19 percent of cases.[294] In the absence of other corroborative evidence, such "flat" responses should not be interpreted as indicative of hypoglycemia, malabsorption, or glucose intolerance. A flat glucose curve may sometimes be indicative of a low renal threshold for glucose (normally at ~170 mg/dl, 9.4 mM); the presence of glucose in urine should then be examined during the test. Also, children and young persons exhibit high rates of tissue glucose uptake with rapid assimilation of the glucose load. An auxiliary testing of other parameters indicative of glucose absorption such as plasma insulin or FFA concentration (a pronounced decrease at 1 to 2 h after glucose administration[295]) may be helpful in the evaluation.

Indications for Glucose Tolerance Testing

In a patient with fasting hyperglycemia, glucose tolerance testing is not necessary (or warranted) for the diagnosis of diabetes. In patients with normal fasting glucose levels, indiscriminate use of the test is also to be avoided. While the glucose tolerance test in itself poses no direct risk to the patient, a variety of hazards of overdiagnosis of diabetes are now recognized. Overzealous diagnosis of diabetes may lead to employment discrimination, denial of insurance, mental anguish to the patient and family, and unnecessary treatment with antidiabetic drugs. The significance of these potential dangers is underscored by the observations that (1) a large proportion (up to 50 percent) of patients with impaired glucose tolerance on first testing revert to normal on subsequent testing and (2) intervention with sulfonylurea agents fails to lower the rate of progression to overt diabetes.[296] Consequently, glucose tolerance testing should not be done as a mass or even individual screening procedure but should be limited to situations in which some intervention is likely to be of benefit.

In obesity, the detection of glucose intolerance may provide a stimulus (to the patient as well as the physician) to implement a weight-reducing diet inasmuch as normalization of body weight generally results in improved metabolism of carbohydrates. In pregnancy (see below), proper management of gestational diabetes with insulin, particularly in patients above the age of 25, leads to improved fetal survival. In patients with a strong genetic predisposition for diabetes (e.g., if both parents have overt diabetes), a normal glucose tolerance test may have prognostic value and relieve anxiety (<2 percent of patients with normal glucose tolerance develop frank diabetes over the ensuing 5 to 10 years). The glucose tolerance test may be useful in evaluating patients with nephrotic syndrome, peripheral neuropathy, or premature arteriosclerosis, since these syndromes may manifest themselves as complications of diabetes prior to the development of fasting hyperglycemia.

THE INTRAVENOUS GLUCOSE TOLERANCE TEST

The IV glucose tolerance test is less widely used than the oral procedure but is preferable in patients who develop nausea after an oral glucose load or who have GI disease with malabsorption. It has recently been used for evaluation of residual beta cell function in persons suspected of developing type I diabetes. Glucose is administered IV as a 50% solution over 2 to 4 min in a standard 25-g dose or in a dose of 0.5 g per kilogram of ideal body weight. Blood samples are then obtained at 10-min intervals until 60 min.

Evaluation of the test is based on the assumption that the curve of glucose disappearance is logarithmic, as described by the equation

$$C_t = C_0 e^{-kt}$$

where C_0 = glucose concentration at time zero
C_t = glucose concentration at time t
k = rate constant or rate of fall of blood glucose concentration, in percent/min

Calculation of k is simplified by determining $t_{1/2}$, or the time necessary for the glucose concentration to fall by one-half, using the formula

$$k = \frac{0.69}{t_{1/2}} \times 100$$

In normal subjects $k > 1.2$. In instances of impaired glucose tolerance, $k < 1.0$.

INSULIN DETERMINATION

Measurements of insulin concentration are frequently obtained during glucose tolerance tests as part of studies concerned with insulin secretion and/or response. In clinical practice, insulin concentration provides little information to facilitate the diagnosis of diabetes or impaired glucose tolerance. This is particularly true because of the heterogeneity of insulin response in type II diabetes and the frequent coexistence in type II patients of obesity, which of itself raises insulin levels. Consequently, insulin determination should be restricted to research, to circumstances in which hypoglycemia due to an islet cell tumor is suspected (see Chap. 20), or when flat glucose tolerance curves are encountered.

URINARY GLUCOSE DETERMINATION

Clinical measurements of urinary glucose are nowadays made with paper strips impregnated with glucose-specific enzymes. The paper strips are quite sensitive, so that the range of concentrations which can be determined is generally from 0.1 to 0.25%; however, false-negative results may be produced when various enzyme inhibitors are present in the urine. The paper strips do not detect other reducing hexoses in urine, so special methods have to be used when nonglucose melliturias (e.g., of galactose or fructose) are suspected.

The urinary glucose concentration does not necessarily reflect the concentration of glucose in the plasma. The glucose in the glomerular filtrate is quantitatively reabsorbed until the maximum capacity of the tubules to remove glucose is exceeded. In normal humans this occurs at a concentration of 160 to 180 mg/dl, the renal threshold. This level varies from one person to another, however, and is also altered by changes in kidney function. In patients with a low renal threshold, glucose may appear in the urine even when the blood glucose concentration is within the normal range; in some patients with kidney disease even high blood glucose concentrations may not be associated with glucosuria. Moreover, the urine in the bladder at any given time reflects the blood concentration at the time the urine was excreted by the kidney and not at the time it is passed from the bladder. Therefore, when patients have not voided for several hours, the degree of glycosuria may bear little relation to the blood glucose concentration at the time of urination. The diagnosis of diabetes should never be established solely on the basis of a single or even multiple urine glucose determinations; diagnosis depends on measurement of plasma or blood glucose concentration. However, in the patient with known diabetes, the urinary glucose concentration provides an index for the assessment of blood glucose control. It is more useful when "second-voided" urine, collected within 30 min of prior voiding, is tested.

GLYCOHEMOGLOBIN

The red cells of diabetic patients have an increased proportion of a component of hemoglobin which elutes on cation exchange chromatography or moves on electrophoresis before the main HbA peak; it is designated *glycohemoglobin* (HbA_{Ic}). This component is structurally identical to HbA except for the presence of hexose residues bound covalently to the terminal valine of the β chain and to the ϵ-amino lysine side chains. The formation of glycohemoglobin represents a posttranscriptional nonenzymatic modification of the hemoglobin protein (Fig. 19-9), which is dependent on the concentration of blood glucose. In poorly regulated diabetics HbA_{Ic} increases to 12 to 15 percent of total Hb compared with 4 to 6 percent in normal subjects (Fig. 19-45). Since the life span of the red cell is 15 weeks, glycated hemoglobin concentration provides a time-averaged index of the blood glucose level over a 5- to 10-week period, rather than just at the time of blood sampling.[297,298] Consequently, measurements of glycohemoglobin should provide a more reliable index of overall plasma glucose control than can be obtained from isolated blood or urine glucose determinations.

Since plasma albumin likewise undergoes glycation during hyperglycemia[31,32] and its half-life is markedly shorter than that of hemoglobin, measurement of glycoalbumin level may provide a weekly integrative assessment of blood glucose control.[299,300] Whereas 1 week of intense insulin treatment of type 1 diabetes has been shown to reduce HBA_{Ic} by <10 percent of the original value, glycoalbumin was found to fall by 18 percent at 1 week and by 40 percent after 17 days.[31]

Certain problems are encountered in routine HbA_{Ic} tests. A labile form of HbA_{Ic} exists, representing glucose bound in aldimine linkage prior to undergoing the Amadori rearrangement to form the stable ketoamine bond. Its presence may affect interpretation of HbA_{Ic} levels. The labile adduct can be eliminated by prior dialysis. HbA_{Ic} can be determined by affinity chromatography, ion exchange chromatography, agarose gel electrophoresis, and high-performance liquid chromatography. Affinity chromatography is widely used; it is simple to apply, using commercially available kits, and has the advantage of being unaffected by associated hemoglobinopathies or the presence of the labile fraction of hemoglobin. Specimens may be stored up to 21 days at room temperature without affecting the HbA_{Ic} value.[301]

A particular advantage of HbA_{Ic} determinations for the assessment of diabetes control is seen in patients with wide fluctuations in plasma glucose concentration or disparities between self-monitored blood glucose levels and laboratory glucose determinations. Furthermore, low HbA_{Ic} levels in insulin-treated patients may suggest the presence of nocturnal and/or asymptomatic hypoglycemia.

SUMMARY OF DIAGNOSTIC CRITERIA AND DIAGNOSTIC TERMS

The diagnosis of diabetes is dependent on the demonstration of fasting hyperglycemia (plasma glucose concentration $>$ 140 mg/dl or $>$ 7.8 mM) on more than one occasion, or a 2-h plasma glucose level (plus one other value) $>$ 200 mg/dl (or $>$ 11.1 mM) during an oral glucose tolerance test. Two-hour values on the oral glucose tolerance test of 140 to 200 mg/dl indicate *impaired glucose tolerance.* Patients with the latter diagnosis develop overt diabetes at a rate of 1 to 5 percent per year and, in the absence of such progression, are not generally at risk of developing microangiopathy. The terms chemical, latent, and asymptomatic or subclinical diabetes, previously used to describe patients with impaired glucose tolerance, should be discarded. *Prediabetes* refers to entirely normal glucose tolerance in an individual who is predisposed to develop overt diabetes. Because of the complexity and heterogeneity of the genetic and environmental factors diagnostically predictive for diabetes, the prediabetic state is hypothetical; presently, it can be identified only in retrospect. *Gestational diabetes* refers to generally transient diabetes or glucose intolerance which has its onset in pregnancy; this is discussed in detail below (see Pregnancy and Diabetes).

Prevalence

The prevalence of diabetes can only be estimated in view of the relatively arbitrary nature of the criteria employed for diagnosis. The overall prevalence of type 2 diabetes is estimated at 5 to 7 percent in the United States and Japan and 25 percent in Europe.[2] However, overt diabetes is present in only 2 to 3 percent of the population. The prevalence of insulin-dependent (type I) diabetes is approximately 0.5 percent.

The frequency with which diabetes is encountered is quite variable among different ethnic groups. Diabetes is virtually never seen in the Inuit (Eskimo). In contrast, the highest reported prevalence is among the Pima, where conventional interpretation of the oral glucose tolerance test results in a diagnosis of dia-

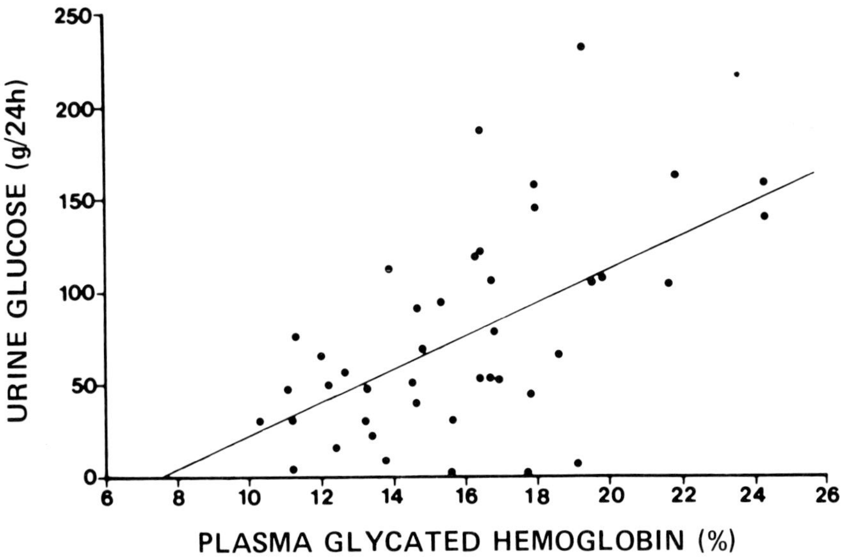

FIGURE 19-45 Correlation of percentage of plasma glycated hemoglobin to antecedent (43 to 70 days prior) urinary glucose levels in a diabetic population. (*From Gabbay KH et al: J Clin Endocrinol Metab 44:859, 1977.*)

betes in 50 percent of the population. This is not a specifically American Indian trait, because the Cocopah have a much lower incidence, in spite of a roughly comparable level of obesity. As noted above, the Pima differ from other population groups by showing a bimodal distribution on glucose tolerance testing; the cutoff between the nondiabetics and diabetics ranges between 200 and 250 mg/dl (11.7 and 13.4 mM).[293]

Pathology

Florid diabetes (with DKA) may exist in the absence of any pathognomonic lesions identifiable by histologic examination. This is particularly true in patients in whom diabetes has been present for a relatively brief period (a few months). However, in most patients dying with diabetes, histologic changes are observed in the islets of Langerhans; with long-standing diabetes pathognomonic lesions are observed in small blood vessels (microangiopathy) and in peripheral nerves (neuropathy).

ISLETS OF LANGERHANS

As discussed above (see Etiology), in patients who succumb to acute-onset type I diabetes a lymphocytic infiltration of the islets (insulitis) is frequently observed on autopsy, providing evidence for an autoimmune and/or viral etiology for type I diabetes (Fig. 19-37). In addition to the infiltrative changes, immunocytochemical studies reveal a reduction in the number of beta cells, while the numbers of alpha and delta cells remain unchanged.[302] By the time diabetes has been established for 5 years or more, the number of islets, the size of the islets, and the number of beta cells are reduced. As the disease progresses, about 40 percent of patients ultimately develop hyaline degeneration, an abnormality manifested by the appearance of amorphous deposits (with staining characteristics suggestive of amyloid) around the blood vessels and between the cells. These changes may be minimal or may completely replace the islet so that only the amorphous deposits and the blood vessels remain. Hyaline degeneration is more common in diabetics over the age of 40 than in younger patients; it occurs in at least half of the patients who have had the disease > 10 years.

Fibrosis occurs in about 25 percent of patients. It begins with thickening of the capsule and invasion of the islet with fibrous tissue; the fibrous tissue ultimately replaces the functioning cells completely. The process also extends outward from the islets, so that the exocrine portion of the pancreas may also be extensively involved. Although hyalinization and fibrosis affect both the alpha and the beta cells, the latter are more heavily involved.

Glycogenosis of the islets occurs in a small percentage of patients. This appears as large vacuolated cells. These findings, formerly termed *hydropic degeneration*, are now unusual; they are generally a reflection of severe, persistent hyperglycemia.

In some patients with type II diabetes histologic examination of the islets reveals minimal or no changes. However, careful determination of islet volume reveals a decrease in the mass of islet cells in virtually all patients with diabetes.[302]

BLOOD VESSELS

Arteriosclerosis occurs with a much greater frequency and at an earlier age in the diabetic compared with the nondiabetic population.[1,2] However, in the case of coronary artery disease as well as large-vessel peripheral vascular disease (the two major areas resulting in clinical disease, myocardial infarction and gangrene), the histologic appearance of the lesions (atheromatous plaque formation) is no different from that observed in the general population.

Diabetic patients are, however, also predisposed to microangiopathy. This term derives from the fact that the earliest lesions involve the capillaries and precapillary arterioles. The characteristic finding in early diabetic microangiopathy is a thickening of the capillary basement membrane (Fig. 19-46). On light microscopy this thickening is due to the accumulation of material which stains positively with periodic acid Schiff (PAS) reagent and is composed of glycoproteins. Basement membrane thickening may be observed in virtually all tissues (including skin and muscle) but is of particular importance when present in the renal glomerulus (diabetic nephropathy) and the retina (diabetic retinopathy). Contrary to initial reports, basement membrane thickening in muscle tissue is related to the duration of clinically overt diabetes; it is absent in unaffected monozygotic twins of individuals with known diabetes.[303]

THE KIDNEY

In newly diagnosed type I diabetes, kidney size is increased (as determined by x-ray examination) and the volume of the glomerular tufts is increased on renal biopsy. A reduction to normal size is observed within a few months of the initiation of insulin treatment.

Thickening of the glomerular basement membrane and of basement membrane-like PAS-positive material in the mesangium (the interstitial tissue lying between gomerular capillaries) is demonstrable on electron microscopic examination of renal biopsy material obtained 2 years after the clinical onset of diabetes.[304] The thickening may progress so that the entire glomerulus is ultimately replaced by a sheet of amorphous material. Alternatively, it may coalesce into nodular masses, as first described by Kimmelstiel and Wilson, which are highly characteristic of diabetes mellitus. The Kimmelstiel-Wilson lesions consist of spherical hyaline masses within the glomerular

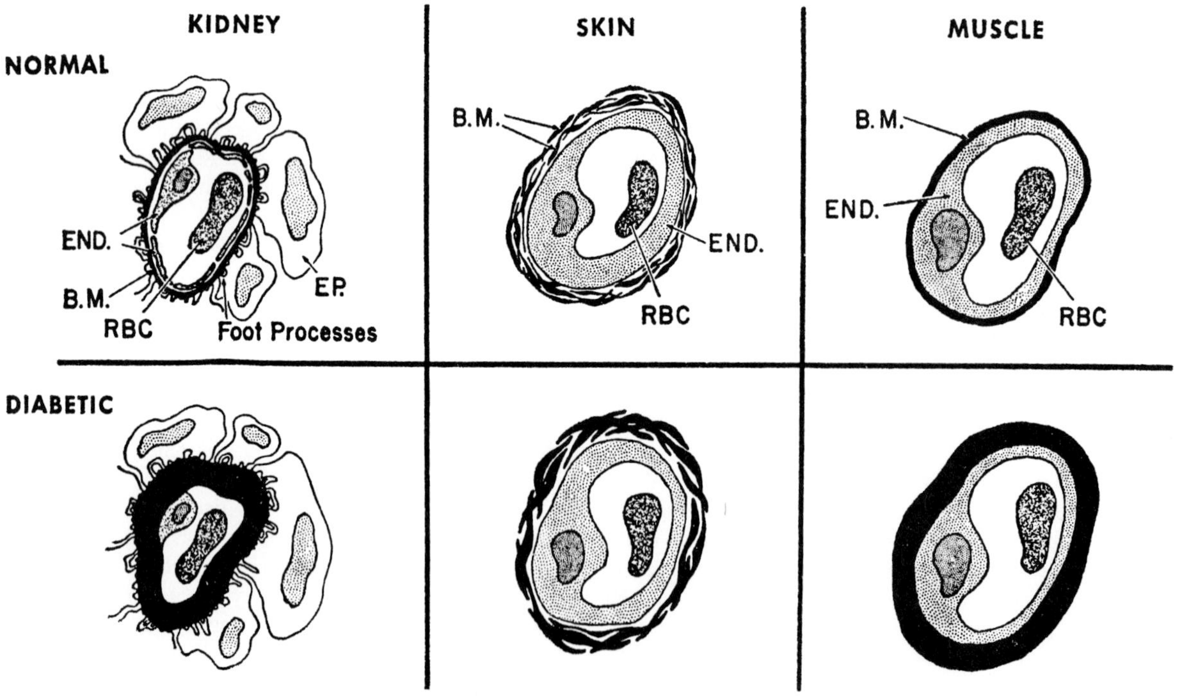

FIGURE 19-46 Schematic representation of capillary basement membrane in the kidney glomerulus, skin, and muscle of normal and diabetic patients. Thickening of the basement membrane is the earliest histologic evidence of diabetic microangiopathy. BM, basement membrane; END, endothelial cell; EP epithelial cell; RBC, red blood cell. (*From Siperstein M: Adv Intern Med* 18:325, 1972.)

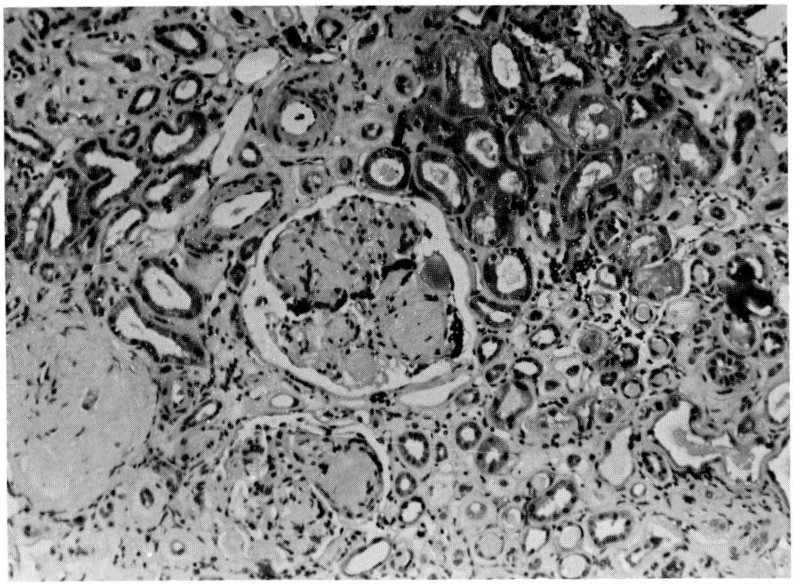

FIGURE 19-47 Section of kidney from a patient with type I (insulin-dependent) diabetes demonstrating the nodular intercapillary glomerulosclerosis (Kimmelstiel-Wilson lesions) characteristic of diabetic nephropathy. (*Courtesy of M Kashgarian.*)

tufts; they are acidophilic and PAS-positive (Fig. 19-47). Similar thickening, but of lesser degree, has been reported in rare instances before clinically detectable diabetes is present. This finding has been cited as evidence that the microvascular lesions are not caused by the carbohydrate defect, but the possibility cannot be excluded that such patients had mild fluctuations in glucose tolerance prior to the development of these lesions. Furthermore, as noted above, patients with overt diabetes show neither light microscopic nor electron microscopic evidence of basement membrane thickening until the metabolic abnormalities (e.g., hyperglycemia) have been present for at least 2 years.

THE EYE

The earliest histologic changes in diabetic retinopathy are *microaneurysms*, globular or fusiform outpouchings of the capillary walls.[305] These lesions are often associated with loss of pericytes (mural cells which normally surround the endothelial cells) and adjacent areas of occluded capillaries; whether the occlusions are a cause or a consequence of the microaneurysms has not been established. The *yellow exudates* observed on funduscopic examination consist of foci of extravasated lipid and protein in the deep layers of the retina. Hemorrhages are also observed in the deep layers (round) or superficial layers (flame-shaped) of the retina. *Proliferative retinopathy* is characterized by *neovascularization*, new vessel formation which undergoes repeated regression and scarring, resulting in a mass of fibrovascular tissue which forms adhesions with the vitreous body. Contraction of this scar tissue results in hemorrhage from these fragile vessels into the vitreous or detachment of the retina, the two major causes of blindness in diabetic retinopathy. Blindness may also occur when intraretinal hemorrhages destroy the macular region.

NERVOUS SYSTEM

In patients with diabetic peripheral polyneuropathy there is segmental demyelination, proliferation of Schwann cells, and an increase in connective tissue elements, while the vasa nervorum remain patent and show no significant disease. In contrast, the pathologic basis of cranial nerve palsies and mononeuritis multiplex associated with diabetes consists of ischemic changes involving the nutrient vessels.[22]

OTHER TISSUES

Hepatomegaly due to marked fatty infiltration of the liver is often observed in poorly regulated diabetes. When accompanied by hypercholesterolemia and (in rare instances) evidence of portal hypertension, the term *Mauriac syndrome* has been applied.[306]

Osteopenia has been reported in diabetes.[307] However, the mechanism of the decrease in bone mass has not been established.

Clinical Manifestations

The symptoms and signs of diabetes may be divided into three groups: (1) those directly related to elevations in plasma glucose concentration (e.g., polydipsia and polyuria), (2) those arising from the specific long-term lesions of diabetes [e.g., microangiopathy (particularly in the eye and kidney) and neuropathy], and (3) those resulting from the acceleration of or increased predisposition to disease processes which occur in the general population (e.g., atherosclerosis and skin and urinary tract infections). In addition, the diabetic syndrome may be clinically silent; its recognition may result from the discovery of hyperglycemia or glucosuria in the course of a routine medical examination or during the evaluation of some other disease process. Occasionally, the premature development of myocardial infarction or peripheral vascular disease calls attention to the presence of diabetes. In rare cases, retinopathy or nephropathy may constitute the first clinical manifestation of diabetes.

SYMPTOMS OF HYPERGLYCEMIA

When hyperglycemia is of sufficient magnitude to result in fairly consistent glucosuria (generally > 180 mg/dl or 10.0 mM throughout the day and night), the "polys" characteristic of diabetes appear: polydipsia, polyuria, and polyphagia. Despite the increase in food intake, such patients lose weight because of the loss of glucose in the urine. In patients with a high renal threshold for glucose (as a consequence of reduced GFR caused by diabetic nephropathy or other forms of renal disease) hyperglycemia may be persistent and moderately severe, yet fail to result in glucosuria. In such circumstances, poor control of diabetes cannot be invoked as the explanation for weight loss irrespective of blood glucose level. The increase in hyperglycemia which occurs in the postprandial period accounts for the lethargy which individuals with poorly controlled diabetes often notice after meals.

The augmentation in gluconeogenesis which contributes to the development of fasting hyperglycemia results in protein wasting and increased urinary nitrogen loss. These changes in protein metabolism contribute to the growth failure observed in children with untreated or poorly regulated insulin-dependent diabetes. Protein wasting may also be responsible for muscle weakness and may contribute to poor wound healing.

Marked swings in blood glucose concentration may cause visual blurring. This is due to changes in the water content of the lens in response to alterations in plasma osmolarity. The visual symptoms may be particularly troublesome when insulin treatment is instituted. Consequently, the patient should be reassured that the visual disturbance is transient and not due to retinopathy. In addition, refraction for the purpose of fitting corrective lenses should not be undertaken until the blood glucose level has been stabilized.

Persistent glucosuria in women is frequently accompanied by vulvovaginitis, which manifests itself as itching and a malodorous vaginal discharge. Recurrent or severe skin infections (furunculosis) and cellulitis may also call attention to the presence of hyperglycemia.

The clinical manifestations of DKA and nonketotic hyperosmolar coma are discussed below.

DIABETIC RETINOPATHY

In addition to refractive errors associated with fluctuations in blood glucose concentration, visual impairment may occur in diabetes as a result of cataracts, glaucoma, and most commonly as a consequence of retinal microangiopathy, generally referred to as diabetic retinopathy. The significance of diabetic retinopathy is underscored by the fact that diabetes is the leading cause of blindness in the United States. Among blind diabetics, 85 percent lose sight as a result of retinopathy.[308] Of those who are legally blind, diabetes is the reported etiology in ~8 percent. The absolute risk of blindness is dependent on the age of onset as well as the duration of diabetes. If diabetes is diagnosed at age 20, the risk of blindness at age 40 is 23 times that of the nondiabetic population. If diagnosis is at age 40, by age 70 the risk of blindness is 15 times the risk for the general population. Among patients who have had type I diabetes for > 30 years, 12 percent are legally blind. An estimated 40 percent of type I and 50 percent of type II patients have proliferative retinopathy. Overall, the rate of blindness among all diabetics is ~2 percent.[305]

Clinical evaluation of diabetic retinopathy is based on ophthalmoscopic examination of the fundus and, where indicated, slit lamp examination and fluorescein angiography of the retina. The retinal changes observed in the diabetic patient are generally divided into *background* retinopathy and *proliferative* retinopathy.[308] This classification has prognostic as well as therapeutic implications. Background retinopathy represents the earliest ophthalmic manifestation of diabetes; it consists of microaneurysms, dot and blot hemorrhages, exudates, and retinal edema (Fig. 19-48). It is often not possible to be certain that small red dots observed on ophthalmoscopic examination in the posterior fundus represent microaneurysms rather than dot hemorrhages. The exudates present in the diabetic may be the "hard" yellow type with discrete borders, or the "fluffy" white "cotton wool" exudates, grayish white lesions with indistinct borders. The cotton wool exudates were previously thought to be a

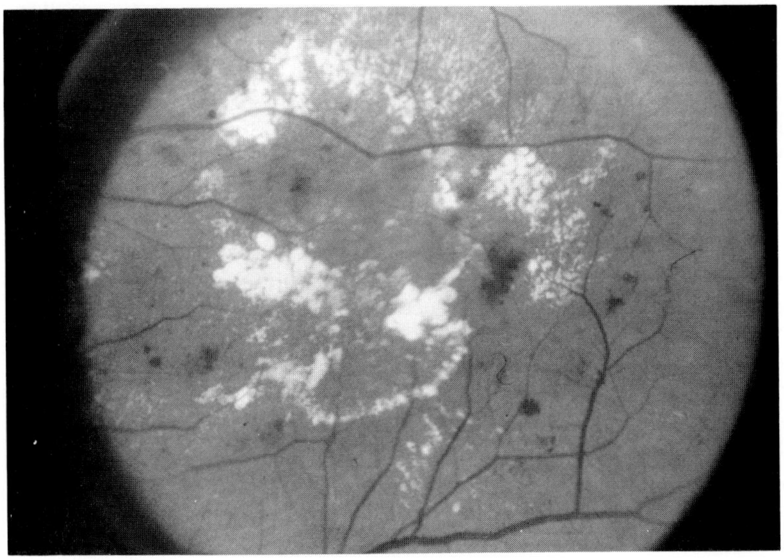

FIGURE 19-48 Fundus photograph demonstrating hemorrhages and exudates characteristic of background retinopathy in diabetes. (*Courtesy of J Puklin.*)

consequence of hypertension but are now recognized in normotensive diabetics. They correspond to areas of microinfarction of the superficial nerve fiber layer.

Background retinopathy generally fails to result in visual impairment unless retinal edema, a plaque of hard exudate, or an intraretinal hemorrhage occurs at the macula (maculopathy). Maculopathy may be more common in NIDDM patients than in the type I population. Background retinopathy is found with increasing frequency both as the patients become older and as the disease progresses. Thus, it occurs very rarely in patients whose diabetes was diagnosed before the age of 30 and who have had the disease < 5 years. On the other hand, the frequency approaches 50 percent in patients who have had diabetes 10 years or more, 65 percent in those with diabetes for 15 years, and over 80 percent in patients who have had diabetes > 30 years, no matter how old they were at the time of diagnosis.[305] The lesions of simple retinopathy are not fixed; when the patient is followed over the course of years, the lesions appear and disappear in an unpredictable fashion.

The more severe and dangerous form of retinal disease is proliferative retinopathy. This consists of neovascularization (see above) (Fig. 19-49). These vessels proliferate outside of the retina (into the vitreous)

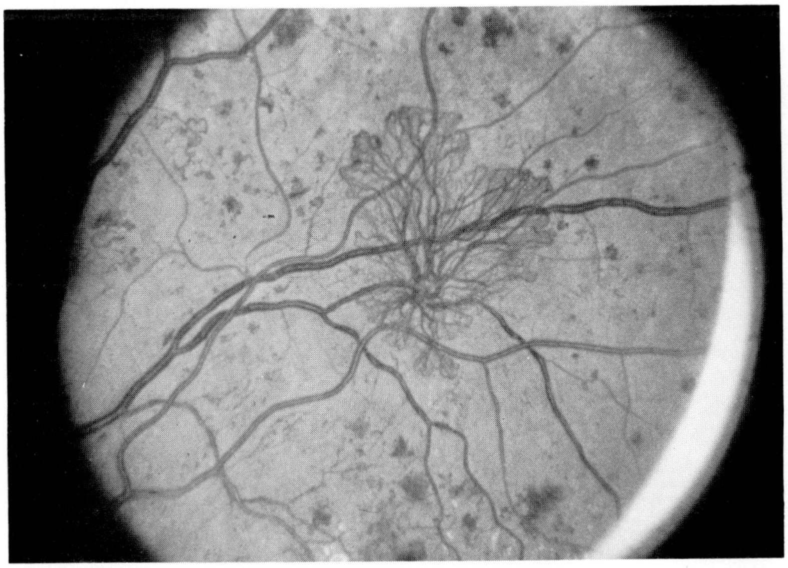

FIGURE 19-49 Fundus photograph demonstrating proliferative retinopathy as indicated by new vessel formation and scar tissue formation. (*Courtesy of J Puklin.*)

and are prone to hemorrhage, particularly when present near the optic disk. This leads to the development of fibrous tissue extending into the vitreous. Vitreous hemorrhages may initially be small and resorbed in days or weeks, causing only partial and temporary impairment of vision. However, severe visual loss occurs with massive hemorrhage or the contraction of fibrous bands leading to retinal detachment. This type of retinopathy occurs predominantly but not exclusively in insulin-dependent diabetes which begins in childhood. Thus, while only 15 percent of all diabetics are type I, ~50 percent of patients referred for treatment of proliferative retinopathy developed diabetes before age 20 and only 15 percent after age 50.[308]

From the standpoint of clinical assessment and management, a major concern is the identification of those patients who are at greatest risk of developing visual loss if left untreated. In some patients intraretinal hemorrhages occur in association with new vessel formation which is either at the disk or is moderate or severe in degree regardless of location; a prospective study has revealed that in such patients the 2-year incidence of severe visual loss is increased from 3 to 4 percent to 25 to 35 percent.[309] These findings underscore the importance of fluorescein angiography in the evaluation of retinopathy, since this technique permits the identification of new vessels which often go undetected on ophthalmoscopic examination. In addition, a more advanced phase of background retinopathy, termed *preproliferative retinopathy*, can be identified by fluorescein angiography.[310] Preproliferative retinopathy consists of large, extensive areas of capillary closure (usually associated with cotton wool exudates) or venous abnormalities in the form of dilated capillary shunt vessels. The presence of these findings suggests early progression to the proliferative state.

The most frequently employed method for the treatment of diabetic retinopathy is *photocoagulation*.[308] The principle underlying this treatment is that absorption of light by pigmented retinal epithelium and its conversion to heat results in protein denaturation and a therapeutic burn (Fig. 19-50). After healing, points of vascular leakage are closed, areas of neovascularization may be obliterated, and further neovascularization is diminished, presumably by lessening the demand for oxygen in tissues where the vascular supply is compromised. The light source employed is either a xenon arc or an argon laser. The latter is two to three times more effective than the xenon arc in raising the temperature of retinal epithelium; it also permits greater safety in treating conditions in high-risk areas, such as neovascularization arising from the optic nerve head and leaking microvascular abnormalities near the macula. A variety of studies have clearly documented the beneficial effects of photocoagulation in the treatment of diabetic retinopathy. In a large multicenter study in which patients with severe proliferative retinopathy received treatment to one eye only, the incidence of legal blindness over a 2-year follow-up was 16.3 percent in untreated eyes and 6.4 percent in treated eyes, a difference of 61 percent. On the basis of these encouraging results, photocoagulation is currently recommended in the following circumstances: (1) moderate or severe neovascularization extending from or close to the optic nerve; (2) mild neovascularization extending from the optic nerve with hemorrhage into the vitreous; (3) moderate peripheral neovascularization with a hemorrhage into

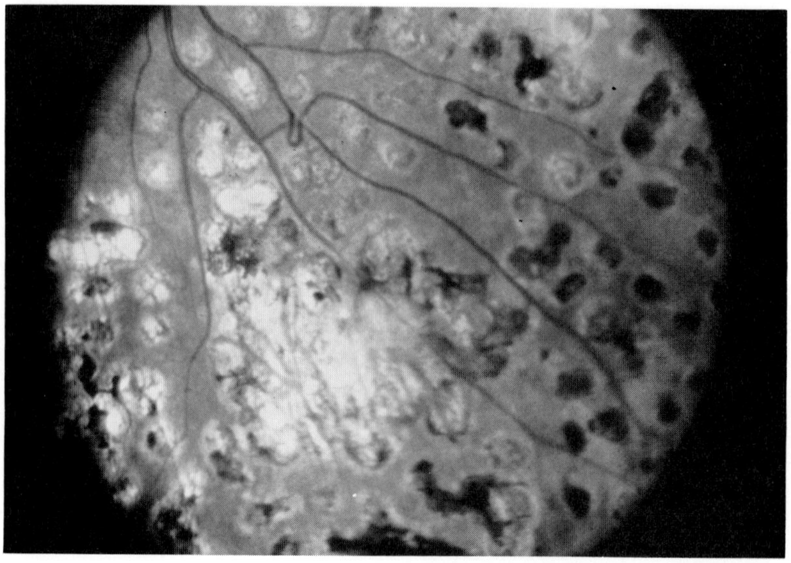

FIGURE 19-50 Fundus photograph demonstrating lesions produced by photocoagulation therapy for diabetic retinopathy. (*Courtesy of J Puklin.*)

the vitreous; (4) diabetic maculopathy; (5) diabetic rubeosis of the iris (proliferation of vessels on the iris or in the angle). Because treatment is most effective, yet not without risk, when started early, current investigation is directed at determining whether treatment is useful in patients with moderate or preproliferative background retinopathy.

A second major advance in the treatment of diabetic retinopathy has been the development of vitrectomy.[308] This procedure involves the surgical excision of the vitreous via an incision in the pars plana behind the lens. The development of tiny rotating cutting instruments which suck in vitreous, cut it off, and replace the lost volume with saline now permits the excision of the vitreous without the corneal and retinal complications which accompanied earlier techniques. Currently, vitrectomy is indicated in patients who have sustained a massive vitreous hemorrhage that fails to clear after 1 year. Prior to vitrectomy, ultrasonography and electroretinography are performed to ensure that the retina is attached and functioning well. The results to date indicate improvement of vision in 50 to 75 percent of cases. Vitrectomy is also frequently indicated for macular detachment since prolonged detachment may result in poor function even if the surgical outcome is good.[311]

The observation that a patient with severe retinopathy underwent remission after spontaneous infarction of the pituitary led to the hypothesis that ablation of the pituitary will bring about improvement or prevent progression of diabetic retinopathy. Hypophysectomy, either surgical or by some form of radiation (implantation of radioactive pellets or heavy-particle beam), and pituitary stalk section had their vogue in the 1960s. Both unoperated controls and patients with varying grades of hypophysectomy were studied. Microaneurysms, neovascularization, and hemorrhages were better controlled in some patients with maximal or severe pituitary destruction than unoperated or mildly hypopituitary controls, but visual acuity was not significantly improved. As compared with photocoagulation, the hazards of hypophysectomy are far greater and the benefits considerably less. Accordingly, hypophysectomy has been virtually abandoned in the management of diabetic retinopathy.

The relationship of control of blood glucose concentration to the progression of diabetic retinopathy is discussed below (see Pathogenesis of Complications). Treatment of coexisting hypertension may be of value equal to blood glucose level control in modifying the development of retinopathy.

Diabetics are prone to the development of glaucoma. This may take the form of narrow-angle glaucoma due to neovascularization of the iris (rubeosis of the iris). In addition, primary open-angle glaucoma is more prevalent in diabetics, particularly in patients who are free of proliferative retinopathy.

The general assumption that cataracts are more common in diabetics than nondiabetics is difficult to document. One particular type of cataract, the "snowflake" cataract, is characteristic of diabetes and is most commonly observed in children or adolescents with "brittle" diabetes. Similar "sugar" cataracts develop in rats with experimentally induced hyperglycemia and can be produced in vitro when rabbit lenses are maintained in organ culture with high concentrations of glucose. These cataracts are believed to be associated with sorbitol accumulation within the lens.

DIABETIC NEPHROPATHY

Microangiopathy involving the kidney (diabetic nephropathy) is a major cause of morbidity and mortality in the diabetic population. Among diabetics, clinically detectable proteinuria develops in 30 to 50 percent of cases after 20 years and renal failure is responsible for 40 to 50 percent of deaths. In most patients with type 2 diabetes, proteinuria is seen early after clinical diagnosis; in type I, on the other hand, it generally occurs after ~15 years of disease. Approximately one-fifth of type 2 patients develop clinically overt diabetic nephropathy. Hypertension, poor glycemia control, and cigarette smoking are associated with a higher prevalence of nephropathy. Diabetes accounts for ~25 percent of new cases of end-stage renal disease in the United States. As noted above, the histologic lesions specific to diabetic renal disease consist of thickening and accumulation of basement membrane material and mesangium, which may form nodular deposits described as Kimmelstiel-Wilson lesions (Fig. 19-47). The functional correlates of these morphologic changes are increased glomerular permeability resulting in proteinuria, followed by a progressive reduction in GFR and overall renal function.

In the earliest stages of type I diabetes both renal size (as assessed by radiographic or ultrasound studies) and GFR are increased.[312,313] The increase in GFR is a consequence of an elevation in renal plasma flow and (based on studies in experimental animals) an increase in the glomerular transcapillary hydraulic pressure difference.[314,315] These changes in intrarenal hemodynamics can be reversed by restoration of normal or near-normal blood glucose concentrations.[316] The increases in glomerular pressure and flow have been proposed to be the basis for the increased glomerular passage of protein, leading to proteinuria. Mesangial protein accumulation occurs as well; this is a postulated forerunner of glomerular sclerosis. Independent of increased perfusion, the increase in renal size and/or changes in the chemical structure of the basement membrane may also be of importance in the pathogenesis of diabetic nephropathy.[317,318] Increase in hydroxylysine and hydroxyproline content, greater amounts of glucose and galactose, decrease in number of sialic acid residues, and reduced sulfation of glycosaminoglycans have been observed in diabetic glomerular basement membrane compared with control material from nondiabetics.[319-321] The reduction in negatively charged sialic acid and sulfate residues may impede the normal charge-dependent barrier to filtration of negatively charged macromolecules (e.g., albumin), thereby leading to proteinuria. The increased hexose content of the basement membrane proteins may alter the tridimensional shape and packaging and affect the membrane permeability. The possibility also exists that nephromegaly, excessive perfusion, and alterations in chemical structure of basement membrane act in concert to produce diabetic nephropathy.

The earliest clinical manifestation of renal disease is the development of proteinuria. Interestingly, histologic evidence of diabetic nephropathy may be present for years prior to the appearance of proteinuria.[322] Although gross proteinuria ($>$500 mg/24 h) has long been recognized as a hallmark of diabetic nephropathy, recent studies have focused on the presence of microalbuminuria which appears earlier in the development of renal disease. Microalbuminuria is defined as an increase in urinary albumin measurable by RIA [20 to 450 mg/24h or 15 to 300 μg/min but undetectable by conventional dipstick assay ($<$500 mg/24 h or 300 μg/min)]. Microalbuminuria (particularly when accompanied by markedly increased perfusion) has predictive significance for clinically overt nephropathy (gross proteinuria) and its possible reversal by the restoration of normal or near-normal blood glucose concentration.[323-325] Consequently, the presence of microalbuminuria has been suggested as identifying a stage of diabetic renal disease designated as *incipient diabetic nephropathy*.[326] Whether further progression from incipient to clinically overt diabetic nephropathy can be prevented or slowed by strict maintenance of euglycemia remains to be established. In 20 to 40 percent of diabetics progression to gross proteinuria occurs. In such patients there is an inexorable deterioration culminating in renal failure within 5 to 7 years. Institution of intensive insulin therapy and restoration of euglycemia generally fail to alter progression at this stage.[327] The proteinuria may reach massive proportions, resulting in the nephrotic syndrome, characterized by hypoalbuminemia and edema. Classically, the diabetic with the nephrotic syndrome also shows hypertension and hyperlipidemia. Patients in whom the level of serum creatinine has reached 8 mg/dl survive (in the absence of treatment with hemodialysis or transplantation) for an average of 7 months. In those patients who develop renal failure the interval from the diagnosis of diabetes to the appearance of an elevation in blood urea nitrogen (BUN) concentration is 12 to 15 years; this interval varies from 8 to 21 years among insulin-dependent diabetic patients and from 2 to 35 years among non-insulin-dependent diabetes patients.[328] Once azotemia is present, progression to frank uremia occurs in 3 to 4 years.

The course of diabetic nephropathy is complicated by the presence of hypertension in over 70 percent of patients. In the large majority of cases the hypertension follows rather than precedes the development of renal insufficiency. Low plasma renin concentration is often observed in diabetics, suggesting that the hypertension is not due to increased activity of the renin-angiotensin system but may be due to increased fluid volume. In addition to hypertension and the nephrotic syndrome, fluid overload is also frequently manifested as recurrent pulmonary edema. Diabetic retinopathy is almost invariably present; it often deteriorates rapidly, perhaps as a consequence of accompanying hypertension and possibly as a result of the use of heparin during hemodialysis treatment. However, patients occasionally display only mild background retinopathy. Severe neuropathy is also frequently present in patients with renal failure. Differentiation of uremic from diabetic neuropathy in such patients is often not possible. *Hyperkalemia* is not uncommonly observed in diabetics in the presence of only moderate azotemia (BUN $<$ 60 mg/dl) and in the absence of acidosis. Several mechanisms have been advanced to account for this syndrome of nonacidotic, nonuremic hyperkalemia of diabetes.[112a] Hyporeninemic hypoaldosteronism, presumably due to interstitial nephritis, is demonstrable in some patients. Alternatively, in view of the importance of basal insulin levels for maintaining potassium homeostasis, hypoinsulinemia per se may predispose to the accumulation of serum potassium in circumstances of compromised renal function.[112]

Since diabetics are susceptible to all the other diseases of the kidney which may afflict nondiabetic individuals, many diabetics have glomerular nephritis, chronic pyelonephritis, and other kidney diseases which may lead to the nephrotic syndrome. Asymptomatic bacteruria is particularly common in diabetics. Renal papillary necrosis, a lesion which is almost never observed in the nondiabetic population, is also only rarely diagnosed among patients with diabetes (in only 1 percent of diabetics with end-stage renal failure). However, it is likely that many cases of papillary necrosis go unrecognized during life, since as many as 10 percent of diabetics show such lesions at autopsy.

Although renal biopsy is the only definitive means of being certain of the presence of diabetic nephropathy, the procedure is rarely necessary in the diabetic patient with severe or end-stage renal disease. Diagnostic procedures should be directed at the detection of reversible lesions, such as bacterial infection or obstructive uropathy, which frequently complicate diabetic nephropathy. Caution should be applied in the use of the IV pyelogram. In diabetic patients with a serum creatinine concentration in excess of 4 to 6 mg/dl, irreversible deterioration of renal function and oliguria may follow IV pyelography or angiography.[329]

A common observation in patients with advanced diabetic nephropathy and uremia is their tendency to require less insulin than before the onset of renal failure. Careful examination of large numbers of patients with this complication, however, shows that as many patients have an increased insulin requirement as have a decreased one; it is therefore impossible to justify a blanket statement that advanced renal disease reduces the insulin requirement. It is quite likely that when the reduced insulin requirement occurs, it is a result of anorexia and decreased caloric intake as well as loss of insulin-degradative function of the kidneys.[161]

Prior to the development of frank uremia, the management of diabetic renal disease is directed at control of blood pressure with antihypertensive agents, use of diuretics for the management of edema, and restriction of dietary salt and, where appropriate, protein. Improved metabolic control may delay or reverse the onset of nephropathy, but once proteinuria has developed, the clinical course is unlikely to be significantly altered. The control of hypertension, however, has been shown to be beneficial in decreasing the rate of decline of GFR.[330,331] Ultimately, consideration must be given to dialysis or transplantation. The 1-year survival rate for patients receiving hemodialysis or transplantation is now reported to exceed 70 percent. Which of the two modalities is the preferred method of treatment and the precise degree of renal impairment (adjudged by serum creatinine concentration or creatinine clearance) at which hemodialysis should be instituted have not been established. Continuous ambulatory peritoneal dialysis has also been shown to be an effective alternative to hemodialysis.[333] It should be noted that histologic changes compatible with diabetic vascular disease have been observed in normal kidneys 2 to 4 years after transplantation into patients with diabetes.[334] However, a functional renal transplant offers improved quality of life when compared with dialysis. As many as 88 percent of renal transplant patients and 82 percent of grafts survive 2 years, regardless of donor source; of those receiving transplants for HLA-identical siblings, 100 percent survive 2 years.[335,336]

The relationship of control of hyperglycemia in diabetes to diabetic nephropathy is discussed below (see Pathogenesis of Complications).

DIABETIC NEUROPATHY

Involvement of the nervous system in diabetes may take the form of clinical syndromes due to lesions specific for diabetes (e.g., symmetrical distal polyneuropathy) or may be a consequence of accelerated atherosclerosis leading to infarction of a spinal or cerebral artery and the resultant focal neurologic deficit (e.g., paraplegia). Those syndromes resulting from disordered function of somatic or autonomic nerves are collectively referred to as *diabetic neuropathy*. The true prevalence of neuropathy in the diabetic population is not known; it depends in part on the criteria employed for diagnosis. For example, on the basis of laboratory examination of nerve conduction velocity, 71 percent of a group of unselected diabetics showed impaired function.[337] The prevalence of clinically overt neuropathy is substantially lower and does not constitute the potentially life-threatening situation observed with diabetic renal disease. Nevertheless, neuropathy may cause severe disability in the form of pain, motor weakness, or abnormal bowel and bladder function. In addition, it may result in repeated trauma to the legs and feet (because of sensory loss), resulting in nonhealing ulcers that ultimately necessitate amputation.

The various forms of neuropathy may be divided into three major categories, depending on whether there is involvement of multiple peripheral nerves in symmetrical fashion (symmetrical peripheral polyneuropathy), one or several specific nerve trunks (mononeuropathy, or mononeuritis multiplex), or the autonomic nervous system (autonomic neuropathy). These syndromes differ with regard to clinical manifestations, histologic findings, and prognosis. A finding common to all forms of diabetic neuropathy is an elevation in the protein content of cerebrospinal fluid, which may, in diabetics, precede the clinically overt neuropathy.

Symmetrical Peripheral Polyneuropathy

Symmetrical peripheral polyneuropathy is the most common form of diabetic neuropathy. It is characterized by the development of symmetrical sensory loss which is most marked in the distal portions of the lower extremities; motor loss and involvement of the upper extremities are less frequently observed. The symptoms, which often begin insidiously, consist of numbness, tingling, and, later, paresthesias, burning, and sharp, shooting pains; the pain is particularly severe at night. In spite of numbness, hyperesthesia is also often present. Consequently, even the light touch of the bedclothes rubbing against the skin may evoke a severe burning sensation. Ambulation may result in clinical improvement; this can be helpful in differentiating neuropathy from vascular insufficiency (claudication). On physical examination the earliest findings are loss of vibratory sensation and absence of the ankle jerk reflex. Ultimately, there may be loss of all sensory modalities (light touch, pain, position) in a stocking type of distribution.

When sensory loss due to polyneuropathy is severe, secondary changes may develop as a result of repeated unrecognized trauma to the feet. *Neuropathic ulcers* may appear in the area of callus formation; they are often deep and penetrating. *Charcot's joints* (neuropathic arthropathy) have also been reported. Painless swelling and deformity of the feet, in association with joint instability, and radiographic evidence of disruption of articular surfaces and bone demineralization are the characteristic findings. Neuropathy also contributes to the disability associated with peripheral vascular disease (see below) because of the greater likelihood of repeated foot trauma in a patient who has lost sensation (e.g., skin burns resulting from the use of excessively hot water for bathing or penetrating infection after stepping on a tack).

The pathogenesis of neuropathy (as well as other diabetic complications), particularly with respect to the polyol pathway and low cellular inositol content is discussed in detail below.[22] As previously noted, the histologic changes consist of segmental demyelination despite intact vasa nervorum. Interestingly, subclinical polyneuropathy in the form of decreased nerve conduction velocity may be present in type I diabetics at the time of diagnosis; it reverts to normal with institution of insulin treatment.[337] However, an effect of insulin treatment on clinically overt neuropathy has not been established. Treatment of polyneuropathy is thus symptomatic, in the form of analgesics. Although high doses of thiamine and phenytoin (Dilantin) have been advocated in the past, neither has proved to be consistently beneficial. Other pharmacologic agents used in the treatment of neuropathy include chlorpromazine, amitriptyline, carbamazepine, and fluphenazine. The use of aldose reductase inhibitors to reduce sorbitol accumulation is currently under investigation.

Mononeuropathy

Disease of the nervous system may involve a single, clinically identifiable nerve trunk or several specific nerve trunks. In the latter circumstance, the term *mononeuritis multiplex* is applied. The peripheral nerves most commonly affected are the femoral, obturator, and sciatic nerves in the lower extremity and the median and ulnar nerves in the upper extremity. The external pressure points are the sites involved, or an entrapment type of syndrome (e.g., the median nerve in the carpal tunnel) may arise. Onset is abrupt, consisting of weakness, pain, and muscle atrophy. The distribution of weakness reflects the nerve trunk involvement (e.g., wrist drop with ulnar nerve involvement). Entrapment syndromes are frequently only remedied by surgical decompression. *Diabetic amyotrophy* is a syndrome affecting the pelvic girdle or, less commonly, the shoulder muscles. In it there is severe weakness, atrophy, fasciculations, and pain, but no clinically overt sensory loss.

Mononeuropathy may also take the form of isolated or multiple cranial nerve palsies. The third, sixth, and fourth nerves (in descending order of frequency) are most commonly affected.

In contrast to the demyelinative changes observed with symmetrical peripheral polyneuropathy, the mononeuropathies are felt to be vascular in origin.[306,338] Attempts to "improve" blood glucose control have had no influence on the course of the disorder. The prognosis is nevertheless generally good, with recovery of function and resolution of pain over 6 to 18 months.

Autonomic Neuropathy

Abnormalities of the autonomic nervous system commonly occur in long-standing diabetes, particularly in patients with peripheral polyneuropathy. Impairment in the regulation of blood pressure and in genitourinary and gastrointestinal function are the consequences of such involvement. A simple bedside test of parasympathetic function involves measuring the heart rate response to deep breathing by comparing the longest RR interval in expiration with the shortest during inspiration. Heart rate can also be determined while performing the Valsalva maneuver or on standing up.[339] Papillary light reflex may also be defective in the presence of autonomic neuropathy.[340] *Orthostatic hypotension* reflects the loss of normal vasomotor tone on assuming the upright posture as well as failure of stimulation of plasma renin release.[341] Decreased sweating in the lower extremities accompanied by excessive sweating in the upper half of the body is another frequent finding.

Urogenital dysfunction takes the form of impotence (present in as many as 40 to 50 percent of diabetics),[342] retrograde ejaculation (reflecting incompetence of the internal vesicle sphincter), urinary incontinence, and failure to empty the bladder fully. The resulting dilated, flaccid bladder may be a contributory factor in the development of chronic urinary tract infections.

GI involvement is manifested as either subclinical or clinical disturbances of motility. Esophageal motility is frequently abnormal; emptying time is delayed and primary esophageal contractions are poor or absent. Retention of gastric contents is also quite common; at times, this complication may cause retention of large volumes of fluid in the dilated stomach (*gastroparesis diabeticorum*). Comparable distention of the gallbladder also occurs quite commonly. These abnormalities of motility are usually asymptomatic, but may be responsible for nausea, vomiting, or dysphagia. Use of the motility-increasing agent metoclopramide may provide symptomatic relief.[343] The small intestine and colon also suffer from abnormalities of motility, but in these organs increased activity associated with diarrhea is the common pattern. Characteristically, the diarrhea is worse at night and may be associated with fecal incontinence. Intestinal stasis permits development of abnormal bacterial flora in the upper jejunum in some patients, and a pattern reminiscent of the "blind loop" syndrome may occur. Steatorrhea is a common problem in association with diabetic diarrhea, but in most cases pancreatic exocrine function is unimpaired, and the histologic appearance of the mucosa and muscular and vascular apparatus is normal. Since diabetic diarrhea is usually associated with malabsorption, vitamin supplementation may be helpful. The use of pancreatic enzymes is not usually helpful. In some patients, administration of a nonabsorbable antibiotic may cause improvement in the diarrhea and the malabsorption. Celiac disease is also more common in the diabetic population resulting from a shared predisposing HLA haplotype.

In occasional patients with combined peripheral and autonomic neuropathy, marked weight loss may be observed. This syndrome, which has been described as *diabetic neuropathic cachexia,* generally is self-limited and may suggest the presence of a malignant tumor. There is usually spontaneous improvement in symptoms and gain in weight after 6 to 18 months.[344]

CORONARY ARTERY DISEASE

Atheromatous disease involving the coronary arteries occurs more frequently and at an earlier stage in diabetics as compared with the general population; studies have shown an excess mortality rate from "sudden death" and myocardial infarction.[345] The risk of a fatal myocardial infarction is also greater in diabetics than in nondiabetics. The greater risk of experiencing a myocardial infarction holds particularly for diabetic women before the age of 40, contrary to the "protection" against coronary disease characteristic of the female gender. It has been suggested that chest pain is less frequent and less intense in diabetics than in nondiabetics at the time of infarction. However, objective evidence documenting a greater prevalence of "silent" myocardial infarction among diabetics has not been reported.

The factors responsible for the accelerated atherosclerosis in the diabetic population have not been entirely identified. As discussed earlier (see Pathophysiology), hypercholesterolemia and hypertriglyceridemia are more common in diabetics, and are associated with increased concentrations of VLDL and LDL and reduced concentrations of HDL. Current theories of the pathogenesis of atherosclerosis ascribe an important role to platelet adherence and aggregation at the site of endothelial damage.[346] Abnormalities in platelet function (increased adhesiveness and sensitivity to aggregating agents) have been observed in diabetics and may contribute to accelerated atherogenesis.[347] Glycation of VLDL, LDL, and HDL apolipoproteins,[33,34] and other compositional changes in lipoproteins[270,271] may result in defective clearance and metabolism of these particles; this would establish a favorable milieu for atherogenesis. As noted previously,[282] glycation can also alter the properties of collagen, thereby contributing to vascular abnormalities by binding LDL and VLDL remnants. Regardless of the precise mechanism, in view of the markedly increased risk for coronary disease, prudence dictates that diabetic patients restrict the cholesterol and saturated fat content of their diets (see Diet, below).

PERIPHERAL VASCULAR DISEASE: THE DIABETIC FOOT

Besides coronary artery disease, the second major site of clinically overt arteriosclerosis in the diabetic is in the vasculature of the lower extremity. The major syndromes resulting from vascular impairment in the leg and/or foot are intermittent claudication, foot ulcer, and gangrene; the last is $>$ 50 times more frequent in diabetics than in nondiabetics. Peripheral vessel disease may lead to intermittent claudication and, in more severe cases, pain at rest and necrosis. The sites of occlusion in the diabetic are often smaller (tibial and popliteal arteries) than in nondiabetics (in whom iliac and femoral arteries are involved) and the affected segments are often longer, making reconstructive surgery more difficult.

Foot ulcers develop as a consequence of ischemia, peripheral polyneuropathy, or, more commonly, a combination of the two. Ulceration may be followed by the development of gangrene and/or infection.

Infected necrotic lesions may show evidence of gas on x-ray examination. Gas does not necessarily signify the presence of clostridia; it may be a result of *Escherichia coli*, anaerobic streptococci, or *Bacteroides* sp. infection. Treatment of septic necrosis consists of bed rest and vigorous use of broad-spectrum antibiotics. Since failure to respond may lead to generalized septicemia and death, it necessitates amputation. The general principle applied in amputation is preservation of as much limb as feasible while ensuring healing of the stump.

In most instances gangrenous lesions and/or ulcers develop as a result of avoidable and (because of accompanying neuropathy) unrecognized episodes of trauma. Vigorous care and protection of the feet thus constitutes an extremely important aspect of the day-to-day management of the diabetic patient. The principles of diabetic foot care to be followed by the patient are: (1) inspect the foot daily for ulceration, discoloration, or cracking of callus; (2) avoid poorly fitting shoes which cause pressure sores; (3) never walk barefoot; (4) apply skin lubricant daily to prevent or reduce callus formation; (5) cut toenails straight across (to avoid ingrown toenails) and, where necessary (e.g., when vision is impaired), have it done by a podiatrist. Patients should be advised to refrain from smoking since this may aggravate the existing vascular disease. The most important principle to be followed by the physician is to be certain to examine the patient's feet at regular office visits.

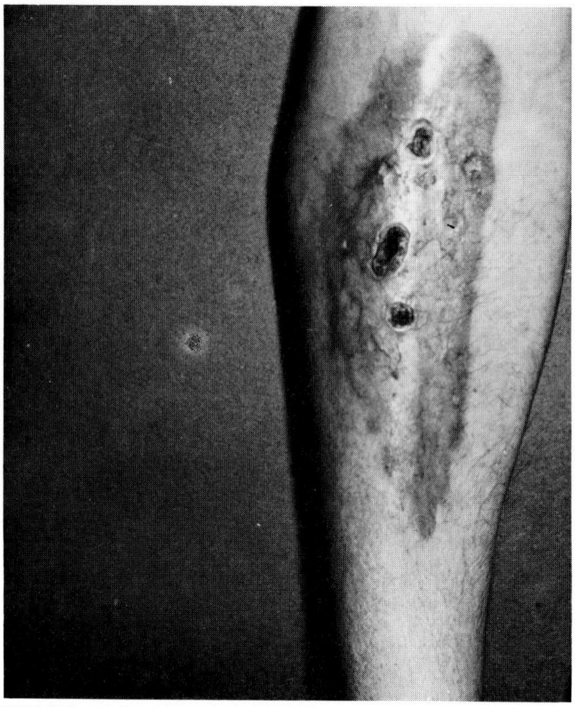

FIGURE 19-51 Necrobiosis lipoidica diabeticorum. The lesions consist of plaquelike areas in the pretibial region with a shiny atrophic surface, a red-brown center that becomes yellow, telangiectatic vessels, and areas of ulceration with crusts. (*Courtesy of I Braverman.*)

THE SKIN

Skin changes may be observed in diabetes as a consequence of large- or small-vessel disease, as a direct result of metabolic abnormalities (e.g., hypertriglyceridemia), and as a result of infection.[349]

Necrobiosis lipoidica diabeticorum is an uncommon but highly characteristic lesion consisting of a sharply demarcated plaque with an erythematous border and a red-brown, shiny center that becomes yellow as lipids (including carotene) are deposited (Fig. 19-51). Ulcerations with crusts and dilated blood vessels frequently occur in the central portions of the lesions. The plaques vary in size from 0.5 to 15 cm and often begin as flat erythematous areas which slowly expand. In $>$ 90 percent of cases the lesions are located in the shin (pretibial) area. They occur three times more often in women than in men. The histopathologic changes accompanying necrobiosis lipoidica diabeticorum are characteristic of the microangiopathy observed in other tissues. There is an accompanying secondary necrosis of collagen. In occasional patients the skin lesions antedate the appearance of clinical diabetes and in rare instances no abnormalities of glucose tolerance are observed.

Diabetic dermopathy or shin spots are circumscribed, atrophic, hyperpigmented, scaly patches which begin as red-brown papules. The lesions are almost always located in the pretibial area. Whether these skin findings are a consequence of microangiopathy remains to be determined.

Eruptive xanthomas may develop in diabetics with marked hypertriglyceridemia. The lesions are no different from those observed in familial or primary hypertriglyceridemic states without diabetes; they consist of red-yellow papules with an erythematous base, located primarily in the elbow, buttocks, and posterior thigh areas. Diabetic patients with these lesions usually have very poor metabolic control (marked hyperglycemia and weight loss) and may display *lipemia retinalis* as a further manifestation of their hypertriglyceridemia. Generally, elevation in plasma cholesterol concentration with normal triglyceride concentrations (e.g., an increase in LDL concentration only) does not give rise to eruptive xanthomas.

INFECTIOUS COMPLICATIONS

Infections of various types come to clinical attention more often in diabetic patients not because invasion by bacteria is more common among diabetics, but because they handle the invaders less well than do nondiabetic individuals. For example, sporadic furuncles occur in most normal individuals, but they do not usually progress to carbuncles or disseminated furunculosis, whereas in diabetics this course is common. The incidence of asymptomatic bacteriuria is no greater in diabetics than in control groups, whether the study is conducted in hospital populations or in otherwise healthy ambulatory subjects, but the most rapidly advancing phase of pyelonephritis, *necrotizing papillitis,* is almost unknown except in diabetics and patients with urinary tract obstruction. Bacteremia is more common as a complication of urinary tract infections in diabetics than in nondiabetic individuals.

Infections with relatively benign organisms may assume progressive and threatening forms in diabetics. For example, *E. coli* may present the picture of gas gangrene. Tuberculosis progresses more rapidly in diabetic than nondiabetic patients, and the course of the tuberculous infection is not greatly altered by the treatment of diabetes as long as ketoacidosis is prevented. In spite of the improved control provided by antituberculous treatment, the prognosis for the diabetic is worse than that for the nondiabetic patient. Malignant otitis externa caused by *Psuedomonas aeruginosa* may be seen in elderly diabetic patients. This can result in osteomyelitis of the base of the skull, cranial nerve paralysis, brain abscess, and meningitis. Cellulitis may be caused by mixed pathogens including *Staphylococcus aureus,* streptococci, and *Proteus* and *Pseudomonas* spp. Gas-forming anaerobes may be involved as well.

Saprophytic fungi of the order Mucorales, which rarely cause disease in normal subjects, may produce a progressive and usually fatal mucormycosis infection in diabetics. The process usually begins in the nasal sinuses and invades the orbit and cranial cavity, causing neurologic disorders and ultimately death. It is associated initially with purulent nasal discharge and gangrene of the nasal mucous membrane; later, unilateral ophthalmoplegia and exophthalmos herald involvement of the orbit. In about one-third of the patients late blood-borne involvement of the heart, kidneys, and other organs occurs. The fungus may also infect the lungs (where it is usually an airborne infection) or the skin. The infection can sometimes be controlled by treatment with amphotericin B and careful control of the diabetes.[350]

With respect to the mechanisms whereby infectious processes may be more severe in diabetes, there is no evidence of defective antibody formation, but mobilization of inflammatory cells is defective, and phagocytosis is clearly impaired in the white cells of diabetics with ketoacidosis.[351] Even in the absence of ketosis, there is defective phagocytosis and killing by diabetic cells; the reason for this impairment is not known. Hyperosmolar solutions interfere in vitro with phagocytosis, but the degree of hyperosmolarity required is do large (~400 mOsm or 700 mg/dl of glucose) that this factor has usually been discounted. Undoubtedly, acidosis and dehydration, when present, also play a part. These observations justify the conclusion that the progression of infection can probably be reduced by careful control of the blood glucose concentration.

Pathogenesis of Diabetic Complications

One of the most important unresolved questions in diabetes mellitus concerns the pathogenesis of the long-term microvascular and neuropathic complications.[352] In general, two schools of thought regarding pathogenesis have emerged. One school holds that microangiopathy and neuropathy are a consequence of hyperglycemia and/or other metabolic abnormalities resulting from insulin lack ("metabolic" hypothesis).[353] The second school holds that these lesions are genetically determined abnormalities that occur independent of elevations in blood glucose concentration and/or insulin deficiency, and may in fact precede any of the metabolic changes ("genetic" hypothesis).[354] This controversy is of more than academic significance because it is intimately related to concepts of the management of diabetes. Proponents of the metabolic theory generally believe that control of hyperglycemia prevents or minimizes diabetic complications; they consequently favor tight control of insulin-dependent diabetes. In contrast, advocates of the genetic theory favor "loose" control, since (by their formulation) the magnitude of hyperglycemia does not influence the development of complications. A host of data have been accumulated in recent years on both sides of the argument based on the investigation of tissue biopsies, metabolic studies in target tissues, and evaluation of the effect of treatment on the development of complications (Table 19-14). On balance, the data presently favor strongly the conclusion that metabolic factors are primarily responsible for the initiation and development of complications in most diabetics. A role for genetic predisposition to certain complications is also suggested but remains to be firmly established.

Table 19-14. Evidence Supporting the Two Major Theories for the Pathogenesis of Diabetic Complications

Study type	Metabolic theory	Genetic theory
Biopsy	Normal glomeruli in first 2 years of diabetes	Basement membrane thickening in "prediabetics"
	Vascular lesions in normal kidneys transplanted in diabetics	Possible lack of specificity of "lesions" in transplanted kidneys
	Glomerulopathy in secondary or acquired diabetes	Rarity of glomerulopathy in secondary diabetes
Metabolic	Increased content of hexose residues on glomerular basement membrane	Normal content of hexose residues on glomerular basement membrane
	Increased glycohemoglobin	Inability to establish causal relation between metabolic changes and functional and histologic abnormalities in target tissues
	Increased sorbitol, decreased myoinositol and low Na^{+},K^{+}-ATPase in diabetic nerve, and other tissues affected with complications	Inconclusive data from clinical studies
Treatment effect	Less retinopathy and glomerulopathy in patients treated with early multiple insulin doses	Lack of direct histologic comparability of lesions in diabetic animals with those in humans
	Prevention of retinopathy in insulin-treated diabetic dogs	
	Amelioration of neuropathy	

BIOPSY STUDIES

As noted previously, basement membrane thickening is present in diabetics in skin and muscle tissue as well as in the target sites of diabetic complications such as the renal glomerulus and retina (Fig. 19-47). The accessibility of muscle tissue for needle biopsy has permitted studies of capillary basement membrane in normal subjects, in patients who are predisposed to the development of diabetes but have normal glucose tolerance, and in diabetics after varying durations of overt hyperglycemia. With this approach Siperstein et al. reported electron micrographic evidence of thickened basement membranes in the offspring of two diabetic parents ("prediabetics") despite normal glucose tolerance in the biopsied subjects.[355] In contrast, Williamson et al. have shown that muscle capillary basement membrane thickening in patients with overt diabetes depends on the duration of hyperglycemia.[356] Furthermore, in monozygotic twin pairs discordant for diabetes, the basement membrane was thickened in the diabetic twin and normal-sized in the nondiabetic twin in most pairs.[357,358] Studies in the Pima also favor the conclusion that muscle capillary basement membrane thickening follows rather than precedes the development of overt diabetes.[359] This view is further supported by a recent report from Siperstein's laboratory concerning individuals who have ingested pyriminil (Vacor).[359a] These hyperglycemic patients exhibited a thickening of muscle capillary basement membrane, to an extent comparable with that of a group of type I diabetics, in frequent association with retinopathy and proteinuria. Thus, hyperglycemia of nongenetic origin can cause microvascular abnormalities.

Regardless of the state of basement membrane in muscle capillaries, it is well recognized that clinical evidence of retinal and glomerular capillary involvement is related to duration of diabetes. Biopsy studies also show that histologic changes in the kidney are absent for at least the first 2 years after the onset of insulin-dependent diabetes.[304,322] Important evidence in favor of the metabolic theory is also derived from studies in patients with secondary diabetes (chronic pancreatitis) and in patients with primary diabetes who have received a kidney transplant from a nondiabetic donor. In patients with chronic pancreatitis and secondary diabetes nodular and diffuse glomerulosclerosis has been observed;[360] in normal kidneys transplanted in diabetics, hyalinosis of arterioles is more common than in nondiabetic transplant recipients.[333]

METABOLIC STUDIES

A second approach to determining the pathogenesis of complications in diabetes involves metabolic studies of target tissues (e.g., basement membrane, peripheral nerve). Such investigations are directed at providing the metabolic link between insulin deficiency and/or hyperglycemia and diabetic complications.[35] As discussed above (see Diabetic Nephropathy), fine polar and configurational changes in the diabetic glomerular basement membrane appear to alter its filtration characteristics, shape, and packing. Furthermore, since the entry of glucose into the kidney cells is not insulin-dependent, these changes, related at least in part to excessive glycosylation, would be expected to depend on substrate concentration and to increase with cellular hyperglycemia. It is pertinent that no complications are seen in tissues with insulin-obligated glucose transport.

Studies have also been conducted on the chemical composition and synthesis of myelin in peripheral nerve tissue from animals with experimentally induced diabetes. As discussed above (see Fig. 19-9 and Carbohydrate Metabolism), an increase in sorbitol content was demonstrated in diabetic nerve tissue[21] and the prevalence of neuropathy may itself be related to the adequacy of glucoregulation.[361] The osmotic theory proposed that accumulation of sorbitol (Fig. 19-52) leads to swelling of Schwann cells, resulting in cell damage and eventual segmental demyelination. In support of sorbitol involvement are data demonstrating that normalization of blood glucose concentration by insulin treatment reduces the sorbitol content of nerve tissue and that inhibitors of aldose reductase can prevent polyol accumulation as well as the slowing of nerve conduction. However, the assumed swelling of Schwann cells has not been substantiated in studies examining the water content of cytoplasmic elements in nerve tissues; sorbitol accumulation is thought to be connected to other cellular abnormalities.

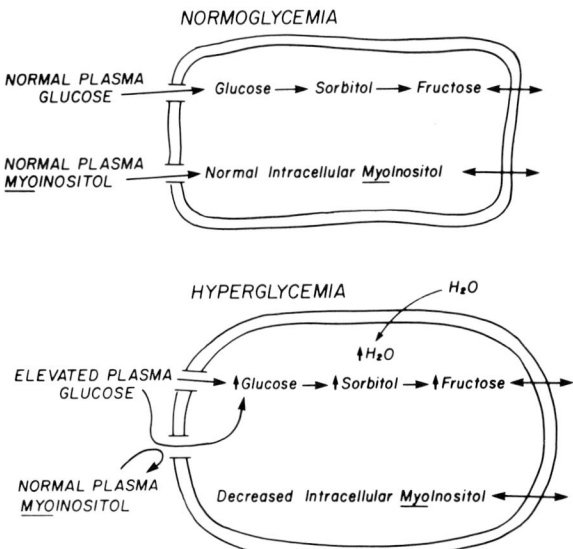

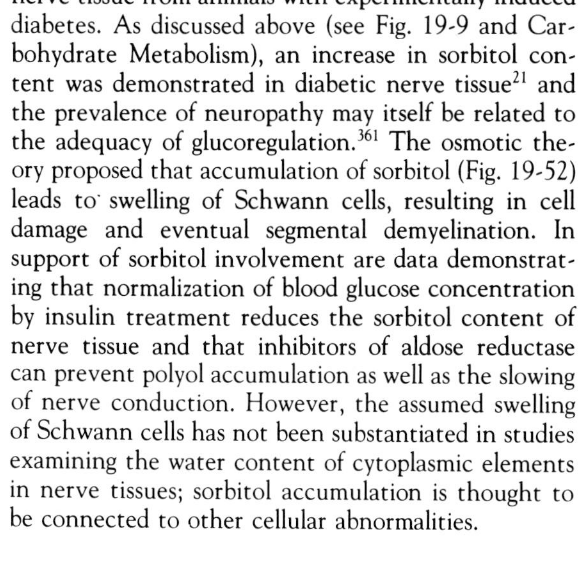

FIGURE 19-52 Schematic representation of proposed mechanisms whereby hyperglycemia leads to diabetic neuropathy. *Upper panel*: Schwann cell exposed to normal plasma glucose and myoinositol levels. *Lower panel*: Elevation in plasma glucose concentration results in high intracellular glucose levels resulting in sorbitol and fructose accumulation. In response to the osmotic effect of intracellular sorbitol, water enters the cell, resulting in swelling of the cell. Also shown is the postulated competitive inhibition (by hyperglycemia) of myoinositol transport into the Schwann cell, resulting in cellular depletion of myoinositol. (*From Clements*.[22])

Recently, Winegrad has proposed a unifying concept that the risks of complications in several susceptible tissues, i.e., peripheral nerve, glomerulus, and retina, are conferred by a common mechanism, the polyol pathway.[362] In these insulin-independent tissues the glucose level in the extracellular fluid is the determinant of intracellular glucose concentration. Thus, in the situation of chronic hyperglycemia, glucose imposes its metabolism on aldose reductase by reaching a concentration near its K_m. Also, the development of irreversible morphologic lesions, characteristic for each of the three tissues, is preceded by similar functional abnormalities, closely connected with the increased metabolism via the polyol pathway, but reversible upon corrective measures.

As shown first in the nerve,[363,364] but also in the glomerulus and retina, the accumulation of sorbitol is associated with a secondary decrease in the cellular myoinositol content (Fig. 19-52), whereas plasma myoinositol concentration is not appreciably affected. The increased operation of the polyol pathway is causally related to the depletion of a small but specific pool of myoinositol within the cell, which is important for the regulation of Na^+,K^+-ATPase activity.[365] Na^+,K^+-ATPase is a membrane transport enzyme, the energy of hydrolysis of an ATP molecule being used to translocate 3 Na^+ ions from and 2 K^+ ions into the cytosol. The activity of Na^+,K^+-ATPase is thus electrogenic and, importantly, contributes to the maintenance of a proper membrane potential. A decrease in ATPase activity was found in the three complication-susceptible tissues, in association with the decline in myoinositol content and the increased flow through the polyol pathway.

In the nerve, the maintenance of an axoplasmic transmembrane ion gradient is essential for the generation of the normal action potential. Decreased ATPase activity, failing to extrude the axoplasmic Na^+, is thus involved in causation of the reduced nerve conduction velocity in diabetes.

In the kidney, the early hemodynamic defect in the afferent/efferent arterioles and the mesangium, rather than metabolic abnormalities, has been proposed as the critical determinant of the initiation of hyperfiltration and its progress to nephropathy (see above). However, the hemodynamic effect which stems from hyperglycemia, appears to be initially associated with elevated intracellular Na^+ concentration, reduced Na^+,K^+-ATPase activity, and low myoinositol content. Treatment with aldose reductase inhibitors, myoinositol-rich diet, or vigorous control of hyperglycemia prevent the increase in GFR, glomerular hypertension, and mesangial permeability, similar to the prevention of the decrease in conduction velocity in the peripheral nerve.[365-368]

In the retina an early functional derangement is likewise demonstrable in human and animal type I diabetes, manifested by vitreous fluorescein retention on IV injection. It is due to the increase in permeability of the pigmented epithelium, a component in the blood-retina barrier regulating the composition of the retinal fluid. This abnormality results from delayed outward transport of ions and metabolites which appear to be responsible for the elevated Na^+ content due to the decreased activity of Na^+,K^+-ATPase, retinal edema, and consequent vascular disease. It is likewise preventable by control of hyperglycemia, inhibition of aldose reductase or dietary myoinositol supplementation.

A novel regulatory system appears to be involved in the modulation of the electrogenic Na^+,K^+-ATPase activity as well as of other cellular processes (Fig. 19-53). The effector arm is phosphatidylinositol (PI) derived from myoinositol and a specific diglyceride by the action of CDP diacylglyceride phosphotransferase. The system also includes products of PI phosphorylation, i.e., phosphatidylinositol phosphate and diphosphate, and of PI hydrolysis, i.e., inositol 1,4,5-triphosphate.[21a] These compounds affect cellular Ca^{2+} concentrations and protein kinase C–catalyzed (cAMP-independent) phosphorylation, the latter of which may be instrumental in maintaining ATPase activity. Winegrad postulates that tissues which are susceptible to hyperglycemia-induced polyol pathway-related lesions are dependent on enrichment with external myoinositol to prevent the depletion at a site at which PI synthesis and ATPase activation take place.[362]

Changes in myelin content and synthesis in diabetic nerves have also been observed. Although the chemical composition of myelin does not deviate from normal, in diabetic animals the total amount of myelin is lower. Loss of myelinated axons is most evident in distal portions of the nerves, together with segmental demyelination in large axons.

The demonstration that diabetics incorporate glucose into hemoglobin and other plasma proteins (Fig. 19-9) may have relevance to the pathogenesis of diabetic complications. Such abnormal, hyperglycemia-induced postsynthetic glycation of valine and lysine residues in proteins produces changes in their configuration generally causing a deterioration in functional performance. While glycohemoglobin concentration may provide a useful basis for the assessment of blood glucose control, glycation results in enhanced oxygen binding,[27,28] evident from the rightward shift in the O_2 dissociation curve. The decreased release of oxygen to the peripheral tissues may not be sufficient to cause local ischemia in normal situations, but may become critical when the oxygen demand is increased in infected, hyperemic, or

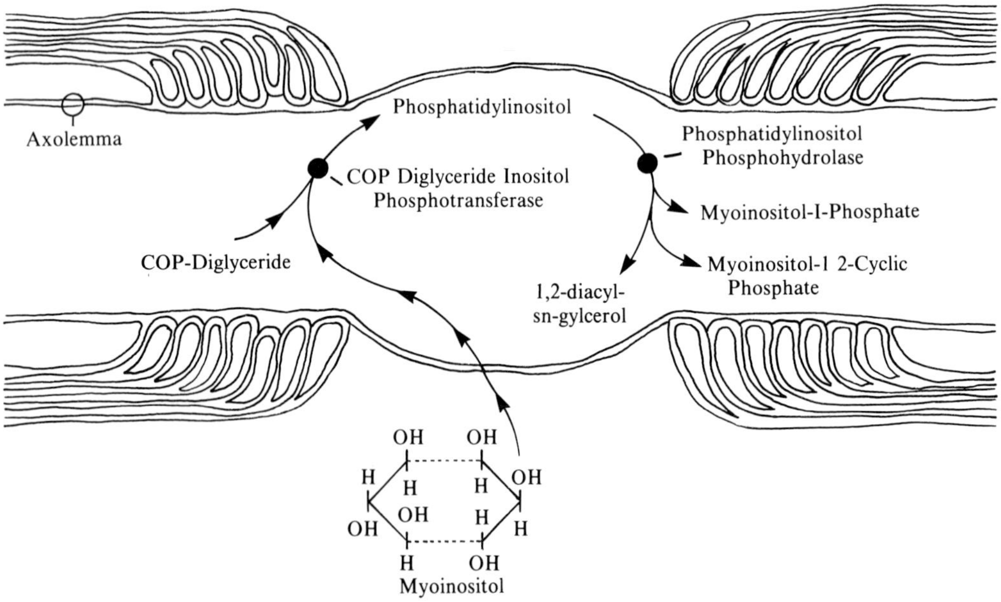

FIGURE 19-53 Scheme representing the metabolism of myoinositol in the peripheral nerve axon. Myoinositol is shown to be actively transported from the endoneural space into the axoplasm. Incorporation of myoinositol into the axolemmal phosphoinositides is mediated by CDP-diglyceride inositol transferase. Following nerve impulse transmission there is a rapid breakdown of the axolemmal phosphoinositides with the production of diacylglycerol and phosphorylated derivatives of myoinositol. (*Reproduced from Clements.*[22])

injured body regions. It may be of importance in the slow wound healing in diabetics.

Glycation of the lysine residues in proteins may interfere with the recognition of glycoproteins by hepatic cells,[369] enhance albumin's passage through the endothelial membranes, and reduce its affinity for small molecules. Glycation of the clotting factor VIII has been shown to be related to the increased tendency toward platelet aggregation in diabetes.[370] Glycation of immunoglobulins may impair their antibody functions.[371] Glycation of lipoproteins alters their biological behavior, decreasing (LDL)[31] or increasing (HDL)[32] their catabolism. Further evidence that protein turnover is altered by glycation is provided by the finding that glycated fibrinogen produces clots that are more resistant to fibrinolysis by the enzyme plasmin.[372] This may be instrumental in producing tissue fibrin deposits in diabetes.[373]

Glycation with or without glycosylation of serine and threonine residues of structural tissue proteins has also been reported to result in untoward functional alterations. The glycated crystalline proteins of the lens[374] seem liable to form cross-linking disulfide bridges. This increases their particle size and renders their structure more compact and less transparent, leading to cataract formation.[28] Glycosylation of tissue collagen, apart from causing basement membrane thickening in kidney glomeruli, may have deleterious effects in other tissues as well. These effects include trapping of lipoproteins in vascular walls and reduction of skin collagen solubility and digestibility by collagenase,[375] thus prolonging its biological turnover time. On the other hand, glycosylation and/or glycation of the cell membrane appears to reduce the life span of red cells.[376] This membrane modification also decreases red cell capability for shape adaptation, resulting in a tendency to sludge in capillaries, which is probably connected to diabetic peripheral ischemia.[377–379]

The typical functions of leukocytes, such as chemotaxis, phagocytosis, and bactericidal potency,[380–382] are adversely affected by membrane rigidity resulting from excessive glycosylation and/or glycation. Finally, glycosylated tissue proteins may present a new, "foreign" epitope to the immunoprotective systems of the body and stimulate the formation of autoantibodies, as demonstrated in the case of glycosylated collagen.[383] This finding is of potential importance. If expanded, it could represent a link between hyperglycemia and the immune complications in diabetes; such complications are evident from the deposition of antibody complexes in diabetic tissues, particularly in the kidney.

An additional metabolic mechanism whereby insulin lack may bring about diabetic complications involves abnormalities in GH secretion. Hypersecretion of GH is observed in poorly controlled diabetes in the resting state and even in moderately controlled diabetes in response to exercise; these changes are reversed when glucose homeostasis is normalized by insulin.[254] Merimee has observed that GH-deficient dwarfs with coexistent diabetes do not develop microangiopathy or neuropathy despite the presence of hyperglycemia.[384] However, in view of the etiologic heterogeneity of diabetes,[199–201] it is unclear whether it is the lack of GH per se or other genetic factors which can protect the diabetic dwarfs from the development of long-term diabetic complications.

EFFECT OF TREATMENT

A major corollary of the metabolic hypothesis is that treatment of diabetes resulting in normalization of blood glucose concentration prevents the vascular and neurologic complications. Although retrospective studies have been published suggesting that, by comparison with long-term insulin therapy, multiple short-acting insulin injections and better control of hyperglycemia are associated with lower incidence of some complications,[385–388] other studies are not conclusively supportive. The failure to demonstrate a consistently beneficial effect of tight glucose control in preventing diabetic complications may not, however, reflect the lack of a causal relationship between hyperglycemia and these complications. It is now recognized that the plasma glucose level in normal humans is an extremely well regulated parameter, rarely varying outside the range of 70 to 120 mg/dl over a 24-h period.[389] Even under the best of circumstances, conventional or even multiple insulin doses fail to reduce the mean plasma glucose concentration or restrict the excursions in plasma glucose concentration to the values observed normally.[390,391] Consequently, the failure to prevent diabetic complications may reflect the inadequacy of conventional management rather than the inexorable progression of genetically determined abnormalities in blood vessels and nerves.

Studies on the beneficial effects of insulin treatment on complications in experimentally diabetic animals have been more consistent than data from humans. In dogs with alloxan-induced diabetes, insulin therapy has been shown to reduce the incidence of retinopathy.[392] In rats with streptozotocin-induced diabetes, renal glomerular lesions regress after islet cell transplants.[393,394] In genetically diabetic *dbdb* mice, metabolic control by several pharmacologic and dietary means results in improvement of glomerular abnormalities.[395] Nerve conduction is also ameliorated in diabetic animals after insulin treatment.[221,396] However, since animals do not develop renal histologic lesions or neurologic disturbances identical to human diabetic patients, the significance of these findings requires a careful comparative evaluation.

The effect of intensive treatment, with self-monitoring of blood glucose levels, on microvascular and neuropathic complications of human diabetes remains to be established. An NIH multicenter, prospective, randomized trial evaluating this very critical issue is in progress. As it takes 10 or more years for complications to develop in most type I diabetics, this study may provide definitive answers only after several years.[397] Data are, however, available on the effect on background retinopathy of continuous subcutaneous insulin infusion (CSII) as a means of achieving optimal metabolic control.[398] These studies suggest that the progression of retinopathy is somewhat greater in the CSII-treated group, largely due to increased numbers of nerve fiber layer infarcts (cotton wool spots). The cause of this paradoxical, possibly transient, worsening of retinopathy during CSII treatment is unknown. Incresed somatomedin secretion[399] upon insulin restoration or reaction to resumption of glucose uptake by the insulin-dependent retinal cells may elicit the proliferative response. The differences between the conventionally and the intensively treated patients were, however, small; visual acuity remained unaffected. The tight control did not arrest or retard progression of already-established retinopathy in type I diabetic patients.[386]

With regard to nephropathy, CSII treatment evoked significant improvement in patients with microalbuminuria of < 500 mg/24 h but failed to produce improvement in renal function in patients with gross proteinuria.[400] Furthermore, beneficial effects of intensified treatment on neuropathy[401] and capillary basement membrane thickening,[402] as well as growth abnormalities in juvenile diabetics, have been reported for CSII treatment.

SUMMARY

A wealth of data indicates that microvascular lesions in the retina and kidney follow (by 3 to 5 years) rather than precede the development of overt diabetes mellitus. Similar lesions occur in secondary diabetes and in normal kidneys transplanted into diabetics.[403] Conversely, function of diabetic kidneys has been observed to improve upon transplantation in normal recipients.[404] A variety of biochemical abnormalities, including nonenzymatic and enzymatic incorporation of glucose into soluble and structural proteins as well as changes in polyol and myoinositol metabolism, may constitute the metabolic link between hyperglycemia with or without insulin deficiency and the development of diabetic complications. Results of a prospective trial evaluating the effect of restoration of normal or near-normal glucose metabolism on the development of complications are needed to confirm this relationship. Thus, while the data strongly support the metabolic theory for the development of complications of diabetes, final proof is still lacking. Perhaps the metabolic and genetic hypotheses are not mutually exclusive. In diabetics followed for 25 to 30 years, microangiopathy progressively increases, reaching a peak prevalence of 80 percent.[405] The 20 percent of patients who escape these complications are no different with respect to clinical control of their diabetes but may differ from other diabetics with respect to HLA haplotype.[199,205] Fortunately, a genetic component necessary for the development of complications may be lacking or a genetic factor conferring protection may be present in these patients. In contrast, in the remaining 80 percent of patients, metabolic changes such as the presence of hyperglycemia and/or other consequences of insulin deficiency may be necessary initial steps for the clinical expression of their genetic predisposition to the development of microangiopathy and neuropathy. Unfortunately, those patients who are protected from the development of complications cannot be identified in advance at the present time. Consequently, in the light of current knowledge, the implication with regard to therapy is to commend the restoration of as normal a metabolic milieu as possible without incurring hypoglycemia or impairing psychosocial adaptation.

Mortality

Over the past 50 to 60 years there has been a striking change in the life expectancy as well as causes of death among diabetic patients. In the preinsulin era, the survival of insulin-dependent diabetics was measured in months after diagnosis, and death in > 40 percent of cases was due to DKA. At present, ketoacidosis and hyperosmolar coma account for < 1 percent of deaths among diabetics; the major causes of death are renal failure in type I diabetics and coronary artery disease in type II diabetics. Ischemic heart disease is involved in ~25 percent. Of deaths related to diabetes, ~75 percent occur at age 65 or older and ~46 percent after the age of 75. The 20-year survival rate after the diagnosis of diabetes is 50 to 80 percent of the expected survival rate in the general population; ~12 percent of individuals with type I diabetes die within 20 years after the onset of the disease.[406]

Treatment

Management of the diabetic patient has as its optimal goals (1) normalization of carbohydrate, fat, and protein metabolism, (2) prevention of long-term systemic complications, (3) normal psychosocial adaptation, and (4) avoidance of hypoglycemia or other complications of treatment. The application of intensive programs of insulin therapy involving self-monitoring of blood glucose concentration (see below) has increased the success rate with which normal or near-normal blood glucose concentrations can be achieved.[407–409]

The principle underlying all forms of treatment of diabetes is the recognition that an imbalance exists between the availability of insulin from endogenous sources (i.e., beta cell secretion) and the amount of insulin required by target tissues to maintain normal disposal and mobilization of glucose, fat, and protein. Normalization of these metabolic processes requires equalization of the supply of and demand for insulin. In type II diabetics, among whom > 80 percent are obese and insulin-resistant, the demand for insulin is increased in the face of a diminished (but not exhausted) beta cell capacity for insulin secretion. Treatment is thus directed at reducing the demand for insulin by dietary management involving a low calorie intake aimed at reducing body weight. If dietary measures fail or are insufficient, stimulation of endogenous insulin secretion by sulfonylurea agents may, in limited cases, be helpful. In contrast, the insulin-dependent, ketosis-prone, non-obese type I diabetic is characterized by virtually absolute secretory deficiency of insulin which is not improved by sulfonylurea administration or mitigated by dietary management. In such patients treatment with insulin is the mainstay of management.

The therapy of the various complications of diabetes (e.g., photocoagulation for retinopathy, hemodialysis for renal failure) has been covered above.

INSULIN THERAPY

Of the total population of diabetic patients only a minority (15 to 25 percent) require insulin treatment. This category includes (1) insulin-dependent, ketosis-prone (type I) diabetics, regardless of age of onset, (2) maturity-onset NIDDM (type II) patients not responsive to dietary measures and/or sulfonylurea agents, (3) type II diabetics during periods of intercurrent stress (e.g., surgery, acute inflammation, etc.) in which a transient deterioration in metabolic homeostasis is observed, and (4) gestational diabetics in whom postprandial or fasting hyperglycemia is present during pregnancy (see Pregnancy and Diabetes, below). Proper management of such patients requires familiarity with the types of insulin preparations available, knowledge of the techniques of intensive management programs, and recognition of the need for individualization of treatment so as to meet the metabolic, psychological, and social needs of the patient.

Insulin Preparations

The most widely used preparations are intermediate-acting isophane insulin suspension (NPH) and insulin zinc suspension (lente insulin) and the rapid-acting regular insulin and (semilente) insulin zinc suspension (Table 19-15). In addition, long-acting (ultralente) insulin zinc suspension is occasionally used to prolong the action of lente insulin. These insulins used singly or in combination can generally provide for the needs of virtually all insulin-dependent diabetics. Protamine zinc suspension and globin insulin, while still commercially available, have little application in current clinical practice. Animal insulin preparations currently available are derived from porcine or bovine sources and are highly purified. Human insulin, manufactured either by recombinant DNA technology or semisynthetically (removal of alanine from porcine insulin), is also available for clinical use. The desired advantage of using human insulin, avoiding immunogenicity (i.e., elicitation of insulin antibodies), has not been borne out.[410] Nevertheless, such preparations guarantee an ongoing supply of insulin irrespective of the availability of animal pancreases.

The approximate time course of activity of the various insulin preparations currently used is shown in Table 19-15. While the values shown apply for most patients, it is not uncommon for some diabetic patients to experience a slower onset and longer duration of action than expected. This effect is at least in part a consequence of the development of insulin antibodies. Thus, the pharmacokinetics of a particular preparation should be evaluated on an individual basis. Furthermore, the duration of action of insulin varies according to the insulin dose employed. The larger the quantity of insulin administered, the longer are critical levels of insulin necessary for stimulation of glucose metabolism present at receptor sites.

Human insulin activity may have a somewhat altered time course. NPH human insulin may be slightly shorter-acting than its animal-derived counterpart and the regular form of human insulin may be more rapid-acting than bovine or porcine regular insulin. This may require a modification of existing insulin regimens when patients are switched to human insulin from bovine or porcine insulins.

Whereas the intermediate-acting insulins are generally capable of preventing marked hyperglycemia through much of the day, their peak action does not coincide with the increases in blood glucose concentration occurring with each meal; they therefore preclude (in most patients) complete elimination of

Table 19-15. Insulin Preparations

Insulin preparation	Action	Peak activity, h	Duration, h	Buffer	Protein
Regular (neutral)	Rapid	1–3	5–7	None	
Semilente	Rapid	3–4	10–16	Acetate	
NPH	Intermediate	6–14	18–28	Phosphate	Protamine
Lente	Intermediate	6–14	18–28	Acetate	
Ultralente	Prolonged	18–24	30–40	Acetate	

postprandial hyperglycemia. Glucoregulation can be improved by the use of insulin mixtures (rapid- plus intermediate-acting insulin), split doses (a morning and evening dose of insulin), or combined split doses (morning and evening doses, each consisting of mixtures of intermediate- and rapid-acting insulin).

Although not yet available commercially, proinsulin may have advantages in the treatment of diabetes due to its unique biological properties. Synthetic human proinsulin, despite its low activity, has a more prolonged hypoglycemic effect than regular insulin. Furthermore, it suppresses hepatic glucose output to a relatively greater extent than it stimulates peripheral glucose disposal. This is important for suppression of hepatic glucose output in patients with fasting hyperglycemia.[411]

Types of Diabetes Control

Treatment of patients with insulin-dependent diabetes can now be defined on the basis of the techniques used to monitor, control, and adjust the dose of insulin, rather than on the basis of therapeutic goals (e.g., tight vs. loose control). Management of the ambulatory patient with diabetes may be characterized as either conventional or intensive. Conventional treatment involves one or two injections of insulin per day. Urinary glucose levels are monitored by the patient and blood glucose and/or glycohemoglobin determinations are made by the physician at various intervals during office visits. Intensive management consists of self-monitoring of blood glucose levels by the patient and adjustment of insulin doses on the basis of the determinations. The insulin is injected manually twice or more per day or administered by CSII with a portable pump.

CONVENTIONAL INSULIN TREATMENT Insulin therapy may be initiated either in the hospital or in an outpatient setting, depending on the severity of the metabolic disorder, the prior medical condition of the patient, and the availability of instructional personnel. There is no way of knowing in advance the necessary dose of insulin; the treatment programs thus must be worked out empirically. Care should be taken to rule out factors which may precipitate diabetes, the correction of which might obviate the need for insulin, e.g., Cushing's disease, pheochromocytoma, acromegaly, and hypokalemia. The renal threshold should also be determined carefully in order to assess the value of urinary glucose concentration measurements as a means of monitoring control (this is particularly important in the elderly). With the advent of capillary blood glucose monitoring (see below), the use of urine testing for determining control of diabetes is less widely employed. Patients with stable hyperglycemia (without acidosis) may be started on a single dose of 15 to 20 U of intermediate-acting insulin (NPH or lente) administered 30 min before breakfast. In patients with severe hyperglycemia or ketosis, supplementary short-acting insulin should be given in the morning and evening until adequate doses of intermediate-acting insulin are reached.

When urine testing is used for glucose monitoring it should be performed before meals and at bedtime (before snack). Ketone monitoring is recommended when significant glucosuria is present and/or when symptoms of ketoacidosis may be present. Patients should wait 30 min after initially emptying their bladders before voiding to provide urine specimens (double-voided specimens). Under these circumstances the urine sample reflects the blood glucose concentration during the previous 30 min. When capillary blood glucose monitoring is performed, measurements must be taken with sufficient frequency during the course of a given week to allow adequate assessment and adjustment in the insulin dosage (see Intensive Insulin Treatment: Self-monitoring of Blood Glucose Concentration, below). In hospitalized patients plasma glucose concentration is measured before breakfast and before the evening meal. The dose of intermediate-acting insulin is increased 4 to 5 U every other day until the urinary glucose levels approach zero and blood glucose values remain consistently in the range of 150 to 200 mg/dl or below. Optimal doses of intermediate-acting insulin are eventually achieved by gradual dosage adjustment at a time when the patient has resumed his or her daily activities (outside the hospital).

When the maximal glucoregulatory effect is achieved during the daytime, it is important to determine whether a single dose of intermediate-acting insulin is capable of sustaining the effect throughout the night. In many patients, nocturnal and early-morning hyperglycemia cannot be controlled by a single dose of intermediate-acting (NPH) or lente insulin without causing afternoon or early-evening hypoglycemic reactions. Such patients should receive a second dose of intermediate-acting insulin at 5 to 6 P.M. or before bedtime. NPH or lente insulin is given before breakfast (65 to 90 percent of the total dose), and the remainder of the dose (10 to 35 percent) is given as a second dose before the evening meal. The need for rapid-acting insulin is based on urinary and blood glucose concentrations in the late morning and early afternoon. Generally, patients without significant residual insulin secretion require a twice-daily schedule of combined rapid- and intermediate-acting insulin. Often the dose of intermediate-acting insulin must be given at bedtime (with a snack) while the short-acting insulin is administered before the evening meal. This is desirable to avert early-morning hyperglycemia, probably due to the dawn phenomenon (see below); during this time excessive secretion of counterregulatory hormones occurs, involving GH in particular.[412,413]

Initiation of insulin therapy is not complete without an effort toward patient education. Instruction by a nurse trained in the technical and medical aspects of diabetes and by a dietitian is particularly useful at this time. Insulin treatment will not be successful if dietary intake is haphazard or if faulty injection techniques are employed. Periodic instruction is strongly advisable, even in those patients who are seemingly knowledgeable.

Once the dose of insulin is established, it is important that the patient continue monitoring (the frequency of testing will depend on the severity of the diabetes and the insulin preparations used) and that glycohemoglobin levels be checked every 2 to 3 months. Generally, the patient's insulin needs are not fixed, so that periodic reevaluation is essential. A variety of factors may induce changes in the patient's insulin requirements over time. The development of anti-insulin antibodies may prolong the duration of action from that observed at initiation of treatment. A marked increase in physical activity may necessitate a reduction in insulin dosage or an increase in snacks to prevent hypoglycemia (see Exercise, below). Normal adolescence is frequently accompanied by a marked increase in insulin requirements. Finally, progressive deterioration in renal function, reducing insulin degradation, may lead to lowering of the insulin dose.[161] Unfortunately, the clinician's ability to assess the adequacy of diabetes control with random urinary and blood glucose concentration measurements can only give small glimpses of the actual metabolic status of the patient. Assays of glycohemoglobin (see above) permit a more complete assessment of glucoregulation and are particularly helpful in the patient with wide fluctuations from day to day (or within a given day) in blood and/or urinary glucose concentration.

Some patients have erratic, unpredictable, and unexplained swings of blood glucose concentration, varying from severe hyperglycemia to normal or even hypoglycemic levels regardless of the insulin regimen employed. It is not clear why this pattern of "brittle" diabetes occurs. In some cases erratic eating habits may produce an unpredictable variation between the amount of insulin available and the amount of carbohydrate entering the blood. In these cases, careful control of the pattern of eating may help. For example, addition of a between-meal snack may eliminate hypoglycemia and subsequent reactive hyperglycemia (Somogyi Phenomenon, see below). Sometimes the lability can be explained by emotional problems which incite excessive secretion of catecholamines. In this situation the use of β-adrenergic blocking agents has been recommended; however, the overall experience with these drugs has been disappointing. One explanation for the "brittle" state derives from the observation that many insulin-dependent diabetics continue to secrete some endogenous insulin, as reflected by plasma levels of C peptide. The lack of or variation in this residual endogenous insulin may contribute to a more brittle state.[230] In some type I diabetics, frequent, severe episodes of hypoglycemia may be a consequence of the loss of normal sympathoadrenal mechanisms for counterregulating insulin-induced hypoglycemia.[412] This predisposition to hypoglycemia may occur in the absence of other evidence of autonomic dysfunction. For whatever reason, some diabetics appear never to reach a stable state; they present very difficult problems in designing proper control regimens. In these patients it may be necessary to accept less rigid control standards than might otherwise be preferred in order to prevent severe hypoglycemic reactions.

INTENSIVE INSULIN TREATMENT: SELF-MONITORING OF BLOOD GLUCOSE CONCENTRATION A major limitation in the conventional management of diabetic patients is the poor correlation between blood and urinary glucose concentration values. This discrepancy is a consequence of the variability of the renal threshold for glucose, the variation in interval over which the urine sample may have accumulated before being voided, and the semiquantitative nature of the urinary glucose determination. Furthermore, at blood glucose concentrations below the renal threshold (~160 mg/dl, 8.9 mM), a zero urinary value cannot distinguish between a normal blood glucose concentration, moderate hyperglycemia, and hypoglycemia. To overcome these deficiencies, the procedure of self-monitoring of blood glucose levels was introduced in the late 1970s.

To monitor the blood glucose level, the patient measures the concentration in a capillary blood sample obtained by pricking the finger or earlobe. A drop of capillary blood is placed on a reagent-treated test strip which is read on a reflectance meter or by visual comparison with a color chart. There is no consensus on the frequency of capillary blood testing needed to optimize diabetic regulation. Some investigators favor obtaining one fasting sample and one other value on 6 days of the week with a complete profile (fasting, pre-, and postprandial determinations, and one at night) determined on the seventh day. Others have suggested six daily measurements. A favored approach consists of four determinations daily (before the main meals and at bedtime) plus occasionally sampling during the night (at about 3 A.M.) to diagnose nocturnal hypoglycemia.[413-415] The practitioner should be aware that patients do not always reliably report results of blood glucose level monitoring.[409] Recommended target fasting and preprandial blood glucose concentration values are between 80 and 110 mg/dl (4.4 and 6.1 mM); target 2-h postprandial level is <150 mg/dl (8.3 mM). Performance of self-monitoring should occasionally be compared with simultaneously obtained laboratory determinations to ensure accuracy in the performance and interpretation of patient-determined values.

Central to all programs of self-monitoring of blood glucose level is the administration of at least two doses of insulin per day and modification of the insulin dose on the basis of the blood glucose determinations. The dose adjustments are carried out through frequent contact with the physician and by providing the patient with instructions or rules to be followed when the blood glucose level falls outside the desired range; for example, if the fasting blood glucose level exceeds 150 mg/dl the evening doses of NPH or lente insulin should be increased by 2 U (Table 19-16). The types of rules used have ranged from relatively simple instructions to complex algorithms. The involvement of the patient in the management of his or her disease is consequently far greater than that in conventional treatment.

The effectiveness of such treatment regimens in lowering the blood glucose level to normal or near-normal concentration and in restoring a normal concentration of glycohemoglobin has been documented in many, but not all, patients. Despite the evidence of metabolic improvement it remains to be established beyond doubt that maintenance of physiologic blood glucose levels is the essential factor responsible for better control of diabetes or whether other aspects of management (such as the use of multiple insulin injections, better dietary compliance, or more frequent contact with health professionals) are equally important.

Intensive management of type I diabetes is not without risk. The hazards include the precipitation of hypoglycemia, adverse psychological effects due to preoccupation with the care of diabetes, and increased cost. Furthermore, as discussed above, its long-term impact in preventing or retarding the microvascular

Table 19-16. Intensive Insulin Treatment: Protocol and Rules for Adjustments

Goal: Fasting, preprandial, and bedtime blood glucose concentration 80 to 110 mg/dl.
Protocol: NPH or lente plus regular insulin in the morning (7:00 to 8:00 A.M.) and evening (5:30 to 6:30 P.M.).
Adjustments:

1. If blood glucose concentration is too high (>150 mg/dl) on two consecutive days,	
Before breakfast:	Increase evening dose of NPH or lente.*
Before lunch:	Increase morning dose of regular insulin.
Before dinner:	Increase morning dose of NPH or lente.
Before bed:	Increase evening dose of regular insulin.
2. If blood glucose concentration is too low (<60 mg/dl),	
Between breakfast and lunch:	Decrease morning dose of regular insulin.†
Between lunch and dinner:	Decrease morning dose of NPH or lente.
Between dinner and bedtime:	Decrease evening dose of regular insulin.
During the night or early morning:	Decrease evening dose of NPH or lente.

*Insulin dose should be increased by 2U; adjust only one insulin type at a time.
†Reduce dose by 2U, depending on severity of reaction.
Source: Felig and Bergman,[416] as modified from Judd S, Sonksen PH: *Diabetes Care* 3:134, 1980.

and/or neuropathic complications of diabetes remains to be established. Consequently, self-monitoring of blood glucose concentration is not indicated for all insulin-treated diabetics. It should be strongly encouraged in the management of diabetes occurring during pregnancy; for growing, adolescent diabetics; for those with brittle diabetes; and in individuals with an abnormal renal threshold for glucose. It should always be employed in patients treated with a portable insulin infusion pump. Capillary blood glucose monitoring can also be useful in diagnosing suspected hypoglycemia. It is unwarranted in patients who already have severe nephropathy and are not undergoing a renal transplant and in patients who are free of microvascular disease but have a limited life expectancy (e.g., those of advanced age or with severe coronary artery disease). For the remainder of the type I diabetic population, self-monitoring of blood glucose concentration together with an intensive program of insulin administration should be offered as a therapeutic option.

Devices for Insulin Delivery

The development of insulin delivery devices for the normalization of blood glucose concentration has involved two types of systems, designated *closed-loop* and *open-loop* devices.[416] The closed-loop types consist of a feedback circuit in which the insulin delivery rate is variable and automatically dictated by continuous monitoring of the blood glucose concentration. Such systems, however, require the continuous withdrawal of small amounts of blood for glucose determination and are bulky; they are thus limited to inpatient use for 24- to 48-h periods. More practical use of closed-loop systems must await the development of an implantable long-lasting glucose sensor, which still remains an elusive goal.

The open-loop systems involve the use of a preprogrammed portable infusion pump which delivers insulin at basal, between-meal rates and which, upon activation by the patient, increases the insulin delivery rate prior to meals (CSII). In addition to eliminating the need for a glucose sensor, they employ a subcutaneous rather than IV access route, thus reducing the possibility of problems with infection and thrombosis. Pickup and colleagues in Great Britain[417] and Tamborlane et al. at Yale[68,418,419] first demonstrated the efficacy of such systems when continuously employed for periods of 2 weeks to several months. Virtually complete normalization of concentrations of plasma glucose, lipids, and branched-chain amino acids have been observed. Furthermore, the exaggerated rise in concentrations of counterregulatory hormones induced by exercise in conventionally treated patients is returned to normal after 1 to 2 weeks of pump treatment.

The diurnal profiles of glycemic control during long-term use of CSII have been shown to approximate closely the upper limits of glucose fluctuation found in normal individuals.[420] Insulin pumps capable of providing variable basal rates of infusion may facilitate control during the overnight period when insulin requirements are increased as a result of the dawn phenomenon.[421,422] Delivery of insulin at a basal rate has also been successfully applied in the management of diabetes during hyperalimentation.[423] Although CSII provides insulin levels that are significantly higher than those found in individuals without diabetes, the concentrations are similar when compared with a conventionally treated diabetic population.[420,423]

As in the case of intensive regimens of insulin therapy involving multiple manual injections, the key to successful treatment with an insulin pump is proper use of self-monitoring of blood glucose concentration (see above). The indications and contraindications for insulin pump therapy are similar to those discussed above for self-monitoring of blood glucose concentration.

CSII therapy may result in a number of complications. The rate of occurrence of DKA may be higher than during conventional insulin therapy and appears to be independent of simple instrument failure; it may be a consequence of needle dislodgement. Other causes, such as minor stress or emotional upset, may be responsible.[424] The frequency of localized infections at infusion sites is greater with CSII than with depot injections. The rate of localized infection is influenced by factors such as hygiene, antiseptic precautions, and the frequency with which infusion sites are changed. Another consideration is the insulin preparation used for CSII. Buffered purified porcine insulin has been shown to cause less infusion-site inflammation and obstruction of the catheter and/or needle than unbuffered bovine-porcine insulin mixture. Chemical changes in the insulin solution may occur as a result of prolonged exposure prior to the infusion.[425–427] However, there is no evidence of excess mortality with CSII when compared with conventional therapy.[428]

Studies on the impact of CSII on the complications of diabetes, compared with conventional treatment, suggest that microalbuminuria, a predictor of clinical nephropathy, may decline.[398,429] On the other hand, gross proteinuria is unaffected by CSII.[327] Furthermore, retinopathy has been found in some studies to deteriorate, although the worsening may be transient and occurs in patients presenting with more severe retinal disease at the start of insulin pump therapy.[388,398,429,430] The results of the current NIH multicenter diabetes control and complications trials are awaited to determine if long-term intensive control results in less microvascular disease than is found in conventionally treated patients.[397]

Implantable pumps for the IV or intraperitoneal administration of insulin have been employed in limited numbers of patients.[416] The use of devices is severely limited at present even for investigational purposes, due to the lack of an implantable glucose sensor, the inability to vary infusion rates, aggregation of insulin in the reservoir or catheter when kept at body temperature, and the potential for leakage of insulin from the device, resulting in more rapid insulin absorption than anticipated.[416]

Complications of Insulin Treatment

HYPOGLYCEMIA The most common and potentially most serious complication of insulin treatment is hypoglycemia. Hypoglycemia may be produced with any dose or preparation of insulin if the amount of insulin administered is excessive relative to the availability of glucose from endogenous and exogenous (e.g., dietary) sources. The time at which hypoglycemia occurs depends on the circumstances precipitating the attack. Overdoses of intermediate-acting insulin usually produce hypoglycemia in the late afternoon or evening; rapid-acting insulin causes this complication about 3 h after administration and with long-acting insulin it is a hazard during the early hours of the morning. Exercise may produce its effect within an hour, although delayed postexercise hypoglycemia may be more common than originally realized. Insulin-induced hypoglycemia is experienced at some time by virtually all type I diabetics. In some series, severe hypoglycemia (necessitating hospitalization or assistance from another person) has been observed in 25 percent of patients over a 1-year period.[432] In addition, hypoglycemia accounts for 3 to 7 percent of deaths in patients with type I diabetes.[432]

The symptoms of hypoglycemia may be divided into two categories: the effect of low blood glucose concentration itself, which results mainly in symptoms in the central nervous system (confusion, bizarre behavior, depression, neurologic manifestations, convulsions, and coma), and the effects of the response of the body to hypoglycemia, which include secretion of epinephrine with resulting vasoconstriction, tachycardia, piloerection, perspiration, and subjective tension or a feeling of impending disaster. A rapid fall of blood glucose concentration is more likely to call forth the typical sympathetic discharge. When hypoglycemia occurs during sleep, the only symptoms may be nightmares, sweating, and a headache on awakening in the morning. Symptomatic nocturnal hypoglycemia (plasma glucose concentration < 36 mg/dl or < 2.0 mM) may occur in as many as 30 to 40 percent of insulin-treated diabetics.[433]

Patients with specific areas of reduced cerebral blood flow (a common problem since diabetics often have atherosclerosis) may experience localized neurologic defects during hypoglycemia, such as hemiplegias, visual disturbances, or temporal or frontal lobe syndromes. These aberrations usually are transient but may persist if the blood glucose concentration remains depressed long enough to cause irreversible damage to certain brain cells. Hypothermia is common during hypoglycemia and may be helpful as a diagnostic hint in a comatose patient. In view of the ability of the heart to subsist on substrates other than glucose, it is not surprising that hypoglycemia may be well tolerated in patients with arteriosclerotic heart disease, although the reactive secretion of epinephrine may precipate arrhythmias, pulmonary edema, angina, or myocardial infarction.

Symptoms subjectively indistinguishable from those caused by absolute hypoglycemia may sometimes occur when the plasma glucose level is not markedly below the normal range (e.g., 60 to 120 mg/dl or 3.3 to 6.7 mM). Presumably, these symptoms result from a rapid rate of fall of blood glucose concentration from high levels. Whereas normal subjects must become frankly hypoglycemic (<50 mg/dl or <2.7 mM) to elicit an adrenergic discharge, in chronically hyperglycemic diabetics plasma catecholamine concentrations rise when plasma glucose concentration rapidly declines to values of 100 mg/dl.[434] It is important to document a fall in plasma glucose concentration if the symptoms are equivocal, since an inappropriate reduction in insulin dose or increase in dietary carbohydrate may make overall control more difficult.

Although a single attack of hypoglycemia is uncomfortable or even hazardous, the major risk is from repeated attacks, which can cause serious, though subtle, cerebral deterioration with reduction of intelligence and a tendency to cerebral dysrhythmias. Unfortunately, data are not available regarding the prevalence of brain damage due to hypoglycemia in insulin-treated diabetics.[352] In animals, hypoglycemia results in brain damage only when of sufficient severity to cause an arrest of brain wave activity.

The occurrence of hypoglycemia in insulin-treated diabetics depends in part on the adequacy of counterregulatory hormone secretion and the intensity of the treatment program. A deficiency of glucagon secretion in response to hypoglycemia is frequently observed in type I diabetes, but does not of itself increase vulnerability to insulin-induced hypoglycemia.[416] However, diabetic patients in whom epinephrine deficiency is combined with glucagon deficiency are severely predisposed to insulin-induced hypoglycemia.[416] Such combined deficiencies are often, but not always, accompanied by clinical evidence of autonomic neuropathy. Other factors which predispose to the development of insulin-induced hypoglycemia include a marked increase in physical activity (i.e., exercise), faulty injection technique, a decrease in food intake (skipped meals, low-calorie diet, or fasting), and a decrease in insulin turnover (e.g., renal failure).

Patients who are prone toward exercise-induced hypoglycemia may be instructed to consume extra carbohydrate before exercise, to use a nonexercised injection site such as the abdomen (see Exercise, below), or to reduce the insulin dose prior to exercise. Faulty injection technique (e.g., failure to agitate the insulin vial properly before use), errors in the preparation of insulin mixtures, accidental injection into muscle, or injection into sites where insulin absorption is irregular may be uncovered when the history is taken and eliminated by instruction by a trained nurse. Insulin infusion techniques for evaluating the adequacy of sympathoadrenal counterregulatory mechanisms have been described,[436] but their practical usefulness has not been established. The sudden onset of frequent hypoglycemic episodes may also result from (1) failure to reduce insulin dosage after resolution of stress or illness, (2) onset of diseases associated with increased insulin sensitivity (e.g., adrenal or pituitary insufficiency), and (3) onset of pregnancy.

The immediate treatment of hypoglycemia is to administer carbohydrate, preferably as a sweetened drink or food or commercially prepared, premeasured glucose tablets; in an emergency IV injection of 50 ml or more of a 50% glucose solution can be used. For occasions when glucose is unavailable or IV injection (e.g., by the patient's spouse) is not feasible, 1 mg of glucagon injected intramuscularly is effective; the small volume in which it is dissolved makes it convenient for inclusion in a physician's bag. If a single dose of glucagon is not effective within 15 min, it is unlikely that a second dose will help. Therefore, if glucagon fails, treatment with IV glucose is mandatory.

Insulin-treated diabetics should be instructed to have at all times immediate access to (or carry) a source of carbohydrate (e.g., candy) and to carry identification noting their diabetic status. They should become familiar with symptoms resulting from the gradual onset of hypoglycemia (loss of ability to concentrate, aberrant behavior, or other mental dysfunction) and the signs of hypoglycemia while asleep (nightmares, morning headache, or bed sheets drenched with sweat), in addition to the more commonly appreciated autonomic symptoms resulting from acute hypoglycemia. The patient's spouse or parent should also be instructed on the symptoms of hypoglycemia and in the use of glucagon in the event of hypoglycemic coma.

SOMOGYI PHENOMENON Hyperglycemia and ketonuria may paradoxically occur after excessive insulin administration. Rebound or reactive hyperglycemia, otherwise known as the *Somogyi phenomenon*, results from the release of catecholamines, cortisol, and GH in response to acute hypoglycemia; this phenomenon may be responsible for worsening of diabetes. Of the various counterregulatory hormones contributing to reactive hyperglycemia, epinephrine appears to be the most important.[437,438] The rebound hyperglycemia may be further aggravated by excessive food intake in response to the symptoms of hypoglycemia. Patients exhibiting the Somogyi phenomenon are usually type I diabetics whose diabetes is difficult to control with single doses of insulin. If the Somogyi phenomenon is suspected, the patient's insulin dose should be reduced under careful supervision and/or additional carbohydrate should be added in the form of a late-evening snack. Improvement in control despite a reduction in insulin dose is strong presumptive evidence of the Somogyi phenomenon.

DAWN PHENOMENON An early-morning increase in blood glucose concentration may, of course, be observed in insulin-treated type I diabetics in the absence of antecedent hypoglycemia. Dissipation of the action of previously injected insulin is by far the most common cause of such early-morning hyperglycemia.[439] On the other hand, in occasional patients there is an early-morning rise in blood glucose concentration despite ongoing CSII; this occurrence has been termed the *dawn phenomenon*. In this circumstance the waning of previously injected insulin cannot be invoked as an explanation.[439a] A nocturnal increase in GH secretion appears to be the mechanism responsible for the dawn phenomenon,[440] raising the possibility that late-evening administration of a long-acting somatostatin analogue (SMS 201-995), which prevents nocturnal increases in GH secretion, may improve blood glucose regulation in some diabetics (see Somatostatin and Its Analogues, below).

INSULIN LIPODYSTROPHY Insulin lipodystrophy is a distressing, although benign, complication of insulin treatment which may take the form of hypertrophy or atrophy of subcutaneous tissues. The fibrous masses that develop are hypesthetic; the problem is therefore often perpetuated (particularly in young diabetics), since these sites are favored for injection. Unfortunately, the absorption of insulin from these sites is often erratic and incomplete, thereby leading to a deterioration in control of diabetes. The development of insulin preparations which are > 98 percent pure has markedly reduced the incidence of this complication. The use of human insulin may also be advantageous in this circumstance. Lipoatrophic areas should be injected gradually from the periphery toward the center of the "crater" until completely filled in.

INSULIN ALLERGY Insulin allergy has been less of a problem since purified animal and human insulins have been introduced. It is thought that intermittent administration of insulin, particularly with bovine-porcine or bovine insulins, might serve as a potent immunogenic stimulus if the same insulin were to be administered again at a later time. Although human insulin of recombinant DNA origin is somewhat less immunogenic than porcine or bovine, low-titer antibody formation may still occur, resulting in insulin allergy in rare patients.

Allergic reactions to insulin may be localized or systemic. Localized allergic reactions are manifested as induration, pruritus, erythema, or pain at the injection site. The symptoms appear 30 min to 4 h or more after the injection. The usual onset is within the first week or month of initiation of insulin treatment. The immediate type of local allergy (within 30 to 120 min) is IgG-mediated. In most patients the reactions disappear spontaneously after several weeks. Improvement may occur by switching to monospecies insulin (e.g., pure porcine), human insulin, or local use of small doses of glucocorticoids.

Systemic allergy may be manifested as generalized pruritus and urticaria, angioedema, or acute anaphylaxis; the last, fortunately, is extremely rare. Sixty percent of patients with systemic allergy have a history of discontinuation of treatment with insulin and recent reinstitution of insulin therapy. The systemic allergic reaction is thought to be mediated by IgE antibody. Treatment consists of desensitization with human or porcine insulin at an initial dose of 0.001 U.

INSULIN RESISTANCE The normal 24-h insulin output from the islets of Langerhans has been estimated at 20 to 40 U per day. Consequently, patients requiring a greater amount of insulin have some degree of insensitivity to insulin. The most common cause of resistance to insulin is obesity; intercurrent stress and illness may also increase insulin requirements, through a variety of mechanisms. From a practical standpoint, clinical insulin resistance has been defined as the requirement for 200 U or more of insulin per day for several days in the absence of ketoacidosis, intercurrent infection, or associated endocrine disease (acromegaly, Cushing's syndrome). In the nonobese patient, various mechanisms may be responsible for clinical insulin resistance: circulating antibodies to insulin, abnormalities of insulin receptors, increased local destruction of insulin, or secretion of abnormal insulin.

Immunogenic insulin insensitivity results from a higher titer of circulating IgG antibodies directed at bovine insulin and, to a lesser extent, porcine or human insulin. While all patients develop antibodies to insulin, in only a small proportion of patients is the titer sufficiently high as to necessitate daily doses of >200 U of insulin. Most patients are adults who have been treated with insulin for long periods (>15 years); however, insensitivity may sometimes arise after several weeks. Insulin allergy usually does not accompany insulin insensitivity. Treatment consists initially of switching to pure porcine insulin or, preferably, human insulin. If the latter fails, systemic steroids (60 to 80 mg of prednisone per day for 10 days) generally result in a marked reduction in insulin requirements.

A rare form of insulin resistance in which titers of circulating insulin antibodies are not increased is that encountered in young women who also have acanthosis nigricans. As discussed earlier, this syndrome has been subdivided into two types, in both of which there appear abnormalities in insulin receptors:[154] in type A there is a decrease in the number of insulin receptors and the patients show virilization and accelerated growth. In type B circulating antibodies to the insulin receptor are demonstrable and evidence of an autoimmune disorder is present.

A limited number of patients have been observed who respond poorly to subcutaneous insulin but are quite sensitive to IV insulin.[440] Localized destruction of insulin has been postulated to account for this unusual disturbance. Neither the use of aprotinin, a nonspecific protease inhibitor, nor lidocaine has been uniformly successful in the treatment of this syndrome. Furthermore, when studied carefully, so-called peripheral insulin resistance has been found, in the majority of patients with this syndrome, to be of factitious origin (e.g., failure to administer insulin). Close attention should be given to this possibility, since true peripheral insulin resistance to peripherally but not intravenously administered insulin has been documented, either IV or intraperitoneal insulin administration can be attempted.[441]

Insulin resistance is also encountered in a rare form of diabetes, lipoatrophic diabetes (see below).

INSULIN-INDUCED EDEMA Edema is a rare complication observed in patients with poorly regulated diabetes in whom glycemic control is restored by insulin. While sodium and fluid retention may, in part, be related to correction of volume reduction induced by glucosuria, insulin may have a direct effect on urinary sodium excretion. Infusions of insulin in the upper physiologic range (without changes in blood glucose concentration) markedly reduce urinary sodium excretion in the absence of changes in the filtered load of glucose, GFR, renal blood flow, or aldosterone concentration.[112] Insulin-induced edema thus may be analogous to the refeeding edema observed in concentration camp survivors after they were placed on a normal caloric intake.

Goals of Insulin Treatment

There is a long-standing controversy between proponents of tight and loose control in the management of type I diabetes,[352,353] which in part lies in differences of opinion as to the pathogenesis of the *onset* of diabetic complications. As discussed above, neither the metabolic nor the genetic hypothesis can be proved at present, although the preponderance of evidence favors a metabolic pathogenesis. Evidence that restoration of a normal or near-normal blood glucose concentration prevents or retards the *progress* of existing complications also remains to be established. Differences of opinion also exist with regard to the frequency and sequelae of hypoglycemia, for which no objective data are available. Despite these difficulties, the overall philosophy, to which virtually all diabetologists subscribe, is that insulin treatment should be directed at restoring the plasma glucose concentration to as close to normal as possible without causing hypoglycemia or impairing the patient's psychosocial adaptation. The real issue is thus not the goal of treatment but the manner of implementation, i.e., whether to employ an intensive program of insulin administration. The indications and contraindications for such programs have already been dsicussed (see Intensive Insulin Treatment: Self-Monitoring of Blood Glucose Concentration, above). It should, however, be recognized that acceptance by the patient of an intensive regimen is likely to be influenced by the enthusiasm and zeal demonstrated by the physician, which in turns derives from the extent to which the metabolic hypothesis is embraced.

DIET THERAPY

Dietary management forms the cornerstone of treatment of all diabetic patients. This is true in circumstances in which insulin or oral hypoglycemic agents are used, as well as in the patients in whom dietary measures are the sole form of therapy. Despite its paramount importance, successful implementation of dietary management is achieved in only occasional patients.[442] The reasons for this frequent failure largely relate to a failure on the part of the physician and the patient to understand the goals, principles, and specific strategies of treatment. Whereas the purpose of insulin and oral agent treatment involves primarily the normalization of blood glucose concentration, the goals of diet therapy are two: normoglycemia and ideal body weight. These aims are achieved on the basis of three principles: (1) regulation of caloric intake, (2) selection of carbohydrate foods less likely to cause marked increases in blood glucose concentration, without reducing total carbohydrate content, and (3) maintenance of frequent food intake in small portions.

Regulation of total caloric intake is directed at achievement of ideal body weight. For type II diabetics (among whom, as already noted, the frequency of obesity is > 80 percent), this generally entails a reduction in caloric intake. The importance of weight reduction in these patients is based upon the fact that obesity results in resistance to endogenous insulin, which is reversed by a return to ideal weight;[443] with restoration to normal weight, the demand for endogenous insulin is reduced and an improvement in glucose tolerance ensues. In contrast to the obese type II diabetic, a high caloric intake is indicated in the wasted type I diabetic, particularly in childhood. Such patients require an increase in calories to restore body fat and protein and permit normal growth.

The total carbohydrate content of the diet should not be disproportionately restricted. There is no compelling evidence that reduction in the carbohydrate content to 30 percent without reducing total caloric intake results in improvement of the diabetic state. Such an approach may, in the long run, be deleterious, since the calories not taken in as carbohydrate are generally made up in the form of fat; a high fat intake may have an adverse effect, by accelerating atherosclerosis. Furthermore, an increase in the proportion of carbohydrate in the diet may improve glucose tolerance.

Once the appropriate caloric intake has been determined, 50 to 60 percent of the calories should be provided in the form of carbohydrate. An exception is the diabetic with a carbohydrate-inducible (type 4 or 5) form of hyperlipidemia, in whom a low-carbohydrate, high-fat intake may be indicated. The classic dietary recommendations for choice of carbohydrate-containing foods have called for avoidance by diabetics of concentrated sweets (e.g., table sugar, candies, pastries). The basis for this recommendation is the notion that foods containing preformed mono- or disaccharides are more likely to cause a marked rise in blood glucose concentration than equivalent amounts of carbohydrate present as a starch (e.g., potato). Studies indicate, however, that such simple rules may not adequately predict the "glycemic index" of foods.[444] For example, the glycemic index of mashed potatoes is substantially greater than that of ice cream, sucrose, or fructose.[444] Sucrose (or fructose)-rich diets are not recommended in general, even if the postprandial glucose and insulin elevations they elicit may be lower in comparison with other carbohydrates.[444a,b] There is a metabolic tendency of fructose to be preferentially converted to lipids, mainly as a result of obligatory hepatic fructose metabolism with consequent hyperlipogenesis.[12] Excessive fructose consumption should, in fact, be considered as an accessory risk factor in diabetes. The emerging data on blood glucose concentration responses to specific foods should thus permit a dietary selection process which contributes substantially to improving overall blood glucose level control.

Day-to-day regularity of food intake both with respect to total consumption of calories and carbohydrates and with regard to the timing of meals and snacks is of importance in insulin-dependent diabetics so as to prevent insulin-induced hypoglycemia. The regularity and frequency of feedings are predicated upon the fact that, in contrast to the normal subject, in whom insulin secretion is dictated by food ingestion, the insulin-dependent diabetic must match food intake to the continuing action of injected insulin. Since insulin is continuously being released from injection sites, ideally the patient should eat sparingly but frequently rather than allow long intervals between large meals. Consistency in the pattern of food ingestion does not apply on those days in which there is a marked increase in caloric expenditure as a consequence of moderate to intense exercise. In normal subjects, exercise causes a fall in endogenous insulin levels, which permits an increase in hepatic glucose output. In the diabetic subject receiving insulin injections, such homeostatic changes in circulating insulin levels do not happen; in fact, rapid insulin mobilization from the injection site may occur in response to exercise (see below). In such circumstances extra food should be taken so as to meet the needs of contracting muscles and to prevent hypoglycemia.

Despite the simplicity of many of these principles, $<$ 50 percent of the diabetic population adheres to the recommended dietary regimen. Poor understanding on the part of the patient as well as the physician with respect to dietary goals and tactics is frequently responsible for failures. Often, the basic prescription is clearly in error and unsuitable for the specific patient. For example, to many physicians a "diabetic diet" almost by definition means an 1800-calorie intake. Such a diet in a vigorous, nonobese, 160-lb (73-kg) type I diabetic is obviously too restricted and is likely to have one of two adverse consequences. Either the patient does not follow the diet and supplements his or her intake, generally with concentrated sweets, resulting in marked swings in the blood glucose concentration, or the patient sticks to the diet but develops hypoglycemic episodes and/or loses weight. An 1800-calorie diet is equally inappropriate in the 180-lb (82-kg), 5-ft 2-in (158-cm), 50-year-old, sedentary type II diabetic woman; in such a patient the major objective should be weight reduction by means of a more limited caloric intake.

Dietary management thus must begin with a precise diet prescription which is meaningful to the dietitian as well as the patient. This necessarily involves tailoring the diet to the individual patient. For example, in type II diabetics the most important consideration is caloric restriction. This should be emphasized to the patient and communicated to the dietitian in terms of total caloric content. In contrast, in the nonobese type I diabetic, regularity of food intake, use of between-meal snacks, and selectivity concerning the types of carbohydrate-containing foods are of greater priority than total caloric intake.

In all forms of diabetes the importance of patient education in implementation of dietary management cannot be overstated. Of great importance is making certain that the patient understands the goals and strategies of the diet and that the dietary prescription takes into account the habits, behavior, and specific requirements of the individual patient. Initial referral and frequent follow-up by a competent dietitian is essential to reinforce the importance of dietary compliance.

Many studies have been performed recently showing that addition to the diet of fiber (nonabsorbable carbohydrate) decreases postprandial hyperglycemia[444,445] and lowers lipid levels.[446] The ingestion of guar gum (a storage polysaccharide obtained from the cluster bean) or pectin (a structural polysaccharide obtained from apples and citrus fruits), together with meals containing absorbable carbohydrates, slows or reduces carbohydrate absorption as well as plasma insulin response[447] in normal and diabetic subjects. Studies of peripheral insulin sensitivity have shown no increase after fiber ingestion, suggesting that its major effect in reducing postprandial hyperglycemia is via effects on the GI handling of carbohydrate-containing foods.[448] Since relatively large amounts of fiber (10 to 15 g per meal) are required to achieve an effect, and inasmuch as the palatability of such diets is poor, the overall practicability and long-term efficacy of high-fiber diets in the routine management of diabetes remain to be established.

ORAL HYPOGLYCEMIC AGENTS

Since the introduction of the sulfonylureas in the 1950s the management of many patients with type II diabetes has included the use of oral hypoglycemic agents. The two classes of hypoglycemic drugs which have been employed are the sulfonylurea and biguanide compounds. These compounds differ with regard to structure, action, and clinical usefulness.

The Sulfonylureas

The sulfonylurea drugs share a basic molecular structure but differ in substituents on the benzene and urea groups. These substitutions account for differences in the potency, metabolism, and duration of action of the sulfonylureas (Table 19-17). Sulfonylureas reduce blood glucose concentration mainly by augmenting the amount of endogenous insulin released by directly affecting the pancreatic islets. IV administration of sulfonylureas produces abrupt release of insulin and the insulin response to feeding is increased after short-term sulfonylurea therapy. This concept is further supported by evidence that these drugs fail to reduce blood glucose concentration in pancreatectomized animals or in type I diabetics without residual endogenous insulin, and produce rapid release of insulin from isolated islet cell systems. The second-generation oral agents glipizide and glyburide are substantially more potent than the first-generation sulfonylureas in facilitating insulin release.[449,449a] While these data convincingly demonstrate that sulfonylureas are effective insulin secretagogues, the persistent hypoglycemic action of these drugs may not be solely mediated via changes in insulin secretion. In fact, insulin secretion is actually reduced after several months of treatment, despite improvement in glucose tolerance. The reduction in insulin secretion may, however, be more apparent than real; it may reflect the lower ambient blood glucose levels and improved metabolic control achieved with the sulfonylurea agents. Thus if plasma glucose level is raised to the pretreatment value, the insulin secretory response is greater than it was prior to treatment.[449a] Additional evidence supporting an extrapancreatic effect of sulfonylureas is provided by studies demonstrating an increase in peripheral sensitivity to insulin.[450] However, those effects may also be secondary to enhanced insulin secretion and improved control of blood glucose concentration, inasmuch as intensive treatment of type II diabetics with sulfonylureas[450a] or exogenous insulin[451] reduces insulin resistance, increases basal insulin levels, and causes a drop in fasting plasma glucose levels, most probably by restraining hepatic glucose production. In a recent comparison of treatments with exogenous insulin and tolazamide,[451a] similar lowering of glycohemoglobin levels and glucose production was obtained. Since no change in insulin binding was seen, these improvements were achieved by increasing the maximal insulin response. All curves were shifted, however, to the right of normal, indicating a residual, postbinding defect in insulin action, which could not be reversed either by tolazamide or insulin. Oral agents should not be regarded, therefore, as more physiologic than exogenous insulin because by augmenting the endogenous insulin secretion they may effect a "normal" portal/peripheral insulin ratio.

SULFONYLUREA PREPARATIONS The various sulfonylurea agents differ primarily with respect to duration of action and potency (Table 19-17). The differences in duration of action reflect differences in drug metabolism.[452–454] Tolbutamide, the shortest-acting drug, is metabolized by the liver to metabolically inert prod-

Table 19-17. Properties of Sulfonylurea Agents

	Relative potency	Duration of activity, h	Metabolite activity	Protein binding	Dose, mg	Disulfiram-like effect	Frequency of hypoglycemia
Tolbutamide	1	6–8	Weak	Ionic	500–3000	No	Rare
Acetohexamide	2.5	8–12	Active	Ionic	250–1500	No	< 1%
Tolazamide	5	12–18	One active, one non-active	Ionic	100–1000	No	< 1%
Chlorpropamide	5	24–72	70% less active; 30% excreted intact	Ionic	100–500 (750)	Yes	2–3%
Glipizide	100	12–18	Inactive	Nonionic	2.5–40	Weak	3–5%
Glyburide	150	16–24	Inactive	Nonionic	1.25–20	Weak	4–6%

Source: Modified from Gerich JE: *Mayo Clin Proc* 60:439, 1985.

ucts. Acetohexamide and tolazamide are also metabolized by the liver, but their metabolic products retain hypoglycemic activity, which may account for the more prolonged action of these drugs. The principal metabolic product of acetohexamide metabolism, hydroxyhexamide, is a particularly potent hypoglycemic agent; like other active metabolites it is removed by the kidney. Chlorpropamide is bound to plasma proteins (a property which likely accounts for its long duration of action) and is excreted either unchanged via the kidney or after hepatic metabolism. Metabolites of chlorpropamide retain some hypoglycemic activity.

The second-generation sulfonylureas glipizide and glyburide differ from the first-generation ones in their structure and potency. In these agents the aliphatic side chains of tolbutamide and chlorpropamide have been replaced by a cyclohexyl group, with another ring structure added to the opposite side. Glipizide and glyburide are 50 to 100 times more potent than chlorpropamide and are effective at nanomolar rather than micromolar blood levels.

CLINICAL EFFECTS The clinical usefulness of the sulfonylureas is limited by the requirement for beta cell reserve to ensure endogenous production of insulin in substantial amounts. This is true whether the agents act solely by enhancing insulin secretion or via an action on insulin sensitivity as well. The drugs are consequently ineffective in type I diabetics. Their chief value is in patients with type II diabetes who have little tendency to develop ketoacidosis. Even in this group, 15 to 40 percent do not respond. Moreover, of those whose diabetes is reasonably well controlled for a month or more, 25 to 40 percent ultimately escape from control (secondary failure), presumably because of progression of beta cell secretory failure. The tendency to develop secondary failure is greater in women than in men and in patients with diabetes for > 1 year before treatment was started as compared with those given treatment within the first year after recognition of the disease. Thus, continuous satisfactory control is exercised in no more than 20 to 30 percent.[452–454] Despite the increased potency of the second-generation agents, their efficacy is no greater than that of the first-generation compounds.[449]

Initial favorable responses to sulfonylureas have been attributed to the following factors: (1) age of onset > 40 years, (2) duration of diabetes < 5 years, (3) normal or excessive weight, and (4) lack of previous treatment with insulin or insulin requirement < 40 U per day. While exhaustion of islet cell function cannot be attributed to sulfonylurea agents, there is also no compelling evidence that prophylactic treatment of asymptomatic glucose intolerance with oral hypoglycemic agents either restores carbohydrate tolerance to normal or prevents its deterioration to overt diabetes.[452]

With tolbutamide it is preferable to give the drug in divided doses because of the short period of effectiveness. If chlorpropamide, tolazamide, glipizide, or glyburide is used, a single dose once a day is adequate. There is no advantage in exceeding the maximum dosage recommended (Table 19-17), since no increase of effect is to be expected from doses larger than the maximum indicated.

TOXICITY Sulfonylureas may, on occasion, induce profound and sustained hypoglycemia. These hypoglycemic episodes are generally associated with a condition which delays the metabolism or excretion of the sulphonylureas. Thus, they must be used with caution in the presence of liver and/or renal dysfunction, the latter being particularly common in elderly diabetic patients. Because of their long duration of action, chlorpropamide and glyburide may be especially prone to cause hypoglycemia. In addition, certain drugs have been shown to potentiate the effects of sulfonylureas by (1) interfering with hepatic metabolism, e.g., sulfisoxazole, dicumarol, (2) reducing urinary excretion, e.g., phenylbutazone or acetohexamide, or (3) possessing an additive hypoglycemic action, e.g., salicylates.[452] In contrast to the first-generation sulfonylureas, the second-generation sulfonylureas are nonionically bound to plasma proteins. Consequently, less variation in their bioavailability because of displacement from plasma proteins by other charged drugs may be expected.[453,454]

Another complication of sulfonylurea treatment is the development of hyponatremia.[455,456] While other sulfonylureas are potentially capable of impairing water excretion, clinically this syndrome is almost exclusively observed with chlorpropamide treatment. This is probably a consequence of its long half-life and the resultant inability to escape from its effects. The hyponatremia is believed to result from chlorpropamide's ability to enhance the action of antidiuretic hormone (ADH). An additional factor may be the failure of ADH secretion in these patients to be completely suppressed in the face of a decline in serum osmolarity.[455] In one study the prevalence of hyponatremia (serum $[Na^+] < 129$ meq/liter) was 6.3 percent in chlorpropamide-treated patients during a mean follow-up period of 7.4 years; in contrast, only 0.6 percent of patients treated with either tolbutamide or glyburide developed this complication. Risk factors for the development of hyponatremia in patients treated with chlorpropamide include older age and coadministration of thiazide diuretics.[456]

In rare instances, patients may develop skin rashes, leukopenia, anemia, thrombocytopenia, jaundice due to allergic hepatitis, or the nephrotic syndrome.[457] In some patients chlorpropamide administration is associated with the development of an intensive flush after the consumption of alcohol (chlorpropamide-alcohol flush, CPAF) which is reminiscent of that observed with disulfiram (Antabuse). Although it has been hypothesized that CPAF may represent a genetic marker for a subtype of type II diabetes,[458] this has been refuted by evidence demonstrating that CPAF may be present in both type I diabetics and nondiabetics with the same frequency as it occurs in type II diabetics.[459] The suggestion that CPAF patients may be protected against developing microvascular complications of diabetes has not been uniformly substantiated. This may be due to the lack of clarity of defining CPAF, since it is affected by a number of variables including plasma chlorpropamide levels, ethanol, dose ambient temperature, basal facial skin temperature, response to ethanol alone, and activity of acetaldehyde dehydrogenase. The combined prevalence of all these complications of sulfonylurea treatment is <5 percent.

The most important question regarding the toxicity of the sulfonylurea drugs relates to the findings of the (UGDP) study.[460] The UGDP study, originally conceived to evaluate the relative effectiveness of tolbutamide, phenformin, and insulin in reducing vascular complications in type II diabetes, led to the unexpected observation that cardiovascular mortality was actually increased in subjects receiving tolbutamide and phenformin when compared with placebo- and insulin-treated groups. These results incited an extensive debate among diabetologists and statisticians who maintained that (1) the mortality was concentrated in only a few of the treatment centers, (2) cardiovascular risk factors were not adequately evaluated (smoking and drug histories were not adequately obtained), (3) the treatment schedule for oral agents was fixed and therefore no attempt was made to adjust the dose of the drug to the prevailing hyperglycemia (as is done in practice), and (4) the standards used to diagnose diabetes were inadequate, thereby including subjects with age-induced glucose intolerance. Arguments have also been made suggesting that the increased incidence of cardiovascular events in the tolbutamide-treated group was related to lowering of plasma HDL levels. Serious questions regarding the validity of the study thus continue to be raised.

INDICATIONS FOR USE Given the uncertainty regarding the UGDP findings it is difficult to delineate the precise indications for sulfonylurea use. Nevertheless, certain considerations hold: (1) the treatment of choice, whether an oral agent or exogenous insulin, should not be based on amelioration of insulin resistance but on the capacity to lower adequately the blood glucose levels, in view of the general noxious effects of hyperglycemia; (2) sulfonylureas are adjuncts to the dietary management of type II diabetes; they are not a replacement for dietary therapy; (3) there is no apparent advantage of adding sulfonylurea to insulin treatment to enhance insulin effectiveness; (4) the continuous satisfactory control rate with these agents is ~30 percent; (5) many patients receiving sulfonylureas for prolonged periods have no improvement in blood glucose concentration; consequently, it is recommended that sulfonylurea agents be administered to type II diabetics only when vigorous attempts to achieve glucose control with dietary measures alone have failed.

The Biguanides

The mechanism of action of the biguanides (phenformin and metformin) is not established, but is clearly independent of altered insulin secretion. An increase in insulin sensitivity has been postulated for metformin as a result of actions at the receptor and/or postreceptor level. It has been suggested that phenformin acts via stimulation of anaerobic glycolysis and inhibition of gluconeogenesis. However, the doses required to produce these effects in vitro generally exceed those used in clinical practice. More recently, it has been demonstrated that phenformin inhibits gastrointestinal absorption of glucose.[461] This effect, coupled with its anorexigenic properties, may largely account for the drug's weak hypoglycemic action.

Phenformin is capable of inducing lactic acidosis in the diabetic patient.[462] This rare but frequently fatal complication of phenformin treatment may derive from the drug's stimulatory effect on anaerobic glycolysis (thereby augmenting the production of lactate), as well as its inhibition of gluconeogenesis (thereby reducing lactate utilization). Lactic acidosis is particularly likely to occur in circumstances leading to reduced drug metabolism. The presence of renal and/or hepatic disease (phenformin is both excreted unchanged in the urine and metabolized by the liver) markedly increases the risk of lactic acidosis. Patients receiving phenformin are also particularly susceptible to lactacidemia in the presence of conditions known to augment lactic acid production (hypoxia) or reduce lactate utilization (alcohol use). Because of the substantial incidence of lactic acidosis, the U.S. Food and Drug Administration has withdrawn phenformin from the market in the United States. Metformin, however, has rarely resulted in lactic acidosis and is available for use in Europe and Canada. A frequent problem associated with the use of metformin is the occurrence of severe diarrhea with incontinence.[463]

EXERCISE

Exercise has long been recommended as part of the overall management of the diabetic patient. Already in the preinsulin era Allen observed that exercise has a blood glucose concentration–lowering effect. In fact, in type I diabetics exercise may provoke hypoglycemia in some circumstances or intensify hyperglycemia, depending in part on the nature of the patient's blood glucose concentration control in the resting state, dietary intake, and the timing of the exercise relative to insulin administration and food intake. In addition, repeated exercise (i.e., physical training) may alter tissue sensitivity to insulin. The overall interaction between exercise and diabetes is understood best in the context of the normal response of body fuel metabolism to exercise.[196,464,465]

Carbohydrate Metabolism During Exercise in Normal Humans

GLUCOSE UTILIZATION In the resting state muscle satisfies most of its fuel requirements by oxidizing fatty acids; glucose accounts for < 10 percent of total oxygen consumption. In contrast, during exercise, muscle glycogen and blood-borne glucose are major fuels for contracting muscle. During the earliest phase of exercise, muscle glycogen constitutes the major fuel consumed. The rate of glycogenolysis in muscle is most rapid in the first 5 to 10 min of exercise. As exercise continues and blood flow to muscle increases, blood-borne substrates become increasingly important sources of energy. During exercise lasting 10 to 40 min, glucose uptake by muscle rises 7- to 40-fold, increasing in proportion to the intensity of the work performed. The rise in glucose utilization is sufficient to account for 30 to 40 percent of the total oxygen consumption by muscle. The dependence of muscle on blood glucose concentration is thus comparable with the dependence on FFA, which provide an additional 40 percent of the oxidizable fuels.

As exercise is continued beyond 40 min, the rate of glucose utilization progressively increases, reaching a peak at 90 to 180 min and then declining slightly. In contrast to this late decline in glucose consumption, FFA utilization progressively increases in prolonged exercise. As a consequence, after 4 h of continuous exercise the relative contribution of FFA to total oxygen utilization is twice that of carbohydrate. This increase in uptake of FFA is in direct proportion to the delivery of FFA, as determined by the product of arterial concentration and plasma flow. Amino acid catabolism also occurs in exercise, but its overall contribution accounts for <5 percent of total energy used.[466]

The overall pattern of fuel use during mild to moderate exercise extending for prolonged periods may thus be characterized as a triphasic sequence in which muscle glycogen, blood glucose, and FFA successively predominate as the major energy-yielding substrate. With exercise at heavy work loads, there is a more persistent dependence on muscle glycogen. This is suggested by the observation that exhaustion coincides with depletion of muscle glycogen but is not accompanied by significant changes in other physiologic parameters such as heart rate, blood pressure, blood level of glucose, and concentrations of lactate or muscle electrolytes. It is unclear, however, why glycogen depletion should coincide with fatigue when large amounts of circulating substrate in the form of FFA are still available. It may be added that, as a result of long-range homeostatic adjustment to physical training in type II diabetics, there is a decrease in concentrations of circulating lipids along with the improvement in glucose tolerance.[467]

BLOOD GLUCOSE CONCENTRATION Despite the marked increase in glucose uptake by muscle, there is little change in blood glucose concentration during exercise of brief duration. With strenuous exercise an increment in blood glucose concentration of 20 to 30 mg/dl may be observed. When exercise is continued for 90 min or more, a decline in blood glucose concentration by 20 to 40 mg/dl is observed. Frank hypoglycemia (< 50 mg/dl) is observed occasionally with very prolonged exercise in normal subjects. However, exercise performance may remain unimpaired in the face of hypoglycemia, nor is it necessarily improved by glucose administration.[464] The asymptomatic hypoglycemia of prolonged exercise in normal subjects contrasts markedly with the severe symptomatic hypoglycemia which may be precipitated by exercise in insulin-treated diabetics (see below).

GLUCOSE PRODUCTION In view of the stimulation of glucose utilization which characterizes exercise, ongoing repletion of the blood glucose pool can be achieved only by an increase in glucose production. During short-term exercise, hepatic glucose output increases two- to fivefold, depending on the intensity of the work performed, and keeps pace with the increment in glucose utilization by muscle tissue. This increase in glucose production is almost entirely a consequence of augmented glycogenolysis, inasmuch as uptake of gluconeogenic precursors remains unchanged from the resting state, save for a transient rise in lactate consumption. The total amount of glucose released from the liver during 40 min of heavy work is estimated to be 18 g, representing 20 to 25 percent of the total hepatic glycogen stores in the postabsorptive state.

As exercise extends beyond 40 min, a slight imbalance between hepatic production and peripheral utilization of glucose and increasing reliance on hepatic gluconeogenesis are observed. During prolonged mild exercise, glucose output doubles in the first 40 min and thereafter remains constant for the ensuing 3 to 4 h. Since glucose utilization continues to rise for 90 min or more, glucose production fails to keep pace with utilization, and a modest decline in blood glucose concentration is observed. The relative contribution from gluconeogenesis to overall hepatic glucose output (as inferred from substrate balances across the splanchnic bed) increases from 25 percent in the basal state to 45 percent during prolonged exercise, representing a threefold rise in the absolute rate of gluconeogenesis. These increments in hepatic uptake of glucose precursors are largely a result of augmented fractional extraction. In the case of alanine, the major gluconeogenic precursor, fractional extraction by the splanchnic bed increases from resting levels of 35 to 50 percent to almost 90 percent in prolonged exercise, a rate which is well in excess of the 50 to 70 percent extraction rates observed in other circumstances of increased gluconeogenesis such as diabetes, obesity, and starvation. The overall importance of gluconeogenesis in prolonged exercise is underscored by the estimation that 50 to 60 g of liver glycogen is mobilized in 4 h of exercise, representing a depletion of 75 percent of total liver glycogen stores.

GLUCOREGULATORY HORMONES The hormonal response to exercise is characterized by a fall in plasma insulin concentration and an increase in plasma glucagon concentration. These findings are especially pronounced in prolonged or severe exercise. The decrease in insulin concentration is particularly noteworthy in intensive exercise, in which circumstance hypoinsulinemia occurs despite a modest rise in blood glucose concentration. These findings suggest an inhibition of insulin secretion, probably mediated via the adrenergic nervous system and/or circulating catecholamines. Other hormonal changes occurring in exercise include elevation in plasma GH, cortisol, epinephrine, and norepinephrine levels.

The stimulatory effect of exercise on glucose uptake in the face of hypoinsulinemia indicates that such enhancement of glucose consumption is not dependent on an increase in insulin secretion. In fact, the presence of even minimal concentrations of insulin may not be necessary for exercise-induced increases in glucose utilization.[468] Experiments with isolated muscles have established that the work-induced increment in glucose uptake is non-insulin-dependent. The physiologic significance of the altered hormonal milieu in exercise relates more to the stimulation of hepatic glucose production than to glucose utilization. The exquisite sensitivity of human hepatic glycogenolysis to the inhibitory action of small increments in insulin concentration has been demonstrated.[196] The importance of the hypoinsulinemia of exercise is thus manifested by its effect on hepatic glycogenolysis. In prolonged or severe exercise, the rises in glucagon, GH, and catecholamine concentrations also contribute to the glycogenolytic and gluconeogenic response. The overall substrate and hormone response to exercise is summarized in Fig. 19-54.

Exercise-Induced Hypoglycemia

For the type I diabetic exercise-induced hypoglycemia is a well-recognized complication of treatment with insulin. The tendency of these patients to develop hypoglycemia derives from the failure of their plasma insulin levels to decrease during exercise. In addition, some patients are deficient in catecholamine as well as in glucagon secretion that is necessary for protection against hypoglycemia.[468] Thus, if exercise occurs at a time when insulin is being released from injection sites in amounts that exceed normal basal plasma levels, hypoglycemia is likely to occur. The presence of insulin levels higher than basal leads to excessive glucose utilization coupled with decreased glucose production. In the presence of deficient catecholamine and glucagon response as well, the patient is unable to overcome the effects of an insulin level inappropriately high for brief exercise.

The factors influencing the occurrence of exercise-induced hypoglycemia include (1) the timing of exercise in relation to the peak action of insulin, (2) the intensity of the exercise, (3) the training status of the patient (see below), (4) the timing and magnitude of meal and/or snack ingestion, (5) the use of pump vs. manual injection of insulin, and (6) the site of insulin injection. Clearly, exercise should be undertaken at times which do not coincide with the peak effect of previously injected rapid- or intermediate-acting insulin. If hypoglycemia is not prevented by appropriately timing the activity, then a snack before or during the exercise should be tried. Avoidance of use of exercised areas as an injection site (e.g., the abdominal wall or legs) helps prevent the accelerated insulin absorption which may occur from these areas.[469] The use of a portable pump has also been shown to lessen somewhat the tendency to develop exercise-induced hypoglycemia. If other approaches fail, insulin

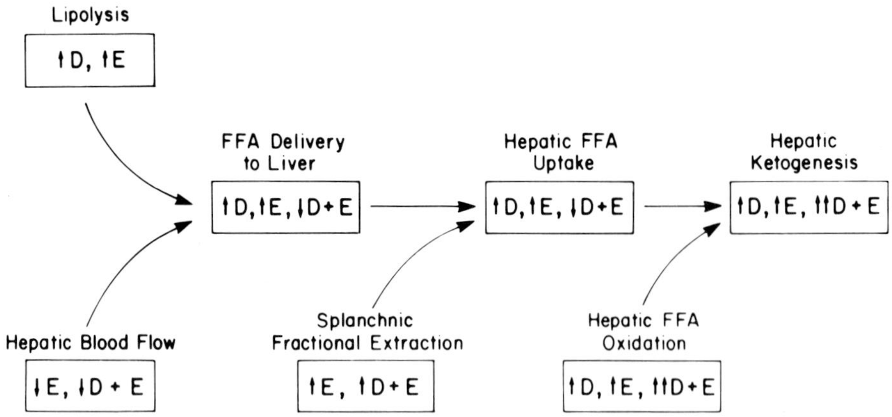

FIGURE 19-54 Regulatory sites in the control of ketogenesis in diabetes (D), with exercise (E), and during exercise in diabetics (D+E). ↑, Increase; ↑↑, marked increase; ↓, decrease. (*From Wahren et al.*[471])

dose should be reduced. Unfortunately, neither the amount of extra dietary carbohydrate nor the amount of insulin to be reduced can be predicted in advance; both must be determined by trial and error.

Despite the potential danger of hypoglycemia, insulin treatment is by no means incompatible with a vigorous life in which exercise is a frequent pastime. In fact, there are a number of professional athletes for whom the treatment of type I diabetes and the associated risk of exercise-induced hypoglycemia has not interfered with their vigorous daily routines and their attainment of superstar status.

Exercise-Induced Hyperglycemia and Hyperketonemia

In some circumstances exercise may actually worsen hyperglycemia and increase ketogenesis in the diabetic.[470,471,471a] This is true in the patient with poorly regulated diabetes. When moderate to severe hyperglycemia (> 300 mg/dl or > 17 mM) and hyperketonemia (> 2 mM) are present in the resting state, acute exercise causes a further rise rather than a fall in blood glucose concentration. Contributing to the rise in blood glucose concentration are inappropriate increments in levels of counterregulatory hormones (GH, epinephrine, and norepinephrine).[254]

An exaggerated ketogenic response to exercise is observed in diabetics, particularly if there is poor diabetic control prior to exercise. This ketogenesis is a result of increased fractional extraction of FFA by the liver as well as a marked increase in intrahepatic conversion of FFA to ketones[471] (Fig. 19-14). Despite the increase in ketogenesis which occurs during exercise, the hyperketonemic effect of exercise is not apparent until the postexercise recovery period. This is because the augmented ketogenesis of the diabetic is accompanied by increased muscle utilization of ketones. However, immediately following exercise, ketone utilization falls abruptly while ketone overproduction is sustained into the recovery period in poorly regulated diabetes.[471,471a] The largest increment in concentrations of circulating ketones observed in poorly regulated diabetes occurs during recovery.[471,471a] The important clinical implication of these observations is that exercise cannot be viewed as an alternative but should rather be viewed as an adjunct to proper control of blood glucose concentration with insulin.

Exercise-Induced Alterations in Insulin Action

In well-trained athletes (e.g., long-distance runners) the plasma insulin response to an IV glucose load is diminished in the face of normal glucose tolerance, suggesting enhanced tissue response to insulin. More direct evidence of increased insulin response is derived from studies involving the insulin clamp procedure. With this technique insulin-mediated glucose uptake has been shown to increase in previously untrained healthy subjects after a 6-week training program. This increment in insulin sensitivity occurs in the absence of changes in body weight.[468]

Despite these findings in normal subjects, in the diabetic population a clinically useful effect of physical training in improving blood glucose concentration control has not been as readily demonstrable. Regular exercise in type II diabetics lowers plasma insulin level and enhances insulin sensitivity. However, a consistent improvement in blood glucose concentration regulation has not been demonstrated.[472] The failure to observe an enhancement of blood glucose level control in type II diabetes may reflect the fact that, while muscle response to insulin is increasing, insulin secretion falls and hepatic sensitivity to insulin fails to increase after physical training.[473] Thus, the net effect is often a reduction in hyperinsulinemia without an accompanying improvement in blood glucose concentration control. Similarly, in type I diabetics physical training results in an increase in sensitivity to insulin without an overall improvement in glucoregulation.[473] Nevertheless, to the extent that hyperinsulinemia may of itself be a risk factor for atherosclerosis, through an effect on concentrations of plasma lipids physical training may be useful in improving longevity.

Summary: Risks and Benefits of Exercise in Diabetes

Exercise produces complex metabolic effects, in part immediately manifested in blood glucose concentration and in part more sustained on tissue response to insulin. The benefits of exercise may be summarized as follows:

1. Decrease in cardiovascular risk factors. Exercise decreases plasma insulin concentration in type II diabetes and the need for exogenous insulin in type I diabetes, increases plasma HDL concentration and lowers LDL levels, increases myocardial vascularity and work efficiency, increases pulmonary function, and decreases both systolic and diastolic blood pressure. These benefits, however, do not persist when training is discontinued.
2. Achievement of weight loss, as an adjunct to diet in type II diabetes. Exercise results in increased energy expenditure but does not by itself usually lead to significant weight loss. Exercise alters body composition by increasing muscle mass and decreasing body fat content. Therefore, by improving self-image this may provide motivation for increasing dietary compliance.
3. Potential improvement in glucose tolerance in some patients due to increased glucose utilization and increased response to insulin. This may result in a reduction in insulin or oral hypoglycemic agent dosage.
4. Increased work capacity.
5. Increased sense of well-being and enrichment of quality of life.

The following risks have been found to be associated with exercise and diabetes:

1. Potentiation of the hypoglycemic effect of insulin or oral hypoglycemic agents in prolonged and/or vigorous exercise
2. Deterioration of metabolic control in poorly controlled diabetes (blood glucose concentration <300 mg/dl)
3. Worsening of musculoskeletal complications associated with neuropathy, retinopathy (e.g., vitreous hemorrhage), and nephropathy (e.g., increased proteinuria with exercise)

These observations indicate that exercise is a useful adjunct but not a substitute for proper glucoregulation with insulin and/or diet. Exercise should be encouraged as a means of decreasing risk factors for cardiovascular disease and possibly improving glucose homeostasis provided that no contraindications exist. The current state of knowledge, however, does not permit the formulation of a precise exercise prescription as part of the management of the diabetic patient.

FUTURE TREATMENT

As noted above, even under optimal conditions complete normalization of blood glucose concentration is difficult to achieve with conventional or intensive therapy. Recognition of the inadequacy or difficulty of implementation of current treatment regimens and, more importantly, their unproven ability to prevent vascular and neurologic complications of diabetes has led to a search for newer approaches to treatment. Current investigative efforts are directed at three possible modalities: (1) immunosuppression as a means of inducing remission or preventing appearance of type I diabetes, (2) transplantation of whole pancreas or islet cells, and (3) use of somatostatin analogues.

Immunosuppression

As discussed above, a variety of findings provide compelling evidence that humoral and cell-mediated autoimmune processes are central to the etiology and pathogenesis of type I diabetes. Such observations make it probable that intervention with immunosuppressive agents may prevent, attenuate, or retard the onset of type I diabetes or induce a remission in patients in whom the disease is already manifest. A definite marker for type I diabetes is not yet available, although vigorous investigations for a predictive indicator are in progress. Consequently, therapeutic intervention can be contemplated at present only for patients soon after the onset of type I diabetes. With advances in identification and characterization of the specific antigenic factor(s) leading to islet cell destruction, a preventive immunosuppressive program may be elaborated. A plausible strategy over the next decade would be to screen newborns for diabetogenic genes or gene products, then to follow the predisposed individuals prospectively, using sensitive tests of insulin secretion capacity and assays for specific islet cell antibodies, up to the point justifying intervention.[473a] In patients with long-standing disease, beta cell destruction is of such an advanced degree that recovery of function and an accompanying clinical remission cannot be expected. Newly discovered type I diabetes often enters a clinical remission or "honeymoon" phase, in which insulin requirements decline and there is a partial, although transient, recovery of endogenous insulin secretion. Based on these findings and the observation that cyclosporine A, a nonmyelotoxic immunosuppressive agent, is capable of preventing diabetes in the BB rat and the NOD mouse,[473b,c] (models of immunogenic type I diabetes), the effects of cyclosporine A on human type I diabetes have recently been investigated. In two independent studies, cyclosporine A was demonstrated to induce complete remissions (defined as normal glycohemoglobin levels in the absence of insulin therapy) in 24 to 37 percent of patients in whom treatment was initiated within a few weeks of clinical recognition of type I diabetes.[221,222] These remissions were accompanied by recovery of endogenous insulin secretory rates which were within the normal range and suppression of anti-beta cell autoimmunity. Since the frequency of spontaneous complete remission in type I diabetes is reported to be <6 percent, the findings suggest that the immunosuppressive treatment was in fact responsible for the recovery of beta cell function in the treated patients.

A number of important issues regarding the role of immunosuppression in type I diabetes remain to be clarified. First, remissions have been maintained for periods of 1 year while immunosuppression is continued, but cessation of cyclosporine A therapy is associated with recurrence of insulin dependence. The observation that autoimmune destruction of beta cells may be retriggered as long as 20 years after initial manifestation of diabetes[474] suggests that lifelong immunosuppression may be required to protect the beta cells, rather than a 1- to 2-year course of therapy. Also, the risk/benefit ratio of long-term cyclosporine A therapy in type I diabetes remains to be established. Although the incidence of tumors in patients receiving cyclosporine A for transplant or other autoimmune indications is extremely low,[475,476] the danger of nephropathy cannot be discounted. Consequently, the use of cyclosporine A in type I diabetes is now limited to investigational trials.

Pancreatic and Islet Cell Transplants

Whole-pancreas transplants have generally been undertaken in type I diabetes in conjunction with renal transplants which would otherwise necessitate the use of immunosuppressive agents. The procedures used in pancreas transplantation involve grafting of the whole pancreas together with the duodenum, the whole pancreas alone, or only a segment of the pancreas; the last is the procedure generally used at present. Cadaver grafts and, to a very limited extent, segmental grafts from living related donors have been employed. A number of approaches also have been used to deal with the exocrine secretions of the pancreas, including cutaneous, ureteral, intraperitoneal, and enteral drainage. The most popular approach involves exocrine suppression by injecting the duct with synthetic polymers.[477] This procedure results in duct occlusion and atrophy of exocrine tissue in the transplant.

In the 16-year period until the end of 1981, 191 pancreas allotransplants were performed in 178 diabetic patients.[478] Most of these transplants were performed in patients with far-advanced complications of diabetes (75 percent of the patients had end-stage renal disease). By March 1982 only 10 percent of these transplants were functioning.[416] In addition to elimination of exogenous insulin, evidence of pancreatic islet function in these patients has included the restoration of normal insulin secretory responses to meal ingestion, normal suppressibility of glucagon secretion by glucose ingestion, and normal glycohemoglobin levels.[416] The causes of failure in 165 transplants with > 1 year of function included rejection and technical problems such as thrombosis (vascular complications), ascites, infection, abscess, and hemorrhage.

Pancreas transplantation requires, of course, the ongoing use of immunosuppressive agents and its attendant risks. Consequently, pancreatic transplantation has generally been restricted to patients requiring immunosuppression for concurrent renal transplantation. The improved success rate of kidney, heart, and liver transplants since the advent of cyclosporine A[479] is likely to result in similar improvement in the success rate of pancreatic transplants in the future.

Islet transplantation has been studied extensively in animals but thus far has been of quite limited application in humans. Islet grafts have the potential advantage of greater safety: they avoid many of the technical complications associated with the more extensive surgery and need for drainage of exocrine secretions which are associated with pancreas grafts. In addition, islets have the potential for manipulation (e.g., in tissue culture), which may reduce antigenicity. A total of 76 islet transplants in 71 diabetic patients were reported to the transplant registry between 1970 and 1981.[478] The donor islets are prepared by dispersion of adult cadaveric pancreas tissue. The transplant method most widely used is intraportal injection. The experience to date clearly indicates that islet transplantation is a safe procedure; no deaths have been attributed to the procedure. However, except in extremely rare instances (perhaps 4 of 76 cases), it has been ineffective in restoring insulin secretion.[478] The problems encountered have included low yield of islets from donor pancreas, lack of viability of the isolated islets, and rejection. Studies with islet transplants in experimental animals have provided possible approaches to preventing the rejection process. Successful transplantation of islet allografts and even xenografts in nonimmunosuppressed rodent recipients has been achieved when the donor islets were cultured at 24°C or in 95% O_2 prior to transplantation. The effectiveness of organ culture in prolonging graft survival is attributed to a loss of stimulator cells or passenger lymphocytes before transplantation. These observations may have implications for improving the success of transplantation of a variety of tissues. On the other hand, studies in nonimmunosuppressed patients receiving live donor segmental pancreatic isografts (i.e., between identical twins) have shown recrudescence of diabetes after transient amelioration. The reappearance of diabetes in the recipients is due to reactivation of an autoimmune process consequent to the presentation of islet cells and their associated antigens.[474] Thus, immunosuppression may be necessary in transplant recipients not ony to prevent rejection but to prevent recurrence of the autoimmune process initially responsible for beta cell destruction and type I diabetes.

In summary, transplantations of whole pancreas and of isolated islets have been performed in a limited number of diabetic patients. The need for immunosuppression and its attendant risks have generally resulted in restricting transplantation to patients requiring immunosuppression on other grounds (e.g., patients requiring kidney transplants). Pancreatic duct occlusion with polymers and use of segmental grafts have reduced some of the technical problems associated with pancreas transplants. The use of cyclosporin A and the development of techniques for manipulation of human islet cells that reduce immunogenicity may result in the more widespread use of transplantation in the management of type I diabetes.

Somatostatin and Its Analogues

The evidence implicating glucagon in the pathogenesis of type I diabetes and GH in causing instability of blood glucose concentration has led to the hope that suppression of glucagon and/or GH secretion would improve control of diabetes. Somatostatin effectively reduces plasma glucagon and GH levels and decreases fasting and postprandial blood glucose levels in the diabetic; this is true whether the diet contains carbohydrate or is carbohydrate-free (consisting of protein and fat).[480] The postprandial effectiveness of somatostatin may, however, be largely a consequence of inhibition of carbohydrate and protein absorption, rather than improvement in glucose disposal.[94,481] On the other hand, the bedtime administration of the long-acting somatostatin analogue SMS 201-995 has a suppressive effect on nocturnal and early-morning GH secretion, which may reduce fasting hyperglycemia due to the dawn phenomenon (see above).[481] The role of somatostatin analogues in the suppression of oversecretion of pancreatic and pituitary hormones[481a] and in the management of diabetes is currently being investigated.

Hyperglycemic-Ketoacidotic Emergencies

Although diabetes mellitus is generally manifested as a chronic disorder, in certain circumstances large increases in concentrations of plasma glucose and/or ketoacids may pose a life-threatening emergency. In clinical practice a spectrum of disorders is observed in which either glucose or ketones or both accumulate, either alone or in combination with lactic acid. Consequently, the major syndromes encountered are DKA (glucose plus ketone accumulation), alcoholic ketoacidosis (ketone accumulation with hyperglycemia), hyperosmolar nonketotic coma (glucose accumulation without ketonemia), and, finally, any of the above plus lactic acidosis. These disorders require special attention because of the need for prompt, accurate diagnosis and treatment lest the condition rapidly progress to death.

DIABETIC KETOACIDOSIS

The most severe clinical manifestation of insulin lack is the development of DKA. Since the advent of insulin therapy $>$ 60 years ago, the importance of DKA as a cause of death in the diabetic population has progressively declined. Nevertheless, this condition is encountered not infrequently. It may be a recurrent disorder, particularly in patients of limited educational background and lower socioeconomic class who are followed in hospital clinics rather than by a personal physician.[482] Furthermore, it is a potentially lethal disorder, particularly in elderly patients; the mortality rate remains at ~5 percent.[484,485]

In most circumstances death is not due to DKA per se but to some intercurrent catastrophic event (e.g., sepsis, myocardial infarction, pancreatitis) which may have precipitated or complicated the course of DKA.

Pathogenesis

From a metabolic standpoint the major findings in DKA are the accumulation of the organic acids acetoacetate and β-hydroxybutyrate, elevation in serum acetone concentration, a marked increase in blood glucose concentration, and a serious cation loss in urine. Clinically, the major life-threatening abnormalities are metabolic acidosis (due to the hyperketonemia), hyperosmolarity (due to hyperglycemia and water loss), and dehydration (due to the osmotic diuresis accompanying hyperglycemia and the vomiting which generally accompanies severe metabolic acidosis). All these abnormalities may be traced directly to an absolute or relative lack of insulin which may develop over a period of several hours or days. A deficiency of insulin may result from failure of endogenous insulin secretion (as in the individual with newly discovered diabetes), inadequate administration of exogenous insulin (in the patient with known, insulin-dependent diabetes), or increased requirements for insulin engendered by the stress associated with an intercurrent infectious, inflammatory, traumatic, or endocrinologic disorder. The increased insulin requirements in such disorders may be attributed to the augmented secretion of hormones with an action antagonistic to insulin (e.g., epinephrine, cortisol, glucagon, and GH).

Severely decreased tissue utilization of glucose and glucose overproduction by the liver (and kidney in this condition) characterize the insulin-deficient state. Whereas glucose is released by the liver at a rate of 150 to 200 mg/min (2 to 3 mg per kilogram of body weight per min) in normal, postabsorptive subjects, in DKA the rate of glucose production may rise to 600 mg/min. The kidney contributes to the hyperglycemia by acidosis-stimulated gluconeogenesis, as discussed earlier. Hyperglycemia thus does not depend on failure to metabolize ingested carbohydrate but is a result of excessive production of glucose from endogenous precursors. Consequently, the diabetic may have had no intake of carbohydrate or other food for 12 to 24 h yet manifest hyperglycemia of 500 mg/dl (28 mM). Since protein-derived amino acids are the major precursors for de novo glucose synthesis, implicit in this increase in gluconeogenesis are dissolution of body protein stores and development of negative nitrogen balance. Massive mobilization of fat from adipose tissue in the form of FFA (ketone precursors) and glycerol (a glucogenic substrate) causes an additional body weight loss. In the juvenile, insulin-dependent diabetic, repeated episodes of DKA may thus interfere with normal growth. A more immediate threat to the patient, however, is the osmotic diuresis which accompanies severe hyperglycemia. This leads to dehydration, as a result of urinary losses of water and sodium, and the development of hyperosmolarity.

Coincident with the increase in blood glucose concentration, acetoacetate, β-hydroxybutyrate, and acetone progressively accumulate in blood, reaching levels of 8 to 15 mM. Insulin deficiency is responsible for the unrestrained FFA outflow from adipose tissue, as discussed earlier. The increased hepatic ketogenesis is the outcome not only of the sheer mass of FFA but is also due to the regulatory adjustments within the liver. As illustrated in Fig. 19-13, the entry of fatty acyl CoA into the mitochondria and the consequent β oxidation is preferred over esterification of fatty acyl CoA with glycerol 3-phosphate because of the decrease in malonyl CoA concentration upon cessation of de novo lipogenesis. The reduction in malonyl CoA concentration removes the inhibition of CAT 1, the enzyme responsible for intramitochondrial transfer of long-chain fatty acyl CoA,[40] resulting in excessive acetyl CoA production. The superfluity in acetyl CoA exceeds the capacity for its oxidation to CO_2 via the Krebs cycle, resulting in condensation of acetyl CoA to ketone acids (Fig. 19-14). An ancillary elevation in glucagon concentration potentiates the hepatic ketogenesis. Hyperglucagonemia increases the level of carnitine, decreases the concentration of malonyl CoA, and increases the activity of CAT in excess of that attributable to insulin deficiency alone. As a consequence, in pancreatectomized patients in whom glucagon as well as insulin is lacking, the magnitude of hyperketonemia is less than that observed in those with spontaneous diabetes.[168] Furthermore, in type I diabetics who have been taken off of insulin therapy and rendered hypoglucagonemic by administration of somatostatin, hyperketonemia is diminished, although not entirely prevented.[93]

In addition to increased ketone production, hyperketonemia in diabetes is a consequence of decreased utilization of the ketoacids by muscle tissue. Even in patients with mild insulin lack, a diminution in the ability to dispose of ketones is demonstrable; this diminished disposal becomes increasingly important as serum ketone levels reach 10 mM.[485]

The ketone acids are generally present in plasma in a ratio of 3:1, favoring β-hydroxybutyrate. Acetone is also formed (by the spontaneous decarboxylation of acetoacetate) and circulates in a concentration which may reach 10 to 15 mM. Because of its low vapor pressure, excretion by the lungs, and characteristic fruity odor, the presence of acetone may be detected on the patient's breath and may serve as a useful diagnostic clue.

In addition to changes in glucose and fat metabolism, DKA is characterized by fluid and electrolyte losses. The severe hyperglycemia causes osmotic diuresis, resulting in large urinary losses of water and electrolytes. (As compared with plasma, the urine in osmotic diuresis is always hypotonic with respect to sodium concentration.) Cation losses are aggravated by the need to neutralize the organic acids before excreting them in urine. Insulin deficiency may of itself (independent of the osmotic diuresis) also contribute to renal sodium losses. Insulin administration has been shown to have an antinatriuretic effect, whereas an acute reduction in insulin concentration results in natriuresis.[112] If fluid intake is reduced, often because of nausea and vomiting, which are early harbingers of DKA, dehydration proceeds rapidly; blood volume drops, peripheral resistance is reduced, blood pressure falls, and renal function is impaired. Loss of water into vomitus and urine dehydrates the intracellular space. In fully developed DKA therefore, all body compartments are dehydrated, and there are absolute deficiencies of water, sodium, potassium, magnesium, chloride, and bicarbonate. The hypovolemia may, in turn, aggravate the ketosis, perhaps by acting as a stimulus for secretion of epinephrine. Contrariwise, if fluids and electrolytes are given to diabetics from whom insulin treatment has been withdrawn, hyperketonemia is delayed or reduced, even in the absence of insulin administration.

The presence of large amounts of ketone bodies, which are moderately strong acids, causes an increase in the hydrogen ion concentration of the body fluids. As a result there is a fall in concentration of serum bicarbonate and an increase in the anion gap (i.e., the difference between the serum sodium concentration and the sum of chloride plus bicarbonate exceeds the normal range of 10 to 12 meq/liter).

Clinical Manifestations

The major symptoms of DKA are nausea, vomiting, labored breathing, and depressed mental function which may vary from mild drowsiness to severe coma. On physical examination the patient appears dehydrated as reflected by dry mucous membranes and decreased skin turgor. There is a characteristic fruity odor on the breath and air hunger (Kussmaul's breathing, rapid deep respiration) is observed. Blood pressure is often reduced and there is an accompanying tachycardia. In some patients the GI symptoms are quite severe and include abdominal pain which may simulate an acute surgical abdomen (e.g., appendicitis).

The characteristic laboratory findings in DKA are an elevation in plasma glucose concentration, reductions in serum bicarbonate concentration and arterial pH, increase in anion gap, and large amounts of ketones in undiluted plasma. Because specific enzymatic techniques are cumbersome, reliance is placed on the semiquantitative reagent strip or tablet (nitroprusside) test for urinary ketone determinations. Unfortunately, the test measures only acetoacetate and acetone but not β-hydroxybutyrate concentration. Consequently, when acetoacetate accounts for $<$ 25 percent of the total ketone acids (as in combined DKA and lactic acidosis or in alcoholic ketoacidosis), the test may give a spuriously low value. Conversely, a spuriously high value is obtained after insulin treatment has been instituted because the β-hydroxybutyrate component falls before any change is observed in acetoacetate concentration.

Elevations in serum amylase concentration and in the amylase/creatinine clearance ratio are not uncommon in DKA. Although in some patients hyperamylasemia may signify accompanying pancreatitis, in most circumstances there is no clinical evidence of pancreatitis. The data suggest that the elevated amylase concentrations in DKA are of salivary rather than pancreatic origin.[486] The mechanism of this change in release and renal clearance of amylase remains to be established.

In dehydration, in addition to the increased hematocrit, the hemogram usually shows leukocytosis, frequently with increased numbers of young polymorphonuclear leukocytes. Sometimes this finding reflects the precipitating cause of acidosis, such as infection, but even in the absence of such a complication leukocytosis may be present, probably as a reflection of the severe hypertonicity of the plasma.

Diagnosis

Prompt diagnosis of DKA requires a high index of suspicion in patients with obfuscation, dehydration, hyperpnea, vomiting, and abdominal pain, or an acetone odor on the breath. The diagnosis can be rapidly established even before the serum bicarbonate concentration is reported, by examining four parameters: (1) blood and/or urinary glucose concentration, (2) urinary ketone concentrations, (3) arterial blood pH and blood gases, and (4) serum ketone concentration. The diagnosis of DKA is established if all the following findings are present: (1) blood glucose concentration $>$ 200 mg/dl and/or 4+ glucosuria, (2) strong reaction for ketones in urine, (3) arterial pH below 7.3 with a P_{CO_2} of 40 mmHg or less, and (4) a strongly positive ketone reaction in serum.

The differential diagnosis includes all types of metabolic acidosis and coma. An accumulation of ketone acids sufficient to cause metabolic acidosis may be seen in the absence of diabetes in poorly nourished alcoholic patients with repeated bouts of vomiting.[487] In such cases of *alcoholic ketoacidosis*, treatment consists of glucose infusion (insulin is not required); blood glucose levels are $<$200 mg/dl (in 30 percent of cases frank hypoglycemia is present), and urine tests do not show a 4+ reaction for glucose. In addition, the plasma ketone reaction is generally only mildly or moderately positive since the ratio of β-hydroxybutyrate to acetoacetate is increased. The change in this ratio reflects the ability of alcohol to increase cellular levels of NADH. Often, it is not possible to separate the effects of ingested alcohol from those of diabetes, and patients may have combined diabetic and alcoholic ketoacidoses.

Acidosis of uremia or of various types of poisoning may present problems, especially since patients with diabetic acidosis may also have impaired renal function due to diabetic nephropathy as well as prerenal azotemia as a consequence of dehydration. Ketosis, however, is not present in uncomplicated uremic acidosis or in methanol toxicity.

Hypoglycemia may also cause coma, but differentiation from DKA with coma is usually not difficult. In DKA the onset is gradual and signs of acidosis are present, including hyperventilation, dehydration, hypotension, and tachycardia. In contrast, hypoglycemia occurs relatively rapidly and the patient is not dehydrated or hyperventilating. In spite of these differences, if there is uncertainty, the physician should draw a blood sample for determination of glucose and electrolyte concentrations and administer IV glucose (25 g) while awaiting the laboratory report. Coma may also occur with severe hyperglycemia without ketoacidosis; this syndrome, *nonketotic hyperosmolar coma,* is discussed below. Severe metabolic acidosis and coma may be present in the absence of ketosis in patients with lactic acidosis. The latter condition (also discussed below) is characterized by a reduction in arterial pH and serum bicarbonate concentration in the absence of a positive plasma ketone determination. However, a mildly positive reaction for ketones in a hyperglycemic patient with anion gap acidosis may signify the coexistence of DKA and lactic acidosis or combined alcoholic and diabetic acidoses.

Treatment

The immediate and long-term therapeutic goals are provision of adequate insulin so as to normalize intermediary metabolism, restoration of water and electrolyte losses, and identification (when possible) of precipitating factors (infection, medication errors, psychosocial stresses, etc.) so as to prevent recurrence of DKA and facilitate the response to management. Coincident with initiation of treatment, a diabetes flow sheet is constructed on which vital signs, laboratory data (blood glucose, ketone, and electrolyte concentrations, pH, urine volume, and content of glucose and ketones, and treatment (insulin, fluids, and electrolytes) are sequentially recorded.

Catheterization of the bladder should not be routinely performed but should be reserved for patients failing to produce a urine sample after 3 to 4 h of treatment. Similarly, gastric lavage and aspiration should be undertaken only in mentally obtunded patients who are repeatedly vomiting or have evidence of gastric dilatation.

INSULIN All patients in DKA have an immediate need for insulin. Accordingly, only rapid-acting insulin should be employed. The time-honored approach has involved intermittent administration of 50 to 100 U of insulin at 2- to 4-h intervals (high-dose insulin). Over the past 10 years studies have shown that the administration of 6 to 10 U of insulin per hour by continuous IV infusion or by intermittent intramuscular or subcutaneous injection (low-dose insulin) is equally effective.[488,489] It is clear that both techniques are successful provided that clinical and laboratory parameters are carefully monitored and treatment is individualized in accordance with the data obtained in monitoring the patient. The low-dose regimens may be more advantageous in that they lead to a lower incidence of hypoglycemia and hypokalemia.[488,489]

Regardless of the insulin dose, it is advantageous to give all insulin IV in the initial phases of treatment, since impaired circulation may prevent absorption of subcutaneously or intramuscularly administered hormone. An initial loading dose of 6 to 10 U by bolus administration, followed by a continuous infusion of 6 U/h until the plasma glucose concentration falls to 250 mg/dl is recommended. In children a dose of 0.1 U per kilogram of body weight per hour may be used. The low-dose continuous insulin infusion procedure as initially introduced involved the use of an infusion pump (to ensure delivery rates) and the use of serum albumin (to prevent adsorption of insulin to tubing or glassware). Subsequent experience has indicated that simpler procedures in which neither the pump nor albumin is employed are equally successful.

The response to treatment is assessed by monitoring the plasma glucose and serum electrolyte concentrations, arterial pH, and urinary glucose and ketone levels at 2- to 4-h intervals. If the plasma glucose level does not decline by 30 percent in the first 2 to 4 h or by 50 percent in 6 to 8 h, the insulin dose should be doubled. If hyperglycemia persists, the rate should be doubled at 2-h intervals. Once the plasma glucose level falls to 250 mg/dl (14 mM) the insulin infusion is discontinued and infusion of a 5% glucose solution is started. Intermittent small doses (10 U) of rapid-acting insulin are administered subcutaneously thereafter as necessary to control glucosuria. The arterial pH and serum bicarbonate level as well as the plasma glucose concentration should be used as indexes to determine when to stop the insulin infusion. If the plasma glucose level has fallen below 250 mg/dl but the arterial pH remains below 7.3, then the serum (or plasma) ketone determination should be repeated. If large or moderate amounts of ketones are present (in undiluted serum), then insulin (6 U/h) together with glucose (200 ml/h of 5% glucose) should be administered. This lag in the clearance of ketones may reflect a slower turnover as compared with glucose. If the ketone reaction is negative or only faintly positive, the findings (euglycemic, nonketotic metabolic acidosis) suggest the development of an accompanying lactic acidosis requiring treatment with sodium bicarbonate.

Intermediate-acting insulin should not be given until the clinical situation has stabilized and the patient is taking food and/or fluids by mouth. However, in patients whose clinical pattern is known to consist of brief episodes of DKA which respond rapidly to small amounts of extra insulin, there may be an advantage in giving intermediate-acting insulin early in the course of treatment.

FLUIDS In most patients the total fluid deficit is ~6 and rarely >10 liters. Since dehydration is a consequence of osmotic diuresis, the loss of water is relatively greater than that of salt. Fluid replacement (in the absence of hypotension) should thus be in the form of hypotonic saline, administered IV as 0.45% sodium chloride (half-isotonic), or, alternatively (to avoid the unlikely possibility of hemolysis from infusion of dilute solutions), sodium-free water may be infused in the form of 2.5% fructose in 0.45% saline. In the first hour of treatment, 1 liter of fluid should be infused; thereafter, fluids should be administered at the rate of 300 to 500 ml/h. In patients in shock the most important goal is expansion of intravascular fluid. Consequently, isotonic saline should be used.

After 4 to 6 h of treatment, or sooner if the blood glucose concentration falls below 250 mg/dl, the IV infusion should be changed from saline to 5% glucose. The importance of administering glucose is not only to prevent hypoglycemia but also to reduce the likelihood of the development of cerebral edema. The latter is a complication (see below) which may accompany rapid, insulin-induced reductions in plasma glucose concentration to levels below 250 mg/dl.[490] In patients with severe fluid depletion or persistent vomiting, 5% glucose in 0.45% saline should be administered. The overall rate of administration and choice of IV fluids is facilitated by placement of a central venous catheter, particularly in elderly persons and in patients with cardiac or renal impairment. Total fluid replacement in the first 12 h generally approximates 5 liters.

BICARBONATE Since acetoacetate and β-hydroxybutyrate are metabolizable anions, their oxidation (in a setting in which further production has been inhibited by insulin administration) results in the production of bicarbonate, resulting in a rise in serum bicarbonate concentration toward normal even in the absence of treatment with alkali-containing solutions. Consequently, infusion of bicarbonate in amounts sufficient to restore as little as 50 percent of the calculated base deficit (estimated on the basis of the reduction in serum bicarbonate concentration and 50 percent of body weight) often results in mild metabolic alkalosis. Theoretical objections to the routine use of bicarbonate may also be raised on the grounds that a rapid elevation in arterial pH may be accompanied by an exaggerated fall in cerebrospinal fluid pH and attendant worsening of CNS function. In addition, the shift to the left in the oxygen dissociation curve brought about by alkalinization may limit tissue oxygen delivery, since red cell 2,3-diphosphoglycerate concentration is reduced in DKA and is not immediately restored by insulin treatment. Furthermore, retrospective analysis has not shown an improved outcome in patients receiving bicarbonate.[491] On the other hand, severe reductions in arterial pH may impair myocardial contractility and may directly contribute to CNS depression. Accordingly, treatment with bicarbonate should be restricted to patients with severe metabolic acidosis as indicated by an arterial pH of 7.1 or less or a bicarbonate level of <5 meq/liter. In such circumstances 88 to 100 meq of sodium bicarbonate (132 meq if pH < 7.0) should be added to the initial liter of hypotonic saline. Additional bicarbonate is given only so long as blood pH (measured 2 h after institution of treatment) remains < 7.25. To avoid the possibility of aggravating cellular dehydration by infusion of a hypertonic solution, it is important to add the bicarbonate to a hypotonic, 0.45% solution of sodium chloride rather than infuse it with isotonic (0.9%) saline. Since blood lactate levels tend to be slightly elevated in ketoacidotic patients, there is no justification for infusion of sodium lactate in preference to bicarbonate.

POTASSIUM As a consequence of the ketonuria, diuresis, and frequent vomiting, body potassium stores are depleted by 5 to 10 meq per kilogram of body weight. Nevertheless, the serum potassium concentration is generally normal or even elevated in DKA because of the shift in potassium from intracellular to extracellular fluid which accompanies an increase in hydrogen ion concentration. With correction of the acidosis and stimulation of cellular uptake of glucose, serum potassium levels decline. Accordingly, potassium chloride should be administered 3 h after initiation of therapy (provided the patient is not anuric), in a dose of 40 meq per liter of IV fluid. A total of 120 to 160 meq is generally infused in the first 12 to 18 h. In rare patients (< 5 percent of cases) in whom hypokalemia is present at the outset, potassium supplements (40 to 60 meq of KCl per liter) are added to the initial IV infusion. Monitoring of the electrocardiogram may be useful in detecting hypokalemia or hyperkalemia but should not replace frequent measurement of serum potassium concentration (at intervals of 2 to 4 h) in determining the need for, and the rate of, administration of potassium supplements.

Since body phosphate stores are reduced in DKA, there may be some theoretical advantage in administering potassium as the phosphate rather than the chloride salt. On the other hand, administration of phosphate fails to accelerate improvement in clinical or biochemical parameters and may precipitate hypocalcemia.[492] In view of the long experience with potassium chloride, this remains the choice for potassium repletion.

Complications

In most cases a fatal outcome in DKA is attributable to a severe underlying illness such as myocardial infarction, overwhelming sepsis, or acute pancreatitis, rather than DKA per se. Three complicating and potentially fatal situations that may occur in the absence of intercurrent illness are *shock, cerebral edema,* and *adult respiratory distress syndrome* (RDS).

Shock may develop as a consequence of severe hypovolemia, reduced myocardial contractility secondary to acidosis, and, possibly, decreased peripheral resistance. In hypotensive patients a central venous catheter should be placed, followed by rapid infusion of large volumes of isotonic (rather than hypotonic) saline. Failure to respond to saline may necessitate treatment with blood or plasma volume expanders. The efficacy of vasoconstrictor drugs (metaraminol and norepinephrine) or dopamine in such patients has not been established.

Attention has been called to the problem of irreversible, fatal cerebral edema complicating DKA. The clinical picture is generally one of an adolescent diabetic with no underlying illness in whom progressive deterioration in consciousness develops after an initial period (3 to 10 h) of treatment characterized by improving laboratory test results. Papilledema, elevated cerebrospinal fluid pressure, dilated pupils of unequal size, hyperpyrexia, and, occasionally, diabetes insipidus may be observed in such cases.

Studies in hyperglycemic dogs and rabbits have shown that a sharp drop in blood glucose concentration to < 250 mg/dl by rapid infusion of saline or administration of insulin results in gross brain edema.[490] The imbibition of water by the brain is due to a disequilibrium between brain and plasma osmolarity. The possibility that glucose-induced injury to brain capillaries may contribute to brain swelling has been suggested.[493] Cerebral edema is not observed in hyperglycemic experimental animals until the blood glucose concentration falls to < 250 mg/dl. Similarly, in the clinical setting cerebral edema generally has not been shown to occur until the plasma glucose concentration has reached normal or near-normal levels. Accordingly, when treating DKA or hyperosmolar coma, insulin treatment should be reduced or discontinued and glucose-containing fluids should be administered when the plasma glucose concentration has fallen to 250 mg/dl.

Although no cases of successful treatment of cerebral edema have been recorded (spontaneous reversal has been noted), the use of mannitol or large doses of corticosteroids may be of some value in reducing cerebral swelling. Fortunately, the overall incidence of clinically overt cerebral edema is quite low; not a single case was recognized in one series of 257 patients.[494] On the other hand, subclinical brain swelling detectable by cranial CT scan is commonly observed during the course of treatment of DKA.[495]

In a recent report, *adult RDS* was observed in patients with DKA as well as hyperosmolar nonketotic coma.[496] The findings are those of dyspnea, hypothermia, chest x-ray pictures suggestive of pulmonary edema, and normal capillary wedge pressures. Mortality is high in such patients.

HYPEROSMOLAR NONKETOTIC COMA

Impaired consciousness may occur in the diabetic as a consequence of severe hyperglycemia, hyperosmolarity, and dehydration in the absence of ketoacidosis. In hyperosmolar nonketotic coma, by definition, blood ketone acid concentrations are normal or only mildly elevated. Typically, this syndrome develops in middle-aged or elderly patients as either the first manifestation of diabetes or in a setting of previously mild type II diabetes. Symptoms of polydipsia and polyuria generally develop over a period of several (usually 7 to 10) days, culminating in disturbances of consciousness which are often the basis for the patient's coming to medical attention. As in DKA, mental obtundation varying from lethargy to coma occurs. However, in contrast to DKA, patients with hyperosmolar coma often have focal or generalized seizures.[497] In many instances the syndrome is temporally (and perhaps causally) related to the prior administration of drugs such as diuretics, glucocorticoids, immunosuppressive agents, or phenytoin. In as many as 25 percent of patients there is clinical and/or autopsy evidence of acute pancreatitis.

The laboratory findings consist of marked hyperglycemia (> 600 mg/dl or 33 mM), hyperosmolarity (generally >310 mOsm), azotemia, and, by definition, the absence of hyperketonemia. The degree of azotemia is on average greater than that observed in DKA (BUN 70 to 90 mg/dl, as compared with 40 mg/dl in DKA).[498] The serum sodium concentration may be normal, elevated, or even reduced. The failure to observe a consistent elevation of serum sodium concentration in the face of marked dehydration is a consequence of the redistribution of body fluids from the intracellular to the extracellular compartment engendered by hyperglycemia. The expected reduction in serum sodium concentration brought about by hyperglycemia may be calculated as 1.6 meq/liter for each 100 mg/dl increment in serum glucose concentration above normal.[499] Thus, in the patient with a markedly elevated blood glucose level and a normal or elevated serum sodium concentration, a severe state of dehydration is likely to be present.

The pathogenesis of the syndrome of nonketotic hyperosmolar coma remains somewhat unclear. Two factors require explanation, the presence of hyperglycemia which exceeds that generally observed in DKA and the absence of ketoacidosis. With respect to the former, the diminution in renal function may limit the extent to which glucose can be excreted in the urine, thereby resulting in the progressive accumulation of glucose in the blood. Supporting this possibility is the observation that alloxan-treated animals develop nonketotic hyperosmolar coma if the ureters are tied and glucocorticoids are administered.[500] The presence of small amounts of insulin sufficient to inhibit lipolysis (but not hyperglycemia) has been postulated to account for the failure to develop ketoacidosis. C peptide levels tend to be higher in hyperosmolar nonketotic coma than in DKA.[501] Hyperosmolarity per se has been shown to interfere with lipolysis and thus may have a role in preventing ketogenesis.[502] Plasma FFA levels tend to stay low in patients with hyperosmolar nonketotic coma.[501] Animal studies have shown that an increase in liver glycogen diminishes ketogenic capacity. The provocative effect of glucocorticoids in the pathogenesis of experimental or spontaneous hyperosmolar coma and the contributory role of excess carbohydrate intake in the experimental syndrome[503] support a role for increased liver glycogen content in the inhibition of ketogenesis.

Treatment consists of continuous IV infusion of insulin in low doses (6 to 10 U/h), together with large amounts of fluids as hypotonic saline (unless the patient is in shock, in which case isotonic saline is infused), and repletion of body potassium.[489]

The mortality rate has been reported to vary from 5 to 40 percent. Many of the fatal cases have accompanying lactic acidosis (see below) as reflected by reduced arterial pH and large anion gap. In many instances death is due to some underlying disease process such as pancreatitis or sepsis.

LACTIC ACIDOSIS

Severe metabolic acidosis due to the accumulation of lactate (and to a much smaller extent pyruvate) may be observed in the diabetic as well as the nondiabetic population.[504] Among diabetics lactic acidosis may develop in a variety of circumstances: (1) in association with DKA (~10 percent of patients with DKA have an accompanying lactic acidosis), (2) in association with hyperosmolar nonketotic coma (as many as 40 to 60 percent of such patients also have lactic acidosis), (3) as a complication of phenformin therapy, (4) in association with inadequate tissue perfusion due to cardiogenic, septic, or hypovolemic shock, and (5) as a spontaneous disorder.

The clinical manifestations are deep, labored breathing, dehydration, abdominal pain, and depression of the sensorium ranging from lethargy to coma. The laboratory diagnosis is based on the presence of an arterial pH < 7.3 in the face of normal or reduced P_{CO_2}, reduction in serum bicarbonate concentration with an increased anion gap not attributable to ketonemia (as reflected by no more than trace amounts of serum ketones), and the absence of uremia or a history of the ingestion of salicylates or methanol. Definitive diagnosis rests on the demonstration of an increase in the plasma lactate concentration, generally to > 5 mM.

The pathogenesis of lactic acidosis in patients with DKA, hyperosmolar coma, or various types of shock probably relates to disturbances in tissue perfusion, resulting in failure of hepatic uptake and metabolism of lactate and, possibly, increased production of lactate in muscle.[504] The basis for the increased tendency to develop spontaneous lactic acidosis among diabetics remains unexplained, however. The association with diabetes is particularly surprising, since hepatic uptake and utilization of lactate for gluconeogenesis is increased in diabetics.[105]

As in all forms of lactic acidosis, treatment consists of the administration of large volumes of saline and bicarbonate. In patients with plasma glucose concentration > 250 mg/dl administration of small doses of insulin may be helpful, even in the absence of ketoacidosis or severe hyperosmolarity.[505]

Pregnancy and Diabetes

The interaction of pregnancy and diabetes requires special consideration because of the increased risks to the well-being of the fetus when the mother is diabetic and because the presence of the conceptus (fetus and placenta) alters substrate and hormone metabolism in the mother. The net result is that various aspects of diagnosis and management of diabetes are either altered or require emphasis when dealing with the pregnant diabetic.[506] Furthermore, it is now recognized that normalization of maternal fuel metabolism, which previously had been emphasized in late pregnancy to prevent perinatal mortality and morbidity, must be attempted at conception and during early pregnancy (i.e., during the earliest stages of embryogenesis) in order to lower congenital malformation rates.

MATERNAL AND FETAL FUEL METABOLISM

The overall metabolic influence of pregnancy in normal subjects is the sum of two seemingly opposite phenomena: (1) the presence of "accelerated starvation," resulting in a tendency to develop fasting hypoglycemia and hyperketonemia,[506a] and (2) the presence of insulin resistance, resulting in a tendency toward postprandial hyperglycemia. Which of these influences predominates depends on the stage of pregnancy (first or second half) and nutritional condition (fasted or fed).

Accelerated Starvation

The impact of pregnancy on metabolism in the postabsorptive or fasted condition is to lower plasma glucose and insulin levels while causing increased concentrations of ketones and FFA. The hormonal and substrate milieu after an overnight, 12- to 14-h fast in pregnancy is thus comparable with that observed after a 24- to 36-h fast in the nongravid state; hence the term "accelerated starvation."[506a] This exaggerated response to fasting occurs in a setting of continuous siphoning of glucose and amino acids from the maternal to the fetal circulation (Fig. 19-55).

The conceptus is an obligate glucose-consuming organism whose utilization of glucose is not dependent on the availability of maternal insulin. In fact, maternal insulin and glucagon fail to cross the placenta, while glucose is readily transferred by a process of facilitated diffusion (Fig. 19-56). The rate of glucose utilization by the fetus at term is estimated at 6 mg per kilogram of body weight per minute, which is two to three times greater than in normal adult subjects. While maternal insulin does not reach the fetus, the fetal islets produce insulin by 12 weeks of gestation; this hormone is a key growth factor in intrauterine life.

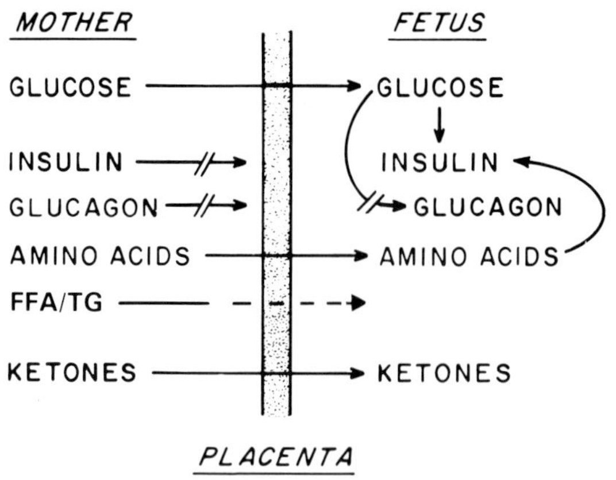

FIGURE 19-55 Maternal-fetal fuel and hormone exchange in normal pregnancy. Glucose readily traverses the placenta and is continuously siphoned by the fetus from the mother. Active transport of amino acids and transfer of ketones to the fetus also occur. Free fatty acids (FFA) and triglycerides (TG) do not cross directly but are retained by the placenta and slowly released on the fetal side. In contrast, maternal insulin and glucagon do not reach the fetal circulation. Excessive fetal levels of glucose and amino acids elicit local hyperinsulinemia in the fetus.

In addition to glucose, amino acids are transferred to the fetus by a process of active transport. Besides their utilization for protein synthesis, amino acids may also be catabolized and serve as an energy-yielding fuel. Regardless of their ultimate metabolic fate, the transfer of amino acids to the fetus results in maternal hypoaminoacidemia and therefore decreased availability of amino acids (particularly alanine) for maternal gluconeogenesis.

The sequence of events resulting in accelerated starvation is thus initiated by fetal glucose utilization. An increase in the maternal glucose dilution space may also contribute to the reduction in maternal plasma glucose concentration.[506] As a consequence, plasma insulin levels fall, resulting in augmented lipolysis and hyperketonemia. Simultaneously, the reduced availability of amino acids in the maternal circulation perpetuates and exaggerates the hypoglycemic state by limiting maternal gluconeogenesis.

FFA and triglycerides cross the placenta indirectly, to a limited extent.[507] The transfer is increased in diabetes[508–510] as a result of maternal hyperlipidemia, producing a steep maternal-fetal triglyceride and FFA gradient. Even in gestational diabetes or in controlled diabetic pregnancy increased transfer to the fetus is evident from a rise in the placental lipid content.[511] However, from a clinical standpoint the important immediate consideration in fasting or diabetes is the elevation in blood ketone concentrations since the ketones cross the placenta freely. On the fetal side they are available for oxidation, even by the fetal liver and brain.[511a] Ketone utilization may, however, have an adverse effect on psychoneurologic development. Maternal ketonemia, whether due to starvation or diabetes, has been shown in some studies to be associated with a significant reduction in IQ in offspring studied at age 3 to 5.[512–514] Consequently, strict attention to management is required during pregnancy to avoid starvation ketosis (by frequent feeding and maintaining an adequate caloric and total carbohydrate intake), and to prevent diabetic hyperketonemia due to inadequate insulinization.

Postprandial Hyperglycemia

In contrast to the tendency of *fasting* plasma glucose levels to be lower, in the *postprandial* condition plasma glucose concentration tends to be higher in pregnant glucose concentration tends to be higher in pregnant as compared with nonpregnant subjects. Large population studies have shown that, unless the criteria for glucose intolerance are adjusted upward (by 25 mg/dl, or 1.4 mM, for the 2-h plasma glucose concentration), an inordinate number of women are diagnosed as having glucose intolerance in pregnancy.[515] Furthermore, even with such adjustment in criteria, a substantial number of pregnant women are observed to have glucose intolerance which reverts to normal after delivery ("gestational diabetes"). The basis for these postprandial elevations in plasma glucose concentration is not a lack of insulin in normal pregnancy but the physiologic development of insulin resistance.

The plasma insulin response to glucose or protein ingestion is exaggerated in pregnancy, particularly in the second and third trimesters. The coexistence of hyperinsulinemia and normal or high glucose levels suggests tissue resistance to insulin. Studies of plasma insulin response to hyperglycemia maintained at a fixed level (glucose clamp technique) have indicated that tissue response to insulin is reduced in normal pregnancy by as much as 80 percent.[516] The basis of this insulin resistance is not entirely established; it may be related to the influence of placental hormones (lactogen, estrogen, progesterone, and prolactin), which antagonize the action of insulin and may have stimulatory effects on insulin secretion as well.

Human placental lactogen (HPL, also referred to as chorionic somatomammotropin) is a polypeptide hormone produced by the syncytiotrophoblast. Chemically and immunologically it is similar to GH. However, HPL circulates at term in a concentration 1000 times that of GH. In addition to having an anabolic effect on protein metabolism and a lipolytic action, it is both mammotropic and luteotropic. A mild but definite impairment in glucose tolerance has been observed following a single infusion of HPL in nonpregnant subjects over periods of 5 to 12 h.[517] This is manifested as a small decrease in the rate of glucose utilization despite an increase in circulating insulin level. Despite the known anti-insulin effects of this hormone, it is noteworthy that a consistent relationship has not been observed between maternal HPL levels and insulin requirements during diabetic pregnancy.[518] Furthermore, maternal HPL levels are not altered by physiologic fluctuations in blood glucose concentration.

Pregnancy is characterized, in addition to increasing levels of HPL, by increasing placental secretion of estrogen and progesterone; these hormones readily enter the maternal circulation. Consensus regarding the effects of estrogen on carbohydrate metabolism is lacking. Synthetic estrogens may well produce greater anti-insulin effects than natural estrogens. Thus, while estradiol administration results in hyperinsulinemia, it is accompanied by improvement rather than deterioration in glucose tolerance. These findings are in agreement with the ameliorative effect of natural estrogen on diabetes in partially pancreatectomized animals. Thus, it is clear that estrogen may contribute to hyperinsulinemia but probably is not a major factor in the insulin resistance of pregnancy. Progesterone may be a more important contributor to the tissue insensitivity to insulin.

Pituitary prolactin concentration also increases markedly during pregnancy. Studies on women with prolactin-producing pituitary adenomas have revealed fasting and glucose-induced hyperinsulinemia, elevation in the glucose tolerance test curve, and augmented suppression of glucagon in response to hyperglycemia, similar to the responses observed in human pregnancy.[519,520]

Pregnancy is regarded as a diabetogenic condition on several grounds. For one, the tissue response to insulin is diminished in the fed state in normal pregnant subjects (as reflected by postprandial hyperinsulinemia). Also, pregnancy (particularly in the second and third trimesters) produces a transient gestational diabetes in some previously healthy women or a transient increase in insulin requirements in women with already-manifest diabetes (see below). However, the presence of increasing insulin resistance in pregnancy cannot be equated with increased brittleness of the diabetic state. Brittleness of diabetes refers to variability and unpredictability of, and hence wide swings in, circulating glucose levels, which render clinical control of glycemia very difficult. In pregnant diabetic individuals brittleness may decline compared to the nonpregnant state, despite the increase in insulin resistance.[521]

DIAGNOSIS

The diagnosis of diabetes requires special emphasis when dealing with pregnancy, because the fetal mortality rate may be increased by glucose intolerance in the absence of overt diabetes and may be improved in such patients by insulin treatment.[522] Thus, there are more indications for performing a glucose tolerance test in the pregnant state as compared with the nonpregnant state. Diagnosis is also especially important in pregnant women because, as discussed above, the criteria for diagnosis of glucose tolerance require adjustment in pregnancy. In addition, the normal tendency to renal glucosuria in pregnancy may lead to overdiagnosis of diabetes.

The classic indications for performing a glucose tolerance test in pregnancy include glucosuria in more than one random sample; a strong family history of diabetes (in one or both parents), particularly in an obese patient; a previous infant weighing > 10 lb (4.5 kg) at birth; polyhydramnios; and a history of recurrent unexplained stillbirths, neonatal deaths, or congenital anomalies. Because gestational diabetes may be present in the absence of such historic factors, it is now recommended to perform a 1-h screening test with a 50-g glucose load at 26 to 28 weeks of gestation *in all pregnant women.* If the serum or plasma glucose level is ≥ 140 mg/dl (7.8 mM), or > 135 mg/dl (7.5 mM) when the test is administered to individuals who have not fasted, a full 100-g, 3-h oral glucose tolerance test should be done. In keeping with the characteristic tendency in pregnancy to develop fasting hypoglycemia together with postprandial hyperglycemia, the upper limit for the fasting plasma glucose concentration is lower (105 vs. 125 mg/dl, or 5.8 vs. 6.9 mM in nonpregnant subjects) and the 2-h value is higher in the gravid state (165 vs. 140 mg/dl or 9.2 vs. 7.8 mM) than in nonpregnant subjects.

CLASSIFICATION

Gestational Diabetes

Gestational diabetes refers to overt diabetes or abnormal glucose tolerance which first appears or is diagnosed during pregnancy. Identification of gestational diabetes is important because the risks of congenital malformations, perinatal death,[522] fetal macrosomia, and neonatal hypoglycemia are higher in these women than in the general population. Furthermore, the diagnosis of gestational diabetes has important prognostic implications for the mother. Although most women with gestational diabetes revert to normal post partum, permanent diabetes develops in ~35 percent within 16 years.[523] Recent evidence suggests that the presence of islet cell antibodies in the plasma of gestational diabetics may predict those cases in which permanent diabetes will later develop or persist after delivery,[524] and that women with antepartum fasting plasma glucose concentrations > 130 mg/dl are extremely likely to have permanent diabetes.

In 1948, Priscilla White introduced a classification system specifically designed for the pregnant diabetic. This system has generally proved useful in predicting the outcome of diabetic pregnancy and in individualizing medical and obstetric care. The various classes take into account the duration as well as severity of diabetes, as indicated by the presence of microangiopathic complications in the form of retinopathy or nephropathy. Class A diabetics, as proposed by White, are the patients with "chemical diabetes only, with abnormal blood glucose levels when tested by a glucose load, but fasting values normal or near normal."[236] A more precise definition, which is preferable, is that class A diabetics are patients with abnormal 100-g oral glucose tolerance tests, and normal fasting plasma glucose level (> 100 mg/dl or > 5.5 mM) and postprandial levels (> 120 mg/dl or > 6.7 mM). Class B includes gestational diabetics with elevated fasting and/or postprandial plasma glucose concentrations (class B_1), and patients with overt diabetes with onset after age 20 and duration > 10 years (class B_2). In class C overt diabetes has been present for >10 years with onset before age 20. In classes D, F, and R there is evidence of, respectively, benign retinopathy, nephropathy, or proliferative retinopathy. In general, the incidence of fetal wastage (stillbirths and neonatal deaths) increases in proportion to the severity of diabetes as indicated by White's classification. In contrast, excessive birth weight (fetal macrosomia) is more common in classes A through C than in classes D through R.

EFFECT OF PREGNANCY ON THE COURSE OF DIABETES

The effect of gestation on the clinical course of diabetes is quite variable, depending primarily on whether pregnancy is in an early or late stage. It is useful to divide pregnancy into first and second halves rather than trimesters in assessing its influence on diabetes.

During the early stages of pregnancy the dominant factor contributing to altered carbohydrate homeostasis is the transfer of maternal glucose to the fetus. This siphoning of glucose by the fetus results in a tendency toward maternal hypoglycemia; the hypoglycemia may be symptomatic and frequently necessitates a reduction in insulin dosage if the diabetes has previously been well controlled. A diminution in food intake as a consequence of the nausea and vomiting of early pregnancy may also contribute to a decrease in insulin requirements. The decreased need for insulin thus does not reflect a change in tissue sensitivity; rather, it is a consequence of lessened availability of circulating carbohydrate.

In the second half of pregnancy, the diabetogenic actions of placental hormones and prolactin outweigh the effects of continuous siphoning of glucose by the fetus. As a consequence, the demand for insulin is increased, necessitating an increase in insulin dosage. Quantitative assessment of the progressive rise in insulin requirement has been particularly feasible with the advent of portable pumps that permit the continuous subcutaneous delivery of insulin and produce normal or near-normal glucose concentrations[525,525a] (Fig. 19-56). Coincident with diminished effectiveness of insulin, the tendency to ketoacidosis is increased. The recognition of DKA in pregnancy is often more difficult because plasma glucose levels are generally not markedly elevated. In addition, ketonuria may reflect starvation ketosis rather than DKA, indicating that glucose rather than insulin is needed. The absence of hyperglycemia suggests the presence of starvation rather than diabetic ketosis.

After delivery, the rapid fall in the concentrations of HPL, prolactin, estrogen, and progesterone, plus the continued suppression of GH secretion, which persists for 1 to 2 days post partum, results in a reduction in maternal insulin requirement, frequently to levels below the prepregnant dose. Some patients experience a remarkable postpartum remission and gradually return to the prepregnancy course over the ensuing 3 to 6 weeks.

Table 19-18. Fetal Mortality and Morbidity in Diabetic Pregnancy

Perinatal mortality
Congenital anomalies
Respiratory distress syndrome
Stillbirths
Fetal morbidity
Congenital anomalies
Respiratory distress syndrome
Macrosomia
Hypoglycemia
Hyperbilirubinemia
Hypocalcemia

EFFECT OF DIABETES ON THE OUTCOME OF PREGNANCY

The presence of diabetes in the mother continues to impose an increased risk for the developing fetus (Table 19-18). Perinatal mortality in diabetic pregnancy has progressively declined from rates of ≥ 30 percent 20 to 30 years ago to current rates of 5 to 10

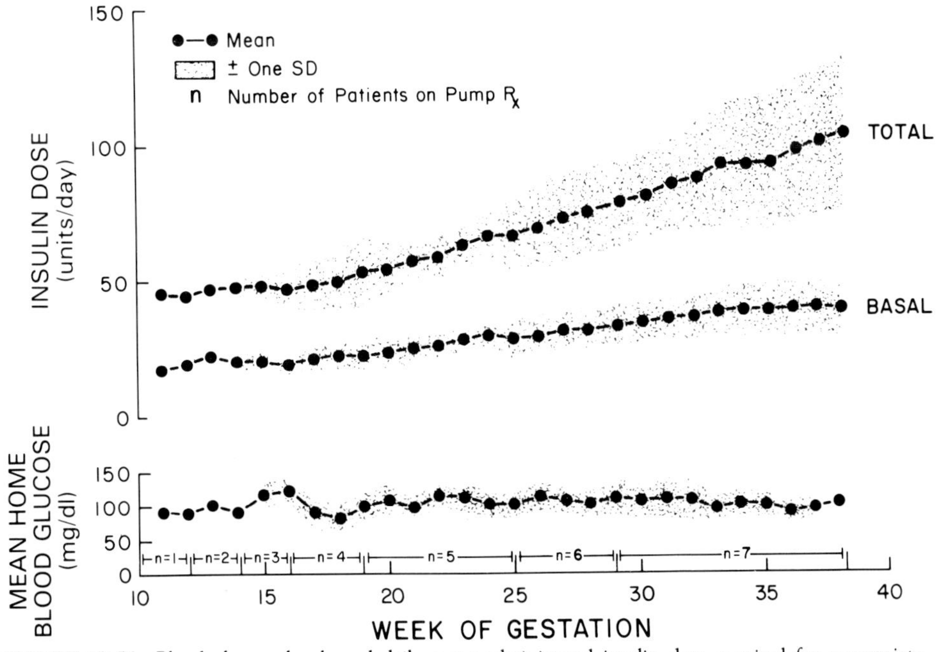

FIGURE 19-56 Blood glucose levels and daily pump-administered insulin dose required for appropriate glucose regulation during the course of gestation. Basal insulin dose represents continuous daily infusion. Total dose includes meal-generated insulin supplement. (*From Rudolf et al.*[525])

percent. Even with ideal management, fetal and neonatal death rates are at least twice those reported in pregnancies uncomplicated by diabetes. The major causes of fetal and neonatal wastage at present fall into three categories: congenital malformations, intrauterine stillbirths, and RDS.

Congenital Anomalies

The single largest perinatal problem remaining in the 1980s has been the two- to threefold-increased incidence of congenital anomalies in infants of diabetic mothers. Birth defects are currently the major cause of perinatal mortality in diabetic pregnancy, accounting for 20,[526,527] 33[528], or 50 percent[529,530] or more of all perinatal losses. Birth defects that occur with increased frequency in the offspring of diabetic mothers most commonly involve the heart and the nervous and skeletal systems.

Studies in experimental animals as well as humans suggest that these abnormalities are a consequence of poor metabolic control during the period of organogenesis in early gestation. High levels of glucose in embryo culture medium have been associated with neural tube malformation,[531] as well as other anomalies.[531–533] Lumbosacral defects occurred in 17 percent of rat fetuses whose streptozotocin-diabetic mothers were not treated, but in only 5 percent of those whose mothers were treated with insulin during the period of organogenesis.[534] When insulin-treated streptozotocin-induced diabetic pregnant rats underwent 2 days of insulin withdrawal during the first 7 days of gestation, increased skeletal malformations resulted in their embryos; however, if insulin was withdrawn for a 2-day period at 8 or more days of gestation, no such anomalies occurred.[535] Human studies also point out the causal role of inadequate metabolic control in teratogenesis. The demonstration that anomalies must have occurred prior to the seventh week of gestation, given the known times during gestation at which organ development occurs,[536] led to a focusing of investigation on the periconceptual period. Elevation in maternal glycohemoglobin at the end of the first trimester has been correlated with an increased incidence of major congenital malformations.[537–539] These observations suggest that any further reduction in perinatal mortality may require the restoration of a normal metabolic milieu in the diabetic mother from the time of conception.

Respiratory Distress Syndrome

Although RDS was previously the major cause of neonatal death, its incidence has been reduced from ~30 percent to current rates of >10 percent of births, mainly due to the use of sophisticated methods of measuring fetal pulmonic maturity. Neonatal death from RDS has become increasingly rare among infants of diabetic mothers because of both the diminished incidence of RDS and because of improvements in the management of this clinical entity.

The pathophysiologic relationship between maternal diabetes and RDS is not yet fully elucidated. Pulmonary maturation in the fetus is largely dependent upon the ability of the fetal lung to synthesize surfactant, a surface-active material which lines the alveoli and lowers surface tension, thereby preventing alveolar collapse (atelectasis). Lecithin is the major surface-active material; in RDS lecithin is deficient. The synthesis of lecithin is dependent, in part, on an elevation in fetal glucocorticoid secretion late in gestation. In diabetic pregnancy, particularly in class A to C diabetics, pulmonary maturation is delayed.[540] Interestingly, insulin has been shown to be an antagonist of cortisol-induced synthesis of lecithin by fetal lung cells.[541] Thus, as in the case of fetal macrosomia (see below), maternal hyperglycemia leading to fetal hyperinsulinism may provide the explanation of the higher incidence of RDS in infants of diabetic mothers. Such an association thus provides impetus for minimizing maternal hyperglycemia during pregnancy and for accurately assessing pulmonary maturation when the timing of delivery is gauged (see below).

Intrauterine Fetal Death

A remarkable reduction in the proportion of stillbirths among pregnant diabetics has occurred in recent years. From 1958 through 1969, in New York State exclusive of New York City, 12.3 percent of pregnancies in diabetics ended with intrauterine fetal death.[542] Recently, large series from tertiary medical centers indicate stillbirth rates ranging from 0 to 4 percent.[543–545] The reasons for this dramatic decline in fetal mortality have not been proved as yet, primarily because the causes of sudden intrauterine fetal death in diabetic pregnancy are poorly understood. Some deaths are due to poorly controlled diabetes with ketoacidosis,[546] and it is probable that intensive metabolic control has contributed greatly to the improvement in outcome. Indeed, it was demonstrated that fetal hyperglycemia and hyperinsulinemia may be associated with hypoxia, lactic acidosis, and fetal death.[547] Similarly, when hypertonic glucose solutions are administered to pregnant diabetic women in preparation for delivery, fetal acidosis may result.[548,549] In addition, placental insufficiency in the diabetic mother with vasculopathy may now be detected with the modern perinatal armamentarium of ultrasound and antepartum monitoring, leading to timely delivery before intrauterine death can occur.

Neonatal Morbidity

In addition to congenital anomalies and RDS, the major factors responsible for neonatal morbidity (Table 19-18) are fetal macrosomia, hypoglycemia, hypocalcemia, and hyperbilirubinemia. Fetal macrosomia refers to excessive fetal size for gestational age; it is much more common in class A to C diabetics than in class D through R diabetics. The increase in body weight is not due to edema; it is a consequence of increased deposition of fat and glycogen as well as visceromegaly. Pedersen in the 1930s was the first to ascribe these findings to maternal hyperglycemia leading to fetal hyperinsulinism and its resultant stimulation of fetal anabolism. Subsequent measurements of fetal insulin levels have substantiated this theory.[550] However, macrosomia is not due solely to the growth-promoting effect of fetal hyperinsulinemia but also to the plethora of glucose, fatty acids, and amino acids in the circulation of diabetic mothers mobilized in excess and reaching the fetus in overabundant amounts.

Neonatal hypoglycemia also stems from persisting fetal hyperinsulinemia, after the glucose source has been cut off at birth. It occurs in as many as 30 to 60 percent of infants of diabetic mothers. Suppression of fetal glucagon secretion during the course of diabetic pregnancy has also been suggested as a contributory factor.[551] In addition to hypoglycemia, hypocalcemia also occurs fairly frequently and may be a consequence of suppression of fetal parathyroid secretion.

Diabetes has an impact on the mother. Diabetic pregnancies are associated with an increased risk of polyhydramnios and hypertensive disorders, including preeclampsia, edema, and pyelonephritis.[506] There is some evidence that preeclampsia is particularly increased in diabetic women with poor metabolic control.[552]

Postnatal Effects

Evidence from experimental animal studies suggests that uncontrolled maternal diabetes may have a protracted modifying effect on the pancreatic function of the offspring.[553] The impact of impaired glucose tolerance during intrauterine life is expressed as retarded growth and glucose intolerance in stressful conditions in adult life. Gestational diabetes is seen in females of the second generation; thus, the defect may be carried over to further generations. No similar data are available in humans, but these findings lend emphasis to the importance of early and dedicated management of glucose intolerance in pregnancy.

Treatment

The principles of management in the pregnant diabetic include (1) frequent evaluation of the patient, (2) close liaison between obstetrician and internist and, at the time of delivery, with the pediatrician, and (3) most importantly, emphasis on intensive metabolic control, which optimally should be initiated prior to conception. The primary medical concern is adequate control of diabetes to minimize the incidence of fetal mortality and morbidity. The major obstetric decision concerns the timing of delivery so as to avoid the risk of intrauterine death while delivering an infant with sufficient pulmonary maturity who will not succumb to RDS.

INSULIN Pregnancy constitutes a major indication for intensive management of diabetes with self-monitoring of blood glucose concentration and either multiple manual injections of insulin or the use of an insulin infusion pump[525,554] (see Intensive Insulin Therapy, above). Ideally, such a treatment program should be instituted prior to conception in women who are contemplating pregnancy. As indicated above, fetal anomalies are the single most important problem facing diabetic women undergoing pregnancy. It is most likely that poor metabolic control during organogenesis is in some way responsible for these anomalies. Recently, a program of intensive preconceptional metabolic control in diabetic women was shown to reduce the birth defect rate to 1.1 percent as opposed to 6.6 percent among diabetic women presenting for their care after the ninth week of gestation.[555] In keeping with those observations, the incidence of fetal anomalies is higher among diabetic pregnancies in which glycohemoglobin is elevated during the first trimester.

CSII has recently become popular for the management of diabetes in pregnancy. However, use of the pump requires a highly motivated individual. In a randomized trial of insulin pump vs. intensive conventional insulin therapy in pregnant diabetic women, there was no distinct advantage of either method.[555]

Although there is little evidence that insulin-induced maternal hypoglycemia has a detrimental effect on the fetus, this possibility has often been cited as a reason to avoid meticulous attempts to achieve euglycemia in the pregnant diabetic. In the Collaborative Perinatal Project, no adverse effect was found of maternal insulin reactions upon subsequent mental and motor function tests of the offspring of diabetic mothers up to the age of 4 years.[556]

In the case of the class A diabetic, management may take the form of strict dietary control or administration of small amounts (15 to 20 U per day) of intermediate- and rapid-acting insulin. The class A diabetic woman should be followed with a weekly set of three circulating glucose determinations. If the fasting plasma glucose concentration exceeds 100 mg/dl or if either of the postprandial values exceeds 120 mg/dl, or both, insulin therapy should be begun (or the previously instituted prophylactic dose increased) and the patient reclassified as class B_1. Class A diabetic women whose circulating glucose concentrations remain below the above thresholds may also benefit from insulin therapy inasmuch as fetal macrosomia and traumatic delivery may be avoided by such treatinsulin treatment in such patients beyond 28 weeks is 20 units of intermediate-acting (NPH) and 10 units of rapid-acting insulin before breakfast. The highly purified animal species or human insulin preparations are preferable in the gestational diabetic, since they are less immunogenic.

DIET Dietary management of normal pregnancy for many years involved emphasis on curtailment of weight gain, generally to no more than 18 to 20 lb (8 to 9 kg). However, studies have shown that an average gain of 27.5 lb (12.5 kg) during the course of pregnancy is associated with the lowest overall incidence of preeclampsia, prematurity, and prenatal mortality. The Committee on Maternal Nutrition of the National Research Council recommends a slightly lower average weight gain, 24 lb (11 kg), and strongly condemns severe caloric restriction or weight reduction programs during normal pregnancy. The importance of avoiding calorie restriction is apparent from the data presented above regarding the acceleration of starvation ketosis in pregnancy and the adverse effects of ketones on fetal development.[557]

In the insulin-dependent pregnant diabetic the principles applying to the nongravid diabetic and those applying to normal pregnancy must be harmonized. This is achieved by recognizing that a weight gain of 24 lb is a physiologic component and a desirable goal of pregnancy in the diabetic as well as the nondiabetic; reduction in body weight to the ideal norm or limitation of weight gain to 20 lb (9 kg) should not be pursued during pregnancy. Accordingly, the recommended diet contains 30 to 35 kcal per kilogram of actual body weight. Of the total number of kcal, 45 percent, equivalent to a minimum of 200 g, is provided in the form of carbohydrate. The daily protein intake is generally 2 g per kilogram of body weight (100 to 120 g total); the remainder of the calories are provided as fat (45 to 60 g total). In patients with marked renal glucosuria, an additional 50 g or more of carbohydrate may have to be provided to make up for urinary losses. As in the nongravid diabetic, regularity and spacing of food intake are essential when insulin is administered.

Although some clinics have found oral hypoglycemic agents useful in pregnancy, patients not responding to dietary control should not be treated with insulin. The administration of sex steroids (estrogen and progesterone) has been recommended by some, but has not been generally adopted inasmuch as the evidence of a gestational hormonal deficiency in diabetes has not been convincing.

Delivery

Classically, the major dilemma in the timing of delivery has been the avoidance of an intrauterine stillbirth, the likelihood of which is increased by delaying delivery too long, while minimizing the risks of RDS (the likelihood of which is increased by delivery prior to the development of pulmonary maturity). With current medical and obstetrical practice the risk of stillbirth is quite low. The advent of biochemical assays of amniotic fluid for fetal lung maturity has added another dimension to the ability to individualize the timing of delivery in these pregnancies. The presence of a mature L/S (lecithin/sphingomyelin ratio) or, better yet, adequate phosphatidylglycerol concentration, assures the obstetrician that RDS is unlikely to develop if the baby is delivered. Furthermore, with intensive management of diabetes, the likelihood of intrauterine death or deterioration of fetal status necessitating early delivery is unusual. Consequently, if the patient's diabetes is in good control, no obstetric or medical complications are present, and fetoplacental function testing indicates good fetal health, amniocentesis should be performed for pulmonic maturity at 38 weeks or beyond, depending on the state of the cervix.

The route of delivery should be vaginal unless obstetrical indications for cesarean section are present. Management of diabetes on the day of delivery depends on the prior state of metabolic control as well as whether labor is to be induced, the patient is in spontaneous labor, or cesarean section is to be performed.[506] If labor is to be induced, insulin may be withheld on the morning of induction and a slow infusion of IV glucose administered. Rapid-acting insulin is infused only if the blood glucose concentration (monitored every 1 to 2 h) is 120 mg/dl. If the patient is in spontaneous labor, a similar approach of constant glucose infusion plus insulin (as necessary) is employed. If an elective cesarean section is to be performed, it should be done at breakfast time. Food is withheld on the morning of surgery and (if the diabetes is well controlled) no insulin is given. IV saline is infused until after delivery.

Lipoatrophic Diabetes

Lipoatrophic diabetes is a rare syndrome characterized by partial or complete absence of body fat, insulin-resistant diabetes, hypermetabolism in association with normal thyroid function, and hepatomegaly which often progresses to cirrhosis.[558,559] The syndrome may be present at birth (congenital lipoatrophy, or the Berardinelli-Seip syndrome), in which circumstance the absence of fat tissue predates the development of diabetes by 10 to 12 years. The congenital variant accounts for ~60 percent of cases of lipoatrophic diabetes. Associated conditions include intracerebral disorders and abnormalities involving the heart, kidneys, and ovaries. Acanthosis nigricans and cirrhosis are usually milder than in the acquired form. Alternatively, in the acquired form (Lawrence syndrome), the diabetes may appear first, the lipoatrophy not becoming manifest until late childhood or adult life, often following an acute viral illness. Associated findings are muscle hypertrophy (which may be more apparent than real, because of the lack of adipose tissue), accelerated growth, acanthosis nigricans, acromegaloid features with thick curly hair, hyperhidrosis, and clitoromegaly. Death is generally due to liver failure, although patients with retinopathy and nephropathy have occasionally been observed. Cirrhosis can progress to portal hypertension with splenomegaly; splenomegaly may, however, occur in the absence of cirrhosis.

The etiology of this syndrome remains unexplained.[558,559] The presence of lipid-mobilizing factor isolated from the urine and abnormalities in pituitary releasing factor have been suggested but remain unproven. An increase in basal metabolic rate, particularly following meals, has been described in lipoatrophic diabetes, although the exact mechanism is not known; thyroid hormone levels are normal. This condition is also characterized by very high basal insulin levels in the postabsorptive state but normal increases in insulin concentration following various beta cell stimuli, with a normal proinsulin/insulin ratio. The pathogenesis of insulin resistance is heterogeneous; it may involve both receptor and postreceptor abnormalities. Glucagon levels in lipoatrophic patients have been reported to be either normal or elevated. Gonadotropin levels are normal, although polycystic ovaries have been described in some cases of congenital lipoatrophic diabetes. Adrenal function is also reported to be normal. Acromegaloid features are present in some patients, but GH concentrations vary.

Radiographic studies show loss of subcutaneous fat and fat surrounding internal organs. Osteosclerosis of long bones appears commonly in this syndrome; it may be related to the replacement of hematopoietic marrow by fat. Marrow fat, in turn, may be transformed into osteogenic cells. Cardiomegaly may occur as a result of increased cardiac output resulting from the chronic hypermetabolic state.

The clinical distinction between lipoatrophic diabetes and poorly regulated, insulin-dependent diabetes with wasting is generally not difficult. Differentiation is based on the lack of ketosis, the requirement for enormous doses of insulin, and the presence of hypermetabolism, as well as the associated findings enumerated above.

Partial lipoatrophy, although rare, is more common than is generalized lipoatrophy. Loss of body fat tends to occur above the waist, but adiposity is normal below it. Partial lipoatrophy may be a variant of the generalized type, with accompanying glucose intolerance, insulin resistance, and hypermetabolism. This condition is associated with an increased incidence of brain tumors and membranoproliferative glomerulonephritis.[559]

Secondary Diabetes

Diabetes may develop as a consequence of destructive lesions or surgical removal of the pancreas (pancreoprival diabetes); it also may result from hypersecretion of hormones with actions antagonistic to insulin or which interfere with insulin secretion (endocrine-associated diabetes). Glucose intolerance is also observed fairly frequently in some nonendocrine disorders (uremia, cirrhosis).

In each of these conditions the possibility that a genetic predisposition to spontaneous diabetes is also playing a role (for example, in increasing the likelihood that a given amount of pancreatic destruction or counterregulatory hormone secretion will result in hyperglycemia) cannot be excluded.

PANCREOPRIVAL DIABETES

The surgical removal of more than two-thirds of the pancreas or pancreatic destruction resulting from chronic relapsing pancreatitis results in the development of diabetes. Clinically, such patients differ from those with spontaneous insulin-dependent diabetes by their greater tendency to develop insulin-induced hypoglycemia, lessened tendency to have ketosis, and requirement (in most instances) of no more than 20 to 40 U of insulin per day.[168,560] These characteristics may be related to the lack of glucagon secretion, which contrasts with the hyperglucagonemia observed in spontaneous diabetes. These patients are of interest from a theoretical standpoint, because they demonstrate that (1) glucagon is not essential for the development of diabetes, but when present, it accentuates the effects of insulin lack; and (2) microangiopathy may occur in the absence of a genetic predisposition to diabetes, thus supporting the metabolic theory with regard to pathogenesis of diabetic complications.[360]

Hemochromatosis is so often associated with diabetes that it is sometimes called "bronze diabetes." In one series of 115 patients, 72 had clinical diabetes and 14 others had abnormal results of glucose tolerance tests.[561] All 86 had an exaggerated insulin response, like that seen in cirrhosis of the liver, which may be one of the causes of the diabetes in this disease. In addition, a family history of diabetes was present in 25 percent of those with diabetes and hemochromatosis. The usual complications of diabetes were quite common in this group of patients. It appears, therefore, that the diabetes of hemochromatosis can be explained as a combination of the effects of inheritance, cirrhosis, and, perhaps, the noxious effects of iron deposits in the pancreas. In this group of patients, 40 percent of the diabetics had some improvement of the carbohydrate abnormality after repeated phlebotomy had depleted the iron stores.[561]

ENDOCRINE-ASSOCIATED DIABETES

Sustained hypersecretion of hormones with actions antagonistic to insulin (e.g., GH, glucocorticoids, epinephrine) or which interfere with insulin secretion (e.g., epinephrine, norepinephrine) is often associated with glucose intolerance of varying degrees of severity.[562] Features common to virtually all forms of such endocrine-associated diabetes are reversibility of the hyperglycemia with cure of the underlying endocrine disorder and absence (in most patients) of ketosis. The latter characteristic probably reflects the ongoing availability of endogenous insulin.

Acromegaly

GH interferes with insulin-mediated glucose uptake while stimulating lipolysis. In most acromegalic patients hyperinsulinemia is present in the basal state and in response to meal ingestion. The hyperinsulinemia may be sufficient to compensate for the insulin resistance so that carbohydrate metabolism remains intact. The prevalence of glucose intolerance in acromegaly is as high as 60 percent. However, fasting hyperglycemia is observed in only 15 to 30 percent of patients and less than 10 percent require insulin therapy. The defect in insulin sensitivity in such patients may be mediated by a reduction in binding of insulin to its receptor.[154]

Cushing's Syndrome

The administration of glucocorticoids in pharmacologic doses results in the development of hyperinsulinemia and insulin resistance in as short a period as 3 days.[563] With more sustained periods of hyperadrenalism, glucose intolerance generally appears. Fasting hyperglycemia is encountered in only 20 to 25 percent of patients with Cushing's syndrome; ketosis is unusual. In addition to stimulating gluconeogenesis, the increase in glucocorticoid concentrations interferes with insulin-mediated glucose uptake. The gluconeogenic action of glucocorticoids may be influenced by concomitant hyperglucagonemia.[564]

Pheochromocytoma

Excessive secretion of catecholamines may interfere with insulin secretion and/or action. In tumors producing primarily norepinephrine, inhibition of insulin secretion is the major factor resulting in glucose intolerance. On the other hand, hypersecretion of epinephrine results in interference with insulin-mediated glucose uptake as well as hypoinsulinemia.[182,183] Glucose load tests tend to show a diabetic pattern with a sudden drop in plasma glucose concentration at 60 to 90 min, probably due to the hyperglycemia-induced breakthrough in insulin secretion, after the initial blockade.[565] The degree of fasting hyperglycemia is usually mild in patients with pheochromocytoma. Abnormal carbohydrate metabolism may persist in some cases for weeks to months after tumor resection because of ongoing resistance to insulin.

Glucagonoma

Glucagon-secreting tumors of the alpha cells of the islets of Langerhans are rare tumors associated with glucose intolerance or fasting hyperglycemia, weight loss, diarrhea, an erythematous bullous skin eruption (necrolytic migratory erythema), anemia, and hypokalemia.[566] Plasma glucagon levels generally are as high as 1000 to 2000 pg/ml, as compared with values of 75 to 100 pg/ml in normal subjects and only moderate elevations (150 to 200 pg/ml) seen in patients with spontaneous diabetes. The increment in immunoreactive plasma glucagon concentration has been shown to be heterogeneous, consisting of four components: BPG, of ~150,000 daltons; "large plasma glucagon," of ~9000 daltons, which corresponds to proglucagon; pancreatic glucagon (~3500 daltons); and "small glucagon" (~2000 daltons). Studies using agents known to stimulate and suppress glucagon secretion have shown parallel changes in levels of the three components other than BPG, which tends to remain constant.[567] Hyperglucagonemia has been observed in clinically unaffected family members of a patient with an alpha cell tumor.[172] However, the elevation in circulating glucagon immunoreactivity in family members was not due to pancreatic glucagon but the larger molecular species, such as proglucagon and BPG.

Plasma insulin concentrations are generally elevated, accounting for the mildness of diabetes and the absence of ketosis despite the severe degree of hyperglucagonemia. The tumors may produce a variety of islet cell hormones (e.g., insulin, somatostatin, pancreatic polypeptide) in addition to glucagon. Furthermore, the glucagonoma syndrome has appeared in patients with a prior history of clinically manifest insulinoma.[568]

Marked reductions in plasma amino acid concentrations are observed in glucagonoma patients. The hypoaminoacidemia is due to the hyperglucagonemia per se as well as the weight loss, diarrhea, and protein loss from the skin lesions. Restoration of normal circulating amino acid levels by IV administration of amino acids has been accompanied by complete clearing of the skin rash.[569] In contrast to insulinomas, alpha cell tumors are often large enough to be detected by diagnostic imaging (i.e., CT scans) by the time they are suspected clinically.[570] Treatment includes surgical resection and, in metastatic disease, administration of streptozotocin. A remarkable improvement in skin lesions has been observed after the administration of somatostatin[571] and SMS 201-995, the long-acting somatostatin analogue.[572]

Multiple Endocrine Deficiency

In some patients diabetes may coexist with adrenal failure and/or hypothyroidism. The simultaneous presence of more than one hormone deficiency state (unrelated to pituitary failure) is referred to as *Schmidt's syndrome* or multiple endocrine deficiency (see Chap. 28). Such patients are characterized by the presence of circulating antibodies to islet cells as well as high titers of thyroid and adrenal antibodies. The diabetes is generally insulin-dependent. Diabetes may antedate or follow the other endocrine deficiencies. It is more commonly observed in women than in men. In contrast to most patients with insulin-dependent diabetes, in whom islet cell antibodies disappear within months to a year after onset of the diabetes, in patients with multiple endocrine deficiency titers of ICA may remain persistently elevated.[216] Clinically, such patients are often difficult to manage because their lack of endogenous adrenal function predisposes them to severe insulin hypoglycemia even in the face of replacement doses of glucocorticoids.

GLUCOSE INTOLERANCE IN NONENDOCRINE DISEASE

The pathogenesis of stress hyperglycemia in association with acute illness such as sepsis or myocardial infarction has been discussed above. In such circumstances tests of glucose tolerance (if indicated) should not be performed until the patient has recovered for several weeks to months after the acute event. In contrast, in certain disease states chronic abnormalities of glucose tolerance are frequently observed even in the absence of acute deterioration in the underlying primary disease process. In *uremia,* postprandial hyperglycemia and mild fasting hyperglycemia occur in a setting of hyperinsulinemia and hyperglucagonemia. Resistance to insulin and hypersensitivity to glucagon are the major pathogenic factors responsible for hyperglycemia.[573] In addition, it is possible that a low-molecular-weight peptide unique to uremia may induce insulin resistance by a protein synthesis–dependent mechanism.[574]

In *cirrhosis,* particularly when accompanied by portal hypertension, glucose intolerance is a frequent occurrence. Hyperinsulinemia as well as hyperglucagonemia have been noted. Decreased hepatic responsiveness to glucagon in cirrhosis suggests that insulin resistance may be the more important pathogenic factor in the derangement in carbohydrate metabolism.[181] Recent evidence suggests that insulin resistance in human cirrhosis may be due to combined receptor and postreceptor defects.[575]

REFERENCES

1. Harris M, Entmacher PS: Mortality from Diabetes, in *Diabetes in America,* NIH Publication 85-1468. U.S. Government Printing Office, 1985.

2. WHO Study Group: *Diabetes Mellitus.* World Health Organization technical report series 727, Geneva, 1985.

3. Lacy PE, Greider MH: Anatomy and ultrastructural organization of pancreatic islets, in DeGroot LJ, Cahill GF Jr et al (eds): *Endocrinology.* New York, Grune & Stratton, 1979, vol 2, p 907.

4. Pearse AGE, Polak JM, Heath CM: Development, differentiation and derivation of endocrine polypeptide cells of the mouse pancreas. *Diabetologia* 9:120, 1973.

5. Hers HG: The control of glycogen metabolism in the liver. *Annu Rev Biochem* 45:167, 1976.

5a. Hers HG, Hue L: Gluconeogenesis and related aspects of glycolysis. *Annu Rev Biochem* 52:617, 1983.

6. DeFronzo R, Ferrannini E, Hendler R, et al: Influence of hyperinsulinemia, hyperglycemia and the route of glucose administration on splanchnic glucose exchange. *Proc Natl Acad Sci USA* 75:5173, 1978.

7. Hutson NJ, Brumley FT, Assimacopoulos FD et al: Studies on the α-adrenergic activation of phosphorylase and gluconeogenesis and inactivation of glycogen synthase in isolated liver parenchymal cells. *J Biol Chem* 251:5200, 1976.

7a. Rosen SG, Clutter WE, Shah SD et al: Direct, α-adrenergic stimulation of hepatic glucose production in postabsorptive man. *Am J Physiol* 245:E616, 1983.

8. Sacca L, Hendler R, Sherwin RS et al: Hyperglycemia inhibits glucose production in man independent of changes in glucoregulatory hormones. *J Clin Endocrinol Metab* 47:1160, 1978.

9. Hers HG, Van Schaftingen E: Fructose 2,6-bisphosphate 2 years after its discovery. *Biochem J* 206:1, 1982.

10. Pilkis SJ, Fox E, Wolfe L et al: Hormonal modulation of hepatic regulatory enzymes in the gluconeogenic/glycolytic pathway. *Ann NY Acad Sci* 478, 1987 (in press).

11. Engstrom I: The regulation of liver pyruvate kinase by phosphorylation-dephosphorylation. *Curr Top Cell Regul* 13:29, 1978.

12. Shafrir E: Effect of sucrose and fructose on carbohydrate and lipid metabolism and the resulting consequences, in Beitner R (ed): *Regulation of Carbohydrate Metabolism.* Boca Raton, CRC, 1985, vol 2, p 96.

13. Owen OE, Felig P, Morgan AP et al: Liver and kidney metabolism during prolonged starvation. *J Clin Invest* 48:574, 1969.

14. Felig P: The glucose-alanine cycle. *Metabolism* 22:179, 1973.

15. Ahlborg G, Wahren J, Felig P et al: Splanchnic and peripheral glucose and lactate metabolism during and after prolonged arm exercise. *J Clin Invest* 77:690, 1986.

16. Granner DK, Andreone TL: Insulin modulation of gene expression, in DeFronzo RA (ed): *Diabetes/Metabolism Reviews* New York, Wiley, 1985, vol 1, p 139.

17. Hod Y, Cook JS, Weldon SL et al: Differential expression of the genes for the mitochondrial and cytosolic forms of P-enolpyruvate carboxykinase. *Ann NY Acad Sci* 478, 1987 (in press).

18. Denton RM, Hughes WA: Pyruvate dehydrogenase and the hormonal regulation of fat synthesis in mammalian tissues. *Int J Biochem* 9:545, 1978.

19. Laker ME, Mayes PA: Investigations into the direct effects of insulin on hepatic ketogenesis, lipoprotein secretion and pyruvate dehydrogenase activity. *Biochim Biophys Acta* 795:4, 1984.

20. Chang TM, Goldberg AL: Leucine inhibits oxidation of glucose and pyruvate in skeletal muscles during fasting. *J Biol Chem* 253:3696, 1978.

21. Gabbay KH: The sorbitol pathway and the complications of diabetes. *N Engl J Med* 295:443, 1976.

21a. Majerus PW, Conolly TM, Deckmyn H et al: The metabolism of phosphoinositide-derived messenger molecules. *Science* 234:1519, 1986.

22. Clements RS Jr: Diabetic neuropathy—new concepts of its etiology. *Diabetes* 28:604, 1979.

23. Simmons DA, Winegrad AI, Martin DB et al: Significance of tissue myo-inositol concentrations in metabolic regulation in nerve. *Science* 217:848, 1982.

24. Page MG, Hutson NJ (eds): Symposium on the effects of sorbinil on the pathophysiology of diabetic complications. *Metabolism* 35(suppl 1):1986.

25. Judzewitsch RG, Jaspan J, Polonsky KS, et al: Aldose reductase inhibition improves nerve conduction velocity in cute streptozotocin diabetes. *N Engl J Med* 308:119, 1983.

26. Greene DA, Lattimer SA: Action of Sorbinil in diabetic peripheral nerve. Relation of polyol (sorbitol) pathway to a myoinositol mediated defect in sodium-potassium ATPase activity. *Diabetes* 33:712, 1984.

27. Fluckiger R, Winterhalter KH: Glycosylated hemoglobins, in Caughey WS (ed): *Biochemical and Clinical Aspects of Hemoglobin Abnormalities.* New York, Academic, 1978, p 205.

28. Cerami A, Stevens VJ, Monnier VM: Role of nonenzymatic glycosylation in the development of the sequelae of diabetes mellitus. *Metabolism* 28 (suppl 1):431, 1979.

29. Dunn PJ, Cole RA, Soeldner JS, et al: Temporal relationship of glycosylated hemoglobin concentrations to glucose control in diabetics. *Diabetologia* 17:213, 1979.

30. Bunn HF: Evaluation of glycosylated hemoglobin in diabetic patients. *Diabetes* 30:613, 1981.

31. Dolhofer R, Brenner R, Wieland OH: Different behavior of hemoglobin A_{1c} and glycosyl-albumin levels during recovery from diabetic ketoacidosis and nonacidotic coma. *Diabetologia* 21:211, 1981.

32. Day JF, Thorpe SR, Baynes JW: Nonenzymatically glucosylated albumin. *In vitro* preparation and isolation from normal human serum. *J Biol Chem* 234:595, 1979.

33. Witztum JL, Mahoney EM, Branks MS et al: Nonenzymatic glucosylation of low-density lipoprotein alters its biological activity. *Diabetes* 31:283, 1982.

34. Witztum JL, Fisher M, Pietro T et al: Nonenzymatic glucosylation of high-density lipoprotein accelerates its metabolism in guinea pigs. *Diabetes* 31:1029, 1982.

35. Spiro RG: Search for a biochemical basis of diabetic microangiopathy. *Diabetologia* 12:1, 1976.

36. Cohen MP, Urdanivia E, Surma M et al: Increased glycosylation of glomerular basement membrane collagen in diabetes. *Biochem Biophys Res Commun* 5:765, 1980.

37. Kohn RR, Schnider SL: Glucosylation of human collagen. *Diabetes* 31 (suppl 3):47, 1982.

38. Rahrbach DH, Hassell JR, Kleinman HK et al: Alterations in the basement membrane (heparan sulfate) proteoglycan in diabetic mice. *Diabetes* 31:185, 1982.

39. Wakil SJ, Stoops JK, Joshi VC: Fatty acid synthesis and its regulation. *Annu Rev Biochem* 52:537, 1983.

40. McGarry JD, Foster DW: Regulation of hepatic fatty acid oxidation and ketone body production. *Annu Rev Biochem* 49:395, 1980.

41. Foster DW: From glycogen to ketones and back. *Diabetes* 33:1188, 1984.

42. Owen OE, Reichard GA Jr: Fuels consumed by man. The interplay between carbohydrates and fatty acids. *Prog Biochem Pharmacol* 6:177, 1971.

43. Shambaugh GE III et al: Fetal fuels II. *Am J Physiol* 233:E457, 1977; Fetal fuels III. *Am J Physiol* 235:E330, 1978.

43a. Kosugi K, Scofield RF, Chandramouli V et al: Pathways of acetone's metabolism in the rat. *J Biol Chem* 261:3952, 1986.

44. Casazza JP, Felver ME, Veech RL: The metabolism of acetone in rats. *J Biol Chem* 259:231, 1984.

45. Hetenyi G Jr, Ferrarotto C: Gluconeogenesis from acetone in starved rats. *Biochem J* 231:151, 1985.

46. Reichard GA Jr, Hoff AC, Skutches CL et al: Plasma acetone metabolism in the fasting human. *J Clin Invest* 63:619, 1979.

47. Ruderman NB, Toews CJ, Shafrir E: The role of free fatty acids in glucose homeostasis. *Arch Intern Med* 123:299, 1968.

48. Rennie MJ, Holoszy JD: Inhibition of glucose uptake and glycogenolysis by availability of oleate in well-oxygenated perfused skeletal muscle. *Biochem J* 168:161, 1977.

49. Randle PT, Garland PB, Hales CN et al: Glucose fatty acid cycle. *Lancet* 1:785, 1963.

50. Felig P, Pozefsky T, Marliss E, Cahill GF Jr: Alanine: Key role in gluconeogenesis. *Science* 167:1003, 1970.

51. Felig P: Amino acid metabolism in man. *Annu Rev Biochem* 44:933, 1975.

52. Felig P, Kim YJ, Lynch V, Hendler R: Amino acid metabolism during starvation in human pregnancy. *J Clin Invest* 51:195, 1972.

53. Haymond MW, Karl IE, Pagliara AS: Ketotic hypoglycemia: An amino acid substrate-limited disorder. *J Clin Endocrinol Metab* 38:521, 1974.

54. Haymond MW, Ben-Galim E, Strobel KE: Glucose and alanine metabolism in children with maple syrup urine disease. *J Clin Invest* 62:398, 1978.

55. Wahren J, Felig P, Hagenfeldt L: Effect of protein ingestion on splanchnic and leg metabolism in normal man and in diabetes mellitus. *J Clin Invest* 57:987, 1976.

56. Buse MG, Reid SS: Leucine. A possible regulator of protein turnover in muscle. *J Clin Invest* 56:1250, 1975.

57. Steiner D: Insulin today. *Diabetes* 26:322, 1977.

58. Goeddel DV, Kleid DG, Bolivar F, et al: Expression in *Escherichia coli* of chemically synthesized genes for human insulin. *Proc Natl Acad Sci USA* 76:106, 1979.

59. Weitzer G, Eisele K, Schulz V, Stock W: Structure and activity of insulin: XII. Further studies on biologically active synthetic fragments of B-chain. *Hoppe Seylers Z Physiol Chem* 354:321, 1973.

60. Chan SJ, Keim P, Steiner DF: Cell-free synthesis of rat preproinsulins: Characterization and partial amino acid sequence determination. *Proc Natl Acad Sci USA* 73:1964, 1976.

61. Bonser AM, Garcia-Webb P: C-peptide measurement: Methods and clinical utility. *CRC Crit Rev Clin Lab Sci* 19:297, 1984.

61a. Polonsky K, Frank B, Pugh W et al: The limitations to and valid use of C-peptide as a marker of the secretion of insulin. *Diabetes* 35:379, 1986.

62. Gerich JE, Charles MA, Grodsky GM: Regulation of pancreatic insulin and glucagon secretion. *Annu Rev Physiol* 38:353, 1976.

63. Villa-Komaroff L, Efstratiadis A, Broome S et al: A bacterial clone synthesizing proinsulin. *Proc Natl Acad Sci USA* 75:3727, 1978.

64. Felig P, Wahren J: Influence of endogenous insulin secretion on splanchnic glucose and amino acid metabolism. *J Clin Invest* 50:1702, 1971.

65. Gabbay KH, DeLuca K, Fisher JN Jr et al: Familial hyperproinsulinemia. An autosomal dominant defect. *N Engl J Med* 294:911, 1976.

66. Robbins DC, Shoelson SE, Rubenstein AH, Tager HS: Familial hyperproinsulinemia: Two families secreting indistinguishable type II intermediates of proinsulin conversion. *J Clin Invest* 73:714, 1984.

67. Robbins DC, Tager HS, Rubenstein AH: Biologic and clinical importance of proinsulin. *N Engl J Med* 310:1165, 1984.

68. Tamborlane WV, Sherwin RS, Genel M, Felig P: Reduction to normal of plasma glucose in juvenile diabetes by subcutaneous administration of insulin with a portable infusion pump. *N Engl J Med* 300:573, 1979.

69. Malaisse-Lagae F, Sener A, Malaisse WJ: Phosphoglucomutase: Its role in the response of pancreatic islets to glucose epimers and anomers. *Biochimie* 64:1059, 1982.

70. Malaisse WJ, Hutton JC, Kawazu S et al: The stimulus-secretion coupling of glucose-induced insulin release: XXXV. The links between metabolic and cationic events. *Diabetologia* 16:331, 1979.

71. Meglasson MD, Matschinsky FM: Pancreatic glucose metabolism and regulation of insulin secretion, in DeFronzo RA (ed): *Diabetes/Metabolism Reviews.* New York, Wiley, 1986, vol 2, p 163.

72. Meglasson MD, Burch PT, Benner DK et al: Identification of glucokinase as an alloxan-sensitive glucose sensor of the pancreatic beta-cell. *Diabetes* 35:1163, 1986.

73. Malaisse WJ, Malaisse-Lagae F, Sener A: The glycolytic cascade in pancreatic cells. *Diabetologia* 23:1, 1982.

74. Hellman B: B-cell cytoplasmic Ca^{2+} balance as a determinant for glucose-stimulated insulin-release. *Diabetologia* 28:494, 1985.

75. Charles MA, Laweck J, Pictet R, Grodsky GM: Insulin secretion. Interrelationships of glucose, cyclic adenosine 3′5′-monophosphate and calcium. *J Biol Chem* 250:6134, 1976.

76. Wollheim CB, Pozzan T: Correlation between cytosolic free Ca^{2+} and insulin release in an insulin-secreting cell line. *J Biol Chem* 259:2262, 1984.

77. Porte D Jr, Pupo AA: Insulin responses to glucose: Evidence for a two-pool system in man. *J Clin Invest* 48:2309, 1969.

78. Permutt MA: Effect of glucose on initiation and elongation rates in isolated rat pancreatic islets. *J Biol Chem* 248:2738, 1974.

79. Moore B, Edie ES, Abram JH: On the treatment of diabetes mellitus by acid extract of duodenal mucous membrane. *Biochem J* 1:28, 1906.

80. Creutzfeldt W: The incretin concept today. *Diabetologia* 16:75, 1979.

81. Ebert R, Creutzfeldt W: Influence of gastric inhibitory polypeptide antiserum on glucose-induced insulin secretion in rats. *Endocrinology* 111:1601, 1982.

82. Anderson DK: Physiological effects of GIP in man, in Bloom SR, Polak JM (eds): *Gut Hormones.* Edinburgh, New York, Churchill Livingstone, 1981, p 256.

83. Mazzaferri EL, Ciofalo L, Waters LA et al: Effects of gastric inhibitory polypeptide on leucine and arginine-stimulated insulin release. *Am J Physiol* 245:E114, 1983.

84. Sener A, Malaisse-Lagae F, Malaisse WJ: Stimulation of pancreatic islet metabolism and insulin release by a nonmetabolizable amino acid. *Proc Natl Acad Sci USA* 78:5460, 1981.

84a. Crespin SR, Greenough WB III, Steinberg D: Stimulation of insulin secretion by long-chain free fatty acids. A direct pancreatic effect. *J Clin Invest* 52:1979, 1973.

85. Owen OE, Reichard GA Jr, Markus H et al: Rapid intravenous sodium acetate infusion in man. Metabolic and kinetic responses. *J Clin Invest* 52:2606, 1973.

86. Porte D Jr, Smith PH, Ensinck JW: Neurohumoral regulaton of the pancreatic islet A and B cells. *Metabolism* 25 (suppl 1):1453, 1976.

87. Hamburg S, Hendler R, Sherwin RS: Epinephrine: Exquisite sensitivity to its diabetogenic effects in normal man. *Clin Res* 27:252A, 1979.

88. Martin JM, Konijnendijk W, Bouman PR: Insulin and growth hormone secretion in rats with ventromedial hypothalamic lesions maintained on restricted food intake. *Diabetes* 23:203, 1974.

89. Lebovitz HE, Feldman JM: Pancreatic biogenic amines and insulin secretion in health and disease. *Fed Proc* 32:1797, 1973.

90. Robertson RP, Chem M: A role for prostaglandin E in defective insulin secretion and carbohydrate intolerance in diabetes mellitus. *J Clin Invest* 60:747, 1977.

91. Metz SA, Murphy RC, Fujimoto W: Effects of glucose-induced insulin secretion of lipoxygenase-derived metabolites of arachidonic acid. *Diabetes* 33:119, 1984.

92. Green IC, Perrin D, Penman E et al: Effect of dynorphin on insulin and somatostatin secretion. Calcium uptake and cAMP levels in isolated rat islets of Langerhans. *Diabetes* 32:685, 1983.

93. Gerich JE, Raptis S, Rosenthal J: Somatostatin symposium. *Metabolism* 27 (suppl 1):1, 1978.

94. Wahren J, Felig P: Influence of somatostatin on carbohydrate disposal and absorption in diabetes mellitus. *Lancet* 2:1213, 1976.

95. Krejs GJ, Orci L, Conlon JM et al: Somatostatinoma syndrome. Biochemical, morphologic and clinical features. *N Engl J Med* 301:285, 1979.

96. Ipp E, Dobbs E, Arimura A, Unger RH: Release of immunoreactive somatostatin from the pancreas in response to glucose, amino acids, pancreozymin-cholecystokinin and tolbutamide. *J Clin Invest* 60:760, 1977.

97. Bjorntorp P, de Jounge C, Sjostrom L: The effect of physical training on insulin production in obesity. *Metabolism* 19:631, 1970.

98. Felig P, Marliss E, Cahill GF Jr: Plasma amino acid levels and insulin secretion in obesity. *N Engl J Med* 281:811, 1969.

99. Felig P, Wahren J, Hendler R: Influence of oral glucose ingestion on splanchnic glucose and amino acid metabolism. *Diabetes* 24:468, 1975.

100. Katz J, McGarry JD: The glucose paradox. Is glucose a substrate for liver metabolism? *J Clin Invest* 74:1901, 1981.

101. DeFronzo RA, Ferrannini E, Hendler R et al: Regulation of splanchnic and peripheral glucose uptake by insulin and hyperglycemia in man. *Diabetes* 32:35, 1983.

101a. Radziuk J: Glucose and glycogen metabolism following glucose ingestion in man: A turnover method, in Cobelli C, Bergman RN (eds): *Carbohydrate Metabolism.* New York, Wiley, 1981, p 239.

102. Newgard CB, Moore SV, Foster DW, McGarry JD: Efficient hepatic glycogen synthesis in refeeding rats requires continued carbon flow through the gluconeogenic pathway. *J Biol Chem* 259:6958, 1984.

102a. Shulman GI, Rothman DL, Smith D et al: Mechanism of liver glycogen repletion in vivo by nuclear magnetic resonance spectroscopy. *J Clin Invest* 76:1229, 1985.

102b. Magnusson I, Chandramouli V, Schumann WC et al: Direct versus indirect pathways of glucose conversion to glycogen in humans. *Clin Res* 34:726A, 1986.

103. Chiasson JL, Liljenquist JE, Finger FE, Lacy WW: Differential sensitivity of glycogenolysis and gluconeogenesis to insulin infusions in dogs. *Diabetes* 25:283, 1976.

104. Bergman RN: Integrated control of hepatic glucose metabolism. *Fed Proc* 36:256, 1977.

105. Wahren J, Felig P, Cerasi E, Luft R: Splanchnic and peripheral glucose and amino acid metabolism in diabetes mellitus. *J Clin Invest* 51:1870, 1972.

106. Bergman RN, Beir JR, Hourigan PM: Intraportal glucose infusion matched to oral glucose absorption. Lack of evidence for "gut factor" involvement in hepatic glucose storage. *Diabetes* 31:27, 1982.

107. Ishida T, Chap Z, Chou J et al: Differential effects of oral peripheral intravenous and intraportal glucose on hepatic glucose uptake and insulin and glucagon extraction in conscious dogs. *J Clin Invest* 72:590, 1983.

108. Felig P, Wahren J, Sherwin RS, Palaiologos G: Protein and amino acid metabolism in diabetes mellitus. *Arch Intern Med* 137:507, 1977.

109. Mayer M, Shafrir E: Glucocorticoid- and insulin-mediated regulation of skeletal muscle protein catabolism, in Shafrir E, Renold AE (eds): *Lessons from Animal Diabetes.* London, Libbey, 1984, p 235.

110. Dahlman B, Schroeter C, Herbertz L, Reinauer H: Myofibrillar protein, degradation and muscle proteinase in normal and diabetic rats. *Biochem Med* 21:33, 1979.

111. Sherwin RS, Hendler RG, Felig P: Effect of diabetes mellitus and insulin on the turnover and metabolic response to ketones in man. *Diabetes* 25:776, 1976.

112. DeFronzo RA, Sherwin RS, Dillingham M et al: Influence of basal insulin and glucagon secretion on potassium and sodium metabolism: Studies with somatostatin in normal dogs and in normal and diabetic human beings. *J Clin Invest* 61:426, 1978.

112a. DeFronzo RA: The effect of insulin on renal sodium metabolism. A review with clinical implications. *Diabetologia* 21:165, 1981.

113. Kahn CR, Crettaz M: Insulin receptors and the molecular mechanism of insulin action, in DeFronzo RA (ed): *Diabetes/Metabolism Reviews.* New York, Wiley, 1985, vol 1, p 5.

114. Hedo JA, Kasuga M, Van Obberghen E et al: Direct demonstration of glycosylation of insulin receptor subunits by biosynthetic and external labeling: Evidence for heterogeneity. *Proc Natl Acad Sci USA* 78:4791, 1981.

115. Kahn CR, Freychet P, Neville DM Jr, Roth J: Quantitative aspects of the insulin-receptor interactions in liver plasma membranes. *J Biol Chem* 249:2249, 1984.

116. DeMeyts P, Bianco AR, Roth J: Site-site interactions among insulin receptors: Characterization of the negative cooperativity. *J Biol Chem* 251:1187, 1976.

117. Olefsky JM, Chang H: Insulin binding to adipocytes. Evidence for functionally distinct receptors. *Diabetes* 27:946, 1978.

118. Pollet RJ, Kampner ES, Standaert ML, Haase BA: Structure of the insulin receptor of cultured human lymphoblastoid cells IM-9: Evidence suggesting that two subunits are required for insulin binding. *J Biol Chem* 257:894, 1982.

119. Massague J, Pilch PF, Czech MP: Electrophoretic resolution of three major insulin receptor structures with unique subunit stoichiometries. *Proc Natl Acad Sci USA* 77:7137, 1980.

120. Crettaz M, Jialal I, Kasuga M, Kahn CR: Insulin receptor regulation and desensitization in rat hepatoma cells: The loss of the oligomeric forms of the receptor correlates with the change in receptor affinity. *J Biol Chem* 259:11542, 1984.

121. Spiegel AM, Grerschik P, Levine MA, Downs AW Jr: Clinical implications of guanine nucleotide-binding proteins as receptor-effector couplers. *N Engl J Med* 312:26, 1985.

122. Hiedenreich KA, Zahniser NR, Berhanu P et al: Structural differences between insulin receptors in the brain and peripheral target tissues. *J Biol Chem* 258:8527, 1983.

123. Jeong-Hyok I, Meezan E et al: Isolation and characterization of human erythrocyte insulin receptors. *J Biol Chem* 258:5021, 1983.

124. King GL, Buzney SM, Kahn CR et al: Differential responsiveness to insulin of endothelial and support cells from micro- and macrovessels. *J Clin Invest* 71:974, 1983.

125. Saucier J, Dube JY, Tremblay RR: Specific insulin binding sites in rat testis: Characterization and variations. *Endocrinology* 190:2220, 1981.

125a. Posner BI: Insulin receptors in human and animal placental tissue. *Diabetes* 23:209, 1974.

126. Hedo JA, Kahn CR, Hayashi M et al: Biosynthesis and glycosylation of the insulin receptors. Evidence for a single polypeptide precursor of the two major subunits. *J Biol Chem* 258:10020, 1983.

127. Carpentier J-L, Gorden P, Freychet P et al: Lysosomal association of internalized ^{125}I-insulin in isolated hepatocytes. Direct demonstration by quantitative electron microscopic autoradiography. *J Clin Invest* 63:1249, 1979.

128. Marshall S: Kinetics of insulin receptor biosynthesis and membrane insertion: Relationship to cellular function. *Diabetes* 32:319, 1983.

129. Marshall S, Olefsky JM: Separate intracellular pathways for insulin receptor recycling and insulin degradation in isolated rat adipocytes. *Cell Physiol* 117:195, 1983.

130. Posner BI, Kahn MN, Bergeron JJM: Internalization of insulin: Structures involved and significance, in Vranic M, Hollenberg CH, Steiner G (eds): *Comparison of Type I and Type II Diabetes.* New York, Plenum, 1985, p 159.

131. Kalant N, Osaki H, Mackubo B et al: Downregulation of insulin binding by human and rat hepatocytes in primary cultures: The possible role of insulin internalization and degradation. *Endocrinology* 114:37, 1984.

132. Kasuga M, Zick Y, Blithe OL et al: Insulin stimulation of phosphorylation of the β-subunit of the insulin receptor: Formation of both phosphoserine and phosphotyrosine. *J Biol Chem* 257:9891, 1982.

132a. Gammeltoft S, Van Obberghen E: Protein kinase activity of the insulin receptor. *Biochem J* 235:1, 1986.

133. Jacobs S, Sahyoun NE, Saltiel AR, Cuatrecasas P: Phorbol esters stimulate the phosphorylation of receptors for insulin and somatomedin C. *Proc Natl Acad Sci USA* 80:6211, 1983.

134. Takayama S, White MF, Lauris V, Kahn CR: Phorbol esters modulate insulin receptor phosphorylation and insulin action in cultured hepatoma cells. *Proc Natl Acad Sci USA* 81:7797, 1984.

135. Cohen S, Ushiro H, Stoscheck C, Chinkers M: A native 170,000 epidermal growth factor receptor-kinase complex from shed plasma membrane vesicles. *J Biol Chem* 257:1523, 1982.

136. Ek B, Heldin CH: Characterization of a tyrosine-specific kinase activity in human fibroblast membranes stimulated by platelet-derived growth factor. *J Biol Chem* 257:10486, 1982.

137. Jacobs S, Kull FC Jr, Earp HS et al: Somatomedin-C stimulates the phosphorylation of the subunit of its own receptor. *J Biol Chem* 258:9581, 1983.

138. Koepfer-Hobelsberger B, Wieland OH: Insulin activates phospholipase C in fat cells: Similarity with the activation of pyruvate dehydrogenase. *Mol Cell Endocrinol* 36:1123, 1984.

139. Sale G, Fujita-Yamaguchi Y, Kahn CR: Evidence that the insulin receptor is associated with phosphatidylinositol kinase activity. *Eur J Biochem* 155:345, 1986.

140. Berridge MJ: Inositol triphosphate and diacylglycerol as second messengers. *Biochemistry* 220:345, 1984.

141. Rozengurt E, Rodriguez-Pena A, Coombs M, Sinnett-Smith J: Diacylglycerol stimulates DNA synthesis and cell division in

mouse 3T3 cells: Role of Ca^{2+}-sensitive phospholipid-dependent protein kinase. *Proc Natl Acad Sci USA* 81:5748, 1984.

142. Levine R: Insulin: The effects and mode of action of the hormone. *Vitam Horm* 39:145, 1982.

143. Larner J: Mediators of postreceptor insulin action. *Am J Med* 74:38, 1983.

144. Gottschalk WK, Jarett L: Intracellular mediators of insulin action, in DeFronzo RA (ed): *Diabetes/Metabolism Reviews.* New York, Wiley, 1985, p. 229.

145. Czech MP, Kim-Tak Y, Lewis RE et al: Insulin receptor kinase and its mode of signaling membrane components, in DeFronzo RA (ed): *Diabetes/Metabolism Reviews.* New York, Wiley, 1985, p 59.

146. Horuk R, Olefsky JM: Postbinding effects of insulin action, in DeFronzo RA (ed): *Diabetes/Metabolism Reviews.* New York, Wiley, 1985, p 33.

147. Susuki K, Kono T: Evidence that insulin causes translocation of glucose transport activity to the plasma membrane from an intracellular storage site. *Proc Natl Acad Sci USA* 77:2542, 1980.

148. Cushman SW, Wardzala LJ: Potential mechanism of insulin action on glucose transport in the isolated rat adipose cell: Apparent translocation of intracellular transport systems to the plasma membrane. *J Biol Chem* 255:4758, 1980.

148a. Cushman SW, Wardzala LJ, Simpson IA et al: Insulin-induced translocation of intracellular glucose transporters of the isolated rat adipose cell. *Fed Proc* 43:2251, 1984.

149. Denton RM, Brownsey RW, Belsham GJ et al: A partial view of the mechanism of insulin action. *Diabetologia* 21:347, 1981.

150. Gabbay RA, Lardy HA: Site of insulin inhibition of cAMP-stimulated glycogenolysis: cAMP-dependent protein kinase is affected independent of cAMP changes. *J Biol Chem* 259:6052, 1984.

150a. Mato JM, Kelly KL, Abler A, Jarett L: Identification of a novel insulin-sensitive glycophospholipid from H35 hepatoma cells. *J Biol Chem* 262, 1987 (in press).

151. Alexander MC, Kowaloff EM, Witters LA et al: Purification of a 123,000 dalton hormone-stimulated ^{32}P-peptide and its identification as ATP-citrate lyase. *J Biol Chem* 254:8052, 1979.

152. Seals JR, Czech MP: Characterization of a pyruvate dehydrogenase activator released by adipocyte plasma membranes in response to insulin. *J Biol Chem* 256:6529, 1981.

153. Roth J et al: Receptors for insulin, NSILA-S and growth hormone: Applications to disease states in man. *Recent Prog Horm Res* 31:95, 1975.

154. Flier JS, Kahn CR, Roth J: Receptors, antireceptor antibodies and mechanisms of insulin resistance. *N Engl J Med* 300:413, 1979.

155. Hedo JA, McElduff A, Taylor SI: Defects in receptor biosynthesis in patients with genetic forms of extreme insulin resistance. *Trans Assoc Am Physicians* 97:151, 1984.

156. Greenberger G, Zick Y, Gorden P: Defect in phosphorylation of insulin receptors in cells from an insulin resistant patient with insulin binding. *Science* 223:932, 1984.

157. Wachslicht-Rodbard H, Gross HA, Rodbard D, Roth J: Increased insulin binding to erythrocytes in anorexia nervosa: Restoration to normal with refeeding. *N Engl J Med* 300:882, 1979.

158. Olefsky JM: The insulin receptor: Its role in the insulin resistance of obesity and diabetes. *Diabetes* 25:1154, 1976.

158a. Ciaraldi TP, Kolterman OG, Scarlet JA, Olefsky JM: Role of glucose transport in the post-receptor defect of non-insulin-dependent diabetes mellitus. *Diabetes* 31:1016, 1982.

159. DeFronzo RA, Soman V, Sherwin RS et al: Insulin binding to monocytes and insulin action in human obesity, starvation and refeeding. *J Clin Invest* 62:204, 1978.

160. Duckworth WC, Stentz FB, Heinemann M, Kitabchi AE: Initial site of insulin cleavage by insulin protease. *Proc Natl Acad Sci USA* 76:635, 1979.

161. Rabkin R, Simon N, Steiner S, Colwell JA: Effect of renal disease on renal uptake and excretion of insulin in man. *N Engl J Med* 282:182, 1970.

162. Orci L: The microanatomy of the islets of Langerhans. *Metabolism* 25:1303, 1976.

163. Moody AJ, Frandsen EK, Jacobson H et al: The structural and immunologic relationship between gut GLI and glucagon. *Metabolism* 25 (suppl 1):1336, 1976.

164. Ravazzola M, Orci L: Glucagon and glicentin immunoreactivity are topographically segregated in the A granule of the human pancreatic cell. *Nature* 284:66, 1980.

165. Unger RH: Glucagon in diabetes, in Alberti KGMM, Krall LP (eds): *The Diabetes Annual.* New York, Elsevier, 1985, p 480.

166. Moody AJ, Thim L: Glucagon, glicentin and related peptides, in Lefebvre PJ (ed): *Glucagon.* Berlin, Springer-Verlag, 1983, p 139.

167. Kuku SF, Jaspan JB, Emmanouel DS et al: Heterogeneity of plasma glucagon. *J Clin Invest* 58:742, 1976.

168. Barnes AJ, Bloom SR, Alberti KGMM et al: Ketoacidosis in pancreatectomized man. *N Engl J Med* 296:1250, 1977.

169. Koranyi F, Peterfy F, Szabo J et al: Evidence for transformation of glucagon-like immunoreactivity of gut into pancreatic glucagon *in vivo. Diabetes* 30:792, 1981.

170. Holst JJ, Holst-Pedersen J, Baldissera F, Stadil F: Circulating glucagon after total pancreatectomy in man. *Diabetologia* 25:396, 1983.

171. Geraud JC, Elroy R, Moody AJ et al: Glucagon-glicentin immunoreactive cells in the lumen of the digestive tract. *Cell Tissue Res* 213:121, 1980.

172. Boden G, Owen OE: Familial hyperglucagonemia—an autosomal dominant trait. *N Engl J Med* 296:534, 1977.

173. Sherwin RS, Felig P: Glucagon physiology in health and disease, in McCann SM (ed): *International Review of Physiology,* vol 16: *Endocrine Physiology.* Baltimore, University Park, 1977, p 151.

174. Unger RH: Glucagon physiology and pathophysiology in the light of new advances. *Diabetologia* 28:574, 1985.

175. Raskin P, Pietri A, Unger RH: Changes in glucagon levels after four to five weeks of glucoregulation by portable insulin infusion pumps. *Diabetes* 28:1033, 1979.

176. Cherrington AD, Chiasson JL, Liljenquist JE et al: The role of insulin and glucagon in the regulation of basal glucose production in the postabsorptive dog. *J Clin Invest* 58:1407, 1976.

177. Fradkin J, Shamoon H, Felig P, Sherwin RS: Evidence for an important role of changes in rather than absolute concentrations of glucagon in the regulation of glucose production in man. *J Clin Endocrinol Metab* 50:698, 1980.

177a. Komjati M, Bratusch-Marrain P, Waldhausl W: Superior efficacy of pulsatile versus continuous hormone exposure on hepatic glucose production in vitro. *Endocrinology* 118:312, 1986.

178. Felig P, Wahren J, Sherwin RS, Hendler R: Insulin, glucagon and somatostatin in normal physiology and diabetes mellitus. *Diabetes* 25:1091, 1976.

179. Sherwin RS, Fisher M, Hendler R, Felig P: Hyperglucagonemia and blood glucose regulation in normal, obese and diabetic subjects. *N Engl J Med* 294:455, 1976.

180. Rodbell M: The actions of glucagon at its receptor: Regulation of adenylate cyclase, in Lefebvre P (ed): *Glucagon.* Berlin, Springer-Verlag, 1983, p 263.

180a. Rodbell M: Programmable messengers: A new theory of hormone action. *Trends Biochem Sci* 10:461, 1985.

181. Sherwin RS, Fisher M, Bessoff J et al: Hyperglucagonemia in cirrhosis: Altered secretion and sensitivity to glucagon. *Gastroenterology* 74:1224, 1978.

182. Deibert DC, DeFronzo RA: Epinephrine-induced insulin resistance in man. *J Clin Invest* 65:717, 1980.

183. Eigler N, Sacca L, Sherwin RS: Synergistic interactions of physiologic increments of glucagon, epinephrine, and cortisol in the dog. A model for stress-induced hyperglycemia. *J Clin Invest* 63:114, 1979.

184. Sacca L, Sherwin R, Felig P: Influence of somatostatin on glucagon- and epinephrine-stimulated hepatic glucose output in the dog. *Am J Physiol* 236:E113, 1979.

185. Brodows RG, Ensinck JW, Campbell RG: Mechanism of plasma cyclic AMP response to hypoglycemia in man. *Metabolism* 25:659, 1976.

186. Olefsky JM: Effect of dexamethasone on insulin binding, glucose transport and glucose oxidation of isolated rat adipocytes. *J Clin Invest* 56:1499, 1975.

187. Merimee TJ, Felig P, Marliss E et al: Glucose and lipid homeostasis in the absence of human growth hormone. *J Clin Invest* 50:574, 1971.

188. Philips LS, Vassilopoulou-Sellin R: Somatomedin. *N Engl J Med* 302:438, 1980.

189. Zapf J, Rinderknecht E, Humbel RE, Froesch ER: Nonsuppressible insulin-like activity (NSILA) from human serum: Recent accomplishments and their physiologic implications. *Metabolism* 27:1803, 1978.

190. Froesch ER, Zapf J: Insulin-like growth factors and insulin: Comparative aspects. *Diabetologia* 28:485, 1985.

191. Merimee TJ, Zapf J, Froesch ER: Dwarfism in the pygmy: An isolated deficiency of insulin-like growth factor 1. *N Engl J Med* 305:965, 1981.

192. Tomita T, Friesen SR, Kimmel JR et al: Pancreatic polypeptide secreting islet-cell tumors. A study of three cases. *Am J Pathol* 113:134, 1983.

193. Felig P, Sherwin RS et al: Hormonal interactions in the regulation of blood glucose. *Recent Prog Horm Res* 35:501, 1979.

194. Lilavivathana V, Campbell RG, Brodows RG: Control of insulin secretion during fasting in man. *Metabolism* 27:815, 1978.

195. Felig P: The metabolic events of starvation. *Am J Med* 60:117, 1976.

196. Felig P, Wahren J: Fuel homeostasis in exercise. *N Engl J Med* 293:1078, 1975.

197. Sacca L, Sherwin R, Hendler R, Felig P: Influence of continuous physiologic hyperinsulinemia on glucose kinetics and counterregulatory hormones in normal and diabetic humans. *J Clin Invest* 63:849, 1979.

198. Mann RJ: Historical vignette. "Honey urine" to pancreatic diabetes: 600 B.C.–1922. *Mayo Clin Proc* 46:56, 1971.

199. Fajans SS, Cloutier MC, Crowther RL: Clinical and etiologic heterogeneity of idiopathic diabetes mellitus. *Diabetes* 27:1112, 1978.

200. Ganda OP, Soeldner JS: Genetic, acquired and related factors in the etiology of diabetes mellitus. *Arch Intern Med* 137:461, 1977.

201. Craighead JE: Current views on the etiology of insulin-dependent diabetes mellitus. *N Engl J Med* 299:1439, 1978.

202. Zonana J, Rimoin DL: Current concepts in genetics. Inheritance of diabetes mellitus. *N Engl J Med* 295:603, 1976.

203. Wolf E, Spencer KM, Cudworth AG: The genetic susceptibility to type 1 (insulin-dependent) diabetes: Analysis of the HLA-DR association. *Diabetologia* 24:224, 1983.

204. Johnston C, Pyke DA, Cudworth AG, Wolf E: HLA-DR typing in identical twins with insulin-dependent diabetes: Difference between concordant and discordant pairs. *Br Med J* 286:253, 1983.

205. Rotter JI, Anderson CE, Rubin R et al: HLA genotypic study of insulin-dependent diabetes. The excess of DR3/DR4 heterozygotes allows rejection of the recessive hypothesis. *Diabetes* 32:169, 1983.

206. Eberhardt MS, Wagener DK, Orchard TJ et al: HLA heterogeneity of insulin-dependent diabetes mellitus at diagnosis, the Pittsburgh IDDM study. *Diabetes* 34:1247, 1985.

207. Srikanta S, Ganda OP, Jackson RA et al: Pre-type 1 (insulin-dependent) diabetes: Common endocrinological course despite immunological and immunogenetic heterogeneity. *Diabetologia* 27 (suppl 1):146, 1984.

208. Lernmark A, Baekkeskov S, Gerling I et al: Immunological aspects of type 1 and 2 diabetes mellitus. *Adv Exp Med Biol* 189:107, 1985.

209. Spencer KM, Tarn A, Dean BM et al: Fluctuating islet-cell autoimmunity in unaffected relatives of patients with insulin-dependent diabetes. *Lancet* 1:764, 1984.

210. Yoon JW, Notkins AL: Virus-induced diabetes in mice. *Metabolism* 32 (suppl 1):37, 1983.

211. Ginsberg-Fellner F, Witt ME, Franklin BH et al: Triad of markers for identifying children at high risk of developing insulin-dependent diabetes mellitus. *JAMA* 254:1469, 1985.

212. Yoon JW, Morishima T, McClintock PR et al: Virus-induced diabetes mellitus: Mengovirus infects pancreatic beta cells in strains of mice resistant to the diabetogenic effect of encephalomyocarditis virus. *J Virol* 50:684, 1984.

213. Barrett-Connor E: Is insulin-dependent diabetes mellitus caused by coxsackievirus B infection? A review of the epidemiologic evidence. *Rev Infect Dis* 7:207, 1985.

214. Yoon JW, McClintock PR, Bachurski CJ et al: Virus-induced diabetes mellitus. No evidence for immune mechanisms in the destruction of beta-cells by the D-variant of encephalomyocarditis virus. *Diabetes* 34:922, 1985.

215. Yoon JW, Austin M, Onodera T, Notkins AL: Virus-induced diabetes mellitus. Isolation of a virus from the pancreas of a child with diabetic ketoacidosis. *N Engl J Med* 300:1173, 1979.

216. Nerup J, Platz P, Ryder LP et al: HLA, islet cell antibodies and types of diabetes. *Diabetes* 27 (suppl 1):247, 1978.

217. Marner B, Ludvigsson J, MacKay P et al: Islet cell antibodies in insulin-dependent (type 1) diabetic children treated with plasmapheresis. *Diabetes Res* 2:231, 1985.

218. Dyrberg T, Poussier P, Nakhooda F et al: Islet cell surface and lymphocyte antibodies often precede the spontaneous diabetes in the BB rat. *Diabetologia* 26:159, 1984.

219. Powers AC, Eisenbarth GS: Autoimmunity to islet cells in diabetes mellitus. *Annu Rev Med* 36:533, 1985.

220. Toguchi Y, Ginsberg-Fellner F, Rubinstein P: Cytotoxic islet cell surface antibodies (ICSA) in patients with type I diabetes and their first-degree relatives. *Diabetes* 34:855, 1985.

221. Stiller CR, Dupre J, Gent M et al: Effects of cyclosporine immunosuppression in insulin-dependent diabetes of recent onset. *Science* 223:1362, 1985.

222. Feutren G, Papoz L, Assan R et al: Cyclosporin increases the rate and length of remissions in insulin-dependent diabetes of recent onset. *Lancet* 2:119, 1986.

223. Huang SW, MaClaren NK: Insulin-dependent diabetes: A disease of autoaggression. *Science* 192:64, 1976.

224. Srikanta S, Ganda OP, Gleason RE et al: Pre-type I diabetes. Linear loss of beta cell response to intravenous glucose. *Diabetes* 33:717, 1984.

225. Rossini AA, Williams RM, Appel MC, Like AA: Complete protection from low dose streptozotocin-induced diabetes in mice. *Nature* 276:182, 1978.

226. Karam JH, Prosser PR, DeWitt PA: Islet-cell surface antibodies in a patient with diabetes mellitus after rodenticide ingestion. *N Engl J Med* 299:1191, 1978.

227. Like AA, Butler L, Williams RM et al: Spontaneous autoimmune diabetes mellitus in the BB rat. *Diabetes* 31 (suppl 1):7, 1982.

228. Baekkeskov S, Dyrberg T, Lernmark A: Autoantibodies to a 64-kilodalton islet cell protein precede the onset of spontaneous diabetes in the BB rat. *Science* 224:1348, 1984.

229. Marliss EB (ed): The JDF workshop on the spontaneously diabetic BB rat. Its potential for insight into human juvenile diabetes. Banff, Alberta, Canada. *Metabolism* 32 (suppl 1), 1983.

230. Felig P: Insulin is the mediator of feeding-related thermogenesis: Insulin resistance and/or deficiency results in a thermogenic defect which contributes to the pathogenesis of obesity. *Clin Physiol* 4:267, 1984.

231. Pfeifer MA, Halter JB, Porte D Jr: Insulin secretion in diabetes mellitus. *Am J Med* 70:579, 1981.

232. Drucker D, Zinman B: Pathophysiology of beta-cell failure

after prolonged remission in insulin-dependent diabetes mellitus. *Diabetes Care* 1:83, 1984.
233. DeFronzo RA, Hendler R, Simonson D: Insulin resistance is a prominent feature of type 1 (juvenile-onset) diabetes mellitus: *Diabetes* 31:795, 1982.
234. Proietto J, Nankervis A, Aitken P et al: Glucose utilization in type 1 (insulin-dependent) diabetes: Evidence for a defect not reversible with acute duration in insulin. *Diabetologia* 25:331, 1983.
235. Pedersen O, Hjolland E: Insulin receptor binding to fat and blood cells and insulin action in fat cells from insulin dependent diabetes. *Diabetes* 31:706, 1982.
236. Caruso G, Proietto J, Calenti A, Alford F: Insulin resistance in alloxan-diabetic dogs: Evidence for reversal following insulin therapy. *Diabetologia* 25:273, 1983.
237. Kipnis DM: Insulin secretion in normal and diabetic individuals. *Adv Intern Med* 16:103, 1970.
238. Efendic S, Cerasi E, Elander I et al: Studies on low insulin responders. *Acta Endocrinol* 90 (suppl 224):5, 1979.
239. Reaven GM, Bernstein R, Davis B, Olefsky JM: Nonketotic diabetes mellitus: Insulin deficiency or insulin resistance. *Am J Med* 60:80, 1976.
240. Halter JB, Graf RJ, Porte D Jr: Potentiation of insulin secretory responses by plasma glucose levels in man: Evidence that hyperglycemia in diabetes compensates for impaired glucose potentiation. *J Clin Endocrinol Metab* 48:946, 1979.
241. Baron AD, Kolterman OG, Bell J et al: Rates of noninsulin-mediated glucose uptake are elevated in type II diabetic subjects. *J Clin Invest* 76:1782, 1985.
242. DeFronzo RA, Deibert D, Felig P, Soman V: Insulin sensitivity and insulin binding to monocytes in maturity onset diabetes. *J Clin Invest* 63:939, 1979.
243. Kolterman OG, Gray RS, Griffin J et al: Receptor and postreceptor defects contribute to the insulin resistance in non-insulin-dependent diabetes mellitus. *J Clin Invest* 68:957, 1981.
244. DeFronzo RA, Gunnarsson R, Björkman O et al: Effect of insulin on peripheral and splanchnic glucose metabolism in non-insulin-dependent (type II) diabetes mellitus. *J Clin Invest* 76:149, 1985.
245. Olefsky JM, Kolterman OG, Scarlett JA: Insulin action and resistance in obesity and noninsulin-dependent type II diabetes mellitus. *Am J Physiol* 243:E15, 1982.
246. Garvey WT, Olefsky JM, Marshall S: Insulin induces progressive insulin resistance in cultured rat adipocytes. Sequential effects at receptor and multiple postreceptor sites. *Diabetes* 35:258, 1986.
247. Scarlett JA, Kolterman OG, Ciaraldi TP et al: Insulin treatment reverses the postreceptor defect in adipocyte 3-O-methylglucose transport in type II diabetes mellitus. *J Clin Endocrinol Metab* 56:1195, 1983.
248. Revers RR, Fink R, Griffin J et al: Influence of hyperglycemia on insulin's in vivo effects in type II diabetes. *J Clin Invest* 73:664, 1984.
249. Bar RS, Muggeo M, Kahn CR et al: Characterization of the insulin receptors in patients with the syndromes of insulin resistance and acanthosis nigricans. *Diabetologia* 18:209, 1980.
250. Bar RS, Gorden P, Roth J et al: Fluctuations in the affinity and concentration of insulin receptors on circulating monocytes of obese patients: Effects of starvation, refeeding, and dieting. *J Clin Invest* 58:1123, 1976.
251. Taylor SI, Sammuels B, Roth J et al: Decreased insulin binding in cultured lymphocytes from two patients with extreme insulin resistance. *J Clin Endocrinol Metab* 54:919, 1982.
252. Gerich JE, Langlois M, Noacco C et al: Lack of glucagon responses to hypoglycemia in diabetes: Evidence for an intrinsic alpha cell defect. *Science* 182:171, 1973.
253. Sherwin R, Fisher M, Hendler R, Felig P: Hyperglucagonemia and blood glucose regulation in normal, diabetic and obese subjects. *N Engl J Med* 294:455, 1976.
254. Tamborlane WV, Sherwin RS, Koivisto V et al: Normalization of the growth hormone and catecholamine response to exercise in juvenile onset diabetics treated with a portable insulin infusion pump. *Diabetes* 28:785, 1979.
255. Felig P, Wahren J, Hendler R: Influence of maturity onset diabetes on splanchnic glucose balance after oral glucose ingestion. *Diabetes* 27:121, 1978.
256. Felig P, Wahren J: Renal substrate exchange in human diabetes. *Diabetes* 24:730, 1975.
257. Owen OE, Felig P, Morgan AP, Wahren J, Cahill GF Jr: Liver and kidney metabolism during prolonged starvation. *J Clin Invest* 48:574, 1969.
258. Kamm DE, Cahill GF Jr: Effect of acid-base status on renal and hepatic gluconeogenesis in diabetes and fasting. *Am J Physiol* 216:1207, 1969.
259. Pagliara AS, Goodman AD: Relation of renal cortical gluconeogenesis, glutamate content, and production of ammonia. *J Clin Invest* 49:1967, 1970.
260. Buse MG, Hertong HF, Wiegand DA: The effect of diabetes, insulin and the redox potential on leucine metabolism by isolated rat hemidiaphragm. *Endocrinology* 98:1166, 1976.
261. Chase PH, Glasgow AM: Juvenile diabetes mellitus and serum lipids and lipoprotein levels. *Am J Dis Child* 130:1113, 1976.
262. Jones AL, Ruderman NB, Emans JB: An electron microscopic study of hepatic lipoprotein synthesis in the rat following anti-insulin serum, nicotinic acid and puromycin administration. *Gastroenterology* 56:402, 1969.
263. Murthy VK, Shipp JC: Regulation of hepatic triglyceride synthesis in diabetic rats. *J Clin Invest* 67:923, 1981.
264. Brunzell JD, Chait A, Bierman EL: Plasma lipoproteins in human diabetes mellitus, in Alberti KGMM, Krall LP (eds): *Diabetes Annual.* New York, Elsevier, 1985, p 463.
265. Garfinkel AS, Nilsson-Ehle P, Schotz MC: Regulation of lipoprotein lipase induction by insulin. *Biochim Biophys Acta* 424:265, 1976.
266. Cryer A, Riley SE, Williams ER, Robinson DS: Effect of nutritional status on rat adipose tissue, muscle and post-heparin plasma clearing factor lipase activities: Their relationship to triglyceride fatty acid uptake by fat-cells and to plasma insulin concentrations. *Clin Sci Mol Med* 50:213, 1976.
267. Lithel H, Boberg J, Hellsing K et al: Lipoprotein lipase activity in human skeletal muscle and adipose tissue in the fasting and fed states. *Atherosclerosis* 30:89, 1978.
268. Nikkila EA, Torsti P, Pentila O: The effect of exercise on lipoprotein lipase activity of rat heart, adipose tissue and skeletal muscle. *Metabolism* 12:863, 1963.
269. Krausz Y, Bar-On H, Shafrir E: Origin and pattern of glucocorticoid-induced hyperlipidemia in rats. Dose-dependent bimodal changes in serum lipids and lipoproteins in relation to hepatic lipogenesis and tissue lipoprotein lipase activity. *Biochim Biophys Acta* 663:69, 1981.
270. Bar-On H, Oschry Y, Levy E et al: Removal defect of very low density lipoproteins from diabetic rats. *Biochim Biophys Acta* 793:115, 1984.
271. Levy E, Shafrir E, Ziv E, Bar-On H: Composition, removal and metabolic fate of chylomicrons derived from diabetic rats. *Biochim Biophys Acta* 834:376, 1985.
272. Taskinen MR, Nikkila EA, Ollas A: Serum lipids and lipoproteins in insulin-dependent diabetic subjects during high-carbohydrate, high-fiber diet. *Diabetes Care* 6:224, 1983.
273. Hollenbeck CB, Connor WE, Riddle MC et al: The effects of a high-carbohydrates, low-fat cholesterol-restricted diet on plasma lipid, lipoproteins, and apoprotein concentrations in insulin-dependent (type 1) diabetes mellitus. *Metabolism* 34:559, 1985.
274. Fraze E, Donner CC, Swislock et al: Ambient plasma free fatty acid concentrations in noninsulin-dependent diabetes mellitus: Evidence for insulin resistance. *J Clin Endocrinol Metab* 61:807, 1985.
275. Nestel PJ, Whyte HM: Plasma free fatty acid and triglyceride

turnover in obesity. *Metabolism* 17:1122, 1968.

276. Birkenhager JC, Tjabbes T: Turnover rate of plasma FFA and rate of esterification of plasma FFA to plasma triglycerides in obese humans before and after weight reduction. *Metabolism* 18:18, 1969.

277. Nikkila EA, Kekki M: Plasma triglyceride transport kinetics in diabetes mellitus. *Metabolism* 22:1, 1973.

278. Taskinen MR, Bogardus C, Kennedy A, Howard BV: Multiple disturbances of free fatty acid metabolism in noninsulin-dependent diabetes. *J Clin Invest* 76:637, 1985.

279. Saudek CD, Brach EL: Cholesterol metabolism in diabetes: I. The effect of diabetic control on sterol balance. *Diabetes* 27:1059, 1978.

280. Barrett-Connor E, Grundy SM, Holdbrook MJ: Plasma lipids and diabetes mellitus. *Am J Epidemiol* 115:657, 1982.

281. Feingold KR, Lear SR, Moser AH: De novo cholesterol synthesis in three different animal models of diabetes. *Diabetologia* 26:234, 1984.

282. Brownlee M, Vlassara H, Cerami A: Nonenzymatic glycosylation products of collagen covalently trap low-density lipoprotein. *Diabetes* 34:938, 1985.

283. Bergman M, Gidez LI, Eder HA: High density lipoprotein subclasses in diabetes. *Am J Med* 81:488, 1986.

284. Bergman M, Gidez LI, Eder HA: The effect of glipizide on HDL and HDL subclasses. *Diabetes Res,* 3:245, 1986.

285. Briones ER, Mao SJT, Palumbo PJ et al: Analysis of plasma lipids and apolipoproteins in insulin-dependent and non-insulin-dependent diabetes. *Metabolism* 33:42, 1984.

285a. Laakso M, Voutilainen E, Pyörälä K, Sarlund H: Association of low HDL and HDL_2 cholesterol with coronary heart disease in noninsulin-dependent diabetics. *Arteriosclerosis* 5:653, 1985.

286. Sherwin RS: Limitations of the oral glucose tolerance test in the diagnosis of early diabetes. *Primary Care* 44:255, 1977.

287. Wilkerson HLC, Hyman H, Kaufman M et al: Diagnostic evaluation of oral glucose tolerance tests in nondiabetic subjects after various levels of carbohydrate intake. *N Engl J Med* 262:1047, 1960.

288. Andres R: Aging and diabetes. *Med Clin North Am* 55:835, 1971.

289. Davidson MB: The effect of aging carbohydrate metabolism: A review of the English literature and a practical approach to the diagnosis of diabetes mellitus in the elderly. *Metabolism* 28:688, 1979.

290. Lohmann D, Liebold F, Heilmann W: Diminished insulin response in highly trained athletes. *Metabolism* 27:521, 1978.

291. O'Sullivan JB, Mahan CM: Prospective study of 352 young patients with chemical diabetes. *N Engl J Med* 278:1038, 1968.

292. Sayegh HA, Jarrett RJ: Oral glucose-tolerance tests and the diagnosis of diabetes: Results of a prospective study based on the Whitehall survey. *Lancet* 2:431, 1979.

293. Bennett PH: Epidemiologic studies of diabetes in the Pima Indians. *Recent Prog Horm Res* 31:333, 1976.

294. Sisk CW, Burnham CE, Stewart J, McDonald GW: Comparison of the 50 and 100 gram oral glucose tolerance test. *Diabetes* 19:852, 1970.

295. Shafrir E, Gutman A: Patterns of decrease of free fatty acids during glucose tolerance tests. *Diabetes* 14:77, 1965.

296. Keen H, Jarrett RJ, Fuller JH: Tolbutamide and arterial disease in borderline diabetics, in Mallaise W, Pirart J (eds): *Diabetes,* International Congress Series. Amsterdam, Excerpta Medica, 1974, no 312, p 588.

297. Koenig RJ, Peterson CM, Jones RL et al: Correlation of glucose regulation and hemoglobin A in diabetes mellitus. *N Engl J Med* 295:417, 1976.

298. Gabbay KH, Sosenko JM, Banuchi GA et al: Glycosylated hemoglobins: Increased glycosylation of hemoglobin A in diabetic patients. *Diabetes* 28:337, 1979.

299. Mehl TD, Wenzel SE, Russell B et al: Comparison of two indices of glycemic control in diabetic subjects: Glycosylated serum protein and hemoglobin. *Diabetes Care* 6:34, 1983.

300. Schleicher ED, Gerbitz KD, Dolhofer R et al: Clinical utility of nonenzymatically glycosylated blood proteins as an index of glucose control. *Diabetes Care* 7:548, 1984.

301. Little RR, England JD, Wiedmeyer HM, Goldstein DE: Glycosylated hemoglobin measured by affinity chromatography: Microsample collection and room temperature storage. *Clin Chem* 29:1080, 1983.

302. Gepts W: Sequential changes in the cytological composition of the pancreatic islets in juvenile diabetes, in Bajaj JS (ed): *Diabetes,* International Congress Series. Amsterdam, Excerpta Medica, 1977, p 299.

303. Karam JH, Rosenthal M, O'Donnell JL et al: Discordance of diabetic microangiopathy in identical twins. *Diabetes* 25:24, 1976.

304. Kalant N: Diabetic glomerulosclerosis: Current status. *Can Med Assoc J* 119:146, 1978.

305. Kohner EM: Diabetic retinopathy. *Clin Endocrinol Metab* 6:345, 1977.

306. Bronstein HD, Kantrowitz P, Schaffner R: Marked enlargement of the liver and transient ascites associated with the treatment of diabetic acidosis. *N Engl J Med* 261:1314, 1959.

307. Levin ME, Boisseau AV, Avioli LV: Effects of diabetes mellitus on bone mass in juvenile and adult onset diabetes. *N Engl J Med* 294:241, 1976.

308. L'Esperance F: Diabetic retinopathy. *Med Clin North Am* 62:767, 1978.

309. The Diabetic Retinopathy Study Group: Four risk factors for severe visual loss in diabetic retinopathy. *Arch Ophthalmol* 97:654, 1979.

310. Patz A: Current concepts in ophthalmology. Retinal vascular diseases. *N Engl J Med* 298:1451, 1978.

311. Charles S: Pars plana vitrectomy for traction retinal detachment, in Little HL et al (eds): *Diabetic Retinopathy.* New York, Thieme-Stratton, 1984, p 305.

312. Christiansen JS, Gammelguard J, Troneir B et al: Kidney function and size in diabetes before and during initial insulin treatment. *Kidney Int* 21:683, 1982.

313. Hostetter TH, Troy JL, Brenner BM: Glomerular hemodynamics in experimental diabetes mellitus. *Kidney Int* 19:410, 1981.

314. Hostetter TH, Rennke HG, Brenner BM: The case for intrarenal hypertension in the initiation and progression of diabetic and other glomerulopathies. *Am J Med* 72:375, 1982.

315. Zatz R, Meyer TW, Rennke HG, Brenner BM: Predominance of hemodynamic rather than metabolic factors in the pathogenesis of diabetic glomerulopathy. *Proc Natl Acad Sci USA* 82:5967, 1985.

316. Wiseman MJ, Saunders AJ, Keen H, Viberti GC: Effect of blood glucose control on increased glomerular filtration rate and kidney size in insulin-dependent diabetes. *N Engl J Med* 312:617, 1985.

317. Mauer SM, Steffes MW, Ellis EN et al: Structural-functional relationship in diabetic nephropathy. *J Clin Invest* 74:1143, 1984.

318. Friedman S, Jones HW, Golbetz HV et al: Mechanism of proteinuria in diabetic neuropathy II: A study of size selective glomerular filtration barrier. *Diabetes* 32 (suppl 2):40, 1983.

319. Beisswenger PJ, Spiro RG: Studies on the human glomerular basement membrane. Composition, nature of the carbohydrate units and chemical changes in diabetes mellitus. *Diabetes* 22:180, 1973.

320. Schober E, Pollak A, Coradello H, Lubec G: Glycosylation of glomerular basement membrane in type I (insulin-dependent) diabetic children. *Diabetologia* 23:485, 1982.

321. Cohen MP, Surma ML: [^{35}S]Sulfate incorporation into glomerular basement membrane glycosaminoglycans is decreased in experimental diabetes. *J Lab Clin Med* 98:715, 1981.

322. Osterby R: Early phases in the development of diabetic glomerulopathy. A quantitative electron microscopic study. *Acta Med Scand* (suppl) 574:3, 1974.

323. Mogensen CE, Christensen CK: Predicting diabetic nephrop-

athy in insulin-dependent patients. *N Engl J Med* 311:89, 1984.

324. Viberti GC, Jarrett RJ, Mahmud U et al: Microalbuminuria as a predictor of clinical nephropathy in insulin-dependent diabetes mellitus. *Lancet* 1:1430, 1982.

325. Parving HH, Oxenboll B, Svensen PA et al: Early detection of patients at risk of developing diabetic nephropathy: A longitudinal study of urinary albumin excretion. *Acta Endocrinol* 100:550, 1982.

326. Mogensen CE, Christensen CK, Vittinghus E: The stages of diabetic renal disease with emphasis on the state of incipient diabetic nephropathy. *Diabetes* 32 (suppl 2):64, 1983.

327. Viberti GC, Bilous RW, Mackintosh D: Long term correction of hyperglycemia and progression of renal failure in insulin dependent diabetes. *Br Med J* 286:598, 1983.

328. Goldstein DA, Massry SG: Diabetic nephropathy. Clinical course and effect of hemodialysis. *Nephron* 20:286, 1978.

329. Kamdar A, Wiedmann P, Makoff DL, Massry SG: Acute renal failure following intravenous use of radiographic contrast dyes in patients with diabetes mellitus. *Diabetes* 26:643, 1977.

330. Parving HH, Smidt UM, Andersen AR, Svendsen PA: Early aggressive anti-hypertensive treatment reduces rate of decline in kidney function in diabetic nephropathy. *Lancet* 1:1175, 1983.

331. Mogensen CE: Long-term antihypertensive treatment inhibiting progression of diabetic nephropathy. *Br Med J* 285:685, 1982.

332. Amair P, Khanna R, Leibel B et al: Continuous ambulatory peritoneal dialysis in diabetics with end-stage disease. *N Engl J Med* 306:625, 1982.

333. Mauer MS, Barbosa J, Vernier RL et al: Development of diabetic vascular lesions in normal kidneys transplanted into patients with diabetes mellitus. *N Engl J Med* 295:916, 1976.

334. Sutherland DER, Morrow CE et al: Improved patient and primary renal allograft survival in uremic diabetic recipients. *Transplantation* 34:319, 1982.

335. Khauli RB, Norick AC, Brawn WE et al: Improved results of cadaver renal transplantation in the diabetic patient. *J Urol* 130:867, 1983.

336. Braddom RL, Hollis JB, Castell DO: Diabetic peripheral neuropathy. A correlation of nerve conduction studies and clinical findings. *Arch Phys Med Rehabil* 58:308, 1977.

337. Ward JD, Fisher DJ, Barnes CG et al: Improvement in nerve conduction following treatment in newly diagnosed diabetics. *Lancet* 1:428, 1971.

338. Winegrad AI, Morrison AD, Greene DA: Late complications of diabetes, in DeGroot LJ, Cahill GF Jr et al (eds): *Endocrinology*. New York, Grune & Stratton, 1979, vol 2 p 1041.

339. Ewing DJ, Campbell IW, Clarke BF: Heart rate changes in diabetes mellitus. *Lancet* 1:183, 1981.

340. Smith SA, Smith SE: Reduced papillary light reflexes in diabetic autoimmune neuropathy. *Diabetologia* 24:330, 1983.

341. Campbell IW, Ewing DJ, Anderson JD: Plasma renin activity in diabetic autonomic neuropathy. *Eur J Clin Invest* 6:381, 1976.

342. Ellenberg M: Importance in diabetes: The neurologic factor. *Ann Intern Med* 75:213, 1971.

343. Longstreth GF, Malagelada JR, Kelly KA: Metoclopramide stimulation of gastric mobility and emptying in diabetic gastroparesis. *Ann Intern Med* 86:195, 1977.

344. Ellenberg M: Diabetic neuropathic cachexia. *Diabetes* 23:418, 1974.

345. Crall FV, Roberts WC: The extramural and intramural coronary arteries in juvenile diabetes mellitus. *Am J Med* 64:221, 1978.

346. Saunders RN: Platelets and atherosclerosis. *Prog Drug Res* 29:49, 1985.

347. Colwell JA, Nair RMG, Halushka PV et al: Platelet adhesion and aggregation in diabetes mellitus. *Metabolism* 28 (suppl 1):394, 1979.

348. Curtiss LK, Witztum JL: Plasma apolipoproteins AI, AII, B, C, and E are glucosylated in hyperglycemic diabetes subjects. *Diabetes* 34:452, 1985.

349. Braverman IM: Cutaneous manifestations of diabetes mellitus. *Med Clin North Am* 55:1019, 1971.

350. Battock DT, Grausz H, Bobrowsky M, Littman ML: Alternate-day amphotericin B therapy in the treatment of rhinocerebral phycomycosis (mucormycosis). *Ann Intern Med* 68:122, 1968.

351. Bagdade JD, Nielson K, Root R, Bulger R: Host defense in diabetes mellitus: The feckless phagocyte during poor control and ketoacidosis. *Diabetes* 19:364, 1970.

352. Ingelfinger FJ: Debates on diabetes. *N Engl J Med* 296:1228, 1977.

353. Cahill GF, Etzwiler DD, Freinkel N: "Control" and diabetes. *N Engl J Med* 294:1004, 1976.

354. Siperstein MD, Foster DW, Knowles HC et al: Control of blood glucose and diabetic vascular disease. *N Engl J Med* 296:1060, 1977.

355. Siperstein MD, Unger RH, Madison LL: Studies of muscle capillary basement membranes in normal subjects, diabetic and prediabetic patients. *J Clin Invest* 47:1973, 1968.

356. Kilo C, Vogler N, Williamson JR: Muscle capillary basement membrane changes related to aging and to diabetes mellitus. *Diabetes* 21:881, 1972.

357. Barnett AH, Spiliopoulos AJ, Pyke DA: Muscle capillary basement membrane in identical twins discordant for insulin-dependent diabetes. *Diabetes* 32:557, 1983.

358. Steffes MW, Sutherland DER, Goetz FC: Studies of kidney and muscle biopsy specimens from identical twins discordant for type I diabetes mellitus. *N Engl J Med* 312:1282, 1985.

359. Bennett PH: The basement membrane controversy. *Diabetologia* 16:280, 1979.

359a. Feingold KR, Lee TH, Chung MY, Siperstein MD: Muscle capillary membrane width in patients with Vacor-induced diabetes mellitus. *J Clin Invest* 78:102, 1986.

360. Ireland JT, Patnaik BK, Duncan LJP: Glomerular ultrastructure in secondary diabetics and normal subjects. *Diabetes* 16:628, 1967.

361. Pietri A, Ehle AL, Raskin P: Changes in nerve conduction velocity after six weeks of glucoregulation with portable insulin infusion pumps. *Diabetes* 29:668, 1980.

362. Winegrad AI: Does a common mechanism induce the diverse complications of diabetes? *Diabetes* 36, 1987 (in press).

363. Simmonds DA, Winegrad AI, Martin DB: Significance of tissue myoinositol concentrations in metabolic regulation in nerve. *Science* 217:848, 1982.

364. Finegold D, Lattimer SA, Nolle S et al: Polyol pathway activity and myo-inositol metabolism. A suggested relationship in the pathogenesis of diabetic neuropathy. *Diabetes* 32:988, 1983.

365. Clements RS Jr, Vourganti B, Kuba T et al: Dietary myo-inostiol intake and peripheral nerve function in diabetic neuropathy. *Metabolism* 28:477, 1979.

366. Gillon RKW, Hawthorne JN, Tomlinson DR: Myo-inositol and sorbitol metabolism in relation to peripheral nerve function in experimental diabetes in the rat: The effect of aldose reductase inhibition. *Diabetologia* 25:365, 1983.

367. Green DA, Lattimer SA: Impaired rat sciatic nerve sodium-potassium adenosine triphosphatase in acute streptozotocin diabetes and its correction by dietary myo-inositol supplementation. *J Clin Invest* 72:1058, 1983.

368. Cohen MP: Aldose reductase, glomerular metabolism, and diabetic nephropathy. *Metabolism* 35(suppl 1):55, 1986.

369. Summerfield JA, Vergalla J, Jones EA: Modulation of a glycoprotein recognition system on rat hepatic endothelial cells by glucose and diabetes mellitus. *J Clin Invest* 69:1337, 1982.

370. Jones RL, Peterson CM: Hematologic alterations in diabetes mellitus. *Am J Med* 70:339, 1981.

371. Dolhofer R, Siess EA, Wieland OH: Nonenzymatic glycation

of immunoglobulins leads to an impairment of immunoreactivity. *Biol Chem Hoppe Seylers* 366:361, 1985.

372. Brownlee M, Vlassara H, Cerami A: Nonenzymatic glycosylation reduces the susceptibility of fibrin to degradation by plasma. *Diabetes* 32:680, 1983.

373. Davies MJ, Woolf N, Carstairs KC: Immunohistochemical studies in diabetic glomerulosclerosis. *J Pathol Bacteriol* 92:441, 1966.

374. Liang JN, Hershorin LL, Chylack LT Jr: Non-enzymatic glycosylation in human diabetic lens crystellins. *Diabetologia* 29:225, 1986.

375. Schnider SL, Kohn RR: Effects of age and diabetes mellitus on the solubility and nonenzymatic glucosylation of human skin collagen. *J Clin Invest* 67:1630, 1981.

376. Petersen CM, Jones RL, Koenig RJ et al: Reversible hematologic sequelae of diabetes mellitus. *Ann Intern Med* 86:425, 1977.

377. Schmid-Schonbein H, Volger E: Red-cell aggregation and red-cell deformability in diabetes. *Diabetes* 25 (suppl 2):897, 1976.

378. McMillan DE, Utterback NG, La Puma J: Reduced erythrocyte deformability in diabetes. *Diabetes* 27:895, 1978.

379. Kohner EM, McLeod D, Marshall J: Diabetic eye disease, in Keen H, Jarrett J, (eds): *Complications of Diabetes.* London, Edward Arnold, 1982, p 19.

380. Mowat AG, Baum J: Chemotaxis of polymorphonuclear leukocytes from patients with diabetes mellitus. *N Engl J Med* 248:621, 1971.

381. Tan JS, Anderson JL, Watanakunakorn C et al: Neutrophil dysfunction in diabetes mellitus. *J Lab Clin Med* 85:26, 1975.

382. Bagdade JD: Phagocytic and microbicidal function in diabetes mellitus. *Acta Endocrinol* 83(suppl 205):27, 1976.

383. Bassiouny AR, Rosenberg H, McDonald TL: Glucosylated collagen is antigenic. *Diabetes* 32:1182, 1983.

384. Merimee TJ: A follow-up study of vascular disease in growth-hormone-deficient dwarfs with diabetes. *N Engl J Med* 298:1217, 1978.

385. Johnsson S: Retinopathy and nephropathy in diabetes mellitus. Comparison of the effects of two forms of treatment. *Diabetes* 9:18, 1960.

386. Pirart J: Diabetes mellitus and its degenerative complications: A prospective study of 4400 patients observed between 1947 and 1973. *Diabetes Care* 1:168, 1:252, 1978.

387. Eschwege E, Job D, Guyot-Argenton C et al: Delayed progression of diabetic retinopathy by divided insulin administration: A further followup. *Diabetologia* 16:131, 1979.

388. Lauritzen T, Larsen HW, Frost-Larsen K, Deckert T, the Steno Study Group: Effect of 1 year of near-normal blood gluose levels on retinopathy in insulin-dependent diabetics. *Lancet* 1:200, 1983.

389. Tasaka Y, Sekine M, Wakatsuki M et al: Levels of pancreatic glucagon, insulin and glucose during twenty-four hours of the day in normal subjects. *Horm Metab Res* 7:205, 1975.

390. Service FJ, Molnar GD, Rosevear JW et al: Mean amplitude of glycemic excursions, a measure of diabetic instability. *Diabetes* 19:644, 1970.

391. Sonksen PH, Judd SL, Lowy C: Home monitoring of blood glucose. Method for improving diabetic control. *Lancet* 1:729, 1979.

392. Engerman R, Bloodworth JMB Jr, Nelson S: Relationship of microvascular disease in diabetes to metabolic control. *Diabetes* 26:760, 1977.

393. Mauer SM, Steffes MW, Sutherland DER: Studies of the rate of regression of glomerular lesion in diabetic rats treated with pancreatic transplantation. *Diabetes* 24:280, 1975.

394. Bretzel RG, Brocks DG, Federlin KF: Reversal and prevention of nephropathy by islet transplantation in diabetic rats, in Shafrir E, Renold AE (eds): *Lessons from Animal Diabetes.* London, Libbey, 1984, p 425.

395. Lee SM: Experimental diabetic nephropathy in the db/db mouse. Dietary and pharmacologic therapy, in Shafrir E, Renold AE (eds): *Lessons from Animal Diabetes.* London, Libbey, 1984, p 419.

396. Clements RS Jr, Stockard CR: Abnormal sciatic nerve myoinositol metabolism in the streptozotocin-diabetic rat. *Diabetes* 29:227, 1980.

397. Protocol for the clinical trial to assess the relationship between metabolic control and early vascular complications of insulin-dependent diabetics. *Diabetes* 31:1132, 1982.

398. The KROC Study Group: Blood glucose control and the evolution of diabetic retinopathy and albuminuria. *N Engl J Med* 31:365, 1984.

399. Tamborlane WV, Hintz RL, Bergman M et al: Insulin infusion pump treatment of diabetes: Influence of improved metabolic control on plasma somatomedin levels. *N Engl J Med* 305:303, 1981.

400. Tamborlane WV, Puklin J, Bergman M et al: Long-term improvement of metabolic control with the insulin pump does not reverse diabetic microangiopathy. *Diabetes Care* 5 (suppl 1):58, 1982.

401. Holman RR, Dornan TL, Mayor-White V et al: Prevention of deterioration of renal and sensory nerve function by more intensive management of insulin-dependent diabetic patients. A two-year randomized prospective study. *Lancet* 1:204, 1983.

402. Raskin P, Pietri AO, Unger R et al: The effect of diabetic control on the width of skeletal-muscle capillary basement membrane in patients with type I diabetes mellitus. *N Engl J Med* 309:1546, 1983.

403. Mauer SM, Miller K, Goetz FC et al: Immunopathology of renal extracellular membranes in kidneys transplanted into patients with diabetes mellitus. *Diabetes* 25:709, 1976.

404. Abouna GM, Kremer GD, Daddah SK et al: Reversal of diabetic nephropathy in human cadaveric kidneys after transplantation into non-diabetic recipients. *Lancet* 2:1274, 1983.

405. Knowles H: Long-term juvenile diabetes treated with unmeasured diet. *Trans Assoc Am Physicians* 85:95, 1971.

406. Dorman JS, LaPorte RE: Mortality in insulin-dependent diabetes, in *Diabetes in America,* NIH publication 85-1468. U.S. Government Printing Office, 1985.

407. Felig P, Bergman M: Insulin pump treatment of diabetes. *JAMA* 250:1045, 1983.

408. Tattersall RB: Self-monitoring of blood glucose 1978–1984, in Alberti KGMM, Krall LP (eds): *Diabetes Annual.* New York, Elsevier, 1985, vol 1.

409. Mazze RS, Shammoon H, Pasmantier R et al: Reliability of blood glucose monitoring by patients with diabetes mellitus. *Am J Med* 77:211, 1984.

410. Fineberg SE, Galloway JA, Fineberg NS et al: Immunogenicity of recombinant DNA human insulin. *Diabetologia* 25:465, 1983.

411. Revers RR, Henry R, Schmeiser L et al: The effects of biosynthetic human proinsulin on carbohydrate metabolism. *Diabetes* 33:762, 1984.

412. Cryer PE, Gerich JE: Glucose counterregulation, hypoglycemia, and intensive insulin therapy in diabetes mellitus. *N Engl J Med* 25:232, 1985.

413. Campbell PJ, Bolli GB, Cryer PE, Gerich JE: Pathogenesis of the dawn phenomenon in patients with insulin-dependent diabetes mellitus. *N Engl J Med* 312:1473, 1985.

414. Bergman M, Felig P: Self-monitoring of blood glucose levels in diabetes. Principles and practice. *Arch Intern Med* 144:2029, 1984.

415. Felig P, Bergman M: Intensive ambulatory treatment of insulin-dependent diabetes. *Ann Intern Med* 97:225, 1982.

416. Felig P, Bergman M: Newer approaches to the control of the insulin-dependent diabetic patient. *Disease-A-Month* 29: No 7, 1983.

417. Pickup JC, White MC, Keen H et al: Long-term continuous subcutaneous insulin infusions in diabetics at home. *Lancet* 2:870, 1979.

418. Tamborlane WV, Sherwin RS, Genel H, Felig P: Restoration

of normal lipid and amino acid metabolism in diabetic patients treated with a portable insulin infusion pump. *Lancet* 1:1258, 1979.

419. Tamborlane WV, Sherwin RS, Genel M, Felig P: Outpatient treatment of juvenile-onset diabetes with a preprogrammed portable subcutaneous insulin infusion system. *Am J Med* 68:190, 1980.

420. Conference on Insulin Pump Therapy in Diabetes: Multicenter Study of Effect on Microvascular Disease. Wilson RN (ed): *Diabetes* 35(suppl 3), 1985.

421. Clarke W, Haymond M, Santiago J: Overnight basal insulin requirements in fasting insulin-dependent diabetes. *Diabetes* 29:78, 1980.

422. Service F, Rizza R, Westand R et al: Considerations for the programming of an open-loop insulin infusion device from the biostator glucose controller. *Diabetes Care* 3:278, 1980.

423. Buysschaert M, Marchand E, Ketelslagers JM, Lambert AE: Comparison of plasma glucose and plasma free insulin during CSII and intensified conventional insulin therapy. *Diabetes Care* 6:1, 1983.

424. Peden NR, Braaten JT, McKendry JBR: Diabetic ketoacidosis during long-term treatment with continuous subcutaneous insulin infusion. *Diabetes Care* 7:1, 1984.

425. Lougheed WD, Woulfe-Flanagan H, Clement JR, Albisser AM: Insulin aggregation in artificial delivery systems. *Diabetologia* 19:1, 1980.

426. Freedman DJ, Wolfe BM, Mascarennas M: Ketoacidosis resulting from precipitation of insulin in syringe used for delivery of constant subcutaneous insulin infusion. *Lancet* 1:828, 1983.

427. Mecklenburg RS, Guinn TS: Complications of insulin pump therapy: The effect of insulin preparation. *Diabetes Care* 8:367, 1985.

428. Teutsch SM, Herman WH, Dweyer DM, Lane JM: Mortality among diabetic patients using continuous subcutaneous insulin infusion. *N Engl J Med* 310:361, 1984.

429. Beck-Neilsen H, Richelson B, Mogensen CE et al: Effect of insulin pump treatment for one year on renal function and retinal morphology in patients with IDDM. *Diabetes Care* 8:585, 1985.

430. Lauritzen T, Frost-Larsen K, Larsen HW, Deckut T, the Steno Study Group: Continuous subcutaneous insulin. *Lancet* 1:1445, 1983.

431. Goldgewicht C, Slama G, Papoz L, Tchobroutsky G: Hypoglycaemic reactions in 172 type I (insulin-dependent) diabetic patients. *Diabetologia* 24:95, 1983.

432. Turnbridge WMG: Factors contributing to deaths of diabetics under fifty years of age. *Lancet* 2:569, 1981.

433. Gale EAM, Tattersall RB: Unrecognized nocturnal hypoglycemia in insulin-treated diabetics. *Lancet* 1:1049, 1979.

434. DeFronzo R, Hendler R, Christensen N: Stimulation of counterregulatory hormonal responses in diabetic man by a fall in glucose concentration. *Diabetes* 29:125, 1980.

435. Bolli GB, De Feo P, De Cosmo S et al: A reliable and reproducible test for adequate glucose counterregulation in type I diabetes mellitus. *Diabetes* 33:732, 1984.

436. Bolli GB, Gottesman IS, Campbell PJ et al: Glucose counterregulation and waning of insulin in the Somogyi phenomenon (posthypoglycemic hyperglycemia). *N Engl J Med* 311:1214, 1984.

437. Cherrington AD, Fuchs H, Stevenson RW et al: Effect of epinephrine on glycogenolysis and gluconeogenesis in conscious overnight-fasted dogs. *Am J Physiol* 247:E362, 1984.

438. Gale EAM, Kurtz AB, Tattersall RB: In search of the Somogyi effect. *Lancet* 2:279, 1980.

439. Porte D Jr: Sympathetic regulation of insulin secretion. Its relations to diabetes mellitus. *Arch Intern Med* 123:252, 1969.

439a. Campbell PJ, Gerich JE: Occurrence of dawn phenomenon without change in insulin clearance in patients with insulin-dependent diabetes mellitus. *Diabetes* 35:749, 1986.

440. Dandona P, Foster M, Healey F et al: Low dose insulin infusions in diabetic patients with high insulin requirements. *Lancet* 2:283, 1978.

441. Schade DA, Drumm DA, Eaton RP, Sterling WA: Factitious brittle diabetes mellitus. *Am J Med* 78:777, 1985.

442. West KM: Diet therapy of diabetes: An analysis of failure. *Ann Intern Med* 79:425, 1973.

443. Archer JA, Gorden P, Roth J: Defect in insulin binding to receptors in obese man. Amelioration with caloric restriction. *J Clin Invest* 55:166, 1976.

444. Jenkins DJA: Lente carbohydrate: A new approach to the dietary management of diabetes. *Diabetes Care* 5:634, 1982.

444a. Crapo PA, Scarlett JA, Kolterman OG: Comparison of the metabolic responses to fructose and sucrose sweetened foods. *Am J Clin Nutr* 36:256, 1982.

444b. Bantle JP, Laine DC, Castle GW et al: Postprandial glucose and insulin responses to meals containing different carbohydrates in normal and diabetic subjects. *N Engl J Med* 309:7, 1983.

445. Anderson JW, Ward K: High carbohydrate, high fiber diets for insulin-treated men with diabetes mellitus. *Am J Clin Nutr* 32:2312, 1979.

446. Anderson JW, Chen WL: Plant fiber carbohydrate and lipid metabolism. *Am J Clin Nutr* 32:346, 1979.

447. Crapo PA, Reaven G, Olefsky J: Post-prandial plasma-glucose and insulin responses to different complex carbohydrates. *Diabetes* 26:1178, 1977.

448. Wahren J, Juhlin-Dannfelt A, Bjorkman O et al: Influence of fibre ingestion on carbohydrate utilization and absorption. *Clin Physiol* 2:315, 1982.

449. Kreisberg RA: The second-generation sulfonylureas: Change or progress? *Ann Intern Med* 102:125, 1985.

449a. Pfeifer MA, Halter JB, Judzewitsch RG et al: Acute and chronic effect of sulfonylurea drugs on pancreatic islet function in man. *Diabetes Care* 7 (suppl 1):25, 1984.

450. Olefsky JM, Reaven GM: Effects of sulfonylurea therapy on insulin binding to mononuclear leukocytes of diabetic patients. *Am J Med* 60:89, 1976.

450a. Judzewitsch RG, Pfeifer MA, Best JD et al: Chronic chlorpropamide therapy of noninsulin-olepeudent diabetes augments basal and stimulated insulin secretion by increasing islet sensitivity to glucose. *J Clin Endocrinol Metab* 55:321, 1982.

451. Scarlett JA, Gray RS, Griffin J et al: Insulin treatment reverses the insulin resistance of type II diabetes mellitus. *Diabetes Care* 5:353, 1982.

451a. Firth RG, Bell PM, Rizza RA: Effects of tolazamide and exogenous insulin on insulin action in patients with non-insulin-dependent diabetes mellitus. *N Engl J Med* 314:1280, 1986.

452. Shen SW, Bressler R: Clinical pharmacology of oral antidiabetic agents. *N Engl J Med* 296:493, 1977.

453. Jackson JE, Bressler R: Clinical pharmacology of sulfonylurea hypoglycemic agents. *Drugs* 22:211, 22:295, 1981.

454. Skillman TG, Feldman JM: The pharmacology of sulfonylureas. *Am J Med* 70:361, 1981.

455. Moses AM, Numann P, Miller M: Mechanism of chlorpropamide-induced antidiuresis in man: Evidence for release of ADH and enhancement of peripheral action. *Metabolism* 22:59, 1973.

456. Kadowaki T, Hagura R, Kajin H et al: Chlorpropamide-induced hyponatremia: Incidence and risk factors. *Diabetes Care* 6:468, 1983.

457. Appel GB, D'Agati V, Bergman M, Pirani CL: Nephrotic syndrome and immune complex glomerulonephritis associated with chlorpropamide therapy. *Am J Med* 74:377, 1983.

458. Johnston C, Wiles PG, Pyke DA: Chlorpropamide-alcohol flush: The case in favour. *Diabetologia* 26:1, 1981.

459. Hillson RM, Hockaday TNR: Chlorpropamide-alcohol flush: A critical reappraisal. *Diabetologia* 26:6, 1984.

460. The University Group Diabetes Program: A study of the effects of hypoglycemic agents on vascular complications in patients with maturity-onset diabetes. *Diabetes* 19 (suppl 2):747, 1970.

461. Natrass M, Todd PG, Hinks L: Comparative effects of phenformin, metformin, and glibenclamide on metabolic rhythms

in maturity-onset diabetics. *Diabetologia* 13:145, 1977.

462. Conlay LA, Karam JH, Matin SB, Lowenstein JE: Serum phenformin-associated lactic acidosis. *Diabetes* 26:628, 1977.

463. Dandona P, Fonseca V, Mier A, Beckett AG: Diarrhea and metformin in a diabetic clinic. *Diabetes Care* 6:472, 1983.

464. Calles-Escandon J, Felig P: Symposium on exercise: Physiology and clinical applications. Fuel-hormone metabolism during exercise and after physical training. *Clin Chest Med* 5, 1984.

465. Bergman M, Felig P: Exercise, in DeGroot L, Cahill GF Jr et al (eds): *Endocrinology*, 2d ed. New York, Grune & Stratton, 1987.

466. Calles-Escandon J, Cunningham JJ, Snyder P et al: Influence of exercise on urea, creatinine, and 3-methylhistidine excretion in normal human subjects. *Am J Physiol* 246:E334, 1984.

467. Ruderman NB, Ganda OP, Johansen K: The effect of physical training on glucose tolerance and plasma lipids in maturity onset diabetes. *Diabetes* 28 (suppl 1):89, 1979.

468. Richter EA, Ploug-Gulbo H: Increased muscle glucose uptake after exercise. No need for insulin during exercise. *Diabetes* 34:1071, 1985.

469. Koivisto V, Felig P: Effects of acute exercise on insulin absorption in diabetic patients. *N Engl J Med* 298:79, 1978.

470. Felig P, Ali-Cherif MS, Minagawa A et al: Hypoglycemia during prolonged exercise in normal man. *N Engl J Med* 306:895, 1982.

471. Wahren J, Sato Y, Ostman J et al: Turnover and splanchnic metabolism of free fatty acids and ketones in insulin-dependent diabetics at rest and in response to exercise. *J Clin Invest* 73:1367, 1984.

471a. Wahren J, Felig P, Hagenfeldt L: Physical exercise and fuel homeostasis in diabetes. *Diabetologia* 14:213, 1978.

472. Wallberg-Henriksson W, Gunnarsson R, Henriksson J et al: Increased peripheral insulin sensitivity and muscle mitochondrial enzymes but unchanged blood glucose control in type I diabetics after physical training. *Diabetes* 31:1044, 1982.

473. Zawalich W, Maturo S, Felig P: Influence of physical training on insulin release and glucose utilization by islet cells and liver glucokinase activity in the rat. *Am J Physiol* 243:E464, 1982.

473a. Stiller JS: Insulin-dependent diabetes, in Kohler PO (ed): *Clinical Endocrinology*. New York, Wiley, 1986, p 491.

473b. Laupacis A, Stiller CR, Gardell C et al: Cyclosporin prevents diabetes in BB Wistar rats. *Lancet* 1:10, 1983.

473c. Mori Y, Suko M, Okudaiva H et al: Preventive effects of cyclosporin on diabetes in NOD mice. *Diabetologia* 29:244, 1986.

474. Sutherland DER, Sibley R, Xu X-Z et al: Twin-to-twin pancreas transportation: Reversal and reenactment of the pathogenesis of type 1 diabetes. *Trans Assoc Am Physicians* 97:80, 1984.

475. Dhein B, Bartell L, Ferguson RM: Infectious complications and lymphomas in cyclosporine patients. *Transplant Proc* 15 (suppl 1/2):3162, 1983.

476. Rosenthal JT, Iwatsuki S, Starzl TE et al: Histiocytic lymphoma in renal transplant patients receiving cyclosporine. *Transplant Proc* 15 (suppl 1/2):2805, 1983.

477. Sutherland DER: Pancreas and islet transplantation. I. Experimental studies. *Diabetologia* 20:161; II. Clinical trials. *Diabetologia* 20:435, 1981.

478. Sutherland DER: Report of international human pancreas and islet transplantation registry cases through 1981. *Diabetes* 31 (suppl 4):112, 1982.

479. Kahan BD (ed): First International Congress on Cyclosporine, Houston. *Transplant Proc* 15 (suppl 1/2), 1983.

480. Raskin P, Unger RH: Hyperglucagonemia and its suppression. Importance in the metabolic control of diabetes. *N Engl J Med* 299:433, 1978.

481. Goldberg DJ, Walesky M, Sherwin RS: Effect of somatostatin on the plasma amino acid response to ingested protein in man. *Metabolism* 28:866, 1979.

481a. Phillips RE, Looareesuwan S, Bloom SR et al: Effectiveness of SMS 201-995, a synthetic, long-acting somatostatin analogue, in treatment of quinine-induced hyperinsulinaemia. *Lancet* 1:713, 1986.

482. Flexner CW, Weiner JP, Saudek CD, Dans PE: Repeated hospitalization for diabetic ketoacidosis. The game of "Sartoris." *Am J Med* 76:691, 1984.

483. Faich GA, Fishbein HA, Ellis SE: The epidemiology of diabetic acidosis: A population-based study. *Am J Epidemiol* 117:551, 1983.

484. Ellemann K, Soerensen JN, Pedersen L et al: Epidemiology and treatment of diabetic ketoacidosis in a community population. *Diabetes Care* 7:528, 1984.

485. Fery F, Balasse EO: Ketone body production and disposal in diabetic ketosis. A comparison with fasting ketosis. *Diabetes* 34:326, 1985.

486. Vinicor F, Lehrner LM, Karn RG, Merritt AD: Hyperamylasemia in diabetic ketoacidosis: Sources and significance. *Ann Intern Med* 91:200, 1979.

487. Levy LJ, Duga J, Girgis M, Gordon EE: Ketoacidosis associated with alcoholism in nondiabetic subjects. *Ann Intern Med* 78:213, 1978.

488. Fisher JN, Shahshahani MN, Kitabchi AE: Diabetic ketoacidosis: Low dose insulin therapy by various routes. *N Engl J Med* 297:238, 1977.

489. Carol P, Matz R: Uncontrolled diabetes mellitus in adults: Experience in treating diabetic ketoacidosis and hyperosmolar nonketotic coma with low-dose insulin and a uniform treatment regimen. *Diabetes Care* 6:579, 1983.

490. Arieff AL, Kleeman CR: Cerebral edema in diabetic comas: II. Effects of hyperosmolarity, hyperglycemia and insulin in diabetic rabbits. *J Clin Endocrinol Metab* 38:1057, 1974.

491. Lever E, Jaspan JB: Sodium bicarbonate therapy in severe diabetic ketoacidosis. *Am J Med* 75:263, 1983.

492. Fisher JN, Kitabchi AE: A randomized study of phosphate therapy in the treatment of diabetic ketoacidosis. *J Clin Endocrinol Metab* 57:177, 1983.

493. Winegrad AL, Kern EFO, Simmons DA: Cerebral edema in diabetic ketoacidosis. *N Engl J Med* 312:1184, 1985.

494. Beigelman PM: Severe diabetic ketoacidosis (diabetic "coma"), 482 episodes in 257 patients; experience of three years. *Diabetes* 20:490, 1971.

495. Krane EJ, Rockoff MA, Wallman JK, Wolfsdorf JI: Subclinical brain swelling in children during treatment of diabetic ketoacidosis. *N Engl J Med* 312:1147, 1985.

496. Carroll P, Matz R: Adult respiratory distress syndrome complicating severely uncontrolled diabetes mellitus. *Diabetes Care* 5:574, 1982.

497. Guisado R, Arieff AL: Neurologic manifestations of diabetic comas: Correlation with biochemical alterations in the brain. *Metabolism* 24:665, 1975.

498. Arieff AL, Carrol JH: Non-ketotic hyperosmolar coma with hyperglycemia: Clinical features, pathophysiology, renal function, acid-base balance, plasma-cerebrospinal fluid equilibria and the effects of therapy. *Medicine* 51:73, 1972.

499. Katz JA: Hyperglycemia-induced hyponatremia. Calculation of expected serum sodium depression. *N Engl J Med* 289:843, 1973.

500. Bavli S, Gordon EE: Experimental diabetic hyperosmolar coma in rats. *Diabetes* 20:92, 1971.

501. Malchoff CD, Pohl SL, Kaiser DL, Carey RM: Determinants of glucose and ketoacid concentrations in acutely hyperglycemic diabetic patients. *Am J Med* 77:275, 1984.

502. Turpin P, Duckworth WC, Solomon SS: Simulated hyperglycemic hyperosmolar syndrome: Impaired insulin and epinephrine effects upon lipolysis in the isolated rat fat cell. *J Clin Invest* 63:403, 1979.

503. Joffe BI, Seftel HC, Goldberg R et al: Factors in the pathogenesis of experimental nonketotic and ketoacidotic diabetic stupor. *Diabetes* 22:653, 1973.

504. Cohen RD: Disorders of lactic acid metabolism. *Clin*

Endocrinol Metab 5:613, 1976.
505. Dembo A, Marliss EB, Halperin ML: Insulin therapy in phenformin-associated lactic acidosis: A case report, biochemical considerations and review of the literature. *Diabetes* 24:28, 1975.
506. Coustan DR, Felig P: Diabetes mellitus, in Burrow GN, Ferris TF (eds): *Medical Complications During Pregnancy,* 3d ed. Philadelphia, Saunders, 1986.
506a. Freinkel N: Of pregnancy and progeny. *Diabetes* 29:1023, 1980.
507. Hull D, Elphick MC: Evidence for fatty acid transfer across the human placenta in Beard RW, Hoet JJ (eds): *Pregnancy Metabolism, Diabetes and the Fetus,* Ciba Foundation Symposium no. 63. New York, Excerpta Medica, 1979, p 71.
508. Szabo AJ, Szabo O: Placental free-fatty-acid transfer and fetal adipose-tissue development: An explanation of fetal adiposity in infants of diabetic mothers. *Lancet* 2:498, 1974.
509. Shafrir E, Khassis S: Maternal-fetal rat transport versus new fat synthesis in the pregnant diabetic rat. *Diabetologia* 22:111, 1982.
510. Shafrir E, Barash V: Placental function in maternal-fetal fat transport in diabetes. *Biol Neonate,* 49, 1987 (in press).
511. Diamant YZ, Metzger GE, Freinkel N, Shafrir E: Placental lipid and glycogen content in human and experimental diabetes mellitus. *Am J Obstet Gynecol* 144:5, 1982.
511a. Shambaugh GE III: Ketone body metabolism in development, in Meisami E, Tamiras PS (eds): *CRC Handbook of Human Growth and Developmental Biology,* vol 2 Boca Raton, CRC, 1987.
512. Churchill JA, Berendes HW, Nemore J: Neuropsychological deficits in children of diabetic mothers. *Am J Obstet Gynecol* 105:257, 1969.
513. Naeye RL, Chez RA: Effects of maternal acetonuria and low pregnancy weight gain on children's psychomotor development. *Am J Obstet Gynecol* 139:189, 1981.
514. Stehbens JA, Baker GL, Kitchell M: Outcome at age 1, 3 and 5 years of children born to diabetic women. *Am J Obstet Gynecol* 127:408, 1977.
515. O'Sullivan JB, Mahan CM: Criteria for the oral glucose tolerance test in pregnancy. *Diabetes* 13:278, 1964.
516. Fisher PM, Sutherland HW, Bewsher PD: Insulin response to glucose infusion in normal human pregnancy. *Diabetologia* 19:15, 1980.
517. Kalkhoff RK, Richardson BL, Beck P: Relative effects of pregnancy, human placental lactogen and prednisone on carbohydrate tolerance in normal and subclinical diabetic subjects. *Diabetes* 18:153, 1969.
518. Spellacy WN, Cohen JE: Human placental lactogen levels and insulin requirements in patients with diabetes mellitus complicating pregnancy. *Obstet Gynecol* 42:330, 1973.
519. Gustafson AB, Banasiak ME, Kalkhoff RK et al: Correlation of hyperprolactinemia with altered plasma insulin and glucagon: Similarity to effects of late human pregnancy. *J Clin Endocrinol Metab* 51:242, 1980.
520. Landgraf R, Landgraf-Leurs MMC, Weissman A et al: Prolactin: A diabetogenic hormone. *Diabetologia* 13:99, 1977.
521. Lev-Ran A, Goldman JA: Brittle diabetes in pregnancy. *Diabetes* 26:926, 1977.
522. O'Sullivan JB, Charles D, Mahan CM, Dandrow RV: Gestational diabetes and perinatal mortality rate. *Am J Obstet Gynecol* 116:901, 1973.
523. O'Sullivan JB, Mahan CM: Insulin treatment and high risk groups. *Diabetes Care* 3:482, 1980.
524. Metzger BE, Bybee DE, Freinkel N et al: Gestational diabetes mellitus: Correlations between the phenotypic and genotypic characteristics of the mother and abnormal glucose tolerance during the first year postpartum. *Diabetes* 34 (suppl 2):111, 1985.
525. Rudolf MCJ, Coustan DR, Sherwin RS et al: Efficacy of the insulin pump in the home treatment of pregnant diabetics. *Diabetes* 30:891, 1981.
525a. Coustan DR, Reece EA, Sherwin RS et al: A randomized trial of the insulin pump and intensive conventional therapy in diabetic pregnancies. *JAMA* 255:631, 1986.
526. Drury MI, Greene AT, Stronge JM: Pregnancy complicated by clinical diabetes mellitus. *Obstet Gynecol* 49:519, 1977.
527. Kitzmiller JL, Cloherty JP, Younger MD et al: Diabetic pregnancy and perinatal morbidity. *Am J Obstet Gynecol* 131:560, 1978.
528. Dooley SL, Depp R, Socol ML et al: Urinary estriols in diabetic pregnancy: A reappraisal. *Obstet Gynecol* 64:469, 1984.
529. Coustan DR: Recent advances in the management of diabetic pregnant women. *Clin Perinatol* 7:299, 1980.
530. Soler NG, Soler SM, Malins JM: Neonatal morbidity among infants of diabetic mothers. *Diabetes Care* 1:340, 1978.
531. Ultrastructural analysis of malformations of the embryonic neural axis induced by *in vitro* hyperglycemic conditions. *Teratology* 32:363, 1985.
532. Eriksson UJ: Congenital malformations in diabetic animal models—a review. *Diabetes Res* 1:57, 1984.
533. Ornoy A, Zusman I, Cohen AM, Shafrir E: Effects of sera from Cohen, genetically determined diabetic rats, streptozotocin diabetic rats and sucrose fed rats on *in vitro* development of early somite rat embryos. *Diab Res* 3:43, 1986.
534. Baker L, Egler JM, Klein SH, Goldman AS: Meticulous control of diabetes during organogenesis prevents congenital lumbosacral defects in rats. *Diabetes* 30:955, 1981.
535. Eriksson UJ, Dahlstrom E, Hellerstrom C: Diabetes in pregnancy: Skeletal malformations in the offspring of diabetic rats after intermittent withdrawal of insulin in early gestation. *Diabetes* 32:1141, 1983.
536. Mills JL, Baker L, Goldman AS: Malformations in infants of diabetic mothers occur before the seventh gestational week. *Diabetes* 28:292, 1979.
537. Leslie RDG, John PN, Pyke SA, White JM: Haemoglobin A_1 in diabetic pregnancy. *Lancet* 2:958, 1978.
538. Miller E, Hare JW, Cloherty JP et al: Elevated maternal hemoglobin A_{1c} in early pregnancy and major congenital anomalies in infants of diabetic mothers. *N Engl J Med* 304:1331, 1981.
539. Ylinen K, Aula P, Stenman UH et al: Risk of minor and major fetal malformations in diabetics with high haemoglobin A1C values in early pregnancy. *Br Med J* 289:345, 1984.
540. Gluck L, Kulovich MV: Lecithin/sphingomyelin ratios in amniotic fluid in normal and abnormal pregnancy. *Am J Obstet Gynecol* 115:539, 1973.
541. Smith BT, Giroud CJP, Robert M, Avery ME: Insulin antagonism of cortisol action on lecithin synthesis by cultured fetal lung cells. *J Pediatr* 87:953, 1975.
542. North AF, Mazumdar S, Logrillo VM: Birth weight, gestational age, and perinatal deaths in 5471 infants of diabetic mothers. *Pediatrics* 90:444, 1977.
543. Jovanovic L, Druzin M, Peterson CM: Effect of euglycemia on the outcome of pregnancy in insulin-dependent diabetic women as compared with normal control subjects. *Am J Med* 71:921, 1981.
544. Olofsson P, Sjoberg NO, Solum T, Svenningsen NW: Changing panorama of perinatal and infant mortality in diabetic pregnancy. *Acta Obstet Gynecol Scand* 63:467, 1984.
545. Tevaarwerk GJM, Harding PGR, Miline KJ et al: Pregnancy in diabetic women: Outcome with a program aimed at normoglycemia before meals. *Can Med Assoc J* 125:435, 1981.
546. Delaney JJ, Ptacek J: Three decades of experience with diabetic pregnancies. *Am J Obstet Gynecol* 106:550, 1970.
547. Widness JA, Susa JB, Garcia JF et al: Increased erythropoiesis and elevated erythropoietin in infants born to diabetic mothers and in hyperinsulinemic rhesus fetuses. *J Clin Invest* 67:637, 1981.
548. Kenepp NB, Kumar S, Shelley WC et al: Fetal and neonatal hazards of maternal hydration with 5% dextrose before cesarean section. *Lancet* 1:1150, 1982.
549. Lawrence GF, Brown VA, Parsons RJ, Cooke ID: Feto-maternal consequences of high-dose glucose infusion during labour.

Br J Obstet Gynaecol 89:27, 1982.
550. Sosenko IR, Kitzmiller JL, Loo SW et al: The infant of the diabetic mother: Correlation of increased cord C-peptide levels with macrosomia and hypoglycemia. *N Engl J Med* 301:859, 1979.
551. Bloom SR, Johnston DI: Failure of glucagon release in infants of diabetic mothers. *Br Med J* 4:453, 1972.
552. Bromham DR: The increased risk of pre-eclampsia in pregnant diabetics. *J Obstet Gynaecol* 3:212, 1983.
553. Aerts L, Van Assche FA: Transmission of experimentally induced diabetes in pregnant rats to their offspring in subsequent generations. A morphometric study of maternal and fetal endocrine pancreases at histological and ultrastructural level, in Shafrir E, Renold AE (eds): *Lessons from Animal Diabetes.* London, Libbey, 1984, p 705.
554. Cohen AW, Liston RM, Mennuti MT, Gabbe SG: Glycemic control in pregnant diabetic women using a continuous subcutaneous insulin infusion pump. *J Reprod Med* 10:651, 1982.
555. Fuhrmann K, Reiher H, Semmler K, Glockner E: The effect of intensified conventional insulin therapy before and during pregnancy on the malformation rate in offspring of diabetic mothers. *J Exp Clin Endocrinol* 83:173, 1984.
556. Churchill JA, Berendes HW: Intelligence of children whose mothers had acetonuria during pregnancy, in *Perinatal Factors Affecting Human Development,* scientific publication no 185. Washington, D.C., Pan American Health Organization, 1969.
557. Felig P: Maternal and fetal fuel homeostasis in pregnancy. *Am J Clin Nutr* 26:998, 1973.
558. Rossini AA, Cahill GF Jr: Lipoatrophic diabetes, in DeGroot LJ, Cahill GF Jr, et al (eds): *Endocrinology.* New York, Grune & Stratton, 1979, vol 2, p 1093.
559. Rossini A: Lipoatrophic diabetes, in Marble A, Krall LP, Bradley RF et al (eds): *Joslin's Diabetes Mellitus.* Philadelphia, Lea and Febiger, 1985, p 834.
560. Bank S: The management of diabetes in the underprivileged, with special reference to pancreatic disease. *S Afr Med J* 40:342, 1966.
561. Dymock IW, Cassar J, Pyke DA, Oakley WG, Williams R: Observations on the pathogenesis, complications and treatment of diabetes in 115 cases of hemochromatosis. *Am J Med* 52:203, 1972.
562. Flier J, Roth J: Diabetes in acromegaly and other endocrine disorders, in DeGroot LJ, Cahill GF Jr et al (eds): *Endocrinology.* New York, Grune & Stratton, 1979, vol 2, p 1089.
563. Perley M, Kipnis DM: Effect of glucocorticoids on plasma insulin. *N Engl J Med* 274:1237, 1966.
564. Wise JK, Hendler R, Felig P: Influence of glucocorticoids on glucagon secretion and amino acid concentrations in man. *J Clin Invest* 52:2774, 1973.
565. Chowers I, Shapiro M, Pfau A, Shafrir E: Serum glucose and free fatty acid responses in pheochromocytoma. *Isr J Med Sci* 2:697, 1966.
566. Leichter SB: Chemical and metabolic aspects of glucagonoma. *Medicine* 59:100, 1980.
567. Tanaka K, Watabe T, Shimizu N et al: Immunologic characterization of plasma glucagon components in a patient with malignant glucagonoma. *Metabolism* 33:8, 1984.
568. D'Arcangues CM, Awoke S, Lawrence GD: Metastatic insulinoma with long survival and glucagonoma syndrome. *Ann Intern Med* 100:233, 1984.
569. Norton JA, Kahn CR, Schiebinger R et al: Amino acid deficiency and the skin rash associated with glucagonoma. *Ann Intern Med* 91:213, 1979.
570. Breatnach ES, Han SY, Rahatzad MT, Stanley RJ: CT evaluation of glucagonomas. *J Comput Assist Tomogr* 9:25, 1985.
571. Elsbor L, Glenth A: Effect of somatostatin in necrolytic migratory erythema and glucagonoma. *Acta Med Scand* 218:245, 1985.
572. Ch'ng JLC, Anderson JV, Williams SI et al: Remission of symptoms during chronic treatment of metastatic endocrine tumours with a long acting somatostatin analogue. *Br Med J* 292:981, 1986.
573. Sherwin RS, Bastl C, Finkelstein FO et al: Influence of uremia and hemodialysis on the turnover and metabolic effects of glucagon. *J Clin Invest* 57:722, 1976.
574. McCaleb ML, Izzo MS, Lockwood DH: Characterization and partial purification of a factor from uremic human serum that induces insulin resistance. *J Clin Invest* 75:391, 1985.
575. Cavallo-Perin P, Cassader M, Bozzo C et al: Mechanism of insulin resistance in human liver cirrhosis. *J Clin Invest* 75:1659, 1985.

Hypoglycemia

Robert S. Sherwin
Philip Felig

Under normal circumstances the circulating plasma glucose concentration is maintained within relatively narrow limits over the course of a 24-h period. In healthy subjects eating mixed meals, the plasma glucose concentration generally remains between 60 and 130 mg/dl throughout the day. Abnormal reductions in plasma glucose concentration may be encountered in a variety of disease states, however, and often represent perplexing problems in diagnosis and management. Hypoglycemia may be the major manifestation of a disease process (e.g., in patients with insulin-producing islet cell tumors), a complication of medical therapy (e.g., insulin treatment for diabetes), a relatively uncommon occurrence (e.g., in Addison's disease), or a mild and asymptomatic condition (e.g., in viral hepatitis). The signs and symptoms of hypoglycemia are relatively nonspecific and may be confused with other organic disturbances (e.g., primary disorders of the central nervous system) or with functional disturbances (e.g., anxiety states and neuroses). Compounding the problem further is the lack of unanimity as to the precise lower limit of normal for the plasma glucose concentration. These uncertainties have generally made physicians feel far less secure in dealing with the question of hypoglycemia as compared with the diagnosis and management of diabetes. Nevertheless, there is sufficient documentation to permit a rigorous approach to the diagnosis as well as treatment of hypoglycemic states.

DEFINITION

Hypoglycemia can more readily be defined in clinical rather than precise quantitative terms. Hypoglycemia is a reduction in plasma glucose concentration to levels which are responsible for symptoms which generally revert upon restoration of a normal glucose concentration. Whether or not a given reduction in plasma glucose concentration will cause hypoglycemic symptoms depends on such factors as (1) the individual subject's glucose threshold, at which a sympathoadrenal response is triggered, (2) the subject's previous glucose control, and (3) the availability of alternative fuels (i.e., ketones) for brain metabolism. Current data indicate that the primary signal triggering the release of catecholamines during hypoglycemia is the absolute glucose level and not the rate at which plasma glucose concentration declines.[1] Furthermore, the glucose threshold below which counterregulatory hormone responses are initiated appears to vary from 50 to 70 mg/dl among healthy individuals. The role of the antecedent glucose concentration is reflected by the observation that abrupt reductions in plasma glucose level to 90 to 100 mg/dl in chronically hyperglycemic diabetic patients may provoke symptoms and a secretory burst of counterregulatory hormones, although these values for plasma glucose level are well within the normal range for healthy subjects.[2] Conversely, intensive insulin treatment of diabetes with accompanying frequent episodes of hypoglycemia appears to diminish both patient perception of hypoglycemia and counterregulatory hormone responses to it.[3] It has also been observed that subjects who have fasted for very prolonged periods (3 weeks or more) tolerate hypoglycemia better. In this circumstance cerebral utilization of ketones reduces the symptomatic effects of insulin-induced hypoglycemia.

The definition of hypoglycemia under fasting conditions must also take into account the sex of the patient. It has been shown that in normal healthy women, the plasma glucose level is 10 to 15 mg/dl lower than in healthy males over the course of a 72-h fast.[4,5] The precise mechanisms for this sex difference are not established, although the difference may be related to a lessened supply of protein-derived glucose precursors (e.g., alanine) in women as compared to men.[6]

Given these variables, a practical definition of hypoglycemia is: (1) in adult males and females after an overnight fast, a plasma glucose value below 60 mg/dl; (2) in males who have fasted for 72 h, a plasma glucose level below 55 mg/dl; (3) in females who have fasted for 72 h, a plasma glucose concentration below 45 mg/dl; and (4) in males and females given a 75- to 100-g oral glucose load, a nadir plasma glucose value below 50 mg/dl.

SIGNS AND SYMPTOMS

The clinical manifestations of hypoglycemia are a consequence of two phenomena: (1) lack of glucose supply to the brain (*neuroglycopenia*) and attendant decrease in cerebral oxygen consumption, and (2) stimulation of the sympathoadrenal system, resulting in increased secretion of catecholamines. The neuroglycopenic symptoms consist of headache, inability to concentrate, fatigue, confusion, bizarre behavior, hallucinations, and, ultimately, convulsions or coma; the convulsions may be generalized or focal in nature. In addition, there may be localized impairment of CNS function such as hemiplegia or aphasia. These symptoms are more likely to occur in older individuals with underlying cerebral vascular disease and may, in fact, mimic a cerebrovascular accident. Repeated, sustained attacks of hypoglycemia may result in chronic brain syndrome with sustained loss in intellectual function.

The symptoms resulting from stimulation of the sympathoadrenal system consist of palpitations, anxiety, sweating, tremulousness, and hunger. These symptoms often constitute early warning signs of an impending hypoglycemic attack, since they are likely to precede impairment of cortical function. The patient can consequently often abort the attack by ingesting glucose. The importance of these symptoms is underscored by the problems encountered by insulin-requiring diabetics who develop autonomic neuropathy or are treated with β-adrenergic-blocking agents. In such patients hypoglycemia may progress to coma without any warning or opportunity for the patient to abort the attack.

The adrenergic symptoms accompanying hypoglycemia appear to be largely mediated by activation of adrenal medullary secretion, although increased sympathetic nervous system activity probably contributes as well. In keeping with this concept, the early symptoms of hypoglycemia normally coincide with the prompt rise in levels of circulating epinephrine and norepinephrine that follows a decline in plasma glucose concentration. The importance of the adrenal medulla in this response is suggested by the substantially greater increment in plasma epinephrine concentration which occurs during hypoglycemia (the norepinephrine rise may also be derived in part from the adrenal medulla) as well as the failure of tissue norepinephrine turnover to increase when animals are made hypoglycemic.[7,8] It is noteworthy that, while the warning symptoms of hypoglycemia in normal subjects are critically dependent on an intact symphathoadrenal system, the physiological mechanisms responsible for endogenous glucose counterregulation are not. This is reflected by the fact that a normal glucose rebound after insulin-induced hypoglycemia is observed in adrenalectomized patients,[9] in normal subjects receiving combined α- and β-adrenergic blockade,[10] as well as in patients with spinal cord transection or thoracolumbar sympathectomy.[11]

The role of counterregulatory hormones in the recovery from hypoglycemia has recently been clarified using insulin as a hypoglycemia stimulus. In this setting, reversal of insulin-mediated suppression of hepatic glucose production is the predominant mechanism leading to glucose recovery. When very small doses of insulin are given, nonhormonal factors (so-called autoregulation) may be sufficient to overcome the hepatic effects of insulin and prevent plasma glucose concentration from falling to levels at which counterregulatory hormone release is triggered.[7] With larger doses of insulin, however, glucose recovery is dependent on the secretion of counterregulatory hormones, which begins once plasma glucose concentration has fallen below a threshold level of approximately 60 mg/dl[1] (Fig. 20-1). Among the counterregulatory hormones, glucagon and epinephrine are of special importance. They tend to be released first;[7,12] more important, they are the only hormones capable of stimulating hepatic glucose production within minutes. This is essential, given that a further decline in plasma glucose concentration may relatively quickly lead to neuroglycopenia. The vital contribution of the glucagon and epinephrine response is underscored by studies showing that combined deficiency of these hormones markedly impairs glucose recovery from hypoglycemia in normal individuals.[10,13] Interestingly, a deficient response of either glucagon or epinephrine alone has only a minor impact on glucose counterregulation. Thus, this critical defense mechanism is not dependent on a single hormone. The benefits of such a redundant control system are readily apparent, considering that most patients with insulin-dependent diabetes fail to secrete glucagon in response to hypoglycemia.[13,14]

A characteristic of hypoglycemic symptoms regardless of their etiology is their *episodic nature.* Although symptoms may recur repeatedly, they generally last for a period of minutes to hours rather than days or weeks. The reason for this relatively brief period is that hypoglycemia results in one of three outcomes within a brief period: (1) plasma glucose

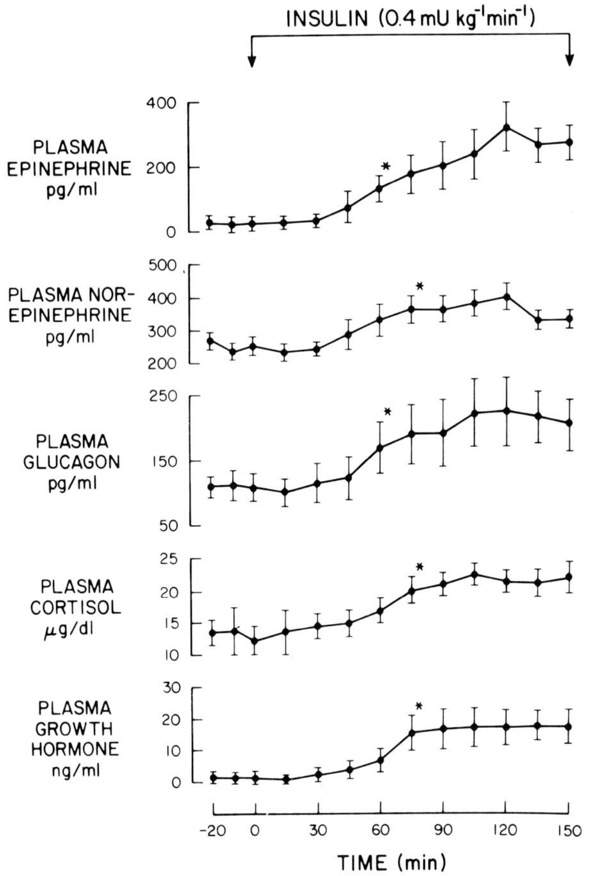

FIGURE 20-1 The counterregulatory hormone response to insulin-induced hypoglycemia. The infusion of insulin resulted in a reduction of plasma glucose concentration to levels of 50 to 55 mg/dl (not shown) and caused an increase in plasma concentrations of epinephrine, norepinephrine, glucagon, cortisol, and growth hormone. The asterisks indicate the first time point at which the rise in plasma hormone concentration was significantly above basal. (*From Sacca et al.*[7])

concentration spontaneously reverts to normal because of counterregulatory mechanisms, (2) ingestion of food results in a return of plasma glucose level to normal, or (3) if both (1) and (2) fail to occur, the plasma glucose concentration continues to fall to levels which will result in either syncope, seizures, or coma. Thus, when a patient complains of such symptoms as fatigue, lassitude, or lack of concentration lasting for days, weeks, or months, without identifiable episodic disability which is of minutes to hours in duration, hypoglycemia is unlikely to be present or responsible for the symptoms.

A second important characteristic of hypoglycemic symptoms concerns the response to ingestion of glucose-containing foodstuffs or beverages: *symptomatic relief associated with glucose ingestion does not constitute a specific sign of hypoglycemia.* A variety of symptoms associated with anxiety states may be relieved by the ingestion of glucose as a placebo (see below). Consequently, if, during the course of an evaluation for hypoglycemia, the patient develops symptoms, the physician should draw a blood sample for glucose determination *before* attempting to relieve the symptoms by administering glucose.

In comatose or severely obtunded patients with hypoglycemia a relatively frequent finding is hypothermia.[15] This is particularly common in patients with alcohol-induced hypoglycemia. While hypothermia is a useful diagnostic clue in the evaluation of the comatose patient, it, too, is not specific for hypoglycemia, since it may be encountered after drug overdose (particularly with barbiturates), following cold exposure, and in myxedema coma (see Chap. 10).

NONHYPOGLYCEMIA

In recent years there has been an increasing tendency for patients to self-refer for evaluation of possible hypoglycemia. This can be attributed in part to a deluge of articles in lay magazines and books written for the lay population which emphasize the "frequency and importance" of hypoglycemia in the causation of a variety of symptoms ranging from poor work or study habits to disturbances of sexual potency. As a result, the classic admonition to medical students to always consider hypoglycemia as a possible cause of neuropsychiatric disease must now be emphasized in reverse: patients with a variety of functional complaints should not be misdiagnosed as hypoglycemic.[16]

The characteristic syndrome of "nonhypoglycemia" is one in which patients complain of anxiety, fatigue, headaches, light-headedness, palpitations, and weakness which may be episodic in nature but often persists for periods of days to weeks. The patients generally report that the frequency of attacks can be prevented and their general sense of well-being can be improved by consuming diets which are severely restricted in carbohydrate. By consuming large amounts of carbohydrate, they can "relieve" symptoms once they do appear. In such patients, nonhypoglycemia is established by obtaining a careful history to determine whether the symptoms are episodic in nature and then by demonstrating normal plasma glucose responses during a fast and/or after glucose or meal administration. The physician should then carefully explain the findings to the patient, emphasizing that symptoms compatible with hypoglycemia may be a result of other causes (e.g., depression, anxiety) and that relief of symptoms by glucose ingestion or prevention of attacks by dietary restriction may reflect a placebo action. Efforts should then be directed at identifying the psychological or organic factors responsible for the patient's symptoms. The importance of proper diagnosis and attribution of symptoms is reflected by the fact that patients may become so incapacitated by their self-diagnosis of hypoglycemia that they will refuse to eat in restaurants lest they inadvertently ingest small amounts of carbohydrate, nor will they be willing to drive an automobile lest they not have carbohydrate immediately available should they begin to have symptoms. Such patients require in-depth counseling to prevent their becoming "dietary cripples."

Nonhypoglycemia may be the appropriate diagnosis even in circumstances in which chemical hypoglycemia has been documented during the course of a 5-h glucose tolerance test. In some patients with episodic postprandial symptoms and a documented hypoglycemic response to a pure glucose load, ingestion of a mixed meal (typical of daily life) may induce typical symptoms yet fail to induce chemical hypoglycemia.[16a] It has been suggested that the disorder demonstrated by such patients should be termed the "idiopathic postprandial syndrome" to avoid the connotation of hypoglycemia.[16a]

CLASSIFICATION

Various efforts to classify hypoglycemia on the basis of pathogenetic mechanisms (i.e., disturbances in glucose production vs. utilization) often fail to permit clear distinctions because of the multiplicity of mechanisms which may contribute in specific disease states. A more useful categorization for the clinician is one in which the circumstance in which hypoglycemia appears is the basis of the classification. In this manner, three major categories of hypoglycemia may be recognized, *fasting* hypoglycemia, *postprandial* hypoglycemia, and *induced* hypoglycemia (Table 20-1). In the fasting hypoglycemias, the reduction in plasma glucose level is most severe when food is withheld; food ingestion is thus not required to provoke hypoglycemic attacks. In contrast, in the postprandial hypoglycemias, fasting does not induce an abnormal reduction in glucose concentration, while meal ingestion is followed (usually within 2 to 5 h) by hypoglycemia. In the induced hypoglycemias, administration of medication (e.g., insulin) or ingestion of substances with toxic properties (e.g., alcohol, the unripe akee nut) is responsible for the fall in glucose concentration.

Table 20-1. Major Categories of Hypoglycemia and Some Frequently Encountered Examples

Fasting hypoglycemia
Insulin-producing islet cell tumor
Ketotic hypoglycemia of infancy
Postprandial hypoglycemia
Spontaneous reactive hypoglycemia
Alimentary hypoglycemia
Induced hypoglycemia
Alcohol hypoglycemia
Insulin overdose
Factitious hypoglycemia

Fasting Hypoglycemia

The fasting hypoglycemias are characterized by a failure to maintain normal glucose homeostasis when food is withheld. In these disorders neither the ingestion of food nor some drug or toxin is required to precipitate hypoglycemia. The pathophysiology, diagnosis, and management of such disorders is best understood in the context of the response to starvation in normal humans.

STARVATION IN NORMAL HUMANS

Under normal circumstances humans feed intermittently; the interval between meals generally varies from 2 to 14 h. Occasionally, however, either because of voluntary cessation of intake, intercurrent disease interfering with feeding, or lack of food availability, humans are faced with more prolonged periods of fasting. The metabolic response to starvation represents an integration of hormonal secretion and fuel use designed to (1) maintain glucose production (glycogenolysis and gluconeogenesis) to meet the needs of obligate glucose-consuming tissues, particularly the brain, (2) maximize utilization of the major storage fuel (i.e., fat), and (3) minimize dissipation of body protein. The normal response to starvation may be viewed as a continuum which can be divided into three phases: the *postabsorptive* state (6 to 12 h after food intake), *short-term starvation* (lasting 12 to 72 h), and *prolonged starvation* (2 weeks or longer).[17]

After an overnight fast (the postabsorptive state), glucose is produced exclusively by the liver and is consumed primarily by the brain. The rate of glucose turnover in an adult is 2 mg per kilogram of body weight per minute. The production of glucose by the liver is a consequence of glycogenolysis (accounting for 75 percent of glucose output) and gluconeogenesis (accounting for 25 percent). The major substrates used by the liver for gluconeogenesis are the glycolytic intermediates lactate and pyruvate; the amino acids, particularly alanine; and glycerol.

Glucose uptake in the postabsorptive state in humans occurs predominantly in insulin-insensitive tissues, particularly the brain. Small amounts of glucose are also taken up by the formed elements of the blood and splanchnic tissues. In marked contrast, insulin-sensitive tissues such as muscle and adipose tissue consume virtually no glucose when subjects fast for 12 h or more. These tissues are dependent on free fatty acids as an energy source.

The major hormonal signal which allows for the orderly transition from a fed to a fasted condition without the development of hypoglycemia is a fall in plasma insulin concentration. While plasma insulin concentration rises to a level of 30 to 100 microunits [(μU)/ml] 1 to 3 h after meal ingestion, it declines to values of 10 to 20 μU/ml in the postabsorptive state. The presence of these basal (rather than postprandial) concentrations of insulin allows for glucagon-mediated stimulation of glycogenolytic and gluconeogenic processes so as to provide the hepatic glucose output necessary to meet the ongoing needs of the brain. Furthermore, the drop in insulin concentration to basal levels signals a cessation of glucose uptake by insulin-sensitive muscle and adipose tissue.

If meal ingestion is withheld for more than 12 to 14 h, further adaptive mechanisms come into play to maintain euglycemia. Since liver glycogen stores are limited to 70 to 90 g after an overnight fast while brain uses glucose at a rate of 125 g per day, liver glycogen is virtually totally depleted within the course of a 24- to 48-h fast. Consequently, maintenance of hepatic glucose production and euglycemia requires a progressive increase in hepatic gluconeogenesis. The latter is in turn dependent on the mobilization of alanine and other amino acids from muscle stores. The uptake and conversion of alanine to glucose by the liver progressively rises as fasting extends beyond 12 h. In addition, the mobilization of fatty acids from adipose tissue also increases (i.e., lipolysis is stimulated), thereby providing an energy-yielding fuel for hepatic gluconeogenesis and for muscle contraction which, in turn, spares glucose for use by the brain. Furthermore, the oxidation of fatty acids by the liver results in ketogenesis and a progressive rise in circulating levels of β-hydroxybutyrate and acetoacetate.

The primary hormonal signal which results in stimulation of amino acid mobilization, gluconeogenesis, lipolysis, and ketogenesis as fasting extends beyond 12 to 14 h is a further decline in concentration of plasma insulin to below 10 μU/ml. This is underscored by the fact that patients with an insulinoma, who do not exhibit absolute hyperinsulinemia, nonetheless experience life-threatening hypoglycemia within 72 h of fasting because their insulin concentrations fail to decline below postabsorptive levels. The rise in plasma glucagon concentration which also occurs during short-term fasting provides an additional stimulus for hepatic gluconeogenesis and ketogenesis and substantially magnifies the effect of insulin deficiency on these processes. Also contributing to the gluconeogenic response is the presence of basal levels of cortisol and growth hormone (GH). With respect to the mechanism for the drop in plasma insulin concentration, the small decline (15 to 20 mg/dl) in plasma glucose level which normally characterizes a 24- to 72-h fast is the major stimulus. However, negative caloric balance may of itself contribute to the drop in insulin secretion. The overall fuel-hormone changes characterizing a 24- to 72-h fast are summarized in Fig. 20-2.

When fasting is extended from periods of days to weeks, the homeostatic mechanisms are concerned not only with the maintenance of euglycemia but also with the conservation of body protein stores. The importance of the latter is indicated by the fact that death in starvation is a consequence of the dissolution of one-third to one-half of body protein mass, at which time there is weakening of respiratory muscles, atelectasis, pneumonia, sepsis, and death. Since protein provides the only source of noncarbohydrate precursors for gluconeogenesis (mammalian liver cannot convert fatty acids to glucose), a decrease in protein catabolism necessitates a reduction in gluconeogenesis. Euglycemia and brain fuel needs are maintained in the face of reduced glucose production in very prolonged fasting because the brain oxidizes ketone bodies as an alternative fuel.[18] The key determinant of brain ketone utilization is the rise in arterial ketone acid concentration. The precise level of ketone acids and duration of fasting at which brain ketone uptake occurs has not been determined, but it is in excess of 3 days and probably less than 14 days.

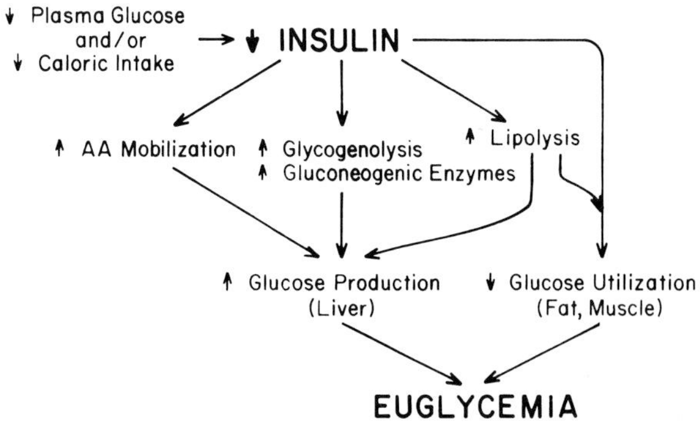

FIGURE 20-2 The hormonal and substrate changes whereby euglycemia is maintained (and hypoglycemia is prevented) in normal subjects during a fast. The fall in plasma insulin concentration is the key hormonal change resulting in increased glucose production and decreased glucose utilization. The decline in plasma insulin level is in turn a result of a small decrease in plasma glucose concentration (5 to 10 mg/dl) and/or a decrease in caloric intake per se.

MECHANISMS AND CLASSIFICATION OF FASTING HYPOGLYCEMIA

From the foregoing discussion it is clear that the maintenance of euglycemia in the fasting state is dependent on three major factors: (1) a hormonal milieu characterized by basal or reduced insulin levels and basal or increased levels of glucagon, GH, and cortisol; (2) intact glycogenolytic and gluconeogenic processes in the liver; and (3) substrate availability to provide the precursors (e.g., alanine) necessary for hepatic gluconeogenesis. Fasting hypoglycemia thus may be categorized as endocrine, hepatic, or substrate in origin (Table 20-2). In addition, occasional miscellaneous causes are observed which must be classified separately (Table 20-2).

INSULIN-PRODUCING ISLET CELL TUMORS

Clinical Characteristics

Hyperinsulinemia resulting in hypoglycemia is the major clinical manifestation of insulin-producing islet cell tumors. These tumors may be either benign or malignant, the latter representing about 10 percent of the total. Multiple tumors occur in approximately 10 percent of cases as well, frequently as part of *multiple endocrine neoplasia type 1* (MEN 1), in which the frequency of multiple tumors is about 50 percent. The tumors are very rare in patients less than 10 years old; about 90 percent of such tumors occur in patients over the age of 20. When these tumors are diagnosed in children, it is critical to search for other endocrine neoplasias (i.e., MEN 1) in the patient as well as family members. Islet cell adenomas may occur in any part of the pancreas, but over 60 percent occur in the body and tail of the gland. The histological appearance is of whorls of typical beta cells. It is impossible to tell whether the tumor is actively secreting insulin by examining the histology of the adenoma itself, but excessive secretion of insulin by the tumor causes degranulation of the islet cells of the adjacent pancreas, which is an indication of activity of the neoplasm. Extracts of the tumor contain large amounts of insulin (0.02 to 60.8 U/g). Neither can the histological appearance of the tumor be used to determine its malignant potential; the presence of metastasis (e.g., liver or regional lymph nodes) is the only reliable marker. Malignant tumors generally measure more than 2 cm in diameter, whereas most benign tumors range in size between 0.5 and 2 cm. However, there is sufficient overlap of the ranges in size of benign and malignant tumors to preclude using size as a diagnostic criterion.

Table 20-2. Classification of Fasting Hypoglycemia

Endocrine
Excess insulin or insulin-like factors
Insulin-producing islet cell tumors
Extrapancreatic tumors causing hypoglycemia
Growth hormone deficiency
Hypopituitarism
Isolated growth hormone deficiency
Cortisol deficiency
Hypopituitarism
Isolated ACTH deficiency
Addison's disease
Hepatic
Glycogen storage diseases
Deficiency of gluconeogenic enzymes
Acute hepatic necrosis
Toxins
Viral hepatitis
Reye's syndrome
Congestive heart failure
Substrate
Fasting hypoglycemia of pregnancy
Ketotic hypoglycemia of infancy
Uremia
Severe malnutrition
Maple syrup urine disease
Miscellaneous
Insulin autoimmune hypoglycemia
Systemic carnitine deficiency

In children, hyperinsulinemic hypoglycemia may occur as a result of hyperplasia of beta cells or in association with *nesidioblastosis,* a histological entity in which there is evidence of transformation of exocrine cells to form endocrine cells. The significance of beta cell nesidioblastosis must, however, be questioned because similar changes have also been found in pancreatic tissue from normal young children.[19] Thus, in some cases hyperinsulinemia may result from a hitherto unidentified defect in islet cell function.

The pathogenesis of hypoglycemia in patients with functioning islet cell tumors or hyperplasia is either an *absolute elevation* of plasma insulin levels in the fasting state or during exercise, or a *failure of insulin levels to decline* as is normally observed in those circumstances. The hyperinsulinemia inhibits glycogenolysis and interferes with gluconeogenic processes both by directly affecting the liver as well as by inhibiting amino acid mobilization and lipolysis. The fall in glucose production in association with ongoing glucose use by the brain results in hypoglycemia. When absolute (rather than relative) hyperinsulinemia is present, the fall in plasma glucose concentration may also be caused by stimulation of glucose utilization by muscle and fat tissue. The hypoglycemic effects of hyperinsulinemia are further intensified during exercise. This reflects the fact that exercise increases the demand for glucose production, inasmuch as glucose is being consumed by muscle as well as brain in such circumstances (see Chap. 19).

Diagnosis

Diagnosis of an insulin-producing islet cell tumor is usually made by finding an abnormally low plasma glucose concentration and an elevated plasma insulin level in the fasting state; but it may sometimes be necessary that the patient fast, in the hospital, for as long as 72 h and engage in moderate exercise before an attack can be produced. In about 50 percent of patients with islet cell tumors, the overnight fasting plasma glucose concentration is less than 60 mg/100 ml and the plasma insulin level exceeds 20 μU/ml.[5] In an additional 25 to 35 percent of patients, hypoglycemia is provoked by merely prolonging the fast for up to 4 h (by withholding breakfast). In only 10 percent of cases or less is a 72-h fast followed by exercise necessary to provoke hypoglycemia. Occasionally, hypoglycemia may be accompanied by a "normal" plasma insulin level. This situation generally reflects a failure of insulin concentration to decline normally in association with a fast. In such circumstances the insulin/glucose (I/G) ratio may be helpful. An I/G ratio in excess of 0.30 is generally indicative of hyperinsulinism.[5] The failure to observe peripheral hyperinsulinemia may also reflect increased hepatic extraction of insulin entering the portal vein or, alternatively, the episodic nature of insulin secretion by islet cell tumors. In addition to insulin, it is important to measure C peptide levels at the time the patient is hypoglycemic. This serves to exclude factitious hypoglycemia due to exogenous insulin administration (see below), a situation where C peptide is suppressed rather than elevated, as in insulinoma.[20]

Further supporting evidence for the presence of an insulinoma may be provided if plasma insulin is fractionated into insulin and proinsulin. Whereas the latter usually represents 20 percent or less of the total circulating fasting insulin in normal individuals, it commonly constitutes a much larger portion of circulating insulin in patients with insulinomas. In some instances it can rise to as high as 70 percent of the total immunoreactive insulin-like material in the plasma.[21] However, proinsulin measurements can rarely be relied on as the sole means of separating patients with marginal elevations in plasma insulin level. It is also noteworthy that proinsulin may bind to C peptide antisera, thereby interfering with the assay of C peptide.

An additional finding which helps distinguish hyperinsulinemic hypoglycemia from other causes (e.g., alcohol-induced hypoglycemia, Addison's disease) is the absence of ketonuria (or ketonemia). The latter finding reflects the inhibitory action of insulin on lipolysis and ketogenesis.

Provocative tests involving the administration of leucine, tolbutamide, glucagon, or calcium have been recommended in the past. However, tumors vary in their responsiveness to these agents and false-negative results are observed in 25 percent or more of cases. Although the tolbutamide test appears to yield the lowest rate of false-negative results, the risk of profound hypoglycemia is sufficient to limit its usefulness as an outpatient screening test. In addition, in rare patients without islet cell tumors, intravenous (IV) tolbutamide may provoke severe hypoglycemia. Suppression tests have also been recommended involving the administration of fish insulin (which does not react with the antiserum used to measure human insulin) or the administration of commercial insulin (0.1 U per kilogram of body weight over 1 h) followed by C peptide determination. In the latter test C peptide levels (an index of endogenous insulin secretion) fall in normal subjects but remain elevated in patients with islet cell tumors.[20] Since C peptide assays are readily available, whereas fish insulin is not, the C peptide suppression test has been adopted for clinical use. It has been suggested that this approach is more reliable than provocative testing and offers the additional advantage of detecting patients with factitious hypoglycemia. Nevertheless, this test probably should be reserved for difficult diagnostic problems where hyperinsulinemia is equivocal. The best diagnostic approach is the repeated determination of the overnight fasting plasma glucose and insulin levels. If this fails to give diagnostic information, the overnight fast should be prolonged for 4 h. If hypoglycemia still is not provoked, the fast is continued for 72 h.

The glucose tolerance test is generally not helpful in the diagnosis of an islet cell tumor; the test result may have a normal or even diabetic pattern. The latter usually occurs when the adenomatous tissue is unresponsive to glucose and there is accompanying atrophy of normal islet tissue. In some patients, in whom the plasma glucose level shows a progressive decline throughout the 5- to 6-h period after glucose ingestion with no rebound increase, an insulinoma should be suspected. This pattern is distinctly different from that normally seen in patients with reactive hypoglycemia, in whom a spontaneous, rebound increase in glucose level occurs between 3 and 6 h after glucose is ingested (see below). In some instances islet cell tumors may be multihormonal, producing not only insulin but also pancreatic polypeptide, gastrin, glucagon, somatostatin, and serotonin, either singly or in various combinations. It is noteworthy that malignant insulinomas commonly secrete human chorionic gonadotropin or its alpha subunit, whereas benign tumors do not. Thus, measurements of the levels of these species can be helpful in the preoperative screening for possible malignancy.

Surgical Therapy

Once a diagnosis of hyperinsulinism caused by islet cell adenoma has been made, the tumor should be excised surgically. It is advantageous to try to locate the tumor before operation by noninvasive techniques [computerized axial tomography (CT)] and/or angiography via the pancreaticoduodenal artery. Celiac artery injection is less effective. Angiography is currently the most accurate detection procedure, detecting adenomas in 70 to 90 percent of cases. Usually, the tumor shows up as a highly vascular mass within the substance of the pancreas, although avascular tumors may be seen. The procedure may help facilitate surgery as well as alert the surgeon to the existence of multiple tumors. CT may be helpful in some cases, although it remains considerably less effective than angiography in detecting these small tumors. Ultrasonography is of limited value, correctly locating tumors in about 25 percent of cases. Nevertheless, the above noninvasive procedures are probably still worth attempting because they may occasionally obviate the need for angiography (with its attendant risks) and may provide evidence for the existence of mestastases. Some investigators have advocated selective percutaneous trans-hepatic venous sampling to detect an increase in insulin concentration in blood draining specific regions of the pancreas. This procedure is probably best reserved for select clinical centers and for secondary operations in which the ability of the surgeon to locate tumors at the time of operation is hampered. Success in locating the tumor(s) at operation may be verified by sequential measurements of plasma glucose concentration (every 15 to 30 min) after surgical resection. Commonly, plasma glucose concentration rises abruptly upon complete removal of all tumor tissue. This procedure is especially useful in patients suspected of having multiple tumors, such as patients with MEN 1.

There is little argument that surgery is the treatment of choice for insulinomas, provided metastatic disease is not clinically evident. In the Mayo Clinic series, 154 patients underwent surgery; 7 operative deaths (5.4 percent) resulted.[22] Fifteen explorations failed to reveal any tumor. Of the remaining 132 tumors, 118 were adenomas; of these, 7 were multiple. In 33 instances, no tumor was identified at surgery, so the decision was made to resect the body and tail of the pancreas blindly in the hope that the tumor was hidden in that portion of the organ. The maneuver was successful in 15 cases, a success rate appropriate to the anatomical distribution already mentioned. Thus, surgery was successful in removing a tumor in 132 of the 154 patients operated on (85 percent) and in 93 percent of those who were diagnosed as having adenomas. The success rate was much lower among the 14 with carcinomas. Only half of these tumors were found at operation; the other half were too small to be discovered at the time of the original surgery, and only manifested themselves as malignant by forming metastases. Among malignant insulinomas, the prognosis appears to be considerably better if spread is confined to regional lymph nodes. The presence of hepatic metastases normally indicates the need for chemotherapy.

Pharmacological Treatment

If the insulin-secreting tumor cannot be found, if the patient refuses operation, or if the tumor is malignant, medical methods of treating hypoglycemia may be useful. Alloxan, which might be expected to help, turns out to be ineffective in humans. Glucagon, adrenocorticosteroids, or GH may be given with temporary benefit, but these modalities are not very effective for long-term care and are not without risk. A much preferred treatment is diazoxide, which reduces the release of insulin and thus minimizes the endocrine effect of the tumor. Diazoxide is effective in about 50 percent of cases. Careful dosage adjustment is required in the initial stages of treatment. The usual starting dosage is 100 to 200 mg per day in three divided doses (every 8 h). Thereafter the dosage is increased by 50 to 100 mg per day up to 600 mg per day. The maintenance dose in children averages 12 mg per kilogram of body weight. Anorexia is common but is relieved by reducing the dose. It is important to avoid this side effect since hypoglycemia may be exacerbated. Most adults and occasional children develop edema, which is treated by adding thiazide diuretics, which reduce the edema and also may enhance the antihypoglycemic effect of diazoxide. Tachycardia is quite common, probably as a result of increased catecholamine secretion. Almost all patients develop hirsutism, which is a minor problem in males but important in women and children. Dermatitis and thrombocytopenia are occasionally seen but do not usually cause difficulty.

The failure of alloxan to help patients with inoperable insulinomas and the need for continuous treatment with diazoxide (a drug that does not affect tumor growth) has led to the use of streptozocin in this situation. Streptozocin is not without danger, since it usually produces nausea and vomiting when given systemically, and adequate doses are often associated with renal tubular damage leading to aminoaciduria, renal glycosuria, and tubular acidosis. Proteinuria is common, and impaired creatinine clearance may persist for many months. Hepatic damage probably also occurs, since the plasma enzyme levels rise. In spite of these disadvantages, it appears justifiable to use the drug in otherwise uncontrollable cases, since a complete (albeit temporary) remission is achieved in nearly 25 percent of patients, as evidenced by regression of the tumor and control of hyperinsulinism. In one large series, 52 patients with metastatic islet cell carcinomas were treated with streptozocin.[23] Of those cases which could be evaluated, partial or complete normalization of plasma insulin and glucose levels was observed in 64 percent. In 50 percent a decrease in measurable tumor (organomegaly, lymph nodes, or masses) was noted. A significant increase in the 1-year survival rate and a doubling of median survival (to 3.5 years) were shown for responders as compared with nonresponders. The dose of streptozocin recommended is 500 mg/m^2 given IV daily for 5 days with repeat cycles at 6-week intervals. The effect of streptozocin may be enhanced by the addition of 5-fluorouracil to the regimen. Generally, the treatment is continued, but at less frequent intervals, if remission occurs. Patients who fail to respond to streptozocin (with or without 5-fluorouracil) may be given doxorubicin (Adriamycin) or dacarbazine; however, their efficacy remains uncertain. Because of the inherent toxicity, streptozocin therapy (or use of other chemotherapeutic agents) should be limited to patients with unresectable or metastatic disease.

Nonadenomatous Hyperinsulinemic Hypoglycemia

As noted above, in infants and children, hyperinsulinemic hypoglycemia not uncommonly occurs in the absence of an identifiable adenoma (or microadenoma). Careful histological evaluation of the pancreas in such cases may reveal nesidioblastosis or simply an increase in islet cell mass. Treatment in these cases consists of subtotal pancreatectomy and, where necessary, diazoxide therapy. Total pancreatectomy should be avoided because some of these children show evidence of clinical improvement after long-term follow-up.

Hyperinsulinemic hypoglycemia in the neonate is observed in *Beckwith's syndrome,* which is characterized by macroglossia, visceromegaly, microcephaly, and umbilical hernia. The hypoglycemia observed in the infant of the diabetic mother is discussed in Chap. 19.

EXTRAPANCREATIC TUMOR HYPOGLYCEMIA

Tumors arising outside the pancreas may cause hypoglycemia, in some instances by secreting an insulin-like material, in others by using glucose at an accelerated rate, and in still others by inhibiting, in some way, the ability of the liver to release glucose. Most commonly these tumors arise from mesenchymal tissue (fibromas, fibrosarcomas, neuromas) and are retroperitoneal or, occasionally, mediastinal in location. Next in frequency are hepatomas, adrenocortical carcinomas, and gastrointestinal malignancies. These tumors are generally very large; they therefore are often evident from examination of the abdomen, chest x-ray, ultrasonography, or CT scans. Current data suggest that about half of the patients with extrapancreatic tumor hypoglycemia have increased circulating levels of insulin-like growth factor (IGF) activity, as determined by radioreceptor assay.[24,24a] The precise nature of the peptide and its role in the development of hypoglycemia remains uncertain. However, it is possible that the peptide (regardless of whether it is identical to one of the two naturally occurring IGFs, IGF-I or IGF-II) may produce hypoglycemia by interacting with the insulin receptor when the peptide is present in large concentrations (see Chap. 19). Only in very rare instances have such tumors been shown to produce radioimmunoassayable insulin. Treatment of hypoglycemia associated with non-islet tumors is directed at the tumor itself; i.e., surgery or chemotherapy is used. Partial surgical removal of the tumor may be helpful in some cases. Since the hypoglycemia in these cases is accompanied by hypoinsulinemia, treatment directed toward suppressing insulin secretion (e.g., diazoxide) is not indicated.

HYPOGLYCEMIA IN ENDOCRINE-DEFICIENCY STATES

As discussed above, in addition to the fall in insulin secretion, maintenance of glucose homeostasis in the fasting state requires intact secretion of GH, cortisol, and glucagon. Clinical hypoglycemia may be observed in patients with hypopituitarism, isolated deficiency of GH or adrenocorticotropic hormone (ACTH), and in Addison's disease. The occurrence of hypoglycemia in these conditions is more common in childhood, perhaps because the relative increase in glucose flux in children places a greater demand on the liver for glucose production.[25] In each of these circumstances the hypoglycemia is accompanied by an appropriate reduction in plasma insulin concentration and the presence of ketosis. Diagnosis depends on evaluation of pituitary and/or adrenal function. Although glucagon is required for the maintenance of glucose production in starvation, clinical hypoglycemia due to deficiency of this hormone has not been convincingly documented.

HYPOGLYCEMIC HEPATIC DISEASE

Hypoglycemia is not uncommon in patients with viral hepatitis, but the degree of hypoglycemia is rarely sufficient to cause symptoms.[26] In patients with very severe liver disease, failure of gluconeogenesis may cause the concentration of plasma amino acids to rise and blood glucose concentration to fall, but this is ordinarily seen only in the terminal phase of hepatic necrosis. In these patients the demand for glucose may be much larger than would be expected if simple replacement of the minimal glucose utilization of fasting were required; it seems likely that an additional problem is the loss of the insulin-inactivating mechanisms which the normal liver possesses. The result is a combined increase of insulin activity and a decrease of gluconeogenesis. Hypoglycemia is also observed in Reye's syndrome, a disorder of childhood characterized by vomiting, encephalopathy, hyperammonemia, and fatty liver. Prodromal viral infection and the ingestion of salicylates have been implicated as contributory (though not causal) factors.[27] Rarely, severe hepatic congestion in chronic congestive heart failure may be associated with hypoglycemia, especially in children. Hypoglycemia may also be observed with congenital liver disorders such as the glycogenoses and deficiencies of gluconeogenic enzymes.

HYPOGLYCEMIA DUE TO SUBSTRATE DEFICIENCY

In addition to a reduction in insulin, the availability of counterregulatory hormones, and an intact hepatic gluconeogenic mechanism, glucose production in fasting requires the availability of precursor substrate, notably alanine. In normal subjects the rate of alanine release from muscle determines the rate of gluconeogenesis in starvation.[28] A physiological reduction in alanine concentration and accentuation of fasting hypoglycemia is observed in normal pregnancy.[29] Alanine deficiency has also been implicated in the pathogenesis of *ketotic hypoglycemia* of infancy and childhood.[30] In this disorder, hypoglycemia and hyperketonemia generally are provoked by a gastrointestinal (GI) upset. Plasma insulin levels are appropriately reduced. The children respond to glucose administration. The long-term prognosis is good, with disappearance of the attacks. In maple syrup urine disease, an enzymatic defect involving decarboxylation of the branched-chain amino acids (valine, leucine, and isoleucine), muscle alanine production is deficient and hypoglycemia due to impaired gluconeogenesis is observed.[31] Decreased availability of alanine may also contribute to the hypoglycemia observed in rare instances in patients with uremia.[31a] In patients with severe wasting associated with kwashiorkor or marasmus, hypoglycemia may be observed (in terminal stages) and is due at least in part to lack of amino acid precursors for gluconeogenesis.

Hypoglycemia occurs in association with muscle weakness, liver dysfunction, and cardiomyopathy in patients with systemic carnitine deficiency.[32a] Carnitine is necessary for the transfer of long-chain fatty acids across the mitochondrial membrane, where they undergo oxidation. A deficiency of carnitine results in diminished fatty acid oxidation, thereby impairing muscle function. The diminution in fatty acid oxidation leads to an increased dependence on glucose utilization by muscle. In addition, fatty acid oxidation in liver is intimately coupled to gluconeogenesis. Acetyl CoA, a major end product of fatty acid oxidation, is an allosteric activator of pyruvate carboxylase, a key enzyme in the gluconeogenic pathway. Thus, the combination of augmented glucose use by muscle and deficient gluconeogenesis by liver results in an inability to maintain euglycemia in the fasting state. Ketogenesis is also impaired in carnitine deficiency (because of the inability to oxidize fatty acids), resulting in the unique circumstance of hypoinsulinemic hypoglycemia without ketosis.

Avoidance of fasting, high-carbohydrate feeding, and the administration of medium-chain triglycerides (whose oxidation does not require carnitine) may decrease the frequency of hypoglycemia.

INSULIN AUTOIMMUNE HYPOGLYCEMIA

A small number of patients have been reported in whom hypoglycemia is associated with circulating antibodies to insulin, despite the absence of a history of insulin treatment.[32] Investigation of these antibodies has shown them to possess the properties of IgG; their light chains were exclusively of K type. The postulated mechanism of hypoglycemia is the sudden release of free insulin from a large pool of antibody-bound insulin. The hypoglycemia may occur in the fasted state or after meals. Antibodies to insulin are also observed in factitious hypoglycemia due to surreptitious insulin injection (see below). Measurements of C peptide may provide a means of distinguishing these disorders. In factitious hypoglycemia C peptide levels are extremely low, reflecting inhibition of endogenous insulin secretion. In contrast, elevated C peptide levels have been observed in autoimmune hypoglycemia, reflecting release of endogenously secreted insulin.

Postprandial Hypoglycemia

Postprandial or "reactive" hypoglycemia is a poorly defined benign clinical syndrome of diverse etiologies, characterized by the development of symptomatic hypoglycemia within a few hours of meal ingestion. By definition, in this type of hypoglycemia the plasma glucose concentration remains normal if food is withheld. Characteristically, hypoglycemia is provoked by ingestion of large amounts of glucose-containing foods and reduced when glucose is eliminated from the diet. There has been considerable debate among physicians as well as the lay public regarding the clinical significance and frequency of the condition. Some suggest that between-meal hypoglycemia sufficient to cause symptoms is very rarely encountered in ordinary daily life. Others have invoked hypoglycemia as a major cause of behavioral disturbance or anxiety. As noted above, the latter view, often expressed in the lay press, has led to self-referral and overdiagnosis by patients as well as physicians. Much of the confusion surrounding this clinical entity is due to the varying criteria used to define hypoglycemia, the nonspecific nature of the symptoms, and the difficulty in obtaining plasma glucose concentration measurements at the time that symptoms develop in the patient's usual environment. The problem is compounded by the fact that chemical hypoglycemia may occur after high-carbohydrate meals in healthy subjects in the absence of any symptoms.

DEFINITION

Postprandial hypoglycemia may be defined as a fall in plasma glucose concentration sufficient to cause symptoms which occurs during the transition period between the fed and the fasted state. The two essential components of the syndrome are (1) chemical hypoglycemia after feeding and (2) the simultaneous onset of symptoms referable to the fall in circulating glucose levels. Neither the presence of hypoglycemia nor symptoms alone is adequate for the diagnosis of the clinical condition.

It is now widely appreciated that the plasma glucose concentration may fall below levels of 60 mg/dl (blood glucose concentration 52 to 53 mg/dl) after glucose ingestion in healthy individuals without eliciting symptoms.[33] In contrast, plasma glucose levels below 50 mg/dl produce symptoms in a significant proportion of (but not all) subjects.[16] Consequently, postprandial chemical hypoglycemia may be defined as a plasma glucose level below 50 mg/dl. It is of clinical significance only if accompanied by symptoms.

SYMPTOMS

In contrast to fasting hypoglycemia, neuroglycopenic symptoms are only rarely encountered in patients with postprandial hypoglycemia. Syncope, seizures, or focal neurologic defects virtually never occur in this syndrome. The usual lack of cerebral symptoms may be related to the nadir to which plasma glucose concentration declines in this syndrome (which is not as low as that seen in the fasting hypoglycemias). A possible additional factor is the much shorter duration of hypoglycemia as compared with fasting hypoglycemia. Adrenergic symptoms (e.g., palpitations, perspiration, pallor, anxiety, hunger, tremor) predominate; these represent the clinical hallmark of the syndrome. These symptoms are transient in nature.

Characteristically, patients with reactive hypoglycemia experience symptoms between meals, particularly after breakfast and/or lunch but rarely after dinner. In contrast, they are able to tolerate prolonged periods of fasting without difficulty. The patient may or may not recognize a relationship between the development of symptoms and prior meal ingestion or the amelioration of symptoms and prior ingestion of carbohydrate-containing foods. The latter is a rather poor marker for the syndrome, since patients without chemical hypoglycemia but with episodic symptoms due to anxiety often report improvement in symptoms after food consumption. It must be emphasized that the vast majority of patients complaining of paroxysmal adrenergic-like symptoms do not, in fact, have postprandial hypoglycemia. Sympathoadrenal stimulation is not specific for hypoglycemia and most commonly occurs in response to anxiety and/or depression.

PREVALENCE AND DIAGNOSIS

The true prevalence of clinical (i.e., symptomatic and chemical) postprandial hypoglycemia has not been established with certainty. Most estimates are based entirely on measurements of plasma glucose concentration during a standard (75- to 100-g) oral glucose tolerance test. This test is performed after an overnight fast; it is generally accepted as the best test available, especially for excluding the diagnosis. To evaluate hypoglycemia, the test should be extended for at least 5 h and blood samples should be obtained every 30 to 60 min. It is particularly important that the patient report any symptoms and that a blood sample be obtained whenever the patient reports symptoms. Using the glucose tolerance test, 24 percent of 4928 men inducted into the U.S. Air Force were observed to have plasma glucose levels below 60 mg/dl 2 h after ingestion of 100 g of glucose.[34] Others have reported rates of "chemical" hypoglycemia (plasma glucose concentration < 60 mg/dl) varying between 15 and 45 percent. However, values below 50 mg/dl occur generally in about 5 to 10 percent of subjects.[35]

Although these data suggest that a postprandial reduction in plasma glucose level to 50 to 60 mg/dl may be a common occurrence, it should be emphasized that values observed in response to the ingestion of 75 to 100 g of pure glucose may not necessarily reflect the biochemical response to ingestion of mixed meals. As already noted (see Nonhypoglycemia), in some patients with chemical hypoglycemia following a glucose load, ingestion of a mixed meal may provoke typical symptoms in the absence of a decline in plasma glucose concentration.[16a] Furthermore, few normal subjects (examined during mass screening programs) report symptoms coincident with the plasma glucose nadir.[16] This is particularly true in the large group of individuals with plasma glucose levels between 50 and 60 mg/dl.[16] As a consequence, probably no more than 2 to 3 percent of subjects actually manifest both chemical hypoglycemia and symptoms (i.e., clinical postprandial hypoglycemia) during the course of a 5-h glucose tolerance test.

Measurements of plasma insulin concentration during the glucose tolerance test are usually of little value in establishing a diagnosis of postprandial hypoglycemia. In normal subjects, the magnitude and pattern of the plasma insulin response are extremely variable following oral glucose ingestion. Furthermore, the plasma insulin levels in patients with postprandial hypoglycemia are often no different from those observed in healthy controls.[16a]

PATHOPHYSIOLOGY

Little is known regarding the mechanisms underlying the development of postprandial hypoglycemia. Nevertheless, important insights may be obtained by examining the physiological response to glucose ingestion in normal subjects.

After glucose ingestion, the rate and magnitude of the rise of circulating glucose concentration is determined by the balance between the rate of glucose absorption from the GI tract and the homeostatic mechanisms which serve to limit extracellular glucose accumulation. With respect to the latter, the elevation in plasma glucose concentration caused by glucose ingestion is minimized by the prompt suppression of endogenous glucose production from the liver and, more important, by the uptake of exogenous glucose from the portal and systemic circulation (Fig. 20-3). These processes are largely regulated by enhanced insulin secretion by the pancreatic islets and the concomitant release of GI hormones. That the route of glucose entry as well as its concentration in blood is an important determinant of insulin release is indicated by the higher levels of circulating insulin observed following an oral glucose load as compared with an equivalent IV dose. This "alimentary augmentation" of insulin secretion is due to the secretion of GI hormones (particularly gastric inhibitory polypeptide) and, possibly, vagal stimulation.

The liver as well as peripheral tissues, particularly muscle, contribute to the uptake of orally ingested glucose.[36,37] When the rate of glucose uptake by hepatic and peripheral tissues exceeds the rate of influx of absorbed glucose from the gut, the plasma glucose concentration declines. Within 2 h after glucose ingestion plasma glucose levels normally approach baseline values and then often fall below postabsorptive levels (between 1 and 4 h) as glucose absorption is completed. Hypoglycemia is prevented in this circumstance by a rapid fall in the rate of glucose removal by hepatic and peripheral tissues and by a rise in hepatic glucose output toward premeal values (Fig. 20-3). These responses are mediated, in part, by the decline in insulin secretion which follows the reduction in circulating glucose concentration. However, postprandial plasma insulin levels may remain as much as fourfold above baseline values at the time plasma glucose concentration returns to baseline.[38] Thus, factors other than a dissipation of insulin are necessary for the prevention of postprandial hypoglycemia. A late rise in plasma GH and epinephrine concentrations as well as a transient decrease in plasma glucagon concentration followed by a rise to baseline are observed after glucose ingestion.[38] Studies using somatostatin (to produce glucagon deficiency) in bilaterally adrenalectomized patients suggest that neither glucagon nor epinephrine alone is critical for postprandial glucose homeostasis, but that combined glucagon and epinephrine deficiency results in postprandial hypoglycemia.[39] In addition to these hormonal factors, neurogenic mechanisms and/or a decline in plasma glucose concentration per se (i.e., glucose autoregulation) may initiate endogenous glucose production, thereby limiting the decline in blood glucose concentration and restoring euglycemia after meal ingestion.[7,40] In contrast to the role of epinephrine and glucagon, plasma concentrations of norepinephrine or cortisol need not change for glucose homeostasis to be normally maintained in the postprandial period.[38]

From these observations it is evident that postprandial hypoglycemia may result either from a failure of glucose uptake to decline appropriately as plasma glucose concentration falls below baseline or from an inadequate rebound rise in hepatic glucose production. Since the liver is an important site of glucose disposal and the only site of glucose production, the major event underlying the normal response is the switch of the liver from an organ of net glucose uptake to one of net glucose output. A number of mechanisms could account for a disturbance in this

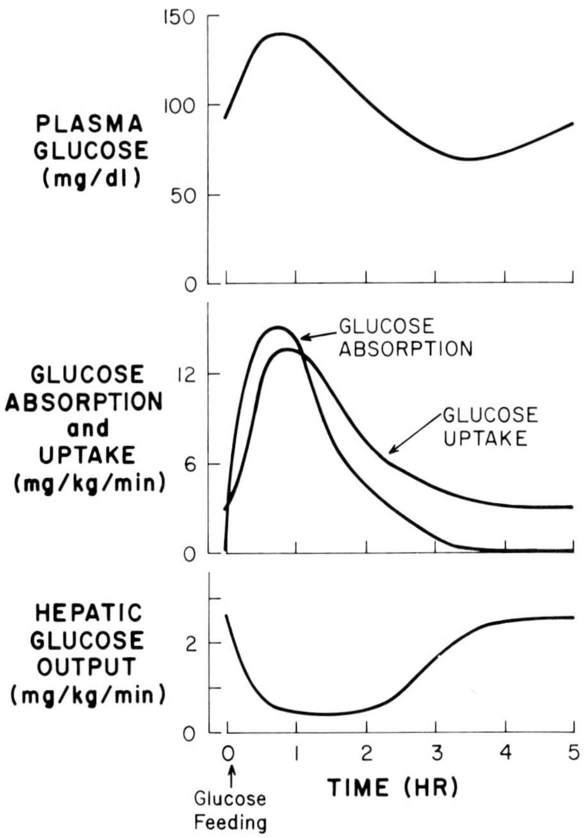

FIGURE 20-3 The effect of glucose feeding (e.g., an oral glucose tolerance test) on plasma glucose concentration, glucose absorption (from the gut), glucose uptake (by liver and peripheral tissues), and hepatic glucose output (glycogenolysis and gluconeogenesis). The initial rise in plasma glucose concentration is a consequence of the fact that glucose absorption initially exceeds the rate of glucose uptake. The subsequent decline in plasma glucose concentration, *generally to below basal levels*, is a result of the rate of glucose uptake exceeding the rate of glucose absorption while hepatic glucose production remains suppressed. The final stabilization of plasma glucose concentration at basal levels is dependent on the return of hepatic glucose production to basal rates and the fall in glucose uptake.

process. Clearly, excessive or inappropriately sustained insulin secretion would be expected to interfere with the hepatic shift from glucose uptake to output. Alternatively, increased insulin action could result from combined deficiency of glucagon and epinephrine secretion.[38] In addition, failure of hepatic autoregulation or of hepatic neurogenic control could result in hypoglycemia.[7,40] Finally, the gut may have a special role via endocrine or neurogenic (vagal) signals which influence insulin secretion or action on the liver. Unfortunately, data are generally not available which permit a determination of the precise mechanism responsible for postprandial hypoglycemia in most cases.

CLASSIFICATION

Postprandial hypoglycemia, unlike hypoglycemia in the fasting state, is rarely a life-threatening medical condition. The clinical forms of this disorder are generally differentiated on the basis of whether the disorder occurs in the absence of other disease or is associated with gastric surgery (alimentary) or in the early stages of insulin-independent (maturity-onset, type II) diabetes.

Idiopathic (Functional) Hypoglycemia

By far the most common form of postprandial hypoglycemia, idiopathic postprandial hypoglycemia is a diagnosis of exclusion. Patients with this disorder appear healthy but often complain of weakness, faintness, or palpitations. Their somatic symptoms may seem out of proportion to their actual physical disability. For this reason, they are frequently characterized as being emotionally labile or having compulsive personalities. The disorder is most commonly seen in women, generally between 25 and 35 years of age. On glucose tolerance testing, the nadir glucose value, and symptoms, are generally observed at 3 to 4 h and are followed by a rebound increment.

The insulin secretory pattern in these patients is heterogeneous. In the majority of cases, neither the peak insulin levels nor the total insulin response is increased.[16a] Some patients exhibit a delayed rise in peak postprandial insulin levels; however, the pathogenetic significance of this finding has not been established. It has been suggested that some patients may have increased vagal tone, which leads to more rapid gastric emptying and enhanced insulin secretion.[33,41] Evidence is lacking, however, for an alteration in gastrointestinal or counterregulatory hormone secretion; hepatic autoregulatory mechanisms, neurogenic mechanisms, and insulin sensitivity have not been quantified in these patients.

Symptoms related to postprandial hypoglycemia tend to wax and wane over many years, without long-term progression. Many patients note improvement with diet therapy (see below). However, it is unclear how much of this improvement is related to correction of hypoglycemia per se. The discovery of an organic explanation for the symptoms and the medical attention directed to the problem may be important factors in the patient's improvement. Frequently, postprandial hypoglycemia and psychological disorders coexist in the same patient.

Alimentary Hypoglycemia

Postprandial hypoglycemia is occasionally observed in patients who have undergone gastric surgery (e.g., gastrectomy, gastrojejunostomy, or vagotomy and pyloroplasty). When evaluated with an oral glucose tolerance test, these patients characteristically exhibit exaggerated early hyperglycemia and hyperinsulinemia, followed by a rapid fall to hypoglycemic levels within 1.5 to 3 h. The onset of hypoglycemia is usually earlier than in patients with the idiopathic form of the disorder and the intensity is greater. Adrenergic symptoms may be particularly severe; in rare cases neurologic disturbances, including syncope and seizures, have been reported. From a therapeutic standpoint, it is important to distinguish hypoglycemic symptoms from those of the "dumping syndrome." The latter usually occurs sooner after feeding (30 to 60 min) and results in gastrointestinal complaints (e.g., epigastric fullness, nausea) as well as adrenergic symptoms.

The observation that in such patients hypoglycemia occurs after oral glucose feeding but not after IV glucose administration has focused attention on a possible gut (rather than islet cell) defect as the primary cause of this disorder.[33] Rapid gastric emptying has been postulated to be the mechanism responsible for excessive glucose absorption, leading secondarily to early hyperglycemia and excessive insulin secretion. While this hypothesis seems attractive, an exaggerated early rise in plasma glucose concentration is observed in patients who have undergone gastric surgery even when the effects of gastric emptying are bypassed and glucose is infused directly into the jejunum.[42] Interestingly, some patients with peptic ulcer disease have an increased rise in plasma insulin concentration after oral glucose feeding and an increased incidence of postprandial hypoglycemia. Thus, it is possible that surgery intensified a preexisting abnormality in glucose absorption or gut hormone release. Whether gastrectomy alters counterregulatory mechanisms, particularly glucagon and epinephrine secretion, has not been established.

Early Diabetes

It has long been recognized that postprandial hypoglycemia may be an early manifestation of insulin-independent (type II, maturity-onset) diabetes mellitus.[43] These patients have normal fasting glucose levels, an exaggerated early rise in plasma glucose concentration due to inadequate insulin release, and late hyperinsulinemia due to hyperglycemia early in the test. Hypoglycemia usually occurs after 3 to 5 h, i.e., later than hypoglycemia of the alimentary variety. It is not known how many of these patients actually go on to develop overt diabetes (i.e., fasting hyperglycemia) or whether some revert to normal on repeat testing. Furthermore, it is not established whether the development of hyperinsulinemia can account entirely for the hypoglycemia. When the plasma insulin responses of patients with early diabetes are examined, no difference is evident between patients with and without hypoglycemia.

Other Causes

Postprandial hypoglycemia has been reported in association with obesity, renal glycosuria, and various endocrine deficiency states (hypopituitarism, Addison's disease, hypothyroidism). In obesity, where hyperinsulinism would seem an obvious factor, the plasma insulin responses to glucose ingestion are not consistently exaggerated when hypoglycemia is present. In renal glycosuria, it is likely that excessive urinary glucose loss is an important contributory factor, whereas in endocrine deficiency diseases alterations in insulin sensitivity and/or hepatic counterregulation may account for this phenomenon.

TREATMENT

It is generally believed that the use of a carbohydrate-restricted diet is of therapeutic benefit in postprandial hypoglycemia. However, controlled studies documenting the efficacy of such a regimen are lacking. From a physiological standpoint this approach makes sense, since the disorder is largely caused by ingestion of glucose-containing foods. Most patients can be managed solely by dietary manipulation; the use of drugs is rarely indicated.

There is lack of agreement regarding how much carbohydrate restriction is required. Some advocate a diet extremely low in carbohydrate ($<$ 100 g per day). These diets lead to ketosis, glucose intolerance, and a decreased ability to dispose of amino acids after oral protein feeding. Curiously, even normal subjects exhibit a tendency to chemical hypoglycemia with large glucose loads after being placed on such diets.[44] As a consequence, it is possible that near-total carbohydrate elimination may lead to the aggravation of symptoms during dietary indiscretions. For these reasons, it is prudent to initiate treatment with a diet only moderately reduced in carbohydrate, i.e., 120 to 150 g per day. Carbohydrate should be given in the form of multiple small feedings, i.e., three meals a day interspersed with three snacks. If mild carbohydrate restriction is unsuccessful, a further decrease in carbohydrate content may then be attempted.

Some patients may not improve after dietary manipulation; in rare circumstances, symptoms may even worsen. The latter finding should alert the physician to the possibility of fasting hypoglycemia or, more likely, may indicate that hypoglycemia is not responsible for the patient's symptoms.

When carbohydrate restriction fails, and there is no question that the symptoms are due to hypoglycemia, various drug treatments have been advocated. Anticholinergic agents may be useful.[33] Since they act by delaying gastric emptying and reducing intestinal motility, they are particularly helpful in patients with alimentary hypoglycemia. While biguanides have been reported to alleviate symptoms in occasional patients, their risks (e.g., lactic acidosis) outweigh their benefits. Some investigators have suggested the use of sulfonylurea drugs in patients with early diabetes. However, there is no convincing evidence of their therapeutic benefit. Diphenylhydantoin, an inhibitor of insulin secretion, may be of some value, but only a few anecdotal accounts of its usefulness have been reported. Finally, propranolol has been suggested as a potentially useful drug. Its use should be discouraged, however, since it has been reported to accentuate hypoglycemia in some patients.[45] Propranolol probably does not block hypoglycemia per se, but rather its symptoms.

Induced Hypoglycemia

Induced hypoglycemia refers to those conditions in which an abnormal reduction in plasma glucose concentration is due to (1) the administration of a drug (e.g., insulin), (2) the ingestion of a toxic substance (e.g., alcohol), or (3) an inborn error in metabolism or unexplained sensitivity that renders a specific nutrient in the diet capable of inducing hypoglycemia (e.g., hereditary fructose intolerance, leucine-induced hypoglycemia). The last form of hypoglycemia is thus a variant of postprandial hypoglycemia. It is considered here, however, because it is not mixed-meal ingestion per se which causes the hypoglycemia but a specific metabolite (e.g., fructose or leucine) in a predisposed population group. The clinical significance of the induced hypoglycemias is underscored by the fact that insulin-induced hypoglycemia (in insulin-treated diabetic patients) and alcohol-induced hypoglycemia are the two most common causes of hypoglycemia encountered in adults.

INSULIN-INDUCED HYPOGLYCEMIA

In view of the relatively small margin in many diabetic patients between optimal blood glucose regulation by insulin and the development of hypoglycemia, it is not surprising that hypoglycemia is greatest in the long-standing, juvenile-onset (type I) diabetic patient without residual insulin secretion. It is less commonly observed in obese, maturity-onset (type II) diabetic patients in whom insulin resistance is invariably present. Insulin-induced hypoglycemia is experienced at some time by virtually all type I diabetic patients and constitutes the most frequent complication of insulin treatment. In some series, severe hypoglycemia (necessitating hospitalization or assistance from another person) has been observed in 25 percent of patients over a 1-year period.[46] In addition, hypoglycemia accounts for 3 to 7 percent of deaths in patients with type I diabetes.[47]

The frequency of hypoglycemia in insulin-treated diabetic patients depends in part on the adequacy of counterregulatory hormone secretion and the intensity of the treatment program. A deficiency of glucagon secretion in response to hypoglycemia is frequently observed in type I diabetes, but does not of itself increase vulnerability to insulin-induced hypoglycemia.[10] However, diabetic patients in whom epinephrine deficiency is combined with glucagon deficiency are severely predisposed to insulin-induced hypoglycemia.[10] Such combined deficiencies are often, but not always, accompanied by clinical evidence of autonomic neuropathy.

Other factors which predispose to the development of insulin-induced hypoglycemia include a marked increase in physical activity (exercise), a decrease in food intake (skipped meals, low-calorie diet, or fasting), and a decrease in insulin turnover (e.g., renal failure).

Faulty injection techniques, e.g., failure to agitate the insulin vial properly before use, errors in the preparation of insulin mixtures, accidental injection into muscle (rather than subcutaneous tissue), leading to more rapid insulin absorption, or injection into sites where insulin absorption is irregular (e.g., lipoatrophic sites), may on occasion be important contributory factors. Severe, recurrent bouts of hypoglycemia may also occur suddenly in patients not usually prone to hypoglycemia. In this circumstance, several possible causes should be considered: (1) development of renal insufficiency, (2) failure to reduce insulin dosage after resolution of some intercurrent stress or illness, (3) onset of other conditions causing hypersensitivity to insulin (e.g., adrenal or pituitary insufficiency), (4) development of autonomic neuropathy, and (5) early pregnancy. In early pregnancy, hypoglycemia may result from a siphoning of glucose by the conceptus and a decrease in the availability of glycogenic amino acids (e.g., alanine) at a time when placental hormones with anti-insulin effects (e.g., progesterone, human placental lactogen) are present in only low concentrations.[48] Overzealous treatment of renal glycosuria (the renal threshold for glucose invariably declines during pregnancy) may also result in hypoglycemia.

The symptoms of insulin-induced hypoglycemia vary, depending in part on whether short-acting or intermediate- and long-acting insulins are the primary offending agents and autonomic neuropathy is present.[10] With the short-acting insulins (regular insulin and an insulin zinc suspension such as Semilente Iletin) adrenergic symptoms predominate. With the intermediate- or long-acting insulins (isophane insulin suspension or insulin zinc suspensions such as lente insulin or Ultralente Iletin), neuroglycopenic rather than adrenergic symptoms are often more prominent, perhaps owing to the very gradual nature of the glucose decline and the longer duration of hypoglycemia. Occasionally, patients may pass from alertness to severe confusion or coma without warning; this is particularly true in patients with autonomic neuropathy.

As noted above, a sharp fall in plasma glucose concentration in the insulin-treated diabetic may lead to the development of symptoms at plasma glucose levels (90 to 100 mg/dl) which are not abnormal in the general population.[2] On the other hand, when a patient has adrenergic-like symptoms in association with plasma glucose levels in excess of 125 to 150 mg/dl, the symptoms cannot be ascribed to a rapid decline in plasma glucose concentration, and a reduction in insulin dosage is not warranted.

SULFONYLUREA-INDUCED HYPOGLYCEMIA

The sulfonylurea agents are in rare instances responsible for hypoglycemia in maturity-onset (type II) diabetic patients when administered in usual therapeutic doses. Many of these cases occur within the first few days of treatment. Occasionally, however, hypoglycemia may develop after long-standing treatment without a change in dose. The hypoglycemic episodes are generally associated with a condition or drug which alters the metabolism of the sulfonylurea agent. Liver disease prolongs the hypoglycemic action of tolbutamide, acetohexamide, and the second-generation sulfonylureas glyburide and glipizide, since these drugs are normally metabolized in the liver. Chlorpropamide and acetohexamide may bring about hypoglycemia in patients with renal insufficiency, since either the drug (chlorpropamide) or its active metabolite (in the case of acetohexamide) is excreted via the kidney. In view of the relatively high incidence of azotemia in the diabetic population and the very prolonged half-life of chlorpropamide under normal circumstances (24 to 60 h), this drug is particularly likely to cause severe hypoglycemia.

In addition to liver or kidney disease, drug interactions may be responsible for the development of hypoglycemia in patients receiving sulfonylurea agents. Certain drugs have been shown to potentiate the effects of sulfonylurea by (1) interfering with hepatic metabolism (e.g., sulfisoxazole and dicumarol), (2) reducing urinary excretion (e.g., phenylbutazone), or (3) possessing an additive hypoglycemia action (e.g., salicylates).

FACTITIOUS HYPOGLYCEMIA

Insulin and Sulfonylureas

Self-induction of hypoglycemia by the surreptitious administration of insulin or sulfonylureas must be considered in all cases of fasting hypoglycemia and hyperinsulinemia, particularly in medical personnel, diabetic patients, or those in contact with diabetic patients. The condition is most common in young females and may be considered a variant of the Munchausen syndrome.[49] These individuals may have no obvious psychological disorder and may give a history which suggests spontaneous hypoglycemia. Diabetic patients may claim that they experience hypoglycemic attacks even when they forgo using insulin. The development of hypoglycemia in the hospital does not preclude the diagnosis of factitious hypoglycemia, since these patients are often ingenious in concealing the offending drug. A careful inspection for needle marks which may be overlooked on a routine examination is quite helpful.

In patients injecting themselves with insulin, the characteristic laboratory finding is intermittent hypoglycemia in conjunction with enormous elevations in plasma insulin level. The finding of insulin antibodies in nondiabetic patients during the course of insulin measurements is an important diagnostic clue. However, antibodies may not be present for several months; therefore, their absence does not exclude factitious hypoglycemia. Furthermore, the presence of antibodies is not pathognomonic. Several patients have been described with spontaneous hypoglycemia associated with insulin antibodies arising on an autoimmune basis (see Insulin Autoimmune Hypoglycemia, above).[32] Factitious hypoglycemia resulting from insulin use is best established by the triad of hypoglycemia, hyperinsulinemia, and suppressed C peptide levels.[20] In contrast to endogenous hyperinsulinemia (e.g., islet cell tumor), which is invariably accompanied by simultaneous elevations of insulin and C peptide levels, exogenous hyperinsulinemia leads to the secondary inhibition of endogenous insulin release and thus reduced C peptide levels.[20]

Factitious hypoglycemia in the insulin-treated diabetic poses an especially difficult problem. In these patients, proinsulin bound to antibodies may lead to spurious increases in C peptide levels and consequently the mistaken diagnosis of an islet cell tumor. This laboratory artifact may be eliminated by using urinary C peptide measurements or methods which precipitate antibody-bound proinsulin before doing the C peptide assay.

In patients ingesting sulfonylurea drugs, the measurement of C peptide is of no value, since endogenous insulin secretion is stimulated by these drugs. Furthermore, sulfonylurea agents accentuate the endogenous insulin response to leucine administration, leading to a false-positive test for insulinoma. For this reason, clandestine abuse of sulfonylureas may be more difficult to diagnose than insulin abuse. Fortunately, assays are available for the measurement of concentrations of sulfonylurea drugs in plasma. In addition, tolbutamide may be detected in the urine, since it forms a white precipitate (carboxytolbutamine) upon acidification.

Other Drugs

A number of drugs or drug combinations have been implicated in hypoglycemia.[50] However, hypoglycemia is an extremely unusual complication of drug therapy in the absence of simultaneous insulin or sulfonylurea administration. In an extensive review of the literature, Seltzer uncovered only 22 such cases out of 300 reports of drug-induced hypoglycemic coma.[50] Among these cases, salicylates were the most common offenders. In virtually all instances of salicylate-induced hypoglycemia, the clinical picture consisted of young children with a severe febrile illness given excessive doses of the drug. Salicylate intoxication leads to acid-base disturbances (respiratory alkalosis and metabolic acidosis) far more frequently than it causes hypoglycemia. Salicylate ingestion has also been associated with the development of Reye's syndrome (see above), in which hypoglycemia is a frequent finding.

The beta-blocking agent propranolol in occasional instances has been implicated in the development of hypoglycemia. This drug has been reported to enhance hypoglycemia in patients with alimentary or idiopathic postprandial hypoglycemia.[45] The mechanism underlying this phenomenon is not firmly established but presumably involves hypersensitivity to insulin by virtue of removal of the insulin-antagonistic effects of epinephrine mediated via beta-adrenergic receptors. The tendency to develop hypoglycemia in association with beta-adrenergic blockade is increased in insulin-treated diabetics during periods of exercise.[51]

ALCOHOL-INDUCED HYPOGLYCEMIA

Undoubtedly the most common cause of hypoglycemia in the nondiabetic population is that related to overindulgence in alcohol. Originally, this syndrome was attributed to contaminants in various illicit preparations of alcoholic beverages rather than ethanol itself. However, this view became untenable when it was shown that pure ethanol can produce the same effect when it is given to poorly nourished subjects or to normal individuals who have fasted for 48 to 72 h.

Alcohol-induced hypoglycemia is most characteristically observed in binge drinkers who have consumed little or no food for one or more days.[52] Hypoglycemia usually develops 6 to 24 h after cessation of alcohol ingestion, and thus the telltale sign of alcohol on the patient's breath may not be present. Generally, the patients are chronic alcoholics who have been drinking for several days and eating poorly. Often, there is a history of repeated vomiting, providing further evidence that few nonalcohol calories have been taken in. Some individuals are more susceptible to the glucose-lowering effects of alcohol. These include (1) young children, who may consume alcohol accidentally, (2) diabetic patients treated with insulin, and (3) patients with disturbances of the adrenopituitary axis (e.g., hypopituitarism, isolated ACTH deficiency, and Addison's disease).

Affected individuals usually lapse into coma without premonitory adrenergic symptoms. Since the breath may not smell of alcohol, the diagnosis may be overlooked. Differentiation from acute alcoholic intoxication is sometimes difficult without laboratory investigation. Important distinguishing clinical signs are the presence of hypothermia (due to hypoglycemia) and tachypnea (due to accompanying lactic acidosis) and the presence of blood alcohol levels below values observed in acute intoxication ($<$ 100 mg/dl). Plasma glucose levels are generally extremely low (below 30 mg/dl) and do not respond to glucagon administration. Plasma insulin concentration is reduced and ketonuria is generally present. An important feature is the presence of severe metabolic acidosis due to the accumulation of lactic acid and, in some patients, accompanying alcoholic ketoacidosis.[53] Tests of liver function are not helpful; liver function is frequently normal.

The diagnosis of alcohol-induced hypoglycemia rests entirely upon the history of alcohol intake and the demonstration of hypoglycemia in conjunction with mild elevations of blood alcohol and lactic acid levels. Once the hypoglycemia has been corrected and the patient has resumed eating, diagnostic tests are of little value. Alcohol provocation usually does not lead to hypoglycemia once glycogen stores have been repleted by refeeding and is of no diagnostic value under conditions of prolonged fasting when glycogen stores have been depleted. Since alcohol consumption is so common and often accentuates hypoglycemia due to other causes, other diagnostic possibilities should not be dismissed, particularly if hypoglycemia is recurrent. Consequently, it may be necessary for the patient to undergo a 72-h fast to exclude other causes of fasting hypoglycemia. Hypoglycemia is not reproduced during fasting if alcohol was the sole cause of hypoglycemia, provided that alcohol intake is prevented during the fast.

The mechanism of alcohol-induced hypoglycemia is dependent on the metabolism of alcohol by the liver and requires a glycogen-depeleted state (Fig. 20-4). The major pathway of ethanol oxidation is via the cytoplasmic enzyme *alcohol dehydrogenase.* This reaction leads to the production of acetaldehyde and the reduction of NAD to NADH. The acetaldehyde thus formed is further oxidized to acetate by *aldehyde dehydrogenase* in the presence of NAD, which acts as a hydrogen acceptor. As a consequence, when large amounts of ethanol are metabolized, excessive amounts of NADH are generated and the ratio of NADH to NAD in the liver cell markedly increases. The accumulation of NADH favors the reduction of pyruvate to lactate. Since the formation of glucose from the major gluconeogenic precursors lactate and alanine requires, as a first step, that they be converted to pyruvate, the reduction of pyruvate to lactate effectively interferes with gluconeogenesis. In addition, the increase in the hepatic ratio of NADH/NAD reduces the contribution of glycerol to gluconeogenesis. This substrate enters the gluconeogenic pathway via the oxidation of α-glycerophosphate to dihydroxyacetone phosphate, a reaction which depends on the reduction of NAD to NADH. The suppressive effect of alcohol on hepatic gluconeogenesis has been confirmed in humans using isotopic techniques. Kreisberg et al.[53] have shown that the oral administration of ethanol to normal humans promptly inhibits incorporation of lactate into glucose, both in the postabsorptive state and after prolonged starvation (48 to 72 h). Furthermore, the conversion of alanine (the principal glycogenic amino acid) into glucose is also reduced by alcohol. Since glucose output by the liver is largely (75 percent) due to glycogenolysis after an overnight fast, the hypoglycemic effect of alcohol is manifest only when glycogen stores have been depleted (i.e., after days of poor food intake), at which point glucose homeostasis is largely dependent on intact mechanisms of gluconeogenesis. This accounts for the fact that alcohol-induced hypoglycemia is seen almost exclusively in poorly nourished patients and/or individuals who have been drinking but eating poorly for several days. The greater vulnerability of children to alcohol-induced hypoglycemia in the absence of prolonged fasting or binge drinking reflects their more rapid glucose turnover (per kilogram of body weight) and, therefore, more rapid depletion of liver glycogen stores than is observed in adults.[25]

Alcohol-induced hypoglycemia is treated by the intravenous administration of glucose. Glucagon should not be used, since glycogen-depleted patients do not respond to this hormone.

LEUCINE SENSITIVITY

Although protein feeding or infusion of amino acids stimulates insulin secretion in normal subjects, only leucine has been reported to cause symptomatic hypoglycemia. Leucine-induced hypoglycemia may occur as a relatively uncommon congenital disorder or may be acquired in patients with hyperinsulinism (insulinoma or nesidioblastosis) or in normal subjects given sulfonylurea drugs.

Congenital leucine sensitivity is generally a familial disorder which affects both sexes equally. Patients usually present in early infancy with recurrent seizures or failure to thrive. Hypoglycemia may be observed in the fasting state but is especially pronounced following ingestion of protein meals with a high leucine content. While metabolites of leucine (isovaleric acid and α-ketoisocaproic acid) and the other branched-chain amino acids (isoleucine and valine) may lower blood glucose concentration in some of these patients, they

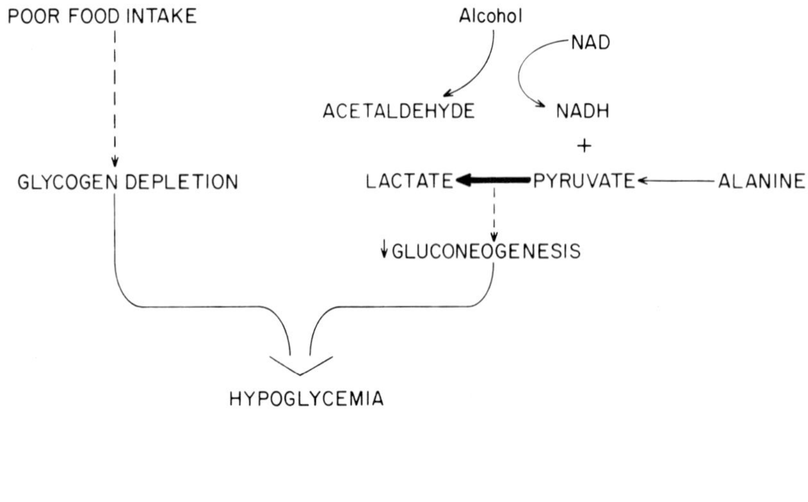

FIGURE 20-4 Mechanism of alcohol-induced hypoglycemia. The metabolism of alcohol results in the accumulation of NADH, thereby shunting pyruvate to lactate. Since gluconeogenesis from alanine or lactate requires their initial conversion to pyruvate, the shunting of pyruvate to lactate interferes with gluconeogenesis. A history of poor food intake is also required, since the inhibitory effect of alcohol on gluconeogenesis is manifest as hypoglycemia only when liver glycogen stores have been depleted.

are not nearly as potent as leucine. With increasing age there is a gradual reduction in hypoglycemic episodes, so that by 6 to 10 years symptomatic hypoglycemia is uncommon. Nevertheless, if the diagnosis goes unrecognized, permanent brain damage may occur.

The diagnosis of leucine sensitivity is best made by studying the response of plasma insulin and glucose concentrations to an oral leucine load (150 mg per kilogram of body weight). In leucine-sensitive children, ingestion of leucine elicits a marked hyperinsulinemic response, which in turn leads to profound hypoglycemia. In contrast, normal individuals demonstrate a much smaller increase in plasma insulin concentration (5 to 10 μU/ml) and only a mild (5 to 10 mg/ml) fall in plasma glucose levels. Neither glucose nor tolbutamide produces an exaggerated insulin rise in these patients.

Treatment is directed toward reducing the leucine (hence, protein) content of the diet. However, it may be difficult to find a diet low enough in leucine to prevent hypoglycemia and at the same time meet the daily requirements of the child for protein. In these cases treatment with diazoxide may be worthwhile. Some patients have responded to treatment with glucocorticoids, but this is inadvisable unless the hypoglycemia is quite severe, because of the danger of impairing growth.

HEREDITARY FRUCTOSE INTOLERANCE

Hereditary fructose intolerance is a rare disorder (sometimes called *fructosemia*) characterized by severe GI symptoms and hypoglycemia following the ingestion of fructose-containing foods (e.g., sucrose in infant formula, candies, fruits). It is inherited as an autosomal recessive trait, affecting males and females equally. The parents of affected offspring are, as a rule, normal. Patients are characteristically asymptomatic until they consume fructose for the first time, i.e., upon weaning from the breast or when fruit juices are added to the infant's diet. The use of infant-feeding formulas containing sucrose has created a special problem for affected infants. Since they are unable to refuse sucrose and thus protect themselves, they get into difficulty immediately. Consequently, the prognosis is much poorer for newborns fed formula containing fructose than for those who are breast-fed and thus avoid fructose early in life. In milder cases, offending foods are eliminated from the diet by trial and error, and the diagnosis may go unrecognized until adulthood.

The clinical picture varies, depending on whether the patient is seen in infancy or later in childhood. In babies, repeated fructose exposure leads to a clinical picture characterized by recurrent vomiting, dehydration, lethargy, seizures, and failure to thrive. The liver enlarges because of accumulation of glycogen and/or fat, resulting in jaundice and abnormal liver function tests in some cases. A series of abnormalities of function of the proximal convoluted tubule of the kidney also occurs. The renal lesion causes aminoaciduria, phosphaturia, glycosuria, and bicarbonate wasting, a pattern similar to that associated with the Fanconi syndrome. Hyperuricemia and lactic acidosis are other characteristic findings. If the cause of the disorder is recognized and fructose is eliminated from the diet, the signs and symptoms rapidly disappear. If not treated, the disease may proceed to death within the first few months of life. If children with fructose intolerance reach the age of 6 to 12 months, their chances of doing well are markedly enhanced, as they become able to avoid sucrose. These children become symptomatic only when fructose is inadvertently ingested. When this happens, severe vomiting and alterations in consciousness occur, the latter due to hypoglycemia.

The diagnosis of fructose intolerance is made by means of an IV fructose tolerance test (3 g per square meter of body surface area). The IV route is preferred, since GI symptoms are avoided. After fructose administration, plasma glucose concentration falls (rather than rises, as in normal subjects), despite a concomitant reduction in circulating insulin level. In addition, there is a profound decrease in serum inorganic phosphate concentration, as well as an increase in urinary phosphate and bicarbonate excretion and blood lactate concentration.

The basic defect is a lack of fructose-1-phosphate aldolase (aldolase B), a cytosolic, genetically distinct isoenzyme expressed in liver, kidney, and intestine.[54] The enzyme *fructose-1,6-diphosphatase* is also reduced in activity (10 to 50 percent of normal), but its activity is sufficient to maintain hepatic gluconeogenesis during prolonged periods of fasting. However, when fructose is administered, fructose-1-phosphate cannot be metabolized and accumulates, leading to inhibition of three enzymes. *Fructokinase* is inhibited, so that fructose is poorly cleared from the circulation. Second, fructose-1-phosphate in conjunction with low intracellular levels of inorganic phosphate inhibits hepatic *phosphorylase,* thus preventing glycogen breakdown. Finally, fructose-1-phosphate competitively inhibits fructose-1,6-diphosphatase. Since all three-carbon gluconeogenic precursors (e.g., lactate, alanine, pyruvate, glycerol) must pass through this enzymatic step, its deficiency seriously impedes gluconeogenesis. Fructose administration thus suppresses glycogenolysis and gluconeogenesis, resulting in hypoglycemia. It is probable that the acute GI symptoms and the renal tubular abnormalities also result from intracellular changes in fructose-1-phosphate and inorganic phosphate in gut mucosa and kidney tissue.

Treatment of hereditary fructose intolerance consists of restriction of dietary fructose intake. Moderate restriction (130 to 160 mg per kilogram of body weight per day) may be sufficient to prevent symptoms of acute intoxication. However, more stringent restriction (40 mg per kilogram of body weight per day) may be necessary to prevent somatic growth retardation due to chronic fructose intoxication.[55]

Hereditary fructose intolerance must be distinguished from two other disorders of fructose metabolism, namely, *benign fructosuria* and *fructose-1,6-diphosphatase* deficiency. Benign fructosuria is a rare familial anomaly caused by a lack of fructokinase. Failure of phosphorylation prevents rapid entry of fructose into cells. As a result, a fructose load produces an exaggerated elevation in plasma fructose concentration as well as fructose in the urine. The latter may be confused with glucose (if nonspecific tests, e.g., Clinitest, are used) and result in an erroneous diagnosis of diabetes mellitus. Benign fructosuria is easily differentiated from fructose intolerance by the fact that fructose ingestion fails to elicit hypoglycemic symptoms. Patients are entirely asymptomatic and thus require no treatment.

In fructose-1,6-diphosphatase deficiency, frank hypoglycemia and lactic acidosis are observed after the ingestion of large fructose loads. However, consumption of smaller amounts of fructose causes neither hypoglycemia nor gastrointestinal symptoms. These patients usually present in early childhood with profound hypoglycemia and lactic acidosis during the course of a febrile illness. Hepatomegaly is characteristic, but there is rarely a history of fructose- or sucrose-induced symptoms. In contrast to fructose intolerance, which is characterized by euglycemia during fasting, a prolonged fast invariably leads to hypoglycemia as glycogen stores are depleted.[56] Glycerol administration also produces hypoglycemia in these patients, but not in those with fructose intolerance. The primary defect is a total lack of fructose-1,6-diphosphatase, one of the rate-limiting enzymes of hepatic gluconeogenesis. Hepatic glucose production remains normal so long as glycogen is present. However, when glycogen is depleted, hypoglycemia occurs.

HYPOGLYCIN

Ingestion of the unripe akee fruit of the tree *Blighia sapida* produces a severe illness characterized by vomiting and hypoglycemic coma. Akee is grown throughout Jamaica, where it is a staple of the diet. Although the tree is distributed throughout the tropics (e.g., west and central Africa and the southern part of Florida), the fruit is not commonly eaten outside of Jamaica; hence, the name "Jamaican vomiting sickness."

The disorder occurs most commonly in young, malnourished children; it is unusual in adults. Whether young children have a metabolic predisposition or simply have not learned to avoid the unripe fruit is not known. Typically, the child suddenly develops severe vomiting and retching. There is severe weakness and in some cases convulsions, which may be followed by death. The most important laboratory finding is severe hypoglycemia. Plasma glucose levels below 20 mg/dl are not uncommon. In addition, metabolic acidosis may be observed, which is not attributable to ketones or lactate. The acidosis is due to the accumulation of organic acids (dicarboxylic acids and short-chain fatty acids), as discussed below. The entire time course of the sickness varies from a few hours to 2 to 3 days.

The offending substance in the unripe akee fruit is *hypoglycin* A (L-α-amino-β-[methylenecyclopropyl]-propionic acid). In the body it is metabolized by deamination and oxidative decarboxylation to methylenecyclopropylacetic acid (MCPA), which is the actual toxic element. This substance is a potent inhibitor of several short-chain acyl CoA dehydrogenases[57] and may also compete with long-chain fatty acids for access to carnitine (which is necessary for the transport of long-chain fatty acids into mitochondria, where they undergo oxidation). As a consequence, MCPA leads to the inhibition of long-chain fatty acid oxidation as well as the accumulation of short-chain fatty acids (e.g., hexanoic, butyric, and isovaleric acids) and unusual medium-chain dicarboxylic acids[57,58] (e.g., glutarate, adipate, superate, sebacate, and ethylmalonate). As in the case of systemic carnitine deficiency (see above), the inhibition of fatty acid oxidation results in a suppression of gluconeogenesis due to reduced availability of acetyl CoA, an allosteric activator of the gluconeogenic enzyme pyruvate carboxylase. The massive elevations in concentrations of dicarboxylic acids (glutarate, ethylmalonate) further depress gluconeogenesis by inhibiting the mitochondrial transport of malate, thereby reducing the availability of oxaloacetate for conversion to phospho*enol*-pyruvate. Since fatty acids cannot be efficiently oxidized for the formation of ATP, increased demands are made on glucose utilization to supply the energy requirements of the body. The interference with glucose production coupled with increased glucose utilization leads to the rapid depletion of liver glycogen and the development of hypoglycemia.

Therapy is directed toward restoring blood glucose levels by administration of glucose. Correction of hypoglycemia may fail to prevent death, however.

Whether the lack of response is due to irreversible changes caused by prolonged hypoglycemia or to the large variety of toxic compounds generated by hypoglycin A has not been established.

DIAGNOSTIC EVALUATION

When a patient presents with symptoms suggestive of hypoglycemia, studies should be initiated to determine whether or not hypoglycemia is actually present and, if so, the etiologic factor responsible. Diagnostic evaluation must proceed in a logical fashion, based on a careful history and physical examination. The indiscriminate use of specialized tests should be avoided.

History and Physical Examination

A detailed history is of critical importance in determining both the extent and order of laboratory testing and the potential causes of hypoglycemia. The primary goal should be establishing the likelihood that symptoms are a consequence of either postprandial or fasting hypoglycemia. Unless the latter can be excluded, more extensive evaluation is usually required. Therefore, it is important that the physician not solely rely on the patient, but question family members and friends as well. Furthermore, many patients are unaware of the relationship between their symptoms and fasting. It is worthwhile to determine specifically if the patient had missed breakfast and/or lunch when symptoms occurred.

Other important diagnostic clues may be obtained by careful questioning. Some of these include (1) a history of seizures (suggestive of fasting rather than postprandial hypoglycemia), (2) recent weight gain or exercise-induced symptoms (suggestive of an insulinoma), (3) symptoms of adrenal or pituitary insufficiency, (4) previous gastric surgery, (5) a family history of diabetes (postprandial hypoglycemia) or hypoglycemia (hepatic enzymatic defect), (6) a medically oriented occupation (suggestive of factitious hypoglycemia), or (7) heavy alcohol intake.

Physical examination is usually less helpful, especially in evaluating postprandial hypoglycemia or if an insulinoma is suspected. However, several diagnoses may be suggested by specific physical findings. For example, signs of endocrine disease, hepatic dysfunction, chronic alcoholism, or extrapancreatic tumor (abdominal mass) may be helpful clues.

Laboratory Tests

The diagnosis of hypoglycemia and its causes is largely based upon laboratory testing. Such testing should be individualized if a specific disease entity is suggested; otherwise the diagnostic approach should vary, depending on whether or not fasting hypoglycemia is suspected on clinical grounds.

If postprandial hypoglycemia is suspected by clinical symptoms and the physician is confident that fasting hypoglycemia is not a diagnostic possibility, generally only a 5-h oral glucose tolerance test is required (Fig. 20-5). Postprandial hypoglycemia may be excluded if hypoglycemia fails to develop or if symptoms do not occur in spite of a fall in plasma glucose concentration below 50 mg/dl. When biochemical or symptomatic hypoglycemia is observed during the oral glucose tolerance test, it is usually unnecessary to proceed with testing for fasting hypoglycemia. It may be useful, however, to evaluate whether hypoglycemia is evoked by usual mixed meals, since the glucose tolerance test is not representative of the ordinary life conditions associated with most patients' symptoms.[16a]

A particular pattern on the glucose tolerance curve should alert the physician that a more serious underlying condition may be present. When hypoglycemia is of the postprandial variety it is only transient, and plasma glucose levels rebound toward basal values by the fourth to sixth hour (i.e., by completion of test). Occasionally, this late rebound fails to occur, resulting in a progressive reduction in glucose concentration. While this pattern may be seen in patients with postprandial hypoglycemia, it is more characteristically observed in patients with insulin-producing islet cell tumors. Consequently, the latter diagnosis should be excluded by a prolonged fast.

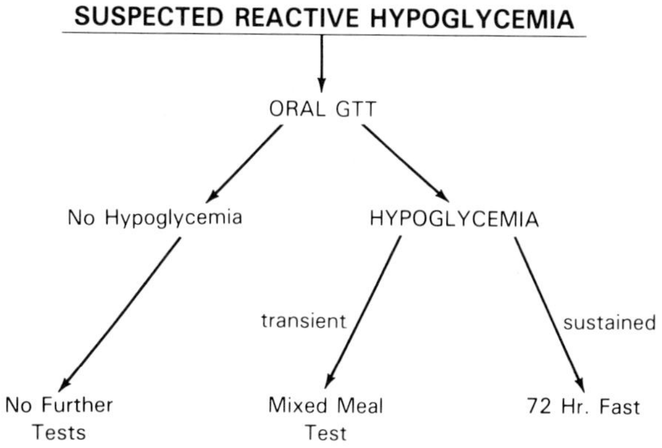

FIGURE 20-5 Flow sheet for the evaluation of a patient with suspected reactive (postprandial) hypoglycemia. "Mixed meal test" refers to determination of response of plasma glucose concentration to mixed meals.

When hypoglycemia is suspected, but neither postprandial nor fasting hypoglycemia can be excluded on the basis of the history, the diagnostic workup is considerably more complicated. The oral glucose tolerance test is once again useful in evaluating whether postprandial hypoglycemia is present. However, this test is of little or no value in the diagnosis of fasting hypoglycemia. As a consequence, if fasting hypoglycemia is considered a serious possibility, it is best to have the patient fast (Fig. 20-6). This can be accomplished best by hospitalizing the patient and withholding food for up to 72 h; in children the fast should be limited to 24 to 36 h, depending on age. The fast serves two very important functions. First, it establishes, with very rare exceptions, whether the patient has a condition which results in hypoglycemia in the fasting state. Second, by permitting measurement of plasma insulin as well as glucose concentration sequentially during the fast, it provides the best means of determining if hypoglycemia is due to excessive insulin secretion or not. In this regard, it is important to note that hyperinsulinism cannot be evaluated by measurements of plasma insulin concentration obtained within a few hours of meals or glucose administration. The plasma insulin response under these circumstances is highly variable in normal subjects, precluding a valid differentiation between normal and excessive insulin levels. Furthermore, when hypoglycemia develops within a few hours of glucose administration (as in postprandial hypoglycemia), the fall in plasma glucose concentration generally precedes the decline in plasma insulin concentration. If blood samples are obtained immediately after a rapid decrease from hyperglycemic to hypoglycemic levels, the plasma insulin level may still be increased, leading the physician to an incorrect diagnosis of inappropriate hyperinsulinemia.

In the patient with hypoglycemia after an overnight fast, simultaneous measurements of plasma glucose and insulin concentrations after the overnight fast will suffice in establishing a diagnosis. Subjecting the patient with documented hypoglycemia after brief fasting to a 72-h fast is unwarranted and extremely dangerous. In some instances in which the history is not very suggestive of hypoglycemia, it may be sufficient for the patient to undergo only an 18-h fast

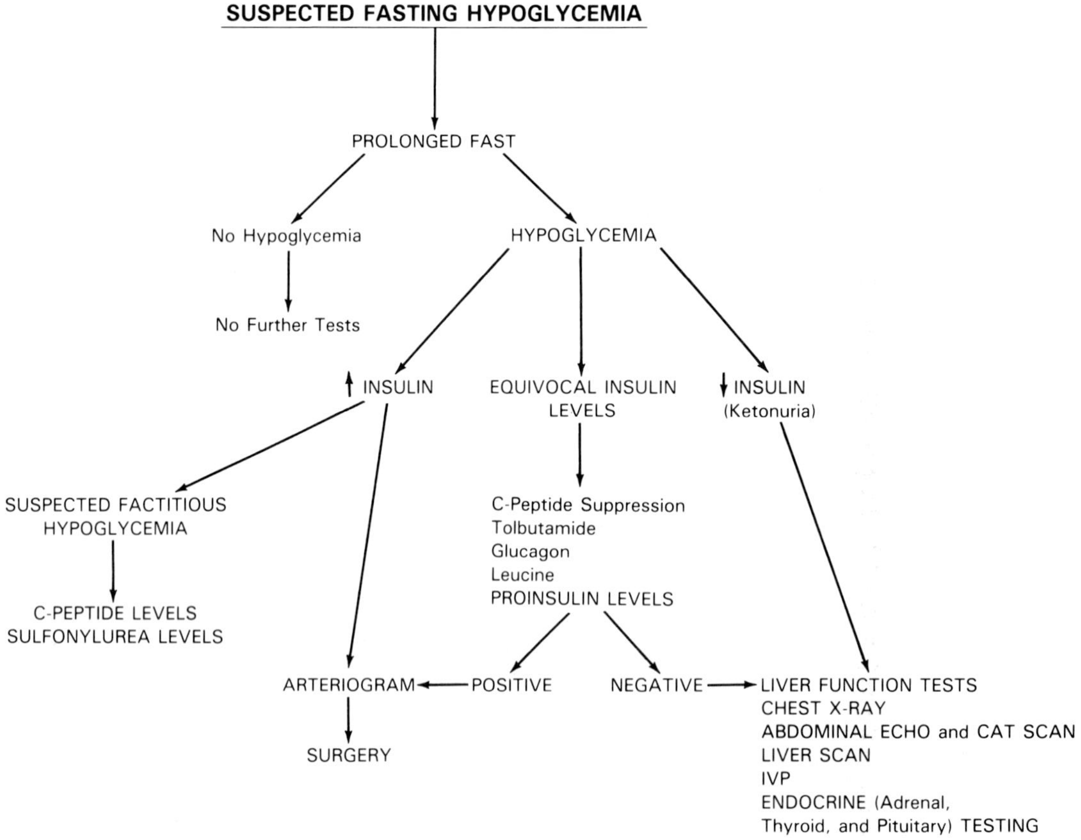

FIGURE 20-6 Flow sheet for the evaluation of a patient with suspected fasting hypoglycemia.

(withhold breakfast) and for simultaneous glucose and insulin levels to be obtained prior to lunch. If the plasma glucose concentration remains above 70 mg/dl, further studies may not be warranted. Obviously, if the physician seriously considers the diagnosis of fasting hypoglycemia, a more prolonged fast is required.

Once fasting hypoglycemia has been established, further diagnostic testing is dependent on the plasma insulin response to the fast (Fig. 20-6). If fasting hyperinsulinemia is unequivocal and factitious hypoglycemia is suspected, C peptide measurements and a search for other hypoglycemic agents should be undertaken before considering surgery. Only in those patients with equivocal hyperinsulinemia is it necessary to perform provocative or suppression tests of insulin secretion or measurements of proinsulin concentration.

When hypoglycemia occurs during fasting but the plasma insulin concentration declines appropriately, a wide variety of disorders must be considered. This situation may be suggested at the bedside by positive urinary ketone measurements (ketonemia virtually rules out the possibility of hyperinsulinemic hypoglycemia), thereby allowing the workup to proceed before insulin values are reported by the laboratory. In most of these cases the cause of hypoglycemia may be discovered by tests designed to detect liver or endocrine disease or the presence of an extrapancreatic tumor. Occasionally, a liver biopsy (hepatic enzymatic defect) or specialized studies of hepatic gluconeogenesis (alanine infusion) are required. Finally, it should be remembered that one of the most common causes of hypoglycemia, alcohol ingestion, is not uncovered by the various testing procedures. This diagnosis is made on the basis of the history of alcohol ingestion and poor food intake and findings of detectable blood levels of alcohol.

REFERENCES

1. Amiel S, Simonson DC, Tamborlane WV, DeFronzo RA, Sherwin RS: Rate of glucose fall does not affect counterregulatory hormone responses to hypoglycemia in normal and diabetic humans. *Diabetes* 36, 1987.
2. DeFronzo RA, Hendler R, Christensen N: Stimulation of counterregulatory hormonal responses in diabetic man by a fall in glucose concentration. *Diabetes* 29:125, 1980.
3. Simonson DC, Tamborlane WV, DeFronzo RA, Sherwin RS: Intensive insulin therapy reduces counterregulatory hormone responses to hypoglycemia in patients with type 1 diabetes. *Ann Intern Med* 103:184, 1985.
4. Merimee TJ, Tyson JE: Stabilization of plasma glucose during fasting. Normal variations in two separate studies. *N Engl J Med* 291:1275, 1979.
5. Fajans S, Floyd JC: Fasting hypoglycemia in adults. *N Engl J Med* 294:766, 1976.
6. Haymond MW, Karl IE, Clarke WL, Pagliara AS, Santiago JV: Differences in circulating gluconeogenic substrates during short-term fasting in men, women, and children. *Metabolism* 31:33, 1982.
7. Sacca L, Sherwin RS, Hendler R, Felig P: Influence of continuous physiologic hyperinsulinemia on glucose kinetics and counterregulatory hormones in normal and diabetic humans. *J Clin Invest* 63:849, 1979.
8. Landsberg L, Greff L, Gunn S, Young JB: Adrenergic mechanisms in the metabolic adaptation to fasting and feeding: Effects of phlorizin on diet-induced changes in sympathoadrenal activity in the rat. *Metabolism* 29:1128, 1980.
9. Brodows RG, Ensinck JW, Campbell RG: Mechanism of plasma cyclic AMP response to hypoglycemia in man. *Metabolism* 25:659, 1976.
10. Cryer PE, Gerich JE: Glucose counterregulation, hyperglycemia and intensive insulin therapy in diabetes mellitus. *N Engl J Med* 313:232, 1985.
11. Palmer JP, Henry DP, Benson JW, Johnson DG, Ensinck JW: Glucagon response to hypoglycemia in sympathectomized man. *J Clin Invest* 57:522, 1976.
12. Garber AJ, Cryer PE, Santiago JV, Haymond MW, Pagliara AS, Kipnis DM: The role of adrenergic mechanisms in the substrate and hormonal response to insulin-induced hypoglycemia in man. *J Clin Invest* 58:7, 1976.
13. Cryer PE: Glucose counterregulation in man. *Diabetes* 30:261, 1981.
14. Gerich JE, Langlois M, Novacco C, Karam JH, Forsham PH: Lack of glucagon response to hypoglycemia in diabetes: Evidence for an intrinsic pancreatic alpha-cell defect. *Science* 182:172, 1973.
15. Strauch B, Felig P, Baxter J, Schimpff S: Hypothermia in hypoglycemia. *JAMA* 210:345, 1969.
16. Cahill GF, Soeldner JS: A non-editorial on non-hypoglycemia. *N Engl J Med* 291:905, 1974.
16a. Charles MA, Hofeldt F, Shackleford A, Waldeck N, Dodson LE Jr, Bunker D, Coggins JT, Eichner H: Comparison of oral glucose tolerance tests and mixed meals in patients with apparent idiopathic postabsorptive hypoglycemia. Absence of hypoglycemia after meals. *Diabetes* 30:465, 1981.
17. Felig P: Starvation, in DeGroot L, Cahill GF Jr, Odell WD, Martini L, Potts JT Jr, Nelson DH, Stenberger E, Winegrad AI (eds): *Endocrinology*. New York, Grune & Stratton, 1979, vol 3, p 1927.
18. Owen OE, Morgan AP, Kemp HG, Sullivan JM, Herrera MG, Cahill GF Jr: Brain metabolism during fasting. *J Clin Invest* 46:1589, 1967.
19. Heitz PV, Kloppel G, Haski WH, Polak JM, Pearse AGE: Nesidioblastosis: The pathologic basis of persistent hyperinsulinemic hypoglycemia in infants. *Diabetes* 26:632, 1977.
20. Bonser AM, Garcia-Webb P: C-peptide measurement: Methods and clinical utility. *CRC Crit Rev Clin Lab Sci* 19:297, 1984.
21. Gorden P, Sherman B, Roth J: Pro-insulin-like component of circulating insulin in the basal state and in patients and hamsters with islet cell tumors. *J Clin Invest* 50:2113, 1971.
22. Laroche GP, Ferris DO, Priestly JT, Scholz DA, Dockerly MR: Hyperinsulinism: Surgical results and management of occult functioning islet cell tumors; review of 154 cases. *Arch Surg* 96:763, 1968.
23. Broder LE, Carter SK: Pancretic islet cell carcinoma. Clinical features of 52 patients. *Ann Intern Med* 79:105, 1973.
24. Kahn CR, Megyesi K, Bar RS, Eastman RC, Flier JS: Receptors for peptide hormones: New insights into the pathophysiology of disease states in man. *Ann Intern Med* 86:205, 1977.
24a. Froesch ER, Schmid C, Schwander J, Zapf J: Actions of insulin-like growth factors. *Annu Rev Physiol* 47:443, 1985.
25. Bier D, Rosemary DL, Haymond MW, Arnold KJ, Gruenke LD, Sperling MA, Kipnis DM: Measurement of "true"glucose production rates in infancy and childhood with 6,6-dideuteroglucose. *Diabetes* 26:1016, 1977.

26. Felig P, Brown WV, Levine RA, Klatskin G: Glucose homeostasis in viral hepatitis. *N Engl J Med* 283:1436, 1970.
27. Partin J: Serum salicylate concentration in Reye's disease. A study of 130 biopsy proven cures. *Lancet* 1:191, 1982.
28. Felig P, Pozefsky T, Marliss E, Cahill GF Jr: Alanine: Key role in gluconeogenesis. *Science* 167:1003, 1970.
29. Felig P, Kim YJ, Lynch V, Hendler R: Amino acid metabolism during starvation in human pregnancy. *J Clin Invest* 51:1195, 1975.
30. Haymond MW, Pagliara AS: Ketotic hypoglycemia. *Clin Endocrinol Metab* 12:447, 1983.
31. Haymond MW, Ben-Galim E, Strobel KE: Glucose and alanine metabolism in children with maple syrup urine disease. *J Clin Invest* 62:398, 1978.
31a. Garber AJ, Bier DM, Cryer PE, Pagliara AS: Hypoglycemia in compensated chronic renal insufficiency: Substrate limitation of gluconeogenesis. *Diabetes* 23:982, 1974.
32. Ichihara K, Shima K, Saito Y, Nonaka K, Tarui S, Nishikawa M: Mechanism of hypoglycemia observed in a patient with insulin autoimmune syndrome. *Diabetes* 26:500, 1977.
32a. Rebouche CJ, Engel AG: Carnitine metabolism and deficiency. *Mayo Clin Proc* 58:533, 1983.
33. Permutt MA: Postprandial hypoglycemia. *Diabetes* 25:719, 1976.
34. Farriss BL: Prevalence of post-glucose-load glycosuria and hypoglycemia in a group of healthy young men. *Diabetes* 23:189, 1974.
35. Lev-Ran A, Anderson RW: The diagnosis of postprandial hypoglycemia. *Diabetes* 30:996, 1981.
36. Felig P, Wahren J, Hendler R: Influence of oral glucose ingestion on splanchnic glucose and gluconeogenic substrate metabolism. *Diabetes* 24:468, 1975.
37. Katz LD, Glickman MG, Rapoport S, Ferrannini E, DeFronzo RA: Splanchnic and peripheral disposal of oral glucose in man. *Diabetes* 32:675, 1983.
38. Tse TF, Clutter W, Shah SD, Miller JP, Cryer PE: Neuroendocrine responses to glucose ingestion in man. Specificity, temporal relationships and quantitative aspects. *J Clin Invest* 72:270, 1983.
39. Tse TF, Clutter WE, Shah SD, Cryer P: Mechanisms of postprandial glucose counterregulation in man. Physiologic roles of glucagon and epinephrine vis-a-vis insulin in the prevention of hypoglycemia late after glucose ingestion. *J Clin Invest* 72:278, 1983.
40. Bolli G, DeFeo P, Perriello G, DeCosvo S, Ventura M, Campbell P, Brunetti P, Gerich JE: Role of hepatic autoregulation in defense against hypoglycemia in humans. *J Clin Invest* 75:1623, 1985.
41. Permutt MA, Kelly J, Bernstein R, Alpers DH, Siegel BA, Kipnis DM: Alimentary hypoglycemia in the absence of gastrointestinal surgery. *N Engl J Med* 288:1206, 1973.
42. Breuer RI, Moses H, Hagen TC, Zuckerman L: Gastric operations and glucose homeostasis. *Gastroenterology* 62:1109, 1972.
43. Seltzer HS, Fajans SS, Conn JW: Spontaneous hypoglycemia as an early manifestation of diabetes mellitus. *Diabetes* 5:437, 1956.
44. Permutt MA, Delmez J, Stenson W: Effects of carbohydrate restriction on the hypoglycemic phase of the glucose tolerance test. *J Clin Endocrinol Metab* 43:1088, 1976.
45. Abramson EA, Arky RA, Woeber KA: Effects of propranolol on the hormonal and metabolic response to insulin-induced hypoglycemia. *Lancet* 2:1386, 1966.
46. Goldgewicht C, Slama G, Papoz L, Tchobroisky G: Hypoglycemic reactions in 172 type I (insulin-dependent) diabetic patients. *Diabetologia* 24:95, 1983.
47. Turnbridge WMG: Factors contributing to deaths of diabetics under fifty years of age. *Lancet* 2:569, 1981.
48. Coustan D, Felig P: Diabetes mellitus, in Burrow G, Ferris TF (eds): *Medical Complications in Pregnancy,* 3d ed. Philadelphia, Saunders, in press.
49. Scarlett JA, Mako ME, Rubinstein AH, Blix PM, Goldman J, Horwitz DL, Tager H, Jaspan JB, Stjernholm MR, Olefsky JM: Diagnosis of factitious hypoglycemia. *N Engl J Med* 297:1029, 1977.
50. Seltzer HS: Drug-induced hypoglycemia. A review based on 473 cases. *Diabetes* 21:955, 1972.
51. Simonson DC, Koivisto V, Sherwin RS, Ferrannini E, Hendler R, Juhlin-Dannfelt A, DeFronzo RA: Adrenergic blockade alters glucose kinetics during exercise in insulin-dependent diabetics. *J Clin Invest* 73:1648, 1984.
52. Williams HE: Alcoholic hypoglycemia and ketoacidosis. *Med Clin North Am* 68:33, 1984.
53. Kreisberg RA, Siegel AM, Owen CW: Glucose-lactate interrelationships: Effect of ethanol. *J Clin Invest* 50:175, 1971.
54. Cox TM, O'Donnell MW, Camilleri M, Burghes AH: Isolation and characterization of a mutant liver aldolase in adult hereditary fructose intolerance. Identification of the enzyme variant by radioassay in tissue biopsy specimens. *J Clin Invest* 72:201, 1983.
55. Mock DM, Perman JA, Thaler MM, Morris RC Jr: Chronic fructose intoxication after infancy in children with hereditary fructose intolerance. A cause of growth retardation. *N Engl J Med* 309:764, 1983.
56. Baker L, Winegrad AI: Fasting hypoglycemia and metabolic acidosis associated with deficiency of hepatic fructose-1,6-diphosphatase activity. *Lancet* 2:13, 1970.
57. Tanaka K, Kean EA, Johnson B: Jamaican vomiting sickness. Biochemical investigation of two cases. *N Engl J Med* 295:461, 1976.
58. Golden KD, Kean EA, Terry SI: Jamaican vomiting sickness: A study of two adult cases. *Clin Chim Acta* 142:293, 1984.

21

The Obesities

Lester B. Salans

Obesity, like fever and anemia, is a symptom rather than a single disease entity; a variety of different causes have been identified in humans and laboratory animals. In humans, the underlying cause of obesity can only occasionally be identified; in the overwhelming majority of patients, the etiology of obesity cannot be determined. Inability to identify underlying cause precludes the development of specific means to prevent and control most forms of human obesity, a fact which is reflected in the uniformly unsatisfactory and discouraging therapeutic experience. This is especially unfortunate because obesity is very common and is associated with shortened life span, increased morbidity from a variety of serious chronic disorders, and considerable economic cost.

Given its magnitude and seriousness, the problem of obesity is a major public health concern in the United States. This situation will prevail until the factors that normally regulate energy balance, body weight, and adiposity are better understood and identification of their derangements in obesity permits the development of specific preventive and therapeutic measures. In the meantime, physicians and other health care deliverers must capitalize on currently available knowledge to develop the most effective treatment programs possible. Indeed, research progress during the past several years has advanced knowledge of the natural history and health consequences of obesity sufficiently to provide the framework on which a more rational approach to the prevention and treatment of obesity and its complications can be developed.

DEFINITION

Obesity, at the simplest level, is defined as an excess of body fat or adipose tissue. Although lean body mass (skeleton and muscle) is also usually increased in the obese individual, the predominant and most characteristic anatomic change is the excessive accumulation of adipose tissue. Thus, the diagnosis of obesity depends, in the strictest sense, on the demonstration of an increased body fat content.

Several sophisticated laboratory methods are available for estimating body fat content, including the determination of cytoplasmic mass from the amount of naturally occurring isotopes such as ^{40}K, measurement of the in vivo dilution of isotopes such as tritiated or deuterated water, underwater weighing to determine body density, and, most recently, measurement of total body electrical conductivity with electromagnetic techniques.[1-3] All of these methods require assumptions which may not always be valid. Moreover, all are time-consuming, require highly specialized skills and laboratories, and cannot, at this time, be applied on a routine clinical basis or in public studies of large populations. Simpler and less direct measures of body fat, therefore, have been used. Determination of skin fold thickness has become the most widely used means of assessing body fatness.[4] While this method is more practical, its accuracy is limited by several factors, including variations in observer skill, lack of standardization and uniformity of technique, variability in skin fold thickness among different adipose depot sites in the body, and restriction to assessment of subcutaneous fat. When assessments are made at multiple sites in the body, including the upper, middle, and lower body segments, skin fold thickness measurements appear to provide a useful indirect index of obesity.

Based on data obtained using these techniques, it is apparent that body fat is continuously distributed in the population, with no clear cutoff between lean and obese individuals. Thus, there is a problem in defining what is a "normal" amount or proportion of body fat and what is obesity. Normal body fat for any individual probably depends on a variety of factors, including the relationship between total body fat, life span, and hazard to health and the genetic predisposition toward obesity-related diseases such as diabetes, coronary heart disease, hypertension, etc. A quantitative evaluation of how much body fat constitutes a health hazard, therefore, is an essential part of the definition of obesity. Other factors such as (1) the nature of the environment, particularly with respect to the likelihood of encountering situations such as caloric deprivation, (2) psychological comfort, and (3) the cultural concept of what constitutes an appropriate body size and shape are also important ingredients in the definitions of normal and obese. At present there are few quantitative data upon which firm conclusions about the "normal" amount of body fat can be based. The definitions of normal and obese are therefore somewhat arbitrary. The proportions of body weight as fat generally accepted as normal are 15 to 20 percent for men and 20 to 25 percent for women. Obesity in males, then, is a proportion of body fat greater than 20 percent; in females obesity is greater than 25 percent body weight as fat. Some massively obese individuals may have as much as 50 percent of their body mass as adipose tissue. However, as previously discussed, measurement of body fat content in humans is impractical and cannot be used to diagnose obesity at this time.

In most clinical settings and in most surveys body weight is used to estimate body fat. Several different body weight tables exist which provide standards or recommended levels of body weight in relation to height and, in some instances, body frame.[5] Obesity is defined as a weight which exceeds the "standard" or recommended level provided in the table for a person of the same sex, height, and frame size. In 1985 a consensus conference sponsored by the National Institutes of Health (NIH) concluded that a modest, even conservative definition of obesity corresponds to body weights 20 percent or more in excess of the standard or recommended levels in these tables.[5–7] It is highly likely that even lesser degrees of overweight, e.g., 10 percent in excess of "desirable" or recommended, represent obesity.

Body weight and fatness can both vary nearly 10-fold over relatively small changes in the remaining fat-free mass; thus weight is to some degree a valid estimator of fatness. The use of body weight tables to assess fatness and obesity is made particularly attractive by the existence of data on longevity provided by these tables. Theoretically, the tables could establish which weight is associated with the best expectation for long survival. However, several problems limit the usefulness of body weight and weight-height tables as valid estimators of body fat and therefore as indexes of obesity and its health consequences.[5]

Obesity and overweight are not always synonomous, as for example in athletes or individuals engaged in heavy manual labor who have an increased amount of lean body mass (muscle). It may be important to differentiate the effects on health of increased body fat from increased lean body mass.

The various reference weight-height tables provide different recommended body weight levels to which a given individual's body weight is compared and on which the diagnosis of overweight and obesity is based. In addition, they use different terms for their weight standards. Some tables use the term "average" body weight, others use "ideal" body weight, and still others "desirable" body weight. Average body weight is generally defined as the average weight of a selected group of individuals within the population, corrected for height and sex. Among the limitations of this approach are the fact that the population selected may not be representative of the population as a whole and the possibility that the average weight of the selected population may already be overweight. Use of the average weight of a selected population as a reference against which to judge overweight and obesity in a given individual, may, therefore, not be appropriate. Ideal body weight is defined as that weight associated with optimal health and life-style. Since the body weight associated with optimal health for a population, much less for individuals within that population, has yet to be determined, ideal weight remains a theoretical term. Originally it was designed to encourage people to keep their weight below the average weight of a population determined from actuarial statistics. Desirable body weight is most often defined as that weight associated with the lowest mortality based on actuarial statistics; the 1959 Metropolitan Life tables (see below) are an example. Those tables set desirable body weight below the average weight for the insured population at that time, since people of below-average weight had the greatest longevity. The use of the average body weight of such a select population to derive desirable standards is inappropriate for the same reasons that it is an invalid standard against which to judge overweight and obesity, as discussed above.

Metropolitan Life Insurance Company Weight Tables

The most commonly used body weight tables have been the 1959 *Metropolitan Life Insurance Company Desirable Weight Tables*.[8] The reference weights promulgated by these tables were based on the body weights which were associated with lowest mortality among insured persons; thus, they are referred to as desirable body weights. Using these tables, an individual is considered to be overweight if he or she exceeds the desirable weight for persons of the same sex, height, and frame size. Obesity is generally defined as a body weight greater than 20 percent above the desirable weight for individuals of the same sex, height, and frame. An individual with a body weight that exceeds the reference weight by less than 20 percent is overweight, but may or may not be obese; some more direct measurement of body fat would be required to establish the absence or presence of obesity in these persons. These tables failed to take into account confounding factors such as cigarette smoking and other risk factors and illnesses, thus limiting their usefulness in assessing the health hazards associated with a given body weight and, hence, presumably a given level of body fatness.

In 1983, Metropolitan Life developed new standard weight and height tables based on data obtained from the 1979 Build Study of more than 4 million insured persons in the United States and Canada collected from 1950 to 1972.[9] The new tables, called the *Metropolitan Height and Weight Tables,* no longer refer to desirable body weight in recognition of the fact that they are derived from a selected sample of individuals and are not representative of the entire United States population. The recommended weights for both males and females at each height and frame size in the new tables are 5 to 15 percent greater than those in the 1959 tables. These new weight recommendations are based on data which show that longevity among those considered in the 1979 Build Study is greatest at these body weights. However, as with the 1959 tables, smoking, behavior, and other risk factors and diseases are confounding variables in the 1983 tables, making them highly suspect. This author prefers the more stringent 1959 tables to the 1983 tables.

Table 21-1. Reasonable Body Weights

Height, ft. and in.*	Weight† Men	Weight† Women
4′10″		92–119
4′11″		94–122
5′0″		96–125
5′1″		99–128
5′2″	112–141	102–131
5′3″	115–144	105–134
5′4″	118–148	108–138
5′5″	121–152	111–142
5′6″	124–156	114–146
5′7″	128–161	118–150
5′8″	132–166	122–154
5′9″	136–170	126–158
5′10″	140–174	130–163
5′11″	144–179	134–168
6′0″	148–184	138–173
6′1″	152–189	
6′2″	156–194	
6′3″	160–199	
6′4″	164–204	

*Height with shoes (men in 1-in heels, woman in 2-in heels).
†Weight in pounds in indoor clothing (approximately 7 lb for men, 4 lb for women).
Source: Adapted from Bray.[10]

The Fogarty Conference Tables

In 1973, the Fogarty International Center Conference on Obesity recommended for general use a modification of the 1959 Metropolitan Life tables;[10] in it, desirable weight was defined as the mean of the lowest to highest ranges of body weight in the Metropolitan tables for medium-frame individuals of each sex. Table 21-1 has been adapted from the recommendations of that conference on obesity; note that recommended values are presented as "reasonable" body weights rather than desirable weights.

National Center for Health Statistics Tables

The National Center for Health Statistics (NCHS) has conducted national surveys of body weight and height from a national probability sample representative of the United States noninstitutionalized civilian population aged 1 through 74 years. The latest NCHS survey, the National Health and Nutrition Examination Survey (NHANES II), conducted from 1976 to 1980, examined approximately 20,000 persons in a carefully selected sample.[11,12] It collected normative data on body weight and height, skin fold thickness, and other anthropometric indexes, and analyzed the consequences to health of various degrees of overweight. Using these data, a "desirable" body weight table has been developed based on the average weight of Americans at age 20 through 29 years. Overweight is identified by comparing the body weight of a given individual, corrected for height, to the "desirable" level observed in this probability sample. The use of average body weight to define desirable body weight and overweight may not be appropriate, since these are normative data. Furthermore, since data from several studies indicate that body weight continuously increases between ages 20 and 29, use of the NCHS table leads to an overestimation of desirable weight and an underestimation of overweight in the population.

NHANÉS II defines obesity on the basis of its skin fold thickness data. Obesity exists when the sum of triceps and subscapular skin fold thickness is at or above the 85th percentile for the 20- to 29-year-old reference group. Severe obesity exists when the sum of triceps and subscapular skin fold thickness is at or above the 95th percentile of the same reference group. In addition to the criticisms of skin fold thickness measurements mentioned above, the use of triceps plus subscapular skin fold thickness alone as an index of obesity and health risk can be criticized in view of recent data showing that the distribution of adipose tissue between upper and lower segments of the body varies among obese people and that this variability in distribution of adiposity has important consequences in terms of risk; e.g., lower segment obesity carries a lower risk of glucose and lipid metabolic abnormalities and hypertension than does upper segment obesity.[13,14] Furthermore, since these are normative data, their use as a standard for the entire population may be inappropriate.

Body Mass Index

As a consequence of the limitations associated with the use of body weight as a means of assessing body fatness, several other measures for obesity have been developed. Among these various indexes the most commonly used is the body mass index (BMI), which is now recommended by several obesity experts as the preferred method for evaluating overweight body fatness and obesity.[6,7] The BMI is calculated by dividing body weight in kilograms (W) by the square of height in meters (H), according to the formula W/H^2. BMI is said to correlate relatively well with body fat, particularly when age is taken into consideration. It tends to be constant for individuals of a given degree of leanness or fatness over a wide range of height; therefore, a change in BMI may provide a useful measure of adiposity independent of height. The BMIs of individuals within populations have been converted into standard tables as a reference against which to judge overweight, obesity, and health risks. The midpoint of the desirable weight-height range of the 1959 Metropolitan Life tables is equal to a BMI of 22. The desirable body weight of the NHANES II tables is also equivalent to a BMI of approximately 22. In the less stringent 1983 Metropolitan tables a BMI of 23 corresponds to the recommended body weight. As previously discussed, data derived from select populations may not be representative of the population as a whole; the standard BMIs derived from such populations may not be an appropriate reference against which to assess overweight, obesity, or health hazard. Nevertheless, definite obesity has been defined as a BMI ≥ 27, based on data which show this degree of fatness to be associated with significant health hazards.[6,7] Since adverse health consequences are likely with even lesser degrees of fatness and obesity, especially when other risk factors are present, treatment should ideally aim for maintaining the BMI at or restoring it to 22. In the opinion of this author, it is uncertain whether BMI provides a major advantage over body weight in relation to height for assessing overweight, body fatness, and obesity. Since overweight and obesity are not always synonymous and since BMI appears to correlate relatively well with body fat, BMI may be preferable.

Summary

Which, if any, particular body weight or BMI table provides the most reliable standard for studying the prevalence of overweight or obesity per se in a population and their influence is uncertain. Ultimately, recommended or desirable body weights should be based on reliable data from studies which assess and quantify the risk of morbidity and mortality associated with body weight and obesity. Data from several recent studies may begin to provide this information (see below). Yet, until a practical and standardized method is developed for reliable and accurate measurement of body fat, comparison of an individual's body weight or BMI with a standard reference will continue to be the most practical and widely used criterion of leanness and fatness. Furthermore, until more definitive information regarding the relationship between obesity, body weight, BMI, and health is forthcoming, overweight or BMI will be used to assess the risk and prevalence of the health consequences of obesity. Although admittedly an arbitrary judgment, body weight shown in Table 21-1 (adapted from the 1973 Fogarty conference), or BMIs calculated from this table, remains the standard reference of choice. However, its limitations must always be recognized, as must the interpretation of data derived from it.

PREVALENCE AND GENERAL CHARACTERISTICS

The bulk of information regarding the prevalence and natural history of obesity in the United States has been derived from cross-sectional studies in which measurement of body weight in relation to height, age, and frame size has been the index of obesity. In light of the preceding discussion and in view of the fact that overweight and obesity may not be synonymous, the data to be discussed should be regarded as more qualitative than quantitative.

Prevalence of Obesity in Adults

Current estimates of the prevalence of obesity vary greatly; the exact frequency of obesity in the population is not known. Nevertheless, the available data indicate that overweight and obesity are highly prevalent at every age and in both sexes. Data derived from NHANES II suggest that 32.6 million American adults are overweight when defined by BMI criteria (see Body Mass Index, above).[12] Of these, approximately 11.5 million are severely overweight (BMI of 31 or higher). Data from the same NCHS survey indicate that approximately 30.6 million Americans are obese on the basis of skin fold measurements (referred to the 20- to 29-year-old age group). Over 10 million Americans are severely obese, as defined by triceps plus subscapular skin fold thickness at or above the 95th percentile of the reference group.

Overweight and obesity appear to increase in frequency throughout the life span of the population. Women have a higher prevalence of overweight and obesity than men. From the NHANES II survey it was estimated that 25.8 percent of American women and 22.8 percent of men are overweight, 8.8 percent of women and 8.4 percent of men are severely overweight, 24 percent of women and 22 percent of men are obese, and 8.6 percent of women and 7.1 percent of men are severely obese. The NCHS data also reveal that the prevalence of overweight among American black women is twice that among white women. The prevalence of overweight among the adult American population appears, therefore, to be alarmingly high. Moreover, when data from the three NCHS surveys (1960 to 1962, 1971 to 1974, and 1976 to 1980) are compared, body weights of both men and women have progressively increased from 1960 to 1980. To the extent to which increased body weight reflects an increased adipose tissue mass, it can be inferred that the prevalence of obesity among adults in this country is increasing.

Prevalence of Obesity in Children

Information concerning the prevalence of overweight and obesity in infancy, childhood, and adolecence is limited. The prevalence of overweight in children in the United States has been reported to be anywhere from 6 to 45 percent, depending on age, sex, and other demographic characteristics of the population studied.[15-17] Clearly, more reliable data are required regarding the prevalence of obesity in childhood.

Some studies suggest that obese infants are likely to become obese children and adults. A study of one population, for example, indicated that 80 percent of obese children became obese adults, and 50 percent of very obese adults had been obese as infants.[18] Another study, which reported an increased risk of adult obesity in those who were obese as infants, also demonstrated an interaction between infant and parental overweight which increased the risk of adult obesity in overweight infants.[19] There are, however, data to the contrary. For example, one study indicates that most obese infants lose their excess fat during childhood and do not become obese adults.[20] Another study indicates that restriction of food intake early in life does not necessarily alter the risk of obesity in adult life.[21] While it appears that infants and children with severe obesity have poor prognoses and are likely to become obese adults, the extent to which obesity of early life is a determinant of adult obesity remains to be clarified. It is an issue of obvious and considerable importance from the standpoint of prevention.

Socioeconomic Aspects of Occurrence

Obesity is a disease of economically developed, industrialized countries; it is almost nonexistent in underdeveloped nations. Data available from epidemiologic studies and surveys in the United States indicate that, in addition to being more prevalent in women than men and more common in black than Caucasian women, obesity is most prevalent in women from lower socioeconomic groups.[6,7,12,17,22,23] Prevalence is inversely related to level of education, and is greater in Americans of eastern European origin than those of western European descent. These observations indicate that environmental factors, e.g., life-style, may contribute significantly to the development and prevalence of obesity. Nevertheless, as discussed below, there is strong evidence that genetic factors are important, perhaps the most important underlying determinants of obesity in the general population, and that obesity is the result of the complex interaction of genetic susceptibility and various environmental factors.

Health Consequences

The development and maintenance of the obese state is accompanied by serious and widespread adverse health consequences.[6,7,12,24] Obese persons tend to have shortened life spans compared to nonobese persons; this is particularly true for those who are 30 percent or more overweight and is also very likely to be the case with lesser degrees of overweight. The obese individual is at increased risk for a variety of disorders: abnormalities in systemic carbohydrate and lipid metabolism are more frequent; the risks of developing diabetes mellitus, cardiovascular disease, hypertension, cholecystitis, and cholelithiasis, among other diseases which significantly affect the quality and length of life, are increased; and obesity may have considerable social, psychological, and economic impact. (Health consequences of obesity are discussed in detail below.)

Resistance to Weight Loss

Another characteristic of human obesity is that most obese individuals, particularly those with severe lifelong obesity, resist weight reduction. Weight loss is either not achieved or is followed by return to previous levels of obesity, even in individuals who appear to be highly motivated. This disturbing fact is one of the most perplexing and frustrating characteristics of the natural history of human obesity. Studies of the cellular character of human adipose tissue may provide some insight into this characteristic.[5,6,25–27] Adipose tissue in humans normally grows through adipose cell hyperplasia (increase in cell number through cell division) and adipose cell hypertrophy (cellular enlargement through increased accumulation of lipid). Severe and lifelong human obesity is characterized by adipose hypercellularity, i.e., the number of adipose cells is increased. It has been demonstrated, both in nonobese and obese humans, that, once established, adipose cell number cannot be decreased. Thus, hypercellularity of the adipose tissue is a permanent, irreversible morphologic abnormality, a phenomenon which might explain the resistance to weight loss and almost inevitable recidivism after weight reduction that occurs in some forms of human obesity.

GROWTH AND DEVELOPMENT OF ADIPOSE TISSUE

Since obesity is defined as the accumulation of excessive adipose tissue, an examination of the growth and development of this tissue in both the normal, nonobese state and the obese state is relevant. A large number of studies in laboratory animals and humans have generated a great deal of information on this subject.[25–51]

In the nonobese rodent, adipose tissue normally grows through adipose cell hyperplasia and hypertrophy. Many, probably most, fat cells are formed in utero and during early life (5 to 6 weeks after birth), although individual adipose cells contain little lipid during this time. There is evidence that a precursor cells or *adipoblast* exists; at present, this cell is indistinguishable from the fibroblast.[52] The factors which stimulate growth and development of these cells is an area of active research. In many cases the adipose tissue expands through increases in both fat cell size and number (in some but not all adipose tissue depots) until approximately 6 months of age. Thereafter, in the female, adipose cell size and number remain relatively constant; in the male, fat cell size remains constant but fat cell number gradually increases.

The total number of adipose cells in rodents can be influenced in a variety of ways. The cellularity of adult adipose tissue can be influenced by early nutritional experiences: under- and overfeeding rats during the first 3 weeks of life results in a decrease or increase in total adipose cell number; this number persists into and throughout adult life, even though these animals are allowed free access to food after the early period of deprivation or overnutrition.[33,38] In adult life, prolonged food restriction (semistarvation) and exposure to cold can prevent the normal modest increase in fat cell number that occurs in some adipose depots of the rat.[42,43] Prolonged intake of diets high in fat and sugar during adult life results in adipose cellular division and proliferation and in adipose hypercellularity.[36,44]

A key new concept regarding the regulation of adipose tissue growth is that adipose cell size influences new cell formation and total adipose cell number.[31,44] It is postulated that achievement of a critical maximum adipose cell size somehow initiates adipocyte proliferation. Thus, feeding adult rats palatable high-fat, high-sugar diets leads to expansion of the adipose tissue mass. Initially, this increased adiposity is achieved by adipose cell enlargement, but once a maximum cell size is attained, further expansion of the adipose tissue is achieved through an increase in cell number. Studies measuring tritiated thymidine incorporation into cellular DNA demonstrate that this increase in cell number is due to new cell formation rather than to filling of preexistent, undetectable fat cells by lipid.[25,31]

While the total number of adipose cells in adult rodents can be increased under the experimental conditions described above, total fat cell number apparently cannot be decreased by any intervention other than surgical extirpation. Weight loss achieved through caloric deprivation and/or exercise is accompanied by a reduction in adipose cell size only; total fat cell number remains constant.[25,32,45,46] Even with surgical extirpation, there is some evidence in rats that regeneration of removed adipose cells or compensatory growth in other adipose depots may occur following lipectomy.[47–49]

Studies of the cellular character of the adipose tissue of obese rodents reveal that the excessive growth of the adipose tissue may be due to an increase in either the number or size of adipose cells.[50] Some forms of obesity in mice and rats are associated with hyperplastic, hypercellular adipose tissue mass (e.g., *obob* and New Zealand obese mice, Zucker fatty rats) and other forms with hypertrophic, normal cellular tissue (e.g., the Danforth or yellow mouse and rats with ventromedial hypothalamic lesions). Since adipose cell number cannot be decreased, adipose hypercellularity and obesity are permanent abnormalities in those animals with hyperplastic obesity.

Normal growth of adipose tissue in humans is achieved through increases in both adipose cell size and number.[25-30,51] It is believed that an adipoblast also exists in humans. Adipose cells first appear around the 15th week of gestation. The adipose tissue then expands during the remainder of gestation, through a combination of active cellular proliferation and enlargement. Nonobese newborns have about 10 to 15 percent of body weight as fat, located mainly in subcutaneous depots; within the first 6 months of infancy, the proportion of body weight which is fat increases to about 25 percent; the proportion of fat then gradually diminishes to normal levels in nonobese individuals. During the first 2 years of life, increases in adipose cell size account for most of the growth in the adipose mass, although some new cell formation (increase in cell number) also occurs after age 6 to 12 months. Cell number remains relatively constant or rises very slowly from 2 years of age until close to the onset of puberty, during which time the adipose tissue expands through the filling of existing adipose cells by lipid (i.e., cellular hypertrophy). During adolescence there is another increase in cell number, which accounts for a second spurt in the growth of the adipose tissue mass. Thereafter, the amount of adipose tissue of nonobese adults maintaining constant body weight remains relatively stable, as do adipose cell size and number.

The size of adipose cells within nonobese individuals can vary considerably from fat depot to fat depot; in a large group of nonobese healthy subjects, cell size in six separate fat depots ranged from 0.14 to 0.68 μg of lipid per cell, with a mean size of 0.41 μg of lipid per cell.[26] The average total cell number in this nonobese population was 39×10^9. Modest increases or decreases in fat cell size occur with modest changes in body weight, but adipose cell number remains constant throughout the adult life of nonobese individuals maintaining constant body weight. When nonobese people lose weight, only the size of the fat cells decreases; adipose cell number does not decline even if weight loss is massive.

Studies of obese humans reveal that the excessive expansion of adipose tissue can be achieved either by an increase in adipose cell size (hypertrophic, normal cellular obesity) or in both adipose cell number and size (hypercellular, hypertrophic obesity). In one study of a large number of obese adults, the mean total adipose cell number in six fat depots was 0.84×10^9.[26] In another study of obese children between 4 months and 19 years of age, beginning after age 1 year the obese subjects had larger fat cells than did subjects of normal weight; this difference persisted throughout the study.[30] The obese children also had significantly greater numbers of adipose cells than nonobese subjects at all ages examined from 2 to 19 years.

The existence of adipose hypercellularity in humans apparently depends on two factors: the age of onset and the severity of obesity. Hypercellular obesity usually, but not always, has its onset in early life, usually before the age of 20 years. Obesity of later onset is usually, but not always, accompanied by adipose cellular enlargement and normal cell number. There appear to be two periods in early life when hypercellularity is most likely to develop: very early, within the first year or two, and later, at or around the time of puberty. The studies of obese children cited above demonstrate, in contrast to the nonobese pattern of adipose tissue growth and cellular development, marked expansion of the adipose depots throughout childhood, accompanied by both cellular enlargement and proliferation, beginning especially during the second year of life.

The relationship between hypercellularity and the severity of obesity is a direct one: the more severe the obesity the greater the number of adipose cells. In the study of obese children noted above, total adipose cell number was markedly increased when body fat constituted greater than 25 percent of body weight.[51] Furthermore, when expansion of the adipose tissue during adult life is massive, increases in cell number and hypercellular obesity can occur. Evidence from studies of rodents also indicates that obesity of adult onset can, under certain circumstances, be accompanied by marked increases in fat cell number.[44] It has also been reported that when adult body weight exceeds 170 percent of ideal, a maximum cell size (1 to 2 μg of lipid per cell) is apparently reached, above which cell number and obesity are highly correlated.[25] Similar observations relating severity of obesity to hypercellularity of adipose tissue have been made in the Pima population of American Indians. Thus, studies in rodents and in humans suggest that attainment of maximum adipose cell size is accompanied by the activation of some factor(s) which can stimulate adipose cell proliferation; whenever a maximum cell size is attained, replication of adipose cells occurs. The nature of this putative signal is unknown.

Although hypercellularity is most often found in those with early-onset obesity, individuals have been observed with increased cell number in whom obesity has apparently developed during adult life; these people usually suffer from massive obesity. On the other hand, adipose hypercellularity is not limited to patients with severe obesity; increased cell number has been observed in some individuals with only moderate degrees of obesity, usually beginning in early life.

The possible relevance of these observations on adipose cellularity to the natural history of human obesity becomes apparent when the effects of weight loss and reduction in adipose tissue mass are considered. In all adult obese patients and in obese children, regardless of age of onset or degree and duration of obesity, loss of weight and reduction in adipose tissue mass have so far been shown to be accompanied by a change in adipose cell size alone;[25-29] cell number remains constant even in the face of massive degrees of weight loss. Thus, adipose hypercellularity appears to inflict a permanent, irreversible abnormality on the patient suffering from this type of obesity.

These morphologic phenomena parallel many aspects of the development and course of human obesity, particularly the well-recognized and frustrating clinical course and natural history of the disorder, which appears to be intractable in the lifelong severely obese patient.[27] These observations also provide a theoretical explanation for the inference that obesity of early onset may provide an important reservoir of adult obesity. However, much more data from humans and laboratory animals are required before final conclusions can be drawn.

ETIOLOGY AND PATHOGENESIS

Obesity has multiple causes and pathophysiological mechanisms which lead to the accumulation of excessive adipose tissue. It is probably best, therefore, to refer to this group of disorders as "the obesities." The study of obesity in laboratory animals has generated and continues to provide extremely valuable information regarding potential causes and pathogenic mechanisms involved in the development and perpetuation of human obesity. Obesity in laboratory animals can be the result of genetic factors, hypothalamic injury, endocrine or metabolic imbalance, nutritional manipulation, physical inactivity, or emotional disturbance.[53,54] Indeed, each of these factors has been shown to be responsible for the development of obesity in humans. Unfortunately, however, in the overwhelming majority of obese patients, neither these nor any other factors can be identified as a specific underlying cause; only in perhaps 5 percent or less of cases can one of these specific causes of obesity be detected.

At the simplest level, obesity is the result of energy imbalance: total energy intake into the body in the form of nutrient calories is in excess of the body's expenditure of energy. Energy intake is derived entirely from ingested food. Energy expenditure by the body has several major components, including that used for maintenance of vital metabolic and physiological functions of the body at rest (basal metabolism or resting metabolic rate), that used for performing work on the environment, i.e., physical activity (exercise), and that expended and released as heat in response to food intake and exercise, i.e., thermogenesis (diet-induced thermogenesis, exercise-induced thermogenesis).[55] The thermogenic response to ingested food has two components: heat generated from the processing of food by the body and heat generated through diet-induced metabolic adaptive changes in the cells of the body. In the rodent, the latter component of thermogenesis is a function of brown adipose tissue, a tissue which is of uncertain importance in humans (see below).

When energy (calorie) intake is excessive relative to caloric expenditure, the surplus calories are stored as triglyceride in the body's major energy storage organ, the adipose tissue; as a consequence, body fat depots increase in size and body weight increases. Positive energy balance and obesity result, therefore, from excessive caloric intake (overeating), decreased expenditure of energy, or a combination of the two. Overeating is extremely important in the etiology and pathogenesis of obesity and even modest increases in intake over time can markedly alter the level of storage. In fact, in the overwhelming majority of obese patients, excessive caloric intake or overeating is probably the primary etiologic factor. Decreased energy expenditure (decreased physical activity, decreased resting metabolic rate, and decreased thermogenesis) may also produce and perpetuate the obese state. Some obese individuals might possess subtle defects in energy expenditure which result in and perpetuate obesity. Moreover, there is abundant evidence that food intake and energy expenditure are coupled so as to maintain a fairly fixed level of energy storage, so it might be expected that the two components would be closely linked in contributing to an expanded adipose tissue mass.[56] Finally, there are a number of so-called futile biochemical cycles in which energy is expended without evident performance of physiological work.[57] As will be discussed below, a decrease in these cycles might lead to enhanced energy efficiency, more ready storage of calories, and hence obesity.

It should be clear, then, that obesity can be the result of different derangements in energy balance. Many factors are involved in the regulation of energy balance and contribute to the loss of control of energy storage, including those of genetic and environmental origin. Genetic influences may be mediated through neural, hormonal, metabolic, and psychological mechanisms, acting alone or in combination. Environmental influences may be mediated through nutritional, psychological, socioeconomic, or other acquired factors. Unfortunately, at present, the underlying derangements in these and other factors regulating energy intake and expenditure, which lead to positive energy balance, excessive accumulation of calories in adipose tissue, and obesity, are not known in the great majority of obese individuals.

Genetic Factors

Genetic factors undoubtedly contribute to some types of human obesity, and although genetic obesity has been well described in laboratory animals, specific genetic defects leading to obesity in humans have not been identified. Theoretically, genetic defects in energy intake or expenditure could lead to obesity by producing overeating or decreased utilization of energy. Genetic defects could be mediated through their influence on central, peripheral, and autonomic nervous system function, endocrine and metabolic factors, adipose tissue growth and development, and behavior. While alterations in each of these have been described in obese humans, none has been directly related to specific genetic factors. On the other hand, genetic abnormalities might confer increased susceptibility to nongenetic, presumably environmental, factors which influence eating or energy expenditure, factors which convert genetic predisposition to obesity into overt clinical disease.

The most direct evidence that genetic factors can produce obesity comes from animal studies. Genetic obesity in laboratory animals has been shown to be the result of the independent action of several different single genes.[53,54] Mutations at four loci, obese (*ob*), diabetes (*db*), agouti (A^{vy}), and fatty (*fa*), cause obesity in mice; one mutation, fatty (*fa*), cause obesity in rats. The obesity of the New Zealand obese (NZO) strain of mice appears to be polygenic. Detailed studies of these gene mutations have led to considerable insight into possible mechanisms by which they might produce obesity in these animals, including effects on appetite regulation, metabolism, and function of the CNS, pituitary, thyroid, and pancreas. One abnormality in the *dbdb* mouse appears to be a defect in the hypothalamic satiety center, which prevents this animal from recognizing satiety cues.[58] In contrast, the *obob* mouse appears to have some defect in the production of sufficient or effective satiety factors, so it remains hyperphagic and becomes obese.[59] Other primary defects appear to involve the adipose cell itself; e.g., a more efficient utilization of calories to produce fat appears to occur in both NZO mice and Zucker fatty rats.[54] Obesity in the Zucker rat is caused by the recessive state of the fatty gene, i.e., *fafa*. The earliest abnormality in this animal so far detected is an increase in lipoprotein lipase activity, which occurs prior to the development of obesity.[60] This enzyme hydrolyzes circulating triglycerides, liberating free fatty acids which are taken up and stored as triglyceride within the adipose cell. A genetically determined increase in the activity of this enzyme could contribute to the excessive accumulation of lipid in adipose cells and the development of obesity in the Zucker fatty rat. In addition to the excessive growth of adipose tissue in this animal, there is decreased growth of skeletal and muscle tissue. Moreover, a variety of CNS derangements have been described in the Zucker fatty rat, including alterations in hypothalamic function.[54,61,62] These abnormalities are associated with alterations in the secretion of insulin and growth hormone (GH), changes which may contribute to the development and maintenance of obesity. Whether these animal models of obesity are applicable to the human condition and the extent to which they so apply remain to be determined.

The genetic contribution to human obesity has been more difficult to assess. Epidemiologic data, including studies on monozygotic and dizygotic twins, clearly indicate that obesity tends to run in families and that genetic influences are important.[23] Yet, a clear-cut contribution has been difficult to establish in humans because of the inability to distinguish between the effects of inherited and environmental factors.

Obese patients tend to generate obese children and obese propositi tend to have obese siblings. In one study it was reported that, whereas offspring of two normal-weight parents had only a 9 percent chance of becoming obese, the probability of obesity in the offspring when one or both parents were obese increased to 41 and 73 percent, respectively.[63] A recent study of a large population in Denmark strongly suggests that body fatness and obesity in humans are hereditable.[64] It was demonstrated that the adiposity of adopted Danes, as assessed by BMI, is more strongly correlated at all levels of leanness and fatness with the BMI of their biologic parents, especially mothers, than with the BMI of adopted parents. A similar relationship was observed for obesity. Although such studies support the concept that there is a strong genetic factor in human obesity, they do not imply that environmental factors are irrelevant. In fact, environmental factors appear to be very important in determining the level of body fatness. For example, it has been reported that exactly the same body weight trends occur in the adopted children of obese parents and the genetically unrelated adopted siblings of obese propositi as occur in the natural offspring.[65] These and many other observations suggest that environmental factors, e.g., peer and parent role models, are also important contributors to human obesity.

Occasionally human obesity is part of an established genetic syndrome. Several rare genetic syndromes in humans have obesity as a clinical manifestation. For example, the Prader-Willi syndrome, characterized by hyperphagia, obesity, diabetes mellitus, and mental retardation, has been associated with a specific genetic defect. The Laurence-Moon-Biedl syndrome is inherited as a recessive genetic trait and is characterized by hyperphagia, obesity, mental retardation, hypogonadism, retinitis pigmentosa, and polydactylism. Recessive inheritance has also been associated with Alström's syndrome. While genetic defects are probably responsible for these obesities, neither an anatomic nor a biologic basis has been identified, although the hypothalamus or a higher center is presumed to be involved.

Observations such as those described in laboratory animals and humans strongly suggest that genetic factors may act as primary determinants of at least some forms of obesity. These genetic factors may influence the processes which regulate energy balance and body weight, including those concerned with eating behavior and/or energy expenditure. Environmental factors related to life-style and cultural and socioeconomic conditions also influence eating behavior and physical activity and thereby produce overt clinical obesity, or may interact with genetic factors to convert an inherited predisposition into obesity. The abundance of, easy accessibility to, and almost constant exposure to food and the sedentary life-style of many populations surely contribute to the cause and maintenance of the obesities just as do genetic factors. The specific genetic defects and the products of genes which lead to alterations in energy balance and obesity have not yet been identified, nor has the nature of the interaction of heredity and the environment in the development and perpetuation of human obesity been defined.

Central Nervous System Factors

The basic mechanisms regulating energy intake or eating reside in the CNS at several levels within the brain.[66–68] At the same time, the CNS regulation of feeding behavior is influenced by a variety of factors which have their origins in the peripheral tissues, as well as by factors in the external environment. Furthermore, both the CNS and the peripheral tissues play a key role in the regulation of the body's energy metabolism through the control of hormone (e.g., insulin) secretion and action, flow of nutrient substrates (e.g., glucose and fatty acids), and, possibly, through the regulation of adaptive thermogenesis via the sympathetic nervous system.[55,68–70]

Although the precise nature of the CNS regulatory process is poorly understood, it involves an extensive, highly encephalized control system with functional units capable of sensing and analyzing alterations in the metabolic and energy state of the internal environment; these functional units must also be capable of reacting to such alterations and to stimuli from the external environment by producing suitable effectors which elicit or inhibit eating, hormone secretion, and substrate flow.

The hypothalamus is the most studied and best understood of the CNS components regulating food intake. It has long been recognized that hypothalamic damage may be associated with obesity. Electrical or chemical destruction of the ventromedial nucleus of the hypothalamus of various laboratory animals causes hyperphagia, hyperinsulinemia, decreased GH secretion, rapid weight gain, and obesity which persists until a new plateau in body weight is achieved. Electrical stimulation of this so-called satiety center leads to cessation of eating. Lesions in an area in the lateral hypothalamus cause cessation of eating, weight loss, and maintenance of reduced body weight. In humans, tumor, inflammation, or injury due to surgery or hemorrhage in the ventromedial nucleus of the hypothalamus may lead to obesity; these, however, are extremely rare causes of this condition.[71] It remains to be established whether more subtle anatomic or functional abnormalities of the hypothalamus, occurring either on a genetic or an acquired basis, are responsible for some types of human obesity.

Although the hypothalamus is crucial to, and indeed may be the seat of, the food intake–regulatory process, it does not operate alone. Both higher and lower brain centers can influence hypothalamic function and affect eating behavior. Destruction of various components of the limbic system, e.g., the frontal and temporal lobes and various regions of the reticular formation and brainstem, has been shown to affect food intake in several species. Lesions in these areas of the brain, induced either by surgery, tumor, or injury, have been associated with obesity in humans, although these are rare. Information is transmitted from these higher centers to the specialized neural receptor cells of the hypothalamus via neural and humoral mechanisms. The ventromedial and lateral hypothalamic nuclei have numerous afferent neural connections with these higher brain structures. Neurotransmitters such as norepinephrine, serotonin (5-hydroxytryptamine), thyrotropin releasing hormone (TRH), and dopamine also provide a humoral link between cells from higher centers and the hypothalamus.[66–68] Norepinephrine may be a particularly important regulator of eating; its effects vary, depending on the hypothalamic site of its release. Norepinephrine applied to the paraventricular region of the ventromedial nucleus of the hypothalamus stimulates food intake, which can be blocked by alpha-adrenergic agents. When applied to the lateral hypothalamus, norepinephrine decreases food intake, an effect which is blocked by beta-adrenergic antagonists. Serotonin and serotonin agonists have been shown to increase food intake when applied to the ventromedial nucleus of rats, and to decrease eating when applied to the lateral hypothalamic region.

Various brain peptides such as cholecystokinin (CCK), endogenous opiates (β-endorphin, dynorphin, and the enkephalins), TRH, and bombesin may influence eating in humans and/or laboratory animals; in some instances specific receptors have been identified (e.g., for CCK).[66-68] Application of β-endorphin to the ventromedial nucleus stimulates eating, an effect which can be inhibited by naloxone. TRH is widely distributed throughout the brain, although its highest concentration is within the hypothalamus. Introduction of TRH into the third ventricle of rats diminishes food and water intake. Similar effects have been observed for some metabolites of TRH. Alterations in any of these or other CNS substances could be associated with abnormal regulation of eating behavior and obesity in humans, but such alterations, and a physiological or pathophysiological role for these substances, have yet to be demonstrated in human obesity.

Regulation of eating behavior by the CNS is influenced by a diversity of neural, chemical, and other factors coming to the brain from the periphery. Information about the intake, utilization, and storage of energy is continuously provided to the CNS from the peripheral tissues, so that control of food intake can be integrated with, and adjusted to, the energy needs of the body. Neural and humoral signals transmitted to the hypothalamic regulatory mechanisms from the GI tract during the ingestion and digestion of food ultimately result in the termination of a meal.[66] Gastrointestinal humoral factors implicated in the regulation of eating behavior include CCK, bombesin, somatostatin, vasoactive inhibitory peptide, pancreatic polypeptide, and gastrin.[66,67] If these are important regulators of food intake, they probably influence short-term eating behavior, i.e., intermeal or postprandial eating, meal size, and satiety. CCK, bombesin, and somatostatin have been isolated from, and are believed to be synthesized in, not only the GI tract but also the brain. CCK and bombesin receptors have also been identified in the brain, especially the hypothalamus.

Whether there is a functional relationship between these peptides of both brain and gut and, if so, how they modulate eating behavior remains to be clarified. It is probable that the gut factors influence eating behavior, in part, through local effects on the stomach and intestine. For example, CCK has been shown to decrease food intake in laboratory animals and humans. Parenteral administration of CCK both to a variety of laboratory animals, including rats, mice, and monkeys, and to humans inhibits food intake; this effect is blocked by vagotomy. One of the ways that CCK may influence food intake, therefore, is through its effects on gastric emptying or upper intestinal function, mediated through neural signals transmitted via afferent fibers of the vagus nerve to centers in the brain. Injection of CCK into the ventromedial nuclei of rats also has been reported by some investigators to inhibit eating, but others have not found this to occur. The presence of CCK and other gut peptides in the brain raises the possibility that these peptides are transmitted to the hypothalamic regulatory mechanisms from the GI tract, but it seems apparent that the brain synthesizes its own CCK; either the carboxy-terminal octapeptide or a pure extract of CCK has been identified in rat brains. It is possible that the influence of endogenous brain CCK as well as other brain peptides on eating behavior is somehow triggered by signals emanating from the gut. Parenteral administration of bombesin decreases eating in rats, an effect which is not abolished by vagotomy. Research on this peptide has, to date, been less extensive than on CCK; therefore, understanding of the role of bombesin is even less complete.

Food absorption and subsequent metabolism produce additional chemical changes in the internal metabolic environment; e.g., changes in the concentrations of glucose, amino acids, various lipids, and other nutrients are transmitted via the circulation to the centers regulating eating behavior in the brain. It has been suggested that such a chemostatic mechanism operating as a feedback system between the peripheral tissues and the brain may be an important contributor to the short-term, postprandial, or intermeal regulation of eating.[67] Abnormalities in any component of this process, whether primary defects in the central nervous sensing system or in peripheral metabolism and the chemical or neural signals generated from it, could theoretically play a role in the development of human obesity.

Changes in concentrations of hormones such as insulin and glucagon are also induced by eating; it has been proposed that insulin itself may be an important regulator of eating, either short- or long-term. Intracranial administration of insulin to rats and baboons has been reported to decrease food intake.[66,67] Indeed, insulin and insulin receptors have been identified in various parts of the brains of rodents, dogs, and some obese patients. Several studies provide evidence that circulating insulin can enter the brain and that brain cells may also synthesize insulin. Thus, the brain may be exposed to both endogenous and exogenous insulin. The role for either of these insulins, if any, in the regulation of eating behavior needs to be clarified.

The amount of adipose tissue in the body may also be an important regulator of eating behavior; it may be especially important to long-term control. Information about the state of energy stores and body weight is apparently provided to the hypothalamus.[66,67] It is postulated that such information permits the regulatory system to correct for errors introduced over time through short-term regulation and, thus, to maintain constant body weight and energy stores over long periods. The nature of the long-term signal, whether a metabolite from the adipose tissue or some other factor, remains to be identified. The primary function of the regulation of eating appears to be to regulate body energy stores, and the major energy storage organ of the body is the adipose tissue. It is therefore not surprising that adipose tissue has been implicated as an important component of the long-term control mechanism for maintaining energy balance. Indeed, it has been suggested that the central regulatory system monitors adipose tissue and in turn is regulated by this tissue. The so-called lipostatic theory postulates that this feedback control of eating is mediated through some circulating biochemical analogue of adipose tissue energy stores; although such a factor has been sought, it has not been found. It is partly on this basis, however, that the adipose cell theory of obesity (discussed below) has developed.[72] Other signals and other tissues, particularly the liver,[73] may be as important as, or more important than, adipose tissue in the long-term regulation of eating and the pathogenesis of obesity.

In addition to regulating body weight through its control of eating behavior, the nervous system regulates body weight through its control of energy metabolism and storage in the tissues of the body. It accomplishes this in many ways, including neural control of substrate flow, substrate metabolism, and endocrine secretion and action.[68] The autonomic nervous system appears to play an especially key role in the control of energy uptake, storage, and expenditure.[74,75] For example, it influences insulin secretion and action, thereby affecting energy storage and utilization in white adipose cells, liver, and muscle; the effect is mediated by the regulation of glucose and lipid metabolism. The autonomic nervous system influences energy (i.e, calorie) utilization through regulation of lipolysis by insulin, catecholamines, and other endocrine and neural factors. In rodents, it is an important regulator of energy expenditure through its control of thermogenesis in brown adipose tissue.[69] As discussed below, alterations in nervous system control of energy metabolism and storage may contribute to some types of obesity. For example, defective sympathetic nervous system control of diet-induced thermogenesis has been detected in some animal models of obesity.

It is clear that the CNS regulation of eating behavior and energy balance requires the integrated action of an extensive network of processes located throughout the body which regulate food intake, nutrient metabolism, and energy expenditure. Superimposed on this internal physiological regulatory system are the modulating effects of factors in the external environment, probably primarily mediated by effects on higher brain centers. An abnormality in any one of these components of the regulatory process could lead to increased energy intake relative to energy expenditure and thus to development of obesity.

Hyperphagia and hyperinsulinemia appear to be two key factors in the development of hypothalamic obesity in laboratory animals.[53] The two are closely intertwined. It is probable that each contributes to the development of the other; both probably contribute to the development and maintenance of obesity in certain laboratory animals. Hyperinsulinemia appears to be essential for the development of the obesity of the animal with a ventromedial hypothalamic lesion.[76] Destruction of the ventromedial nuclei in rats may produce hyperinsulinemia and enhance lipid synthesis in the adipose tissue, even in the absence of hyperphagia. Moreover, in some other laboratory animal models of obesity, hyperinsulinemia precedes hyperphagia and obesity. For example, studies in the Zucker obese rat demonstrate that, before obesity can be detected, i.e., at age 17 days (when body weight is identical to normal), animals destined to become obese secrete excessive amounts of insulin as well as decreased amounts of GH in response to intravenous arginine.[61,62] It is postulated that these hormonal abnormalities are the result of genetically determined abnormalities in CNS function, including hypothalamic function. Increased vagal tone, with increased parasympathetic nervous system activity and decreased sympathetic nervous system activity, has been detected in these animal models of obesity. The imbalance between parasympathetic and sympathetic nervous system activity has been proposed to be responsible not only for hyperinsulinemia and decreased GH secretion, but also increased lipogenesis and decreased lipolysis in white adipose tissue and decreased expenditure of energy through sympathetic nervous system–mediated diet-induced thermogenesis in brown adipose tissue.[69] Whether these derangements in experimental animal models of obesity parallel any form of human obesity remains conjectural. These observations, however, have renewed interest in the possibility that excessive secretion and action of insulin due to a primary hypothalamic defect, with or without alterations in GH secretion, may be the underlying cause of some forms of human obesity.

Endocrine Factors

A possible explanation for some human obesity lies in some primary hormonal imbalance which, by affecting eating behavior and/or energy expenditure, could lead to positive energy balance and consequent excessive caloric storage in the adipose tissue. Indeed, several changes in endocrine function have been observed in many obese patients; in most instances, however, these alterations appear to be a consequence rather than a cause of obesity.[77-79]

ADRENAL CORTICAL HORMONES

Studies in *dbdb* and *obob* obese mice and *fafa* rats demonstrate that obesity does not occur if adrenalectomy is performed; food intake decreases and energy expenditure increases in these animals after adrenalectomy.[80] Administration of cortisol reverses these changes and permits the obesity to occur. Thus, in these animal models of obesity, cortisol appears to be a permissive hormone. In humans, cortisol may play a similar permissive role, but only rarely is hypercortisolism the cause of human obesity. Cortisol secretion rates and 24-h urinary excretion of 17-hydroxycorticosteroids (uncorrected for body weight) are increased in obese patients, but are restored to normal after weight reduction. Cushing's syndrome can cause obesity, but is a rare cause; when it does cause obesity, the obesity tends to be mild in degree and reversible after definitive treatment of the underlying cause of the hypercortisolism. Of course, Cushing's syndrome and obesity of another etiology may coexist, in which case the obesity persists even after correction of the hypercortisolism.

THYROID HORMONES

In most obese patients, thyroid function is normal, at least as measured by standard tests. More sensitive indicators of thyroid function demonstrate that subtle changes in thyroid hormone metabolism may occur in obesity and in response to both over- and underfeeding.[70,81,82] Plasma thyroxine (T_4), reverse triiodothyronine (rT_3), and TRH-stimulated thyroid stimulating hormone (TSH) concentrations have been found to be similar in obese and nonobese persons at stable weight. On the other hand, plasma T_3 concentrations have been found to be greater in weight-stable obese persons compared to nonobese control individuals. Weight loss in both obese humans and rodents has been reported to be accompanied by a decrease in plasma T_3 concentration and an increased conversion of T_4 to the calorically inert T_3 as part of the adaptation to restricted food intake. Theoretically, these adaptations in thyroid function to caloric restriction and weight loss might contribute to regain of weight and adipose tissue mass. In contrast, plasma T_3 concentration has been reported to increase and rT_3 concentration to decrease after overfeeding.

These observations suggest that adaptations in the obese individual and in response to overfeeding are directed toward preventing excess energy storage in adipose cells, whereas after weight reduction this "protective" adaptation is removed. It appears, therefore, that altered thyroid function is not usually responsible for the origin of human obesity, but it may contribute to recidivism after weight loss.

In those rare instances in which hypothyroidism is the cause of obesity, the obesity is usually mild and treatment of the hormonal dysfunction is accompanied by restoration of normal body weight. As with Cushing's syndrome, obesity of another etiology and hypothyroidism may coexist, in which case the obesity persists after correction of the hypothyroidism.

GROWTH HORMONE

While decreased GH secretion and action may be a factor contributing to the obesity of certain laboratory animals, in humans alterations in this hormone appear to be a consequence rather than a cause of obesity.[83] GH secretion in response to glucose and arginine is markedly decreased in obese compared to nonobese patients, but weight reduction is associated with a restoration to normal of hormone secretion and plasma GH level.

OTHER HORMONES

The role and character of such potentially important hormones as those of gonadal origin has not been well studied. Hormones of GI origin have been discussed earlier. A role for these gut hormones in the development and perpetuation of human obesity has not been identified.

INSULIN

The possible etiologic role of hyperinsulinemia in obesity has become the subject of increasing research attention. It is now well established that hyperinsulinemia is present in most, if not all, experimental animal models of obesity studied to date; plasma insulin concentration is usually, but not always, increased in human obesity. Moreover, development of hyperphagia and obesity in several rodents appears to be preceded by hyperinsulinemia (see above). A rise in serum insulin concentration has also been observed within the first few days of hypothalamic injury in humans;[71] this sequential relationship has not yet been demonstrated for other types of human obesity. It has been postulated, therefore, that hyperinsulinemia may produce hyperphagia and consequent obesity.

The underlying mechanisms responsible for the hypersecretion of insulin in obese laboratory animals and humans are still poorly understood. Abnormal hypothalamic function and alterations in the relative activities of the parasympathetic and sympathetic nervous systems (i.e., decreases in sympathetic activity) have, as discussed earlier, been postulated to lead to hyperinsulinemia in the Zucker obese rat, but no such changes have been found in human obesity. One or more primary abnormalities in pancreatic beta cells could also lead to hyperinsulinemia and, secondarily, to hyperphagia, increased lipogenesis, decreased lipolysis, and obesity.

Pancreatic insulin-secreting tumors are a rare cause of human obesity. Investigations aimed at identifying which factors trigger the hypersecretion of insulin and whether these reside in- or outside of the pancreas are in progress. The possibility that some obese patients suffer a genetically determined or acquired dysfunction of hypothalamic or higher brain centers concerned with the regulation of pancreatic insulin secretion requires careful study.

Metabolic Factors

A metabolic basis for the human obesities has long been sought, but, except in extremely rare instances, has not been demonstrable. The fact that metabolic defects have been demonstrated in obese laboratory animals, however, suggests that similar abnormalities could exist in humans.

An underlying metabolic abnormality theoretically might operate to increase storage of energy in adipose tissue in the form of triglycerides in several ways, including: (1) preferential shunting of nutrient energy into lipid-producing pathways due to some enzymatic, hormonal, or other metabolic alteration or imbalance favoring lipogenesis; (2) inhibition of mobilization of energy that is stored as triglyceride in adipose cells, due to some alteration in the metabolic regulation of lipolysis; (3) subtle defects in energy expenditure. The last might involve increased efficiency in extracting energy from nutrients with resulting reduced energy expenditure or increased efficiency at performing physiological and/or physical work, also resulting in decreased energy expenditure, or decreased futile biochemical cycles.[57] Indeed, some of these abnormalities have been demonstrated in laboratory animal models of obesity.

METABOLIC DEFECTS IN LABORATORY ANIMALS

The Zucker fatty rat and New Zealand obese mouse display a metabolic alteration in which ingested calories are preferentially shunted into triglyceride formation in adipose tissues;[53,71] in the Zucker fatty rat there is a concomitant decrease in lean body mass. An increase in lipoprotein lipase activity has been observed prior to the development of obesity in the Zucker fatty rat.[60] The increased activity of this enzyme, in concert with the previously described hyperinsulinemia, decreased GH levels, and hyperphagia, might be responsible for the obesity of this animal by shunting nutrient calories into the adipose tissue.

The *obob* mouse has been demonstrated to lack thyroid-dependent Na^+,K^+-ATPase in kidney, liver, and muscle cells.[84] It is of interest that adrenalectomy normalizes Na^+,K^+-ATPase activity in these animals.[80] It has been proposed that this metabolic defect results in an increase in the efficiency with which ATP energy is used, a decreased requirement for ATP, and, thus, reduced expenditure of energy. However, others have found no reduction in Na^+,K^+-ATPase activity in some tissues from *obob* mice.[85] There is evidence that Na^+,K^+-ATPase activity varies from tissue to tissue; activity may be decreased in one tissue while it is normal in other tissues.

Of particular interest is the recent demonstration of defective diet-induced thermogenesis in several obese rodents.[69,86,87] In rodents energy expenditure for heat production (thermogenesis) in brown adipose tissue plays an important role not only in the regulation of body temperature but also in the regulation of body weight; thermogenesis in brown adipose may also figure in the development of some forms of animal obesity. Thermogenesis by brown adipose tissue in rodents is normally stimulated by overeating (diet-induced thermogenesis), physical activity (exercise-induced thermogenesis), and exposure to cold (cold-induced nonshivering thermogenesis). These forms of adaptive thermogenesis by brown adipose tissue in rodents are regulated by the sympathetic nervous system, which also increases the growth and metabolic activity of these cells. There is extensive innervation of brown adipose tissue by the sympathetic nervous system. When stimulated electrically or by exposure to cold or overeating, sympathetic nerves release norepinephrine, which binds to beta-adrenergic receptors on brown adipose cells. Binding of hormone to receptor triggers a variety of biochemical events which lead to, among other things, the uncoupling of mitochondrial substrate oxidation from ATP production and, hence, to increased heat production. Thus, adaptive thermogenesis makes the animal metabolically less energy efficient.

Adaptive thermogenesis in brown adipose tissue appears to play an important role in the regulation of total energy expenditure in rats and mice. For example, cold-acclimated normal rats become hyperphagic, but much of the increased energy intake is converted to heat in the enlarged and hypermetabolic brown adipose tissue; thus, these animals remain lean in spite of increased energy intake. Overfeeding certain genetic strains of normal rats highly palatable diets produces obesity. However, these animals do not gain as much weight as would be expected on the basis of the excess calories consumed. The explanation for this apparent wasting of calories is believed to reside in diet-induced adaptive thermogenesis. The increased metabolic rate in an enlarged mass of brown adipose tissue leads to dissipation of energy as heat and, therefore, to decreased metabolic efficiency.

Several rodent models of obesity have been shown to have defective adaptive thermogenesis.[69,86,87] Thermogenesis in brown adipose tissue is decreased in *obob* and *dbdb* mice in response to both cold exposure and overeating, due to a defect in which brown adipose tissue is unresponsive to norepinephrine. In the Zucker fatty rat brown adipose tissue thermogenesis is not activated after overeating, but is activated on exposure to cold. It appears in this animal model of obesity that overeating does not stimulate sympathetic nervous system activity; the brown adipose tissue itself appears to be normal. Hypothalamic obesity in the mouse produced by gold thioglucose or in the rat due to a lesion in the ventromedial hypothalamic nucleus has been reported to be associated with an inability to activate thermogenesis in brown adipose tissue in response to overeating; the defect appears to be in the hypothalamus, which is unresponsive to the effects of overeating and unable to regulate diet-induced thermogenesis in brown adipose tissue through the sympathetic nervous system. It has been proposed that because these animals normally stimulate thermogenesis in brown adipose tissue there is decreased energy expenditure and increased energy efficiency which contribute to the development of obesity.

Thus, a variety of metabolic defects have been observed to be associated with obesity in experimental animals; it seems both attractive and reasonable to consider that similar metabolic defects may be responsible for human obesity.

METABOLIC DEFECTS IN HUMANS

Metabolic differences between obese and nonobese humans certainly do exist, but the etiologic significance of these differences remains to be established. Most of the demonstrated differences between obese and nonobese patients appear to represent metabolic adaptations to obesity rather than underlying causes. Occasionally, a metabolic defect has been reported which appears to cause obesity. For example, a kindred has been described in which three obese family members appear to have a defect in lipolysis as reflected by decreased in vitro mobilization of glycerol from their adipose tissue.[88] An inability of cyclic AMP to activate adipose cell triglyceride lipase has been observed; the responsible defect appears to lie at the level of the protein kinase–dependent phosphorylation which activates inactive triglyceride lipase. Although this defect appears to have been responsible for the obesity of these individuals, no such abnormality in this or any other aspect of lipolysis has been described in the adipose cells of most obese patients studied. Quite to the contrary, lipolytic activity in the adipose cells from obese patients has generally been observed to be increased compared to cells from nonobese subjects; this alteration appears to be an adaptive response to obesity.[89]

The past few years have witnessed an intensive effort to detect metabolic defects that result in decreased energy expenditure which, in the face of normal energy intake, could cause obesity. Although there has been a resurgence of interest in and willingness to consider this possibility, the data do not yet seem to support this concept. This, however, may only reflect the limitations of current methodologies for studying energy expenditure in humans.

Energy expenditure by humans comprises three major components: (1) energy used to perform the vital metabolic and physiological functions of the body at rest, i.e., resting or basal metabolic rate; (2) energy expended through thermogenesis (thermic response to food and exercise); and (3) energy spent in performing work on the environment, i.e., physical activity (exercise).

Evidence for the existence of meaningful differences in basal energy expenditure between the obese and the nonobese at the biochemical level is sparse. Most studies reveal that the resting or basal metabolic rate of obese humans is greater than in nonobese individuals.[70,75,90] Moreover, it has been demonstrated that in the obese state, total energy need (resting plus physical activity plus thermogenesis) or expenditure per unit of active metabolic mass is not deficient. Biochemical evidence for the existence of meaningful differences in basal metabolic efficiency between obese and nonobese humans, whether in the efficiency with which usable energy is generated and captured as ATP; the efficiency with which energy-requiring processes such as biosynthesis, transport, and contraction are conducted; or the regulation of these processes by hormonal factors such as thyroid hormone, is also lacking.

The activity of Na^+,K^+-ATPase in erythrocytes has been reported to be decreased in obese compared to lean individuals in the resting state.[91] The finding suggests that the obese may be metabolically more efficient; some have postulated that this defect may be a primary etiologic factor in some forms of human obesity since, in their studies, it is not reversed with weight loss. It is proposed that the energy not used by the Na^+,K^+ pump could be stored as triglyceride in adipose cells, resulting in weight gain and obesity even in the individual who is not overeating. Moreover, since insulin stimulates Na^+,K^+-ATPase, it has been postulated that the insulin resistance of obesity might further contribute to a reduction in energy expenditure. There are, however, serious problems with this hypothesis. For example, one study has reported finding increased Na^+,K^+-ATPase activity in red cells from obese patients; another found no difference between obese and nonobese patients in Na^+,K^+-ATPase activity in fibroblasts.[92,93] The theory that reduced erythrocyte Na^+,K^+-ATPase activity contributes to or is responsible for obesity in humans is based on an assumption that the energy used by the erythrocyte Na^+,K^+-ATPase pump makes the same significant contribution to the total amount of energy expended by a human individual as it apparently does in rodents. This assumption has not been validated. Na^+,K^+-ATPase activity in other tissues, such as white and brown adipose, which are likely to contribute more significantly than red blood cells, has not been systematically studied in humans; defects have not been demonstrated in human obesity. Na^+,K^+-ATPase activity has been reported to be decreased in erythrocytes from obese subjects compared to nonobese controls, but has been found to be increased in the liver.[94] It remains necessary, therefore, to clarify not only the role of the Na^+,K^+ pump in the metabolic rate, but also to identify which tissues might contribute significantly to reduced energy expenditure. Some workers have reported that the reduction in erythrocyte Na^+,K^+-ATPase activity in obese humans is not reversed with weight loss, suggesting that a primary metabolic defect exists;[91] others, however, have found that weight reduction restores the activity of this enzyme to normal, indicating that this defect in the red blood cell is a metabolic alteration which is secondary to obesity.[93] Finally, resting or basal metabolic rate in obese humans appears to be greater than that in the nonobese; this finding seems inconsistent with the concept that decreased erythrocyte Na^+,K^+-ATPase activity leads to decreased energy expenditure in obese compared to nonobese individuals.

One of the strongest lines of evidence that individual human beings may differ significantly enough in the efficiency with which they use nutrient energy to influence weight gain and adiposity comes from the overfeeding experiments of the Vermont study.[78] In this study, nonobese volunteers were subjected to excessive caloric intake over several months in an attempt to experimentally induce obesity. One of the most interesting findings was that not all subjects gained the amount of weight predicted from the number of excess calories presumed to have been ingested; some individuals gained weight more readily than others. Another observation was that subjects made obese through voluntary overeating had an energy requirement for maintenance of body weight and adiposity which was considerably more than that required by spontaneously obese individuals (1800 $kcal/m^2$ vs. 1200 $kcal/m^2$). These results have been interpreted to suggest that the spontaneously obese patients used food energy more efficiently than the experimentally obese subjects. However, it is not certain that the subjects were always identically physically active; thus, the role of metabolic efficiency in these differences cannot be assessed with certainty. Moreover, it remains to be determined whether obesity induced over a period of months is comparable to that which develops over, and has existed for, several years. The metabolic adaptation to short-term overeating may be sufficiently different from that due to persistent overeating and continually excessive adiposity as to make such comparisons less meaningful. Thus, while individuals may differ somewhat in their metabolic efficiency, it remains to be demonstrated that these variations are primary determinants of human obesity.

The demonstration of defective adaptive thermogenesis in brown fat in laboratory animals has led several investigators to propose that some forms of human obesity are the result of similar abnormalities in thermogenesis.[55,69,70,75,82,87,90,95–101] This is a highly attractive hypothesis, since it could explain the obesity in some patients who deny overeating: increased energy efficiency due to decreased thermogenesis frees calories, which are stored as triglyceride in an expanded adipose tissue mass. Subtle defects in the thermogenesis leading to small degrees of positive energy balance could lead to obesity over many years if not accompanied by a reduction in caloric intake. In this regard, it is of interest that when the body's caloric reservoir, the adipose tissue mass, is reduced by caloric restriction, the reduction in oxygen consumption is greater than can be accounted for by loss of body mass.[55] This adaptive increase in energy efficiency is consistent with diminished thermogenesis.

Unfortunately, the evidence from currently available studies in humans does not support the hypothesis that human obesity is the result of an underactivity of brown adipose tissue or defective thermogenesis. In the first place, it is uncertain whether brown fat exists in humans and, if so, in what amount. Although it appears that brown adipose tissue may be present at birth, there is little evidence to support the view that adult humans possess significant amounts of this tissue; much less evidence exists for differences between obese and nonobese individuals. However, it must be pointed out that detection of brown fat in humans is technically extremely difficult; failure to demonstrate its existence now does not preclude success in the future.

An additional problem with the hypothesis that defective thermogenesis may play a role in the etiology of some forms of human obesity is the lack, to date, of conclusive evidence that the capacity for adaptive thermogenesis differs between lean and obese humans; the evidence, in fact, has been conflicting. Some have observed a small reduction in diet-induced thermogenesis in obese women, some found no differences in diet-induced thermogenesis between obese and nonobese individuals, and others reported increased diet-induced thermogenesis in obese women.[87,96-99] Exercise-induced thermogenesis has been reported to be both decreased and normal in obese compared to nonobese individuals.[87,98-100] Moreover, even when a reduction in adaptive thermogenesis has been observed in obese patients, measurement of *total* energy expenditure (resting metabolic rate plus thermogenesis plus energy expended on the environment) has demonstrated that obese individuals expend an equal or greater amount of energy compared to nonobese individuals throughout the day, regardless of whether metabolic rate is expressed per unit of body weight or per unit of fat-free mass.[87,90,99] Put another way, under conditions of equal physical activity, obese patients require more calories to maintain contant body weight than nonobese controls. Using the best techniques currently available, therefore, these investigators found no evidence that the obese individuals they studied are more energy-efficient than nonobese controls.

Nevertheless, the role of sympathetic nervous system control of energy metabolism and diet-induced obesity may be important. A potentially important recent finding in this regard is the demonstration that some formerly obese individuals whose body composition becomes normal or near normal after weight loss have a decreased thermogenic response to glucose and require fewer calories for energy balance than subjects who had never been obese.[97,101] It has been postulated that this defect in energy metabolism, i.e., the diminished expenditure of energy via thermogenesis by obese individuals after weight reduction, might play a role in the almost inevitable post-weight-reduction weight gain and recurrence of obesity. Before this conclusion can be accepted, however, it must be shown that diet-induced thermogenesis is decreased to a greater degree in obese patients who have lost weight than in nonobese patients whose weight has reduced.

The possibility that obese are more efficient than nonobese persons at performing work on the external environment, i.e., physical activity, is not supported by the existing evidence. Just the opposite appears to be true: the energy cost of physical activity increases as body weight increases; for a given activity energy expenditure is greater in the obese than in the nonobese individual.[102]

Other metabolic defects have been proposed as possible underlying factors in the etiology of obesity, including alterations in protein turnover and the low flux of biochemical cycles such as glucose to glucose phosphate or the fructose phosphate shuttle.[57] The evidence, however, is very weak for a role for any of these cycles sufficient to disturb energy metabolism in humans so as to produce obesity.

At present, then, conclusive evidence for the existence in obese humans of an underlying metabolic defect causing increased efficiency of caloric use or storage is lacking. Nevertheless, metabolic abnormalities have been demonstrated to contribute to the development of obesity in certain experimental animals; this, together with the present limited understanding of the complex processes regulating energy balance and body weight in humans and the limitations on the technology for studying the processes, makes this an important area of continued research.

Nutritional Factors

Obesity results from the ingestion of more nutrient (food) energy than the body needs. The great majority of obese people probably *become* obese because they overeat; to be sure, once obesity develops other factors such as physical inactivity and metabolic, hormonal, and adipose tissue morphologic changes may contribute to its *perpetuation* and aggravation, but only rarely are these factors the underlying causes of obesity. Overeating can occur at any stage of life, but overeating in early life has received particular attention as a possible mechanism for inducing a permanent biologic change and the development of irreversible obesity.

MATERNAL NUTRITION

Maternal nutrition prior to and during pregnancy may be an important determinant of body weight at birth and during adult life. Studies of infants born to mothers exposed to severe undernutrition clearly indicate that maternal undernutrition can markedly lower birth weight.[103] The effects of maternal overnutrition on body weight at birth and in adult life are, however, less well documented; some studies report little or no correlation while others find that both maternal weight and weight gain during pregnancy are highly correlated with the development of childhood obesity.[103,104] Several studies have reported an increased frequency of obesity in infants of obese diabetic mothers, while others have not.[105,106] Even in those studies in which a positive correlation was observed, however, the degree of obesity in diabetic mothers did not correlate with the degree of obesity in their offspring. The evidence for a correlation between birth weight of normal newborns and subsequent obesity is also weak. It may be tempting to postulate a relationship between maternal overnutrition, excessive weight gain during pregnancy, and obesity in the offspring; such a relationship seems probable. Yet, the data currently available are not sufficient to permit this conclusion. Moreover, if maternal nutrition does influence the birth weight and body composition of the offspring, it is likely a complex process depending on, among other factors, the timing and duration of the overnutrition, placental function, hormonal and substrate milieu, and perhaps even the carbohydrate, fat, and protein composition of the maternal diet.

NUTRITION DURING INFANCY

Nutritional status during infancy has been postulated to play a significant role in the subsequent development of obesity. The classic rodent studies of McCance and Widdowson clearly demonstrated that nutritional experiences during the earliest stages of a rat's life can have a profound and lasting effect on adult body weight.[107] There is abundant evidence in laboratory animals that undernutrition limited to the very earliest days of life can lead to a permanent reduction in body weight, body size, body fat content, and adipose cell number.[33] Evidence is also available which demonstrates that overfeeding rats during the first 3 weeks of life results in a permanent increase in adipose cell number, and adipose tissue mass.[34]

A causal relationship between early nutritional experiences and adult obesity has also been proposed to exist for humans. A study of adult men born during the Dutch famine of 1944 to 1945 indicates that those whose earliest days of life were during famine suffered less obesity as adults than those who escaped such severe undernutrition.[108] In contrast, adults who were infants during the immediate postwar period when calories were more plentiful were approximately three times more likely to become obese than adults who had been born to famine. In another population, infant birth weight was shown to correlate quite highly with obesity in adult life;[19] those whose body weight was over the 97th percentile as infants were more than three times as likely to become obese adults as were normal-weight infants.

The introduction of solid food into the diets of infants at progressively earlier ages and a tendency to feed infants diets containing more calories and protein than the recommended dietary allowances have been observed.[109] It has been postulated that such practices may contribute to the growing prevalence of obesity in the United States. A similar contention has been made regarding the increasing tendency in some societies toward bottle-feeding of infants and away from breast-feeding.[110] It has been suggested that the ability to regulate energy balance is greater in the breast-fed compared to the bottle-fed infants; the mechanisms responsible for this, whether related to (1) differences in total caloric intake or density or in carbohydrate, lipid, and protein composition, (2) variations in other substances, or (3) behavioral changes, are unknown. The extent to which any of these nutritional factors in early life contributes to the development of obesity in childhood and adult life remains to be determined.

CHILDHOOD NUTRITION

Although there clearly is a group of obese children who become obese adults, most children do not. Evidence from several studies fails to confirm a long-term correlation between obesity in infancy or childhood and obesity in adult life.[20,21] Attempts to use a number of different measures such as birth weight, rate of weight gain early in life, or weight attained at 6 to 12 months of age have not been successful in predicting adult obesity. Restriction of food intake early in life has been shown in one study not to alter risk of obesity.[21] In spite of this lack of conclusive evidence, it has been proposed that the prevention of obesity requires drastic alteration in eating habits during the earliest stages of life. Such changes in nutritional practice have the potential for harmful long-term health consequences. Before major alterations in infant-feeding practices are initiated, it seems desirable to have additional information from carefully designed and controlled studies to establish whether, and to what extent, early nutritional environment may contribute to the development of human obesity.

ADULT NUTRITION

Clearly, early life is not the only period when nutritional experiences can influence the development of obesity in adult life. Many individuals begin to overeat and become obese only as adults. It is of interest, therefore, that excessive caloric intake by rats and mice during adult life, through the consumption of highly palatable diets, induces adipose cellular hyperplasia (i.e., new cell formation) and obesity; obesity established for a sufficient period of time tends to persist even after the animals return to standard chow.[41,42,44] Thus, overeating, even in adult life, may induce a permanent biologic change and persistent obesity in the rat. A similar situation could exist in humans since adult humans, like laboratory animals, tend to overeat when highly palatable food is freely available, particularly when either the fat or sugar content is high. The abundance and ease of availability, indeed the all-pervasiveness, of food in developed societies compounds this situation. With excessive caloric intake the rate of fat synthesis is greatly enhanced, surplus calories are stored as triglyceride in adipose tissue, and obesity results.

Whether the frequency of eating contributes to increased lipogenesis and calorie storage in humans is unknown. It is a frequent clinical observation that obese individuals eat fewer and larger meals than do the nonobese.[111,112] Some studies suggest that adipose tissue lipogenesis in vitro may be increased under such conditions.[113] Rats allowed to eat one 2-h meal per day rather than ad libitum show increased lipogenesis in their adipose tissue once adapted to this regimen; men eating one or two meals per day were shown to weigh more and to have thicker skin folds than men eating three or more meals per day.

Adaptive hyperlipogenesis in adipose tissue and liver has been observed upon refeeding obese individuals who had lost weight. This may be a contributing factor to rapid regain of adipose tissue upon refeeding in such persons. Increased synthesis and storage of fat in adipose tissue and resultant weight gain and obesity, however, depend primarily on the intake of excessive calories; that caloric excess, in turn, depends on the total number, not the kind (i.e., carbohydrate, fat, or protein) of calories consumed relative to calories expended. The frequency of eating and the nature of the food being ingested may influence total caloric intake and, thus, contribute to the development of obesity.

Physical Activity

Decreased physical activity in the face of constant caloric intake leads to positive energy balance, storage of excess calories as triglyceride in adipose cells, and expansion of the adipose tissue mass. Advancing technology has encouraged a more sedentary life-style; combined with the abundance and ease of availability of food, this has certainly contributed to the trend in the United States population toward increasing body weight and obesity. Excessive caloric intake (i.e., overeating) is, however, still the major factor responsible for obesity in the majority of individuals who become obese.

Studies of some obese and nonobese adolescent and adult populations have shown that the level of physical activity in obese individuals may be less than that in the nonobese.[114,115] Some of these studies revealed that these less-active obese individuals ingested fewer calories per day than the nonobese, an observation which has led to the concept that obesity in some individuals is the result of decreased physical activity rather than excessive caloric intake. The demonstration of an association between decreased physical activity and obesity does not, however, establish the inactivity to be the cause of the obesity; physical inactivity may be a consequence of the obesity: obesity limits spontaneous physical activity.[116] Studies of lean humans made obese through overeating demonstrate that weight gain and increased adiposity is associated with a spontaneous reduction in, and motivation to perform, physical activity. In addition, the energy expended to perform equivalent levels of physical activity is greater in the obese than the nonobese. Furthermore, some investigators have reported that obese children are no more prone to hypoactivity than normal-weight children.[117]

Based on the evidence currently available, the explanation most likely in the great majority of cases for the decreased physical activity in obese persons is that increased adiposity leads to a voluntary inhibition of physical activity. In most cases, the process of becoming obese involves ingestion of excess calories (i.e., overeating), but once the obesity is established, inactivity may contribute to the aggravation and *perpetuation* of the obesity.

Adipose Cell Hypothesis

It has been postulated that adipose tissue cellularity, i.e., fat cell size and/or number, may regulate eating behavior and/or caloric storage in adipose tissue; some alteration in the morphology of the adipose tissue is proposed to play a role in the etiology and/or perpetuation of some forms of human obesity, by somehow stimulating excess food intake or excess storage of energy as triglyceride in adipose cells. This has been referred to as the *adipose cell hypothesis*.[72]

One proposal that has been advanced is that the increased number of adipose cells in hyperplastic obesity somehow leads to or perpetuates obesity. In some forms of obesity, adipocyte differentiation and proliferation are abnormally stimulated early in life, causing adipose hypercellularity, excessive expansion of the adipose tissue, and obesity; the hypercellularity, once established, is irreversible. It is postulated that this persistent hypercellularity either stimulates excess food intake or energy storage as triglyceride in adipose cells. A further postulate of the adipose cell hypothesis is that body fat, and therefore body weight, can always increase but, except under extreme conditions, cannot decrease below a minimum level set by the total number of adipose cells. This hypothesis has led to a great deal of attention to early life and factors such as early nutritional experience which may produce adipose cell proliferation, hypercellularity of the adipose tissue, and persistent obesity. Earlier data suggested that total adipocyte number is determined early in life and that increases in cell number, and therefore adipose hypercellularity, could occur only during certain "critical periods," e.g., in utero, during infancy, and around puberty. However, more recent information indicates that cell number may be increased in laboratory animals and humans at any time during life, given an appropriate stimulus such as excessive caloric intake. Rats, mice, and humans have been described in whom adipose hypercellularity appears to be associated with the onset of obesity in adult life. Moreover, as discussed earlier, the correlation between obesity in early life and adulthood is, in most studies, weak. Thus, the validity of an adipose cell hypothesis which focuses only on early life experiences has been questioned.

Studies in experimental animals suggest that adipose cell size may influence food intake. Lipectomized Osborne-Mendel rats and rats which underwent sham operations were fed highly palatable high-fat diets; they were found to overeat and their body fat and adipose cell size increased.[47–49] Initially, caloric intake by the control and lipectomized animals was equal; since the lipectomized animals have fewer fat cells, however, their adipose tissue expanded by increasing the amount of lipid stored in existing fat cells (i.e., increasing adipose cell size) to a greater degree than the adipose tissue in animals who had undergone sham operations. Lipectomized animals, with larger fat cells, then began to overeat to a lesser degree than control animals. After 9 weeks of high-fat feeding, lipectomized animals had overeaten less and had gained less body fat than control animals, but by that time adipose cell size was similar in the two groups. At that time, hyperphagia also decreased in control rats. It appears, then, that in these animals eating was altered in response to adipose cellular enlargement.

Studies in obese humans add further support to the possibility that adipose cell size may influence food intake. Obese individuals losing weight through caloric restriction were observed to have increasing difficulty adhering to their diets the closer their adipose cells approached normal size.[27] Further weight reduction appeared to be restricted as adipose cell size fell to below normal. These and other studies in laboratory animals and humans have been interpreted to suggest an adipose cell size–food intake relationship.

As previously discussed, adipose cell size may also influence total adipose cell number. Studies in experimental animals suggest that attainment of a maximum fat cell size somehow results in a stimulus of adipose cellular proliferation and, hence, increased cell number. Thus, according to the adipose cell theory of obesity, adipose cell size could influence eating behavior and energy storage either directly or indirectly through its influence on total cell number, and hence coud contribute to the development and/or perpetuation of obesity. This is an attractive hypothesis but it remains highly theoretical; the mechanism(s) by which adipose cell number and/or size might act to produce or perpetuate obesity remains speculative at this time. One possibility is that increased cell number or some cell-size-associated phenomenon somehow stimulates the CNS centers regulating eating behavior. The lipostatic theory of regulation of food intake postulates that this central mechanism controls, and in turn is regulated by, the body's stores of energy as triglyceride in adipose tissue.[67] This feedback could be mediated through some chemical or neural mechanism associated with fat cell number and/or size. It must be emphasized, however, that no hormonal or neural relationship has yet been identified which relates adipose cell size or number to eating behavior or energy expenditure.

Psychological Factors

It is clear that human eating behavior can be affected by a wide variety of nonphysiological, nonnutritional factors. One of the longest-standing and most popular explanations for some types of human obesity is that psychological factors cause overeating and obesity. It is postulated that these factors influence eating behavior through their ability to modulate and override the internal physiological CNS mechanisms which normally regulate food intake. Such psychological factors may be of emotional, perceptual, or social origin.

Emotional disturbance is a frequent precipitant of overeating in humans and often accompanies human obesity.[118,119] Almost every imaginable negative feeling has been observed in obese individuals, including anxiety, guilt, frustration, boredom, depression, and feelings of rejection and vulnerability, to name but a few. Yet, no characteristic personality or psychiatric disturbance has been described in obesity; only rarely has a specific factor been documented to be etiologic. Nevertheless, it is apparent that emotional factors may contribute to the development and maintenance of at least some forms of human obesity. Under these conditions it is presumed that eating assumes a symbolic value rather than satisfying nutritional needs: e.g., food intake relieves anxiety or depression. It should, however, be noted that normal-weight individuals suffer the same psychopathologies and often use food for other than fulfillment of nutritional requirements; yet they do not become obese. This suggests that psychological influences may be contributing rather than primary factors in the development of most human obesity.

Perceptual factors have also been implicated in the development and cause of obesity. It has been suggested that obese subjects are more responsive and reactive to food-related stimuli or cues in their external environment (appearance, form, and smell of food, social setting, time of day, etc.) than nonobese individuals, and are less able to perceive or respond to the normal internal physiological mechanisms regulating feeding.[120,121] It is postulated that this hyperresponsiveness to nonphysiological, external cues ("externality") leads to obesity in these individuals. The concept that externally cued eating behavior is a primary determinant of obesity has, however, been challenged. Several studies cast doubt on the postulated differences in the ability of nonobese and obese individuals to detect and respond to internal and external cues. It has been demonstrated, for example, that some obese patients can show appropriate internal control while some nonobese individuals do not.[122]

It appears that, although psychological factors may contribute to the development and perpetuation of human obesity, and may occasionally cause obesity, most obese individuals are not obese as a result of psychological problems. The psychopathology associated with obesity appears more often to be the result rather than the cause of obesity. The emotional burden of being obese in a society that rewards leanness but stigmatizes and discriminates against fat people can be enormous. It is no wonder that obese persons frequently suffer a variety of psychological disturbances.

Bulimia or bulimia nervosa is a condition in which gorging of excessive amounts of food occurs on a recurrent basis.[123] Its underlying cause is not known, but it might be a phase of anorexia nervosa. Affected patients are usually not obese, but like those with anorexia nervosa have an exaggerated fear of becoming obese. After overeating, the patient induces vomiting and/or diarrhea. This can lead to severe dehydration, hypokalemia, hyponatremia, and hypochloremic alkalosis. Muscular weakness, seizures, and electrocardiographic abnormalities due to chronic potassium deficiency can be observed. Treatment includes hospitalization when recurrent emesis results in hypokalemic alkalosis, and long-term combined behavioral therapy and psychotherapy.

Other Nonphysiological Factors

Epidemiologic data indicate that the prevalence and cause of human obesity is strongly influenced by social, economic, racial, and life-style factors.[6,7] These data demonstrate that obesity is far from being uniformly distributed within a society; it is, for example, much more prevalent among middle-aged women of lower socioeconomic status and in certain racial and ethnic groups. It is possible that this uneven distribution of obesity is a reflection more of life-style, i.e., of different underlying attitudes toward eating, physical activity, and body weight and configuration, than of genetic, metabolic, or other physiological factors.

Certainly, the level of fatness and therefore the proportion of obese individuals in a population is determined by food availability up to a point. Economically advanced countries have an abundant and readily accessible food supply to which their populations are continuously exposed via the various mass media. The almost constant exposure to high-calorie foods, the easy accessibility of these foods, and the relatively sedentary life-style of members of these populations all seem to foster the development of obesity. Available evidence indicates that factors other than food availability, such as those of economic, social, and cultural origin, may also be important contributors to the development and course of the human obesities.

The level of adiposity appears to be influenced by socioeconomic factors.[22,23,124] Obesity is relatively uncommon in both impoverished and highly affluent adults of both sexes. As the socioeconomic status of the population rises through the lower and median United States levels, females appear to get leaner and males fatter. Thus, there tends to be an inverse relationship between socioeconomic status and obesity in both black and white middle-aged women; on the other hand, lower income levels are associated with less obesity in older women and in both black and white males.

A change in socioeconomic status tends to be reflected in body weight: upward socioeconomic mobility is associated with a decreasing prevalence and downward mobility with an increasing prevalence of obesity in both sexes. An explanation for these relationships, whether reflective of diet, physical activity, education, or other factors, is not available. Of interest, however, is the observation that prevalence of obesity among those of low socioeconomic class has been reported not to be excessive in individuals actively engaged in heavy manual labor.[125] Thus, physical activity appears to be able to override the socioeconomic factors contributing to obesity.

A correlation between body weight and level of education has been reported.[126] In general, the prevalence of obesity is lowest among the most-educated and highest among the least-educated individuals. To what extent this reflects recognition and understanding of the importance of nutrition and exercise, as opposed to other social and economic factors associated with educational status, is not known.

A relationship between race and obesity has also been reported.[23] For example, various surveys in the United States indicate that black women have the highest prevalence of obesity at all ages, while the prevalence of obesity in males does not differ between the races. It has been contended, however, that correction for socioeconomic status restores the level of fatness in the black population to that observed among whites.[126] Several American Indian populations have an extraordinarily high prevalence of obesity, e.g., the Pima of southwestern Arizona.[127] The explanation for this, whether genetic, socioeconomic, or life-style-related, remains to be identified.

Cultural factors can also be important determinants of eating and physical activity. Certain groups place heavy emphasis on a pattern of eating and physical activity which may predispose people toward obesity. Cultural attitudes about specific foods and physical size may also contribute to a higher incidence of obesity in certain populations.

It is apparent that obesity is related to several socioeconomic and cultural factors. These latter forces do not appear to act in a uniform manner throughout the population. Much of the epidemiologic data in this regard are frankly contradictory. One explanation may be that genetic and environmental factors interact; certain life-style factors may convert a genetic susceptibility to obesity into overt disease. On the other hand, certain types of obesity may be genetically transmitted while others are more the consequence of learning and life-style patterns. Whether, and the extent to which, life-style factors are primary determinants of human obesity cannot be ascertained now. The evidence available suggests that, while genetic factors may be preeminent determinants, life-style can be an important contributing factor. The identification of factors leading to obesity in a given patient provides an opportunity to develop a therapeutic approach tailored to a patient's background and needs.

CLASSIFICATION OF OBESITY

In the preceding discussion it was pointed out that in most obese patients the underlying cause cannot be determined. It is therefore not surprising that a satisfactory classification of human obesity has not been developed, although several classifications of obesity have been advanced. Classification of obesity into that of known etiology (perhaps less than 5 percent of patients) and idiopathic obesity contributes little to the understanding of this disorder and precludes the development of specific therapy aimed at its treatment, control, and prevention. The classification shown in Table 21-2 suffers from limitations similar to many others, but it attempts to present those elements recognized to be important either as primary or as contributors to the development and/or maintenance of the obese state; upon such a classification, it is hoped, a more rational approach to the obese patient can be developed.

HEALTH CONSEQUENCES OF OBESITY

That obesity is associated with widespread and serious health consequences is well recognized.[6,7,79,128] The nature of this relationship, however, has, in most cases, not been fully defined. In particular, it has been difficult to distinguish between obesity as a *cause* of a given condition and obesity as a phenomenon *associated* with the condition. Moreover, it has not been possible to determine whether the adverse health consequences associated with excess body weight reflect the role of obesity per se or other factors associated with increased body weight. Nevertheless, whatever the nature of these relationships, a large body of evidence clearly indicates that the risk of morbidity, and probably the risk of mortality, from a variety of illnesses is increased in the overweight/obese population.

Mortality

In the past it was generally accepted that overweight and obesity confer an increased risk of mortality.[5,129,130]

Table 21-2. Classifications of Human Obesity

Etiologic
Genetic
Inherited predisposition to obesity
Genetic syndromes associated with obesity:
Prader-Willi syndrome
Alström's syndrome
Laurence-Moon-Biedl syndrome
Stewart-Morel-Morgagni syndrome (hyperostosis frontalis internal)
Down's syndrome
Pseudo- and pseudo pseudohypoparathyroidism
Central nervous system–hypothalamic function
Tumors
Inflammation
Trauma and surgical injury
Increased intracranial pressure
? Functional changes causing hyperinsulinemia
Endocrine
Glucocorticoid excess (Cushing's syndrome)
Thyroid hormone deficiency (hypothyroidism)
Hypopituitarism
Gonadal deficiency (primary and secondary hypogonadism)
Hyperinsulinism (insulinoma, excess exogenous insulin)
Metabolic
Enzyme abnormality
? Increased energy efficiency
Nutritional
? Maternal nutritional factors
? Infant-feeding practices
Excess caloric intake during adult life
Drugs
Phenothiazines
Insulin
Corticosteroids
Cyproheptadine
Tricyclic antidepressants
Anatomic
Hypercellular, hypertrophic: early-onset, severe
Hypertrophic, normal-cellular: adult-onset, milder
Contributory factors
Familial influences
Physical inactivity
Dietary factors:
Eating patterns
Type of diet
Socioeconomic
Educational
Cultural-ethnic
Psychological

Excess mortality was believed to be associated with all degrees of obesity in all age groups, although mortality risk is greatest in the most severely obese and during early and middle age. This view has recently been challenged.[6,7,79,131] Using actuarial statistics from a variety of populations, some have concluded that there is no evidence that obesity is associated with excess mortality except in those who are greater than 30 percent overweight (according to the 1959 Metropolitan Life weight tables) or who have a BMI greater than 25. These investigators have concluded that persons who are somewhat overweight have a reduced risk of mortality compared to those who are at average or "desirable" weight or who are underweight. However, these investigators failed to adjust the life insurance statistics for the effects of cigarette smoking or the existence of other risk factors, diseases, or factors associated with insurability.[132] There is abundant evidence that persons who smoke tobacco or who suffer from other diseases are likely to be below average weight. Failure to adjust for the effects of smoking or coexistent disease exaggerates the risk of being underweight and underestimates the risk of being overweight.

The 1983 Metropolitan Life height and weight tables, in which recommended body weight for a given height and frame size has been significantly increased over that presented in the 1959 tables, also fail to adjust for smoking behavior and other confounding factors. Thus, use of these tables to assess risk of mortality associated with obesity is also flawed.

In 1982, a workshop on body weight, health, and longevity was held at NIH; it was attended by expert physicians, researchers, anthropologists, statisticians, and public health workers.[5] One of the conclusions of this group was

> In the United States, studies based on life insurance data (e.g., the Build and Blood Pressure Study, 1959; Build Study, 1979; Provident Mutual Life Study; the American Cancer Society; and other long-term studies such as the Framingham Heart Study and Manitoba Study) indicate that below-average weights tend to be associated with the greatest longevity, if such weights are not associated with concurrent illness or a history of significant medical impairment. Overweight persons tend to die sooner than average-weight persons, particularly those who are overweight at younger ages. The effect of obesity on mortality is delayed, so that it is not seen in short-term studies. . . . Furthermore, the concept of "desirable weight" developed by the Metropolitan Life Insurance Company in 1959 has been validated by a recent long-term study.

Overweight individuals with hypertension, cardiovascular disease, or a family history of cardiovascular disease are at an increased mortality risk compared to those of normal weight with similar conditions. Death rates from a variety of diseases are significantly greater in the overweight population than expected on the basis of normal mortality rate;[6,7,128] e.g., coronary artery disease carries an excess mortality of 40 percent, in renal disease excess death is more than 50 percent, and in diabetes mortality rate is more than four times the expected.[132] Other causes of death are found more frequently among overweight individuals, including cerebral vascular accidents, biliary tract disorders, and cirrhosis of the liver.

It seems apparent, then, that obesity has adverse effects on longevity. A consensus conference sponsored by NIH in 1985 using data derived from NHANES II concluded that the adverse effects of obesity on longevity occurred in Americans with a body weight 20 percent above "desirable" or a BMI of 26 or 27, and that even lesser degrees of obesity are likely to increase mortality risk.[6,7] At the same time, however, existing evidence suggests that the relationship between body weight and mortality is neither clear-cut nor simple.

Diabetes Mellitus

The association between obesity, abnormal carbohydrate metabolism, and maturity-onset diabetes is well recognized. Most patients with non-insulin-dependent (type II) diabetes mellitus (NIDDM), approximately 80 percent in most populations studied, are obese. Many obese patients have frank NIDDM as defined by the criteria of the National Diabetes Data Group (NDDG): (1) not ketosis-prone under basal conditions; (2) not requiring exogenous insulin for short-term survival; and (3) having a fasting plasma glucose concentration (FPG) $\geq$ 140 mg/dl or a sustained elevation of plasma glucose concentration of $\geq$ 200 mg/dl 2 h after an oral glucose load of 75 g, with one other value between zero time and 2 h $\geq$ 200 mg/dl. Many other obese patients have impaired glucose tolerance (IGT) as defined by the NDDG as: (1) FPG $<$ 140 mg/dl; (2) one plasma glucose concentration value $\geq$ 200 mg/dl between zero time and 2 h after receiving 75 g of oral glucose; and (3) glucose concentration 2 h after receiving oral glucose of 140 to 199 mg/dl. Still other obese individuals have lesser degrees of glucose intolerance classified as "nondiagnostic" by the NDDG; i.e., levels of plasma glucose between normal and IGT. While NIDDM and these other types of glucose intolerance are relatively uncommon in nonobese populations, they are very frequently observed in obese populations and their prevalence increases strikingly in populations undergoing changes in life-style that lead to obesity.

Weight gain may precede and precipitate the development of maturity-onset diabetes, or may coincide with its development. The onset of diabetes in the Pima, a group in which the prevalence of diabetes may reach as high as 50 to 60 percent, is characteristically preceded by a 10- to 15-lb weight gain over several months.[127] Weight gain can aggravate preexisting diabetes, resulting in the need to initiate treatment with insulin or oral sulfonylurea drugs or to increase the dosage of such agents to control hyperglycemia and ketonemia.

Weight loss results in an improvement in the metabolic aspects of the diabetic state in the great majority of, if not all, obese individuals with diabetes. In many patients, glucose, lipid, and protein metabolism and insulin secretion and action are restored to normal and all evidence of diabetes disappears after weight reduction. In others, the state of these metabolic parameters improves, but remains somewhat abnormal even after weight loss; these metabolic effects are, however, well controlled by diet. In still others, weight loss improves the diabetic state, but the remaining degree of metabolic derangement requires that insulin continue to be administered, albeit in reduced amounts.

Although obesity is an important, perhaps the most important, risk factor for diabetes mellitus, the relationship between obesity and diabetes is neither simple nor straightforward. For example, while many NIDDM patients are obese, not all are; approximately 20 percent of Americans with NIDDM are lean.[134] Moreover, while many obese patients have NIDDM, in most populations studied only a portion of them (40 to 60 percent) do.[134] Even in the Pima population the high incidence of NIDDM cannot be entirely attributed to obesity. The prevalence of NIDDM is reported to be low in some populations in which obesity is common, e.g., the Inuit.[134] The studies of Asian and Oceanic populations have demonstrated that obesity has little relationship to the prevalence of NIDDM in some populations, while in others it is important.[135] Such observations suggest that, while obesity is a very important risk factor, it may not, by and of itself, be enough to produce NIDDM. A genetic susceptibility to diabetes may be necessary for obesity to induce clinical disease. It is clear from the studies of Asian and Oceanic populations that, even in the genetically susceptible individual, obesity may not induce NIDDM; there are other environmental risk factors for NIDDM. Among the risk factors which have received the most attention are total caloric intake, dietary composition, physical activity, stress, drug use, and the intrauterine environment. There is some evidence that each of these factors can be important and that, while a diabetes gene (or genes) is necessary in most individuals, it is not sufficient.

Even when an association between obesity and NIDDM is demonstrated, the nature of the relationship is not obvious. It is not clear at what level of obesity the genetically susceptible individual is at increased risk. Whether the risk for NIDDM increases with increasing duration of obesity is not known. When obesity can be linked to NIDDM, it is uncertain what it is about obesity that is diabetogenic. The presence of an excess adipose tissue mass has generally been accepted to be the primary diabetogenic factor. However, caloric restriction improves hyperglycemia in obese NIDDM patients before a significant amount of body fat is lost, suggesting that excessive caloric intake rather than the increased adiposity per se may be most important.[136] On the other hand, refeeding of these obese patients whose caloric intake is restricted and weight is modestly reduced restores the prior hyperglycemia. Physical training has also been shown to improve hyperglycemia in the obese diabetic in the absence of significant loss of adipose tissue, suggesting that decreased physical activity, a characteristic of obese individuals, may be more important than increased adiposity per se.[137] Moreover, some studies suggest that maximum oxygen uptake, an estimate of physical fitness, correlates with glucose tolerance to a greater degree than adiposity per se in obese individuals.[138] Much attention has been focused on the role of diet composition in the diabetogenicity of obesity, especially on the carbohydrate, fat, and fiber content of the diet. In the view of this author there is no convincing evidence that changes in dietary composition or of specific dietary constituents are responsible for the diabetogenic effect of obesity. Several recent reports indicate that the distribution of the excess adipose tissue in obesity may be an important factor in determining risk for NIDDM.[13,14,128,139,140] Thus, an abdominal or "spare tire" fat distribution in men and women is associated with a greater risk for NIDDM than when the excess fat is located in other regions of the body. Interestingly, a similar relationship exists in nonobese individuals with an abdominal distribution of adipose tissue. This association also appears to be true for hypertriglyceridemia and hypertension.

While obesity and NIDDM are closely related, it is by no means certain that all obese patients with the various abnormalities of glucose tolerance described above have or will ever have NIDDM. Moreover, in many obese individuals the glucose, insulin, and lipid abnormalities disappear completely after weight reduction and all currently recognized evidence of diabetes is lost. Furthermore, most obese patients do not develop the specific microangiopathies characteristic of diabetes, even when followed for prolonged periods. In such patients the diagnosis of NIDDM rests solely on the presence of arbitrarily established criteria of glucose intolerance. Since it is well recognized that glucose intolerance and diabetes mellitus are not always synonymous, and given the well-known observation that glucose intolerance occurs in conditions other than diabetes, it may be more appropriate to consider that some, perhaps many, of these obese individuals with obesity-induced abnormalities of glucose metabolism suffer a condition which is distinct from true NIDDM. Unfortunately, at present a definitive answer to this question is not possible because a specific marker for NIDDM is lacking. Moreover, many obese patients develop neither NIDDM, IGT, nondiagnostic glucose intolerance, nor any other identifiable abnormality of glucose metabolism, insulin action, or insulin secretion. Thus, obesity does not guarantee the development of deranged glucose metabolism, and even when the latter does occur it might not represent true NIDDM.

Such observations suggest that, while obesity may be a very important risk factor for NIDDM, it is not, by and of itself, sufficient to produce this disease. A genetic susceptibility for NIDDM may be necessary for obesity to induce clinical disease. The studies on Asian and Oceanic populations also indicate that, even in genetically susceptible individuals, obesity may not induce NIDDM; other risk factors appear to be operating.[135] Thus, obesity is not necessary for the development of NIDDM and it does not guarantee that NIDDM will occur.

Nevertheless, there is a relationship between obesity and NIDDM. Most clinicians and investigators believe that obesity can somehow induce NIDDM, i.e., that obesity is diabetogenic. Indeed, most diabetologists consider obesity to be the greatest risk factor for the development of NIDDM. As such, obesity can be viewed to be acting as an environmental factor which converts genetic susceptibility to NIDDM into overt clinical disease. The mechanisms responsible for the diabetogenic effect of obesity have been the subject of intensive investigation. Several mechanisms may be involved.

PLASMA INSULIN LEVELS IN OBESITY

One of the most characteristic metabolic features of obesity is the existence of hyperglycemia in the face of hyperinsulinemia, most often observed after an oral glucose challenge or a meal, but in some instances in the fasting state.[141-145] This has been interpreted as reflecting the fact that insulin's ability to influence glucose metabolism is impaired in obesity, a condition which has been referred to as *insulin resistance.*

However, not all obese persons with abnormal glucose tolerance are hyperinsulinemic; some have normal plasma insulin levels and those with severe fasting hyperglycemia may be hypoinsulinemic.[141,145] The explanation for this variation in plasma insulin levels among obese individuals is not known, although some have postulated the existence of two defects in obese diabetic individuals: one in insulin action and the other in insulin secretion. Studies of large numbers of nonobese patients ranging widely in fasting plasma glucose concentration from mild to severe hyperglycemia reveal a pattern in which the mean plasma insulin response during an oral glucose tolerance test is excessive (hyperinsulinemia) at FPG levels up to approximately 160 mg/dl, after which the insulin response is diminished and hypoinsulinemia exists.[145] This has been interpreted to reflect the existence of defects in both insulin action and insulin secretion in NIDDM, but whether a similar situation exists in obese nondiabetic persons is not known. In any case, it is clear that insulin resistance is a major factor responsible for the diabetogenic effect of obesity, and it is this aspect of the relationship that is the subject of the present discussion.

INSULIN RESISTANCE

There is abundant in vivo and in vitro evidence that insulin's ability to regulate glucose metabolism in its target tissues, i.e., skeletal muscle, liver, and adipose tissue, is impaired in obese humans and laboratory animals.[138,141–148]

The insulin resistance of obesity could be the result of one or more of the following tissue abnormalities: (1) impaired glucose uptake by peripheral tissues (skeletal muscle and adipose tissue), (2) impaired glucose uptake by the liver, or (3) increased hepatic glucose production. While many studies have been undertaken to evaluate these possibilities, in the opinion of this author the available data do not permit definitive conclusions on which of these defects is involved or on their relative importance to the insulin resistance associated with obesity. This is a consequence of, among other things, methodological limitations of the clamp technique; differing definitions of obesity, diabetes, and insulin resistance among studies; and patient selection, especially failure to satisfactorily control for the presence of confounding factors such as NIDDM, making it difficult to tell whether one is studying the effects of obesity or those of NIDDM.

There is general agreement that obesity is accompanied by an impaired ability of insulin to stimulate glucose uptake and metabolism and to decrease lipolysis in peripheral tissues (peripheral insulin resistance). This resistance to insulin action also occurs in the peripheral tissues of patients with NIDDM independent of obesity, i.e., in lean individuals with NIDDM;[145] thus, peripheral tissue insulin resistance is characteristic of NIDDM per se and obesity is not required to produce it.

In vitro studies of isolated adipose cells also show an impairment of insulin's ability to stimulate glucose transport and metabolism in fat cells from obese persons and those with NIDDM compared to lean diabetics.[138,143,145–149] Adipocytes from obese diabetics show a greater impairment than those from nondiabetic individuals of equal obesity.[138] Nonobese NIDDM patients have insulin-resistant fat cells; thus obesity is not essential for insulin resistance in adipose fat cells, but it makes it worse.[138,145] As discussed below, evidence is emerging that the defect responsible for the insulin resistance in this cell type may be different in obesity and NIDDM.

The picture is less clear in the liver than in the peripheral tissues. There appears to be little or no evidence for a decreased ability of insulin to stimulate hepatic glucose uptake in either obesity or NIDDM when this function is studied under the conditions of the standard euglycemic clamp technique.[141,145]

Some investigators have found the basal rate of hepatic glucose output to be increased in obesity, but others, using the same technique of euglycemic clamp and the same insulin steady-state conditions, observed no difference in basal hepatic glucose output between nonobese and obese subjects. Part of the explanation for this discrepancy could be that in the former study the obese patients had glucose intolerance or NIDDM while in the latter study the obese patients had normal glucose tolerance. There is general agreement that in NIDDM, basal hepatic glucose output is increased with or without accompanying obesity, i.e., overproduction of glucose by the liver in the basal state is characteristic of NIDDM per se.

The picture is even less clear regarding insulin's effect on hepatic glucose output in obesity and NIDDM. Some investigators reported a diminished ability of insulin to inhibit hepatic glucose output in obese patients with NIDDM or lesser degrees of glucose intolerance using euglycemic clamping and steady-state insulin conditions, while others found no resistance to this action of insulin on the livers of obese patients without NIDDM or NIDDM patients with or without obesity under these same experimental conditions.[138,141,145] Recently, the euglycemic clamp technique has been modified to permit kinetic as well as steady-state studies of the effects of insulin on glucose disposal and hepatic glucose output.[144] These investigators believe that non-steady-state studies of insulin action may be more physiological than studies of insulin action during steady state as performed with the standard euglycemic clamp, since insulin is normally secreted in a phasic manner and steady-state biologic effects of this hormone are probably not achieved under physiological circumstances. Using this approach they observed decreased steady-state effects of insulin on glucose disposal in peripheral tissues and glucose output from the liver and, in addition, kinetic alterations in the rates of insulin action on the peripheral tissue glucose clearance and glucose production from the liver in obese nondiabetic subjects compared to normal individuals. The rate of activation of insulin-stimulated glucose disposal in these obese patients was lower and the rate of deactivation was higher than in the normal controls at comparable insulin infusion rates, supporting the existence of peripheral tissue insulin resistance observed at steady state. The kinetic studies of insulin action on the liver were less clear-cut. The rate of suppression of hepatic glucose output was equal in normal and obese subjects, but the rate of recovery of glucose production by the liver was faster in the obese subjects, indicating that a hepatic defect may exist but is not as well established as that in the periphery. Furthermore, the resistance of the liver to insulin suppression of glucose output was quantitatively mild compared to the insulin resistance in the peripheral tissues.

Taken together, the available evidence seems to indicate that obesity unaccompanied by NIDDM is associated with resistance to the action of insulin to dispose of glucose in the peripheral tissues and may be associated with an increased production of glucose from the liver in the absence and presence of insulin. When both of these defects are observed in obese nondiabetics the insulin resistance in the peripheral tissues is more severe than in the liver and appears to be relatively more important in the diabetogenic effects of obesity. Resistance to the action of insulin on glucose disposal is also present in NIDDM independent of obesity, and basal hepatic glucose production is increased; whether or not an impairment exists in insulin suppression of hepatic glucose output (hepatic insulin resistance) in NIDDM is uncertain.

While increased glucose output from the liver may be the source of fasting hyperglycemia in NIDDM or obesity, it might not account for postprandial hyperglycemia. Furthermore, even if the liver is delivering excess glucose into the circulation in the basal and insulin-stimulated state, it is not necessarily the site of the primary defect in the key insulin-resistant tissue in either obesity or NIDDM. The reduced ability of insulin to stimulate glucose disposal in the peripheral tissues, i.e., skeletal muscle and adipose tissue, may be primary. According to this concept, the increased hepatic glucose output reflects increased delivery of gluconeogenic substrates, i.e., pyruvate, lactate, glycerol, free fatty acids, amino acids, to the liver from the insulin-resistant peripheral tissues and, hence, increased gluconeogenesis.

At this time the bulk of the evidence documents the existence of insulin resistance in obesity and the presence of insulin resistance at least in the peripheral tissues of the body. Most investigators believe that the diabetogenicity of obesity is due to this insulin resistance. One hypothesis is that NIDDM itself is associated with an inherited predisposition to insulin resistance (and probably to abnormal pancreatic beta cell insulin secretion). Obesity-induced insulin resistance superimposed on NIDDM susceptibility produces overt hyperglycemia in NIDDM, an example of the interaction of genetic and environmental factors.

MECHANISMS RESPONSIBLE FOR INSULIN RESISTANCE

A definitive understanding of the mechanism(s) responsible for the insulin resistance of obesity is not yet available. A variety of defects could and probably do exist, e.g., mutations in the insulin gene, producing insulin with reduced biologic activity; circulating antibodies or antagonists to insulin; antibodies to the insulin receptor; and defects in the mechanism of insulin action on its target cells.[145,147,148] The bulk of the evidence indicates that the first three defects are rare and that in most instances the problem is at or within insulin's target cells. Thus, research has focused on how insulin normally acts to regulate glucose metabolism in these cells and what is changed in obesity.

A thorough review of the mechanism of insulin action and of the abnormalities observed in obesity is beyond the scope of this discussion; for this the reader is referred to Chap. 19 of this book. Suffice it to say that much has been learned about the normal mechanism of insulin action and that several defects in insulin action have been described in the tissues of obese humans and laboratory animals, which may eventually help to explain the mechanism of insulin resistance in obesity.[147]

Defects in insulin action have been classified into two broad categories: receptor and postreceptor defects. Some studies indicate that in certain types of obesity the number of cell membrane–localized specific insulin receptors is decreased in adipose, muscle, and liver cells (or their isolated plasma membranes) and in circulating monocytes; an abnormality which is reversed through caloric restriction and weight reduction. This defect could certainly lead to insulin resistance. Most studies report that an impairment of the effect of insulin on glucose metabolism in cells from obese patients and animals is not due to a decrease in insulin binding or number of insulin receptors, but rather, blunted insulin action is associated with alterations in postbinding events. These alterations could be due to defects in the insulin receptor unrelated to insulin binding or to postreceptor abnormalities. A postbinding receptor abnormality has been demonstrated in peripheral tissues from the obese diabetic mouse (*obob*), specifically a decreased ability of insulin to activate tyrosine kinase activity and autophosphorylation.[150] While it has been proposed that these biochemical activities are essential for normal insulin action, this remains to be proven. Furthermore, defective insulin receptor tyrosine kinase activity or autophosphorylation has not been demonstrated in the cells from obese humans. Other as yet unidentified postbinding receptor events might be defective in obesity and/or NIDDM, and thus produce insulin resistance.

Studies in insulin-resistant obese rodents and humans demonstrate the existence of defects in insulin action at postreceptor sites in the absence of defects in the insulin receptor. For example a decreased ability of insulin to stimulate glucose uptake into cells, independent of insulin binding, has been observed in some obese rats and humans; this defect is reversed by weight reduction.[143] Studies in rats have identified a specific defect in glucose transport by adipose and skeletal muscle cells, an impairment in insulin's ability to translocate glucose transport molecules which reside inside the cell to the plasma membrane, where they can bind and transport glucose into the cell.[151] Other alterations in the intracellular metabolism of glucose have been identified. Different defects in insulin action may exist among different obese patients; a given patient may also possess more than one defect in insulin action. The meaning of this variability is unknown; it could reflect the expression of different types of obesity. However, there is no evidence that the various deficiencies of insulin action reflect different genetic defects; rather, the evidence suggests that these alterations in insulin action are the result of the influence of various environmental actions on the cell, such as increased total caloric intake, dietary composition, and physical inactivity.

It should be noted that chronic hyperglycemia per se may adversely influence glucoregulatory processes and thereby induce insulin resistance through mechanisms which are independent of defects in the specific actions of insulin.[152] Reduction of hyperglycemia in obese nondiabetics and obese diabetics through caloric restriction or insulin administration results in a reduction in insulin resistance, but so far it has not been possible to determine whether this beneficial effect is the result of the decreased hyperglycemia or the changes in plasma insulin level associated with these treatments.[136,145] Increased lipolysis and consequent increased availability and utilization of free fatty acids might also induce insulin resistance in obesity, especially in the key peripheral tissue utilizer of glucose, skeletal muscle.[145] Any or all of these defects might cause insulin resistance in obesity. A given obese individual may have more than one defect leading to insulin resistance and different defects may lead to insulin resistance in different obese patients.

Recently, some evidence has suggested that the defects responsible for insulin resistance in the peripheral tissues in obesity may be different than those operating in NIDDM.[146] In vitro studies of adipose cells isolated from nondiabetic obese individuals demonstrate a decreased sensitivity of glucose transport *and* antilipolysis to insulin in the face of normal insulin binding. These defects in the sensitivity of glucose transport and antilipolysis presumably reflect changes early in the action of insulin, possibly at the level of insulin receptor autophosphorylation. On the other hand, adipocytes isolated from obese NIDDM patients display decreased sensitivity of glucose transport but not antilipolysis to insulin in the face of normal insulin binding. These differences between the defects in insulin action on glucose transport and antilipolysis observed between fat cells from obese nondiabetic individuals and NIDDM patients suggest that the underlying cellular mechanisms responsible for insulin resistance in obesity and NIDDM may be different. Further support for this concept comes from the observation that while the capacity of maximally insulin-stimulated glucose disposal and transport is only slightly reduced in NIDDM, it is even much less impaired in the nondiabetic obese state, suggesting the presence of different postreceptor defects as well.

OVEREATING

While many have postulated that the hyperglycemia and hyperinsulinemia of obesity is the result of insulin resistance, as described in the preceding paragraphs, it has also been suggested that the hyperglycemia and hyperinsulinemia of obesity might be the direct result of overeating, with the insulin resistance only an adaptive response.[153] It has been postulated that ingestion of excess calories, particularly in the form of carbohydrate, leads to increased pancreatic insulin secretion and secondarily to insulin resistance; the insulin resistance is a protective adaptation of the insulin-sensitive tissues, particularly the liver, to prolonged exposure to high levels of insulin. Indeed, some investigators have reported that chronic hyperinsulinemia exerts negative feedback on the cell membrane–localized specific receptors, reducing the ability of insulin to bind to these cells (so-called down regulation of insulin receptors).[148]

FAT DISTRIBUTION

An additional factor which has been proposed to play a role in the relationship between NIDDM and obesity is the distribution of the excess adipose tissue between the upper and lower body.[13,14,128,139,140] Thus, an abdominal or "spare tire" distribution of excess adipose tissue is associated with a greater risk for NIDDM than when the excess fat is located in other regions of the body (buttocks, thigh). This association also appears to be true for hypertriglyceridemia and hypertension. The relationship is equally applicable to nonobese individuals with an abdominal distribution of adipose tissue. The mechanism responsible for the increased risk for NIDDM is not known. Some have suggested that it might be related to the fact that adipocytes located in the abdomen are more sensitive to lipolytic stimuli than adipose cells elsewhere in the body. It has been proposed that the delivery of lipolytic products, e.g., glycerol and fatty acids, directly to the liver enhances gluconeogenesis; thus, the risk of hyperglycemia increases. A similar phenomenon could explain the association between abdominal obesity and hypertriglyceridemia. Interpretation of these relationships must, however, be made with great care, especially with respect to conclusions about the causal role of body fat distribution in these risk factors. If body fat distribution is genetically determined, as has been suggested, the etiologic factors may be genetic and not related to the location of the adipose tissue in the body.

INSULIN SECRETION

Not all obese diabetic patients are hyperinsulinemic; decreased plasma insulin response to oral glucose has been reported. Thus, an additional mechanism through which obesity exerts its diabetogenic effects may involve defective insulin secretion. Two recent observations are of interest in this regard. In obese diabetic patients with a decreased insulin response to an acute oral glucose challenge, insulin levels in response to actual meals have been observed to be normal or above normal.[154] This suggests that, while such patients may have abnormal insulin-secretory responses to glucose when it is administered orally, ambient concentrations of circulating insulin are actually not decreased; their cells are not insulin deficient. Secondly, the decreased plasma insulin response to oral glucose in such obese diabetic patients can often be improved by caloric restriction and weight loss.[136,145,155]

Whatever the mechanism, it is clear that obesity imposes a burden on glucose metabolism and insulin secretion; i.e., obesity is a diabetogenic factor. The ultimate effect of this burden depends on the degree of insulin resistance and the ability of the pancreatic beta cells to respond to the continuing demand for insulin.

Hyperlipoproteinemia

Obesity can be associated with hypertriglyceridemia and, to a lesser extent, hypercholesterolemia, two abnormalities considered to be important risk factors for atherosclerosis and coronary heart disease.[156,157] The nature of these relationships and the factors responsible have yet to be fully identified.

Elevation of plasma triglyceride levels is commonly observed in obese individuals; weight loss tends to restore them to normal. This relationship between obesity and hypertriglyceridemia appears to be the result of an increased influx of nutrient substrates (glucose, glycerol, fatty acids) into the liver in obese patients; the consequent production of triglyceride-containing very low density lipoproteins (VLDLs) occurs faster than peripheral tissues can hydrolyze and utilize such triglycerides.[158] The appearance of hypertriglyceridemia, then, is a function of both hepatic production rates and the rate of peripheral VLDL clearance. That an increased flux of substrate into the liver and hepatic overproduction of VLDLs appear to occur in most obese patients, but that not all of these patients exhibit hypertriglyceridemia, might be explained on the basis of the individual's capacity to clear VLDLs; persons without hypertriglyceridemia are able to increase the rate of clearance sufficiently, while those who cannot develop hypertriglyceridemia. A role for insulin in the hypertriglyceridemia of obesity is suggested by studies demonstrating that the hyperinsulinemia which accompanies obesity accelerates hepatic triglyceride synthesis and consequently elevates the level of plasma triglycerides as VLDL.[159] The increased flux of substrate for hepatic VLDL production is said to be the result of insulin resistance in the peripheral tissues. The risk for hypertriglyceridemia in obese patients is, however, greater among those whose excess adiposity is primarily located in the abdomen compared to those whose obesity is primarily in the upper segment of the body. Because adipose cells in the abdomen and surrounding abdominal tissues appear to be more sensitive to lipolytic stimuli, an alternative explanation for the increased flux of substrate through the liver and increased synthesis of VLDL has been proposed: increased delivery of glycerol and fatty acids from abdominal adipocytes into the adjacent liver may contribute to the greater frequency of hypertriglyceridemia observed in individuals with upper segment obesity.[13,14,139]

A relationship between body weight and plasma cholesterol level has been established.[156] Generally, plasma cholesterol concentrations appear to increase with increasing body weight. Total body cholesterol synthesis increases with increasing body weight and weight loss is often accompanied by a reduction in plasma cholesterol level, but not always into the normal range. The biochemical mechanisms responsible for the increased cholesterol synthesis remain to be elucidated. Increased hepatic cholesterol production has been advanced as the explanation for the increased risk of development of cholesterol gallstones in the obese.[160] Whether the explanation for the absence or presence of hypercholesterolemia lies in a given individual's ability to clear cholesterol-containing lipoproteins, as might be the case with triglycerides and VLDLs, is not known, nor has the relationship between body fat distribution and risk of hypercholesterolemia been elucidated. The relationship of obesity to high-density lipoproteins (HDLs), HDL-cholesterol levels, and the HDL-cholesterol/LDL-cholesterol ratio, factors which are believed to protect against atherosclerosis, is not yet clear.

Cardiovascular Consequences

Epidemiologic studies indicate that the risk of mortality and morbidity from cardiovascular disease increases with increased body weight. The Framingham heart study provided evidence that obesity, as assessed by Metropolitan Life relative weight, is directly related to differences in 26-year incidence of coronary heart disease, congestive heart failure, and coronary death in men, and of coronary disease, stroke, congestive heart failure, and coronary death in women.[161] The Framingham data further indicate that the risk of these cardiovascular events in the obese is independent of age, cholesterol level, systolic blood pressure, cigarette smoking, left ventricular hypertrophy, and glucose intolerance. Since obesity is associated with, and probably directly contributes to, the development of other cardiovascular risk factors such as diabetes mellitus, hypertriglyceridemia, hypercholesterolemia, and hypertension, these factors undoubtedly also contribute to the increased cardiovascular mortality and morbidity associated with obesity. But the Framingham study demonstrates that obesity per se is an independent risk factor and long-term predictor of cardiovascular disease in humans. Although correction of existing obesity per se has not been established to confer direct protection from atherosclerotic cardiovascular disease, it is well documented that weight loss ameliorates such risk factors as hyperglycemia, hypertriglyceridemia, and hypercholesterolemia.

Obesity places an increased demand on the heart; hence, it increases cardiovascular work.[162] Left ventricular hypertrophy and elevated left ventricular end-diastolic pressure have been observed both at rest and with exercise in massively obese patients. Indeed, congestive heart failure is said to be a common cause of death in the markedly obese. There is only limited information on the effects of more mild degrees of obesity on cardiovascular function. Most of these alterations are reversed by weight loss, although it has been reported that elevated left end-diastolic pressure may persist, suggesting that severe obesity may induce permanent cardiac dysfunction.

Hypertension

A clear association between obesity and hypertension has been demonstrated; the relationship is most dramatic among women.[128,163,164] The relationship between hypertension and obesity appears to be linear and is similar across all adult age groups. Weight reduction is often accompanied by blood pressure reduction. The factors responsible for the increased risk of hypertension in obesity are not known. It appears that obesity's influence on blood pressure can be mediated independently from the effects of sodium. Since hypertension is a serious disease in itself, and an important risk factor for atherogenesis, prevention and reversal of obesity constitute important treatments for hypertension and cardiovascular disease. The risk of coronary heart disease is greater in patients having both hypertension and obesity than in those having hypertension alone, lending further support to this concept.

Endocrine Consequences

A number of alterations in endocrine function have been observed in obese individuals, including changes in sex steroid metabolism and menstrual abnormalities, changes in thyroid hormone metabolism and adrenal function, disturbances of growth hormone secretion, and changes in insulin action and secretion.[79,128] Most often these appear to be secondary to the obesity rather than a primary characteristic of it. The alterations in insulin action and secretion have already been discussed.

SEX STEROID ABNORMALITIES

The onset of menarche tends to be earlier in obese compared to nonobese girls, and obese women often suffer from a variety of menstrual cycle abnormalities including hypermenorrhea, oligomenorrhea, amenorrhea, irregular or anovulatory cycles, infertility, and premature menopause. Obesity also appears to be associated with polycystic ovarian disease, hyperandrogenism, and hirsutism. While the explanation for these abnormalities in obese women is not known, several possibilities exist. One possible explanation lies in alterations in hypothalamic-pituitary function, specifically in the secretion of follicle stimulating hormone (FSH), luteinizing hormone (LH), and their releasing factors. Reduction of plasma levels of FSH, elevation of plasma LH levels, and increased plasma LH/FSH ratios have been reported in some obese women. Obesity could also produce menstrual abnormalities by inducing changes in the synthesis and/or secretion of estrogen and/or androgens from the ovaries and the adrenals. Elevation of circulating levels of estrogens and androgens has been observed in some but not all obese women studied. These elevations may be of either ovarian or adrenal origin. Prolonged elevation of plasma estrogen levels could suppress FSH levels sufficiently to prevent follicle maturation and subsequent LH-mediated ovulation. Chronic elevation of circulating androgen levels might contribute to the hyperandrogenism and hirsutism often associated with obesity, as well as to the menstrual cycle abnormalities. Alterations in sex steroid metabolism may also play a role in some of these obesity-associated abnormalities as well as the increased prevalence of breast cancer observed in obese women.[6,7,165] Increased conversion of androstenedione of adrenal origin to estrone and its metabolites by non-steroid-producing peripheral tissues might be one mechanism by which obesity alters sex steroid metabolism. In contrast, increased conversion of estrogen to androgen by peripheral tissues, particularly the excess adipose tissue, has been postulated to be a factor contributing to these problems.[166] Most of these changes are reversed by weight loss.

THYROID FUNCTION

In most obese patients thyroid function is normal, but subtle changes in thyroid hormone metabolism may occur.[82–84,167] As previously discussed, plasma T_3 levels are increased and rT_3 levels are decreased in many obese patients compared to nonobese individuals, while T_4 and TSH levels are normal; obese patients are almost always euthyroid by ordinary clinical indices. The T_3 and rT_3 changes are reversed by weight loss, indicating that these changes are secondary to obesity. Occasionally, however, hypothyroidism is a cause of obesity and, thus, this diagnosis should always be considered and ruled out; the obesity is usually mild, and restoration to euthyroidism eliminates the problem. Of course, hypothyroidism and obesity of another etiology can coexist, in which case the obesity will persist even after correction of the hypothyroidism.

ADRENAL FUNCTION

Cortisol secretion rates are increased in obesity, but, in contrast to Cushing's syndrome, plasma cortisol concentration is normal and diurnal variation in secretion and response to dexamethasone suppression are normal.[77,78] Total urinary 24-h 17-hydroxycorticosteroid level is generally increased in obese patients, but is normal when expressed per kilogram of body weight. Total 24-h 17-ketosteroid level is also increased in obese patients, although to a lesser degree than are the 17-hydroxycorticosteroids. Weight reduction restores cortisol secretion rate and levels of urinary 17-hydroxycorticosteroids and 17-ketosteroids to normal, indicating that these changes are secondary to obesity. It should be recognized, however, that hypercortisolism can cause obesity; thus, it should always be considered and ruled out in a given obese person. As with hypothyroidism, when Cushing's syndrome is the cause of obesity, the obesity tends to be mild and reversible after definitive treatment. Cushing's syndrome and obesity of another etiology can coexist, in which case the obesity will persist even after correction of the hypercortisolism.

GH responses to glucose and arginine are decreased in obese compared to nonobese patients, but weight reduction usually restores GH secretion and plasma GH level to normal, suggesting again that this alteration is secondary to obesity.[83]

The strongest evidence that these endocrine abnormalities are the consequence of overeating and/or obesity comes from observations made on normal volunteers, in whom obesity was experimentally induced by prolonged overeating.[78] The data from those studies indicate that when lean individuals overeat and become obese, they develop endocrine and metabolic changes which, with few exceptions, are in the same direction as those observed in spontaneous obesity.

Pulmonary Consequences

An association between obesity and pulmonary dysfunction has also been observed.[168] Dyspnea is the most common clinical complaint. The most characteristic functional change is alveolar hypoventilation, as evidenced by decreased Pa_{O_2} and elevated Pa_{CO_2}. The most striking clinical example of this is seen in the Pickwickian syndrome, in which a severe degree of alveolar hypoventilation with marked hypercapnia and respiratory acidosis is accompanied by somnolence, lethargy, and cyanosis. The Pickwickian syndrome is, however, relatively rare; hypoventilation associated with obesity is usually less severe than this.

Other abnormalities of respiratory function have been observed in severely obese patients, including reductions in expiratory reserve volume and vital capacity. The mechanisms responsible for these abnormalities are not known. The presence of massive obesity of the abdomen and thorax with resultant diminished chest wall compliance and uneven air flow may be partially responsible for some of these changes. In the Pickwickian syndrome, diminished CNS sensitivity to CO_2 has also been reported to be present. While such alterations in pulmonary function have been observed in many obese individuals, many obese patients appear to have perfectly normal respiratory function.

Miscellaneous Consequences

Obesity has been found to be associated with an increased risk for some malignancies, particularly of the breast, uterus, and ovaries for females and the colon, rectum, and prostate for males.[6,7,165,169] An explanation for these associations is not available, although it has been postulated that the sex hormone changes induced by obesity discussed above and/or the increased intake of fat in the diet of obese persons may be involved.

The prevalence of cholecystitis and cholelithiasis appears to increase as adiposity increases.[170] The prevalence of cholesterol gallstones is threefold greater in the massively obese compared to the nonobese population; this association is probably related to the increased hepatic synthesis and secretion of cholesterol in obesity, supersaturation of the bile with cholesterol, and cholesterol crystallization.[160]

Obesity and osteoarthritis, both of the hands and, particularly, the knees and feet, have been reported to be related. This may be attributable to the increased burden placed on the joints by the massively expanded adipose tissue. In one study, the occurrence of nonspecific arthritis was reported to be 55 percent greater in women who are 85 percent or more above "desirable" body weight compared to those 10 percent or less overweight.[163] Weight reduction often reduces symptoms, especially when the involved joints are weight-bearing. The risk and prevalence of gout increase as relative body weight increases. The mechanisms responsible for these associations are not known.

Obstetrical problems occur more commonly in obese than nonobese women. The most common complications associated with obesity are eclampsia, toxemia, hypertension, prolonged labor, fetal loss, postpartum hemorrhage, increased fetal weight, and failure of lactation.[104]

TREATMENT OF OBESITY

Given the widespread and serious health consequences of obesity, there is a need to intervene to prevent and treat this disorder. However, since in most cases of obesity an underlying cause cannot be determined and specific therapy and preventive measures usually cannot be introduced, it is a difficult disorder to prevent or treat successfully.

Preventive measures are probably best focused on children who are at risk by virtue of family history, with particular attention to weight control through diet and exercise during childhood and adolescence. In view of the risk of disrupting normal growth and development that is associated with severe restriction of food intake in infancy and childhood, this approach should be avoided.

Those individuals who are already obese and in whom a specific aggravating or etiologic factor can be identified, e.g., hypothyroidism, hyperadrenalism, hyperinsulinism, hypopituitarism, or brain tumors, should receive specific treatments. Although these disorders only rarely cause obesity, it is important to at least consider them in every patient who is already obese, since treatment will be curative. Thus, if there is a reasonable degree of suspicion, diagnostic laboratory evaluation is indicated to confirm or rule out their presence. Specific therapy, e.g., administration of thyroid hormone or treatment of Cushing's syndrome, is indicated, however, *only* when a specific diagnosis has been established.

In the great majority of obese patients, a specific underlying cause or aggravating factor cannot be determined and treatment must be nonspecific. Under these circumstances, intervention is usually unsuccessful over the long term and may be associated with certain hazards. Although many varied therapies have been advanced for the treatment of those who are already obese, none has had much success in achieving the ultimate objective: for the patient to lose weight and keep it off. While short-term weight loss can often be achieved, most obese patients who lose weight regain their lost weight over time; at best, only approximately 20 percent of obese patients maintain weight loss over a 5- to 15-year period after initial treatment. In addition, in the frustrating process of repeated unsuccessful attempts at weight loss, certain psychological and other disorders may develop.

For individuals who are already obese, weight reduction should be regarded as a medical rather than a cosmetic issue and should be initiated in those with a BMI equal to or greater than 27. Treatment should also be initiated with even lesser degrees of obesity in those with associated disorders such as hyperglycemia or NIDDM; hyperlipidemia or arteriosclerotic disease;

hypertension; pulmonary or cardiovascular diseases; gout; and severe osteoarthritis. In these individuals treatment should aim for restoring the BMI to and maintaining it at 22. Until additional research sheds new information on the underlying causes of obesity and permits more specific, efficacious, and safe therapeutic and preventive measures to be developed, this general approach is recommended. However, the conventional therapeutic approach currently employed by most physicians, i.e., prescription of a diet and periodic follow-up, is inadequate. New approaches that extend beyond the narrow confines of traditional medical settings are required. While the diagnosis of obesity and the formulation of a therapeutic plan are the responsibility of the physician, a contemporary treatment program of this complex disorder requires the active involvement and participation of various nonphysician resources in the community. In this way an attempt can be made to provide an environment conducive to the development of more healthy lifestyles with respect to eating and physical activity.

Diet

The cornerstone of the treatment of obesity is diet, specifically, caloric restriction. Weight loss depends on engendering a caloric deficit, which, in turn, depends on the total number (not the kind) of calories consumed relative to calories expended. Many different types of calorie-restricted diets have been advanced for the treatment of obesity, some of which are in the form of liquid formulas, others which use bizarre combinations of foods or nutrients based on unfounded theories and which may be hazardous. None of these fad diets appears to offer any inherent advantages over a calorie-restricted diet of normal foods, balanced to provide the conventional distribution of carbohydrate (50 percent of total calories), fat (35 percent of total calories), and protein (15 percent of total calories). A particular unbalanced diet may on occasion be more suitable and effective on a short-term basis in a given patient, but in the opinion of this author unbalanced diets should be recommended only rarely, and certain diets (e.g., liquid protein, total starvation) should be avoided in all patients for the reasons discussed below.

Generally, two phases of weight loss are observed with caloric restriction: an initial period of rapid weight loss, primarily reflecting loss of body sodium and water, is followed by a slower phase of weight reduction due predominantly to fat catabolism. The rapid loss of weight often achieved during the first few weeks of treatment with fad or unbalanced diets is usually due to the loss of sodium and water (and body protein) rather than body fat. The slower phase of weight reduction is accompanied by a decrease in resting or basal metabolism, an adaptation to caloric restriction that is observed in both lean and obese patients; it makes them more energy-efficient and more resistant to weight loss.[172] Patients frequently become discouraged during this slower phase of weight loss, particularly with the monotony of a given diet. It is at this time that the introduction of the other modalities of therapy (discussed below) may be particularly helpful.

The extent to which caloric intake is to be restricted in a given patient depends on the degree of obesity, age, sex, physical activity, and general health. Unless the obesity is associated with severe metabolic abnormalities, there appears to be little need or justification for a program of rapid weight loss; therefore, drastic reduction in caloric intake is usually unnecessary. Loss of approximately 2 lb per week is a reasonable goal in most patients and can be accomplished by inducing a daily caloric deficit of approximately 1000 kcal. Restriction to 800 to 1200 kcal per day is generally appropriate for a moderately active woman; 1000 to 1400 kcal per day is appropriate for a man of similar activity. Adjustments must be made for variations in physical activity, the coexistence of other risk factors, or conditions such as diabetes mellitus, pregnancy, and certain acute illnesses. All patients losing weight on such hypocaloric diets must receive close medical supervision. If the obesity is associated with severe debilitating or life-threatening disease, e.g., the Pickwickian syndrome, severe congestive heart failure, or severe hyperglycemia, a more drastic reduction in caloric intake may be indicated in order to achieve more rapid weight loss; under such circumstances even closer medical supervision will be required.

Calorie-restricted diets can be balanced to provide the conventional distribution of fat, carbohydrate, and protein, or unbalanced so as to specifically limit or emphasize a particular nutrient. A balanced, hypocaloric diet in which caloric restriction is emphasized and the degree of reduction specified is, in the opinion of this author, preferable; the distribution of calories among carbohydrate, fat, and protein should be 50:35:15 as percent of total caloric intake. Others prefer to use unbalanced diets which may or may not actually stipulate caloric reduction, but manipulate dietary composition such that spontaneous reduction in caloric intake ensues. The low-carbohydrate, high-fat diet is perhaps the best example of this approach. These diets are "ketogenic"; their effectiveness may be attributable to the postulated hunger-suppressing action of ketosis. While the rate of weight loss is often more rapid during the first few weeks of treatment with a hypocaloric, low-carbohydrate, high-fat, ketogenic diet than a hypocaloric, balanced diet, this is due to greater loss of sodium, water, and body protein, not loss of fat. Furthermore, after the rapid initial weight loss, the rate of weight loss is usually disappointing. Because low-carbohydrate, high-fat, ketogenic diets are not palatable, patient compliance over the long run is likely to be poor. Hypocaloric, low-carbohydrate, ketogenic diets can be associated with various side effects, including weakness, fatigue, apathy, nausea, and postural hypotension.[12] Since the long-term effects of ketosis are not known, this approach should be employed with caution, especially in patients with insulin-dependent, ketoacidosis-prone diabetes mellitus, renal disease, or other acidotic conditions; it should not be used during pregnancy or during infancy, childhood, or adolescence. The use of the low-carbohydrate, high-fat, ketogenic diet is not recommended, except when compelling reasons exist. Finally, ingestion of these unbalanced diets does nothing to modify the patient's eating habits or to develop sound and healthy long-term nutritional practices, an essential component of the successful long-term management of obesity.

Another approach that has been advanced for weight reduction is the use of low-calorie diets comprising only or primarily protein. The *protein-sparing modified fast* (PSMF) is the most widely used such diet.[173] The diet contains 1.25 to 1.4 g of protein per kilogram of ideal body weight per day, and less than 10 g of carbohydrate and 50 g of fat per day. Supplementation with a multivitamin preparation containing folate, iron, potassium (25 mg per day), and calcium carbonate and liberal water intake (6 to 8 oz per day) are essential. Such a regimen has been shown to restore nitrogen balance after 2 to 3 weeks. Ketosis is reported to be less than occurs with low-carbohydrate, high-fat diets. Significant weight loss with a high degree of satiety and an unusual degree of feeling of well-being has been reported.

Certain hazards and contraindications to the PSMF regimen have, however, been noted.[12,174] Levels of plasma uric acid and cholesterol tend to rise in many patients. Menstrual abnormalities have frequently been observed. An increased tendency toward cholelithiasis and cholecystitis has been reported. The development of postural hypotension is not uncommon. The PSMF should not be used in patients with hypertension, congestive heart failure, coronary heart disease, and ketoacidosis-prone diabetes mellitus, or in those under treatment with diuretics, drugs affecting vascular responses, insulin, or oral hypoglycemic agents. Patients suffering from cholelithiasis, cholecystitis, liver disease, severe renal failure, or gout should not be placed on this diet. Furthermore, there is no experience with this diet in children and adolescents; since childhood and adolescence are periods of active growth and development dependent on adequate supplies of a broad range of nutrients, the PSMF should not be used to achieve weight reduction in obese children.

A number of sudden cardiovascular deaths have been reported in patients using the PSMF, particularly when low-quality protein (usually hydrolyzed gelatin) in the form of a "liquid protein diet" has been used. While the cause appears to have been ventricular arrhythmia, the underlying pathophysiology remains unclear. *Use of the liquid protein diets containing low-quality protein for weight reduction is not justified under any circumstances.*

The PSMF fails to modify eating habits and lifestyle and thus, by itself, is of limited value in the long-term management of obesity, especially since it is associated with significant and serious side effects. This author does not recommend the use of the PSMF. If, however, it is to be used, it must be undertaken under extremely close medical supervision, it must contain at least 55 g of high-quality protein, and it must include adequate potassium supplementation and liberal water intake.

High-fiber diets have been advocated for weight reduction, based on the premise that fiber reduces appetite.[12,174] While ingestion of diets with a high fiber content may indeed lead to decreased appetite, weight loss, and improvement in glucose tolerance and plasma lipid concentration, achievement of these effects requires an amount of fiber that renders diets unpalatable to the majority of patients; prolonged adherence cannot be expected in most individuals. Moreover, the improvements in rate of weight loss and blood glucose and lipid concentrations are only slightly greater than those achieved through balanced hypocaloric diets; thus the negative aspects of such diets outweigh the benefits. One potential risk in ingesting a diet containing very large amounts of fiber is that it could lead to trace mineral deficiencies. Americans, obese and nonobese alike, probably should increase the amount of fiber in their diets compared to current average United States intake, but in moderate amounts.

Total starvation has also been used in the treatment of obesity. Obese humans can tolerate fasting for prolonged periods of time and, in general, starvation as a treatment for obesity has met with only a few difficulties. Adherence to fasting is generally good and initial weight loss is quite rapid compared to that observed with calorie-restricted diets. The benefits of starvation are, however, short-lasting. Weight loss over the long run is similar to that achieved with hypocaloric, balanced diets. Long-term results using starvation have not been particularly impressive; in one study not more than one-third of patients treated in this way had maintained their weight reduction after 2 years.[174] A variety of problems have been observed during the course of therapeutic starvation in obese patients:[12,174] lean body mass is lost to a significantly greater degree during total starvation than calorie restriction;[175] hypotension; severe cardiovascular disturbances, including arrhythmia and death; electrolyte imbalance; and ketoacidosis have been observed to accompany prolonged starvation. And, as is the case with fad or unbalanced diets, total starvation does not modify the patient's eating habits or develop sound and healthy nutritional practices essential to the successful long-term management of obesity. For these reasons, calorie-restricted diets are clearly preferable to total starvation regimens. The author does not recommend total starvation for the treatment of obesity. If total starvation is to be used, it should not be undertaken in the absence of close medical supervision, it should not be prolonged, and it should be restricted to the rare, selected patient with severe obesity in whom rapid weight loss is vital. Patients should be hospitalized; fluid, electrolyte, and acid-base balances should be carefully monitored and adjusted; and vitamins should be administered as appropriate. After the patient has been on the regimen for a short period, a more conventional program of therapy should be reintroduced.

There is little current evidence to support the idea that any particular fad or formula diet has an advantage over a calorie-restricted balanced diet in achieving weight reduction; some of these diets may even be hazardous. On the other hand, a given individual may prefer one type of caloric restriction to another for reasons of taste, habit, and socioeconomic or cultural factors, and therefore be more likely to adhere to it. If taken under proper supervision, if not used in the face of contraindications, and if coupled to a broader program directed toward modifying eating behavior and developing sound and healthy long-term nutritional attitudes and practices, such diets may be of value for certain persons. The basis for recommending any hypocaloric weight-reduction diet for an individual patient and determining the pattern in which it is to be administered lies in recognizing its potential hazards and defining its potential advantages for that person in terms of motivation, adherence, and development of sound and healthy long-term nutritional practices.

Exercise

A daily exercise program is an important adjunct to caloric restriction in achieving and especially in maintaining reduced weight.[176] However, exercise is not an effective means of inducing weight loss unless combined with reduction of calorie intake; exercise appears to potentiate the effects of caloric restriction. When combined with a hypocaloric diet, a daily exercise program, carefully planned and tailored to the patient's abilities and physical condition, is an important component of a long-term weight reduction program. During the period of slow weight loss due to caloric restriction, when resting metabolic rate is decreased and energy efficiency is increased, exercise increases energy expenditure and the degree of negative energy balance.

Although the combination of decreased caloric intake and increased physical activity leads to more negative energy balance than does dieting alone, the rate of weight loss is probably not greatly enhanced by the amount and type of physical activity that obese people can and will do. It is not often that an obese patient can or should undertake the kind of strenuous exercise program required to make an impact on weight loss; indeed, such a program may be hazardous. On the other hand a daily exercise program of low levels of aerobic physical activity such as walking, swimming, or cycling, tailored to the patient's physical condition, ability, and environment, can be associated with other important benefits. Exercise has been reported to shift body composition in the direction of increasing lean body mass at the expense of adipose tissue. Plasma glucose and insulin concentrations decrease, the sensitivity to insulin in the tissues of the body increases, and plasma cortisol and triglyceride levels decrease. Cardiovascular function may improve during carefully planned, prolonged physical training. Successful participation in an exercise program can have considerable psychological benefit, particularly with respect to improved self-esteem.

Exercise is not without its hazards, especially in an individual unaccustomed to physical activity. A sudden increase in physical activity is contraindicated, particularly in individuals with evidence of atherosclerotic disease. For this reason, if an exercise program is to be added to the dietary treatment of obesity, it should be introduced very gradually and with great care, and tailored to the individual's physical condition and ability. Physical activity should be gradually incorporated into the daily schedule so that it becomes part of the patient's routine. Walking appears to be the best activity to start with. Later on, different activities can be introduced, depending on the progress of the individual. Once again, however, exercise alone is not an effective means of weight reduction; reduced calorie intake is essential.

Behavior Modification

A critically important component of the management of obesity is the institution of a program aimed at changing or modifying the individual's attitudes, beliefs, and behavior with respect to eating and physical activity. Only through such life-style changes can long-term success be achieved. Various behavioral techniques and programs have, therefore, been introduced into the treatment of obesity.[22,176] Since patterns of and attitudes toward eating behavior and physical activity vary considerably among obese people, the particular behavioral approach used for a given patient must be individualized. Furthermore, as with exercise, a program of behavior modification must be viewed as an adjunct to the primary form of treatment, restriction of caloric intake.

A program of behavior modification is usually initiated after significant weight reduction has already been achieved and is administered over a long period, with emphasis on the positive, rewarding aspects of self-control rather than on an aversive approach, and with frequent positive reinforcement. Behavior modification aimed at stopping a behavior, e.g., hyperphagia, is apt not to be as successful as behavior modification introducing or reinforcing a new behavior, e.g., physical activity. In certain obese persons, an individualized behavioral modification program combined with a program of diet and exercise appears to offer considerable advantage for short-term weight loss. Many obese patients derive short-term benefit from the various self-help groups currently in existence; these groups may be of considerable help in the modifying of eating behavior and physical activity, in addition to bolstering motivation. The problem, however, is that the goal is not merely to lose weight, but to keep it off for a lifetime. It is in achieving this long-term goal that even the best behavioral modification techniques and programs have not yet been successful in most obese persons.

Psychotherapy

Many obese individuals suffer from emotional problems. While occasionally these may be the cause of obesity, most often they are the consequence of obesity or weight reduction. When obesity is associated with emotional disturbance of such magnitude that it significantly interferes with an individual's ability to function, or when psychological disturbances can be identified as being etiologic of or contributory to the development and maintenance of obesity, psychotherapy may be indicated. Severe emotional disturbance resulting from weight loss may also be an indication for psychotherapeutic intervention and for termination of a weight reduction program. In most instances, however, obese patients do not require special psychiatric treatment; general emotional support by the physician and other members of the therapeutic team during the course of weight reduction is usually sufficient.

Drug Therapy

At present drug therapy in the treatment of obesity is of limited usefulness. The evidence presently available indicates that pharmacologic therapy is ineffective as the sole approach to the treatment of obesity, and it is unclear whether the benefits of adding drugs to calorie restriction, exercise, and behavioral modification outweigh their adverse effects.

If there is any role for appetite-suppressing drugs in this disorder, it is as part of a larger treatment program comprising caloric restriction and exercise. Although there is evidence to suggest that appetite-suppressing drugs can increase the weight loss achieved by caloric restriction, these data have been derived from short-term studies;[177,178] more long-term trials with drug therapy are required before the efficacy of these agents can be established.

The principles advanced by the Fogarty task force on obesity in 1977 provide useful guidelines for the use of appetite-suppressant drugs in the treatment of obesity.[178] The use of some drugs, e.g., the amphetamines, is associated with a high risk of addiction and abuse. Since the available data indicate that a similar degree of effectiveness pertains to the various appetite-suppressant drugs, those with less potential for addiction and abuse appear to be preferable. Injectable forms of these drugs have no place in the treatment of obesity.

Intermittent use of these drugs, i.e., periodic discontinuation of drug therapy, may produce as satisfactory results as, and fewer problems than, continuous drug use. Therapy should not be prolonged if weight loss cannot be achieved or continued. Appetite suppressants should not be used in the treatment of obesity unless the patient is clinically obese (more than 30 percent overweight or BMI ≥ 27) or has an associated condition for which weight loss would be beneficial. Pharmacologic intervention may be most helpful during the beginning of the slow phase of weight loss, when patients tend to be most discouraged.

A variety of drugs other than appetite suppressants, including thyroid hormone, diuretics, digitalis, and human chorionic gonadotropin (HCG), have been widely used in the treatment of obesity. Digitalis, diuretics, and thyroid hormones should be employed only when specific indications exists, i.e., congestive heart failure, edema, and hypertension for digitalis and the diuretics and clinically and laboratory-documented hypothyroidism in the case of thyroid hormone. There is no place for the use of HCG in the treatment of obesity.

There is reason to be optimistic that in the future effective pharmacologic agents may be developed which will prove useful adjuncts to dietary therapy in the management of obesity.[177] Increasing knowledge, gained through research, about the factors which regulate eating and caloric expenditure provides a potential basis for the development of drugs which can specifically influence energy input or output. For example, current research in neuroendocrinology has demonstrated a role for several CNS neurotransmitters and their metabolites in the regulation of appetite and eating behavior in humans and laboratory animals.[66,67,177] The effects of the catecholaminergic, serotoninergic, dopaminergic, and opioid systems on eating are being elucidated and new pharmacologic agents which influence these systems are being developed and tested. Furthermore, new knowledge about the nature of thermogenesis and its role in energy balance provides a potential basis for the development of thermogenic agents which increase energy expenditure.

Gastrointestinal Surgery

Failure of the traditional conservative therapies for obesity has provided the rationale for gastrointestinal surgery as a treatment. Two forms of surgery are now fairly widely used in the treatment of obesity, particularly in patients suffering severe forms of this disorder: jejunoileal bypass, which reduces intestinal energy absorption, and gastroplasty, which has no known influence on intestinal absorption but decreases stomach size.[179–181]

Two major types of jejunoileal bypass are employed: in one, the end of the distal segment of the jejunum is attached to the side of the ileum near the ileocecal valve; in the other, the distal portion of the jejunum is anastomosed to the end of the ileum. Both procedures have been observed to be effective means of achieving and maintaining weight loss. The amount and rate of weight loss are related to the length of anastomosed intestine, the patient's initial body weight, the type of surgery, and postoperative caloric intake. Weight reduction apparently occurs primarily as a result of malabsorption, but decreased food intake is also observed in many patients.

It is of interest that long-term postoperative experience with such patients indicates that both caloric intake and intestinal absorption gradually increase over time; the levels of both activities, however, remain less than those observed prior to surgery. In addition to achieving permanent weight loss, jejunoileal bypass surgery is associated with several other effects. The most striking of these is an improvement in psychosocial function in many, but not all, obese patients.[180] In addition, improvement in obesity-associated health risk factors such as diabetes, hyperlipoproteinemia, hypertension, respiratory problems, and symptoms of arthritis is observed.

Jejunoileal bypass surgery is, however, also associated with significant and serious complications. The mortality from this form of therapy far exceeds that from all other forms of treatment; the overall mortality following jejunoileal bypass has been reported to be as high as 11 percent with an average of approximately 3 percent. Diarrhea and malnutrition, particularly with respect to vitamins (B_{12}, A, and E), proteins, albumin, electrolytes (Ca^{2+},K^{+}), and carbohydrates, are among the most prominent postoperative complications. With careful and frequent monitoring and appropriate treatment these can usually be managed satisfactorily. More serious are problems related to hepatic failure and the development of urinary calculi. Liver function tests and liver biopsies are usually abnormal during the early postoperative period; although liver function tests usually return toward normal, abnormal liver histology often persists. In 2 to 4 percent of cases, liver deterioration and hepatic failure have been observed. Urinary calculi have been reported with a frequency varying between 3 and 10 percent; the mechanism appears to reside, at least in part, in the increased absorption of oxalates.

Other major complications reported with jejunoileal bypass include polyarthritis, peptic ulcer, acute cholecystitis, and intestinal obstruction. Most of these problems can be completely reversed with reanastomosis, a procedure which, unfortunately, also restores the obesity.

In view of these problems, jejunoileal bypass surgery seems justified as a therapeutic procedure in obesity only for selected, massively obese patients who are faced with life-threatening medical problems or who are severely impaired in psychosocial life. When used as a form of treatment in such patients, this procedure should be conducted in a setting in which short- and long-term follow-up can be very carefully maintained.

Gastroplasty is associated with significantly fewer complications than jejunoileal bypass; as a consequence, it is in widespread and increasingly common use in the treatment of morbid obesity. Since gastroplasty has no known influence on intestinal energy absorption, it should be regarded only as an adjunct to dietary therapy.

Community Involvement

Involvement of community resources in the treatment of obesity is based on the premise that life-style factors contribute to the development and maintenance of obesity and that these influences are more likely to be effected through the broader resources of the community than the narrower confines of traditional medical settings. Places of employment, schools, supermarkets, community centers, churches, and the home, as well as traditional health care settings, may be important resources for support and educational efforts. Various nonprofit organizations as well as mass media outlets may also be enlisted in this effort. The cooperation and coordination of all health workers and allied health personnel of the community should be enlisted; frequent patient follow-up by the physician, dietitian, and behavioral therapist is essential not only during weight reduction but after the desired goal has been achieved.

MANAGEMENT OF ASSOCIATED PROBLEMS

In view of the adverse effects of obesity on health and the generally unsuccessful and frustrating treatment of this disorder, every reasonable attempt ought to be made to address those components of obesity amenable to therapy in order to increase the quality of life.

When obesity and hypertension coexist, the hazards to health are greater than when either is present alone; therefore, in addition to a program of weight reduction, pharmacologic treatment of significant degrees of hypertension should be instituted.

Treatment of the obese diabetic patient is especially difficult since such patients are insulin-resistant; reduction of blood glucose concentration toward normal requires doses of insulin which may stimulate appetite and lipogenesis, thus acting counter to the primary goal of weight reduction. For this reason, treatment of the obese diabetic is primarily dietary; reduced caloric intake and weight loss frequently improve the diabetic state sufficiently to eliminate or at least reduce the requirement for insulin or oral hypoglycemic therapy. If the dietary approach is unsuccessful and if the obese patient suffers from the clinical symptoms of marked hyperglycemia and glycosuria, oral sulfonylureas should be administered in doses sufficient to eliminate these symptoms. If these oral hypoglycemic agents fail to lower blood glucose concentration and relieve symptoms, insulin should be administered in doses sufficient to eliminate symptoms, but not necessarily to restore normoglycemia. Of course, if the obese patient suffers severe metabolic abnormalities such as ketoacidosis or hyperosmolarity syndrome, insulin treatment is indicated; this type of diabetes also improves with weight loss. Although the need for insulin may not be entirely eliminated in all patients, insulin requirements can be markedly decreased.

Hyperlipoproteinemia associated with obesity responds to caloric restriction and weight reduction. Only when this approach fails is manipulation of dietary composition or drug therapy indicated.

When the coexistence of other disorders with obesity can be established, e.g., congestive heart failure, severe edema, endocrine dysfunction, or psychiatric illness, treatment with specific agents is important in improving the quality of the patient's life.

REFERENCES

1. Powers PS: *Obesity. The Regulation of Weight.* Baltimore, Williams and Wilkins, 1980, p 1.
2. Forbes GB, Gallup J, Hirsch JB: Estimation of total body fat from ^{40}K content. *Science* 133:1, 1961.
3. Presta E, Wang J, Harrison GG, Bjorntorp P, Houker WH, Van Itallie TB: Measurement of total body electrical conductivity: A new method for estimation of body composition. *Am J Clin Nutr* 37:735, 1983.
4. Durnin JVGA, Womersly J: Body fat assessed from total body density and its estimation from skinfold thickness: Measurements of 481 men and women aged 17 to 72 years. *Br J Nutr* 32:77, 1974.
5. Simopoulos AM, Van Itallie TB: Body weight, height and longevity. *Ann Intern Med* 100:285, 1984.
6. Burton BT, Foster WR, Hirsch J, Van Itallie TB: *Proceedings, NIH Consensus Development Conference, Health Implications of Obesity. Int J Obesity* 9:155, 1985.
7. Foster WR, Burton BT (eds): *NIH Consensus Development Conference, Health Implications of Obesity. Ann Intern Med* 103(suppl 6, pt 2):981, 1985.
8. New weight standards for men and women. *Metropolitan Life Insurance Company Statistical Bulletin,* 40:1, 1959.
9. 1983 Metropolitan Height and Weight Tables. *Metropolitan Life Insurance Company Statistical Bulletin* 64:3, 1983.
10. Bray GA (ed): Obesity in Perspective. *Fogarty International Center Series on Preventive Medicine.* U.S. DHEW Publication NIH 75-708, 1975, vol 2, pt 1, p 72.
11. Abraham S, Carroll M, Naijar MF: Trends in obesity and overweight among adults age 20–74 years: United States 1960–1962, 1971–1974, 1976–1980, in *Vital and Health Statistics,* ser 11. Hyattsville, MD, National Center for Health Statistics, 1985.
12. Van Itallie TB: Hazards of obesity and hazards of treatment, in Hirsch J, Van Itallie TB (eds): *Proceedings of the 4th International Congress on Obesity.* London, Libbey, 1983.
13. Kissebah AH, Vydelingum N, Murray R, Evans DJ, Mariz AJ, Kalkhoff RK, Adam PK: Relation of body fat distribution to metabolic consequences of obesity. *J Clin Endocrinol Metab* 54:524, 1982.
14. Kalkhoff RK, Hartz AH, Rupley D, Kissebah AH, Kelber J: Relationship of body fat distribution to blood pressure, carbohydrate tolerance and plasma lipids in healthy obese women. *J Lab Clin Med* 102:61, 1983.
15. National Center for Health Statistics: Skinfold thickness of youths 12–17 years in the United States. Vital and Health Statistics, U.S. DHEW, no. 120, Washington, DC, US Government Printing Office, 1972.
16. Bray GA: The obese patient, in Smith LI Jr (ed): *Major Problems in Internal Medicine.* Philadelphia, Saunders, 1976.
17. U.S. DHEW: Ten State Nutrition Survey 1968–1970. DHEW Publication (HSM) 72-8134. Atlanta, Centers for Disease Control, 1972.
18. Abraham S, Nordsieck M: Relationship of excess weight of children and adults. *Public Health Rep* 75:263, 1960.

19. Charney E, Goodman HC, McBride M, Lyon B, Pratt R: Childhood antecedents of adult obesity. Do chubby infants become obese adults? *N Engl J Med* 295:6, 1976.

20. Poskitt EM, Cole TJ: Do fat babies stay fat?, in *Diet Related to Killer Diseases II. Hearings before the Select Committee on Nutritional Human Needs of the U.S. Senate.* 95th Cong, 1st Sess, 1977, p 72.

21. Peckham CS, Stark O, Simonite V, Wolff OH: Prevalence of obesity in British children born in 1946 and 1958. *Br Med J* 286:1237, 1983.

22. Stunkard AJ: Obesity and the social environment: Current status, future prospects, in Bray G (ed): *Obesity in America.* U.S. DHEW Publication NIH 79-359, 1979, p 206.

23. Goldblatt P, Moore ME, Stunkard A: Social factors in obesity. *JAMA* 192:1038, 1965.

24. Seltzer CC: Some reevaluations of the Build and Blood Pressure Study of 1959 as related to ponderal index, somatotype and mortality. *N Engl J Med* 274:254, 1966.

25. Hirsch J, Batchelor B: Adipose tissue cellularity in human obesity. *Clin Endocrinol Metab* 5:299, 1976.

26. Salans LB, Cushman S, Weismann RE: Studies of human adipose tissue: Adipose cell size and number in nonobese and obese patients. *J Clin Invest* 52:929, 1973.

27. Krotkiewski M, Sjostrom L, Bjorntorp P, Carlgren G, Garellick G, Smith U: Adipose tissue cellularity in relation to prognosis for weight reduction. *Int J Obesity* 1:395, 1977.

28. Hirsch J, Gallian E: Methods for determination of adipose cell size in man and animals. *J Lipid Res* 9:110, 1968.

29. Hirsch J, Knittle JL: Cellularity of obese and nonobese human adipose tissue. *Fed Proc* 29:1516, 1970.

30. Knittle JL, Ginsberg-Fellner F, Braun R: Adipose tissue development in man. *Am J Clin Nutr* 30:762, 1977.

31. Greenwood MRC, Johnson PR, Hirsch J: Postnatal development of adipocyte cellularity in the normal rat. *J Lipid Res* 15:474, 1974.

32. Hirsch J, Han P: Cellularity of rat adipose tissue: Effects of growth, starvation and obesity. *J Lipid Res* 10:77, 1969.

33. Knittle JL, Hirsch J: The effect of early nutrition on the development of rat epididymal fat pads: Cellularity and metabolism. *J Clin Invest* 47:2091, 1968.

34. Johnson PR, Stern JS, Greenwood MRC, Zucker LM, Hirsch J: Effect of early nutrition on adipose cellularity and pancreatic insulin release in the Zucker rat. *J Nutr* 103:738, 1973.

35. Salans LB, Horton ES, Sims EAH: Experimental obesity in man: Cellular character of the adipose tissue. *J Clin Invest* 50:1005, 1971.

36. Lemmonier D: Effects of age, sex and weight on cellularity of the adipose tissue in mice rendered obese by a high fat diet. *J Clin Invest* 51:2907, 1972.

37. Stiles J, Francendese AA, Masoro J: Influence of age on size and number of fat cells in the epididymal depot. *Am J Physiol* 229:1561, 1975.

38. Johnson PR, Stern JS, Greenwood MRC, Zucker LM, Hirsch J: Effect of early nutrition on adipose cellularity and pancreatic insulin release in the Zucker rat. *J Nutr* 103:738, 1973.

39. Greenwood MRC, Hirsch J: Postnatal development of adipocyte cellularity in the normal rat. *J Lipid Res* 15:474, 1974.

40. Bertrand HA, Masoro EJ, Yu BP: Increasing adipocyte number as the basis for perirenal depot growth in adult rats. *Science* 201:1234, 1978.

41. Faust IM, Miller WM Jr: Effects of diet and environment on adipocyte development. *Int J Obesity* 5:593, 1981.

42. Bertrand HA, Lynd FT, Masoro EJ, Yu BP: Changes in adipose mass and cellularity through the adult life of rats fed *ad libitum* or a life-prolonging restricted diet. *J Gerontol* 35:827, 1980.

43. Miller WH, Faust IM: Alterations in rat adipose tissue morphology induced by a low temperature environment. *Am J Physiol* 242:E93, 1982.

44. Faust IM, Johnson PR, Stern JS, Hirsch J: Diet-induced adipocyte number increase in adult rats. A new model of obesity. *Am J Physiol* 235:E279, 1978.

45. Miller WH, Faust IM, Goldberger AC, Hirsch J: Effects of severe long-term food deprivation and refeeding on adipose tissue cells in the rat. *Am J Physiol* 245:E74, 1983.

46. Despres JP, Bouchard C, Savard R, Temblay A, Marcotte M, Theriaut G: The effect of a 20-week endurance training program on adipose tissue morphology and lipolysis in men and women. *Metabolism* 33:235, 1984.

47. Faust IM, Johnson PR, Hirsch J: Adipose tissue regeneration following lipectomy. *Science* 197:391, 1977.

48. Faust IM, Johnson PR, Hirsch J: Adipose regeneration in adult rats. *Proc Soc Exp Biol Med* 161:111, 1979.

49. Faust IM, Johnson PR, Hirsch J: Surgical removal of adipose tissue alters feeding behavior and the development of obesity in rats. *Science* 197:393, 1977.

50. Johnson PR, Hirsch J: Cellularity of adipose depots in six strains of genetically obese mice. *J Lipid Res* 13:2, 1972.

51. Knittle JL: Adipose tissue development in man, in Faulkner F, Tanner JM (eds): *Postnatal Growth in Human Growth.* New York, Plenum, 1978, vol 2, p 295.

52. Bjorntorp P, Karlson M, Pertoft H, Pettersson P, Sjostrom L, Smith V: Isolation and characterization of cells from rat adipose tissue developing into adipocytes. *J Lipid Res* 19:36, 1978.

53. Jeanrenaud B, Assimocopoulos-Jeannet F, Crettaz M, Berthood HR, Bereiter DA, Jeanrenaud FR: Experimental obesities: A progressive pathology with reference to the potential importance of the CNS in hyperinsulinemia, in Bjorntorp P, Cairella M, Howard AN (eds): *Recent Advances in Obesity Research.* London, Libbey, 1981, p 159.

54. Bray GA, York DA: Genetically transmitted obesity in rodents. *Physiol Rev* 51:598, 1971.

55. Garrow JS: The regulation of energy expenditure in man, in Bray GA (ed): *Recent Advances in Obesity Research.* London, Libbey, 1978, vol 2, p 200.

56. Hirsch J, Leibel RL: What constitutes a sufficient psychobiologic explanation for obesity?, in Stunkard AJ, Stellar E (eds): *Eating and Its Disorders.* New York, Raven, 1984, p 121.

57. Newshome EA: A possible metabolic basis for the control of body weight. *N Engl J Med* 302:400, 1980.

58. Coleman DL, Hummel KP: Effects of parabiosis of normal with genetically diabetic mice. *Am J Physiol* 217:1298, 1969.

59. Coleman DL: Effects of parabiosis of obese with diabetic and normal mice. *Diabetologia* 9:294, 1973.

60. Gruen RK, Hietanen E, Greenwood MRC: Increased adipose tissue lipoprotein lipase activity during the development of the genetically obese rat (fa/fa). *Metabolism* 27:1955, 1978.

61. Rohner-Jeanrenaud F, Jeanrenaud B: A role of the vagus nerve in the etiology and maintenance of the hyperinsulinemia of genetically obese fa/fa rats, in Hirsch J, Van Itallie TB (eds): *Proceedings of the 4th International Congress on Obesity.* London, Libbey, 1983.

62. Martin RJ, Jeanrenaud B: Growth hormone in obesity and diabetes: Inappropriate hypothalamic control of secretion, in Hirsch J, Van Itallie TB (eds): *Proceedings of the 4th International Congress on Obesity.* London, Libbey, 1983.

63. Bawkin H: Obesity in children. *J Pediatr* 54:392, 1952.

64. Stunkard AJ, Thorkild MD, Sorenson IA, Hanis C, Teasdale TW, Ranajit-Chakrabort MA, Schullin J: An adoption study of human obesity. *N Engl J Med* 314:193, 1986.

65. Garn SH, Bailey SM, Cole PE: Similarities between parents and their adopted children. *Am J Phys Anthropol* 45:539, 1976.

66. Schneider BS, Friedman JM, Hirsch J: Feeding behavior, in Krieger DT, Brownstein MJ, Martin JB (eds): *Brain Peptides.* New York, Wiley, 1983, p 251.

67. Morley JE, Levine AS: The central control of appetite. *Lancet*

1:392, 1983.
68. Frohman LA: The central nervous system and metabolic regulation, in Katzen HM, Mahler RJ (eds): *Diabetes, Obesity and Vascular Disease, Advances in Modern Nutrition*. Washington, DC, Hemisphere, 1978, p 493.
69. Himms-Hagen J: Brown adipose tissue thermogenesis in obese animals. *Nutr Rev* 41:261, 1983.
70. Acheson K, Jequier E, Burger A, Danforth E: Thyroid hormones and thermogenesis: The metabolic cost of food and exercise. *Metabolism* 33:262, 1984.
71. Bray GA, Gallagher RF: Manifestations of hypothalamic obesity in man: A comprehensive investigation of eight patients and a review of the literature. *Annu Rev Med* 54:301, 1974.
72. Hirsch J: The adipose cell hypothesis. *N Engl J Med* 294:389, 1976.
73. Nijima A: Afferent impulse discharges from glucoreceptors in the liver of the guinea pig. *Ann NY Acad Sci* 157:690, 1969.
74. Young JB, Landsberg L: Catecholamines and a sympathoadrenal system: Regulation of metabolism, in Ingbar SH (ed): *Contemporary Endocrinology*. New York, Plenum, 1979, vol 1, p 245.
75. Acheson K, Jequier E, Wahren J: Influence of beta adrenergic blockade on glucose induced thermogenesis in man. *J Clin Invest* 72:981, 1981.
76. Goldman JK, Bernardis LL, Frohman L: Food intake in hypothalamic obesity. *Am J Physiol* 277:88, 1974.
77. Rabinowitz D: Some endocrine and metabolic aspects of obesity. *Annu Rev Med* 21:241, 1970.
78. Sims E, Danforth AH, Horton ES, Bray GA, Glennon J, Salans LB: Effects of experimental obesity in man. *Recent Prog Horm Res* 29:457, 1972.
79. Bray GA: Complications of obesity. *Ann Intern Med* 103:1052, 1983.
80. Shimomura Y, Bray GA, York DA: Effects of thyroid hormone and adrenalectomy on [Na^+,K^+]ATPase in the ob/ob mouse. *Horm Metab Res* 13:578, 1981.
81. Scriba PC, Baver M, Emmert D: Effects of obesity, total fasting and realimentation on L-thyroxine (T_4), 3,5,3′-L-triiodothyronine (T_3), 3,5,3′-triiodothyronine (rT_3), thyroxine-binding globulin (TBG), cortisol, thyrotropin, cortisol-binding globulin (CBG), transferrin, alpha-2 haptoglobin and complement in serum. *Acta Endocrinol* 91:629, 1979.
82. Sims EAH: Experimental obesity, dietary-induced thermogenesis and their clinical implications. *Clin Endocrinol Metab* 5:377, 1976.
83. Londono JH, Gallagher TF, Bray GA: Effect of weight reduction, triiodothyronine, and diethyl-stilbestrol on growth hormone in obesity. *Metabolism* 18:986, 1969.
84. York DA, Bray GA, Yukimura Y: An enzymatic defect in the obese (ob/ob) mouse: Loss of thyroid-induced sodium and potassium dependent adenosine triphosphatase. *Proc Natl Acad Sci USA* 75:497, 1978.
85. Clausen T, Hansen O: The Na^+,K^+-pump, energy metabolism and obesity. *Biochem Biophys Res Commun* 104:357, 1982.
86. Rothwell NJ, Stock MJ: A role for brown adipose tissue in diet-induced thermogenesis. *Nature* 281:31, 1979.
87. Bjorntorp P, Horton ES, Danforth E Jr (eds): *Regulation of energy expenditure. Proceedings of an International Symposium on the Regulation of Energy Expenditure*, Sept-Oct 1983. *Int J Obesity* 9(suppl 2):1, 1985.
88. Galton DJ, Gilbert C, Reckless JPD: Triglyceride storage disease: A group of inborn errors of triglyceride metabolism. *Q J Med* 43:63, 1974.
89. Salans LB, Cushman SW: The roles of adiposity and diet in the carbohydrate and lipid metabolic abnormalities of obesity, in Katzen HM, Mahler RJ (eds): *Diabetes, Obesity and Vascular Disease, Advances in Modern Nutrition*. Washington, DC, Hemisphere, 1978, p 267.
90. Jequier E, Schutz Y: Long-term measurements of energy expenditure in humans using a respiration chamber. *Am J Clin Nutr* 38:989, 1983.
91. Deleuise M, Blackburn GL, Flier JS: Reduced activity of the red-cell sodium-potassium pump in human obesity. *N Engl J Med* 303:107, 1980.
92. Mir MA, Charalambous BM, Morgan K: Erythrocyte sodium-potassium-ATPase and sodium transport in obesity. *N Engl J Med* 305:1264, 1981.
93. Klimes I, Howard BV, Mott DM: Sodium-potassium pump in cultured fibroblasts from obese donors: No evidence for an inherent decrease of basal or insulin-stimulated activity. *Metabolism* 33:317, 1984.
94. Bray GA, Kral JG, Bjorntorp P: Hepatic sodium-potassium dependent ATPase in obesity. *N Engl J Med* 304:1580, 1981.
95. Rothwell NJ, Stock MJ: A role for brown adipose tissue in diet-induced thermogenesis. *Nature* 281:31, 1979.
96. Schwartz RS, Halter JB, Bierman EL: Reduced thermic effect of feeding in obesity: Role of norepinephrine. *Metabolism* 32:114, 1983.
97. Bressard T, Schutz Y, Jequier E: Energy expenditure and postprandial thermogenesis in obese women before and after weight loss. *Am J Clin Nutr* 38:680, 1983.
98. Jequier E, Schutz Y: Does a defect in energy balance play a role in favoring human obesity, in Hirsch J, Van Itallie TB (eds): *Proceedings of the 4th International Congress on Obesity*. London, Libbey, 1983.
99. Ravussin E, Burnand B, Schutz Y, Jequier E: 24 Hour energy expenditure and resting metabolic rate in obese, moderately obese and control subjects. *Am J Clin Nutr* 35:566, 1982.
100. Segal KR, Gutin B: Thermic effects of food and exercise in lean and obese women. *Metabolism* 32:581, 1983.
101. Leibel RL, Hirsch J: Diminished energy requirements in reduced-obese patients. *Metabolism* 33:64, 1984.
102. Atkinson RL, Bray GA: Energy balance in obesity and its relationship to diabetes mellitus, in Katzen MH, Mahler RJ (eds): *Diabetes, Obesity and Vascular Disease, Advances in Modern Nutrition*. Washington, DC, Hemisphere, 1978, p 373.
103. Weis W, Jackson EC: Maternal factors affecting birthweight, in: *Perinatal Factors Affecting Human Development*. Washington, DC, Pan American Health Treaty Organization, 1969.
104. Peckham CH: The relationship between pregnancy weight and certain obstetrical factors. *Am J Obstet Gynecol* 111:1, 1971.
105. Farquhar J: Programs for babies born to diabetic mothers in Edinburgh. *Arch Dis Child* 44:36, 1969.
106. Ginsburg-Fellner F, Knittle J: Maternal diabetes as a factor in the development of childhood obesity. *Pediatr Res* 41:197, 1971.
107. McCance RA, Widdowson DM: Early nutrition and later development. *Proc R Soc Lond (Biol)* 156:326, 1962.
108. Revielli GP, Stein ZA, Susser MW: Obesity in young men after famine exposure in utero and early infancy. *N Engl J Med* 295:349, 1976.
109. Jelliffe DB, Jelliffe EF: Fat babies prevalence, perils and prevention. *J Trop Peds* and *Environ Child Health* 21:123, 1975.
110. Fomon SJ, Thomas LN, Filer LJ, Ziegler EE, Leonard MT: Food consumption and growth of normal infants fed milk based formulas. *Acta Pediatr Scand (Suppl)* 223:1, 1971.
111. Metzner HL, Lamphiear E, Wheller NC, Larkin FA: The relationship between frequency of eating and adiposity on adult men and women in the Tecumseh community health study. *Am J Clin Nutr* 30:722, 1977.
112. Fabry P, Fodor J, Hejl Z, Braun T, Zvolantlova K: The frequency of meals; its relationship to overweight, hypercholesterolemia and decreased glucose tolerance. *Lancet* 2:614, 1964.
113. Bray GA: Lipogenesis in human adipose tissue. Some effects of nibbling and gorging. *J Clin Invest* 51:537, 1972.
114. Bullen BA, Reed RB, Mayer J: Physical activity of obese and

nonobese adolescent girls appraised by motion picture sampling. *Am J Clin Nutr* 14:211, 1964.
115. Durnin JVGA: Body weight, body fat and the activity factor in energy balance, in Apfelbaum M (ed): *Energy Balance in Man.* Paris, Masson, 1973, p 141.
116. Bray GA, Whipp BJ, Kayla SN, Wasserman K: Some respiratory and metabolic effects of exercise in moderately obese men. *Metabolism* 26:402, 1977.
117. Brownell KD, Stunkard AJ: Physical activity in the development and control of obesity, in Stunkard AJ (ed): *Obesity.* Philadelphia, Saunders, 1980, p 300.
118. Jordan HA: Psychological factors associated with obesity, in Bray GA (ed): *Obesity in Perspective.* U.S. DHEW Publication 75-708, 1973, vol 2, pt 2, p 50.
119. Rodin J: Psychological factors in obesity, in Bjorntorp P, Cairella M, Howard AN (eds): *Recent Advances in Obesity Research.* London, Libbey, 1981, vol 3, p 106.
120. Schacter S: Obesity and eating. *Science* 161:751, 1968.
121. Rodin J, Bray GA, Atkinson RL, Dahms WT, Greenway FL, Hamilton K, Molitch M: Predictors of successful weight loss in an out-patient obesity clinic. *Int J Obesity* 1:40, 1976.
122. Grinker JA: Obesity and taste: Sensory and cognitive factors in food intake, in Bray GA (ed): *Obesity in Perspective.* U.S. DHEW Publication 75-708, 1973, vol 2, pt 2, p 73.
123. Russell GFM: Bulimia nervosa: An ominous variant of anorexia nervosa. *Psychol Med* 9:429, 1979.
124. Garn SM: Trends in fatness and the origins of obesity. *Pediatrics* 57:4, 1976.
125. Silverstone JT, Gordon PR, Stunkard A: Social factors in obesity in London. *Practitioner* 202:682, 1969.
126. Garn SM, Bailey M, Cole PE, Higgens TT: Levels of education, income and fatness in adults. *Am J Clin Nutr* 30:721, 1977.
127. Bennett PH, Rushforth NB, Miller M, Lecompre P: Epidemiological studies of diabetes in the Pima Indian. *Recent Prog Horm Res* 108:497, 1978.
128. Vague J, Bjorntorp P, Guy-Grand B, Rebuffe-Scrive M, Vauge P (eds): *Metabolic Consequences of Human Obesities.* Amsterdam, Excerpta Medica, 1985.
129. Chicago Society of Actuaries: *Build and Blood Pressure Study.* Chicago, 1959.
130. Hutchinson JJ: Clinical implications of extensive actuarial study of build and blood pressure. *Ann Intern Med* 54:190, 1961.
131. Andres R: Effect of obesity on total mortality. *Int J Obesity* 4:381, 1980.
132. Garrison RJ, Feinleib M, Castelli WP, McNamara PM: Cigarette smoking as a confounder of the relationship between relative weight and long-term mortality. *JAMA* 249:2199, 1983.
133. National Diabetes Data Group: Classification and diagnosis of diabetes mellitus and other categories of glucose intolerance. *Diabetes* 28:1039, 1979.
134. West KM (ed): *Epidemiology of Diabetes and Its Vascular Complications.* New York, Elsevier, 1978.
135. Zimmet P: Epidemiology of diabetes, in Ellenberg M, Rifkin H (eds): *Diabetes Mellitus, Theory and Practice.* New York, Medical Examination Publishing, 1981, p 451.
136. Greenfield M, Kolterman O, Olefsky JM, Reaven GM: The effect of ten days of fasting on various aspects of carbohydrate metabolism in obese diabetic subjects with significant fasting hyperglycemia. *Metabolism* 27:(suppl 2):1839, 1978.
137. Kovisto VA, Felig PF: Exercise in diabetes: Clinical implications, in Rykin H, Raskin P (eds): *Diabetes Mellitus.* American Diabetes Association, Bowie MD, R.J. Brady, 1981, vol 5, p 137.
138. Bogardus C, Lillioja S, Mott D, Reaven GM, Kashiwagi A, Foley JE: Relationship between obesity and maximal insulin stimulated glucose uptake in vivo and in vitro in Pima Indians. *J Clin Invest* 73:800, 1984.
139. Kortiewski M, Bjorntorp P, Sjostrom L, Smith U: Impact of obesity on metabolism in men and women: Importance of regional adipose tissue distribution. *J Clin Invest* 72:1150, 1983.
140. Wisniewski C, Silbert CK: Relationship of fat distribution to glucose tolerance: Results of computer tomography in male participants of the normative aging study. *Diabetes* 35:411, 1986.
141. Bogardus C, Lillioja S, Howard BV, Reaven GM, Mott D: Relationship between plasma glucose concentration in nondiabetic and noninsulin-dependent diabetic subjects. *J Clin Invest* 71:1238, 1985.
142. Karam JH, Grodsky GM, Forsham PH: Excessive insulin response to glucose in obese subjects. *Diabetes* 12:196, 1963.
143. Olefsky J, Kolterman O: Mechanisms of insulin resistance in obesity and noninsulin-dependent (type II) diabetes. *Am J Med* 70:151, 1981.
144. Prager R, Wallace P, Olefsky JM: In vivo kinetics of insulin action on peripheral glucose disposal and hepatic glucose output in normal and obese subjects. *J Clin Invest* 78:471, 1986.
145. Reaven GM: The role of insulin resistance in the pathogenesis and treatment of noninsulin dependent diabetes mellitus. *Am J Med* 74:1, 1983.
146. Foley JE, Thuillez P, Lillioja S, Zawadzki J, Bogardus C: Insulin sensitivity in adiposity from subjects with varying degrees of glucose tolerance. *Am J Physiol* 14:E306, 1986.
147. Kahn CR: Mechanism of insulin action. *Recent Prog Horm Res* 40:429, 1984.
148. Roth J, Kahn CR, Lesniask MA, Gorden P, De Meyts P, Megyesi K, Meville DM, Gavin JR, Soll AH, Freychet P, Goldine I, Barr RS, Archer JA: Receptors for insulin NSILA-S and growth hormone. *Recent Prog Horm Res* 31:95, 1975.
149. Salans LB, Knittle JL, Hirsch J: The role of adipose cell size and adipose tissue insulin sensitivity in the carbohydrate intolerance of obesity. *J Clin Invest* 47:153, 1968.
150. LeMarchand-Brustel Y, Gremeaux T, Ballotti R, Van Obberghen E: Insulin receptor tyrosine kinase is defective in skeletal muscle of insulin-resistant obese mice. *Nature* 315:676, 1985.
151. Cushman SW, Wardzala L, Karnieli E, Hissin PJ, Simpson I, Salans LB: Regulation of glucose transport by insulin: Reversible translocation of intracellular glucose transport systems to the plasma membrane, in Bjorntorp P, Cairella M, Howard AN (eds): *Recent Advances in Obesity Research.* London, Libbey, 1981, p 273.
152. Rosetti L, Papachristou D, Shulman G, Smith D, DeFronzo R: Insulin resistance in partially pancreatectomized rats (PX): Reversal with phlorizin therapy. *Diabetes (Suppl)* 35:38A, 1986.
153. Grey N, Kipnis DM: Effect of diet composition on the hyperinsulinemia of obesity. *N Engl J Med* 285:837, 1975.
154. Liu G, Coulston A, Chen YDI, Reaven GM: Does day-long absolute hypoinsulinemia characterize the patient with noninsulin dependent diabetes mellitus? *Metabolism* 32:754, 1983.
155. Hadden DR, Montgomery DAD, Skeely RJ: Maturity onset diabetes mellitus: Response to intensive dietary management. *Br Med J* 3:276, 1975.
156. Nestel P, Goldrick RB: Obesity: Changes in lipid metabolism and the role of insulin. *Clin Endocrinol Metab* 5:313, 1976.
157. Bierman EL, Brunzell JD: Interrelation of atherosclerosis, abnormal lipid metabolism and diabetes mellitus, in Katzen MM, Mahler RJ (eds): *Diabetes, Obesity and Vascular Disease, Advances in Modern Nutrition.* Washington, DC, Hemisphere, 1978, p 187.
158. Grundy SM, Mok HYI: Chylomicron clearance in normal healthy and hyperlipidemic man. *Metabolism* 25:1225, 1976.
159. Reaven GM, Lerner RL, Stern ML, Farquhar JW: Role of insulin in endogenous hypertriglyceridemia. *J Clin Invest* 46:1756, 1967.
160. Mabee TM: The mechanism of increased gallstone formation in obese human subjects. *Surgery* 79:460, 1976.
161. Hubert HB, Feinleib M, McNamara PM, Castelli WP: Obesity as an independent risk factor for cardiovascular disease: A 26-year follow-up of participants in the Framingham heart study. *Circula-*

tion 67:698, 1983.
162. Alexander JK: Effects of weight reduction on the cardiovascular system, in Bray GA (ed): *Obesity in Perspective.* U.S. DHEW Publication 75-708, 1973, vol 2, pt 2, p 233.
163. Rimm AA, Werner LG, Van Yserloo B, Bernstein RA: Relationship of obesity and disease in 73,532 weight-conscious women. *Public Health Rep* 90:44, 1975.
164. Chiang BN, Pearlman LV, Epstein FHP: Overweight and hypertension: A review. *Circulation* 39:403, 1969.
165. Garfield L: Overweight and cancer. *Ann Intern Med* 103:1034, 1985.
166. Nimrod A, Ryan KJ: Aromatization of androgens by human abdominal and breast fat tissue. *J Clin Endocrinol Metab* 40:367, 1975.
167. Danforth E Jr: Adaptive thermogenesis and thyroid hormones, in Bjorntorp P, Cairella M, Howard AN (eds): *Recent Advances in Obesity Research.* London, Libbey, 1980, vol 3, p 228.
168. Buskrik ER, Bartlett HL: Obesity and pulmonary function, in Bray GA (ed): *Obesity in Perspective.* U.S. DHEW Publication 75-708, 1973, vol 2, pt 2, p 225.
169. Blitzer PH, Blitzer EC, Rimm AA: Association between teenage obesity and cancer in 56,111 women. *Prev Med* 5:20, 1976.
170. Bernstein RA, Werner LH, Rimm AA: Relationship between gallbladder disease, parity, obesity and age in 62,739 weight conscious women. *Health Serv Reps* 88:925, 1973.
171. Drenick E: The prognosis of conventional treatment in severe obesity, in Bjorntorp P, Cairella M, Howard AN (eds): *Recent Advances in Obesity Research.* London, Libbey, 1981, vol 3, p 80.
172. Bray GA: Effect of caloric restriction on energy expenditure in obese patients. *Lancet* 2:397, 1969.
173. Lindner PG, Blackburn GL: Multidisciplinary approach to obesity utilizing fasting modified by protein-sparing therapy. *Obes Bariatr Med* 5:198, 1976.
174. Van Itallie TB: Dietary management of obesity. *Am J Clin Nutr* 31:543, 1978.
175. Yang MU, Barbosa-Saldivar JL, Pisunyer FX, Van Itallie TB: Metabolic effects of substituting carbohydrate for protein in a low-calorie diet: A prolonged study in obese patients. *Int J Obesity* 5:231, 1981.
176. Van Itallie TB: Conservative approaches to treatment, in Bray GA (ed): *Obesity in America.* U.S. DHEW Publication 79-359, 1979, p 164.
177. Sullivan AC, Garattini S (eds): Novel approaches and drugs for obesity, a satellite symposium. *4th International Congress on Obesity, October 1983. International Monographs on Obesity Series.* London, Libbey, 1983, no. 1.
178. Bray GA: Treatment of obesity with drugs and invasive procedures, in Bray GA (ed): *Obesity in America.* U.S. DHEW Publication 79-359, p 179.
179. Gomez CA: Gastroplasty in morbid obesity. *Surg Clin North Am* 59:1113, 1979.
180. Solow C, Silberfarb PM, Swift K: Psychosocial effects of intestinal bypass surgery for severe obesity. *N Engl J Med* 290:300, 1974.
181. Kral JG: Morbid obesity and related health risks. *Ann Intern Med* 103:1043, 1985.

22

Disorders of Lipid Metabolism*

D. Roger Illingworth
William E. Connor

Hyperlipidemia warrants special concern and interest because it is found with exceptional frequency in the American population. Ten percent of children and at least 25 percent of adults in the United States are hyperlipidemic. While most affected individuals have hyperlipidemia secondary to dietary factors or other metabolic disorders, some have genetic hyperlipidemia. This is estimated to be the most common genetic defect seen in adult medical practice. Thus asymptomatic hyperlipidemia may be detected both in so-called healthy people and in patients seeking medical attention for a variety of other problems. Hyperlipidemia is especially noted today because plasma cholesterol and triglyceride concentrations are so frequently determined in the course of routine chemical screening.

Hyperlipidemia involves an elevation of plasma lipid levels, cholesterol, and triglyceride, singly or in

*This work was supported by Public Health Service Research Grants HL 28399, HL 32271, HL 25687, and HL 20911, National Heart, Lung and Blood Institute, and by the General Clinical Research Centers Program (RR-334) of the Division of Research Resources, National Institutes of Health. DRI is the recipient of a Research Career Development Award (HL 00953) from the National Institutes of Health.

combination. Because these lipids are transported in the plasma as components of lipoprotein molecules, hyperlipidemia implies an associated lipoprotein abnormality as well.

There are four important clinical reasons for concern about the correct diagnosis and treatment of hyperlipidemia. The first reason is the strong causative relation between hyperlipidemia and atherosclerotic vascular disease: coronary heart disease, stroke, visceral atherosclerosis, and peripheral vascular disease. The second reason is the direct correlation of hyperlipidemia with the occurrence of xanthomas in the skin and tendons, which should be regarded as external manifestations of lipid deposits in tissues that are analogous to similar deposits occurring internally in the arteries. Xanthomas present cosmetic problems and because of their unique characteristics may be of value in the differential diagnosis of the exact type of hyperlipidemia. Both atherosclerosis and xanthomas will be the subject of more extensive discussions in subsequent sections of this chapter.

The third reason for concern relates to the diagnosis of obscure abdominal distress and even acute abdominal pain. In some patients, the episode of abdominal pain may progress to acute pancreatitis. Many hyperlipidemic patients with abdominal pain on the basis of a lipemic state have even been explored for the possibility of an acute abdomen. Thus hyperlipidemia should be considered as a possible cause of both acute pancreatitis and obscure abdominal pain.

The fourth reason for clinical concern is that the occurrence of hyperlipidemia may point to another disease to which the hyperlipidemia is secondary. While the primary condition may be obvious, in some instances hyperlipidemia may alert one to the possibility of hypothyroidism, for example.

THE PLASMA LIPOPROTEINS

The plasma of all vertebrates, including human beings, contains lipids which are transported as soluble complexes called *lipoproteins*. Individually such lipids have very limited solubility in aqueous environments, whereas as lipoprotein complexes they are readily held in solution. It is the lipid moieties with hydrated densities of 0.8 to 0.9 g/ml which give lipoproteins a unique density range that is lighter than that of the other plasma proteins. Notable landmarks in the separation of lipoproteins have been the development of ultracentrifugal flotation by Gofman and coworkers[1] and the development of electrophoretic separation techniques by Lees and Hatch.[2]

Lipoprotein Classification

The separation of different lipoproteins has been achieved by means of two principal techniques—electrophoresis and ultracentrifugation in salt solutions—and their classification is most commonly expressed in operational terms. On the basis of ultracentrifugal separation of plasma, four lipoprotein classes are recognized: chylomicrons, very-low-density lipoproteins (VLDL), low-density lipoproteins (LDL), and high-density lipoproteins (HDL). The relation between this ultracentrifugal classification and the size and electrophoretic mobility of lipoproteins is shown in Fig. 22-1. Further refinements in these density classes have been made and are a topic of considerable current interest. Low-density lipoproteins may be separated into two fractions: LDL_1 [also commonly referred to as intermediate-density lipoprotein, IDL; density (d) 1.006 to 1.019] and LDL_2 (d 1.019 to 1.063). High-density lipoproteins may be similarly divided into HDL_2 (d 1.063 to 1.125) and HDL_3 (d 1.125 to 1.21).

In addition to this operational classification, Alaupovic[3] has proposed a concept of lipoprotein families each of which is distinguished by its apoprotein moiety. These moieties are designated alphabetically as apo-A, apo-B, apo-C, apo-D, and apo-E. The apo-A family in turn contains two separate apoproteins designated A-I and A-II, whereas the C family has three: C-I, C-II, and C-III. The distribution of these apoproteins within the four operational density classes is shown in Table 22-1. It is evident that when lipoproteins are classified according to their density, each class represents a polydisperse system of particles which differ in size, hydrated density, and constituent

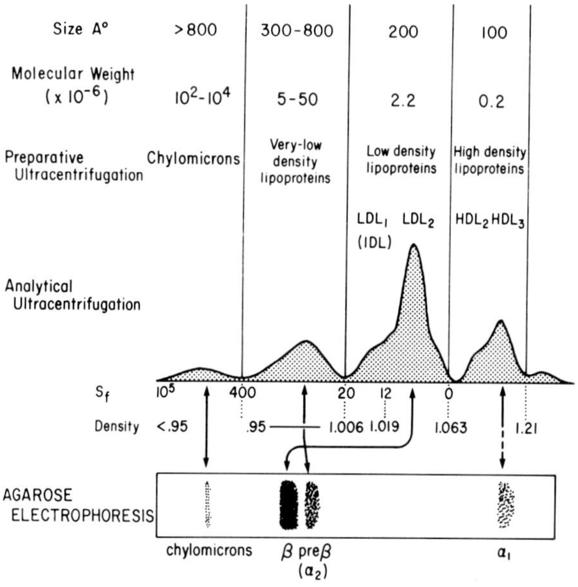

FIGURE 22-1 Diagrammatic representation of the major classes and properties of human lipoproteins separated by electrophoresis and ultracentrifugation.

Table 22-1. Apoprotein Content of Human Plasma Lipoproteins

Chylomicrons	VLDL	LDL	HDL
Major apoproteins			
Apo B-48	Apo B-100	Apo B-100	Apo A-I
Apo C-I	Apo C-I		Apo A-II
Apo C-II	Apo C-II		
Apo C-III	Apo C-III		
Apo E	Apo E		
Minor apoproteins			
Apo A-I	Apo D		Apo C-I
Apo A-II			Apo C-II
Apo A-IV			Apo C-III
Apo D			Apo D
			Apo E

Note: Apoproteins A-I, A-II, and A-IV each constitute 5 to 10 percent of the apoproteins in lymph chylomicrons but are minor components of the chylomicron particles present in plasma.

apoproteins. In contrast, the lipoprotein family classification[4] defines five families, each of which consists of a polydisperse system of lipid-apoprotein associations characterized by the presence of a single distinct apoprotein or its constituent polypeptides. We shall rely on the operational definition in this review. For further discussion of the lipoprotein-family concept, the reader is referred to the review by Osborne and Brewer.[4]

Lipoprotein Composition

CHYLOMICRONS

Chylomicrons are the largest of the lipoprotein particles whose primary role in the transport of exogenously derived fat from the intestine is well defined. Their size varies from 800 to 10,000 Å, with larger particles being produced under conditions of high dietary fat intake. The larger particles contain relatively more triglycerides and less polar phospholipids and free cholesterol than their smaller counterparts. Typical values for the composition of plasma chylomicrons are shown in Table 22-2. Following a lipid-rich meal, the fatty acid composition of chylomicron triglycerides generally resembles that of consumed dietary fat, although with lower fat intakes the proportions of linoleic acid, which is derived from biliary lecithin, are higher. The large size and high triglyceride content of chylomicrons are responsible for the lactescent appearance of plasma with a high content of these particles. When present, a chylomicron layer will float to the surface of plasma stored overnight at 4°C. Despite their low content of protein, the A, B, and C apoproteins all appear to be integral components of chylomicrons. Recent research[5,6] has shown that the apoprotein B secreted from the intestine differs from that secreted from the liver of most mammalian species. The two proteins appear to be closely related immunologically, but the intestinal protein, which is termed *B-48*, has a lower apparent molecular weight and a primary structure distinct from that of the hepatogenous protein, which is termed B-100. Because of apoprotein transfer reactions, the C-apoprotein content of chylomicrons isolated from plasma is higher

Table 22-2. Composition of Human Plasma Lipoproteins

	Chylomicrons	VLDL	LDL	HDL
Protein	2	8	21	50
Phospholipid	7	19	22	23
Cholesterol-free	2	7	8	4
Cholesterol ester	5	13	37	18
Triglyceride	84	51	11	4
Nonesterified fatty acid		2	1	1

Note: Values are expressed as percent total dry weight of the lipoprotein.

than that of similar particles isolated from thoracic-duct lymph. The reverse situation is true for apoproteins A-I, A-II, and A-IV, whose concentrations are higher in chylomicron particles isolated from lymph compared with their plasma counterparts. As will be discussed later, such a transfer is physiologically important in the activation of lipoprotein lipase and subsequent hydrolysis of chylomicron triglycerides.

VERY-LOW-DENSITY LIPOPROTEINS

Very-low-density lipoproteins (VLDL), which are the major transport vehicle for endogenous triglycerides in plasma, are smaller than chylomicrons and constitute a heterogeneous series of particles ranging in diameter from 300 to 800 Å. Typical values for VLDL composition are shown in Tables 22-1 and 22-2. The size of VLDL particles is sufficient to scatter transmitted light and gives plasma containing these particles a turbid appearance. However, in contrast to lipemia due to chylomicrons, the turbidity due to VLDL does not separate after storage of plasma for 12 to 18 h at 4°C. Various methods have been used to show that the size heterogeneity of VLDL particles is paralleled by variations in both their lipid and their protein composition. Larger particles contain relatively more of the nonpolar triglycerides and less phospholipid and cholesterol than their smaller counterparts. Thus, as a VLDL particle gets smaller, its relative content of both free and esterified cholesterol is increased. The proportion of C peptides present is also directly related to the size and triglyceride content of the VLDL particle, whereas the B-protein content shows an inverse relation with these parameters. VLDL particles contain the higher-molecular-weight form of apoprotein B termed *B-100*, which is the same apoprotein B present in LDL but is different from the B-48 protein present in chylomicrons.[7]

LOW-DENSITY LIPOPROTEINS

Low-density lipoproteins (β-lipoproteins) are the major carrier of cholesterol, cholesterol ester, and phospholipid in human plasma. The LDL molecule has a molecular weight of 2.2×10^6 and is composed of 20 to 25 percent protein and 75 to 80 percent lipid (Tables 22-1 and 22-2). Apo-B (B-100) constitutes more than 95 percent of the protein content of LDL, with trace quantities of A, C, and E apoproteins also being present. Lower-density fractions of LDL do, however, contain higher proportions of apo-E and the C peptides, but apo-B still contributes more than 90 percent of the total protein.

HIGH-DENSITY LIPOPROTEINS

High-density lipoproteins (α-lipoproteins) are the heaviest (*d* 1.063 to 1.21) and smallest (diameter 90 to 120 Å) of the human lipoproteins and contain about equal proportions of lipid and protein (Table 22-2). Apo-A-I (55 percent) and A-II (30 percent) constitute the major apoproteins in HDL, with smaller quantities of apo-C, apo-D, and apo-E also being present. The lipoproteins isolated in the HDL density range have frequently been further separated into HDL_2 (*d* 1.063 to 1.125) and HDL_3 (*d* 1.125 to 1.21). The latter are smaller and contain relatively more apo-A-I and apo-A-II and less apo-C and apo-E. Although the significance of HDL_2 and HDL_3 in physiological terms remains unclear, the concentration of HDL_2 is some three times higher in premenopausal women than in men. Perturbations in HDL levels caused by factors such as increased exercise also seem to specifically increase the concentrations of HDL_2 in plasma.

ABNORMAL LIPOPROTEINS

Certain pathological conditions may be associated with the presence of abnormal lipoprotein particles in plasma. This is most commonly seen in patients with cholestasis in which an abnormal cholesterol-rich lipoprotein termed lipoprotein X (LPX) is present in plasma.[8,9] Lipoprotein X appears as bilamellar discoidal structures measuring 40 to 60 nm in diameter and 10 nm in thickness when studied under electron microscopy. Lipoprotein X contains phospholipid and free cholesterol in a 1:1 molar ratio and albumin and apoproteins C-I, C-II, and C-III as the protein moieties. The cholesterol ester content is low. The lecithin contained in LPX contains fatty acid moieties of similar composition to those of biliary lecithin, and this lipoprotein is believed to contain phospholipid and cholesterol which are transported into plasma when their normal route of excretion in bile is impaired. Similar lipoprotein particles also occur in the plasma of patients with lecithin cholesterol acyltransferase deficiency.[10]

The Apoproteins

STRUCTURE

The apoprotein moieties of plasma lipoproteins have in common the requirement that they bind and transport lipid in the bloodstream. During the past decade, major advances have occurred which have delineated the synthesis, structure, and function of these unique proteins. Seven apoproteins—apo-A-I, apo-A-II, apo-A-IV, apo-C-I, apo-C-II, apo-C-III, and apo-E—have been extensively purified, and their complete amino acid sequences have been determined.[11-13] All these apoproteins have one common structural feature: a domain containing an amphipathic helix.[14] The amino acid sequences of these regions of the protein are such that hydrophobic amino acids are arranged on one side of the helix and hydrophilic polar amino acids form the other side. The hydrophobic face of the helix is thought to interact with the acyl chains of phospholipids, whereas the hydrophilic region faces the polar region of phospholipid head groups. With the exception of apoprotein B, all the apoproteins appear capable of dissociating from one lipoprotein particle and moving to another. This movement of apoproteins between lipoproteins not only serves to enhance metabolic processing of given lipoprotein particles, it also prolongs the residence time of the apoproteins in plasma. Despite its high concentration in plasma, apoprotein B remains the least well characterized of the major apoproteins, a fact that is attributable in large part to the marked insolubility of the delipidated apoprotein in aqueous solutions. The Lp(a) lipoprotein contains a second incompletely characterized protein, apo(a), in association with apoprotein B. The structure and function of Lp(a) are not known.

Studies of the biosynthesis of several apoproteins have indicated that the apoproteins are initially synthesized as preapolipoproteins or preproapolipoproteins, with pre and pro segments of the apolipoprotein being cleaved posttranslationally within the cell or following secretion of the proapolipoprotein into plasma.[15-18] The cDNA and genomic clones for apoproteins A-I, C-III, E, and C-II have been isolated and characterized.[19-22] The genes for apolipoproteins A-I and C-III have been localized to chromosome 11, whereas the genes for apoprotein C-II, apoprotein E, and the low-density lipoprotein receptor are known to be localized on chromosome 19. Application of the techniques of modern molecular biology to plasma apolipoproteins has resulted in the identification of regulatory and structural mutations in the genes for these apoproteins, several of which appear to predispose individuals to dyslipoproteinemias and the premature development of atherosclerosis. Different allelic forms of apoprotein E resulting from amino acid substitutions in the receptor-binding region of this apoprotein have been described and underlie susceptibility to type III hyperlipoproteinemia. A variety of apolipoprotein A-I isoproteins resulting from amino acid substitutions have also been described, and it is likely that many more variations will be identified in the future. In addition to variations in apoprotein composition caused by amino acid substitutions resulting from structural gene mutations, differences in the sialic acid content of apoproteins also contribute to the apparent variations detected on isoelectric focusing. For example, three forms of apoprotein C-III can be resolved by means of isoelectric focusing; apoprotein C-III_0 contains no sialic acid, apoprotein C-III_1 has 1 mol of sialic acid per mole of protein, and apoprotein C-III_2 has 2 mol.[23] Various dietary and hormonal manipulations have been shown to alter the degree of sialation of apo-C-III.[24]

The major sites of biosynthesis of apolipoproteins are the liver and the intestinal mucosal cells; both organs appear to contribute to the plasma pool of apoproteins of the A and C families as well as apoprotein E. Current data[7] indicate that the biosynthesis of human apoprotein B-48 occurs exclusively in the intestine, whereas apoprotein B-100 appears to be exclusively of hepatic origin. Recent studies have also indicated that the biosynthesis of apoprotein E occurs in many nonhepatic tissues, including muscle and macrophages.[25] Muscle tissue also appears capable of synthesizing apolipoprotein A-I.[26]

FUNCTION

In addition to their structural role in maintaining lipoprotein stability, several apolipoproteins are known to play distinct roles in the intravascular metabolism and cellular uptake of lipoproteins (Table 22-3). Apolipoprotein C-II serves as a cofactor for lipoprotein lipase, the enzyme which hydrolyzes the triglycerides on plasma chylomicrons and VLDL,[27] and a deficiency of apo-C-II is associated with severe hypertriglyceridemia.[28] The infusion of normal plasma or isolated apo-C-II fractions dramatically reduces the hypertriglyceridemia seen in patients with apo-C-II deficiency.[28,29] Apolipoprotein A-I, the major apoprotein in HDL, is a cofactor for lecithin cholesterol acyltransferase (LCAT), a plasma enzyme that catalyzes the conversion of cholesterol and phosphatidylcholine to cholesterol esters and lysophosphatidylcholine.[30] Apo-C-I may also serve as an activator of LCAT.

Distinct roles for apoprotein E and apoprotein B-100 in the cellular uptake of lipoprotein particles have been well established. The uptake of chylomicron and VLDL remnant particles is dependent on a specific hepatic receptor which recognizes apoprotein E contained in these lipoprotein particles and facilitates its removal from plasma.[31] A single amino acid substitution between residues 140 and 160 of the 299 amino acid sequence of apoprotein E can profoundly affect receptor binding, and a substitution of cysteine for arginine at residue 158 is primarily responsible for the decreased receptor binding which is believed to underlie the clinical development of type III hyper-

Table 22-3. Metabolic Functions of Plasma Apoproteins

Apoprotein	Molecular weight	Metabolic role
A-I	28,000	Activates LCAT
A-II	17,500	Activates hepatic lipase; may inhibit LCAT
A-IV	46,000	Unknown
B-48	210,000	Transport of lipids from the gut as chylomicrons
B-100	350,000	Transport of lipids from the liver as VLDL and LDL; recognized by cellular LDL receptors
C-I	7,000	Activates LCAT
C-II	9,000	Activates lipoprotein lipase
C-III	9,000	May inhibit activation of lipoprotein lipase by apo C-II
D	22,000	May be involved in lipid transfer between lipoproteins
E	34,000	Recognized by hepatic apo E receptors and cellular LDL receptors; recognition facilitates hepatic uptake of chylomicron and VLDL remnants
Transfer proteins	Variable	Facilitate the transfer of triglycerides, phospholipids, and cholesterol esters between lipoproteins

lipoproteinemia.[31] The synthesis of apoprotein B-48 within intestinal mucosal cells and of apoprotein B-100 within the liver appears necessary for the normal formation of chylomicron and VLDL-LDL particles, respectively. Although the hepatic uptake of chylomicron remnants does not apparently require an interaction of apoprotein B-48 with hepatic receptors, the removal of LDL from plasma is facilitated by specific receptors which recognize a region of the apoprotein B-100 contained in LDL. Chemical modification of LDL with agents that block the charge on lysine or arginine residues inhibits the recognition of LDL by specific high-affinity LDL receptors and blocks this receptor-mediated pathway of cellular LDL uptake without having an apparent effect on receptor-independent pathways.[32]

Lipoprotein Structure

When viewed under the electron microscope, all normal lipoproteins appear as spherical particles without any discernible subunit structure.[11] The nonpolar triglycerides and cholesterol esters are found in the central core of the lipoprotein particle, and the more polar phospholipids and free cholesterol are found at the surface. The apoproteins are also thought to be primarily located in an alpha-helical arrangement at the surface, although apolar regions of the protein chain may extend into the milieu of the lipid core. This lipid-core model is consistent with the greater exchange of phospholipids and free cholesterol compared with the exchange of triglyceride and cholesterol esters between lipoproteins.[11]

SYNTHESIS AND CATABOLISM OF LIPIDS AND LIPOPROTEINS

Lipids

CHOLESTEROL

In the schemata for the cholesterol balance of the body (see Table 22-4), cholesterol is synthesized from acetate by the liver and intestinal mucosa and released into the plasma in lipoproteins. Cholesterol biosynthesis is regulated in the liver by the enzyme 3-hydroxy-3-methylglutaryl coenzyme A reductase (HMG CoA reductase). This enzyme catalyzes the production of mevalonic acid, which is converted to

Table 22-4. The Cholesterol Balance of the Body

	Milligrams per day
Input	
From synthesis	500–1000
Absorbed from the diet	0– 400
	500–1400
Output	
Excretion in the bile (cholesterol and bile acids) and subsequently in the feces	400–1300
Skin excretion	80– 100
Synthesis of steroid hormones	Variable
Losses during pregnancy and lactation	Variable
Storage in the tissues	Variable
	500–1400

cholesterol. Cholesterol absorbed from the diet also enters the body pool of cholesterol and thus provides a second major source of cholesterol which circulates in the plasma. Only about 40 percent of dietary cholesterol is absorbed by the intestine. While all cells in the body have the capacity to synthesize cholesterol, in most cells cholesterol is utilized for membrane formation within the cell and does not contribute en masse to the plasma cholesterol concentration.

A variety of circumstances favor cholesterol biosynthesis, including excessive calories in the diet, saturated fat in the diet, and perhaps the total fat content of the diet. Cholesterol synthesis is depressed with hypocaloric and starvation diets. As will be indicated in Pharmaceutical Agents, some of these agents act by altering cholesterol biosynthesis, although in general the earlier agents such as triparanol, which inhibited a late stage in cholesterol biosynthesis, proved too toxic for therapeutic use.

Cholesterol synthesis may also be inhibited by the presence of cholesterol in the liver cells; this is known as *feedback inhibition*. Likewise, the presence of bile acids through feedback inhibition tends to inhibit the synthesis of further bile acids from cholesterol. In humans, however, the inhibition of cholesterol biosynthesis is never sufficient such that a rise in plasma cholesterol concentration will not occur if a sufficient quantity of cholesterol is present in the diet.

Besides the efflux of cholesterol from the plasma as carried by LDL to supply cholesterol for membranes in growing cells, cholesterol from the plasma may be utilized for the synthesis of the steroid hormones and bile acids.

The primary route of excretion of cholesterol from the body begins in the liver, where it is secreted directly into the bile and where bile acids are synthesized from cholesterol and excreted in the bile. Thus the chief pathway of excretion of cholesterol from the body ultimately occurs via the feces, where this steroid nucleus appears either as cholesterol or as its bacterially altered products coprosterol (coprostanol) and coprostanone and as bile acids. The bile acids in the stool represent the small fraction excreted in the bile and not absorbed by the enterohepatic circulation. The usual output of cholesterol from the body is approximately 600 to 1000 mg per day. About 60 percent of the output is as cholesterol (or coprostanol), and the other 40 percent is as the secondary bile acids.

Cholesterol ester is the predominant circulating form of cholesterol, with some 70 to 80 percent of the total plasma cholesterol being esterified through the action of the LCAT enzyme, as will be discussed subsequently. The predominant cholesterol ester is cholesterol linoleate, followed by cholesterol oleate, cholesterol palmitate, and cholesterol stearate. Some arachidonic acid is also transported as a cholesterol ester. The cholesterol of the bodily tissues is largely in the free form, except for the storage of cholesterol ester in the adrenal glands and other steroid-synthesizing endocrine glands, where it becomes readily available for synthesis of steroid hormones under conditions of rapid need. Some cholesterol ester is also present in the liver, but in general normal tissues contain only free cholesterol, which is present primarily in cell membranes; of course, cholesterol ester predominates in atheroma and xanthoma. Finally, it must be appreciated that cholesterol is unique in that once it is present in the body, it remains until it is excreted. The steroid nucleus cannot be broken down by the tissues, unlike lipids such as triglyceride.

TRIGLYCERIDE

Like cholesterol, the triglyceride of the plasma lipoproteins is synthesized either by the intestinal tract (from absorbed fatty acids) or by the liver from both acetate and fatty acids and enters the plasma in the form of one of the four major lipoprotein classes: chylomicrons, VLDL, LDL, and HDL. The plasma triglyceride constitutes a readily available source of energy for the body, again through the action of lipoprotein lipase at the cellular level. The free fatty acid produced from the hydrolysis of triglyceride is then taken up by the cells of the body either for storage, as in adipose tissue, or for oxidation by muscle cells. Thus hypertriglyceridemia can result from oversynthesis or impaired catabolism or a combination of both circumstances. Caloric excess and adiposity apparently favor both increased synthesis of triglycerides in liver and gut and impaired removal by the peripheral tissues.

PHOSPHOLIPIDS

The plasma phospholipids are derived almost entirely from synthesis in the liver and intestinal mucosa but can be synthesized by most body tissues. Dietary phospholipids are not absorbed as such and undergo hydrolysis by phospholipases in the intestinal juices with formation of both lysophosphatides and the basic constituent phosphorus-containing amine, 2 mol of fatty acids, and glycerol. Phospholipids are catabolized as components of their respective lipoproteins and also readily exchange between lipoproteins and cell membranes. Catabolism of individual phospholipids may proceed to their basic constituents or may undergo deacylation-reacylation reactions during which the fatty acid composition is altered. Lysolecithin may be formed by tissue phospholipases or may be formed in plasma by LCAT, and this somewhat toxic molecule is rapidly metabolized.

Enzymes Active in Lipoprotein Metabolism

Two enzymes—lipoprotein lipase (LPL) and lecithin cholesterol acyltransferase (LCAT)—the activity of which may be measured in plasma, are of physiological importance in lipoprotein metabolism.

LECITHIN CHOLESTEROL ACYLTRANSFERASE

The enzyme LCAT catalyzes the transfer of fatty acid from the 2 position of phosphatidylcholine to cholesterol with the formation of cholesterol ester and lysophosphatidyl choline[33] (Fig. 22-2). Current evidence suggests that this enzyme is responsible for the formation of most of the esterified cholesterol present in plasma, although lesser amounts of cholesterol ester also enter plasma as native constituents of VLDL and probably as chylomicrons. Phosphatidylcholine and free cholesterol present on HDL are the preferred substrate for LCAT, for which apo-A-I, the major apoprotein of HDL, and apo-C-I act as specific activators. The enzyme itself is secreted by the liver and is present in plasma, lymph, and cerebrospinal fluid. LCAT shows fatty acid specificity, which results in the preferential formation of cholesterol linoleate. The absence of LCAT has been described in a rare disease which will be discussed later.

LIPOPROTEIN LIPASE AND HEPATIC LIPASE

Lipoprotein lipase is an important tissue enzyme that is responsible for clearance of the triglyceride-rich lipoproteins, chylomicrons, and VLDL. Distinct forms of LPL appear to be present in adipose tissue and muscle, but their physiological functions are similar. Both enzymes are present on capillary endothelial cells, where they hydrolyze lipoprotein triglycerides, liberating fatty acids which are picked up by the peripheral tissues. Classically, when LPL is absent, familial type I hyperchylomicronemia occurs. This enzyme may be functionally inactive in type V hyperlipidemia and in other hypertriglyceridemia states. It is reduced in starvation and in diabetes. A second distinct enzyme, hepatic lipase, is present on liver cell membranes and may play a role in the catabolism of chylomicron and VLDL remnants as well as in the hepatic uptake of HDL.[34]

Not normally present in the blood, LPL is released into the plasma after the parenteral administration of heparin and can be specifically identified as such. Since hepatic lipase is also released into the plasma after heparin, these two triglyceride-splitting enzymes must be separately measured, as discussed in Laboratory Tests, before LPL deficiency can be specifically identified.

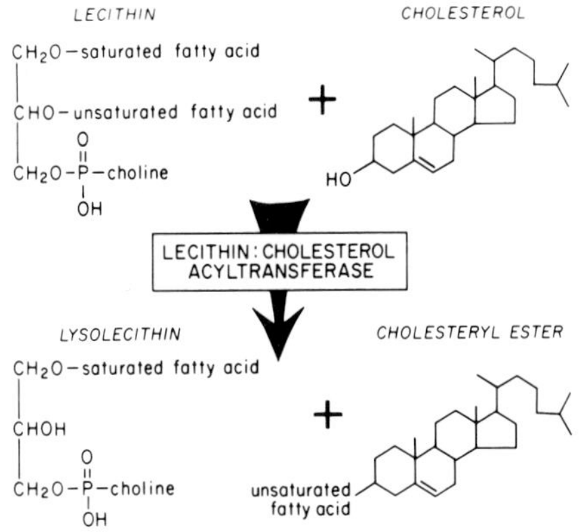

FIGURE 22-2 Lipid reactants in the plasma lecithin cholesterol acyltransferase reaction. (*Reproduced from Glomset et al.*[33] *with permission.*)

Lipoprotein Metabolism

CHYLOMICRONS

Chylomicrons are synthesized by the small intestine, principally the jejunum, in response to the absorption of dietary fat. Following a fat-rich meal, lipids are hydrolyzed in the intestinal lumen; the digestive products are then absorbed and utilized in the synthesis of triglycerides, cholesterol esters, and phospholipids within the mucosal cell. Synthesis of apoproteins A-I, A-II, A-IV, and B-48, and possibly some C and E apoproteins, occurs concurrently, and the resultant chylomicron particle is subsequently released from the mucosal cell into the lacteals, from where it progresses to enter the systemic circulation via the thoracic duct. Fatty acids with a chain length less than 12 carbon atoms are transported in the portal blood.

Upon entry into the systemic circulation, chylomicrons are metabolized rapidly with a half-life of 5 to 15 min. Transfer of apo-A-I and A-II to HDL and reciprocal transfers of C and E apoproteins from HDL serve to enhance the hydrolysis of chylomicron triglycerides by lipoprotein lipase and provide a source of chylomicron surface components which act as a precursor of nascent HDL particles. Hydrolysis of chylomicron triglycerides by this enzyme occurs at the endothelial cell surface and results in chylomicron remnants that are relatively enriched in cholesterol. These particles are taken up by the liver via specific apo-E receptors (and possibly the apo-B or LDL receptor), where they are catabolized. As previously discussed, apo-E is the apoprotein responsible for receptor-mediated clearance of chylomicron (and VLDL) remnants by the liver. Such uptake results in an increased hepatic cholesterol content and is associated with a decrease in de novo cholesterol synthesis.

VERY-LOW-DENSITY LIPOPROTEINS

The liver is the major site of synthesis of VLDL, with a minor contribution being derived from the intestine. Transport of endogenous triglyceride from the liver to peripheral tissues is probably the principal function of VLDL, but it also serves as the major precursor of LDL (Fig. 22-3). Many factors, including the basal diet; time of day; levels of insulin, glucagon, and epinephrine in plasma; and degree of adiposity, appear to modulate the rate of secretion of hepatic VLDL. Apo-B-100 appears essential for VLDL synthesis. Like chylomicrons, newly secreted VLDL rapidly acquires some C and possibly E apoproteins from HDL in plasma; this gain in apo-C-II in turn increases their susceptibility to hydrolysis by lipoprotein lipase. Clearance of VLDL is slower than that of chylomicrons, and their half-life in plasma is 6 to 12 h. Hydrolysis of VLDL triglycerides and phospholipids by lipoprotein lipase and hepatic lipase results in a progressively smaller particle with lower S_f but with a constant content of apoprotein B. The content of C and E apoproteins in VLDL, however, decreases as the particle is metabolized and these proteins are transferred back to HDL. Hepatic apo-E receptors facilitate the removal and catabolism of VLDL remnants; this process is abnormal in patients with apo-E variants (e.g., E-2) that have reduced receptor binding. HDL functions as a reservoir for the C apoproteins, and such transfer reactions between VLDL and HDL serve an economical role and prolong the half-life of the C apoproteins in plasma. In normolipidemic humans, virtually all the B apoprotein that enters plasma as a constituent of VLDL is preserved as the particle is metabolized to intermediate-density lipoproteins (IDL) and eventually to LDL. In contrast, in patients with severe hypertriglyceridemia, most of the VLDL particles are removed prior to conversion to LDL, and LDL concentrations are low. In addition to apo-B, a considerable proportion of the phospholipid, free cholesterol, and some of the cholesterol esters of the plasma VLDL are retained during metabolism of the latter to LDL. This precursor-product relation between VLDL and LDL may be seen clinically in patients with type IV hyperlipidemia who are treated with either diet or drugs. In such cases, initial falls in VLDL are not uncommonly accompanied by reciprocal rises in LDL.

LOW-DENSITY LIPOPROTEINS

In humans, most of the LDL in plasma are derived from the intravascular catabolism of VLDL; LDL may therefore be regarded as the end product of VLDL metabolism (Fig. 22-3). Catabolism of LDL occurs in both peripheral cells and the liver (the liver is the major site of removal) and is facilitated by both receptor-mediated and non-receptor-mediated pathways.[35,36] The turnover of LDL is considerably slower than that of VLDL; the half-life in normal humans is from 3 to 4 days and is prolonged in patients with familial hypercholesterolemia. Based largely on the elegant studies of Goldstein and Brown,[35,36] a variety of cells have been shown to contain specific receptors for LDL. The uptake of LDL by cells results in suppression of endogenous cholesterol biosynthesis, an enhanced rate of intracellular cholesterol esterification, and a reduction in the number of high-affinity LDL receptors expressed on the cell surface (Fig. 22-4).

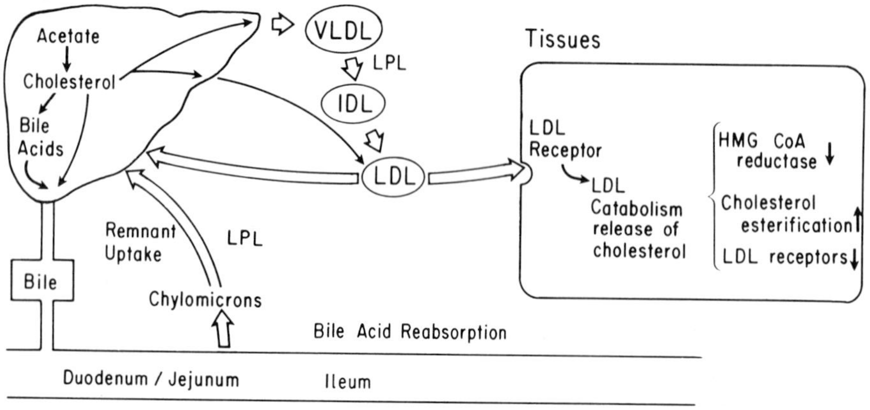

FIGURE 22-3 Metabolism and transport of lipoproteins in humans and the cellular changes that result from receptor-mediated uptake of low-density lipoproteins.

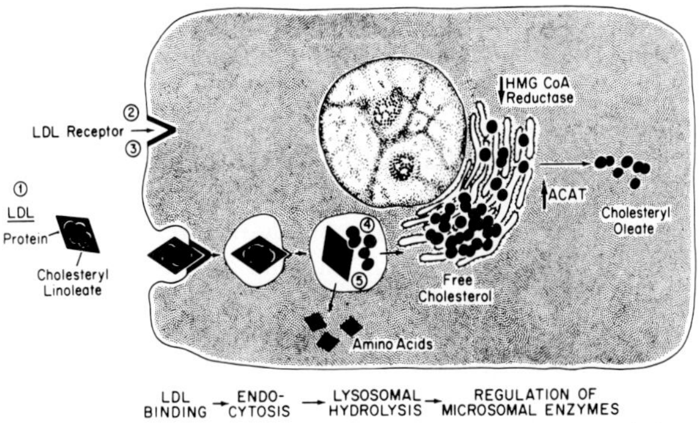

FIGURE 22-4 Sequential steps in the pathway of LDL metabolism in cultured human fibroblasts. The numbers indicate the sites in the pathway in which mutations have been identified (see text): (1) abetalipoproteinemia, (2) familial hypercholesterolemia, receptor-negative type, (3) familial hypercholesterolemia, receptor-defective type, (4) Wolman's syndrome, and (5) cholesterol ester storage disease. The central role of the LDL receptor in controlling the binding, uptake, lysosomal hydrolysis, and regulation of cholesterol synthesis and cholesterol ester formation is illustrated. (*Reproduced from Fredrickson, Goldstein, and Brown*[45] *with permission.*)

Functional high-affinity LDL receptors are absent from the cells of most patients with homozygous familial hypercholesterolemia. Although the liver is quantitatively the most important organ for removal of LDL from plasma, the *relative* rate of uptake is greatest in certain endocrine tissues (e.g., adrenal cortex and corpus luteum of the ovary) which have a high capacity for the synthesis of steroid hormones for which cholesterol contained in LDL serves as an important precursor.[37,38] Clinical and epidemiologic studies have shown a strong positive relation between elevated levels of LDL cholesterol and an increased risk of cardiovascular morbidity and mortality.

HIGH-DENSITY LIPOPROTEINS

The synthesis and secretion of HDL from the liver are well documented.[39] In addition, some HDL particles are also derived from the surface components of chylomicrons and VLDL particles during lipolysis (Fig. 22-5). This dual etiology for HDL explains the inverse correlation between plasma triglycerides and HDL as well as the known presence of HDL in patients with abetalipoproteinemia (who do not form chylomicrons and VLDL). Newly secreted HDL appears as flat, disk-shaped structures containing predominantly protein, phospholipid, and free cholesterol. When exposed to the action of LCAT, these particles are converted to spherical particles that are enriched in cholesterol esters. Indeed, the formation of cholesterol esters in plasma catalyzed by LCAT appears to be an important function of HDL. HDL also provides a reservoir for C apoproteins which transfer to chylomicrons and VLDL during alimentary lipemia and which subsequently move back to HDL with clearance of the larger fat-rich particles from plasma. The half-life of HDL, as assessed by that of apo-A-I and A-II, is from 4 to 6 days and is influenced by both diet and drugs. Thus diets high in carbohydrate which raise VLDL cause a lowering of HDL and an enhanced HDL turnover. Similarly, nicotinic acid, which depresses VLDL synthesis, raises HDL levels and prolongs the half-life. Both effects on HDL metabolism probably are a consequence of primary changes in VLDL synthesis and flux and support the general view that VLDL and HDL levels change reciprocally. On the basis of animal experiments, it has been concluded that the major site of HDL catabolism is the liver, although evidence to support this view in humans is not available. Glomset and Norum[10] have proposed that an additional major function of HDL is to transport cholesterol from peripheral tissues back to the liver. Thus high levels of HDL may enhance removal of cholesterol from tissues, including the arterial wall, and protect against the development of atherosclerosis. Several factors have been shown to increase the concentrations of HDL in plasma,[40] and fluctuations in total HDL concentrations are usually due to alterations in the levels in the ligher HDL_2 subfraction. Variations in the concentration of HDL_2 also show the strongest inverse correlation with cardiovascular risk; thus increased concentrations of HDL_2 are viewed as protective, whereas low concentrations may be detrimental. Factors which have been shown to increase the concentrations of HDL include moderate ethanol consumption,[41] sustained regular exercise, correction of hypertriglyceridemia, and certain drugs including phenobarbital, phenytoin, clofibrate, estrogens, nicotinic acid, and gemfibrozil. Decreases in the

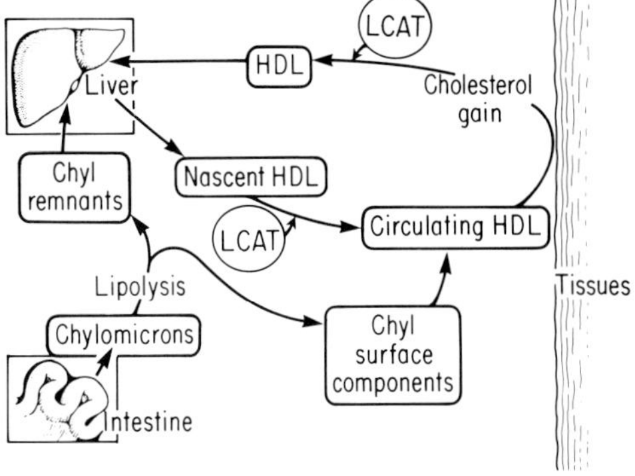

FIGURE 22-5 Diagrammatic representation of the origin and intravascular metabolism of high-density lipoproteins.

plasma concentrations of HDL may be seen in association with weight gain, cigarette smoking, hypertriglyceridemia, and the use of probucol.

FREE FATTY ACIDS

Free fatty acids (FFA) constitute the fifth class of lipoproteins. They consist of long-chain fatty acids bound to albumin, occupying up to two tight binding sites on the albumin molecule; if FFA levels are elevated, additional looser binding sites are then occupied. FFA constitute a major metabolic fuel of the body. They are derived from lipolysis of triglycerides stored in the adipose-tissue cell. The tissue lipase in these cells is under neuroendocrine control and operates through the adenyl cyclase system. A second origin of FFA is through the hydrolysis of plasma triglyceride present in chylomicrons and VLDL through the action of lipoprotein lipase.

FFA have a very short half-life of 4 to 8 min and are readily taken up from plasma by the muscle cells of the body. A second pathway for their catabolism is uptake by the liver and resynthesis into triglyceride, which then may be transported from the liver in VLDL, or oxidation to acetyl CoA. Physiologically, FFA levels may rise and fall in the blood with great rapidity in order to meet the body's needs for this form of energy. Levels tend to be low after the absorption of carbohydrate and resulting insulin secretion but rise postprandially as the blood glucose falls. In the fasting state, levels of 400 to 600 μeq per liter are common; with a prolonged fast of 24 to 72 h, the levels of FFA may range from 1000 to 1500 μeq per liter. Glucagon, epinephrine, growth hormone, and adrenocorticotropic hormone (ACTH) may also increase FFA levels. The major physiological regulators of the plasma FFA are insulin and epinephrine.

The chief fatty acids of the plasma FFA fraction are oleic, palmitic, linoleic, and stearic acids, which reflect in most instances the composition of the adipose-tissue triglyceride. Three of these four fatty acids (oleic, palmitic, and stearic acids) may be synthesized by the body from acetate. Linoleic acid is unique in being an essential fatty acid which cannot be synthesized in humans but is necessary for the body's growth and for membrane formation. The syndrome of essential fatty acid deficiency results when linoleic acid accounts for less than 1 percent of the total calories in the diet, as occurs after prolonged total parenteral nutrition. Linoleic acid is of special importance as the precursor substance for arachidonic acid, which in turn has multitudinous functions, of which a most important one is as a precursor for prostaglandin formation.

Atherogenicity of Individual Lipoprotein Particles

The lipoprotein particles in human plasma all contain cholesterol, but the extent to which elevated levels of each of these particles may contribute to the development of atherosclerosis differs widely (Table 22-5). Whereas elevated levels of LDL and cholesterol-rich remnant particles, as occur in familial hypercholesterolemia and type III hyperlipoproteinemia, respectively, are highly atherogenic, increased levels of HDL cholesterol appear to afford protection from atherosclerosis.

Plasma concentrations of the major LDL apoprotein (apoprotein B) may provide a better prediction of the risk of coronary artery disease than measurement of LDL cholesterol. Similarly, plasma concentrations of the major HDL apoproteins (A-I and A-II) may be better discriminators for cardiovascular risk associated with low concentrations of HDL particles than are measurements of HDL cholesterol.[42–44] Hyperchylomicronemia as an isolated entity (e.g., that seen in patients with LPL deficiency) does not appear to be associated with an increased risk of atherosclerosis,[45] but concurrent or isolated elevations of VLDL do appear to be moderately atherogenic, as do lipoprotein particles produced from the intravascular hydrolysis of triglycerides from VLDL and chylomicrons.[46]

Table 22-5. Relative Atherogenicity of Individual Lipoprotein Particles

Lipoprotein	Atherogenicity	Typical associated dyslipoproteinemia
Chylomicrons (lipoprotein lipase deficiency)	0	Type I
VLDL	+	Type IV (familial hypertriglyceridemia)
Chylomicron and VLDL remnants	+++	Type III (dysbetalipoproteinemia)
LDL	++++	Type II (familial hypercholesterolemia)
HDL	Negatively correlated with atherosclerosis	Familial hyperalphalipoproteinemia

Table 22-6. Classification of Hyperlipidemias Based on Lipoprotein Concentrations

Type	Lipoprotein abnormality	Lipid profiles	Typical values, mg/dl
I	Chylomicrons markedly ↑, VLDL and LDL both normal or low	Chol ↑	320
		Tg ↑↑	4000
IIa	LDL ↑, VLDL normal	Chol ↑	370
		Tg N	90
IIb	LDL ↑, VLDL ↑	Chol ↑	350
		Tg ↑	400
III	Abnormal cholesterol-enriched VLDL present in excess	Chol ↑	500
		Tg ↑	700
IV	VLDL ↑, LDL normal	Chol N	220
		Tg ↑	400
V	Chylomicrons markedly ↑, VLDL ↑, LDL normal or low	Chol ↑	700
		Tg ↑↑	5000

Source: Based on Fredrickson, Levy, and Lees[47] and the WHO committee.[48]

THE HYPERLIPIDEMIAS

Classification of Hyperlipidemias

Classification of hyperlipidemias on the basis of plasma lipoprotein patterns, as originally proposed by Fredrickson, Levy, and Lees[47] and modified by the WHO,[48] is the most widely used system of nomenclature. As shown in Table 22-6, the six types are classified with respect to increased levels of chylomicrons, VLDL, and LDL. Although this classification provides a simple way in which to categorize increases in the concentrations of given lipoproteins, it does not provide any information about the etiology of the abnormality. Thus a given phenotype may occur as a primary genetic disorder or may be secondary to a variety of associated conditions. Similarly, this classification system does not consider variations in HDL concentrations as an independent variable. Despite these limitations, the Fredrickson classification provides a useful basis for describing most hyperlipoproteinemias.

Determination of the plasma concentrations of cholesterol and triglyceride constitutes the basic lipid profile in most patients. In discussing hyperlipoproteinemic states as they pertain to a given patient, we shall use the basic cholesterol and triglyceride determinations as a starting point and divide the discussion of hyperlipoproteinemias into three categories: (1) hypercholesterolemia with normal triglyceride concentrations (type IIa phenotype), (2) combined elevations of cholesterol and triglyceride in which the triglyceride levels are one to two times higher than the cholesterol values (phenotypes IIb and III), and (3) conditions that are associated with a primary elevation in the concentrations of triglyceride-rich lipoproteins and in which cholesterol levels are nearly normal (type IV phenotype) or are increased to a much smaller extent than are the triglyceride levels (type I and type V phenotypes). Disorders associated with variations in the concentrations of HDL will be discussed as separate entities.

Criteria for the Diagnosis of Hyperlipoproteinemia

The accurate determination of cholesterol and triglyceride represents the basic testing necessary for the diagnosis of most hyperlipidemias. Plasma concentrations of triglycerides increase postprandially, and for this reason the accurate determination of triglycerides requires the patient to have fasted 12 to 16 h before venipuncture. In contrast, cholesterol levels are minimally affected by eating, and casual blood samples are quite satisfactory if only cholesterol is to be determined. Patients with elevated levels of both cholesterol and triglyceride often require further characterization in order to distinguish between a type IIb and a type III phenotype, and in most other patients it is desirable to determine the concentrations of LDL and HDL cholesterol. In evaluating the results of lipid determinations, it is important to consider the age of the patient and have an idea of the appropriate normal values for that individual (with the caveat that values which are classed as "normal" in western societies may in fact be too high). Data from the Lipid Research Program[49] which document the mean and 95th percentile values of plasma lipids and lipoproteins are shown in Table 22-7. Although precise cutoffs for the designation of hyperlipidemia remain somewhat

Table 22-7. Normal Values for Lipids and Lipoproteins in American Men and Women*

Age	Total plasma cholesterol	LDL cholesterol	HDL cholesterol	Total plasma triglyceride
		Men		
20–24	162 (212)	103 (147)	45 (63)	89 (165)
25–29	179 (234)	117 (165)	45 (63)	104 (204)
30–34	193 (258)	126 (185)	46 (63)	122 (253)
35–39	201 (267)	133 (189)	43 (62)	141 (316)
40–44	205 (260)	136 (186)	44 (67)	152 (318)
45–49	213 (275)	144 (202)	45 (64)	143 (279)
50–54	213 (274)	142 (197)	44 (63)	154 (313)
		Women		
20–24	162	98	52	68
25–29	174 (222)	106 (151)	56 (81)	71 (128)
30–34	174 (220)	109 (148)	55 (75)	74 (138)
35–39	186 (251)	119 (173)	56 (82)	89 (174)
40–44	196 (253)	125 (174)	57 (87)	92 (179)
45–49	205 (267)	130 (188)	58 (86)	105 (192)
50–54	222 (292)	145 (214)	60 (89)	112 (214)
55–59	231 (296)	150 (212)	60 (86)	132 (280)

*Data obtained from 11 communities across the United States.[49] Values given in milligrams per deciliter are means and 95th percentiles (in parentheses) for white men and women.

arbitrary, patients in whom these values exceed the 75th and especially the 90th percentiles for age and sex constitute the group in which further evaluation and therapy is clearly indicated.[50,51]

Secondary Hyperlipidemias

DIETARY

In regard to secondary hyperlipidemias[52] (Table 22-8), the most common cause is dietary. Dietary hypercholesterolemia afflicts an appreciable proportion of the American population and begins early in life, as witness the much higher plasma cholesterol concentrations in American children than in children of other cultures (e.g., the Mexican Tarahumara Indians) in good health. American children have mean plasma cholesterol levels of 168 mg/dl, compared with the Tarahumara children, who consume a low-fat diet and have cholesterol levels of 118 mg/gl.[53] Tarahumara adults have values only a little higher (136 mg/dl), whereas in Americans there is a much greater rise with age to 230 mg/dl (Fig. 22-6) which continues to age 55 to 60 years.[54] This rise of plasma cholesterol with age is believed to be caused by a functional impairment of the LDL receptor.[55] The parallel rise of plasma triglyceride with age is related more to the age increase in obesity.

The dietary factors important in this environmental hyperlipidemia include the following: dietary

Table 22-8. Primary versus Secondary Hyperlipidemias

1. Primary: genetic
2. Secondary:
   a. Diet; excessive cholesterol, saturated fat, or calories
   b. Uncontrolled diabetes
   c. Alcohol
   d. Hypothyroidism
   e. Nephrotic syndrome
   f. Chronic renal failure
   g. Biliary obstruction; primary biliary cirrhosis
   h. Dysglobulinemia; autoimmune disease
   i. Glycogen storage disease
   j. Acute intermittent porphyria
   k. Cushing's syndrome
   l. Anorexia nervosa
   m. Hepatoma
   n. Drug-induced: corticosteroids, estrogens, thiazides, beta blockers, 13-*cis*-retinoic acid (isotretinoin, Accutane)

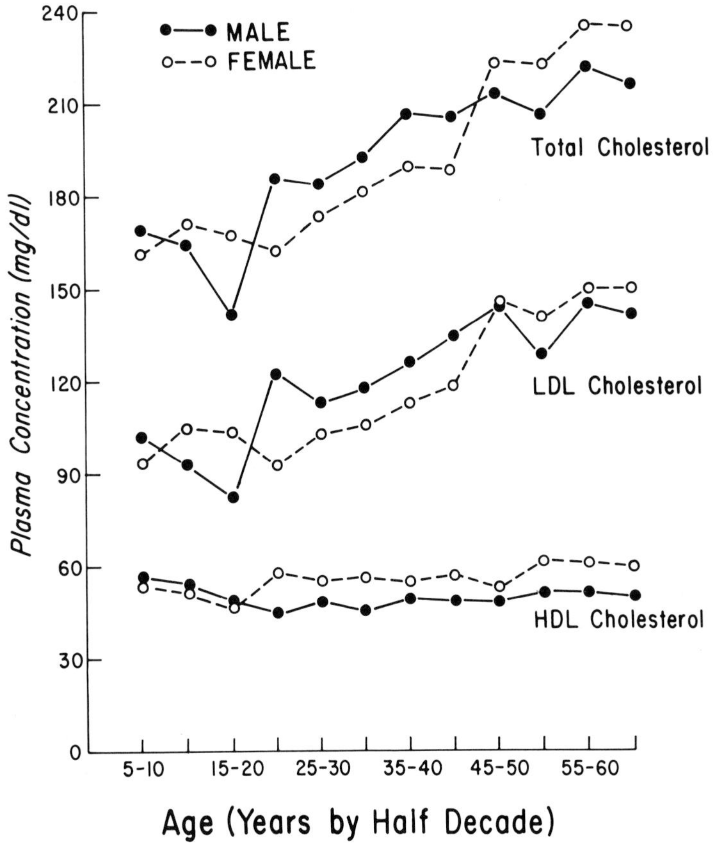

FIGURE 22-6 Age-related changes in the plasma concentrations of total, high-density, and low-density lipoprotein cholesterol in men and women aged 6 to 65 years. Data derived from lipid analyses on 619 subjects residing in Portland, Oregon. (*Reproduced from Connor et al.*[53] *with permission.*)

cholesterol, total fat intake, saturated fat, and excessive calories. Contributing also to this hyperlipidemia for various reasons may be deficiencies of unrefined carbohydrate, starch, fiber, and vegetable protein. How each of these nutritional substances affects the plasma cholesterol will be dealt with in Dietary Treatment of Hyperlipidemia, below.

DIABETES

The next most common form of secondary hyperlipidemia occurs in diabetic patients. Their hyperlipidemia may be associated with either diabetes mellitus per se or the prediabetic state, or it may coexist in the same patient with two primary defects: one of lipid metabolism and the other of carbohydrate metabolism. Diabetic patients with hyperlipidemia may be divided into the following groups:

1. The diabetic patient in ketoacidosis. Such an individual has impaired clearing of chylomicrons and VLDL, which results in elevated levels of triglyceride and, to a lesser extent, cholesterol and a type IV or V phenotype. Correction of the acidotic state by insulin will promptly ameliorate the hyperlipidemia, and since this is a temporary state, it does not present a long-term management problem. One reason for the hyperlipidemia of diabetic acidosis is that the enzyme lipoprotein lipase, which is responsible for the clearance of triglyceride from VLDL and chylomicrons, is deficient when insulin is insufficient at the cellular level. Increased production of hepatic VLDL also occurs in diabetic acidosis because of the extremely high circulating FFA levels derived from lipolysis of adipose-tissue triglyceride. FFA concentrations are always higher (800 to 1600 meq per liter) in poorly controlled diabetes and correlate directly with the blood glucose levels. When glucose cannot enter the cells because of absolute or relative insulin deficiency, the endocrine and biochemical effects are those of starvation. Triglyceride in adipose-tissue cells undergoes lipolysis, and plasma FFA levels increase greatly to provide this alternative energy source of the working cells of the body. FFA elevations may also promote vascular damage and platelet aggregation, although the clinical significance of this tendency to thrombosis has not been elucidated.

2. The second cause of hyperlipidemia in diabetes is relatively poor diabetic control. This is usually seen in overweight maturity-onset diabetics. The reason for the hyperlipidemia relates both to insulin deficiency at the cellular level, with impaired lipoprotein lipase action and reduced clearance of VLDL triglyceride, and to increased production of triglyceride, the latter propagated both by elevated concentrations of free fatty acids and by excessive caloric intake. Increased synthesis of cholesterol and its accumulation in low-density lipoproteins also occurs in such patients.[56]

3. The third cause of hyperlipidemia which relates more to hypercholesterolemia is the typical diet of high fat, high saturated fat, high cholesterol, and relatively low carbohydrate still in use in some diabetic patients. While there has been some moderation of this dietary approach, there still is a tendency to shun carbohydrate in the diet and to prefer a diet high in animal fat. This may lead to increased LDL production and levels. The underlying etiology of the profound atherosclerotic complications of diabetes is thus not appropriately recognized.

4. A fourth cause of hyperlipidemia in diabetics is the coexistence with diabetes of primary genetic hyperlipidemias, the most common of which are familial hypertriglyceridemia and familial combined hyperlipidemia.

Thus the lipoprotein abnormalities which may be found in diabetic patients run the gamut. Increases in chylomicrons, VLDL and their remnants, LDL, and FFA may occur, and concurrently HDL levels are frequently decreased.

HYPOTHYROIDISM

Apart from diabetes, hypothyroidism constitutes the most frequently seen endocrine disorder associated with secondary hyperlipidemia. Any of the lipoprotein phenotypes may occur in hypothyroidism, but elevations of plasma cholesterol in the range of 250 to 600 mg/dl with or without associated triglyceride elevation occurs most commonly, i.e., a IIa or IIb pattern. Types IV, III, and V occur with decreasing frequency. The degree of hyperlipidemia shows a positive correlation with the severity of hypothyroidism and in one study[57] was noted to occur only in patients with TSH levels $> 40\ \mu U/ml$ and T_4 levels $< 3.5\ \mu g/dl$. Hypothyroidism may also occur concurrently with familial hyperlipidemia, and in such cases plasma lipid elevations are more extreme. Indeed, young patients with the heterozygous form of familial hypercholesterolemia and hypothyroidism may present with lipid values and xanthomas resembling those seen in homozygous familial hypercholesterolemia.[58]

The mechanisms responsible for the hyperlipidemia of hypothyroidism include reduced high-affinity receptor-mediated catabolism of LDL, lower biliary excretion of cholesterol and bile acids, and decreased LPL activity. These factors more than counteract a concomitant decrease in cholesterol biosynthesis.

The hypolipidemic response which accompanies thyroid replacement is particularly gratifying. Plasma cholesterol values frequently return to normal within 3 to 6 weeks of full-replacement doses of thyroxine and begin to decline within days of the initiation of therapy. It is the authors' practice and recommendation to screen most hyperlipidemic patients for hypothyroidism in order not to overlook this rewarding diagnosis.

RENAL DISEASE

Hyperlipidemia is common in renal disease and may be manifested by a variety of lipid and lipoprotein abnormalities.[52] Three categories of hyperlipidemic renal patients may be observed: uremic patients undergoing dialysis, renal-transplant patients under immunosuppressive therapy with corticosteroids and azathioprine, and nephrotic patients. The characteristic abnormality in patients undergoing dialysis is hypertriglyceridemia with an increase in VLDL and a type IV pattern. These patients have reduced clearing of triglyceride from the plasma, presumably because LPL activity is reduced. Transplant patients most frequently have an elevation of LDL with hypercholesterolemia and a IIa pattern but commonly also show elevated levels of VLDL and triglycerides with a IV or IIb phenotype. Rarely, patients with type V hyperlipidemia have been observed after transplantation. While no mechanism for transplant hyperlipidemia has been described, it presumably is related to increased appetite, weight gain, and use of steroids.

Patients with the nephrotic syndrome frequently have a mixed form of hyperlipidemia with elevation of both plasma cholesterol and triglyceride levels (type IIb being the most common). The hyperlipidemia is roughly related to the hypoalbuminemia characteristic of this syndrome. Remission of the nephrotic state invariably brings about correction of the hyperlipidemia.

The numbers of patients with renal hyperlipidemia have dramatically increased in the past decade with the development of dialysis and transplantation programs and enhanced survival of patients with end-stage kidney disease. The major cause of death in these patients is atherosclerotic coronary heart disease. Carotid and aortoileofemoral atherosclerosis is also common and emphasizes the fact that therapeutic attention to the hyperlipidemic state is of great importance. Our observations are that the same principles of dietary management should be applied to patients with secondary renal hyperlipidemia, especially to the transplant population. Hyperlipidemic transplantation patients should be offered the maximum in dietary treatment. In those with normal renal function in whom control of hyperlipidemia has not been achieved, the use of hypolipidemic drugs is appropriate.

BILE-DUCT OBSTRUCTION, $ALPHA_1$ ANTITRYPSIN DEFICIENCY

Hyperlipidemia invariably occurs with impairment of bile flow. This secondary hyperlipidemia is always seen in biliary cirrhosis and biliary atresia in which the hyperlipidemia is profound, with plasma cholesterol values over 1500 mg/dl not being unusual. Eruptive and planar xanthomas frequently occur as a result of the intense hyperlipidemia. Less strikingly, a similar hyperlipidemia is also seen in biliary obstruction from other causes, such as obstruction of the common bile duct by a stone or tumor. This secondary hyperlipidemia invariably remits as hepatocellular function becomes progressively impaired. Hyperlipidemia has also occurred in a child with severe liver disease present at birth and $alpha_1$ antitrypsin deficiency.[59] Lipoprotein X was present, but the bilirubin was only mildly elevated. Thus liver disease per se in the absence of biliary obstruction may be a rare cause of the same lipoprotein abnormality seen with biliary obstruction.

The lipoprotein abnormality of biliary obstruction is a characteristic one termed *lipoprotein X*. This lipoprotein has beta mobility upon electrophoresis but has an unusual composition in that most of the cholesterol is transported in the free form with greatly reduced cholesterol esters. Although not routinely determined, plasma phospholipid is also greatly increased, whereas plasma triglyceride is only moderately elevated. Lipoprotein X can be characterized by immunological techniques and is diagnostic of biliary obstruction.

The cause of this hyperlipidemia relates to the impairment of bile acid and probably to cholesterol excretion into bile. Serum bile acids increase, and there is decreased conversion of cholesterol to bile acids in the liver. The activity of the enzyme LCAT is also reduced and probably contributes to the reduced cholesterol ester level in plasma. Abnormal HDL particles which appear as disks instead of spheres under electron microscopy are present; the changed shape is believed to be due to the reduced cholesterol ester content. While cholestyramine may be used to control the itching these patients invariably have and may reduce plasma lipid levels, therapy is primarily aimed at the underlying hepatic disease or biliary obstruction. Plasmapheresis may be useful to remove cholesterol in patients with xanthomatous neuropathy.

ALCOHOL

A common cause of hyperlipidemia in western societies is excessive alcohol intake.[52] Considerable variation exists in the plasma lipid response of a given individual to alcohol, as is discussed later, and only about 10 percent of patients who habitually abuse alcohol will develop hyperlipidemia, usually with a type IV phenotype. Combined elevations of cholesterol and triglycerides (type IIb) occur also, as do cases with more severe hypertriglyceridemia and a type V phenotype. The latter pattern is most apt to occur in chronic alcohol abusers during periods of high fat intake and may lead to pancreatitis.

The mechanisms of alcoholic hyperlipidemia are complex and are related in part to caloric content. When alcohol is taken with food, the magnitude and duration of alimentary lipemia are increased; this increase appears to be due to an enhanced secretion of VLDL which occurs concomitantly with postprandial hyperchylomicronemia and results in a prolonged clearance of both particles. In the fasting state, alcohol also enhances hepatic synthesis and secretion of VLDL and is the main factor responsible for development of the type IV phenotype. This occurs because the increased levels of nicotinamide adenine dinucleotide (NADH) which are produced during the metabolism of ethanol by alcohol dehydrogenase inhibit oxidation of free fatty acids and result in an enhanced synthesis of triglycerides and VLDL. Alcohol may also promote induction of hepatic microsomal enzymes with a separate stimulatory effect on lipoprotein synthesis.

DRUG-INDUCED HYPERLIPOPROTEINEMIA

A number of drugs and hormones have been reported to have an adverse effect on plasma lipoprotein concentrations in humans. In the case of glucocorticoids,[60] estrogens,[61] and 13-*cis*-retinoic acid (isotretinoin, Accutane),[62] the primary effect appears to be stimulation of VLDL production and an increase in the concentrations of triglyceride-rich lipoproteins. In patients with underlying familial hypertriglyceridemia or familial combined hyperlipidemia, use of these agents may result in profound elevations in concentrations of serum triglycerides and clinical symptoms of abdominal pain or development of eruptive xanthomas. The thiazide diuretics have also been reported to increase the concentrations of cholesterol and triglyceride, an effect that is attributable to increased concentrations of VLDL and LDL particles in plasma.[63] Beta-blocking agents such as propranolol may also cause plasma triglyceride concentrations to increase and may concurrently reduce HDL cholesterol levels.[64] Combined therapy with thiazide diuretics and beta blockers should be avoided in patients with known hypertriglyceridemia if other avenues of therapy are available.

Hypercholesterolemia

Elevated levels of plasma cholesterol in the setting of normal triglyceride concentrations are usually attributable to an increased number of LDL particles in plasma. Less commonly, hypercholesterolemia reflects cholestasis in which an abnormal lipoprotein (LPX) accumulates or is seen in the occasional patient with an atypically high level of HDL cholesterol; in this case, no treatment is indicated (see Familial Hyperalphalipoproteinemia under Disorders of High-Density Lipoproteins). The causes of hypercholesterolemia may be divided into primary (genetic) etiologies, secondary causes, and a combination of two of these. Evaluation of a patient with hypercholesterolemia should therefore include satisfactory exclusion of secondary factors and a detailed family history. The potential value of identifying asymptomatic children and young adults with primary hypercholesterolemia cannot be overemphasized if preventive therapeutic measures to minimize the future development of atherosclerosis are to be successful. Increased concentrations of LDL cholesterol with normal triglycerides can be seen in patients with familial hypercholesterolemia, familial combined hyperlipidemia, and so-called polygenic hypercholesterolemia. Polygenic hypercholesterolemia is a poorly characterized disorder of unknown etiology in which affected adults display moderate hypercholesterolemia (220 to 280 mg/dl) without evidence of tendon xanthomas. Whether it is a distinct disorder has not been established.

FAMILIAL HYPERCHOLESTEROLEMIA

Definition

This condition (synonyms: familial xanthomatous hypercholesterolemia, type IIa and IIb hyperlipoproteinemia, hyperbetalipoproteinemia) is characterized by increased LDL, or β-lipoproteins, which are the chief carriers of cholesterol and cholesterol ester in the plasma. Consequently, the plasma cholesterol concentration is always moderately to profoundly elevated, with plasma triglyceride levels usually normal or low (type IIa) but at times elevated (type IIb). The cause of the hypercholesterolemia is related to a deficiency of low-density lipoprotein receptors in the cells of the body, with the result that there is impairment of LDL removal from the plasma. Of all the hyperlipidemias, familial hypercholesterolemia especially is characterized clinically by premature artherosclerosis and coronary heart disease as well as by the occurrence of tuberous and tendon xanthomas.[65]

Clinical Characteristics

The heterozygous form of familial hypercholesterolemia represents one of the most common causes of moderate to severe hypercholesterolemia in North America.[65] The disorder may be found at any age in either sex and may be diagnosed in the homozygous state during intrauterine life.[66] The chief clinical manifestations of this disease are the occurrence of xanthomatous deposits in the skin and tendons and greatly accelerated rates of atherosclerosis. The homozygous form of familial hypercholesterolemia is usually detected in childhood; affected patients have planar, tuberous, and tendon xanthomas during the first 5 years of life and in some cases may even be born with these skin manifestations. Plasma cholesterol concentrations in these patients are generally in excess of 600 to 700 mg/dl. Because of their inherently lower levels of total (240 to 450 mg/dl) and LDL cholesterol (160 to 400 mg/dl), children and young adults with heterozygous familial hypercholesterolemia frequently have no physical abnormalities.[67] Small planar xanthomas (slightly raised yellow lesions) may occasionally be seen in the digital webs or behind the knees. Recurrent episodes of Achilles tendonitis, usually exercise-related, occur in 50 to 75 percent of heterozygotes and frequently have their onset in the patient's late teens or early twenties.[68] These episodes are a reflection of the insidious deposition of LDL cholesterol in the tendons of patients with familial hypercholesterolemia and often precede clinical evidence of thickening or xanthomatous deposits in the Achilles tendons. These nodular lipid-rich lesions have a mild inflammatory tissue reaction and an associated collagen accumulation. Tendon xanthomas, which are the hallmark of familial hypercholesterolemia, become more prominent as the patient gets older, and their development is often accelerated by local trauma. In adult patients with heterozygous familial hypercholesterolemia who are over 30 to 35, tendon xanthomas are usually detectable by means of clinical examination. Tendon xanthomas characteristically involve the extensor tendons of the hands (Figs. 22-7 and 22-8), the olecranon tendon, the patellar tendon, and the Achilles tendon (Fig. 22-9). An

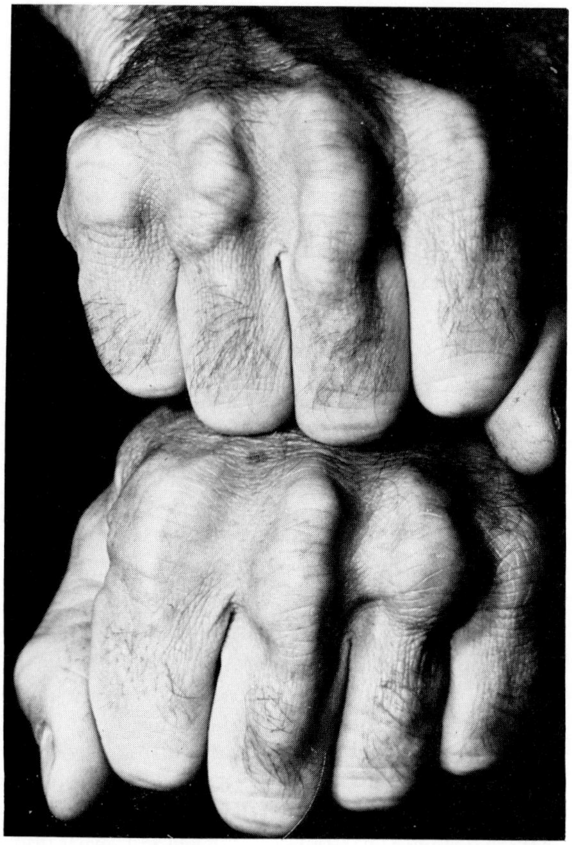

FIGURE 22-7 Tendon xanthomas in a patient with heterozygous familial hypercholesterolemia.

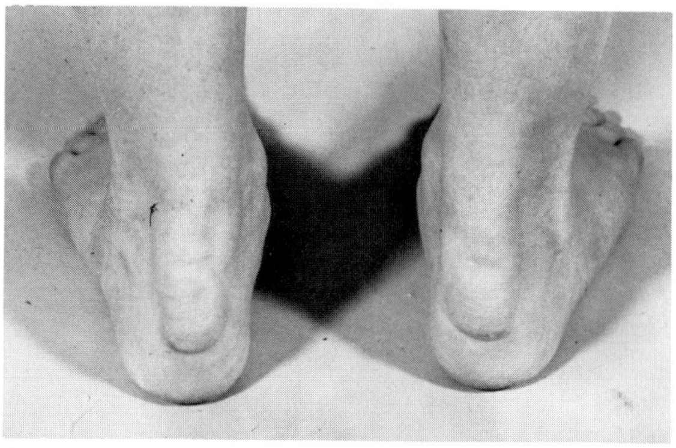

FIGURE 22-9 Xanthomas of the Achilles tendons in a patient with heterozygous familial hypercholesterolemia.

increased thickening and nodularity of the Achilles tendon is often noted on palpation. Xanthelasmas (Fig. 22-10) are present in less than 20 percent of older patients[67] but are not specific for familial hypercholesterolemia, occurring frequently in patients with normal lipid values.[69] The presence of a corneal arcus in patients under age 35 years constitutes another external hallmark of familial hypercholesterolemia[67] but is surprisingly absent in some patients with severe hypercholesterolemia. In many patients, however, a long latent period with only hypercholesterolemia precedes clinical manifestations of cholesterol accumulation in the tendons, skin, and arterial walls. Lipid accumulation in these tissues, however, tends to proceed in parallel, and manifestations of cardiovascular disease are more likely to be present in patients with prominent tendon xanthomas than in patients in whom such lesions are less conspicuous.[70]

The high incidence of premature coronary artery disease in patients with familial hypercholesterolemia

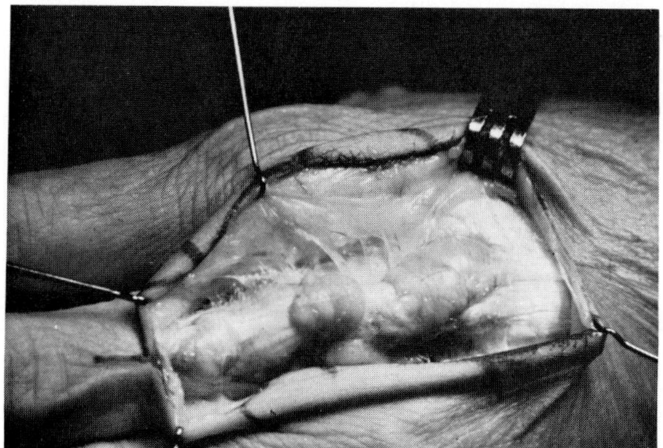

FIGURE 22-8 The appearance of tendon xanthomas prior to surgical removal in a patient with heterozygous familial hypercholesterolemia.

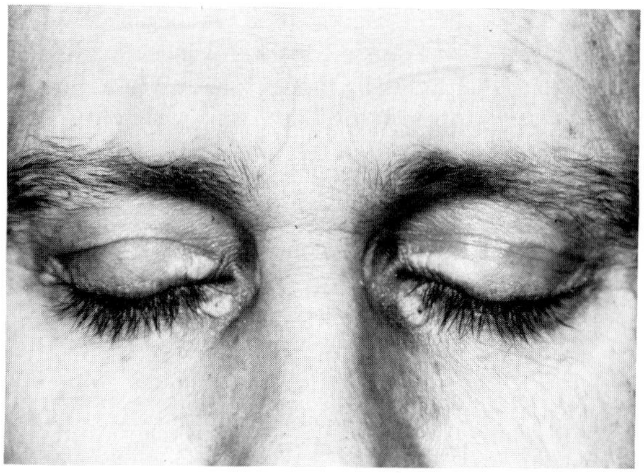

FIGURE 22-10 Xanthelasma in a patient with heterozygous familial hypercholesterolemia.

has been well documented.[36,65,67,71–73] Homozygotes are the most severely affected individuals and develop symptoms of coronary atherosclerosis by 10 to 15 years of age.[36] Myocardial infarction has been reported at 1½ and 3 years of age.[74,75] In addition to precocious coronary artery disease, patients with homozygous familial hypercholesterolemia are also predisposed to both valvular and supravalvular aortic stenosis[76,77] and to atherosclerosis of the carotid and femoral arteries. Premature coronary artery disease is also a hallmark of heterozygous familial hypercholesterolemia. Unlike the situation in homozygotes, among whom vascular complications appear to be similar in men and women, the predilection for atherosclerosis is greater in men. The average age of onset for symptomatic coronary artery disease is 40 to 45 years in men and 50 to 60 years in women with heterozygous familial hypercholesterolemia (Table 22-9). Angiographic studies have also disclosed a higher than expected incidence of proximal lesions of the coronary arteries, including left main coronary artery disease, in patients with familial hypercholesterolemia.[78,79]

Diagnostic Laboratory Features

It must be stressed that many individuals with hypercholesterolemia resulting from elevated plasma levels of LDL will not have a distinctly definable genetic disorder and will have hypercholesterolemia on the basis of dietary or other secondary factors. These patients in general have plasma cholesterol concentrations which are lower than those of the genetically affected individuals, although severe hypercholesterolemia may be seen in association with both hypothyroidism and renal disease. Patients with familial hypercholesterolemia in the heterozygous form usually present with elevated levels of total and LDL cholesterol and normal levels of plasma triglycerides. Concentrations of HDL cholesterol are infrequently reduced by 5 to 10 mg/dl in heterozygotes and are even lower in homozygotes.[36,80] Plasma cholesterol levels in heterozygous patients generally range from 280 to 550 mg/dl in adults, and in homozygous patients they generally exceed 600 mg/dl during childhood. These increases correlate with increased concentrations of LDL cholesterol. Although not associated with other metabolic disorders, the concurrent presence of familial hypercholesterolemia with obesity, diabetes, or renal disease often results in increased triglyceride levels and the expression of a type IIb phenotype. Similarly, the coexistence of heterozygous familial hypercholesterolemia and another primary disorder of lipid metabolism (e.g., familial combined hyperlipidemia),[81] type III hyperlipoproteinemia,[82] or a secondary disorder such as hypothyroidism or the nephrotic syndrome may lead to more profound elevations of total cholesterol (often exceeding 500 to 600 mg/dl) than are usually seen in patients with heterozygous familial hypercholesterolemia alone.

Pathophysiology

Major insights into the biochemical basis of familial hypercholesterolemia have been provided by the elegant studies of Goldstein and Brown. These investigators have proceeded from the initial demonstration of specific membrane receptors for LDL on normal cultured fibroblasts and their absence in cells cultured from patients with homozygous familial hypercholesterolemia to delineation of the molecular heterogeneity of the cellular abnormalities in familial hypercholesterolemia[83] and, most recently, delineation of the precise gene defects in cells from different patients with homozygous familial hypercholesterolemia.[84] As previously discussed, specific high-affinity LDL receptors appear to be present on virtually all cells, including hepatocytes and mononuclear leukocytes. From the pathophysiological point of view, the inability of cells in the body to incorporate LDL via the specific receptor pathway has a number of consequences, including an elevation in the concentration of LDL in plasma and an inappropriately higher rate of cellular cholesterol biosynthesis and LDL production from the liver. A number of different mutations at the LDL receptor locus have been identified, and these result in a variety of cellular defects in the binding, internalization, and cellular processing of the LDL molecule.[83,84] Patients with familial hypercholesterolemia show a

Table 22-9. Coronary Artery Disease in Familial Hypercholesterolemia*

	Mean age for onset of coronary artery disease	Chance of myocardial infarction before		
		Age 30, %	Age 50, %	Age 60, %
Men	40	5	50	85
Women	55	<1	15	50

*Data from Refs. 67, 71, 72, and 73.

decrease in the fractional rate of catabolism of LDL which is most marked in the homozygous state.[85] The biosynthesis of LDL, however, is normal or only modestly increased in heterozygotes but is two to three times greater than normal in homozygous patients.[85,86] Although genetic defects which reduce the number or functional capacity of LDL receptors explain the marked hypercholesterolemia in patients with familial hypercholesterolemia, the high rate of atherosclerosis which occurs in these patients clearly indicates that other non-receptor-mediated pathways must exist in which LDL cholesterol can be incorporated into cells. Such non-receptor-mediated pathways may be more important for the entry of LDL into certain cells (including macrophages)[87] and may contribute to the deposition of lipid in the arterial wall.

Genetics

Familial hypercholesterolemia is transmitted by an autosomal dominant mode of inheritance. Because this disorder is seldom lethal in the heterozygous form until after or during the child-bearing period, the passage of the disorder from one generation to the next readily explains the large pedigrees of the disorder which have been described. Care must be taken to differentiate familial hypercholesterolemia from familial combined hyperlipidemia and from the characteristically environmentally and dietarily induced hypercholesterolemia and other forms of secondary hyperlipidemia. The homozygous form may be diagnosed in utero by tissue-culture studies of the LDL receptor in cells derived from the amniotic fluid[66] as well as in children and adults by means of skin biopsies and skin fibroblast studies of the LDL receptor mechanism.[65] However, in most patients, this technique is not necessary; the diagnosis can be made on the basis of clinical and usual laboratory features. Only in the homozygote is such precise characterization desirable from the point of view of the demonstration of deficient LDL receptors.

To facilitate the detection of couples at risk for having a child with homozygous familial hypercholesterolemia, it is advisable to check lipid values in the spouses or future spouses of all young patients with known familial hypercholesterolemia. The incidence of heterozygous familial hypercholesterolemia is about 1 in 500 in Europe and North America but appears to be higher in certain other population groups, most notably in the Afrikaans (Dutch) population of South Africa,[88] in Quebec, and in Lebanon.[89]

Treatment

Because of the severe predilection for coronary heart disease, individuals with familial hypercholesterolemia should have intensive treatment to lower plasma LDL and cholesterol concentrations. It is the responsibility of the physician to identify other affected family members. The treatment in all patients should initially consist of the low-cholesterol, low-fat diet described in Dietary Treatment of Hyperlipidemia. If the plasma cholesterol concentrations are below 250 to 300 mg/dl, the response to dietary treatment may be most gratifying. The combination of intensive dietary treatment and pharmaceutical agents is almost always necessary if xanthomas are present and plasma cholesterol concentrations are 300 mg/dl or above.

The bile acid–binding resins cholestyramine (Questran) and colestipol (Colestid) are the drugs of choice for the initial therapy of most patients with heterozygous familial hypercholesterolemia. Notable exceptions include patients with a concurrent elevation of plasma triglyceride levels, in whom these drugs often cause a further increase in triglycerides, and patients with a history of severe constipation, which is often exacerbated by bile acid sequestrants. Because they are not absorbed, cholestyramine and colestipol remain the only drugs the authors consider safe for use in children; such therapy should not be begun before 5 to 6 years of age except in severe cases. The dose-response curves for both cholestyramine and colestipol are nonlinear, and 15 to 20 percent decreases in the concentration of LDL are often seen with 5 g of colestipol or 4 g of cholestyramine twice daily. In adult patients, the dose is usually increased to 10 g of colestipol twice daily; maximal doses of 15 g twice daily should be used in severe cases, but the benefits from the additional 5 to 10 percent decrease in LDL cholesterol must be balanced against the poorer patient compliance and greater incidence of gastrointestinal side effects observed with this dose. The mechanism by which bile acid–binding resins lower LDL cholesterol is discussed in Pharmaceutical Agents for the Treatment of Hyperlipidemia. Nicotinic acid is the second-choice drug for the treatment of patients with heterozygous familial hypercholesterolemia and is probably the first-choice agent for patients with concurrent hypertriglyceridemia. The drug is taken three or four times daily with food; initial therapy should start with 100 to 250 mg per day with a gradual increase to 3 to 4.5 g per day taken in divided doses. Liver function tests and serum uric acid levels must be monitored in patients treated with this drug. Used by itself, nicotinic acid in doses of 3 to 8 g daily results in 15 to 40 percent decreases in the concentrations of LDL cholesterol, with a modest increase in HDL cholesterol levels. Probucol (Lorelco) 500 mg twice daily is moderately effective in some patients but has no effect in others. On the average, probucol results in 8 to 12 percent decreases in LDL cholesterol levels, often with a concurrent decrease in HDL. Parenthetically, probucol appears to be more effective in patients with homozygous familial hypercholesterolemia than it is in heterozygotes.[90] Gemfibrozil (Lopid) and clofibrate (Atromid-S) are minimally effective in most patients with familial hypercholesterolemia when used as single-drug therapy. Because of the higher incidence of adverse cardiovascular effects noted in the Coronary Drug Project,[91] the use of dextrothyroxine sodium 4 to 6 mg per day should be reserved for young adult patients with familial hypercholesterolemia who are unable to take other agents. Such therapy results in 10 to 18 percent decreases in the concentrations of LDL cholesterol.[92] Although currently limited to investigational use, mevinolin (lovastatin), which is an inhibitor of the rate-limiting enzyme of cholesterol biosynthesis (HMG CoA reductase) is an extremely effective hypocholesterolemic agent in patients with familial hypercholesterolemia. In doses of 20 to 40 mg twice daily, mevinolin lowers LDL cholesterol concentrations 35 to 40 percent; this reduction appears to be sustained during long-term therapy.[93]

Combined drug therapy with a bile acid–binding resin and nicotinic acid constitutes the most effective regimen currently available for maximally reducing LDL levels in patients with familial hypercholesterolemia.[94–96] Decreases of 40 to 60 percent in the concentrations of LDL cholesterol, often paralleled by a small increase in HDL, are attained with this regimen. Prolonged use of nicotinic acid plus colestipol has been shown to result in the regression of xanthomas[95] and to arrest the progression of angiographically defined lesions in the coronary arteries.[96] Combined therapy with a bile acid sequestrant and probucol[97] or gemfibrozil may also be of use in patients who are unable to take nicotinic acid; however, the efficacy of this combination is unpredictable, and some patients show no additional decreases in LDL cholesterol upon the addition of the second drug. Combined drug therapy with mevinolin and colestipol is more effective than the use of mevinolin as a single agent, and this regimen is capable of reducing LDL cholesterol concentrations 40 to 60 percent in patients with heterozygous familial hypercholesterolemia.[98,99]

A number of surgical techniques have been used to treat patients with familial hypercholesterolemia, but none can be generally recommended. In heterozygous patients, resection of the distal 200 cm of the ileum effectively reduces reabsorption of bile acid and lowers concentrations of LDL cholesterol 30 to 40 percent.[100] Side effects including diarrhea and abdominal pain are common.[101] The operation is not effective in homozygotes, and combined drug therapy is more efficacious in heterozygotes. This operation cannot be recommended and should be considered only in selected severe heterozygous patients who are unable to take cholestyramine or colestipol.[102] With the potential availability of mevinolin, the number of such patients is, in the authors' experience, likely to be very small. Portacaval shunts may be effective in both heterozygotes and homozygotes with familial hypercholesterolemia; by reducing the synthesis of LDL, these shunts can lower LDL concentrations 25 to 40 percent.[81,103] As with distal ileal bypass, this procedure should be reserved for refractory patients in whom all other pharmaceutical measures have failed; even then an effective LDL-lowering effect cannot be guaranteed.

Repetitive plasmapheresis every 2 to 3 weeks[104–106] with or without the use of an affinity column to which LDL is selectively bound[106] has been successfully applied to the treatment of the rare patient with homozygous familial hypercholesterolemia. Liver transplantation is also an effective therapeutic means of lowering LDL cholesterol concentrations in patients with this disorder.[107]

FAMILIAL COMBINED HYPERLIPIDEMIA

Definition

Familial combined hyperlipidemia is an autosomal dominant inherited disorder in which affected family members may display different phenotypic forms of hyperlipidemia. The disorder appears to be due to an inherent overproduction of VLDL and LDL by the liver and results in the expression of increased levels of LDL cholesterol (type IIa phenotype), combined elevations of VLDL and LDL cholesterol (type IIb phenotype), or singular elevation in the concentrations of VLDL (type IV phenotype).

Clinical Characteristics

There are no typical physical findings associated with the underlying presence of familial combined hyperlipidemia. Tendon xanthomas are usually but not invariably[108] absent in patients with this disorder, and the absence of tendon xanthomas in patients with primary hypercholesterolemia serves as a useful distinction between this disorder and familial hypercholesterolemia. Severe hypertriglyceridemia with the development of eruptive xanthomas may occur in patients with familial combined hyperlipidemia who concurrently develop diabetes, whereas patients who are homozygous for apoprotein E-2 may present clinically with tuberous xanthomas and a type III phenotype. In patients with familial combined hyperlipidemia who have elevated levels of LDL cholesterol, total plasma cholesterol concentrations usually range from 250 to 350 mg/dl, with LDL cholesterol ranging from 180 to 300 mg/dl. Because familial combined hyperlipidemia shows incomplete penetration in children and young adults, lipid values in affected patients often increase substantially during the third and fourth decades of life. This, together with the lower absolute lipid values usually seen in familial combined hyperlipidemia compared with familial hypercholesterolemia, may explain the lower incidence of premature coronary artery disease in familial combined hyperlipidemia. The typical age of onset for symptomatic coronary artery disease in men with familial combined hyperlipidemia is approximately 50; it occurs some 10 to 15 years later in women patients.[109]

Genetics

Familial combined hyperlipidemia is inherited as an autosomal dominant trait which shows incomplete penetration in children and young adults. It is not uncommon; the gene frequency has been estimated to be approximately 1 in 200 in North America.[109] Because no specific marker for familial combined hyperlipidemia exists, it is likely that many patients with moderate hypercholesterolemia who do not have tendon xanthomas have familial combined hyperlipidemia but that this disorder is itself quite heterogeneous.

Diagnostic Laboratory Features

Patients with familial combined hyperlipidemia may present with primary hypercholesterolemia, primary hypertriglyceridemia, or combined elevations of cholesterol and triglyceride. Because expression of this disorder appears to be exacerbated by factors such as weight gain and increasing age, the diagnosis of familial combined hyperlipidemia rests on demonstration of multiple different lipoprotein phenotypes in different family members. Some patients with familial combined hyperlipidemia appear to have proportionally higher levels of LDL apoprotein B than would be expected from their LDL cholesterol concentrations.[110] Studies by Sniderman and colleagues[111] suggest that these patients also have an increased incidence of premature cardiovascular disease.

Pathophysiology

Lack of a specific marker for familial combined hyperlipidemia has hindered investigations of the biochemical causes of this disorder(s). Kinetic studies in which radioiodinated lipoproteins have been injected into patients with familial combined hyperlipidemia have shown an inherently high production rate of VLDL and LDL in these patients. In contrast to the low fractional catabolic rate of LDL seen in patients with familial hypercholesterolemia, the rate of catabolism of LDL is normal in patients with familial combined hyperlipidemia, and the expression of LDL receptors in cells from these patients is also normal.[112] By current diagnostic criteria, familial combined hyperlipidemia undoubtedly represents a heterogeneous group of disorders in which the hepatic production of apoprotein B-100 is increased. Further insights into the causes of this defect should be rapidly forthcoming now that the gene for apoprotein B has been cloned.[113,114]

Treatment

Treatment of patients with familial combined hyperlipidemia is intended to reduce the levels of LDL cholesterol in plasma as the primary goal of therapy. Because hepatic production of VLDL and LDL is increased by secondary factors such as obesity, type II diabetes, and excessive alcohol intake, correction of secondary predisposing factors should be attempted in all patients with this disorder. Knowledge about the pathophysiology of familial combined hyperlipidemia suggests that those hypolipidemic agents which primarily inhibit the synthesis of VLDL and LDL may be the most effective in patients with this disorder. We regard nicotinic acid as the drug of choice for patients with familial combined hyperlipidemia; the bile acid–binding resins cholestyramine and colestipol are second-choice agents. Gemfibrozil and probucol are variably effective in this disorder, but their efficacy is often enhanced when they are used in combination with a bile acid sequestrant. Preliminary results indicate that mevinolin 20 mg twice daily is also an effective hypolipidemic agent in patients with familial combined hyperlipidemia.

THRESHOLDS FOR THE DRUG TREATMENT OF HYPERCHOLESTEROLEMIA

The question What level of plasma cholesterol warrants therapy with drugs? is of considerable importance. Although no absolute values can be given, a more aggressive approach is warranted in men, young people with a strong family history of early death from coronary artery disease, and patients with concurrent other risk factors or atypically low HDL cholesterol levels. Patients with concentrations of total and LDL cholesterol which exceed the 75th percentile for age should receive dietary advice and, in selected cases, pharmaceutical therapy, whereas patients with total and LDL cholesterol exceeding the 90th to 95th percentiles should be strongly considered for drug treatment if diet does not substantially reduce the magnitude of hypercholesterolemia.[51] A recently reported randomized clinical trial demonstrated that reduction in LDL cholesterol by means of diet plus cholestyramine can reduce the incidence of fatal and nonfatal coronary heart disease in a primary prevention trial (the Lipid Research Clinics Coronary Primary Prevention Trial).[115,116] A second study (the NHLBI Type II Coronary Intervention Study) showed reduction in the angiographic progression of coronary artery disease in hypercholesterolemic patients with preexisting coronary artery disease.[117] These studies support the view that if the premature development of coronary atherosclerosis in patients with primary hypercholesterolemia is to be prevented, patients who remain significantly hypercholesterolemic on optimal dietary therapy should be treated with hypolipidemic drugs. General guidelines for the institution of drug therapy are cholesterol values in excess of 240 to 250 mg/dl in children over age 6 with heterozygous familial hypercholesterolemia and cholesterol values of 250 to 260 mg/dl in patients up to age 45 to 50. Among adults between the ages of 45 and 65 drug therapy should be considered in patients whose cholesterol values remain above 260 to 280 mg/dl on diet therapy, whereas a less aggressive approach is probably warranted in older (over 65 to 70 years) patients without clinical evidence of atherosclerosis. Especially aggressive treatment is warranted in patients who have already developed clinical expressions of atherosclerosis, e.g., overt coronary heart disease.

Combined Hypercholesterolemia and Hypertriglyceridemia

Combined elevations of cholesterol and triglyceride can be due to the presence of an increased number of VLDL and LDL particles of normal composition (type IIb phenotype) or may reflect the presence of abnormal chylomicron and VLDL remnant particles that are typical of dysbetalipoproteinemia (type III hyperlipoproteinemia). It is in this group of patients with total plasma cholesterol values ranging between 280 and 700 mg/dl and concurrent triglyceride values ranging between 300 and 1500 mg/dl that more detailed studies to precisely define the lipoprotein phenotype should always be undertaken. Differentiation between patients with increased concentrations of VLDL and LDL (type IIb phenotype) and patients with type III hyperlipoproteinemia requires ultracentrifugal separation of VLDL in order to document the abnormal cholesterol-rich particles which are present in the plasma of patients with type III hyperlipoproteinemia.

Increased concentrations of LDL in the presence of concurrent hypertriglyceridemia (phenotypic type IIb) may occur on the basis of secondary disorders (Table 22-8) or may be attributable to familial hypercholesterolemia, familial combined hyperlipidemia, or other genotypically less well defined causes. The elevated levels of VLDL present in the plasma of these patients are commonly accompanied by reduced levels of HDL cholesterol.[80] In many patients with phenotypic type IIb hyperlipidemia, the presence of the primary genetic disorder is exacerbated by concurrent secondary disorders such as adult-onset diabetes mellitus, obesity, and excessive alcohol intake. Thus attainment of ideal weight and restricted use of alcohol should be strongly encouraged in these patients. The presence of tendon xanthomas and/or primary hypercholesterolemia in children within a given family indicates an underlying genotypic diagnosis of familial hypercholesterolemia, whereas in a family with multiple different phenotypes the genotypic diagnosis is most likely to be familial combined hyperlipidemia. The risk of premature cardiovascular disease in patients with these hereditary disorders and a type IIb phenotype is increased and appears to parallel that seen in similar patients with elevated concentrations of LDL cholesterol but normal triglyceride levels.

As discussed elsewhere, we favor a single dietary approach to the treatment of hyperlipidemia; however, in patients with hypertriglyceridemia, particular attention must be paid to total caloric intake, alcohol, and restriction of saturated fats. Drug therapy should be aimed primarily at reducing the elevated levels of LDL cholesterol. Nicotinic acid is the most effective single agent in most patients and results in decreases in the concentrations of both VLDL (30 to 75 percent) and LDL (10 to 35 percent) with concurrent rises in plasma concentrations of HDL cholesterol. Combined drug therapy with colestipol or cholestyramine may produce further decreases in the concentrations of LDL; if used alone, however, these agents frequently cause an elevation in VLDL levels and an increase in total plasma triglycerides.[118] Gemfibrozil or to a lesser extent clofibrate may be effective in reducing the VLDL levels in these patients, but single-drug treatment with these drugs often results in a reciprocal rise in the concentrations of LDL cholesterol so that overall total plasma cholesterol values may remain relatively unchanged.[119] Subsequent addition of a bile acid sequestrant may reduce LDL levels 15 to 25 percent, but overall these combinations are less effective than the nicotinic acid–bile acid sequestrant regimen.[95] Combined therapy with an inhibitor of HMG CoA reductase such as mevinolin and a hypotriglyceridemic agent such as gemfibrozil or nicotinic acid may also constitute an effective drug regimen for patients with combined elevations of VLDL and LDL levels.

PRIMARY TYPE III HYPERLIPOPROTEINEMIA

Definition

Type III hyperlipoproteinemia, also referred to as broad-beta or floating beta disease or dysbetalipoproteinemia, is a relatively uncommon disorder characterized by the presence of abnormal very-low-density and intermediate-density lipoprotein (*d* 1.006 to 1.019) particles with an abnormally high ratio of cholesterol to triglyceride and with beta mobility on electrophoresis. Patients with this disorder are usually homozygous for one allelic form of apoprotein E (E-2). Plasma lipid values vary widely but generally reveal cholesterol levels in the range of 300 to 600 mg/dl with triglyceride levels of 400 to 800 mg/dl.

Clinically, patients with type III hyperlipidemia commonly have palmar and tuberous xanthomas and display an increased incidence of both coronary and peripheral vascular disease.

Clinical Characteristics

The initial recognition of type III hyperlipidemia was as "xanthoma tuberosum" by Goffman and colleagues[120] over 30 years ago. Although the physical findings in patients with type III vary widely, certain features are strongly suggestive of this diagnosis.[121] The most characteristic and common[122] xanthomas seen in type III, termed xanthoma striatum palmeris, are present on the hands. These lesions, which may be the only skin manifestation of the disorder, vary from a yellow-orange discoloration of the palmar creases of both hands to more advanced lesions with planar elevation of the skin and eventually, in the most severe form, to raised tuberous xanthomas on the palms and fingers (Fig. 22-11).

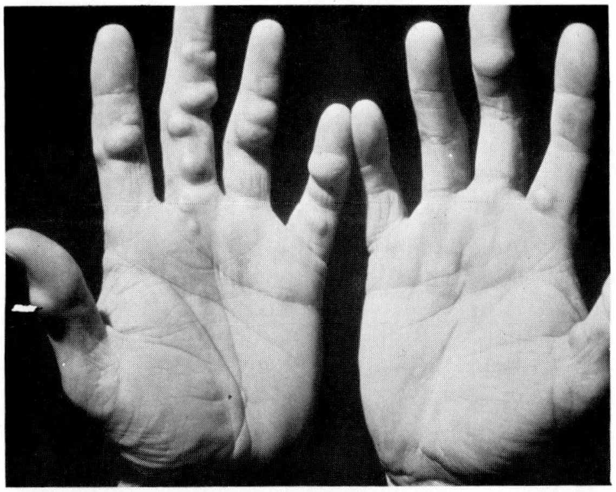

FIGURE 22-11 Tuberous palmar xanthomas in a patient with type III hyperlipoproteinemia.

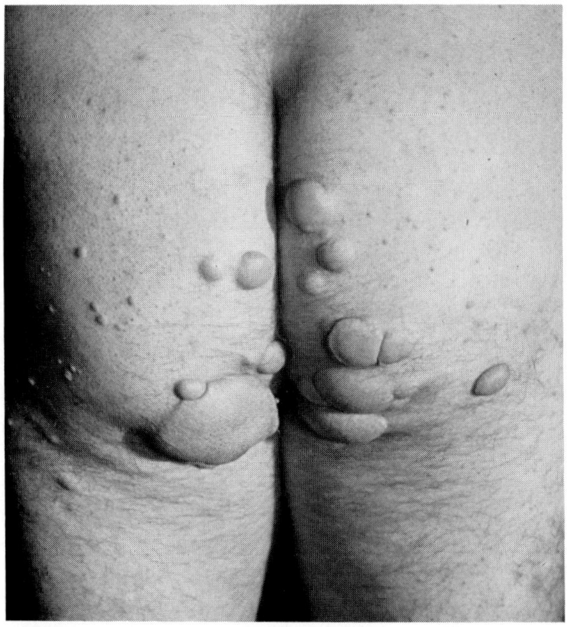

FIGURE 22-12 Tuberoeruptive xanthomas on the buttocks of a patient with type III hyperlipoproteinemia. The lesions regressed with hypolipidemic therapy.

Tuberoeruptive xanthomas (Fig. 22-12), which consist of raised erythematous nodular lesions 0.5 cm or greater in diameter which commonly coalesce into larger lesions, are also typical of type III. They have a tendency to occur in areas of pressure, most notably the extensor surface of the elbows and knees and on the buttocks. Tuberous xanthomas were present in 51 percent of the patients studied by Morganroth and associates,[122] whereas in other series their incidence has varied from 35 to 100 percent. Xanthelasmas and corneal arcus are uncommon, but tendon xanthomas are present in about 10 percent of patients with type III. Patients with type III have an increased incidence of premature coronary and peripheral vascular disease, both of which have been present in 20 to 40 percent of the patients studied in most reports.[121] The likelihood of both these complications is higher in patients who present with advanced tuberous xanthomas than in those with less severe skin lesions.

To date, fewer than 10 cases of phenotypic type III have been described in patients under 20 years of age, and these have frequently been associated with coexisting hypothyroidism. Phenotypic expression of the type III disorder in older patients is also commonly associated with obesity, hypothyroidism, diabetes mellitus, or a coexistent separate familial hyperlipidemia. By far the most common of these factors is obesity, which is present in up to 75 percent of cases. To date, no convincing evidence for the secondary occurrence of the type III phenotype in patients with obesity or hypothyroidism who do not have abnormal apoprotein E has been presented. Thorough screening of the family members of a patient with type III hyperlipidemia is extremely rewarding and should be a mandatory part of the evaluation. Phenotypic expression of the type III disorder is more common in men than in women and ranges from 60 to 80 percent of the total in most series. The prevalence of the type III phenotype is not known but has been estimated at 0.01 to 0.04 percent of the population.[120]

Genetics

Prior to 1977, studies to delineate the inheritance of type III were hindered by the lack of a specific marker for this disorder. When the diagnosis was based on the presence of beta-migrating VLDL and a VLDL cholesterol/plasma triglyceride ratio greater than 0.3, three separate studies[122–124] concluded that the type of inheritance was autosomal dominant.

Delineation of the hereditary nature of type III hyperlipoproteinemia has been clarified by the recognition that apoprotein E exists in three common allelic forms—apoproteins E-2, E-3, and E-4—and that the vast majority of patients with this disorder are homozygous for apoprotein E-2.[31] The different allelic forms of apoprotein E can be separated by means of isoelectric focusing, and the biochemical difference is due to specific amino acid substitutions in the apoprotein E molecule. The gene frequency of homozygotes for apoprotein E-2 has been estimated at 1 percent of the population,[125] whereas heterozygotes have a gene frequency of approximately 15 percent of the population. As discussed below, however, less than 5 percent of patients who are homozygous for E-2 actually develop hyperlipidemia, but all these individuals do show an abnormal ratio of VLDL cholesterol to triglyceride and the accumulation of abnormal beta VLDL in plasma.

Diagnostic Laboratory Features

Lipid values in patients with the type III phenotype vary widely but frequentlly show cholesterol levels in the range of 300 to 600 mg/dl with triglycerides of 400 to 800 mg/dl. These parameters alone, however, are not diagnostic, since similar values may occur in patients with type IIb hyperlipidemia. Determination of the ratio of VLDL cholesterol to the total plasma triglyceride concentration is the most readily available method for the diagnosis of type III hyperlipoproteinemia.[126] A ratio greater than 0.30 is regarded as diagnostic, whereas values of 0.25 to 0.30 should be considered suggestive. This method is reliable at triglyceride values of 150 to 1000 mg/dl, above which spuriously low ratios may be obtained because of the contribution of chylomicrons to the calculated ratio. An older and less optimal criterion for the diagnosis of type III is based on the demonstration of a beta-migrating band on agarose gel electrophoresis of isolated VLDL. The presence of such a slow-moving band in VLDL is, however, not specific and may be seen in patients with the type IV phenotype.

Although still available primarily in research laboratories, separation of the apoprotein E isoproteins by means of isoelectric focusing constitutes the most precise method for the diagnosis of most patients with type III hyperlipoproteinemia.[31,125] These studies have disclosed that the vast majority of patients with type III hyperlipoproteinemia are homozygotes for one of the three common allelic forms of apoprotein E (apoprotein E-2) and lack apoproteins E-3 and E-4. This disorder may also occur in patients with a complete deficiency of apoprotein E[127] and is likely to be found in patients with aberrant hepatic receptors for apoprotein E[125] and patients with other amino acid substitutions in the apoprotein E receptor-binding domain which do not affect the isoelectric point of the variant.

Pathophysiology

Type III hyperlipoproteinemia represents an inherited disorder whose phenotypic expression is modified by such factors as obesity, hypothyroidism, and concomitant familial hyperlipidemia. Studies on the binding of apoprotein E–containing lipoproteins to the apoprotein B,E (LDL) receptor of various cells have shown why patients who are homozygous for apoprotein E-2 have the potential to develop type III hyperlipoproteinemia. The normal interaction of apoprotein E with its receptor depends on the presence of specific lysine and arginine residues situated between amino acids 140 and 160 in the apoprotein E molecule. Lipoproteins containing only apoprotein E-2 have a markedly reduced binding affinity to the B,E receptor and are presumed also to have a reduced binding affinity to the specific hepatic apoprotein E receptor. This decrease in binding affinity is known to be due to a specific amino acid substitution at residue 158 in the apoprotein E molecule, which in apoprotein E-2 contains cysteine instead of the positive charged amino acid arginine which is present in apoprotein E-3. The difference in isoelectric point between apoproteins E-3 and E-4 reflects a substitution of cysteine for arginine at residue 112; however, this does not affect receptor binding, and the affinity of apoproteins E-3 and E-4 for the receptor is similar. In patients with type III hyperlipoproteinemia who are homozygous for apoprotein E-2, the reduced binding affinity of chylomicron and VLDL remnant particles to the hepatic apoprotein E receptor results in delayed clearance of these particles from plasma. This leads to the accumulation of remnant lipoproteins (e.g., beta-VLDL) which are relatively enriched in cholesterol. Such remnant lipoproteins accumulate in the plasma of all patients who are homozygous for apoprotein E-2, but the development of clinically apparent hyperlipidemia necessitates the concurrent presence of an impaired hepatic clearance of chylomicron and VLDL remnants together with an overproduction of VLDL (Fig. 22-13). Subjects who are homozygous for apoprotein E-2 but do not overproduce VLDL have beta-VLDL particles detectable in plasma and tend to have low levels of total and LDL cholesterol. This is presumably attributable to the impaired conversion of VLDL to LDL and to possible increases in the rate of catabolism of LDL.[31,125] The concurrent presence of an enhanced rate of production of VLDL as seen in patients with familial combined hyperlipidemia or in obesity leads to attenuation of the accumulation of beta-VLDL remnant particles and the development of clinical type III hyperlipoproteinemia. The accelerated atherosclerosis which develops in patients with type III hyperlipoproteinemia is believed to be due to the uptake of cholesterol-rich beta-VLDL particles by macrophages and possibly by smooth muscle cells in the arteries.

Treatment

Patients with type III respond very well to therapy. As with all forms of hyperlipidemia, elimination of secondary causes is mandatory if a coexistent disorder is not to be overlooked. Thus appropriate studies to evaluate the percentage of ideal body weight and to exclude hypothyroidism, excessive alcohol consumption, diabetes mellitus, and a concomitant second familial hyperlipidemia should be undertaken in all patients. Reduction of caloric intake in order to achieve ideal body weight in obese patients is extremely rewarding and by itself was successful in achieving normal lipid values in 25 of 39 patients treated by Morganroth and associates.[122] As discussed later, we favor a unified approach to dietary treatment of hyperlipidemias and encourage a low-fat (20 percent), 100-mg cholesterol diet together with caloric restriction to achieve ideal body weight.

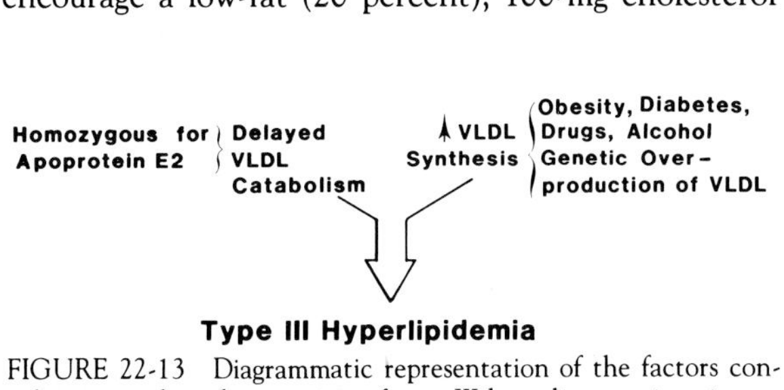

FIGURE 22-13 Diagrammatic representation of the factors contributing to clinical expression of type III hyperlipoproteinemia.

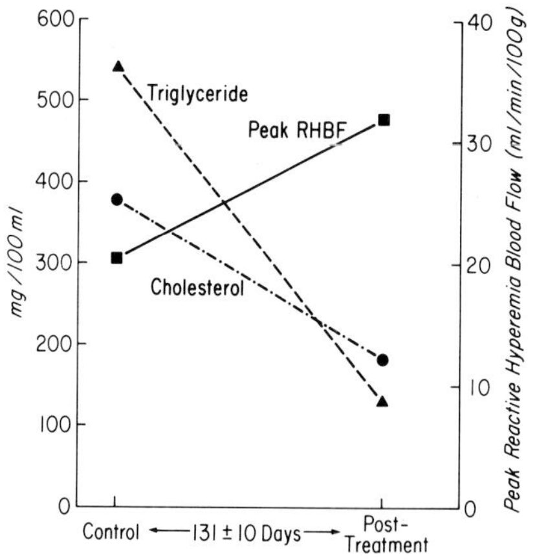

FIGURE 22-14 The effects of an isocaloric < 300 mg cholesterol diet plus clofibrate (2 g per day) on the plasma cholesterol, triglyceride, and peak reactive hyperemic blood flow (RHBF) in six patients with type III hyperlipoproteinemia. (*Adapted from Zelis et al.*[129])

In patients whose response to diet is less than adequate, drug therapy is usually extremely effective. Despite reservations about the use of clofibrate as therapy for other disorders of lipid metabolism, this drug is extremely effective in patients with type III hyperlipoproteinemia, for which it is the drug of choice. Therapy with 1 g twice daily usually results in rapid decreases in the concentrations of cholesterol and triglyceride (Fig. 22-14), and in some cases patients can be maintained on lower doses (e.g., 500 mg twice daily) with equal efficacy. Nicotinic acid 3 to 6 g per day and gemfibrozil 600 mg twice daily are also effective. Refractory patients, particularly those in whom the expression of type III hyperlipoproteinemia occurs as a consequence of underlying familial combined hyperlipidemia, may be treated with a combination of clofibrate and nicotinic acid. Women patients who are unable to take any of these medications may also respond to treatment with ethinyl estradiol (1 μg per kilogram per day).[128] Although this paradoxical effect of estrogen may in part explain the higher prevalence of type III hyperlipoproteinemia in men, such therapy is not generally advocated and probably should be reserved for selected women patients in whom dietary treatment alone is unsuccessful and who are unable to take clofibrate or nicotinic acid. The bile acid–binding resins and probucol are contraindicated in patients with type III hyperlipidemia, and the use of bile acid–binding resins will exacerbate this disorder, as will distal ileal bypass surgery.

Response to diet and drug therapy is usually dramatic, and, as occurred with the patient shown in

Figs. 22-11 and 22-12, regression of xanthomas frequently occurs in less than 1 year. Marked improvement from symptoms of angina pectoris and intermittent claudication have also been noted and suggest that regression of xanthomas may be paralleled by similar changes in lesions of the arterial wall. Objective evidence of such changes was obtained by Zelis and associates[129] (Fig. 22-14), who noted a 55 percent improvement in maximal blood flow after hyperlipidemic treatment of six patients with type III. The excellent therapeutic response found in patients with type III hyperlipidemia justifies an aggressive approach to both the diagnosis and the treatment of this interesting disorder.

HEPATIC LIPASE DEFICIENCY

Combined hyperlipidemia with elevated plasma concentrations of cholesterol (260 to 1500 mg/dl) and triglyceride (395 to 8200 mg/dl) have been ascribed to a deficiency of hepatic lipase in two Canadian patients.[34] Clinically, the index patient had palmar and tuberoeruptive xanthomas and was noted to have a corneal arcus at age 38. Lipoprotein studies demonstrated the accumulation of small VLDL particles with beta mobility, but no abnormality in apoprotein E could be demonstrated. After intravenous injection of heparin, concentrations of hepatic lipase in plasma were less than 5 percent of normal whereas LPL activity was not reduced. The ratio of VLDL cholesterol to total plasma cholesterol (which is generally greater than 0.3 in patients with type III hyperlipoproteinemia) ranged between 0.16 and 0.22 in patients with hepatic lipase deficiency, whereas analysis of the composition of LDL disclosed a characteristic enrichment of these particles with triglyceride (28 percent of LDL by weight; normal, 6 percent). Dietary restriction of calories, total fat, and cholesterol was effective in reducing plasma lipid values in this disorder, but clofibrate appeared to be ineffective.

Hypertriglyceridemia

HYPERCHYLOMICRONEMIA: TYPES I AND V HYPERLIPOPROTEINEMIA, FAMILIAL APOPROTEIN C-II DEFICIENCY

Definition

An abnormal accumulation of chylomicrons in plasma is characteristic of both type I and type V hyperlipidemia and justifies discussing them together. In type I hyperlipidemia, chylomicronemia is detectable in plasma obtained after an overnight (12 to 16 h) fast, and levels of VLDL are normal; in the type V phenotype, chylomicronemia is accompanied by a concomitant increase in concentrations of VLDL. Both phenotypes may occur either as primary familial disorders or secondary to a variety of associated conditions. The biochemical defect in type I is due to a functional deficiency or absence of the enzyme lipoprotein lipase; in type V, impaired clearance of chylomicrons has not been correlated with lipolytic activity, and the nature of the deficit or deficits is not known. In familial apoprotein C-II deficiency, the clearances of both chylomicrons and VLDL are impaired since C-II is a cofactor for LPL activation. The clinical aspects of this rare apoprotein disorder are identical to those of the type I and type V phenotypes.[130]

Clinical Features

Both the type I and type V phenotypes may occur as primary familial disorders or may be secondary to a number of associated underlying conditions (Table 22-8). In children the disorder is most likely to be familial, whereas in adults secondary causes constitute the most common etiology. In many cases, however, secondary factors are the provoking stimulus which exacerbates the expression of an underlying familial hyperlipidemia and brings it to clinical attention. The clinical features of both type I and type V are similar and are attributable to the presence of hyperchylomicronemia.[131-133] The age of presentation, however, is different, and in most cases type I is detected in childhood. In a review of 32 cases, Fredrickson and Levy[131] noted that the diagnosis was made before age 10 in 22 of these, and was made prior to age 1 in 7. In contrast, patients with type V usually, although not invariably,[134] are detected after age 20 and generally do not have severe hyperchylomicronemia in childhood.

Abdominal pain is the most frequent symptom which brings the patient to medical attention. The pain may be mild to severe and may mimic an "acute abdomen." The pain may be generalized or localized to the upper abdomen and frequently radiates to the back. Associated tenderness of the liver or spleen is common and is accompanied by hepatomegaly, splenomegaly, or both in over 50 percent of cases. The abdominal pain may proceed to acute pancreatitis. In the series of 32 patients with type I reported by Fredrickson and Levy,[131] 24 reported abdominal pains and 12 had episodes of pancreatitis, with the latter being responsible for four fatalities. Similarly, in reports of patients with type V hyperlipidemia, abdominal pain has been noted in up to 70 percent, with pancreatitis seen in 50 percent.[135,136] Because chylomicrons may interfere with the chemical determination of amylase and result in falsely low readings, such assays should be performed on diluted or chylomicron-free plasma, or alternatively, the amylase creatinine clearance ratios should be determined on urine samples.[137] Values over 0.04 are suggestive of pancreatitis. The mechanism(s) by which hyperchylomicronemia produces abdominal pain and pancreatitis remains an enigma. Stretching of the hepatic and splenic capsule secondary to enlargement of these organs and occlusion of the pancreatic microvasculature by aggregates of chylomicrons with resultant ischemia and local release of pancreatic enzymes remain attractive but unproven hypotheses.

Two physical findings—lipemia retinalis and eruptive xanthomas—are diagnostic of severe hyperchylomicronemia. Eruptive xanthomas appear as 1- to 5-mm yellow papules on an erythematous base. The lesions are nonpruritic and characteristically appear on the trunk and the extensor surfaces of the arms, buttocks, and thighs (Figs. 22-15 and 22-16) over a period of several weeks. Their presence implies severe hyperchylomicronemia (triglycerides usually greater than 4000 mg/dl). After therapeutic reduction of the hyperchylomicronemia, eruptive xanthomas gradually disappear over a 4- to 12-week period. In lipemia retinalis, the other hallmark of hyperchylomicronemia, the retinal arteries and veins have a salmon-pink color on fundoscopic examination.

The type I phenotype is rarely associated with hyperglycemia or abnormal glucose tolerance, and affected patients are usually of normal body weight. In contrast, patients with the type V phenotype have a high incidence of hyperglycemia with hyperinsulinism and are frequently above ideal body weight. Although the relation between these abnormalities is unclear, a positive correlation has been documented between the degree of hypertriglyceridemia and both body weight and hyperglycemia.[135] Type I hyperlipidemia does not appear to be associated with an increased incidence of atherosclerotic vascular disease.[131,133] In type V patients, atherosclerotic coronary heart disease is certainly observed.

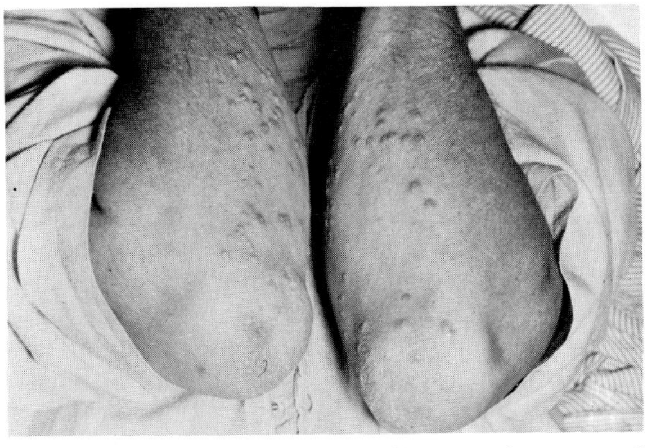

FIGURE 22-15 Eruptive xanthomas on the arms of a patient with severe hypertriglyceridemia and phenotypic type V hyperlipoproteinemia.

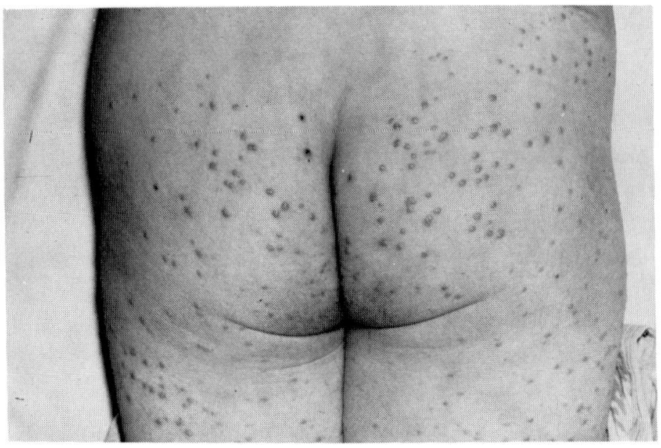

FIGURE 22-16 Eruptive xanthomas on the buttocks of a patient with severe hypertriglyceridemia and phenotypic type V hyperlipoproteinemia.

Genetics

Familial lipoprotein lipase deficiency (type I hyperlipoproteinemia) is inherited as an autosomal recessive trait for which affected individuals are homozygous. Obligate heterozygotes usually have normal lipid values but appear to have reduced levels of adipose-tissue lipoprotein lipase.[138] Family members of an index patient with phenotypic type V hyperlipoproteinemia show a high incidence of both the type IV and type V phenotypes, the frequencies of which both increase with age. In the largest study to date,[135] the distribution of lipoprotein phenotypes in 181 first-degree relatives from 32 patients with familial type V revealed 57 percent to be normal, 11 percent with type II phenotype, 15 percent with type IV, and 16 percent with type V. Fallat and Glueck[136] noted an even higher incidence of type IV and type V phenotypes in first-degree relatives and concluded that the inheritance was consistent with an autosomal dominant mode of transmission. These studies are consistent with the view that patients with the type V phenotype represent a heterogeneous population in which most appear to have familial hypertriglyceridemia or familial combined hyperlipidemia as the underlying genetic disorder.[133] Familial apoprotein C-II deficiency is inherited as an autosomal recessive trait.[28,130]

DIAGNOSTIC LABORATORY FEATURES

The determinations of cholesterol and triglyceride in plasma obtained after a 12- to 14-h fast, together with the visual inspection of a plasma sample that has been allowed to stand for 12 to 18 h at 4°C for the presence of chylomicronemia, will permit diagnosis of the type I or type V phenotype in most cases. In type I hyperlipidemia, increases in triglyceride are paralleled by a much smaller rise in cholesterol such that the triglyceride/cholesterol ratio is usually greater than 10:1 (e.g., triglyceride 4200 mg/dl, cholesterol 320 mg/dl). Upon refrigeration, the chylomicron layer is seen to overlay a clear subnatant which does not contain increased concentrations of VLDL. The levels of both LDL and HDL in type I are low, typically averaging 50 percent of normal. Lipid values in the type V phenotype reflect the combined increase in both VLDL and chylomicrons; the triglyceride/cholesterol ratio is therefore lower than in type I and usually ranges from 5:1 to 8:1 (e.g., triglyceride 4800 mg/dl, cholesterol 730 mg/dl). Concentrations of LDL and HDL in type V are 50 percent or more lower than normal and reflect the impaired catabolism of both VLDL and chylomicrons to smaller particles in this disorder. As previously discussed, hyperglycemia frequently coexists in patients with the type V phenotype but rarely occurs in patients with the type I disorder. Documentation of very low or absent levels of lipoprotein lipase either in adipose tissue or in plasma after intravenous injection of heparin remains the sine qua non for the diagnosis of type I hyperlipidemia. In contrast, the activity of both hepatic lipase and lipoprotein lipase is usually normal in patients with type V hyperlipidemia.

Pathophysiology

The biochemical defect(s) in type I hyperlipidemia involves an abnormality in the synthesis, the storage, or, less likely, the release of lipoprotein lipase, but the molecular nature of this defect remains unknown. Abnormalities in chylomicrons obtained from patients with type I have not been demonstrated, and such particles are metabolized at a normal rate when infused into control subjects or used as a substrate for lipoprotein lipase in vitro. The profound impairment in chylomicron metabolism which occurs in patients with type I clearly illustrates the key role of lipoprotein lipase in normal chylomicron metabolism. It is also not clear why only chylomicrons accumulate in patients with type I, when in fact both chylomicrons and VLDL are thought to require lipoprotein lipase for hydrolysis of their triglycerides. Although the etiologic factor or factors responsible for the development of phenotypic type V hyperlipidemia remain poorly understood. Most patients have an underlying hereditary disorder associated with enhanced VLDL production (familial hypertriglyceridemia or familial combined hyperlipidemia) plus a secondary factor which concurrently stimulates triglyceride synthesis (e.g., diabetes or estrogen therapy).[133] The activities of both lipoprotein lipase and hepatic lipase are normal in most patients with type V[139] and do not explain the impaired triglyceride clearance found in this disorder. Enhanced production of VLDL has been demonstrated in some patients with type V and may, in the presence of a high fat intake, lead to overload of the normal lipolytic pathway, with resultant elevation of both VLDL and chylomicrons. Impaired chylomicron and VLDL catabolism occurs concomitantly and is responsible for the low levels of LDL and HDL which typically occur. A deficiency of apo-C-II, the apoprotein activator of lipoprotein lipase, has recently been reported in several families, with one family member being originally diagnosed as type V.[28,29,130]

Treatment

In both the type I and the type V phenotypes, elimination of secondary factors is important if a readily treatable etiology is not to be overlooked (Table 22-8). Lipid values in first-degree relatives should also be determined and are valuable both for verification of a familial pattern and to detect other hyperlipidemic family members. Therapy of both type I and type V hyperlipidemia is primarily aimed at reduction or elimination of hyperchylomicronemia so that episodes of abdominal pain and pancreatitis can be prevented. Correction of hyperchylomicronemia is accomplished by means of a reduction in dietary fat, as described in Dietary Treatment. Fish oils and fatty fish may be useful in the type V disorder, as will be amplified later. Hypolipidemic drugs have no place in the therapy of type I. In the authors' experience, gemfibrozil (Lopid) is especially helpful in patients with type V hyperlipidemia. Niacin is of some value; other drugs have not been useful. Infusions of normal plasma containing apoprotein C-II will temporarily correct the defect in familial apoprotein C-II deficiency.[28,29] This may be helpful during episodes of acute pancreatitis.

TYPE IV HYPERLIPOPROTEINEMIA

Definition

Type IV hyperlipidemia, also called hyperprebetalipoproteinemia, is characterized by an increased concentration of VLDL in plasma without the concomitant presence of chylomicrons or increased levels of LDL. The disorder may be secondary to a number of associated conditions or may result from primary familial disorders, most notably familial hypertriglyceridemia and familial combined hyperlipidemia. Lipid values obtained after a 12- to 14-h fast characteristically reveal elevated triglyceride levels greater than 140 mg/dl, usually above 200 mg/dl and under 1000 mg/dl without chylomicronemia. Cholesterol levels are average or only mildly elevated.

Clinical Characteristics

The clinical presentation of type IV hyperlipidemia varies markedly. The disorder may be primary or, more commonly, secondary.[140] Most patients are asymptomatic, and the abnormality is frequently detected on a routine multichannel chemistry screen. Xanthomas are seldom seen. Xanthelasmas are likewise uncommon; their presence in patients with increased triglycerides is more suggestive of the type IIb phenotype. Vascular disease, particularly coronary heart disease, is a frequent complication in patients over age 45 with type IV hyperlipidemia, particularly those with genotypic familial combined hyperlipidemia. Peripheral vascular disease is less common. The importance of type IV hyperlipidemia as a risk factor in coronary heart disease was illustrated in a study of 500 survivors of myocardial infarction,[141] among whom this phenotype was present in 15 percent. Secondary causes should be sought in all patients who present with a type IV phenotype. Obesity, chronic renal failure or nephrotic syndrome, diabetes mellitus, and hypothyroidism together with excessive consumption of alcohol are the most commonly associated conditions. It must be stressed that the vast majority of patients with type IV are overweight. Only in families with endogenous familial hypertriglyceridemia or familial combined hyperlipidemia is obesity not common. In this group are children and slender individuals with type IV. A variety of medications, most notably estrogen-containing oral contraceptives and thiazide diuretics, have also been implicated.

Genetics

In addition to secondary causes, the type IV phenotype may occur in patients with endogenous familial hypertriglyceridemia and in familial combined hyperlipidemia. The distinction between the two is dependent on the lipid values in first-degree family members.[109] In the former, the proband comes from a family in which all affected relatives have isolated hypertriglyceridemia with increased levels of VLDL. In familial combined hyperlipidemia, the affected relatives are heterogeneous and may have isolated hypercholesterolemia (IIa), hypertriglyceridemia (IV or V), or both (IIb).[109] Both disorders appear to be inherited as an autosomal dominant trait which frequently shows penetrance in the first two decades of life.

Diagnostic Laboratory Features

The hallmark of type IV hyperlipidemia is an elevation of endogenously synthesized VLDL. The criteria for the diagnosis of this disorder are not absolute and are influenced by the race, age, sex, and diet of the patient and by the reliability of the available lipid determinations. For North American adults over age 45, the combination of a plasma cholesterol level lower than 240 mg/dl with a triglyceride level higher than 200 mg/dl without chylomicrons present may be considered diagnostic. Visualization of turbid plasma without chylomicrons together with an increased triglyceride level and a slightly elevated cholesterol level is all that is required in the diagnosis of type IV (see Laboratory Tests). Frequently, HDL will be low; this is probably partly responsible for the vascular disease in these patients. Associated laboratory abnormalities commonly seen in patients with type IV include hyperuricemia, hyperglycemia, and an abnormal glucose tolerance test.

Pathophysiology

The accumulation of endogenously synthesized VLDL may result from enhanced synthesis of this lipoprotein with overload of the normal removal mechanism or, alternatively, from impaired removal in the presence of normal rates of synthesis. In some cases, both mechanisms may be operative together. The secondary forms of hypertriglyceridemia, particularly those associated with obesity and hyperinsulinism, excessive alcohol intake, and the use of oral contraceptives, are associated with enhanced synthesis of VLDL; this seems to be the primary factor responsible for the type IV phenotype. In contrast, both increased synthesis and decreased catabolism may occur in obese patients and in poorly controlled insulin-dependent diabetics. The primary mechanism underlying VLDL accumulation in the familial hypertriglyceridemias has not been clearly established but may involve increased synthesis of VLDL. Enhanced hepatic VLDL and triglyceride synthesis, possibly mediated by an increased responsiveness to insulin, has been proposed to explain the lipid abnormalities in patients with endogenous familial hypertriglyceridemia.[142]

Treatment

Because of the common association of the type IV phenotype with obesity, adult-onset diabetes mellitus, and excessive alcohol intake, correction of secondary predisposing factors should be attempted in all patients. Thus the attainment of ideal weight and restricted use of alcohol should be strongly encouraged;

caloric restriction is essential if the patient is overweight. Estrogens, unless prescribed for a compelling medical reason, should be withdrawn from all patients with type IV. As discussed elsewhere, we favor a single dietary approach to the treatment of hyperlipidemias and recommend a low-cholesterol (100-mg) diet in which the fat content is reduced to 20 percent of total calories, with an emphasis on restriction of saturated fat.

Drug therapy for type IV should be reserved for patients in whom an adequate trial of dietary therapy (6 to 8 months) and correction of secondary factors have failed to reduce the elevated VLDL levels. Drug therapy should be regarded as an adjunct to, rather than a substitute for, dietary therapy. Gemfibrozil 600 mg twice daily is the most widely accepted and most tolerated drug for therapy of type IV (see Pharmaceutical Agents). Gemfibrozil is successful in reducing triglyceride and VLDL levels in most patients. Clofibrate is no longer the drug of choice for type IV hyperlipidemia because of possible long-term, ill-defined adverse effects (see Pharmaceutical Agents, below). In some cases, however, decreases in VLDL are not paralleled by reductions in total cholesterol, which may actually increase.[119] This paradox is attributable to enhanced conversion of VLDL to LDL and to mild increases in HDL and may on occasion convert a type IV phenotype to a mild type IIa pattern. Strict control of dietary cholesterol and saturated fat will frequently correct the latter, but if this does not occur, serious thought should be given to the discontinuation of gemfibrozil or the addition of a second drug effective in type IIa. Nicotinic acid is probably more effective than gemfibrozil in reducing VLDL triglyceride and apoprotein B levels and rarely produces a paradoxical increase in LDL. As discussed in Pharmaceutical Agents, side effects are much more common with this medication and result in much poorer patient compliance. Bile acid sequestrants (cholestyramine and colestipol) and probucol (Lorelco) have no place in the therapy of type IV hyperlipidemia.

DISORDERS OF HIGH-DENSITY LIPOPROTEINS

A number of epidemiologic studies conducted over the last three decades[143,144] have established a strong inverse relation between the concentrations of HDL cholesterol in plasma and the incidence of coronary heart disease observed in western populations. Although these studies support the view that HDL may facilitate the transport of cholesterol from peripheral tissues back to the liver, the precise role of HDL in the pathogenesis of the atherosclerotic process has not been clarified. Thus it is not clear whether high levels of HDL are themselves protective or whether they are simply a marker for other, more fundamental differences in lipoprotein metabolism (for example, more efficient lipolysis and hepatic uptake of triglyceride-rich lipoproteins) which occur in patients with high levels of HDL cholesterol. Concentrations of HDL cholesterol are low (25 to 30 mg/dl) in some societies not habituated to a typical Western diet, in which the incidence of coronary heart disease is also very low.[54] Notably, concentrations of LDL are also low in these populations, suggesting that the inverse correlations noted between low concentrations of HDL cholesterol and high rates of coronary heart disease in Western societies may require the concurrent presence of a permissive level of LDL cholesterol (e.g., $>$ 120 mg/dl) which is not normally present in more "primitive" societies. Despite strong epidemiologic associations between low levels of HDL cholesterol and an increased incidence of coronary heart disease, it is not clear whether therapeutic measures to increase HDL cholesterol levels in individuals in whom these are low are of therapeutic benefit.[50] The use of pharmaceutical agents or alcohol which are intended *solely* to increase HDL cholesterol levels cannot therefore be recommended. In contrast, the use of other measures (e.g., diet, weight loss, increase in exercise, and cessation of cigarette smoking) which may raise HDL cholesterol levels as a secondary phenomenon should be encouraged, as should the use of pharmaceutical agents which concurrently reduce elevated levels of VLDL and LDL cholesterol (e.g., nicotinic acid and gemfibrozil) but which are themselves prescribed *for that purpose.*

Reduced levels of HDL cholesterol may occur in association with several secondary factors, including hypertriglyceridemia, obesity, cigarette smoking, and physical inactivity, and are 10 mg/dl lower in men than in premenopausal women.[41] Reductions in plasma concentrations of HDL cholesterol may also be seen in patients receiving probucol[145] and during the administration of anabolic steroids. A number of secondary factors have been shown to increase concentrations of HDL cholesterol in human plasma.[41] These include exercise, moderate consumption of alcohol, cessation of cigarette smoking, and correction of hypertriglyceridemia. Several medications, including estrogens, phenytoin, and barbiturates, are also known to increase plasma concentrations of HDL cholesterol.

A number of familial syndromes in which HDL cholesterol levels are reduced below the 10th percentile in the absence of severe hypertriglyceridemia or LCAT deficiency have been described. These disorders include familial apo-A-I and -C-III deficiency,[146,147] Tangier disease,[30] HDL deficiency with planar xanthomas,[148,149] fish eye disease,[150,151] apo-A-I Milano,[152] and familial hypoalphalipoproteinemia.[153,154] In addition to these disorders, reduced concentrations of HDL cholesterol have been observed in several families that have been shown to have single amino acid substitutions in apoprotein A-I, whereas increased plasma concentrations of HDL cholesterol have been described in familial hyperalphalipoproteinemia.[155] In the following section, we shall briefly review the salient features of these disorders, which have also been the subject of a recent review by Schaefer.[156] Distinguishing clinical and biochemical features of the familial HDL deficiency disorders are outlined in Table 22-10.

Familial Apolipoprotein A-I and C-III Deficiency

Three patients from two separate kindreds have been described with a marked reduction in the concentrations of HDL cholesterol (1 to 6 mg/dl) and a virtual absence of apoproteins A-I and C-III from plasma.[146,147] Corneal opacification was noted in all three patients, and prominent planar xanthomas were present on the trunk, neck, and eyelids of the two sisters from the second family. Coronary atherosclerosis was present in one patient by age 40 years and was present in the other two by their late twenties. Reduced concentrations of HDL cholesterol (25 to 35 mg/dl) were found in obligate heterozygotes from both kindreds, but of 17 heterozygotes in one kindred, none developed premature coronary artery disease before age 40 and only two did so before age 60. Thus the heterozygous form of this disorder does not appear to be associated with a marked increase in premature coronary artery disease. The defect in this disease appears to be an inability to synthesize apoproteins A-I and C-III because of a DNA insertion in the coding region of the apo-A-I gene. Although this is of unproven efficacy in this rare disorder, it would seem prudent to attempt to reduce LDL cholesterol concentrations with a view to reversing the tendency for accelerated atherosclerosis and possibly causing regression of the cutaneous xanthomas.

HDL Deficiency with Planar Xanthomas

This disorder of unknown etiology[148,149] has been described in one Swedish woman who presented with an HDL cholesterol of 3 mg/dl and extensive cutaneous planar xanthomas. The patient developed coronary artery disease in her late forties, and apoprotein analyses disclosed a marked decrease in the concentrations of apo-A-I with concentrations of apo-C-III that were slightly above normal. Corneal opacification was also observed, but the patient's tonsils were normal. The molecular defect responsible for this disorder has not been determined.

Fish Eye Disease

Severe corneal opacification and low concentrations of HDL cholesterol (7 mg/dl) have been reported in two Swedish kindreds, and this abnormality has been

Table 22-10. Clinical and Biochemical Findings in Familial HDL Deficiency Disorders

	Familial apo A-I, C-III deficiency	Tangier disease	HDL deficiency with planar xanthomas	Apo A-I Milano	Fish eye disease	Familial hypoalphalipoproteinemia
Corneal opacities	+	+	+	−	+++	−
Planar xanthomas	+	−	+	−	−	−
Abnormal tonsils	−	+	−	−	−	−
Neuropathy	−	+	−	−	−	−
Hepatosplenomegaly	−	+	+	−	−	−
Premature CAD*	+++	+	++	−	−	+++
Plasma cholesterol (mg/dl)						
Total	110–156	70	260	208	207	165
LDL	106–120	20	134	171	199	115
HDL	1–6	2	3	11	7	26
Plasma triglycerides (mg/dl)	62	200	290	243	424	113

*Coronary artery disease.
For premature CAD, +++ indicates onset before age 40, ++ before age 50, and + before age 60. Patients with Apo A-I Milano and familial hypoalphalipoproteinemia are heterozygotes, whereas for the other disorders the description refers to homozygotes.
Source: Modified from Schaefer.[156]

termed *fish eye disease* because of the ocular findings.[150,151] Despite modest elevations in the concentrations of LDL cholesterol and modest hypertriglyceridemia, the reported patients did not develop coronary artery disease prior to the sixth decade of life. Concentrations of apo-A-I and A-II were reduced in the homozygous patients, and concentrations of HDL cholesterol were approximately 50 percent of normal in heterozygotes. The metabolic defect in this disorder has not been determined.

Apo-A-I Milano

Low levels of HDL cholesterol (11 mg/dl) were reported in an Italian man with no clinical evidence of coronary artery disease in whom the low concentrations of HDL cholesterol were due to a substitution of cysteine for arginine in apo-A-I; this resulted in an enhanced rate of catabolism of these lipoprotein particles from plasma.[152,157] Corneal opacification, xanthomas, and hepatosplenomegaly were not reported in this patient, and there was no family history of premature coronary artery disease.

Familial Hypoalphalipoproteinemia

Familial hypoalphalipoproteinemia is an autosomal dominant inherited trait which is associated with concentrations of HDL cholesterol below the 10th percentile (less than 30 mg/dl in men; less than 35 mg/dl in women) and an accelerated rate of premature coronary artery disease.[154,155] There are no specific clinical findings, and corneal opacities are not characteristic of this disorder. Recent studies suggest that familial hypoalphalipoproteinemia may have a gene frequency as common as 1 in 400 in the United States. Although the cause of this disorder is not known, patients with familial hypoalphalipoproteinemia appear to have a 15-fold increase in the frequency of a restriction-enzyme polymorphism following DNA digestion with the restriction enzyme PstI.[158] Familial hypoalphalipoproteinemia has also been associated with an increased incidence of strokes in children.[159] Therapy for patients with familial hypoalphalipoproteinemia should aim to minimize other potential risk factors for cardiovascular disease and maintain LDL cholesterol below 100 mg/dl. Whether pharmaceutical measures which raise HDL cholesterol levels have any benefit in this disorder is not known, but therapy with nicotinic acid would be an attractive strategy to reduce LDL and increase HDL cholesterol levels.

Tangier Disease

DEFINITION

Tangier disease is a rare disorder characterized by severe deficiency of normal HDL in plasma and by the accumulation of cholesterol esters in many tissues throughout the body, including the characteristic deposition in the tonsils. The disorder takes its name from Tangier Island, Virginia, where the first cases were reported. To date, fewer than 50 cases have been reported in the United States, Europe, and Australia.[30]

CLINICAL FEATURES

Suspicion of Tangier disease is most commonly aroused by the unique appearance of the tonsils. Oral pharyngeal examination reveals large lobulated tonsils which have a distinctive orange or yellow color that is attributable to deposits of cholesterol esters within the tissue. Deposition of this lipid in other tissues frequently results in splenomegaly (80 percent), hepatomegaly (30 percent), and lymphadenopathy (20 percent) and may provoke suspicion of a malignancy. Cholesterol esters are also deposited in the rectal mucosa, which shows 1- to 2-mm orange and brown spots on proctosigmoidoscopic examination. Rectal biopsy reveals foamy cholesterol ester–laden histiocytes in the mucosa and submucosa. Corneal infiltration is usually detectable by means of slit-lamp examination in patients over age 40 years but does not impair vision. A variety of neurological symptoms occur in patients with Tangier disease, and these symptoms may constitute the initial reason for seeking medical attention. Symptoms include weakness, paresthesias, diplopia, and increased sweating. Objectively, reduced muscle strength with wasting, decreased tendon reflexes, occular palsies, and selective loss of pain and temperature sensation have been described. Electromyography (EMG) reveals signs of denervation in affected muscles, but nerve conduction is normal. No episodes of premature coronary artery disease or cerebral vascular disease have been noted in homozygous or heterozygous patients with Tangier disease before age 40. However, among eight homozygotes over age 40, five had evidence of coronary artery disease or cerebral vascular disease[160] whereas the other three are alive and well in their fourth and fifth decades. Thus, although patients homozygous for Tangier disease may be at increased risk for the premature development of atherosclerosis, this risk is clearly lower than in several other disorders which are associated with a similar marked deficiency of HDL but in which LDL cholesterol concentrations are generally higher.

GENETICS

Full expression of Tangier disease occurs in patients homozygous for this disorder and is consistent with an autosomal dominant mode of transmission.[30] Heterozygous patients frequently have reduced levels of HDL cholesterol (25 to 30 mg/dl) and reduced concentrations of apoprotein A-I but do not have any of the tonsillar or neuropathic findings noted in the homozygous form and remain asymptomatic. Because of their reduced concentration of HDL cholesterol, heterozygous patients may be at increased risk for the premature development of coronary artery disease.[161]

DIAGNOSTIC LABORATORY FEATURES

The plasma lipid profile of patients who are homozygous for Tangier disease is characterized by a low concentration of cholesterol (60 to 100 mg/dl) with moderately increased triglyceride levels (100 to 300 mg/dl). Lipoprotein fractionation discloses reductions in the concentrations of HDL cholesterol, apo-A-I, and apomately 35 percent of normal, and a marked reduction in the concentration of HDL cholesterol (1 to 3 mg/dl). Plasma concentrations of apoprotein A-I and A-II are reduced to 1 percent and 9 percent of normal, respectively, and concentrations of other major apoproteins are 50 to 80 percent of normal. Patients who are heterozygous for Tangier disease have plasma concentrations of HDL cholesterol, apo-A-I and apo-A-II that are approximately 50 percent of normal. The laboratory findings taken in conjunction with the usual clinical picture permit a definitive diagnosis of Tangier disease to be made in virtually all cases.

PATHOPHYSIOLOGY

The biochemical defects underlying the lipoprotein abnormalities and presumed secondary storage of cholesterol esters in Tangier disease have not been fully elucidated. Studies utilizing apoprotein A-I isolated from the plasma of patients with Tangier disease have demonstrated an increased content of proapo-A-I,[162] which has a reduced affinity to associate with HDL particles.[161] The amino acid composition of apo-A-I Tangier may also differ slightly from that of normal apoprotein A-I.[163] Kinetic studies have indicated an enhanced fractional catabolic rate for proapoprotein A-I in patients with Tangier disease, but the activity of the converting enzyme responsible for the formation of apo-A-I from proapo-A-I is normal. Thus, despite considerable progress and the application of the newer tools of molecular biology, the precise defects responsible for the apparent hypercatabolism of apoprotein A-I in this disorder remain unknown. The increased catabolism of apoprotein A-I is, however, presumably responsible for the uptake of cholesterol ester–rich chylomicron remnants by macrophages of the reticuloendothelial system, which results in the selective storage of this lipid in these tissues from homozygous patients with Tangier disease.

TREATMENT

There is no treatment for Tangier disease. Dietary restriction of fat in order to minimize formation of chylomicron remnants has been advocated by some authors; although of unproven benefit, such a regimen would seem prudent until further evidence becomes available.

Familial Hyperalphalipoproteinemia

Familial hyperalphalipoproteinemia is characterized by distinct elevations in the concentrations of HDL cholesterol in association with normal levels of LDL and VLDL cholesterol and normal plasma triglyceride concentrations.[155] When adjusted for age and sex, total cholesterol concentrations are mildly elevated and typically lie in the range of 230 to 280 mg/dl. The condition is of interest largely because it is the only known hyperlipidemia which actually appears to be beneficial to the patient. As with familial hypobetalipoproteinemia, patients with this disorder have a low incidence of cardiovascular disease and show increased longevity. Familial hyperalphalipoproteinemia should be suspected when there are HDL cholesterol levels in excess of 70 mg/dl in male patients and levels in excess of 85 to 90 mg/dl in female patients in whom secondary causes of HDL elevation have been excluded. Genetic studies by Glueck and associates[164] have indicated that familial hyperalphalipoproteinemia is inherited as an autosomal dominant trait with full penetrance in neonates and children. The incidence of this condition in the general population is not known but is probably greater than 1 in 3000. The condition is benign, and no treatment is indicated.

OTHER LIPOPROTEIN DISORDERS

Abetalipoproteinemia

DEFINITION

The term *abetalipoproteinemia* refers to a group of disorders characterized by a complete absence of apoprotein B-100, the protein essential for the formation of

LDL and VLDL, from plasma.[30] To date, three distinct genetic conditions have been described in which there is a complete absence of VLDL and LDL from plasma. In classic abetalipoproteinemia and homozygous hypobetalipoproteinemia there is a concurrent absence of apoprotein B-48–containing chylomicron particles from plasma, whereas in normotriglyceridemic abetalipoproteinemia the intestinal production of apoprotein B-48–containing chylomicron particles is normal and hepatic production of apoprotein B-100 in VLDL and LDL is impaired.[165,166] Patients with these disorders have profound hypocholesterolemia (20 to 40 mg/dl), which in classic abetalipoproteinemia and homozygous hypobetalipoproteinemia is accompanied by marked hypotriglyceridemia (5 to 10 mg/dl).

CLINICAL CHARACTERISTICS

Patients with phenotypic abetalipoproteinemia due to the classic form of this disorder or to homozygous hypobetalipoproteinemia show similar clinical features. Such patients manifest steatorrhea from birth which is attributable to the block in mucosal formation of chylomicron particles, with a resulting impairment of fat absorption. There is concomitantly an impairment of the absorption of the fat-soluble vitamins (A, D, E, and K) and of essential fatty acids and cholesterol. Biopsies of intestinal mucosal cells show intense engorgement of fat within the enterocytes, and in at least one patient[167] there was a concurrent absence of immunofluorescence for apoprotein B. Because of the malabsorption of fat-soluble vitamins, patients with abetalipoproteinemia may manifest vitamin A and vitamin K deficiency at a young age[168] and clearly develop profound vitamin E deficiency.[169,170] This results from two factors. First, absorption of vitamin E is impaired, as is absorption of all other fat-soluble vitamins, because of the blockade of chylomicron formation. Second, plasma transport of vitamin E is greatly disturbed because the chief transport form, LDL, is not present at all. Thus, vitamin E deficiency in humans may be most clearly seen in patients with abetalipoproteinemia.

Steatorrhea and, in patients who remain undiagnosed, a general failure to thrive may be the only manifestations of the disease for the first 5 to 7 years of life. Subsequent to this, in untreated patients, there is progressive development of neurological and retinal dysfunction, which if unrecognized ultimately will prove profoundly disabling. Initially, deep tendon reflexes disappear and there is mild impairment of sensation. Signs of abnormal cerebellar, posterior column, and peripheral nerve function together with muscle weakness progress if the disease is not recognized, and in untreated patients severe ataxia is present by the second decade of life. Retinal dysfunction is manifested by the insidious development of retinitis pigmentosa with loss of night vision and progressive visual impairment. Although some of the visual loss may reflect vitamin A deficiency, treatment with vitamin A alone does not halt further progression of disease, suggesting that vitamin E deficiency may be the primary insult responsible for these retinal abnormalities.

The abnormal lipoprotein environment also affects the erythrocytes, and the peripheral smear reveals large numbers of acanthocytes, which form because of the abnormal cholesterol and phospholipid composition of the erythrocyte membranes. These patients do not, however, generally develop anemia as a result of the abnormal red cell membranes.

Because of the important role of LDL in delivering cholesterol to steroid-hormone-producing tissues, the question of whether corticosteroid or progesterone production may be impaired in abetalipoproteinemia has been addressed. Studies of the adrenal response to prolonged ACTH infusion have documented a modest impairment in corticosteroid production which is probably not of clinical significance.[171,172] Reduced progesterone levels were reported in one patient with homozygous hypobetalipoproteinemia[173] followed through pregnancy. Although pregnancy proceeded normally in this patient without the need for exogenous progesterone, such a supplement may be necessary in other patients.

Recognition of the key role of vitamin E deficiency in the pathogenesis of the neurological abnormalities in abetalipoproteinemia has radically changed the prognosis for patients with this disorder. Current data strongly suggest that with appropriate therapy the disabling neurological and visual deterioration can be totally prevented.[174,175]

Reported findings in normotriglyceridemic abetalipoproteinemia have included hypocholesterolemia (25 mg/dl) with plasma triglyceride concentrations of 25 to 35 mg/dl, a lack of significant steatorrhea, and the presence of acanthocytes on peripheral blood smears.[165,166] The older of the two reported patients[165] was obese and had neurological symptoms of ataxia at age 8 years.

GENETICS

The inherited pattern of phenotypic abetalipoproteinemia takes two forms. The most common disorder (classic abetalipoproteinemia) is inherited as an autosomal recessive trait for which affected patients are homozygotes. Obligate heterozygous parents have normal concentrations of plasma lipids and lipoproteins, and the carrier state cannot be identified. In the second form, phenotypic abetalipoproteinemia represents the homozygous form of hypobetalipoproteinemia, which is inherited as an autosomal dominant trait. Fewer than 10 cases of homozygous hypobetalipoproteinemia have been reported, and obligate heterozygotes show LDL cholesterol concentrations ranging from 15 to 40 mg/dl.[176] Normotriglyceridemic abetalipoproteinemia appears to be inherited as an autosomal recessive trait, and obligate heterozygous parents have normal plasma lipid values.[166]

LABORATORY FINDINGS

Patients with phenotypic abetalipoproteinemia show extremely low levels of plasma cholesterol (20 to 30 mg/dl), and their levels of triglycerides are generally lower than 10 mg/dl. Lipoprotein fractionation studies disclose a total absence of chylomicrons, VLDL, and LDL, and plasma concentrations of HDL are reduced approximately 50 percent. A fatty meal does not result in the appearance of chylomicrons in the blood or elevation of the plasma triglyceride concentrations. In untreated patients, plasma concentrations of carotene and vitamin A are very low whereas vitamin E levels are usually undetectable. Because of vitamin K deficiency, the vitamin K–dependent coagulation factors may be reduced, resulting in a prolonged prothrombin time; hemorrhagic bleeding has been the initial presentation in several cases.[168] The synthesis of vitamin D in the skin appears to be adequate to compensate for the presumed decrease in the absorption of vitamin D, and rickets is not described as a complication of abetalipoproteinemia. The content of linoleic acid in plasma lipids is reduced, and this is also reflected in reduced levels of this essential fatty acid in adipose tissue and erythrocytes. Mild elevations in alkaline phosphatase, lactic acid dehydrogenase (LDH), and serum glutamic oxaloacetic transaminase (SGOT) have been observed in some patients and are presumed to reflect hepatic steatosis.

PATHOPHYSIOLOGY

The biochemical disorders responsible for all three genotypic forms of abetalipoproteinemia are not known. A recent study[177] indicated that the gene for apoprotein B was present in liver and intestine of one patient with classic abetalipoproteinemia in whom messenger RNA for apoprotein B was also detectable. This suggests that in this particular case the disorder resulted from a posttranslational defect in the assembly or secretion of apoprotein B from hepatocytes. Current data[174,175] strongly support the view that the acquired neurological and retinal degeneration which occurs in untreated patients with abetalipoproteinemia represents a manifestation of vitamin E deficiency. A current hypothesis suggests that the formation of peroxides in the face of low levels of vitamin E may create damage to certain tissues (the retina and the posterior columns of the spinal cord) which are rich in long-chain polyunsaturated fatty acids. Symptoms of deficiency of essential fatty acids have not been reported in patients with abetalipoproteinemia despite profound fat malabsorption and low concentrations of linoleic acid in plasma and adipose tissues.

TREATMENT

Steatorrhea in patients with phenotypic abetalipoproteinemia can be readily controlled with a very-low-fat diet (5 to 10 percent of total calories as fat). The degree of fat restriction necessary to prevent steatorrhea is greater in infants and children than in adults, in whom a diet with 15 to 20 percent of calories derived from fat is usually well tolerated. Deficiencies of fat-soluble vitamins can be completely corrected by the administration of water-soluble forms of vitamin A (Aquasol A) 10,000 to 25,000 U daily and vitamin K (Synkayvite) 5 mg weekly. Plasma levels of vitamin E can never be restored to normal, but high-dose vitamin E therapy has been shown to result in normal tissue concentrations of vitamin E in both adults and children[178,179] and clinical improvement and lack of further deterioration in newly diagnosed patients. We recommend that vitamin E be administered at 200 mg per kilogram of body weight per day in single or divided doses.[170] Treatment of patients with normotriglyceridemic abetalipoproteinemia aims at providing adequate intake of the fat-soluble vitamins, particularly vitamin E, but the ability of these patients to form chylomicrons allows the use of lower doses (400 U per day). Use of medium-chain triglycerides should be regarded as contraindicated in all patients with abetalipoproteinemia.[180] In the face of defective hepatic triglyceride secretion, medium-chain triglycerides may result in the accumulation of two-carbon fragments in the liver and may lead to the development of cirrhosis.

Hypobetalipoproteinemia

Reduced plasma concentrations of LDL cholesterol in the absence of hypertriglyceridemia (less than 40 mg/dl) can be seen in association with hyperthyroidism, malabsorption, and resection of the ileum and can be seen also in patients with autoantibodies directed against apoprotein B.[181] Low plasma concentrations of LDL may also be due to an inherited condition, heterozygous familial hypobetalipoproteinemia, which is inherited as an autosomal dominant trait with full phenotypic expression in childhood.[182,183] Heterozygous familial hypobetalipoproteinemia has an estimated gene frequency of 1 in 1000 to 1 in 2000,[184] and because of the low risk of coronary heart disease, it is associated with an overall increase in longevity.[185] Patients with heterozygous familial hypobetalipoproteinemia have no clinical abnormalities and do not require specific treatment or vitamin supplementation. In a family where two patients with heterozygous hypobetalipoproteinemia are to marry, the risk of having a child homozygous for this disorder will be one out of four, and such a child will have the clinical features of abetalipoproteinemia.

Familial Lecithin Cholesterol Acyltransferase Deficiency

Absence of the enzyme LCAT is a rare disorder characterized by moderately increased total cholesterol and triglyceride levels with markedly reduced levels of cholesterol ester and lysolecithin and an increased level of free cholesterol in plasma. Clinically, patients have corneal opacities and normochromic anemia and develop progressive renal insufficiency.[33]

CLINICAL FEATURES

Corneal opacities which develop in early childhood and consist of numerous gray dots in the corneal stroma, and especially in the periphery, resembling an arcus senilis are the most consistent and sometimes the only abnormal physical findings in patients with LCAT deficiency. The disorder is associated with premature atherosclerosis and progressive renal dysfunction, both of which are commonly present in the third and fourth decades.

GENETICS

Familial LCAT deficiency appears to be an autosomal recessive disorder, the clinical expression of which occurs only in homozygotes. Obligate heterozygotes have normal levels of both plasma LCAT and esterified cholesterol and do not develop corneal opacities.

DIAGNOSTIC LABORATORY FEATURES

The plasma lipid profile in patients with LCAT deficiency is variable but generally reveals total cholesterol of 250 to 400 mg/dl and triglycerides of 250 to 800 mg/dl. Chromatographic separation of plasma lipids reveals 85 to 90 percent of the cholesterol to be in the free form, with only 10 to 15 percent esterified. Various lipoprotein abnormalities can be demonstrated; paper electrophoresis reveals a prominent beta band with faint or absent prebeta and alpha bands, whereas ultracentrifugal separation shows reduced HDL levels. Documentation of the absence of LCAT remains the key to diagnosis. Some other disorders, notably obstructive jaundice, primary biliary cirrhosis, and $alpha_1$ antitrypsin deficiency, may be associated with marked elevations in free cholesterol and the presence of an abnormal low-density lipoprotein, termed LPX, similar to that seen in LCAT deficiency. Such conditions, however, are usually evident clinically and are not associated with a total deficiency of LCAT. Laboratory findings in patients with LCAT deficiency frequently include a normochromic anemia with hemoglobin concentrations of 10 g/dl and target cells visible on peripheral smear. Proteinuria of 1 to 2 g/24 h is also commonly seen and increases as renal function deteriorates. Bone marrow aspiration has revealed foam cells which stain as sea-blue histiocytes on Giemsa stain.

PATHOPHYSIOLOGY

The primary defect of this disease is a failure in the hepatic synthesis or secretion of the enzyme LCAT. This in turn leads to above-normal concentrations of free cholesterol and phosphatidylcholine in plasma and is manifested by a variety of abnormal lipoproteins. Although the precise pathophysiological mechanisms by which these lipids affect blood vessels and the renal glomerulus and are responsible for the pathological features of LCAT deficiency are not known, this may be mediated by an enhanced transfer of free cholesterol from plasma lipoproteins to cell plasma membranes, or alternatively, by a reduction in the normal egress of this lipid from the cells to the plasma.

TREATMENT

At present, there is no specific therapy for patients with LCAT deficiency. Restriction of fat and cholesterol has been advocated and seems efficacious in lowering both cholesterol and triglyceride levels. Progressive renal disease has been managed with hemodialysis and transplantation, but both maneuvers must be regarded as palliative rather than curative.

STEROL STORAGE DISEASES

Atherosclerosis

The common atherosclerotic lesions of the coronary arteries, the extracranial arteries of the head, and the distal aorta and arteries of the lower extremities represent fundamentally a biochemical storage disease with a tremendous accumulation of cholesterol, particularly cholesterol ester. This great storage of sterol occurs intracellularly initially but later occurs mainly extracellularly. There is associated proliferation of smooth muscle cells and macrophages which become foam cells as a result of the storage of cholesterol ester. A second biochemical event is the synthesis of collagen, which occurs as a reaction to the presence of cholesterol in the arterial intima. Thrombosis and platelet aggregation are important late events occurring after the endothelial surface of the growing atheromatous plaque has been disrupted.

This storage of cholesterol ester and free cholesterol in the intima of the arteries has its counterpart in only a few other conditions. A similar storage occurs in xanthomatous lesions, whose chemistry will be discussed later. An accumulation of free cholesterol clearly occurs in cholesterol gallstones, with the cholesterol content being 60 to 80 percent by weight. Large quantities of cholesterol ester under physiological circumstances are stored in the steroid-secreting endocrine glands as precursors for hormonal synthesis. Cholesterol ester, of course, circulates physiologically in the blood as a vital constituent of lipoproteins. In only the latter two circumstances is the presence of cholesterol ester other than pathological.

The origin of the cholesterol in the atherosclerotic plaque has been well worked out both in animal and in human lesions. While the arterial wall has a small capacity to synthesize cholesterol, its synthetic rate is insufficient to account for the tremendous mass of cholesterol present. Isotopic studies have shown that most of the cholesterol of the plaque originates from the blood plasma. It enters the arterial wall as a part of the LDL molecule, which is taken up by bulk endocytosis as it is by other tissues. Indeed, the LDL molecule has been identified immunologically in atherosclerotic plaques along with some VLDL. When one considers the high percentage of the LDL molecule—roughly 50 percent by weight—that is cholesterol or cholesterol ester, the atherogenicity of this lipoprotein particle becomes clear.

With hypercholesterolemia and concomitant increases in LDL cholesterol, the arterial wall picks up the LDL molecule and its cholesterol load at a rate which is greater than the amount of cholesterol which is exchanged back into the plasma and picked up by the HDL molecule for transport to the liver. Thus the physiological disposal system for excess cholesterol in any tissue, but particularly in the arterial intima, becomes overloaded when the plasma LDL cholesterol concentration is high. An abnormally low concentration of HDL would similarly affect the situation in favoring storage of cholesterol in the arterial wall.[40]

This concept of cholesterol transport and storage in the artery has been greatly clarified by tissue-culture experiments in which a variety of cells from animals and humans have been incubated with both LDL and HDL. When LDL is in high concentration, there is a tremendous uptake of cholesterol, particularly cholesterol ester. The resultant mass accumulation within the cell may be reversed by incubation of the cells in a medium containing HDL.

After the uptake of LDL by cultured cells, there is intracellular digestion of the LDL molecule, and its load of cholesterol, especially cholesterol ester, is left within the cell in a storage from which the cell is unable to excrete as long as the medium contains a high content of LDL (Fig. 22-4). Some internal rearrangement with further esterification of free cholesterol taken up by the cell may also be occurring.[35] It has been suggested that there is a relative enzymatic deficiency of cholesterol ester hydrolase in the arterial wall which would tend to promote the accumulation of cholesterol ester which has come into the wall carried by LDL. This cellular uptake of cholesterol ester from the medium may be considered as a model system for the uptake of cholesterol and cholesterol ester by the arterial wall in atherosclerosis and by the skin and tendons in xanthomatosis. Thus the lifetime accumulation of cholesterol in countless numbers of smooth muscle cells and macrophages and in the extracellular milieu brings about the atherosclerotic process.

The pathogenicity of other lipoproteins for the development of atherosclerosis varies greatly (see Table 22-5). Epidemiologically, except in older women, there is a lack of association between VLDL and triglyceride levels and the development of coronary heart disease. Clinically, however, premature coronary heart disease has been observed in families with type IV hyperlipidemia. The VLDL molecule, unlike HDL, can be picked up by tissue-culture cells and does contain apoprotein B. Furthermore, it carries a considerable amount of cholesterol, albeit less than LDL. Thus a moderate view would acknowledge that VLDL in excess is associated with an increased risk for coronary heart disease. IDL, which is found in type III hyperlipoproteinemia, has an undisputed relation with both atherosclerosis and xanthomatosis. Both coronary heart disease and especially peripheral atherosclerosis occur at an accelerated rate with IDL elevation.

Chylomicrons would appear to have a minimum of atherogenicity because of the large size of the particle. Atherosclerosis is reportedly rare in type I hyperlipoproteinemia with an absence or deficiency of lipoprotein lipase. However, there is considerable evidence that the chylomicron remnant, which is produced during the action of the tissue enzyme lipoprotein lipase on chylomicron triglycerides, is very atherogenic. This chylomicron remnant is less rich in triglyceride and richer in cholesterol and cholesterol ester than the original chylomicron. In type V hyperlipidemia, with poor clearing of chylomicrons, with a great accumulation of remnants and VLDL, and with low HDL, atherosclerosis and coronary heart disease certainly do occur. The remnant of chylomicron metabolism may be analogous to the remnant, IDL, from VLDL metabolism.

However, HDL, or α-lipoprotein, has a negative relation to atherosclerosis.[143,144] The data from all sources place HDL as having a protective role against the development of atherosclerosis. This applies particularly to American women before menopause, who have an attack rate for coronary heart disease much lower than that for similarly aged men and in whom HDL levels are 10 to 15 mg/dl higher. As has already been stressed,[39,40] the current thinking about HDL in this connection is that HDL may be a transport mechanism to carry cholesterol from the tissues back to the liver. Animals, for example, that have high HDL levels are relatively resistant to atherosclerosis, e.g., the rat and the dog. In tissue-culture systems, HDL does not induce deposition of cholesterol ester. Instead, its presence in the medium seems to prevent this occurrence and to actually produce regression of cholesterol esters in cells previously incubated in LDL. Both autopsy and, more recently, coronary angiographic evidence afford further confirmation of these concepts about the atherogenicity of various lipoproteins and plasma lipids.

Xanthomas

In the discussions of the various types of hyperlipidemia, considerable emphasis has been placed on xanthomas as one of the chief and cardinal clinical manifestations. In this section, emphasis will be placed on their collective characteristics, particularly as representing another disorder of lipid storage. Tendon and tuberous xanthomas represent sterol (ester) storage, but in eruptive xanthomas of the skin, triglyceride (from chylomicrons) is the chief constituent.

Ordinarily xanthomas represent a clinical manifestation of severe hyperlipidemia. The more severe the hyperlipidemia, the earlier in life the xanthomas appear. This concept is expressed most fully in the homozygote of familial hypercholesterolemia when the xanthomas appear in the first decade of life or at birth.

While the appearance of xanthomas is usually related to the duration and level of hypercholesterolemia, important exceptions occur. These include several other sterol storage diseases: cerebrotendinous xanthomatosis (the CTX syndrome) and "sitosterolemia and xanthomatosis." The presence of other sterols in the blood and in the tissues, cholestanol (CTX syndrome) and the plant sterols (sitosterolemia and xanthomatosis), potentiates greatly the development of xanthomas, particularly tendon xanthomas, as will be discussed subsequently.

Xanthomas may be regarded as the outward manifestation of sterol and lipid storage, analogous to the internal sterol storage occurring in developing atherosclerotic lesions. These two manifestations generally can be correlated, and when xanthomas are present, suspicion of underlying latent atherosclerosis must always be entertained. Xanthomas may also provide a clue to the diagnosis of a particular hyperlipidemia. Eruptive xanthomas indicate the presence of type I or type V hyperlipidemia with chylomicrons. Tuberous xanthomas may indicate type II familial hypercholesterolemia or type III. Tendon xanthomas are also found in these two conditions. Xanthelasmas have no absolute predilection for a given form of hyperlipidemia, although they are most commonly seen in association with hypercholesterolemia. The fact that many patients with severe familial hypercholesterolemia may not have xanthelasmas at all is also puzzling. The appearance of corneal arcus, another lipid storage entity, is certainly not predictable on the basis of hyperlipidemia. It may or may not be present. However, when found early in life without there having been injury to the eye, the presence of a profound corneal arcus is highly suggestive of severe hypercholesterolemia.

As is the case with early atherosclerotic plaques, xanthomas are composed principally of foam cells laden with cholesterol esters, a mild inflammatory reaction with the presence of Touton giant cells, and some increased collagen. Cholesterol ester is the chemical constituent most characteristically increased.[186] It is presumed that LDL (or IDL) is taken up by the cells of the tendons and skin, much in the same way that these lipoproteins are taken up from the plasma into the atherosclerotic plaque.

It is worth emphasizing the potential reversibility of all xanthomas in response to decreases in plasma lipid concentrations. Reversibility has occurred most dramatically with regard to the eruptive xanthomas of types I and V hyperlipidemia. These lesions may disappear completely in a month. Xanthelasmas and tuberous xanthomas have been observed to disappear over a period of 1 to 2 years with pronounced plasma lipid lowering. Tendon xanthomas are slower to regress, and significant changes take 2 or more years of effective therapy to become evident.

The surgical removal of xanthomatous lesions,

usually for cosmetic reasons, is almost invariably succeeded by their recurrence unless attention is paid to concomitant lowering of plasma lipids. This has occurred especially in regard to xanthelasma but also for surgically removed tendon and tuberous xanthomas.

Acid Cholesterol Ester Hydrolase Deficiency

Two other sterol storage diseases—Wolman's disease and cholesterol ester storage disease—in which cholesterol esters and triglycerides accumulate in lysosomes have been described[187] and appear to be allelic. In both inherited disorders, the biochemical defect involves the deficiency of a lysosomal esterase which at optimal acidic pH is capable of the hydrolysis of both cholesterol esters and triglycerides. Etiologically, both diseases appear to be similar to other lysosomal storage diseases associated with catabolic enzyme deficiencies, such as the sphingolipidoses and gangliosidoses.

WOLMAN'S DISEASE

Wolman's disease is usually detected within the first few weeks of life. Symptoms include vomiting, abdominal distention, steatorrhea, and a general failure to thrive.[187] Examination reveals hepatosplenomegaly with normal tonsils. Calcification of the adrenal glands is usually apparent on x-ray, and the plasma lipids are normal or low. Bone marrow aspiration reveals foam cells laden with cholesterol esters and triglycerides; at autopsy, increased concentrations of these lipids are found throughout the body, most notably in the liver, spleen, and lymph nodes. Definitive diagnosis is based on the clinical picture together with a demonstrable absence of acid cholesterol esterase in cultured fibroblasts or peripheral leukocytes. Studies of the known cases suggest that the disorder is inherited as an autosomal recessive trait; obligate heterozygotes may have reduced acid esterase activity but are clinically normal. Treatment is supportive, and the disease is fatal within the first year of life.

CHOLESTEROL ESTER STORAGE DISEASE

Clinically less severe than Wolman's disease, cholesterol ester storage disease is usually but not invariably detected in childhood.[187] Affected infants are usually asymptomatic, and the only consistent finding on physical examination has been hepatomegaly, which may be associated with splenomegaly in older subjects. Adrenal calcification is unusual in children but may occur in older subjects. Portal hypertension and esophageal varices have been reported secondary to hepatic fibrosis and cirrhosis in 3 of the 10 reported cases. Plasma lipid values have shown moderate hypercholesterolemia (250 to 400 mg/dl) with increased levels of VLDL and LDL and low levels of HDL. Xanthomas have not been reported, but there is autopsy evidence for premature atherosclerosis in two subjects.

The diagnosis of this autosomal recessive disorder is based on clinical findings together with enzyme studies similar to those in Wolman's disease, which reveal a virtual absence of lysosomal cholesterol esterase. In the absence of a specific treatment, dietary restriction of fat and cholesterol would seem a prudent but unproven recommendation.

FAMILIAL DISEASES WITH STORAGE OF STEROLS OTHER THAN CHOLESTEROL

This section describes two lipid storage diseases characterized by the accumulation of unusual sterols in the blood and tissue. In cerebrotendinous xanthomatosis (CTX syndrome), cholestanol (dihydrocholesterol) accumulates in the blood and tissues. The second disease, sitosterolemia and xanthomatosis, involves accumulation of plant sterols, particularly β-sitosterol, in the blood and tissues, notably in the tendons. Xanthomas occur in the absence of hypercholesterolemia in both disorders.[188,189]

Cerebrotendinous Xanthomatosis

Cerebrotendinous xanthomatosis is a rare familial disease characterized by xanthomas of the tendons, lungs, and brain in spite of normal or low plasma cholesterol levels.[188,189] The other clinical manifestations include cataracts, subnormal intelligence, progressive cerebellar ataxia, dementia, and spinal cord paresis. Cholestanol accumulates in the white matter of the cerebrum and cerebellum and in xanthomas. The plasma cholestanol concentration is increased. The disease appears to be inherited according to an autosomal recessive mode; the basic inheritable defect is not yet known.

CLINICAL MANIFESTATIONS

The onset of CTX is insidious and unpredictable. Dementia has been observed at age 10 years, cataracts by age 15, tendon xanthomas at age 15, and ataxia by age 18 years.

The course may be divided into several time phases. The initial stage usually begins in childhood, when borderline intelligence, mental retardation, mental deterioration, or even dementia may be found. This is not invariable, however, and in some patients mentation has been found to be normal even in the third and fourth decades of life.

During adolescence and young adulthood, spasticity and at times ataxia develop and become progressively more severe. Juvenile cataracts and tendon xanthomas are frequently observed in this second stage of disease and are usually well developed by young adulthood. The Achilles tendon is the most common site of xanthoma formation, but xanthomas also may occur in the triceps, the tibial tuberosities, and the extensor tendons of the fingers. These lesions are similar in appearance to those seen in familial hypercholesterolemia. Tuberous xanthomas and xanthelasmas (palpebral xanthomas) may also be present.

In the third stage of CTX, enlargement of xanthomas and neurological deterioration with spasticity, ataxia, difficulties of speech, tremors, and atrophy of the distal musculature become prominent. There may be bilateral Babinski signs and loss of pain and vibratory sensation. The disease follows a deteriorating course characterized by cerebellar ataxia, systemic spinal cord involvement, and finally a phase of pseudobulbar paresis leading to death. Four of the ten deaths reported so far, however, resulted from acute myocardial infarction. In the others, death presumably resulted from neurological dysfunction. Death has usually occurred between the fourth and sixth decades.

LABORATORY AND PATHOLOGICAL FINDINGS

In most patients, the plasma cholesterol and triglyceride levels have been within normal range, i.e., 117 to 220 mg/dl. The plasma cholestanol (5α-cholestan-3β-ol) is elevated (i.e., to 4 mg/dl vs. a normal level of less than 0.6 mg/dl). Cholestanol is a saturated sterol which differs from cholesterol in the absence of the 5,6 double bond. Cholestanol is normally present in small amounts in tissues and plasma and occurs in both the free and the ester forms.

Cholestanol is normally excreted in trace amounts in the bile, but in the CTX syndrome its excretion is greatly increased (4 to 11 percent of total sterols). Abnormalities of the secretion of bile acid occur concomitantly and reveal decreased concentrations of chenodeoxycholic acid with an increase in cholic acid, to about 80 percent of the total bile acids. Allocholic acid, which is formed from cholestanol, is also increased and represents the other bile acid abnormality.

In the CTX syndrome, large quantities of cholestanol are found in the tissues throughout the body. This phenomenon is particularly manifest in the nervous system, where cholestanol may constitute up to 25 percent of the total sterols. Although in the tendon xanthomas cholestanol may constitute up to 11 percent of the total sterols, cholesterol is still the predominant steroid present. Considerable amounts of cholestanol may be found in any tissue examined, including that of the skin, lung, liver, spleen, adipose tissue, and muscle. Large ectopic xanthomas that are particularly rich in cholestanol may be found internally, particularly in the lung and brain.

PATHOPHYSIOLOGY

The metabolic defect responsible for the great accumulation of cholestanol in tissues, particularly in the nervous system and tendons, is not known. The origin of tissue cholestanol hypothetically includes increased local synthesis, influx from the blood after synthesis elsewhere, absorption from the diet, or a block in catabolism or excretion from the tissues. One view is that cholestanol is stored in the tissue because of a transport problem in its removal. HDL levels in the plasma are low. Presumably, the functional derangements of the nervous system result from the accumulation of cholestanol in the myelin of nerve tissue.

Another unifying hypothesis has developed from the finding that the primary bile acid, chenodeoxycholic acid, is markedly deficient in CTX patients. This defect in the synthesis of chenodeoxycholic acid is accompanied by the appearance of bile acid precursors as alcohols in the bile. Thus the underlying biochemical defect may be a deficiency in a hepatic enzyme involved in the synthesis of bile acids from cholesterol. With the deficiency of bile acid synthesis, there is believed to be increased hepatic synthesis of both cholesterol and cholestanol.[189]

TREATMENT

Since cholestanol is present in certain foods of animal origin, mainly eggs and dairy products, reduction in or elimination of their consumption in a very-low-cholesterol diet has led to a lowering of plasma cholestanol levels.[8] The logical drug treatment has been chenodeoxycholic acid administered orally. This treatment has increased the bile acid pool and produced normal concentrations of chenodeoxycholic acid in bile. The abnormally present bile acid precursors disappear from bile, and levels of cholestanol in the plasma are reduced. Whether this treatment will ultimately change the course of this progressively deteriorating disorder is not yet certain, but the prospect is certainly exciting.[190]

Sitosterolemia and Xanthomatosis

This rare familial disease was initially described in two sisters[188] and has now been verified in a number of other patients.[189] It is characterized by the accumulation of plant sterols, particularly sitosterol, in the blood and tissues. The prominent clinical manifestations of the disease reported to date are xanthomas of tendons and skin, which appear in childhood despite normal or only slightly elevated plasma cholesterol concentrations.

The metabolic defects causing the disease are twofold: greatly increased intestinal absorption of all dietary sterols, including sitosterol and other plant sterols which are normally absorbed only in minute amounts, and impaired excretion of sitosterol from the body. The exact nature of these metabolic defects is not known. The disease appears to be inherited as an autosomal recessive trait.

CLINICAL FEATURES

In the patients in the initial report, xanthomas were first noted in childhood in the extensor tendons of both hands; over the years, they subsequently developed in the patellar, plantar, and Achilles tendons. Aside from the xanthomas, findings on physical examination and in extensive laboratory tests in the two sisters were within normal limits. A subsequent patient had a bruit over the abdominal aorta; others have had coronary heart disease.[191] The plant sterols—sitosterol, campesterol, and stigmasterol—are present in high concentrations in the blood and tissues. Cholestanol levels are also increased.

CHEMISTRY, ABSORPTION, AND METABOLISM OF PLANT STEROLS IN HUMANS

The three plant sterols—sitosterol, campesterol, and stigmasterol—are usually found only in the lipids of plants and thus are particularly plentiful in vegetable oils, nuts, and fat-rich vegetables and fruits. In chemical structure, the three plant sterols resemble cholesterol except for minor differences in their side chains.

Plant sterols are habitually consumed by human beings in the usual diet. A typical American diet may contain up to 250 mg of these sterols per day, of which sitosterol makes up to 75 percent of the total, with lesser proportions of campesterol and stigmasterol.

Intestinal absorption of plant sterols in humans is normally less than 5 percent of the amount in the diet and is responsible for their low plasma concentration (0.3 to 1.73 mg/dl). However, during infancy considerable amounts of sitosterol can be found in the blood (up to 9 mg/dl) and also in the aortas of infants fed vegetable oil–rich formulas. Twenty percent of the absorbed dietary sitosterol is converted to bile acids, and the remainder is excreted in the bile as free sterol. As discussed later, large quantities of plant sterols inhibit cholesterol absorption and have had limited use in the treatment of hypercholesterolemia.

LABORATORY ABNORMALITIES

High concentrations of sitosterol and the other two plant sterols in the plasma are the chief characteristic of sitosterolemia and xanthomatosis. Sitosterol predominates in concentrations ranging between 12 and 27 mg/dl. The campesterol concentration is 6 to 10 mg/dl, while less than 1 mg/dl of stigmasterol is present. About 60 percent of the plasma sitosterol and campesterol is esterified. The plasma plant sterols are distributed between the low-density (about 70 percent of the total) and high-density lipoproteins. The very-low-density lipoproteins carry only trace amounts. Hypercholesterolemia is a variable feature that is most prominent in children with sitosterolemia who are also consuming and hyperabsorbing a high-cholesterol diet.

Erythrocytes also contain unesterified plant sterols. The ratio of cholesterol to sitosterol in these cells is similar to that in the plasma and suggests that free exchange of both sterols occurs.

Considerable accumulation of plant sterols, mainly unesterified sitosterol, occurs in the tendon xanthomas. However, despite the high content of plant sterols, cholesterol is still the predominant sterol, constituting 73 to 88 percent of the total. Histologically, these xanthomatous lesions are indistinguishable from the tendon xanthomas found in hyperlipoproteinemia and cerebrotendinous xanthomatosis.

The subcutaneous adipose tissue and the skin of patients also have been found to contain plant sterols. Other tissues of the body also probably contain them in abnormal amounts, but no autopsy data are available for this recently described disease.

PATHOPHYSIOLOGY

The principal metabolic defect in sitosterolemia and xanthomatosis appears to be the greatly increased intestinal absorption of dietary sitosterol and other sterols including cholesterol, but the exact mechanism is not known. One hypothesis is that the esterification of plant sterols is abnormally enhanced and that this in turn promotes absorption. It is also possible that biliary excretion of sitosterol as neutral sterol or as bile acid may be critically limited, resulting in slow turnover of sitosterol.

The accumulation of sitosterol and the other two plant sterols in smaller amounts in the tendons implies that the plant sterols probably produce the major manifestations of the disease and initiate xanthoma formation. Analogously to the situation in cerebrotendinous xanthomatosis, it is noteworthy that despite high concentrations of sitosterol in the xanthomas, the increase in the xanthoma cholesterol is quantitatively more important. It has been hypothesized that perhaps the incorporation of the plant sterols into the plasma lipoproteins affects the stability of the lipoprotein complexes, thereby favoring deposition of sterols generally into the tissues.

In this context, a potential role of plant sterols in the development of atherosclerotic vascular disease should also be considered. It is possible that plant sterols may favor deposition of cholesterol in the arterial wall and lead to premature atherosclerotic lesions. The development of overt coronary disease and an aortic bruit in patients with sitosterolemia and xanthomatosis provides evidence in support of this view.

DIAGNOSIS

Sitosterolemia and xanthomatosis should be considered in every patient who has developed xanthomas in childhood and does not have either familial hypercholesterolemia or the CTX syndrome. The diagnosis of this disease can be established by analyzing the sterols of the plasma by means of gas-liquid chromatography. The variable hypercholesterolemia which some of these patients manifest is noteworthy. There should be a high index of suspicion that sitosterolemia may be the underlying diagnosis in any young person with xanthomas whose cholesterol level is normal or elevated in the range of 300 to 500 mg/dl. Some of these hypercholesterolemic sitosterolemia patients have been termed pseudohomozygotes of hypercholesterolemia because their parents were completely normal.[65] Restudied with plasma sterols determined, they were found to have sitosterolemia.[192]

TREATMENT

The logical treatment for this sterol storage disease is a diet low in or devoid of plant sterols, since the excessive plant sterols in the body originate from the diet. The results of such treatment in two patients revealed a 29 percent decrease in the level of plasma sitosterol. Presumably the great stores of plant sterols in the tissues are in equilibration with the plant sterols of plasma, and prolonged dietary treatment is required to reduce the plasma β-sitosterol level to normal.

The guiding principles in the formulation of a diet with a low content of plant sterol are to (1) eliminate all sources of vegetable fats such as vegetable oil, shortenings, and margarines, (2) eliminate all plant foods with a high fat content such as nuts, seeds, chocolate, olives, and avocado, and (3) use only refined cereal products which have the germ (rich in fat and plant sterols) removed. In general, foods which have a high content of vegetable fat will also have a high content of plant sterols. The detailed composition of such a diet has been published elsewhere.[188]

Theoretically, drugs that may interfere with the intestinal absorption of plant sterols may prevent the expression of sitosterolemia and xanthomatosis. No such drug trial has been conducted. However, the use of bile acid–binding resins (e.g., cholestyramine) has consistently lowered the total sterol levels in plasma and appears to be the treatment of choice in addition to the dietary measures described above.[189]

DIETARY TREATMENT OF HYPERLIPIDEMIA

The cornerstone in the treatment of hyperlipidemia is dietary alteration. This is true regardless of the degree to which primary genetic abnormalities are partly or completely responsible for the development of the hyperlipidemia. Dietary factors in the American population inevitably exacerbate any genetic abnormality when this is largely responsible for the hyperlipidemic state. Dietary treatment will almost always result in some improvement of the condition. Therapy has been simplified by the concept that a single basic diet may be used initially in the treatment of all forms of hyperlipidemia.[193] This single diet is low in cholesterol and low in total and saturated fat; it is high in complex carbohydrate. It is of low caloric density and provides calories only sufficient to achieve and maintain ideal body weight.

The aim of the dietary treatment of hyperlipidemia is straightforward: the achievement of "normal" plasma cholesterol and triglyceride concentrations. Dietary treatment should be initiated when the plasma cholesterol concentration is above 220 mg/dl in older adults and 200 mg/dl in young adults and children; the upper limit for plasma triglyceride concentration is 140 mg/dl.

The recommended dietary treatment is appropriate and safe for both adults and children. Such treatment must clearly answer all the nutritional needs of the body and at the same time have beneficial effects on the elevated plasma lipid and lipoprotein concentrations. These criteria have been satisfied both theoretically and practically.[193]

The Effects of Specific Nutrients on the Plasma Lipids and Lipoproteins

Historically and to the present time, a vast amount of evidence in both humans and animals has pointed to certain dietary factors which have hyperlipidemic effects (Table 22-11). Some have a hypolipidemic action. Many other factors have no or minimal effects. These nutritional factors will be discussed briefly to provide a theoretical and practical basis for dietary prescription in the treatment of hyperlipidemia.

CHOLESTEROL

Cholesterol in the diet has important effects on lipid metabolism.[194] Cholesterol-rich diets have regularly caused hypercholesterolemia, atherosclerosis, and even, at times, myocardial infarction in a large number of species of experimental animals, including primates.[195,196] Dietary cholesterol enters the body by way of the chylomicron pathway and is removed from the plasma by the liver as a component of chylomicron remnants. Only about 40 percent of ingested cholesterol is absorbed; the remaining 60 percent passes out in the stool. Dietary cholesterol is thus added to the cholesterol synthesized by the body, since feedback inhibition of cholesterol biosynthesis in the body only partially occurs in humans, even when a large amount of dietary cholesterol is ingested.[197]

Table 22-11. Dietary Effects on Plasma Lipids and Lipoproteins in Humans

Hyperlipidemic dietary factors
1. Dietary cholesterol
2. Saturated fat
3. Total fat
4. Total calories with adiposity
5. Alcohol (in some individuals)
Hypolipidemic dietary factors
6. Polyunsaturated fat: omega-6-rich vegetable oils* and omega-3-rich fish and fish oils
7. Some fibers (pectin, guar gum)
8. Carbohydrate as starches replacing fat
9. Possibly vegetable protein or other substances from vegetables
Dietary factors with no discrete long-term effects
10. Protein generally
11. Vitamins and minerals
12. Lecithin

*Very high amounts of polyunsaturated vegetable fat, while resulting in a hypocholesterolemic effect overall, would produce postprandial hypertriglyceridemia and increased remnant formation.

Because the ring structure of the sterol nucleus cannot be broken down by the tissues of the body, as occurs with fat, protein, and carbohydrate, it must be either excreted or stored. Thus it is easy to see how the body or a particular tissue (i.e., a coronary artery) can become overloaded with cholesterol if there are limitations in cholesterol excretion from the body. Cholesterol is excreted in the bile and ultimately in the stool, either as cholesterol or as bile acids synthesized in the liver from cholesterol. Both pathways of excretion are limited, and furthermore, much of what is excreted is returned to the body by the very efficient enterohepatic reabsorption and circulation.

Dietary cholesterol does not directly enter into the formation of the very-low-density lipoproteins and low-density lipoproteins synthesized in the liver because it is removed by the liver as a component of the chylomicron remnants. It can, however, profoundly affect the catabolism of LDL as mediated through the LDL receptor. Because dietary cholesterol ultimately contributes to the total amount of hepatic-cell cholesterol, it can affect the biosynthesis of both cholesterol and LDL receptors in the liver. In particular, an increase in hepatic-cell cholesterol will decrease the number of LDL receptors and subsequently, as in other conditions that decrease LDL receptors, will cause an *increase* in the plasma level of LDL cholesterol.[198,199] Conversely, a drastic decrease in dietary cholesterol will increase the number of LDL receptors in the liver, will enhance LDL removal, and hence will lower plasma LDL levels. The effects of dietary cholesterol follow.

1. Increased chylomicrons and remnants
2. Increased hepatic-cell cholesterol, which has the following consequences:
    a. Decreased cholesterol biosynthesis
    b. Partial compensation in excretion of biliary cholesterol and bile acids to lessen hepatic cholesterol
    c. Decreased synthesis of LDL receptors
    d. Increased plasma LDL
3. Increased plasma LDL and deposition of cholesterol into the arterial wall

Over the past 25 years 26 separate metabolic experiments involving 196 human subjects have demonstrated that dietary cholesterol exerts decisive effects on plasma cholesterol and LDL levels.[200–202] However, as pointed out years ago, the doubling or tripling of the amount of dietary cholesterol will not necessarily increase the plasma levels if the initial amount of dietary cholesterol is already substantial (e.g., an increase in intake from 475 mg per day to 950 mg per day).[201] Despite this earlier literature, such attempts are still being carried out and are highly touted as showing that dietary cholesterol has no effect on plasma cholesterol levels. For those who wish to explore the subject more fully, a fairly recent review exists.[203]

The effects on the plasma cholesterol levels as the amount of dietary cholesterol is gradually increased are depicted in Fig. 22-17. These data are supported by both animal and human experiments. With a baseline cholesterol-free diet, the amount of dietary cholesterol necessary to produce an increase in the plasma cholesterol concentration is referred to as the *threshold amount.* Then, as the amount of dietary cholesterol is increased, the plasma cholesterol increases until the second important point on this curve—the *ceiling amount*— is reached. Further increases in dietary cholesterol do not lead to higher levels of plasma cholesterol, even though phenomenally high amounts may be ingested. Each animal or human being probably has its own distinctive threshold and ceiling amounts. Generally speaking, however, and again based on the experimental literature, we suggest that an average threshold amount for human beings is 100 mg per day; an average ceiling amount of dietary cholesterol is in the neighborhood of 300 to 400 mg per day. Further experiments are necessary to provide more precise information about the ceiling. Thus a baseline dietary cholesterol intake of 500 mg per day from two eggs would already exceed the ceiling for most individuals. The addition of two more egg yolks, for a total dietary cholesterol intake of 1000 mg per day, would not then further increase the plasma cholesterol concentration. Yet beginning with a baseline very-low-cholesterol diet under 100 mg per day and

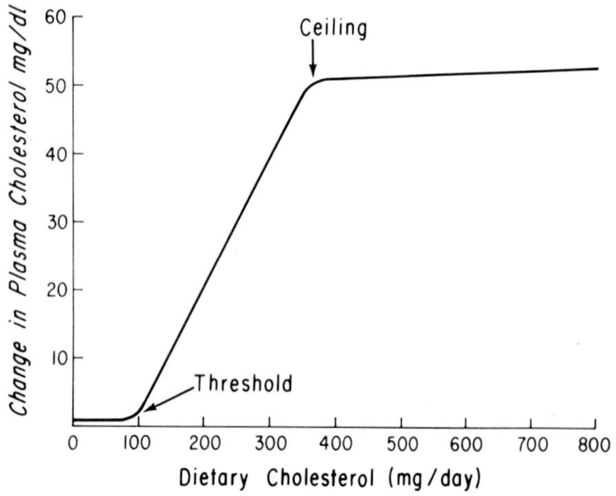

FIGURE 22-17 The effects of gradually increasing amounts of dietary cholesterol on the plasma cholesterol levels of human subjects whose background diet is very low in cholesterol content. (See text for a discussion of threshold and ceiling concepts.)

adding the equivalent of two egg yolks, or 500 mg, to this baseline amount would produce a striking change in plasma cholesterol concentrations, perhaps, as shown in many experiments, to 60 mg/dl.

Recent dietary surveys indicate that the average American intake of dietary cholesterol is about 400 mg per day for women and 500 mg per day for men.[204] Decreasing these amounts of dietary cholesterol, as would take place in the therapeutic and preventive diets, would then have a profound effect on plasma cholesterol concentrations, because, as shown in Fig. 22-17, operationally one would be on the descending limb of the curve.

DIETARY FAT, AMOUNT AND SATURATION, KINDS OF POLYUNSATURATION

The amount and kind of fat in the diet have a well-documented effect on plasma lipid concentrations. The *total* amount of dietary fat is important because the formation of chylomicrons in the intestinal mucosa and their subsequent circulation in the blood are directly proportional to the amount of fat that has been consumed in the diet. A fatty meal will result in the production of large numbers of chylomicrons and will impart the characteristic lactescent appearance to postprandial plasma that is observed some 3 to 5 h after meal consumption. A typical American diet containing 110 g of fat will produce 110 g of chylomicron triglyceride per day. *Remnant* production from chylomicrons is proportional to the number of chylomicrons synthesized. Chylomicron remnants are considered to be atherogenic particles. Fat is important in cholesterol metabolism because cholesterol is absorbed in the presence of dietary fat and is transported in chylomicrons.

However, the most important effect of dietary fat on the plasma cholesterol level relates to the *type* of fat. Fats may be divided into three major classes identified by saturation and unsaturation characteristics. Long-chain saturated fatty acids have no double bonds, are not essential nutrients, and may be readily synthesized in the body from acetate. Dietary saturated fatty acids have a profound hypercholesterolemic effect and increase the concentrations of LDL. All animal fats are highly saturated, except those which occur in fish and shellfish, which are in contrast highly polyunsaturated.

The second class of dietary fats consists of the characteristic monounsaturated fatty acids that are present in all animal and vegetable fats. For practical purposes, oleic acid, which has one double bond at the omega-9 position, is the only significant dietary monounsaturated fatty acid. In general, the effects of dietary monounsaturated fatty acids on the plasma lipids are neutral, neither raising nor lowering their concentrations. Olive oil is the most characteristic monounsaturated fat. Because it has such a low content of saturated fat, it has a hypocholesterolemic effect when substituted for "saturated" fat in a diet. Monounsaturated fatty acids are not essential and are readily synthesized by the body.

Polyunsaturated fatty acids, the third class of fatty acids, are vital constituents of cellular membranes and serve as prostaglandin precursors. Because they cannot be synthesized by the body and are obtainable only from dietary sources, they are *essential* fatty acids. The two classes of polyunsaturated fatty acids we shall discuss are omega-6 and omega-3 fatty acids (Fig. 22-18). The most common examples of omega-6 fatty acids are linoleic acid, which is found in food, and arachidonic acid, 20 carbons in length with four double bonds, which is usually synthesized from linoleic acid by the liver. Because the basic structure of omega-6 fatty acids cannot be synthesized by the body, in order to meet the body's requirements for the omega-6 structure, as much as 2 to 3 percent of total energy must be supplied as lineolic acid, that is, as an essential fatty acid.

Omega-3 fatty acids differ in the position of the first double bond, counting from the methyl end of the molecule. This particular structure is also an essential nutrient for human beings because the body is unable to synthesize omega-3 fatty acids. Omega-6 and omega-3 fatty acids are not interconvertible. The dietary sources of omega-3 fatty acids are some but not all vegetable oils, leafy vegetables, and in particular, fish and shellfish. Linolenic fatty acid, C18:3, is obtained from vegetable products. Eicosapentaenoic acid, C20:5, and docosahexaenoic acid, C22:6, are derived from fish and shellfish and phytoplankton (the plants of the ocean) and are highly concentrated in fish oils. Once either the omega-3 or the omega-6 structure comes into the body as linoleic or linolenic acid, the body can synthesize the longer-chain and more highly polyunsaturated omega-6 and omega-3 fatty acids.

It appears that there are different functions in the body for omega-3 and omega-6 fatty acids. Both serve as a substrate for the formation of different prostaglandins and are rich in phospholipid membranes.[205] Both are particularly concentrated in nerve tissue. Omega-3 fatty acids are concentrated in the retina, spermatozoa, gonads, and many other organs. Omega-6 fatty acids are concentrated in the different plasma lipid classes (cholesterol esters, phospholipids, and so forth) and are concerned with lipid transport.

Polyunsaturated fatty acids of either the omega-6 structure or the omega-3 structure depress plasma cholesterol concentrations and the concentration of LDL.[206] Omega-3 fatty acids have an additional action in lowering plasma triglyceride concentrations and, in particular, VLDL[207] (see Fig. 22-19). Dietary omega-3 fatty acids have an additional advantage in that they are definitely antithrombotic.[205] These fatty acids inhibit the synthesis of thromboxane A_2 and enhance the synthesis of prostacyclin, with the former inducing platelet aggregation and the latter opposing platelet aggregation. Thus the omega-3 fatty acids present in fish have two potent activities: they are hypolipidemic, and they inhibit the thrombotic process.

Many but not all of the currently marketed

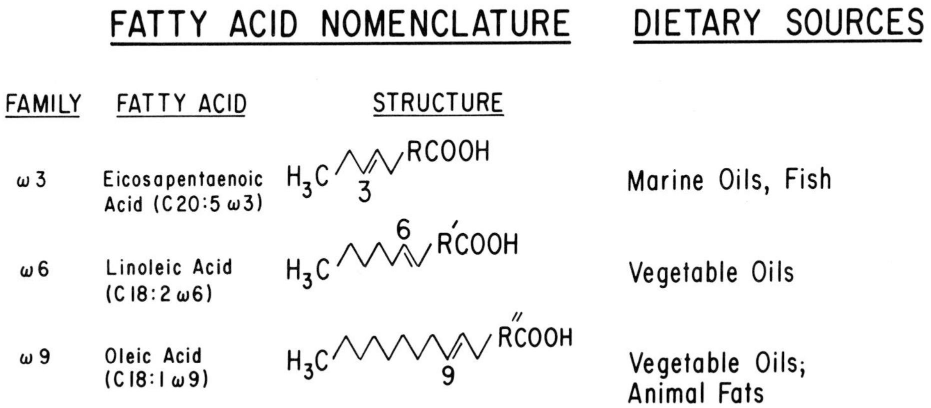

FATTY ACID NOMENCLATURE
DIETARY SOURCES
FAMILY
FATTY ACID
STRUCTURE
ω3
Eicosapentaenoic Acid (C20:5 ω3)
H3C
RCOOH
3
Marine Oils, Fish
ω6
Linoleic Acid (C18:2 ω6)
H3C
6
RCOOH
Vegetable Oils
ω9
Oleic Acid (C18:1 ω9)
H3C
RCOOH
9
Vegetable Oils; Animal Fats

FIGURE 22-18 The structure and sources of dietary fatty acids. Fatty acids can be organized into families according to the position of the first double bond from the terminal methyl group. The omega-3 fatty acids all have three carbons between the methyl end and the first double bond. Fatty acids in this family include eicosapentaenoic acid (C20:5), linolenic acid (C18:3), and docosahexaenoic acid (C22:6). Linoleic acid (C18:2) and arachidonic acid (C20:4) are the most important omega-6 fatty acids, while oleic acid (C18:1) is the most common fatty acid in the omega-9 family.

vegetable oils, shortenings, and margarines are only partially hydrogenated and thus retain the basic unsaturated characteristics of vegetable oils. Coconut oil, cocoa butter (the fat of chocolate), and palm oil are common "saturated" vegetable fats that are consumed in quantities; they have a hypercholesterolemic effect. The ratio of polyunsaturated to saturated fatty acids in a given fat or oil is termed the *P/S value*. Fats with a high P/S value of 2 and above, compared with 0.4 and less, are generally recognized as being hypocholesterolemic. The typical American diet has a P/S value of 0.4. In the suggested alternative diet to prevent coronary disease, the P/S value is above 1.0.

Most comparisons of the effects of saturated and polyunsaturated fat on the plasma lipids have indicated that gram for gram, saturated fat is up to two times greater at raising plasma cholesterol than are polyunsaturated fats in depressing it. The equations are as follows:

$$\Delta \text{ cholesterol} = 2.74\ \Delta S - 1.31\ \Delta P \quad \text{(Keys et al.}^{208}\text{)}$$

$$\Delta \text{ cholesterol} = 2.16\ \Delta S - 1.65\ \Delta P + 6.77\ \Delta C - 0.53 \quad \text{(Hegsted et al.}^{209}\text{)}$$

In these equations, *S* and *P* represent the percentage of dietary calories derived from saturated and polyunsaturated fat and C is the dietary cholesterol content in units of 100 mg.

CALORIES AND OBESITY

Excessive caloric intake from any source (fat, carbohydrate, protein, or alcohol) promotes hyperlipidemia (especially hypertriglyceridemia) in some individuals. Plasma triglyceride levels rise, and levels of high-density lipoprotein fall. The immediate metabolic consequence of excessive calories is an increased substrate for triglyceride synthesis in the liver, with subsequent elevated plasma VLDL triglyceride.[210] Furthermore, reduced clearance of VLDL triglyceride from the blood may in part be responsible for the hypertriglyceridemia of obesity. The enlarged adipose-tissue cells, because of their lessened sensitivity to the circulating insulin that activates lipoprotein lipase, the clearing factor enzyme, may have a reduced capacity to remove circulating triglyceride from the plasma.

In hypertriglyceridemic overweight patients, there is usually an associated hypercholesterolemia, partly

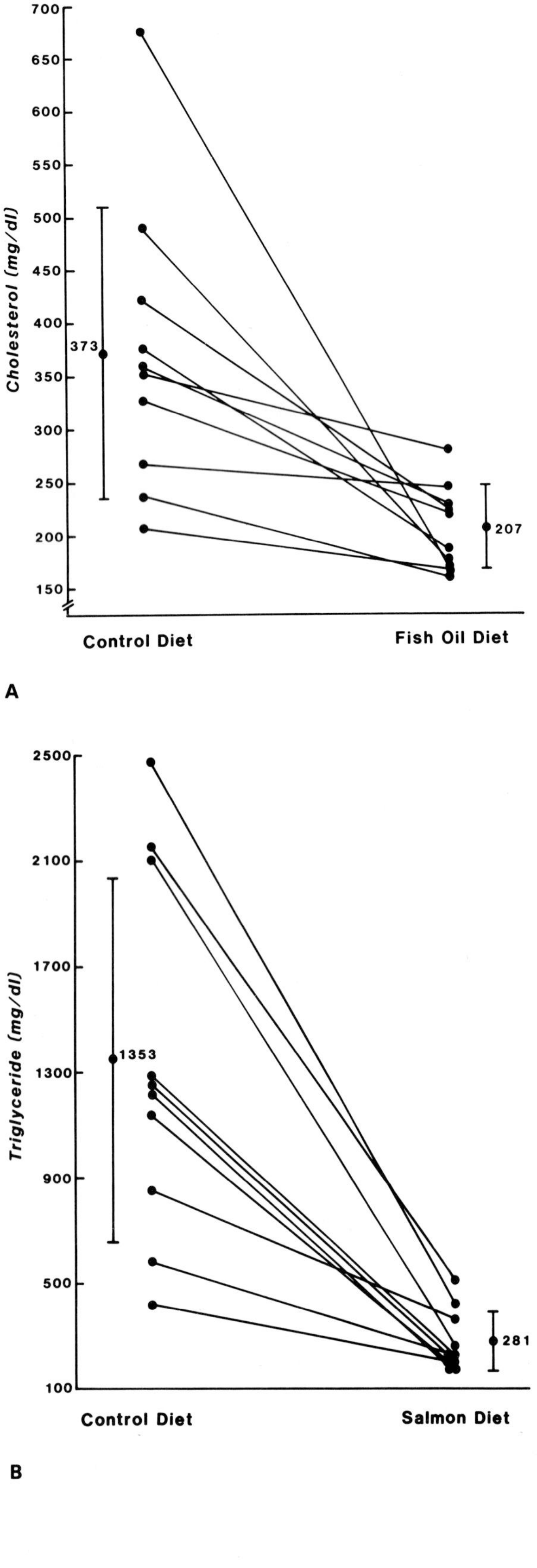

FIGURE 22-19 The hypocholesterolemic and hypotriglyceridemic effects of fish oils rich in omega-3 fatty acids in patients with phenotypic type V hyperlipoproteinemia. Changes in the plasma concentrations of total cholesterol, $\Delta = -166$ mg/dl, $p < 0.01$ (A) and triglyceride, $\Delta = -1072$ mg/dl, $p < 0.001$ (B) from 10 patients fed a fish oil-supplemented diet containing 20 to 30 g of omega-3 fatty acids. (*Reproduced from Phillipson et al.*[207] *with permission.*)

because of the increased intake of dietary cholesterol and saturated fat that occurs in the obese but also because the VLDL that carries the increased triglyceride content transports cholesterol as well. The lower HDL concentrations apparently reflect the shunting of HDL apoproteins into the VLDL molecule. Moderate reduction of caloric intake in hypertriglyceridemic overweight patients and the subsequent loss of adiposity invariably lead to lower plasma triglyceride levels, often to a normal range. Plasma cholesterol levels concomitantly fall; HDL levels reciprocally rise.[210,211]

While caloric control is the most important consideration for these hypertriglyceridemic patients, the source of the calories in weight-loss diets is of some importance in the establishment of patterns of food consumption that will be useful when a more ideal weight has been achieved. Many patients have combined hyperlipidemia (i.e., type IIb), and whatever hypercholesterolemia remains after both body weight and plasma triglyceride stabilize at lower levels will require attention in regard to the reduction of dietary cholesterol and saturated fat. Furthermore, the pattern of food intake should then be such that future weight gain will be avoided. The low-cholesterol or alternative-diet concept can be useful for both the period of weight reduction and the subsequent period of stabilization of body weight.

CARBOHYDRATE

From all the evidence available, it may now be said that the amount and type of carbohydrate consumed in natural diets has little or no long-term effect on plasma lipid levels. The effect of a sudden increase in the amount of carbohydrate in the diet does, however, produce an initial temporary elevation of plasma triglyceride concentration, so-called carbohydrate-induced hyperlipidemia. This short-term phenomenon is well established in both normal and hyperlipidemic Americans who have been given high-carbohydrate diets (65 to 90 percent of total calories). This hypertriglyceridemia usually lasts 2 to 4 weeks but may last up to 20 weeks before returning to baseline or upper normal values. The response of normal and diabetic Americans to increased dietary carbohydrate over long periods of time has actually been a lowering of serum lipid levels provided that dietary cholesterol and fat have been concurrently lowered.[193]

Studies in rats indicate that in contrast to starch and glucose, sucrose and fructose have a hypertriglyceridemic effect.[212] The evidence in humans that even very large amounts of sucrose (over 50 percent of total calories) produce hyperlipidemia is not completely convincing.[212] However, even if large quantities of sucrose have a mild hypertriglyceridemic and perhaps also a hypercholesterolemic effect, this does not bear particularly upon the dietary design of the low-cholesterol, low-fat, high-carbohydrate diet as envisioned. In the alternative diet the vast majority of the carbohydrate is in the form of cereals and legumes rather than sucrose. Americans commonly consume about 20 percent of their total calories as sucrose, which is about one-half of their carbohydrate intake. In the dietary changes being suggested, sucrose would fall to 10 to 15 percent of the total calories; thus any effect from sucrose would be diminished rather than accentuated by the dietary change.

FIBER

Dietary fiber is a broad, nondescriptive term which includes several carbohydrates thought to be indigestible by the human gut. These include cellulose, hemicelluloses, lignin, and pectin, which are commonly found in cereals, legumes, vegetables, and fruits. Dietary fiber contributes considerable bulk to the human diet but adds little to the caloric content. There is little evidence that most dietary fibers are hypocholesterolemic, although when certain fibers are taken as pharmaceutical agents, such as pectin and guar gum, some lowering of plasma cholesterol is achieved.

The probable major importance of dietary fiber in hyperlipidemic states is indirect. Foods high in fiber and low in caloric density have, in the customary American diet, been replaced with foods of high caloric density which also have a high content of cholesterol and saturated fat. Likewise, when dietary fiber is added to the diet through the use of foods which are naturally high in fiber and low in cholesterol and saturated fat, the intake of these hypercholesterolemic food factors usually decreases concomitantly.

ALCOHOL

Confusion about the effects of alcohol on the plasma lipids exists because on the one hand experienced clinicians have long recognized the association between alcohol ingestion and hypertriglyceridemia, while on the other hand there have been well-documented epidemiologic observations that alcohol intake is related to both higher HDL levels and reduced mortality from coronary heart disease.[213,214] Confounding the problem are the low HDL concentrations found in hypertriglyceridemic, overweight, alcohol-ingesting patients. Metabolic studies do indicate that alcohol substituted for dietary carbohydrate has an elevating effect on plasma triglyceride levels in certain individuals.[215,216] The caloric content of alcohol may in itself have a hypertriglyceridemic effect. Four drinks per day will contribute 560 calories. When it is considered that adult Americans consume 5 to 8 percent of their total calories as alcohol, the magnitude of alcohol-related hypertriglyceridemia may be considerable. The mechanisms by which alcohol may affect the plasma lipid levels include impairment of plasma triglyceride removal and increased synthesis of triglyceride-rich lipoproteins.[217]

Most patients can consume 1 to 3 oz of alcohol as part of the total diet and avoid hyperlipidemia, provided that weight gain is avoided. However, if such a trial produces hyperlipidemia, the use of alcohol should be completely discontinued. The use of alcohol is clearly precluded in types I and V patients who have had pancreatitis. If liver disease and hyperlipidemia occur together, alcohol should not be used in any circumstances. The use of alcohol as a means of elevating HDL concentrations is not to be recommended. Evidence that benefit would result is flimsy, and the diseases and social calamities that can result from excessive alcohol consumption are problems that are just as serious as hyperlipidemia.

PROTEIN

Dietary protein has been studied extensively for possible effects on plasma lipid concentrations. These studies have utilized both single protein sources and mixtures of different proteins with ranges of protein intake from 25 to 150 g per day. No changes in the plasma cholesterol and triglyceride concentrations have resulted from these different amounts of protein, provided that at least the minimum amounts of essential amino acids were ingested. It has been suggested on the basis of animal studies that animal protein (such as casein from milk) is hypercholesterolemic and that vegetable protein (such as soybean protein) has a hypocholesterolemic effect. Well-designed experiments in humans to test the differential effects of casein and soy protein have not been conclusive. However, the rabbit experiments are not completely translatable to humans. Many human studies have used formula diets with casein as the sole protein source. Since these diets were also free of cholesterol, plasma lipid levels fell greatly; this suggests that casein is probably not hypercholesterolemic. While the single-diet concept makes extensive use of proteins from vegetable sources, it does contain casein and is not a vegetarian diet. Thus the inclusion of more protein from vegetable sources may confer some benefit to hyperlipidemic patients.

LECITHIN

This phospholipid derived from soybeans is commonly sold in health food stores and is widely publicized as a popular remedy for hypercholesterolemia. Aside from its high content of linoleic acid, the consumption of lecithin is irrational, since this lipid is not absorbed as such from the digestive tract but is hydrolyzed into its constituent fatty acids, glycerol and choline. A higher content of linoleic acid in the diet can therefore be obtained much more inexpensively from a liquid polyunsaturated vegetable oil. There are no practical or theoretical reasons for the discrete use of lecithin, but no harm occurs.

MINERALS AND VITAMINS

Assuming that the minimum daily requirements for minerals and vitamins have been met in the diet, there is no information to indicate that additional vitamins and minerals will have any effect on the plasma lipid concentrations. This comment applies equally to vitamin C and vitamin E, again popularly consumed by the public without any proof of benefit. Excessive amounts of vitamin D cause hypercalcemia and hence would promote atherogenesis. The one exception is niacin, vitamin B_3, which, when given as a drug in a dose 50 times its requirement as a vitamin, does have a hypolipidemic effect. In this instance, niacin is used as a pharmaceutical preparation, not as a nutrient.

Implementation of the Single-Diet Concept for the Treatment of Hyperlipidemia

Instead of multiple diets, each for a different form of hyperlipidemia, we favor a "single-diet" concept for the treatment of hyperlipidemia. The chemical formulation of the single diet, termed the *alternative diet,* is presented in terms of major components, as follows. Of course, the ultimate and optimal objectives in terms of a diet to produce maximal plasma lipid lowering will be achieved in a series of phases which have been fully described in detail with appropriate menu planning and recipes in recent publications.[193,218,219]

Dietary cholesterol is reduced from the usual American intake of 500 mg per day to 100 mg per day. This change will lower LDL cholesterol, which is elevated in types IIa and IIb hyperlipidemia, and also both VLDL and intermediate-density lipoproteins in types IV and III hyperlipidemias, respectively (Table 22-11). In many patients with "diet-induced" IIa or IIb hypercholesterolemia, a reduction of dietary cholesterol to 100 mg per day will lower the plasma lipids to "normal" values (plasma cholesterol level below 220 mg/dl). Frequently, hyperlipidemic patients are also overweight. For overweight patients, the same diet at a hypocaloric level should be prescribed initially until the patient attains optimum weight. At that time, the alternative diet at a eucaloric level is prescribed.

In patients with genetically determined severe hypercholesterolemia, normal plasma cholesterol levels cannot be achieved by means of diet alone; combined diet plus drug therapy is needed. Restrictions on dietary cholesterol and saturated fat are nevertheless critically important in severe type IIa patients.

Dietary fat content is lowered to 20 percent of total calories compared with the usual American fat intake of 40 percent of total calories. Most of this decrease is in saturated fat, which is reduced to no more than 5 percent of total calories. This change in total fat content and composition has a beneficial effect in all forms of hyperlipidemia for reasons already discussed but especially in type II and types I and V hyperlipidemia (Table 22-12). In the latter two cases, when dietary fat is reduced to a minimum, the chylomicrons present in the blood gradually clear and the plasma triglycerides fall. Plasma cholesterol levels also decline, and HDL and LDL, both very low, rise. This "minimum" of dietary fat varies from patient to patient with hyperchylomicronemia; the exact level necessary for chylomicron clearance can be ascertained only by means of a trial of several diets with fat contents varying from 5 to 20 percent.[220] In the 5 to 10 percent fat diets, a small quantity of medium-chain triglycerides (MCT) which are handled metabolically as carbohydrates can be incorporated to enhance palatability.

In some patients with extreme chylomicronemia who are in danger of acute pancreatitis, a 1 percent fat or fat-free formula diet (protein, glucose, minerals, and vitamins) can be employed to promote maximal chylomicron lowering. Another simple but effective approach is the use of fruit juices for a few days of initial therapy. In both cases, triglyceride levels fall rapidly (Fig. 22-20).

While the basic problem in types I and V hyperlipidemia is not an excess of dietary cholesterol and while the suggested diets need not restrict cholesterol per se, they are lower in cholesterol content because most foods containing cholesterol are also high in fat. However, shellfish, which are relatively high in cholesterol content, are low in fat content and in saturated fat. Consequently, they and fish can be freely used by patients with types I and V hyperlipidemia.

Omega-3 fatty acids derived from fish may be added to the low-fat diet in order to achieve a specific hypolipidemic effect over and above what can be obtained from the dietary measures suggested in the single-diet concept. The omega-3 fatty acids from fatty fish, or even fish oil used experimentally, will have a pronounced plasma triglyceride (VLDL)–lower-

Table 22-12. Dietary Factors in the Causation and Correction of Lipoprotein Abnormalities

Lipoprotein abnormality	Cause	Dietary factor increasing lipoprotein synthesis	Dietary correction
Lipoprotein increased			
Chylomicrons (types I and V)	Impaired removal	Fat, regardless of relative saturation	Reduction of dietary fat to 5–10% of total calories*
VLDL (types IV and IIb) and IDL (type III)	Impaired removal (obesity) and/or increased synthesis	Excessive calories from any source Dietary cholesterol and saturated fat	A hypocaloric 20% fat diet to induce loss of excess adiposity; reduction of dietary cholesterol and saturated fat
LDL (types IIa and IIb)	Increased synthesis and impaired removal	Dietary cholesterol, saturated fat, and total fat	Reduction of dietary cholesterol to 100 mg, saturated fat to 5% of total calories, and total fat to 20%
Lipoprotein decreased			
HDL	Utilization of HDL apoproteins in triglyceride-carrying lipoproteins in types I, V, IV, IIb, and III hyperlipidemias	Excessive calories with adiposity	Correction of obesity as noted above

*All overweight hyperlipidemic patients should have the appropriate dietary factor modified as above and should be provided with a hypocaloric diet to help in the attainment of normal body weight. For an insulin-dependent diabetic, appropriate use of insulin may also aid in the correction of the hyperlipidemia.

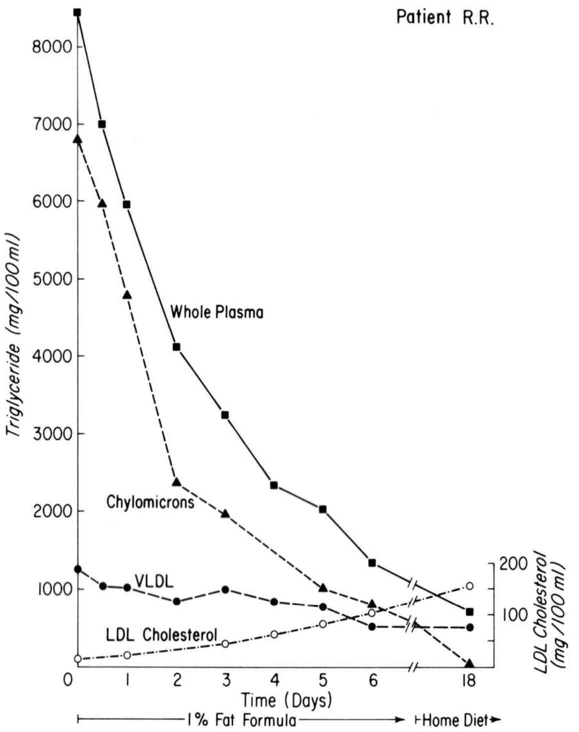

FIGURE 22-20 Reduction in chylomicronemia by means of a 1 percent fat formula diet plus insulin replacement in a patient with adult-onset diabetes mellitus and phenotypic type V hyperlipoproteinemia. Note that the fall in chylomicron and VLDL levels is associated with a reciprocal rise in LDL cholesterol. Concentrations of HDL cholesterol also rose (not shown).

ing action in hypertriglyceridemic patients with an exaggerated synthesis of VLDL. The result of giving omega-3 fatty acids to type V patients is illustrated in Fig. 22-19.[207] Polyunsaturated vegetable oil, as is well known, raises triglyceride levels in type V patients, and its use is therefore contraindicated. Fatty fish such as salmon, mackerel, and sardines may be particularly effective. Fish oil in doses of 15 g per day or more may also be used in type V patients.

Saturated fat in the diet is reduced greatly to maximize the lowering of LDL in types IIa and IIb. The polyunsaturated fat content remains little changed from the usual American intake of 6 to 8 percent of total calories. Because the saturated fat content is decreased, the *P/S* value of the dietary fat increases from 0.4 to 1.3. Most of the reduction of the total fat from 40 percent of total calories to 20 percent is accomplished by cutting down on foods which are rich in saturated fatty acids.

THE CHOLESTEROL–SATURATED FAT INDEX OF FOODS

The major plasma cholesterol–elevating effects of a given food reside in its content of cholesterol and saturated fat. To help understand the contribution of these two factors in a single food item and to compare one food with another, we have computed a cholesterol–saturated fat index (CSI)[220a] for selected foods (Table 22-13). This index is based on a modification of the regression equation used earlier to calculate the cholesterol index of foods.[221] Because the objective of the alternative diet is to maintain but not to increase the current intake of polyunsaturated fat, we chose not to include the polyunsaturated fat component of the equation when assessing an individual food item. The cholesterol index of foods was thus modified and called the cholesterol–saturated fat index: CSI = (1.01 × g saturated fat) + (0.05 × mg cholesterol), where the amounts of saturated fat and cholesterol in a given amount of a food item are entered into the equation.

In this context it is particularly instructive to compare the CSI of fish with that of moderately fat beef. A 100-g portion of cooked fish contains 66 mg of cholesterol and 0.20 g of saturated fat. This contrasts to a 96-mg cholesterol content and 8.1 g of saturated fat in beef that contains 20 percent fat. The CSI for 100 g (3.5 oz) of fish is 4, while that of beef is 13. The caloric value of these two portions also differs greatly (91 for fish and 286 for beef). The CSI of cooked chicken and turkey (without the skin) is also preferable to that of beef and other red meats. Again, the total fat content is quite a bit lower, and the saturated fat per 100 g is 1.3 with 87 mg of cholesterol. The CSI of poultry is 6. Table 22-13 lists the CSI index for various foods.

Shellfish have low CSI indexes because their saturated fat content is extremely low despite the fact that their cholesterol or total sterol content is 1.5 to 2 times higher than that of fish, poultry, or red meat. This means that, considering both cholesterol and saturated fat, shellfish have a CSI of 6, very much like poultry, and thus constitute a better choice than even the leanest red meats. Salmon also has a low CSI and is preferred to meat.

The *protein* intake is kept at an amount similar to what Americans commonly eat: about 15 percent of total calories. The decrease in fat content is thus offset by a reciprocal increase in dietary *carbohydrate*, ultimately to 65 percent of total calories. This is provided primarily in terms of complex carbohydrate ordinarily associated with protein. Other constituents of the diet are not reduced or even are enhanced in terms of nutritional adequacy.

Caloric control is vitally important in overweight patients for decreasing the VLDL of types IIb and IV and the IDL of type III hyperlipidemia and in improving the chylomicron clearance in type V hyperlipidemia (Table 22-11). These overweight patients have elevated plasma triglyceride levels, often with

Table 22-13. The Cholesterol–Saturated Fat Index and Kilocalorie Content of Selected Foods (100 g or 3½ oz)

	CSI	Kilocalories
Fish, poultry, red meat		
Whitefish: snapper, perch, sole, etc.	4	91
Shellfish	6	104
Salmon	5	149
Poultry, no skin	6	171
Beef, pork, and lamb		
10% fat (ground sirloin, flank steak)	9	214
15% fat (ground round)	10	258
20% fat (ground chuck, pot roast)	13	286
30% fat (ground beef, pork, and lamb; steaks; ribs; pork and lamb chops; roasts)	18	381
Eggs		
White	0	51
Egg substitute	1	91
Whole	29	163
Fats		
Most vegetable oils	13	884
Soft vegetable margarines	16	720
Soft shortenings	26	884
Bacon grease	39	902
Butter	54	716
Coconut oil, palm oil, cocoa butter (chocolate)	78	884
Cheeses		
Count-down, dry-curd cottage cheese, tofu (bean curd), pot cheese, low-fat cottage cheese, St. Otho	1	98
Cottage cheese, Lite-Line, Lite'n Lively, part-skim ricotta	6	139
Cheezola, Scandic or Min Chol, Hickory Farm Lyte, Pizza Pal, Saffola American*	6	317
Green River (lower-fat cheddar), part-skim mozzarella, Neufchâtel (lower-fat cream cheese), Keil Kase, Skim American, Olympia Low Fat	12	256
Cheddar, roquefort, Swiss, brie, jack, American, cream cheese, Velveeta, cheese spreads (jars), etc.	26	386
Frozen desserts		
Water ices or sorbets	0	105
Sherbet or frozen yogurt	1	119
Ice milk	4	152
Ice cream, 10% fat	9	193
Milk		
Skim milk (0.1% fat) or buttermilk	< 1	36
1% milk	1	47
2% milk	2	59
Whole milk (3.5% fat)	4	65
Liquid nondairy creamers: store brands, Cereal Blend, Coffee Rich	9	141
Liquid nondairy creamers: Mocha Mix, Poly Rich	3	154

*Cheeses made with skim milk and vegetable oils

concomitant adult-onset diabetes. Such hyperlipidemias are particularly sensitive to the state of caloric balance. Dietary factors operate indirectly but crucially in supplying the substrate for triglyceride synthesis. Type III hyperlipidemia is rare, and because its dietary treatment is similar to that for type IV, it will not be referred to specifically in the subsequent comments other than to emphasize the extreme importance of weight control.

Reduction of excess body weight is the most important measure for the correction of type IV hyperlipidemia. We stress gradual rather than sudden weight loss so that the weight-loss diet will be balanced in nutrients and will not have untoward effects. For the overweight patient, the caloric content of the diet can be reduced to one-third or two-fifths of the patient's caloric requirements. We then expect a gentle weight loss of about 2 lb per week.

The plasma triglyceride response to caloric restriction and weight loss is prompt and dramatic. Within 1 to 2 weeks, the plasma triglyceride level decreases, and it remains lower as long as weight loss continues. With the achievement of normal weight, the plasma triglyceride level usually is in the normal range. Glucose intolerance and the associated diabetic state may also disappear with the hypertriglyceridemia.

The special case of overweight type IIb patients warrants further comment. After the excessive plasma triglyceride levels are corrected by means of weight loss, such patients will be left with some hypercholesterolemia carried by LDL. Particular attention will have to be directed toward the restriction of dietary cholesterol and fat when the eucaloric diet to maintain weight is initiated.

Table 22-14. Summary of the Suggested Dietary Changes in the Different Phases of the Alternative Diet

Phase I
Avoid foods very high in cholesterol and saturated fat:
Delete egg yolk, butterfat, lard, and organ meats
Substitute soft margarine for butter, vegetable oils and shortening for lard, skim milk for whole milk, egg whites for whole eggs
Phase II
Gradually use less meat and more fish, chicken, and turkey:
No more than 6–8 oz a day
Use less fat and cheese
Acquire new recipes
Phase III
Eat mainly cereals, legumes, fruit, and vegetables:
Use meat as a condiment
Use low-cholesterol cheeses
Save these foods for use only on special occasions: extra meats, regular cheese, chocolate, candy, and coconut

The Alternative Diet: A Phased Approach to the Dietary Treatment of Hyperlipidemia

A realistic view is that even well-motivated patients have difficulty making abrupt changes in their dietary habits. It may take many months and even years to change patterns of food consumption. Therefore, the changes recommended from the current American diet of most hyperlipidemic patients should be approached in a gradual manner, with each of three phases introducing more changes toward the "alternative dietary" pattern, ultimately required for maximal therapy.

The goal of phase I is to modify the customary consumption of foods very high in cholesterol and saturated fat (Table 22-14). This can be accomplished by deleting egg yolk, butterfat, lard, and organ meats from the diet and by using substitute products when possible: soft margarine for butter, vegetable oils and shortening for lard, skim milk for whole milk, and egg whites for whole eggs.

In phase II, a reduction in meat consumption is the goal, with a gradual transition from the presumed American ideal of up to a pound of meat a day to no more than 6 to 8 oz per day (Table 22-14). Meat can no longer be the center of the meal, particularly for two or three meals a day. Some ideas for lunch with and without sandwiches have been detailed in sample menus and recipes.[193,219,220] In addition, in phase II we propose the use of less fat and cheese.

Substitute recipes have been developed to replace recipes which are centered on meat or high-fat dairy products (cream cheese, butter, sour cream, cheese) as the principal ingredients. Since these foods are to be eaten in smaller amounts or even omitted (butterfat), the patient needs to find recipes which use larger amounts of grains, legumes, vegetables, and fruits. Examples of such recipes are included in Refs. 193, 219, and 220.

In phase III, the maximal diet for the treatment of hyperlipidemia is attained (Table 22-14). The cholesterol content of the diet is reduced to 100 mg per day, and saturated fat is lowered to 5 to 6 percent of total calories. Since cholesterol is contained only in foods of animal origin, these changes mean that meat consumption in particular must be further reduced. Meat, fish, and poultry should be used as "condiments" rather than "aliments." With this philosophy, the meat dish will no longer occupy the center of the table. Instead, meat in smaller quantities will spice up dishes based on vegetables, rice, cereal, and legumes much as Asian, Indian, and Mediterranean cookery has been doing for eons. The total of meat and poultry should average 3 to 4 oz per day, but the use of poultry should be stressed because of its lower content of saturated fat. The use of fish is also preferred. Note the low cholesterol–saturated fat index of fish in Table 22-13, shared also by shellfish, as alluded to subsequently. Because of a low CSI, up to 6 oz of fish can be used in place of meat during phase III of the alternative diet. All fish contain omega-3 fatty acids.

Shellfish are divided into two groups: high-cholesterol shellfish (shrimp, crab, and lobster) and low-cholesterol shellfish (oysters, clams, and scallops). Both contain omega-3 fatty acids and have a low fat content. Because of these differences, high-cholesterol shellfish are more restricted in the daily diet than are low-cholesterol shellfish, i.e., 3 oz vs. 6 oz per day. The low-cholesterol shellfish contain other sterols (e.g., brassicasterol) that are more analogous to plant sterols. These are poorly absorbed by humans.

The use of special low-cholesterol cheeses is an important component of phase III. The sample menus in Refs. 193, 219, and 220 give some idea about the eating pattern in phase III.

THE CHEMICAL COMPOSITION OF THE ALTERNATIVE DIET

The American diet contains approximately 750 mg cholesterol per day. This is decreased in phase I to 450 mg, in phase II to 300 mg, and in phase III to 100 mg. The fat content decreases from 40 percent of calories in the American diet to 35 percent in phase I, 25 percent in phase II, and 20 percent in phase III, with special consideration given to the decrease in saturated fat. In order to provide sufficient calories to meet body needs, the carbohydrate content should be increased as the fat content is decreased, with emphasis on the use of the fiber-containing complex carbohydrates contained in whole grains, cereal products, and legumes. The carbohydrate content increases from 45 percent of the calories in the American diet to 50 percent in phase I, 60 percent in phase II, and 65 percent in phase III. The bulk or fiber in the diet is enhanced considerably, a feature which induces satiety sooner per unit of calories and helps promote weight loss. The crude-fiber content of the alternative diet increases from 4 to 12 g per day.

PREDICTED PLASMA CHOLESTEROL LOWERING FROM THE THREE PHASES OF THE ALTERNATIVE DIET

As has been emphasized, both dietary cholesterol and saturated fat elevate plasma cholesterol levels, whereas polyunsaturated fat has a mild depressing effect. In stepwise fashion, the cholesterol and saturated fat of each phase of the alternative diet are successively reduced, with phase III providing for the lowest intakes. According to calculations derived from Hegsted and coworkers,[209] phase III of the alternative diet would provide for maximal plasma cholesterol lowering, an estimated change of 77 mg/dl. Phase II would produce a lowering of 49 mg/dl; and phase I, 28 mg/dl. These plasma cholesterol changes for all phases offer the possibility of improved plasma lipids, depending on the amount of dietary modifications, with phase III as the ultimate goal.

THE USE OF THE ALTERNATIVE DIET IN DIABETIC PATIENTS, PREGNANT PATIENTS, CHILDREN, AND HYPERTENSIVE PATIENTS

The approach to diabetic patients who are also hyperlipidemic involves the same dietary considerations for the treatment of the hyperlipidemia. Phase III of the alternative diet has been used successfully in both juvenile-onset and maturity-onset diabetic patients, insulin-dependent and non-insulin-dependent. Clearly involved in this treatment is the appropriate control of carbohydrate as well as lipid metabolism by means of adequate amounts of insulin and weight reduction when the patient is overweight. The great propensity of diabetic patients to atherosclerotic vascular disease makes control of their hyperlipidemia of particular importance. The principles we have outlined can be utilized fully with benefit to the patient.

Pregnancy constitutes a particularly difficult situation, because in most pregnant women there will be a 40 to 50 percent increase in plasma lipids and lipoproteins (chiefly LDL) in physiological circumstances. A hyperlipidemic patient who becomes pregnant should continue on the same diet advised previously for the treatment of her hyperlipidemia, supplemented by vitamins and minerals as is usual in pregnancy. In patients with familial hypercholesterolemia, the phase III diet is utilized as before, with some increase in calories to permit the desired weight gain. In the type I or V hypertriglyceridemic pregnant patient, there is apt to be a profound augmentation of the usual hyperchylomicronemia, and strict adherence to the 5 to 10 percent fat diet is often necessary to avoid pancreatitis.

The single-diet concept for the treatment of hyperlipidemic children can be applied as for adults with the exception that a child up to 4 years of age is allowed less cholesterol than an older child. Above age 4 years, no more than 3 oz of meat per day is the goal. Egg yolk, organ meat, and butterfat are eliminated from the diet, even for infants. Dietary iron is supplemented from fortified cereals. Human breast milk or whole cow's milk is recommended prior to weaning or until the infant eats sufficient table food to provide adequate calories for growth. This is usually from 1 to 2 years. From that time on, the child should drink skim milk.

For the rare infant with type I hyperlipidemia, the fat content of the usual human breast or cow's milk is much too high. A basic skim milk formula will have to be used to avoid the abdominal pain and episodes of pancreatitis to which these patients are so prone. The main objective of such therapy is the provision of sufficient amounts of essential fatty acid, which can be prescribed separately as safflower or sunflower seed oil, to yield at least 1 to 2 percent of the total calories. In this way most of the fat intake will be from linoleic acid, and very little other fat will be taken in. Success in several infants with the type I disorder has been achieved using this dietary approach, resulting in the abolition of episodes of abdominal pain.

Special attention must be given to hypertensive, hyperlipidemic patients for several reasons. First, coronary heart disease and atherosclerotic brain disease are common causes of death in hypertensive patients. Second, some diuretic agents (thiazides) are hyperlipidemic in themselves so that the usual hypertensive patient will have an increase in plasma lipids from the use of these agents alone. Thus hypertensive individuals given thiazides should have additional dietary therapy in the form of the alternative-diet or single-diet approach. Finally, in the alternative diet, a salt-restriction program can readily be incorporated to provide for the additional treatment of the essential hypertension as this is desired by the physician. The correction of obesity may also have a blood-pressure-lowering effect. In order to combine the dietary treatment of hypertension and that of hyperlipidemia in a single diet, a stepwise reduction in salt use is also advocated and incorporated into the different phases.[219]

PHARMACEUTICAL AGENTS FOR THE TREATMENT OF HYPERLIPOPROTEINEMIA

The rationale for the treatment of hyperlipoproteinemia is based on the premise that successful reduction in lipid levels will lead to slowing of the rate of progression of atherosclerosis or, potentially, a reversal of this process with a subsequent reduction in cardiovascular morbidity and mortality. Recent results from the Lipid Research Clinics Primary Prevention Trial[115,116] and the NHLBI Coronary Angiographic Trial[117] support this view with respect to elevated concentrations of LDL cholesterol. Treatment of patients with severe hypertriglyceridemia is aimed at the prevention of medical complications (abdominal pain and pancreatitis) resulting from severe hyperchylomicronemia and concurrently at a reduction of the long-term risks of atherosclerosis. Because hyperlipoproteinemia is a lifelong disorder, the decision to begin drug therapy should be made only after satisfactory exclusion of secondary factors and after an adequate trial of diet has failed to achieve satisfactory lipid levels. It must be emphasized that once drugs are used to treat hyperlipoproteinemia, dietary therapy should be stressed again at the same time. The response to therapy generally will be maximized when this twofold approach is employed. A limited number of drugs are available, and their clinical indications will be reviewed in this section. Several reviews have been published recently.[222-225]

Bile Acid Sequestrants

Two products are currently available: cholestyramine (Questran) and colestipol (Colestid). Both are high-molecular-weight polymers to which anionic bile acids are ionically bound in exchange for chloride ions. These bile acid–binding resins are not absorbed, and their activities are based entirely on sequestration of bile acids in the intestinal lumen. The bile acid–resin complex is excreted in the stools.

MECHANISM OF ACTION

The primary action of both cholestyramine and colestipol is to bind bile acids in the intestinal lumen. This in turn results in an interruption of the enterohepatic circulation of bile acids and a markedly increased excretion of these steroids in the feces. The size of the bile acid pool is decreased, and this reduction stimulates increased hepatic synthesis of bile acids from cholesterol. Depletion of the hepatic pool of cholesterol results in two compensatory changes: an increase in cholesterol biosynthesis and an increase in the number of specific high-affinity receptors for LDL on the hepatocyte membrane.[226,227] The increased number of hepatic LDL receptors stimulates the rate of LDL catabolism from plasma and thereby lowers the concentration of this lipoprotein. The selective stimulation of hepatic LDL receptors explains why concentrations of LDL are selectively reduced during therapy with a bile acid sequestrant. Bile acid sequestrants are ineffective in patients with homozygous familial hypercholesterolemia who lack the ability to make more high-affinity LDL receptors. The increase in hepatic cholesterol biosynthesis which occurs during therapy with a bile acid sequestrant may be paralleled by an increase in hepatic VLDL production and often results in a slight increase in plasma concentrations of triglyceride and VLDL.

SIDE EFFECTS

The most common side effects of cholestyramine and colestipol consist of changes in bowel function including constipation, bloating, epigastric fullness, nausea, and flatulence. Constipation, which is the most frequent side effect, may be relieved with stool softeners, but the gritty nature of these medications may exacerbate hemorrhoids. Patients frequently complain that these medications are bulky, and some find the sandy or gritty texture unpleasant. Rare side effects have included intestinal obstruction and the development of hyperchloremic acidosis. Decreased absorption of fat-soluble vitamins and folic acid may occur with prolonged high doses of both medications, and oral supplementation with these vitamins may be advisable in children. Because of their avidity for anionic molecules, cholestyramine and colestipol may interfere with the absorption of other drugs, and it is advisable to take other medications 1 h before or 4 h after taking the resin. Such effects have been reported with digoxin, thyroxine, warfarin, and thiazides and may occur with any anionic drug. Biochemical side effects include a modest increase in plasma triglyceride concentrations in many patients; mild increases in alkaline phosphatase and transaminases have also been reported.

INDICATIONS AND DOSAGE

Cholestyramine is available in 9-g packets (which contain 4 g of cholestyramine and 5 g of orange flavoring) and in cans that contain 378 g. Colestipol is available in 5-g packets and 500-g bottles; this formulation contains no additives. The cholesterol-lowering effects of 4 g of cholestyramine appear to be equivalent to those obtained with 5 g of colestipol. Both medications must be mixed with water or juice and are taken in two (or occasionally three) divided doses with or just after meals. The total daily dose of cholestyramine is 8 to 24 g a day, and the daily dose of colestipol is 10 to 30 g; however, the benefits of increasing the dose above 16 g of cholestyramine or 20 g of colestipol per day must be balanced against the high incidence of gastrointestinal side effects and poorer patient compliance at these higher doses.

As discussed in Hypercholesterolemia, bile acid sequestrants are the drugs of choice for patients with primary elevations in the concentrations of LDL cholesterol who do not have concurrent hypertriglyceridemia. These agents have no place in the therapy of other hyperlipidemias and may in fact aggravate the hypertriglyceridemia seen in patients with type III hyperlipoproteinemia and patients with chylomicronemia. The response to therapy in patients with primary hypercholesterolemia is variable, but 15 to 25 percent reductions in concentrations of LDL cholesterol may be achieved with 16 g a day of cholestyramine or 20 g of colestipol.[181-184] The addition of nicotinic acid to this regimen may result in further decrements of 20 to 25 percent, and this combination remains the most effective for patients with severe type IIa hypercholesterolemia.[94-96] This is illustrated in Fig. 22-21. As discussed in Hypercholesterolemia, combined drug therapy with a bile acid sequestrant and probucol[97] or gemfibrozil is sometimes effective in patients who are unable to take nicotinic acid. Combined drug therapy with an inhibitor of HMG CoA reductase plus a bile acid sequestrant is the most consistently effective regimen available, resulting in a greater than 50 percent reduction in the concentrations of LDL cholesterol in patients with familial hypercholesterolemia.[98,99]

Cholestyramine was the drug used in the Lipid Research Clinics Primary Prevention Trial. The results from this large clinical trial have established the long-term safety and efficacy of bile acid sequestrants and have provided conclusive proof that reduction of LDL cholesterol reduces morbidity and mortality from cardiovascular disease. Because they are not absorbed, bile acid sequestrants are the only drugs safe for use in the treatment of children with heterozygous familial hypercholesterolemia; if clinically indicated, these drugs can also be used for the treatment of patients with severe type II hypercholesterolemia during pregnancy.

Nicotinic Acid

The hypolipidemic action of nicotinic acid, or niacin, has been recognized for 30 years[228] and appears to be

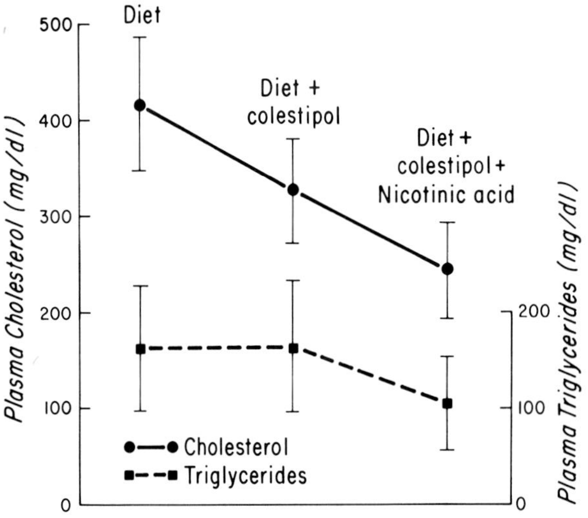

FIGURE 22-21 The effects of sequential therapy with diet, colestipol, and colestipol plus nicotinic acid on the plasma concentrations of cholesterol and triglycerides in 13 patients with heterozygous familial hypercholesterolemia. (*Redrawn from Illingworth et al.*[94])

unrelated to its action as a coenzyme in intermediary metabolism. It is well absorbed from the gastrointestinal tract and is excreted in the urine.

MECHANISM OF ACTION

The precise mechanism of action of nicotinic acid at the cellular level that is responsible for reducing plasma concentrations of VLDL and LDL is not known. Considerable evidence, however, points to an effect in reducing the hepatic synthesis of VLDL,[229] which in turn leads to a reduction in LDL synthesis. Factors responsible for the decreased hepatic production of VLDL include inhibition of lipolysis with a concomitant decrease in FFA levels in plasma, decreased hepatic esterification of triglycerides, and possible effects on the hepatic production of apoprotein B.

SIDE EFFECTS

The main side effects of nicotinic acid involve the skin and gastrointestinal tract. Cutaneous flushing occurs 15 min to 2 h after a patient takes the medication, but the duration and magnitude usually diminish with prolonged therapy and can be minimized by starting at a low dose and always taking the medication after the ingestion of food. The flushing appears to mediated by prostaglandins and can be reduced by means of concurrent administration of 150 to 325 mg of aspirin.[230] Nausea, abdominal discomfort, and diarrhea constitute the most common gastrointestinal side effects, and the drug is contraindicated in patients with active liver disease, peptic ulcer disease, or hyperuricemia. Less common side effects include itching, development of rash, hyperpigmentation of the skin with development of acanthosis nigricans, and blurred vision due to macular edema; the latter is not common but will necessitate discontinuation of therapy. Other side effects have included activation of peptic ulcer disease and exacerbation of both hyperuricemia and diabetes. Laboratory disturbances noted in patients on nicotinic acid are more common with higher doses (> 3 g per day) and include increases in alkaline phosphatase and transaminases and elevation of uric acid and glucose. The incidence of elevated transaminases and alkaline phosphatase may be higher in patients receiving time-release forms of niacin.[231] Liver function tests and uric acid should be monitored during the initiation of nicotinic acid and should be checked periodically once an appropriate dosage regimen has been established.

INDICATIONS AND DOSAGE

Nicotinic acid is available in tablets containing 100, 250, or 500 mg and in time-release preparations containing 125, 250, or 500 mg. The authors do not recommend the time-release forms of nicotinic acid for the treatment of hyperlipidemia. Therapy with nicotinic acid is best initiated with a low-dose regimen (e.g., 100 to 250 mg once to three times daily with or just after meals), with the dosage then being gradually increased at 7- to 14-day intervals to a total dose of 3 g per day. Lipid values as well as tests of liver function and uric acid should be assessed at this point; if a satisfactory reduction in plasma lipids has not been achieved, the dose should be increased a further 1.5 g per day. Periodic increases in dosage up to a maximum of 7.5 to 8 g per day may be administered, but the increased hypolipidemic effect of such higher doses must be balanced against the higher incidence of side effects noted at doses above 4.5 g per day. Nicotinic acid is useful in the treatment of all hyperlipoproteinemias except those due to familial lipoprotein lipase deficiency. The drug is used chiefly in the treatment of primary hypercholesterolemia; when used by itself, it results in 15 to 30 percent decreases in concentrations of LDL cholesterol with a concurrent 10 to 20 percent rise in HDL levels.[232] Forty to eighty percent reductions in the concentrations of plasma triglycerides may be obtained with nicotinic acid, and this drug is effective in reducing both VLDL and LDL levels in patients with phenotypic type IIb hyperlipidemia. Nicotinic acid is the second-choice drug for patients with type III hyperlipoproteinemia (clofibrate is the drug of choice) and is a good second-choice drug for patients with severe hypertriglyceridemia (type V phenotype), in whom gemfibrozil is currently the drug of choice. As discussed previously, combined therapy with nicotinic acid and a bile acid sequestrant provides particularly effective therapy for patients with severe hypercholesterolemia and LDL concentrations greater than 300 mg/dl.

Probucol

Probucol (Lorelco) is a second-line drug for the treatment of primary hypercholesterolemia. Less than 10 percent of probucol is absorbed in the intestinal tract, and the hydrophobic nature of this drug contributes to its prolonged storage in adipose tissue. When used as a single agent, probucol has been shown to reduce plasma LDL cholesterol concentrations 8 to 15 percent and concurrently to lower HDL levels up to 25 percent.[145]

MECHANISM OF ACTION

The mechanism by which probucol influences plasma lipoprotein levels has not been completely defined. The drug has been shown to increase the fractional rate of clearance of LDL[233] and to increase biliary secretion of cholesterol. The increased removal of LDL may be due to an increase in non-receptor-mediated pathways, and this would explain the modest efficacy of probucol in patients with homozygous familial hypercholesterolemia who lack LDL receptors.[90] The decrease in HDL levels seen with probucol is due to a decrease in apoprotein A-I synthesis and a decrease in lipoprotein lipase.[233,234]

SIDE EFFECTS

Probucol is well tolerated and appears to have minimal side effects; in order of decreasing frequency, these include diarrhea (10 percent of patients), flatulence, abdominal pain, and nausea and vomiting. Less common side effects have included hyperhidrosis, fetid sweat, and angionecrotic edema. With the possible exception of mild eosinophilia, no consistent biochemical abnormalities have been reported. Probucol causes prolongation of the QT interval, and although no arrhythmias have been attributed to its use in humans, the drug should probably be regarded as contraindicated in patients with electrocardiographic (ECG) findings suggestive of ventricular irritability.[225] Probucol is stored in adipose tissue, and blood levels fall slowly after therapy is discontinued. For this reason, the drug should not be given to women who plan to have children in the near future or to children.

INDICATIONS AND DOSAGE

Probucol is available in 250-mg tablets. The recommended dose is 500 mg twice daily with the morning and evening meals. Probucol should be regarded as a second-line drug for the treatment of primary hypercholesterolemia, and 8 to 15 percent reductions in plasma concentrations of LDL can be expected. The drug concurrently lowers HDL levels up to 25 percent and may adversely affect the ratio of LDL to HDL. Combined drug therapy with probucol and a bile acid sequestrant may be of use in patients who are unable to take nicotinic acid.[97] Probucol has no role in the treatment of hypertriglyceridemia.

Clofibrate

Clofibrate (Atromid-S) is the ethyl ester of *p*-chlorophenoxyisobutyrate and is well absorbed from the gastrointestinal tract. In plasma, the ester bond is hydrolyzed and the free acid is transported bound to albumin. The plasma half-life is 12 to 15 h. The drug is excreted in the urine, and its clearance is decreased in patients with chronic renal failure.

MECHANISM OF ACTION

The mechanism of action of clofibrate at the molecular level is not known. The most important effect, however, is to increase the rate of metabolism of triglyceride-rich lipoproteins, as a result of increases in the activity of lipoprotein lipase.[235,236] Small and variable reductions in the synthesis and/or secretion of hepatic VLDL into plasma may also occur; these may be mediated by a number of mechanisms, including decreases in the hepatic synthesis of cholesterol and fatty acids and enhanced biliary excretion of cholesterol.

SIDE EFFECTS

Clofibrate is generally well tolerated and has a low incidence of side effects. Nausea, abdominal discomfort, and in men decreased libido and breast tenderness are the most commonly reported. Less common side effects include dry skin, alopecia, and the development of a myositis-like syndrome with muscle tenderness and increased creatine phosphokinase (CPK).[237] The latter syndrome is more likely to occur in patients with hypoalbuminemia or impaired renal function. Rarely, ventricular arrhythmias and a lupus-like syndrome have been associated with clofibrate therapy. Biochemical abnormalities have included a decrease in alkaline phosphatase and transient increases in transaminases. Two long-term clinical trials, The Coronary Drug Research Project[238] and the WHO Primary Prevention Trial,[239] have provided data concerning the long-term safety and efficacy of clofibrate. In both studies there was an increased incidence of gallstones, whereas in the WHO study clofibrate-treated patients had a higher noncardiac mortality rate than control subjects. This was mainly attributable to an increased incidence of malignant neoplasms and complications resulting from cholecystectomy. The increased incidence of noncardiac deaths did not persist after discontinuation of clofibrate therapy.[240] Drug interactions may occur with clofibrate and other albumin-bound drugs, most notably warfarin (Coumadin).

INDICATIONS AND DOSAGE

Clofibrate is available in 500-mg capsules; the usual dose is 1 g twice daily. Clofibrate is the drug of choice for patients with type III hyperlipoproteinemia and should be regarded as a second-choice drug for patients with severe hypertriglyceridemia (type V phenotype) who are unable to take gemfibrozil or nicotinic acid. In patients with type III hyperlipoproteinemia, clofibrate therapy frequently reduces cholesterol and triglyceride concentrations 50 to 80 percent and leads to the regression of xanthomas. When given to patients with primary hypertriglyceridemia, clofibrate lowers VLDL cholesterol and plasma triglyceride concentrations up to 50 percent but frequently results in increased concentrations of LDL cholesterol. The drug is generally ineffective in patients with primary hypercholesterolemia and has no role in the therapy of disorders associated with increased plasma concentrations of LDL cholesterol. The drug is contraindicated in patients with chronic renal disease or the nephrotic syndrome; use in this population frequently results in the development of muscle tenderness and a myositis-like syndrome.

Gemfibrozil

Gemfibrozil (Lopid) is a fibric acid derivative that is structurally related to clofibrate. The drug is well absorbed from the intestinal tract and is transported, in part, bound to albumin. Although gemfibrozil undergoes enterohepatic circulation, the primary route of excretion is in urine.[225]

MECHANISM OF ACTION

The hypotriglyceridemic effect of gemfibrozil results primarily from a reduction in VLDL triglyceride and, to a lesser extent, apoprotein B synthesis with a concurrent increase in the rate of removal of triglyceride-rich lipoproteins from plasma.[235] The latter effect is believed to result from an increased activity of lipoprotein lipase, but the ability of gemfibrozil to inhibit VLDL triglyceride production appears to be much greater than that seen with clofibrate. Although gemfibrozil has also been shown to reduce the rate of synthesis of LDL apoprotein B,[241] this may simply be a reflection of a reduced rate of synthesis of VLDL, the precursor for LDL, in plasma.

SIDE EFFECTS

Gemfibrozil is well tolerated in most patients; the most frequent side effects are changes in bowel function, abdominal pain, diarrhea, and occasionally nausea. These occur in 3 to 5 percent of patients and may necessitate the discontinuation of gemfibrozil. Less common side effects include muscle tenderness and skin rash. Biochemical changes are uncommon; they include eosinophilia, decreases in the plasma concentration of alkaline phosphatase, and occasionally rises in transaminases. Like clofibrate, gemfibrozil potentiates the effects of oral anticoagulants and may increase biliary lithogenicity, with a predicted long-term increase in the incidence of gallstones.

INDICATIONS AND DOSAGE

Gemfibrozil is available in 300-mg capsules; the usual dose is 600 mg twice daily. Gemfibrozil is the drug of choice for patients with severe hypertriglyceridemia (type V phenotype) and in the authors' experience is superior to clofibrate in treating this disorder. Reductions of 75 to 90 percent in plasma concentrations of triglycerides may be seen in patients with severe hypertriglyceridemia; in this population, the drug may be effective in reducing the risk of pancreatitis and, on a long-term basis, the risk of atherosclerosis. Gemfibrozil should be regarded as a second-choice drug for patients with type III hyperlipoproteinemia, but it is inconsistently effective in patients with primary hypercholesterolemia and elevated concentrations of LDL cholesterol.[225] In the latter group of patients, particularly those unable to take nicotinic acid, combined drug therapy with gemfibrozil and a bile acid sequestrant is often quite effective. In the authors' experience, 25 to 45 percent reductions in concentrations of LDL cholesterol can be achieved in some patients on this regimen whereas in other patients no additional LDL-lowering effect is seen with the addition of gemfibrozil. Concentrations of HDL cholesterol increase 10 to 20 percent during therapy with gemfibrozil, and even greater increases may be seen in patients with severe hypertriglyceridemia.

Neomycin

Neomycin is a nonabsorbable aminoglycoside antibiotic with hypocholesterolemic effects that appear to be mediated by a reduction in the absorption of cholesterol from the small intestine.[242] This drug should be regarded as a second-line agent for patients with primary hypercholesterolemia who are unable to take bile acid sequestrants.

MECHANISM OF ACTION

Metabolic studies have indicated that neomycin increases the fecal excretion of neutral steroids (cholesterol and metabolites) but does not change the fecal secretion of bile acids. The hypocholesterolemic effect is therefore believed to result from reduced absorption of exogeneous and endogenous cholesterol owing to an effect of neomycin on the intestinal flora and possibly the integrity of interluminal micelles in the gastrointestinal tract.[242] It is presumed that the increased biliary loss of cholesterol results in compensatory increases in the number of high-affinity LDL receptors present on hepatic cell membranes and that this in turn stimulates an increase in the rate of catabolism of LDL.

SIDE EFFECTS

Side effects are common with neomycin, and one-third to one-half of patients treated with this drug have significant changes in bowel function, including diarrhea and abdominal cramps.[242] The drug should be regarded as contraindicated in patients with impaired renal function and those with gastrointestinal disorders associated with a potential for increased absorption of neomycin. Neomycin can cause serious ototoxicity and nephrotoxicity, and periodic hearing tests and assessments of renal function are mandatory in patients maintained on this drug for the therapy of hypercholesterolemia, even though the incidence of changes in these parameters appears to be low.[243]

INDICATIONS AND DOSAGE

Neomycin is available in 500-mg tablets, and the usual dose is 1 g twice daily. The drug is indicated as a second-line agent in the treatment of primary hypercholesterolemia and has no role in therapy for hypertriglyceridemic states. Neomycin reduces LDL concentrations 15 to 20 percent in patients with primary hypercholesterolemia[242,243] but has no effect on HDL levels. The hypocholesterolemic effect of neomycin can be potentiated by means of combined therapy with a bile acid sequestrant[244] or nicotinic acid; when neomycin was used in combination with the latter drug, 45 percent reductions in concentrations of LDL cholesterol were reported.[245]

Dextrothyroxine

Dextrothyroxine (D-thyroxine), the optical isomer of L-thyroxine, has a modest hypocholesterolemic effect in patients with primary hypercholesterolemia but achieves this effect at the expense of making the patients moderately hyperthyroid.[92]

MECHANISM OF ACTION

D-Thyroxine lowers the concentrations of LDL cholesterol by stimulating high-affinity LDL receptor activity in hepatocytes, thus promoting an increased rate of LDL catabolism.[246]

SIDE EFFECTS

Side effects occur more frequently at doses of D-thyroxine above 4 to 6 mg per day and consist of an increased incidence of cardiac arrhythmias and hypermetabolic effects consistent with mild hyperthyroidism, such as nervousness, increased sweating, and fine tremor. Because of the higher incidence of adverse cardiovascular effects noted in the Coronary Drug Project,[91] the use of dextrothyroxine should be reserved for selected young adult patients with familial hypercholesterolemia who are unable to take other effective lipid-lowering agents.

INDICATIONS AND DOSAGE

Dextrothyroxine (Choloxin) is available in tablets of 1, 2, 4, and 6 mg. The usual starting dose is 2 mg per day, and the dose should be increased by 1-mg increments until a maximum dose of 4 to 6 mg is achieved. This drug is contraindicated in older patients who may have latent coronary atherosclerosis and in patients with known cardiovascular disease. D-Thyroxine lowers concentrations of LDL cholesterol 10 to 20 percent but has little effect on plasma triglycerides or concentrations of HDL cholesterol.[92]

Miscellaneous Agents

A number of other drugs may be of value in specific situations, but these agents are not recommended for general use and will be discussed only briefly.

ANABOLIC STEROIDS

The anabolic steroid oxandrolone 7.5 mg per day has been shown to reduce VLDL and chylomicron levels and to increase postheparin lipolytic activity.[247] Oxandrolone concurrently reduces the concentrations of HDL cholesterol. The drug may be potentially useful in certain male patients with severe hypertriglyceridemia who have not responded to conventional therapy.

PROGESTATIONAL AGENTS

The use of norethindrone acetate (Norlutate) 5 mg per day has been shown to reduce triglyceride levels in women patients with severe hypertriglyceridemia and the type V phenotype.[248] The drug appears to increase postheparin lipolytic activity and results in an enhanced clearance of triglyceride-rich lipoproteins from plasma. Norethindrone acetate may be useful in women patients with severe hypertriglyceridemia who fail to respond to other therapeutic regimens.

ESTROGENS

With the possible exception of postmenopausal women patients with type III hyperlipoproteinemia in whom clofibrate, nicotinic acid, or gemfibrozil has failed to normalize plasma lipid values, estrogens have no role in the drug therapy of hyperlipoproteinemias. In the Coronary Drug Project,[249] the use of both 2.5-mg and 5-mg dosages of Premarin was associated with an increased incidence of morbid cardiovascular events, and the study was terminated prematurely. Although estrogens increase concentrations of HDL cholesterol, they also stimulate VLDL synthesis and may lead to severe hypertriglyceridemia in patients with preexistent hypertriglyceridemia.

Future Advances

FIBRIC ACID DERIVATIVES

Two fibric acid derivatives—clofibrate and gemfibrozil—have been approved for clinical use in the United States, and several other derivatives are currently undergoing clinical trials or have been approved for general use in Europe. These drugs, which include bezafibrate,[250] fenofibrate,[251] and ciprofibrate,[252] are considerably more effective than either clofibrate or gemfibrozil in reducing LDL concentrations in patients with primary hypercholesterolemia. Fenofibrate and ciprofibrate seem to be the most effective, and both have been shown to reduce levels of LDL cholesterol 20 to 25 percent in patients with heterozygous familial hypercholesterolemia. The hypocholesterolemic effects of these drugs appear to be mediated by an enhanced rate of receptor-mediated clearance of LDL from plasma.[253,254]

HMG CoA Reductase Inhibitors: Lovastatin (Mevinolin) and Related Compounds

Two specific competitive inhibitors of the rate-limiting enzyme in cholesterol biosynthesis (HMG CoA reductase) have been discovered, and analogues of the parent compounds have been synthesized. The two parent compounds, mevastatin (compactin)[255] and lovastatin (mevinolin),[256] are fungal metabolites which are effective in milligram quantities when given to normal human volunteers and patients with primary hypercholesterolemia. Clinical use of compactin has

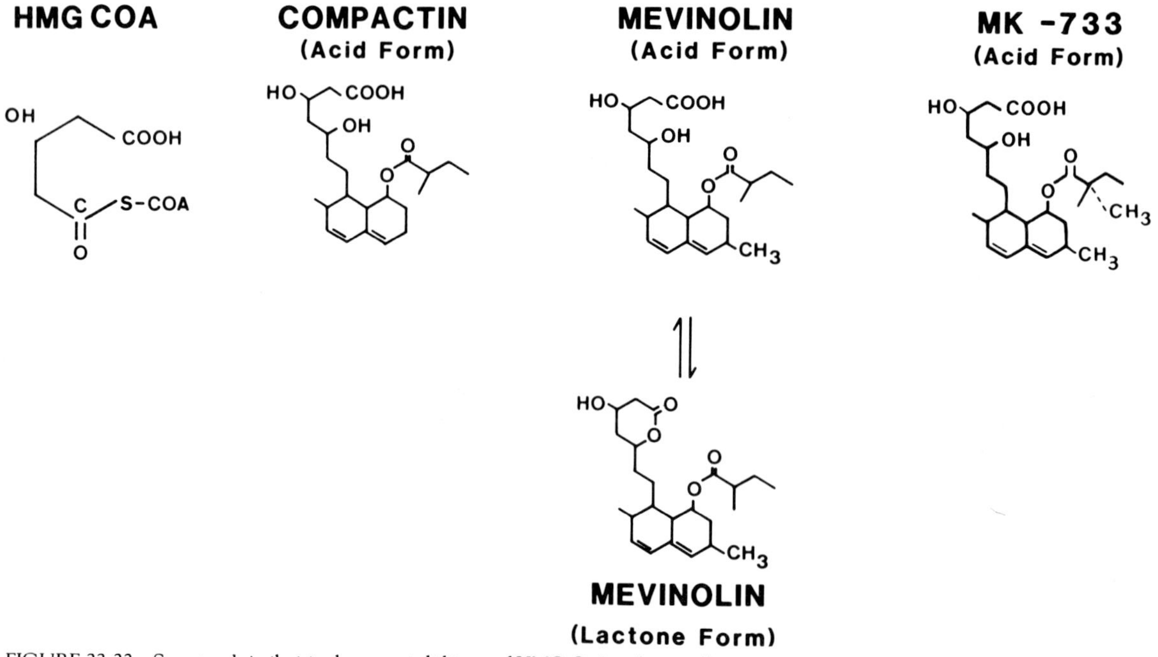

FIGURE 22-22 Structural similarities between inhibitors of HMG CoA reductase [lovastatin (mevinolin), mevastatin (compactin), and MK-733] and HMG CoA.

been limited to investigational studies in Japan, whereas mevinolin and a related compound, MK-733, are undergoing clinical trials in the United States and Canada.

The structures of mevinolin, compactin, and MK-733 are illustrated in Fig. 22-22, in which the structure of HMG CoA is also shown. The open-acid form of mevinolin has a ring structure similar to that of HMG CoA and is presumed to be the active part of this drug in terms of its ability to inhibit HMG CoA reductase. The hypocholesterolemic effects of mevinolin and related compounds result primarily from an enhanced rate of receptor-mediated catabolism of LDL from plasma together with a small and less consistent reduction in the rate of LDL synthesis.[99,257] At the cellular level, mevinolin reduces hepatic cholesterol biosynthesis and promotes a compensatory increase in the number of high-affinity LDL receptors expressed on the hepatocyte membrane; this increase in receptor numbers stimulates an enhanced rate of LDL catabolism from plasma.

Mevinolin 20 to 40 mg twice daily has been shown to reduce plasma concentrations of LDL cholesterol 35 to 38 percent in patients with heterozygous familial hypercholesterolemia.[93] This drug is also effective in patients with familial combined hyperlipidemia and may be of use in therapy for patients with hypercholesterolemia resulting from the nephrotic syndrome. The hypocholesterolemic effects of mevinolin are potentiated when it is combined with a bile acid sequestrant.[98,99] The efficacy of this combined therapy is illustrated in Fig. 22-23. Mevinolin is also an effective adjunct to therapy in patients who remain hypercholesterolemic after distal ileal bypass surgery.[258]

Mevinolin 20 to 40 mg twice daily is well tolerated, and short-term side effects have been minimal. These have included changes in bowel function, headache, insomnia, nausea, and fatigue. Biochemical changes have included increases in alkaline phosphatase, transaminases, and CPK in less than 5 percent of patients. Mevinolin does not reduce whole-body cholesterol synthesis[259] or impair adrenal steroidogenesis during ACTH stimulation.[260] Although current data indicate that mevinolin and its analogues represent a major development in the treatment of hypercholesterolemia, the long-term safety of these agents has not been established and their use is currently limited to investigational studies in patients with primary hypercholesterolemia.

THE SURGICAL TREATMENT OF HYPERLIPOPROTEINEMIA

A variety of surgical procedures have been performed on patients with familial hypercholesterolemia in an attempt to reduce plasma concentrations of total and LDL cholesterol. The distal ileal bypass operation is the most widely used surgical procedure for the treatment of severe hypercholesterolemia but is less effective than combined drug therapy in lowering LDL cholesterol concentrations; thus this surgical procedure cannot be generally recommended. The operation bypasses 200 cm of the distal ileum, leaving a blind loop, and in experienced hands has an operative mortality rate under 1 percent. This surgical procedure interrupts the normal enterohepatic circulation of bile acids; the mechanism of action is similar to that of the bile acid–binding resins discussed earlier. In patients with heterozygous familial hypercholesterolemia, reductions of 30 to 40 percent in concentrations of LDL cholesterol can be attained.[100–102] In a 10-year follow up of 27 patients treated with this operation,[261] only 2 patients achieved normal lipid values, indicating that even in patients who undergo distal ileal bypass surgery, other medical measures are necessary to achieve optimal lipid values. Mevinolin appears particularly well suited for this purpose.[99,258] Complications of distal ileal bypass surgery include diarrhea, bowel obstruction, vitamin B_{12} deficiency, and an increased risk of hyperoxaluria and oxalate kidney stones. Patients frequently need to take bile

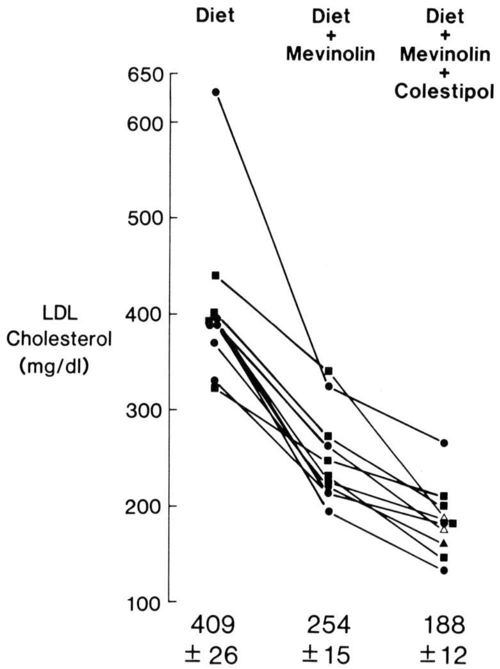

FIGURE 22-23 Changes in concentrations of low-density lipoprotein cholesterol in 10 patients with heterozygous familial hypercholesterolemia during sequential therapy with diet, lovastatin (mevinolin) (80 mg per day), and lovastatin (mevinolin) plus colestipol (15 to 20 g per day). (*Reproduced from Illingworth[98] with permission.*)

acid sequestrants in order to control diarrhea, which is caused by increased fecal excretion of unbound bile acids, and they require lifelong injections of vitamin B_{12}. Because of unknown effects on growth and development, distal ileal bypass surgery should not be considered for children. The operation has no role in other forms of hyperlipoproteinemia, nor is it effective in patients with homozygous familial hypercholesterolemia.

Portacaval shunt surgery has also been performed in patients with heterozygous familial hypercholesterolemia,[262] but in these patients the operation must be regarded as an investigational procedure and cannot be recommended.

Surgical Procedures in Homozygous Familial Hypercholesterolemia

A variety of surgical procedures have been performed in patients with homozygous familial hypercholesterolemia in an attempt to reduce their markedly elevated LDL cholesterol concentrations. Distal ileal bypass surgery and total biliary diversion do not work in these patients because of compensatory increases in cholesterol biosynthesis which nullify the increased excretion of bile acid. Portacaval shunt surgery has been shown to be effective in some patients,[103] but the 25 to 40 percent decrease in LDL cholesterol concentrations achieved following this procedure still leaves these patients markedly hypercholesterolemic. Liver transplantation has been successful in one patient.[107] By providing a liver which is able to express high-affinity LDL receptors, this operation is physiologically the most attractive. At the present time, however, all surgical procedures employed in patients with homozygous familial hypercholesterolemia must be regarded as experimental.

LABORATORY TESTS IN THE DIAGNOSIS OF HYPERLIPIDEMIAS

The accurate determination of cholesterol and triglyceride remains the cornerstone for the diagnosis of hyperlipidemia. In this section, we shall briefly discuss factors which can interfere with determinations as well as the indications and methods available for lipoprotein quantification. Mention will also be made of provocative tests which may aid in the diagnosis of hyperlipidemias. Detailed reviews have been published.[263,264]

COLLECTION AND HANDLING OF THE SAMPLE

Lipid and lipoprotein determinations may be performed on serum or plasma, but plasma is preferable, since it allows for more rapid cooling and separation of plasma and red cells. Ethylenediaminetetraacetic acid (EDTA) is the preferred anticoagulant. Lipid values in plasma are about 3 percent lower than in similar samples of serum obtained simultaneously from the same subject. Because of increases in the plasma volume which occur when subjects change from a standing to a recumbent posture, lipid values may be 5 to 10 percent lower when taken from patients in a supine position. Much smaller changes occur with sitting, and this is the position we recommend for venipuncture. Fluid shifts may also occur with prolonged venous occlusion and result in erroneously increased lipid values.

Separation of red cells should occur promptly; in the interim, the sample should be stored at 4°C. For determinations of total cholesterol and triglyceride, plasma samples can be frozen or stored at 4°C for up to a week. When lipoproteins are to be separated, the plasma should not be frozen and the samples should be handled promptly. Addition of SH inhibitors to such samples is advisable to minimize lipid changes which may occur before lipoprotein separation. Plasma triglyceride concentrations increase postprandially, and for this reason accurate determinations of triglyceride require the patient to have fasted 12 to 16 h before venipuncture. In contrast, cholesterol levels are minimally affected by eating, and casual blood samples are quite satisfactory if only cholesterol is to be determined.

LIPID DETERMINATIONS

Multichannel automated systems constitute the most commonly available methods for cholesterol and triglyceride determination by either enzymatic or colorimetric methods. Extraction of the samples with isopropanol prior to colorimetric assay of cholesterol is more tedious; this was the method used by the Lipid Research Clinics.

Lipoprotein Separations

INDICATIONS

Determination of plasma concentrations of LDL cholesterol and HDL cholesterol provides more detailed information about cardiovascular risk in patients with normal concentrations of plasma triglycerides (less than 200 mg/dl) and plasma cholesterol values in excess of 220 to 240 mg/dl. Determination of LDL and HDL concentrations is also appropriate in patients with premature cardiovascular disease (before age 50) and in any patient with skin lesions suggestive of an underlying lipid abnormality. In patients with elevated levels of both cholesterol and triglyceride in whom the distinction between phenotypic type IIb and type III hyperlipoproteinemia cannot be made, ultracentrifugal flotation of VLDL with determination of the ratio of VLDL cholesterol to total triglycerides is the method of choice. This will indicate that an abnormal cholesterol-rich VLDL particle is present in the plasma of patients with type III hyperlipoproteinemia. This method is more specific and is preferable to the electrophoretic demonstration of a beta-migrating band, which has also been considered diagnostic of type III hyperlipidemia.

Demonstration of chylomicronemia does not generally require lipoprotein separations and can be visually documented by means of inspection of plasma which has been stored for 12 to 18 h at 4°C or has been centrifuged for 20 min at 3000 g in a refrigerated centrifuge. It is the authors' belief that current indications for electrophoresis of whole plasma are minimal and that the usefulness of this procedure is small. With the growing awareness of apoprotein abnormalities as causal factors in the pathogenesis of dyslipoproteinemias, it is likely that apoprotein determinations will become more readily available in the coming years. At the present time, however, commercial assays for apoproteins are not available and patients with suspected dyslipoproteinemias due to apoprotein abnormalities should be referred to centers with a specialized interest in lipid disorders where these assays are routinely performed on a research basis.

AVAILABLE METHODS

Three methods are available for lipoprotein separation: electrophoresis, ultracentrifugation, and precipitation. Electrophoresis is usually carried out on paper, cellulose acetate, or agarose, but the method is imprecise and not easily quantitated in terms of the lipid content of a given lipoprotein. Ultracentrifugal separation of plasma is the most precise method but is time-consuming and requires an ultracentrifuge. Detailed information on the methods used for isolation of VLDL, LDL, and HDL have been published[264] and are beyond the scope of this chapter. Precipitation methods which rely on the interaction between lower-density lipoproteins (VLDL and LDL), sulfated polysaccharides, and divalent cations have gained in acceptance and are widely used. For example, the supernatant obtained after precipitation of VLDL and LDL by heparin-manganese contains only HDL and may be used for determination of the cholesterol content of the lipoprotein. Two additions to this method have been used to provide extra data. In the first, VLDL is removed by ultracentrifugation from the *d* 1.006 subnatant containing LDL and HDL. Determination of the lipid content of whole plasma, the heparin-manganese supernatant from whole plasma (HDL), and the VLDL and LDL plus HDL fractions from ultracentrifugation allows for quantification of VLDL, LDL, and HDL. A second, simpler method which does not require an ultracentrifuge has been used and gives indirect values for VLDL and LDL and direct values for HDL. This procedure relies on the assumption that the total plasma triglycerides divided by 5 approximates the value for VLDL cholesterol. Lipid values for whole plasma and for the heparin-manganese supernatant (HDL) are determined, and concentrations are calculated as follows:

$$\text{HDL cholesterol} = \text{cholesterol in heparin-manganese supernatant} \quad (22\text{-}1)$$

$$\text{VLDL cholesterol} = \text{total plasma triglyceride} \div 5 \quad (22\text{-}2)$$

$$\text{LDL cholesterol} = \text{total plasma cholesterol} - (\text{HDL cholesterol} + \text{VLDL cholesterol}) \quad (22\text{-}3)$$

This method is not reliable at triglyceride concentrations greater than 400 mg/dl or in the presence of either chylomicrons or the intermediate-density lipoproteins seen in type III.

Additional Laboratory Tests

A number of additional laboratory tests may aid in the precise characterization of patients with rare disorders of lipoprotein metabolism. Specific assays for LCAT, lipoprotein lipase, and hepatic lipase are available in several research laboratories but are not commercially available, and it is probably preferable to send samples to centers where these assays are performed regularly. Reliable commercial assays for apoproteins are not available, and accurate diagnosis of the major HDL deficiency disorders and apoprotein C-II deficiency or confirmation of apoprotein E-2 homozygosity in a patient with suspected type III hyperlipoproteinemia depends on the availability of assays in medical centers which specialize in lipoprotein metabolism. The precise diagnosis of homozygous familial hypercholesterolemia requires the determination of high-affinity LDL receptor activity on cultured fibroblasts, which can be obtained by means of amniocentesis in the case of prenatal diagnosis[66] or skin biopsy in a suspected case.[65,107] Determination of the number of high-affinity LDL receptors requires culture of the fibroblasts and subsequent measurement of the binding, internalization, and degradation of radiolabeled low-density lipoprotein. Consultation with a medical center or research laboratory that routinely performs this assay should be obtained prior to obtaining the fibroblast sample so that the cells will remain viable and the assay will be run with appropriate controls.

REFERENCES

1. Goffman JW, Lindgren FT, Elliot M: Ultracentrifugal studies of lipoproteins of human plasma. *J Biol Chem* 179:973, 1949.
2. Lees RS, Hatch FT: Sharper separation of lipoprotein species by paper electrophoresis in albumin containing buffer. *J Lab Clin Med* 61:418, 1963.
3. Alaupovic P: Apoproteins and lipoproteins. *Atherosclerosis* 13:141, 1971.
4. Osborne JC Jr, Brewer HB Jr: The plasma lipoproteins. *Adv Protein Chem* 31:253, 1977.
5. Kane JP, Hardman DA, Pauleus HE: Heterogeneity of apolipoprotein B isolation of a new species from human chylomicrons. *Proc Natl Acad Sci USA* 77:2465, 1980.
6. Krishnaiah DV, Walker LF, Borensztajn J, Getz GS: Apolipoprotein B variant derived from rat intestine. *Proc Natl Acad Sci USA* 77:3806, 1980.
7. Kane JP: Apolipoprotein B structural and metabolic heterogeneity. *Annu Rev Physiol* 45:637, 1983.
8. Hamilton RL, Havel RJ, Kane JP, Blaurock AE, Sata T: Cholestasis: Lamellar structure of the abnormal human serum lipoprotein. *Science* 172:475, 1971.
9. Sabesin SM: Cholestatic lipoproteins: Their pathogenesis and significance. *Gastroenterology* 83:704, 1982.
10. Glomset JA, Norum KR: The metabolic role of lecithin cholesterol acyltransferase: Perspective from pathology. *Adv Lipid Res* 11:1, 1973.
11. Jackson RL, Morrisett JD, Gotto AM Jr: Apoprotein structure and metabolism. *Physiol Rev* 56:259, 1976.
12. Schonfeld G: Disorders of lipid transport, update 1983. *Prog Cardiovasc Dis* 26:89, 1983.
13. Hospattankar AV, Fairwell T, Ronan R, Brewer HB Jr: Amino acid sequence of human plasma apolipoprotein CII from normal and hyperlipoproteinemic subjects. *J Biol Chem* 259:318, 1984.
14. Segrest JP: A molecular theory of lipid protein interactions in the plasma lipoproteins. *FEBS Lett* 38:247, 1974.
15. Zannis VI, Kurnit DM, Breslow JL: Hepatic apo A1, apo E and intestinal apo A1 are synthesized in precursor isoprotein forms by organ cultures of human fetal tissues. *J Biol Chem* 257:5367, 1982.
16. Gordon JI, Sims HF, Lentz SR, Edelstein C, Scanu AM, Strauss AW: Proteolytic processing of human preproapolipoprotein A1. *J Biol Chem* 258:4037, 1983.
17. Gordon JI, Bisgaier CL, Sims HF, Sachdev OP, Glickman RM, Strauss AW: Biosynthesis of human preapolipoprotein AIV. *J Biol Chem* 259:468, 1984.
18. Blaufuss MC, Gordon JI, Schonfeld G, Strauss AW, Alpers DH: Biosynthesis of apolipoprotein CIII in rat liver and small intestinal mucosa. *J Biol Chem* 259:2452, 1984.
19. Bruns GAP, Karathanasis SK, Breslow JL: Human apolipoprotein AI, CIII gene complex is located on chromosome 11. *Arteriosclerosis* 4:97, 1984.
20. Cheung P, Kao FT, Law ML, Jones C, Puck TT, Chen L: Localization of the structural gene for the human apolipoprotein AI on the long arm of chromosome 11. *Proc Natl Acad Sci USA* 81:508, 1984.
21. Fojo SS, Law SW, Brewer HB Jr: Human apolipoprotein CII: Complete nucleic acid sequence of preapolipoprotein CII. *Proc Natl Acad Sci USA* 81:6354, 1984.
22. Zannis VI, MacPherson J, Goldberger G, Karathanasis SK, Breslow JL: Synthesis, intracellular processing, and signal peptide of human apolipoprotein E. *J Biol Chem* 259:5495, 1984.
23. Vaith P, Hassman G, Uhlenbreck G: Characterization of the oligosaccharide side chain of apolipoprotein CIII from human plasma very low density lipoproteins. *Biochim Biophys Acta* 541:234, 1978.
24. Patsch W, Schonfeld G: Degree of sialation of apo CIII is altered by diet. *Diabetes* 30:530, 1981.
25. Basu SK, Goldstein JL, Brown MS: Independent pathways for secretion of cholesterol and apolipoprotein E by macrophages. *Science* 219:871, 1983.
26. Shackelford JE, Lebherz HG: Synthesis and secretion of apolipoprotein AI by chick breast muscle. *J Biol Chem* 258:7175, 1983.
27. Jackson RL, Pattus F, deHaas G: Mechanism of action of milk lipoprotein lipase at substrate interphases: Effects of apolipoproteins. *Biochemistry* 19:373, 1980.
28. Breckenridge WC, Little JA, Steiner G, Chow A, Poast M: Hypertriglyceridemia associated with a deficiency of apolipoprotein CII. *N Engl J Med* 298:1265, 1978.
29. Miller NE, Rao SN, Alaupovic P, Noble N, Slack J, Brunzell JD, Lewis B: Familial apolipoprotein CII deficiency: Plasma lipoproteins and apolipoproteins in heterozygous and homozygous subjects and the effects of plasma infusion. *Eur J Clin Invest* 11:69, 1981.
30. Herbert PN, Assman G, Gotto AM Jr, Fredrickson DS: Familial lipoprotein deficiency: Abetalipoproteinemia, hypobetalipoproteinemia and Tangier disease, in Stanbury JB, Wyngaarden JB, Fredrickson DS, Goldstein JL, Brown MS (eds): *The Metabolic Basis of Inherited Disease,* 5th ed. New York, McGraw-Hill, 1983, p 589.
31. Mahley RW, Angeline B: Type III hyperlipoproteinemia: Recent insights into the genetic defect of familial dysbetalipoproteinemia. *Adv Intern Med* 29:395, 1984.
32. Mahley RW, Innerarity TL, Pitis RE, Weisgraber KH, Brown JH, Gross E: Inhibition of lipoprotein binding to cell surface receptors of fibroblasts following selective modification of arginyl residues in arginine rich and B apoproteins. *J Biol Chem* 252:7279, 1977.
33. Glomset JA, Norum KR, Gjone E: Familial lecithin cholesterol acyl transferase deficiency, in Stanbury JB, Wyngaarden JB, Fredrickson DS, Goldstein JL, Brown MS (eds): *The Metabolic Basis of Inherited Disease,* 5th ed. New York, McGraw-Hill, 1983, p 643.
34. Breckenridge WC, Little JA, Alaupovic P, Wang CS, Kuksis A, Lundgren A, Gardiner G: Lipoprotein abnormalities associated with a familial deficiency of hepatic lipase. *Atherosclerosis* 45:161, 1982.
35. Goldstein JL, Brown MS: Low density lipoprotein pathway and its relationship to atherosclerosis. *Annu Rev Biochem* 46:897, 1977.
36. Goldstein JL, Brown MS: The LDL receptor defect in familial hypercholesterolemia: Implications for pathogenesis and therapy. *Med Clin North Am* 66:355, 1982.
37. Carr BR, Simpson ER: Lipoprotein utilization and cholesterol synthesis by the human fetal adrenal gland. *Endocr Rev* 2:306, 1981.
38. Gwynne JJ, Strauss JF III: The role of lipoproteins in steroidogenesis and cholesterol metabolism in steroidogenic glands. *Endocr Rev* 3:299, 1982.
39. Nicoll A, Miller NE, Lewis B: High density lipoprotein metabolism. *Adv Lipid Res* 17:54, 1980.
40. Krauss RM: Regulation of high density lipoprotein levels. *Med Clin North Am* 66:403, 1982.

41. Camargo CA, Williams PT, Vranizan KM, Albers JJ, Wood PD: The effect of moderate alcohol intake on serum apolipoproteins AI and AII: A controlled study. *JAMA* 253:2854, 1985.

42. Avogaro P, Pittlo BG, Cazzolato G: Are apolipoproteins better discriminators than lipids for atherosclerosis? *Lancet* 1:901, 1979.

43. Vergani C, Trovato G, Dioguardi N: Serum total lipids and lipoproteins, cholesterol apoproteins A and B in cardiovascular disease. *Clin Chim Acta* 87:127, 1978.

44. Noma A, Yokosuka T, Kitamura K: Plasma lipids and apolipoproteins as discriminators for presence and severity of angiographically defined coronary artery disease. *Atherosclerosis* 49:1, 1983.

45. Fredrickson DS, Goldstein JL, Brown MS: The familial hyperlipoproteinemias, in Stanbury JD, Wyngaarden JB, Fredrickson DS (eds): *The Metabolic Basis of Inherited Disease,* 3d ed. New York, McGraw-Hill, 1978, p 604.

46. Zilversmit DB: Atherogenesis: A postprandial phenomenon. *Circulation* 60:473, 1979.

47. Fredrickson DS, Levy RI, Lees RS: Fat transport in lipoproteins: An integrated approach to mechanisms and disorders. *N Engl J Med* 276:32, 94, 148, 215, 273, 1967.

48. Beaumont JL, Carlson LA, Cooper GR, Fejfar Z, Fredrickson DS, Strasser T: Classification of hyperlipidemias and hyperlipoproteinemias. *Bull WHO* 43:891, 1970.

49. Lipid Research Program: *The Lipid Research Clinics Population Studies Data Book,* Bethesda, NIH Publication No. 80:1527, vol 1, 1980.

50. Havel RJ: Treatment of hyperlipidemia: Where do we stand? *Am J Med* 73:301, 1982.

51. Consensus Conference: Lowering blood cholesterol to prevent heart disease. *JAMA* 253:2080, 1985.

52. Lewis B: *The Hyperlipidemias: Clinical and Laboratory Practise.* Oxford, Blackwell Scientific Publications, 1976, p 292.

53. Connor SL, Connor WE, Sexton G, Calvin L, Bacon S: The effects of age, body weight and family relationships on plasma lipoproteins and lipids in men, women and children of randomly selected families. *Circulation* 65:1290, 1982.

54. Connor WE, Cerqueira MT, Connor RW, Wallace RB, Malinow MR, Casdorph HR: The plasma lipids, lipoproteins and diet of the Tarahumara Indians of Mexico. *Am J Clin Nutr* 31:1131, 1978.

55. Grundy SM, Vega GL, Bilheimer DW: Kinetic mechanism determining variability in low density lipoprotein levels and rise with age. *Arteriosclerosis* 5:623, 1985.

56. Bennion LJ, Grundy SM: Effects of diabetes mellitus on cholesterol metabolism in man. *N Engl J Med* 296:1365, 1977.

57. Kutty KM, Bryant DG, Farid NR: Serum lipids in hypothyroidism—a re-evaluation. *J Clin Endocrinol Metab* 46:55, 1978.

58. Illingworth DR, McClung MR, Connor WE, Alaupovic P: Familial hypercholesterolemia and primary hypothyroidism: Coexistence of both disorders in a young woman with severe hypercholesterolemia. *Clin Endocrinol* 14:145, 1981.

59. DeLiberti JH, McMurry MP, Connor WE, Alaupovic P: Hypercholesterolemia associated with alpha-1 antitrypsin deficiency and hepatitis: Lipoprotein and apoprotein determinations, sterol balance and treatment. *Am J Med Sci* 288:81, 1984.

60. Shaboury AM, Hayes TM: Hyperlipidemia in asthmatic patients receiving long term steroid therapy. *Br Med J* 1:85, 1973.

61. Molitch ME, Oill P, Odell WD: Massive hyperlipidemia during estrogen therapy. *JAMA* 227:522, 1974.

62. Katz RA, Jorgensen H, Nigra TP: Elevation of serum triglyceride levels from oral isotretinoin in disorders of keratinization. *Arch Dermatol* 116:1369, 1980.

63. Schiffel H, Weidmann P, Mordasini R, Riesen W, Bachmann C: Reversal of diuretic induced increases in serum low density lipoprotein cholesterol by the beta blocker, pindolol. *Metabolism* 31:411, 1982.

64. Johnson BF: The emergent problem of plasma lipid changes during antihypertensive therapy. *J Cardiovasc Pharmacol* 4(suppl 2):S213, 1982.

65. Goldstein JL, Brown MS: Familial hypercholesterolemia, in Stanbury JB, Wyngaarden JB, Fredrickson DS, Goldstein JL, Brown MS (eds): *The Metabolic Basis of Inherited Disease,* 5th ed. New York, McGraw-Hill, 1983, p 672.

66. Brown MS, Kovanen PT, Goldstein JL, Eeckles R, Vandenberg K, Vandenberg H, Fryns JP, Cassiman JJ: Prenatal diagnosis of homozygous familial hypercholesterolemia. *Lancet* 1:526, 1978.

67. Gagne C, Moorjani S, Brun D, Doussaint M, Lupen PJ: Heterozygous familial hypercholesterolemia: The relationship between plasma lipids, lipoproteins, clinical manifestations, and ischemic heart disease in men and women. *Atherosclerosis* 34:13, 1979.

68. Shapiro JR, Fallet RW, Tsang RC, Glueck CJ: Achilles tendonitis and tenosinovitis: A diagnostic manifestation of familial type II hyperlipoproteinemia in children. *Am J Dis Child* 128:486, 1974.

69. Watanabe A, Yoshimura A, Wacasugi T, Tatami R, Takada R: Serum lipids, lipoproteins, and coronary heart disease in patients with xanthelasma palpebrarum. *Atherosclerosis* 38:283, 1981.

70. Mabuchi M, Ito S, Haba T: Achilles tendon thickness and ischemic heart disease in familial hypercholesterolemia. *Metabolism* 27:1672, 1978.

71. Jensen D, Blankenhorn DH, Kornerup V: Coronary disease in familial hypercholesterolemia. *Circulation* 36:77, 1967.

72. Stone NY, Levy RI, Fredrickson DS, Verter J: Coronary artery disease in 116 kindred with familial type II hypercholesterolemia. *Circulation* 49:476, 1974.

73. Slack J: Risks of ischemic heart disease in familial hypercholesterolemia. *Lancet* 2:1380, 1969.

74. Coetze GA, VanderWesthuyzen DR, Berger JMB, Henderson HE, Gevers W: Low density lipoprotein metabolism in cultured fibroblasts from a new group of patients presenting clinically with homozygous familial hypercholesterolemia. *Arteriosclerosis* 2:303, 1982.

75. Rose V, Wilson G, Steiner G: Familial hypercholesterolemia: Report of coronary death at age 3 in a homozygous child and prenatal diagnosis in a heterozygous sibling. *J Pediatr* 100:757, 1982.

76. Allen JM, Thompson GR, Myant MB, Steiner R, Oakley MC: Cardiovascular complications of homozygous familial hypercholesterolemia. *Br Heart J* 44:361, 1980.

77. Forman MB, Kinsley RH, Duplessis JP, Danskey R, Milner S, Levine SE: Surgical correction of combined supravalvular and valvular aortic stenosis in homozygous familial hypercholesterolemia. *S Afr Med J* 61:579, 1982.

78. Bloch A, Dinsmore RE, Lees RS: Coronary angiographic findings in type II and type IV hyperlipoproteinemia. *Lancet* 1:928, 1976.

79. Sugrue DD, Thompson GR, Oakley CM, Trainer IM, Steiner RE: Contrasting patterns of coronary atherosclerosis in normocholesterolemic smokers and patients with familial hypercholesterolemia. *Br Med J* 283:1358, 1981.

80. Streja D, Steiner G, Kwiterovich PO: Plasma high density lipoproteins in ischemic heart disease: Studies in a large kindred with familial hypercholesterolemia. *Ann Intern Med* 89:871, 1978.

81. Ginsberg H, Davidson N, Le NA, Gibson J, Ahrens EH, Brown WV: Marked overproduction of low density lipoprotein apoprotein B in a subject with heterozygous familial hypercholesterolemia. *Biochim Biophys Acta* 712:250, 1982.

82. Hazzard WR, Albers JJ, Baron P, Lewis B: Association of isoapolipoprotein EIII deficiency with heterozygous familial hypercholesterolemia: Implications for lipoprotein physiology. *Lancet* 1:298, 1981.

83. Tolleshaug H, Hopgood KK, Brown MS, Goldstein JL: The LDL receptor locus in familial hypercholesterolemia: Multiple mutations disrupt transport and processing of a membrane receptor. *Cell* 32:941, 1983.

84. Lehrman MA, Goldstein JL, Brown MS, Russell DW, Schneider WJ: Internalization of defective LDL receptors produced by genes with nonsense and frame shift mutations that truncate the cytoplasmic domain. *Cell* 41:735, 1985.
85. Bilheimer DW, Stone NJ, Grundy SM: Metabolic studies in familial hypercholesterolemia: Evidence for a gene dosage effect in vivo. *J Clin Invest* 64:524, 1979.
86. Soutar AK, Myant NB, Thompson GR: Simultaneous measurement of apoprotein B turnover in very low and low density lipoproteins in familial hypercholesterolemia. *Atherosclerosis* 28:247, 1977.
87. Fogelman AM, Hokam MM, Haberland ME, Tanaka RD, Edwards PA: Lipoprotein regulation of cholesterol metabolism in macrophages derived from human monocytes. *J Biol Chem* 257: 14081, 1982.
88. Seftel HC, Baker CG, Sundler MP: A host of hypercholesterolemic homozygotes in South Africa. *Br Med J* 281:633, 1980.
89. Khachadurian AK, Uthman SM: Experiences with homozygous cases of hypercholesterolemia: A report of 52 patients. *Nutr Metab* 15:132, 1973.
90. Baker SG, Joffe BI, Mendelsohn D, Seftel HC: Treatment of homozygous familial hypercholesterolemia with probucol. *S Afr Med J* 62:7, 1982.
91. Coronary Drug Project: Findings leading to further modifications of its protocol with respect to dextrothyroxin. *JAMA* 220:996, 1972.
92. Bantle JP, Oppenheimer JH, Schwartz HL, Hunninghake DB, Probstfield JL, Hansom RL: TSH response to TRH in euthyroid hypercholesterolemic patients treated with graded doses of dextrothyroxine. *Metabolism* 30:63, 1981.
93. Illingworth DR, Sexton GJ: Hypocholesterolemic effects of mevinolin in patients with heterozygous familial hypercholesterolemia. *J Clin Invest* 74:1972, 1984.
94. Illingworth DR, Phillipson BE, Rapp JH, Connor WE: Colestipol plus nicotinic acid in treatment of heterozygous familial hypercholesterolemia. *Lancet* 1:296, 1981.
95. Kane JP, Malloy MJ, Tun P, Phillips NR, Freeman D, Williams MC, Rowe JS, Havel RJ: Normalization of low density lipoprotein levels in heterozygous familial hypercholesterolemia with a combined drug regimen. *N Engl J Med* 304:251, 1981.
96. Kuo PT, Kostis JB, Moreyra A, Hayes JA: Familial type II hyperlipoproteinemia with coronary heart disease: Effects of colestipol plus nicotinic acid. *Chest* 79:286, 1981.
97. Dujovne CA, Krehbiel P, Decoursey S, Jackson B, Chernoff SB, Pitteman A, Garty M: Probucol with colestipol in the treatment of hypercholesterolemia. *Ann Intern Med* 100:477, 1984.
98. Illingworth DR: Mevinolin plus colestipol in therapy for severe heterozygous familial hypercholesterolemia. *Ann Intern Med* 101:598, 1984.
99. Grundy SM, Vega GL, Bilheimer DW: Influence of combined therapy with mevinolin and interruption of bile acid reabsorption on low density lipoproteins in heterozygous familial hypercholesterolemia. *Ann Intern Med* 103:339, 1985.
100. Miettinen TA, Lampinen M: Cholestyramine and ileal bypass in the treatment of familial hypercholesterolemia. *Eur J Clin Invest* 7:509, 1977.
101. Russell D, Fritz V, Mieny L, Mendlesohn D, Joffe BI, Seftel HC: Treatment of familial hypercholesterolemia by partial ileal bypass. *S Afr Med J* 55:237, 1979.
102. Spengel FA, Jadhav A, Duffield RGM, Wood CB, Thompson GR: Superiority of partial ileal bypass over cholestyramine in reducing cholesterol in familial hypercholesterolemia. *Lancet* 2:768, 1981.
103. Forman MB, Baker SG, Many CJ: Treatment of homozygous familial hypercholesterolemia with portacaval shunt. *Atherosclerosis* 41:349, 1982.
104. King MEE, Breslow JL, Lees RS: Plasma exchange therapy of homozygous familial hypercholesterolemia. *N Engl J Med* 302:1457, 1980.
105. Thompson GR, Myant MB, Kilpatrick D, Oakley CM, Raphael MJ, Steiner RE: Assessment of long term plasma exchange for familial hypercholesterolemia. *Br Heart J* 43:680, 1980.
106. Lupien PJ, Moorjani S, Lon M: Removal of cholesterol from blood by affinity binding to heparin-agarose: Evaluation of treatment of homozygous familial hypercholesterolemia. *Pediatr Res* 14:113, 1980.
107. Bilheimer DW, Goldstein GL, Grundy SM, Starzl TE, Brown MS: Liver transplantation to provide low density lipoprotein receptors and lower plasma cholesterol in a child with homozygous familial hypercholesterolemia. *N Engl J Med* 311:1658, 1984.
108. Vega GL, Illingworth DR, Grundy SM, Lindgrun FT, Connor WE: Normocholesterolemic tendon xanthomatosis with overproduction of apolipoprotein B. *Metabolism* 32:118, 1983.
109. Goldstein JL, Schrott HG, Hazzard WR: Hyperlipidemia in coronary heart disease: Genetic analysis of lipid levels in 176 families and delineation of a new inherited disorder combined hyperlipidemia. *J Clin Invest* 52:1544, 1973.
110. Sniderman AD, Shapiro S, Marpole D, Skinner B, Tang G, Kwiterovich PO Jr: Association of coronary atherosclerosis with hyperapobetalipoproteinemia. *Proc Natl Acad Sci USA* 77:604, 1980.
111. Sniderman AD, Wolfson C, Tang B, Franklin FA, Bachorik PS, Kwiterovich PO Jr: Association of hyperapobetalipoproteinemia with endogenous hypertriglyceridemia and atherosclerosis. *Ann Intern Med* 97:833, 1982.
112. Janus ED, Nicoll AM, Turner PL, Lewis B: Kinetic basis of the primary hyperlipoproteinemias: Studies of apolipoprotein B turnover in genetically defined subjects. *Eur J Clin Invest* 10:161, 1980.
113. Deeb SS, Motulsky AG, Albers JJ: A partial cDNA clone for human apolipoprotein B. *Proc Natl Acad Sci USA* 82:4983, 1985.
114. Knott TJ, Rall SC, Inerarity TL, Jacobson SF, Urdea MS, Wilson BL, Powell LM, Pease RJ, Eddy R, Nakei H, Byers M, Priestly LM, Robertson E, Rall LB, Betz C, Sows TV, Mahley RW, Scott J: Human apolipoprotein B: Structure of carboxyterminal domains, cytogenic expression and chromosomal localization. *Science* 230:37, 1985.
115. Lipid Research Clinics Program: The lipid research clinics program coronary primary prevention trial results: I. Reduction in incidence in coronary heart disease. *JAMA* 251:351, 1984.
116. Lipid Research Clinics Program: The lipid research clinics coronary primary prevention trial results: II. The relationship of reduction in incidence of coronary heart disease to cholesterol lowering. *JAMA* 251:365, 1984.
117. Brensike JF, Levy RI, Kelsy SF: Effects of therapy with cholestyramine on progression of coronary arteriosclerosis: Results of the NHLBI type II coronary intervention study. *Circulation* 69:313, 1984.
118. Hunninghake DB, Probtsfield JB: Drug treatment of hyperlipoproteinemia, in Rifkind BM, Levy RI (eds): *Hyperlipidemia: Diagnosis and Therapy*. New York, Grune & Stratton, 1977, p 327.
119. Wilson DE, Lees RS: Metabolic relationships among the plasma lipoproteins: Reciprocal changes in the concentrations of very low and low density lipoproteins in man. *J Clin Invest* 51:1051, 1972.
120. Goffman JW, Dipalla O, Glazier F, Freeman NK, Linguen FT, Nichols AV, Strisower EH, Tamplan AR: The serum lipoprotein transport system and health, metabolic disorders, atherosclerosis and coronary heart disease. *Plasma* 2:413, 1954.
121. Hazzard WR: Primary type III hyperlipidemia, in Rifkind BM, Levy RI (eds): *Hyperlipidemia: Diagnosis and Therapy*. New York, Grune & Stratton, 1977, p 137.
122. Morganroth J, Levy RI, Fredrickson DS: The biochemical,

clinical and genetic features of type III hyperlipoproteinemia. *Ann Intern Med* 82:158, 1975.
123. Vessby B, Headstand H, Lundin LG, Olsen U: Inheritance of type III hyperlipoproteinemia: Lipoprotein patterns in first degree relatives. *Metabolism* 26:225, 1977.
124. Hazzard WR, O'Donnell TF, Lee YL: Broad beta disease (type III hyperlipoproteinemia) in a large kindred: Evidence for a monogenic mechanism. *Ann Intern Med* 82:141, 1975.
125. Havel RJ: Familial dysbetalipoproteinemia: New aspects of pathogenesis and diagnosis. *Med Clin North Am* 66:441, 1982.
126. Fredrickson DS, Morganroth J, Levy RI: Type III hyperlipoproteinemia: An analysis of two contemporary definitions. *Ann Intern Med* 82:150, 1975.
127. Ghiselli G, Schaffer EJ, Gascon P, Brewer HB Jr: Type III hyperlipoproteinemia associated with apolipoprotein E deficiency. *Science* 214:1239, 1981.
128. Kushwaha RS, Hazzard WR, Gagne C, Chait A, Albers AA: Type III hyperlipoproteinemia: Paradoxical hypolipidemic response to estrogen. *Ann Intern Med* 87:517, 1977.
129. Zelis R, Mason DT, Bronwald E, Levy RI: Effects of hyperlipoproteinemias and their treatment on the peripheral circulation. *J Clin Invest* 49:1007, 1970.
130. Nikkila EA: Familial lipoprotein lipase deficiency and related disorders of chylomicron metabolism, in Stanbury JB, Wyngaarden JB, Fredrickson DS, Goldstein JL, Brown MS (eds): *The Metabolic Basis of Inherited Disease,* 5th ed. New York, McGraw-Hill, 1983, p 622.
131. Fredrickson DS, Levy RI: Familial hyperlipoproteinemia, in Stanbury JB, Wyngaarden JB, Fredrickson DS (eds): *The Metabolic Basis of Inherited Disease,* 3d ed. New York, McGraw-Hill, 1972, p 545.
132. Brown WV, Baginsky ML, Ehnholm C: Primary type I and V hyperlipoproteinemia, in Rifkind BM, Levy RI (eds): *Hyperlipidemia: Diagnosis and Therapy.* New York, Grune & Stratton, 1977, p 93.
133. Brunzell JD, Bierman EL: Chylomicronemia syndrome: Interaction of genetic and acquired hypertriglyceridemia. *Med Clin North Am* 66:455, 1982.
134. Kwiterovich PO, Farah JR, Brown WV, Bachorik PS, Baylin SB, Neill CA: The clinical, biochemical, and familial presentation of type V hyperlipoproteinemia in childhood. *Pediatrics* 59:513, 1977.
135. Greenberg BM, Blackwelder WC, Levy RI: Primary type V hyperlipoproteinemia. *Ann Intern Med* 87:526, 1977.
136. Fallat RW, Glueck CJ: Familial and acquired type V hyperlipoproteinemia. *Atherosclerosis* 23:41, 1976.
137. Lesser PB, Warshaw AL: Diagnosis of pancreatitis masked by hyperlipidemia. *Ann Intern Med* 82:795, 1975.
138. Harlan WR, Winesett PS, Wasserman AJ: Tissue lipoprotein lipase in normal individuals and in individuals with exogenous hypertriglyceridemia and the relation of this enzyme to the assimilation of fat. *J Clin Invest* 46:239, 1967.
139. Sigurdson G, Nicoll A, Lewis B: Metabolism of very low density lipoproteins in hyperlipidemia: Studies of apoprotein B kinetics in man. *Eur J Clin Invest* 6:167, 1976.
140. Mishkel MA, Stein EA: Primary type IV hyperlipoproteinemia, in Rifkind BM, Levy RI (eds): *Hyperlipidemia: Diagnosis and Therapy.* New York, Grune & Stratton, 1977, p 177.
141. Goldstein JL, Hazzard WR, Schrott HG, Bierman EL, Motulsky AG, Levinski MJ, Campbell ED: Hyperlipidemia in coronary heart disease: I. Lipid levels in 500 survivors of myocardial infarction. *J Clin Invest* 52:1533, 1973.
142. Brunzell JD, Bierman EL: Plasma triglyceride and insulin levels in familial hypertriglyceridemia. *Ann Intern Med* 87:198, 1977.
143. Barr DP, Russ EM, Eder HA: Protein lipid relationships in human plasma. *Am J Med* 11:480, 1951.
144. Gordon T, Castelli WP, Hjortland MC, Kannel WM: High density lipoprotein as a protective factor against coronary heart disease: The Framingham study. *Am J Med* 62:707, 1977.
145. Mellies MJ, Gartside PS, Galtfelter L, Glueck CJ: Effect of probucol on plasma cholesterol high and low density lipoprotein cholesterol and apolipoprotein A1 and A2 in adults with primary familial hypercholesterolemia. *Metabolism* 29:956, 1980.
146. Schaefer EJ, Heaton WH, Wetzel MG, Brewer HB Jr: Plasma apolipoprotein A1 absence associated with a marked reduction of high density lipoproteins and premature coronary artery disease. *Arteriosclerosis* 2:16, 1982.
147. Norum RA, Lakier JB, Goldstein S, Angel A, Goldberg RB, Block WD, Noffze DK, Dolphin PJ, Bogorad DD, Edelglass J, Alaupovic P: Familial deficiency of apolipoproteins A1 and C3 and precocious coronary artery disease. *N Engl J Med* 306:1513, 1982.
148. Lindeskog GR, Gustafson A, Enerback L: Serum lipoprotein deficiency and diffuse planar xanthoma. *Arch Dermatol* 106:529, 1972.
149. Gustafson A, McCounathy W, Alaupovic P, Curry MD, Persson B: Identification of apoprotein families in a variant of human plasma apolipoprotein A deficiency. *Scand J Clin Lab Invest* 39:377, 1979.
150. Carlson LA, Phillipson B: Fish eye disease: A new familial condition associated with massive corneal opacities and dyslipoproteinemia. *Lancet* 2:921, 1979.
151. Carlson LA: Fish eye disease: A new familial condition with massive corneal opacities and dyslipoproteinemia. *Eur J Clin Invest* 12:41, 1982.
152. Weisgraber KH, Bersot TP, Mahley RW, Francheschini G, Sirtori CR: AI Milano apoprotein: Isolation and characterization of cysteine containing variant of the A1 apoprotein from human high density lipoproteins. *J Clin Invest* 66:901, 1980.
153. Vergani C, Bettale A: Familial hypoalphalipoproteinemia. *Clin Chim Acta* 114:45, 1981.
154. Glueck CJ, Daniels SR, Bates S, Benton C, Tracey T, Third JLHC: Pediatric victims of unexplained stroke and their families: Familial lipid and lipoprotein abnormalities. *Pediatrics* 69:308, 1982.
155. Glueck CJ, Fallet RW, Millet F, Gottside P, Elston RC, Go RCP: Familial hyperalphalipoproteinemia: Studies in 18 kindreds. *Metabolism* 24:1243, 1975.
156. Schaefer EJ: Clinical, biochemical and genetic features in familial disorders of high density lipoprotein deficiency. *Arteriosclerosis* 4:303, 1984.
157. Francheschini G, Sirtori CR, Capurso A, Weisgraber KH, Mahley RW: AI Milano apoprotein: Decreased high density lipoprotein cholesterol levels with significant lipoprotein modifications and with clinical atherosclerosis in an Italian family. *J Clin Invest* 66:892, 1980.
158. Glueck CJ: Familial hypoalphalipoproteinemia, in Frohlich J, Angel A (eds): *Proceedings of the International Conference on Lipoprotein Deficiency Syndromes.* Vancouver, BC, May 1985, in press.
159. Daniels SR, Bates S, Lukin RR, Benton C, Third JLHC, Glueck CJ: Cerebral vascular arteriopathy (arteriosclerosis) and ischemic childhood stroke. *Stroke* 13:360, 1982.
160. Schaefer EJ, Zech LA, Schwartz DS, Brewer HP Jr: Coronary heart disease prevalence and other clinical features in familial high density lipoprotein deficiency (Tangiers disease). *Ann Intern Med* 93:261, 1980.
161. Schmitz G, Assmann G, Rall SE Jr, Mahley RW: Tangier disease: Defective recombination of a specific Tangier apolipoprotein A1 isoform (proapo A1) with high density lipoproteins. *Proc Natl Acad Sci USA* 80:6081, 1983.
162. Zannis VI, Lees AM, Lees RS, Breslow JL: Abnormal apo A1 isoprotein composition in patients with Tangier disease. *J Biochem* 257:4978, 1982.
163. Kay L, Ronan R, Schaefer EJ, Brewer HB Jr: Tangier disease: A structural defect in apolipoprotein A1. *Proc Natl Acad Sci USA* 79:2485, 1982.
164. Glueck CJ, Kostis PM, Tsang RC, Mellies MJ, Steiner PM:

Neonatal familial hyperalphalipoproteinemia. *Metabolism* 26:469, 1977.
165. Malloy MJ, Kane JP, Hardman DA, Hamilton RL, Dalal KB: Normotriglyceridemic abetalipoproteinemia: Absence of the B100 apolipoprotein. *J Clin Invest* 67:1441, 1981.
166. Takashimo Y, Kodama T, Lida H, Kawamura M, Aburatani H, Itakura H, Akanuma Y, Takaku F, Kawade M: Normotriglyceridemic abetalipoproteinemia in infancy: An isolated apolipoprotein B100 deficiency. *Pediatrics* 75:541, 1985.
167. Glickman RM, Green PHR, Lees RS, Lux SE, Kilgore A: Immunofluorescent studies of apolipoprotein B in intestinal mucosa: Absence of abetalipoproteinemia. *Gastroenterology* 76:288, 1979.
168. Caballero FM, Buchanan GR: Abetalipoproteinemia presenting as severe vitamin K deficiency. *Pediatrics* 65:161, 1980.
169. Muller DPR, Lloyd JK, Bird AC: Long term management of abetalipoproteinemia: Possible role for vitamin E. *Arch Dis Child* 52:209, 1977.
170. Illingworth DR, Connor WE, Miller RG: Abetalipoproteinemia: Report of two cases and review of therapy. *Arch Neurol* 37:659, 1980.
171. Illingworth DR, Kenny TA, Orwoll ES: Adrenal function in heterozygous and homozygous hypobetalipoproteinemia. *J Clin Endocrinol Metab* 54:27, 1982.
172. Illingworth DR, Kenny TA, Connor WE, Orwoll ES: Corticosteroid production in abetalipoproteinemia: Evidence for an impaired response to ACTH. *J Lab Clin Med* 100:115, 1982.
173. Parker CR Jr, Illingworth DR, Bissonnette J, Carr BR: Endocrinology of pregnancy in abetalipoproteinemia: Studies in a patient with homozygous familial hypobetalipoproteinemia. *N Engl J* Med, 314:557, 1986.
174. Muller DPR, Lloyd JK: Effect of large oral doses of vitamin E on the neurological sequelae of patients with abetalipoproteinemia. *Ann NY Acad Sci* 393:133, 1982.
175. Hegele RA, Angel A: Arrest of neuropathy and myopathy in abetalipoproteinemia with high dose vitamin E therapy. *Can Med Assoc J* 132:41, 1985.
176. Illingworth DR, Connor WE, Buist NRM, Jhaveri DJ, Lin DS, McMurray MP: Sterol balance in abetalipoproteinemia: Studies in a patient with homozygous familial hypobetalipoproteinemia. *Metabolism* 28:1152, 1979.
177. Lackner KJ, Monge JC, Law SW, Gregg RE, Brewer HB Jr: Abetalipoproteinemia analysis of the hepatic mRNA and gene coding for apolipoprotein B100 (abstract). *Circulation* 72:10, 1985.
178. Bieri JG, Hoeg JM, Schaefer EJ, Zech LA, Brewer HB Jr: Vitamin A and vitamin E replacement in abetalipoproteinemia. *Ann Intern Med* 100:238, 1984.
179. Kayden HJ, Hatem LJ, Traber MG: The measurement of nanograms of tocopherol from needle aspiration biopsies of adipose tissue: Normal and abetalipoproteinemic subjects. *J Lipid Res* 24:652, 1983.
180. Partin JS, Partin JC, Schubert WK, McAdams AJ: Liver ultrastructure in abetalipoproteinemia: Evolution of micronodular cirrhosis. *Gastroenterology* 67:107, 1974.
181. Noseda G, Riesen W, Schlumph E, Morell A: Hypobetalipoproteinemia associated with autoantibodies against betalipoproteins. *Eur J Clin Invest* 2:342, 1972.
182. Cottrill C, Glueck CJ, Leuba V, Millett F, Puppione D, Brown WV: Familial homozygous hypobetalipoproteinemia. *Metabolism* 23:779, 1974.
183. Salt HB, Wolff OH, Lloyd JK, Fosbrooke AS, Cameron AH, Hubble DV: On having no betalipoprotein: A syndrome comprising abetalipoproteinemia, acanthocytosis, and steatorrhea. *Lancet* 2:325, 1960.
184. Andersen GE, Brokhatting NK, Lous P: Familial hypobetalipoproteinemia in nine children diagnosed as the result of core blood screening for hypolipoproteinemia in 10,000 Danish newborns. *Arch Dis Child* 54:691, 1979.
185. Glueck CJ, Gartside PS, Steiner PM, Miller M, Todd-Hunter T, Haaf J, Puck EM, Terrana M, Fallet RW, Kashyap ML: Hyperalpha and hypobetalipoproteinemia in octogenarian kindreds. *Atherosclerosis* 27:387, 1977.
186. Bhattacharyya AK, Connor WE, Mausolf FA, Flatt AE: Turnover of xanthoma cholesterol in hyperlipoproteinemic patients. *J Lab Clin Med* 87:503, 1976.
187. Assmann G, Fredrickson DS: Acid lipase deficiency: Wolman's disease and cholesterol ester storage disease, in Stanbury JB, Wyngaarden JB, Fredrickson DS, Goldstein JL, Brown MS (eds): *The Metabolic Basis of Inherited Disease,* 5th ed. New York, McGraw-Hill, 1983, p 803.
188. Bhattacharyya AK, Connor WE: Familial diseases with storage of sterols other than cholesterol (cerebrotendinous xanthomatosis and β-sitosterolemia and xanthomatosis), in Stanbury JB, Wyngaarden JB, Fredrickson DS (eds): *The Metabolic Basis of Inherited Disease,* 4th ed. New York, McGraw-Hill, 1978, p 656.
189. Salen G, Shefer S, Berginer VN: Familial disease with storage of sterols other than cholesterol: Cerebrotendinous xanthomatosis and sitosterolemia with xanthomatosis, in Stanbury JB, Wyngaarden JB, Fredrickson DS, Goldstein JL, Brown MS (eds): *The Metabolic Basis of Inherited Disease,* 5th ed. New York, McGraw-Hill, 1983, p 713.
190. Berginer VN, Salen G, Shefer S: Longterm treatment of cerebrotendinous xanthomatosis with chenodeoxycholic acid. *N Engl J Med* 311:1649, 1984.
191. Salen G, Horak I, Rothkopf M, Cohen J, Speck J, Tint JS, Shore V, Dayal B, Chen T, Shefer S: Lethal atherosclerosis associated with abnormal plasma and tissue sterol composition in sitosterolemia with xanthomatosis. *J Lipid Res* 26:1126, 1985.
192. Connor WE: Unpublished observations.
193. Connor WE, Connor SL: Dietary treatment of hyperlipidemia, in Rifkind BM, Levy RI (eds): *Hyperlipidemia: Diagnosis and Therapy.* New York, Grune & Stratton, 1977, p 281.
194. Connor WE, Connor SL: The key role of nutritional factors in the prevention of coronary heart disease. *Prev Med* 1:49, 1972.
195. Taylor CB, Patton DE, Cox GE: Atherosclerosis in rhesus monkeys: VI. Fatal myocardial infarction in a monkey fed fat and cholesterol. *Arch Pathol* 76:404, 1963.
196. Armstrong ML, Warner ED, Connor WE: Regression of coronary atheromatosis in rhesus monkeys. *Circ Res* 27:59, 1970.
197. Lin DS, Connor WE: The long-term effects of dietary cholesterol upon the plasma lipids, lipoproteins, cholesterol absorption, and the sterol balance in man: The demonstration of feedback inhibition of cholesterol biosynthesis and increased bile acid excretion. *J Lipid Res* 21:1042, 1981.
198. Kovanen PT, Brown MS, Basu SK, et al: Saturation and suppression of hepatic lipoprotein receptors: A mechanism for the hypercholesterolemia of cholesterol-fed rabbits. *Proc Natl Acad Sci USA* 78:1396, 1981.
199. Mahley RW, Hui DY, Innerarity TL, et al: Two independent lipoprotein receptors on hepatic membranes of dog, swine and man. *J Clin Invest* 68:1197, 1981.
200. Becker N, Illingworth DR, Alaupovic P, et al: Effects of saturated, monounsaturated, and omega-6 polyunsaturated fatty acids on plasma lipids, lipoproteins and apoproteins in humans. *Am J Clin Nutr* 37:355, 1983.
201. Connor WE, Hodges RE, Bleiler RE: The serum lipids in men receiving high cholesterol and cholesterol-free diets. *J Clin Invest* 40:894, 1961.
202. Connor WE, Stone DB, Hodges RE: The interrelated effects of dietary cholesterol and fat upon the human serum lipid levels. *J Clin Invest* 43:1691, 1964.
203. Roberts SL, McMurry M, Connor WE: Does egg feeding (i.e. dietary cholesterol) affect plasma cholesterol levels in humans? The results of a double-blind study. *Am J Clin Nutr* 34:2092, 1981.
204. Gordon T, Fisher M, Ernst M, et al: Relation of diet to LDL cholesterol, VLDL cholesterol and plasma total cholesterol and

triglycerides in white adults. *Atherosclerosis* 2:502, 1982.
205. Goodnight SH Jr, Harris WS, Connor WE, Illingworth DR: Polyunsaturated fatty acids, hyperlipidemia and thrombosis. *Arteriosclerosis* 2:87, 1982.
206. Harris WS, Connor WE, McMurry MP: The comparative reductions of the plasma lipids and lipoproteins by dietary polyunsaturated fats: Salmon oil versus vegetable oils. *Metabolism* 32:179, 1983.
207. Phillipson BE, Rothrock DW, Connor WE, Harris WS, Illingworth DR: The reduction of plasma lipids, lipoproteins, and apoproteins in hypertriglyceridemic patients by dietary fish oils. *N Engl J Med* 312:1210, 1985.
208. Keys A, Anderson JT, Grande F: Prediction of serum-cholesterol responses of man to changes in fats in the diet. *Lancet* 2:959, 1957.
209. Hegsted DM, McGandy RB, Myers ML, Stare FJ: Quantitative effects of dietary fat on serum cholesterol in man. *Am J Clin Nutr* 17:281, 1965.
210. Olefsky J, Reaven GM, Farquhar JW: Effects of weight reduction on obesity. *J Clin Invest* 53:64, 1974.
211. Schwartz RS, Brunzell JD: Increase of adipose tissue lipoprotein lipase activity with weight loss. *J Clin Invest* 67:1425, 1981.
212. Nikkila EA, Ojala K: Induction of hypertriglyceridemia by fructose in the rat. *Life Sci* 4:937, 1965.
213. Castelli WP, Gordon T, Hjortland MC, et al: Alcohol and blood lipids. *Lancet* 2:153, 1977.
214. St Leger AS, Cochrance AL, Moore F: Factors associated with cardiac mortality in developed countries with particular reference to the consumption of wine. *Lancet* 1:1017, 1979.
215. Fry MM, Spector AA, Connor SL, et al: Intensification of hypertriglyceridemia by either alcohol or carbohydrate. *Am J Clin Nutr* 26:798, 1973.
216. Kudzma DJ, Schonfeld G: Alcoholic hyperlipidemia: Induction by alcohol but not by carbohydrate. *J Lab Clin Med* 77:384, 1970.
217. Ginsberg H, Olefsky J, Farquhar JW, et al: Moderate ethanol ingestin and plasma triglyceride levels—a study in normal and hypertriglyceridemic persons. *Ann Intern Med* 80:143, 1974.
218. Connor WE, Connor SL: The dietary treatment of hyperlipidemia: Rationale, technique and efficacy, in Havel RJ (ed): Lipid disorders. *Med Clin North Am* 66:485, 1982.
219. Connor SL, Connor WE: The New American Diet. New York, Simon & Schuster, 1986.
220. Connor WE, Brown HB, Fredrickson DS, Steinberg C, Connor SL, Bickel JH: *A Maximal Approach to the Dietary Treatment of the Hyperlipidemias* (five manuals). Subcommittee on Diet and Hyperlipidemia, Council on Arteriosclerosis, American Heart Association, 1973.
220a. Connor SL, Artand-Wild SM, Classick-Kohn CJ, Gustafson JR, Flavell DP, Hatcher LF, Connor WE: The cholesterol/saturated fat index: An indication of the hypercholesterolemic and atherogenic potential of food. *Lancet* 1:1229, 1986.
221. Zilversmit DB: Cholesterol index of foods. *J Am Diet Assoc* 74:562, 1979.
222. Kane JP, Malloy MJ: Treatment of hypercholesterolemia. *Med Clin North Am* 66:537, 1982.
223. Brown WV, Goldberg IJ, Ginsberg HN: Treatment of common lipoprotein disorders. *Prog Cardiovasc Dis* 27:1, 1984.
224. Schaefer EJ, Levy RI: Pathogenesis and management of lipoprotein disorders. *N Engl J Med* 312:1300, 1985.
225. Brown MS, Goldstein JL: Drugs used in the treatment of hyperlipoproteinemias, in Gilman AG, Goodman AS, Rall TW, Murad F (eds): *The Pharmacological Basis of Therapeutics,* 7th ed. New York, Macmillan, 1985, p 827.
226. Shepherd J, Packard CJ, Bicker S, Laurie TDV, Morgan HG: Cholestyramine promotes receptor mediated low density lipoprotein catabolism. *N Engl J Med* 302:1029, 1980.
227. Kovanen PT, Bilheimer DW, Goldstein JL, Jaramillow JJ, Brown MS: Regulatory role for hepatic low density lipoprotein receptors in vivo in the dog. *Proc Natl Acad Sci USA,* 78:194, 1981.
228. Altschul R, Hoeffer A, Stephen JD: Influence of nicotinic acid on serum cholesterol in man. *Arch Biochem Biophys* 54:558, 1955.
229. Grundy SM, Mok HYI, Zack L, Berman M: The influence of nicotinic acid on metabolism of cholesterol and triglycerides in man. *J Lipid Res* 22:24, 1981.
230. Olsson AG, Carlson LA, Anggard E, Ciabattoni G: Prostacyclin production augmented in the short term by nicotinic acid. *Lancet* 2:565, 1983.
231. Knopp RH, Ginsberg J, Albers JJ, Hoff C, Oglivie JT, Warnick GR, Burrows E, Retzliff B, Poole M: Contrasting effects of unmodified and time released forms of niacin on lipoproteins in hyperlipidemic subjects: Clues to mechanism of action of niacin. *Metabolism* 34:642, 1985.
232. Carlson LA: Effect of nicotinic acid on serum lipids and lipoproteins, in Carlson LA, Olsson AG (eds): *Treatment of Hyperlipoproteinemia.* New York, Raven, 1984, p 115.
233. Nestel PJ, Billington T: Effects of probucol on low density lipoprotein removal and high density lipoprotein synthesis. *Atherosclerosis* 38:203, 1981.
234. Miettinen TA, Huttenen LK, Kusi T: Effect of probucol on the activity of post heparin plasma lipoprotein lipase and hepatic lipase. *Clin Chim Acta* 113:59, 1981.
235. Kesaniemi YA, Grundy SM: Influence of gemfibrozil and clofibrate on metabolism of cholesterol and plasma triglycerides in man. *JAMA* 251:2241, 1984.
236. Boberg J, Boberg M, Gross R: The effect of treatment with clofibrate on hepatic triglyceride and lipoprotein lipase activities of post heparin plasma in male patients with hyperlipidemia. *Atherosclerosis* 27:499, 1977.
237. Langer T, Levy RI: Acute muscular syndrome associated with administration of clofibrate. *N Engl J Med* 279:856, 1968.
238. Coronary Drug Project Research Group: Clofibrate and niacin in coronary heart disease. *JAMA* 231:360, 1975.
239. Committee of Principal Investigators: A cooperative trial in the primary prevention of ischemic heart disease using clofibrate. *Br Heart J* 40:1069, 1978.
240. Committee of Principal Investigators: WHO cooperative trial on primary prevention of ischemic heart disease using clofibrate to lower cholesterol: Final mortality follow-up. *Lancet* 2:600, 1984.
241. Vega GL, Grundy SM: Gemfibrozil therapy in primary hypertriglyceridemia associated with coronary heart disease: Effects on metabolism of low density lipoproteins. *JAMA* 253:2398, 1985.
242. Samuel P: Treatment of hypercholesterolemia with neomycin: A time for reappraisal. *N Engl J Med* 301:595, 1979.
243. Hoeg JM, Schaefer EJ, Romano CA, Bou E, Pikus AM, Zeck LA, Bailey KR, Gregg RE, Wilson PWF, Sprecher EL, Grimes AM, Febring NG, Ayres EJ, John CE, Brewer HB Jr: Neomycin and plasma lipoproteins in type II hyperlipoproteinemia. *Clin Pharmacol Ther* 36:555, 1984.
244. Miettinen TA: Effects of neomycin alone and in combination with cholestyramine on serum cholesterol and fecal steroids in hypercholesterolemic subjects. *J Clin Invest* 64:1485, 1979.
245. Hoeg JM, Maher MB, Bou E, Zeck LA, Bailey KR, Gregg RE, Sprecher EL, Susser JK, Pikus AM, Brewer HB Jr: Normalization of plasma lipoprotein concentrations in patients with type II hyperlipoproteinemia by combined use of neomycin and niacin. *Circulation* 70:1004, 1984.
246. Thompson GR, Soutar AV, Spengel FA: Defects of receptor mediated low density lipoprotein catabolism in homozygous familial hypercholesterolemia and hypothyroidism in vivo. *Proc Natl Acad Sci USA* 78:2591, 1981.
247. Glueck CJ: Effects of oxandrolone on plasma triglycerides and postheparin lipolytic activity in patients with types III, IV and V familial hyperlipoproteinemia. *Metabolism* 20:691, 1971.
248. Glueck CJ, Levy RI, Fredrickson DS: Norethindrone acetate,

post heparin lipolytic activity and plasma triglycerides in familial types I, III, IV and V hyperlipoproteinemia: Studies in 26 patients and 5 normal patients. *Ann Intern Med* 75:345, 1971.

249. Coronary Drug Project: Findings leading to discontinuation of the 2.5 mg/day estrogen group. *JAMA* 226:652, 1973.

250. Mordasani R, Reisen W, Oster P: Reduced LDL and increased HDL apoproteins in patients with hypercholesterolemia under treatment with bezafibrate. *Atherosclerosis* 40:153, 1981.

251. Rossner S, Oro L: Fenofibrate therapy of hyperlipoproteinemia—a dose response study and comparison with clofibrate. *Atherosclerosis* 38:273, 1981.

252. Illingworth DR, Olsen GD, Cook SF, Sexton GJ, Wendell HA, Connor WE: Ciprofibrate in the therapy of type II hypercholesterolemia: A double blind trial. *Atherosclerosis* 44:211, 1982.

253. Stewart JM, Packard CJ, Lorimer AR, Boag DE, Shepard J: Effects of bezafibrate on receptor mediated and receptor-independent low density lipoprotein catabolism in type II hyperlipoproteinemia subjects. *Atherosclerosis* 44:355, 1982.

254. Malmendier CL, Delcroix C: Effects of fenofibrate on high and low density lipoprotein metabolism in heterozygous familial hypercholesterolemia. *Atherosclerosis* 55:161, 1985.

255. Endo A, Tsujita Y, Kuroda M, Tanazawa K: Inhibition of cholesterol synthesis in vivo by ML236B, a competitive inhibitor of 3-hydroxy 3-methyl glutaryl coenzyme A reductase. *Eur J Biochem* 87:313, 1977.

256. Alberts AW, Chen J, Kuron G: Mevinolin: A highly potent competitive inhibitor of hydroxy methyl glutaryl coenzyme A reductase and a cholesterol lowering agent. *Proc Natl Acad Sci USA* 77:3957, 1980.

257. Bilheimer BW, Grundy SM, Brown MS, Goldstein JL: Mevinolin and colestipol stimulate receptor mediated clearance of low density lipoprotein from plasma in familial hypercholesterolemia heterozygotes. *Proc Natl Acad Sci USA* 80:4124, 1983.

258. Illingworth DR, Connor WE: Hypercholesterolemia persisting after distal ileal bypass: Response to mevinolin. *Ann Intern Med* 100:850, 1984.

259. Grundy SM, Bilheimer DW: Inhibition of 3-hydroxy 3-methyl glutaryl CoA reductase by mevinolin in familial hypercholesterolemia heterozygotes: Effects on cholesterol balance. *Proc Natl Acad Sci USA* 81:2538, 1984.

260. Illingworth DR, Corbin D: Influence of mevinolin on the adrenocortical response to corticotropin in heterozygous familial hypercholesterolemia. *Proc Natl Acad Sci USA* 82:6291, 1985.

261. Koivisto P, Miettinen TA: Long term effects of ileal bypass on lipoproteins in patients with familial hypercholesterolemia. *Circulation* 70:290, 1984.

262. Madras PN: Portocaval shunt for familial heterozygous hypercholesterolemia. *Surg Gynecol Obstet* 152:187, 1981.

263. Bachorik PS, Wood PDS: Laboratory considerations in diagnosis and management of hyperlipoproteinemia, in Rifkind BM, Levy RI (eds): *Hyperlipidemia: Diagnosis and Therapy.* New York, Grune & Stratton, 1977, p 41.

264. Lipid Research Clinics Program: *Manual of Laboratory Operations:* vol 1: *Lipid and Lipoprotein Analysis.* Bethesda, MD, NIH, DHEW Publication (NIH) 75-628, 1974.

PART VII

CALCIUM AND BONE METABOLISM

23

Mineral Metabolism*

Andrew F. Stewart
Arthur E. Broadus

Chapters 23, 24, and 25 are devoted to disorders of mineral metabolism, disorders of skeletal homeostasis, and nephrolithiasis, respectively. This chapter contains a detailed description of systemic mineral homeostasis as well as the biochemistry and physiology of the hormones responsible for regulating the systemic balance of these ions. This description is designed to serve as the physiological introduction to the disorders discussed in all three chapters. The clinical sections of this chapter are confined to disorders which principally affect serum calcium, phosphorus, and magnesium and mineral ion balance; disorders primarily affecting skeletal homeostasis are discussed in their entirety in Chap. 24. Each of the three chapters contains a final section on routine and specialized testing relevant to the conditions described in the text.

CELLULAR AND EXTRACELLULAR MINERAL METABOLISM

General Considerations

The normal adult contains approximately 1000 g of calcium (Table 23-1). About 99 percent of this calcium is present in the skeleton, largely in the form of hydroxylapatite, a crystalline structure composed of calcium, phosphate, and hydroxyl ions.[1] Although only about 1 percent of the calcium in the skeleton is freely exchangeable with extracellular calcium, this exchangeable pool represents an important storehouse or buffer of some 5000 to 10,000 mg of calcium. Approximately 1 percent of total body calcium is contained in the soft tissues and extracellular fluids. The concentration of calcium ions in intracellular fluids is low (about 10^{-6} M).

The physiological importance of calcium falls into two broad categories. The *calcium salts* in bone provide the *structural* integrity of the skeleton. The *calcium ion* (Ca^{2+}) present in cellular and extracellular fluids is critically important to the normal function of a number of *biochemical processes*, including neuromuscular excitability, blood coagulation, membrane integrity and function, and cellular enzymatic and secretory activity. The biochemical importance of Ca^{2+} requires that its extracellular and cellular concentrations be maintained with constancy, and this is achieved by means of an elaborate system of hormonal controls.

Table 23-1. Content and Distribution of Calcium, Phosphorus, and Magnesium in Human Tissues

	Total body content, g	% in skeleton	% in soft tissues
Calcium	1000	99	1
Phosphorus	600	85	15
Magnesium	25	65	35

Source: Adapted from Krane.[1]

*Mrs. Nancy Canetti provided superb secretarial assistance. A portion of the work described was supported by Grants RR 125, AM 31998, and AM 30102 from the National Institutes of Health.

The normal human contains approximately 600 g of phosphorus. Some 85 percent of this phosphorus is present in crystalline form in the skeleton and plays a structural role. About 15 percent is present in the extracellular fluids, largely in the form of inorganic phosphate ions, and in the soft tissues, almost totally in the form of phosphate esters. Intracellular phosphate esters and phosphorylated intermediates are involved in a number of important biochemical processes, including the generation and transfer of cellular energy. Intracellular and extracellular concentrations of phosphorus are less rigidly maintained than are concentrations of calcium and magnesium.

The normal human adult contains approximately 25 g, or 2000 meq, of magnesium. About two-thirds of this is present in the skeleton in crystalline form. The magnesium in bone is not an integral part of the crystalline lattice of hydroxylapatite but appears to be located on the crystal surface. However, only a minor fraction of the magnesium in bone is freely exchangeable with extracellular magnesium. A relatively large portion of magnesium is present in the soft tissues, and it is the most abundant intracellular divalent cation. Cellular magnesium is important as a cofactor in a number of enzymatic reactions and in the regulation of neuromuscular excitability. Approximately 1 percent of total body magnesium is contained in the extracellular fluid compartment. This point is of clinical importance, since it suggests that measurement of the plasma magnesium concentration may provide a rather poor index of total body magnesium content, a prediction which has proved to be accurate. Cellular and extracellular magnesium concentrations are rigidly controlled.

Cellular Mineral Metabolism

A detailed review of the protean metabolic functions of calcium, phosphorus, and magnesium is beyond the scope of this chapter. The following section attempts only to summarize important aspects of the involvement of these ions in cellular physiology.

Life appears to have begun in a primordial sea rich in potassium and magnesium and poor in sodium and calcium, and it is speculated that the present composition of intracellular fluids, rich in potassium and magnesium and poor in sodium and calcium, is derived from this heritage.[2] With the passage of time, geological changes altered the composition of the oceans to one rich in sodium and calcium. Thus the development of membrane pumps and cellular systems for maintaining the asymmetries of these ions may be viewed as among the most *fundamental evolutionary developments* in cell biology. The maintenance of transmembrane potassium/sodium and magnesium/calcium ratios is critically important in the control of cell excitation and the regulation of intracellular metabolism. In general, more active tissues such as nerve tissue, liver, and muscle have a higher ratio of potassium/sodium and magnesium/calcium than do inactive tissues such as skin and erythrocytes. In addition, more active tissues have a higher phosphorus content than inactive tissues, in keeping with the role of phosphate esters in cellular energy metabolism.

CELLULAR CALCIUM METABOLISM

The extracellular and intracellular distributions of calcium, phosphorus, and magnesium are shown in Table 23-2, and cellular calcium metabolism in an idealized mammalian cell is depicted in Fig. 23-1.

The control of cellular calcium homeostasis is quite complex, and the regulation of the concentration of the calcium ion in the cytosol is as rigidly maintained as its concentration in extracellular fluids.[2-5] Cells are bathed in extracellular fluids containing approximately 10^{-3} M calcium ion. The concentration of calcium ions in the cytoplasm is approximately 10^{-6} M, or one one-thousandth of that in the extracellular fluids. Cytosolic calcium is to some extent buffered by binding to other cytoplasmic constituents, such as phospholipids and dicarboxylic acids. Certain cells contain a specific calcium-binding protein, which may serve as a buffer and/or a calcium transport protein within the cytosol. The mitochondria and microsomes contain 90 to 99 percent of the intracellular calcium, bound largely to organic and inorganic phosphates. The calcium content of these organelles is sufficient to replenish cytosolic calcium some 500 times.

The low cytosolic calcium concentration is maintained by three calcium *pump-leak transport systems:* an "external" system located in the plasma membrane and two "internal" systems located in the microsomal

Table 23-2. Estimated Ion Activities in a Typical Mammalian Cell

Fluid phase	Ca^{2+}	HPO_4^{2-}	Mg^{2+}
Extracellular fluid	5×10^{-4}	2×10^{-4}	5×10^{-4}
Cytosol	2.5×10^{-7}	1×10^{-4}	5×10^{-4}
Mitochondria (soluble)	0.2×10^{-4}	5×10^{-4}	$\sim 1 \times 10^{-3}$ (soluble and insoluble)
Mitochondria (insoluble)	1.5×10^{-3}	1×10^{-3}	

Source: Adapted from Rasmussen and Bordier.[2]

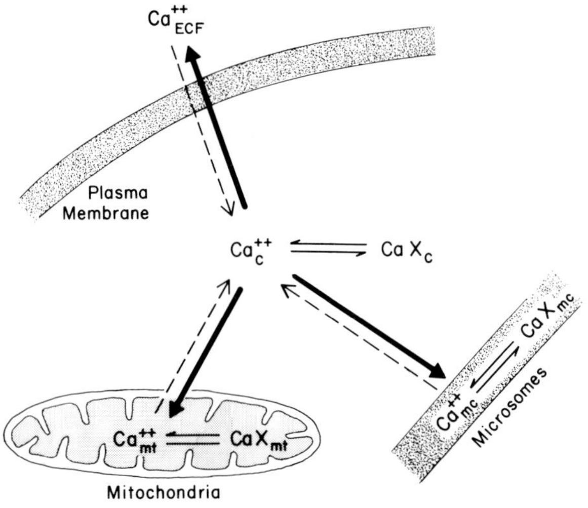

FIGURE 23-1 Schematic representation of the distribution of calcium ions (Ca^{2+}) in a typical mammalian cell. Three pump-leak systems located in the plasma, mitochondrial (mt), and microsomal (mc) membranes control the concentration of calcium in the cytosol (Ca_c^{2+}). The dashed arrows depict diffusion; the heavy, solid arrows depict active transport. Note that all three pumps are directed away from the cytosolic calcium pool. A substantial amount of the calcium in the cytosolic, mitochondrial, and microsomal pools is bound (Ca X_c, Ca X_{mt}, and Ca X_{mc}). (*Adapted from Rasmussen and Bordier.*[2])

membrane and the inner mitochondrial membrane. Calcium "leaks" into the cytosol by diffusing across these three membranes. Each of the three pumps is oriented in a direction of calcium egress from the cytosol, each requires energy, and each shares a high affinity for calcium ($K_m \cong 10^{-6}$ M). Thus, cellular calcium homeostasis is maintained by a complex series of external and internal transport systems designed either for calcium transport out of the cell or for calcium storage in intracellular organelles.

The importance of these three calcium transport systems in integrating cellular calcium metabolism varies considerably from cell to cell, depending on the function of a particular cell type. Table 23-3 lists a number of important biological functions mediated or modulated by the calcium ion, and several examples illustrate how the details of maintenance of cellular calcium homeostasis have been adapted to subserve the specific physiological function of a given cell type.

Calcium ion is the coupling factor linking excitation and contraction in all forms of skeletal and cardiac muscle.[4] In striated muscle, the microsomes are extensively developed as the sarcoplasmic reticulum, a series of microtubules ramifying throughout the sarcoplasm. The sarcoplasmic reticulum is the principal storehouse of intracellular calcium in muscle and is the most highly developed calcium transport system known. Depolarization of the plasma membrane is accompanied by the entry of a small amount of extracellular calcium into the cell, which acts as a trigger to release large quantities of calcium stored in the sarcoplasmic reticulum. The abrupt increase in cytosolic calcium interacts with troponin, a specific calcium-binding protein, leading to a conformational change and the actin-myosin interaction which is muscle contraction. The reticulum vesicles are capable of reaccumulating the large quantity of cytosolic calcium with the extreme speed required by the relaxation process. This is produced by active transport and perhaps also by the binding of calcium to specific calcium-binding proteins in the reticulum.

In most mammalian cells other than muscle, the principal internal calcium pump-leak system is that of the inner mitochondrial membrane, and the mitochondria serve as the major storehouse of intracellular calcium. The calcium ion may serve a number of functions in such cells (Table 23-3). For example, calcium has been implicated as an important coupling factor in neurotransmitter release as well as in the release of exocrine (e.g., amylase) and endocrine (e.g., insulin) secretions. In each case, calcium induces the secretion by exocytosis of preformed cell products stored in secretory vesicles. In these systems, cytoplasmic calcium mediates secretion by binding to the vesicle membranes and causing their association with the plasma membrane and/or by regulating the mechanical activity of the microfilament-microtubule system which links the secretory vesicles to the plasma membrane. The mitochondria appear to be the source of the cytosolic calcium involved in the secretion of these cellular products.

In a number of cell types, calcium serves as a second messenger, mediating the effects of membrane signals on both acute-phase and sustained-phase

Table 23-3. Functions of Calcium Ion

1. Extracellular
   a. Maintenance of normal ion product for mineralization
   b. Cofactor for prothrombin factors VII, IX, and X
   c. Maintenance of plasma membrane stability and permeability
2. Cellular
   a. Skeletal and cardiac muscle contraction
   b. Cellular secretion
      (1) Exocrine
      (2) Endocrine
      (3) Neurotransmitter
   c. Neural excitation and light transmission
   d. Regulation of membrane ion transport
   e. Enzyme regulation (gluconeogenesis, glycogenolysis)
   f. Cell growth and division

release of secretory products such as insulin and aldosterone.[4] The calcium messenger system is quite complex and involves a flow of information along several branches, including a calmodulin branch and a C-kinase branch. It is now recognized that in many cells the several branches of the calcium messenger system and the cyclic adenosine monophosphate (cAMP) messenger system are intimately related and that these systems are integrated in such a way that the net cellular response to a given stimulus is determined by a complex interplay between these systems.[4] The details of the calcium messenger system are beyond the scope of this chapter; they are presented in Chap. 5 and in an excellent recent review.[4]

Specialized bone, kidney, and intestinal cells are primarily concerned with the transcellular translocation of calcium. The best studied of these cell types is the cultured kidney cell.[5] In this cell, the pump-leak systems in the plasma membrane and inner mitochondrial membrane are predominant, and the mitochondria contain over 60 percent of the intracellular calcium. Parathyroid hormone influences this cell in two ways: (1) by increasing the influx of calcium across the plasma membrane into the cell and (2) by stimulating adenylate cyclase and the formation of cAMP. cAMP increases the efflux of calcium from the mitochondria in such a manner that the net effect of both actions of parathyroid hormone is an increase in cytosolic calcium. This results in an increase in the rate of calcium transport across the contralateral cell membrane and net calcium translocation.

CELLULAR PHOSPHORUS AND MAGNESIUM METABOLISM

The details of cellular and subcellular phosphorus and magnesium metabolism are not well understood, in large part owing to technological limitations. Both ions are asymmetrically distributed in cells (Table 23-2).

The transport of phosphate ions across the plasma membrane and the membranes of intracellular organelles proceeds passively but is determined by the movement of cations, in particular calcium. The phosphate content is high in mitochondria (Table 23-2), where it is largely in the form of calcium salts which serve as a storehouse of both calcium and phosphorus. The cytoplasmic concentration of free phosphate ions is estimated to be quite low, and the remaining portion of intracellular phosphate is either bound or in the form of organic phosphate esters. These phosphate esters play a variety of critically important roles in cellular metabolism: purine nucleotides provide the cell with stored energy; phosphorylated intermediates are concerned with energy conservation and transfer; nucleic acids are phosphate polymers; phospholipids are major constituents of cell membranes; and the phosphorylation of proteins is an important means of regulating their function.

Magnesium is the most abundant intracellular divalent cation and is the second most abundant intracellular cation after potassium. Approximately 60 percent of cellular magnesium is contained in the mitochondria, and it is estimated that only 5 to 10 percent of intracellular magnesium exists as free ions in the cytoplasm. Whether calcium and magnesium share common transport systems is not clear, but the cellular metabolism of these ions appears to be independently regulated. Magnesium regulates or is an essential cofactor in the function of a wide variety of key enzymes, including essentially all enzymes concerned with the transfer of phosphate groups, all reactions that require adenosine triphosphate (ATP), and each of the steps concerned with the replication, transcription, and translation of genetic information.

Extracellular Mineral Metabolism

CALCIUM

The state of calcium in serum has long been recognized to be complex, and our modern understanding of the physiological importance of these fractions dates from the classic work of McLean and Hastings.[6] There are three definable fractions of calcium in serum: ionized calcium (about 50 percent), protein-bound calcium (about 40 percent), and calcium which is complexed to other constituents in serum, mostly citrate and phosphate (about 10 percent).[7] Both complexed and ionized calcium are ultrafilterable so that about 60 percent of the total calcium in serum crosses semipermeable membranes. About 90 percent of the protein-bound calcium is bound to albumin, and the remainder is bound to globulins. Calcium appears to be bound largely to carboxyl groups in albumin, and this binding is pH-dependent. Acute acidosis decreases binding and increases ionized calcium, and acute alkalosis increases binding with a consequent decrease in ionized calcium.

It is the ionized fraction of calcium which is physiologically important and which is maintained at a remarkably constant level by means of a complex series of hormonal controls. Ionized calcium plays an important role in mineralization, coagulation, and membrane function (Table 23-3). The calcium ion stabilizes or lends rigidity to plasma membranes, probably by binding to phospholipids in the lipid monolayer, and influences permeability and excitability. A reduction in ionized calcium increases sodium permeability and enhances the excitability of all excitable tissues; an increase in ionized calcium has the opposite effect.

PHOSPHORUS

Serum inorganic phosphate also exists as three fractions: ionized, protein-bound, and complexed (Table 23-4). Protein binding is relatively insignificant for phosphate, representing some 10 percent of the total, but about 35 percent is complexed to sodium, calcium, and magnesium. Thus, approximately 90 percent of the inorganic phosphate in serum is ultrafilterable. The major ionic species of phosphate in serum is the divalent anion (HPO_4^{2-}).

In contrast to calcium, the serum phosphorus concentration varies widely and is influenced by age, sex, diet, pH, and a variety of hormones. An adequate serum phosphate concentration is critical in maintaining a sufficient ion product for normal mineralization and independently influences bone resorption.

MAGNESIUM

Less magnesium than calcium is protein-bound (Table 23-4), and about two-thirds of the total is ultrafilterable. Only a minor fraction is complexed. The protein-bound fraction is largely bound to albumin and is influenced by pH in a fashion analogous to that for calcium. It is the ionized magnesium fraction which is physiologically important and is rather rigidly maintained.

PARATHYROID HORMONE

Embryology, Anatomy, and Histology of the Parathyroid Glands

The adult human possesses two pairs of parathyroid glands. Each gland is a flattened ellipsoid of a tan or reddish-tan hue, measures 6 by 4 by 2 mm, and weighs 30 to 50 mg. Thus, the aggregate parathyroid mass in a normal adult is about 130 to 140 mg. Supernumerary parathyroids (totaling six to eight glands) are estimated to occur in 2 to 5 percent of individuals, but rarely if ever does an individual possess fewer than four parathyroid glands.[8]

The parathyroids arise as paired entodermal structures from the third (parathyroids III) and fourth (parathyroids IV) branchial pouches. Parathyroids III, which migrate to become the inferior glands, form in close association with the thymus and are commonly associated with thymic remnants. As the heart descends into the thorax, the thymus is drawn caudally. Parathyroids III normally pinch off just inferolateral to the lower pole of the thyroid. The anatomy of the inferior glands, however, is quite variable, and one or both glands may occur as far caudad as the anterior mediastinum at the level of the pericardium.

Parathyroids IV form in close association with the ultimobranchial body or lateral thyroid primordium. These glands remain relatively stationary and normally pinch off from the ultimobranchial body as it is incorporated into the thyroid. The anatomy of the superior glands is quite constant, and they typically lie dorsolateral to the thyroid at the level of the thyroid isthmus, close to the point where the middle thyroid artery crosses the recurrent laryngeal nerve. Uncommonly, these glands (or abnormal parathyroid tissue derived from them) may be attached to the posterior capsule of the thyroid, may actually be embedded in thyroid tissue, or may lie in the laryngeal-esophageal groove or posterior to the esophagus.

Each gland is surrounded by an ill-defined fibrous capsule and is supplied by a generous capillary plexus derived from the hilar vessels. The chief cell, the principal parenchymal parathyroid cell, is responsible for the synthesis and secretion of parathyroid hormone (PTH). The chief cell has the typical appearance of an active synthetic and secretory cell, with a prominent Golgi apparatus and rough endoplasmic reticulum and many secretory granules. Chief cells are usually ar-

Table 23-4. State of Calcium, Phosphate, and Magnesium in Normal Human Plasma

	Calcium		Phosphate		Magnesium	
	mg/dl	% total	mg/dl	% total	mg/dl	% total
Total	10.0	100	3.5	100	2.4	100
Ionized	4.8	48	1.9	55	1.3	55
Protein-bound	4.4	44	0.4	11	0.7	30
Complexed or unidentified	0.8	8	1.2	34	0.4	15

Source: Adapted from Marshall.[7]

ranged in cords or nests but may have a follicular arrangement.

The oxyphil cells are fewer in number and are usually scattered as single cells among the cords of chief cells. The oxyphil cells have prominent mitochondria and a poorly developed rough endoplasmic reticulum and Golgi apparatus, suggesting that they are not normally important secretory cells. Their precise function is unknown. In hyperplastic or adenomatous parathyroid glands, oxyphil cells may occasionally have a very different appearance and may be actively involved in PTH synthesis and secretion.

Water-clear cells are large polygonal cells with a striking lack of cytoplasmic staining. These cells are few in number in normal parathyroid tissue. Water-clear cells may be prominent in a small percentage of hyperplastic parathyroid glands.

The fat cell content of the glands increases throughout life and may account for two-thirds of the volume of the glands in old age.

Biosynthesis and Secretion of PTH

In recent years a great deal has been learned about the biosynthesis, sequence, control of secretion, metabolism, and mechanism of action of PTH. As knowledge has increased, it has become clear that each of these aspects of PTH physiology is complex and that these complexities may have important biological and clinical implications.

SEQUENCE AND BIOSYNTHESIS OF PARATHYROID HORMONE

PTH is a single-chain polypeptide composed of 84 amino acids. The molecular weight of the hormone is 9500, and it has no intrachain disulfide linkages.

In 1925, Collip extracted an active principle from bovine parathyroid glands using hot hydrochloric acid.[9] The work of Aurbach and of Rasmussen and coworkers in the 1950s and early 1960s produced increasingly purified preparations of the hormone, and complete purification was achieved in the 1970s.[9] The amino acid sequences of bovine, porcine, rat, and human PTH have been determined and/or deduced from gene sequences, and the genes for bovine, rat, and human PTH have been cloned.[10,11] In humans there is a single PTH gene, which is located on the short arm of chromosome 11. Knowledge about the sequence of the hormone has enabled the synthesis of both active fragments of the peptide and inactive fragments or derivatives which may act as competitive inhibitors of hormone binding and action in vitro and in vivo (see below).

PTH is produced by means of two sequential enzymic cleavages from a larger precursor polypeptide, as illustrated in Fig. 23-2. This precursor or prehormone is the synthetic product that is actually encoded in the gene for PTH and is termed *prepro-PTH.* Prepro-PTH is short-lived, being rapidly cleaved to a smaller peptide, *pro-PTH.* Pro-PTH is subsequently cleaved to PTH, the final stored and secreted product.

The primary structure of bovine prepro-PTH and its cleavage products is shown in Fig. 23-3. Prepro-PTH is a polypeptide of 115 amino acids and has a molecular weight of 13,000. It consists of the structure of pro-PTH with a 25-amino acid peptide extension at the amino terminus of the molecule. This peptide extension is particularly rich in uncharged, or hydrophobic, amino acids, and it is this *leader* or *signal* sequence which in essence defines the PTH gene product as a secretory peptide.[9-12] The signal recognition particle, docking protein, and other features of the pathway of biosynthesis and processing of a secretory peptide are discussed in detail in Chap. 5. The synthe-

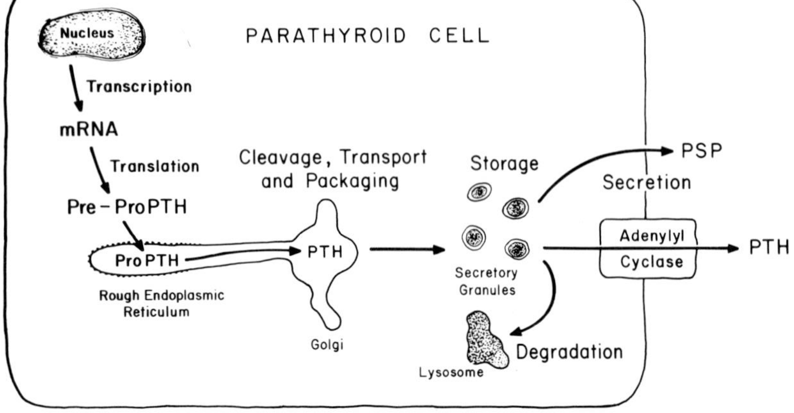

FIGURE 23-2 Schema showing the biosynthetic sequence of events in the production and secretion of parathyroid hormone.

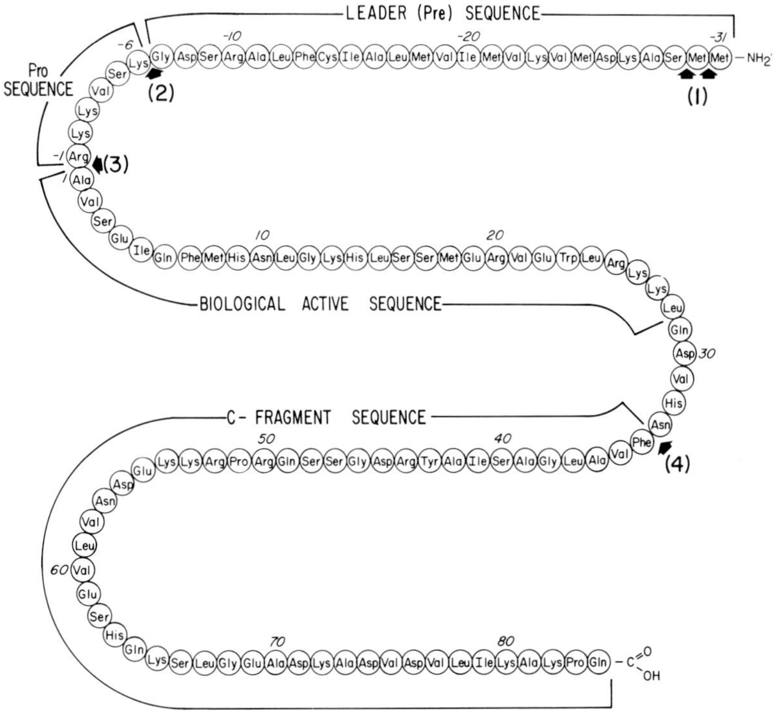

FIGURE 23-3 Primary structure of bovine preproparathyroid hormone. The arrows indicate sites of specific peptide-bond cleavages which occur in the sequence of biosynthesis and peripheral metabolism of the hormone. The biologically active sequence is enclosed in the center of the native biosynthetic product. (*Courtesy of JF Habener.*)

sis and processing of PTH is a classic example of this pathway.[9,10,12] The peptide extension at the amino terminus is the initial portion of the molecule to be translated on the ribosomes of the endoplasmic reticulum, and the hydrophobic nature of the signal sequence is considered important in guiding the nascent peptide across the reticular membrane into the intracisternal space.[9,10,12] Immediately upon entry into the intracisternal space, the leader sequence is cleaved from the peptide by a specific enzyme, yielding pro-PTH.

Pro-PTH is a peptide composed of 90 amino acids and has a molecular weight of 10,200. It consists of the structure of PTH with a 6-amino acid extension at the amino terminus of the molecule. Four of the six amino acids of the peptide extension are charged, and so the entire hexapeptide sequence is highly charged. The exact function of pro-PTH is not known, but it may be involved in the transport of the polypeptide through the membrane channels of the endoplasmic reticulum of the Golgi apparatus. On arrival in the Golgi apparatus, the hexapeptide extension is cleaved from the molecule to yield PTH. The conversion of pro-PTH to PTH occurs about 15 min after the initiation of translation of the messenger RNA in the rough endoplasmic reticulum. In the Golgi apparatus, PTH is packaged into secretory granules for storage and subsequent secretion. In some circumstances, PTH may be degraded intracellularly rather than stored (see below).

The prehormone and prohormone precursors appear to function entirely as intermediates in the biosynthetic sequence leading to the final hormonal product. Studies in vivo and in vitro have produced no evidence that either precursor is secreted by normal or abnormal tissue.[12] Pro-PTH has been found in vitro to have little biological activity, and prepro-PTH is probably entirely devoid of biological activity.[12]

The strategy employed by Rosenblatt and associates in developing PTH analogues is outlined in detail in a recent review.[12] This strategy has been based entirely on knowledge of structure-function relations. The most widely used competitive inhibitor in vitro is [Nle^{8},Nle^{18},Tyr^{34}]bPTH-(3-34) amide.[12] This analogue contains the receptor-binding domain (with a carboxy-terminal substitution to improve binding) but lacks the short but critical "message" domain (positions 1 and 2). The norleucine residues are substituted for methionines so that the analogue is resistant to oxidation. This analogue inhibits PTH binding in a number of systems and has also been shown to inhibit at least some of the actions of the peptide which appears to be responsible for the syndrome of humoral hypercalcemia of malignancy (see Hypercalcemia). A more recently developed analogue has been shown to inhibit the effects of PTH in vivo, but this analogue does not appear to have sufficient intrinsic inhibitory activity to merit consideration as an antihypercalcemic agent.[13]

Parathyroid secretory protein (PSP) is a large acidic glycoprotein synthesized by the chief cells.[9] It is formed as a preprotein, with an amino-terminal extension of 18 amino acids, which is converted to PSP.[14] There appears to be no pro-PSP intermediate. The protein normally exists as a dimer of identical subunits with a molecular weight of 70,000 each. It has been identified in secretory granules in the chief cell and is cosecreted with PTH. The exact function of PSP is not known, but it has been suggested that it binds electrostatically to the highly charged pro-PTH and serves a transport or carrier role within the cisternal space of the endoplasmic reticulum. PSP has been reported to be very similar structurally to chromogranin A from the adrenal medulla.[15]

CONTROL AND MECHANISM OF PARATHYROID HORMONE SECRETION

There is no convincing evidence that a trophic factor influences PTH secretion or that innervation of the parathyroid glands is important in the control of secretion. The major regulator of PTH synthesis and secretion is the concentration of ionized calcium in the extracellular fluids. This fact was established by a number of early studies of parathyroid physiology. For example, Copp et al.[16] demonstrated in dogs that perfusion of the parathyroid glands in situ with blood containing a low calcium concentration led to systemic hypercalcemia, and clinical states associated with chronic hypocalcemia were noted to be associated with gross hyperplasia of the parathyroid glands. With the introduction of the radioimmunoassay for PTH and the development of in vitro methods for studying parathyroid slices, organ cultures, and isolated parathyroid cells, the inferences of these early studies have been confirmed and considerably expanded.

It has been estimated from studies in cows that the reserve content of PTH is sufficient to maintain a normal rate of secretion for approximately 7 h and a maximal rate of secretion for only 1½ h.[12] Thus the parathyroid glands do not contain a large store of hormone, and so a sustained stimulus must be accompanied by synthesis as well as secretion of the hormone.

Figure 23-4 illustrates the relation between serum calcium and the secretion rate of PTH.[17] Within the normal range of serum calcium, approximately 9.0 to 10.5 mg/dl, there is a linear inverse relation between PTH secretion and serum calcium (slope C in Fig. 23-4). As the serum calcium dips below 9.0 mg/dl, there is a sharp increase in the PTH secretory rate, which becomes maximal at approximately five times the normal secretion rate at a calcium concentration of about 8.0 mg/dl (slope B). Acutely, further decreases in serum calcium below 8.0 mg/dl are not accompanied by a further increase in the PTH secretion rate (slope A). Chronic hypocalcemia, however, is associated with gross parathyroid hyperplasia and an aggregate parathyroid mass which can generate maximal rates of secretion 50 times greater than the basal rate.

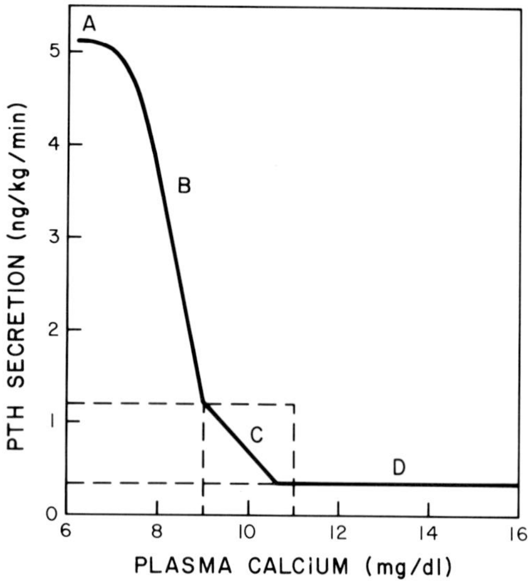

FIGURE 23-4 The relation between the extracellular concentration of calcium and the secretion rate of parathyroid hormone in cows. The broken lines enclose the approximate normal ranges of total serum calcium and the PTH secretion rate, and the letters A through D identify the slopes of PTH secretion at various levels of serum calcium. (*Modified from Habener JF and Potts JT, Handbook of Physiology, sec 7: Endocrinology, vol. 7, American Physiological Society, 1976.*)

The gradual gradation of PTH secretion within the range of normal calcium concentrations and the steep slope of secretion in the slightly hypocalcemic range constitute a homeostatic mechanism which provides optimal protection against hypocalcemia. Although the exact nature of the calcium "sensor" in the parathyroid cell is not known, this sensor is unique among the cell types of the organism in its exquisite sensitivity to small changes in the concentration of ionized calcium. It is implied that the specific details of this sensing mechanism are unique to the parathyroid chief cell.

There is general agreement based on both in vivo[12] and in vitro[16,18] data that there exists a calcium-independent or nonsuppressible portion of PTH secretion, which represents about 15 percent of the normal secretion rate (slope D in Fig. 23-4). For example, sustained hypercalcemia in the range of 16 to 18 mg/dl for up to 35 h in cows does not completely abolish the secretion of the hormone.[17] As will be discussed later in this chapter, this calcium-independent component of PTH secretion may have a number of important clinical implications.

It is clear from both clinical and experimental evidence that magnesium can influence PTH secretion.[9,12,18,19] Hypomagnesemia may be associated with an impairment in PTH secretion in vivo and in vitro. Thus, a finite concentration of magnesium appears to be required for normal PTH secretion.[9,19] Increasing concentrations of magnesium above the physiological range also inhibit PTH secretion in a parallel fashion to the inhibition produced by calcium.[9,18] On a molar basis, however, about 2½ times as much magnesium as calcium is required to produce an equivalent inhibition of hormone secretion, and high magnesium concentrations produce only a partial inhibition of PTH secretion.[9,18,19] Most studies suggest that the effects of magnesium and calcium are additive, and so the PTH secretion rate is a function of the net divalent cation concentration.

Although the evidence is not conclusive, it is doubtful that variations in magnesium concentrations within the physiological range exert a significant influence on PTH secretion, and PTH is not regarded as an important regulator of magnesium homeostasis in a classic negative feedback sense. Thus, magnesium appears to play an important role in PTH secretion only at the extremes of magnesium concentrations. The impairment in the secretion of PTH observed in severe hypomagnesemia is the most important clinical example of the influence of magnesium on parathyroid function (see Hypocalcemia).

Beta-adrenergic receptors have been identified in parathyroid cells in vitro,[20] and isoproterenol and epinephrine have been shown to stimulate PTH secretion in vivo[21,22] and in vitro.[19] These catecholamine effects can be blocked by administration of the beta-blocking agent propranolol and are also abolished by an increase in extracellular calcium concentrations. Epinephrine and hypocalcemia potentiate each other as stimuli to PTH secretion but appear to influence PTH function by means of independent mechanisms.[21] Although propranolol administration has been reported to reduce basal serum PTH levels in humans,[22] the importance of the catecholamines in regulating parathyroid secretion in physiological circumstances remains unclear. Hypercalcemia has been reported in several patients with pheochromocytoma, but a number of mechanisms may explain this association (see Hypercalcemia). Serotinin, histamine, and serotonin have been reported to influence the secretion rate of parathyroid cells in vitro and/or receptors for these agents have been demonstrated on these cells.[9] None of these agents appears to be physiologically important in regard to PTH secretion.

The available data concerning the influence of the various vitamin D metabolites on PTH secretion are fragmentary and inconsistent.[9,12,23-26] A number of lines of evidence suggest that one or more of these metabolites may modulate parathyroid function.

1. The specific binding protein and receptor system for vitamin D have been identified in both avian and human parathyroid tissue.[23]
2. Avian parathyroid tissue accumulates the active vitamin D metabolite 1,25-$(OH)_2D_3$ to a concentration some four times that present in blood.
3. In some species, a vitamin D–inducible calcium-binding protein has been detected in parathyroid tissue.[26]
4. Several of the vitamin D metabolites have been reported to stimulate or suppress PTH secretion in vitro and in vivo.[9,24,25]

However, studies of the influence of various vitamin D metabolites on PTH secretion have led to somewhat conflicting data: 24,25-$(OH)_2D_3$ has been reported to suppress PTH secretion,[24] but 1,25-$(OH)_2D_3$ has been reported both to stimulate and to inhibit PTH secretion.[9,24,25] In none of these studies is it clear that physiological concentrations of the vitamin D metabolites were employed. Thus, although one or more of the vitamin D metabolites may influence parathyroid function in certain circumstances, the PTH–1,25-$(OH)_2D_3$ axis does not appear to function as a classical short-loop feedback system in physiological conditions.[12]

Both calcitonin and glucagon have been reported to stimulate PTH secretion. However, pharmacological doses of both agents are required to produce a significant effect on parathyroid function, and in each case the effect appears to be indirectly mediated by the systemic hypocalcemia associated with these large doses.

Inorganic phosphorus has no direct influence on PTH secretion; the effects on parathyroid function produced by alterations of serum phosphorus in vivo are mediated by the phosphorus-induced changes in the concentration of serum ionized calcium. Somatostatin does not influence parathyroid function.

The integrated control of PTH secretion in vivo may be briefly summarized as follows. The parathyroid chief cell is exquisitely sensitive to the extracellular concentration of ionized calcium, and this constitutes the fundamental control mechanism of PTH secretion. In certain circumstances this fundamental mechanism may be modulated positively or negatively by other ionic or hormonal influences, but even in these circumstances the level of ionized calcium appears to exert primary control over the secretion of the hormone.

The details of the mechanism of PTH secretion and the regulation of hormone biosynthesis are not well understood. It is not clear, for example, whether secretion and biosynthesis are separately regulated or are subject to the same controls, as is generally assumed on the basis of only modest evidence.[12,27] It is also not clear whether the events governing PTH secretion and/or synthesis occur primarily at the cell surface or are more dependent on changes in free calcium in the cytosol. It is clear that the calcium sensor in the parathyroid chief cell, however ill defined, is unique in its exquisite sensitivity to changes in ionized calcium concentrations. Any hypothesis concerning the mechanism of PTH secretion must explain this sensitivity as well as the nearly instantaneous release of the hormone on stimulation and the other features of secretion noted above.

A high adenylate cyclase activity has been observed in human and animal parathyroid tissue, and dibutyryl cAMP and theophylline administration have been reported to stimulate PTH secretion. The enzyme has an absolute requirement for magnesium, is stimulated by hypocalcemia and beta-adrenergic agonists, and is inhibited by high concentrations of calcium and magnesium.[19] Although calcium has been shown to inhibit adenylate cyclase activity in a wide variety of tissues, the enzyme in the parathyroid cell has been estimated to be some 100 to 200 times more sensitive to calcium inhibition than the adenylate cyclase systems in other cell types.[19] Elements of the calcium messenger system (calmodulin and C-kinase) have also been identified in parathyroid tissue but have not been extensively studied.[12,28] Similarly, the role of the high-affinity calcium-binding protein, if any, in controlling PTH secretion is not known.[26] It is possible that this protein buffers intracellular calcium or participates in intracellular calcium transport in such a way as to provide a mechanism for modulating PTH synthesis and/or secretion.

PTH and PSP are believed to be cosecreted by means of exocytosis. In most tissues exocytosis is a calcium-mediated process, but calcium inhibits the process in parathyroid cells.[12]

An intracellular calcium-sensitive degradative pathway for PTH has been identified in the parathyroid cell (Fig. 23-3). This pathway may function in regulating the quantity of stored hormone. For example, at high concentrations of calcium, up to 50 percent of the PTH synthesized appears to be degraded rather than stored in secretory granules.[9,12] This degradation may proceed by general proteolysis, but there is evidence that it may also be mediated by cathepsin B,[9] an enzyme that has been shown to cleave PTH between residues 36 and 37 and which could therefore account for the secretion of carboxy-terminal fragments of the hormone (see Circulating Fragments). Alterations in calcium concentration have been shown to have no effect in the conversion of pro-PTH to PTH,[18] so that the synthetic pathway of the hormone does not represent a site of negative feedback regulation.

Circulating Fragments and Metabolism of Parathyroid Hormone

In 1968, Berson and Yalow[29] reported that parathyroid hormone in peripheral human plasma was heterogeneous and differed immunochemically from the material extracted from human parathyroid glands. This observation gave birth to an area of investigation with profound implications regarding PTH physiology and the design and interpretation of results of immunoassays for the hormone. It rapidly became clear that the traditional view of hormone secretion, receptor interaction, inactivation, and clearance could not be applied to PTH and that the details of secretion and metabolism of the hormone were complex. Current concepts concerning the circulating fragments and metabolism of the hormone are presented in Table 23-5 and Fig. 23-5.

The intact, biologically active hormone has a short circulating half-life and represents only about 10 percent of the immunoreactivity detected in peripheral human plasma. Amino-terminal fragments of the hormone, also with a short circulating half-life and possibly biologically active, may represent 5 to 10 percent of the circulating immunoreactivity. Carboxy-terminal fragments of the peptide constitute approximately 80 percent of the immunoreactivity in peripheral human plasma; these fragments are biologically inactive and have a long circulating half-life. Inactive midregion fragments of the peptide may also be present in the circulation. The major unsettled issues in this area do not concern the acknowledged heterogeneity of the circulating forms of PTH but rather (1) the sources of these forms or fragments and (2) their biological significance.

An understanding of the potential physiological importance of the heterogeneity of the circulating forms of PTH requires a knowledge of the structure-function characteristics of the hormone. The 84-amino acid peptide secreted by the parathyroid glands contains complete biological activity. This biological activity resides in the amino-terminal third of the molecule; the middle and carboxy-terminal portions of the peptide are biologically inert (Fig. 23-3). The minimum length required for demonstrable biological

Table 23-5. Features of Immunoreactive Fragments of Parathyroid Hormone in the Peripheral Circulation

Fragment	Molecular weight	Source	Biologically active	Target organs	% total immuno-reactivity	Circulating half-life	Site of clearance
Intact PTH	9500	Parathyroids	Yes	Kidney Bone	~10	~10 min	Kidney (interstitial) Liver Kidney (filtration)
Amino terminal	3000–4000	Kidney Liver	? Yes	? Kidney ? Bone	~10	~10 min	Kidney (interstitial) ? Bone Kidney (filtration)
Carboxy terminal	6000–7000	Kidney Liver ? Parathyroids	No		~80	≥1 h	Kidney (filtration)

activity is the continuous amino-terminal sequence of approximately 27 amino acids, and the 1–34 amino acid sequence has been shown to possess full biological activity.[9,10,12] Preliminary evidence suggests that amino acid residues 3–34 are responsible for receptor binding and that residues 1 and 2 are responsible for adenylate cyclase activation. Thus, the secretion or peripheral generation of amino-terminal fragments of sufficient length could lead to multiple active circulating forms of the hormone. Conversely, the secretion or peripheral generation of carboxy-terminal fragments of the peptide would lead to the accumulation of inactive forms of the hormone in the circulation.

As noted under Biosynthesis and Secretion of PTH, the intact 84-amino acid peptide is the major hormonal secretory product of the parathyroid glands. Whether the glands may also secrete lower-molecular-weight forms of the peptide is a point of controversy. This question has been evaluated by examining the secretory products of parathyroid tissue maintained in vitro and also by examining the peptide forms present in parathyroid venous effluent from patients with primary hyperparathyroidism. Both approaches have generated conflicting data.[30] Several recent studies have reported that although the intact hormone is the major secreted species of the peptide, the parathyroid glands also secrete inactive carboxy-terminal and midregion fragments of the peptide and that the secretion of these fragments is particularly evident at elevated ambient calcium concentrations.[31] Taken together with the known facts concerning the calcium-independent component of PTH secretion and the long circulating half-life of carboxy-terminal fragments of the peptide, these data suggest that the para-

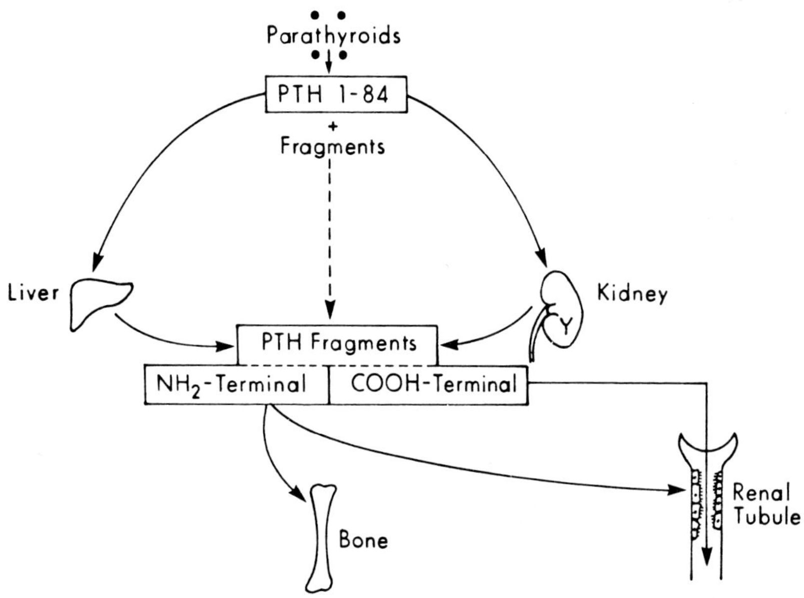

FIGURE 23-5 Schema of the peripheral metabolism of parathyroid hormone. (*By permission of Martin KJ, Freitag TJ, Conrades MB, Hruska KA, Klahr S, and Slatopolsky E, J Clin Invest 63:256, 1978.*)

thyroid glands may be, at least in some circumstances, a source of the heterogeneous forms of PTH in the peripheral circulation.

There is abundant evidence that metabolism of the intact parathyroid hormone molecule by peripheral organs constitutes a major source of the smaller circulating forms of the peptide. Following secretion or injection of the intact hormone, the profile of circulating immunoreactivity rapidly changes from predominantly intact hormone to a mixture of intact hormone and amino- and carboxy-terminal hormone fragments and finally to carboxy-terminal fragments alone. The initial site of cleavage has been localized to the amino acid region 33 to 37, thus potentially resulting in the generation of a biologically active amino-terminal fragment. The specificity of this initial cleavage has been shown in several ways experimentally, including the demonstration that the process can be competitively inhibited by a synthetic peptide containing the amino acid sequence of the region of cleavage.[32] The organs principally responsible for the peripheral metabolism of parathyroid hormone are the kidney and liver and, possibly, bone.

The kidney is a major target organ for PTH and plays several important roles in the metabolism of the hormone.[12,30] Interaction with interstitial tubular sites (peritubular uptake) results in cleavage of the intact peptide into amino- and carboxy-terminal fragments indistinguishable from those in the peripheral circulation. Peritubular uptake can also be demonstrated for amino-terminal fragments but not for carboxy-terminal fragments, suggesting that this process may be limited to forms of the peptide that possess biological activity. Carboxy-terminal fragments are filtered at the glomerulus and presumably are reabsorbed and degraded by the tubules, since minimal immunoreactive material appears in the urine. Glomerular filtration is the major route of elimination of carboxy-terminal fragments of PTH from the peripheral circulation, and this accounts for the disproportionate accumulation of these fragments in the blood of patients with renal impairment. Glomerular filtration of intact and amino-terminal forms of PTH can also be demonstrated but is of relatively minor importance in the overall elimination of these peptide forms from the circulation.

Although not regarded as a major target organ for PTH, the liver is capable of cleaving the intact PTH molecule into amino- and carboxy-terminal fragments similar or identical to those in the peripheral circulation.[30] In contrast to the kidney, the liver does not appear to take up or metabolize the amino- or carboxy-terminal fragments of the peptide. Thus the liver may serve as a source of the circulating fragments of the hormone but does not appear to play a role in their elimination from blood. The Kupffer cells rather than the hepatocytes are responsible for the cleavage process.[33]

The role of bone in the metabolism of PTH is somewhat unclear. The intact hormone is generally regarded as the peptide species which is active in bone, and the intact peptide has been shown to possess full biological activity in certain experimental bone systems.[34] However, several studies have reported that bone exhibits a preferential uptake of and response to amino-terminal fragments of the peptide.[30] These findings have led to speculation regarding a possible specific biological function in bone for the circulating amino-terminal forms of the peptide derived from renal and hepatic cleavage of the intact hormone; this is an interesting but unproven concept requiring further study.[30]

In summary (Table 23-5 and Fig. 23-5), the intact, biologically active PTH molecule is the major secretory product of the parathyroid glands. The intact peptide has a circulating half-life measured in minutes and is cleaved into amino- and carboxy-terminal fragments by the kidney and liver; in addition, a small amount of the intact hormone is filtered and degraded by the kidney. Amino-terminal fragments of the peptide, presumably possessing biological activity, are derived from cleavage of the intact hormone by the kidney and liver; these amino-terminal fragments have a circulating half-life measured in minutes and are taken up by the kidney and bone and, to a lesser extent, are filtered and degraded by the kidney. Carboxy-terminal fragments of the peptide are derived from hepatic and renal cleavage of the intact hormone, and to some extent carboxy-terminal and midregion fragments may be derived from the parathyroid glands themselves. These fragments are biologically inactive, have a circulating half-life measured in hours, and appear to be eliminated from the circulation solely by means of glomerular filtration and degradation.

Biological Effects and Mechanism of Action of Parathyroid Hormone

The parathyroid glands, through the integrated actions of PTH, are primarily responsible for the regulation of mineral homeostasis in humans. This control results from (1) direct effects of PTH on calcium and phosphorus transport in the kidney, (2) effects of PTH on mineral mobilization from bone, and (3) stimulation by PTH of 1,25-dihydroxyvitamin D synthesis in the kidney, with resultant indirect control of the intestinal absorption of calcium and phosphorus. This section discusses the mechanism of action of PTH and its specific effects on tissues; systemic mineral homeostasis is presented in a later section (see Integrated Control).

HISTORY

In the latter part of the nineteenth century, it was recognized that an extract of the parathyroid glands could reverse the tetany which followed experimental parathyroidectomy. By about 1910 it was known that this effect was due to the influence of the parathyroid principle on serum calcium. The full spectrum of the biological effects of PTH was discovered sequentially over the next half century.[35] The phosphaturic effect of PTH had been well documented by the 1930s. For a time, it was widely held that this was the only major effect of the hormone, and it was believed that the effect of PTH on serum calcium was indirectly mediated by its influence on the serum phosphorus concentration. That is, the serum calcium × phosphorus product was regarded as a biological constant so that any alteration in serum phosphorus levels would automatically result in an opposite adjustment in the concentration of serum calcium. By 1950, however, it had become clear that PTH could directly stimulate both bone resorption and renal tubular calcium reabsorption, and by 1960 it was known that the hormone increased intestinal calcium absorption. The metabolic sequence of activation of vitamin D and the indirect nature of the influence of PTH on intestinal calcium absorption were not established until the late 1960s. Thus, a detailed picture of the control of phosphorus and calcium metabolism exerted by PTH has evolved only in the past 15 years.

EFFECTS OF PARATHYROID HORMONE ON BONE

The discussion below of bone function and skeletal homeostasis is simplified and presents only sufficient detail to allow for an understanding of how this complex tissue participates in the hormonal control of mineral homeostasis.[3,35–37] Bone cell physiology is currently an active area of investigation, and a number of recent developments appear to be of importance in regard to bone turnover and homeostasis. These developments include the characterization of bone-derived proteins which seem to be involved in the mineralization process (osteocalcin and osteonectin) and that of other bone-derived peptides which probably serve a paracrine function in coordinating the activities of osteoblasts and osteoclasts (bone-derived growth factors and/or coupling factors). Further details concerning these bone cell products and their roles in skeletal homeostasis are presented in Chap. 24.

Bone has two major components: a highly organized *bone matrix,* which is composed of collagen fibrils rich in lysine, proline, and hydroxyproline residues, and *bone mineral,* which is composed largely of calcium and phosphorus in the form of hydroxyapatite crystals deposited in the matrix. The adult skeleton is composed of two distinct types of bone (Fig. 23-6). The shafts of long bones and the surfaces of flat bones are made up of *cortical* (compact) bone. The bone in the metaphyseal areas of long bones and between the cortical surfaces of flat (e.g., pelvis) and short (e.g., vertebra) bones is *trabecular* (cancellous) bone.

Cortical bone has a periosteal surface and an endosteal surface and is often referred to as *haversian bone* because it is made up of an organized group of haversian systems (osteons). Each haversian system has a microcirculation running through the central haversian canal and is composed of dense bone organized in a lamellar arrangement around the central canal. Lacunae containing mature osteocytes are interspersed throughout the dense bone, and a weblike arrangement of canaliculi contains cytoplasmic extensions which interconnect the osteocytes. These cytoplasmic extensions also connect the osteocytes to the cells lining the internal endosteal surface so that the entire cellular network of haversian bone forms a part of the so-called bone membrane.

Trabecular bone is formed by a spongy network of interlacing bone spicules. The bone substance contains scattered mature osteocytes but is avascular and lacks the highly organized haversian arrangement. The two endosteal surfaces of trabecular bone combine to give this type of bone a very large total surface area, and it is metabolically far more active than cortical bone. The endosteal surfaces are lined by a variety of cell types: active osteoclasts and osteoblasts and a large number of undifferentiated mesenchymal cells termed *lining cells* (Fig. 23-6, detail B).

The endosteal surfaces of trabecular and cortical bone are covered or lined at all times by a syncytial arrangement of cells having cytoplasmic interconnections with underlying osteocytes in the bone substance. This complex syncytial network is termed the *bone membrane* or *bone envelope,* and it is viewed in the aggregate as forming an anatomical structure which physically separates bone surfaces from the extracellular fluids. This cellular and membranous barrier is presumed to play an important role in ion fluxes into and out of bone.

Osteoclasts are large multinucleated cells which participate in bone resorption. The origin of these cells remains unclear; they were previously regarded as arising from primitive local mesenchymal cells, but recent evidence suggests that they are derived from circulating mononuclear cells.[38,39] The multiple nuclei

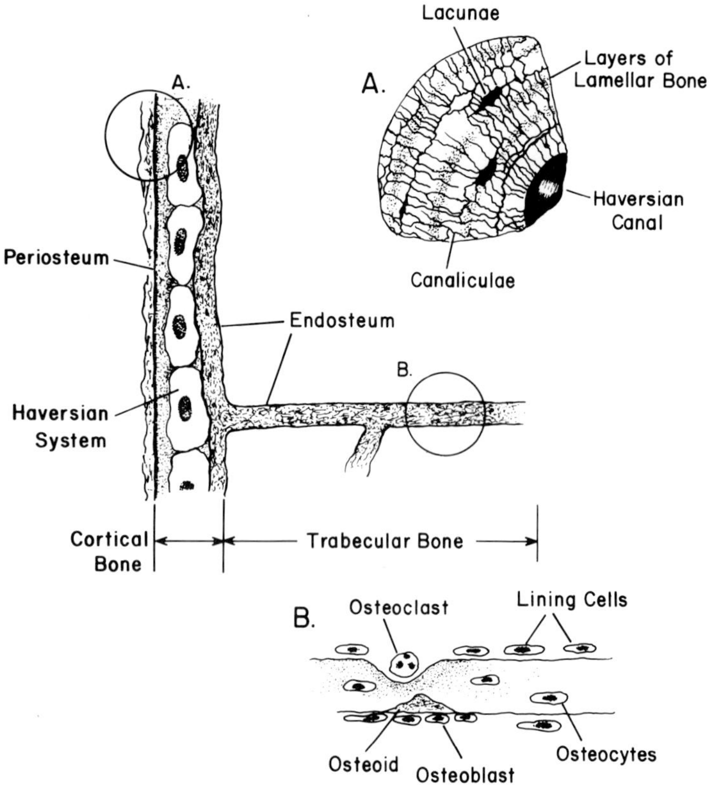

FIGURE 23-6 Schematic section of adult bone showing areas of both cortical (compact) and trabecular (cancellous) bone. The histological details of a portion of a haversian system (osteon) and a small area of trabecular bone undergoing active bone formation and resorption are also shown.

result from cell fusion rather than nuclear division. The cells have an extensive ruffled or brush border in intimate contact with the resorbing bone surface and an abundant supply of mitochondria containing dense granules of amorphous calcium phosphate. Osteoclasts act on mineralized bone and do not resorb unmineralized matrix (osteoid). *Osteoblasts* are derived from local mesenchymal cells and are the principal cells of bone formation. The cells contain an abundant rough endoplasmic reticulum and an extensive Golgi apparatus, in keeping with their role in collagen synthesis. Osteoblasts also synthesize osteocalcin (bone Gla protein) and osteonectin, bone-derived proteins which may play important roles in the mineralization process.[36] Active osteoblasts line the surface of newly synthesized, unmineralized matrix, known as *osteoid.* As osteoblasts are surrounded by newly synthesized osteoid, they become osteocytes and are replaced by a new layer of osteoblasts which form a new layer of matrix. Cytoplasmic extensions connect these new osteocytes with the next layer of bone-forming cells. The new osteocytes in unmineralized osteoid are often referred to as *osteoid osteocytes* to distinguish them from the mature osteocytes in mineralized bone. *Osteocytes* are the mature bone cells and are derived from osteoblasts. Osteocytes vary in microscopic appearance depending, to some extent, on their age. Older osteocytes are larger and reside in enlarged lacunae with irregular margins, suggesting that these may be the cells responsible for internal bone resorption (osteocytic osteolysis). In some circumstances, osteocytes may be capable of metabolic and functional changes which enable them to remodel bone internally in a sequence similar to that which occurs on the endosteal bone surface.[2]

Bone is continuously metabolically active. The activity of bone can be considered in two categories, related to the structural and storehouse roles of the skeleton, respectively. *Skeletal homeostasis* refers to the process of bone remodeling and renewal necessary to maintain the integrity of the skeleton. Bone also participates in *systemic mineral homeostasis* by supplying bone mineral to the organism in response to systemic stimuli. In some circumstances (e.g., Paget's disease), striking abnormalities of skeleton homeostasis may exist without influencing systemic mineral homeostasis; in other circumstances (e.g., vitamin D deficiency), both skeletal homeostasis and systemic mineral homeostasis are profoundly disturbed in an interdependent fashion.

Bone remodeling is normally a highly coordinated or coupled process which produces no net change in either skeletal or systemic mineral balance.[3,37] The term *coupling* emphasizes the orderly sequence of events which constitutes the remodeling process (Fig. 23-7). Following *activation* (e.g., by PTH or local stimuli), precursor cells differentiate into osteoclasts which resorb a localized area of mineralized bone. The exact biochemical basis of bone resorption remains unknown, but osteoclasts secrete a large number of enzymes, and the resorption process results in the destruction and removal of both bone mineral and bone matrix. There follows an *intermediate,* or reversal, phase during which large mononuclear cells line the surface of resorbed bone. It is not clear whether these cells represent postosteoclasts or preosteoblasts. Following this intermediate phase, new osteoid is laid down by osteoblasts (the *formation* phase). Finally, this new osteoid is *mineralized* to complete the remodeling sequence. The net result is the formation of new bone in a localized area. The remodeling process is most easily visualized as it occurs on the highly active endosteal surfaces of trabecular bone (Fig. 23-6); however, a basically similar sequence of events occurs in haversian bone. On the average, completion of the remodeling sequence requires about 4 months in humans. Although the remodeling process may be modulated by systemic influences, the primary role of this process is the renewal of bone and maintenance of the structural integrity of the skeleton.

In response to systemic needs, bone mineral is made available by the combined process of osteocytic osteolysis and osteoclastic bone resorption. *Osteocytic osteolysis* refers to the mobilization of bone mineral by the lacunar osteocytes in haversian bone; there is some evidence that this type of mineral mobilization may occur without actual resorption or destruction of bone. *Osteoclastic resorption* refers to the resorptive process described above. Although both processes are important in mineral homeostasis, the exact quantitative importance of each process in serving systemic needs is not clear. In fact, it is likely that the participation of the two processes in mineral mobilization

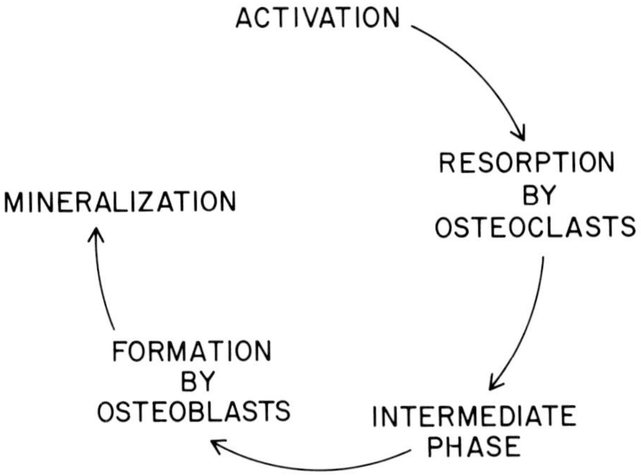

FIGURE 23-7 Coupled sequence of events in normal bone remodeling.

differs depending on the degree and duration of the stimulus to bone resorption, as discussed below.

PTH is an important regulator of bone metabolism, and its actions on bone are complex. Since the secretion rate of PTH is a function of the ambient extracellular concentration of ionized calcium, it is intuitively apparent that this hormone is primarily concerned with mineral homeostasis rather than skeletal homeostasis. Nevertheless, the hormone has important influences on both aspects of bone metabolism and function.

Experimentally, a variety of responses to PTH can be demonstrated in bone, and the response observed appears to reflect the concentration of PTH employed as well as elapsed time following hormonal stimulation. That is, both rapid and long-term effects of PTH can be demonstrated, and results differ with high and low hormone concentrations (Table 23-6). PTH can be shown to (1) stimulate osteocytic osteolysis and the resorption of bone by preexisting osteoclasts, (2) stimulate the activation process leading to the formation of new osteoclasts, and (3) inhibit acutely osteoblastic

Table 23-6. Features of the Early and Late Responses of Bone to Stimulation by Parathyroid Hormone

Feature	Early response	Late response
Time of onset	Minutes	Hours to days
Cells affected	Osteocytes and osteoclasts	Preosteoclasts
Major result of effect	Mineral mobilization	Bone resorption, formation of new bone cell pools
Matrix resorption	Little	Great
Sensitivity to PTH	Sensitive	Relatively insensitive
Magnitude of response	Limited	Potentially unlimited
Constant presence of PTH	Necessary	Unnecessary

function and collagen biosynthesis. Late effects of the hormone include an increase in osteoblastic activity, resulting from the coupling of bone remodeling which follows as a matter of course from the hormone-induced formation of new osteoclasts.

In both in vivo and in vitro systems of study, the first observed response to PTH is a transient decrease in the extracellular concentration of calcium. This phenomenon is thought to represent an initial stimulation of calcium influx into bone cells by PTH, which may be an important aspect of the mechanism of action of the hormone. Within minutes, there follows an increase in calcium mobilization from bone, which persists as long as PTH is present but wanes almost immediately following removal of the hormone. The early response is not accompanied by a significant increase in hydroxyproline mobilization from bone, indicating that little actual bone resorption with matrix digestion has occurred. In addition, the response is limited in magnitude and plateaus at relatively low PTH concentrations. The cellular basis of this rapid response appears to be the stimulation by PTH of osteocytic osteolysis by mature osteocytes together with a small amount of osteoclastic bone resorption produced by preformed osteoclasts. The rapid response to the hormone cannot be blocked by inhibitors of either protein or RNA synthesis. Synthesis of collagen by osteoblasts is also acutely inhibited by PTH.

The late response to PTH (Table 23-6) is observed approximately 12 h after exposure to the hormone and may persist for many days after hormonal stimulation. The response is concentration-dependent and is relatively insensitive; a significant late response occurs only after exposure of bone to a large or prolonged stimulation with PTH. The mobilization of bone mineral during the late response is accompanied by dissolution of bone matrix, as evidenced by increased hydroxyproline released from bone, and the late response can be blocked by inhibition of either protein or by RNA synthesis. The response does not plateau, and its magnitude is potentially unlimited. The cellular basis of the late response appears to be dependent entirely on PTH-induced formation of a new active pool of osteoclasts, with recruitment of a larger bone surface into the resorption process. In usual circumstances this resorptive effect of the hormone occurs primarily in trabecular and haversian bone, but with time the periosteal area is also affected, leading to the characteristic picture of *subperiosteal resorption* noted in primary hyperparathyroidism. Because of the coupled nature of bone remodeling, the PTH-induced formation of a new osteoclast pool ultimately leads to a stimulation of all aspects of the remodeling sequence, and evidence of increased osteoblastic activity is noted several days after initiation of the late response.

Thus the *biphasic* response of bone to PTH stimulation consists of a rapid or immediate phase in which the hormone stimulates the activity of existing bone cells and a delayed or late phase in which the hormone stimulates the formation of new pools of active bone cells. The rapid phase may be viewed as important in maintaining systemic mineral homeostasis on a minute-to-minute basis, whereas the late phase represents a recruitment phenomenon which is important in serving more extreme systemic needs in addition to its importance in remodeling and skeletal homeostasis. To a greater or lesser extent, depending on the nature of the stimulus, the two phases proceed together.

All three major cell types of bone are target cells for PTH action: PTH stimulates the activity of osteocytes and osteoclasts and inhibits osteoblast function. In addition, the hormone activates precursor cells to differentiate into resorbing osteoclasts. The influence of PTH on these various bone cells may not be direct. For example, osteoblasts bear specific PTH receptors, but osteoclasts may not, and it has been proposed that the stimulation of at least certain osteoclastic functions by PTH may be mediated by a local osteoblast-derived paracrine product.[40,41] The preparation of specific bone cell populations for detailed study in vitro remains a difficult problem; this has limited progress in understanding the effects of PTH in individual cells as well as its mechanism of action. Both the cAMP and calcium messenger systems appear to be involved in mediating PTH effects in bone cells,[12,36] and it is envisioned that the specific biochemical processes modulated by these messengers differ from cell type to cell type, depending on the role of each cell in bone metabolism.

EFFECTS OF PARATHYROID HORMONE ON THE KIDNEY

PTH has two principal effects on renal ion transport: (1) It decreases proximal tubular phosphate reabsorption, and (2) it increases calcium reabsorption in the distal nephron. Both effects are important in the minute-to-minute regulation of the serum concentrations of phosphorus and calcium. The third major renal effect of the hormone is to increase 1-hydroxylase activity and the conversion of 25-hydroxyvitamin D to 1,25-dihydroxyvitamin D; this effect is described in detail in Formation, Transport, Metabolic Sequence of Activation, and Metabolism of Vitamin D. In this section, the renal handling of phosphate and calcium and the effects of PTH on these processes are presented at the organ and single nephron level. The many complex variables determining the rates of phosphate and calcium excretion in the whole organism are discussed in later sections.

Phosphate Transport

A schema of phosphate and calcium transport in the nephron is shown in Fig. 23-8. Approximately 10 percent of the phosphate ions in serum are protein-bound, but a number of fortuitous counterbalancing influences result in a phosphate concentration in the glomerular filtrate which is essentially identical to the concentration in serum.[42] Therefore, the filtered load of phosphate at the glomerulus is computed simply as the product of the serum phosphorus concentration and the glomerular filtration rate. The total rate of phosphate excretion in urine is always less than the filtered load of phosphate so that net reabsorption of phosphate by the kidney can always be demonstrated. The proximal tubule plays the dominant, and perhaps the only, role in phosphate reabsorption in humans. The evidence for more distal reabsorptive sites or for tubular secretion of phosphate is fragmentary and inconclusive.[43] In the proximal tubule, the phosphate transport system is pH- and sodium-dependent, active, and saturable.[43,44] The system appears to be a cotransport system which facilitates the electroneutral transport of sodium and phosphate ions. The rate of phosphate transport is maximal in the early portion of the proximal tubule and falls off progressively as the tubular fluid traverses the proximal tubule from the glomerulus to the pars recta of the proximal tubule.[43]

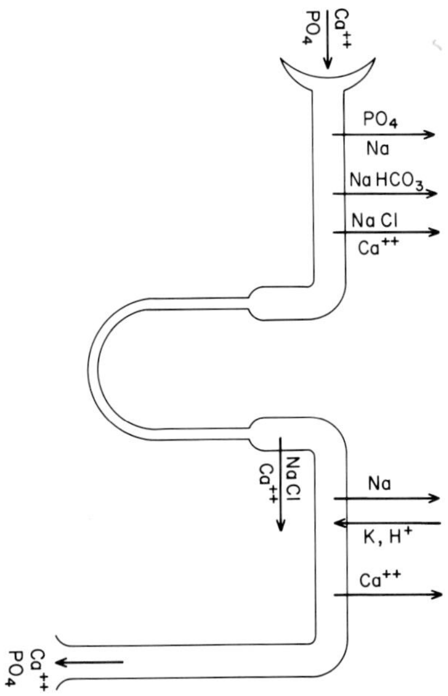

FIGURE 23-8 Schematic representation of the transport of phosphate and calcium in the mammalian nephron.

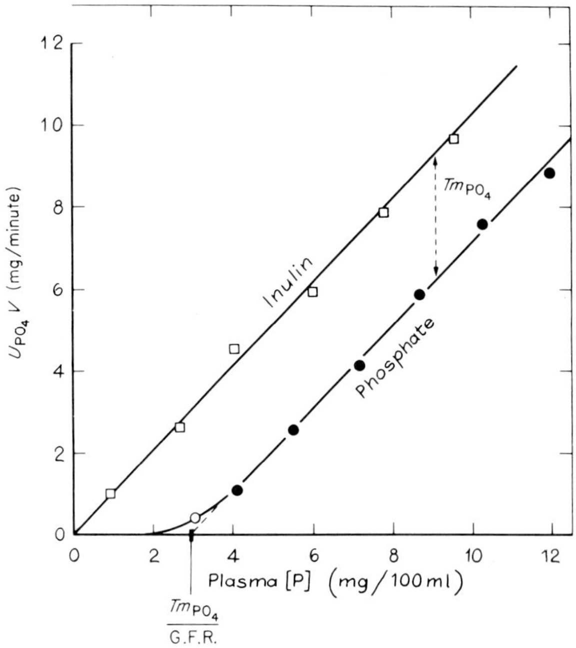

FIGURE 23-9 The relation between the plasma phosphorus concentration (mg/dl) and the urinary excretion rate of phosphate (mg/min) in a normal individual while fasting (○) and during an intravenous infusion of phosphate (●). Also shown is the relation between the urinary excretion rate and plasma concentraton of inulin when inulin was simultaneously infused. The slopes of the lines through the inulin and phosphate data are identical and are numerically equal to the glomerular filtration rate. The vertical distance between the two lines is the maximum rate of tubular reabsorption of phosphate (TmP, in mg/min). The intercept of the extrapolated line through the closed circles with the abscissa is the maximum tubular reabsorption of phosphate per 100 ml of glomerular filtrate (TmP/GFR, in mg/dl). (*By permission of Bijvoet OLM, Clin Sci 37:23, 1969.*)

The saturability of the proximal reabsorptive system for phosphate is illustrated in Fig. 23-9. The figure contrasts the excretion rates of inulin and phosphate over a wide range of plasma concentrations of both substances. Since inulin is filtered at the glomerulus and is neither reabsorbed nor secreted, the excretion rate of inulin factored by the plasma concentration of inulin always equals the glomerular filtration rate. That is, the slope of the line relating inulin excretion to the plasma inulin concentration is numerically equal to the glomerular filtration rate. At any given serum phosphorus concentration, the phosphate excretion rate is always lower than the filtered load of phosphate by a value which is equal to the vertical distance between the inulin and phosphate lines in Fig. 23-9. Initially, at serum phosphorus concentrations close to the fasting serum phosphorus level (designated by the open circle in Fig. 23-9), the phosphate line is splayed or curved, indicating an increasing rate of phosphate reabsorption as the serum phosphorus concentration is raised. The reabsorption rate rapidly reaches a constant maximum value, and any further increment in the filtered load that is due to an increment in serum phosphorus concentration is excreted entirely, yielding a line which is parallel to the inulin line. At this point, the proximal tubular reabsorption system for phosphate is saturated, and the maximal rate of phosphate reabsorption is the distance between the inulin and phosphate lines. This constant maximum reabsorption rate is designated the *tubular maximum* for phosphate (TmP). If this line is extrapolated backward, it intercepts the abscissa at a point called the *phosphate threshold*. This threshold is the serum phosphorus concentration at which tubular phosphate reabsorption proceeds at its maximal rate and at which the filtered load of phosphate equals the maximal reabsorptive rate. Expressed as a function of the glomerular filtration rate (TmP/GFR), this phosphate threshold provides an extremely useful measurement of phosphate reabsorptive capacity per unit of renal mass. In both a conceptual and a practical sense, the TmP/GFR may be regarded as the "set point" of renal phosphate reabsorption. At a serum phosphorus concentration below the TmP/GFR, most of the filtered phosphate is reclaimed by the proximal tubule and little phosphate is excreted. At plasma phosphorus concentrations progressively above the TmP/GFR, increasing quantities of the filtered phosphate are rejected by the proximal tubule and excreted. Thus, the kidney plays a primary role in regulating the serum phosphorus concentration and tends to maintain this concentration at a value close to the TmP/GFR. Most of the variation in the fasting serum phosphorus concentration in humans appears to result from variations in TmP/GFR,[42] and it is particularly useful to consider the many factors which influence serum phosphorus concentrations and phosphate excretion in humans in terms of how these factors influence TmP/GFR.

As noted previously, by the 1930s a number of lines of evidence had clearly established the influence of PTH on the renal handling of phosphate, and for many years this was considered to be the principal action of the hormone. This action of PTH is often referred to as its *phosphaturic* effect. An abrupt increase in phosphate excretion is noted within minutes in response to an acute injection or infusion of PTH; thus in such conditions the term *phosphaturia* is descriptively accurate. PTH functions in this regard by decreasing the proximal tubular reabsorption of phosphate; in effect, the hormone resets TmP/GFR at a lower level. Therefore, a prolonged infusion of PTH or a clinical state of hyperparathyroidism results in a new steady state in which a reduction in TmP/GFR and the serum phosphorus concentration occurs but in which an actual increased rate of phosphate excretion is not observed. In such circumstances, the term *phosphaturia* is somewhat of a misnomer, even though the degree of phosphate excretion is clearly inappropriate for the ambient level of serum phosphorus. As will become clear in later sections, this distinction is far more than a matter of semantics. The determination of TmP/GFR is a powerful investigative and clinical tool, whereas the measurement of urinary phosphate excretion is of limited use.

The mechanism by which PTH decreases proximal tubular phosphate reabsorption is illustrated in Fig. 23-10. The hormone binds to its receptors in the contraluminal (basal-lateral) membrane of the proximal tubular cell,[45] leading to an activation of the membrane-bound adenylate cyclase system.[45,46] This activation results in the conversion of ATP to cAMP and an increase in the cytosolic concentration of the second messenger. The cAMP-dependent protein kinase in the proximal tubular cell is highly concentrated in the luminal (brush-border) membranes of the cell.[47] cAMP binds to the regulatory subunit of the protein kinase, leading to the dissociation of the regulatory and catalytic subunits of the enzyme. The activated catalytic moiety of the kinase phosphorylates specific membrane-bound proteins in the brush-border membrane, resulting in an inhibition of the sodium-phosphate cotransport system and a decrease in phosphate transport into the cell. The exact biochemical details concerning the protein phosphorylation step and how this influences the mechanism of phosphate transport are not known. A decrease in phosphate transport can be demonstrated in brush-border vesi-

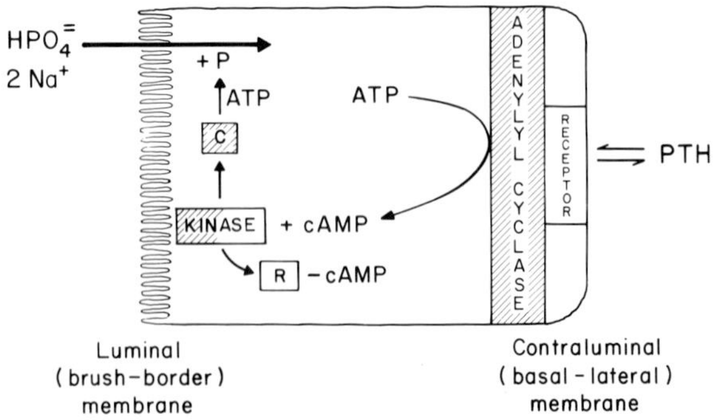

FIGURE 23-10 Mechanism of action of parathyroid hormone in the proximal renal tubular cell. The hormone interacts with its receptors in the contraluminal membrane, activating the membrane-bound adenylate cyclase. cAMP binds to the regulatory (R) subunit of the cAMP-dependent protein kinase in the region of the luminal membrane, liberating the catalytic (C) subunit of the enzyme. Luminal membrane proteins are phosphorylated, resulting in an inhibition of the cotransport of phosphate and sodium.

cles prepared from animals pretreated in vivo with either PTH or dibutyryl cAMP, but neither agent when added directly in vitro influences phosphate transport by these vesicles.[44] Whether a modulation of the cytosolic concentration of ionized calcium by PTH and cAMP is involved in the mechanism of action of PTH in the proximal tubular cell is not known.

Calcium Transport

Approximately 60 percent of the serum calcium is ultrafilterable so that at a normal glomerular filtration rate, the filtered load of calcium is approximately 10,000 mg per day.[42,48–50] In normal circumstances, the tubular reabsorption of calcium is extremely efficient; 97 to 99 percent of the filtered load of calcium is reabsorbed, and only 100 to 300 mg is excreted in urine. There is no convincing evidence that tubular secretion of calcium occurs in the mammalian kidney. In contrast to the tubular handling of phosphate, calcium is reabsorbed at multiple sites along the nephron. Approximately two-thirds of the filtered load of calcium is reabsorbed in the proximal tubule, one-fourth in the loop of Henle, and the remaining 10 percent in the distal elements of the tubule (Fig. 23-11). The characteristics of the proximal and distal sites for calcium reabsorption differ markedly and will be discussed separately.[42,48–51]

Taken together, the calcium reabsorptive sites in the proximal tubule and the ascending loop of Henle account for the reabsorption of approximately 90 percent of the filtered load of calcium. These sites share certain characteristics and for simplicity will be referred to in the aggregate as the *proximal* process of calcium reabsorption. The characteristics of proximal calcium reabsorption are as follows:

1. The reabsorptive process is essentially isotonic and is strongly linked to the tubular reabsorption of sodium.
2. It is not saturable or Tm-limited so that the rate of calcium reabsorption varies directly with the concentration of calcium in the tubular urine.
3. It is insensitive to PTH.

Reabsorption of calcium and sodium is so tightly coupled in the proximal sites that the reabsorption of these two ions cannot be dissociated, and micropuncture studies have revealed that an identical percentage of the filtered load of sodium and calcium is reclaimed by the tubules down to the level of the distal nephron. Thus, factors which enhance the delivery of sodium to the distal tubules (e.g., a high dietary intake of sodium, saline infusion, or the administration of furosemide) lead to a corresponding increase in the distal delivery of calcium. The proximal reabsorption of sodium and calcium appears to be in part passive and in part active,[51] but an actual sodium-calcium cotransport system has not been identified. Since proximal reabsorption proceeds in an essentially isotonic fashion, the actual concentration of calcium in the tubular urine is largely unaffected by the reabsorption process and remains approximately the same from the glomerulus to the distal tubule.

The fact that proximal calcium reabsorption is not saturable means that the total quantity of calcium

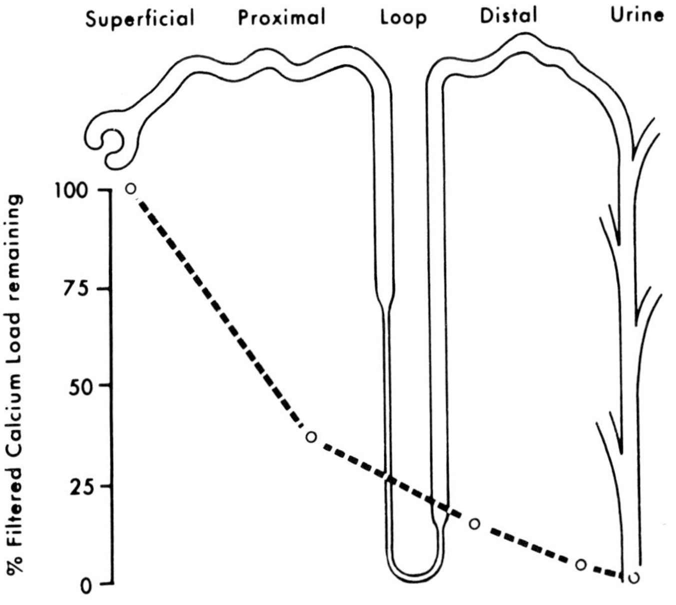

FIGURE 23-11 Fraction of the filtered load of calcium remaining at successive sites in the rat nephron. (*From Sutton and Dirks,*[49] *by permission of Federation Proceedings.*)

reclaimed by this process is a function of the calcium concentration in the glomerular filtrate and the influence of local factors, particularly the filtered load of sodium, on the transport process. The net quantitative result of proximal calcium reabsorption is not easily visualized and can best be considered in terms of how the process influences several interrelated aspects of the calcium content in the urine delivered to the distal tubule: (1) the calcium concentration, (2) the absolute quantity of calcium delivered, and (3) the fraction of the filtered load of calcium reaching the distal nephron. Several illustrations will make clear the necessity of considering these various quantitative aspects of the proximal reabsorptive process. For example, although an increased filtered load of calcium (e.g., in a hypercalcemic patient) is associated with an increased concentration-dependent rate of proximal calcium reabsorption, the fraction of the filtered load of calcium which is reabsorbed is unaltered, and the urine presented to the distal tubule contains both an increased concentration of calcium and an increased absolute amount of calcium. However, an increased filtered load of sodium (e.g., during a saline infusion) decreases both the quantity and the fraction of filtered calcium which is reabsorbed proximally without actually affecting the calcium concentration at any level. In this case, the distal tubule is presented with urine containing an increased fraction of the filtered load of calcium and an increased total quantity of calcium but at a "normal" calcium concentration.

PTH has no direct influence on proximal calcium reabsorption. In fact, by inhibiting the proximal cotransport of phosphate and sodium, the hormone may actually increase slightly the distal delivery of sodium, with a corresponding increase in the distal delivery of calcium.

The distal nephron is the final arbiter of the rate of calcium excretion, and it is the distal calcium reabsorption process which is regulated to subserve systemic needs.[42,48–50] Although only approximately 10 percent of the filtered load of calcium reaches the distal tubule, this percentage is the equivalent of approximately 1000 mg of calcium daily. The characteristics of distal calcium reabsorption are as follows:

1. The process is independent of sodium transport.
2. In some respects it appears to behave in a saturable or Tm-limited fashion.
3. It is sensitive to PTH.

The distal calcium transport sites appear to reside in the terminal segments of the distal convoluted tubule and also in a portion of the collecting duct.[48–50]

Calcium and sodium transport in the distal nephron are clearly dissociable. For example, sodium-retaining steroids increase distal tubular sodium reabsorption without affecting calcium reabsorption, whereas PTH enhances distal calcium reabsorption without influencing sodium transport. These and other findings provide strong evidence that the reabsorption of calcium and sodium in the distal nephron proceeds by two completely independent transport processes (Fig. 23-8). The net increase in urinary calcium excretion which accompanies a saline diuresis results entirely from the fact that the sodium-induced increase in the distal delivery of calcium overwhelms the reabsorptive capacity for calcium in the distal nephron.

Because of the many complexities of the system, direct data concerning the saturability of calcium transport in the distal nephron are unavailable. However, a tubular maximum (TmCa) for distal calcium reabsorption can be estimated,[42] and it is conceptually useful to regard the process as Tm-limited. Thus, analogous to the reabsorption of phosphate in the proximal tubule, the distal tubule either rejects or reclaims a variable amount of the calcium presented to it based on whether the calcium content in the tubular urine exceeds or is less than the "set point" or TmCa. In this case the TmCa is a function of the circulating concentration of PTH, meaning that the set point for distal calcium reabsorption is determined by the parathyroid glands on the basis of systemic calcium requirements.

In all experimental and clinical conditions, PTH leads to an increase in the percentage of the filtered load of calcium which is reabsorbed. Infusion of the hormone systemically or directly into the renal artery causes an abrupt decrease in the fractional excretion of calcium before the serum calcium concentration begins to rise.[52] Conversely, acute experimental parathyroidectomy leads to a marked increase in calcium excretion before a detectable fall in serum calcium occurs.[52] In rats, acute parathyroidectomy virtually eliminates calcium reabsorption in the distal nephron and results in an overall threefold increase in urinary calcium excretion.[48] Studies in normal and hypoparathyroid humans have led to a similar quantitative estimate of the importance of PTH in eliminating calcium loss into the urine.[53] That is, at a serum calcium concentration between 9 and 10 mg/dl, calcium excretion is about threefold higher in hypoparathyroid patients than in normal individuals.These and other considerations make it clear that PTH-mediated calcium reabsorption in the distal nephron is the dominant quantitative process that governs the control of the serum concentration of ionized calcium on a minute-to-minute basis. For example, the approximately 1000 mg per day of filtered calcium which reaches the distal tubule is some fourfold to fivefold greater than the net quantity of calcium which is normally absorbed by the intestine on a daily basis. As discussed in later sections, the system is so finely tuned that even an overnight fast constitutes a state of physiological "hyperparathyroidism," whereas a normal calcium-containing meal may suppress "normal" parathyroid function by as much as one-third. The fine tuning of this system is largely subserved by the influence of PTH on the functional TmCa in the distal nephron.

The cellular mechanism by which PTH increases calcium transport in the cells of the distal tubule and collecting duct has not been firmly established, but there is evidence that this process is mediated by the cAMP messenger system.[5,49]

PTH Effects on Other Ions

PTH has been reported to influence the renal tubular handling of a number of ions other than calcium and phosphate. Acute pharmacological doses of PTH lead to a transient increase in the glomerular filtration rate, but this effect is of no importance in physiological or pathophysiological conditions. PTH increases the delivery of sodium to the distal tubule by inhibiting the cotransport of sodium and phosphate in the proximal tubule. This sodium is reabsorbed by the exchange mechanism in the distal tubule, and this may result in a slight increase in potassium excretion. PTH inhibits bicarbonate reabsorption in the proximal tubule by an unknown mechanism. This bicarbonate is reclaimed in the distal tubule, resulting in little net influence of PTH on urinary bicarbonate excretion or urinary pH. Clinically, frankly hyperchloremic acidosis is noted almost exclusively in patients with hyperparathyroidism and coincident renal impairment. Thus the actual significance of the *proximal renal tubular acidosis* that is often ascribed to clinical states of hyperparathyroidism is not clear. Although the renal handling of magnesium is not well defined, some evidence suggests that magnesium is reabsorbed by a Tm-limited process (see Systemic Magnesium Homeostasis). PTH has been reported to decrease the fractional excretion of magnesium, but this effect of the hormone has not been carefully studied. PTH stimulates renal gluconeogenesis, which may be of importance in generating cellular energy to meet the demands of the transport effects of the hormone.[2]

EFFECTS OF PARATHYROID HORMONE ON OTHER TISSUES

PTH plays a critically important role in controlling the rate of calcium and phosphate absorption in the small intestine. Current evidence indicates that this control is entirely mediated by 1,25-dihydroxyvitamin D, and the hormonal control of intestinal calcium reabsorption is described in detail in a later section. The wide variety of symptoms and findings in clinical hyperparathyroidism have suggested to some observers that PTH may influence the function of many tissues, including nerve and muscle. However, these suggestions are not supported by convincing direct evidence, and many of the symptoms of hyperparathyroidism may reflect the tissue influences of the coincident hypercalcemia and/or hypophosphatemia.

CALCITONIN

Historical Introduction

The brief history of calcitonin is remarkable. Less than a decade elapsed between the earliest suspicions of the existence of a hypocalcemic principle, based on the studies of Copp and coworkers in the early 1960s,[16] and the isolation, purification, sequencing, and actual synthesis of the human hormone in 1968. A large number of laboratories participated in this rapid and elegant work.[54,55] The cell of origin of calcitonin was identified as the parafollicular or C cell of the thyroid; its principal action was found to be an inhibition of bone resorption, and its mechanism of action was found to be mediated by cAMP.[54–56] In addition, calcitonin has proved to be an important hormonal marker for the detection of *medullary carcinoma of the thyroid* and is a useful pharmacological agent in the treatment of Paget's disease. However, its precise role in the regulation of mineral and/or skeletal homeostasis in humans remains unclear.

The next and in many ways the most fascinating chapter in the history of calcitonin began in the early 1980s. The calcitonin gene (or the calcitonin/CGRP gene as it is currently known) actually generates two discrete mRNAs, which encode the precursor peptides for calcitonin and calcitonin gene-related peptide (CGRP). The choice between these mRNAs is made by a process of *alternative RNA processing*, a post-transcriptional event that is tissue-specific. The calcitonin pathway predominates in the C cells of the thyroid and the CGRP pathway in the nervous system. Each of these mRNAs in turn encodes cryptic peptides which are presumed or known to be expressed in their tissues of origin. These developments may or may not be germane to the hormonal control of mineral metabolism, but they certainly represent elegant biology. Details are provided in Chemistry and Biosynthesis, below.

Embryology, Anatomy, and Histology

Calcitonin is formed by the parafollicular or C cells of the thyroid. In the adult human, C cells are unevenly distributed and are concentrated in the middle third of the lateral lobes of the thyroid, deep within the thyroid parenchyma. The cells occur as isolated individual cells and are present in both intrafollicular and parafollicular locations, with the latter predominating. C cells constitute only a few percent of the total number of thyroid cells in humans. Similar or identical cells have been identified in very small numbers in the parathyroid glands and in the thymus. C cells are morphologically distinct from the follicular cells of the thyroid. The cells are larger than follicular cells and have a large clear nucleus, prominent mitochondria, a well-developed Golgi apparatus, and numerous fine granules. The granules can be demonstrated to contain calcitonin by means of immunochemical techniques, and the cells rapidly degranulate in response to a hypercalcemic stimulus.

C cells are derived from the ventral portion of the last branchial pouch, which migrates and fuses with the substance of the thyroid early in embryologic development. In all jawed vertebrates except mammals, the ventral portion of the last branchial pouch remains as a separate gland known as the *ultimobranchial body*. In these species, the ultimobranchial body serves as a rich source of calcitonin (e.g., the *salmon* calcitonin employed clinically is prepared from this source), and the thyroid is devoid of C cells. The ultimobranchial body is an older structure phylogenetically than the parathyroid glands.

C cells are actually neuroendocrine cells which originate in the neural crest. The neural crest cells colonize the ventral portion of the last branchial pouch before its migration caudad. C cells are included in the APUD cell family (amine precursor uptake and decarboxylation), which may explain the association of medullary carcinoma of the thyroid with tumors of other APUD cell types in *multiple endocrine neoplasia type II* as well as the potential of malignant C cells for the "ectopic" production of hormones of other APUD cell types.

Chemistry and Biosynthesis of Calcitonin

In all species studied to date, calcitonin has been found to be a 32-amino acid polypeptide with an amino-terminal disulfide bridge linking positions 1 and 7 and with an amide group on the carboxy-terminal proline residue (Fig. 23-12). The molecular weight of the calcitonin monomer (calcitonin M, Fig. 23-12) is 3400. Human thyroid tissue contains less stored calcitonin than does the thyroid (or ultimobranchial) tissue from other species so that many studies of the human hormone have employed human medullary carcinoma tissue. This tissue contains approximately 5000 times more calcitonin on a weight basis than normal thyroid tissue, and the hormonal product appears to be structurally identical to native human calcitonin. The amino acid sequences of the calcitonin molecule from a variety of species (human, bovine, porcine, ovine, rat, and salmon) reveal close homologies for only 9 of the 32 amino acid residues.[54,55] All sequences share the carboxy-terminal prolinamide and have close homologies in the amino-terminal seven-membered ring but show marked heterogeneity in the central three-fourths of the molecule. This heterogeneity is sufficient that most radioimmunoassays which have been developed for calcitonin are relatively species-specific: that is, the antisera generated to the calcitonin molecule of one species cross-react poorly with the calcitonin molecules of other species.

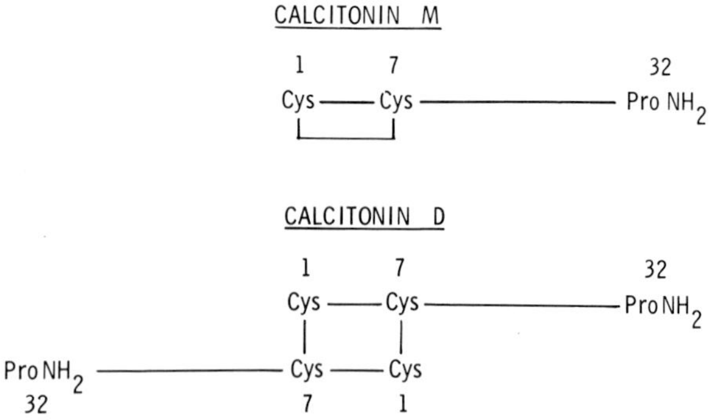

FIGURE 23-12 Human calcitonin monomer (calcitonin M) and calcitonin dimer (calcitonin D). (*From Foster, Byfield, and Gudmundsson, Clin Endocrinol Metab 1:93, 1972.*)

The close homologies in the amino-terminal region of the calcitonin molecule initially suggested that this region of the peptide might be responsible for biological activity in a fashion analogous to that noted in the parathyroid hormone molecule. However, detailed studies have revealed that the entire 32-amino acid sequence of calcitonin is required for biological activity and that even single amino acid deletions at either end of the molecule result in virtually complete loss of biological activity.[54,55]

Salmon calcitonin is a more potent hypocalcemic agent than the mammalian calcitonins when tested in a variety of species, including the mouse, rat, and human. For example, in humans, salmon calcitonin is approximately 10 times more potent than human calcitonin on a weight basis. The increased potency of salmon calcitonin appears to result both from a prolonged circulating half-time and from an increased affinity for and/or an increased duration of binding to calcitonin receptors in the target tissues of the hormone.[54-56] Both the decrease in metabolic clearance and the receptor binding characteristics of the salmon peptide are presumably a function of its primary structure. To date, more potent analogues of calcitonin have not been introduced.

The details of calcitonin biosynthesis are illustrated in Fig. 23-13. These details actually evolved from observations in a serially transplanted rat medullary carcinoma of the thyroid which largely lost its ability to synthesize calcitonin but was found to be producing a new and larger cytoplasmic RNA which encoded a different peptide: calcitonin gene-related peptide. This peptide does not contain immunoreactive calcitonin. Using the nucleotide sequence of CGRP as a probe, its mRNA was detected in neural tissues of the rat. Complementary sequences to the mRNAs encoding calcitonin and CGRP were used to identify the calcitonin/CGRP gene in a rat genomic library, and the model of tissue-specific alternative splicing was worked out.[57]

The rat calcitonin/CGRP gene contains six exons (Fig. 23-13). In the C cells of the thyroid, the first three exons are spliced to the fourth calcitonin-coding exon to generate the mature calcitonin mRNA. In the nervous system, in the pituitary, and to a lesser extent in the thyroid C cell, the first three exons are spliced to the fifth and sixth exons, the latter contain-

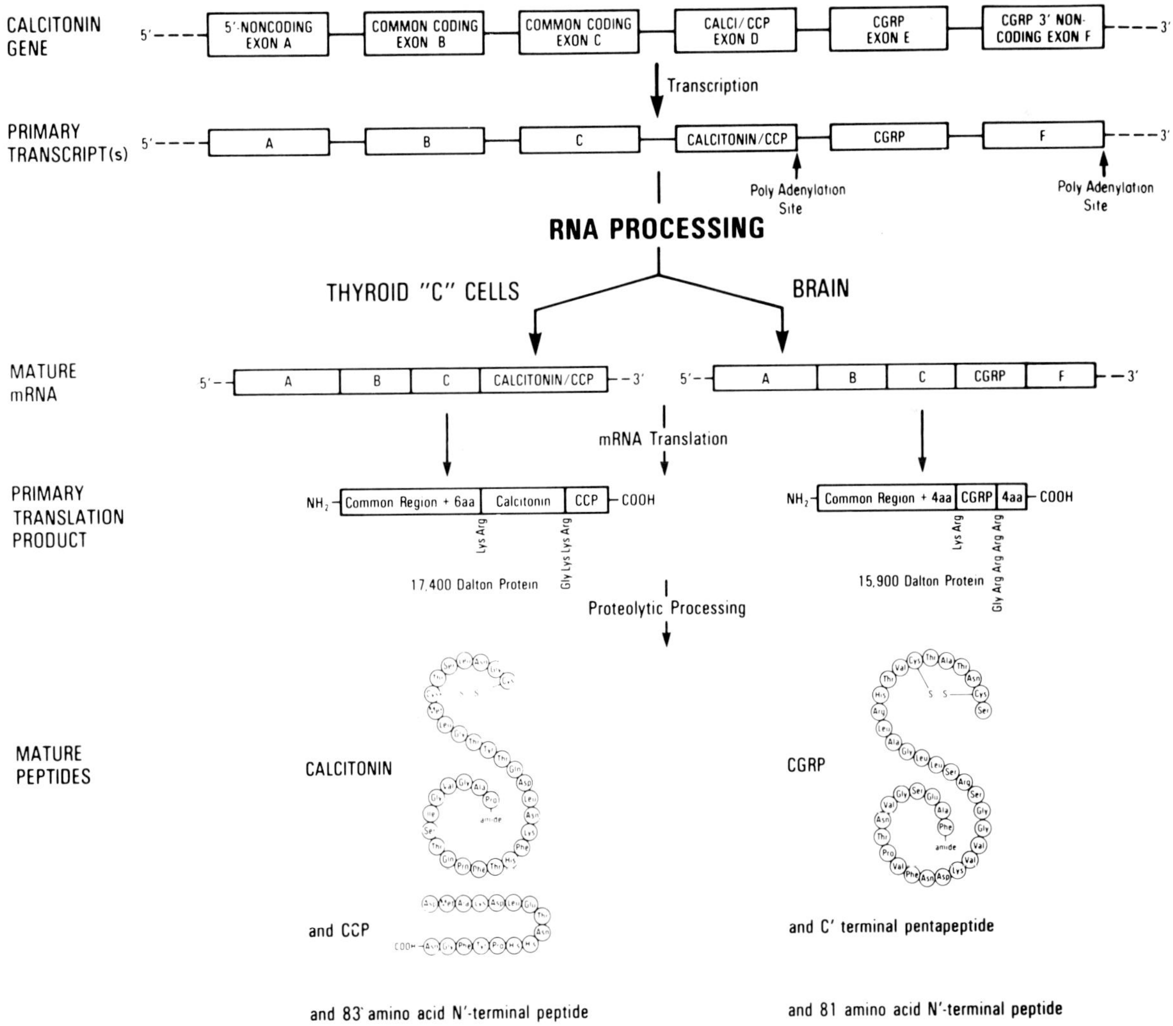

FIGURE 23-13 Model of alternative RNA processing involved in the tissue-specific expression of the calcitonin/CGRP gene. The calcitonin pathway predominates in the C cells of the thyroid, and the CGRP pathway predominates in the nervous system. (By *permission of Rosenfeld MG, Amara SG, Birnberg NC, Mermod JJ, Murdoch GH, Evans RM, Recent Prog Horm Res 39:305, 1983.*)

ing the polyadenylation signal used specifically with this peptide. In these tissues, the fourth (calcitonin-coding) exon is excised and is not expressed. The tissue specificity of this endonucleolytic cleavage, or alternative splicing, determines the pattern of expression of calcitonin and CGRP in their respective tissues of origin. At present, calcitonin is regarded as a calcium regulating hormone and CGRP as a neuropeptide, but physiological studies concerning CGRP and other calcitonin/CGRP gene-encoded peptides (see below) are in their infancy. Exactly the same sequence of events has been demonstrated for the human calcitonin/CGRP gene,[58] and human CGRP has been isolated and sequenced.[59]

The mature calcitonin mRNA encodes preprocalcitonin, a 136-amino acid peptide from which the hydrophobic pre sequence is removed cotranslationally to yield procalcitonin, a 111-amino acid peptide. Posttranslational processing of this peptide results in the removal of the pro sequence and the generation of four different peptides: (1) calcitonin from the middle region, (2) a 16-amino acid carboxy-terminal calcitonin adjacent peptide (C-CAP) from the carboxy terminus, and both (3) an amino-terminal peptide (NTP) and (4) an amino-terminal calcitonin adjacent peptide (N-CAP) from the amino terminus.[60] In humans, preprocalcitonin includes 141 amino acids, and C-CAP has 21 amino acids. C-CAP is also referred to as katacalcin; it is known to be cosecreted by medullary carcinoma tissue and is reported to have calcium-lowering effects in large doses.[61,62] Little is known about the two amino-terminal peptides.

CGRP is a unique 37-amino acid peptide which shares greater homology with salmon calcitonin than with either rat or human calcitonin.[59,63] The sequence of human CGRP is shown in Fig. 23-14; it will be noted that CGRP, like calcitonin, contains an intrachain disulfide bridge and is amidated at the carboxy terminus. The close homology of CGRP to salmon calcitonin has invited speculation as to the potential origin of the calcitonin and CGRP exons from a common primordial gene. This homology has also been invoked to explain putative effects of calcitonin in the nervous system, especially for the salmon peptide, although this point has been disputed.[63] Binding sites for human CGRP have been demonstrated in the nervous system, with the most enriched sites being in the dorsal spinal cord and the pituitary.[63] CGRP has been reported to have prominent cardiovascular and central effects, and it may also inhibit bone resorption at extremely high concentrations. The expression of CGRP mRNA in a variety of different medullary carcinomas of the thyroid has been shown to vary from a few percent of the level of the expression of calcitonin mRNA to a virtually identical level of expression; this observation may explain in part the heterogeneity of circulating calcitonin or calcitonin-like peptides observed in these patients. The amino-terminal peptides encoded by the two mRNAs are derived from common exons and are presumably expressed to an equivalent degree in tissues which synthesize both calcitonin and CGRP.

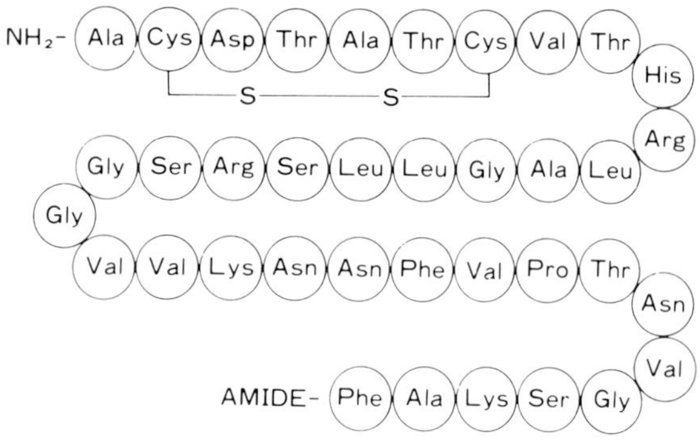

FIGURE 23-14 Sequence of human calcitonin gene-related peptide. (*From Morris, Panico, Etienne, Tippins, Girgis, and MacIntyre,*[59] *by permission of Nature.*)

Secretion and Metabolism of Calcitonin

The primary stimulus for calcitonin synthesis and secretion is an increase in the concentration of serum ionized calcium.[54–56] The rate of calcitonin secretion is a direct function of the level of serum calcium above 9 mg/dl (Fig. 23-15). Calcitonin secretion appears to proceed at a low basal rate within the normal range of serum calcium and is reduced to undetectable levels during hypocalcemia. In certain circumstances, calcitonin synthesis and secretion can be dissociated. For example, prolonged experimental or clinical hypocalcemia results in the accumulation of calcitonin in the C cells at a time when calcitonin secretion is essentially nonexistent; that is, synthesis and storage of the hormone appear to proceed without being linked to a stimulus for calcitonin secretion. In this circumstance, a calcium challenge leads to an exaggerated calcitonin secretory response. High magnesium levels have been shown experimentally to increase calcitonin secretion. However, the range of magnesium concentrations required to elicit a calcitonin response far exceeds the physiological or pathophysiological range.[54–56]

A large body of literature has evolved concerning the potential influence of a variety of endocrine factors on calcitonin secretion.[54–56] Calcitonin secretion has been found to be uninfluenced by parathyroid hormone, 25-hydroxyvitamin D, thyroid stimulating

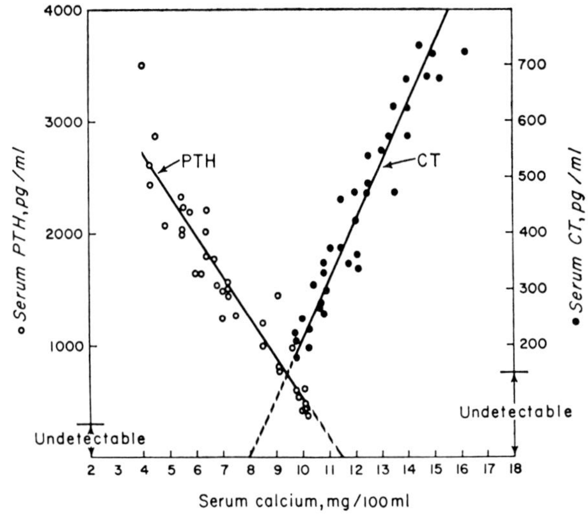

FIGURE 23-15 The concentrations of immunoreactive PTH and calcitonin in pig serum in response to alterations in serum calcium produced by calcium or EGTA infusion. [*By permission of Arnaud CD, Littledike T, Tsao HS: in Taylor S, Foster GV (eds): Proceedings of the Symposium on Calcitonin and C Cells. London, Heinemann, 1969.*]

hormone (TSH), thyroxine, somatostatin, prostaglandin E, and secretin.[54-56] Calcitonin secretion is stimulated by gastrin, cholecystokinin, glucagon, and beta-adrenergic agents.[54-56,64] Calcitonin secretion is inhibited by somatostatin.[64]

Full biological activity for the stimulation of acid secretion as well as calcitonin secretion resides in the carboxy-terminal tetrapeptide amide of the gastrin molecule.[64] This carboxy-terminal sequence is homologous in the cholecystokinin molecule, accounting for the ability of this hormone to stimulate calcitonin secretion also, and is included in the synthetic pentapeptide pentagastrin, an agent widely used in physiological and clinical testing. The infusion of isoproterenol into normal humans increases calcitonin levels to approximately the same degree as is noted in response to a standard calcium infusion, and the infusion of the beta blocker propranolol decreases baseline calcitonin levels by roughly 50 percent. The potential physiological significance of this effect is not known.

The available information is insufficient to allow for a clear picture of the integrated control of calcitonin secretion in vivo. It seems clear that the level of ionized calcium is the principal regulator of calcitonin secretion, and it is conceptually useful to regard this calcium regulation as the basic mechanism of secretory control upon which hormonal effects may be superimposed as modulating influences.

Calcitonin secretion in vitro can be stimulated by treatment with theophylline or dibutyryl cAMP. These data suggest that cAMP may be involved in the calcium-mediated control of calcitonin secretion in a fashion similar to the proposed calcium-cAMP interaction in the parathyroid cell and/or that cAMP may be mechanistically involved in the modulation of calcitonin secretion by gastrin and beta-adrenergic agents.

Calcitonin distributes into a space equivalent to the extracellular fluid volume and is cleared from the circulation with a half-time of 2 to 30 min, depending on both the species studied and the species source of the hormone. In humans, the half-time for human calcitonin monomer is about 10 min.[54] In all species, salmon calcitonin is cleared from the circulation more slowly than the mammalian calcitonins. The principal site of calcitonin clearance and metabolism appears to be the kidney, and the metabolic clearance rate of calcitonin is markedly reduced in patients with renal insufficiency.[54] This process appears to result from filtration of calcitonin, with tubular reabsorption and degradation. Very little calcitonin appears in the urine.

Circulating calcitonin has been reported to be heterogeneous in patients with medullary carcinoma of the thyroid, in patients with nonthyroid malignancies (e.g., bronchogenic carcinoma), and to a lesser extent in normal subjects.[56,65] For example, in many patients with medullary carcinoma of the thyroid, only 20 to 50 percent of the circulating immunoreactive calcitonin appears to be calcitonin monomer, and from one to as many as four additional immunoreactive peaks may be obtained by means of gel filtration.[56] These additional peaks range in estimated size from 7000 to 60,000 daltons. There are several potential explanations for this heterogeneity, including dimerization of calcitonin and the secretion by tumors of incompletely processed, higher-molecular-weight forms of calcitonin. In addition, since the reactive determinants of individual antisera differ, the detection of different circulating forms of calcitonin may vary from assay to assay.

The reactivity of the disulfide linkage of the calcitonin molecule can give rise to dimeric or possibly even polymeric forms of the hormone. The calcitonin dimer (calcitonin D, Fig. 23-12) consists of two monomers covalently linked in an antiparallel fashion by interchain disulfide bridges. The dimer appears to be metabolically inactive. High-molecular-weight forms of calcitonin, which appear to include dimers and/or polymers of the hormone, constitute a major fraction of the immunoreactive material secreted by medullary carcinoma tissue in vitro.[66] The sequence of events illustrated in Fig. 23-13 certainly makes the secretion of higher-molecular-weight species of calcitonin a plausible additional explanation for the immunoheterogeneity of calcitonin, especially in patients with nonthyroid malignancy. This mechanism has not been demonstrated.

An extraction method for determining calcitonin monomer has recently been reported.[65] Based on this assay, the normal circulating level of calcitonin is < 20 pg/ml, a figure which is clearly lower than that reported from many other assays.[56,65] Additional details concerning the measurement of calcitonin are provided in Biochemical and Immunoassay Determinations and in Chap. 28.

Biological Effects and Mechanisms of Action of Calcitonin

The acute intravenous administration of calcitonin to experimental animals produces a prompt reduction in the serum calcium and serum phosphorus concentrations. Both effects result largely from the influence of the hormone on bone, although in pharmacological doses, calcitonin also affects the renal handling of calcium and phosphorus. With the initial discovery of calcitonin came the postulate that the hormone might play an important counterregulatory role, buffering the effects of PTH and aiding the organism in the fine control of ionized serum calcium. As discussed below, detailed study has not confirmed this postulate, and the hormone is currently viewed as having limited significance in normal adult human physiology. The term *antihypercalcemic,* introduced by Copp, is more descriptively appropriate to the presumptive role of calcitonin than is the more frequently used term *hypocalcemic hormone.*[55]

EFFECTS OF CALCITONIN ON BONE

Calcitonin directly, rapidly, and profoundly inhibits bone resorption and bone-resorbing cells. There is little evidence to suggest that calcitonin has any direct influence on bone formation or mineralization or on bone growth in growing animals.[36] The inhibition of bone resorption by calcitonin has been demonstrated in a variety of in vivo and in vitro systems of study, and the hormone inhibits the resorption of both the mineral and the matrix phases of bone, as evidenced by a reduction in serum calcium and hydroxyproline mobilization and excretion.[54,55] In vivo, the reduction in hydroxyproline excretion is a more sensitive index of the effect of calcitonin than the decrease in serum calcium.

The net influence of calcitonin on serum calcium and calcium mobilization from the skeleton depends on the rate of preexisting bone resorption.[54,55] The greatest effects of the hormone are seen in circumstances in which bone resorption is increased, as in (1) young animals with a rapid bone remodeling rate, (2) bone which has been previously stimulated by PTH or vitamin D, or (3) disease states associated with an increase in bone resorption and bone turnover (e.g., Paget's disease, primary hyperparathyroidism, and Graves' disease). For example, relatively small doses of calcitonin produce hypocalcemia in young, growing rats, whereas large doses of the hormone in older animals have only a slight influence on serum calcium; a reduction in serum calcium is regularly observed in patients with Paget's disease in response to calcitonin, yet the hormone has no demonstrable effect on serum calcium in normal adult humans.

Calcitonin inhibits both osteoclastic bone resorption and osteocytic osteolysis. Histological changes are noted in the osteoclast within minutes of calcitonin administration: The expanse of the ruffled border of the osteoclast decreases, and the cells begin to withdraw physically from bone-resorbing surfaces.[3] The number of active osteoclasts decreases within an hour of calcitonin treatment, presumably owing to both an inhibition of osteoclast formation from precursor cells and a dedifferentiation of preformed osteoclasts. Although calcitonin affects both osteoclastic bone resorption and osteocytic osteolysis, its influence on the former process is probably quantitatively the more important. In humans, there is a direct correlation between the number of active osteoclasts and the fall in serum calcium produced by calcitonin in a variety of metabolic disorders of bone.[2] Since osteocytic osteolysis appears to be of central importance in the minute-to-minute regulation of serum calcium by PTH, these findings indicate a putative role for calcitonin in more extreme conditions of bone resorption, in which osteoclastic bone resorption predominates. In this sense, calcitonin would predictably have little influence on minute-to-minute calcium homeostasis in humans. Because of the coupled nature of bone turnover, chronic exposure to calcitonin leads ultimately to a decrease in all aspects of bone turnover, including osteoblast number and function. Bone chronically exposed to calcitonin may be aptly described as "asleep." In intact animals, the hypocalcemia associated with calcitonin administration may elicit a rebound increase in parathyroid hormone secretion, which can alter both the histological and the chemical pattern of the direct bone response to calcitonin.

An *escape* phenomenon to large, prolonged doses of calcitonin has been described. For example, in bone systems stimulated with PTH or 1,25-$(OH)_2D$, calcitonin initially inhibits bone resorption, but this effect is lost with time despite the continued presence of biologically active calcitonin. Studies by Tashjian and coworkers[67] have shown this escape phenomenon to be the result of "down regulation," or a reversible loss of specific calcitonin-binding sites in bone. In the case of calcitonin, down regulation appears to be due in large part to continuous receptor occupancy by tightly bound, poorly dissociable hormone. Although "escape" is probably of limited importance in physiological conditions, the phenomenon may be of clinical relevance and may explain, for example, the lack of a sustained hypocalcemic effect of pharmacological doses of calcitonin employed in the treatment of hypercalcemia associated with malignant disease.

Although details are limited by the difficulties in preparing homogeneous bone cell populations for study in vitro, the cAMP messenger system appears to mediate the action of calcitonin in bone.[56]

EFFECTS OF CALCITONIN ON THE KIDNEY

Infused in sufficient doses into humans and experimental animals, calcitonin leads to a transient increase in the excretion of calcium, phosphorus, sodium, potassium, and magnesium.[42,54,55] These effects are observed in hypoparathyroid patients and parathyroidectomized animals and therefore are due to direct effects of the hormone rather than secondary changes brought about by rebound increases in PTH secretion. The calciuric and phosphaturic effects of calcitonin participate in or potentiate the hypocalcemia and hypophosphatemia which result from the actions of the hormone on bone. The increase in phosphorus excretion caused by calcitonin is associated with a reduction in TmP/GFR. In response to a continuous infusion of calcitonin, the transient increase in calcium excretion is followed by a period during which calcium excretion falls because of the calcitonin-induced hypocalcemia and a reduced filtered load of calcium. However, even during the latter period an increased fractional excretion of calcium can be demonstrated.[42]

Although the initial studies of the effects of calcitonin on electrolyte excretion resulted in conflicting data and conclusions, there is now agreement that the renal tubular effects of calcitonin described above can be reproducibly demonstrated.[42] Most of these effects appear to derive from an influence of the hormone on proximal tubular ion transport. In contrast to the fundamental and potentially long lasting effects of calcitonin on bone, all the renal tubular effects are transient and limited in time to the actual period of hormonal stimulation. Thus, a single daily injection of calcitonin (e.g., in the treatment of Paget's disease) with a half-time measured in minutes produces no discernible effect on 24-h electrolyte excretion in humans.

The major issue concerns whether any of these effects of calcitonin on renal tubular ion transport are of physiological relevance or can be demonstrated in response to physiological doses of the hormone. Although there are differences of investigative opinion, there is little evidence to suggest that the renal effects of calcitonin are of physiological or even pathophysiological (e.g., in patients with medullary carcinoma of the thyroid) relevance. The importance of the renal effects of calcitonin therefore appears to be limited to circumstances in which pharmacological doses of the hormone are employed. cAMP mediates the actions of calcitonin in the renal tubule.[46] The distribution of calcitonin-reactive sites in the tubule differs from that described for PTH,[46] and calcitonin has no influence on nephrogenous cAMP excretion.

Physiological Significance of Calcitonin

Classical endocrinology has traditionally developed around the discovery of hormonal mechanisms responsible for hypofunctioning and hyperfunctioning endocrine states in humans. In this sense, the history of calcitonin is distinctly unusual, since the metabolic consequences of clinical calcitonin deficiency or excess are unknown. Total thyroidectomy in humans is not associated with a tendency to hypercalcemia or any identifiable alteration in mineral balance. Conversely, the extremely high circulating levels of calcitonin (up to 20,000 times normal) in patients with medullary carcinoma of the thyroid do not result in hypocalcemia, hypophosphatemia, or other definable abnormalities in mineral balance. Bone biopsies in patients with medullary carcinoma of the thyroid reveal a markedly reduced bone turnover rate,[2] indicating a skeletal effect of the high circulating titers of calcitonin, yet there are no clear alterations in systemic mineral homeostasis in these patients. The lack of metabolic states of calcitonin deficiency or excess in humans is taken by some investigators as prima facie evidence that calcitonin has no identifiable role in human physiology. This assessment may or may not be premature. However, there have been interesting findings in subhuman mammalian species which indicate a potential role for calcitonin in these species, at least in certain circumstances.

Studies in the pig have revealed that an oral dose of calcium produces a prompt severalfold increase in calcitonin secretion at a time when the serum calcium is not demonstrably altered.[64] Cooper and associates[64] have provided evidence that calcitonin secretion during these experiments is stimulated by gastrin released as a consequence of feeding. These and other findings have led to a postulated antral–C cell axis in which gastrin-mediated calcitonin secretion serves to conserve efficiently the calcium absorbed from a calcium-containing meal. Such an axis is viewed as particularly relevant in extreme physiological conditions of calcium demand, for example, in a lactating animal or suckling pup. In both circumstances, the rates of intestinal calcium absorption are extremely high and there are pressing physiological requirements for calcium conservation and for milk production and rapid skeletal growth, respectively. The antral–C cell axis does not appear to be of physiological importance in humans.

There is general agreement that both basal and stimulated calcitonin concentrations are lower in women than in men.[65,68] These data have been interpreted to mean that the integrated secretion rate of calcitonin in women is lower than the rate in men and that women also have a decreased calcitonin "reserve." It has been proposed that this relative decrease in circulating calcitonin in women may predispose them to osteopenia,[68] but this proposition has not been proved.

VITAMIN D

Historical Introduction

Scarcely more than 15 years ago, the complex role of vitamin D in regulating mineral metabolism in humans was almost entirely unknown. Historically, the compound has been regarded for many years as a fat-soluble vitamin necessary for the prevention of rickets.[69-71] Although initially described clinically more than three centuries ago, vitamin D–deficiency rickets did not become a major clinical problem until the industrial revolution, when large populations migrated to urban areas and experienced a combination of poor nutrition and limited exposure to sunlight. Cod liver oil was employed as a folk remedy for treating rickets from the early eighteenth century, but the medical community remained largely ignorant of its efficacy until the early twentieth century. By the 1920s, it was appreciated that clinical rickets could be cured either by the administration of cod liver oil or by exposure to sunlight and that experimental rickets in animals could be cured just as readily by irradiating the animals' food as by irradiating the animals themselves.[70] Vitamin D was isolated in about 1930 and thereafter became available as a dietary supplement. Vitamin D–deficiency rickets virtually disappeared in the United States. The exact metabolic function of vitamin D remained unknown, however, and there was little investigative progress for a quarter century.

During the past 15 years, a series of elegant studies in the laboratories of DeLuca, Norman, Fraser, Haussler, and many other investigators has unraveled the complex details of vitamin D metabolism and physiology.[69-71] Whether vitamin D is regarded as a "vitamin" or as a "hormone" is a semantic issue of limited importance; in fact, it may be regarded as either or as both. Vitamin D serves as a "vitamin" only when sunlight exposure is inadequate to ensure its endogenous synthesis in the skin; in this case, a finite supply of the steroid nucleus via the diet is necessary to prevent vitamin D deficiency. Whether derived from endogenous synthesis or from the diet, the basic steroid nucleus is essentially devoid of metabolic activity and serves as a *prohormone.* This prohormone is "activated" by a series of hydroxylation steps in the liver and kidney to produce the monohydroxy and dihydroxy vitamin D metabolites of physiological importance in humans. By virtue of its endogenous production, the metabolic and feedback regulation of its synthesis, its distribution by the bloodstream to target tissues remote from its site of production, and its mechanism of action, vitamin D is a classical steroid hormone.

Knowledge of this sequence of activation has led to an uncovering of the details of pathogenesis of two rare rachitic syndromes. Vitamin D–dependent rickets type I results from deficient 1-hydroxylase activity in the kidney. Vitamin D–dependent rickets type II results from absent or defective receptors for 1,25-dihydroxyvitamin D in its target tissues. Both syndromes are described in detail in Chap. 24.

Chemistry

The antirachitic sterols are a group of closely related compounds which resemble cholesterol. The structures of the biologically important precursors, metabolites, and analogues of vitamin D are shown in Fig. 23-16. Chemically, these sterols and their precursors are known as secosteroids because the B ring of cholesterol has undergone fission. The term *calciferol* refers collectively to two sterols: cholecalciferol (vitamin D_3)—the form of the vitamin found in animal tissues, fish liver oils, and irradiated milk—and ergocalciferol (vitamin D_2)—the form of vitamin D found in plants and irradiated yeast and bread. The calciferols are not widely distributed in nature. Most foodstuffs from either plant or animal sources contain only inactive vitamin D precursors and require ultraviolet irradiation for the conversion of these precursors to the calciferols. Calciferol dosages are expressed in USP units (which are identical to international units); 1 mg of calciferol is equivalent to 40,000 USP units. The adult requirement for calciferol is considered to be 400 USP units daily; this requirement is also regarded as adequate during periods of physiological stress such as

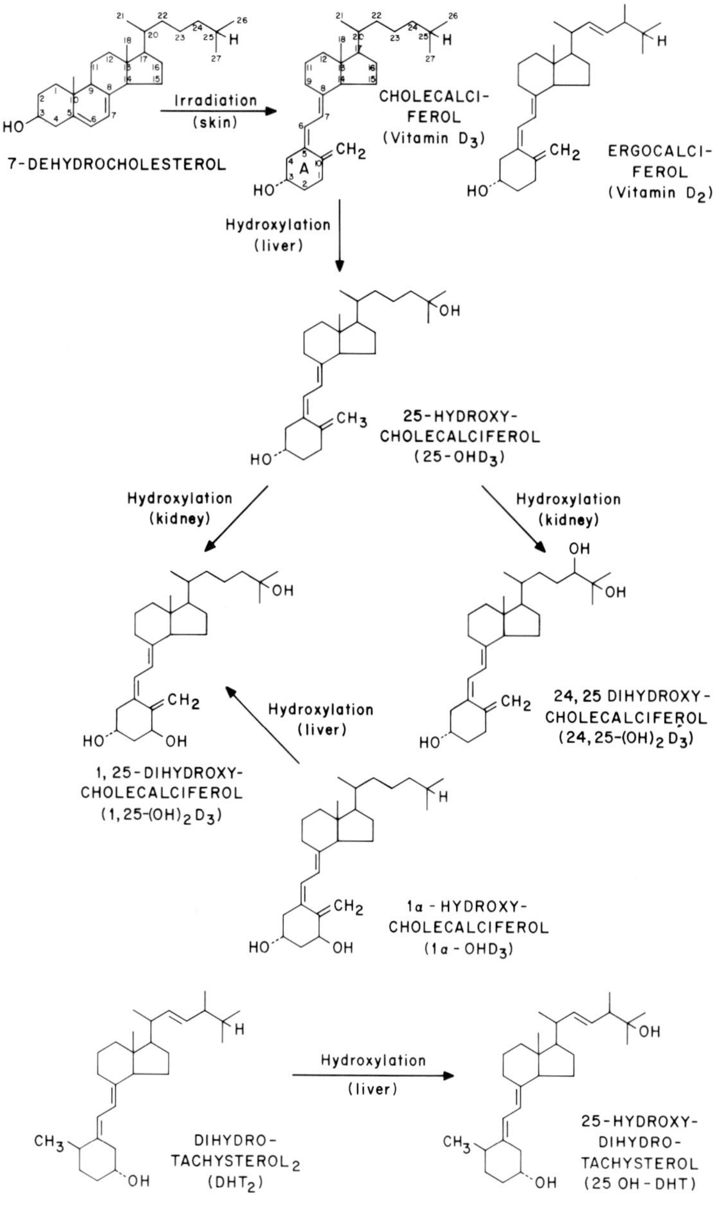

FIGURE 23-16 Chemical structures of the major vitamin D metabolites and analogues. The numbering system is based on that of cholesterol, and the A ring of cholecalciferol is so designated.

growth, pregnancy, and lactation. In the United States, vitamin D additives are present in a number of foods, including milk and milk products and cereals. Most commercial vitamin D preparations contain vitamin D_2.

Vitamin D_3 and vitamin D_2 are produced nonenzymatically by ultraviolet irradiation of animal skin and plants, respectively. The precursor of vitamin D_3 in skin is 7-dehydrocholesterol, sometimes referred to as provitamin D. Ultraviolet irradiation results in the cleavage of carbon bonds of 7-dehydrocholesterol to yield cholecalciferol, and the relation between the two compounds accounts for the somewhat unusual numbering system employed for vitamin D (Fig. 23-16). A similar cleavage results in the production of ergocalciferol from the plant precursor sterol ergosterol. In humans, the storage, transport, metabolism, and potency of vitamin D_2 and vitamin D_3 are identical, and the net biological activity of vitamin D in vivo results from the combined effects of the hydroxylated derivatives of vitamin D_2 and vitamin D_3. That is, the percentage of 1,25-dihydroxyvitamin D [1,25-$(OH)_2$D] derived from vitamin D_2 and vitamin D_3 may differ depending on the relative dietary and endogenous sources of the common vitamin D_2—vitamin D_3 prohormone pool, but the net 1,25-dihydroxyvitamin D activity results from the combined effects of 1,25-$(OH)_2D_2$ and 1,25-$(OH)_2D_3$, which are of equivalent potency. The equivalent potency of vitamin D_2 and vitamin D_3 and their metabolites has been noted in a number of species, including the human being and the rat, but it does not hold for all species. For example, the chick appears to discriminate against all C-24–substituted vitamin D forms, and so vitamin D_2 has only one-tenth the potency of vitamin D_3 in this species.[69] Unless otherwise specified, the discussion of human physiology below will employ the terms vitamin D, 25-OHD, 1,25-$(OH)_2$D, and 24,25-$(OH)_2$D as generic terms for both vitamin D_2 and vitamin D_3 and their metabolites.

All forms of vitamin D circulate bound to a specific vitamin D–binding protein (Fig. 23-17). Vitamin D, the biologically inactive prohormone, is transported to the liver, where it is hydroxylated at C-25 to form 25-OHD, a partially active product. 25-OHD is transported to the kidney, where it is hydroxylated either at C-1 to produce 1,25-$(OH)_2$D, a potent steroid hormone, or at C-24 to produce 24,25-$(OH)_2$D, a less active compound of unclear biological significance. Although there is evidence of regulation at both the level of cholecalciferol production in the skin and the initial hydroxylation of vitamin D in the liver, the hydroxylase reactions in the kidney are the key points of biological regulation of the metabolic activation of vitamin D.

Figure 23-16 also shows the structures of several important synthetic vitamin D analogues. 1α-Hydroxyvitamin D_3 (1α-OHD_3) may be conveniently produced from cholesterol and has been widely employed in physiological and clinical studies. When studied in vitro, 1α-OHD_3 is several orders of magnitude less potent than 1,25-$(OH)_2D_3$, whereas it is effective in microgram doses in vivo. Current evidence suggests that 1α-OHD_3 undergoes an obligatory 25-hydroxylation in vivo to produce native 1,25-$(OH)_2D_3$. Crystalline dihydrotachysterol (DHT) is an A-ring analogue of vitamin D in which the A ring is rotated so that the C-3 hydroxyl group occupies a pseudo 1-hydroxyl position. Thus, DHT sterically resembles 1α-OHD_3 and 1,25-$(OH)_2D_3$. DHT is prepared as a reduction product from calciferol (DHT_2 from ergocalciferol and DHT_3 from cholecalciferol) and was the active principle in AT-10 and other early impure preparations of variable potency which have been replaced by pure crystalline DHT. In the treatment of hypoparathyroidism and other conditions, DHT has approximately three times the potency of the calciferols (1 mg of DHT is equivalent to about 3 mg or 120,000 USP units of calciferol). DHT is rapidly hydroxylated in vivo to 25-OHDHT (Fig. 23-16). Both 1α-OHD_3 and DHT bypass the renal 1-hydroxylation step, and this appears to explain their rapidity of action and potency in syndromes classically considered to be "vitamin-resistant" (e.g., hypoparathyroidism and chronic renal insufficiency). In addition, the polarity of both compounds and lower dosage requirements limit their storage in fat and make them theoretically less likely to produce significant or prolonged vitamin D intoxication.

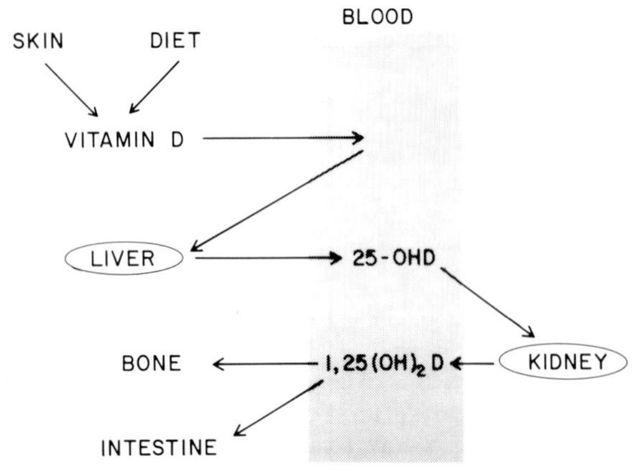

FIGURE 23-17 Transport and metabolic sequence of activation of vitamin D in humans.

Formation, Transport, Metabolic Sequence of Activation, and Metabolism of Vitamin D

The sequence of synthesis, transport, storage, and activation of vitamin D is a model of biological elegance. The sequence embodies an elaborate set of inherent checks and balances designed at the proximal end to ensure an adequate supply of the steroid nucleus and at the distal end to guard against excessive production of the final, potent steroid hormone.

Studies by Holick and associates[72] have revealed that photolytic conversion of provitamin D (7-dihydrocholesterol) to cholecalciferol in the skin proceeds via an additional intermediate termed previtamin D_3. Ultraviolet irradiation photolytically converts provitamin D_3 to previtamin D_3, and the latter compound slowly transforms to vitamin D_3 at body temperature. The vitamin D–binding protein in blood has a thousandfold higher affinity for vitamin D_3 than for previtamin D_3 so that vitamin D_3 is preferentially transported from the skin into the circulation. The vitamin D_3 removed into the circulation is replaced by slow thermal conversion of previtamin D_3 to vitamin

D_3. This series of steps appears to constitute an important mechanism which by relatively brief exposure to ultraviolet irradiation may lead to a continuous supply of vitamin D for days to weeks. Vitamin D_3 is produced in the stratum granulosum of the skin; its production is less efficient in dark-skinned races and also appears to decline with age.[70,72]

Adipose tissue and muscle are the major storage sites for vitamin D. The quantity of the vitamin stored in these sites is not regulated in any way and is simply a function of the state of vitamin D repletion of the organism. Dietary vitamin D_2 and vitamin D_3 are absorbed into the lymphatic channels from the duodenum and jejunum, incorporated loosely into chylomicrons. This absorption may fail in circumstances of fat malabsorption. The absorbed vitamin D admixes with endogenous vitamin D and becomes a part of the total pool of circulating and stored prohormone. The concentration of vitamin D in human serum is approximately 1 to 10 ng/ml, and it disappears with a biological half-time of about 24 h.

The circulating *vitamin D–binding protein* in humans is a single protein with the electrophoretic mobility of an α-globulin and a molecular weight of 56,000.[73] The protein has a single binding site which is shared by all vitamin D metabolites, and it serves as the transport protein for all vitamin D sterols. The protein has a greater affinity for 25-OHD than for vitamin D or 1,25-$(OH)_2D$ and, with prior purification of the sample, can be employed in ligand assays for 25-OHD. The protein circulates at a concentration of about 6 μM (350 mg per liter), far in excess of requirements for vitamin D transport, and it is only 1 to 3 percent saturated by physiological circulating levels of the vitamin D sterols. Because of its large net capacity for vitamin D binding, some investigators view the vitamin D–binding protein as possibly serving a circulating storage as well as a transport function analogous to the relation between thyroxine-binding globulin and the thyroid hormones. This analogy is conceptually appealing in another sense, in that the relative affinity of the vitamin D–binding protein for 25-OHD and 1,25-$(OH)_2D$ is similar to the relative affinity of the thyroxine-binding globulin for thyroxine and triiodothyronine; in both cases, the most active hormonal product is the most freely dissociable. The concentration of the vitamin-binding protein is the same in men and women but its concentration is increased in pregnancy and by estrogen administration. The circulating level of the protein is unaltered in states of vitamin D deficiency or excess. The synthesis of the protein may be reduced in cirrhosis, and it may be lost into the urine in patients with the nephrotic syndrome, but in neither case does frank vitamin D deficiency necessarily ensue.[74,75]

25-OHD constitutes the major circulating form of vitamin D in humans, with an average serum concentration in the range of 30 ng/ml. The circulating biological half-time of 25-OHD is approximately 15 days, and the circulating pool of this metabolite is presumably in equilibrium with a storage pool of 25-OHD in muscle and fat. The size and/or significance of this storage pool of 25-OHD is not known. Although extrahepatic sites of 25-hydroxylation of vitamin D have been identified in the chick, in mammals the liver is the principal site of 25-hydroxylation.[69,71] The 25-hydroxylation of vitamin D in the liver proceeds rapidly; by 4 h after administration of radioactive vitamin D to vitamin D–deficient animals, approximately one-third of the administered material has been converted to 25-OHD, and by 48 h, practically all of it is in the form of 25-OHD. In all species studied, the 25-hydroxylase is a mixed-function monooxygenase located exclusively in the microsomes. This enzyme system has been solubilized and shown to be composed of two enzymes, neither of which has been purified.[69] Prior vitamin D administration reduces hepatic 25-hydroxylase activity, and this has been regarded as evidence for feedback or product inhibition of the enzyme by 25-OHD. However, in normal circumstances, this "autoregulation" of the 25-hydroxylase is of limited significance, and the production of 25-OHD appears to be a direct function of the quantity of circulating vitamin D substrate. Measured circulating levels of 25-OHD correlate strongly with exposure to sunlight and the dietary intake of vitamin D, and this determination is regarded as a good index of the state of vitamin D repletion (or depletion) of the organism. Isolated hepatic mitochondria are capable of converting vitamin D to polar hydroxylated compounds dissimilar to 25-OHD; the mitochondrial enzymes are not of apparent physiological significance. Systemic calcium and phosphorus status does not influence hepatic 25-hydroxylase activity, and this enzyme has not been regarded as a site of biological, ionic, or hormonal control in the organism. However, the hepatic production of 25-OHD has recently been reported to be inhibited by 1,25-$(OH)_2D$ administration in normal humans.[76] The potential physiological importance of this observation is not known. Anticonvulsants and a number of other drugs are known to induce hepatic microsomal mixed-oxidase enzymes which can convert a variety of steroid hormones to polar hydroxylated biologically inactive products. This mechanism has been implicated as a partial explanation for the occurrence of reduced circulating 25-OHD levels and/or clinical osteomalacia in patients receiving prolonged, high-dose anticonvulsant therapy (see Chap. 24).

It was initially thought that 25-OHD was the

final biologically active metabolite of vitamin D. However, it was subsequently recognized that 25-OHD has limited biological activity so that at physiological circulating levels it appears to account for only a minor proportion of the net effect of vitamin D in its target tissues. 25-OHD is transported to the kidney, where it is further metabolized to form the two major dihydroxylated metabolites of vitamin D (Fig. 23-17). The discovery in the early 1970s of 1,25-$(OH)_2D$ and the renal regulation of the production of the dihydroxy-vitamin D metabolites is a particularly exciting chapter in vitamin D physiology which resulted from simultaneous studies in the principal vitamin D laboratories in Wisconsin, California, and England.[69-71] These studies demonstrated that 1,25-$(OH)_2D$ is a potent steroid hormone several orders of magnitude more active than 25-OHD and that the kidney is the key site of biological control in the sequence of activation of vitamin D.

In normal humans, 24,25-$(OH)_2D$ is the major quantitative dihydroxyvitamin D product and circulates at levels of approximately 1 to 5 ng/ml. 1,25-$(OH)_2D$ circulates at levels in the range of 20 to 50 pg/mL ($\sim 10^{-10}$ M), similar to the low circulating titers of aldosterone and in keeping with its role as a potent steroid hormone. The circulating half-time of 1,25-$(OH)_2D$ in normal humans is approximately 15 h; the half-time of 24,25-$(OH)_2D$ is approximately 6 h.[77,78] The two dihydroxyvitamin D metabolites are produced in the kidney by separate enzymes, the 24-hydroxylase and the 1-hydroxylase, which hydroxylate 25-OHD at either C-24 or C-1, respectively. The kidney is the primary and most important source of 1,25-$(OH)_2D$ and 24,25-$(OH)_2D$ in the organism in a quantitative sense, although 1-hydroxylase activity and 24-hydroxylase activity have also been demonstrated in other tissues (see below). Both enzymes are concentrated in the proximal convoluted tubule, and 1-hydroxylase activity appears to be controlled by the cAMP messenger system.[79] The renal hydroxylase reactions are largely analogous to steroidogenesis systems in the adrenal cortex.[69] The 1-hydroxylase is a mixed-function monooxygenase in the mitochondria and has been shown to have three components, the first two of which can be substituted for by the corresponding bovine adrenal proteins.[69] The 24-hydroxylase is also a mitochondrial enzyme system and has very similar characteristics.

In certain circumstances, 24-hydroxylase activity has been demonstrated in intestine, cartilage, and bone; 1-hydroxylase activity has been demonstrated in bone, intestine, and placenta.[69,70] In addition, low circulating levels of the dihydroxyvitamin D metabolites have recently been reported in anephric humans.[80] The significance of these extrarenal sites of 1,25-$(OH)_2D$ and 24,25-$(OH)_2D$ production is a matter of controversy.[69,70,80] In general, the collective enzyme activities in these sites are not regarded as sufficient to generate physiologically important circulating concentrations of dihydroxyvitamin D metabolites, but the synthesis of either metabolite could be physiologically important in a given tissue in a local sense. The synthesis of 1,25-$(OH)_2D$ by the placenta and by granulomatous tissue is a special case that is discussed below and in Hypercalcemia.

The activities of the renal hydroxylases are separately and reciprocally regulated such that conditions which favor the synthesis of one dihydroxylated metabolite inhibit the synthesis of the other dihydroxy metabolite. A number of factors participate in this reciprocal regulation, including PTH, phosphate, 1-25$(OH)_2D$ itself, and possibly the calcium ion.

Figure 23-18 illustrates the relation between serum calcium and the renal production of 1,25-$(OH)_2D$ and 24,25-$(OH)_2D$ in rats whose serum calcium was manipulated by dietary means. At a normal serum calcium in the range of 9.2 mg/dl, both 1,25-$(OH)_2D$ and 24,25-$(OH)_2D$ are produced, and 24,25-$(OH)_2D$ is the major circulating dihydroxy metabolite. With even slight degrees of hypocalcemia, there is a sharp rise in 1,25-$(OH)_2D$ synthesis, and 24,25-$(OH)_2D$ production declines. Conversely, a modest increase in serum calcium is associated with suppression of 1,25-$(OH)_2D$ synthesis and an increase in the rate of the 24-hydroxylation reaction. The system is finely tuned around a serum calcium level in the midnormal range in a fashion reminiscent of the influence of serum calcium on PTH secretion. The similarity of the effects of the serum calcium on PTH secretion and 1,25-$(OH)_2D$ synthesis is more than

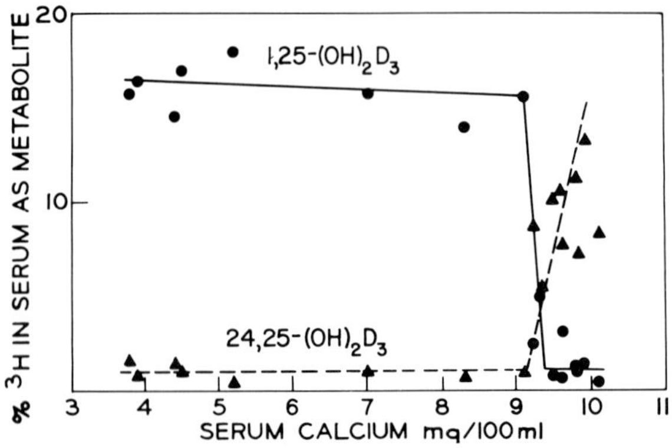

FIGURE 23-18 Relation between serum calcium and the accumulation of radioactive 1,25-$(OH)_2D$ and 24,25-$(OH)_2D$ in rat serum. Serum calcium was manipulated by dietary means. [*By permission of Boyle IT, Gray RW, Deluca HF: in Taylor S (ed): Endocrinology 1971. London, Heinemann, 1972.*]

fortuitous; the renal hydroxylase response to calcium demand in vivo is entirely mediated by PTH stimulation of 1-hydroxylase activity. Parathyroidectomy eliminates 1,25-$(OH)_2D$ synthesis in the face of pronounced hypocalcemia, and only 24,25-$(OH)_2D$ is formed. In parathyroidectomized animals, the synthesis of 1,25-$(OH)_2D$ is restored by means of PTH administration. In vivo, the influence of PTH on renal 1-hydroxylase and 24-hydroxylase activity is not immediate; maximal stimulation and inhibition of the hydroxylases is observed some hours after administration of the hormone. Once synthesized, the renal hydroxylases have survival half-times of only several hours.[71] This and a number of other findings suggest that the major influence of PTH on renal hydroxylase activity occurs at the level of induction or inhibition of the biosynthesis of the enzymes. The inhibition of 24-hydroxylase activity observed in response to PTH is probably indirectly mediated by the effect of 1,25-$(OH)_2D$ on the synthesis of the enzyme (see below).

The manipulation of dietary calcium at the high and low extremes of a normal calcium intake has a pronounced influence on circulating 1,25-$(OH)_2D$ levels in normal humans.[81] Severe restriction of dietary calcium is associated with a 50 percent rise in plasma 1,25-$(OH)_2D$, and oral calcium loading produces a 50 percent fall in the circulating level of hormone. Both effects are observed within 24 h and are maximal by 48 h. These studies further revealed a strong negative correlation between plasma 1,25-$(OH)_2D$ concentrations and urinary calcium excretion in a large group of normal subjects, suggesting that the quantity of calcium absorbed from the diet is a key determinant of 1,25-$(OH)_2D$ synthesis in normal circumstances. In all circumstances, the induced changes in the circulating levels of 1,25-$(OH)_2D$ were found to be strongly correlated with alterations in PTH secretion.[81]

Figure 23-19 shows the relation between serum phosphorus levels and the synthesis of the dihydroxy-vitamin D metabolites in thyroparathyroidectomized rats in which serum phosphorus was altered by means of dietary phosphorus restriction and supplementation. There is a clear inverse relation between serum phosphorus and 1,25-$(OH)_2D$ synthesis. Thus at a low serum phosphorus concentration 1,25-$(OH)_2D$ synthesis proceeds preferentially, and at higher serum phosphorus concentrations 1,25-$(OH)_2D$ production is inhibited and the synthesis of 24,25-$(OH)_2D$ is observed. Since phosphorus deprivation stimulates the production of 1,25-$(OH)_2D$ in the absence of the parathyroid glands, it is apparent that the organism contains a "sensing" mechanism which is capable of detecting a low level of serum phosphorus and influencing 1-hydroxylase activity. Taken together

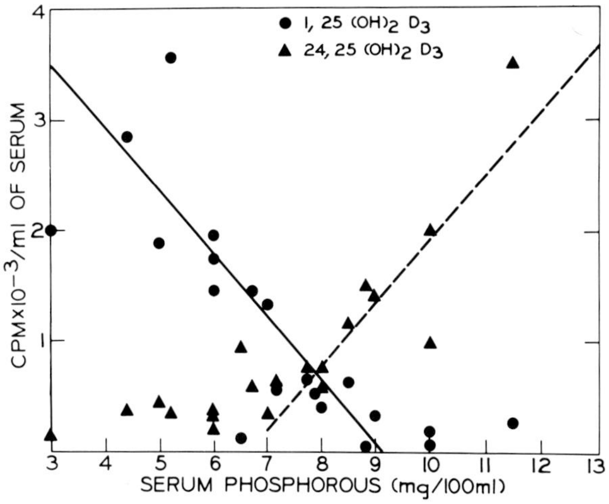

FIGURE 23-19 Relation between serum phosphorus and the accumulation of radioactive 1,25-$(OH)_2D$ in the serum of thyroparathyroidectomized rats in which serum phosphorus was manipulated by variations in phosphorus intake. The high level of "normal" serum phosphorus in these studies reflects both the effects of parathyroidectomy and the fact that serum phosphorus is normally considerably higher in rats than in humans. (*By permission of Tanaka Y, DeLuca HF, Arch Biochem Biophys 154:566, 1973.*)

with the ability of 1,25-$(OH)_2D$ to stimulate phosphorus mobilization from bone and to enhance the absorption of phosphorus in the intestine, this mechanism provides the organism with a classical feedback loop system for regulating serum phosphorus which is entirely independent of the calcium–PTH–1,25-$(OH)_2D$ loop. The detailed mechanism mediating this phosphorus effect and the cellular location of the presumed "phosphostat" remain unknown. Most investigators favor the view that the specific renal tubular cell in which hydroxylase activity is concentrated may be capable of sensing and responding to a reduction either in serum phosphorus or in inorganic or organic phosphate in some critical subcellular compartment. An alternative hypothesis holds that an extrarenal cell type may be sensitive to phosphorus levels and that renal tubular phosphorus retention and/or 1-hydroxylase activity may be stimulated by an unidentified hormone elaborated by this extrarenal cell.

Experimental dietary phosphorus deprivation increases the production of 1,25-$(OH)_2D$ in normal human subjects.[82,83] An increase in circulating 1,25-$(OH)_2D$ is detectable within 24 h, and a maximal mean rise of about 40 percent is achieved by 72 h.[82] The conditions of these experiments are rather extreme in that phosphate-binding gels and a rigidly restricted phorphorus intake are required in order to demonstrate a significant effect on 1,25-$(OH)_2D$ production. This observation, together with the generally acknowledged fact that the serum phosphorus concentration is not rigidly maintained, has suggested to investigators that the phosphopenic stimulus is less important than PTH in controlling 1,25-$(OH)_2D$ synthesis in most physiological conditions. Nevertheless, the control of 1,25-$(OH)_2D$ production by phosphorus is clearly of major clinical importance. For example, in children with only moderate renal impairment, variations in dietary phosphorus at the extremes of a normal intake have a pronounced effect on circulating 1,25-$(OH)_2D$.[84]

Experimental vitamin D deficiency is associated with high basal 1-hydroxylase activity and negligible renal 24-hydroxylase activity. The administration of physiological doses of 1,25-$(OH)_2D$ to vitamin D–deficient animals produces a concomitant disappearance of 1-hydroxylase activity together with a stimulation of 24-hydroxylase activity. Both effects can be largely blocked by inhibitors of transcription and protein synthesis. The available evidence suggests that the influence of 1,25-$(OH)_2D$ on both enzymes is not mediated by a direct influence of the steroid on enzyme activity. Rather, 1,25-$(OH)_2D$ appears to regulate renal hydroxylase activity at the level of enzyme biosynthesis or, possibly, by inducing the synthesis of a protein or some other factor which directly inhibits 1-hydroxylase activity.[71] In spite of the unknown mechanistic details, the influence of 1,25-$(OH)_2D$ on the activities of the two hydroxylases appears to be the key element in the reciprocal control of these enzymes. That is, implicit in any stimulus of 1-hydroxylase activity appears to be a secondary induction of 24-hydroxylase biosynthesis as well as a feedback inhibition of 1-hydroxylase biosynthesis, both of which effects buffer the net renal production of 1,25-$(OH)_2D$.

In vitro, the calcium-ion concentration can be shown either to stimulate or to inhibit 1-hydroxylase activity, depending on experimental conditions. This influence can be demonstrated in mitochondrial preparations but not with solubilized enzyme, suggesting that the effect results from altered mitochondrial structure or function. The available data suggest that a critical range of calcium-ion concentration is required for maximal 1-hydroxylase activity but that this influence does not constitute a classical feedback system of physiological relevance.

Pregnancy, lactation, and to a lesser extent growth are associated with an exaggerated systemic requirement for calcium. A physiological increase in intestinal calcium absorption has been observed during the second and third trimesters of pregnancy as well as during lactation, and increased circulating concentrations of 1,25-$(OH)_2D$ have been demonstrated in pregnant and lactating animals and humans.[71,85,86] The hormonal mechanisms responsible for these increases in plasma 1,25-$(OH)_2D$ levels are not entirely understood and may include PTH, prolactin, and/or estrogen. There is disagreement as to whether a state of mild secondary hyperparathyroidism accompanies pregnancy.[85,86] Probably the most important source of 1,25-$(OH)_2D$ during pregnancy is the placenta itself.[87] For years, the prevailing view has been that pregnancy is a state of potentially negative maternal calcium balance because of the mineral demands of the developing fetus. In fact, this view may be incorrect, and placenta-derived 1,25-$(OH)_2D$ may lead to a state of physiological hyperabsorption of calcium which persists throughout pregnancy and is more than adequate to meet fetal mineral requirements.[86]

There are conflicting data concerning the effects of growth hormone and insulin on 1,25-$(OH)_2D$ synthesis, but recent studies indicate that neither hormone appears to influence 1-hydroxylase activity appreciably. Glucocorticoids may interfere with the biological effects of 1,25-$(OH)_2D$ but appear to have little or no effect on renal hydroxylase activity. Both strontium and high-dose diphosphonate (EHDP) administration have been noted to inhibit 1-hydroxylase activity, which may provide a partial explanation for the osteomalacia or rickets which may be observed with the use of these agents.

A synthesis of the data presented above into an integrated picture of the regulation of the renal production of 1,25-$(OH)_2D$ and 24,25-$(OH)_2D$ in vivo reveals that PTH, 1,25-$(OH)_2D$, and phosphate are the key determinants of renal hydroxylase activity, probably in that order. In all circumstances, the *critical point of biological control* and the rate-limiting step is the activity of the 1-hydroxylase. 24-hydroxylase activity appears to be largely if not entirely modulated by changes in the local concentration of 1,25-$(OH)_2D$ which result from alterations in 1-hydroxylase activity. The regulation of 1-hydroxylase activity by PTH is of prime importance in normal calcium homeostasis, and the parathyroid-renal axis has been considered by some investigators to be largely analogous to the pituitary-adrenal axis. That is, PTH is regarded as the major tropic hormone which controls the synthesis of 1,25-$(OH)_2D$ in its primary endocrine organ, the kidney. More extreme alterations in serum phosphorus appear to be required to exert a prominent influence on renal hydroxylase activity, yet this mechanism is of great potential homeostatic importance. Obviously, at any moment in time, net activity of the renal hydroxylases and the relative production rates of 1,25-$(OH)_2D$ and 24,25-$(OH)_2D$ are an integral function of the influence of all three factors on the activity of the enzymes.

A total of 20 metabolites of vitamin D have been

characterized chemically.[69–71] Nineteen of these metabolites have been identified in vivo in one or another species.[70] 25,26-$(OH)_2D$ is produced by a 26-hydroxylase which utilizes 25-OHD as a substrate. The enzyme is present in both the kidney and extrarenal tissues, and its function may be regulated by the vitamin D status of the organism. 25,26-$(OH)_2D$ does not appear to be metabolically active and has not been isolated from target tissues for vitamin D. The trihydroxy metabolite, 1,24,25-$(OH)_3D$, can be produced either by the hydroxylation of C-1 of 24,25-$(OH)_2D$ by the 1-hydroxylase or by the hydroxylation of C-24 of 1,25-$(OH)_2D$ by the 24-hydroxylase. In vivo, the synthesis of 1,24,25-$(OH)_3D$ from 1,25-$(OH)_2D$ is probably the more important pathway, since 1,25-$(OH)_2D$ induces the 24-hydroxylase which can use 1,25-$(OH)_2D$ as substrate. The functional significance of 1,24,25-$(OH)_3D$ is unclear. 1,24,25-$(OH)_3D$ has approximately one-third the activity of 1,25-$(OH)_2D$ in the intestine, and it is only marginally active in bone resorption; in both tissues, the effects of 1,24,25-$(OH)_3D$ are relatively short-lived. Many investigators favor the view that the hydroxylation of the vitamin D nucleus at C-24 represents a step in the direction of inactivation rather than activation, so that 24-hydroxylase activity in all tissues may constitute an important initial step in inactivation of the hormone.[69] An alternative view is that the hydroxyl group at C-24 may confer specific biological activity to the steroid nucleus, which differs from the activity inherent in 1,25-$(OH)_2D$.[70] The continuing debate concerning this issue is considered in the next section. Most of the remaining metabolites identified to date are products of side chain cleavage, lack vitamin D–like activity in conventional biological assays, and are regarded as intermediate or final degradation products.[69,71]

The kinetics and metabolism of the hydroxylated metabolites of vitamin D in vitro have been recently reviewed.[77] In normal individuals, 1,25-$(OH)_2D$ circulates with a half-time of approximately 12 to 15 h, has a metabolic clearance rate of about 35 ml/min, and is produced at a rate of approximately 2 μg per day.[77,78] The principal mechanisms of 1,25-$(OH)_2D$ clearance are side chain oxidation in its target tissues and hepatic metabolism and/or biliary excretion.[70,72] Biliary excretion of polar and substituted metabolites may account for as much as one-quarter of the total clearance of a tracer dose of 1,25-$(OH)_2D$ in humans.[77] Metabolites present in bile include vitamin D glucuronides and sulfates. There is an active enterohepatic circulation of vitamin D metabolites and biliary excretion products in humans, with some 20 percent of these metabolites and products normally being reabsorbed. This process may fail in patients with malabsorption syndromes and thus may contribute to the low levels of circulating vitamin D metabolites observed in these patients.[77] 24,25-$(OH)_2D$ circulates with a half-time of about 6 h and has a production rate of approximately 25 μg per day.[77] It is also cleared and metabolized by a combination of side chain oxidation and hepatic metabolic and biliary excretion.

Biological Effects and Mechanism of Action of Vitamin D

The classical target tissues for vitamin D action are the intestine, bone, and kidney. The regulation of intestinal mineral absorption by vitamin D is the most completely studied effect of vitamin D in the organism. There is general agreement that 1,25-$(OH)_2D$ is the principal metabolite of vitamin D which regulates intestinal absorption and bone resorption. Whether other hydroxylated metabolites of vitamin D, particularly 24,25-$(OH)_2D$, may have physiologically important actions in bone or kidney remains unclear. Because of the importance of the effects of 1,25-$(OH)_2D$ on intestinal absorption, the initial portion of this section is given to a complete description of intestinal mineral absorption.

INTESTINAL ABSORPTION OF CALCIUM AND PHOSPHORUS

The ultimate source of calcium and phosphorus required for normal metabolic and structural mineral homeostasis is the diet. The absorption of these elements is controlled by highly regulated mechanisms in the specialized absorptive cells of the intestine.[88,89] These cells have a distinct polarity: Their luminal surfaces are covered by an extensive brush border, their basal-lateral membranes are relatively smooth, and the cells are locked together by tight junctions in the apical areas of adjacent cells. The microvilli on the luminal surfaces of the cells are continuously covered by an anionic mucopolysaccharide coat, the glycocalyx. The discussion below is confined to the absorption of calcium and phosphorus at the cellular and organ level; overall mineral balance is discussed in the subsequent section.

Calcium is absorbed throughout the intestinal tract by the combined processes of passive diffusion and active transport (Fig. 23-20). The net absorption of calcium in the intestinal segments proceeds in the following quantitative sequence: ileum (60 percent) > jejunum (20 percent) > duodenum (10 percent) > colon (8 percent) > stomach (2 percent). The *rate* of calcium absorption (quantity absorbed/length) is actually highest in the duodenum, and the greater length

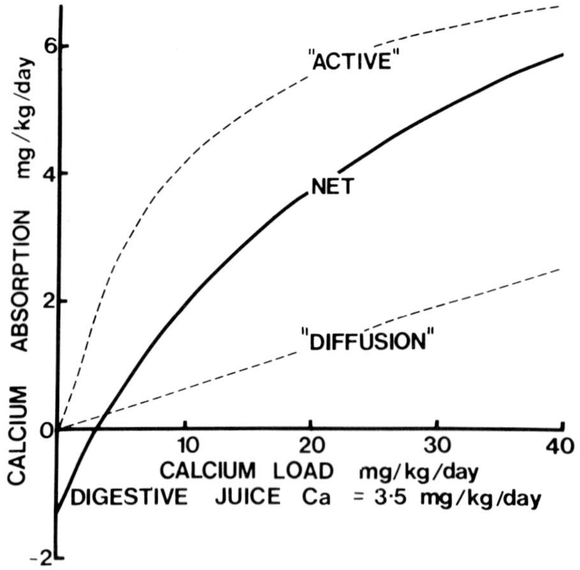

FIGURE 23-20 The active and diffusional components of true calcium absorption in normal humans. The data are derived from balance studies in normal subjects, and the curves are generated from computerized models. Net calcium absorption is true absorption minus endogenous fecal calcium (digestive juice calcium). [*By permission of Marshall DH, in Nordin BEC (ed): Calcium, Phosphate and Magnesium Metabolism. London, Churchill Livingstone, 1976.*]

of the ileum accounts for its major role in calcium absorption. Peak calcium absorption in humans occurs approximately 3 to 4 h after oral calcium administration.

The diffusional component of calcium absorption is concentration-dependent, nonsaturable, and of limited quantitative importance at physiological levels of calcium intake. There is a downhill concentration gradient for calcium across the brush-border membrane, but a transcellular downhill gradient for calcium exists only at very high concentrations of calcium in the intestinal contents (Fig. 23-21). At a normal calcium intake of approximately 1000 mg per day, only about 15 percent of the true calcium absorption in a normal individual proceeds by passive diffusion (Fig. 23-20). In the absence of the active component of calcium absorption, the diffusional component is inadequate to subserve systemic demands for calcium. Phosphate (as HPO_4^{2-}) normally accompanies calcium during diffusion.

The active component of calcium absorption is saturable, carrier-mediated, and the dominant calcium transport process at physiological concentrations of calcium in the intestinal contents (Fig. 23-20). At a cellular level, the active transport of calcium can be subdivided into several interrelated constituent parts: (1) transport at the brush-border membrane, (2) movement and/or storage of calcium within the cell, and (3) transport at the basal-lateral membrane (Fig. 23-21). The initial step in calcium transport is probably the attraction of calcium to the anionic glycocalyx. In all circumstances, the transport of calcium at the brush-border membrane is the rate-limiting step in the overall transport sequence. The exact nature of the transport step in the brush-border membrane is not known, but it is this process which is finely and ultimately regulated by 1,25-$(OH)_2$D. Both alkaline phosphatase and calcium-dependent ATPase activities can be detected in the brush-border membrane of

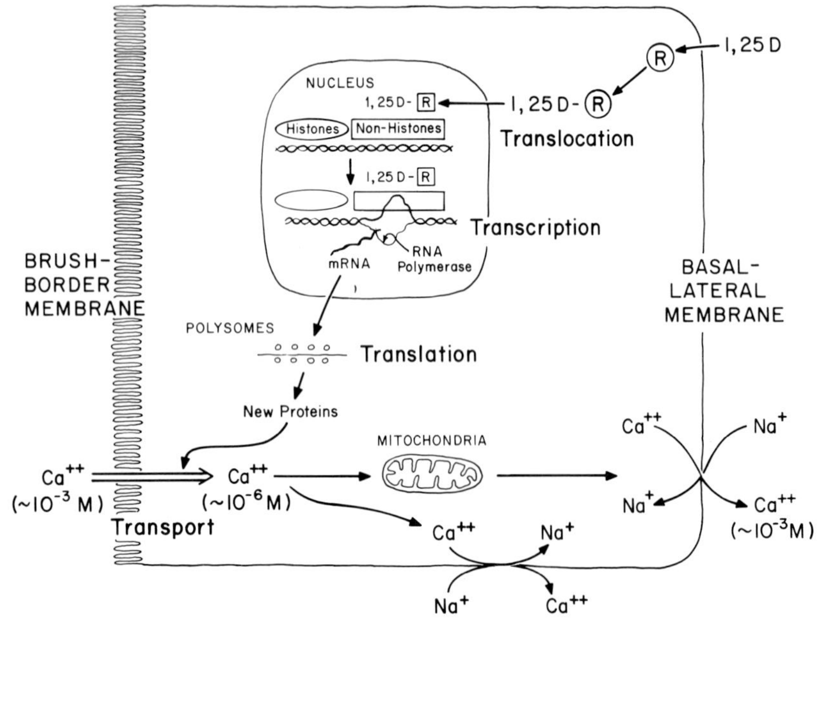

FIGURE 23-21 Mechanism of action of 1,25-$(OH)_2$D in the intestinal mucosa cell. Ⓡ represents the cytosol receptor for 1,25-$(OH)_2$D, and 1,25D-R represents the 1,25-$(OH)_2$D chromatin–associated receptor. The approximate molar concentrations of free calcium ions in the cytosol and at the luminal and basal surfaces of the cell are indicated in parentheses. (*Modified from Haussler and McCain.*[71])

intestinal cells, but current evidence suggests that these activities can be dissociated from calcium transport. A vitamin D–dependent or inducible high-affinity *calcium-binding protein* has been identified in intestinal cells of a wide variety of species. The calcium-binding protein in human intestinal cells has a molecular weight of approximately 15,000 and possesses four high-affinity calcium-binding sites (affinity constant about 10^{-6} M) per molecule. It was initially thought that this protein might associate with the brush-border membrane and serve as the actual carrier mediating calcium transport. However, it is now known that the calcium-binding protein is primarily a cytosolic rather than a membrane-associated protein. Experimental changes in its concentration can be dissociated from induced changes in calcium transport, and so it is unlikely that the protein functions in exactly this fashion.[70] Nevertheless, there is much experimental evidence which indicates that the calcium-binding protein plays a significant role in vitamin D–mediated calcium transport.[70,89] One such role may be to serve as a buffer or "shuttle" in the complex system of cytosolic transfer of calcium. The cytosolic concentration of calcium ions has been estimated to be in the range of 10^{-6} M, or several orders of magnitude lower than the concentration of ionized calcium at the luminal and intestinal surfaces of the cell. Thus, the bulk of cytosolic calcium must be sequestered and/or bound. The principal site of sequestration of calcium within the intestinal cell is the mitochondrion, and the principal binding component in the cytosol appears to be the calcium-binding protein. It is likely that the mitochondria and the calcium-binding protein combine to provide an orderly system of cytosolic transfer of calcium between the luminal and basal-lateral membranes; this accomplishes translocation of calcium without perturbing the delicate cytosolic concentration of free calcium ions. At the basal-lateral membrane, calcium is actively transported against an uphill calcium concentration gradient by means of a calcium-sodium cotransport system (Fig. 23-21). This system does not appear to be biologically regulated. The transmembrane sodium gradient at the basal-lateral membrane is maintained by a separate Na/K-dependent ATPase in the basal membrane. Although calcium can be shown to be translocated across the intestinal cell independently of phosphorus transport, phosphate (as HPO_4^{2-}) is the anionic species which normally accompanies calcium.

The ultimate quantitative result of intestinal calcium absorption requires the consideration of several variables and can be expressed as several different quantities. *True* calcium absorption is the sum of the diffusional and active components of calcium transport across the intestine. Calcium is actively secreted into the intestinal lumen in the digestive secretions of the gastrointestinal tract, and this quantity, termed the *endogenous fecal calcium,* can be estimated by the appearance of intravenously administered radiocalcium in the feces. Therefore, the *net* calcium absorption is the *total* calcium absorption minus the *endogenous fecal calcium* (Fig. 23-20). Any of these quantities can be expressed either as a fractional or a percentage absorption or as an absolute quantity or rate. Obviously, the net calcium absorption is also equivalent to the dietary intake of calcium minus the fecal excretion of calcium. In a normal individual consuming 1000 mg of calcium daily, true calcium absorption is approximately 300 mg per day, endogenous fecal calcium is approximately 125 mg per day, and net calcium is approximately 175 mg per day. Thus, net calcium absorption normally averages about 20 percent of calcium intake.

The absorption of *phosphorus* from the diet is less rigidly regulated than the absorption of calcium, and net intestinal absorption of phosphorus in humans is a linear function of dietary phosphorus intake.[89] Approximately 60 percent of ingested phosphorus is absorbed over the normal range of dietary phosphorus intake. Thus, there are two distinctive differences in the way the intestine handles dietary calcium and phosphorus: (1) The percentage net absorption of phosphorus is approximately three times higher than is that of calcium, and (2) an apparently nonsaturable process plays the dominant role in phosphorus absorption, whereas calcium absorption is rigidly regulated by a dominant, saturable transport process. The efficiency of intestinal phosphorus absorption, together with the ubiquitous occurrence of inorganic and organic phosphates in foodstuffs, explains the relative rarity of dietary deficiency as a cause of phosphorus depletion in humans. The linear relation between net phosphorus absorption and dietary phosphorus intake also accounts for the wide fluctuations in the serum phosphorus concentration which accompany feeding. Peak phosphorus absorption in humans occurs approximately 3 h after oral phosphorus administration. The terms *true phosphorus absorption, net phosphorus absorption,* and *endogenous fecal phosphorus* represent the same conceptual and quantitative relations described above for calcium. In a normal individual consuming 1400 mg of phosphorus daily, true phosphorus absorption is approximately 1100 mg per day, endogenous fecal phosphorus is approximately 200 mg per day, and net phosphorus absorption is approximately 900 mg per day. Phosphorus is absorbed from the intestinal contents mostly as orthophosphate. The phosphorus present in foodstuffs as phosphoproteins, phospholipids, and phosphosugars is absorbed following hydrolysis of these dietary constituents.

Phosphorus is transported throughout the intestinal tract in the following quantitative sequence: ileum (38 percent) > duodenum (29 percent) > jejunum (25 percent) > colon (8 percent). As is the case with calcium, the rate of phosphorus transport is highest in the duodenum, but a greater quantity of phosphorus is absorbed in the ileum because of its greater length.

Phosphorus absorption can be considered to be similar to calcium absorption in that it proceeds by means of the combined processes of passive diffusion and active transport. The linear relation between phosphorus intake and phosphorus absorption initially suggested that passive diffusion was the dominant process in phosphorus absorption, but recent studies do not support this conclusion. The active transport component of phosphorus absorption is concentrative, energy-dependent, and carrier-mediated. This component is both a high-affinity and a high-capacity system so that, considered in absolute terms or on a molar concentration basis, the net absorption of phosphate is two to three times greater than net calcium absorption at any given concentration of the two ions in the luminal contents. Stated in another fashion, the capacity of the active phosphate component and the concentration required for half saturation are much greater than is the case with calcium. The phosphate diffusional system is a low-affinity system which is only of quantitative importance at high mucosal phosphate concentrations. It is the active transport system for phosphorus which is responsive to 1,25-$(OH)_2D$.

The intimate details of phosphate transport at the cellular level are largely unknown. Although calcium absorption and phosphorus absorption tend to accompany each other to an extent, each transport system can be demonstrated and/or manipulated independently of the other system. Phosphorus is transported as orthophosphate, which appears to be translocated across the cell in a directed fashion and does not admix with the total cellular pool of inorganic phosphate. The active system is sodium-dependent and inhibitable by ouabain, suggesting that the process may be a brush-border system similar to the phosphate-sodium cotransport system in the proximal renal tubule. No specific phosphate-binding protein has been identified. Intestinal alkaline phosphatase activity can be shown to vary in parallel with phosphorus absorption, but the exact involvement of this enzyme in phosphate transport remains unknown.

Magnesium absorption is considered in Systemic Magnesium Homeostasis, below.

EFFECTS OF VITAMIN D IN THE INTESTINE

A wide variety of effects of vitamin D in the intestine have been demonstrated. It was from its target cells in the intestinal mucosa that 1,25-$(OH)_2D$ was initially isolated. The hormone increases the absorption of calcium and phosphorus, stimulates the formation of the high-affinity calcium-binding protein, and leads to increased activities of alkaline phosphatase and calcium-dependent ATPase in the mucosal cell. All these effects can be blocked by inhibitors of transcription or protein synthesis. Maximal effects are observed approximately 20 h after administration of calciferol and approximately 2 to 4 h after administration of 1,25-$(OH)_2D$. The prolonged time lag following calciferol administration is a reflection of the sequential steps required for its "activation," and the time lag noted after 1,25-$(OH)_2D$ administration is in keeping with the mechanism of action of 1,25-$(OH)_2D$ as a steroid hormone.

The proposed mechanism of 1,25-$(OH)_2D$ action in the intestinal mucosal cell is illustrated in Fig. 23-21. After it crosses the basal-lateral membrane, the initial step in 1,25-$(OH)_2D$ action is binding to a high-affinity vitamin D receptor protein in the cytosol.[69-71] The cytosol receptor protein in human intestine sediments at 3.5 S on sucrose gradients and has a molecular weight of approximately 70,000. It has a low capacity and a high affinity ($K_d \cong 10^{-10}$ M) for 1,25-$(OH)_2D$. Competition studies have revealed an excellent correlation between the biological potency of the vitamin D metabolites and their relative ability to bind to the receptor protein. Compared with 1,25-$(OH)_2D$, the relative affinities of these metabolites for receptor binding are approximately 1:3 for 1,24,25-$(OH)_3D$, 1:1000 for 25-OHD, 1:1500 for 24,25-$(OH)_2D$, and 1:1,000,000 for the parent vitamin D. The 1,25-$(OH)_2D$–receptor complex is *translocated* to the nucleus of the mucosal cell, where it associates with nonhistone chromatin proteins. The nuclear binding is saturable and proceeds rapidly, reaching a half-maximal level 30 min after 1,25-$(OH)_2D$ is added to in vitro systems. The nuclear binding of the receptor complex leads to the stimulation of DNA-dependent RNA polymerase II, the enzyme responsible for synthesis of messenger RNA. The net result is the *transcription* of specific messenger RNAs which code for the particular vitamin D–dependent proteins induced by the hormone. The *translation* of these protein products is maximal 2 to 3 h after 1,25-$(OH)_2D$ administration. These protein products include calcium-binding protein, alkaline phosphatase, the calcium-dependent ATPase, and a number of membrane-associated proteins.[70]

As described previously, the exact biochemical events leading to a stimulation of the rate-limiting calcium transport in the brush-border membrane are not known. The proposed mechanism above implies that 1,25-$(OH)_2D$ may induce the synthesis of a membrane protein or an enzyme which phosphorylates or otherwise alters the transport function of a membrane-bound protein. Recent data, however, indicate that 1,25-$(OH)_2D$ stimulates calcium transport at the brush border by a mechanism which is independent of protein synthesis and may result from an alteration in membrane lipid structure.[90] There are other effects of 1,25-$(OH)_2D$ in the mucosal cell which are considered to be too rapid to be mediated by transcription.[70] How the various 1,25-$(OH)_2D$–sensitive subcellular steps are integrated into the final process of cellular calcium translocation has not been clarified.

There is general agreement that the active transport component of calcium absorption is entirely under the control of 1,25-$(OH)_2D$. PTH and calcitonin have no direct influence on intestinal calcium absorption. In the absence of 1,25-$(OH)_2D$, active calcium transport cannot be demonstrated, and calcium is absorbed in the intestine only by means of simple diffusion. There are conflicting data as to whether 1,25-$(OH)_2D$ also stimulates the diffusional component of calcium absorption, but the predominance of the active component of calcium absorption limits the quantitative importance of such a potential effect. In essence, 1,25-$(OH)_2D$ is the key hormonal link in calcium homeostasis vis-à-vis the environment, and the absence of the effects of vitamin D in the intestine leads to calcium malabsorption and a state of negative calcium balance. In the aggregate, the PTH–1,25-$(OH)_2D$ axis represents the "endogenous factor" postulated in the 1940s to account for the ability of the organism to adjust the efficiency of intestinal calcium absorption to meet systemic needs for calcium.

1,25-$(OH)_2D$ also leads to an increase in active phosphate transport in the intestine, but at all levels this process is less well understood than are the effects of the hormone on calcium transport. The process is clearly independent of active calcium transport, although a certain quantity of orthophosphate appears to be cotransported with calcium. The general mechanism of 1,25-$(OH)_2D$ action in the mucosal cell presumably leads to a protein product or an alteration in membrane structure which increases phosphate-sodium cotransport in the brush-border membrane. Whether the enhanced intestinal alkaline phosphatase activity noted in response to 1,25-$(OH)_2D$ treatment is important in this regard is not known. Vitamin D deficiency is associated with an impairment in intestinal phosphorus absorption, which is readily reversed by means of vitamin D repletion. However, the net absorption of phosphorus in the intestine appears to be less strictly dependent on the transport effects of 1,25-$(OH)_2D$ than is the case with calcium; thus, even in vitamin D deficiency, phosphorus absorption may proceed at 50 percent or more of the normal rate.

EFFECTS OF VITAMIN D ON BONE

The cellular and physiological aspects of bone resorption, formation, and mineralization and the tight coupling of these events in normal bone were described in a previous section. Historically, vitamin D was discovered as a consequence of the bone disease caused by its deficiency. The histological hallmark of rickets and osteomalacia is an increase in unmineralized osteoid; that is, the principal defect in vitamin D deficiency is a failure of normal mineralization.[3,36,37,91] Prolonged vitamin D deficiency is also associated with a reduction in bone formation and linear growth. Attempts to demonstrate direct effects of vitamin D or its metabolites on the mineralization process, however, have been largely unsuccessful, in contrast to the readily demonstrable effects of vitamin D on intestinal calcium and phosphorus absorption and mineral mobilization from bone. Thus, the classical view has evolved that vitamin D [as 1,25-$(OH)_2D$] participates with PTH in regulating bone resorption but that bone mineralization is a passive phenomenon which proceeds normally given an adequate calcium $\times$ phosphate product in the extracellular fluids. Simply stated, this viewpoint holds that the key role of vitamin D in skeletal homeostasis is indirect and is a consequence of the influence of vitamin D on systemic calcium and phosphorus homeostasis. A number of lines of evidence have been marshaled in support of this classical viewpoint:

1. Rachitic cartilage will mineralize in vitro when incubated in buffers containing adequate concentrations of calcium and phosphate.
2. The infusion of calcium and phosphate into vitamin D–deficient humans sufficient to normalize the mineral ion product is associated with remineralization of bone.
3. The administration of vitamin D to experimental animals made deficient in both vitamin D and calcium leads to mineral mobilization from old bone and mineralization of new osteoid even in the absence of calcium repletion.

The major unsettled issues concerning the influence of vitamin D on bone do not threaten the foundation of the classical viewpoint but rather raise certain questions as to whether this relatively simple concept is adequate to explain all aspects of the effects of the hormone on bone metabolism. The relevant issues are basically two: (1) whether the hydroxylated metabolites of vitamin D directly influence bone formation and mineralization as well as bone resorption and (2) whether vitamin D metabolites other than 1,25-$(OH)_2D$ are important in skeletal metabolism.

In organ cultures and other in vitro systems, both 25-OHD and 1,25-$(OH)_2D$ possess bone resorptive activity, with 1,25-$(OH)_2D$ being 100 to several thousand times more potent than 25-OHD, depending on the system employed.[36,69] The older literature concluded that effects of vitamin D on bone mineral mobilization in vivo could not be demonstrated in the absence of PTH. More recent studies, however, have conclusively demonstrated that 1,25-$(OH)_2D$ administration leads to bone resorption both in vitro and in parathyroidectomized animals, and the older negative findings may have resulted from an inadequate pool of bone mineral for mobilization. Nevertheless, PTH and 1,25-$(OH)_2D$ clearly potentiate each other in bone resorption, and a maximal rate of resorption is observed only in response to the combined effects of both hormones. One proposal to explain these findings is that 1,25-$(OH)_2D$ may stimulate osteocytic osteolysis and bone resorption by preformed osteoclasts but that the recruitment of new osteoclasts with the involvement of a larger bone surface in the resorptive process is exclusively the domain of PTH. This proposal is supported by the observation that the administration of 1,25-$(OH)_2D$ to patients with hypoparathyroidism does not result in an increase in osteoclast numbers in bone.[91] However, 1,25-$(OH)_2D$ receptors have been identified in cells of monocyte-macrophage lineage, and it has been proposed that 1,25-$(OH)_2D$ may stimulate bone resorption by these cells and/or lead to their fusion to form new osteoclasts.[38,39] Clearly, the intimate details of the exact roles of PTH and 1,25-$(OH)_2D$, as well as their synergism, in controlling bone resorption have not been worked out.

From a strictly clinical viewpoint, the importance of 1,25-$(OH)_2D$–mediated bone resorption in a given patient or condition may be to some extent dose-related. For example, modest elevations in circulating 1,25-$(OH)_2D$ in the range of 70 pg/ml (e.g., in a patient with absorptive hypercalciuria) are not associated with hypercalcemia, whereas marked elevations of the hormone in the range of 125 pg/ml (e.g., in a patient with sarcoidosis) are regularly associated with hypercalcemia.

Whether the hydroxylated vitamin D metabolites directly influence bone formation and/or mineralization is not clear. By definition, bone formation outstrips mineralization in vitamin D deficiency, but the rate of bone formation is also retarded in vitamin D–deficient states. The histological appearance of osteoblasts is decidedly abnormal in vitamin D–deficient humans.[91] Vitamin D repletion in humans is accompanied by an increase in serum alkaline phosphatase activity as well as histological evidence of increased bone formation.[91] It has been noted that the mineralization which occurs with an adequate mineral ion product but in the absence of vitamin D is patchy and disordered, in contrast to the orderly mineralization process which occurs with vitamin D repletion.[91] It has therefore been postulated that mineralization may be a cell-directed event, perhaps resulting from the effects of an unknown vitamin D metabolite on osteoid osteocytes or chondrocytes. Osteoblasts and osteoblast-like cells contain receptors for 1,25-$(OH)_2D$.[36,69,70] 1,25-$(OH)_2D$ appears to stimulate osteocalcin synthesis by these cells, but it also inhibits the synthesis of collagen and alkaline phosphatase in vitro.[36] These latter findings are difficult to reconcile with the reported effects of vitamin D in vivo and are among several observations that have led investigators to suggest that if indeed there is a direct vitamin D effect on bone formation and mineralization, it is likely to be mediated by a metabolite other than 1,25-$(OH)_2D$.

One candidate for such a role is 24,25-$(OH)_2D$. The putative role of 24,25-$(OH)_2D$ in the aggregate effects of vitamin D in the organism is as hotly debated as any issue in the vitamin D field.[36,69,70] Receptors for 24,25-$(OH)_2D$ have been reported in bone,[36,70] and anabolic effects in cultured chondrocytes have been demonstrated in response to concentrations of 24,25-$(OH)_2D$ in the range of 10^{-12} M.[70] It has also been reported that a combination of 1,25-$(OH)_2D$ and 24,25-$(OH)_2D$ is required to achieve normal or nearly normal mineralization of bone in vitamin D–deficient humans and patients with renal osteodystrophy and that a similar combination is needed to confer normal hatchability to eggs from vitamin D–deficient chickens.[70] However, analogues of vitamin D which are fluorinated at ^{24}C and therefore incapable of being 24-hydroxylated have been reported to be fully active in mobilizing bone mineral, preventing rickets, and maintaining growth in vivo. These findings have been taken as conclusive evidence that the presence of a hydroxyl group at the C-24 position confers no specific biological effects on the steroid nucleus of vitamin D.[69] Additional details concerning this debate are available in several recent reviews.[69,70]

EFFECTS OF VITAMIN D ON THE KIDNEY

When administered to rachitic animals, vitamin D leads to an increase in the renal tubular reabsorption of phosphorus and calcium.[42] In these circumstances, the vitamin D–induced increase in TmP/GFR results, at least in part, from a reversal of the state of secondary hyperparathyroidism which accompanies rickets, but the reduction in calcium excretion appears to occur before a significant readjustment in serum calcium is observed. In the treatment of hypoparathyroidism, vitamin D reduces TmP/GFR from elevated to normal values. In this setting, the reduction in TmP/GFR is largely the result of vitamin D–induced increases in serum calcium concentrations, since an increase in serum calcium to normal levels directly reduces proximal tubular phosphorus reabsorption.

Vitamin D and its metabolites do not appear to directly influence TmP/GFR.[44] However, 1,25-$(OH)_2D$ may affect the inherent ability of the kidney to adapt to alterations in phosphorus intake. As noted previously and in subsequent sections, even in the absence of PTH, the renal tubule appears to be capable of adjusting the TmP/GFR as an inverse function of phosphorus intake; this process is a slow (days) but important mechanism for maintaining normal phosphorus homeostasis. This adaptive process appears to proceed more efficiently in vitamin D–replete than in vitamin D–deficient animals.[44,92]

The evidence for an influence of vitamin D on renal tubular calcium excretion is convincing. In experiments in which all variables were controlled except the vitamin D status of the animals, the fractional excretion of calcium was higher in vitamin D–deficient than in vitamin D–replete rats.[93] Furthermore, the vitamin D–deficient animals were relatively resistant to the hypocalciuric effects of PTH so that an entirely normal pattern of control of fractional calcium excretion appeared to require both vitamin D and PTH.[93] These observations fit nicely with the recent demonstration of the vitamin D–inducible calcium-binding protein exclusively in the distal convoluted tubule and collecting duct, the known sites of PTH-mediated calcium reabsorption.[70]

It should be noted that the effects of vitamin D or its metabolites on renal tubular phosphate and calcium reabsorption have been demonstrated only in an experimental setting of vitamin D–deficient vs. vitamin D–replete animals. It follows that such effects may be relevant to the syndromes of vitamin D deficiency or resistance, but it is not implied that vitamin D metabolites are involved in the fine tuning of the renal tubular handling of phosphate and calcium on a minute-to-minute basis in normal physiological conditions.

EFFECTS OF VITAMIN D ON OTHER TISSUES

The most remarkable development in vitamin D research in recent years has been the demonstration of 1,25-$(OH)_2D$ receptors in a wide variety of tissues and cell types not regarded as classical target sites for vitamin D action. 1,25-$(OH)_2D$ receptors have been identified in the colon, pancreas, pituitary, ovary, testes, parotid gland, skin, breast, uterus, and thymus, as well as in a variety of cultured cell lines, mostly transformed cells.[69,70,76] These receptors have been identified by chemical means (e.g., sucrose density gradient analysis) as well as by the autoradiographic demonstration of specific localization of tritium-labeled 1,25-$(OH)_2D$ of high specific radioactivity in these same tissues.[69,70] In addition, a tight correlation between the presence of 1,25-$(OH)_2D$ receptors and the vitamin D–dependent calcium-binding protein has been observed.[70] Thus the biological effects of vitamin D are envisioned as extending well beyond its conventional role in regulating mineral metabolism. This area of investigation is beyond the scope of this chapter.

INTEGRATED CONTROL OF MINERAL HOMEOSTASIS

Previous sections have described mineral metabolism at the cellular and organ level and the regulation of these processes by PTH, calcitonin, and vitamin D. The discussion below integrates these processes at the level of the intact organism and describes the fine set of checks and balances which regulates mineral homeostasis in vivo.

Normal Mineral Homeostasis and Balance

Balance refers to the state of mineral homeostasis in the organism vis-à-vis the environment. In zero balance, mineral intake and accretion exactly match mineral losses. In positive balance, mineral intake and accretion exceed mineral losses; for example, a growing child is in positive mineral balance. In negative balance, mineral intake and accretion are less than mineral losses; for example, an immobilized patient is in negative mineral balance.

Figure 23-22 is a schematic representation of calcium, phosphorus, and magnesium metabolism in a normal adult who is consuming an average diet and is in zero mineral balance.

The total extracellular pool of calcium is approximately 900 mg. This pool is in dynamic equilibrium, with calcium entering and exiting via the intestine, bone, and renal tubule. In zero balance, bone resorption and formation are equivalent, and the net quantity of calcium absorbed by the intestine, approximately 175 mg per day, is quantitatively excreted into the urine. Therefore, in normal circumstances net calcium absorption provides a surplus of calcium which considerably exceeds systemic requirements. At middle age and beyond, normal adults lose approximately 1 percent of their skeletons yearly; this is the equivalent of a calcium loss of approximately 25 mg per day.

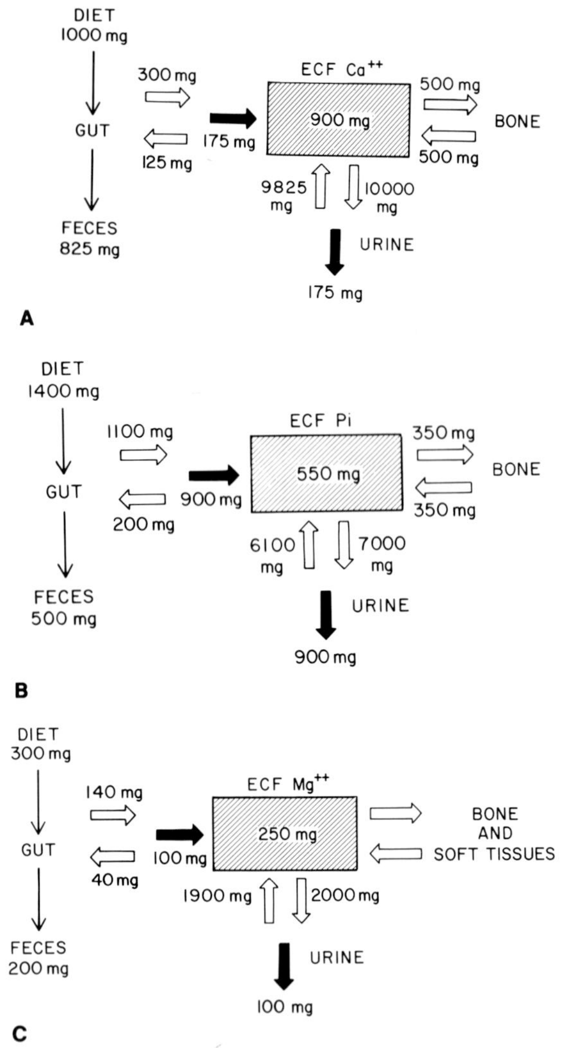

FIGURE 23-22 Schemata of (*A*) calcium, (*B*) phosphorus, and (*C*) magnesium metabolism in a normal human adult in zero mineral balance. The open arrows denote unidirectional mineral fluxes, and the solid arrows denote net fluxes.

The extracellular pool of orthophosphate is approximately 550 mg (Fig. 23-22*B*). This pool is in dynamic equilibrium with phosphorus entry and exit via the intestine, bone, kidney, and soft tissues (not depicted in the figure). In zero balance, fractional net phosphorus absorption is about two-thirds of phosphorus intake; this amount represents a vast excess over systemic requirements and is quantitatively excreted into the urine.

The extracellular pool of magnesium is approximately 250 mg and is in bidirectional equilibrium with magnesium fluxes across the intestine, kidney, bone, and soft tissues (Fig. 23-22C). In zero balance, the magnesium derived from net intestinal absorption, approximately 100 mg per day, represents a considerable systemic surplus and is quantitatively excreted.

In aggregate, the schemata in Fig. 23-22 emphasize two major points: (1) the dominant quantitative role played by the renal tubules in the maintenance of normal mineral homeostasis and (2) the fact that in normal circumstances, hormonal and/or intrinsic mechanisms of mineral absorption provide the organism with a mineral supply which considerably exceeds systemic mineral needs. Within this framework, minor fluctuations in systemic mineral requirements are easily met by the surfeit of normal mineral absorption and do not require hormonal adjustments.

Systemic Calcium Homeostasis

MAINTENANCE OF A NORMAL SERUM CALCIUM

The parathyroid glands are exquisitely sensitive to minor changes in serum ionized calcium (Fig. 23-4). The integrated actions of parathyroid hormone on bone resorption, distal tubular calcium reabsorption, and 1,25-$(OH)_2$D–mediated intestinal calcium absorption are responsible for the fine regulation of serum ionized calcium in humans (see Figs. 23-8 and 23-20, respectively). The precision of this integrated control is such that in a normal individual, ionized serum calcium probably fluctuates by no more than 0.1 mg/dl in either direction from its "set" normal value throughout the day. The "acute" phases of bone resorption and distal tubular calcium reabsorption are the major control points in minute-to-minute serum calcium homeostasis; of these two processes, the effect of PTH on the distal tubule is quantitatively the most important. Together, these effects constitute a classical "short-loop" feedback system. Adjustments in the rate of intestinal calcium absorption via the PTH–1,25-$(OH)_2$D axis require approximately 24 to 48 h to become maximal. This axis represents a classical "long-loop" feedback system.

DEFENSE AGAINST HYPOCALCEMIA

Figure 23-23 illustrates the sequence of events which is initiated in response to a hypocalcemic challenge. Several examples of such a challenge will be discussed: (1) a minor, transient challenge, (2) a moderate challenge, and (3) a severe, prolonged challenge.

A 12- to 15-h fast in a normal individual represents a minor physiological hypocalcemic challenge which requires only subtle hormonal readjustments for correction. The total quantity of calcium lost into the urine during this time is in the range of 50 to 75

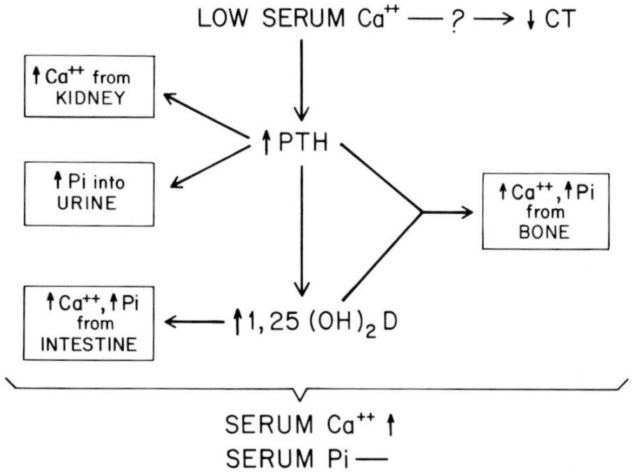

FIGURE 23-23 The sequence of adjustments initiated in response to hypocalcemia.

mg. An unmeasureable fall in serum calcium occurs, leading to a slight increase in PTH secretion. The dip in serum calcium is corrected by an increased efficiency of calcium reclamation in the distal tubule and by the rapid resorptive response to PTH in bone; by 12 h, only minor increases in 1,25-$(OH)_2D$ synthesis will have occurred.

An abrupt reduction in dietary calcium intake to less than 100 mg per day or the administration of 80 mg of furosemide daily to a normal individual represent moderate hypocalcemic challenges; in each case, the initial balance deficit of calcium is in the range of 100 to 150 mg per day.[81] A series of adjustments occurs, leading to a new steady state by 48 h. A moderate increase in the secretion rate of PTH results in (1) increased calcium reabsorption from the distal tubule, (2) increased mobilization of calcium and phosphorus from bone, and (3) increased synthesis of 1,25-$(OH)_2D$, which participates with PTH in bone resorption and increases the efficiency of calcium and phosphorus absorption in the intestine. The increased circulating concentration of PTH resets TmP/GFR at a lower level so that the increased amount of phosphorus mobiized from bone and absorbed from the intestine is quantitatively excreted into the urine. In the new steady state, serum calcium has returned to normal, serum phosphorus is unchanged or slightly reduced, and a state of mild secondary hyperparathyroidism and efficient intestinal mineral absorption exists. At this point, the initial requirement for calcium mobilization from the skeleton is largely replaced by the enhanced absorption of calcium in the intestine.

Complete calcium malabsorption represents a severe, prolonged hypocalcemic challenge. Assuming adequate exposure to sunlight, vitamin D deficiency does not necessarily accompany intestinal malabsorption. The sequence of events described above would ensue, but the malabsorption would prevent the compensation of calcium losses by the stimulation of calcium absorption by the PTH–1,25-$(OH)_2D$ axis. At this point, the compensatory sequence would include (1) a maximal PTH secretion rate of approximately five times normal, (2) a maximal rate of 1,25-$(OH)_2D$ synthesis, and (3) a maximal "rapid" phase and the initiation of the "late" phase of bone resorption in response to the combined effects of PTH and 1,25-$(OH)_2D$. Continued hypocalcemia would ultimately lead to gross hyperplasia of the parathyroid glands, with increases in the PTH secretion rate up to 10 to 50 times normal. The high circulating concentrations of PTH would result in the recruitment of an increasingly large pool of osteoclasts and the incorporation of a substantial bone surface into the resorption process. In the final steady state, serum calcium would be maintained in the range of 8.5 mg/dl at the expense of the skeleton, and clinical osteomalacia would ultimately ensue. This example represents a circumstance in which the integrity of skeletal mineral homeostasis is sacrificed in an attempt to compensate for systemic mineral deficits.

DEFENSE AGAINST HYPERCALCEMIA

The systemic mechanisms for the prevention of hypercalcemia consist largely of a reversal of the sequence just described, namely, an inhibition of PTH and 1,25-$(OH)_2D$ synthesis, with a reduction in calcium mobilization from bone, absorption from the intestine, and reclamation from the distal renal tubules. Whether the putative effects of calcitonin are of pathophysiological importance in humans remains unclear.

The bottleneck in the defense against hypercalcemia is the limited capacity of the kidneys to excrete calcium. In theory, normal kidneys can excrete a calcium load of 1000 mg or more per day. In practice, calcium excretion rates in this range are rarely seen. Limitations in the theoretical ability of the kidney to combat hypercalcemia include (1) the fact that abnormalities in distal tubular reabsorption are actually involved in the genesis of hypercalcemia in a number of conditions (e.g., familial hypocalciuric hypercalcemia, primary hyperparathyroidism, and thiazide-associated hypercalcemia), (2) the fact that a degree of renal impairment frequently accompanies many hypercalcemic conditions (in part, this may result from the effects of hypercalcemia per se), and (3) the fact that an increased calcium concentration inhibits the ability of the renal tubule to conserve water, which may lead to a vicious cycle of dehydration, prerenal azotemia, and worsening hypercalcemia. The importance of each of these limitations in the ability of the kidney to excrete calcium varies considerably, depending on the specific hypercalcemic condition, but one or more of these limitations can usually be demonstrated in any given patient with hypercalcemia.

Several examples of a hypercalcemic challenge will be discussed: (1) a trivial, transient challenge, (2) a moderate challenge, and (3) a severe, prolonged challenge.

A normal individual in zero calcium balance absorbs 50 to 75 mg of calcium over a 4- to 6-h period following a normal calcium-containing meal (approximately 300 mg of calcium). Although this rate of absorption is associated with a change in serum ionized calcium concentration $\leq$ 0.1 mg/dl, parathyroid function is suppressed by 30 percent or more.[94] The principal result of this suppression is a decrease in distal tubular calcium reabsorption so that the postprandial increase in the filtered load of calcium is "spilled" into the urine. This example is an excellent illustration of the exquisite sensitivity of the calcium-parathyroid axis in normal circumstances.

Patients with active clinical sarcoidosis often have associated hypercalciuria and, occasionally, frank hypercalcemia. In these patients, an increase in circulating 1,25-$(OH)_2D$ results from an unregulated conversion of 25-OHD to 1,25-$(OH)_2D$ in diseased macrophages; the "normal" PTH–1,25-$(OH)_2D$ axis is appropriately suppressed. The average patient of this type may absorb 400 mg of calcium daily from the intestine and mobilize an additional 100 mg of calcium daily from the skeleton; this load of calcium is filtered and quantitatively excreted, leading to hypercalciuria without the development of hypercalcemia. Hypercalcemia ensues only if the net absorbed and mobilized load of calcium exceeds the threshold of the kidney for calcium excretion and/or if there is associated nephrocalcinosis, which reduces this threshold. Patients with moderate to severe "absorptive" hypercalciuria present a relatively similar pathophysiological picture; in both conditions, mild postprandial hypercalcemia may be demonstrated in hypercalciuric patients with fasting normocalcemia.

A patient with advanced breast carcinoma metastatic to bone represents a severe hypercalcemic challenge. In such a patient, calcium is mobilized from bone by local osteolytic mechanisms; parathyroid function and 1,25-$(OH)_2D$ synthesis are appropriately suppressed, and the normal mechanisms of bone resorption, intestinal calcium absorption, and distal tubular calcium reabsorption are virtually eliminated. Initially, these adjustments may lead to a compensated steady state in which approximatley 800 to 1000 mg per day of mobilized calcium is excreted, with a serum calcium which is high-normal or only slightly elevated. With advancing disease or, as often occurs, with immobilization resulting from the basic disease process or an intercurrent illness, the quantity of mobilized calcium overwhelms the renal capacity for calcium excretion, and the spiral of hypercalcemia, dehydration, azotemia, and worsening hypercalcemia begins. In such conditions, the serum calcium may climb from 10.5 to 15 mg/dl within 48 h.

Systemic Phosphorus Homeostasis

MAINTENANCE OF A NORMAL SERUM PHOSPHORUS

The kidney plays the dominant role in systemic phosphorus homeostasis and maintains the serum phosphorus concentration at a value close to the tubular phosphorus threshold or TmP/GFR (Fig. 23-9). Because of the normal efficiency and lack of fine regulation of phosphorus absorption in the intestine, only in unusual circumstances (e.g., prolonged use of phosphate-binding antacids) is the systemic supply of phosphorus a limiting factor in phosphorus homeostasis. Thus, most disorders associated with chronic hypophosphatemia and/or phosphorus depletion in humans result from either intrinsic (e.g., familial hypophosphatemic rickets) or extrinsic (e.g., primary hyperparathyroidism) alterations in TmP/GFR. Acute hypophosphatemia most commonly results from the flux of extracellular phosphate ions into soft tissues.

DEFENSE AGAINST HYPOPHOSPHATEMIA

Figure 23-24 shows the sequence of events initiated in response to a hypophosphatemic challenge. The effects of hypophosphatemia per se include (1) stimulation of 1,25-$(OH)_2D$ synthesis in the kidney, (2) enhanced mobilization of phosphorus and calcium from bone, and (3) an "intrinsic" increase in TmP/GFR (see below). The increased circulating concentration of 1,25-$(OH)_2D$ leads to increases in phosphorus and calcium absorption in the intestine and provides an additional stimulus to phosphorus and calcium mobilization from bone. The increased flow of calcium from bone and the intestine results in an inhibition of PTH secretion, which diverts the systemic flow of calcium into the urine and further increases TmP/GFR. The net result of this sequence of adjustments is a return of the serum phosphorus concentration to normal without change in the serum calcium concentration (Fig. 23-24). Since the new steady state includes a reduction in PTH secretion, the initial hypophospha-

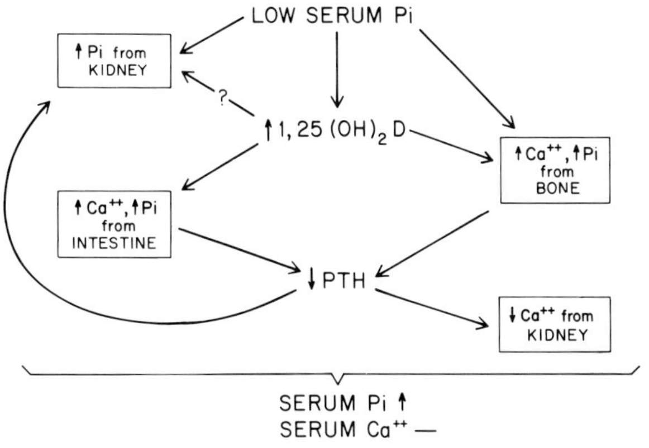

FIGURE 23-24 The sequence of adjustments initiated in response to hypophosphatemia.

temia- and 1,25-$(OH)_2D$–induced mobilization of bone mineral is largely replaced by the subsequent increase in mineral flow from the intestine.

Alterations in 1,25-$(OH)_2D$ synthesis sufficient to cause significant increases in the circulating level of the hormone probably occur only in response to a hypophosphatemic challenge of some magnitude. Thus, the key variables which constitute the major systemic defense against hypophosphatemia are those factors which influence TmP/GFR. As shown in Fig. 23-24, these factors are at least two in number: (1) the suppression of PTH secretion and (2) the hypophosphatemia-associated "intrinsic" increase in TmP/GFR. As noted in previous sections, the renal tubule possesses a seemingly innate ability to adjust its phosphorus reabsorptive capacity to systemic phosphorus requirements by a mechanism which is largely independent of PTH. This process is not a rapid adjustment and requires a matter of days to become maximal; however, when maximal, it is extremely efficient and virtually eliminates phosphorus from the urine. The efficiency of this tubular adjustment can be readily demonstrated in normal or parathyroidectomized humans and experimental animals, as can the time required for the initiation or dissipation of this adjustment. For example, if phosphorus-deprived rats are abruptly placed on a normal phosphorus intake, the animals die with profound hyperphosphatemia and hypocalcemia because of the failure of the mechanism to adjust rapidly. Whether this adjustment is a local tubular phenomenon or results from the tubular effects of an unidentified humoral substance released by a phosphorus-sensitive tissue is not known. Experimental data indicate that 1,25-$(OH)_2D$ is required for a maximal "intrinsic" alteration in tubular phosphorus threshold to occur and suggest that local concentrations of 1,25-$(OH)_2D$ may be mechanistically involved in this process.[92]

DEFENSE AGAINST HYPERPHOSPHATEMIA

As is the case with clinical states of hypophosphatemia, most conditions of chronic hyperphosphatemia in humans result from intrinsic (e.g., renal impairment) or extrinsic (e.g., hypoparathyroidism) abnormalities in the renal threshold for phosphorus. The defense against hyperphosphatemia consists largely of a reversal of the sequence of adjustments shown in Fig. 23-24. The principal humoral factor which combats hyperphosphatemia is PTH. An acute rise in the serum phosphorus concentration produces a transient fall in the concentration of serum ionized calcium and a stimulation of PTH secretion, which reduces TmP/GFR and leads to a readjustment in serum phosphorus and calcium concentrations. A sustained rise in serum phosphorus leads to the progressive development of secondary hyperparathyroidism. If the hyperphosphatemia is of sufficient magnitude and is prolonged, as it is in many patients with chronic renal failure, the secondary hyperparathyroidism ultimately produces the typical osteitic bone lesion of hyperparathyroidism.

The second major defense mechanism against hyperphosphatemia is the "intrinsic" adjustment in TmP/GFR in the renal tubules. Acute parathyroidectomy leads to an immediate and marked reduction in the fractional excretion of phosphorus. However, the TmP/GFR slowly adapts over the next 48 h, achieving a final level which is approximately 50 percent lower than the initial level and resulting in a partial correction of the state of hyperphosphatemia and phosphorus retention. Although important, this adaptive mechanism only partially corrects the capacity for phosphorus transport in the renal tubule; a complete normalization in TmP/GFR requires the presence of PTH. As discussed above, the intimate mechanistic details of this tubular adjustment remain unknown.

Systemic Magnesium Homeostasis

The understanding of systemic magnesium homeostasis remains at a relatively primitive state compared with that of calcium and phosphorus. Unlike these latter minerals, there appears to be no important systemic or hormonal regulation of the magnesium concentration in the extracellular fluids. Instead, maintenance of the serum magnesium concentration appears to result from the combined fluxes of magnesium at the levels of the intestine, kidney, intracellular fluids, and perhaps the skeleton. The kidney is primarily responsible for the regulation of the serum magnesium concentration. The direction and magnitude of the fluxes which occur at these sites are depicted schematically in "black box" form in Figure 23-22c. Several recent reviews address these areas in detail.[95–97]

INTESTINAL ABSORPTION OF MAGNESIUM

Magnesium is abundant in a variety of foodstuffs. The normal diet contains approximately 300 mg (24 meq) of magnesium. Approximately 30 percent of this is absorbed. In conditions of dietary magnesium excess a smaller proportion may be absorbed, and conversely, in conditions of dietary magnesium deficiency a higher proportion may be absorbed. Magnesium absorption occurs predominantly in the small intestine and has been demonstrated in the duodenum, jejunum, and ileum in varying experimental conditions.[98–100] The relative importance of these portions of the small intestine to net magnesium absorption in normal conditions remains undefined. Colonic magnesium absorption may occur, as evidenced by case reports of hypermagnesemia following colonic irrigation with magnesium-containing enemas.[95] Intestinal secretion of magnesium also occurs, as evidenced by (1) the appearance of ^{28}Mg in the feces after intravenous infusion of the isotope, (2) the presence of magnesium in the feces during complete, prolonged dietary magnesium restriction, and (3) the discrepant values for *net* intestinal magnesium absorption obtained using balance techniques (30 percent) and for unidirectional magnesium absorption using oral ^{28}Mg tracer studies (50 to 70 percent).[95–97] The source of this obligate intestinal magnesium secretion (stomach, small intestine, large intestine, bile, and pancreas) remains uncertain, but it assumes clinical relevance in patients with nutritional or intestinal disorders. These obligate losses amount to approximately 1 meq (12 mg) per day.[95,101]

The cellular mechanisms mediating magnesium absorption are poorly defined, but evidence would suggest elements of both passive and facilitated (but not active) transport. In some experimental systems, calcium appears to compete with magnesium for absorption, but this competition, if it exists, is not regarded as being of physiological or pathophysiological importance.

As indicated above, there appears to be no important systemic or hormonal regulation of intestinal magnesium absorption by PTH, calcitonin, or vitamin D or its metabolites, although some evidence suggests that jejunal magnesium absorption may be increased by means of the administration of $1,25\text{-}(OH)_2D$.[100] Therefore, the net quantity of magnesium absorbed appears to be primarily a function of magnesium intake.

RENAL TUBULAR HANDLING OF MAGNESIUM

The filtered load of magnesium is approximately 2400 mg (200 meq) per day, or 10 percent of the total body magnesium stores.[95–97] In the proximal tubule, approximately 30 percent of this filtered load is reabsorbed. The major site of magnesium reabsorption is the thick ascending loop of Henle, where approximately one-half to two-thirds of filtered magnesium is reabsorbed. Approximately 5 percent is reabsorbed in the distal tubule. Normal urinary magnesium excretion is in the range of 100 mg (8 meq) per day. Thus, of the 2400 mg filtered per day, 96 percent is reabsorbed along the nephron and approximately 4 percent is excreted in the urine (fractional magnesium excretion). The mechanisms of magnesium reabsorption along the nephron at a cellular level are poorly understood, but evidence suggests that magnesium transport is sodium-linked. It seems likely that calcium and magnesium compete for a common carrier in the proximal tubule and thick ascending limb of the loop of Henle. As is the case with calcium and phosphorus, it is possible to define a renal magnesium threshold or tubular maximum for magnesium (TmMg). Rude and colleagues[102] demonstrated that the TmMg in humans is approximately 1.4 mg/dl when expressed as a function of the ultrafilterable serum magnesium concentration. When expressed in terms of total serum magnesium, this value would be in the range of 2.0 mg/dl, which is very close to the normal serum magnesium concentration. The TmMg represents the net effects of magnesium reabsorption at different sites along the nephron.

As in the intestine, renal magnesium handling does not appear to be regulated by systemic or humoral mechanisms in any important way. Although a variety of effects on magnesium transport by PTH can be demonstrated in various nephron subsegments in experimental conditions, PTH, calcitonin, and vitamin D do not appear to have important regulatory effects in vivo.

Magnesium excretion may be influenced by nonhormonal factors in pathological conditions. Examples would include the enhanced renal magnesium excretion which accompanies hypercalcemia, expansion of extracellular fluid volume, and the magnesuria induced by loop diuretics.

INTRACELLULAR FLUID AND THE SKELETON

Little is known regarding the rates of magnesium flux into and out of the intracellular fluids, nor is there substantial information regarding the factors, if any, which regulate these fluxes. Nonetheless, these fluxes must occur and must be regulated in some manner, as evidenced by the fact that severe magnesium deficiency may be associated with relatively normal serum magnesium concentrations and the fact that hypomagnesemia may occur in conditions where total body magnesium content is judged to be normal.

Similarly, skeletal magnesium fluxes must exist but have not been carefully quantitated. Insofar as the vast bulk of total body magnesium content is present in the skeleton, one might predict that in conditions of rapid bone mineralization or rapid osteolysis, significant skeletal magnesium fluxes would occur. However, clinical examples reflecting these fluxes are unusual; one example would appear to be the hypomagnesemia that accompanies the "hungry bones syndrome" after parathyroidectomy.

In summary, systemic magnesium homeostasis does not appear to be hormonally regulated and therefore reflects largely the quantitative interplay of net magnesium absorption in the intestine and the fractional excretion of magnesium by the kidney. The fractional excretion of magnesium functions as a Tm-limited process and is primarily responsible for maintaining the serum magnesium concentration within rather narrow limits. The fine regulation of the serum magnesium concentration in the absence of hormonal controls provides an excellent example of the biological power of a Tm-limited transport process.

Influence of Other Hormones on Mineral Homeostasis

Although PTH, calcitonin, and vitamin D are the principal hormones concerned with the maintenance of normal mineral homeostasis, a number of other hormones are known to influence directly or indirectly either skeletal homeostasis or various aspects of systemic mineral homeostasis in humans. Several examples of hormonal influences of physiological relevance, such as the hormonal adjustments which accompany pregnancy and lactation, have been discussed previously. Most other examples are of clinical rather than physiological relevance and are discussed in detail in the clinical sections in this chapter and in Chap. 24. For example, the osteopenia which may accompany hyperthyroidism, endogenous or exogenous hypercortisolism, and estrogen or insulin lack are described in Chap. 24, and the mechanisms of the occasional occurrence of hypercalcemia in hyperthyroidism and Addison's disease are discussed below. Other effects, such as the influence of growth hormone and insulin on Tm/GFR and plasma phosphorus homeostasis, are presented in appropriate sections of this chapter.

CHEMICAL AND BIOCHEMICAL ANALYSES RELATED TO MINERAL METABOLISM

The final section of this chapter (see Testing) describes in detail the proper collection of samples and the performance of specialized tests in patients with disorders of mineral metabolism. This section describes the analytical basis and interpretation of results of both routine chemical analyses and the more sophisticated biochemical determinations often required for accurate diagnosis.

Routine Chemical Determinations in Serum

CALCIUM

The complex state of calcium in serum and the factors which influence the ionized (50 percent), protein-bound (40 percent), and complexed (10 percent) fractions were described previously. In most conditions, the determination of total serum calcium is adequate for routine clinical purposes. In other circumstances, the value for total serum calcium may require correction or adjustment as a result of alterations in serum protein concentration and/or pH, or the ionized calcium concentration may be calculated or actually measured. Calcium concentration data throughout this chapter are presented in milligrams per deciliter (mg/dl); these data may be converted to molar units (mmol per liter or mM) simply by dividing by 4 (e.g., 5 mg/dl converts to 1.25 mM).

The timing, technique of venipuncture, and analytic method employed are of critical importance to the proper interpretation of results for total serum calcium. Only values determined after an overnight fast should be regarded as reliable. The determination of total serum calcium in random, rather than fasting, specimens appears to be a common error in clinical practice. Depending on the nature of the meal, postprandial changes in total serum calcium in either direction may be observed. Although significant postprandial changes are typically confined to patients with an identifiable disorder of calcium metabolism, these induced changes may nevertheless form the basis for serious interpretative error (e.g., the suspicion of subtle primary hyperparathyroidism in a patient with "absorptive" hypercalciuria based on random high-normal values for total serum calcium).

Prolonged application of the tourniquet leads to venostasis, hemoconcentration, and spurious elevations in total serum calcium. The increases in total serum calcium resulting from venostasis correlate well with the increases in serum specific gravity. This problem is a continuous and frequent source of error, particularly in samples derived from a "difficult" venipuncture. Similar but smaller increases in total serum calcium occur with prolonged standing. Autoanalyzer techniques are employed by most clinical laboratories for the routine determination of total serum calcium. With adequate care, these techniques provide reliable data, yet the results are clearly less accurate than those determined by means of atomic absorption spectrophotometry. With scrupulous attention to detail, the results of atomic absorption spectrophotometry for total serum calcium are reproducible within ± 0.1 mg/dl.

There are important age and sex differences in values for total serum calcium. Total serum calcium declines slightly but progressively from the third (mean concentration approximately 9.6 mg/dl) to the ninth (mean concentration approximately 9.3 mg/dl) decade in men, whereas it remains constant in women.[103] Until age 60, mean values for total serum calcium are approximately 0.2 mg/dl lower in women than in men; thereafter, the mean values are identical. The actual normal range for total serum calcium is laboratory-specific. It must be recalled that this range is conventionally established as 95 percent confidence limits (mean ± 2 standard deviations of the mean) so that 2.5 percent of the population would be regarded as "hypercalcemic" by statistical definition. This approach is obviously inadequate in a day when "hypercalcemia" is being diagnosed at a nearly epidemic rate. Based on 95 percent confidence limits, typical normal limits in the United States would be approximately 9.0 to 10.6 mg/dl. The normal upper limit for total serum calcium is of crucial importance, yet various laboratories continue to report upper limit values ranging anywhere between 10.2 and 11.0 mg/dl. As emphasized by Keating and coworkers,[103] many such limits are inappropriately high, and an upper limit value of approximately 10.2 mg/dl (mean ± 2SD) is obtained with scrupulous attention to blood drawing and analytical technique. Probably the most useful approach is to establish the upper limit for total serum calcium on the basis of 99 percent confidence limits (mean ± 3SD), thus eliminating all but 0.5 percent of the normal population from the hypercalcemic category. Based on the results of atomic absorption spectrophotometry, this upper limit should be approximately 10.5 mg/dl for women and 10.6 mg/dl for men. There is no significant diurnal variation in the level of total serum calcium.

Most recent series conclude that none of the available algorithms for correcting total serum calcium for alterations in serum protein concentration and/or pH or for calculating "free" calcium concentrations provide precise values compared with actual measurements of the free calcium concentration.[104] This conclusion is warranted if precise data are required, but a number of algorithms are adequate for routine clinical interpretation of serum calcium results. Alterations in serum albumin constitute the major variable which significantly influences results for total serum calcium; at pH 7.4, each gram per deciliter of albumin binds approximately 0.8 mg/dl of calcium. For this correction, the simplest calculation is

$$\text{Total serum calcium (mg/dl)} - \text{albumin (g/dl)} + 4.0 = \text{corrected total serum calcium}$$

For example, with values for total serum calcium of 7.5 mg/dl and albumin of 2.0 g/dl, the corrected serum calcium is 9.5 mg/dl.

The ionized fraction is the biologically important component of serum calcium, and there is general agreement that measurements of ionized or free calcium should provide the most physiologically meaningful assessment of the extracellular concentration of calcium. This determination, however, has proved to be technically difficult, as demonstrated by the multiple divergent normal ranges for ionized calcium which have been reported in the literature. An average of many of these series provides a normal range for ionized serum calcium of about 4.4 to 5.1 mg/dl (mean ± 2SD). Age and sex differences in the direction of those noted for total serum calcium have been reported, but these differences have been less well studied than the values for total serum calcium. Acute increases and decreases in blood pH produced parallel increases and decreases in calcium binding to the carboxyl groups of albumin, leading to inverse changes in the concentration of ionized calcium. The alkalosis-induced reduction in the concentration of serum ionized calcium is responsible for the tetanic symptoms of acute hyperventilation. During prolonged acidosis or alkalosis, however, compensatory mechanisms result in a normalization of the serum ionized calcium concentration. The equipment currently available measures ionized calcium at ambient pH in samples which must be collected anaerobically. If not analyzed immediately, samples must be stored anaerobically. There are differences of opinion as to the exact utility of measurements of serum ionized calcium in clinical diagnosis.

The "ultrafilterable" calcium concentration may be determined by measuring the quantity of calcium which penetrates a semipermeable filter cone; this quantity represents the ionized fraction and the bulk of the complexed fraction.

PHOSPHORUS

Only approximately 10 percent of the inorganic phosphate in serum is protein-bound; the remaining 90 percent exists as free and complexed monovalent and divalent anions. Although measured in serum as orthophosphate, results are expressed as milligrams per deciliter of elemental phosphorus by convention. It is for this reason that certain purists insist on the use of the term *serum phosphorus* rather than *serum phosphate.*

The concentration of phosphorus in serum is not rigidly controlled, and increases or decrements of 1.0 mg/dl or more may be observed following phosphorus-rich or carbohydrate-rich meals, respectively. Therefore, meaningful results can be obtained only from samples drawn after an overnight fast. The serum should be promptly separated from the cells, since prolonged standing of whole blood leads to spurious reductions in the serum phosphorus concentration. The determination of phosphorus in heparinized plasma yields results that are slightly lower than those in serum.

As described in the section on clinical abnormalities of phosphorus metabolism, a vast number of influences other than diet directly or indirectly affect the concentration of phosphorus in serum (see Hypophosphatemia and Hyperphosphatemia). In general, these influences can be classified into those factors which affect the extracellular–soft-tissue distribution of phosphate ions and those which modulate TmP/GFR. For example, acute respiratory alkalosis and an abrupt increase in insulin and glucose concentrations in blood drive phosphate ions into the soft tissues and can profoundly lower the serum phosphorus concentration. In addition to the regulation of TmP/GFR by the conventional mineral hormones described previously, a number of other humoral influences on TmP/GFR are of physiological relevance. For example, growth hormone increases TmP/GFR, and estrogen decreases TmP/GFR; these influences appear to explain the high values for serum phosphorus and TmP/GFR noted in growing children and postmenopausal women, respectively. Although alterations in TmP/GFR are noted even with mild degrees of renal impairment, statistical increases in serum phosphorus concentrations are not observed until the glomerular filtration rate has fallen into the range of 30 ml/min or below.

There are important age and sex differences in serum phosphorus concentrations. The serum phosphorus concentration is quite high in growing children of both sexes, averaging about 4.5 to 5.0 mg/dl during the first 15 years of life and falling to normal adult levels shortly after puberty. In males, the concentration of phosphorus in serum falls progressively throughout adult life; representative normal ranges for serum phosphorus in males are approximately 2.5 to 4.5 mg/dl at age 20, 2.4 to 4.4 mg/dl at age 50, and 2.3 to 4.3 mg/dl at age 70. In females, the normal ranges for serum phosphorus correspond to those in males until the time of menopause, when the serum phosphorus concentration begins to rise progressively as a function of age. Representative normal ranges in females are 2.7 to 4.4 mg/dl at age 50 and 2.8 to 4.8 mg/dl at age 70. As is the case with calcium, the normal range for serum phosphorus concentrations and the statistics employed to develop these limits are laboratory-specific. Few laboratories, however, report serum phosphorus values in the appropriate context of age- and sex-matched control data.

MAGNESIUM

Approximately one-third of the magnesium in serum is protein-bound, and the remainder exists as free or complexed divalent cations (Table 23-4). As is the case with calcium, the binding of magnesium to albumin is pH-dependent, and algorithms exist for the correction of total serum magnesium for alterations in albumin concentration and pH and for the calculation of ionized magnesium. In clinical practice, the use of these algorithms is seldom necessary. The actual measurement of ionized magnesium in serum remains an investigative technique. The normal limits (mean $\pm$ 2SD) for total serum magnesium are approximately 1.7 to 2.4 mg/dl, and age, sex, and diurnal variation are not important considerations. One millimole of magnesium is equal to 24 mg, and 1 meq is equal to 12 mg. Data given as milligrams per deciliter can be converted to millimoles per liter by dividing by 2.4 and to milliequivalents per liter by dividing by 1.2 (e.g., 2.4 mg/dl converts to 2 meq per liter).

ALKALINE PHOSPHATASE

Alkaline phosphatase activity in serum is measured by the capacity of alkaline phosphatase to hydrolyze phosphate esters in an alkaline medium. Alkaline phosphatase activity is widely distributed in tissues, with high levels of activity occurring in the placenta, the small intestine, renal tubular cells, leukocytes, certain malignant tumors, bone, and the hepatobiliary system.[105] Two enzymes—"hepatic" alkaline phosphatase and "bile" alkaline phosphatase—are derived from the hepatobiliary system, and it is the latter enzyme which circulates in patients with hepatobiliary disease. The major interpretive limitations associated with the measurement of serum alkaline phosphatase activity are (1) the difficulties associated with defining the tissue sources of the aggregate circulating activity of the enzyme and (2) imprecise knowledge about the exact function of the skeletal alkaline phosphatase in bone metabolism.

Circulating alkaline phosphatase activity in normal adults consists of a mixture of skeletal and nonskeletal enzymes. Approximately 60 percent of the circulating alkaline phosphatase activity in normal adults is of skeletal origin, and 20 percent is of hepatobiliary-intestinal origin; the source of the remaining 20 percent of activity remains unclear. The skeletal enzyme can be identified by its electrophoretic mobility and by its heat lability ("bone burns"), and both approaches have become standard techniques for fractionating total serum alkaline phosphatase activity according to its apparent tissue source. Such fractionation techniques are of use only in the setting of an elevation of total serum alkaline phosphatase activity and are unlikely to identify a "hidden" high skeletal or intestinal component in a serum with normal total enzyme activity. An additional approach in a patient with an elevated total serum alkaline phosphatase activity is to determine the circulating activity of another enzyme, such as 5′-nucleotidase, regarded as being derived specifically from the hepatobiliary tract.

The presence of alkaline phosphatase activity in skeletal tissue and the high circulating activity in patients with certain skeletal disorders have been known for a half century,[105] yet the exact metabolic function of the enzyme in bone remains unknown. The "calcification" hypothesis was initially proposed in the 1920s and exists in modified form today. In essence, this hypothesis holds that the activity of the enzyme in bone alters the local milieu with respect to the concentration of orthophosphate and/or inhibitors of calcification such that normal mineralization of osteoid proceeds. The merits and demerits of modifications of this basic theory continue to be debated without a consensus.[105] Osteoblasts and osteocytes are rich sources of alkaline phosphatase, but osteoclasts have negligible activity of the enzyme. In general, circulating skeletal alkaline phosphatase activity is regarded as a reflection of osteoblastic activity and the turnover rate of bone. However, this reflection is very crude and insensitive and correlates poorly with other parameters of osteoblastic activity in individual patients. Interpretation of results in patients with various disorders of bone is discussed in further detail in Chap. 24.

Depending on the analytic method employed, serum alkaline phosphatase activity is expressed in various units (and normal ranges, as mean ± 2SD): Bodansky units (1.5 to 4.0 U/dl), King-Armstrong units (4 to 20 U/dl), or international units (6 to 110 IU per liter). Results are laboratory-specific, and each laboratory may report normal limits which differ slightly from those listed above because of minor methodological modifications. Alkaline phosphatase activity is identical in serum and heparinized plasma, but ethylenediaminetetraacetic acid (EDTA) irreversibly inactivates skeletal alkaline phosphatase. Alkaline phosphatase activity tends to increase slightly in serum samples stored at room temperature or at 4°C but is stable in frozen samples. Normal children and adolescents of both sexes have mean levels of serum alkaline phosphatase activity which are two- to threefold higher than normal adult levels. A "pubertal spurt" in serum alkaline phosphatase activity is noted in some but not all children. Between the ages of 20 and 50 years, mean serum alkaline phosphatase activity is approximately 30 percent higher in normal males than in normal females. After age 50, mean serum alkaline phosphatase activity rises slightly in both sexes. Whether this rise reflects an increased incidence of subclinical Paget's disease and/or osteomalacia in this older population is not known.

Routine Chemical Determinations in Urine

CALCIUM

The approach to sample collection and the interpretation of results for urinary calcium excretion are described in detail in the section on hypercalciuria in Chap. 25. The present discussion will be limited to the conditions of sample collection and relevant normal ranges.

Fasting calcium excretion refers to the determination of the rate of calcium excretion in a spot or timed urine sample after an overnight fast. The normal upper limit for fasting calcium excretion is influenced by antecedent calcium and sodium intake and by the length of the fast before sample collection; the most reliable results are obtained after several days of a low-normal (~400 mg per day) calcium intake and a 12- to 15-h fast. Results should be expressed as a function of the glomerular filtration rate (milligrams of calcium per 100 ml GF, where GF represents glomerular filtrate) rather than as a function of creatinine excretion (milligrams of calcium per milligram of creatinine). The normal range for fasting calcium excretion differs between laboratories but is approximately 0.03 to 0.15 mg Ca per 100 ml GF. The lower limit is such that an actual statistical decrease in fasting calcium excretion, as in a patient with familial hypocalciuric hypercalcemia, is difficult to define. Increased values for fasting calcium excretion reflect either an increase in bone resorption and the filtered load of calcium or a decrease in the renal tubular reabsorption of calcium or both. Distinguishing between these two conditions and further defining the renal tubular handling of calcium can be achieved only by actually measuring the free or ultrafilterable serum calcium concentration and calculating the fractional excretion of calcium.

Because of the large number of dietary factors and other variables which influence calcium excretion, precise normal ranges for 24-h calcium excretion have been difficult to establish. Conventional upper normal limits for 24-h calcium results determined on a "free" or undefined diet are $\leq$ 300 mg per day for males, $\leq$ 250 mg per day for females, or $\leq$ 4 mg per kilogram of body weight per day for either sex. A diagnosis of "hypercalciuria" as defined by samples collected on a free diet does not necessarily imply the presence of a systemic disorder of calcium metabolism, and the implications of such a diagnosis must be viewed with a degree of caution. More precise and readily interpretable data for calcium excretion are obtained from patients who are consuming "metabolic" diets. These diets are defined in terms of all dietary factors which may influence calcium absorption and/or excretion (e.g., protein and sodium intake) so that hypercalciuria detected on such a controlled diet almost always signifies the presence of an underlying disorder of mineral metabolism. The two dietary approaches most widely employed by investigators in the United States are the low-normal (400 mg) calcium intake and the high-normal (1000 mg) calcium intake. Upper normal limits for calcium excretion determined on the 400-mg calcium intake are $\leq$ 200 mg per day. On the 1000-mg calcium intake, the limits are $\leq$ 250 mg per day in females, $\leq$ 300 mg per day in males, and/or $\leq$ 4 mg per kilogram of body weight per day in either sex and in children. The weight-adjusted upper-normal limit (4 mg/kg per day) is the single most useful definition of hypercalciuria. As discussed in Chap. 25, the choice between these dietary approaches is entirely dependent on the clinical information desired. Use of the 1000-mg diet provides the most sensitive and accurate screening approach for defining the presence and degree of hypercalciuria in any patient in whom the abnormality in calcium excretion is based, entirely or in part, on an increase in intestinal calcium absorption.

PHOSPHORUS

In steady-state conditions, the quantity of phosphorus excreted in the urine is a direct reflection of dietary phosphorus intake. Thus, normal quantitative limits for phosphorus excretion have little meaning. An average individual may consume 1400 mg of phosphorus daily and excrete 900 mg daily in the urine. There is normally a diurnal rhythm in the rate of phosphorus excretion, with the nadir occurring at approximately 11 A.M. This rhythm is determined in part by phosphorus intake and possibly also by variables such as muscular exercise.[42] Phosphorus excretion is low or undetectable in spot or timed urine specimens from phosphorus-depleted patients and inappropriately high in urine specimens from patients with one of the disorders associated with abnormal renal tubular phosphorus reabsorption. In all circumstances, however, simply measuring the phosphorus excretion rate provides rather limited information, and clinical assessment should always aim at the calculation of TmP/GFR.

A massive body of literature has developed concerning various indices of renal phosphorus reabsorption. The merits and demerits of the determination of phosphorus clearance, tubular reabsorption of phosphorus (TRP), fractional excretion of phosphorus (C_{P_i}/C_{creat}), phosphorus excretion index (PEI), and other such indices have been reviewed by Bijvoet and will not be discussed in detail.[42] Of the available indices of renal tubular phosphorus reabsorption, the TmP/GFR is the soundest conceptually, and it is the only index which expresses phosphorus reabsorption as a function of *both* the serum phosphorus concentration and the glomerular filtration rate. Both variables are key influences on the rate of tubular phosphorus reabsorption and/or the appropriateness of this rate. The TmP/GFR appears to define a fundamental property of renal tubular reabsorptive capacity which at levels of GFR above 40 mg/min largely defines the ambient serum phosphorus concentration. The concept of a Tm-limited reabsorptive system and the rigorous measurement of the TmP/GFR by coinfusions of phosphate and inulin were presented in Fig. 23-9. From such studies, a nomogram has been derived (Fig. 23-25) which allows the TmP/GFR to be calculated from simple routine measurements. The use of the nomogram is described in the legend of Fig. 23-25, and sampling and calculation of the fractional excretion of phosphorus and/or TRP are presented in Testing, below. Optimum results are obtained from the simultaneous determination of the concentrations of phosphorus and creatinine in serum and urine in early morning to midmorning samples collected after an overnight fast. The urine sample may be a spot collection or a timed collection of 1 to 2 h.

An extensive data base for TmP/GFR has been published only for normal adults, in whom the normal range is 2.5 to 4.2 mg/dl (mean $\pm$ 2SD). In growing

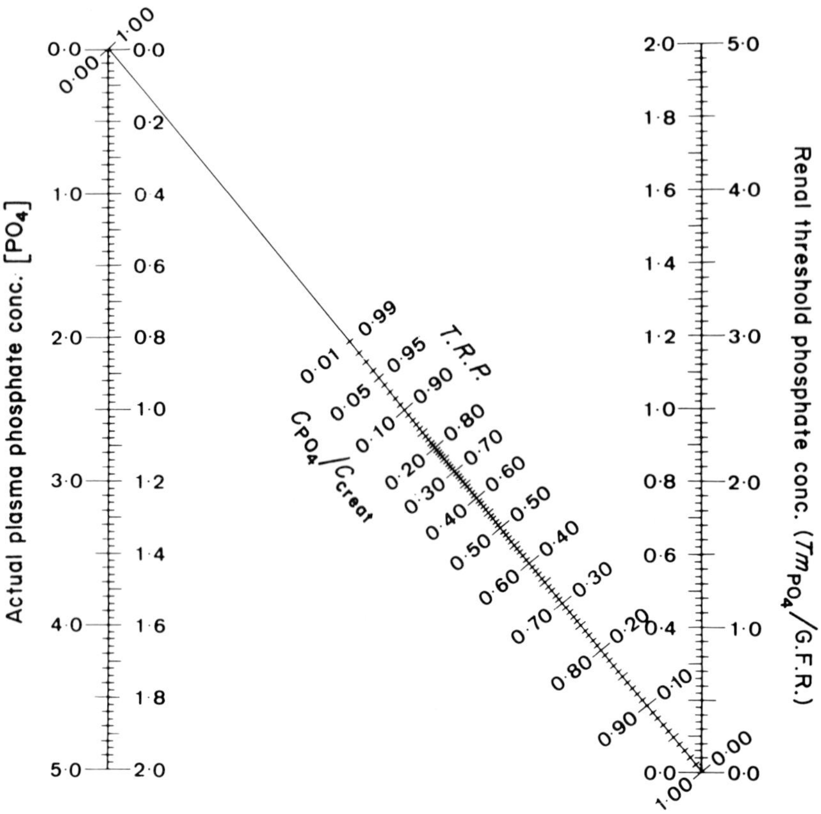

FIGURE 23-25 Nomogram for deriving TmP/GFR from known values for serum phosphorus and the fractional excretion of phosphorus (C_{P_i}/C_{creat}) or TRP. The estimation of C_{P_i}/C_{creat} and TRP is described in the section on testing. The outer scale on each ordinate represents units as mg/dl, and the inner scale on each ordinate represents units as mmol/l. The diagonal connecting the two ordinates has a scale for values for TRP to the right and a scale for values for C_{P_i}/C_{creat} to the left. A straight line through the appropriate values for serum phosphorus concentration and C_{P_i}/C_{creat} (or TRP) intersects the TmP scale at the appropriate value for TmP/GFR. The scales used (mg/dl or mmol/l) must be the same. All data in the text are presented as mg/dl. For example, at a serum phosphorus concentration of 2.5 mg/dl and a C_{P_i}/C_{creat} of 0.14, the TmP/GFR is 2.3 mg/dl. (*By permission of Walton RJ, Bijvoet OLM, Lancet, i:309, 1975.*)

children, TmP/GFR is considerably higher, averaging about 4.5 to 5.0 mg/dl until age 15 years. This finding reflects, at least in part, the effects of growth hormone on renal tubular phosphorus reabsorption. In premenopausal women, the TmP/GFR is probably slightly higher (estimated normal limits 2.6 to 4.3 mg/dl) than in normal men. In postmenopausal women, TmP/GFR is increased above both normal male and premenopausal levels, with approximate normal limits of 2.8 to 4.5 mg/dl. Estrogen replacement in postmenopausal women decreases TmP/GFR to normal male levels. It is likely that there is a significant diurnal variation in TmP/GFR, but this question has not been carefully evaluated. Calculated values for TmP/GFR can be reliably interpreted on the basis of age- and sex-matched control values down to levels of glomerular filtration rate in the range of 40 ml/min. Values for TmP/GFR in patients with more advanced renal insufficiency appear to be uninterpretable.

MAGNESIUM

In steady-state conditions, the urinary excretion of magnesium is a direct function of magnesium intake, and normal quantitative limits for magnesium excretion have little meaning. The range of magnesium excretion rates in normal adults is approximately 50 to 225 mg per day, and the average excretion rate is approximately 100 mg per day in men and 90 mg per day in women. In conditions of magnesium depletion, an individual with normal renal tubular function can reduce the magnesium excretion rate to < 10 mg per day.

Intestinal Calcium Absorption

There are two general methods for quantitating intestinal calcium absorption in humans: (1) the measurement of net calcium absorption as the difference between the dietary intake and the fecal excretion of calcium and (2) the measurement of fractional or percentage calcium absorption from an orally administered calcium solution under standardized conditions. Both methods are research techniques which require specialized facilities. In general, it may be stated that there is no ideal technique for measuring calcium absorption; available methods are either difficult or fraught with some degree of inaccuracy, or both.

As described in Mineral Balance, the time-honored measurement of net calcium absorption is laborious and relatively insensitive. Initially, techniques for measuring fractional calcium absorption involved the oral administration of a standard dose of radioactive calcium together with a suitable amount of nonradioactive "carrier" calcium and the quantitation of the appearance of the isotope in blood, urine, or feces or its retention in the whole body or some representative portion of the body. The major limitation of these techniques is the assumption that the rate of calcium appearance in body fluids or excreta or its retention is a reflection solely of the rate of intestinal calcium absorption. For example, in a patient whose bones "hunger" for calcium and who has a rapid clearance of calcium into the skeleton, the measurement of isotope retention or its appearance in the feces would overestimate the fractional absorption of calcium, and the measurement of the isotope in blood or urine would underestimate fractional calcium absorption. In order to avoid some of these problems, *double-isotope* methods for measuring fractional calcium absorption were introduced. These techniques involve the administration of two isotopes (e.g., ^{47}Ca and ^{45}Ca) by separate intravenous and oral routes or the administration of the same isotope by each route following a time lag sufficient for isotope decay (several days to a week). The data obtained from the intravenous administration of isotope reflect the clearance of calcium into the bone, urine, and intestine and are used to "correct" the data obtained from the oral administration of isotope for these influences. Although the double-isotope techniques are currently the most reliable methods for measuring fractional calcium absorption, even these techniques may be subject to error.

The *oral calcium tolerance test* is described in detail in Chap. 25. This test involves the oral administration of a standardized nonradioactive dose of calcium and utilizes the appearance of calcium in the urine as an index of intestinal calcium absorption. The assumption that the "calciuric" response to this test is an accurate reflection of the rate of intestinal calcium absorption may not be valid in certain circumstances (see above), but the test is simple and rapid and can be performed with routine facilities. At present, the use of this test should be confined to clinical situations in which its validity has been documented.

Mineral Balance

Because of the labor and time involved and the advent of more modern diagnostic techniques, mineral balance studies are rarely performed today. Yet with these techniques and little else, Fuller Albright and his colleagues in Boston launched the modern era of investigative mineral metabolism in the middle part of this century. Indeed, the *concept* of external mineral balance is as important and vital today as it was over three decades ago when Albright and Reifenstein's classic work, *The Parathyroid Glands and Metabolic Bone Disease,* was published.

The measurement of mineral balance involves the preparation and consumption of a carefully defined diet and the precise analysis of the mineral content in urine, feces, and diet rejects. The accurate collection of feces is the limiting factor in balance studies. Nonabsorbable "markers" such as chromium or carmine are generally used to correct for variations in intestinal emptying, and the feces are collected in approximately 4-day periods. A typical balance study requires sample collections for 14 days or more to ensure accuracy. Figure 23-26 illustrates the method of graphing balance data advocated by Albright; the data in the figure are derived from the study of a historic patient with primary hyperparathyroidism.

The state of mineral balance can often be calculated or inferred from a data base less rigorous than an actual formal balance study. Approximate calcium balance figures can be calculated on the basis of known values for calcium intake, fractional calcium absorption, and urinary calcium excretion. It requires no calculation to recognize that a patient who excretes 400 mg of calcium per day while on a rigidly restricted calcium intake is in profoundly negative calcium balance (see periods 3 to 5, Fig. 23-26).

Hormonal Measurements

PARATHYROID HORMONE

The biosynthesis and secretion of parathyroid hormone (PTH) and the biological activity and sources of the circulating fragments of the peptide were described in detail in previous sections. A clear grasp of these complexities of PTH physiology is of particular relevance to an understanding of existing assay systems for the hormone. The intact PTH peptide normally circulates at a concentration in the range of 10^{-12} M.

Bioassays for PTH were introduced as early as 1925. In vivo bioassays for PTH have typically been based on the hypercalcemic response to graded doses of the hormone and remain in use for defining official pharmacological units of commercial and experimental PTH preparations. USP and Medical Research Council (MRC) units are identical, and 2000 to 4000 USP or MRC units are the equivalent of 1 mg of purified intact bovine PTH. A number of in vitro bioassays for PTH have been developed. These assays are based on

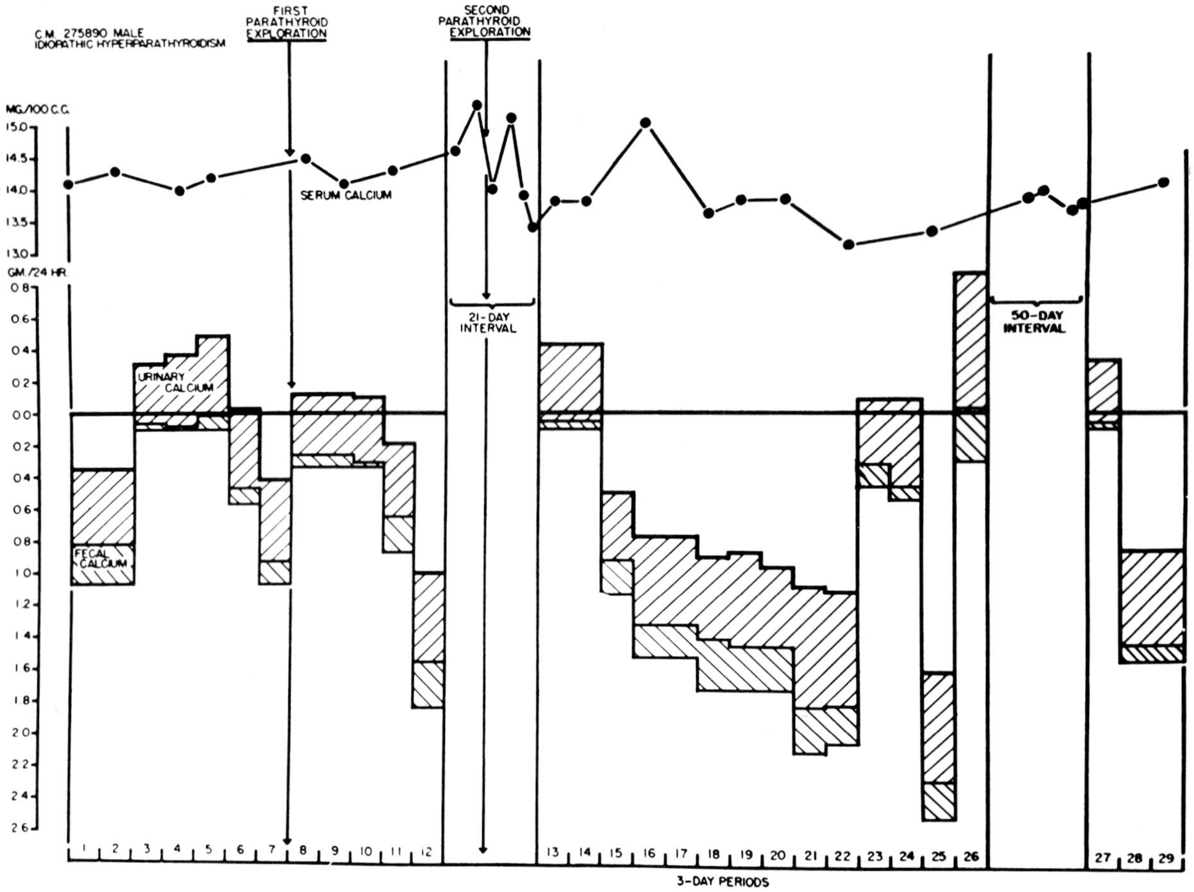

FIGURE 23-26 Method of graphing metabolic balance data according to Albright. By convention, the chart is constructed as follows: (1) The scale for intake and balance in grams per 24 h is shown on the ordinate, (2) the time scale is shown on the abscissa, (3) the heavy horizontal line at ordinate point 0 is the baseline to which intake and balance are referred, and (4) excretion in feces and urine is plotted as hatched areas extending upward from the bottom of the diagram (which defines the intake) toward the top. If the total excretion does not reach the baseline, a white area remains which represents positive balance. If the total excretion reaches the baseline, zero balance exists. If the total excretion exceeds the baseline, a state of negative balance exists.

The actual data shown are from metabolic studies performed in a historic patient, Captain Charles Martell, who ultimately succumbed to complications of his final, successful operation. The two procedures noted in the figure were unsuccessful. The studies plotted show the influence of calcium intake on calcium balance in a patient with severe hyperparathyroidism. At low levels of calcium intake, the patient was in negative calcium balance (e.g., periods 3 to 5), and at high levels of calcium intake, the patient was in positive calcium balance (e.g., periods 15 to 22). *(By permission of Albright F, Reifenstein EC: The Parathyroid Glands and Metabolic Bone Disease. Baltimore, Williams & Wilkins, 1948.)*

the generation of cAMP in bone or kidney preparations or the release of radiocalcium from bone preparations in response to the hormone.[106] The most widely used method is the stimulation of canine renal cortical adenylate cyclase activity by PTH, and this technique can also be used to standardize PTH preparations. None of the conventional bioassays for the hormone is sufficiently sensitive to serve as an experimental or clinical method for determining PTH activity in the peripheral circulation.

Because of the lack of direct measurements for PTH, various indices of renal tubular phosphorus reabsorption were introduced as "endogenous bioassays" of circulating PTH activity and were widely used in the 1950s and 1960s. The massive literature which developed concerning the diagnostic use of these indices, with or without calcium infusion, has been justly regarded as both confusing and controversial.[42] This controversy has resulted in an unfortunate and widespread lack of interest in clinical measurements of tubular phosphorus reabsorption in favor of more modern diagnostic techniques. Properly performed and interpreted, however, the TmP/GFR is an extremely useful tool in differential diagnosis, and reduced values for TmP/GFR are noted in 80 percent or more of patients with primary hyperparathyroidism compared with age- and sex-matched normal values. Although a reduction in TmP/GFR is clearly not specifically confined to patients with primary hyperparathyroidism, the determination is routinely available, and results may be obtained within 24 h.

The *radioimmunoassay for PTH* was introduced by Berson and Yalow in 1963. The development of a direct method for measuring circulating PTH has been a major factor in the burst of new basic and clinical information in the past two decades. However, as assays for PTH began to be established in different laboratories, widely divergent assay results began to appear in the literature. It rapidly became clear that the immunoassay of PTH presented far more complex problems than the routine immunoassays which had been established for the measurement of insulin, growth hormone, and other peptide hormones. The three basic difficulties involved in the assay of PTH are now well understood: (1) the heterologous nature of many assay systems, (2) the heterogeneity of circulating forms or fragments of PTH, and (3) the lack of standardized assay procedures between laboratories.[106–108] The key reagents and, therefore, the key variables distinguishing different radioimmunoassays are the choice of antiserum, radioligand, and standard employed in the assay. There is also a substantial "serum effect" in the assay, which is called "damage" by some investigators and "nonspecific binding" by others. This effect can be controlled for by setting up the standard curve in hypoparathyroid serum and by running "damage" (nonantiserum) tubes with each sample. Assays which do not include these safeguards suffer from substantial "noise," and this is a major problem with many commercial assays.

Because of the general unavailability of human PTH (hPTH), the anti-PTH antisera which were initially developed were against peptides from other species, mostly bovine PTH (bPTH). Cross-reactivity between anti-bPTH antisera and the human peptide forms is imperfect so that the major limitation of such heterologous assays is a loss in sensitivity. This issue is less of a problem in many assays in current use because of the fortuitous generation of antisera of great sensitivity as well as the increased availability of antisera generated against hPTH.

As noted in previous sections, the species of PTH in the circulation include the intact biologically active hormone, carboxy-terminal fragments of the peptide derived from peripheral catabolism, midregion and/or carboxy-terminal fragments secreted by the parathyroid glands themselves, and possibly amino-terminal cleavage products. The inactive carboxy-terminal and midregion forms of the peptide constitute 80 to 90 percent of the immunoreactive material in normal serum. These fragments are cleared by glomerular filtration and pile up in the circulation in patients with renal insufficiency. There is also evidence that patients with primary hyperparathyroidism may have a relatively greater proportion of inactive fragments in the circulation than normal subjects; this appears to result in part from the disproportionate secretion of midregion and/or carboxy-terminal fragments by the abnormal parathyroid tissue in these patients.[31,106]

The problem of the immunoheterogeneity of the circulating forms of PTH cannot be solved technologically because it is basically a biological problem. The problem has been approached by means of the development of region-specific assays. Most of the original PTH antisera established were "multivalent," meaning that they contained a family of antibodies that recognized different regions of the peptide. "Carboxy-terminal" antisera have reactive determinants in the carboxy terminus of the peptide. These antisera tend to be more sensitive than multivalent antisera and provide good clinical results even though they detect almost exclusively degradation products of the peptide.[106] "Midregion" antisera have reactive determinants in the middle portion of the PTH molecule.[31] These antisera are also sensitive, and many assays established with these antisera also employ radioiodinated fragments as ligand to further increase sensitivity.[31] Carboxy-terminal and midregion antisera are not useful for dynamic testing, particularly suppression testing, because of the long circulating half-time of these inactive fragments. Initial attempts to develop "amino-terminal" antisera did not yield assays of sufficient sensitivity to be clinically useful.[106] However, very sensitive amino-terminal antisera have recently been developed,[107] and this assay system appears to be useful for dynamic testing and seems to provide more biologically meaningful results in patients with renal insufficiency than those provided by other assay systems.

The lack of a standardized interlaboratory technique for assaying PTH is a major cause of the divergent assay results which have appeared and continue to appear in the literature. The region specificity of the antiserum employed in a given assay is an important determinant of the characteristics of that assay, but it is only one of the important variables in this regard, the others being the choice of radioligand and standard and the methods employed to control for the "serum effect." By far the most systematic assessment of the impact of the choice of these reagents on assay results has been provided by the European PTH Study Group.[108] This assessment was derived from the measurement of coded normal, hypoparathyroid, and hyperparathyroid sera in 12 different assay systems in

Europe and the United States.[108] The characteristics of the assay systems differed widely, with a variety of combinations and permutations of antisera, radioligands, and standards. The study concluded that agreement between laboratories by direct comparison of assay results was poor but that agreement was substantially improved when results were expressed as a function of a single serum standard. The standards most frequently employed in assays are purified bPTH, hPTH extracted from abnormal human parathyroid tissue, and graded dilutions of a single "hyperparathyroid" serum or serum pool, often obtained from a patient with chronic renal failure. Results are typically expressed as mass or volume equivalents to these standards (e.g., ng equiv/ml or μl equiv/ml). The choice of standards by which displacement of radioligand by unknown samples is judged is obviously of crucial importance, but this variable has been less emphasized in the American literature than the influence of the region specificity of the antiserum. An international standard (WHO 79/500) has been introduced by the World Health Organization.[109] It is reasonable to expect that published results as well as commercial assay values will be expressed in these units or at least cross-referenced to this standard in the near future.

The essential conclusion to be drawn is that an intelligent interpretation of radioimmunoassay results for PTH requires a knowledge of the characteristics of the assay from which the results are derived. This is particularly true of the commercially available PTH assays, with which there has been considerable dis-

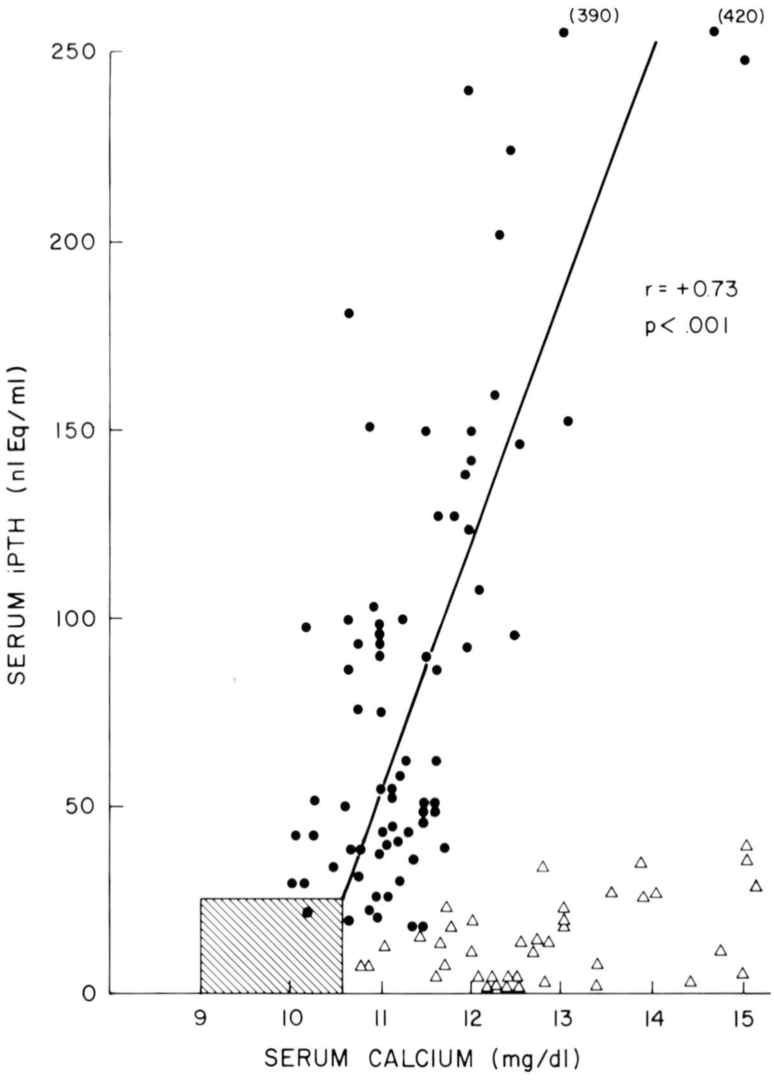

FIGURE 23-27 Serum immunoreactive parathyroid hormone plotted as a function of the serum calcium concentration in 75 patients with primary hyperparathyroidism and 40 patients with malignancy-associated hypercalcemia. Note the strong positive correlation ($r = 0.73$, $p < 0.001$) between the serum calcium and immunoassay results in the patients with hyperparathyroidism. The borderline-high to slightly elevated values for immunoreactive PTH in a small minority of patients with malignancy-associated hypercalcemia are thought to result from the finite nonsuppressible component of PTH secretion (Fig. 23-4) in the face of renal impairment. The immunoassay is a midregion method and has been cross-referenced with WHO standard 79/500, in which units the upper-normal limit is 525 μU/ml.

pleasure.[110] The limitations of these assays are not entirely a function of suboptimal reagents. There is an emphasis on turnaround time in many commercial laboratories which translates into a reduction in incubation time and other methodological modifications that result in both noise and insensitivity. It is common practice to plot PTH assay results graphically on a nomogram as a function of the serum calcium concentration (Fig. 23-27). The pathophysiological rationale for such a nomogram is self-evident, for primary hyperparathyroidism can be viewed in a pragmatic, interpretive sense as a dose-related disease (see legend of Fig. 23-27). However, such nomographic results derived from insensitive assay systems which show the bulk of clinical assay results in the "inappropriate" range should be interpreted with extreme caution. The most meaningful assay result is one which is statistically clearly outside the normal range.

The normal range for serum immunoreactive PTH is laboratory-specific. Diurnal variation is probably not an important consideration in the interpretation of results from carboxy-terminal and midregion assays, but it may be important in the interpretation of results from amino-terminal assays. Immunoreactive PTH has been reported to increase with age in both sexes.[111] In part this age-related increase is a function of a decreasing glomerular filtration rate, and in part it appears to be real, perhaps reflecting a decrease in calcium intake and/or absorption with age.[111] Recent data reveal a remarkable degree of parathyroid suppressibility in certain patients with primary hyperparathyroidism; thus optimal results are obtained when patients are evaluated on a restricted calcium diet[112] (see Hyperparathyroidism).

A cytochemical assay for PTH based on the activation of glucose 6-phosphate dehydrogenase activity in distal tubular cells from guinea pig kidney has been developed.[113,114] Although laborious, the technique is exquisitely sensitive and detects $bPTH_{1-84}$ in the femtogram per milliliter range ($\sim 10^{-14}$ M). This assay has been used to characterize the biological activity of circulating forms of PTH,[114] and it is also capable of detecting the factor which appears to be responsible for humoral hypercalcemia of malignancy (see Malignancy-Associated Hypercalcemia). The cytochemical bioassay is not commercially available.

Figure 23-28 is a schematic representation of the mechanism of renal plasma clearance and the sources of cAMP in human urine.[94] cAMP in plasma is filtered at the glomerulus and excreted by means of a process of simple glomerular filtration. To this filtered load of the nucleotide is added a quantity of cAMP produced de novo in the kidney and excreted directly into the tubular urine. The contribution of the nucleotide by the kidney is termed *nephrogenous* cAMP in order to

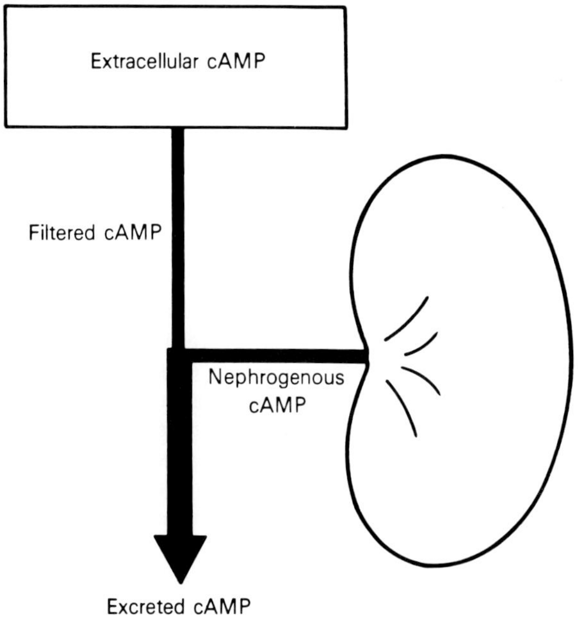

FIGURE 23-28 Schematic representation of the mechanism of renal plasma clearance and of the sources of cAMP in human urine.

emphasize that the mechanism of renal clearance of cAMP in humans is not renal tubular secretion according to conventional clearance terminology. Thus, the total quantity of cAMP excreted in humans is simply a sum of the filtered and nephrogenous components. In normal subjects, each component accounts for approximately 50 percent of the total excretion rate of the nucleotide.

At all levels of glomerular filtration rate above 20 ml/min, the filtered load of cAMP is relatively constant. Because of the rapid turnover and wide distribution of the nucleotide in the extracellular pool, the concentration of cAMP in plasma provides a very insensitive reflection of altered rates of cAMP production in tissues in equilibration with this pool, and physiological quantities of agents (e.g., glucagon) which interact with these tissues do not produce discernible increases in plasma cAMP or total cAMP excretion. Therefore, the filtered component provides a rather constant "background" of excreted nucleotide, and variations in nephrogenous cAMP are primarily responsible for alterations in the total excretion rate of the nucleotide in humans. The proximal tubular effects of PTH are mediated by cAMP, and the proximal tubule appears to be the major, if not the only, source of the nephrogenous component of the nucleotide. Other agents, such as calcitonin and antidiuretic hormone, which influence cAMP synthesis in kidney preparations in vitro have no effects on nephrogenous cyclic production and excretion in vivo in either physiological or pharmacological amounts. Thus, the proximal tubular effects of PTH have been estimated to account for 80 to 100 percent of the nephrogenous contribution of cAMP in humans.[94]

Clinically, measurements of nephrogenous cAMP are employed as a sensitive "in vivo bioassay" of the effects of circulating *active* PTH. Elevated levels of nephrogenous cAMP are noted in over 90 percent of patients with primary hyperparathyroidism, and values near zero are found in patients with hypoparathyroidism (Fig. 23-29). The determination is useful for dynamic testing, particularly suppression testing. For example, the oral administration of the amount of calcium in a normal calcium-containing meal results in a 30 percent suppression of nephrogenous cAMP in normal subjects.[94] These features are discussed in more detail in Chap. 25. The measurement of nephrogenous cAMP provides a valid index of parathyroid function at levels of glomerular filtration rate down to 20 ml/min; the validity of results in patients with more severe renal impairment is not known. The measurement of plasma cAMP is technically somewhat difficult so that currently the determination of nephrogenous cAMP is largely confined to research laboratories. However, the determination of the total cAMP excretion rate by radioimmunoassay or protein-binding assay is technically simple, and such assays are available. Because of the relatively constant background of the filtered component of excreted cAMP, the simple determination of total cAMP excretion is, in most circumstances, almost as useful clinically as the technically more demanding measurement of nephrogenous cAMP.

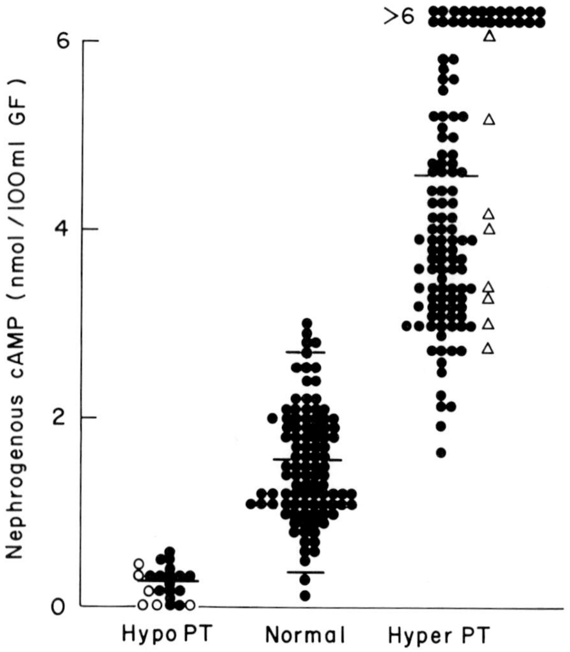

FIGURE 23-29 Values for nephrogenous cAMP in normal subjects and patients with hypoparathyroidism (HypoPT), nonparathyroid hypercalcemia (○), primary hyperparathyroidism (HyperPT), and nonazotemic secondary hyperparathyroidism (△). The marginated bars represent mean ± 2SD in the normal subjects and mean values in the patients with hypoparathyroidism and hyperparathyroidism. (*By permission of Broadus AE, Nephron 23:136, 1978.*)

Details of sample collection, preservation, and computation of cAMP results are presented in Testing, as in the coupling of the determination with PTH infusion in the diagnosis of pseudohypoparathyroidism. Depending on the information desired, spot, timed, or 24-h urine samples may be obtained. Because of the sensitivity of cAMP measurements, it is important that hypercalcemic patients be evaluated on a restricted calcium intake.[112] Spot or timed tasting specimens are preferred in hypercalcemic patients. The manner in which the data are computed and expressed is of critical importance. Both nephrogenous cAMP and the filtered component of the nucleotide are functions of the glomerular filtration rate, and results for both nephrogenous cAMP and total cAMP excretion *must* be expressed on a filtration rate basis (nanomoles per 100 ml GF, where GF is glomerular filtrate). The use of other units (e.g., micromoles per day, nanomoles per milligram of creatinine) has no physiological basis and is associated with serious interpretive error. At present, the importance of the mode of data expression has escaped the attention of commercial laboratories, some of which continue to report results in meaningless units. Normal limits for nephrogenous cAMP are 0.34 to 2.70 nmol per 100 ml GF, and for total cAMP excretion they are 1.83 to 4.50 nmol per 100 mg GF.[94] Diurnal variation of the several components of cAMP excretion does not appear to be an important consideration. Elevated values for nephrogenous cAMP are observed in patients with primary and secondary hyperparathyroidism and in patients with humoral hypercalcemia of malignancy. In normocalcemic patients with a pheochromocytoma, results for total cAMP excretion may be elevated, but nephrogenous cAMP is normal.

CALCITONIN

Induced hypocalcemia in the rat was initially employed as a bioassay for calcitonin and was the method by which MRC units were initially defined.[54,55] One milligram of synthetic human calcitonin is equivalent to 90 MRC units. Bioassays are not sufficiently sensitive for measurement of circulating calcitonin in humans.

The determination of circulating human calcitonin (hCT) by radioimmunoassay is less complex than is the case for PTH. Current methods are homologous assay systems employing antisera generated against synthetic hCT, synthetic hCT as standard, and [^{131}I]hCT as radioligand.[56,65,68] Earlier assay systems lacked sensitivity, but higher-affinity antisera and improved techniques have resulted in assays which can detect the low circulating levels of the hormone in 90 percent or more of normal individuals. Gel filtration studies have revealed that plasma calcitonin is heterogeneous in patients with medullary carcinoma of the thyroid and patients with "ectopic" calcitonin production and possibly also in normal subjects.[56,65] As discussed in Calcitonin, this heterogeneity appears to result from dimeric or polymeric forms of calcitonin and may also be due to the secretion of incompletely processed larger forms of the hormone. The nature, relative quantities, and exact sources of the circulating forms of calcitonin are not well defined. The heterogeneity of plasma calcitonin does not appear to interfere appreciably with the use of the assay for diagnosis of medullary carcinoma of the thyroid.

Many laboratories report a normal range for plasma calcitonin of 20 to 75 pg/ml,[56] but the extractable calcitonin monomer in normal plasma appears to be less than 20 pg/ml.[65] At all ages, men have basal calcitonin levels about 30 percent higher than those in women, and provocative tests elicit larger calcitonin responses in men than in women.[56,65,68] The mean basal calcitonin concentration has been reported to decline in both sexes with age.[68] Whether the sex and age differences are of physiological importance is not known. Both elevated and normal calcitonin levels have been reported in hypercalcemic patients; thus, the role of calcitonin as an "antihypercalcemic hormone" in humans has not been clearly defined.[56,115] Heparinized plasma samples are preferred in most assay systems.

The major clinical utility of the calcitonin radioimmunoassay is in the diagnosis and management of patients with medullary carcinoma of the thyroid (Chap. 28). Elevated values for plasma calcitonin have also been reported in patients with a variety of malignancies (Chaps. 28 and 29) and in patients with chronic renal failure, in whom the metabolic clearance of circulating calcitonin is decreased.

VITAMIN D

Reliable radioligand, spectral, and/or bioassays are currently available for the determination of each of the physiologically important vitamin D metabolites in human plasma. Accurate quantitation of metabolites by many of these methods requires extensive purification in order to separate the metabolites from each other and from other interfering substances. The purification steps are far more laborious and time-consuming than the actual assays; often these steps include lipid extraction of plasma, one or more preparative column chromatographic steps, and final separation of the metabolites on high-performance liquid chromatography (HPLC) equipment prior to assay. Assays for plasma 25-OHD and 1,25-$(OH)_2D$ are commercially available and are quite reliable. Kits for the measurement of 1,25-$(OH)_2D$ using several techniques are also available.

The calciferols circulate in normal individuals at a concentration ranging from 1 to 10 ng/ml, with the actual concentration depending on sunlight exposure and the amount of vitamin D in the diet. Vitamin D_2 and vitamin D_3 can be quantitated by ultraviolet absorption after extensive purification. Ligand assays employing rat serum vitamin D–binding protein have also been introduced for measurement of vitamin D_2 and vitamin D_3 in purified samples. Since determination of the plasma concentration of 25-OHD provides a good index of systemic vitamin D status, there are a few clinical circumstances in which measurements of the calciferols are of particular interest.

25-OHD may be measured by ligand assays employing either the human or rat serum vitamin D–binding protein or the 6-S cytosolic binding protein and also by ultraviolet absorption in purified samples.[71,116] The ligand assays do not discriminate between 25-OHD_2 and 25-OHD_3, but these metabolites can be separated by HPLC and quantitated independently. Ligand techniques for the determination of 25-OHD in raw plasma have been described, but 24,25-$(OH)_2D$, and perhaps other substances such as the calcidol lactone, have been found to compete in these assays. Therefore, such assays may provide a general index of vitamin D status but do not yield accurate data as to actual 25-OHD concentrations. In normal adults, the mean plasma concentration of 25-OHD is approximately 30 ng/ml, with a range of 10 to 80 ng/ml, depending on sunlight exposure and diet. In the absence of vitamin supplements, approximately 80 percent of the circulating material is 25-OHD_3. Seasonal variations in plasma 25-OHD concentration have been observed, with maximal values in September and minimal values in midwinter.[71] Plasma levels of 25-OHD in Great Britain are approximately one-third of those noted in sun-rich parts of the United States. The determination of plasma 25-OHD concentration may be used to confirm a diagnosis of vitamin D intoxication or to detect states of dietary-, disease-, or drug-related vitamin D deficiency. Reductions in plasma 25-OHD have also been reported in patients with cirrhosis and patients with the nephrotic syndrome.[74,75] A plasma concentration of 25-OHD less than 5 ng/ml is compatible with vitamin D deficiency.

The plasma content of 24,25-$(OH)_2D$ can be determined in purified samples by ligand assays using the serum or cytosolic binding proteins or by ultraviolet absorption. The average plasma concentration of 24,25-$(OH)_2D$ in normal adults is approximately 1.5 ng/ml and ranges from about 0.5 to 5 ng/ml. The plasma concentration of 24,25-$(OH)_2D$ correlates positively with the plasma concentration of 25-OHD but not with the plasma concentration of 1,25-$(OH)_2D$. Circulating 24,25-$(OH)_2D$ is reduced in patients with renal insufficiency.[80] Specific syndromes associated with an increase or a decrease in the plasma level of 24,25-$(OH)_2D$ have not been reported.

A variety of bioassay and ligand techniques have been developed for the measurement of 1,25-$(OH)_2D$ in plasma. These techniques include the use of the hormone-cytosol receptor-chromatin complex from chick intestine as a radioreceptor assay,[71] the use of the receptor from chick intestine in a protein-binding assay,[116,117] a bioassay employing cultured fetal rat bones,[118] radioimmunoassay,[119] a protein-binding assay using receptor from calf thymus,[120] and a cytoreceptor assay using cultured rat osteosarcoma cells.[121] The last two techniques require only minimal purification of samples prior to assay. Improvements in sensitivity and technique have reduced the volume of plasma required from 20 ml to 2 to 5 ml. The normal ranges reported by different laboratories have varied, but typical normal adult values are approximately 20 to 65 pg/ml (48 to 155 pmol per liter). Values expressed as picograms per milliliter can be converted to picomoles per liter by multiplying by a factor of 2.4. The plasma concentration of 1,25-$(OH)_2D$ does not correlate with the plasma concentration of 25-OHD or 24,25-$(OH)_2D$. Very low values for plasma 1,25-$(OH)_2D$ have been observed in patients with renal failure.[80] Diurnal variation is not an important consideration in interpreting assay results,[122] but circulating 1,25-$(OH)_2D$ may be quite sensitive to dietary calcium intake in hypercalcemic and/or hypercalciuric patients; thus, the most readily interpretable results are obtained from patients evaluated on a restricted calcium diet.[112,123] There is some disagreement as to a reported reduction in circulating 1,25-$(OH)_2D$ in elderly and/or osteoporotic patients, but such patients do appear to display a decrease in the 1,25-$(OH)_2D$ "reserve" in response to infused PTH.[76] Mean values for both serum iPTH and plasma 1,25-$(OH)_2D$ have been reported to be higher in obese and nonobese black subjects than in lean white individuals, and these findings have been interpreted as a physiological adjustment by which the increased skeletal mass in obese and black individuals is maintained.[76] DHT is converted in vivo to a metabolite which cross-reacts in the 1,25-$(OH)_2D$ assay.[124] The measurement of plasma 1,25-$(OH)_2D$ has proved to be a key tool in differential diagnosis and in dissecting out the details of pathogenesis of a wide variety of disorders of mineral and skeletal metabolism, as described in the clinical sections of this chapter and in Chaps. 24 and 25. Heparinized plasma is generally preferred for the determination of all vitamin D metabolites.

Assessment of Bone Metabolism and Skeletal Homeostasis

The elements of this chapter are primarily concerned with mineral metabolism and homeostasis. The assessment of bone metabolism by chemical, biochemical, radiographic, and histological techniques is described in detail in Chap. 24. Abnormalities of skeletal homeostasis which occur in specific systemic disorders of mineral metabolism are presented in the clinical sections below.

HYPERCALCEMIA

The systemic mechanisms for preventing hypercalcemia were presented in an earlier section. It was emphasized that hypercalcemia develops only when the rate of calcium entry into the extracellular pool exceeds the renal capacity for calcium excretion. This renal capacity is quantitatively limited and is actually altered in a number of hypercalcemic conditions. It is always useful to think of the sources and mechanisms of calcium entry into the extracellular pool in any hypercalcemic patient or condition, and pure examples of "bone," "intestinal," and "renal" mechanisms of hypercalcemia can be readily identified. For example, in immobilized patients and those with osseous metastases, bone is the sole source of the calcium entering the extracellular pool; in the milk-alkali syndrome, calcium entry via the intestine is largely responsible for the hypercalcemia; and in patients with familial hypocalciuric hypercalcemia, hypercalcemia develops primarily as a result of an abnormally efficient renal tubular reabsorption of calcium. In other conditions, such as primary hyperparathyroidism, elements of calcium entry into the extracellular pool from all three sources can be identified, and the quantitative importance of these sources may vary from patient to patient. The consideration of hypercalcemia by source and mechanism has diagnostic and therapeutic as well as theoretical significance.

Table 23-7 lists the hypercalcemic conditions by category in decreasing order of approximate clinical frequency. The table is organized so that the thrust of differential diagnosis is largely confined to the first

Table 23-7. Hypercalcemic Conditions Arranged by Category in Descending Order of Approximate Frequency

1. Primary hyperparathyroidism
   a. Sporadic
   b. Clinical variants
   c. Familial endocrine neoplasia and familial hypocalciuric hypercalcemia
2. Malignancy-associated hypercalcemia
   a. Local osteolytic hypercalcemia
   b. Humoral hypercalcemia of malignancy
   c. Lymphoma-associated hypercalcemia
3. Endocrinopathies
   a. Thyrotoxicosis
   b. Adrenal insufficiency
   c. Pheochromocytoma
   d. VIP-oma syndrome
4. Medications
   a. Thiazide diuretics
   b. Vitamins A and D
   c. Milk-alkali syndrome
   d. Lithium
   e. Estrogens and antiestrogens
5. Sarcoidosis and other granulomatous diseases
6. Miscellaneous conditions
   a. Immobilization
   b. Acute renal failure
   c. Idiopathic hypercalcemia of infancy
   d. Serum protein abnormalities

five categories; hypercalcemia developing in the setting of the conditions grouped in category 6 is usually diagnostically self-evident. The outline provided by the table will be followed in the discussion below. Each condition will be described in detail in terms of clinical presentation, pathophysiology, and specific diagnosis and therapy. The final portions of this section will describe a unified approach to differential diagnosis and medical therapy for hypercalcemia.

Primary Hyperparathyroidism

HISTORY

The history of hyperparathyroidism has been recounted in detail by several investigators involved in the early studies of the disorder, most notably Fuller Albright.[125] When originally described in Vienna and Boston in the mid-1920s, primary hyperparathyroidism was regarded as a rare and severe disease of bone, *osteitis fibrosa cystica.* Subsequently, Albright's group recognized a different clinical presentation of primary hyperparathyroidism in patients with renal stones but without evidence of overt bone disease. The "stone" and "bone" presentations of the disorder impressed these investigators as sufficiently distinctive that they referred to their patients with primary hyperparathyroidism as those "with" and those "without" clinical bone disease. Thinking in terms of classical external calcium balance, Albright proposed that bone disease developed in primary hyperparathyroidism when dietary calcium intake was inadequate to meet systemic calcium losses, whereas stone disease developed when dietary calcium intake was excessive. This hypothesis was disproved by Dent's dietary survey in patients with primary hyperparathyroidism, but the English group was also impressed by the distinctive clinical spectrum of the disorder and proposed that the parathyroid glands might produce two hormones, with the classical parathyroid principle being pathogenetically related to stone formation and with a combined hormonal abnormality being responsible for bone disease.[126] As further details of pathophysiology have become clear, there is a certain irony associated with both the balance and the dual hormone hypotheses. As described in detail below, clinical bone disease in primary hyperparathyroidism most often occurs in patients with a severe and aggressive disease process, and stone disease typically occurs in patients with a milder and somewhat more indolent disease process. There are exceptions, for some patients present with both bone and stone involvement, and other patients are identified with neither of these classical presentations. In the end, although mechanistically oversimplified, Albright's conceptual viewpoint appears to have been typically prescient.

INCIDENCE AND NATURAL HISTORY

Primary hyperparathyroidism was initially regarded as rare. During the past several decades, however, estimated incidence figures for primary hyperparathyroidism have been steadily climbing, and the disorder is now recognized as being quite common. These increased incidence figures reflect (1) enhanced physician awareness of the varied clinical presentations of the disorder, (2) routine screening of serum calcium by automated clinical chemistry techniques, and (3) improved methods for specific diagnosis. Recent estimates of the incidence of primary hyperparathyroidism in the United States and England are on the order of 25 cases per 100,000 population per year.[127,128] This corresponds to 35,000 to 85,000 new cases per year in the United States. Primary hyperparathyroidism is an adult disease and is discovered in over 85 percent of diagnosed patients after age 30. At all ages, women with primary hyperparathyroidism outnumber men by a ratio of 2:1. Postmenopausal women constitute the single population at greatest risk, with an incidence some five times that of the general adult population.[127]

Of the three variables which have contributed to the increased rate of detection of hyperparathyroidism in the population, the routine screening of serum calcium has clearly had the greatest impact.[127] Since the determination of total serum calcium is the most important routine tool for detection of primary hyperparathyroidism, it is crucial that normal ranges for serum calcium be carefully established and results be interpreted intelligently (see Routine Chemical Determinations in Serum, above). The clinical discovery of hypercalcemia in an asymptomatic patient or one who suffers from vague, nonspecific symptoms has been termed the *serendipity syndrome.* With the discovery of an increasingly large population of such patients has come an awareness that the natural history of primary hyperparathyroidism is largely unknown. A generation ago, when primary hyperparathyroidism was regarded as rare, it was also regarded as severe and rapidly progressive. Although such aggressive presentations of the disorder continue to be observed, it is now these cases which are uncommon in comparison with the number of patients who present with an apparently indolent basic disease process. Attempts to define further the natural history of primary hyperparathyroidism in patients lacking specific complications of the disorder have been initiated in the past decade, but these studies have not been reported in detail. Lacking this important information, the present therapeutic approach toward patients with the serendipity syndrome must remain largely judgmental.

PATHOLOGY AND ETIOLOGY

In most series, a single parathyroid adenoma is found in more than 80 percent of patients with primary hyperparathyroidism (Table 23-8). In several series, the reported incidence of primary chief cell hyperplasia has been higher than shown in Table 23-8, and there is a suspicion that this lesion is more frequently identified today than a decade ago. However, primary chief cell hyperplasia is probably present in no more than 15 percent of representative patients with primary hyperparathyroidism. As is the case with other endocrine tissues, histological criteria for reliably distinguishing contiguous members of the histological sequence normal-hyperplasia-adenoma-carcinoma have been difficult to establish. The major clinical problem lies in distinguishing adenoma from primary chief cell hyperplasia.[129,130]

Table 23-8. Pathological Classification of Parathyroid Lesions in 1076 Patients with Primary Hyperparathyroidism (in %)

Adenoma:	
Single	84
"Double"*	2
Hyperplasia:	
Chief cell	9
Clear cell	2
Carcinoma	3

*Nodular hyperplasia as an alternate pathological diagnosis was not definitely excluded in all cases.
Source: Data derived from Habener and Potts[129] and from Watson *Clin Endocrinol Metab* 3:215, 1974.

The typical parathyroid adenoma is smooth, ovoid, and reddish brown, resembling normal liver tissue in color. The darker color of the adenoma, in contrast to the yellowish-brown hue of normal parathyroid tissue, is due to its decreased fat content. In some series, inferior parathyroid glands have been reported to be involved more frequently than the superior glands; in other series, the inferior and superior glands have been involved with similar frequency. Approximately 6 to 10 percent of parathyroid adenomas are found in unusual or "ectopic" locations, such as behind the esophagus, within the thyroid capsule or parenchyma, or within the thymus or other mediastinal structures. The inferior glands are more frequently ectopic than the superior glands, as would be predicted from the embryologic development of the two parathyroid pairs. Hyperfunctioning supernumerary parathyroid glands occur rarely and are usually mediastinal in location.[131] Typical parathyroid adenomas weigh between 0.5 and 5 g; rarely, they are as large as 10 to 25 g, and the largest reported adenoma was 120 g. Older series reported larger weights for parathyroid surgical specimens than do modern series. There is a crude but clear correlation between the aggregate parathyroid mass and the severity of disease as judged clinically, chemically, or biochemically.[129,132–134] Each 1 mg/dl increase in total serum calcium above normal corresponds to roughly 1 g of abnormal parathyroid tissue. Thus a patient with a serum calcium of approximately 11 mg/dl typically harbors a parathyroid adenoma weighing in the range of 1 g, and a patient with a serum calcium of 15 mg/dl typically harbors 5 to 8 g of abnormal parathyroid tissue. Average tumor weights are higher in patients with the more severe "bone" presentation of the disorder (mean 3.3 to 5.9 g) than in patients with the more indolent "stone" presentation (mean 1.1 to 1.4 g).[132–134]

Histologically, an adenoma is usually made up of sheets or cords of cells with the ultrastructural appearance of active protein synthetic cells. In the vast majority of adenomas, these cells are chief cells; less commonly, they are oxyphil cells or cells of mixed microscopic appearance. There is a reduction in fat content in the adenomatous tissue, and the adenoma may be surrounded by a clearly defined capsule with an external rim of compressed normal parathyroid tissue. Uninvolved glands in a patient with a parathyroid adenoma are often described as "atrophic," but typically these glands have a fat content and cellularity which are indistinguishable from normal.

There are two gross and histological variants of *primary parathyroid hyperplasia.* In *clear cell hyperplasia,* all four glands are grossly involved. Histologically, the cells have a monotonously empty-looking appearance. The normal cell type from which clear cells are derived is not known. The lesion is rare and has not been observed in familial disease or in states of secondary hyperparathyroidism. *Primary chief cell hyperplasia* is more common and represents a far more difficult problem. A single hyperplastic gland cannot be distinguished grossly or histologically from an adenomatous gland, and this, coupled with the fact that the four parathyroid glands are frequently unequally involved by the hyperplastic process, defines the nature of the clinical problem. The term *pseudoadenomatous hyperplasia* has been introduced to emphasize (1) the fact that gland involvement may be sufficiently uneven to suggest grossly to the surgeon that a single parathyroid adenoma exists together with three normal parathyroid glands and (2) the pseudoencapsulation which may be observed histologically, erroneously suggesting the presence of a single adenoma. Other investigators prefer the term *nodular hyperplasia* to emphasize that the hyperplastic tissue frequently contains nodules of hyperplastic cells and that occasionally these nodules contain oxyphil cells rather than chief cells. Regardless of the nomenclature employed, the differentiation between a parathyroid adenoma and chief cell hyperplasia constitutes a major challenge in regard to the proper surgical management of the disease. "Double" parathyroid adenomas are rarely reported today, and it is thought that the increased frequency of this pathological diagnosis in the older literature probably reflected unappreciated chief cell hyperplasia. Whether multiple adenomas can be defined as a distinct histopathological entity is a matter of opinion.

Both clear cell hyperplasia and chief cell hyperplasia occur sporadically. Chief cell hyperplasia is the predominant, if not the only, lesion which occurs in patients with multiple endocrine neoplasia types I and II. It is also the typical lesion in patients with familial hyperparathyroidism without other demonstrable elements of the multiple glandular syndromes, although first-degree relatives are occasionally observed who, possibly by chance occurrence, harbor a single parathyroid adenoma. All such patients require subtotal parathyroidectomy, with or without parathyroid autotransplantation.

Parathyroid carcinoma is rare (Table 23-8). More than 90 percent of parathyroid carcinomas are functional and are associated with the clinical diagnosis of primary hyperparathyroidism. The lesion typically grows and invades slowly and metastasizes by means of local lymphatic spread. Rarely, the lesion is nonfunctional and/or pursues a fulminant course in a conventional carcinomatous sense, with widespread hematogenous metastases. The clinical presentation of hyperparathyroidism is often but not invariably more severe and rapidly progressive than is noted in the average patient with primary hyperparathyroidism.[135,136] The lesion is recognized grossly by adherence to surrounding tissue and/or by local metastases and histologically by the presence of fibrosis, mitotic figures, and capsular or blood vessel invasion by the malignant cells.[130,135] Not infrequently, the nature of the process goes unrecognized, and the patient is subjected to multiple neck explorations for "recurrent" primary hyperparathyroidism.

The etiology of primary hyperparathyroidism in patients with sporadic parathyroid adenomas and primary hyperplasia is unknown. Evidence for a multicellular origin of parathyroid adenomas based on the distribution of isoenzymes for glucose-6-phosphate dehydrogenase in neoplastic parathyroid cells has been reported.[137] An increasing number of reports in the literature suggest that prior head and neck irradiation is associated with an increased incidence of primary hyperparathyroidism, largely due to a parathyroid adenoma.[138] Parathyroid carcinoma in this setting has not been reported. The etiology of chief cell hyperplasia in patients with familial hyperparathyroidism, multiple endocrine neoplasia type I, and multiple endocrine neoplasia type II remains unclear, as described in Chap. 28. A major difficulty with the APUD hypothesis with respect to the parathyroid lesion is the lack of evidence that parathyroid cells are neuroectodermal in origin.

CLINICAL PRESENTATION AND PATHOPHYSIOLOGY

Figure 23-30 illustrates the presenting features in 1205 patients with primary hyperparathyroidism reported in various clinical series between 1954 and 1971. It is clear that the patients populating these series, which antedated the routine measurement of serum calcium and were reported from referral centers, suffered from the complications that have long been the clinical hallmarks of primary hyperparathyroidism: renal stones and bone disease. It is equally clear from more recent surveys based on the detection of hypercalcemia by means of routine screening in general outpatient and inpatient populations that the clinical presentation of

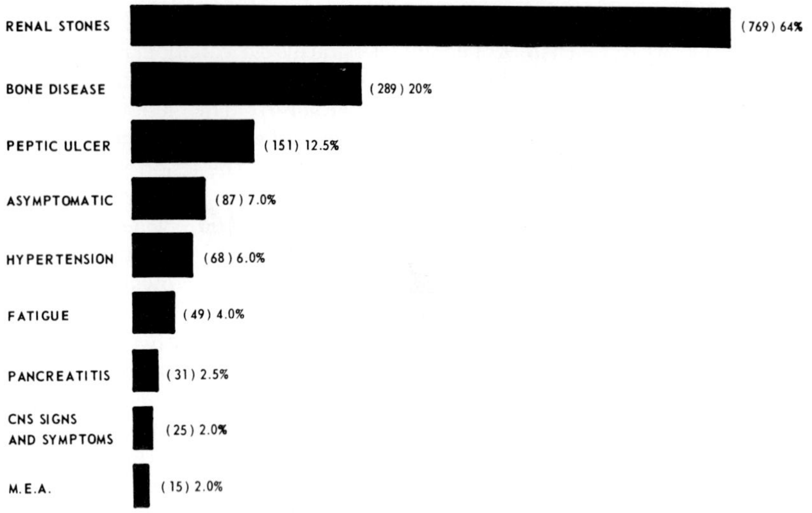

FIGURE 23-30 Clinical manifestations in 1205 patients with primary hyperparathyroidism. [*By permission of Mazzaferri EL: in Mazzaferri EL (ed): Endocrinology. Flushing, NY, Medical Examination Publishing Company, 1974.*]

primary hyperparathyroidism has changed dramatically.[127,128] Stone and bone complications each appeared to be present in less than 10 percent of the patients described in these series, and one-half or more of the patients had no apparent sequelae or manifestations of the disease.[127,128] That is, fully 50 percent of patients with primary hyperparathyroidism presenting today have the serendipity syndrome. Whether such patients are truly asymptomatic and at no serious risk is a matter of debate.

In the discussion below, only bone disease and renal stones will be classified as *specific* complications of primary hyperparathyroidism. The other signs and symptoms shown in Fig. 23-30, although possibly disease-related, will be classified as *nonspecific.* In this context, the term *nonspecific* is used to indicate that the sign or symptom occurs commonly in conditions other than hyperparathyroidism and may not be necessarily attributable to the disease in individual patients.

The clinical presentation of primary hyperparathyroidism can be conveniently remembered by considering the six "moans of hyperparathyroidism": (1) stones, (2) bones, (3) groans (abdominal symptoms), (4) ions (the serendipity syndrome), (5) neurons (the neuromuscular and psychiatric presentations), and (6) hormones (to emphasize the occurrence of primary hyperparathyroidism as part of the multiple endocrine neoplasia syndromes). Although convenient and a means for recalling clinical circumstances requiring consideration of a possible diagnosis of hyperparathyroidism, the "moans" approach fails to emphasize certain important features of the disorder.

A more meaningful approach is to consider the *spectrum* of the disease of primary hyperparathyroidism, as shown in Table 23-9. The table serves to emphasize certain known features of natural history and pathophysiology and, most important, provides a framework for consideration of certain difficult aspects of clinical differential diagnosis and decision making. The "stone," "groan," and "bone" categories listed in the table are somewhat artificial and are designed to describe the framework within which typical patients with primary hyperparathyroidism present clinically; the disease is clinically and pathophysiologically a continuous spectrum, and a number of patients present

Table 23-9. Spectrum of Primary Hyperparathyroidism

	Stones	Groans	Bones
History	Chronic	Indeterminate	Subacute
Serum calcium	Mild	11–12 mg/dl	Severe
iPTH, NcAMP	1+	1+ to 2+	3+ to 4+
Parathyroid mass	1 g	Indeterminate	5 g
Differential diagnosis	Idiopathic hypercalciuria	Multiple	Cancer

Note: iPTH = immunoreactive PTH; NcAMP = nephrogenous cAMP; 1+ to 4+ = increasing quantitative degrees of abnormality.

with features included in more than one of these categories.

The *typical* patient with primary hyperparathyroidism complicated by renal stones presents with a history of chronicity (often years), mild hypercalcemia, mildly to moderately abnormal parathyroid function tests, and a modest parathyroid mass at surgery.[132–134,139] The chief clinical problem within this category is that of differential diagnosis between patients with subtle forms of primary hyperparathyroidism and those with idiopathic hypercalciuria. The *typical* patient with overt hyperparathyroid bone disease has a more subacute history, moderate to severe hypercalcemia, markedly abnormal parathyroid function tests, and a large mass of abnormal parathyroid tissue. The major clinical problem within this category is that of differential diagnosis between patients with severe hyperparathyroidism and those with malignancy and hypercalcemia. The *typical* patient with the "groan," or nonspecific, presentation is in all ways intermediate in the spectrum of primary hyperparathyroidism. The main clinical problems within this category do not have to do with confirmation of diagnosis, which is usually readily achievable with modern diagnostic techniques, but with the requirement that the diagnosis be considered in so many clinical settings (e.g., hypertension, fatigue) and insecurities regarding the recommendation of neck exploration on the basis of such nonspecific manifestations of the disorder. Although there is clearly overlap between the "stone" and "groan" categories and between the "groan" and "bone" categories, patients with a history or clinical findings of both renal stones and overt bone disease are unusual, and the natural history of primary hyperparathyroidism is not one of evolution or progression from left to right in the table. Rather, patients tend to present and remain predominantly within one category when followed over time.

In the discussion below, the specific stone and bone complications of primary hyperparathyroidism will be initially described, followed by a discussion of the nonspecific manifestations of the disease.

PRIMARY HYPERPARATHYROIDISM AND RENAL STONES

Albright's group initially described the occurrence of primary hyperparathyroidism among patients presenting with *renal stones*.[125] The incidence of renal stones in 1317 patients with primary hyperparathyroidism in nine clinical series published between 1961 and 1979 was 55 percent, with a range of 39 to 78 percent.[139] The incidence of primary hyperparathyroidism in 3084 patients with renal stones in eight clinical series published between 1960 and 1978 was 7.2 percent, with a range of 2.9 to 13.3 percent. The dilution of the former incidence figure by patients presenting with the serendipity syndrome was noted above,[127,128] yet renal stones remain the most common single presenting complaint in symptomatic patients,[91,140–142] and the pathogenesis of this complication is well understood. In the older literature, patients with primary hyperparathyroidism were reported to have an increased frequency of pure calcium phosphate stones as well as an increase in the calcium phosphate composition of mixed calcium stones.[91] Today, the most common stone in these patients is the "garden variety" calcium oxalate or mixed calcium oxalate–calcium phosphate stone.

It is important to distinguish between *nephrolithiasis*, which by definition denotes stone formation in the collecting system of the kidneys, and *medullary nephrocalcinosis*, which denotes calcification in the renal parenchyma. Patients with renal stones typically do not display nephrocalcinosis, whereas patients with more severe and/or prolonged hypercalcemia may display nephrocalcinosis without nephrolithiasis, often in the setting of moderate renal impairment. It is unusual for a patient with primary hyperparathyroidism to present with both parenchymal and collecting system calcifications. The pathogenetic mechanisms responsible for these two types of renal calcifications are incompletely understood, but it is likely that nephrolithiasis and nephrocalcinosis result from distinctly different mechanisms, and the terms will be used specifically in the following discussion.

As is the case with all clinical forms of renal stone disease, the pathogenesis of stone formation in primary hyperparathyroidism is complex. Risk factors which have been proposed to be of pathogenetic importance in the formation of stones by patients with primary hyperparathyroidism include (1) proximal renal tubular acidosis related to the tubular effects of PTH, (2) physicochemical factors, and (3) the presence and degree of hypercalciuria. Among these factors, hypercalciuria appears to be the most important.

An increase in urinary pH decreases calcium phosphate solubility. Patients with classic, distal renal tubular acidosis form pure calcium phosphate stones. The increased percentage of calcium phosphate composition reported in stones from patients with primary hyperparathyroidism initially suggested that the effects of PTH on proximal bicarbonate handling may be an important influence on stone formation in this disorder. The reported frequency of an actual systemic hyperchloremic acidosis in primary hyperparathyroidism has varied widely; some series have noted reduced serum bicarbonate concentrations in upwards of 20 percent of patients,[134] and other series report that systemic acidosis is rare in primary hyperparathyroidism and correlates poorly with circulating PTH.[143] A clear-cut systemic acidosis is most frequently observed in patients with coincident renal impairment,[139,143] usually in the absence of stones but sometimes in the presence of nephrocalcinosis. Such patients may also display glucosuria and aminoaciduria. In addition, there are important pathophysiological differences between the proximal and distal forms of renal tubular acidosis such that the effects of PTH on the proximal tubular handling of bicarbonate are associated with little influence on the final urinary pH.[139,142,144] Thus, acidification disturbances in primary hyperparathyroidism must currently be viewed as a possible but unproved risk factor for stone formation in the disorder.

The physicochemical aspects of stone formation in primary hyperparathyroidism have not been extensively studied. The techniques and terminology employed in such studies are described in Chap. 25. The urine of patients with primary hyperparathyroidism has been reported to be supersaturated with respect to stone-forming constituents, a finding attributed to increased urinary calcium concentrations.[144] In addition, the urine from these patients displayed an unexplained propensity for crystallization and crystal growth, a finding compatible with either a decrease in "inhibitors" or an increase in "promoters" of crystallization and growth. The chemical nature of such positive and negative influences on stone formation is not known.[139]

The occurrence of hypercalciuria in primary hyperparathyroidism has been recognized as a risk factor for stone formation since Albright's era, yet the exact relation between hypercalciuria and stone formation and the pathogenesis of hypercalciuria in primary hyperparathyroidism has remained largely unexplained. Approximately two-thirds of patients with primary hyperparathyroidism have demonstrable hypercalciuria, but statistical relations between the quantity of calcium excreted and stone formation in hyperparathyroid patients with and without stones have been and remain difficult to establish. The history of chronicity and the mild hypercalcemia typically noted in patients with primary hyperparathyroidism complicated by renal stones and the balance and dual hormone hypotheses of Albright and Dent, respectively, were discussed previously. Albright's conceptualization was subsequently confirmed in that it was found that patients with primary hyperparathyroidism, mild hypercalcemia, and stone disease were in zero or slightly positive external calcium balance, whereas patients with severe hypercalcemia were usually in negative calcium balance (Fig. 23-31). Other observations came to be generally appreciated: (1) that patients with severe hypercalcemia do not often display a proportionate degree of hypercalciuria and (2) that certain patients with mild hypercalcemia present with disproportionate hypercalciuria.[139–141] Although the first observation appeared to be explicable by virtue of the renal impairment often noted in such patients and the effects of the markedly elevated circulating concentrations of PTH on distal tubular calcium reabsorption, the second observation represented a paradox when considered in terms of the classical relation between the filtered load of calcium and urinary calcium excretion and the known renal effects of PTH. This issue can best be visualized by considering two patients with primary hyperparathyroidism. Each has a fasting serum calcium of 11.0 mg/dl, but the first has a urinary calcium of 500 mg per day and a history of stones and

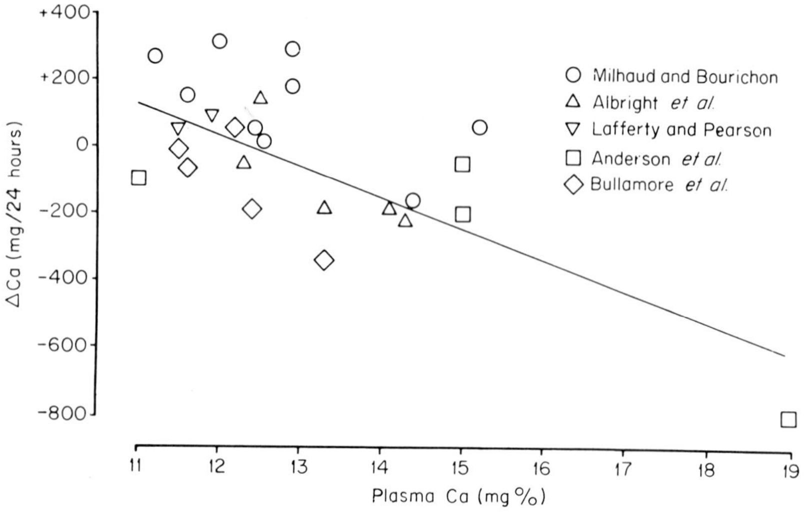

FIGURE 23-31 Net calcium balance plotted as a function of the serum calcium concentration in 25 patients with primary hyperparathyroidism reported in various series according to the symbols in the figure. The data are strongly correlated ($r = -0.67$, $p = 0.001$) and support the view that patients with mild hyperparathyroidism are in zero or positive balance, whereas patients with severe hyperparathyroidism are in negative balance. [By permission of Parsons JA: in Bourne GH (ed): *The Biochemistry and Physiology of Bone*, vol 4. New York, Academic Press, 1976.]

the second has a urinary calcium of 250 mg per day and no history of stones. The obvious pathophysiological difference between these two patients is the marked hypercalciuria in the first patient.

The initial key to this paradox was provided by Peacock's studies of fractional intestinal calcium absorption in a large series of patients with primary hyperparathyroidism.[145] He found that patients presenting with a history of renal stones uniformly displayed an increase in calcium absorption, whereas patients with "other" (nonstone) presentations displayed widely varying patterns of calcium absorption (Fig. 23-32). The implications of these studies have recently been confirmed by determinations of circulating concentrations of 1,25-$(OH)_2D$ in patients with primary hyperparathyroidism (Fig. 23-33). Although the data for circulating 1,25-$(OH)_2D$, calcium absorption, and calcium excretion in primary hyperparathyroidism represent a continuous spectrum, the patients with marked elevations in serum 1,25-$(OH)_2D$, intestinal hyperabsorption of calcium, and resultant hypercalciuria are those who are most prone to stone disease (Fig. 23-33). The major source of the calcium excreted by these patients is therefore the diet, and the pattern of absorption and excretion of calcium is remarkably similar to that observed in patients with "absorptive" hypercalciuria (Chap. 25). These findings provide a clear pathophysiological explanation for the often observed disproportionality between the level of serum calcium and the rate of calcium excretion in patients with primary hyperparathyroidism.[139–141] Why certain patients with hyperparathyroidism have normal or nearly normal circulating levels of 1,25-$(OH)_2D$ while others have marked elevations in the circulating level of the active metabolite remains unexplained.[139,141] It has recently been recognized that the PTH–1,25-$(OH)_2D$ axis may be remarkably sensitive to dietary calcium intake in patients with primary hyperparathyroidism.[112] The suppressibility of circulating 1,25-$(OH)_2D$ was such that a majority of values were well within normal range if patients were placed on an unrestricted calcium diet.[112] It follows that a clear appreciation of the pathophysiological importance of circulating 1,25-$(OH)_2D$ in these patients requires that they be evaluated on a restricted calcium diet.

The foregoing discussion is not intended to imply direct causality between hypercalciuria and stone formation in primary hyperparathyroidism, for a number of hypercalciuric patients with this disorder are observed who have not formed stones, and occasional patients with hyperparathyroidism present with renal stones and are found not to be hypercalciuric. These points explain such apparent interpretive discrepancies as exist in the recent literature; these discrepancies are a function of patient classification and the

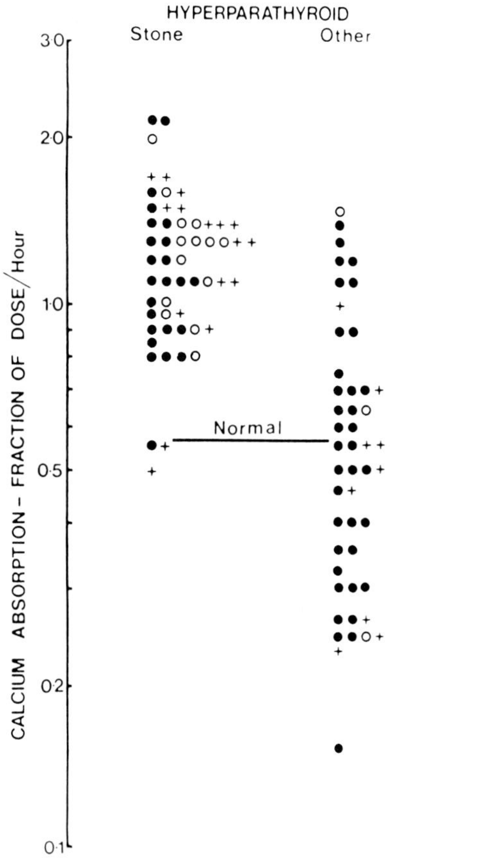

FIGURE 23-32 Fractional isotopic calcium absorption in 111 patients with primary hyperparathyroidism. The symbols correspond to male (+), premenopausal female (○), and postmenopausal female (●) patients with (stone) or without (other) renal stone disease. The mean calcium absorption in normal control subjects is indicated. [*By permission of Peacock M, in Talmadge RV, Owen M, Parsons JA (eds): Calcium Regulating Hormones. Amsterdam, Excerpta Medica, 1975.*]

statistical correlations attempted rather than a result of disagreement about the pathophysiological mechanisms leading to hypercalciuria in patients with hyperparathyroidism.[141,142] In essence, hypercalciuria should be viewed as a risk factor for stone formation in patients with primary hyperparathyroidism, just as it is in the general population of patients with stone disease, and it should be recognized that marked hypercalciuria confers a definite statistical risk for stone-related complications in individual patients with the disorder. In this context, it is of interest to note the virtual absence of renal stone disease in patients with familial hypocalciuric hypercalcemia (see below). Although the previous discussion emphasized the fact that the typical patient with primary hyperparathyroidism complicated by stones has a mean total serum calcium in the range of 11 mg/dl, patients with stones

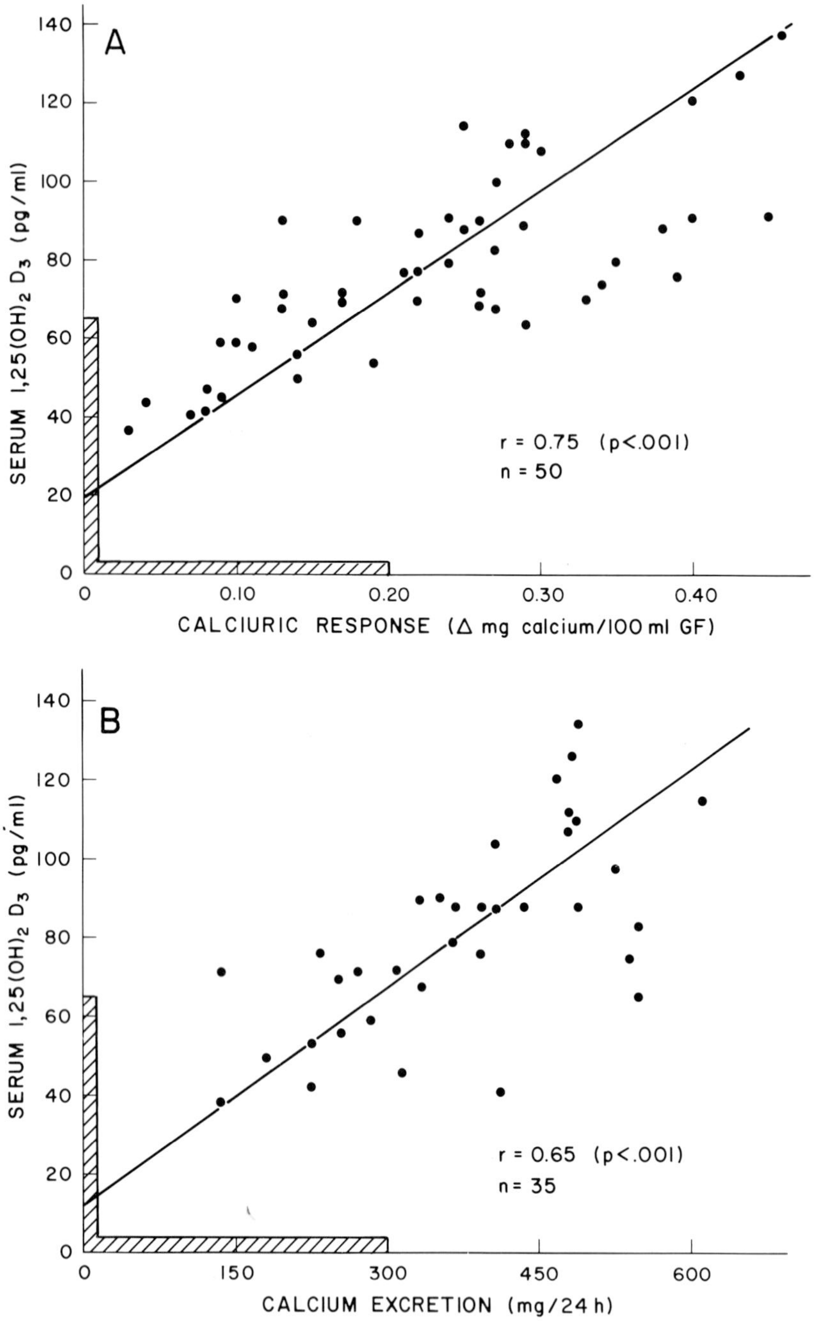

FIGURE 23-33 Correlations between circulating 1,25-$(OH)_2D$ and the calciuric response to an oral calcium tolerance test (*A*) and 24-h calcium excretion on a 1000-mg calcium intake (*B*) in patients with primary hyperparathyroidism. The number of patients studied and the correlation coefficients are indicated on the figures. The normal ranges are designated by the crosshatched bars adjoining the abscissa and ordinate. Approximately two-thirds of the patients with an abnormal calciuric response to the calcium tolerance test and elevations in circulating 1,25-$(OH)_2D$ and calcium excretion had a history of one or more renal stone events. (*By permission of Broadus AE, Horst RL, Lang R, Littledike ET, Rasmussen H, N Engl J Med 302:421, 1980.*)

and serum calcium values in the range of 12 to 13 mg/dl may also be observed. The differential diagnosis between patients with "subtle" primary hyperparathyroidism and those with various subtypes of hypercalciuria is presented in the hypercalciuria section of Chap. 25.

HYPERPARATHYROID BONE DISEASE

Just as the effects of PTH on bone are complex, so are the skeletal manifestations of primary hyperparathyroidism. The ill-defined nature of the term *hyperparathyroid bone disease* relates to many difficulties: (1)

imperfect knowledge regarding pathogenesis and natural history, (2) the largely unknown present-day incidence of clinically relevant bone "disease" in the disorder, (3) overlap in the osteitic and osteopenic varieties of bone involvement, and (4) imprecise definitions for separating clinical or overt bone disease from subclinical skeletal findings of unknown significance. For example, histological or isotopic evidence of an increase in bone turnover rate can be demonstrated in virtually 100 percent of patients with primary hyperparathyroidism, yet this finding is physiologically predictable and of little clinical significance if bone remodeling remains tightly coupled. Attempts to understand bone involvement in primary hyperparathyroidism must include an appreciation of the complex interplay of the elements controlling both skeletal homeostasis and systemic mineral homeostasis.

The classical bone disease of primary hyperparathyroidism is osteitis fibrosa cystica. The history of primary hyperparathyroidism began in the 1920s with the clinical description of this form of the disease. Clinically, severe osteitis fibrosa cystica is characterized by bone pain, pathological fractures of long bones and crush fractures of the spine, and skeletal deformities. Radiologically, it is characterized by demineralization, erosion of outer and inner cortical surfaces, fractures and deformities, locally destructive lesions, chondrocalcinosis, and soft-tissue calcifications. The demineralization is patchy rather than homogeneous, as typified by the moth-eaten or ground-glass appearance of the skull. The outer cortical erosions are referred to as subperiosteal resorption and may be demonstrable in the pelvis, the medial surfaces of the tibia and humerus, the outer ends of the clavicles, the superior borders of the ribs, and the metacarpal and phalangeal bones in the hand. Whenever subperiosteal resorption is detected in any portion of the skeleton, it is also evident in the hands.[146] The radial aspect of the middle phalanges is the most sensitive site for detection of subperiosteal resorption; in this region, the degree of erosion may be graded on a semiquantitative scale of 0 to 5 using fine-detailed radiography and optical magnification (Fig. 23-34). On routine hand radiographs, subtle erosions can be better appreciated if the films are examined with a 5X or 10X lens from an ordinary microscope. The locally destructive lesions comprise two types of cystic lesions: true bone cysts and "brown tumors." The former are true fluid-filled cysts, and the latter are composed largely of osteoclasts intermixed with poorly mineralized woven bone and are sometimes referred to as osteoclastomas. These two lesions have the same radiological appearance, but bone cysts remain indefinitely after successful surgery whereas brown tumors resolve and remineralize. A brown tumor in the mandible or maxilla (epulis) is a rare presenting complaint in severe hyperparathyroidism. Loss of the lamina dura of the teeth may be observed but is a far less specific and sensitive finding than is subperiosteal resorption. Apart from the true bone cysts, virtually all radiographic findings of osteitis fibrosa cystica are reversible. Osteosclerosis is rarely seen in primary hyperparathyroidism, in contrast to its relatively frequent occurrence in renal osteodystrophy. Classic radiographic findings of osteitis fibrosa cystica are considered to be diagnostic of hyperparathyroidism.

The histological hallmarks of osteitis fibrosa cystica are (1) increased rates of bone formation and resorption with a marked increase in the number of active osteoclasts, (2) a loss of cortical and trabecular bone together with a loss of normal trabecular architecture, (3) an increase in unmineralized osteoid, and (4) extensive fibrosis, with replacement of normal marrow and bone cell elements. Although there remains some degree of coupling, quantitative morphometric or other techniques reveal that the rate of bone resorption considerably exceeds the rate of bone formation.

The incidence of symptomatic and/or radiologically apparent osteitis fibrosa cystica has been estimated to have been as high as 50 percent in patients with primary hyperparathyroidism diagnosed between 1925 and 1950.[129,132] Thereafter, the reported percentage of patients with significant osteitic bone involvement has steadily fallen to approximately 20 percent by 1960 and to 10 percent or less today.[127,128] It is doubtful that these figures reflect an alteration in the basic disease process; rather, they are regarded as indicative of a wider appreciation of the disease, improved diagnostic methods, and the reported frequency of the serendipity syndrome.[127,128] What today constitutes a clinically relevant diagnosis of osteitis fibrosa cystica is a matter of opinion; most authorities would accept the finding of unequivocal radiological subperiosteal resorption as evidence of clinical bone involvement, and all would accept subperiosteal resorption together with manifest demineralization. Such a patient may or may not complain of bone pain or have demonstrable bone tenderness on physical examination. Whereas the radiological diagnosis of osteitis fibrosa cystica may be made in 5 to 10 percent of patients with primary hyperparathyroidism today, less than 5 percent of patients with the disorder present with bone-related symptoms as the chief complaint.

The pathogenesis of osteitis fibrosa cystica has not been clearly defined. A number of series have stressed the subacute clinical history, marked hypercalcemia, and large aggregate parathyroid mass typically noted in patients with osteitis fibrosa cystica. Current opinion

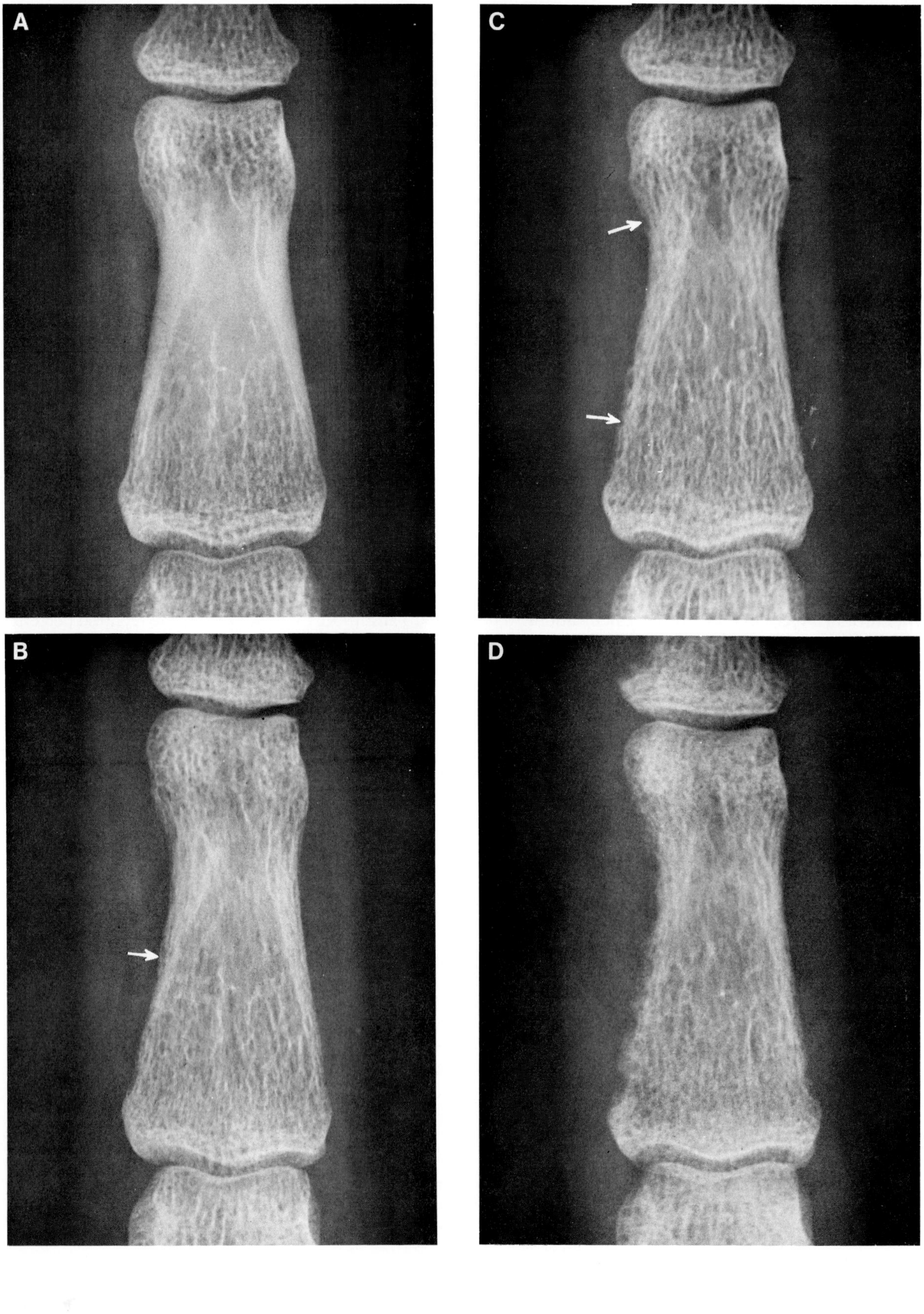
A
B
C
D

favors the view that osteitis fibrosa cystica is a complication of severe and rapidly progressive primary hyperparathyroidism that is due largely to the growth potential of the parathyroid lesion. Indeed, such a presentation is typical of patients harboring a parathyroid carcinoma.[135,136] This view is also supported by the biochemical-histological correlates from the studies of Bordier and associates,[147] who noted that the osteoclast count correlated well with immunoreactive PTH only at high circulating concentrations of the hormone. In terms of mineral homeostasis, most patients with osteitis fibrosa cystica are in negative calcium balance, and often this negative balance is profound (Fig. 23-31). Nephrocalcinosis is demonstrable in approximately 25 percent of such patients, and moderate renal impairment is frequent.[132] Measurements of calcium absorption and/or circulating levels of 1,25-$(OH)_2D$ in patients specifically defined as having osteitis fibrosa cystica have not been reported, but the balance data imply that systemic calcium losses considerably outstrip net intestinal calcium absorption. It will be recalled that Dent's dietary survey did not support Albright's proposal that dietary calcium deficiency might be a causal factor in the development of osteitis fibrosa cystica.[126]

Several recent series have emphasized the frequency of radiological evidence of osteopenia rather than osteitis fibrosa cystica in patients with primary hyperparathyroidism. Radiologically this osteopenia is diffuse and resembles osteoporosis. In a series reported in 1973, osteopenia of the spine was noted in 20 percent and of the hands in 36 percent of patients with primary hyperparathyroidism.[148] This series antedated the routine measurement of serum calcium and therefore might have been enriched for symptomatic patients. The study of patients with primary hyperparathyroidism by modern densitometric techniques (^{125}I bone densitometry and photon absorptiometry) has also provided evidence of decreased bone mineral density in one-third or more of patients with the disorder, and osteopenia has been reported to be particularly prevalent among postmenopausal women.[149–151] The demineralization apparent on detailed hand films has the appearance of intracortical resorption and can be graded on a semiquantitative scale of 0 to 4 (Fig. 23-34). There is disagreement as to whether cortical or trabecular bone is most at risk and, correspondingly, as to which detection techniques applied to what part of the skeleton provide the most reliable means of diagnosing osteopenia in patients with primary hyperparathyroidism.[150,151] The major and critical unsettled issues regarding this osteopenia are (1) unknown aspects of pathogenesis and natural history, (2) the specificity of its relation to primary hyperparathyroidism, and (3) its potential reversibility after parathyroidectomy and/or its progression in untreated patients. Practically all such patients lack actual bone symptoms.

FIGURE 23-34 Fine-detail radiographs of the middle phalanx: (*A*) normal; (*B*) intracortical resorption (arrow), grade 2 on a scale of 4; (*C*) subperiosteal resorption (arrows), grade 2 on a scale of 4; (*D*) grade 4 subperiosteal resorption. (*Courtesy of P.S. Jensen.*)

←

As studied by quantitative morphometric or isotopic techniques, the average patient with primary hyperparathyroidism is estimated to have a severalfold increase in bone turnover rate. If the resorption and formation rates remain firmly coupled, this increase in bone turnover will not ultimately affect skeletal homeostasis and bone mineral content.[37,152–154] However, if the resorption rate exceeds formation rate, even by a slight margin, loss of bone mineral and osteopenia will ultimately ensue. Employing quantitative morphometry of iliac crest biopsies, Meunier and coworkers[152] reported evidence of increased osteoclastic resorption surfaces and increased osteocytic osteolysis in 40 patients with primary hyperparathyroidism. Conceptually, these biopsy findings are equivalent to a fully activated "acute" resorptive effect of PTH in bone, together with a modest "late" resorptive response. It is therefore tempting to speculate that osteopenia in primary hyperparathyroidism is a mild and perhaps subclinical skeletal manifestation of the disease, in contrast to osteitis fibrosa cystica, which may be regarded as a somewhat extreme example of the "late" response to the hormone.

Details of pathogenesis in osteopenic patients are entirely unknown. It is also unknown whether the osteopenia is predictably progressive and merges imperceptively with mild osteitis fibrosa cystica with time. Existing studies of patients with osteitis fibrosa cystica and/or osteopenia have not provided essential details regarding mineral balance and hormonal correlates. Multiple variables are probably of pathogenetic importance in all degrees of bone involvement in primary hyperparathyroidism. For example, hypophosphatemia per se increases bone resorption, and normal skeletal balance is restored by means of phosphorus repletion. In addition, patients with primary hyperparathyroidism and predominant osteomalacia have been described in the setting of simple vitamin D deficiency or anticonvulsant drug therapy or as a result of intestinal malabsorption.

In the final analysis, bone involvement in primary hyperparathyroidism must be regarded as a spectrum, with variable clinical, radiological, and histological findings depending on both the aggressiveness of the basic disease process and elements of systemic mineral homeostasis. The key question to be resolved in the coming decade relates to the clinical relevance of osteopenia in primary hyperparathyroidism; at present, this radiological finding is reported with approximately four times the frequency of classical findings of osteitis fibrosa cystica.

NONSPECIFIC FEATURES OF PRIMARY HYPERPARATHYROIDISM

The nonspecific symptoms and findings in primary hyperparathyroidism will be treated in considerably less detail than the specific stone and bone complications of the disorder. The literature purporting to establish pathogenetic relations between hyperparathyroidism and these various symptoms is massive, but in the aggregate the direct evidence supplied is hardly compelling. These various symptoms and findings may or may not occur with increased frequency in primary hyperparathyroidism; they may or may not be related to abnormalities in serum calcium, phosphorus, PTH, or vitamin D levels; and they may or may not respond to successful parathyroidectomy. The physician should be cautious in recommending surgery to middle-aged or elderly patients with hypertension, depression, or other nonspecific symptoms and should be particularly circumspect with regard to communicating expected operative results to such patients.

The initial clear neurological description of *neuromyopathic* symptoms and findings in primary hyperparathyroidism appeared in 1949,[155] and the importance of these findings was reemphasized in the mid-1970s.[147] Although neuromuscular symptoms were noted with some frequency in older series of patients with primary hyperparathyroidism, they were not emphasized and were largely attributed to systemic consequences of the severe disease process typifying patients in those series. In Patten's studies,[156] 14 of 16 patients with primary hyperparathyroidism of varying severity had clear-cut symptoms, physical findings, and/or laboratory evidence of neuromyopathic involvement. These symptoms frequently constituted the patient's presenting complaints and in some patients even suggested primary neuromuscular disease to the examining physicians. The most common symptoms were weakness and fatigability, most particularly in the proximal muscles of the lower extremity. Physical findings variably included muscular weakness, muscle atrophy, hyperreflexia, and peculiar fine fasciculations of the tongue. Sensory abnormalities were rare. Detailed evaluation of the patients by electromyography, determination of nerve conduction time, and muscle biopsies revealed findings similar to those seen in experimental denervation, indicating that the process is neuropathic rather than myopathic in nature.[156] Neuropathic symptoms and findings showed no correlation with the serum or cerebrospinal fluid content of calcium, phosphorus, or magnesium. Serum levels of muscle enzymes were normal. The most important feature of the neuropathic symptoms of primary hyperparathyroidism is their apparent complete reversibility following successful neck exploration.[156] These studies are impressive and await confirmation in a larger series of patients. It is certainly implied that patients should be carefully questioned and examined before being delegated to the "asymptomatic" category, and it may be the alleviation of just such symptoms that contributes to the improved sense of well-being noted by certain patients following parathyroidectomy. A similar symptom complex has been described in various states of secondary hyperparathyroidism.[155] The pathogenesis of the neuropathic process in these hyperparathyroid states is not known, but its occurrence in both primary and secondary hyperparathyroidism suggests that alterations in PTH and/or phosphorus levels may be of pathogenetic importance.

Central nervous system symptoms in primary hyperparathyroidism and other hypercalcemic states can be considered in several categories. A sequence of mild lethargy–confusion–obtundation is the predictable consequence of increasing degrees of hypercalcemia. However predictable, the quantitative relation between the level of serum calcium and the degree of mental impairment is very crude; some patients are perfectly lucid at a serum calcium of 17 mg/dl, whereas others are markedly confused at a serum calcium of 13 mg/dl. Other variables which may influence the ultimate degree of mental impairment are the rate of development of hypercalcemia, the amount of attendant dehydration, and the mental substrate on which the hypercalcemia is superimposed. The importance of these variables has been clearly defined in the series of Mundy et al.[128] In this series, 14 percent of patients with primary hyperparathyroidism in a general hospital setting were described as presenting with dehydration and confusion, and all but one of these patients was beyond the age of 70 years. In the absence of prolonged coma and actual central nervous system damage, calcium-induced alterations in mental status are readily reversible.

The potential relation between hypercalcemia and psychoneurotic or actual psychiatric symptoms represents a particularly difficult problem. Such symptoms may include depression, personality change, memory loss, and overtly psychotic behavior. A mild subclinical depression may accompany the neuropathic symptoms described above and may or may not resolve with successful parathyroidectomy. Psychoneurotic symptoms often are not influenced by curative surgery. There are a number of existing anecdotes relating dramatic improvement in overtly psychotic symptoms after parathyroidectomy. Although these anecdotes may be widely circulated, they do not appear to be representative of the more typical negative experience with such patients. Contemplation of surgery in a patient with coincident primary hyperparathyroidism and psychiatric symptoms requires consideration of the manifest severity of the hyperparathyroidism together with a detailed psychiatric opinion regarding the possible "toxic" or organic nature of the psychiatric symptoms.

Several *gastrointestinal* symptom complexes require consideration in patients with primary hyperparathyroidism: (1) peptic ulcer disease, (2) pancreatitis, and (3) diffuse, nonspecific abdominal pain. The association of all three of these complexes with primary hyperparathyroidism has become standard medical teaching, yet significant questions regarding pathogenesis and the specificity of the relation of these abdominal complications to hyperparathyroidism remain unresolved.

Whether peptic ulcer disease occurs with an increased frequency in primary hyperparathyroidism has been repeatedly debated and reviewed.[129,157,158] A combination of the series summarized by Barreras together with the NIH series indicates that findings of peptic ulcer disease were noted in approximately 14 percent of 985 patients with primary hyperparathyroidism.[134,157] This is presumed to be a higher frequency than that found in the general adult population, although precise prevalence figures for ulcer disease in the general population are largely unavailable and have been estimated to be as low as 2 to 3 percent or as high as 5 to 10 percent.[157,158] Thus, the frequency of peptic ulcer disease in primary hyperparathyroidism has been considered to be approximately equal to or as much as fivefold higher than that in the general population. In the absence of a gastrinoma, peptic ulcer disease in primary hyperparathyroidism appears to be of the "garden variety" in terms of location and recurrence. However, several series have reported an increased gastric to duodenal ulcer ratio in men and a disproportionately increased frequency of duodenal ulcers in women. In the published series of the 1980s, ulcer disease was reported in less than 10 percent of patients with primary hyperparathyroidism.[127,128]

It is clear that endogenous and/or induced hypercalcemia can increase gastrin levels and gastric acid secretion in normal subjects, patients with primary hyperparathyroidism, and patients with the Zollinger-Ellison syndrome.[129,157] Conversely, hypocalcemia has been shown to inhibit or abolish gastric acid secretion. It is also known that oral administration of the "antacid" calcium carbonate increases gastrin secretion and gastric output without an attendant change in serum calcium and that the calcium ion stimulates parietal cell secretion in the absence of gastrin. Basal and stimulated gastric secretion and basal and stimulated serum gastrin levels in preoperative and postoperative patients with primary hyperparathyroidism have been reported by several groups, with conflicting data and interpretations. Increases in basal acid output and/or fasting serum gastrin concentrations have been noted in one-quarter to one-third of patients with primary hyperparathyroidism and have been reported either to normalize or to remain largely unchanged postoperatively.[129,157–159] A careful review of these various series shows a poor correlation between the acid studies and serum gastrin levels and actual clinical ulcer findings in patients with primary hyperparathyroidism. Although symptoms and objective findings of acid-peptic disease are generally said to improve after parathyroidectomy, this impression is based on surprisingly little systematic evidence.

Patients with the Zollinger-Ellison syndrome represent a special case. Gastrinomas may coexist with primary hyperparathyroidism in multiple endocrine neoplasia type I. It has been reported that the elevations in gastrin levels and acid output in some patients with this syndrome improve after parathyroid surgery, occasionally to such a degree that an actual improvement in ulcer symptoms and findings is noted.[157] Rare patients have been reported in whom parathyroidectomy essentially reversed striking preoperative findings of acid output, gastrin concentrations, and the ulcer diathesis, and these cases have been interpreted as examples of a pseudo-Zollinger-Ellison syndrome. This interpretation has been questioned. Typically, the basal elevations and/or stimulability of serum gastrin concentrations observed in patients with primary hyperparathyroidism are not in the range noted in patients with a gastrinoma, in whom basal levels of serum gastrin are rarely lower than 150 pg/ml. If serious questions exist in a rare individual case, neck exploration should be undertaken before consideration of gastrin surgery.

Acute or chronic pancreatitis occurs in approximately 2 percent of patients with primary hyperparathyroidism. The frequency of pancreatitis is much higher in patients with severe hyperparathyroidism or "parathyroid crisis," in whom an incidence of 30 percent or more has been reported.[129] In their review, which remains the best published to date, Mixter and coworkers[160] identified all the clinical forms of pancreatitis in patients with primary hyperparathyroidism and classified the pancreatitis into five types: (1) acute, (2) acute postoperative (any surgical procedure), (3) recurrent, (4) chronic with pain, and (5) chronic without pain. The chronic types may present with or without a history of recurrent acute episodes and with or without evidence of pancreatic insufficiency. Chronic pancreatitis with pain was the most common type noted, occurring in 26 of the 62 (42 percent) cases reviewed.[160] Typically, other contributing factors, such as alcohol abuse, were not identified in the patients. Pancreatic calculi were noted radiologically or pathologically with great frequency, regardless of the clinical presentation. Symptoms of pancreatitis preceded the diagnosis of hyperparathyroidism in the majority of patients. Patients presenting with pancreatitis were virtually absent in the recent series of Heath and coworkers[127] and Mundy and associates.[128]

The pathogenesis of pancreatitis as it occurs in primary hyperparathyroidism is unknown. There is a presumptive relation between the hypercalcemia and pancreatitis, as evidenced by the frequency of pancreatitis in patients with severe hyperparathyroidism and reports of the occurrence of pancreatitis in other hypercalcemic conditions. Pathogenetic proposals include (1) pancreatic obstruction and/or injury due to ductal calculi and parenchymal calcifications and (2) direct effects of PTH and/or the calcium ion on pancreatic enzyme activation. Neither proposal is supported by direct experimental evidence.

It is often noted that the total serum calcium may be reduced during severe, acute episodes of pancreatitis or in chronic pancreatitis associated with malabsorption such that coincident primary hyperparathyroidism may be "missed." However, the hypercalcemia is usually readily apparent at all times. A presumptive diagnosis of primary hyperparathyroidism must be confirmed by standard methods, since other hypercalcemic conditions appear also to be associated with pancreatitis. Mixter and coworkers[160] noted substantial clinical improvement in abdominal symptoms following successful parathyroidectomy in their personal and reviewed cases.

In the absence of pancreatitis, hypercalcemia and/or hyperparathyroidism may influence insulin secretion and diabetic management. The exact nature of this influence has been the subject of conflicting reports and remains unclear.[161]

Diffuse, ill-defined abdominal pain is the presenting complaint in a small percentage of patients with primary hyperparathyroidism. The pain may be intermittent or relatively persistent and is poorly described and localized. A thorough abdominal evaluation is usually negative. The pain tends to resolve quite dramatically following curative parathyroidectomy. Other gastrointestinal symptoms which may accompany hypercalcemia of any cause are constipation, anorexia, weight loss, and nausea and vomiting. In older series, these various symptoms were reported in 20 to 30 percent of patients. These symptoms are clearly calcium-related, increasing in severity with the degree of hypercalcemia and rapidly resolving with restoration of normocalcemia.

An increased frequency of cholelithiasis has been reported in primary hyperparathyroidism, and the association was particularly striking among young patients.[162] A disproportionate number of radiopaque gallstones was noted. This presumed relation between primary hyperparathyroidism and cholelithiasis has not been stressed in previous large series of patients with primary hyperparathyroidism or in more recent series.

In a recent and careful case-control comparison of the prevalence of *hypertension* in patients with hyperparathyroidism vs. the prevalence in sex-, age-, and race-matched control patients, the prevalence figures were 48 percent and 35 percent, respectively.[127] This difference was statistically significant, but the authors chose not to regard hypertension as a specific consequence of hyperparathyroidism for rather obvious reasons. As defined in categories of mild, moderate, and severe hypertension, the pattern of hypertension is similar in the general adult and hyperparathyroid populations.[128,134] Pathogenic proposals to explain the presumed relation of hypertension and primary hyperparathyroidism include (1) effects of the calcium ion on peripheral vascular resistance, mediated either by direct ionic effects on vascular smooth muscle or by local catecholamine release, (2) associated abnormalities of the renin-angiotensin system, (3) an increased frequency of renal impairment in primary hyperparathyroidism, and (4) coexistent pheochromocytoma and primary hyperparathyroidism in patients with multiple endocrine neoplasia type II.[163,164] The latter association should be considered in any hypertensive patient with primary hyperparathyroidism but is rare. In Hellstrom's series,[164] there was a strong correlation between severe hypertension and coexistent renal impairment, and it was noted in this and subsequent series that the severe hypertension associated with renal impairment was unlikely to improve following successful parathyroidectomy. The reported influence of surgical correction of primary hyperparathyroidism on blood pressure has been widely and puzzlingly divergent, with several series reporting a high incidence of normalization of blood pressure and others reporting little influence of surgery on preexisting hypertension.[163] Clearly, direct causality between primary hyperparathyroidism and associated hypertension cannot be assumed in individual patients.

Hypercalcemia is associated with a reversible shortening of the QT interval and a prolongation of the PR interval. Occasionally first-degree heart block is observed, but the cardiographic manifestations of hypercalcemia are rarely of actual clinical significance.

A variety of *articular* manifestations are observed in patients with primary hyperparathyroidism. Skeletal fractures and/or deformity are commonly associated with degenerative osteoarthritis in contiguous weight-bearing joints. Both uric acid and calcium crystal deposition diseases have been reported to occur with increased frequency in primary hyperparathyroidism. The renal clearance of uric acid is reduced in the disorder, and mild hyperuricemia is reasonably common. Attacks of acute gouty arthritis are not common, occurring in a few percent of patients.[134] Chronic chondrocalcinosis, with or without acute attacks of pseudogout, is the more characteristic crystal deposition disease in primary hyperparathyroidism and affects approximately 5 percent of patients; both manifestations occur more frequently in patients with severe than in those with mild hyperparathyroidism. The knee is by far the most common joint involved, and the typical course is one of degenerative arthropathy interspersed with episodes of acute inflammation. X-rays reveal calcification of articular cartilage, and definitive diagnosis is made by demonstrating the characteristic rhomboidal calcium pyrophosphate dihydrate crystals in joint fluid. The great toe is far less frequently involved than in urate gout. Chondrocalcinosis has been found in a wide variety of metabolic disorders other than hyperparathyroidism so that the association of the two disorders is by no means specific. Acute attacks of both urate gout and pseudogout may occur following parathyroidectomy,[165] and both types of crystals may be simultaneously identified in joint fluid from an occasional patient in this setting. Salicylates are employed in the treatment of chronic symptomatic chondrocalcinosis, and indomethacin and phenylbutazone are the drugs of choice in acute pseudogout. Occasionally, resorption of bone in articular areas and/or periarticular calcifications can produce a polyarticular syndrome superficially resembling rheumatoid arthritis.

CLINICAL VARIANTS OF PRIMARY HYPERPARATHYROIDISM

Acute hyperparathyroidism and *parathyroid crisis* are terms used in reference to particularly severe and emergent presentations of the disorder. Such cases are typified by subacute histories, extreme hypercalcemia, clinical bone disease, renal impairment, and severe systemic manifestations of hypercalcemia.[166] Without expert medical and surgical management, the usual end result in these patients is death. Parathyroid carcinoma should be suspected in such circumstances,[135,136] but large and apparently rapidly growing parathyroid adenomas and parathyroid hyperplasia may lead to the same presentation. These patients represent the extreme end of the spectrum shown in Table 23-9, and the usual and erroneous clinical diagnosis is malignancy-associated hypercalcemia. The parathyroid lesion is not infrequently palpable and may often be visualized by computerized tomography or other routine radiological techniques. Parathyroid function tests are usually dramatically elevated in these patients, readily distinguishing them from patients with a malignancy. However, intervention may be required before laboratory confirmation is available.

Patients with "normocalcemic" hyperparathyroidism represent the opposite extreme of the spectrum of the disorder. In many ways, this term is unfortunate, but it appears to be well ingrained in medical usage. There are several clinical circumstances in which patients with primary hyperparathyroidism may present with true normocalcemia or with only mild, intermittent hypercalcemia.

Patients with coincident malabsorption and/or simple or disease- or drug-related vitamin D deficiency may present with clinical bone disease and normal values for serum calcium. The bone lesion may be osteitis fibrosa cystica variably admixed with osteomalacia. The diagnosis is usually "missed" but becomes chemically obvious with successful treatment of the concomitant disorder or vitamin D deficiency. Such patients are frequently reported as examples of "tertiary" hyperparathyroidism, but it is equally likely that the parathyroid lesion is primary and is simply obscured by the associated clinical abnormalities.[167]

Patients with subtle hyperparathyroidism complicated by renal stone disease represent a far more frequent clinical and diagnostic problem. Only rarely are such patients continuously normocalcemic; typically they display a rather characteristic pattern of mild, intermittent hypercalcemia.[168] These patients represent a striking example of disproportionality between serum calcium levels and the rate of urinary calcium excretion and uniformly display marked elevations in circulating concentrations of $1,25\text{-}(OH)_2D$ and gastrointestinal calcium absorption. Modern techniques have simplified diagnosis in this patient group; these techniques are described in detail in Chap. 25. Less commonly, patients with borderline serum calcium values present without hypercalciuria, stones, or other definable symptoms of primary hyperparathyroidism. These patients are usually older than the patients described above and probably have very mild disease together with normal or nearly normal circulating levels of $1,25\text{-}(OH)_2D$. Diagnosis can be achieved with the same techniques, but therapeutic intervention may not be warranted.

Primary hyperparathyroidism during pregnancy is associated with a high rate of fetal loss and neonatal morbidity and mortality. Reviews estimate a 50 to 80 percent incidence of serious fetal or neonatal complications resulting from maternal primary hyperparathyroidism and stress that such patients can and should be managed surgically.[169,170] Calcium penetrates the placenta, and neonates born of hypercalcemic mothers predictably have functional hypoparathyroidism, with hypocalcemia, hyperphosphatemia, and moderate to severe tetany lasting weeks to months. Patients with very mild hypercalcemia may be carried through pregnancy without surgery, but their risk of developing stone complications appears to be substantial.

Primary hyperparathyroidism in infancy and childhood is rare.[129,170] The majority of reported pediatric cases of hyperparathyroidism presented with severe hypercalcemia complicated by overt bone disease, and only a handful of patients presenting with renal stones have been described. Primary hyperparathyroidism in the pediatric age group should be managed surgically, but only after the syndrome of familial hypocalciuric hypercalcemia has been excluded by careful evaluation and family screening.

"Tertiary" hyperparathyroidism refers to the development of hypercalcemia and biochemical hyperparathyroidism following a prolonged period of secondary hyperparathyroidism. Tertiary hyperparathyroidism is observed most commonly in patients having a successful renal transplant after years of progressive renal failure and dialysis management.[171] The most important factor relating to the occurrence, severity, and persistence of tertiary hyperparathyroidism after transplantation appears to be the success with which the patient's mineral homeostasis and secondary hyperparathyroidism were managed prior to transplantation, as defined by the aggregate parathyroid mass at the time of renal transplantation. The hypercalcemia is typically mild and transient, regressing over a period of months and normalizing in less than a year. In occasional patients, the hypercalcemia is moderate to severe and is associated with systemic symptoms or may actually threaten the integrity of the transplanted kidney; in other patients, the hypercalcemia is mild but persists for years after the transplant procedure. The histopathological correlate of tertiary hyperparathyroidism is chief cell hyperplasia, indistinguishable from that which occurs sporadically or that which is associated with secondary hyperparathyroidism.[130] The term *autonomy* was used for many years in connection with tertiary hyperparathyroidism, but it is now clear that virtually all abnormal parathyroid tissue is responsive to alterations in the ambient concentration of ionized calcium.[17] Most investigators currently view the biochemical hyperparathyroidism in tertiary hyperparathyroidism as resulting from a "mass effect," that is, a large functional parathyroid mass together with a finite nonsuppressible rate of PTH synthesis and secretion (Fig. 23-4). Patients with tertiary hyperparathyroidism of sufficient severity and/or persistence to merit surgical intervention require subtotal parathyroidectomy or parathyroid autotransplantation. Patients with a single parathyroid adenoma in this setting are rarely described, and the adenoma is variously interpreted as having developed from adenomatous transformation of previously hyperplastic cells or as being due to primary adenomatous hyperparathyroidism occurring in a patient with coincident chronic renal disease. Tertiary hyperparathyroidism has also been described following correction of intestinal malabsorption or various states of vitamin D deficiency, and the finding of a single parathyroid adenoma in such a patient is subject to the same varied interpretations noted above.[167]

Rarely, abnormal parathyroid tissue outgrows its blood supply and spontaneously infarcts. This infarction is usually associated with transient hypocalcemia, which can be pronounced if significant bone demineralization was previously present. Whether transient or permanent remission of the hyperparathyroid state occurs depends on the quantity of tissue infarcted. Several patients have been reported in whom hemorrhage into a parathyroid adenoma resulted in an acute exacerbation of hypercalcemia, together with a painful, palpable neck mass.

FAMILIAL ENDOCRINE NEOPLASIA AND FAMILIAL HYPOCALCIURIC HYPERCALCEMIA

There are three familial hypercalcemic syndromes which are genetically distinct in that certain features of each syndrome virtually never occur in the other two syndromes. The syndromes are *multiple endocrine neoplasia type I* (MEN I), *multiple endocrine neoplasia type II* (MEN II), and *familial hypocalciuric hypercalcemia.* Hypercalcemia and an autosomal dominant pattern of inheritance are the only features shared by all three syndromes. The features of MEN I and MEN II and the principal theories proposed to account for these polyendocrine syndromes are presented in detail in Chap. 28. The discussion below is primarily concerned with hyperparathyroidism in the MEN syndromes, familial hyperparathyroidism in the apparent absence of other elements of MEN I or MEN II, and a thorough description of the recently recognized syndrome of familial hypocalciuric hypercalcemia.

MEN I consists of neoplasms of the pituitary, parathyroids, and pancreas ("the three P's").[172] The usual pituitary lesion is a chromophobe adenoma, although associated Cushing's disease and acromegaly have been rarely reported. As anticipated, prolactinomas are currently being reported with some frequency in this setting.[173] The usual pancreatic lesion is a gastrinoma, although insulinomas, glucagonomas, and mixed islet cell tumors with multiple secretory products have been described. In 100 patients reported in nine series between 1964 and 1975, the incidence of pituitary tumors was 10 percent; pancreatic tumors, 25 percent; and parathyroid involvement, 95 percent. Very similar percentages have been reported in recent series.[174] Approximately 15 percent of patients have associated lipomas, and a small percentage of patients have bronchial adenomas. There is no set pattern or predictable natural history of glandular involvement in individual patients or families, and patients may present with multiple features of the syndrome, may develop multiple features sequentially, or may display only a single feature for prolonged periods. Peptic ulcer disease is noted in approximately 30 percent of patients with MEN I, and approximately one-half to two-thirds of these patients are found to have the Zollinger-Ellison syndrome.[175]

The parathyroid lesion is pseudoadenomatous chief cell hyperplasia. The hyperparathyroidism is otherwise clinically and biochemically indistinguishable from sporadic hyperparathyroidism, with a similar reported frequency of bone involvement, stone disease, and other systemic manifestations.[176] The average age at the time of diagnosis is somewhat younger than in sporadic hyperparathyroidism, and pediatric and even neonatal cases of hyperparathyroidism have been described. However, such cases are infrequent, and the diagnosis is usually established during the third to fifth decades. The striking frequency of hyperparathyroidism in involved patients makes the measurement of serum calcium a convenient tool for screening families for affected members.[174]

There are two variants of MEN II: MEN IIA and MEN IIB.[177–180] These variants are distinctive hereditary entities. The key features of MEN IIA, in order of frequency in involved patients, are medullary carcinoma of the thyroid, hyperparathyroidism, and pheochromocytoma.[177,178] Medullary carcinoma of the thyroid is the dominant lesion, occurring in three-quarters or more of affected individuals. In familial medullary carcinoma of the thyroid, disease is typically bilateral and/or multicentric and has an early onset, with a mean age at the time of diagnosis of approximately 20 years. The disease process evolves through a sequence from hyperplasia to carcinoma. As described in Chap. 28, the radioimmunoassay for calcitonin, together with techniques for stimulating calcitonin secretion, has revolutionized the diagnosis and management of this tumor, and the disorder can be diagnosed in a premalignant phase amenable to curative surgical therapy.

Histological or biochemical evidence of hyperparathyroidism occurs in approximately 50 percent of patients. In some families, the hyperparathyroidism appears to be quite indolent and is only infrequently associated with systemic manifestations or complications.[177] The parathyroid lesion is pseudoadenomatous chief cell hyperplasia, and the glands are often very unevenly involved. Pheochromocytomas occur in approximately 40 to 50 percent of patients.[177,178] Adrenal medullary involvement is bilateral in approximately two-thirds of these patients, and the tumors may be malignant and/or secrete other hormonal products such as ACTH. Several patients have been reported in whom hypercalcemia and/or hyperparathyroidism appeared to resolve following curative adrenalectomy for pheochromocytoma, and several mechanisms have been proposed to explain this occurrence (see Pheochromocytoma, below). In patients with MEN II and a pheochromocytoma, with or without other features of the syndrome, bilateral adrenalectomy is always the initial surgical procedure attempted.

The key features of MEN IIB are mucosal neuromas, skeletal deformities, medullary carcinoma of the thyroid, and pheochromocytomas.[179,180] Medullary carcinoma of the thyroid and pheochromocytomas are present in about 95 and 50 percent of affected individuals, respectively, and the pattern and natural history of these tumors are identical in the MEN IIA and MEN IIB syndromes. The neuromas are uniformly present in patients with MEN IIB and frequently affect the conjunctiva and oral cavity; in about two-thirds of patients, the neuromas are present in other regions of the gastrointestinal tract, and gastrointestinal symptoms may dominate the clinical picture. Marfanoid or other skeletal deformities are noted in approximately 85 percent of patients. Hyperparathyroidism is rare, being definitely present in only 1 of the 41 patients reviewed by Khairi and associates.[179]

Familial hyperparathyroidism in the absence of other features of MEN I or MEN II has been reported.[181] These kindreds are clearly less common than those with MEN I and MEN II, and the latter can be excluded only by means of careful family screening and/or prolonged follow-up. The mode of inheritance in familial hyperparathyroidism appears to be autosomal dominant, and available evidence suggests that the parathyroid lesion is pseudoadenomatous chief cell hyperplasia.[181] The clinical manifestations in these patients are indistinguishable from those in patients with sporadic disease. Primary adenomatous hyperparathyroidism is occasionally observed in first-degree relatives, but no large kindreds with this parathyroid lesion have been reported. One kindred has been reported in which affected patients had a solitary parathyroid adenoma and the mode of inheritance appeared to be autosomal recessive.[182]

Familial hypocalciuric hypercalcemia (FHH) and *familial benign hypercalcemia* are synonymous terms.[183–185] As shown in Table 23-10, a number of features

Table 23-10. Distinctive Features of Familial Hypocalciuric Hypercalcemia

1. Early age of onset
2. Benign course, absence of renal stone disease
3. Absence of features of multiple endocrine neoplasia
4. Reduced fractional excretion of calcium and magnesium
5. Disproportionately low indices of parathyroid function
6. Poor response to subtotal parathyroidectomy

characterize FHH and serve to distinguish this syndrome from both classical sporadic hyperparathyroidism and other familial hyperparathyroid states. The mode of inheritance is autosomal dominant, and the age of onset is distinctly earlier than that of the other familial syndromes. The prevalence of hypercalcemia approaches a theoretical limit of 50 percent within the first two decades of life, and it is thought that affected individuals express the disorder at a very early age, perhaps from birth. The typical complications of primary hyperparathyroidism, renal stones, and bone involvement do not occur in FHH, and the only clear clinical complications which have been reported in the syndrome are neonatal severe hyperparathyroidism and pancreatitis in adults.[183–185] Neonatal severe hyperparathyroidism is a rare presentation rather than the expected presentation in affected offspring; neonates usually have hypercalcemia which is mild and clinically benign. There also appears to be an increased incidence of chondrocalcinosis.[183,184] Patients may complain of fatigue, abnormal mentation, arthralgias, headache, and other nonspecific symptoms, but the majority of affected individuals are without complaints.[183–185] Features of MEN I or MEN II have not been observed in patients with FHH. A key pathogenic feature in FHH is a clear-cut reduction in the fractional excretion of both calcium and magnesium, and so these patients display a roughly proportional degree of hypermagnesemia and hypercalcemia. Results for both fasting and 24-h calcium excretion are characteristically low in patients with FHH, and values for 24-h calcium excretion greater than 250 mg per day on a 400-mg calcium intake are unusual.[183,184] In spite of the relative hypocalciuria which characterizes FHH, there is substantial overlap between the values for 24-h calcium excretion observed in these patients and the values in patients with sporadic primary hyperparathyroidism.[184] Results for serum immunoreactive PTH, plasma 1,25-$(OH)_2D$, and nephrogenous or urinary cAMP are usually in the mid- to high-normal range in patients with FHH, in contrast to the findings in the great majority of patients with classical primary hyperparathyroidism.[183–185] TmP/GFR is also less frequently reduced than in true primary hyperparathyroidism. Finally and most important, operative experience has been miserable. Of 27 patients with FHH evaluated by the NIH group after one or multiple neck explorations, 21 remained hypercalcemic, 5 were hypocalcemic, and only 1 was normocalcemic.[184] The nature of the parathyroid lesion is debated; it appears to be chief cell hyperplasia or some histologically similar variant.[183–185] The mass of parathyroid tissue in patients with FHH is typically very small.[186]

The pathogenesis of FHH is puzzling, and no single biochemical lesion is apparent which might explain the syndrome in its entirety. It is clear that the renal tubular reabsorption of divalent cations is abnormally efficient, and this abnormality presumably resides in the distal nephron. A reduction in fractional calcium excretion can even be demonstrated in patients with FHH who have been rendered surgically aparathyroid.[187] The parathyroid glands are also clearly involved, as evidenced by the biochemical and pathological findings as well as the hypocalcemia which results from total parathyroidectomy. The circulating PTH levels and urinary cAMP data are quantitatively comparable and do not suggest a generalized state of hyperresponsiveness to PTH. Current pathogenetic speculation involves an undefined abnormality in the manner in which multiple cell types in the organism perceive and/or handle divalent cations. It is of interest that lithium induces a rather similar pattern of parathyroid cell and renal tubular abnormalities[183] (see Lithium-Induced Hypercalcemia, below). Diagnosis is achieved by means of maintenance of a high index of suspicion, together with a demonstration of multiple features of the syndrome as listed in Table 23-10, most particularly hypercalcemia in first-degree relatives. Given the pathogenesis of hypercalciuria in typical hyperparathyroidism as described previously and the normal circulating levels of 1,25-$(OH)_2D$ and absence of calcium hyperabsorption in patients with FHH, one would anticipate a better segregation of values for 24-h calcium if patients were routinely screened on an unrestricted rather than a restricted calcium diet, and it is our practice to do so. However, a substantial data base employing this approach has not been published. Medical and/or surgical therapy is not recommended in typical patients with FHH. In the rare patients with neonatal hypercalcemia and severe pancreatitis in whom intervention is clearly necessary, the recommended approach is total parathyroidectomy or parathyroidectomy plus autotransplantation.[183]

In the aggregate, the familial hypercalcemic syndromes are by no means uncommon, and they are of tremendous pathophysiological and clinical interest. It is estimated that several thousand large kindreds with these disorders exist in the United States and also that as many as 5 to 10 percent of patients diagnosed as harboring hyperparathyroidism may suffer from one of the familial syndromes. In units specializing in parathyroid reexploration, such patients may constitute one-third or more of referrals. Some investigators urge that the families of all patients with primary hyperparathyroidism be screened, and such screening is clearly mandatory if the patient in question is found surgically to have chief cell hyperplasia. There may be key suggestive features in a patient's family history, but experience with multiple index cases has taught that the family history is often vague. How extensive the evaluation of a given patient with primary hyperparathyroidism should be in order to rule out other features of the familial syndromes is a matter of judgment. The surgical management of all such patients is very difficult, as evidenced by their disproportionate frequency in referral centers for parathyroid reexploration.

PHYSICAL FINDINGS

The general physical examination may provide important information regarding systemic manifestations of hyperparathyroidism, but few physical findings are of assistance in differential diagnosis. Hypertension is frequent. As shown in Fig. 23-35, band keratopathy is occasionally grossly visible in patients with primary hyperparathyroidism and must be distinguished from the limbic girdle, which is frequently mistaken for band keratopathy in older patients. In modern series, band keratopathy is observed in only a few patients with primary hyperparathyroidism and is usually visualized by slit-lamp examination but not by direct vision. Subtle neuromuscular findings can be demonstrated in many patients with primary hyperparathyroidism but usually will go unappreciated by the casual examiner. The most frequent findings are proximal muscle weakness in the lower extremities and peculiar fine fasciculations in the tongue. Bone tenderness should be specifically searched for and is most readily appreciated when one applies moderate thumb pressure to the patient's distal tibia. Tibial tenderness is not observed in osteoporosis, and its presence is firm physical evidence of bone involvement in a patient with primary hyperparathyroidism.

LABORATORY FINDINGS AND DEFINITIVE DIAGNOSIS

A discussion of the laboratory findings in primary hyperparathyroidism outside the context of the clini-

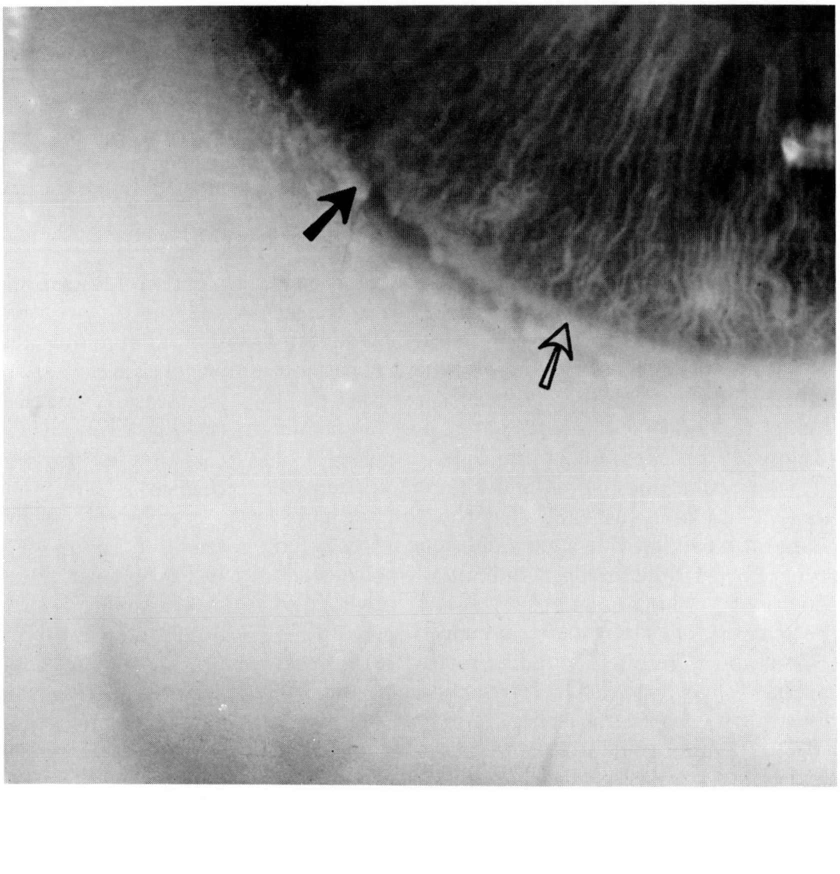

FIGURE 23-35 Corneal photograph in a hypercalcemic patient. The open arrow identifies the linear calcification known as a limbic girdle; this finding is entirely nonspecific. The solid arrow identifies the moth-eaten, irregular calcium deposits of band keratopathy, a finding which may be observed in patients with severe and/or prolonged hypercalcemia. Both types of deposit are composed of calcium phosphate, and both are apparent at the medial and lateral limbic margins. These locations are presumably the result of diffusion of carbon dioxide from the air-exposed portions of the cornea, with resultant local alkalosis and precipitation of calcium phosphate crystals.

cal spectrum of the disorder is of limited use. This section will begin with a description of the general laboratory findings in hyperparathyroidism, followed by a specific discussion of laboratory abnormalities and diagnosis in the patient categories presented in Table 23-9.

The classical laboratory findings in primary hyperparathyroidism are hypercalcemia and hypophosphatemia. Both determinations require attention to technical detail and interpretation based on age- and sex-matched control ranges. Serum phosphorus concentrations in postmenopausal female patients with primary hyperparathyroidism are often in the range of 2.5 to 3.0 mg/dl, and modern series frequently underestimate the incidence of hypophosphatemia in the disorder by failing to employ properly defined control ranges. In the absence of renal impairment and employing age- and sex-matched control ranges, hypophosphatemia is demonstrable in approximately 70 percent of patients with primary hyperparathyroidism. The determination of TmP/GFR is a far more powerful diagnostic tool in that it represents a direct measure of renal phosphorus threshold expressed as a function of the glomerular filtration rate. Based on age- and sex-matched control ranges, reduced values for TmP/GFR are observed in 80 percent or more of patients with primary hyperparathyroidism, and values above 3.0 mg/dl are rare.

An increase in serum alkaline phosphatase activity is found in approximately one-fourth of patients with primary hyperparathyroidism and is positively correlated with the degree of hypercalcemia.[126] Alkaline phosphatase activity does not correlate well with x-ray evidence of bone involvement except in patients with severe disease. Hypomagnesemia is observed in 10 to 15 percent of patients and is of little consequence. Modest hyperuricemia is frequent. The frequency of actual hyperchloremic acidosis in primary hyperparathyroidism has been debated, but it is clear that patients with hyperparathyroidism have a tendency toward metabolic acidosis, whereas patients with chronic hypoparathyroidism or suppressed parathyroid function have a tendency toward metabolic alkalosis.[134,139,143] Because of the divergent effects of PTH on serum phosphorus and chloride concentrations, it has been suggested that the chloride/phosphate ratio may provide a good discriminant between primary hyperparathyroidism and other hypercalcemic conditions.[188] Ratios greater than 33 were observed in the majority of patients with primary hyperparathyroidism and were rarely found in patients with other causes of hypercalcemia.[188] These findings and the utility of the chloride/phosphate ratio have been challenged.[189] Although debate continues, it appears to be clear that the chloride/phosphate ratio is of little use in attempting to establish a diagnosis in a patient suspected of having primary hyperparathyroidism, whereas it is reasonably useful as a nonspecific front-line test in the differential diagnosis of patients with moderate to severe hypercalcemia. Hypokalemia is found in about 5 percent of patients with primary hyperparathyroidism. An increase in the sedimentation rate is observed in one-half of patients with primary hyperparathyroidism and correlates roughly with the severity of the disease process.[134] Mild, nonspecific anemia is noted in 20 percent of patients and resolves following surgical correction of the disorder.[134] Occasionally, iron deficiency anemia is found in a patient with coincident peptic ulcer disease and gastrointestinal bleeding.

The definitive diagnosis of primary hyperparathyroidism rests on the simultaneous demonstration of hypercalcemia and an index of abnormal or inappropriate parathyroid function. The chronicity of primary hyperparathyroidism is an extremely useful diagnostic consideration, and attempts to obtain previously determined values for serum calcium should be made in any hypercalcemic patient. The demonstration of known hypercalcemia for 12 months or more together with a reduction in TmP/GFR constitutes definitive evidence of primary hyperparathyroidism, which requires no further laboratory confirmation. In the absence of this demonstrated history of chronicity or in a severely ill patient who may harbor a malignancy or some other cause of hypercalcemia, more definitive laboratory methods are required. The laboratory findings and diagnostic approach to patients with mild, moderate, and severe hypercalcemia will be discussed below; these categories correspond in general to the clinical spectrum of primary hyperparathyroidism shown in Table 23-9. As noted previously, there is a reasonable correlation between the mass of abnormal parathyroid tissue and both the level of serum calcium and the quantitative degree of abnormality of parathyroid function tests such that specific laboratory diagnosis becomes progressively easier as the spectrum of disease is traversed from left to right in the table (see Fig. 23-27). It is important to recall that parathyroid function in patients with primary hyperparathyroidism is not predictably autonomous and that a spectrum of parathyroid suppressibility has been observed both in vivo and in vitro in these patients and/or in their abnormal parathyroid cells.[17,112,190] This suppressibility is such that it may even influence the results of parathyroid function tests obtained on an unrestricted calcium diet (Fig. 23-36). The optimal interpretation of laboratory studies is therefore provided by samples obtained on a restricted calcium diet, and this is of particular importance in patients with mild disease.[112]

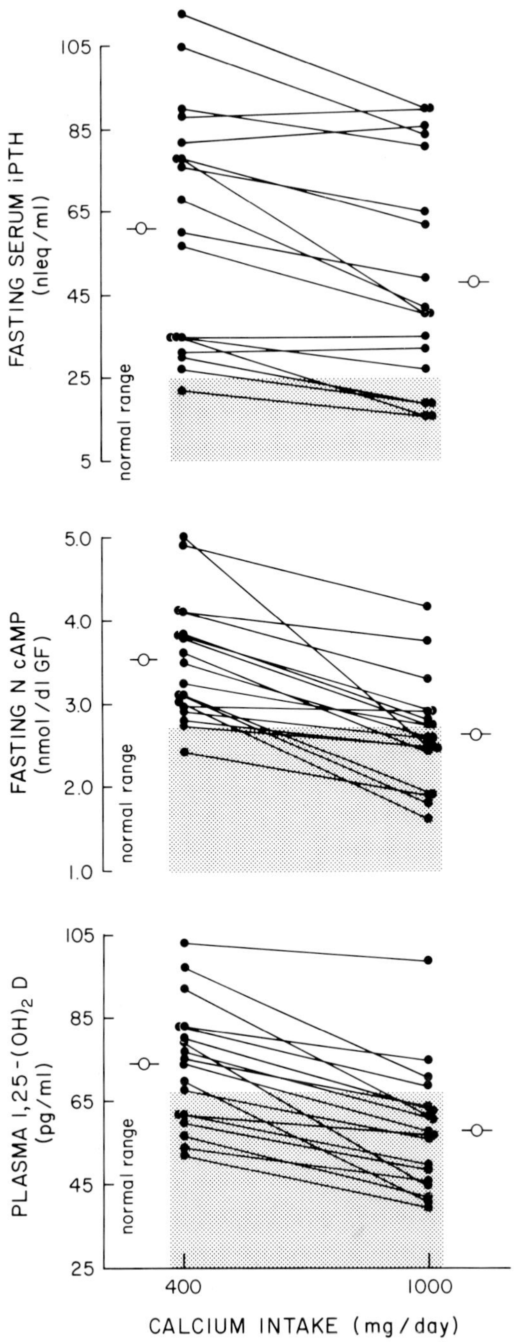

FIGURE 23-36 Serum immunoreactive parathyroid hormone, nephrogenous cAMP, and plasma 1,25-$(OH)_2D$ in 18 patients with primary hyperparathyroidism studied on a restricted (400-mg) calcium diet and again 3 days after being placed on an unrestricted (1000-mg) calcium diet. The hatched areas depict normal ranges, and the open circles indicate values. Note that each determination was significantly suppressed by the increase in calcium intake and that the mean values for nephrogenous cAMP and plasma 1,25-$(OH)_2D$ were suppressed into the normal range. (*From Insogna, Mitnick, Stewart, Burtis, Mallette, and Broadus,*[112] *by permission of the New England Journal of Medicine.*)

Patients with mild hypercalcemia in the range of 11 mg/dl typically have normal serum alkaline phosphatase activity and normal x-ray studies. Hypercalciuria occurs frequently in these patients, and a large minority present with renal stone disease. In patients with well-established hypercalcemia, diagnosis is usually straightforward and can be confirmed by reduced values for TmP/GFR in a patient with a chronic history or by elevated values for serum immunoreactive PTH and/or nephrogenous cAMP or total cAMP excretion. As described previously, mild hypercalcemia is the rule rather than the exception in patients presenting with renal stone disease, and a minority of patients display only intermittent hypercalcemia. This intermittent pattern is quite characteristic and is typified by swings in serum calcium of $\pm$ 0.5 to 1.0 mg/dl around a mean value in the range of 10.1 to 10.2 mg/dl.[139,168] This pattern can be appreciated only by means of repeated measurements of serum calcium, and the diagnosis of subtle primary hyperparathyroidism must be seriously considered in any patient presenting with renal stones who demonstrates a mean value for serum calcium greater than 10.0 mg/dl on three determinations performed while fasting and with scrupulous technique. Definitive diagnosis in these patients may require more sophisticated laboratory techniques, as described in Chap. 25. Other patients with mild or borderline serum calcium values in the absence of stone disease may be observed, particularly in older age groups. Expensive laboratory procedures are difficult to justify in such patients unless the physician clearly intends to base a therapeutic decision on the results of such tests; a reasonable clinical alternative is simply to measure TmP/GFR and follow the patient, thereby achieving diagnosis by virtue of demonstrating chronicity.

Patients with moderate hypercalcemia in the range of 11.5 to 12.5 mg/dl frequently present with a nonspecific history and findings. The degree of hypercalciuria is roughly proportional to the level of serum calcium in these patients. Other laboratory abnormalities such as anemia, hyperuricemia, and borderline to slightly elevated values for serum alkaline phosphatase activity are variously observed, and radiological evidence of mild skeletal demineralization is present in one-third or more of such patients, particularly in postmenopausal women. Specific laboratory diagnosis is usually readily achievable in this patient group, and the major clinical problem relates to therapeutic decision making. This decision is generally based on the patient's age and general medical condition, together with the physician's assessment of the relation between the hyperparathyroidism and the patient's symptoms.

Patients with severe hypercalcemia in the range of 13 mg/dl or greater usually present with systemic symptoms of hypercalcemia and frequently demonstrate one or more complications of hyperparathyroidism. These patients are often quite ill in a general medical sense and display a constellation of laboratory findings including anemia, moderate renal impairment, and elevated levels of serum alkaline phosphate activity. Urinary calcium excretion may or may not be absolutely elevated but is disproportionately low in comparison with the degree of hypercalcemia. Nephrocalcinosis is demonstrable in one-third or more of patients, but nephrolithiasis is infrequent. Radiological evidence of mild to moderate demineralization is present in the majority of patients, and approximately one-third of patients display findings of subperiosteal resorption or frank osteitis fibrosa cystica. The differential diagnosis usually lies between severe primary hyperparathyroidism and malignant disease complicated by hypercalcemia. Although superficially confusing, this differential diagnosis is rather easily achieved on the following grounds:

1. Hypercalcemia complicating malignant disease is a poor prognostic sign and correlates with extensive disease which is generally readily apparent.
2. Radiological evidence of osteitis fibrosa cystica is rare in patients with a malignancy.
3. Patients with malignancy and hypercalcemia tend to be slightly alkalotic, whereas patients with severe primary hyperparathyroidism and some degree of renal impairment are particularly likely to display a metabolic acidosis.
4. Although detectable or occasionally slightly elevated serum levels of immunoreactive PTH are variously reported by different laboratories in patients with malignant disease and hypercalcemia, these levels are usually discordant with the degree of hypercalcemia (Fig. 23-27).

Patients with the humoral syndrome of malignancy-associated hypercalcemia display reduced values for TmP/GFR and elevations in nephrogenous cAMP, whereas patients with malignancy-associated hypercalcemia based on a local osteolytic mechanism tend to have normal results for TmP/GFR and values for nephrogenous cAMP that are near zero. Circulating $1,25\text{-(OH)}_2D$ is generally markedly reduced in patients with malignancy-associated hypercalcemia, and this determination is therefore useful in differential diagnosis. Diagnostic difficulties may be encountered in patients with malignant disease and coincident primary hyperparathyroidism, patients with familial hypocalciuric hypercalcemia and moderate to severe hypercalcemia, and patients with sarcoidosis. Sarcoidosis should be suspected in any patient presenting with systemic symptoms, moderate to severe hypercalcemia, and moderate renal impairment. Additional details concerning the pathogenesis of malignancy-associated hypercalcemia and other hypercalcemic syndromes and the approach to differential diagnosis are given in the relevant sections below.

PREOPERATIVE LOCALIZATION STUDIES

Two types of information are desirable preoperatively in a patient with primary hyperparathyroidism: (1) whether the patient is likely to have a parathyroid adenoma or primary parathyroid hyperplasia and (2) the location of the abnormal parathyroid tissue. A variety of noninvasive and invasive techniques have been introduced in an attempt to provide one or both types of information.

It was initially reported that parathyroid adenomas and primary parathyroid hyperplasia could be differentiated by the degree of suppressibility in circulating PTH levels observed in response to calcium infusion and that both adenomatous and hyperplastic parathyroid tissue could be localized by measuring increases in peripheral circulating levels of the hormone following neck massage.[191] Neither of these observations has been confirmed.[17,190,192] Although hyperplastic parathyroid cells are generally more responsive to alterations in the extracellular calcium concentration than are adenomatous cells, the degree of parathyroid suppressibility observed in vivo in response to calcium infusion is sufficiently variable that there is no response which clearly distinguishes adenomatous from hyperplastic tissue.[190] At present, there are no reliable noninvasive techniques for distinguishing between these two categories of parathyroid lesion. Patients with familial disease can be assumed to have parathyroid hyperplasia and must be managed accordingly.

Noninvasive techniques for localization of abnormal parathyroid tissue include [^{75}Se]selenomethionine scanning, thermography, ultrasonography, cervical esophagography, computerized tomography, and thallium/technetium subtraction scanning.[193] Of these techniques, the best and most recent experience has been achieved with high-resolution sonography and subtraction scanning.[193] Given the crude but definite correlation between the severity of disease and the aggregate mass of abnormal parathyroid tissue, all these findings would be anticipated to provide better localizing information in patients with moderate to severe disease than in patients with mild disease. However, the techniques are innocuous and relatively inexpensive and may reasonably be attempted on the basis of institutional availability of equipment and expertise. Localizing information provided by these methods should form the basis for deciding which side of the neck to explore initially and must not be taken to mean that disease is necessarily unilateral.

Invasive techniques for differentiating adenomatous and hyperplastic disease and for localizing parathyroid lesion(s) include digital subtraction angiography, arteriography, venography, and venography with thyroid venous sampling.[194,195] Arteriography and venography are sufficiently low-yield procedures that they should not be attempted as localizing techniques in and of themselves. However, venography (and sometimes arteriography) is performed in conjunction with venous sampling, and large parathyroid lesions may be visualized with one of these techniques in about 15 percent of patients. Occasionally, a parathyroid adenoma visualized by arteriography can be embolized, leading to palliation or even cure of the patient. Initial attempts to localize parathyroid lesions by sampling for PTH gradients in large (i.e., the innominate and jugular) cervical veins provided inconsistent results, and selective thyroid venous sampling was found to be required for reliable localizing information. Proper performance of this technique requires a great deal of angiographic skill and experience, and it should not be attempted in institutions where it is not regularly performed.

The thyroid venous bed is an anastomosing venous plexus usually made up of paired superior, middle, and inferior thyroid veins. Venous drainage is directed inferiorly and is usually ipsilateral so that the key localizing samples to be obtained during catheterization are inferior thyroid vein samples reflecting right-sided and left-sided drainage. The thyroid venous anatomy is quite variable; the two most common patterns of inferior venous drainage are illustrated in Fig. 23-37. Inferior thyroid veins draining separately into the innominate vein must be selectively catheterized and sampled. If the inferior thyroid veins join to form a common inferior thyroid vein, this vessel must be entered in order to sample the two inferior thyroid veins selectively above their site of merger. The most common cause of failure in selective venous catheterization is the inability to obtain representative inferior thyroid vein samples. The inferior thyroid venous anatomy is anomalous in approximately 15 percent of patients and is often markedly distorted in patients who have undergone previous neck exploration. In patients to be catheterized prior to parathyroid reexploration, cervical arteriography is initially performed in order to outline the distorted venous anatomy prior to attempted selective venous catheterization.

Examples of successful catheterization studies are illustrated in Fig. 23-37. In both studies, samples obtained from the inferior thyroid veins differentiated between parathyroid hyperplasia and adenoma and localized the parathyroid pathology. A fourfold "step-up" in PTH concentrations over peripheral circulating levels is regarded as significant. Accurate differential and localizing information is obtained by experienced angiographers in approximately 80 percent of patients who have not undergone prior neck exploration and in approximately 70 percent of patients who have been previously explored.[194,195] Mediastinal parathyroid tissue may not be localized because of anomalous venous drainage.

Because of the expense and the limited number of angiographers widely experienced in its performance, selective venous catheterization is not routinely performed in newly diagnosed patients with primary

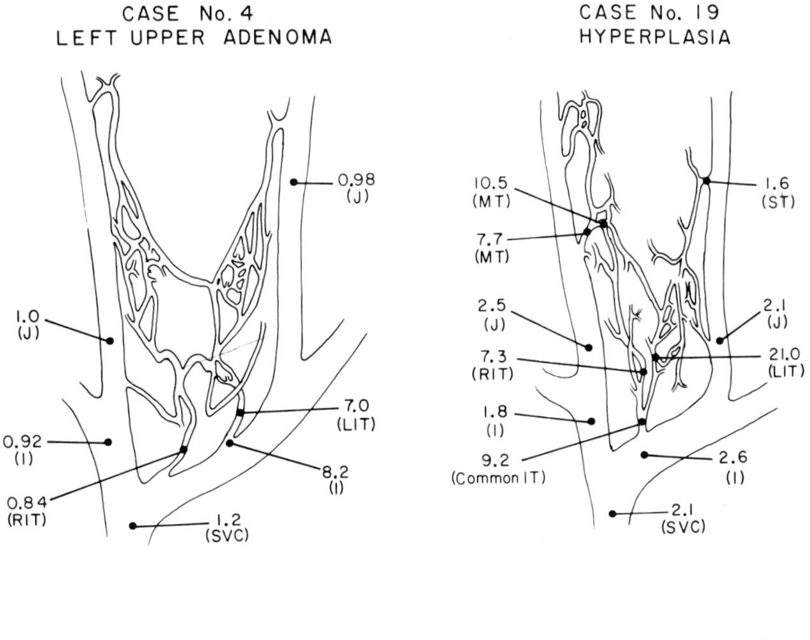

FIGURE 23-37 Results of selective venous catheterization in a patient with a parathyroid adenoma (*left*) and in a patient with primary parathyroid hyperplasia (*right*). Note that although the adenoma was located in the left upper gland, it was lateralized by an inferior thyroid vein sample. Note also that the bilaterality of disease in the patient with hyperplasia was reflected in the inferior thyroid vein samples. (*By permission of Powell D, Shimkin PM, Doppman JL, Wells S, Aurbach GD, Marx SJ, Ketcham AS, Potts JT, N Engl J Med 286:1169, 1972.*)

hyperparathyroidism and is not recommended in such patients. The technique is most commonly indicated in (1) patients with prior unsuccessful neck exploration, (2) patients in poor general medical condition with hyperparathyroidism of sufficient severity to require surgery and in whom an expeditious exploration is desired, and (3) patients with known malignant disease suspected of having coincident primary hyperparathyroidism. The first of these would appear to be the only reasonably compelling indication, and these patients particularly should be entrusted to skilled and experienced hands. The technique should not be performed in patients with familial disease, since the results will have no influence on proper surgical management. In addition, the technique cannot be employed for the diagnosis of patients suspected of having subtle primary hyperparathyroidism in that significant PTH gradients may be noted in neck vein specimens obtained from nonhypercalcemic individuals.

If a thorough neck exploration results in complete failure to identify a parathyroid lesion, thyroid veins may be sampled intraoperatively in an attempt to localize the lesion for future reference.

PARATHYROID EXPLORATION AND PERIOPERATIVE MANAGEMENT

The principal surgical challenges of parathyroid exploration are (1) finding the parathyroid lesion(s) and (2) differentiating chief cell hyperplasia from a parathyroid adenoma. Patients must be entrusted to a skilled neck surgeon, and optimal results are obtained when patients are managed by an experienced internist-surgeon-pathologist team.

Conventional operative therapy for a parathyroid adenoma consists of removal of the adenoma, together with gross identification of all remaining parathyroid glands, with or without biopsy evidence of normality of one grossly normal-appearing gland. More aggressive surgery is performed in a few centers, but it is generally regarded as unnecessary.

Primary parathyroid hyperplasia is managed by means of subtotal parathyroidectomy, the extent of which varies from center to center.[196,197] By definition, this procedure is palliative and difficult. Recurrent or persistent hyperparathyroidism occurs in 50 percent of patients with chief cell hyperplasia after both an initial operation and reoperation.[197] Chronic hypocalcemia occurs in 10 percent of these patients after an initial neck exploration and in 25 percent after reoperation.[197] These figures are to be contrasted with an estimated "cure" rate exceeding 90 percent in patients with a single adenoma.[196] The approaches to subtotal parathyroidectomy employed by different surgical teams include (1) removal of three parathyroid glands and all but approximately 50 mg of the fourth gland, (2) removal of only grossly abnormal glands, and (3) removal of all but an estimated 100 mg of parathyroid tissue, which may constitute one or more glands. There is no clear consensus as to which procedure should be preferentially employed, but there is evidence that the results following the removal of three or more glands are better than those following the removal of two and a half glands or less.[197] There is no debate regarding several rather clear-cut rules of thumb:

1. The surgeon must have an established plan of action and must not deviate from this plan in the heat of a difficult procedure.
2. All parathyroid tissue should be removed from one side of the neck so that any subsequent operative procedure is unilateral.
3. Remaining parathyroid tissue must be clipped for purposes of future identification.

Because of the inherent difficulties in subtotal parathyroidectomy, complete cervical parathyroidectomy with autotransplantation of parathyroid fragments into the forearm musculature has been introduced as a technique for managing patients with primary parathyroid hyperplasia and patients with severe hyperparathyroidism in the setting of renal osteodystrophy.[196,198] Techniques for maintaining frozen parathyroid tissue in a viable state have been developed,[196] and this tissue can be autografted into the forearm at a time distant from the initial cervical procedure. Following single- or two-stage autotransplantation, patients require substitution vitamin D therapy for variable periods of time, and autograft function can be monitored by measuring PTH concentrations in antecubital vein specimens above the transplant.[196,198] Tissue can be removed from or implanted into the forearm under local anesthesia. These techniques are elegant and have begun to replace conventional subtotal parathyroidectomy in centers experienced in their use. Autotransplantation may also be employed in patients undergoing reoperation whose sole remaining parathyroid tissue is an adenoma. Additional details concerning indications, surgical and cryopreservation techniques, and postoperative follow-up can be found in an extensive recent review.[196]

Parathyroid carcinoma is managed by means of a wide excision together with a local node dissection or a more extensive dissection, depending on the extent of disease.

If inadequate parathyroid tissue is found during an initial or repeat neck exploration, the mediastinal fat pad and thymus are routinely mobilized and pulled up into the operative field and explored. If thorough neck exploration is negative, a unilateral thyroidectomy is commonly performed in hopes of removing a parathyroid lesion in the thyroid capsule or parenchyma. Parathyroid reexploration is a difficult procedure but can be performed with a very high percentage of success in experienced hands.[199] Preoperative localization studies may be very helpful. Although an increased frequency of multiglandular, carcinomatous, or ectopic parathyroid lesions is noted in these patients, the majority of these lesions are found in the neck rather than the mediastinum.[199] Sternotomy and exploration of the anterior mediastinum is generally not done at the same time as a negative neck exploration but is performed as a separate procedure.

Operative complications are uncommon in skilled hands and include damage to the recurrent laryngeal nerves, partial or complete hypoparathyroidism, and rare wound infections. All these complications are more frequently observed following reexploration. Unilateral recurrent nerve damage results in transient or permanent hoarseness. Bilateral nerve damage has disastrous consequences: The cords close in the midline, rendering the patient aphonic and stridorous. Reparative techniques are available but provide only marginally successful results.

Postoperative management in uncomplicated patients with primary hyperparathyroidism is usually a relatively simple matter. Serum calcium and phosphorus levels should be monitored twice daily until stable. Typically, the serum calcium falls into the range of 8.0 mg/dl, with the nadir occurring within 3 days but occasionally being observed 6 to 7 days postoperatively. In this range, patients may experience modest tingling in the circumoral area or fingertips but are not truly uncomfortable. Patients may note symptoms only after inducing respiratory alkalosis by using blow bottles or other respiratory therapy. In general, the rule of thumb is to treat the patient, not the laboratory result. Such patients generally require no treatment. If the patient is moderately uncomfortable, oral calcium supplements of 1 to 2 g per day may be administered in four to six divided doses (the calcium elixir marketed as Neocalglucon contains 23 mg elemental calcium per milliliter and is preferred by most patients). Dairy products should be avoided because of their high phosphorus content. Intravenous calcium should be employed only for moderate to severe symptoms.

More difficult management problems may be anticipated in patients following subtotal parathyroidectomy and in patients with severe hyperparathyroidism and significant bone disease. The majority of patients having a subtotal parathyroidectomy follow a course similar to that described above, but a minority of patients display transient and partial or permanent and complete hypoparathyroidism. The rate of fall of the serum calcium is similar to that noted above, but the degree of hypocalcemia and hyperphosphatemia is more marked. Again, the patient's symptoms rather than laboratory values should be treated, and oral and/or intravenous calcium should be administered to maintain the patient's serum calcium in the range of 8.0 mg/dl. At this level, parathyroid remnants are continuously stimulated to function, and parathyroid function tests may be obtained and interpreted with confidence. In such a patient, TmP/GFR should be measured each morning and more specific parathyroid function tests should be determined as required. All efforts should be made to avoid vitamin D therapy for as long as possible and to reach a definite conclusion regarding quantitative parathyroid status before the patient is discharged on chronic vitamin D substitution therapy.

Patients with significant preoperative bone disease may develop a "hungry bones syndrome" of varying severity postoperatively; this sequence of events is also referred to as "recalcification tetany." This syndrome develops as a consequence of (1) removal of the source of the greatly elevated circulating quantities of PTH together with a degree of suppression of residual parathyroid tissue and (2) rapid remineralization of bone. The serum calcium may fall to 6.0 mg/dl within 48 h. In occasional patients with preoperative systemic acidosis, the acidosis may inexplicably worsen postoperatively and mask tetanic symptoms at serious levels of hypocalcemia. These patients must be monitored very closely, and intravenous calcium therapy should be initiated promptly. Patients with severe bone disease may require oral vitamin D and calcium therapy for months before bone remineralization is complete. In the hungry bones syndrome, the serum phosphorus concentration remains low, and the rapid return of parathyroid function can be monitored by measurements of TmP/GFR or more specific parathyroid function tests. Hypomagnesemia develops postoperatively in a small minority of such patients, presumably as a result of magnesium deposition in mineralizing bone, and magnesium replacement may be required in order to relieve the symptoms of tetany and/or hypocalcemia (see Hypomagnesemia, below).

MEDICAL MANAGEMENT OF PRIMARY HYPERPARATHYROIDISM

The final portion of this section is devoted to the medical management of hypercalcemia in general, and the brief discussion below is confined to medical management as it specifically relates to primary hyperparathyroidism.

Patients with primary hyperparathyroidism presenting with severe, symptomatic hypercalcemia may require acute antihypercalcemic therapy while awaiting definitive laboratory results and in preparation for surgery. As is the case with the acute management of hypocalcemia, the rule of thumb in managing hypercalcemia is to treat the patient, not the laboratory result. Many patients are stable and relatively symptom-free at a serum calcium in the range of 15 mg/dl, and more harm than good may result from an aggressive attempt to lower the serum calcium. The front-line medical measures include rehydration, mobilization, intravenous saline, and intravenous or oral furosemide. The net result of these measures is usually a reduction in serum calcium of about 3 mg/dl, which is sufficient in the vast majority of patients. After the patient is stabilized, small oral doses of phosphate (approximately 1000 mg elemental phosphorus daily) may be employed in the short term. Oral phosphates should not be employed in large doses or in the long term in patients with severe hypercalcemia, and intravenous phosphate administration should be avoided.

Because of patient refusal, age, general medical condition, or lack of apparent specific complications of the disorder, many patients with primary hyperparathyroidism do not undergo neck exploration and are simply observed in follow-up. Reasonable general measures in such patients would include instructions to maintain adequate hydration and remain physically active.[200] Thiazide diuretics should probably be avoided. Whether to advise a restricted or an unrestricted calcium intake has been the subject of considerable debate, but there are few data; recent short-term findings indicate that patients may be individualized in this regard, but these findings require confirmation in a longer-term study before they can be regarded as grounds for individualized dietary recommendations.[112] The fasting serum calcium should be monitored at 6-month intervals, and renal function, bone mineral density, and plain x-rays of the kidney may reasonably be followed at 12- to 18-month intervals. More elaborate follow-up may not be cost-effective. Criteria for surgical intervention in patients being followed medically have been proposed, but these indications do not represent a clear consensus.[201]

Estrogen therapy has been recommended in postmenopausal women with primary hyperparathyroidism, and a recent careful study documented significant reductions in the serum calcium concentration, urinary calcium excretion, serum alkaline phosphatase activity, and hydroxyproline excretion in women followed for a year or more on therapy.[202] Serum immunoreactive parathyroid hormone and plasma 1,25-$(OH)_2D$ were not influenced by therapy. The average dose was 1.25 mg of conjugated estrogen per day.[202] It seems clear that the mechanism of estrogen action in this and similar previous studies was an inhibition of bone resorption,[202,203] and estrogens would appear to constitute a viable therapeutic option in postmenopausal women, particularly those with existing evidence of bone loss.

Chronic oral phosphate therapy has been employed in patients with mild hypercalcemia and has been successful in controlling renal stone disease.[201] In a more recent series, patients were selected for phosphate therapy on the basis of a pretreatment "hyperabsorptive" pattern of abnormalities, and it was shown that circulating 1,25-$(OH)_2D$, intestinal hyperabsorption of calcium, and hypercalciuria could be largely controlled by means of therapy.[204] Phosphate treatment had little influence on the serum calcium concentration, but there was a modest reduction in indices of bone turnover.[204] The principal indication for phosphate therapy in patients with primary hyperparathyroidism would appear to be hypercalciuria and/or stone complications, and this therapy can best be viewed as antihypercalciuric rather than antihypercalcemic.[201,204] Oral phosphate therapy is specifically contraindicated in patients with primary hyperparathyroidism and (1) serum calcium levels higher than 12 mg/dl, (2) glomerular filtration rates lower than 75 ml/min, and (3) serum phosphorus concentrations and/or TmP/GFR values higher than 3.0 mg/dl. Doses higher than approximately 1500 mg per day of elemental phosphorus should not be employed. All published examples of extraskeletal calcification and complications resulting from oral phosphorus therapy in patients with primary hyperparathyroidism have violated one or more of these principles of therapy and are explicable in terms of induced increases in the mineral ion product. Patients generally prefer oral phosphorus tablets to preparations requiring dissolution prior to consumption.

In short-term studies, dichloromethylene diphosphonate has been shown to reduce serum calcium concentration, urinary calcium excretion, and hydroxyproline excretion in patients with primary hyperparathyroidism.[205] This agent appears to inhibit osteoclastic bone formation and was regarded as particularly promising because, unlike etidronate disodium, it does not inhibit the mineralization process. Unfortunately, it has been removed from trials because of reported toxicity. Other diphosphonates are undergoing evaluation in Europe.

In spite of initial reports, propranolol and cimetidine appear to be without consistent effect in patients with primary hyperparathyroidism.[200]

Malignancy-Associated Hypercalcemia

INTRODUCTION

Malignancy-associated hypercalcemia (MAHC) is the most common variety of hypercalcemia encountered among hospitalized patients[206] and is second in frequency only to primary hyperparathyroidism among outpatients.[127] Hypercalcemia generally occurs late in the natural history of malignancy, and its occurrence therefore constitutes a grave prognostic sign. Without successful antitumor therapy, most patients with malignancy-associated hypercalcemia die within 3 to 6 months of the onset of hypercalcemia.[207] While tumors of essentially every variety have been associated with hypercalcemia,[207–209] this disorder rarely accompanies certain common tumors (e.g., colon, prostate, and gastric carcinomas). In contrast, it is a frequent complication of other tumors (renal and urothelial carcinomas, breast carcinomas, squamous carcinomas, ovarian neoplasms, and multiple myeloma).[206–208]

Malignancy-associated hypercalcemia can be broadly divided into two mechanistic categories: *local osteolytic hypercalcemia* (LOH) and *humoral hypercalcemia of malignancy* (HHM). As the terms imply, the hypercalcemia in patients wtih LOH is envisioned as resulting from the effects of primary or metastatic malignant cells in direct contact with bone and/or bone-resorbing cells, whereas the hypercalcemia in patients with HHM is envisioned as resulting from the secretion of a bone-resorbing factor(s) by malignant cells remote from bone. Recently, a subgroup of patients with lymphoma-associated hypercalcemia and an apparent humoral mechanism has been described. Because of their unusual clinical and pathophysiological characteristics, these patients will be treated as a third mechanistic subtype of MAHC. Occasional patients are encountered who do not appear to fit into any of these three categories. These patients will be discussed in Uncommon Variants of Malignancy-Associated Hypercalcemia.

LOCAL OSTEOLYTIC HYPERCALCEMIA

This group includes patients with widespread skeletal metastases as well as those with extensive bone marrow involvement by a primary hematologic malignancy. The tumors most commonly associated with this type of MAHC are breast cancer, multiple myeloma, and lymphomas.[207,210] Biochemically, patients with LOH are characterized by evidence of bone resorption (marked fasting hypercalciuria) and parathyroid suppression [normal to reduced immunoreactive PTH, reduced nephrogenous cAMP excretion, and reduced plasma 1,25-$(OH)_2D$].[211,212] Serum phosphorus concentrations and results for TmP/GFR in the absence of renal impairment are in the normal to low-normal range.

Although the precise mechanisms responsible for the accelerated bone resorption which occurs in these patients are incompletely understood, several mechanisms have been invoked. In the case of breast carcinoma, it is known that cultured breast carcinoma lines are capable of directly resorbing irradiated, devitalized (i.e., osteoclast-depleted) bone.[213] It has also been demonstrated in experimental animals with metastatic mammary carcinoma that skeletal metastases are surrounded by areas of bone with increased numbers of active osteoclasts.[214] The latter finding would suggest that a locally acting secretory product of the tumor or surrounding inflammatory cells serves to activate osteoclasts. Prostaglandin E_2 (PGE_2) has been implicated in this process in that (1) it can be synthesized by cultured breast carcinoma cells, (2) it is a potent activator of osteoclastic bone resorption, and (3) such a mechanism would explain the sensitivity of breast cancer–associated hypercalcemia to glucocorticoid therapy.[210,215–217] A role for osteoclast activating factor (see below), produced not by the breast carcinoma cells themselves but by adjacent inflammatory cells, has been postulated and would also explain the observed sensitivity to glucocorticoids.[210]

Multiple myeloma has been more carefully studied from a pathogenetic standpoint. Bone biopsies from patients with multiple myeloma and hypercalcemia display marked osteoclastic activity.[218,219] Mundy and colleagues[218] have shown that tissue culture medium exposed to bone marrow aspirates from hypercalcemic patients with multiple myeloma or lymphoma contains a substance (or substances) which stimulates osteoclastic bone resorption and which has been termed *osteoclast activating factor* (OAF). OAF is not considered to be a single protein but appears to comprise a family of bone-resorbing cytokines. Production of OAF is prostaglandin-dependent and can be accomplished by plasma cells as well as by macrophages and lymphocytes.[210] These cells are also capable of synthesizing PGE_2.[210] As is the case in breast cancer, the precise scenario in which plasma cells, lymphocytes, macrophages, and osteoclasts interrelate to result in bone resorption is not clear. Which cells are primarily responsible for OAF and PGE_2 production in vivo, which of these two osteoclast stimulators is more important in vivo, and whether additional myeloma-related bone-resorbing factors remain to be identified are all open questions. The striking sensitivity of myeloma- and lymphoma-associated hypercalcemia to glucocorticoids may reflect the inhibition of OAF and PGE_2 production by these agents.[210]

HUMORAL HYPERCALCEMIA OF MALIGNANCY

Some patients with MAHC have few or no bone metastases.[207–212] In instances where tumor resection can be accomplished, hypercalcemia may be dramatically reversed.[209] Bone biopsies from such patients display a striking increase in the number of osteoclasts in the absence of marrow involvement by tumor.[220] These patients are typically hypophosphatemic, and virtually all display an increase in nephrogenous cAMP excretion.[211,212] These observations collectively suggest that certain tumors are capable of secreting a systemic bone-resorbing phosphaturic substance. Affected individuals typically have squamous carcinomas (of the larynx, oral pharynx, lung, esophagus, vulva, cervix, or skin), renal carcinomas, bladder carcinomas, or ovarian carcinomas.[207–212]

The relative frequency of this humoral syndrome compared with the local osteolytic syndrome is a matter of debate, with some authors viewing it as uncommon[221] and others considering it to be the most common variety of MAHC.[211,212] This debate centers primarily on the definition of the syndrome and, in particular, on the role bone metastases play in this definition. Historically, patients who have had even a single bone metastasis have been considered to have local osteolytic hypercalcemia. Most current investigators view this as a dated and restrictive criterion for patient classification in view of (1) the imprecision of available techniques for detecting foci of bone involvement, (2) the frequency with which bone metastases occur in certain tumors which are only very rarely associated with hypercalcemia (e.g., oat cell carcinoma of the lung),[222] (3) the unlikelihood that one or a few small bone metastases represents an adequate mechanism to produce hypercalcemia, and (4) the fact that patients with HHM (defined biochemically), whether they have skeletal metastases or not, displayed dramatic increases in osteoclastic bone resorption in areas of the skeleton uninvolved by tumor.[220] It has been the authors' practice, therefore, to classify patients biochemically, with an increase in nephrogenous cAMP excretion being the key biochemical marker for the humoral syndrome in vivo. Patients with MAHC who display increased nephrogenous cAMP excretion have proved to constitute a rather homogeneous population. Most have squamous, renal, bladder, or ovarian carcinomas, and most have little or nothing in the way of skeletal metastases.[211,212] In contrast, patients with MAHC and suppressed nephrogenous cAMP excretion typically have breast cancer, lymphoma, or myeloma, and without exception these patients have extensive skeletal tumor involvement.[211,212] Based on this biochemical scheme of classification, 80 percent of patients with MAHC appear to have the humoral syndrome.[211,212]

Prior to the advent of accurate means of assessing parathyroid function, it was assumed that parathyroid hormone was the "humor" responsible for HHM, and terms such as *ectopic hyperparathyroidism* and *pseudohyperparathyroidism* were commonly used. It is now clear that parathyroid hormone is rarely if ever involved in this syndrome and that such terminology is dated and mechanistically inaccurate. Patients with HHM are characterized biochemically by hypercalcemia, hypophosphatemia (if renal function is normal), increased fractional excretion of calcium, reduction in TmP/GFR, normal to unmeasurable circulating levels of immunoreactive PTH, reduction in circulating $1,25\text{-}(OH)_2D$, and elevation in nephrogenous cAMP excretion (Figs. 23-38 and 23-39).[209,211,212,221,223] Bone histomorphometry reveals a marked increase in osteoclastic activity but reduced osteoblastic activity, indicating that bone resorption and bone formation have become uncoupled and providing an explanation for the enormous net losses of skeletal calcium which occur in these patients (Fig. 23-40).[220]

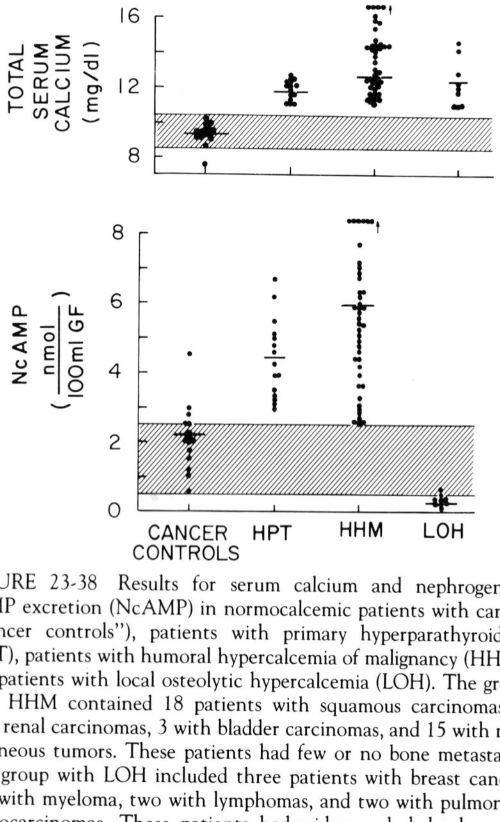

FIGURE 23-38 Results for serum calcium and nephrogenous cAMP excretion (NcAMP) in normocalcemic patients with cancer ("cancer controls"), patients with primary hyperparathyroidism (HPT), patients with humoral hypercalcemia of malignancy (HHM), and patients with local osteolytic hypercalcemia (LOH). The group with HHM contained 18 patients with squamous carcinomas, 5 with renal carcinomas, 3 with bladder carcinomas, and 15 with miscellaneous tumors. These patients had few or no bone metastases. The group with LOH included three patients with breast cancer, two with myeloma, two with lymphomas, and two with pulmonary adenocarcinomas. These patients had widespread skeletal metastases. (*From Stewart, Horst, Deftos, Cadman, Lang, and Broadus,*[211] *by permission of the New England Journal of Medicine.*)

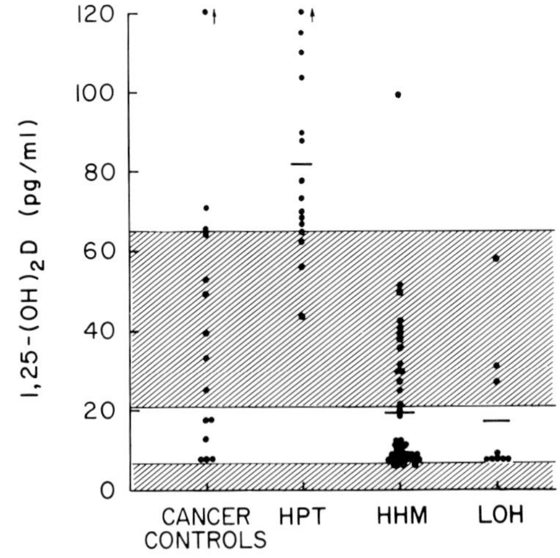

FIGURE 23-39 Values for plasma 1,25-$(OH)_2D$ in the patients described in Fig. 23-38. Note that 1,25-$(OH)_2D$ values are elevated in patients with HPT but are normal or reduced in patients with HHM and LOH. (*From Stewart, Horst, Deftos, Cadman, Lang, and Broadus,*[211] *by permission of the New England Journal of Medicine.*)

Table 23-11. Proposed Mediators of Humoral Hypercalcemia of Malignancy

1. Osteolytic phytosterols: sitosterol, β-sitosterol, stigmasterol, β-stigmasterol
2. Prostaglandin E_2
3. Parathyroid hormone
4. PTH-like adenylate cyclase–stimulating factors
5. Tumor-derived growth factors
6. 1,25 Dihydroxyvitamin D (associated with certain lymphomas)
7. Other unidentified substances

The nature of the circulating factor(s) responsible for HHM remains an area of active investigation. Candidates for the responsible mediator are listed in Table 23-11.

Osteolytic phytosterols were suggested as potential mediators by Gordan in the 1960s, but other investigators subsequently have shown that such sub-

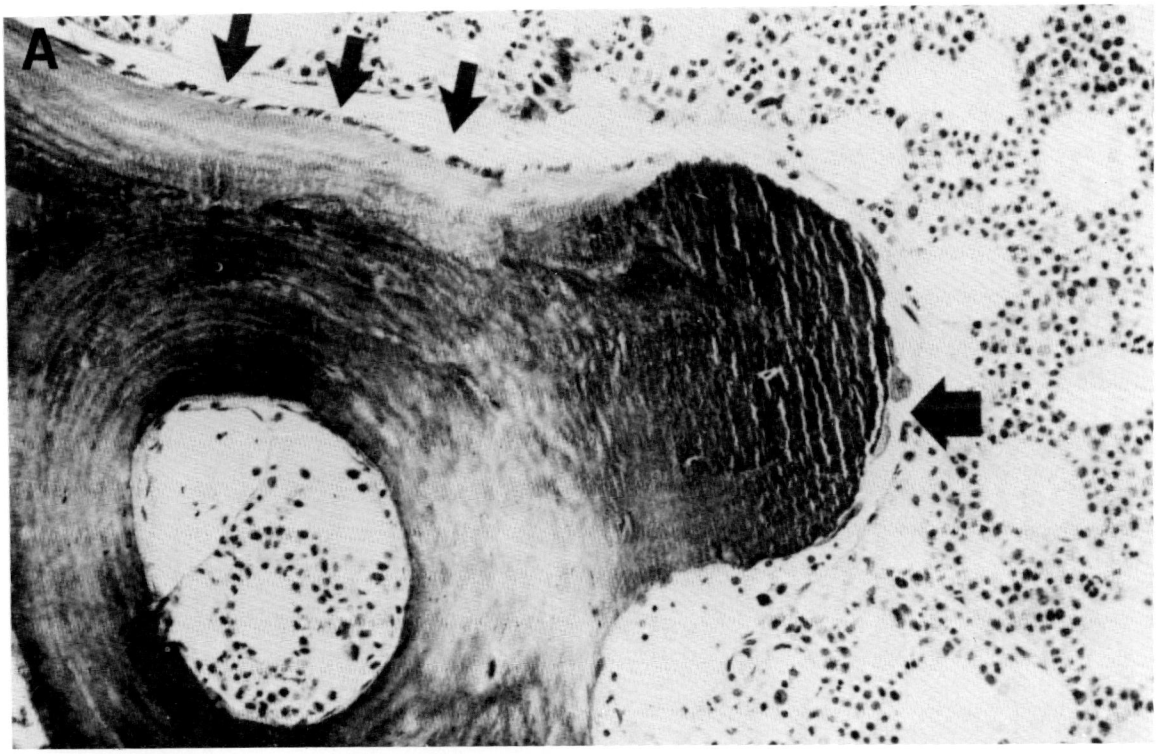

FIGURE 23-40 Bone histology in patients with primary hyperparathyroidism and both subtypes of malignancy-associated hypercalcemia. (A) This demonstrates increased numbers of osteoclasts (large arrows) and osteoblasts and osteoid (small arrows) on the trabecular bone surface of a patient with primary hyperparathyroidism. (B) This demonstrates dramatically increased numbers of osteoclasts and absent osteoblasts and osteoid lining on the trabeculae of two patients with HHM. Note the absence of tumor cells in the adjacent marrow. (C) This shows a biopsy from a patient with multiple myeloma. Note that the marrow space is replaced by plasma cells and that adjacent osteoclasts are increased in number. [*(A) and (B) are from Stewart, Vignery, Silverglate, Ravin, Livolsi, Broadus, and Baron,*[220] *by permission of the Journal of Clinical Endocrinology and Metabolism. (C) is from Mundy, Raisz, Cooper, Schechter, and Salmon,*[218] *by permission of the New England Journal of Medicine.*]

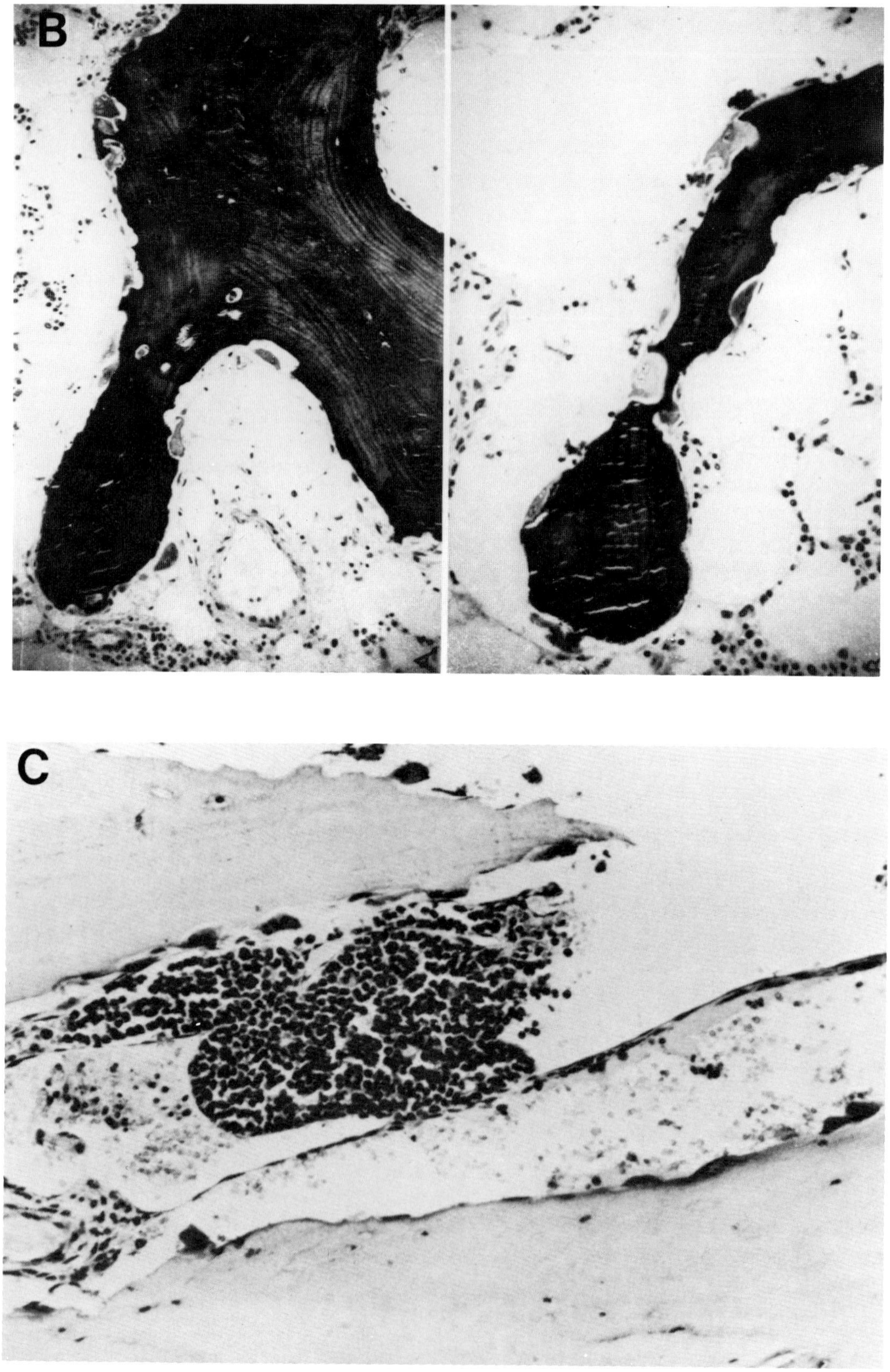

FIGURE 23-40 (*Continued*).

stances are also present in the plasma of healthy individuals.[224]

Prostaglandins of the E series have been implicated by some investigators in a few patients with HHM and in two animal models of HHM.[210] Other investigators, however, have shown that circulating prostaglandin levels are not differentially elevated in hypercalcemic patients compared with normocalcemic patients with cancer.[225] In addition, therapy with prostaglandin synthetase inhibitors rarely influences hypercalcemia in patients with HHM.[226] Thus, a current consensus would hold that "ectopic prostaglandin secretion" is an unusual cause of HHM.

Parathyroid hormone has been implicated by (1) the humoral nature of this syndrome, (2) the accompanying decrease in TmP/GFR and hypophosphatemia, and (3) immunoassay data which have been interpreted by some investigators as "inappropriate" to the level of hypercalcemia in patients with MAHC.[227] This interpretation is no longer considered mechanistically meaningful in that normal or marginally elevated values for immunoreactive PTH are seen with equal frequency in patients with LOH and HHM,[110,209,211,212,221] and these results are generally regarded as reflecting the continued nonsuppressible component of PTH secretion in the face of retained hormone fragments in patients with moderate renal impairment (see Fig. 23-27). In addition, patients with HHM are typified by marked reductions in circulating 1,25-$(OH)_2D$, a striking mean increase in fractional calcium excretion, and a pattern of uncoupled bone turnover; these features are very different from those observed in primary hyperparathyroidism.[211,212,220] Finally, human and animal tumors associated with HHM do not contain detectable messenger RNA for PTH,[228] suggesting that active transcription of the PTH gene does not occur in these tumors. This observation provides evidence not only against the participation of PTH in the humoral syndrome but also against the possible participation of unprocessed PTH precursors in the syndrome.

At the time of this writing, two types of substances are under intensive investigation as potential mediators of the humoral syndrome. One hypothesis holds that this factor is a substance which is unrelated to parathyroid hormone or its gene products but is able to bind to and stimulate certain PTH-sensitive target tissues; the other hypothesis holds that the HHM-factor is a tumor-derived growth factor with bone-resorbing capability.

Evidence in favor of the first hypothesis can be summarized under the heading of three categories of data obtained in vivo and/or in vitro. First, there is good evidence that patients with HHM produce a systemic factor which is in a limited sense "PTH-like." These patients display elevations in nephrogenous cAMP and reductions in TmP/GFR, findings which indicate the activation of the proximal tubular PTH-sensitive adenylate cyclase.[211,212] Furthermore, plasma from patients with HHM contains a substance which activates the PTH-sensitive renal tubular cytochemical bioassay for PTH; this bioactivity is reduced in plasma from patients with LOH.[229] The bioactivity is present despite the absence of immunoreactive PTH and behaves chromatographically as if it were larger than PTH.[229] Second, extracts of tumors obtained from patients and animals with HHM as well as tissue culture media in which such tumor cells have been grown contain a substance which stimulates PTH-sensitive adenylate cyclases in a variety of systems (including a canine renal cortical PTH-sensitive adenylate cyclase, an intact-cell rat osteosarcoma PTH-sensitive adenylate cyclase, and the cytochemical bioassay for PTH) (Fig. 23-41).[229-232] In extracts and conditioned medium from tumors and cell lines associated with HHM, this activity can be regularly and completely inhibited in these assay systems by means of incubation with truncated, substituted PTH analogues which function as competitive inhibitors of PTH binding; these observations provide direct evidence of the interaction of the factor in question with PTH receptors (Fig. 23-42).[230,231] In contrast, preincubation with a variety of anti-PTH antisera, including those which recognize the amino terminus of the molecule, has no appreciable effect on activity in these assay systems (Fig. 23-42).[212,230] Extracts from control tumors contain little or no activity of this sort. Third, in vitro bone-resorbing activity as well as adenylate cyclase-stimulating activity has been demonstrated in extracts of tumors associated with HHM, and these activities have been shown to copurify in a variety of chromatographic systems.[233,234] In essence, the "PTH agonist" or "PTH-like" hypothesis holds that the HHM factor is a protein which is larger than PTH or its precursors and is derived from a gene distinct from that for PTH. This factor, for reasons which are uncertain, appears to interact with certain but not all PTH receptors in a fashion analogous to somatomedin binding and stimulation of insulin receptors. It is assumed that the presence of this HHM factor in the systemic circulation is related to disordered or excessive production of the factor by malignant tissue and that a normal role exists for this material in certain undefined tissues. Preliminary evidence suggests that normal squamous epithelia such as skin may be such a tissue.[235]

The second hypothesis holds that the HHM factor is a tumor-derived growth factor. This theory is derived from the observations that epidermal growth factor (EGF) is a potent stimulator of in vitro bone

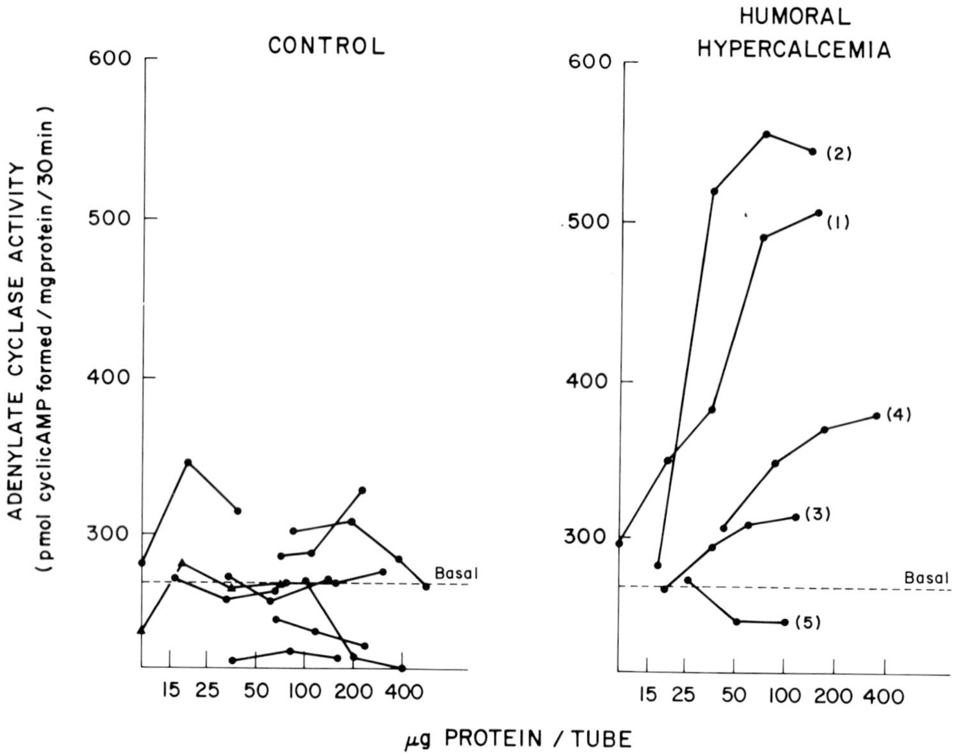

FIGURE 23-41 Adenylate cyclase–stimulating activity (ACSA) in extracts of tumors derived from normocalcemic patients ("control") and patients with HHM. Four of five HHM-associated extracts contained definite ACSA, while the control patients were negative. ACSA is measured by the conversion of ATP to cAMP by canine renal cortical membranes. (*From Stewart, Insogna, Goltzman, and Broadus,*[230] *by permission of Proceedings of the National Academy of Science, USA.*)

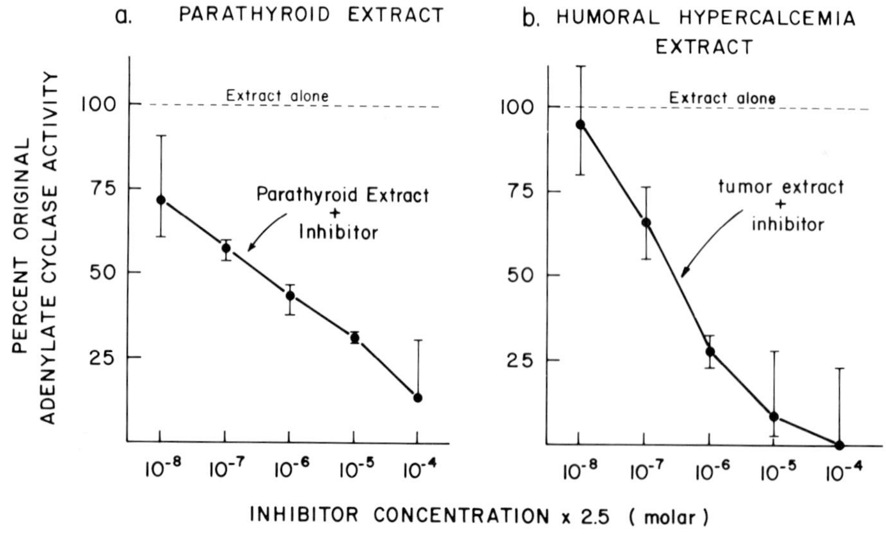

FIGURE 23-42 Inhibition by the PTH analogue and inhibitor [$Nle^{8,18}$, Tyr^{34}]bPTH-(3-34)amide of adenylate cyclase stimulation induced by a human parathyroid adenoma extract and by a human HHM-associated tumor extract. The PTH receptor–binding analogue inhibited the ACSA in both extracts, indicating that the factor in the HHM extract is operating through the PTH receptor. (*From Stewart, Insogna, Goltzman, and Broadus,*[230] *by permission of Proceedings of the National Academy of Science, USA.*)

resorption systems. Although immunoreactive EGF cannot be demonstrated in HHM-derived tissues, it is possible that tumor-derived growth factors (TGFs), which bind to and activate EGF receptors in bone, may be responsible for HHM. Evidence which would support the notion that the HHM-factor is a TGF includes the following:

1. Tumor extracts and conditioned medium derived from three HHM-associated tumors (one human and two animal) contain bone-resorbing activity.
2. These extracts and media also contain transforming growth factors, as evidenced by their ability to competitively displace EGF from its receptors, stimulate mitogenesis in osteosarcoma cells, and stimulate anchorage-independent growth of mouse fibroblasts in soft agar.
3. It has been shown that growth factor activities and bone-resorbing activity from these tumors copurify on gel filtration, suggesting that both activities may be the result of a single substance (Fig. 23-43).[236–238]

It is possible that both the "PTH-like" and the "growth factor–like" theories of HHM are correct. For example, it is possible that the mediator in question is a tumor-derived growth factor which binds selectively to certain PTH receptors. Alternatively, both factors may be produced by HHM-associated tumors and thus act in a concerted fashion.[238] The resolution of this question will have to await the complete purification of the HHM factor from one or multiple sources.

LYMPHOMA-ASSOCIATED HYPERCALCEMIA

Historically, lymphomas have been viewed as an unusual cause of hypercalcemia. When hypercalcemia has occurred in individuals with a lymphoma, it has most often occurred in patients with extensive skeletal involvement.[239,240] The mechanism of these patients' hypercalcemia appears to be similar to that described above in patients with multiple myeloma, and it is likely that this mechanism continues to apply in most instances. Recently, however, two observations have been made which suggest that alternative mechanisms may exist in occasional patients with lymphoma.

First, two groups have demonstrated that some patients with a lymphoma and hypercalcemia have

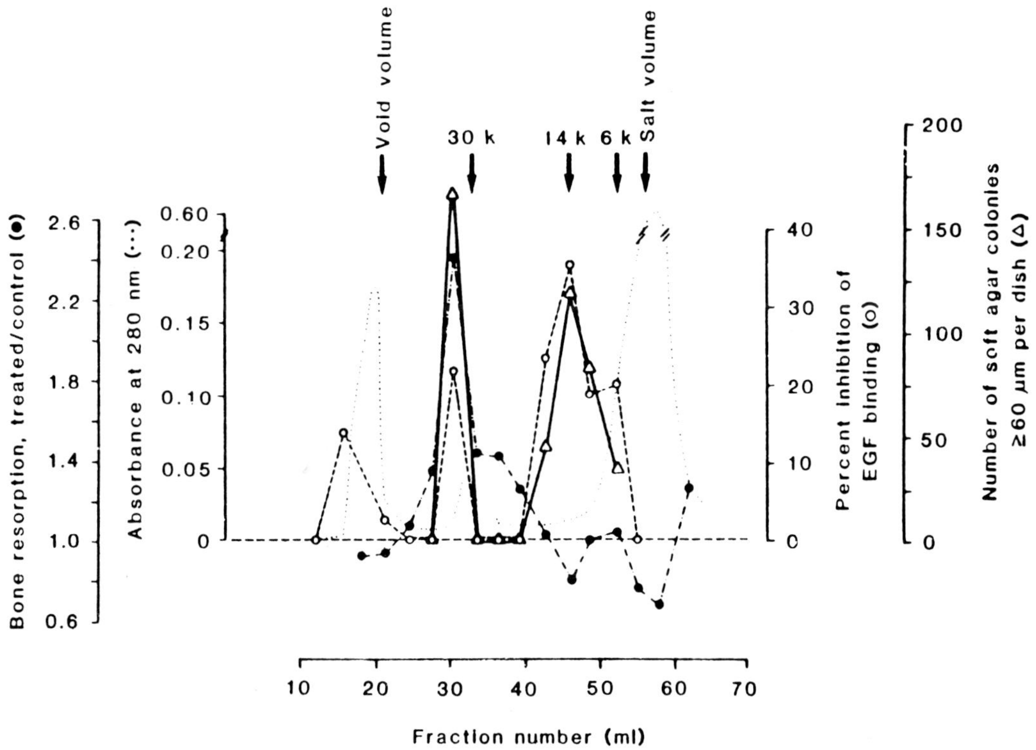

FIGURE 23-43 Comigration of bone-resorbing (●), EGF-displacing (○), and growth factor (△) activities from a rat HHM-associated tumor on a gel filtration column. These findings indicate that the three activities are due to a protein or proteins of similar molecular weight. (*From Ibbotson, D'Souza, Ng, Osborne, Niall, Martin, and Mundy,*[237] *by permission of Science.*)

elevations in circulating 1,25-$(OH)_2D$.[223,241] These reports have suggested that 1,25-$(OH)_2D$ can be produced by lymphomas, as it is by sarcoid granulomas (see below), and that it can cause intestinal calcium hyperabsorption and bone resorption. Four of the six patients described with this syndrome had diffuse histiocytic lymphomas using the Lukes-Collins classification. Using the more recently described functional or immunological classification of Rappaport, no clear histological distinctions could be made in these patients compared with normocalcemic patients with lymphoma. Since the availability of 1,25-$(OH)_2D$ measurements is comparatively recent, it is possible that this syndrome is more common than is currently appreciated. These findings are all the more interesting in view of recent observations which indicate that a variety of cell types in the immune system contain receptors for, produce, and functionally respond to 1,25-$(OH)_2D$.[242]

A second recent phenomenon of interest is the striking association of the retrovirus-associated human T-cell lymphoma with hypercalcemia. This type of lymphoma was initially described as occurring endemically in southwestern Japan and then in the Caribbean. More recently, descriptions of similar patients in the United States have appeared.[243] Ninety percent of these patients have been hypercalcemic. Some have had widespread skeletal involvement, but others have had none, suggesting that local skeletal invasion may be important in some instances but that humoral mechanisms may be operative in others. Alternatively, a single bone-resorbing substance could be operative in both instances, acting both locally and systemically. Whether this substance is 1,25-$(OH)_2D$ or some other bone-resorbing substance is not known.

UNCOMMON VARIANTS OF MALIGNANCY-ASSOCIATED HYPERCALCEMIA

The foregoing categories include the vast majority of patients with MAHC. A small minority of patients, however, appear to represent different mechanisms. For example, the authors have reported a patient with an ovarian dysgerminoma who had no evidence of skeletal metastases and whose hypercalcemia was reversed by means of tumor excision.[244] Her immunoreactive PTH, nephrogenous cAMP, and 1,25-$(OH)_2D$ values were all suppressed prior to therapy, and all rose into the normal range following successful tumor removal. Thus, although she clearly had a "humoral" type of hypercalcemia, the unusual tumor histology and suppression of nephrogenous cAMP separate her mechanistically from the bulk of patients with HHM. A second example is a patient with a malignant melanoma metastatic to inguinal lymph nodes.[245] This patient also had surgically reversible hypercalcemia. Although biochemical measurements were not available from this patient in vivo, studies in vitro suggest that hypercalcemia occurred through tumor production of a bone-resorbing protein distinct from that usually associated with HHM. Again, surgical reversibility suggested that this was a "humoral" variety of MAHC, but the unusual histology and in vitro data separate this patient's humoral hypercalcemia from the mainstream. Another example may be the unusual patient, as described above, who would appear to have bona fide prostaglandin-mediated hypercalcemia. Examples of such patients have been described.[225,246,247] These uncommon variants of MAHC are rare.

PATHOPHYSIOLOGY AND DIAGNOSIS

In both HHM and LOH, the primary abnormality in systemic mineral homeostasis is accelerated and uncoupled bone resorption. That is, the hypercalcemia is purely "resorptive" in both syndromes, and the PTH–1,25-$(OH)_2D$ axis is appropriately suppressed, with attendant reductions in intestinal calcium absorption and distal tubular calcium reabsorption. Patients with either syndrome can be observed to pass through a "prehypercalcemic" stage during which the suppression of the PTH–1,25-$(OH)_2D$ axis and their ability to clear the resorbed load of calcium into the urine compensate, and frank hypercalcemia does not develop. This compensated state is often short-lived because of coincident inanition, vomiting, diarrhea, immobilization, and ultimately a hypercalcemia-induced inability to concentrate the urine. Also, most patients with hypercalcemia have a degree of prerenal or renal azotemia at the time of presentation. At this point, the vicious cycle of dehydration, hypercalcemia, worsening dehydration, and worsening hypercalcemia has begun.

In patients with lymphoma-associated 1,25-$(OH)_2D$–mediated hypercalcemia, intestinal calcium absorption and bone resorption appear to be increased.[223,241] PTH secretion is reduced, and patients are markedly hypercalciuric until renal insufficiency supervenes.

In most patients with a malignancy and hypercalcemia, the hematologic malignancy or solid tumor is clinically obvious and the diagnosis is self-evident. Significant problems in differential diagnosis may occur in unusual patients with a malignancy in an occult location or in a patient with coincident primary hyperparathyroidism and either a history of malignancy or a tumor which is clinically apparent on presentation. In virtually 100 percent of patients, the differential diagnosis can be achieved biochemically, as described in Differential Diagnosis, below.

TREATMENT

The management of emergent hypercalcemia is described in detail in the final portion of Hypercalcemia. The vicious spiral of hypercalcemia, dehydration, immobilization, and worsening hypercalcemia is particularly common in patients with malignant disease. Initial steps in management include rehydration, calciuretic therapy, and mobilization of the patient, and these steps usually lead to a reduction in serum calcium to nonemergent levels. Many oncologists employ mithramycin or other agents as soon as significant hypercalcemia is detected in a patient with cancer, but it may be useful to withhold these agents until the results of the front-line measures are apparent and/or until the nature of the malignancy is known, if it has not previously been diagnosed. A patient with a serum calcium in the range of 12 to 13 mg/dl may be clinically stable and can often be managed by some combination of (1) mobilization, (2) forced oral fluids with a high sodium intake, (3) oral furosemide, and/or (4) small doses of oral phosphates while specific surgical, radiation, or chemical therapy is being initiated. In patients requiring further antihypercalcemic therapy, mithramycin, steroids, calcitonin, and oral phosphates are variously employed as agents which inhibit bone resorption. Steroids are particularly useful in patients with hematologic malignancies and in a large minority of patients with breast carcinoma.[207] Estrogen and antiestrogen therapy may be associated with a rapid and transient or persistent hypercalcemic "flair" in a minority of patients with breast carcinoma (see below).

In patients who are clearly terminal, it is sometimes elected not to treat severe hypercalcemia; the patient is allowed to succumb to the central effects of the hypercalcemia as a form of endogenous morphinization.

Endocrinopathies

THYROTOXICOSIS

Mild hypercalcemia occurs in approximately 20 percent of patients with hyperthyroidism. The serum albumin concentration is often modestly reduced in hyperthyroid patients so that increases in ionized serum calcium or corrected total serum calcium may be seen in as many as 50 percent of patients.[248] The hypercalcemia is usually in the range of 11 mg/dl, and seurm calcium values greater than 11.5 mg/dl are rarely observed. Calcium excretion rates are elevated in one-third to one-half of patients, but an increased frequency of renal stone disease has not been reported in hyperthyroidism. Values for serum phosphorus and TmP/GFR are either high-normal or slightly increased.[248] The degree of the abnormality in the circulating quantities of the thyroid hormones is strongly correlated with measured abnormalities in serum and urinary calcium and TmP/GFR.[248]

The major, if not the only, mechanism responsible for abnormalities in mineral and skeletal homeostasis in hyperthyroidism is the direct influence of the thyroid hormones on bone resorption and bone turnover.[249] The increased bone turnover in hyperthyroidism is reflected by increases in serum alkaline phosphatase activity, urinary hydroxyproline excretion, and osteoclastic and osteoblastic activity in bone biopsy specimens. The thyroid hormones stimulate osteoclastic bone resorption and, to some extent, osteocytic osteolysis, and the histological findings on bone biopsy may closely resemble the findings in patients with mild hyperparathyroidism.[250] Bone resorption outstrips bone formation, leading to net loss of both bone mineral and bone matrix. In vitro, the stimulation of bone resorption by the thyroid hormones is slower and less marked than that produced by PTH and 1,25-$(OH)_2D$ and can be inhibited by calcitonin, cortisol, and propranolol but not by indomethacin.[249] A reduction in bone mineral density may be demonstrated in a majority of patients by sensitive densitometric and other techniques, but radiologically apparent and significant bone demineralization is usually confined to postmenopausal female patients and patients with very severe hyperthyroidism. The bone loss in hyperthyroidism is generally considered to be reversible but may be partially irreversible in the latter group of patients. The radiological findings in hyperthyroidism are diffuse and resemble those of osteoporosis.

Patients with hyperthyroidism are characteristically in negative calcium balance, with reduced fractional and net intestinal calcium absorption and increased urinary and fecal calcium excretion. Although the initial reports contain conflicting data, parathyroid function is significantly suppressed in hyperthyroidism.[248] The high-normal or increased TmP/GFR reflects the suppression in parathyroid function; the quantitative importance of a putative direct influence of the thyroid hormones on tubular phosphorus threshold remains unclear. Circulating levels of 1,25-$(OH)_2D$ are markedly reduced in patients with hyperthyroidism.[251] These findings corroborate the previously documented decreases in intestinal calcium absorption in hyperthyroidism and presumably reflect the suppression in parathyroid function and increased TmP/GFR in the disorder, although altered rates of vitamin D metabolism are also possible. In essence, the pathophysiological picture in hyperthyroidism appears to be one of "pure" bone resorption, with attendant negative calcium balance and suppression of the hormonal network associated with calcium mobilization and absorption. The administration of pharmacological quantities of PTH to hyperthyroid patients has been reported to result in exaggerated calcemic and urinary cAMP responses vis-à-vis those noted in normal subjects. However, hypercalcemia can be demonstrated in parathyroidectomized animals treated with excessive doses of thyroid hormone, and so the apparent hyperresponsiveness to PTH in hyperthyroidism is probably of limited pathophysiological importance.

Diagnosis generally presents no difficulties, and the hypercalcemia is usually noted as an incidental laboratory finding in an obviously hyperthyroid patient. The TmP/GFR is often in the range of 4.0 mg/dl in hyperthyroidism and is a useful confirmatory measurement. The increased total cAMP excretion rate reported in earlier studies of hyperthyroid patients represents an error in data expression; properly expressed, nephrogenous cAMP and total cAMP excretion are normal in hyperthyroidism.[94] A large number of patients with coincident hyperthyroidism and primary hyperparathyroidism have been reported, and this combination should be suspected in a hyperthyroid patient with a serum calcium greater than 11.5 mg/dl, a TmP/GFR lower than 3.0 mg/dl, or frank elevations in parathyroid function tests. In such a patient, the serum calcium will be reduced but not normalized by antithyroid therapy.

Antithyroid therapy reverses the abnormalities in mineral homeostasis associated with hyperthyroidism in a matter of weeks. The elevated serum alkaline phosphatase activity is actually further increased by antithyroid therapy and remains high until the rebound increase in bone formation rate subsides, which usually requires several months. This increase in bone formation is sufficient to restore a normal bone mass in most but not all patients (see above). Propranolol has been reported to reduce serum calcium levels in hypercalcemic patients with hyperthyroidism, presumably by directly inhibiting the effects of the thyroid hormone on osteoclastic bone resorption.

ADRENAL INSUFFICIENCY

Significant hypercalcemia may be observed in acute adrenal insufficiency.[252] A variety of proposals to explain this hypercalcemia have been offered, including hemoconcentration, reduced urinary calcium excretion, and the lack of the oppositional effects of cortisol on vitamin D action on bone resorption and intestinal calcium absorption. Systematic biochemical studies have not been performed in patients with acute adrenal insufficiency and hypercalcemia, however, and the pathogenesis of the hypercalcemia remains obscure.[129,252] Once the diagnosis of adrenal insufficiency is achieved, the basis of the associated hypercalcemia is readily apparent, and the hypercalcemia resolves rapidly with steroid replacement therapy.

PHEOCHROMOCYTOMA

Hypercalcemia is an unusual but well-documented occurrence among patients with pheochromocytoma. Most often, hypercalcemia proves to be due to coexisting primary hyperparathyroidism (parathyroid hyperplasia) in a patient with multiple endocrine neoplasma type IIA. These patients typically have family histories of hyperparathyroidism, pheochromocytoma, and/or medullary carcinoma of the thyroid. The existence of primary hyperparathyroidism can be documented by the elevations in serum calcium and immunoreactive PTH which persist following surgical excision of the pheochromocytoma.

Occasionally, hypercalcemia appears to occur as a direct result of the pheochromocytoma, as evidenced by the prompt reversal of hypercalcemia following resection of the adrenal tumor. Several hypotheses have been put forward to explain these events:

1. Hypercalcemia may be due to ectopic secretion of PTH by the pheochromocytoma.
2. Hypercalcemia occurs as a result of a catechol-mediated increase in bone resorption.
3. Hypercalcemia occurs as a result of catechol-induced PTH secretion from the parathyroid glands.
4. Hypercalcemia results from secretion by the pheochromocytoma of the same adenylate cyclase–stimulating bone-resorbing factor which has been described in tumors derived from patients with humoral hypercalcemia of malignancy.

The most recent and detailed data support the last hypothesis.[253]

In patients with pheochromocytoma and hypercalcemia, resection of the pheochromocytoma(s) should be performed prior to attempted parathyroidectomy. This approach minimizes the surgical risks associated with pheochromocytoma and surgery/anesthesia and allows one to exclude the possibility of pheochromocytoma-dependent hypercalcemia.

VIP-OMA SYNDROME

Hypercalcemia was recorded in 7 of 16 patients with the VIP-oma (watery diarrhea, hypokalemia and achlorhydria, or WDHA) syndrome reviewed by Verner and Morrison in 1974.[254] The mechanism responsible for this hypercalcemia has not been examined carefully. Coexisting primary hyperparathyroidism may be present in some patients, but reversal of hypercalcemia following resection of an islet cell tumor has been reported.[254] Thus, secretion of PTH secretagogues and secretion of bone-resorbing agents by the tumor are possible explanations. Whether VIP is such a bone-resorbing agent is not known.

Medications

The potential involvement of medications in a hypercalcemic patient should be apparent in the patient's medication history, but this is not always the case. Because of habitual and/or surreptitious use, patients may not accurately relate their medication intake, and a patient with an apparently obscure hypercalcemic syndrome must be carefully and repeatedly questioned.

THIAZIDE DIURETICS

The thiazides and related diuretics (e.g., chlorthalidone) can induce or exacerbate hypercalcemia in any patient with an increased rate of calcium entry into the extracellular pool. In this regard, the thiazides differ from most other diuretics, which are calciuretic as well as natriuretic. The thiazides may produce mild, intermittent hypercalcemia in individuals with otherwise normal mineral homeostasis, but sustained hypercalcemia suggests the presence of an underlying disorder of calcium homeostasis.

The literature concerning the mechanism of thiazide-induced alterations in serum and urinary calcium is massive, conflicting, and inconclusive.[255] Thiazides have been variously reported to (1) reduce the fractional excretion of calcium, (2) induce volume contraction and hemoconcentration, (3) increase net intestinal calcium absorption, (4) increase bone resorption, and/or (5) stimulate parathyroid hyperplasia and hormone secretion; the latter effect has never been confirmed in humans. The hypocalciuric effect of the thiazides can be readily demonstrated in normal individuals and in patients with a wide variety of disorders of mineral metabolism. The drugs initially induce an increase in both sodium and calcium excretion, and the maximal hypocalciuric effect is observed on the third or fourth day of treatment, after the acute natriuresis has subsided. On the average, urinary calcium excretion is reduced to approximately 60 percent of its pretreatment rate.[255] The hypocalciuria appears to result from a combination of volume depletion and the effects of the thiazides on distal tubular reabsorption,[256] and it can be largely reversed by sodium administration.[255] Notwithstanding frequent statements to the contrary, the thiazides produce a reduction in fractional calcium excretion in patients with chronic hypoparathyroidism,[256] but the hypocalciuric effect of the agents may be obscured in these patients by the concomitant increases in the serum level and filtered load of calcium.

The hypercalcemic influence of the thiazides is demonstrable in anephric patients, indicating that effects of the agents on organ systems other than the kidney must participate in the net calcemic response. The reports in the literature are conflicting, but the thiazides are generally regarded as having a modest stimulatory influence on both intestinal calcium absorption and bone resorption. It is impossible to sort out the quantitative importance of these various thiazide effects in the integrated calcemic response observed in vivo. The agents are associated with a clear tendency toward a positive calcium balance, which appears to spill over into frank hypercalcemia only in patients with an increased input of calcium into the extracellular pool.[255] Thiazide treatment regularly increases total serum calcium by 0.5 to 1.0 mg/dl or more in patients with primary hyperparathyroidism and those with chronic hypoparathyroidism on vitamin D replacement therapy. This response in hypoparathyroid patients is so regularly observed that the agents have been proposed as a therapeutic alternative for the treatment of chronic hypoparathyroidism.

Given an accurate medication history, the potential involvement of thiazides is diagnostically self-evident, and the usual course of action in a patient with persistent hypercalcemia on repeated determinations is to discontinue or substitute diuretic therapy and to investigate the patient further with standard techniques. The proposed use of thiazide provocation in an attempt to diagnose subtle primary hyperparathyroidism is to be avoided because of the nonspecificity and unpredictability of the response;[255] far more sensitive and reliable diagnostic techniques are available (Chap. 25). Frank elevations in parathyroid function tests in a hypercalcemic patient in thiazide therapy are diagnostic of underlying primary hyperparathyroidism.

VITAMINS A AND D

Vitamin D intoxication is usually noted as an unpredictable complication of long-term therapy in patients with hypoparathyroidism, renal osteodystrophy, hypophosphatemic rickets, or intestinal malabsorption. Occasionally, self-induced intoxication is discovered in an individual surreptitiously taking large doses of a vitamin D preparation. Following the introduction of crystalline preparations of the calciferols in the 1930s, these agents were empirically employed in the unsuccessful treatment of a variety of medical disorders, and severe vitamin D intoxication was observed with some frequency.[257] It was during this time that the "sensitivity" of patients with sarcoidosis to vitamin D was initially described.

The calcemic effects of all vitamin D preparations are due to their combined stimulatory effects on intestinal calcium absorption and bone resorption, and intoxication has been observed in response to all vitamin D analogues and metabolites. Intoxication is usually noted only in patients consuming large quantities of vitamin D (100,000 U or more of calciferol daily or equivalent doses of the more recently introduced vitamin D preparations). Typically and inexplicably, hypercalcemia develops suddenly in a patient successfully managed for months to years on a stable dosage of vitamin D. Early signs include polyuria and lassitude, and complications of more prolonged hypercalcemia are extraskeletal calcification, nephrocalcinosis, and renal impairment, which are only partially reversible. Because of extensive storage in fat, intoxication with the calciferols may persist for weeks to months, and many clinicians prefer DHT or other vitamin D analogues for long-term therapy for this reason (see Treament under Hypocalcemia). A more subtle form of "intoxication" consisting of hypercalciuria, nephrolithiasis, and/or nephrocalcinosis may be observed in patients with hypoparathyroidism treated with slightly excessive doses of vitamin D sufficient to maintain a chronic serum calcium concentration in the range of 10 mg/dl.

The diagnosis is usually self-evident by history and/or by the high-normal or elevated values for serum phosphorus and TmP/GFR, the tendency to a metabolic alkalosis, and suppressed parathyroid function tests. The diagnosis can be confirmed by the rapid reduction in serum calcium in response to steroids (the cortisone suppression test) or by measuring serum levels of total 25-OHD, which usually exceed 350 ng/ml in patients intoxicated with calciferol.[258] Interestingly, serum levels of 1,25-$(OH)_2$D are normal in these patients, indicating that the intoxication results from the aggregate effects of the massive circulating levels of the less active vitamin D metabolites.[258] Vitamin D intoxication has also been observed in anephric patients treated with calciferol. Treatment consists of discontinuing vitamin D and calcium supplements, fluid and diuretic therapy as required, and steroids in initial doses of 100 to 200 mg hydrocortisone daily. The steroids are rapidly tapered as the hypercalcemia comes under control.

Hypervitaminosis A is rare and is observed only in individuals consuming 10 or more times the minimum adult requirement of 5000 IU daily. The hypercalcemia may be severe, and in addition to the usual symptoms of hypercalcemia, patients usually complain of vague, diffuse musculoskeletal discomfort. Patients intoxicated with vitamin A frequently have nephrocalcinosis and renal impairment, and the diagnosis may be suggested by peculiar, fine periosteal calcifications along the shafts of the metacarpals and proximal phalanges.[259] Similar radiographic findings have been reported in patients treated with retinoic acid or its derivatives.[260] The pathogenesis appears to be based on vitamin A–induced osteoclastic bone resorption. Vitamin A is available on an over-the-counter basis, in some preparations in combination with vitamin D, and combined hypervitaminoses have been described.[259] Vitamin A and retinoic acid derivatives are increasingly employed in the treatment of miscellaneous skin disorders. The diagnosis should be suspected in any obscure hypercalcemic syndrome and can be confirmed by the history of vitamin A intake, measurements of excessive vitamin A levels in serum, or rapid response to the cortisone suppression test. The treatment is identical to that of vitamin D intoxication.

MILK-ALKALI SYNDROME

The milk-alkali syndrome results from an excessive intake of milk and an absorbable alkali, such as calcium carbonate, sodium carbonate, or sodium bicarbonate. Because of the substitution of nonabsorbable antacids for the soluble alkalies in the treatment of peptic ulcer disease, the syndrome is uncommon today. Development of the syndrome requires the ingestion of 4000 mg or more of elemental calcium per day.[260,261] Both acute and chronic syndromes have been described, but it is the chronic syndrome which is of clinical importance.[260,261] Patients present with nonspecific symptoms of hypercalcemia, nephrocalcinosis and extraskeletal calcification, renal impairment, alkalosis, and hyperphosphatemia. Hypercalciuria is usually absent because of the renal impairment, and nephrolithiasis is not observed. The diagnosis may not be obvious in a patient who fails to mention his or her large intake of over-the-counter antacids (e.g., Tums). Treatment consists of the usual acute antihypercalcemic measures and elimination of milk and soluble antacid intake. The hypercalcemia resolves rapidly, and the band keratopathy and other signs of extraskeletal calcification are often also reversible. The renal impairment, however, is typically only partially reversible.[260,261]

LITHIUM

Lithium is a relatively recent addition to the list of medications which may be associated with hypercalcemia.[262,263] Series have described patients on long-term lithium who have had associated mild hypercalcemia, hypermagnesemia, osteopenia, and biochemical hyperparathyroidism together with normophosphatemia and relative hypocalciuria.[262] Small parathyroid adenomas have been removed in some reported cases.[263] Specific complications of primary hyperparathyroidism are reportedly absent. The pattern of abnormalities in patients on long-term lithium has been likened to that observed in patients with familial hypocalciuric hypercalcemia.[183] This analogy has also been suggested by reports that lithium decreases the fractional excretion of calcium and magnesium in humans in vivo[264] and increases the set point of PTH secretion by bovine parathyroid cells in vitro.[265] The latter effect has not been demonstrable in humans studied in vivo after short-term lithium administration.[266] Management of such patients should be conservative pending more complete information regarding the clinical relevance of the associated hypercalcemia. Parathyroidectomy has not altered the course of the basic psychiatric disturbance.

ESTROGENS AND ANTIESTROGENS

Both estrogens (e.g., diethylstilbestrol) and antiestrogens (e.g., tamoxifen) have been reported to produce hypercalcemia in some patients with breast carcinoma.[267,268] Patients typically have widespread skeletal metastases. Interestingly, following an initial hypercalcemic "flare," hypercalcemia may eventually reverse despite continued or resumed therapy; this flare may even indicate the likelihood of an eventual tumor response to these hormonal agents. The mechanism of the hypercalcemic flare induced by these agents is not known.

Sarcoidosis and Other Granulomatous Diseases

In modern series, hypercalcemia is observed in 10 percent or less of patients with active sarcoidosis, and hypercalciuria is noted in approximately 40 percent of these patients. These figures are lower than those in older reports and presumably reflect improved diagnosis and earlier institution of effective steroid treatment.[269,270] It is probable that an increase in intestinal calcium absorption is present in the majority of patients with active sarcoidosis, but systematic data on this point are unavailable.

Although severe hypercalcemia may occur in sarcoidosis, a pattern of mild, intermittent, and unpredictable hypercalcemia is more commonly observed. Significant and sustained hypercalcemia correlates with chronic, advanced sarcoidosis, and renal impairment due to hypercalcemic nephropathy usually limits the hypercalciuria in these patients. Hypercalciuria and mild hypercalcemia are more frequently observed in patients with stage 1 or stage 2 sarcoidosis. These patients are predisposed to nephrolithiasis and may represent a difficult problem in differential diagnosis, since the radiological and other manifestations of sarcoidosis may be easily missed or may not be apparent. A diagnosis of sarcoidosis in such patients has occasionally been made on the basis of examination of lymph node specimens removed during neck exploration for a presumed diagnosis of primary hyperparathyroidism.[129]

Hypercalcemia in sarcoidosis was initially and erroneously regarded as resulting from bone involvement by the granulomatous process. The pattern of calcium abnormalities in sarcoidosis is virtually identical to that observed in mild to moderate hypervitaminosis D, and the abnormal sensitivity of patients with sarcoidosis to vitamin D has long suggested an association between vitamin D and the pathogenesis of the calcium abnormalities in the disorder. Patients with active sarcoidosis were found to develop toxicity to daily doses as low as 10,000 IU of calciferol, whereas doses in the range of 150,000 IU could be tolerated by most other adults.[269] In a number of series, spontaneous hypercalcemia has been reported to occur more frequently during the summer than the winter months.

Patients with sarcoidosis and abnormalities in calcium metabolism display increased rates of intestinal calcium absorption and bone resorption. The degree of hypercalciuria and/or hypercalcemia observed depends on the quantitative abnormalities in intestinal calcium absorption and bone resorption as well as the dietary calcium intake and the integrity of renal function. Subtle manifestations resemble those in patients with "absorptive" hypercalciuria, and more advanced abnormalities are similar to those of moderately severe vitamin D intoxication. The pathogenesis of these abnormalities has recently been clarified and involves an abnormal rate of conversion of 25-OHD to 1,25-$(OH)_2D$ rather than an abnormal "sensitivity" to 1,25-$(OH)_2D$. An initial clue that the granulomatous tissue may be involved in this conversion was provided by a case report of a hypercalcemic anephric patient with sarcoidosis and increased circulating 1,25-$(OH)_2D$.[271] Production of 1,25-$(OH)_2D$ has since been demonstrated in both lymph node homogenates and alveolar macrophages from patients with sarcoidosis.[272,273] These macrophages lack 24-hydroxylase activity, and the enzyme mediating the conversion of 25-OHD to 1,25-$(OH)_2D$ is not sensitive to feedback inhibition by 1,25-$(OH)_2D$, although it is exquisitely sensitive to inhibition by glucocorticoids. As might be anticipated, the production of 1,25-$(OH)_2D$ in hypercalcemic patients with sarcoidosis appears to be completely autonomous in vivo and does not appear to be subject to any known regulation.[123] The production of and response to 1,25-$(OH)_2D$ in normal immune cells was noted in an earlier section, and it has been speculated that the excessive synthesis of 1,25-$(OH)_2D$ in certain patients with sarcoidosis, lymphoma, or other granulomatous diseases may actually represent the disordered production of what is normally a local "lymphokine." The chemical identity of the circulating vitamin D metabolite in hypercalcemic patients with sarcoidosis has recently been questioned,[274] although there is no debate as to the pathogenetic importance of this metabolite, if not of 1,25-$(OH)_2D$ itself, in mediating the hypercalciuria and/or hypercalcemia in affected patients.

The clinical diagnosis of sarcoidosis is based on conventional radiographic, chemical, and biopsy evidence of the disease. Parathyroid function tests are suppressed in hypercalcemic and many hypercalciuric patients, and circulating 1,25-$(OH)_2D$ is elevated, usually markedly. The plasma concentration of 25-OHD is normal. The serum phosphorus concentration is usually normal or low-normal. Values for TmP/GFR are usually normal but may be reduced in azotemic patients, in whom such results are best viewed as uninterpretable. Increases in serum alkaline phosphatase activity are usually a reflection of liver rather than bone involvement. Steroids are the mainstay of therapy, and the cortisone suppression test may be used to corroborate the diagnosis in patients who present a problem in differential diagnosis. The increased plasma concentration of 1,25-$(OH)_2D$ falls with the half-time of the hormone in response to steroids in such patients, and a reduction in circulating 1,25-$(OH)_2D$ from over 100 pg/ml to undetectable values may be observed in a matter of 3 to 4 days. The acute and chronic steroid dosages are determined by the degree of hypercalcemia as well as by other manifestations of the disease. Primary hyperparathyroidism and sarcoidosis may coexist, and the hyperparathyroidism can be diagnosed by demonstrating (1) elevations in parathyroid function tests in a hypercalcemic patient and/or (2) hypercalcemia which is nonsuppressible in response to the cortisone suppression test.

Hypercalcemia has been reported in conjunction with active and/or disseminated tuberculosis, coccidioidomycosis, berylliosis, histoplasmosis, eosinophilic granuloma, candidiasis, and silicone-induced granulomas.[275-279] The pathogenesis of the hypercalcemia in these conditions is unclear and may relate to bone involvement and/or abnormalities in vitamin D metabolism similar to those in sarcoidosis.[277,279] Where measured, parathyroid function has been normal or suppressed and serum phosphorus concentrations have been normal. The hypercalcemia has usually been discovered as an incidental laboratory finding in patients presenting with a severe systemic infection and is steroid-suppressible. The treatment is that of the basic disease process.

Miscellaneous Conditions

IMMOBILIZATION

Complete immobilization, as occurs in patients with spinal cord injury, poliomyelitis, or femoral fractures with extensive plaster casts or in normal volunteers confined to bed rest, is commonly associated with hypercalcemia, hypercalciuria, and the rapid appearance of demineralization.[280,281] The affected individuals are typically children, adolescents, or young adults. The syndrome has never been described in the elderly (e.g., patients immobilized by stroke). The association with younger age groups reflects the higher skeletal turnover rate in these groups. Immobilization may lead to or exacerbate hypercalcemia in patients with increased bone turnover of other types (e.g., Paget's disease or hyperparathyroidism) or with increased resorption alone (e.g., multiple myeloma and breast cancer with bone metastases). A similar syndrome has been described in astronauts during periods of weightlessness.[282] If allowed to continue, hypercalciuria leads to an increase in the incidence of calcium oxalate nephrolithiasis. In patients with urinary tract infection and/or an indwelling catheter, there is also a high incidence of magnesium ammonium phosphate stones.[283] Hypercalcemia is usually mild but may be severe, leading to obtundation, coma, and/or renal failure. Parathyroid function as measured by immunoreactive PTH, nephrogenous cAMP, and plasma 1,25-$(OH)_2D$ is suppressed.[284] Serum phosphorus and results for TmP/GFR are usually high or high-normal. Bone biopsies reveal an increase in osteoclastic bone resorption and a reduction in bone formation.[285] The pathogenesis of this increase in osteoclast activity and the uncoupling of osteoclast and osteoblast activities are poorly understood. Urinary hydroxyproline excretion is increased, reflecting the increased osteoclastic activity.[286]

If left untreated, the hypercalciuria, hypercalcemia, and accelerated bone resorption normally reverse within 12 to 18 months despite continued immobilization.[286] In the interim, hypercalcemia can be rapidly and completely reversed by means of resumption of active weight bearing when this is possible. In patients with spinal cord injury or other neurological disorders, this may be impossible. In these patients, saline, furosemide, calcitonin, glucocorticoids, mithramycin, and diphosphonates have been used with varying success.[287,288]

Remineralization may occur upon resumption of active weight bearing, but it is unlikely that this remineralization will be complete. Episodes of prolonged immobilization in childhood or young adulthood may constitute a risk factor for the subsequent development of osteoporosis and pathological fracture.

ACUTE RENAL FAILURE

Hypercalcemia is occasionally observed in patients with acute renal failure, usually during the first or second week of the diuretic, or recovery, phase. In most patients, the acute renal failure has been associated with extensive soft-tissue injury and rhabdomyolysis, and the hypercalcemia noted late in the patient's course was preceded by pronounced hyperphosphatemia and hypocalcemia during the oliguric phase.[289–291] The hypercalcemia is mild to moderate and persists for 1 to 3 weeks, resolving with the return of normal renal function. Recorded values for serum phosphorus, renal phosphorus handling, and serum PTH during the hypercalcemic phase have been inconsistent and difficult to interpret; serum alkaline phosphatase activity and urinary calcium excretion are usually increased, and the calcium × phosphate mineral ion product is always elevated, often exceeding 100. The elevated mineral ion product may result in extraskeletal calcification, with symptoms of conjunctivitis or severe tissue damage. The pathogenesis of the hypercalcemia may involve a combination of excessive PTH secretion and/or $1,25\text{-}(OH)_2D$ production.[290,291] Recommended therapy includes hydration, mobilization, dialysis against a low calcium concentration, and steroids.

IDIOPATHIC HYPERCALCEMIA OF INFANCY

There are several rare syndromes of hypercalcemia of infancy. Neonatal hypercalcemia resulting from familial hypocalciuric hypercalcemia was discussed in a previous section. Williams syndrome refers to a constellation of infantile hypercalcemia, supravalvular aortic stenosis or other congenital cardiac abnormalities, mental retardation, elfin facies, and a variety of other systemic anomalies.[292] The cardiac lesions are the dominant clinical manifestation and usually require surgical correction. In many cases, the hypercalcemia has been reported to ameliorate or disappear with time. In other patients, the hypercalcemia persists into the second or third decade,[292] and biochemical hyperparathyroidism has been documented in several unpublished cases. 1,25-Dihydroxyvitamin D has recently been implicated in the hypercalcemia of Williams syndrome,[293] but substantial unpublished experience from several centers does not support this report. A familial pattern of idiopathic hypercalcemia of infancy lacking the other somatic features of Williams syndrome has also been reported.[170,294]

SERUM PROTEIN ABNORMALITIES

Artifactual "hypercalcemia" may result from hyperalbuminemia or hyperglobulinemia. Hyperalbuminemia may occur in extreme dehydration, with an attendant increase in protein-bound calcium and the total serum calcium concentration. The ionized serum calcium concentration is normal. The "hypercalcemia" is promptly reversed by means of rehydration.

An increase in the total serum calcium concentration with a normal ionized serum calcium concentration has also been reported in occasional patients with multiple myeloma due to calcium binding by the myeloma protein.[295,296] This mechanism must be considered in apparently hypercalcemic patients with myeloma and can be distinguished from true local osteolytic hypercalcemia in these patients by the measurement of the ionized serum calcium concentration.

Differential Diagnosis of Hypercalcemia

The differential diagnosis of hypercalcemia is usually not difficult. The most important diagnostic tool is clinical experience and the confident and intelligent use and interpretation of laboratory data that comes with this experience. The second most important tool is the clinical history, together with attempts to obtain previously measured laboratory values. Often the specific hormonal determinations serve only to confirm a clinical diagnosis which has already been made with confidence. The "diagnosis by exclusion" approach of the past, and all too frequently of the present, is expensive, time-consuming, and unnecessary.

The key elements of specific diagnosis and certain difficult problems of differential diagnosis were presented in previous sections. Difficult diagnostic problems usually fall into one of four categories: (1) patients with subtle sarcoidosis, (2) patients with an occult malignancy, (3) patients with an obscure and/or surreptitious medication intake, and (4) patients with several coincident causes of hypercalcemia. Other diagnostic and/or management challenges include patients with familial hypocalciuric hypercalcemia and the other familial hypercalcemic syndromes, patients with subtle primary hyperparathyroidism, and patients with an isolated pheochromocytoma and hypercalcemia. The latter patient groups require a high index of suspicion.

As noted in the section Hypercalcemia, the crux of differential diagnosis usually lies in differentiating the conditions listed in the first five categories of Table 23-7. The conditions listed under category 6 are usually diagnostically self-evident and/or the circumstances in which these mechanisms must be considered are confined to very discrete clinical populations. Although the immobilization syndrome per se is not common in a general medical population, immobilization may contribute to the net hypercalcemia in patients with other primary hypercalcemic mechanisms (e.g., malignancy-associated hypercalcemia).

The medication history should not be approached casually. Rather, patients should be specifically questioned about their use of the agents listed in Table 23-7. Patients tend not to regard an over-the-counter preparation such as calcium carbonate as a "medication" and may not volunteer details about its use. In instances where the medication history is unreliable or unobtainable, lithium and 25-(OH)D levels can be measured if appropriate, as can urinary thiazide levels.

The hypercalcemia observed in association with hyperthyroidism, Addisonian crisis, or a VIP-oma is usually noted as an incidental laboratory finding in a patient in whom the primary diagnosis has already been established. This may also be the case in individuals with an isolated pheochromocytoma and hypercalcemia, but this diagnosis requires a particularly high index of suspicion. We routinely measure urinary catecholamine excretion in patients prior to surgery for presumed primary hyperparathyroidism.

Patients with hypercalcemia due to sarcoidosis or other granulomatous diseases are usually systemically ill and have mild-moderate renal impairment on presentation, findings which are not typically observed in patients with uncomplicated primary hyperparathyroidism. The granulomatous process is almost always clinically or radiographically apparent, and the circulating concentration of 1,25-$(OH)_2D$ is often markedly increased ($\geq$100 pg/ml). The steroid suppression test remains a diagnostic mainstay in such patients, and both the hypercalcemia and the increase in circulating 1,25-$(OH)_2D$ tend to respond in a matter of a few days, often dramatically. The standard hydrocortisone suppression test employs 100 to 200 mg of hydrocortisone daily in four divided doses for 7 to 10 days. Hydrocortisone is recommended over other steroid preparations because of anecdotal reports of abnormalities in hepatic steroid conversion in rare patients with hepatic involvement by their basic disease process. A full 10-day course of hydrocortisone is frequently not required for diagnosis and should be approached with some caution in a patient suspected of harboring a fungal disease or tuberculosis. In patients who require maintenance therapy, the steroid suppression test should be rapidly translated into an alternate-day program, employing the lowest clinically effective dose of steroids. The circulating concentration of 1,25-$(OH)_2D$ may provide a convenient and very sensitive gauge of disease activity in such patients. Occasional hypercalcemic patients are encountered who have the biochemical hallmarks of sarcoidosis, including steroid responsiveness, but in whom there is no evidence of a granulomatous process or a lymphoma despite a meticulous search. Such patients must be classified as "idiopathic"; they may require steroid therapy for control of hypercalcemia and should be periodically reevaluated in a search for the primary disease process.

Given the frequency with which primary hyperparathyroidism and malignancy-associated hypercalcemia occur, the differential diagnosis of hypercalcemia most often rests between these two entities. It should be emphasized that primary hyperparathyroidism and malignancy may coexist, and so hypercalcemia in a patient known to have cancer may be due to coincident primary hyperparathyroidism. Can the hypercalcemia be documented to have been present for some months? If so, has the level of the serum calcium been stable? Does the patient have a history of nephrolithiasis suggesting the presence of long-standing hypercalciuria? Chronicity and relatively stable hypercalcemia are the clinical hallmarks of primary hyperparathyroidism and greatly favor this diagnosis in any clinical setting.

In contrast, patients with malignancy-associated hypercalcemia are generally in the late stages of the disease. Their tumor burdens are correspondingly large and are apparent on preliminary clinical screening. Small or occult laryngeal, renal, gynecological, pulmonary, and breast neoplasms do not cause hypercalcemia. Similarly, patients with hypercalcemia resulting from hematologic malignancies generally have advanced disease which is clinically and biochemically obvious. Thus, the absence of evidence for a tumor after a thorough history and physical examination targeted at the oropharynx, hematopoietic system, gastrointestinal tract, breasts, skeleton, kidneys and bladder, skin, and gynecological systems would favor a diagnosis of primary hyperparathyroidism. The findings of normal hematologic indices, serum and urine protein electrophoresis, urinalysis, intravenous pyelogram or renal ultrasound examination, bone scan, and chest x-ray also provide strong evidence against MAHC and favor primary hyperparathyroidism. Exceptions to these general clinical rules of thumb exist but are collectively rare. One example would be the occasional patient with a large retroperitoneal neoplasm which may remain occult for a prolonged period. Another would be a patient with severe primary hyperparathyroidism, not infrequently due to parathyroid carcinoma, who presents with severe hypercalcemia, systemic signs and symptoms, moderate renal impairment, and an aggregate clinical picture which is indistinguishable from the typical picture observed in MAHC.

Even though we have emphasized the clinical approach to this differential diagnosis, parathyroid function test results may be invaluable, particularly when the differential diagnosis is clinically difficult. Three general points with respect to the use and interpretation of these results should be reemphasized.

1. Primary hyperparathyroidism is in effect a dose-related disease (Fig. 23-27).
2. The PTH–1,25-$(OH)_2D$ axis may be quite sensitive to exogenous calcium so that improper study conditions may lead to interpretive difficulties (Fig. 23-36).
3. As a tool for differential diagnosis, the plasma concentration of 1,25-$(OH)_2D$ is probably underutilized (Fig. 23-39).

Patients with both the humoral and the local osteolytic forms of MACH demonstrate marked increases in fasting calcium excretion, normal to reduced circulating 1,25-$(OH)_2D$, and normal to borderline-high values for immunoreactive PTH. Occasional patients with lymphoma appear to have 1,25-$(OH)_2D$–mediated hypercalcemia (Fig. 23-44), but their remaining parathyroid function tests are normal or suppressed. Patients with the humoral and local osteolytic syndromes of MAHC can be distinguished by their results for nephrogenous cAMP or total cAMP excretion (Fig. 23-38).

The differential diagnostic difficulties which may be encountered within the patient populations classified under "primary hyperparathyroidism" in Table 23-7 are basically three: (1) distinguishing those patients with severe primary hyperparathyroidism from those with MAHC or other severe hypercalcemic syndromes, (2) identifying patients with "subtle" primary hyperparathyroidism among the large pool of hypercalciuric patients with stone disease, and (3) distinguishing between primary hyperparathyroidism and familial hypocalciuric hypercalcemia. The first differential is best made by measuring serum immunoreactive PTH and plasma 1,25-$(OH)_2D$ (see above). The second differential is described in more detail in Chap. 25; in general, this differential is less difficult than is generally assumed. The third differential is best considered by attempting to demonstrate the features of FHH summarized in Table 23-10. If parathyroid function test results are unimpressive and/or if multiple hypercalcemic first-degree relatives cannot be identified, this differential diagnosis may be difficult if not impossible to achieve.

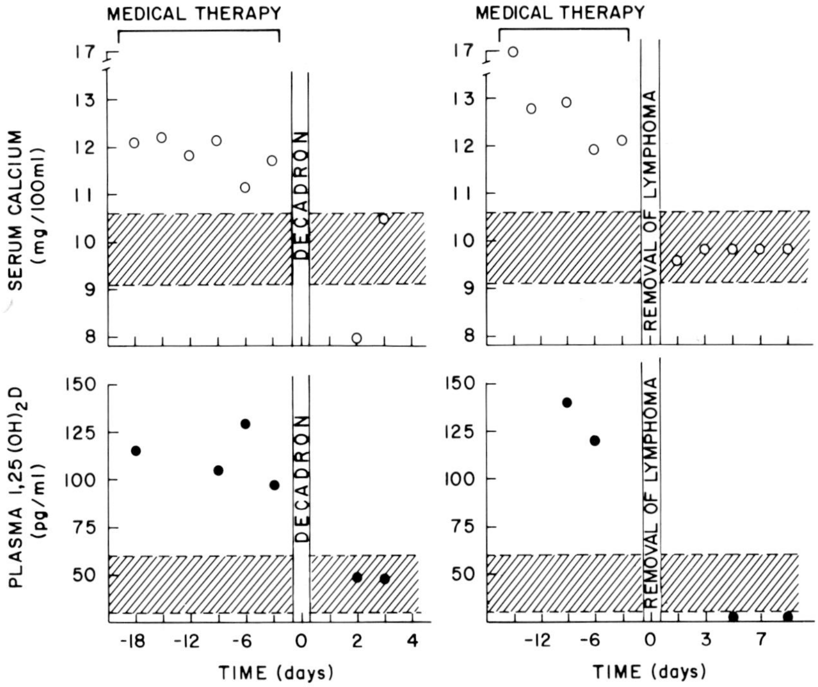

FIGURE 23-44 Results for serum calcium and plasma 1,25-$(OH)_2D$ in two patients with histiocytic lymphomas and hypercalcemia. Note that the serum calcium and circulating 1,25-$(OH)_2D$ fell dramatically following glucocorticoid therapy (*left*) or surgical excision of a solitary splenic lymphoma (*right*). (*From Rosenthal, Insogna, Godsall, Smaldone, Waldron, and Stewart,*[241] *by permission of the Journal of Clinical Endocrinology and Metabolism.*)

Medical Therapy

The acute and subacute medical measures for controlling moderate to severe hypercalcemia are described in this section; chronic medical therapy for certain specific hypercalcemic disorders was discussed previously. Emergent hypercalcemia is most commonly encountered in patients with a malignancy, and rapid treatment may be lifesaving. If there is a lesion of care in these patients, it is a tendency toward overtreatment, and the most useful rule of thumb is to treat the patient rather than the laboratory value. The initial therapeutic goal is to reduce the serum calcium to safe but not necessarily normal levels.

GENERAL MEASURES

General measures include rehydration, attempts to mobilize the patient, and dietary restrictions or supplementation. Dehydration is common in severe hypercalcemia because of the impairment in renal concentrating ability and the frequency of associated nausea and vomiting. In a severely ill patient, rehydration alone may reduce the serum calcium by 2 mg/dl or more. Immobilization increases the rate of bone resorption in any patient and is of particular importance in patients with preexisting high rates of bone resorption. Mobilization requires weight bearing to be effective, and quiet standing or assisted walking is far more beneficial than exercise programs in a bed- or chair-confined patient. A restriction in oral calcium intake to 200 to 400 mg daily is commonly employed but is useful only in patients with the milk-alkali syndrome, sarcoidosis, and hypervitaminosis D. Calcium should be eliminated from intravenous fluids (e.g., hyperalimentation solutions).

Following the stabilization of the serum calcium concentration by front-line rehydration and calciuretic measures, a program of forced oral fluids (3 or more liters daily) and high oral sodium intake (200 to 300 meq of sodium daily), with or without oral doses of furosemide, may allow discontinuance of intravenous saline therapy, assisting in the complete mobilization of the patient.

CALCIURETIC MEASURES

The most commonly employed front-line calciuretic measures are the intravenous infusion of isotonic saline together with intravenous doses of furosemide. The induced natriuresis inhibits proximal tubular calcium reabsorption, and the increased calcium delivery to the distal nephron overwhelms distal tubular calcium reabsorption. The quantity of calcium excreted per day by a given patient depends on the degree of hypercalcemia, the renal status, and the quantities of saline and furosemide employed, but excretion rates of 1000 to 2000 mg per day can be regularly achieved in most patients.[297]

The initial rate of saline infusion is determined by the degree of dehydration and the patient's cardiovascular status but is usually in the range of 200 to 300 ml/h. The initial doses of furosemide are 80 to 100 mg every 2 h, with a reduction in dosage and spacing of doses to every 4 h as the calcium level begins to stabilize. Patients with renal impairment may require much larger diuretic doses.[297] A patient with a delicate cardiovascular system should be initially rehydrated, and the subsequent rate of saline infusion should be carefully monitored by central venous pressure recordings and adjusted to correspond to the rate of the furosemide-induced diuresis. Serum calcium, phosphorus, and electrolytes are measured twice daily, and losses of potassium and magnesium must be rapidly corrected. These front-line measures usually lead to a reduction in serum calcium of approximately 3 mg/dl within 24 h.

Both hemodialysis and peritoneal dialysis against calcium-free solutions have been successfully employed in patients with emergent hypercalcemia and severe renal impairment.[298,299]

MEASURES WHICH INHIBIT BONE RESORPTION

A number of agents inhibit bone resorption, and the choice among these therapies rests in large part on the patient's specific diagnosis.

Mithramycin is a cytotoxic antibiotic which inhibits RNA synthesis and is useful as a chemotherapeutic agent in testicular tumors. This agent effectively inhibits osteoclastic bone resorption in doses of 25 μg/kg, approximately one-tenth of the chemotherapeutic dosage.[300] The hypocalcemic effect is usually maximal 48 h after a single intravenous dose and persists for approximately 1 week, although the duration of response is variable. The hypocalcemic response is accompanied by hypophosphatemia and a reduction in excretion of hydroxyproline. Thrombocytopenia is the principal toxicity of mithramycin and may limit its use in patients whose hematologic status is already compromised. The agent is also nephrotoxic and hepatotoxic. Mithramycin is uniformly effective in reducing serum calcium levels, and doses every 1 to 2 weeks have been successfully employed in the long-term management of patients with severe hypercalcemia.

Steroids are effective in sarcoidosis, hypervitaminosis A or D, myeloma and the other hematologic malignancies, and in a large minority of patients with breast carcinoma.[207] The initial dose employed is 100 to 200 mg of hydrocortisone daily (or equivalent amounts of other steroid preparations), and a clear-cut response is usually apparent within 48 to 72 h. In addition to inhibiting vitamin D– and vitamin A–induced osteoclastic bone resorption and the direct effects of breast carcinoma cells on bone resorption, steroids inhibit the effects of vitamin D on intestinal calcium absorption and may be cytotoxic in the hematologic malignancies. The steroid dosage is tapered according to the clinical response and merges into a maintenance dosage schedule in patients requiring long-term therapy.

Phosphate administered either orally or intravenously is effective in reducing serum calcium levels in all hypercalcemic conditions.[301] Phosphate both inhibits bone resorption and promotes bone mineral accretion, and the antihypercalcemic effect persists several days after discontinuation of phosphate therapy. The principal concern associated with the use of phosphates is the potential complication of extraskeletal calcification. This complication appears to be a predictable consequence when a normal calcium × phosphate mineral ion product is exceeded. For this reason and because of the availability of other effective measures, the use of intravenous phosphate should be avoided in severely hypercalcemic patients unless hypophosphatemia is severe (e.g., less than 1.5 mg/dl) and oral replacement is impossible. Parenteral phosphorus is available as a potassium phosphate solution containing 93 mg of elemental phosphorus per milliliter.[302] Daily doses should not exceed 600 mg elemental phosphorus per day. Urine flow, serum calcium, and creatinine and/or blood urea nitrogen (BUN) should be monitored closely when parenteral phosphorus is employed. Oral phosphates should also be avoided or used cautiously in patients with severe hypercalcemia, azotemia, or pretreatment levels of serum phosphorus above 3.0 mg/dl. However, in nonazotemic hypophosphatemic patients who have been initially stabilized to moderate levels of hypercalcemia by front-line measures, modest doses of oral phosphate (1000 to 1500 mg elemental phosphorus daily in four divided doses) may be very useful in maintaining the serum calcium at acceptable levels. The mineral ion product should not exceed 35 to 40 and can be monitored by fasting serum chemistries as well as determinations performed 4 h following a representative oral dose of phosphate. Long-term phosphate therapy should be limited to nonazotemic hypophosphatemic patients with a stable serum calcium less than 12 mg/dl and should be carefully monitored by serial measures of renal function, slit-lamp examinations, and soft-tissue x-rays for vascular and soft-tissue calcifications.

Calcitonin is a potent inhibitor of osteoclastic bone resorption, and porcine, salmon, and synthetic human calcitonin have been employed in the treatment of the hypercalcemia associated with a variety of conditions.[207,303] The usual dose is 2 to 8 MRC units per kilogram of body weight per day, given as a continuous intravenous infusion or as two to four intramuscular injections daily. The hypocalcemic effect of a single intravenous or intramuscular injection is detectable by 2 h, and a maximal reduction of approximately 2 mg/dl is observed by 6 to 10 h; the serum calcium rebounds by 20 to 24 h, often to pretreatment levels. The acute hypocalcemic response to calcitonin is usually accompanied by hypophosphatemia. Experience with calcitonin has been somewhat disappointing because of its transient effectiveness and the unpredictable loss of a sustained response to the hormone in some patients, a finding presumably reflecting the "escape" phenomenon (see Effects of Calcitonin on Bone). The use of calcitonin in conjunction with oral phosphate therapy has been recommended, but no large experience has been reported. Similarly, calcitonin has been used in conjunction with glucocorticoids, but no long-term results are available.[304]

Intravenous ethylenediaminetetraacetic acid (EDTA) forms a stable excretable chelate with calcium but is seldom employed today because of the transient effects, nephrotoxicity, and severe intravenous pain associated with its use.

Intravenous etidronic acid [ethane-1-hydroxy-1,1-diphosphonic acid (EHDP)],[305] dichloromethylenediphosphonate,[306] and aminopropylidine diphosphonate[307] have each been demonstrated in clinical trials to be highly effective in lowering serum calcium in patients with malignancy-associated hypercalcemia. Unfortunately, none of these agents is currently available in the United States. Oral EHDP is poorly absorbed and ineffective in treating hypercalcemia. Three other experimental agents—WR-2721,[308] thionapthene-2-carboxylic acid,[309] and gallium nitrate[310]—have shown promise but are not available for clinical use at the time of this writing.

Finally, long-term therapy of hypercalcemia in patients with malignancy-associated hypercalcemia can be accomplished only by eradication of tumor through the use of chemotherapy, surgery, or radiotherapy. Attempts at antitumor therapy should be begun promptly in patients with malignancy-associated hypercalcemia, since responses to the various medical regimens described above are usually transient or are associated with cumulative toxicity. Thus, these agents are best used to buy time while waiting for a tumor to respond to specific antitumor therapy.

HYPOCALCEMIA

The systemic mechanisms which defend against hypocalcemia were described in an earlier section. The exquisite sensitivity of the parathyroid glands to alterations in ionized calcium, the importance of distal tubular calcium reabsorption and the "acute" phase of bone resorption in the minute-to-minute maintenance of calcium homeostasis, and the more subacute defense mechanism represented by the PTH–1,25-$(OH)_2D$ axis were emphasized.

This section is organized into an initial description of the clinical symptoms and signs of hypocalcemia, followed by a thorough discussion of the various conditions associated with PTH deficiency or resistance (Table 23-12) and a brief description of other hypocalcemic conditions (Table 23-13). Renal osteodystrophy and the syndromes of vitamin D–deficiency rickets and/or osteomalacia are by far the most important conditions in the second category; the clinical manifestations of these disorders primarily involve abnormalities in skeletal homeostasis, and they are described in their entirety in Chap. 24. Differential diagnosis and acute and chronic treatment of hypocalcemia are discussed in the final portions of the section. Several excellent reviews of hypocalcemia and/or hypoparathyroidism are available.[311–313]

Clinical Manifestations of Hypocalcemia

Tetany is the classical expression of the increased neuromuscular irritability which is associated with hypocalcemia. The tetany may be latent or overt, and the symptoms in overt tetany range from mild muscle cramps to frank seizures. Latent tetany may be demonstrated clinically by eliciting Chvostek's sign or Trousseau's sign. *Chvostek's sign* is a twitching of the muscles at the margin of the lips which is produced by tapping the facial nerve about 1 in in front of the ear. The twitching can be crudely rated on a scale of 1+ to 4+, with 1+ being a barely visible response and 4+ being a clear drawing of the facial muscles. A 1+ response is demonstrable in approximately 10 percent of normal individuals. *Trousseau's sign* is elicited by inflating a blood pressure cuff to 20 mmHg above systolic blood pressure for 3 min. A positive response is the classical "obstetrical hand" of frank tetany, in which the wrist and metacarpophalangeal joints are flexed, the interphalangeal joints are extended, and the fingers and thumb are adducted. Trousseau's sign is based on local ischemia and irritation of nerves in the region of the cuff rather than ischemia to the limb. This can be demonstrated by inflating a second blood pressure cuff distal to the initial cuff and immediately deflating the first cuff. The positive sign will subside, to recur several minutes later. In addition to its time-honored role in roundsmanship, this "double

Table 23-12. Hypoparathyroidism

1. Postoperative hypocalcemia and hypoparathyroidism
2. Idiopathic hypoparathyroidism
   a. Isolated
   b. Associated with atrophic polyendocrine failure
3. Other acquired forms of functional hypoparathyroidism
   a. Nonsurgical parathyroid damage
   b. Parathyroid infiltration
   c. Hypomagnesemia
4. Pseudohypoparathyroidism
5. Neonatal hypocalcemic syndromes
   a. Early and late neonatal hypocalcemia
   b. Secondary hypoparathyroidism
   c. DiGeorge's syndrome and idiopathic hypoparathyroidism

Table 23-13. Nonhypoparathyroid Hypocalcemia

1. Renal insufficiency
   a. Reduced 1,25-$(OH)_2D$
   b. Hyperphosphatemia
2. Vitamin D disorders
   a. Vitamin D deficiency
   b. Intestinal malabsorption
   c. Hepatic and biliary disorders
   d. Anticonvulsant therapy
   e. Vitamin D–dependent rickets
   f. Vitamin D–resistant (hypophosphatemic) rickets or osteomalacia
3. Acute pancreatitis
4. Rapid or excessive skeletal mineralization
   a. Hungry bones syndrome
   b. Osteoblastic metastases
   c. Vitamin D therapy for vitamin D disorders
5. Hypoalbuminemia
6. Hyperphosphatemia
   a. Parenteral phosphorus administration
   b. Phosphate-containing enemas
   c. Excessive oral phosphorus administration
   d. Renal failure
   e. Crush injuries
   f. Rapid tumor lysis
7. Hypomagnesemia
8. Toxic shock syndrome
9. Medications
   a. Mithramycin
   b. Calcitonin
   c. Citrated blood
   d. Fluoride intoxication

cuff" test will usually fool the occasional patient who is malingering with tetanic symptoms. A positive Trousseau's sign is rarely demonstrable in normal individuals. Both Chvostek's sign and Trousseau's sign are regularly but not invariably positive in patients with a significant reduction in serum ionized calcium.

The symptom complex associated with overt tetany is by no means diagnostically obvious, and pediatric and adult patients with hypoparathyroidism often escape diagnosis for many years and/or may be misdiagnosed as suffering from seizures or other neurological disorders. Predominant symptoms may occur in the form of "spells" or "attacks," precipitated by emotional or physical stress, vomiting, or respiratory alkalosis. Symptoms in female patients predictably worsen during pregnancy and lactation. Alkalosis influences the binding of the calcium ion to albumin and reduces the extracellular concentration of ionized calcium. In addition, alkalosis and the calcium ion concentration appear to influence neuromuscular excitability synergistically.[314] It has been suggested that a reduction in the concentration of ionized calcium in the cerebrospinal fluid sensitizes the respiratory center and that chronic hypocalcemia predisposes a patient to hyperventilation and respiratory alkalosis.[314] Taken together with the tendency of many patients toward metabolic alkalosis, this sensitization may set the stage for a vicious cycle in which mild symptoms induce anxiety and hyperventilation and initiate a spiral of worsening symptoms and respiratory alkalosis leading to a frank "attack."

The most typical symptoms of tetany are muscle cramps and paresthesias. The paresthesias consist of a tingling sensation in the circumoral region and in the fingertips and toes. The cramps are usually noted in the lower back, calves, or feet. In severe tetany, the cramps give way to frank contraction of muscle groups, as typified by the characteristic tonic contraction of the muscles of the forearm and hand. Laryngospasm and bronchospasm occur infrequently. Smooth muscle contraction rarely leads to abdominal cramps and urinary frequency.

The central nervous system manifestations of hypocalcemia are many and varied. The most frequent misdiagnosis in pediatric patients with hypoparathyroidism is an idiopathic seizure disorder. The seizures may be "hypocalcemic" seizures, consisting of syncopal episodes or "gray out" periods lacking the other features of classical seizures, or typical petit mal, grand mal, or focal seizure patterns. Whether the typical seizure patterns are due solely to hypocalcemia or represent a reduced seizure threshold in patients with an inherent seizure disorder is a matter of debate.[311] However, both "hypocalcemic" and typical seizures are improved and/or eliminated by restoration of normocalcemia, and the substitution of a specific diagnosis of hypoparathyroidism for the clinical diagnosis of "idiopathic seizure disorder" may dramatically influence the prospects of a patient so mislabeled. The electroencephalographic findings in hypocalcemia are high-voltage slow waves, which correlate with the degree of hypocalcemia.[312] There have been rare reports of pseudotumor cerebri with papilledema and increased cerebrospinal fluid pressure in patients with idiopathic and postoperative hypoparathyroidism.[311]

Mental symptoms associated with hypocalcemia range from irritability, lassitude, and impaired memory and cognitive function to psychoneurotic or frankly psychotic behavior. Poor performance in school is a predictable historical finding in children with hypoparathyroidism. These symptoms are usually dramatically improved by correction of the hypocalcemia. Extrapyramidal symptoms resembling parkinsonism, choreoathetosis, or other abnormal posturing occur rarely in patients with hypoparathyroidism.[311] These symptoms are usually confined to patients with calcification of the basal ganglia. These calcifications are observed in approximately 50 percent of patients with untreated idiopathic hypoparathyroidism and pseudohypoparathyroidism and are irreversible, but their progression may be halted by replacement therapy. The extrapyramidal symptoms may or may not improve with the restoration of normocalcemia.

Reversible congestive heart failure may be seen in severe hypocalcemia, and the response to calcium replacement therapy is dramatic.[315,316] The classical ECG correlate of hypocalcemia is prolongation of the QT interval, which results from a lengthened ST segment rather than an altered QRS complex.[317]

Subcapsular cataracts are frequent in hypoparathyroidism and are usually visible with the naked eye or an ophthalmoscope.[318] Cataracts are a consequence of prolonged untreated hypoparathyroidism, and their frequency and density are directly correlated with the duration of hypocalcemia.[318] The pathogenesis of the cataracts in hypoparathyroidism is obscure. They are irreversible, but their progression is limited by replacement therapy.

The skin is often dry and flaky in hyperparathyroidism, and the nails and hair may be coarse and brittle. The eyebrows may be sparse. Hypocalcemia may precipitate the appearance of a particularly virulent dermatological syndrome known variously as impetigo herpetiformis or pustular psoriasis of von Zumbusch.[319] Mucocutaneous candidiasis may be associated with idiopathic hypoparathyroidism. Dental hypoplasia and delayed eruption are frequent in pediatric patients with hypoparathyroidism, and these abnormalities can be used to date the presumed onset of the disorder retrospectively.[311]

The skeletal findings which dominate the clinical picture in renal osteodystrophy, rickets, and osteomalacia are described in Chap. 24. Osteosclerosis and/or thickened calvaria may be observed in chronic hypoparathyroidism. Patients with pseudohypoparathyroidism occasionally present with radiological evidence of frank osteitis fibrosa cystica (see below).

Hypoparathyroidism

The clinical forms and variants of hypoparathyroidism will be described in the sequence presented in Table 23-12. Clinical hypoparathyroidism from any cause is uncommon. However, prolonged periods of misdiagnosis are frequent in both pediatric and adult patients with hypoparathyroidism, and a high index of suspicion is required for early and accurate diagnosis. In addition, the syndromes of idiopathic hypoparathyroidism and pseudohypoparathyroidism command a position of biological importance and interest which far outweighs their frequency in the population.

POSTOPERATIVE HYPOCALCEMIA AND HYPOPARATHYROIDISM

Postoperative hypoparathyroidism is a complication of parathyroid, thyroid, and other forms of cervical (e.g., laryngeal) surgery. Postoperative hypoparathyroidism is not an all-or-none phenomenon; it may be clinically latent or overt, partial or complete, transient or permanent. Significant hypocalcemia may be apparent during the immediate postoperative period or may occur many years afterward. This clinical variability is based on the amount of remaining functional parathyroid tissue and the natural history of its regrowth or demise. Postoperative hypocalcemia and/or tetanic symptoms must not be equated with the clinical diagnosis of permanent, complete hypoparathyroidism, and a great many patients with this misdiagnosis can be demonstrated to have adequate parathyroid reserve and can be weaned from vitamin D replacement therapy. After the immediate postoperative period, there is a reasonably close correlation between the degree of hypoparathyroidism and the untreated level of serum calcium: A serum calcium concentration in the range of 8 mg/dl suggests partial hypoparathyroidism, and a concentration in the range of 5 to 6 mg/dl suggests functional aparathyroidism.

The postoperative course following *parathyroid exploration* was described in a previous section. The most important variables which influence the postoperative serum calcium level are the quantity of remaining functional parathyroid tissue and preexisting clinical bone disease, which is associated with postoperative recalcification tetany, or the "hungry bones syndrome." The hungry bones syndrome may affect magnesium as well as calcium (see Hypomagnesemia). There is surprisingly little published information regarding the frequency of significant long-term hypoparathyroidism following parathyroid surgery.[311] This complication is most frequently observed following subtotal parathyroidectomy for primary parathyroid hyperplasia or after parathyroid reexploration,[197] and it correlates inversely with the skill and experience of the surgeon. As emphasized previously, the differential diagnosis and management of postoperative hypocalcemia are usually straightforward, and an accurate assessment of parathyroid reserve is essential in all patients prior to discharge.

There are several postoperative hypocalcemic and/or tetanic syndromes which may follow *thyroid surgery*. The postoperative course following subtotal thyroidectomy for thyrotoxicosis is a special case and illustrates the distinction between *transient postoperative tetany* and *postoperative hypoparathyroidism*. Hyperthyroidism is regularly associated with bone resorption and demineralization, parathyroid suppression, and negative calcium balance, and these abnormalities correlate well with the severity of the hyperthyroidism (see Hyperparathyroidism). The serum calcium falls by an average of 1.0 mg/dl following subtotal thyroidectomy, and many patients experience mild tetanic symptoms.[320] The fall in serum calcium is rapid, and levels in the hypocalcemic range are observed in approximately one-third of patients within 24 to 48 h.[320] The pathogenesis of the postoperative hypocalcemia is related to (1) the preoperative suppression of parathyroid function and (2) the remineralization tetany, or hungry bones syndrome, which predictably follows correction of the hyperthyroidism. Although most patients are rendered medically euthyroid prior to subtotal thyroidectomy, the period of euthyroidism is usually insufficient to restore normal bone mineralization.[311] Assuming that parathyroid injury is avoided during the thyroid procedure, the postoperative course in hyperthyroidism classically defines the use of the term *postoperative tetany*, and the hypocalcemia is mild and transient and resolves when bone remineralization is complete. In nonthyrotoxic patients undergoing thyroid or other surgical procedures in the neck, postoperative tetany and hypocalcemia are relatively infrequent.[311]

Long-term hypocalcemia occurs in approximately 2 percent of patients following thyroid surgery. The frequency with which postoperative hypoparathyroidism is observed depends on a number of variables, including the extent of the operative procedure and the operative technique and experience of the surgeon. Postoperative hypoparathyroidism is extremely rare after hemithyroidectomy, occurs more frequently following subtotal thyroidectomy, and may be observed in as many as 25 percent of patients having a "total" thyroidectomy for carcinoma.[311] In most patients, postoperative hypoparathyroidism results from interruption of the blood supply to the end arteries of the parathyroid glands rather than actual removal of parathyroid tissue.

As emphasized by Parfitt,[321] chronic postoperative hypoparathyroidism is a continuous spectrum, ranging from a nearly compensated loss of parathyroid reserve to complete functional hypoparathyroidism similar in severity to that observed in idiopathic hypoparathyroidism. A number of tests for assessing parathyroid reserve and diagnosing latent hypoparathyroidism have been described,[311] but the serial determination of serum calcium provides a reasonable quantitative assessment of the degree of functional parathyroid impairment and serves as a guide for medical management. The presence of a modest degree of parathyroid function can be demonstrated in an untreated patient with a serum calcium in the range of 8 mg/dl by recording a midnormal range result for nephrogenous cAMP; available assays for PTH lack sufficient sensitivity to quantitate parathyroid function accurately in this range.

The management of postoperative hypoparathyroidism is based on the degree of parathyroid impairment; many patients can be maintained on small doses of vitamin D or on oral calcium supplements alone (see Treatment, below).

IDIOPATHIC HYPOPARATHYROIDISM

Idiopathic hypoparathyroidism is rare. Classifications based on the time of onset, the presence or absence of associated endocrinopathies, and sporadic or familial occurrence have been proposed, but none is entirely satisfactory.

Most isolated cases of idiopathic hypoparathyroidism are sporadic. The majority of cases present before age 15. The usual delay between the onset of symptoms and the time of diagnosis is estimated to be approximately 5 years.[311] Virtually all patients are functionally aparathyroid at the time of diagnosis, as evidenced by mean serum calcium and phosphorus values of 5.4 and 7.7 mg/dl, respectively.[311] Parathyroid antibodies can be demonstrated in about one-third of cases.[322] Familial cases are sufficiently rare that no clear mendelian pattern of inheritance is recognized.

Idiopathic hypoparathyroidism occurring together with other autoimmune polyendocrine disorders may be sporadic but is familial in about 50 percent of cases, usually with an autosomal recessive inheritance pattern.[311] The pathogenesis and other features of these polyendocrine syndromes are described in detail in Chap. 28. Associated features variably include mucocutaneous candidiasis, Addison's disease, autoimmune thyroid disease (Graves' disease or Hashimoto's disease), ovarian failure, pernicious anemia, alopecia and/or vitiligo, primary biliary cirrhosis, myasthenia gravis, and steatorrhea. Most patients present during the first decade of life. The term *HAM syndrome* has been used to emphasize the three features which are clinically dominant: hypoparathyroidism, Addison's disease, and moniliasis.[311] The pattern of organ involvement is variable, but approximately one-third of patients have the complete HAM syndrome. The sequence usually begins with severe, intractable monilial infections of the skin, mucous membranes, and nails followed by hypoparathyroidism and Addison's disease in that order. Rare cases have been reported in which the tendency to hypercalcemia associated with Addison's disease "masked" underlying hypoparathyroidism. Steatorrhea is not described in some series but appears to be an associated feature in a large minority of patients.[311] The pathogenesis of the steatorrhea is unknown, but it often improves with restoration of normocalcemia. A wide assortment of parathyroid, thyroid, parietal cell, ovarian, and other antibodies are demonstrable in a large percentage of patients.[322]

The hypoparathyroidism is severe, with mean calcium and phosphorus values at diagnosis similar to those described above for isolated idiopathic hypoparathyroidism. In essence, all patients with idiopathic hypoparathyroidism tend to have complete parathyroid destruction or atrophy, as has been demonstrated pathologically in the few cases examined.[311] The patients require full replacement doses of vitamin D. Because of the complete absence of parathyroid function, management is frequently much more complex than in patients with postoperative hypoparathyroidism. Although vitamin D "resistance" is rare, most reported examples have been in patients with idiopathic hypoparathyroidism.

OTHER ACQUIRED FORMS OF FUNCTIONAL HYPOPARATHYROIDISM

Parathyroid tissue is quite radioresistant, and fewer than 10 cases of hypoparathyroidism following ^{131}I therapy for thyrotoxicosis have been reported.[311,313] Whether there is an identifiable loss of parathyroid reserve in a significant minority of patients after ^{131}I treatment is a matter of debate.[311] Hypoparathyroidism following head and neck irradiation has not been described; rather, an apparent increase in the incidence of hyperparathyroidism has been suggested (see

Pathology and Etiology under Primary Hyperparathyroidism).

Metastases to the parathyroids are noted in approximately 10 percent of patients with widely metastatic cancer, but functional hypoparathyroidism due to malignant infiltration of the parathyroids is very rare and has been limited to a handful of reported cases.[323] Iron deposition in the parathyroids is frequent in primary and secondary hemochromatosis, but actual hypoparathyroidism is uncommon.[311] Amyloid deposits are demonstrable in the parathyroids in systemic amyloidosis, but hypoparathyroidism has not been reported.

Hypocalcemia, hyperphosphatemia, and a state of functional hypoparathyroidism and/or PTH resistance may be observed in patients with magnesium depletion and hypomagnesemia. Significant abnormalities in serum calcium and phosphorus are usually confined to patients with severe hypomagnesemia (serum magnesium < 1.2 mg/dl). The pathogenesis of the abnormalities in mineral homeostasis associated with magnesium depletion is somewhat controversial. As pointed out in Biosynthesis and Secretion of PTH, a finite concentration of magnesium is required for normal PTH secretion, and there is clear evidence that PTH synthesis and/or secretion is impaired in severely hypomagnesemic patients.[324,325] In most such patients, circulating PTH levels are undetectable or inappropriately low in the face of chronic hypocalcemia.[311,324] Intravenous injections of magnesium produce rapid bursts in PTH secretion,[324] and long-term magnesium repletion results in a normalization of PTH secretion and a restoration of normocalcemia and normophosphatemia (Fig. 23-45). In addition, hypomagnesemia may be associated with resistance to the actions of parathyroid hormone on its target organs. Subnormal calcemic, phosphaturic, cAMP, and 1,25-$(OH)_2D$ responses to PTH infusion have been reported in patients with hypomagnesemia.[324,326] Circulating 1,25-$(OH)_2D$ has been reported to be reduced in hypomagnesemic patients.[327]

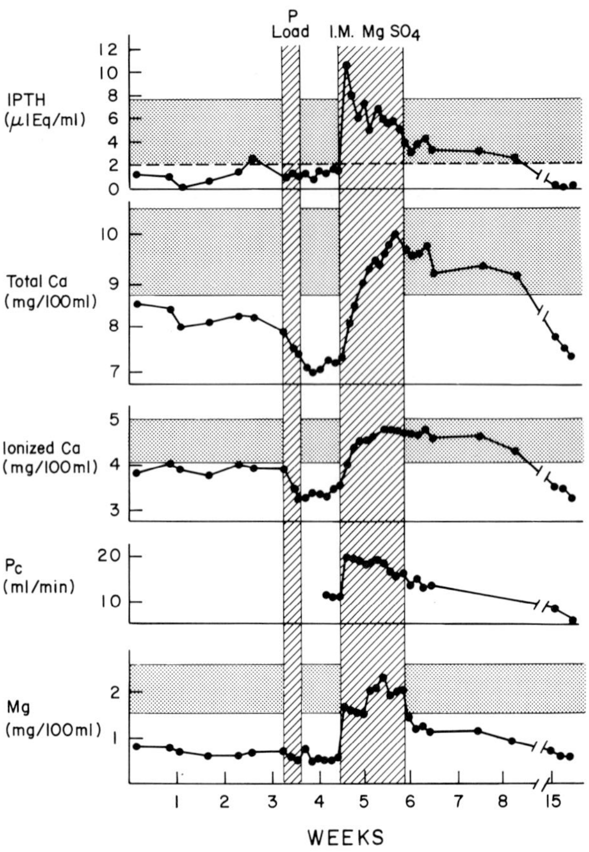

FIGURE 23-45 Response of serum calcium, parathyroid hormone, and phosphorus clearance (P_c) to magnesium replacement in a patient with severe hypomagnesemia. The hypocalcemia produced by an oral phosphorus challenge prior to magnesium replacement did not result in an increase in PTH secretion. The shaded areas represent the normal ranges, and the dotted line represents the detection limit of the PTH assay. (*Adapted from and by permission of Anast CS, Mohs JM, Kaplan SL, Burns TW, Science 177:606, 1972.*)

PSEUDOHYPOPARATHYROIDISM

Introduction and Clinical Features

Pseudohypoparathyroidism (PHP) consists of a group of syndromes which share the presence of hypocalcemia, hyperphosphatemia, and elevated circulating levels of immunoreactive PTH. The pathogenesis of each of these syndromes is incompletely understood and continues to evolve. The classification and terminology of these syndromes are therefore also evolving, and the terminology is sometimes confusing. The term *pseudopseudohypoparathyroidism* (PPHP) is used in connection with patients who have some of the typical phenotypic features but none of the chemical and biochemical features of PHP. Patients with PHP and PPHP can coexist within a single family.

Albright described the first three patients with the syndrome in 1942 and believed that the syndrome was due to "resistance" to the actions of PTH, since infusion of exogenous parathyroid extract had no effect on either the hypocalcemia or renal phosphorus excretion and since surgical exploration of the neck revealed normal parathyroid glands.[328] He termed the syndrome the *Seabright bantam syndrome* by analogy to a species of cockerel which has female tail feathers on the basis of androgen resistance. The appreciation that PHP might be due to PTH resistance was particularly prescient in that it antedated the description of other hormone resistance syndromes such as testicular feminization and nephrogenic diabetes insipidus. The constellation of phenotypic abnormalities present in Albright's patients is now commonly referred to as *Albright's hereditary osteodystrophy* (AHO) (see Table 23-14 and Fig. 23-46).

Patients are typically short (5 ft tall or shorter) and have a stocky build and a round face (Fig. 23-46). The short stature is usually not obvious in comparison with peers until the preteenage years and is not related to the mineral abnormalities in that it is not a feature of idiopathic hypoparathyroidism. Most patients are somewhat dull mentally but are not severely retarded. There is an impression that early diagnosis and replacement therapy improves serial intelligence scores, but the occurrence of mental retardation in PPHP and the increased frequency of subnormal intelligence in PHP compared with idiopathic hypoparathyroidism indicates that this abnormality is largely genetically determined rather than acquired.

Short metacarpals (brachymetacarpia), short metatarsals (brachymetatarsia), and calvarial thickening are frequent. Foreshortening of the fourth and fifth metacarpals and metatarsals is the most typical pattern and may be apparent on gross inspection or on x-rays (Fig. 23-46). When the hand is made into a fist, dimples rather than knuckles appear at the distal ends

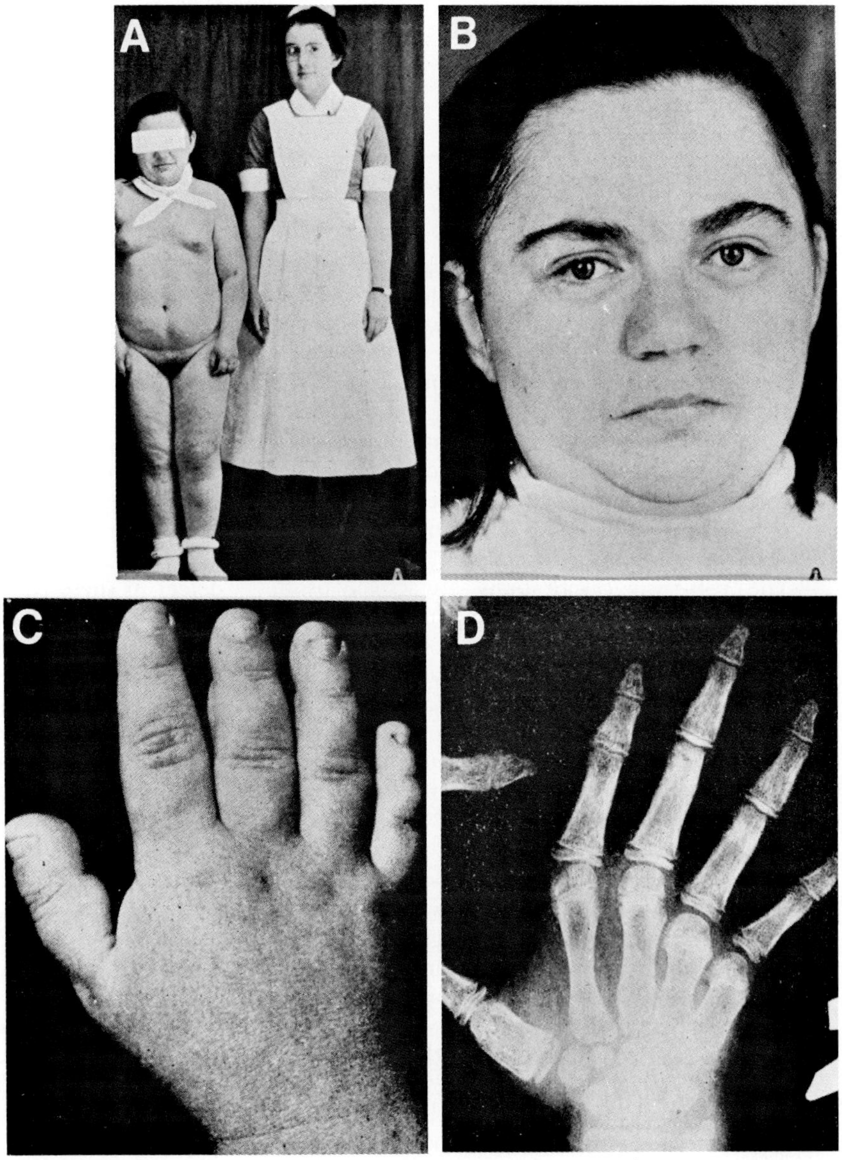

FIGURE 23-46 Phenotypic abnormalities in pseudohypoparathyroidism: (*A*) short, stocky habitus; (*B*) round face; and (*C* and *D*) short metacarpals. [*(A), (B), and (C) by permission of Albright F, Burnett CH, Smith PH, Parson W, Endocrinology 30:922, 1942. (D) by permission of Kolb FO, Steinbach HJ, J Clin Endocrinol Metab 22:59, 1962.*]

Table 23-14. Symptoms and Signs in Pseudohypoparathyroidism

Symptom or sign	% incidence
1. Somatotype	
a. Short stature	80
b. Round face	92
c. Stocky or obese habitus	50
2. Mental retardation	75
3. Dystrophic changes in bone	
a. Short metacarpals	68
b. Short metatarsals	43
c. Calvarial thickening	62
4. Ectopic ossification	56
5. Symptoms or signs of hypocalcemia	
a. Tetany	86
b. Seizures	59
c. Cataracts	44
d. Calcification of the basal ganglia	45
e. Dental abnormalities	55

Source: Adapted from Nagant de Deuxchaisnes and Krane.[311]

of affected metacarpals. A straightedge held against the distal ends of the fourth and fifth metacarpals during flexion of the metacarpophalangeal joints should normally pass distal to the end of the third metacarpal. If the edge intersects the third metacarpal, the "metacarpal sign" is positive, indicating a short fourth metacarpal. This sign is nonspecific and is positive in approximately 10 percent of normal individuals. Other skeletal anomalies observed with less frequency include short phalanges, radius curvus, and abnormal angles at the elbow, hip, and knee joints.[311]

The "soft-tissue calcifications" are actually ossifications and have the histological appearance of organized bone.[311] Apart from calcification of the basal ganglia, dystrophic calcification of soft tissues as such does not occur in PHP, and the ossifications are observed in both PHP and PPHP. Ectopic ossifications are usually present early in life and are most frequent in the extremities and in the region of the large joints, where they may be palpable and/or visible as hard, nontender nodules.

The typical symptoms of chronic hypocalcemia are noted in the majority of patients with PHP. Cataracts, calcification of the basal ganglia, and dental abnormalities are observed in approximately one-half of patients. In contrast to idiopathic hypoparathyroidism of "early onset," symptomatic hypocalcemia occurs infrequently in infancy in patients with PHP, and the average age at onset of symptoms is 8½ years. In addition, the hypocalcemia and hyperphosphatemia in PHP are somewhat less pronounced than in idiopathic hypoparathyroidism.[311] The onset of symptoms during childhood and the milder hypocalcemia are important aspects of the natural history of PHP and probably result from the fact that peripheral "resistance" to PTH is incomplete such that a partially compensated state is maintained until stressed by the mineral demands of childhood growth.

Pathogenesis

In 1968, Lee and coworkers[329] demonstrated that circulating immunoreactive PTH levels were elevated in patients with PHP and interpreted this finding as lending support to the PTH-resistance concept. In 1969, Chase, Melson, and Aurbach[330] demonstrated that patients with the syndrome fail to demonstrate a rise in urinary cAMP excretion following infusion of exogenous parathyroid extract (Fig. 23-47). Thus, by 1969 the syndrome appeared to include a homogeneous group of patients with AHO, hypocalcemia, hyperphosphatemia, elevated immunoreactive PTH, and absent or minimal rises in urinary cAMP excretion in response to exogenous PTH. The etiology of the disorder was felt to involve a defect at the level of the renal PTH receptor–adenylate cyclase complex and perhaps also to include similar defects in other PTH-responsive tissues.

In 1973, Drezner and colleagues[331] described a subgroup of patients with PHP who, like the classical patients with PHP, had deficient phosphaturic responses to PTH but, unlike the classical patients, displayed normal urinary cAMP responses. These patients were designated as having PHP type II to distinguish them from the more common patients with "classical" PHP, who were referred to as having PHP type I. The defect in these patients is believed to be "distal" to the PTH receptor–adenylate cyclase complex. Only a handful of such patients have been described to date.

In 1975, Kooh and associates[332] suggested that renal conversion of 25-OHD to 1,25-$(OH)_2D$ was impaired in a patient with PHP, based on the observation that physiological doses of 1,25-$(OH)_2D$ reversed this patient's hypocalcemia and normalized her intestinal calcium absorption. Subsequent studies have documented the presence of low or low-normal circulating 1,25-$(OH)_2D$ despite elevations in immunoreactive PTH in patients with PHP.[333,334] It has also been demonstrated that 1,25-$(OH)_2D$ levels rise in response to infusions of exogenous dibutyryl cAMP in patients with PHP type I.[334]

In 1978, Drezner and Burch[335] demonstrated that the K_m for ATP in a renal membrane preparation from a patient with PHP type I was abnormally high, indicating that a defect in the regulatory subunit (termed the G or *N protein*) of the adenylate cyclase

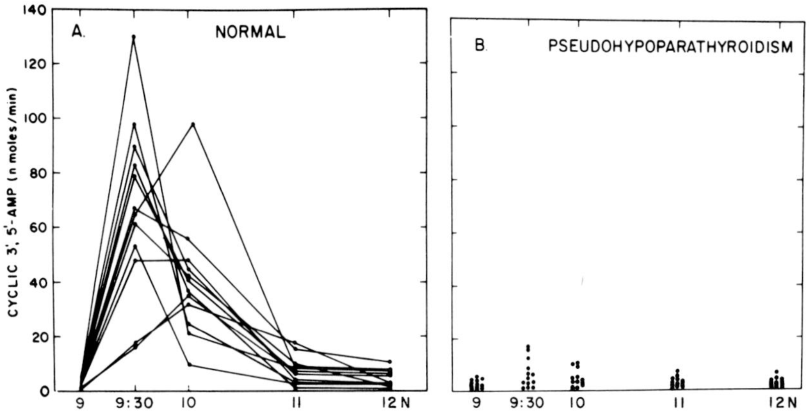

FIGURE 23-47 Urinary cAMP response to parathyroid hormone administration in normal subjects and patients with pseudohypoparathyroidism. (*From Chase, Melson, and Aurbach,*[330] *by permission of the Journal of Clinical Investigation.*)

complex was present in this patient and that the PTH receptor and the catalytic subunit of adenylate cyclase were "partially uncoupled." Direct examination of erythrocyte G or N protein in normal subjects and patients with PHP type I was reported in 1980 by Farfel and coworkers,[336] who demonstrated that the erythrocyte regulatory subunit activity was reduced 50 percent in patients with PHP type I but was normal in patients with PHP type II and patients with idiopathic and surgical hypoparathyroidism. This was confirmed by Levine and coworkers.[337] Subsequently, regulatory subunit deficiency has been documented in fibroblasts, lymphoblasts, platelets, and thyroid membranes from patients with PHP type I.[338-341] Downs and associates[342] also demonstrated deficiency of the regulatory subunit in renal membranes derived from the same patient Drezner and Burch[335] had studied. Most recently, this group has shown that the defect is present in the stimulatory regulatory subunit ("Ns" or "Gs") but not in its inhibitory counterpart ("Ni" or "Gi").[343]

The presence of a defect in the adenylate cyclase regulatory subunit in patients with PHP as described above would predict, since this protein is common to all adenylate cyclases and since the defect is present in all tissues examined, that resistance to multiple hormones in addition to PTH should be present. Multiple endocrinopathies (e.g., gonadal failure, hypothyroidism, prolactin deficiency, and nephrogenic diabetes insipidus) have long been known to be present in certain patients and kindreds with PHP. In 1983, Levine and coworkers[344] examined the relation between the phenotypic syndrome (AHO), the presence or absence of multiple hormone resistance, and the activity of the regulatory subunit in 29 patients with PHP. In general, patients with regulatory subunit deficiency were the same patients who had both AHO and multiple hormone resistance. A second, smaller group of patients with PHP (i.e., hypocalcemia, hyperphosphatemia, and elevated iPTH) had normal regulatory subunit activity. These patients had normal phenotypes (i.e., were AHO-negative), and in most there was no evidence of endocrine dysfunction other than hypoparathyroidism. Thus, it appears that PHP type I can be further divided into two subgroups which have been termed types Ia and Ib,[345] with type Ia being characterized by AHO, multiple hormone resistance, and widespread regulatory subunit deficiency. Patients with PHP type Ib generally have normal regulatory subunits, normal phenotypes, and normal endocrine profiles, with the exception of their hypoparathyroidism. The findings in PHP type Ib are consistent with a defect in the PTH receptor.[346]

The findings in type Ia are consistent with a widespread defect in the regulatory subunit which leads to hypoparathyroidism as well as phenotypic abnormalities and multiple hormone resistance. This hypothesis leaves a number of unanswered questions. For example, it (1) fails to account for the fact that hypoparathyroidism is far more severe and more common than the other endocrinopathies, (2) does not explain why some patients who have AHO do not have the regulatory subunit deficiency, and (3) does not explain the absence of defects in nonendocrine tissues (e.g., erythrocytes, platelets, and fibroblasts) which have been demonstrated to display the biochemical abnormality. Thus, it is possible that the regulatory subunit deficiency may be widely present in the tissues of patients with PHP Ia but that another defect leads to their hypoparathyroidism.

Two other major etiologic possibilities have been implicated to explain this functional hypoparathyroidism. Nagant de Deuxchaisnes and coworkers[347] and Mitchell and Goltzman[348] demonstrated that while immunoreactive PTH values are elevated in PHP, biologically active PTH values are normal or low. This dissociation between immunoreactive PTH and bioactive PTH is consistent with a defect in the primary or tertiary structure of PTH (the "defective PTH" hypothesis) or with the presence of circulating inhibitors of PTH in patients with PHP (the "circulating inhibitor" hypothesis).

Despite the failure of PTH to induce phosphaturic and nephrogenous cAMP responses in patients with PHP, there is evidence that PTH is capable of displaying its expected actions on bone metabolism and on renal calcium reabsorption. For example, in 1962 Kolb and Steinbach[349] described two patients with AHO, hypocalcemia, and hyperphosphatemia (type Ia PHP) who had evidence of severe osteitis fibrosa cystica. More recently, Breslau and coworkers[350] demonstrated that patients with PHP have lower bone mineral density and higher urinary hydroxyproline excretion compared with patients with idiopathic and surgical hypoparathyroidism. Both groups displayed an increase in urinary hydroxyproline in response to injections of parathyroid extract. Thus, patients with PHP may display skeletal evidence of hyperparathyroidism. The incidence and prevalence of skeletal abnormalities among patients with PHP and the relation of these abnormalities to the proposed subtypes of PHP require further investigation. Nonetheless, one of the goals of therapy in patients with PHP should be normalization of iPTH values in an effort to prevent the skeletal effects of excessive circulating PTH.

Urinary calcium excretion may be relatively lower in patients with PHP than in patients with surgical or idiopathic hypoparathyroidism at a comparable serum calcium concentration,[311] suggesting that the increase in circulating PTH may be able to stimulate distal tubular calcium reabsorption in at least certain patients with PHP. The responsiveness to PTH in the distal nephron may not be normal,[351] and the relative hypocalciuria reported in these patients may reflect marked increases in circulating PTH. This point has not been examined as a function of the specific subtypes of PHP.

PHP and PPHP may occur sporadically or in families, in which they may be variously admixed. Whether PHP and PPHP should be viewed as biochemically distinct syndromes is not clear, and a reduction in regulatory subunit activity has been demonstrated in certain patients with PPHP.[344] Conversely, unusual patients with PHP have been observed to achieve normocalcemia spontaneously.[352,353] This phenomenon remains unexplained.

The incidence of the various PHP and PPHP syndromes is not known. All appear to be rare, although precise incidence figures are unavailable. Women are affected more commonly than men. As indicated above, both sporadic and familial forms exist, although again, the relative incidences are uncertain. The mode of inheritance has varied in different families, with evidence for autosomal dominant, autosomal recessive, and x-linked patterns being present in different kindreds.

Diagnosis

Because of the variable expression of phenotypic abnormalities, PHP should be suspected in any patient with nonsurgical hypoparathyroidism. Diagnosis can be achieved by means of (1) detection of increased circulating levels of PTH, together with an increase in TmP/GFR and/or disproportionately low basal values for nephrogenous cAMP or total cAMP excretion, (2) demonstration of a blunted or absent nephrogenous or urinary cAMP and/or phosphaturic response to acute exogenous PTH administration, in the format of the Ellsworth-Howard test or minor modifications thereof, and/or (3) demonstration of abnormal calcemic, phosphaturic, and cAMP responses to a more prolonged protocol, involving intramuscular PTH administration for a period of 3 to 6 days (each procedure is described under Testing, below). Some investigators have suggested that these diagnostic maneuvers are best carried out once patients have been adequately replaced with vitamin D and calcium supplements, but it is clear that certain patients will regain a degree of calcemic and phosphaturic responsiveness when so treated and tested.[311] Because of diurnal variation and other factors which influence the phosphorus excretion rate, protocols based on PTH-induced changes in phosphorus excretion must be performed with great care, and borderline responses are not infrequent. In all circumstances, the demonstration of an abnormal urinary cAMP response to PTH is the single most reliable diagnostic technique in both untreated and treated patients. In the format employed by Chase and Aurbach and subsequently by others, the infusion of 300 U of purified PTH or parathyroid extract over 15 min produces a maximal 20-fold increase in cAMP excretion in normal subjects, whereas increases greater than two- to fivefold are rarely observed in patients with PHP.[311,330] An average 15-fold response is seen in patients with PPHP.[330] Hypomagnesemia should be ruled out in all patients prior to testing.[311]

NEONATAL HYPOCALCEMIC SYNDROMES

Neonatal hypocalcemia is relatively common, but the syndromes associated with long-term hypoparathyroidism are rare (Table 23-12).

"Early" neonatal hypocalcemia refers to hypocalcemia which is manifest within the first 72 h of life.[170] Physiological hypocalcemia occurs at birth, and limits of pathological hypocalcemia are usually set below 8.0 mg/dl for full-term infants and below 7.0

mg/dl for premature infants. Serum calcium values below these limits are observed in one-third of premature infants, one-third of infants with birth asphyxia, and one-half of babies born of insulin-dependent diabetic mothers.[170] Symptoms may be absent or there may be associated irritability, muscular twitching, or frank seizures. The hypocalcemia tends to resolve spontaneously during the first week. Treatment consists of oral and/or intravenous calcium, depending on the severity of the hypocalcemia and symptoms. Early neonatal hypocalcemia appears to be simply an extreme example of the transient hypoparathyroidism at birth, which is variously attributed to parathyroid immaturity and/or physiological maternal hyperparathyroidism.[311] Spontaneous resolution is associated with the assumption of normal parathyroid function. Long-term sequelae are the complications associated with asphyxia and the other conditions predisposing to the hypocalcemia.

"Late" neonatal hypocalcemia refers to hypocalcemia, which is noted at about 1 week of life and always within the first 2 weeks.[170,311] This form of neonatal hypocalcemia occurs in large full-term infants; symptoms ranging from irritability to convulsions may or may not occur, and the long-term prognosis is excellent. Hyperphosphatemia and a tendency to hypomagnesemia are regularly observed.[170] Functional hypoparathyroidism is not a feature in these infants. The pathogenesis of late neonatal hypocalcemia appears to relate to (1) intake of formulas with a higher phosphorus/calcium ratio than that of breast milk, together with (2) immaturity of renal tubular phosphorus handling and/or the renal adenylate cyclase system.[311] The hypomagnesemia is presumed to result from phosphate-induced interference with intestinal magnesium absorption; it is usually mild and probably is of limited importance in the pathogenesis of the hypocalcemia. Treatment is self-evident. Current recommendations for milk formulas suggest a calcium/phosphorus ratio more closely resembling that of mother's milk.[170]

As noted in the discussion of primary hyperparathyroidism occurring during pregnancy, the placental transfer of calcium is predictably associated with neonatal secondary hypoparathyroidism and hypocalcemia. The fetal and neonatal sequelae of this association are often severe, and protracted neonatal hypocalcemia has occasionally led to the diagnosis of primary hyperparathyroidism in a previously undiagnosed mother. Hypocalcemia in the infant tends to occur somewhat later than in the syndromes described above, and medical therapy is often required for several months before normal parathyroid function is restored.[311] All major vitamin D metabolites also cross the placenta, and transient hypocalcemia has been rarely described in neonates born of mothers on chronic vitamin D therapy. Untreated maternal hypocalcemia is associated with fetal and neonatal secondary hyperparathyroidism, and rare cases manifesting frank osteitis fibrosa cystica at birth have been reported.[311]

DiGeorge's syndrome (otherwise known as the third-fourth pharyngeal pouch syndrome or branchial dysembryogenesis) is a rare congenital syndrome which variously includes agenesis of the parathyroids and thymus, cardiac anomalies, unusual facies, and a number of other congenital anomalies.[311,312] The syndrome is not familial. Functional aparathyroidism is present at birth. Immunological deficiencies usually dominate the clinical course.

Other patients with "early-onset" hypoparathyroidism (i.e., within the first year of life) appear to be examples of parathyroid hypoplasia or aplasia or simply represent very early presentations of idiopathic hypoparathyroidism and related syndromes.[311]

Other Hypocalcemic Conditions and Tetanic Syndromes

The conditions listed in Table 23-13 are usually but not invariably associated with secondary hyperparathyroidism. The pathogenesis of the abnormalities in skeletal homeostasis in renal osteodystrophy and the various syndromes of rickets and osteomalacia are described in detail in Chap. 24.

The principal pathogenetic factors responsible for hypocalcemia in renal insufficiency are phosphorus retention and impaired $1,25\text{-}(OH)_2D$ production. Secondary hyperparathyroidism is regularly observed, and extreme elevations in circulating PTH immunoreactivity are common. However, the bulk of this circulating material results from the inability to excrete carboxy-terminal fragments of the PTH peptide, and immunoassay results are difficult to interpret in a quantitative sense in severely azotemic patients (see Parathyroid Hormone under Hormonal Measurements, above).

Mild to moderate hypocalcemia accompanies most clinical forms of rickets and osteomalacia. In the majority of these syndromes, however, hypophosphatemia is more regularly observed and is more pronounced than hypocalcemia. Some degree of secondary hyperparathyroidism is usually noted in the first five syndromes listed in this category in Table 23-13; parathyroid function is variably normal or slightly increased in vitamin D–resistant rickets.

Hypocalcemia and tetanic symptoms may be observed in patients with acute pancreatitis. Significant hypocalcemia correlates with severe pancreatitis and is a poor prognostic sign. In spite of a relatively large literature on the subject, the pathogenesis of hypocalcemia in acute pancreatitis is largely unknown. Proposed mechanisms include saponification of calcium in the region of inflammation, associated hypomagnesemia, hypoparathyroidism due to the destruction of PTH by circulating proteases, and the hypocalcemic effects of glucagon-mediated calcitonin secretion.[312,354–356] None of these mechanisms has been conclusively demonstrated. In the authors' view, the incorporation of calcium into intra- and retroperitoneal free fatty acid complexes seems the most likely mechanism. The causal relation between primary hyperparathyroidism and other hypercalcemic conditions and acute and chronic pancreatitis was described in an earlier section.

Rapid or excessive skeletal mineralization may rarely lead to hypocalcemia. This has occurred in patients with breast or prostate cancer with extensive osteoblastic skeletal metastases[357] and is the explanation for the hungry bones syndrome of postparathyroidectomy hypocalcemia. Rapid healing of severe vitamin D–deficient osteomalacia may lead to hypocalcemia following the initiation of therapy with vitamin D.

Hypoalbuminemia results in a reduction in total but not ionized serum calcium. Such findings are common in patients with cirrhosis, nephrotic syndrome, malnutrition, cancer, burns, and other chronic illnesses.

Hyperphosphatemia due to parenteral, oral, or rectal (Phospho-Soda enema) phosphorus administration, particularly in patients with renal compromise, regularly leads to hypocalcemia. Similarly, the release of endogenous intracellular phosphorus may lead to severe hyperphosphatemia and hypocalcemia in patients with extensive "crush injuries" and patients with leukemia and lymphoma following successful chemotherapy.[358]

Hypomagnesemia, either through inhibition of PTH release or by producing resistance to the action of PTH, may lead to hypocalcemia, as discussed in Hypoparathyroidism.

Mild hypocalcemia has been reported in patients with the toxic shock syndrome. The reduction in total serum calcium is due in part to a reduction in the ionized calcium concentration.[359]

Hypocalcemia is often observed when mithramycin is used overzealously, and this complication can and should be avoided. Hypocalcemia may also occur following the administration of large doses of calcitonin in patients with increased bone turnover. The rapid infusion of citrated whole blood chelates calcium and lowers the serum ionized calcium concentration. Since citrate is metabolized by the liver, patients with hepatic dysfunction are particularly prone to accumulate citrate and experience a significant reduction in ionized calcium. Each unit of citrated blood creates an extracellular deficit of approximately 150 mg of calcium, and this amount of elemental calcium can be administered per unit in order to prevent a decrease in the extracellular concentration of ionized calcium.[312] Acute fluoride intoxication is associated with marked symptomatic hypocalcemia due to the formation of an insoluble precipitate with calcium. The hypocalcemia should be vigorously treated; however, the ingestion of more than 2 g of sodium fluoride usually results in cardiopulmonary death.

Tetanic symptoms regularly accompany hyperventilation, occasionally to the extent of frank carpopedal spasm. Tetany is uncommon in conditions associated with chronic metabolic alkalosis, such as primary hyperaldosteronism. Signs of tetany may be expressed during a conversion reaction. A vague syndrome of normocalcemic tetany which occurs predominantly in women has been described as "idiopathic tetany" or "spasmophilia." The basis of this nonspecific syndrome is not clear, and it is rarely reported in the United States.[311]

Differential Diagnosis

Severe hypocalcemia is not a common problem in clinical practice. When it is observed, the cause is usually immediately apparent or can be easily ascertained through "exclusion" by eliminating the items in Tables 23-12 and 23-13 on clinical grounds. Usually, hypocalcemia is mild and is most often attributable to hypoalbuminemia. Correction formulas for normalizing total serum calcium values in hypoalbuminemic patients are reasonably useful clinically but have not proved to be particularly accurate. Thus, the direct measurement of ionized calcium, which is now widely available, should be performed in hypoalbuminemic, hypocalcemic patients if there is any question as to whether clinically significant hypocalcemia exists.

Most instances of hypocalcemia are accompanied by *hypo*phosphatemia. The hypophosphatemia may result from (1) secondary hyperparathyroidism, (2) inadequate phosphorus intake (e.g., malabsorption, chronic illness, pancreatitis), (3) excessive renal losses independent of PTH (e.g., intravenous saline, diuretics), or some combination of these factors. Thus, the presence of *hyper*phosphatemia should bring to mind parathyroid failure (Table 23-12), renal failure, or those disorders associated with endogenous or exogenous phosphate loads (Table 23-13, items 1 and 6).

The major diagnostic difficulty posed by hypoparathyroidism is a failure to suspect the diagnosis in a pediatric or adult patient with vague neuromuscular or other symptoms; chemical or biochemical confirmation of the diagnosis is usually a simple matter. The serum magnesium must be measured in any hypocalcemic patient, and pseudohypoparathyroidism should be suspected and tested for in any nonazotemic patient with hypocalcemia and hyperphosphatemia in whom the basis for the hypoparathyroidism is not clear. The neonatal hypocalcemic syndromes usually define themselves by virtue of their natural course.

Vitamin D disorders are considered separately in Chap. 24. Vitamin D deficiency, whether due to dietary causes or to gastrointestinal disorders, is accompanied by reductions in circulating 25-OHD and marked elevations in circulating PTH. Diet-related vitamin D deficiency is rare in the United States as a result of the widespread supplementation of milk products and other foodstuffs with this vitamin. Anticonvulsant therapy and hepatobiliary disorders should be apparent from the history and clinical examination. Similarly, renal failure is typically advanced, with glomerular filtration rates below 15 ml/min, before hypocalcemia occurs; most of these patients are on chronic hemodialysis. Hypocalcemia of pancreatitis occurs in patients with severe pancreatitis. Vitamin D and magnesium deficiency may occur in these patients and should be specifically sought and corrected. Hypocalcemia due to excessive skeletal mineralization occurs only in specific clinical settings: in patients with widespread osteoblastic metastases, following thyroidectomy or parathyroidectomy in patients with Graves' disease or primary or tertiary hyperparathyroidism, and following initiation of vitamin D therapy in severely vitamin D–deficient individuals. Medication-induced hypocalcemia and hypocalcemia related to the toxic shock syndrome are clinically obvious.

Treatment

ACUTE HYPOCALCEMIA

Acute hypocalcemia with frank tetany requires intravenous calcium therapy. Available solutions include calcium chloride (272 mg elemental calcium per 10-ml ampul), calcium gluceptate (90 mg calcium per 5-ml ampul), and calcium gluconate (90 mg calcium per 10-ml ampul). Initial therapy consists of the intravenous administration of approximately 200 mg of elemental calcium. Concentrated calcium solutions are irritating to veins and may cause extensive inflammation if they extravasate into soft tissues, and so it is preferable to dilute the calcium solutions into 50 to 100 ml of dextrose and administer the required dose over 5 to 10 min by a secure intravenous route. Calcium should be administered very cautiously in digitalized patients, since hypercalcemia predisposes to digitalis intoxication and arrhythmias. Persistent or recurrent severe symptomatic hypocalcemia may be treated with repeated intravenous doses at 6- to 8-h intervals or by a constant intravenous infusion of a dilute calcium solution, with the exact dosage determined by serial measurements of serum calcium. If it is clear that long-term replacement therapy will be required, oral calcium supplements and a vitamin D preparation should be begun immediately. Whether vitamin D therapy should be initiated with a "loading" dose (e.g., 2 mg DHT four times daily for 2 to 3 days) or by simply commencing an estimated maintenance dose (e.g., 0.5 to 1 mg DHT daily) is a matter of opinion. Some physicians prefer to initiate therapy with 1,25-$(OH)_2D$ because of its rapid action; it is also reasonable to institute therapy with both 1,25-$(OH)_2D$ and DHT (or some other vitamin D preparation), eliminating the 1,25-$(OH)_2D$ as the serum calcium concentration stabilizes over a matter of days. Acute hypocalcemia in the range of 8 mg/dl with or without mild neuromuscular symptoms can usually be managed with oral calcium supplements alone (1 to 2 g elemental calcium daily in four divided doses).

Magnesium replacement should be given not only to patients with known magnesium deficiency but also to patients with severe hypocalcemia in whom hypomagnesemia is suspected (see Hypomagnesemia, below).

CHRONIC HYPOCALCEMIA

The approach to chronic replacement therapy described below refers specifically to the treatment of hypoparathyroidism; the therapeutic approach in patients with renal osteodystrophy and other chronic hypocalcemic conditions is similar, but the regimens differ, based on the specific disorder being treated.

The therapeutic goals in the chronic management of hypoparathyroidism are to (1) alleviate all but the mildest symptoms, (2) avoid predictable complications of modest, chronic overdosage, and (3) avoid episodes of vitamin D intoxication insofar as this is possible. These goals translate into a regimen which maintains the serum calcium in the range of 8.5 to 9.0 mg/dl and includes the minimal possible dosage of vitamin D. At this level of serum calcium, the vast majority of patients are symptom-free; hypercalciuria is minimized, and episodes of intoxication are relatively infrequent. At serum calcium concentrations between 9 and 10 mg/dl, calcium excretion is approximately threefold higher in patients with idiopathic and severe postoperative hypoparathyroidism than in normal individuals,[53] and these patients are predisposed to renal stone formation; hypercalciuria is usually absent or less marked in patients with pseudohypoparathyroidism. Symptoms may predictably worsen owing to alterations in the total and/or ionized serum calcium following vomiting-induced metabolic alkalosis or hyperventilation-induced respiratory alkalosis, during periods of emotional or physical stress, or during menstruation or estrogen administration, presumably because of an effect of estrogen on bone resorption. Patients should be educated to anticipate these vagaries and participate in their management. In general, patients should be instructed to maintain a constant dosage of vitamin D and to manage acute or subacute symptoms by increasing the quantity of calcium supplements. If symptoms persist, the patient should be seen and the regimen altered based on serum chemistry determinations. Chronic management regimens frequently require alteration during pregnancy and lactation or when anticonvulsants or thiazide diuretics are introduced. In all circumstances, however, the three goals stated above are the principal guidelines for therapy.

Oral calcium supplements are available as the gluconate, lactate, chloride, carbonate, and citrate salts. Calcium lactate tablets dissolve poorly, and the chloride and carbonate preparations may induce acid-base alterations which are undesirable. Calcium gluconate is available in tablets of 325, 500, 650, and 1000 mg, containing 30, 46, 60, and 92 mg of elemental calcium, respectively. These tablets should be chewed into fine particles rather than swallowed whole. Calcium glubionate syrup contains 23 mg of elemental calcium per milliliter (115 mg per teaspoon). Calcium carbonate contains 39 percent elemental calcium by weight and is widely available in a variety of preparations, usually containing 200 to 500 mg of elemental calcium per tablet. Calcium citrate has been advocated for use in patients with achlorhydria.[360,361] Calcium supplements are taken as four divided doses daily, and many patients prefer to use the syrup while at home and the tablets for the midday dose. Milk products have an approximately equivalent calcium and phosphorus content. Many physicians prescribe calcium supplementation in the form of a high intake of milk products, but others regard the high phosphorus content in these products as unphysiological and employ a moderate (about 500 mg) calcium diet, with approximately 1000 mg of elemental calcium daily added in the form of calcium supplements.

Crystalline ergocalciferol and DHT are the forms of vitamin D most widely employed in chronic therapy. Ergocalciferol contains 40,000 USP units or IU per milligram and is available in gelatin capsules of 25,000 U (625 μg) and 50,000 U (1.25 mg) and as a solution in vegetable oil containing 50,000 U/ml. DHT contains approximately 120,000 U equiv/mg and is available in tablets of 0.125, 0.2, and 0.4 mg, in capsules of 0.125 mg, and as a solution in oil containing 0.25 mg/ml. 25-OHD_3 is available commercially in Europe and for investigational use in the United States in capsules of 20 and 50 μg and as a solution in oil containing approximately 50 μg/ml. The doses used in hypoparathyroid patients have ranged from 25 to 200 μg per day. 1,25-$(OH)_2D_3$ has approximately 50 to 100 times the activity of 25-OHD_3 and is available commercially in 0.25- and 0.5-μg gelatin capsules. Long-term doses of 1,25-$(OH)_2D_3$ in hypoparathyroidism have ranged from 0.5 to 5.0 μg per day.[311,362] 1α-OHD_3 is available on an investigational basis only and has been used in doses equivalent to those of 1,25-$(OH)_2D_3$. If an arbitrary value of unity is assigned to the biological potency of calciferol, the relative potencies of the other vitamin D metabolites and analogues are DHT = 3:1, 25-OHD_3 = 10:1 to 15:1, and 1,25-$(OH)_2D_3$ and 1α-OHD_3 = 1000:1 to 1500:1.[311] However, these relative potencies are no more than approximate, and therapeutic substitutions must be carefully monitored empirically. Although the vitamin D solutions in oil are marketed for oral use, they may be administered intramuscularly if necessary. All vitamin D preparations should be protected from exposure to heat, direct light, and moisture.

The efficacy of the vitamin D preparations in long-term replacement therapy is based on their aggregate effects on intestinal calcium absorption and bone resorption. Which of these effects is predominant and whether the various vitamin D preparations influence these two processes to an equivalent extent is not clear and may in fact differ from one patient to another. In patients with functional aparathyroidism calciferol appears to exert its major effects through conversion to 25-OHD, whereas in patients with mild or partial hypoparathyroidism it is likely that an entire profile of vitamin D metabolites is produced. Both DHT and 1α-OHD_3 undergo 25-hydroxylation and bypass the bottleneck of the renal 1-hydroxylase reaction. It is doubtful that renal tubular effects constitute an important action of any of the vitamin D forms, and the reduction in serum phosphorus concentrations and TmP/GFR which occurs in response to vitamin D therapy is regarded as resulting from a direct calcium-mediated effect on tubular phosphorus handling. A similar reduction is observed in response to intravenous calcium administration in hypoparathyroid patients in the absence of administered vitamin D. The hydroxylated vitamin D metabolites have certain theoretical advantages and have been shown to be efficacious in chronic treatment in small series of patients with hypoparathyroidism. Reservations concerning the use of these metabolites are associated with their expense and imperfect knowledge regarding whether the complete biological effectiveness of vitamin D is implicit in the structure of each of these metabolites. Certainly, there are no clear-cut indications for altering therapy in patients who have been successfully managed with calciferol or DHT. Most experienced clinicians regard DHT as the drug of choice.

Patients with mild postoperative hypoparathyroidism can often be managed with oral calcium supplements alone (1 to 2 g of elemental calcium daily), and a significant number of such patients ultimately recover sufficient parathyroid function to be weaned from all therapy.[321] Patients with moderate to severe hypoparathyroidism require calciferol in an average dose of approximately 80,000 U per day (usual range of 50,000 to 100,000 U daily) or DHT in an average dose of 0.75 mg per day (usual range of 0.5 to 1.0 mg daily). A small minority of patients require doses above these ranges, but episodes of intoxication frequently accompany the use of higher doses of vitamin D.[311] In the average patient maintained on a dose of 0.75 mg of DHT and 1000 to 1500 mg of elemental calcium daily, episodes of intoxication are relatively infrequent. Serum calcium and phosphorus should be checked at weekly intervals when therapy is initiated. Once a regimen is established, serum calcium and phosphorus and urinary calcium excretion should be determined at monthly intervals until a reproducible pattern of results is obtained and at 3- to 6-month intervals thereafter. Patients requiring higher vitamin D doses require closer monitoring than those on average doses. Patients with pseudohypoparathyroidism can usually be managed with modest doses of vitamin D, and serum PTH levels may serve as an additional guide to therapy.

Episodes of vitamin D intoxication typically occur in a totally unpredictable fashion, often in a patient who has been on a stable regimen for a prolonged period. Mild episodes usually pass unnoticed and are revealed only by periodic testing. Severe, symptomatic episodes are less frequent and are managed as described previously. Whether patients are more "sensitive" to vitamin D following episodes of intoxication is a matter of debate, but therapy should be closely monitored for 4 to 6 months following such an episode. Intoxication has been observed with all available vitamin D preparations and is a function of the narrow therapeutic-toxic range rather than the form of the vitamin employed.

"Resistance" to vitamin D is observed rarely in patients with severe hypoparathyroidism, usually of the idiopathic variety. Patients may be initially resistant to large doses of vitamin D preparations, may acquire resistance after months to years of stable treatment, or may be intermittently resistant. Patients may be resistant to calciferol but responsive to DHT or one of the hydroxylated vitamin D preparations or may variably express resistance to all vitamin D preparations. Patients have been described in whom the resistance has been "broken" by magnesium supplementation, cortisone administration, or small parenteral doses of parathyroid extract;[311] other patients appear to reacquire responsiveness in spite of rather than because of therapeutic alterations.

Phosphate-binding gels have only a small role in the chronic therapy of hypoparathyroidism. While their use in patients with renal osteodystrophy and hyperphosphatemia was once considered essential, the potential role of phosphate-binding gels in aluminum-related bone disease has prompted a reconsideration of their routine use in this setting (see Chap. 24). Thiazide diuretics have been suggested as adjunctive therapy, but these agents exacerbate the tendency to metabolic alkalosis in hypoparathyroidism and are not widely used. These agents may be particularly useful in limiting hypercalciuria and preventing nephrolithiasis in selected patients.[363] The addition of a thiazide to the regimen of a patient with hypoparathyroidism regularly increases the fasting serum calcium concentration, and so the antihypercalciuric effect of the agent may go unappreciated until the regimen is readjusted to achieve an identical prethiazide serum calcium concentration.

HYPOPHOSPHATEMIA AND HYPERPHOSPHATEMIA

The systemic mechanisms which regulate phosphorus homeostasis and the importance of the renal tubular phosphorus threshold in this regulation have been discussed (see Systemic Phosphorus Homeostasis under Integrated Control of Mineral Homeostasis). The mechanisms, pathophysiological consequences, and treatment of hypophosphatemia and hyperphosphatemia are described in the following sections.

Hypophosphatemia

PATHOGENESIS

Clinical hypophosphatemia can be classified (1) as acute or chronic, (2) as moderate (serum phosphorus 1.0 to 2.5 mg/dl) or severe (serum phosphorus < 1.0 mg/dl), (3) according to whether it is associated with systemic phosphorus depletion, and/or (4) into mechanistic categories of deficient intake, increased excretion, or altered extracellular-tissue distribution of phosphate ions. The latter format is used in the classification in Table 23-15. Most chronic forms of hypophosphatemia are due to intrinsic or extrinsic abnormalities in TmP/GFR and are associated with moderate rather than severe hypophosphatemia. Most examples of severe hypophosphatemia are acute and result from extracellular–soft tissue fluxes of phosphate. The serum phosphorus concentration is frequently a poor index of systemic phosphorus stores, since extracellular phosphorus represents only a small fraction of total body phosphorus stores (Tables 23-1 and 23-2). Treatment must always be guided empirically.

Because of the ubiquitous occurrence of phosphorus in foodstuffs and the normal efficiency of intestinal phosphate absorption, phosphorus depletion resulting from a deficient intake is rare. Hypophosphatemia may accompany prolonged diarrhea and/or nasogastric suctioning and can also occur in patients with intestinal or pancreatic malabsorption. In these latter disorders, hypophosphatemia is largely the result of secondary hyperparathyroidism due to the malabsorption of calcium and vitamin D. Many nonabsorbable antacids bind phosphate ions and limit their absorption. A phosphorus-depletion syndrome consisting of hypophosphatemia, hypercalciuria, and symptoms of anorexia, weakness, bone pain, and malaise can be produced experimentally in humans by the combination of a rigidly restricted phosphorus intake and phosphate-binding antacids, and a very similar clinical syndrome has been reported.[364,365] The hypercalciuria associated with this syndrome results from hypophosphatemia-induced increases in bone resorption and from increased synthesis of 1,25-$(OH)_2D$, with consequent effects on bone resorption and intestinal calcium absorption. However, the syndrome is not induced by conventional clinical doses of antacids because an ample phosphorus intake overwhelms the phosphate-binding capacity of these doses and results in a normal phosphorus balance. In the experimental and/or clinical syndrome, phosphorus is eliminated from the urine and TmP/GFR is elevated owing to the suppression in parathyroid function and the intrinsic adjustment in renal tubular phosphorus reabsorption.

Moderate chronic hypophosphatemia occurs regularly in primary hyperparathyroidism, all nonazotemic forms of secondary hyperparathyroidism (except pseudohypoparathyroidism), the various renal tubular syndromes of rickets and osteomalacia (Chap. 24), and in a minority of patients with idiopathic hypercalciuria (Chap. 25). Hypophosphatemia is the rule in patients with humoral hypercalcemia of malignancy, provided that renal function is not severely compromised.[211,212] Moderate or severe hypophosphatemia may be observed in tumor-associated osteomalacia (Chap. 24). In all these disorders, TmP/GFR is reduced, and the rate of phosphorus excretion is inappropriate for the level of the serum phosphorus. Hypercalcemia in and of itself appears to lower TmP/GFR and may lead to hypophosphatemia,[366] an observation which limits its usefulness in the differential diagnosis of hypercalcemia. Increases in circulating 1,25-$(OH)_2D$ are commonly observed in primary and secondary hyperparathyroidism and in idiopathic hypercalciuria, but low or low-normal levels occur in the renal tubular disorders, tumor-associated osteomalacia, and malignancy-associated hypercalciuria and are partially responsible for the osteomalacia in the first two disorders. Neuromuscular symptoms relating to the hypophosphatemia are variably present in patients with chronic, moderate hypophosphatemia but may be difficult to distinguish from the symptoms because of coincident hypercalcemia, hypocalcemia, or other associated abnormalities. Chronic diuretic therapy, saline infusion, glucose-induced osmotic diuresis, and calcitonin therapy are all phosphaturic but are uncommon causes of chronic hypophosphatemia.

Acute, severe hypophosphatemia is most commonly observed in patients receiving intravenous hyperalimentation without adequate phosphorus supplements and following glucose and/or insulin therapy in patients with diabetic ketoacidosis or chronic alcoholism.[367] The time course of development of severe hypophosphatemia in these various disorders differs (Fig. 23-48), and the mechanisms responsible for the hypophosphatemia are complex, often including an element of chronic phosphorus depletion. Most important, the morbidity and mortality associated with the

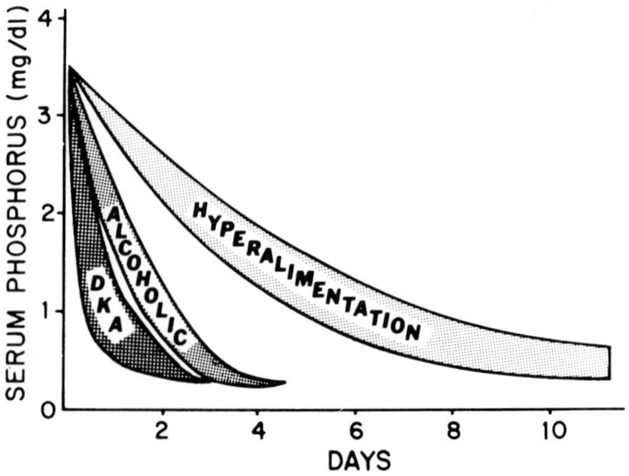

FIGURE 23-48 Approximate time course of development of severe hypophosphatemia in patients with diabetic ketoacidosis, in chronic alcoholics, and in patients receiving intravenous hyperalimentation without phosphorus supplementation. (*From Knochel,*[367] *by permission of the Archives of Internal Medicine.*)

severe hypophosphatemia in these conditions are partially iatrogenic and are preventable. Severe hypophosphatemia may also be induced by extreme hyperventilation and respiratory alkalosis.[368] The presumed mechanism of this effect is diffusion of carbon dioxide from cells, with activation of glycolysis and a trapping of phosphorus intracellularly in the form of phosphorylated intermediates.[367] Although hyperventilation of this severity is uncommon clinically, respiratory alkalosis may contribute to the hypophosphatemia in many conditions, most particularly in chronic alcoholism. Only minor changes in serum phosphorus concentrations accompany metabolic alkalosis.[368]

The occurrence of significant phosphorus depletion and hypophosphatemia during hyperalimentation is uncommon at present, owing to the supplementation of modern hyperalimentation solutions with phosphorus. However, serum phosphorus concentrations in the range of 1 mg/dl are still occasionally observed in patients receiving prolonged intravenous feedings without phosphorus supplementation (Fig. 23-48). The responsible mechanisms are phosphorus depletion and the glucose- and insulin-mediated uptake and trapping of phosphorus in soft tissues in the form of phosphorylated intermediates.

The pathogenesis and time course of phosphorus depletion and hypophosphatemia in diabetic ketoacidosis are largely analogous to the more widely recognized potassium depletion and hypokalemia in these patients. A degree of phosphorus depletion accompanies diabetic ketoacidosis because of the acidosis-induced mobilization of phosphorus from bone and soft tissues. In untreated patients, serum phosphorus concentrations are usually normal or high-normal and phosphaturia is prominent in spite of significant deficits in phosphorus stores. With the institution of therapy and correction of the ketoacidosis, phosphate ions accompany the transport of glucose and potassium into soft tissues; the serum phosphorus concentration plummets, and phosphorus is eliminated from the urine (Fig. 23-48).

Hypophosphatemia may occur in patients following parathyroidectomy for primary or secondary hyperparathyroidism in the setting of severe osteitis fibrosa cystica. These patients may be hypocalcemic and hypophosphatemic, in contrast to the hypocalcemia and hyperphosphatemia observed in patients who are rendered surgically hypoparathyroid. Patients with extensive osteoblastic metastases and patients receiving vitamin D therapy for vitamin D–deficient osteomalacia may also demonstrate hypocalcemia and hypophosphatemia. In all these circumstances, a degree of secondary hyperparathyroidism is predictably present so that the net hypophosphatemia observed has both "bone" and "renal" components.

Significant hypophosphatemia occurs in approximately one-half of patients hospitalized with chronic alcoholism. Various mechanisms are responsible for the hypophosphatemia, including malnutrition, frequent antacid use, acidosis, hypomagnesemia, and intravenous glucose therapy.[367] The serum phosphorus concentration is usually normal or low-normal on admission, and the decline in serum phosphorus concentrations parallels that in diabetic ketoacidosis but occurs somewhat later (Fig. 23-48). Other rare causes of severe hypophosphatemia are the anabolic-diuretic state that follows severe burns, overfeeding of patients with severe starvation, and the combination of antacids and a phosphate-poor dialysate in patients with chronic renal failure.[367]

As noted in Table 23-15 and observed clinically, many hypophosphatemic patients have combinations of the disorders and/or causes of hypophosphatemia listed in the table. An example would be a patient with humoral hypercalcemia of malignancy who is treated with saline, furosemide, and calcitonin, whose oral intake is restricted, and who is receiving antacids.

Table 23-15. Causes of Hypophosphatemia

1. Disorders of phosphorus intake and absorption
   - *a.* Dietary deficiency
   - *b.* Malabsorption, diarrhea
   - *c.* Continuous nasogastric suction
   - *d.* Phosphorus-binding antacids
2. Renal phosphorus losses
   - *a.* Diuresis (saline infusion, loop and thiazide diuretics, osmotic diuresis)
   - *b.* 1°, 2°, 3° hyperparathyroidism
   - *c.* Humoral hypercalcemia of malignancy
   - *d.* Oncogenic osteomalacia
   - *e.* Vitamin D–resistant rickets
   - *f.* Acquired renal tubular disorders
   - *g.* Hypercalcemia
   - *h.* Calcitonin therapy
3. Extracellular-intracellular shifts
   - *a.* Respiratory alkalosis
   - *b.* Diabetic ketoacidosis
   - *c.* Glucose and insulin therapy
4. Shifts into bone
   - *a.* Osteoblastic metastases
   - *b.* Hungry bones syndrome
5. Miscellaneous conditions
   - *a.* Alcoholism
   - *b.* Burns
   - *c.* Dialysis against phosphorus-poor dialysate
6. Combinations of the above

PATHOPHYSIOLOGICAL CONSEQUENCES OF HYPOPHOSPHATEMIA

Moderate hypophosphatemia may or may not lead to identifiable symptoms or tissue dysfunction, but severe hypophosphatemia is life-threatening. Severe hypophosphatemia is associated with a depletion of erythrocyte ATP and 2,3-diphosphoglycerate, which impairs oxygen release and decreases red cell survival.[367] Frank hemolysis is rare. A similar depletion of ATP occurs in leukocytes and platelets and may interfere with their function. A spectrum of central nervous system symptoms accompanies severe hypophosphatemia, ranging from irritability, weakness, paresthesias, and confusion to seizures, progressive obtundation, coma, and death.[367] These symptoms may be erroneously attributed to attendant diabetic ketoacidosis or delirium tremens, but the syndrome has been well characterized in patients receiving hyperalimentation and patients who lack other reasons for metabolic encephalopathy. The progression of symptoms closely resembles that of ascending paralysis, and the usual neurological misdiagnosis is the Guillain-Barré syndrome. The biochemical basis of the syndrome is not known, but it is presumed to be related to depletion of ATP and phosphorylated intermediates in the nervous system and/or associated anoxia. The syndrome may be reversed by means of prompt diagnosis and replacement therapy, but delayed diagnosis and treatment usually results in death. Myopathic symptoms and rhabdomyolysis have also been described, particularly in chronic alcoholics, and may be accompanied by increased concentrations of muscle enzymes in serum.[367] Other complications of severe hypophosphatemia have not been well characterized, but it is likely that few tissues are not affected by such a fundamental threat to oxygenation and energy production.

TREATMENT

Because of the multitude of variables responsible for significant clinical hypophosphatemia and the generally poor correlation of the serum phosphorus concentration and tissue phosphorus stores, treatment is empirical and must be guided by serial determinations of the phosphorus level in serum.[367,369] Prevention and early diagnosis are extremely important.

A wide variety of commercial preparations of phosphate salts are available for oral or intravenous use (each millimole of phosphate is equivalent to 31 mg of elemental phosphorus). This array of preparations and their content of elemental phosphorus have been summarized in a review.[369] Severe hypophosphatemia should always be treated with intravenous phosphorus administration, with an initial dose of approximately 2.5 mg elemental phosphorus per kilogram of body weight infused over 6 h.[369] Subsequent 6-h doses are guided by phosphorus determinations at the fifth or sixth hour of each dose. Requirements of more than 600 mg of parenteral elemental phosphorus per 24 h are unusual, and even this amount should be used and monitored with great care. Potassium salts are most commonly employed at the authors' institution. It should be noted that 10 ml of the common commercial potassium phosphate preparations contains 930 mg of elemental phosphorus but only 44 meq of potassium.[369] Thus, an attempt to use such a preparation as a source of potassium replacement would involve the coadministration of an enormous and dangerous quantity of phosphorus. Potassium in the chloride form should therefore be used as the principal source of potassium in patients requiring potassium replacement. Specific recommendations in diabetic ketoacidosis are given in Chap. 19. Current guidelines call for the administration of approximately 1000 mg of elemental phosphorus daily to adults receiving intravenous hyperalimentation.

Milk contains approximately 1 mg/ml of elemental phosphorus and is the form of oral phosphorus supplementation preferred by most patients. Sodium, potassium, and combined phosphate salts are available in tablet or capsule form (each containing 250 mg of elemental phosphorus); the latter require dissolution in liquid prior to consumption and are somewhat cumbersome. Phosphorus therapy should be used very cautiously in azotemic patients and those with significant hypercalcemia. Large doses of oral phosphate salts are cathartic, but moderate doses (e.g., 1500 mg of elemental phosphorus daily) are usually well tolerated.

Hyperphosphatemia

Clinically relevant hyperphosphatemia occurs in only a handful of conditions. The hyperphosphatemia of childhood and adolescence and the tendency to elevated values for serum phosphorus and TmP/GFR in postmenopausal women are physiological. Acute hyperphosphatemia may follow rapid cell lysis induced by chemotherapy, is rarely seen in children or adults receiving toxic quantities of commercial sodium phosphate laxative preparations (e.g., Phospho-Soda), and is a complication of the overzealous use of intravenous phosphate preparations. The pathogenesis of the hyperphosphatemia which commonly accompanies lactic acidosis is not known; hyperphosphatemia is uncommon in other types of metabolic acidosis.[370]

Chronic hyperphosphatemia occurs in patients with chronic renal insufficiency, hypoparathyroidism, and hyperthyroidism. Of these, chronic renal failure is the most common and important. Significant increases in the serum phosphorus concentration appear at glomerular filtration rates in the range of 30 ml/min, and phosphorus retention progresses as the glomerular filtration rate falls. Calculated values for TmP/GFR are usually low in patients with moderate renal insufficiency, but an extensive data base in patients with severe renal impairment has not been published. TmP/GFR is elevated in patients with hypoparathyroidism and hyperthyroidism.

In acute hyperphosphatemia, treatment consists of elimination of the phosphorus source and the cautious administration of intravenous calcium if clinically significant hypocalcemia coexists. The hyperphosphatemia of hyperthyroidism is a mild, incidental laboratory finding. The hyperphosphatemia of chronic hypoparathyroidism corrects with adequate vitamin D and calcium therapy and does not require additional measures. The use of a low phosphorus intake and phosphate-binding gels is discussed under the management of patients with chronic renal insufficiency (Chap. 24).

HYPOMAGNESEMIA AND HYPERMAGNESEMIA

As summarized in detail under Systemic Magnesium Homeostasis above, the normal serum magnesium concentration and normal body magnesium stores are maintained by the balance of magnesium ingestion and magnesium excretion. Renal tubular magnesium reabsorption appears to be a Tm-limited process and is the principal determinant of the ambient serum magnesium concentration in normal circumstances. No classical feedback loop systems are recognized, and the principal causes of hypomagnesemia and hypermagnesemia in humans are general medical conditions which influence magnesium absorption and/or excretion.

Hypomagnesemia and Magnesium Depletion

PATHOGENESIS

Obligate renal and intestinal magnesium losses (see Systemic Magnesium Homeostasis) are small, collectively equaling less than 1 meq (12 mg) per day when conditions of dietary magnesium deficiency exist. Thus, over the short term, conditions associated with inadequate magnesium intake do not lead to hypomagnesemia. If inadequate magnesium intake is prolonged, however, hypomagnesemia and total body magnesium deficiency will occur. Similarly, renal magnesium wasting can be tolerated over the short term without the appearance of hypomagnesemia. If renal magnesium wasting is prolonged or severe and exceeds intestinal absorption, hypomagnesemia and systemic magnesium deficiency will occur. Disorders which may lead to hypomagnesemia or magnesium deficiency are outlined in Table 23-16. It is useful conceptually to group these disorders into renal, intestinal, and miscellaneous categories. It should be recalled that magnesium is the dominant intracellular divalent cation, that the correlation between the extracellular magnesium concentration and intracellular stores is poor, and that substantial magnesium deficits may occur in the presence of a normal or nearly normal serum magnesium concentration.

Table 23-16. Causes of Hypomagnesemia and Magnesium Depletion

1. Decreased intake or absorption
   - *a.* Dietary deficiency; protein-calorie malnutrition
   - *b.* Vomiting, diarrhea, nasogastric suction
   - *c.* Malabsorption syndromes, pancreatic and intestinal
   - *d.* Parenteral hyperalimentation without adequate magnesium
   - *e.* Primary hypomagnesemia
2. Renal disorders
   - *a.* Osmotic diuresis: mannitol, glucose, urea
   - *b.* Following relief of obstructive uropathy and resolution of acute tubular necrosis
   - *c.* Post renal transplant
   - *d.* Drug-induced: loop diuretics, cisplatin, gentamicin, amphotericin, digoxin, capreomycin, viomycin, tobramycin, amikacin
   - *e.* ECF expansion, hyperaldosteronism, Bartter's syndrome
   - *f.* Congenital, hereditary renal magnesium wasting
3. Miscellaneous disorders
   - *a.* Alcoholism
   - *b.* Diabetes mellitus/diabetic ketoacidosis
   - *c.* Primary hyperparathyroidism
   - *d.* Postparathyroidectomy
   - *e.* Thyrotoxicosis
   - *f.* Syndrome of inappropriate ADH
   - *g.* Chronic hypoparathyroidism
   - *h.* Hypoalbuminemia
   - *i.* Dialysis against a magnesium-deficient dialysate
   - *j.* Excessive lactation
   - *k.* Pancreatitis
4. Combinations of the above

The magnesium depletion which has been described in severe protein-calorie malnutrition (kwashiorkor) in children appears to result from multiple mechanisms.[95] Excessive losses of magnesium-containing intestinal fluids, as occurs with prolonged diarrhea or nasogastric suction, may lead to magnesium depletion, particularly in patients receiving only parenteral fluids lacking magnesium supplements. Patients with a wide variety of intestinal disorders associated with small bowel malabsorption and steatorrhea may develop magnesium depletion. The responsible mechanisms are the formation of magnesium soaps with unabsorbed fatty acids and the losses of magnesium in intestinal fluids.[95] In some series, hypomagnesemia, with or without related symptoms, has been reported in up to one-third of patients with malabsorption.[371] Correction of steatorrhea improves magnesium absorption in these patients. Primary infantile hypomagnesemia is a rare autosomal recessive disorder which appears to be based on a specific abnormality in intestinal magnesium absorption.[372] Affected children present with tetany and/or seizures in the neonatal period or early infancy and have a combination of hypocalcemia and severe hypomagnesemia, both of which are corrected by means of magnesium replacement therapy.

Osmotic diuretics (mannitol, glucose, urea) all enhance renal magnesium excretion, and hyperosmolar states regularly lead to hypomagnesemia and magnesium deficiency. Common examples are chronic hyperglycemia (diabetes mellitus) and the combination of uremia with normal or normalizing renal function. Examples of the latter include the hypomagnesemia observed during the diuretic phase of acute tubular necrosis,[95,96] following relief of ureteral or urethral obstruction,[373] and following renal transplantation[373] as well as that observed in patients with renal tubular acidosis, pyelonephritis, hydronephrosis, and other predominantly nonazotemic renal disorders.[95,96] Impaired magnesium reabsorption and hypomagnesemia have been observed as part of the nephrotoxicity of gentamicin and all other members of the aminoglycoside family,[374] during amphotericin therapy,[375] and during cisplatin chemotherapy.[376] Virtually all diuretics increase magnesium excretion, but symptomatic hypomagnesemia is rare.[95] Magnesium depletion predisposes to digitalis intoxication in experimental animals and is of theoretical concern in diuretic-treated digitalized patients.[95] Cardiac glycosides have also been implicated in renal magnesium wasting.[377] Aldosterone increases both urinary and fecal excretion of magnesium, and a tendency to hypomagnesemia occurs in patients with primary aldosteronism and those with various states of secondary aldosteronism, including Bartter's syndrome.[95,96] Mild hypomagnesemia is seen in approximately one-half of patients with primary aldosteronism and may be partially responsible for tetanic symptoms in these patients. Ethanol also increases renal magnesium excretion (see below). Finally, rare inherited defects in renal magnesium reabsorption have been described.[378,379] These are usually accompanied by other tubular defects (associated with hypokalemia, renal tubular acidosis, etc.).

Hypomagnesemia is noted in approximately 50 percent of hospitalized alcoholics.[380] Predisposing mechanisms include (1) poor diet, (2) vomiting, diarrhea, and/or malabsorption, (3) secondary aldosteronism, and (4) direct effects of ethanol on magnesium excretion.[95] The tubular mechanism mediating the latter effect is unknown. The similarity of the symptoms of hypomagnesemia to those of delirium tremens has long suggested a relation between magnesium depletion and ethanol withdrawal, but the evidence in support of this relation is variable and inconclusive.[95] The osmotic diuresis of diabetic ketoacidosis is associated with significant urinary losses of magnesium. The time course of the development of hypomagnesemia in response to treatment of ketoacidosis resembles the pattern of changes in serum potassium and phosphorus in these patients, with normal pretreatment values which may fall to less than 1 mg/dl during the first 24 h of therapy. Treatment-associated hypomagnesemia occurs in approximately 50 percent of patients, and magnesium supplementation is now included in the routine fluid and electrolyte replacement in diabetic ketoacidosis in many centers.[380] Significant hypomagnesemia is unusual in patients with untreated primary hyperparathyroidism but may develop postoperatively in a small minority of patients.[381,382] This course of events is usually confined to patients with significant preoperative hyperparathyroid bone disease and appears to result from a hungry bones syndrome which affects magnesium as well as calcium. In this setting, both magnesium and calcium must be replaced in order to relieve the symptoms of tetany. Hyperthyroidism is associated with hypermagnesuria, negative magnesium balance, and a tendency to hypomagnesemia.[383] The hypomagnesemia reported in patients with the syndrome of inappropriate ADH secretion appears to be largely dilutional.[95] Patients with hypoparathyroidism on chronic vitamin D replacement therapy rarely develop hypomagnesemia and apparent vitamin D "resistance," which resolves with magnesium replacement. The mechanism responsible for the magnesium losses in these patients is unknown but may be related to the hypercalciuria which often accompanies vitamin D therapy for hypoparathyroidism. Hypoalbuminemia may lead to mild hypomagnesemia, since one-third of circulating magnesium is protein-bound. Dialysis against a magnesium-deficient dialysate has been reported to cause hypomagnesemia. A single report of hypomagnesemia occurring in a postpartum woman serving as a wet nurse in addition to nursing her own child has appeared.[384] Finally, pancreatitis may be associated with hypomagnesemia. Possible mechanisms include vomiting, inadequate intake, hypoalbuminemia, nasogastric suctioning, formation of insoluble peritoneal magnesium-free fatty acid soaps, concomitant diabetes mellitus, and coexisting alcoholism.

SYMPTOMS

Neuromuscular symptoms clinically indistinguishable from those of hypocalcemia have been described in hypomagnesemic patients. The symptoms result from increased neuronal excitability and neuromuscular transmission, although the exact mechanism by which magnesium deficiency leads to abnormal neuromuscular function remains unknown.[95] Associated symptoms and signs may include latent or overt tetany, muscle weakness, tremors, dysphagia, nystagmus, cerebellar signs, various degrees of confusion and obtundation, seizures, depression, personality changes, and frankly psychotic behavior. The electrocardiographic changes of hypomagnesemia differ from those of hypocalcemia and consist of ST-segment depression and flattened or inverted T waves in the precordial leads. Although these symptoms and signs have been described in magnesium-deficient experimental animals and in several human syndromes of apparently isolated magnesium depletion, in the usual clinical setting the relation between demonstrable hypomagnesemia and potentially related symptoms is often difficult to establish. The difficulties are two: (1) the poor quantitative relation and unpredictability with which symptoms accompany varying degrees of hypomagnesemia and (2) the frequency of hypokalemia, hypocalcemia, alkalosis, and other potentially symptomatic chemical abnormalities in many hypomagnesemic patients.[95,380]

Symptoms of hypomagnesemia do not usually occur at serum levels of magnesium above 1.5 mg/dl, and most patients with overt symptoms have serum magnesium concentrations below 1.0 mg/dl.[95,380] However, even at serum magnesium levels below 1.0 mg/dl, overt symptoms are not observed in all patients. In part, this poor quantitative relation may reflect the inaccurate assessment of tissue magnesium stores provided by the determination of serum magnesium, and some authorities recommend the measurement of erythrocyte magnesium content for this reason.

The mechanism(s) of the hypocalcemia frequently noted in severely hypomagnesemic patients has been discussed (see Other Acquired Forms of Functional Hypoparathyroidism, above). Hypokalemia is also common in these patients and results from both impaired renal tubular potassium reabsorption and soft-tissue wasting of potassium. The basis of these abnormalities in potassium transport is not clear, but it has been suggested that significant magnesium deficiency may lead to a generalized disorder of ion transport.[95] Alkalosis is variably noted in hypomagnesemic patients and predisposes to symptoms by virtue of its effects on serum ionized magnesium and calcium and perhaps also by potentiating the effects of reductions in ionized divalent cations on excitable tissues.[314]

In a given patient, therefore, neuromuscular symptoms depend on the sum of these various influences on neuromuscular excitability. In a patient with severe symptoms, abnormalities in serum magnesium, calcium, and electrolytes are usually treated simultaneously, and so the exact role of the hypomagnesemia is never entirely clear. With less severe and/or prolonged symptoms, a trial of magnesium replacement alone may be warranted.

DIAGNOSIS AND TREATMENT

Hypomagnesemia should be suspected in any patient with latent or overt symptoms in the clinical settings described above. Laboratory confirmation is provided by measures of the serum magnesium concentration and urinary magnesium excretion, expressed either as milligrams or milliequivalents per 24 h or as a fractional excretion (see appendix on Testing). More sophisticated measures, such as measurement of red cell or muscle biopsy magnesium content or of urinary magnesium retention following an intravenous magnesium infusion (the percent retention increases in magnesium deficiency), have been proposed, but each has associated technical problems and none has been uniformly accepted as a "gold standard" in the diagnosis of magnesium deficiency. Serum calcium, phosphorus, and electrolytes should be obtained in all magnesium-deficient patients. Urinary magnesium is low or undetectable in hypomagnesemic patients with chronic magnesium depletion or altered extracellular–soft-tissue magnesium distribution.

Overt symptoms should be treated with parenteral magnesium administration. Magnesium sulfate is the most widely used preparation and is available in aqueous solutions of 10, 25, and 50 percent [containing 98 mg (8.1 meq) elemental magnesium per gram of magnesium sulfate, $MgSO_4 \cdot 7H_2O$]. Intramuscular and intravenous administration are equally effective. Intramuscular injection is painful. Recommended initial doses are approximately 600 mg (48 meq) of elemental magnesium during the first 3 to 4 h, followed by a total of approximately 900 mg (72 meq) of elemental magnesium administered as 4-h divided intramuscular doses or as a continuous intravenous infusion throughout the remainder of the first day.[385] In emergent situations, a "loading dose" of approximately 500 mg (40 meq) of elemental magnesium may be administered intravenously, but the rate of administration should not exceed 15 mg/min. The quantity of magnesium administered on the second day approximates one-half of the total dose during the initial 24 h, and subsequent doses are determined empirically. The doses recommended above regularly achieve mean serum magnesium concentrations in the range of 2.5 to 3.5 mg/dl, and induced hypermagnesemia is avoided. Magnesium should be administered cautiously to patients with coincident renal impairment (see below). Magnesium acetate and other magnesium salts are equally effective.[385]

Chronic oral magnesium supplements may be useful in certain patients. Many antacids and laxatives contain magnesium, but these preparations are relatively inert and are variably absorbed. Preferred preparations are magnesium oxide and magnesium chloride in two or three divided doses as needed. Magnesium oxide contains approximately 60 percent elemental magnesium by weight, magnesium chloride approximately 25 percent, and magnesium sulfate as the hydrate approximately 10 percent. Oral magnesium replacement may be limited by the cathartic effects of magnesium, and patients with large magnesium requirements may have to receive chronic intramuscular magnesium therapy.

Hypermagnesemia

Clinically significant hypermagnesemia is rare. Magnesium retention accompanies progressive renal impairment, with statistical increases in serum magnesium concentrations being apparent at levels of glomerular filtration rate in the range of 20 ml/min.[95] However, because of the efficiency of the Tm-limited process in eliminating excessive magnesium and/or glomerulotubular adjustments, the fractional excretion of magnesium is increased in renal insufficiency; thus serum magnesium levels above 3 to 4 mg/dl are unusual. Patients with chronic renal insufficiency are intolerant of even small doses of magnesium, however, and magnesium-containing antacids, laxatives, and other preparations should be avoided in these patients. Hypermagnesemia is also noted during the oliguric phase of acute renal failure. Significant hypermagnesemia is rarely observed in nonazotemic patients consuming extraordinary doses of magnesium preparations[386] or following excessive parenteral magnesium administration, as may occur in eclamptic patients. Patients with familial hypocalciuric hypercalcemia, Addison's disease, and hypothryodism have a tendency toward hypermagnesemia, but the degree of hypermagnesemia is of no clinical consequence.

Pharmacological doses of magnesium lead to a curare-like impairment of neuromuscular transmission, accounting for the occasional previous use of parenteral magnesium as an anesthetic-anticonvulsant agent and its continued use in eclampsia.[95] Serum magnesium levels in the range of 6 to 12 mg/dl impair atrioventricular and intraventricular conduction and are associated with a prolonged PR interval and a widened QRS complex; extreme hypermagnesemia leads to asystole. Serum magnesium levels in the range of 12 to 18 mg/dl may produce muscular flaccidity and/or respiratory paralysis. The modest hypermagnesemia observed in chronic renal failure is not generally regarded as sufficient to account for central nervous system symptoms in these patients.[95]

In patients with extreme hypermagnesemia, with or without coincident renal failure, magnesium may be removed by dialysis against a magnesium-free dialysate. In patients intoxicated as a result of consumption of magnesium preparations, treatment consists simply of eliminating the source of exogenous magnesium.

TESTING

This section describes the collection and preservation of samples, calculations, and the performance of certain specialized tests in patients with disorders of mineral metabolism. Analytic details and normal ranges were presented in detail in Chemical and Biochemical Analyses Related to Mineral Metabolism.

Serum Chemistries

1. Calcium, phosphorus, magnesium, and alkaline phosphatase activity are measured in fresh serum. Serum calcium and phosphorus determinations *must* be performed in the fasting state. Spurious elevations in serum calcium are produced by venostasis and hemoconcentration, and spurious reductions and elevations in serum phosphorus levels result from prolonged standing of whole blood and hemolysis, respectively.
2. Most instruments currently available for the measurement of ionized calcium require heparinized blood or serum which is handled anaerobically and must be analyzed immediately. The quantity of heparin may be an important variable, and most laboratories have specific instructions for sample collection.

Urine Determinations

1. Twenty-four-hour urinary calcium, phosphorus, and magnesium may be collected into plain urine containers or into jugs containing 20 ml of 6 *N* HCl. Results are expressed as milligrams per day or as milligrams per kilogram of body weight per day. All three determinations are influenced by diet, and the interpretation of results for calcium excretion is particularly diet-dependent (Chap. 25).

2. Fasting calcium excretion is determined in a "spot" or timed specimen after a 12- to 15-h or overnight fast. Distilled water can be given to promote urine flow. Urinary calcium and creatinine and serum creatinine are determined simultaneously. Results are calculated and expressed as milligrams of calcium per 100 ml of glomerular filtrate (GF):

$$\begin{aligned} \text{Urine calcium} &= 10 \text{ mg/dl} \\ \text{Urine creatinine} &= 100 \text{ mg/dl} \\ \text{Serum creatinine} &= 0.8 \text{ mg/dl} \end{aligned}$$

$$\begin{aligned} \text{Fasting calcium excretion} &= \frac{U_{\text{Ca}}}{U_{\text{creat}}} \times S_{\text{creat}} \\ &= \frac{10}{100} \times 0.8 \\ &= 0.08 \text{ mg Ca/100 ml GF} \end{aligned}$$

3. Total hydroxyproline is measured in 24-h urine samples collected into 20 ml of 6 *N* HCl or into plain containers, with acidification of the sample at the time it is aliquoted. Results are expressed as milligrams per day. Patients should be on a diet containing limited amounts of meat and gelatin.

4. TmP/GFR is obtained from simultaneous measurements of serum and urinary phosphorus and creatinine in fasting early morning specimens, calculation of C_{P_i}/C_{creat} (or TRP), and use of a nomogram (see legend of Fig. 23-25):

$$\begin{aligned} \text{Urine phosphorus} &= 30 \text{ mg/dl} \\ \text{Urine creatinine} &= 60 \text{ mg/dl} \\ \text{Serum phosphorus} &= 2.5 \text{ mg/dl} \\ \text{Serum creatinine} &= 0.8 \text{ mg/dl} \end{aligned}$$

$$\begin{aligned} \frac{C_{P_i}}{C_{\text{creat}}} &= \frac{S_{\text{creat}} \times U_{P_i}}{S_{P_i} \times U_{\text{creat}}} \\ &= \frac{0.8 \times 30}{2.5 \times 60} = 0.16 \\ \frac{\text{TmP}}{\text{GFR}} &= 2.1 \text{ mg/dl} \quad \text{(from Fig. 23-25)} \\ \text{TRP} &= 1 - \frac{C_{P_i}}{C_{\text{creat}}} \\ &= 0.84 \\ \frac{\text{TmP}}{\text{GFR}} &= 2.1 \text{ mg/dl} \quad \text{(from Fig. 23-25)} \end{aligned}$$

5. Urinary magnesium may be expressed as milligrams or milliequivalents per 24 h or as the fractional excretion. The latter can be calculated as

$$\frac{U_{\text{Mg}}}{U_{\text{creat}}} \times \frac{S_{\text{creat}}}{S_{\text{Mg}}} \times 100 = \text{FE}_{\text{Mg}}$$

Magnesium concentration units may be either milligrams per deciliter or milliequivalents per liter as long as both serum and urine units are the same. The fractional excretion of a substance is the percentage of the filtered load of the substance which appears in the final urine, and the equation above can also be used to calculate the fractional excretion of calcium, using the measured value for serum ionized calcium. All fractional excretion determinations assume a steady state and must be performed in fasting patients, using spot or timed urine specimens. The normal limits for the fractional excretion of magnesium and calcium are less than 4 percent and less than 2.5 percent, respectively. Twenty-four-hour magnesium excretion is diet-dependent but is typically in the range of 100 mg (8 meq) per day.

Biochemical and Immunoassay Determinations

As emphasized in previous sections and demonstrated in patients with primary hyperparathyroidism in Fig. 23-36, the dietary calcium intake can have a marked influence on biochemical measurements of the PTH–1,25-$(OH)_2D$ axis in patients with a variety of disorders of mineral metabolism. This is particularly true for determinations which reflect circulating PTH bioactivity, such as nephrogenous cAMP and plasma 1,25-$(OH)_2D$.[112,123] It is imperative that attention be paid to antecedent calcium intake, and it is recommended that whenever possible biochemical measurements be performed on fasting specimens obtained from patients on a restricted (about 400 mg) calcium diet for 3 or more days. The dietary intake of phosphorus and sodium may also be important, but only limited data are available.

1. Immunoreactive PTH is usually determined in serum; heparin variably interferes with many assay systems. Most laboratories require that samples be collected on ice, centrifuged at 4°C, and stored frozen until assay. Results are reported in a variety of units, depending on the standards employed in the assay.

2. Immunoreactive calcitonin is determined in serum, processed as described above. Heparinized samples are satisfactory in certain assay systems. Results are reported as picograms per milliliter.

3. Total cAMP excretion may be determined in spot,

timed, or 24-h urine collections. Samples are collected into acid (1 ml of 6 *N* HCl per estimated hour of collection or a conventional catecholamine jug containing 20 ml of 6 *N* HCl for a 24-h collection). Fasting spot or timed specimens are preferable for differential diagnosis in hypercalcemic patients, and urine creatinine and serum calcium and creatinine are determined simultaneously. Results *must* be expressed as a function of the glomerular filtration rate (nanomoles per 100 ml GF):

$$\text{Urinary cAMP} = 4.0 \text{ nmol/ml } (\mu\text{mol per liter})$$
$$\text{Urinary creatinine} = 60 \text{ mg/dl } (0.6 \text{ mg/ml})$$
$$\text{Serum creatinine} = 0.8 \text{ mg/dl}$$

$$\text{Total urinary cAMP} = \frac{U_{\text{cAMP}}}{U_{\text{creat}}} \times S_{creat} = \frac{4.0}{0.6} \times 0.8 = 5.34 \text{ nmol/100 ml GF}$$

4. Nephrogenous cAMP is determined from values for plasma cAMP and results for total cAMP excretion, determined and expressed as described above. Blood is collected into an EDTA tube at room temperature (preferably lavender top vacutainer tubes containing EDTA in liquid form, in that solid EDTA may dissolve poorly). The patient should be unstressed and sitting or supine for 10 to 15 min prior to venipuncture. The blood sample is centrifuged at 1500 g (or full speed in a conventional tabletop clinical centrifuge) for 10 min, and the plasma is removed with care to leave the buffy coat undisturbed. Results are expressed as nanomoles per 100 ml GF:[94]

$$\text{Total cAMP excretion} = 5.34 \text{ nmol/100 ml GF}$$
$$\text{Plasma cAMP} = 15 \text{ nmol per liter } (1.5 \text{ nmol/100 ml})$$
$$\text{Nephrogenous cAMP} = \text{total cAMP excretion} - \text{filtered load of cAMP}^{*} = 5.34 - 1.5 = 3.84 \text{ nmol/100 ml GF}$$

5. All vitamin D metabolites are measured in serum or heparinized plasma. Results for calciferol, 25-OHD, and 24,25-$(OH)_2D$ are reported in units of nanograms per milliliter, and 1,25-$(OH)_2D$ is reported in units of picograms per milliliter. Some laboratories report values in molar units (see Vitamin D under Hormonal Measurements, above).

Testing for Pseudohypoparathyroidism

Preparations of parathyroid extract or synthetic PTH fragments are currently unavailable for testing in humans in the United States. The diagnosis of pseudohypoparathyroidism can usually be achieved quite simply by measuring serum immunoreactive PTH and/or by demonstrating an increase in circulating PTH together with a reduced value for nephrogenous cAMP or total cAMP excretion. It is hoped that a PTH preparation will become available for human use, and the classical tests for pseudohypoparathyroidism are described in detail below.

The Ellsworth-Howard test involves the administration of 200 USP units of purified PTH or parathyroid extract over 15 min, with the determination of phosphorus excretion in three 1-h control urine specimens and in three to four 1-h specimens collected after hormone administration. Patients should be fasting, supine except for voiding, and hydrated with 200 ml of distilled water hourly beginning 2 h before the control urine collections. Spontaneous and diurnal variations in phosphorus excretion may cause interpretive difficulties, and it is variously advised that patients be on a low (approximately 400 mg) phosphorus intake for 3 days prior to testing, that the test be performed in the midafternoon (when diurnal variation is minimized), that a control day without hormone administration be performed in each patient tested, and/or that the test be routinely validated in a control subject or patient with idiopathic hypoparathyroidism with each lot of commercial material employed.[311] Results are expressed as absolute or fold increase in phosphorus excretion (milligrams of phosphorus per hour or milligrams of phosphorus per milligram of creatinine) or as induced alterations in the various measures of renal tubular phosphorus handling. Normal individuals usually display a two- to fourfold, patients with idiopathic hypoparathyroidism a four- to tenfold, and patients with pseudohypoparathyroidism less than a twofold increase in phosphorus excretion.[311]

The protocol introduced by Chase, Melson, and Aurbach[330] involves the intravenous administration of 300 U purified PTH or parathyroid extract from 9 to 9:15 A.M., with the collection of one or more control urine specimens before 9 A.M. and experimental urine specimens from 9 to 9:30, 9:30 to 10, 10 to 11, and 11 to 12. Patients are fasting, supine except for voiding, and hydrated with 250 ml of distilled water hourly from 6 A.M. to noon. Results are expressed as nanomoles of cAMP per milligram of creatinine or, preferably, as nanomoles per 100 ml GF. It is recommended that each lot of hormone preparation be validated by testing in a normal individual. Responses in normal subjects and patients with pseudohypoparathyroidism and pseudopseudohypoparathyroidism were discussed above and are shown in Fig. 23-47.

Bone responsiveness to PTH is assessed by mea-

*Equivalent to the cAMP content in 100 ml of plasma.

suring the calcemic response to prolonged intramuscular or intravenous administration of the hormone. It is recommended that 600 U per day be administered for an initial 3-day period, followed by 900 to 1200 U per day for an additional 3-day period.[311] Normal subjects usually demonstrate approximately a 2-mg rise in serum calcium. Proportionately smaller doses are employed in pediatric patients.

Miscellaneous Determinations

Balance techniques and the various isotopic measures of intestinal calcium absorption are described in standard references. Performance of the oral calcium tolerance test is described in Chap. 25.

REFERENCES

1. Krane SM: Calcium, phosphate and magnesium, in Rasmussen H (ed): *International Encyclopedia of Pharmacology and Therapeutics.* Oxford, Pergamon Press, 1970, pp 19–59.
2. Rasmussen H, Bordier P: *The Physiologic and Cellular Basis of Metabolic Bone Disease.* Baltimore, Williams & Wilkins, 1974.
3. Humes HD: Regulation of intracellular calcium. *Semin Nephrol* 4:117, 1984.
4. Rasmussen H: Calcium messenger system. *N Engl J Med* 314:1094,1164, 1986.
5. Borle AB: Control, modulation and regulation of cell calcium. *Rev Physiol Biochem Pharmacol* 90:13, 1981.
6. McLean FC, Hastings AB: A biological method for the estimation of calcium ion concentration. *J Biol Chem* 107:337, 1934.
7. Marshall RW: Plasma fractions, in Nordin BEC (ed): *Calcium, Phosphate and Magnesium Metabolism.* London, Churchill Livingstone, 1976, pp 162–185.
8. Roth SI, Schiller AL: Comparative anatomy of the parathyroid glands, in Aurbach GD (ed): *Handbook of Physiology,* sec 7: *Endocrinology,* vol 7. Washington, D.C., American Physiological Society, 1976, pp 281–311.
9. Cohn DV, MacGregor RR: The biosynthesis, intracellular processing, and secretion of parathormone. *Endocr Rev* 2:1, 1981.
10. Potts JT, Kronenberg HM, Rosenblatt M: Parathyroid hormone: Chemistry, biosynthesis, and mode of action. *Adv Protein Chem* 35:323, 1982.
11. Vasicek TJ, McDevitt BE, Freeman MW, Fennick BJ, Hendy GH, Potts JT, Rich A, Kronenberg HM: Nucleotide sequence of the human parathyroid hormone gene. *Proc Natl Acad Sci USA* 80:2127, 1983.
12. Habener JF, Rosenblatt M, Potts JT: Parathyroid hormone: Biochemical aspects of biosynthesis, secretion, action, and metabolism. *Physiol Rev* 64:985, 1984.
13. Horiuchi N, Holick MF, Potts JT, Rosenblatt M: A parathyroid hormone inhibitor *in vivo:* Design and biological evaluation of a hormone analog. *Science* 220:1053, 1983.
14. Majzoub JA, Kronenberg HM, Potts JT, Rich A, Habener JF: Identification and cell-free translation of mRNA coding for a precursor of parathyroid secretory protein. *J Biol Chem* 254:7449, 1979.
15. Cohn DV, Zangerle R, Fisher-Colbrie R, Chu LLH, Elting JS, Hamilton JW, Winkler H: Similarity of secretory protein I from parathyroid gland to chromogranin A from adrenal medulla. *Proc Natl Acad Sci USA* 79:6056, 1982.
16. Copp DH: Parathyroids, calcitonin and control of plasma calcium. *Recent Prog Horm Res* 20:59, 1964.
17. Brown EM: Four-parameter model of the sigmoidal relationship between parathyroid hormone release and extracellular calcium concentration in normal and abnormal parathyroid tissue. *J Clin Endocrinol Metab* 56:572, 1983.
18. Habener JF, Potts JT: Relative effectiveness of magnesium and calcium on the secretion and biosynthesis of parathyroid hormone in vitro. *Endocrinology* 98:197, 1976.
19. Rodriguez HJ, Morrison A, Slatopolsky E, Klahr S: Adenylate cyclase of human parathyroid gland. *J Clin Endocrinol Metab* 47:319, 1978.
20. Brown EM, Hurwitz S, Aurbach GD, Woodard CJ: Direct identification of beta adrenergic receptors on isolated bovine parathyroid cells. *Endocrinology* 100:1703, 1977.
21. Blum JW, Fischer JA, Hunziker WH, Binswanger U, Picotti GB, Da Prada M, Guillebeau A: Parathyroid hormone responses to catecholamines and to changes in extracellular calcium in cows. *J Clin Invest* 61:1113, 1978.
22. Kukreja SC, Hargis GK, Bowser EN, Henderson WJ, Fisherman EW, Williams GA: Role of adrenergic stimuli in parathyroid secretion in man. *J Clin Endocrinol Metab* 40:478, 1978.
23. Brumbaugh PF, Hughes MR, Haussler MR: Cytoplasmic and nuclear binding components for 1,25-dihydroxyvitamin D_3 in chick parathyroid glands. *Proc Natl Acad Sci USA* 72:4871, 1975.
24. Canterbury JM, Lerman S, Claflin AJ, Henry H, Norman A, Reiss E: Inhibition of parathyroid hormone secretion by 25-hydroxycholecalciferol and 24,25-dihydroxycholecalciferol in the dog. *J Clin Invest* 61:1375, 1978.
25. Madsen S, Olgaard K, Ladefoged J: Suppressive effect of 1,25-dihydroxyvitamin D_3 on circulating parathyroid hormone in acute renal failure. *J Clin Endocrinol Metab* 53:823, 1981.
26. Oldman SB, Fischer JA, Shen LH, Arnaud CD: Isolation and properties of a calcium-binding protein from porcine parathyroid glands. *Biochemistry* 13:4790, 1974.
27. Russell J, Lettieri D, Sherwood LM: Direct regulation by calcium of cytoplasmic messenger ribonucleic acid coding for preproparathyroid hormone in isolated bovine parathyroid cells. *J Clin Invest* 72:1851, 1983.
28. Brown EM, Dawson-Hughes BF, Wilson RE, Adragna N: Calmodulin in dispersed human parathyroid cells. *J Clin Endocrinol Metab* 53:1064, 1981.
29. Berson SA, Yalow RS: Immunochemical heterogeneity of parathyroid hormone in plasma. *J Clin Endocrinol Metab* 28:1037, 1968.
30. Martin KJ, Hruska KA, Freitag JJ, Klahr S, Slatopolsky E: The peripheral metabolism of parathyroid hormone. *N Engl J Med* 301:1092, 1979.
31. Marx SJ, Sharp ME, Krudy A, Rosenblatt M, Mallette LE: Radioimmunoassay for the middle region of human parathyroid hormone: Studies with a radioiodinated synthetic peptide. *J Clin Endocrinol Metab* 53:76, 1981.
32. Segre GV, Niall HD, Habener JF, Potts JT: Metabolism of parathyroid hormone. Physiologic and clinical significance. *Am J Med* 56:774, 1974.
33. Bringhurst FR, Segre GV, Lampman GW, Potts JT: Metabolism of parathyroid hormone by Kupffer cells: Analysis by reverse-phase high-performance liquid chromatography. *Biochemistry* 21:4252, 1982.
34. Goltzman D: Examination of the requirement of metabolism of parathyroid hormone in skeletal tissue before biological action. *Endocrinology* 102:1555, 1978.
35. Robinson CJ: The physiology of parathyroid hormone. *Clin Endocrinol Metab* 3:389, 1974.
36. Raisz LG, Kream BE: Regulation of bone formation. *N Engl J Med* 309:29, 83, 1983.
37. Meunier PJ, Bressot C: Endocrine influences on bone cells and

bone remodeling evaluated by clinical histomorphometry, in Parsons JA (ed): *Endocrinology of Calcium Metabolism.* New York, Raven Press, 1982, pp 445–465.

38. Mundy GR: Monocyte-macrophage system and bone resorption. *Lab Invest* 49:119, 1983.

39. Provvedini DM, Tsoukas CD, Deftos LJ, Manolagas SC: 1,25-dihydroxyvitamin D_3 receptors in human leukocytes. *Science* 221: 1181, 1983.

40. Rodan GA, Martin TJ: Role of osteoblasts in the hormonal control of bone resorption—a hypothesis. *Calcif Tissue Int* 33:349, 1981.

41. Wong G: Paracrine interactions in bone-secreted products of osteoblasts permit osteoclasts to respond to parathyroid hormone. *J Biol Chem* 259:4019, 1984.

42. Bijvoet OLM: Kidney function in calcium and phosphate metabolism, in Avioli LV, Krane SM (eds): *Metabolic Bone Disease,* vol. 1. New York, Academic Press, 1977, pp 49–140.

43. Knox FG, Osswald H, Marchand GR, Spielman WS, Haas JA, Berndt T, Youngberg SP: Phosphate transport along the nephron. *Am J Physiol* 233:F261, 1977.

44. Mizgala CL, Quamme GA: Renal handling of phosphate. *Physiol Rev* 65:431, 1985.

45. Chase LR, Aurbach GD: Parathyroid function and the renal excretion of 3′,5′-adenylic acid. *Proc Natl Acad Sci USA* 58:518, 1967.

46. Morel F: Sites of hormone action in the mammalian nephron. *Am J Physiol* 240:F159, 1981.

47. Kinne R, Shlatz LJ, Kinne-Saffran E, Schwartz IL: Distribution of membrane-bound cyclic AMP-dependent protein kinase in plasma membranes of the kidney cortex. *J Membr Biol* 24:145, 1975.

48. Agus ZS, Chiu PJS, Goldberg M: Regulation of urinary calcium excretion in the rat. *Am J Physiol* 232:F545, 1977.

49. Sutton RAL, Dirks JH: Renal handling of calcium. *Fed Proc* 37:2112, 1978.

50. Suki WN: Calcium transport in the nephron. *Am J Physiol* 237:F1, 1979

51. Ng RCK, Rouse D, Suki WN: Calcium transport in the rabbit superficial proximal convoluted tubule. *J Clin Invest* 74:834, 1984.

52. Talmadge RV, Kraintz FW: Progressive changes in renal phosphate and calcium excretion in rats following parathyroidectomy or parathyroid administration. *Proc Soc Exp Biol Med* 87:263, 1954.

53. Nordin BEC, Peacock M: Role of kidney in regulation of plasma calcium. *Lancet* ii:1280, 1969.

54. Foster GV, Byfield PGH, Gudmundsson TV: Calcitonin. *Clin Endocrinol Metab* 1:93, 1972.

55. Munson PL: Physiology and pharmacology of thyrocalcitonin, in Aurbach GD (ed): *Handbook of Physiology,* sec 7: *Endocrinology,* vol 7. Washington, D.C., American Physiological Society, 1976, pp 443–464.

56. Austin LA, Heath H: Calcitonin physiology and pathophysiology. *N Engl J Med* 304:269, 1981.

57. Amara SG, Jonas V, Rosenfeld MG, Ong EJ, Evans RM: Alternative RNA processing in calcitonin gene expression generates mRNAs encoding different polypeptide products. *Nature* 298:240, 1982.

58. Steenbergh PH, Hoppener JWM, Zandberg J, Van De Ven WJM, Jansz HS, Lips CJM: Calcitonin gene related peptide coding sequence is conserved in the human genome and is expressed in medullary carcinoma of the thyroid. *J Clin Endocrinol Metab* 59:358, 1984.

59. Morris HR, Panico M, Etienne T, Tippins J, Girgis SI, MacIntyre I: Isolation and characterization of human calcitonin gene-related peptide. *Nature* 308:746, 1984.

60. Birnbaum RS, O'Neil JA, Muszynski M, Aron DC, Roos BA: A noncalcitonin secretory peptide derived from preprocalcitonin. *J Biol Chem* 257:241, 1982.

61. Roos BA, Huber B, Birnbaum RS, Aron DC, Lindall AW, Lips K, Baylin SB: Medullary thyroid carcinomas secrete a noncalcitonin peptide corresponding to the carboxy-terminal region of preprocalcitonin. *J Clin Endocrinol Metab* 56:802, 1983.

62. Hillyard CJ, Myers C, Abeysekera G, Stevenson JC, Craig RK, MacIntyre I: Katacalcin: Measurement in man of a calcium-lowering hormone. *Lancet* i:846, 1983.

63. Tschopp FA, Henke H, Petermann JB, Tobler PH, Janzer R, Hokfelt T, Lundberg JM, Cuello C, Fischer JA: Calcitonin gene-related peptide and its binding sites in the human central nervous system and pituitary. *Proc Natl Acad Sci USA* 82:248, 1985.

64. Cooper CW, Bolman RM, Linehan WM, Wells SA: Interrelationships between calcium, calcemic hormones and gastrointestinal hormones. *Recent Prog Horm Res* 34:259, 1978.

65. Body JJ, Heath H: Estimates of circulating monomeric calcitonin: Physiological studies in normal and thyroidectomized man. *J Clin Endocrinol Metab* 57:897, 1983.

66. Goltzman D, Tischler AS: Characterization of the immunochemical forms of calcitonin released by a medullary thyroid carcinoma in tissue culture. *J Clin Invest* 61:449, 1978.

67. Tashjian AH, Wright DR, Ivey SL, Pont A: Calcitonin binding sites in bone: Relationships to biological response and escape. *Recent Prog Horm Res* 34:285, 1978.

68. Deftos LJ, Weisman MH, Williams GW, Karpf DB, Frumar AM, Davidson BJ, Parthemore JG, Judd HL: Influence of age and sex on plasma calcitonin in human beings. *N Engl J Med* 302:1351, 1980.

69. DeLuca HF, Schnoes HK: Vitamin D: Recent advances. *Annu Rev Biochem* 52:411, 1983.

70. Norman AW, Roth J, Orci L: The vitamin D endocrine system: Steroid metabolism, hormone receptors, and biological response. *Endocr Rev* 3:331, 1982.

71. Haussler MR, McCain TA: Basic and clinical concepts related to vitamin D metabolism and action. *N Engl J Med* 297:974, 1977.

72. Holick MF, MacLaughlin JA, Doppelt SA: Factors that influence the cutaneous photosynthesis of previtamin D_3. *Science* 211:590, 1981.

73. Haddad JG: Nature and functions of the plasma binding protein for vitamin D and its metabolites, in Kumar R (ed): *Vitamin D: Basic and Clinical Aspects.* Boston, Martinus Nijhoff, 1984, pp. 383-396.

74. Korkor A, Schwartz J, Bergfeld M, Teitelbaum S, Avioli L, Klahr S, Slatopolsky E: Absence of metabolic bone disease in adult patients with the nephrotic syndrome and normal renal function. *J Clin Endocrinol Metab* 56:496, 1983.

75. Bouillon R, Auwerx J, Dekeyser L, Fevery J, Lissens W, DeMoor P: Serum vitamin D metabolites and their binding protein in patients with liver cirrhosis. *J Clin Endocrinol Metab* 59:86, 1984.

76. Bell NH: Vitamin D-endocrine system. *J Clin Invest* 76:1, 1985.

77. Kumar R: Metabolism of 1,25-dihydroxyvitamin D_3. *Physiol Rev* 64:478, 1984.

78. Insogna KL, Broadus AE, Dreyer BE, Ellison AF, Gertner JM: Elevated production rate for 1,25-dihydroxyvitamin D in patients with absorptive hypercalciuria. *J Clin Endocrinol Metab* 61:490, 1985.

79. Kawashima H, Torikai S, Kurokawa K: Localization of 25-hydroxyvitamin D_3 1 α-hydroxylase and 24-hydroxylase along the rat nephron. *Proc Natl Acad Sci USA* 78:1199, 1981.

80. Lambert PW, Stern PH, Avioli RC, Brackett NC, Turner RT, Greene A, Fu IY, Bell NH: Evidence for extrarenal production of 1,25-dihydroxyvitamin D in man. *J Clin Invest* 69:722, 1982.

81. Adams ND, Gray RW, Lemann J: The effects of oral $CaCO_3$ loading and dietary calcium deprivation on plasma 1,25-dihydroxyvitamin D concentrations in healthy adults. *J Clin Endocrinol Metab* 48:1008, 1979.

82. Insogna KL, Broadus AE, Gertner JM: Impaired phosphorus

conservation and 1,25 dihydroxyvitamin D generation during phosphorus deprivation in familial hypophosphatemic rickets. *J Clin Invest* 71:1562, 1983.
83. Portale AA, Halloran BP, Murphy MM, Morris RC: Oral intake of phosphorus can determine the serum concentration of 1,25-dihydroxyvitamin D by determining its production rate in humans. *J Clin Invest* 77:7, 1986.
84. Portale AA, Booth BE, Halloran BP, Morris RC: Effect of dietary phosphorus on circulating concentrations of 1,25-dihydroxyvitamin D and immunoreactive parathyroid hormone in children with moderate renal insufficiency. *J Clin Invest* 73:1580, 1984.
85. Gray TK, Lowe W, Lester GE: Vitamin D and pregnancy: The maternal-fetal metabolism of vitamin D. *Endocr Rev* 2:264, 1981.
86. Gertner JM, Coustan DR, Kliger AS, Mallette LE, Ravin N, Broadus AE: Pregnancy is a state of physiological absorptive hypercalciuria *Am J Med* 81:451, 1986.
87. Delvin EE, Arabian A, Glorieux FH, Mamer OA: In vitro metabolism of 25-hydroxycholecalciferol by isolated cells from human decidua. *J Clin Endocrinol Metab* 60:880, 1985.
88. Wilkinson R: Absorption of calcium, phosphorus and magnesium, in Nordin BEC (ed): *Calcium, Phosphate and Magnesium Metabolism.* London, Churchill Livingstone, 1976, pp 36–112.
89. Wasserman RH: Intestinal absorption of calcium and phosphorus. *Fed Proc* 40:68, 1981.
90. Matsumoto T, Fontaine O, Rasmussen H: Effect of 1,25-dihydroxyvitamin D on phospholipid metabolism in chick duodenal mucosal cell. *J Biol Chem* 256:3354, 1981.
91. Rasmussen H, Bordier P: Vitamin D and bone. *Metab Bone Dis Relat Res* 1:7, 1978.
92. Bonjour JP, Preston C, Fleish H: Effect of 1,25-dihydroxyvitamin D_3 on the renal handling of P_i in thyroparathyroidectomized rats. *J Clin Invest* 60:1419, 1977.
93. Yamamoto M, Kawanobe Y, Takahashi H, Shimazawa E, Kimura S, Ogata E: Vitamin D deficiency and renal calcium transport in the rat. *J Clin Invest* 74:507, 1984.
94. Broadus AE: Nephrogenous cyclic AMP. *Recent Prog Horm Res* 37:667, 1981.
95. Wacker WEC, Parisi AF: Magnesium metabolism. *N Engl J Med* 278:658, 712, 772, 1968.
96. Agus ZS, Wasserstein A, Goldfarb S: Disorders of calcium and magnesium homeostasis. *Am J Med* 72:473, 1982.
97. Dirks JH: The kidney and magnesium regulation. *Kidney Int* 23:771, 1983.
98. Brannon PG, Vergene-Marini P, Pak CYC, Hull AR, Fordtran JS: Magnesium absorption in the human small intestine. *J Clin Invest* 57:1412, 1976.
99. Petith MM, Schedl HP: Effects of magnesium deficiency on duodenal and magnesium absorption and secretion. *Dig Dis Sci* 1:1, 1978.
100. Krejs GJ, Nicar MJ, Zerwekh JE, Norman DA, Kane MG, Pak CYC: Effect of 1,25 dihydroxyvitamin D_3 on calcium and magnesium absorption in the healthy human jejunum and ileum. *Am J Med* 75:973, 1983.
101. Shils ME: Experimental human magnesium depletion. *Medicine (Baltimore)* 48:61, 1969.
102. Rude RK, Bethune JE, Singer FR: Renal tubular maximum for magnesium in normal, hyperparathyroid and hypoparathyroid man. *J Clin Endocrinol Metab* 51:1425, 1980.
103. Keating FR, Jones JD, Elveback CR, Randall RV: The relation of age and sex to distribution of values in healthy adults of serum calcium, inorganic phosphorus, magnesium, alkaline phosphatase, total proteins, albumin, and blood urea. *J Lab Clin Med* 73:825, 1969.
104. Ladenson JH, Lewis JW, Boyd JC: Failure of total calcium corrected for protein, albumin, and pH to correctly assess free calcium status. *J Clin Endocrinol Metab* 46:986, 1978.
105. Posen S, Cornish C, Kleerekoper M: Alkaline phosphatase and metabolic bone disorders, in Avioli LV, Krane SM (eds): *Metabolic Bone Disease.* New York, Academic Press, 1977, vol. 1, pp 141–181.
106. Fischer JA: Parathyroid hormone, in Bronner F, Coburn JW (eds): *Disorders of Mineral Metabolism.* New York, Academic Press, 1982, vol. 2 pp 272–358.
107. Chost IN, Steinberg SF, Tropper PJ, Fox HE, Segre GV, Bilizekian JP: The influence of hypermagnesemia on serum calcium and parathyroid hormone levels in human subjects. *N Engl J Med* 310:1221, 1984.
108. European PTH Study Group: Interlaboratory comparison of radioimmunological parathyroid hormone determination. *Eur J Clin Invest* 8:149, 1978.
109. Zanelli IM, Gaines-Das RE: The first international reference preparation of human parathyroid hormone for immunoassay: Characterization and calibration by international collaborative study. *J Clin Endocrinol Metab* 57:462, 1983.
110. Raisz LG, Yajnik CH, Bockman RS, Bower BF: Comparison of commercially available parathyroid hormone immunoassays in the differential diagnosis of hypercalcemia due to primary hyperparathyroidism or malignancy. *Ann Intern Med* 91:739, 1979.
111. Marcus R, Madvig P, Young G: Age-related changes in parathyroid hormone and parathyroid hormone action in normal humans. *J Clin Endocrinol Metab* 58:223, 1984.
112. Insogna KL, Mitnick ME, Stewart AF, Burtis WJ, Mallette LE, Broadus AE: Sensitivity of the parathyroid hormone—1,25 dihydroxyvitamin D axis to variations in calcium intake in patients with primary hyperparathyroidism. *N Engl J Med* 313:1126, 1985.
113. Chambers DJ, Dunham J, Zanelli JM, Parsons JA, Bitensky L, Chaven J: A sensitive bioassay of parathyroid hormone in plasma. *Clin Endocrinol (Oxf)* 9:375, 1978.
114. Goltzman D, Henderson B, Loveridge N: Cytochemical bioassay of parathyroid hormone. *J Clin Invest* 65:1309, 1980.
115. Parthemore JG, Deftos LJ: Calcitonin secretion in primary hyperparathyroidism. *J Clin Endocrinol Metab* 49:223, 1979.
116. Horst RL, Shepart RM, Jorgensen NA, DeLuca HF: The determination of the vitamin D metabolites on a single plasma sample: Changes during parturition in dairy cows. *Arch Biochem Biophys* 192:512, 1979.
117. Eisman JA, Hamstra AJ, Kream BE, DeLuca HF: 1,25-Dihydroxyvitamin D in biological fluids: A simplified and sensitive assay. *Science* 193:1021, 1976.
118. Stern PH, Hamstra AJ, DeLuca HF, Bell NH: A bioassay capable of measuring 1 picogram of 1,25-dihydroxyvitamin D_3. *J Clin Endocrinol Metab* 46:891, 1978.
119. Clemens TL, Hendy GN, Papapoulos SE, Fraher LJ, Care AD, O'Riordan JLH: Measurement of 1,25-dihydroxycholecalciferol in man by radioimmunoassay. *Clin Endocrinol (Oxf)* 11:225, 1979.
120. Reinhardt TA, Horst RL, Orf JW, Hollis BW: A microassay for 1,25-dihydroxyvitamin D not requiring high performance liquid chromatography: Application to clinical studies. *J Clin Endocrinol Metab* 58:91, 1984.
121. Manolagas SC, Culler FL, Howard JE, Brickman AS, Deftos JH: The cytoreceptor assay for 1,25-dihydroxyvitamin D and its application to clinical studies. *J Clin Endocrinol Metab* 56:751, 1983.
122. Halloran BP, Portale AA, Castro M, Morris RC, Goldsmith RS: Serum concentration of 1,25-dihydroxyvitamin D in the human: Diurnal variation. *J Clin Endocrinol Metab* 60:1104, 1985.
123. Broadus AE, Insogna KL, Lang R, Ellison AF, Dreyer BE: Evidence for disordered control of 1,25-dihydroxyvitamin D production in absorptive hypercalciuria. *N Engl J Med* 311:73, 1984.
124. Gray RW, Adams ND, Caldas AE, Lemann J: The effects of dihydrotachysterol therapy on the measurement of plasma 1,25-$(OH)_2D$-vitamin D in humans. *J Lab Clin Med* 93:1031, 1979.
125. Albright F: A page out of the history of hyperparathyroidism. *J Clin Endocrinol Metab* 8:637, 1948.
126. Dent CE: Some problems of hyperparathyroidism. *Br Med J* 2:1419, 1495, 1962.

127. Heath H, Hodgson SF, Kennedy MA: Primary hyperparathyroidism: Incidence, morbidity and potential economic impact in a community. *N Engl J Med* 302:189, 1980.
128. Mundy GR, Cove DH, Fisken R: Primary hyperparathyroidism: Changes in the pattern of clinical presentation. *Lancet* i:1317, 1980.
129. Habener JF, Potts JT: Parathyroid physiology and primary hyperparathyroidism, in Avioli LV, Krane SM (eds): *Metabolic Bone Disease.* New York, Academic Press, 1978, vol. 2, pp 1–147.
130. Roth SI: Recent advances in parathyroid gland pathology. *Am J Med* 50:612, 1971.
131. Russell CF, Grant SC, van Heerden JA: Hyperfunctioning supernumerary parathyroid glands. *Mayo Clin Proc* 57:121, 1982.
132. Lloyd HM: Primary hyperparathyroidism: An analysis of the role of the parathyroid tumor. *Medicine (Baltimore)* 47:53, 1968.
133. Purnell DC, Smith LH, Scholz DA, Elveback LR, Arnaud CD: Primary hyperparathyroidism: a prospective clinical study. *Am J Med* 50:670, 1971
134. Mallette LE, Bilezikian JP, Heath DA, Aurbach DG: Primary hyperparathyroidism: Clinical and biochemical features. *Medicine (Baltimore)* 53:127, 1974.
135. Schantz A, Castleman B: Parathyroid carcinoma. *Cancer* 31:600, 1973.
136. Shane E, Bilezikian JP: Parathyroid carcinoma: A review of 62 patients. *Endocr Rev* 3:218, 1982.
137. Jackson CE, Cerny JC, Block MA, Fialkow PJ: Probable clonal origin of aldosteronomas versus multicellular origin of parathyroid adenomas. *Surgery* 92:875, 1982.
138. Rao SD, Frame B, Miller MJ, Kleerekoper M, Block MA, Parfitt AM: Hyperparathyroidism following head and neck irradiation. *Arch Intern Med* 140:205, 1980.
139. Broadus AE: Nephrolithiasis in primary hyperparathyroidism, in Coe FL, Brenner BM, Stein JH (eds): *Contemporary Issues in Nephrology.* Edinburgh, Churchill Livingstone, 1980, vol. 5, pp 59–85.
140. Parks J, Coe F, Favus M: Hyperparathyroidism in nephrolithiasis. *Arch Intern Med* 140:1479, 1980.
141. Broadus AE, Horst RL, Lang R, Littledike ET, Rasmussen H: The importance of circulating 1,25-dihydroxyvitamin D in the pathogenesis of hypercalciuria and renal stone formation in primary hyperparathyroidism. *N Engl J Med* 302:421, 1980.
142. Pak CYC, Nicar MJ, Peterson R, Zerwekh JE, Synder W: A lack of unique pathophysiologic background for nephrolithiasis of primary hyperparathyroidism. *J Clin Endocrinol Metab* 53:536, 1981.
143. Coe FL: Magnitude of metabolic acidosis in primary hyperparathyroidism. *Arch Intern Med* 134:262, 1974.
144. Pak CYC, Holt K: Nucleation and growth of brushite and calcium oxalate in urine of stone formers. *Metabolism* 25:665, 1976.
145. Peacock M: Renal stone disease and bone disease in primary hyperparathyroidism and their relationship to the action of parathyroid hormone on calcium absorption, in Talmage RV, Owen M, Parsons JA (eds): *Calcium Regulating Hormones.* Amsterdam, Excerpta Medica, 1975, pp 78–81.
146. Jensen PS, Klinger AS: Early radiographic manifestations of secondary hyperparathyroidism associated with chronic renal disease. *Radiology* 125:645, 1977.
147. Bordier C, Arnaud C, Hawker C, Tun-Chot S, Hioco D: Relationship between serum immunoreactive parathyroid hormone, osteoclastic and osteocytic bone resorptions and serum calcium in primary hyperparathyroidism and osteomalacia. *Excerpta Med Int Congr Ser* 270:222, 1970.
148. Genant HK, Heck LL, Lanzl LH, Rossman K, Vander Horst J, Paloyan E: Primary hyperparathyroidism: A comprehensive study of clinical, biochemical, and radiological manifestations. *Radiology* 109:513, 1973.
149. Pak CYC, Stewart A, Kaplan R, Bone H, Notz C, Browne R: Photon absorptiometric analysis of bone density in primary hyperparathyroidism. *Lancet* ii:7, 1975.
150. Dalen N, Hjern B: Bone mineral content in patients with primary hyperparathyroidism without radiologic evidence of skeletal changes. *Acta Endocrinol (Copenh)* 75:297, 1974.
151. Seeman E, Walner HW, Offord KP, Kumar R, Johnson WJ, Riggs BL: Differential effects of endocrine dysfunction on the axial and appendicular skeleton. *J Clin Invest* 69:1302, 1982.
152. Meunier P, Vignon G, Bernard J, Edouard C, Courpron P: Quantitative bone histology as applied to the diagnosis of hyperparathyroid states, in Frame B, Parfitt AM, Duncan H (eds): *Clinical Aspects of Metabolic Bone Disease.* Amsterdam, Exerpta Medica, 1973, pp 215–221.
153. Charhon SA, Edouard CM, Arlot ME, Meunier PJ: Effects of parathyroid hormone on remodeling of iliac trabecular bone packets in patients with primary hyperparathyroidism. *Clin Orthop* 162:255, 1982.
154. Tam CS, Bayley A, Cross EG, Murray TM, Harrison JE: Increased bone apposition in primary hyperparathyroidism: Measurements based on short internal tetracycline labeling of bone. *Metabolism* 31:759, 1982.
155. Vicale CT: Diagnostic features of muscular syndrome resulting from hyperparathyroidism, osteomalacia owing to renal tubular acidosis and perhaps to related disorders of calcium metabolism. *Trans Am Neurol Assoc* 74:143, 1949.
156. Patten BM, Bilezikian JP, Mallette LE, Prince A, Engel WK, Aurbach GD: Neuromuscular disease in primary hyperparathyroidism. *Ann Intern Med* 80:182, 1974.
157. Barreras RF: Calcium and gastric secretion. *Gastroenterology* 64:1168, 1973.
158. Ostrow JD, Blandshard G, Gray SJ: Peptic ulcer in primary hyperparathyroidism. *Am J Med* 24:769, 1960.
159. Wilson SD, Singh RB, Kalkhoff RK, Go VLW: Does hyperparathyroidism cause hypergastrinemia? *Surgery* 80:231, 1976.
160. Mixter CG, Keynes WM, Chir M, Cope O: Further experience with pancreatitis as a diagnostic clue to hyperparathyroidism. *N Engl J Med* 266:265, 1962.
161. Ljunghall S, Palmer M, Akerstrom G, Wide L: Diabetes mellitus, glucose tolerance and insulin response to glucose in patients with primary hyperparathyroidism before and after parathyroidectomy. *Eur J Clin Invest* 13:373, 1983.
162. Selle JG, Altemeier WA, Fullen WD, Goldsmith RE: Cholelithiasis in hyperparathyroidism. *Arch Surg* 105:369, 1972.
163. Scholz DA: Hypertension and hyperparathyroidism. *Arch Intern Med* 137:1123, 1977.
164. Hellstrom J, Birke G, Edvall CA: Hypertension in hyperparathyroidism. *Br J Urol* 30:13, 1958.
165. Bilezikian JP, Connor TB, Aptekar R, Freijanes J, Aurbach GD, Pachas WN, Wells SA, Decker JL: Pseudogout after parathyroidectomy. *Lancet* i:445, 1973.
166. Yeager RM, Krementz ET: Acute hyperparathyroidism. *South Med J* 64:797, 1971.
167. Broadus AE, Hanson TAS, Bartter FC, Walton J: Primary hyperparathyroidism presenting as anticonvulsant-induced osteomalacia. *Am J Med* 63:298, 1977.
168. Broadus AE, Horst RL, Littledike ET, Mahaffey JE, Rasmussen H: Primary hyperparathyroidism with intermittent hypercalcemia: Serial observations and simple diagnosis by means of an oral calcium tolerance test. *Clin Endocrinol (Oxf)* 12:225, 1980.
169. Delmonico FL, Neer RM, Cosimi AB, Barnes AB, Russell PS: Hyperparathyroidism during pregnancy. *Am J Surg* 131:328, 1976.
170. Tsang RC, Donovan EF, Steichen JJ: Calcium physiology and pathology in the neonate. *Pediatr Clin North Am* 23:611, 1976.
171. Avioli LV: Renal osteodystrophy, in Avioli LV, Krane SM (eds): *Metabolic Bone Disease.* New York, Academic Press, 1978, vol. 2, pp 149–215.
172. Wermer P: Genetic aspects of adenomatosis of endocrine glands. *Am J Med* 16:363, 1954.
173. Hershon KS, Kelly WA, Shaw CM, Schwartz R, Bierman EL:

Prolactinomas as part of the multiple endocrine neoplastic syndrome type 1. *Am J Med* 74:713, 1983.
174. Oberg K, Walinder O, Bostrom H, Lundqvist G, Wide L: Peptide hormone markers in screening for endocrine tumors in multiple endocrine adenomatosis type 1. *Am J Med* 73:619, 1982.
175. Jensen RT, Gardner JD, Raufman JP, Pandol SJ, Doppman JL, Collen MJ: Zollinger-Ellison syndrome: Current concepts and management. *Ann Intern Med* 98:59, 1983.
176. Lamers CBHW, Froeling PGAM: Clinical significance of hyperparathyroidism in familial multiple endocrine adenomatosis type 1. *Am J Med* 66:422, 1979.
177. Keiser HR, Beaven MA, Doppman J, Wells S, Buja LM: Sipple's syndrome: Medullary thyroid carcinoma, pheochromocytoma, and parathyroid disease. *Ann Intern Med* 78:561, 1973.
178. Sizemore GW, Heath H, Carney JA: Multiple endocrine neoplasia type 2. *Clin Endocrinol Metab* 9:299, 1980.
179. Khairi MR, Dexter RN, Burzynski NJ, Johnston CC: Mucosal neuroma, pheochromocytoma and medullary thyroid carcinoma: Multiple endocrine neoplasia type 3. *Medicine (Baltimore)* 54:89, 1975.
180. Carney JA, Sizemore GW, Hayles AB: Multiple endocrine neoplasia, type 2b. *Pathobiol Annu* 8:105, 1978.
181. Goldsmith RE, Sizemore GW, Chen IW, Zalme E, Altemeier WA: Familial hyperparathyroidism. *Ann Intern Med* 84:36, 1976.
182. Law WM, Hodgson SF, Heath H: Autosomal recessive inheritance of familial hyperparathyroidism. *N Engl J Med* 309:650, 1983.
183. Marx SJ, Spiegel AM, Levine MA, Rizzoli RE, Lasker RD, Santora AC, Downs RW, Aurbach GD: Familial hypocalciuric hypercalcemia. *N Engl J Med* 307:416, 1982.
184. Marx SJ, Attie MF, Levine MA, Spiegel AM, Downs RW, Lasker RD: The hypocalciuric or benign variant of familial hypercalcemia: Clinical and biochemical features in fifteen kindreds. *Medicine (Baltimore)* 60:397, 1981.
185. Law WM, Heath H: Familial benign hypercalcemia (hypocalciuric hypercalcemia). *Ann Intern Med* 102:511, 1985.
186. Law WM, Carney JA, Heath H: Parathyroid glands in familial benign hypercalcemia (familial hypocalciuric hypercalcemia). *Am J Med* 76:1021, 1984.
187. Attie MF, Stock JL, Spiegel AM, Downs RW, Levine MA, Marx SJ: Urinary calcium excretion in familial hypocalciuric hypercalcemia. *J Clin Invest* 72:667, 1983.
188. Palmer FJ, Nelson JC, Bacchus H: The chloride-phosphate ratio in hypercalcemia. *Ann Intern Med* 80:200, 1974.
189. Pak CYC, Townsend J: Chloride-phosphorus in primary hyperparathyroidism. *Ann Intern Med* 85:830, 1976.
190. Brown EM, Broadus AE, Brennan MF, Gardner DG, Marx SJ, Spiegel AM, Downs RW, Attie M, Aurbach GD: Direct comparison in vivo and in vitro of suppressibility of parathyroid function by calcium in primary hyperparathyroidism. *J Clin Endocrinol Metab* 48:604, 1979.
191. Reiss E, Canterbury JM: Primary hyperparathyroidism: Application of radioimmunoassay to differentiation of adenoma and hyperplasia and to preoperative localization of hyperfunctioning parathyroid glands. *N Engl J Med* 280:1381, 1969.
192. Spiegel AM, Doppman JL, Marx SJ, Brennan MF, Brown EM, Downs RW, Gardner DG, Attie M, Aurbach GD: Preoperative localization of abnormal parathyroid: Neck massage versus arteriography and selective venous sampling. *Ann Intern Med* 89:935, 1978.
193. Winzelberg GG, Hydovitz JD, O'Hara KR, Anderson KM, Turbiner E, Danowski TS, Lippe RD, Melada GA, Harrison AM: Parathyroid adenomas evaluated by Tl-201/Tc-99m pertechnetate subtraction scintigraphy and high-resolution ultrasonography. *Radiology* 155:231, 1985.
194. Mallette LE, Gomez L, Fisher RG: Parathyroid angiography: A review of current knowledge and guidelines for clinical application. *Endocr Rev* 2:124, 1981.
195. Eisenberg H, Pallotta JA: Special localizing techniques for parathyroid disease, in DeGroot LJ, Cahill GF, Odell WD, Martini L, Potts JT, Nelson DH, Steinberger E, Winegrad AI (eds): *Endocrinology*, New York, Grune & Stratton, 1979, vol. 2, pp 717–724.
196. Niederle B, Roka R, Brennan MF: The transplantation of parathyroid tissue in man: Development, indications, techniques, and results. *Endocr Rev* 3:245, 1982.
197. Rizzoli R, Green J, Marx SJ: Primary hyperparathyroidism in familial multiple endocrine neoplasia type 1. *Am J Med* 78:467, 1985.
198. Wells SA, Ellis GJ, Gunnells JC, Schneider AB, Sherwood LM: Parathyroid autotransplantation in primary parathyroid hyperplasia. *N Engl J Med* 295:57, 1976.
199. Wang C: Parathyroid re-exploration: A clinical and pathological study of 112 cases. *Ann Surg* 186:140, 1977.
200. Bilezikian JP: The medical management of primary hyperparathyroidism. *Ann Intern Med* 96:198, 1982.
201. Purnell DC, Scholz DA, Smith LH, Sizemore GW, Black BM, Goldsmith RS, Arnaud CD: Treatment of primary hyperparathyroidism. *Am J Med* 56:800, 1974.
202. Marcus R, Madvig P, Crim M, Pont A, Kosek J: Conjugated estrogens in the treatment of postmenopausal women with hyperparathyroidism. *Ann Intern Med* 100:633, 1984.
203. Gallagher JC, Wilkinson R: The effect of ethinyloestradiol on calcium and phosphorus metabolism of post-menopausal women with primary hyperparathyroidism. *Clin Sci Mol Med* 45:785, 1973.
204. Broadus AE, Magee JS, Mallette LE, Horst RL, Lang R, Jensen PS, Gertner JM, Baron R: A detailed evaluation of oral phosphate therapy in selected patients with primary hyperparathyroidism. *J Clin Endocrinol Metab* 56:953, 1983.
205. Shane E, Baquiran DC, Bilezikian JP: Effects of dichloromethylene diphosphonate on serum and urinary calcium in primary hyperparathyroidism. *Ann Intern Med* 95:23, 1981.
206. Fisken RA, Heath DA, Bold AM: Hypercalcemia—a hospital survey. *Q J Med* 49:405, 1980.
207. Rodman JS, Sherwood LM: Disorders of mineral metabolism in malignancy, in Avioli LV, Krane SM (eds): *Metabolic Bone Disease*. New York, Academic Press, 1978, vol. 2, pp 577–631.
208. Lafferty FW: Pseudohyperparathyroidism. *Medicine (Baltimore)* 45:247, 1966.
209. Powell D, Singer FR, Murray TM, Minkin C, Potts JT: Nonparathyroid humoral hypercalcemia in patients with neoplastic diseases. *N Engl J Med* 289:176, 1973.
210. Mundy GR, Ibbotson KJ, D'Souza SM, Simpson EL, Jacobs JW, Martin TJ: The hypercalcemia of cancer. *N Engl J Med* 310:1718, 1984.
211. Stewart AF, Horst R, Deftos LJ, Cadman EC, Lang R, Broadus AE: Biochemical evaluation of patients with cancer-associated hypercalcemia. *N Engl J Med* 303:1377, 1980.
212. Godsall JW, Burtis WJ, Insogna KL, Broadus AE, Stewart AF: Nephrogenous cyclic AMP, adenylate cyclase-stimulating activity, and humoral hypercalcemia of malignancy. *Recent Prog Horm Res* 42:705, 1986.
213. Eilon G, Mundy GR: Direct resorption of bone by breast cancer cells in vitro. *Nature* 276:726, 1978.
214. Galasko CSB: Mechanisms of bone destruction in the development of skeletal metastases. *Nature* 263:507, 1976.
215. Martin TJ, Partridge NC: Prostaglandins, cancer, and bone. *Metab Bone Dis Relat Res* 2:167, 1980.
216. Watson L, Moxham J, Fraser D: Hydrocortisone suppression test and discriminant analysis in differential diagnosis of hypercalcemia. *Lancet* i:1320, 1980.
217. Mannheimer IH: Hypercalcemia of breast cancer: Management with corticosteroids. *Cancer* 18:679, 1965.
218. Mundy GR, Raisz LG, Cooper RA, Schechter GP, Salmon SE: Evidence for the secretion of an osteoclast stimulating factor in myeloma. *N Engl J Med* 291:1041, 1974.

219. Valentin-Opran A, Charon S, Meunier PJ, Edouard CM, Arlot ME: Quantitative histology of myeloma-induced bone changes. *Br J Haematol* 52:602, 1982.
220. Stewart AF, Vignery A, Silverglate A, Ravin ND, LiVolsi V, Broadus AE, Baron R: Quantitative bone histomorphometry in humoral hypercalcemia of malignancy. *J Clin Endocrinol Metab* 55:219, 1982.
221. Rude RK, Sharp CF, Fredericks RS, Oldham SB, Elbaum N, Link J, Irwin L, Singer FR: Urinary and nephrogenous cyclic AMP excretion in the hypercalcemia of malignancy. *J Clin Endocrinol Metab* 52:765, 1981.
222. Cramer SF, Fried L, Carter KJ: The cellular basis of metabolic bone disease in patients with lung cancer. *Cancer* 48:2649, 1981.
223. Breslau NA, McGuire JL, Zerwekh JE, Frenkel EP, Pak CYC: Hypercalcemia associated with increased serum calcitriol levels in three patients with lymphoma. *Ann Intern Med* 100:1, 1984.
224. Haddad JG, Couranz SJ, Avioli LV: Circulating phytosterols in normal females, lactating mothers, and breast cancer patients. *J Clin Endocrinol Metab* 30:174, 1970.
225. Brenner DE, Harvey HA, Lipton A, Demers L: A study of prostaglandin E_2, parathormone, and response to indomethacin in patients with hypercalcemia of malignancy. *Cancer* 49:556, 1982.
226. Tashjian AH: Prostaglandins, hypercalcemia, and cancer. *N Engl J Med* 293:1317, 1975.
227. Benson RC, Riggs BL, Pickard BM, Arnaud CD: Immunoreactive forms of circulating parathyroid hormone in primary and ectopic hyperparathyroidism. *J Clin Invest* 54:175, 1974.
228. Simpson EL, Mundy GR, D'Souza SM, Ibbotson KJ, Bockman R, Jacobs JW: Absence of parathyroid hormone messenger RNA in non-parathyroid tumors associated with hypercalcemia. *N Engl J Med* 309:325, 1983.
229. Goltzman D, Stewart AF, Broadus AE: Malignancy-associated hypercalcemia: Evaluation with a cytochemical bioassay for parathyroid hormone. *J Clin Endocrinol Metab* 53:899, 1981.
230. Stewart AF, Insogna KL, Goltzman D, Broadus AE: Identification of adenylate cyclase-stimulating activity and cytochemical glucose-6-phosphate dehydrogenase-stimulating activity in extracts of tumors from patients with humoral hypercalcemia of malignancy. *Proc Natl Acad Sci USA* 80:1454, 1983.
231. Strewler GJ, Williams RD, Nissenson RA: Human renal carcinoma cells produce hypercalcemia in the nude mouse and a novel protein recognized by parathyroid hormone receptors. *J Clin Invest* 71:769, 1983.
232. Rodan SB, Insogna KL, Vignery AM, Stewart AF, Broadus AE, D'Souza SM, Bertolini DR, Mundy GR, Rodan GA: Factors associated with humoral hypercalcemia of malignancy stimulate adenylate cyclase in osteoblastic cells. *J Clin Invest* 72:1511, 1983.
233. Klein R, Strewler GJ, Nissenson RA, Williams RD, Leung SC: PTH-like protein from human carcinoma cells stimulates bone resorption. *Clin Res* 32:410A, 1985.
234. Stewart AF, Insogna KL, Burtis WJ, Weir EC, Aminiafshar A, Wu T, Broadus AE: Prevalence and characterization of the adenylate cyclase-stimulating activity in tumors associated with humoral hypercalcemia of malignancy *J Bone Min Res* 1:267, 1986.
235. Merendino JS, Insogna KL, Milstone LM, Broadus AE, Stewart AF: Cultured human keratinocytes produce a parathyroid hormone-like protein. *Science* 231:388, 1986.
236. D'Souza SM, Ibbotson K, Smith DD, Mundy GR: Production of a macromolecular bone-resorbing factor by the hypercalcemic variant of the Walker rat carcinosarcoma. *Endocrinology* 115:1746, 1984.
237. Ibbotson KJ, D'Souza SM, Ng KW, Osborne CK, Niall M, Martin JJ, Mundy GR: Tumor-derived growth factor increases bone resorption in a tumor associated with humoral hypercalcemia of malignancy. *Science* 221:1292, 1983.
238. Mundy GR, Ibbotson KJ, D'Souza SM: Tumor products and the hypercalcemia of malignancy. *J Clin Invest* 76:391, 1985.
239. Cannellos GP: Hypercalcemia in malignant lymphoma and leukemia. *Ann NY Acad Sci* 230:240, 1974.
240. Mundy GR, Luben RA, Raisz LG, Oppenheim JJ, Buell DN: Bone-resorbing activity in supernatants from lymphoid cell lines. *N Engl J Med* 290:867, 1974.
241. Rosenthal ND, Insogna KL, Godsall JW, Smaldone L, Waldron JW, Stewart AF: 1,25 dihydroxyvitamin D-mediated humoral hypercalcemia in malignant lymphoma. *J Clin Endocrinol Metab* 60:29, 1985.
242. Tsoukas CD, Provvedini DM, Manolagas SC: 1,25-dihydroxyvitamin D_3: A novel immunoregulatory hormone. *Science* 224:1438, 1984.
243. Blaney DW, Jaffe ES, Fisher RJ, Schechter GP, Gossman J, Robert-Guroff M, Kalyanaraman VS, Blattner WA, Gallo RC: The human T-cell leukemia-lymphoma virus, lymphoma, lytic bone lesions, and hypercalcemia. *Ann Intern Med* 98:144, 1983.
244. Stewart AF, Broadus AE, Schwartz PE, Kohorn EI, Romero R: Hypercalcemia in gynecologic neoplasms. *Cancer* 49:2389, 1982.
245. Bringhurst FR, Bierer BE, Godeau F, Neyhard N, Varner V, Segre GV: Humoral hypercalcemia of malignancy: Release of a prostaglandin-stimulating bone-resorbing factor in vitro by human transitional carcinoma cells. *J Clin Invest* 77:456, 1986.
246. Seyberth HW, Segre GV, Morgan JL, Sweetman BJ, Potts JT, Oates JA: Prostaglandins as the mediators of hypercalcemia associated with certain types of cancer. *N Engl J Med* 293:1278, 1975.
247. Robertson RP, Baylink DJ, Marini JJ, Adkison HW: Elevated prostaglandins and suppressed parathyroid hormone associated with hypercalcemia and a renal cell carcinoma. *J Clin Endocrinol Metab* 41:164, 1975.
248. Mosekilde L, Christensen MS: Decreased parathyroid function in hyperthyroidism: Interrelationships between parathyroid hormone, calcium-phosphorus metabolism and thyroid function. *Acta Endocrinol (Copenh)* 84:566, 1977.
249. Mundy GR, Shapiro JL, Bandelin JG, Canalis EM, Raisz LG: Direct stimulation of bone resorption by thyroid hormones. *J Clin Invest* 58:529, 1976.
250. Mosekilde L, Melson F, Bagger JP, Myhre-Jensen O, Sorensen NS: Bone changes in hyperthyroidism: Interrelationships between bone morphometry, thyroid function and calcium-phosphorus metabolism. *Acta Endocrinol (Copenh)* 85:515, 1977.
251. Bouillon R, Muls E, DeMoor P: Influence of thyroid function on the serum concentration of 1,25-dihydroxyvitamin D. *J Clin Endocrinol Metab* 51:793, 1980.
252. Mahler R, Hayes TM: A case of diabetes. *Br Med J* 2:1398, 1977.
253. Stewart AF, Hoecker JL, Mallette LE, Segre GV, Amatruda TT: Hypercalcemia in pheochromocytoma. *Ann Intern Med* 102:776, 1985.
254. Verner JV, Morrison AB: Endocrine pancreatic islet disease with diarrhea. *Arch Intern Med* 133:492, 1974.
255. Jorgensen FS: Effect of thiazide diuretics upon calcium metabolism. *Dan Med Bull* 23:223, 1976.
256. Costanzo LS, Moses AM, Rao KJ, Weiner IM: Dissociation of calcium and sodium clearances in patients with hypoparathyroidism by infusion of chlorothiazide. *Metabolism* 24:1367, 1975.
257. Anning ST, Dawson J, Dolby DE, Ingram JT: The toxic effects of calciferol. *Q J Med* 27:203, 1948.
258. Hughes MR, Baylink DJ, Jones PG, Haussler MR: Radioligand receptor assay for 25-hydroxyvitamin D_2/D_3 and 1,25-dihydroxyvitamin D_2/D_3: Application to hypervitaminosis D. *J Clin Invest* 58:61, 1976.
259. Frame B, Jackson CE, Reynolds WA, Umphrey JE: Hypercalcemia and skeletal effects in chronic hypervitaminosis A. *Ann Intern Med* 80:44, 1974.
260. McMillan DE, Freeman RB: The milk alkali syndrome: A study of the acute disorder with comments on the development of the chronic condition. *Medicine (Baltimore)* 44:485, 1965.

261. Orwoll ES: The milk-alkali syndrome: Current concepts. *Ann Intern Med* 97:242, 1982.
262. Christiansen C, Baastrup PC, Lindgreen P, Transbol I: Endocrine effects of lithium: Primary hyperparathyroidism. *Acta Endocrinol (Copenh)* 88:528, 1978.
263. Christiansen TAT: Lithium, hypercalcemia, and hyperparathyroidism. *Lancet* ii:144, 1976.
264. Miller PD, Dubovsky SL, McDonald KM, Arnaud C, Schrier RW: Hypocalciuric effect of lithium in man. *Min Elect Metab* 1:3, 1978.
265. Brown EM: Lithium induces abnormal calcium-regulated PTH release in dispersed bovine parathyroid cells. *J Clin Endocrinol Metab* 52:1046, 1981.
266. Spiegel AM, Rudorfer MV, Marx SJ, Linnoila M: The effect of short term lithium administration on suppressibility of parathyroid hormone secretion by calcium in vivo. *J Clin Endocrinol Metab* 59:354, 1984.
267. Legha SS, Powell K, Buzdar AU, Blumenschein GR: Tamoxifen-induced hypercalcemia in breast cancer. *Cancer* 47:2803, 1981.
268. Villalon AH, Tattersall MH, Fox RM, Woods RL: Hypercalcemia after tamoxifen for breast cancer: A sign of tumour response? *Br Med J* 125:1329, 1979.
269. Winnacker JL, Becker KL, Katz S: Endocrine aspects of sarcoidosis. *N Engl J Med* 278:427, 1968.
270. Goldstein RA, Israel HL, Becker KL, Moore CF: The infrequency of hypercalcemia in sarcoidosis. *Am J Med* 51:21, 1971.
271. Barbour GL, Coburn JW, Slatopolsky E, Norman AW, Horst RL: Hypercalcemia in an anephric patient with sarcoidosis: Evidence for extrarenal generation of 1,25-dihydroxyvitamin D. *N Engl J Med* 305:440, 1981.
272. Mason RS, Frankel TI, Chan Y-L, Lisseur D, Posen S: Vitamin D conversion by sarcoid lymph node homogenate. *Ann Intern Med* 100:59, 1984.
273. Adams JS, Singer FR, Gacad MA, Sharma OP, Hayes MJ, Vouvos P, Holick MF: Isolation and structural identification of 1,25-dihydroxyvitamin D_3 produced by cultured alveolar macrophages in sarcoidosis. *J Clin Endocrinol Metab* 60:960, 1985.
274. Cohen MS, Gray TK: Phagocytic cells metabolize 25-hydroxyvitamin D_3 in vitro. *Proc Natl Acad Sci USA* 81:931, 1984.
275. Murray JT, Heim CR: Hypercalcemia in disseminated histoplasmosis. *Am J Med* 78:881, 1985.
276. Jurney TM: Hypercalcemia in a patient with eosinophilic granuloma. *Am J Med* 76:527, 1984.
277. Kozeny GA, Barbato AL, Bansal VK, Vertuno LL, Hano JE: Hypercalcemia associated with silicone-induced granulomas. *N Engl J Med* 311:1103, 1984.
278. Kantarjian HM, Saad MF, Estey EH, Sellin RV, Samaan NA: Hypercalcemia in disseminated candidiasis. *Am J Med* 74:721, 1983.
279. Gkonos PJ, London R, Hendler ED: Hypercalcemia and elevated 1,25-dihydroxyvitamin D levels in a patient with end stage renal disease and active tuberculosis. *N Engl J Med* 311:1683, 1984.
280. Bergstrom WH: Hypercalciuria and hypercalcemia complicating immobilization. *Am J Dis Child* 132:553, 1978.
281. Lockwood DR, Vogel JM, Schneider VS, Hulley SB: Effect of the diphosphonate EHDP on bone mineral metabolism during prolonged bed rest. *J Clin Endocrinol Metab* 41:533, 1975.
282. Bones in space, editorial. *Br Med J* 280:1288, 1980.
283. DeVivo MJ, Fine PR, Cutter GR, Maetz HM: The risk of bladder calculi in patients with spinal cord injuries. *Arch Intern Med* 145:428, 1985.
284. Stewart AF, Adler M, Byers CM, Segre GV, Broadus AE: Calcium homeostasis in immobilization: An example of resorptive hypercalciuria. *N Engl J Med* 306:1136, 1982.
285. Minaire P, Meunier P, Edouard C, Bernard J, Courpron P, Bourret J: Quantitative histological data on disuse osteoporosis. *Calcif Tissue Res* 17:57, 1974.
286. Bergmann P, Heilporn A, Schoutens A, Paternot J, Tricot A: Longitudinal study of calcium and bone metabolism in paraplegic patients. *Paraplegia* 15:147, 1978.
287. Minaire P, Depassio J, Meunier P, Edouard C, Kanis JA, Caulin F, Pilonchery G: Treatment of acute osteoporosis due to paraplegia with calcitonin. *Clin Sci* 62:1, 1981.
288. Minaire P, Berard E, Meunier PJ, Edouard C, Goedert G, Pilonchery G: Effects of disodium dichloromethylene diphosphonate on bone loss in paraplegic patients. *J Clin Invest* 68:1086, 1981.
289. deTorrente A, Berl T, Cohn PD, Kawamoto E, Hertz P, Schrier RW: Hypercalcemia of acute renal failure. *Am J Med* 61:119, 1976.
290. Llach F, Felsenfeld AJ, Haussler MR: The pathophysiology of altered calcium metabolism in rhabdomyolysis-induced renal failure. *N Engl J Med* 305:117, 1981.
291. Knochel JP: Serum calcium derangements in rhabdomyolysis. *N Engl J Med* 305:161, 1981.
292. Hutchins GM, Mirvis SE, Mendelsohn G, Buckley BH: Supravalvular aortic stenosis with parafollicular cell (C-cell) hyperplasia. *Am J Med* 64:967, 1978.
293. Garabedian M, Jacoz E, Guillozo H, Grimberg R, Guillot M, Gagnadoux MF, Broyer M, Lenoir G, Balsan S: Elevated plasma 1,25-dihydroxyvitamin D concentrations in infants with hypercalcemia and elfin facies. *N Engl J Med* 312:948, 1985.
294. Kenny FM, Aceto T, Purisch M, Harrison HE, Harrison HC, Blizzard RM: Metabolic studies in a patient with idiopathic hypercalcemia of infancy. *J Pediatr* 62:531, 1963.
295. Annesley TM, Burritt MF, Kyle RA: Artifactual hypercalcemia in multiple myeloma. *Mayo Clin Proc* 57:572, 1982.
296. Jaffe JP, Mosher DF: Calcium binding by a myeloma protein. *Am J Med* 67:343, 1979.
297. Suki WN, Yium JJ, Von Minden M, Saller-Hebert C, Eknoyan G, Martinez-Maldonado M: Acute treatment of hypercalcemia with furosemide. *N Engl J Med* 283:836, 1970.
298. Heyburn PL, Selby PL, Peacock M, Sandler LR, Parsons FM: Peritoneal dialysis in the management of severe hypercalcemia. *Br Med J* 280:525, 1980.
299. Cardella CJ, Birkin BL, Roscoe M, Rapoport A: Role of dialysis in the treatment of severe hypercalcemia. *Clin Nephrol* 12:285, 1979.
300. Kiang DT, Loken MK, Kennedy BJ: Mechanism of the hypocalcemic effect of mithramycin. *J Clin Endocrinol Metab* 48:341, 1979.
301. Goldsmith RS, Ingbar SH: Inorganic phosphate treatment of hypercalcemia of diverse etiologies. *N Engl J Med* 274:1, 1966.
302. Lentz RD, Brown DM, Kjellstrand CM: Treatment of severe hypophosphatemia. *Ann Intern Med* 89:941, 1978.
303. Vaughn CB, Vaitkevicius VK: The effects of calcitonin in hypercalcemia in patients with malignancy. *Cancer* 34:1268, 1974.
304. Binstock ML, Mundy GR: Effect of calcitonin and glucocorticoids in combination on the hypercalcemia of malignancy. *Ann Intern Med* 93:269, 1980.
305. Jung A: Comparison of two parenteral diphosphonates in hypercalcemia of malignancy. *Am J Med* 72:221, 1982.
306. Siris ES, Sherman WH, Baquiran DC, Schlatterer JP, Osserman EF, Canfield RE: Effect of dichloromethylene diphosphonate on skeletal mobilization of calcium in multiple myeloma. *N Engl J Med* 302:310, 1980.
307. van Breukelen FJM, Bijvoet OLM, van Osterom AT: Inhibition of osteolytic bone lesions by (3-amino-1-hydroxypropylidine)-1 bisphosphonate. *Lancet* i:803, 1979.
308. Glover DJ, Shaw L, Glick JH, Slatopolsky E, Weiler C, Attie M, Goldfarb S: Treatment of hypercalcemia in parathyroid cancer with WR 2721, S-2-(3-aminopropylamino)ethyl-phosphoro-thiotic acid. *Ann Intern Med* 103:55, 1985.
309. Johannesson AJ, Onkelink C, Rodan GA, Raisz LG: Thionapthene-2-carboxylic acid: A new antihypercalcemic agent. *Endocrinology* 117:150, 1985.

310. Warrell RP, Bockman RS, Coonley CJ, Isaacs M, Staszewski H: Gallium nitrate inhibits calcium resorption from bone and is effective treatment for cancer-related hypercalcemia. *J Clin Invest* 73:1487, 1984.
311. Nagant de Deuxchaisnes C, Krane SM: Hypoparathyroidism, in Avioli LV, Krane SM (eds): *Metabolic Bone Disease.* New York, Academic Press, 1978, vol. 2, pp 217–445.
312. Schneider AB, Sherwood LM: Pathogenesis and management of hypoparathyroidism and other hypocalcemic disorders. *Metabolism* 24:871, 1975.
313. Nusynowitz ML, Frame B, Kolb FO: The spectrum of the hypoparathyroid states: A classification based on physiologic principles. *Medicine (Baltimore)* 55:105, 1976.
314. Edmondson JW, Brashear RE, Li T: Tetany: Quantitative interrelationships between calcium and alkalosis. *Am J Physiol* 228:1082, 1975.
315. Connor TB, Rosen BL, Blaustein MP, Appelfeld MM, Doyle LA: Hypocalcemia precipitating congestive heart failure. *N Engl J Med* 307:869, 1982.
316. Levine SN, Rheams CN: Hypocalcemic heart failure. *Am J Med* 78:1033, 1985.
317. Nierenberg DW, Ransil BJ: Q-aTc interval as a clinical indicator of hypercalcemia. *Am J Cardiol* 44:243, 1979.
318. Ireland AW, Hornbrook JW, Neale FC, Posen S: The crystalline lens in chronic surgical hypoparathyroidism. *Arch Intern Med* 122:408, 1968.
319. Stewart AF, Battaglini-Sabetta J, Milstone LM: Hypocalcemia-induced psoriasis of von Zumbusch: New experience with an old syndrome. *Ann Intern Med* 100:677, 1984.
320. Michie W, Duncan T, Hamer-Hodges DW, Bewsher PD, Stowers JM, Pegg CAS, Hems G, Hedley AJ: Mechanism of hypocalcemia after thyroidectomy for thyrotoxicosis. *Lancet* i:508, 1971.
321. Parfitt AM: The spectrum of hypoparathyroidism. *J Clin Endocrinol Metab* 34:152, 1972.
322. Blizzard RM, Chee D, Davis W: The incidence of parathyroid and other antibodies in the sera of patients with idiopathic hypoparathyroidism. *Clin Exp Immunol* 1:119, 1966.
323. Horwitz CA, Myers WPL, Foote FW: Secondary malignant tumors of the parathyroid glands. *Am J Med* 52:797, 1972.
324. Rude RK, Oldham SB, Sharp CF, Singer FR: Parathyroid hormone secretion in magnesium deficiency. *J Clin Endocrinol Metab* 47:800, 1978.
325. Chase LR, Slatopolsky E: Secretion and metabolic efficacy of parathyroid hormone in patients with severe hypomagnesemia. *J Clin Endocrinol Metab* 38:363, 1974.
326. Estep H, Shaw WA, Watlington C, Hobe R, Holland W, Tucker St G: Hypocalcemia due to hypomagnesemia and reversible parathyroid hormone unresponsiveness. *J Clin Endocrinol Metab* 29:842, 1969.
327. Rude RK, Adams JS, Ryzen E, Endres DB, Niimi H, Horst RL, Haddad JG, Singer FR: Low serum concentrations of 1,25 dihydroxyvitamin D in human magnesium deficiency. *J Clin Endocrinol Metab* 61:933, 1985.
328. Albright F, Burnett CH, Smith PH, Parson W: Pseudohypoparathyroidism—an example of "Seabright-Bantam syndrome." *Endocrinology* 30:922, 1942.
329. Lee JB, Tashjian AM, Streeto JM, Frantz AG: Familial pseudohypoparathyroidism. *N Engl J Med* 279:1179, 1968.
330. Chase LR, Melson GL, Aurbach GD: Pseudohypoparathyroidism: Defective excretion of 3′,5′-AMP in response to parathyroid hormone. *J Clin Invest* 48:1832, 1969.
331. Drezner MK, Neelon FA, Lebovitz HE: Pseudohypoparathyroidism type II: A possible defect in the reception of the cyclic AMP signal. *N Engl J Med* 289:1056, 1973.
332. Kooh SW, Fraser D, DeLuca HF, Holick MF, Belsey RE, Clark B, Murray TM: Treatment of hypoparathyroidism and pseudohypoparathyroidism with metabolites of vitamin D. *N Engl J Med* 293:840, 1975.
333. Drezner MK, Neelon FA, Haussler M, McPherson HT, Lebovitz HE: 1,25-dihydroxycholecalciferol deficiency, the probable cause of hypocalcemia and metabolic bone disease in pseudohypoparathyroidism. *J Clin Endocrinol Metab* 42:621, 1976.
334. Yamaoka K, Seino Y, Ishida M, Ishii T, Shimotsuji T, Tanaka Y, Kurose H, Matsuda S, Satomura K, Yabuuchi H: Effect of dibutyryl adenosine 3′,5′-monophosphate administration on plasma concentration of 1,25 dihydroxyvitamin D in pseudohypoparathyroidism type 1. *J Clin Endocrinol Metab* 53:1096, 1981.
335. Drezner MK, Burch WM: Altered activity of the nucleotide regulatory site in the parathyroid hormone-sensitive adenylate cyclase from the renal cortex of a patient with pseudohypoparathyroidism. *J Clin Invest* 62:1222, 1978.
336. Farfel Z, Brickman AS, Kaslow HR, Brothers VM, Bourne HR: Defect in receptor-cyclase coupling protein in pseudohypoparathyroidism. *N Engl J Med* 303:237, 1980.
337. Levine MA, Downs RW, Singer M, Marx SJ, Aurbach GD, Spiegel AM: Deficient activity of guanine nucleotide regulatory protein in erythrocytes from patients with pseudohypoparathyroidism. *Biochem Biophys Res Commun* 94:1319, 1980.
338. Levine MA, Eil C, Downs RW, Spiegel AM: Deficient guanine nucleotide regulatory subunit activity in cultured fibroblast membranes from patients with pseudohypoparathyroidism type 1. *J Clin Invest* 72:316, 1983.
339. Farfel Z, Abood ME, Brickman AS, Bourne HR: Deficient activity of receptor-cyclase coupling protein in transformed lymphoblasts of patients with pseudohypoparathyroidism type 1. *J Clin Endocrinol Metab* 55:113, 1982.
340. Farfel Z, Bourne HR: Deficient activity of receptor-cyclase coupling protein in platelets of patients with pseudohypoparathyroidism. *J Clin Endocrinol Metab* 51:1202, 1980.
341. Mallet E, Carayon P, Amr S, Brunelle P, Ducastelle T, Basuyau JP, Hellouin de Minibus C: Coupling defect of thyrotropin receptor and adenylate cyclase in a pseudohypoparathyroid patient. *J Clin Endocrinol Metab* 54:1028, 1982.
342. Downs RW, Levine MA, Drezner MK, Burch WM, Spiegel AM: Deficient adenylate cyclase regulatory protein in renal membranes from a patient with pseudohypoparathyroidism. *J Clin Invest* 71:231, 1983.
343. Downs RW, Sekura RD, Levine MA, Spiegel AM: The inhibitory adenylate cyclase coupling protein in pseudohypoparathyroidism. *J Clin Endocrinol Metab* 61:351, 1985.
344. Levine MA, Downs RW, Moses AM, Breslau NA, Marx SJ, Lasker RD, Rizzoli RE, Aurbach GD, Spiegel AM: Resistance to multiple hormones in patients with pseudohypoparathyroidism. *Am J Med* 74:545, 1983.
345. Heinsimer JA, Davies AO, Downs RW, Levine MA, Spiegel AM, Drezner MK, DeLean A, Wresgett KA, Caron MG, Lefkowitz RJ: Impaired formation of B-adrenergic receptor nucleotide regulatory protein complexes in pseudohypoparathyroidism. *J Clin Invest* 73:1335, 1984.
346. Spiegel AM, Gierschick P, Levine MA, Downs RJ: Clinical implications of guanine nucleotide-binding proteins as receptor-effector couplers. *N Engl J Med* 312:26, 1985.
347. Nagant de Deuxchaisnes C, Fischer JA, Dambucher MA, Devogelaer JP, Arber CE, Zanelli JM, Parsons JA, Loveridge N, Bitensky L, Chayen J: Dissociation of parathyroid hormone bioactivity and immunoreactivity in pseudohypoparathyroidism type 1. *J Clin Endocrinol Metab* 53:1105, 1981.
348. Mitchell J, Goltzman D: Examination of circulating parathyroid hormone in pseudohypoparathyroidism. *J Clin Endocrinol Metab* 61:328, 1985.
349. Kolb FO, Steinbach HL: Pseudohypoparathyroidism with secondary hyperparathyroidism and osteitis fibrosa. *J Clin Endocrinol Metab* 22:59, 1962.

350. Breslau NA, Moses AM, Pak CYC: Evidence for bone remodeling but lack of calcium mobilization response to parathyroid hormone in pseudohypoparathyroidism. *J Clin Endocrinol Metab* 57:638, 1983.
351. Moses AM, Breslau NA, Coulson R: Renal responses to PTH in hormone-resistant (pseudo) hypoparathyroidism. *Am J Med* 61:184, 1976.
352. Breslau NA, Notman DD, Canterbury JM, Moses AM: Studies on the attainment of normocalcemia in patients with pseudohypoparathyroidism. *Am J Med* 68:854, 1980.
353. Drezner MK, Haussler MR: Normocalcemic pseudohypoparathyroidism. *Am J Med* 66:503, 1979.
354. Edmondson HA, Fields IA: Relation of calcium and lipids to acute pancreatic necrosis. *Arch Intern Med* 69:177, 1942.
355. Stewart AF, Longo W, Kreutter D, Jacob R, Burtis WJ: Hypocalcemia associated with calcium soap formation in a patient with a pancreatic fistula. *N Engl J Med* 315:496, 1986.
356. Robertson GM, Moore EW, Switz DM, Sizemore GW, Estep HL: Inadequate parathyroid response in acute pancreatitis. *N Engl J Med* 214:512, 1976.
357. Raskin P, McClain CJ, Medsger TA: Hypocalcemia associated with metastatic bone disease. *Arch Intern Med* 132:539, 1973.
358. Cadman EL, Lundberg WB, Bertino JR: Hyperphosphatemia and hypocalcemia accompanying rapid cell lysis in a patient with Burkett's lymphoma and Burkitt cell leukemia. *Am J Med* 62:283, 1977.
359. Chesney RW, McCarron DM, Haddad JG, Hawker CD, DiBella FP, Chesney PJ, Davis JD: Pathogenic mechanisms of the hypocalcemia of the staphylococcal toxic shock syndrome. *J Lab Clin Med* 101:576, 1983.
360. Nicar MJ, Pak CYC: Calcium bioavailability from calcium carbonate and calcium citrate. *J Clin Endocrinol Metab* 61:391, 1985.
361. Recker R: Calcium absorption and achlorhydria. *N Engl J Med* 313:70, 1985.
362. Markowitz ME, Rosen JF, Smith CE, DeLuca HF: 1,25-Dihydroxyvitamin D_3-treated hypoparathyroidism: 35 patient-years in 10 children. *J Clin Endocrinol Metab* 55:727, 1982.
363. Porter RH, Cox BG, Heaney D, Hostetter TH, Stinebaugh BJ, Suki WN: Treatment of hypoparathyroid patients with chlorthalidone. *N Engl J Med* 298:577, 1978.
364. Lotz M, Zisman E, Bartter FC: Evidence for a phosphorus-depletion syndrome in man. *N Engl J Med* 278:409, 1968.
365. Godsall JW, Baron R, Insogna KL: Vitamin D metabolism and bone histomorphometry in a patient with antacid-induced osteomalacia. *Am J Med* 77:747, 1984.
366. Schussler GC, Verso MH, Nemoto T: Phosphaturia in hypercalcemic breast cancer patients. *J Clin Endocrinol Metab* 35:497, 1972.
367. Knochel JP: The pathophysiology and clinical characteristics of severe hypophosphatemia. *Arch Intern Med* 137:203, 1977.
368. Mostellar ME, Tuttle EP: The effects of alkalosis on plasma concentration and urinary excretion of inorganic phosphate in man. *J Clin Invest* 43:138, 1964.
369. Lentz RD, Brown DM, Kjellstrand CM: Treatment of severe hypophosphatemia. *Ann Intern Med* 89:941, 1978.
370. O'Connor LR, Klein KL, Bethune JE: Hyperphosphatemia in lactic acidosis. *N Engl J Med* 297:707, 1977.
371. Booth CC, Babouris N, Hanna S, MacIntyre I: Incidence of hypomagnesemia in intestinal malabsorption. *Br Med J* 2:141, 1963.
372. Suh SM, Tashjian AH, Matsuo N, Parkinson DK, Fraser D: Pathogenesis of hypocalcemia in primary hypomagnesemia. *J Clin Invest* 52:153, 1973.
373. Davis BB, Preuss HG, Murdaugh HV: Hypomagnesemia following the diuresis of post-renal obstruction and renal transplant. *Nephron* 14:275, 1975.
374. Zaloga GP, Chernow B, Pock A, Wood B, Zaritsky A, Zucker A: Hypomagnesemia is a common complication of aminoglycoside therapy. *Surg Gynecol Obstet* 158:561, 1984.
375. Barton CH, Pahl M, Vaziri ND, Cesario T: Renal magnesium wasting associated with amphotericin therapy. *Am J Med* 77:471, 1984.
376. Stewart AF, Keating T, Schwartz PE: Magnesium homeostasis following chemotherapy with cisplatin: A prospective study. *Am J Obstet Gynecol* 153:660, 1985.
377. Kupfer S, Kosovsky JD: Effects of cardiac glycosides on renal tubular transport of calcium, magnesium, inorganic phosphate, and glucose in the dog. *J Clin Invest* 44:1132, 1965.
378. Spencer RW, Voyce MA: Familial hypokalemia and hypomagnesemia. *Acta Paediatr Scand* 65:505, 1976.
379. Manz F, Scharer K, Janka P, Lombeck J: Renal magnesium wasting, incomplete tubular acidosis, hypercalciuria, and nephrocalcinosis in siblings. *Eur J Pediatr* 128:67, 1978.
380. Martin HE: Clinical magnesium deficiency. *Ann NY Acad Sci* 162:891, 1969.
381. King RG, Steinbury SW: Magnesium metabolism in primary hyperparathyroidism. *Clin Sci* 39:287, 1970.
382. Heaton FW, Pyrah LN: Magnesium metabolism in patients with parathyroid disorders. *Clin Sci* 25:475, 1963.
383. Jones E, Desper PC, Shane SR, Flink EB: Magnesium metabolism in hyperthyroidism and hypothyroidism. *J Clin Invest* 45:891, 1966.
384. Greenwald JH, Dubin A, Cardon L: Hypomagnesemic tetany due to excessive lactation. *Am J Med* 35:854, 1963.
385. Flink EF: Therapy of magnesium deficiency. *Ann NY Acad Sci* 162:901, 1969.
386. Mordes JP, Swartz R, Arky RA: Extreme hypermagnesemia as a cause of refractory hypotension. *Ann Intern Med* 83:657, 1975.

24

Metabolic Bone Disease

Frederick R. Singer

A *metabolic bone disease* may best be defined as a skeletal disorder which is generalized in extent.[1] This may not always be clinically apparent, as in patients with osteoporosis, in whom the vertebral lesions are often the clinical focus of attention. However, more subtle abnormalities of a generalized nature can be demonstrated in these patients by bone biopsy or bone densitometry.

Metabolic bone diseases may arise from excessive or deficient hormone secretion, from deficiency of vitamin D, from impaired metabolism of vitamin D or resistance to vitamin D, from other nutritional deficiencies, from heritable abnormalities of connective tissue, from immobilization, and from failure of normal bone stem cell differentiation. In addition, osteoporosis is associated with a number of unrelated primary disorders, such as rheumatoid arthritis, in which the pathogenetic relationship between the bone loss and the primary disorder is ill defined. Finally, there are instances of "idiopathic" bone disease in which no clues to the pathogenesis are apparent.

CLINICAL EVALUATION OF METABOLIC BONE DISEASE

History and Physical Examination

Patients with a metabolic bone disease may have a prolonged asymptomatic course during which time only appropriate laboratory tests will reveal an abnormality. Such a situation is typical of postmenopausal osteoporosis before bone mass has decreased enough to allow a compression fracture of a vertebral body to occur.

The most common symptoms which occur in adult patients with bone disease are pain and deformity. Pathological fractures of the vertebral bodies or femoral neck are sometimes the first indication of underlying disease. In children, failure of normal growth is a common feature. Rarely, neurological deficits may develop as a consequence of abnormal remodeling of bone; for example, optic and auditory nerve compression may complicate osteopetrosis. In patients with hypocalcemia, tetany and seizures may be present. In vitamin D–deficient and phosphate-deficient states, muscle weakness and tenderness may be striking features of physical examination.

It is particularly important to ascertain the dietary history, the family history, and whether there was any period of prolonged immobilization in the past, since these are important determinants of normal skeletal development.

Clinical Chemistry

Important information concerning the type and underlying etiology of metabolic bone disease can be obtained from several routine blood and urine analyses. These have been discussed in detail in Chap. 23 and will be only briefly reviewed.

The fasting serum calcium, phosphorus, and alkaline phosphatase concentrations, usually a part of screening chemistry panels, are simple but valuable parameters in assessing metabolic bone disease.

The serum calcium concentration may be normal, high, or low in patients with bone disease. An elevated concentration suggests that bone resorption is increased, and a low concentration may indicate a failure of adequate release of bone mineral to maintain a normocalcemic state. The presence of a normal serum calcium concentration should not be taken as evidence of normal bone metabolism, since crippling bone disease may be present in normocalcemic patients with osteoporosis, osteomalacia, and renal osteodystrophy.

The serum phosphorus concentration is almost always reduced in osteomalacia and rickets, excluding patients with chronic renal failure. Patients with osteoporosis usually have a normal serum phosphorus concentration. It should be stressed that the serum phosphorus is best measured after an overnight fast to avoid dietary influences and diurnal variation.

The serum alkaline phosphatase activity can be used as an index of osteoblastic activity in the absence of a concomitant disorder which raises extraskeletal enzyme activity. As stressed in Chap. 23, this parameter is a rather insensitive measure of osteoblastic activity, and mild degrees of bone disease in which increased osteoblasts are found on bone biopsy may be associated with normal circulating alkaline phosphatase activity.

A new biochemical test reflecting bone metabolism is measurement of the vitamin K–dependent bone protein osteocalcin (also termed *bone GLA protein*) in the circulation.[2] This γ-carboxyglutamic acid–containing protein is synthesized in cortical and trabecular bone,[3] and its production has also been demonstrated in osteoblast-like cultured rat osteosarcoma cells.[4] Its synthesis is stimulated by 1α,25-dihydroxyvitamin D_3, but its physiological role remains elusive. The protein binds calcium avidly and is first observed in bone with the onset of mineralization, yet in humans vitamin K antagonists such as warfarin do not reduce bone density.[5] In patients with increased bone turnover (and osteoblastic activity), serum or plasma osteocalcin is often increased but does not always correlate with serum alkaline phosphatase activity.[2] Levels may decrease with administration of therapeutic agents such as calcitonin,[6] but patients with inherited rickets treated with 1α,25-dihydroxyvitamin D_3 demonstrate increased levels of serum osteocalcin in response to successful therapy.[7] Factors such as sex, age, renal function, and time of day may influence the levels of osteocalcin in the circulation,[2,8–10] although all studies have not been in complete agreement. Further understanding of the physiological and possible pathological role of this bone matrix protein is needed before it can be considered a standard clinical test of bone metabolism.

Acid-base status, renal function, and liver function tests may be useful in the differential diagnosis of bone disease but are secondary tests.

Twenty-four-hour urinary calcium and phosphorus excretion have commonly been measured in the evaluation of patients with disturbed mineral homeostasis. These measurements, particularly phosphorus excretion, are often of little use when obtained under uncontrolled conditions, since urinary excretion of these substances is influenced by a variety of factors. More relevant information can be obtained by spot urine collections after an overnight fast. The fasting calcium excretion (expressed as milligrams Ca per 100 ml glomerular filtrate) provides an indirect index of bone mineral resorption. Occasionally, fasting calcium excretion may be increased as a result of impaired renal tubular reabsorption of calcium. The best index of phosphorus excretion is the maximum tubular reabsorption of phosphate (TmP) expressed as a function of the glomerular filtration rate (GFR), or TmP/GFR (Chap. 23). This test can be used as an indicator of the level of parathyroid hormone concentration, but it must be kept in mind that a markedly reduced TmP/GFR is typical of various states of primary renal phosphorus wasting unrelated to parathyroid hormone secretion.

The development of radioimmunoassays for parathyroid hormone has provided a more specific test for parathyroid function. Measurements of circulating parathyroid hormone are helpful in determining the pathogenesis of bone disease in patients with primary and secondary hyperparathyroidism. Simultaneous measurement of calcium and parathyroid hormone concentration is necessary for proper interpretation of the hormone assay result. Patients with primary hyperparathyroidism usually have elevated levels of parathyroid hormone, but with some assays there is a significant group of patients with normal levels. In secondary hyperparathyroidism of all types, the parathyroid hormone concentration is almost always above normal in association with a low or normal calcium concentration.

Urinary cAMP or nephrogenous cAMP measurements are a sensitive index of parathyroid hormone activity. They are particularly useful in patients in whom parathyroid hormone resistance is suspected. These patients fail to exhibit a normal increase in cAMP production after the administration of parathyroid extract.

Hydroxyproline is an amino acid which occurs almost exclusively in the collagen molecule.[11] Hydroxyproline-containing peptides and free hydroxyproline are found in plasma and urine.[12] The peptides in urine are primarily of low molecular weight and represent degradation products of bone matrix. About 10 percent of hydroxyproline-containing peptides are larger than 5000 daltons and appear to reflect recently synthesized collagen fragments.[13] Urinary free hydroxyproline excretion is insignificant, since free hydroxyproline is metabolized by the enzyme hydroxyproline oxidase. Because hydroxyproline released from bone matrix is not reutilized for collagen biosynthesis, urinary hydroxyproline excretion has been used clinically as an index of bone matrix resorption.[12] In normal persons, there is a correlation between age and urinary total hydroxyproline excretion. In growing children, the upper limit of normal excretion may be as high as 150 mg per 24 h; this high level occurs at the time of the adolescent growth spurt.[12] In adults the normal range is approximately 20 to 40 mg per 24 h on a low-gelatin diet. A fasting spot urine to determine the ratio of hydroxyproline to creatinine excretion may provide a simpler and more meaningful estimate of bone resorption than 24-h samples. The use of this test after an overnight fast avoids, for the most part, the influences of dietary collagen and careless urine collection. The upper limit of normal is approximately 0.02 in adults.[14] Hydroxyproline excretion may be increased five- to tenfold in patients with severe metabolic bone disease but may be within the normal range in patients with mild disease. Increased hydroxyproline excretion is also associated with extensive dermatoses and burns.[12]

Measurement of urinary hydroxylysine has also been proposed as an index of bone matrix resorption.[15] Although not widely evaluated, this parameter may be superior to urinary hydroxyproline measurements, since hydroxylysine and its glycosides are less extensively metabolized. Another advantage is that skin and bone collagen contain different ratios of the various glycosides, so that the tissue source of urinary hydroxylysine can be estimated if desired.[15–17]

Calcium balance studies, as devised by Albright and Reifenstein, have been extensively used as a research tool in the investigation of bone disease but can be carried out only in a research ward. Various isotopic studies of intestinal calcium absorption have more recently been devised but also have not been widely applied to patients outside of research centers.

Radiology and Nuclear Medicine

Radiological evaluation of the skeleton is a valuable noninvasive means of determining the extent, severity, and nature of bone disease. The "metabolic bone survey" usually consists of a lateral skull x-ray, hand x-rays, lateral thoracic and lumbar x-rays, and a pelvic x-ray. In most patients with a generalized bone disease, an abnormal radiological finding will be apparent in one or more of these sites. If hyperparathyroidism is in the differential diagnosis, films of the clavicles or lamina dura may prove revealing. If osteomalacia is suspected, a search for pseudofractures in the long bones and scapulae is worthwhile, if they are not discovered in other areas.

The types of radiological abnormality which should be sought are a reduction in bone density, unusual bone texture, widening of the epiphyseal cartilage growth plate, thinning or thickening of the cortex, periosteal new bone formation, endosteal scalloping, fractures, pseudofractures, and abnormalities in the size and shape of a bone. These types of abnormality are illustrated in subsequent sections.

Quantitative assessment of bone mineral is of particular importance in view of the high incidence of osteoporosis. Numerous techniques have been devised to assess this. These include visual assessment of lateral radiographs of the spine, radiogrammetry, photodensitometry, single energy photon absorptiometry, dual energy photon absorptiometry, neutron activation analysis, study of Compton scattering, and quantitative computed tomography.[18] Single energy photon absorptiometry of the radius, dual energy photon absorptiometry of the spine, and quantitative computed tomography of the spine have been widely applied in clinical studies.[18–20] These techniques have greatly improved the definition of the osteopenic state.

The development of high-resolution bone scanners and the use of technetium-labeled bisphosphonates have brought about major improvements in the quality of bone scans in recent years. The bone scan provides a visual display of the metabolic activity in different regions of the skeleton. At the present time, scans are primarily used to detect occult bone metastases in patients with cancer. Approximately 4 h after receiving an intravenous injection of the radiolabeled bone-seeking agent, the patient is scanned in the supine position. An example of the scan of a patient with metastatic breast carcinoma is seen in Fig. 24-1. The asymmetry of radioisotopic activity is thought to reflect both increased osteoblastic activity adjacent to metastatic tumor and an increased blood flow in the involved region. Patients with purely osteolytic lesions such as those in multiple myeloma, often have normal bone scans unless pathological fractures are present. There is a developing literature concerning the use of bone scans in patients with metabolic bone disease.[21] It has been suggested that estimation of total isotope uptake by the skeleton would be a valuable parameter of skeletal metabolic activity. This possibility deserves further evaluation.

Bone Biopsy

The bone biopsy may provide valuable information which is not supplied by other techniques. This is particularly true in patients with milder forms of meta-

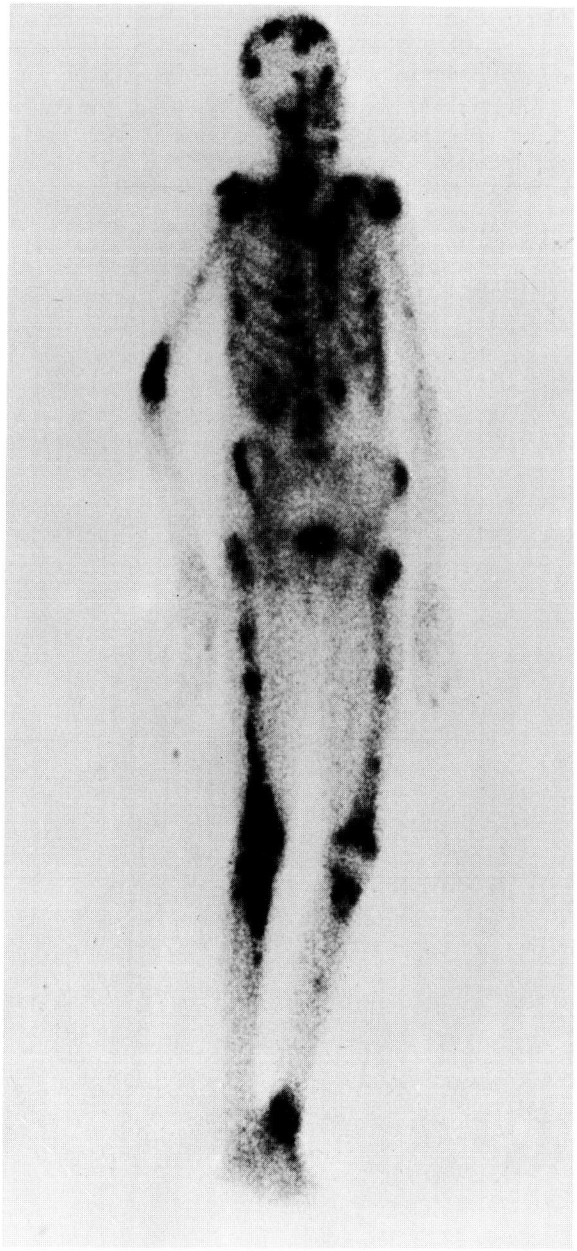

FIGURE 24-1 Technetium-labeled bis-phosphonate bone scan of a patient with widespread metastases from a breast carcinoma. Note the numerous foci of increased radioisotope uptake.

bolic bone disease, in whom the radiological and biochemical parameters are near normal or are not specific for a particular disease entity. Unfortunately, the application of bone biopsies and appropriate histological techniques to clinical problems in the United States has been quite limited. The lack of a sufficient number of physicians trained in obtaining bone biopsies and the limited number of routine pathology laboratories which have experience in the proper processing of bone specimens account for the underutilization of this important technique.

In the past, bone biopsy material was obtained by resecting part of a rib and required the services of a surgeon. A major advance in bone biopsy technique was made possible by the design of a trocar by Bordier and colleagues[22] which made it possible to obtain an iliac crest biopsy specimen in an outpatient setting. After infiltration of the skin, soft tissues, and marrow cavity with xylocaine, a biopsy can be obtained from the iliac crest adjacent to the anterior superior spine with minimal discomfort in most cases. A repeat biopsy after therapeutic intervention can be carried out on the opposite iliac crest.

In most pathology departments, the bone biopsy is fixed in formalin, decalcified, and embedded in paraffin prior to staining with hematoxylin and eosin (H&E). Examination of the bone specimen prepared in this manner allows identification of the number and types of bone cells present and of the overall structure of the bone. Unfortunately, the H&E stain of decalcified bone sections does not allow consistent identification of the unmineralized osteoid which may be present in increased amounts in a variety of disorders. This requires the preparation of undecalcified bone sections. The bone specimen is fixed and then embedded in plastic before sectioning with a special microtome. Several stains can be used to delineate the amount of unmineralized osteoid in the sections. In laboratories which do not have the appropriate equipment to prepare undecalcified sections, an alternative technique can be used to demonstrate unmineralized osteoid.[23] After appropriate demineralization of the specimen, an Azan stain of the section will produce a blue color at sites of previously unmineralized osteoid and a red color in normally mineralized bone.

Quantitative histomorphometry of bone biopsies is available in a few centers and is the most sophisticated approach to analyzing histological sections.[24] Utilizing a variety of specialized microscopes as well as computerized instrumentation, precise quantitation of many parameters can be achieved. These include assessment of the bone volume, the percentage of bone surface covered by osteoid, the average thickness of osteoid, the surface of bone undergoing resorption and formation, the number of osteoclasts, and the average size of the periosteocytic lacunae. Another technique used to assess bone formation and resorption surfaces is quantitative microradiography.[24] Undecalcified sections of bone are examined radiographically. This technique demonstrates the variable density of bone mineral and is particularly useful in demonstrating the low density of partially calcified osteoid.

The discovery that the antibiotic tetracycline localizes at the sites of mineralization in bone led to the development of a dynamic test of bone metabolic activity.[25] A patient receives 500 mg of tetracycline on 2 consecutive days, nothing for 10 days, and 500 mg daily for 3 days; a bone biopsy is done the next day. The iliac crest bone specimen is processed and the sections are evaluated by fluorescent microscopy. Two types of tetracycline which fluoresce differently can be used. In a normal subject two bands of tetracycline fluorescence will be found on the surfaces of bone at which new bone was formed during the period of tetracycline labeling. The inner tetracycline band represents the initial course and the outer band the second course of the antibiotic. The rate of bone formation can then be calculated by measuring the average width between the bands and by dividing this by the number of days between tetracycline administrations. In normal adults, this approaches 1 μm per day.[26] In patients with osteomalacia, in whom the principal defect is in mineralization, tetracycline uptake by bone is impaired.

The indications for bone biopsy are still evolving, but in general a biopsy is indicated when there is a need to establish a diagnosis in patients in whom noninvasive parameters of bone disease are not definitive. Patients with subclinical osteomalacia particularly require bone biopsies for confirmation of the diagnosis. The bone biopsy may also be used to monitor the results of therapy in patients with disorders such as osteoporosis and renal osteodystrophy. It is likely that as more effective therapies become available for these problems, sequential bone biopsies will be more widely used to confirm the efficacy of therapy.

OSTEOMALACIA AND RICKETS

Osteomalacia is characterized by an excess of unmineralized bone which results from an impairment of bone mineralization. It is a disorder of diverse etiology which can be subdivided into two main categories: those disorders associated with a reduction in circulating vitamin D metabolites and those associated with hypophosphatemia.

In children, the term *rickets* is used to indicate a disorder characterized by epiphyseal dysplasia, retardation of longidutinal growth, and a variety of skeletal deformities. Osteomalacia is the predominant histological lesion. Rickets arises from etiologic factors similar to those which produce osteomalacia in adults.

Clinical Presentation

Symptoms and Signs

The manifestations of rickets depend not only upon the severity and duration of the underlying disorder but to a great extent upon the patient's age, because rickets affects the areas of bone which are growing most rapidly, and these vary at different ages.[27] Short stature reflects the epiphyseal dysplasia at the ends of the long bones of the lower extremities. The types of skeletal deformity associated with rickets include craniotabes, frontal bossing, thickening of the rib ends (rachitic rosary), lateral indentation of the chest wall (Harrison's groove), bowing of long bones, and knock-knee (Fig. 24-2).

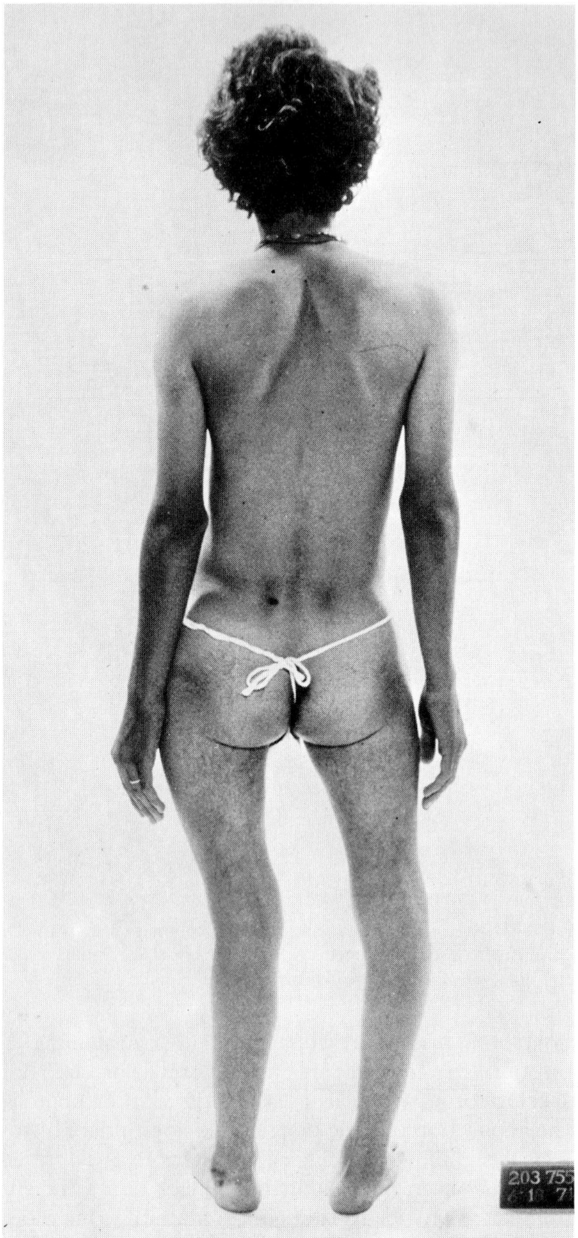

FIGURE 24-2 Bowing and knock-knee deformities in a 19-year-old male with familial X-linked hypophosphatemic rickets.

In adult-onset disease, skeletal deformities are seldom encountered except in the most severe cases. Abnormal spinal curvature, a bell-shaped thorax, or pelvic deformity may develop.

Bone pain is common in both children and adults. It is often experienced in the pelvis, the lower extremities, the spine, and the ribs. The pain is worsened by activity in weight-bearing regions. In severe cases, bone tenderness is present upon palpation. This is best elicited by thumb pressure on the distal tibia.

Muscle weakness and tenderness, particularly of the proximal musculature of the lower extremities, may be the dominant features in some patients. This is much more likely to occur in vitamin D–deficient patients than in hypophosphatemic patients.

In the vitamin D–deficient patient, hypocalcemia may be reflected by the presence of paresthesias, tetany, seizures, and impaired mentation.

Radiological Features

Radiological examination of the skeleton can provide information of a highly specific nature with regard to the diagnosis of rickets or osteomalacia.[28] The radiological signs of advanced rickets include widening of the epiphyseal growth plates, a frayed appearance of the metaphyses, and cupping and widening of the metaphyses (Fig. 24-3). These abnormalities are most readily detected at the metaphyseal sites which are growing most rapidly. Up to the age of 1 year both the upper and the lower extremities are likely to exhibit these findings. After 1 year the lower extremities are more likely to reveal the abnormalities of rickets. Within several weeks of the initiation of appropriate therapy, mineralization of the epiphyseal cartilage can be discerned as a radiodense line adjacent to the metaphyses. In subsequent years, Harris lines, which are transverse radiodense lines across the shafts of long bones, may be noted in patients who have had a fluctuating degree of activity of their disease.

Gross deformity of the skeleton is more likely to occur in children than in adults. Kyphoscoliosis, a bell-shaped thorax, a triangular configuration of the pelvic lumen, and bowing of the upper and lower extremities are abnormalities that may be encountered in patients with severe long-standing disease.

In the adult, the radiological findings in patients with osteomalacia often mimic those found in osteoporosis. A generalized loss of bone density with thinning of the cortex may be impossible to distinguish from that found in patients with osteoporosis. Expansion of intervertebral disk spaces and pathological compression fractures of the vertebral bodies may be observed. Occasionally the trabecular pattern of bone is thickened, and mottled radiolucencies may be discerned. Osteosclerosis may rarely occur in isolated bones, most often affecting vertebral bodies. This unexpected finding remains unexplained. It is much more likely to be seen in the healing phase of the disease when the mineralization defect is corrected.

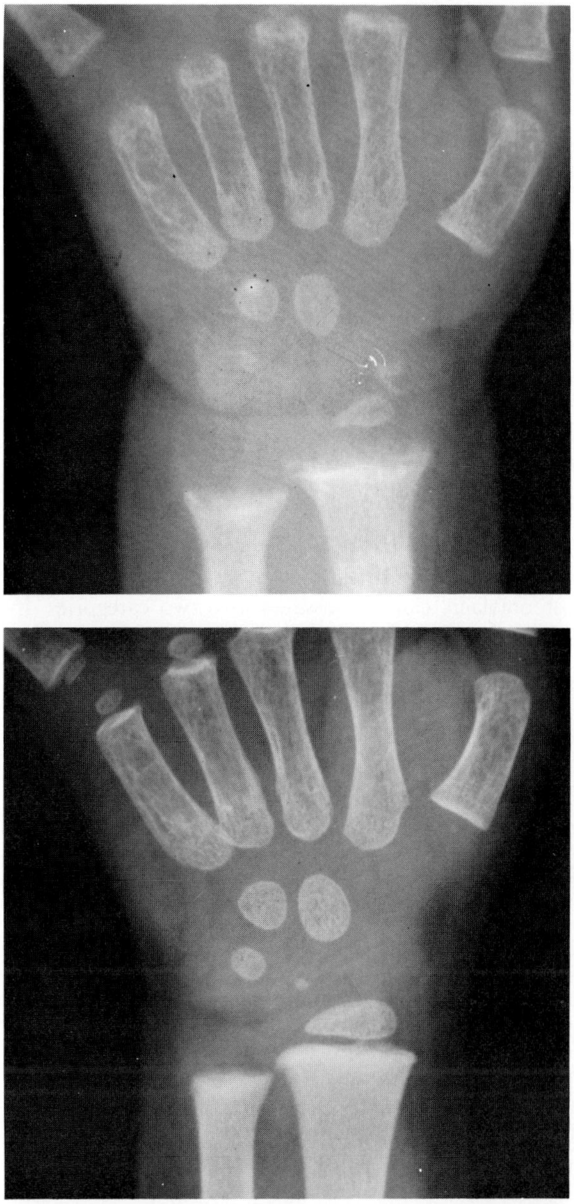

FIGURE 24-3 (*Top*) Roentgenograms of the wrist of a 13-month-old child with rickets due to vitamin D deficiency. Note the frayed appearance associated with widening and cupping of the metaphyses. A pseudofracture is present at the distal radius. (*Bottom*) Nearly total healing of the rickets after 5 months of treatment with vitamin D_2.

In osteomalacic patients who have vitamin D deficiency, secondary hyperparathyroidism may be reflected by subperiosteal resorption of the phalanges, loss of the lamina dura, widening of the spaces at the symphysis pubis and sacroiliac joints, and the presence of brown tumors or bone cysts. These abnormalities rarely if ever occur in hypophosphatemic patients.

The pathognomonic radiological feature of osteomalacia is the presence of pseudofractures, also known as Looser zones or Milkman fractures (Fig. 24-4). These narrow zones of rarefaction are often bilateral and symmetrical. Common sites at which they may be found include the femoral neck and shaft, ulna and radius, pubic and ischial rami, clavicle, ribs, scapula, and metacarpals, metatarsals, and phalanges. The origin of these lesions is not certain. There is an underlying excess of unmineralized osteoid which may reflect healing of a microfracture. In severe longstanding cases the borders of a pseudofracture may appear sclerotic.

Laboratory Findings

Biochemical abnormalities in patients with rickets and osteomalacia can be classified into two categories. In patients whose disorder develops as a consequence of vitamin D lack or abnormal vitamin D metabolism, the concentrations of serum calcium and phosphorus are usually reduced and the serum alkaline phosphatase activity elevated.[29] Patients who develop bone disease on the basis of chronic hypophosphatemia also have elevated serum alkaline phosphatase activity but have a normal serum calcium concentration.[27] The hypocalcemic state of the vitamin D–deficient patients is associated with elevated serum parathyroid hormone levels.[30] The state of secondary hyperparathyroidism is further manifested by a decreased renal phosphate threshold,[29] elevated urinary cAMP excretion,[31] and generalized aminoaciduria,[29] including hydroxyprolinuria.[12] The hypophosphatemic group have seldom been reported to have elevated serum parathyroid hormone levels,[32] but a lowered renal phosphate threshold is usually present, and renal wasting of a single amino acid may be found.[27] Urinary calcium excretion is markedly reduced in hypocalcemic patients but may be less so in the hypophosphatemic patient.[27]

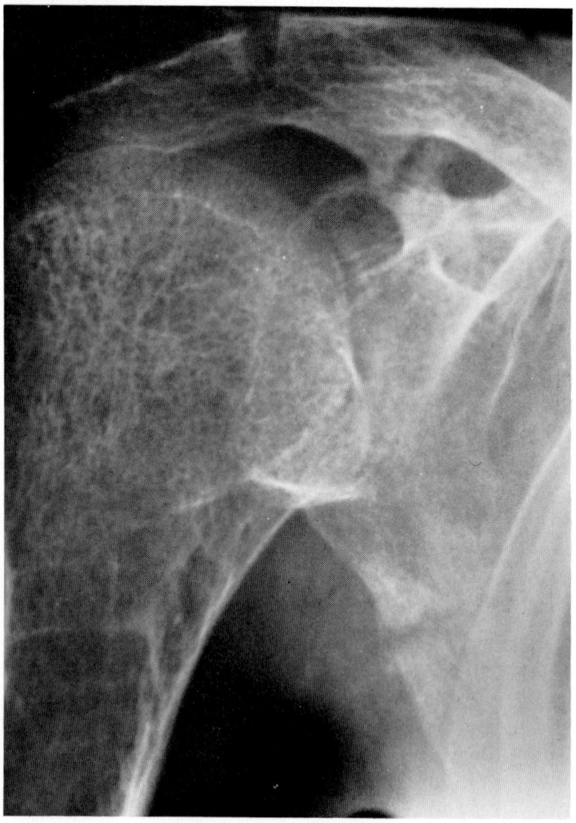

FIGURE 24-4 Pseudofractures of the medial border of the scapula and acromion in a 52-year-old man with malabsorption syndrome.

Assays of vitamin D metabolites have also been applied to the assessment of patients with rickets and osteomalacia.[33] The best measure of vitamin D status is the serum 25-hydroxyvitamin D concentration, since it is the major vitamin D metabolite in the circulation (Chap. 23). As expected, 25-hydroxyvitamin D and 24,25-dihydroxyvitamin D are found in low concentrations in the circulation of patients with classical vitamin D deficiency. Levels of serum 1α,25-dihydroxyvitamin D may be within the normal range in such patients,[34] but in the context of hypocalcemia these "normal" levels reflect inadequate synthesis of the renal vitamin D metabolite. Other quantitative abnormalities of circulating vitamin D metabolites have been described and are discussed under Classification and Pathogenesis, below.

Bone Pathology

To allow for a better understanding of the pathological features of rickets, the histology of endochondral ossification at the epiphyseal growth plate is briefly described here.

Longitudinal bone growth occurs at the epiphyseal growth plate, a cartilaginous band separating the epiphysis from the metaphyseal region of the shaft.[28] In the proliferative zone of the growth plate hypertrophic cartilage cells form orderly columns extending toward the shaft. These cell columns are then penetrated by blood vessels extending from the marrow and subsequently are destroyed by chondroclasts.

Simultaneously, calcification of the cartilage matrix occurs, and osteoblasts arise around the blood vessels. They synthesize the bone matrix adjacent to the calcified cartilage, and this is rapidly mineralized.

In rickets, replication of cartilage cells in the proliferative zone proceeds in a normal fashion. However, the proliferating cells fail to form orderly columns advancing toward the shaft.[28] The marrow vessels also fail to penetrate the cartilage, and the cartilage cells are only partially removed. Thus the zone of proliferating cartilage widens. Inadequate mineralization of cartilage and osteoid is noted as well as penetration of this zone by vessels from the perichondrium and adjacent resting cartilage. The weakened structure at the cartilage shaft junction and the proliferation of cartilage account for the deformities which become apparent by radiological and clinical examination.

Biopsy of the growth plate of a long bone is not recommended, since future bone growth may be impaired. Biopsy of the iliac apophysis can be carried out with less likelihood of skeletal distortion.

The hallmark of osteomalacia is the accumulation of unmineralized osteoid.[35] This occurs as a result of impairment of matrix mineralization and despite a reduction in the rate of bone matrix formation. The increase in osteoid volume is reflected by a greater extent of osteoid seams covering both cortical and trabecular bone surfaces and by an increased width of the osteoid seams. Because excess osteoid may also be a feature of such disorders as thyrotoxicosis, primary hyperparathyroidism, and Paget's disease, it may be necessary to label the bone with tetracycline to establish definitively whether an osteomalacic state is present. In osteomalacic patients the percentage of osteoid seams labeled with tetracycline is reduced; tetracycline uptake, when present, may be diffuse rather than concentrated at the calcification front; bone matrix formation is reduced; and there is an increased mineralization lag time.[35] In states of high bone turnover, tetracycline labels most osteoid seams, and bone matrix formation and mineralization rates are increased. The width of the osteoid seams is usually normal.

Numerous active osteoblasts are usually found lining trabecular bone surfaces in most types of osteomalacia. These are not found in patients with adult hypophosphatasia, in patients with bone disease associated with total parenteral nutrition, and in a small minority of patients with renal osteodystrophy.

Patients with vitamin D deficiency exhibit features of secondary hyperparathyroidism, including increased numbers of osteoclasts and a fibrovascular marrow. Evidence of secondary hyperparathyroidism is generally not found in patients with osteomalacia associated with hypophosphatemic states. The latter patients exhibit increased osteoid volume and a mineralization defect indistinguishable from that found in simple vitamin D deficiency. A partially reversible decrease in mineral surrounding osteocyte lacunae has been reported in hypophosphatemic patients. This may reflect abnormal osteocyte function.[36]

Classification and Pathogenesis

Osteomalacia or rickets may develop as an isolated pathological state or as a complication of another disorder. Table 24-1 contains a classification of osteomalacia and rickets. In the majority of patients, the pathogenesis can be ascribed to either an abnormality of vitamin D supply, metabolic activation or action, or chronic hypophosphatemia. The patients who have an abnormality of vitamin D metabolism are unable to absorb sufficient calcium and phosphorus from their diets to allow normal mineralization of osteoid. A direct effect of vitamin D metabolites on bone mineralization has not been demonstrated convincingly. Patients who develop osteomalacia or rickets as a result of hypophosphatemia probably do so because phosphorus is an essential constituent of hydroxyapatite.

Vitamin D Abnormalities

Vitamin D Deficiency

Classic vitamin D deficiency can develop only in a subject whose skin exposure to ultraviolet light is inadequate *and* whose diet contains insufficient vitamin D.[37] Vitamin D–deficiency rickets has been considered an extremely uncommon disorder since vitamin D supplementation of dairy products and other foods in the United States became a national policy. However, recent reports have indicated a recrudescence of rickets in infants of mothers who follow certain dietary practices. Children who are breast-fed but not given vitamin D supplements and those on vegetarian diets without vitamin D supplementation are susceptible to rickets.[38,39] These recent "outbreaks" of rickets have occurred in northern cities where air pollution may reduce ultraviolet exposure. Dressing in long garments and the use of hoods and veils were contributing factors in one group.[38]

Fraser and Scriver have described three stages in the pathogenesis of human rickets.[32] In stage I, hypo-

Table 24-1. Classification of Causes of Osteomalacia and Rickets

- I. Reduction of circulating vitamin D metabolites
  - A. Inadequate ultraviolet light exposure and inadequate dietary vitamin D
  - B. Vitamin D malabsorption
    - 1. Small intestine disease
    - 2. Pancreatic insufficiency
    - 3. Insufficient bile salts
  - C. Abnormal vitamin D metabolism
    - 1. Liver disease
    - 2. Chronic renal failure
    - 3. Drugs (anticonvulsants, glutethimide)
    - 4. Mesenchymal tumors, prostatic cancer
    - 5. Vitamin D–dependent rickets type I (25-hydroxyvitamin D–1α-hydroxylase deficiency)
  - D. Renal loss
    - 1. Nephrotic syndrome
- II. Peripheral resistance to vitamin D
  - A. Vitamin D–dependent rickets, type II
  - B. Anticonvulsant drugs
  - C. Chronic renal failure
- III. Hypophosphatemia
  - A. Renal phosphate wasting
    - 1. Hypophosphatemic rickets
      - a. Familial X-linked
      - b. Autosomal recessive
      - c. Sporadic
    - 2. Hypophosphatemic osteomalacia
      - a. Familial X-linked
      - b. Sporadic
    - 3. Familial renal phosphate leak with hypercalciuria, nephrolithiasis, and osteomalacia and rickets
    - 4. Fanconi syndrome
    - 5. Mesenchymal tumors, fibrous dysplasia, epidermal nevus syndrome, prostatic cancer
    - 6. Primary hyperparathyroidism
  - B. Malnutrition
  - C. Malabsorption due to gastrointestinal disease or phosphate-binding antacids
  - D. Chronic dialysis
- IV. Miscellaneous
  - A. Inhibitors of calcification
    - 1. Sodium fluoride
    - 2. Disodium etidronate
  - B. Calcium deficiency
  - C. Hypoparathyroidism
  - D. Hypophosphatasia
  - E. Fibrogenesis imperfecta ossium
  - F. Systemic acidosis
  - G. Total parenteral nutrition

calcemia is the sole significant biochemical abnormality. In stage II, the calcium concentration returns to the normal range and hypophosphatemia is apparent, presumably because of secondary hyperparathyroidism. Stage III is associated with severe clinical manifestations of rickets and the return of hypocalcemia.

Vitamin D Malabsorption

Malabsorption of vitamin D may occur in patients with small intestine disease, pancreatic insufficiency, and/or inadequate bile salts.[40] Since osteomalacia may develop in malabsorption states despite adequate ultraviolet light exposure, it is possible that malabsorption of 25-hydroxyvitamin D also occurs after the latter is excreted into the small intestine as a constituent of bile.[41] Evidence for and against this proposal has been obtained.[42] The pathogenesis of bone disease in malabsorption syndromes may be more complex than simply malabsorption of dietary vitamin D and its liver metabolite, since other important nutrients such as proteins may be poorly absorbed.

Abnormal Vitamin D Metabolism

Patients with severe parenchymal liver disease (particularly cholestatic) may develop osteomalacia and secondary hyperparathyroidism.[43] These patients have low levels of 25-hydroxyvitamin D in the circulation. This may occur as a consequence of reduced hydroxylation of vitamin D because of hepatocellular dysfunction and/or because of vitamin D deficiency due to poor nutrition and inadequate ultraviolet light exposure. Oral vitamin D supplementation can be used to delineate patients with vitamin D deficiency from those with a hydroxylation defect or cholestasis-induced malabsorption of vitamin D.[44] The vitamin D–binding protein may be reduced in patients with liver disease[44] and conceivably could confuse interpretation of assays of vitamin D metabolites. In the only study reporting free 25-hydroxyvitamin D levels in sera of patients with liver disease, those levels were normal in association with reduced serum vitamin D–binding protein and total 25-hydroxyvitamin D levels.[45]

In patients with chronic renal failure, there is a reduction in both 1α,25-dihydroxyvitamin D and 24,25-dihydroxyvitamin D in the circulation.[33,46] The pathogenesis of renal osteodystrophy will be discussed later.

Patients who are treated with anticonvulsant drugs are at risk of developing rickets and/or osteomalacia,[47] although a recent study of 20 patients revealed only a modest increase in osteoid volume and no impairment of mineralization rate.[48] The development of bone disease has been attributed to increased liver metabolism of 25-hydroxyvitamin D to more polar metabolites,[49] but not all anticonvulsant-treated patients have low levels of this metabolite,[48] and in some patients inadequate vitamin D intake or ultraviolet light exposure appears to account for reduced levels.[50] While low levels of 24,25-dihydroxyvitamin D have also been found,[51,52] normal, elevated, or low levels of circulating 1α,25-dihydroxyvitamin D have been reported.[52,53] Therefore it is difficult to be certain that anticonvulsant-induced bone disease is attributable solely to impaired vitamin D metabolism. Anticonvulsant-induced bone disease has been prevented with 3000 units of vitamin D_3 per week,[49] but exposure to sunlight may be more effective.[50]

The association of osteomalacia with a variety of mesenchymal tumors has been observed in more than 40 patients.[54] In most patients, a marked reduction in circulating 1α,25-dihydroxyvitamin D levels has been found. The patients were normocalcemic and often markedly hypophosphatemic because of renal phosphate wasting. Complete excision of the neoplasm generally produces resolution of the biochemical abnormalities and osteomalacia. An identical syndrome has also been observed in patients with prostatic cancer,[55] oat cell carcinoma of the lung,[56] and, perhaps, cholangiocarcinoma of the liver.[57] No tumor factor has been isolated as yet which could account for the syndrome.

Vitamin D–dependent rickets type I is a rare autosomal recessive disorder which is thought to be due to a deficiency of renal 25-hydroxy-1α-hydroxylase.[58] This has been deduced from the finding of low circulating levels of 1α,25-dihydroxyvitamin D in affected children even when receiving high doses of vitamin D[59] and from demonstration of radiological healing of the bone lesions with physiological amounts of 1α,25-dihydroxyvitamin D_3.[58]

Renal Loss

Subtle degrees of osteomalacia and secondary hyperparathyroidism may develop in patients with the nephrotic syndrome, presumably on the basis of renal losses of vitamin D–binding protein and 25-hydroxyvitamin D.[60,61] However, in the absence of renal failure bone disease may not develop.[62]

Peripheral Resistance to Vitamin D

Since 1978 it has been recognized that a subset of patients with early-onset rickets, termed *vitamin D–dependent rickets type II,* develop this disorder as a consequence of tissue insensitivity to 1α,25-dihydroxyvitamin D.[63] These patients characteristically have hypocalcemia, secondary hyperparathyroidism, elevation of circulating 1α,25-dihydroxyvitamin D, and a normal intake of vitamin D as well as adequate exposure to sunshine. In some patients, alopecia is a striking clinical feature.[64] A poor response to high doses of 1α,25-dihydroxyvitamin D_3 has also been reported.[65] The syndrome is often found in siblings whose parents have no detectable biochemical or skeletal abnormalities. In all patients thus far evaluated, immunoassayable 1α,25-dihydroxyvitamin D_3 receptors have been found in cultured skin fibroblasts in a concentration similar to that in fibroblasts from normal subjects.[66] However, by the use of a ligand-binding assay to estimate receptor function and nuclear uptake, a variety of biochemical abnormalities have been found in cultured skin fibroblasts[67] and bone cells.[68] These include unmeasurable receptor binding and nuclear uptake of [^{3}H]1α,25-dihydroxyvitamin D_3, decreased capacity with normal affinity for receptor binding and nuclear uptake, and absence of detectable nuclear uptake despite normal or near normal receptor binding. Normal receptor binding and nuclear uptake have also been observed, which suggests an undefined abnormality distal to the nuclear uptake of 1α,25-dihydroxyvitamin D_3. Thus it appears that the vitamin D–resistant state in many patients arises from structural variations in the receptor molecule, not from diminished receptor synthesis. The above biochemical abnormalities have not been found to correlate with the clinical findings of alopecia and poor responsiveness to 1α,25-dihydroxyvitamin D_3 therapy.[65] However, defective induction of 25-hydroxyvitamin D_3-24-hydroxylase by 1α,25-dihydroxyvitamin D_3 in cultured skin fibroblasts has been shown to predict the in vivo response to calciferol therapy. In addition, profound resistance to 1α,25-dihydroxyvitamin D appears to be present in the alopecic patients.

Since patients with anticonvulsant drug–associated rickets and osteomalacia may have normal or elevated 1α,25-dihydroxyvitamin D levels, it is possible that peripheral resistance to this metabolite is a factor in the pathogenesis of the bone disease in those patients.[48,53] In vitro studies have demonstrated impairment of the action of 25-hydroxyvitamin D_3 on bone and a reduction of calcium transport by the intestine in the presence of diphenylhydantoin.[69,70]

Patients with chronic renal failure require supraphysiological doses of 1α,25-dihydroxyvitamin D_3 to increase intestinal calcium absorption.[71] This suggests that peripheral resistance to vitamin D is a factor in the impaired calcium absorption found in patients with chronic renal failure.

Hypophosphatemia

It is generally thought that chronic hypophosphatemia produces metabolic bone disease as a consequence of decreased body stores of phosphorus. A chronic hypophosphatemic state may arise from either inadequate dietary phosphorus, reduced intestinal absorption of dietary phosphorus, or renal wasting of phosphorus. The last is the mechanism most commonly encountered clinically.

Renal Phosphate Wasting

The commonest cause of rickets in the United States is the dominantly inherited genetic disorder termed *familial X-linked hypophosphatemic* or *vitamin D–resistant rickets.* This entity was first recognized by Albright in 1937.[72] The phenotypic trait of hypophosphatemia is transmitted on the X chromosome. Bone disease and short stature are usually more severe in males who carry the abnormal genotype, whereas heterozygous females exhibit a more variable penetrance of these somatic traits.[73]

Hypophosphatemia develops as a consequence of a reduction in TmP/GFR. The exact nature of the abnormality in renal transepithelial phosphorus transport is not known. It cannot be attributed to excessive secretion of parathyroid hormone, since hormone levels in blood are usually normal[32] or only modestly elevated.[74] In one study, an increased phosphaturic response to exogenous parathyroid hormone was found and led the investigators to speculate that an increased responsiveness to normal levels of the hormone might be a factor.[75] However, in a careful study of one patient with idiopathic hypoparathyroidism and familial X-linked hypophosphatemic rickets, a marked renal tubular phosphorus leak was present when the serum calcium was restored to normal by calcium and 1α,25-dihydroxyvitamin D_3 therapy.[76] A few patients have been reported to have reduced intestinal phosphorus absorption,[77] but this is not an invariable finding.

Studies of vitamin D metabolites in the circulation of patients with hypophosphatemic rickets have raised questions concerning the pathogenesis of the bone disease in these patients. It would be expected that chronic hypophosphatemia would raise the level of circulating 1α,25-dihydroxyvitamin D. Instead, normal or frankly reduced levels of this metabolite have been reported by several laboratories.[78–80] Low levels of the metabolite are usually found in patients treated with vitamin D.[78,80] Further evidence of an abnormality in renal hydroxylation of vitamin D was provided by a study which demonstrated a subnormal rise in serum 1α,25-dihydroxyvitamin D levels in untreated patients in response to parathyroid hormone infusion.[81] Impaired synthesis of 1α,25-dihydroxyvitamin D might explain the diminished rate of intestinal calcium absorption found in some patients,[72] but the normocalcemic state which is typical of the disorder suggests that significant 1α,25-dihydroxyvitamin D deficiency is not present. The low levels of 1α,25-dihydroxyvitamin D do not account for the hypophosphatemic state, since physiological doses of the metabolite do not correct the abnormality.[82]

At least two inherited forms of hypophosphatemic rickets other than the X-linked type have been described. Two families with autosomal recessive inheritance patterns have been evaluated.[83,84] An unusual clinical aspect noted in these patients was gross osteosclerosis. A single family with a probable autosomal recessive inheritance pattern has been described in which striking hypercalciuria appeared to develop as a consequence of marked elevation of 1α,25-dihydroxyvitamin D levels.[85]

Sporadic hypophosphatemic rickets may occur in the absence of hypophosphatemia and/or bone disease in any other family member. This form of rickets is clinically indistinguishable from familial X-linked hypophosphatemic rickets and presumably arises from the same mutation responsible for the latter disorder.

Hypophosphatemic osteomalacia in adults occurs most commonly as a sporadic condition,[86] but a familial syndrome has been described in a single large kindred.[87] The inheritance of the disorder is X-linked. The biochemical findings in this syndrome are similar to those of familial X-linked hypophosphatemic rickets, but untreated adults have no stigmata of rickets and hypophosphatemic children demonstrate no radiological evidence of epiphyseal dysplasia.

Osteomalacia and rickets may develop as a complication of a variety of generalized renal tubular disorders.[27] These have been classified under the general term *Fanconi syndrome.* Not only renal phosphate wasting but excessive renal loss of bicarbonate, glucose, uric acid, and amino acids may be detected in affected patients. The bone disease may then be a manifestation of chronic hypophosphatemia and/or systemic acidosis. Acquired renal tubular disorders of phosphate transport differ in one major respect from X-linked hypophosphatemia. Muscle pain and weakness often are prominent features of the acquired disorders but are seldom a problem in X-linked hypophosphatemia. Distal renal tubular acidosis also may cause bone disease in the absence of hypophosphatemia.[27] Rarely, hypophosphatemic rickets may be associated with reversible renal tubular acidosis.[88]

Patients with a variety of benign or malignant mesenchymal tumors,[54] fibrous dysplasia,[88a,89] epidermal nevus syndrome,[90] and prostatic cancer[55] may develop rickets and/or osteomalacia in association with hypophosphatemia. In most of these patients there is renal phosphate wasting, normal or slightly low serum calcium concentrations, normal serum parathyroid hormone concentrations, and reversal of the syndrome after removal of the pathological lesions. It is likely that the lesions secrete a phosphaturic substance, and in one study an extract of a fibroangioma produced a phosphaturic response in dogs.[90] As discussed previously, the significance of low levels of 1α,25-dihydroxyvitamin D in these patients is uncertain, although therapy with 1α,25-dihydroxyvitamin D_3 is often effective.[54]

Primary hyperparathyroidism is associated with hypophosphatemia in approximately 70 percent of cases. It is conceivable that osteomalacia could develop in certain patients with severe hypophosphatemia. In one study, quantitative histomorphometry of bone biopsies revealed a reduction of calcification rate in some patients, but there was no increase in the width of osteoid seams.[91] At present, it does not appear that uncomplicated primary hyperparathyroidism produces significant osteomalacia. However, the patient with primary hyperparathyroidism may more readily develop osteomalacia in the presence of risk factors such as inadequate exposure to sunshine and anticonvulsant therapy. Also, during the postoperative period following parathyroid surgery, osteomalacia might develop as a consequence of the increased need for phosphorus and calcium in the process of healing of osteitis fibrosa.

Malnutrition and Malabsorption

An isolated deficiency of phosphorus due to malnutrition or malabsorption is distinctly uncommon. It is more likely that a combination of vitamin D deficiency and inadequate supplies of calcium and phosphorus would be responsible for osteomalacia or rickets. Persistent use of phosphate-binding antacids is rarely associated with clinical osteomalacia.[92]

Chronic Dialysis

Hypophosphatemia may occur during the course of chronic dialysis in patients with chronic renal failure.[93] Presumably this occurs as a consequence of excessive loss of phosphorus from the extracellular fluid into the dialysate. The use of phosphate-binding antacids to control hyperphosphatemia may also contribute. Osteomalacia may be severe in the hypophosphatemic patient on dialysis but is promptly reversible with appropriate therapy. The involvement of aluminum in the production of osteomalacia in certain patients with renal failure is described in a later section.

Miscellaneous

INHIBITORS OF CALCIFICATION Fluoride is a potent inhibitor of bone mineralization and may cause severe rickets and osteomalacia in areas of endemic fluorosis[94] and in patients treated with pharmacological doses of sodium fluoride. The latter patients usually receive sodium fluoride, 40 mg or more daily, for the treatment of osteoporosis. Osteomalacia will not develop if at least 1 g of elemental calcium is also taken orally each day.[95]

Disodium etidronate, a bisphosphonate used to treat Paget's disease and prevent heterotopic ossification, is an inhibitor of mineralization at doses of 10 to 20 mg per kilogram of body weight.[96] Fortunately, at a dose of 5 mg/kg, Paget's disease can be suppressed without diffuse impairment of mineralization. However, focal osteomalacia has been found in bone biopsies of patients treated with low doses of disodium etidronate.[97]

CALCIUM DEFICIENCY Radiological evidence of rickets has been observed in a child with severe dietary calcium restriction in the presence of normal vitamin D intake and normal circulating 25-hydroxyvitamin D levels.[98] Hypocalcemia, hypophosphatemic secondary hyperparathyroidism, and elevated alkaline phosphatase were biochemical features in this patient. A group of South African children with poor calcium intake were also found to have a similar ricketslike syndrome which was corrected by increasing dietary calcium intake.[99] However, the latter children inexplicably had normal serum calcium and phosphorus levels. Histological evidence of osteomalacia in three South African children on calcium-deficient diets has been reported.[100] Each of these patients was hypocalcemic. It is not known whether isolated calcium deficiency can produce osteomalacia in adults.

HYPOPARATHYROIDISM Rickets and/or osteomalacia have been reported in a few patients with hypoparathyroidism.[101,102] The pathogenesis is unclear, but successful treatment of the hypocalcemia produced healing of the bone disease.

HYPOPHOSPHATASIA Hypophosphatasia is a rare cause of rickets and osteomalacia.[103] It is usually inherited as an autosomal recessive trait. The milder adult form of the disorder may be inherited as an autosomal dominant trait. The biochemical abnormalities which are characteristic of this disorder are (1) low serum alkaline phosphatase activity, (2) elevated serum and urine inorganic pyrophosphate and phosphorylethanolamine levels, and (3) frequently, hypercalcemia in children. Since inorganic pyrophosphate and phosphorylethanolamine are substrates for alkaline phosphatase, it is likely that the high levels of these substances reflect decreased alkaline phosphatase activity in bone and perhaps other organs. Inorganic pyrophosphate may be an important intermediary in the initiation of bone mineralization by extracellular matrix vesicles. It is not known whether phosphorylethanolamine has any function in bone mineralization. The pathogenesis of hypercalcemia in hypophosphatasia is unknown, although one report suggests parathyroid hormone levels may be elevated in infantile hypophosphatasia.[104]

A study of bone histology in a kindred of patients with adult hypophosphatasia demonstrated a paucity of osteoblasts despite the excess of osteoid.[105] The authors proposed that osteoblast dysfunction might be manifested first by mineralization defects and later by a reduction in the numbers of osteoblasts.

FIBROGENESIS IMPERFECTA OSSIUM Fibrogenesis imperfecta ossium is a rare disorder which affects previously healthy males over the age of 50.[106] Skeletal pain and tenderness may be so severe as to cause total incapacitation. Pseudofractures may be seen on roentgenograms, but, unexpectedly, there is a generalized increase in bone density with a lack of trabeculation and a mottled appearance. Bone histology reveals an increased amount of osteoid, impaired uptake of tetracycline, and absence of a normal lamellar pattern of the collagen fibers. The latter finding suggests an underlying defect in collagen synthesis. Consistent with this hypothesis are the findings of normal plasma calcium and phosphorus concentrations. Plasma alkaline phosphatase activity is increased.

SYSTEMIC ACIDOSIS Systemic acidosis due to isolated renal tubular acidosis, Fanconi syndrome, or chronic renal failure may be an important factor in the pathogenesis of osteomalacia associated with these disorders.[27] Normal levels of vitamin D metabolites have been found in the circulation of patients with renal tubular acidosis[107] and in volunteers with induced metabolic acidosis.[108] Therefore, the mineralization defect associated with chronic acidosis remains unexplained.

TOTAL PARENTERAL NUTRITION Long-term use of total parenteral nutrition has been associated with bone pain, patchy osteomalacia, low serum levels of parathyroid hormone and 1α,25-dihydroxyvitamin D, hypercalciuria, and intermittent hypercalcemia.[109,110] In patients receiving casein hydrolysate, inadvertent infusion of aluminum has been implicated as the factor responsible for the syndrome. Such patients have been demonstrated to have aluminum localized to the surface of mineralized bone from which tetracycline uptake was absent.[111] However, the syndrome has also been found in patients infused with free amino acids which are relatively devoid of aluminum.[109]

Treatment

The treatment of osteomalacia and rickets is as heterogeneous as are the underlying causes. Knowledge of the pathogenesis of the disease is critical in assuring an optimum result of therapy, particularly in infants.

Classic vitamin D deficiency can be prevented by the ingestion of 400 IU (10 μg) of vitamin D_2 daily by children and 100 IU daily by adults. These amounts of vitamin D_2 may be used to treat patients with established bone disease, but doses as much as two- to tenfold greater have been used in order to produce a more rapid clinical recovery.[35] Patients also must receive adequate calcium and phosphorus from their diets or, if necessary, from supplementation. In most patients the recommended normal daily intake is adequate.

The earliest biochemical response to vitamin D therapy is a rise in serum phosphorus concentration, which typically occurs within 4 days.[35] Initially, serum calcium may actually decline and alkaline phosphatase rise, but both move toward normal levels within weeks. Vitamin D intoxication can be avoided or minimized by measuring the plasma calcium concentration every 2 to 4 weeks. The dose should be reduced, if pharmacological, when the biochemical parameters approach the normal range and when radiological healing of rickets is apparent.

Patients with vitamin D malabsorption require only short-term vitamin D therapy if the underlying disorder can be effectively treated. This is particularly true in patients with celiac disease, in whom a gluten-free diet will produce a complete remission of the malabsorptive state and concomitant vitamin D deficiency. If the disorder is irreversible, pharmacological doses of vitamin D are required. The dose of vitamin D varies widely, but up to 100,000 IU per day by the oral route may be necessary. In some patients parenteral administration of smaller doses is required. Greater than usual amounts of calcium and phosphorus also may be needed to overcome the inefficiency of intestinal absorption.

In patients with impaired vitamin D metabolism, vitamin D_2 therapy in pharmacological amounts is usually effective in preventing or reversing rickets and osteomalacia. Up to 15,000 IU daily has been used to induce healing of established bone disease. Lower doses of 25-hydroxyvitamin D_3 have been effective in these patients.[112] In patients with low circulating levels of 1α,25-dihdyroxyvitamin D, near physiological doses of this metabolite can produce healing of bone lesions. This has been demonstrated in patients with vitamin D–dependent rickets[58] and in some patients with chronic renal failure. The role of 1α,25-dihydroxyvitamin D_3 in the treatment of renal osteodystrophy is discussed further under Renal Osteodystrophy, below.

The main principle in the treatment of hypophosphatemic bone disease is restoration of the serum phosphorus concentration to the normal range. This may prove difficult if administration of vitamin D_2 or a vitamin D analogue is the sole therapy given to patients with renal phosphate wasting. Pharmacological doses of vitamin D_2 or dihydrotachysterol were the earliest forms of treatment for patients with familial X-linked hypophosphatemic rickets. These drugs often were administered at toxic levels and caused hypercalciuria and hypercalcemia. Despite this high dosage, the rickets was not uniformly healed and there was seldom a significant reversal of short stature. A major improvement in treatment occurred when it was demonstrated that supplemental oral phosphate produced dramatic clinical improvement.[113] If the serum phosphorus concentration can be held within the normal range during the day and night, a marked increase in linear growth velocity will result. In addition, if optimum treatment is begun early in the course of the disease, dwarfism and rachitic deformities can be reversed or prevented. The dosage of oral phosphate in a given patient is empirical and should be adjusted on the basis of serum phosphorus and alkaline phosphatase determinations, radiological changes, and growth rate. To avoid the side effects of diarrhea, initial treatment should be with smaller doses of a buffered phosphate solution. Fraser and Scriver[32] recommend the following schedule in 1-year-old children: 0.125 g elemental phosphorus three times on day 1, 0.25 g three times on day 2, 0.25 g four times on day 3, and 0.25 g five times on day 4 and each succeeding day.[32] The requirement of frequent ingestion of phosphate is dictated by the observation that the peak phosphorus concentration is reached 1½ h after a dose and that the baseline level is restored 4 h later. The doses may need to be adjusted to provide up to 5 g of elemental phosphorus daily to achieve optimum control of the disease. The great difficulty with this therapy is compliance. The cooperation of the parents is critical in assuring that the late evening dose as well as the other doses are taken.

If phosphate therapy alone is administered to the patient with hypophosphatemic bone disease, an increased rate of bone mineralization often will produce hypocalcemia and a state of secondary hyperparathyroidism. This can be corrected or prevented by the daily administration of 50,000 IU or more of vitamin D_2.[19] However, long-term therapy with vitamin D_2 is not fully effective in healing the osteomalacic lesions in these patients,[112–114] whereas 1α,25-dihydroxyvitamin D_3 in combination with phosphorus supplementation not only improves metabolic balance[115] but corrects the mineralization defect in trabecular bone.[116,117] Hypomineralization of periosteocytic lesions was not completely corrected in one study,[36] but it is not certain whether this represents an irreversible defect in osteocytic function or if higher doses of 1α,25-dihydroxyvitamin D_3 are required to produce complete healing of the lesions.[117] Careful observation of these patients during therapy is necessary, since hypercalcemia may intervene as the bone healing continues.[116] The short half-life of 1α,25-dihydroxyvitamin D_3 minimizes the duration of hypercalcemia when the dose is reduced. Equal attention must be given to preventing chronic hypocalcemia secondary to phosphate therapy, since hypercalcemic hyperparathyroidism may be a consequence of long-term therapy.[118] The issue of how long to continue therapy is unresolved, although it is clear that the patient's full growth should be achieved before discontinuance of treatment is considered. Since many adults with X-linked hypophosphatemic rickets (healed) are asymptomatic and have normal serum alkaline phosphatase activity despite persistent hypophosphatemia, it is difficult to convince them of the need for lifelong therapy. Bone biopsies in untreated adults reveal persistent osteomalacia of a similar degree in symptomatic and asymptomatic persons.[119] However, calcified bone volume was normal or increased in all the specimens. Until the benefits of continuing treatment of asymptomatic adults can be shown, it is probably reasonable to discontinue or reduce drug therapy several years after growth has ceased if serum alkaline phosphatase activity is normal and bone pain is absent.

Surgical intervention to correct skeletal deformities may be needed in patients who have not received appropriate medical therapy. Procedures such as osteotomy and epiphyseal stapling may increase the mobility of the patient and prevent the long-term complication of degenerative joint disease.

Patients with autosomal recessive hypophosphatemic rickets, sporadic hypophosphatemic rickets or osteomalacia, and Fanconi syndrome with hypophosphatemia all respond well to phosphate–vitamin D regimens.[20]

In patients with hypophosphatemia due to mesenchymal tumors, treatment with 1α,25-dihydroxyvitamin D_3 and phosphate is generally effective if the tumor is not resectable.[54]

No effective treatment program for hypophosphatasia has been developed. Infusion of alkaline phosphatase–rich plasma in several patients failed to produce any clinical benefit despite increasing the circulating alkaline phosphatase activity into the normal range during a 2-month period.[120] Recently, a patient with fibrogenesis imperfecta ossium and a monoclonal gammopathy experienced an impressive remission when treated with melphalan and prednisolone.[121]

Correction of systemic acidosis with oral alkali therapy can fully heal the osteomalacic lesions. Vitamin D therapy is not necessary.

OSTEOPOROSIS

Osteoporosis is the most common metabolic bone disease and is responsible for significant morbidity in the elderly female and male, and in patients who are treated chronically with glucocorticosteroids in pharmacological doses.

The disorder is not a single entity but rather a pathological state which can arise from a variety of disturbances of skeletal homeostasis. It is characterized in all instances by a decreased mass of bone which is normally mineralized.

Clinical Presentation

Symptoms and Signs

In the clinical evolution of osteoporosis there is a long subclinical phase which occurs in most patients before recognition of the disorder. During this time no symptoms or signs may be detected, but radiological and histological abnormalities would be noted if sought. The term *osteopenia* is sometimes used to describe the existence of a reduced bone mass in the absence of symptoms or signs of osteoporosis.[122]

The initial complaint often experienced by patients is back pain. This may occur suddenly without warning and be of great intensity. It frequently results from lifting a heavy object. The pain is sharp or burning in quality, aggravated by movement or weight bearing, and reflects an underlying compression fracture of a vertebral body. The twelfth thoracic and first lumbar vertebrae are most often affected. After healing of the bone, back pain may completely resolve. More commonly residual pain reflects spasm of the paravertebral muscles.

Spinal deformity may develop after repeated acute episodes of compression fracture or may slowly evolve in the absence of severe back pain. A progressive loss in stature occurs as a result of reduction in the height of multiple vertebral bodies. Dorsal kyphosis is typical of long-standing spinal osteoporosis. In the most severely affected persons the spinal curvature may be so great as to cause the lower ribs to touch the iliac crests.

Osteoporosis does not produce deformities of the extremities unless fractures occur. The common sites of extremity fractures are the femoral neck and the distal radius.

Radiological Features

The radiological feature most characteristic of osteoporosis is a decreased density of bone. This is best visualized with routine films of the spine. Cortical thinning and loss of tranverse trabeculation are common findings. If the latter feature dominates, a paradoxical accentuation of cortical density and vertical trabeculation may result. The weakened vertebral bodies allow ballooning of the nuclei pulposi into the classical biconcave "codfish" deformities of the intervertebral disk spaces (Fig. 24-5). A localized herniation of a

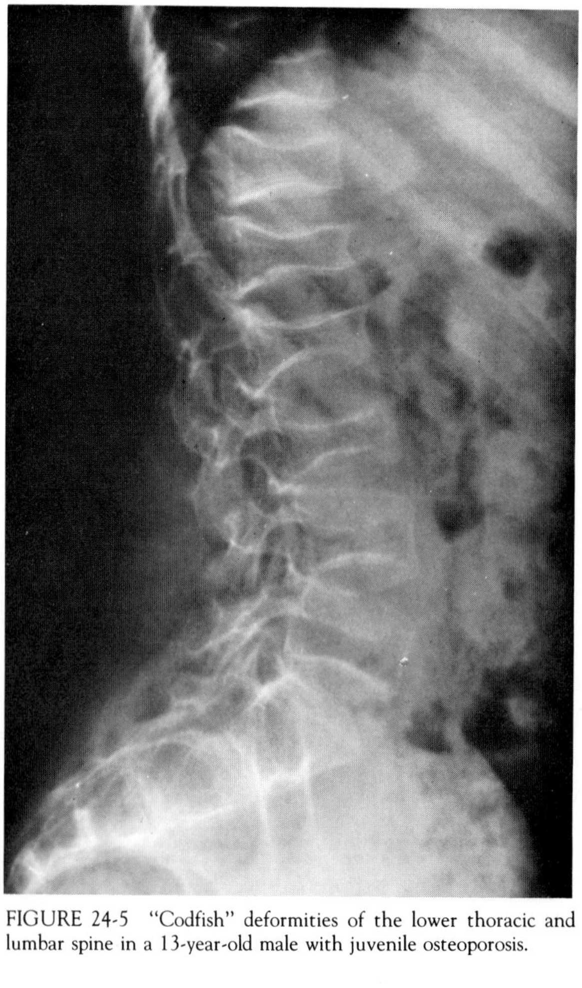

FIGURE 24-5 "Codfish" deformities of the lower thoracic and lumbar spine in a 13-year-old male with juvenile osteoporosis.

nucleus pulposus into a vertebral body, a *Schmorl's node*, may occasionally occur. Anterior wedging of vertebral bodies is usually a sign of marked decrease in bone density but may arise at an earlier stage as a complication of trauma.

Radiological manifestations of osteoporosis at sites other than the spine include a patchy loss of density of the calvarium, decreased cortical density of phalanges and long bones, and vertical striation of long bones. Bowing of the bones of the lower extremity is not typical of osteoporosis but does occur in patients with osteogenesis imperfecta.

Quantitative assessment of trabecular bone mineral in the spine by computed tomography or dual photon absorptiometry has revolutionized the assessment of the patient with osteoporosis. Previously used routine radiographs of the spine could not detect the presence of osteopenia until a 30 to 50 percent deficit of bone mineral was present. The new techniques provide great sensitivity in diagnosis and in follow-up after therapeutic intervention. The possibility of assessing vertebral fracture risk has been suggested by studies utilizing quantitative computed tomography.[123] Vertebral mineral values above 110 mg/cm^3 were generally associated with no vertebral fractures or wedging, whereas below 65 mg/cm^3 almost all patients had fractures (Fig. 24-6).

Cortical bone density also has been assessed by a variety of techniques. Visual examination of radiographs of the hands and shafts of long bones is commonly used but is only semiquantitative. Single energy photon absorptiometry of the radius provides a reproducible quantitative means of measuring cortical bone mineral. However, it has been demonstrated that bone mineral density of the axial skeleton cannot be reliably predicted from measurements of radial cortical bone.[124]

Laboratory Findings

In the great majority of patients, there are no significant abnormalities of the calcium, phosphorus, or alkaline phosphatase concentrations in the circulation. A subset of patients who have thyrotoxicosis may have elevated concentrations of all three parameters,[125] and patients with primary hyperparathyroidism may be hypercalcemic, hypophosphatemic, and hyperphosphatasemic (Chap. 23).

The concentration of immunoreactive parathyroid hormone in the circulation of osteoporotic

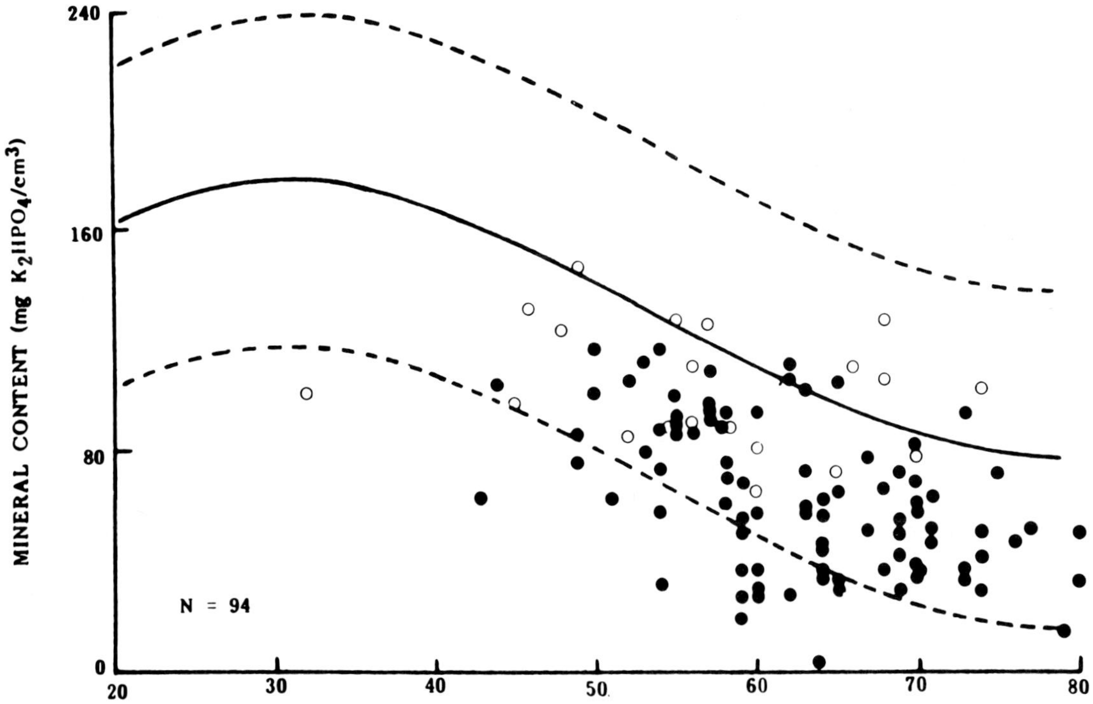

FIGURE 24-6 Vertebral mineral content in osteoporotic (●, with vertebral fractures) and osteopenic (○) females superimposed on mean and 95 percent confidence interval for control women. None of the osteoporotic women with fractures had values higher than 110 mg/cm^3. Only 1 of 23 women with osteopenia but no fracture had a mineral value below 65 mg/cm^3. (*From Cann CE, Genant HK, Kolb FO, Ettinger B, Bone 6:1, 1985.*)

women has been reported to be normal, low, or elevated. In one large series of patients, the hormone levels increased significantly with age in both control subjects and osteoporotic subjects, but the parathyroid hormone concentration was generally lower in patients with postmenopausal osteoporosis.[126] A small group of patients in this study had elevated levels.

Studies of total immunoreactive calcitonin concentrations in the circulation indicate that men have higher levels than women[127] and that the levels in women decline with age.[128] Comparison of total immunoreactive calcitonin levels in untreated postmenopausal women and those receiving estrogen replacement therapy has produced conflicting results. In two studies, estrogen therapy increased calcitonin levels,[129,130] but in one long-term study baseline and calcium-stimulated levels were indistinguishable in untreated and treated women.[131] In two other studies, baseline calcitonin levels also failed to increase after estrogen therapy.[132,133] The concept that estrogens stimulate calcitonin secretion has also been challenged by studies of circulating monomeric calcitonin, in which levels of this biologically active form of calcitonin have been similar in premenopausal and postmenopausal women.[134] Conflicting results have also been obtained in studies comparing calcitonin levels in osteoporotic and normal postmenopausal women. Decreased and normal baseline total immunoreactive calcitonin levels have been reported in osteoporotic women,[135,136] and in one study total immunoreactive calcitonin levels after calcium infusion failed to increase significantly.[137] However, monomeric calcitonin levels after calcium infusion in normal postmenopausal and osteoporotic women were indistinguishable.[138]

Intestinal calcium absorption decreases with aging.[139,140] This has been attributed to a reduction of 1α,25-dihydroxyvitamin D in the circulation of the elderly[140,141] due to an impaired ability of the aging kidney to synthesize 1α,25-dihydroxyvitamin D. Indirect evidence for this interpretation has been provided by the observation that the rise in serum 1α,25-dihydroxyvitamin D levels in response to parathyroid hormone infusion is blunted in elderly women.[141] In countries where there is minimal ultraviolet light exposure and no dietary vitamin D supplementation, calcium malabsorption may also commonly develop as a consequence of vitamin D deficiency, as evidenced by low levels of 25-hydroxyvitamin D in the circulation.[142] There is controversy as to whether elderly patients with osteoporosis have lower levels of 1α,25-dihydroxycholecalciferol in the circulation than subjects of similar age without clinical bone disease, as has been found in some studies[141,142] but not all.[143] In one study it was suggested that resistance to the action of vitamin D metabolites on the intestine was a factor in the pathogenesis of calcium malabsorption.[142]

In patients with evolving osteoporosis, urinary calcium excretion may be significantly elevated, a reflection of an increased rate of bone resorption.[144] This is most likely to be found in patients with hyperthyroidism or in the completely immobilized patient. Urinary hydroxyproline excretion is also elevated in the same patients because of increased bone matrix resorption.[144]

The renal handling of phosphorus has been reported to be abnormal in women with postmenopausal osteoporosis. The TmP/GFR was significantly higher in 24 patients as compared with 18 age-matched normal subjects.[126] This may reflect the modest decrease in serum parathyroid hormone levels found in these patients.

Bone Pathology

The histological features of osteoporosis are quite heterogeneous and, in some respects, still controversial. Two findings are universally agreed upon: (1) bone volume is decreased, and (2) existing bone is normally mineralized.

The rates of bone formation and bone resorption in women with postmenopausal osteoporosis have been estimated by quantitative histomorphometry of iliac crest bone biopsies in several laboratories. Jowsey and colleagues reported that resorptive surfaces were greater than normal and bone-forming surfaces were usually normal in postmenopausal osteoporosis.[145] A similar conclusion was reached more recently in an English study.[146] The former study utilized quantitative microradiography, a technique which measures the density of the mineral phase of bone, and the latter study evaluated the extent of osteoid-covered surfaces and the fraction of surfaces occupied by resorption cavities. The conclusions of these studies have been challenged by other investigators who have demonstrated with tetracycline labeling that in many patients bone formation in the iliac crest is reduced.[147–150] A decrease in the mean wall thickness and duration of formation periods of trabecular bone in women with postmenopausal osteoporosis has also been stressed as indicative of impaired osteoblast function.[151] The reasons for the discrepancies among these histological studies is not entirely clear, but the concept has developed that there is considerable heterogeneity of bone histology in postmenopausal osteoporosis.[149,150,152,153] Biopsy parameters could be classified as indicative of high, low, or normal turnover. Uncoupling of bone resorption and formation is undoubtedly an important factor in determining bone loss and apparently can occur in either a high or a low turnover state. Unfortunately, it has not been possible to consistently correlate biochemical parameters with the histological indices. This may relate to the observation that the skeleton does not respond in a homogeneous manner to the influences of hormones[124] and perhaps other influences. Thus it should not be surprising if local parameters of bone turnover do not correlate with overall skeletal metabolism.

The heterogeneity of the bone pathology of osteoporosis is further reflected by studies of patients with adrenal glucocorticosteroid excess and hyperthyroidism. Cushing's syndrome, spontaneous or iatrogenic, is associated with a marked reduction in bone volume. Studies utilizing either quantitative microradiography or quantitative histomorphometry have demonstrated evidence of increased bone resorption and decreased bone formation in these patients.[154–156] The latter abnormality appears to be the dominant process responsible for the reduced bone mass.

The histology of hyperthyroidism is characterized by a marked increase in bone remodeling.[125] Numerous osteoclasts and osteoblasts are present as well as a fibrous bone marrow. The percentage of trabecular bone covered with osteoid is increased, but there is no widening of the osteoid seams, and the mineralization rate is normal. Decreased cortical and trabecular bone volume must ensue if the rate of bone resorption exceeds that of bone formation. Bone disease induced by hyperthyroidism may be difficult to distinguish from that produced by hyperparathyroidism. It has been reported that the two disorders can be distinguished by measuring the size of the periosteocytic lacunae.[125] There is no increase in this parameter in hyperthyroidism, unlike hyperparathyroidism.

Osteoporosis associated with prolonged immobilization has not been studied extensively. In one study, osteoclastic bone resorption was increased and osteoblastic activity was decreased.[157]

Three studies of bone histology in patients with idiopathic juvenile osteoporosis have been reported.[158–160] In a study utilizing quantitative microradiography there was an increase in bone resorption surfaces, and bone formation surfaces were normal.[158] Quantitative histomorphometry revealed normal osteoclast numbers and a reduced osteoblast surface.[159] In the only study utilizing tetracycline labeling, a single patient was observed to have normal bone formation and resorption.[160]

The histological findings in patients with osteogenesis imperfecta are unique.[161] There is persistence of primitive woven bone and an absence of well-organized haversian systems. Osteoclasts are not present in excessive numbers, and the osteoblasts which are present are spindle-shaped and flattened, like those of inactive cells.

Classification and Pathogenesis

Osteoporosis is associated with aging, hormonal deficiencies and excess, nutritional deficiencies, genetic disorders, hematologic malignancy, immobilization, and a variety of other unrelated disorders (Table 24-2). The pathogenesis of bone disease in many of these states is not completely understood, but modern biochemical and histological techniques have increased our knowledge to a great extent in the past two decades.

Aging

The incidence of osteoporosis and fractures rises with advancing age in women and men. It has recently

Table 24-2. Classification of Causes of Osteoporosis

1. Aging
2. Endocrine abnormality
   a. Estrogen deficiency
   b. Testosterone deficiency
   c. Cushing's syndrome
   d. Thyrotoxicosis
   e. Primary hyperparathyroidism
   f. Diabetes mellitus
3. Immobilization or weightlessness
4. Genetic
   a. Osteogenesis imperfecta
   b. Ehlers-Danlos syndrome
   c. Homocystinuria
   d. Marfan's syndrome
   e. Menkes' syndrome
5. Juvenile osteoporosis
6. Chronic hypophosphatemia
7. Chronic alcoholism
8. Nutritional abnormality
   a. Vitamin C deficiency
   b. Protein deficiency
9. Systemic mastocytosis
10. Heparin therapy
11. Rheumatoid arthritis
12. Chronic liver disease
13. Hematologic malignancy
    a. Multiple myeloma
    b. Leukemia
    c. Lymphoma
14. Idiopathic

been suggested that two distinct syndromes of osteoporosis may occur in the aging population.[162] Type I osteoporosis is thought to occur in a small group of women aged 51 to 65 years and result in fractures in bones in which trabecular bone is dominant, i.e., vertebral bodies. Type II osteoporosis is believed to affect a high proportion of men and women over 75 years of age and produce fractures involving areas containing large amounts of cortical and trabecular bone. Type I osteoporosis may be accounted for in women in large part by gonadal hypofunction, as discussed below, but epidemiological studies indicate that a variety of other factors may contribute to the pathogenesis of osteoporosis. Recently implicated risk factors include cigarette smoking and alcohol intake of moderate degree.[163–165] Decreased exercise as a consequence of degenerative arthritis in weight-bearing joints, poor nutrition, impaired intestinal calcium absorption, and reduced renal function are additional factors which may contribute to abnormal skeletal homeostasis in the elderly and the development of type II osteoporosis. Obesity and black ancestry seem to confer protection against osteoporosis in both sexes.[164,166]

Although symptomatic osteoporosis in the elderly may arise as a consequence of a slowly progressive pathological process, there is another viewpoint. Its proponents suggest that a major factor leading to osteoporosis in the elderly is the failure to acquire a normal skeletal mass during childhood and adolescence.[167] This may result from poor nutrition, severe illness, inadequate exercise, or genetic influences controlling bone matrix synthesis. The "physiological" loss of bone mass which is a universal finding in aging people[122] may lead to symptomatic disease in those who never achieved a normal bone mass during the critical years of growth and development.

Estrogen and Testosterone Deficiency

The incidence of osteoporosis is highest in the postmenopausal female. Evidence has accumulated which implicates estrogen deficiency as a major factor in the pathogenesis of the disorder in these persons, although there is no clear evidence that estrogen levels are lower in osteoporotic subjects. Estrogens may interact at several areas in the control of calcium homeostasis. Estrogens appear to modulate the action of parathyroid hormone on bone, since physiological doses of estrogens reduce serum calcium, urinary calcium, and hydroxyproline levels in postmenopausal women with primary hyperparathyroidism.[168] Classical steroid hormone receptors which bind estrogen have not been found in bone,[169] so it is unclear whether these findings reflect a direct estrogen effect on bone cells. A second interaction of estrogens in calcium homeostasis may be that on vitamin D metabolism and/or action. Postmenopausal women have a mild impairment in intestinal calcium absorption which may be linked to reduced circulating levels of 1α,25-dihydroxyvitamin D.[140] Treatment with estrogen has been reported to reverse both abnormalities.[170] However, in one study, the rise in total plasma 1α,25-dihydroxyvitamin D levels induced by estrogen therapy could be accounted for entirely by an increase in vitamin D–binding protein levels.[132] A direct effect of estrogen on intestinal absorption of calcium could account for improvement in the efficiency of calcium absorption in estrogen-treated postmenopausal women. Although it has been proposed that estrogen stimulation of calcitonin secretion accounts for the estrogen effect on inhibition of bone resorption, studies of monomeric calcitonin in the circulation indicate that calcitonin secretion is similar in normal and osteoporotic postmenopausal women.[138] Therefore, while it may be true that low circulating levels of calcitonin in women account for their lower bone mass than that in men, it is unlikely that impaired calcitonin secretion is a major factor in the pathogenesis of osteoporosis in postmenopausal women.

Since the ovary is a source of both estrogens and androgens, several investigators have examined blood androgen levels as a factor in normal and osteoporotic postmenopausal women. Both androstenedione and testosterone blood production rates were reduced in osteoporotic subjects in one study.[171] Serum dehydroepiandrosterone was somewhat reduced in osteoporotic women in another study.[172] The significance of these data with respect to the pathogenesis of osteoporosis remains unclear.

The central issue of the mechanism of the bone loss in postmenopausal osteoporosis is still unsettled. Albright proposed that this occurred as a consequence of diminished osteoblastic activity.[173] This view is supported by quantitative histological analyses of bone biopsies and by dynamic studies utilizing tetracycline labeling. However, consideration of a variety of biochemical characteristics of postmenopausal patients suggests a different mechanism, i.e., increased bone resorption. Urinary calcium and hydroxyproline are increased,[144] and radiocalcium kinetic studies are compatible with accelerated bone resorption in these patients.[174] These findings are unlikely to be explained by a combination of reduced osteoblastic function and normal osteoclastic activity. A full understanding of the pathogenesis of postmenopausal osteoporosis awaits future studies. In addition, the pathogenesis of decreased bone density found in young female marathon runners, hyperprolactinemic amenorrheic women, and women with anorexia nervosa deserves careful scrutiny.[175–177] Estrogen deficiency of a reversible type may be an important common determinant in these women.

Osteoporosis is less common in the elderly male, and studies of its pathogenesis are rare. Bone loss with aging is not found to the same degree in males as in females.[18] Gonadal hypofunction may be a factor in the bone loss found in elderly males, since a positive correlation has been found between the percentage of cortical area of the second phalanx and plasma levels of testosterone, androstenedione, and estrone in a group of 60- to 90-year-old males.[178] Reports of bone histology utilizing modern technology appear limited to one patient, a 30-year-old hypogonadal male who had iliac crest biopsies before and after testosterone therapy.[179] The linear extent of osteoid surface and of bone formation increased markedly after correction of the hypogonadism.

Cushing's Syndrome

Chronic therapy of such disorders as rheumatoid arthritis, systemic lupus erythematosus, and asthma with glucocorticosteroids often produces a virulent form of osteoporosis. The morbidity resulting from the bone disease may approach or even surpass that of the primary disease being treated. Spontaneous Cushing's syndrome may also cause a severe form of osteoporosis, but spontaneous Cushing's syndrome is a rare finding in the osteoporotic population.

The pathogenesis of glucocorticosteroid-induced osteoporosis is complex and probably involves both direct and indirect effects of glucocorticoids on bone. There is evidence that glucocorticosteroids can inhibit bone formation by existing osteoblasts[180] as well as interfere with mesenchymal cell differentiation into osteoblasts.[181] In children, steroids produce both osteoporosis and decreased linear bone growth[182] as a consequence of inhibition of cartilage growth.[183] The moderate increase in bone resorption found in bone biopsies has been explained by the presence of secondary hyperparathyroidism,[155] although elevated serum parathyroid hormone levels have not been found in all studies.[184–187] The sequence of events that may lead to parathyroid stimulation is unclear, since frank hypocalcemia has not been observed in these patients. It may be that the anti-vitamin D actions of glucocorticosteroids are involved. Pharmacological doses of steroids inhibit intestinal calcium absorption,[188] and it is possible that minimal hypocalcemia is the initial stimulus to parathyroid secretion. Studies of the interaction of glucocorticosteroids with vitamin D metabolism and action have produced confusing results. In animals, steroids have been reported to be without effect on the hepatic hydroxylation step[189] and to variably inhibit,[190] stimulate,[191] or be without effect[189] on the renal 1α-hydroxylation step. In humans, both normal and decreased levels of 25-hydroxyvitamin D have been found in the circulation of patients receiving steroids.[186,192] In two pediatric studies, reduced levels of 1α,25-dihydroxyvitamin D were reported in steroid-treated children with nephritis or systemic lupus erythematosus.[193,194] However, in two studies in adults normal baseline levels were found.[187,195] It has also been suggested that end organ resistance is a major factor in the impairment of intestinal calcium absorption produced by glucocorticosteroids. Administration of 1α,25-dihydroxyvitamin D_3 failed to completely restore calcium transport to normal in cortisone-treated rats.[196] However, near physiological doses of 1α,25-dihydroxyvitamin D_3 significantly increased calcium absorption in five patients receiving high-dose prednisone therapy for rheumatological disorders.[192] The conflicting results which have been reported may, in part, be explained by species differences and experimental design. It may be expected that future studies will better define the exact nature of the interaction of vitamin D and glucocorticosteroids, and that this will significantly improve the therapy of osteoporosis in patients with exogenous and endogenous Cushing's syndrome.

Thyrotoxicosis

Thyrotoxicosis is an uncommon cause of osteoporosis. Clinically apparent bone disease is most likely to develop in the severely affected patient after a long period of untreated disease. Thyroid hormone has been shown to stimulate bone resorption in vitro.[197] Radioactive calcium turnover studies[198] and bone histology[125] indicate that the rates of both bone resorption and bone formation are increased in thyrotoxicosis. The loss of bone in patients with this "high turnover" type of osteoporosis must reflect a dominance of bone resorption, but the factors which account for a relative uncoupling of resorption from formation are not known. The role of reduced intestinal calcium absorption, probably due to low levels of 1α,25-dihydroxyvitamin D in the circulation, is uncertain, but this may also contribute to the reduced bone mass found in thyrotoxicosis.[199,200]

Primary Hyperparathyroidism

Decreased bone density is a recognized abnormality in a significant percentage of patients with primary hyperparathyroidism. Surprisingly, most patients do not have symptoms. This problem is discussed in Chap. 23.

Diabetes Mellitus

Decreased bone density has been found in association with diabetes mellitus,[201] particularly in young insulin-dependent patients. Despite this, the incidence of fractures in diabetic subjects does not appear to be high.[202] Since insulin promotes amino acid uptake by bone cells and stimulates bone collagen synthesis, it is possible that insulin deficiency or resistance reduces bone formation directly. Alternatively, the hypercalciuria associated with poor diabetic control or impaired vitamin D metabolism may be important factors.[201,203,204] In rats, experimental diabetes mellitus produces a reduction in serum 1α,25-dihydroxyvitamin D levels,[204] but this has not been found in humans[205] except in young insulin-dependent diabetic patients[206] and in patients with severe diabetic ketoacidosis.[207]

Immobilization and Weightlessness

Osteoporosis is a serious complication in patients confined to bed for prolonged periods as a consequence of spinal trauma or neuromuscular disorders. Bone loss appears to arise from a combination of increased osteoclastic activity and diminished osteoblastic activity.[156] Patients under 30 years of age may become hypercalcemic and hypercalciuric. The absence of weight bearing and of muscular activity, rather than hormonal abnormalities, is responsible for the derangement in skeletal homeostasis. A related loss of bone density occurs during space flight and is not influenced by exercise in the weightless state.

Genetic Disorders

A variety of rare genetic disorders are associated with osteoporosis. Osteogenesis imperfecta, Ehlers-Danlos syndrome, homocystinuria, Menkes' syndrome, and Marfan's syndrome all appear to be examples of specific defects in bone matrix synthesis.[208]

Juvenile Osteoporosis

Juvenile osteoporosis is a rare disorder which is characterized by a rapid loss of bone in prepubertal children of both sexes.[209] Multiple fractures of long bones, ribs, and vertebral bodies may occur in the absence of any apparent abnormality of skin, sclera, joints, or endocrine function. With the onset of puberty, most patients go into remission. The explanation for the remarkable spontaneous improvement in bone density is not known, but in one patient low serum 1α,25-dihydroxyvitamin D levels were found before puberty and the patient showed clinical improvement when treated with 1α,25-dihydroxyvitamin D_3.[210] Following puberty and discontinuation of this therapy, the blood level of this vitamin D metabolite was normal.

Chronic Hypophosphatemia

Osteoporosis has been demonstrated in the bone biopsies of 19 adults with chronic hypophosphatemia due to renal tubular wasting of phosphate.[211] This was associated with hypercalciuria, increased urinary hydroxyproline excretion, and low levels of serum immunoreactive parathyroid hormone. How this syndrome relates to the more common problems of hypophosphatemic rickets and osteomalacia is unclear.

Chronic Alcoholism

Bone density and histomorphometric measurements in eight middle-aged males with a history of high alcohol intake for at least 10 years revealed a significant degree of osteoporosis.[212] The patients were otherwise generally in good health and had no evidence of cirrhosis of the liver. The pathogenesis of the bone disease is uncertain, but a direct toxic effect of alcohol on bone cells is one possibility.

Miscellaneous

The pathogenesis of osteoporosis associated with a variety of disorders such as systemic mastocytosis, rheumatoid arthritis, and chronic liver disease, as well as heparin therapy, is not known. Vitamin C deficiency may impair bone collagen synthesis. Hematologic malignant disease may cause bone loss by local production of osteoclast-activating factors. Idiopathic osteoporosis in premenopausal adults is an uncommon problem for which there is no explanation.

Treatment

The treatment of osteoporosis should be based upon knowledge of the pathogenesis of the disorder in an individual patient and often involves a program including physical therapy, exercise, diet, and drugs.

By far the most common group of patients who seek care are postmenopausal women. Those who believe that osteoporosis in these patients reflects inadequate development of skeletal mass during childhood and adolescence stress the concept that prevention would have been the most effective therapy. Proper nutrition and exercise are regarded as the most likely means to prevent future bone disease.

At the menopause there are several approaches to

retarding the expected bone loss and preventing symptomatic osteoporosis. Estrogen replacement therapy has been conclusively demonstrated to diminish the loss of bone mass in women who undergo either spontaneous or artificial menopause.[213-216] This can be achieved with relatively modest doses of estrogens (0.2 mg ethinyl estradiol, 0.625 mg conjugated equine estrogens, or 5 mg diethylstilbestrol daily for 25 days each month). Bone resorption is reduced, as indicated by reduction of urinary calcium and hydroxyproline excretion,[173] calcium balance becomes more positive,[217] and intestinal calcium absorption is improved.[180,217] During the initial 6 months of treatment bone mass may actually increase, but subsequently bone formation decreases and no additional major gain in mass is demonstrable.[218] There is now ample evidence that estrogen replacement therapy in postmenopausal women not only inhibits bone loss but reduces the fracture rate as compared with that in untreated women.[216,219] However, it should be noted that the bone-sparing effect may not be equal throughout the skeleton. The vertebral trabecular bone appears to be conserved to a greater degree than cortical bone in the radius and metacarpals.[216]

Estrogen therapy may produce a variety of disturbing complications, including uterine carcinoma, fluid retention, hypertension, and vascular thrombosis. The likelihood of inducing uterine carcinoma is reduced markedly by the daily administration of 10 mg of medroxyprogesterone acetate during the last 10 days of estrogen therapy each month. The other complications are found in low incidence when replacement doses of natural estrogens are used. Despite the relative safety of the estrogen-progestin therapy, the monthly withdrawal bleeding which many women experience remains a significant negative feature of this therapy.

A possible alternative means of inhibiting bone loss in postmenopausal women is manipulation of calcium intake. Correction of negative calcium balance and inhibition of bone loss (Fig. 24-7) by raising calcium intake to 1400 to 1500 mg daily has been reported by two groups.[217,220] These data suggest that an absolute increase in net calcium absorption may be achieved in postmenopausal women in whom the efficiency of intestinal calcium absorption is impaired and that this can result in reduced bone turnover and conservation of bone. However, more studies over a longer term are needed to definitively establish the role of calcium supplementation in postmenopausal women, since studies from Denmark suggest that calcium is not as effective as estrogen in postmenopausal women.[221,222]

A third means of attempting to prevent bone loss is administration of physiological doses of 1α,25-dihydroxyvitamin D_3 in order to reverse the defect in intestinal calcium absorption commonly present in postmenopausal women. Calcium absorption has been improved with doses of 0.25 to 0.75 μg daily.[223,224]

In association with this effect on calcium absorption, there was a decrease in urinary hydroxyproline excretion and alkaline phosphatase. However, with the higher doses and particularly with the use of calcium supplements, hypercalciuria and occasionally hypercalcemia develop. Theoretically, bone mass would be preserved with an appropriate regimen of low-dose 1α,25-dihydroxyvitamin D_3 and a normal calcium intake, but this was not the case in one study.[221] Once more, more studies are needed to demonstrate the safety and efficacy of long-term 1α,25-dihydroxyvita-

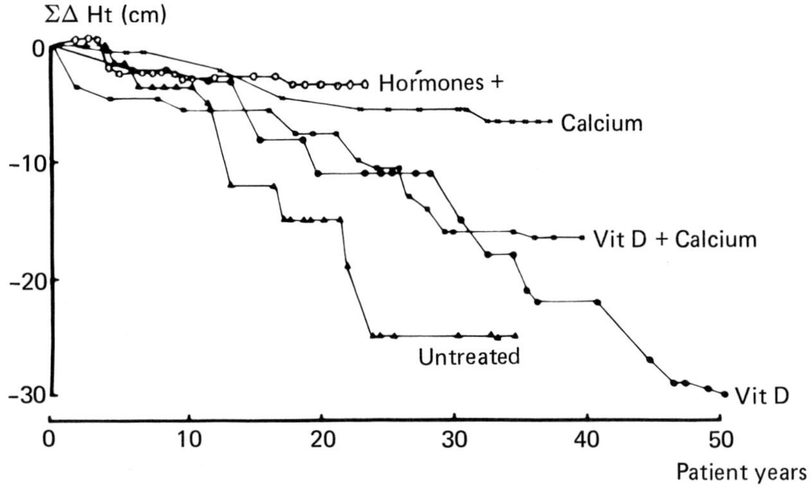

FIGURE 24-7 Cumulative plot of sequential changes in height in groups of women with postmenopausal osteoporosis who were treated with various regimens. Note that oral calcium therapy alone was as effective as estrogens in preventing loss of height. (*From Nordin BEC, Horsman A, Marshall DH, Simpson M, Waterhouse GM, Clin Orthop 140:216, 1979.*)

min D_3 therapy in the prevention of postmenopausal fractures.

In several studies, the administration of salmon calcitonin has been reported to produce a small increase in total body calcium and/or an increase in bone mineral content at specific skeletal sites.[225–227] Bone histomorphometry carried out in one study revealed an increase in percent of total bone area and a reduction in the percent of resorbing surface as compared with control subjects.[225] In no study was the number of patients great enough to permit the conclusion that fracture incidence was reduced by the treatment. Future studies should determine whether fracture incidence is reduced by calcitonin and whether the drug should be considered preventive therapy only or is also effective in treating a severe deficit of bone mass.

In patients who are already symptomatic, simply prescribing estrogens or calcium supplements will not produce major clinical improvement. A carefully planned program of physical therapy and exercise may alleviate much of the perivertebral muscle spasm which is responsible for residual back pain after compression fractures are healed. Analgesic therapy should be kept to a minimum. Estrogens and/or calcium supplementation may prevent further bone loss. However, long-term improvement mainly depends on utilizing an agent which can stimulate new bone formation and thereby strengthen the weakened skeleton. At present, the only drug which can produce a major positive effect on bone formation is sodium fluoride.[228] In doses of approximately 50 to 90 mg daily, with an intake of at least 1000 mg of elemental calcium daily, a positive calcium balance, an increase in trabecular bone, and a reduction in vertebral fracture incidence have been observed.[229–232] In some patients, pharmacological doses of vitamin D or an analogue and phosphorus supplements have been added in an attempt to ensure that normal mineralization of bone occurs. There is no strong evidence that these measures are necessary, but certainly strict adherence to calcium supplementation is critical in the prevention of osteomalacia. Unfortunately, sodium fluoride appears to have no beneficial effect on cortical bone, and side effects may be bothersome. Epigastric distress and peptic ulcers, with possible hemorrhage and arthralgias, may develop in as many as 40 percent of treated patients. These symptoms generally resolve with a decrease in dose or cessation of therapy. The duration of treatment must be individualized. If bone density is markedly diminished, treatment may be necessary for years. It has been suggested that serum fluoride concentrations should be maintained between 0.20 and 0.25 μg/ml by adjusting the fluoride dosage if necessary.[231]

Thiazide diuretics, anabolic steroids, and low-dose human parathyroid hormone (1–34) have all been evaluated as potential agents for the control of osteoporosis.[233–235] Results are too fragmentary to permit any definitive conclusions concerning their possible future role in the therapy of this difficult problem. Other recent research concerns the bioavailability of calcium from different sources such as milk and calcium carbonate supplements. It has been reported that absorption of calcium carbonate by achlorhydric patients is lower than that of calcium citrate in normal subjects, although if the calcium carbonate is given with meals the absorption is normal.[236] It has also been suggested that milk may be a better source of calcium than calcium carbonate, because it may not suppress bone remodeling as severely as calcium carbonate.[237]

Glucocorticoid-induced osteoporosis is second in clinical importance only to postmenopausal osteoporosis. The management of this problem has proved difficult, particularly if it is not possible to discontinue or reduce the dose of steroid. In one study, changing from daily to alternate day use of glucocorticosteroids did not seem to reduce the degree of bone loss in arthritic patients.[238] Possibly newer analogues of cortisol may have less deleterious effects on bone metabolism, as suggested by a study in which deflazacort, a prednisolone derivative, produced approximately one-third less bone loss than prednisone in equipotent anti-inflammatory doses.[239,240]

Because of the known anti-vitamin D effect of glucocorticosteroid therapy, most regimens for therapy of glucocorticoid-induced osteoporosis have included vitamin D and calcium supplementation. Doses of vitamin D_2 ranging from a few thousand to 50,000 IU daily have been administered in combination with 1000 to 1500 mg of dietary and/or supplemental calcium. There is little rigorous documentation of the efficacy of such a therapeutic program. If undertaken, serum and urinary calcium levels should be monitored carefully, since hypercalciuria and hypercalcemia are frequent complications of such therapy. If urinary calcium excretion exceeds 300 mg per day, the calcium intake should be reduced to a level which maintains calcium excretion below this amount. In general, doses of vitamin D_2 above 10,000 IU daily should be avoided because of a greater chance of complications. Recent studies with vitamin D metabolites have suggested a future role for these agents in the patient receiving glucocorticosteroid therapy. In one study, near physiological doses of 1α,25-dihydroxyvitamin D_3 (0.4 μg daily) produced a significant increase in intestinal calcium absorption in patients receiving high-dose steroids.[192] In a second study, treatment with 25-hydroxyvitamin D_3 also increased calcium absorption and prevented a decrease in bone density.[239] A third study reported on a double-blind controlled trial of 2 μg of 1α-hydroxyvitamin D_3 in glucocorticosteroid-treated patients.[241] It was concluded that over a 6-month period the drug inhibited bone resorption without suppressing bone formation in iliac crest bone biopsies. No difference in radial bone mineral content was demonstrated between the control and the treated groups. The total number of patients evaluated in these three studies was relatively small, and at present the vitamin D metabolites have not been approved for general use in steroid-treated patients.

In patients with other endocrine abnormalities which produce osteoporosis, treatment of the underlying abnormality is of greatest value. Resolution of thyrotoxicosis results in an increase in bone mass, although this is less evident in postmenopausal women.[242] Insulin therapy in juvenile-onset diabetes mellitus appears to exert a protective effect on the skeleton.

The osteoporosis of immobilization is best managed by early mobilization of the patient, if this is possible. Although calcitonin is effective in controlling associated hypercalcemia,[243] there is no evidence that osteoporosis can be prevented or corrected by this drug.

The treatment of the osteoporoses associated with genetic disorders has been disappointing. Although several studies suggested a beneficial effect of calcitonin in patients with osteogenesis imperfecta, the most recent study shows no benefits.[244]

A recent study of a boy with juvenile osteoporosis demonstrated a dramatic effect of the bisphosphonate (3-amino-1-hydroxypropylidene)-1,1-bisphosphonate on the clinical course of the disease.[245] A rapid reduction in bone resorption followed by signs of sclerosis near the growth plates of affected metaphyses and at the end plates of the vertebrae was observed over a period of 3 months of treatment with this experimental drug.

OSTEOPETROSIS

Osteopetrosis (*Albers-Schönberg disease, marble bone disease, osteosclerosis fragilis generalisata*) is a rare heritable disorder of bone which is characterized by increased skeletal density.[246] The pattern of inheritance is either autosomal recessive or autosomal dominant. Patients with recessive inheritance usually have a more severe form of clinical involvement. Common abnormalities include an enlarged skull, hearing loss, optic atrophy, pathological fractures, osteomyelitis, retarded growth, leukoerythroblastosis, anemia, thrombocytopenia, lymphadenopathy, and hepatosplenomegaly. Patients often do not survive past age 20 and usually die as a consequence of infection, anemia, or hemorrhage. In approximately 50 percent of patients with an autosomal dominant pattern of inheritance, osteopetrosis is asymptomatic. Fractures, osteomyelitis, and cranial nerve palsies may occur in some patients. Serum calcium, phosphorus, and alkaline phosphatase concentrations are generally normal in both types of osteopetrosis. Serum acid phosphatase is often increased. Occasionally a patient with infantile osteopetrosis will be found to have hypocalcemia, hypophosphatemia, and an elevated alkaline phosphatase. A rare recessive syndrome of osteopetrosis, type I renal tubular acidosis, and basal ganglia calcification has been found to be associated with erythrocyte carbonic anhydrase II deficiency.[247,248]

The radiological features of osteopetrosis are often quite striking. A generalized increase in skeletal density may be associated with a diminution or absence of marrow cavities, clublike deformities of the long bones, and a "bone within a bone" appearance of the vertebral bodies (Fig. 24-8).

Bone biopsies in patients with osteopetrosis may prove difficult to obtain because of increased bone density. Histological examination of the bone reveals an increased density of bone, often with obliteration of the marrow cavities. The bone may be woven in character in the adult, and remnants of fetal calcified cartilage are a characteristic feature. Numerous osteoclasts may be present, but there is an absence of Howship's lacunae, a finding indicative of inactivity of the osteoclasts. This is probably explained by the poorly developed ruffled borders of the osteoclasts observed by electron microscopy.[249] In children, features of rickets may be apparent.[250]

The studies of Walker in osteopetrotic mice have dramatically increased our understanding of the pathogenesis of osteopetrosis.[251] He demonstrated that impaired bone resorption in osteopetrotic mice could be restored by transplanting normal bone marrow or splenic cells and that infusions of splenic cells from osteopetrotic mice to lethally irradiated normal littermates could produce osteopetrosis. These elegant studies have provided strong evidence for the hematopoietic origin of osteoclasts and have stimulated clinical studies of a similar nature. In several institutions, bone marrow transplantations have been attempted in children with the lethal form of osteopetrosis. Remarkable radiological and histological improvement in bone and amelioration of hematologic abnormalities have been reported.[252] In one 5-month-old girl who received a marrow transplant from her normal twin brother, anemia, thrombocytopenia, and leukoerythroblastosis were corrected within 12 weeks.[252] Bone biopsy after transplantation indicated

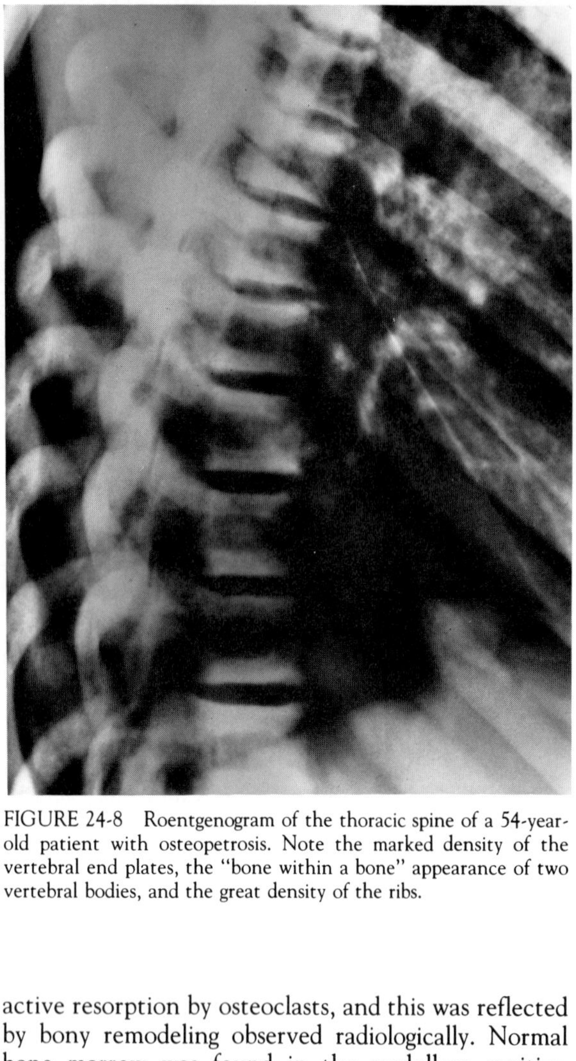

FIGURE 24-8 Roentgenogram of the thoracic spine of a 54-year-old patient with osteopetrosis. Note the marked density of the vertebral end plates, the "bone within a bone" appearance of two vertebral bodies, and the great density of the ribs.

active resorption by osteoclasts, and this was reflected by bony remodeling observed radiologically. Normal bone marrow was found in the medullary cavities. Utilizing fluorescent Y-body analysis, it was demonstrated after transplantation that 22 to 67 percent of the osteoclast nuclei were of male origin. None of the osteoclast nuclei had Y bodies prior to transplantation. Such studies are consistent with the hypothesis that a normal hematopoietic stem cell is not present in osteopetrotic subjects and that transplantation of normal marrow leads to fusion of the putative osteoclast precursor with the recipient's defective osteoclasts and restoration of normal osteoclast function. More studies will be necessary in order to determine whether this form of treatment can be applied to all patients with severe infantile osteopetrosis or whether other abnormalities of bone cell differentiation can be responsible for the pathogenesis of osteopetrosis in some patients. The latter possibility is suggested by the marked heterogeneity of osteoclast populations in a variety of osteopetrotic mutations in mice and rats.[253]

An alternative approach to the treatment of severe infantile osteopetrosis has been the administration of massive doses of 1α,25-dihydroxyvitamin D_3.[254] An increase in bone resorption was noted both biochemically and histologically in one child.

RENAL OSTEODYSTROPHY

Renal osteodystrophy is the general term used in connection with the variety of skeletal abnormalities which may complicate the clinical course of patients with chronic renal failure. Osteomalacia, secondary hyperparathyroidism, osteoporosis, and osteosclerosis may be encountered in a given patient, either as isolated abnormalities or in combination.

Clinical Presentation

Symptoms and Signs

Bone pain, muscle weakness and tenderness, and rarely, gangrene of the fingers or toes are dramatic complications in patients with renal osteodystrophy.[255] In children, short stature and rachitic deformities are additional features.

Soft tissue calcification often can be detected in the corneas and conjunctivas and gives rise to "red eye." Calcinosis cutis may be associated with generalized pruritus. Calcium deposits may occur around large joints and in muscle. Cardiac and pulmonary calcification may cause congestive heart failure and pulmonary insufficiency.

Radiological Features

The radiological findings in patients with renal osteodystrophy are highly variable and reflect the presence of osteomalacia, secondary hyperparathyroidism, osteoporosis, or osteosclerosis in adults and rickets in children.[255] Pseudofractures and rachitic deformities, subperiosteal bone resorption and other lesions of hyperparathyroidism, and uncommonly, generalized osteopenia may be observed. Osteosclerosis is a common finding, primarily in the spine. A "rugger jersey spine" is characterized by sclerosis of the inferior and superior borders of the vertebral bodies. Sclerosis of the skull and long bones is less common.

Laboratory Findings

Serum calcium concentrations may be low, normal, or even elevated.[256] Serum magnesium is normal or moderately elevated. Serum phosphorus is usually elevated but may fall within the normal range. Alkaline phosphatase activity is often elevated. Serum immunoreactive parathyroid hormone concentrations may be markedly elevated, but this is partly dependent on the type of antiserum used. Antisera with carboxy-terminal specificity will measure biologically inactive fragments of parathyroid hormone which are cleared at a reduced rate by diseased kidneys.[257] A small group of dialysis patients will have normal or suppressed levels of immunoreactive parathyroid hormone, even when measured with carboxy-terminal assays.[258] Serum 1α,25-dihydroxyvitamin D and 24,25-dihydroxyvitamin D levels are low,[33,46] but 25-dihydroxyvitamin D is normal if vitamin D intake or sun exposure is adequate.[259] Impaired intestinal calcium absorption is a common finding in severe renal failure.[256] Urinary calcium excretion is low as a consequence of a decreased filtered load of calcium. In patients with elevated serum parathyroid hormone, urinary cAMP excretion is increased and the renal TmP/GFR is reduced. However, the measurement of urinary cAMP and TmP/GFR may not provide a reliable measure of parathyroid function if the GFR is less than 20 to 30 ml/min.

Bone Pathology

The dominant histological abnormalities of renal osteodystrophy are those of osteomalacia and hyperparathyroidism.[260] Patients who develop osteomalacia as the dominant lesion exhibit all the characteristic features of osteomalacia, including widened osteoid seams which cover an increased percentage of the trabecular bone surface and impaired uptake of tetracycline. There is usually evidence of some degree of secondary hyperparathyroidism as manifested by increased osteoclasts and marrow fibrosis. A small percentage of dialysis patients with aluminum excess have osteomalacic histological features but no features of secondary hyperparathyroidism in the bone biopsy.[258] Serum parathyroid hormone concentrations are not significantly elevated in these patients.

When hyperparathyroidism is dominant, a marked increase in osteoclastic bone resorption, severe marrow fibrosis, and osteocytic osteolysis are present.[261] The rate of bone formation in these patients may be increased, in contrast to the osteomalacic type of renal osteodystrophy.

Osteosclerosis is characterized by increased bone density. Widened osteoid seams may be seen, but the amount of mineralized bone is greater than normal. Amorphous calcium phosphate may be deposited rather than hydroxyapatite. This may be a consequence of an abundance of woven bone in the osteosclerotic lesions.[255]

Decreased bone volume is rarely found in patients with chronic renal failure. This complication is always accompanied by the histological features of osteomalacia and/or secondary hyperparathyroidism.

Pathogenesis

Although there has been great progress in unraveling the complex pathogenesis of renal osteodystrophy, a full understanding has not been achieved. Major aspects of this problem remain unresolved or controversial.

The pathogenesis of osteomalacia in patients with renal osteodystrophy is multifactorial and appears to involve some factors which have only recently been implicated. Although circulating levels of 1α,25-dihydroxyvitamin decrease as the functional renal mass decreases,[262,263] this may not be the critical determinant of osteomalacia, since it is a very common finding, yet only a relatively small proportion of patients with end-stage renal failure develop full-blown osteomalacia. It is likely that factors such as aluminum content of bone, prior parathyroidectomy, metabolic acidosis, and dialysis-induced hypophosphatemia are additional important risk factors in producing clinically relevant defects in bone mineralization.[93,264–266]

The syndrome of aluminum-induced osteomalacia in hemodialysis patients has received considerable attention because of the severity of the symptoms and the potential for reversal of the problem. As previously discussed, these patients exhibit osteomalacia without evidence of secondary hyperparathyroidism. They may develop hypercalcemia despite modest parathyroid hormone levels,[267] probably as a consequence of the failure of bone to take up calcium from the extracellular fluid. If vitamin D of any type is administered in even small doses to treat the osteomalacic state, severe hypercalcemia may ensue because of increased intestinal calcium absorption,[258] together with the defective mineralization.

Secondary hyperparathyroidism in chronic renal failure has been attributed to a variety of factors. Phosphate retention, impaired vitamin D metabolism, and skeletal resistance to parathyroid hormone all have been implicated in the genesis of hyperparathyroidism.[256] Dietary phosphate restriction can prevent development of secondary hyperparathyroidism in uremic dogs,[268] and the same result has been convincingly confirmed in humans.[269] At the same time, phosphate restriction produces a rise in 1α,25-dihydroxyvitamin D levels in patients with moderate renal failure.[269] Administration of 1α,25-dihydroxyvitamin D_3 can partially restore responsiveness to parathyroid hormone in uremic dogs, and the administration of both 1α,25-dihydroxyvitamin D_3 and 24,25-dihydroxyvitamin D_3 restores full responsiveness to parathyroid hormone.[270] The relevance of this study to human disease is not established.

The pathogenesis of osteosclerosis in patients with chronic renal failure is unknown. It has been suggested that osteosclerosis is more likely to occur in patients with severe secondary hyperparathyroidism and may reflect an anabolic action of parathyroid hormone.[255]

Treatment

Successful renal transplantation restores vitamin D metabolism to normal and usually produces healing of osteomalacia within 1 year. Resolution of secondary hyperparathyroidism may take longer because the glomerular filtration rate frequently remains slightly reduced. Persistence of elevated parathyroid hormone levels and long-term posttransplant hypercalcemia are well documented.[256] Other complications of renal transplantation affecting the skeleton include steroid-induced osteoporosis, growth retardation in children, and aseptic necrosis of bone.

Measures which are likely to be helpful in the prevention of renal osteodystrophy are outlined in Table 24-3. Maintenance of normal serum calcium and phosphorus concentrations usually can be achieved by providing an adequate calcium intake, as high as 1500 mg daily, and by restricting dietary phosphorus to 1000 mg daily. Phosphate-binding antacids should be used cautiously because of their aluminum content. Calcium carbonate supplements have also been shown to be effective phosphate binders.[271] Dialysis patients should be dialyzed with a dialysate calcium concentration of 6 to 6.5 mg/dl. Careful use of alkali will correct systemic acidosis. Vitamin D, dihydrotachysterol, or the potent metabolites of vitamin D may be needed to achieve a normocalcemic state, but the long-term efficacy of these agents in preventing bone disease is not well established, although short-term therapy with 1α,25-dihydroxyvitamin D_3 in early renal failure can reverse resistance to parathyroid hormone and other metabolic abnormalities.[272] The institution of a prophylactic regimen to prevent renal osteodystrophy requires close follow-up in order to avoid hypophosphatemia, hypercalcemia, and extraskeletal calcification.

Table 24-3. Prevention of Renal Osteodystrophy

1. Maintain normal serum phosphorus concentration
2. Calcium intake of 1500 mg daily
3. Maintain normal acid-base status
4. Prophylactic use of vitamin D or analogue

The treatment of renal osteodystrophy with 25-hydroxyvitamin D_3, 1α,25-dihydroxyvitamin D_3, and 1α-hydroxyvitamin D_3 has received intensive scrutiny in recent years because of the greater potency and shorter half-life of these agents.[256] The 1α derivatives of vitamin D have been demonstrated to be particularly effective in the hypocalcemic patient with secondary hyperparathyroidism. Chronic therapy with 2 μg or less daily produces normocalcemia, suppression of the parathyroid hormone concentration, and a decrease in alkaline phosphatase activity (Fig. 24-9), as well as reversal of the histological lesions of secondary hyperparathyroidism.[273] Relief of bone pain and muscle weakness and an increased growth rate in children have been documented in numerous clinical trials. Less consistent results have been reported in respect to improvement of bone mineralization. In some studies, 1α,25-dihydroxyvitamin D_3 has been reported to produce healing of histological lesions of osteomalacia,[274] but other investigators have reported incomplete healing with this metabolite.[275] It has been claimed that 25-hydroxyvitamin D_3 is a more effective agent in healing osteomalacia.[276] It is not known at present whether 25-hydroxyvitamin D_3 or the induction of 24,25-dihydroxyvitamin D_3 synthesis is responsible for superior healing or whether inadequate doses of 1α,25-dihydroxyvitamin D_3 in some trials account for the above observations. If these potent agents are used, the physician must be aware of the danger of hypercalcemia as a complication. A previously normocalcemic patient often becomes hypercalcemic shortly after a significant fall in alkaline phosphatase activity is observed. Hypercalcemia is also likely to occur early in the course of treatment in patients with severe secondary hyperparathyroidism who are normocalcemic or have borderline hypercalcemia before therapy. These patients may require subtotal parathyroidectomy because of massive parathyroid hyperplasia.[256] Symptomatic hypercalcemia, intractable pruritus, bone pain, fractures, extraskeletal calcifications, and cutaneous gangrene are indications for parathyroid surgery. The studies of Wells suggest that total parathyroidectomy with transplantation of parathyroid tissue in a forearm is the surgery of choice.[277]

A particularly difficult group of patients to treat is the subset of dialysis patients with aluminum excess

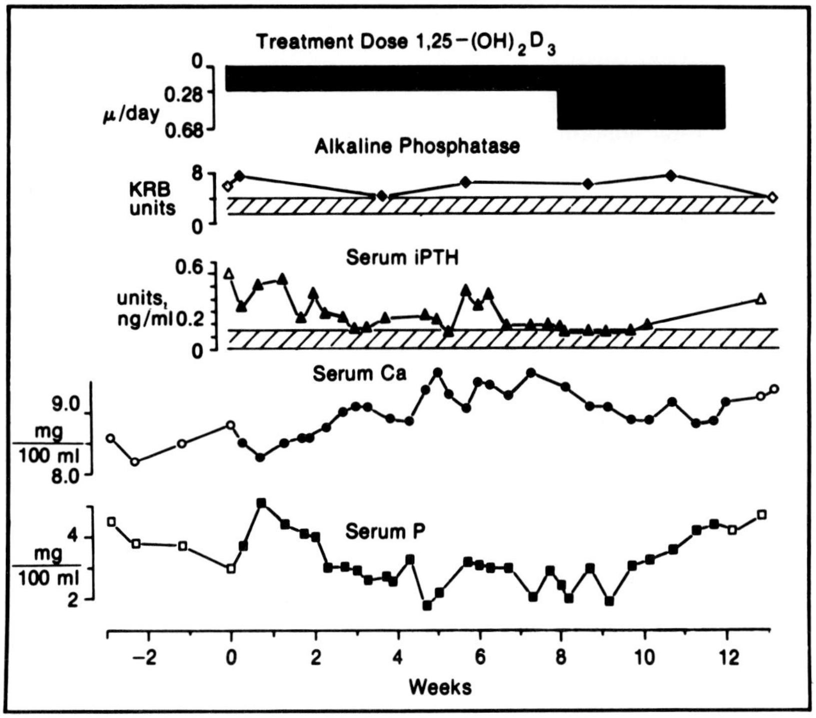

FIGURE 24-9 The effect of 1α,25-dihydroxycholecalciferol therapy in a patient with chronic renal failure. The cross-hatched areas indicate the normal range for serum alkaline phosphatase and immunoreactive parathyroid hormone (iPTH). (*From Brickman AS, Sherrard DJ, Jowsey J, Singer FR, Baylink DJ, Maloney N, Massry SG, Norman AW, Arch Intern Med 134: 883, 1974.*)

who have severe osteomalacia in the absence of biochemical or histological evidence of secondary hyperparathyroidism.[258,264] These patients often do not respond adequately to treatment with 1α,25-dihydroxyvitamin D_3. Preliminary studies suggest that deferoxamine infusions may remove aluminum from bone and reverse the osteomalacic lesion.[278]

HEREDITARY HYPERPHOSPHATASIA

Hereditary hyperphosphatasia is a rare autosomal recessive disorder which usually presents during infancy.[279] This condition has been described by a variety of eponyms, including chronic idiopathic hyperphosphatasia, hyperostosis corticalis deformans juvenilis, osteochalasia desmalis familiaris, familial osteoectasia, chronic progressive osteopathy with hyperphosphatasia, hereditary bone dysplasia with hyperphosphatasemia, and juvenile Paget's disease. Enlargement of the skull and facial bones and bowing of the extremities are common features of the disease. Skin temperature may be increased over affected bones. Bone pain and pathological features are common.

The radiological features of hereditary hyperphosphatasia include loss of the normal cortical architecture, disruption of the corticomedullary border, expansion of the diaphysis, and strikingly increased density of the calvarium with a patchy "cotton-wool" pattern. The latter abnormality is quite similar to the radiological appearance of the skull in patients with advanced Paget's disease of bone.

The laboratory characteristics of this disorder are identical to those of polyostotic Paget's disease of bone. Serum calcium and phosphorus concentrations are normal. Serum alkaline phosphatase activity and urinary hydroxyproline excretion may be markedly elevated.

The reported histological findings in patients with hereditary hyperphosphatasia have been heterogeneous, an indication that classification of patients may be imperfect. There is agreement that the bone is laid down in a chaotic manner indistinguishable from the mosaic pattern of bone characteristic of Paget's disease. Numerous osteoblasts and a fibrovascular bone marrow are present. There is disagreement as to whether woven or lamellar bone is the dominant type of bone formed. Another point of controversy concerns which bone cells are responsible for the increased rate of bone resorption. In one study of several patients,[279] numerous osteoclasts were present in bone biopsies, but in another study osteoclasts were rarely observed.[280] Instead, the investigators found a marked degree of osteocytic osteolysis and concluded that the osteocytes were responsible for the accelerated rate of bone resorption. They also described ultrastructural abnormalities in both the osteocytes and the osteoblasts of their patients.[281] Intramitochondrial microcrystalline bodies thought to represent calcium deposits were observed. The significance of these intracellular deposits is unknown, but they have been reported to disappear after calcitonin therapy.

The pathogenesis of hereditary hyperphosphatasia is unknown. The disease is clearly not a childhood form of Paget's disease, since it is generalized in its distribution and the characteristic nuclear and cytoplasmic inclusions found in the osteoclasts of Paget's disease are not present.

Despite the lack of understanding of the pathogenesis of hereditary hyperphosphatasia, remarkable progress has been made in treating this disorder. Chronic treatment with calcitonin is associated with dramatic clinical improvement of both subjective and objective parameters.[280–284] Reduction in bone pain and in incidence of pathological fractures has been reported. The rate of bone turnover is decreased, as manifested by reduction of alkaline phosphatase activity and urinary hydroxyproline excretion. Improvement of radiological abnormalities has been observed, as well as improvement of the histological abnormalities in bone biopsies. These improvements in skeletal structure and metabolism appear to be maintained during years of therapy.

FIBROUS DYSPLASIA

Fibrous dysplasia of bone (Albright's syndrome, Albright-McCune-Sternberg syndrome) is a rare disorder of unknown etiology which may be monostotic or polyostotic in distribution. It is clearly not a metabolic bone disease, but because of numerous associated endocrinopathies it seems appropriate to include this entity in a discussion of metabolic bone disease.

The disorder was lucidly described by Albright and colleagues in 1937,[285] but Albright subsequently pointed out that the first cases in the medical literature were reported by von Recklinghausen in 1891.[286] Cases 5 and 6 of von Recklinghausen's monograph were mistakenly believed to be examples of osteitis fibrosa generalisata.[287]

Fibrous dysplasia is usually recognized between the ages of 3 and 10. There is no evidence of genetic transmission. A triad of abnormalities is often present: bone lesions, sexual precocity (primarily in girls), and café au lait skin lesions which have serrated edges.[285] The bone lesions most often affect the femur, tibia, pelvis, hand, rib, humerus, and skull.[288] In patients with polyostotic fibrous dysplasia, there is a tendency to unilateral distribution of the disease. Skeletal deformity, pain, and pathological fractures are the main manifestations of the bone lesions. Sarcomas may rarely arise in a lesion of fibrous dysplasia.[289] A great variety of endocrinopathies have been described in patients with fibrous dysplasia since the initial reports of sexual precocity. These include acromegaly, gigantism, hyperthyroidism, hyperparathyroidism, Cushing's syndrome, hypothalamic hypogonadism, and hypophosphatemic rickets.[290–292] The skin pigmentation occurs most frequently over the sacrum, buttocks, and cervical spine.

The characteristic radiological feature of fibrous dysplasia is a ground-glass appearance of the lesions. Focal cortical thinning, expansion of the diaphysis, and a multilocular configuration of the lesions are also features (Fig. 24-10). Gross deformities of the skeleton are often apparent. Shepherd's-crook deformity of the femur, coxa vara, tibial bowing, protrusio acetabuli, and enlarged facial bones are common abnormalities. Increased radiodensity of the base of the skull and thickening of the occiput may be observed.

Serum calcium and phosphorus determinations are usually normal except in the few patients who have associated hyperparathyroidism or hypophosphatemic rickets. Serum alkaline phosphatase activity and urinary hydroxyproline excretion may be increased, a refletion of accelerated bone turnover. The turnover of fibrous connective tissue in bone lesions may also contribute to the level of hydroxyproline excretion.

Pathologically, fibrous dysplasia is dominated by the dense fibrous connective tissue which surrounds the trabeculae[288] (Fig. 24-11). The bone is woven in character, and the randomly oriented collagen fibers appear to extend into the adjacent fibrous tissue. Numerous fibroblasts and osteoblasts may be present in areas of new bone formation. Widened osteoid seams occasionally are noted at sites where there are few osteoblasts. Osteoclasts may be present in areas adjacent to those in which there is increased osteoblastic activity. Islands of cartilage may represent remnants of the epiphysis or abortive callus formation. Callus formation after trauma may be inadequate. Fluid-filled cysts sometimes develop in areas of previous trauma or surgery. Pathological examination of the endocrine glands in patients with endocrine disease has revealed hyperplasia and adenomas of the pituitary, thyroid, parathyroid, and adrenal glands.[290] The ovaries of girls with sexual precocity have not shown evidence of ovulation in the few such patients who have been studied.

The pathogenesis of fibrous dysplasia, its associated endocrinopathies, and skin lesions remains a

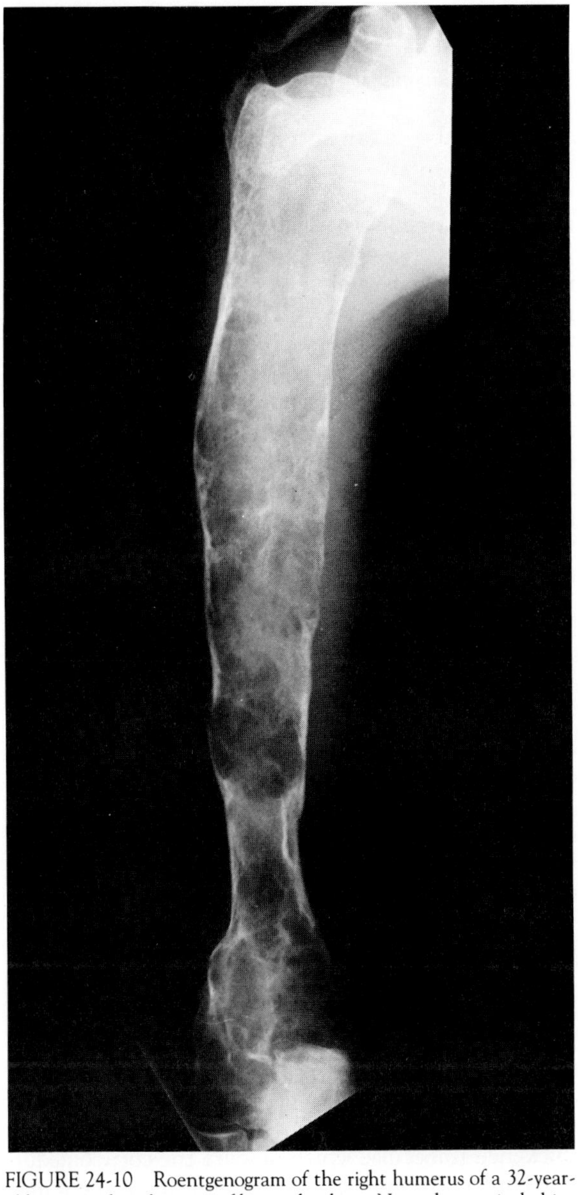

FIGURE 24-10 Roentgenogram of the right humerus of a 32-year-old man with polyostotic fibrous dysplasia. Note the cortical thinning, diaphyseal expansion, and multiloculated appearance of the lesions.

complete mystery. Although it has been suggested that skull involvement might be responsible for stimulation of hypothalamic hormones, it is clear that endocrine disorders can occur in the absence of skull lesions. The resolution of associated hypophosphatemic bone disease after resection of lesions of fibrous dysplasia in one patient does suggest that a phosphaturic factor may be secreted by the bone lesions.[88a]

No satisfactory treatment of fibrous dysplasia is known. Radiation therapy may lead to sarcomatous degeneration. Because of the finding of osteoclasts in bone biopsies, calcitonin has been administered to several patients;[88a,293] no significant improvement has been demonstrated. No specific treatment for sexual precocity has been discovered. In one patient who had an ovarian cyst, treatment with an analogue of luteinizing hormone releasing hormone failed to suppress cyclical ovarian function.[294] Regular menstrual periods and normal fertility usually follow in these patients. Standard treatments of the other endocrinopathies are usually successful.

PAGET'S DISEASE OF BONE

Paget's disease of bone is a common localized disorder of bone which is often included in a consideration of metabolic bone diseases because, in its polyostotic form, the level of metabolic activity of the skeleton is as great as that in any bone disease.

Sir James Paget provided a brilliant description in 1876 of a crippling bone disorder he termed *osteitis*

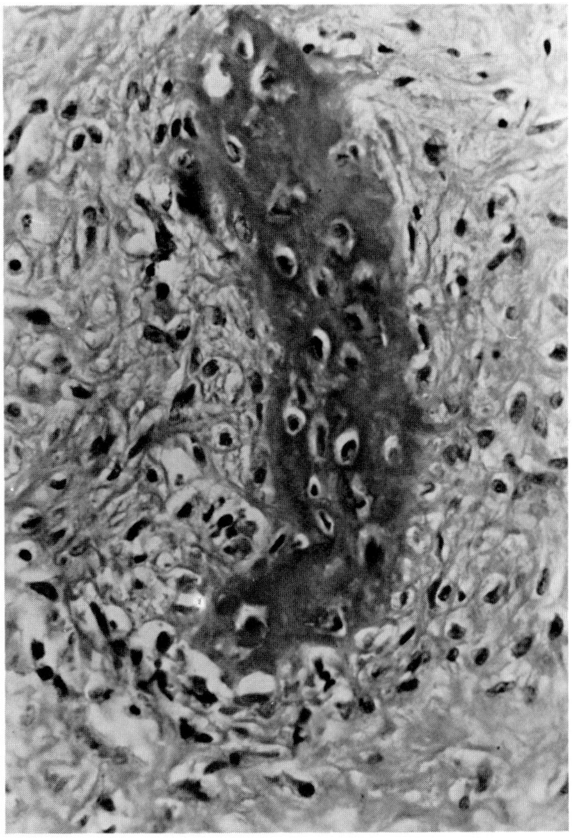

FIGURE 24-11 A trabecula of bone surrounded by dense fibrous connective tissue from a patient with fibrous dysplasia. Decalcified, H&E.

deformans.[295] Although he thought it to be a rare disorder, the advent of roentgenograms revealed it to be a common albeit often asymptomatic affliction. An incidence of 3 percent in persons over age 40 has been found in regions of the world where there are large concentrations of people of Anglo-Saxon origin.[296] The disease is rare in the Orient, India, and Scandinavia. Males and females are almost equally affected. A positive famiy history of Paget's disease has been reported in up to 25 percent of patients.

Clinical Presentation

Symptoms and Signs

A significant proportion of patients with Paget's disease do not have symptoms of the disease. In these patients the disease is discovered because of screening blood chemistry or chance findings on radiological examinations.

Pain and skeletal deformity are the most common presenting complaints in patients with symptomatic Paget's disease. The pain may arise in bones or joints or from spinal cord or nerve impingement.[297] Bone pain is usually not severe and is only slightly worsened by weight bearing if present in the spine, pelvis, or lower extremities. There is a puzzling lack of correlation between the degree of pain and the severity of skeletal deformity. Patients with polyostotic disease, associated with marked deformity, may never experience bone pain, whereas moderate pain may arise in a lesion which is demonstrable only by radiological examination. Joint pain due to degenerative arthritis is usually more severe than bone pain. The most common sites are the hip and knee joints. Weight bearing typically increases the severity of the joint pain. The most excruciating pain occurs as a consequence of impingement by deformed vertebrae on the spinal cord or nerve roots. This pain is often felt in the back and/or lower extremities. Some patients experience pain as a result of a combination of Paget's involvement, degenerative changes, and nerve impingement, and it may be difficult to judge the relative contributions of each type of pain in these patients.

The deformities which may appear in patients with long-standing Paget's disease are most readily appreciated by examining the skull, clavicles, and long bones. The involved bones are generally both increased in size and of an abnormal contour. An increase in skin temperature over affected long bones is a typical finding and is explained by soft tissue vascularity surrounding the bones.[298]

Loss of auditory acuity occurs in approximately 50 percent of patients with skull involvement. A combined conductive and sensorineural hearing deficit is common.

In about 15 percent of patients disruptions of Bruch's membrane produce cracks in the retina which are termed *angioid streaks*. They rarely produce visual impairment.

A variety of other complications may occur in patients with Paget's disease. Pathological fractures of the femur, tibia, and vertebral bodies are not uncommon.[296] Nonunion is usually not a major problem. Bone tumors present with an increase in pain and/or a rapidly growing mass at sites of Paget's disease. Sarcomas are most common but fortunately occur in less than 1 percent of patients.[296] Benign giant-cell tumors may arise in skull and facial lesions. Multiple myeloma and metastatic carcinoma appear to be chance associations. Gout has been reported to affect males with great frequency, but this has not been a uniform finding.[297] An increase in cardiac output may be found in patients whose disease involves 20 percent or more of the skeleton,[299] but intractable high-output cardiac failure is seldom encountered.

Radiological Features

The earliest lesions of Paget's disease which can be detected radiologically are osteolytic in nature. In the skull, these early lesions have been termed *osteoporosis circumscripta* (Fig. 24-12). Osteolytic lesions in the extremities are usually found at either end of the affected bone and advance as a V-shaped osteolytic front at an average rate of 1 cm per year.

The evolution of osteolytic lesions into an osteoblastic phase may require years or even decades. In the skull, there is thickening of the calvarium with a loss of definition of the inner and outer tables. A "cotton wool" appearance due to a patchy increase in bone density is common (Fig. 24-13). Platybasia or basilar invagination may occur in far advanced disease. In the long bones, the osteolytic lesions are replaced by thickened trabeculae which obscure the corticomedullary border. Anterior and lateral bowing of the femur and tibia may develop. Incomplete fissure fractures can be seen on the convex surface of the femur. Pathological fractures of the lower extremity produce a "chalk stick" rather than spiral disruption of the bone. Osteoblastic lesions of the vertebrae may produce a "picture frame" appearance because of sclerosis of the vertebral borders, or they may produce a homogeneous increase in density.

Narrowing of the joint spaces of the hip and knee is observed in patients with Paget's disease and degenerative arthritis.[297] Osteophyte formation may be present at these sites and in the spine. Protrusio acetabuli may occur with extensive Pagetic involvement of the pelvis.

Radiological features of a sarcoma include cortical

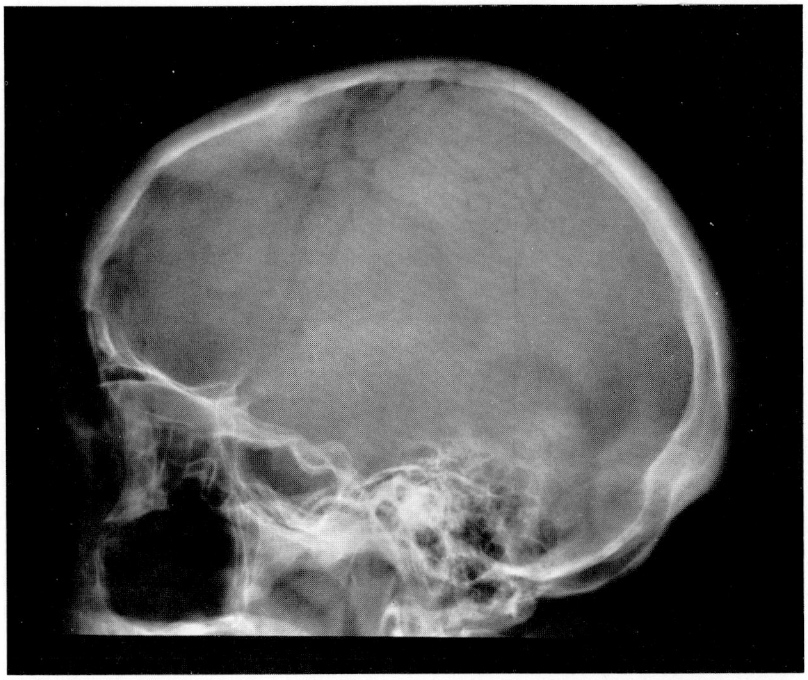

FIGURE 24-12 Roentgenogram of the skull of a 48-year-old patient with osteoporosis circumscripta due to Paget's disease.

destruction and a soft tissue mass which may exhibit patchy calcification.

Computerized tomography of the spine is a valuable technique for demonstrating lesions such as spinal stenosis and is extremely useful in the evaluation of patients with severe back pain.

The metabolic activity of the lesions of Paget's disease is most easily assessed by nuclear medicine techniques (Fig. 24-14). The administration of bone-seeking radioisotopes such as technetium-labeled bisphosphonates to patients with localized disease may be the only noninvasive means of demonstrating disease

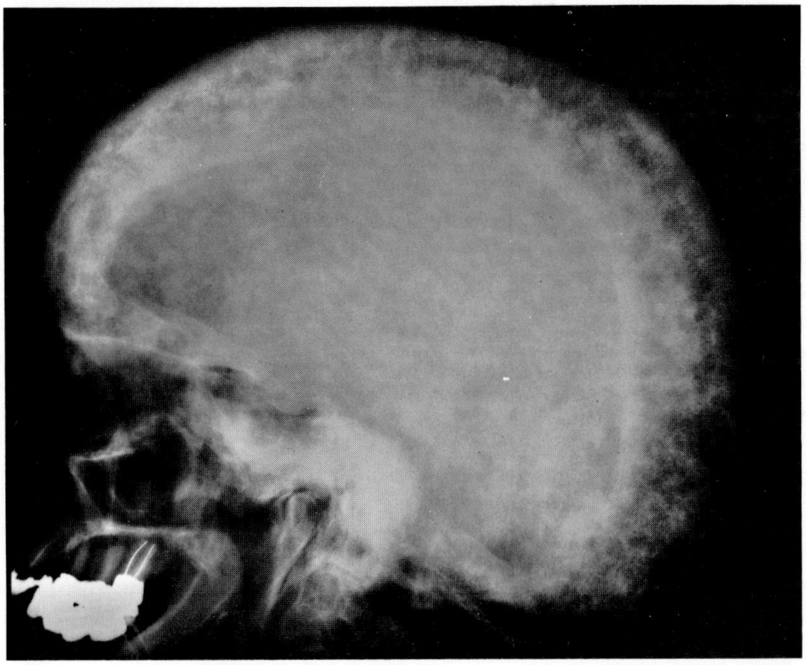

FIGURE 24-13 Roentgenogram of the skull of a 63-year-old patient with the osteoblastic phase of Paget's disease.

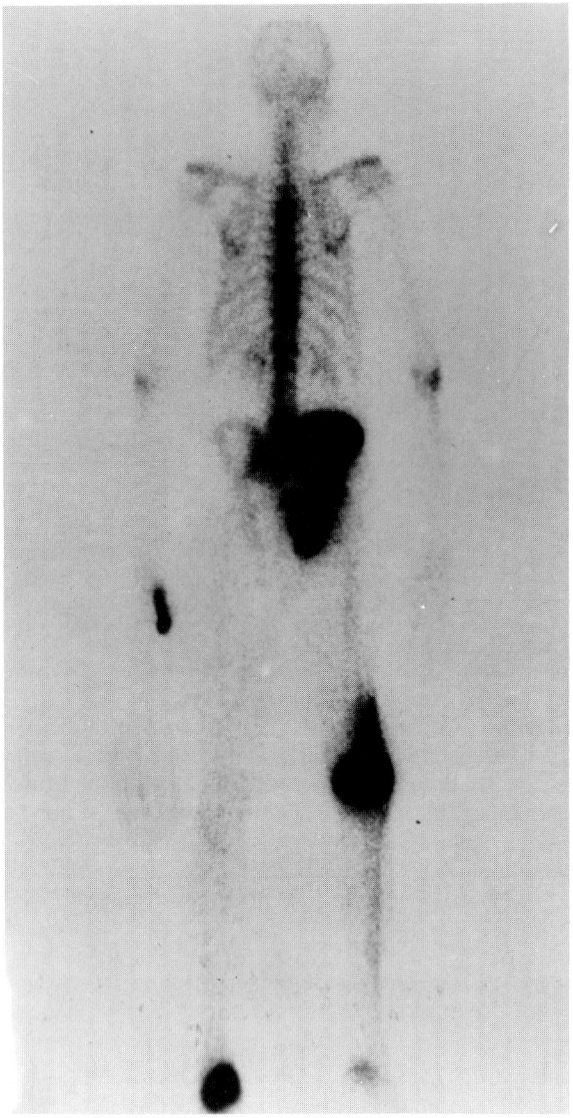

FIGURE 24-14 Bone scan of a 73-year-old patient with Paget's disease involving the left hemipelvis, the distal left femur, the right hand, and the right foot.

activity, since biochemical parameters may be normal in monostotic cases.[300] Bone scans also can detect early lesions of Paget's disease before there is a discernible radiological abnormality.[301] During treatment of Paget's disease with a variety of agents, bone scans can reflect suppression of disease activity. In one study,[302] gallium scans were found to correlate better with suppression of biochemical parameters than technetium bisphosphonate bone scans. Since gallium is thought to localize within cells, the gallium scan may be a better index of the action of drugs on the abnormal cells of Paget's disease.

Laboratory Findings

The serum calcium and phosphorus concentrations are usually normal in the ambulatory patient with Paget's disease. Immobilization because of neurological complications or after a fracture may cause serious hypercalcemia.[303] Hypercalcemia also may reflect the presence of associated primary hyperparathyroidism, and it has been suggested that there is an increased incidence of hyperparathyroidism in patients with Paget's disease.[304] Control studies of an age-matched population have not been adequate to establish this association convincingly.

Radiocalcium kinetic studies have revealed a markedly increased rate of bone turnover in patients with polyostotic Paget's disease.[303] This is more easily demonstrated by the elevated serum alkaline phosphatase activity and increased urinary hydroxyproline excretion found in these patients. In patients with monostotic disease involving a small bone such as a vertebra, all the above studies may be normal.

Urinary calcium excretion is usually normal, although hypercalciuria may be present if the rate of bone resorption exceeds that of bone formation.[303] This occurs primarily in immobilized patients. In ambulatory patients, even with extensive active Paget's disease, the resorption and formation rates are usually closely coupled.

Bone Pathology

The earliest lesion of Paget's disease is a localized area of osteolysis which is produced by an increased number of osteoclasts.[305] The osteoclasts of Paget's disease are heterogeneous in size; some may have up to 100 nuclei in a single cross section (Fig. 24-15). Giant osteoclasts of this size are rarely found in metabolic bone diseases.

Most bone biopsies or surgical specimens show a combination of intensive osteoclastic bone resorption and large numbers of active osteoblasts which are forming bone at sites of previous osteoclastic resorption (Fig. 24-15). The marrow will also be found to contain dense fibrovascular tissue containing numerous fibroblasts and osteoprogenitor cells.

In the quiescent, or "burned-out," phase of Paget's disease, the number of bone cells is markedly reduced and the bone marrow consists mainly of fat cells. A single bone may harbor an advancing osteolytic front, a trailing mixed osteoclastic-osteoblastic pattern, and a burned-out stage of the disease.

The intense cellular activity of Paget's disease produces a characteristic chaotic pattern of bone matrix termed the *mosaic pattern*. The bone is primar-

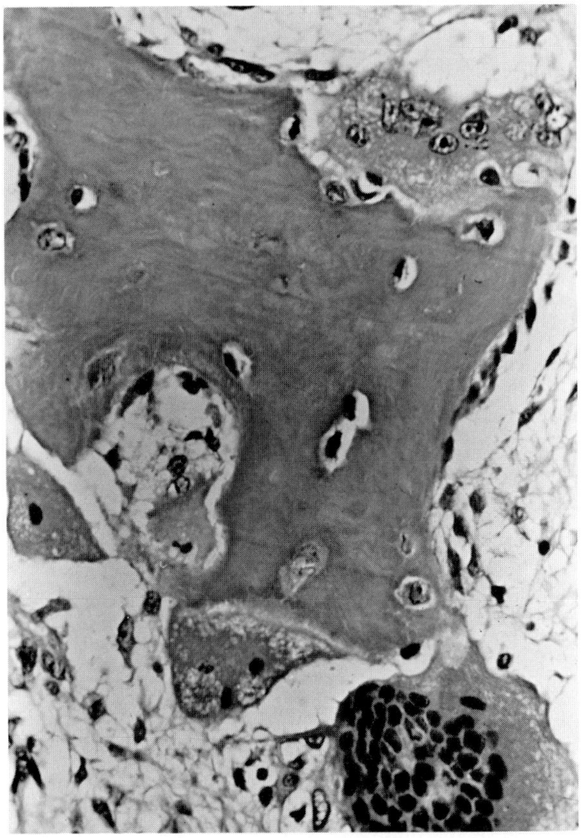

FIGURE 24-15 Several large multinucleated osteoclasts in Howship's lacunae. More than 50 nuclei are present in the osteoclast at the bottom. Note the numerous osteoblasts at the far right of the bone matrix. Decalcified, H&E.

ily lamellar in character, with woven bone interspersed between incomplete osteons. A high percentage of bone surface is covered by osteoid, but mineralization is usually normal. The rate of bone formation as determined by double labeling with tetracycline is often increased.

Studies of the ultrastructure of bone cells in Paget's disease have demonstrated characteristic nuclear and cytoplasmic inclusions in the osteoclasts of all patients whose cells have been examined.[306,307] These inclusions consist of numerous microfibrillar structures which are similar in appearance to viral nucleocapsids of paramyxoviruses and pneumoviruses (Fig. 24-16). The inclusions have not been found in the osteoblasts or osteocytes of Paget's disease or in bone cells from normal subjects.

Pathogenesis

Sir James Paget believed that Paget's disease was inflammatory in nature—hence, the term *osteitis deformans*.[295] Because no infectious agent could be recovered from pathological specimens, this hypothesis was discarded early in this century. The uniform finding of nuclear and cytoplasmic inclusions in the osteoclasts of Paget's disease has revived the search for an infectious cause of the disorder. It is now appreciated that viruses may produce chronic indolent disorders of the nervous system, termed *slow virus infections,* which share many clinical and pathological features with Paget's disease.[308] These shared features include involvement of a single organ, a prolonged latent period, absence of fever and an acute inflammatory process, giant cells, and intracellular inclusions. Recent immunocytologic evidence indicates that measles and/or respiratory syncytial virus antigens are present in the osteoclasts of Paget's disease,[309,310] and that mRNA of measles virus is in a variety of bone and marrow cells.[309,310,310a] Definitive identification of a virus requires that it be isolated from affected tissue. This has yet to be accomplished, although long-term cultures of cells from Paget's bone lesions have been

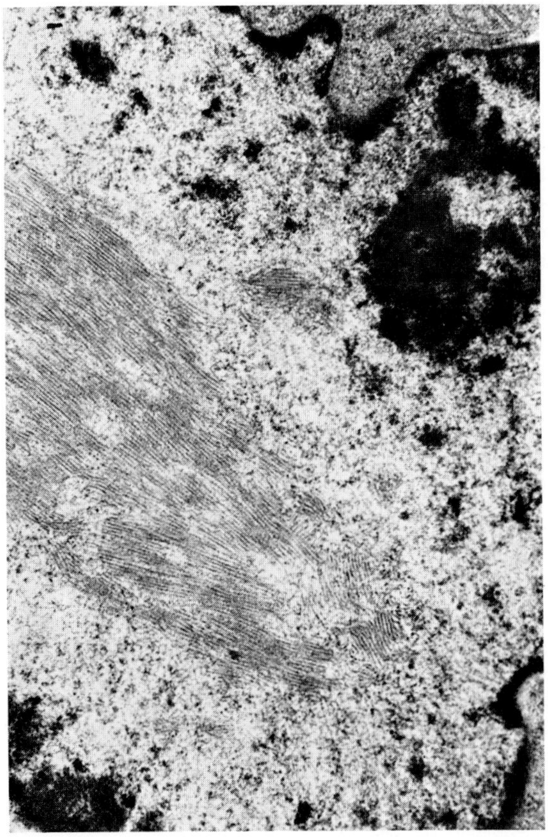

FIGURE 24-16 Characteristic microfibrillar nuclear inclusion found in osteoclasts of patients with Paget's disease. × 32,000. (*Courtesy of BG Mills.*)

established.[311] There has been great difficulty in isolating virus from the lesions of such disorders as subacute sclerosing panencephalitis (postmeasles encephalitis) because of the defective nature of the virus. Successful isolations have been achieved only after multiple passages of cultured cells. The proof of a viral etiology of Paget's disease will require not only isolation of an infectious agent but demonstration that the pathological process is induced by this agent in experimental animals.

A variety of other hypotheses have been proposed to explain the pathogenesis of Paget's disease.[305] It has been suggested that the disease results from an autoimmune process, from an inborn error of connective tissue metabolism, from an abnormality of hormone secretion, from an abnormality of the vascular supply of bone, and from neoplastic transformation of bone cells. Little evidence has been marshaled in support of any of these hypotheses.

Treatment

A variety of medical and surgical therapies can now be offered to patients with Paget's disease who previously would have had little chance for relief of their symptoms.

Before 1970, no safe and effective drugs were available for the treatment of Paget's disease. Clinical trials with calcitonin began at that time. This agent was chosen because of its known inhibitory effect on osteoclastic bone resorption. Within 30 min after injection of calcitonin, osteoclasts appear to detach from trabeculae and lose their well-defined ruffled borders and are reduced in number.[312] Simultaneously, patients with Paget's disease experience a reduction in serum calcium, phosphorus, and serum and urinary hydroxyproline levels, biochemical reflections of an inhibition of bone mineral and matrix resorption. During chronic administration of calcitonin, both histological and biochemical parameters indicate inhibition of bone formation as well as bone resorption, so that the agent ultimately produces a reduced rate of coupled bone turnover.[305]

Salmon and human calcitonin are currently approved for general use in the United States. Salmon calcitonin is administered by subcutaneous injection at a dose of 50 to 100 MRC units daily until symptoms are improved. Subsequently, the dose usually can be reduced to 50 MRC units three times a week with maintenance of clinical benefit. Occasionally a dose of more than 100 MRC units daily is required to induce maximal radiological improvement. Relief of bone pain and a reduction in skin temperature over affected extremities are usually observed after 2 to 6 weeks of treatment. Therapy with salmon calcitonin also has been reported to improve neurological disability, stabilize auditory acuity, decrease cardiac output, decrease the complications of orthopedic surgery, and induce healing of osteolytic bone lesions.[305] Human calcitonin at a dose of 0.5 mg daily produces similar clinical benefit.

Treatment with calcitonin produces an average reduction of 50 percent in both serum alkaline phosphatase activity and urinary hydroxyproline excretion within 3 to 6 months (Fig. 24-17). Urinary hydroxyproline excretion decreases during the first day of treatment and serum alkaline phosphatase activity only after 1 or 2 weeks. This suggests that the effect of calcitonin on osteoblastic activity is indirect and a consequence of inhibition of bone resorption.

Side effects occur in approximately 20 percent of patients treated with salmon calcitonin but seldom require discontinuing treatment. Side effects are surprisingly more common in patients treated with human calcitonin and are more likely to be intolerable. Nausea, facial flushing, and a metallic taste sensation are most common. Abdominal pain, vomiting, diarrhea, and tetany are rare. Allergic reactions also are rare. The transient hypocalcemia which occurs after each injection in patients with polyostotic disease produces a transient rise in serum parathyroid hormone concentration. There is no evidence that this leads to the development of a persistent state of secondary hyperparathyroidism.[305]

Since salmon calcitonin is a foreign protein, it is not surprising that more than 50 percent of patients who are treated with this agent develop circulating antibodies.[313] In the largest series of patients studied, 22 of 85 patients (26 percent) became resistant to salmon calcitonin treatment after an initial biochemical remission was produced. Nineteen of these patients had high titers of antibodies to salmon calcitonin, and three had no detectable antibodies. The development of neutralizing antibodies appears to be a common cause of resistance to salmon calcitonin. In such patients, therapy with salmon calcitonin should be stopped. Human calcitonin therapy has been uniformly effective in these patients.[313] Bisphosphonates and mithramycin can also be used if warranted. The reason for resistance to salmon calcitonin in patients who have no antibodies is unknown but is apparently not related to the foreign nature of salmon calcitonin, since resistance to human calcitonin can also occur in the absence of antibodies.[313]

The indications for treatment with calcitonin are still evolving. Bone pain, neurological deficits, and immobilization hypercalcemia are indications for initiating treatment. The use of calcitonin in preparing patients for orthopedic surgery is reviewed in a later

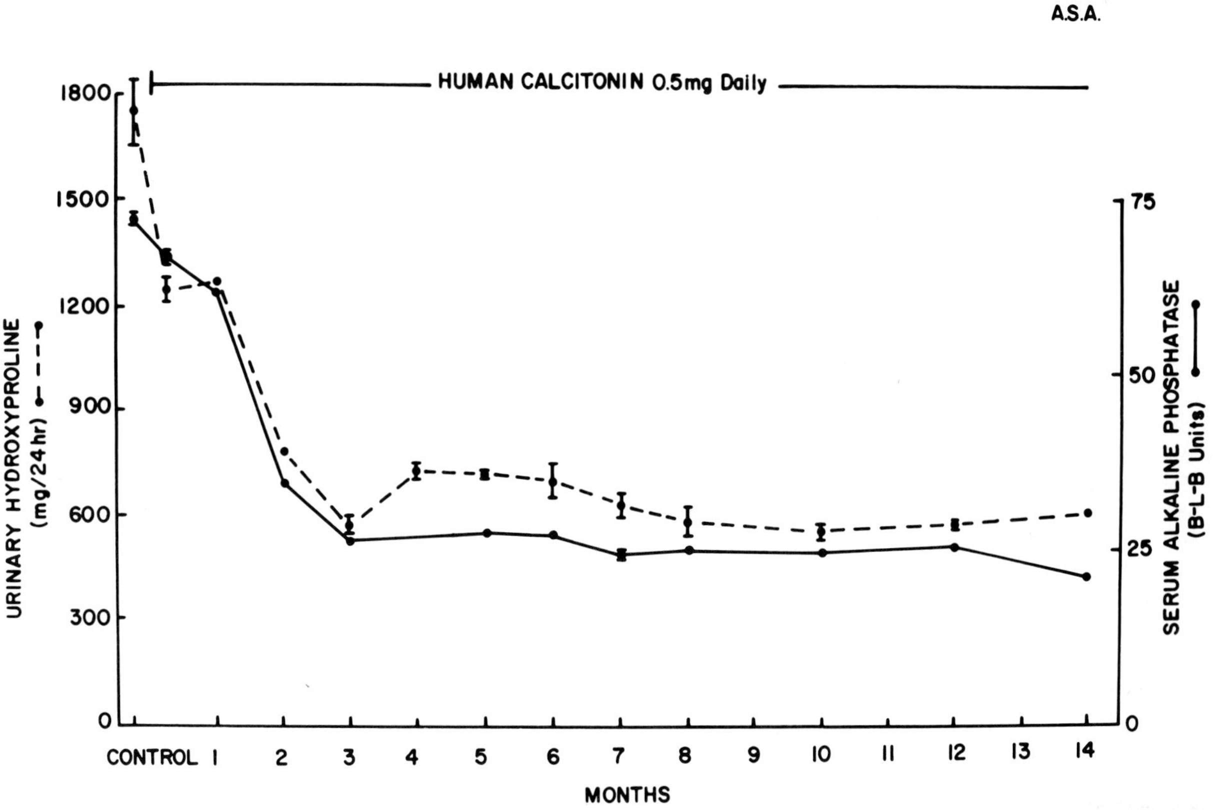

FIGURE 24-17 The effect of long-term treatment with subcutaneous injections of human calcitonin on the biochemical parameters of a patient with polyostotic Paget's disease. Serum alkaline phosphatase activity (normal, 1 to 3 Bessey-Lowrey-Brock units) and urinary hydroxyproline excretion (normal < 40 mg per 24 h) both decreased by more than 50 percent of baseline values.

section. The prevention of future complications of Paget's disease has not been studied but should be considered in relatively young patients whose disease affects the skull or weight-bearing bones.

The optimum duration of treatment with calcitonin has not been established. In patients treated for an average of 22 months, biochemical parameters of Paget's disease remained suppressed for at least 1 year after calcitonin was discontinued.[314] However, in patients with a healed osteolytic lesion, reactivation of the osteolytic front occurred within several months of discontinuing therapy.[315] It may be appropriate to continue such patients on treatment indefinitely. Patients whose lesions are predominantly osteoblastic may do well on a regimen of 1 or 2 years, followed by a treatment-free period. If symptoms return, the drug can be reinstituted.

A second group of compounds which have proved useful in the treatment of Paget's disease are the bisphosphonates. These agents are analogues of pyrophosphate (POP), a substance in bone believed to influence calcification and bone cell metabolism.[316] Bisphosphonates have been shown to suppress bone resorption and formation in experimental animals and humans,[316] although the exact mode of action is not known. Disodium etidronate (disodium ethane-1-hydroxyl-1,1-bisphosphonate) has been approved for the treatment of Paget's disease and the prevention of heterotopic ossification in the United States. Dichloromethylene bisphosphonate and disodium 3-amino-1-hydroxy-propylidene-1,1-bisphosphonate are under current investigation in Europe and South America.

Disodium etidronate is administered orally, although gastrointestinal absorption of the drug is variable. After absorption, it localizes mainly in the skeleton or is excreted by the kidney. The clinical effects of the drug are similar to those of calcitonin, but there are some differences. In general, greater suppression of biochemical parameters is achieved with the bisphosphonates than with calcitonin.[317] This is most often achieved at doses of 10 to 20 mg per kilogram of body weight. Unfortunately, high doses of disodium etidronate cause a mineralization defect which may predispose to osteomalacia and pathological fractures.[318] Since doses of 5 mg per kilogram of body weight usually suppress the disease without producing a mineralization defect, it is best to begin therapy with this lower dose. Should the patient not respond, perhaps because of inadequate intestinal absorption of the drug, a higher dose can be tried. The experimental bisphosphonates are effective in suppressing disease activity without inducing a mineralization defect.[319] Another unusual feature of disodium etidronate therapy is the heterogeneity of the pain response. Most patients are relieved of bone pain, but in about 10 percent of patients there is a paradoxical increase in pain. The severity of pain decreases after the drug is stopped and may not return if treatment is resumed. Another difference between the effects of disodium etidronate and calcitonin is observed in the healing of osteolytic lesions. Roentgenograms of osteolytic lesions seldom have been reported to demonstrate healing after disodium etidronate therapy. In one study, osteolytic lesions progressed despite improvement of biochemical parameters. However, the second-generation bisphosphonates have been shown to induce healing of osteolytic lesions.[320]

The incidence of side effects in patients who receive disodium etidronate is low. Loose bowel movements may occur, and asymptomatic hyperphosphatemia may be observed in patients given high doses.

A major advantage of disodium etidronate is that a 6-month course of treatment may produce a prolonged biochemical remission of 1 year or more duration (Fig. 24-18). If symptoms recur, the drug can be readministered for another 6-month period.

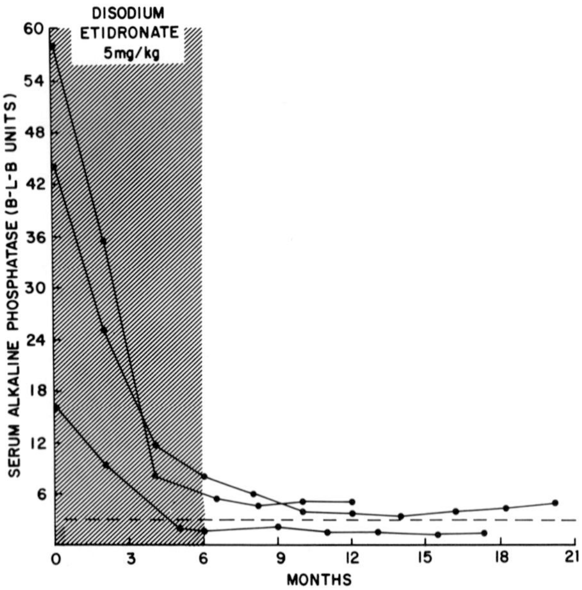

FIGURE 24-18 The effect of 6 months of therapy (hatched lines) with disodium etidronate on serum alkaline phosphatase activity in three patients with Paget's disease. The interrupted line indicates the upper limit of normal. Note the prolonged suppression of the disease after treatment was discontinued.

An alternative therapy of Paget's disease is with the cytotoxic antibiotic mithramycin. This drug is a potent inhibitor of RNA synthesis and acutely inhibits osteoclast activity. It is approved in the United States for the treatment of cancer and severe hypercalcemia but not for Paget's disease.

Mithramycin is administered by intravenous injection or infusion. It has been used at a dose of 15 to 50 μg per kilogram of body weight with a variety of treatment schedules. Early studies employed daily infusions of up to 10 days.[321] More recently weekly infusions have been used.[322] Relief of bone pain and marked suppression of biochemical parameters have been reported. However, side effects and toxicity are more likely to occur during treatment with mithramycin than with other agents. Nausea and malaise may persist for days. Platelet abnormalities leading to hemorrhage, transient elevation of liver enzymes, and impairment of renal function are other toxic effects of mithramycin. Because of this, mithramycin therapy should be reserved for patients who fail to respond to calcitonin and disodium etidronate.

Another proposed therapy is the use of oral calcium supplementation with chlorthalidone.[323] This combination has been given in an attempt to stimulate endogenous calcitonin secretion and thereby suppress disease activity. This inexpensive regimen can produce modest decreases in serum alkaline phosphatase activity and urinary hydroxyproline excretion and has been reported to reduce bone pain in most patients. Healing of osteolytic lesions has not been demonstrated.

Elective surgery is required in the management of certain patients with Paget's disease and may produce benefits which cannot be achieved by medical means. Occipital decompression may be needed in patients with neurological deficits secondary to basilar impression. Neurosurgery also may be necessary in patients with vertebral disease. Total hip replacement in the patient with severe degenerative arthritis may permit pain-free normal ambulation. Patients with severe bowing of the tibia may have difficulty in ambulation not only because of deformity but because of painful degenerative arthritis of the knee. Tibial osteotomy can correct the anatomic abnormality as well as reduce the pain resulting from the arthritis, greatly improving ambulation.

In a series of patients undergoing tibial osteotomy, treatment with calcitonin appeared to prevent excessive hemorrhage and postoperative hypercalcemia.[324] It is likely that any patient with Paget's disease requiring orthopedic surgery would benefit from treatment with a drug which suppresses the activity of the disease. Ideally, the treatment should be administered for a minimum of 2 to 3 months before surgery.

NEW CONCEPTS IN LOCAL REGULATION OF BONE METABOLISM

In the past great attention has been given to studying the influence of parathyroid hormone, vitamin D, and calcitonin as well as other hormones on bone and mineral homeostasis. With the major increase in knowledge concerning the systemic effects of hormones on bone, it has become apparent also that regulation of bone resorption and formation are not solely dependent on the direct effect of a circulating hormone on a bone cell. Recent studies have provided strong evidence of important cell-cell interactions among bone and bone marrow cells and of the existence of bone cell and matrix factors which may influence bone cell function. While these new observations have yet to be placed in a definitive physiological and pathological framework of bone metabolism in humans, these emerging areas of investigation should permit a better understanding of metabolic bone disease in the near future.

Cell-Cell Interactions

As discussed in Chap. 23, there is now excellent evidence that many of the systemic factors that stimulate osteoclastic bone resorption do so through an initial interaction with osteoblasts. This surprising concept was initially proposed on the basis of the observation that parathyroid hormone and 1α,25-dihydroxyvitamin D_3 do not affect osteoclastic activity in vitro unless osteoblasts are present[325] and the demonstration of receptors for parathyroid hormone, 1α,25-dihydroxyvitamin D_3, and prostaglandins in osteoblasts but not in osteoclasts.[326] As yet, the signal which is transmitted from the osteoblast to the osteoclast has not been identified. Presumably this osteoblastic factor not only produces activation of mature osteoclasts but also is likely to induce fusion of mononuclear hematopoietic precursors to form new osteoclasts.

The importance of bone marrow cells in the local regulation of bone resorption developed from studies which demonstrated osteoclast-activating factors from activated lymphocytes[327] and from malignant hematopoietic cells isolated from hypercalcemic patients.[328] One of the osteoclast-activating factors appears to be interleukin-1,[329] but it is likely that there are multiple osteoclast-activating factors which are synthesized by hematopoietic cells. At present, it is reasonably certain that such factors are involved in the pathological bone resorption of diseases such as multiple myeloma, but their physiological role remains unestablished.

Bone Cell and Matrix Factors

A variety of studies have demonstrated that conditioned medium from bone cultures and extracts of bone matrix contain potent factors which induce bone cell differentiation or proliferation. The first of these to be appreciated was bone morphogenetic protein,[330] a bone matrix factor which induces differentiation of perivascular mesenchymal-type cells into osteoprogenitor cells. This protein has been used in clinical studies to repair major skeletal defects.

A skeletal growth factor (83,000 kilodaltons in initial studies, 11,000 subsequently) isolated from human bone increases proliferation of cultured chick calvarial cells and enhances the growth rate of cultured embryonic chick bones.[331] It has been suggested that this factor may be the "coupling" factor which links bone resorption to formation.

Two other bone-derived growth factors have been derived from the conditioned medium of fetal rat calvariae in culture.[332] One factor (10,000 kilodaltons) maximally stimulates collagen synthesis and closely resembles somatomedin C. The other factor (25,000 to 30,000 kilodaltons) produces maximal stimulation of DNA synthesis, a characteristic shared with platelet-derived growth factor.

It is conceivable that one or more of the above factors may be utilized in the future treatment of disorders such as osteoporosis, although no experimental studies have demonstrated that these factors can produce an effect on bone formation when administered systemically. Once the structures have been determined, sufficient material should become available for such studies.

Osteonectin, bone proteoglycan, and bone sialoprotein are produced by fetal bone cells in vitro[333] and account for 1 to 2.5 percent of the protein content of cortical bone. Knowledge of the role of these bone-specific noncollagenous proteins in bone metabolism should lead to greater insights into the pathophysiology of metabolic bone disease.

REFERENCES

1. Albright FA, Reifenstein EC Jr: *The Parathyroid Glands and Metabolic Bone Disease.* Baltimore, Williams & Wilkins, 1948, p 81.
2. Price PA, Parthemore JG, Deftos LJ: New biochemical marker for bone metabolism. *J Clin Invest* 66:878, 1980.

3. Nishimoto SK, Price PA: Proof that the γ-carboxyglutamic acid–containing bone protein is synthesized in calf bone. *J Biol Chem* 254:437, 1979.

4. Price PA, Baukol SA: 1,25-dihydroxyvitamin D_3 increases synthesis of the vitamin K–dependent bone protein by osteosarcoma cells. *J Biol Chem* 255:11660, 1980.

5. Piro LD, Whyte MP, Murphy WA, Birge SJ: Normal cortical bone mass in patients after long term coumadin therapy. *J Clin Endocrinol Metab* 54:470, 1982.

6. Deftos LJ, Parthemore JG, Price PA: Change in plasma bone GLA protein during treatment of bone disease. *Calcif Tissue Int* 34:121, 1982.

7. Gundberg CM, Cole DEC, Lian JB, Reade TR, Gallop PM: Serum osteocalcin in the treatment of inherited rickets with 1,25-dihydroxyvitamin D_3. *J Clin Endocrinol Metab* 56:1063, 1983.

8. Epstein S, Poser J, McClintock R, Johnston CC Jr, Bryce G, Hui S: Differences in serum bone GLA protein with age and sex. *Lancet* 1:307, 1984.

9. Delmas PD, Wilson DM, Mann KG, Riggs BL: Effect of renal function on plasma levels of bone GLA-protein. *J Clin Endocrinol Metab* 57:1028, 1983.

10. Grundberg CM, Markowitz ME, Mizruhi M, Rosen JF: Osteocalcin in human serum: A circadian rhythm. *J Clin Endocrinol Metab* 60:736, 1985.

11. Adams E: Metabolism of proline and of hydroxyproline. *Int Rev Connect Tissue Res* 5:1, 1970.

12. Kivirikko KI: Urinary excretion of hydroxyproline in health and disease. *Int Rev Connect Tissue Res* 5:93, 1970.

13. Krane SM, Munoz AJ, Harris ED Jr: Urinary polypeptides related to collagen synthesis. *J Clin Invest* 49:716, 1970.

14. Aaron J: Diagnostic procedures, in Nordin BEC (ed): *Calcium, Phosphate and Magnesium Metabolism.* London, Churchill Livingstone, 1976, p 469.

15. Cunningham LW, Ford JD, Segrest JP: The isolation of identical hydroxylysyl glycosides from hydroxylysates of soluble collagen and from human urine. *J Biol Chem* 242:2570, 1967.

16. Pinnell SR, Fox R, Krane SM: Human collagens: Differences in glycosylated hydroxylysines in skin and bone. *Biochim Biophys Acta* 229:119, 1971.

17. Askenasi R: Urinary excretion of free hydroxylysine, peptide-bound hydroxylysine and hydroxylysyl glycosides in physiological conditions. *Clin Chim Acta* 59:87, 1972.

18. Richardson ML, Genant HK, Cann CE, Ettinger B, Gordan GS, Kolb FO, Reiser UJ: Assessment of metabolic bone diseases by quantitative computed tomography. *Clin Orthop* 195:224, 1985.

19. Cameron JR, Mazess RB, Sorenson JA: Precision and accuracy of bone mineral determination by direct photon absorptiometry. *Invest Radiol* 3:141, 1968.

20. Mazess RB, Peppler WW, Chesney RW, Lange TA, Lindgren U, Smith E Jr: Total body and regional bone mineral by dual-photon absorptiometry in metabolic bone disease. *Calcif Tissue Int* 36:8, 1984.

21. Fogelman I, Bessent RG, Turner JG, Citrin DL, Boyle IT, Greig WR: The use of whole-body retention of Tc-99m diphosphonate in the diagnosis of metabolic bone disease. *J Nucl Med* 19:270, 1978.

22. Bordier P, Matrajt H, Miravet L, Hioco D: Mésure histologique de la masse et de la résorption des travées osseuses. *Pathol Biol* 12:1238, 1964.

23. Rális ZA, Rális HM: A simple method for demonstration of osteoid in paraffin sections. *Med Lab Technol* 32:203, 1975.

24. Jowsey J: *The Bone Biopsy.* New York, Plenum, 1977, p 79.

25. Harris WH, Jackson RH, Jowsey J: The in vivo distributions of tetracyclines in canine bone. *J Bone Joint Surg [Am]* 44A:1308, 1962.

26. Epker BN, Hattner R, Frost HM: Radial sites of osteon closure. *J Lab Clin Med* 64:643, 1964.

27. Dent CE, Stamp TCB: Vitamin D, rickets and osteomalacia, in Avioli LV, Krane SM (eds): *Metabolic Bone Disease.* New York, Academic, 1977, vol 1, p 237.

28. Mankin H: Rickets, osteomalacia and renal osteodystrophy. *J Bone Joint Surg [Am]* 56A:101, 1974.

29. Fraser D, Kooh SW, Scriver CR: Hyperparathyroidism as the cause of hyperaminoaciduria and phosphaturia in human vitamin D deficiency. *Pediatr Res* 1:425, 1967.

30. Arnaud CD, Glorieux F, Scriver CR: Serum parathyroid hormone levels in acquired vitamin D deficiency. *Pediatrics* 49:837, 1972.

31. Vainsel M, Manderlier T, Otten J: Urinary excretion of adenosine 3′,5′-monophosphate in vitamin D deficiency. *Eur J Clin Invest* 6:127, 1976.

32. Fraser D, Scriver CR: Disorders associated with hereditary or acquired abnormalities in vitamin D function: Hereditary disorders associated with vitamin D resistance or defective phosphate metabolism, in De Groot LJ (ed): *Endocrinology.* New York, Grune & Stratton, 1979, vol 2, p 797.

33. Haussler MR, McCain TA: Basic and clinical concepts related to vitamin D metabolism and action. *N Engl J Med* 297:1041, 1977.

34. Eastwood JB, DeWardener HE, Gray RW, Lemann JL Jr: Normal plasma 1,25-$(OH)_2$-vitamin D concentrations in nutritional osteomalacia. *Lancet* 1:1377, 1979.

35. Frame B, Parfitt AM: Osteomalacia: Current concepts. *Ann Intern Med* 89:966, 1978.

36. Marie PJ, Glorieux FH: Relation between hypomineralized periosteocytic lesions and bone mineralization in vitamin D–resistant rickets. *Calcif Tissue Int* 35:443, 1983.

37. Loomis WF: Rickets. *Sci Am* 223:77, 1970.

38. Bachrach S, Fisher J, Parks JS: An outbreak of vitamin D deficiency rickets in a susceptible population. *Pediatrics* 64:871, 1979.

39. Dwyer JT, Dietz WH Jr, Hass G, Suskind R: Risk of nutritional rickets among vegetarian children. *Am J Dis Child* 133:134, 1979.

40. Thompson GR, Lewis B, Booth CC: Absorption of vitamin D_3-^3H in control subjects and patients with intestinal malabsorption. *J Clin Invest* 45:94, 1966.

41. Arnaud SB, Goldsmith RS, Lambert PW, Go VLW: 25-Hydroxyvitamin D_3: Evidence of an enterohepatic circulation in man. *Proc Soc Exp Biol Med* 149:570, 1975.

42. Clements MR, Chalmers TM, Fraser DR: Enterohepatic circulation of vitamin D: A reappraisal of the hypothesis. *Lancet* 1:1376, 1984.

43. Dibble JB, Sheridan P, Hampshire R, Hardy GJ, Losowsky MS: Evidence for secondary hyperparathyroidism in the osteomalacia associated with chronic liver disease. *Clin Endocrinol* 15:373, 1981.

44. Imawari M, Akanuma Y, Itakura H, Muto Y, Kosaka K, Goodman De WS: The effects of the liver on serum 25-hydroxyvitamin D and on the serum binding protein for vitamin D and its metabolites. *J Lab Clin Med* 93:171, 1979.

45. Bikle DD, Halloran BP, Gee E, Ryzen E, Haddad JG: Free 25-hydroxyvitamin D levels are normal in subjects with liver disease and reduced total 25-hydroxyvitamin D levels. *J Clin Invest* 78:748, 1986.

46. Horst RL, Jorgensen NA, DeLuca HF: The determination of 24,25-dihydroxyvitamin D and 25,26-dihydroxyvitamin D in plasma from normal and nephrectomized man. *J Lab Clin Med* 93:277, 1979.

47. Richens A, Rowe DJF: Disturbance of calcium metabolism by anticonvulsant drugs. *Br Med J* 4:73,1970.

48. Weinstein RS, Bryce GF, Sappington LJ, King DW, Gallagher BB: Decreased serum ionized calcium and normal vitamin D metabolite levels with anticonvulsant drug treatment. *J Clin Endocrinol Metab* 58:1003, 1984.

49. Hahn TJ: Drug-induced disorders of vitamin D and mineral metabolism. *Clin Endocrinol Metab* 9:107, 1980.

50. Morijiri Y, Sato T: Factors causing rickets in institutionalized handicapped children on anticonvulsant therapy. *Arch Dis Child* 56:446, 1981.

51. Weisman Y, Fattal A, Eisenberg Z, Harel S, Spirer Z, Harell A: Decreased serum 24,25-dihydroxyvitamin D concentrations in children receiving chronic anticonvulsant therapy. *Br Med J* 2:521, 1979.

52. Christensen CK, Lund B, Lund BJ, Sorensen OH, Nielsen HE, Mosekilde L: Reduced 1,25-dihydroxyvitamin D and 24,25-dihydroxyvitamin D in epileptic patients receiving chronic combined anticonvulsant therapy. *Metab Bone Dis Rel Res* 3:17, 1981.

53. Jubiz W, Haussler MR, McCain TA, Tolman KG: Plasma 1,25-dihydroxyvitamin D levels in patients receiving anticonvulsant drugs. *J Clin Endocrinol Metab* 44:617, 1977.

54. Ryan EA, Reiss E: Oncogenous osteomalacia. *Am J Med* 77:501, 1984.

55. Lyles KW, Berry WR, Haussler M, Harrelson JM, Drezner MK: Hypophosphatemic osteomalacia: Association with prostatic carcinoma. *Ann Intern Med* 93:275, 1980.

56. Taylor HC, Fallon MD, Velasco ME: Oncogenic osteomalacia and inappropriate antidiuretic hormone secretion due to oat-cell carcinoma. *Ann Int Med* 101:786, 1984.

57. Eulderink F: Adenomatoid changes in Bowman's capsule in primary carcinoma of the liver. *J Pathol* 87:251, 1964.

58. Fraser D, Kooh SW, Kind HP, Holick MF, Tanaka Y, DeLuca HF: Pathogenesis of hereditary vitamin-D-dependent rickets. An inborn error of vitamin D metabolism involving defective conversion of 25-hydroxyvitamin D to 1α,25-dihydroxyvitamin D. *N Engl J Med* 289:817, 1973.

59. Delvin EE, Glorieux FH, Marie PJ, Pettifor JM: Vitamin D dependency: Replacement therapy with calcitriol. *J Pediatr* 99:26, 1981.

60. Schmidt-Gayk H, Schmitt W, Grawunder C, Ritz E, Tschoepe W, Pietsch V, Andrassy K, Bouillon R: 25-Hydroxy-vitamin D in nephrotic syndrome. *Lancet* 2:105, 1977.

61. Malluche HH, Goldstein DA, Massry SG: Osteomalacia and hyperparathyroid bone disease in patients with nephrotic syndrome. *J Clin Invest* 63:494, 1979.

62. Korkor A, Schwartz A, Bergfeld M, Teitelbaum S, Avioli L, Klahr S, Slatopolsky E: Absence of metabolic bone disease in adult patients with the nephrotic syndrome and normal renal function. *J Clin Endocrinol Metab* 56:496, 1983.

63. Brooks MH, Bell NH, Love L, Stern PH, Orfei E, Queener SF, Hamstra AJ, DeLuca HF: Vitamin-D dependent rickets type II. Resistance of target organs to 1,25-dihydroxyvitamin D. *N Engl J Med* 298:996, 1978.

64. Liberman UA, Samuel R, Halabe A, Kauli R, Edelstein S, Weisman Y, Papaplos SE, Clemens TL, Fraher LJ, O'Riordan JLH: End-organ resistance to 1,25-dihydroxycholecalciferol. *Lancet* 1:504, 1980.

65. Gamblin GT, Liberman UA, Eil C, Downs RW Jr, DeGrange DA, Marx SJ: Vitamin D–dependent rickets type II: Defective induction of 25-hydroxyvitamin D_3-24-hydroxylase by 1,25-dihydroxyvitamin D_3 in cultured skin fibroblasts. *J Clin Invest* 75:954, 1985.

66. Pike JW, Dokoh S, Haussler MR, Liberman UA, Marx SJ, Eil C: Vitamin D_3–resistant fibroblasts have immunoassayable 1,25-dihydroxyvitamin D_3 receptors. *Science* 224:879, 1984.

67. Liberman UA, Eil C, Marx SJ: Resistance to 1,25-dihydroxyvitamin D: Association with heterogeneous defects in cultured skin fibroblasts. *J Clin Invest* 71:192, 1983.

68. Liberman UA, Eil C, Holst P, Rosen JF, Marx SJ: Hereditary resistance to 1,25-dihydroxyvitamin D: Defective function of receptors for 1,25-dihydroxyvitamin D in cells cultured from bone. *J Clin Endocrinol Metab* 57:958, 1983.

69. Jenkins MV, Harris M, Wills MR: The effect of phenytoin on parathyroid extract and 25-hydroxycholecalciferol–induced bone resorption: Adenosine 3',5'-cyclic monophosphate production. *Calcif Tissue Res* 16:163, 1974.

70. Corradino RA: Diphenylhydantoin: Direct inhibition of the vitamin D_3-mediated calcium absorptive mechanism in organ cultured duodenum. *Biochem Pharmacol* 25:863, 1976.

71. Brickman AS, Coburn JW, Massry SG: 1,25-Dihydroxyvitamin D_3 in normal man and patients with renal failure. *Ann Intern Med* 80:161, 1974.

72. Albright F, Butler AM, Bloomberg E: Rickets resistant to vitamin D therapy. *Am J Dis Child* 54:529, 1937.

73. Winters RW, Graham JB, Williams TF, McFalls VW, Burnett CH: A genetic study of familial hypophosphatemia and vitamin D resistant rickets with a review of the literature. *Medicine* 37:97, 1958.

74. Reitz RE, Weinstein RL: Parathyroid hormone secretion in familial vitamin-D-resistant rickets. *N Engl J Med* 289:941, 1973.

75. Short E, Morris RC Jr, Sebastian A, Spencer M: Exaggerated phosphaturic response to circulating parathyroid hormone in patients with familial X-linked hypophosphatemic rickets. *J Clin Invest* 58:152, 1976.

76. Lyles KW, Burkes EJ Jr, McNamara CR, Harrelson JM, Pickett JP, Drezner MK: The concurrence of hypoparathyroidism provides new insights to the pathophysiology of X-linked hypophosphatemic rickets. *J Clin Endocrinol Metab* 60:711, 1985.

77. Condon JR, Nassim JR, Rutter A: Defective intestinal phosphate absorption in familial and non-familial hypophosphatemia. *Br Med J* 3:138, 1970.

78. Chesney RW, Mazess RB, Rose P, Hamstra AJ, DeLuca HF: Supranormal 25-hydroxyvitamin D and subnormal 1,25-dihydroxyvitamin D: Their role in X-linked hypophosphatemic rickets. *Am J Dis Child* 134:140, 1980.

79. Seino Y, Shimotsuji T, Ishii T, Ishida M, Ikehara C, Yamaoka K, Yabwichi H, Dokoh S: Treatment of hypophosphatemic vitamin D–resistant rickets with massive dose of 1α-hydroxyvitamin D_3 during childhood. *Arch Dis Child* 55:49, 1980.

80. Delvin EE, Glorieux FH: Serum 1,25-dihydroxyvitamin D concentration in hypophosphatemic vitamin D–resistant rickets. *Calif Tissue Int* 33:173, 1981.

81. Lyles KW, Drezner MK: Parathyroid hormone effects on serum 1,25-dihydroxyvitamin D levels in patients with X-linked hypophosphatemic rickets: Evidence for abnormal 25-hydroxyvitamin D-1-hydroxylase activity. *J Clin Endocrinol Metab* 54:638, 1982.

82. Brickman AS, Coburn JW, Kurokawa K, Bethune JE, Harrison HE, Norman AW: Actions of 1,25-dihydroxycholecalciferol in patients with hypophosphatemic, vitamin D–resistant rickets. *N Engl J Med* 289:495, 1973.

83. Stamp TCB, Baker LRI: Recessive hypophosphatemic rickets, and possible etiology of the "vitamin D–resistant" syndrome. *Arch Dis Child* 51:360, 1976.

84. Perry W, Stamp TCB: Hereditary hypophosphatemic rickets with autosomal recessive inheritance and severe osteosclerosis. *J Bone Joint Surg [Br]* 60B:430, 1978.

85. Tieder M, Modai D, Samuel R, Arie R, Halabe A, Bab J, Gabizon D, Liberman UA: Hereditary hypophosphatemic rickets with hypercalciuria. *N Engl J Med* 312:611, 1985.

86. Nagant de Deuxchaisnes C, Krane SM: The treatment of adult phosphate diabetes and Fanconi syndrome with neutral sodium phosphate. *Am J Med* 43:508, 1967.

87. Frymoyer JW, Hodgkin W: Adult-onset vitamin D–resistant hypophosphatemic osteomalacia: A possible variant of vitamin D–resistant rickets. *J Bone Joint Surg [Am]* 59A:101, 1977.

88. Minari M, Castellani A, Garella S: Renal tubular acidosis associated with vitamin D–resistant rickets. Role of phosphate depletion. *Mineral Electrolyte Metab* 10:371, 1984.

88a. Dent CE, Gertner JM: Hypophosphatemic osteomalacia in fibrous dysplasia. *Q J Med* 45:411, 1976.

89. McArthur RG, Hayles AB, Lambert PW: Albright's syndrome

with rickets. *Mayo Clin Proc* 54:313, 1979.

90. Aschinberg LC, Solomon LM, Zeis PM, Justice P, Rosenthal IM: Vitamin D–resistant rickets associated with epidermal nevus syndrome: Demonstration of a phosphaturic substance in the dermal lesions. *J Pediatr* 91:56, 1977.

91. Bressot C, Courpron P, Edouard C, Meunier P: *Histomorphometrie des ostéopathies endocriniennes.* Lyon, Association Corporative des Étudiants en Médecine de Lyon, 1976, p 117.

92. Dent CE, Winter CE: Osteomalacia due to phosphate depletion from excessive aluminum hydroxide ingestion. *Br Med J* 1:551, 1974.

93. Ahmed KY, Varghese Z, Wills MR, Meinhard E, Skinner RK, Baillod RA, Moorhead JE: Persistent hypophosphatemia and osteomalacia in dialysis patients not on oral phosphate binders: Response to dihydrotachysterol therapy. *Lancet* 2:439, 1976.

94. Teotia SPS, Teotia M: Secondary hyperparathyroidism in patients with endemic skeletal fluorosis. *Br Med J* 1:637, 1973.

95. Jowsey J: The long-term treatment of osteoporosis with fluoride, calcium and vitamin D, in Barzel US (ed): *Osteoporosis II.* New York, Grune & Stratton, 1979, p 123.

96. Khairi MRA, Altman RD, DeRosa GP, Zimmerman J, Schenk RK, Johnston CC: Sodium etidronate in the treatment of Paget's disease of bone: A study of long-term results. *Ann Intern Med* 87:656, 1977.

97. Boyce BF, Smith L, Fogelman I, Johnston E, Ralston S, Boyle IT: Focal osteomalacia due to low dose diphosphonate therapy in Paget's disease. *Lancet* 1:821, 1984.

98. Kooh SW, Fraser D, Reilly BJ, Hamilton JR, Gall DG, Bell L: Rickets due to calcium deficiency. *N Engl J Med* 297:1264, 1977.

99. Pettifor JM, Ross FP, Travers R, Glorieux FH, DeLuca HF: Dietary calcium deficiency: A syndrome associated with bone deformities and elevated serum 1,25-dihydroxyvitamin D concentrations. *Metab Bone Dis Rel Res* 2:301, 1981.

100. Marie PJ, Pettifor JM, Ross FP, Glorieux FH: Histological osteomalacia due to dietary calcium deficiency in children. *N Engl J Med* 307:584, 1982.

101. Albright F: Hypoparathyroidism as a cause of osteomalacia. *J Clin Endocrinol Metab* 16:419, 1956.

102. Schutt-Aine JC, Young MA, Pescovitz OH, Chrousos GP, Marx SJ: Hypoparathyroidism: A possible cause of rickets. *J Pediatr* 106:255, 1985.

103. Rasmussen H: Hypophosphatasia, in Stanbury JB, Wyngaarden JB, Fredrickson DS, Goldstein JL, Brown MS (eds): *The Metabolic Basis of Inherited Disease,* 5th ed. New York, McGraw-Hill, 1983, p 1497.

104. Maesaka H, Niitsu N, Suwa S, Fujita T: Neonatal hypophosphatasia with elevated serum parathyroid hormone. *Eur J Pediatr* 12:71, 1977.

105. Whyte MP, Teitelbaum SL, Murphy WA, Bergfeld MA, Avioli LV: Adult hypophosphatasia: Clinical, laboratory, and genetic investigation of a large kindred with review of the literature. *Medicine* 58:329, 1979.

106. Frame B, Frost HM, Pak CYC, Reynolds W, Argen RJ: Fibrogenesis imperfecta ossium: A collagen defect causing osteomalacia. *N Engl J Med* 285:769, 1971.

107. Chesney RW, Kaplan BS, Phelps M, DeLuca HF: Renal tubular acidosis does not alter circulating values of calcitriol. *J Pediatr* 104:51, 1984.

108. Kraut JA, Gordon EM, Ransom JC, Horst R, Slatopolsky E, Coburn JW, Kurokawa K: Effect of chronic metabolic acidosis on vitamin D metabolism in humans. *Kidney Int* 24:644, 1983.

109. Shike M, Harrison JE, Sturtridge WC, Tam CS, Bobechko PE, Jones G, Murray TM, Jeejeebhoy KN: Metabolic bone disease in patients receiving long-term total parenteral nutrition. *Ann Int Med* 92:343, 1980.

110. Klein GL, Targoff CM, Ament ME, Sherrard DJ, Bluestone R, Young JH, Norman AW, Coburn JW: Bone disease associated with total parenteral nutrition. *Lancet* 2:1041, 1980.

111. Ott SM, Maloney NA, Klein GL, Alfrey AC, Ament ME, Coburn JW, Sherrard DJ: Aluminum is associated with low bone formation in patients receiving chronic parenteral nutrition. *Ann Int Med* 98:910, 1983.

112. Stamp TCB, Round MM, Rowe DJF, Haddad JG: Plasma levels and therapeutic effect of 25-hydroxycholecalciferol in epileptic patients taking anticonvulsant drugs. *Br Med J* 4:9, 1972.

113. Glorieux FH, Scriver CR, Reade TM, Goldman H, Roseborough A: Use of phosphate and vitamin D to prevent dwarfism and rickets in X-linked hypophosphatemia. *N Engl J Med* 287:481, 1972.

114. Lyles KW, Harrelson JM, Drezner MK: The efficacy of vitamin D and oral phosphorus therapy in X-linked hypophosphatemic rickets and osteomalacia. *J Clin Endocrinol Metab* 54:307, 1982.

115. Kirschman GH, DeLuca HF, Chan JCM: Hypophosphatemic vitamin D–resistant rickets: Metabolic balance studies in a child receiving 1,25-dihydroxyvitamin D_3, phosphate, and ascorbic acid. *Pediatrics* 61:451, 1978.

116. Glorieux FH, Marie PJ, Pettifor JM, Delvin EE: Bone response to phosphate salts, ergocalciferol, and calcitriol in hypophosphatemic rickets. *N Engl J Med* 303:1023, 1980.

117. Harrell RM, Lyles KW, Harrelson JM, Friedman NE, Drezner MK: Healing of bone disease in X-linked hypophosphatemic rickets/osteomalacia: Induction and maintenance with phosphorus and calcitriol. *J Clin Invest* 75:1858, 1985.

118. Firth RG, Grant CS, Riggs BL: Development of hypercalcemic hyperparathyroidism after long-term phosphate supplementation in hypophosphatemic osteomalacia. *Am J Med* 78:669, 1985.

119. Marie PJ, Glorieux FH: Bone histomorphometry in asymptomatic adults with hereditary hypophosphatemic vitamin D resistant osteomalacia. *Metab Bone Dis Rel Res* 4:249, 1982.

120. Whyte MP, McAlister WH, Patton LS, Magill HL, Fallon MD, Lorentz WB Jr, Herrod HG: Enzyme replacement therapy for infantile hypophosphatasia attempted by intravenous infusions of alkaline phosphatase–rich Paget plasma: Results in three additional patients. *J Pediatr* 105:926, 1984.

121. Stamp TCB Byers PD, Ali SY, Jenkins MV, Willoughby JMT: Fibrogenesis imperfecta ossium: Remission with melphalan. *Lancet* 1:582, 1985.

122. Thomson DL, Frame B: Involutional osteopenia: Current concepts. *Ann Intern Med* 85:789, 1976.

123. Cann CE, Genant HK, Kolb FO, Ettinger B: Quantitative computed tomography for prediction of vertebral fracture risk. *Bone* 6:1, 1985.

124. Seeman E, Wahner HW, Offord KP, Kumar R, Johnson WJ, Riggs BL: Differential effects of endocrine dysfunction on the axial and appendicular skeleton. *J Clin Invest* 69:1302, 1982.

125. Meunier PJ, Bianchi GGS, Edouard CM, Bernard JC, Coupron P, Vignon GE: Bony manifestations of thyrotoxicosis. *Orthop Clin North Am* 3:745, 1975.

126. Gallagher JC, Riggs BL, Jerpbak CM, Arnaud CD: The effect of age on serum immunoreactive parathyroid hormone in normal and osteoporotic women. *J Lab Clin Med* 95:373, 1980.

127. Heath H, Sizemore GW: Plasma calcitonin in normal man: Differences between men and women. *J Clin Invest* 60:1135, 1977.

128. Shamonki IM, Frumar AM, Tataryn IV, Meldrum DR, Davidson BH, Parthemore JG, Judd HL, Deftos LJ: Age-related changes of calcitonin secretion in females. *J Clin Endocrinol Metab* 50:437, 1980.

129. Morimoto S, Tsuji M, Okada Y, Omishi T, Kumahara Y: The effect of oestrogens on human calcitonin secretion after calcium infusion in elderly female subjects. *Clin Endocrinol* 13:135, 1980.

130. Stevenson JC, Abeyasekera G, Hillyard CJ, Phang K-G, MacIntyre I, Campbell S, Lane G, Townsend PT, Young O, Whitehead MI: Regulation of calcium-regulating hormones by exogenous sex steroids in early postmenopause. *Europ J Clin Invest* 13:481, 1983.

131. Leggate J, Farish E, Fletcher CD, McIntosh W, Hart DM,

Sommerville JM: Calcitonin and postmenopausal osteoporosis. *Clin Endocrinol* 20:85, 1984.
132. Selby PL, Peacock M, Barkworth SA, Brown WB, Taylor GA: Early effects of ethinyloestradiol and norethisterone treatment in post-menopausal women on bone resorption and calcium regulating hormones. *Clin Sci* 69:265, 1985.
133. Lobo RA, Roy S, Shoupe D, Endres DB, Adams JS, Rude RK, Singer FR: Estrogen and progestin effects on urinary calcium and calciotropic hormones in surgically-induced postmenopausal women. *Horm Metab Res* 17:370, 1985.
134. Body JJ, Heath H III: Estimates of circulating monomeric calcitonin: Physiologic studies in normal and thyroidectomized man. *J Clin Endocrinol Metab* 57:897, 1983.
135. Milhaud G, Benezech-Leferre M, Moukhtar MS: Deficiency of calcitonin in age related osteoporosis. *Biomedicine* 29:272, 1978.
136. Chestnut CH III, Baylink DJ, Sisom K, Nelp WB, Roos BA: Basal plasma immunoreactive calcitonin in postmenopausal osteoporosis. *Metabolism* 29:559, 1980.
137. Taggart HM, Chestnut CH III, Ivey JL, Baylink DJ, Sisom K, Huber MB, Roos BA: Deficient calcitonin response to calcium stimulation in postmenopausal osteoporosis. *Lancet* 1:475, 1982.
138. Tiegs RD, Body JJ, Wahner HW, Barta J, Riggs BL, Heath H III: Calcitonin secretion in postmenopausal osteoporosis. *N Engl J Med* 312:1097, 1985.
139. Avioli LV, McDonald JE, Lee SW: The influence of age on the intestinal absorption of ^{47}Ca absorption in postmenopausal osteoporosis. *J Clin Invest* 44:1960, 1965.
140. Gallagher JC, Riggs BL, Eisman J, Hamstra A, Arnaud SB, De Luca HF: Intestinal calcium absorption and serum vitamin D metabolites in normal subjects and osteoporotic patients: Effect of age and dietary calcium. *J Clin Invest* 64:729, 1979.
141. Tsai K-S, Heath H III, Kumar R, Riggs BL: Impaired vitamin D metabolism with aging in women: Possible role in pathogenesis of senile osteoporosis. *J Clin Invest* 73:1668, 1984.
142. Francis RM, Peacock M, Taylor GA, Storer JH, Nordin BEC: Calcium malabsorption in elderly women with vertebral fractures: Evidence for resistance to the action of vitamin D metabolites on the bowel. *Clin Sci* 66:103, 1984.
143. Christiansen C, Rodbro P: Serum vitamin D metabolites in younger and elderly postmenopausal women. *Calcif Tissue Int* 36:19, 1984.
144. Gallagher JC, Nordin BEC: Oestrogens and calcium metabolism. *Front Horm Res* 2:98, 1973.
145. Jowsey J, Kelly PJ, Riggs BL, Bianco AL Jr, Scholz DA, Gershon-Cohen J: Quantitative microradiographic studies of normal and osteoporotic bone. *J Bone Joint Surg [Am]* 47A:785, 1965.
146. Nordin BEC, Aaron J, Speed R, Crilly RB: Bone formation and resorption as the determinants of trabecular bone volume in postmenopausal osteoporosis. *Lancet* 2:77, 1981.
147. Meunier P, Courpron P, Edouard C, Bernard J, Bringuier J, Vignon G: Physiological senile involution and pathological rarefaction of bone. *Clin Endocrinol Metab* 2:239, 1973.
148. Rasmussen H, Bordier P: *The Physiological and Cellular Basis of Metabolic Bone Disease.* Baltimore, Williams & Wilkins, 1974, p 272.
149. Arlot M, Edouard C, Meunier PJ, Neer RM, Reeve J: Impaired osteoblast function in osteoporosis: Comparison between calcium balance and dynamic histomorphometry. *Br Med J* 289:517, 1984.
150. Johnston CC, Norton J, Khairi MRA, Kernek C, Edouard C, Arlot M, Meunier PJ: Heterogeneity of fracture syndromes in postmenopausal women. *J Clin Endocrinol Metab* 61:551, 1985.
151. Darby AJ, Meunier PJ: Mean wall thickness and formation periods of trabecular bone packets in idiopathic osteoporosis. *Calcif Tissue Int* 33:199, 1981.
152. Lips P, Netelenbos JC, Jongen MJM, van Ginkel FC, Althuis AL, van Schaik CL, van der Vijgh WJF, Vermeiden JPW, van der Meer C: Histomorphometric profile and vitamin D status in patients with femoral neck fracture. *Metab Bone Dis Rel Res* 4:85, 1982.
153. Whyte MP, Bergfeld MA, Murphy WA, Avioli LV, Teitelbaum SL: Postmenopausal osteoporosis: A heterogeneous disorder as assessed by histomorphometric analysis of iliac crest bone from untreated patients. *Am J Med* 72:193, 1982.
154. Riggs BL, Jowsey J, Kelly PJ: Quantitative microradiographic study of bone remodeling in Cushing's syndrome. *Metabolism* 15:773, 1966.
155. Jowsey J, Riggs BL: Bone formation in hypercortisonism. *Acta Endocrinol* 63:21, 1970.
156. Bressot C, Meunier PJ, Chapuy MC, Lejeune E, Edouard C, Darby AJ: Histomorphometric profile, pathophysiology and reversibility of corticosteroid-induced osteoporosis. *Metab Bone Dis Relat Res* 1:303, 1979.
157. Minaire P, Meunier P, Edouard C, Bernard J, Courpron P, Bouret J: Quantitative histological data on disuse osteoporosis: Comparison with biological data. *Calcif Tissue Res* 17:57, 1974.
158. Jowsey J, Johnson KA: Juvenile osteoporosis: Bone findings in seven patients. *J Pediatr* 81:511, 1972.
159. Smith R: Idiopathic osteoporosis in the young. *J Bone Joint Surg [Br]* 62-B:417, 1980.
160. Evans RA, Dunstan CR, Hills E: Bone metabolism in idiopathic juvenile osteoporosis: A case report. *Calcif Tissue Int* 35:5, 1983.
161. Jaffe HL: *Metabolic, Degenerative, and Inflammatory Diseases of Bones and Joints.* Philadelphia, Lea & Febiger, 1972, p 162.
162. Riggs BL, Melton LJ III: Evidence for two distinct syndromes of involutional osteoporosis. *Am J Med* 75:899, 1983.
163. Daniell HW: Osteoporosis of the slender smoker: Vertebral compression fractures and loss of metacarpal cortex in relation to postmenopausal cigarette smoking and lack of obesity. *Arch Intern Med* 136:298, 1976.
164. Seeman E, Melton LJ III, O'Fallon WM, Riggs BL: Risk factors for spinal osteoporosis in men. *Am J Med* 75:977, 1983.
165. Aloia JF, Cohn SH, Vaswani A, Yeh JK, Yuen K, Ellis K: Risk factors for postmenopausal osteoporosis. *Am J Med* 78:95, 1985.
166. Melton LJ, Riggs BL: Epidemiology of age-related fractures, in Avioli LV (ed): *The Osteoporotic Syndrome: Detection, Prevention and Treatment.* New York, Grune & Stratton, 1983, p 45.
167. Morgan DB: *Osteomalacia, Renal Osteodystrophy, and Osteoporosis.* Springfield, Ill, Charles C Thomas, 1973, p 248.
168. Gallagher JC, Wilkinson R: The effect of ethinylestradiol on calcium and phosphorus metabolism of postmenopausal women with primary hyperparathyroidism. *Clin Sci Mol Med* 45:785, 1973.
169. Nutik G, Cruess RL: Estrogen receptors in bone: An evaluation of the uptake of estrogen into bone cells. *Proc Soc Exp Biol Med* 146:265, 1974.
170. Gallagher JC, Riggs BL, DeLuca HF: Effect of estrogen on calcium absorption and serum vitamin D metabolites in postmenopausal osteoporosis. *J Clin Endocrinol Metab* 51:1359, 1980.
171. Longcope C, Baker RS, Hui SL, Johnston CC Jr: Androgen and estrogen dynamics in women with vertebral crush fractures. *Maturitas* 6:309, 1984.
172. Nordin BEC, Robertson A, Seamark RF, Bridges A, Philcox JC, Need AG, Horowitz M, Morris HA, Deam S: The relation between calcium absorption, serum dehydroepiandrosterone, and vertebral mineral density in postmenopausal women. *J Clin Endocrinol Metab* 60:651, 1985.
173. Albright F, Bloomberg E, Smith PH: Postmenopausal osteoporosis. *Trans Assoc Am Physicians* 55:305, 1940.
174. Heaney RP, Recker RR, Saville PD: Menopausal changes in bone remodelling. *J Lab Clin Med* 92:964, 1978.
175. Marcus R, Cann C, Madvig P: Menstrual function and bone mass in elite women distance runners: Endocrine and metabolic features. *Ann Int Med* 102:158, 1985.
176. Koppelman MCS, Kurtz DW, Morrish KA, Bau E, Susser JK, Shapiro JR, Loriaux DL: Vertebral body bone mineral content in hyperprolactinemic women. *J Clin Endocrinol Metab* 59:1050, 1984.
177. Rigotti NA, Nussbaum SR, Herzog DB, Neer RM: Osteoporo-

sis in women with anorexia nervosa. *N Engl J Med* 311:1601, 1984.
178. Foresta C, Ruzza G, Mioni R, Guarnieri G, Gribaldo R, Meneghello A, Mastrogiacomo I: Osteoporosis and decline of gonadal function in the elderly. *Hormone Res* 19:18, 1984.
179. Baran DT, Bergfeld MA, Teitelbaum SL, Avioli VL: Effect of testosterone therapy on bone formation in an osteoporotic hypogonadal male. *Calcif Tissue Res* 26:103, 1978.
180. Peck WA, Brandt J, Miller I: Hydrocortisone-induced inhibition of protein synthesis and uridine incorporation in isolated bone cells in vitro. *Proc Natl Acad Sci USA* 57:1599, 1967.
181. Jett S, Wu K, Duncan H, Frost HM: Adrenalcorticosteroid and salicylate actions on human and canine haversian bone formation and resorption. *Clin Orthop* 68:301, 1970.
182. Blodgett FM, Burgin L, Jezzoni D, Gribetz D, Talbot NB: Effects of prolonged cortisone therapy on the statural growth, skeletal maturation and metabolic status of children. *N Engl J Med* 254:636, 1956.
183. Barrett AJ, Sledge CB, Dingle JT: Effect of cortisol on the synthesis of chondroitin sulfate by embryonic cartilage. *Nature* 221:83, 1966.
184. Fucik RF, Kukreja SC, Hargis GK, Bowser EN, Henderson WJ, Williams GA: Effects of glucocorticoids on function of the parathyroid glands in man. *J Clin Endocrinol Metab* 49:152, 1975.
185. Lukert BP, Adams JS: Calcium and phosphorus homeostasis in man. *Arch Intern Med* 136:1249, 1976.
186. Slovik DM, Neer RM, Ohman JL, Lowell FC, Clark MB, Segre GV, Potts JT Jr: Parathyroid hormone and 25-hydroxyvitamin D levels in glucocorticoid-treated patients. *Clin Endocrinol* 12:243, 1980.
187. Findling JW, Adams ND, Lemann J Jr, Gray RW, Thomas CJ, Tyrell JB: Vitamin D metabolites and parathyroid hormone in Cushing's syndrome: Relationship to calcium and phosphorus homeostasis. *J Clin Endocrinol Metab* 54:1039, 1982.
188. Harrison HE, Harrison HC: Transfer of Ca^{45} across intestinal wall in vitro in relation to action of vitamin D and cortisol. *Am J Physiol* 199:265, 1960.
189. Kimberg DV, Baerg RD, Gershon E, Graudusius RT: Effect of cortisone treatment on the active transport of calcium by the small intestine. *J Clin Invest* 50:1309, 1971.
190. Edelstein S, Noff D: The functional metabolism of vitamin D in rats treated with cortisol. *FEBS Lett* 82:115, 1977.
191. Spanos E, Colston KW, MacIntyre I: Effect of glucocorticoids on vitamin D metabolism. *FEBS Lett* 75:73, 1977.
192. Klein RG, Arnaud SB, Gallagher JC, DeLuca HF, Riggs BL: Intestinal calcium absorption in exogenous hypercortisonism. *J Clin Invest* 60:253, 1977.
193. Chesney RW, Mazess RB, Hamstra AJ, DeLuca HF, O'Reagan S: Reduction of serum 1,25-dihydroxyvitamin D_3 in children receiving glucocorticoid. *Lancet* 2:1123, 1978.
194. O'Reagan S, Chesney RW, Hamstra A, Eisman JA, O'Gorman AM, DeLuca HF: Reduced serum 1,25-$(OH)_2$-vitamin D_3 levels in prednisone-treated adolescents with systemic lupus erythematosus. *Acta Paediatr Scand* 68:109, 1979.
195. Rickers H, Deding A, Christiansen C, Rodbro P, Naestoft J: Corticosteroid-induced osteopenia and vitamin D metabolism: Effect of vitamin D_2, calcium phosphate and sodium fluoride administration. *Clin Endocrinol* 16:409, 1982.
196. Favus MJ, Walling MW, Kimberg DV: Effects of 1,25-dihydroxycholecalciferol on intestinal calcium transport in cortisone treated rats. *J Clin Invest* 52:1680, 1973.
197. Mundy GR, Shapiro JL, Bardelin JG, Canalis EM, Raisz LG: Direct stimulation of bone resorption by thyroid hormones. *J Clin Invest* 58:529, 1976.
198. Krane SM, Brownell GL, Stanbury JB, Corrigan H: The effect of thyroid disease on calcium metabolism in man. *J Clin Invest* 35:874, 1956.
199. Singhelakis P, Alevizaka CC, Ikkos DG: Intestinal calcium absorption in hyperthyroidism. *Metabolism* 23:311, 1974.
200. Bouillon R, Muls E, DeMoor P: Influence of thyroid function on the serum concentration of 1,25-dihydroxyvitamin D_3. *J Clin Endocrinol Metab* 51:793, 1980.
201. McNair P, Madsbad S, Chistensen MS, Christiansen C, Faber OK, Binder C, Transbol I: Bone mineral loss in insulin-treated diabetes mellitus: Studies on pathogenesis. *Acta Endocrinol* 90:463, 1979.
202. Heath H III, Melton LJ III, Chu C-P: Diabetes mellitus and risk of skeletal fracture. *N Engl J Med* 303:567, 1980.
203. Raskin P, Stevenson MRM, Barilla DE, Pak CYC: The hypercalciuria of diabetes mellitus: Its amelioration with insulin. *Clin Endocrinol* 9:329, 1978.
204. Schneider LE, Schedl HP, McCain T, Haussler MR: Experimental diabetes reduces circulating 1,25-dihydroxyvitamin D in the rat. *Science* 196:1452, 1977.
205. Heath H III, Lambert PW, Service FJ, Arnaud SB: Calcium homeostasis in diabetes mellitus. *J Clin Endocrinol Metab* 49:462, 1979.
206. Frazer TE, White NH, Hough S, Santiago JV, McGee BR, Bryce G, Mallon J, Avioli LV: Alterations in circulating vitamin D metabolites in the young insulin-dependent diabetic. *J Clin Endocrinol Metab* 53:1154, 1981.
207. Storm TL, Sorensen OH, Lund B, Lund B, Christiansen JS, Andersen AR, Lumholtz IB, Parving H-H: Vitamin D metabolism in insulin-dependent diabetes mellitus. *Metab Bone Dis Rel Res* 5:107, 1983.
208. Prockop DJ, Kivirikko KK: Heritable diseases of collagen. *N Engl J Med* 311:376, 1984.
209. Smith R: Idiopathic juvenile osteoporosis. *Am J Dis Child* 133:889, 1979.
210. Marder KH, Tsang RC, Hug G, Crawford AC: Calcitriol deficiency in idiopathic juvenile osteoporosis. *Am J Dis Child* 136:914, 1982.
211. de Vernejoul MC, Marie P, Kuntz D, Gueris J, Miravet L, Ryckewaert A: Non-osteomalacic osteopathy associated with chronic hypophosphatemia. *Calcif Tissue Int* 34:219, 1982.
212. Bikle DD, Genant HK, Cann C, Recker RR, Halloran BP, Strewler GJ: Bone disease in alcohol abuse. *Ann Int Med* 103:42, 1985.
213. Meema S, Bunker ML, Meema HE: Preventive effect of estrogen on postmenopausal bone loss. *Arch Intern Med* 135:1436, 1975.
214. Recker RR, Saville PD, Heaney RP: Effects of estrogens and calcium carbonate on bone loss in postmenopausal women. *Ann Intern Med* 87:649, 1977.
215. Aitken JM, Hart DM, Lindsay R: Oestrogen replacement therapy for prevention of osteoporosis after oophorectomy. *Br Med J* 3:515, 1973.
216. Ettinger B, Genant HK, Cann CE: Long-term estrogen replacement therapy prevents bone loss and fractures. *Ann Int Med* 102:319, 1985.
217. Heaney RP, Recker RR, Saville PD: Menopausal changes in calcium balance performance. *J Lab Clin Med* 92:953, 1978.
218. Riggs BL, Jowsey J, Goldsmith RS, Kelly PJ, Hoffman DL, Arnaud CD: Short- and long-term effects of estrogen and synthetic anabolic hormone in postmenopausal osteoporosis. *J Clin Invest* 51:1659, 1972.
219. Gordan GS, Picchi J, Roof BS: Antifracture efficacy of long-term estrogens for osteoporosis. *Trans Assoc Am Physicians* 86:326, 1973.
220. Nordin BEC, Horsman A, Marshall DH, Simpson M, Waterhouse GM: Calcium requirement and calcium therapy. *Clin Orthop* 140:216, 1979.
221. Jensen GF, Christiansen C, Transbol I: Treatment of postmenopausal osteoporosis: A controlled therapeutic trial comparing oestrogen/gestagen, 1,25-dihydroxyvitamin D_3 and calcium. *Clin Endocrinol* 16:515, 1982.
222. Nilas I, Christiansen C, Rodbro P: Calcium supplementation and post-menopausal bone loss. *Br Med J* 289:1103, 1984.

223. Need AG, Horowitz M, Philcox JC, Nordin BEC: 1,25-dihydroxycholecalciferol and calcium therapy in osteoporosis with calcium malabsorption. *Mineral Electrolyte Metab* 11:35, 1985.
224. Riggs BL, Nelson KI: Effect of long term treatment with calcitriol on calcium absorption and mineral metabolism in postmenopausal osteoporosis. *J Clin Endocrinol Metab* 61:457, 1985.
225. Gruber HE, Ivey JL, Baylink DJ, Matthews M, Nelp WB, Sisom K, Chestnut CH III: Long-term calcitonin therapy in postmenopausal osteoporosis. *Metabolism* 33:295, 1984.
226. Aloia JF, Vaswani A, Kapoor A, Yeh JK, Cohn SH: Treatment of osteoporosis with calcitonin, with and without growth hormone. *Metabolism* 34:124, 1985.
227. Gennari C, Chierichetti SM, Bigazzi S, Fusi L, Gonelli S, Ferrara R, Zacchei F: Comparative effects on bone mineral content of calcium and calcium plus salmon calcitonin given in two different regimens in postmenopausal osteoporosis. *Curr Ther Res* 38:455, 1985.
228. Baylink DJ, Bernstein DS: The effects of fluoride therapy on metabolic bone disease: A histologic study. *Clin Orthop* 55:51, 1967.
229. Briancon D, Meunier PJ: Treatment of osteoporosis with fluoride, calcium and vitamin D. *Orthop Clin North Am* 12:629, 1981.
230. Riggs BL, Seeman E, Hodgson SF, Taves DR, O'Fallon WM: Effect of the fluoride/calcium regimen on vertebral fracture occurrence in postmenopausal osteoporosis. *N Engl J Med* 306:446, 1982.
231. van Kesteren RG, Duursma SA, Visser WJ, van der Sluysveer J, Dirks OB: Fluoride in serum and bone during treatment of osteoporosis with sodium fluoride, calcium and vitamin D. *Metab Bone Dis Rel Res* 4:31, 1982.
232. Charles P, Mosekilde L, Jensen FT: The effects of sodium fluoride, calcium phosphate, and vitamin D_2 for one to two years on calcium and phosphorus metabolism in postmenopausal women with spinal crush fracture osteoporosis. *Bone* 6:201, 1985.
233. Transbol I, Christensen MS, Jensen GF, Christiansen C, McNair P: Thiazide for the postponement of postmenopausal bone loss. *Metabolism* 31:383, 1982.
234. Chestnut CH III, Ivey JL, Gruber HE, Mathews M, Nelp WB, Sisom K, Baylink DJ: Stanozolol in postmenopausal osteoporosis: Therapeutic efficacy and possible mechanisms of action. *Metabolism* 32:571, 1983.
235. Slovik DM, Rosenthal DI, Doppelt SH, Potts JT Jr, Daly MA, Campbell JA, Neer RM: Restoration of spinal bone in osteoporotic men by treatment with human parathyroid hormone (1-34) and 1,25-dihydroxyvitamin D. *J Bone Mineral Res* 1:377, 1986.
236. Recker RR: Calcium absorption and achlorhydria. *N Engl J Med* 313:70, 1985.
237. Recker RR, Heaney RP: The effect of milk supplements on calcium metabolism, bone metabolism and calcium balance. *Am J Clin Nutr* 41:254, 1985.
238. Gluck OS, Murphy WA, Hahn TJ, Hahn B: Bone loss in adults receiving alternate day glucocorticoid therapy: A comparison with daily therapy. *Arthritis Rheum* 24:892, 1981.
239. Hahn TJ, Halstead LR, Teitelbaum SL, Hahn BH: Altered mineral metabolism in glucocorticoid-induced osteopenia: Effect of 25-hydroxyvitamin D administration. *J Clin Invest* 64:655, 1979.
240. LoCascio V, Bonucci E, Imbimbo B, Ballanti P, Tartarotti D, Galvanini G, Fuccella L, Adami S: Bone loss after glucocorticoid therapy. *Calcif Tissue Int* 36:435, 1984.
241. Braun JJ, Birkenhager-Frenkel DH, Rietveld AH, Juttmann JR, Visser TJ, Birkenhager JC: Influence of 1α-$(OH)D_3$ administration on bone and bone mineral metabolism in patients on chronic glucocorticoid treatment: A double blind controlled study. *Clin Endocrinol* 18:265, 1983.
242. Mosekilde L, Melsen F: Effect of antithyroid treatment on calcium-phosphorus metabolism in hyperthyroidism: II. Bone histomorphometry. *Acta Endocrinol* 87:751, 1978.
243. Rosen JF, Wolin DA, Finberg L: Immobilization hypercalcemia after single limb fractures in children and adolescents. *Am J Dis Child* 132:560, 1978.
244. Pedersen V, Charles P, Hansen HH, Elbrond D: Lack of effects of human calcitonin in osteogenesis imperfecta. *Acta Orthop Scand* 56:260, 1985.
245. Hoekman K, Papapoulos SE, Peters ACB, Bijvoet OLM: Characteristics and bisphosphonate treatment of a patient with juvenile osteoporosis. *J Clin Endocrinol Metab* 61:952, 1985.
246. Jaffe HL: *Metabolic, Degenerative, and Inflammatory Diseases of Bones and Joints.* Philadelphia, Lea & Febiger, 1972, p 178.
247. Whyte MP, Murphy WA, Fallon MD, Sly WS, Teitelbaum SL, McAlister WH, Avioli LV: Osteopetrosis, renal tubular acidosis and basal ganglia calcification in three sisters. *Am J Med* 69:64, 1980.
248. Sly WS, Whyte MP, Sundaram V, Tashian RE, Hewett-Emmett D, Geribaud P, Vainsel M, Baluarte HJ, Gruskin A, Al-Mosawi M, Sakati N, Ohlsson A: Carbonic anhydrase II deficiency in 12 families with the autosomal recessive syndrome of osteopetrosis with renal tubular acidosis and cerebral calcification. *N Engl J Med* 313:139, 1985.
249. Shapiro F, Glimcher MJ, Holtrop ME, Tashjian AH Jr, Brickley-Parsons D, Kenzora JE: Human osteopetrosis: A histological, ultrastructural and biochemical study. *J Bone Joint Surg [Am]* 62-A: 384, 1980.
250. Milgram JW, Jasty M: Osteopetrosis: A morphological study of twenty-one cases. *J Bone Joint Surg [Am]* 64-A:912, 1982.
251. Walker DG: Bone resorption restored in osteopetrotic mice by transplants of normal bone marrow and spleen cells. *Science* 190:784, 1975.
252. Coccia PF, Krivit W, Cervenka J, Clawson C, Kersey J, Kim TH, Nesbit ME, Ramsay NKC, Warkentin PI, Teitelbaum SL, Kahn AJ, Brown DM: Successful bone-marrow transplantation for infantile malignant osteopetrosis. *N Engl J Med* 302:701, 1980.
253. Marks SC Jr: Congenital osteopetrotic mutations as probes of the origin, structure, and function of osteoclasts. *Clin Orthop* 189:239, 1984.
254. Key L, Carnes D, Cole S, Holtrop M, Bar-Shavit Z, Shapiro F, Arceci R, Steinberg J, Gundberg C, Kahn A, Teitelbaum S, Anast C: Treatment of congenital osteopetrosis with high-dose calcitriol. *N Engl J Med* 310:409, 1984.
255. Avioli LV: Renal osteodystrophy, in Avioli LV, Krane SM (eds): *Metabolic Bone Disease.* New York, Academic, 1978, vol II, p 149.
256. Coburn JW, Kurokawa K, Llach F: Altered divalent ion metabolism in renal disease and renal osteodystrophy, in Maxwell MH, Kleeman CR (eds): *Clinical Disorders of Fluid and Electrolyte Metabolism.* New York, McGraw-Hill, 1980, p 1153.
257. Freitag J, Martin KJ, Hruska KA, Anderson C, Conrades M, Ladenson J, Klahr S, Slatopolsky E: Impaired parathyroid hormone metabolism in patients with chronic renal failure. *N Engl J Med* 298:29, 1978.
258. Hodsman AB, Sherrard DJ, Wong EGC, Brickman AS, Lee DBN, Alfrey AC, Singer FR, Norman AW, Coburn JW: Vitamin D–resistant osteomalacia in hemodialysis patients lacking secondary hyperparathyroidism. *Ann Int Med* 94:629, 1981.
259. Eastwood JB, Harris E, Stamp TCB, DeWardener HE: Vitamin D deficiency in the osteomalacia of chronic renal failure. *Lancet* 2:1209, 1976.
260. Sherrard DJ, Baylink DJ, Wergedahl JE, Maloney N: Quantitative histological studies on the pathogenesis of uremic bone disease. *J Clin Endocrinol Metab* 39:119, 1974.
261. Bressot C, Courpron P, Edouard C, Meunier P: *Histomorphométrie des ostéopathies endocriniennes.* Lyon, Association Corpotative des Etudiants en Médecine de Lyon, 1976, p 85.
262. Mason RS, Lissner D, Wilkinson M, Posen S: Vitamin D metabolites and their relationship to azotaemic osteodystrophy. *Clin Endocrinol* 13:375, 1980.
263. Portale AA, Booth BE, Tsai HC, Morris RC Jr: Reduced plasma concentration of 1,25-dihydroxyvitamin D in children with moderate renal insufficiency. *Kidney Int* 21:627, 1982.
264. Hodsman AB, Sherrard DJ, Alfrey AC, Ott S, Brickman AS,

Miller NL, Maloney NA, Coburn JW: Bone aluminum and histomorphometric features of renal osteodystrophy. *J Clin Endocrinol Metab* 54:539, 1982.
265. Teitelbaum SL, Bergfeld MA, Freitag J, Hruska KA, Slatopolsky E: Do parathyroid hormone and 1,25-dihydroxyvitamin D modulate bone formation in uremia? *J Clin Endocrinol Metab* 51:247, 1980.
266. Weinstein RS: Decreased mineralization in hemodialysis patients after subtotal parathyroidectomy. *Calcif Tissue Int* 34:16, 1982.
267. Sherrard DJ, Ott SM, Andress DL: Pseudohyperparathyroidism: Syndrome associated with aluminum intoxication in patients with renal failure. *Am J Med* 79:127, 1985.
268. Slatopolsky E, Caglar S, Gradowska L, Canterbury JM, Reiss E, Bricker NS: On the prevention of secondary hyperparathyroidism in experimental chronic renal disease using "proportional reduction" of dietary phosphorus intake. *Kidney Int* 2:147, 1972.
269. Portale AA, Booth BE, Halloran BP, Morris RC Jr: Effect of dietary phosphorus on circulating concentrations of 1,25-dihydroxyvitamin D and immunoreactive parathyroid hormone in children with moderate renal insufficiency. *J Clin Invest* 73:1580, 1984.
270. Massry SG, Tuma S, Dua S, Goldstein DA: Reversal of skeletal resistance to parathyroid hormone in uremia by vitamin D metabolites: Evidence for the requirement of $1,25(OH)_2D_3$ and $24,25(OH)_2D_3$. *J Lab Clin Med* 94:152, 1979.
271. Mak RHK, Turner C, Thompson T, Powell H, Haycock GB, Chantler C: Suppression of secondary hyperparathyroidism in children with chronic renal failure by high dose phosphate binders: Calcium carbonate versus aluminum hydroxide. *Br Med J* 291:623, 1985.
272. Wilson L, Felsenfeld A, Drezner MK, Llach F: Altered divalent ion metabolism in early renal failure: Role of $1,25(OH)_2D$. *Kidney Int* 27:565, 1985.
273. Brickman AS, Sherrard DJ, Jowsey J, Singer FR, Baylink DJ, Maloney N, Massry SG, Norman AW, Coburn JW: 1,25-Dihydroxycholecalciferol: Effect on skeletal lesions and plasma parathyroid hormone levels in uremic osteodystrophy. *Arch Intern Med* 134:883, 1974.
274. Massry SG: Requirements of vitamin D metabolites in patients with renal disease. *Am J Clin Nutr* 33:1530, 1980.
275. Bordier P, Zingraff J, Gueris J, Jungers P, Marie P, Pechet M, Rasmussen H: The effect of $1\alpha(OH)D_3$ and $1\alpha,25(OH)_2D_3$ on the bone in patients with renal osteodystrophy. *Am J Med* 64:101, 1978.
276. Eastwood JB, Stamp TCB, DeWardener HE, Bordier PJ, Arnaud CD: The effect of 25-hydroxyvitamin D_3 in the osteomalacia of chronic renal failure. *Clin Sci Mol Med* 52:499, 1977.
277. Wells SA Jr, Ross AJ III, Dale JK, Gray RS: Transplantation of the parathyroid glands: Current status. *Surg Clin North Am* 59:167, 1979.
278. Malluche HH, Smith AJ, Abreo K, Faugere M-C: The use of deferoxamine in the management of aluminum accumulation in bone in patients with renal failure. *N Engl J Med* 311:140, 1984.
279. Thompson RC Jr, Gaull GE, Horwitz SJ, Schenk RK: Hereditary hyperphosphatasia: Studies of three siblings. *Am J Med* 47:209, 1969.
280. Whalen JP, Horwith M, Krook L, MacIntyre I, Mena A, Viteri F, Town B, Nunez EA: Calcitonin treatment in hereditary bone dysplasia with hyperphosphatasemia: A radiographic and histologic study of bone. *Am J Roentgenol* 129:29, 1977.
281. Nunez EA, Horwith M, Krook L, Whalen JP: An electron microscopic investigation of human familial bone dysplasia: Inhibition of osteocytic osteolysis and induction of osteocytic formation of elastic fibers following calcitonin treatment. *Am J Pathol* 94:1, 1979.
282. Doyle FH, Woodhouse NJY, Glen CA, Joplin GF, MacIntyre I: Healing of the bones in juvenile Paget's disease treated by human calcitonin. *Br J Radiol* 47:9, 1974.
283. Blanco O, Stivel M, Mautalen C, Schajowicz F: Familial idiopathic hyperphosphatasia. A study of two siblings treated with porcine calcitonin. *J Bone Joint Surg [Br]* 59B:421, 1977.
284. Dunn V, Condon VR, Rallison ML: Familial hyperphosphatasemia: diagnosis in early infancy and response to human thyrocalcitonin therapy. *Am J Roentgenol* 132:541, 1979.
285. Albright F, Butler AM, Hampton AO, Smith P: Syndrome characterized by osteitis fibrosa disseminata, areas of pigmentation and endocrine dysfunction, with precocious puberty in females: Report of five cases. *N Engl J Med* 216:727, 1937.
286. Albright F: Polyostotic fibrous dysplasia: A defense of the entity. *J Clin Endocrinol* 7:307, 1947.
287. von Recklinghausen F: Die Fibrose oder deformirende Ostitis, die Osteomalacie und die osteoplastische Carcinose in ihren gegenseitigen Beziehungen, in *Festschrift für Rudolf Virchow.* Berlin, G Reimer, 1891.
288. Harris WH, Dudley HR Jr, Barry RJ: The natural history of fibrous dysplasia: An orthopaedic, pathological and roentgenographic study. *J Bone Joint Surg [Am]* 44A:207, 1962.
289. Schwartz DT, Alpert M: The malignant transformation of fibrous dysplasia. *Am J Med Sci* 247:35, 1964.
290. Benedict PH: Endocrine features in Albright's syndrome (fibrous dysplasia of bone). *Metabolism* 11:30, 1962.
291. McArthur RG, Hayles AB, Lambert PW: Albright's syndrome with rickets. *Mayo Clin Proc* 54:313, 1979.
292. Shires R, Whyte MP, Avioli LV: Idiopathic hypothalamic hypogonadotropic hypogonadism with polyostotic fibrous dysplasia. *Arch Inter Med* 139:1187, 1979.
293. Bell NH, Avery S, Johnston CC: Effects of calcitonin in Paget's disease and polyostotic fibrous dysplasia. *J Clin Endocrinol Metab* 31:283, 1970.
294. Comite F, Shawker TH, Pescovitz OH, Loriaux DLL, Cutler GB Jr: Cyclical ovarian function resistant to treatment with an analogue of luteinizing hormone releasing hormone in McCune-Albright syndrome. *N Engl J Med* 311:1032, 1984.
295. Paget J: On a form of chronic inflammation of bones (osteitis deformans). *Med Chir Trans* 60:27, 1877.
296. Barry HC: *Paget's Disease of Bone.* Baltimore, Williams & Wilkins, 1969.
297. Franck WA, Bress NM, Singer FR, Krane SM: Rheumatic manifestations of Paget's disease of bone. *Am J Med* 56:592, 1974.
298. Heistad DD, Abboud FM, Schmid PG, Mark AL, Wilson WR: Regulation of blood flow in Paget's disease of bone. *J Clin Invest* 55:69, 1975.
299. Arnalich F, Plaza I, Sobrino JA, Oliver J, Barbado J, Pena JM, Vazquez JJ: Cardiac size and function in Paget's disease of bone. *Int J Cardiol* 5:491, 1984.
300. Waxman AD, Ducker S, McKee D, Siemsen JK, Singer FR: Evaluation of ^{99m}Tc diphosphonate kinetics and bone scans in patients with Paget's disease before and after calcitonin treatment. *Radiology* 125:761, 1977.
301. Khairi MRA, Wellman HN, Robb JA, Johnston CC Jr: Paget's disease of bone (osteitis deformans): Symptomatic lesions and bone scan. *Ann Intern Med* 79:348, 1973.
302. Waxman AD, McKee D, Siemsen JK, Singer FR: Gallium scanning in Paget's disease of bone: The effects of calcitonin. *Am J Roentgenol* 134:303, 1980.
303. Nagant de Deuxchaisnes C, Krane SM: Paget's disease of bone: Clinical and metabolic observations. *Medicine* 43:233, 1964.
304. Posen S, Clifton-Bligh P, Wilkinson M: Paget's disease of bone and hyperparathyroidism: Coincidence or causal relationship? *Calcif Tissue Res* 26:107, 1978.
305. Singer FR: *Paget's Disease of Bone.* New York, Plenum, 1977.
306. Rebel A, Malkani K, Baslé M, Bregeon C: Osteoclast ultrastructure in Paget's disease. *Calcif Tissue Res* 20:187, 1976.
307. Mills BG, Singer FR: Nuclear inclusions in Paget's disease of bone. *Science* 194:201, 1976.

308. Singer FR: Paget's disease of bone: A slow virus infection? *Calcif Tissue Int* 31:185, 1980.
309. Rebel A, Baslé M, Pouplard A, Kouyoumdjian S, Filmon R, Lepatezour A: Viral antigens in osteoclasts from Paget's disease of bone. *Lancet* 2:344, 1980.
310. Mills BG, Singer FR, Weiner LP, Suffin SC, Stabile E, Holst P: Evidence for both respiratory syncytial virus and measles virus antigens in the osteoclasts of patients with Paget's disease of bone. *Clin Orthop* 183:303, 1984.
310a. Baslé MF, Fournier JG, Rozenblatt S, Rebel A, Bouteille M: Measles virus RNA detected in Paget's disease bone tissue by in situ hybridization. *J Gen Virol* 67:907, 1986.
311. Mills BG, Singer FR, Weiner LP, Holst PA: Long term culture of cells from bone affected by Paget's disease. *Calcif Tissue Int* 29:79, 1979.
312. Singer FR, Melvin KEW, Mills BG: Acute effects of calcitonin on osteoclasts in man. *Clin Endocrinol* 5:333s, 1976.
313. Singer FR, Fredericks RS, Minkin C: Salmon calcitonin therapy for Paget's disease of bone: The problem of acquired clinical resistance. *Arthritis Rheum* 23:1148, 1980.
314. Avramides A, Flores A, DeRose J, Wallach S: Paget's disease of bone: Observations after cessation of long-term synthetic salmon calcitonin treatment. *J Clin Endocrinol Metab* 42:459, 1976.
315. Nagant de Deuxchaisnes C, Rombouts-Lindemans C, Huaux JP, Devogelaer JP, Malghem J, Maldague B: The action of the main therapeutic regimes of Paget's disease of bone, with a note on the effect of vitamin D deficiency. *Arthritis Rheum* 23:1215, 1980.
316. Fleisch H: Bisphosphonates: Mechanisms of action and clinical applications, in Peck WA (ed): *Bone and Mineral Research Annual 1.* Amsterdam, Elsevier, 1983, p 319.
317. Khairi MRA, Altman RD, DeRosa GP, Zimmerman J, Schenk RK, Johnston CC: Sodium etidronate in the treatment of Paget's disease of bone: A study of long-term results. *Ann Intern Med* 87:656, 1977.
318. Canfield R, Rosner W, Skinner J, McWhorter J, Resnick L, Feldman F, Kammerman S, Ryan K, Kunigonis M, Bohne W: Diphosphonate therapy of Paget's disease of bone. *J Clin Endocrinol Metab* 44:96, 1977.
319. Delmas PD, Chapuy MC, Vignon E, Charhon S, Briancon D, Alexandre C, Edouard C, Meunier PJ: Long-term effects of dichloromethylene diphosphonate in Paget's disease of bone. *J Clin Endocrinol Metab* 54:837, 1982.
320. Vellenga CJLR, Mulder JD, Bijvoet OLM: Radiological demonstration of healing in Paget's disease of bone treated with APD. *Br J Radiol* 58:831, 1985.
321. Ryan WG, Schwartz TB, Northrop G: Experiences in the treatment of Paget's disease of bone with mithramycin. *J Am Med Assoc* 213:1153, 1970.
322. Lebbin D, Ryan WG, Schwartz TB: Outpatient treatment of Paget's disease of bone with mithramycin. *Ann Intern Med* 81:635, 1974.
323. Evans RA, Dunstan CR, Wong SYP, Hills E: Long-term experience with a calcium-thiazide treatment for Paget's disease of bone. *Mineral Electrolyte Metab* 8:325, 1982.
324. Meyers M, Singer FR: Osteotomy for tibia vara in Paget's disease under cover of calcitonin. *J Bone Joint Surg [Am]* 60A:810, 1978.
325. Chambers TJ, Dunn CJ: The effect of parathyroid hormone, 1,25-dihydroxycholecalciferol and prostaglandins on the cytoplasmic activity of isolated osteoclasts. *J Pathol* 137:193, 1982.
326. Rodan GA, Rodan SB: Expression of the osteoblastic phenotype, in Peck WA (ed): *Bone and Mineral Research Annual 2.* Amsterdam, Elsevier, 1984, p 244.
327. Horton JE, Raisz LG, Simmons HA, Oppenheim JJ, Mergenhagen SE: Bone resorbing activity in supernatant fluid from cultured human peripheral leucocytes. *Science* 177:793, 1972.
328. Mundy GR, Luben RA, Raisz LG, Oppenheim JJ, Buell DN: Bone-resorbing activity in supernatants from lymphoid cell lines. *N Engl J Med* 290:867, 1974.
329. Gowen M, Wood DD, Ihrie EJ, McGuire MKB, Russell RGG: An interleukin 1 like factor stimulates bone resorption in vitro. *Nature* 306:378, 1983.
330. Urist MR, DeLange RJ, Finerman GAM: Bone cell differentiation and growth factors. *Science* 220:680, 1983.
331. Farley JR, Baylink DJ: Purification of a skeletal growth factor from human bone. *Biochemistry* 21:3502, 1982.
332. Canalis E: The hormonal and local regulation of bone formation. *Endocr Rev* 4:62, 1983.
333. Whitson SW, Harrison W, Dunlap MK, Bowers DE Jr, Fisher LW, Robey PG, Termine JD: Fetal bovine bone cells synthesize bone-specific matrix proteins. *J Cell Biol* 99:607, 1984.

25

Nephrolithiasis

Karl L. Insogna
Arthur E. Broadus

Nephrolithiasis is not usually given separate status in textbooks on endocrinology and metabolism. This lapse is not based on tradition, for eminent endocrinologists were among the first investigators to study conditions associated with renal stone formation. Indeed, the subject is not exclusively within the domain of any medical subspecialty, a fact often cited to account for the rather slow and faltering growth of knowledge in the area. An unfortunate consequence of this slow growth and dissemination of knowledge is that the present level of care of many patients with recurrent stone disease is poor by modern standards.

Recent developments have altered the rather dismal clinical and investigative outlook in patients with nephrolithiasis. Ten years ago, the term "idiopathic" was used in connection with the majority of patients with recurrent stone disease; today, this term is appropriately used to describe no more than 10 to 20 percent of such patients. New information has increasingly identified metabolic bases for stone formation, so that the care of patients with stone disease by physicians who are accustomed to relying on the laboratory for diagnosis and whose thinking on metabolism is sound is increasingly appropriate.

This chapter is not written as an endocrinologist's view of renal stone disease. Rather, it is intended to be a complete and free-standing treatment of the subject, which should allow physicians of any persuasion to deliver high-quality care to patients with stones. These patients will be found to represent an extremely gratifying clinical and intellectual component of the physician's practice.

The *risk factor* concept is a central and recurring theme of this chapter. The concept is useful in considering the basis of stone formation in patients with all types of stone disease and is particularly useful in constructing a sound clinical approach to patients with calcium stone disease. The implied analogy to coronary artery disease is fully intended; in both coronary disease and stone disease statistical risk factors, rather than a single cause-and-effect relationship, are recognized. Further, as in patients with coronary disease, multiple risk factors are found in many patients with recurrent stone disease.

GENERAL CONSIDERATIONS

Some 12 percent of males and 5 percent of females in the American population experience a renal stone event at some time in life.[1] The incidence in males is approximately 125 per 100,000 per year, and appears to be increasing.[1] Stones account for 1 in each 1000 hospital admissions in the United States, or approximately 200,000 admissions yearly. Impressive as these figures are, they clearly underestimate the morbidity and economic impact of stone disease, for the majority of stone events do not require hospitalization.[1] In the southeastern United States, which is referred to as a "stone belt" because of the unusual frequency of stone disease, renal stones account for almost 15 percent of new office visits to urologists.

The term *nephrolithiasis* is used with specific reference to kidney stones or stones which form in the pelvis or calyces of the upper urinary tract. Such stones represent 90 to 95 percent of the urinary tract stones encountered in industrialized countries; they are responsible for the ureteral colic which gives stone disease its well-deserved infamy. Upper tract stones may grow or coalesce to mold the collecting system of the kidney; such stones are aptly termed *staghorn calculi.* Staghorn stones are usually a result of infection. They are commonly composed of *struvite* (magnesium ammonium phosphate, MAP), but are occasionally composed of uric acid or cystine. Under conditions of extreme supersaturation, uric acid, cystine, or calcium phosphate crystals may form copious amorphous, semisolid precipitates which produce bilateral intrarenal or extrarenal obstruction; these may cause acute renal failure. The most classic example of this process is the rapid cell lysis and massive uricosuria which may attend the initiation of chemotherapy in patients with leukemia or a lymphoma. Such an episode may or may not be associated with colicky pain, depending upon the principal site of obstruction.

Nephrocalcinosis refers to calcification within the renal parenchyma and is an uncommon radiological finding in a patient with nephrolithiasis. Nephrocalcinosis is usually bilateral and, in the vast majority of instances, involves the medullary or corticomedullary areas of the kidneys. Cortical nephrocalcinosis (e.g., in acute cortical necrosis or chronic glomerulonephritis) is rare. Medullary nephrocalcinosis is often an example of dystrophic soft tissue calcification related to local tissue injury; examples are renal tuberculosis, infarction, mercury poisoning, and tumor. Rarely, a calcified papilla may dislodge and masquerade as a renal stone by producing classic colic in a patient with renal papillary necrosis. Nephrocalcinosis and nephrolithiasis coexist in only a handful of conditions, including medullary sponge kidney (MSK), renal tubular acidosis (RTA), the primary hyperoxalurias, and a small minority of patients with primary hyperparathyroidism and other hypercalcemic conditions. The radiological demonstration of nephrocalcinosis in a patient with clinical stone disease is highly suggestive of one of these conditions.

Bladder stones account for 5 percent or less of urinary tract stones in the United States. They occur principally in elderly men with prostatic obstruction. Approximately 60 percent of bladder stones are calcium oxalate or mixed calcium stones, 40 percent are struvite stones, and less than 10 percent are uric acid. Only a small minority of these men have a history of nephrolithiasis. Bladder stone disease is endemic in children in southern Asia, southern Europe, and the Middle East. These stones are composed predominantly of ammonium acid urate admixed with various proportions of calcium oxalate, a stone composition which is virtually never encountered in industrialized nations. Although the pathogenesis of endemic bladder stones is unknown, diet appears to play a major role; these are sometimes referred to as "malnutrition" stones.[2] These same stones were common in young boys in the western world a century ago, but disappeared with industrialization.[2,3]

The reason(s) for the disproportionate frequency of upper urinary tract stones in the west is unknown. Intuitively, crystalline precipitates would be assumed to tend to occur in areas of stasis, such as the bladder, rather than in the papillary regions of the kidney where urinary flow rates are high; yet, this is not the case. It is clear that the urinary concentration of stone-forming constituents peaks in the distal nephron, but this peak concentration is maintained in the lower urinary tract as well. In the 1930s, Randall proposed that stone growth was initiated on calcified microscopic subendothelial plaques of the renal papillae.[4] Although stones are often asymmetric and occasionally bear a distinct papillary imprint on their surfaces, modern studies have not supported the "Randall's plaque" hypothesis, in that such plaques appear to be relatively uncommon and are found no more frequently in stone-bearing than in normal kidneys.[2] The predominant calyceal location of urinary tract stones therefore remains one of the major enigmas of stone disease. As is stressed below, there is no predictable temporal relationship between the actual formation of a stone in the upper tract and its subsequent dislodgement into the collecting system with attendant symptoms.

The principal clinical consequences of renal stones are obstruction, pain, hematuria, and predisposition to infection. Impairment of renal function is not a natural or predictable consequence of stone disease; it results from stone-related complications, such as chronic obstruction, infection, surgical scarring, or the necessity for partial or complete nephrectomy.

Ureteral colic is pain of incredible intensity. Women who have experienced both labor and colic almost invariably describe the latter in more awesome terms. Patients with recurrent stone disease are unusually compliant and diligent with regard to physician instructions concerning testing procedures and treatment programs, a fact probably attributable to their memories of previous suffering. The term "colic" is actually somewhat of a misnomer, for the pain typically begins as a vague discomfort and builds up over an hour or so to reach a constant maximum intensity, rendering the patient incapable of lying or sitting still. Obstruction in the region of the ureteropelvic junction produces pain in the flank and is often associated with nausea and vomiting. Obstruction lower in the ureter causes pain that radiates from the flank in a downward, anteromedial fashion toward the pelvis. A stone near the ureterovesicle junction produces pain that radiates into the ipsilateral testicle or labium; stones in this region or that have passed into the bladder often also cause urgency and dysuria which perfectly mimics cystitis. All these symptoms resolve promptly with the passage of stone material, but a minority of patients experience a vague, milder discomfort reminiscent of obstructive symptoms for days to weeks after an acute stone event. The basis of these prolonged symptoms is unknown, but they may be related to spasm and/or scarring. Stones too large to negotiate the ureteropelvic junction may produce intermittent upper ureteral obstruction in a ball-valve fashion, ultimately necessitating pyelolithotomy. Staghorn stones, stones which remain adherent to the renal papillae, and nephrocalcinosis usually produce no chronic symptoms, although microscopic hematuria and/or pyuria and episodes of gross hematuria are relatively common. A small minority of such patients, however, experience chronic, nagging flank discomfort which may be so invidious as to threaten seriously their capacity to function, and some patients become drug-dependent. The basis for these persistent symptoms is unknown; serial pyelograms do not usually reveal evidence of obstruction.

The term *gravel* is used to describe the gritty, sandlike material passed by many stone-forming patients. Gravel passage is usually accompanied by symptoms of local bladder or urethral irritation but not colic.

The assessment of stone-related morbidity is an important consideration in defining the natural history of stone disease, in considering individual patients or patient groups as candidates for medical treatment, and in evaluating the efficacy of therapeutic programs. This seemingly simple assessment is, in fact, quite complex. For example, a staghorn calculus is counted as but a single stone, yet its natural history is growth and local invasion, in a fashion reminiscent of tumor invasion, and damage of renal function. One individual may experience hundreds of stone events without ever requiring instrumentation or surgery, whereas another patient may lose a kidney to complications resulting from a single stone. Patients often experience a cluster of rapid-fire clinical stone events related to single or multiple passed stones or gravel; other patients may have one to many years of apparent quiescence between clinical stone events. Many investigators tend to regard a cluster of stone occurrences as a single event in enumerating stones and/or stone complications in individual patients. If the mechanism of such clusters is obstruction-induced reverse pressure which dislodges other stones adherent to the papillary surface, a circumstance which can sometimes be documented radiographically, then it is clearly more accurate to regard the cluster as consisting of more than a single stone.

A number of terms and concepts have been introduced in the attempt to clarify and standardize the assessment of the morbidity of stone disease. The Mayo Clinic group employs the term *metabolic activity* to define clinical and/or radiographic evidence of new stone formation or stone growth; a patient lacking such evidence over a 12-month period is considered to have stone disease which is metabolically inactive.[5] Similarly, the term *surgical activity* is employed to describe the necessity for surgical intervention as a function of time. Coe[3,6] has described five interrelated characteristics of stone disease which, in the aggregate, define stone morbidity: (1) the stone "burden" or the number of stones present radiographically, (2) the rate of formation of new stones, (3) the rate of growth of existing stones, (4) the number and extent of morbid episodes (infections, surgical procedures, and hospitalizations), and (5) the extent of renal or urinary tract damage caused by stones. An example may clarify the necessity for considering these interrelated characteristics separately: a patient with primary hyperparathyroidism may be cured surgically yet be left with four stones in each kidney after parathyroidectomy. This stone burden does not reflect an ongoing tendency for new stone formation but can certainly serve as the basis for future morbid episodes. Regardless of semantics, the importance of careful attention to historical details and examination of serial radiographs in evaluating individual patients is clear. Patients with recurrent stones intuitively understand the need for such attention to detail; less scrupulous evaluation and follow-up seriously erodes patients' confidence.

Renal stones are not simply amorphous precipitates but have an organized, complex architecture.[7] Crystalline substances constitute approximately 90 percent of the mass of a typical stone, and water and protein each account for about 5 percent. The protein is a major constituent of the stone matrix; it is thought by some to be involved in the pathogenesis of stone formation.

Stones are classified into five major types by crystallographic analysis. The term *mixed* is employed when the second-largest crystalline component contributes more than 15 percent of stone mass. Table 25-1 shows the relative frequency of the five stone types in series of analyses published in the last three decades; the table also contains the recent experience of a large ambulatory renal stone clinic.[3] The marked difference in the reported frequency of struvite stones probably reflects a true decline in the incidence of these stones as well as a bias, in that infection stones would constitute a larger percentage of surgical specimens than those derived from a diagnostic clinic. Similarly, the patients most likely to form uric acid stones may not be frequently referred to a diagnostic clinic. Nevertheless, it is clear that calcium oxalate or mixed calcium stones constitute the vast majority of the stones presently encountered and that the other principal stone types are individually uncommon. Patients

Table 25-1. Frequency of Five Types of Renal Stones: Percentages among Patients in Two Different Series

Number of stone patients	Calcium oxalate or mixed	Calcium phosphate	Uric acid	Struvite (MAP)	Cystine
1870*	63.2	7.4	5.4	21.5	2.5
519†	88.6	2.1	1.5	3.0	0.6

*Data derived from four large series of stone analyses published between 1949 and 1967.
†Data derived from the recent experience of a referral renal stone clinic. This series also reported that 4.2 percent of stones were composed of a mixture of calcium salts and uric acid, a finding not noted in previous series.[3]
Source: Modified from Coe.[3]

with calcium stone disease or struvite stones typically present during midlife, whereas patients with uric acid stones tend to be somewhat older and those with cystine stones somewhat younger (Fig. 25-1).

The classification of stones by crystallographic type serves three major purposes: (1) it provides a convenient and logical means for considering stone pathogenesis, particularly as regards the physical chemical aspects of stone formation, (2) it may be diagnostically important in individual patients, and (3) it defines general and/or specific approaches to medical therapy. In fact, the stone analysis is diagnostically useful only when it reveals one of the less common stone types, in which case the analysis either makes the diagnosis (struvite and cystine stones) or limits diagnostic considerations to a handful of associated conditions (calcium phosphate and uric acid stones).

THEORIES AND PHYSICAL CHEMICAL ASPECTS OF RENAL STONE PATHOGENESIS

The pathogenesis of stone disease can be considered at a number of levels. To many, the question appears to be simple enough: the urinary tract is responsible for the elimination of waste products in a predominantly aqueous solution; some of these products are only sparingly soluble and therefore prone to precipitate and form stones. The more waste products, the more stones. To others, the answer lies in solving a series of lengthy equations by computer, in an attempt to understand the complex interplay between ionic species in aqueous solution and stone salts in a solid phase. A sound clinical approach to stone disease comprises elements of both these views, the one pragmatic and the other entirely chemical. The section below describes the concepts, terminology, and methodology of various approaches to stone patho-

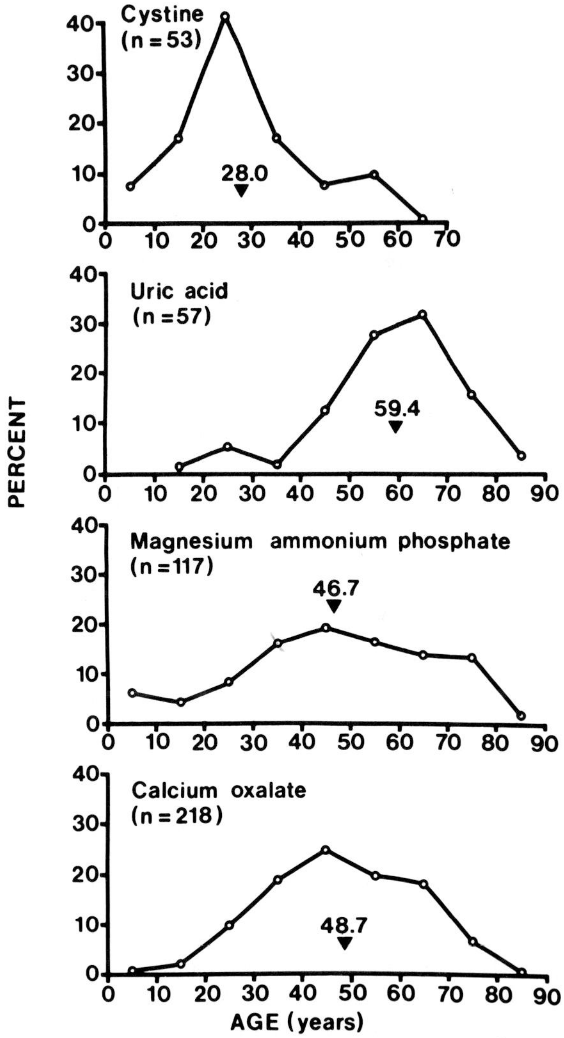

FIGURE 25-1 Age distribution of four major types of renal stones. The mean age signified by the arrow specifies the age at which the patients first sought medical care for stone symptoms, which is assumed to correspond largely to the onset of stone disease. (*From Hodgkinson A, Nordin BEC, in Coggins CH, Cummings NB (eds): Prevention of Kidney and Urinary Tract Diseases. Washington, U.S. Government Printing Office, 1978, by permission.*)

genesis only in sufficient detail to provide the basis for an informed clinical approach to stone disease. More scholarly and detailed reviews of these subjects are available in a number of excellent recent references.[3,6,8]

Theories of Stone Pathogenesis

There are three classic theories of stone pathogenesis: the *matrix theory*, the *inhibitor theory*, and the *crystalloid theory*. Each has undergone a series of modifications since initially proposed; each has its present-day proponents, but none is entirely exclusive of the others. Indeed, much recent evidence is interpreted as indicating that stone pathogenesis should be viewed in the context of a balance of forces, those which tend to cause the precipitation of stone salts and those which inhibit this process.[3]

The matrix theory holds that the high-molecular-weight compounds which constitute the organic matrix present in all stones are causally related to stone formation. The process is considered analogous to the mineralization of the organized organic matrix (osteoid) of bone (Chap. 23). Matrix proteins (mostly mucoproteins) in urine and stone material have been studied most extensively by Boyce.[9] Critics of the theory point out that the matrix substance is similar or identical in stones of all crystalline types as well as in concretions which are artificially precipitated from urine, suggesting that the material is being trapped as an "innocent bystander" rather than causing stone formation.[2] In essence, the central tenets of the matrix theory remain largely unproven, but the theory survives. An unintended extension of the theory which is well-recognized is that stone-related or surgical scarring in the urinary tract may serve as a focus for mineralization and thereby promote stone formation.

The inhibitor theory holds that stone formation results from a deficiency in urine of substances which normally inhibit crystallization and crystal growth and/or aggregation. This theory became attractive over two decades ago when Thomas and Howard reported that urine from stone-forming patients readily calcified rachitic rat cartilage, whereas urine from normal individuals did not.[10] The authors introduced the terms "good" and "evil" urine; they attributed their findings to a relative absence of inhibitor substances in "evil" urine, preliminarily identified as low-molecular-weight peptides. The alternative view, that "evil" urine might be more supersaturated with respect to mineralizing substances, was not critically tested. Other natural inhibitors of crystallization or crystal growth, including pyrophosphate, citrate, magnesium, and other poorly defined substances, have been identified and implicated by various investigators in stone pathogenesis.[2,3,5,8] Such substances are viewed by some as perhaps more important in preventing crystals from growing and aggregating into a significant stone mass than in preventing crystallization per se. The essential issue, however, does not concern the acknowledged presence of multiple inhibitor substances in human urine, but rather whether a relative deficiency of one or more of these substances contributes to stone pathogenesis in affected individuals. At present, this issue is unsettled, and the central theme of the inhibitor theory must be considered unproven. Several clinical examples of stone formation which appear to reflect alterations in inhibitor substances in urine, as well as more recent physical chemical data concerning an unexplained propensity for stone formation in the urine of certain patients, are described below.

The crystalloid (or precipitation-crystallization) theory considers stone formation in strictly physical chemical terms. The central theme of the theory relates crystallization and growth of concretions in urine to supersaturation with respect to stone-forming constituents. Of the three classic theories of stone pathogenesis, the crystalloid theory has the most experimental support; it also provides a conceptual framework on which a sound clinical approach to stone disease can be based. All four of the "minor" stone types (see below) can be readily understood on the basis of relatively straightforward physical chemical principles; the formation of cystine stones in cystinuria is the simplest single example of stone pathogenesis as a function of supersaturation chemistry.

Physical Chemical Aspects of Stone Formation

Figure 25-2 illustrates the relative zones of saturation and the ranges of saturation of the five major stone-forming constituents in normal urine. There are three zones of saturation: *undersaturated*, *metastably supersaturated*, and *oversaturated* (the labile region). These zones are segregated by two limits, the *solubility product* and the *formation product*. The physical chemical meaning of these various terms is best understood by means of several illustrations. If an excess of solid material such as calcium oxalate is added to distilled water and allowed to dissolve for a prolonged period, the solution and remaining solid phase eventually reach a stable equilibrium. This equilibrium defines the solubility of the material in aqueous solution, which at this point is saturated; the solubility product is the product of the concentration of the calcium

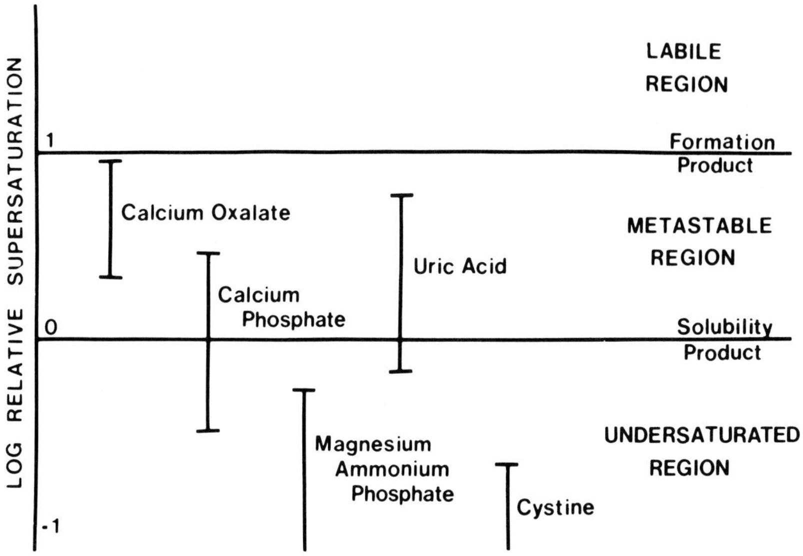

FIGURE 25-2 The three zones of saturation in urine: undersaturation, metastable supersaturation, and oversaturation (labile region). The ranges of saturation of the five major crystalline stone constituents in normal urine are shown. (*From Hodgkinson A, Nordin BEC, in Coggins CH, Cummings NB (eds): Prevention of Kidney and Urinary Tract Diseases. Washington, U.S. Government Printing Office, 1978, by permission.*)

and oxalate ions in solution.* The solid material is now removed, leaving a saturated solution of calcium oxalate without a solid phase. If a concentrated solution of calcium, oxalate, or both is added to the saturated solution, the solution remains clear and free of a solid phase to a critical point, the formation product. At that point, the solution clouds as solid calcium oxalate crystals form and begin to grow. The region between the solubility product and the formation product defines a solution which is supersaturated with the ionic species in question but does not spontaneously precipitate (the metastable region in Fig. 25-2). At and above the formation product, spontaneous precipitation inevitably occurs (the labile or oversaturated region in Fig. 25-2). An undersaturated solution does not lead to crystallization or support crystal growth. A supersaturated solution leads to crystallization under some circumstances (see below) and supports crystal growth. An oversaturated solution produces both spontaneous precipitation and crystal growth.

The term *nucleation* rather than precipitation is used to define the initiation of a crystalline solid phase in aqueous solution. The illustration given above is an example of *homogeneous nucleation* of simple ion pairs in an oversaturated solution. In complex solutions, the stability of the solution with respect to formation of a solid phase may be influenced by the interaction between different types of crystal nuclei or between such nuclei and other particulate material. For example, in the illustration above, if the glass container had been scratched or "seed" particulate matter had been added in the middle of the metastable region, the nucleation and growth of calcium oxalate crystals would have been induced. This is an example of *heterogeneous nucleation.* Heterogeneous nucleation is again a physical phenomenon; it requires only that there be structural similarities between the lattice pattern of the crystal and the "foreign" substance in question. The term *epitaxy* is often used to describe this phenomenon. The term can be taken to mean a cross-species physical marriage of crystals formed on the basis of facets of similar crystalline lattice structure. In essence, although a metastably supersaturated solution will not initiate homogeneous nucleation, it can support both heterogeneous nucleation and homogeneous or epitaxial crystal growth.

Although related, crystal nucleation and crystal growth are considered as separate phenomena. Crystal nuclei of the sort considered above comprise only approximately 100 atoms and could occur without clinical sequelae during transient periods of oversaturation. It is the enlargement of these nascent particles into a solid phase of significant mass that produces clinical consequences. This enlargement requires a persistently supersaturated solution. It is envisioned as occurring by the combined processes of homogeneous crystal growth, epitaxial crystal growth, and crystal aggregation or agglomeration. The aggregation of a large number of small crystals into a smaller number of large crystals decreases total surface area; this is a

*This example deals with a simple aqueous solution. In a complex solution such as urine, a proportion of the ions is complexed rather than free, so that the concentration product is not a good measure of the saturation of the ionic species. In such a solution, a concentration or *activity* of free ions must be measured or calculated, and the term *activity product* rather than saturation product is used.

process which proceeds naturally on the basis of free energy considerations. Obviously, either or both types of crystal growth as well as aggregation can occur together in a supersaturated solution; the rapidity of all three processes would be a function of the relative degree of supersaturation. In addition, any of these growth processes might be subject to inhibition by forces which do not affect nucleation or the other processes of crystal growth. The net result of these various growth processes is the macroscopic stone.

The crystalloid theory can be readily applied to an understanding of the four "minor" types of stones, cystine, uric acid, struvite, and pure calcium phosphate. Each of these stone types is explicable in relatively straightforward terms of urine supersaturation with respect to ionic stone constituents. Calcium oxalate is extremely insoluble in aqueous solution and lies closer to its formation product in normal urine than any of the other stone-forming constituents (Fig. 25-2). This presumably accounts for the overall frequency of calcium oxalate stones in the population. It also provides a conceptual framework by which the formation of calcium oxalate stones may be understood on the basis of one or multiple risk factors; some of these risk factors may have no direct bearing on abnormalities of calcium or oxalate metabolism.

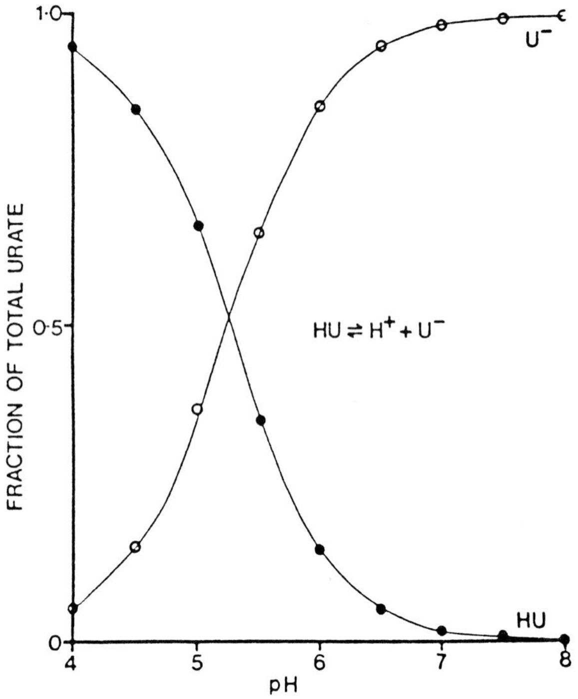

FIGURE 25-3 The fraction of total uric acid in urine as the undissociated acid (HU) and as the urate ion (U^-) as a function of urine pH. (*From Nordin,*[2] *by permission of Churchill Livingstone.*)

CYSTINE STONES

Cystine is the least-soluble naturally occurring amino acid, with a maximum solubility in normal urine of approximately 300 mg/l. Cystine stones are formed by patients with homozygous cystinuria, who commonly excrete 600 to 1400 mg of cystine daily as a result of their genetic defect in renal tubular amino acid reabsorption. The stones form as a direct consequence of urine oversaturation. Although pH has a modest influence on cystine solubility and vigorous alkalinization is a front-line measure in the therapy of cystinuric patients, abnormalities in urine acidification per se play no causative role in the formation of cystine stones.

URIC ACID STONES

Uric acid stones form as a result of oversaturation of urine with undissociated uric acid. Uric acid is far less soluble than its urate salt, which is rarely found in stone material. Uric acid is a weak acid, with a pK_a of 5.35 (in urine at 37°C). The degree of ionization of uric acid as a function of pH is shown in Fig. 25-3. In acid urine with a pH of 5.0 or less, approximately 90 percent of uric acid is undissociated; at pH 6.5 or above, more than 90 percent exists in the form of urate. Thus, the ambient urinary pH is the dominant factor which determines the concentration of the free acid. For example, given a urinary uric acid excretion rate of 1000/mg/day at pH 6.0, the calculated amount of free acid is 360 mg, whereas at pH 5.0 an excretion rate one-half as great, 500 mg/day, results in a greater quantity of free acid, 425 mg.[11] The interplay of pH and the solubility characteristics of the uric acid and urate species determine the ultimate solubility of uric acid in urine, which is estimated to be about 100 mg/l at pH 5.0 and 1500 mg/l at pH 7.0. The clinical risk factors which are responsible for uric acid stones are hyperuricosuria, elaboration of acid urine, and/or dehydration with the excretion of concentrated urine. Of these, persistently acid urine is the most important; it may be the only demonstrable abnormality in some patients with uric acid stones.

MAGNESIUM AMMONIUM PHOSPHATE STONES

Magnesium ammonium phosphate stones are composed of struvite ($MgNH_4PO_4{\cdot}6H_2O$) admixed with minor amounts of carbonate-apatite [$Ca_{10}(PO_4)_6CO_3$]. The solubility product and formation product of struvite lie relatively close together and are never exceeded in sterile normal or stone-forming urine.

Pathological supersaturation of urine with MAP stone constituents occurs only in the presence of infection with bacteria that produce urease; the presence of urease initiates the following sequence of reactions:

$$H_2N{-}\overset{\displaystyle O}{\overset{\|}{C}}{-}NH_2 + H_2O \xrightarrow{\text{urease}} 2NH_3 + CO_2$$

$$2NH_3 + 2H_2O \rightleftharpoons 2NH_4^+ + 2OH^-$$

$$CO_2 + H_2O \rightleftharpoons H_2CO_3$$

$$\rightleftharpoons H^+ + HCO_3^-$$

$$\overset{2OH^-}{\rightleftharpoons} CO_3^{2-} + 2H_2O$$

This sequence leads to a pathological combination of an alkaline urine together with increased concentrations of ammonium, carbonate, and multiply charged phosphate ions which are relatively insoluble. This combination oversaturates the urine with respect to both MAP and carbonate-apatite, and struvite stones both form and grow rapidly.

CALCIUM PHOSPHATE STONES

Pure calcium phosphate stones form in sterile alkaline urine. Variations in urinary pH within the physiological range have little influence on calcium oxalate solubility, but the concentration of HPO_4^{2-} rises markedly with increasing pH, thereby reducing both the solubility and formation products for calcium phosphate (Fig. 25-4). The major crystalline form of calcium phosphate in both pure and mixed stones is hydroxyapatite $[Ca_{10}(PO_4)_6(OH)_2]$. Brushite ($CaHPO_4{\cdot}2H_2O$) is not commonly identified in calculi, but it may serve as an early nidus of calcium phosphate crystals, which later develop into the more mature, hydroxyapatite crystalline form. Pure calcium phosphate stones suggest an underlying disorder of urine acidification associated with persistently alkaline urinary pH.

CALCIUM OXALATE AND MIXED CALCIUM STONES

The solution chemistry of calcium oxalate is far more complex than the rather straightforward solubility concepts described above for the minor stone types. This complexity can be appreciated by simply considering the activity of calcium ions in a complex solution such as urine. At a given pH, calcium may form soluble complexes with citrate, oxalate, sulfate, and four species of phosphate ions. These anions, in turn, form soluble complexes with cations other than calcium, so that their activities are also variable. The computation of calcium ion activity in such a system requires solving approximately a dozen equations of nine or more unknowns each.[3]

In spite of its complexity, the importance of the calcium oxalate system has led to its investigation by a number of workers, including Finlayson, Pak et al., and Robertson et al.[12–15] Although techniques and interpretations differ somewhat, the general implications of the findings of these laboratories regarding saturation and predisposition to crystal formation and growth in stone-forming urine are similar.

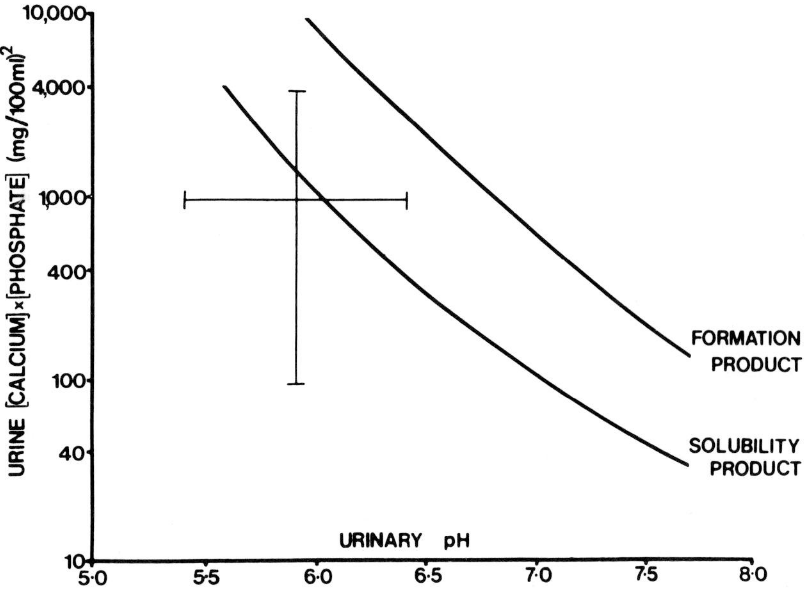

FIGURE 25-4 The relationship between urine pH and the calculated solubility and formation products of octocalcium phosphate. The cross represents the approximate range of normal urine. (*From Nordin,*[2] *by permission of Churchill Livingstone.*)

The *activity product ratio* (APR) describes the state of saturation of urine with respect to calcium oxalate (or calcium phosphate). An APR of unity indicates a saturated urine, a value less than unity is undersaturated, and values progressively greater than unity define increasing degrees of supersaturation. There is agreement among laboratories that patients with recurrent calcium stones typically have values for the APR of calcium oxalate which exceed those of normal individuals. Although not readily translated into pathophysiological abnormalities, these results are generally attributable to increased calcium concentrations in the urine of stone formers, together with a variable tendency toward increased oxalate concentrations. Similar observations have been made for brushite, suggesting that the calcium phosphate system may be an important crystal nidus, particularly in alkaline urine.[8,12]

The *formation product ratio* (FPR) is the lowest supersaturated state at which spontaneous nucleation occurs. In practice, it is measured by adding calcium to urine and noting the activity product at which cloudiness appears. The FPR is normally approximately eight to ten times the APR.[12–15] Several laboratories have reported that the FPR (or an equivalent parameter) in a large percentage of patients with recurrent calcium stones is less than normal, indicating an unexplained predisposition to crystallization in stone-forming urine. This predisposition has been attributed variously to the process of heterogeneous nucleation (e.g., of crystals of calcium oxalate and monosodium urate or uric acid), a deficiency of unidentified inhibitors in stone-forming urine, or the presence of "promoters" of crystallization in stone-forming urine, an ill-defined term suggesting the existence of substances which contribute to crystal formation in a physical sense. Relatively similar data have been derived from systems designed to study crystal growth in stone-forming urine.[8]

Although the specifics of interpretation vary, particularly as regards evidence for inhibitors, promoters, or heterogeneous nucleation, the general thrust of the findings is clear. Patients with recurrent calcium stones tend to excrete urine which is significantly supersaturated with calcium salts and which is also curiously unstable, having a lower limit of metastability than normal urine. Stone formation, therefore, appears to result from an imbalance of those forces which cause and those forces which prevent the crystallization and growth of calcium salts in urine. These concepts are embodied in the saturation-inhibition index proposed by Robertson et al.[13] (Fig. 25-5) and the FPR-APR discriminant score proposed by Pak et al.[15]

Recent experimental findings indicate that the

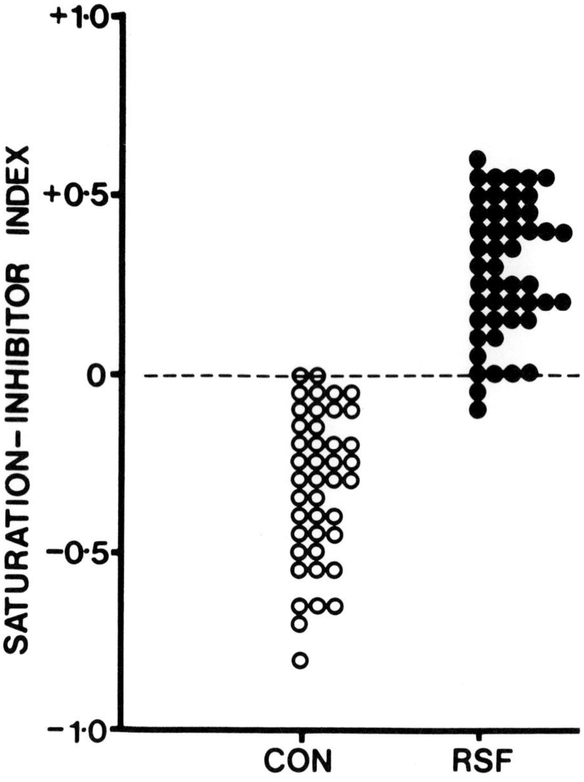

FIGURE 25-5 Values for the saturation-inhibition index in control subjects (CON) and in patients with recurrent calcium oxalate stones (RSF). The index is a discriminant score taken from data for urine supersaturation and inhibitory activity. (*From Robertson et al,*[13] *by permission of the New England Journal of Medicine.*)

postprandial determination of physical chemical parameters and/or crystalluria as compared to measurement of fasting values may be particularly discriminating, but this approach has yet to be applied to patients.[16]

The physical chemical methods described above are not available as clinical tools for the evaluation of patients with stone disease and will remain unavailable in the foreseeable future. Nevertheless, the principles are clinically useful; when presented in straightforward terms they may be very helpful in patient education.

ANATOMICAL CONSIDERATIONS

Anatomical abnormalities which produce obstruction or urinary stasis predispose to stone formation; they must be sought in all patients with stone disease. Representative examples include congenital malformations at all levels of the urinary tract, calyceal or ureteral scarring and stenosis following instrumentation or infection, extrinsic ureteral compression by fibrosis or tumor, and prostatic hypertrophy with stasis and bladder stone formation. Ureteral reflux, instrumentation, and ileal conduits predispose to infection and MAP stones. Papillary necrosis associated with analgesic abuse, diabetes mellitus, or other conditions may occasionally mimic stone disease when a calcified papilla dislodges and produces obstruction, as noted previously. The level of suspicion of an anatomical lesion is determined to some extent by the patient's age and history; a history of recurrent *unilateral* stone disease is particularly suggestive of an underlying anatomical abnormality. The essential screening study is the intravenous pyelogram (IVP). This study should specifically be performed under nonobstructing conditions, since obstruction causes a loss of anatomical detail.

MEDULLARY SPONGE KIDNEY

Medullary sponge kidney is an uncommon but important cause of recurrent stone disease.[17,18] The condition should not be confused with medullary cystic disease, which is a distant relation bearing no clinical resemblance to MSK. The prevalence of MSK in the general population is unknown, but is generally regarded as being less than 1 percent. The prevalence of MSK in patients being evaluated for stone disease is probably between 1 and 5 percent, although recent series in which radiographically more subtle cases have been included have reported frequencies of up to 13 percent.[19–21] Since the stones are typically small (≤ 5 mm), the presence of MSK is suggested by a history of multiple episodes of stone passage not requiring instrumentation.

MSK is a congenital anomaly involving cyst formation and dilatation of collecting ducts in the renal pyramids. The ectasia never extends beyond the corticomedullary junction, and involved kidneys are usually normal in size. On occasion, MSK occurs together with other congenital anomalies of the urinary tract (horseshoe kidney, malrotation, bifid ureter, etc.). Although MSK has been reported in a few families, the lesion almost always occurs sporadically. The sexes are affected equally.

The diagnosis of MSK is made radiographically. Mild degrees of tubular ectasia appear as radial papillary striations or a "papillary blush" following contrast agent administration (Fig. 25-6, panels C and *D*). This pattern is more apparent following ureteral compression or during obstruction; subtle changes merge imperceptibly with normalcy as a function of the technique and imagination of the examining radiologist. Such subtle findings are sometimes referred to as "benign tubular ectasia" and are of limited clinical importance.[17] More extensive involvement presents as medullary nephrocalcinosis on plain films and dilated tubules and communicating cysts which "light up" following contrast agent administration (Fig. 25-6, panels *A* and *B*). The lesions are bilateral in approximately 80 percent of cases; they may involve only a few pyramids or essentially all. Nephrocalcinosis is observed in about two-thirds of patients. The calcifications are densely radiopaque and are usually small, multiple, and confined to the dilated ducts and cysts. These calcifications may erode through the thin cystic walls or escape from ectatic tubules and present as free "stones" in the collecting system. The radiographic pattern tends to remain constant in a given patient on serial examinations.

Uncomplicated MSK produces no symptoms and may be noted as an incidental radiographic finding. Complications of MSK include ureteral colic (occurring in about two-thirds of patients), urinary tract infections ranging from simple cystitis to frank or persistent pyelonephritis (25 percent of patients), and gross hematuria (15 percent of patients). A small minority of patients experience chronic flank pain which defies explanation. The pain may be so persistent and disabling as to force partial or complete nephrectomy. Stone events may be limited to one or several discrete occurrences or may number in the dozens. Passed stones are usually calcium phosphate, calcium oxalate, or mixed calcium stones; in a minority of patients with infection, MAP stones form.

Although renal function is usually grossly normal, detailed study has revealed evidence of mild medullary dysfunction in many patients with MSK. The most common finding is impaired concentrating ability.[17,18] Patients with MSK and coincident complete or incomplete RTA have been described, but in most patients the ability to acidify urine is normal.[17] Recent series have demonstrated that the incidence of metabolic abnormalities predisposing to renal calculi is substantial in stone-forming patients with MSK. Hypercalciuria occurs with a frequency similar to that seen in the general stone-forming population, with a prevalence of about 50 percent in two recent studies.[20,22] Hyperuricosuria has also been reported. As indicated, urinary tract infection is a common complication of MSK; this is particularly true for females, who tend to have a higher incidence of urinary tract infection in the presence of MSK than males.[22] A small number of patients with MSK and primary hyperparathyroidism have been described; presumably, the coincidence of the two conditions arises on the basis of chance.

The natural history of MSK is usually one of intermittent episodes of stone passage, infection, and hematuria without progressive loss of renal function.[23] Whether or not medical therapy materially alters this

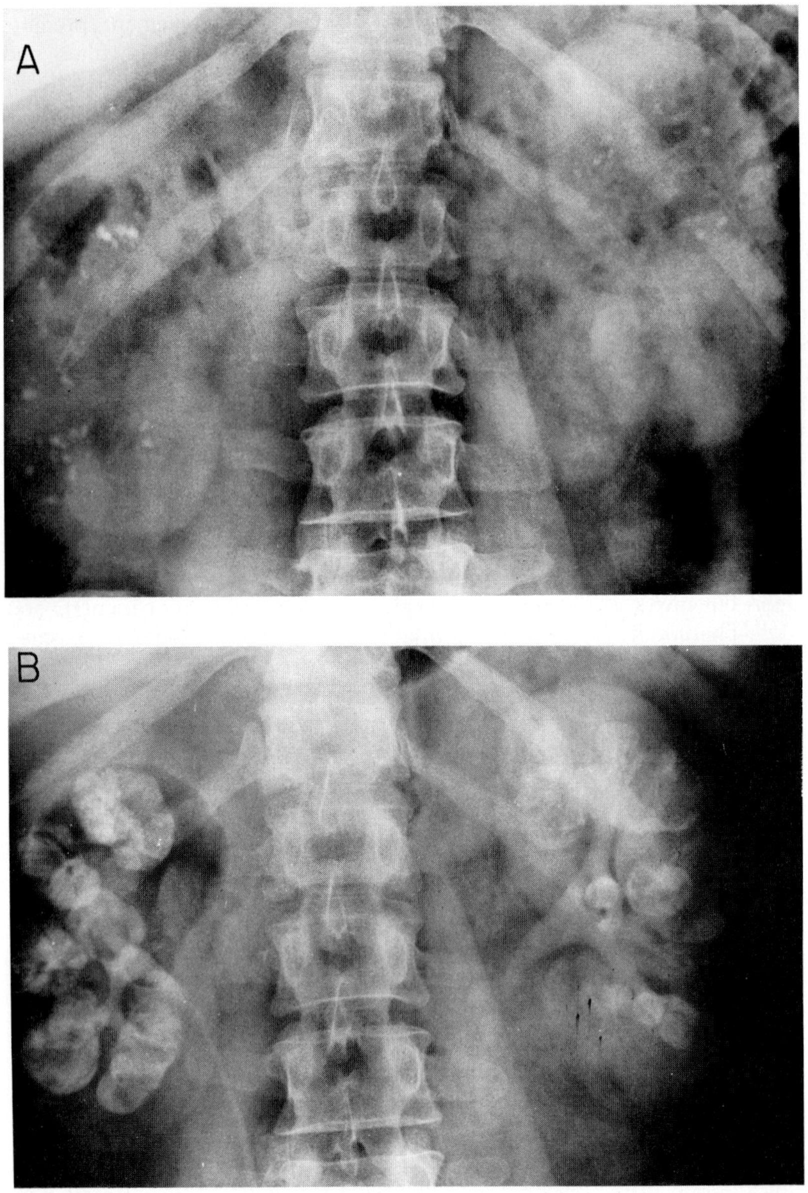

FIGURE 25-6 Medullary sponge kidney. Panels *A* and *B* demonstrate an extreme example and panels C and *D* a borderline example. (*A*) Plain films reveal extensive bilateral nephrocalcinosis. (*B*) Contrast administration causes cysts and dilated ducts to light up all the medullary pyramids are involved in this patient.

natural history is unknown. Acute infection should be identified and treated with bactericidal drugs, and recurrent or persistent infections treated with long-term suppressive agents. Episodes of uncomplicated hematuria are usually transient and resolve spontaneously. It is recommended that all patients with MSK be carefully screened for metabolic risk factors that predispose to calcium stone formation and that these risk factors be treated, if identified. However, assessing clinical response or improvement (by serial radiography or counting stone episodes) may be difficult or impossible in a patient with extensive pretreatment nephrocalcinosis. Partial or complete nephrectomy should be reserved for those few patients whose course defies all conventional measures.

CYSTINURIA

Cystinuria is an inborn error of cystine, ornithine, lysine, and arginine (COLA) transport in the mucosa of the renal tubules and small intestine. It is an autosomal recessive disorder with complex genetic heterogeneity. Clinically, the only recognized manifesta-

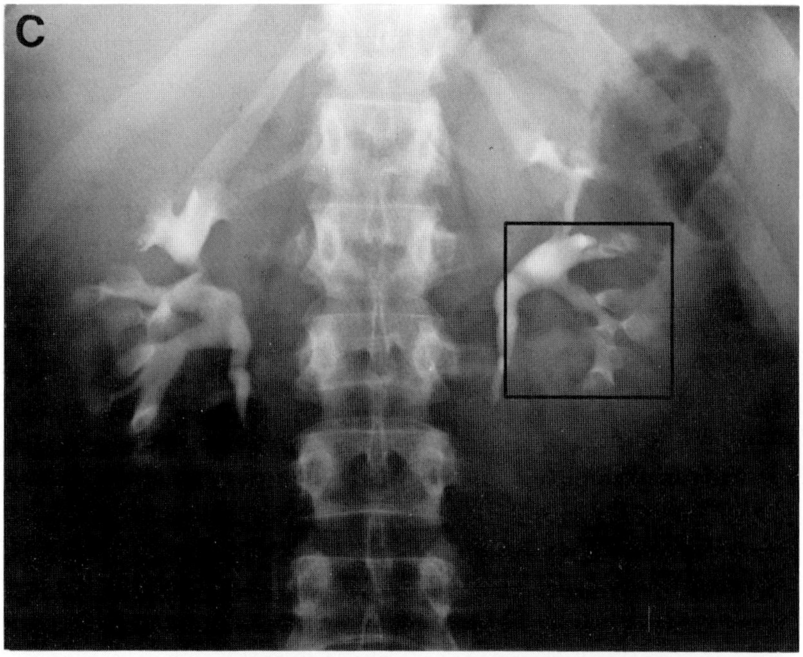

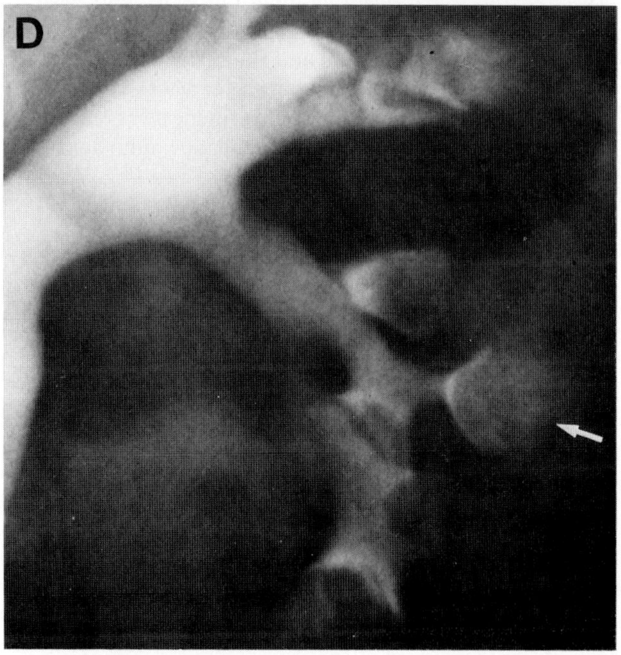

FIGURE 25-6 (*Continued*). (C) An example of a papillary blush. Whether this change is diagnostic of MSK is controversial. (*D*) Enlargement shows fine capillary striations reflective of tubular ectasia.

tion of cystinuria is the formation of cystine stones, owing to the insolubility of cystine in aqueous solution.

Cystine stones were recognized as a distinctive stone type in 1810, and their familial occurrence was described shortly thereafter.[24,25] The relationship between excessive rates of cystine excretion and cystine stones was established as early as 1855, and the familial and clinical aspects of the disorder were well-described by the latter part of the nineteenth century. However, nearly a century passed before the fundamental basis of the disorder became clear. The associated increased rates of ornithine, lysine, and arginine excretion in cystinuric patients were reported in the

1940s. In 1951, Dent and Rose synthesized their classic transport hypothesis from the available information.[26] They pointed out that each of the involved amino acids had two amino or guanidine groups; they suggested that one reabsorptive mechanism in the renal tubule is common to these structurally related amino acids, and that this mechanism is defective in cystinuria. Genetic transport disorders, as a subclass of inborn errors of metabolism, had been previously unrecognized. It was later discovered that cystine and the dibasic amino acids are also malabsorbed in the small intestine in patients with cystinuria. In vitro studies confirming the presence of an amino acid transport system common to cystine and dibasic amino acids in animal tissues and verifying that this system is impaired in intestinal and renal tissue from cystinuric patients have appeared only in the past 20 years.[24,25]

Genetics and Occurrence

Cystinuria has long been regarded as a classic example of simple autosomal recessive inheritance. In homozygotes, excretion rates of cystine and the dibasic amino acids are markedly increased and the incidence of cystine stones is extremely high; heterozygotes can be detected biochemically by virtue of modest increases in the excretion of cystine and the dibasic amino acids but are at negligible risk for cystine stones (Fig. 25-7).[27] Although conventional genetic concepts and parlance are adequate for clinical purposes, in that only homozygous patients are clinically affected, the pattern of inheritance of cystinuria is actually heterogeneous and complex. Three distinct genetic patterns or mutations can be appreciated by studying both intestinal transport and urinary amino acid excretion in cystinuric pedigrees. These patterns differ by the presence and/or degree of abnormal transport of the four amino acids in the intestine and by the presence or absence of abnormal rates of amino acid excretion in heterozygotes.[24] The essential conclusion of these studies is that some "homozygous" patients are actually "double heterozygotes," in that they bear two different allelic mutations rather than a double dose of a single mutant gene. Clinically, "double heterozygotes" and "homozygotes" cannot be clearly distinguished; the latter term is used indiscriminately in the discussion below. The exact frequency of homozygous cystinuria and the frequency of the mutant genes in the general population are unknown. Estimates suggest that homozygous cystinuria occurs with a frequency of about 1 in 18,000, corresponding to a heterozygote frequency as high as 1:60 or 1:70.[24] Patients with homozygous cystinuria constitute only about 1 percent of patients with renal stone disease (Table 25-1).

Pathophysiology and Clinical Manifestations

Five group-specific amino acid transport systems are presently recognized, each mediating the transport of a group of structurally related amino acids. The

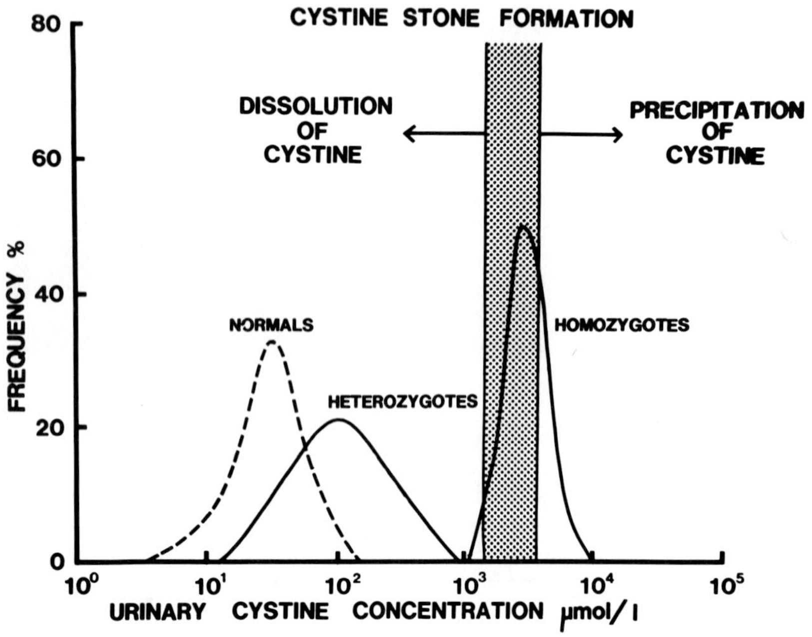

FIGURE 25-7 Urinary concentrations of cystine in normal subjects and in patients with heterozygous and homozygous cystinuria. Regions of cystine solubility and spontaneous precipitation are indicated. (*Courtesy of WG Robertson.*)

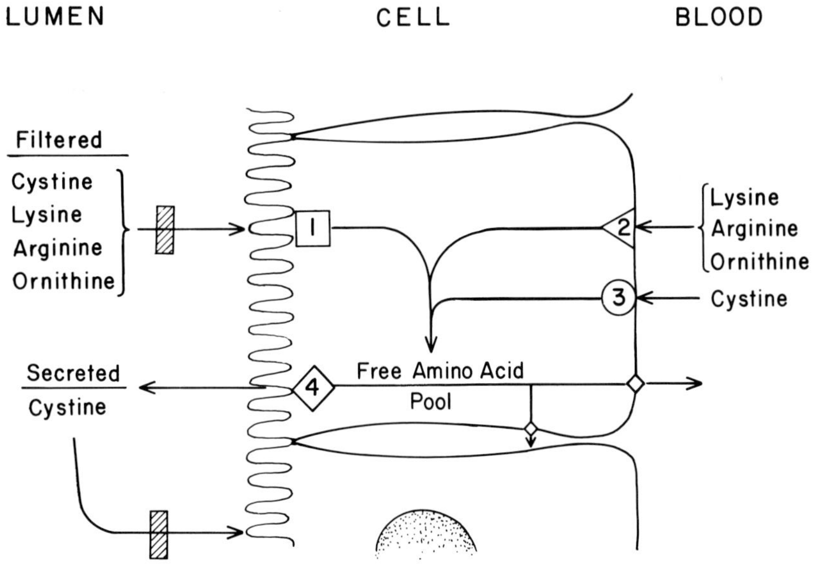

FIGURE 25-8 Schematic representation of the proposed transport systems for cystine, ornithine, lysine, and arginine in the nephron. The cross-hatched bars identify the apparent defect in the brush border transport system in patients with cystinuria. See text for details. (*From Broadus and Thier*[85] *by permission of the New England Journal of Medicine.*)

mutant genes in cystinuria code for an abnormality in the specific transport system for cystine and the dibasic amino acids; the other transport systems are unaffected. Transport in the intestinal mucosa appears to be a single and relatively simple process with striking substrate specificity for COLA. This transport system is either absent or impaired in the vast majority of patients with cystinuria.

The free amino acids in plasma are freely filtered at the glomerulus. Normally, 97 to 99 percent of the filtered load of amino acids is reabsorbed by the group-specific transport systems in the proximal tubule, and negligible quantities appear in the urine. A variety of clinical and experimental observations indicate that the transport of cystine and dibasic amino acids in the renal tubule is more complex than the single shared transport system in the intestine. Figure 25-8 is a schematic representation of the proposed transport systems for cystine and the dibasic amino acids in the nephron and the apparent defect in cystinuria. There appear to be at least three transport systems. The major system is located in the luminal or brush border membrane; it is shared by all four amino acids and is normally responsible for the near-quantitative reabsorption of the filtered load of cystine and related amino acids. It is this system that is defective in cystinuria. In addition, two other systems exist in the basilateral membrane of the cell, one specific for cystine and the other specific for the dibasic amino acids. These systems appear to be largely unaffected in cystinuric patients; they are of importance only to the extent that the cystine which is translocated (probably largely as cysteine) across the cell and into the tubular urine represents an added quantity of the amino acid over and above the filtered load, which cannot be reabsorbed by the defective system in the brush border membrane.[28] This view of cystine and dibasic amino acid renal transport has been refined even further by recent studies employing isolated renal tubule preparations and renal brush border membrane vesicles.[25,28-30] These new data help explain the variability in the occurrence of dibasic aminoaciduria in some cystinuric patients.

In cystinuric patients, who malabsorb dietary cystine, cystine is produced endogenously by the hepatic metabolism of dietary methionine. The filtered load of cystine may be spilled in its entirety by patients with homozygous cystinuria, in whom the renal clearance of cystine may equal or exceed the glomerular filtration rate (GFR). The rate of cystine excretion in cystinuric patients exceeds 400 mg daily and is usually in the range of 600 to 1300 mg/day. Since the maximum solubility of cystine in urine is 300 mg/liter, the predisposition of cystinuric patients to cystine stone formation is self-evident. Indeed, the pathogenesis of cystine stones is the prototype of the application of the concepts of supersaturation chemistry to the understanding of stone formation.

The vast majority of patients with homozygous cystinuria form one or more cystine stones during life; a minority of patients do not form stones, for reasons which are inapparent. Cystine stones may occur initially at any time from infancy to the eighth decade,[31] but the average age of onset is about 20 years (Fig. 25-1). The average time of specific diagnosis lags some 10 years behind the onset of symptoms; occasional patients with recurrent stone disease escape diagnosis well into adulthood. The sexes are affected equally, but males appear to have an unexplained accentuation in stone morbidity. Approximately one-half of patients give a family history of stone disease.

The stones in cystinuric patients are usually multiple and bilateral and frequently require surgical intervention. A particularly characteristic pattern is one of unilateral or bilateral staghorn calculi with multiple small "satellite" stones (Fig. 25-9). Cystine stones are radiopaque with a density that varies but is less than that of contiguous vertebrae. A somewhat vexing clinical observation is that a significant minority of patients with homozygous cystinuria may form stones of mixed composition or may alternately form cystine and either calcium oxalate, pure calcium phosphate, or MAP stones.[24,31] This observation is explained by the occasional coincidence of cystinuria with another stone-forming state, the possible influence of alkali treatment on calcium phosphate solubility and predisposition to apatite stone formation, and infection resulting from instrumentation. It is but one of several reasons why screening for cystinuria is recommended in all patients with recurrent stone disease.

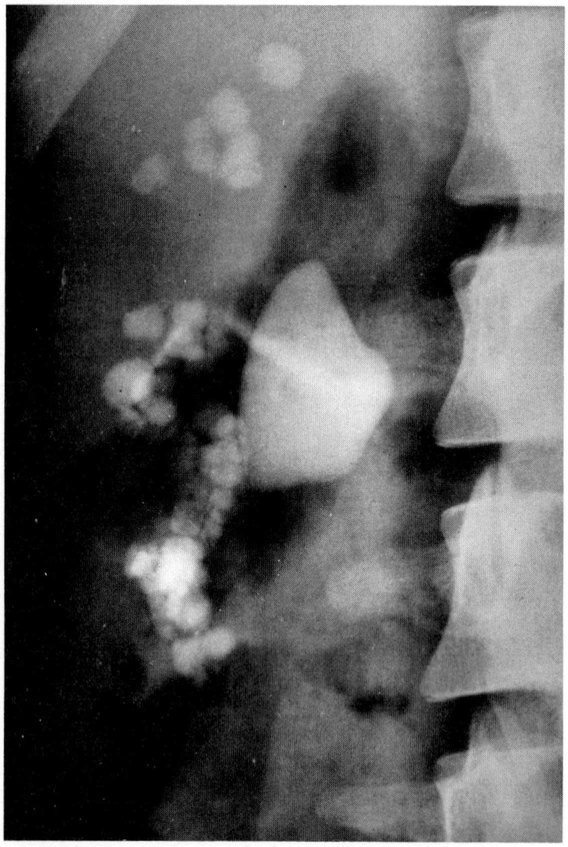

FIGURE 25-9 Multiple cystine stones assuming a characteristic pattern of a staghorn calculus and multiple satellite stones. (*Courtesy of CJ Hodson.*)

The loss of amino acids into the urine in cystinuria appears to be of negligible nutritional significance. Homozygous cystinuria has been reported with an increased frequency in patients with mental illness, an observation which remains unexplained and requires further study.[24] Children with cystinuria have normal intellects and physical development.[32]

Diagnosis

Cystinuria should be considered in any patient with recurrent renal calculi. The diagnosis is suggested by early onset of stone disease or by a characteristic radiological stone pattern (Fig. 25-9). A family history of stones is so common in the general stone-forming population that this finding is not a useful clue to the diagnosis.

The diagnosis of cystinuria can be achieved by stone analysis, demonstration of cystine crystalluria, chemical screening, and/or quantitative urinary amino acid analysis. Cystine crystals are unmistakable flat, hexagonal crystals which are best observed in a cooled, concentrated, acidified urinary specimen. The demonstration of cystine crystals is virtually pathognomonic, but they may not be detected in a dilute urine specimen. The cyanide-nitroprusside test is the simplest and most useful screen for cystinuria. The test is based on the alkaline reduction of cystine to cysteine and a colorimetric reaction of free sulfhydryl groups with nitroprusside. A positive test signifies the presence of 75 to 125 mg of cystine per gram of creatinine and may be observed in heterozygotes as well as in rare dehydrated, oliguric, but genetically normal individuals. Conversely, the test may be negative in a heterozygote with a minimal increase in cystine excretion. A positive nitroprusside test is followed by quantifying urinary amino acid excretion. Column chromatographic techniques provide quantitative information for each of the four related amino acids but are extremely expensive. Cystine excretion can be measured by simpler and less expensive techniques which are adequate for clinical purposes. Column and other techniques for quantitating cystine excretion are commercially available.

There are few differential diagnostic considerations. No other disease is characterized by a selective excessive excretion of COLA. Ketonuria, the generalized aminoacidurias, cystinosis, and homocystinuria, may give a positive nitroprusside test but are not associated with stone disease or cystine crystalluria; these conditions can be differentiated on simple clinical grounds.[24,25]

Treatment

Treatment of cystinuria is guided by quantitative measures of the cystine excretion rate and the foreknowledge that the maximum solubility of cystine is 300 mg/l at physiological pH. Therapeutic measures include hydration, alkalinization, diet, and solubilizing drugs.

Forced hydration is an important aspect of the treatment of all stone disease, but in cystinuria it is the cornerstone of treatment. Patients should be carefully educated regarding the solubility principles involved. Often this is best achieved in a motivated patient by providing actual laboratory results and going through a personalized exercise in saturation chemistry. The urine volume should be sufficient to ensure a cystine concentration less than 250 mg/liter. A definite plan of forced fluids should be designed, specifically to include 8 oz of water at bedtime, again in the early morning hours, and immediately upon arising. All periods of thirst are to be avoided. Patients or physicians may choose to set a minimum total urine volume to be achieved each day (usually 4 liters or more), but this should not replace the emphasis given to continuous daytime and nocturnal hydration.

The pK_a of cystine is 8.4; the slope of the curve of cystine ionization and solubility as a function of pH (Fig. 25-10) is far less steep than is the case with uric acid (Fig. 25-3). Variations in urinary pH within the usual physiological range (pH 5.0 to 7.0) have little influence on cystine solubility, but maximal urine alkalinization (pH 7.5 to 7.8) increases cystine solubility by a factor of two to three. Maximum alkalinization requires sufficient alkali to buffer the daily production rate of hydrogen ions, or approximately 60 to 100 meq/day. This dosage is given as bicarbonate or citrate salts in four divided doses; many physicians prefer citrate because it is metabolized to bicarbonate in the liver and appears to produce a somewhat smoother course of alkalinization. (Table 25-2 lists some of the commonly employed alkali preparations.) A single bedtime dose of acetazolamide (350 to 500 mg) is advocated by some physicians, but is discouraged by others on the grounds that the induced RTA may further increase the risk of calcium phosphate stones or may cause the deposition of calcium phosphate salts on preexisting cystine stones.[31]

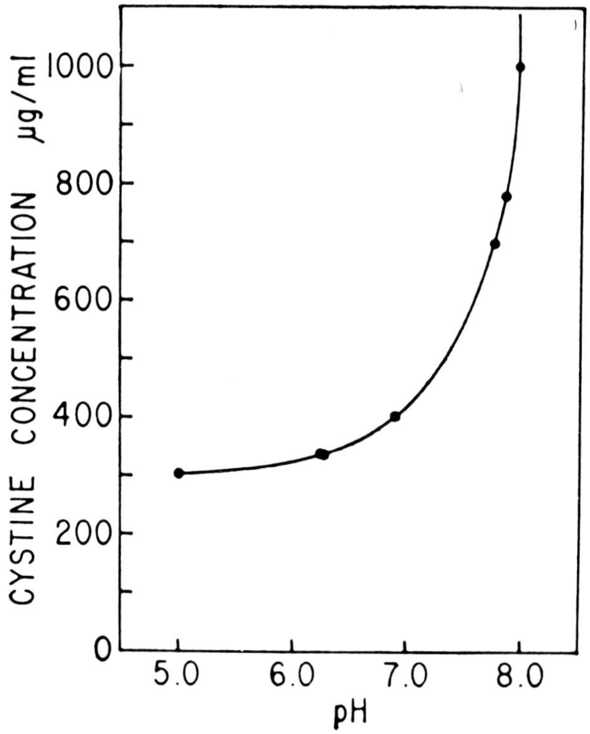

FIGURE 25-10 Effect of urinary pH on solubility of cystine. (*From Rosenberg and Scriver,*[24] *by permission of WB Saunders Co.*)

Patients should be instructed to moderate their protein intake. Diets sufficiently restricted in methionine to reduce cystine excretion significantly are unpalatable and are not a reasonable approach to the treatment of a lifelong disease.

Table 25-2. Commonly Used Preparations of Oral Alkali

Name	Preparation	Base equivalents
Sodium bicarbonate	Tablet (325 mg, 650 mg).	325 mg = 4 meq base
Shohl's solution	1000 ml contains 140 g citric acid and 90 g hydrated crystalline sodium citrate.	1 ml = 1 meq base.
Bicitra	Solution: 5 ml contains 500 mg sodium citrate and 334 mg citric acid.	1 ml = 1 meq base.
Polycitra	Solution: 5 ml contains 550 mg potassium citrate, 500 mg sodium citrate, and 334 mg citric acid.	1 ml = 2 meq base.
Polycitra K	Solution: 5 ml contains 1100 mg potassium citrate and 334 mg citric acid.	1 ml = 2 meq base.

Note: Bicitra, Polycitra, and Polycitra K are trade names for systemic alkalizers.

D-Penicillamine (β,β-dimethylcysteine) is the prototype of a group of sulfhydryl compounds introduced as cystine-complexing agents. Thiols dissociate to form active anions that can undergo disulfide exchange reactions:

$$PSH \rightleftharpoons PS^- + H^+$$
$$CSSC + PS^- \rightleftharpoons CS^- + PSSC$$

where PSH represents penicillamine and CSSC is cystine. The mixed disulfide cysteine-penicillamine (PSSC) is approximately 50 times more soluble in aqueous solution than cystine. Administered in four divided doses totaling 1 to 3 g/day, D-penicillamine reduces the excretion of free cystine to the range of 100 to 200 mg/day.[24,25,31] It is important to employ a quantitative technique that distinguishes free cystine from the mixed disulfide in monitoring the effects of treatment.

D-Penicillamine is an effective agent in preventing cystine stones and has also been reported to dissolve preexisting stones partially or completely.[24,25,31] Unfortunately, the drug is associated with toxic side effects in as many as one-half of patients. The most common toxicity is a syndrome of fever and rash which typically occurs within the first several weeks of treatment. Other reactions include bone marrow depression, hypogeusia, impaired collagen synthesis with poor wound healing and epidermolysis, a Goodpasture-like syndrome, and proteinuria which may progress to frank nephrotic syndrome.[24,25,31,33] A portion of these reactions may be based on vitamin B_6 antagonism, so that 50 mg of pyridoxine is coadministered with penicillamine. In some patients, the side effects are clearly dose-related, resolve rapidly after penicillamine is discontinued, and may not reappear when the drug is reintroduced at a lower dose. Conversely, side effects may appear when the penicillamine dosage is increased after many treatment months previously free of toxicity. Although its use has been reported in pregnancy, avoidance of D-penicillamine during pregnancy seems advisable, particularly in the first trimester.

Because of its toxicity, penicillamine should be used selectively in patients with cystinuria. Approximately 30 to 50 percent of patients can be maintained in a stone-free state with vigorous hydration and alkalinization; the rate of stone complications is diminished in many remaining patients by these measures. Representative indications for penicillamine include (1) inability to control stones with conservative measures (such patients frequently excrete > 1000 mg of cystine daily), (2) cystine stones in a single functioning kidney, and (3) a massive stone burden; in patients with the last indication the drug is used for a finite period in an attempt to dissolve the stones. The stone burden can be diminished or eliminated in approximately two-thirds of patients in this group within a period of approximately 12 months.[31]

Because of the frequently encountered side effects with the use of D-penicillamine, there has been interest in the use of other sulfhydryl compounds. Several recent reports have described the use of mercaptopropionylglycine (MPG) in the treatment of cystinuria. Because of its higher oxidation-reduction potential, this drug may be more efficient than D-penicillamine in undergoing thio-disulfide exchange with cystine. Experience in Europe and Japan has suggested that the use of this drug is associated with fewer serious side effects than are encountered in the use of D-penicillamine.[34] Reported side effects have included skin rash, fever, nausea, and soft feces. Significant proteinuria has been rarely reported. Unfortunately, frequent cross-reactivity may exist between MPG and D-penicillamine. Preliminary results from a multicenter trial in the United States in which MPG therapy was offered to patients who had clear-cut toxicity to D-penicillamine has suggested that up to 45 percent of such patients develop toxicity to MPG.[35]

N-Acetyl-D-penicillamine has been reported to be effective in reducing free cystine concentration in patients with cystinuria and may have fewer side effects than D-penicillamine. However, experience with this drug is limited.[24]

The administration of glutamine has recently been reported to reduce cystine excretion in a single patient,[36] but attempts to confirm this finding in 14 additional patients have been unsuccessful.[37,38]

Renal transplantation (from a noncystinuric donor) has been successfully performed in a handful of patients with cystinuria. The procedure "cures" the cystinuria but is employed only in patients with end-stage renal failure.

Genetic counseling can be effectively performed in cystinuric kindreds but requires careful interpretation of screening studies in the context of the complex genetics of the disorder.[24,25]

Approximately 15 percent of the stones formed by cystinuric patients either do not contain cystine or contain cystine as a minor constituent of mixed stones.[31] MAP stones result from infection, usually introduced by urological instrumentation. Alkalinization poses a risk for calcium phosphate stone formation; this has been reported as a complication of alkali treatment in cystinuric patients.[24,25,31] Some investigators regard this complication as more likely to occur in a patient with coincident hypercalciuria or another risk factor for calcium stone formation; they therefore carefully screen cystinuric patients for such risk factors before initiating alkali treatment.

Resnick et al. have reported that 17 of 126

patients (13 percent) with recurrent calcium stones were heterozygotes for cystinuria,[39] a frequency some 10 times greater than that expected by chance alone. It was concluded that a modest increase in cystine excretion represented a risk factor for calcium stone formation, possibly by a mechanism similar to that invoked to explain the risk posed by hyperuricosuria. The prevalence of heterozygous cystinuria reported in two additional series of patients with calcium oxalate stones has ranged from 1.4 to 7.8 percent.[40,41] Thus, whether this putative relationship and mechanism is generalized or peculiar to certain localized populations remains to be established.

URIC ACID CALCULI

The general term *urate nephropathy* refers to a variety of renal lesions and complications which result from the deposition of uric acid or its salts. *Chronic urate nephropathy* is a slowly progressive form of renal impairment which has been noted in a minority of patients with primary or secondary gout. The process is associated with deposition of monosodium urate in the interstitium of the pyramids and produces a classic histological picture of interstitial nephritis. Whether chronic hyperuricemia and/or hyperuricosuria is pathogenetically related to the renal insufficiency noted in these patients is unclear. Two recent series have suggested that azotemia attributable solely to hyperuricemia or hyperuricosuria rarely occurs in the modern era.[42,43] Chronic urate nephropathy and uric acid stone formation appear to be pathogenetically unrelated. *Acute uric acid nephropathy* is a complication more closely related to the process of stone formation. It is a particularly malignant form of supersaturation-induced precipitation of solid-phase uric acid. Classically, this complication is noted in patients with lymphoproliferative and myeloproliferative disorders following the initiation of chemotherapy. The drug-induced cell lysis leads to a rapid release of large quantities of nucleoprotein, which is metabolized to uric acid, producing massive uricosuria. Rarely, the complication results from the use of uricosuric drugs, such as the diuretic and uricosuric agent tienilic acid. In either case, the acute uricosuria produces a degree of oversaturation of uric acid which so exceeds the formation product as to cause a rapid and extensive precipitation of solid-phase uric acid. The solid-phase material is far less organized than a discrete calculus; it consists of an amorphous, semisolid sludge in the collecting ducts and/or pelvis and ureters.

Although patients may pass "sand" in their urine, the acute nephropathy is usually unaccompanied by classic colic. It typically presents as acute renal shutdown with oliguria or anuria. If promptly recognized and treated vigorously with intravenous (IV) fluids, alkalinization with bicarbonate and acetazolamide administration, and the institution of allopurinol therapy, the course is usually that of the oliguric and diuretic phases of acute tubular necrosis. Lacking prompt recognition and therapy, the outcome is uniformly poor. Acute uric acid nephropathy can be avoided by institution of a preventive program of hydration, alkalinization, and allopurinol administration; the use of these measures in the appropriate clinical settings has greatly reduced the frequency of this complication.

Uric acid lithiasis is the most common form of uric acid deposition in the urinary tract. Uric acid stones are usually pure, affect predominantly middle-aged males (Fig. 25-1), and constitute only some 5 percent of stone disease in western countries (Table 25-1). Pure uric acid stones are the only urinary tract stones which are truly radiolucent. In some countries, such as Israel, uric acid stones are common and may be responsible for as much as 40 percent of clinical stone disease. The pathogenesis of uric acid stones is well-understood, and preventive treatment is highly effective. The subject has been treated in detail by several excellent reviews.[11,44–46] The relationship between hyperuricosuria and calcium oxalate stone formation is discussed below.

Purine Metabolism and Uric Acid Excretion

Uric acid is the final degradation product of purine metabolism in humans. A schema of purine metabolism and the disposition and mechanism of renal clearance of uric acid is presented in Fig. 25-11. Both dietary and endogenous purines contribute to the metabolic purine pool. Under normal circumstances, the rate of metabolism of endogenous purines remains relatively constant, so alterations in purine intake are largely responsible for variations in the uric acid production rate. It is estimated that approximately 50 percent of the nucleic acid purines in the diet are ultimately recoverable as urinary uric acid.[44]

Uric acid is disposed of by two main routes. Approximately one-quarter to one-third of the uric acid produced per day enters the enteric secretions and is destroyed by the intestinal flora (intestinal uricolysis). The remaining two-thirds to three-quarters is excreted into the urine. Uric acid circulates almost entirely as the monovalent anion at pH 7.4 (Fig. 25-3). The protein-bound fraction of circulating urate is thought to be less than 5 percent, so that for all practical purposes serum uric acid may be regarded as

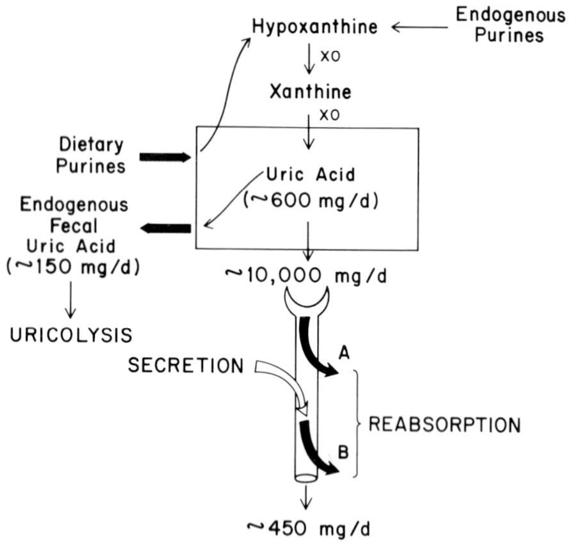

FIGURE 25-11 Schematic representation of purine metabolism and uric acid excretion in normal humans. Exogenous and endogenous purines are oxidized by xanthine oxidase (XO) to uric acid. Some 95 percent of the filtered load of urate is reabsorbed in the proximal tubule. Both secretion and reabsorption of urate occur in the remainder of the tubule. Net reabsorption is the dominant process, so that only about 5 percent of the filtered load of uric acid is excreted.

freely filterable at the glomerulus. At a serum uric acid concentration of 6 mg/dl, the filtered load of uric acid is about 10 g/day. The fractional excretion of uric acid (uric acid clearance divided by creatinine clearance) averages approximately 0.08 in normal individuals, so that only 5 to 10 percent of the filtered load is excreted in the final urine. Thus, tubular reabsorption is clearly the dominant process governing uric acid excretion.

The intimate details of uric acid clearance are complex; they have been the subject of controversy for many years.[44-47] The schema in Fig. 25-11 depicts a modern consensus regarding the mechanisms of uric acid clearance. It includes three transport mechanisms: proximal tubular reabsorption, tubular secretion, and postsecretory reabsorption. Approximately 95 to 98 percent of the filtered load of urate is thought to be actively reabsorbed in the proximal tubule (mechanism A in Fig. 25-11). Many lines of evidence indicate that tubular secretion of uric acid also occurs in humans; this evidence includes the biphasic effects of salicylates on uric acid clearance and the fractional excretion of uric acid clearly exceeding unity in occasional hypouricemic patients. The site of uric acid secretion is not firmly established in humans but is thought to be the proximal tubule. Estimates of the quantity of uric acid secreted vary, but experimental evidence indicates that the rate of secretion may approximate or even exceed the filtered load.[44-47] Thus, postsecretory reabsorption (mechanism B in Fig. 25-11) must occur; this mechanism is presumed to be the major determinant of the final rate of uric acid excretion.[47] An alternative model to that in Fig. 25-11 proposes that both secretion and reabsorption of uric acid occur simultaneously along a substantial length of the renal tubule.

Regardless of the mechanistic details, it is clear that net tubular reabsorption is quantitatively the dominant process which determines the amount of uric acid excreted. The quantitative dominance of the renal tubule in uric acid homeostasis is vaguely reminiscent of the quantitative aspects of calcium, phosphorus, and magnesium clearance (described in Chap. 23). The essential differences are that the renal tubular handling of uric acid is neither systemically regulated nor T_m-limited and that uric acid reabsorption serves no apparent useful purpose in a teleologic sense, unless it is to limit the excretion of a relatively insoluble substance into the urine.

Pathogenesis of Uric Acid Stones and Clinical Populations at Risk

The physical chemical aspects of uric acid solubility in urine provide a clear understanding of the pathogenesis of uric acid stones. The importance of pH in determining the concentration of the free acid in urine and other quantitative considerations were already presented in detail (see Physical Chemical Aspects of Stone Formation, above). Clinically, these solubility considerations translate into the three risk factors for uric acid stone formation: hyperuricosuria, urinary acidity, and dehydration with concentrated urine. Several of these risk factors are often identified in individual patients with uric acid stone disease.

Based on figures for the frequency of stone disease in the general population and the percentage of these stones which are composed of uric acid, the prevalence of uric acid stones in the population is estimated to be approximately 0.01 percent.[11,44,45] The patient populations at statistical risk for uric acid stones are listed in Table 25-3.

Approximately 20 percent of patients with primary gout form one or more uric acid stones, a frequency 1000 times or more that in the general population.[11,44,45] Ninety percent of gouty patients with stones are males. In one-half of affected patients the stone disease is recurrent. Stone symptoms precede articular symptoms in some 40 percent of patients, occasionally by more than 10 years.[11] This is particularly true in patients under age 50.

The gouty population has a combination of risk

Table 25-3. Patient Populations at Risk for Uric Acid Stones

Primary gout
Inborn errors of metabolism:
HPRT deficiency
PRPP synthetase overactivity
Glucose-6-phosphatase deficiency
Secondary gout
Receiving uricosuric drugs
Inflammatory bowel disease and/or ileostomy
Idiopathic uric acid stone formation

factors for uric acid stone formation: hyperuricosuria and undue urine acidity. The gout subpopulation regarded as "overproducers" is at principal risk; there is a strong correlation between the excretion rate of uric acid and the frequency of uric acid stones. This relationship is clearly evident in the data in Table 25-4, which indicate that almost 50 percent of patients with a uric acid excreton rate greater than 1000 mg/day form uric acid stones. Overproducers incorporate a disproportionate percentage of purine nitrogen into uric acid, so that they usually display a proportionate degree of hyperuricemia and hyperuricosuria (i.e., the fractional excretion of uric acid in this subpopulation is normal). Since both exogenous and endogenous purines contribute to the metabolic pool of purine bases, a high purine intake exacerbates the hyperuricemia and hyperuricosuria in these patients.

Approximately 20 percent of the gouty population forms uric acid stones in the absence of hyperuricosuria (Table 25-4), a striking association which was initially baffling. The principal abnormality in this predominantly nonoverproducing population is a persistently acid urinary pH. In fasting morning specimens, the urinary pH is 5.0 or less in about one-half of these patients, in comparison with 15 percent of normal subjects.[45] The abnormality is also manifested by a loss of the normal alkaline tide in the gout population. In spite of a relatively large literature on the subject, the basis of this tendency to excrete persistently acid urine remains unclear.[11,44,45] The aggregate data indicate that patients with gout excrete relatively more titratable acidity and relatively less ammonia than do normal subjects, but it is unclear whether the defect in ammonia production is primary or is dependent on a primary abnormality in the excretion of titratable acid; or, both abnormalities may reflect an unknown fundamental defect in acid-base regulation.[45] The defect is observed in the entire population of gouty patients; it is an added risk factor for stone formation in overproducers and the only identifiable abnormality in normouricosuric patients.

Table 25-4. Relationship Between Rate of Uric Acid Excretion and Frequency of Uric Acid Stones (1319 Patients with Primary Gout)

Urinary uric acid, mg/day	Percentage of gout population	Percentage of patients with stones
<400	12	24
400–599	36	24
600–799	30	32
800–999	16	31
1000–1600	6	49

Source: Modified from Yü.[11]

Several rare inborn errors of metabolism are associated with marked overproduction of uric acid and a particularly fulminant diathesis of articular gout and uric acid stone disease. The three disorders listed in Table 25-3 are hypoxanthine-guanine pyrophosphoribosyl transferase (HPRT) deficiency (the Lesch-Nyhan syndrome), phosphoribosyl pyrophosphate (PRPP) synthetase overactivity, and glucose-6-phosphatase deficiency (type 1 glycogen storage disease). A detailed discussion of these disorders is beyond the scope of this chapter. Affected patients have extreme rates of uric acid overproduction and usually display a serum uric acid concentration in excess of 10 mg/dl and a uric acid excretion rate greater than 1000 mg/day. Approximately three-quarters of patients form uric acid stones, often before the age of 20 years. In about one-half of patients, stone symptoms are the initial manifestation of the underlying disorder.[11,44,45]

Patients with polycythemia, myeloid metaplasia, and myelocytic leukemia frequently display hyperuricemia and hyperuricosuria because of an increased rate of nucleoprotein turnover. Secondary articular gout occurs in only about 10 percent of patients with these myeloproliferative disorders, but as many as 50 percent of patients form uric acid stones, a frequency equal to that of the overproducing subpopulation of patients with primary gout (Table 25-4). The stones tend to be recurrent and may occasionally be the initial clinical manifestation which leads to the diagnosis of the underlying disorder. These are the same patients who are at risk for acute uric acid nephropathy.

A number of drugs (probenecid, salicylates, ascorbic acid, x-ray contrast agents, etc.) produce an acute uricosuria by inhibiting net uric acid reabsorption and increasing the fractional excretion of uric acid. The continual administration of these agents, however, results in a new steady state, in which the rate of uric acid excretion should be no greater than the pretreatment rate. Nevertheless, initiation of probenecid treatment has been reported to be associated with an apparent increased frequency of stone formation in patients with primary gout.[48] Clearly, uricosuric drugs should be avoided in patients with uric acid overproduction, some of whom are also potentially at risk for acute uric acid nephropathy.

Patients with inflammatory bowel disease appear to have an increased frequency of uric acid stones.[11,45] The association is particularly strong in patients with an ileostomy, in whom losses of both bicarbonate and volume via the ileostomy lead to persistently acid, concentrated urine. The excretion rate of uric acid is usually normal in these patients. Patients with inflammatory bowel disease are also at increased risk for calcium stone formation (see Calcium Oxalate and Mixed Calcium Stones, below).

Idiopathic uric acid lithiasis is a term used to describe uric acid stone formation in normouricemic and normouricosuric patients in whom the most consistent abnormality is persistently acid urine. The frequency of such patients in the United States is unknown, but they have seemed to constitute a large minority of patients with pure uric acid stones. A recent report from Europe suggests that the prevalence of this "syndrome" may be as high as 11 percent of the general stone-forming population.[49] The patients in this series were predominantly males of middle age or beyond, and they had a liberal intake of alcohol. The term idiopathic uric acid lithiasis should not be used in connection with that segment of the gout population which displays hyperuricemia and normouricosuria. An unusual hereditary form of idiopathic uric acid lithiasis with dominant inheritance and a particularly malignant stone diathesis has been described.[11]

Dehydration is regarded by some investigators as an independent risk factor for uric acid stone formation and has been invoked as an explanation for the increased prevalence of uric acid stones in certain arid regions, such as Israel. However, this explanation is probably overly simplistic, in that there is little reason to suppose that a concentrated urine would selectively predispose to formation of uric acid as opposed to calcium oxalate stones (see Fig. 25-2).

Diagnosis

Crystallographic analysis of stone material is the most certain means of arriving at a specific diagnosis. Uric acid stones are radiolucent and can be identified radiographically only by a pattern of relief following contrast agent administration, a pattern which may also be produced by a clot, a tumor, or, rarely, a sloughed papilla. Renal ultrasound and computed tomography (CT) have been found to be useful in establishing the correct diagnosis.[50] A presumptive diagnosis may be made in a patient known to be at risk who experiences classic symptoms and signs of a stone event when no stone is visible or stone material recoverable. All patients with uric acid stones should be carefully screened for the three risk factors which predispose to uric acid stone formation; in such patients the underlying disorders listed in Table 25-3 must be strongly suspected. It is important to recall that stone disease precedes articular symptoms in a large minority of patients with primary gout, the largest single patient group at risk for uric acid stones. In addition, patients with hyperuricosuria are at increased risk for calcium stones, and occasional patients are encountered who have sequentially formed both uric acid and calcium stones (see Calcium Oxalate and Mixed Calcium Stones, below).

The *uricase* method provides the most reliable technique for measuring the concentration of uric acid in serum and urine. Urine samples are routinely alkalinized in the laboratory before being divided into aliquots for uric acid determination; the alkalinization solubilizes uric acid precipitates that may have formed during urine collection or upon standing. The collection of urine in containers with acid preservatives may lead to spuriously low results unless great care is taken to alkalinize thoroughly and mix the specimen. The use of uricosuric agents may complicate the interpretation of screening data; the most common error in this regard is the collection of urine samples shortly after the administration of contrast material, which produces a brisk uricosuria. Nitrazine paper provides quite an accurate measure of urine pH within the physiological range and is a convenient means of determining urinary pH during outpatient visits and/or for monitoring urinary pH throughout the day.

Other purine bases or metabolites are sparingly soluble in urine and may form stones under unusual circumstances. *Xanthine* stones occur in patients with xanthinuria, a rare autosomal recessive disorder caused by a deficiency of xanthine oxidase; xanthinuria is associated with hypouricemia and hypouricosuria. Xanthine stones have also been described in occasional patients with the specific inborn errors listed in Table 25-3 following allopurinol administration.[5,44,45] *2,8-Dihydroxyadenine* stones have been reported in a few patients with deficient adenine phosphoribosyl transferase activity.[11] *Oxypurinol*, the principal metabolite of allopurinol, is quite insoluble, but oxypurinol stones have not been a significant complication of allopurinol therapy.[11,45] Individually and in the aggregate, these stone types are extremely rare. Specific diagnosis is achieved by crystallographic stone analysis.

Therapy

Patient management is based upon the presence or absence of a specific underlying disorder, the assessment of risk factors, and a knowledge of stone recurrence or estimate of the likelihood of recurrence. Available modalities include forced hydration, restriction in purine intake, alkalinization, and allopurinol administration. Probenecid should not be used.

A diet rigidly restricted in purines and protein is unpalatable and an unrealistic form of therapy. Moderation in purine intake, however, should be part of the therapeutic program in patients who chronically overproduce uric acid. Alcohol can increase uric acid production and excretion. Further, a high alcohol intake has been associated with uric acid lithiasis, at least in some patients.[49] It therefore seems reasonable to recommend a moderation in alcohol intake.

Alkalinization with sodium bicarbonate (0.6 to 1.2 g orally four times daily) or other alkali (Table 25-2) has long been a mainstay of therapy in patients with persistently acid urine. These patients not infrequently have severe stone disease, and improvement may be dramatic. Patients are provided with nitrazine paper and the dosage of alkali is adjusted to maintain the urine pH between 6.0 and 6.5 throughout the day. Because of the ionization and solubility characteristics of uric acid, dosages and the degree of alkalinization required are less rigid than is the case in patients with cystinuria (compare Figs. 25-3 and 25-10). Acetazolamide is not in general use at present because of concern regarding the associated risk for calcium phosphate stone formation.

Allopurinol has become the agent of choice in many patients in recent years. The drug is an analogue of hypoxanthine, and both allopurinol and its principal metabolite, oxypurinol, are competitive inhibitors of xanthine oxidase, thus leading to a shunting of the metabolic purine pool toward xanthine and hypoxanthine (Fig. 25-11). Allopurinol decreases uric acid production and excretion in a dose-dependent fashion; it also reduces total oxypurine excretion as a result of both oxypurine reutilization and feedback inhibition of de novo purine biosynthesis. Although the circulating half-life ($t_{1/2}$) of allopurinol is on the order of only several hours, its biological effect persists for the better portion of the day, in part because of the long $t_{1/2}$ of oxypurinol. This allows for a single daily dose in most patients, which greatly increases patient compliance. Dosage ranges from 200 to 600 mg/day in the majority of patients and should be initially individualized and monitored by measurements of the uric acid excretion rate. The drug is available in both 100- and 300-mg scored tablets. Allopurinol is generally well-tolerated and has a rather low toxicity, consisting mostly of reversible hypersensitivity reactions involving the skin and blood.[11,45] Oxypurinol has been successfully administered for the treatment of both hyperuricemia and hyperuricosuria to patients who are allergic to allopurinol. The incidence of cross-reactivity in preliminary studies has been approximately 30 percent. [The drug is available only through an Investigational New Drug authorization (IND) held by the Burroughs Wellcome Company.]

Indications for allopurinol therapy include recurrent uric acid stone disease and/or substantial overproduction of uric acid. Patients with a single uric acid stone event without marked overproduction of uric acid or articular symptoms can often be successfully managed with conservative measures.

MAGNESIUM AMMONIUM PHOSPHATE STONES

A variety of synonymous terms, including *struvite stone, infection stone,* and *triple phosphate stone,* are used in connection with MAP stones. The term *triple phosphate* is descriptive of the early recognition that MAP stones are composed of three different cations (magnesium, ammonium, and calcium) together with the predominant phosphate anion. The term *infection stone* is common in urological parlance, in which the remaining four types of stones are often referred to generally as *metabolic stones.*

MAP stones are an ancient affliction. Hippocrates recognized the association between renal abscesses and large masses of stone material.[51] Bladder stones composed of MAP have been found in Egyptian mummies dating from 5000 B.C.[51] In the presurgery, preantibiotic era, the outlook for affected patients was miserable. Both surgical and medical advances have dramatically altered this outlook, and both the prevalence and the recurrence rate of MAP stones have clearly decreased in the past two decades, perhaps by as much as 75 percent.[51,52]

There are three peaks of MAP stone prevalence in the population: in young boys, middle-aged women, and elderly patients of both sexes (Fig. 25-1). The true frequency of MAP stones is unknown, but they probably represent no more than a few percent of total stones (Table 25-1). Patients with MAP stones represent 4 percent of the patient population in the Yale Renal Stone Clinic. Nevertheless, because of the morbidity and mortality implicit in the natural history of untreated MAP stones and the difficulties of medical and surgical management, these stones continue to command a position of importance which far outweighs their general frequency. A coordinated multidisciplinary approach is helpful in managing patients with all types of stone disease but is absolutely essential for optimum care of patients with MAP stones.

Pathogenesis

MAP stones form as a result of supersaturation of urine with magnesium ammonium phosphate and carbonate-apatite (see Physical Chemical Aspects, above). This supersaturation occurs only in the presence of infection with urea-splitting bacteria; sterile urine or urine infected with non-urease-producing organisms is invariably undersaturated with respect to the constituents of MAP stones. The stoichiometry is such that the essential physical chemical conditions responsible for MAP stone formation can be reproduced in vitro simply by adding purified urease to normal urine.[51]

The matrix phase of MAP stones may be of more importance than appears to be the case with other stone types. *Matrix concretions* are large, soft, gel-like masses composed of bacteria, inflammatory cells, mucoid debris, and scattered crystals of MAP and carbonate-apatite. Such "stones" may mineralize rapidly, to assume the appearance of a classic staghorn calculus within a matter of weeks.[53] Based on an in vitro model, it has been suggested that urease-producing bacteria, such as *Proteus* spp., adhere to renal epithelial cells and form small colonies enclosed in a glycocalyx coat.[54] This glycocalyx coat then serves to trap struvite and apatite crystals which form in the infected alkaline urine, as well as urinary mucoproteins. The glycocalyx coat may also offer some resistance to antimicrobial agents. These crystal-encrusted microcolonies then enlarge into mature calculi.

Approximately 90 percent of clinical isolates of *Proteus* spp., *Staphylococcus aureus*, and *Bacteroides* spp. produce urease, and some 30 percent of *Klebsiella* and *Pseudomonas* isolates are urease-positive.[53] It is notable that *Escherichia coli* rarely, if ever, produces urease. Although all the urea-splitting bacterial strains have been implicated clinically in series of patients with MAP stones, *Proteus* species are the principal culprits, having been identified in almost 90 percent of patients.[52] Colony counts are frequently less than 100,000/ml, a finding which must be appreciated for proper diagnosis and management.

Populations at Risk

There are two major categories of patients at risk for MAP stones: (1) those with anatomical and/or functional abnormalities of the urinary tract which predispose to infection and (2) those with antecedent metabolic stones, in whom persistent infection is established in the foreign body focus of a preexisting stone or results from urologic manipulation, or both. The first category includes patients with megaloureter, ureteral reflux or obstruction, ileal conduits, nephrostomy drainage, MSK, or a neurogenic bladder requiring either intermittent catheterization or an indwelling catheter. Bladder stones composed of MAP most commonly result from prostatic obstruction or an indwelling catheter. The second category includes patients with any of the other four stone types, but particularly those patients who have required frequent instrumentation for stone disease. The stone disease in these patients ultimately becomes a vicious cycle of stones predisposing to infection and infection predisposing to stone formation. Which aspect of the cycle is of pathophysiological primacy in such a patient becomes an issue which is academic; all patients with MAP stones deserve a careful and complete metabolic evaluation. In the reported experience of Smith, over 60 percent of patients with MAP stones were found to have abnormalities which predispose to metabolic stone formation.[52]

Clinical Manifestations

The clinical manifestations of MAP stones include flank pain, gross hematuria, recurrent urinary tract infections, and renal colic; each of these four manifestations is the presenting complaint in approximately one-quarter of patients.[52] The relatively infrequent history of renal colic is explained by the large size of the typical MAP stone as well as the fact that the stones are usually well-anchored in the pyelocaliceal system. The flank pain is usually dull, presumably resulting from chronic, partial obstruction. The infections usually present as recurrent episodes of cystitis, with or without concurrent signs and symptoms of pyelonephritis. If pyelonephritis is complicated by a high degree of obstruction, pyonephrosis and sepsis may occur, representing an immediate threat to life. This type of obstruction is often due to a matrix concretion; it must be relieved on an emergency basis. An untreated staghorn calculus grows and invades locally, in a fashion similar to that of a neoplasm. Implicit in this natural history is a threat to renal function in patients who are not successfully managed; untreated patients stand an approximately 50 percent chance of losing the involved kidney within 5 years.[51] The renal impairment associated with a unilateral staghorn stone is usually insufficient to greatly alter renal function tests but can be appreciated by the visualization of a shrunken and/or scarred cortical outline during the nephrogram phase of the IVP. Patients with a staghorn calculus in a single functioning kidney or with bilateral staghorn stones can have manifest azotemia. About 25 percent of patients with bilateral staghorn stones die within 5 years.[53] The mortality associated with unilateral staghorn calculi is unknown but has certainly been reduced by modern medical and surgical therapy.

Bladder stones usually manifest themselves by symptoms of recurrent cystitis, hematuria, or vague suprapubic discomfort.

Diagnosis

The identification of MAP stones usually presents no difficulties. Diagnosis is achieved by the characteristic radiological configuration of the stone and/or by crystallographic analysis. The apatite content confers radiopacity on MAP stones, which are less dense than oxalate stones but, with the exception of occasional matrix concretions, can usually be visualized in their entirety on plain radiographs.

The bacteriologic aspect of diagnosis may be less straightforward. The colony count of the urease-producing bacteria is < 100,000/ml in 50 percent of affected patients and is < 10,000/ml in 20 percent of patients.[52] Mixed infections are common, and there is a tendency to overlook the importance of the urea-splitting organisms in the presence of a quantitatively more impressive mixed infection (e.g., with *E. coli*). However, regardless of the colony count or presence of mixed infection, urease-producing organisms can be cultured from stone material in 100 percent of patients.[52] It follows that surgical specimens should be cultured in all patients in whom a clear bacteriologic diagnosis has not been established. The problem of low colony counts must also be appreciated in monitoring the effectiveness of antimicrobial therapy.

The other aspects of diagnosis relate to metabolic screening and the pyelographic and urological search for structural or functional abnormalities of the urinary tract. Associated metabolic abnormalities are identified in more than 50 percent of patients.[52] In such patients, it is sometimes possible to document a historical sequence of stones with differing compositions or to document prospectively a recurrence of a metabolic stone in a patient with MAP stones whose underlying disorder has been overlooked. Metabolic screening should be complete; this requires consideration of all categories of stone disease. A carefully performed IVP is the essential anatomical diagnostic tool. Films obtained when there is significant obstruction often do not provide sufficient anatomical detail for detection of subtle abnormalities, and the frequent omission of postvoiding films, oblique views, or other relevant aspects of the study in this setting reduces diagnostic accuracy. Cystoscopy and retrograde pyelography are performed when indicated in individual cases.

Treatment

The prognosis for patients with MAP stones has improved considerably with better-coordinated and more sophisticated medical and surgical approaches to the disease. In a recent series of patients with pure MAP stones, a meticulous medical-surgical approach rendered over 90 percent of patients stone- and infection-free after a mean follow-up period of 7 years.[55] This optimistic report is tempered by the fact that the general experience has been for stone recurrence rates to average 30 percent, with 40 percent of patients experiencing recurrent infections.[51]

For patients with MAP stones complicating a metabolic stone diathesis, less specific data are available. In Smith's experience, in which 50 percent of patients with MAP stones were found to have an underlying metabolic disorder, the prognosis was good when all stone material was removed at the time of surgery; 81 percent of such patients remained stone-free.[52]

The management of underlying metabolic disorders in patients with MAP stones does not differ from that in patients lacking infection-stone complications. Metabolic screening and institution of appropriate therapy should be performed before surgical removal of stone material is attempted.

Antimicrobial therapy should be individualized; the approach differs at different times in a given patient's course. Short-term antibiotic administration virtually never eliminates infection in the continued presence of an MAP stone.[53] In preparation for surgery, culture-specific bactericidal drugs are begun 24 to 48 h before the procedure and continued for 10 to 14 days after all urological devices are removed. Patients considered to be free of stone material and infection after surgery are generally maintained on either low-dose bactericidal agents or broad-spectrum drugs for 6 to 12 months, with serial 1- to 3-month urine cultures during treatment. However, in one recent series, stopping antibiotics after only two weeks in stone-free patients had no adverse consequences.[55] Careful follow-up after antimicrobial drugs are discontinued is essential. Patients with retained MAP stone material postoperatively and those in whom surgery cannot be attempted are treated with long-term antimicrobial therapy. Low-dose, culture-specific bactericidal agents are preferred to broad-spectrum agents by most authorities.[51,53] The attempt in these patients is to render the urine sterile *during* therapy and limit both the growth of stones and the frequency of symptoms of infection; therapy is continued indefinitely. If, in fact, the urine is successfully and permanently sterilized, most recent reports have suggested that patients will remain stable.[56–58] Occasionally, long-term antimicrobial treatment is associated with a reduction in stone mass.[51,53]

Complete removal of all stone material is the goal of surgical therapy and represents the only reliable method of cure in patients with MAP stones. The success of this approach depends in large part on meticulous attention to detail in the immediate peri- and intraoperative periods. The large variability in reported frequency of postoperative stones that persist and/or recur attests to this.

Preoperative antibiotics are essential, as indicated above. The operative approach is individualized based on the anatomy of the patient's collecting system and the configuration of the stone. The major difficulties confronted in attempting complete removal are the typical friability of MAP stones and their tendency to mold to inaccessible areas of the collecting system. These difficulties have led to the introduction of a variety of surgical techniques which are beyond the scope of this chapter. Coagulum lithotomy, irrigation of the renal pelvis and collecting system, nephroscopy, and intraoperative radiographs are all important adjuncts to the surgical procedure. Despite such efforts, up to one-quarter of patients have remaining stone fragments after surgery. For this reason, postoperative plain-film tomography is critically important, and routine placement of a nephrotomy tube at the time of surgery has been advocated to permit postoperative irrigation with solutions designed to dissolve remaining stone fragments.[55] Particularly difficult procedures may result in a partial or complete nephrectomy.

The recent application of percutaneous and extracorporeal lithotripsy to upper urinary tract stones (see below) may totally change the surgical management of patients with MAP stones. It is possible that a combination of these two procedures may become the treatment of choice in the not too distant future.[59,60]

Medical approaches designed to limit the growth of MAP stones or to attempt dissolution of stone material include the *Shorr regimen* and the use of *urease inhibitors*. Except perhaps in the setting of MAP stone formation complicated by chronic renal failure, the Shorr regimen is little used today.[53]

Since the production of urease by the offending organism is the key pathogenic event in MAP stone formation, there has been long-standing interest in the development of enzyme-specific inhibitors. Acetohydroxamic acid, a potent urease inhibitor, has recently been approved for use in this country. In a series of nonrandomized studies, the drug has been reported to stabilize or decrease the size of preexisting MAP stones and prevent formation of stones in some patients with chronic urinary tract infections due to urease-producing organisms.[58,61,62]

In a recently completed randomized trial in which 20 patients took the drug for an average of 20 months, no patient in the drug-treatment group showed a doubling of stone size, while 7 of 19 placebo-treated patients did.[63] The drug has been associated with several side effects, including phlebitis, thromboembolism, hemolytic anemia, and iron deficiency anemia, as well as headache and nervousness. The usual dosage is 10 to 15 mg per kilogram of body weight divided into three or four oral doses. The maximal daily dose is 1.5 g. Patients with mild renal insufficiency require lower doses, and patients with significant renal failure should not receive the drug.

CALCIUM PHOSPHATE STONES

Although calcium phosphate in the form of hydroxyapatite is a common minority constituent in the "garden-variety" mixed calcium stone, pure calcium phosphate stones represent only a few percent of all stones (Table 25-1). Calcium phosphate stones are given separate status here in order to emphasize certain unique aspects of their pathogenesis and because their identification by crystallographic analysis often provides an important diagnostic clue in the search for the basis of stone formation in an individual patient.

The importance of an alkaline pH in producing calcium phosphate supersaturation was discussed under Physical Chemical Aspects and is illustrated in Fig. 25-4. The physical chemical milieu favoring calcium phosphate stone formation can be reproduced in vitro simply by alkalinization of a normal, sterile urine specimen. This physical chemical milieu differs from that which leads to the formation of MAP stones (see preceding section). Therefore, the discovery of a pure calcium phosphate stone suggests that an underlying disorder exists which is associated with a sterile but persistently alkaline urine.

Pathogenesis

The process of renal acidification normally maintains the pH of the extracellular fluids within the physiological range in two ways: by reclaiming the filtered load of bicarbonate in its entirety and by excreting a quantity of acid equal to the daily systemic production of nonvolatile acid.[3,64] The proximal tubular reabsorptive mechanism is a high-capacity system which reabsorbs some 90 percent of the filtered bicarbonate. The distal tubular mechanism is a low-capacity, high-gradient system which reabsorbs the remaining quantity of bicarbonate and fixes the final urinary pH. The gradient of the distal process is sufficient to achieve a pH of 5.0 or less; it enables the kidney to excrete ammonium and titratable acid in quantities sufficient to balance the systemic production of acid and regenerate the bicarbonate consumed in buffering the daily production of nonvolatile acid.

Renal tubular acidosis is a rare but important cause of pure calcium phosphate stone formation.[3,64,65] There are several types of RTA, but only patients with the distal (classic or type 1) form are at appreciable risk for stones. Patients with complete distal RTA typically present with systemic hyperchloremic acidosis and persistently alkaline urine. Calcium phosphate nephrolithiasis and/or nephrocalcinosis has been reported to occur in over 50 percent of patients;[65] nephrocalcinosis is more common than nephrolithiasis. Rickets or osteomalacia occurs with severe or long-standing disease, although evidence of bone disease was uncommon in a recent series.[65]

The exact nature of the defect in distal tubular acidification is unknown, but affected patients are only rarely capable of generating a urinary pH less than 5.5. Patients with proximal (type 2 or bicarbonate-losing) RTA typically present with systemic hyperchloremic acidosis and osteopenia, rickets, or osteomalacia. The distal acidification mechanism is normal in these patients, and stones do not occur. Proximal RTA is also frequently associated with aminoaciduria, glycosuria, and other elements of the Fanconi syndrome, features which are lacking in patients with distal RTA.

The pathogenesis of distal RTA remains largely unknown. A familial form with an autosomal dominant pattern of inheritance presents in childhood as growth retardation, rickets, and nephrocalcinosis or nephrolithiasis. Eighth-nerve deafness and RTA in association with an autosomal recessive pattern of inheritance has also been reported. Sjögren's syndrome and other hyperglobulinemic states are prominent causes of acquired distal RTA in adults. Rare causes include MSK, amphotericin B administration, obstructive uropathy, and a wide variety of miscellaneous conditions.[3] No pathogenetic unifying link between these various disorders and the distal acidification defect in RTA is apparent.

Patient Populations at Risk

Patients with distal RTA usually display multiple risk factors for calcium phosphate stone formation. The most consistent and obvious abnormality is the persistently alkaline urinary pH, which is usually relatively fixed at 5.5 or above. Acidosis inhibits the production of citrate in the renal cortex, so that a reduced citrate excretion rate is regularly observed in patients with RTA.[66] Citrate is normally responsible for binding a significant fraction of urinary calcium in the form of soluble complexes. The majority of patients are also hypercalciuric. At least two mechanisms contribute to the hypercalciuria. The systemic acidosis is buffered to some extent in bone, leading to bone mineral dissolution and the mobilization of both calcium and phosphate ions. In addition, renal tubular calcium reabsorption is reduced in patients with distal RTA, possibly as a result of an acidosis-induced defect in calcium reabsorption in the distal nephron.[3] Intestinal calcium absorption is usually normal or decreased in patients with RTA. Mild hypophosphatemia with a reduced renal phosphate threshold (TmP/GFR) is common in patients with RTA for reasons which are not entirely clear; parathyroid function tests have been variously reported to be depressed, normal, or elevated in these patients. Thus, the principal risk factors for stone formation in distal RTA are alkaline urine, reduced citrate excretion, and hypercalciuria.

RTA is described as *complete* when systemic acidosis accompanies the acidification defect and *incomplete* when the process is not of sufficient severity to produce systemic acidosis. Incomplete distal RTA is far more common in stone-forming patients than is complete RTA; it can be identified by acid-loading studies in approximately 5 percent of patients with recurrent stones. A recent Swedish series of 518 consecutive patients with stone disease reported a prevalence of incomplete distal RTA of 7 percent.[67] Several other smaller series have emphasized the association of incomplete distal RTA and recurrent calcium phosphate stone formation.[68–70] In some patients, the defect appears to be a result of tubular damage resulting from severe stone disease, MSK, staghorn calculi, or associated pyelonephritis. In other patients, the tubular acidification defect is not associated with structural abnormalities and appears to be the primary cause for renal stone formation.[67,71]

The mechanisms by which this partial defect contributes to the formation of kidney stones appear to be qualitatively similar to, although quantitatively less severe than, those observed in patients with the complete syndrome. Thus, relatively alkaline urine, hypercalciuria, and hypocitraturia are all commonly observed in patients with incomplete RTA.[67–72]

Acetazolamide is a noncompetitive carbonic anhydrase inhibitor now used primarily in the treatment of glaucoma. The principal action of the drug is to inhibit bicarbonate reabsorption in the proximal tubule, but it also inhibits citrate production, decreases excretion of ammonia and titratable acid, and raises urinary pH, producing, in essence, an "exogenous" RTA.[73] The proximal tubular action is associated both with lowering of TmP/GFR and acute phosphaturia, but the rate of steady-state phosphate excretion is unaltered. Approximately 5 to 10 percent of patients receiving acetazolamide develop pure calcium phosphate stones. Patients with other risk factors for calcium stone formation, such as coincident hypercalciuria, are presumably at greater risk, but this has not been established by prospective study.

"Alkali abuse" is a rare cause of calcium phosphate stone formation. The milk-alkali syndrome (see Chap. 23) is associated with nephrocalcinosis and azotemia, although on occasion nephrolithiasis has been reported.[74] Prolonged, low-dose ingestion of calcium carbonate or sodium bicarbonate can predispose to calcium phosphate nephrolithiasis; several examples of this association have been observed.

Patients with primary hyperparathyroidism, sarcoidosis, and vitamin D intoxication may form pure calcium phosphate stones. Although patients with primary hyperparathyroidism appear, as a group, to form stones with an increased percentage of calcium phosphate, calcium oxalate and mixed stones are the usual finding in these patients.[75] The putative relationship between the effects of parathyroid hormone (PTH) on proximal tubular bicarbonate handling and predisposition to calcium phosphate stone formation is discussed in Chap. 23.

There are no large reported series of patients with pure or predominantly calcium phosphate stones. Of 363 consecutive patients seen in a renal stone clinic, 5 percent formed pure calcium phosphate stones. As a whole, these patients tended to have higher fasting urinary pH values on presentation as well as a higher minimal urinary pH on serial testing. In one-half of the patients, a specific etiology could be established: five patients had distal RTA, two were ingesting absorbable alkali, one patient was taking acetazolamide, and one patient had primary hyperparathyroidism.

Diagnosis and Treatment

Calcium phosphate stones are specifically identifiable only by crystallographic analysis. Radiographically, pure calcium phosphate, pure calcium oxalate, and mixed calcium oxalate–calcium phosphate stones cannot be distinguished. Calcium phosphate stones should be suspected particularly in patients with coincident nephrocalcinosis and in pediatric patients with radiopaque calculi. Eliciting the medication history in patients with stone disease should always include specific questioning regarding acetazolamide or antacid intake.

Clinically, measuring urinary pH is the front-line screening test for predisposition to calcium phosphate stone formation. In the presence of a urea-splitting infection, pH results are uninterpretable. If, in a spot early morning check, urinary pH is 5.5 or less, complete RTA can be ruled out. Patients with a pH of 6.0 or greater on initial evaluation may be given a roll of nitrazine paper in order to record serially their urinary pH. This simple maneuver documents a normal acidification ability in the vast majority of patients and avoids acid-loading studies in all but a small percentage of patients. Serum electrolytes should be measured in patients with initial urine pH values of 6.0 or greater.

The principal goal of diagnosis is to identify patients with complete RTA, a destructive but eminently treatable disorder. The diagnosis is usually straightforward on clinical and routine laboratory grounds. Borderline laboratory results require acid-loading studies for clarification. The "acute" acid load is most commonly used; this consists of the oral administration of 0.1 g of ammonium chloride per kilogram of body weight, with baseline and hourly measurements of urinary pH, venous blood pH, and P_{CO_2} for 6 h.[3] A nonabsorbable antacid should be coadministered to prevent gastric irritation and vomiting. The induced acidosis normally reduces the urinary pH to less than 5.3. Incomplete RTA is diagnosed on the basis of normal serum electrolyte concentrations and inability to acidify the urine maximally on acid loading. Borderline acid-loading results are, unfortunately, not uncommon. In those patients who cannot tolerate the abrupt acid load and/or in those who give equivocal results in response to this test, a "long" acid loading test over three consecutive days can be employed.[71] This test can be performed on an outpatient basis.

The diagnosis of the other conditions associated with calcium phosphate stone formation is achieved by routine clinical and laboratory means. As noted above, crystallographic stone analysis may provide the initial clue that initiates the search for the appropriate underlying disorder.

Patients with complete distal RTA are treated with alkali in quantities sufficient to normalize the serum bicarbonate concentration. In adults, this quantity is usually approximately 1 meq per kilogram of body weight daily, equivalent to the production rate of nonvolatile acid. In children, the acid production rate and dosage requirements are several times higher.[76] The alkali is administered in four to six divided doses daily. Sodium bicarbonate tablets are inexpensive and effective, but many physicians and some patients prefer Shohl's solution or other citrate preparations (Shohl's solution is an equimolar mixture of citric acid and citrate, providing 1 meq of base per ml). Potassium citrate salts are also available (see Table 25-2).

Alkalinization has a dramatic effect on bone involvement and can restore a normal growth rate in children.[76] When present, hypercalciuria is reduced or eliminated, and the excretion of citrate is normalized. Recent evidence indicates that prompt diagnosis and treatment can prevent the development of nephrocalcinosis and stones in children. Renal complications in adults can also probably be reduced by alkalinization. In a recent small series of patients with distal RTA, oral potassium citrate therapy was shown to prevent new stone formation during a 34-month trial period.[70] However, extensive bilateral nephrocalcinosis and stone disease are quite common at the time of diagnosis; this stone burden may complicate the assessment of response to therapy. It is extremely important to emphasize this point to the patient, in order to prevent discouragement and noncompliance. Patients with distal RTA do not display the degree of renal potassium wastage that characterizes proximal RTA. However, many patients with distal RTA require potassium supplements when alkali therapy is initiated, and serum potassium concentration must be closely monitored.

CALCIUM OXALATE AND MIXED CALCIUM STONES

General Considerations

Approximiately 75 percent of upper tract stones in industrialized countries are calcium stones (Table 25-1). About one-half of these stones are composed of pure calcium oxalate, and one-half are mixed calcium oxalate–calcium phosphate stones. The calcium oxalate crystals may exist as either the monohydrate (whewellite) or the dihydrate (weddellite) species; more commonly, a mixture of the two is present.

The relative importance of the calcium oxalate and calcium phosphate components in mixed stones with regard to crystal nucleation and/or growth is unknown, but the calcium phosphate content of these stones appears to be a reflection of the ambient pH in stone-forming urine.[2,77] The percentage of all calcium stones which are pure calcium phosphate stones as well as the percentage calcium phosphate content in mixed calcium stones appear to have fallen in recent years;[78] this has been attributed to altered dietary habits, particularly a change in the intake of animal protein (see below).[79] Affected males outnumber females by three or four to one. There is a broad peak of calcium stone occurrence covering the middle four decades of life (Fig. 25-1).

Calcium stones are predominantly an affliction of industrialized nations. The incidence of calcium stone disease in western populations appears to have been increasing steadily during the past several decades.[1,79] Males are bearing the brunt of this increase, such that the male/female ratio of affected patients has changed from 1.8:1.0 in 1954 to 3.8:1.0 in 1970.[1] Some 12 percent of males experience one or more stone events by age 70, whereas the comparable figure in females is less than 5 percent.[1]

The reason(s) for the increasing incidence of calcium stones in the population in general and in men in particular is unknown, but there is evidence that dietary habits are playing a major role.[79] Surveys in the United Kingdom have emphasized the intake of animal protein (meat, poultry, and fish) as the primary dietary variable related to the increased incidence of calcium oxalate stones; the intake of calcium, oxalate, magnesium, and carbohydrate appears to be relatively unimportant.[79] The putative importance of the intake of animal protein in this regard is supported by several additional observations: (1) the amount of animal protein in the diet is a direct function of affluence, thereby explaining the frequency of calcium stone disease in the west, and (2) dietary protein is known to increase calcium, uric acid, and, possibly, oxalate excretion and also to lead to reduced urinary pH, all factors which would tend to predispose to calcium oxalate stones rather than other stone types.[79] An additional dietary factor which may be important in at least a subpopulation of hypercalciuric patients is sodium (see Hypercalciuria, below).

Although the epidemiological and other evidence marshalled in support of this dietary hypothesis for the predominance and increasing incidence of calcium oxalate stones in the west should not be viewed as having established firm cause-and-effect relationships, the hypothesis clearly has merit and should be kept in mind while considering the risk factors for calcium oxalate stone formation (see below).

The concept of high-prevalence "stone belts" in the United States derives largely from the survey of Boyce et al.[80] This survey covered nationwide hospital admissions for stone disease for the years 1948 through 1952. The authors concluded that the prevalence of stone disease in the population varied by as much as fivefold in different geographic regions, with the southeastern United States being the principal stone belt. A more recent study of similar design yielded a somewhat different distribution of high-prevalence regions,[81] although both studies pinpointed the eastern half of the country as a generalized stone belt.[80,81]

The natural history of calcium stone disease is

complex. It appears to be widely assumed that the majority of patients do not experience a stone recurrence and are therefore single-stone formers; even in recurrent stone formers, stone disease is believed to improve in untreated patients with the passage of time. Both these assumptions are probably incorrect.

The published frequency of stone recurrence in patients after an initial stone episode appears to be largely a function of the length of patient follow-up. Several studies have reported that 40 to 50 percent of males and some 20 percent of females experience stone recurrence within 5 years of the initial stone episode and that the percentage recurrence steadily increases with the length of follow-up.[1,3,82] In one series in which patients were followed for more than 20 years, stone recurrence approached 100 percent.[82] In addition, diagnostic findings and patterns of abnormalities in several recent studies of single-stone formers have been very similar to those observed in patients with recurrent stone disease. The authors were led to conclude that single-stone formers were simply being seen early in the course of an inherently active disease.[83,84] This does not necessarily mean that all patients should be treated in the same fashion (see below).

As effectively argued by Coe, the frequency of stone recurrence in the population at risk is a somewhat misleading statistic as regards the natural history of stone disease in recurrent stone formers.[3] In patients with recurrent stone disease, estimates of the recurrence rate (e.g., stones per patient-year) or intervals between stone recurrences provide a more meaningful clinical assessment of the natural history of stone formation. This distinction is hardly a matter of statistical semantics, for when patients with recurrent stone disease are assessed on the basis of the time interval between stone recurrences, stone disease appears to worsen rather than improve with time.[3] The usual method of plotting the percentage recurrence of stones hides this fact because patients with recurrent stone disease are eliminated from the population at risk at the time of their first recurrent stone episode.[3]

Thus, it appears that the majority of patients with calcium stone disease experience at least one stone recurrence during life and that the subset of patients with recurrent stone disease has an inherently active basic disease process. Both these aspects of natural history are germane to (1) the consideraton of metabolic screening in patients with a single stone event, (2) the initiation of treatment in patients with one or more stone recurrences, and (3) the proposed duration of therapy in patients with recurrent stone disease. At present, there are no absolute rules concerning these three issues. Rather it is preferable to approach patients individually, on the basis of age and the assessment of stone-related morbidity. This assessment is best achieved by considering the five criteria described early in this chapter.

The term *recurrent stone former* is itself somewhat vague and is not defined by an absolute number or rate of stone recurrences. A portrait of the typical patient with recurrent calcium stone disease is perhaps more useful than is any attempt at a standardized definition. The usual patient is male and the onset of stone disease came in his midthirties. He has experienced four stone episodes at a rate of 45 stones per 100 patients per year.[3] Each 100 stone episodes necessitates 25 hospitalizations, 15 cystoscopies, and 15 surgical procedures.[3] One-third of patients have a family history of stone disease, so stone disease may have afflicted one or more first-degree relatives of the typical patient. The patient has been told to drink fluids and avoid dairy products. He may or may not be receiving empirical treatment for stone disease. His compliance has been reasonable, but he has been poorly educated with respect to the principles of therapy. Often, he is discouraged by an apparent lack of therapeutic efficacy, and is searching for expert advice and management. He will be found to be an unusually cooperative and grateful patient. In approximately 80 to 90 percent of such patients, a meticulous evaluation reveals one or more risk factors which predispose to calcium stone formation. The outlook for prevention of further stone recurrences is excellent.

The concepts of saturation chemistry clearly apply to calcium stone formation, but a single discrete biochemical abnormality, such as defines cystine oversaturation and the disease cystinuria, is not observed in patients with calcium stone disease. The essential physical chemical feature of calcium oxalate requiring emphasis is its extreme insolubility in aqueous solution (Fig. 25-2). As already emphasized, this fact is presumably responsible for the overall frequency of calcium stones in the population and may, in general, provide an intuitive framework for considering calcium stone formation as the end result of the interplay of a variety of risk factors, some of which have no direct bearing on calcium or oxalate metabolism.

The risk factors which predispose to calcium stone formation are listed in Table 25-5. They may be broken down into two categories: (1) those which are of general importance but which are poorly understood and/or confer only a vague statistical risk for stone formation in individual patients (e.g., a family history) and (2) the "big four" treatable risk factors, most of which have been extensively studied and which confer a definite risk for stone formation in individual patients in a quantitative fashion (e.g., hypercalciuria, see Fig. 25-12). These risk factors are

Table 25-5. Risk Factors for Calcium Stone Formation

A. General issues and/or risk factors
   1. Positive family history
   2. Medications
   3. Urinary pH
   4. Diet
B. Specific, treatable risk factors
   1. Low urine volume
   2. Hypercalciuria
   3. Hyperoxaluria
   4. Hyperuricosuria
   5. ? Hypocitraturia

discussed individually below. The thrust of the discussion is toward the evaluation and treatment of individual patients.[85] However, the risk factor concept applies equally well to the statistical analysis of data from populations of stone-forming patients.[77]

Family History

A family history of renal stones in one or more first-degree relatives (parents, siblings, offspring) is found in 35 to 50 percent of patients with calcium stone disease.[86,87] The most striking associaton is noted in male first-degree relatives of both male and female patients, in whom the risk for stone formation may be five to ten times that of the general population. Indeed, the lifetime risk for brothers of propositi approaches 50 percent.[86] The history of calcium stone disease in kindreds does not appear to differ from that in the stone-forming population as a whole, with a similar mix of single- and recurrent stone-forming individuals.

This striking familial tendency to form calcium stones is almost entirely unexplained. The large survey of Resnick et al. provided evidence for a polygenic pattern, suggesting that multiple hereditary and/or environmental factors might be involved.[86] Specific disorders with an autosomal dominant or recessive inheritance pattern, such as RTA, the familial forms of hyperparathyroidism, and the primary hyperoxalurias are far too rare to account for more than a small percentage of affected family members. There have been no other reported kindreds similar to that described by Buckalew et al.,[88] in which there were patients with hypercalciuria, some with renal tubular acidosis, and some with both disorders.

Coe et al. screened the families of nine patients presenting with hypercalciuria and calcium stone disease.[87] Of 44 first-degree relatives, 19 (43 percent) were found to be hypercalciuric, suggesting an autosomal dominant mode of inheritance. A history of renal stones was also frequent in these first-degree relatives, but the history of stone disease and the presence of hypercalciuria were curiously unrelated; essentially equal percentages of normocalciuric and hypercalciuric relatives reported a history of stones.[87] Another interesting feature of this study was the clear age-association of a history of stones: only one of nine first-degree relatives less than 20 years of age had a stone history, as compared to 18 of 35 adults.[87]

Renal stones are uncommon in the pediatric age group; this subject is not treated separately in this

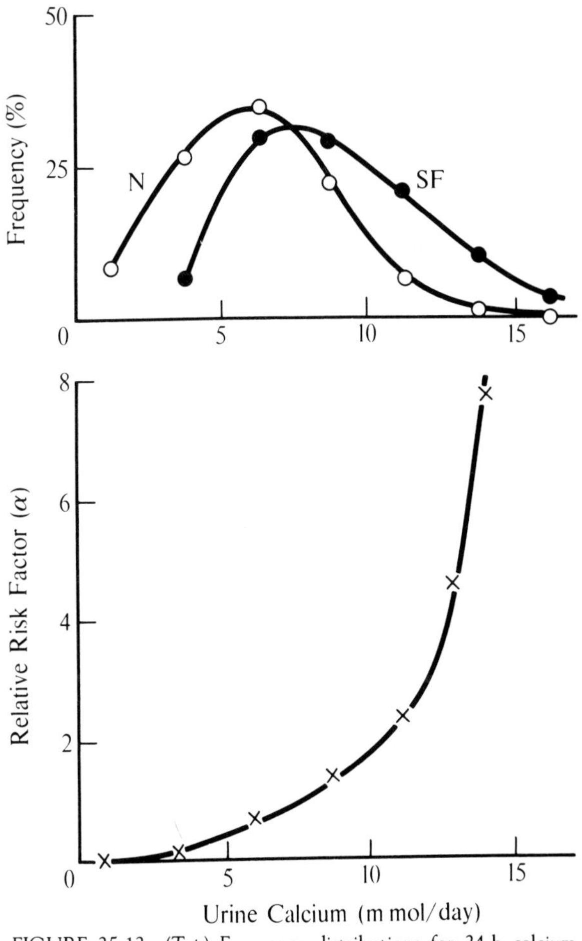

FIGURE 25-12 (*Top*) Frequency distributions for 24-h calcium excretion in normal subjects (N) and patients with recurrent calcium stones (SF) are shown in the top panel. Although the curves for both populations appear to be skewed to the right, the upper ranges are, in fact, normally distributed; it is the paucity of low excretion rates which distorts the curves. (*Bottom*) Plot of relative risk factor or ratio (α) as a function of increasing calcium excretion rates (α is the ratio of the frequency of stone patients divided by the frequency of normal subjects at each level of calcium excretion). This plot reveals a clear quantitative and statistical risk for stone formation as a function of the degree of hypercalciuria. (*From Robertson et al,*[77] *by permission of the British Journal of Urology.*)

chapter. One recent study, however, merits review. In this study, 23 of 83 children presenting with gross or microscopic hematuria were found to be hypercalciuric; mean values for calcium excretion rates in the hypercalciuric and normocalciuric subgroups of these 83 children were 5.8 mg per kilogram of body weight per day and 1.6 mg/kg per day, respectively (vs. an upper limit of normal of 4.0 mg/kg per day).[89] A striking family history of stone disease was found in the hypercalciuric, but not normocalciuric, children. Further, an individual child with both gross hematuria and a family history of stones on presentation had an 86 percent likelihood of being found to be hypercalciuric. Only 2 of the 23 hypercalciuric children had actual stone disease, so that a definite cause-and-effect relationship between the hematuria and hypercalciuria could not be established. Nevertheless, the implications of this study are interesting, in view of the family history relationships and the age-related findings of Coe et al. noted above.

The family history information from patients seen at the renal stone clinic at Yale has recently been summarized. This experience included 206 patients with common calcium stone disease (i.e., patients with primary causes of stones were excluded from analysis). The information was obtained by direct patient contact with first-degree relatives rather than simply by patient recall (perhaps accounting for the rather high percentages noted below).

A history of stone disease in one or more first-degree relatives was found in 104 (50 percent) of these patients. It is of particular interest to analyze this information as a function of identified risk factors for stone formation in individual patients, the three principal risk factors being low urine volume, hyperuricosuria, and hypercalciuria. This was done by isolating subpopulations of patients who displayed a single risk factor and excluding patients who displayed a combination of risk factors. A family history was found in 17 (71 percent) of 24 patients with low urine volume, 13 (62 percent) of 21 patients with hyperuricosuria, 25 (50 percent) of 50 patients with hypercalciuria, and 24 (41 percent) of 58 patients in whom no risk factor could be identified. These findings complement those of Resnick et al. concerning a putative polygenic pattern of inheritance; they indicate that the inherited and/or environmental risks are both multifactorial and complex.[86]

Medications

Vitamin A and vitamin D intoxication and the milk-alkali syndrome are described in detail in Chap. 23. All three conditions are characterized by hypercalcemia, nephrocalcinosis, and azotemia and are only rarely associated with actual renal stone formation. Patients with chronic hypoparathyroidism maintained on vitamin D and calcium supplements are at definite risk for calcium stones and should be managed according to the principles outlined in Chap. 23 in order to prevent this complication. The potential for calcium phosphate stone formation associated with acetazolamide use was already described (see Calcium Phosphate Stones).

Ascorbic acid is oxidized in the liver to yield oxalate (see Hyperoxaluria, below). Large doses of ascorbic acid (4 g or more daily) have been reported to lead to an increase in urinary oxalate excretion, although there is considerable disagreement as to both the reproducibility and significance of this effect.[90,91] There is little evidence that vitamin C intake poses a threat for calcium oxalate stone formation in individuals without a history of stone disease, but there have been reports of exacerbation of calcium oxalate stone disease in patients with a history of stones.[90,91] It is probably prudent to discourage the use of vitamin C in any amount in patients with clearly active stone disease or a significant stone burden. Large doses of ascorbic acid are also uricosuric, but whether this effect potentiates the risk for uric acid or calcium stone formation is unknown.

Urinary pH

The solubility of calcium oxalate in aqueous solution is not influenced by alterations in pH over the physiological range, so that urinary acidity or alkalinity confers no risk for pure calcium oxalate stone formation. The impact of urinary alkalinity on calcium phosphate solubility and stone formation was described in Calcium Phosphate Stones, above. Robertson et al. have reported that the 24-h urinary pH is significantly higher in patients with mixed calcium oxalate–calcium phosphate stones than in normal subjects or patients with pure calcium oxalate stones,[77] suggesting that alkaline urine poses an additional risk for the formation and/or growth of mixed stones. Whether or not a significant number of patients with mixed calcium stones have an underlying defect in urinary acidification is unknown. Acidification measures are not generally advocated in patients with mixed stones and are certainly contraindicated in any patient in whom incomplete RTA has not been carefully excluded. As noted above, the frequency of pure calcium phosphate stones as well as the percentage of calcium phosphate in mixed calcium stones has fallen in the past several decades; this has been attributed to changing dietary patterns and may reflect, in part, a reduction in urinary pH.[78,79]

Diet

The diet history is a potentially important part of the evaluation of a patient with calcium stone disease.[92] There are two relevant aspects of this history: (1) the search for eating habits which may actually contribute to stone formation and (2) attention to dietary details during metabolic screening so that results can be properly interpreted. An example of the former would be high oxalate intake in a patient with enteric hyperoxaluria; an example of the latter would be failure to detect significant hypercalciuria in a hypercalciuric patient because of a rigidly restricted calcium intake on the day of sample collection. The most important recent developments concerning dietary habits and calcium oxalate stone disease include the animal protein intake hypothesis to explain the increasing frequency of calcium oxalate stones (see above), recent data concerning sodium-induced hypercalciuria (see Hypercalciuria, below), and the hyperuricosuria which results from a high-purine diet (see Hyperuricosuria, below).

Low Urine Volume

Dehydration poses an obvious risk for all types of stone formation and has been implicated in the frequency of stone formation in arid regions.[2,3,5,6,8] Low urine volume has long been recognized as a factor contributing to stone formation in certain clinical settings (e.g., in a patient with an ileostomy and uric acid stones). Most authorities, however, have not recognized or emphasized low urine volume as an independent risk factor for the formation of calcium stones. This appears to have been an important omission.

In screening 282 consecutive patients with common calcium stones, an initial urine volume less than 1 l/day (an arbitrary limit) was observed in 51 patients (18 percent). The average urine volume in these 51 patients was 805 ml/day, less than half the mean volume (1783 ml/day) observed in the remaining patients; urine volumes in the 400 to 600 ml/day range were not uncommon. The male/female ratio (about 3:1) was the same as that in the general population of patients with calcium stone disease. Thirty-one of these patients, or 11 percent of the 282 patients screened, had no other identifiable risk factor for stone formation. In these 31 patients, the mean values for calcium and uric acid excretion on a "free" (i.e., chosen ad libitum) diet were 159 mg/day and 516 mg/day, respectively. These values are impressively normal; by inference, they support the importance of low urine volume as an independent risk factor for stone formation. Although there were a few patients with low urine volume whose occupations might be associated with prolonged periods without fluid intake (e.g., long-distance truckers), most patients simply seemed to avoid fluids habitually for reasons which were inapparent. Virtually 100 percent of these patients recalled having been previously instructed to force fluids.

The fact that the calcium oxalate system lies close to its formation product in normal urine (Fig. 25-2) provides a reasonable explanation for why low urine volume might have a particular impact on calcium stone formation. Pak et al. demonstrated that dilution both decreases the APR and increases the FPR of calcium stone constituents in urine,[93] providing additional physical chemical support for viewing a low urine volume as an independent risk factor for calcium stone disease.

The identification of and therapeutic approach to such patients are self-evident. Unfortunately, the subgroup of patients that habitually avoids fluids tends to be very resistant to repeated instructions regarding hydration. Failure to increase urine volume has been shown to be predictive of stone recurrence.[94]

Hypercalciuria

An association between hypercalciuria and calcium stone formation was initially reported by Flocks in 1939.[95] He noted that a group of patients with calcium stone disease exhibited higher rates of calcium excretion than did normal subjects on both calcium-restricted and high-calcium intakes, a finding that has since been reproduced by numerous investigators. The term *idiopathic hypercalciuria* was introduced by Albright in 1953,[96] and the clinical population so defined was reported in detail by Henneman et al. in 1958.[97] The latter paper is a key historical reference, in that it both defined the descriptive or operational use of the term idiopathic hypercalciuria and broached the question of pathogenesis, thus initiating a controversy that has continued to the present day. The term idiopathic hypercalciuria was used to describe patients with calcium stone disease and a triad of apparent abnormalities: normocalcemic hypercalciuria, a tendency to hypophosphatemia, and frequent urinary tract infections. The latter finding was spurious (*Staphylococcus albus* was the organism frequently "identified") but was a central feature of Henneman and coworkers' pathogenetic argument. They reasoned that the primary abnormality in their patients was a pyelonephritis-induced defect in renal tubular calcium reabsorption, leading to hypercalciuria, secondary hyperparathyroidism, and a consequent tendency to hypophosphatemia. They also presented evidence for increased intestinal calcium absorption in these patients but interpreted this finding as a secondary response to the renal "leak" of calcium. It is of particular interest to note that 11 of the 35 patients reported had previously undergone a parathyroid exploration with negative results, so that central to the description of idiopathic hypercalciuria as a distinct entity was the fact that the investigators were convinced that the patients did not have subtle primary hyperparathyroidism. In essence, therefore, the Henneman et al. paper introduced the key elements of the controversy which has continued unabated for the subsequent 25 years concerning the pathogenetic primacy and criteria for diagnosis of "renal" hypercalciuria, "absorptive" hypercalciuria, and subtle or "normocalcemic" primary hyperparathyroidism.

Hypercalciuria is a difficult subject; the literature cannot be summarized in a truly harmonious fashion. In part, this reflects the complexity of the putative pathogenetic mechanisms responsible for hypercalciuria, and, in part, it reflects the fact that many published series are flawed in terms of design, methodology, and/or interpretation. Nevertheless, there has been substantial progress in the past 5 years, and cause-and-effect relationships in more than 90 percent of hypercalciuric patients evaluated in the renal stone clinic at Yale can be established. These relationships include not only such well-characterized syndromes as absorptive hypercalciuria but also more recently described categories of hypercalciuria such as "dietary" hypercalciuria and "constitutional" hypercalciuria (see below). In the following discussion, particular attention should be paid to: (1) the limits employed in defining hypercalciuria and the fact that the limits established for calcium excretion expressed on an absolute basis (mg/day) are not necessarily interchangeable with those expressed on a weight basis (mg per kilogram of body weight per day) in individual patients, (2) the impact of dietary influences on both the detection and definition of hypercalciuria, the most critical influences in this regard being calcium and sodium, (3) the failure of certain widely used criteria for differential diagnosis to stand up under scrutiny (e.g., classification based on results for fasting calcium excretion), and (4) the importance of conditions of study to the collection and interpretation of metabolic data in hypercalciuric patients. Together, these four points explain much of the controversy which has plagued the literature.

DEFINITION, DETECTION, AND INCIDENCE OF HYPERCALCIURIA

The seemingly simple issue of defining hypercalciuria and estimating its frequency in patients with calcium stone disease has been a matter of some consternation. The problems and variables involved are many; they include (1) the use of multiple arbitrary and inconsistent definitions of hypercalciuria in the literature, (2) reported differences in the pattern of calcium excretion in the population from one locale to another, (3) the influence of dietary factors other than calcium on the rate of calcium excretion, and (4) the difficulty of assigning a statistical upper limit of calcium excretion in the normal population because of an apparent upward skew of values in this population (Fig. 25-12).[2,3,5,6,8,77,85,98–103] Of these various issues, dietary influences are by far the most important, as discussed in detail below.

In general, the literature consists of reports of studies confined to outpatients and employing almost exclusively a free diet for metabolic screening and reports of inpatient studies in which rigidly defined "metabolic" diets are employed. Each of these approaches reflects a bias. Those evaluating outpatients on an ad libitum diet regard this as the only clinically relevant approach, since (1) patients develop their stone disease on their habitual diets and (2) dietary factors may play some role in the causation of hypercalciuria and/or stones. Those employing metabolic diets and performing predominantly inpatient studies point out that only controlled studies are likely to generate consistent data in an area as complex to study as hypercalciuria. In fact, the biases inherent in both approaches are quite reasonable, even on intuitive grounds; these two approaches should not be regarded as mutually exclusive. Rather, a clear understanding of the hypercalciurias requires that elements of both approaches be employed: patients should be screened on a free diet, but they should also be screened under more defined conditions, and studies aimed at elucidating the details of pathogenesis must be conducted under carefully controlled conditions.

During the past 8 years in the renal stone clinic at Yale, the results of the metabolic screening of outpatients on unregulated diets have been systematically compared with those from patients on a defined metabolic diet (containing 1 g of calcium, 1 g of protein per kilogram of body weight, and 100 meq of sodium per day).[104] Patients were asked to arrive for their first visit armed with the urine specimen collected while on a free diet together with diet history forms corresponding to this collection. During this first visit, the patients were instructed to follow a defined diet containing a high normal amount of calcium. Twenty-four-hour urine specimens were collected while patients were on this diet on an outpatient basis over the next several days. The defined diet is easily constructed (see Testing, below) and is designed to maximize the ability to detect hypercalciuria in patients with a true

Table 25-6. Definition, Diagnosis, and Study of Hypercalcemia

Definitions
Calcium excretion in excess of conventional upper limits of normal:*
Absolute excretion rate: 300 mg/day in males, 250 mg/day in females.
Weight-adjusted excretion rate: 4 mg per kilogram of body weight per day in either sex and in children.
Excretion of 4 mg of calcium per kilogram of body weight per day is the single most useful limit.
Approaches to Diagnosis
Free (undefined) diet:
Maximizes ability to appreciate dietary hypercalciuria.
Most useful for detection of low urine volume and hyperuricosuria.
Defined diet with high normal calcium intake (1000 mg/day):
Permits identification of a substantial minority of hypercalciuric patients who would be missed on a free diet.
Hypercalciuria on this diet highly correlated with presence of true underlying abnormalities in calcium metabolism.
Study
Detailed metabolic study of hypercalciuric patients should be preceded by a week or more of a diet restricted in calcium (about 400 mg/day) and sodium (about 100 meq/day).

*These limits may not be interchangeable in individual patients (see text).

underlying defect in calcium metabolism and to minimize other dietary influences.[85,104–106] Certain of these data and their implications for metabolic screening are given in Tables 25-6 and 25-7. A more detailed analysis of these data is included under Classification, below.[104]

As shown in Table 25-7, some patients were hypercalciuric only when on the free diet (group A); some patients were hypercalciuric on both the free and defined diets but demonstrated a moderate to marked reduction in calcium excretion on the defined diet, even though their calcium intake had increased on this diet (group B); some patients displayed an essentially equivalent degree of hypercalciuria on both diets (group C), and some patients were hypercalciuric only on the defined diet (group D). It is readily apparent that dietary factors other than calcium must be contributory to, if not entirely responsible for, the hypercalciuria on the free diet in the first two groups and, conversely, that the hypercalciuria in group D patients would have been missed entirely had they not also been screened on the defined, unrestricted-calcium diet. Only a small minority (< 20 percent) of patients found to be hypercalciuric only on the free diet displayed true abnormalities in mineral metabolism on more detailed investigation, whereas approximately 80 percent of patients found to be hypercalciuric on the defined diet (regardless of results on the free diet) had clear-cut abnormalities (see Classification, below). Hence, hypercalciuria detected on the defined diet is highly correlated with the presence of an underlying systemic error in calcium metabolism.[85,104–106]

Simply stated, to maximize the appreciation of hypercalciuria as a risk factor in all patients with calcium stone disease irrespective of mechanism, patients must be screened on *both* a free diet *and* a defined diet high with normal calcium content. The reasons for this statement are implicit in Table 25-7; they can be restated as follows:

1. The free intake specimen is the critical specimen for screening patients for a number of risk factors for calcium stone formation, including low urine volume, hyperuricosuria, and hypercalciuria.[104] This specimen maximizes the appreciation of dietary hypercalciuria, which would go unnoticed if patients were screened

Table 25-7. Results of Screening 122 Hypercalciuric Patients for Hypercalciuria on a Free or Defined Diet

Diet on which hypercalciuria was detected	Calcium excretion on free diet, mg/day*	Calcium excretion on defined diet, mg/day†	Number of patients
A. Free diet only	334	236	27
B. Both free and defined diets: Calcium excretion fell > 50 mg/day on defined diet	422	331	17
C. Both free and defined diets	354	365	41
D. Defined diet only	224	328	37

*Mean values for sodium excretion on the free diet in the four groups were 190, 214, 172, and 121 meq/day, respectively.
†Defined diet contained 1000 mg of calcium, 100 meq of sodium, and 1 g of protein per kilogram of body weight per day.

only on a defined diet. As shown in Table 25-7, some 22 percent of the total hypercalciuric population was found to express hypercalciuria only on the free diet, and dietary factors other than calcium appeared to play an important role in as many as one-third of all patients (groups A and B in Table 25-7). However, free diet conditions are clearly not optimal for the purposes of detailed study of hypercalciuric patients, in that (1) a large majority of patients found to be hypercalciuric only on their habitual diets appear to be quite normal metabolically on detailed study,[104] and (2) such conditions are entirely undefined, making the interpretation of hormonal or other data very difficult. Stated in another fashion, screening patients on a free diet for hypercalciuria is clinically very important, but constructing a study population solely on the basis of such data and regarding such a population as metabolically homogeneous is a clear-cut deficiency in study design.

2. The defined 1000-mg-calcium diet is designed to maximize the detection of patients with a true underlying defect in calcium metabolism and to minimize dietary influences other than calcium.[85,98,99,104-106] As shown in Table 25-7, as many as 30 percent of all hypercalciuric patients would have escaped detection if screened only on a free diet because they were adhering to a restricted calcium intake at the time of screening. The essential point is straightforward: patients should be screened for hypercalciuria under circumstances which allow their abnormality to be expressed. This point is made in an even more telling fashion in Fig. 25-13. The data in this figure were obtained from normal subjects and hypercalciuric patients on defined diets which differed *only* in the quantity of calcium ingested.[85] In normal individuals, increasing calcium intake from low normal (400 mg/day) to high normal (1000 mg/day) has a modest impact on calcium excretion, with a slope of calcium excretion on calcium intake averaging only about 6 percent (i.e., an increase in 6 mg in the excretion of calcium per 100 mg increase in dietary calcium intake). This modest increment reflects the normally tight control of fractional intestinal calcium absorption exerted by circulating 1,25-dihydroxyvitamin D (1,25-$(OH)_2D$).[85,106] In contrast, the slope of calcium excretion vs. calcium intake is steep in the majority of patients with hypercalciuria and stone disease (about 20 percent). The segregation of these patients from normal subjects therefore tends to be far more clear-cut when they are evaluated on an unrestricted rather than a calcium-restricted intake (Fig. 25-13).[85,99,100,106] This steep slope reflects an increase in fractional intestinal calcium absorption, an abnormality which tends to be demonstrable in most hypercalciuric patients irrespective of pathogenesis. This increase in calcium absorption appears usually to reflect an increase in circulating 1,25-$(OH)_2D$ concentration.[106]

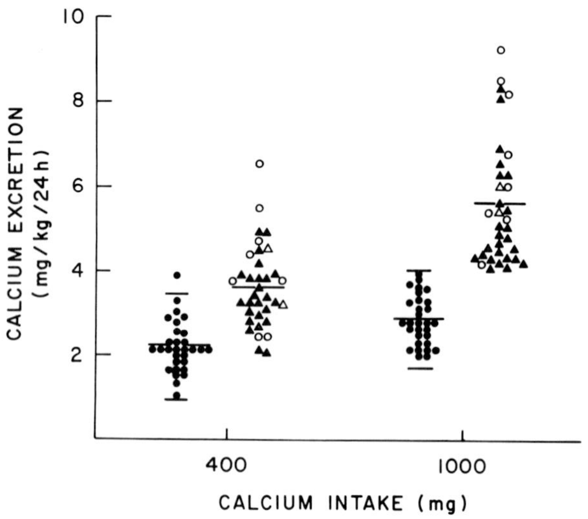

FIGURE 25-13 Urinary calcium excretion determined on both 400- and 1000-mg calcium diets in 30 normal subjects (●), 25 patients with absorptive hypercalciuria (▲), 2 patients with renal hypercalciuria (△), and 8 patients with subtle primary hyperparathyroidism (○). Except for calcium intake, the diets were identical and contained 800 to 1000 mg of phosphorus, 1 g of protein per kilogram of body weight, and 69 to 109 meq of sodium daily. Increasing calcium intake from 400 to 1000 mg had a minimal effect on urinary calcium excretion in the normal subjects but a marked effect in the patients with the various subtypes of idiopathic hypercalciuria. Correspondingly, although the results in the two groups showed considerable overlap when calcium intake was restricted, the segregation between normocalciuria and hypercalciuria was essentially complete when calcium intake was 1000 mg. (*From Broadus and Thier,*[85] *by permission of the New England Journal of Medicine.*)

Several other points deserve mention concerning the approach to screening for hypercalciuria and the study of hypercalciuric patients. First, the defined, high normal calcium diet used to screen outpatients is the same diet employed in inpatient studies and gives essentially equivalent results: in 46 patients initially screened on this diet as outpatients and subsequently studied in detail as inpatients, the mean (± SD) results for calcium excretion on this diet were 352 ± 90 mg/day and 331 ± 78 mg/day, respectively. Given these findings and the ease with which this diet can be administered to outpatients (see Testing below), a sophisticated metabolic ward is unnecessary for the construction of a well-defined study population of hypercalciuric patients. Second, the conditions of study are critically important to the interpretation of metabolic data in hypercalciuric patients; the high normal calcium diet is not optimal for this purpose, since certain abnormalities such as the circulating concentration of 1,25-$(OH)_2D$ are extremely diet-sensitive in these patients (see Table 25-6 and Fig. 25-22).[107] Third, the "normocalciuria" demonstrated by a large subpopulation of hypercalciuric patients on their self- or physician-imposed calcium-restricted diet (group D in Table 25-7) should not mislead the physician into assuming that dietary measures are all that are necessary in such patients and that further screening is unnecessary; this population is highly enriched for patients with absorptive hypercalciuria, a complex disorder in which the hyperabsorption of calcium is but one of several features which appear to predispose to stone formation.[16]

The conventional definitions of hypercalciuria are given in Table 25-6. The most commonly used upper limits for calcium excretion in absolute terms are 300 mg/day in males and 250 mg/day in females.[100,102,106] When expressed on a weight-adjusted basis, the upper limit for calcium excretion is 4 mg per kilogram of body weight per day in either sex and in children. These absolute and weight-adjusted upper limits are not mutually interchangeable, as modest clinical experience quickly teaches. For example, a 50-kg female with a calcium excretion rate of 220 mg/day would be regarded as normocalciuric in absolute terms but hypercalciuric on a weight-adjusted basis (4.4 mg per kilogram of body weight per day), whereas a 100-kg male with a calcium excretion rate of 350 mg/day would be regarded as hypercalciuric in absolute terms but normocalciuric on a weight-adjusted basis (3.5 mg/kg per day). Further, on detailed testing, the female patient would likely represent a classic example of absorptive hypercalciuria, and the male patient would likely be metabolically normal [representing an example of "constitutional" hypercalciuria (see below)]. Thus, for the operational definition of hypercalciuria, it is best to employ both absolute and weight-adjusted limits and to regard a patient exceeding either limit as hypercalciuric. The single most useful definition is 4 mg per kilogram of body weight per day, in that sex, age, and weight are eliminated as variables.

Employing the screening approaches and limits described above, approximately 40 percent of patients with calcium stone disease are found to be hypercalciuric.[2,3,5,6,8,98,100,102,104,108,109] The data in Table 25-7 are from 122 patients, representing 43 percent of 283 consecutive patients with common calcium stone disease screened in the renal stone clinic at Yale.[104] Although hypercalciuria represents the single most common risk factor identified in patients with calcium stone disease, the statistical relationship between calcium excretion and calcium stone formation is far less clear than the relationship between cystine excretion and cystine stone formation (compare the upper panel of Fig. 25-12 with Fig. 25-7). In large part this finding is a reflection of the fact that many patients with calcium stone disease are not hypercalciuric. Nevertheless, as illustrated in the bottom panel of Fig. 25-12, both the presence and degree of hypercalciuria are statistically related to the risk of calcium stone formation. The relative risk is substantial at a calcium excretion rate of 300 mg/day (7.5 mmol/day) and rises sharply at an excretion rate of 400 mg/day (10 mmol/day) or greater.

Some investigators continue to employ a calcium-restricted diet in screening patients for hypercalciuria and regard a calcium excretion rate > 200 mg/day on a metabolic 400-mg-calcium diet as abnormal.[8,109–112] The continued use of a calcium-restricted diet is based, in part, on tradition, for many early investigators employed such a diet in performing calcium balance studies in hypercalciuric patients. However, such an approach is clearly not optimal for purposes of metabolic screening, from either a specificity or a sensitivity perspective (Fig. 25-13). A restricted calcim intake is sometimes employed in an attempt to implicate a nonintestinal basis for hypercalciuria, as, for example, in the resorptive hypercalciuria of the immobilization syndrome.[113] A diet restricted in both calcium and sodium is required for the optimal interpretation of metabolic data in hypercalciuric patients (see Table 25-6) and should be followed for 10 to 14 days before such detailed studies are attempted.[85,105–107,109,112] Twenty-four-hour urine samples may be collected on diets both restricted and unrestricted in calcium as a means of measuring the impact of calcium intake and absorption on calcium excretion (Fig. 25-13) or as a means of assessing the benefit of a therapeutic restriction in calcium intake in hypercalciuric patients (see Fig. 25-13 and the last group in Table 25-6).

Coe has observed that less than 5 percent of normal subjects excrete more than 140 mg of calcium per gram of creatinine on a free diet.[3] He has employed this limit to define "marginal" hypercalciuria.

PHYSIOLOGY OF NORMAL AND ABNORMAL CALCIUM EXCRETION

All aspects of calcium and phosphorus homeostasis which are germane to a consideration of the pathophysiology of hypercalciuria are presented in Chap. 23. The most pertinent sections in that chapter to review are those which deal with the control of bone mineral exchange, proximal and distal processes of calcium reabsorption in the renal tubule, sequence of activation and metabolism of vitamin D, mechanisms and control of intestinal calcium absorption, and calcium and phosphorus homeostasis and balance at the level of the intact organism.

Figure 25-14 illustrates calcium homeostasis in a normal individual in net calcium balance. As emphasized in Chap. 23, the normal hormonal controls are such that net intestinal calcium absorption provides a surplus of calcium which considerably exceeds systemic requirements and is quantitatively excreted in the urine. The scheme in Fig. 25-14 also illustrates several additional straightforward points. First, there are relatively few fundamental mechanisms which could produce hypercalciuria, those being a defect in renal tubular calcium reabsorption, increase in net calcium absorption, increase in bone resorption, or some combination of these processes. In addition, regardless of the basic mechanism, the calcium excreted in the urine must ultimately be derived from dietary calcium or bone mineral, or both. Second, the mechanisms which normally control the rate of calcium excretion are delicate, so that a rather subtle abnormality would be sufficient to produce hypercalciuria. For example, an approximately 1 to 2 percent error in the renal tubular handling of calcium would result in significant hypercalciuria.

The variables governing the rate of calcium excretion can be reduced to two: the filtered load of calcium and renal tubular calcium reabsorption. The renal tubular reabsorption of calcium is a function of the integrity of the tubular reabsorptive mechanism and the influence of circulating PTH on calcium reabsorption in the distal nephron. The filtered load of calcium is a function of GFR and the concentration of ultrafilterable calcium in plasma, the latter ultimately having come from the diet and/or bone mineral.

CLASSIFICATION OF HYPERCALCIURIA

A classification of the hypercalciurias is given in Table 25-8. Several of the categories of hypercalciuria listed, such as dietary hypercalciuria and constitutional hypercalciuria, are not widely recognized; the data supporting these descriptive entities are given in some detail below. The authors' experience is drawn on heavily in the following sections, starting with the patient population and subgroups shown in Table 25-7. An understanding of the pathophysiological and/or pathogenetic mechanism leading to hypercalciuria was sought in every patient in this population who was available for more detailed investigation. The minimum such evaluation was the performance of the oral calcium tolerance test on an outpatient basis under controlled dietary conditions; the full evaluation was a 5-day inpatient protocol.[105–107]

Table 25-8. Classification of Hypercalciuria

Secondary hypercalciuria due to:
Primary hyperparathyroidism
Sarcoidosis
Distal renal tubular acidosis
Vitamin D excess
Immobilization, rapidly progressive osteoporosis, malignant osteolysis
Uncontrolled diabetes mellitus
Glucocorticoid excess
Thyrotoxicosis
Acromegaly
Furosemide administration
Constitutional hypercalciuria
Idiopathic hypercalciuria:
Resorptive hypercalciuria
Subtle primary hyperparathyroidism
Renal hypercalciuria
Absorptive hypercalciuria

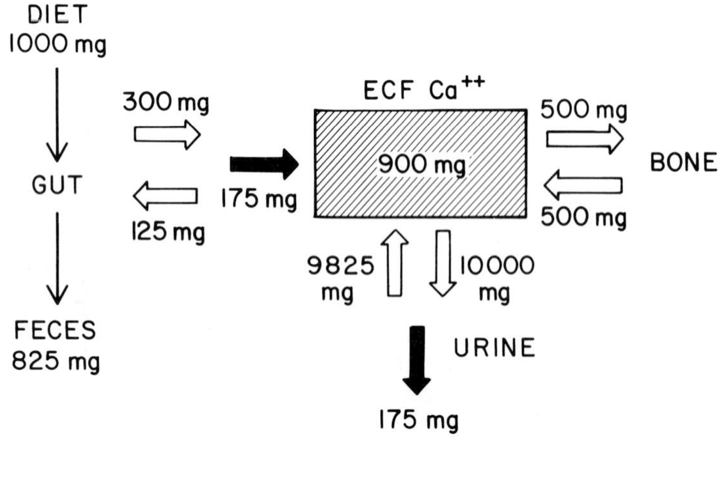

FIGURE 25-14 Schema of calcium metabolism in a normal individual in calcium balance. Open arrows denote unidirectional fluxes; solid arrows denote net fluxes.

Secondary Hypercalciuria

Of the secondary hypercalciurias listed, only the first four are likely to be encountered with any frequency in an adult population with stone disease (each of these conditions is described in detail elsewhere in this chapter or in Chap. 23). Primary hyperparathyroidism is the most important of the secondary hypercalciurias; it was identified, on average, in 7.2 percent of 3084 patients with calcium stone disease reported in eight large series.[75] The "subtle" variety of this disease is easily overlooked and is given separate emphasis below.

In the Yale Renal Stone Clinic, patients with primary hyperparathyroidism, complete RTA, and sarcoidosis accounted for 5 percent, 2 percent, and 0.5 percent of patients presenting with calcium oxalate or calcium phosphate stones. When considered as a percentage of patients presenting with hypercalciuria, patients with primary hyperparathyroidism accounted for 9 percent, those with RTA 2 percent, and those with sarcoidosis 1 percent of patients, so that the secondary hypercalciurias combined accounted for some 12 percent of hypercalciuric patients. As noted previously, the predominant stone type in RTA is the pure calcium phosphate stone; patients with primary hyperparathyroidism form predominantly calcium oxalate or mixed calcium stones. None of these patients is included in the basic population given in Table 25-7.

Constitutional Hypercalciuria

The term "constitutional" hypercalciuria is used in a descriptive sense in connection with patients of large size who appear to be hypercalciuric on an absolute excretion rate basis but not on a weight-adjusted basis, and who also appear to be metabolically normal on detailed evaluation.[104] The principal issue here has to do with the definition of hypercalciuria, particularly as it relates to the predictability of finding metabolic abnormalities in patients on detailed evaluation.

Of the 122 patients in Table 25-7, 95 were hypercalciuric on the defined, 1000-mg-calcium diet (all but group A). Of these 95 patients, 74 were evaluated in detail, and 58 (78 percent) proved to have absorptive hypercalciuria on calcium tolerance testing.[105,106] Based on these data, 16 of the 74 patients would have been regarded as unclassifiable. Scrutiny of this "unclassifiable" population revealed a typical phenotype in 10 of the 16 patients: they were usually males of large size whose calcium excretion was normal when expressed on a weight-adjusted basis.

The patient groups summarized in Table 25-9 include patients considered to have constitutional hypercalciuria, patients of similar large size who proved to have absorptive hypercalciuria on calcium tolerance testing, and patients of small size who proved to have absorptive hypercalciuria on calcium tolerance testing. Note that the mean weight of the first two groups and that of the third group differ by a factor of two and that the first two groups are almost exclusively male and the last group almost exclusively female. The essential message of these data appears to be that expressing calcium excretion on a weight-adjusted basis is the only means of normalizing for the large range of body size encountered in the patient population, particularly the difference in size between the sexes; weight-adjusted values for calcium excretion also correlate far better with metabolic findings than do values for calcium excretion expressed in absolute terms (Table 25-9). If this descriptive definition of constitu-

Table 25-9. Description of Patients with Constitutional Hypercalciuria

Patient population	Weight, kg	Calcium excretion on 1000-mg-calcium diet: Absolute, mg/day	Calcium excretion on 1000-mg-calcium diet: Weight-adjusted, mg/kg per day	Calciuric response to calcium tolerance test*	Plasma [1,25-$(OH)_2D$], pg/ml†	M/F Ratio
Constitutional hypercalciuria	101	363	3.6	0.12	44	9:1
Patients of large size with absorptive hypercalciuria	94	411	4.4	0.25	66	11:1
Patients of small size with absorptive hypercalciuria	52	252	4.6	0.29	66	2:15

*In mg calcium/dl glomerular filtrate. Normal calciuric response to the calcium tolerance test is a change < 0.20 mg calcium/dl glomerular filtrate.

†Upper limit of normal plasma concentration of 1,25-dihydroxyvitamin D = 65 pg/ml.

tional hypercalciuria is accepted at face value, then of the 74 patients evaluated in detail, 58 had absorptive hypercalciuria (78 percent), 10 had constitutional hypercalciuria (14 percent), and 6 fell between the cracks and were unclassifiable (8 percent). If only patients whose calcium excretion exceeded 4.0 mg per kilogram of body weight per day on the defined diet were regarded as truly hypercalciuric, then some 90 percent of the patients evaluated had clear-cut absorptive hypercalciuria.[104–106]

The data in Table 25-9 appear to be germane to patient classification, particularly in metabolic terms, yet they should not be taken to imply that constitutional hypercalciuria is necessarily different from any other type of hypercalciuria as a risk factor for calcium stone formation. The volume of urine excreted by patients with large body size is not proportionately larger than that excreted by patients of small size. The hypercalciuria in patients with constitutional hypercalciuria should therefore, presumably, be treated medically as it is in other patients. Moderation in calcium intake is, however, unlikely to be of particular benefit in patients with constitutional hypercalciuria.

Dietary Hypercalciuria

The 24-h calcium excretion on both the free diet and the high normal calcium diet in patients in groups A and B from Table 25-7 are plotted in Fig. 25-15. Although the calcium intake was several hundred mg/day higher on the defined diet than the free diet, mean calcium excretion in the 44 patients in this combined group *fell* on the defined diet almost 100 mg/day.[106] It is evident that some dietary factor(s) other than calcium must have contributed to the hypercalciuria expressed by these patients on the free diet.

A number of dietary constituents other than calcium influence calcium absorption and/or excretion. Calcium excretion has been reported to be increased by dietary protein, sodium, and carbohydrate and decreased by dietary oxalate and phosphate.[2,3,5,6,8,100] Of these factors, dietary carbohydrate, oxalate, and phosphate appear to be relatively unimportant.

Protein ingestion can have a pronounced influence on calcium excretion: increasing protein ingestion from 0.5 g per kilogram of body weight per day (a restricted intake) to 2 g/kg per day (a liberal intake) doubles calcium excretion in normal individuals. This effect appears to result from the metabolism of protein to fixed acid, which decreases distal tubular calcium reabsorption.[100] However, protein-induced hypercalciuria is not a recognized clinical entity, and there are no direct clinical data bearing on this question apart from the epidemiological dietary surveys noted above (see General Considerations).

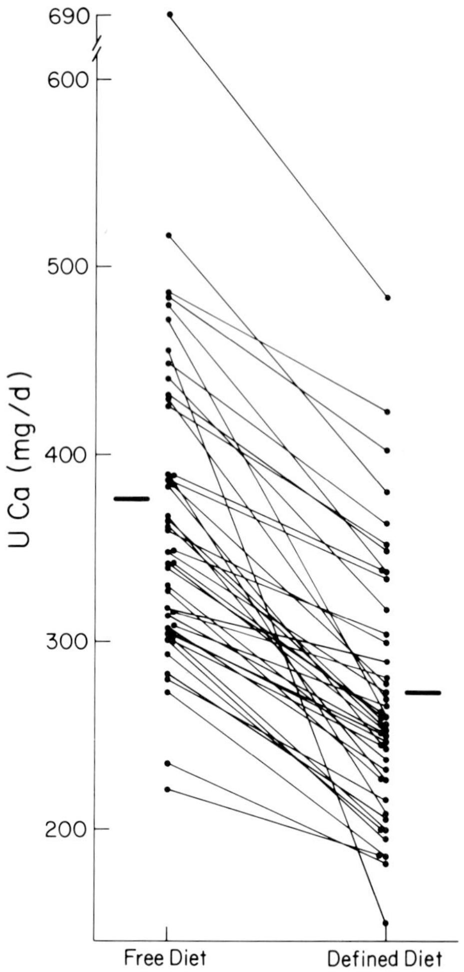

FIGURE 25-15 Calcium excretion on a free diet and on a defined diet with 1000 mg calcium in patients from groups A and B in Table 25-6. Patients in first group were found to be hypercalciuric only on their free diet. Patients in group B were hypercalciuric on both diets but exhibited a fall in calcium excretion of 50 mg/day or more (mean 91 mg/day) on the defined diet compared to the free diet.

It now appears that the principal culprit is sodium. It has been commonly stated that an increase in sodium intake increases calcium excretion by only some 25 mg per 100 meq of sodium in normal subjects, implying that wide swings in sodium intake would be required to have a significant impact on calcium excretion.[100] There is actually considerable disagreement concerning this figure;[100,114–116] some series have reported that the influence of sodium intake on calcium excretion may be as great as 60 to 100 mg of calcium per 100 meq of sodium in normal (non-stone-forming) individuals.[115,116] Strong correlations between sodium excretion and calcium excretion have been observed in both normal individuals and hypercalciuric patients, and it has even been suggested that rea-

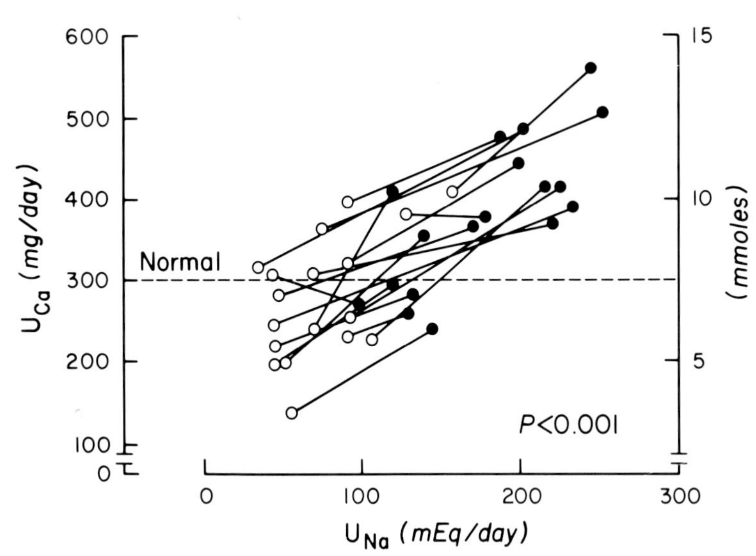

FIGURE 25-16 Twenty-four-hour calcium excretion plotted as a function of sodium excretion in 18 patients initially defined as hypercalciuric on a free diet. These patients were allowed 500 to 700 mg/day calcium; their sodium intake varied from 80 meq/day (open circles) to 200 meq/day (closed circles). The dashed line defines the upper limit for calcium excretion (300 mg/day) in males in this study. (*From Muldowney et al,*[103] *by permission of Kidney International.*)

sonable limits for calcium excretion cannot be defined without close attention to sodium intake and/or excretion.[115,116] Further, several series have reported a pattern of apparent sodium-dependent hypercalciuria in patients with calcium stone disease, meaning that hypercalciuria appeared and disappeared as a function of sodium intake.[103,117] The results in one such series are shown in Fig. 25-16. In this study, 18 patients previously defined as hypercalciuric on an unrestricted diet were placed on a diet containing 500 to 700 mg of calcium per day, and the sodium intake was varied from 80 meq to 200 meq per day.[103] As can be seen, the increase in sodium intake increased calcium excretion by an average of about 100 mg/day, so that the dependence of calcium excretion on sodium intake was approximately 100 mg of calcium per 100 meq of sodium. About one-half of the patients who were hypercalciuric on the 200-meq-sodium diet were normocalciuric on the 80-meq-sodium diet (Fig. 25-16). Complete metabolic evaluations were not performed in the 18 patients in this study, so that it was unclear whether other mechanisms of hypercalciuria, such as absorptive hypercalciuria, might have been at play in certain patients. The sodium effect was considered to be renal in nature (see below).

The data in Table 25-7 and Fig. 25-15 complement those cited above. First, of the various dietary constituents (calcium, protein, sodium) considered as possibly explaining the pattern observed in Fig. 25-15, the strongest single correlation was between sodium excretion and calcium excretion.[104] Second, the data in Table 25-7 suggest that dietary hypercalciuria is common, contributing to if not entirely accounting for the hypercalciuria observed in as many as one-half of patients found to be hypercalciuric on a free diet (groups A, B, and C in Table 25-7). Third, detailed metabolic studies were performed in a majority of the patients reported in Table 25-7, giving a sense of what the patient groups represented in metabolic or pathophysiological terms.[104–106] Seventeen patients in group A were studied in detail, and 14 of these patients were found to be metabolically normal [normal calcium tolerance test results with a mean plasma concentration of 1,25-$(OH)_2D$ of 51 pg/ml]. Twelve patients in group B were studied in detail, and eight patients appeared to have classic examples of absorptive hypercalciuria [elevated calciuric responses to the calcium tolerance test and a mean circulating 1,25-$(OH)_2D$ concentration of 70 pg/ml]. These findings suggest that (1) sodium-induced hypercalciuria can occur in individuals who appear to be otherwise metabolically normal and (2) a sodium-induced component can be superimposed upon another well-established mechanism of hypercalciuria.[104]

Sodium inhibits the reabsorption of calcium in the proximal tubule, and possibly in more distal segments of the nephron; the available evidence suggests that sodium-induced hypercalciuria is renal in nature.[103,114,115,118] This evidence includes the fact that hypercalciuric patients studied on a low-calcium, high-sodium diet are in calcium deficit as well as the observation that the imposition of a high sodium intake increases fasting calcium excretion.[103,115] Indeed, it has been argued that failure to control sodium intake has been a frequent cause of misclassification of patients as having renal hypercalciuria, "renal" in this sense being taken to mean having a primary renal calcium leak.[103] In the study shown in Fig. 25-16, the increase in dietary sodium was not accompanied by an increase in parathyroid function, so that the usual criteria for the diagnosis of a primary renal calcium leak were not fulfilled.[103]

It is likely that the data summarized in this section are as important clinically as any developments in the hypercalciuria field in recent years. Yet there remain a number of unresolved issues. For example, not all individuals with high sodium excretion (e.g., > 200 meq/day) on a free diet are hypercalciuric, so that it is unclear whether certain patients are more susceptible to sodium-induced hypercalciuria than others. Several studies have reported a defect in the proximal tubular reabsorption of multiple ions, including sodium and calcium, in hypercalciuric patients and have suggested that the syndrome of idiopathic hypercalciuria is primarily the result of disordered proximal tubular function.[108,119] Perhaps these patients could be more sensitive than normal subjects to variations in sodium intake. However, the pathogenetic importance of the observations in these series has been questioned on the grounds that a similar defect can be induced in normal individuals by a high sodium intake.[120] It is also unclear whether the slope of the calcium excretion vs. sodium intake curve is steeper in patients considered to be "hypercalciuric" than in nonhypercalciuric patients with stone disease and/or normal individuals, as has been suggested by several series.[116,117,120] This point must be addressed by a systematic study of the effects of variations in sodium intake in well-characterized hypercalciuric patients classified by independent means. Although all of the series summarized above imply a link between a high sodium intake, hypercalciuria, and stone formation, this sequence of events remains unproven.

These important issues notwithstanding, certain simple points are abundantly clear. Urinary sodium output should be routinely measured in the process of screening patients with calcium stone disease, and a moderation in sodium intake should be prescribed to patients who appear to have sodium-induced hypercalciuria. Many patients also require additional therapy, but this does not obviate the apparent usefulness of a moderated sodium intake. It is probably also worth measuring urinary sodium excretion in patients being followed on one or another antihypercalciuric regimen, in that anecdotal experience indicates that the wide swings in calcium excretion observed in some of these patients may be the result of variations in sodium intake.

Idiopathic Hypercalciuria

As noted above, the term idiopathic hypercalciuria has been used to describe patients with normocalcemic hypercalciuria and a tendency to hypophosphatemia.[96,97] Given this operational definition, the abnormalities in all 122 patients included in Table 25-7 could be considered to be examples of idiopathic hypercalciuria. The thrust of this chapter, however, has been to attempt to subdivide hypercalciuric patients according to the mechanism(s) responsible for their hypercalciuria. According to this classification scheme, the idiopathic category in Table 25-7 is exclusive of patients with dietary and constitutional hypercalciuria. In operational terms, the "idiopathic" classification is used in connection with patients who harbor syndromes which may be viewed as representing true endogenous errors in mineral homeostasis.

The four categories or subtypes of idiopathic hypercalciuria listed in Table 25-8 are somewhat unconventional and are intended solely to emphasize the mechanisms of disease; it is of crucial importance to recognize that all diagnostic classifications are based on operational assumptions and definitions. Pathogenetic mechanisms are of far greater importance than the semantics used to describe them; indeed, the semantics may sometimes impede rather than foster pathophysiological reasoning. For example, the single most classic illustration of a "renal leak" of calcium occurs in chronic hypoparathyroidism, yet the term *renal leak* seems oddly misapplied when used in this connection. In addition, a "renal" component can be implicated in the final common pathway of hypercalciuria in a number of syndromes, such as resorptive hypercalciuria and absorptive hypercalciuria; in both of these examples, however, the increased fractional excretion of calcium is due to parathyroid suppression and should not be viewed as of primary pathogenetic significance. In a complex syndrome such as primary hyperparathyroidism, a multiplicity of components (e.g., resorptive and absorptive) may contribute to the net hypercalciuria and/or a given component may predominate in individual patients. Referring to primary hyperparathyroidism simply as resorptive hypercalciuria is therefore an oversimplification.

In each of the examples given above, the intent has been to encourage consideration of physiological mechanisms. This same intent is implicit in Fig. 25-14, which depicts the interplay of bone, kidney, and intestine in maintaining quantitative systemic calcium homeostasis in a normal individual in net calcium balance, and in Fig. 25-17, which represents a summary of the pathophysiological features which perturb this system and which lead to hypercalciuria in the four categories of patients discussed below. Resorptive hypercalciuria and subtle primary hyperparathyroidism are discussed initially, followed by a more detailed summary of the ongoing controversy concerning the criteria for diagnosis and the frequency of renal and absorptive hypercalciuria.

RESORPTIVE HYPERCALCIURIA Patients with resorptive hypercalciuria have a primary disorder associated

	CALCIUM ABSORPTION	BONE RESORPTION	EXTRACELLULAR CALCIUM	PT FUNCTION	CALCIUM EXCRETION FL	CALCIUM EXCRETION Reab	1,25 (OH)$_2$ D$_3$	SERUM P$_I$
RESORPTIVE HC	↓	[↑]	N, ↑	↓	↑	↓	↓	N, ↑
SUBTLE 1° HPT	↑	↑	N, ↑	[↑]	↑	↑	↑	N, ↓
RENAL HC	↑	N, ↑	N, ↓	↑	↓	[↓]	↑	N, ↓
ABSORPTIVE HC	[↑]	N, ↑	N, ↑	N, ↓	↑	↓	[N, ↑]	N, [↓]

FIGURE 25-17 Pathophysiologic features of four categories or subtypes of hypercalciuria. The features enclosed in the rectangle in each subtype denote the known or putative primary pathogenetic defect. Note that increases in intestinal calcium absorption and circulating 1,25-(OH)$_2$D concentrations and a tendency to hypophosphatemia are common to the three main hypercalciuric subtypes. HC, hypercalciuria; 1°HPT, primary hyperparathyroidism; PT, parathyroid; FL, filtered load; Reab, tubular calcium reabsorption; P_i, inorganic phosphorus.

with an increased rate of resorption of bone mineral. As used in Table 25-8, "resorptive hypercalciuria" refers almost exclusively to secondary hypercalciuria. The increase in calcium mobilization from the skeleton increases the ambient concentration of calcium in the extracellular fluids, which suppresses parathyroid function, 1,25-(OH)$_2$D synthesis, and intestinal calcium absorption, increases the filtered load of calcium, and is associated with an increase in fractional calcium excretion; this last, the "renal" component, is a consequence of the parathyroid suppression (Fig. 25-17). The best-studied example of resorptive hypercalciuria to date is the *immobilization syndrome;* the sequence of events described above corresponds exactly to what has been observed in these patients and is in perfect accord with what would be anticipated physiologically.[113] Other rather "pure" examples of resorptive hypercalciuria are rapidly progressive osteoporosis, malignancy-associated osteolysis, and hyperthyroidism; all of these examples are forms of secondary hypercalciuria which do not figure prominently in the differential diagnosis of idiopathic hypercalciuria (Table 25-8). However, there may be a resorptive component to the net hypercalciuria observed in patients with complete distal RTA, primary hyperparathyroidism, glucocorticoid excess, sarcoidosis, and, possibly, absorptive and/or renal hypercalciuria (see below).

SUBTLE PRIMARY HYPERPARATHYROIDISM The term subtle primary hyperparathyroidism is used to describe the disorder in patients who present with subtle abnormalities of serum calcium concentration together with marked hypercalciuria and stone disease. It has been recognized for many years and by many investigators that patients with primary hyperparathyroidism and renal stone complications typically display only mild fasting hypercalcemia and that in a minority of such patients the degree of hypercalcemia is minimal.[75,121–124] The term "normocalcemic" primary hyperparathyroidism is frequently used in the older literature in connection with such patients, but this term has been avoided here because it is descriptively inaccurate: these patients usually present with a fairly characteristic pattern of intermittent hypercalcemia, with swings of ± 0.5 mg/dl around the upper normal limit and a mean fasting serum calcium concentration in the range of 10.2 to 10.3 mg/dl.[75,121–123] A mean serum calcium concentration in this range should not be considered normal in an ambulatory, healthy young adult with hypercalciuria and stone disease.[125]

Recent studies have clarified the pathophysiological features leading to hypercalciuria in patients with primary hyperparathyroidism in general and in those with subtle primary hyperparathyroidism in particular.[121,126] Consider patients A and B in Table 25-10: these two patients have a nearly identical fasting serum calcium concentration, but patient A displays marked hypercalciuria on an unrestricted-calcium diet and has a history of stones, whereas patient B is normocalciuric and has no stone history. The essential question raised by these findings is how to account for the disproportionate hypercalciuria in patient A. The answer to this question is provided by the circulating concentration of 1,25-(OH)$_2$D in these two patients: the concentration is markedly elevated in patient A and within the normal range in patient B (Table 25-10). The disproportionate hypercalciuria in patient A is therefore predominantly absorptive in nature; the pattern of calcium absorption and excretion in this

Table 25-10. Pathophysiological Features in Three Patients with Primary Hyperparathyroidism

	Patient		
Feature	A	B	C
Fasting serum calcium concentration, mg/dl	11.0	11.3	10.2
24-h calcium excretion, mg	439	275	452
History of renal stones	yes	no	yes
Plasma 1,25-$(OH)_2D$ concentration, pg/ml	90	57	90

Source: These three patients are not hypothetical; the values shown are mean data from Broadus et al.[121,126]

patient is remarkably similar to that observed in patients with the syndrome of absorptive hypercalciuria, except that the primary pathogenetic abnormality in patient A is parathyroid hyperfunction.[121,126]

Consider next patient C in Table 25-10; this patient is very similar to patient A except that the mean fasting serum calcium concentration is 10.2 mg/dl. If this patient were followed with serial measurements of fasting serum calcium concentration over several months' time, representative values would be 10.1, 10.3, 10.7, 10.1, and 10.0 mg/dl. Like patient A, patient C has a marked increase in circulating 1,25-$(OH)_2D$ concentration, absorbs excessive calcium from the GI tract, and is hypercalciuric on this basis. In essence, patient C represents a forme fruste of the typical case of primary hyperparathyroidism, hypercalciuria, and stone disease; as such, this patient simply represents an extreme example of the disproportionate hypercalciuria which characterizes these patients.[121,124,126]

The diagnosis of subtle primary hyperparathyroidism should be strongly suspected in any hypercalciuric patient with a mean fasting serum calcium concentration $\geq$ 10.0 mg/dl on three determinations performed with scrupulous care in blood-drawing and analytical technique. The differential diagnosis includes sarcoidosis and, rarely, absorptive hypercalciuria of sufficient severity to spill over into frank mild and/or intermittent hypercalcemia (see below). Although there are a number of ways of approaching this differential diagnosis (see Diagnosis, below), the oral calcium tolerance test is ideally suited for this purpose, in that its very design takes advantage of the extreme hyperabsorption of calcium which typifies patients with subtle primary hyperparathyroidism.[121] In this setting, the tolerance test serves as a classic endocrine suppression test, and the combination of induced hypercalcemia (calcium "intolerance") and inappropriate suppression of nephrogenous cAMP or total cAMP excretion makes diagnosis a relatively simple matter (Fig. 25-18).

RENAL CALCIUM LEAK Patients with a renal leak of calcium (renal hypercalciuria) are envisioned as having a primary renal tubular defect in calcium absorption. The increase in fractional calcium excretion in these

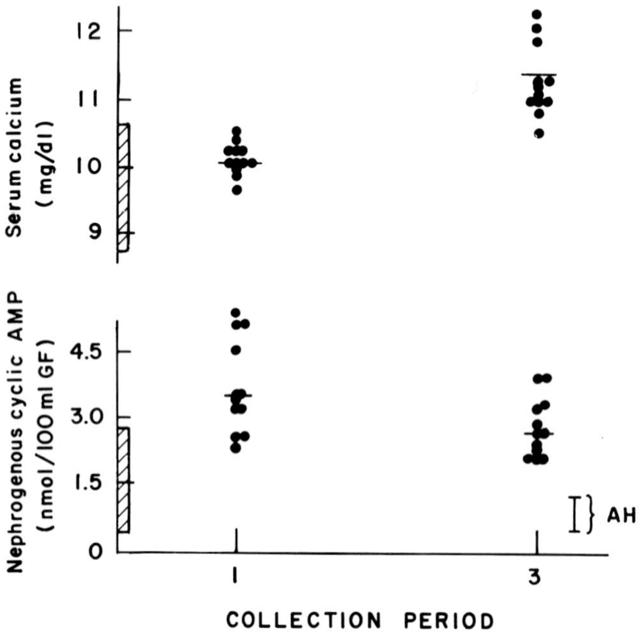

FIGURE 25-18 Results of calcium tolerance testing in 12 patients with subtle primary hyperparathyroidism. The normal ranges are depicted by the cross-hatched bars adjoining the ordinate. Also shown for comparison in the bottom panel is the range of results for nephrogenous cAMP excretion (NcAMP) in 13 patients with absorptive hypercalciuria who developed mild hypercalcemia during the test. Mean data from 30 patients with subtle hyperparathyroidism studied to date: 24-h calcium excretion on a diet unrestricted in calcium: 420 mg/day; plasma 1,25-$(OH)_2D$ concentration: 87 pg/ml; fasting serum calcium concentration: 10.3 mg/dl; calcemic response: 11.5 mg/dl; fasting NcAMP excretion: 3.8 nmol/dl glomerular filtrate; NcAMP excretion during the experimental collection period: 2.6 nmol/dl glomerular filtrate. (*Modified from Broadus et al,*[121] *by permission of Clinical Endocrinology.*)

233-4511 VA

1-800-444-8932

497

patients causes a reduction in the ambient concentration of ionized calcium, which leads to the predictable sequence of secondary hyperparathyroidism, reduction in TmP/GFR and serum phosphorus concentration, stimulation of 1,25-$(OH)_2D$ synthesis, and increase in intestinal calcium absorption (Fig. 25-17). In one study, histomorphometric findings of typical "early" PTH effects in bone were reported, compatible with the state of relatively mild secondary hyperparathyroidism.[127] Thus, under steady-state conditions in near balance for calcium, the net hypercalciuria in patients with renal hypercalciuria would have a combination of renal, absorptive, and resorptive components. The tubular site of the putative defect in calcium reabsorption is unknown.

It should be recalled that the renal leak hypothesis dates from the 1950s and was Henneman's favored pathogenetic formulation at that time.[97] Considerable evidence was generated in support of this hypothesis in the mid-1970s.[110–112,127,128] The most important of these references historically is that of Coe et al., who reported an increase in circulating immunoreactive PTH in two-thirds of hypercalciuric patients and showed that both the hypercalciuria and secondary hyperparathyroidism could be reversed by thiazide administration.[128] In addition, a model of renal hypercalciuria was created in normal subjects by furosemide administration.[128] Pak et al. introduced additional diagnostic criteria for renal hypercalciuria, including an increase in fasting calcium excretion together with abnormal or inappropriate values for serum immunoreactive PTH and/or total cAMP excretion, and also reported that these abnormalities could be partially reversed by thiazide administration.[110–112]

Considerable doubt concerning the frequency of renal hypercalciuria and the validity of criteria for its diagnosis has crept into the literature in the past 5 years or so; the latter concern is the crux of the issue. There is little if any theoretical debate as to what the diagnostic criteria should be: patients should be studied on a calcium-restricted diet to maximize the ability to detect the calcium leak and secondary hyperparathyroidism, and they should display evidence for *both* a decrease in renal calcium reabsorption *and* secondary hyperparathyroidism. In practice, this debate has largely come to focus on the interpretation of fasting calcium excretion (or fasting fractional calcium excretion) values in hypercalciuric patients. This point is treated in some detail below.

It has been appreciated since the earliest descriptive studies of Flocks that hypercalciuric patients exhibit higher rates of calcium excretion than do normal subjects at all levels of calcium intake.[95] This observation also holds for the fasting state; each of 14 laboratories which has published values for fasting calcium excretion has reported a mean increase in excretion in patients with idiopathic hypercalciuria.[89,105,106,108,111,112,119,129–137] More recently, two laboratories have reported an actual increase in fasting fractional calcium excretion in hypercalciuric patients, data which represent prima facie evidence of a renal calcium leak.[106,129] The uniformity of these findings from so many laboratories leaves little doubt that an increase in fasting calcium excretion and/or fasting fractional calcium excretion is common in hypercalciuric patients, yet there are marked differences in interpretation as to whether such a "calcium leak" is of primary or secondary pathogenetic importance. Several points bear directly on this controversy.

First, a renal calcium leak can be induced in normal subjects in whom experimental absorptive hypercalciuria is produced by the administration of 1,25-$(OH)_2D$ (Fig. 25-19). The sequence of events in this model is 1,25-$(OH)_2D$-induced hyperabsorption of calcium from the intestine, parathyroid suppression which persists into the fasting period, and an increase in fasting fractional calcium excretion.[138,139] In this model, the renal leak of calcium is clearly secondary; these findings have led one group of investigators to flatly state that fasting calcium excretion is uninterpretable in an individual with an increased plasma concentration of 1,25-$(OH)_2D$.[139]

Second, exactly the same data and presumed sequence of events have been observed in 45 patients who appeared to have well-characterized examples of the naturally occurring syndrome of absorptive hypercalciuria.[106] In these patients, there was a strong statistical correlation between the degree of parathyroid suppression in the fasting state and fasting fractional calcium excretion (Fig. 25-20). Perhaps the most telling point in this series was the fact that the most "severe" examples of absorptive hypercalciuria displayed the most marked depression in parathyroid function and the highest values for fasting fractional calcium excretion.[106] It should be recalled in this regard that patients who excessively absorb calcium do so at all levels of calcium intake, so that even on a diet restricted to 400 mg of calcium their net calcium absorption and excretion is approximately twice normal.[105,106] Prolonged parathyroid suppression would be the expected consequence of this long-term increase in net calcium absorption.

Third, although there is a consensus that an increase in fasting calcium excretion is observed in something like one-half of hypercalciuric patients studied on a restricted calcium intake, parathyroid function tests have been reported to be normal[89,106,108,119,132–137,140,141,142] or even significantly reduced[129,130,143] in the vast majority of such patients in recent series. It is these patients, in particular, with an

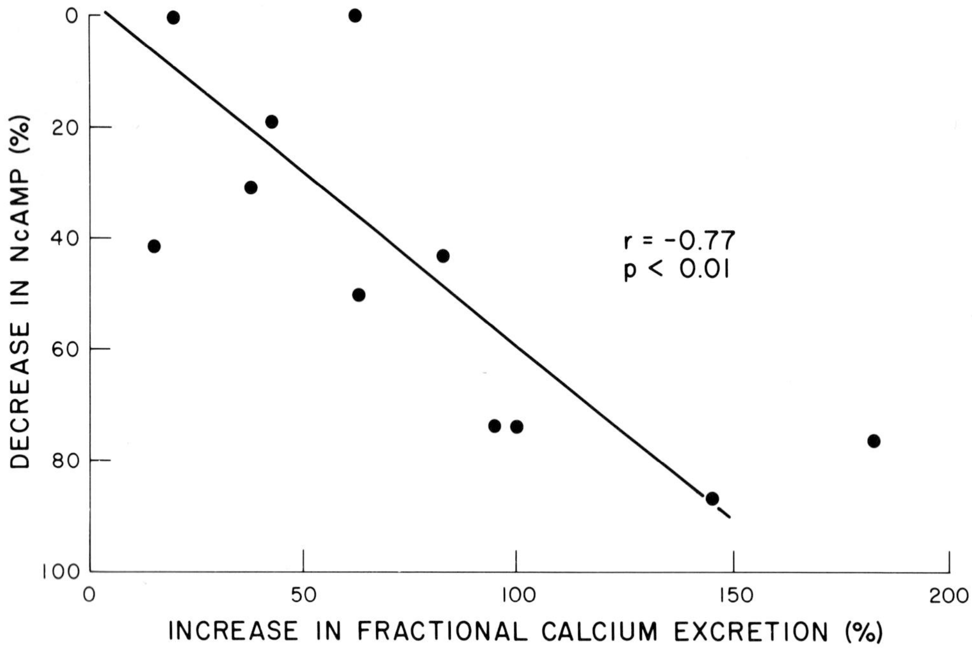

FIGURE 25-19 Correlation between 1,25-$(OH)_2D$-induced decrease in fasting nephrogenous cAMP excretion and fasting fractional calcium excretion in normal subjects in whom a model of absorptive hypercalciuria was created by the administration of 1,25-$(OH)_2D$. The subjects were on a 400-mg calcium diet and had fasted for 10 to 12 h on both occasions of study. Note the strong correlation between the degree of parathyroid suppression and the increase in the fraction of the filtered load of calcium excreted in the fasting state. *(From Broadus et al,*[138] *by permission of the Journal of Clinical Endocrinology and Metabolism.)*

increase in fasting calcium excretion but with normal or reduced parathyroid function, who have become the primary focus of disagreement as to interpretation. Given the sensitivity of modern parathyroid function tests and data such as those shown in Fig. 25-20, it would appear to be irrational to regard such patients as being physiologically pure examples of a primary renal calcium leak.

Finally, an increase in sodium intake has been reported to increase fasting excretion.[103] Although dietary sodium is the least extensively studied of the factors that can influence fasting calcium excretion, only a minority of published series have controlled sodium as well as calcium intake as part of their study design,[89,106,112] and a great many other series could be subject to interpretive error on this basis.[103] As noted in the discussion of dietary hypercalciuria, sodium-induced hypercalciuria did not appear to lead to a state of secondary hyperparathyroidism, so the accepted criteria for diagnosis of renal hypercalciuria were not fulfilled.[103]

A number of laboratories have reported that a substantial percentage of hypercalciuric patients are thrown into negative calcium balance when placed on a diet severely restricted in calcium content; this has been interpreted as evidence for underlying renal hypercalciuria.[130] This experiment has recently been repeated by Coe et al., with the observation of apparent calcium deficit in a majority of patients; these patients in general were those who also displayed an increase in fasting calcium excretion. It was also noted that parathyroid function was significantly reduced in these patients on both a free and a rigidly calcium-restricted diet,[130] a point which clearly does not favor a primary renal mechanism and which is compatible with parathyroid suppression persisting through the period of the low-calcium diet. An alternative possibility is that hypercalciuria represents a continuum of renal and absorptive abnormalities whose sufferers cannot be separated into distinct patient subpopulations.[130]

The prevailing view at present appears to be that a reduction in renal tubular calcium reabsorption can be frequently demonstrated in hypercalciuric patients but that only rarely is this calcium leak of primary pathogenetic importance. Certainly, the demonstration of an increase in fasting calcium excretion in the absence of other diagnostic criteria does not establish a diagnosis of primary renal hypercalciuria. Recent terminology reflects this prevailing view, in that a number of authors are using the term "fasting" hypercalciuria or "unclassifiable" hypercalciuria in connection with such patients.[108,119,144] Based on the requirement of *both* an increase in fasting calcium excretion and evidence of secondary hyperparathyroidism, one group estimates that renal hypercalciuria accounts for some 10 percent of hypercalciuric patients encountered and "unclassifiable" hypercalciuria accounts for about 15 percent.[109,144] Among patients considered to have primary renal hypercalciuria, females outnumber males. There frequently is a history of previous urinary tract infection, suggesting that the renal leak could be acquired.[109,144] In our own experience, patients who appear to fulfill the criteria for primary renal hypercalciuria are exceedingly rare.[104–106]

ABSORPTIVE HYPERCALCIURIA In absorptive hypercalciuria, the excessive intestinal absorption of calcium leads to a postprandial increase in the extracellular calcium concentration, which both increases the filtered load of calcium and suppresses parathyroid function; the absorbed load of calcium is spilled directly into the urine (Fig. 25-17). The suppression of parathyroid function adds a secondary renal component to the net hypercalciuria in these patients, as described above (see also Fig. 25-20). In patients with a severe form of absorptive hypercalciuria[106] and/or in patients who are placed on a rigidly calcium-restricted diet,[145] there may also be a resorptive component, but this component is not thought to be quantitatively significant nor is it a particular threat to bone in most patients. Although there appears to be a growing consensus among current investigators that absorptive hypercalciuria is by far the most common of the causes of idiopathic hypercalciuria listed in Table 25-8, the details of pathogenesis are not entirely clear. Postulated mechanisms of absorptive hypercalciuria include: (1) hyperabsorption of calcium due to a primary intestinal defect, (2) an increase in circulating 1,25-$(OH)_2D$ concentration due to a primary renal phosphate leak, and (3) an increase in circulating 1,25-$(OH)_2D$ concentration due to disordered control of its production. A modification of the third proposal holds that patients with absorptive hypercalciuria may have a fundamental proximal tubular abnormality which is expressed by a

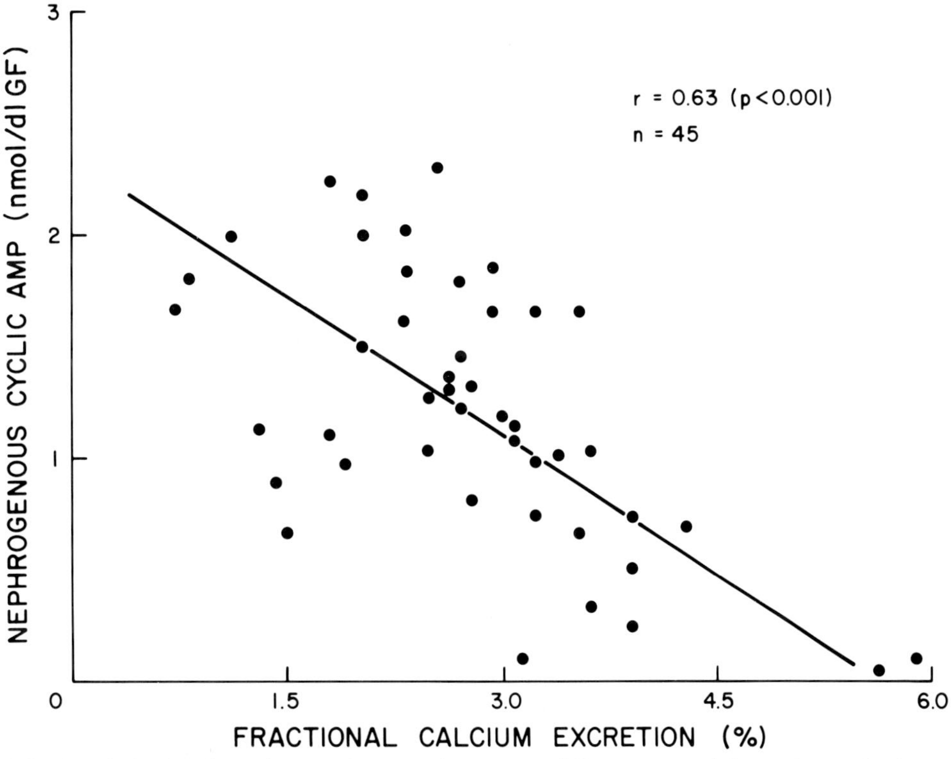

FIGURE 25-20 Correlation between fasting nephrogenous cAMP excretion and fasting fractional calcium excretion in 45 patients with absorptive hypercalciuria. The patients were on a calcium-restricted (400 mg), sodium-restricted (69 to 109 meq) intake and had fasted for 10 to 12 h prior to study. The interpretation is identical to that of the data in Fig. 25-19: patients with absorptive hypercalciuria have a "renal" component to their hypercalciuria due to parathyroid suppression. (*From Broadus et al,*[106] *by permission of the Journal of Clinical Endocrinology and Metabolism.*)

number of presumably related abnormalities, including decreased reabsorption of phosphate and other ions and an increase in 1,25-$(OH)_2D$ production. These hypotheses need not be viewed as mutually exclusive; it is entirely possible that the group of patients defined operationally as having absorptive hypercalciuria may be pathogenetically heterogeneous.

Most of the evidence in support of a primary intestinal abnormality in calcium absorption in patients with absorptive hypercalciuria has been provided by Pak and coworkers.[110,144,146,147] The most direct evidence comes from intestinal perfusion studies which revealed a pattern of selective jejunal hyperabsorption of calcium in patients with absorptive hypercalciuria.[146] This pattern differs from that observed in response to exogenous 1,25-$(OH)_2D$, which produces an increase in calcium absorption in both the jejunum and ileum and which stimulates magnesium as well as calcium uptake in the jejunum.[147] One prediction of this hypothesis is that affected patients should display low normal or frankly low values for circulating 1,25-$(OH)_2D$ concentration as well as increases in serum phosphorus concentration and TmP/GFR. Although a spectrum of values for circulating 1,25-$(OH)_2D$ concentration has been reported in hypercalciuric patients by a number of laboratories (see below), a subpopulation with low or low normal values has not been identified in these series.

The frequency with which an increase in the plasma concentration of 1,25-$(OH)_2D$ has been observed in undefined patients with hypercalciuria and/or in patients considered to have absorptive hypercalciuria is a matter of some controversy.[106,107,130,132,140,141,143,148,149] In our own experience, upwards of 80 percent of patients with absorptive hypercalciuria have been found to display frank elevations in circulating 1,25-$(OH)_2D$ concentration; high normal values are seen in the remaining 20 percent of patients (Fig. 25-21).[106] There are two critical issues of study design which together probably account for most of the disagreement in the literature concerning the role of 1,25-$(OH)_2D$ in hypercalciuria in general and in absorptive hypercalciuria in particular: patient selection and the conditions under which patients are studied.

Most of the series of 1,25-$(OH)_2D$ determinations in hypercalciuric patients published to date were designed such that patients were both selected and studied on a free diet,[130,132,140,143,149] and one series included patients with calcium stone disease without regard to calcium excretion.[141] On average, these series reported an increase in circulating 1,25-$(OH)_2D$ concentration in approximately 40 to 50 percent of the patients studied. Quite apart from the issue of the influence of conditions of study on results obtained on

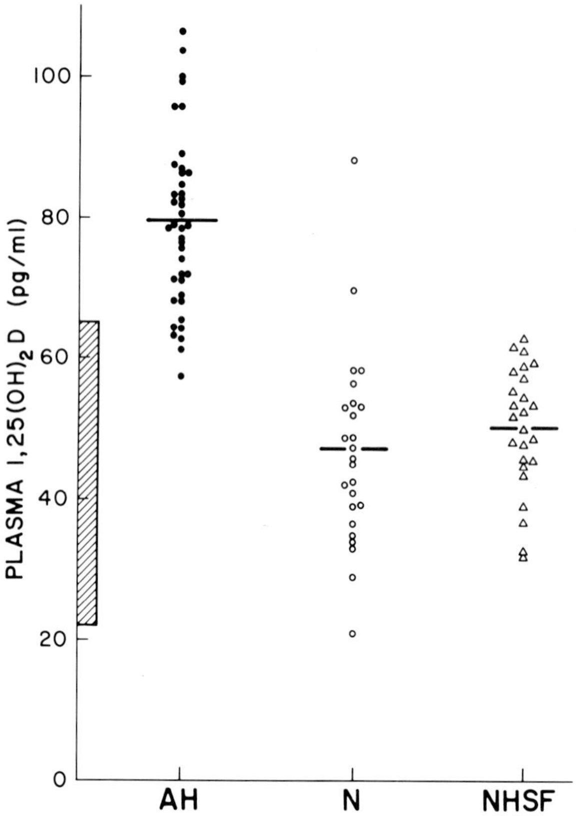

FIGURE 25-21 Plasma 1,25-$(OH)_2D$ concentrations in 50 patients with absorptive hypercalciuria (AH), 25 normal subjects (N), and 25 nonhypercalciuric patients with stone disease (NHSF). All samples were obtained after at least 10 days on a calcium-restricted (400 meq), sodium-restricted (about 100 meq) diet. The horizontal bars represent mean values; the hatched bar defines the normal range for the plasma 1,25-$(OH)_2D$ concentration. (*From Broadus et al,*[106] *by permission of the Journal of Clinical Endocrinology and Metabolism.*)

an undefined diet (see below), the selection of a study population on the basis of calcium excretion on a free diet would include a substantial number of patients with dietary and constitutional hypercalciuria, thereby considerably diluting the population with respect to patients with true idiopathic hypercalciuria (as the term is used here) (Table 25-8). In our series, patients had to fulfill each of three statistically based criteria for purposes of inclusion: (1) hypercalciuria on a defined, high normal calcium intake, (2) hyperabsorption of calcium as demonstrated by calcium tolerance testing, and (3) normal or low results for serum immunoreactive PTH and nephrogenous cAMP concentrations.[105,106] Taken together, these criteria are presumably sufficiently rigorous not only to enrich a study population for patients with true "metabolic" idiopathic hypercalciuria but also to select for clear-cut rather than borderline examples of such patients. Further, a subpopulation of severely affected patients could be identified simply by selecting patients whose circulating 1,25-$(OH)_2D$ concentrations were greater than 4 SD from the normal mean. All measured abnormalities were abnormal in the extreme in this "severe" subpopulation, and several patients, with plasma 1,25-$(OH)_2D$ concentrations in excess of 100 pg/ml, even exhibited mild fasting hypercalcemia.[106]

The dietary conditions under which patients are studied turn out to be a critically important determinant of the circulating concentration of 1,25-$(OH)_2D$ in hypercalciuric patients. The data which form the basis of this statement were unanticipated; they were obtained during a series of studies in which the working hypothesis was that 1,25-$(OH)_2D$ production might be relatively autonomous in patients with absorptive hypercalciuria. That is, given the frequency with which an elevated or high normal plasma level of 1,25-$(OH)_2D$ was observed in patients with absorptive hypercalciuria (Fig. 25-21), it was postulated that a suppression test could be fashioned which might highlight this abnormality.[107] This suppression test took the form of challenging patients who had been on a restricted (400-mg-calcium) diet with the high normal calcium (1000 mg) diet for a 3-day period, with a simple before-and-after design. The findings were compared to those in a group of nonhypercalciuric patients with calcium stone disease.[108] What was observed was quite the opposite of what was anticipated: the circulating concentration of 1,25-$(OH)_2D$ proved to be remarkably diet-sensitive in patients with absorptive hypercalciuria, such that the mean value on the high normal calcium diet was suppressed well into the normal range in these patients (Fig. 25-22). In addition, whereas there was an essentially complete segregation of values for plasma 1,25-$(OH)_2D$ concentration in the hypercalciuric and the nonhypercalciuric patients on the calcium-restricted diet, there was virtually complete overlap of these values on the high normal calcium diet (Fig. 25-22). Even though the short-term data from these studies should not necessarily be equated with what might be observed in hypercalciuric patients under steady-state conditions,[107] it is clear that studying patients under undefined conditions is likely to lead to misinterpretation in a substantial number of instances. As a related issue, whether sodium intake has any influence on circulating 1,25-$(OH)_2D$ concentration in any category of hypercalciuric patient is unknown. The marked suppressibility of circulating 1,25-$(OH)_2D$ concentration in patients with absorptive hypercalciuria also has implications for pathogenesis (see below).

As summarized previously, when selected on the basis of weight-adjusted results for calcium excretion on a defined, high normal calcium diet and studied under the conditions specified, some 90 percent of hypercalciuric patients have the syndrome of absorp-

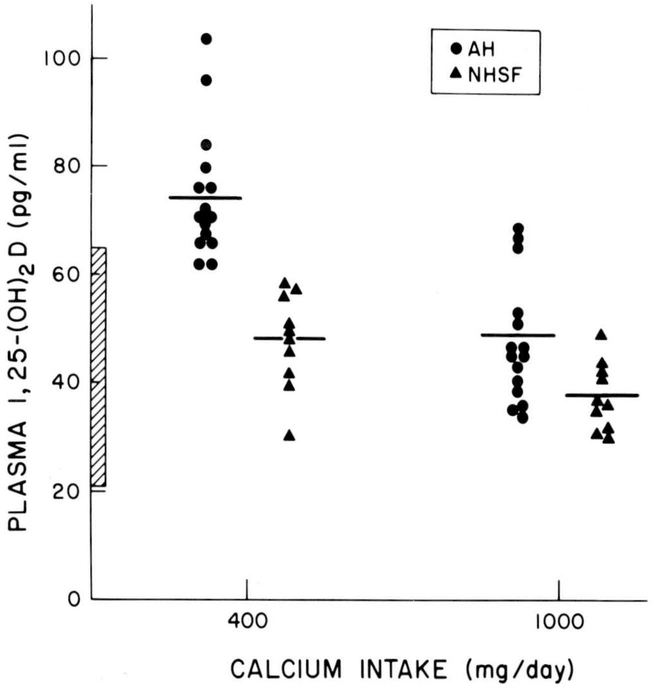

FIGURE 25-22 Values for circulating 1,25-$(OH)_2D$ in 15 patients with absorptive hypercalciuria (circles) and 10 nonhypercalciuric patients with stone disease (triangles) studied on a 400-mg calcium diet and again 3 days after being placed on a 1000-mg calcium diet. Sodium intake was controlled at approximately 100 meq/day throughout the study. The horizontal bars represent mean values and the cross-hatched bar represents the normal range for plasma 1,25-$(OH)_2D$ concentration. Note the marked suppressibility of plasma 1,25-$(OH)_2D$ concentrations in the patients with absorptive hypercalciuria as well as the extensive overlap of values between the two groups on the 1000-mg calcium diet. (*From Broadus et al,*[107] *by permission of the New England Journal of Medicine.*)

tive hypercalciuria.[105–107] The data in Fig. 25-21 come from an otherwise unselected group of these patients; it follows that absorptive hypercalciuria in the vast majority of patients may be viewed as a 1,25-$(OH)_2D$-mediated syndrome. It has also been shown that the increase in circulating 1,25-$(OH)_2D$ concentrations in these patients is the consequence of an increased production rate of the hormone.[150] The next level of questioning therefore has to do with the mechanism(s) leading to an increase in 1,25-$(OH)_2D$ production in patients with absorptive hypercalciuria.

The *phosphate leak* hypothesis holds that the primary pathogenetic abnormality in patients with absorptive hypercalciuria is a renal tubular leak of phosphate, with consequent hypophosphatemia, stimulation of 1,25-$(OH)_2D$ synthesis, and the ensuing sequence of events shown in Fig. 25-17. It will be recalled that a tendency to hypophosphatemia has been repeatedly reported in patients with idiopathic hypercalciuria since the initial descriptive series of Henneman et al.[97] and that phosphorus depletion and/or hypophosphatemia is a well-established stimulus of 1-hydroxylase activity.[151]

The evidence cited in favor of the phosphate leak hypothesis includes: (1) the often-reported tendency to hypophosphatemia and/or a decreased TmP/GFR in hypercalciuric patients,[97,108,141,149] (2) the increase in circulating 1,25-$(OH)_2D$ concentration observed in normal subjects in response to a phosphopenic stimulus,[141,152] (3) a significant inverse correlation between the plasma concentration of 1,25-$(OH)_2D$ and the serum phosphorus concentration and/or TmP/GFR in hypercalciuric patients as compared to normal subjects,[141,143,149] and (4) a partial reversal of elements of the syndrome in patients treated with oral phosphate.[140,143,153] If there is indeed a phosphate leak in these patients, it does not appear to be a fixed abnormality, in that the serum phosphorus concentration in such patients exhibits a normal diurnal variation; values in the early afternoon approach those in normal subjects.[133] The recently described syndrome of *hereditary hypophosphatemic rickets with hypercalciuria*[154] is not directly pertinent to this hypothesis as it might apply to adult patients with hypercalciuria and stone disease, but does represent perhaps the best-studied single example of a phosphate leak in human disease. This syndrome is inherited as an autosomal recessive trait and is dominated clinically by the onset of rickets at an early age.[154]

Evidence cited against the phosphate leak hypothesis includes the comparative rarity with which actual hypophosphatemia and/or frankly reduced values for TmP/GFR are observed in hypercalciuric patients,[119,130,153,155] the fact that the tendency of patients with stone disease to hypophosphatemia is not confined to patients with hypercalciuria but is seen with equal frequency in patients with other risk factors for calcium stone formation as well as in patients with no identifiable metabolic abnormality,[104,106,109,133,134,136,155] and the observation that the response to phosphate treatment does not appear to be a function of pretreatment values for serum phosphorus concentration and/or TmP/GFR.[140,143,154,156] As shown in Fig. 25-23, there is a significant inverse correlation between TmP/GFR and circulating 1,25-$(OH)_2D$ concentration in patients with absorptive hypercalciuria, compared to normal subjects (Fig. 25-23*A*), but this correlation disappears when nonhypercalciuric patients are substituted for normal subjects for purposes of this comparison (Fig. 25-23*B*). This results from the aforementioned observation that values or TmP/GFR in the range of 2.5 mg/dl or less are observed with approximately equal frequency in hypercalciuric and nonhypercalciuric patients; it follows that there is no predictable relationship between the serum phosphorus concentration and/or TmP/GFR and the circulating concentration of 1,25-$(OH)_2D$ in patients with calcium stone disease taken as a whole.[104,106]

The aggregate data may be interpreted in any of three ways: (1) the relationship of serum phosphorus concentration with hypercalciuria in general and 1,25-$(OH)_2D$ production in particular is a classic example of "guilt by association"; there is no direct pathogenetic link between these abnormalities; (2) absorptive hypercalciuria is pathogenetically heterogeneous; certain patients have hypophosphatemic absorptive hypercalciuria and others an increase in 1,25-$(OH)_2D$ production on some other basis; or (3) there is no direct cause-and-effect relationship between abnormalities in phosphate metabolism and the increase in 1,25-$(OH)_2D$ production in patients with absorptive hypercalciuria, but rather there is a fundamental proximal tubular lesion in these patients to which both of these abnormalities might be attributed. In broad terms, this last proposal fits under the heading of the *disordered control of 1,25-$(OH)_2D$ production* hypothesis.

The disordered control hypothesis has only received attention in the past several years. In a sense, the extreme sensitivity of circulating 1,25-$(OH)_2D$ concentration to variations in calcium intake in patients with absorptive hypercalciuria suggests such an abnormality (Fig. 25-22). More direct evidence is provided by the responses in these patients when a high normal calcium diet is continued for several weeks, in which case an apparent "escape" phenomenon is observed, with a rebound increase in circulating 1,25-$(OH)_2D$ level and a pronounced fall in TmP/GFR (Fig. 25-24).[107] As noted above, it has been

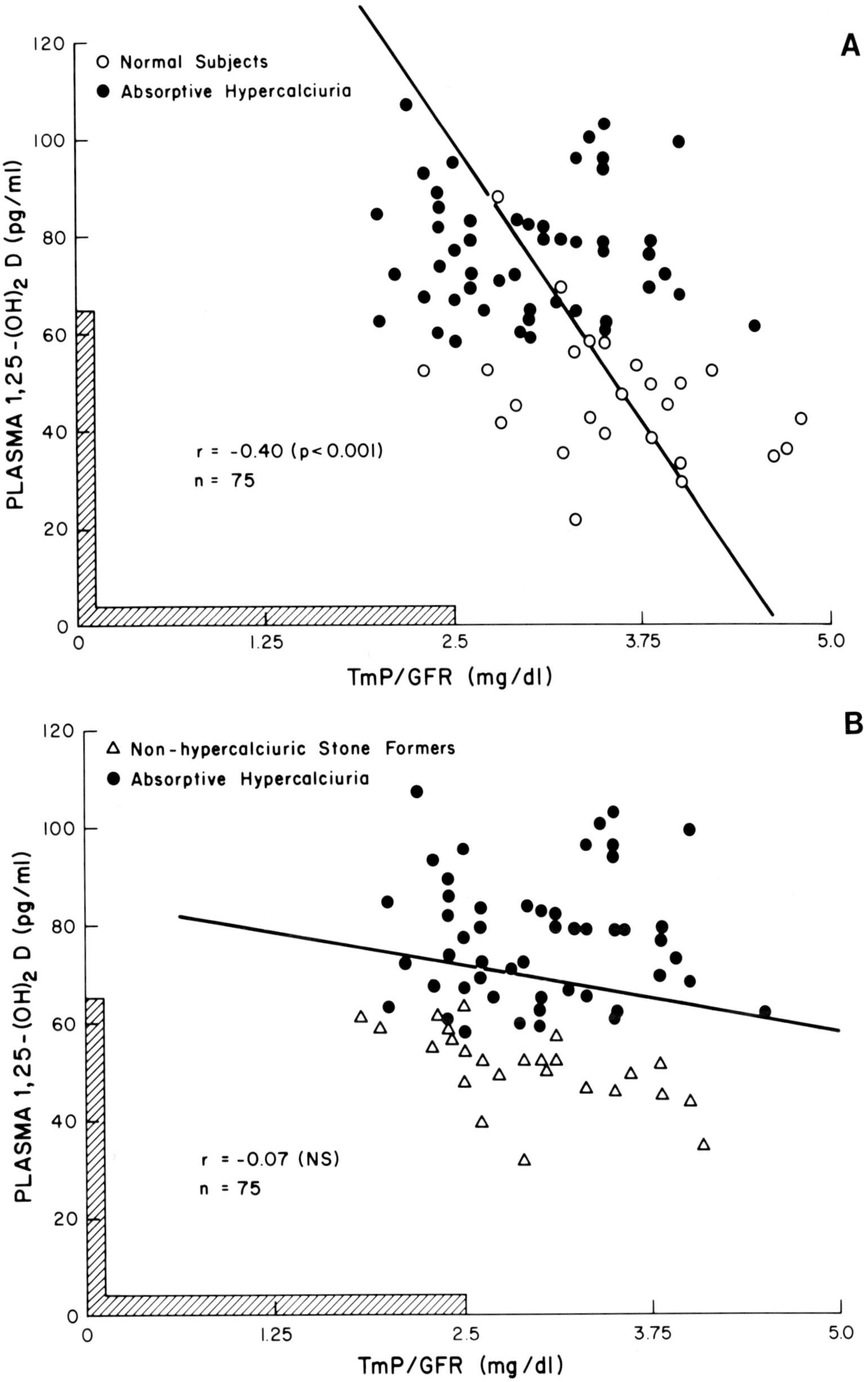

FIGURE 25-23 (A) Correlation between plasma concentration of 1,25-$(OH)_2D$ and renal phosphate threshold (TmP/GFR) in 50 patients with absorptive hypercalciuria (closed circles) and 25 normal subjects (open circles). (B) Correlation in 50 patients with absorptive hypercalciuria (solid circles) and 25 nonhypercalciuric patients with stone disease (open triangles). The hatched area on the ordinate depicts the normal range for plasma 1,25-$(OH)_2D$ concentrations and the hatched area on the abscissa represents abnormally low ($<$ 2.5 mg/dl) results for TmP/GFR in both panels. Note that the significant inverse correlation between plasma 1,25-$(OH)_2D$ concentration and TmP/GFR observed when patients with absorptive hypercalciuria and normal subjects are compared (A) disappears when the nonhypercalciuric patients are substituted for purposes of this comparison (B). *(From Broadus et al,[106] by permission of the Journal of Clinical Endocrinology and Metabolism.)*

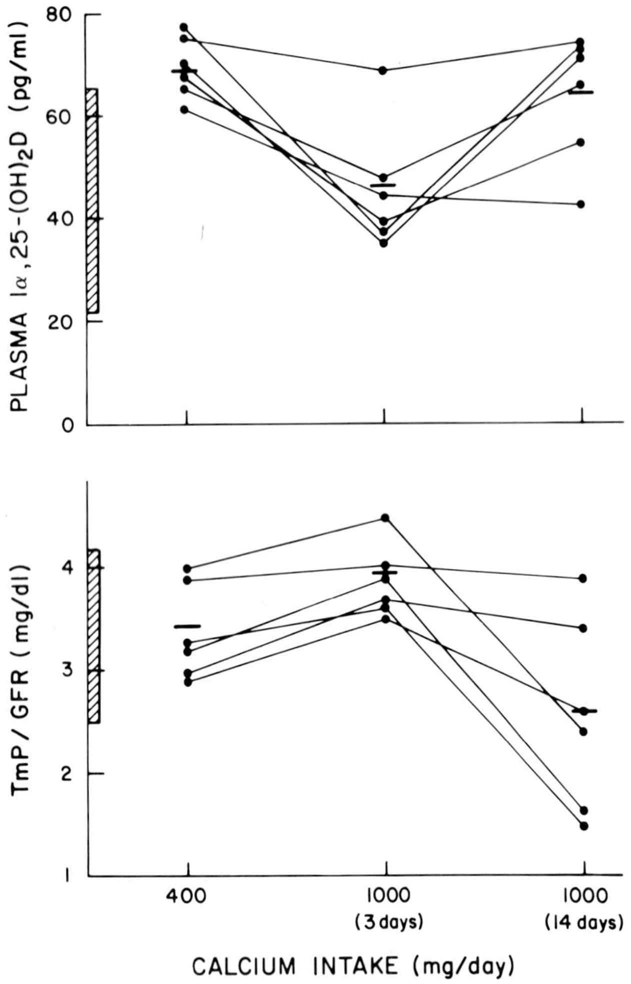

FIGURE 25-24 Plasma concentration of 1,25-$(OH)_2D$ and TmP/GFR in six patients with absorptive hypercalciuria studied sequentially (1) on a diet with 400 mg/day calcium for 7 to 10 days, (2) after 3 days on a 1000-mg/day-calcium diet, and (3) after 14 days on the 1000-mg/day-calcium diet. The hatched areas along the ordinates depict normal ranges and the horizontal bars show mean values. Note that on the prolonged high normal calcium diet, the circulating 1,25-$(OH)_2D$ concentration tends to rebound toward the initial values observed, and TmP/GFR tends to fall, in some individuals quite strikingly. (*From Broadus et al,*[107] *by permission of the New England Journal of Medicine.*)

reported by several laboratories that hypercalciuric patients may display a number of abnormalities in proximal tubular function, including defective reabsorption of calcium, phosphate, sodium, magnesium, and fluid.[108,119,132,157,158] One formulation of the disordered control hypothesis therefore holds that the syndrome of absorptive hypercalciuria is the surface manifestation of a fundamental and multifaceted deficit in proximal tubular function.[108,119,159] However, there remains some debate as to the specificity of these findings in hypercalciuric vs. nonhypercalciuric patients, the exact nature of the patient populations included in individual studies, and the rigor with which diet was controlled in some series.[120,132,160] In recent preliminary studies, a blunted, if not entirely absent, 1,25-$(OH)_2D$ response to a phosphopenic stimulus was observed in patients with absorptive hypercalciuria. If confirmed in a larger series, such a finding would be evidence of a frank, qualitative defect in these patients.[160] Another hypothesis, which has some intuitive appeal and which would explain many of the observations recorded to date in patients with absorptive hypercalciuria (i.e., the increase in 1,25-$(OH)_2D$ production, the tendency to hypophosphatemia, and the marked sensitivity to dietary calcium intake), is that these patients harbor a hypersensitivity to the proximal tubular effects of PTH.[107] This hypothesis is also under active investigation.

In summary, the disordered control hypothesis of the pathogenesis of absorptive hypercalciuria is suggested by a number of recent observations and is favored, in one formulation or another, by a number of current investigators in the field. Whether this hypothesis will stand up under scrutiny any better than its predecessors remains to be seen.

Besides the importance of hypercalciuria as a risk factor for calcium stone formation, there is considerable evidence that individuals who absorb excessive calcium also have a secondary tendency to overly absorb oxalate and that the associated mild hyperoxaluria considerably accentuates their risk for stone formation. This evidence is reviewed under Hyperoxaluria, below; it forms the basis for the therapeutic recommendation of restricting both calcium and oxalate intake in these patients.

Normal pregnancy has recently been shown to be a state of physiological absorptive hypercalciuria.[161] Whether pregnancy is a stone-forming state per se is unknown; the data on this subject are conflicting and not particularly systematic.[161,162] Nevertheless, these data call into question the routine obstetrical practice of administering calcium supplements to all pregnant women, and they would certainly appear to represent grounds for moderating calcium intake in pregnant women with an antecedent history of stone disease.

Bone Involvement in Hypercalciuria

Overt bone disease with fractures, bone pain, or deformity is extremely rare in hypercalciuric patients. The only clearly established link between hypercalciuria and frank clinical bone disease is the recently described syndrome of hereditary hypophosphatemic rickets and hypercalciuria, in which rickets dominates the clinical picture.[154] Evidence of subclinical bone involvement in hypercalciuric patients has been reported, including abnormal bone histomorphometry,[127,163] a decrease in bone mineral density in a variable percentage of patients as measured by absorptiometry,[164,165] an increase in bone turnover rate, based on calcium kinetic data,[166] and an increase in hydroxyproline excretion in a small percentage of patients.[106,127] The data in these various series are difficult to summarize because the selection criteria varied from series to series. Histomorphometric abnormalities have been observed in patients considered to be examples of absorptive hypercalciuria[127,163] as well as those whose cases are considered to be examples of renal hypercalciuria.[127] Secondary hyperparathyroidism, hypophosphatemia, an increase in circulating 1,25-$(OH)_2D$ concentration, or some combination of these variables would be expected to exert at least physiological effects at the level of the skeleton; however, the pathophysiological importance of such effects and/or the quantitative significance of any consequent "resorptive" component to the net hypercalciuria remain unknown. In general, the reported abnormalities at the level of bone in hypercalciuric patients can be viewed as having pathophysiological interest but not as providing evidence of bone disease per se. It follows that clinical bone disease is not the predictable consequence of any of the common forms of hypercalciuria; routine radiological assessment of bone density is not merited in these patients.

DIAGNOSIS

In order to adequately screen patients for hypercalciuria, samples must be collected on both a free and a high normal calcium diet (see Table 25-7 and Definition and Detection of Hypercalciuria, above). This approach maximizes the appreciation of hypercalciuria as a risk factor in individual patients and also provides some information with respect to pathogenesis, certainly in the case of dietary hypercalciuria. The high normal calcium diet is easily constructed in office or clinic practice by providing patients with instructions limiting the intake of calcium, protein, and sodium and by providing calcium supplements in tablet form (see Testing, below).

Hypercalciuria is defined as a calcium excretion rate $>$ 300 mg/day in males, $>$ 250 mg/day in females, or $>$ 4 mg per kilogram of body weight per day in either sex and in children. Clinically, the use of either the absolute excretion rate limits or the weight-adjusted limit, or both, is reasonable, but the weight-adjusted limit is the single most useful definition. When this limit is exceeded on a defined high normal calcium diet, the patient has a very high likelihood of harboring a true systemic defect in calcium metabolism.

The secondary hypercalciurias (Table 25-8) demand a high index of suspicion, but diagnosis is usually straightforward on the basis of routine clinical techniques. Together, the secondary hypercalciurias account for about 10 percent of hypercalciuria in adult patients. These syndromes are described in more detail elsewhere in this chapter and in Chap. 23.

In strictly clinical terms, the entity of dietary hypercalciuria is probably the most important addition to the hypercalciuria literature in recent years. As defined above, dietary hypercalciuria is envisioned as the actual cause of hypercalciuria in a substantial percentage of patients and contributing to, but not necessarily causing, the net hypercalciuria in another substantial percentage of patients (see Table 25-7). Together, these two groups constitute something like one-third of the hypercalciuric patients summarized in Table 25-7 and some one-half of patients whose hypercalciuria was detected on a free diet. The strongest statistical link in these patients is to sodium intake and sodium excretion, but other dietary factors or some combination of factors such as sodium, protein, and calcium may be at work.[104] Dietary hypercalciuria is most easily detected by having patients collect specimens on both a free and a high normal calcium diet (see Table 25-7). Sodium should be measured in the free intake specimen; it is high in the great majority of such patients. It should be recalled that the exact cause-and-effect relationships between high sodium intake and hypercalciuria remain to be established and that occasional patients with a high sodium excretion are encountered who are not hypercalciuric. Dietary hypercalciuria probably also accounts for the wide swings in calcium excretion sometimes observed in a minority of both untreated and treated "hypercalciuric" patients; sodium excretion should also be measured in such patients as a clue to what is an otherwise perplexing pattern of laboratory values.

The entity of so-called constitutional hypercalciuria merits distinguishing on metabolic grounds but probably not in strictly clinical terms. As summarized above, these patients call into question defining hypercalciuria on the basis of absolute excretion rate vs. the weight-adjusted values. These patients are almost exclusively male; they may present with dietary hypercalciuria and/or be found to be hyperuricosuric. There is no reason to suppose that the "hypercalciuria" in these patients is any less important as a risk factor than that in other patients, and they should be so treated.

An essential goal of diagnosis is to avoid overlooking patients with subtle primary hyperparathyroidism. This diagnosis requires serious consideration in any patient with a mean total fasting serum calcium concentration above 10.0 mg/dl on three or more carefully made determinations. The diagnosis can be confirmed in approximately 80 to 90 percent of patients so defined on initial screening. Conversely, the diagnosis does not require serious consideration in patients with a mean total serum calcium concentraton on initial screening of about 9 mg/dl to 10 mg/dl.

The diagnosis of primary hyperparathyroidism in any patient rests on the simultaneous demonstration of hypercalcemia together with a measure of parathyroid function which is frankly elevated or clearly inappropriate. Although the pattern of intermittent hypercalcemia characteristically displayed by these patients is a highly suggestive feature, the abnormalities in serum calcium concentration and parathyroid function under basal conditions are often quite subtle and must be interpreted with great care. Unfortunately, history continues to repeat itself in the form of needless and inappropriate neck explorations in patients in whom this diagnosis is suspected, but in whom confirmatory biochemical evidence is lacking. The most reliable approaches to differential diagnosis include careful measurement of serum total or ionized serum calcium concentration together with a sensitive immunoassay for PTH[123] and performance of the calcium tolerance test (see Fig. 25-18).[75,121] The problem faced by the practicing physician is access to sensitive laboratory techniques; the commercial assays for PTH generally lack sensitivity, and the cAMP assays are not widely available and/or are reported by many (but not all) commercial laboratories in meaningless units. The calcium tolerance test is favored because this test is physiologically based, in the sense of being a fairly classic endocrine suppression test. Also, the pattern of induced abnormalities is usually clear-cut in these patients. Reliable results for cAMP excretion are available commercially and are almost as sensitive clinically as the technically more demanding measurement of nephrogenous cAMP. The *thiazide challenge* test, an attempt to induce sustained hypercalcemia in patients with subtle primary hyperparathyroidism, is both unpredictable and nonspecific.[167] Scanning, venous sampling, and other such techniques are localization rather than diagnostic techniques per se and are rarely useful in confronting this differential diagnosis.

If this point in the differential diagnosis has been reached, having excluded the secondary hypercalciurias, dietary hypercalciuria, and subtle primary hyperparathyroidism, is it worth pursuing diagnosis further? Specifically, do clinical considerations merit distinguishing between renal and absorptive hypercalciuria? Although there is ample disagreement in the literature on this point, the pragmatic answer is probably not. First, there is increasingly compelling evidence that absorptive hypercalciuria constitutes the lion's share of idiopathic hypercalciuria and that primary renal hypercalciuria is quite rare. Second, clinical bone disease does not appear to be a predictable consequence of either renal hypercalciuria or absorptive hypercalciuria. In addition, the differential points are quite subtle, and may require techniques which are not generally available in order to establish a specific diagnosis with certainty. The argument that most physicians are already committed to an empirical treatment plan of personal preference which is not dependent upon this differential diagnosis does not have intellectual appeal; it is based largely on cost-benefit reasoning. The first point above assumes that the classification scheme in Table 25-8 and the interpretation of the data presented in the section on idiopathic hypercalciuria are accepted. If an increase in fasting calcium excretion continues to be regarded as pathogenetically meaningful and therapy is based on the presence or absence of this finding, then some amount of additional testing will be needed.

The conditions of study are crucial to the accuracy of the data obtained in pursuing the differential diagnosis of idiopathic hypercalciuria. All detailed testing should be preceded by 7 to 10 days on a diet restricted in both calcium (about 400 mg/day) and sodium (about 100 meq/day). Compliance with this diet should not be assumed; intake should be monitored by a 24-h urine collection and determination of both calcium and sodium excretion on the day prior to the performance of detailed testing.

The diagnosis of a primary renal calcium leak requires the demonstration of an increase in fasting calcium excretion (or fasting fractional calcium excretion) together with an elevation in serum immunoreactive PTH concentration and/or nephrogenous cAMP or total cAMP excretion. An increase in fasting calcium excretion in the absence of evidence for secondary hyperparathyroidism does not establish this diagnosis, various interpretations in the literature notwithstanding. Significant hypercalciuria on a calcium- and sodium-restricted diet is a contributory point but also does not, in itself, establish a diagnosis of renal hypercalciuria.

The diagnosis of absorptive hypercalciuria requires some evidence that the patient excessively absorbs calcium and has normal or depressed parathyroid function. The measurement of fractional intestinal calcium absorption by isotopic means is a research technique. Available means of demonstrating excessive GI absorption of calcium include performing some version of the calcium tolerance test and/or collecting 24-h urine samples on both a calcium-restricted and an unrestricted diet, with the foreknowledge that the normal regression of calcium excretion on calcium intake is only about 6 percent.[99,100,105,106,168] These same samples can be collected in reverse order and the decrement in calcium excretion used as a gauge of the therapeutic benefit to be derived from a restriction in dietary calcium intake in individual patients. Perhaps the single simplest approach in establishing a diagnosis of absorptive hypercalciuria is to demonstrate significant hypercalciuria ($>$ 4.0 mg calcium excreted per kilogram of body weight per day) and low or low normal total cAMP excretion ($<$ 3.5 nmol per deciliter of glomerular filtrate) in the 24-h urine sample which was collected with the patient on a defined, high normal calcium diet.[168] This serves as a sort of "poorman's" calcium tolerance test.

The calcium tolerance test was introduced by Peacock et al. in 1968;[131] the original version was modified by Pak et al. in 1975,[112] further modified by our group in 1978,[105] and subsequently used and/or further modified by a number of groups.[136,137,154,169-171] Some of the modifications introduced over the years have merit, whereas others appear to be more idiosyncratic and less meaningful. Given adequate patient selection, careful dietary preparation in terms of both calcium and sodium intake, and attention to detail in the performance of the test, the calcium tolerance test is very useful; it provides a diagnosis in some 90 percent of hypercalciuric patients (see above). If patients are selected on the basis of results for calcium excretion on a free diet without attention to the entities of dietary hypercalciuria and constitutional hypercalciuria, if sodium and calcium intake are not carefully controlled, and if undue emphasis is placed on the interpretation of fasting calcium excretion, the test is of marginal diagnostic value, as has been repeatedly reported.[136,137,169-171] As summarized above, if only those patients who were hypercalciuric on a free diet were tested, but patients with dietary hypercalciuria and constitutional hypercalciuria were included in the denominator, diagnostic results would have been obtained in only some 60 percent of patients. Clearly, the working assumption that the hypercalciuria in 100 percent of patients screened on a free diet should have a metabolic explanation is misguided and should not be the grounds for judging the usefulness, or lack thereof, of any test used in pursuing a differential diagnosis.

Plasma 1,25-$(OH)_2D$ concentration and TmP/GFR may be measured selectively in hypercalciuric patients but are not particularly useful in the diagnostic distinction between subtle primary hyperparathyroidism, renal hypercalciuria, and absorptive hypercalciuria. Commercial assays for plasma 1,25-$(OH)_2D$ appear to be quite reliable. Sampling requirements, the performance of the calcium tolerance test, and other relevant techniques are described under Testing and in Chap. 23.

TREATMENT

The therapy of the hypercalciurias is presented here according to the outline in Table 25-8. In many ways, general concepts are far more important than the details of a given regimen, and the reader is referred to General Principles of Therapy, below, for guidelines regarding therapeutic decision-making, therapeutic programs, and the monitoring of patients during therapy.

The secondary hypercalciurias should be treated specifically, as outlined above and in Chap. 23. Patients with subtle primary hyperparathyroidism should undergo neck exploration and should be managed during the perioperative period as described in Chap. 23. Approximately 80 percent of these patients harbor a single, small parathyroid adenoma, in keeping with the view that their disorder simply represents a mild form of primary hyperparathyroidism. Because of the small mass of abnormal parathyroid tissue typically identified in patients with subtle primary hyperparathyroidism, these patients, particularly, should be entrusted to the hands of a skilled neck surgeon. The postoperative course is generally very smooth, and significant postoperative hypocalcemia is rare. Bordier et al. have reported some fascinating postoperative observations in several patients presumed before surgery to have subtle primary hyperparathyroidism.[127] These observations suggested that the patients' parathyroid lesions developed as a consequence of adenomatous transformation of secondarily hyperplastic parathyroid tissue in patients with renal hypercalciuria, that is, that the patients had "tertiary" hyperparathyroidism. The frequency of this putative sequence of events in patients with subtle primary hyperparathyroidism is unknown; Parks et al. identified long-term hypercalciuria in only 1 of 52 patients with mild primary hyperparathyroidism during postoperative follow-up.[124] An equally plausible explanation for the findings reported by Bordier et al. is that the patients described had primary chief cell hyperplasia, with disease recurrence after subtotal parathyroidectomy. This sequence of events is quite predictable in some patients, since subtotal parathyroidectomy is but a palliative procedure. It must be recalled that patients with a significant stone burden at the time of parathyroidectomy may experience stone-related complications after surgery without implications for the success of the operative procedure.

Patients judged not to be good candidates for neck exploration or who have persistent hyperparathyroidism following exploration can be managed successfully with oral phosphorus therapy. In short-term studies, oral phosphorus supplements in a dosage of approximately 1500 mg/day have been shown to reduce circulating 1,25-$(OH)_2D$, calcium absorption and excretion, and the rate of stone formation in patients with primary hyperparathyroidism.[172] This therapy is basically antihypercalciuric rather than antihypercalcemic and is not recommended in patients with moderate to severe hypercalcemia.[172]

As emphasized below (see General Principles of Therapy), the treatment of patients with any form of stone disease is a program, not simply a pill. This treatment program consists of (1) specific and repeated instructions to force fluids,[93,173,174] (2) guidelines concerning dietary moderation,[173–175] and, in some patients, (3) an agent targeted at reducing the excretion rate of a stone-forming constituent. It is the net effect of this program, not of any single component thereof, which can change the amount of the stone-forming constituent and the urinary volume in such a way as to prevent stone progression or recurrence. The therapeutic literature has recently been taken to task in this regard,[173,176] with specific criticism aimed at the 10 trials of thiazide therapy reported in the English language to date.[176] These criticisms appear to be equally valid when applied to most reports concerning the efficacy of other agents, so that the thiazide literature should not be regarded as being peculiarly lax in terms of study design. One specific criticism, implied above, is that of "cointervention," meaning that patients are placed on a multifaceted program but all beneficial effects are attributed to the drug component of this program.[176] This and other issues are described in more detail below.

A second general point of conceptual importance is that the approach to a given patient with stone disease should be considered as consisting of four interdependent phases: (1) the diagnostic phase, (2) the initial therapeutic phase, (3) the prolonged therapeutic phase, and, possibly, (4) discontinuance of therapy. These phases should be explained in sufficient detail to permit the patient to understand the concepts involved and become an active participant in his or her own care. (These phases and the common deficiencies of care associated with them are also covered in General Principles of Therapy.)

Patients with dietary hypercalciuria are managed with a program of forced fluids and moderations in sodium intake (to approximately 100 meq/day), calcium intake (to approximately 400 to 600 mg/day), and protein intake (to approximately 120 g/day).[103,117,175] Most of these patients are male, and some are also hyperuricosuric. The effects of fluid and dietary therapy can be monitored during the initial therapeutic phase (phase II); measurement of sodium excretion provides a convenient indicator of patient compliance. A large minority of these patients appear to have underlying absorptive hypercalciuria, on which a dietary component is superimposed (see Table 25-7 and accompanying text), and these patients may require additional medical therapy to achieve normocalciuria.

There is a substantial literature which argues for specific therapy in patients with renal hypercalciuria and absorptive hypercalciuria. This literature reports that thiazide diuretics partially or completely reverse the pattern of abnormalities associated with renal hypercalciuria,[128,177] and oral phosphate therapy partially reverses the pattern of abnormalities associated with absorptive hypercalciuria; this is true whether or not patients had hypophosphatemia before treatment.[140,143,178] If the data in these reports are examined closely, the biochemical changes reported are found to be statistically significant but in general quite subtle; it is difficult to know whether the recommendations for specific therapy are justified based on the data provided.[128,140,143,177,178] This is particularly true given the diagnostic criteria used for patient selection in some of these series. The antihypercalciuric effects of the thiazides and oral phosphates have been shown to be roughly equivalent, both in large series of hypercalciuric patients not further defined[179–183] and in patients with absorptive hypercalciuria,[156] so that the response to these agents is not necessarily dependent upon the underlying mechanism leading to the hypercalciuria.

Given adequate grounds for a diagnosis of primary renal hypercalciuria, the agents of choice are clearly the thiazide diuretics.[128,177] Additional general measures include the fluid and dietary instructions summarized above. Thiazides are also regarded as the agents of choice in hypercalciuric patients with coincident hypertension.

Patients with absorptive hypercalciuria are instructed to follow a program of forced fluids and dietary moderation, specifically to include a restricted oxalate intake (see Table 25-11 for guidelines, including the availability of specific guidelines). Additional measures may include administration of either oral phosphates or a thiazide diuretic, which appear to have an equivalent antihypercalciuric effect in these patients.[156,179-183] Thiazides do not appear to substantially reverse the fundamental pathophysiological features of absorptive hypercalciuria, at least in the short term,[156,177] leaving a question of where the calcium which continues to be hyperabsorbed is being deposited. However, dystrophic calcification has not been observed in several large series of hypercalciuric patients on thiazide diuretics for prolonged periods, and it is assumed that these series contained many patients with absorptive hypercalciuria.[179,180]

Sodium cellulose phosphate is a special case. This agent is a nonabsorbable cation exchange resin which binds calcium and prevents its absorption from the intestinal contents.[184,185] Sodium cellulose phosphate has only recently been released in the United States and is specifically intended for use in patients with absorptive hypercalciuria. Patients receiving this agent must be on magnesium supplements and must also follow an oxalate-restricted diet;[184,185] some patients experience gastrointestinal side effects.[185] The effects and required dosage of sodium cellulose phosphate can be rather easily monitored by serial measurements of urinary calcium excretion, and the agent does not induce secondary hyperparathyroidism or negative calcium balance.[184] The drug is expensive and not particularly easy to use.[174] It may be of particular benefit, by itself or in combination, in patients with severe absorptive hypercalciuria, who may be difficult to manage by any other means.

Table 25-11. Oxalate Content of Some Foods and Beverages

High		
Rhubarb	Sweet potatoes	Tea
Spinach	Dill	Some instant coffee
Beet greens	Nuts	Grapefruit juice
Swiss chard	Unripe bananas	Orange juice
Turnip greens	Chocolate	Cranberry juice
Beets	Cocoa	Grape juice
Sorrel	Ovaltine	Pepper
Parsley		
Low		
Meats	Peas	Melons
Fish	Turnips	Peaches
Dairy products	Lettuce	Pears
Eggs	Radishes	Pineapples
Cereals	Apples	Plums
Cabbage	Ripe bananas	Raspberries
Asparagus	Apricots	Margarine
Cauliflower		

Source: From Smith.[190]
Note: A booklet entitled the "Low Oxalate Diet Book" can be requested from the Oxalate Research Program, Clinical Research Center, H-203, University of California Hospital, 225 West Dickinson Street, San Diego, California 92103. A check for $2 made payable to the Regents of the University of California should be enclosed.

By far the most extensive experience with either thiazides or phosphorus therapy has been gained in the empirical treatment of hypercalciuric patients not further defined as to pathophysiological subtype. Each form of treatment has its staunch proponents; each appears to result in an approximately equivalent decrease in the rate of calcium excretion, and each has been reported to eliminate or greatly reduce stone formation in 90 percent or more of treated patients in most, but not all, series.[2,3,5,6,8,174,178-183] The reduction in calcium excretion produced by these agents is thought to be only partially responsible for their apparent efficacy in stone prevention. Long-term therapy with thiazides may also decrease oxalate excretion,[186] although this point has been questioned.[187] Oral phosphate therapy has been reported to increase the excretion of pyrophosphate, an inhibitor of crystallization and crystal growth.[181,182]

Conventional antihypertensive doses of the thiazides are used in patients with stone disease. The hypocalciuric effect of the thiazides results from a combination of volume contraction and direct action to increase calcium reabsorption in the distal nephron.[188] This effect is shared by all thiazide congeners and related diuretics (e.g., chlorthalidone); there is no clear agent of choice. Trichlormethiazide is commonly used in a dosage of 2 mg twice daily without potassium supplementation by other than dietary means. On average, full doses of the thiazides reduce the calcium excretion rate to approximately 60 percent of the pretreatment rate.[109,128,167,179,180] A high salt intake can largely overcome the antihypercalciuric effect of the drug. The most common side effect is a feeling of lassitude, which is usually transient and which does not appear to be related to hypokalemia. As noted above, dystrophic calcification has not been observed in hypercalciuric patients on thiazide therapy.[179,180] Triamterene-containing agents are not used in patients with stone disease because triamterene and/or its products have been identified in stone material obtained from such patients.[189]

Oral phosphorus is administered as 1500 to 2000 mg of elemental phosphorus daily in three or four divided doses. The neutral, rather than the acid, phosphorus preparations are most commonly employed,[178,181-183] and pure potassium salts are available. Patients tend to prefer tablets of the phosphate salts to those forms which require suspension prior to consumption. All phosphate salts are cathartic, and this side effect limits the dosage in a small minority of treated patients. Dystrophic calcification and treatment-induced secondary hyperparathyroidism do not appear to be realistic concerns.[178,181,182] However, the frequent dosage schedule may reduce patient compliance. Although there are no data to support it, avoidance of oral phosphates appears reasonable in patients whose stones contain a high percentage of calcium phosphate.

Some 10 percent of patients treated with either thiazides or phosphates do not display the anticipated hypocalciuric response. In patients on thiazides, this lack of response may be due to a coincident high salt intake. In other patients seemingly unresponsive to thiazides or phosphorus, the reason(s) for the poor chemical response is inapparent. A trial of alternative therapy may be warranted in such a patient. Smaller doses of thiazides or phosphates than those described above are employed in the treatment of certain patients because of side effects or other considerations, but these are regarded as less effective than the conventional doses.[179,182]

Hyperoxaluria

Although oxalate is the major anionic constituent in the great majority of calcium stones, disorders of oxalate metabolism per se are only rarely identified in patients with calcium stone disease. However, relatively subtle abnormalities in oxalate metabolism and/or excretion could easily pass undetected, for available methods for measuring oxalate are imprecise, and the metabolic pathways leading to the production of oxalate are imperfectly understood. Such subtle abnormalities could have a major impact on the tendency to form calcium stones because of the extreme insolubility of oxalate in aqueous solution. Clearly, the development of a means of inhibiting oxalate production in a fashion analogous to the inhibition of uric acid synthesis by allopurinol would have profound implications for treatment of patients with calcium stone disease, even in the absence of defined abnormalities of oxalate production.

ABSORPTION, PRODUCTION, AND RENAL CLEARANCE OF OXALATE

Oxalate is a metabolic end product and serves no known biochemical function. Oxalic acid is a simple two-carbon dicarboxylic acid. It is a relatively strong organic acid, with a pK_a of 1.2. Oxalate forms a number of complexes and salts in complex solution, but it is the insolubility of its calcium salt which defines the clinical relevance of oxalate. In a simple aqueous solution, the maximum solubility of the calcium salt is 0.67 mg/dl; solubility is little influenced by variations in pH over the physiological range.[190,191]

The metabolic pool of oxalate is derived from two sources: intestinal absorption and endogenous production.[190,191] Solubility considerations limit the intestinal absorption of oxalate, so that in normal individuals endogenous oxalate production accounts for some 85 percent of the daily excretion rate of oxalate.

Oxalate is absorbed throughout the small and large intestine by diffusion.[190-193] This process was initially thought to be simple, passive diffusion, but more recent evidence indicates that it is facilitated diffusion, occurring via an anion exchange mechanism in both small and large bowel.[193] When a simple isotopic solution of oxalate is administered in the fasting state, approximately 15 percent of the administered oxalate is normally absorbed.[190-192] Estimates of oxalate absorption from foodstuffs, however, indicate that only some 5 to 10 percent of ingested oxalate is absorbed. The calcium salt is just as insoluble in the luminal contents of the intestine as in other complex solutions, and dietary calcium is a major determinant of oxalate absorption. This fact may have important implications regarding both the pathogenesis and the therapy of patients with calcium stone disease. Methodological difficulties have limited knowledge of the oxalate content in foodstuffs; reported estimates in various diet tables vary widely. Foodstuffs considered to have high and low oxalate content are listed in Table 25-11. Little is known concerning the soluble and insoluble proportions of oxalate in these foods and beverages, and therefore the biological availability of oxalate for absorption. Depending on dietary habits and the particular food table employed, the typical adult intake of oxalate has been estimated to be as low as 100 mg/day and as high as 900 mg/day.[190]

The details of endogenous oxalate metabolism are poorly understood (Fig. 25-25). The two principal metabolic sources of oxalate are ascorbic acid and glyoxylate.[190,191,194] The metabolism of ascorbic acid accounts for approximately 30 percent of the daily oxalate production and excretion rates, but the exact metabolic pathway responsible for the oxidation of ascorbic acid is unknown. The oxidation of glyoxylate

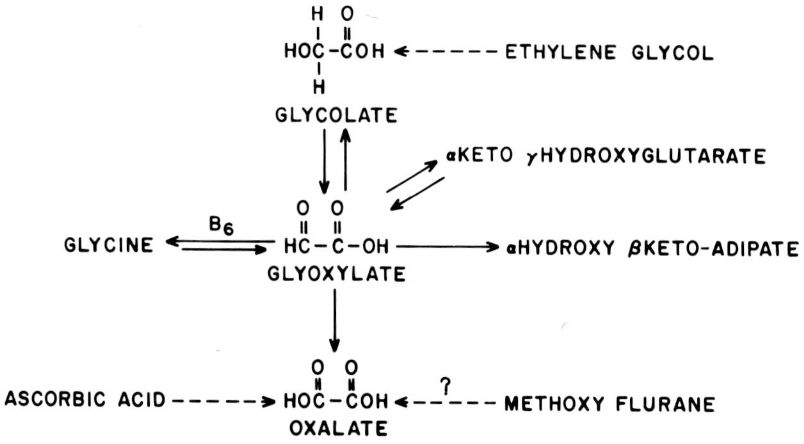

FIGURE 25-25 Pathways of oxalate biosynthesis. (*From Dobbins and Binder,*[192] *by permission of Grune & Stratton.*)

accounts for the bulk of the remaining production of oxalate. Lactic dehydrogenase appears to be the most important enzyme in the conversion of glyoxylate to oxalate. A major portion of the metabolic pool of glyoxylate is also transaminated to glycine by an enzyme that requires pyridoxine as a cofactor (Fig. 25-25). An additional important pathway in glyoxylate metabolism is the formation of α-hydroxy-β-keto-adipate from α-ketoglutarate and glyoxylate. A deficiency of this enzyme (2-oxoglutarate:glyoxylate carboligase) occurs in primary hyperoxaluria type 1.[190,191,194]

Although there is a small amount of oxalate present in bile and in intestinal secretions, the excretion of oxalate into the urine is the principal route of its elimination from the extracellular pool. Circulating oxalate is freely filtered at the glomerulus. In all species studied, the fractional excretion of oxalate exceeds unity, indicating net tubular secretion of oxalate.[190,191,195] In the rat, the principal site of tubular secretion is the proximal tubule, and net transport of oxalate along the remainder of the nephron does not appear to occur.[195] The proximal tubular system differs from the classic organic acid secretory system which transports *p*-aminohippuric acid and is uninfluenced by probenecid.[195] Abnormalities in oxalate clearance in humans are unknown.

CLASSIFICATION OF HYPEROXALURIC STATES

Hyperoxaluria is conventionally classified into those disorders associated with an increased endogenous production of oxalate and those conditions associated with an increase in oxalate intake and/or absorption (Table 25-12).

The *primary hyperoxalurias* are rare inborn errors of oxalate metabolism and are the most malignant crystal deposition diseases known.[190,191,194] Type 1 hyperoxaluria (glycolic aciduria) is inherited as an autosomal recessive trait. It results from a deficiency of the soluble carboligase which converts glyoxylate to α-hydroxy-β-ketoadipate (Fig. 25-25). This deficiency results in an accumulation of glyoxylate and increased production and excretion of glyoxylate, oxalate, and glycolate. Heterozygotes are unaffected clinically and cannot be detected by chemical screening. Type 2 hyperoxaluria (L-glyceric aciduria) results from a deficiency in D-glyceric dehydrogenase, an enzyme in the gluconeogenic pathway of serine metabolism.[190,191,194] The mechanism by which a deficiency of this enzyme leads to an increased production of oxalate is unknown. Affected patients display increased rates of L-glyceric acid and oxalate excretion and diminished rates of glyoxylate and glycolate excretion.[190,191,194] Only a handful of patients with the type 2 syndrome have been described to date; the mechanism of inheritance is unknown but is presumed to be autosomal recessive.

Patients with type 1 hyperoxaluria typically present with calcium oxalate stones in early childhood, usually before the age of 6 years.[190,191,194] In addition to

Table 25-12. Classification and Causes of Hyperoxaluria

Increased endogenous oxalate production
Primary hyperoxaluria, types 1 and 2
Administration or increased intake of oxalate precursors:
Ethylene glycol
Methoxyflurane
Ascorbic acid
Pyridoxine deficiency
Increased oxalate intake and/or absorption
Excessive oxalate ingestion
Enteric hyperoxaluria
Influence of calcium intake and absorption

the particularly virulent pattern of recurrent stone formation, patients usually also develop deposits of oxalate (oxalosis) in soft tissues, including the heart, blood vessels, central nervous system, bone marrow, and kidney. The majority of untreated patients die before the age of 20 years as a result of renal insufficiency produced by stone complications, infection, and oxalosis-induced interstitial nephritis.[190,191,194] Patients with type 2 hyperoxaluria present with recurrent calcium oxalate stones at an early age, but definitive evidence of soft tissue oxalosis in these patients has not been reported.[194] Fortunately, the grim natural history of the primary hyperoxalurias may be altered in many patients by appropriate therapy. Occasional hyperoxaluric patients presenting with calcium oxalate stones in adulthood have been described; it is speculated that such patients may have a mild form of primary hyperoxaluria.

Ethylene glycol is metabolized to oxalate by a metabolic sequence which is initiated by its oxidation by alcohol dehydrogenase (Fig. 25-25). The agent is a common ingredient in antifreeze preparations and industrial solvents and is a rare cause of poisoning due to accidental or purposeful ingestion. Ethylene glycol poisoning produces massive hyperoxaluria and oxalosis, which commonly results in acute renal failure and death.

The anesthetic agent *methoxyflurane* is partially metabolized to oxalate in the liver (Fig. 25-25). Occasional cases of acute renal failure following methoxyflurane anesthesia have been reported; they appear to have resulted from hyperoxaluria and renal oxalosis.[190,191]

The oxidation of *ascorbic acid* accounts for a significant proportion of the endogenous production rate of oxalate under normal circumstances. "Megavitamin" doses of ascorbic acid have been reported to increase endogenous oxalate production and excretion, although there is some disagreement as to the reproducibility or clinical significance of this effect.[90] The ingestion of vitamin C has been reported to possibly exacerbate stone formation in patients with antecedent stone disease, and its use is discouraged in such patients.[91] The potential effects and/or risks of the conventional 500- to 1000-mg/day dosage in such widespread use in the general population is unknown, but is probably quite small.[90]

Pyridoxine is a cofactor in the transamination of glyoxylate to glycine (Fig. 25-25), and *pyridoxine deficiency* has been reported to lead to increased oxalate production and excretion in humans and experimental animals.[190,191] Clinical examples of this association, however, are exceedingly rare. The therapeutic use of pharmacological doses of pyridoxine in patients with calcium stone disease represents an attempt to force this transamination reaction toward glycine, thereby decreasing the conversion of glyoxylate to oxalate.

Because of the poor net intestinal absorption of oxalate from foodstuffs, frank hyperoxaluria as a result solely of excessive oxalate intake is very rare. Massive ingestion of one or more of the foodstuffs considered to be high in oxalate content (Table 25-11) requires very unusual dietary habits and is usually readily identified by even a relatively casual dietary history. Rhubarb gluttony is often cited as an example of dietary hyperoxaluria.[190]

Enteric hyperoxaluria is by far the most common and clinically important of the hyperoxaluric states. It is identified in some 2 to 5 percent of patients presenting with calcium oxalate stones.[2,3,5,6,8,190–192] An increased prevalence of nephrolithiasis in patients with a variety of chronic GI disorders was initially recognized in the late 1930s, and it was later noted that such patients are prone to both calcium oxalate and uric acid stone formation. The frequency of stone disease in patients with chronic inflammatory bowel disease is estimated to be about double that of the general population.[190–192] Although calcium stones outnumber uric acid stones by 3 to 1 in patients with gastrointestinal disease, this ratio remains considerably lower than the approximately 12 to 1 ratio noted in the general stone-forming population (Table 25-1). Patients with an ileostomy are at particular risk for uric acid stones because of the frequent combination of low urine volume and acid urinary pH (see Uric Acid Calculi, above).

Enteric hyperoxaluria was described as a distinct entity by the Mayo Clinic group in the early 1970s;[196] this report was rapidly confirmed and extended by a number of laboratories.[190–192,197] It was recognized that hyperoxaluria and a predisposition to calcium stone disease were associated with a variety of GI conditions, including regional enteritis, nontropical sprue, chronic pancreatic and biliary tract disease, the blind loop syndrome, and ileal resection or jejunoileal bypass postoperatively. Calcium oxalate stones were noted to be particularly common in patients following jejunoileal bypass for obesity, with reported frequencies ranging from 17 to 32 percent.[190] Ulcerative colitis is notably absent from the list of disorders associated with enteric hyperoxaluria.

A number of hypotheses were initially proposed to explain the pathogenesis of enteric hyperoxaluria, but by 1973 it was appreciated that the principal abnormality in affected patients is an increase in intestinal oxalate absorption.[197] Again, this observation was rapidly confirmed, and further studies suggested a direct correlation between the degree of fat malabsorption and steatorrhea and the absorption and excretion of oxalate. These studies also pinpointed the colon as the major site of oxalate absorption.[190–192] The importance of the colon in the hyperabsorption of dietary oxalate in patients with enteric hyperoxaluria is supported by a number of lines of evidence, including the presence of the syndrome in patients who lack all but a small percentage of their small intestinal absorptive surface because of jejunoileal bypass.[192] Thus, the terms "colonic hyperoxaluria" or "absorptive hyperoxaluria" could serve as equally descriptive synonyms for the disorder.

As noted in the preceding section, the absorption of oxalate throughout the intestine is known to occur via facilitated diffusion.[192,194] Therefore, the absorption of oxalate is dependent upon the concentration of unbound oxalate in the intestinal contents. Two hypotheses have been advanced to explain the increased colonic absorption of oxalate in patients with enteric hyperoxaluria. The *solubility theory* holds that malabsorbed fatty acids bind calcium in the intestinal contents, thus decreasing the quantity of insoluble calcium oxalate and making more free oxalate available for passive absorption. The *permeability theory* holds that exposure of the colonic mucosa to unabsorbed bile acids and fatty acids produces a nonspecific increase in the permeability of the mucosa with a resultant increase in the diffusion of oxalate. There is considerable evidence in support of each of these hypotheses, and it is likely that both mechanisms apply to one extent or another in most patients with enteric hyperoxaluria.[190–192]

Actual stone formation is considerably less frequent than is the presence of detectable hyperoxaluria in patients with the various GI disorders noted above. Smith has emphasized that hyperoxaluria is but one of a number of potential risk factors for calcium stone formation in patients with intestinal disease and has stressed the importance of carefully assessing patients for other factors which may bear on stone formation.[190] These factors include intestinal losses of fluids with low urine volume, malabsorption of magnesium with hypomagnesuria, reduction in pyrophosphate excretion, and hypocitraturia.[190,198] Hypocitraturia, the most recently described of these risk factors, was initially reported in patients with active steatorrhea.[198] The basis of the hypocitraturia in these patients appeared to be multifactorial; it was in part the consequence of citrate malabsorption and in part secondary to a hypomagnesuria-associated increase in the renal tubular reabsorption of citrate.[198] The importance of hypomagnesuria and/or hypocitraturia as risk factors for stone formation in patients in whom steatorrhea is controlled is unknown.

A number of laboratories have reported small but significant increases in oxalate excretion in a variable percentage of patients with calcium stone disease who lack evidence of primary or enteric hyperoxaluria.[190,199–202] Reported excretion rates in these patients have been only slightly elevated, in the 50 to 80 mg/day range, and have been interpreted with some caution because of the methodological uncertainties in the measurement of oxalate concentration. Nevertheless, oxalate is considered to have a relatively greater impact on urine supersaturation than calcium, so that such modest increases in oxalate excretion could represent an important risk factor for stone formation.[77,190,199] There are several mechanisms which might account for the variable and modest increases in oxalate excretion which have been observed. First, patients with recurrent calcium stone disease are almost invariably instructed to avoid dietary calcium, and it is possible that this restriction in calcium intake influences the biological availability of dietary oxalate and results in an increase in oxalate absorption. Second, several laboratories have recently reported that patients with increased intestinal calcium absorption and hypercalciuria display a coincident increase in oxalate absorption and that these two abnormalities are strongly correlated.[201,202] Again, the mechanism responsible for this association is presumed to be a reduced concentration of calcium in the intestinal contents because of the hyperabsorption of calcium, with a consequent increase in the amount of unbound, absorbable oxalate.[190,199,201,202] This mechanism has been demonstrated directly in normal subjects in whom a model of absorptive hypercalciuria was created by the administration of 1,25-$(OH)_2D$.[16] As might be anticipated, in both the aforementioned model and in patients with the naturally occurring syndrome of absorptive hypercalciuria, the increases in oxalate absorption and excretion are particularly evident when the patients are on a calcium-restricted diet.[16,201,202] The importance of these apparent abnormalities in oxalate absorption and excretion in hypercalciuric patients or those with idiopathic calcium stone disease is not entirely clear; certainly, the evidence is strong enough to merit instructing patients to moderate their intake of both calcium and oxalate.

DIAGNOSIS

Available methods for measuring oxalate concentration include colorimetric, isotope dilution, and enzymatic techniques.[190] The most difficult and demanding aspects of the measurement are sample extraction and purification; without attention to detail any of the methods may be associated with variable recoveries and poor reproducibility. Normal limits for oxalate excretion vary from one laboratory to another but are usually reported to be approximately 15 to 50 mg/day, with a mean of about 30 mg/day.[190] No sex difference in the oxalate excretion rate has been observed. Accurate diagnosis lies in the demonstration of *persistent* hyperoxaluria, and abnormal results should always be followed by one or more repeat determinations.

Calcium stones are rare in patients less than 15 years of age (Fig. 25-1); the diagnosis of primary hyperoxaluria should be considered in any pediatric patient presenting with calcium stones. The diagnosis is confirmed by demonstrating an oxalate excretion rate greater than 60 mg per 1.73 square meters of body surface per day.[190,194] Affected patients usually excrete more than 100 mg/1.73 m^2 per day of oxalate.[190,191,194] If renal failure has already supervened, the oxalate excretion rate may be normal or near-normal in patients with primary hyperoxaluria, thus complicating diagnosis and/or a quantitative appraisal of the biochemical severity of the process. Methods for determining oxalate concentration in plasma are not widely available. Siblings of affected patients should be routinely screened. The type 1 and type 2 syndromes can be distinguished by the different patterns of excretion of glyoxylate, glycolate, or L-glyceric acid in the two syndromes; these determinations can presently be performed only by research laboratories.

In general, the pattern of stone formation and complications in patients with enteric hyperoxaluria does not differ significantly from that observed in patients with other forms of calcium stone disease. However, occasional patients have been reported to develop progressive renal insufficiency and/or distal RTA following jejunoileal bypass; both complications appear to be related to renal oxalosis.[190] The diagnosis of enteric hyperoxaluria usually suggests itself in a patient with stone disease in the setting of one of the chronic GI disorders listed above and can be confirmed by demonstrating an increase in oxalate excretion. In these patients, the urinary oxalate excretion rate is heavily dependent on oxalate intake but usually exceeds 60 mg/day.[190–192] In addition to the measurement of oxalate excretion, patients should be completely screened for other risk factors for stone formation.[190] Patients with enteric hyperoxaluria are frequently found to be relatively hypocalciuric; this may be an important chemical clue to the correct diagnosis if the manifestations of the intestinal disease are subtle.[109,190,198] If not previously documented and quantified, steatorrhea should be assessed by fecal fat determinations. In affected patients, all these determinations provide important baseline information against which the effects of therapy can be judged. Hyperoxaluria can be demonstrated in many patients with chronic intestinal disease in the absence of stone disease, and the detection of significant abnormalities in these patients may constitute grounds for instituting simple preventive measures such as hydration and a low-oxalate diet. Patients with an ileostomy and/or ulcerative colitis are not at risk for enteric hyperoxaluria but may form uric acid or calcium stones because of other risk factors for stone formation.

The potential role of oxalate measurements in the evaluation of the average patient with calcium stone disease is a matter of clinical judgment and the availability of a precise method for determining urinary oxalate excretion. The measurement is warranted in relatively young patients with particularly severe stone disease and/or in the small percentage of patients with significant stone disease in whom other risk factors for stone formation are not identified by metabolic screening. Ongoing research efforts aimed at the development of more precise methodology may make the determination of far more clinical relevance than is presently the case.

The other potential secondary causes of hyperoxaluria listed in Table 25-12 are usually diagnostically self-evident and are of limited clinical importance. Ethylene glycol and methoxyflurane toxicity are not stone-forming states in a conventional sense, and stone formation on the basis of pyridoxine deficiency has not been convincingly described. As noted previously, gluttony for foodstuffs with a high oxalate content is unusual, and the intake of oxalate is of clear-cut importance only in patients with enteric hyperoxaluria.

TREATMENT

Patients with primary hyperoxaluria are given particularly detailed instructions regarding forced hydration, similar to those employed in patients with cystinuria. They are also usually placed on a low-oxalate diet, even though the quantity of urinary oxalate derived from the diet is small. Large doses of pyridoxine (200 to 400 mg/day) have been reported to decrease variably the oxalate excretion rate in patients with primary hyperoxaluria, presumably by increasing the conversion of glyoxylate to glycine (Fig. 25-25). In a recent small series, much smaller doses of pyridoxine were found to be effective in some patients, and it was also suggested that the correct diagnosis could be masked in such patients if they were initially screened in a pyridoxine-replete state.[203] In addition to pyridoxine, one of several agents is administered in an attempt to alter the physical chemical environment in the urine. Magnesium is thought to form a soluble complex with oxalate in urine, and the administration of magnesium supplements has been reported to control stone formation in several small series of patients.[190,194] The most commonly used preparations are magnesium oxide (450 mg/day) and magnesium hydroxide (210 mg/day). Oral phosphorus therapy, in quantities of 1500 to 2500 mg of elemental phosphorus in four divided doses daily, has also been reported to prevent stone formation effectively in patients with primary hyperoxaluria.[190,194] The beneficial effects of phosphorus therapy are thought to result from both a decrease in supersaturation, due to the treatment-induced reduction in calcium excretion, and an increase in inhibitory substances in urine, most notably pyrophosphate.[190,194] Both magnesium and phosphorus should be used very cautiously if at all in patients with moderate or advanced renal insufficiency. Early diagnosis and therapy is extremely important in patients with primary hyperoxaluria, and management is very difficult once renal insufficiency has supervened. Dialysis does not effectively control progressive systemic oxalosis, and primary hyperoxaluria is currently viewed as a contraindication for renal transplantation.[190,194]

The therapeutic approach to patients with enteric hyperoxaluria is an excellent example of the importance of viewing treatment in terms of a program, rather than a prescription, and of constructing and monitoring this program according to the phases of care discussed in General Principles of Therapy, below. The management of individual patients ranges from quite straightforward to extremely difficult. Frontline measures include (1) hydration, (2) controlling steatorrhea, and (3) administering an oxalate-restricted diet.[190–192,204] Patients with a short bowel have difficulty consuming large quantities of fluids and maintaining an adequate urine output. A low-fat diet may improve steatorrhea, but a diet rigidly restricted in fat is unpalatable, and many patients prefer to use medium-chain triglycerides.[204] A low-oxalate diet can be constructed around the guidelines given above or using the low-oxalate diet booklet (Table 25-11). In many patients, these general measures suffice; in others, hyperoxaluria and/or other risk factors cannot be controlled, and other measures are required. A number of agents have been used in the attempt to bind oxalate in the intestinal contents and limit its biological availability. These agents include calcium, magnesium, aluminum, cholestyramine, and colestipol.[204] Fortuitously, many of these agents also bind bile acids and fatty acids. Calcium is probably the agent of choice. There is usually a considerable margin of safety in terms of calcium dosage because many patients absorb calcium poorly and are relatively hypocalciuric prior to therapy. The antacid Camalox is a useful combination agent, in that it contains calcium carbonate, aluminum hydroxide, and magnesium hydroxide; a typical starting dosage is 15 ml (or three tablets) three times daily with meals. Long-term trials have yet to be reported with any of these binding agents. Significant stone complications are regarded as an indication for restoring intestinal continuity in patients with a jejunoileal bypass.[190]

Hyperuricosuria

An apparent association between calcium stone disease and clinical gout and/or hyperuricemia was initially reported in the late 1960s.[7,205,206] It was subsequently recognized that hyperuricosuria, rather than hyperuricemia, confers risk for calcium stone formation, and the term *hyperuricosuric calcium oxalate nephrolithiasis* was introduced to describe this clinical syndrome.[3,6,207,208] Although the exact mechanism by which hyperuricosuria predisposes to calcium stone formation remains unsettled, hyperuricosuria appears to be a common and important risk factor in patients with stone disease.

The actual crystallographic identification of mixed calcium–uric acid stones in these patients is unusual; less than 5 percent of patients with clinical stone disease present with such mixed stones or with a history of passage of both calcium oxalate and uric acid stones.[209] Rather, the garden-variety calcium oxalate or mixed calcium oxalate–calcium phosphate stone is the typical finding in patients with hyperuricosuric calcium oxalate nephrolithiasis, and the stone analysis is of limited diagnostic usefulness. Diagnosis is based on demonstrating hyperuricosuria in a patient with calcium stone disease. Treatment with allopurinol has been reported to be extremely effective in preventing stone formation in these patients. Indeed, the effectiveness of allopurinol constitutes perhaps the strongest single line of evidence implicating hyperuricosuria as an independent risk factor for calcium stone formation.[208,210]

URIC ACID METABOLISM AND DEFINITION OF HYPERURICOSURIA

The details of purine metabolism and uric acid clearance were discussed previously (see Uric Acid Calculi and Fig. 25-11). The key variables determining the uric acid excretion rate are the fractional excretion of uric acid and the metabolic production rate of uric acid. Under steady-state conditions, the production rate is the most important variable and is determined by a combination of dietary purine intake and endogenous purine turnover. Approximately 50 percent of dietary purine bases are ultimately recoverable in the urine as uric acid.[45]

Statistically, precise normal limits for uric acid excretion have not been established. Among the difficulties in establishing such limits is the fact that results are extremely diet-sensitive and the uric acid excretion rate on a given day may vary by as much as several hundred mg depending on purine intake.[46] Similarly, precise limits determined in individuals on metabolic purine diets have little relevance to outpatient results determined on free or undefined diets.

The excretion rate of uric acid in normal subjects and patients with calcium stone disease does not have a bimodal distribution. What has been observed is a clear tendency toward elevated values in a subgroup of patients with stone disease, in a fashion reminiscent of the patterns of calcium excretion in normal subjects and patients with calcium stone disease (compare Fig. 25-26 and the upper panel of Fig. 25-12). The major physiological difference between systemic calcium and purine metabolism is that the intestinal absorption of calcium is rigidly regulated, whereas the absorption of purines is not. The principal consequence of this difference is that "dietary hyperuricosuria" is common, whereas "dietary hypercalciuria," as a reflection solely of overconsumption of calcium, is rare.

Gutman and Yü,[205] Coe and Raisen,[207] and Coe[208] have suggested upper normal limits for uric acid excretion of 800 mg/day for males and 750 mg/day for females. By these criteria, some 10 percent of normal males and 5 percent of normal females are hyperuricosuric.[208] Pak employs an upper limit of 600 mg/day in both sexes, regarding this limit as a "functional definition" of hyperuricosuria based on the quantity of uric acid usually required to supersaturate the urine with respect to monosodium urate.[109] This definition is unusually lax, in that some 60 percent of normal men would thereby be considered to be hyperuricosuric.[208] Weight-adjusted limits for uric acid excretion have not been developed.

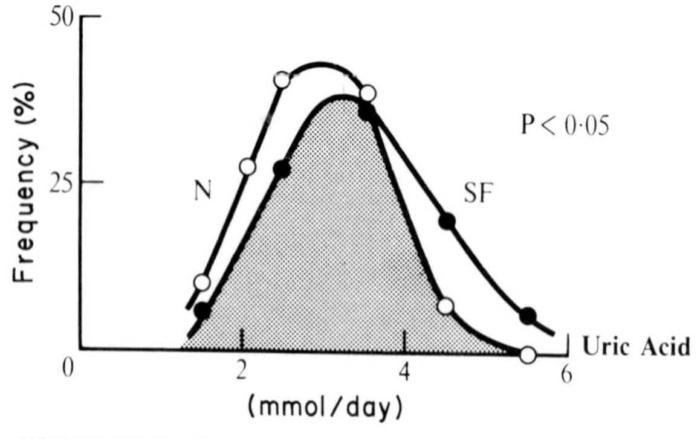

FIGURE 25-26 Frequency distributions of 24-h uric acid excretion in normal subjects (N) and patients with recurrent calcium stone disease (SF). (The molecular weight of uric acid is 168.1.) (*From Robertson et al.*[77] *by permission of the British Journal of Urology.*)

PATHOGENESIS

Approximately one-third of patients with calcium stones are found to be hyperuricosuric, based on the limits proposed by Coe.[3,6,104,207,208] Males outnumber females by about 3 to 1.[104,207,208] In some 35 to 50 percent of these patients, one or more additional risk factors for calcium stone formation can be identified.[104,208] In patients in whom hyperuricosuria is the only risk factor identified, the male preponderance is very striking: this population is 90 percent male.[104] In the majority of hyperuricosuric patients with calcium stone disease, the hyperuricosuria is mild; only some 15 percent of patients excrete more than 1000 mg/day of uric acid. In addition, patients with mild hyperuricosuria frequently display this abnormality only intermittently, presumably as a result of variation in purine intake.

There are three potential mechanisms which could account for the hyperuricosuria in patients with calcium stone disease: (1) endogenous uric acid overproduction, (2) "gluttony" for a purine-rich animal protein diet, and (3) an increase in the fractional excretion of uric acid. To date, there is little evidence to suggest that the third mechanism applies in patients with calcium stones; fasting fractional uric acid excretion is almost always less than 10 percent in hyperuricosuric patients. Approximately 40 percent of hyperuricosuric patients with calcium stone disease present with coincident fasting hyperuricemia, and 60 percent are normouricemic. These findings suggest that patients with hyperuricosuric calcium oxalate nephrolithiasis represent an admixture of two subpopulations: those with endogenous uric acid overproduction and those with purine overconsumption. These two subgroups are separated by a fine line; clearly, a high purine intake would contribute to the hyperuricosuria in both subpopulations. Coe has emphasized the importance of excessive purine intake in patients with hyperuricosuric calcium oxalate nephrolithiasis.[3,208] He found by diet survey that purine intake was approximately 70 percent higher in hyperuricosuric calcium stone formers than in a control population. In addition, he observed that a rigid restriction in purine intake eliminated the hyperuricosuria in all but 30 percent of patients, suggesting that only some one-third of patients with hyperuricosuric calcium oxalate nephrolithiasis have a true underlying overproduction of uric acid.[3,208] A definite history of clinical gout is found in only some 15 percent of patients with hyperuricosuria and calcium stones.

Coe has also reviewed the natural history of hyperuricosuric calcium oxalate nephrolithiasis. He observed a slightly later age of onset and a more severe and protracted course, in terms of stone recurrence rate and the frequency of hospitalization and instrumentation, than in patients with hypercalciuria or idiopathic calcium stone disease.[3,208] Roughly one-third of hyperuricosuric patients were found to have one or more additional risk factors for calcium stone formation, but combined abnormalities did not appear to influence the natural history substantially in terms of severity.[3,208]

Several hypotheses have been proposed to explain the pathogenetic relationship between hyperuricosuria and calcium stone formation. Lonsdale initially reported that there were similarities in lattice structure between crystals of calcium oxalate monohydrate, calcium oxalate dihydrate, uric acid, and monosodium urate, and suggested that epitaxy might occur between any of these crystal pairs.[211] Experimental evidence for the induction of heterogeneous nucleation and/or crystal growth of the calcium oxalate system in aqueous solution by both uric acid and monosodium urate has been reported.[3,6,208,212] There remains some controversy as to which of the two ionic species of uric acid is of most importance in physical chemical terms in vivo. In part, this controversy arises because there is some disagreement as to the ambient urinary pH in patients with hyperuricosuric calcium oxalate nephrolithiasis.[109,208,209] The consumption of a purine-rich, high-protein diet not only increases uric acid excretion but also decreases urinary pH because of the quantity of fixed acid that must be excreted. This point favors uric acid as being the more important of the two ionic species, at least in patients who overconsume purines.[79,213]

An alternative pathogenetic proposal is that uric acid or monosodium urate may adsorb or otherwise interfere with certain normally occurring macromolecular inhibitors of calcium oxalate crystallization.[178,184] Pak et al. have reported that oral purine loading is associated with a reduction of the formation product of calcium oxalate toward that which is observed in a simple aqueous solution.[214] Allopurinol treatment was found to retard calcium oxalate crystallization and crystal growth.[214] These data add further credibility to the thesis that hyperuricosuria represents an independent risk factor for calcium stone formation, but they do not directly bear on the details of pathogenesis, in that the findings are compatible with either the epitaxial or inhibitor hypothesis.

Although the fine points of pathogenesis in patients with hyperuricosuric calcium oxalate nephrolithiasis continue to be debated, there is one extremely important clinical point that has been repeatedly emphasized in recent series: these patients *do not* display the fixed, low urinary pH which typifies many patients with uric acid stone disease.[104,109,209] Low urinary pH is the predominant risk factor identified in patients with uric acid stones or a mixture of uric acid and calcium stone disease; it should be carefully sought in these patients (see Uric Acid Calculi, above).

DIAGNOSIS

Hyperuricosuria is best demonstrated in an outpatient setting, with patients consuming their customary diets. Coincident fasting hyperuricemia and hyperuricosuria suggest that the patient is an overproducer of uric acid, whereas the combination of normouricemia and hyperuricosuria suggests that the patient is a "purine glutton." A careful diet history can identify overconsumption of a purine-rich animal protein diet in many patients and may provide the basis for subsequent instructions regarding a moderated purine intake. The patient should be questioned for a history of clinical gout. The stone analysis is helpful diagnostically only in the small percentage of patients with mixed calcium oxalate–uric acid stones or with a history of forming both uric acid and calcium stones.

As noted previously, a pattern of intermittent hyperuricosuria is quite common in patients with calcium stone disease, so that screening is best accomplished by having patients collect two or more urine specimens as outpatients. Uricosuric agents, particularly x-ray contrast material, may produce spuriously elevated results, and the collection of specimens in acidified containers may produce spuriously low results (see Uric Acid Calculi, above). The uricase method is the most precise analytical technique available. Since one or more risk factors in addition to hyperuricosuria are commonly identified in individual patients with calcium stone disease, all patients should be thoroughly screened. Concurrent hypercalciuria and hyperuricosuria are observed in approximately 10 percent of patients with calcium stone disease, particularly in males.[3,6,104,180,208,209] This means that as many as one-third to one-half of hyperuricosuric patients will also be found to be hypercalciuric.[104,180,208] Not surprisingly, the hypercalciuria in these patients is frequently dietary in nature, or a prominent dietary component is superimposed on underlying absorptive hypercalciuria (see Hypercalciuria, above, and Table 25-7).

TREATMENT

Patients with hyperuricosuric calcium oxalate nephrolithiasis are treated with a program of high fluid intake, a moderate purine diet, and, frequently, allopurinol. The principle of dietary moderation rather than restriction is emphasized to the patient because compliance with a truly purine-restricted diet is poor. Purine moderation is best achieved by providing the patient with a list of purine-rich foods (e.g., glandular meats, meat extracts and gravies, dried legumes, sardines, and shrimp) to be avoided. In patients who appear to have coincident dietary hypercalciuria, sodium restriction is also employed. In some patients, these general measures appear to be sufficient.[173,210] Certainly, these conservative measures are a reasonable alternative in a patient with a single stone event or with a minimal history of stone disease.

Allopurinol has been shown to be very effective in preventing stone recurrences in patients with hyperuricosuric calcium oxalate stone disease (Fig. 25-27),[3,6,207,208,210,214] and its efficacy has been recently demonstrated in a double-blind therapeutic trial.[210] Details concerning the mechanism of action, dosage, and toxicity of allopurinol were presented above (see Uric Acid Calculi). The drug should be given in a dosage sufficient to reduce uric acid excretion into the middle of the normal range. This dosage varies between 200 and 600 mg/day in individual patients, with an average of approximately 300 mg daily. A single daily dose provides adequate coverage in most patients, and compliance is high. Alkalinization plays no role in the therapy of patients with calcium stone disease.

As noted above, coincident hypercalciuria and hyperuricosuria are noted in approximately 10 percent of patients with calcium stone disease.[3,6,104,180,208] Coe advocates treating such patients with combined allopurinol and thiazide therapy and has reported good control of stone recurrences with this regimen.[180,208] An alternative approach in a young patient or one with minimal to moderate stone disease would be to treat the quantitatively dominant abnormality with medication and attempt to manage the associated abnormality with dietary moderation. The nature of the hypercalciuria (dietary vs. absorptive, vs. a combination of the two) appears to be an important consideration in this regard.

Hypocitraturia

RENAL METABOLISM OF CITRATE

Citric acid, in the form of citrate, is the most abundant organic acid found in urine. It is extensively metabolized by the kidney. Although the average American diet contains approximately 4 g of citrate, dietary citrate appears to have little immediate influence on the final urinary citrate content. Thus, normal individuals on a citrate-free diet show no significant increase in urinary citrate levels when placed on a diet containing 4.5 g of citrate per day.[215]

Citrate circulates in blood at a concentration ranging between 1 and 6 mg/dl, almost entirely in the form of the triply charged citrate ion, which is freely filtered at the glomerulus. Approximately 2400 mg is filtered per day, of which 1800 mg is reabsorbed, principally in the proximal renal tubule; roughly 600 mg appears in the final urine. An additional 400 mg is extracted by the kidney from peritubular blood, so that a total of approximately 2000 mg/day of citrate is metabolized by the kidney.[216]

Citrate binds calcium in the urine, thereby preventing the precipitation of calcium salts. It is princi-

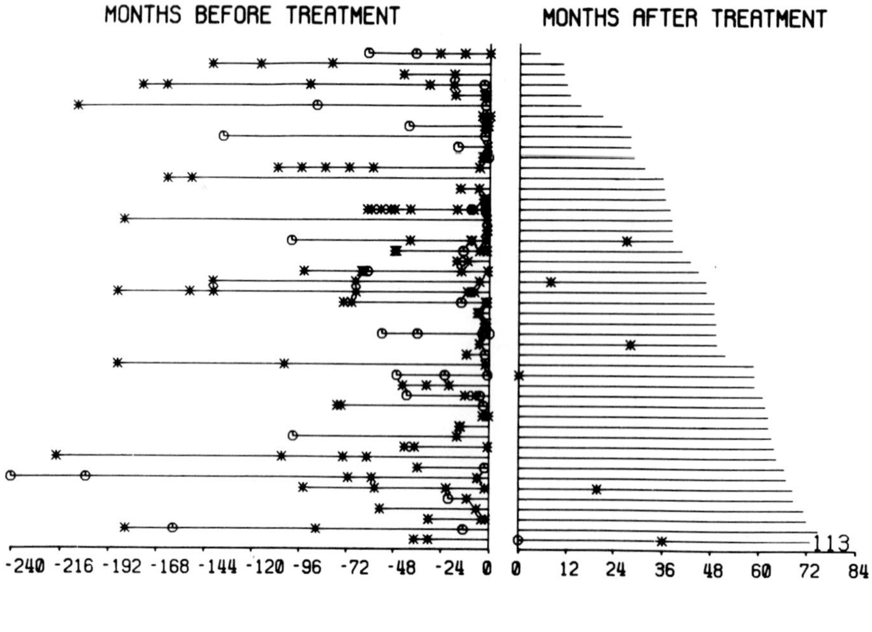

FIGURE 25-27 The influence of allopurinol therapy on recurrent stone events in patients with hyperuricosuric calcium oxalate nephrolithiasis. Each of the 48 patients is represented by a horizontal line; the symbols correspond to single (*) or a cluster (o) of stone events. (*From Coe FL: Ann Intern Med 87:404, 1977, by permission.*)

pally through its effect of reducing the ionic activity of calcium in urine that citrate is thought to act as an inhibitor of calcium stone formation and/or growth. Up to 70 percent of urinary calcium may be bound by citrate.[217]

ACID-BASE STATUS AND CITRATE EXCRETION

A number of conditions are known to influence citrate excretion.[216] In relation to stone formation, the most important and well-established such condition is an alteration in systemic acid-base status. The mechanism by which disturbances in acid-base status alter citrate excretion has been a source of considerable investigative interest. Metabolic alkalosis induces a prompt and dramatic increase in citrate excretion. This is accompanied by an increase in citrate content in the renal cortex. Although several processes contribute to this effect, the primary mechanism appears to be an inhibition of citrate metabolism in renal tubular cells. Conversely, systemic acidosis is associated with a decrease in renal cortical citrate content as well as a decrease in citrate excretion, findings which suggest an increased rate of renal citrate metabolism.[216]

The major site of intracellular citrate metabolism is the mitochondrion. Mitochondrial citrate oxidation is extremely sensitive to changes in pH. Citrate is actively transported into mitochondria; it has been hypothesized that the pH gradient which exists across the mitochondrion is critical to this transport process. Under normal circumstances, the matrix of the mitochondrion is alkaline with respect to the outer membrane. Thus, a rise in extramitochondrial bicarbonate concentration induced by systemic alkalosis would reduce the mitochondrial pH gradient and inhibit citrate transport. This in turn would lead to elevated intracellular citrate levels and impaired renal tubular citrate reabsorption, which would cause citrate excretion to rise (Fig. 25-28). Conversely, acidosis would stimulate mitochondrial citrate uptake, lower the intracellular citrate concentration, increase citrate reabsorption, and thereby decrease citrate excretion (Fig. 25-28).

HYPOCITRATURIA AND NEPHROLITHIASIS IN PATIENTS WITH ACID-BASE ABNORMALITIES

A variety of conditions associated with disturbances in acid-base balance are accompanied by hypocitraturia.

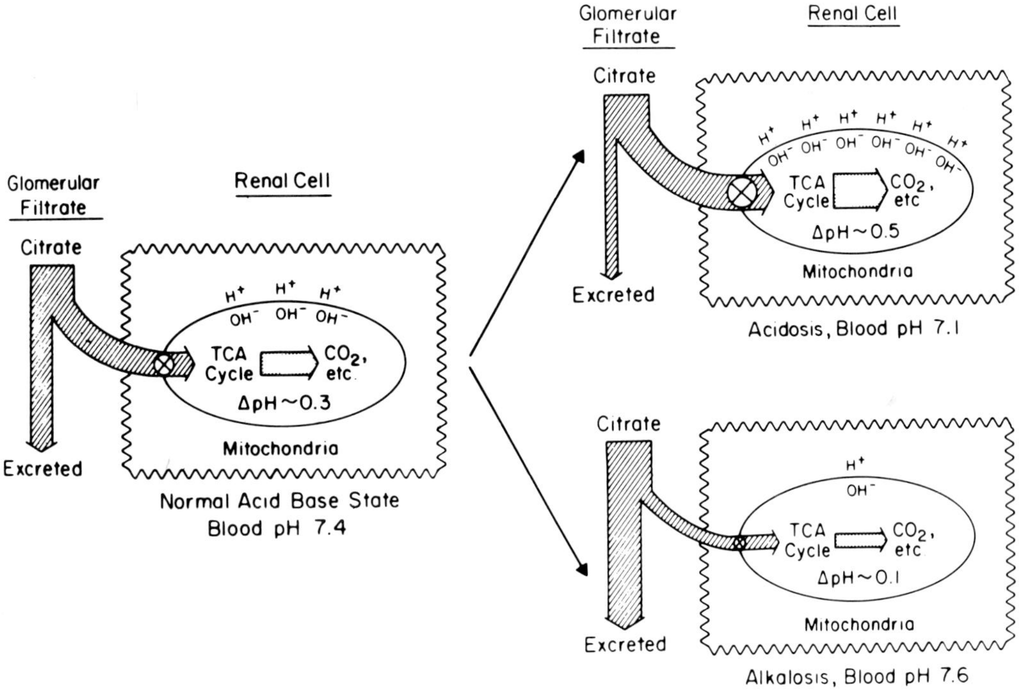

FIGURE 25-28 Schematic representation of the effect of changes in acid-base status on renal tubular cell citrate metabolism. With acidosis (upper right), the pH gradient across the mitochondrial membrane (Δ pH) increases, enhancing citrate uptake and metabolism, and thereby increasing tubular reabsorption. In alkalosis (lower right), the reverse occurs. (*From Simpson,*[216] *by permission of the American Journal of Physiology.*)

The two conditions which have received the most attention are distal RTA and enteric hyperoxaluria.

In distal RTA, the renal tubular dysfunction leads to systemic acidosis and hypocitraturia.[218] In enteric hyperoxaluria, multiple factors have been implicated as contributing to the hypocitraturia. Many patients have metabolic acidosis due to bicarbonate wasting in the GI tract. In others, a combination of factors, including hypocitratemia with a reduced renal filtered load and increased renal citrate reabsorption due to hypomagnesuria, may contribute to the hypocitraturia.[198] In both distal RTA and enteric hyperoxaluria, hypocitraturia is regarded as an important risk factor for calcium stone formation, and treatment directed at correcting this abnormality is felt to be effective. (Both conditions were treated in detail above.)

Acetazolamide induces an "exogenous" RTA, accompanied by hypocitraturia (see Calcium Phosphate Stones above).[217] Potassium depletion appears to lead to intracellular metabolic acidosis in the renal cortex and is attended by hypocitraturia as well.[216,219]

HYPOCITRATURIA AND NEPHROLITHIASIS IN PATIENTS WITHOUT ACID-BASE DISTURBANCES

Since the 1930s there have been many reports of hypocitraturia in patients with calcium oxalate nephrolithiasis who have normal acid-base status and no GI disease. The prevalence, basis, and importance of this finding as a contributing factor to calcium oxalate stone disease remain uncertain. In two recent series of consecutive patients with calcium oxalate nephrolithiasis and no obvious cause for hypocitraturia, the prevalence of hypocitraturia ranged between 15 and 30 percent.[220,221] In the larger of these two series, no relationship was demonstrated between 24-h citrate excretion and the severity of stone disease.[221] Further, urinary citrate excretion was found to vary: in 15 of 22 patients in this series in whom several urinary citrate excretion measurements were made, at least one was normal. In this same study, urinary citrate excretion in normal individuals was found to increase with age, but citrate excretion remained unchanged in patients with stone disease. Significant differences in citrate excretion between normal and stone-forming patients were therefore confined to males greater than 49 years of age and females greater than 40 years of age.

One of the major difficulties in attempting to assess the importance of hypocitraturia as a risk factor for calcium stone formation has been the failure of most studies to control for a host of dietary factors that might influence citrate excretion. However, in one small study in which dietary factors were carefully controlled, it appeared that patients with calcium oxalate nephrolithiasis had an elevated tubular reabsorption of citrate as compared to normal individuals.[215]

Recently, there has been interest in the treatment of patients with hypocitraturia and calcium oxalate nephrolithiasis with oral alkali. None of the studies reported to date has been well-controlled. In one study of 89 patients treated with potassium citrate for periods ranging from 1 to 4 years, stone formation rate was decreased in almost all patients. This series included a heterogeneous group of patients with calcium oxalate stone disease associated with a variety of metabolic abnormalities; however, even in those patients without diarrheal syndromes or RTA the response to treatment was impressive.[222] A substantial minority of the patients lacking evidence for RTA or enteric hyperoxaluria were found to be hypocitraturic,[222] a finding also reported by the same group in a larger series of such patients.[223] In a separate study, 13 patients with hypercalciuria which appeared to be refractory to thiazide therapy were found to be hypocitraturic and appeared to respond clinically to potassium citrate supplementation.[224] Incomplete RTA was present in one of these patients and was not tested for in eight.

Based on these studies, a sustained-release potassium citrate preparation has recently been released by the U.S. Food and Drug Administration for the treatment of patients with calcium stone disease. The drug is marketed in wax matrix and contains 5 meq of citrate per tablet. This preparation purportedly leads to a more sustained increase in citrate excretion than other forms of oral alkali. In addition, its potassium content might be useful in correcting thiazide-induced potassium depletion in patients receiving these agents. At present, the exact role of potassium citrate therapy in patients with calcium stone disease remains uncertain, and more carefully controlled studies will be required to determine its efficacy in various clinical settings.

Whether all patients with calcium stone disease should be screened for hypocitraturia is unclear. Certainly, it is reasonable practice to determine citrate excretion in patients without obvious metabolic abnormalities during routine screening and in patients who are refractory to conventional therapy. The measurement of citrate is not difficult, and commercial assays are regarded as reliable.

Idiopathic Calcium Stones

The term *idiopathic calcium stone disease* is used in connection with patients who form calcium oxalate or mixed calcium stones but in whom no clinical risk factors for stone formation can be identified. In the older literature, the term was frequently used as a synonym for calcium stone disease in general, presumably because the pathogenesis of stone formation was viewed as enigmatic in all patients. However, a meticulous evaluation should identify one or more risk factors for stone formation in approximately 80 to 90 percent of patients with recurrent calcium stone disease, and the term is appropriately used only to describe patients without evident risk factors for stone formation.

The natural history and morbidity of stone formation in patients with idiopathic calcium stone disease does not differ appreciably from what is observed in patients with well-recognized risk factors for stone formation. In occasional patients with apparent idiopathic calcium stone disease, a history of antecedent immobilization or some other secondary cause for stone formation can be elicited, and it is possible that the stone burden in such a patient reflects active stone formation at a time remote from the actual time of evaluation. In other patients, the process remains totally enigmatic. Whether or not intermittent abnormalities which predispose to stone formation occur with any frequency in these patients is unknown. It is certainly reasonable to measure urinary oxalate and citrate excretion in patients with idiopathic stone disease and to attempt to treat either abnormality if it is identified.

Idiopathic calcium stone disease is a diagnosis of exclusion. The decision to treat such an individual is based, as it is in any patient with stone disease, on the assessment of stone-related morbidity. Virtually all agents used to treat patients with calcium stones were initially introduced on empirical grounds and have been reported to be of benefit in patients with idiopathic calcium stone disease or in patients whose potential risk factors for stone formation were not described. Efficacy has been reported for oral phosphates,[181,182] thiazides,[179] thiazides together with allopurinol,[180] magnesium oxide and pyridoxine,[225] and oral methylene blue.[226] In general, double-blind or comparison studies have not been performed, and the choice of therapy must be based on clinical judgment and experience. Routine hydration instructions are also given. The potential benefit of dietary restrictions in this specific patient group is unknown.

TESTING AND GENERAL PRINCIPLES OF THERAPY

General Considerations

The management of patients with stone disease can be subdivided into several phases. Phase I involves the diligent evaluation necessary to identify all risk factors predisposing a given patient to stone formation. A part of this evaluation is the careful radiological identification of the number, location, and size of preexisting (old) stones. Phase II is the initial therapeutic period, in which the adequacy of the therapeutic regimen is demonstrated by documenting on several occasions the elimination or amelioration of the risk factors associated with stone formation. The end result of this phase is the choice of a final regimen for long-term treatment. In some patients, this regimen consists of fluids and dietary restrictions alone; in others it consists of these measures plus an agent chosen to reduce the excretion rate of a stone-forming constituent. Phase III is the long-term treatment period during which the desired result of prevention of new stone formation is monitored. In a patient without preexisting stones, this assessment is a simple matter of clinical follow-up and a yearly x-ray. In patients with preexisting stones, the differentiation of clinical stone events as being due to old versus new stones must be made by careful x-ray assessment with each stone event and/or by yearly x-rays. Only new stones have implications for therapeutic success or failure. Phase IV involves the consideration of discontinuing all or parts of a therapeutic regimen in a patient who appears to have responded well to therapy. For most conditions associated with stone formation, whether or when phase IV should be attempted remains unknown.

Testing

The meticulous evaluation necessary to delineate the risk factors responsible for stone formation requires attention to detail on the part of both physician and patient. Individuals with recurrent stone disease are as compliant and cooperative as any patients encountered in the practice of medicine. The physician can request and expect such patients to arrive for their initial visit armed with previous x-rays and all relevant historical and analytical data provided by referring physicians. Internists should make clear from the outset that their role in the care of the patient differs from that of the urologist and that the patient should maintain continuity with the referring urologist. Patients should be made aware that they are important participants in their own care. Empirical therapy should be discontinued several weeks before analytical screening. Collapsible 24-h urine collection containers and instructions for urine collection may be mailed to patients, so that the initial urine specimen collected on a free diet accompanies the patient on the initial visit. Patients should be instructed to arrive fasting.

INITIAL EVALUATION

The history and physical examination should be complete ones, with particular care given to the history of stone events, family history of stones, and medication and diet histories. The number, composition, location, and result (e.g., passed, nephrolithotomy) of stone events should be recorded in a chronological fashion, to serve as the basis for judging stone morbidity. Patients are encouraged to summarize their family history of stones by direct contact with first-degree relatives. The physician can obtain a brief diet history, but a detailed, quantitative history is best obtained by a trained nutritionist by use of diet diaries and questionnaires.

An IVP should be carefully examined for anatomical abnormalities which predispose to stone formation. The study should preferably have been performed within the previous year and in the absence of a high degree of obstruction. The study should be repeated if renal, pelvicalyceal, or ureteral surgery has been performed since the most recent available films. The plain films preceding the IVP are usually not performed with the care necessary to delineate clearly the number, size, and location of existing stones and are a notorious source of misinformation in this regard.

Results of previous stone analyses should be examined and a representative recent stone, if available, sent for crystallographic analysis. Simple chemical stone analysis is inadequate.

The initial fasting blood determinations should include calcium, phosphorus, bicarbonate, chloride, creatinine, uric acid, and albumin concentrations. More extensive chemical screening is optional.

The initial 24-h urine specimen should be collected on a free or undefined diet and analyzed for creatinine, calcium, sodium, and uric acid concentrations. Optional determinations include phosphorus and oxalate and the cystine screen. The urine volume should be carefully noted. The excretion of creatinine serves as an index of the completeness of collection.

A clean-voided, spot, fasting urine sample should be obtained for culture and pH determination by nitrazine paper or pH meter. The cystine screen can be conveniently performed on this specimen, and it may also be acidified and examined for cystine crystals. Optional analyses are creatinine, phosphorus, and calcium, which, together with the blood analyses, allow the calculation of fasting calcium excretion and TmP/GFR.

SUBSEQUENT EVALUATION

Fasting serum calcium, phosphorus, and uric acid determinations should be repeated on at least one occasion.

If the initial urinary pH was >5.5, serum electrolyte concentrations should be determined again, and the patient should be given a roll of nitrazine paper to record serially urinary pH and/or to document on several occasions that urinary pH is less than 5.5. If there is any suspicion that the patient may be suffering from uric acid stone disease and the initial fasting urinary pH is low, serial monitoring of the urinary pH is indicated, in search of the low and relatively fixed pH which is seen in many of these patients. Such a fixed, low urinary pH may be the only identifiable risk factor for uric acid stone formation.

The conditions for subsequent 24-h urine collections vary depending on the results of the initial collection. If hyperuricosuria was initially noted, an additional specimen should be obtained on the free diet, and the specimen analyzed for creatinine, calcium, and uric acid excretion. If indicated, oxalate excretion may also be measured in this specimen. The presence and degree of hypercalciuria should be evaluated by instructing patients to collect at least one specimen on a diet unrestricted in calcium and lacking excessive quantities of protein and sodium. One relatively simple means of structuring such a diet is to instruct the patient to (1) limit protein intake to approximately 1 g per kilogram of body weight per day, (2) limit sodium intake to approximately 100 meq/day, (3) eliminate dairy products from the diet (thereby limiting dietary calcium intake to approximately 400 to 500 mg daily), and (4) supplement the diet with calcium gluconate tablets, 2 g three times daily with meals (thereby adding approximately 600 mg of elemental calcium to the dietary intake). The tablets should be chewed carefully before swallowing. The net daily calcium intake of approximately 1000 mg is maintained for several days, with one or more urine collections performed after at least 1 day of equilibration on the diet. The specimen(s) should be analyzed for calcium and creatinine and, in selected patients, sodium excretion. If cAMP is to be determined, the specimen should be collected into 20 ml of 6 *N* hydrochloric acid. The use of dairy products rather than the calcium tablets is not recommended because the protein content of milk may have a pronounced effect on calcium excretion, and no normative data are available.

The 24-h excretion of oxalate and/or citrate should be measured selectively. Different laboratories have differing requirements with respect to preservatives for these collections.

The number, size, and location of existing stones should be documented by careful plain x-rays. Patients should be prepared by diet instructions and laxatives as for an IVP, and oblique and cone-down views should be performed in addition to the routine abdominal plain film. Patient preparation is important if stone material is to be adequately seen. The usual IVP is no substitute for these films. Conversely, serial IVPs play no role in defining the stone burden and/or response to therapy; serial IVPs represent a common form of poor care, associated with an unacceptable radiation exposure in predominantly young patients. The implications of an existing stone burden with regard to the clinical assessment of response to therapy should be carefully and repeatedly explained to the patient. The diet and laxative instructions in preparation for x-ray are usually followed for 24 h before the films are obtained and will influence the results of 24-h urine collections, which are not performed during this period.

EVALUATION OF THE PATIENT WITH A SINGLE STONE EVENT

There are no clear-cut and accepted rules of thumb as to which patients with a single clinical stone event should be evaluated and how extensive this evaluation should be. As already noted, risk factors for stone formation are identified in patients with a single stone event with roughly the same frequency as in patients with recurrent stone disease, and the prevailing view is that patients with a single stone are simply being seen early in the course of a chronic process.[83,84] The minimum evaluation is a careful plain x-ray, in order to detect the presence of additional "silent" stones, and a crystallographic stone analysis. A reasonable chemical screen would consist of measures of fasting serum calcium bicarbonate concentrations, determination of urinary pH, and measurement of 24-h urine volume and calcium and uric acid excretion. Additional evaluation is performed on a patient-specific basis.

ORAL CALCIUM TOLERANCE TEST

Figure 25-29 contains a flow diagram of the calcium tolerance test and lists the data which can be derived from this test. The extensive data base listed is that which may be obtained for research purposes; the analytical base required for diagnostic purposes is quite simple (see below).

Patients are prepared for the tolerance test by following a calcium-restricted (approximately 400 mg/day) and sodium-restricted (approximately 100 meq/day) diet for 7 to 10 days prior to testing and by fasting except for distilled water for 10 to 12 h before the test begins. Patients are hydrated with 8 oz of distilled water hourly beginning 1 h before the initial urine is voided and discarded ($t = 0$) and ending 1 h before the test is completed. Milk replaces the distilled water at the end of the initial collection period. With appropriate patient preparation, outpatient and inpatient test results are diagnostically equivalent.

The test consists of three consecutive 2-h urine collections with midpoint blood specimens drawn during the first and third collection periods. An oral dose of approximately 1000 mg of elemental calcium (administered as 35 ml of calcium glubionate syrup

I. FLOW DIAGRAM

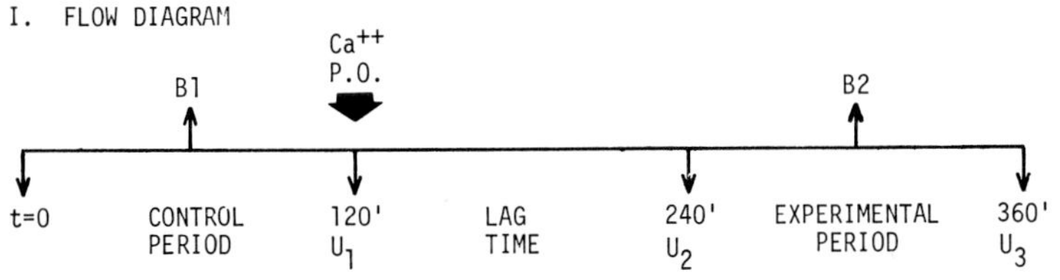

II. DATA BASE

A. STATIC MEASUREMENTS (CONTROL PERIOD)

1. BASAL SERUM CALCIUM & PHOSPHORUS
2. FASTING CALCIUM EXCRETION
3. FASTING TMP/GFR
4. BASAL NEPHROGENOUS OR TOTAL cAMP EXCRETION
5. BASAL VITAMIN D METABOLITES

B. DYNAMIC MEASUREMENTS (EXPERIMENTAL VS CONTROL PERIOD)

1. CALCEMIC RESPONSE AS INDEX OF "CALCIUM TOLERANCE"
2. CALCIURIC RESPONSE (Δ mg CALCIUM/100 ML GF) AS INDEX OF GI ABSORPTION
3. SUPPRESSIBILITY OF NEPHROGENOUS OR TOTAL cAMP EXCRETION

FIGURE 25-29 Flow diagram and data base derived from the oral calcium tolerance test.

plus 8 oz of milk) is given promptly after closing the initial collection period. Lactase-treated milk or synthetic liquid meal preparations can be used instead of milk in patients with lactose intolerance. The three collection periods represent, respectively, a fasting control period, a 2-h lag period required for peak calcium absorption to occur, and an experimental period demonstrating the maximal systemic and physiological effects of the absorbed calcium. The control period can be lengthened or shortened for patient convenience, but the timing of the subsequent blood and urine specimens must be precise. No data are derived from the second or lag-time urine specimen; this specimen can be discarded.

The calcemic response serves as an index of calcium "tolerance," the calciuric response is an index of intestinal calcium absorption, and induced changes in nephrogenous cAMP or total cAMP excretion provide an index of parathyroid suppressibility. The measurement of nephrogenous cAMP excretion provides an index of parathyroid suppressibility which is approximately twice as sensitive as that provided by the simple determination of total cAMP excretion, but the latter determination is adequate for diagnostic purposes in the vast majority of patients. The test embodies a number of modifications from similar techniques which were described previously.[112,131] The most important of these modifications are (1) the expression of the calciuric response as the induced increase in calcium excretion over the wide range of fasting control results, (2) the expression of data on a GFR basis rather than as a function of creatinine excretion, and (3) determination of the calcemic response.[105,121]

The minimum data base derived from the tolerance test is obtained from measurements of serum calcium, phosphorus, and creatinine concentrations and urinary calcium, phosphorus, creatinine, and cAMP excretion. The phosphorus determinations are performed only on the control blood and urine specimens and are used to calculate TmP/GFR. There is no diurnal variation in the plasma cAMP concentration during the morning hours, so that a single determination of plasma cAMP concentration during the control period may be used for calculating nephrogenous cAMP throughout the test.[105] Similarly, if the serum creatinine determination is known to be highly reproducible in the laboratory performing the analysis, only an initial determination is required. Data are computed and expressed as described in the testing section of Chap. 23. The calciuric response is computed by subtracting the rate of calcium excretion during the control period from that during the experimental period (e.g., if the rate of calcium excretion during the experimental period is 0.38 mg calcium per 100 ml of glomerular filtrate (GF) and fasting calcium excretion is 0.11 mg calcium per 100 ml GF, the calciuric response is 0.27 mg calcium per 100 ml GF). The upper normal limit (mean + 2 SD) for the calciuric response is 0.20 mg calcium per 100 ml GF.[105] As noted in Chap. 23, use of the calciuric response as an index of intestinal calcium absorption has not been validated in all circumstances, and the calcium tolerance test should be used only to evaluate conditions in which the assumptions underlying the test have been systematically validated. The calcemic response in normal individuals is usually less than 0.4 mg/dl.

General Principles of Therapy

Patients should be educated and enrolled as active participants in their own care. Specific goals of therapy and the continuity of follow-up are clearly spelled out. It is often useful to stress the general principles of supersaturation chemistry and to put the patient through a personalized exercise in saturation chemistry. This is done within the context of a specific therapeutic *program* consisting of forced hydration, dietary moderation, and drug therapy. For example, a hyperuricosuric patient with a uric acid excretion rate of 1000 mg/day and a 24-h urine volume of 1000 ml/day can easily comprehend that the concentration of uric acid in the urine is 1000 mg/liter. The patient can readily see that if urine volume is doubled, the concentration of uric acid is halved. If the physician can reduce the uric acid excretion rate to 500 mg/day, the uric acid concentration is halved again, yielding a final uric acid concentration of 250 mg/liter.

As simple as these principles are, only some 10 to 15 percent of patients with recurrent stone disease have been properly instructed when initially seen in consultation, and poor patient education appears to be a major deficiency in office practice care. Failure to inform patients of the implications of a preexisting stone burden and the importance of distinguishing old and new stones is another major failing and is responsible for discouragement and poor compliance in many patients.

General instructions regarding fluid intake are described under Cystinuria, above, and specific therapeutic programs are presented in the appropriate preceding sections of this chapter. In general, a urine output of 2 liters per day is the desired goal. This requires the intake of some 3 liters of fluid per day, in the absence of accelerated fluid losses via skin or GI tract. The initial therapeutic period (phase II) consists of documenting the patient's response to treatment by urine and/or blood determinations on several occasions, preferably about 6 weeks apart. Both the chemical and urine volume responses are noted, and the patient is given feedback in specific *concentration* terms. These samples serve either to reinforce or to alter the treatment program. After the initial therapeutic period, the patient is seen at 6-month or yearly intervals, depending upon the preexisting activity of the stone disease and the perceived need for supervision and/or reinforcement of the program (phase III). Appropriate analyses and plain x-rays with multiple views are performed at these times but at least on a yearly basis.

As noted above (see Hypercalciuria), the literature concerning the putative efficacy of thiazide treatment in hypercalciuric patients and/or those with idiopathic calcium stone disease has been criticized on the grounds of study design.[176] It was also noted that the thiazide literature is not peculiar in this regard and that these same criticisms could be leveled at the general literature concerning various therapies for stone disease of all types. There are many issues which merit consideration in reviewing this literature, but there are three which are of particular importance, inasmuch as they are issues which are as germane to the self-critical physician as they are to an intelligent reader of the literature.

First, the natural history of stone events is such that it has been likened to the mathematics of radioisotope decay; in essence, the events in question are statistically random. Many patients seek care and are entered into treatment programs soon after one or a cluster of stone events. This is entirely reasonable, since it is in response to the patient's motivation in seeking care in the first place. Yet, it also creates an enormous treatment bias in favor of apparent efficacy, given the usual method of plotting stone events before and after the beginning of therapy (i.e., stones per patient-year).

Second, patients typically begin a *program* of fluids, dietary measures, and a therapeutic agent simultaneously, and it is the drug which is given the credit (cointervention). This is true of both the assessment of stone events and, in many cases, of the chemical response to the program.[176]

Third, the radiological assessment of the stone burden and the differentiation of new versus old stones are the most difficult aspects of the follow-up of a patient with recurrent stone disease; obviously, they are critical in determining the efficacy of any therapeutic literature or is glossed over as though it pose are not routine; they must be specifically requested, and the patient must be properly prepared. In general, this point is either not mentioned in the therapeutic iterature or is glossed over as though it were a relatively simple matter. Since stone formation on the papillary surface of the kidney and the dislodging of this stone in the clinical episode which ensues do not occur close together in time, series which simply enumerate episodes and which make no mention of radiological assessment are extremely lax in design.

In the end, it is likely that none of the published therapeutic programs is quite as effective as many authors would like to believe. It is also likely that specific drugs are given more credit than is their due. Nevertheless, if therapeutic goals are properly established and assessed, most patients with recurrent stone disease can be helped substantially. They will be found to represent an intellectually challenging and rewarding component of the physician's practice.

Many patients are wary of an apparent lifelong commitment to treatment and inquire as to the proposed length of therapy (phase IV). Present information regarding the natural history of most forms of recurrent stone disease is inadequate to allow an objective answer to this question. Patients are best advised that the initial goal of therapy is to gain control of stone formation for a period of years and that consideration of discontinuing part or all of the therapeutic program must be based on assessment of individual responses and further knowledge regarding the natural history of recurrent stone disease.

Recent Advances in the Surgical Treatment of Nephrolithiasis

Although recent developments in the surgical treatment of nephrolithiasis, such as anatrophic nephrolithotomy,[227] coagulum pyelolithotomy,[53] and chemolysis for certain types of stones,[228] have made important contributions to the urological management of patients with stone disease, the recent introduction of lithotripsy for upper urinary tract stone disease represents a major advance in the treatment of renal and ureteral calculi.

The transurethral destruction of bladder stones by ultrasound or electrohydraulic shock waves has been practiced for some time. Only recently, however, have new techniques permitted application of these methods to upper urinary tract stones. The use of ultrasonic destruction of renal calculi has been possible only since the advent of techniques for percutaneous renal puncture. The technique involves percutaneous nephrostomy, dilation of the nephrostomy channel, and endoscopic stone destruction by means of a rigid ultrasound lithotrite.[229] The procedure can be performed with peridural anesthesia. This, in addition to the reduced postoperative recovery time, is the major advantage of the approach. In a recent series of 250 consecutive patients, the procedure was

97 percent successful in removing the targeted stone.[230] This technique is also applicable to destruction of ureteral stones, for which a special lithotrite is used.

Electrohydraulic lithotripsy involves the generation of a shock wave by a high-voltage condenser spark discharge, which causes explosive evaporation of the surrounding fluid and the generation of shock waves. This technique has been applied to ureteral stones by means of a rigid ureteroscope.[231,232] Recently, an extracorporeal method of shock-wave destruction of kidney stones has been developed.[233-235] The patient is submerged in a water bath and anesthetized, and a focused, high-energy shock wave is directed at the kidney stone. European studies suggest that when patients are properly selected, morbidity is low and the need for surgery following treatment is under 1 percent. Generally 1000 to 1500 individual shock waves are required to destroy a stone. Although to date this method has been used principally in patients with noninfected renal calculi, the technique has also been applied to small or partially fragmented MAP stones after antibiotic sterilization of the urine. Permission for premarketing evaluation of this technique in the United States has been granted by the U.S. Food and Drug Administration and a half-dozen clinical centers now have lithotripters.

These techniques have been the focus of considerable publicity, leading a substantial segment of the public to regard them as having revolutionized the care of patients with stone disease. However, these advances specifically relate only to the urological management of patients with stone disease and should in no way influence the top priority in the long-term care of these patients, which is prevention.

Acknowledgments

We are particularly indebted to the other members of the Renal Stone Clinic at Yale: Mrs. Alice Ellison, Mrs. Linda Gay, and Drs. William Burtis, Mort Glickman, Alan Kliger, Robert Lang, and Dan Oren. Mrs. Nancy Canetti provided superb secretarial assistance. A portion of the work described was supported by grants RR 125 and AM 31998 from the National Institutes of Health.

REFERENCES

1. Johnson MS, Wilson DM, O'Fallon WM, Malek RS, Kurland LT: Renal stone epidemiology: A 25-year study in Rochester, Minnesota. *Kidney Int* 16:624, 1979.
2. Nordin BEC: *Metabolic Bone and Stone Disease,* 2d ed. London, Churchill Livingstone, 1984.
3. Coe FL: *Nephrolithiasis.* Chicago, Year Book Medical Publishers, 1978.
4. Randall A: The origin and growth of renal calculi. *Ann Surg* 105:1009, 1937.
5. Smith LH: Urolithiasis, in Earley LE, Gottschalk CW (eds): *Strauss and Welt's Diseases of the Kidney,* 3d ed. Boston, Little, Brown, 1979, p 893.
6. Coe FL, Brenner BM, Stein JH (eds): *Current Issues in Nephrology: Nephrolithiasis.* London, Churchill Livingstone, 1980, vol 5.
7. Prien EL, Prien EL Jr: Composition and structure of urinary stone. *Am J Med* 45:654, 1968.
8. Pak CYC: *Calcium Urolithiasis.* New York, Plenum, 1978.
9. Boyce WH: Organic matrix of human urinary concretions. *Am J Med* 45:673, 1968.
10. Thomas WC, Howard JE: Studies in the mineralizing propensity of urine from patients with and without renal calculi. *Trans Assoc Am Physicians* 72:181, 1959.
11. Yü T: Uric acid nephrolithiasis, in Kelley WN, Weiner IM (eds): *Uric Acid.* New York, Springer-Verlag, 1978, p 397.
12. Pak CYC, Holt K: Nucleation and growth of brushite and calcium oxalate in urine of stone-formers. *Metabolism* 25:665, 1976.
13. Robertson WG, Peacock M, Marshall RW, Marshall DH, Nordin BEC: Saturation-inhibition index as a measure of the risk of calcium oxalate stone formation in the urinary tract. *N Engl J Med* 294:249, 1976.
14. Finlayson B: Physiochemical aspects of urolithiasis. *Kidney Int* 13:344, 1978.
15. Pak CYC, Galosy RA: Propensity for spontaneous nucleation of calcium oxalate. *Am J Med* 69:681, 1980.
16. Erickson SB, Cooper K, Broadus AE, Smith LH, Werness PG, Binder HJ, Dobbins JW: Oxalate absorption and postprandial urine supersaturation in an experimental human model of absorptive hypercalciuria. *Clin Sci* 67:131, 1984.
17. Kuiper JJ: Medullary sponge kidney, in Gardner KD (ed): *Cystic Diseases of the Kidney.* New York, Wiley, 1976, p 151.
18. Ekström T, Engfeldt B, Lagergren C, Lindvall N: *Medullary Sponge Kidney.* Stockholm, Almqvist and Wiksell, 1959.
19. Yendt ER, Jarzylo S, Finnis WA, Cohanim M: Medullary sponge kidney (tubular ectasia) in calcium urolithiasis, in Smith LH, Robertson WG, Finlayson B (eds): *Urolithiasis: Clinical and Basic Research.* New York, Plenum, 1981, p 105.
20. Parks JH, Coe FL, Strauss AL: Calcium nephrolithiasis and medullary sponge kidney in women. *N Engl J Med* 306:1988, 1982.
21. Sage MR, Lawson AD, Marshall UR, Ryall RL: Medullary sponge kidney and urolithiasis. *Clin Radiol* 33:435, 1982.
22. O'Neill M, Breslaw NA, Pak CYC: Metabolic evaluation of nephrolithiasis in patients with medullary sponge kidney. *JAMA* 245:1233, 1981.
23. Harrison R, Rose AG: Medullary sponge kidney. *Urol Res* 7:197, 1979.
24. Rosenberg LE, Scriver CR: Disorders of amino acid metabolism, in Bondy PK, Rosenberg LE (eds): *Metabolic Control and Disease.* Philadelphia, Saunders, 1980.
25. Segal S, Thier SO: Cystinuria, in Stanbury JB, Wyngaarden JB, Frederickson DS (eds): *The Metabolic Basis of Inherited Disease.* New York, McGraw-Hill, 1983, p 1774.
26. Dent CE, Rose GA: Amino acid metabolism in cystinuria. *Q J Med* 20:205, 1951.
27. Crawhall JC, Purkiss P, Watts WE, Young EP: The excretion of amino acids by cystinuric patients and their relatives. *Ann Hum Genet* 33:149, 1969.
28. Segal S, McNamara PD, Pepe LM: Transport interaction of cystine and dibasic amino acids in renal brush border vesicles. *Science* 197:169, 1977.
29. McNamara PD, Pepe LM, Segal S: Cystine uptake by renal brush border vesicles. *Biochem J* 194:443, 1981.
30. Foreman JW, Hwang SM, Segal S: Transport interactions of cystine and dibasic amino acids in isolated rat renal tubules. *Metabolism* 29:53, 1980.

31. Dahlberg PJ, Van Den Berg CJ, Kurtz SB, Wilson DM, Smith LH: Clinical features and management of cystinuria. *Mayo Clin Proc* 52:533, 1977.

32. Smith A, Yu JS, Brown DA: Childhood cystinuria in New South Wales. *Arch Dis Child* 54:676, 1979.

33. Halperin EC, Thier SO, Rosenberg LE: The use of D-penicillamine in cystinuria: Efficacy and untoward reactions. *Yale J Biol Med* 54:439, 1981.

34. Rizzoni G, Pavanello L, Dussini N, Chiandetti L, Zachello G: Nephrotic syndrome during treatment with alpha-mercaptopropionylglycine. *J Urol* 122:381, 1979.

35. Denneberg T, Jeppsson J-O, Stenberg P: Alternative treatment of cystinuria with α-merkaptopropionylglycine, thiola. *Proc Eur Dial Transplant Assoc* 20:427, 1983.

36. Miyagi K, Nakade F, Ohshiro S: Effect of glutamine on cystine excretion in a patient with cystinuria. *N Engl J Med* 301:196, 1979.

37. Skovby F, Rosenberg LE, Thier SO: No effect of L-glutamine on cystinuria. *N Engl J Med* 302:236, 1980.

38. Van Den Berg CJ, Jones JD, Wilson DM, Smith LH: Glutamine therapy of cystinuria. *Invest Urol* 18:155, 1980.

39. Resnick MI, Goodman HO, Boyce WH: Heterozygous cystinuria and calcium oxalate urolithiasis. *J Urol* 122:52, 1979.

40. Thomas WC, Malagodi MH, Rennert M: Amino acids in urine and blood of calculous patients. *Invest Urol* 19:115, 1981.

41. Carpenter PJ, Kurth KH, Blum W, Huijmans JG: Heterozygous cystinuria and calcium oxalate urolithiasis. *J Urol* 130:302, 1983.

42. Fessel WJ: Renal outcomes of gout and hyperuricemia. *Am J Med* 67:74, 1979.

43. Yü TF, Berger L, Dorph DJ, Smith H: Renal function in gout V. Factors influencing the renal hemodynamics. *Am J Med* 67:766, 1969.

44. Levinson DJ, Sorensen LB: Uric acid stones, in Coe FL (ed): *Nephrolithiasis.* Chicago, Year Book Medical Publishers, 1978, p 172.

45. Holmes EW: Uric acid nephrolithiasis, in Coe FL, Brenner BM, Stein JH (eds): *Contemporary Issues in Nephrology: Nephrolithiasis.* Edinburgh, Churchill Livingstone, 1980, vol 5, p 188.

46. Wyngaarden JB, Kelley WN: *Gout and Hyperuricemia.* New York, Grune & Stratton, 1976.

47. Steele TH: Urate excretion in man, normal and gouty, in Kelley WN, Weiner IM (eds): *Uric Acid.* New York, Springer-Verlag, 1978, p 254.

48. Gutman A, Yü TF: Uric acid nephrolithiasis. *Am J Med* 45:756, 1968.

49. Zechner O, Pfluger Scheiber V: Idiopathic uric acid lithiasis: Epidemiologic and metabolic aspects. *J Urol* 128:1219, 1982.

50. Resnick M, Kursh E, Cohen A: Use of computerized tomography in the delineation of uric acid calculi. *J Urol* 131:9, 1984.

51. Griffith DP: Struvite stones. *Kidney Int* 13:372, 1978.

52. Smith LH: Renal lithiasis and infection, in Thomas WC Jr (ed): *Renal Calculi.* Springfield, Ill., Charles C. Thomas, 1976, p 77.

53. Griffith DP, Bruce RR, Fishbein WN: Infection (urease)-induced stones, in Coe FL, Brenner BM, Stein JH (eds): *Contemporary Issues in Nephrology: Nephrolithiasis.* Edinburgh, Churchill Livingstone, 1980, vol 5, p 231.

54. McLean RJ, Nickel JC, Noakes VC, Costerton JW: An in vitro ultrastructural study of infectious kidney stone genesis. *Infect Immun* 49:805, 1985.

55. Silverman DE, Stamey TA: Management of infection stones: The Stamford experience. *Medicine* 62:44, 1983.

56. Chinn RH, Maskell R, Mead JA, Polak A: Renal stones and urinary infection: A study of antibiotic treatment. *Br Med J* 2:1411, 1976.

57. Feit R, Fair W: The treatment of infection stones with penicillin. *J Urol* 122:592, 1979.

58. Griffith DP, Moskowitz PA, Carlton CE: Adjunctive chemotherapy of infection-induced staghorn calculi. *J Urol* 121:711, 1979.

59. Smith L: New treatment for struvite stones. *N Engl J Med* 311:792, 1984.

60. Krieger JN, Rudd TG, Mayo E: Current treatment of infection stones in high risk patients. *J Urol* 132:874, 1984.

61. Griffith DP, Gibson JR, Clinton CW, Musher DM: Acetohydroxamic acid: Clinical studies of a urease inhibitor in patients with staghorn renal calculi. *J Urol* 119:9, 1978.

62. Martelli A, Buli P, Curtecchia V: Acetohydroxamic acid therapy in infected renal stones. *Urology* 17:320, 1981.

63. Williams J, Rodman J, Peterson C: A randomized double-blind study of acetohydroxamic acid in struvite nephrolithiasis. *N Engl J Med* 311:760, 1984.

64. Cogan MG, Rector FC, Seldin DW: Acid-base disorders, in Brenner BM, Rector RC (eds): *The Kidney,* 2d ed. Philadelphia, Saunders, 1981, p 841.

65. Brenner RJ, Spring AB, Sebastian A, McSherry EM, Genant HK, Palubinskas AJ, Morris RC: Incidence of radiographically evident bone disease, nephrocalcinosis and nephrolithiasis in various types of renal tubular acidosis. *N Engl J Med* 307:217, 1982.

66. Simpson DP: Regulation of renal citrate metabolism by bicarbonate ion and pH; observations in tissue slices and mitochondria. *J Clin Invest* 46:225, 1967.

67. Danielson BG, Backman U, Fellstrom B, Johansson G, Ljunghall S, Wikstrom B: Experience with the short ammonium chloride test, in Smith LH, Robertson WG, Finlayson B (eds): *Urolithiasis: Clinical and Basic Research.* New York, Plenum, 1981, p 71.

68. Tannen RL, Falls WF, Brackett NC: Incomplete renal tubular acidosis: Some clinical and physiological features. *Nephron* 15:111, 1975.

69. Konnak J, Kogan B, Lau K: Renal calculi associated with incomplete distal renal tubular acidosis. *J Urol* 128:900, 1982.

70. Preminger GM, Sakhaee K, Skurla C, Pak CYC: Prevention of recurrent calcium stone formation with potassium citrate therapy in patients with distal renal tubular acidosis. *J Urol* 134:20, 1985.

71. Batlle DC, Kurtzman HA: Distal renal tubular acidosis, in Coe F (ed): *The Hypercalciuric States: Pathogenesis Consequences and Treatment.* Orlando, Grune & Stratton, 1984, p 239.

72. Backman U, Danielson G, Fellstrom B, Johansson G, Ljunghall S, Wikstrom B: The clinical importance of renal tubular acidosis in recurrent renal stone formers, in Smith LH, Robertson WG, Finlayson B (eds): *Urolithiasis: Clinical and Basic Research.* New York, Plenum, 1981, p 67.

73. Parfitt AM: Acetazolamide and sodium bicarbonate induced nephrocalcinosis and nephrolithiasis. *Arch Intern Med* 124:736, 1969.

74. Pyrah L: *Renal calculus.* New York, Springer-Verlag, 1979.

75. Broadus AE: Nephrolithiasis in primary hyperparathyroidism, in Coe FL, Brenner BM, Stein JH (eds): *Contemporary Issues in Nephrology: Nephrolithiasis.* Edinburgh, Churchill Livingstone, 1980, vol 5, p 59.

76. McSherry E, Morris RC: Attainment and maintenance of normal stature with alkali therapy in infants and children with classic renal tubular acidosis. *J Clin Invest* 61:509, 1978.

77. Robertson WG, Peacock M, Heyburn PJ, Marshall DH, Clark PB: Risk factors in calcium stone disease of the urinary tract. *Br J Urol* 50:449, 1978.

78. Hodgkinson A, Marshall RW: Changes in the composition of urinary tract stones. *Invest Urol* 13:131, 1975.

79. Robertson WG, Peacock M: The pattern of urinary stone disease in Leeds and in the United Kingdom in relation to animal protein intake during the period 1960–1980. *Urol Int* 37:394, 1982.

80. Boyce WH, Garvey FK, Strawcutter HE: Incidence of urinary calculi among patients in general hospitals, 1948 to 1952. *JAMA* 161:1437, 1956.

81. Sierakowski RL, Finlayson B, Landes RR, Finlayson CD, Sierakowski NA: The frequency of urolithiasis in hospital discharge diagnoses in the U.S. *Invest Urol* 15:438, 1978.

82. Williams RE: Long term survey of 538 patients with upper urinary tract stone. *Br J Urol* 35:416, 1963.

83. Strauss AL, Coe FL, Parks JH: Formation of a single stone of renal origin. *Arch Intern Med* 142:504, 1982.

84. Pak CYC: Should patients with single renal stone occurrence undergo diagnostic evaluation? *J Urol* 127:855, 1982.

85. Broadus AE, Thier SO: Metabolic basis of renal stone disease. *N Engl J Med* 300:839, 1979.

86. Resnick M, Pridgen DB, Goodman HO: Genetic predisposition to formation of calcium oxalate renal calculi. *N Engl J Med* 278:1313, 1968.

87. Coe FL, Parks JH, Moore ES: Familial idiopathic hypercalciuria. *N Engl J Med* 300:337, 1979.

88. Buckalew VM, Purvis ML, Shulman MG, Herndon CN, Rudman D: Hereditary renal tubular acidosis. Report of a 64 member kindred with variable clinical expression including idiopathic hypercalciuria. *Medicine* 53:229, 1974.

89. Stapleton FB, Roy S, Noe NH, Jerkins G: Hypercalciuria in children with hematuria. *N Engl J Med* 310:1345, 1984.

90. Sestili MA: Possible adverse health effects of vitamin C and ascorbic acid. *Semin Oncol* 10:299, 1983.

91. Smith LH: Risk of oxalate stone from large doses of vitamin C. *N Engl J Med* 298:856, 1978.

92. Smith LH, Van Den Berg CJ, Wilson DM: Nutrition and urolithiasis. *N Engl J Med* 298:87, 1978.

93. Pak CYC, Sakhaee K, Crowther C, Brinkley L: An objective evidence for the beneficial effect of a high fluid intake in the management of nephrolithiasis. *Ann Intern Med* 93:36, 1980.

94. Strauss AL, Coe FL, Deutsch L, Parks JH: Factors that predict relapse of calcium nephrolithiasis during treatment. *Am J Med* 72:17, 1982.

95. Flocks RH: Calcium and phosphorus excretion in the urine of patients with renal or ureteral calculi. *JAMA* 113:1466, 1939.

96. Albright F, Henneman P, Benedict PH, Forbes AP: Idiopathic hypercalciuria. *Proc R Soc Med* 46:1077, 1953.

97. Henneman PH, Benedict PH, Forbes AP, Dudley HR: Idiopathic hypercalciuria. *N Engl J Med* 259:802, 1958.

98. Nordin BEC, Peacock M, Wilkinson R: Hypercalciuria and calcium stone disease. *Clin Endocrinol Metab* 1:169, 1972.

99. Peacock M, Hodgkinson A, Nordin BEC: Importance of dietary calcium in the definition of hypercalciuria. *Br Med J* 3:469, 1967.

100. Lemann J, Adams ND, Gray RW: Urinary calcium excretion in human beings. *N Engl J Med* 301:535, 1979.

101. Hodgkinson A, Pyrah LN: The urinary excretion of calcium and inorganic phosphate in 344 patients with calcium stone of renal origin. *Br J Surg* 48:10, 1958.

102. Lemann J: Idiopathic hypercalciuria, in Coe FL, Brenner BM, Stein JH (eds): *Contemporary Issues in Nephrology: Nephrolithiasis.* Edinburgh, Churchill Livingstone, 1980, vol 5, p 86.

103. Muldowney FP, Freaney R, Moloney MF: Importance of dietary sodium in the hypercalciuria syndrome. *Kidney Int* 22:292, 1982.

104. Burtis WJ, Oren DA, Insogna KL, Lang R, Kliger AS, Sartori L, Gay L, Ellison AF, Broadus AE: Metabolic evaluation of 363 consecutive patients in a renal stone clinic. (Submitted for publication.)

105. Broadus AE, Dominguez M, Bartter FC: Pathophysiological studies in idiopathic hypercalciuria: Use of an oral calcium tolerance test to characterize distinctive hypercalciuric subgroups. *J Clin Endocrinol Metab* 47:751, 1978.

106. Broadus AE, Insogna KL, Mallette LE, Oren DA, Gertner JM, Kliger AS, Ellison AF: A consideration of the hormonal basis and phosphate leak hypothesis of absorptive hypercalciuria. *J Clin Endocrinol Metab* 58:161, 1984.

107. Broadus AE, Insogna KL, Lang R, Ellison AF, Dreyer BE: Evidence for disordered control of 1,25-dihydroxyvitamin D production in absorptive hypercalciuria. *N Engl J Med* 311:73, 1984.

108. Lau YK, Wasserstein A, Westby GR, Bosanac P, Grabie M, Mitnick P, Slatopolsky E, Goldfarb S, Agus ZS: Proximal tubular defects in idiopathic hypercalciuria: Resistance to phosphate administration. *Min Elect Metab* 7:237, 1982.

109. Pak CYC, Britton F, Peterson R, Ward D, Northcutt C, Breslau NA, McGuire J, Sakhaee K, Bush S, Nicar M, Norman D, Peters P: Ambulatory evaluation of nephrolithiasis: Classification, clinical presentation and diagnostic criteria. *Am J Med* 69:19, 1980.

110. Pak CYC: Physiological basis for absorptive and renal hypercalciuria. *Am J Physiol* 237:F415, 1979.

111. Pak CYC, Galosy RA: Fasting urinary calcium and adenosine 3′,5′-monophosphate: A discriminant analysis for the identification of renal and absorptive hypercalciurias. *J Clin Endocrinol Metab* 48:260, 1979.

112. Pak CYC, Kaplan R, Bone H, Townsend J, Waters O: A simple test for the diagnosis of absorptive, resorptive, and renal hypercalciurias. *N Engl J Med* 292:497, 1975.

113. Stewart AF, Adler M, Byers CM, Segre GV, Broadus AE: Calcium homeostasis in immobilization: An example of resorptive hypercalciuria. *N Engl J Med* 306:1136, 1982.

114. Breslau NA, McGuire JL, Zerwekh JE, Pak CYC: The role of dietary sodium on renal excretion and intestinal absorption of calcium and on vitamin D metabolism. *J Clin Endocrinol Metab* 55:369, 1982.

115. Phillips MJ, Cooke JNC: Relation between urinary calcium and sodium in patients with idiopathic hypercalciuria. *Lancet* 2:1354, 1967.

116. Sabto J, Powell MJ, Breidahl MJ, Gurr FW: Influence of urinary sodium on calcium excretion in normal individuals. *Med J Aust* 140:354, 1984.

117. Silver J, Friedlaender MM, Rubinger D, Popovtzer MM: Sodium-dependent idiopathic hypercalciuria in renal stone formers. *Lancet* 2:484, 1983.

118. Agus ZS, Chiu PJS, Goldberg M: Regulation of urinary calcium excretion in the rat. *Am J Physiol* 1:F545, 1977.

119. Sutton RAL, Walker VR: Responses to hydrochlorothiazide and acetazolamide in patients with calcium stones. *N Engl J Med* 302:709, 1980.

120. Colussi G, Surian M, DeFerrari ME, Pontoriero G, Rombola G, Brando B, Malberti F, Cosci P, Aroldi A, Castelnovo C, Minetti L: Relationship between sodium intake, proximal tubular function and calcium excretion in normal subjects and in idiopathic hypercalciuria. *Proc Eur Dial Transplant Assoc* 20:455, 1983.

121. Broadus AE, Horst RL, Mahaffey JE, Rasmussen H: Primary hyperparathyroidism with intermittent hypercalcemia: Serial observations and simple diagnosis by means of an oral calcium tolerance test. *Clin Endocrinol* 12:225, 1980.

122. Yendt ER, Gagne RJA: Detection of primary hyperparathyroidism, with special reference to its occurrence in hypercalciuric females with normal or borderline serum calcium. *Can Med Assoc J* 98:331, 1968.

123. Muldowney FP, Freaney R, McMullin JP, Towers RP, Spillane A, O'Connor P, O'Donohue P, Moloney M: Serum ionized calcium and parathyroid hormone in renal stone disease. *Q J Med* 45:75, 1976.

124. Parks J, Coe FL, Favus M: Hyperparathyroidism in nephrolithiasis. *Arch Intern Med* 140:1479, 1980.

125. Keating FR, Jones JD, Elveback CR, Randall RV: The relation of age and sex to distribution of values in healthy adults of serum calcium, inorganic phosphorus, magnesium, alkaline phosphatase, total proteins, albumin, and blood urea. *J Lab Clin Med* 73:825, 1969.

126. Broadus AE, Horst RL, Lang R, Littledike ET, Rasmussen H: The importance of circulating 1,25-dihydroxyvitamin D in the pathogenesis of hypercalciuria and renal stone formation in primary hyperparathyroidism. *N Engl J Med* 302:421, 1980.

127. Bordier P, Ryckewart A, Gueris J, Rasmusen H: On the

pathogenesis of so-called idiopathic hypercalciuria. *Am J Med* 63:398, 1977.
128. Coe FL, Canterbury JM, Firpo JJ, Reiss E: Evidence for secondary hyperparathyroidism in idiopathic hypercalciuria. *J Clin Invest* 52:134, 1973.
129. Muldowney FP, Freaney R, Ryan JG: The pathogenesis of idiopathic hypercalciuria: Evidence for renal tubular calcium leak. *QJ Med* 49:87, 1980.
130. Coe FL, Favus MJ, Crockett T, Strauss AL, Parks JH, Porat A, Gantt CL, Sherwood LM: Effects of low-calcium diet on urine calcium excretion, parathyroid function and serum $1,25(OH)_2D_3$ levels in patients with idiopathic hypercalciuria and normal subjects. *Am J Med* 72:25, 1982.
131. Peacock M, Knowles F, Nordin BEC: Effect of calcium administration and deprivation on serum and urine calcium in stone-forming and control subjects. *Br Med J* 2:729, 1968.
132. Ulmann A, Aubert J, Bourdeau A, Cheynel C, Bader C: Effects of weight and glucose ingestion on urinary calcium and phosphate excretion: Implications for calcium urolithiasis. *J Clin Endocrinol Metab* 54:1063, 1982.
133. Tschope W, Ritz E, Schmidt-Gayk H: Is there a renal phosphate leak in recurrent renal stone formers with absorptive hypercalciuria? *Eur J Clin Invest* 10:381, 1980.
134. Schwille PO, Scholz D, Schwille K, Engelhardt W, Schreiber B, Goldberg I, Sigel A: Parathyroid gland function in subgroups of metabolically mediated urolithiasis as evaluated by serum parathyroid hormone, and urinary and nephrogenous cyclic nucleotides. *Klin Wochenschr* 69:229, 1982.
135. Lilienfeld-Toal H, Bach D, Hesse A, Franck H, Issa S: Parathyroid hormone is normal in renal stone patients with idiopathic hypercalciuria and high fasting urinary calcium. *Urol Res* 10:205, 1982.
136. Lien J, Keane P: Urinary cAMP and calcium excretion in the fasting state and their response to oral calcium loading in patients with calcium urolithiasis. *J Urol* 129:401, 1983.
137. Hymes LC, Warshaw BL: Idiopathic hypercalciuria. *Am J Dis Child* 138:176, 1984.
138. Broadus AE, Erickson SB, Gertner JM, Cooper K, Dobbins JW: An experimental human model of 1,25-dihydroxyvitamin D-mediated hypercalciuria. *J Clin Endocrinol Metab* 59:202, 1984.
139. Adams ND, Gray RW, Lemann J, Cheung HS: Effects of calcitriol administration on calcium metabolism in healthy men. *Kidney Int* 21:90, 1982.
140. Van Den Berg CJ, Kumar R, Wilson DM, Heath H, Smith LH: Orthophosphate therapy decreases urinary calcium excretion and serum 1,25-dihydroxyvitamin D concentrations in idiopathic hypercalciuria. *J Clin Endocrinol Metab* 51:998, 1980.
141. Gray RW, Wilz DR, Caldas AE, Lemann J: The importance of phosphate in regulating plasma $1,25\text{-}(OH)_2$-vitamin D levels in humans: Studies in healthy subjects, in calcium-stone formers and in patients with primary hyperparathyroidism. *J Clin Endocrinol Metab* 45:299, 1977.
142. Burckhardt P, Jaeger P: Secondary hyperparathyroidism in idiopathic hypercalciuria: Fact or theory? *J Clin Endocrinol Metab* 53:550, 1981.
143. Shen FH, Ivey JL, Sherrard DJ, Nielsen RL, Haussler MR, Baylink DJ: Further evidence supporting the phosphate leak hypothesis of idiopathic hypercalciuria. *Adv Exp Med Biol* 103:217, 1978.
144. Pak CYC: Pathogenesis, consequences, and treatment of the hypercalciuric states. *Semin Nephrol* 1:356, 1981.
145. Maierhofer WJ, Gray RW, Cheung HS, Lemann J: Bone resorption stimulated by elevated serum $1,25\text{-}(OH)_2$-vitamin D concentrations in healthy men. *Kidney Int* 24:555, 1983.
146. Brannan PG, Morawski S, Pak CYC, Fordtran J: Selective jejunal hyperabsorption of calcium in absorptive hypercalciuria. *Am J Med* 66:425, 1979.
147. Kreis GJ, Nicar MJ, Zerwekh JE, Normann DA, Kane MG, Pak CYC: Effect of 1,25-dihydroxyvitamin D on calcium and magnesium absorption in the healthy human jejunum and ileum. *Am J Med* 75:973, 1983.
148. Kaplan RA, Haussler MR, Deftos LJ, Bone H, Pak CYC: The role of 1α, 25-dihydroxyvitamin D in the mediation of intestinal hyperabsorption of calcium in primary hyperparathyroidism and absorptive hypercalciuria. *J Clin Invest* 59:756, 1977.
149. Shen FH, Baylink DJ, Nielsen RL, Sherrard DJ, Ivey JL, Haussler MJ: Increased serum 1,25-dihydroxyvitamin D in idiopathic hypercalciuria. *J Lab Clin Med* 90:955, 1977.
150. Insogna KL, Broadus AE, Dreyer BE, Ellison AF, Gertner JM: Elevated production rate for 1,25-dihydroxyvitamin D in patients with absorptive hypercalciuria. *J Clin Endocrinol Metab* 61:490, 1985.
151. Tanaka Y, DeLuca HF: The control of 25-hydroxyvitamin D metabolism by inorganic phosphorus. *Arch Biochem Biophys* 154:566, 1973.
152. Insogna KL, Broadus AE, Gertner JW: Impaired phosphorus conservation and 1,25-dihydroxyvitamin D generation during phosphorus deprivation in familial hypophosphatemic rickets. *J Clin Invest* 71:1562, 1983.
153. Barilla DE, Zerwekh JE, Pak CYC: A critical evaluation of the role of phosphate in the pathogenesis of absorptive hypercalciuria. *Min Elect Metab* 2:302, 1979.
154. Tieder M, Modai D, Samuel R, Arie R, Halabe A, Bab I, Gabizon D, Lieberman UA: Hereditary hypophosphatemic rickets with hypercalciuria. *N Engl J Med* 312:611, 1985.
155. Edwards NA, Hodgkinson A: Phosphate metabolism in patients with renal calculus. *Clin Sci* 29:93, 1965.
156. Insogna KL, Burtis WJ, Lang R, Sartori L, Ellison AF, Broadus AE: A short-term prospective comparison of the effects of trichlormethiazide and oral phosphate therapy in patients with absorptive hypercalciuria. (Submitted for publication.)
157. Ulmann A, Dard S, Lacour B, Rieu M, Roullet JB, Gueris J, Funck-Brentano JL: Idiopathic hypercalciuria: Effect of an acute reduction in phosphorus. *Nouv Presse Med* 8:3619, 1979.
158. Lemann J, Gray RW, Wilz DR: Evidence for a renal phosphate leak in patients with calcium nephrolithiasis. *Adv Exp Med Biol* 103:225, 1978.
159. Coe FL, Bushinsky DA: Pathophysiology of hypercalciuria. *Am J Physiol* 247:F1, 1984.
160. Insogna KL, Lang R, Ellison A, Broadus A: Qualitative abnormality in 1,25-dihydroxyvitamin D response to phosphorus deprivation in patients with absorptive hypercalciuria. *Clin Res* 33:433A, 1985.
161. Gertner JM, Coustan DR, Kliger AS, Mallette LE, Ravin N, Broadus AE: Pregnancy is a state of physiological absorptive hypercalciuria. *Am J Med* 81:451, 1986.
162. Coe FL, Parks JH, Lindheimer MD: Nephrolithiasis during pregnancy. *N Engl J Med* 298:324, 1978.
163. Malluche HH, Tschoepe W, Ritz E, Meyer-Sabellek W, Massry SG: Abnormal bone histology in idiopathic hypercalciuria. *J Clin Endocrinol Metab* 50:654, 1980.
164. Lawoyin S, Sismilich S, Browne R, Pak CYC: Bone mineral density in patients with calcium urolithiasis. *Metabolism* 28:1250, 1979.
165. Alhava EM, Juuti M, Karjalainen P: Bone mineral density in patients with urolithiasis. *Scand J Urol Nephrol* 10:154, 1976.
166. Lieberman UA, Sperling O, Atsmon A, Frank M, Modan M, deVries A: Metabolic and calcium kinetic studies in idiopathic hypercalciuria. *J Clin Invest* 47:2580, 1968.
167. Jorgensen FS: Effect of thiazide diuretics upon calcium metabolism. *Dan Med Bull* 23:223, 1976.
168. Broadus AE, Lang R, Kliger AS: The influence of calcium intake and the status of intestinal calcium absorption on the diagnostic utility of measurements of 24-hour cyclic adenosine 3′,5′-monophosphate excretion. *J Clin Endocrinol Metab* 52:1085, 1981.

169. Kraiem Z, Schotland Y, Bernheim J, Embon O, Lurie A, Sheinfeld M, Gonda M: Assessment of the calcium loading test in differentiating between various forms of idiopathic hypercalciuria. *Isr J Med Sci* 19:596, 1983.
170. Walker VR, Sutton RAL: Urinary adenosine 3′,5′-monophosphate in idiopathic calcium stone formers: Response to an oral calcium load. *Clin Sci* 66:193, 1984.
171. Lein JW, Keane PM: Limitations of the oral calcium loading test in the management of the recurrent calcareous renal stone former. *Am J Kidney Dis* 3:76, 1983.
172. Broadus AE, Magee JS, Mallette LE, Horst RL, Lang R, Jensen PS, Gertner JM, Baron R: A detailed evaluation of oral phosphate therapy in selected patients with primary hyperparathyroidism. *J Clin Endocrinol Metab* 56:953, 1983.
173. Hosking DH, Erickson SB, Van Den Berg CJ, Wilson DM, Smith LH: The stone clinic effect in patients with idiopathic calcium urolithiasis. *J Urol* 130:1115, 1983.
174. Insogna KL, Broadus AE: Nephrolithiasis, in Krieger DR, Bardin CW (eds): *Current Therapy in Endocrinology and Metabolism.* St. Louis, Mosby, 1985, p 353.
175. Pak CYC, Smith LH, Resnick MI, Weinerth JL: Dietary management of idiopathic calcium urolithiasis. *J Urol* 131:850, 1984.
176. Churchill DN, Taylor DW: Thiazides for patients with recurrent calcium stones: Still an open question. *J Urol* 133:749, 1985.
177. Zerwekh JE, Pak CYC: Selective effects of thiazide therapy on serum 1,25-dihydroxyvitamin D and intestinal calcium absorption in renal and absorptive hypercalciurias. *Metabolism* 29:13, 1980.
178. Heyburn PJ, Robertson WG, Peacock M: Phosphate treatment of recurrent calcium stone disease. *Nephron* 32:314, 1982.
179. Yendt ER, Cohanim M: Prevention of calcium stones with thiazides. *Kidney Int* 13:397, 1978.
180. Coe FL: Treated and untreated recurrent calcium nephrolithiasis in patients with idiopathic hypercalciuria, hyperuricosuria, or no metabolic disorder. *Ann Intern Med* 87:404, 1977.
181. Smith LH, Thomas WC, Arnaud CD: Orthophosphate therapy in calcium renal lithiasis, in Cifuentes DL, Rapado A, Hodgkinson A (eds): *Urinary Calculi: Recent Advances in Aetiology, Stone Structure and Treatment.* Basel, Karger, 1973, p 188.
182. Thomas WC: Use of phosphates in patients with calcareous renal calculi. *Kidney Int* 13:390, 1978.
183. Ettinger B: Recurrent nephrolithiasis: Natural history and effect of phosphate therapy. *Am J Med* 61:200, 1976.
184. Pak CYC: A cautious use of sodium cellulose phosphate in the management of calcium nephrolithiasis. *Invest Urol* 19:187, 1981.
185. Backman U, Danielson BG, Johansson G, Ljunghall S, Wikstrom B: Treatment of recurrent calcium stone formation with cellulose phosphate. *J Urol* 123:9, 1980.
186. Cohanim M, Yendt ER: Reduction of urine oxalate during long-term thiazide therapy in patients with calcium urolithiasis. *Invest Urol* 18:170, 1980.
187. Scholz D, Schwille PO, Sigel A: Double-blind study with thiazide in recurrent calcium lithiasis. *J Urol* 128:903, 1982.
188. Costanzo LS, Windhager EE: Calcium and sodium transport by the distal convoluted tubule of the rat. *Am J Physiol* 235:F492, 1978.
189. Ettinger B: Risk of kidney stones. *JAMA* 248:1971, 1982.
190. Smith LH: Enteric hyperoxaluria and other hyperoxaluric states, in Coe FL, Brenner BM, Stein JH (eds): *Contemporary Issues in Nephrology: Nephrolithiasis.* Edinburgh, Churchill Livingstone, 1980, vol 5, p 136.
191. Williams HE: Oxalic acid and the hyperoxaluric syndromes. *Kidney Int* 13:410, 1978.
192. Dobbins JW, Binder HJ: Derangements of oxalate metabolism in gastrointestinal disease and their mechanisms, in Glass GBJ (ed): *Progress in Gastroenterology.* New York, Grune & Stratton, 1977, p 505.
193. Knickelbein RG, Aronson PS, Dobbins JW: Oxalate transport by anion exchange across rabbit ileal brush border. *J Clin Invest* 77:170, 1986.
194. Williams HE, Smith LH: Primary hyperoxaluria, in Stanbury JB, Wyngaarden JB, Frederickson DS, Goldstein JL, Brown MS (eds): *The Metabolic Basis of Inherited Disease,* 5th ed. New York, McGraw-Hill, 1983, p 204.
195. Weinman EJ, Frankfurt SJ, Ince A, Sansom S: Renal tubular transport of organic acids. *J Clin Invest* 61:801, 1978.
196. Smith LH, Fromm H, Hoffmann AF: Acquired hyperoxaluria, nephrolithiasis, and intestinal disease. *N Engl J Med* 286:1371, 1972.
197. Chadwick VS, Modha K, Dowling RH: Mechanism for hyperoxaluria in patients with ileal dysfunction. *N Engl J Med* 289:172, 1973.
198. Rudman D, Dedonis JL, Fountain MT, Chandler JB, Gerron GG, Fleming GA, Kutner MH: Hypocitraturia in patients with gastrointestinal malabsorption. *N Engl J Med* 303:657, 1980.
199. Hodgkinson A: Evidence of increased oxalate absorption in patients with calcium-containing renal stones. *Clin Sci Mol Med* 54:291, 1978.
200. Galosy R, Clarke L, Ward DL, Pak CYC: Renal oxalate excretion in calcium urolithiasis. *J Urol* 123:320, 1980.
201. Marangella M, Fruttero B, Bruno M, Linari F: Hyperoxaluria in idiopathic calcium stone disease: Further evidence of intestinal hyperabsorption of oxalate. *Clin Sci* 63:381, 1982.
202. Jaeger P, Portmann L, Jacquet AF, Burckhardt P: Influence of the calcium content of the diet on the incidence of mild hyperoxaluria in idiopathic renal stone formers. *Am J Nephrol* 5:40, 1985.
203. Yendt ER, Cohanim M: Response to a physiologic dose of pyridoxine in type I primary hyperoxaluria. *N Engl J Med* 312:953, 1985.
204. Dobbins JW: Nephrolithiasis and intestinal disease. *J Clin Gastroenterol* 7:21, 1985.
205. Gutman AB, Yü T: Uric acid nephrolithiasis. *Am J Med* 45:756, 1968.
206. Smith MJV, Hunt LD, King JS, Boyce WH: Uricemia and urolithiasis. *J Urol* 101:637, 1969.
207. Coe FL, Raisen L: Allopurinol treatment of uric acid disorders in calcium-stone formers. *Lancet* 1:129, 1973.
208. Coe FL: Hyperuricosuric calcium oxalate nephrolithiasis. *Kidney Int* 13:418, 1978.
209. Coe FL: Uric acid and calcium oxalate nephrolithiasis. *Kidney Int* 24:392, 1983.
210. Ettinger B, Tang A, Citron J, Livermore B, Williams T: Allopurinol prevents calcium oxalate stone recurrence in hyperuricosuric normocalciuric subjects. *N Engl J Med* 315:1386, 1986.
211. Lonsdale K: Epitaxy as a growth factor in urinary calculi and gallstones. *Nature* 217:56, 1968.
212. Meyer JL, Bergert JH, Smith LH: The epitaxially induced crystal growth of calcium oxalate by crystalline uric acid. *Invest Urol* 14:115, 1976.
213. Fellstrom B, Danielson RG, Karlstrom B, Lithell H, Ljunghall S, Vessby B: The influence of a high dietary intake of purine-rich animal protein on urinary urate excretion and supersaturation in renal stone disease. *Clin Sci* 64:399, 1983.
214. Pak CYC, Barilla DE, Holt K, Brinkley L, Tolentino R, Zerwekh JE: Effect of oral purine load and allopurinol on the crystallization of calcium salts in urine of patients with hyperuricosuric calcium urolithiasis. *Am J Med* 65:593, 1978.
215. Rudman D, Kutner MH, Redd SC, Waters WC, Gerron GG, Bleier J: Hypocitraturia in calcium nephrolithiasis. *J Clin Endocrinol Metab* 55:1052, 1982.
216. Simpson DP: Citrate excretion: A window on renal metabolism. *Am J Physiol* 244:F223, 1983.
217. Gordon EE, Sheps SG: Effect of acetazolamide on citrate excretion and formation of renal calculi. Report of a case and study of five normal subjects. *N Engl J Med* 256:1215, 1957.

218. Morrissey JF, Ochoa M, Lotspeich W, Waterhouse C: Citrate excretion in renal tubular acidosis. *Ann Intern Med* 58:159, 1963.
219. Fourman P, Robinson JR: Diminished urinary excretion of citrate during deficiencies of potassium in man: A preliminary communication. *Lancet* 2:656, 1953.
220. Menon M, Mahle CJ: Urinary citrate excretion in patients with renal calculi. *J Urol* 129:1158, 1983.
221. Hosking D, Wilson J, Liedtke R, Smith L, Wilson D: Urinary citrate excretion in normal persons and patients with idiopathic calcium nephrolithiasis. *J Lab Clin Med* 106:682, 1985.
222. Pak CYC, Fuller C, Sakhaee K, Preminger GM, Britton F: Long-term treatment of calcium nephrolithiasis with potassium citrate. *J Urol* 134:11, 1985.
223. Nicar MJ, Shurla G, Sakhaee K, Pak CYC: Low urinary citrate excretion in nephrolithiasis. *Urology* 21:8, 1983.
224. Pak CYC, Peterson R, Sakhaee K, Fuller C, Preminger G, Reisch J: Correction of hypocitraturia and prevention of stone formation by combined thiazide and potassium citrate therapy in thiazide-unresponsive hypercalciuric nephrolithiasis. *Am J Med* 79:284, 1985.
225. Prien EL, Gershoff SF: Magnesium oxide-pyridoxine therapy for recurrent calcium oxalate calculi. *J Urol* 112:509, 1974.
226. Wein AJ, Benson GS, Raezer DM, Mulholland SG: Oral methylene blue and the dissolution of renal calculi. *J Urol* 116:140, 1976.
227. Redman JF, Bissada NK, Harper DL: Anatrophic nephrolithotomy: Experience with a simplification of the Smith and Boyce technique. *J Urol* 122:595, 1979.
228. Sheldon CA, Smith AD: Chemolysis of calculi. *Urol Clin North Am* 9:121, 1982.
229. Alken P: Percutaneous ultrasonic destruction of renal calculi. *Urol Clin North Am* 9:145, 1982.
230. Brannen GE, Bush WH, Correa RJ, Gibbons RP, Elder J: Kidney stone removal: Percutaneous versus surgical lithotomy. *J Urol* 133:6, 1985.
231. Reuler HJ: Electronic lithotripsy: Transurethral treatment of bladder stones in 50 cases. *J Urol* 104:834, 1970.
232. Reuler HJ, Kern E: Electronic lithotripsy of ureteral calculi. *J Urol* 110:181, 1973.
233. Chaussy C, Schmiedt E, Jochan D, Brendel W, Forssmann B, Walther V: First clinical experience with extracorporeally induced destruction of kidney stones by shock wave. *J Urol* 127:417, 1982.
234. Chaussy C, Schmiedt E: Shock wave treatment for stones in the upper urinary tract. *Urol Clin North Am* 10:743, 1983.
235. Finlayson B, Thomas W: Extracorporeal shock-wave lithotripsy. *Ann Intern Med* 101:387, 1984.

PART VIII

MISCELLANEOUS DISORDERS

Disorders of Growth and Development

Margaret H. MacGillivray

The growth of the human organism from the zygote stage to its culmination in adult stature is a highly complex phenomenon involving a multitude of regulatory mechanisms which control tissue differentiation, generation, and maturation. In practical terms, growth is the net of mass produced and retained less that destroyed or lost. The word "growth" implies a continuum of harmonious metabolic generation and degradation.[1] Terminal or mature size represents an equilibrium between the incremental and decremental processes, while aging signifies an imbalance, in which more tissue is lost than is replaced. Tissue differentiation and maturation, although not explicit in this definition, are essential components of growth.

Throughout childhood and adolescence, gains in height and weight are sensitive and reasonably accurate indexes of the health and well-being of an individual. In general, stature or height is a more accurate basis for evaluating the overall growth process because healthy children show wide variability in weight. However, in chronically malnourished children, weight is the more sensitive indicator of disease; linear growth is disturbed to a lesser degree.

This chapter discusses the mechanisms which control the overall growth processes of healthy children as well as the many factors which disturb or enhance growth, and provides criteria for differentiating children with pathologic growth from those with short or tall stature at either limit of the normal growth channels. Practical information on diagnostic procedures and therapy is also given.

BIOLOGIC STAGES OF GROWTH

The growth of all tissues consists of an initial, critical phase of rapid cell division (hyperplasia). During this period, diseases that interfere with DNA replication may have a permanent stunting effect because tissues are denied their full complement of cells. The second phase is attributable to both hyperplasia and increased cell size (hypertrophy). In the final stage, cellular enlargement is responsible for the attainment of full organ size.[2,3] Maturity is a period of equilibrium. It is followed by the process of aging which is characterized by more tissue degeneration than regeneration (Fig. 26-1). Most studies support the hypothesis that tissues grow first by cellular multiplication and later by cellular size increase; a notable exception is the report by Sands and colleagues,[4] who observed that cell size increased during the early phase of tissue growth and that cellular multiplication continued throughout all the stages.

The phases of cellular hyperplasia, hyperplasia plus hypertrophy, and lastly hypertrophy alone, do not occur simultaneously in all organs; also, the length of time in each of these stages varies from one tissue to another (Fig. 26-2). Hence, growth in terms of cellular behavior is not the homogeneous process suggested by external body measurements.[2,5] Nevertheless, the adult state is achieved by virtue of smooth integration of these growth phenomena.

A comparison of brain growth with musculoskeletal growth illustrates the individualistic growth characteristics of different tissues. The greatest rates of DNA synthesis in the brain take place prior to birth. After birth, there is gradual reduction in mitotic rates; by 6 to 8 months of life the critical period of brain growth is completed and the infant possesses the total number of brain cells needed for the remainder of its life. In contrast, the critical phase of growth for the musculoskeletal system lasts for 15 to 20 years and extends from fetal life to early adulthood.

The long-range impact of disease on the growth process depends upon the timing, duration, and severity of the insult. In general, the prognosis for recovery is better if the injury occurs during the stage of hypertrophy rather than that of hyperplasia. The risk of irreparable damage to the growth process is especially high if prolonged injury occurs during both stages; e.g., microcephaly due to fetal alcohol syndrome or viral infections of the CNS.

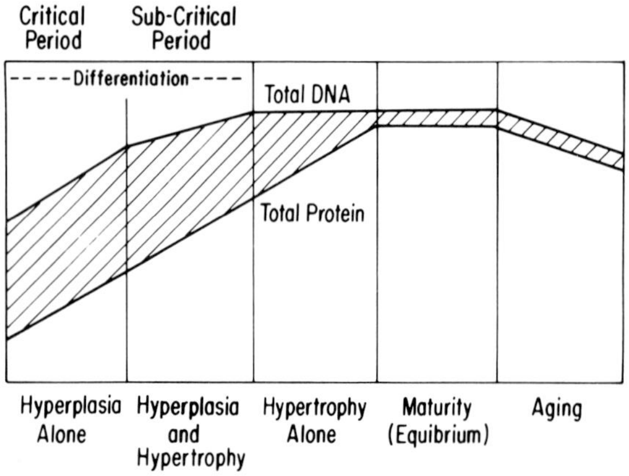

FIGURE 26-1 Representation of the various stages of organ growth and differentiation. During the phase of hyperplasia, growth is due entirely to cellular multiplication, which is represented by the steepness of the DNA slope. In the next phase, the rate of DNA synthesis is less rapid, but the rate of protein synthesis is unchanged; consequently, tissue growth is now the result of both cellular multiplication and enlargement. This is followed by a stage of growth due to hypertrophy alone as DNA synthesis plateaus but protein synthesis persists at its previous rate. At maturity, constancy of size is due to equilibrium between tissue gained and lost. During the aging process, tissue loss exceeds replacement. (*From Weiss and Kavanau*[1] *and Smith.*[93])

CONTROL OF GROWTH PROCESSES

Normal growth is controlled by a number of interacting forces which include genetic mechanisms, tissue-specific factors, hormone regulators, responsiveness of tissues, and nutritional influences.

Genetic Factors

Two aspects of growth are influenced by genetic mechanisms which are polygenic in nature: the first is regulation of the rate of cellular multiplication and, therefore, overall size, and the second is control of the pace of maturation. Studies indicate that birth size does not correlate with midparental height (mean height of parents) or with paternal size or subsequent adult stature but does correlate with maternal size (pre-pregnancy weight of mother). On this basis, it has been concluded that genetic factors may not play a dominant role in the growth of the fetus.[6,7] However, during the first 12 to 18 months of postnatal life, genetic influences become increasingly apparent. In this period the linear growth curves of two-thirds of infants shift; the direction of the change correlates best with the mean height of parents. Approximately one-half drift upward and the remainder downward in growth percentile. From the age of 2 years to adulthood, genetic mechanisms play a dominant role; thus, a close correlation exists between midparental height and the child's stature.[8,9] Genetic controls also regulate the pace of biologic maturation in children, which is best illustrated by familial patterns of delayed or early sexual maturation and age of attainment of adult stature.

Both the X and Y chromosomes contain growth-regulating genes. The special influence of the X chromosome is inferred from growth studies in females. As a rule, girls develop two years earlier than boys, and sisters are more similar in pattern of osseous maturation than are brothers.[10] Also, girls with total or partial loss of the X chromosome are short in stature. A recent study revealed a possible influence of Yq heterochromatin on attainment of body height; i.e., the length of the heterochromatic band Y(q12) was found to correlate with height.[11]

Genetic factors are also known to influence size by race. Although black infants at birth are smaller than white infants, their stature and pace of osseous maturation during the childhood years are equal to or even a little ahead of white children from families of comparable income.[12] Japanese children raised in the United States and Chinese children raised in the United Kingdom are taller than Japanese and Chinese children raised in Japan and Hong Kong, respectively. However, final heights of the Asian emigrés are somewhat less than adult Americans and Europeans.[13,14]

Tissue-Specific Factors

The precise mechanisms which control cellular multiplication, differentiation, and organ development dur-

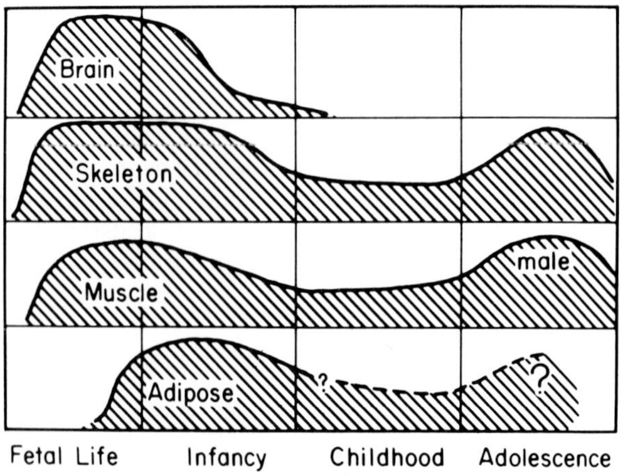

FIGURE 26-2 Critical periods of high mitotic rate with increasing cell number for various tissues. By 6 to 8 months of postnatal life, cellular multiplication in the brain is completed. In contrast, rapid rates of DNA synthesis persist for years in muscle, skeleton, and adipose tissues. (*From Smith and Bierman.*[5])

ing the embryonic period of fetal life remain a mystery. Studies of hepatic organogenesis indicate that mitotic rates are stimulated by tissue-specific growth factors and that organ size is limited by an antimitotic humoral substance. This putative antimitotic protein factor, which has a negative feedback effect on the tissue from which it originates, is called a *chalone*.[15] The function of this regulator is believed to be maintenance of appropriate proportions in organ size relative to the whole individual.

The concept that classic hormones directly regulate growth and maturation has been largely replaced by the hypothesis that growth is controlled by a variety of growth factors whose production is stimulated by the classic hormones. These growth factors can be considered "mediatory hormones" because they mediate some of the biologic actions of the classic hormones. Table 26-1 lists some of the presumed interrelationships between growth factors and hormones. The specific contributions of many of these growth factors to the overall growth process in children are still unproven.[16]

Hormonal Regulation

In healthy children, statural growth is controlled by the action of circulating hormones on the skeletal system.[17] Growth hormone (GH) and thyroid hormone (T_4) are the major determinants of growth rate during the childhood years. The growth spurt and skeletal maturation of adolescence are primarily dependent on gonadal steroids in conjunction with GH and T_4. Insulin and glucocorticoids influence carbohydrate, fat, and protein metabolism, provide sources of energy needed for growth, and exert a permissive influence on the anabolic actions of GH. Whether insulin acts only permissively or whether it also functions as a growth factor is still unsolved because of the inseparable link between insulin and nutrition. The growth

Table 26-1. Interrelationships between Growth Factors and Classic Hormones

Growth factor*	Sources	Properties	Hormone regulators
Somatomedin	Synthesized by liver, fetal lung, kidney, heart, limb, mesenchyme.	See text.	GH, placental lactogen, prolactin(?), insulin(?)
Epidermal growth factor	First isolated from male mouse submaxillary gland. Urogastrone in human urine may be equivalent of mouse EGF.	In mice, stimulates early eyelid opening and incisor eruption. Role in humans unclear.	Androgens, thyroxine.
Nerve growth factor	First isolated from male mouse submaxillary gland.	Regulates growth of sensory and sympathetic neurons; stimulates axon outgrowth; regulates levels of peptide neurotransmitters. May play a role in peripheral neurofibromatosis, familial dysautonomia, MEN 2b.	Thyroxine.
Fibroblast pneumonocyte factor	Secreted by human fetal lung fibroblasts. Present in human amniotic fluid.	Stimulates surfactant synthesis by type 2 pneumonocytes in vitro.	Glucocorticoids.
Erythropoietin		Mitogen for proerythrocytes.	GH, androgens.
Fibroblast growth factor	First isolated from bovine pituitary gland.	Mol wt 13,400. Mitogen for endodermal, mesodermal, amniotic fluid–derived cells.	?
Platelet-derived growth factor	Released by human platelets during blood coagulation in vivo.	May influence connective tissue response to injury and development of atherosclerotic lesions.	?
Thymic hormone		Controls development of mature thymocytes.	?

*See Refs. 16, 189.
Abbreviations: EGF, epidermal growth factor; MEN 2b, multiple endocrine neoplasia, type 2b.

excess of hyperinsulinemic obese children appears to result from increased insulin concentration coupled to increased nutrient intake. Conversely, poor growth in insulin-deficient (type 1) diabetic youngsters is associated with intracellular undernutrition. Skeletal growth and ossification are dependent on parathyroid hormone (PTH), the vitamin D metabolites, and, possibly, calcitonin.

GROWTH HORMONE

Growth hormone, secreted by the somatotrophs of the anterior pituitary gland, is a single-chain polypeptide (mol wt 22,000) containing 191 amino acid residues. Its configuration depends upon two intrachain disulfide bridges. Approximately 4 to 10 percent of the wet weight of the human pituitary gland is GH (5 to 15 mg per gland). Although GH shares structural homology with prolactin and chorionic mammosomatotropin (placental lactogen), it is the only member of this family of peptides which exhibits postnatal growth-promoting activity in humans.[18]

GH secretion is regulated primarily by two hypothalamic hormones: *somatostatin*, which inhibits, and *growth hormone releasing factor* (GRF), which stimulates GH secretion. Current hypotheses concerning the mechanisms which regulate GH secretion are illustrated in Fig. 26-3. Somatostatin, a tetradecapeptide isolated from ovine hypothalamic tissue in 1973, is present in high concentrations in the preoptic basal area of the hypothalamus, CNS, and GI tract, particularly the pancreas.[19,20] Somatostatin suppresses the GH response to insulin hypoglycemia, arginine infusion, levodopa ingestion, and deep sleep. Somatostatin also blocks thyrotropin releasing hormone (TRH)-induced thyroid stimulating hormone (TSH) release, but does not block the prolactin rise following TRH stimulation. The extrapituitary effects of somatostatin include suppression of glucagon and insulin secretion by the pancreas. GH secretion is also inhibited by *somatomedin* C (Sm C, also called insulin-like growth factor 1, IGF 1) and by GH itself; both appear to act directly on the pituitary gland as well as the hypothalamic regulatory centers (i.e., by stimulating somatostatin production and suppressing GRF release) (Fig. 26-3).

The main areas of the hypothalamus which secrete GRF are the arcuate nucleus and adjacent ventromedial nucleus (VMN).[21] Final proof of the

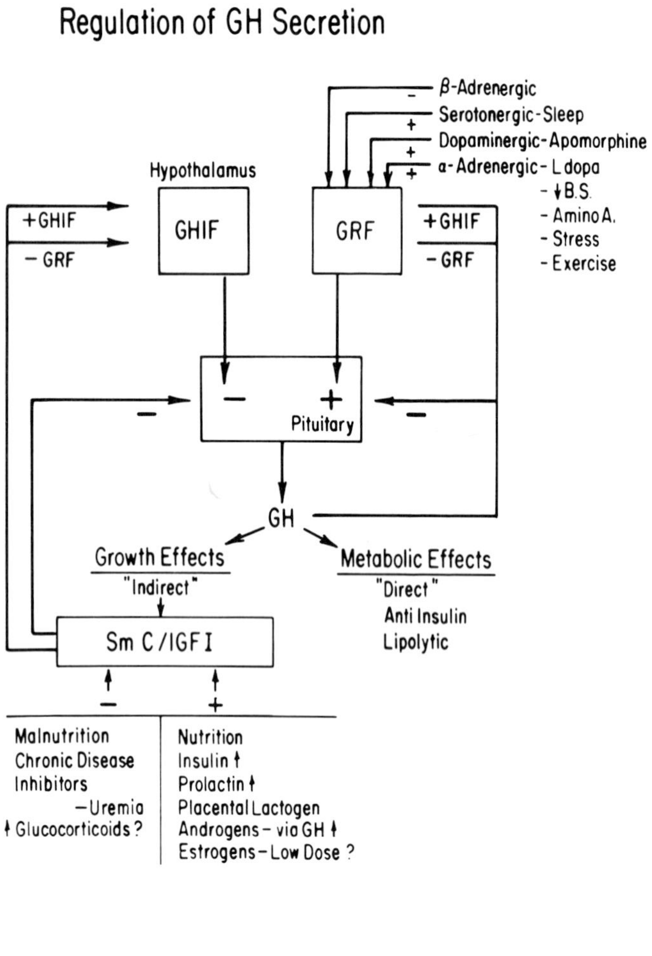

FIGURE 26-3 Regulation of GH secretion. Current hypothesis: GH secretion is regulated by hypothalamic hormones: somatostatin inhibits and growth hormone releasing hormone (GRH) stimulates GH secretion. GRH production is enhanced by α-adrenergic, dopaminergic and serotoninergic neurons and suppressed by β-adrenergic tracts. GH and Sm C/IGF 1 inhibit GRF secretion and enhance somatostatin production. These phenomena indirectly suppress GH secretion. GH production at the pituitary level is directly suppressed by the negative feedback effects of Sm C/IGF 1 and GH. GH acts directly on carbohydrate and lipid metabolism and indirectly on growth (via Sm C/IGF 1). Sm C/IGF 1 production is enhanced by nutrition, insulin, prolactin, placental lactogen, and androgens. Sm C/IGF 1 production is suppressed by malnutrition, chronic diseases, glucocorticoids (?), and high doses of estrogen. Inhibitors of Sm C/IGF 1 have been documented in uremia.

existence of GRF was provided when the hormone was isolated from the pancreatic tumors of two patients who had developed acromegaly as a result of tumor-derived GRF.[22,23] The structure of human hypothalamic GRF is identical to GRF isolated from the pancreatic tumors.[24,25] Isolation of GRF from the pancreatic tumors culminated many years of frustrating research. Its existence had been suggested by animal studies carried out over two decades ago, and later by clinical and laboratory documentation of acromegaly due to hypersecretion of biologically active GRF from pancreatic tumors.[26] The two human GRF peptides which have been recently purified and synthesized contain 40 and 44 amino acid residues; they have similar properties in vivo and in vitro. Synthetic GRF administration to normal subjects [1 to 10 μg per kilogram of body weight, intravenously (IV)] results in rapid and large increments in serum GH concentration; peak GH concentration occurs 30 to 60 minutes after IV bolus injection. Synthetic GRF also stimulates modest elevations of serum GH and Sm C/IGF 1 concentrations in many patients with idiopathic hypopituitarism.[27,28] Accelerated growth rates have been reported recently in GH-deficient children who received pulses of GRF by infusion pump.[29,29a]

Synthetic human GRF (hGRF) appears to be highly specific for the somatotroph: no change has been observed in serum concentrations of glucose, gonadotropins [follicle stimulating hormone (FSH) or luteinizing hormone (LH)], TSH, prolactin, or hydrocortisone.[23] The only side effect observed to date is slight facial flushing. A recent report suggests that rat GRF (rGRF) and, to a lesser degree, hGRF stimulate amylase secretion from exocrine pancreatic cells in vitro. This is the only extrapituitary effect of GRF noted to date.[30]

Release of the hypothalamic hormones GRF and somatostatin is in turn regulated by biogenic amines derived from neurosecretory neurons in the CNS.[31–33] In general, secretion of GRF is enhanced by alpha-adrenergic, dopaminergic, and serotoninergic neurons, and suppressed by beta-adrenergic tracts. The exact interplay between the biogenic amines and somatostatin production is not known. Alpha-adrenergic pathways (norepinephrine and alpha-adrenergic receptors) are primary regulators of GRF release. Drugs which mimic the action of norepinephrine (alpha-adrenergic agonists, e.g., clonidine) enhance GRF production; those which block the alpha receptors (e.g., phentolamine) inhibit GRF release. Dopaminergic receptor stimulation (e.g., by apomorphine) also enhances GRF release. However, oral administration of levodopa appears to enhance GRF release via alpha-adrenergic rather than dopaminergic pathways. Evidence for this was derived from studies which reported that phentolamine prevents levodopa-induced GH release. The normal somatotroph has no demonstrable dopamine receptor. However, GH-secreting pituitary adenomas paradoxically possess a dopamine receptor which inhibits GH secretion when stimulated. This accounts for the suppression of plasma GH levels in approximately 80 percent of acromegalic patients treated either with levodopa or the dopaminergic agent bromocriptine. The actual significance of the serotoninergic pathways in the control of GH is less well understood. Administration of 5-hydroxytryptophan, a serotonin precursor, enhances GH release, and cyproheptadine, a serotonin antagonist, decreases GH responses to exercise, hypoglycemia, and 5-hydroxytryptophan. Beta-adrenergic blocking agents (e.g., propranolol) augment GH responses to levodopa, glucagon, and antidiuretic hormone (ADH), and the beta-adrenergic agonist isoproterenol inhibits GH release.

Under physiologic conditions, the pituitary gland secretes approximately eight discrete peaks of GH each day, with very low basal levels between the episodic bursts.[33] In children and young adults approximately 50 to 75 percent of the daily production of GH occurs during the early nighttime hours that follow the onset of deep sleep; in contrast, prolactin and cortisol concentrations rise progressively during the later hours of sleep. GH secretion is stimulated by exercise, emotional stress, high-protein meals, rapid onset of hypoglycemia, and prolonged fasting; it is suppressed by elevated glucose levels in healthy nondiabetic subjects. Most investigators have reported that the pituitary gland secretes greater amounts of GH during the adolescent growth spurt than it does throughout childhood or adulthood.[34,35]

GH in circulation is unbound. It comprises a family of peptides which can be distinguished according to mass or charge. The major physiologic component of GH has a molecular weight of 22,000 (22-K form); the minor components are a 20-K isomer and a 45-K variant, formed from aggregation of 22-K molecules. Two genes (*N* and *V*), located on chromosome 17, are involved in GH biosynthesis.[36]

The precise mechanism of action of GH has yet to be fully clarified. In general terms, GH is an anabolic hormone which stimulates postnatal growth, antagonizes the action of insulin, and possesses lipolytic activity. Direct influences of GH on isolated extraskeletal tissues (e.g., heart muscle, diaphragm, adipocytes, hematopoietic cells, hepatocytes) and on perfused organs (e.g., liver) have been documented.[18] GH also plays an important role in carbohydrate, fat, protein, and mineral metabolism (Table 26-2).

Opinions differ about how GH regulates the

Table 26-2. Metabolic Effects of Growth Hormone

Increases DNA, RNA, protein synthesis; mitosis; sulfate incorporation.
Lowers urinary nitrogen concentration and BUN; raises urinary hydroxyproline concentration.
Fat: stimulates lipolysis, liberates free fatty acids.
Carbohydrate:
Early: insulin-like effect.
Late: insulin antagonism.
Prolonged GH excess causes carbohydrate intolerance and diabetes mellitus.
Mineral: decreases urinary phosphorus excretion, increases urinary calcium excretion.
Electrolyte: permits retention of K^+, Na^+, Cl^-, Mg^+.

growth of skeletal and extraskeletal tissues. One hypothesis proposes that GH acts directly on cartilage.[37] The alternative explanation, which has much wider acceptance, states that GH indirectly controls linear growth via its ability to regulate the production of serum growth factors which in turn stimulate bone growth (*somatomedin hypothesis*). The modern era of research pertaining to the mode of action of GH began in the 1950s with the discovery that GH stimulates the in vivo uptake of sulfate into cartilage and continued later with the historic evidence from in vitro experiments that a serum factor (*sulfation factor*) and not GH itself was responsible for this phenomenon.[38] The term sulfation factor proved to be too restrictive; it has been replaced by two terms, somatomedin (Sm) and "insulin-like growth factor," which are used synonymously to designate the family of GH-dependent serum growth factors. The term somatomedin was given by investigators whose research emphasis was in the area of growth. Its derivation implies "mediator of growth hormone." Similarly, the name insulin-like growth factor (formerly called non-suppressible insulin-like activity, NSILA) originated with investigators whose interest was in the field of insulin research. IGFs, by definition, are polypeptides with insulin-like structural and biologic properties which are not neutralized by the presence of excess anti-insulin antibodies.[39–41]

Two major types of Sm/IGF in human serum are Sm C/IGF 1 (basic Sm) and IGF 2 (neutral Sm). The evidence that somatomedin C and IGF 1 are identical peptides was derived from experiments which compared their behavior in radioligand assays and analyzed the similarities of their primary amino acid sequences.[42] Sm C/IGF 1 has greater post-natal growth-promoting potency than IGF 2, based on in vivo and in vitro experiments; it is the peptide whose potential role in health and disease has received the most attention. A possible third type of Sm/IGF is Sm A, a neutral peptide, which has structural and functional similarities to Sm C/IGF 1.[43–45]

The Sm/IGF family of growth factors possesses many unique characteristics which influence their biologic activity. Of particular importance is the finding that Sm C/IGF 1 and IGF 2 are small polypeptides (mol wt 7649 and 7471, respectively) which are noncovalently bound to specific carrier proteins.[44–46] Eighty percent of the total immunoreactive Sm C/IGF 1 and IGF 2 is recovered in a "gamma globulin–sized fraction" (mol wt 150,000 to 200,000) following neutral Sephadex G-200 gel filtration of serum; the remainder is contained in a second protein fraction (mol wt 50,000), which elutes after the albumin peak (albumin-sized IGF peak).

Although a vast amount of data exists on the biologic properties of the free form of the Sm/IGF peptides, information concerning the properties of the complexed or *native* peptides is scant. This problem exists because serum is the only source of the Sm/IGF peptides; during the extraction and purification procedures serum must be treated with either acid-ethanol or acidic gel filtration; this removes the carrier proteins and yields only the free Sm/IGF peptides, which are used exclusively in basic and clinical investigations. The complexed forms of Sm/IGF differ in many ways from the free peptides: the carrier protein abolishes the insulin-like actions of the free hormones, inhibits their permeation through capillaries and access to target tissues, and prevents their interaction with membrane receptors. If it is true that the Sm C/IGF 1 complexes are metabolically inactive, then how can they act as growth factors? Several explanations have been proposed: (1) Albumin-sized complexes have been shown to cross the capillary barrier and reach the IGF receptors of target tissues, which extract free IGF by equilibrium exchange. The albumin-sized carrier may then return to the vascular space to be reloaded with IGF obtained from the gamma globulin–sized IGF complexes. (2) Specific IGF receptors on vascular endothelial cells may facilitate the transport of free Sm/IGF to target tissues (receptor-mediated transport of IGF). (3) Small amounts of free Sm/IGF which cannot be detected by present assay techniques may exist in serum, freely cross capillary barriers, and reach the IGF receptors of target tissues. Although the validity of the somatomedin hypothesis has not been proved, recent studies provide strong support for this concept. Hypophysectomized rats infused with purified Sm C/IGF 1 exhibited increased width of tibial epiphyses and enhanced thymidine uptake by costal cartilages; infusions with purified IGF 2 had less pronounced effects.[44] These findings do not negate the possibility that GH also exerts a direct effect on the growth plate.

In addition to the effects on skeletal tissues, free Sm C/IGF 1 and IGF 2 possess insulin-like properties (enhanced glucose transport and short-term antilipolytic activities) when administered to experimental animals. However, the native IGF complexes, whose concentrations are 2000 to 3000 times greater than that of pancreatic insulin, have no such effect. Hence, most complexed IGF is inactive because (1) the carrier protein interferes with the biologic activity of bound IGF and (2) the IGF receptor is 8000 daltons smaller than the insulin receptor, which makes each a functionally and physically distinct receptor molecule.[44,47]

Recent studies indicate that GH regulates the production of the gamma globulin–sized carrier protein but does not appear to control the albumin-sized moiety.[44] When Sm/IGF was infused into hypophysectomized rats, it appeared only in the albumin-sized complex. Treatment of hypophysectomized rats with GH infusions resulted in the reappearance of the gamma globulin–sized complex.

The major site of production of Sm C/IGF 1 appears to be the liver; however, many tissues (e.g., fibroblasts) are also capable of synthesizing Sm C/IGF 1. This observation has formed the basis for the theory that the Sm/IGF family of peptides may exert their influence on cellular growth not only by classical endocrine means but also by autocrine and paracrine mechanisms.[16,48]

Measurements of Sm/IGF concentrations are most commonly performed by radioimmunoassay (RIA) of unextracted or extracted serum. Bioassay and receptor techniques are more difficult and less practical for clinical purposes.[49,50]

Numerous factors influence the concentration of Sm C/IGF 1 in serum.[45] Immunoreactive Sm C/IGF 1 serum concentrations are low in the fetus and remain low during the first few years of life. Thereafter, the levels rise progressively, reaching peak values during the second stage of puberty and gradually declining in adulthood (Fig. 26-4).

During childhood and adolescence, girls tend to have levels of Sm C/IGF 1 which are 10 to 20 percent higher than boys; a similar relationship exists for adult females and males (Fig. 26-4). Unlike plasma GH, which is secreted periodically, the Sm C/IGF 1 levels are stable throughout the day except for a modest 30 percent fall which occurs during deep sleep. The nocturnal Sm C/IGF 1 concentration and GH secretion are inversely related; Sm C level falls during the sleep-associated bursts of GH secretion. The GH status of the subject has a significant effect on Sm C/IGF 1 concentration. Hypopituitary children have low circulating levels of Sm C/IGF 1; however, some of these

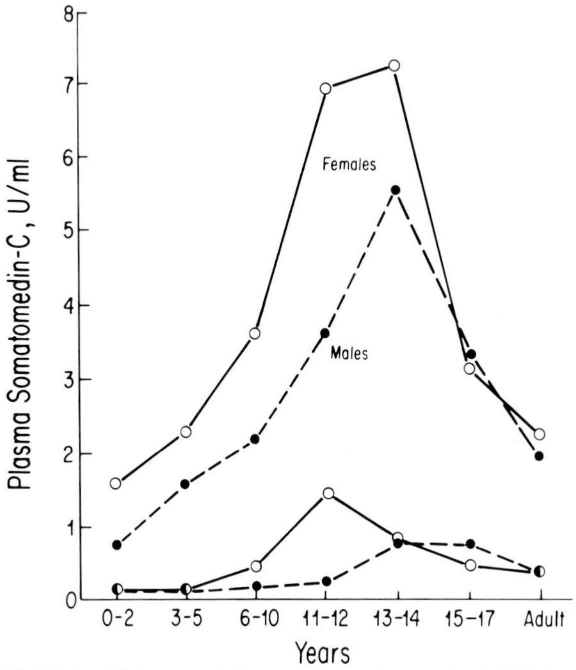

FIGURE 26-4 Range of plasma concentrations of Sm C/IGF 1 in boys and girls based on chronologic age. Levels are low in both sexes during the first years of life and gradually rise to reach peak values during midpuberty. Girls have levels which are 10 to 20 percent higher than boys throughout childhood and adolescence and their peak Sm C/IGF 1 concentration is reached at an earlier chronologic age. Adult men and women have lower Sm C/IGF 1 levels than pubertal boys and girls; with aging, the Sm C/IGF 1 concentration further declines. (*Data derived from Nichols Laboratory and Underwood, D'Ercole and Van Wyk.*[49])

children have values that overlap with the normal range. Sm C/IGF 1 levels are far more GH-dependent than those of IGF 2; thus GH status is more accurately assessed if specific RIA measurements of Sm C/IGF 1 are used instead of radioreceptor assays or bioassays. It was expected that changes in Sm C/IGF 1 after GH administration would predict which GH-deficient children would benefit from prolonged GH treatment. This expectation has not become a reality: some children with persistently low Sm C/IGF 1 concentrations have responded to GH treatment; many have not shown a correlation between the degree of rise of Sm C/IGF 1 and the growth response to prolonged GH treatment. In still others with idiopathic growth failure and normal basal Sm C/IGF 1 concentration, growth has accelerated following GH administration.[51,52] In untreated acromegaly, Sm C/IGF 1 values are elevated, reaching levels 10 times that of the normal population; IGF 2 concentrations are not increased by GH excess. The RIA for Sm C/IGF 1 gives more definitive diagnostic information in patients with acromegaly than in patients with hypopituitarism because the factors which can depress Sm C/IGF 1 are numerous whereas GH excess is the main cause of Sm C/IGF 1 elevations.

Nutritional state has a profound effect on Sm C/IGF 1 level. Protein-calorie malnutrition or prolonged fasting causes a pronounced fall in Sm C/IGF 1 concentrations. Restoration of a normal value with refeeding requires that the diet have adequate protein content as well as caloric value. In states of malnutrition, plasma GH levels are elevated while Sm C/IGF 1 values are low and fail to rise following GH administration. Thus, fasting and protein-calorie malnutrition impair the ability of GH to stimulate Sm C/IGF 1 production.[53,54]

Hypothyroidism results in reduced levels of Sm C/IGF 1 and also impairs GH responsiveness to provocative stimuli. Treatment with thyroxine or GH results in a rise in Sm C/IGF 1 value.[55]

Pharmacologic doses of estrogens suppress Sm C/IGF 1 concentration as measured by RIA or bioassay.[56] When very small doses (100 ng per kilogram of body weight) are administered, accelerated linear growth is observed in patients with Turner's syndrome, even though Sm C/IGF 1 level does not rise. When standard doses of estrogen are given to these patients, Sm C/IGF 1 levels increase but bone growth is suppressed.[57] More studies are required to clarify the relationships between estrogens, Sm C/IGF 1, and bone growth.

Androgen therapy raises Sm C/IGF 1 level in children with intact pituitary glands but not in hypopituitary children. The data suggest that androgens work indirectly by enhancing GH secretion, which increases the level of Sm C/IGF 1; androgens do not appear to increase Sm C/IGF 1 levels directly.[58]

Cortisol excess has been reported to suppress bioassayable somatomedin. However, Sm C/IGF 1 levels measured by RIA are normal or elevated in patients receiving cortisol therapy. This observation suggests that hypercortisolemia interferes with the action of Sm on peripheral tissue but does not suppress its production. Further studies are required to resolve the contradictory results obtained by bioassay versus RIA.[59,60] Somatomedin inhibitors have been documented in patients with chronic renal failure and diabetes mellitus.[61]

In contrast to the considerable gains made in understanding how GH regulates postnatal growth, understanding of its influence on fetal growth is poor.[16,62] It is generally believed that neither GH nor T_4 has a significant effect on fetal somatic growth because infants with congenital hypopituitarism or hypothyroidism are of normal or near-normal size at birth.[63] However, it is important to recognize that the glands in a majority of these infants function poorly but are not absent; precise information is lacking on the contribution of both GH and T_4 to growth of the fetus. Also, the influences of androgens, estrogens, and cortisol have not been precisely evaluated. Insulin has been hypothesized to be a fetal growth factor because intrauterine hyperinsulinemia leads to fetal gigantism and obesity; conversely, insulin deficiency or insulin resistance during fetal life results in growth retardation.[64] Although insulin is secreted by the fetal pancreas at approximately 12 weeks of gestation and fetal tissues exhibit increased incorporation of amino acids and protein synthesis when exposed to insulin, it is still not known (1) whether insulin is actually a growth factor, (2) whether it acts permissively to maintain a favorable homeostatic environment, or (3) whether it augments fetal growth through stimulation of somatomedin production. Normal somatomedin levels have recently been documented in hyperinsulinemic infants of diabetic mothers;[65] this suggests that fetal somatomedin production may not be controlled by insulin.

It is almost impossible to evaluate the effect on fetal growth of each of the placental hormones, many of which have structural homology with pituitary and hypothalamic hormones. Of the many hormones synthesized by the placenta [placental lactogen, chorionic gonadotropin (hCG), prolactin, luteinizing hormone releasing hormone (LHRH), nerve growth factor (NGF), steroids], the one which has been reported to be anabolic for the fetus and neonate is placental lactogen. Also, there is active investigation into the possibility that placental lactogen or prolactin may have an indirect effect on fetal growth via regulation of fetal somatomedin production.[66-68]

Conflicting opinions exist concerning the role of the somatomedins during fetal life. The main evidence against somatomedin having an influence on fetal growth is the presence of low levels of somatomedin in fetal and cord serum (measured by both bioassay and RIA) compared to adult and maternal serum. Despite these suppressed somatomedin concentrations, positive correlations exist in human newborns between Sm C/IGF 1 concentration and birth length, birth weight, and placental weight.[69] Also, it is theoretically possible that circulating levels of somatomedin do not reflect tissue concentrations because somatomedin may be produced locally and act in an autocrine and paracrine manner. Furthermore, fetal tissues may be unusually sensitive to low circulating concentrations of somatomedin. Fetal somatomedin production appears to be under the control of hormones from the placenta rather than the fetal pituitary; somatomedin level does not fall after hypophysectomy of fetal rabbits, whereas concentrations of biologically active somatomedin decline in pregnant rats after delivery of the fetoplacental unit.[70]

THYROID HORMONE

Thyroid hormone by itself does not fulfill the criteria needed to classify it as a true growth-promoting hormone because it is unable to directly stimulate cellular multiplication if GH is absent. Nevertheless, the importance of the synergism between these hormones has been demonstrated in studies which show that maximal GH stimulation of tissues requires the presence of T_4. Furthermore, primary hypothyroidism causes a reduction in both the number of somatotrophs and the GH content of the anterior pituitary; it also leads to GH unresponsiveness to stimulation by insulin hypoglycemia or L-arginine.[71,72] The growth spurt which follows thyroid replacement therapy is accompanied by a return of normal pituitary gland GH content and response to stimuli.

It has been suggested that, during fetal life, somatic growth is not dependent on T_4, because infants with congenital hypothyroidism due to thyroid dysfunction or pituitary-hypothalamic disorders are of normal body size at birth. This conclusion requires reexamination, since a majority of congenitally hypothyroid infants have lingual or hypoplastic glands and those with anencephaly or other types of hypopituitarism have variable degrees of thyroid function.[73] Evidence that thyroid hormone may influence fetal somatic growth is derived from experiments, which documented that growth in three animal species (rat, sheep, and monkey) is impaired after fetal thyroidectomy.[74-76]

In contrast to the uncertainties pertaining to the role of T_4 in fetal somatic growth, it is evident that T_4 is essential for normal brain development, specifically, neuronal and neuroglial cell growth in the cerebrum and cerebellum, nerve terminal maturation, axonal and dendritic proliferation, and normal myelinization. Recent studies suggest that T_4 increases the production of nerve growth factor, which stimulates axon outgrowth and increased neuron cell size and plays a crucial role in the development and survival of sympathetic and sensory neurons. If these data are confirmed, thyroid hormone may have an indirect rather than a direct influence on brain development.[77]

Acquired hypothyroidism in childhood usually delays puberty, but, rarely, a child exhibits precocious sexual development, ovarian cysts, galactorrhea, diabetes insipidus, and a large sella without bony erosion; all abnormalities regress with thyroid replacement.

GONADAL STEROIDS: ANDROGENS, ESTROGENS, AND THE PUBERTAL GROWTH SPURT

The growth spurt of puberty is dependent mainly on gonadal steroids, GH, and T_4; adrenal steroids are probably not essential. Recent studies indicate that males experience rapid growth during puberty because of androgen-mediated enhancement of GH secretion; this, in turn, stimulates increased production of Sm C/IGF 1 and accounts for the elevated levels observed in adolescence.[58] Growth rates in males with isolated GH deficiency do not accelerate sufficiently during puberty, yet osseous maturation progresses and epiphyseal fusion occurs. Consequently, their adult height is compromised. Treatment of these individuals with GH during puberty is essential. Normal thyroid function is a fundamental requirement of the pubertal growth process. Hypothyroid children usually have delayed adolescence; those who experience puberty do not exhibit a growth spurt.

The precise mechanisms which control the onset of puberty have not been fully defined. In human and nonhuman primates, the pituitary gland releases increased quantities of FSH and LH at three times of life: during fetal life, during the first 6 months of infancy, and during adolescence and adulthood. Suppression of gonadotropin production during the decade of "childhood," between infancy and adolescence, has been attributed to two mechanisms: (1) intrinsic CNS inhibitory influences operating independently of sex steroids, which accounts for the diphasic pattern of gonadotropin secretion seen during childhood in patients with gonadal dysgenesis; and (2) increased sensitivity of the hypothalamic-pituitary regulatory centers (the "gonadostat") to the negative feedback effects of low childhood levels of gonadal steroids.[78] Coincident with the onset of puberty, the arcuate nucleus of the hypothalamus becomes progressively less sensitive to the inhibitory effects of the sex steroids and the intrinsic CNS inhibitory influences gradually are suppressed. Removal of these restraints on gonadotropin releasing hormone (GnRH) secretion allows the pulsatile production of GnRH in increasing amounts, which in turn stimulates augmented secretion of pituitary gonadotropins.[78-83] A model of the mechanisms which control gonadal sex steroid production is shown in Fig. 26-5.

Two separate processes, *gonadarche* and *adrenarche,* account for the increased production of sex steroids in the peripubertal and pubertal periods. Gonadarche, the final activation and maturation of the hypothalamic-pituitary-gonadal axis, is the sine qua non of puberty. It is responsible for the adolescent growth spurt, development of secondary sexual char-

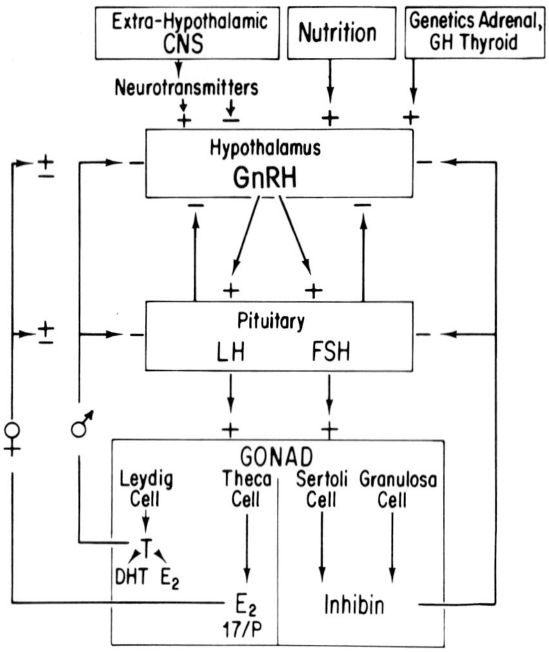

FIGURE 26-5 Schematic representation of the CNS-hypothalamic-pituitary-gonadal axis in males and females. Stimulatory effects are represented by +; inhibition is shown by −. Gonadotropin releasing hormone GnRH from the hypothalamus stimulates pituitary secretion of luteinizing hormone (LH) and follicle stimulating hormone (FSH), which have a negative feedback effect on GnRH via a short-loop mechanism. In males, LH stimulates the Leydig cell to produce testosterone (T), subsequently converted to dihydrotestosterone (DHT) and estradiol (E_2), which inhibit hypothalamic and pituitary production of LH. In females, LH stimulates E_2 and progesterone (P), which have both stimulatory and inhibitory effects on hypothalamic and pituitary control of gonadotropin production. In both sexes, inhibin, produced by the Sertoli cell in males and the granulosa cell in females, is the hormone which is presumed to inhibit FSH secretion. (*Adapted from Odell and Swerdloff.*[96])

acteristics, and eventual attainment of fertility. Adrenarche signifies increased androgen production from the zona reticularis of the adrenal gland; it occurs about 2 years prior to gonadarche. Serum concentration of dehydroepiandrosterone (DHEA) usually begins to increase by 8 years of age in boys and girls; this serves as a biochemical marker of adrenal androgenesis. The temporal relationship between adrenarche and gonadarche had suggested that adrenal androgen might have a regulatory influence on the timing of puberty; it is now evident that adrenarche is not essential for the onset of gonadarche and that the two events are independent processes. The mechanisms responsible for adrenarche have not been fully defined; hypotheses include (1) an intrinsic alteration in the activity of the enzymes involved in adrenal androgen synthesis ("*escalator*" *theory*), (2) a pituitary androgen stimulating hormone (ASH) may be produced, although ASH has yet to be isolated (*zonal theory*), and (3) an extrapituitary stimulating factor such as estrogen.[78,84] The role of adrenal androgens in puberty is not clearly understood, other than stimulation of sexual hair growth in females.

During puberty the Leydig cells of the testes secrete increasing amounts of testosterone, which circulates either bound to protein (i.e., sex hormone-binding globulin, SHBG) or in biologically active free form. Testosterone stimulation of DNA, RNA, and protein synthesis and cell mitosis requires entrance of free hormone into the cytoplasm of androgen-sensitive cells, where it is metabolized to either 5α- or 5β-dihydrotestosterone (DHT) by 5α- or 5β-reductase. Both testosterone and DHT form complexes with the cytoplasmic receptor which enter the nucleus; there they interact with nuclear acceptor sites and stimulate cellular multiplication. The relative importance of testosterone as compared to DHT in stimulation of statural growth during puberty is not fully understood. In adult males and females, DHT is not present in skeletal muscle; it thus appears that testosterone may directly promote muscular growth during sexual maturation.[85–87]

During early fetal life in males, conversion of testosterone to DHT via the action of 5α-reductase in the external genital tissues is essential for complete sexual differentiation of male external genitalia. The wolffian duct system develops normally in XY individuals who lack 5α-reductase. Therefore, it can be concluded that the internal genital duct system is testosterone- rather than DHT-dependent. During adolescence, XY subjects with 5α-reductase deficiency develop muscular, virile physiques even though they were phenotypic females during their prepubertal years.[87] These observations support the hypothesis that testosterone directly contributes to musculoskeletal growth in adolescence.

The characteristic actions of androgens on the skeletal system involve augmentation of bone length and acceleration of bone maturation. Because of the latter, the width of the growth plate is gradually reduced throughout the period of rapid statural growth until epiphyseal fusion occurs and adult height is attained.

There is suggestive evidence that androgens increase GH responses to hypoglycemic stimulation, enhance responsiveness to GnRH stimulation, and promote the onset of puberty.[88,89]

In the female, the onset of the adolescent growth spurt coincides with breast development and ovarian production of estrogens. The magnitude of the growth spurt is less than in the male. Estrogens increase the width of the pelvic bones and hips, which are characteristic features of sexually mature women. Increased adiposity and body weight in pubertal girls are estrogen-mediated. Estrogens have less growth-promoting capacity than androgens, yet are capable of accelerating the pace of osseous maturation. As described previously, estrogens appear to have a biphasic effect on statural growth.[56,57]

Nutrition

The rate of growth and sexual maturation in children is influenced by their nutritional state.[90] Frisch and McArthur have proposed that the onset of menses in healthy girls occurs at a critical weight which approximates the 10th percentile.[91] Improved nutrition and freedom from chronic infections are factors which have contributed to the taller stature and earlier puberty of European and American children. In countries where malnutrition is prevalent, poor linear growth and delayed adolescence are common. In this country, anorexia nervosa and chronic inflammatory bowel disease are examples in which malnutrition interferes with normal growth because of both inadequate availability of substrates for cell replication and suppression of gonadotropin and somatomedin production. Recommended nutrient intakes based on age are given in Table 26-3.

Table 26-3. Daily requirement of nutrients

	Energy, kcal	Protein, g
Infants:		
<6 months	117 × kg	2.2
6–12 months	108 × kg	2.0
Children:		
1–3 years	1360	16
4–6 years	1830	20
7–9 years	2190	25
Male adolescents:		
10–12 years	2600	30
13–15 years	2900	37
16–19 years	3070	38
Female adolescents:		
10–12 years	2350	29
13–15 years	2490	31
16–19 years	2310	30

Source: *WHO Monograph Series*, no. 61, 1974.

PHYSIOLOGY OF SKELETAL GROWTH

Skeletal growth, which is the determinant of stature, is achieved by means of two types of ossification. First, transformation of cartilage into bone, defined as *endochondral ossification,* is responsible for the growth of the long bones, cuboid bones, base of the skull, vertebral bodies, and parts of the pelvis. Second, bone formation directly from fibrous membrane, or *membranous ossification,* occurs in the calvaria, clavicles, body of the mandible, vertebral spinous processes, and parts of the pelvis.

Elongation of long bones is responsible for statural growth. In the growth plate, chondrocytes produce the cartilaginous matrix consisting of type 2 collagen, mucopolysaccharides, and core proteins. The matrix undergoes an initial period of calcification followed by a stage of breakdown and chondrocyte degeneration. Finally, there is a phase of inward osteoblast migration via vascular channels from the metaphyses; bone is deposited on the remaining calcified cartilage, which is gradually resorbed and replaced by true bone. Disturbances in chondrocyte proliferation, matrix formation, calcification, or ossification cause short stature.

Endochondrial ossification is hormonally controlled. An excess of glucocorticoids disturbs the protein matrix and causes osteoporosis. Vitamin D deficiency or PTH excess leads to abnormalities in mineralization and osteomalacia.

Bone width is determined by the thickness of the diaphyseal cortex, which is formed by membranous ossification directly from the periosteum.

The fetus develops primary centers of ossification in the cartilaginous anlage of long bones at 7 weeks. By the third fetal month, the process of ossification extends to the metaphyses, and the growth plate begins to contain chondrocytes. In early fetal life, the epiphyseal ends of long bones exist mainly as cartilage; later in gestation, secondary centers of ossification convert the cartilaginous epiphyses to bone. Bone age or biologic age is defined by the size and appearance of these secondary centers of epiphyseal ossification.

DEVELOPMENTAL STAGES

Intrauterine Life

The initial growth period of the fetus is one of rapid cellular generation, differentiation, and organogenesis. During this embryonic period the fetus grows primarily by a process of cellular multiplication. Extraordinary linear growth rates are observed during fetal life. Peak velocities of 10 to 11 cm/month occur at 4 to 5 months of gestation; growth rate gradually declines during the last trimester as uterine constraints become a limiting force. However, even this growth rate is spectacular: 2 cm/month (Fig. 26-6). In the last tri-

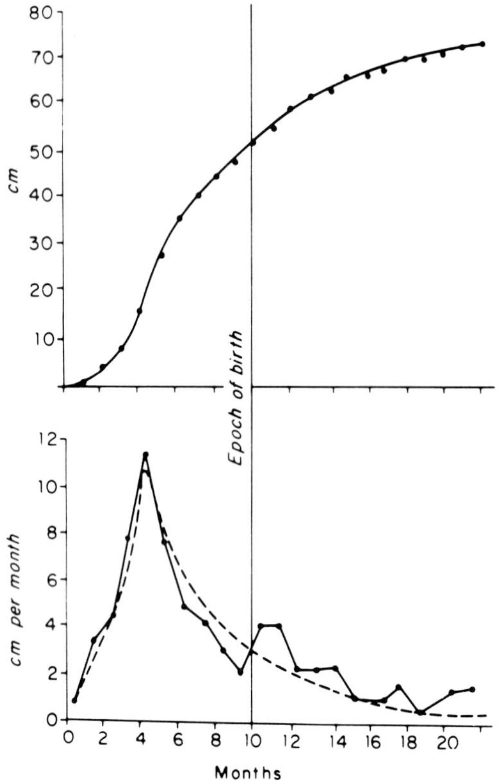

FIGURE 26-6 Linear growth by lunar months during fetal life and in the first postnatal year. The slowing of late fetal growth rate is compatible with the concept of constraints to growth by the uterus and is followed postnatally by a brief period of accelerated "catch-up" growth. (*From Smith.*[93])

mester, adipose tissue is formed at an increasing rate; fetal weight doubles during the last 2 months of pregnancy.

The size of the full-term newborn is mainly dependent on the size of the mother, not the father. In controlled animal studies, the offspring of large mothers and small fathers are larger than the products of matings between small mothers and large fathers.[92] This observation indicates that lifelong adequate nutrition is essential for girls in order to enhance their own adult height and the size of their offspring.

An additional factor which influences fetal growth is uterine size in the late gestational period. In women with twins or triplets, uterine constraints may limit fetal size.

The placenta is yet another determinant of fetal growth and well-being since it is the portal for delivery of nutrients and removal of metabolic wastes. The placenta is a fetal organ which grows by cellular multiplication until the 35th week of gestation; thereafter, it enlarges by cellular hypertrophy until full size is achieved at the 38th to 40th week. Any disturbance of early placental growth due to embryologic abnormalities, infections, or vascular insults may cause permanent growth retardation.[2]

Gender plays a minor role in determining fetal growth rate. Males grow faster after 32 weeks of gestation and at birth are more muscular and have less adipose tissue than females. Newborn boys have a slightly larger head circumference and are, on average, 0.9 cm longer and 150 g heavier than girls.[93] However, osseous maturation is more rapid in girls than in boys after 30 weeks of gestation. At birth, bone age in females is 2 weeks ahead of that in males; by 1 year, this difference has increased to 8 weeks.

Infancy: Birth to 2 Years of Age

In the first year of life, linear growth and weight gain continue at a rate which is still remarkable although less spectacular than during fetal life. The fastest gains in length occur in the first months after birth, when uterine constraints are no longer present. By 1 year, the infant has accumulated generous stores of adipose tissue, has tripled its birth weight, and has grown 25 additional cm (an increase of 50 percent of birth length). Male infants continue to grow slightly faster in length, weight, and head circumference during the first 3 to 6 months after birth. These phenomena have been attributed to increased testosterone production in males, which gradually diminishes by 6 months of postnatal age.[94] In the second year, there is continued deceleration of linear growth rates; by the age of 2 years, linear growth has stabilized at a rate which is characteristic of the childhood years (Fig. 26-7).

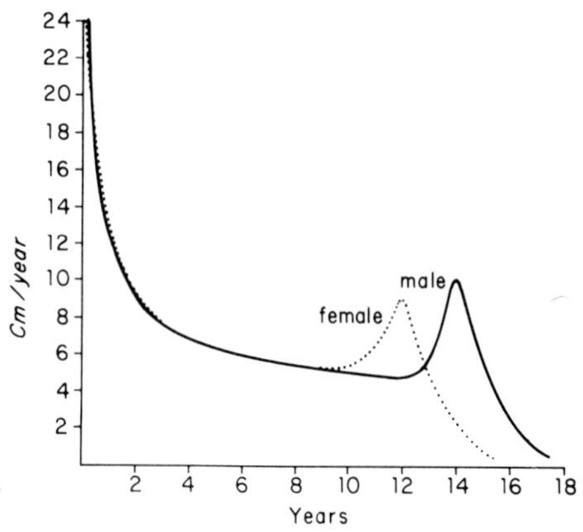

FIGURE 26-7 Velocity curves for length (<2 years) and height (2 to 28 years) for females and males show deceleration of growth rate from infancy until the onset of adolescence. (*From Smith*[93] *and Tanner et al.*[99,187])

Childhood

The period of childhood, which extends from the age of 2 years to the onset of puberty, is characterized by relatively stable rates of gain in height (5 to 7.5 cm/year) and weight (2 to 2.5 kg/year). Throughout these years, there is a slight deceleration in linear growth rate (Fig. 26-7) and acceleration in weight gain (Fig. 26-8). The major period of brain growth has already been completed, and cellular multiplication in the musculoskeletal and adipose systems continues at a lesser pace than is evident during infancy or adolescence. In the years prior to puberty, there is an increased gain in adipose tissue. During this period, lymphoid tissue reaches its maximum size relative to body size.

Adolescence

Adolescence is the last period of major growth; in it, there is attainment of adult stature, sexual maturation, and reproductive function.

Among healthy children, chronologic age at the onset of puberty and rate of sexual maturation are highly variable. These differences are largely dependent on genetic factors. The individual's sex also plays a role; the average girl enters and completes pubertal development 1 to 2 years ahead of the average boy. The most accurate criterion for assessment of adolescence is not chronologic age but the individual's biologic age (bone age) and his or her physical stage of sexual maturation, based on Tanner's criteria.[95]

The sequence of physiologic and hormonal events during adolescence in girls is shown in Fig. 26-9. The first signs of puberty in females are the appearance of breast buds and the beginning of the adolescent

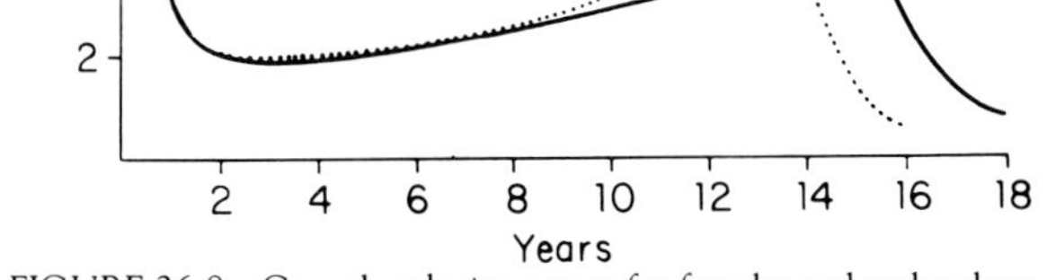

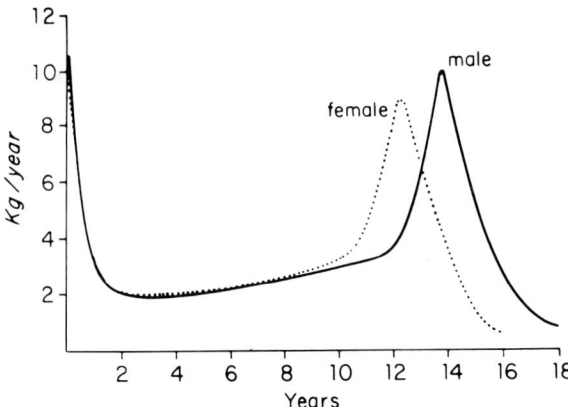

FIGURE 26-8 Growth velocity curves for females and males show gradual increases in rates of weight gain from 2 years until adolescence. (*From Smith*[93] *and Tanner et al.*[99,187])

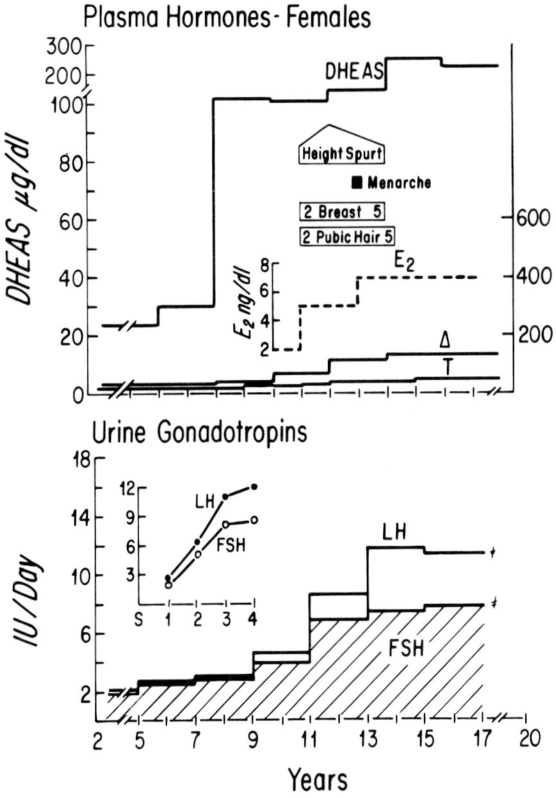

	FSH excretion, IU/day	LH excretion, IU/day
S1 (completely prepubertal, t1)	1–5	1–5
S2 (only breast tissue, t2 to t3)	4–9	4–9
S3 (breasts and sexual hair, t3 to t4)	5–11	6–16
S4 adult breasts and hair, t4 to t5)	5–12	7–28
Midcycle peak	39–49	108–122

Not shown in the diagram is the sleep-associated increase in LH secretion during early and midpuberty. (*Tanner criteria from Tanner;*[95] *hormonal events of puberty from Grumbach et al,*[81] *Kelch et al,*[86] *Penny et al.*[189])

FIGURE 26-9 Relationship between the stages of pubertal development in girls based on Tanner (t) criteria and the hormonal events of puberty. Increased plasma levels of DHEA sulfate from the adrenal gland (adrenarche) are detected before increased secretion of gonadotropins or gonadal steroids (gonadarche). E_2 = estradiol, Δ = androstenedione, T = testosterone. Based on chronologic age, urinary gonadotropin levels appear to increase prior to average age of breast development. However, when urinary gonadotropin excretion is based on stage of sexual maturation (S), a positive correlation exists with stages 2 and 3.

growth spurt; for the average girl, these events occur at 11 years of age. They are followed by the appearance of pubic hair, at 11.5 years, peak growth rates (approximately 9 cm/year) at 12 years, appearance of axillary hair at 12.5 to 13 years, and menarche at 12.5 years. Almost invariably, menarche occurs after the attainment of peak growth velocity. Slower rates of linear growth continue after menarche until 16 to 17 years, when epiphyseal fusion occurs; this information has relevance to the management of girls who are concerned about genetic tall stature. Adolescence in females is also associated with widening hips due to fat deposition and a general increase in body adipose tissue. The normal ranges in chronologic age for each pubertal event in girls are listed in Table 26-4.

In boys, the first signs of adolescence are axillary sweat, body odor, testicular enlargement, and thinning of the scrotal skin. The average boy gains 20 cm and 20 kg during adolescence.[95] The mechanisms of gonadotropin action on testicular growth and function have not been fully clarified. FSH is primarily responsible for growth of the seminiferous tubules and, thereby, increments in testes size in addition to sperm development. LH is the regulator of androgen, primarily testosterone, production by the Leydig cells. Evidence suggests that optimal sexual maturation depends upon interaction of FSH and LH in the testes.[96]

The sequence of physiologic events and their relationship to the hormonal changes in adolescent boys are depicted in Fig. 26-10. Unlike girls, who simultaneously exhibit increased growth velocity and breast buds at the outset of puberty, boys begin their growth spurt approximately 1 year after the first signs of testicular enlargement and achieve greater peak rates of linear growth (mean 10.3 cm/year) at age 14, as compared to age 12 in girls. The male adolescent growth spurt is largely due to the increased secretion of testosterone, which enhances production of GH; deficiencies of either of these hormones or lack of T_4

Table 26-4. Range of Chronological Ages for Pubertal Events in Healthy Girls

Event	Age, years: Onset	Age, years: Completion
Height spurt	9½–14½	12–17½
Breast bud*	8–13	10½–16
Pubic hair	8–14	11–17½
Menarche	10–16†	

*Asymmetry when breast = Tanner 5; will not resolve spontaneously.
†9 to 16 years in other series.
Source: Based on Tanner.[95]

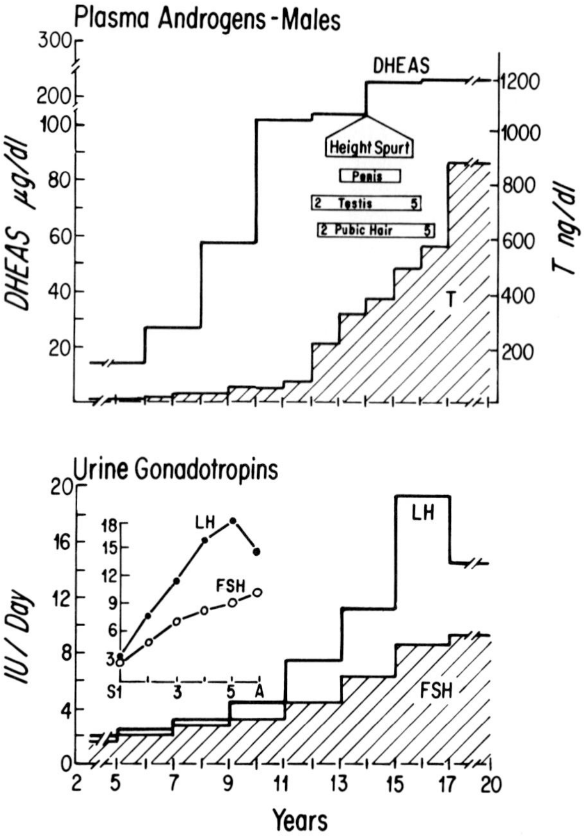

	FSH excretion, IU/day	LH excretion, IU/day
S1 (prepubertal)	0.5–5	0.5–6
S2 (testes ≥ 2 cm, scrotal changes)	2–9	2–13
S3 (penis > 7 cm)	3–12	5–23
S4 (further penis and testes growth)	3–14	9–29
S5 (prostate palpable, sexual hair)	5–16	9–39
SA [adult testes (> 4 cm) and penis (> 13 cm stretched)	5–16	8–24

Sleep-associated increases in LH secretion have been documented in early and midpuberty. After adolescence, daytime and nighttime excretion of LH are equal. (*From Grumbach et al,*[81] *Tanner,*[95] *Reiter et al,*[188] *Penny et al.*[190])

FIGURE 26-10 Relationship between the stages of pubertal development in boys and the hormonal events during adolescence. As noted in girls, DHEA sulfate levels are increased prior to any evidence of sexual maturation. Based on chronologic age, increased gonadotropin excretion appears to precede the onset of testicular enlargement. However, when gonadotropin excretion is related to stages of sexual maturation (S), there is a positive correlation between increased gonadotropin output and stages 2, 3, and 4. Positive correlations also exist for increases in LH excretion, testes enlargement, and testosterone concentration (T).

impair the adolescent growth spurt. Males achieve greater growth velocities, muscular development, and statural height than do females, because of augmented androgen production.

In the average male, testicular size increases at age 12 years. This is followed 1 year later by the onset of penis enlargement. The first ejaculation of seminal fluid and nocturnal emissions occur at approximately 14 years of age. Pubic hair growth begins at approximately 12.5 to 13 years; the first signs of axillary and facial hair occur 2 years later (i.e., 14.5 to 15 years). Acne and apocrine sweat are characteristic features of adolescence. The male physique undergoes striking changes as a result of androgen action: shoulder width increases, facial bone structure enlarges, vocal cords expand to deepen the voice, muscle cell number doubles, and muscle mass and strength show striking gains. Early developers are athletically superior with regard to strength and coordination than late developers. However, the later onset of adolescence may contribute to the tall stature seen in some adult males.[95]

Approximately one-half of boys develop a small amount of breast tissue (2 to 3 cm in diameter) midway through adolescence. Usually this lasts for 12 to 18 months and resolves completely. Progressive breast enlargement over a period of 1 to 2 years is not likely to resolve spontaneously, and mastectomy via a periareolar incision should be considered before excessive stretching of breast skin develops. In most instances, these boys have idiopathic gynecomastia; however, the possibility of Klinefelter's syndrome, true hermaphroditism, choriocarcinoma, or estrogen-producing lesions must be considered.

Adult height in males is usually attained by age 18; growth cessation occurs first in the hands and feet, followed by the legs, trunk, and shoulder girdle. The ranges in age for the events of male adolescence are shown in Table 26-5.

Table 26-5. Range of Chronologic Ages for Pubertal Events in Healthy Boys

	Age, years	
Event	Onset	Completion
Testis enlargement	10–13½	14½–18
Height spurt	10½–16	2½–3*
Penis enlargement	11–14½	13½–17
Pubic hair	10–15	14–18

*Years after onset.
Source: Based on Tanner.[95]

SHORT STATURE

Clinical Approach to Short Stature

Anxiety due to teasing is the usual reason short children are brought for medical evaluation. Throughout the childhood years, emotional stresses increase; they peak during adolescence, when striking differences in stature and sexual maturation are seen among individuals. The medical consultation usually results in one of three outcomes. The most frequent (40 to 50 percent of cases) is reassurance that the child is growing normally, albeit along a lower channel because of genetic short stature or slow rate of maturation.[97] The other possibilities include diagnosis of a treatable growth disorder, e.g., one of the endocrinopathies (Table 26-6), or confirmation that pathologic growth exists but medical help is not available at present, e.g., the chondrodystrophies. Successful management of growth problems depends upon an appreciation of the importance of the physical and emotional needs of short children. Early professional counseling of parents and patients helps to ensure that children are treated appropriately for age, rather than size, lessens their frustrations, and channels their energies into activities which foster emotional maturation and self-confidence. Small children should not be held back a grade in school solely on the basis of size. Teachers must encourage these children to be assertive and assume their share of classroom responsibilities. Gym instructors play a key role by keeping these children involved in the many physical activities which do not require a large physique, e.g., tennis, judo, karate, wrestling, swimming, skiing, skating, gymnastics, and baseball.

Prior to the first examination, it is advisable to ask parents to send in previous heights and weights obtained from school health records, personal physicians, or clinics. Annual school photographs are particularly valuable in growth problems which are associated with changing facial appearance, e.g., hypothyroidism or Cushing's syndrome. The initial medical evaluation involves taking the patient's history and performing a physical examination and laboratory and radiographic studies.

HISTORY

A complete history includes details of the child's health from conception to the time of examination; specifics of maternal health, including drug use and diseases prior to and during the pregnancy; information on height, weight, rate of maturation, and health

Table 26-6. Differential Diagnosis of Short Stature

- Causes of normal short stature
  - Genetic or familial short stature
  - Constitutional growth delay with or without delayed adolescence
- Pathologic growth
  - Intrauterine disturbances:
    - Placental dysfunction
    - Maternal factors
      - Malnutrition
      - Disease
      - Drug use
    - Fetal disease
      - Infections
      - Congenital abnormalities
      - Chromosomal abnormalities
    - Premature delivery
    - Genetic syndromes: Bloom's, Hallermann-Streiff-François, Russell-Silver, Seckel's Donahue's, Dubowitz', progeria, Cornelia de Lange's, Williams
  - Postnatal malnutrition
    - Poverty, ignorance, neglect
    - Mechanical gastrointestinal disorders
      - Esophageal stenosis, web, reflux
      - Pyloric stenosis
      - Duodenal atresia, stenosis, bands, annular pancreas
      - Malrotation, volvulus
      - Foreign body
      - Aganglionosis (Hirschsprung's)
      - Short-bowel syndrome
    - Digestive diseases
      - Enzyme deficiencies:
        - Proteolytic enzymes: trypsin, cystic fibrosis
        - Disaccharidases: sucrase, isomaltase, lactase
        - α_1-Antitrypsin: liver cirrhosis
      - Intolerance: milk-protein allergy
      - Chronic infection: *Escherichia coli,* salmonella, giardiasis, shigella, staphylococcus, etc.
      - Inflammatory bowel disease: ulcerative colitis, granulomatous ileocolitis
      - Tumor: neural crest tumors
      - Miscellaneous: celiac disease, gluten sensitivity, immunologic disorders, acrodermatitis enteropathica, abetalipoproteinemia
- Endocrine causes
  - Hypothyroidism: congenital or acquired; primary, secondary (TSH), or tertiary (TRH)
  - GH deficiency (also assess anterior pituitary function: TSH, ACTH, prolactin, FSH-LH) (see Table 26-7)
  - Cushing's syndrome: glucocorticoid excess
  - Short adult stature due to precocious sexual maturation
- Metabolic disorders:
  - Glycogen storage disease
  - Cystinosis
  - Fructose intolerance
  - Galactosemia
  - Mucopolysaccharidoses
  - Diabetes insipidus: vasopressin-resistant, vasopressin-sensitive
- Bone disorders (skeletal dysplasias):
  - Chondrodystrophies: achondroplasia, hypochondroplasia
  - Rickets: hypophosphatemia, vitamin D deficiency or resistance
  - Epiphyseal dysplasia
  - Metaphyseal dysplasia
  - Spondyloepiphyseal dysplasia, metaphyseal dysplasia
  - Osteogenesis imperfecta
  - Multiple exostoses syndrome
- Chromosomal abnormalities:
  - X chromosome abnormalities: gonadal dysgenesis, Turner's syndrome
  - Trisomy syndromes
- Environmental deprivation syndrome: emotional(?), parental(?), nutritional(?)
- Anoxemia:
  - Pulmonary disease: cystic fibrosis, hypoplastic lung, fibrous dysplasia(?)
  - Hemoglobinopathies
  - Cardiovascular disease
- Chronic disease in a major organ:
  - Kidney: renal insufficiency, acidosis
  - Neurologic system: microcephaly, hydrocephalus, diencephalic syndrome, degenerative disease, neurofibromatosis
  - Hepatic cirrhosis
  - Malignancy
- Primordial dwarfism
- Drugs: daily cortisone therapy for asthma, collagen disease, nephrotic syndrome, rheumatoid arthritis, aplastic anemia, malignancy (leukemia, Hodgkin's, etc.)

of family members; and assessment of emotional stresses within the family.

PHYSICAL EXAMINATION

A thorough examination either indicates excellent health or provides clues to an endocrinopathy or an underlying chronic disease in a major organ (GI tract, kidney, heart, lungs, CNS) or stigmata of one of the many growth-deficiency syndromes.[98]

Measurements

The body measurements listed below must be recorded. Disproportionate short stature points to the chondrodystrophies and other skeletal dysplasias; normal body proportions characterize most of the remaining growth disorders (Table 26-6).

1. Length: From birth to 1½ to 2 years, measure infant on a flat, horizontal board which has one vertical, immovable end to brace the feet, the other vertical end slides along a track until it touches the vertex of the head. Place the infant supine and hold knees flat.[93]
2. Height: For children > age 2, stand child with buttocks and heels (remove shoes and socks) against a vertical rule which has a movable device at right angles to the rule that can be lowered until it touches the top of the cranium.
3. Weight: Measure with a minimum of clothing.
4. Head circumference: Place nonstretchable tape over maximal occipital prominence and just above eyebrows.
5. Body proportions:
   a. Lower segment length (L) is the distance from the upper level of the pubic bone to the point where the medial aspect of the heel touches the floor.
   b. Derive upper segment length (U) by subtracting L from height (H); i.e., $U = H - L$.
   c. Calculate the U/L ratio. At birth, $U/L = 1.7$; it decreases as leg length increases until it equals 1.0 at 7 to 10 years of age. The U/L ratio for adult white males (0.95) is greater than that for adult black males (0.85), who tend to have longer leg length. The current standards for U/L ratio have many deficiencies.
6. Span: Stand patient flat against wall with arms outstretched at shoulder height. With nonstretchable tape held against wall (i.e., behind patient), measure the widest distance between extended fingers. Usually, span and height measurements are similar. Marked discrepancies point to disproportionate growth of limb versus trunk.
7. Other measurements: *sitting height* measures trunk length; *triceps skinfold thickness* estimates subcutaneous adipose tissue (use calipers and measure at midpoint between shoulder and elbow posteriorly); *testis length* and *width* or *volume* (latter measured with Prader orchidometer); *penis* stretched *length, width,* and *circumference.*

Plotting Growth Data on Standard Growth Curves

The graphic display of the child's growth characteristics (this can be prepared prior to the first visit) either informs the physician that a steady, normal rate of growth exists or documents the nature and time of onset of pathologic growth.

The most recently developed growth curves for American children are based on cross-sectional measurements of middle-class, well-nourished Caucasians; they do not make allowances for genetic and ethnic influences on height or for the variability of age of onset of adolescence in normal children. The Tanner-Whitehouse growth charts,[99] based on data collected in English children, are the ones most widely used internationally. The disadvantages of the available charts are not serious if the physician is aware that children whose growth follows the 3d percentile and whose parents are short are growing normally based on midparental height. Growth curves which are adjusted to correct for parental height have been developed by Tanner et al.[99]

The physical measurements (height, weight, etc.) of an individual can be expressed either in terms of percentiles for chronologic age, with the range of normal being the 3d to 97th percentiles, or in terms of standard deviations (SD) above or below the mean. One SD extends from the 16th to 84th percentile; 2 SD extends from the 2½th to 97½ percentile, approximating the 3d and 97th percentiles on the growth curve. The use of SD provides information on the magnitude of the growth disorder and is particularly helpful in quantifying growth abnormalities in children whose height and weight fall above the 97th or below the 3d percentile. An increase in the number of SD away from the mean indicates the growth problem is worsening; a decrease in the number of SD from the mean is synonymous with improved growth in small children being treated for GH deficiency or hypothyroidism or tall children with precocious sexual development.

The growth curves also allow for expression of an individual's size in terms of height age (HA) and weight age (WA). HA is defined as the chronologic age at which the patient's height would fall at the 50th percentile. This is calculated by drawing a horizontal line from the patient's position on the growth curve to the 50th percentile and dropping a vertical line to age in years. It does not take into account genetic influences on stature and pace of maturation. Nevertheless, it is extremely valuable when used to compare an individual's stature with his or her biologic age (i.e., bone age). For example, a healthy 15-year-old male with delayed adolescence and a height age of 11 and bone age of 11 has a much better prognosis for adult height than a 15-year-old sexually maturing young man with genetic short stature whose height age is 13 and bone age is 15.

The method for calculating WA is similar to that for HA but is more subject to error. The relationship between chronologic age, HA, WA, and bone age in a patient helps delineate the etiology of the growth disorder; e.g., a 2-year-old with HA = 18 months and WA = 6 months is likely to have a nutritional problem which impairs weight gain more seriously than linear growth. Conversely, a 6-year-old child with HA = 3, WA = 4, and a bone age of 3 may have GH or thyroid deficiency.

The other practical use of these relationships is in the context of counseling the patient and family concerning the risks and benefits of prescribing anabolic therapy for patients with genetic short stature or delayed adolescence. Many families who understand the significance of the relationship between height age and bone age prefer to avoid anabolic therapy, as it may compromise adult stature.

RADIOGRAPHIC STUDIES

Skeletal maturation (bone age) is based on the size, shape, and number of the secondary centers of ossification in the epiphyses. To minimize x-ray exposure, the left hand and wrist, and occasionally the knee, are most commonly used for radiographic study. The carpal, metacarpal, and phalangeal epiphyses are compared with standards obtained on healthy children at different ages. When there is variation in the maturation of these epiphyses, more weight is given to the metacarpal and phalangeal centers than to the carpal epiphyses. The standard in the Greulich and Pyle *Radiographic Atlas* which most closely approximates that of the child indicates his or her bone age.[100] Bone age is of great value in children with significant growth disorders due to endocrine disturbances. In situations where a problem in mineralization exists or bone growth is disordered (skeletal dysplasia), cautious interpretation of bone age is advisable.

Prediction of estimated adult height based on present height and bone age can be made from the Bayley and Pinneau predictive tables[101] in the Greulich and Pyle atlas. This requires consideration of midparental height. Height prediction cannot be made accurately in children with pathologic growth but is useful in healthy children with normal types of short stature. However, patients must be advised that these estimations do not make allowances for rapid progress in sexual maturation, which may accelerate bone age disproportionately to height gain and result in stature which is less than predicted.

LABORATORY STUDIES

Additional laboratory tests may be ordered on the basis of evidence obtained during the history, physical, growth-curve, and radiographic evaluations. Further information concerning hormone determinations, hematologic tests, chromosome analyses, blood chemistry determinations, and elaborate radiologic procedures (e.g., CT scan) is discussed in the sections below dealing with specific growth disorders.

Causes of Short Stature

INTRODUCTION

Precise terminology and the ability to distinguish normal from abnormal growth have never been more important that at present because of the increasing pressure to administer GH to children whose heights are within the low normal range. Two examples of normal short stature discussed below are genetic short stature and constitutional growth delay. In both entities, growth rate is normal, height is within 2.5 SD of the mean, body proportions are normal, and general health is good. These children are different from the subgroups of pathologically short patients who have been recently classified as having *normal-variant short stature* (NVSS) or simple "short stature."[102–104] The characteristics of the children in the latter subgroups are heights greater than 2.5 SD from the mean and abnormally low growth rates. GH responses to provocative stimuli are normal and Sm C/IGF 1 levels low or normal in many. GH treatment was beneficial for a majority. There is evidence to support the concept that many of these children may have atypical forms of GH deficiency (biologically inactive GH or GH neurosecretory dysfunction).[105,106] An alternative nomenclature, *idiopathic growth failure,* has been recommended to differentiate these pathologically short children from the groups of normal children with genetic short stature or constitutional growth delay. However, even the most well-informed physician will be challenged and frustrated by a child whose growth is neither clearly normal nor distinctly abnormal.

CAUSES OF NORMAL SHORT STATURE

Genetic or Familial Short Stature

Throughout childhood and adolescence, growth in children with genetic short stature remains consistently at lower percentiles, with rates equal to or greater than 5 cm/year. These childrens' heights are in the normal range based on midparental stature, and they are healthy, well-proportioned young individuals. Bone age based on radiologic examination of the left wrist is usually within 2 SD of chronologic age. Occasionally, a child inherits both short stature and constitutional growth delay (Table 26-6). This combination increases the severity of the growth problem. The greatest burden to these families is the emotional stress which results from teasing, feelings of inadequacy, and parental guilt. Diagnostic studies can usually be kept to a minimum (bone age determination, T_4 assay) if the history, physical, and growth data implicate genetic short stature.

The ultimate height of these children can be estimated directly from midparental height or calculated, either using predictive data which include allowances for midparental height or the unadjusted predictive tables of Bayley and Pinneau.[101] There is no effective treatment for genetic short stature. Androgen therapy is contraindicated because of the risk of acceleration in bone maturation, which further compromises adult height. Oxandrolone, a synthetic androgen, when given during adolecence, has not enhanced the ultimate heights of genetically short boys. There is considerable interest in determining whether pharmacologic doses of GH might increase the adult height of these children; at present such evidence is lacking. The potential adverse effects of such treatment (eliciting antibodies to GH, generating glucose intolerance, etc.) and the enormous costs are reasons why most endocrinologists advise against this therapy. At present, the management of genetic short stature consists mainly of supportive counseling, career planning, and encouraging the child to engage in appropriate physical activities which build self-confidence.

Constitutional Growth Delay with or without Delayed Adolescence

Children with constitutional growth delay have a more gradual rate of biologic aging. The slow growth pattern starts at about 2 years of age. By kindergarten, the child is shorter and younger-appearing than the majority of his or her schoolmates, although health is good and body proportions are normal. Bone age is less than chronologic age and is equal or close to height age. Growth rates are 5 cm or more per year; linear growth, with height at a lower percentile, is a characteristic feature. A dip in growth rate before starting puberty is usually seen. The family has a history of slow maturation and delayed onset of adolescence. Parental heights are average to tall, although an occasional family with genetic short stature has the added burden of familial slow maturation. Males are more often affected than females; most such boys are also delayed in sexual maturation, although an occasional patient enters puberty at age 12 years. Those with delayed adolescence continue to grow at approximately 5 cm/year and do not have a growth spurt until age 15 to 16; in contrast, the average boy's growth velocity accelerates at 13 years. This is the chronologic age when all growth charts show a steeper slope, representative of the mean increase in growth velocity during puberty. Consequently, the growth curve of the delayed developer often falls below the 5th percentile at around age 13 and steepens later as puberty begins. As long as the linear growth rate is over 5 cm/year, there is usually no need for concern. These young men reach their adult height at 20 to 21 years of age instead of the usual age of 18; they may not begin shaving regularly until aged 20 years or more.

The criteria for diagnosing delayed adolescence include absence of testicular enlargement at 14 years, pubic hair at 15¼ years, penis enlargement at 15½ years, and growth spurt at 16 years.[95]

The management of delayed adolescence in a boy depends on his chronologic age when first seen, his history and physical characteristics. If a young man of 14 to 15 is healthy but has no evidence of testicular enlargement or sexual hair, the management can be limited to determining his bone age, plotting his growth curve, and giving him reassurance. Alternatively, the assessment may be extended to include a complete blood count (CBC) and sedimentation rate, biochemical profile, T_4 assay, and urinalysis. These tests exclude the possibility that chronic diseases such as renal insufficiency, hypothyroidism, and chronic inflammatory bowel disease are present. If the data support the clinical diagnosis of delayed adolescence, the patient is reassured and examined every 6 months. Most boys enter puberty within the following 12 to 18 months and agree to allow sexual maturation to proceed without androgen supplementation. If, however, the patient is very emotionally distressed, modest doses of androgens may be used for 3 to 6 months in conjunction with psychological counseling.

The patient who presents at 16 years without any evidence of puberty may still have an innocent delay of adolescence; however, a search for organic disease is indicated before making this diagnosis. Boys who grow less than 4.5 cm/year or who have an abnormal physical sign or symptom (small penis, hypoplastic testes, pallor, dry skin, cushingoid features, headaches, visual disturbances, or anosmia) require thorough investigation. The differential diagnoses of delayed adolescence include (1) gonadotropin deficiency (either idiopathic or due to organic disease in the hypothalamus or pituitary, i.e., GnRH or FSH-LH deficiency, respectively), (2) primary testicular disease (hypoplastic testes, Leydig cell deficiency or dysfunction), (3) sex chromosome defects (Klinefelter's syndrome), (4) hypothyroidism (primary hypothyroidism or TSH or TRH deficiency), (5) Cushing's syndrome or disease (glucocorticoid treatment of asthma, rheumatoid arthritis, etc., or lesions in the hypothalamic, pituitary, or adrenal gland), and (6) chronic disease (chronic inflammatory bowel disease, cystic fibrosis, cardiac disease, CNS lesions, renal insufficiency, etc.).

The extent of the diagnostic evaluation must be individualized for each patient. The following are diagnostic procedures which aid in confirming or excluding diseases listed in the differential diagnoses:

1. CBC, sedimentation rate, biochemical profile.
2. Assays for TSH, T_4 (RIA), T_3 (RIA), free T_4; TRH stimulation test (optional).
3. Assays of urine and/or plasma FSH and LH concentrations.
4. GnRH testing (optional; may not differentiate hypothalamic from pituitary dysfunction with a single injection or infusion).
5. Measurement of plasma GH and cortisol responses to insulin hypoglycemia and L-arginine infusion.
6. Plasma testosterone and DHEA sulfate assays.
7. Determinations of diurnal patterns of plasma cortisol and urinary 17-ketosteroid, 17-hydroxycorticosteroid, and free cortisol levels before and after low- and high-dose dexamethasone administration for suspected Cushing's syndrome.
8. Chromosome analysis for Klinefelter's syndrome.
9. hCG stimulation to test Leydig cell function.
10. Radiologic studies: bone age, skull x-rays. (Optional: CT scan of head, skeletal survey for bone disease, GI series, chest x-ray for heart or lung disease, kidney studies.)
11. Visual acuity, fields, and fundoscopic examinations and visual evoked response for suspected organic lesions in the hypothalamic-pituitary axis.

One of the following treatment programs may be used in healthy boys with delayed adolescence who need treatment for psychological reasons. If chronic disease (e.g., Crohn's disease) is discovered to be the cause of delayed adolescence, these treatment programs are not applicable because they may advance bone age without promoting linear growth or sexual maturation.

1. Testosterone enanthate, 100 mg every 3 weeks for 3 to 6 months. This treatment may trigger the onset of puberty. If a permanent lack of androgens exists and satisfactory height has been achieved, the full virilizing dose is 200 mg intramuscularly (IM) every 2 to 3 weeks. Bone age is measured at the beginning and every 6 months if the effect of therapy on osseous maturation is an important factor.
2. Fluoxymesterone, 2 to 3 mg per m^2 of body surface per day for 3 to 6 months (fluoxymesterone is an oral synthetic androgen with potent androgenic and anabolic properties).
3. Oxandrolone, 0.05 to 0.1 mg per kilogram of body weight per day for 3 to 6 months (oxandrolone is an oral synthetic androgen with potent anabolic and weak androgenic properties). Oxandrolone is used in situations in which the priority is linear growth and sexual maturation can be postponed.
4. hCG, 500 to 1000 units (U) IM three times weekly for 1 to 2 months; plasma testosterone concentration is monitored and dose adjusted accordingly. hCG is useful only if Leydig cell function is intact.

Delayed adolescence in girls is present when breast tissue and/or sexual hair have not appeared by 14 years of age. Usually, menarche occurs 2.3 years after the onset of breast development, but it can occur as late as 4.5 years after breast budding.[95]

The differential diagnoses of delayed menarche in girls include (1) emotional disorders (e.g., anorexia nervosa), (2) gonadotropin deficiency, (3) primary ovarian disease (embryologic defects or acquired disease, e.g., agenesis, polycystic ovarian disease, or torsion of the ovary), (4) chronic disease, (5) absence of the uterus, (6) X chromosome abnormalities (Turner's syndrome), (7) XY male pseudohermaphrodism (androgen insensitivity, 17α-hydroxylase deficiency, embryologic defects in the testes, e.g., agenesis or absence of Leydig cells).

On the initial evaluation, the history and physical examination guide the extent to which the patient is investigated. A healthy-appearing girl who presents at 15 years without breast tissue and with normal height and growth rate probably will begin puberty in the following 6 to 12 months and only needs reexamination and reassurance. However, if she is short or if her growth rate is 4.5 cm or less per year, a search must be initiated for chromosomal abnormalities, pituitary-hypothalamic disorders, and chronic diseases. On rare occasions, girls have presented with excellent breast growth, normal sexual hair, and primary amenorrhea due to congenital absence of the uterus; the vaginal examination shows an absence of the cervix. Pelvic sonogram and peritoneoscopic examination are indicated if a normal female karyotype and elevated gonadotropin concentrations are discovered or if absence of the uterus is suspected. Laparotomy and gonadectomy must be performed in females who possess a Y chromosome, because of the increased risk of gonadal malignancy.

Estrogen therapy for simple delayed adolescence in girls is unnecessary except for psychological reasons.

PATHOLOGIC SHORT STATURE (TABLE 26-6)

Intrauterine Growth Disturbances

Abnormal intrauterine growth must be considered in any newborn whose birth weight is inappropriately low for gestational age. These babies are usually referred to as "small-for-date" infants; the prognosis for their recovery depends upon the timing, severity, and duration of the intrauterine insult. As a rule, small-for-date infants whose growth accelerates and achieves a normal channel by 6 months of postnatal age grow normally thereafter. If they show persistence of an abnormal growth rate at 2 years of age, they are likely to be short throughout childhood and adulthood.

A careful evaluation of the health of the mother, the placenta, and the fetus is needed to determine the likely cause of the fetal growth abnormality.

PLACENTA Abnormal embryologic development of the placenta or injuries from infection or vascular accidents interrupt the supply of essential nutrients to the fetus. The size and gross appearance as well as the histologic characteristics of the placenta should be documented in all cases of intrauterine growth failure.

MOTHER Many factors related to maternal health and well-being influence fetal growth. Chronic malnutrition throughout the childhood and early adult years of prospective mothers places their infants in jeopardy physically and intellectually. Maternal diseases such as toxemia, hypertension, compromised cardiac status, or renal insufficiency may impair fetal growth because of placental dysfunction.

Drugs ingested by pregnant women are a potential hazard to fetal growth and well-being. The teratogenic effects to the fetus of excessive alcohol ingestion (*fetal alcohol syndrome*)[107] include (1) intrauterine growth failure, (2) microcephaly (and possibly hydrocephalus), (3) mental retardation, which may be mild or severe (IQ range 15 to 105; in 16 of 20 infants the IQ was $<$ 80), (3) facial abnormalities, including small midface, strabismus, ptosis, short palpebral fissures, epicanthal folds, thin upper lip, short nose, micrognathia, and maxillary hypoplasia, (4) minor joint and limb abnormalities, including limited range of movement and altered palm creases; and (5) behavioral problems, mainly hyperactivity, short attention span, and learning difficulties, but not rebelliousness, negativism, or psychosis.[107] Narcotic (heroin and morphine) addiction during pregnancy causes intrauterine growth failure in half the offspring and also increases the risk of prematurity and intrauterine infection. Anticoagulants (e.g., warfarin) used in mothers with prosthetic mitral valves have resulted in infants with mental retardation, hypotonia, seizures, optic atrophy, flat facies, hypoplastic nose, and stippled epiphyses. Anticonvulsants (e.g. phenytoin) have caused intrauterine growth failure, mental retardation, hypertelorism, cleft lip and palate, and hypoplastic distal phalanges with small nails. Aminopterin used for abortion in the first trimester causes poor fetal growth, microcephaly, craniofacial abnormalities, and shortness of limbs. Heavy cigarette smoking is associated with an increased incidence of prematurity as well as smaller-sized offspring.

FETUS The fetal diseases which interfere most frequently with growth are intrauterine infections which are maternally transmitted, congenital abnormalities of major organ systems, chromosomal defects, and a variety of growth-deficiency syndromes of genetic or unknown origin.

Maternally transmitted infections include (1) rubella, which causes microcephaly, mental retardation, deafness, cataracts, chorioretinitis, microphthalmus, congenital heart disease (patent ductus arteriosus, pulmonic stenosis, septal defects, etc.), (2) toxoplasmosis, caused by a protozoan agent, which causes fetal growth retardation, hepatosplenomegaly, microcephaly or hydrocephalus, retinal pigmentation, mental retardation, and intracranial calcification, (3) cytomegalovirus, which causes poor fetal growth, hepatosplenomegaly, jaundice, retinopathy, mental retardation, and intracranial calcification, and (4) syphilis, which is associated with small fetal size, brain and bone abnormalities, and nasal mucous membrane lesions.

Congenital malformations of the brain, lung, etc., may interfere with fetal growth. Many chromosomal defects cause intrauterine growth failure: trisomy 18, trisomy 13, Down's syndrome (trisomy 21), etc. The phenotypic characteristics of these and many other syndromes of unknown etiology are fully described by Smith.[98]

Postnatal Malnutrition

Malnutrition due to inadequate food supplies is the major cause worldwide of poor growth in infancy and childhood. In this country, poverty and parental neglect or ignorance are the usual reasons for growth failure due to malnutrition. Poor weight gain or actual weight loss are the main findings. A careful history with particular emphasis on caloric intake and a thorough physical examination are essential. Characteristically, these infants are hungry and have very little subcutaneous fat and muscle mass. They are prone to develop gastroenteritis and dehydration, which further compromise their nutritional state. The cachexia, dehydration, and electrolyte abnormalities in these infants may mimic salt loss due to Addison's disease or adrenogenital syndrome, but can be easily differentiated by documenting stress elevations of plasma cortisol and aldosterone concentrations.

Management consists of hospitalizing the child in a clean area, avoiding unnecessary diagnostic tests, and providing optimal nutrition. Weight gain on this simple regimen is adequate proof of the diagnosis. The need for cultures, blood chemistry studies, and hormone determinations (plasma cortisol and 17-hydroxyprogesterone and urinary 17-ketosteroid, allopregnanetriol, aldosterone, etc. concentrations) must be individualized. Dietary counseling and psychological support for the mother, plus home supervision after discharge by a visiting nurse, suffice if the maternal-child relationship is a healthy one. The prognosis for catch-up growth and subsequent normal stature is good if the duration and severity of the period of malnutrition are not excessive. If parental neglect has placed the infant in jeopardy, removal to a good foster home is advisable.

Gastrointestinal diseases which compromise growth in infants and young children include esophageal reflux, obstructive lesions of the bowel, and deficiencies of the digestive enzymes. Cystic fibrosis of the pancreas produces malabsorption due to insufficiency of pancreatic enzymes (trypsin, lipase, amylase). It also causes chronic pulmonary disease because of airway obstruction from abnormally thick mucus, combined with bacterial superinfection. Persistent elevation of sweat sodium concentration above 70 meq/liter is diagnostic for this disorder; concentrations above 50 meq/liter should elicit suspicion. Children with disaccharidase enzyme abnormalities need the expertise of a pediatric gastroenterologist who is skilled in performing endoscopic biopsies of the proximal small bowel for histology and quantitative enzyme determinations. Diarrheal stools which are acidic (pH < 6) and contain reducing substance by Clinitest Reagent tablet ($>$ 0.25 percent) strongly suggest this disorder.

Chronic inflammatory bowel disease (Crohn's disease) occurs most frequently (78 percent of cases) between the ages of 10 and 29 years. Growth failure and delayed sexual maturation result from decreased caloric intake and increased fecal losses of nutrients. Hypoalbuminemia occurs in 50 percent of patients; anemia (iron and folate deficiencies) is also a frequent complication. Improved growth has occurred in prepubertal children treated with nutritional support (hyperalimentation for periods of 8 weeks or more) or by surgical resection of the diseased bowel. If bone age is greater than 13 years, surgery may not result in catch-up growth. Androgens should be used with extreme caution because they do not enhance growth in the absence of adequate protein and caloric intake and may compromise adult height.

Endocrine Causes of Short Stature

HYPOTHYROIDISM *Congenital Hypothyroidism* Congenital hypothyroidism occurs in approximately 1 of 5000 newborns; the female/male ratio is 4:1. Data from screening programs indicate that 84 percent of congenitally hypothyroid infants have thyroid dysgenesis or agenesis, 8 percent have enzymatic defects in hormonogenesis, and 8 percent have either TSH or TRH deficiency. Early recognition and treatment afford the best hope of ameliorating or reversing the harmful effects of hypothyroidism on the brain. The placenta is relatively impermeable to maternal thyroid hormones; thus, the factors which influence the infant's prognosis for intelligence are the severity of intrauterine hypothyroidism, (postnatal) age at diagnosis and adequacy of treatment.

After birth, linear growth is poor in hypothyroid infants. The diagnosis of congenital primary hypothyroidism is confirmed by low serum T_4, low free T_4, and high TSH concentrations. Additional criteria include absence or dysgenesis of the tibial epiphysis on knee x-ray and absence, hypoplasia, or maldescent of the thyroid gland by technetium scan. Breast-fed infants were once believed to be partially protected by breast milk because of its thyroid hormone content. This concept is no longer considered valid because breast milk contains insignificant amounts of thyroid hormone.

Early signs of congenital hypothyroidism include large posterior fontanel, suture separation, feeding difficulties, prolonged unconjugated hyperbilirubinemia, and hypothermia. These subtle features usually go unnoticed by most physicians; therefore, the advantage of screening is detection of these infants prior to the development of obvious signs such as cretinous facies, myxedematous protruding tongue, hypotonia, umbilical hernia, mottling, lethargy, and constipation. The benefits of early detection and treatment justify the approximate cost of $5000 per case identified: approximately 80 percent of congenitally hypothyroid infants treated before 3 months of age have IQs > 90, whereas only 45 percent of infants treated before 6 months have IQs > 90.[108–110]

Management consists of administering L-thyroxine, 6 to 10 μg per kilogram of body weight per day for the first year.[111,112] The thyroxine tablet is crushed and mixed in a teaspoon of formula or cereal. The criteria for judging response to treatment include improvements in the infant's behavior and appearance, increased growth rate, assessment of developmental milestones, and serum T_4 and TSH concentrations. In a few infants, TSH elevations have persisted even though the clinical response was excellent and the serum T_4 concentration normal for age; therefore, TSH concentrations have not been relied on exclusively.[113] Initially, these infants must be seen every 4 to 6 weeks in order to monitor growth and T_4 levels and to adjust thyroid hormone dosage. From age 6 months to 1 year, they are examined at 2- to 3-month intervals and then every 6 months until the age of 4 to 5 years. Thereafter, yearly examinations are sufficient to monitor progress and adjust dosage. Assessment of developmental progress and intelligence must be made prior to the child's entry into kindergarten in order to identify whether there is a need for special educational support.

Acquired Hypothyroidism The onset of acquired hypothyroidism in childhood can be readily diagnosed from the linear growth curve. Deceleration or complete cessation of growth is the earliest sign. The myxedematous physical findings seen in adults are usually absent. Features of acquired hypothyroidism include pallor, stocky physique, coarseness of facial features and puffiness about the eyes, delayed dental development, cool hands and feet, constipation, and sluggish behavior; occasionally, muscle hypertrophy is present. Scalp hair may be normal or sparse and dry. Rarely, children with hypothyroidism exhibit precocious sexual development and ovarian cysts which regress after thyroid replacement is begun. A goiter, usually due to thyroiditis, may be present or there may be no palpable thyroid tissue. These children tend to socialize with inappropriately young playmates and by nature are quiet and studious. School performance is usually satisfactory until thyroid hormone is prescribed, after which there is frequently an adjustment period characterized by deterioration in school performance, rebelliousness, and "acting-out" behavior. Gradual increments in thyroid dosage have been tried but have not significantly altered this difficult transition period. Family members and school authorities should be informed of the changes in personality which follow the patient's discovery of new energies and interests. With time, there is return to behavior patterns which are appropriate for chronologic age. The intelligence of these children is not adversely affected by the period of hypothyroidism.

The possible etiologies of acquired hypothyroidism include embryologic defects (thyroid hypoplasia), maldescent (lingual thyroid), chronic lymphocytic thyroiditis (Hashimoto's disease), acute and subacute thyroiditis, and pituitary hypothalamic disease. Lingual thyroid, when present, may be seen as a mass in the midline posterior portion of the extended tongue. Hypothyroidism develops in 40 to 50 percent of children who clinically have a goiter due to chronic lymphocytic thyroiditis. Primary hypothyroidism is characterized by elevated serum concentrations of TSH and low serum T_4, free T_4, and T_3 levels. In secondary hypothyroidism, the TSH concentration is low or normal and fails to increase after TRH stimulation. In tertiary hypothyroidism, the disease is in the hypothalamus; TRH stimulation elevates serum TSH levels.

The thoroughness of the diagnostic evaluation depends on the suspected etiology; it should include construction of a growth curve, measurement of serum T_4, free T_4, T_3, and TSH concentrations, determinations of thyroid antibody titers against thyroglobulin and microsomal antigens, and a ^{99m}Tc or ^{123}I thyroid scan. Measurement of bone age gives valuable data concerning the patient's biologic age, the estimated age of onset of disease, and remaining growth potential. Skull x-rays (anteroposterior and lateral views) are useful for evaluating sella size and detecting bony erosion. Long-standing primary hypothyroidism may result in pituitary hypertrophy and sella enlargement; the sella is free of erosion and returns to normal size with thyroid replacement. Electrocardiograms show low voltage; they are not essential. Anemia is a common finding, which disappears with thyroid medication. Pituitary function tests (e.g., TRH stimulation, GH responses) and special radiologic (CT scan of brain), neurologic, and ophthalmologic studies must be considered in children with hypothyroidism and low serum TSH concentrations.

Treatment consists of oral L-thyroxine, 0.1 mg per square meter of body surface (3 to 4 μg per kilogram of body weight) per day, given as a single dose. The whole dose may be administered at the outset.

The clinical response to treatment in primary hypothyroidism consists of a catch-up growth spurt, disappearance of the abnormal physical stigmata, and improvement in facial features, including loss of puffiness and pallor. The most valuable laboratory data are serum T_4, TSH, and hemoglobin concentrations and hematocrit; these indexes should be monitored every 2 months for the first 6 months. Bone age x-rays (at 6 to 12 months) are optional during the growth spurt and are not needed after the patient resumes growth at a normal percentile. After the patient is stabilized, the growth response and serum T_4 and TSH concentrations can be evaluated every 6 to 12 months to be certain of compliance. The prognosis for adult height is excellent if the patient is compliant and if the bone age is young. In cases where noncompliance is persistent, the entire weekly dose can be administered by a visiting nurse or school nurse once each week.[114] This therapy cannot safely be used in adults or in children with compromised cardiac or adrenal function. Excessive daily doses of thyroid should be avoided, because it causes disproportionate acceleration of bone maturation and aggravates behavioral problems.

The thyroid treatment dosages for patients with secondary or tertiary hypothyroidism are slightly lower than for primary hypothyroidism. Usually, two-thirds or even one-half of the normal dose provides satisfactory serum thyroxine concentrations. It is especially important to avoid overtreatment in these children because undue acceleration of osseous maturation shortens the period of responsiveness if GH therapy is also needed. The prognosis for normal intelligence is excellent in children who acquire hypothyroidism after the first 1 to 2 years of age.

GH DEFICIENCY The clinical features of patients with GH deficiency vary with the etiology, age at onset, and severity of the disorder. Those with congenital GH deficiency have characteristic growth patterns which distinguish them from children with acquired disease. In general, the idiopathic form is more common than the organic variety (disease due to tumor, trauma, embryologic defect, etc.).

The prevalence of GH deficiency has been estimated to be as low as 1 in 30,000 births or as high as 1 in 4018 in two studies carried out in Great Britain.[115,116] It is possible that identification of the milder forms of GH deficiency will result in a disease frequency which is greater than 1 in 4000.

A classification of the causes of GH deficiency and GH resistance is outlined in Table 26-7. No attempt is made to distinguish whether the defect in GH secretion is due to disease in the hypothalamus or the pituitary gland.

Congenital GH Deficiency Infants with congenital GH deficiency usually have normal birth length and weight. They grow normally for 3 to 6 months, but linear growth rates decelerate thereafter. Their linear growth curves deviate progressively from the mean. The severity of the growth disorder is not usually appreciated by parents, relatives, and even family physicians until the child is 2 to 5 years of age, at which time it is obvious that a marked height discrepancy exists between the patient and peers. Growth failure is the primary concern which prompts families to seek medical consultation. After 3 years of age, growth rates in affected children are almost always less than 4 or 5 cm/year. Characteristically, these patients have normal body proportions for chronologic age. Most, but not all, children with GH deficiency are overweight for height; some are frankly obese. Excessive accumulation of fat occurs predominantly in the chest and abdominal areas and the overlying skin has a grossly ripply or bosselated appearance. The general appearance of the child is always younger than is appropriate for chronologic age. In early childhood, the facies are frequently cherubic, infantile, or doll-like and the voice may be high-pitched. Frontal bossing, a common feature, is due to undergrowth of facial bones. Eruption and shedding of primary teeth usually are delayed. The permanent teeth also may appear late and are often crowded and irregularly positioned. Muscle mass is diminished. The hair is thin and nail growth is poor. Skeletal age in the prepubertal hypopituitary patient is always delayed and the degree of retardation of bone maturation is proportional to that of height age. Head circumference is within the normal range for age but the sella turcica is often small. Closure of the anterior fontanel is usually very delayed.

During early infancy and childhood, patients with GH deficiency may experience recurring episodes of fasting hypoglycemia and convulsions which, untreated, may result in mental retardation, a seizure disorder, and even death. Therapy with GH is highly effective. Some of these infants have a concomitant deficiency of ACTH; their treatment includes maintenance doses of hydrocortisone [10 to 15 mg per square meter of surface per day in 2 or 3 divided doses (PO)] in addition to GH (0.05 to 1 mg per kilogram of body weight IM or SC on Monday, Wednesday, and Friday, or daily if necessary to prevent hypoglycemia). During illnesses, stress doses of hydrocortisone given orally (60 mg/m^2 in 3 divided doses) or parenterally (60 mg/m^2 IM or IV given in 2 or 3 divided doses) are required. Glucose-containing electrolyte solutions must frequently be used IV when oral intake is curtailed in these children. The tendency to fasting hypoglycemia usually disappears by 5 years of age, but may reappear if severe illnesses prevent oral intake for prolonged periods. Apart from the problems of hypoglycemia and seizures during the early childhood years, children with idiopathic GH deficiency are generally healthy and have normal intelligence. Emotional problems are more frequent, however, in this population, because patients are perceived to be much younger than their chronologic age and are treated accordingly. Excessive teasing and social isolation are common complaints.

GH-deficient boys with microphallus and hypoplastic testes are likely to also have gonadotropin deficiency which may be partial or complete. Usually, the gonadotropin status cannot be accurately assessed until their adolescent years. Small doses of androgen should be prescribed during infancy and early childhood to bring the penis size into the normal range for age. During the adolescent and adult years, testicular growth and enhanced virilization can be facilitated in gonadotropin-deficient hypopituitary males by the use of hCG in combination with human menopausal gonadotropin (HMG).[117] In children with isolated idiopathic GH deficiency who are treated with GH from an early age, pubertal maturation is likely to begin normally whereas puberty is often delayed in those who begin treatment late in childhood. Hypopituitarism of organic origin (birth trauma, embryologic brain defects, etc.) carries a high risk of multiple pituitary hormone deficiencies.

There are several possible causes of congenital GH deficiency (see Table 26-7). *Idiopathic hypopituitarism* is the most common type of hypopituitarism. By definition, no organic lesion or etiologic factor can be identified. Males are affected more frequently than females. The disorder may involve only GH (*isolated GH deficiency*) or may be associated with deficiencies of TSH and/or gonadotropins and/or ACTH (*idiopathic multiple pituitary deficiencies*). Prepubertal children with GH plus TSH or ACTH deficiency are likely to exhibit gonadotropin deficiency (partial or complete) in their adolescent years. Hypothalamic regulation of the pituitary is believed to be defective in a majority of individuals with idiopathic hypopituitarism.

Genetic transmission of GH deficiency has been documented in six types of single-gene disorders. The modes of inheritance are autosomal recessive, autosomal dominant, and x-linked. Genetic types of GH deficiency have been caused by two mechanisms: (1) mutations within or close to the GH gene cluster on the long arm of chromosome 17, which lead to underproduction of normal GH or synthesis of biologically inactive GH or (2) mutations within the regulatory gene loci which are distant from the GH gene cluster, which cause an underproduction of biologically normal GH.[118]

A unique genetic disorder with GH deficiency, *isolated GH deficiency, type 1A,* was described by Illig and colleagues. This entity is characterized by familial occurrence of early, extremely severe dwarfism. Patients have a typical appearance; they respond well initially to GH therapy, but then develop anti-GH antibodies and resistance to GH therapy. These

Table 26-7. Causes of GH Deficiency or Defective GH Action

Congenital GH Deficiency	
Decreased GH secretion	
Idiopathic	
Hereditary: autosomal recessive, autosomal dominant	
Embryologic defects:	
Aplasia, hypoplasia, ectopia	
Anencephaly, arrhinencephalia	
Septo-optic dysplasia	
Midline facial dysplasia	
Empty sella syndrome	
Miscellaneous syndromes	
Biologically inactive GH	
Neurosecretory defects	
GH resistance:	
Laron dwarfism	
Pygmy	
Acquired GH Deficiency	
Idiopathic	
Neurosecretory defects	
CNS tumors:	
Craniopharyngioma	Dysgerminoma
Optic glioma	Hamartoma
Trauma:	
Perinatal insult: breech deliveries, hypoxemia, asphyxia, difficult forceps delivery, intracranial hemorrhage, precipitate or prolonged delivery, twin pregnancy	
Child abuse	
Accidental trauma	
Inflammatory diseases	
Viral encephalitis	
Bacteria, group B streptococcal meningitis, etc.	
Fungal	
Granulomatous: tuberculosis, syphilis, sarcoidosis, unknown etiology	
Autoimmunity: lymphocytic hypophysitis	
Irradiation: CNS radiation for brain tumors, leukemia	
Vascular lesions:	
Aneurysms, pituitary vessels	
Infarction	
Hematologic disorders:	
Hemochromatosis	
Sickle cell disease	
Thalassemia	
Histiocytosis	
Transient defects in GH secretion or action:	
Peripuberty (secretion)	
Primary hypothyroidism (secretion, action)	
Psychosocial stress (secretion, action)	
Malnutrition (action)	
Glucocorticoid excess (?)	
Drug use	

patients are believed to have a total absence of GH during prenatal life, which causes them to lack immune tolerance to exogenous GH. The mechanism of inheritance is autosomal recessive.[118a]

Patients with other forms of inherited GH deficiency continue to respond to exogenous GH therapy and present with variable degrees of growth failure. Those with X-linked recessive forms of GH deficiency have two distinct clinical phenotypes; this suggests that at least two loci on the X chromosome influence GH production.

Embryologic defects include aplasia, hypoplasia, or ectopic location of the pituitary. These may occur as isolated, congenital defects or in association with anencephaly or arrhinencephalia. The latter comprises a spectrum of embryologic abnormalities which interfere with midline cleavage of the forebrain and cause midline dysplasia of the face.

The syndrome of septo-optic dysplasia (De Morsier's syndrome) consists of optic nerve and optic disc hypoplasia with or without abnormalities of the septum pellucidum and corpus callosum. Growth failure and hypopituitarism occur in 60 percent of cases. Other features include median facial cleft, hyperprolactinemia, and diabetes insipidus. Septo-optic dysplasia may represent a mild form of arrhinencephalia.[119–121]

An increased incidence of hypopituitarism has been documented in patients with cleft lip and palate.[122]

Extension of the subarachnoid space into the sella turcica is responsible for the *empty sella syndrome.* It is presumed to result from an incompetent sella diaphragm and an increase in CSF pressure.[123–125] In the absence of surgery or radiation, the condition is called *primary* empty sella syndrome. Familial cases are rare. In most patients, pituitary function is normal and the sella turcica is diffusely enlarged. Empty sella syndrome is seen most frequently in obese, middle-aged women; it is rarely recognized during childhood. The disorder can be readily distinguished from pituitary tumor by CT. Most of the reported cases have associated cranial defects. One kindred has been described in which empty sella syndrome was transmitted as an autosomal dominant trait in association with Rieger's anomaly of the anterior chamber of the eye.[126]

Children with *biologically inactive* GH present with growth failure and have the following characteristics: height that is below the mean by > 3 SD, abnormal growth rate (< 4 cm/year), apparent good health, normal body proportions, normal plasma GH responses by RIA, but abnormally low ratios of radioreceptor-measured/RIA measured GH concentrations, low Sm C concentrations which improve following 3 to 10 daily injections of GH, and improvement of linear growth when given GH therapy.[105] The assumption is made that the endogenous GH in these children has reduced biologic activity but is immunologically reactive. Biologically inactive GH is thought to be one of the etiologic factors in NVSS.[102]

Neurosecretory dysfunction has been identified in children with heights below the 1st percentile, growth velocity < 4 cm/year, peak GH concentration > 10 ng/ml after provocative testing, but low Sm C levels and abnormally low diurnal frequency and amplitude of GH pulses.[106] Sm C levels have been reported to double after GH administration daily for 5 days. Both number and amplitude of GH secretory pulses during a 24-h period are significantly below those observed in healthy children but greater than those documented in classic GH deficiency. Treatment with exogenous GH enhances linear growth in all subjects. The data suggest that these children have defective neuroregulation of GH secretion and suffer from a less severe form of GH deficiency. They may be overlooked because of their normal GH responses to provocative tests. Identification of this disorder is somewhat difficult because it requires blood sampling at 20-min intervals for 24 h.

Defective GH action is another cause of congenital GH deficiency. The clinical characteristics of children with Laron-type dwarfism are identical to those observed in GH-deficient children. In contrast, however, they exhibit very elevated basal levels of GH and exaggerated GH responses to provocative testing. The endogenous GH in these children is biologically active and binds normally in standard GH receptor assays. Laron dwarfs are short at birth and have low Sm C levels which do not rise after GH therapy. Administration of GH does not enhance growth or stimulate nitrogen retention. Adults rarely exceed 130 cm in height and are presumed to be fertile. This growth disorder results from cellular unresponsiveness to GH, or possibly an abnormal GH receptor. The disease is seen most commonly in the products of consanguinous marriages involving Jewish parents of middle eastern extraction. It is transmitted by autosomal recessive inheritance. Affected children may benefit from somatomedin therapy when it becomes available.[127,128]

Pygmies represent another example of individuals with GH resistance in whom IGF 1 levels are low and IGF 2 levels are normal. Treatment with exogenous GH fails to correct the IGF 1 deficiency. Merimee and colleagues postulate that pygmies have isolated deficiencies of IGF 1 due to either a defect in a complex carrier protein system or an abnormal GH receptor.[129,130] Malnutrition is an alternative explanation for the low IGF 1 in pygmies.[130a]

Acquired GH Deficiency Children with acquired GH deficiency by definition grow normally during early childhood and then fail to grow because they develop GH deficiency. It is essential that organic disease be excluded. The causes of acquired GH deficiency are discussed briefly here.

CNS tumors: Craniopharyngioma is the most common CNS tumor to cause GH deficiency in childhood. The tumor is believed to rise from embryonic squamous cell rests located at the junction of the adenohypophysis and neurohypophysis. Because of its location, expansion may cause permanent injury to the hypothalamus, optic nerves, and pituitary gland. The only complaint may be growth failure. Other clinical features include visual field defects, signs and symptoms of increased intracranial pressure, and multiple pituitary endocrine deficiencies. Following surgical extirpation of the tumor, a majority of children have panhypopituitarism. Destruction of the satiety center may result in uncontrolled hyperphagia and obesity. Normal or excessive growth has been observed after surgery in some hyperphagic patients who have abnormally low GH responses and normal somatomedin levels.[131] Recent studies suggest that hyperprolactinemia or hyperinsulinism may account for the normal IGF 1 levels and sustained growth in these children.[132–134] Other CNS tumors which cause hypopituitarism in childhood are optic gliomas, germinomas, ependymomas, meningiomas, colloid cysts of the third ventricle, and, rarely, chromophobe adenomas.

Trauma may also produce GH deficiency. Perinatal injury to the pituitary and/or hypothalamus may account for a significant number of childhood cases of presumed congenital idiopathic GH deficiency. A careful review of the birth histories of these children has shown that 50 to 65 percent of cases had one or more significant perinatal insults. Birth size is generally normal. The male/female ratio is 4:1. Perinatal risk factors included intrapartum hypoxemia or asphyxia, breech deliveries, difficult forceps deliveries, intracranial hemorrhage, precipitate or prolonged labor, twin pregnancies, and postnatal seizures. Other risk factors include bleeding during pregnancy and toxemia.[135,136] Throughout childhood, accidental head trauma or child abuse may result in hypopituitarism.

Inflammatory diseases, including bacterial meningitis, viral encephalitis, and fungal infections of the CNS, may cause permanent injury to the pituitary and hypothalamus. Giant-cell granuloma of the pituitary gland is a rare cause of hypopituitarism. Its presentation may be indistinguishable from that of pituitary adenoma;[137] the diagnosis is usually made at autopsy or by obtaining pituitary tissue for histologic examination. The disease is usually of unknown etiology but has been seen in association with tuberculosis, syphilis, and sarcoidosis.

Lymphocytic hypophysitis is considered an *autoimmune disorder,* clinical characteristics of which resemble those of pituitary tumors; hypopituitarism is frequently present. The disease has been described most frequently in women who are or were recently pregnant.[138–140]

Irradiation for tumors of the head and neck carries a high risk for impaired pituitary function.[141–143] The doses of radiation usually exceed 4000 rads. GH deficiency is the most common abnormality; TSH and ACTH secretion usually are preserved. Less is known about the gonadotropin status of these children. Primary thyroid dysfunction due to radiation injury of the thyroid gland is not uncommon. Usually, the patient appears euthyroid and has an elevated TSH level with normal T_4 and T_3 concentrations. Clinical hypothyroidism with low T_4 and T_3 levels has also been observed in these children.

Aneurysms of the pituitary vessels or infarction of the pituitary gland due to vascular malformations are extremely rare causes of hypopituitarism in childhood.[144]

Impaired hypothalamic-pituitary function may be observed in patients with *thalassemia major* who have iron overload. Normal GH responses and low somatomedin levels have been documented.[145–147]

Permanent vasopressin deficiency and diabetes insipidus is the most common CNS complication of *disseminated histiocytosis.* Many affected children have inadequate GH responses to provocative tests but grow satisfactorily and do not require treatment. Those with growth failure and abnormal GH responses benefit from GH therapy. Usually TSH, ACTH, FSH, and LH secretion remain normal.[148]

Transient Defects in GH Secretion or Action Transient or functional hypopituitarism has been documented in prepubertal males; it has been called "lazy pituitary syndrome."[148a] Therapy with GH or androgens accelerates growth velocity. Normal GH responses to provocative stimuli have been observed after the onset of puberty.[149,150]

Hypopituitarism has been documented in young children with growth failure who come from hostile home environments. Psychological stress and nutritional factors are the probable causes of the entity known as *psychosocial dwarfism.* These patients have delayed onset of speech, are withdrawn, and have abnormal sleep patterns and bizarre eating habits. After these children are placed in foster homes or after the home stresses are resolved, pituitary function returns to normal, growth accelerates, and they exhibit improved behavior and normal dietary habits.[151–154]

Transient GH deficiency due to depletion of pituitary GH has been documented in primary hypothyroidism. Treatment with thyroid hormone is associated with catch-up growth and normal GH responses to provocative stimuli. It is standard practice to postpone GH testing in hypothyroid children until they have received 1 or 2 months of thyroxine replacement; the results of tests of GH secretion cannot be interpreted accurately if children are evaluated while hypothyroid.

Diagnosis of GH Deficiency The diagnostic evaluation and treatment of GH deficiency depends upon the age of the child and the presence or absence of hypoglycemia. Small infants with hypoglycemia require immediate evaluation and treatment but are able to undergo only limited diagnostic studies. The most practical test involves measurement of glucose, plasma cortisol, GH, and insulin concentrations every 15 min for 1 h during a documented episode of hypoglycemia. The latter is readily provoked by a 3- to 6-h fast. Serum T_4 and TSH concentrations should be determined. Insulin-induced hypoglycemia is a hazardous diagnostic test in small infants. L-Arginine stimulation is safe but requires an infusion and six or more blood samples. The diagnosis of GH and ACTH deficiency is based on a plasma GH level < 4 ng/ml and plasma cortisol concentration < 5 μg/dl during fasting hypoglycemia or L-arginine challenge. Frequent feedings at 3- to 4-hour intervals coupled with GH and hydrocortisone treatment usually restore carbohydrate homeostasis. With advancing age, the tendency to hypoglycemia lessens. The ability of each child to tolerate a fast of 6 or more hours must be evaluated and the frequency of the feeding schedule adjusted accordingly. During illness, therapy with stress doses of hydrocortisone (see above) may be needed to protect the patient from hypoglycemia and seizures. Parents can also be taught to give rectal glucose (25 ml of 50 percent glucose diluted in equal parts with tap water and dispensed from a pediatric Fleet's enema container which has been emptied of enema solution).

Opinions differ concerning the appropriate age for conducting pituitary function tests beyond infancy. If growth failure is the child's only problem it is preferable to wait until 3 or 4 years of age; other centers recommend diagnostic evaluation be performed as early as possible. No child should undergo GH testing while hypothyroid, because the results are unreliable. Treatment with T_4 for 1 or 2 months prior to assessment of GH responsiveness is recommended.

The usual indications for evaluation of GH deficiency include (1) pathologic short stature in a child with normal body proportions (height > 2.5 SD below the mean; some centers require height be > 3 SD below the mean), (2) abnormal growth rate for chronologic age (< 7 cm/year prior to age 3, < 4 to 5 cm/year from age 3 to onset of puberty, and < 5.5 to 6 cm/year during the pubertal years), (3) delayed skeletal maturation (bone age > 2 SD below the mean for chronologic age), (4) special clinical considerations (e.g., microgenitalia, prior hypoglycemia, history of head trauma, CNS tumor, hypoxemia, or intracranial hemorrhage). In addition, tests of pituitary function are necessary when linear growth in children with suspected acquired hypopituitarism decelerates or ceases, even if height is within the normal range.

Valuable information is obtained from the following: construction of growth curves, serum T_4 and TSH assays (T_3 and TRH stimulation tests are optional), insulin hypoglycemia challenge for GH and cortisol secretion (if GH deficiency is suspected, use only 0.05 U regular insulin per kilogram of body weight as an IV bolus and take the precautions noted in Table 26-12), L-arginine stimulation test for GH, prolactin determination, urine specific gravity and/or osmolality (on the second voided urine after an overnight water-deprivation test to assess vasopressin secretion), CBC, urinalysis, biochemical profile, bone age determination, anteroposterior and lateral skull x-rays for sella size and shape, examinations of visual fields and acuity, fundoscopic examination, and CT scan (in selected cases only). Preliminary studies confirm that GRF administration is a reliable test of pituitary GH reserves in short children; it is likely to become a valuable diagnostic test of hypothalamic-pituitary disorders.

Traditionally, diagnosis of GH deficiency has been based on a peak plasma GH concentration less than 4 ng/ml on two stimulation tests. Partial GH deficiency is suspected if the peak plasma GH level is between 4 and 8 ng/ml. A normal GH response is a GH concentration greater than 9 ng/ml (10 ng/ml, according to some investigators) at any time during the studies. It is generally believed that these criteria may be too rigid, because they exclude many children who would benefit from GH treatment. The evidence for this opinion comes from investigations which have demonstrated that GH treatment is beneficial not only to patients with classic GH deficiency (complete or partial) but also to those with idiopathic growth failure who have normal GH responses to provocative stimuli and low somatomedin levels.

Treatment At present, hypopituitary children are being treated exclusively with recombinant DNA–derived human GH. The dose is 0.05 to 0.1 mg per kilogram of body weight given IM on Monday, Wednesday, and Friday of each week. Subcutaneous administration is probably equally efficacious.[155] Daily injections or pulsatile infusions of GH have not been evaluated sufficiently to assess the long range benefits of these regimens. The currently approved preparation of biosynthetic GH has an extra methionine residue, hence its name, met-GH. Methionine-free or natural sequence biosynthetic GH is being developed for clinical use. A higher frequency of GH antibodies has been observed in patients treated with met-GH than has been seen in children given pituitary–derived monomeric GH.

Up until 1985, the standard GH used for treatment was purified GH extracted from human pituitary glands. This preparation was withdrawn from human use in 1985 because four young adults who had received GH in the late 1960s and early 1970s died of Creutzfeldt-Jakob disease (CJD).[155a,b,c] CJD is a slow degenerative disease of the central nervous system caused by a transmissable unconventional ("slow") virus. It has been classified as one of the subacute spongiform encephalopathies. Clinically, the disease is characterized by progressive truncal ataxia, tremors of the head and extremities, speech disturbances, involuntary movements, dementia and death. Seldom is CJD seen in patients prior to the age of 30 years. Whether the preparations of pituitary–derived GH contained the CJD agent is still unknown. The future use of human GH from pituitary glands is uncertain at present.

During the first treatment periods, the growth response is 9 to 12 cm/year; subsequently, it is 7 to 8 cm/year. Within a few months of starting therapy there is a loss of subcutaneous fat and the children lose their cherubic, babyish facial appearance and look more mature.

Small doses of androgens given simultaneously with GH during the prepubertal years enhance linear growth responses.[156,157] A regimen of oxandrolone, 0.05 to 0.1 mg per kilogram of body weight per day PO, plus GH increases growth rates without significant enlargement of the phallus. When microphallus is present, GH combined with fluoxymesterone, 2 mg per square meter of surface per day PO, enlarges the penis and also increases growth velocity. Androgen therapy should never be used without concurrent GH administration, because bone maturation usually accelerates without compensatory increases in height and ultimate stature may be compromised. Bone age must be evaluated at both the start and completion of each treatment period in order to assess the effects of therapy on bone maturation relative to height gain. Lastly, androgens should not be combined with GH if the bone age has moved significantly ahead of height age during the previous treatment period. In these circumstances, it is safer to use only GH treatment. Thyroid hormone determination should be performed at 6- to 12-month intervals because hypopituitary children with previously normal serum T_4 levels have been known to develop hypothyroidism during GH treatment. This may be due to a stimulation of somatostatin release by GH which, in turn, suppresses TSH secretion. In this situation, thyroid replacement must be administered concurrently to ensure an optimal growth response to administered GH. At present, GH therapy should be continued until the epiphyses close or the patient ceases to respond to therapy.

Assessment of gonadotropin secretion is usually postponed until the adolescent years. In a male who has reached the age of 14 years and has no increase in testicular size, 24-h urinary FSH and LH excretion (by RIA) and plasma testosterone concentration should be determined. Stimulation of pituitary FSH and LH by GnRH is now being standardized. Unfortunately, a single GnRH injection may not differentiate whether dysfunction exists in the pituitary or the hypothalamus. Absence of a rise in plasma and/or urinary FSH and LH concentration is indicative of either pituitary disease or prolonged endogenous lack of GnRH. Repeated GnRH stimulation has been used to differentiate pituitary versus hypothalamic dysfunction.

The treatment of gonadotropin deficiency depends on the height and bone age of the patient. If the patient is 14 years old, bone age is < 14 years, and height is approximately 5 ft, GH plus fluoxymesterone (2 to 3 mg per square meter of surface per day PO) or testosterone 17β-cypionate or testosterone enanthate (50 to 100 mg every 3 to 4 weeks), results in increased growth velocity as well as penis and sexual hair growth. After the patient has achieved a height of 5 ft 4 in or has begun epiphyseal fusion (bone age = 16 years), larger doses of testosterone (200 mg every 2 to 3 weeks IM) are needed to promote sexual maturation. For reasons which are poorly understood, many gonadotropin-deficient hypopituitary males do not achieve satisfactory beard growth or muscular development. An alternative treatment program for gonadotropin-deficient males involves simultaneous administration of HMG and hCG to promote testicular maturation, virilization, and fertility. The treatment of pituitary hormone deficits is summarized in Table 26-8.

CUSHING'S SYNDROME Obesity, linear growth failure, and delayed adolescence may be the only signs of Cushing's syndrome in childhood. In contrast to obese normal children who grow rapidly, those with Cushing's syndrome exhibit linear growth deceleration and subtle or obvious cushingoid facial features. Annual school photographs often document the onset of a cushingoid facial appearance. The diagnostic protocol includes measurement of diurnal plasma cortisol concentrations; plasma ACTH concentration; 24-h excretion of 17-hydroxycorticosteroids, 17-ketosteroids, and cortisol; low-dose dexamethasone suppression test (20 μg per kilogram of body weight per day divided into 4

Table 26-8. Treatment of Hormone Deficits and Monitoring Schedule for **Hypopituitary** Patients

Hormone deficit	Treatment	Monitoring system
TRH-TSH	1. L-Thyroxine, 0.05–0.1 mg/m^2 per day PO *or* 2. USP thyroid, 90–120 mg/m^2 per day PO	Growth rate, serum T_4 concentration
GH	hGH, 0.05–0.1 mg IM or SC on Monday, Wednesday, and Friday (three times each week)	Linear growth rate, bone age, clinical appearance, somatomedin T_4
ACTH	1. Oral hydrocortisone or cortisone acetate, 10–15 mg/m^2 per day divided into 2 or 3 doses, *or* 2. IM cortisone acetate maintenance dose, 10–15 mg/m^2 per day; stress dose, 60–75 mg/m^2 per day	Fasting blood sugar, plasma cortisol concentrations
FSH-LH	1. Testosterone, 100–200 IM every 2–4 weeks after completion of GH therapy, *or* 2. hCG, 1000–2000 U in 0.2–0.4 ml diluent, IM, three times weekly; Pergonal menotropins, one vial in 1 ml diluent, IM, three times weekly; hCG and Pergonal menotropins may be combined in single syringe	1. Plasma testosterone concentration, penis size, sexual hair growth 2. Plasma testosterone concentration, penis and testis size, sexual hair and beard growth, sperm analysis
Vasopressin	1. DDAVP,* 50 μl at bedtime, 25–50 μl every morning, *or* 2. Pitressin in oil, 0.5–1.0 ml IM every 1–3 days	Clinical response (↓ thirst, etc.), specific gravity ↑, volume of urine ↓, serum Na, Cl, and osmolality in normal range

*DDAVP, desmopressin (1-desamino-8-D-arginine vasopressin)

doses and given at 6-h intervals); high-dose dexamethasone suppression test (80 μg/kg per day given in 4 doses); ACTH stimulation test; skeletal x-rays for osteoporosis and bone age; and CT scans of the head and abdomen. Abdominal ultrasonography may also aid in detection of an adrenal lesion. These less-invasive diagnostic tests have almost entirely replaced adrenal arteriography and/or angiography, which were once the only means for localizing an adrenal tumor.

The treatment of Cushing's syndrome due to adenoma or carcinoma is unilateral adrenalectomy and supportive glucocorticoid therapy during and after surgery until function is restored in the contralateral adrenal gland. Bilateral adrenalectomy is necessary for Cushing's syndrome due to micronodular adrenal disease, a non-ACTH-dependent form of glucocorticoid excess. The choices of therapy for bilateral adrenal hyperplasia (Cushing's disease) include (1) transsphenoidal pituitary microadenectomy, (2) pituitary irradiation, or (3) bilateral adrenalectomy. A recent study documented the presence of pituitary microadenoma in 14 of 15 children with Cushing's disease.[158] Only three displayed radiographic evidence of an abnormal sella turcica. In the hands of an experienced neurosurgeon, pituitary microadenectomy has been reported to cause rapid amelioration of glucocorticoid excess, resumption of growth, and progression through puberty; other pituitary functions generally improve or remain unchanged. Jennings and coworkers have reported favorable results following cranial irradiation for childhood Cushing's disease.[159] However, the long-range impact of cranial irradiation on pituitary function and behavior is unknown. Bilateral adrenalectomy has been widely used as therapy in children with Cushing's disease. Unfortunately, 25 to 45 percent of patients develop hyperpigmentation and enlargement of the sella turcica due to Nelson's syndrome. Glucocorticoid (hydrocortisone, 25 mg per square meter of body surface per day PO, or cortisone acetate, 30 mg/m^2 per day PO) and mineralocorticoid replacement (9α-fluorocortisone, 0.1 mg/day PO) also are needed following bilateral adrenalectomy. These patients also require stress doses of hydrocortisone (60 to 75 mg per square meter of body surface per day) with febrile illness, trauma, anesthesia, etc. Careful periodic evaluation for Nelson's syndrome is mandatory. Cyproheptadine, bromocriptine, metyrapone, and mitotane are agents which are seldom used in childhood Cushing's disease.

Short Adult Stature Due to Precocious Sexual Maturation

During the early childhood years, children who have had precocious puberty or who secrete excessive amounts of androgens, as in non-salt-losing congenital virilizing adrenal hyperplasia (CVAH), are at risk for short stature in their adult years. Prior to epiphyseal fusion, these children are tall, but their markedly accelerated pace of bone maturation without compensatory increases in height results in epiphyseal fusion and growth cessation at an inappropriately young age.

Bone Disorders (Chondrodystrophies or Skeletal Dysplasias)

Disproportionate short stature is the distinguishing characteristic of the chondrodystrophies, a heterogeneous group of bone diseases which disturb, to various degrees, the length and shape of long bones, trunk, and skull. The 50 or more chondrodystrophies have been classified by clinical, radiographic, and pathophysiologic criteria.

One clinical classification divides the chondrodystrophies into those with predominantly short limbs (e.g., achondroplasia) versus those with predominantly short trunk (e.g., spondyloepiphyseal dysplasia). Other clinical features used to classify these patients include age of onset; location of the defect, i.e., in proximal, medial, or distal segments of limbs; and presence of associated physical abnormalities, e.g., polydactylism in Ellis-van Creveld syndrome (chondroectodermal dysplasia) or fine hair in cartilage-hair hypoplasia.

The radiographic classifications are based on the location of the abnormality in the long bones, e.g., epiphyses (epiphyseal dysplasia), metaphyses (metaphyseal dysplasia), or diaphysis (Fig. 26-11). When both the spine and long bones have disordered growth, the terms *spondyloepiphyseal* or *spondylometaphyseal* dysplasia have been used. Further subdivision of these groups has been based on other distinguishing abnormalities. The clinical and radiographic classifications are descriptive only and do not provide information on the cellular abnormalities responsible for abnormal bone growth.

The pathophysiologic classification is based on the histochemical and ultrastructural characteristics of cartilage and bone; it thus gives more detailed information on the possible pathogenesis of many of these disorders. Examples include abnormal chondrocyte metabolism (mucopolysaccharidosis), chondrocyte proliferation (achondroplasia), chondrocyte maturation and degeneration (metaphyseal dysplasia), and epiphyseal ossification (epiphyseal dysplasia).[160]

None of the present methods of grouping the chondrodystrophies is perfect because the precise biochemical defect in many of these disorders is unknown, and there is much overlap in their clinical and radiographic features. Nevertheless, more order now exists because of the progress made in classifying the skeletal dysplasias.

This group of disorders is characterized by poor linear growth from early life, abnormal body proportions, distinguishing physical and radiographic data, bone age close to chronologic age (and ahead of height age), normal sexual maturation, and appropriate age of epiphyseal fusion. Detailed endocrine evaluation is seldom needed. Gonadal dysgenesis in girls may resemble the milder forms of chondrodystrophy, in which case chromosome analysis is advisable. The genetic implications must be shared with the patients as adulthood approaches. No specific therapy is available; the major investment of energy is in supportive counseling and career planning.

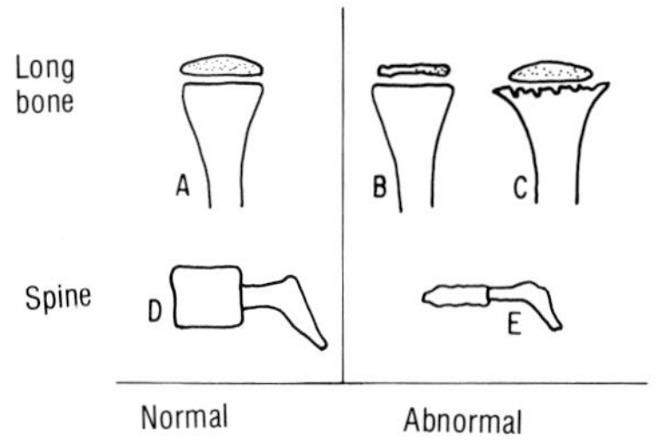

Involvement	Classification
A + D	Normal
B + D	Epiphyseal dysplasia
C + D	Metaphyseal dysplasia
B + E	Spondyloepiphyseal dysplasia
C + E	Spondylometaphyseal dysplasia

(*From Rimoin.*[160])

FIGURE 26-11. Classification of the chondropdystrophies based on radiographic abnormalities in the long bones.

Chromosome Abnormalities

The phenotypic and genotypic diversity of patients with X chromosome abnormalities and gonadal dysgenesis is of such magnitude that any girl with undiagnosed pathologic short stature should have a peripheral leukocyte chromosome analysis. A buccal smear examination for Barr body size and number will not detect subtle forms of mosaicism or small structural defects in the X chromosome.

Small size at birth is a frequent but not diagnostic feature of X chromosome abnormalities. In infancy, the only clues may be multiple loose skin folds in the posterior neck region (Bonnevie-Ullrich syndrome) which later form pterygium colli (webbed neck), pitting lymphedema on the dorsum of the feet and hands, increased carrying angle, and various nail abnormalities; the most common nail abnormalities are rudimentary dysplastic nails or nails surrounded by abundant soft tissue.

Throughout early childhood, the growth of most girls with Turner's syndrome is slow and steady, 3 to 4 SD from the mean; this is followed by deceleration of growth velocity to approximately 3 cm/year after the age of 9 to 11 years. All lack the adolescent growth spurt. A few patients may actually grow along the 3d or 10th percentile during childhood; others may exhibit marked growth retardation from infancy. The range of adult height is 125 to 150 cm (50 to 60 in) with a mean of 140 cm (55 in). The precise cause of this growth problem is unknown, but the presumed etiology is a defect at the cellular level. GH and somatomedin concentrations are usually adequate. The X chromosome abnormality is known to cause loss of growth-regulating genes.

Physical stigmata of this disorder range from minimal to extremely severe. Short stature may be the only finding, or there may be various combinations of physical abnormalities: pterygium colli, low posterior occipital hairline, short neck, ptosis, multiple nevi, increased carrying angle, nail abnormalities, short third and fourth metacarpals and metatarsals, broad chest, and nipples widely set apart. The main health problems include hypertension, coarctation of the aorta, renal abnormalities, diabetes mellitus, otitis media, and thyroiditis. The laboratory studies of greatest value are chromosome analysis, plasma or urine gonadotropin measurements, thyroid function tests, vaginal smear for maturation index, and bone age determination.

There is no uniform treatment for the growth problem of Turner's syndrome. In the past, androgen therapy with oxandrolone, 0.05 to 0.1 mg per kilogram of body weight per day, was used intermittently (6 months on, 6 months off) or continuously. Fluoxymesterone, 2 or 3 mg per square meter of body surface per day, has also been prescribed.[161,163] Both hormones gave temporary improvements in growth velocity followed by declining responsiveness. The use of anabolic drugs was usually restricted to girls whose bone age was retarded by 2 or more years and whose chronologic age was 10 or more years. In a recent collaborative study sponsored by the National Hormone and Pituitary Program, approximately 50 girls with Turner's syndrome received 0.2 U of pituitary GH per kilogram of body weight three times weekly. The equivalent dose for biosynthetic GH is approximately 0.1 mg per kilogram of body weight. The patients grew at a rate of approximately 6 cm/year during the first 12 months.[163a] The long-range impact of this treatment protocol and the potential risks are not known. An alternative treatment program involves administration of 0.125 mg biosynthetic GH per kilogram of body weight three times weekly in combination with 0.1 mg of oxandrolone per kilogram of body weight per day. During one year of combined therapy the mean growth rate was approximately 9 cm/year.[163b] Minute doses of estradiol (5 μg/day) have also been recommended for these patients on the premise that enhanced growth will result if the dose of estrogen used is very small.

The age at which sex hormone therapy is begun in order to stimulate breast development and menstruation varies with the individual patient's level of emotional maturity and her attitudes concerning the importance of height versus sexual maturation. During the first 21 to 24 days of each calendar month, estrogen is administered daily (0.02 mg of estradiol or 1.25 mg of Premarin). Progesterone (medroxyprogesterone), 10 mg, is given on the last 7 to 10 days of the estrogen cycle. When adequate sexual maturation has occurred, maintenance estrogen therapy should be kept at the lowest possible therapeutic level. Rare patients with gonadal dysgenesis fail to develop breasts on sex hormone therapy and need information concerning augmentation mammoplasty. Although unusual, some girls with Turner's syndrome have spontaneous breast growth and menstruation associated with high or normal gonadotropin concentrations. Fertility has been reported in rare patients. Menses usually become less regular with time and finally cease. Thus the extent of the gonadal abnormality varies from "streak" gonads to hypoplastic tissue to "normal" ovarian function. The usual pattern, however, is near-normal ovarian development during early fetal life followed rapidly by ovarian degeneration. Laparotomy is no longer justified as a routine procedure to inspect and biopsy the ovaries.

Although intellectual development is normal in girls with Turner's syndrome, there is an increased incidence of deficits in space-form perception and a tendency to do less well in mathematics. Starting at age 8 to 10, these patients should be given sex education. Gradually, they must be told that the majority of girls with Turner's syndrome have underdeveloped ovaries and, as a result, need hormone therapy in order to menstruate and have breast growth. Also, they will, in all likelihood, be able to have children only by adoption, though, pregnancy by in vitro fertilization is theoretically feasible. Genetic transmission of Turner's syndrome is remotely possible in spontaneously sexually mature women with structural deletions of the X chromosome; therefore, genetic counseling is advisable.

Many of the phenotypic abnormalities which characterize Turner's syndrome are present also in Noonan's syndrome, a familial growth disorder with an autosomal dominant mode of inheritance.[164] Approximately 70 percent of males with Noonan's syndrome have cryptorchism and hypogonadism, whereas gonadal function tends to be normal in affected females; hence transmission usually occurs through the affected female. The cardiovascular defects include pulmonic stenosis, peripheral branch stenosis, and asymmetric septal hypertrophy. In contrast, the cardiovascular lesions of Turner's syndrome are extracardiac, mainly coarctation of the aorta or renal arteries. The main features of Noonan's syndrome are short stature; triangular facies with micrognathia; prominent, low-set ears; hypertelorism; ptosis; epicanthal folds; antimongoloid slant of eyes; low posterior hairline; pterygium colli; shield-shaped chest with hypoplastic, widely spaced nipples; cubitus valgus; lymphedema of dorsum of hands and feet; clinodactylism; scoliosis; kyphosis; pectus excavatum (funnel chest); pigmented nevi; dystrophic nails; and tendency to keloid formation. The karyotype is normal in affected individuals. Varied incidences of mental retardation have been reported. Genetic counseling is essential because this is a heritable growth disorder.

Environmental Deprivation Syndrome (Psychosocial Dwarfism and Emotional, Maternal, and Parental Deprivation Syndromes)

Environmental deprivation syndrome is a growth disorder which occurs in young infants and children from infancy to early childhood whose family life is filled with turmoil. Usually, one child exhibits "psychosocial dwarfism" and the others are not affected. Previous studies implicated disturbed maternal-child interaction, but the problem may result from conflict between the child and either or both parents or be due to entire family pathology. The importance of emotional stress vs. malnutrition in a particular child with deprivation syndrome is not readily evident from the history. These children are said to have large appetites and their eating behavior is abnormal, e.g., they may have pica, eat from garbage cans or toilet bowl, or eat animal food. Foul, bulky stools may occur. Restless sleep patterns have been described. These children are developmentally delayed and frequently display temper tantrums. The physical features resemble those seen in hypopituitarism; a fraction of these patients actually have laboratory evidence of GH, TSH, and ACTH deficiencies. In addition, they exhibit abdominal protuberance, body hypertrichosis, and sparse scalp hair, all signs of long-standing malnutrition.[151-154]

The management of these children consists of placing them in a happy environment and providing optimal nutrition; improvement in growth and behavior may then be observed. Usually, this can be achieved with hospitalization, but the child should be protected from infection, and diagnostic studies should be avoided or postponed in order to minimize the stresses during this recuperative period. Blood count, serum T_4 determination, biochemical profile, and urinalysis are usually adequate at the start. The behavioral changes in the child should be recorded along with the daily caloric intake and changes in stool character. At the outset, a psychologist or health worker should follow the child and work with the parents. If the child is sent home, home visits should be regularly carried out and the growth progress of the child monitored every 1 to 2 months. If weight loss or lack of progress in growth are observed, attempts should be made to move the child to a secure and supportive foster home.

Anoxemia

Optimal cellular growth requires an adequate supply of oxygen. Poor linear growth, weight gain, and delayed adolescence are frequently seen in patients who have severe anoxemia due to chronic pulmonary disorders (cystic fibrosis of pancreas), cardiovascular deficits (right-to-left shunts), or red blood cell diseases (hemoglobinopathies, sickle cell or Cooley's anemias, aplastic anemia, etc.). Marked improvement in growth has resulted from prolonged transfusion programs aimed at correcting anemia in children with sickle cell disease or Cooley's anemia. Unfortunately, the risk of hemosiderosis due to iron overload limits the length of time transfusion programs can be used at present.

GROWTH EXCESS

The normal and abnormal causes of excessive growth during childhood and adolescence are listed in Table 26-9.

Normal Variants

FAMILIAL, GENETIC, OR CONSTITUTIONAL TALL STATURE

Healthy girls and boys with extremely tall predicted adult height may seek medical help to slow or arrest linear growth. The only treatment available at present is sex steroids. This presents a dilemma for the physician who must decide whether the risks of treatment with high-dose estrogens or androgens are greater or less than the psychosocial traumas of very tall stature. These hormones can suppress the hypothalamic-pituitary-gonadal axis, and they have carcinogenic potential. In addition, there is always the possibility of error in height prediction. Some children show ex-

Table 26-9. Causes of Growth Excess in Childhood and Adolescence

Normal variants
Familial, genetic, or constitutional tall stature
Familial early maturation
Abnormal overgrowth
Endocrine causes:
Congenital virilizing hyperplasia
Precocious sexual maturation (puberty, etc.)
Acromegaly
Hyperthyroidism
Chromosome abnormalities
XYY
XXY Klinefelter's syndrome
Tumor: granulosa cell tumor of ovary, interstitial cell tumor of testis
Miscellaneous
Marfan's syndrome
Homocystinuria
Cerebral gigantism (Sotos's syndrome)
Obesity
Beckwith-Weidemann syndrome
Infant of diabetic mother
Gigantism and lipodystrophy

tremely rapid rates of sexual maturation and may have adult heights which are shorter than predicted. Despite these shortcomings, useful information can be obtained from the patient's growth curve, and from estimations of bone age and adult height.

The indications for treating genetic tall stature in healthy girls (predicted height > 183 cm or 6 ft) are psychosocial only. Treatment is nonphysiologic and should be undertaken only after careful estimation of predicted final height and evaluation of the physical and mental health of the patient. Girls exposed to stilbestrol during fetal life must not be placed at risk with pharmacologic doses of sex steroids. Mean height reduction is 6 cm if treatment is begun when the chronologic and bone ages are less than 13 years; the earlier treatment is begun, the greater is the curtailment of predicted adult stature. Treatment schedules vary considerably; ethinyl estradiol, 0.15 to 0.3 mg/day continuously, and 10 mg of medroxyprogesterone or 5 mg of norethindrone on the first 7 to 10 days of each calendar month are examples. Curtailment of adult height is due to estrogen-mediated reduction of somatomedin concentration and growth velocity coupled with acceleration of bone maturation. Hormone therapy is usually prescribed for 18 months to 2 years and is discontinued after linear growth has ceased for three consecutive monthly measurements. Careful follow-up of these patients includes menstrual history and determination of reproductive capacity and changes in vaginal cytology. If a young woman is postmenarcheal and has a bone age of 14 years, estrogen treatment provides negligible benefits and should not be used.[165,166]

Similarly, in tall boys whose predicted adult height is 195 to 200 cm (approximately 6 ft 6 in), testosterone treatment (500 mg per square meter of body surface of long-acting testosterone per month IM given at 2- to 3-week intervals) reduces estimated adult stature by about 8 cm if the starting bone age is 12 to 14 years. At a later bone age, the benefits of treatment are insufficient to justify the risks. Normal testicular function has been reported in a series of 29 boys after cessation of treatment.[167]

In summary, reduction in adult height can only be accomplished if pharmacologic doses of sex hormones are used to promote early adolescence and rapid maturation of bone age. Physicians who prescribe these steroids must advise parents that the long-term effects to patients and their offspring are still unknown.

FAMILIAL EARLY MATURATION

Children with familial early maturation are different from patients with genetic tall stature because they grow physically and biologically at a rapid pace during childhood and achieve adolescence and adult height at the earliest limits of normal. During childhood, they are tall and look more mature than their chronologic age; unfortunately, they are expected to behave accordingly. Their bone age and height age are proportionately advanced ahead of their chronologic age. Usually, parents are of average height, and there is a family history of early development. The predicted adult height is compatible with parental height, and medical therapy is not needed. Psychological support and sex education should be offered to these children and their families to help them understand and accept the psychosocial stresses which accompany early development.

Pathologic Overgrowth

CONGENITAL VIRILIZING ADRENAL HYPERPLASIA

CVAH is caused by a biochemical error in the synthesis of cortisol from steroid precursors in the adrenal cortex. The most common form of the disease is due to a deficiency of the enzyme 21-hydroxylase with or without salt loss; less common defects are deficiencies of 11β-hydroxylase or 3β-hydroxysteroid dehydrogenase. In patients with deficient cortisol synthesis there is overproduction of ACTH, adrenal cortical hyperplasia, and excessive production of intermediary steroid metabolites with androgenic activity. In the rare patients with 17α-hydroxylase deficiency, gonadal and adrenal sex steroids cannot be synthesized; thus, genetic males have a female phenotype, and genetic females do not become sexually mature. The disease follows an autosomal recessive pattern of inheritance[168] (see Chap. 12).

Exposure of the female fetus to excessive amounts of adrenal androgens results in varying degrees of masculinization of the external genitalia, manifested by labioscrotal fusion, a urogenital sinus, and clitoral hypertrophy. The vaginal orifice and urinary meatus frequently are located within the perineal opening of the urogenital sinus. Since müllerian duct development is not suppressed by excesses of adrenal androgen, the fallopian tubes, uterus, and upper vagina are normal, as are the ovaries.

The external genitalia of the male fetus are not affected significantly by the overproduction of adrenal androgens and are structurally normal, but scrotal hyperpigmentation may be present. There are exceptions: in boys born with 3β-hydroxysteroid dehydrogenase deficiency synthesis of fetal testicular hormones is defective; they cannot achieve full virilization of the external genitalia. XY male pseudohermaphrodites with a 17α-hydroxylase deficiency totally lack sex steroid production and are hypertensive, phenotypic females with no müllerian structures.

Females with non-salt-losing CVAH usually are diagnosed and treated in the newborn period because of their genital abnormalities. Failure to make an early diagnosis and provide cortisone therapy results in excessive androgen production, which causes heterosexual precocious development with masculinization and clitoromegaly. The problem is often not suspected in boys with the non-salt-losing form of the disease until several years have passed because their genitalia are normal at birth. By then, the continued overproduction of androgens has caused acceleration in the rate of somatic growth, accompanied by even more rapid osseous maturation, virilization with acne, deepening of the voice, increased musculature, growth of sexual hair, and enlargement of the penis. The testes usually remain prepubertal in size, however, because of the absence of gonadotropin stimulation.

Both males and females with the salt-losing variety of CVAH have a normal early neonatal course, but after 7 days of age are at risk for developing vomiting, diarrhea, severe dehydration, and shock, with the clinical and biochemical features of classic addisonian crisis. Patients with the 11β-hydroxylase defect develop hypertension due to overproduction of deoxycorticosterone.

Diagnosis

Nearly all individuals with CVAH excrete excessive amounts of 17-ketosteroids in their urine. In addition, patients with 21-hydroxylase deficiency have increased amounts of plasma 17-hydroxyprogesterone and its metabolite, pregnanetriol. In the hypertensive form of the disease, the urinary excretion of tetrahydro compounds derived from 11-deoxycortisol is high. Following adequate administration of cortisol, the levels of these hormones in blood and urine are normal.

Patients with the salt-losing form of the disease who have not been treated characteristically present with metabolic acidosis, low serum sodium concentration, and high serum potassium level. They can be easily differentiated from infants with dehydration due to pyloric stenosis, who present with hypochloremic metabolic alkalosis and normokalemia.

Treatment

The principle of therapy in CVAH is to provide physiologic doses of cortisol, which inhibits ACTH overproduction and accumulation of adrenal steroid metabolites with androgenic or hypertensive properties. Patients with the salt-losing form of the disorder also must receive deoxycorticosterone or a synthetic mineralocorticoid as a substitute for aldosterone, in order to prevent excessive urinary losses of sodium. With treatment, the concentrations of steroids and their metabolites in plasma and urine fall to the normal range; progressive virilization ceases, and a normal growth rate ensues.

Physiologic doses of glucocorticoid may be prescribed as follows: (1) cortisone acetate, 45 mg per square meter of body surface IM every 3 days for the first 6 to 12 months of life, or (2) oral hydrocortisone, 25 mg/m^2 per day, in three divided doses. Use of longer-acting glucocorticoid preparations is not recommended during childhood because of their adverse effects on growth. In postmenarcheal girls with irregular menses, 0.25 to 0.75 mg of dexamethasone daily has been used because it provides greater adrenal suppression. Salt-retaining hormone may be administered initially as 2 to 4 mg of deoxycorticosterone acetate (DOCA) per day IM, until a DOCA pellet (125 to 250 mg) can be implanted subcutaneously near the scapula. These pellets need to be replaced every 6 to 12 months. Alternatively, a long-acting IM preparation of deoxycorticosterone (e.g., Percorten pivalate) can be administered in doses of 25 to 37.5 mg every month. Older children prefer to be treated with an oral mineralocorticoid, 9α-fludrocortisone, 0.05 to 0.1 mg/day. A sodium chloride supplement to the diet of 2 to 4 g/day (½ to 1 tsp of table salt) may be needed early in infancy, but is usually discontinued by 6 to 12 months of age. In times of stress (high fever, anesthesia, etc.), the daily glucocorticoid dose must be increased approximately three times.

Occasionally, a child develops hypoglycemic seizures when an episode of gastroenteritis causes oral food intake to be curtailed. Prompt use of IV glucose-containing electrolyte solutions (5 to 10% dextrose in half-normal saline) during periods of starvation and illness protects these children from hypoglycemia.

In addition to steroid therapy, most affected girls need perineal surgery. Usually, a clitoridectomy or, preferably, clitoral recession is performed between 6 and 12 months of age together with exteriorization of the urinary meatus and vaginal orifice. Vaginal reconstruction may be needed during adolescence if the entroitus is hypoplastic and dilation is unsuccessful or if the vagina enters a urogenital sinus. Psychological support, sex education, and sympathetic medical care in an atmosphere of privacy and confidentiality are essential to the emotional health of these young women.

PRECOCIOUS SEXUAL MATURATION

A classification of the causes of sexual precocity is given in Table 26-10. True or complete precocious puberty is defined as activation of the hypothalamic-pituitary-gonadal axis at an abnormally early age. In girls, breast enlargement, sexual hair, accelerated rates of linear growth, and menstruation prior to the age of eight years are seen. Boys with precocious puberty exhibit progressive enlargement of the testes and penis, development of sexual hair, and growth spurt prior to the age of 10 years. Early onset of acne is common. Precocious puberty occurs more frequently in girls than in boys. Seventy-five percent of the females have no identifiable organic lesion; they are classified as having idiopathic or constitutional precocious puberty. The long-range prognosis for health is good; fertility and age of menopause are normal. The major physical abnormality is eventual short stature. The prognosis for adult height is especially poor if precocious puberty begins in the first years of life and if bone age advances rapidly without compensatory gains in height.

It is possible that newer and more sensitive neuroradiologic techniques will identify congenital or acquired lesions in girls with presumed idiopathic precocious puberty. In contrast to girls, boys are at greater risk of having a space-occupying lesion (over 50 percent of boys in some series are thus affected). Careful neuroradiologic and endocrine evaluation are required to rule out CNS tumors, especially in boys.

Table 26-10. Classification of Precocious Sexual Maturation

- True Precocious Puberty
  - Complete
    - Idiopathic
      - Sporadic (more common in females)
      - Familial:
        - Autosomal recessive
        - Autosomal dominant (males)
    - Organic lesions of the hypothalamic-pituitary region
      - Congenital: hydrocephalus, cysts
      - Acquired
        - Tumors: pinealoma, glioma, hamartoma, teratoma, ependymoma, chorioepithelioma
        - Trauma
        - Inflammation: meningitis, encephalitis
        - Hydrocephalus
    - Associated with other conditions:
      - Neurofibromatosis
      - McCune-Albright syndrome
      - Primary hypothyroidism
  - Incomplete
    - Premature thelarche
    - Premature adrenarche (pubarche)
    - Premature menarche
- Precocious pseudopuberty
  - Isosexual
    - Ectopic gonadotropin production: hepatoblastoma, choriocarcinoma
    - Ovarian tumors, testicular tumors
    - Boys with non-salt-losing congenital adrenal hyperplasia or virilizing tumors
    - McCune-Albright syndrome
    - Iatrogenic
    - Primary Leydig cell hyperplasia (testitoxicosis)
  - Heterosexual
    - Girls with congenital adrenal hyperplasia, adrenal virilizing tumors, ovarian virilizing tumors
    - Boys with feminizing tumors (adrenal or testicular), gynecomastia
    - Iatrogenic

The most common CNS tumors are hamartomas, teratomas, ependymomas, and, less frequently, optic gliomas, astrocytomas, chorioepitheliomas, and neurofibromas. These tumors tend to be located in the posterior hypothalamus, pineal gland, median eminence, or floor of the third ventricle. Conditions which may be associated with true precocious puberty include prenatal anoxia, microcephaly, hydrocephalus, head trauma, CNS infections, severe primary hypothyroidism, poorly controlled CVAH and McCune-Albright syndrome. Precocious puberty also may be transmitted by either autosomal recessive or autosomal dominant inheritance; the latter occurs only in males and may be transmitted by an affected father or unaffected mother.[79]

Incomplete or partial precocious puberty is the early appearance of one of the characteristics of complete puberty, e.g., isolated breast development (premature thelarche), isolated sexual hair growth (premature pubarche or adrenarche), or isolated premature menarche.

Premature thelarche is seen only in girls, usually is bilateral and is not accompanied by estrogenization of the vaginal mucosa, growth of pubic or axillary hair, or acceleration of linear growth or bone maturation. Most commonly, it presents in the second year of life, persists for a variable period, and regresses within 2 years. Subsequently, puberty occurs at the appropriate age in a majority of cases. These children and their families need reassurance and psychological support; medications should be avoided. Careful follow-up every 6 months by a single observer is advisable because early breast development may be the first sign of complete puberty. Should this be the case, the child will exhibit progressive changes, including appearance of sexual hair, rapid linear growth, etc. Premature thelarche is presumed to result from a transient elevation of gonadotropin concentrations; however, its precise etiology is unknown.

Premature adrenarche (or pubarche) is the isolated early appearance of sexual hair. Pubic hair alone may appear (pubarche) or hair in both the pubic and axillary areas may appear. It occurs more frequently in healthy girls than boys and also is seen with severe CNS dysfunction. Increased production of adrenal androgens (e.g., DHEA, DHEA sulfate) from the zona reticularis has been reported in these children. Linear growth and bone maturation may accelerate slightly in some children; however, they never exhibit the features of intense androgen stimulation. In affected children, height age and hormone levels (plasma DHEA sulfate, testosterone, 17-hydroxyprogesterone, urinary 17-ketosteroids) are appropriate for bone age. Management consists of reassurance and psychological support. Careful follow-up examinations every 4 to 6 months are advisable because premature pubarche may be the first sign of precocious puberty, androgen-producing tumors, or adrenal dysfunction (late onset congenital adrenal hyperplasia).

Isolated premature menarche presents as vaginal spotting or frank menstruation without other signs of sexual maturation. The phenomenon is poorly understood. It is most frequently seen in children with McCune-Albright syndrome and may precede the appearance of the bony lesions. An ultrasound examination of the pelvis may document the presence of an ovarian cyst.

Precocious pseudopuberty is present when children exhibit physical changes similar to those present in true puberty but their sexual maturation is due to autonomous production of sex steroids (ovarian, testicular, or adrenal hormones) or to gonadotropin-like hormones (e.g., hCG). The hypothalamic-pituitary axis is suppressed in these children, so gonadotropin excretion is low. In patients who have ectopic production of hCG, care must be taken to use specific antisera which distinguish hCG from LH; the antisera used in routine RIAs cross-react with hCG and give falsely elevated levels of LH.

In girls, the ovarian lesions include granulosa cell tumors, thecal lipoid tumors, and functional ovarian cysts. The mass is frequently palpable by abdominal and rectal examination and is readily confirmed by pelvic ultrasound or CT. In boys with autonomously functioning testicular tumors (embryonal testicular carcinomas) or ectopic tumors that secrete androgens or hCG (dysgerminomas, hepatoblastomas), the clinical picture mimics true puberty. Testicular tumors usually cause unilateral testicular enlargement. Boys with untreated or poorly managed CVAH exhibit sexual precocity; their testes remain prepubertal in size, in contrast to the generous testicular volumes observed in boys with true puberty.

Precocious pseudopuberty is also observed in a majority of girls who have McCune-Albright syndrome, a poorly understood disease which is characterized by many large areas of skin hyperpigmentation (café au lait spots), bony lesions (polyostotic fibrous dysplasia), and sexual precocity.[169] Gonadotropin production is suppressed in a majority of these patients who usually have autonomously functioning ovarian follicular cysts. Rarely, a child with McCune-Albright syndrome may present with isolated menses prior to the appearance of skin or bone lesions. The variable presentation of patients with McCune-Albright syndrome requires that this diagnosis be considered in all children with atypical sexual precocity, and that careful physical examinations, skeletal x-rays, and endocrine diagnostic tests be repeated at regular intervals. A unique syndrome of precocious pseudopuberty has been described in males with gonadotropin-independent familial primary Leydig cell hyperplasia (testitoxicosis). GnRH analogue therapy fails to suppress testosterone hypersecretion in these boys; greater androgen suppression and clinical improvement were noted with ketoconazole therapy.[170,170a]

Children who exhibit precocious sexual maturation which is not compatible with their phenotype are said to have *heterosexual precocity*. Examples include girls who are masculinized because of CVAH (noncompliance or untreated non-salt losers) or androgen-producing tumors; feminizing tumors may similarly cause heterosexual precocity in boys. Heterosexual precocity is pathologic and requires immediate investigation and treatment.[171]

The diagnostic approach to precocious puberty should be individualized. In general, a personal and family history should be obtained for each patient, with previous and current growth data; each child should undergo ophthalmologic examination, complete physical examination, bone age determination, and (in females) vaginal cytology for maturation index. In select patients it is necessary to obtain a 24-h urine collection for FSH, LH, hCG, 17-ketosteroids, and pregnanetriol determinations and measure the serum concentrations of FSH, LH, hCG, alpha fetoprotein, testosterone, estradiol, and 17-hydroxyprogesterone. CT scans of the head, abdomen, and pelvis are indicated if a tumor in one of these areas is suspected. Pelvic and/or abdominal ultrasound examination aids in the detection of cysts or tumors in abdominal or pelvic organs. The extent of the diagnostic evaluation depends upon the nature of the clinical problem. For example, a 3-year-old girl with a one-year history of isolated, nonprogressive breast enlargement probably needs minimal testing, e.g., bone age determination and vaginal cytology for maturation index. The same holds true for an 8-year-old girl with a 6-month history of breast enlargement, growth of sexual hair, and accelerated linear growth. However, patients with rapid appearance of complete puberty in the first years of life should have a thorough endocrine and radiologic evaluation, especially boys. The diagnosis of idiopathic constitutional precocious puberty can only be made after a thorough evaluation has excluded the presence of organic disease.

The treatment of precocious sexual maturation depends upon the etiology of the disorder. Surgery with or without radiation and chemotherapy may be required if a tumor is found. Precocious thelarche or adenarche does not need treatment. The aims of treatment for idiopathic precocious puberty are suppression of sexual maturation (in girls: regression of breast size, cessation of menses, return to normal rate of linear growth and bone maturation; in boys: cessation of erections, curtailment of phallic growth, reduction of testicular volume, return to normal rate of linear growth and bone maturation). The oldest and most commonly used drug in the United States is medroxyprogesterone acetate; 100 to 300 mg is given IM every 2 weeks. Medroxyprogesterone acetate administration usually suppresses menstruation and curtails breast growth. However, its effects on linear growth, bone maturation, and adult height are variable and controversial. Currently, clinical studies are being carried out with a long-acting analogue of GnRH, which is being administered subcutaneously each day (4 to 8 μg per kilogram of body weight per day) to children with precocious puberty.[172] This drug is believed to suppress gonadotropin production by suppressing the pituitary receptors for GnRH. Preliminary reports indicate that the drug causes regression of breast size and pubic hair growth and slowing of linear growth and rate of bone maturation. However, proof that the drug will eventually lead to taller adult height is lacking at present. A recent report indicates that approximately one-quarter of patients receiving prolonged treatment with a GnRH analogue have subnormal growth rates, similar to those observed in hypopituitary patients. Whether the GnRH analogue may have long-range adverse effects on the pituitary, gonads, or other endocrine tissues is unknown.[173] Outside of the United States, cyproterone acetate (70 to 150 mg per square meter of body surface per day PO) has been widely used as treatment for precocious puberty. In children whose bone age was less than 11 years, the drug reduced both growth velocity and rate of osseous maturation.[174] Among the potential side effects of medroxyprogesterone and cyproterone acetate is mild adrenal suppression. The long-term effects of these agents have also not been carefully evaluated.

Children with precocious puberty need supportive counseling and sex education in order to adjust to the extra demands encountered because of their mature appearance. Emotional and social development of these children have been reported to be between the chronologic age and physical age, depending upon the patient's range of experience. Their emotional adjustment is generally satisfactory and their verbal IQs are higher than their performance IQs, which tend to be average.[175]

ACROMEGALY AND GIGANTISM

Gigantism in childhood is a rare disease which is characterized by rapid linear growth in the presence of normal rates of osseous maturation. Therefore, the patient is at risk for extraordinarily tall stature in adulthood (7 ft or more).[176] Acromegalic features usually accompany the excessive growth velocity. Extremely large hands and feet, overgrowth of the mandible and supraorbital ridges, coarse facies, splanchnomegaly, joint discomfort, and weakness are common features. Radiologic examination of the skull may reveal thick calvaria, enlargement of the sella with erosion, and increased size of the sinuses. Cortical thickening of bones with tufting of the terminal phalanges and overgrowth of soft tissues are additional characteristic radiologic findings. Long-standing, active acromegaly may cause diabetes mellitus and cardiac decompensation. In most patients, excessive GH secretion can be demonstrated. Fasting GH levels may be elevated and nonsuppressible, or GH concentration may paradoxically increase during a glucose tolerance test. However, deficiencies of other pituitary hormones may result from intrasellar pressure from the tumor. In rare cases all the clinical features of acromegaly are present and GH concentration is normal or low. Sm C concentration is elevated in active acromegaly. The usual lesion is an eosinophilic adenoma or, less commonly, a chromophobe adenoma of the pituitary. Rare causes include pancreatic malignancies which produce ectopic GRF or ectopic GH.[22,23,26,177] Treatment consists mainly of surgical removal of the tumor; radiation and/or chemotherapy may also be necessary. Pharmacologic doses of estrogen are palliative; newer agents, such as the somatostatin analogue SMS 201-995, require additional evaluation.[56,176,178]

HYPERTHYROIDISM

Hyperthyroidism during fetal life and in early childhood causes acceleration in linear growth and osseous maturation. Early closure of the fontanels and craniosynostosis have been reported in young infants. However, hyperthyroidism in late childhood is not likely to compromise adult stature because there is proportional advancement of height and osseous maturation, which return to normal after therapy has been initiated.[179]

CHROMOSOME ABNORMALITIES

XYY Genotype

The distinguishing feature of adult males with XYY syndrome is their tendency to have tall stature which is not caused by overproduction of androgens. Chromosome analysis confirms the diagnosis; endocrine testing and therapy usually are not needed. Surprisingly, during childhood, boys with XYY genotype are not taller than their XY peers.[180] A large-scale prospective study of growth of XYY males is needed to clarify the true incidence of excessive height and the growth characteristics of asymptomatic patients. A recent evaluation of XYY males in a general population has shown that they are not more aggressive than height-matched XY males, although, as a group, they have significantly lower mean intelligence scores; the increased crime rate previously reported for the XYY population was mainly accounted for by property offenses rather than acts of violence. Criminal behavior by this group correlates only with low intelligence and not with height or an inherent tendency to overaggressiveness. A similar explanation has been offered for the increased frequency of XYY individuals in penal mental institutions. Psychological support and career counseling should be offered to these patients.

Klinefelter's Syndrome

The XXY genotype is associated with tall stature, eunuchoid appearance, and arm span greater than height. Gynecomastia during the adolescent and adult years often is present. If Leydig cell function is intact, phallic size is normal. However in patients with a deficiency of testosterone, penile growth is inadequate. The testes are small because of tubular dysgenesis, and facial and body hair are sparse. Infertility is almost always present. Confirmation of the diagnosis depends on chromosome analysis. Elevated plasma and urinary concentrations of the gonadotropins and low to normal levels of plasma testosterone are characteristic. During adolescence, especially after the age of 14, boys with high gonadotropin and low plasma testosterone levels should receive long-acting testosterone preparations (testosterone enanthate or testosterone 17β-cypionate, 200 to 400 mg/month, given at 2- or 4-week intervals) in order to increase penis size, sexual hair growth, and muscle mass, and to enhance psychosocial well-being. Androgen treatment for emotionally disturbed patients with personality disorders should be undertaken only if approved by the patient's psychotherapist and provided there is close supervision.

In the general population, young men with XXY genotype have mean intelligence scores which are substantially lower than height-matched XY controls. The increased frequency of XXY males in penal mental institutions is attributable to psychosocial pathology which correlates with low intelligence in specific patients and not to a genotypic or height-determined tendency to criminality or overaggressiveness in the group as a whole.[181]

MISCELLANEOUS SYNDROMES

Marfan's Syndrome and Homocystinuria

The tall, slender stature which characterizes both Marfan's and the homocystinuria syndromes is associated with a generalized disease of connective tissue which involves the eye, cardiovascular system, and skeletal system. The etiology of Marfan's syndrome is unknown, but a defect in mucopolysaccharide metabolism is suspected. In homocystinuria, the enzyme activity of cystathionine synthetase is decreased, causing an accumulation of homocystine and methionine and a deficiency of cystathionine and cystine. Mental retardation is present in more than 50 percent of patients with homocystinuria, whereas normal intelligence is characteristic of Marfan's syndrome. The similarities and differences of these two phenotypically similar diseases are listed in Table 26-11.

Skovby and McKusick[182] have reported impressive benefits from the use of conjugated estrogens (Premarin, 10 mg/day), or ethinyl estradiol, 0.15 mg/day in young girls with Marfan's syndrome, age 4½ to 9½ years. The final height ranged from 156 to 165 cm, a reduction of 12.5 to 17 cm of predicted height. Treatment lasted from 33 to 78 months and was not discontinued until bone age was 16 and growth had ceased for 12 months. There was no benefit of estrogen treatment in girls with Marfan's syndrome after spontaneous menarche had occurred. The authors concluded that estrogen treatment must be started before or early in the growth spurt, preferably when the bone age is less than 10 years.

Cerebral Gigantism (Sotos's Syndrome)

Children with Sotos's syndrome are large from birth and have accelerated osseous maturation. The most common findings are gigantism, prominent forehead, hypertelorism, dolichocephalus, large hands and feet, pointed chin, poor coordination, delayed development early in infancy, and mental retardation (IQ range 18 to 119, mean 72). No chromosomal abnormalities have been found, and numerous investigations have failed to show any endocrine abnormalities (GH and somatomedin levels are normal). When compared with healthy children, glucose intolerance is more frequently found; 14 percent of affected children are glucose intolerant. At birth, these children are large (mean weight 3400 g, 75th percentile) and long (55.2 cm, 97th percentile). Growth is most rapid in the first 3 to 4 years, followed by normal rates during childhood; stature in adulthood is variably tall. The major handicaps are intellectual retardation and emotional disorders. Genetic mechanisms, either an autosomal recessive or dominant mode of inheritance, are presumed to be the cause of this syndrome.[183]

Obesity

Obese boys and girls are taller by 6 cm or more than normal weight children of comparable age, and they have a larger bony frame.[184] Bone age, height age, and dental maturation are advanced during childhood. Usually, obese children reach adolescence early and are of average height as adults. Occasionally, the diagnosis of Cushing's syndrome is considered, but it can be readily disproved because these children are tall and have normal growth rates and pubertal development, features which are not seen in states of glucocorticoid excess. Psychological stress, especially in late childhood and adolescence, is the main problem of obese children; as a rule, they are otherwise healthy. Metabolic and endocrine testing may cause un-

Table 26-11. Comparison of Marfan's Syndrome with Homocystinuria

	Marfan's syndrome	Homocystinuria
Intelligence	Normal	60% of patients retarded
Skeletal	Tall, slender stature	Tall, slender stature
	Long limbs, arachnodactyly	Osteoporosis, collapsed vertebrae
	Span > height	Scoliosis (variably present)
	Scoliosis, kyphosis	Pectus excavatum or carinatum
	Pectus excavatum or carinatum	Increased fractures
	Hypotonic muscles	
Joints	Hyperextensible	Asymmetric spasticity (variable)
Eye	Lens subluxation—upward	Lens subluxation—downward
	Myopia, blue sclerae	Myopia, occasional cataracts
		Retinal detachment (variable)
Cardiovascular	Dilation of ascending aorta with or without dissecting aneurysm	Medial degeneration of aorta
	Aortic regurgitation	Irregular inner surface of vessels due to fibrosis and hyperplasia
		Frequent thromboses
Other	Hernias	Hernias
Inheritance	Autosomal dominant	Autosomal recessive
Biochemical defect	Unknown disease of connective tissue, abnormal mucopolysaccharide metabolism(?)	Connective tissue disease due to cystathionine synthetase deficiency

necessary concern. Glucose intolerance with elevated insulin levels may be a result of the obesity; they usually return to normal with weight reduction. Increased urinary 17-hydroxycorticosteroid excretion and poor GH responses to stimulation tests have been reported in obese subjects. Treatment consists of restricted caloric intake and vigorous physical activities. Only highly motivated patients have long-term success in controlling their weight.

Beckwith-Wiedemann Syndrome

This syndrome (omphalocele, macroglossia, and gigantism) was first recognized in 1963. Splanchnomegaly, hemihypertrophy, earlobe malformation, and port-wine nevus (nevus flammeus) may occur. Hypoglycemia has been observed in the majority of patients.[185]

Infant of a Diabetic Mother

Gigantism is a common finding in infants born of mothers with poorly controlled diabetes and in some infants born many years preceding the diagnosis of maternal diabetes. The excess tissue is mostly fat resulting from increased fetal adipogenesis. Hypoglycemia due to hyperinsulinism and respiratory disease are commonly found in the newborn period.

Gigantism and Lipodystrophy

Total and partial lipodystrophy have been reported in children. In addition to partial or generalized fat loss, affected individuals may have increased height, advanced bone age, hirsutism, muscle hypertrophy, abdominal protuberance, penile or clitoral enlargement, liver and renal disease, hyperglycemia, hyperlipemia, and hypermetabolism. No specific treatment is available.[186]

APPENDIX: DETAILS OF TESTING PROCEDURES IN CHILDREN

Pituitary-Hypothalamic Evaluation

GROWTH HORMONE

Preparation of Patient

Do not evaluate GH responses to stimuli while patient is hypothyroid. Administer L-thyroxine, 3 to 4 μg per kilogram of body weight per day PO, 1 to 2 months before performing GH stimulation tests if patient is hypothyroid.
Nothing by mouth after 10 P.M.
Keep patient at rest and fasting except for water throughout test.
Insert a no. 21 butterfly needle which is kept patent by flushing with dilute heparinized saline (0.1 ml heparin added to 30 ml saline) after each sample is obtained, or use a slow saline infusion to prevent the needle from clogging.

Diagnostic Tests for GH

See Table 26-12.

Interpretation of GH Tests

Severe GH deficiency: peak GH concentration < 4 ng/ml on two of the above tests.
Partial GH deficiency: peak GH concentration > 4 and < 8 ng/ml.
Normal response: peak GH concentration > 9 ng/ml on any test at any time.

Factors which Modify GH Stimulation Tests

Food (suppresses)
Obesity (suppresses)
Hypothyroidism (suppresses)
Glucocorticoids (suppress)
Puberty (enhances)
Estrogens (enhance)
Androgens (enhance)

ACTH RESERVE

See Table 26-13.

TSH RESERVE

See Table 26-14.

FSH AND LH CONCENTRATIONS

The reported plasma FSH and LH concentrations in normal children and adolescents vary greatly depending on the source of the standards [Second International Reference Preparation/Human Menopausal Gonadotropin (IRP/HMG) or pituitary FSH-LH] and the definition of international unit (IU). The normal range for the laboratory performing the assay must be the basis for interpreting basal gonadotropin values in plasma or urine and for evaluating FSH and LH responses to GnRH.

Table 26-12. Diagnostic Tests for Growth Hormone

Test	Method	Comment
Insulin hypoglycemia	Give regular insulin, 0.05–0.1 U/kg IV. Glucose nadir <40 mg/dl at 20–30 min. Take samples at −15,0,+15,30,45,60,90,120 min.	Peak GH concentration at 45–75 min. Peak cortisol >15 μg/dl. Requires constant supervision.
Arginine	L-Arginine monohydrochloride (10%), 0.5 g/kg IV over 30 min. Same sampling times as for insulin.	No discomfort. May cause hypoglycemia in hypopituitary children.
Arginine-insulin	Same dosages as in above two tests. Give arginine from 0 to +30 min; give insulin at +60 min.	Same precautions as insulin hypoglycemia test
Clonidine	0.075–0.15 mg/m^2 PO. Take samples at 0, +30,45,60,90,120 min. (25 μg PO also used.)	Peak GH concentration at 60–90 min. Somnolence and fall in blood pressure result. Dose-related side effects.
Levodopa	10 mg/kg PO; maximum dose = 500 mg. Take samples at 0,+30,60,90,120 min. Crush tablet or open capsule.	Keep patient recumbent. Nausea, vomiting result. Peak GH concentration at 45–120 min.
Propranolol	Give 0.75 mg/kg PO 30–60 min before glucagon, insulin, or arginine (20 mg for patients who weigh <20 kg; 40 mg for all others).	Do not use in asthmatic or cardiac patients. Weakness, pallor, sweating, confusion result.
Glucagon	Give 0.03 mg/kg IM or subcutaneously. Sample times same as insulin, plus 150 and 180 min.	Nausea, vomiting result. Peak GH at 45–120 min.
Sleep	Take samples at 60 and 90 min after onset of deep sleep.	Questionable reliability.
Exercise	Have patient exercise strenuously for 20 min. Take samples at 0,+20,40,60 min.	Questionable reliability.
Diurnal GH profile	Take samples at 20 min intervals over 24 h.	Requires special staff and diagnostic unit. Interpretation based on number and amplitude of GH pulses.
Sm C generation test	Take baseline sample. Give GH, 0.1 mg/kg qd for 5 days. Sample 12 h after last GH injection.	Sm C levels should double and post-Sm C level should be in normal range for age. Of questionable value.

Table 26-13. Test for ACTH Reserve

Test	Dose and sampling times	Comments and Results
Insulin hypoglycemia	Give insulin dose (see Table 26-12). Measure plasma cortisol concentration at 0, 30, 60, 90, and 120 min.	Normal response: Basal cortisol concentration = 10–25 μg/dl; Peak concentration > 15 μg/dl

Table 26-14. Test for TSH Reserve

Test	Dose and sampling times	Comments and Results
TRH	Give 10 μg/kg IV or 200 μg/1.7 m^2 IV. Measure plasma TSH concentration at 0, +30, and 60 min.	Normal response: Basal = 4.5 ± 3.6 μU/ml (varies with assay). Peak TSH = 20-40 μU/ml (increment in TSH exceeds 10 μU/ml). Peak at 15–30 min.

PROLACTIN CONCENTRATION

Basal prolactin concentration < 20 ng/ml.
Peak prolactin concentration after TRH administration = 10 to 150 ng/ml, in prepubertal child.

VASOPRESSIN

See Table 26-15.

Adrenal Function Tests

BASAL HORMONE LEVELS

Urinary 17-hydroxycorticosteroid Excretion

Age 6 months to 15 years: 3.1 ± 1.0 mg per square meter of body surface per 24 h.
Adult males: 3 to 9 mg/24 h.
Adult females: 2 to 8 mg/24 h.

Urinary 17-ketosteroid Excretion

Age 0 to 1 month: < 2.5 mg/24 h.
1 month to 5 years: < 0.5 mg/24 h.
6 to 9 years: 1 to 2 mg/24 h.
Puberty: progressive increase to adult values.
Adult males: 7 to 17 mg/h.
Adult females: 5 to 15 mg/24 h.

Plasma Cortisol Concentration

8 A.M.: 10 to 25 μg/dl.
8 P.M.: 1 to 8 μg/dl.

ACTH SUPPRESSION TESTS

1. Days 1 and 2: obtain control 24-h urine collections.

2. Days 3 and 4 (and possibly day 5): give low-dose dexamethasone, 20 μg per kilogram of body weight per day (in four doses per day, every 6 h).

3. Days 6 and 7 (and possibly day 8): give high-dose dexamethasone, 80 μg/kg per day (in four doses per day, every 6 h).

4. Obtain 24-h urine collection on days 1, 2, 4, (possibly day 5), 6, 7, (and possibly day 8) for 17-hydroxycorticosteroids and creatinine determinations (17-ketosteroids and free cortisol determinations optional).

5. Measure plasma cortisol concentration every 12 to 24 h on days 1, 4, and 7.

Normal response: by day 4, urinary 17-hydroxycorticosteroid excretion is less than 2 mg/24 h or less than 1 mg per gram of creatinine, and plasma cortisol concentration is less than 5 μg/dl.

Abnormal values: Cushing's syndrome is diagnosed if 17-hydroxycorticosteroid excretion is greater than 2 mg/24 h on days 4 and 5. If Cushing's syndrome is due to bilateral adrenal hyperplasia, urinary 17-hydroxycorticosteroid excretion is less than 2 mg/24 h by days 7 and 8, except if hyperplasia is due to an autonomous ACTH-producing tumor or to adrenal carcinoma; then, urinary 17-hydroxycorticosteroid excretion exceeds 2 mg/24 h on days 7 and 8. Rarely, a hypothalamic tumor is not suppressed.

Table 26-15. Vasopressin Tests

Test	Dose and sampling times	Comments and Results
Water deprivation, overnight test, 8 P.M.–8 A.M.	Void and discard 7 A.M. urine. Void and record 8 A.M. specific gravity.	Use if no history of polydipsia or polyuria. Normal response: specific gravity > 1.020.
Daytime	At 0 time, record body weight, serum Na^+, Cl^-, and osmolality, and urine specific gravity and volume. Recheck these indexes every 2 h.	Use when polydipsia or polyuria present. Criteria for vasopressin-sensitive diabetes insipidus: Weight loss > 5% of body weight Serum osmolality > 290 mOsm Serum [Na^+] > 150 meq/l Urine specific gravity < 1.005 Plasma vasopressin < 2 pg/ml Positive response to vasopressin Constant supervision necessary, especially for infants and small children. Stop test if weight loss exceeds 5%.

ACTH STIMULATION TESTS

Intravenous Synthetic ACTH (Cosyntropin) Bolus

Use a dose of 0.25 mg IV.

Measure plasma cortisol concentration at 0, 30, 60, and 90 min. A normal response is a peak plasma cortisol concentration exceeding 20 μg/dl.

IV Infusion of ACTH

Administer 0.25 mg cosyntropin in 250 ml saline over 6 h. Measure plasma cortisol concentration at 0 and 6 h. A normal response is a plasma cortisol concentration exceeding 30 μg/dl at 6 h.

Unresponsiveness occurs in patients with Addison's disease or Cushing's syndrome due to adrenal carcinoma. The test is unreliable in patients with prolonged adrenal suppression.

IM Injection of ACTH Gel (Corticotropin)

Collect two control 24-h urine samples for 17-hydroxycorticosteroids (with or without 17-ketosteroids) determination. Administer 20 mg of corticotropin per square meter of body surface every 12 h for 3 to 6 days (40 mg/m^2 per day). Measure plasma cortisol concentration at 0 and 48 h and then every 24 h. Collect a 24-h urine sample for 17-hydroxycorticosteroids (with or without 17-ketosteroids) determination on days 3 to 6.

A normal response is an increase in urinary 17-hydroxycorticosteroid excretion to 5 to 10 times the normal basal value.

Use 4 to 6 days of stimulation in states associated with long-standing ACTH deficiency and adrenal suppression. Inadequate response is seen in some patients with Cushing's syndrome.

REFERENCES

1. Weiss P, Kavanau JL: A model of growth and growth control in mathematical terms. *J Gen Physiol* 41:1, 1957.
2. Winick M: Fetal malnutrition and growth processes. *Hosp Pract* 34:33, 1970.
3. Winick M: Nutrition, growth and development, in Freinkel N (ed): *The Year in Metabolism.* New York, Plenum, 1977, p 379.
4. Sands J, Dobbing J, Gratrix C: Cell number and cell size: Organ growth and development and the control of catch-up growth in rats. *Lancet* 2:503, 1979.
5. Smith DW, Bierman EL: *The Biologic Ages of Man.* Philadelphia, Saunders, 1973.
6. Tanner JM, Healy MJR, Lockhart RD, MacKenzie JD, Whitehouse RH: The prediction of adult body measurements from measurements taken every year from birth to 5 years. *Arch Dis Child* 31:372, 1956.
7. Garn SM, Pesick SD: Relationship between various maternal body mass measures and size of the newborn. *Am J Clin Nutr* 36:664, 1982.
8. Smith DW, Truog W, Rogers JE, Greitzer LJ, Skinner AL, McCann JJ, Harvey MS: Shifting linear growth during infancy: Illustration of genetic factors in growth from fetal life through infancy. *J Pediatr* 89:225, 1976.
9. Tanner JM: Regulation of growth in size of mammals. *Nature* 199:845, 1963.
10. Garn SM, Rohmann CG: X-linked inheritance of developmental timing in man. *Nature* 196:695, 1962.
11. Yamada K, Ohta M, Yoshimura K, Hasekura H: A possible association of Y chromosome heterochromatin with stature. *Hum Genet* 58:268, 1981.
12. Wingerd J, Solomon IL, Schoen EJ: Parent-specific height standards for preadolescent children of three racial groups. *Pediatrics* 52:555, 1973.
13. Wheeler E, Tan SP: Trends in the growth of ethnic Chinese children living in London. *Ann Hum Biol* 10:441, 1983.
14. Barr GD, Allen CM, Shinefield HR: Height and weight of 7500 children of three skin colors. Pediatric multiphasic program: Report 3. *Am J Dis Child* 124:866, 1972.
15. Bullough WS: Chalone control mechanisms. *Life Sci* 16:323, 1975.
16. Underwood LE, D'Ercole AJ: Insulin and insulin-like growth factors/somatomedins in fetal and neonatal development. *Clin Endocrinol Metab* 13:69, 1984.
17. Daughaday WH, Herington AC, Phillips LS: The regulation of growth by endocrines. *Annu Rev Physiol* 37:211, 1975.
18. Daughaday WH: Growth hormone and the somatomedins, in Daughaday WH (ed): *Endocrine Control of Growth.* New York, Elsevier, 1981.
19. Brazeau P, Vale W, Burgus R, Ling N, Butcher M, Rivier J, Guillemin R: Hypothalamic peptide that inhibits the secretion of immunoreactive pituitary growth hormone. *Science* 179:77, 1973.
20. Guillemin R, Gerich JE: Somatostatin: Physiological and clinical significance. *Annu Rev Med* 27:379, 1976.
21. Bernardis LL, Frohman LA: Plasma growth hormone responses to electrical stimulation of the hypothalamus in the rat. *Neuroendocrinology* 7:193, 1971.
22. Rivier J, Spiess J, Thorner M, Vale W: Characterization of a growth hormone-releasing factor from a human pancreatic islet tumour. *Nature* 300:276, 1982.
23. Guillemin R, Brazeau P, Bohlen P, Esch F, Ling N, Wehrenberg W: Growth hormone-releasing factor from a human pancreatic tumor that caused acromegaly. *Science* 218:585, 1982.
24. Bloch B, Brazeau P, Ling N, Bohlen P, Esch F, Wehrenberg WB, Benoit R, Bloom F, Guillemin R: Immunochemical detection of growth hormone-releasing factor in brain. *Nature* 301:607, 1983.
25. Bohlen P, Brazeau P, Bloch B, Ling N, Gaillard R, Guillemin R: Human hypothalamic growth hormone-releasing factor (GRF): Evidence for two forms identical to tumor derived GRF-44-NH2 and GRF 40. *Biochem Biophys Res Commun* 114:930, 1983.
26. Frohman LA, Szabo M, Berelowitz M, Stachura ME: Partial purification and characterization of a peptide with growth hormone-releasing activity from extrapituitary tumors in patients with acromegaly. *J Clin Invest* 65:43, 1980.
27. Borges JLC, Blizzard RM, Evans WS, Furlanetto R, Rogol AD, Kaiser DL, Rivier J, Vale W, Thorner MO: Stimulation of growth hormone (GH) and somatomedin C in idiopathic GH-deficient subjects by intermittent pulsatile administration of synthetic human pancreatic tumor GH-releasing factor. *J Clin Endocrinol Metab* 59:1, 1984.
28. Schriock EA, Lustig RH, Rosenthal SM, Kaplan SL, Grumbach MM: Effect of growth hormone (GH)-releasing hormone (GRH) on plasma GH in relation to magnitude and duration of GH deficiency in 26 children and adults with isolated GH deficiency or multiple pituitary hormone deficiencies: Evidence for hypothalamic GRH deficiency. *J Clin Endocrinol Metab* 58:1043, 1984.

29. Thorner MO, Reschke J, Chitwood J, Rogol AD, Furlanetto RW, Rivier J, Vale J, Blizzard RM: Acceleration of growth in two children treated with human growth hormone-releasing factor. *N Engl J Med* 312:4, 1985.

29a. Gelato MC, Ross JL, Malozowski S, Pescovitz OH, Skerda M, Cassorla F, Loriaux DL, Merriam GR: Effects of pulsatile administration of growth hormone (GH)-releasing hormone on short term linear growth in children with GH deficiency. *J Clin Endocrinol Metab* 61:444, 1985.

30. Pandol SJ, Seifert H, Thomas MW, Rivier J, Vale W: Growth hormone-releasing factor stimulates pancreatic enzyme secretion. *Science* 225:326, 1984.

31. Frohman LA: Neurotransmitters as regulators of endocrine function, in Krieger D, Hughes J (eds): *Neuroendocrinology*. New York, HP Publishing Co, 1980.

32. Martin JB, Reichlin S, Brown G: Neuropharmacology of anterior pituitary control, in: *Clinical Neuroendocrinology*. Philadelphia, Davis, 1977, p 45.

33. Martin JB, Reichlin S, Brown G: Regulation of growth hormone secretion and its disorders, in *Clinical Neuroendocrinology*. Philadelphia, Davis, 1977, p 147.

34. Plotnick LP, Thompson RC, Kowarski A, DeLacerdo L, Migeon CJ, Blizzard RM: Circadian variation of integrated concentration of growth hormone in children and adults. *J Clin Endocrinol Metab* 40:240, 1975.

35. Finkelstein JW, Roffwarg WHP, Boyar RM, Kream J, Hellman J: Age-related change in the twenty-four-hour spontaneous secretion of growth hormone. *J Clin Endocrinol Metab* 35:665, 1972.

36. Chawla RK, Parks JS, Rudman D: Structural variants of human growth hormone: Biochemical, genetic and clinical aspects. *Annu Rev Med* 34:519, 1983.

37. Isaksson OGP, Jansson JO, Gause IAG: Growth hormone stimulates longitudinal bone growth directly. *Science* 216:1237, 1982.

38. Salmon WD, Daughaday WH: A hormonally controlled serum factor which stimulates sulfate incorporation by cartilage in man. *J Lab Clin Med* 49:825, 1957.

39. Daughaday WH, Hall K, Raben MS, Salmon WD, Van den Brande JL, Van Wyk JJ: Somatomedin: Proposed designation for sulfation factor. *Nature* 235:107, 1972.

40. Rinderknecht E, Humbel RE: Primary structure of human insulin-like growth factor I and its structural homology with proinsulin. *J Biol Chem* 253:2769, 1978.

41. Rinderknecht E, Humbel RE: Primary structure of human insulin-like growth factor II. *FEBS Lett* 89:283, 1978.

42. Klapper DC, Svoboda ME, Van Wyk JJ: Sequence analysis of somatomedin C: Confirmation of identity with insulin-like growth factor I. *Endocrinology* 112:2215, 1983.

43. Hall K, Sara VR: Somatomedin levels in childhood, adolescence and adult life. *Clin Endocrinol Metab* 13:91, 1984.

44. Zapf J, Schmid CH, Froesch ER: Biological and immunological properties of insulin-like growth factors. *Clin Endocrinol Metab* 13:3, 1984.

45. Clemmons DR, Van Wyk JJ: Factors controlling blood concentrations of somatomedin C. *Clin Endocrinol Metab* 13:113, 1984.

46. Hintz RL: Plasma forms of somatomedin and the binding protein phenomenon. *Clin Endocrinol Metab* 13:31, 1984.

47. Stuart CA, Pietrzyk R, Siu AKQ, Furlanetto RW: Size discrepancy between somatomedin C and insulin receptor. *J Clin Endocrinol Metab* 58:1, 1984.

48. Clemmons DR, Underwood LE, Van Wyk JJ: Hormonal control of immunoreactive somatomedin production by cultured human fibroblasts. *J Clin Invest* 67:10, 1981.

49. Underwood LE, D'Ercole AJ, Van Wyk JJ: Somatomedin C and the assessment of growth. *Pediatr Clin North Am* 27:771, 1980.

50. Kemp SF, Rosenfeld RG, Liu F, Gaspich S, Hintz RL: Acute somatomedin response to growth hormone: Radioreceptor assay versus radioimmunoassay. *J Clin Endocrinol Metab* 52:616, 1981.

51. Van Vliet G, Styne DM, Kaplan SL, Grumbach MM: Growth hormone treatment for short stature. *N Engl J Med* 309:1016, 1983.

52. Plotnick LP, Van Meter QL, Kowarski AA: Human growth hormone treatment of children with growth failure and normal growth hormone levels by immunoassay: Lack of correlation with somatomedin generation. *Pediatrics* 71:324, 1983.

53. Clemmons DR, Klibanski A, Underwood LE, McArthur JW, Ridgway EC, Beitins IZ, Van Wyk JJ: Reduction of plasma somatomedin C during fasting in humans. *J Clin Endocrinol Metab* 53:1247, 1981.

54. Hintz RL, Suskind R, Amatayakul K, Thanagkul O, Olson R: Plasma somatomedin and growth hormone values in children with protein-calorie malnutrition. *J Pediatr* 92:153, 1978.

55. Chernausek SD, Underwood LE, Utiger RD, Van Wyk JJ: Growth hormone secretion and plasma somatomedin-C in primary hypothyroidism. *Clin Endocrinol* 19:337, 1983.

56. Clemmons DR, Underwood LE, Ridgway EC, Kliman B, Kjellberg RN, Van Wyk JJ: Estradiol treatment of acromegaly. *Am J Med* 69:571, 1980.

57. Ross JL, Cassorla FG, Skerda MC, Valk IM, Loriaux DL, Cutler GB: A preliminary study of the effect of estrogen dose on growth in Turner's syndrome. *N Engl J Med* 309:1104, 1983.

58. Parker MW, Johanson AJ, Rogol AD, Kaiser DL, Blizzard RM: Effect of testosterone on somatomedin-C concentrations in prepubertal boys. *J Clin Endocrinol Metab* 58:87, 1984.

59. Kilgore BS, McNah ML, Meadors S: Alterations of glycosaminoglycan protein acceptor by somatomedin and inhibition by cortisol. *Pediatr Res* 13:96, 1979.

60. Gourmelen M, Girard F, Binoux M: Serum somatomedin/insulin like growth factor (IGF) and IGF carrier levels in patients with Cushing's syndrome or receiving glucocorticoid therapy. *J Clin Endocrinol Metab* 54:884, 1982.

61. Phillips LS, Fusco AC, Unterman TG, del Greco F: Somatomedin inhibitor in uremia. *J Clin Endocrinol Metab* 59:764, 1984.

62. Cooke PS, Nicoll CS: Hormonal control of fetal growth. *Physiologist* 26:317, 1983.

63. Lovinger RD, Kaplan SL, Grumbach MM: Congenital hypopituitarism associated with neonatal hypoglycemia and microphallus: Four cases secondary to hypothalamic hormone deficiencies. *J Pediatr* 87:1171, 1975.

64. Blethen SL, White NH, Santiago JV, Daughaday WH: Plasma somatomedins, endogenous insulin secretion and growth in transient neonatal diabetes mellitus. *J Clin Endocrinol Metab* 52:144, 1981.

65. Susa JB, Widness JA, Hintz R, Liu F, Sehgal P, Schwartz R: Somatomedins and insulin in diabetic pregnancies: Effects of fetal macrosomia in the human and rhesus monkey. *J Clin Endocrinol Metab* 58:1099, 1984.

66. Francis MJO, Hill DJ: Prolactin-stimulated production of somatomedin by rat liver. *Nature* 255:167, 1975.

67. Hurley TW, D'Ercole AJ, Handwerger S: Ovine prolactin induces somatomedin: A possible role in fetal growth. *Endocrinology* 101:1635, 1977.

68. Furlanetto RW, Underwood LE, Van Wyk JJ, Handwerger S: Serum immunoreactive somatomedin C is elevated late in pregnancy. *J Clin Endocrinol Metab* 47:695, 1978.

69. Gluckman PD, Brinshead MW: Somatomedin in cord blood: Relationship to gestational age and birth size. *J Clin Endocrinol Metab* 43:1378, 1976.

70. Hill DJ, Davidson P, Milner RDG: Retention of plasma somatomedin activity in the fetal rabbit following decapitation in utero. *J Endocrinol* 81:93, 1979.

71. MacGillivray MH, Aceto T, Frohman LA: Plasma growth hormone response and growth retardation of hypothyroidism. *Am J Dis Child* 115:273, 1969.

72. Peake GT, Birge CA, Daughaday WH: Alterations of radioimmunoassayable growth hormone and prolactin during hypothyroidism. *Endocrinology* 92:487, 1973.

73. Mosier HD Jr: Thyroid hormone, in Daughaday WH (ed):

Endocrine Control of Growth. New York, Elsevier, 1981, p 25.
74. Hamburgh M, Lynn E, Weiss EP: Analysis of the influence of thyroid hormone on prenatal and postnatal maturation of the rat. *Anat Rec* 150:147, 1964.
75. Hopkins PS, Thorburn GD: The effects of foetal thyroidectomy on the development of the ovine foetus. *J Endocrinol* 54:55, 1972.
76. Kerr GK, Tyson IB, Allen JR, Wallace JH, Scheffler G: Deficiency of thyroid hormone and development of the fetal rhesus monkey. *Biol Neonate* 21:282, 1972.
77. Walker P, Weichsel ME, Fisher DA, Guo SM: Thyroxine increases nerve growth factor concentration in adult mouse brain. *Science* 204:427, 1979.
78. Reiter EO, Grumbach MM: Neuroendocrine control mechanisms and the onset of puberty. *Annu Rev Physiol* 44:595, 1982.
79. Ducharme JR, Collu R: Pubertal development: Normal, precocious and delayed. *Clin Endocrinol Metab* 11:57, 1982.
80. Ducharme JR, Forest MG, De Peretti E, Sempe M, Collu R, Bertrand J: Plasma adrenal and gonadal sex steroids in human pubertal development. *J Clin Endocrinol Metab* 42:468, 1976.
81. Grumbach MM, Roth JC, Kaplan SL, Kelch RP: Hypothalamic pituitary regulation of puberty: Evidence and concepts derived from clinical research, in Grumbach MM et al (eds): *The Control of the Onset of Puberty.* New York, Wiley, 1974, p 115.
82. Lee PA, Jaffe RB, Midgley AR Jr: Serum gonadotropin, testosterone and prolactin concentrations throughout puberty in boys. A longitudinal study. *J Clin Endocrinol Metab* 39:664, 1974.
83. Lee PA, Xenakis T, Winer J, Matsenbaugh S: Puberty in girls; correlation of serum levels of gonadotropins, prolactin, androgens, estrogens and progestins with physical changes. *J Clin Endocrinol Metab* 43:775, 1976.
84. Anderson DC: The adrenal androgen-stimulating hormone does not exist. *Lancet* 2:454, 1980.
85. Mainwaring WIP: The mechanism of action of androgens, in *Monographs on Endocrinology.* New York, Springer-Verlag, 1977, vol 10.
86. Kelch RP, Lindolm UB, Jaffe RB: Testosterone metabolism in target tissues: 2. Human fetal and adult reproductive tissues, perineal skin and skeletal muscle. *J Clin Endocrinol Metab* 32:449, 1971.
87. Peterson RE, Imperato-McGinley J, Gautier T, Sturla E: Male pseudohermaphroditism due to steroid 5α-reductase deficiency. *Am J Med* 62:170, 1977.
88. Martin LG, Clark JW, Conner TB: Growth hormone secretion enhanced by androgens. *J Clin Endocrinol Metab* 28:425, 1968.
89. Rosenfeld RG, Northcraft GB, Hintz RL: A prospective, randomized study of testosterone treatment of constitutional delay of growth and development in male adolescents. *Pediatrics* 69:681, 1982.
90. Marshall WA, Tanner JM: Puberty, in David JA, Dobbing J (eds): *Scientific Foundations of Paediatrics.* Philadelphia, Saunders, 1974.
91. Frisch RE, McArthur JW: Menstrual cycles: Fatness as a determinant of minimum weight for height necessary for their maintenance or onset. *Science* 185:949, 1974.
92. Walton A, Hammond J: The maternal effects of growth and conformation in shire-horse-Shetland pony crosses. *Proc R Soc London (Biol)* 125:311, 1938.
93. Smith DW: Growth and its disorders, in: *Major Problems in Clinical Pediatrics.* Philadelphia, Saunders, 1977, vol 15.
94. Forest MG: Plasma androgens in normal and premature newborns and infants: Evidence for maturation of the gonadostat's regulation. *Proceedings of the Fourteenth International Congress of Pediatrics.* Buenos Aires, 1974.
95. Tanner JM: *Growth at Adolescence,* 2d ed. Oxford, Blackwell, 1955.
96. Odell WD, Swerdloff RS: Etiologies of sexual maturation. A model system based on the sexually maturing rat. *Recent Prog Horm Res* 32:245, 1976.
97. Brasel JA, Blizzard RM: The influence of the endocrine glands upon growth and development, in Williams RH (ed): *Textbook of Endocrinology,* 5th ed. Philadelphia, Saunders, 1974, p 1030.
98. Smith DW: Recognizable patterns of human malformation, in: *Major Problems in Clinical Pediatrics,* 2d ed. Philadelphia, Saunders, 1976, vol 7.
99. Tanner JM, Whitehouse RH, Marshall WA, Carter BS: Prediction of adult height, from height, bone age, and occurrence of menarche at ages 4 to 16 with allowance for mid parent height. *Arch Dis Child* 50:14, 1975.
100. Greulich WW, Pyle SE: *Radiographic Atlas of Skeletal Development of the Hand and Wrist,* 2d ed. Stanford, Stanford University Press, 1959.
101. Bayley N, Pinneau S: Tables for predicting adult height from skeletal age. *J Pediatr* 40:432, 1952.
102. Rudman D, Kutner MH, Blackston RD, Cushman RA, Bain RP, Patterson JH: Children with normal-variant short stature: Treatment with human growth hormone for six months. *N Engl J Med* 305:123, 1981.
103. Van Vliet G, Styne DM, Kaplan SL, Grumbach MM: Growth hormone treatment for short stature. *N Engl J Med* 309:1016, 1983.
104. Gertner JM, Genel M, Granfredi SP, Hintz RL, Rosenfeld RG, Tamborlane WV, Wilson DM: Prospective clinical trial of human growth hormone in short children without growth hormone deficiency. *J Pediatr* 104:172, 1984.
105. Kowarski AA, Schneider J, Ben-Galim E, Weldon VV, Daughaday WH: Growth failure with normal serum RIA-GH and low somatomedin activity: Somatomedin restoration and growth acceleration after exogenous GH. *J Clin Endocrinol Metab* 47:461, 1978.
106. Spiliotis BE, August GP, Hung W, Sonis W, Mendelson W, Bercu BB: Growth hormone neurosecretory dysfunction. *JAMA* 251:2223, 1984.
107. Clarren SK, Smith DW: The fetal alcohol syndrome. *N Engl J Med* 298:1063, 1978.
107a. Streissguth AP, Harmon CS, Smith DW: Intelligence, behavior, and dysmorphogenesis in fetal alcohol syndrome: A report on 20 patients. *J Pediatr* 92:363, 1978.
108. Klein AH, Melner S, Kenny FM: Improved prognosis in congenital hypothyroidism treated before three months. *J Pediatr* 81:912, 1972.
109. Glorieux J, Dussault JH, Letarte J, Guyda H, Morissette J: Preliminary results on the mental development of hypothyroid infants detected by the Quebec Screening Program. *J Pediatr* 102:19, 1983.
109a. New England Congenital Hypothyroidism Collaborative: Characteristics of infantile hypothyroidism discovered on neonatal screening. *J Pediatr* 104:539, 1984.
110. Smith DW, Blizzard RM, Wilkins L: The mental prognosis in hypothyroidism of infancy and childhood. *Pediatrics* 19:1011, 1957.
111. Abbassi V, Aldige C: Evaluation of sodium L-thyroxine (T4) requirement in replacement therapy of hypothyroidism. *J Pediatr* 90:298, 1977.
112. Rezvani I, DiGeorge AM: Reassessment of the daily dose of oral thyroxine for replacement therapy in hypothyroid children. *J Pediatr* 90:291, 1977.
113. Schultz RM, Glassman MS, MacGillivray MH: Elevated threshold for thyrotropin suppression in congenital hypothyroidism. *Am J Dis Child* 134:19, 1980.
114. Sekadde CB, Slaunwhite WR Jr, Aceto T Jr, Murray KA: Administration of thyroxine once a week. *J Clin Endocrinol Metab* 39:759, 1974.
115. Vimpani GV, Vimpani AF, Lidgard GP, Cameron EHD, Farquhar JW: Prevalence of severe growth hormone deficiency. *Br Med J* 2:427, 1977.

116. Parkin JM: Incidence of growth hormone deficiency. *Arch Dis Child* 49:905, 1974.

117. Clopper RR, Mazur T, MacGillivray MH, Peterson RE, Voorhees ML: Data on virilization and erotosexual behavior in male hypopituitarism during gonadotropin and androgen treatment. *J Androl* 4:303, 1983.

118. Phillips JA III: The growth hormone (hGH) gene and human disease, in *Banbury Report 14: Recombinant DNA Applications to Human Disease.* Cold Spring Harbor, N.Y., Cold Spring Laboratory, 1983.

118a. Illig R, Prader A, Ferrandez A: Hereditary prenatal growth hormone deficiency with increased tendency to growth hormone antibody formation ("A-type" of isolated growth hormone deficiency). *Acta Paediatr Scand* 60:607, 1971.

119. Kaplan SL, Grumbach MM, Hoyt WF: A syndrome of hypopituitary dwarfism, hypoplasia of optic nerves and malformation of the prosencephalon. *Pediatr Res* 4:480, 1970.

120. Patel H, Tze WJ, Crichton JU, McCormick AQ, Robinson GC, Dolman CL: Optic nerve hypoplasia with hypopituitarism. *Am J Dis Child* 129:175, 1975.

121. Stewart C, Castro-Magana M, Sherman J, Angulo M, Collipp PJ: Septo-optic dysplasia and median cleft face syndrome in a patient with isolated growth hormone deficiency and hyperprolactinemia. *Am J Dis Child* 137:484, 1983.

122. Rudman D, Davis GT, Priest JH, Patterson JH, Kutner MH, Heymsfield SB, Bethel RA: Prevalence of growth hormone deficiency in children with cleft lip or palate. *J Pediatr* 93:378, 1978.

123. Berke JP, Buxton LF, Kokmen E: The empty sella. *Neurology* 25:1137, 1975.

124. Jordan RM, Kendall JW, Kerber CW: The primary empty sella syndrome: Analysis of the clinical characteristics, radiographic features, pituitary function and cerebrospinal fluid adenohypophysial hormone concentrations. *Am J Med* 62:569, 1977.

125. Onur K, Lala V, Zimmer J, Juan CS, AvRuskin TW: The primary empty sella syndrome in a child. *J Pediatr* 90:425, 1977.

126. Kleinmann RE, Kazarian EL, Raptopoulos V, Braverman LE: Primary empty sella and Rieger's anomaly of the anterior chamber of the eye. *N Engl J Med* 304:90, 1981.

127. Laron Z, Pertzelan A, Karp M, Kowaldo A, Daughaday WH: Administration of growth hormone to patients with familial dwarfism with high plasma immunoreactive growth hormone: Measurement of sulfation factor, metabolic and linear growth responses. *J Clin Endocrinol Metab* 33:332, 1971.

128. Golde DW, Bersch N, Kaplan SA, Rimoin DL, Li CH: Peripheral unresponsiveness to human growth hormone in Laron dwarfism. *N Engl J Med* 303:1156, 1980.

129. Merimee TJ, Zapf J, Froesch ER: Dwarfism in the pygmy. *N Engl J Med* 305:965, 1981.

130. Merimee TJ, Zapf J, Froesch ER: Insulin-like growth factors (IGFs) in pygmies and subjects with the pygmy trait: Characterization of the metabolic actions of IGF I and IGF II in man. *J Clin Endocrinol Metab* 55:1081, 1982.

130a. Bode H, Bailey RC, Underwood LE: Somatomedin C in EFE pygmy of the Ituri forest. *Pediatr Res* 20:211a, 1986.

131. Thomsett MJ, Conte FA, Kaplan SL, Grumbach MM: Endocrine and neurologic outcome in childhood craniopharyngioma. Review of effect of treatment in 42 patients. *J Pediatr* 97:728, 1980.

132. Clemmons DR, Underwood LE, Ridgway EC, Kliman B, Van Wyk JJ: Hyperprolactinemia is associated with increased immunoreactive somatomedin C in hypopituitarism. *J Clin Endocrinol Metab* 52:731, 1981.

133. Blethen SL, White NH, Santiago JV, Daughaday WH: Plasma somatomedins in children with hyperinsulinism. *J Clin Endocrinol Metab* 52:748, 1981.

134. Bucher J, Zapf J, Torresani T, Prader A, Froesch ER, Illig R: Insulin-like growth factors I and II, prolactin, and insulin in 19 growth homrone-deficient children with excessive, normal, or decreased longitudinal growth after operation for craniopharyngioma. *N Engl J Med* 309:1142, 1983.

135. Rona RJ, Tanner JM: Aetiology of idiopathic growth hormone deficiency in England and Wales. *Arch Dis Child* 52:197, 1977.

136. Craft WH, Underwood LE, Van Wyk JJ: High incidence of perinatal insult in children with idiopathic hypopituitarism. *J Pediatr* 96:397, 1980.

137. Del Pozo JM, Roda JE, Montoya JG, Iglesias JR, Hurtado A: Intrasellar granuloma. *J Neurosurg* 53:717, 1980.

138. Bottazzo GF, McIntosh C, Stanford W, Preece M: Growth hormone cell antibodies and partial growth hormone deficiency in a girl with Turner's syndrome. *Clin Endocrinol* 12:1, 1980.

139. Portocarrero CJ, Robinson AG, Taylor AL, Klein I: Lymphoid hypophysitis. *JAMA* 246:1811, 1981.

140. Asa SL, Bilbao JM, Kovacs K, Josse RG, Kreines K: Lymphocytic hypophysitis of pregnancy resulting in hypopituitarism: A distinct clincopathologic entity. *Ann Intern Med* 95:166, 1981.

141. Richards GE, Wara WM, Grumbach MM, Kaplan SL, Sheline GE, Conte FA: Delayed onset of hypopituitarism: Sequelae of therapeutic irradiation of central nervous system, eye and middle ear tumors. *J Pediatr* 89:553, 1976.

142. Samaan NA, Bakdash MM, Caderao JB, Cangir A, Jesse RH, Ballantyne AJ: Hypopituitarism after external irradiation: Evidence for both hypothalamic and pituitary origin. *Ann Intern Med* 83:771, 1975.

143. Duffner PK, Cohen ME, Anderson SW, Voorhees ML, MacGillivray MH, Panahon A, Brecher ML: Long-term effects of treatment on endocrine function in children with brain tumors. *Ann Neurol* 14:528, 1983.

144. Russell JD, Wise PH, Rischbieth HG: Vascular malformation of the hypothalamus: A cause of isolated growth hormone deficiency. *Pediatrics* 66:306, 1980.

145. Saenger P, Schwartz E, Markenson AL, Graziano JH, Levine LS, New MI, Hilgartner MW: Depressed serum somatomedin activity in beta-thalassemia. *J Pediatr* 96:214, 1980.

146. Costin G, Kogut MD, Hyman CB, Ortega JA: Endocrine abnormalities in thalassemia major. *Am J Dis Child* 133:497, 1979.

147. McIntosh N: Endocrinopathy in thalassaemia major. *Arch Dis Child* 51:195, 1976.

148. Braunstein GD, Kohler PO: Pituitary function in Hand-Schuller-Christian disease. Evidence for deficient growth hormone release in patients with short stature. *N Engl J Med* 286:1225, 1972.

148a. Underwood LE, Van Wyk JJ: Hormones in normal and aberrant growth, in Williams RH (ed): *Textbook of Endocrinology.* Philadelphia, Saunders, 1981, p 1177.

149. Penny R, Blizzard RM: The possible influence of puberty on the release of growth hormone in 3 males with apparent growth hormone deficiency. *J Clin Endocrinol Metab* 34:82, 1972.

150. Gourmelen M, Pham-Huu-Trung MT, Girard F: Transient partial hGH deficiency in prepubertal children with delay of growth. *Pediatr Res* 13:221, 1979.

151. Patton RG, Gardner LI: Influence of family environment on growth: The syndrome of "maternal deprivation." *Pediatrics* 30:957, 1962.

152. Powell GF, Brasel JA, Blizzard RM: Emotional deprivation and growth retardation simulating idiopathic hypopituitarism. I. Clinical evaluation of the syndrome. *N Engl J Med* 276:1271, 1967.

153. Powell GF, Brasel JA, Raiti S, Blizzard RM: Emotional deprivation and growth retardation simulating idiopathic hypopituitarism. II. Endocrinologic evaluation of the syndrome. *N Engl J Med* 276:1279, 1967.

154. Krieger I, Mellinger RC: Pituitary function in the deprivation syndrome. *J Pediatr* 79:216, 1971.

155. Russo L, Moore WV: A comparison of subcutaneous and intramuscular administration of human growth hormone in the

therapy of growth hormone deficiency. *J Clin Endocrinol Metab* 82:103, 1982.

155a. Gibbs CJ Jr, Joy A, Heffner R, Franko M, Miyazaki M, Asher DM, Parisi JE, Brown PW, Gajdusek DC: Clinical and pathological features and laboratory confirmation of Creutzfeldt-Jakob disease in a recipient of pituitary-derived human growth hormone. *N Engl J Med* 313:734, 1985.

155b. Koch TK, Berg BO, De Armond SJ, Gravina RF: Creutzfeldt-Jakob disease in a young adult with idiopathic hypopituitarism. Possible relation to the administration of cadaveric human growth hormone. *New Engl J Med* 313:731, 1985.

155c. Powell-Jackson J, Kennedy P, Whitcombe EM, Weller RO, Preece MA, Newsom-Davis J: Creutzfeldt-Jakob disease after administration of human growth hormone. *Lancet* 3:244, 1985.

156. Raiti S, Trias E, Levitsky L, Grossman MS: Oxandrolone and human growth hormone. Comparison of growth stimulating effects in short children. *Am J Dis Child* 126:597, 1973.

157. MacGillivray MH, Kolotkin M, Munschauer RW: Enhanced linear growth responses in hypopituitary dwarfs treated with growth hormone plus androgen versus growth hormone alone. *Pediatr Res* 8:103, 1974.

158. Styne DM, Grumbach MM, Kaplan SL, Wilson CB, Conte FA: Treatment of Cushing's disease in childhood and adolescence by transsphenoidal microadenomectomy. *N Engl J Med* 310:899, 1984.

159. Jennings AS, Liddle GW, Orth DN: Results of treating childhood Cushing's disease with pituitary irradiation. *N Engl J Med* 297:957, 1977.

160. Rimoin DL: The chondrodystrophies. *Adv Hum Genet* 5:1, 1975.

161. Johanson AJ, Brasel JA, Blizzard RM: Growth in patients with gonadal dysgenesis receiving fluoxymesterone. *J Pediatr* 75:1015, 1969.

162. Urban MD, Lee PA, Dorst JP, Plotnick LP, Migeon CJ: Oxandrolone therapy in patients with Turner syndrome. *J Pediatr* 94:823, 1979.

163. Moore DC, Tattoni DS, Ruvalcava RHA, Limbeck GA, Kelly VC: Studies of anabolic steroids: Effects of prolonged administration of oxandrolone on growth in children and adolescents with gonadal dysgenesis. *J Pediatr* 90:462, 1977.

163a. Raiti S and the Committee on Growth Hormone Usage: Growth stimulating effects of human growth hormone therapy in Turner's syndrome, in Raiti S and Tolman RA (eds). New York, 1986, p 109.

163b. Rosenfeld RG, Hintz RL, Johanson AJ: One year results of recombinant methionyl human growth hormone and/or oxandrolone in Turner syndrome. *Pedia Res* 20:221a, 1986.

164. Collins E, Turner G: The Noonan syndrome—a review of the clinical and genetic features of 27 cases. *J Pediatr* 83:941, 1973.

165. Crawford JD: Excessively tall stature in adolescent girls, in Gellis S, Kagan B (eds): *Current Pediatric Therapy* 6. Philadelphia, Saunders, 1973, p 306.

166. Crawford JD: Treatment of tall girls with estrogens. *Pediatrics* 62:1189, 1978.

167. Zachman M, Ferrandez A, Murset G, Guehn HE, Prader A: Testosterone treatment of excessively tall boys. *J Pediatr* 88:116, 1976.

168. New MI, Levine LS: Congenital adrenal hyperplasia. *Pediatr Ann* 3:27, 1974.

169. Foster CM, Ross JL, Shawker T, Pescovitz OH, Loriaux DL, Cutler GB Jr, Comite F: Absence of pubertal gonadotropin secretion in girls with McCune Albright syndrome. *J Clin Endocrinol Metab* 58:1161, 1984.

170. Schedewie HK, Reiter EO, Beitins IZ, Seyed S, Wooten VD, Jimenez JF, Aiman EJ, DeVane GW, Redman JF, Elders MJ: Testicular Leydig cell hyperplasia as a cause of familial sexual precocity. *J Clin Endocrinol Metab* 52:271, 1981.

170a. Holland FJ, Fishman L, Bailey JD, Fazekas ATA: Ketoconazole in the management of precocious puberty not responsive to LHRH-analogue therapy. *N Engl J Med* 312:1023, 1985.

171. Winters JS, Faiman C, Reyes FI: Normal and abnormal pubertal development. *Clin Obstet Gynecol* 21:67, 1978.

172. Mansfield MJ, Beardsworth DE, Loughlen JS, Crawford JD, Bude HH, Rivier J, Vale W, Kushner DC, Crigler JF, Crowley WF: Long-term treatment of central precocious puberty with a long-acting analogue of luteinizing hormone-releasing hormone. *N Engl J Med* 309:1286, 1983.

173. MacGillivray MH: Treatment of idiopathic precocious puberty. *N Engl J Med* 306:1109, 1982.

174. Kauli R, Pertzelan R, Prager-Lewin R, Grunebaum M, Laron Z: Cyproterone acetate in treatment of precocious puberty. *Arch Dis Child* 51:202, 1976.

175. Solyom AE, Austad CC, Sherick I, Bacon GG: Precocious sexual development in girls: The emotional impact on the child and her parents. *J Pediatr Psychol* 5:385, 1980.

176. Spence HJ, Trias EP, Raiti S: Acromegaly in a 9½ year old boy. *Am J Dis Child* 123:504, 1972.

177. Melmed S, Ezrin C, Kovacs K, Goodman RS, Frohman LA: Acromegaly due to secretion of growth hormone by an ectopic pancreatic islet-cell tumor. *N Engl J Med* 312:9, 1985.

178. Plewe G, Krause U, Beyer J, Neufeld M: Long-acting and selective suppression of growth hormone secretion by somatostatin analogue SMS 201-995 in acromegaly. *Lancet* 2:782, 1984.

179. Schlesinger S, MacGillivray MH, Munschauer RW: Acceleration of growth and bone maturation in childhood thyrotoxicosis. *J Pediatr* 83:233, 1973.

180. Higurashi M, Iijima K, Ikeda Y, Egi S, Ohzeki T: Anthropometric study of cases with Turner's syndrome and XYY, in *Birth Defects: Original Article Series.* New York, Alan R. Liss, 1982, vol 18, p 155.

181. Watkin HA, Mednick LSA, Schulsinger F, Bakkestrom E, Christensen KO: Criminality in XYY and XXY men. *Science* 193:547, 1976.

182. Skovby F, McKusick VA: Estrogen treatment of tall stature in girls with Marfan's syndrome, in *Birth Defects: Original Article Series.* New York, Alan R. Liss, 1977, vol 13, p 155.

183. Sotos JF: Cerebral gigantism. *Am J Dis Child* 131:625, 1977.

184. Garn SM, Clark DC: Nutrition, growth, development and maturation. Findings from the ten state nutrition survey of 1968–70. *Pediatrics* 56:306, 1975.

185. Filippi G, McKusick VA: The Beckwith-Wiedemann syndrome. *Medicine* 49:279, 1970.

186. Senior B, Geillis SS: The syndrome of total lipodystrophy and of partial lipodystrophy. *Pediatrics* 33:593, 1964.

187. Tanner JM, Whitehouse RH, Takaishi M: Standards from birth to maturity for height, weight, height velocity and weight velocity. British children. *Arch Dis Child* 41:613, 1966.

188. Reiter EO, Fuldauer VG, Root AW: Secretion of adrenal androgen, dehydroepiandrosterone during normal infancy, childhood and adolescence in sick infants and in children with endocrinologic abnormalities. *J Pediatr* 90:766, 1977.

189. Penny R, Goldstein IP, Frasier SD: Overnight gonadotropin excretion in normal females. *J Clin Endocrinol* 44:780, 1977.

190. Penny R, Goldstein IP, Frasier SD: Overnight follicle stimulating hormone (FSH) and luteinizing hormone (LH) excretion in normal males. *J Clin Endocrinol* 43:1394, 1976.

Gastrointestinal Hormones and Carcinoid Tumors and Syndrome*

Guenther Boden
John J. Shelmet

Gastrointestinal hormones have had a long and varied history. At the end of the nineteenth century, Pavlov's opinion that the nervous system controls most bodily activities, including gastrointestinal functions, dominated the thinking of most physiologists. The discovery of secretin in 1902 by Bayliss and Starling destroyed the concept of exclusive nervous control over gastrointestinal functions. More importantly, Bayliss and Starling recognized that they had discovered a system of chemical coordination of bodily functions. Secretin and the previously discovered adrenaline (epinephrine) and renin were substances produced in one organ and carried by the blood to distant targets where they exerted their effects. They could thus be considered chemical messengers.[1] The name *hormone* (from the Greek verb meaning "to set in motion") was proposed by W.B. Hardy and adopted by Bayliss in 1905 to characterize this new concept.[2] Thus, the discovery of the first intestinal hormone may be viewed as the beginning of endocrinology. During the years following the discovery of secretin, gastrointestinal hormones attracted a great deal of scientific interest. Later on, however, they faded into oblivion while pituitary, pancreatic, thyroid, adrenal, and gonadal hormones captured the limelight. In recent years, however, gastrointestinal endocrinology has experienced a renaissance brought about by the availability of gut hormones in pure form, the discovery of many new hormonally active peptides in the gut, and the recognition that human disorders such as the Zollinger-Ellison, WDHA (Verner-Morrison), and somatostatinoma syndromes can be caused by excess production of gastrointestinal hormones.

*Supported by U.S. Public Health Service grants AM 19397, 5T32, AM 07162 and RR 349.

THE GUT AS AN ENDOCRINE ORGAN

The intestinal tract can be looked at as a large endocrine organ, containing many hormonally active peptides. Intestinal endocrine cells, like other endocrine cells, contain secretory granules. These can be discharged into adjacent blood vessels in response to stimuli delivered from luminal contents, from nerves, or through the blood. There are, however, important differences between the endocrine gut and other endocrine organs. Endocrine cells in the intestinal tract do not occur as clusters of cells forming separate organs. Instead, single endocrine cells are dispersed among other mucosal cells, forming what has been called a *diffuse endocrine system.* This arrangement can be rationalized teleologically. Gastrointestinal endocrine cells are primarily concerned with detecting and reacting to substrates or hydrogen ions. This cannot be accomplished by detecting substrate concentrations at a single location because of their uneven distribution in the gut. The intestinal endocrine system, with its wide distribution of sensory-secretory cells, is uniquely qualified to sense and react to the total amount of food to be digested and absorbed.

Several of the gastrointestinal hormones are also found outside the gastrointestinal tract, notably in the central and peripheral nervous systems, where they may have neurotransmitter, neuroendocrine, and perhaps paracrine actions in addition to their endocrine activities (Table 27-1). The scattering of endocrine cells throughout the entire gastrointestinal (GI) tract and their occurrence outside the GI tract has made it impossible to apply the classical endocrine approach to the study of hormonal actions, i.e., to create hormonal deficiency by ablation of the endocrine organ under study. It is equally difficult for complete loss of GI hormones to occur on the basis of a disease process. Consequently, no deficiency states are known for any of the gastrointestinal hormones. This has made it

Table 27-1. Modes of Actions of Gastrointestinal Peptides

Endocrine (established)	Peptide secreted into the blood from specific endocrine cells exerting biologic actions on distant target cells
Paracrine (hypothetical)	Peptide secreted into the interstitial space by specific endocrine cells exerting biologic effects on contiguous target cells
Neuroendocrine (hypothetical)	Peptide secreted into the blood by nerve cells or endings exerting biologic actions on distant target cells
Neurotransmission or modulation (hypothetical)	Peptide released from nerve endings into the synaptosomal space exerting biologic actions on nearby neurons

difficult to establish physiological roles for many intestinal hormones.

The number of currently known gut hormones and hormone-like peptides has grown confusingly large. In order to keep the following discussion as simple and as pertinent as possible, emphasis will be placed on human data and on hormonal actions of physiological or pathological relevance. Not discussed are peptides which have not been completely sequenced; those which, although present in the gastrointestinal tract, are not considered gastrointestinal hormones (glucagon, thyrotropin releasing hormone, enkephalin, etc.); and various biologic effects of crude gastrointestinal extracts (villikinin, enterocrinin, gastrone effects, etc.).

GUT HORMONES AND HORMONE-LIKE PEPTIDES

Gastrin

History

In 1905, Edkins found that intravenous infusion of extracts of gastric antral mucosa stimulated gastric acid secretion in anesthetized cats. He named the active principle *gastrin.*[3] In 1955, Zollinger and Ellison described what was later termed the *gastrinoma,* or *Zollinger-Ellison syndrome.* In 1964, Gregory and Tracy isolated and purified gastrin from hog antral mucosa. The amino acid sequence and complete synthesis of gastrin were reported by the same group in the same year. In 1968, McGuigan published the first radioimmunoassay for gastrin.

Chemistry and Structure-Activity Relationships

Human gastrin cDNA, derived by transcription of mRNA obtained from a gastrinoma, has been reported.[4] The coding region of the human gastrin mRNA consists of 303 nucleotides. The primary translation product contains 101 amino acids (molecular weight of 11,381). Cleavage at two pairs of basic amino acid residues (Arg-Arg and Lys-Lys) yields the two major forms of gastrin which are found in the circulation and in gastrin-producing tissues, namely, "big" gastrin (G34) and "little" gastrin (G17). Big gastrin (G34) (Table 27-2) is a straight-chain polypeptide containing 34 amino acids. It has a molecular weight of 3839. Little gastrin (G17) consists of the 17 carboxy-terminal amino acids of big gastrin and has a molecular weight of 2096. "Minigastrin" (G14), one of several minor forms, consists of the 14 carboxy-terminal amino acids of big gastrin. These forms have all been chemically characterized. All occur in sulfated and nonsulfated forms. For instance, gastrin II (G17-II) is little gastrin (G17) sulfated at the tyrosine residue, and gastrin I (G17-I) is the nonsulfated G17. Approximately 50 percent of G17 is sulfated. Sulfation of gastrins does not appear to affect biologic activity, which is confined to the carboxy-terminal end of the molecule. Equivalent blood concentrations of human big gastrin (hG34) and of human little gastrin and minigastrin (hG17 and hG14) have comparable potencies with respect to stimulation of gastric acid secretion.[3,5] The carboxy-terminal tetrapeptide (Trp-Met-Asp-Phe-NH_2) is one-sixth as bioactive as G17 on a molar basis. Pentagastrin, which consists of the carboxy-terminal tetrapeptide plus β-alanine and an amino-terminal blocking group, also has about one-sixth the bioactivity of G17. In addition, there are larger forms of gastrin ("big-big" gastrin) which have not been chemically or biologically characterized.

Distribution

Gastrin is produced by the G cells in the gastric antrum and the duodenum. The concentration of G cells is greater in the antrum than in the duodenum (Fig. 27-1). However, because of the large duodenal mass in humans, substantial amounts of gastrin are released from the duodenum. Therefore, gastrin responses to feeding are not eliminated after antrectomy. Gastrin released from the duodenum has been

Table 27-2. Sequences of Gastrin and Gastrin-Related Peptides

Gastrin 34, human (mol wt 3839)	Pyroglu-Leu-Gly-Pro-Gln-Gly-His-Pro-Ser-Leu-Val-Ala-Asp-Pro-Ser-Lys-Lys-Gln-Gly-Pro-Trp-Leu-Glu-Glu-Glu-Glu-Glu-Ala-Tyr-Gly-Trp-Met-Asp-Phe-NH_2
Gastrin 17-I, human (mol wt 2096)	Pyroglu-Gly-Pro-Trp-Leu-Glu-Glu-Glu-Glu-Glu-Ala-Tyr-Gly-Trp-Met-Asp-Phe-NH_2
Gastrin 14-I, human (mol wt 1759)	Trp-Leu-Glu-Glu-Glu-Glu-Glu-Ala-Tyr-Gly-Trp-Met-Asp-Phe-NH_2
Pentagastrin	t-Boc-B-Ala-Trp-Met-Asp-Phe-NH_2
CCK 33, human (mol wt 3918)	Lys-Ala-Pro-Ser-Gly-Arg-Val-Ser-Met-Ile-Lys-Asn-Leu-Gln-Ser-Leu-Asp-Pro-Ser-His-Arg-Ile-Ser-Asp-Arg-Asp-Tyr(SO_3H)-Met-Gly-Trp-Met-Asp-Phe-NH_2
Caerulein (mol wt 1352)	Pyroglu-Glu-Asp-Tyr(SO_3H)-Thr-Gly-Trp-Met-Asp-Phe-NH_2

Note: Identical amino acid sequences are boxed.

reported to consist predominantly of G34.[6] Microscopically, the G cells are pearlike structures with secretory granules at the base and microvilli at the mucosal surface. The microvilli are possible sensors of stimulatory and inhibitory impulses (Fig. 27-2). Small amounts of immunoreactive gastrin have also been found in the pituitary gland and in vagal nerves.[7] The quantitative contribution of central nervous system gastrin to circulating gastrin is probably negligible. Its function is probably that of a local neurotransmitter.

Measurement

Sensitive and specific radioimmunoassays for gastrin are commercially available. Normal values range from 20 to 200 pg/ml and vary with the affinities of different antisera for the various molecular forms of gastrin. Radioimmunological measurements of gastrin do not always correlate well with bioactivity. The reason may be that antisera recognize several heterogeneous forms of gastrin, some of which are bioactive (G17, G34, and G14) while others may not be (big-big gastrin, amino-terminal G13, deaminated gastrins). Under most circumstances, however, use of an antiserum which recognizes the carboxy-terminal end of the gastrin molecule and measures the two major equipotent forms (G34 and G17) equally will produce values reflecting acid stimulatory activity.[5]

Release

Protein-containing meals and large peptides are well-established stimuli for gastrin release in humans. Among amino acids, phenylalanine and tryptophan are potent releasers of gastrin when given intragastri-

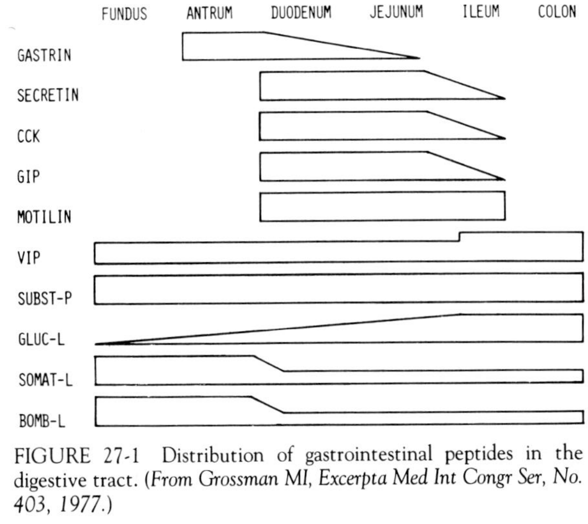

FIGURE 27-1 Distribution of gastrointestinal peptides in the digestive tract. (*From Grossman MI, Excerpta Med Int Congr Ser, No. 403, 1977.*)

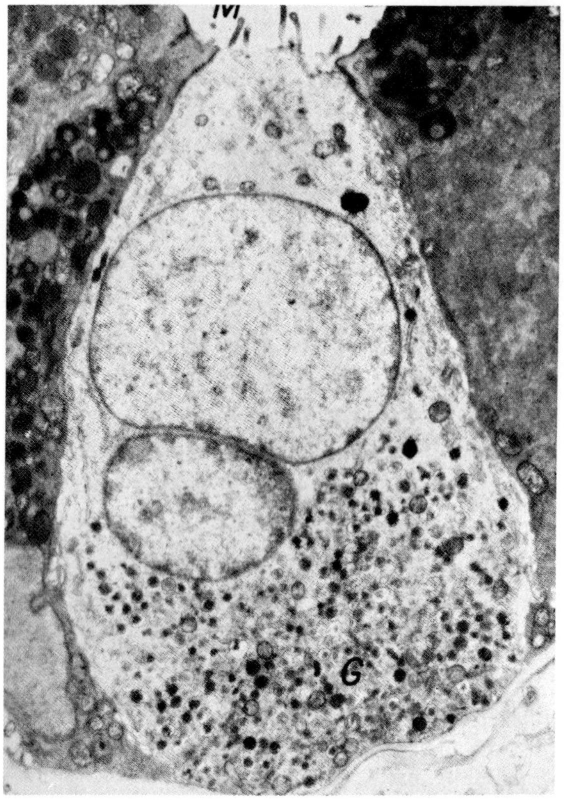

FIGURE 27-2 Electron micrograph of a single human G cell, demonstrating basal storage granules (G) and microvillous (M) structures at the luminal surface. (*From Walsh JH, Grossman MI, N Engl J Med 292:1324, 1975.*)

cally, while others, including glycine, alanine, serine, and arginine, are only weak stimulants. Casein hydrolysate, a mixture of amino acids, has approximately 60 percent of the gastrin-releasing activity of a meat meal. Water extracts of cooked or partially hydrolyzed protein are potent gastrin releasers. It is doubtful whether their activities are fully explained by their amino acid and peptide content, as dietary amines such as ammonia, methylamine, and ethylamine, which can be generated by hydrolysis from dietary proteins, can also release gastrin.[8] Nonprotein food and caffeine have little or no effect on gastrin release. Beer and wine, but not whiskey and ethanol, have been reported to stimulate gastrin release.[9]

Hypercalcemia appears to enhance gastrin release only if associated with hyperparathyroidism, particularly in patients who also have a gastrinoma. Vagal (cholinergic) impulses release gastrin in dogs. In humans, the effects of cholinergic stimulation are less clear. On one hand, sham feeding increases gastrin release, but this effect cannot be suppressed consistently with atropine. Doses of atropine too low to affect gastric emptying have been shown to decrease gastrin release, suggesting that cholinergic mechanisms may facilitate meal-stimulated gastrin release.[10] On the other hand, selective proximal vagotomy increases food-stimulated gastrin release; and atropine, instead of inhibiting, increases gastrin release after insulin-induced hypoglycemia. On the basis of animal experiments, it has been suggested that atropine-sensitive cholinergic neurons stimulate gastrin release indirectly by inhibiting the release of somatostatin and that noncholinergic atropine-insensitive neurons stimulate gastrin release via unidentified mediators (possibly bombesin-like substances).[11] Adrenergic impulses (catecholamines) have been proposed as gastrin releasers during insulin-induced hypoglycemia. Patients with pheochromocytomas secreting excessive amounts of epinephrine have been reported to have increased basal and meal-stimulated gastrin concentrations which decreased after tumor resection.[12] Gastric distention stimulates gastric acid secretion, but its effect on gastrin release in humans is uncertain. It has recently been found that large amounts of gastrin (G17) are secreted intraluminally into the gastric juice. The function of this luminal gastrin, however, remains unknown.

Inhibition of Release

At a gastric pH of less than 1, gastrin release in response to all stimuli is maximally inhibited. At a gastric pH of 2.5, the inhibition is still about 80 percent. Acid or alkali per se, however, has little or no acute effects on unstimulated gastrin levels; they only potentiate or attenuate gastrin responses to other stimuli. In contrast, long-term hypoacidity (achlorhydria, pernicious anemia) causes antral G cell hyperplasia associated with increased basal and stimulated gastrin release. Acidification sharply decreases the elevated gastrin concentrations in these conditions. Oral administration of therapeutic doses of lithium and infusion of somatostatin, secretin, glucagon, or prostaglandin E suppress gastrin release. The physiological significance of these inhibitors, however, has not been established.

Actions

The only actions of gastrin seen with blood levels such as occur after a meal are stimulation of gastric acid and pepsin secretion and increase in gastric antral motility. Increased pepsin release, however, may be a result of stimulation of gastric acid secretion rather than of gastrin. Elevated levels of gastrin in patients with Zollinger-Ellison syndrome are frequently associated with marked hyperplasia of the gastric mucosa, and there is evidence suggesting that gastrin may exert important trophic actions on the intestinal mucosa. In addition, there is a long list of biologic actions of gastrin which are unlikely to have physiological significance. This list includes stimulation of water and electrolyte secretion from the stomach, pancreas, liver, and small intestine; stimulation of smooth muscle tone in the lower esophageal sphincter, stomach, gallbladder, and small intestine; stimulation of insulin release; inhibition of water, electrolyte, and glucose absorption in the small intestine; and inhibition of tone in pyloric muscle and the ileocecal sphincters.

Metabolism

The metabolic half-life of G17 in humans is estimated to be about 8 min; that of G34 is about 40 min. Big-big gastrin probably has an even longer half-life (90 min in dogs). The major sites of degradation are the kidneys, while the liver and the intestinal tract play minor roles. Concordantly, hypergastrinemia is found in nephrectomized patients and in patients with chronic renal failure.

Gastrin and Human Disease: Gastrinoma

Gastrinomas (Zollinger-Ellison syndrome) are non-beta-cell islet cell tumors which secrete excessive amounts of gastrin.[13] The peak incidence is during the fifth decade. Most gastrinomas are found in the pancreas; they rarely originate from the duodenal wall or from the stomach (about 10 percent of cases). They are frequently small (less than 1 cm) and multifocal (in over 80 percent of cases), and they metastasize early, particularly to the liver. The frequent occurrence of tubular and ductal structures in and around gastrinomas and other endocrine pancreatic tumors suggests that they originate from undifferentiated pancreatic cells. This hypothesis is supported by the finding that these tumors frequently produce several hormones. Histologically, gastrinomas resemble carcinoid tumors and other islet cell tumors, from which they are difficult to differentiate by light microscopy. Electron microscopy is usually of little diagnostic help, particularly in malignant tumors, where the shape and size of the secretory granules are commonly atypical. A more reliable method of identification is by extraction and measurement of gastrin from the tumor. The diagnosis of malignancy rests on the demonstration of infiltrative and metastatic growth rather than microscopic appearance.

SYMPTOMS AND SIGNS The hallmarks of the Zollinger-Ellison syndrome (ZES) are recurrent and intractable peptic ulcers and diarrhea (Table 27-3). The ulcers are caused by hypersecretion of gastric acid. More than 75 percent of them are located in or around the duodenal bulb. Distal ulcers are relatively rare, but if present, they are suggestive of the diagnosis. More than one-third of patients with gastrinoma have diarrhea and/or steatorrhea caused by delivery of excessive gastric acid into the lower gut. Other important diagnostic signs are the finding on x-ray of hypertrophic gastric folds and the dilution of barium by excessive gastric acid.

DIAGNOSIS The diagnosis should be considered in all patients with duodenal ulcer, since the symptoms caused by gastrinomas and by ordinary duodenal ulcers may be indistinguishable. More specific clues to the presence of a gastrinoma are (1) duodenal ulcer associated with diarrhea (which is uncommon in ordinary peptic ulcer disease), (2) ulcer recurring after vagotomy or gastric resection, (3) a family history of peptic ulcer, or (4) a history of pancreatic, parathyroid, or pituitary endocrine tumor in ulcer patients or their relatives (multiple endocrine adenomatosis type 1, or MEA-1). It has been reported that about two-thirds of ZES patients have so-called sporadic gastrinomas, i.e., have no family history of peptic ulcer disease or MEA-1. The other one-third have some features of MEA, are frequently younger, and tend to have a more benign course.[14] If the presence of a gastrinoma is suspected, an upper gastrointestinal series and/or endoscopy, gastric analysis, and a serum gastrin measurement should be obtained. Suggestive findings on x-ray are multiple duodenal ulcers, ulcers in the distal duodenum or jejunum, and hypertrophic gastric folds. Gastric basal acid output is usually more than 15 meq/h, ($>$5 meq/h in patients who have had previous gastric surgery), and the ratio of basal/maximal acid output (BAO/MAO) is 0.6 or greater. However, because of considerable overlap in BAO and BAO/MAO between patients with peptic ulcer and those with gastrinoma, gastric analysis has not been very helpful to determine whether an ulcer patient has a gastrinoma.[15] In many institutions, gastric analysis is therefore no longer part of the initial workup. A basal gastrin concentration of more than 500 pg/ml in a patient with acid hypersecretion strongly suggests a

Table 27-3. Summary of Diagnosis and Therapy of Gastrinoma

1. Clinical features
   a. Recurrent and/or therapy-resistant peptic ulcer, particularly if located in the distal duodenum or lower (but remember that 75 percent are found in the proximal duodenum, the typical location of ordinary duodenal ulcers)
   b. Diarrhea and/or steatorrhea
   c. Hypertrophic gastric mucosal folds
   d. Presence of parathyroid, pituitary, adrenal, or other islet cell tumors (MEA-I) in the patient or in relatives
2. Initial workup
   a. Upper GI series and/or endoscopy (positive if peptic ulcers or large gastric mucosal folds are demonstrated)
   b. Gastric analysis (positive if BAO $\geqq$ 15 meq/h, BAO/MAO $\geqq$ 0.6)
   c. Basal (overnight fasting) plasma gastrin level (positive if more than 250 pg/ml, highly suspicious if more than 500 pg/ml)
3. Provocative tests
   a. IV secretin test. After an overnight fast give two clinical units per kilogram of secretin (available from Kabi Group Inc. Greenwich, Conn.) as bolus intravenously. Take blood samples before and 2, 5, 10, 20, and 30 min after injection. The test is positive if gastrin concentration rises by 200 pg/ml or more within 30 min of secretin injection. False-negative but no false-positive results have been reported
4. Therapy
   a. Tumor resection (presently possible in less than 10 percent of cases)
   b. Histamine H_2 receptor blockers (cimetidine or ranitidine)
   c. Total gastrectomy (when medical therapy is unsatisfactory)
   d. Chemotherapy for metastatic tumors (combination therapy with streptozocin, 5-fluorouracil, and doxorubicin)

gastrinoma. Provocative testing is usually necessary if the basal serum gastrin concentration is normal or only moderately elevated (between 250 and 500 pg/ml) and gastrinoma is suspected. The preferred test is the secretin test (Fig. 27-3), in which two clinical units of secretin per kilogram of body weight is administered intravenously as a bolus. In normal subjects, there is either no change or a decrease in serum gastrin concentration in response to this procedure. In patients with gastrinoma, gastrin concentration increases by at least 200 pg/ml within 2 to 10 min (Table 27-3 and Fig. 27-3). Another useful but more cumbersome provocative test is the slow infusion of calcium gluconate (4 mg/kg hourly over a 3-h period). A positive response is a 400 pg/ml or greater increase of the serum gastrin concentration during the 3-h cal-

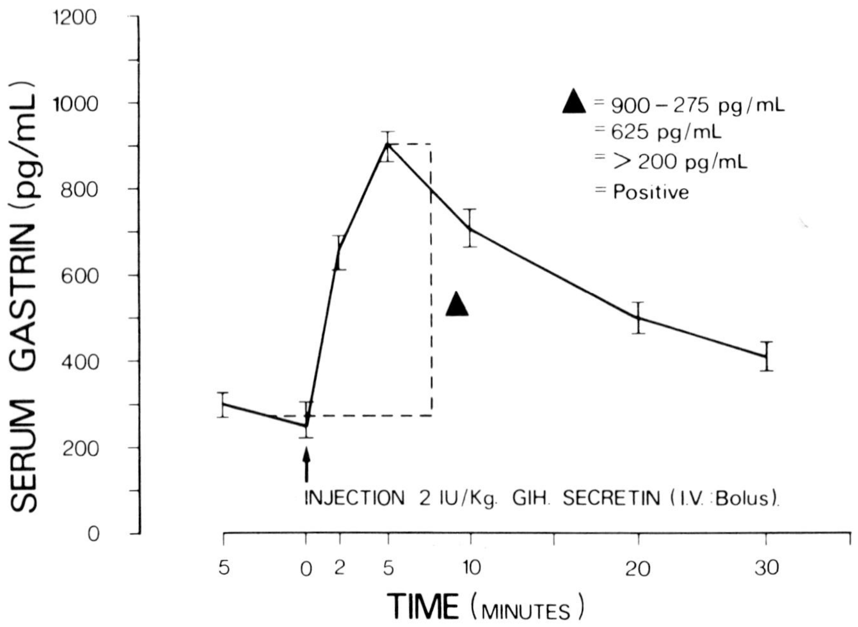

FIGURE 27-3 Gastrin response to IV secretin in a patient with ZES. The filled triangle ▲ indicates the peak change in concentration from basal. An increase of more than 200 pg/μl is considered positive. (*From McCarthy DM, Jensen RT: Hormone Producing Tumors of the Gastrointestinal Tract. New York, Churchill Livingston, p 30, 1985.*)

cium infusion. Both tests have been reported to have occasional false-negative and rarely false-positive results.

Once a gastrinoma has been diagnosed, precise localization of the tumor should be attempted. Visualization of gastrinomas is possible in less than half the cases by selective angiography (gastroduodenal and/or splenic artery), pancreatic computed axial tomography, or ultrasound studies. The detection rate may be higher when the three methods are combined, but this has not been established. Small tumor size (0.5 cm or less) is the main reason for the low detection rate. In some patients, transhepatic portal catheterization of the pancreatic veins with gastrin measurements has allowed localization of the gastrinoma and resection of the part of the pancreas containing the tumor. Recently, dynamic computed tomography (CT) scanning has been found to be a useful adjunct to routine angiographic and CT workup of patients with gastrinomas and other islet cell tumors.[16] Hepatic and bone scanning or ultrasound studies are useful to determine the presence of metastatic disease.

In the differential diagnosis of gastrinoma, the following conditions in which increased basal gastrin concentrations and increased basal acid output occur should be considered (Table 27-4):

1. Duodenal ulcer associated with moderately elevated gastrin levels and gastric acid output. The differentiation of these cases from gastrinomas depends on the demonstration of absence of abnormal serum gastrin increases after IV secretin or calcium.
2. Isolated retained antrum. This is a rare condition occurring in patients who have undergone a partial gastrectomy and gastroduodenostomy (Billroth II) but in whom part of the gastric antrum remains attached to the duodenal stump. The reason for the hypergastrinemia is the persistence, in the duodenal stump, of G cells which oversecrete gastrin because they are no longer under the inhibitory influence of gastric acid. The diagnosis of retained antrum can be verified by scanning with ^{99m}Tc-pertechnetate, which is concentrated in gastric tissue. In contrast to patients with gastrinoma, patients with retained antrum show a decrease in gastrin levels with IV secretin.
3. Gastric outlet obstruction is occasionally caused by duodenal ulcer and results in increased gastric acid secretion and hypergastrinemia. In this case, hypergastrinemia may be caused by chronic gastric distention. The presence of gastric outlet obstruction can be documented by a gastric emptying study. Gastric outlet obstruction, however, can be associated with gastrinoma. To exclude this possibility, it has been suggested that the effects of continuous gastric aspiration or pharmacological stimulation of gastric emptying on serum gastrin levels be assessed.
4. Renal insufficiency commonly results in moderate (200 to 300 pg/ml) increases in gastrin levels and is occasionally associated with increased gastric acid secretion and duodenal ulcer disease.
5. Antral G cell hyperplasia is a rare condition in which it has been postulated that the primary antral G cell hyperplasia causes elevated basal and postprandial gastrin levels and basal acid output and peptic ulcers. A negative secretin or calcium infusion test may help in differentiating this condition from gastrinoma.
6. Antral G cell hyperfunction is characterized by hypergastrinemia and an elevated basal acid output but a normal number of antral G cells. In some patients, it is associated with hyperpepsinogenemia I and autosomal dominant inheritance. A negative secretin test or a marked rise in serum gastrin after a test meal can help to differentiate this condition from gastrinoma.

Table 27-4. Conditions Associated with Hypergastrinemia

Conditions with hypergastrinemia and increased acid output:
Duodenal ulcer
Isolated retained antrum
Gastric outlet obstruction
Renal insufficiency
Antral G cell hyperplasia
Antral G cell hyperfunction
Conditions with hypergastrinemia and normal or low acid output:
Pernicious anemia
Atrophic gastritis without pernicious anemia
Gastric malignant disease (sparing the antrum)

Hypergastrinemia without peptic ulcer and associated with low or normal gastric acid output is commonly found in patients with pernicious anemia, atrophic gastritis without pernicious anemia, and gastric cancer in which the antral area is spared. The cause of the hypergastrinemia is chronic achlorhydria, which is common to all three conditions. If atrophic gastritis extends into the antral area, gastrin levels are usually not elevated. This is seen in approximately 25 percent of patients with pernicious anemia. Hypergastrinemia has also been reported in a few patients with pheochromocytoma. Gastrin levels returned to normal in these patients after phenoxybenzamine administration or after resection of the tumor. Some patients with rheumatoid arthritis and others with hyperthyroidism have high gastrin levels for unknown reasons.

THERAPY Significant changes have occurred in gastrinoma therapy during the past several years. Total gastrectomy is no longer the therapy of choice. Instead, it has been shown that the histamine H_2 receptor blocking agent cimetidine, alone or used in combination with either anticholinergic agents or highly selective vagotomy, can control pain, diarrhea, and gastric acid hypersecretion and allow healing of peptic ulcers. In some cases, progressively more cimetidine is needed for control of acid hypersecretion (from a starting dose of 2.4 to 6.0 g per day and more). Aside from mild and transient liver dysfunction, the most serious side effects observed with cimetidine have been impotence, gynecomastia, and breast tenderness occurring in male patients. Ranitidine, a newer H_2 antagonist, appears to be free of these adverse effects and is probably the drug of choice in male patients. Omeprazole, a new benzimidazole inhibitor of gastric acid secretion currently undergoing clinical trials, has been shown to be effective in patients whose peptic ulcer disease is relatively resistant to treatment with H_2 receptor antagonists.[17]

Total gastrectomy is still needed for those patients (10 percent or less) in whom drug therapy is unsatisfactory because of noncompliance or insufficient suppression of gastric acid. It can be expected that the number of patients requiring total gastrectomy will decline further as more efficient and longer-acting drugs become available.

Medical therapy, however, does not eliminate the tumor, which, although usually slow-growing, is frequently malignant and can eventually cause death. In one large study, overall survival after total gastrectomy was 55 percent after 5 years and 42 percent after 10 years, indicating that a large number of patients will eventually die from their tumors. Presently available data suggest that curative surgery is possible in less than 10 percent of cases. Presence of metastatic disease at the time of diagnosis, multiple tumors, tumors inoperable because of location (e.g., head of pancreas), and technical difficulties with enucleation of tumors were the main reasons. However, surgical therapy of gastrinoma is continually evolving and the disease is now detected earlier. As a result, it is hoped that in the future the rate of surgical cures will increase. At the present time it appears reasonable to recommend surgical exploration for all patients with gastrinoma who have no serious medical contraindications to major surgery and in whom preoperative workup, including angiography, CT scans, ultrasound studies, liver-spleen scans, and endoscopy, have failed to reveal metastatic disease. Tumors located near the head of the pancreas should not be operated on because they require total pancreatectomy, duodenectomy, splenectomy, and hemigastrectomy with reconstruction of the bile duct (Whipple procedure), which frequently has a worse prognosis than untreated gastrinoma.

Chemotherapy for metastatic gastrinoma remains problematic, because the drugs used (streptozocin, 5-fluorouracil, and doxorubicin) are only modestly effective and rather toxic. On the other hand, some patients have lived for several decades with untreated metastatic gastrinoma. A reasonable approach to this problem is to use chemotherapy combining all three agents in only those patients with proven metastatic disease and evidence of rapidly progressing tumor size.

Cholecystokinin

History

Since the middle of the nineteenth century, it had been known that HCl, fatty acids, and soaps introduced into the stomach or the duodenum are potent stimuli for bile secretion. However, it was not until 1928 that Ivy and coworkers provided proof that a humoral substance different from secretin caused emptying of the gallbladder. They named this substance *cholecystokinin* (CCK).[3,18] Recently, it has become apparent that the enzyme-releasing activity of duodenal extracts, which had been named *pancreozymin* by Harper and Raper in 1943, is also caused by cholecystokinin.

Chemistry and Structure-Function Relationships

The amino acid sequence of porcine cholecystokinin was elucidated by Mutt and Jorpes in 1971. Cholecystokinin contains 33 amino acid residues and has a molecular weight of 3918. The tyrosine residue in position 27 is sulfated. The sulfate group appears to be essential for the biologic activity of the molecule. Mutt and Jorpes also isolated and purified another CCK containing 39 amino acids. This larger form consists of the 33-amino acid CCK enlarged on the amino terminus by a hexapeptide (Tyr-Ile-Glu-Glu-Ala-Arg). Both forms are equally bioactive. Subsequently, additional molecular forms, including the carboxy-terminal octo- and tetrapeptide (CCK 8 and CCK 4, respectively) of CCK have been identified. CCK 8 has been found to be a major CCK component in intestinal mucosa, brain, and plasma extracts. A large CCK molecule (CCK 58), which may be a CCK precursor, has been isolated from dog brain and intestines. The carboxy-terminal pentapeptide of CCK is identical with that of gastrin and caerulein (Table 27-2). The last is a polypeptide extracted from the skin of the Australian bullfrog.

The determinants for bioactivity are located in the carboxy-terminal end of the CCK molecule. Interestingly, CCK 8 is two to ten times more bioactive and CCK 10 about 10 to 15 times more bioactive than CCK 33.

Measurement

CCK has been determined by bioassay, using the contracting effect of this hormone on the gallbladder or on isolated strips of gallbladder musculature. These assays are not sensitive enough to detect CCK in biologic fluids. Recently, a very sensitive bioassay has been described which is based on the ability of CCK to stimulate amylase release from isolated rat pancreas.[18a] Radioimmunological methods for CCK have been reported by several laboratories. They suffer, however, from several problems. First, iodination of CCK with chloramine-T results in sulfoxidation of methionine and loss of immunoreactivity. Second, antibodies directed against the carboxy terminal of CCK cross-react heavily with gastrin because both peptides have identical COOH-terminal sequences. On the other hand, antibodies directed against the NH_2 terminal do not recognize the smaller but bioactive forms CCK 4 and CCK 8. To circumvent these problems, Walsh et al. fractionated plasma CCK with high-performance liquid chromatography and measured CCK in individual elution fractions with two antibodies, one of which detected gastrin and CCK equally while the other was specific for gastrin.[19] CCK was obtained by subtraction.

Distribution

CCK has been found in the mucosa of the small intestine, mostly in the duodenum and the proximal jejunum (Fig. 27-1). There, it is secreted from endocrine cells (I cells). In addition, significant amounts of CCK have been found in brain tissues, with the highest concentrations occurring in the cortex and striatum. The major form of CCK in rat brain appears to be sulfated CCK 8. The cerebral CCK is localized in neurons. It has been suggested that it may act as neurotransmitter and/or modulator.

Release

It has been reported that unstimulated CCK concentration in human plasma, measured with a sensitive bioassay, was about 1 pmol and rose about sixfold after a liquid mixed meal and after oral ingestion of fat, amino acids, and, to a lesser extent, glucose (Fig. 27-4).[18a] Infusions of CCK 8, resulting in plasma concentrations similar to those seen after a meal, were associated with gallbladder contraction.

Measured by radioimmunoassay, CCK concentrations were usually less than 0.2 pmol per liter after an overnight fast and rose severalfold after a meal.[19] About two-thirds of the CCK immunoreactivity consisted of material eluting together with CCK 8. Moreover, postprandial CCK levels were lower than those required to stimulate pancreatic enzyme release. This suggested that CCK alone could not stimulate pancreatic enzyme secretions and that the CCK effect was potentiated either by other hormones or by neural influences. However, a different group, using a COOH-terminal specific antiserum with minimal cross-reactivity with gastrin reported that the amount of CCK released after a meal was sufficient to account for postprandial pancreatic trypsin secretion.[19a] Thus, the question as to whether CCK is the only or the major regulator of pancreatic enzyme secretion and gallbladder contraction has not been settled unequivocally.

Actions

Effects of CCK which are probably of physiological significance are contraction of the gallbladder and stimulation of pancreatic enzyme secretion. Other actions that can be achieved with comparable doses of CCK are inhibition of gastric emptying and potentiation of the bicarbonate-secretory action of secretin. In addition, CCK may inhibit gastric acid secretion after a meal (enterogastrone effect).[20] It is also of interest that CCK 33 is at least as potent as GIP in potentiating glucose or amino acid–stimulated insulin release (incretin effect).[21] Moreover, there is increasing evidence suggesting that postprandial release of CCK represents an intestinal satiety signal and that deficient CCK release may result in overfeeding and obesity. The evidence for this, however, is not conclusive. CCK administered systemically has also been shown to antagonize opiate analgesia.[22]

Clinical Use

CCK or its carboxy-terminal octapeptide is occasionally administered by gastroenterologists together with secretin as a pancreatic function test. It has been used by radiologists to accelerate intestinal transit time and to contract the gallbladder and by gastrointestinal surgeons for the treatment of postsurgical ileus.

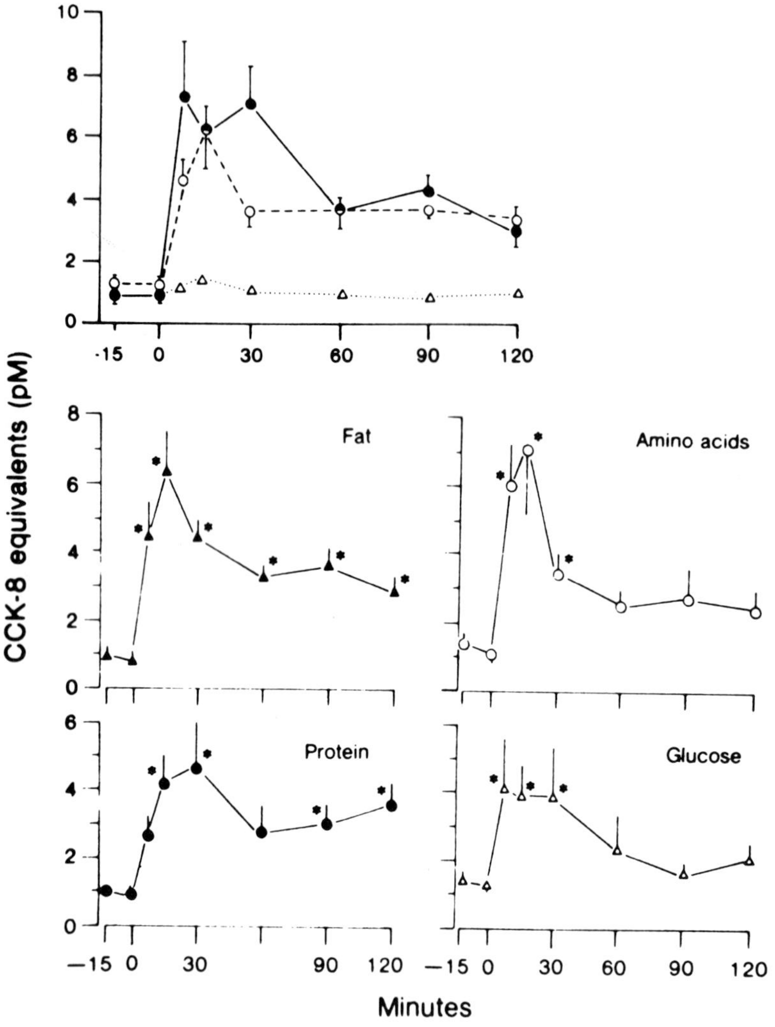

FIGURE 27-4 (*Upper panel*) Plasma CCK responses to feeding of saline (△) or a mixed liquid meal to overnight-fasted normal male (●) and female (○) subjects. (*Lower four panels*) Plasma CCK responses to feeding of 100 g of fat (corn oil), protein (casein), mixed amino acids, or glucose to normal subjects. Asterisks denote statistically significant increments in CCK concentrations. (*From Liddle et al.*[18a])

Vasoactive Intestinal Polypeptide

History and Chemistry

Vasodilatory actions of crude gut extracts prompted Said and Mutt in 1970 to isolate a vasoactive substance from hog intestinal mucosa which they named *vasoactive intestinal polypeptide* (VIP).[3,23]

Human VIP has been found to be identical to porcine and bovine VIP. It is a highly basic 28-amino acid polypeptide with a molecular weight of 3326 which has been completely synthesized. VIP has many amino acid homologies with glucagon, secretin, and gastric inhibitory polypeptide (GIP) (Table 27-5). A precursor molecule with a molecular weight of 17,500 (pro-VIP) and the primary translation product of the mRNA for VIP with a molecular weight of 20,000 (prepro-VIP) have been identified.

Measurement and Distribution

VIP can be measured by sensitive and specific radioimmunoassays. A bioassay for VIP is based on the ability of this hormone to relax isolated nonvascular smooth muscle.

It was originally believed that VIP occurred in endocrine cells (H cells) throughout the entire gastrointestinal tract from the lower esophagus to the rectum as well as in the brain and in peripheral nervous tissues. Recent immunohistochemical and radioimmunoassay studies with COOH-terminal specific antibodies against VIP suggest that VIP is localized exclusively in nerve fibers and nerve cells. The highest VIP concentrations in brain were in the cerebral cortex, hypothalamus, amygdaloid nucleus, and corpus striatum. In these locations, immunocytochemical techniques showed VIP immunofluorescence in nerve

Table 27-5. Sequences of VIP, Secretin, Glucagon, and GIP

VIP (porcine) 28AA (mol wt 3326)	His-Ser-Asp-Ala-Val-Phe-Thr-Asp-Asn-Tyr-Thr-Arg-Leu-Arg-Lys-Gln-Met-Ala-Val-Lys-Lys-Tyr-Leu-Asn-Ser-Ile-Leu-Asn-NH_2
Secretin (porcine) 27 AA (mol wt 3055)	His-Ser-Asp-Gly-Thr-Phe-Thr-Ser-Glu-Leu-Ser-Arg-Leu-Arg-Asp-Ser-Ala-Arg-Leu-Gln-Arg-Leu-Leu-Gln-Gly-Leu-Val-NH_2
Glucagon (porcine) 29 AA (mol wt 3484)	His-Ser-Gln-Gly-Thr-Phe-Thr-Ser-Asp-Tyr-Ser-Lys-Tyr-Leu-Asp-Ser-Arg-Arg-Ala-Gln-Asp-Phe-Val-Gly-Trp-Leu-Met-Asp-Thr-NH_2
GIP (porcine) 43 AA (mol wt 5104)	Try-Ala-Glu-Gly-Thr-Phe-Ile-Ser-Asp-Tyr-Ser-Ile-Ala-Met-Asp-Lys-Ile-Arg-Gln-Gln-Asp-Phe-Val-Asn-Trp-Leu-Leu-Ala-Gln-Gln-Lys-Gly-Lys-Lys-Ser-Asp-Trp-Lys-His-Asn-Ile-Thr-Gln-NH_2

terminals and neurons. Subcellular fractionation of cerebral cortex, hypothalamus, or striatum revealed that synaptosomal fractions (isolated presynaptic nerve terminals) of these tissues contained the highest VIP levels. VIP was also found in the peripheral autonomic nervous system, especially in the superior and inferior mesenteric ganglia and the submucosal (Meissner's) and myenteric (Auerbach's) plexus of the intestinal wall, in cerebrovascular nerves, and in nerves of female and male genital organs. The latter observation suggests that VIP may play a physiological role in promoting blood flow to male and female reproductive organs. Other organs containing VIP include the heart, lungs, eyes, kidneys, skin, blood, and lymphatic vessels, as well as chromaffin granules of the adrenal medulla.

Release and Metabolism

VIP circulates in human plasma in low concentrations (usually less than 10 pg/ml). Its concentration does not rise after a meal. Release of VIP has been reported in pigs upon electrical stimulation of the vagus and in dogs upon intraduodenal administration of hypertonic saline, phenylalanine, or dilute HCl and following intravenous infusions of calcium gluconate. Increases in VIP have been reported in humans after intraduodenal administration of HCl, fat, and ethanol. Work in pigs suggests that VIP release is a consequence of activation of postganglionic vagal fibers and can be inhibited by α-adrenergic impulses.

VIP has been found to bind to specific binding sites (receptors) in the CNS, the GI tract, and many other organs. In enterocytes from rabbit ileum and rat jejunum these receptors were located in the basolateral (contraluminal) wall. Binding of VIP is followed by activation of adenylate cyclase and intracellular accumulation of cAMP.

VIP is rapidly cleared from the circulation (with a half-life of approximately 1 min); the liver appears to be a major degrading site.

Actions

A physiological role for VIP has not been established. The peptide may have important functions as a local or paracrine hormone and as a mediator/modulator of blood flow, smooth muscle relaxation, and exocrine secretions. Actions of VIP achieved with supraphysiological doses are diverse. It is a potent vasodilator, an action which led to its discovery. Like secretin, VIP stimulates pancreatic bicarbonate and water secretion. In birds, VIP is a more potent pancreatic secretagogue than secretin. Like glucagon, VIP stimulates glycogenolysis, resulting in hyperglycemia; like GIP, it stimulates release of insulin and inhibits gastric acid secretion. VIP also stimulates small intestinal water and electrolyte secretion, an action important for its pathogenetic role in the WDHA syndrome (see below).

VIP in Human Disease

VIP EXCESS: WDHA SYNDROME Plasma VIP concentrations are elevated in many patients with the watery diarrhea-hypokalemia-achlorhydria (WDHA) syndrome (also called *Verner-Morrison syndrome* or *pancreatic cholera;* Table 27-6).[24-26] This syndrome is characterized by chronic profuse watery diarrhea leading to dehydration and hypokalemia. During attacks, daily fecal losses may exceed 6 to 10 liters of water and 200 to 400 meq of potassium. Plasma potassium levels frequently decrease to values below 2 meq per liter, and massive intravenous infusions of potassium may be required. Fecal losses of bicarbonate frequently lead to metabolic acidosis. Azotemia results from dehydration and hypokalemic nephropathy. About half the patients with WDHA syndrome have diminished glucose tolerance. Some have overt fasting hyperglycemia. The reason for the glucose intolerance has not been established. Possible causes are the adverse effects of hypokalemia on glucose tolerance and the glycogenolytic effect of elevated VIP levels. Normalization of glucose tolerance has been reported in patients after successful tumor resection. Hypercalcemia is present in about half the patients, but parathyroid adenomas are rarely found. Steathorrhea is rare. Gastric acid secretion is often suppressed in the presence of a normal number of gastric parietal cells. Occasionally it is only slightly suppressed or normal. In fact, most patients are hypochlorhydric, not achlorhydric as the name WDHA suggests. Absence of peptic ulcers and diminished or normal gastric acid secretion are important features which differentiate patients with WDHA syndrome from those with Zollinger-Ellison syndrome who have diarrhea. Less frequent features of this syndrome are hypotension and episodes of flushing and tetany. WDHA syndrome is occasionally part of the familial multiple endocrine adenomatosis syndrome (MEA-I).

The pathophysiological abnormality in this entity is markedly stimulated intestinal secretion. VIP and prostaglandins have been demonstrated to promote secretory diarrhea by inhibiting NaCl absorption and by stimulating chloride secretion throughout the intestinal tract via stimulation of adenylate cyclase activity in enterocytes.

There is strong evidence that VIP can cause the WDHA syndrome. First, many patients with this syndrome have tumors secreting excessive amounts of VIP, resulting in chronically elevated plasma VIP levels. Moreover, Kane et al. have produced profuse watery diarrhea and large fecal sodium and bicarbonate losses, resulting in hyperchloremic metabolic acidosis, in five out of five healthy volunteers, by infusing VIP and raising their plasma VIP concentrations to levels similar to those seen in patients with WDHA syndrome.[27] On the other hand, there is evidence that VIP is not the only mediator able to produce this syndrome. First, some patients have elevated plasma concentrations of other diarrheagenic substances together with normal or elevated VIP concentrations. For instance, some patients were reported to have elevated plasma and tumor concentrations of VIP and prostaglandin E_1 and E_2, while others had elevated prostaglandin but normal VIP levels.[28] Like VIP, prostaglandin E compounds can provoke the symptoms and signs of WDHA syndrome. In addition, serotonin can cause diarrhea, hypochlorhydria, and flushing. Lastly, plasma concentrations of PHI (peptide, histidine, and isoleucine), a 27-amino acid peptide sharing many sequence homologies with VIP,[29] have been reported elevated in 22 of 24 patients with VIP-secreting tumor.[30] Infused into normal volunteers, PHI induced secretion of chloride and sodium and stimulated water and potassium excretion. Therefore, it appears that the WDHA syndrome is a heterogeneous mix of diarrhea syndromes in which VIP, prostaglandin E, serotonin, PHI, and perhaps other substances may be involved alone or in combination.

The tumors associated with this syndrome are pancreatic islet cell tumors or islet cell hyperplasia in the majority, ganglioneuroblastomas and pheochromocytomas in some, and bronchogenic carcinoma in rare cases. About half the islet cell tumors found in these patients have been malignant.

The diagnosis of WDHA syndrome requires determination of stool electrolytes and volume. Secretory diarrhea in patients with WDHA syndrome is characterized by high volume (>1 liter per day) and isotonicity with plasma. In addition, stool cultures, x-ray studies of the upper and lower gastrointestinal tract, and proctosigmoidoscopy are needed to rule out infection, inflammation, and villous tumors of the colon (Table 27-6). Most importantly, chronic laxative and diuretic abuse has to be excluded. Sometimes laxative abuse can be demonstrated by alkalinizing the stool to a pH of greater than 10; red discoloration indicates the presence of phenolphthalein-containing laxatives. Selective angiography and CT scanning are helpful in identifying pancreatic and adrenal tumors. Demonstration of elevated (over 200 pg/ml) plasma VIP levels supports the diagnosis of a VIP-secreting tumor. Small bowel ischemia and severe shock can be associated with elevated VIP levels and have to be

Table 27-6. Summary of Diagnosis and Therapy of WDHA Syndrome

1. Clinical features
   a. Chronic watery diarrhea associated with hypokalemia, dehydration, azotemia, and metabolic acidosis
   b. Hypochlorhydria
   c. Glucose intolerance
   d. Hypercalcemia
   e. Flushing
   f. Tetany
2. Diagnostic workup
   a. Confirm presence of secretory diarrhea (24-h stool volume and electrolytes)
   b. Rule out bowel infection, inflammation, and villous tumors by examination of stools for ova and parasites, WBC (methylene blue stain), stool culture
   c. Proctosigmoidoscopy
   d. X-rays (upper GI series, small-bowel follow-through, barium enema)
   e. Exclude laxative or diuretic abuse (history, room search, alkalinization of stools)
   f. Plasma VIP and prostaglandin E levels*
   g. Selective pancreatic arteriography, CT scans
   h. Exploratory laparoscopy if previous tests were inconclusive
3. Therapy
   a. Correction of water and electrolyte imbalance
   b. Somatostatin analogue (SMS 201-995)
   c. Tumor resection or debulking
   d. Chemotherapy (streptozocin, chlorozocin, 5-FU, alone or in combination)

*If the clinical picture is compatible and the VIP and/or PGE levels are in the tumor range (more than 1000 pg/ml) but pancreatic angiography is negative, look for bronchial cancer (chest films, tomograms, bronchoscopy).

excluded. If no pancreatic tumor can be found in patients with the WDHA syndrome, it is important to search carefully for a thoracic neoplasm.

Treatment The first goal of treatment is to replace fluid and electrolyte losses. Surgical resection of a benign pancreatic islet cell tumor or ganglioneuroblastoma is possible in about half the patients. Another 20 percent of patients have diffuse islet cell hyperplasia and may be helped by partial or complete pancreatectomy. Patients with large inoperable tumors can benefit from debulking operations and from chemotherapy with streptozocin, chlorozocin, and 5-fluorouracil (5-FU), given alone or in combination.

Several pharmacological agents, including indomethacin, lithium carbonate, opiates, and β-adrenergic and calcium-channel blockers, have been used with varying success in an effort to control diarrhea in small numbers of patients. Recently, a long-acting somatostatin analogue (SMS 201-995) has been reported to control the diarrhea in patients with WDHA syndrome[31] as well as other symptoms caused by gastrinomas, glucagonomas, insulinomas, and carcinoid tumors.[32] This analogue can be given by subcutaneous injection (100 μg once or twice daily) and has not produced significant side effects even after use for many months. Moreover, it has been suggested that SMS 201-995 may shrink the size of these endocrine tumors and their metastases.[33]

VIP DEFICIENCY Lack of VIP-containing nerves has been reported in the aganglionic segments of the colon in patients with Hirschsprung's disease[34] and in esophageal smooth muscle in patients with achalasia,[35] suggesting that the lack of VIP may be at least partially responsible for these conditions.

Gastric Inhibitory Polypeptide

History and Chemistry

The key to the discovery of GIP was the observation by Brown that crude CCK (10 percent pure) inhibited gastric acid secretion more than a purified CCK preparation (40 percent pure). He interpreted this as meaning that purification had removed an agent which inhibited gastric acid secretion. Subsequently, Brown isolated, purified, and sequenced GIP.[36] The structure of GIP has recently been revised.[37] It is a straight-chain 42-amino acid polypeptide with a molecular weight of 5104. A shorter form (GIP 3–42), lacking the first two amino-terminal amino acid residues of GIP, has been isolated from porcine upper intestinal tissues.[37] GIP has many amino acid homologies with glucagon, secretin, and VIP and thus is considered a member of the glucagon-secretin family of hormones (Table 27-5).

Distribution, Measurement, and Release

GIP is found in decreasing concentrations in the mucosa of the duodenum, the proximal and mid jejunum, and the ileum (Fig. 27-1). A particular cell type (K cell) which contains GIP has been identified immunohistochemically.

GIP concentrations in biologic fluids can be measured by radioimmunoassay. Most antisera recognize the 5000-mol wt GIP and a larger (8000 mol wt) molecule. One antiserum has been reported which reacts with the COOH-terminal tripeptide of GIP and detects only the 5000-mol wt species.[38] Resting GIP concentrations increase severalfold in response to oral and intraduodenal but not parenteral administration of carbohydrate, fat, some amino acids, and a mixed meal.[3,36,38] GIP concentrations have also been reported to increase during starvation, after intraduodenal infusion of HCl,[39] and in response to β-adrenergic stimulation with isoproterenol.[40] GIP's half-life in plasma is about 20 min, resulting in prolonged elevations of hormone levels after meals.[41]

Actions

GIP's enterogastrone effect (inhibitory action on gastric acid secretion and gastric motility), which led to its discovery, is probably of little physiological significance.[42] Peripheral GIP concentrations needed to reproduce these effects are severalfold greater than those observed after a meal. On the other hand, GIP's insulinotropic action appears to be of physiological importance. GIP when given alone in physiological doses has no effect on insulin release. However, when given together with intravenous glucose, GIP potentiates insulin release and improves glucose tolerance.[42] This potentiation of glucose-stimulated insulin release can also be demonstrated with endogenously released GIP, provided the plasma glucose concentration is normal or elevated. In addition, recent studies with rats suggest that GIP may also potentiate amino acid–mediated insulin release.[43]

Incretin Effect

It is well established that considerably more insulin is released after oral than after parenteral administration of carbohydrates or amino acids, suggesting the presence of an enteropancreatic axis (Fig. 27-5). It has been postulated that a humoral substance or substances (*incretin*) is released after oral substrate administration. This substance then primes the pancreatic beta cells, which in turn respond to the postprandial rise of circulating substrate levels with enhanced insulin release. GIP meets these criteria. There is, however, evidence to suggest that it is not the only incretin: CCK is probably another incretin.[21] In addition, there may be other as yet unidentified substances with similar activities.[44,45] It has therefore been suggested that a more appropriate name for GIP would be *glucose-dependent insulinotropic polypeptide*.

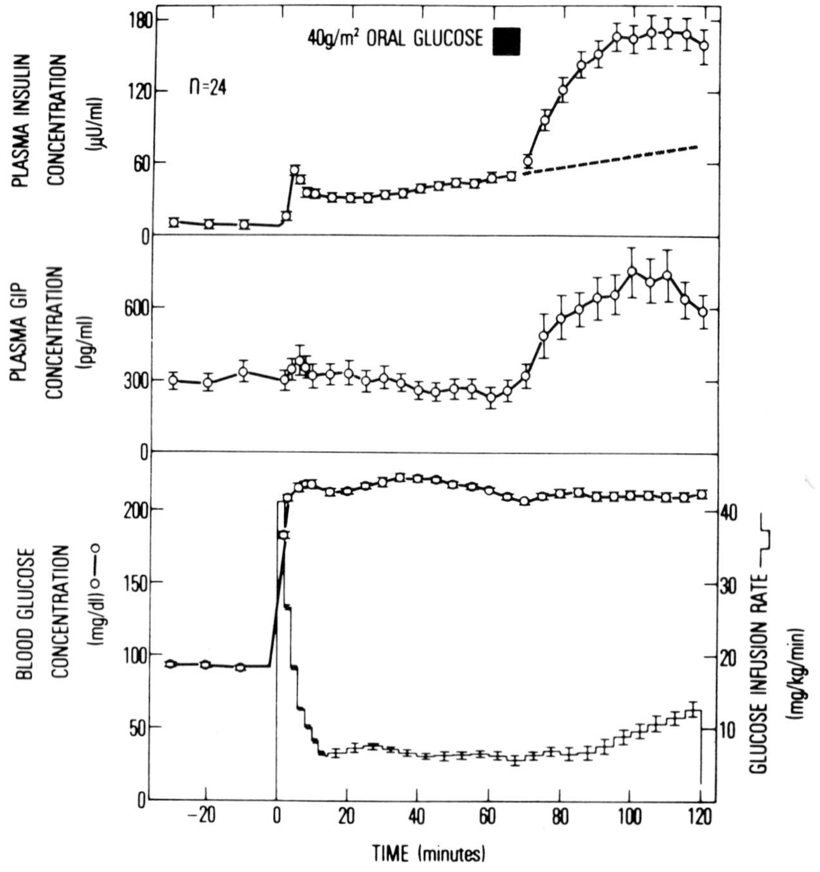

FIGURE 27-5 Hyperglycemic clamp with oral glucose. Plasma insulin, plasma GIP, and blood glucose concentrations are shown for 24 subjects (means ±1 SEM). The dashed line represents the plasma insulin concentration that would have been expected for these subjects had oral glucose not been given. (*From Anderson DK, Elahi D, Brown JC, Tobin JD, Andres R, J Clin Invest 62:152, 1978.*)

GIP in Human Disease

Although several conditions have been reported to be associated with abnormal plasma GIP concentrations, a pathophysiological role for this peptide has not been definitively demonstrated. Pancreatic beta cells of patients with non-insulin-dependent diabetes mellitus (NIDDM) contain insulin secretory granules, but it appears that the release of this insulin is defective. It was therefore suspected that deficient GIP release may be responsible for this defect. It has been found, however, that basal and glucose-stimulated GIP concentrations in patients with NIDDM are usually higher than normal.[46] Similarly, no causal relationship has been found between beta cell function and GIP in patients with insulin-dependent diabetes mellitus.[47] Elevated GIP levels have been reported in obese subjects and in patients with chronic pancreatitis.[48] The cause for the elevated GIP levels in these conditions is unknown. Elevated GIP concentrations have also been reported in patients with duodenal ulcer and may be caused by accelerated gastric emptying.[49] Recently it has been proposed that increased secretion of GIP may be responsible for the postprandial hypoglycemia in certain patients with idiopathic reactive hypoglycemia.[50]

Secretin

History

In 1902, in a classical experiment, Bayliss and Starling introduced dilute HCl into a denervated jejunal loop of a dog, then scraped off the mucosa and boiled and neutralized it. Intravenous injection of the mucosal filtrate prompted the pancreas to secrete copious amounts of water and bicarbonate. They named the active principle *secretin.*

Chemistry and Structure-Activity Relationship

Porcine secretin has been purified and sequenced,[51] and its amino acid sequence has been confirmed by complete synthesis.[52] It is a strongly basic polypeptide consisting of 27 amino acids and has a molecular weight of 3055. Larger molecular forms have been reported but have not been further characterized. Secretin has many amino acid homologies with glucagon, GIP, and VIP (Table 27-5). The entire secretin molecule is needed for bioactivity. Removal of only one amino acid from either the amino- or the carboxy-terminal end results in almost complete loss of bioactivity. Immunoreactivity is located in the carboxy-terminal end and is not affected by removal of as many as four amino-terminal amino acid residues.

Distribution, Measurement, and Release

Secretin has been localized immunohistochemically in the S cells which are located between crypts and villi of the upper intestinal mucosa in decreasing concentrations from the proximal duodenum to the distal ileum (Fig. 27-1). In addition, secretin has been detected in the central nervous systems of rats and pigs.[53]

Secretin can be measured by radioimmunoassay. Most antisera reported are directed against the COOH terminus of the secretin molecule. Normal values in humans are usually less than 10 pg/ml. Bioassays measuring pancreatic bicarbonate output in anesthetized dogs or cats are available but are much less sensitive and specific.

Intestinal acidification is the only well-established stimulus for secretin release. After gastric emptying, the duodenal pH decreases below the pH threshold for the release of secretin (pH 4.0 to 4.5) only briefly and only in the proximal parts of the duodenum. The resulting postprandial increases in blood secretin concentrations are very small[54,55] but in concert with simultaneously released CCK or other substances appear to be sufficient to stimulate pancreatic bicarbonate secretion. The release of secretin is inhibited by somatostatin.[56]

Metabolism

The half-life of secretin in the blood is approximately 3 min.[57] The kidneys appear to be major catabolic sites, and increased secretin concentrations have been found in patients with chronic renal failure.

Actions

Important physiological actions of secretin are stimulation of pancreatic water and bicarbonate secretion and potentiation of the effects of CCK on pancreatic enzyme release. On the other hand, many of secretin's biologic actions, including its insulin-, parathyroid hormone-, and calcitonin-releasing activity, its effect on pancreatic blood flow, and its trophic effects on acinar tissue are probably nonphysiological. Moreover, secretin is unlikely to play a physiological role as an inhibitor of gastric acid secretion.[58]

Secretin in Human Disease

Elevated plasma concentrations of secretin have been reported in patients with chronic renal failure, cystic fibrosis, and Zollinger-Ellison syndrome. The cause for the hypersecretinemia in chronic renal failure is reduced hormone metabolism. Increased gastric acid secretion and intestinal acidification are responsible for hypersecretinemia in patients with Zollinger-Ellison syndrome.[59] Secretin concentrations in patients with duodenal ulcer are usually normal except in patients with basal acid outputs of more than 15 meq/h, who may have elevated secretin levels.

Use in Clinical Practice

Secretin is used in a provocative test for the diagnosis of gastrinoma (Zollinger-Ellison syndrome; see Gastrin, above). It is also used as a stimulatory agent in the evaluation of exocrine pancreatic function. Recently, secretin has been reported to partially protect against some forms of experimentally induced acute pancreatitis in rats.[60] So far, however, beneficial effects of secretin in the treatment of acute pancreatitis in humans have not been documented.

Gastrointestinal Glucagon

History, Chemistry, Distribution, and Release

In 1948, Sutherland and deDuve first suggested extrapancreatic production of glucagon on the basis of their findings of hyperglycemic and glycogenolytic activities in gut extracts.[61,62] Subsequently, A cells were identified in the fundic mucosa of dogs and other experimental animals. They were also found, albeit in much smaller numbers, in the fundic and duodenal mucosa of human subjects, where they were irregularly dispersed among other cells. Extracts of fundic mucosa of dogs and other animals were shown to contain and to synthesize a material which was immunologically, biologically, and chemically identical with pancreatic glucagon. In addition, it was shown that plasma concentrations of immunoreactive glucagon (IRG) remained normal or rose after complete pancreatectomy in experimental animals and in some human subjects. The greater part of this IRG consisted of high-molecular-weight material. However, some IRG with a molecular weight of 3500 (IRG^{3500}) could be detected in most pancreatectomized patients. The amounts of IRG^{3500} varied considerably and ranged from barely detectable to low-normal concentrations. Thus, the presence of significant amounts of extrapancreatic glucagon has been established in dogs and in some other animal species. Present evidence suggest that, compared with that of dogs, human gastrointestinal tissues contain much less glucagon. It has been demonstrated that glucagon, isolated from canine fundic mucosa and purified to homogeneity, has biologic activity identical with that of pancreatic glucagon with respect to glycogenolysis and ureagenesis. Whether this is also true for extrapancreatic human glucagon is not known, and further work is needed to clarify the role of extrapancreatic glucagon in human physiology and pathophysiology.

Release of IRG from extrapancreatic A cells has been found to be qualitatively different from its release from pancreatic A cells. In most pancreatectomized patients who are adequately treated with insulin, IRG release cannot be stimulated by IV arginine, whereas in normal human subjects plasma IRG rises predictably in response to IV arginine. The reason for the difference in IRG release from fundic and from pancreatic A cells is not clear. Conceivably, paracrine effects exerted within the pancreatic islets, where B and D cells are contiguous with A cells, may modulate the stimulus-secretion process. Such effects are likely to be absent or attenuated in the stomach, where A cells are dispersed in acinar tissue and B cells are lacking. A high-molecular-weight IRG has been extracted from human salivary and submaxillary glands. Its contribution to circulating extrapancreatic IRG, as well as its biochemical identity and physiological role, are unknown.

Gut Glucagon-like Immunoreactants

The gut also contains substances which are similar to pancreatic glucagon but not identical. Collectively, they have been named *gut glucagon-like immunoreactive substances* (gut GLI).[63] By definition, they are gastrointestinal peptides which react with antibodies directed against the NH_2 terminal end or the midportion of the glucagon molecule but not with antibodies directed against the COOH-terminal end. To determine gut GLI in a sample by radioimmunoassay, an NH_2-terminal specific antiglucagon serum is used to determine total GLI, and a COOH-terminal antiglucagon serum is used to specifically measure glucagon. Gut GLI is obtained by subtracting the glucagon from the total GLI measurements.

Gut GLI substances are found in low concentrations in the human duodenum and jejunum, with tissue concentrations rising to peak levels in the lower ileum and the ascending colon. Basal plasma gut GLI concentrations are elevated in infants and in pancreatectomized and insulin-dependent diabetic patients, in whom they are normalized by adequate insulin treatment. In normal adults, plasma gut GLI concentrations rise after oral glucose administration and after large mixed meals. Lipids appear to be weaker stimulants than glucose. Larger than normal increases have been reported under conditions of accelerated intestinal transit, suggesting that release of GLI depends on the amount of nutrients reaching the jejunum and colon. Gleeson et al. have reported a patient with a renal tumor containing large amounts of GLI, elevated plasma gut GLI levels, severe intestinal stasis, and hypertrophy of the small intestine mucosa.[64] These abnormalities disappeared after resection of the tumor. The observations suggest that gut GLI may control intestinal motor function and may be an enterotrophin.

Several of these GLI substances have been isolated, purified, and chemically identified. Porcine glicentin is a 69-amino acid polypeptide containing within its structure the full sequence of glucagon (the glicentin sequence 33–61 is identical with glucagon; Fig. 27-6). The peptide was named *glicentin* because it was originally believed that it consisted of 100 amino acids (*glicentin* = *GLI* plus *cent*, 100).

Glicentin has amino acid homologies with secretin, with VIP, GIP, and α- and β-endorphin, with bovine pancreatic polypeptide, and with somatostatin. It has been suspected that proglucagon is either identical with or contains glicentin. Supporting this hypothesis is the observation that the main fragments of glicentin, namely, glucagon (glicentin 33–61) and glicentin-related pancreatic peptide (GRPP, identical with glicentin 1–30; Fig. 27-6) are stored in secretory granules of A cells and are secreted together with glucagon in equimolar amounts, comparable to the secretion of insulin and C peptide.

A specific radioimmunoassay for the measurement of glicentin has been developed. Glicentin-like immunoreactivity is present in human intestinal L cells as well as in pancreatic A cells. It is found in increasing concentrations from the duodenum to the colon.

Glicentin has minimal or no glucagon-like effects; however, when infused at low doses (370 pmol/kg hourly) it inhibits gastrin-stimulated gastric acid release in rats.

Oxyntomodulin, corresponding to glicentin 33–69, is glucagon extended at the COOH terminus by the COOH-terminal octapeptide of glicentin (Table 27-6). Oxyntomodulin is 20 times more potent than glucagon in stimulating the activity of adenylate cyclase in plasma membrane fractions of the gastric oxyntic mucosa. This action provided the basis for its name.

The physiological role of gut GLI is uncertain. Elevated levels in human infants and increases after feeding suggest that gut GLI may modify development and function of the gastrointestinal tract. The glucagonoma syndrome is discussed in Chap. 19.

Pancreatic Polypeptide

History and Chemistry

Pancreatic polypeptide (PP)[3,65] was discovered in 1971 by Kimmel et al. as a contaminant of chicken insulin. It is a straight-chain peptide containing 36 amino acids. Subsequently, Chance and Lin identified similar peptides from bovine, porcine, sheep, and human pancreas. Human and bovine PP differ in two amino acids (Table 27-7).

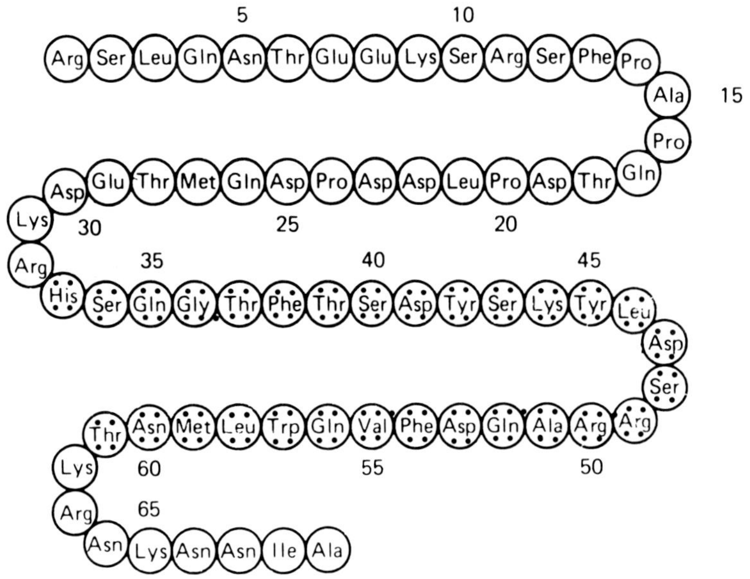

FIGURE 27-6 The amino acid sequence of porcine glicentin. Sequence 1–30 is identical with GRPP, sequence 33–61 (stippled circles) is identical with glucagon, and sequence 33–69 is identical with oxyntomodulin. (*From Moody and Thim.*[63])

Table 27-7. Sequences of Pancreatic Polypeptide, PYY, and NPY

	1	2	3	4	5	6	7	8	9	10	11	12	13	14	15	16	17	18
Bovine PP	Ala	Pro	Leu	Glu	Pro	Glu	Tyr	Pro	Gly	Asp	Asn	Ala	Thr	Pro	Glu	Gln	Met	Ala
Human PP	Ala	Pro	Leu	Glu	Pro	Val	Tyr	Pro	Gly	Asp	Asn	Ala	Thr	Pro	Glu	Gln	Met	Ala
PYY	Tyr	Pro	Ala	Lys	Pro	Glu	Ala	Pro	Gly	Glu	Asn	Ala	Ser	Pro	Glu	Glu	Leu	Ser
NPY	Tyr	Pro	Ser	Lys	Pro	Asp	Asn	Pro	Gly	Glu	Asp	Ala	Pro	Ala	Glu	Asp	Leu	Ala

	19	20	21	22	23	24	25	26	27	28	29	30	31	32	33	34	35	36
Bovine PP	Gln	Tyr	Ala	Ala	Glu	Leu	Arg	Arg	Tyr	Ile	Asn	Met	Leu	Thr	Arg	Pro	Arg	Tyr-NH_2
Human PP	Gln	Tyr	Ala	Ala	Asp	Leu	Arg	Arg	Tyr	Ile	Asn	Met	Leu	Thr	Arg	Pro	Arg	Tyr-NH_2
PYY	Arg	Tyr	Tyr	Ala	Ser	Leu	Arg	His	Tyr	Leu	Asn	Leu	Val	Thr	Arg	Gln	Arg	Tyr-NH_2
NPY	Arg	Tyr	Tyr	Ser	Ala	Leu	Arg	His	Tyr	Ile	Asn	Leu	Ile	Thr	Arg	Gln	Arg	Tyr-NH_2

Distribution

Pancreatic polypeptide has been extracted in the greatest amounts from the pancreas. Smaller amounts have been found in the stomach and the upper small intestine. The F cell has been identified, by immunohistochemical means, as the PP-containing cell. Some of these cells are found in the islets of Langerhans, but most are scattered throughout the exocrine pancreas. There, they are particularly abundant in the uncinate process and the pancreatic head, in contrast to the A cells, which are more concentrated in the body and the tail.

Measurement and Release

Human, bovine, and porcine PP can be measured by highly sensitive and specific radioimmunoassays. Rat PP does not cross-react well with antibovine or antiporcine PP antisera and requires an antirat-PP antiserum for measurement. Peripheral venous human PP (hPP) concentration rises with age. Floyd reported basal PP concentrations in normal subjects as rising from 54 ± 28 pg/ml during the third decade to 207 ± 129 pg/ml during the seventh decade. PP also increases after acute hypoglycemia, exercise, or prolonged fasting; after oral ingestion of fat, protein, or mixed meals; and after parasympathetic stimulation.[65-67] The observation that plasma PP rises within minutes after oral but not after IV administration of nutrients suggests that PP release is mediated by direct effects on intestinal mucosa rather than by stimulation of pancreatic PP cells via blood-borne digestive products. In addition, injection of supraphysiological amounts of secretin, CCK, pentagastrin, and bombesin results in PP release, which can, in most instances, be blocked with atropine, suggesting cholinergic mediation of hormone release.

Actions and Metabolism

Given in pharmacological doses to dogs, PP has a variety of biological actions, including enhancement of intestinal motility, gallbladder tone, and choledochal resistance and inhibition of pancreatic secretion. Given in physiological amounts, it has been shown to inhibit pancreatic secretion of bicarbonate and protein in dogs[68] and trypsin and bilirubin output in humans.[69] These actions of PP on pancreas and gallbladder are directly opposite to those of CCK. Also in contrast to CCK, PP levels remain elevated for many hours after meals. Thus, they may help to conserve pancreatic enzymes and bile late in the interprandial period.[69] Nevertheless, the physiological role of PP remains undefined.

The half-life of hPP in plasma is approximately 6 min. The kidneys but not the liver are important sites for hPP metabolism. As a result, plasma hPP concentrations are elevated in patients with renal but not with hepatic insufficiency.[70]

PP in Human Disease

Some insulin-dependent diabetic patients have high antibody titers against PP caused by contamination of insulin preparations with PP. Other diabetic patients who have never received insulin may also have elevated plasma hPP concentrations for unknown reasons. High plasma hPP concentrations are frequently found in patients with insulinomas, glucagonomas, VIP-secreting tumors, gastrinomas, and carcinoid tumors. In addition, several pancreatic tumors containing or secreting excessive amounts of hPP exclusively have been reported.[71,72] However, the chronically elevated blood levels of PP in these patients were not associated with a clearly identifiable clinical "PPoma" syndrome. It has been suspected, therefore, that many of the so-called nonfunctional endocrine tumors of the pancreas may be PP-secreting tumors.[72]

Other Members of the PP Family

Using a novel method of detecting peptides with COOH-terminal α-amides, Tatemoto has discovered several new bioactive peptides, including peptide YY (PYY) and neuropeptide Y (NPY).[73,74] Those peptides share major sequence homologies with PP and are considered members of an emerging PP family (Table 27-7).

Peptide YY has been isolated from porcine intestinal extracts. It is linear 36-amino acid peptide and has been completely sequenced. The name is derived from its NH_2- and COOH-terminal amino acid residues, i.e., the peptide (P) having an NH_2-terminal tyrosine (Y) and a COOH-terminal tyrosine (Y). PYY has been found in the intestinal mucosa of several species, including humans and rats. In rats, the PYY immunoreactivity was about 100-fold higher in the colon than in the duodenum.[75] In dogs, plasma PYY rises after a meat meal and following intraduodenal administration of oleic acid. PYY infused in doses which simulate postprandial plasma PYY concentrations causes a decrease in basal and in CCK- and secretin-stimulated bicarbonate and protein secretion by the pancreas. Intraarterial administration of PYY in cats causes intestinal vasoconstriction, a rise in systemic arterial blood pressure, and inhibition of jejunal and colonic motility.

Neuropeptide Y has been isolated from porcine brain.[74] It is also a straight 36-amino acid peptide and has many sequence homologies with PYY (70 percent) and with PP (50 percent). Immunohistochemistry shows NPY cell bodies and fibers to be most prevalent in corticoid, limbic, and hypothalamic regions. Concentrations of NPY were higher than those of any other peptide so far discovered in mammalian brain.[76]

Neither the physiological nor the pathophysiological role (if any) of PYY or NPY has as yet been established.

Somatostatin

History and Chemistry

In 1972, when searching for a growth hormone releasing factor, Guillemin et al. instead found growth hormone release inhibiting activity in sheep hypothalamic extracts. The substance responsible for this action was isolated and purified and was found to be a cyclic tetradecapeptide. It was named *somatotropin release inhibiting factor* (SRIF), or *somatostatin.*[77] An NH_2-terminal extended somatostatin (somatostatin-28) has been isolated and sequenced from porcine intestine. In addition, the sequence of a human preprosomatostatin has been identified, using mRNA obtained from a somatostatinoma.[78] Somatostatin-14 and -28 as well as many of their analogues have been synthesized.

Measurement and Distribution

Somatostatin can be measured by sensitive and specific radioimmunoassays. Nonspecific interference of human plasma in the assay necessitates deproteinization of the plasma before measuring somatostatin. The inhibitory activities of somatostatin on hormone release are the basis for several bioassays. For instance, somatostatin-like bioactivity can be determined by measuring inhibition of insulin release from beta cells or growth hormone release from anterior pituitary cells.

Somatostatin has been extracted from many areas of the brain as well as from the pancreas and the gut mucosa, where it is found in decreasing concentrations from the antrum of the stomach to the colon (Fig. 27-1). In the nervous system, somatostatin has been found in many areas, including nerve cell bodies of the cerebral cortex and periventricular region of the hypothalamus and nerve endings in the medial eminence, pituitary stalk, and posterior pituitary. In addition, somatostatin has been found in many sensory neurons, as well as in the retina and the auditory, optic, and many sympathetic nerves. In the gut and pancreas, an endocrine-like cell, the D cell, has been identified as a source of somatostatin. The sulfhydryl drug cysteamine causes a rapid but reversible loss of somatostatin immunoactivity and bioactivity from tissues and plasma. The exact nature of this loss has not been identified, but it seems to be related to a chemical modification of the disulfide bond of the somatostatin molecule.

Release

The concentration of basal somatostatin-like immunoreactive substances (SLI) in animals and humans, when measured in extracted blood, ranges from about 10 to 80 pg/ml in peripheral blood and is approximately three to seven times higher in portal venous blood.[79] Small increases in peripheral SLI concentration after mixed meals have been reported. Evidence accumulated from animal experiments and perfusion of isolated organs (mainly pancreas and stomach) and isolated cells (islet cells) indicates that glucose, amino acids, free fatty acids, and several hormones, including gastrin, secretin, and CCK, as well as tolbutamide and theophylline stimulate SLI release. Metenkephalin and substance P inhibit SLI release. Starvation reduces and obesity increases SLI release. Isoproterenol increases SLI release, and this effect is abolished by propranolol, suggesting adrenergic control of somatostatin release.

Metabolism

The half-life of SLI after exogenous administration of somatostatin-14 is less than 3 min in humans and dogs. In patients with chronic renal failure the half-life is increased by about 50 percent.[79] Moreover, somatostatin is excreted in the urine. These observations and a large portal-peripheral venous somatostatin gradient suggest that the liver and the kidneys participate in the metabolism of SLI.

Actions

Besides its inhibitory action on growth hormone release, somatostatin suppresses the release of a large number of polypeptide and glycoprotein hormones, including insulin, glucagon, thyroid stimulating hormone (TSH), gastrin, secretin, and renin. However, it is not a universal inhibitor of hormone release. For instance, somatostatin has little or no inhibitory effect on the release of follicle stimulating hormone (FSH), luteinizing hormone (LH), prolactin, and parathyroid hormone (PTH). In addition, a number of nonendocrine effects of somatostatin have been described. These include inhibition of gastric acid and pepsin secretion, of pancreatic water, bicarbonate, and enzyme secretion, and of splanchnic blood flow and intestinal motility. These effects have all been produced with pharmacological doses of somatostatin. Whether any of these actions has physiological significance is presently unknown.

Strong support for a tonic inhibitory role of somatostatin on the release of several hormones has come from experiments in which antisomatostatin antibodies were infused into experimental animals or isolated organs. Infusion of these antibodies has been shown to result in increases in concentrations of growth hormone, TSH, glucagon, and gastrin. In addition, it has provided evidence that somatostatin may play a physiological role in the regulation of the rate at which ingested nutrients enter the circulation.[80] The observation that somatostatin concentration rises in the circulation after a meal suggests that it may exert biologic actions on distant target organs (hormonal actions). In addition, it may have a role as a local hormone, exerting its effects on neighboring cells (paracrine actions). The best evidence for a paracrine action has been found in the isolated perfused rat stomach. There stimulation of somatostatin release was associated with decreased gastrin secretion, while suppression of somatostatin release was associated with increased gastrin secretion (Fig. 27-7).[81] The finding that gastric D cells have long extensions which touch on the surfaces of neighboring G cells strongly supports this concept.[82] The presence of somatostatin in the central nervous system suggests that it may function as a neurotransmitter or modulator.

To initiate its various actions, somatostatin has been shown to bind to receptors localized on surface membranes of pituitary and pancreatic islet cells and on brain synoptosomal membranes. Little is known about the postreceptor events leading to the bioeffects.

Somatostatin in Human Disease and Clinical Use

SLI concentration has been reported to be markedly reduced in brains of patients with senile dementia of the Alzheimer type.[83] SLI concentrations were elevated in the cerebrospinal fluid of patients with various CNS disorders, including brain tumors, spinal cord compression, and metabolic encephalopathy, probably indicating leakage of somatostatin from damaged tissue into the cerebrospinal canal.[84]

Somatostatin has been used in the medical treatment of acromegaly, insulinoma, and gastrinoma and in the management of acute gastrointestinal bleeding and acute pancreatitis. Because of its glucagon-suppressing effect, it has also been proposed as therapy for insulin-dependent diabetes mellitus, together with insulin. It has, however, become clear that the many extraendocrine effects of somatostatin, together with its short half-life, preclude long-term medical use. Recently, a long-acting octapeptide somatostatin analogue (SMS-201-995) has been used successfully for prolonged periods (several months) to control diarrhea in patients with WDHA syndrome.[31] Somatostatin

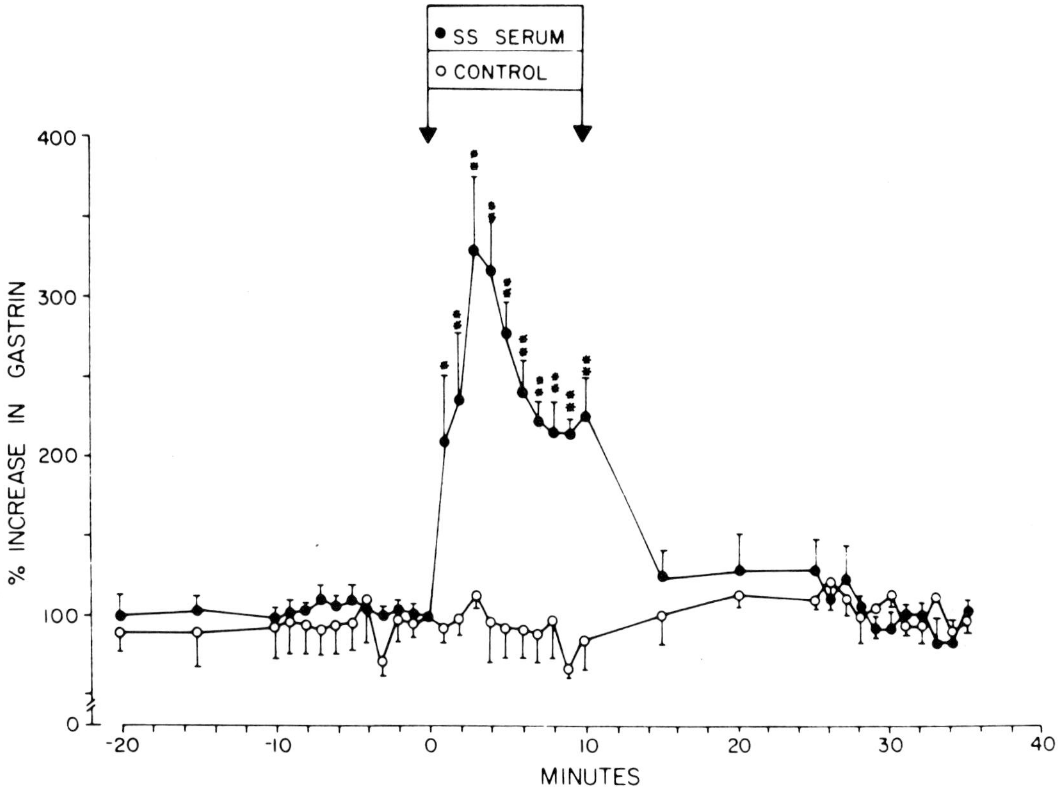

FIGURE 27-7 Concentration of gastrin in the venous effluent of isolated, perfused rat stomach before, during, and after a 10-min infusion of control serum (open circles) or somatostatin (SS) antiserum (closed circles). Each point represents the mean SEM± of three experiments. Single asterisk, $P<0.05$, double asterisk, $P<0.01$, for significance of difference from corresponding control values. (*From Saffouri et al.*[81])

and its octapeptide analogue are also currently being investigated for the management of upper gastrointestinal tract bleeding.

SOMATOSTATINOMA In 1977, Ganda et al. and Larsson et al. independently reported the first two cases of somatostatinoma, i.e., a tumor containing or secreting excessive amounts of somatostatin.[85,86] On the basis of these reports, Unger tentatively proposed a clinical somatostatinoma syndrome consisting of mild diabetes, gallbladder disease, weight loss, and anemia. Diarrhea, steatorrhea, and hypochlorhydria became additional features as more cases were discovered. In a recent review of 20 somatostatinomas, most were large solitary tumors; 75 percent were located in the pancreas, 20 percent in the duodenum or jejunum.[87] At the time of diagnosis, 80 percent had metastasized to the liver or regional lymph nodes or both.

Somatostatinomas contain large amounts of two molecular forms of somatostatin, somatostatin-14 and a somatostatin-like immunoreactive substance with an apparent molecular weight of between 10,000 and 15,000, possibly a somatostatin precursor. Several somatostatinomas contained in addition other hormones, including insulin, glucagon, gastrin, VIP, calcitonin, substance P, and motilin. The peak age of patients with a somatostatinoma was the fifth decade. Males and females were affected equally. Clinical features in patients with somatostatinoma (Table 27-8) were diabetes mellitus, gallbladder disease, diarrhea and steatorrhea, hypochlorhydria, weight loss, anemia, and elevated plasma SLI concentrations ranging from 160 to 107,000 pg/ml (mean, 15,500 pg/ml). Approximately half the patients with somatostatinoma had other endocrinopathies, including insulinoma, gastrinoma, Cushing's syndrome, pheochromocytoma, and goiter. Most of these somatostatinomas were discovered accidentally, many during cholecystectomy. Of 18 patients for whom this information was provided, 12 had had surgical treatment, 4 chemotherapy, and 2 surgery plus chemotherapy. The malignant nature of this disorder is underlined by the fact that 8 of the 20 patients died at intervals ranging from 1 week to 14 months after diagnosis.

Table 27-8. The Clinical Somatostatinoma Syndrome

Diabetes mellitus (nonketotic)
Gallbladder disease
Diarrhea/steatorrhea
Hypochlorhydria
Weight loss
Anemia
Elevated plasma SLI

Bombesin and Gastrin-Releasing Peptide

Chemistry, Distribution, and Measurement

Bombesin, a tetradecapeptide (molecular weight 1620; Table 27-9), is one of several biologically active peptides extracted from amphibian skin by Erspamer.[3] Recently, McDonald et al. have isolated a peptide with gastrin-releasing activity from porcine nonantral gastric and intestinal tissues which was named *gastrin-releasing peptide* (GRP).[88] GRP is a 27-amino acid peptide. Of its 10 COOH-terminal amino acid residues, 9 are identical with the COOH-terminal decapeptide of bombesin (Table 27-9). This homology and similarities in biologic responses between bombesin and GRP suggested that GRP may be a mammalian bombesin.[89] A bombesin-like immunoreactive substance (BLI) has been found in the brain and gut of rats and in the gastrointestinal mucosa and fetal lung tissue of humans. In rats and humans, BLI appears to be confined to the mucosa, submucosa, and myenteric nerve fibers, while in frogs and birds it has been demonstrated in intestinal endocrine-like cells. BLI can be measured by radioimmunoassay, using antisera which recognize mostly the COOH-terminal end of the molecule.

Actions

Infusion of bombesin causes a variety of biologic responses, including stimulation of the release of gastrin, CCK, pancreatic polypeptide, and gastric acid; pancreatic enzyme secretion; and gallbladder contraction. In addition, it inhibits gastric motor activity and causes renal arterial vasoconstriction and hypertension in dogs. Administered intracisternally to rats, bombesin causes hypothermia, analgesia, hyperglucagonemia, and hyperglycemia; injected into the ventromedial or the lateral hypothalamic area, it causes sustained hyperglycemia.[90] In vitro, bombesin results in contraction of smooth muscle. Bombesin and GRP have been found in normal human bronchial cells and in small cell lung cancer. In these cells they exert mitogenic actions.[91–93] It has been suggested, therefore, that bombesin and GRP may be important growth-regulating factors.

Table 27-9. Sequences of Porcine Gastrin Releasing Peptide (GRP) and Bombesin

	1	2	3	4	5	6	7	8	9	10	11	12	13	14	15	16	17	18	19	20	21	22	23	24	25	26	27
Porcine gastrin releasing peptide	Ala	Pro	Val	Ser	Val	Gly	Gly	Gly	Thr	Val	Leu	Ala	Lys	Met	Tyr	Pro	Arg	Gly	Asn	His	Trp	Ala	Val	Gly	His	Leu	Met-NH_2
Bombesin														Pyr	Gln	Arg	Leu	Gly	Asn	Gln	Trp	Ala	Val	Gly	His	Leu	Met-NH_2

Note: Identical amino acid sequences are boxed.

Table 27-10. Sequences of Substance P and Related Peptides (Tachykinin Family of Peptides)

Substance P (bovine)	Arg-Pro-Lys-Pro-Gln-Gln-Phe-Phe-Gly-Leu-Met-NH_2
Eledoisin	Gln-Pro-Ser-Lys-Asp-Ala-Phe-Ile-Gly-Leu-Met-NH_2
Kassinin	Asp-Val-Pro-Lys-Ser-Asp-Gln-Phe-Val-Gly-Leu-Met-NH_2
Substance K (neurokinin α)	His-Lys-Thr-Asp-Ser-Phe-Val-Gly-Leu-Met-NH_2
Neurokinin K (neurokinin β)	Asp-Met-His-Asp-Phe-Phe-Val-Gly-Leu-Met-NH_2

Substance P

History and Chemistry

Substance P (SP)[3,94] was originally identified in equine brain and intestine by von Euler and Gaddum in 1931 and later by Leeman and Carraway as a substance causing salivary flow in anesthetized rats. In 1971, Chang et al. isolated SP in pure form from bovine hypothalamus and determined its amino acid sequence. SP is a polypeptide consisting of 11 amino acids and has a molecular weight of 1348 (Table 27-10). SP belongs to the tachykinin family of peptides, which are characterized by the COOH-terminal sequence Phe-X-Gly-Leu-Met-NH_2. The molluscan salivary gland peptide eledoisin and the amphibian peptide kassinin are members of this family, as are two recently identified mammalian peptides, neuromedin K and substance K (Table 27-10).[95]

Distribution

SP has been found in many organs, including gut, brain, and most peripheral tissues. It is distributed throughout the intestinal tract, with the highest concentrations occurring in the duodenum. Most of the extractable gut SP is localized in nerves. A smaller part is found in mucosal enterochromaffin (EC) cells, some of which also contain serotonin. SP is distributed in more than 30 areas of the brain, including cell bodies in the brainstem and the spinal cord, particularly in the dorsal horns of the spinal column at all levels. SP-containing nerve fibers have been found in most peripheral tissues.

Measurement and Release

Several radioimmunoassays for determination of SP in unextracted plasma have been reported. It appears, however, that unextracted plasma may produce falsely elevated values. Some reports have postulated that SP is released into the circulation by a test meal. Others, however, have failed to confirm this observation.

Actions

Biologic actions of SP include direct effects on vascular smooth muscle resulting in vasodilatation and hypotension, decreased pulmonary vascular resistance, intense dermal erythema, stimulation of intestinal peristalsis, and increases in lower esophageal sphincter and circular gut muscle pressure. In addition, SP stimulates salivation and produces many of the tissue changes of acute inflammation, including vasodilatation, increased vascular permeability, stimulation of phagocytosis by leucocytes, and histamine release by mast cells. Moreover, it has recently been shown to bind to and stimulate proliferation of blood T lymphocytes, providing a mechanism for modulation of immune processes by neuropeptides.[96]

Physiology and Pathology

A physiological role for SP has not been established. It has been speculated that SP may act as a neurotransmitter-modulator, may be involved in the transmission of pain signals (nociception), may participate in axon reflexes causing cutaneous vasodilatation, and may exacerbate inflammatory reactions, including arthritis.[97] Diminished concentrations of SP have been demonstrated in the aganglionic colon segments in patients with Hirschsprung's disease and in the atrophic areas of the brain in patients with Huntington's chorea. Some carcinoid tumors and medullary carcinomas of the thyroid contain SP, and some patients with carcinoid syndrome have elevated levels of SP.[98] The significance of these findings, however, remains uncertain.

Neurotensin

History and Chemistry

Neurotensin (NT) is a linear 13-amino acid peptide. It was discovered accidentally because of its vasoactive properties and was isolated, purified, and sequenced from bovine hypothalamic extracts and later synthesized completely by Leeman and Carraway. It has the amino acid sequence Glu-Leu-Tyr-Glu-Asn-Lys-Pro-Arg-Arg-Pro-Tyr-Ile-Leu-OH.[3,99,100]

Actions

NT has many pharmacological actions. Infused intravenously it causes systemic hypotension, increased vascular permeability, hyperglycemia, hyperglucagonemia, hypoinsulinemia, and increased plasma concentrations of human gonadotropic hormone, prolactin, adrenocorticotropic hormone, LH, and FSH. In addition, it inhibits pentagastrin-stimulated gastric acid and pepsin secretion and delays gastric emptying. In dogs, it also inhibits gastric motor activity. It is not known which, if any, of these actions are physiologically relevant.

Distribution

NT has been identified in the brain and the gastrointestinal tract. In the rat, about 10 percent of total extractable NT is found in nerve fibers in the brain, with the highest concentrations occurring in hypothalamic and pituitary tissues. The remaining 90 percent is found in endocrine-type cells in the intestinal mucosa (N cells), with the highest concentrations found in the distal ileum and lesser concentrations in the colon, jejunum, duodenum, and stomach. The apex of the N cell, like the G cell, is in contact with the gut lumen.

Measurement and Release

Neurotensin-like immunoreactive substance (NTLI) can be measured in biologic fluids by radioimmunoassay. NTLI has been reported to increase in humans after mixed meals and after oral intake of fat but not after oral administration of glucose or amino acids. However, it is not clear to what extent NTLI in plasma represents true NT. For instance, fractionation of plasma samples obtained after a fat meal demonstrates the presence of several amino-terminal fragments of neurotensin (NT 1–8, 1–10, 1–11) similar to those found in fasted rat plasma after infusion of synthetic neurotensin. Thus it is likely that a considerable portion of the NTLI detected in plasma by amino-terminally directed antisera consists of metabolized neurotensin whose biologic activity has not been demonstrated.

The physiological role of NT remains unknown. Like other peptides occurring in the brain and gastrointestinal tract, it is seen as a putative neurotransmitter or neuromodulator. It has also been suggested that NT may be an enterogastrone, i.e., a substance released from the distal small intestine in response to an oral fat load which suppresses gastric acid secretion. No known pathological conditions are associated with neurotensin hyper- or hyposecretion.

Motilin

History and Chemistry

In 1966, Brown et al. reported that duodenal alkalinization in dogs stimulated motility in transplanted pouches of the fundic portion of the stomach. He identified the agent responsible for this action as a 22-amino acid polypeptide with a molecular weight of 2699 which has since been completely synthesized. Its amino acid sequence is Phe-Val-Pro-Ile-Phe-Thr-Tyr-Gly-Glu-Leu-Gln-Arg-Met-Gln-Glu-Lys-Glu-Arg-Asn-Lys-Gly-Gln. Motilin has been extracted from duodenal, jejunal, and upper ileal mucosa. It appears to be produced by EC cells.[3,101]

Actions and Physiology

Motilin has a number of effects on intestinal smooth muscle. Infused intravenously at low doses, it increases the lower esophageal sphincter pressure in fasting dogs, accelerates gastric emptying of meals, and stimulates colonic motility in humans.

Several radioimmunoassays have been described which can be used to measure motilin-like immunoreactivity (MLI) in human blood. MLI has been reported to increase after gastric distention with water, after oral intake of fat, and, to a much lesser extent, after mixed meals. In conscious and fasting dogs but not in fed dogs, plasma MLI increases two- to threefold at cyclic intervals (every 90 to 120 min). These cyclic increases coincide closely with the onset of enteric interdigestive myoelectric complexes, i.e., contractile waves advancing from the stomach through the small intestine. Similar interdigestive myoelectric complexes can be produced by intravenous infusion of motilin into fasting dogs. Food intake abolishes the cyclic increases in plasma MLI as well as the myoelectric complexes. On the basis of this evidence, it has been suggested that the cyclic release of motilin could initiate interdigestive myoelectric complexes. This effect, however, has been questioned, since interdigestive myoelectric complexes can be initiated even when plasma motilin concentrations are suppressed.

CARCINOID

Historical Background

The term *carcinoid* was coined in 1907 by Oberndorfer. He described several small intestinal neoplasms which he believed were nonmalignant and had a tendency to grow slowly. Similar tumors had been reported earlier by others, including Merling (1808), Langhens (1867), Beger (1882), and Lubarsch (1888). In 1914, Gosset and Masson described the silver-staining (argentaffinic) properties of these tumors and postulated that they originated from the Kultschitzsky (also known as *enterochromaffin*) cells of the crypts of Lieberkühn.[102–104]

In 1954, Thorson et al. described the clinical carcinoid syndrome and its relation to intestinal tumors. At about the same time, it was discovered that many carcinoid tumors contained large amounts of serotonin (5-hydroxytryptamine) and that some patients with the carcinoid syndrome had elevated serum serotonin levels and excreted in the urine large amounts of 5-hydroxyindoleacetic acid (5-HIAA), the major metabolite of serotonin. In 1958, Sandler and Snow reported an "atypical" carcinoid tumor of the stomach. This tumor had different staining properties (argyrophilic rather than argentaffinic), caused a different type of flush (bright red rather than cyanotic or livid), and was associated with markedly elevated urinary levels of histamine and 5-hydroxytryptophan (5-HTP), a precursor of serotonin. Further evidence for the heterogeneity of carcinoid tumors was provided by Oates in 1966, who demonstrated elevated serum concentrations of bradykinin in several patients with the carcinoid syndrome. Subsequently, it became clear that carcinoid tumors can secrete a wide variety of amines and peptides, which makes it difficult to classify them on the basis of their secretory products. Williams and Sandler classified carcinoid tumors in 1963 according to their differing staining properties (argentaffinic versus argyrophilic) and embryological sites of origin (foregut, midgut, or hindgut). Soga and Tazawa expanded the classification in 1972 by dividing carcinoid tumors into five categories on the basis of their light-microscopic appearance.

Prevalence

Carcinoid tumors are relatively uncommon but not rare. Berge and Linell found 199 cases of carcinoid tumor in 16,294 autopsies (1.22 percent). This study comprised 62.6 percent of all deaths occurring over a 12-y period in one Swedish community. On the basis of these data, the authors calculated an annual incidence rate of 8.4 cases per 100,000 population.[105] MacDonald reported 254 cases of carcinoid among 26,401 autopsies (0.96 percent) (as cited in Ref. 103). By comparison, a Mayo Clinic autopsy series of 10,314 patients revealed islet cell tumors to be present in 0.43 percent. Overall, carcinoid tumors make up 0.4 to 1 percent of gastrointestinal tumors and 0.05 to 0.2 percent of all neoplasms.[106,106a]

Size

Primary carcinoid tumors of the gastrointestinal tract are usually small. In a review of 209 surgical and autopsy cases from the Mayo Clinic, 73 percent of all tumors were less than 1.5 cm in diameter and the largest tumor was 3.5 cm in diameter.[107] Similarly, Bates reported that 76 percent of 307 rectal carcinoids were less than 1 cm in diameter.[108] Exceptions are ovarian carcinoids, in that most are larger than 5 cm (diameters of up to 20 cm and weights of up to 12 kg have been reported).

Multiple Tumors

Large autopsy series have reported multiple tumors in 29 percent[107] and 32.9 percent of cases.[109] This is lower than rates reported for gastrinomas (55 percent) but higher than rates reported for insulinomas (10 percent) and glucagonomas (10 to 15 percent).[106a]

Malignancy and Metastases

Contrary to Oberndorfer's impression, malignancy, defined as local infiltrative or destructive growth and/or metastatic spread, is not rare among carcinoid tumors. Several investigators have noted a strong correlation between tumor size and metastatic disease (Table 27-11). Tumors of less than 1 cm in diameter are rarely metastatic, whereas tumors larger than 2 cm are almost always metastatic. Common metastatic sites are regional lymph nodes and liver. Pulmonary metastases predominate among the more unusual metastatic sites that include bone, skin, ovary, brain, breast, pancreas, heart, spleen, adrenals, bone marrow, kidney, thyroid, bladder, pleura, testes, epididymus, prostate, and cervix.[110]

Table 27-11. Relation of GI Carcinoid Tumor Size to Metastatic Rate

No. of patients	Metastatic rate, %			Reference no.
	<1 cm	1–2 cm	>2 cm	
139	0	50	100	110
86	0	29	88	121
307	0	10	82	108
102	0		86	109
209	0	50	80	107

Table 27-12. Anatomic Distribution of Carcinoid Tumors

Tumor site	Surgical/clinical (6965 cases)*	Autopsy (201 cases)†
Stomach	2.8	2.5
Duodenum	2.9	0.0
Jejunoileum	25.5	75.6
Appendix	36.2	3.5
Colon	6.0	6.5
Rectum	16.4	1.5
Bronchus	9.9	9.0
Ovary	0.5	0.0
Miscellaneous	0.2	0.0
Unknown primary	3.3	1.0

*Refs. 110, 112, 121, 123.
†Ref. 105.

Anatomic Distribution

Data from postmortem studies and data from clinical or surgical studies show considerable disparity in the distribution of carcinoid tumors (Table 27-12). Among 6965 patients from seven surgical series, the appendix was by far the most frequent site of origin for a primary tumor (36.2 percent). The jejunoileum (25.5 percent), rectum (16.4 percent), bronchi (9.9 percent), and colon (6.0 percent) are other relatively common sites. Duodenal and gastric carcinoids each occurred in less than 3 percent and ovarian carcinoids in only 0.5 percent of cases. Rarer sites of occurrence (less than 1 percent) include the esophagus, biliary tract, pancreas, Meckel's diverticulum, testes, larynx, thymus, breast, and skin.[111] In contrast, postmortem findings revealed a marked predominance of jejunoileal tumors (75.6 percent), while appendiceal and rectal tumors together make up only 5 percent of all tumors. The difference between surgical and autopsy data can probably be explained by the fact that jejunoileal tumors remained undetected during life because they were frequently asymptomatic and were inaccessible to noninvasive examinations, while accidental discovery of carcinoids during rectal examinations and appendectomies may account for the high prevalence of tumors at these sites in the clinical-surgical series.

Histology and Staining Characteristics

The initial and still most widely used classification of carcinoid tumors is that of Williams and Sandler, which is based on the embryological origin and silver-staining properties of tumor cells (Table 27-13). In this classification, carcinoid tumors are divided into foregut, midgut, and hindgut tumors. Foregut tumors arise between the oral cavity and the mid duodenum and include tumors of the stomach, pancreas, biliary tract, and bronchial tree. These tumors are argyrophilic, i.e., they accept silver stain only in the presence of another reducing agent. Midgut tumors are found between the mid duodenum and the mid transverse colon and are argentaffinic, i.e., they stain with silver salts in the absence of other reducing agents. Jejunoileal, appendiceal, and ascending colon carcinoids are included in this group, which is commonly associated with the classical carcinoid syndrome. Hindgut tumors are found from the mid transverse colon to the anus and are neither argentaffinic nor argyrophilic. Tumors in this group are rarely associated with the carcinoid syndrome. Tumor histology provides the basis for the classification scheme of Soga and Tazawa (Table 27-13).

Age and Sex of Patients

The peak incidence of carcinoid tumors of all sites except the appendix occurs in the fifth to sixth decades of life. However, tumors have been reported at patient ages from less than 1 year to 98 years old. There is no significant sex predominance in most series if appendiceal tumors, which appear to be more common in females (ratio of 10:3), are excluded. This may be due to a greater number of appendectomies in conjunction with pelvic or gallbladder surgery in women. Age-adjusted rates of incidence have been

Table 27-13. Carcinoid Tumor Cell Characteristics

	Foregut	Midgut	Hindgut
Silver-staining characteristics	Argyrophilic	Argentaffinic	Nonreactive
Histology	Type B (Soga)	Type A (Soga)	Mixed (Soga)
Secretory granules	Uniformly round Variably dense 150–250 nm	Pleomorphic Uniformly dense 75–500 nm	Round Variably dense 165–235 nm

Source: Adapted from Soga J, Tazawa K, *Cancer* 28:990, 1971.

reported to be slightly higher in blacks than in whites (2.0 to 1.47 per 100,000 a year), for unknown reasons.[112]

Association with Other Neoplasms

Carcinoid tumors are frequently associated with other neoplasms. Among 390 patients from four autopsy series, 37 percent had another primary neoplasm, as did 18 percent of 374 patients in four surgical series.[107] The reason for these findings is unknown.

Secretory Products

A wide variety of secretory products have been identified in the circulation or extracted from carcinoid tumors or their metastases (Table 27-14). Serotonin was most frequently found. However, the prevalence of serotonin or any of the other compounds remains uncertain. Serotonin, 5-hydroxytryptophan, bradykinin, histamine, and prostaglandins have frequently been implicated in the pathophysiology of different aspects of the malignant carcinoid syndrome. However, there is no conclusive evidence to prove involvement of any one of these compounds.

Clinical Features

The large majority of carcinoid tumors are small (less than 2 cm) and asymptomatic and are found at autopsy or during unrelated surgical procedures. They can cause biliary obstruction and jaundice when located at or near the ampulla of Vater. Larger carcinoids (more than 2 cm), which are usually located in the ileum, can produce diarrhea, bleeding, infarction and intermittent jaundice; moreover, larger carcinoids are usually malignant (see above).

Table 27-14. Secretory Products of Carcinoid Tumors or Metastases

Serotonin	} relatively common	Dopamine
5-Hydroxytryptophan		Norepinephrine
Histamine		Vasointestinal peptide
Bradykinin		MSH
5-HIAA		PTH
		ADH
ACTH		Neurotensin
Kallikrein		Enteroglucagon
Prostaglandins		Glucagon
Calcitonin		Insulin
Growth hormone		Gastrin
Motilin		HCG-α
Substance P		Pancreatic polypeptide

Table 27-15. Clinical Manifestations of the Carcinoid Syndrome

Manifestation	Percent of patients affected*
Cutaneous flushing	84
GI hypermotility	79
Signs of heart disease	37
Bronchoconstriction	17
Abnormal pigmentation (pellagra-like)	5

*Total: 282 patients.
Source: Data from Kahler HJ: *Das Karzinoid*. Berlin, Springer-Verlag, 1967; Thorson AH, *Acta Med Scand (Suppl)* 344, 1958; Davis Z, *Surg Gyn Obstet* 137: 637, 1973.

The Clinical Carcinoid Syndrome

Classical symptoms of this syndrome include episodic cutaneous flushing, gastrointestinal disturbances such as diarrhea and cramps, bronchoconstriction, and right-sided valvular heart disease. The syndrome is a rare complication occurring in only about 5 percent of patients with carcinoid tumors. Ileal tumors are much more likely to be associated with the syndrome than rectal and appendiceal tumors.[109,110]

It has generally been accepted that the carcinoid syndrome associated with gastrointestinal carcinoids requires the presence of hepatic metastases. The most likely reason for the absence of symptoms in most patients is hepatic inactivation of tumor products released into the portal circulation. Hepatic metastases, on the other hand, secrete their products directly into the peripheral circulation. Bronchial and ovarian carcinoids also secrete their products into the peripheral circulation and have been known to be associated with the carcinoid syndrome in the absence of liver metastases.

Tumor mass may also play a role in the development of the carcinoid syndrome. Gastrointestinal carcinoids are generally small tumors and may require the additional tumor mass supplied by hepatic metastases to produce sufficient humoral material.

Cutaneous flushing is the most commonly reported finding (about 84 percent of cases; Table 27-15). It consists of a diffuse, erythematous flush in the face, neck, and anterior chest. The flush usually lasts from 3 to 10 min and may recur as often as 30 times a day. The flushing may be spontaneous or triggered by food intake, emotion, liver palpation, or administration of catecholamines, reserpine, alcohol, calcium, pentagastrin, or isoproterenol. A variant of the carcinoid flush has been reported, consisting of a more cyanotic skin discoloration. It may last longer and result in the development of facial telangiectases, conjunctival injection, and lacrimation.[103] This may, however, be simply a more severe form of the ordinary carcinoid flush.

Intestinal symptoms have been reported in about 79 percent of patients with the carcinoid syndrome. Explosive and watery diarrhea, with as many as 20 stools daily, is the most common manifestation. This is often accompanied by cramping, bloating, and borborygmi. These symptoms may or may not occur together with flushing. Whether the diarrhea is secretory or due to hypermotility or both is not clear.

Signs of cardiac involvement have been reported in about 37 percent of patients with carcinoid syndrome. It is likely that with the use of modern diagnostic tests, such as echocardiography and CT scanning, the incidence of heart disease will be found to be even higher.

Cardiac lesions are primarily right-sided valvular lesions, most commonly tricuspid regurgitation. Pulmonary stenosis also occurs, but rarely in the absence of concomitant tricuspid valve involvement. The anatomic basis for carcinoid heart disease is the carcinoid plaque, a thick, whitish material covering the surfaces of the right heart valves, right atrium, and interior surfaces of vessels draining into the right side of the heart. These plaques consist of smooth muscle cells (myofibroblasts) embedded in a stroma of reticulum fibers and acid mucopolysaccharides. The cause of the plaque formation remains obscure.[113] Tricuspid regurgitation occurs secondary to valvular leaflet deformity caused by plaque accumulation. Chordae tendiniae thickened by plaque may also contribute to regurgitation.[114] Rigidity of the plaque-covered leaflets most likely accounts for tricuspid or pulmonic stenosis. Predilection for right-sided structures is best explained by the fact that whatever substance is responsible for the production of plaque is present in higher concentrations in the right than in the left side of the heart. Left-sided cardiac involvement is sometimes seen with bronchial or ovarian carcinoid tumors, probably because of release of products from these tumors directly into the systemic circulation.

Bronchoconstriction and asthmalike symptoms are reported in about 17 percent of patients with the carcinoid syndrome. Wheezing and hyperventilation are prominent symptoms. Bronchoconstriction related to carcinoid syndrome should not be treated with catecholamines because of the risk of further mediator release.

Skin lesions resembling those of pellagra are seen in about 5 percent of patients. It has been speculated that these may be due to the shunting of tryptophan away from niacin production to provide for increased serotonin synthesis (Fig. 27-8). Darkening of the facial skin and development of telangiectases secondary to repeated flushing have also been noted.

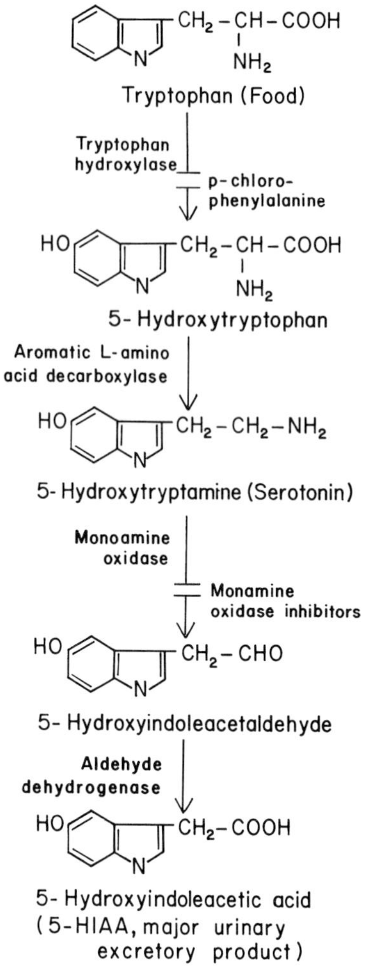

FIGURE 27-8 Synthesis and metabolism of serotonin.

Pathophysiology and Biochemistry

Tryptophan hydroxylase is the rate-limiting enzyme in the formation of serotonin from tryptophan (Fig. 27-8). Serotonin is subsequently deaminated by monoamine oxidase and aldehyde dehydrogenase to yield 5-HIAA, the major urine-excreted metabolite. Although initially thought to be responsible for most of the symptoms of malignant carcinoid syndrome, the role of serotonin appears to be limited to the gastrointestinal, respiratory, and cardiac manifestations. There is evidence that serotonin plays no important part in the flush mechanism. For instance, intravenous administration of serotonin does not reliably reproduce typical flushing in carcinoid patients; there is little correlation between free blood serotonin levels and flushing; and catecholamine infusion, which *does* provoke flushing, is not accompanied by changes in serotonin levels, nor do inhibitors of serotonin action (parachlorophenylalanine and methysergide) inhibit flushing. On the other hand, serotonin's role in gastrointestinal hypermotility is supported by the ability of serotonin inhibitors to decrease diarrhea and cramping (see Treatment). Also, serotonin given intravenously to healthy volunteers causes diarrhea. Serotonin's possible role in the formation of the carcinoid plaque is supported by the finding that similar lesions can be induced in guinea pigs fed diets rich in serotonin and that certain African populations who eat large amounts of plantain, a rich source of serotonin, frequently develop endomyocardial fibrosis.[115]

In 1966, Oates et al. provided evidence supporting bradykinin's participation in the carcinoid flush.[116] Carcinoid tumors and their metastases are known to synthesize kallikrein, which catalyzes the conversion of kininogen to bradykinin. When given intravenously to normal volunteers, bradykinin causes arteriolar vasodilation and reflex venoconstriction and generally provokes a typical carcinoidlike cutaneous flush. Bradykinin concentrations have been found to be elevated in the blood of most patients with carcinoid tumors. Catecholamine-induced release of kallikrein is thought to be a major mechanism in increased blood levels of bradykinin and flushing. Bradykinin is also a prime candidate for the pulmonary symptoms of carcinoid syndrome because of its ability to constrict bronchiolar smooth muscle.

It appears likely that other as yet unidentified gastrointestinal peptides or amines may be involved in the carcinoid flush. This belief is supported by the finding that somatostatin, a potent inhibitor of peptide release, inhibits carcinoid flushing provoked by the intravenous administration of pentagastrin.[117] Inhibition of carcinoid flushing with clonidine, suggesting involvement of the α-adrenergic system in flush-mediator release or action, has been reported.[118]

Diagnosis

Measurement of urinary 5-HIAA is probably the most reliable diagnostic test in the evaluation of a suspected carcinoid tumor.[102,103,119] Normal excretion of urinary 5-HIAA is less than 10 mg in 24 h. Most patients with the carcinoid syndrome excrete more than 50 mg per 24 h. Several days of urine collection are recommended because of the fluctuating nature of urinary 5-HIAA excretion. Increased urinary 5-HIAA excretion may be seen after the ingestion of serotonin-containing foods such as bananas, pineapples, walnuts, and chocolate and after administration of phenothiazines, glyceryl guaiacolate, mandelamine, and reserpine. Direct measurement of circulating serotonin levels may aid in the diagnosis (see Table 27-16).

Provocation of the carcinoid flush with intravenous injection of epinephrine has been reported useful in patients with equivocal biochemical profiles (Table 27-16). The test is positive when patients experience a flush which is similar to their spontaneous flushes. However, provocation of flushing may be hazardous, particularly in patients with cardiac disease or asthma. In addition, the incidence of false-positive or false-negative results with flush provocation is not known, further limiting the usefulness of this test.

LOCALIZATION CT scanning and ultrasonography have been used to detect abdominal, retroperitoneal, or hepatic tumors. Liver scintigraphic studies are useful in delineating metastases and may guide biopsy attempts. Upper gastrointestinal series are occasionally helpful by revealing an intraluminal filling defect in the esophagus, stomach, or proximal small bowel. Multiple filling defects in the esophagus, stomach, or

Table 27-16. Suggested Workup of Patients with Suspected Carcinoid Tumors or Carcinoid Syndrome

Biochemical evaluation:

1. Urine collection (24 h) for 5-HIAA (see text for details); urinary 5-hydroxytryptophan if foregut tumor suspected
2. Blood serotonin determination (normal range 30–200 ng/ml). Tagari et al. (*Clin Chem* 30:131, 1984) reported levels 25 times normal in patients with carcinoid syndrome. Same pre-test dietary restrictions as urinary 5-HIAA assay
3. Liver function tests. Generally elevated with hepatic metastases. No specific pattern reported
4. Flush provocation—protocol of Levine and Sjoerdsma, *Ann Intern Med* 58:818 1963—may be helpful in patients with equivocal biochemical profiles

Tumor Localization (as dictated by clinical situation; no pathognomonic findings; most GI carcinoids too small for contrast study detection):

1. CT scanning
2. Ultrasonography
3. Liver scan
4. Upper GI series
5. Barium enema
6. Chest x-ray
7. Endoscopy
8. Bronchoscopy
9. Angiography—selective celiac and/or superior mesenteric artery
10. Echocardiography—early evidence of valve leaflet thickening

proximal small bowel or in the ileum on small bowel follow-through examinations strongly suggest carcinoid.

Selective superior mesenteric and/or celiac angiography with or without contrast material has been used to visualize carcinoid tumors, particularly ileal tumors. Enhancement of the tumor stain is sometimes possible by administration of small doses of epinephrine (16 μg) prior to infusion of the contrast material.

Echocardiography has emerged as an invaluable aid in the diagnosis of carcinoid heart disease. Early involvement of the tricuspid valve can be detected as thickening of the leaflets while normal chamber size and leaflet motion is maintained. As the disease progresses, right ventricular hypertrophy and abnormal septal motion develop. In addition, the tricuspid valve becomes more thickened and begins to retract, until eventually the leaflets remain in a semiopen position throughout the cardiac cycle. Similar thickening and retraction may involve the pulmonic valve.[120] Characteristic is the absence of left-sided structural abnormalities except for occasional cases of left-sided disease accompanying ovarian or bronchial carcinoids.

Carcinoid Variants

GASTRIC CARCINOIDS Gastric carcinoids are rare. An average of 2.8 percent of close to 7000 patients with carcinoid tumors (Table 27-12) had gastric carcinoid tumors. Unique features of gastric carcinoids include a distinctive flush, an increased incidence of peptic ulcer disease,[121] and variations in tumor biochemistry. The flush associated with the gastric carcinoid syndrome has a bright red and geographic appearance and usually involves the base of the neck.[103] Histamine is a likely candidate as mediator of this flush and may also be responsible for the increased incidence of peptic ulceration (up to 25 percent) in patients with gastric carcinoid. Flushing in gastric carcinoid patients can be blocked by prophylactic administration of diphenhydramine and cimetidine to block H_1 and H_2 receptors.[115] Gastric carcinoid tumors, like most foregut tumors, lack aromatic L-amino acid decarboxylase (Fig. 27-8). This prevents conversion of 5-hydroxytryptophan to serotonin and results in the elevated levels of 5-hydroxytryptophan which are typically seen in the serum and urine of such patients. The lack of serotonin production by these tumors has been suggested as the explanation for their low rate of cardiac involvement.

BRONCHIAL CARCINOIDS Bronchial carcinoids account for about 10 percent of all carcinoid tumors (Table 27-12). There are ultrastructural similarities between this type of carcinoid tumor and small cell carcinoma of the lung. The two entities may, in fact, be difficult to distinguish histologically. Okike et al. have reviewed 203 cases of bronchial carcinoids and found the average age of patients to be 48.[122] Symptoms of bronchial obstruction occurred in 61.5 percent. There was a 5 percent incidence of metastatic spread to many organs, with bony lesions being most common. Unique features of the bronchial carcinoid variant include a distinctive flush, a predominance of left-sided cardiac involvement, and an association with other endocrine disorders. The bronchial carcinoid flush often lasts for hours or even days, may involve the entire body, and is frequently accompanied by lacrimation, conjunctival suffusion, and facial edema. As with other foregut tumors, 5-hydroxytryptophan may be a more reliable biochemical marker than serotonin and may be measured in the urine.

Treatment and Prognosis

LOCALIZED DISEASE Small tumors (less than 1 cm in diameter), which are usually discovered incidentally, require nothing more than local resection, which results in cure rates approaching 100 percent. Large tumors (2 cm or more) are likely to be metastatic (>80 percent). They require aggressive surgery to resect the primary tumor, involved nodes, and surrounding tissue. In a recent series, this form of localized debulking resulted in a 71 percent 5-year survival. The surgical approach to tumors ranging from 1 to 2 cm in diameter lies somewhere between these two extremes and is based on several considerations, including tumor size, patient age, operative risk, and degree of tumor invasion.[118,123]

METASTATIC DISEASE Distant metastases are usually hepatic. Resection of hepatic metastases in selected patients with isolated solitary lesions or well-demarcated clusters of lesions may relieve the symptoms of the carcinoid syndrome. Hazards of this approach include the surgical risk of the procedure, the propensity of patients with carcinoid tumors to the formation of peritoneal adhesions postoperatively, and life-threatening hypotension during surgery or anesthesia secondary to stress-induced mediator release. Because of the small number of reported cases, the efficacy of this procedure remains uncertain. Hepatic artery occlusion for metastatic disease limited to the liver has been proposed. In a recent series of 10 patients, this procedure resulted in more than a 50 percent reduction in postoperative urinary 5-HIAA levels in all, a marked reduction in symptoms in eight, and one postoperative death. The median duration of response, however, was only 5 months.

Chemotherapy for metastatic carcinoid tumor remains disappointing. It should probably be reserved for those patients with symptoms that significantly interfere with daily activities or to patients with a poor prognosis, including those with carcinoid heart disease (median survival 14 months) or urinary 5-HIAA excretion of more than 150 mg per 24 h (median survival 11 months). A wide variety of single-agent and combination regimens have been employed. A recent large series of 200 patient treatments revealed adriamycin to be the most effective single agent and streptozotocin-5FU the most effective drug combination, producing an objective response in 33 percent, which lasted for a median of 7 months. Thus it would appear that the chemotherapeutic regimens have little or no beneficial effect when the median survival data are compared.

MALIGNANT CARCINOID SYNDROME Various pharmacological agents have been utilized to control the symptoms of the carcinoid syndrome.[115,118] None have been shown to be reliably effective. Parachlorophenylalanine (1 to 4 g per day), an inhibitor of serotonin synthesis through inhibition of tryptophan-5-hydroxylase (Fig. 27-8), has been shown to control gastrointestinal symptoms in some patients. Its effect on flushing has been minimal in most cases. Moreover, its use is complicated by serious side effects, including confusion, ataxia, and hallucinations. Methysergide (6 to 24 mg PO daily in divided doses) acts by blocking peripheral serotonin receptors. It has also been shown to be fairly effective in relieving diarrhea. Cyproheptadine (12 to 40 mg daily) acts as a peripheral antagonist of serotonin and histamine and relieves diarrhea. It also inhibits the flushing associated with gastric carcinoids, believed to be caused by histamine. Methyldopa inhibits the conversion of 5-hydroxytryptophan to serotonin (Fig. 27-8), but side effects secondary to the large doses needed (4 to 6 g daily) usually preclude its use. α-Adrenergic blockers such as clonidine and phenoxybenzamine have been used with some success to control flushing, presumably through blocking of catecholamine-mediated activation of the kallikrein-bradykinin system. Antihistaminic agents, including cimetidine, have been used in controlling the histamine-induced flush of gastric carcinoid. Prednisone, presumably acting as a lysosomal membrane stabilizer, has been shown to suppress bradykinin release and may help with carcinoid flushing. Somatostatin, an investigational drug, has been shown to inhibit the carcinoid flush if used prophylactically. Somatostatin has also been shown to reverse bronchoconstriction in a carcinoid patient. The somatostatin analogue SMS 201-995 has also been used successfully for the treatment of diarrhea in the carcinoid syndrome.

REFERENCES

1. Bayliss WM, Starling EH: Croonian lecture: The chemical regulation of the secretory process. *Proc R Soc Lond* 73:310, 1904.
2. Bayliss WM: *Principles of General Physiology*. London, Longmans, 1915, p 706.
3. Walsh JH: Endocrine cells of the digestive system, in Johnson LR (ed): *Physiology of the Gastrointestinal Tract*. New York, Raven, 1981, p 59.
4. Boel E, Vuust J, Norris F, Norris K, Wind A, Rehfeld JF, Marcker KA: Molecular cloning of human gastrin cDNA: Evidence for evolution of gastrin by gene duplication. *Proc Natl Acad Sci USA* 80:2866, 1983.
5. Eysselein VE, Maxwell V, Reedy T, Wunsch E, Walsh JH: Similar acid stimulatory potencies of synthetic human big and little gastrins in man. *J Clin Invest* 73:1284, 1984.
6. Lamers CB, Walsh JH, Jansen JB, Harrison AR, Ippoliti AF, van Tongeren JH: Evidence that gastrin 34 is preferentially released from the human duodenum. *Gastroenterology* 83:233, 1982.
7. Larsson L-I, Rehfeld JF: Pituitary gastrins occur in corticotrophs and melanotrophs. *Science* 213:768, 1981.
8. Lichtenberger LM, Graziani LA, Dubinsky WP: Importance of dietary amines in meal-induced gastrin release. *Am J Physiol* 243:G341, 1982.
9. Singer MV, Eysselein V, Goebell H: Beer and wine but not whisky and pure ethanol do stimulate release of gastrin in humans. *Digestion* 26:73, 1983.
10. Schiller LR, Walsh JH, Feldman M: Effect of atropine on gastrin release stimulated by an amino acid meal in humans. *Gastroenterology* 83:267, 1982.
11. Schubert ML, Bitar KN, Makhlouf GM: Regulation of gastrin and somatostatin secretion by cholinergic and noncholinergic intramural neurons. *Am J Physiol* 243:G442, 1982.
12. Tatsuta M, Baba M, Itoh T: Increased gastrin secretion in patients with pheochromocytoma. *Gastroenterology* 84:920, 1983.
13. Jensen RT: Zollinger-Ellison syndrome: Current concepts and management. *Ann Int Med* 98:59, 1983.
14. McCarthy DM, Jensen RT: Zollinger-Ellison syndrome, in Cohen S, Soloway RD (eds): *Contemporary Issues in Gastroenterology: Hormone-Producing Tumors of the Gastrointestinal Tract*. New York, Churchill Livingstone, 1985, p 25.
15. Malagelada J-R, Davis CS, O'Fallon WM, Go VLW: Laboratory diagnosis of gastrinoma: I. A prospective evaluation of gastric analysis and fasting serum gastrin levels. *Mayo Clin Proc* 57:211, 1982.
16. Krudy AG, Doppman JL, Jensen RT, Norton JA, Collen MJ, Shawker TH, Gardner JD, McArthur K, Gorden P: Localization of islet cell tumors by dynamic CT: Comparison with plain CT, arteriography, sonography, and venous sampling. *Am J Roentgenol* 143:585, 1984.
17. Lamers CBHW, Lind T, Moberg S, Jansen JBMJ, Olbe L: Omeprazole in Zollinger-Ellison syndrome: Effects of a single dose and of long-term treatment in patients resistant to histamine H_2-receptor antagonists. *N Engl J Med* 310:758, 1984.
18. Dockray GJ: Cholecystokinin, in Bloom SR, Polak JM (eds): *Gut Hormones*. Edinburgh, Churchill Livingstone, 1981, p 228.

18a. Liddle RA, Goldfine ID, Rosen MS, Taplitz RA, Williams JA: Cholecystokinin bioactivity in human plasma: Molecular forms, responses to feeding, and relationship to gallbladder contraction. *J Clin Invest* 75:1144, 1985.

19. Walsh JH, Lamers CB, Valenzuela JE: Cholecystokinin-octapeptide–like immunoreactivity in human plasma. *Gastroenterology* 82:438, 1982.

19a. Beglinger C, Fried M, Whitehouse I, Jansen JB, Lamers CB, Gyr K: Pancreas enzyme response to a liquid meal and to hormonal stimulation: Correlation with plasma secretin and cholecystokinin levels. *J Clin Invest* 75:1471, 1985.

20. Renny A, Snape WJ Jr, Sun EA, London R, Cohen S: Role of cholecystokinin in the gastrocolonic response to a fat meal. *Gastroenterology* 85:17, 1983.
21. Szecowka J, Lins PE, Efendic S: Effects of cholecystokinin, gastric inhibitory polypeptide, and secretin on insulin and glucagon secretion in rats. *Endocrinology* 110:1268, 1982.
22. Faris PL, Komisaruk BR, Watkins LR, Mayer DJ: Evidence for the neuropeptide cholecystokinin as an antagonist of opiate analgesia. *Science* 219:310, 1983.
23. Said SI: Vasoactive intestinal polypeptide (VIP): Current status. *Peptides* 5:143, 1984.
24. O'Dorisio TM, Mekhjian HS: VIPoma syndrome, in Cohen S, Soloway RD (eds): *Contemporary Issues in Gastroenterology: Hormone Producing Tumors of the Gastrointestinal Tract.* New York, Churchill Livingstone, 1985, p 101.
25. Welbourn RB, Wood SM, Polak JM, Bloom SR: Pancreatic endocrine tumours, in Bloom SR, Polak JM (eds): *Gut Hormones.* Edinburgh, Churchill Livingstone, 1981, p 547.
26. Yamaguchi K, Abe K, Otsubo K, Haniuda C, Suzuki M, Shimada A, Kimura S, Adachi I, Kameya T, Yanaihara N: The WHDA syndrome. Clinical and laboratory data on 28 Japanese cases. *Peptides* 5:415, 1984.
27. Kane MG, O'Dorisio TM, Krejs GJ: Production of secretory diarrhea by intravenous infusion of vasoactive intestinal polypeptide. *N Engl J Med* 309:1482, 1983.
28. Jaffe BM, Kopen DF, DeSchryver-Kecskemeti K, Gingerich RL, Greider M: Indomethacin-responsive pancreatic cholera. *N Engl J Med* 297:817, 1977.
29. Tatemoto K, Mutt V: Isolation and characterization of the intestinal peptide porcine PHI (PHI-27), a new member of the glucagon secretin family. *Proc Natl Acad Sci USA* 78:6603, 1981.
30. Bloom SR, Christofides ND, Delamarter J, Buell G, Kawashima E, Polak JM: Diarrhoea in VIPoma patients associated with cosecretion of a second active peptide (peptide histidine isoleucine) explained by a single coding gene. *Lancet* 2:1163, 1983.
31. Maton PN, O'Dorisio TM, Howe BA, McArthur KE, Howard JM, Cherner JA, Malarkey TB, Collen MJ, Gardner JD, Jensen RT: Effect of a long-acting somatostatin analogue (SMS 201-995) in a patient with pancreatic cholera. *N Engl J Med* 312:17, 1985.
32. Wood SM, Kraenzlin ME, Bloom SR: New somatostatin analogue for home treatment of endocrine tumours. *Gut* 24:A984, 1983 (abstract).
33. Kraenzlin ME, Ch'ng JC, Wood SM, Bloom SR: Can inhibition of hormone secretion be associated with endocrine tumour shrinkage? *Lancet* 2:1501, 1983 (letter).
34. Tsuto TH, Okamura K, Fukui HL, Obata H, Terubayashi N, Iwai S, Marijima N, Yanaihara N, Ibata Y: An immunohistochemical investigation of vasoactive intestinal polypeptide in the colon of patients with Hirschsprung's disease. *Neurosci Lett* 34:57, 1982.
35. Aggestrup S, Uddman R, Sundler F, Fahrenkrug J, Hakanson R, Sorensen R, Hambraeus G: Lack of vasoactive intestinal polypeptide nerves in esophageal achalasia. *Gastroenterology* 84:924, 1983.
36. Brown JC, Dryburgh JR, Ross RA, Dupré J: Identification and actions of gastric inhibitory polypeptide. *Recent Prog Horm Res* 31:487, 1975.
37. Jornvall H, Carlquist M, Kwauk S, Otte SC, McIntosh CHS, Brown JC, Mutt V: Amino acid sequence and heterogeneity of gastric inhibitory polypeptide (GIP). *FEBS Lett* 123:205, 1981.
38. Krarup T, Madsbad S, Moody AJ, Regeur L, Faber OK, Holst JJ, Sestoft L: Diminished immunoreactive gastric inhibitory polypeptide response to a meal in newly diagnosed type I (insulin-dependent) diabetics. *J Clin Endocrinol Metab* 56:1306, 1983.
39. Ebert R, Illmer K, Creutzfeldt W: Release of gastric inhibitory polypeptide (GIP) by intraduodenal acidification in rats and humans and the abolishment of the incretin effect of acid by GIP-antiserum in rats. *Gastroenterology* 76:515, 1979.
40. Flaten O, Sand I, Myren J: Beta-adrenergic stimulation and blockade of the release of gastric inhibitory polypeptide and insulin in man. *Scand J Gastroenterol* 17:283, 1982.
41. Sarson DL, Hayter RC, Bloom SR: The pharmacokinetics of porcine glucose-dependent insulinotropic polypeptide (GIP) in man. *Eur J Clin Invest* 12:457, 1982.
42. Anderson DK: Physiological effects of GIP in man, in Bloom SR, Polak JM (eds): *Gut Hormones.* Edinburgh, Churchill Livingstone, 1981, p 256.
43. Mazzaferri EL, Ciofalo L, Waters LA, Starich GH, Groshong JC, DePalma L: Effects of gastric inhibitory polypeptide on leucine- and arginine-stimulated insulin release. *Am J Physiol* 245:E114, 1983.
44. Lauritsen KB, Lauritzen JB, Christensen KC: Gastric inhibitory polypeptide and insulin release in response to oral and intravenous glucose in coeliac disease. *Scand J Gastroenterol* 17:241, 1982.
45. Ebert R, Creutzfeldt W: Influence of gastric inhibitory polypeptide antiserum on glucose-induced insulin secretion in rats. *Endocrinology* 111:1601, 1982.
46. Ross SA, Brown JC, Dupré J: Hypersecretion of gastric inhibitory polypeptide following oral glucose in diabetes mellitus. *Diabetes* 26:525, 1977.
47. Krarup T, Madsbad S, Moody AJ: Immunoreactive gastric inhibitory polypeptide response to a meal during the first eighteen months after diagnosis of type 1 (insulin dependent) diabetes mellitus. *J Clin Endocrinol Metab* 60:120, 1985.
48. Ebert R, Creutzfeldt W, Brown JC, Frerichs H, Arnold R: Response of gastric inhibitory polypeptide (GIP) to test meal in chronic pancreatitis: Relationship to endocrine and exocrine insufficiency. *Diabetologia* 12:609, 1976.
49. Cataland S, O'Dorisio TM, Brooks R, Mekhjian HS: Stimulation of gastric inhibitory polypeptide in normal and duodenal ulcer patients. *Gastroenterology* 73:19, 1977.
50. Hadji-Georgopoulos A, Schmidt MI, Elahi D, Hershcopf R, Kowarski AA: Increased gastric inhibitory polypeptide levels in patients with symptomatic postprandial hypoglycemia. *J Clin Endocrinol Metab* 56:648, 1983.
51. Mutt V, Jorpes JE: Secretin: Isolation and determination of structure. *Proc 4th Int Sympos Chem Natural Products, Stockholm, Sweden, 1966,* sec 2C-3.
52. Bodansky M, Ondetti MA, Levine SD, Marajam VC, von Saltza JT, Williams NJ, Sabo ET: Synthesis of a heptacosapeptide amide with the hormonal activity of secretin. *Chem Industry* 42:1757, 1966.
53. O'Donohue TL, Charlton CG, Miller RL, Boden G, Jacobowitz DM: Identification, characterization, and distribution of secretin immunoreactivity in rat and pig brain. *Proc Natl Acad Sci USA* 78:5221, 1981.
54. Schaffalitzky de Muckadell OB, Fahrenkrug J: Secretion pattern of secretin in man: Regulation by gastric acid. *Gut* 19:812, 1978.
55. Yang RK, Li HR, Eng J, Greenstein R, Straus E, Yalow RS: Secretin responses to feeding and acid load. *J Lab Clin Med* 102:17, 1983.
56. Boden G, Sivitz MC, Owen OE, Essa-Koumar N, Landor J: Somatostatin suppresses secretin and pancreatic exocrine secretion. *Science* 190:163, 1975.
57. Boden G, Essa N, Owen OE, Reichle FA: Effect of intraduodenal administration of HCl and glucose on circulating immunoreactive secretin and insulin concentrations. *J Clin Invest* 53:1185, 1974.
58. Kleibeuker JH, Eysselein VE, Maxwell VE, Walsh JH: Role of endogenous secretin in acid-induced inhibition of human gastric function. *J Clin Invest* 73:526, 1984.
59. Straus E: Radioimmunoassay of gastrointestinal hormones. *Gastroenterology* 74:141, 1978.
60. Renner IG, Wisner JR Jr, Rinderknecht H: Protective effects

of exogenous secretin on ceruletide-induced acute pancreatitis in the rat. *J Clin Invest* 72:1081, 1983.

61. Boden G: Extrapancreatic glucagon in human subjects, in Unger RH, Orci L (eds): *Glucagon: Physiology, Pathophysiology, and Morphology of the Pancreatic A-cells.* New York, Elsevier, 1981, p 349.

62. Lefebvre PJ, Lyckx AS: Extrapancreatic glucagon and its regulation, in Lefebvre PJ (ed): *Handbook of Experimental Pharmacology,* vol 66-II, *Glucagon.* New York, Springer Verlag, 1983, p 205.

63. Moody AJ, Thim L: Glucagon, glicentin, and related peptides, in Lefebvre PJ (ed): *Handbook of Experimental Pharmacology,* vol 66-I, *Glucagon.* New York, Springer Verlag, 1983, p 139.

64. Gleeson MH, Bloom SR, Polak JM, Henry K, Dowling RH: Endocrine tumor in kidney affecting small bowel structure, motility, and absorptive function. *Gut* 12:773, 1971.

65. Floyd JC, Vinik AI: Pancreatic polypeptide, in Bloom SR, Polak JM (eds): *Gut Hormones.* New York, Churchill Livingstone, 1981, p 195.

66. Wilson RM, Boden G, Owen OE: Pancreatic polypeptide responses to a meal and to intraduodenal amino acids and sodium oleate. *Endocrinology* 102:859, 1978.

67. Schwartz TW, Holst JJ, Fahrenkrug J, Lindkaer Jensen S, Nielsen OV, Rehfeld JF, Schaffalitzky de Muckadell OB, Stadil F: Vagal, cholinergic regulation of pancreatic-polypeptide secretion. *J Clin Invest* 61:781, 1978.

68. Taylor IL, Solomon TE, Walsh JH, Grossman MI: Pancreatic polypeptide metabolism and effect on pancreatic secretion in dogs. *Gastroenterology* 76:525, 1979.

69. Adrian TE, Greenberg GR, Bloom SR: Actions of pancreatic polypeptide in man, in Bloom SR, Polak JM (eds): *Gut Hormones.* Edinburgh, Churchill Livingstone, 1981, p 206.

70. Boden G, Master RW, Owen OE, Rudnick MR: Human pancreatic polypeptide in chronic renal failure and cirrhosis of the liver: Role of kidneys and liver in pancreatic polypeptide metabolism. *J Clin Endocrinol Metab* 51:573, 1980.

71. Strodel WE, Vinik AI, Lloyd RV, Glaser B, Eckhauser FE, Fiddian-Green RG, Turcotte JG, Thompson NW: Pancreatic polypeptide-producing tumors. *Arch Surg* 119:508, 1984.

72. O'Dorisio TM, Vinik AI: Pancreatic peptide and mixed peptide producing tumors of the gastrointestinal tract, in Cohen S, Soloway RD (eds): *Contemporary Issues in Gastroenterology: Hormone Producing Tumors of the Gastrointestinal Tract.* New York, Churchill Livingstone, 1985, p 117.

73. Tatemoto K: Isolation and characterization of peptide YY (PYY), a candidate gut hormone that inhibits pancreatic exocrine secretion. *Proc Natl Acad Sci USA* 79:2514, 1982.

74. Tatemoto K: Neuropeptide Y: Complete amino acid sequence of the brain peptide. *Proc Natl Acad Sci USA* 79:5485, 1982.

75. Lundberg JM, Tatemoto K, Terenius L, Hellstrom PM, Mutt V, Hokfelt T, Hamberger B: Localization of peptide YY (PYY) in gastrointestinal endocrine cells and effects on intestinal blood flow and motility. *Proc Natl Acad Sci USA* 79:4471, 1982.

76. Allen YS, Adrian TE, Allen JM, Tatemoto K, Crow TJ, Bloom SR, Polak JM: Neuropeptide Y distribution in the rat brain. *Science* 221:877, 1983.

77. Reichlin S: Somatostatin. *N Engl J Med* 309:1495, 1983.

78. Shen LP, Pictet RL, Rutter WJ: Human somatostatin I: Sequence of the cDNA. *Proc Natl Acad Sci USA* 79:4575, 1982.

79. Sheppard M, Shapiro B, Pimstone B, Kronheim S, Berelowitz M, Gregory M: Metabolic clearance and plasma half-disappearance time of exogenous somatostatin in man. *J Clin Endocrinol Metab* 48:50, 1979.

80. Schusdziarra V, Zyznar E, Rouiller D, Boden G, Brown JC, Arimura A, Unger RH: Splanchnic somatostatin: A hormonal regulator of nutrient homeostasis. *Science* 207:530, 1980.

81. Saffouri B, Weir G, Bitar K, Makhlouf G: Stimulation of gastrin secretion from the perfused rat stomach by somatostatin antiserum. *Life Sci* 25:1749, 1979.

82. Larson LI: Gastrointestinal cells producing endocrine, neurocrine and paracrine messengers. *Clin Gastroenterol* 9:485, 1980.

83. Davies P, Katzman R, Terry RD: Reduced somatostatin-like immunoreactivity in cerebral cortex from cases of Alzheimer disease and Alzheimer senile dementia. *Nature* 288:279, 1980.

84. Patel YC, Rao K, Reichlin S: Somatostatin in human cerebrospinal fluid. *N Engl J Med* 296:529, 1977.

85. Ganda OP, Weir GC, Soeldner JS, Pegg MA, Chick WL, Patel YC, Ebeid AM, Gabbay KH, Reichlin S: 'Somatostatinoma': A somatostatin-containing tumor of the endocrine pancreas. *N Engl J Med* 296:963, 1977.

86. Larsson L-I, Holst JJ, Kuhl C, Lundquist G, Hirsch MA, Ingemansson S, Lindkaer Jenson S, Rehfeld JF, Schwartz TW: Pancreatic somatostatinoma: Clinical features and physiological implications. *Lancet* 1:666, 1977.

87. Boden G, Shimoyama R: Somatostatinoma, in Cohen S, Soloway RD (eds): *Contemporary Issues in Gastroenterology: Hormone Producing Tumors of the Gastrointestinal Tract.* New York, Churchill Livingstone, 1985, p 85.

88. McDonald TJ, Jornvall H, Nilsson G, Vagne M, Ghatei M, Bloom SR, Mutt V: Characterization of a gastrin releasing peptide from porcine non-antral gastric tissue. *Biochem Biophys Res Commun* 90:227, 1979.

89. Brown M, Marki W, Rivier J: Is gastrin releasing peptide mammalian bombesin? *Life Sci* 27:125, 1980.

90. Iguchi A, Matsunaga H, Nomura T, Gotoh M, Sakamoto N: Glucoregulatory effects of intrahypothalamic injections of bombesin and other peptides. *Endocrinology* 114:2242, 1984.

91. Willey JC, Lechner JF, Harris CC: Bombesin and the C-terminal tetradecapeptide of gastrin-releasing peptide are growth factors for normal human bronchial epithelial cells. *Exp Cell Res* 153:245, 1984.

92. Moody TW, Pert CB, Gazdar AF, Carney DN, Minna JD: High levels of intracellular bombesin characterize human small cell lung carcinoma. *Science* 214:1246, 1981.

93. Weber S, Zuckerman JE, Bostwick DG, Bensch KG, Sikic BI, Raffin TA: Gastrin releasing peptide is a selective mitogen for small cell lung carcinoma in vitro. *J Clin Invest* 75:306, 1985.

94. Pernow B: Substance P. *Pharmacol Rev* 35:85, 1983.

95. Buck SH, Burcher E, Shults CW, Lovenburg W, O'Donohue TL: Novel pharmacology of substance K–binding sites: A third type of tachykinin receptor. *Science* 226:987, 1984.

96. Payan DG, Brewster DR, Missirian-Bastian A, Goetzl EJ: Substance P recognition by a subset of human T lymphocytes. *J Clin Invest* 74:1532, 1984.

97. Levine JD, Clark R, Devor M, Helms C, Moskowitz MA, Basbaum AI: Intraneuronal substance P contributes to the severity of experimental arthritis. *Science* 226:547, 1984.

98. Powell D, Skrabanek P: Substance P, in Bloom SR, Polak JM (eds): *Gut Hormones.* Edinburgh, Churchill Livingstone, 1981, p 396.

99. Leeman SE, Carraway RE: Neurotensin: Discovery, isolation, characterization, synthesis and possible physiologic roles. *Ann NY Acad Sci* 400:1, 1982.

100. Hammer RA, Leeman SE: Neurotensin: Properties and actions, in Bloom SR, Polak JM (eds): *Gut Hormones.* Edinburgh, Churchill Livingstone, 1981, p 290.

101. Christofides ND, Bloom SR: Motilin, in Bloom SR, Polak JM (eds): *Gut Hormones.* Edinburgh, Churchill Livingstone, 1981, p 271.

102. Modlin IM: Carcinoid syndrome. *J Clin Gastroenterol* 2:349, 1980.

103. Grahame-Smith DG: The carcinoid syndrome. *Am J Cardiol* 21:376, 1968.

104. Soga J: Carcinoids: Their changing concepts and a new histologic classification, in Fujita T (ed): *Gastro-Entero-Pancreatic Endo-*

crine System. Baltimore, Williams & Wilkins, 1974, p 101.
105. Berge T and Linell F: Carcinoid tumors—frequency in a defined population during a 12-year period. *Acta Pathol Microbiol Scand* 84:322, 1976.
106. Moertel CG: Small intestine, in Holland JF, Frei E III (eds): *Cancer Medicine.* Philadelphia, Lea & Febiger, 1982, p 1808.
106a. Mengel CE: The carcinoid syndrome, in Holland JF, Frei E III (eds): *Cancer Medicine.* Philadelphia, Lea & Febiger, 1982, p 1818.
107. Moertel CG, Sauer WG, Dockerty MB, Baggenstoss AH: Life history of the carcinoid tumor of the small intestine. *Cancer* 14:901, 1961.
108. Bates HR Jr: Carcinoid tumors of the rectum: A statistical review. *Dis Colon Rectum,* 9:90, 1966.
109. Beaton H, Homan W, Dineen P: Gastrointestinal carcinoids and the malignant carcinoid syndrome. *Surg Gynecol Obstet* 152:268, 1981.
110. Wilson H, Cheek RC, Sherman RT, Storer EH: Carcinoid tumors, in Ravitch MM (ed): *Current Problems in Surgery.* Chicago, Yearbook, p 1, 1970.
111. DeLellis RA, Dayal Y, Wolfe HJ: Carcinoid tumors: Changing concepts and new perspectives. *Am J Surg Pathol* 8:295, 1984.
112. Godwin JD II: Carcinoid tumors: An analysis of 2837 cases. *Cancer* 36:560, 1975.
113. Strickman NE, Rossi PA, Massumkhani GA, Hall RJ: Carcinoid heart disease: A clinical pathologic and therapeutic update. *Curr Prob Cardiol* 6:1, 1982.
114. Davies MK, Lowry PJ, Littler WA: Cross sectional echocardiographic feature in carcinoid heart disease. *Br Heart J* 51:355, 1984.
115. Gillin JS, Winawer SJ: Malignant carcinoid syndrome: Manifestations and management. *Drug Ther* 13 (June):149, 1983.
116. Oates JA, Pettinger WA, Doctor RB: Evidence for the release of bradykinin in carcinoid syndrome. *J Clin Invest* 45:173, 1966.
117. Frolich JC, Bloomgarden ZT, Oates JA, McGuigan JE, Rabinowitz D: The carcinoid flush: Provocation by pentagastrin and inhibition by somatostatin. *N Engl J Med* 299:1055, 1978.
118. Moertel CG: Treatment of the carcinoid tumor and the malignant carcinoid syndrome. *J Clin Oncol* 1:727, 1983.
119. Strodel WE, Vinik AI, Thompson NW, Edkhauser FE, Talpos GB: Small bowel carcinoid tumors and the carcinoid syndrome, in Thompson NW, Vinik AI (eds): *Endocrine Surgery Update.* New York, Grune & Stratton, 1983, p 277.
120. Callahan JA, Wroblewski EM, Reeder GS, Edwards WD, Seward JB, Tajik AJ: Echocardiographic features of carcinoid heart disease. *Am J Cardiol* 50:762, 1982.
121. Dawes L, Schulte WJ, Condon RE: Carcinoid tumors. *Arch Surg* 119:375, 1984.
122. Okike N, Bernatz PE, Woolner LB: Carcinoid tumors of the lung. *Ann Thorac Surg* 22:270, 1976.
123. Wareing TH, Sawyers JL: Carcinoids and the carcinoid syndrome. *Am J Surg* 145:769, 1983.

28

Multiglandular Endocrine Disorders*

Leonard J. Deftos
Bayard D. Catherwood
Henry G. Bone III

MULTIPLE ENDOCRINE NEOPLASIA TYPE 1

Definition and History

Since early in this century, multiglandular neoplastic changes have been observed in the endocrine organs of certain individuals. Over time, consistent patterns of such tumors were found to occur in several members of affected families. From these observations have emerged certain widely recognized hereditary syndromes of multiple endocrine neoplasia. These include multiple endocrine neoplasia type 1 (MEN 1), also known as the *multiple endocrine adenomatosis* (MEA)–*peptic ulcer syndrome*, or *Wermer's syndrome,* and the two variants of *Sipple's syndrome,* medullary thyroid carcinoma and pheochromocytoma (known as MEN 2a and 2b). It should be understood that not every example of polyglandular endocrine neoplasia fits one of these well-defined hereditary syndromes.

*Supported by the National Institutes of Health, the American Cancer Society, and the Veterans Administration.

As knowledge advances, it may be possible to delineate additional distinct genetic disorders manifested by various combinations of tumors of endocrine glands beyond the classic syndromes described in this chapter.

Components of the Syndrome

MEN 1 is an autosomal dominant disorder with a high degree of penetrance and some variability of expression. Affected individuals typically have tumors of the parathyroid and pituitary glands and the endocrine pancreas; they may have other tumors as well. The early reports which led to the recognition of this syndrome were based on autopsy studies. Erdheim appears to have been the first to describe the appearance of more than one endocrine tumor in a single individual, in his report of autopsy studies published in 1903.[1] In a subsequent autopsy study, Cushing and Davidoff reported thyroid, parathyroid, and adrenal hyperplasia in four acromegalic patients.[2] Lloyd described a case of "hypophyseo-parathyreo-insular syndrome" in 1929.[3] An early premortem description of patients with what would probably now be recognized as MEN 1 was published by Rossier and Dressler in 1939.[4] They reported sisters with multiple endocrine disorders whose brothers had peptic ulcer disease. These authors were apparently the first to recognize the familial nature of multiple endocrine neoplasia. The specific association among adenomas of the parathyroid glands, the pituitary, and pancreatic islets was recognized by Underdahl et al.[5] in 1953 and by Moldawer et al.[6] in 1954. Current understanding of the syndrome is largely attributable to Wermer,[7] who, in 1954, described the familial aggregation of multiple adenomas of these glands and proposed that this constituted a distinct syndrome inherited as an autosomal dominant disorder. He noted the association with peptic ulcer disease in these patients and suggested the possibility of a genetic relationship between the ulcer disease and the endocrine adenomatosis. In 1955, an independent investigation led Zollinger and Ellison to the recognition of the syndrome that bears their names.[8] They described the association of severe peptic ulcer disease and gastric hypersecretion with non-insulin-producing islet cell tumors of the pancreas. It was subsequently recognized that the same syndrome may also be manifested by malabsorption or watery diarrhea.[9,10] It was gradually appreciated that the Zollinger-Ellison syndrome was produced by gastrin-secreting pancreatic neoplasms and could occur as a component of MEA syndrome along with insulinomas and parathyroid and pituitary tumors.[11–13]

The approximate relative frequencies of the various glandular tumors constituting the MEN 1 syndrome are indicated in Table 28-1. This table is based on a large number of reports and reviews; it should be understood that generally uncommon associations may be quite frequent within particular pedigrees. As shown in the table, primary hyperparathyroidism is the most common manifestation of the syndrome. Next most common among the adenomas are those occurring in the pancreas. The two kinds of pancreatic lesions generally recognized in this syndrome are insulinomas arising from the beta cells of the islets of Langerhans and gastrinomas of delta cell origin, which produce the Zollinger-Ellison syndrome. Both types of pancreatic adenoma are often multiple; either may appear as areas of hyperplasia rather than well-localized nodular adenomas. Pituitary adenomas may be slightly less common. In the past, these were thought to be nonfunctional in the majority of cases, although functional tumors were recognized, especially those causing acromegaly. More recently, it has been

Table 28-1. Approximate Relative Frequencies of Elements of the MEN 1 Syndrome

	Frequency, percent of patients
Hyperparathyroidism	80
Pancreatic tumors:	
Gastrinomas	
Benign	20
Malignant	30
Insulinomas	
Benign	20
Malignant	5
Nonfunctioning	
Benign	<5
Malignant	<5
Pituitary tumors:	
Chromophobe or nonfunctioning	
Benign	40
Malignant	<5
Eosinophilic or acromegalic (benign)	15
Cushing's disease, basophilic	5
Mixed and other types (benign)	<5
Prolactin-secreting	15(?)
Other tumors:	
Carcinoid and bronchial adenoma	<5
Lipoma/liposarcoma	5
Adrenal cortical adenoma	10
Thyroid adenomas	5

Note: These figures are based on the reviews cited in the text but are adjusted to reflect modern diagnostic criteria and to reduce ascertainment bias.

recognized that some of the pituitary adenomas are prolactin-producing.[14-17] As Table 28-1 indicates, adenomas of the other endocrine glands are much less common. Their etiologic relationship to the genetic disorder is uncertain. Lipomas occur regularly in affected members of certain pedigrees.[18]

PRIMARY HYPERPARATHYROIDISM

Primary hyperparathyroidism is the single most common feature of MEN 1, occurring in 80 to 90 percent of cases. It has become clear that, although one or more of the parathyroid glands may appear at surgery to be normal, all the glands have the potential for neoplastic enlargement. If only one or two enlarged glands are removed at the time of the original operation, the likelihood of persistent or recurrent hyperparathyroidism is great. This has led to the recommendation of subtotal parathyroidectomy.[19,20]

There has been considerable difference of opinion as to the proper description of the pathologic process in these parathyroid glands. Although the contemporaneous enlargement of multiple glands has prompted some authors to use the term *hyperplasia,* others have preferred to use the term *multiple adenomas.* The latter term carries the implication that the neoplastic changes are primary processes which may arise concurrently but independently in the different glands; it is more in keeping with current theories of pathogenesis. From a pragmatic standpoint, the use of the term *multiglandular primary hyperparathyroidism* has considerable appeal.[19] Histologically, these glands are usually dominated by chief cells, but clear-cell dominance may also be seen, as well as a mixed picture. Parathyroid carcinoma is not a feature of typical MEN 1, although a case has been reported in association with familial primary hyperparathyroidism and a suspect family history.[21] Patients with primary multiglandular hyperparathyroidism are fairly often found to have relatives with either familial primary hyperparathyroidism or MEN 1, but sporadic instances of isolated primary multiglandular parathyroid disease occur as well.[22-24] (See Note Added in Proof.)

PANCREATIC TUMORS

Malignant Potential

The pancreatic tumors differ markedly from the other elements of the MEN 1 syndrome in that both the insulin- and gastrin-producing tumors may take a malignant course, with invasion and metastasis in as many as half of affected individuals in some series.[12,13,25]

Insulinoma

Insulinoma is a fairly common and often clinically striking feature of the MEN 1 syndrome. This tumor arises from the beta cells of the islets of Langerhans; it secretes excessive amounts of insulin. The clinical presentation is similar to that seen with sporadic insulinomas; the principal features are hypoglycemia and its associated symptoms. These may include seizures, loss of consciousness, or symptoms associated with the counterregulatory response. Typically, patients have a constant sensation of hunger, and the hypoglycemia may be masked by a constant carbohydrate intake. Often, such patients have nightmares or other nocturnal symptoms when their carbohydrate intake is interrupted by sleep. Such patients are frequently affected by marked weight gain and may have hypoglycemic symptoms when they attempt to restrict their caloric intake in order to lose weight. Insulinomas may be single or multiple and may be poorly demarcated. The common occurrence of multiple insulinomas or nodular hyperplasia of the beta cells makes selective resection extremely difficult, so subtotal pancreatectomy is frequently required. Of all the components of the MEN 1 syndrome, insulinoma probably constitutes the most severe hazard to the patient because of the neurologic effects of hypoglycemia.

Gastrinoma

Gastrin-producing tumors, derived from the delta cells of the islets of Langerhans, may occur in patients with insulin-producing tumors; more often, though, patients are afflicted with only one or the other pancreatic tumor. Although for some time the Zollinger-Ellison syndrome was treated as a completely separate entity, it is now recognized that individual patients may have the gastrinoma syndrome alone or as a feature of MEA. The Zollinger-Ellison syndrome is quite likely to be diagnosed because of the severe symptoms of the ulcer diathesis, with gastric hypersecretion and/or secretory diarrhea and malabsorption. For this reason, it is often the presenting complaint of the index case in an affected family. It should be borne in mind that hyperparathyroidism may mimic or unmask the Zollinger-Ellison syndrome.[26,27]

Glucagonoma and Somatostatinoma

There have been several reports of pancreatic alpha cell tumors which secrete glucagon, usually in association with a distinctive rash.[28-30] A kindred has been reported with glucagonoma and MEN 1.[31] There have also been reports of pancreatic tumors which secrete somatostatin.[31-33] While these somatostatinomas have not yet been described in association with typical MEN 1, it may be that with further investigation such an association will be noted. The relatively mild and nonspecific symptoms that might be associated with these tumors may cause underrecognition of cases of glucagonoma and somatostatinoma. As the clinical features of glucagonoma and somatostatinoma are more completely described and radioimmunoassays (RIAs) for glucagon and somatostatin are made more widely available, a better understanding of these disorders and their possible relationship to MEN 1 may be achieved.

PITUITARY TUMORS

Chromophobe Adenomas

A variety of functional and histological types of pituitary tumors have been described in association with multiple endocrine neoplasia. Historically, the most commonly described tumor type appears to be the nonfunctioning chromophobe adenoma.[12,13,34] While these tumors do not produce hormones themselves, they may cause significant endocrine effects when their mass impinges upon the normal pituitary cells and interferes with the hypothalamic-pituitary axis. It now appears that a number of the reported "nonfunctional" tumors may well have been prolactinomas.[35–38] Patients from the family originally studied by Wermer have been reevaluated and found to have evidence of prolactinomas.[39]

Functioning Adenomas

In addition to the reports of chromophobe adenomas, there have been a substantial number of reports of acromegaly, which is associated with eosinophilic pituitary adenomas.[13] There have also been reports of Cushing's syndrome in MEN 1, perhaps due to pituitary disease, although pancreatic tumor cells also may secrete adrenocorticotropic hormone (ACTH).[40] Although precocious puberty has been described in endocrine polyneoplasia,[41,42] gonadotropin-secreting pituitary adenomas have not been demonstrated in the MEN 1 syndrome.

Recent reports indicate that prolactinomas occur fairly commonly in the MEN 1 syndrome.[35–38] The possibility that hyperprolactinemia was caused by the tumor mass interfering with transfer of hypothalamic prolactin inhibitory factor to the appropriate pituitary cells has not been rigorously excluded in every case. In several cases, however, it has been demonstrated by immunohistology and electron microscopy that the pituitary tumor cells contain prolactin.[16,17]

For the most part, the pituitary adenomas recognized in multiple endocrine neoplasia have been associated with enlargement of the sella turcica; the frequency and clinical significance of microadenomas have not been established. Presumably, early detection of pituitary tumors as microadenomas would permit surgical removal with improved preservation of pituitary function. Whether additional adenomas might form subsequently is as yet unknown.

OTHER ASSOCIATIONS

Lipomas

In certain kindreds,[13,34] lipomas are closely associated with the more typical features of parathyroid, pituitary, and pancreatic tumors. The lipomas may be small and few in number or may be large and quite prominent.[18] In those kindreds in which lipomas occur, they are often a useful sign, indicating which members will be affected by the other features of the syndrome.[42]

Bronchial Adenomas and Carcinoid Tumors

Rarely, bronchial adenomas and intestinal carcinoid tumors have been reported in association with the fully expressed MEN 1 syndrome.[42–44] In a few other cases, these tumors have been associated with individual components of the MEN 1 syndrome, as reviewed by Amano et al.[44] These patients may have the typical carcinoid syndrome or may be found to have carcinoid tumors incidentally.

Adrenal Cortical Adenomas

Although there have been case reports of steroid-producing adrenal cortical adenomas and hyperplasia in association with the MEN 1 syndrome,[13,43,44] these are extraordinarily rare. Somewhat more commonly, small adrenal cortical nodules are discovered at autopsy.[2,13,44] Such nodules may be found in as many as half of autopsied adults;[45] thus, they may be only incidental findings in patients with MEN 1. Generally, these do not appear to have caused any clinical symptoms and are thought to have been nonfunctional.

Thyroid Adenomas

Some patients with MEN 1 have been noted to have thyroid hyperplasia or follicular adenomas.[2,12,13] These are nonfunctioning lesions which may occur in as many as 50 percent of carefully examined autopsy specimens from unselected subjects.[46] Therefore, the significance of these findings in MEN 1 is questionable. Hyperthyroidism has only rarely been associated with cases of MEA, and its etiologic relationship to MEN 1 is uncertain.

Other Associated Tumors

Renal adenomas and leiomyomas[13,47] have been reported as incidental findings in patients with other endocrine tumors. It is particularly important to interpret the older reports with care because of the uncertain relationship of many of those cases to what is now recognized as classic MEN 1 syndrome.

Clinical Evaluation

PATIENT EVALUATION

There are two principal settings in which diagnostic studies are likely to be undertaken. A patient may appear with clinical features of one or more of the component disorders and therefore be evaluated for other features of the syndrome, or asymptomatic subjects may be investigated because of their familial relationship to a patient with the disorder. Patients may present such common problems as nephrolithiasis or other features of hyperparathyroidism, peptic ulcer disease, or symptoms of hypoglycemia. They may have such manifestations of pituitary tumors as headaches, visual field disturbances, amenorrhea, impotence, secondary hypothyroidism, or evidence of pituitary hyperfunction as in acromegaly. The diagnostic yield is great enough to justify investigation of such patients in order to determine whether other components of the MEN 1 syndrome are present. Fortunately, such an assessment is fairly easily carried out. Determination of the serum calcium level should be made in order to detect hyperparathyroidism. An x-ray examination of the sella turcica is generally a satisfactory method of ascertaining whether pituitary enlargement has occurred. Tomographic studies in order to detect microadenomas are probably necessary only if there is other evidence of pituitary dysfunction or if the patient is known to have MEA. Prolactin levels should be checked in both men and women. Hypergastrinemia is usually symptomatic, and determination of the serum gastrin level or gastric acid secretion, perhaps employing a secretin test, helps to exclude or confirm the diagnosis of Zollinger-Ellison syndrome. The diagnosis of Zollinger-Ellison syndrome may be problematical in occasional patients with hyperparathyroidism because hypercalcemia may cause hypergastrinemia and increased gastric acid secretion, mimicking gastrinoma (see Chap. 23). For this reason, it has been recommended that definitive evaluation for gastrinoma be carried out *after* parathyroidectomy in such cases.[26] Some investigators have found that a secretin test generally provides adequate discrimination between gastrinoma and the effects of hyperparathyroidism,[48] although others have disagreed.[31,49] Most reports indicate that extremely high gastrin levels can usually be attributed to gastrinoma, although hypercalcemia causes amplification of gastrin secretion.

Evaluation of the adrenal glands is called for only in rare cases in which there appears to be abnormal adrenal function. Thyroid nodules may be detected by palpation of the gland. The benign nature of the thyroid lesions reported with MEN 1 should not distract the physician from proper evaluation of any thyroid nodule for possible malignancy. It is generally not necessary to screen patients or relatives for disorders only rarely associated with this syndrome unless there is a specific reason for suspecting such abnormalities.

FAMILY EVALUATION

Initial Evaluation

Once it has been ascertained that the proband has two or more of the typical components of the MEA syndrome, family studies should be carried out; family studies may also be indicated in patients with multiglandular parathyroid disease alone[22,23] or multifocal insulinoma.[50] It should be realized that thorough family evaluation is a detailed and often difficult process. Repeated evaluation is required because individuals may appear to be normal when first studied but may develop abnormalities some years later. The siblings, parents, and children of the index patients should be evaluated.

The first step is a meticulous review of the family members' medical histories, searching for manifestations that the family may be able to recall, such as kidney stones, peptic ulcers, low blood sugar, and premature menopause. Considerations of compliance, time, and cost require that screening be performed simply, quickly, and cheaply: physical examination, determinations of serum calcium and prolactin concentrations and fasting blood sugar level, and x-ray examination of the sella turcica, together with the review of the medical history, should generally be an adequate screening examination. Further studies should be undertaken if there are specific indications for them. Although many affected individuals do not manifest the complete syndrome, the degree of penetrance in this disorder is high. Therefore, it is generally sufficient to study first-degree relatives of affected individuals. More distant relatives require investigation if there are historical or clinical findings suggestive of the disorder, or if findings indicating MEN 1 are present in intermediate relatives.

Further Evaluation

Once the diagnosis of MEN 1 is established in a family, the occurrence of any one feature of this disorder in an individual family member is presumptive evidence of the genetic disease. It is important that relatives of the propositus understand that negative tests at the time of their initial evaluation do not exclude the possibility of future development of features of the disease. Furthermore, members of such families should understand that often the adenomas do not develop concurrently and that another organ may be affected some years after the treatment of the initial tumor.

Epidemiology

All studies of MEN 1 have indicated that the inheritance follows an autosomal dominant pattern; thus, approximately equal numbers of males and females are affected. The degree of penetrance is quite high, although the expression is variable; the pattern, or combination, of adenomas may differ between family members. Therefore, the family history is usually strongly positive and screening of relatives of affected individuals is highly productive. This disorder has been found in both white and black families in North America and in families from Europe and Central America as well.[51]

The prevalence of MEN 1 in the general population is not known. Its apparent prevalence has been steadily increasing owing to the increased awareness of this syndrome and the improvement of diagnostic methods. The frequency of MEN 1 appears to be sufficient to warrant a screening investigation in patients presenting with any of the typical features.

MEN in Other Species

Endocrine polyneoplasia of a pattern similar to that of MEN 1 in humans has been observed in a variety of species, but spontaneously occurring examples are extremely rare.[52] Quite a high incidence has been observed in irradiated rats,[53,54] suggesting that multiple somatic mutations are present in the irradiated animals.

Pathogenesis

THEORIES OF PATHOGENESIS

Autosomal Dominance

In his landmark paper in 1954, Wermer[7] demonstrated the autosomal dominant inheritance of the syndrome. He postulated that the heritable abnormality was in a gene responsible for regulation of growth of the affected glands. The generalized character of the defect was inferred from the multiple parathyroid adenomas and multiple islet cell tumors found in his patients.

"Nesidioblastosis" Theory

The "nesidioblastosis" theory of pathogenesis was proposed later. This theory held that "the genetic defect in the familial MEA syndrome involves only the cytogenesis of the totipotential pancreatic ductal cell, resulting in the excessive production of insulin, glucagon, and/or gastrin which stimulates the changes in other endocrine glands."[41] The potential of islet cell tumors to produce a variety of hormones is compatible with this hypothesis, but the apparent occurrence of parathyroid and pituitary disease in individuals without demonstrable pancreatic lesions argues against it.

"Two-Hit" Mutation Model

A hypothesis with greater current acceptance is the "two-hit" mutation model for tumor formation.[55,56] This model proposes that mutations must occur in both members of a pair of allelic genes within a single cell in order to produce a neoplastic change, in both hereditary and nonhereditary tumors. In nonhereditary tumors, two independent somatic mutations must occur at precisely corresponding gene loci. In the absence of an intense mutagenic stimulus, such an event is relatively improbable. Furthermore, the occurrence of such a somatic mutation in more than one organ would be almost vanishingly improbable, except in such cases as irradiated rats.[53,54] In hereditary cases, including individuals in whom there is a new mutation in a parent's germ cell, the inherited factor is thought to be a mutation, which is present in all cells, at one of the critical loci. All that is then required is a somatic mutation at the corresponding allele, which would result in neoplastic change in the tissues for which that particular gene is critical. While this is a relatively improbable event in any individual cell, the probability of such an event occurring in one of the many cells of a gland is relatively high. (See Note Added in Proof.)

One implication of this model is that even individuals in whom the syndrome appears to have occurred sporadically should be regarded as possibly having the capacity for genetic transmission of the disorder to their progeny. The nature of the defect in mutant cells is unknown. A variety of possible defects could be postulated to be involved; they might involve the genes responsible for regulation of DNA synthesis or cell division, or abnormalities of cell surface receptors which serve to regulate the metabolic, synthetic, or secretory activity of the cell.[57,58] The deletion of an inhibitory gene results in the curiosity of a "recessive" gene disorder inherited in a dominant pattern. The terms *oncogenes* and *antioncogenes* have been used to describe genes at which mutations result in malignant growth due to excessive production of growth-promoting gene products, lack of growth inhibition, or loss of differentiation due to deletion of a regulatory gene. Multiple oncogenes may be required for neoplastic changes to occur. The presence of known oncogenes has not been demonstrated in MEN 1.

APUD Concept

It has been suggested that cells which carry out amine precursor uptake and decarboxylation (i.e., APUD cells) may have a common or closely related embryologic progenitor cell or site of origin in the neural crest. This grouping of cells from various neuroendocrine tissues was the outgrowth of investigations demonstrating common biochemical and electrophysiological features in cells of the adenohypophysis, chromaffin cells, paraganglionic cells, parafollicular cells of the thyroid gland, pancreatic islet cells, and others.[59,60] Because these are the tissues principally involved in the MEN syndromes, it is tempting to suggest that an abnormality in a common progenitor cell is a factor in the pathogenesis of these syndromes. Either a somatic mutation very early in embryonic life or a hereditary mutation affecting some regulatory process in the growth of the particular affected cell line could cause the adenomas. Some authors have suggested that there are two lines of APUD cells: (1) the entodermal cell line, which gives rise to carcinoid tumors, pituitary tumors, and tumors of the parathyroid glands and the pancreatic islet, and (2) the neuroectodermal line, which is thought to give rise to neuromas, neurofibromas, medullary carcinoma of the thyroid, and pheochromocytomas. The evidence for the dual cell origin hypothesis is reviewed by Ellison and Neville.[61]

Mixed Cases

A small number of cases have been reported in which patients had elements associated with MEN 1 and other elements associated with MEN 2.[62,63] In some of these cases, the findings reported were not definite diagnostic features of the syndrome to which they were ascribed. In other cases, certain major features of both categories of MEN were present. However, these reports do not describe concurrence of two or more of the *distinguishing* diagnostic features of each syndrome (e.g., a patient with medullary thyroid carcinoma and pheochromocytoma as well as an islet cell tumor and a pituitary adenoma). The concurrence of elements associated with each of the two classes of MEN has been invoked as support for the single progenitor cell theory. The lack of concurrence of the fully expressed syndromes, however, suggests that this inference should be drawn with caution. Furthermore, the lack of evidence of inheritance of these atypical combinations is consistent with sporadic occurrence. The basic principle of pathogenesis suggested by the two-hit proposal would be applicable to either a single or dual cell line hypothesis.

Management

The management of the component disorders of MEN is presented in detail in the relevant chapters. There are, however, some special considerations when these disorders occur in cases of MEN 1. In general, surgical treatment is the basis of management.

PARATHYROID

When parathyroidectomy is undertaken, it must be borne in mind that the patient has (or will have) multiglandular involvement.[64] In general, a subtotal parathyroidectomy is the preferred procedure, even though gross enlargement may not be obvious in all parathyroid glands. If a less extensive procedure is performed, the likelihood of persistence or recurrence of hyperparathyroidism is great. Should the patient with a small remnant of one gland again develop hyperparathyroidism, completion of a total parathyroidectomy and medical management of hypocalcemia is generally satisfactory. Autografting of parathyroid tissue (e.g., to the forearm) may prove to be useful,[65] but concern exists because of the neoplastic nature of the tissue and the potential risk of recurrent hyperparathyroidism as observed in an autografted adenoma.[66]

PITUITARY

The rebirth of transsphenoidal hypophysectomy[67,68] has inaugurated a new era in the management of pituitary neoplasms and has made the surgery of the pituitary gland by an experienced neurosurgeon much safer and more reliable than was previously the case. Suprasellar extension of the pituitary gland, even to the extent of affecting visual fields, does not necessarily preclude a satisfactory result from transsphenoidal surgery. Such a surgical approach permits the resection of small tumors that are entirely within the sella turcica and permits more complete removal of the intrasellar tumor than is possible by the transcranial approach. The early detection of pituitary adenomas by advanced radiologic techniques combined with microsurgery of the hypophysis may well permit early resection of adenomas in patients in whom their occurrence can be anticipated owing to positive family history or the presence of other features of MEN 1. This may permit preservation of pituitary function that might otherwise be lost. Only experience will determine whether such tumors will recur.

GASTRINOMA

Current management of the Zollinger-Ellison syndrome is largely based on total gastrectomy by such improved methods as the Hunt-Lawrence[69] and modified Roux-19[70] gastrectomies. The gastrinoma may be resected if it is apparent; however, as gastrinomas are often multiple or obscure, resection is an adjunctive part of the management. Histamine-2 antagonists are of considerable value in the preoperative management of Zollinger-Ellison syndrome and in the long-term management of selected cases.[71] Streptozocin has also been useful.[72]

INSULINOMA

Insulinomas are often multiple in the MEN 1 syndrome, usually requiring a subtotal or near-total pancreatectomy for adequate resection. In cases of metastatic insulinomas and other instances in which adequate resection is not possible, or for interim management, diazoxide may be useful,[73] as may streptozocin[74] in the case of unresectable tumors.

In both gastrinoma and insulinoma, resection of the tumor is important, if it can be accomplished, because of the malignant potential of the pancreatic tumors as well as their endocrine effects.

The most important general considerations in the management of MEN 1 are recognition of other elements of the syndrome in patients who present with one of its components, and awareness of the implications for the families of patients with this heritable disease.

MULTIPLE ENDOCRINE NEOPLASIA TYPE 2 (MEN 2)

During the last three decades a second clinical syndrome involving tumors of multiple endocrine glands has been defined.[75] This syndrome can be clearly distinguished from MEN 1; it has been designated MEN 2. The signal tumor of MEN 2 is *medullary thyroid carcinoma* (MTC), a neoplasm of the calcitonin-secreting cells (C cells) of the thyroid gland.[76] In the early reports of MTC as part of a multiple endocrine disorder, the associated lesions were pheochromocytomas, hyperparathyroidism, and a syndrome consisting of multiple mucosal neuromas (MMN) and marfanoid habitus.[75] More experience with MEN 2 has led to the appreciation that two distinct clinical syndromes of associated endocrinopathies can be defined: MEN 2a and MEN 2b. Both involve MTC; this tumor thus remains the signal neoplasm of both syndromes.

MEN 2a consists of MTC, pheochromocytoma, and hyperparathyroidism (Sipple's syndrome); MEN 2b consists of MTC and pheochromocytoma with MMN and marfanoid habitus. The component tumors of MEN 2a and MEN 2b vary in their incidence and prevalence. In MEN 2a the frequency of pheochromocytoma is less than 50 percent and the frequency of hyperparathyroidism ranges from 10 to 60 percent. In MEN 2b the prevalence of pheochromocytoma exceeds 50 percent and hyperparathyroidism is rare or nonexistent; MMN syndrome is part of MEN 2b only.[76,77] In addition to these clinical differences, there are other features that distinguish these two syndromes. MEN 2a seems to be transmitted as an autosomal dominant characteristic. MEN 2b may also exhibit this genetic pattern, but a number of sporadic cases have also been described.[78]

With one exception, the clinical behavior of the component tumors in both syndromes seems to be similar; the exception is the clinical behavior of the MTC. In patients with MEN 2a, the MTC may run an indolent course, whereas in MEN 2b it is likely to be more aggressive.[79] There are, however, dramatic exceptions to these generalities, and patient management must be individualized.

There is an embryologic as well as a genetic basis for the association of MTC with these other tumors. The cells of MTC, pheochromocytomas, and the neurogangliomas are all of neural crest origin.[80] The associated hyperparathyroidism does not fit into this unitary concept of embryogenesis, since parathyroid cells are not classically considered to be of neural crest origin. However, some authorities have suggested that the parathyroid gland is of neural crest origin.[81] An alternative explanation for the hyperparathyroidism is a functional relationship between it and MTC. According to this hypothesis, the abnormal concentrations of calcitonin produce hyperparathyroidism that is a consequence of the hypocalcemic actions of the calcitonin.[82] Although this type of functional relationship between the neoplasias may exist, the most convincing evidence supports a genetic relationship between MTC and hyperparathyroidism.[83]

There are important clinical consequences of the association of MTC with other tumors. When they occur, the mucosal neurogangliomas may be the first manifestation of the MEN syndrome. These lesions thus may provide an early warning of the presence of two potentially lethal tumors, MTC and pheochromocytoma. Additionally, the existence of either pheochromocytoma or MTC should suggest that the other may coexist. Hyperparathyroidism can be similarly regarded. It is therefore important for physicians to recognize that the presence of MTC in their patients should stimulate a search for other tumors in the patients' families. If diagnosed early, all the serious features of MEN 2 are treatable and even curable.

Medullary Thyroid Carcinoma

In contrast to the follicular cells of the thyroid, the presence of C cells within the human thyroid gland has been established only recently. This population of cells had attracted little attention until the discovery of (thyro)calcitonin in the early 1960s. Williams[84] suggested in 1966 that C cells might be the cells of origin of MTC. This tumor had been recognized by Hazard and his colleagues[85] as a distinct pathological entity that could be distinguished from other thyroid tumors. Williams' hypothesis was proved correct when several investigators demonstrated by bioassay the presence of calcitonin in MTC.[86-89] These findings were later confirmed by specific RIAs of human calcitonin in tumor and blood[90] and by histochemical studies.[91] Subsequently, the tumor was also shown to produce a wide variety of other bioactive substances.[92] The unique histological and biochemical features of MTC were soon embellished by its unique clinical associations with other endocrine and nonendocrine neoplasms (Table 28-2), most of which share with MTC a common embryologic origin, the neural crest.[81,93]

EMBRYOLOGY

Thyroidal C cells, which become neoplastic in MTC, are now generally accepted to be of neural crest origin.[93] These cells migrate to the ultimobranchial bodies from the neural crest. In nonmammalian species the cells form a distinct organ, the ultimobranchial organ, which becomes the residence of the C cells and their secretory product, calcitonin. In mammals, the C cells become incorporated into the thyroid gland and perhaps other sites. The neural crest origin of C cells offers an explanation for the association of MTC with other tumors of neural crest origin; it also appears to explain the production by these tumors of a wide variety of bioactive substances.[81]

Table 28-2. Endocrine and Nonendocrine Neoplasms Associated with MEN 2a and 2b

MEN 2a	MEN 2b
Medullary thyroid carcinoma	Medullary thyroid carcinoma
Pheochromocytoma	Pheochromocytoma
Hyperparathyroidism	Multiple mucosal neuromas with marfanoid habitus

PATHOLOGY

MTC is usually a firm, rounded tumor located in the middle or upper lobes of the thyroid gland.[84] It is commonly bilateral and multifocal, especially in familial cases. The histological features of the tumor vary, and in general cannot be used for prognosis. However, immunohistochemical studies suggest that cellular heterogeneity of calcitonin production may indicate a grave prognosis.[94] The cells usually are polyhedral or polygonal in shape and are arranged in a variety of patterns.[95] The arrangement of the cells can be influenced by the distribution of stromal elements, which can be scanty or predominant. Calcification is commonly found in the tumor; the calcifications are more dense and irregular than the homogeneous psammoma bodies which occur in other thyroid cancers. Dense calcifications may be visible on x-ray. A common feature of MTC is the presence of amyloid. The amyloid has the histochemical characteristics of the immune amyloids, but immunochemical and immunohistological studies suggest that it is also secreted by the C cells and is structurally related to calcitonin. Although the presence of amyloid has long been considered to be important in the diagnosis of medullary thyroid carcinoma, the diagnosis is best established by the use of specific immunohistochemical procedures for calcitonin which demonstrate the abnormal C cells.[96,97] Specimens collected by needle biopsy are usually not adequate for diagnosis, even with immunohistology.[75] However, immunohistological evaluation of sputum may demonstrate pulmonary metastases.[98] Mixed tumors containing malignant elements of thyroid follicles are rare.[99]

C Cell Hyperplasia

Wolfe and his colleagues defined C cell hyperplasia as a distinct pathological entity.[100] This had been preceded by the description of increased C cell populations in animals[84] and humans[95] with MTC. Wolfe and his colleagues[100] were studying three patients at risk for MTC because of their family history. These patients had small but progressive increases in plasma calcitonin concentration during calcium infusion; they consequently underwent thyroidectomy. The extirpated thyroid glands did not display the presence of MTC, but did show clusters of hyperplastic parafollicular cells which were calcitonin-positive by immunohistological studies. The presence of increased calcitonin levels in these cells was confirmed by bioassay and immunoassay. These hyperplastic parafollicular cells were found to be localized to the areas where C cells are usually most prominent, the upper and middle portions of the lateral thyroid lobes. These cells exhibited no nuclear atypia or invasive tendencies. These observations suggest that, at least in familial cases of MTC, the frank malignancy is preceded by progressive hyperplasia of C cells.

This predecessor of MTC can become manifest in early childhood or as late as the second decade.[100–102] These early stages of MTC are of fundamental importance to cancer pathogenesis; detection of them is of considerable clinical significance. The early stages of MTC, when the neoplastic process is confined to the thyroid gland, are the most amenable to surgery; C cell hyperplasia and even more subtle histological changes are below the threshold of clinical detection but may be identifiable with the calcitonin assay. Such early identification offers the best hope for effective therapy and even cure. Provocative testing is especially valuable in such patients, who may have normal basal levels of plasma calcitonin.[103]

C Cell Adenoma

Several instances of C cell adenoma have been reported.[104,105] These results must be considered as only preliminary evidence for the existence of such an adenoma. Definitive evidence will have to be provided by specific immunohistochemical studies which demonstrate the presence of calcitonin in tumor and perhaps in peripheral blood.

OCCURRENCE

MTC has been reported to comprise 4 to 12 percent of all thyroid cancer; it is a relatively uncommon tumor.[106] The ratio of affected females to males is closer to unity than in other thyroid tumors. Although the majority of cases reported in the earlier literature appeared to occur sporadically, an appreciation of the familial incidence of the tumor is resulting in an increasing identification of inherited cases,[92] especially in patients with MEN 2a. Despite its rarity, the tumor has acquired a clinical importance that far outweighs its prevalence. This has occurred because the tumor commonly exists in a familial distribution with an autosomal dominant pattern, its presence can be established by measuring the concentration of calcitonin, and it is associated with an intriguing constellation of clinical features (Table 28-2). Since the tumor is often inherited as an autosomal dominant characteristic, screening the family of an affected individual is often fruitful. In fact, by biochemical testing, the tumor can be diagnosed even when there has been no clinical evidence of its presence.[107]

NATURAL HISTORY

The natural history of MTC can vary greatly; this may make decisions regarding therapy difficult. The tumor is generally regarded as intermediate between the aggressive behavior of anaplastic thyroid carcinoma and the more indolent papillary and follicular thyroid carcinoma. However, it can be rapidly progressive and widely metastatic, and can lead to death within weeks of diagnosis. By contrast, it can be indolent and compatible with decades of life.[106] In patients with MEN 2b, MTC develops at an earlier age, metastasizes earlier, and has a higher mortality rate.[79] MTC commonly spreads via regional lymphatics; local metastases have been present in the majority of tumors reported. Distant metastases can involve any organ; lung, liver, bone, and adrenal gland are relatively common sites.[108] The most common presentation is a thyroid nodule and the most common symptom is diarrhea.[75]

SECRETORY PRODUCTS

Calcitonin and Related Peptides and Proteins

Since MTC is a neoplastic disorder of the C cells of the thyroid gland, the tumor produces abnormally high amounts of calcitonin. The calcitonin content of the tumor can exceed that of the normal thyroid by orders of magnitude. As a result, patients with this tumor have elevated concentrations of calcitonin in peripheral blood and urine. In most patients, basal concentrations of the hormone are sufficiently elevated to be diagnostic of the presence of the tumor. Therefore, the RIA for calcitonin can be used to diagnose the presence of MTC with an exceptional degree of accuracy and specificity when applied to measurements in random plasma samples. However, in a small but increasing percentage of patients with this tumor, basal levels of the hormone are indistinguishable from normal.[109] Many of these cases represent early stages of C cell neoplasia, or perhaps even hyperplasia; these early stages are most amenable to surgical cure. Thus, provocative tests have been developed for the diagnosis of MTC and its histological antecedents.[83] These tests have led to the identification of the tumor in patients in whom the diagnosis could have been missed by basal calcitonin determinations.[75]

It has been recently shown that the calcitonin gene encodes other peptides, among them a 37-amino-acid peptide termed *calcitonin gene–related peptide* (CGRP) and a 21-amino-acid peptide termed *katacalcin*.[110,111] Although the function of these peptides is unknown, they are secreted by MTC and may thus serve as tumor markers. C cells also secrete chromogranin A (Chr A), a high-molecular-weight protein originally discovered in the secretory granules of pheochromocytomas and now appreciated to be present in other endocrine tissues, among them the parathyroid, pancreas, and pituitary.[112] This protein could thus be a marker for each of the endocrine neoplasias of both MEN 1 and MEN 2.[113]

PROVOCATIVE TESTING *Calcium* The intravenous (IV) infusion of calcium has been the most widely used technique for stimulating calcitonin secretion in MTC. In early studies, calcium was infused at doses ranging from 3 to 5 mg per kilogram of body weight per hour for periods varying from 2 to 4 h. The increase in serum calcium concentration produced by such infusions, usually several mg/dl, consistently produced an abnormal increase in plasma calcitonin concentration in patients with MTC.[107] The abnormal increase in plasma calcitonin concentration occurred even in patients who had basal concentrations of the hormone that were indistinguishable from normal.[109]

Prolonged calcium infusions have several disadvantages. The length of the procedure is inconvenient and the dose of calcium used often produces untoward effects such as hypertension, nausea, and even vomiting. This necessitates hospitalization in research wards under constant professional supervision. For these reasons, shorter infusions of calcium have been developed which are more convenient and safer than the longer procedures and yet seem to be reliable in stimulating calcitonin secretion.[114] In these procedures, the increase in plasma calcium concentration usually is less than 1 mg/dl, but calcitonin secretion is reliably stimulated. The procedure can be completed in several minutes, and it is generally well-tolerated.[114]

Pentagastrin Pentagastrin is another widely used provocative agent for calcitonin secretion in patients with MTC.[114] When administered IV at a dose of 0.5 μg per kilogram of body weight, pentagastrin produces a rapid increase in plasma calcitonin concentration. This pattern of calcitonin response, however, probably is a function of the dose and rapidity of administration of pentagastrin rather than any innate properties of this secretagogue. When calcium is given in a similar intravenous manner over a few seconds, a calcitonin response similar to that seen with pentagastrin infusion is observed; when pentagastrin is infused over several minutes, a response similar to that produced by calcium infusion is seen.[92]

Although the rapidity of the pentagastrin infusion is advantageous, this provocative test does have some drawbacks. The administration of pentagastrin produces an unpleasant (but poorly described) sensation in the recipient which is commonly called "burning" or "flushing." Also, the use of pentagastrin as a diagnostic test for suspected MTC is not currently approved by the U.S. Food and Drug Administration; therefore, an institutionally approved protocol may be required for its administration.

Wells and his colleagues[116] have described interesting modifications of the pentagastrin test. They administered the peptide to patients with MTC while an indwelling catheter was located in the inferior thyroid veins to permit plasma sampling for calcitonin assay. During this procedure, they were able to demonstrate a dramatic increase in thyroidal vein as well as peripheral calcitonin concentration. In some patients, however, there was a diagnostic increase in thyroid vein calcitonin concentration, while the increase in peripheral calcitonin concentration was not diagnostic. However, such procedures cannot be considered routine, and they require considerable competence. Not only is the normal concentration of thyroidal venous calcitonin not well established, but it can be influenced by a small change in the position of the indwelling catheter used to collect the sample for assay. The improved diagnostic potential of these catheterization procedures is certainly diminished by their technical difficulty and may be obviated by the increased sensitivity of newer calcitonin RIAs. These newer assays have better-defined normal and abnormal ranges of both basal as well as stimulated calcitonin concentrations in peripheral human plasma.[117] Accordingly, patients in whom provocative testing was previously necessary for establishing the diagnosis of MTC can now often be identified by basal calcitonin measurements with assays of improved sensitivity.

A more practical use of selective venous catheterization is in the evaluation of the location and extent of MTC or an ectopic calcitonin-producing tumor.[116] This procedure may be able to localize a recurrence of MTC precisely and thus may result in more effective treatment.[117a] However, considerable skill is also necessary for these procedures; even when they are technically successful, a calcitonin gradient from the tumor may be obscured by high basal circulating concentrations of hormone.

Pentagastrin vs. Calcium Differences of opinion have appeared in the literature regarding the relative clinical value of pentagastrin and calcium infusion in the diagnosis of MTC.[116] The most important point to keep in mind is that most tumors respond to either agent and that both infusion procedures have a small incidence of false-negative results; i.e., some tumors (or hyperplasia) respond to calcium but not to gastrin and vice versa.[75] Therefore, if one procedure gives negative results in a patient suspected of having MTC, the alternative procedure should be considered before the diagnosis is excluded.[92] There is, however, some preliminary evidence to suggest that calcium infusion may be more valuable in diagnosing early forms of the tumor.[103] In general, both the sensitivity and specificity of the calcitonin assay are probably just as important as the choice between calcium and pentagastrin in provocative testing of suspected MTC. With a sensitive assay (of the appropriate specificity), either pentagastrin or calcium will identify the patient with tumor in most instances. Preliminary results of combined calcium-pentagastrin infusions have not been consistent.[103,116]

Whiskey Another agent recently introduced as a provocative test for calcitonin is Scotch whiskey.[118] When 50 ml is administered orally to a patient with MTC, there is an increase in plasma calcitonin concentration comparable to that produced by some calcium infusions. The diagnostic increase usually occurs within 15 min. Whiskey has the advantage of oral administration over other provocative agents and is therefore more convenient, especially in testing patients in nonhospital settings. However, as with the other provocative agents, false-negative results have been observed. Thus, more experience is necessary to establish the reliability of whiskey. In addition, amounts recommended for use in testing may produce side effects: alcohol can produce diarrhea and flushing in patients with MTC, perhaps by stimulating the secretion of humors produced by the tumor which are responsible for these symptoms.[118]

Magnesium In experimental animals and normal humans, magnesium infusion increases circulating calcitonin concentration.[75] In contrast, magnesium infusion has been observed by Anast and colleagues[119] to suppress the secretion of calcitonin in three patients with MTC. These results may reflect a basic difference between normal and malignant C cells in their secretory response to magnesium.

Glucagon Although glucagon can stimulate calcitonin secretion, it is not widely used as a diagnostic agent in suspected cases of MTC. Glucagon is not a reliable calcitonin secretagogue, since its effects can vary.[75] Also, glucagon can release catecholamines, and since patients with MTC may have associated pheochromocytomas, an adrenergic crisis can be precipitated by its administration.[115]

VENOUS CATHETERIZATION PROCEDURES The presence as well as the location of MTC can be established by calcitonin assay in conjunction with selective venous catheterization. A gradient of hormone concentration in a specific vein may localize the tumor to the site draining that vein. This procedure requires accurate catheter placement and confirmation of location by appropriate venography studies. Several factors limit the usefulness of catheterization procedures. The high incidence of bilaterality in familial MTC mandates bilateral neck surgery, so that the procedure has limited use in primary diagnosis and preoperative localization. If recurrence or persistence after surgical treatment is being evaluated, catheterization must be done in an area in which the venous anatomy has been distorted by prior surgery.[120] Therefore, accurate correlation between venous samples and anatomical sites necessitates preliminary arteriography studies to establish blood flow patterns. Such studies add considerable risk, time, and expense to venous catheterization. Therefore, the greatest potential value of catheterization studies is probably in the location of tumor metastases (or ectopic calcitonin production). Prior knowledge of the presence of metastatic (or ectopic) disease can greatly influence therapy.[117]

CALCITONIN MEASUREMENTS IN THE EVALUATION OF THERAPY The effectiveness of therapy in patients with calcitonin-producing tumors can be monitored by serial measurements of plasma calcitonin concentration.[75] This application of the calcitonin assay pertains to surgical as well as chemotherapeutic treatment. In addition to determining the relatively immediate effects of a given treatment regimen, periodic surveillance with appropriate provocative testing can be conducted for recurrence of the tumor.[121]

IMMUNOCHEMICAL HETEROGENEITY There are multiple immunochemical forms of calcitonin in tumor tissue and in plasma.[122,123] When plasma or tumor extracts from a patient with MTC are immunoassayed after gel filtration chromatography, multiple peaks of immunoreactive calcitonin are observed. The number of peaks can be influenced by the size of the column, the nature of the matrix gel, and the elution conditions. Under such influences, calcitonin auto- or homoaggregation (dimerization or polymerization) or heteroaggregation (with other proteins) may influence its elution profile. Thus, only some of the peaks may actually reflect the biosynthesis, secretion, and metabolism of calcitonin. Biosynthetic precursors for calcitonin have been described and these species may be represented in plasma.[124] And, since calcitonin is metabolized after secretion and perhaps also inside cells, such metabolic derivatives may also be represented in plasma. Therefore, the multiple forms of immunoassayable plasma calcitonin represent a complex mixture of actual as well as operatively created species of calcitonin, its biosynthetic precursors, and its metabolites.

The immunochemical profile of calcitonin may vary among certain disease states. This variation has been demonstrated for calcitonin-producing tumors and for renal disease.[92,125] The differing species of plasma calcitonin seen in renal disease and malignancy are produced in part by the abnormalities in hormone metabolism as well as secretion. While there is a significant peak of calcitonin monomer in MTC plasma, in renal disease most of the calcitonin elutes at or near the void volume of the column used.[125] This also appears to be true in some instances of ectopic calcitonin production, where the hormone may also elute at or near the position of the biosynthetic precursor(s) of calcitonin.[111] In other malignancies, calcitonin monomer may predominate.[123] Therefore, it may be possible to use the immunochemical pattern of plasma calcitonin in the differential diagnosis of hypercalcitoninemic states. Because of this, specificity as well as sensitivity must be considered in evaluating the diagnostic value of a calcitonin assay system.

Certain characteristics of the immunochemical heterogeneity of plasma calcitonin are also conferred by the immunochemical specificity of the antiserum used to make hormone measurements. Antibodies of a given specificity for the calcitonin molecule react with (and therefore detect) preferentially species of the hormone which have that specificity. For example, if calcitonin is metabolized to a fragment which contains a carboxy-terminal peptide, an antiserum with specificity for the carboxy-terminal region of calcitonin will detect that fragment, whereas an antiserum with specificity for another region of the molecule may not. Therefore, immunochemical heterogeneity is a function of the hormone species being measured as well as the assay procedure employed.

Assessment of the immunochemical heterogeneity of plasma calcitonin can provide fundamental information about C cell function as well as information of clinical importance. Perhaps the most important clinical implication of calcitonin heterogeneity will be in screening patients for the early diagnosis of MTC or other calcitonin-producing tumors. Some assay procedures may identify better than other assay systems the slightly increased basal concentrations of calcitonin which occur in early MTC. Furthermore, different provocative agents may stimulate the secretion (or release) of different species of calcitonin.[124] Thus, the optimal diagnostic combination may depend on the correct provocative test for a given assay system and the correct assay system for a given provocative test. Clearly, optimum results are provided by sensitive assay systems which have been well characterized and extensively applied.

SERIAL CALCITONIN MEASUREMENTS Patients at risk for MTC should be evaluated periodically for the manifestations of the tumor. Sensitive and specific assays for calcitonin should be applied at frequent intervals.[126] In general, screening should begin no later than age 5 and continue until at least age 35 at intervals of approximately 6 to 9 months; more aggressive screening might be indicated in some patients.[113] Since other endocrine tumors occur later, screening procedures for them should be conducted indefinitely.[75]

Other Secretory Products

In addition to calcitonin, MTC produces other substances, nonpeptides as well as peptides (Table 28-3). This unusual biosynthetic capacity of MTC may be related to the neural crest origin of C cells.[127,128]

PROSTAGLANDINS Abnormal concentrations of prostaglandins (PGs) are present in the tumor and blood of some patients with MTC. The excess PGs have been implicated in the pathogenesis of the diarrhea

Table 28-3. Products of Medullary Thyroid Carcinoma

Calcitonin
Calcitonin gene–related peptide
PDN21 (katacalcin)
L-Dopa decarboxylase
Histaminase
Serotonin
Prostaglandins
Kallikrein and kinins
Adrenocorticotropin
Melanocyte stimulating hormone
Somatostatin
β-Endorphin
Substance P
Vasoactive intestinal polypeptide
Corticotropin releasing hormone
Prolactin releasing factor
Nerve growth factor
Amyloid
Carcinoembryonic antigen
Melanin
Neuron-specific enolase
Chromogranin A

commonly seen in patients with this tumor. It is known that PGs can stimulate intestinal smooth muscle, and diarrhea seems to be a more prominent symptom in patients with an extensive tumor burden. Furthermore, diarrhea may be decreased by surgical removal of the tumor and treatment with PG inhibitors. However, patients with diarrhea and MTC may have normal PG levels, and patients with elevated PG levels may not have diarrhea. Furthermore, excess PG production occurs in a variety of other tumors which are not associated with diarrhea.

SEROTONIN MTC can be associated with abnormal serotonin production and the carcinoid syndrome. In some patients, the carcinoid syndrome is uncovered by procedures, such as calcium infusion, which stimulate the secretory activity of MTC. The tumor can also produce peptides such as bradykinin and kallikrein which are integral to the carcinoid syndrome. As with prostaglandins, serotonin and its metabolites may contribute to the diarrhea commonly seen in the patients with MTC.

HISTAMINASE Elevated levels of histaminase, an enzyme which catalyzes the deamination of histamine, are commonly found in the tumor and serum of patients with MTC. This may play some role in the abnormal result of a histaminase test observed in some patients with this tumor, although alternative explanations are possible. Unlike PGs and serotonin and like calcitonin, abnormal histaminase production seems to be somewhat specific for MTC as opposed to other tumors. Thus, the measurement of histaminase level may have some clinical value in the diagnosis and management of the patient with MTC. Although histaminase is generally not as sensitive a marker for MTC as is calcitonin, it may be useful in identifying patients with metastatic MTC.

PEPTIDE HORMONES In addition to calcitonin, MTC can produce a variety of other peptide hormones, including ACTH, melanocyte stimulating hormone (MSH), somatostatin, and β-endorphin. This group of peptides, including calcitonin, is also commonly represented in other tumors of neural crest origin, notably oat-cell carcinoma of the lung. It has also been reported that pituitary cells produce calcitonin or a substance immunochemically related to calcitonin. The concurrent production of this variety of peptide hormones may be an independent expression of the malignant state. However, it has been postulated that the production of some of these peptide hormones may be regulated by closely related genes, and that there may even be a precursor molecule common to some of them.

Pheochromocytoma

In 1961, Sipple presented evidence for an association between pheochromocytoma and thyroid tumor.[129] He reported the case of a 33-year-old male with bilateral pheochromocytomas and a poorly differentiated invasive thyroid tumor thought to be a follicular adenocarcinoma. Sipple reviewed the literature and presented five other cases with pheochromocytoma and thyroid tumor. The pheochromocytomas were bilateral in four of the cases. The thyroid tumors were variously described as follicular adenocarcinoma, papillary adenocarcinoma, adenocarcinoma, and anaplastic carcinoma.

In the early 1960s there were additional case reports of the simultaneous occurrence of pheochromocytomas and thyroid carcinomas (reviewed in Ref. 92). In 1967, Williams reported two cases of pheochromocytomas and thyroid cancer; he reviewed 15 others.[130] He was able to establish that at least 11 of the total of 17 cases of thyroid tumor actually were MTC. In the same year, Schimke and Hartmann[131] also reviewed the previous reports of the simultaneous occurrence of pheochromocytoma and MTC and added studies of their own of two families in which these two tumors occurred simultaneously in each of five patients.[131] Thus, the association between pheochromocytomas and MTC has become well established only in the past 15 years.[92]

OCCURRENCE

Since different reports have emphasized different aspects of the MEN syndrome, it is difficult to determine how commonly pheochromocytomas occur in association with MTC. It has become apparent that the frequency of pheochromocytomas is much higher than previously appreciated. In MEN 2b, the prevalence of pheochromocytomas usually approaches 50 percent,[132] whereas in MEN 2a it usually is less than 20 percent.[105] However, it is likely that these represent underestimates, especially in MEN 2b, since most recent studies suggest a much higher frequency.[92]

There are several distinct features of pheochromocytomas occurring in association with MTC. In this circumstance, bilateral and multifocal pheochromocytomas are very common and have a prevalence of greater than 70 percent; this contrasts with a prevalence of bilateral pheochromocytoma of usually less than 10 percent for sporadic MTC. Pheochromocytomas are much more likely to occur in patients with familial rather than sporadic MTC.[132,133] When pheochromocytomas and MTC occur together in the same patient, the MTC is likely to be diagnosed first.[106,132,133] The thyroid tumor may antedate the pheochromocytomas by as much as 21 years. Furthermore, a second pheochromocytoma may become manifest after removal of the first.[106] This sequence of events results in a greater incidence of pheochromocytomas in older patients with MTC. Less often, the thyroid and adrenal tumors may be discovered contemporaneously; in some cases, pheochromocytomas may be diagnosed before MTC. If hyperparathyroidism also exists, it, too, is likely to be diagnosed before the pheochromocytoma.[106,132,133]

ADRENAL MEDULLARY HYPERPLASIA

Adrenal medullary hyperplasia may be a predecessor of the pheochromocytomas seen with MTC, just as C cell hyperplasia may be a predecessor of MTC.[95,134] Although cases of adrenal medullary hyperplasia had been reported previously in the literature, none of them occurred in patients with MTC.[75] DeLellis and colleagues described the adrenal glands of 10 patients from a large kindred with familial MTC.[135] There was an increase in the medullary volume of adrenal glands when compared with controls. The increase in medullary mass resulted from diffuse and/or multifocal proliferation of adrenal medullary cells, primarily those found within the head and body of the glands. Multifocal proliferation can give an adenomatous appearance.[95] There is hypertrophy as well as hyperplasia of the cells, and they show increased mitotic activity and increased total catecholamine content.[134] In addition, the ratio of epinephrine to norepinephrine was increased in the tumor.[135] These findings suggest that a sequence of events similar to that postulated for MTC and hyperparathyroidism takes place in the development of pheochromocytomas: hypertrophy develops into hyperplasia; multifocal hyperplasia develops into nodularity; nodularity undergoes neoplastic transformation to pheochromocytomas. This transformation is the final stage of the sequence in most tumors, but malignant transformation can also be seen.

Hyperparathyroidism

Cushman described the simultaneous occurrence of a parathyroid adenoma in a patient with MTC who also had a pheochromocytoma.[136] Additional reports of the association of hyperparathyroidism and MTC subsequently appeared, and the two additional cases of Steiner et al. in 1968 brought the literature total to 13 at that time.[133] In the ensuing years other reports have clearly established the association between MTC and hyperparathyroidism.

OCCURRENCE

It is difficult to establish the exact prevalence of hyperparathyroidism in patients with MTC. Melvin and colleagues made the diagnosis of hyperparathyroidism in 10 of 12 patients of a kindred with MTC,[83] whereas Hill et al. could establish the diagnosis of hyperparathyroidism in only 2 of 73 patients with MTC.[106] The most recent literature suggests that hyperplasia is more common than adenoma.[92] There are several possible explanations for this disparity. For one, there is disagreement regarding the criteria necessary to distinguish between a normal and an abnormal parathyroid gland as well as the criteria used to classify parathyroid abnormalities.[75] Another possible explanation involves the developing appreciation that hyperparathyroidism is considerably more common in MEN 2a than in MEN 2b. Despite these differences, the concurrence of hyperparathyroidism and MTC is well established; although the frequency with which they occur together cannot be specified, the presence of one tumor should always arouse suspicion of the presence of the other.

PATHOLOGY

Steiner and his colleagues reviewed the literature on MEN 2a in 1968 and recorded 10 cases with parathyroid adenoma and 3 cases with parathyroid hyperplasia.[133] In later reports, the prevalence of parathyroid hyperplasia in patients with MTC has increased and has even approached 100 percent.[102,137] The controversy regarding parathyroid pathology in patients with MTC is only reflective of the general difficulties in this area of histological diagnosis.[102,138]

RELATIONSHIP TO MTC

Two hypotheses prevail regarding the link between hyperparathyroidism and MTC. One possibility is that the hyperparathyroidism is a functional disorder representing a compensatory response of the parathyroid glands to a hypocalcemic effect of calcitonin. This view does have some clinical and experimental support.[82] There are, however, equally convincing data that the hyperparathyroidism is an inherited rather than a functional component of the syndrome.[92] The genetic view would be more attractive if the embryologic origin of the parathyroid gland were the neural crest, in keeping with the embryologic origin of the other prominent features of the syndrome, i.e., pheochromocytoma, MTC, and mucosal neuromas. Most evidence suggests that the parathyroid glands are of entodermal origin, arising from the third and fourth branchial pouches. However, if the data which suggest that the parathyroid glands are of neural crest origin[81] are confirmed, a more unifying genetic basis for MEN 2a and 2b would be provided.

Multiple Mucosal Neuromas

In 1966, Williams and Pollock described two patients with MTC and pheochromocytomas who had neuromas involving the mucous membranes of the lips, tongue, and eyes.[139] In 1968, Schimke and colleagues described three additional patients with this syndrome; they recorded the presence of megacolon in each patient.[140] In one patient, rectal biopsy was consistent with ganglioneuromatosis of the submucous and myenteric plexuses. In the same year, Gorlin and coworkers reemphasized the association between MMNs, pheochromocytomas, and MTC by reviewing 17 published cases.[141] In several patients, the neuromas were either congenital or noticed within the first few years of life, thus becoming manifest before the other features of the syndrome. These authors also commented on the presence of marfanoid habitus, intestinal ganglioneuromatosis, and medullated corneal nerve fibers in this group of patients and thus articulated the features of this syndrome as it is currently appreciated: MTC, pheochromocytomas, diffuse neurogangliomatosis involving the mucosa of the gastrointestinal tract, and marfanoid habitus.[132]

MUCOSAL NEUROMAS

The presence of neuromas with a centrofacial distribution is the most consistent component of the MMN syndrome. The most prominent microscopic feature of the neuromas is an increase in the size and number of nerves. The nerves are tortuous and highly branched and are often surrounded by a thickened perineurium; both medullated and unmedullated fibers are involved. Ganglion cells and connective tissue may be present, but the latter often is not prominent. This latter feature usually distinguishes these neuromas from the neurofibromas of von Recklinghausen's neurofibromatosis.

The most common location of neuromas is in the oral cavity. The lips, tongue, and buccal mucosa are the most common sites for the oral mucosal neuromas. The oral lesions usually are the first components of the syndrome to appear. They are almost invariably present by the first decade and can even be present at birth.[132] The mucosal neuromas, along with ocular findings described below, give the affected patients a very characteristic facial appearance. Because of this, there is striking similarity in appearance of different subjects with the syndrome, even though they may be unrelated and of the opposite sex.

Mucosal neuromas can be present in the eyelids, conjunctiva, and cornea. The tarsal neuromas result in thickened eyelids and retracted eyelashes, which give the eye a hooded, sleepy look. In addition to the neuromas, a variety of other ocular abnormalities have been reported. The medullated corneal nerves are thickened; they traverse the cornea and anastomose in the pupillary area. These hypertrophied nerve fibers are seen readily with the slit lamp but occasionally may be evident on direct fundoscopic examination.[132]

GASTROINTESTINAL ABNORMALITIES

One of the most prominent features of MEN 2a and 2b is the presence of GI abnormalities.[101,106] Diarrhea is a common symptom in affected patients.[106] Its etiology is multifactoral. The diarrhea seen in these patients often can be ascribed to one of the many humors produced by MTC.[92] Most of these agents have been variably described to increase GI motility, either directly or indirectly. Some of the GI symptoms of diarrhea and constipation additionally can be ascribed to those gastrointestinal abnormalities that are part of the mucosal neuroma syndrome. The most common of these is gastrointestinal ganglioneuromatosis. The lesions of GI ganglioneuromatosis are reminiscent of those that occur in the facial mucosal neuromas. In fact, all cases of diffuse GI ganglioneuromatosis occur in association with mucosal neuromas; isolated intestinal ganglioneuromatosis is not associated with MTC. The ganglioneuromatosis is best observed in the small and large intestine but has also been noted in the esophagus and stomach.[101] There is a proliferation of the neural elements of the myenteric and submucosal plexuses. The anatomic lesions can be associated with functional difficulties in swallowing, megacolon, diarrhea, and constipation.[132] Another common GI finding which may contribute to the diarrhea is the presence of diverticulosis.

MARFANOID HABITUS

A marfanoid habitus is seen commonly in the MMN syndrome.[132] The marfanoid habitus refers to a tall, slender body with an abnormal upper- to lower-body-segment size ratio and poor muscle development. The extremities are thin and long; there may be lax joints and hypotonic muscles. Associated with the marfanoid habitus may be dorsal kyphosis, pectus excavatum (funnel chest), pectus carinatum (pigeon breast), pes cavus, and high-arched palate. In contrast to patients with true Marfan's syndrome, no patients

Table 28-4. Types of Immunologic Tissue Injury

1. IgE-mediated immediate hypersensitivity
2. Complement-dependent direct humoral cytotoxicity
3. Antigen-antibody complex deposition
4. T-cell-mediated immunity
5. Anti-receptor antibody binding (blocking or stimulating)
6. Antibody-dependent cell-mediated cytotoxicity

with MMN have been reported to have aortic abnormalities, ectopia lentis, homocystinuria, or mucopolysaccharide abnormalities.

PLURIGLANDULAR ENDOCRINE INSUFFICIENCY SYNDROMES

Physicians have noted the coincidence of diabetes mellitus and Addison's disease in the same patient since the nineteenth century.[151] In 1926, Schmidt described a "biglandular illness" in two patients with nontuberculous Addison's disease and lymphocytic thyroiditis. In 1964, Carpenter et al.[152] reviewed Schmidt's syndrome and found coexisting diabetes mellitus in 10 out of 15 patients with Addison's disease and thyroiditis. They expanded the definition of the syndrome to nontuberculous Addison's disease associated with either of these other endocrinopathies. It has since become apparent that there are multiple associations among presumed autoimmune diseases of endocrine organs, including the adrenals, endocrine pancreas, thyroid, parathyroids, ovaries, and, probably, testes and adenohypophysis. Schmidt's syndrome, as defined by Carpenter et al.[152] (and as used in this chapter), is characteristic of but one subset of patients with pluriglandular endocrine failure. In addition, these endocrine disorders are frequently associated with other disorders of tissue-specific autoimmunity, notably pernicious anemia and vitiligo. The clinical and immunologic relationships among the autoimmune endocrinopathies are reviewed here.

Immunologic tissue injury can result from six mechanisms (Table 28-4). The primary agents in autoimmune reactions are immunoglobulins, effector T cells (thymus-dependent lymphocytes which become sensitized to specific antigens and release soluble non-immunoglobulin mediators), and monocytes (which possess receptors for the Fc region of immunoglobulins and cytotoxic capabilities in the presence of tissue-specific antibody). Table 28-5 shows some of the methods which have been used to detect tissue-specific immunity and the mechanism of injury implied. The indirect immunofluorescence technique for autoantibodies to cytoplasmic microsomal antigens has been especially versatile; a pathogenetic role for these antibodies is suggested by observations that they also react with cell-surface antigens of living cells.[153] The pathogenesis of autoimmune endocrine disease has been most extensively studied in Hashimoto's thyroiditis and Graves' disease and has been the subject of several recent reviews.[154–156] T-cell-mediated immunity and antibody-dependent cell-mediated cytotoxicity (ADCC) have received the greatest attention as mechanisms of target organ destruction in Hashimoto's thyroiditis. In addition, in vitro evidence for T cells specifically sensitized against other endocrine tissues exists.[151,156–159] Although immune complexes are present in the sera of some patients with Hashimoto's thyroiditis (and Graves' disease), the pathological significance of this finding is unclear.[160] Volpe[156] has proposed a unifying theory of pathogenesis of autoimmune thyroid disease based on a defect in immunoregulation by suppressor T cells (thymus-dependent lymphocytes which suppress immune responses, possibly including recognition of autoantigens); evidence to support this hypothesis is building.[161,162]

Pluriglandular Autoimmunity with Addison's Disease

For several reasons Addison's disease has provided a good focus for investigation of the pluriglandular endocrine insufficiency syndromes. First, the clinical impact of this disease is such that few of these

Table 28-5. Tests of Tissue-Specific Immunity

Antibody determinations	Tests for cell-mediated immunity (type 4)
Immunoprecipitation (gel counterdiffusion)	Direct lymphocytotoxicity
Complement fixation	Lymphocyte blast transformation
Indirect immunofluorescence	Leukocyte migration inhibition
Demonstration of direct serum cytotoxicity (type 2)	Intradermal skin testing
Facilitation of cell-mediated cytotoxicity (type 6)	

patients should escape medical attention. This is confirmed by the low prevalence of subclinical antiadrenal autoimmunity as detected serologically. Second, tuberculous destruction of the adrenal glands provides a natural control group for clinical and immunologic comparison.

Some variation in criteria for making a diagnosis of idiopathic Addison's disease exists in the literature. Pulmonary tuberculosis and radiographic evidence of adrenal calcification allow a presumptive diagnosis of tuberculous Addison's disease to be made; idiopathic Addison's disease is diagnosed when there is no evidence of tuberculosis or another reasonable etiology. In patients with tuberculous disease on the x-ray film of the chest but without adrenal calcification, no definitive assignment of etiology can be made (i.e., etiology is indeterminate). Age of onset does not permit distinction between idiopathic and tuberculous Addison's disease except that tuberculous Addison's disease is uncommon under the age of 10. However, there is an approximate 2:1 female predominance in idiopathic Addison's disease, whereas the sex ratio in tuberculous Addison's disease is approximately unity. Table 28-6 shows the high frequency of one or more second diseases in patients with idiopathic Addison's disease and notes the much lower prevalence of associated disorders in tuberculous Addison's disease. Cumulation of five series shows that 39 percent of 419 patients with idiopathic Addison's disease had an associated tissue-specific autoimmune disease, compared with only 8 percent of patients with tuberculous Addison's disease. The diseases found with tuberculous Addison's disease have generally been diabetes and thyroid disease.[151] Additionally, in 90 patients with tuberculous Addison's disease (as defined above), none had adrenal antibodies, whereas the prevalence of adrenal antibodies in idiopathic Addison's disease ranges from 48 to 74 percent.[151] In vitro evidence of cell-mediated immunity to adrenal antigens is present in many patients with idiopathic Addison's disease but not in patients with tuberculous Addison's disease.[159] The above findings reinforce the conclusion that idiopathic Addison's disease is part of an autoimmune endocrine syndrome and that the in vitro immunologic abnormalities found in idiopathic Addison's disease (and by inference in the other disorders) are not simply a result of tissue destruction.

Nerup[163] has studied the frequency of associated endocrine disorders and antibodies in the group of patients with Addison's disease of indeterminate etiology. He detected adrenal antibodies in 39 percent of patients in this group by indirect immunofluorescence, compared with 74 percent in idiopathic Addison's disease and none in tuberculous Addison's disease patients. Five percent of these patients had an associated endocrinopathy, compared with 5 percent of tuberculous Addison's disease patients and 39 percent of idiopathic Addison's disease patients. These results suggest that this group is mixed with respect to etiology. Some studies of idiopathic Addison's disease have included these patients and other studies have excluded them. If found, mineralocorticoid deficiency with partial if not complete preservation of glucocorticoid secretory reserve may suggest idiopathic Addison's disease.[164] Testing of adrenal medullary function[165] also discriminates between tuberculous and idiopathic Addison's disease, but this has not become a generally accepted procedure.

Adrenal antibodies in blood, detected most commonly by indirect immunofluorescence and precipitation, correlate with the presence of clinical Addison's disease and associated diseases. Table 28-7 shows the frequency of adrenal antibody by immunofluorescence according to sex of the patient or the age of onset of adrenal insufficiency in patients with and without associated disease. Adrenal antibodies may disappear in patients studied later than 1 to 5 years after the onset of Addison's disease.[163,166] The higher prevalence

Table 28-6. Frequencies of Other Disorders in Idiopathic Addison's Disease

Ref.	Number of patients	Diabetes	Hyperthyroidism	Hashimoto's myxedema	Pernicious anemia	Hypogonadism	Hypoparathyroidism	One or more
196	23	3 (13)	1 (4)	4 (17)	1 (4)	7 (30)	0	9 (40)
197	46	4 (10)	5 (10)	4 (10)	1 (3)	2 (5)	0	18 (45)
198	18	1 (6)	1 (6)	2 (12)	0	3 (18)	3 (18)	8 (44)
163	71	13 (18)	7 (10)	4 (5)	2 (2)	8 (11)	0	28 (39)
151	261	21 (8)	19 (7)	23 (9)	12 (5)	47 (18)	16 (6)	101 (39)
Total	419	42 (10)	33 (8)	37 (9)	16 (4)	67 (16)	19 (5)	164 (39)

Note: Among 114 patients with tuberculous Addison's disease in the five series, 9 (8 percent) had one or more other disorders.
Source: Modified from Irvine and Barnes.[151]

Table 28-7. Frequency* of Anti-Adrenal Antibodies in Patients with Idiopathic Addison's Disease Alone and with Other Disorders Classified by Sex and Age at Onset of Addison's Disease

	Sex			Age at onset†		
	Female	Male	Total	<17	≥17	Total
Addison's alone	14/27 (52)	7/40 (18)	21/67 (31)	4/26 (15)	16/36 (44)	20/62 (32)
Addison's + other disease	23/30 (77)	13/21 (62)	36/51 (71)	15/21 (71)	20/28 (71)	35/49 (71)
		Total	57/118 (48)			55/111 (50)

*Fraction of patients of sex or age category with anti-adrenal antibodies; percentages in parentheses.
†Of patients whose age at onset of Addison's disease was known.
Source: Modified from Blizzard et al.[167]

of antibodies in Addison's disease associated with other disorders is particularly striking; conversely, the association of a second autoimmune disease is 2.5 to 2.7 times greater in antibody-positive compared with antibody-negative patients.[159,167] Most investigators[151,167] have found adrenal antibodies to be more frequent in women, although this has not been uniformly reported.[163] Patients with Addison's disease alone who are male or whose adrenal insufficiency began prior to age 20 have adrenal antibodies much less frequently. Adrenal antibodies have been found in 12 of a total of 95 patients with idiopathic hypoparathyroidism in three separate studies.[151,163,168] Such antibodies are found rarely in patients with Cushing's disease, Hashimoto's thyroiditis, or diabetes alone, or first-degree relatives of patients with idiopathic Addison's disease.[151,163] The prevalence of adrenal antibodies in the general population is < 1/1000.[163]

Many investigators have also found an increased frequency of other tissue-specific antibodies in patients with antibody-positive Addison's disease, including antibodies to parathyroid, islet cell, and thyroid tissue, in the absence of clinical disease of these tissues.[151,163,167,168] Nerup[163] found a sixfold increase in prevalence of thyroid antibodies and a tenfold increase in frequency of parietal cell antibodies in patients with adrenal antibody-positive Addison's disease compared to age- and sex-matched controls, but no difference was observed between Addison's disease patients without adrenal antibodies and controls. A group of 118 patients with idiopathic Addison's disease was studied by Blizzard et al.,[167] for associated autoimmune diseases and presence of three extraadrenal antibodies; the prevalence of one of these abnormalities was 84 percent in patients who were adrenal antibody-positive compared with 44 percent of patients who were adrenal antibody-negative. The prevalence of at least one additional autoimmune disease or extraadrenal antibody was 82 percent in females with Addison's disease and 46 percent in males.

The above findings suggest that (1) idiopathic Addison's disease is not a homogeneous disorder with a random coincidence of other autoimmune endocrine disease and (2) those patients with pluriglandular endocrine insufficiency might also be heterogeneous. Figure 28-1 supports this thesis, showing the distribution of age of onset or diagnosis for each sex for isolated Addison's disease and Addison's disease with other endocrine disorders. Differences in percentage of childhood-onset patients between the two series shown are probably attributable to the pediatric orientation of one set of investigators. It is clear that the Addison's disease associated with hypoparathyroidism has a much younger age of onset than the other two major groups; in all three groups a trend toward earlier onset of disease in males may be noted. Spinner et al.[168,169] analyzed 140 families containing 182 patients with idiopathic Addison's disease, idiopathic hypoparathyroidism, or both disorders. They found evidence for genetic as well as clinical heterogeneity among these patients. They divided their patients into four groups: Addison's disease with hypoparathyroidism, isolated hypoparathyroidism, isolated Addison's disease, and Schmidt's syndrome. Immunologic findings in the patients with isolated Addison's disease or isolated hypoparathyroidism suggest that the abnormality in some of these patients may represent a forme fruste of pluriglandular endocrine insufficiency. Furthermore, evidence discussed below indicates that diabetes and autoimmune thyroid disease frequently coexist in the absence of adrenal autoimmunity. Thus, pluriglandular endocrine autoimmunity can be divided into the major types and variations shown in Fig. 28-2.

ADDISON'S DISEASE WITH HYPOPARATHYROIDISM

As shown in Fig. 28-1, the group of patients with Addison's disease plus hypoparathyroidism is distinguished by a much earlier onset of Addison's disease in

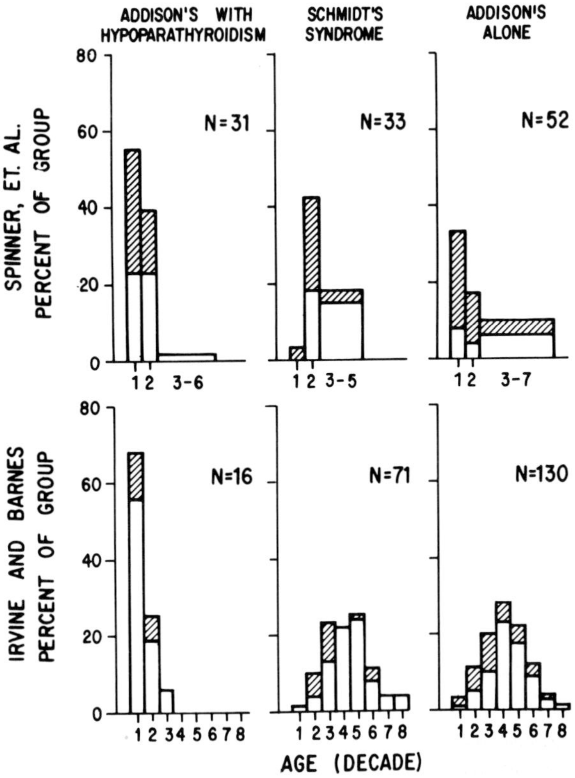

FIGURE 28-1 Clinical heterogeneity of Addison's disease. Distribution of age of onset (*top*) or age of diagnosis (*bottom*) of Addison's disease alone, or Addison's disease with hypoparathyroidism or Schmidt's syndrome. The open area represents females; the closed area represents males. (*Data from Spinner et al.*[169] *and Irvine and Barnes.*[151])

both sexes. Taken together, the two series shown in Fig. 28-1 demonstrate only a slight excess of female patients in this category. Chronic mucocutaneous candidiasis occurs frequently in this group; in 84 percent of patients with this infection and an associated endocrinopathy the endocrine disorder is hypoparathyroidism.[170] The onset of candidiasis and hypoparathyroidism (usually in that order) is even earlier than that of Addison's disease: hypoparathyroidism occurs before age 10 in 88 percent of patients[169] (Fig. 28-3). Addison's disease follows within 2 years in half the patients and within 9 years in three-fourths. These patients are occasionally afflicted by a third endocrine disorder, including thyroid disease, diabetes, pernicious anemia, or ovarian failure.

Addison's disease with hypoparathyroidism is frequently familial; the probability is estimated to be 0.35 that the sibling of an affected person will have Addison's disease, hypoparathyroidism, or any one of the above-mentioned secondary disorders.[169] It is relatively uncommon, however, for the sib to have both Addison's disease and hypoparathyroidism. Spinner et al.[169] found, among the families of probands with both endocrinopathies, 10 siblings with either Addison's disease or hypoparathyroidism but only two with both disorders. It is, of course, likely that some siblings with only one of the two disorders will eventually develop the second.

Antibodies to parathyroid tissue demonstrated by indirect immunofluorescence occur in 38 percent of patients with idiopathic hypoparathyroidism;[171] in addition, they are found in 26 percent of patients with idiopathic Addison's disease without hypoparathyroidism (see below). Among patients with Addison's disease and hypoparathyroidism there is also an increased frequency of thyroid and parietal cell antibodies.[168]

A variety of immunologic defects have been

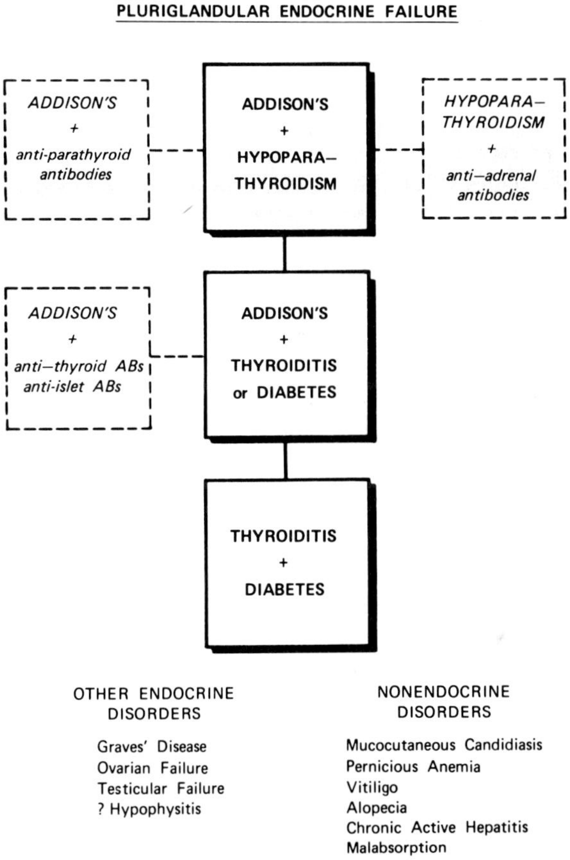

FIGURE 28-2 The three major clinical categories of pluriglandular autoimmune endocrinopathy (center column), with forme fruste variants (dashed boxes) and less frequently associated endocrine disorders and nonendocrine disorders. Graves' disease may substitute for thyroiditis. Gonadal failure is associated with a pan-steroid cell antibody in Addison's disease; candidiasis is strongly associated with hypoparathyroidism.

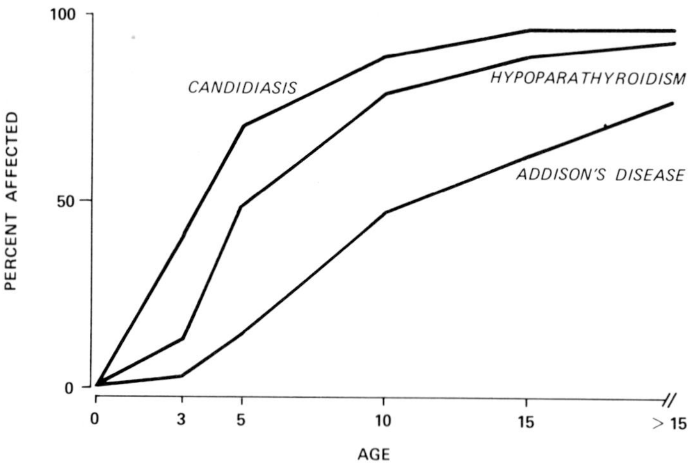

FIGURE 28-3 Typical sequence of childhood onset of chronic mucocutaneous candidiasis, autoimmune hypoparathyroidism, and Addison's disease. Patients with hypoparathyroidism may not develop Addison's, but frequent adrenal antibodies suggest the polyendocrine diathesis is still present. (*Data from Neufeld et al: Medicine 60:355, 1981.*)

reported in patients with chronic mucocutaneous candidiasis with or without endocrinopathies, including impaired blast transformation, impaired macrophage migration inhibition, and impaired lymphocytotoxicity.[172] The pathogenetic relationship between these defects and those responsible for immune sensitization to endocrine tissue is unclear.

HYPOPARATHYROIDISM WITHOUT ADDISON'S DISEASE

Patients with hypoparathyroidism but no Addison's disease have an early onset of hypoparathyroidism (73 percent prior to age 10) and chronic candidiasis, similar to those with Addison's disease. In the group of patients reported by Spinner et al.,[169] the time elapsed after the onset of hypoparathyroidism was sufficient to make it unlikely that many of these patients would later develop Addison's disease. Familial aggregation is infrequent, although a few patients or their sibs have developed thyroid disease or pernicious anemia. The prevalence of parathyroid antibodies in this group is similar to that of the group with Addison's disease and hypoparathyroidism.[171] In hypoparathyroid patients there is a 7 percent rate of immunofluorescent adrenal antibody detection,[168] but in hypoparathyroidism with candidiasis subclinical antiadrenal autoimmunity may occur in greater than half.[173] The occurrence of adrenal antibodies and candidiasis in this group suggests that this subset may represent a forme fruste of pluriglandular endocrine insufficiency. Thyroid and parietal cell antibodies do not appear to be significantly more prevalent than in control subjects.

ISOLATED ADDISON'S DISEASE

As noted above, isolated idiopathic Addison's disease is associated with a lower prevalence of adrenal antibodies than in patients who have other endocrinopathies associated with their Addison's disease. However, this group still has an increased frequency of thyroid, parathyroid, and islet cell antibodies compared with control populations.[167,168] Although these patients do not have clinically evident involvement of any other endocrine glands, the immunologic findings suggest that they should not be excluded from the spectrum of pluriglandular endocrine disease, and some may ultimately develop an associated endocrinopathy. Patients with isolated Addison's disease may have one or more affected siblings, especially if the onset was before 20 years of age.[169]

SCHMIDT'S SYNDROME

Schmidt's syndrome (Addison's disease with diabetes mellitus and/or chronic thyroiditis) has a predominantly adult age of onset and a 2:1 female predominance[169] (Fig. 28-1). In half the cases there is familial aggregation; the probability that a given sibling will also be affected is estimated to be 0.25. Table 28-6 shows that the overall frequency of diabetes mellitus in idiopathic Addison's disease is 10 percent and that of Hashimoto's thyroiditis and primary myxedema is 9 percent. Diabetes mellitus in these patients may begin in either childhood or adulthood, but most of the patients have been treated with insulin.[151] The onset of Hashimoto's thyroiditis or diabetes is not closely linked to the Addison's disease; they start an average of 7 years later. Schmidt's syndrome is frequently associated with additional disorders, including ovarian failure and pernicious anemia. As mentioned above, some patients with idiopathic Addison's disease without associated endocrinopathies may be at risk for the later development of Schmidt's syndrome. In the absence of a sibling with established Schmidt's syndrome, these individuals cannot be clinically identified.

As might be expected, patients with Schmidt's syndrome have a higher prevalence of thyroid antibodies than any other group of patients with Addison's disease. Assays for antibodies against thyroglobulin and thyroid cytoplasmic antigens are widely available; the latter antibody is the more prevalent in Hashimoto's thyroiditis and appears to be more discriminative.[154] The presence of thyroid antibodies in Addison's disease indicates an increased risk for thyroid failure. McCarthy-Young et al.[174] found elevated serum TSH concentrations in 10 of 13 patients with idiopathic Addison's disease and thyroid antibodies compared with 3 of 14 patients without thyroid antibodies. Parents and siblings of patients with Schmidt's syndrome have a significantly greater prevalence of thyroid antibodies (50 and 18 percent, respectively) compared with age- and sex-matched controls.[168]

Islet cell antibodies may also be a feature of Schmidt's syndrome. Bottazzo et al.[175] and MacCuish et al.[158] originally detected islet cell antibodies by immunofluorescence in a group of 18 patients with diabetes and other tissue-specific autoantibodies: one-half had Addison's disease. Subsequent studies have shown such antibodies to be present in 60 percent of patients with insulin-dependent diabetes when tested within 1 year of diagnosis, irrespective of the presence of autoimmune disease.[176] Islet cell antibodies disappear with time in those patients with isolated diabetes; however, among patients in whom islet cell antibodies persist for 3 to 5 years after the diagnosis of diabetes, another autoimmune disease occurs in 29 percent[176] and 67 percent have thyroid or parietal cell antibodies.[177] Islet cell antibodies were present in 16 percent of nondiabetic patients with Addison's disease plus another autoimmune disease.[176]

ADDISON'S DISEASE WITH OTHER ENDOCRINOPATHIES

There is a striking incidence of ovarian failure in women with idiopathic Addison's disease. In the large series of Irvine and Barnes,[151] 24 percent of women whose menstrual history was known had amenorrhea and an additional 6 percent had oligomenorrhea. Abnormal menstrual function is not related to deficiency of adrenal corticosteroids, since it persists after replacement therapy and is uncommon in tuberculous Addison's disease. Figure 28-4 shows the age of diagnosis of amenorrhea compared with the age of diagnosis of idiopathic Addison's disease in a group of these patients. Many patients with childhood onset of Addi-

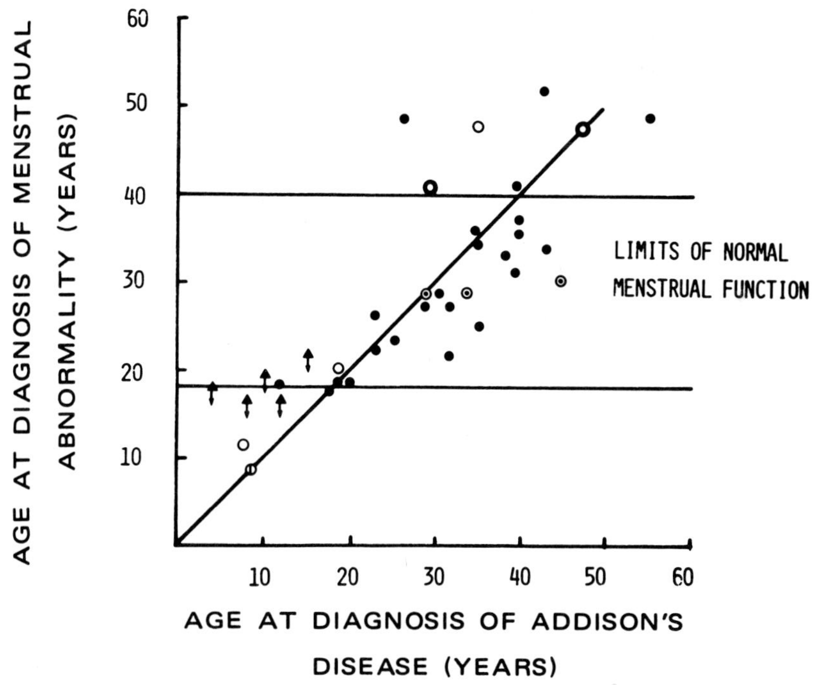

FIGURE 28-4 Correlation between age at diagnosis of menstrual abnormality and age of diagnosis of Addison's disease in patients with steroid cell antibodies (△ = primary amenorrhea, ● = secondary amenorrhea or normal menopause, ⊙ = oligomenorrhea, ○ = menorrhagia, ○ = normal menses, ⦶ = prepubertal). (*From Irvine and Barnes.*[151])

son's disease developed primary amenorrhea; in the patients with secondary amenorrhea the ages of diagnosis of the two disorders were close, with ovarian failure usually preceding Addison's disease by a few years.

Ovarian failure in Addison's disease is associated with a special type of antibody against multiple steroid-producing cells, including Leydig cells and cells of the theca interna, corpus luteum, placenta, and adrenal cortex.[178,179] Absorption studies with these tissues distinguish between those antibodies to common antigens and others which react only with adrenal cortex. Sera containing steroid cell antibodies possess direct cytotoxicity for granulosa cells in monolayer cell culture. These steroid cell antibodies are found in 20 percent of women with Addison's disease but only 4 percent of men.[151] The frequency of amenorrhea or other menstrual disorders in women with Addison's disease is significantly greater in those with steroid cell antibodies (Table 28-8). In a small number of patients with idiopathic Addison's disease, steroid cell antibodies, and gonadal failure, ovarian biopsy has shown lymphocytic infiltration or, in some cases, streak gonads. This type of antibody also indicates more active autoimmune disease, as shown by a higher frequency of other components of the pluriglandular endocrine insufficiency syndrome (Table 28-8). Steroid cell antibodies occur only rarely in other autoimmune diseases and have not been demonstrated in nonaddisonian patients with menstrual disorders. Although steroid cell antibodies are uncommon in men with Addison's disease, two cases of testicular failure associated with Addison's disease have been reported.[151,180]

Although most autoimmune disorders of the endocrine glands cause decreased function or failure, Graves' disease is intimately associated with these disorders. Thyrotoxicosis occurs in about 8 percent of patients with Addison's disease. In patients with idiopathic Addison's disease, pernicious anemia may occur with or without diabetes, thyroid disease, hypoparathyroidism, or ovarian failure. The prevalence of pernicious anemia in Addison's disease is approximately 4 percent (Table 28-3). (The association of thyroid disease, diabetes, and pernicious anemia is discussed below.)

Thyroid Disease and Diabetes Mellitus without Addison's Disease

The greater prevalence of diabetes and thyroid disease in the general population makes the quantitative study of an association between these disorders difficult. Nevertheless, many authors have cited an increased frequency of autoimmune thyroid disease in diabetics; pernicious anemia is also associated. This is confirmed by studies of tissue-specific autoantibodies in diabetics compared with age- and sex-matched controls (Fig. 28-5). Table 28-9 summarizes representative studies of the interrelationships of autoimmune sensitivities to these three tissues.

Other Disorders

Vitiligo may occur with any of the above pluriglandular endocrine insufficiency syndromes. The suspicion that this disorder represents another tissue-specific autoimmune disease is supported by the recent identification of antibodies to melanin-producing cells.[185]

A dozen cases of lymphocytic infiltration of the adenohypophysis have been reported. All of these cases have been temporally related to pregnancy and have presented as sellar masses or sudden collapse; half were associated with autoimmune diseases, particularly lymphocytic thyroiditis and atrophic gastritis. In several cases, the adrenals were atrophic and the patient appeared to have died in adrenal crisis; however, hypopituitarism was diagnosed during life in at least one of these patients.[186] This entity may represent

Table 28-8. Occurrence of Associated Disorders in Idiopathic Addison's Disease Patients with and without Steroid Cell Antibodies

	Amenorrhea or oligomenorrhea*	Other associated disorders	No associated disorder
Steroid cell antibody-positive ($n = 40$)	27†	9‡	4
Steroid cell antibody-negative ($n = 221$)	20	45	156

*Of women with known menstrual histories (36 antibody-positive, 121 antibody-negative).
†Statistically significant difference between seropositive and seronegative groups, $p < 0.00025$.
‡$p < 0.0005$; independent risk of associated autoimmune disorder, excluding oligomenorrhea and Addison's disease.
Source: Modified from Irvine and Barnes.[151]

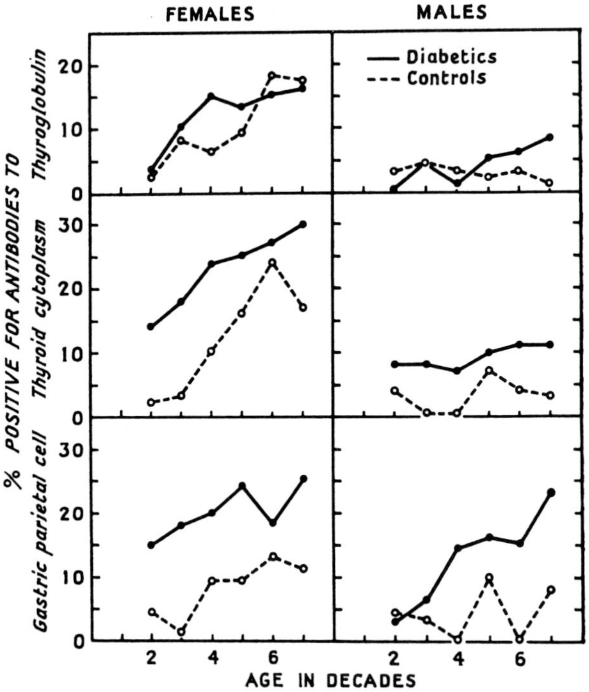

FIGURE 28-5 Frequency of antibodies to thyroglobulin, thyroid cytoplasm, and parietal cell cytoplasm in diabetics over 10 years of age and in age- and sex-matched controls. (*From Irvine et al.*[181])

"autoimmune hypophysitis." One case of diabetes insipidus associated with Addison's disease and hypoparathyroidism has been reported, but the pathogenesis of the diabetes insipidus is unclear.[187]

Diagnosis, Complications, and Surveillance

The signs, symptoms, diagnostic testing, and therapy of the individual endocrinopathies discussed in this section are generally the same as when these disorders occur individually (see the appropriate chapters elsewhere in this text). Some observed or theoretically possible pitfalls in diagnosis due to hormonal interactions are discussed in this section.

The most serious possible error in diagnosis of multiple endocrine failure would be to attribute adrenal, thyroid, and ovarian failure solely to hypopituitarism. This is easily avoided, as the diagnosis of autoimmune primary end organ failures should be considered in every case, and integrity of pituitary function should be proved by detecting elevated blood levels of TSH, luteinizing hormone (LH), or ACTH. The coexistence of hypoparathyroidism or diabetes is an obvious indicator of autoimmune endocrinopathy. Conversely, the entity of lymphocytic hypophysitis should be kept in mind in the setting of pregnancy.

Failure to effect normal regulation because of glucocorticosteroid deficiency in Addison's disease may alter the secretion and action of other hormones. Lack of the suppressive effect of glucocorticosteroids on TSH release can result in elevated TSH levels in the absence of intrinsic thyroid disease.[188] TSH levels are therefore unreliable indicators of thyroid failure in untreated Addison's disease and should be reevaluated after adrenal steroid replacement. Adrenal insufficiency could theoretically also mask the development of glucose intolerance during early insulitis, but this has not been documented clinically. Calcium is an important controller of stimulus-secretion coupling in many endocrine cell types, but clinically important effects of hypocalcemia on secretion of other hormones have not been observed.

A number of interactions with thyroid hormone status must be kept in mind in the diagnostic evaluation of untreated patients with pluriglandular failure. Hypothyroidism can cause a macrocytic anemia, especially in children,[189] but also in adults. This should be

Table 28-9. Interrelationship of Thyroid, Gastric, and Islet Cell Autoimmunity

Index disease	Associated finding	Frequency, %	Ref.
Diabetes	Thyroid antibodies	16	181
	↑ TSH (males)	6	182
	↑ TSH (females)	17	182
	Parietal cell antibodies	17	181
Thyroiditis	Islet cell antibodies	9	168
	Intrinsic factor antibodies	2	183
	Pernicious anemia	9	183
Hyperthyroidism	Islet cell antibodies	3	168
	Intrinsic factor antibodies	3	183
	Pernicious anemia	3	183
Pernicious anemia	Islet cell antibodies	11	168
	Thyroid antibodies	38	184
	Hypothyroidism	12	184
	Hyperthyroidism	9	184

differentiated from pernicious anemia by clinical assessment of other effects of B_{12} deficiency, response to thyroid hormone replacement, and Schilling test, as indicated. Hypothyroidism can also cause a blunted adrenal response to ACTH and abnormal menses. Conversely, low serum T_4 and T_3 concentrations can be caused by a variety of acute and chronic nonthyroid illnesses ("euthyroid sick syndrome"). This phenomenon could lead to the suspicion of associated hypothyroidism in poorly controlled diabetes.

In surveillance for development of new endocrine gland involvement, emphasis should go to the patients with Addison's disease, as these individuals are at greater risk. Hypothyroidism and pernicious anemia may have a prolonged, insidious onset; the physician should be highly suspicious that these problems are present, especially in patients with Addison's disease. Hypothyroidism should be considered in children with sudden deceleration of growth, but poorly controlled diabetes may be a more frequent cause.[190] Determination of serum TSH concentration, anti-thyroid antibody assay, complete blood count, and serum B_{12} assay are useful laboratory screens. Elevated serum TSH concentration alone is not a good predictor of future clinical hypothyroidism; but, in patients in whom elevated TSH level is combined with a positive test for anti-thyroid antibodies, the incidence of clinical hypothyroidism is 4 percent per year. When antibody titers are markedly elevated the incidence may be as high as 26 percent per year.[191]

Therapeutic implications of pluriglandular endocrine failure are less well characterized. It is known that cortisol antagonizes the intestinal calcium transport effects of vitamin D and its metabolites, which are used to treat hypoparathyroidism. The subsequent development of adrenal insufficiency can result in sudden vitamin D intoxication in these patients.[192]

Genetics of Pluriglandular Endocrine Insufficiency Syndromes

Early genetic analyses of the pluriglandular endocrine insufficiency syndromes attempted to estimate the probability that the sib of a proband would be affected. With the assumption of complete ascertainment (no affected sibs unknown owing to mild disease), one study[169] gave probabilities of 0.25 to 0.35 for Schmidt's syndrome and Addison's disease with hypoparathyroidism. More recently, the application of human histocompatibility (HLA) typing has provided new information. Histocompatibility antigens are expressions of a gene complex located on chromosome 6. Antigens of the HLA-A and -B loci are detected by cytotoxicity to patient lymphocytes of a panel of test sera (i.e., are serologically defined, or SD). Other antigens are detected by the ability of patient lymphocytes to stimulate a panel of test lymphocytes (lymphocyte-defined, LD). The presumed defect in immune regulation resulting in sensitization to autoantigens in these disorders may reside in a gene near the HLA region and be genetically linked to certain alleles. An increased incidence of some HLA antigens has been noted in patients with diabetes (antigens HLA-B8 and -Bw15) and those with Addison's disease (antigen HLA-B8). Disorders linked to HLA-B8 may be even more closely linked to LD antigens.[175,193] Studies of HLA typing in insulin-dependent diabetes have suggested that only the HLA-B8-linked diabetogenic gene is associated with persistent islet cell antibodies and with other autoimmune disease.[176] Several investigations have found that homozygosity for HLA-B8 confers no increased risk for the development of diabetes,[193] although not all studies agree.[194] The hypothesis of a dominant HLA-B8-linked diabetogenic gene correlates with results of HLA typing reported in a kindred with pluriglandular endocrine insufficiency studied for SD antigens (Fig. 28-6). In this kindred, the possession of an HLA-B8 haplotype appeared to impart susceptibility to autoimmune disease with a high degree of penetrance. The one family member with the same haplotype without disease was only 17 years old and still at risk. Although this study appears to suggest a dominant pattern of inheritance, it is possible that further HLA typing studies will demonstrate genetic heterogeneity in these disorders.

Nonautoimmune Pluriglandular Dysfunction

Bardwick et al.[195] have recently reviewed a syndrome which had previously been reported mostly in Japan. Seventy-five percent of these patients are male; they have plasma cell dyscrasias occurring in the fourth or fifth decade, usually sclerotic plasmacytomas. This has been given the acronym POEMS syndrome (polyneuropathy, organomegaly, endocrinopathy, M protein, and skin changes). Hypogonadism, gynecomastia, and diabetes mellitus are frequent endocrine disorders, while adrenal failure is uncommon. In one of the cases of Bardwick et al., fasting hyperglycemia requiring insulin resolved with radiotherapy of the patient's plasmacytoma, recurred three years later with the appearance of a new bone lesion, and resolved again with radiation treatment. Neither the polyneuropathy nor the endocrinopathy appears to be explainable on the basis of infiltration by amyloid protein, nor were the investigators able to demonstrate tissue-specific endocrine antibodies as are present in many patients with the autoimmune endocrinopathies. The mechanism of this interesting syndrome remains obscure.

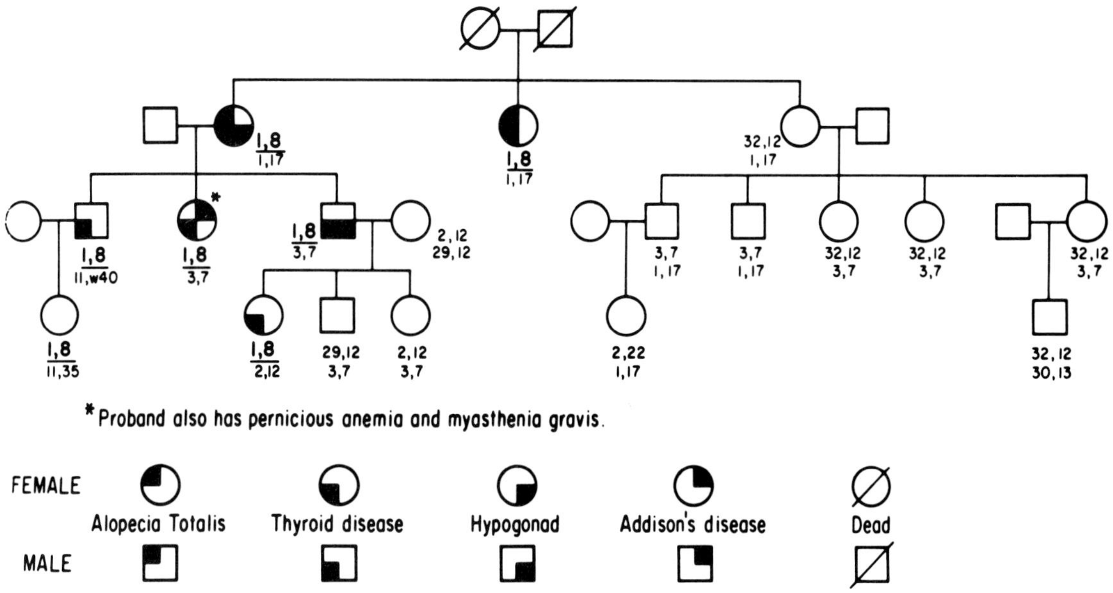

FIGURE 28-6 HLA typing of a kindred with pluriglandular endocrine insufficiency syndrome. The proband is indicated by the asterisk. HLA haplotypes are shown one above the other; the A1/B8 haplotype is underlined. (*From Eisenbarth et al: N Engl J Med* 298:92, 1978.)

REFERENCES

1. Erdheim J: Zur normalen und pathologischen histologie der glandula thyreodea, parathyreoidea, und hypophysis. *Beitr Pathol Anat* 33:158, 1903.

2. Cushing H, Davidoff LM: The pathological findings in four autopsied cases of acromegaly with a discussion of their significance. The Rockefeller Institute for Medical Research Monograph 22, 1927.

3. Lloyd PC: Hypophyseo-parathyreo-insular syndrome. *Bull Johns Hopkins Hosp* 45:1, 1929.

4. Rossier PH, Dressler M: Familare Erkrankunginnersekretorischer Drusen kombiniert mit Ulcuskrankheit. *Schweiz Med Wochenschr* 20:985, 1939.

5. Underdahl LO, Woolner LB, Black BM: Multiple endocrine adenomas. Report of eight cases in which parathyroids, pituitary, and pancreatic islets were involved. *J Clin Endocrinol* 13:20, 1953.

6. Moldawer MP, Nordi GL, Raker W: Concomitance of multiple adenomas of the parathyroids and pancreatic islets with tumor of the pituitary: A syndrome with familial incidence. *Am J Med Sci* 228:190, 1954.

7. Wermer P: Genetic aspects of adenomatosis of endocrine glands. *Am J Med* 16:363, 1954.

8. Zollinger RM, Ellison EH: Primary peptic ulceration of the jejunum associated with islet cell tumors of the pancreas. *Ann Surg* 142:709, 1955.

9. Verner JF, Morrison AB: Islet cell tumor and a syndrome of refractory watery diarrhea and hypokalemia. *Am J Med* 25:374, 1958.

10. Spencer SS, Summerskill WHJ: Malabsorption induced by gastrin hypersecretion due to ectopic islet cell adenoma. *Am J Gastroenterol* 39:26, 1963.

11. Schmid JR, Labhart A, Rossier PH: Relationship of multiple endocrine adenomas to syndrome of ulcerogenic islet cell adenomas (Zollinger-Ellison): Occurrence of both syndromes in one family. *Am J Med* 31:343, 1961.

12. Huizenga KA, Goodrick WIM, Summerskill WHJ: Peptic ulcer with islet cell tumor. *Am J Med* 37:564, 1964.

13. Ballard HS, Frame B, Harstock RJ: Familial multiple endocrine adenoma–peptic ulcer complex. *Medicine* 43:481, 1964.

14. Vanderweghe M, Schutyser J, Braxer K, Vermeulen A: A case of multiple endocrine adenomatosis with primary amenorrhea. *Postgrad Med J* 54:618, 1978.

15. Carlson HE, Levine JA, Goldberg NJ, Hershman JM: Hyperprolactinemia in multiple endocrine adenomatosis, type 1. *Arch Intern Med* 138:1807, 1978.

16. Tourniaire J, Trouillas J, Maillet P, David L, Pallo D, Tran Minh V, Pressot C: Polyadénomatose endocrinienne associant un adénome hypophysaire à prolactine et un adénome parathyroïdien intrathyroïdien. *Ann Endocrinol* 38:1, 1977.

17. Levine JH, Sagel J, Rosebrock GL Jr, Gonzalez J: Hyperprolactinemia in the multiple endocrine adenomatosis type 1 (MEA-1) syndrome. *Arch Intern Med* 38:1777, 1977.

18. Wermer P: Endocrine adenomatosis and peptic ulcer in a large kindred. Inherited multiple tumors and mosaic pleotropism in man. *Am J Med* 35:205, 1963.

19. Paloyan E, Lawrence AM: Laboratory diagnosis of parathyroid tumors. *Ann Clin Lab Sci* 4:241, 1974.

20. Block MA, Frame B: The extent of operation for primary hyperparathyroidism. *Arch Surg* 109:798, 1974.

21. Mallete LE, Bilezikian JP, Ketcham AS, Aurbach GD: Parathyroid carcinoma in familial hyperparathyroidism. *Am J Med* 57:642, 1974.

22. Marx SJ, Spiegel AM, Brown EM, Aurbach GD: Family studies in patients with primary parathyroid hyperplasia. *Am J Med* 62:698, 1977.

23. Jung RT, Davie M, Grant AM, Jenkins D, Chalmers TM: Multiple endocrine adenomatosis (type I) and familial hyperparathyroidism. *Postgrad Med J* 54:92, 1978.

24. Scholz DA, Purnell DC, Edis AJ, van Heerden JA, Woolner LB: Primary hyperparathyroidism with multiple parathyroid gland enlargement. Review of 53 cases. *Mayo Clin Proc* 53:792, 1978.

25. Isenberg JI, Walsch JH, Grossman MI: Zollinger-Ellison syndrome. *Gastroenterology* 65:140, 1973.

26. McGuigan JE, Colwell JA, Franklin J: Effect of parathyroidectomy on hypercalcemic hypersecretory peptic ulcer disease. *Gastroenterology* 66:269, 1974.

27. Gogel HK, Buckman MT, Cadieux D, McCarthy DM: Gastric secretion and hormonal interactions in multiple endocrine neoplasia type I. *Arch Intern Med* 145:855, 1985.

28. McGavaran MH, Unger RH, Recant L, Polk HC, Kilo C, Levin ME: A glucagon-secreting alpha-cell carcinoma of the pancreas. *N Engl J Med* 274:1408, 1966.

29. Mallinson CN, Bloom SR, Warin AP, Salmon PR, Cox B: A glucagonoma syndrome. *Lancet* 2:1, 1974.

30. Stacpoole PW, Jaspan J, Kasselberg AG, Halter SA, Polonsky K, Gluck FW, Liljenquist JE, Rabin D: A familial glucagonoma syndrome. *Am J Med* 70:1017, 1981.

31. Krejs GJ, Orci L, Conlon JM, Ravazzola M, Davis GR, Raskin P, Collins SM, McCarthy DM, Baetens D, Rubenstein A, Aldor TAM, Unger RH: Somatostatinoma syndrome. *N Engl J Med* 301:285, 1979.

32. Ganda OP, Weir GC, Soeldner JS, Legg ML, Chick WL, Patel YC, Ebeid AM, Gabbay KH, Reichlin S: "Somatostatinoma": A somatostatin-containing tumor of the endocrine pancreas. *N Engl J Med* 296:963, 1977.

33. Larsson L-I, Hirsch MA, Holst JJ, Ingemansson S, Kuhl C, Jensen SL, Lundqvist G, Rehfeld JF, Schwartz TW: Pancreatic somatostatinoma: Clinical features and physiological implications. *Lancet* 1:666, 1977.

34. Rimoin DL, Schimke RN: *Genetic Disorders of the Endocrine Glands.* St. Louis, Mosby, 1971.

35. Prosser PR, Karam JH, Townsend JJ, Forsham P: Prolactin-secreting pituitary adenomas in multiple endocrine adenomatosis, type-I. *Ann Intern Med* 91:41, 1979.

36. Stabile BE, Passaro E, Carlson HE: Elevated serum prolactin level in the Zollinger-Ellison syndrome. *Arch Surg* 116:449, 1981.

37. Farid NR, Buehler S, Russell NA, Maroun FB, Allerdice P: Prolactinomas in familial multiple endocrine neoplasia syndrome type I. *Am J Med* 69:874, 1980.

38. Veldhuis JD, Green JE, Kovacs E, Worgul TJ, Murray FT, Hammond JM: Prolactin-secreting pituitary adenomas. *Am J Med* 67:830, 1979.

39. Goldman M, Holub D: Prolactinomas and the multiple endocrine adenomatosis type-I complex. *Ann Intern Med* 91:791, 1979.

40. O'Neal LW, Kipnis DM, Luse SA, Lacy PE, Jarrett L: Secretion of various endocrine substances by ACTH-secreting tumors—gastrin, melanotropin, norepinephrine, serotonin, parathormone, vasopressin, glucagon. *Cancer* 21:1219, 1968.

41. Vance JE, Stoll RW, Kitabachi AE, Williams RH, Wood FC Jr: Nesidioblastosis in familial endocrine adenomatosis. *JAMA* 207:1679, 1969.

42. Snyder N III, Scurry MT, Deiss WP: Five families with multiple endocrine adenomatosis. *Ann Intern Med* 76:53, 1972.

43. Williams ED, Celestin LR: The association of bronchial carcinoid and pluriglandular adenomatosis. *Thorax* 17:120, 1962.

44. Amano S, Hazama F, Haebara H, Tsurusawa M, Kaito H: Ectopic ACTH-MSH producing carcinoid with multiple endocrine hyperplasia in a child. *Acta Pathol Jpn* 28:721, 1978.

45. Sommers SC: Adrenal glands, in Anderson WAD (ed): *Pathology.* St. Louis, Mosby, 1971, pp 1464–1487.

46. Mortensen JD, Woolner LB, Bennett WA: Gross and microscopic findings in clinically normal thyroid glands. *J Clin Endocrinol Metab* 15:1270, 1955.

47. Friedman NB: Chronic hypoglycemia: Report of two cases with islet adenoma and changes in the hypophysis. *Arch Pathol* 27:994, 1939.

48. Lamers CB, Buis JT, van Tongeren J: Secretin-stimulated serum gastrin levels in hyperparathyroid patients from families with multiple endocrine adenomatosis. *Ann Intern Med* 86:719, 1977.

49. Selking O, Johansson H, Lundqvist G: Serum gastrin and its response to secretin in hyperparathyroid patients. *Acta Chir Scand* 147:649, 1981.

50. Service FJ, Dale AJD, Elveback LR, Jiang N-S: Insulinoma. Clinical and diagnostic features of 60 consecutive cases. *Mayo Clin Proc* 51:417, 1976.

51. Goldstein JL: Multiple endocrine adenoma–peptic ulcer syndrome, in *Medical Grand Rounds, Parkland Memorial Hospital.* Jan. 30, 1975, p 1.

52. Effron M, Griner L, Benirschke K: Nature and rate of neoplasia found in captive wild mammals, birds, and reptiles at necropsy. *JNCI* 59:185, 1977.

53. Berdjis CC: Pluriglandular syndrome. I. Multiple endocrine adenomas in irradiated rats. *Oncologia* 13:441, 1960.

54. Rosen VJ Jr, Castanera TJ, Jones DC, Kimeldorf DJ: Islet-cell tumors of the pancreas in the irradiated and non-irradiated rat. *Lab Invest* 10:608, 1961.

55. Knudson AG: Genetics and etiology of human cancer, in Harris H, Hirschhorn K (eds): *Advances in Human Genetics.* New York, Plenum, 1977, vol 8, pp 1–66.

56. Knudson AG: Hereditary cancer, oncogenes, and antioncogenes. *Cancer Res* 45:1437, 1985.

57. Stoker MGP: Signals and switches: A summary, in Clarkson B, Baserga R (eds): *Control of Proliferation in Animal Cells.* Cold Spring Harbor, Cold Spring Harbor Laboratory, 1974, pp 1009–1013.

58. Oseroff AR, Robbins PW, Burger MM: The cell surface membrane. *Annu Rev Biochem* 42:647, 1973.

59. Pearse AGE: Common cytochemical properties of cells producing polypeptide hormones, with particular reference to CT and the thyroid C-cells. *Vet Rec* 79:587, 1966.

60. Tischler AS, Dichter MA, Biales B, Greene LA: Neuroendocrine neoplasms and their cells of origin. *N Engl J Med* 296:919, 1977.

61. Ellison EH, Neville AM: Neoplasia and ectopic hormone production, in Raven RW (ed): *Modern Trends in Oncology.* London, Butterworths, 1973, vol 1, pt 1, pp 163–181.

62. Hansen OP, Hansen M, Hansen HH, Rose B: Multiple endocrine adenomatosis of mixed type. *Acta Med Scand* 200:327, 1976.

63. Berg B, Biorklund A, Grimelius L, Ingemansson S, Larsson L-I, Stenram U, Akerman M: A new pattern of multiple endocrine adenomatosis. *Acta Med Scand* 200:321, 1976.

64. Wells SA Jr, Ellis GJ, Gunnells JC, Schneider AB, Sherwood LM: Parathyroid autotransplantation in primary parathyroid hyperplasia. *N Engl J Med* 295:57, 1976.

65. van Heerden JE, Kent RB, Sizemore GW, Grant CS, Remine WH: Primary hyperparathyroidism in patients with multiple endocrine neoplasia syndromes. *Arch Surg* 118:533, 1983.

66. Brennan MF, Brown EM, Marx SJ, Spiegel AM, Broadus AE, Doppman JL, Webber B, Aurbach GD: Recurrent hyperparathyroidism from an autotransplanted parathyroid adenoma. *N Engl J Med* 299:1057, 1978.

67. Guiot G: Transsphenoidal approach in surgical treatment of pituitary adenomas: General principles and indications in nonfunctioning adenomas, in Kohler PO, Ross GT (eds): *Diagnosis and Treatment of Pituitary Tumors.* New York, American Elsevier, 1973, pp 159–178.

68. Hardy J: Transsphenoidal surgery of hyper-secreting pituitary tumors, in Kohler PO, Ross GT (eds): *Diagnosis and Treatment of Pituitary Tumors.* New York, American Elsevier, 1973, pp 179–194.

69. Scott HW Jr, Gobbel WG Jr, Law DH IV: Clinical experience with a jejunal pouch (Hunt-Lawrence) as a substitute stomach after total gastrectomy. *Surg Gynecol Obstet* 121:1231, 1965.

70. Turner WW, McLelland RN, Fry WJ: Roux-19 esophagojejunostomy following total gastrectomy. *Curr Surg* 35:64, 1978.

71. McCarthy DM: Report on the United States experience with cimetidine in Zollinger-Ellison syndrome and other hypersecretory states. *Gastroenterology* 74:453, 1978.

72. Cryer PE, Hill GJ: Pancreatic islet cell carcinoma with

hypercalcemia and hypergastrinemia. Response to streptozotocin. *Cancer* 38:2217, 1976.

73. Graber AL, Porte D Jr, Williams RH: Clinical use of diazoxide and mechanism for its hyperglycemic effects. *Diabetes* 15:143, 1966.

74. Schein PS: Chemotherapeutic management of the hormone-secreting malignancies. *Cancer* 30:1616, 1972.

75. Deftos LJ: *Medullary Thyroid Carcinoma.* Basel, Karger, 1983.

76. Sizemore GW, Carney JA, Heath H: Epidemiology of medullary carcinoma of the thyroid gland. *Surg Clin North Am* 57:633, 1977.

77. Chang GC, Beahrs O, Sizemore GW, Woolner CH: Medullary carcinoma of the thyroid gland. *Cancer* 35:695, 1975.

78. Carney JA, Sizemore GW, Hayles AB: C-cell disease of the thyroid gland in multiple endocrine neoplasia, type 2b. *Cancer* 44:2173, 1979.

79. Norton JA, Froome LC, Farrell RE, Wells SA: Multiple endocrine neoplasia type IIb: The most aggressive form of medullary thyroid carcinoma. *Surg Clin North Am* 59:109, 1979.

80. Pearse AGE: Common cytochemical and ultrastructural characteristics of cells producing polypeptide hormones (the APUD series) and their relevance to thyroid and ultimobranchial C-cells and calcitonin. *Proc R Soc Lond* 170:71, 1968.

81. Pearse AGE, Takor TT: Neuroendocrine embryology and the APUD concept. *Clin Endocrinol* 5:299, 1976.

82. Deftos LJ, Parthemore JG: Secretion of parathyroid hormone in patients with medullary thyroid carcinoma. *J Clin Invest* 54:416, 1974.

83. Melvin KEW, Tashjian AH Jr, Miller HH: Studies in familial thyroid cancer. *Trans Assoc Am Physicians* 84:144, 1971.

84. Williams ED: Medullary carcinoma of the thyroid. *J Clin Pathol* 19:114, 1966.

85. Hazard JB, Hawk WA, Crile G: Medullary (solid) carcinoma of the thyroid—a clinicopathologic entity. *J Clin Endocrinol Metab* 19:152, 1959.

86. Cunliffe WJ, Black MM, Hall R, Johnston IDA, Hudgson P, Shuster S, Gudmundsson TV, Joplin GF, Williams ED, Woodhouse NJY, Galante L, MacIntyre I: A calcitonin-secreting thyroid carcinoma. *Lancet* 2:63, 1968.

87. Melvin KEW, Tashjian AH Jr: The syndrome of excessive thyrocalcitonin produced by medullary carcinoma of the thyroid. *Proc Natl Acad Sci USA* 59:1216, 1968.

88. Meyer JS, Abdel-Bari W: Granules and thyroidcalcitonin-like activity in medullary carcinoma of the thyroid. *N Engl J Med* 278:523, 1968.

89. Milhaud G, Tubiana M, Parmentier C, Coutris G: Epithelioma de la thyroide secretant de la thyrocalcitonine. *C R Seances Acad Sci* 266:608, 1968.

90. Clark MB, Byfield PGH, Boyd GW, Foster GV: A radioimmunoassay for human calcitonin M. *Lancet* 2:74, 1969.

91. Kalina M, Foster GV, Clark MB, Pearse AGE: C-cells in man, in Taylor S, Foster G (eds): *Calcitonin, 1969.* New York, Heinemann, 1970, pp 268–273.

92. Deftos LJ: Calcitonin in clinical medicine, in Stollerman GH (ed): *Advances in Internal Medicine.* New York, Year Book, 1978, pp 159–193.

93. LeDourain N, LeLievre C: Demonstration de l'origine neural des cellules a calcitonine du corps ultimobranchial chez l'embryon de poulet. *C R Seances Acad Sci* 270:2857, 1970.

94. Lippman SM, Mendelsohn G, Trump DL, Wells SA, Baylin SB: The prognostic and biological significance of cellular heterogeneity in medullary thyroid carcinoma: A study of calcitonin, L-dopa decarboxylase, and histaminase. *J Clin Endocrinol Metab* 54:233, 1982.

95. Ljungberg O: On medullary carcinoma of the thyroid: A clinicopathologic entity. *Acta Pathol Microbiol Scand* 231:1, 1972.

96. Livolsi VA, Feind CR, LoGerfo P, Tashjian AH Jr: Demonstration by immunoperoxidase staining of hyperplasia of parafollicular cells in the thyroid gland in hyperparathyroidism. *J Clin Endocrinol Metab* 37:550, 1973.

97. McMillan PJ, Hooker WM, Deftos LJ: Distribution of calcitonin-containing cells in human thyroid. *Am J Anat* 140:73, 1974.

98. Hamilton CW, Bigner SH, Wells SA, Johnston WW: Metastatic medullary thyroid carcinoma in sputum. *Acta Cytol* 27:49, 1983.

99. Lamberg BA, Reissel P, Stenman S, Koivuniemi A, Ekblom M, Makinen J, Franssila K: Concurrent medullary and papillary thyroid carcinoma in the same lobe and in siblings. *Acta Med Scand* 209:421, 1981.

100. Wolfe HJ, Melvin KEW, Cervi-Skinner SJ, Al Saadi AA, Juliar JF, Jackson CE, Tashjian AH Jr: C-cell hyperplasia preceding medullary thyroid carcinoma. *N Engl J Med* 289:437, 1973.

101. Carney AJ, Sizemore GW, Lovestedt SA: Mucosal ganglioneuromatosis, medullary thyroid carcinoma, and pheochromocytoma: MEN, type 2B. *Oral Surg* 41:739, 1976.

102. Keiser JR, Beaven MA, Doppman J, Wells S, Buja LM: Medullary thyroid carcinoma, pheochromocytoma, and parathyroid disease. *Ann Intern Med* 78:561, 1973.

103. McKenna TJ, McLean D, Lorber DL, Bone HG, Parthemore JG, Deftos LJ: Comparison of calcitonin stimulation tests used in screening for medullary carcinoma of the thyroid, *Proceedings of the 60th Annual Meeting of the Endocrine Society,* 1978, p 370.

104. Beskid M: Thyroid C-cells in normal and goitrous gland: A histochemical study. *Acta Histochem* 54:313, 1975.

105. Milhaud G, Calmettes C, Jullienne A, Tharaud D, Bloch-Michel H, Cavaillon JP, Colin R, Moukhtar MS: A new chapter in human pathology: Calcitonin disorders and therapeutic use, in Talmage RV, Munson PL (eds): *Calcium, Parathyroid Hormone, and the Calcitonins.* Amsterdam, Excerpta Medica, 1972, pp 56–70.

106. Hill CS Jr, Ibanez ML, Samaan NA, Ahearn MJ, Clark RL: Medullary (solid) carcinoma of the thyroid gland: An analysis of the M.D. Anderson Hospital experience with patients with the tumor, its special features, and its histogenesis. *Medicine* 52:141, 1973.

107. Tashjian AH Jr, Howland BG, Kenneth BA, Melvin KEW, Hill CS Jr: Immunoassay of human calcitonin. (Clinical measurement, relation to serum calcium and studies in patients with medullary thyroid carcinoma.) *N Engl J Med* 283:890, 1970.

108. Ibanez ML, Cole VW, Russell WO, Clark RI: Solid carcinoma of the thyroid gland. *Cancer* 20:706, 1967.

109. Deftos LJ: Radioimmunoassay for calcitonin in medullary thyroid carcinoma. *JAMA* 227:403, 1974.

110. MacIntyre I, Hillyard CJ, Murphy PK, Reynolds JJ, Gaines RE, Craig RK: A second plasma calcium-lowering peptide from the human calcitonin precursor. *Nature* 300:460, 1982.

111. Roos BA, O'Niel JA, Muszynski M, Birnbaum RS: Noncalcitonin secretory products of calcitonin gene expression. Proceedings of the International Conference on Calcium Regulating Hormones, Japan, 1983, in Cohn PV, Fujita T, Potts JT Jr, Talmage RV (eds): *Endocrine Control of Bone and Calcium Metabolism.* Amsterdam, Elsevier, 1984, pp 169–175.

112. O'Connor DT, Burton D, Deftos LJ: Immunoreactive human chromagranin A in diverse polypeptide hormone producing human tumors and normal endocrine tissues. *J Clin Endocrinol Metab* 57:1084, 1983.

113. O'Connor DT, Burton D, Deftos LJ: Chromagranin A: Immunohistology reveals its universal occurrence in normal polypeptide hormone producing endocrine glands. *Life Sci* 33:1657, 1983.

114. Parthemore JG, Bronzert D, Roberts G, Deftos LJ: A short calcium infusion in the diagnosis of medullary thyroid carcinoma. *J Clin Endocrinol Metab* 39:108, 1974.

115. Hennessey JF, Wells SA, Ontjes DA, Cooper CW: A comparison of pentagastrin injection and calcium infusion as provocative agents for the detection of medullary thyroid carcinoma. *J Clin Endocrinol Metab* 39:487, 1974.

116. Wells SA Jr, Ontjes DA, Cooper CW, Hennessey JF, Ellis GJ, MacPherson HT, Sabiston DC Jr: The early diagnosis of medullary carcinoma of the thyroid gland in patients with multiple endocrine neoplasia, type II. *Ann Surg* 182:362, 1975.

117. Parthemore JG, Deftos LJ: Calcitonin secretion in normal human subjects. *J Clin Endocrinol Metab* 47:184, 1978.

117a. Wells SA Jr, Baylin SB, Leight GS, Dale JK, Dilley WG, Farndon JR: The importance of early diagnosis in patients with hereditary medullary thyroid carcinoma. *Ann Surg* 195:595, 1982.

118. Cohen SL, MacIntyre I, Grahame-Smith D, Walker JG: Alcohol-stimulated calcitonin release in medullary carcinoma of the thyroid. *Lancet* 2:1172, 1973.

119. Anast C, David L, Winnacker J, Glass R, Baskin W, Brubaker L, Burns T: Serum calcitonin-lowering effect of magnesium in patients with medullary thyroid carcinoma. *J Clin Invest* 56:1615, 1975.

120. Norton JA, Doppman JL, Brennan MF: Localization and resection of clinically inapparent medullary carcinoma of the thyroid. *Surgery* 87:616, 1980.

121. Silva OL, Becker KL, Primack A, Doppman JL, Snider RH: Hypercalcitoninemia in bronchogenic cancer. *JAMA* 234:183, 1975.

122. Deftos LJ, Roos BA, Bronzert D, Parthemore JG: Immunochemical heterogeneity of calcitonin in plasma. *J Clin Endocrinol Metab* 40:407, 1975.

123. Sizemore GW, Heath H: Immunochemical heterogeneity of calcitonin in plasma of patients with medullary thyroid carcinoma. *J Clin Invest* 55:111, 1975.

124. Amara SG, Jonas V, Rosenfeld MG: Alternative RNA processing in calcitonin gene expression. *Nature* 298:240, 1982.

125. Lee JC, Parthemore JG, Deftos LJ: Calcitonin secretion in renal disease. *Calcif Tissue Res* 22S:154, 1977.

126. Bigner SH, Mendelsohn G, Wells SA, Cox EB, Baylin SB, Eggleston JC: Medullary carcinoma of the thyroid in the multiple endocrine neoplasia IIA syndrome. *Am J Surg Pathol* 5:459, 1981.

127. Lloyd RV, Sisson JC, Marangos PL: Calcitonin, carcinoembryonic antigen and neuron-specific enolase in medullary thyroid carcinoma. *Cancer* 51:2234, 1982.

128. Marcus JN, Dise CA, Livolsi VA: Melanin production in a medullary thyroid carcinoma. *Cancer* 49:2518, 1982.

129. Sipple JH: The association of pheochromocytoma with carcinoma of the thyroid gland. *Am J Med* 31:163, 1961.

130. Williams ED: Medullary carcinoma of the thyroid. *J Clin Pathol* 20:395, 1967.

131. Schimke RN, Hartmann WH: Familial amyloid-producing medullary thyroid carcinoma and pheochromocytoma. A distinct genetic entity. *Ann Intern Med* 63:1027, 1965.

132. Khairi MRA, Dexter RN, Burzynski NJ, Johnston CC Jr: Mucosal neuroma, pheochromocytoma, and medullary thyroid carcinoma: MEN, type III. *Medicine* 54:89, 1975.

133. Steiner AL, Goodman AD, Powers SR: Study of kindred with pheochromocytoma, medullary thyroid carcinoma, hyperparathyroidism, and Cushing's disease: MEN, type II. *Medicine* 47:371, 1968.

134. Carney AJ, Sizemore GW, Tyce GM: Bilateral adrenal medullary hyperplasia in MEN, type 2. *Mayo Clin Proc* 50:3, 1975.

135. DeLellis RA, Wolfe HJ, Gagel RF, Feldman ZT, Miller HH, Gang DL, Reichlin S: Adrenal medullary hyperplasia. *Am J Pathol* 83:177, 1976.

136. Cushman P Jr: Familial endocrine tumors: Report of two unrelated kindred affected with pheochromocytomas, one also with multiple thyroid carcinomas. *Am J Med* 32:352, 1962.

137. Melvin KEW, Miller HH, Tashjian AH Jr: Early diagnosis of medullary thyroid carcinoma of the thyroid gland by means of calcitonin assay. *N Engl J Med* 285:1115, 1971.

138. Potts JT Jr, Deftos LJ: Parathyroid hormone, thyrocalcitonin, vitamin D, and diseases of bone and bone mineral metabolism, in Bondy PK, Rosenberg LE (eds): *Duncan's Diseases of Metabolism*, 6th ed. Philadelphia, Saunders, 1969, pp 904–1082.

139. Williams ED, Pollock DJ: Multiple mucosal neuromata with endocrine tumors: A syndrome allied to von Recklinghausen's disease. *J Pathol Bacteriol* 91:71, 1966.

140. Schimke RN, Hartmann WH, Prout TE, Rimoin DL: Syndrome of bilateral pheochromocytoma, medullary thyroid carcinoma, and multiple neuromas. *N Engl J Med* 279:1, 1968.

141. Gorlin RJ, Sedano HO, Vicker RA, Cervenka J: Multiple mucosal neuromas, pheochromocytomas, and medullary carcinoma of the thyroid—a syndrome. *Cancer* 22:293, 1968.

142. Russell CF, van Heerden JA, Sizemore GW, Edis J, Taylor WF, Remine WH, Carney JA: The surgical management of medullary thyroid carcinoma. *Ann Surg* 197:42, 1982.

143. Block MA: Management of carcinoma of the thyroid. *Ann Surg* 185:133, 1977.

144. Jones BA, Sisson JC: Early diagnosis and thyroidectomy in multiple endocrine neoplasia, type 2b. *J Pediatr* 102:219, 1983.

145. Block MA, Horn RC Jr, Miller JM, Barrett JL, Brush BE: Familial medullary carcinoma of the thyroid. *Ann Surg* 166:403, 1967.

145a. Block MA, Xavier A, Brush BE: Management of primary hyperparathyroidism in the elderly. *J Am Geriatr Soc* 23:385, 1975.

146. Nusynowitz ML, Pollard E, Benedetto AR, Leckitner ML, Ware RW: Treatment of medullary carcinoma of the thyroid with I-131. *J Nucl Med* 23:143, 1981.

147. Saad M, Guido JJ, Samman NA: Radioactive iodine in the treatment of medullary carcinoma of the thyroid. *J Clin Endocrinol Metab* 57:124, 1983.

148. Gottlieb JA, Hill CS Jr: Adriamycin (NSC-123127) therapy in thyroid carcinoma. *Cancer Chemother Rep* 6:283, 1975.

149. Gautvik KM, Svindahl K, Skretting A, Stenberg B, Aas M, Myhre L, Johannesen JV: Uptake and localization of I-labeled anticalcitonin immunoglobulins in rat medullary thyroid carcinoma tissue. *Cancer* 50:1107, 1982.

150. Shimoaka K: Adjunctive management of thyroid cancer. *Chemotherapy* 15:283, 1980.

151. Irvine WJ, Barnes EW: Addison's disease, ovarian failure and hypoparathyroidism. *Clin Endocrinol Metab* 4:379, 1975.

152. Carpenter CCJ, Solomon N, Silverberg SG, Bledsoe T, Northcutt RC, Klinenberg JR, Bennett IL Jr, Harvey AM: Schmidt's syndrome (thyroid and adrenal insufficiency): A review of the literature and a report of fifteen new cases including ten instances of coexistent diabetes mellitus. *Medicine* 43:153, 1964.

153. Khoury EL, Hammond L, Bottazzo GF, Doniach D: Surface reactive antibodies to human adrenal cells in Addison's disease. *Clin Exp Immunol* 45:48, 1981.

154. Doniach D: Humoral and genetic aspects of thyroid autoimmunity. *Clin Endocrinol Metab* 4:287, 1975.

155. Calder EA, Irvine WJ: Cell-mediated immunity and immune complexes in thyroid disease. *Clin Endocrinol Metab* 4:379, 1975.

156. Volpe R: The role of autoimmunity in hypoendocrine and hyperendocrine function with special emphasis on autoimmune thyroid disease. *Ann Intern Med* 87:86, 1977.

157. Nerup J, Andersen OO, Bendixen G, Egeberg J, Poulsen JE: Antipancreatic cellular hypersensitivity in diabetes mellitus. *Diabetes* 20:424, 1971.

158. MacCuish AC, Jordan J, Campbell CJ, Duncan LJP, Irvine WJ: Cell-mediated immunity to human pancreas in diabetes mellitus. *Diabetes* 23:693, 1974.

159. Nerup J, Bendixen G: Anti-adrenal cellular hypersensitivity in Addison's disease: II. Correlation with clinical and serological findings. *Clin Exp Immunol* 5:341, 1969.

160. Calder EA, Penhale WJ, Barnes EW, Irvine WJ: Evidence for circulating immune complexes in thyroid disease. *Br Med J* 2:30, 1974.

161. Okita N, Row VV, Volpe R: Suppressor T-lymphocyte deficiency in Graves' disease and Hashimoto's thyroiditis. *J Clin Endocrinol Metab* 52:528, 1981.

162. Sridama V, Pacini F, DeGroot L: Decreased suppressor T-

lymphocytes in autoimmune thyroid diseases detected by monoclonal antibodies. *J Clin Endocrinol Metab* 54:316, 1982.

163. Nerup J: Addison's disease. *Acta Endocrinol* 76:127, 1974.

164. Marieb NJ, Melby JC, Lyall SS: Isolated hypoaldosteronism associated with idiopathic hypoparathyroidism. *Arch Intern Med* 134:424, 1974.

165. Wegienka LC, Grasso SG, Forsham PH: Estimation of adrenomedullary reserve by infusion of 2-deoxy-D-glucose. *J Clin Endocrinol* 26:37, 1966.

166. Wuepper KD, Wegienka LC, Fudenberg HH: Immunologic aspects of adrenocortical insufficiency. *Am J Med* 45:206, 1969.

167. Blizzard RM, Chee D, Davis W: The incidence of adrenal and other antibodies in the sera of patients with idiopathic adrenal insufficiency (Addison's disease). *Clin Exp Immunol* 2:19, 1967.

168. Spinner MW, Blizzard RM, Gibbs J, Abbey H, Childs B: Familial distribution of organ specific antibodies in the blood of patients with Addison's disease and hypoparathyroidism and their relatives. *Clin Exp Immunol* 5:461, 1969.

169. Spinner MW, Blizzard RM, Childs B: Clinical and genetic heterogeneity in idiopathic Addison's disease and hypoparathyroidism. *J Clin Endocrinol* 28:795, 1968.

170. Blizzard RM, Gibbs JH: Candidiasis: Studies pertaining to its association with endocrinopathies and pernicious anemia. *Pediatrics* 42:231, 1968.

171. Blizzard RM, Chee D, Davis W: The incidence of parathyroid and other antibodies in the sera of patients with idiopathic hypoparathyroidism. *Clin Exp Immunol* 1:119, 1966.

172. Dwyer JM: Chronic mucocutaneous candidiasis. *Annu Rev Med* 32:491, 1981.

173. Krohn K, Perheentupa J, Heinonen E: Precipitating anti-adrenal antibodies in Addison's disease. *Clin Immunol Immunopathol* 3:59, 1974.

174. McCarthy-Young S, Lessof MH, Maisey MN: Serum TSH and thyroid antibody studies in Addison's disease. *Clin Endocrinol* 1:45, 1972.

175. Bottazzo GF, Florin-Christensen A, Doniach D: Islet-cell antibodies in diabetes mellitus with autoimmune polyendocrine deficiencies. *Lancet* 2:1279, 1974.

176. Irvine WJ, McCallu CJ, Gray RS, Campbell CJ, Duncan LJP, Farquhar JW, Vaughn H, Morris PJ: Pancreatic islet-cell antibodies in diabetes mellitus correlated with the duration and type of diabetes, coexistent autoimmune disease, and HLA type. *Diabetes* 26:138, 1977.

177. Bottazzo GF, Mann JI, Thorogood M, Baum JD, Doniach D: Autoimmunity in juvenile diabetics and their families. *Br Med J* 2:165, 1978.

178. de Moraes Ruehsen M, Blizzard RM, Garcia-Bunuel R, Seegar Jones G: Autoimmunity and ovarian failure. *Am J Obstet Gynecol* 112:693, 1972.

179. Irvine WJ, Chan MMW, Scarth L, Kolb FO, Hartog M, Bayliss RIS, Drury MI: Immunological aspects of premature ovarian failure associated with idiopathic Addison's disease. *Lancet* 2:883, 1968.

180. Weinberg U, Kraemer FB, Kammerman S: Coexistence of primary endocrine deficiencies: A unique case of male hypergonadism [*sic*] associated with hypoparathyroidism, hypoadrenocorticism, and hypothyroidism. *Am J Med Sci* 272:215, 1976.

181. Irvine WJ, Scarth L, Clarke BF, Cullen DR, Duncan LJP: Thyroid and gastric autoimmunity in patients with diabetes mellitus. *Lancet* 2:164, 1970.

182. Gray RS, Borsey DQ, Seth J, Herd R, Brown NS, Clarke BF: Prevalence of subclinical thyroid failure in insulin-dependent diabetes. *J Clin Endocrinol Metab* 50:1034, 1980.

183. Ardeman S, Chanarin I, Krafchik B, Singer W: Addisonian pernicious anemia and intrinsic factor antibodies in thyroid disorders. *Q J Med* 35:421, 1965.

184. Carmel R, Spencer CA: Clinical and subclinical thyroid disorders associated with pernicious anemia. *Arch Intern Med* 142:1465, 1982.

185. Hertz KC, Gazze LA, Kirkpatrick CH, Katz SI: Autoimmune vitiligo: Detection of antibodies to melanin-producing cells. *N Engl J Med* 297:634, 1971.

186. Asa SL, Bilbao JM, Kovacs K, Josse RG, Kreines K: Lymphocytic hypophysitis of pregnancy resulting in hypopituitarism: A distinct clinicopathologic entity. *Ann Intern Med* 95:166, 1981.

187. Clifton-Bligh P, Lee C, Smith H, Posen S: The association of diabetes insipidus with hypoparathyroidism, Addison's disease and mucocutaneous candidiasis. *Aust NZ J Med* 10:548, 1980.

188. Topliss DJ, White EL, Stockigt JR: Significance of thyrotropin excess in untreated primary adrenal insufficiency. *J Clin Endocrinol Metab* 50:52, 1980.

189. Chu J-Y, Monteleone JA, Peden VH, Graviss ER, Vernava AM: Anemia in children and adolescents with hypothyroidism. *Clin Pediatr* 20:696, 1981.

190. Court S, Parkin JM: Hypothyroidism and growth failure in diabetes mellitus. *Arch Dis Child* 57:622, 1982.

191. Gordin A, Lamberg B-A: Spontaneous hypothyroidism in symptomless autoimmune thyroiditis. A long-term follow-up study. *Clin Endocrinol* 15:537, 1981.

192. Walker DA, Davies M: Addison's disease presenting as a hypercalcemic crisis in a patient with idiopathic hypoparathyroidism. *Clin Endocrinol* 14:419, 1981.

193. Rotter J, Rimoin DL: Heterogeneity in diabetes mellitus—update 1978. *Diabetes* 27:599, 1978.

194. Rubinstein P, Suciu-Foca N, Nicholson F: Genetics of juvenile diabetes mellitus, a recessive gene closely linked to HLA D and with 50 percent penetrance. *N Engl J Med* 297:1036, 1977.

195. Bardwick PA, Zvaifler NJ, Gill GN, Newman D, Greenway GD, Resnick DL: Plasma cell dyscrasia with polyneuropathy, organomegaly, endocrinopathy, M protein, and skin changes: The POEMS syndrome. *Medicine* 59:311, 1980.

196. Turkington RW, Lebovitz HE: Extra-adrenal endocrine deficiencies in Addison's disease. *Am J Med* 43:449, 1967.

197. Maisey MN, Lessof MH: Addison's disease: A clinical study. *Guy's Hosp Rep* 118:363, 1969.

198. Males JL, Spitler AL, Townsend JL: Addison's disease: A review of 32 cases. *Okla Med J* 64:298, 1971.

Noted Added in Proof

Recently, plasma specimen from a number of subjects with MEN 1 have been found to contain mitogenic activity for parathyroid cells. This activity is apparently not of parathyroid gland origin.

Brandi ML, Aurbach GD, Fitzpatrick LA, et al: Parathyroid mitogenic activity in plasma for patients with familial multiple endocrine neoplasia type 1. *N Engl Med* 314:1287, 1986.

Ectopic Hormone Production*

David N. Orth

The mere physical presence of a tumor in a specific anatomic site often does not provide an explanation for all the patient's symptoms. Tumors synthesize and secrete a variety of hormones that are carried by the circulation to distant target tissues, where they can act to produce systemic effects.[1] These systemic metabolic effects may be a more immediate threat to the patient's health than the tumor itself; such patients may rightly be considered to have "biochemical malignancy."

Ectopic hormone secretion is the term used in clinical practice to denote secretion of a hormone by a tumor arising from tissue other than the endocrine gland that normally produces the hormone.[1] *Eutopic hormone secretion,* on the other hand, refers to secretion of a hormone by the gland or by a tumor of the gland that normally secretes the hormone.[2] Thus, production of calcitonin by medullary thyroid carcinoma, which arises from parafollicular C cells that normally secrete calcitonin, is not ectopic, but production of adrenocorticotropic hormone (ACTH) by this same tumor is. Without exception, ectopic hormones are peptides or glycopeptides, not steroids, iodothyronines, or biogenic amines. It is true that a number of tumors and a variety of normal tissues are capable of metabolizing steroid hormones, iodothyronines, and biogenic amines. In some cases, this may alter biologic activity and even cause clinical syndromes, but it does not represent ectopic secretion. Prostaglandins can be synthesized by so many normal tissues that it is not clear whether prostaglandin production can ever be regarded as truly ectopic.

The concept of ectopic hormone production presumes that all normal sites of synthesis for each hormone are known. However, many hormones appear to be widely distributed outside what was previously thought to be their sole tissue of origin. Somatostatin, originally isolated from the hypothalamus, is found in the pancreatic islet D cells, adrenal medulla, and gastrointestinal tract, and most of the peptide hormones originally identified in the gastrointestinal tract are distributed in the central nervous system, where they presumably function as neurotransmitters. ACTH, once thought to be synthesized exclusively by the anterior pituitary, is but one of several products cleaved from a large glycopeptide precursor molecule, proopiomelanocortin (POMC), that is also synthesized in the intermediate lobe of the pituitary; probably in the normal brain, pancreatic islets, adrenal medulla, testis, and placenta; quite possibly in the lung and C cells of the thyroid;[3] and perhaps in other tissues.[4] Thus, secretion of ACTH by medullary thyroid carcinoma, the example used earlier to distinguish ectopic from eutopic secretion, may not, in fact, be ectopic. However, *inappropriate* is not a useful term, because eutopic hormone secretion can also be inappropriate. *Paraneoplastic,* a term used to describe syndromes associated with malignancy, does not differentiate between those associated with nonendocrine and with endocrine tumors, nor does it necessarily implicate hormone secretion as the cause of the syndrome—although this is an appropriate heuristic assumption. Thus, for operational purposes it remains useful to classify secretion of a particular hormone by a specific tumor as ectopic, but this should not be construed to reflect certain knowledge that the hormone in question is never synthesized by the nonneoplastic cells from which the tumor arose.

Study of tumor hormone synthesis has provided valuable new insights into normal biosynthetic mechanisms by which peptide hormones are produced. It has, in the case of ectopic hormone secretion, provided an exceptionally useful model for studying the more general phenomenon of aberrant or atavistic synthesis of proteins by tumors and its relationship to malignant transformation. From a clinical point of view, it has revealed causal mechanisms for previously

*The author gratefully acknowledges the support of National Cancer Institute Research Grant 5-R01-CA11685, the constructive review of the manuscript by Dr. C. Rowan DeBold and Dr. William J. Kovacs, and the assistance of Ms. Linda D. D'Errico in preparing the manuscript for this chapter.

unexplained paraneoplastic syndromes and thus rationales for their treatment. It has held promise—probably not to be fulfilled—of offering sensitive assays for specific tumor markers with which to detect tumor presence and to monitor results of antitumor therapy. Some of the earliest insights into the function of hormones such as growth hormone were provided by the clinical caricatures of normal physiology caused by functioning tumors of endocrine glands. More recently, the structure of growth hormone releasing hormone was first determined with peptide purified from pancreatic islet cell tumors in patients with acromegaly[5] and only later was shown to be identical to the hypothalamic peptide.[6] Characterization of the peptide responsible for many cases of the humoral hypercalcemia of malignancy appears to be imminent. The peptide presumably also is a product of normal cells, as are other ectopic hormones. It is likely that studies of still unexplained paraneoplastic syndromes may reveal new hormones or new actions of known hormones.

Several excellent reviews have dealt with the subject of ectopic hormone secretion.[2,7-9] This chapter addresses the following issues: criteria for diagnosing ectopic hormone secretion; incidence of ectopic hormonal syndromes; hypotheses concerning the mechanisms of ectopic hormone secretion; individual ectopic hormonal syndromes and their clinical presentations, associated tumors, diagnosis, and treatment; biologic, immunologic, and physical characteristics of individual ectopic hormones; and usefulness of ectopic hormones as tumor markers.

CRITERIA FOR DIAGNOSIS OF ECTOPIC HORMONE SECRETION

Progressively vigorous criteria for establishing ectopic hormone synthesis are listed in Table 29-1. Some must be satisfied to justify the clinical diagnosis and to undertake rational therapy; all the criteria have never been satisfied in even the most carefully studied tumor.

Table 29-1. Criteria for Establishing Ectopic Hormone Secretion

Clinical criteria:
Association of a neoplasm with an endocrine syndrome
Association of a neoplasm with inappropriately elevated plasma or urine hormone levels
Failure of plasma or urine hormone levels to respond to normal homeostatic suppression
Absence of other possible causal mechanisms
Fall in hormone levels after tumor-specific therapy
Arteriovenous step-up gradient across the tumor capillary bed
Presence of hormone in tumor tissue
Investigative criteria:
In vitro hormone synthesis and release by tumor tissue
Presence of hormone-specific messenger RNA in tumor tissue
Absence of hormone in normal cells of the type from which the tumor arose
Absence of hormone-specific messenger RNA in normal cells of the type from which the tumor arose

Association of a Neoplasm with an Endocrine Syndrome

Ectopic hormones can circulate without causing any clinical abnormality, but it is usually only when an endocrine syndrome and a coexistent tumor are found that the diagnosis of ectopic hormone secretion is entertained. The frequency with which physicians make the clinical diagnosis is directly proportional to their index of suspicion. For example, the only manifestation of acute ectopic ACTH secretion, despite extremely high plasma cortisol concentrations, may be minimal hypokalemic alkalosis. Conversely, the association of the tumor and the syndrome does not demonstrate cause and effect. Thus, patients with bronchogenic carcinoma and hypercalcemia may have primary hyperparathyroidism.[10]

Association of a Neoplasm with Inappropriately Elevated Plasma or Urine Hormone Levels

The presence of elevated plasma or urine hormone levels is a necessary but insufficient criterion for confirming the clinical diagnosis. Hormone secretion by normal glands and tumors is episodic, with brief bursts of secretory activity. This and the short circulating half-life of most peptide hormones means that plasma concentration at any moment may not accurately reflect the overall rate of hormone secretion. Furthermore, secretion by tumors tends to vary more from one day to another than that by normal endocrine glands and is occasionally frankly periodic, with cycles up to several days in length.[11] Therefore, more than one specimen may often be required to demonstrate increased hormone levels. Conversely, secretion of hormones such as prolactin, growth hormone, and ACTH (and, consequently, cortisol) are exquisitely responsive to stressful stimuli, so care must be taken to obtain specimens under appropriate conditions to avoid obtaining misleading data.

Failure of Plasma or Urine Hormone Levels to Respond to Normal Homeostatic Suppression

A characteristic feature of ectopic hormone secretion is its apparent autonomy: ectopic gonadotropin secretion is seldom inhibited by estrogen, and ectopic ACTH secretion is almost never suppressed by high doses of glucocorticoid. The molecular basis for this phenomenon is still poorly defined but may prove central to our understanding of malignancy. One explanation is that the necessary regulatory effector mechanism, such as the intracellular glucocorticoid receptor in the case of POMC secretion, is defective or absent in the ectopic POMC-producing cell.[12] Another explanation is that apparently autonomous function by some endocrine tumors may actually be the result of promiscuous membrane receptors, whereby adenylate cyclase is activated by a variety of inappropriate hormones.[13] If tissue hyperplasia also depends upon binding of trophic hormones to specific cell surface or cytoplasmic receptors, the response to inappropriate stimuli via promiscuous receptors might also result in unrestrained growth. In fact, an exciting recent discovery about cancer is that tumor growth may be stimulated by expression of genes encoding growth factor receptors or growth factors themselves.

Absence of Other Possible Causal Mechanisms

In the clinical setting, exclusion of other causes for the metabolic abnormality is usually the last criterion that must be satisfied before proceeding with a trial of appropriate therapy, and it is an essential criterion. Thus, coincident primary hyperparathyroidism must be excluded in the patient who has hypercalcemia and a tumor,[10] and the possibility must be considered that plasma cortisol is elevated in a woman with small cell carcinoma of the lung because she is also taking estrogens and has elevated cortisol-binding globulin.

Fall in Hormone Levels after Tumor-Specific Therapy

A fall or normalization of inappropriately elevated hormone levels after successful surgery, radiotherapy, or chemotherapy has been documented for a number of ectopic hormones and forms one rationale for their usefulness as tumor markers. If the syndrome is caused by tumor hormone secretion, remission should likewise follow. Remission of the syndrome with drugs that specifically block the synthesis or action of the hormone (e.g., inhibitors of prostaglandin synthesis in certain unusual cases of tumor-associated hypercalcemia[14] or inhibitors of adrenal steroid biosynthesis in the ectopic ACTH syndrome[1,15]) is strong evidence for a causal effect of the hormone but offers no direct evidence that its secretion is ectopic.

Arteriovenous Step-up Gradient of Hormone Concentration across the Tumor Capillary Bed

The previous criteria are compatible not only with ectopic hormone secretion but also with tumor production of a substance that stimulates eutopic hormone secretion by the normal endocrine gland. However, demonstration of an arteriovenous step-up hormone gradient across the tumor capillary bed provides definitive in vivo evidence for ectopic hormone secretion.

The episodic nature of peptide hormone secretion must be considered when attempting to demonstrate an arteriovenous gradient. This means that simultaneous paired samples must be obtained both from a vein draining the tumor and from an artery supplying the tumor during surgery or, more often in practice, from a central or peripheral venous source remote from the tumor. Otherwise a gradient will not actually have been demonstrated, and an apparent increase in hormone concentration in an isolated sample of tumor venous blood may simply reflect a general increase in circulating hormone resulting from episodic secretion by a distant source, usually the normal endocrine gland.

Furthermore, the short circulating half-life of peptide hormones requires that the catheter be placed in a vein actually draining the ectopic tumor source to avoid dilution with hormone-poor peripheral venous blood. Unfortunately, many tumors associated with ectopic hormone secretion are drained by the pulmonary or splanchnic venous system, making selective percutaneous catheterization of veins draining these tumors difficult or impossible.

Presence of Hormone in Tumor Tissue

Demonstration of immunoreactive or bioactive hormone in tumor tissue extracts provides reasonable proof of hormone production by the tumor[1] and has been the most stringent evidence provided for individual reports of a number of the syndromes discussed in this chapter. However, tumor hormone concentrations vary widely and are often very low (1 to 10 ng per gram of wet tumor tissue, sometimes less than 0.01 percent of those in the normal endocrine tissue of origin).[16] In order to be considered evidence of hormone production, tumor hormone content must at least be greater than that which might be accounted for by the elevated hormone concentration in contained blood. Furthermore, other tumors may contain similar concentrations of immunoreactive hormone without evidence of any endocrine abnormality or, for that matter, release of detectable quantities of hormone into the circulation.[17] Possible explanations for such observations include synthesis of immunoreactive but biologically inactive hormone precursors, intracellular metabolism of the hormones to biologically inactive but immunoreactive fragments, faulty packaging of the hormone into secretory granules for exocytosis, and secretion of too little hormone to increase plasma levels appreciably or to produce significant metabolic effects. Conversely, hormone may be present in the tumor in a form not detected by either immunoassay or bioassay or may be released so rapidly that its concentration in the tumor remains low. In addition, degradation of hormonal peptides, due either to tumor necrosis prior to removal or to autolysis afterwards, can be a problem even with specimens obtained at the time of surgery. Thus, failure to demonstrate the hormone does not entirely exclude the possibility of its production by the tumor.

Immunohistochemical techniques have provided further evidence for ectopic hormone production and can localize hormone within individual tumor cells. Hormone may be present in most of the tumor cells, as in the case of ectopic ACTH in bronchial carcinoid adenoma,[18] or in only scattered cells, as in the case of the same hormone in adenocarcinoma of the lung[19] or medullary thyroid carcinoma.[20] This finding is reflected by the range of ACTH concentrations in extracts of these tumor types and has a corollary in the presence of secretory granules in most cells in bronchial carcinoids but in only scattered cells in small cell carcinomas[19] and few if any in squamous cell carcinomas of the lung.

The ultimate goal is to demonstrate the structural identity of the ectopic and eutopic hormones. However, most tumors causing ectopic hormonal syndromes are relatively small, and the hormone concentration usually seems to be inversely proportional to their size. Thus, the total amount of hormone available from any single tumor for purification and analysis has almost always been too small for complete sequence analysis. Efficient purification and sequencing techniques are overcoming this obstacle.[21]

In Vitro Hormone Synthesis and Release by Tumor Tissue

At this point we pass beyond those criteria which deserve consideration for confirming the clinical diagnosis to those which are primarily of research interest. These represent systems in which the structure of the ectopic hormonal gene, the regulation of its expression, and the structure and secretion of its products can be studied.

A number of tumors have now been studied in short-term incubation systems, prolonged primary cultures, or continuous clonal cell cultures.[22] Synthesis of hormones has been demonstrated by continued production in vitro or by incorporation of labeled amino acids into identifiable hormone products. The effects of various humoral stimuli on ectopic hormone synthesis and release have been studied, and the biologic, immunologic, and structural characteristics of the hormones and their related peptides (precursors, subunits, biosynthetic companions, and fragments) continue to be the subject of investigation in a number of laboratories.[23] Short-term incubations are often justifiably subject to criticism as being "dying cell" systems. In continuous cell culture systems, the possibility of in vitro transformation and selection of atypical clones must be acknowledged. Nevertheless, uniquely valuable information can be obtained by studying tumors in a variety of culture systems.

Presence of Hormone-Specific Messenger RNA in Tumor Tissue

Techniques for extracting total messenger RNA (mRNA) from cells, purifying individual mRNA species, translating mRNA in cell-free systems, generating complementary DNA (cDNA) to the mRNA, amplifying the cDNA by cloning techniques, and sequencing nucleotides make it possible to analyze the molecular events involved in the synthesis of peptide hormones by nonendocrine tumors.

Ectopic hormone-specific mRNA can be isolated from tumor tissue or cultured cells and translated in the rabbit reticulocyte lysate or wheat germ system and the hormone product identified and characterized, using techniques that have been widely applied to the study of eutopic hormones. A major impediment to studies of ectopic hormones is the limited amount of tissue available from any single tumor and the relatively low concentrations of ectopic hormone-specific mRNA in many tumors. Continuous tumor cell lines may provide the means by which this problem can be overcome.

Cloned cDNA fragments or synthetic oligonucleotides can be hybridized to hormone-specific mRNA in fixed sections of tumor tissue.[24] These labeled probes are usually derived from mRNA from the eutopic source or from genomic DNA or are synthesized on the basis of the peptide sequence of the eutopic hormone. Demonstration of hormone-specific mRNA in the tissue by in situ hybridization is more compelling evidence for synthesis of the hormone than mere demonstration of the presence of hormone, because mRNA is not exported from one cell to another, whereas the possibility remains that the hormone may have been synthesized elsewhere and taken up from the circulation by the tumor cell.[25] Furthermore, stringency conditions can be adjusted whereby the specificity of cDNA–mRNA hybridization may be greater than that of antibody-peptide binding. Studies of this type are lacking thus far but are needed to demonstrate hormone synthesis in tumors and specific tumor cell types and to determine whether the hormone is synthesized in the normal cells from which the tumor arose.

In situ hybridization studies can be complemented by the Northern blot technique, in which mRNA is extracted from tumor tissue, separated by electrophoresis on sizing gels, transferred to nitrocellulose filter paper, and hybridized with hormone-specific labeled cDNA or synthetic oligonucleotide probe and its size compared with that of mRNA from the normal endocrine tissue source. This may sometimes reveal differences reflecting altered gene transcription or mRNA processing.[26,27]

The ultimate demonstration that the authentic hormonal gene is being expressed in tumor cells is determination of the sequence of the hormone-specific mRNA extracted from tumor tissue. The sequence has been determined for a major portion of POMC mRNA from a thymic carcinoid tumor, that which codes for β-melanotropin and β-endorphin (see Ectopic ACTH Syndrome), the noncoding 3′ region, and the poly(A) tail.[26] A shorter sequence of the same portion of POMC mRNA from a medullary thyroid carcinoma was subsequently determined.[27] Both were identical to human POMC genomic DNA, demonstrating that ectopic POMC and, presumably, other ectopic hormones are products of normal genes.

Absence of Hormone in Normal Cells from which the Tumor Arose

Synthesis of peptide hormones is a normal activity of many cells other than those which make up the classical endocrine glands. Consequently, while evidence for nonendocrine tumor synthesis of hormones has been adduced for a number of peptides in a variety of tumors, it is now necessary to exclude the possibility that normal cells of the type from which the tumor arises can synthesize the same hormone. Unfortunately, it is easier to demonstrate hormone presence than to exclude it, because of the possibility that the level of expression is below the detection limit of the technique, that the peptide exists in a nonimmunoreactive or nonbioactive form, that there is rapid release and little storage of the peptide, or that the hormonal gene is expressed in the normal cell only at a certain stage of differentiation or only in response to certain stimuli, such as chronic inflammation.[9,28]

Absence of Hormone-Specific Messenger RNA in Normal Cells from which the Tumor Arose

In situ hybridization and Northern blot techniques are very sensitive and can be made highly specific. They are useful adjuncts to methods for detecting hormone in an effort to exclude hormone synthesis by normal cells and provide persuasive evidence for lack of hormone production.[29]

INCIDENCE OF ECTOPIC HORMONAL SYNDROMES

The actual incidence of ectopic hormone production is not known. Estimates differ widely, ranging from the obvious lower limit, which is that "there are many paraneoplastic endocrinopathies but no ectopic hormones,"[30] to the other extreme, which is that peptide hormone secretion is a "universal concomitant of cancer."[31] The true incidence presumably lies somewhere between, and the reported incidence of clinically diagnosed ectopic hormonal syndromes is certainly less than 10 percent of all cancer patients. However, the list of hormones and hormone precursors reported to have been produced by tumors (Table 29-2) is long and growing ever longer.

Some of the factors that may obscure the actual incidence of ectopic hormone production are listed in Table 29-3. The first nine represent factors that may obscure the true incidence of clinical syndromes resulting from ectopic hormone secretion; they relate primarily to the physicians or clinical investigators who care for the patient, the likelihood that they will suspect the diagnosis, their interest in confirming it, and the resources they have available to do so. The last four factors tend to obscure the true incidence of ectopic hormone secretion that is not associated with recognized clinical syndromes. Estimates of the actual incidence in this category differ as much as those for the first category and appear to depend largely upon the bias and interest of the investigators and the extent and reliability of the laboratory resources available to them. Examples of this are the widely divergent estimates of the incidence of ectopic ACTH secretion and humoral hypercalcemia of malignancy, both discussed later in this chapter.

Although the incidence of any one of the recognized paraneoplastic endocrine syndromes appears to be less than 2 percent, the incidence of ectopic hormone secretion is actually much higher when assiduously sought in association with specific tumor types. Thus, increased plasma concentrations of a high-molecular-weight form of ACTH, presumably POMC or a biosynthetic intermediate form, have been reported in 78 percent of patients who were

Table 29-2. Hormones and Hormone Precursors That Have Been Reported to be Produced Ectopically by Tumors*

Parathyroid hormone
Humoral hypercalcemia of malignancy factor
Osteoclast-activating factor
Prostaglandins
1,25-Dihydroxyvitamin D
Growth factors: epidermal growth factor, platelet-derived growth factor, transforming growth factors α and β
Proopiomelanocortin, intermediate biosynthetic forms and hormone products: NH_2-terminal fragment, γ-melanocyte stimulating hormone, ACTH, α-MSH, corticotropin-like intermediate lobe peptide, β-lipotropin, γ-LPH, β-MSH 1–18, β-MSH 1–22, and β-endorphin
Propressophysin and its products: arginine vasopressin (antidiuretic hormone) and neurophysin II
Oxytocin and neurophysin I
Chorionic gonadotropin and its α and β subunits
Follicle-stimulating hormone
Insulin
Insulin-like growth factors: IGF-I (somatomedin C) and IGF-II (multiplication-stimulating activity)
Tumor-associated hypophosphatemic factor
Procalcitonin and calcitonin
Progrowth hormone and growth hormone
Growth hormone releasing hormone
Corticotropin releasing hormone
Thyrotropin releasing hormone
Somatostatin
Gastrin-releasing peptide
Erythropoietin
Placental lactogen or somatomammotropin
Prolactin
Prorenin and renin
Gut-brain peptides: cholecystokinin, enkephalins, enteroglucagon, gastric-inhibitory polypeptide, gastrin, glucagon, motilin, neurotensin, pancreatic polypeptide, secretin, substance P, vasoactive intestinal polypeptide
Others: tumor angiogenesis factor, tumor necrosis factor (cachectin), interleukins, eosinophilopoietic factor, granulocytopoietic factors, osteoblast-stimulating factor, leukocyte chemotactic factor, hypotensive factor

*Listed in the order in which they are discussed in this chapter.

subsequently shown to have carcinoma of the lung,[32] and hypercalcemia was documented in 15 percent of patients with squamous cell carcinoma of the lung who were followed until death.[33]

The facts are that the incidence is significant, that the syndromes can appear at any time during the course of a variety of malignant conditions, that the presenting signs and symptoms are often subtle, and that the consequences of the metabolic disturbance, if undetected and untreated, may be serious and even fatal for the patient. Since the screening diagnostic tests (serum calcium, plasma cortisol, serum sodium

Table 29-3. Factors That May Obscure the Actual Incidence of Ectopic Hormone Secretion

Factor	Examples
Inadequate clinical suspicion	Minimal hypokalemic alkalosis in ectopic ACTH syndrome; minimal hyponatremia in ectopic AVP syndrome
Inadequate clinical follow-up of cancer patients	Higher incidence of hypercalcemia when patients are followed until death; late development of obvious syndromes in patients with known tumors
Bias of clinician-investigator	Higher incidence of specific ectopic syndromes in centers that study them
Inadequate laboratory resources	Higher incidence of ectopic ACTH syndrome in centers that have a sensitive and reliable ACTH assay
Ectopic hormone with chronic effects but short duration of illness	Growth hormone releasing hormone, ACTH, humoral hypercalcemia of malignancy factor
Ectopic hormone secretion replacing normal hormone secretion (physiological negative feedback)	ACTH (cortisol), AVP (osmolarity)
Ectopic hormonal syndrome obscured by other paraneoplastic syndromes and effects	Catabolic state obscuring Cushing's obesity in ectopic ACTH syndrome; ectopic ACTH syndrome obscuring signs of coincident ectopic AVP secretion
Ectopic secretion of as yet unidentified hormones	Until recently, corticotropin releasing hormone and growth hormone releasing hormone
Inadequate representation in literature	All well-known (and therefore "uninteresting") ectopic hormonal syndromes
Ectopic hormone without overt or recognized clinical effect	Gastrin-releasing peptide, calcitonin, endorphin, lipotropins, oxytocin
Ectopic hormone precursor with insignificant bioactivity	POMC, pro-CG α-subunit, pro-CG β-subunit, prorenin
Ectopic hormone subunits with insignificant bioactivity	α and β subunits of CG
Ectopic hormone fragments with altered or insignificant bioactivity	Corticotropin-like intermediate lobe peptide, POMC NH_2-terminal fragment

Source: Adapted in part from Rees.[7]

and/or osmolality) for the most serious syndromes are readily available and relatively inexpensive, they should be applied to confirm a reasonable clinical suspicion at any time during the course of the patient's often prolonged illness.

HYPOTHESES CONCERNING THE MECHANISM OF ECTOPIC HORMONE SECRETION

A variety of mechanisms have been proposed to explain the phenomenon of ectopic hormone synthesis. Any unifying hypothesis must explain all the observed phenomena (Table 29-4). Unfortunately, none of the hypotheses advanced thus far appears to explain fully all these observations. The hypotheses, discussed below, have had to be modified or discarded as our knowledge about peptide hormone synthesis, malignant transformation, and the molecular biology of eukaryotic cells has expanded.

The 'Sponge' Hypothesis

This hypothesis suggests that ectopic hormones are not synthesized by tumors but that eutopic hormones are absorbed from the circulation and released upon tumor cell death.[25] An improbable hypothesis from the beginning, it has been challenged on a variety of theoretical and clinical grounds. For example, there are a number of well-documented cases in which patients have had total hypophysectomy for Cushing's syndrome without reduction in their plasma ACTH levels or amelioration of the syndrome. Months later, a previously unsuspected nonpituitary neoplasm, such as a bronchial or thymic carcinoid tumor, has been discovered and removed, reducing plasma ACTH to undetectable concentrations and curing the Cushing's syndrome, the tumor being found to contain high levels of ACTH. This sequence of events is incompatible with the 'sponge' hypothesis, which has also been disproved by in vitro studies of the synthesis of hormones by tumor cells. Nevertheless, this hypothesis has been slow to die in some quarters.

The Derepression Hypothesis

Among the earliest and most attractive hypotheses, the derepression hypothesis suggests that ectopic hormone synthesis is the result of random derepression in tumor cells of those portions of the genome

Table 29-4. Observations Concerning Ectopic Hormone Secretion

1. Tumors synthesize and secrete ectopic peptide and glycopeptide hormones but not ectopic steroids, iodothyronines, or biogenic amines.
2. Ectopic hormones appear to be identical to eutopic hormones in structure and biologic activity.
3. Tumors synthesize and secrete hormone precursors, glycopeptide hormone subunits, and subunit precursors, alone and in every possible combination with the hormones themselves.
4. Individual tumors secrete multiple, apparently unrelated hormones.
5. Ectopic hormones generally appear to fall into four groups:
   a. Gut-brain hormones (e.g., POMC peptides; vasopressin, oxytocin and their neurophysins; hypothalamic releasing hormones and somatostatin; calcitonin; gastrin; gastrin-releasing peptide; vasoactive intestinal polypeptide; and glucagon and, rarely, insulin). These peptides are produced most frequently by nonsquamous cell lung carcinoma; bronchial, thymic, and pancreatic carcinoid tumors; and medullary thyroid carcinoma.
   b. Fetoplacental hormones (i.e., chorionic gonadotropin and placental lactogen). These peptides are associated most frequently with lung carcinoma and hepatoma.
   c. Growth factors (e.g., IGF-I, or somatomedin C; IGF-II, or multiplication-stimulating activity; and erythropoietin). These peptides are usually produced by mesodermal tumors, hepatomas, renal cell tumors, and gastrointestinal carcinoids and carcinomas.
   d. Hormones associated with the hypercalcemia of malignancy (e.g., humoral hypercalcemia of malignancy factor, a peptide that acts like parathyroid hormone on renal tubular adenylate cyclase and is most often associated with squamous cell carcinoma of the lung, renal carcinoma, bladder carcinoma, and carcinoma of the ovary; parathyroid hormone itself; osteoclast-activating factor, a peptide that is associated with multiple myeloma; 1,25-dihydroxyvitamin D_3; and a lymphokine associated with adult T cell lymphoma).
6. Tumors can produce hormone fragments not detected in the normal endocrine tissue.
7. Ectopic hormone secretion is usually "autonomous" and unresponsive to normal physiological negative feedback control.
8. Ectopic hormone secretion can occur early or late in the history of a tumor's growth.
9. Specific ectopic hormones tend to be associated with specific tumor types.
10. Specific hormones can be secreted by a wide variety of tumor types.
11. Some hormones (e.g., all the anterior pituitary hormones except POMC peptides, which are, unlike the others, also produced in other tissues) are almost never produced ectopically.
12. Tumors of certain types rarely if ever appear to secrete ectopic hormones.

that code for a variety of peptides, among them hormones.[34] This theory correctly predicts that ectopic hormones are identical to normal ones and is compatible with the observations that only peptide hormones are ectopically secreted (because of the complex enzyme systems required for steroid, iodothyronine, and biogenic amine biosynthesis), that precursors are commonly secreted (because of nonderepression of processing enzymes), that isolated hormone subunits are sometimes synthesized, that secretion is autonomous (beause of nonderepression of genes for cellular mediators or inhibitors of synthesis and secretion), that ectopic hormone synthesis can begin at any time a tumor cell clone becomes derepressed, and that ontogeny is recapitulated by synthesis of fetoplacental hormones, often in association with other fetoplacental peptides.

The derepression hypothesis does not explain, however, why certain hormones are rarely synthesized, why specific hormones are associated with specific tumors, or why the phenomenon is not universal, occurring in all types of tumors. Thus, simple random derepression is no longer a viable hypothesis.

The Dedifferentiation Hypothesis

In contrast to random derepression, the dedifferentiation hypothesis presumes that tumor cells can undergo a specific, highly ordered process of gene repression and derepression that retraces the normal process of cell differentiation to earlier and earlier progenitor cell types.[35] There is no convincing evidence to support this presumption. The evidence, in fact, suggests that the process of differentiation can move only forward toward the terminally differentiated state.[36] This hypothesis also implies that the hormonal gene was expressed at one stage of differentiation of the normal cell and was later repressed. There is little direct evidence to support this notion, either, which is a feature also of the dysdifferentiation hypothesis.[9] Thus, dedifferentiation no longer appears to be a useful concept for explaining most aspects of tumor biology.

The Dysdifferentiation Hypothesis

This provocative model presumes that all the cells of a normal epithelial surface, such as the bronchial or intestinal mucosa, including a small number of hormone-secreting endocrine or paracrine cells, are derived from a single precursor cell type.[9] There is experimental evidence that this presumption is correct.[37] The process of differentiation is presumed to move forward from the progenitor cell, influenced and directed by cell-cell interactions, other factors in the local environment, and possibly hormones. It further postulates that, in adult epithelial tissues, genes for different proteins are expressed at different rates at different stages of differentiation. Thus, fetoplacental peptides such as carcinoembryonic antigen, chorionic gonadotropin, and α-fetoprotein are expressed most actively by rapidly proliferating progenitor cells in their early "fetal" stage of differentiation, less actively in less rapidly proliferating cells in their later "adult" stage of differentiation, and least actively in the various cell types that constitute the nonproliferative terminally differentiated epithelium. Genes for other proteins, such as L-dopa decarboxylase, an essential enzyme of APUD cells (defined in following section), are expressed least actively or not at all during the fetal stage, most actively during the adult proliferative stage, and, among terminally differentiated epithelial cells, only in those which synthesize peptide hormones and biogenic amines. Genes for still other proteins, such as certain peptide hormones, are expressed least actively or not at all in the fetal stage of differentiation, to only a small extent in progenitor cells in the adult stage of differentiation, and most actively only in those terminally differentiated cells committed to peptide hormone synthesis. Malignancy is viewed as being the result of a transforming event in a single cell that is not yet terminally differentiated.[38] The histological appearance of the tumor and the nature of its protein products depends upon the stage of differentiation at which the proliferating progenitor cell is transformed, the rate of tumor cell proliferation and turnover (very rapidly dividing cells might not achieve any terminally differentiated function before dying), and possibly other local factors and postmutational events.

This hypothesis has explanatory power with respect to how ectopic hormone-secreting tumors can arise from epithelium that consists mostly of cells without endocrine function; how different histological types of tumor from the same tissue can produce ectopic hormones;[16,17,19,32,39,40] how tumors can be heterogeneous with respect to morphology and hormone production;[19] how a tumor metastasis, which represents the progeny of a subpopulation of cells from the primary tumor, can differ markedly from the primary tumor in appearance and hormone production; and how specific hormones can be associated with specific tumors. It can also offer an explanation for why hormones such as ACTH and arginine vasopressin can sometimes be expressed under conditions of rapid cell proliferation other than neoplasia, such as chronic inflammation.[28,40,41] It does not readily explain some of the other characteristics of ectopic hormone secretion, however, and its basic assumptions have not yet been proved. Nevertheless, it is a useful heuristic model.

The Endocrine (APUD) Cell Hypothesis

This hypothesis, which probably has enjoyed more widespread acceptance than any other, attempts to explain why only certain types of tumors are capable of ectopic peptide hormone production. It proposes that ectopic hormone-secreting tumors are derived from cells that are embryologically related to the precursors of normal endocrine tissues and are themselves capable of secreting hormones.[42,43] These cells, which are proposed to derive from neural crest ectoderm, have common histochemical and ultrastructural characteristics[44–47] which define them as APUD (*a*mine *p*recursor *u*ptake and *d*ecarboxylation) cells that have the ability to take up and, via the action of L-dopa decarboxylase, decarboxylate biogenic amine precursors (5-hydroxytryptamine and dopamine). The large number of cell types allegedly sharing these characteristics gave rise to the concept of a widely dispersed system of neuroendocrine cells,[48] tumors of which are capable of secreting peptide hormones characteristic of the normal APUD cells from which they arise. However, it appears probable that the APUD cells of the pancreatic islets and gut are of endodermal origin[49–51] and may derive either from fetal endodermal APUD cells[52] or, together with other epithelial cells in the gut, from common precursor cells present in the adult.[53] Thus it seems that cells other than those derived from neural crest can have APUD functional characteristics. Furthermore, non-APUD tumors clearly can produce peptide hormones,[16,17,19,32,39,40] although they may not secrete sufficient quantities of biologically active peptide to cause a clinical syndrome.

The concept of "APUDomas" arising from the dispersed neuroendocrine system does not explain all the observations about ectopic hormone secretion, but the essential element for proper posttranslational processing and secretion of peptide hormones is the same as that which identifies the APUD cell: the neurosecretory-type granule. This cellular organelle is pinched off from the Golgi apparatus and contains, together with the Golgi apparatus and rough endoplasmic reticulum, the necessary posttranslational processing enzymes. Thus the main contribution of the APUD, or endocrine, cell hypothesis may be to emphasize the importance of these granules and their biosynthetic properties to the ability of a tumor, whatever its origin, to synthesize and secrete a mature, biologically active peptide hormone.[9]

The Variable State of DNA Repression Hypothesis

A provocative hypothesis has been briefly sketched which proposes that DNA exists in four operational states: (1) actively transcribing mRNA, (2) easily derepressed by the appropriate "effector" metabolite, (3) not available for derepression by the normal effector but not irreversibly repressed, and (4) repressed and virtually inaccessible to the normal cell.[54] The most common ectopic hormone-producing tumors, including APUD tumors, presumably are those in which type 3 hormone-specific DNA is converted to type 1 or type 2 DNA as a consequence (or a necessary concomitant) of neoplastic transformation, whereas tumors that only rarely produce ectopic hormones represent transformed progeny of cells in which type 4 hormone-specific DNA had been converted to type 1 or type 2 DNA. The molecular biologic mechanisms underlying this hypothesis have not been explained, however, nor has evidence been adduced to support it.

The Oncogene Hypothesis

There is strong circumstantial evidence that normal cellular genes are involved in the development of human cancer.[55] This constitutes a conceptual revolution concerning the pathogenesis of human malignancy. One can no longer propose mechanisms for ectopic hormone secretion without taking into account this concept.

About twenty "cancer genes" (oncogenes) have now been described in normal cells, and many of them have been sequenced. These cellular oncogenes (c-onc) or protooncogenes have extensive sequence homology with the transforming genes (v-onc) of acute transforming retroviruses but have no transforming activity of their own. It is theorized that protooncogenes were at some point in evolution picked up by previously nontransforming retroviruses. The protooncogenes are highly conserved[56] and are found in mammals, amphibians, fish, insects, and perhaps yeasts. It is reasonable to presume, therefore, that their expression regulates some essential cellular process, such as proliferation[57] or differentiation.[58] There is evidence that growth factors, which stimulate cell proliferation, also stimulate protooncogene expression.[59]

How oncogenes cause cancer is not yet clear. Specific oncogenes appear to be expressed in specific types of tumor.[60] It seems that two oncogenes must cooperate to cause cell transformation, presumably because they act in different ways upon cell function. These two actions apparently correspond to the separate promoter and activator events required for malignant transformation. The protooncogene may be activated by a variety of mechanisms,[56] including chromosomal translocation. The break points in chromosomal translocations associated with a number of human malignant diseases are at the precise location of protooncogenes.[61] Expression of oncogenes alone may not be sufficient to cause transformation; rather, a point mutation in the coding sequence, causing a single amino acid substitution, may be involved in the transforming capacity of some oncogenes, presumably by altering their dependence on normal physiological stimuli or feedback regulation.

The function of some oncogenes may be closely related to endocrine function, since their products resemble growth factors, growth factor receptors, or the functional subunits of growth factor receptors, a special case of promiscuous receptor synthesis.[13] For example, the protooncogene c-*sis* encodes a protein similar or identical to platelet-derived growth factor (PDGF) and may be the normal gene for the B-chain of that factor;[62,63] the PDGF A-chain can be expressed independently by tumor cells.[63a] A viral oncogene, v-*erb-B*, which has a protooncogene counterpart, encodes a protein similar to part of the epidermal growth factor (EGF) receptor;[64] and the product of v-*src* is a tyrosine kinase,[65] as are the protein kinase subunits of PDGF, EGF, insulin, and somatomedin C receptors. As discussed in Chap. 5, these protein kinases may function primarily as inositol phospholipid kinases,[66] eventually leading to formation of 1,2-diacylglycerol and inositol triphosphate, which activate protein kinase C and mobilize intracellular calcium ions, respectively. Moreover, tumors of many kinds produce and secrete peptide transforming growth factors (TGFs), one of which, TGF-α, is structurally related to EGF,[67] binds to the EGF receptor, and activates its protein kinase catalytic subunit. Other TGFs are structurally unrelated to EGF and bind to other receptors, and one, TGF-β, enhances or inhibits the responses of a wide variety of cells to other hormones and growth factors.[68] Thus, either by increasing their growth factor receptor number, thereby enhancing their response to normal growth factors, or by secreting growth factors for which they have receptors, thereby stimulating their own growth in an autocrine fashion, tumor cells are thought to escape normal restrictions on continued proliferation.

The relationship of oncogene activation to ectopic hormone secretion is uncertain. Perhaps it simply provides the proliferative stimulus to a progenitor cell, which then behaves as envisioned in the dysdifferentiation hypothesis.[9,58] On the other hand, it may have a more direct bearing. For example, c-*myc*, which is found on chromosome 8 in humans and 15 in mice, is translocated to the immunoglobulin heavy-chain locus on chromosome 14 in human Burkitt's lymphoma and chromosome 12 in mouse plasmacytoma.[61] The transposed oncogene may not only transform the lymphocyte precursor cell but may also activate expression of the immunoglobulin gene. Activation of a cellular oncogene by transposition or other mechanisms could also activate expression of a hormonal gene. This might explain ectopic production of hormones by "unusual" (i.e., non-APUD) tumors and the association of certain hormones with so many different tumors.

Other Hypotheses

The theory that ectopic hormone synthesis represents gene mutation is not supported by accumulating data that ectopic hormones and other peptides are identical to their eutopic counterparts.[21,26] The cell hybridization hypothesis proposes that malignant nonneuroectodermal cells acquire their ability to synthesize hormones by fusing with normal neuroectodermal cells.[69] This hypothesis has little direct support, and analysis of isoenzymes in tumors of heterozygotes indicates that most tumors derive from a single cell, arguing against it.[70]

One possibility that appears not to have received serious consideration is that ectopic peptide secretion may have survival value for the tumor cell. Secretion of osteolytic substances by breast carcinoma cells may ensure the survival of skeletal metastases. Tumor cells appear to produce growth factors which stimulate their own proliferation in an autocrine manner. Thus the survival of transformed cells may depend upon their producing factors that stimulate their own growth or that favorably modify their environment. It may be worthy of note, in this context, that the fetoplacental unit is a highly successful obligate parasite whose interface with its host is the syncytiotrophoblast, an invasive, proliferative, and immunologically protected tissue. The trophoblast is richly endowed with EGF receptors and elaborates a substance similar or identical to the tumor angiogenesis factor of invasive neoplasms and other hormones, such as chorionic gonadotropin (which may mediate its immunologically protected state), human placental lactogen, POMC, and other fetoplacental proteins often associated with malignancy. Therefore, it is possible that one of the genes derepressed by activation of a protooncogene is the normal trophoblastic gene, or *trophogene*, expressed inappropriately in nontrophoblastic progenitor cells and conferring upon them certain aspects of their malignant behavior. The variable expression of ectopic synthesis of individual hormones might then depend upon the structural or functional proximity of the particular hormonal gene to the trophogene (those for fetoplacental hormones being most frequently expressed, those for non-POMC anterior pituitary hormones essentially not at all), the normal hormonal potential of the transformed progenitor cell, and the degree of its differentiation.

Finally, returning to the problems in defining

ectopic hormone secretion, hormone-secreting cells appear to be much more widely distributed than was originally thought, and even fetoplacental hormones, or closely related peptides, are found in normal adult male and female tissues.[71–73] Thus hormonal genes may not be completely repressed in nonendocrine cells. Furthermore, cells such as the Kultschitsky cell—which is thought to share a common stem cell with bronchial and thymic carcinoid tumors and small cell carcinomas of the lung, although even this dogma has recently been challenged[74]—may normally secrete peptide hormones. Hormone secretion by tumors related to these cells may not be ectopic, only exaggerated or inappropriate. This chapter is not concerned with a case-by-case examination of whether secretion of a particular hormone by a particular tumor type is truly ectopic or is merely inappropriate. Rather, it uses the term *ectopic* in an operational sense to discuss the clinical syndromes associated with secretion of hormones by tumors of tissues other than those with which their production is currently generally associated.

HYPERCALCEMIA OF MALIGNANCY

The most common cause of hypercalcemia, when clinical criteria alone are used to suggest the diagnosis, is osteolytic metastasis of a malignant tumor, usually breast carcinoma, to bone;[75] it is found in approximately 2 percent of all hospitalized patients. Primary hyperparathyroidism is the second most common cause, and hypercalcemia associated with nonmetastatic malignancy is only slightly less frequent than hyperparathyroidism.[75] On the basis of chemical criteria that have been developed as the result of widespread application of screening serum chemistry tests, hypercalcemia has been found to be much more common than previously suspected, and hypercalcemia associated with metastases to bone appears to account for a majority of the cases of hypercalcemia of malignancy. Significant hypercalcemia develops in at least 10 percent of patients with advanced cancer and is probably the most common clinical endocrine manifestation of malignancy.

The association of hypercalcemia and malignancy was first reported by Zondek, Petow, and Siebert in 1924.[76] Fuller Albright first speculated in 1941 that a nonparathyroid tumor might secrete a factor similar to parathyroid hormone (PTH) after studying a patient with hypercalcemia and hypophosphatemia associated with a renal cell carcinoma and a solitary bone metastasis.[77] Tumors most often associated with hypercalcemia in the absence of skeletal metastases are squamous cell carcinoma of the lung, renal adenocarcinoma, bladder carcinoma, and carcinoma of the ovary, but a wide variety of other tumors have been implicated.* Conversely, certain common types of tumor (e.g., small cell lung carcinoma, adenocarcinoma of the colon, and gastric and prostatic carcinoma) are rarely associated with hypercalcemia.

There are probably several causes of the hypercalcemia of malignancy, and it is important to establish some definitions at the outset. Introduction of the term "*pseudohyperparathyroidism*" by Lafferty[75] has not served a useful purpose. It suggests a syndrome that is the converse of pseudo*hypo*parathyroidism (i.e., target tissue *hypo*sensitivity to PTH), which it is not. Furthermore, PTH is probably not involved in the great majority of cases of the hypercalcemia of malignancy. The most accurate generic term is simply *hypercalcemia of malignancy*. In the presence of focal osteolytic metastases, local production of osteoclast-activating factor, prostaglandins, or other agents may be the mediator of local bone resorption. In the absence of demonstrable metastases to bone, coincident primary hyperparathyroidism,[10] or other causes of hypercalcemia (e.g., immobilization, dehydration, thiazide diuretics—see Chap. 24), the syndrome can be presumed to be humoral hypercalcemia of malignancy. The term *ectopic PTH syndrome* should be reserved for those rare cases of humoral hypercalcemia of malignancy in which the criteria for ectopic secretion of PTH by the tumor have been satisfied convincingly. The causes of the humoral hypercalcemia of malignancy may include tumor elaboration of humoral hypercalcemia of malignancy factor, EGF, transforming growth factor-α (TGF-α) and perhaps other, as yet unidentified osteolytic substances. When their ectopic secretion and/or causal roles in the hypercalcemia are convincingly established, further specific categories of humoral hypercalcemia of malignancy may be defined. Other, rarer forms of hypercalcemia of malignancy include the increased production of 1,25-dihydroxyvitamin D in some patients with lymphomas.

Clinical Presentation

The clinical features of hypercalcemia of malignancy are similar to those of acute hypercalcemia of any other etiology. The patient may be asymptomatic, or the hypercalcemia may cause gastrointestinal effects such as anorexia, nausea, vomiting, cramping abdomi-

*Others include carcinoma of the pharynx, floor of the mouth, nasal sinuses, parotid, tonsils, larynx, thyroid, esophagus, endometrium, cervix, vagina, vulva, adrenal, prostate, penis, testis, breast, liver, gallbladder, pancreas, colon, and renal pelvis; small cell carcinoma of the lung and pancreas; pheochromocytoma; nephroblastoma; melanoma; myeloma; acute lymphoblastic leukemia and chronic lymphocytic leukemia; lymphoma; and lymphosarcoma, reticulum cell sarcoma, hemangiosarcoma, fibrosarcoma, rhabdomyosarcoma, and leiomyosarcoma.

nal pain, and constipation; cerebral dysfunction manifested by lethargy, drowsiness, headache, confusion, stupor, and coma; renal manifestations including polyuria, polydipsia, and dehydration; and cardiac idioventricular arrhythmias which, if allowed to persist, may be the cause of death. Renal calculi, nephrocalcinosis, hypertension, osteitis fibrosa cystica, and band keratopathy are much less common than in primary hyperparathyroidism, presumably because the hypercalcemia is of shorter duration. However, the osteopenia associated with most cases of humoral hypercalcemia of malignancy is more severe than in primary hyperparathyroidism with a similar degree of hypercalcemia. The development of hypercalcemia in patients with malignant disease is usually a grave prognostic sign; a majority of the patients die within 6 months. As with other paraneoplastic syndromes, the clinical features of hypercalcemia may be masked or complicated by other manifestations of malignancy, including syndromes caused by other metabolically active substances secreted by the tumor. Tumors producing osteolytic factors may not always cause sustained hypercalcemia; this may be manifested only when the patient's calcium homeostasis is stressed, as by restriction of physical activity or fluid intake.

The differential diagnosis of hypercalcemia is discussed in detail in Chap. 24. All other causes of hypercalcemia must be considered, even in the patient with demonstrated malignant disease. In particular, coexistent primary hyperparathyroidism must be excluded.[10] A history of hypercalcemia of more than 1 year's duration, recurrent renal stones, or radiographic evidence of subperiosteal bone resorption is essentially diagnostic of primary hyperparathyroidism,[75] although exceptions due to secretion of humoral hypercalcemia of malignancy factor by indolent tumors[78] do rarely occur. Any patient who has a malignant tumor, hypercalcemia, and a clearly elevated plasma NH_2-terminal or midportion immunoreactive PTH concentration must be considered to have primary hyperparathyroidism until proved otherwise. Evidence for extensive nonsymptomatic metastases to bone must be sought by such means as x-ray survey of the skeleton, radionuclide scans, and histological examination of the bone marrow, but a few small bone metastases do not exclude humoral hypercalcemia of malignancy. Even tumors that metastasize extensively to bone, such as breast carcinoma, may produce local osteolytic factors, such as prostaglandin E_2.

Tumor Osteolytic Factors

Parathyroid Hormone

Immunoreactive PTH-like components have been extracted from renal adenocarcinomas, squamous cell carcinomas of the lung, breast carcinomas, and a variety of other tumors but are not found in extracts of normal nonparathyroid tissue or tumors not associated with hypercalcemia. Arteriovenous step-up gradients of immunoreactive PTH have been measured across the capillary beds of a hepatoma[79] and two renal adenocarcinomas associated with hypercalcemia. PTH has been demonstrated by immunocytochemistry in tissue sections of several tumors associated with the ectopic PTH syndrome.[80,81] Furthermore, a renal adenocarcinoma has been reported to secrete both PTH and pro-PTH-like immunoreactive materials in tissue culture,[82] and in vitro production of immunoreactive PTH by acute myeloblastic leukemia cells has also been described.[83] In no instance, however, has the immunoreactive PTH—like material been demonstrated to have PTH biologic activity.

Parathyroid hormone is synthesized as a high-molecular-weight polypeptide, prepro-PTH, which is almost immediately converted into pro-PTH (90 amino acids, mol wt 10,200) by removal of the NH_2-terminal leader sequence. Pro-PTH is rapidly converted to PTH (84 amino acids, mol wt 9500) in the Golgi apparatus by removal of six more NH_2-terminal amino acids.

Despite the evidence that certain nonparathyroid tumors are capable of synthesizing PTH-like polypeptides, the percentage of tumors causing humoral hypercalcemia of malignancy by producing ectopic PTH is probably very small.[84] It is true that confusion reigned for several years because of conflicting results obtained by investigators using different PTH radioimmunoassays (see Chap. 24). One group used an antiserum directed at the biologically inactive COOH-terminal portion of PTH and found abnormal immunoreactive PTH levels in 95 percent of such patients,[84] whereas another group used an NH_2-terminal PTH antiserum and found elevated IR-PTH in almost none.[85] The greater part of the immunoreactive PTH in parathyroid tissue extracts appears to be intact PTH, but both PTH and five- to tenfold greater concentrations of biologically inactive COOH-terminal fragments of PTH are found in peripheral plasma. Some of these fragments apparently result from peripheral metabolism of PTH, but others may be secreted, along with PTH, by the parathyroid glands.[86] In either case, once formed, they appear to be cleared more slowly from circulating plasma. Secretion of PTH is not completely suppressed by hypercalcemia.[87] These two phenomena may provide at least a partial explanation for the different results obtained with different PTH radioimmunoassays in humoral hypercalcemia of malignancy: PTH continues to be secreted despite the hypercalcemia, and COOH-terminal PTH fragments tend to accumulate because of their slower clearance, especially in the presence of renal insufficiency.

Peripheral plasma immunoreactive PTH values tend to be lower for a given serum calcium concentration in humoral hypercalcemia of malignancy, in which PTH is not the cause, than in primary hyperparathyroidism, in which PTH is the cause.[88] Therefore, an absolute increase in peripheral NH_2-terminal or midportion immunoreactive PTH strongly favors primary hyperparathyroidism as the cause of the hypercalcemia. In true ectopic PTH secretion, the metabolic abnormalities and chemical findings are similar, if not identical, to those in primary hyperparathyroidism. Thus, demonstrating absence of an arteriovenous immunoreactive PTH gradient across the parathyroid gland capillary bed or presence of an arteriovenous gradient across the tumor capillary bed may be the only definitive method of establishing the diagnosis prior to therapy.

Humoral Hypercalcemia of Malignancy Factor

The weight of current evidence appears to indicate that a peptide factor or factors other than PTH is responsible for most cases of humoral hypercalcemia of malignancy. One of the leading candidates is humoral hypercalcemia of malignancy factor (HHMF), a basic, heat-stable peptide with a proposed molecular weight of about 25,000 that stimulates adenylate cyclase and glucose-6-phosphate dehydrogenase in proximal renal tubular cells[89] and adenylate cyclase in osteoblasts[90] by binding to PTH receptors. However, HHMF is different from PTH in that a 9500-molecular weight form has an amino acid composition different from that of PTH or proPTH,[90a] it does not react with antibodies to PTH and does not appear to stimulate distal renal tubular reabsorption of calcium or renal 1α-hydroxylation of 25-hydroxyvitamin D_3, whereas it does appear to uncouple bone cell activity, resulting in relatively more osteoclastic bone resorption than osteoblastic bone formation.[91] It is not yet clear how a factor that binds to the PTH receptor can mimic some but not all of the actions of PTH. Messenger RNA from tumors associated with humoral hypercalcemia of malignancy has been shown to direct the synthesis of a HHMF-like secretory peptide in *Xenopus* oocytes.[91a]

Nephrogenous cyclic AMP excretion is elevated in both primary hyperparathyroidism and this form of humoral hypercalcemia of malignancy, but fasting and fractional calcium excretion are greater (although calcium reabsorption may still be stimulated),[92] serum 1,25-dihydroxyvitamin D_3 levels (and intestinal calcium absorption) are lower, and skeletal calcium losses are greater in humoral hypercalcemia of malignancy.[93] This factor appears to be produced by the tumors that most commonly cause this syndrome, including renal carcinoma and squamous carcinomas of the lung, head, neck, and female reproductive tract.[94] Like many other factors produced by tumors, it appears that HHMF may also be a product of normal cells.[94a]

Growth Factors

Tumors produce a variety of growth factors, including EGF, PDGF, TGF-α, and TGF-β, as has already been mentioned. EGF and PDGF stimulate bone resorption in vitro, apparently by a prostaglandin-mediated mechanism,[95,96] as does TGF-α,[97] which binds to EGF receptors. A rat Leydig-cell tumor has been reported to secrete a bone-resorbing peptide that binds to EGF receptors and has TGF activity[98] but whose actions are not inhibited with indomethacin. The same or another factor produced by the same tumor binds to fibroblast PTH receptors and stimulates cyclic AMP production.[97] Possibly related peptides with molecular weights of 17,000 and 28,000 have been extracted from a human renal cell carcinoma and synthesized by injecting tumor mRNA into *Xenopus* oocytes, leading to the hypothesis that one mechanism of humoral hypercalcemia of malignancy is tumor cell production of growth factors.[99] TGF-β, which is structurally unrelated to TGF-α and does not bind to EGF receptors, is also a potent bone-resorbing peptide.[99a] Others have described bone-resorbing activity extracted from renal, ovarian, lung, and liver carcinomas that was inhibited by prostaglandin synthesis inhibitors.[100] Squamous cell carcinomas associated with hypercalcemia and granulocytosis, perhaps caused by a colony-stimulating factor, which also appears to act by a prostaglandin-mediated mechanism, have also been described.[101]

Prostaglandins

Following the demonstration that PGE_2 stimulates bone resorption in vitro,[102] two animal tumors were described that caused hypercalcemia by producing PGE_2.[103] Tumors, like many normal tissues, are capable of synthesizing prostaglandins, and local release of PGE_2 may be the mechanism by which breast carcinoma metastases exert their osteolytic effect.[104] Antiestrogens and estrogens may stimulate its release;[105] this may explain why some patients with advanced breast cancer treated with these steroids develop acute hypercalcemia. The question is whether nonmetastatic tumors release sufficient PGE_2 into the circulation to mobilize calcium from distant bone. Despite an early report that a rather large percentage of patients with humoral hypercalcemia of malignancy had elevated levels of the major metabolite of PGE_2 in their urine and that prostaglandin synthesis inhibitors corrected their hypercalcemia,[14] subsequent series failed to confirm this finding.[106] Most investigators now agree that systemic levels of PGE_2 are rarely, if ever, the cause of this syndrome.

Osteoclast-Activating Factor

Osteoclast-activating factor (OAF) is a bone-resorbing lymphokine secreted into culture medium by normal peripheral blood T and B lymphocytes[107] activated by phytohemagglutinin or other mitogens and by cultured malignant cells from patients with hematologic malignant disease such as myeloma, acute blastic leukemia, chronic lymphocytic leukemia, Burkitt's lymphoma, lymphosarcoma, and possibly adult T cell lymphoma.[99,108] There is a direct relationship between the degree of bone destruction and the in vitro rate of production of OAF.[109] The production of OAF depends upon prostaglandin synthesis,[110] and its action on bone is inhibited by glucocorticoids, calcitonin, and phosphate.[111] OAF may be involved, as may PGE_2, in the bone resorption that accompanies chronic inflammation in diseases such as rheumatoid arthritis and periodontal disease.

The structure of OAF has not been defined, although it is clearly not PTH, a prostaglandin, or a vitamin D analogue. It appears to be a relatively small polypeptide (mol wt 1500) that can aggregate or bind noncovalently to a carrier protein to form "big" OAF (mol wt 18,000);[112] molecular weights as high as 60,000 have been estimated.[113] A lymphokine with characteristics of interleukin-1 has been reported to have bone-resorbing activity in vitro.[114] It may be that this is (one form of) OAF.

OAF is an important locally active osteolytic factor that is involved in the hypercalcemia associated with hematologic tumors that have extensive contact with bone. It is not thought to play a role in systemic humoral hypercalcemia of malignancy.[115]

Vitamin D and Its Metabolites

Increased circulating levels of 1,25-dihydroxyvitamin D_3 can cause hypercalcemia. It was thought that only the kidney could hydroxylate 25-hydroxyvitamin D_3, but cultured normal keratinocytes, fibroblasts, and placental cells, as well as alveolar macrophages from patients with sarcoidosis and, perhaps, granulomas of other etiologies, can also produce 1,25-dihydroxyvitamin D_3.[116,117] A report of increased plasma phytosterol vitamin D analogues in breast cancer patients with hypercalcemia was later refuted.[118] However, an adolescent boy with a benign intrathoracic plasma cell granuloma producing 1,25-dihydroxy vitamin D_3 and humoral hypercalcemia of malignancy has been reported,[118a] and adult patients with rare T cell leukemia/lymphoma or histiocytic lymphoma frequently have humoral hypercalcemia of malignancy and have been reported to have markedly increased serum 1,25-dihydroxyvitamin D_3, normal serum phosphate, suppressed serum PTH, low urinary PGE excretion, hypercalciuria, increased fractional intestinal absorption of calcium, and significant renal impairment;[119] nephrogenous cyclic AMP excretion is suppressed, either absolutely or in relation to the degree of azotemia.[120] Both the hypercalcemia and the elevated serum 1,25-dihydroxyvitamin D_3 levels return to normal in response to glucocorticoid therapy (60 to 100 mg prednisone or 24 mg dexamethasone per day) but do not respond to indomethacin. Normal umbilical cord blood lymphocytes transformed with human T cell lymphotrophic virus type I (HTLV-I), which has been found in an adult T cell lymphoma, metabolize 25-hydroxyvitamin D_3 to 1,25-dihydroxyvitamin D_3.[120a] A 1,24(R)-dihydroxyvitamin D_3–like material has also been suggested as a hypercalcemic factor in malignancy.[121]

Treatment

The treatment of hypercalcemia is discussed in detail. in Chap. 24 and includes calcium restriction, hydration, avoidance of immobilization, and administration of sodium chloride and furosemide, mithramycin, and/or oral or intravenous phosphate. A trial of prostaglandin synthesis inhibitors may be considered in those occasional patients with tumor-associated hypercalcemia who have low nephrogenous cyclic AMP excretion and low serum immunoreactive PTH; elevated serum PGE_2 and increased PGE_2 metabolite in urine would provide additional support for this mode of therapy. Indomethacin may cause acute gastrointestinal ulceration and hemorrhage; aspirin (1.8 to 4.8 g per day) may be a safer effective drug. If they are going to respond, patients without skeletal metastases will do so within 3 to 5 days; those with metastases to bone will respond only partially.[14] High-dose glucocorticoids or the combination of calcitonin and glucocorticoid may be effective in patients with hematologic malignant disease and impaired renal function.[120–122] Chloroquine phosphate, which may act by blocking the conversion of 25-hydroxyvitamin D_3 to 1,25-dihydroxyvitamin D_3, may also be useful when given at a dose of 500 mg per day with ophthalmologic surveillance for retinopathy.[122a] The radioprotective agent WR-2721 [S-2,2-(3-aminopropylamino)-ethylphosphorothioic acid] inhibits PTH secretion as well as PTH-independent tubular reabsorption of calcium[122b] and corrected the hypercalcemia in an animal model of humoral hypercalcemia of malignancy.[122c] Dichloromethylene diphosphonate or more effective oral or intravenous diphosphonate preparations may provide useful adjunctive therapy when they become available. Finally, continuous infusion of a relatively low dose of gallium nitrate, an antitumor drug, was reported to have corrected hypercalcemia within 4 to 7 days in 10 patients with advanced cancers, probably by inhibiting calcium release from bone.[124] At this dose, there was no nausea or marrow suppression and only a minor, transient decrease in renal function in 4 of the patients; renal function improved in all 10 patients after the hypercalcemia was corrected.

ECTOPIC ACTH SYNDROME

The syndrome caused by hypercortisolemia secondary to nonpituitary tumor secretion of ACTH was the first in which ectopic hormone secretion was proved[125] and is one of the most extensively studied. Nevertheless, 25 years since its description, its true incidence, the complete structures of the hormones involved, the normal biologic significance of some of the hormones, and the precise derangements in molecular mechanisms that initiate hormone secretion and render it independent of glucocorticoid negative feedback control are still for the most part unknown.

Even before Cushing's syndrome was defined, Brown described a patient with diabetes, hirsutism, hypertension, adrenal hyperplasia, and an undifferentiated small cell (oat cell) carcinoma of the lung; no causal association was inferred.[126] About half of all cases of ectopic ACTH syndrome are caused by small cell lung carcinoma; 10 percent by thymic carcinoid tumors (epithelial thymomas);[127] 10 percent by bronchial carcinoids; 5 percent by carcinoid tumors of the esophagus, stomach, duodenum, pancreas, and appendix; 5 percent by pancreatic islet cell tumors; and another 5 percent by medullary carcinoma of the thyroid.[*;128] The frequent association with small cell lung carcinoma reflects mostly the high incidence of the tumor itself; actually, the great majority of patients with small cell lung carcinoma do not have the ectopic ACTH syndrome. However, all these tumors are thought to arise from normal neuroectodermal or endodermal foregut APUD precursor cells, as discussed earlier. Thus, about 85 percent of all cases of ectopic ACTH syndrome are due to tumors of this type.[8] Many of these tumors secrete calcitonin,[129] gastrin-releasing peptide,[130,131] and arginine vasopressin[132] as well.

The majority of tumors of the lung, regardless of their histological type, contain immunoreactive POMC, usually the precursor form itself, despite the fact that there may be no detectable increase in immunoreactive POMC peptides in plasma or evidence of hypercortisolism.[17,39,133] As discussed earlier in this chapter, cells that produce POMC peptides appear to be widely dispersed in normal tissues that may include the thyroid, lung, pancreatic islets, gastrointestinal tract, adrenal medulla,[3,134–136] and, according to some investigators, "all normal . . . extrapituitary tissues."[4] The immunoreactive POMC in these normal tissues is reported to be almost entirely POMC itself, present at concentrations (2.5 to 25 fmol per milligram of protein)[4] which, in terms of ACTH, are equal to about 1 to 10 ng per gram of wet tissue, 20 to 200 times greater than the mean plasma immunoreactive ACTH concentration and equal to that observed in many tumors causing the ectopic ACTH syndrome,[16] but less than 1 percent of that found in the normal pituitary gland. The significance of these observations remains to be determined, but it seems clear that POMC production by some nonpituitary tumors is not ectopic, merely inappropriate. From a clinical standpoint, however, the syndrome and its diagnosis and treatment are the same.

Clinical Presentation

Most patients with ectopic ACTH-producing tumors do not have the classical physical changes of Cushing's syndrome caused by chronic glucocorticoid excess. The duration of the disease is usually brief, hypercortisolemia is often extreme, and the clinical picture may be complicated by other manifestations of malignancy. Thus, the acute metabolic consequences of severe cortisol excess may predominate in both glucocorticoid effects (glucose intolerance) and mineralocorticoid effects (hypokalemia, edema and, occasion-

*Others include pheochromocytoma, ganglioma, paraganglioma, and neuroblastoma; papillary adenocarcinoma of the thyroid; hemangiopericytoma; anaplastic, non-islet-cell adenocarcinoma and small cell carcinoma of the pancreas; squamous cell laryngeal carcinoma; squamous cell carcinoma, large cell undifferentiated carcinoma, papillary bronchiolar-alveolar cell adenocarcinoma, and bronchogenic adenocarcinoma of the lung; parotid carcinoma, palatine adenocarcinoma, and submandibular adenoid cystadenocarcinoma of the salivary glands; squamous cell and small cell undifferentiated carcinoma of the esophagus; undifferentiated mediastinal carcinoma; gastric adenocarcinoma; poorly differentiated adenocarcinoma of the gallbladder; hepatoma and hepatoblastoma; adenocarcinoma of the appendix and colon; hypernephroma and nephroblastoma (Wilms' tumor); adenocarcinoma and poorly differentiated small cell (oat cell) and anaplastic carcinoma of the prostate; ovarian carcinoma; testicular carcinoma; carcinoid and small cell carcinoma of the cervix; melanoma; plasmacytoma; and acute myeloblastic leukemia and lymphosarcoma–acute leukemia.

ally, hypertension); the chronic effects of cortisol on fat and protein metabolism are usually minimal or absent. Even these demonstrable metabolic abnormalities may be minimal for the degree of hypercortisolemia. A patient may have a serum potassium concentration of 3.5 meq per liter with a plasma cortisol greater than 100 μg/dl (upper limit of normal about 25 μg/dl). When severe, however, hypokalemia may cause profound muscle weakness. The patient usually has not gained weight and may have lost some. The incidence is greater among males than among females at present, but the rapidly increasing incidence of lung cancer among women because of cigarette smoking is fast changing this ratio. The majority of patients are over 50 years old, although occasional cases in young children are also reported, reflecting the bimodal age distribution of malignant disease.

Occasional patients with benign or indolent malignant tumors may present with classical features of Cushing's syndrome because of the chronicity of their disease and the relative lack of other effects of malignancy.[137] However, the diagnosis is usually made on the basis of minimal clinical or laboratory clues and is probably never suspected in most patients with the ectopic ACTH syndrome, despite the fact that the metabolic consequences of hypercortisolism complicate the disease course and may be the immediate cause of their death.

The diagnosis is confirmed by demonstrating (1) elevated basal plasma cortisol and/or urinary 17-hydroxycorticosteroids (17-OHCS), 17-ketogenic steroids (17-KGS), or free cortisol, (2) lack of normal diurnal rhythm in plasma cortisol, (3) failure to suppress plasma and/or urinary steroids after either low- or high-dose dexamethasone administration, and (4) high levels of plasma ACTH without diurnal variation. The use of pituitary-adrenal function tests in the differential diagnosis of hypercortisolism is discussed in detail in Chap. 12.

Laboratory clues may help with the more difficult differential diagnostic problems.

Ectopic ACTH Syndrome vs. Adrenal Tumor

In ectopic ACTH syndrome, the ratio of 17-ketosteroids (17-KS) to 17-OHCS is usually similar to that in normal persons or in patients with Cushing's disease: about 2:1 to 3:1. If the ratio is much lower (i.e., if 17-OHCS are distinctly elevated but 17-KS are normal), the likelihood of an adrenal adenoma is increased; if the ratio is much higher (i.e., disproportionate elevation of 17-KS), an adrenal carcinoma is more likely. A normal ratio has no differential diagnostic significance.[138] Adrenal tumors cause chronic hypercortisolism, chronic suppression of normal pituitary ACTH secretion, loss of pituitary ACTH secretory reserve, and atrophy of the normal adrenal cortices; adrenal carcinomas are almost never responsive to ACTH, and half of adrenal adenomas fail to respond.[138] In contrast, ectopic ACTH syndrome is usually associated with acute hypercortisolism, incomplete loss of pituitary ACTH reserve, and bilateral adrenocortical hyperplasia, with hyperresponsiveness to ACTH. Consequently, urinary 17-OHCS fall after metyrapone administration in virtually all patients with Cushing's syndrome due to adrenal tumors but are unchanged or rise in most patients with ectopic ACTH syndrome. For the same reasons, most patients with ectopic ACTH syndrome respond briskly to exogenous ACTH, whereas most patients with adrenal tumors do not. However, the only absolute functional test is to measure plasma ACTH, which is high (usually > 100 pg/ml) in ectopic ACTH syndrome but suppressed (usually to < 10 pg/ml) by adrenal tumors. These functional tests should be complemented by anatomic evidence, such as computerized axial tomography, which is very efficient at demonstrating adrenal masses, less accurate in detecting adrenocortical hyperplasis and unreliable in confirming adrenocortical atrophy. Nuclear magnetic resonance scanning, also called magnetic resonance imaging, is a more sensitive method for detecting adrenal tumors that are not large enough to alter the cross-sectional outline of the gland. Neither of these methods can differentiate primary from metastatic tumor; therefore they should be used in addition to functional tests rather than in place of them.

Ectopic ACTH Syndrome vs. Pituitary ACTH Excess (Cushing's Disease)

Certain tumors are associated with chronic secretion of ectopic ACTH and may thus cause classical Cushing's syndrome. Hypercortisolemia caused by some of these tumors also appears to be suppressed by high-dose dexamethasone. The most common of these are bronchial carcinoid tumors, about 50 percent of which suppress,[139,140] and thymic carcinoids and hepatomas, which can behave similarly. Careful computerized tomographic examination of the lungs and anterior mediastinum is indicated in all patients with dexamethasone-suppressible hypercortisolemia. Plasma ACTH is usually higher (> 100 pg/ml) in ectopic ACTH syndrome. Assay of plasma ACTH in samples obtained by selective percutaneous venous catheterization, including the petrosal, internal jugular, azygos, other mediastinal, and hepatic veins, with simultaneous peripheral control samples being obtained from the right atrium or a peripheral vein for each central sample, is usually definitive in proving Cushing's disease and is occasionally helpful in locating ectopic tumors.[141,142] It has been suggested that response to corticotropin releasing hormone (CRH) is a reliable way to differentiate patients with Cushing's disease, who respond to CRH, from patients with ectopic ACTH syndrome, who do not.[143] It probably has about the same reliability—and reflects the same pathophysiology—as the metyrapone test: patients with chronic ectopic ACTH excess and more classical manifestations of Cushing's syndrome will fail to respond to either and patients with acute ectopic ACTH syndrome will respond to metyrapone and, if their basal plasma cortisol levels are not too elevated, to CRH as well.

Ectopic ACTH Syndrome vs. Stress

Patients who are terminally ill may have elevated, nonsuppressible ACTH and cortisol secretion. There is no clinically useful method to differentiate this physiological response to severe stress from the ectopic ACTH syndrome other than an assessment of the setting in which it occurs (e.g., bacterial infection, high fever, severe pain, extreme respiratory distress). Retrospectively, tumor tissue will be found not to contain ACTH.

Tumor Peptide Products

Normal Biosynthesis of Proopiomelanocortin Peptides

These hormones are synthesized as a common glycopeptide precursor molecule, which in humans consists of 241 amino acid residues (mol wt 26,681) plus a single carbohydrate side chain (Fig. 29-1). The precursor has been called *proopiolipomelanocortin* (pro-OLMC), POMC, *proopiocortin, pro-ACTH,* and, prior to elucidation of its structure, *big ACTH.*[144] In the Golgi apparatus and secretory granules, POMC is subjected to posttranslational processing into a variety of different peptides. In the anterior lobe of the pituitary, this consists of cleavage of Lys-Arg bonds to form a 76-amino acid NH_2-terminal glycopeptide (NT), the function of which is unknown but which may be an adrenocortical growth factor;[145] 39-amino acid ACTH; β-lipotropic hormone (β-LPH), which consists of 89 amino acids and is a weak steroidogenic and lipolytic peptide but which may have potent melanocyte-stimulating activity;[146] γ-LPH, or β-LPH 1–56, the function of which is unknown; and β-endorphin (β-END), or β-LPH 58–89, which is a potent opioid peptide in the central nervous system but whose function in peripheral plasma is unknown. In the intermediate pituitary lobe of adult subprimates, human fetuses, and pregnant women, these five peptides are further processed by cleavage of Lys-Lys and Arg-Arg bonds, acetylation, and amidation to form γ-melanocyte stimulating hormone (γ-MSH), a weak steroidogenic and melanotropic peptide; α-MSH, or acetyl ACTH 1–13 NH_2, a potent melanotropin; corticotropin-like intermediate lobe peptide (CLIP), or ACTH 18–39, an insulin secretagogue; β-MSH, a moderately potent melanotropin; and β-END metabolites, including acetyl β-END, which has little opiate activity, and α-END.

These ectopic tumor peptides are discussed in greater detail in the sections that follow.

Proopiomelanocortin

An immunoreactive POMC-like component was first described in a thymoma[144] and has since been described in many tumors, including some that were not associated with hypercortisolism,[17] and in nontumorous lung tissue.[17,133] It is, as expected, a glycopeptide[147] from which bioactive ACTH can be cleaved with trypsin.[148] Biosynthetic intermediate forms are also regularly observed.[149] POMC has also been identified in the medium in which continuous lines of small cell lung carcinoma cells were cultured,[150,151] and the sequence of a major portion of POMC mRNA from this cell line[151a] and a carcinoid tumor has been determined.[26] In addition, the POMC mRNA in two normal pituitaries and several pituitary and nonpituitary tumors has been found to be qualitatively similar, except for a second, larger mRNA in a thymic carcinoid tumor.[151b]

Although immunoreactive POMC-like materials are found in many tumors and some would suggest that "all carcinomas . . . synthesize and secrete ACTH,"[152] most would agree that elevated immunoreactive ACTH is detected in the plasma of less than a third of patients with small cell lung carcinoma[153] and of far fewer patients with other tumors. Bioactive ACTH is found in only a small percentage even of patients with small cell lung carcinoma, mostly those who have the clinical syndrome.[153] Problems of patient stress, chronic bronchial inflammatory disease, inappropriate time of day for sampling, failure to demonstrate dexamethasone nonsuppressibility, and the known interference of plasma proteins in radioimmunoassays and radioreceptor assays of unextracted plasma make some studies difficult to evaluate.[31,40]

Anterior Lobe POMC Peptides

NH_2-TERMINAL PEPTIDE Immunoreactive NT–like materials have been found in the plasma of patients

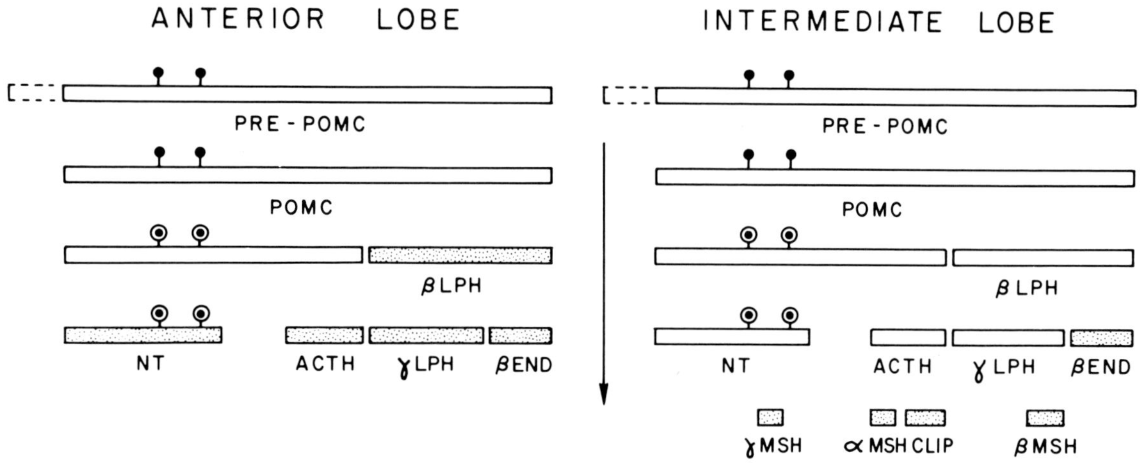

FIGURE 29-1 Diagrammatic representation of the different normal posttranslational processing of human proopiomelanocortin (POMC) (241 amino acid residues) by the anterior and intermediate lobes of the pituitary gland. [_ , Signal peptide (26 residues); •, mannose-rich carbohydrate side-chain; ◉, higher-molecular-weight mannose-poor carbohydrate side chain; ▨, major hormone products that are secreted: NT, NH_2-terminal peptide (76 residues); ACTH, adrenocorticotropin (39 residues); β-LPH, β-lipotropin (89 residues); γ-LPH (56 residues); β-END, β-endorphin (31 residues); γ-MSH, γ-melanocyte stimulating hormone (12 residues); α-MSH (13 residues); CLIP, corticotropin-like intermediate lobe peptide (22 residues); and β-MSH (18 residues). In POMC, each of the major products is flanked by basic dipeptides.

with ectopic ACTH syndrome and Cushing's disease and appear to be primarily NT, rather than the smaller γ-MSH fragments.[154] Allowing for the different plasma half-life of the various POMC peptides, their plasma concentrations indicate that they are secreted in equimolar quantities by pituitary and nonpituitary tumors. The clinical result of hypersecretion of NT is unclear, although, if it is an adrenal growth factor, it may contribute to the adrenal hyperplasia observed in ectopic ACTH syndrome and pituitary Cushing's disease. In addition to NT–like peptide, lesser amounts of materials intermediate in size between NT and γ_3-MSH were found in five ectopic POMC-secreting tumors.[151b]

ADRENOCORTICOTROPIN Tumor ACTH has been shown to be identical to pituitary ACTH in a wide variety of biologic, immunologic, and chemical systems,[1,16] although a molecule that appeared to be ACTH 2–38 was extracted from one tumor.[155] Both melanoma and small cell lung carcinoma cell lines have been shown to secrete immunoreactive ACTH into culture medium in vitro.[150,151,156]

β-LIPOTROPIN AND γ-LIPOTROPIN Immunoreactive components the size of β-LPH and γ-LPH have been found in tumor extracts and plasma of patients with ectopic ACTH syndrome, as have high-molecular-weight immunoreactive LPH materials that coelute with POMC.[157,158] Similar components are secreted by small cell lung carcinoma cells in culture, and the high-molecular-weight immunoreactive LPH materials are part of the same molecule, presumably POMC, as immunoreactive ACTH.[151]

The melanotropic potency of β-LPH is still in doubt. It was originally thought to have less than 1 percent of the activity of β-MSH, but some have found it to be of equal or greater potency.[146] This would explain the otherwise inexplicable report that immunoreactive β-MSH, presumably representing mostly β-LPH and γ-LPH, accounted for the melanotropic bioactivity of most tumor extracts.[159] Neither the exact structure nor the bioactivity of the LPH-like peptides produced in ectopic ACTH syndrome has been defined, but the ectopic β-LPH 38–89 sequence predicted from analysis of POMC mRNA from a carcinoid tumor is identical to that of human pituitary β-LPH.[26]

One group of investigators suggested that the ratio of plasma immunoreactive LPHs measured with two LPH antisera, one of which was somewhat more specific for γ-LPH, differentiated patients with Cushing's disease from those with ectopic ACTH syndrome.[160] It would not be too surprising if cleavage of β-LPH to γ-LPH and β-END were inefficient in an ectopic ACTH-secreting tumor, because of either deficient cleavage enzyme activity or inadequate time for processing due to a deficient storage mechanism. There is considerable overlap in the ratios among individual patients, however, and these antisera are not generally available. The phenomenon does not, therefore, appear to be clinically useful.

Other than their possible role in causing the hyperpigmentation observed in some patients with ectopic ACTH syndrome, high plasma concentrations of the LPHs have no known clinical effects.

ENDORPHINS Immunoreactive β-END has been found in tumor extracts[161] and in culture medium from a continuous small cell lung carcinoma cell line that also secretes other POMC peptides.[151] Its predicted sequence is identical to that of the pituitary peptide.[26] Immunoreactive β-END, which includes β-LPH in reports that do not separate β-END from β-LPH by gel filtration, immunoaffinity chromatography, high-performance liquid chromatography, or other means, is elevated in the plasma of patients with ectopic ACTH syndrome in proportion to the elevation of other POMC peptides.[162]

The physiological significance of plasma β-END is as yet unclear. Although very small amounts of endorphins administered intrathecally have a marked opiate effect, massive dosages given intravenously have little effect. Therefore, secretion by primary or metastatic intracerebral tumors might exert a significant opiate effect, but the clinical manifestations of systemic β-END excess, if any, remain to be defined.

Intermediate Lobe POMC Peptides

γ-MELANOCYTE STIMULATING HORMONE The γ-MSH peptides are cleavage products of NT. They have not often been looked for in the ectopic ACTH syndrome, but materials the size of γ-MSH have been observed.[163] γ-MSH does not have the adrenal weight-maintaining activity of NT. Although γ-MSH, like β-LPH, has been claimed to stimulate aldosterone secretion,[164] there is no evidence that either of these peptides stimulates inappropriate plasma aldosterone concentrations in the ecoptic ACTH syndrome.

α-MELANOCYTE STIMULATING HORMONE Very little α-MSH, the most potent pigmentary hormone known (three to four times as potent as β-MSH and 100 times as potent as ACTH), is found in normal human pituitary (except possibly in early fetal life and during pregnancy) or tumor tissue.[165] Even the low concentrations of immunoreactive α-MSH found in tumor extracts may have been largely due to cross-reaction in the α-MSH radioimmunoassay of ACTH and NH_2-terminal ACTH fragments. If α-MSH were secreted in sufficient amounts, it could contribute to hyperpigmentation.

CORTICOTROPIN-LIKE INTERMEDIATE LOBE PEPTIDE High concentrations of a COOH-terminal ACTH fragment, relative to those of ACTH, are sometimes found in tumor extracts and plasma.[16] Fragments in the tumor may represent CLIP,[166] a peptide which has neither steroidogenic nor melanotropic activity but which may be an insulin secretagogue in pancreatic islets and may stimulate amylase and protein secretion by the exocrine pancreas. The exact origin of the fragments in plasma is less clear; they may either be secreted by the tumor or produced by peripheral metabolism of ACTH, or both.[16] There is no evidence that these fragments have any biologic effect in patients with ectopic ACTH syndrome.

β-MELANOCYTE STIMULATING HORMONE Early studies of immunoreactive β-MSH-like peptides in tumor tissue and plasma did not assess their molecular size.[159] Therefore, the radioimmunoassays may have been measuring γ-LPH and β-LPH, although the melanotropic bioactivity of the extracts was greater than would have been expected, if this were the case. β-MSH-like peptides are present in some tumor extracts[157,158,167] and appear to represent both 18- and 22-residue COOH-terminal cleavage products of γ-LPH,[168] the sequence of which is identical to that of the same region of pituitary γ-LPH.[26] β-MSH is a moderately potent melanotropin and may contribute to hyperpigmentation.

Association with Other Hormones

In addition to the POMC peptides, arginine vasopressin, calcitonin, and gastrin releasing peptide, the ectopic ACTH syndrome has been associated with simultaneous eutopic or ectopic production of a variety of other hormones, including oxytocin, prolactin, insulin, gastrin, glucagon, PTH, somatostatin, vasoactive intestinal polypeptide, norepinephrine, and serotonin. If two or more of these hormones are secreted in amounts sufficient to cause metabolic effects, the composite clinical syndrome can be quite confusing.

Treatment

The best treatment for ectopic ACTH syndrome is complete removal of the tumor.[1,15] However, most tumors causing ectopic ACTH syndrome are nonresectable when discovered. Combination chemotherapy offers limited benefit in treating small cell lung carcinoma, and streptozotocin is useful in some pancreatic islet cell carcinomas. When antitumor therapy is unsuccessful or more rapid control of hypercortisolism is required, therapy should be directed at the adrenal glands.[15] In patients with indolent but nonresectable tumors, total bilateral adrenalectomy should be seriously considered. It is always effective and obviates the need for frequent monitoring of the response to antisteroidogenic drugs. If the patient's hypercortisolism suddenly worsens, especially without a concomitant rise in plasma ACTH, metastasis to the adrenal cortex causing high local ACTH levels should be suspected and may be an indication for adrenalectomy. A "medical adrenalectomy" can be carried out by administering the adrenocorticolytic drug *o,p'*-DDD (mitotane). However, adequate control of cortisol synthesis may take several weeks to months, and the drug has unpleasant gastrointestinal and central nervous system side effects for which individual patients have variable tolerance. Inhibitors of steroid biosynthesis such as aminoglutethimide or metyrapone, used alone, together, or in combination with *o,p'*-DDD, are usually effective in controlling hypercortisolism, because in ectopic ACTH syndrome, unlike Cushing's disease, there is no compensatory increase in tumor ACTH secretion as plasma cortisol falls. Lower doses of the drugs can generally be used when they are given in combination; side effects are usually less, and control of excess steroidogenesis is usually more rapid. In fact, frank adrenal insufficiency may be produced within a few days, so patients should be followed closely. The use of these drugs is discussed in greater detail in Chap. 12.

ECTOPIC SECRETION OF ANTIDIURETIC HORMONE

The association of hyponatremia with a lung carcinoma was first described in 1938,[169] but it was not until 1957 that inappropriate secretion of antidiuretic hormone (ADH; the human ADH is arginine vasopressin) was postulated by Schwartz et al.[170] Amatruda and coworkers were the first to demonstrate an ADH-like substance in an extract of a lung carcinoma.[171] The syndrome is usually associated with small cell lung carcinoma, although other tumors have been associated with the syndrome of inappropriate ADH secretion (SIADH), including adenocarcinoma and large cell undifferentiated carcinoma of the lung; bronchial carcinoid adenoma; carcinoma of the thymus and duodenum; small cell carcinoma of the esophagus and pancreas; carcinoma of the adrenal cortex, ureter, prostate, and bladder; and Hodgkin's and non-Hodgkin's lymphomas.

Clinical Presentation

SIADH is defined as the existence of serum hypoosmolality and hyponatremia in the presence of less than maximally dilute urine and normal renal, adrenal, and thyroid function.[172] As many as 50 percent of all cases of SIADH appear to be associated with ectopic ADH secretion, usually by small cell lung carcinoma,[173] and as many as 30 percent of all patients with small cell lung carcinoma may have SIADH,[174] although a recent study of 250 patients reported an incidence of 7 percent.[175]

SIADH results in water intoxication. As discussed in detail in Chap. 9, ADH increases the permeability of the renal distal convoluted tubule and collecting duct to water. In the distal convoluted tubule, ADH action allows dilute urine delivered from the loop of Henle to become isosmolar with respect to plasma. In the collecting duct, which traverses the hypertonic environment of the renal medulla, ADH action allows the urine to become hyperosmolar with respect to plasma. These portions of the nephron are constantly permeable to water in SIADH, resulting in water retention, urine hyperosmolality, and serum hypoosmolality.

Unless water intake is sufficiently high (about 3 liters a day) to decrease serum sodium concentrations to less than about 120 meq per liter, the patient may be asymptomatic. Subsequent symptoms and their severity reflect both the degree of body fluid dilution and the rate at which serum sodium declines. If it falls slowly, over a period of days to weeks, the symptoms may include only the gradual onset of vague headache, generalized muscle weakness, apathy, lethargy, somnolence, and confusion. If the fall in serum sodium is more precipitous, anorexia, nausea, and vomiting may be the initial symptoms. As the serum sodium falls below about 110 meq per liter, the syndrome may progress to coma, convulsions, hypothermia, hyporeflexia, and death. The clinical features of the syndrome, including the frequent association with hypouricemia,[176] and its differential diagnosis are reviewed in detail[172,173] in Chap. 9.

Tumor Peptide Products

Propressophysin

Arginine vasopressin (AVP) and neurophysin II are synthesized in the hypothalamus as parts of a common glycopeptide precursor molecule (mol wt 20,000) called pro-AVP or propressophysin.[177] Propressophysin-like immunoreactive materials have been found in extracts of the medium in which small cell lung carcinoma cells were incubated and in the plasma of patients with SIADH due to small cell lung carcinoma.[178] Human small cell lung carcinoma cells also incorporate [^{35}S]-cysteine into a molecule that, by several criteria, appears to be propressophysin.[179] As with POMC, propressophysin appears to be present in higher concentrations, relative to its hormone products, when its secretion is ectopic. Propressophysin presumably has little antidiuretic activity.

Arginine Vasopressin

Increased concentrations of bioactive and immunoreactive AVP have been found in the plasma and urine of patients with SIADH; they are not suppressed appropriately by water loading, alcohol, phenytoin, or vagus nerve blockade, all of which inhibit hypothalamic AVP secretion (see Chap. 9). Nude mice to which tumor from a patient with SIADH and a small cell lung carcinoma was transplanted developed inappropriate plasma AVP and neurophysin levels.[180]

The ADH extracted from tumor tissue is biologically, immunologically and chemically indistinguishable from AVP,[181,182] although its precise structure has not been determined. Fresh tumor tissue from a patient with SIADH and small cell carcinoma of the lung incorporated [^{3}H]-phenylalanine into a polypeptide that behaved like authentic AVP under a variety of conditions;[181] limited trypsin treatment of [^{35}S]-cysteine-labeled propressophysin generated an AVP-like peptide,[178] and immunoreactive AVP has been detected in medium from cultures of lung tumor cells.[183] Thus it appears that these tumors are capable of secreting AVP. A number of other conditions are also associated with SIADH, however, including chronic granulomatous pulmonary disease. In one patient with advanced pulmonary tuberculosis, a substance with ADH bioactivity was extracted from the granulomatous tissue.[40] Furthermore, as with other ectopic hormonal products, AVP may be found in tumors of patients who do not exhibit clinical or chemical manifestations of SIADH,[182] although it is seldom found in lung tumors other than small cell carcinoma. It may also be detected in tumor-associated pleural effusion.[184]

Oxytocin

AVP and oxytocin (OT) differ by only two amino acid residues. They appear to be synthesized in the hypothalamus as separate precursors: propressophysin, which contains AVP and neurophysin II, and prooxyphysin, which contains OT and neurophysin I (see Chap. 9).[185] Although immunoreactive OT has been described in rare small cell lung carcinomas[186,187] and a pancreatic tumor[188] and has been reported to have bioactivity,[185] some have found that the OT bioactivity of several tumor extracts was neutralized by specific AVP antiserum but not by OT antiserum.[182] The OT milk-ejection activity reported appeared, therefore, to be due to the intrinsic oxytocin bioactivity of AVP.

If OT is ectopically secreted, this occurs only rarely. The marked difference in the frequency of AVP secretion and that of OT secretion is another of the unexplained phenomena characteristic of ectopic hormone secretion. Ectopic OT secretion, if it exists, would be associated with no symptoms in men or in nonpregnant, nonlactating women.

Neurophysins

One would anticipate that production of AVP would always be associated with neurophysin production, because of their common precursor. Although this is usually the case,[187,189] at least one exception has been reported.[183] The reported exception would suggest either alteration in gene structure or transcription, abnormal mRNA processing or translation, or rapid posttranslational metabolism of neurophysin. Neurophysin has no known metabolic action, thus its overproduction results in no overt clinical abnormalities.

Treatment

Complete removal of the tumor is the treatment of choice, but small cell lung carcinoma is usually nonresectable. The metabolic disturbances associated with SIADH of any etiology can be successfully treated simply by restricting fluid intake to less than insensible water loss. In patients whose serum sodium is above 120 meq per liter, treatment is often unnecessary, but the patient should be followed carefully because of the danger of excessive fluid intake. If the serum sodium falls to less than about 110 meq per liter and life-threatening cerebral dysfunction is present, slow infusion of hypertonic saline may be considered. However, this is usually ineffective, resulting in only a small, transient increase in serum sodium. Furthermore, it aggravates preexisting hypervolemia and is never justified in the patient with cardiac insufficiency. The most effective therapy in such patients is to induce diuresis rapidly by administering furosemide, then determine urinary sodium and potassium losses on an hourly basis and replace them during the diuresis.[173] The use of oral or intravenous urea (80 to 90 g per day) has been recommended as an alternative means for inducing water diuresis.[190] Too rapid a correction of hyponatremia has been reported to cause pontine myelinolysis[191] and should be avoided. Although regulation of aldosterone secretion appears to be normal in SIADH, administration of the synthetic mineralocorticoid fludrocortisone (9α-fluorohydrocortisone), in pharmacological doses (up to 4 mg per day) during fluid restriction may hasten recovery from hyponatremia; development of hypokalemia must be avoided.

For chronic management of the ambulatory patient who cannot sufficiently restrict fluid intake, administration of demethylchlortetracycline (demeclocycline), which inhibits renal concentrating ability, in oral doses of 150 to 300 mg four times per day appears to be a safe and effective treatment.[192] In ambulatory patients who cannot be controlled by water restriction or the use of demeclocycline or urea, furosemide 40 mg per day may be tried,[193] but sodium, potassium, and water balance must be carefully monitored. It should also be noted that appropriate combination chemotherapy for small cell lung carcinoma can rapidly and dramatically lower serum AVP levels during the time that it remains effective against the tumor.[175]

ECTOPIC SECRETION OF GONADOTROPINS

In 1959, Reeves et al. demonstrated a bioactive gonadotropin in an extract of a hepatic carcinoma from a boy with precocious puberty.[194] Since that time, precocious puberty in children and gynecomastia in adults have been described in association with secretion of gonadotropins, almost always chorionic gonadotropin (CG), by a variety of nonpituitary, nontrophoblastic tumors.

Ironically, the problem of defining secretion as ectopic is now perhaps as difficult for CG, a placental hormone, as for any other hormone. Only a few years ago, CG and other placental hormonal and nonhormonal peptides were thought to be ideal tumor markers, virtually diagnostic of malignancy in males and nonpregnant females. Now, CG-like materials have been described in the urine of normal males and postmenopausal females and in a variety of normal tissues.[71-73] Thus, in order to classify CG production as ectopic, one must exclude not only metastases of tumors arising from intrauterine trophoblastic tissues (hydatidiform mole and choriocarcinoma) or "burned out" primary testicular trophoblastic tumors, seminomas, and ovarian dysgerminomas but also tumors arising from extrauterine, extragonadal foci of germinal or trophoblastic cells, tumors described as germinomas, embryonal carcinomas, teratocarcinomas, ectopic pinealomas, and choriocarcinomas. In some cases, it may be difficult to distinguish between an anaplastic large cell carcinoma of the lung and choriocarcinoma itself.[195] Clinically, the distinction is only semantic, because the tumor that is the source of the circulating gonadotropin must be located and treated.

Ectopic gonadotropin secretion has been reported in as many as 84 percent of patients with lung tumors,[196] 75 percent of patients with pancreatic islet cell tumors,[197] 50 percent of patients with breast cancer,[198] and 20 percent of those with gastric adenocarcinoma (who may have immunoreactive CG levels similar to those of first-trimester pregnancy),[199] hepatoma, or colorectal cancer, as well as in patients with many other tumors.[*;199,200] Plasma levels must be interpreted with care, depending upon radioimmunoassay specificity, because of cross-reactivity with luteinizing hormone (LH) at midcycle and in postmenopausal women.[200]

Clinical Presentation

Two syndromes are associated with ectopic CG production, isosexual precocious puberty in children and gynecomastia in the adult male. These syndromes are said to be very rare, having been reported less than 50 times.[201] About 20 cases of boys with precocious puberty, high levels of a CG-like gonadotropin, and hepatoblastoma have been reported.[202] These patients presented with accelerated linear growth, virilization, clubbing, and hepatomegaly. In addition they had congenital anomalies, such as spina bifida occulta and hemihypertrophy of the tongue and extremities. Histological examination revealed Leydig cell hyperplasia and prostatic glandular hyperplasia. A 3-year-old boy with isosexual precocious development and enlarged testes due to ectopic CG production by an adrenocortical carcinoma has also been reported.[203] Only one case of isosexual precocious puberty associated with tumor CG production has been described in a girl, a 5-year-old with an ectopic pinealoma.[204]

In adult males, the only endocrine abnormality resulting from ectopic CG production is gynecomastia, which is usually bilateral and sometimes painful. There is no good evidence that CG acts directly on the breast, but serum estradiol levels are elevated in these patients and correlate with gonadotropin production and tumor mass. The tumor itself produces the estrogen by conversion of circulating dehydroepiandrosterone sulfate to estradiol,[205] a function performed by normal placental tissue. Parenthetically, this does not represent ectopic steroid production; only normal or neoplastic adrenal and gonadal tissues are capable of synthesizing steroids from cholesterol, but many normal and neoplastic tissues, such as adipose tissue, the placenta, and small cell lung carcinoma, are capable of further modification and metabolism of the steroid molecule.

*Among them: carcinoma of the breast, esophagus, mediastinum, biliary tract, liver, exocrine pancreas, adrenal cortex, kidney, renal pelvis, fallopian tube, bladder, prostate, and cervix; melanoma; thymoma; gastric carcinoid; hepatoblastoma; testicular liposarcoma; and osteogenic sarcoma and leiomyosarcoma.

Although CG has weak thyroid-stimulating activity, hyperthyroidism occurs only when circulating CG levels are extremely high, as in hydatidiform mole or gestational choriocarcinoma. Ectopic human placental lactogen may also be secreted by the same tumors that produce ectopic CG, but galactorrhea has not been described as part of the clinical syndrome.

Confirmation of the clinical diagnosis consists of demonstration of elevated plasma or urinary levels of CG and estradiol; testosterone levels are usually normal, suggesting that the testes of these patients are for some reason refractory to CG stimulation. Since these tumors frequently produce disproportionately large quantities of CG subunits,[199] it has been suggested that perhaps the subunits interfere with binding of the biologically active CG heterodimer to the cell membrane receptors of testicular and ovarian target cells. Leydig cell hyperplasia may or may not be observed in testicular biopsy material. Plasma "LH" may also be increased in radioimmunoassays that are not specific for the CG β subunit. Ectopic secretion of CG is not suppressed by administration of androgens, estrogens, or progestogens.

Tumor Peptide Products

Except in one case, in which an arteriovenous step-up gradient of immunoreactive follicle-stimulating hormone (FSH) and, less convincingly, immunoreactive LH across the capillary bed of a lung tumor was documented,[206] all reported cases have either been demonstrated by specific radioimmunoassays to involve ectopic production of CG and/or its subunits or have been studied with relatively nonspecific radioimmunoassays in which cross-reaction with CG could not be excluded. Not only have CG and its subunits been extracted from a variety of tumor tissues, but they have been demonstrated immunohistochemically in tumor tissue sections and produced by several tumor cell lines transplanted into nude mice or maintained in tissue culture. These tumors have included bronchogenic carcinoma, gastric carcinoma, epidermoid cervical carcinoma, and the ubiquitous HeLa cell, which was derived from a cervical carcinoma and, at 30 years of age, is the oldest continuously cultured human cell line.[207] Thus there is unequivocal evidence for the production of CG and its subunits by nontrophoblastic tumor cells. Ectopic production of CG may be unique, in that it requires coordinate expression of two separate genes, one for its α subunit and the other for its β subunit, which are located on the long arms of chromosomes 6 and 19, respectively.

Like the other glycopeptide hormones, FSH, LH, and thyroid-stimulating hormone (TSH), CG is a noncovalently bound heterodimer composed of two dissimilar glycosylated subunits (see Chap. 4). The α subunits of all the glycopeptide hormones are almost identical[208] and are capable, when dissociated from their native β subunits, of combining with the β subunits of the others. The β subunits, on the other hand, are structurally different and confer biologic specificity on the complete heterodimer molecule. Combination of the two subunits is required for effective receptor binding and thus for bioactivity. The β subunit of CG differs from that of LH in having a unique 30-amino acid COOH-terminal sequence extension. Thus, antisera directed at this sequence are specific for CG and do not cross-react with LH.

The carbohydrate side chains present on both the α and β subunits are not necessary for immunoreactivity, heterodimerization, or receptor binding, but the carbohydrate side chains on the α subunit are necessary for transduction of the stimulating signal via activation of adenylate cyclase by CG[209] and thus for its biologic activity in vitro. They also greatly prolong the circulating half-life of the hormone in vivo.

These structure-function relationships are important for consideration of current evidence about synthesis of CG-related substances by normal and neoplastic tissues and the presence or absence of associated clinical syndromes. Secretion of isolated CG subunits or of nonglycosylated CG may be useful as a tumor marker but produces no clinical abnormality.

A CG-like material was found in normal human testes[71] and later in normal human pituitary gland and in a gonadotropin preparation from the urine of postmenopausal women (Pergonal) and a male patient with Klinefelter's syndrome.[72] Subsequently, CG-like material was reported to be present in all normal tissues examined,[73] and an immunoprecipitable CG-like material has been synthesized by normal tissues in vitro, leading certain investigators to the conclusion that "all normal human tissues . . . [and] all carcinomas . . . synthesize and secrete a CG-like protein."[152] Isolated β subunit may also sometimes be secreted, but it is more common for the free α subunit to be secreted, alone or together with the CG heterodimer.[199] Ectopic CG may lack a portion of the COOH-terminal sequence of the β subunit,[210,211] but the ectopic α subunit appears to be intact[212] except, in the case of an ectopic α subunit purified from a patient's urine and sequenced, a single amino acid substitution.[212a] There is disagreement about glycosylation of ectopic CG. One group, observing decreased binding to concanavalin A, drew the global conclusion that "all normal tissues and all carcinomas elaborate CG which has reduced carbohydrate content and is probably carbohydrate-free."[213] Others, using exoglycosidase digestion, concluded that there is considerable heterogeneity but that the tissue, serum, and urinary forms of ectopic CG are glycosylated to about the same degree as placental CG.[212] This difference may be explained by the report that binding to concanavalin A may be inhibited by the presence of extra sugar moieties rather than a lack of them.[214] Perhaps as a result of the differences in glycosylation or changes in tertiary structure due to amino acid substitutions in the ectopic CG α subunit or truncation or extension of the COOH-terminus of the β-subunit,[214a,214b] the ectopic CG subunits appear less able than the normal subunits to combine to form a heterodimer capable of binding to testicular membrane receptors[215] and therefore of exerting a biologic effect.

The precise structure of ectopic CG, like most of the other ectopic hormones, remains to be elucidated.

Treatment

Therapy is directed at the tumor, although the prognosis in most cases is poor. The painful gynecomastia can, if necessary, be treated by reductive mammoplasty.

HYPERTHYROIDISM ASSOCIATED WITH NONPITUITARY TUMORS

Since the initial report by Kupperman and Epstein of a patient with hydatidiform mole and hyperthyroidism,[216] a number of patients with nonpituitary tumors causing secondary hyperthyroidism have been described. In no case, however, has the tumor been of other than trophoblastic origin (i.e., hydatidiform mole or choriocarcinoma). Furthermore, since a material with thyroid-stimulating activity has been extracted from normal human placenta,[217] this is an instance in which the term *ectopic hormonal syndrome* is not appropriate.

Clinical Presentation

The syndrome itself is quite rare. It has the interesting feature that some patients have minimal overt clinical signs of hyperthyroidism and no goiter, despite increased thyroidal iodine uptake, circulating thyroid hormone levels, and basal metabolic rate.[218] Other patients have typical thyrotoxicosis with diffuse goiter, however, and in one instance, thyroid storm appeared to occur following a surgical procedure.[219] The syndrome differs from Graves' disease in that it is not associated with exophthalmos or pretibial myxedema; but the lid retraction, stare, lid lag, and other manifestations of increased circulating thyroxine may be present. Male patients may have gynecomastia due to increased conversion by the trophoblastic tumor cells of dehydroepiandrosterone sulfate or other C_{19} steroids to estradiol.[206]

Tumor Peptide Product

The thyrotropin in the tumors and plasma of patients with trophoblastic tumors and thyroid hyperfunction does not cross-react in the human TSH radioimmunoassay, and basal immunoreactive TSH levels are normal or low and do not increase after administration of thyrotropin releasing hormone. In the McKenzie mouse bioassay (see Chap. 10), the response to trophoblastic thyrotropin is more prolonged (9 h) than that to TSH (2 h) but shorter than the response to the thyroid-stimulating immunoglobulin of Graves' disease (24 h).[219] Its bioactivity is not neutralized by antiserum to human pituitary TSH. Trophoblastic thyrotropin bioactivity is inseparable from CG in a variety of physicochemical systems,[219,220] and it now seems certain that it is due to the weak intrinsic thyroid-stimulating activity of CG,[221] which binds to the TSH receptor.[222]

There are at least three possible reasons why hyperthyroidism is not observed more frequently in patients with trophoblastic tumors, with other tumors that secrete CG, or even in normal pregnancy. The first is that CG is a very weak thyrotropin, so that extremely high levels of circulating CG, levels usually associated only with hydatidiform mole or choriocarcinoma, are required to cause clinical hyperthyroidism. The second is that CG itself or some other principle elaborated in association with it may interfere with the peripheral action of thyroxine, although there is no direct evidence supporting this hypothesis. The third is that the carbohydrate side chains in trophoblastic CG differ from those of normal chorionic CG,[223] reducing its bioactivity without affecting its immunoreactivity. As already noted, there is evidence that hyperglycosylation of CG may affect lectin binding, heterodimer formation, and possibly bioactivity; this may account, at least in part, for the infrequent occurrence of hyperthyroidism with these tumors.

Treatment

The treatment of trophoblastic hyperthyroidism is the same, except for measures directed at removing or inhibiting the tumor itself, as that for other forms of secondary hyperthyroidism (see Chap. 10).

HYPOGLYCEMIA ASSOCIATED WITH NON-ISLET-CELL TUMORS

The association of symptomatic hypoglycemia with a nonpancreatic tumor was first reported by Nadler and Wolfer in 1929.[224] It has since been described in almost 200 patients harboring a wide variety of tumors, most often large mesenchymal tumors, two-thirds of which arise in the abdomen and most of the remainder in the thorax.[225] These tumors, which include fibrosarcomas, mesotheliomas, liposarcomas, rhabdomyosarcomas, leiomyosarcomas, and hemangiopericytomas, account for about half of all reported cases; another 20 percent are associated with primary hepatomas, 10 percent with gastrointestinal carcinomas, and 5 to 10 percent with adrenocortical carcinomas. The remainder are associated with a variety of tumors, including bronchogenic carcinoma; carcinoid tumors of the pancreas, lung, liver, ileum, and jejunum; and breast carcinoma, reticulum cell sarcoma, neurilemoma, neuroblastoma, neurofibrosarcoma, malignant pheochromocytoma, renal-cell carcinoma, Wilms' tumor, hepatoblastoma, pancreatic adenocarcinoma, carcinoma of the cervix, and Hodgkin's lymphoma.[226–228] Hypoglycemia is found in about 4 percent of patients with fibrous mesotheliomas.[229] Although hypoglycemia due to insulin secretion by a benign mediastinal teratoma has been described,[230] the tumor, like many other mediastinal and sacrococcygeal teratomas, contained pancreatic islet cell tissue and thus is not strictly an ectopic source.

Clinical Presentation

The symptoms are those of prolonged hypoglycemia, with headache, confusion, syncope, seizures, somnolence, coma, and a variety of psychiatric symptoms. The hypoglycemia is often profound and unresponsive to any therapy other than resection of the tumor; it is often the primary cause of death. The differential diagnosis of hypoglycemia is discussed in Chap. 20. The most common causes of this rare syndrome are misuse of drugs such as insulin, sulfonylureas, and alcohol; insulin-secreting pancreatic islet cell tumors; and non-islet-cell tumors. Other causes include adrenal insufficiency, pituitary insufficiency, hepatic dysfunction, and the presence of circulating antibodies against insulin or its receptor.

Tumor Hypoglycemic Factors

The cause of hypoglycemia is still unclear in the majority of these tumors.[231] It is possible that the tumor consumes glucose because of its size and constant metabolic activity. However, although arteriovenous gradients across tumor capillary beds and increased in vitro consumption by tumor slices have been reported and the tumors are often large, it seems unlikely that glucose utilization by most of these tumors could exceed the tremendous capacity of the liver for glucose production or account for the failure of massive intravenous infusions of glucose to correct the hypoglycemia in some patients. Early reports of increased glycogen deposition in these tumors, which provided one basis for the hypothesis, have not been confirmed.

It is unlikely that the tumors produce a substance that stimulates insulin release by pancreatic islet cells or inhibits insulin degradation, because serum insulin levels are not elevated and pancreatic beta cells, when examined, are neither hypertrophied nor degranulated. The suggestion that the tumors release tryptophan or other amino acids into the circulation, inhibiting lipolysis and hepatic gluconeogenesis,[232] lacks adequate data to support it. It is therefore generally assumed that these tumors secrete insulin or insulin-like factors.

Insulin

Immunoreactive or bioactive insulin has been extracted from tumor tissue in only about a dozen cases, which include the spectrum of mesothelial and carcinoid tumors with which the syndrome has been associated as well as occasional tumors unassociated with symptomatic hypoglycemia.[227,233,234] Membrane-bound secretory granules have been observed in at least one tumor.[227] Tumor concentrations of immunoreactive insulin are low, usually far less than 1 percent of that found in the normal pancreas, but insulin concentrations in the normal pancreatic tissue appear to be suppressed,[233] a phenomenon reminiscent of the suppressed pituitary ACTH concentrations in the ectopic ACTH syndrome.[1] It is clear that the majority of cases of tumor hypoglycemia are caused by factors other than ectopic insulin secretion.

It is in a sense curious that this syndrome is not more common and that it is not usually caused by inappropriate insulin secretion, because insulin, like POMC and CG-like materials, has been said to be found in all normal tissues.[235] If this is true, then significant synthesis and secretion of these normal hormonal peptides by tumors appears to be a relatively unusual and highly selective phenomenon.

Insulin-like Growth Factors

Serum nonsuppressible insulin-like activity (NSILA-s) consists mainly of insulin-like growth factor I (IGF-I), also known as *somatomedin* C, and IGF-II, also known as *multiplication-stimulating activity*.[236] These two polypeptides are synthesized by the liver, IGF-I in response to stimulation by growth hormone, and share several biologic activities with insulin (see Chaps. 5 and 8). The characteristics of the hypoglycemic principle from a number of the tumors associated with hypoglycemia suggested that IGFs might be the responsible agents.[237] NSILA-s, measured by rat liver membrane radioreceptor assay, was elevated in 19 of 52 patients,[238] and IGF-II, measured by rat placental membrane radioreceptor assay, was found to be elevated in 10 of 14 of these patients.[239] However, using the rat liver radioreceptor assay for IGF-II and radioimmunoassays specific for IGF-I and IGF-II, another group found slightly decreased serum IGF-II and markedly suppressed IGF-I in 9 of the same patients and in 22 additional patients with tumor-associated hypoglycemia.[240] Thus the role of IGFs in tumor-associated hypoglycemia remains controversial.[241]

Other Factors

A promyelocytic leukemia cell line has been reported to produce a potent hypoglycemic peptide that is immunologically distinct from insulin, does not bind to the insulin receptor, has a major component with a molecular weight of about 10,000 and a minor component of about 50,000, and may have growth factor activity.[242] A factor that may have been responsible for a three- to fivefold increase in insulin receptor number in liver, muscle, and mononuclear leukocytes has been implicated in the intractable hypoglycemia of a patient with colon carcinoma.[242a]

Treatment

The only effective treatment usually is removal of the tumor. Fortunately, these tumors are frequently benign. In nonresectable tumors, administration of diazoxide (to inhibit insulin release), glucocorticoids (to stimulate gluconeogenesis), or glucagon (to stimulate hepatic glucose production) is usually ineffective, and blood glucose levels can be maintained only with intravenous glucose infusion. Even then, it is sometimes impossible to meet the enormous glucose requirements.

TUMOR-ASSOCIATED OSTEOMALACIA

The first patient with this uncommon condition was reported in 1947 by McCance,[243] but the possible causal relationship was not recognized until 1959.[244] Only about 50 cases have been reported,[245] but the actual incidence is probably greater than this paucity of reports would suggest. The syndrome is associated with benign or, rarely, malignant mesenchymal tumors, including hemangiopericytoma, hemangioma, fibroangioma, osteoblastoma, neuroma, giant cell tumors of bone, and osteosarcoma. The tumors are usually highly vascular and have prominent giant cells and spindle cells. The syndrome has also been reported in two patients with prostatic carcinoma[246] and in one case of small cell lung carcinoma that was associated also with SIADH.[247] It may also be associated with von Recklinghausen's neurofibromatosis.[248]

Clinical Presentation

Patients are usually young adults and complain of diffuse or low back bone pain and muscle weakness that may be profound. Because of pain and weakness, they are often unable to walk. The course is chronic, and the tumor is often small and may not be discovered until years after the metabolic disturbance is documented. In patients with adult-onset osteomalacia and phosphaturia and without a history of familial rickets, heavy metal exposure, or Fanconi syndrome, tumor-associated osteomalacia is the most likely cause.[245] Their serum phosphorus is low, about 1.5 mg/dl, serum calcium is normal, and serum alkaline phosphatase is markedly elevated. There is profound phosphaturia despite severe hypophosphatemia. Aminoaciduria and glucosuria in the absence of hyperglycemia are found in about 25 and 50 percent of patients, respectively. Serum PTH and calcitonin concentrations are generally normal, as is serum 25-hydroxyvitamin D. However, the concentrations of serum 1,25-dihydroxyvitamin D are decreased in almost all patients. These findings indicate that the most likely defect is in the proximal convoluted tube of the kidney, leading to impaired phosphate, glucose, and amino acid transport and defective 1α-hydroxylation of 25-hydroxyvitamin D.

Tumor Hyperphosphaturic Factor

The factor responsible for the metabolic abnormality remains elusive. None of the tumors examined by electron microscopy has shown evidence of secretory granules, and only once was a tumor extract able to produce phosphaturia in an experimental animal, a result that could not later be duplicated.[249] PTH and HHMF are unlikely to be involved, because their serum concentrations are normal when measured, nephrogenous cyclic AMP is normal, and hypercalcemia is absent. Calcitonin is also unlikely to be involved for the same kinds of reason. However, a factor which, like PTH and HHMF, stimulates renal adenylate cyclase has been described in extracts of tumors from three patients with this syndrome.[249a]

Treatment

Most of these tumors are benign, and removal results in rapid and dramatic reversal of all the metabolic abnormalities and clinical symptoms. In those patients in whom the tumor cannot be completely excised, partial resection or treatment with 1,25-dihydroxyvitamin D, 1α-hydroxyvitamin D, or dihydrotachysterol (but not vitamin D or 25-hydroxyvitamin D) and oral phosphate supplements may ameliorate but seldom completely corrects the hypophosphatemia. However, the clinical response may be more impressive than the biochemical response would predict.[245]

ECTOPIC SECRETION OF OTHER HORMONES

Calcitonin

Secretion of human calcitonin (CT) by medullary carcinoma of the thyroid, a tumor of the parafollicular C cells of the thyroid which normally secrete CT (see Chaps. 11 and 28), is a well-known example of eutopic tumor hormone secretion. It is only rarely associated with hypocalcemia. Diarrhea is the major clinical manifestation but affects only a small percent of patients with medullary thyroid carcinoma; its exact pathogenesis is unknown.

Ectopic secretion of CT was first described in a patient with a carcinoid tumor.[250] Since that time it has been described in association with a wide variety of tumors.* Increased immunoreactive CT levels were found in the plasma and tumor tissues of up to half of several series of patients with cancers of varying types.[129,251,252] Serum immunoreactive CT is increased in about 60 percent of patients with small cell carcinoma and 15 percent of patients with large cell or adenocarcinoma of the lung;[251,253,254] urine CT levels are also increased.[255] Even when basal serum CT concentration is normal, it may increase abnormally after pentagastrin stimulation.[256] A large percentage of patients with breast cancer and leukemia also have elevated serum CT levels.[252,257,258]

There appears to be no clinical manifestation of ectopic CT excess; diarrhea has yet to be described with ectopic CT secretion, possibly because serum CT levels are much lower than in medullary thyroid carcinoma. It has been suggested that the hypocalcemia rarely associated with bone metastases might be caused by CT or that CT might be the agent responsible for osteoblastic responses to skeletal metastases, but there is no substantial experimental evidence for these hypotheses as yet. Nor is there evidence that CT is involved in the hypocalcemia and hyperphosphatemia observed as the result of effective chemotherapy for acute and chronic leukemia and, rarely, prostatic carcinoma. The nature of the abnormality in these patients is unknown.

The differential diagnosis of medullary carcinoma of the thyroid versus ectopic CT secretion is complicated by the fact that patients with either may have raised basal immunoreactive CT levels and abnormal increases after calcium or pentagastrin infusion.

Calcitonin has been demonstrated by immunocytochemistry in tumor tissue sections whose cells contain secretory granules.[19] Immunoreactive CT has been extracted from tumor tissues and identified in the medium in which a line of poorly differentiated bronchial carcinoma cells was grown, appearing as a biologically inactive high-molecular-weight form that could be converted to bioactive CT by brief exposure to trypsin. Messenger RNA extracted from these cells was identical in size to mRNA from human medullary thyroid carcinoma and produced a single immunoprecipitable peptide in an in vitro translation system.[259] The peptide product had a molecular weight of 17,000, like that of the translation product of mRNA extracted from human medullary thyroid carcinoma, but was not processed to 3500 molecular weight CT by the lung tumor cells.

Growth Hormone

Evidence for ectopic secretion of growth hormone has been sought most often in patients with lung carcinoma and osteoarthropathy. In the first reported case, elevated immunoreactive GH levels fell and osteoarthropathy improved after tumor resection.[260] However, there is no clear association of elevated plasma GH and osteoarthropathy. Immunoreactive GH has been extracted from small cell carcinoma, large cell undifferentiated carcinoma, squamous cell carcinoma, and adenocarcinoma of the lung and from bronchial carcinoid tumor, gastric adenocarcinoma, and endometrial carcinoma. In vitro incorporation of [^{14}C]-leucine into material with the chromatographic characteristics of GH was reported for lung carcinoma cells that also released immunoreactive GH into the culture medium.[260] In only one of these reports was the possibility excluded that the secreted material was

*Among them: breast carcinoma; small cell carcinoma, adenocarcinoma, and squamous cell carcinoma of the lung; pheochromocytoma; melanoma; bronchial, thymic, gastric, and small intestinal carcinoid tumors; papillary and follicular thyroid carcinoma; pancreatic islet B and D cell carcinomas; non-islet-cell pancreatic carcinoma; esophageal squamous cell carcinoma; carcinomas of the maxillary sinus, colon, uterus, bladder, and prostate; acute monocytic and myeloblastic leukemia and chronic myelocytic leukemia; and Hodgkin's and non-Hodgkin's lymphoma.

placental lactogen, a structurally and immunologically closely related hormone.

A recent thorough study of acromegaly caused by an intramesenteric ectopic pancreatic islet cell tumor included demonstration of an arteriovenous gradient of GH, high GH and lack of growth hormone releasing hormone (GRH) in plasma, fall in serum GH to normal within hours of tumor excision, and normal responses to gluçose and GRH after surgery.[261] The tumor contained a high concentration of GH but barely detectable GRH and incorporated [^{3}H]-leucine into immunoprecipitable GH material, most of it the size of GH but some much larger. The immunoreactive GH in plasma, tumor extract, and culture medium was the size of GH. GH was demonstrated by immunocytochemistry in secretory granules in tumor cells. Hybridization with a human GH cDNA probe revealed GH mRNA in the tumor extract. Thus there is no doubt that this tumor secreted GH. What is surprising, in light of the report of material in a wide variety of normal human tissues that reacts with GH antisera, binds to hepatocyte GH receptors, and has the apparent molecular size of GH,[262] is that ectopic GH secretion is such an exceedingly rare event.

Hypothalamic Hormones

Growth Hormone Releasing Hormone

Some tumors, most often carcinoid or pancreatic islet cell tumors,[263–270] are associated with elevated plasma immunoreactive GH and immunoreactive GRH levels,[270–272] sometimes with an enlarged sella turcica, and with acromegaly that is cured by resection of the nonpituitary tumor. These tumors contain GRH, which was, in fact, first extracted from a pancreatic islet cell tumor from a patient with acromegaly due to somatotroph hyperplasia,[267] isolated, sequenced,[5] and only later shown to be identical to the hypothalamic peptide.[6] The sequence of the GRH mRNA in this tumor was also determined.[273] Immunoreactive GRH can be demonstrated in a wide variety of tumors, especially small cell lung carcinoma, removed from patients who have no evidence of GH hypersecretion.[274,275]

Ectopic GRH secretion is a rare cause of acromegaly[271,272] that should be excluded, if possible, before unnecessary pituitary irradiation or surgery is performed. However, as in acromegalic patients without ectopic GRH secretion, plasma GH may be nonsuppressible or may rise paradoxically after glucose administration and may increase after insulin-induced hypoglycemia and TRH administration.[268,270] Furthermore, some acromegalic patients with long-standing pituitary adenomas may have elevated plasma GRH levels.[272] It is not clear whether these patients have, as the source of GRH, a dysfunctional hypothalamus; an occult, indolent, nonpituitary tumor ectopically secreting GRH; or an occult hypothalamic gangliocytoma, which can be present in patients with acromegaly of many years' duration.[276] Thus, it may be difficult to differentiate the cause of acromegaly in individual patients. In at least one patient with a GRH-secreting pancreatic carcinoid tumor, serum GH concentration did not increase after GRH administration,[270] whereas it does so in virtually all patients with acromegaly due to primary pituitary adenomas. Thus, responsiveness to GRH may be an important differential diagnostic test in patients with acromegaly. Hypothalamic gangliocytomas or extracranial tumors should be sought in acromegalic patients with high plasma GRH levels. In nonresectable tumors, long-acting somatostatin agonists may inhibit the secretion or block the action of GRH.

Corticotropin Releasing Hormone

Adrenocortical steroid secretion is suppressible by high-dose dexamethasone (8 mg per day) in about 50 percent of patients with hypercortisolism caused by bronchial carcinoid tumors[139,140] and in some patients with thymic carcinoid tumors or hepatomas. One may postulate that these tumors produce ACTH which is subject to glucocorticoid negative feedback inhibition; this would require that the tumors have functional glucocorticoid receptors. Alternatively, these carcinoid tumors may produce corticotropin releasing hormone (CRH), a 41-amino acid residue polypeptide, the action of which on normal pituitary corticotrophs is blocked by dexamethasone (see Chaps. 7 and 8). Several tumors with biologic CRH-like activity have been reported.[277–279] In most instances, however, the issue is clouded by the fact that ACTH is found in the same tumors.

Five patients with hypercortisolemia apparently caused by ectopic CRH secretion have now been reported. One had widely metastatic small cell prostatic carcinoma with metastasis to the infundibulum, median eminence, and pituitary stalk.[280] CRH released from the tumor cells presumably reached the pituitary by way of the hypothalamic-hypophysial portal circulation. There was marked corticotroph hyperplasia. Peripheral plasma CRH and ACTH concentrations were elevated. The tumor had CRH bioactivity and immunoreactivity that coeluted with synthetic human CRH on reverse-phase high-performance liquid chromatography (ACTH was not measured), and tumor sections immunostained for CRH but not ACTH. The second patient had medullary thyroid carcinoma metastatic to the liver but apparently not to the brain.[281] Plasma ACTH was increased, and the tumor metastases immunostained for CRH but not ACTH (neither plasma concentration nor tumor content of CRH was determined). Two of the patients had bronchial carcinoid tumors that contained both ACTH and CRH by immunohistochemical staining; the hormones were present in the same cells in one tumor, but in distinct cell populations in the other.[281a,281b] An arteriovenous gradient of both ACTH and CRH was demonstrated in one patient.[281b] Cushing's syndrome persisted after removal of a pituitary chromophobe adenoma that did not stain for ACTH in the other. The fifth patient had a pheochromocytoma that contained both ACTH and bioactive CRH; an arteriovenous CRH gradient was demonstrated.[281c]

Interestingly, ACTH secretion was not suppressed by high-dose dexamethasone in four of these patients. The reason for this phenomenon is unclear, in view of the fact that concentrations of dexamethasone similar to those achieved in plasma during high-dose dexamethasone administration inhibit the ACTH-releasing action of maximally stimulating doses of CRH (W. E. Nicholson and D.N. Orth, unpublished observations). In those patients with ectopic CRH secretion who exhibit this phenomenon, it will readily distinguish them from patients with Cushing's disease. Except by measuring plasma CRH levels, however, it may be difficult to differentiate ectopic CRH from ectopic ACTH secretion. From a clinical standpoint this is probably unimportant, because the therapeutic options—other than hypophysectomy in certain instances of ectopic CRH syndrome, perhaps—would be the same. Cushing's syndrome due to presumably eutopic secretion of CRH by a gangliocytoma[282] appears to be an extremely rare occurrence.

Other Hypothalamic Hormones

Ectopic secretion of arginine vasopressin, another hypothalamic hormone, was discussed earlier. Gonadotropin releasing hormone (see Chap. 7) has not been described in tumor tissue, but TRH (see Chap. 7) was found in all seven tumors of various types that were studied.[283] The highest concentrations, which were about 0.1 percent of those in normal hypothalamus and about equal to those in placenta, were found in a melanoma, two small cell carcinomas, and one adenocarcinoma of the lung. None of these patients had evidence of hyperthyroidism.

The last of the known hypothalamic peptide hormones, somatostatin (somatotropin release inhibiting hormone, SRIH) is widely distributed in the central nervous system as well as in the C cells of the thyroid, thymus, gastroenteropancreatic D cells, and adrenomedullary cells. In addition to its eutopic production by tumors of these cells, SRIH secretion was reported in 8 of 11 small cell lung carcinoma lines,[284] and SRIH was found in four small cell lung carcinomas, in bronchial and thymic carcinoid tumors,[284,285] and in one of three adenocarcinomas of the lung, in which it was present alone and in combination with calcitonin in individual tumor cells.[19] In none of these patients was the clinical syndrome of SRIH excess (see Chap. 27) observed; presumably, plasma SRIH concentrations were normal or only modestly elevated.[285] It should be noted, however, that eutopic SRIH-secreting pancreatic D cell tumors (somatostatinomas) have been associated with ectopic secretion of other hormones.

Gastrin Releasing Peptide

Gastrin releasing peptide (GRP) is a 27-amino acid residue peptide, the carboxy-terminus of which has 64 percent sequence homology with the 14-residue amphibian peptide bombesin.[286] Human GRP shares 22 residues with porcine and canine GRP. The carboxy-terminal portion of GRP has all the known bioactivity in the molecule. GRP has a variety of actions on the central nervous system and gastrointestinal tract, including induction of satiety; release of gastrin, cholecystokinin, and pancreatic polypeptide; and stimulation of intestinal motility. Immunoreactive GRP is widely distributed in normal human brain, spinal cord, gastrointestinal nerve fibers, Kultschitsky-type neuroendocrine cells of the fetal and adult lung, and C cells of the thyroid. It is not surprising, then, that GRP is produced by neuroendocrine lung tumorlets, bronchial carcinoids, and small cell lung carcinoma,[287–290] all of which are considered to be derived from pulmonary Kultschitsky cells or their precursors. GRP has been described in a variety of other tumors, including hepatic, ileal, appendiceal, cecal, and rectal carcinoids; medullary carcinoma of the thyroid; large cell carcinoma, squamous cell carcinoma, and adenocarcinoma of the lung; and pheochromocytoma.[130,131,289] Perhaps in none of these tumors can GRP secretion be termed truly ectopic. Plasma levels of immunoreactive GRP are increased in some patients from normal fasting levels of about 4 pg/ml to 30 to 330 pg/ml.[131] Analysis of GRP mRNA in small cell lung carcinoma reveals three forms produced by alternative processing of the primary transcript that would be predicted to code for three different GRP precursors.[290a]

No known clinical syndrome is associated with GRP secretion, although the diarrhea associated with some tumors and the anorexia associated with others might be considered possible manifestations. Despite its name, it is not associated with peptic ulcer disease. It was claimed that Cushing's syndrome was caused in one patient by ectopic secretion of GRP by a medullary thyroid carcinoma,[290] presumably because of the synergistic effect of GRP, which has little ACTH-releasing activity of its own, on CRH action.[291] This seems an unlikely explanation on three counts: first, ectopic GRP production appears to be a relatively common phenomenon,[130,131,289] with elevated plasma levels in many of those patients who have been tested,[131] yet the ectopic ACTH syndrome is relatively uncommon and is almost always associated with tumors that secrete ACTH or, rarely, CRH; second, arginine vasopressin is at least as potent a synergist of CRH action as GRP, yet Cushing's syndrome is not associated with SIADH; and third, it is difficult to explain why the normal secretion and action of CRH would not be inhibited by the elevated plasma cortisol concentration induced by the synergistic effect of GRP, leaving no CRH with which GRP could synergize. Thus the clinical effects, if any, of ectopic GRP secretion remain unclear. It is of interest, however, that GRP receptors are found on small cell lung carcinoma cells[292] and that GRP is a growth-stimulating factor for both normal bronchial epithelial cells and small cell lung carcinoma cells.[293] It is possible, therefore, that neuroendocrine lung tumors stimulate their own growth.

Immunoreactive GRP is found in individual tumor cells, alone[19] or in combination with other peptides (calcitonin, for example) in some medullary thyroid carcinoma cells.[294] GRP and a carboxy-terminal GRP ~14–27 fragment have been found in varying proportions in a number of tumors,[130,131,288] and a complementary amino-terminal fragment was identified in one of them.[288] The secretion of GRP by some small cell lung carcinoma cells is stimulated by dibutyryl cyclic AMP, calcium ion, and cholinergic agonists.[295]

Erythropoietin

Erythrocytosis has been reported in association with a variety of tumors. About 3 percent of adult patients with renal cell carcinoma, 7 percent of patients with hepatoma, and 18 percent of those with cerebellar hemangioblastoma have erythrocytosis.[296] Conversely, about half of all cases of tumor-associated erythrocytosis are due to renal cell carcinomas, 20 percent to cerebellar hemangioblastomas, 15 percent to benign renal tumors and cysts, another 5 percent to uterine leiomyomas, and the remainder to hepatomas, small cell lung carcinomas, thymic carcinoid tumors, pheochromocytomas, and rarely other tumors, such as dermoid cysts and lipid cell tumors of the ovary.[297–300] Although adrenocortical carcinoma and virilizing ovarian tumors have been associated with erythrocytosis, the effect of steroids, particularly androgenic steroids, on erythropoietin production[301] suggests that tumor production of steroids, not erythropoietin,[298,299] may be the mechanism involved in these tumors. Prostaglandins also appear to cause erythrocytosis, both by stimulating erythropoietin production and by augmenting erythropoietin stimulation of responsive marrow precursor cells. This may be the mechanism by which some uterine fibroid tumors cause erythrocytosis, although some clearly produce erythropoietin.[297] Because β-adrenergic agonists are known to increase erythropoietin production, this mechanism must be considered in pheochromocytomas associated with erythrocytosis. Thus, there are several possible causes of tumor-associated erythrocytosis other than ectopic erythropoietin secretion. Furthermore, before concluding that the tumor is the cause of the erythrocytosis, primary erythrocytosis (polycythemia vera), secondary erythrocytosis, and relative polycythemia (stress erythrocytosis) must be excluded.[301]

Patients with tumor-associated erythrocytosis can be distinguished from most patients with polycythemia vera by the lack of leukocytosis, thrombocytosis, and splenomegaly and from patients with secondary erythrocytosis by the absence of diminished arterial oxygen concentrations; lesions that might cause renal hypoxia and resultant renal erythropoietin secretion must be excluded.

Erythropoietin is a 166-residue glycopeptide that has two or more carbohydrate chains which contribute almost half of its apparent molecular weight of about 39,000; it apparently has at least one internal disulfide bond and perhaps two.[302] Erythropoietin is synthesized in the liver of fetuses and neonates and in the kidney and liver of adults. It acts on responsive precursor cells in adult bone marrow and spleen to stimulate proliferation and differentiation into mature erythrocytes.

Bioactive or immunoreactive erythropoietin has been measured in tumor tissue, cyst fluid, and plasma from patients with a variety of tumors associated with erythrocytosis,[296–299,303–306] but the bioactive material sometimes appears to be immunologically distinct from erythropoietin.[304] A human mixed testicular germ cell tumor that consisted of embryonal and yolk sac carcinoma cells apparently produced not only α-fetoprotein and erythropoietin, but hemoglobin as well;[307] this tumor may have been stimulating its own erythroid differentiation. Messenger RNA from a renal tumor removed from a polycythemic patient produced a material with the biologic and physicochemical properties of erythropoietin when translated by microinjection into *Xenopus* oocytes.[308]

Erythropoietin concentrations in plasma, measured as an index of erythropoietin production, have been difficult to interpret. For example, serum erythropoietin levels, measured by a standard bioassay, were closely correlated with the presence of active disease in 36 patients with Wilms' tumor, despite the fact that Wilms' tumor is not associated with erythrocytosis,[309] but were not consistently elevated in patients with tumor-associated erythrocytosis.[310] Serum erythropoietin concentrations in patients with polycythemia vera are reported to be low when measured by bioassay[310] but normal when measured by radioimmunoassay,[311,312] while most patients with secondary polycythemia have elevated serum erythropoietin levels when measured by either assay.[310-312] Development of more sensitive and specific radioimmunoassays using antisera raised to synthetic fragments of erythropoietin[313] will, it is hoped, improve the ability of serum erythropoietin assays to establish the etiology of erythrocytosis.

Clinically, the major importance of tumor-associated erythrocytosis is as a clue to the presence of an otherwise occult tumor. Treatment of this syndrome is directed at the tumor. The polycythemia rarely needs treatment unless it is severe, in which case phlebotomy may be indicated.[301]

Placental Lactogen

The first case of ectopic secretion of placental lactogen (PL), or chorionic somatomammotropin, was described in 1966.[314] In a retrospective study of 295 patients with nontrophoblastic, nongonadal tumors,[315] about 9 percent had detectable PL in their plasma; most had lung carcinoma, but plasma PL has also been described in patients with carcinoma of the oropharynx, thyroid, breast, gastrointestinal tract, liver, kidney, ovary, testis, uterus, cervix, and vagina and with pheochromocytoma, carcinoid tumors, leukemia, lymphoma, and lymphosarcoma.[316,317]

As with other ectopic hormones, the frequency of PL detection depends upon where and how vigorously it is sought. Thus, in retrospective studies, plasma PL was elevated in only 14 percent of patients with breast cancer[318] and in only 16 percent of 135 patients with a variety of tumors,[317] whereas PL was detected by immunohistochemistry in tissue sections of 82 percent of a variety of tumors.[319] In any study, the frequency with which plasma PL is detected increases with increasing assay sensitivity. Also, the incidence may be lower in unbiased prospective studies than in biased retrospective ones. Furthermore, although PL is thought to be entirely absent from the plasma and tissues of nonpregnant women and normal men,[316] discovery of CG-like peptides in nontrophoblastic tissues suggests that caution is advisable in designating PL a specific tumor marker, as CG was previously thought to be.

Human placental lactogen has rather strong lactogenic activity but weak growth hormone activity. The plasma levels of immunoreactive PL in the plasma of patients with ectopic PL production are generally less than 5 percent of the levels of immunoreactive prolactin (PRL) in patients with galactorrhea due to PRL-secreting pituitary tumors. Galactorrhea has not been described in association with ectopic PL secretion, perhaps because ectopic PL may also be secreted in a high-molecular-weight, biologically inactive form. Gynecomastia is frequently observed but is probably due to tumor conversion of dehydroepiandrosterone to estradiol.

Prolactin

Increased serum bioactive PRL levels have been described in two patients, one with an undifferentiated lung carcinoma and the other with a renal carcinoma associated with galactorrhea.[320] Serum PRL fell after therapy in both patients, and medium in which renal carcinoma explants were grown in vitro contained bioactive PRL that was neutralized by a specific anti-PRL antibody. A small cell carcinoma of the lung has also been described in which PRL, six other hormones, and neurophysin were extracted from primary and metastatic tumor tissues from a patient in whom no clinical manifestations of PRL secretion were observed.[321] PRL has been demonstrated by immunocytochemistry in epithelial cells of the normal breast and prostate and in prostatic adenocarcinoma and infiltrating ductal carcinoma of the breast but not in colon carcinoma.[322] Since breast and prostate have receptors for PRL, this may represent another instance of autostimulation of tumor growth. There have been no reports of galactorrhea or increased plasma PRL levels in patients with these common tumors, despite the fact that an extensive effort has been made to implicate PRL in the etiology of breast cancer.

Renin

Renin is not a hormone but a renal enzyme that cleaves angiotensin I from circulating renin substrate or angiotensinogen (see Chap. 14). Renovascular hypertension is caused by increased renin production as a result of segmental or unilateral renal ischemia and is, therefore, the inappropriate result of a perfectly normal physiological response. The patients have increased peripheral plasma renin activity and secondary hyperaldosteronism. Hypertension caused by renin-secreting benign renal hemangiopericytomas (juxtaglomerular cell tumors), Wilms' tumors,[323] and clear cell renal carcinoma[324] has been recognized since 1967.[325] In fact, the association of Wilms' tumor and hypertension was first reported by Pincoffs and Bradley in 1937.[326] Most of these patients are young and have secondary hyperaldosteronism and hypokalemia. Renin production by most, if not all, renal tumors is probably best considered eutopic; immunocytochemical evidence has been reported for the presence of renin in normal brain, anterior pituitary, adrenal cortex, Leydig cells in the testis, follicular thyroid cells, and epithelial cells in the prostate.[327]

The first extrarenal tumor reported to contain renin was from a 38-year-old man with small cell lung carcinoma who had increased plasma renin activity and hypokalemic alkalosis without hypertension; there was no evidence of ectopic ACTH secretion.[328] In 1975, Genest et al. reported a 37-year-old woman with severe hypertension, a large, widely metastatic glandular adenocarcinoma of the lung, and severe hypokalemia; there was elevated plasma renin activity, 11-deoxycorticosterone, and aldosterone, as well as high renin activity in the primary tumor and its metastases, decreased renal cortical renin activity, and a decreased number of juxtaglomerular cells, which were devoid of granules.[329] Ectopic renin secretion has subsequently been reported in paraovarian carcinomas[330,331] and a pancreatic adenocarcinoma.[332] The levels of plasma renin activity can be extraordinarily high in patients with ectopic renin production, and, as in other hormone-secreting tumors, an unusually large proportion of the circulating peptide may be in the form of its precursor, which in this case is prorenin.[331] Both tumor prorenin and renin appear to be biologically, immunologically, and biochemically similar to the normal renal products.[331,333]

Ectopic renin production is a rare cause of hypertension. Treatment should be directed at the tumor, but captopril and other drugs useful in treating high-renin hypertension may be of value in controlling the hypertension and hypokalemia in these patients.

Gut-Brain Peptides

Gut-brain peptides are widely distributed in the gastrointestinal tract and brain. They include POMC, cholecystokinin, enkephalins, enteroglucagon, gastric inhibitory polypeptide, gastrin, glucagon, GRP, motilin, neurotensin, pancreatic polypeptide (PP), secretin, SRIH, substance P, and vasoactive intestinal polypeptide (VIP); insulin should probably also be included. The chemical structures, posttranslational modifications, and actions of these peptides are known, but the physiological significance of all but a few of them in either gastrointestinal or central nervous system function is unknown.

The syndromes of eutopic hypersecretion of gastrin (Zollinger-Ellison syndrome), glucagon (glucagonoma syndrome), somatostatin, and VIP (Verner-Morrison syndrome, pancreatic cholera, or the watery diarrhea-hypokalemia-achlorhydria or WDHA syndrome) are discussed elsewhere in this volume. These syndromes are also occasionally caused by ectopic secretion of the relevant peptides. The Zollinger-Ellison syndrome, which is due to pancreatic islet or, much less commonly, gastric or duodenal G cell tumors, has also been associated with duodenal carcinoid tumor,[334] hyperplastic parathyroid glands,[335] ovarian cystadenomas,[336] and pancreatic cystadenocarcinomas.[337] Islet cell tumors can be extrapancreatic and extraintestinal, but gastrin production by them is eutopic.[338] As in other ectopic hormonal syndromes, tumors of many patients without clinical symptoms also stain for gastrin.[18,339,340] The WDHA syndrome has been associated with elevated plasma or tumor concentrations of VIP in patients with squamous cell lung carcinoma, pancreatic islet cell tumors, ganglioneuromas, ganglioneuroblastomas, and pheochromocytomas,[21,341,342] although the tumors that were called pheochromocytomas were not associated with hypertension and were probably ganglioneuromas. VIP can also be found in many tumors, such as bronchogenic carcinomas, from patients who do not have the WDHA syndrome. The sequence of tumor VIP has been determined.[21]

Hypersecretion of most of the other gut-brain peptides has not been associated with specific clinical syndromes, but most if not all of these peptides have been found in some tumor (see, for example, Refs. 18, 19, and 340). A patient with hypersalivation apparently due to ectopic secretion of substance P by a laryngeal carcinoid tumor has been described,[343] although this symptom was not observed in other patients with elevated plasma substance P levels due to metastatic midgut carcinoids.[344] Fasting hyperglycemia in a cachectic man with a neurotensin-secreting bronchial adenocarcinoma has also been reported.[345] Eutopic PP-producing pancreatic islet cell tumors are thought to be clinically silent,[346] but a patient with PP-producing gastric tumor had flushing, tachycardia, lacrimation, and headache that may have been caused by extremely high plasma PP levels.[347] It is possible that, as other patients with pure gut-brain peptide–secreting tumors are observed, distinct clinical syndromes associated with elevated plasma levels of these peptides will be defined.

Other Humoral Factors

A variety of other humors, such as tumor angiogenesis factor, tumor necrosis factor, interleukins, an eosinophilopoietic factor, granulocytopoietic factors, an osteoblast-stimulating factor, a leukocyte chemotactic factor, and a hypotensive factor (perhaps prostaglandin A), have been described.[348–351] The exact nature of these humoral factors and their normal tissues of origin remain to be fully elucidated.

Other Paraneoplastic Syndromes

The mechanisms for a number of syndromes associated with neoplasia have not been defined, including the anorexia so frequently observed with even small tumors. An animal model for this syndrome is the rat, in which it appears that estrogen may be the responsible factor.[352] Tumor necrosis factor, which is also called cachectin, may cause the weight loss accompanying many malignant tumors by inhibiting the expression of lipogenic enzymes in adipocytes.[352a] Gastrin releasing peptide (GRP) is a possible candidate in other tumors. Fever is associated with a number of tumors, including breast cancer;[353] its cause is unknown. The mechanisms responsible for the hypertrichosis, polyneuropathy, edema, and hyperpigmentation associated with various tumors, most often myeloma, are also unknown,[354,355] although it has been suggested that malignant plasma cells are capable of accelerated conversion of androgen to estrogen.[356] Hypocalcemia and hypophosphatemia associated with malignant tumors is extremely rare but may be severe;[356a] it may be caused by osteoblast–stimulating factor.[351] It is possible that these and other syndromes are clinical caricatures caused by inappropriate secretion of known humoral factors or are caused by factors yet to be discovered.

Multiple Ectopic Hormones

Certain hormones are secreted in concert, both eutopically and ectopically, because they derive from common precursor molecules (e.g., POMC for ACTH, LPHs, MSHs, and endorphins; propressophysin for AVP and neurophysin II). Others appear to be secreted together frequently because their genetic expression is normally closely linked (e.g., the placental hormones and glycopeptide hormone subunits). Still others are often produced concomitantly for reasons that are not yet altogether clear (e.g., ACTH, AVP, CT, and GRP). However, synthesis of multiple hormones, both ectopic and, if the tumor is of neuroendocrine cell origin, eutopic, and of other nonhormonal proteins (e.g., carcinoembryonic antigen, α-fetoprotein, and placental alkaline phosphatase) by single tumors appears to be the rule rather than the exception.

ECTOPIC HORMONES AS TUMOR MARKERS

The reasonable assumption that early detection of the presence of a tumor might allow it to be located and eradicated by excision or other treatment and the clinical requirement for some quantitative, noninvasive means to evaluate the results of antitumor therapy and to detect tumor recurrence have led to a vast effort to identify specific tumor markers. The possibility of measuring circulating concentrations of hormones produced by tumors to achieve this purpose has historical precedents. Measurement of serum calcitonin under basal conditions and after provocative testing with calcium and pentagastrin infusions has permitted the identification of patients with medullary microcarcinomas of the thyroid and even premalignant C cell hyperplasia in kindreds affected by MEN 2 (see Chap. 28). These patients are cured of their disease by total thyroidectomy, in contrast to the inevitably malignant course of extrathyroidal medullary carcinoma. The measurement of plasma chorionic gonadotropin (CG) in patients with choriocarcinoma has made it possible to follow the results of therapy.[357] With the use of automated radioimmunoassays for CG and CG β-subunit, it has been estimated that as few as 1×10^6 cells (1 mm^3 of tumor mass) can be detected, since each tumor cell secretes about 1 pg of CG every 24 h and the circulating half-life of CG is several hours. At least 1×10^9 cells (1 cm^3 of tumor mass) are required for detection by the usual clinical or radiologic examination. Thus, measurement of ectopic hormones in plasma as a method for cancer screening, early detection, localization, and evaluation of therapy has undeniable appeal. However, it should be apparent that no known hormone has all the characteristics of an ideal tumor marker, as summarized in Table 29-5.

General Characteristics

No known hormone or hormone analogue seems to be secreted only by tumor cells, so one must always also consider normal endocrine tissue, nonendocrine tissue affected by a nonneoplastic process, or some other normal tissue as the possible source of immunoreactive peptide detected in the circulation. It was assumed, for example, that fetoplacental hormones

Table 29-5. Characteristics of an Ideal Tumor Marker

General:	
	Uniquely secreted or shed by tumor cells
	Measurable in circulating plasma
	Detectable in plasma when tumor mass is small
Screening:	
	Secreted by a wide variety of tumor types
	Secreted constantly by tumor cells
	Amenable to inexpensive, specific, accurate, large-scale, routine laboratory measurement
Localization:	
	Secreted by a single tumor type or a limited number of tumor types
	Detectable in high concentrations in tumor venous effluent plasma
	Detectable in tumor tissue by external sensors
Evaluation of therapy:	
	Secreted in amounts directly proportional to viable tumor cell number
	Rate of secretion by each cell constant throughout the course of disease
	Presence or onset of secretion has unique prognostic significance

and other polypeptides constituted ideal tumor markers, since they would presumably be totally absent in normal men and nonpregnant women. However, as discussed earlier, this appears not to be true; CG or CG-like material has been identified in endocrine and nonendocrine tissues in normal subjects. This is reminiscent of the experience with carcinoembryonic antigen (CEA), which was originally considered to be a specific marker for carcinoma of the colon. With early, insensitive plasma CEA assays there were few false-positive results, but many patients with proven colonic cancer had undetectable plasma CEA. However, as ever more sensitive assays were developed to identify these patients, patients with other neoplasms were found to have CEA in their plasma, patients with nonneoplastic gastrointestinal diseases were found to have detectable CEA, and, finally, CEA was found in the plasma of apparently normal subjects. Another example is α-fetoprotein, which is normally produced by fetal yolk sac endodermal cells. It was originally thought to be a specific marker for hepatic carcinomas and those pancreatic, gastric, and pulmonary adenocarcinomas that arose from tissues derived from yolk sac endoderm, but it has now been found in the serum of patients with other tumors and in that of normal subjects. Thus, although GRP or some other peptide may appear to be a specific tumor marker at present,[358] history tends to repeat itself, and caution is indicated.

Although all the hormones discussed can be assayed in plasma, most of them have a very short circulating half-life, usually measured in minutes, unlike CG in choriocarcinoma. Thus, either a much higher secretory rate or a much greater tumor mass is necessary to produce detectable levels in peripheral plasma.

Screening

No single hormone appears to be secreted ectopically with great frequency by a wide variety of tumors in quantities detectable in peripheral plasma; detection of immunoreactive or bioactive hormone in tumor tissue extracts is not equivalent to finding the hormone in measurable concentrations in circulating blood. This disadvantage theoretically could be overcome by using panels of several hormone radioimmunoassays, and there is evidence that this is useful,[2] but it increases the cost and complexity of the screening process.

Further complicating the screening process is the fact that the rate of tumor hormone synthesis tends to be more erratic than the rate of synthesis of normal endocrine tissue, and it may be frankly periodic.[11] Multiple samples may therefore be required to screen patients effectively.

Ironically, the hormones involved in the most frequently encountered ectopic hormonal syndromes—ACTH and other POMC peptides and AVP—have been among the most difficult for which to establish sensitive, specific, and reliable routine radioimmunoassays.

Localization

There is, as already noted, a tendency for certain types of tumor to secrete a specific hormone or related group of hormones. Unfortunately, this proclivity is not so constant as to allow definition of the site of origin of a tumor on the basis of hormone levels in peripheral blood.

The anatomic site of ectopic secretion of some hormones has been localized by assaying plasma obtained during percutaneous venous catheterization.[141,142] As in the case of the normal endocrine gland, secretion appears to be episodic and the half-life of peptide hormones is short, so care should be taken to obtain a simultaneous peripheral venous blood sample for each catheter sample. This will reduce the chance of misinterpreting as evidence of local secretion a transient general increase in circulating hormone level secondary to a secretory episode at a site remote from the catheter tip. It is also of paramount importance to place the catheter tip as close to the tumor as possible. Obviously, tumors drained by the pulmonary or splanchnic venous system may be inaccessible to percutaneous catheterization. Nevertheless, pancreatic tumors can sometimes be localized by left adrenal vein catheterization because of normal pancreatic venous anastomoses with the left adrenal venous circulation.

It may be possible to inject ^{131}I-labeled antibodies to ectopic hormones and localize tumors by external radionuclide photoscanning (radioimmunolocalization). This technique was employed in 17 patients with elevated plasma CEA due to a variety of tumors, using ^{131}I-labeled purified goat anti-CEA immunoglobulin.[359] It is not clear whether antibodies to hormones would be similarly effective, since CEA is presumably displayed on the surface of the tumor cell, accessible to injected antibody, but the hormone might not be. Alternatively, if promiscuous peptide hormone receptors exist on tumor cell membranes,[13] it might be possible to use labeled antihormone receptor immunoglobulin or even hormones themselves for the same purpose, the latter a diagnostic variation on the "sponge" hypothesis.[25]

Evaluation of Therapy

As with CEA, when a tumor produces a hormone in amounts detectable in peripheral plasma, measurement of plasma concentrations can be used to monitor the results of treatment. However, a direct relationship between tumor mass and peripheral hormone concentration rarely exists, perhaps reflecting variable hormone release as the result of intermittent tumor ischemia and necrosis on the one hand and tumor degradation of the hormone on the other. Furthermore, recurrent or metastatic tumors may not produce detectable levels of hormone, presumably reflecting ascendance of a nonproductive clone. When ectopic secretion is reduced by antitumor therapy, one can expect a period of recurrence during which ectopic secretion is masked by the background of eutopic secretion once again. Tumors sometimes even begin producing new hormones late in their course, and there is no evidence for constant long-term production of any tumor peptide. Thus, recurrent production of a tumor hormone marker after a remission is a useful qualitative indicator of tumor recurrence; failure to detect the hormone in plasma does not guarantee, however, that there is no regrowth of tumor.

It has been suggested, on the basis of immunocytochemistry studies, that absence of PL and another "pregnancy-specific" protein from the tumor tissue sections of breast cancer patients implied a significantly longer survival time than presence of these proteins.[360] This kind of correlation has not yet generally been sought in careful studies measuring peripheral blood hormone levels. However, it has already been noted that development of hypercalcemia is an ominous sign and that ectopic hormone secretion may begin late in the clinical course, both perhaps indicative of a more malignant phase of tumor behavior. It has also been reported that immunoreactive PL is found in the plasma of only those patients with malignant pancreatic islet cell tumors, not those with benign diseases. Thus, it is possible that detection of specific hormonal markers in the plasma of patients with certain tumors may offer a prognostic index of value in deciding, for example, how aggressive the therapeutic approach should be.

For all its limitations, measurement of ectopic hormones as tumor markers appears to be useful if the upper limits of normal are carefully defined, if specimens are obtained under conditions in which eutopic secretion is minimal, and if the technique is applied only as an intermediate screening procedure for high-risk patients, as a diagnostic test in selected patients, or as a localizing or monitoring procedure in patients whose tumors are known to secrete the peptides.

REFERENCES

1. Liddle GW, Nicholson WE, Island DP, Orth DN, Abe K, Lowder SC: Clinical and laboratory studies of ectopic humoral syndromes. *Recent Prog Horm Res* 25:283, 1969.

2. Blackman MR, Rosen SW, Weintraub BD: Ectopic hormones. *Adv Intern Med* 23:85, 1978.

3. Clements JA, Funder JW, Tracy K, Morgan FJ, Campbell DJ, Lewis P, Hearn MTW: Adrenocorticotropin, β-endorphin, and β-lipotropin in normal thyroid and lung: Possible implications for ectopic hormone secretion. *Endocrinology* 111:2097, 1982.

4. Saito E, Odell WD: Corticotropin/lipotropin common precursor–like material in normal rat extrapituitary tissues. *Proc Natl Acad Sci USA* 80:3792, 1983.

5. Rivier J, Spiess J, Thorner M, Vale W: Characterization of a growth hormone–releasing factor from a human pancreatic islet tumour. *Nature* 300:276, 1982.

6. Ling N, Esch F, Böhlen P, Brazeau P, Wehrenberg WB, Guillemin R: Isolation, primary structure, and synthesis of human hypothalamic somatocrinin: growth hormone–releasing factor. *Proc Natl Acad Sci USA* 81:4302, 1984.

7. Rees LH: Concepts in ectopic hormone production. *Clin Endocrinol* 5(suppl):363, 1976.

8. Imura H: Ectopic hormone syndromes. *Clin Endocrinol Metab* 9:235, 1980.

9. Baylin SB, Mendelsohn G: Ectopic (inappropriate) hormone production by tumors: Mechanisms involved and the biological and clinical implications. *Endocrine Rev* 1:45, 1980.

10. Samaan NA, Hickey RC, Sethi MR, Yang KP, Wallace S: Hypercalcemia in patients with known malignant disease. *Surgery* 80:382, 1976.

11. Bailey RE: Periodic hormonogenesis—a new phenomenon. *J Clin Endocrinol Metab* 32:317, 1971.

12. Garroway NW, Orth DN, Harrison RW: Binding of cytosol receptor–glucocorticoid complexes by isolated nuclei of glucocorticoid-responsive and nonresponsive cultured cells. *Endocrinology* 98:1092, 1976.

13. Katz MS, Kelly TM, Dax EM, Pineyro MA, Partilla JS, Gregerman RI: Ectopic β-adrenergic receptors coupled to adenylate cyclase in human adrenocortical carcinomas. *J Clin Endocrinol Metab* 60:900, 1985.

14. Seyberth HW, Segre GV, Hamet P, Sweetman BJ, Potts JT Jr, Oates JA: Characterization of the group of patients with the hypercalcemia of cancer who respond to treatment with prostaglandin synthesis inhibitors. *Trans Assoc Am Physicians* 89:92, 1976.

15. Orth DN, Liddle GW: Results of treatment in 108 patients with Cushing's syndrome. *N Engl J Med* 285:243, 1971.

16. Orth DN, Nicholson WE, Mitchell WM, Island DP, Liddle GW: Biologic and immunologic characterization and physical separation of ACTH and ACTH fragments in the ectopic ACTH syndrome. *J Clin Invest* 52:1756, 1973.

17. Ratcliffe JG, Knight RA, Besser GM, Landon J, Stansfeld AG: Tumour and plasma ACTH concentrations in patients with and without the ectopic ACTH syndrome. *Clin Endocrinol* 1:27, 1972.

18. Yang K, Ulich T, Taylor I, Cheng L, Lewin KJ: Pulmonary carcinoids: Immunohistochemical demonstration of brain-gut peptides. *Cancer* 52:819, 1983.

19. Kameya T, Shimosato Y, Kodama T, Tsumuraya M, Koide T, Yamaguchi K, Abe K: Peptide hormone production by adenocarcinomas of the lung: Its morphologic basis and histogenetic considerations. *Virchows Arch [Pathol Anat]* 400:245, 1983.

20. Charpin C, Andrac L, Monier-Faugere MC, Hassoun J, Cannoni M, Vagneur JP, Toga M: Calcitonin, somatostatin and ACTH immunoreactive cells in a case of familial bilateral thyroid medullary carcinoma. *Cancer* 50:1806, 1982.

21. Bunnett NW, Reeve JR Jr, Dimaline R, Shively JE, Hawke D, Walsh JH: The isolation and sequence analysis of vasoactive intestinal peptide from a ganglioneuroblastoma. *J Clin Endocrinol Metab* 59:1133, 1984.

22. Tashjian AH Jr, Weintraub BD, Barowsky NJ, Rabson AS, Rosen SW: Subunits of human chorionic gonadotropin: Unbalanced synthesis and secretion by clonal cell strains derived from a bronchogenic carcinoma. *Proc Natl Acad Sci USA* 70:1419, 1973.

23. Sorenson GD, Pettengill OS, Brinck-Johnsen T, Cate CC, Maurer LH: Hormone production by cultures of small-cell carcinoma of the lung. *Cancer* 47:1289, 1981.

24. Brahic M, Haase AT: Detection of viral sequences of low reiteration frequency by *in situ* hybridization. *Proc Natl Acad Sci USA* 75:6125, 1978.

25. Unger RH, Lochner JDeV, Eisentraut AM: Identification of insulin and glucagon in a bronchogenic metastasis. *J Clin Endocrinol Metab* 24:823, 1964.

26. DeBold CR, Schworer ME, Connor TB, Bird RE, Orth DN: Ectopic pro-opiolipomelanocortin: Sequence of cDNA coding for β-melanocyte-stimulating hormone and β-endorphin. *Science* 220:721, 1983.

27. Steenburgh PH, Höppener JWM, Zandberg J, Roos BA, Jansz HS, Lips CJM: Expression of proopiomelanocortin gene in human medullary thyroid carcinoma. *J Clin Endocrinol Metab* 58:904, 1984.

28. DuPont AG, Somers G, van Steirteghem AC, Warson F, VanHaelst L: Ectopic adrenocorticotropin production: Disappearance after removal of inflammatory tissue. *J Clin Endocrinol Metab* 58:654, 1984.

29. Simpson EL, Mundy GR, D'Souza SM, Ibbotson KJ, Bockman R, Jacobs JW: Absence of parathyroid hormone messenger RNA in nonparathyroid tumors associated with hypercalcemia. *N Engl J Med* 309:325, 1983.

30. Skrabanek P: "Ectopic" hormones in cancer: A reappraisal. *Irish J Med Sci* 149:181, 1980.

31. Odell WD, Wolfsen AR, Yoshimoto Y, Weitzman R, Fisher D, Hirose FM: Ectopic peptide synthesis: A universal concomitant of neoplasia. *Trans Assoc Am Physicians* 90:204, 1977.

32. Wolfsen AR, Odell WD: ProACTH: Use for early detection of lung cancer. *Am J Med* 66:765, 1979.

33. Azzopardi JG, Whittaker RS: Bronchial carcinoma and hypercalcemia. *J Clin Pathol* 22:718, 1969.

34. Gellhorn A: The unifying thread. *Cancer Res* 23:961, 1963.

35. Shields R: Gene derepression in tumours. *Nature* 269:752, 1977.

36. Quesenberry P, Levitt L: Hematopoietic stem cells. *N Engl J Med* 301:755, 819, 868, 1979.

37. Ponder BAJ, Schmidt GH, Wilkinson MM, Wood MJ, Monk M, Reid A: Derivation of mouse intestinal crypts from single progenitor cells. *Nature* 313:689, 1985.

38. Mackillop WJ, Ciampi A, Till JE, Buick RN: A stem cell model of human tumor growth: Implications for tumor cell clonogenic assays. *J Natl Cancer Inst* 70:9, 1983.

39. Gewirtz G, Yalow RS: Ectopic ACTH production in carcinoma of the lung. *J Clin Invest* 53:1022, 1974.

40. Ayvazian LF, Schneider B, Gewirtz G, Yalow RS: Ectopic production of big ACTH in carcinoma of the lung. *Am Rev Respir Dis* 111:279, 1975.

41. Vorherr H, Massry SG, Fallett R, Kaplan L, Kleeman CR: Antidiuretic principle in tuberculous lung tissue of a patient with pulmonary tuberculosis and hyponatremia. *Ann Intern Med* 72:383, 1970.

42. Azzopardi JG, Williams ED: Pathology of non-endocrine tumors associated with Cushing's syndrome. *Cancer* 22:274, 1968.

43. Weichert RF III: The neural ectodermal origin of the peptide-secreting endocrine glands. *Am J Med* 49:232, 1970.

44. Pearse AGE: The cytochemistry and ultrastructure of polypeptide hormone-producing cells of the APUD series and the embryologic, physiologic and pathologic implications of the concept. *J Histochem Cytochem* 17:303, 1969.

45. Pearse AGE, Takor Takor T: Neuroendocrine embryology and the APUD concept. *Clin Endocrinol* 5 (suppl):229, 1976.

46. Lloyd RV, Wilson BS: Specific endocrine tissue marker defined by a monoclonal antibody. *Science* 222:628, 1983.

47. Lehto V-P, Miettinen M, Dahl D, Virtanen I: Bronchial carcinoid cells contain neural-type intermediate filaments. *Cancer* 54:624, 1984.

48. Pearse AGE, Takor Takor T: Embryology of the diffuse neuroendocrine system and its relation to the common peptides. *Fed Proc* 38:2288, 1979.

49. Andrew A: An experimental investigation into the possible neural crest origin of pancreatic APUD (islet) cells. *J Embryol Exp Morphol* 35:577, 1976.

50. Pictet RL, Rall LB, Phelps P, Rutter WJ: The neural crest and the origin of the insulin-producing and other gastrointestinal hormone-producing cells. *Science* 191:191, 1976.

51. Fontaine J, Le Douarin NM: Analysis of endoderm formation in the avian blastoderm by the use of quail-chick chimeras: Problem of the neuroectodermal origin of the cells of the APUD series. *J Embryol Exp Morphol* 41:209, 1977.

52. Andrew A: APUD cells in the endocrine pancreas and the intestine of chick embryos. *Gen Comp Endocrinol* 26:485, 1975.

53. Cheng H, Leblond CP: Origin, differentiation and renewal of the four main epithelial cell types in the mouse intestine: V. Unitarian theory of the origin of the four epithelial cell types. *Am J Anat* 141:537, 1974.

54. Williams ED: Tumours, hormones, and cellular differentiation. *Lancet* 2:1108, 1969.

55. Bishop JM: Cancer genes come of age. *Cell* 32:1018, 1983.

56. Persson H, Hennighausen L, Taub R, DeGrado W, Leder P: Antibodies to human c-*myc* oncogene product: Evidence of an

evolutionarily conserved protein induced during cell proliferation. *Science* 225:687, 1984.

57. Leder P, Battey J, Lenoir G, Moulding C, Murphy W, Potter H, Stewart T, Taub R: Translocation among antibody genes in human cancer. *Science* 222:765, 1983.

58. Slamon DJ, Cline MJ: Expression of cellular oncogenes during embryonic and fetal development in the mouse. *Proc Natl Acad Sci USA* 81:7141, 1984.

59. Buick RN, Pollak MN: Perspective on clonogenic tumor cells, stem cells, and oncogenes. *Cancer Res* 44:4909, 1984.

60. Slamon DJ, deKernion JB, Verma IM, Cline MJ: Expression of cellular oncogenes in human malignancies. *Science* 224:256, 1984.

61. Rowley JD: Human oncogene locations and chromosome aberrations. *Nature* 301:290, 1983.

62. Chiu IM, Reddy EP, Givol D, Robbins KC, Tronick SR, Aaronson SA: Nucleotide sequence analysis identifies the human c-*sis* proto-oncogene as a structural gene for platelet-derived growth factor. *Cell* 37:123, 1984.

63. Josephs SF, Ratner L, Clarke MF, Westin EH, Reitz MS, Wong-Staal F: Transforming potential of human c-*sis* nucleotide sequences encoding platelet-derived growth factor. *Science* 225:636, 1984.

63a. Betsholtz C, Johnsson A, Heldin C-K, Westermark B, Lind P, Urdea MS, Eddy R, Shows TB, Philpott K, Mellor AL, Knott TJ, Scott J: cDNA sequence and chromosomal localization of human platelet-derived growth factor A-chain and its expression in tumour cell lines. *Nature* 320:695, 1986.

64. Downward J, Yarden Y, Mayes E, Scrace G, Totty N, Stockwell P, Ullrich A, Schlessinger J, Waterfield MD: Close similarity of epidermal growth factor receptor and v-*erb-B* oncogene protein sequences. *Nature* 307:521, 1984.

65. Levinson AD, Oppermann H, Varmus HE, Bishop JM: The purified product of the transforming gene of avian sarcoma virus phosphorylates tyrosine. *J Biol Chem* 255:11973, 1980.

66. Sugimoto Y, Whitman M, Cantley LC, Erikson RL: Evidence that the Rous sarcoma virus transforming gene product phosphorylates phosphatidylinositol and diacylglycerol. *Proc Natl Acad Sci USA* 81:2117, 1984.

67. Marquadt H, Hunkapillar MW, Hood LE, Twardzik DR, De Larco JE, Stephenson JR, Todaro GJ: Transforming growth factors produced by retrovirus-transformed rodent fibroblasts and human melanoma cells: Amino acid sequence homology with epidermal growth factor. *Proc Natl Acad Sci USA* 80:4684, 1983.

68. Sporn MB, Roberts AB, Wakefield LM, Assoian RK: Transforming growth factor-β: Biological function and chemical structure. *Science* 233:532, 1986.

69. Warner TFCS: Cell hybridization: An explanation for the phenotypic diversity of certain tumours. *Med Hypotheses* 1:51, 1975.

70. Fialkow PJ, Denman AM, Jacobson RJ, Lowenthal MN: Origin of some lymphocytes from leukemic stem cells. *J Clin Invest* 62:18, 1978.

71. Braunstein GD, Rasor J, Wade ME: Presence in normal human testes of a chorionic-gonadotropin-like substance distinct from human luteinizing hormone. *N Engl J Med* 293:1339, 1975.

72. Chen H-C, Hodgen GD, Matsuura S, Lin LJ, Gross E, Reichert LE Jr, Birken S, Canfield RE, Ross GT: Evidence for a gonadotropin from nonpregnant subjects that has physical, immunological, and biological similarities to human chorionic gonadotropin. *Proc Natl Acad Sci USA* 73:2885, 1976.

73. Yoshimoto Y, Wolfsen AR, Odell WD: Human chorionic gonadotropin-like substance in non-endocrine tissues of normal subjects. *Science* 197:575, 1977.

74. Ruff MR, Pert CB: Origin of human small cell lung cancer. *N Engl J Med* 229:680, 1985.

75. Lafferty FW: Pseudohyperparathyroidism. *Medicine* 45:247, 1966.

76. Zondek H, Petow H, Siebert W: Die Bedeutung der Calciumbestimmung im Blute für die Diagnose der Niereninsuffizienz. *Z Klin Med* 99:129, 1924.

77. Albright F: Case records of the Massachusetts General Hospital (Case 27461). *N Engl J Med* 225:789, 1941.

78. Loveridge N, Kent GN, Heath DA, Jones EL: Parathyroid hormone-like bioactivity in a patient with severe osteitis fibrosa cystica due to malignancy: Renotropic actions of a tumour extract as assessed by cytochemical bioassay. *Clin Endocrinol* 22:135, 1985.

79. Knill-Jones RP, Buckle RM, Parsons V, Calne RY, Williams R: Hypercalcemia and increased parathyroid-hormone activity in a primary hepatoma: Studies before and after hepatic transplantation. *N Engl J Med* 282:704, 1970.

80. Palmieri GMA, Nordquist RE, Omenn GS: Immunochemical localization of parathyroid hormone in cancer tissue. *J Clin Invest* 53:1726, 1974.

81. Mayes LC, Kasselberg AG, Roloff JS, Lukens JN: Hypercalcemia associated with immunoreactive parathyroid hormone in a malignant rhabdoid tumor of the kidney (rhabdoid Wilms' tumor). *Cancer* 54:882, 1984.

82. Greenberg PB, Martin TJ, Sutcliffe HS: Synthesis and release of parathyroid hormone by a renal carcinoma in cell culture. *Clin Sci Mol Med* 45:183, 1973.

83. Zidar BL, Shadduck RK, Winkelstein A, Zeigler Z, Hawker CD: Acute myeloblastic leukemia and hypercalcemia. *N Engl J Med* 295:692, 1976.

84. Benson RC Jr, Riggs BL, Pickard BM, Arnaud CD: Radioimmunoassay of parathyroid hormone in hypercalcemic patients with malignant disease. *Am J Med* 56:821, 1974.

85. Powell D, Singer FR, Murray TM, Minkin C, Potts JT Jr: Nonparathyroid humoral hypercalcemia in patients with neoplastic diseases. *N Engl J Med* 289:176, 1973.

86. Flueck JA, Di Bella FP, Edis AJ, Kehrwald JM, Arnaud CD: Immunoheterogeneity of parathyroid hormone in venous effluent serum from hyperfunctioning parathyroid glands. *J Clin Invest* 60:1367, 1977.

87. Mayer GP, Habener JF, Potts JT Jr: Parathyroid hormone secretion in vivo: Demonstration of a calcium-independent, nonsuppressible component of secretion. *J Clin Invest* 57:678, 1976.

88. Riggs BL, Arnaud CD, Pickard BM, Smith LH: Immunologic differentiation of primary hyperparathyroidism from hyperparathyroidism due to non-parathyroid cancer. *J Clin Invest* 50:2079, 1971.

89. Stewart AF, Insogna KL, Goltzman D, Broadus AE: Identification of adenylate cyclase–stimulating activity and cytochemical glucose-6-phosphate dehydrogenase-stimulating activity in extracts of tumors from patients with humoral hypercalcemia of malignancy. *Proc Natl Acad Sci USA* 80:1454, 1983.

90. Rodan SB, Insogna KL, Vignery AM-C, Stewart AF, Broadus AE, D'Souza SM, Bertolini DR, Mundy GR, Rodan GA: Factors associated with humoral hypercalcemia of malignancy stimulate adenylate cyclase in osteoblastic cells. *J Clin Invest* 72:1511, 1983.

90a. Rabbani SA, Mitchell J, Roy DR, Kremer R, Bennett HPJ, Goltzman D: Purification of peptides with parathyroid hormone-like bioactivity from human and rat malignancies associated with hypercalcemia. *Endocrinology* 118:1200, 1986.

91. Stewart AF, Vignery A, Silverglate A, Ravin ND, LiVolsi V, Broadus AE, Baron R: Quantitative bone histomorphometry in humoral hypercalcemia of malignancy: Uncoupling of bone cell activity. *J Clin Endocrinol Metab* 55:219, 1982.

91a. Broadus AE, Goltzman D, Webb AC, Kronenberg HM: Messenger ribonucleic acid from tumors associated with humoral hypercalcemia of malignancy directs the synthesis of a secretory parathyroid-like peptide. *Endocrinology* 117:1661, 1985.

92. Ralston SH, Fogelman I, Gardner MD, Dryburgh FJ, Cowan RA, Boyle IT: Hypercalcemia of malignancy: Evidence of a nonparathyroid humoral agent with an effect on renal tubular handling of calcium. *Clin Sci* 66:187, 1984.

93. Stewart AF, Horst R, Deftos LJ, Cadman EC, Lang R, Broadus AE: Biochemical evaluation of patients with cancer-associated hypercalcemia: Evidence for humoral and nonhumoral groups. *N Engl J Med* 303:1377, 1980.

94. Stewart AF, Romero R, Schwartz PE, Kohorn EI, Broadus AE: Hypercalcemia associated with gynecologic malignancies: Biochemical characterization. *Cancer* 49:2389, 1982.

94a. Merendino JJ Jr, Insogna KL, Milstone LM, Broadus AE, Stewart AF: A parathyroid hormone-like protein from cultured human keratinocytes. *Science* 231:388, 1986.

95. Tashjian AH Jr, Levine L: Epidermal growth factor stimulates prostaglandin synthesis and bone resorption in cultured mouse calvaria. *Biochem Biophys Res Commun* 85:966, 1978.

96. Tashjian AH Jr, Hohmann EL, Antoniades HN, Levine L: Platelet-derived growth factor stimulates bone resorption via a prostaglandin-mediated mechanism. *Endocrinology* 111:118, 1982.

97. Ibbotson KJ, Harrod J, Gowen M, D'Souza S, Smith DD, Winkler ME, Derynck R, Mundy GR: Human recombinant transforming growth factor α stimulates bone resorption and inhibits formation *in vitro*. *Proc Natl Acad Sci USA* 83:2228, 1986.

98. Ibbotson KJ, D'Souza SM, Ng KW, Osborne CK, Niall M, Martin TJ, Mundy GR: Tumor-derived growth factor increases bone resorption in a tumor associated with humoral hypercalcemia of malignancy. *Science* 221:1292, 1983.

99. Mundy GR, Ibbotson KJ, D'Souza SM: Tumor products and the hypercalcemia of malignancy. *J Clin Invest* 76:391, 1985.

99a. Tashjian AH Jr, Voelkel EF, Lazzaro M, Singer FR, Roberts AB, Derynck R, Winkler ME, Levine L: α and β human transforming growth factors stimulate prostaglandin production and bone resorption in cultured mouse calvaria. *Proc Natl Acad Sci USA* 82:2535, 1985.

100. Minkin C, Fredericks RS, Pokress S, Rude RK, Sharp CF Jr, Tong M, Singer FR: Bone resorption and humoral hypercalcemia of malignancy: Stimulation of bone resorption *in vitro* by tumor extracts is inhibited by prostaglandin synthesis inhibitors. *J Clin Endocrinol Metab* 53:941, 1981.

101. Sato K, Mimura H, Han DC, Kakiuchi T, Ueyama Y, Ohkawa H, Okabe T, Kondo Y, Ohsawa N, Tsushima T, Shizume K: Production of bone-resorbing activity and colony-stimulating activity in vivo and in vitro by a human squamous cell carcinoma associated with hypercalcemia and leukocytosis. *J Clin Invest* 78:145, 1986.

102. Klein DC, Raisz LG: Prostaglandins: Stimulation of bone resorption in tissue culture. *Endocrinology* 86:1436, 1970.

103. Tashjian AH Jr: Role of prostaglandins in the production of hypercalcemia by tumors. *Cancer Res* 38:4138, 1978.

104. Dowsett M, Easty GC, Powles TJ, Easty DM, Neville AM: Human breast tumour–induced osteolysis and prostaglandins. *Prostaglandins* 11:447, 1976.

105. Valentin-Opran A, Eilon G, Saez S, Mundy GR: Estrogens and antiestrogens stimulate release of bone resorbing activity by cultured human breast cancer cells. *J Clin Invest* 75:726, 1985.

106. Brenner D, Harvey HA, Lipton A, Demers L: A study of prostaglandin E_2, parathormone, and response to indomethacin in patients with hypercalcemia and malignancy. *Cancer* 49:566, 1982.

107. Horton JE, Raisz LG, Simmons HA, Oppenheim JJ, Mergenhagen SE: Bone resorbing activity in supernatant fluid from cultured human peripheral blood leukocytes. *Science* 177:793, 1972.

108. Mundy GR, Raisz LG, Cooper RA, Schechter GP, Salmon SE: Evidence for the secretion of an osteoclast stimulating factor in myeloma. *N Engl J Med* 291:1041, 1974.

109. Durie BGM, Salmon SE, Mundy GR: Relation of osteoclast activating factor production to the extent of bone disease in multiple myeloma. *Br J Haematol* 47:21, 1981.

110. Josse RG, Murray TM, Mundy GR, Jez D, Heersche JNM: Observations on the mechanism of bone resorption by multiple myeloma marrow culture fluids and partially purified osteoclast-activating factor. *J Clin Invest* 67:1472, 1981.

111. Raisz LG, Luben RA, Mundy GR, Dietrich JW, Horton JE, Trummel CL: Effect of osteoclast activating factor from human leukocytes on bone metabolism. *J Clin Invest* 56:408, 1975.

112. Mundy GR, Raisz LG: Big and little forms of osteoclast activating factor. *J Clin Invest* 60:122, 1977.

113. Nimberg RB, Humphries DE, Lloyd WS, Badger AM, Cooperband SR, Wells H, Schmid K: Isolation of a bone-resorptive factor from human cancer ascites fluid. *Cancer Res* 38:1983, 1978.

114. Gowen M, Wood DD, Ihrie EJ, McGuire MKB, Russell RGG: An interleukin 1 like factor stimulates bone resorption *in vitro*. *Nature* 306:378, 1983.

115. Mundy GR, Martin TJ: The hypercalcemia of malignancy: Pathogenesis and management. *Metabolism* 31:1247, 1982.

116. Adams JS, Singer FR, Gacad MA, Sharma OP, Hayes MJ, Vouros P, Holick MF: Isolation and structural identification of 1,25-dihydroxyvitamin D_3 produced by cultured alveolar macrophages in sarcoidosis. *J Clin Endocrinol Metab* 60:960, 1985.

117. Kozeny GA, Barbato AL, Bansal VK, Vertuno LL, Hano JE: Hypercalcemia associated with silicone-induced granulomas. *N Engl J Med* 311:1103, 1984.

118. Haddad JG, Couranz SJ, Avioli LV: Circulating phytosterols in normal females, lactating mothers, and breast cancer patients. *J Clin Endocrinol Metab* 30:174, 1970.

118a. Helikson MA, Havey AD, Zerwekh JE, Breslau NA, Gardner DW: Plasma-cell granuloma producing calcitriol and hypercalcemia. *Ann Intern Med* 105:379, 1986.

119. Breslau NA, McGuire JL, Zerwekh JE, Frenkel EP, Pak CYC: Hypercalcemia associated with increased serum calcitriol levels in three patients with lymphoma. *Ann Intern Med* 100:1, 1984.

120. Rosenthal N, Insogna KL, Godsall JW, Smaldone L, Waldron JA, Stewart AF: Elevations in circulating 1,25-dihydroxyvitamin D in three patients with lymphoma-associated hypercalcemia. *J Clin Endocrinol Metab* 60:29, 1985.

120a. Fetchick DA, Bertolini DR, Sarin PS, Weintraub ST, Mundy GR, Dunn JF: Production of 1,25-dihydroxyvitamin D_3 by human T cell lymphotrophic virus-I-transformed lymphocytes. *J Clin Invest* 78:592, 1986.

121. Shigeno C, Yamamoto I, Dokoh S, Hino M, Aoki J, Yamada K, Morita R, Kameyama M, Torizuka K: Identification of 1,24(R)-dihydroxyvitamin D_3–like bone-resorbing lipid in a patient with cancer-associated hypercalcemia. *J Clin Endocrinol Metab* 61:761, 1985.

122. Binstock ML, Mundy GR: Effects of calcitonin and glucocorticoids in combination on the hypercalcemia of malignancy. *Ann Intern Med* 93:269, 1980.

122a. O'Leary TJ, Jones G, Yip A, Lohnes D, Cohanim M, Yendt ER: The effects of chloroquine on serum 1,25-dihydroxyvitamin D and calcium metabolism in sarcoidosis. *N Engl J Med* 315:727, 1986.

122b. Glover D, Shaw L, Glick JH, Slatopolsky E, Weiler C, Attie M, Goldfarb S: Treatment of hypercalcemia in parathyroid cancer with WR-2721, S-2-(3-aminopropylamino)-ethyl-phosphorothioic acid. *Ann Intern Med* 102:55, 1985.

122c. Hirschel-Scholz S, Caverzasio J, Rizzoli R, Bonjour J-P: Normalization of hypercalcemia associated with a decrease in renal calcium reabsorption in Leydig cell tumor-bearing rats treated with WR-2721. *J Clin Invest* 78:319, 1986.

123. Jung A, Chantraine A, Donath A, van Ouwenaller C, Turnill D, Mermillod B, Kitler ME: Use of dichloromethylene diphosphonate in metastatic bone disease. *N Engl J Med* 308:1499, 1983.

124. Warrell RP Jr, Bockman RS, Coonley CJ, Isaacs M, Staszewski H: Gallium nitrate inhibits calcium resorption from bone and is effective treatment for cancer-related hypercalcemia. *J Clin Invest* 73:1487, 1984.

125. Meador CK, Liddle GW, Island DP, Nicholson WE, Lucas CP, Nuckton JG, Luetscher JA: Cause of Cushing's syndrome in patients with tumors arising from "nonendocrine" tissue. *J Clin Endocrinol Metab* 22:693, 1962.

126. Brown WH: A case of pluriglandular syndrome: "Diabetes of bearded women." *Lancet* 2:1022, 1928.

127. Salyer WR, Salyer DC, Eggleston JC: Carcinoid tumors of the thymus. *Cancer* 37:958, 1976.

128. Keusch G, Binswanger U, Dambacher MA, Fischer JA: Ectopic ACTH syndrome and medullary thyroid carcinoma. *Acta Endocrinol* 86:306, 1977.

129. Abe K, Adachi I, Miyakawa S, Tanaka M, Yamaguchi K, Tanaka N, Kameya T, Shimosato Y: Production of calcitonin, adrenocorticotropic hormone, and β-melanocyte-stimulating hormone in tumors derived from amine precursor uptake and decarboxylation cells. *Cancer Res* 37:4190, 1977.

130. Yamaguchi K, Abe K, Kameya T, Adachi I, Taguchi S, Otsubo K, Yanaihara N: Production and molecular size heterogeneity of immunoreactive gastrin-releasing peptide in fetal and adult lungs and primary lung tumors. *Cancer Res* 43:3932, 1983.

131. Price J, Nieuwenhuijzen Kruseman AC, Doniach I, Howlett TA, Besser GM, Rees LH: Bombesin-like peptides in human endocrine tumors: Quantitation, biochemical characterization, and secretion. *J Clin Endocrinol Metab* 60:1097, 1985.

132. Hansen M, Hammer M, Hummer L: Diagnostic and therapeutic implications of ectopic hormone production in small cell carcinoma of the lung. *Thorax* 35:101, 1980.

133. Bloomfield GA, Holdaway IM, Corrin B, Ratcliffe JG, Rees GM, Ellison M, Rees LH: Lung tumours and ACTH production. *Clin Endocrinol* 6:95, 1977.

134. Orwoll ES, Kendall JW: β-Endorphin and adrenocorticotropin in extrapituitary sites: Gastrointestinal tract. *Endocrinology* 107:438, 1980.

135. Evans CJ, Erdelyi E, Weber E, Barchas JD: Identification of proopiomelanocortin-derived peptides in the human adrenal medulla. *Science* 221:957, 1983.

136. Suda T, Tomori N, Tozawa F, Demura H, Shizume K, Mouri T, Miura Y, Sasano N: Immunoreactive corticotropin and corticotropin-releasing factor in human hypothalamus, adrenal, lung cancer, and pheochromocytoma. *J Clin Endocrinol Metab* 58:919, 1984.

137. Rosenberg EM, Hahn TJ, Orth DN, Deftos LJ, Tanaka K: ACTH-secreting medullary carcinoma of the thyroid presenting as severe idiopathic osteoporosis and senile purpura: Report of a case and review of the literature. *J Clin Endocrinol Metab* 47:255, 1978.

138. Bertagna C, Orth DN: Clinical and laboratory findings and results of therapy in 58 patients with adrenocortical tumors admitted to a single medical center (1951 to 1978). *Am J Med* 71:855, 1981.

139. Strott CA, Nugent CA, Tyler FH: Cushing's syndrome caused by bronchial adenomas. *Am J Med* 44:97, 1968.

140. Mason AMS, Ratcliffe JG, Buckle RM, Mason AS: ACTH secretion by bronchial carcinoid tumours. *Clin Endocrinol* 1:3, 1972.

141. Schteingart DE, Conn JW, Orth DN, Harrison TS, Fox FE, Bookstein JJ: Secretion of ACTH and MSH by an adrenal medullary paraganglioma. *J Clin Endocrinol Metab* 34:676, 1972.

142. Rees LH, Bloomfield GA, Gilkes JJH, Jeffcoate WJ, Besser GM: ACTH as a tumor marker. *Ann NY Acad Sci* 297:603, 1977.

143. Chrousos GP, Schulte HM, Oldfield EH, Gold PW, Cutler GB Jr, Loriaux DL: The corticotropin-releasing factor stimulation test: An aid in the evaluation of patients with Cushing's syndrome. *N Engl J Med* 310:622, 1984.

144. Yalow RS, Berson SA: Size heterogeneity of immunoreactive human ACTH in plasma and in extracts of pituitary glands and ACTH-producing thymoma. *Biochem Biophys Res Commun* 44:439, 1971.

145. Lowry PJ, Silas L, McLean C, Linton EA, Estivariz FE: Pro-γ-melanocyte-stimulating hormone cleavage in adrenal gland undergoing compensatory growth. *Nature* 306:70, 1983.

146. Carter RJ, Shuster S, Morley JS: Melanotropin potentiating factor is the C-terminal tetrapeptide of human β-lipotropin. *Nature* 279:74, 1979.

147. Orth DN, Nicholson WE: High molecular weight forms of human ACTH are glycoproteins. *J Clin Endocrinol Metab* 44:214, 1977.

148. Gewirtz G, Schneider B, Krieger DT, Yalow RS: Big ACTH: Conversion to biologically active ACTH by trypsin. *J Clin Endocrinol Metab* 38:227, 1974.

149. Orth DN, Nicholson WE: Different molecular forms of ACTH. *Ann NY Acad Sci* 297:27, 1977.

150. Ellison ML, Hillyard CJ, Bloomfield GA, Rees LH, Coombes RC, Neville AM: Ectopic hormone production by bronchial carcinomas in culture. *Clin Endocrinol* 5(suppl):397, 1976.

151. Bertagna XY, Nicholson WE, Sorenson GD, Pettengill OS, Mount CD, Orth DN: Corticotropin, lipotropin, and β-endorphin production by a human nonpituitary tumor in tissue culture: Evidence for a common precursor. *Proc Natl Acad Sci USA* 75:5160, 1978.

151a. Schworer ME, DeBold CR, Orth DN: Sequence of mRNA encoding ectopic proopiomelanocortin from a human small cell lung carcinoma maintained in tissue culture. *Endocrinology* 116(suppl): 163, 1985.

151b. de Keyzer Y, Bertagna X, Lenne F, Girard F, Luton J-P, Kahn A: Altered proopiomelanocortin gene expression in adrenocorticotropin-producing nonpituitary tumors. *J Clin Invest* 76:1892, 1985.

152. Odell WD, Wolfsen AR: Humoral syndromes associated with cancer: Ectopic hormone production. *Prog Clin Cancer* 8:57, 1982.

153. Ratcliffe JG, Podmore J, Stack BHR, Spilg WGS, Gropp C: Circulating ACTH and related peptides in lung cancer. *Br J Cancer* 45:230, 1982.

154. Hale AC, Ratter SJ, Tomlin SJ, Lytras N, Besser GM, Rees LH: Measurement of immunoreactive γ-MSH in human plasma. *Clin Endocrinol* 21:139, 1984.

155. Lowry PJ, Rees LH, Tomlin S, Gillies G, Landon J: Chemical characterization of ectopic ACTH purified from a malignant thymic carcinoid tumor. *J Clin Endocrinol Metab* 43:831, 1976.

156. Orth DN: Establishment of human malignant melanoma clonal cell lines that secrete ectopic adrenocorticotropin. *Nature* 242:26, 1973.

157. Hirata Y, Matsukura S, Imura H, Nakamura M, Tanaka A: Size heterogeneity of β-MSH in ectopic ACTH-producing tumors: Presence of β-LPH-like peptide. *J Clin Endocrinol Metab* 42:33, 1976.

158. Tanaka K, Nicholson WE, Orth DN: The nature of the immunoreactive lipotropins in human plasma and tissue extracts. *J Clin Invest* 62:94, 1978.

159. Abe K, Nicholson WE, Liddle GW, Island DP, Orth DN: Radioimmunoassay of β-MSH in human plasma and tissues. *J Clin Invest* 46:1609, 1967.

160. Gilkes JJH, Rees LH, Besser GM: Plasma immunoreactive corticotrophin and lipotrophin in Cushing's syndrome and Addison's disease. *Br Med J* 1:996, 1977.

161. Orth DN, Guillemin R, Ling N, Nicholson WE: Immunoreactive endorphins, lipotropins and corticotropins in a human nonpituitary tumor: Evidence for a common precursor. *J Clin Endocrinol Metab* 46:849, 1978.

162. Bertagna XY, Stone WJ, Nicholson WE, Mount CD, Orth DN: Simultaneous assay of immunoreactive β-lipotropin, γ-lipotropin, and β-endorphin in plasma of normal human subjects, patients with ACTH/lipotropin hypersecretory syndromes, and patients undergoing chronic hemodialysis. *J Clin Invest* 67:124, 1981.

163. Tanaka I, Nakai Y, Nakao K, Oki S, Yoshimasa T, Imura H: γ_1-Melanotropin-like immunoreactivity in bovine and human adrenocorticotropin-producing tissues. *J Clin Endocrinol Metab* 56:1080, 1983.

164. Pederson RC, Brownie AC, Ling N: Pro-adrenocorticotropin/endorphin–derived peptides: Coordinate action on adrenal steroidogenesis. *Science* 208:1044, 1980.

165. Abe K, Island DP, Liddle GW, Fleischer N, Nicholson WE: Radioimmunologic evidence for α-MSH (melanocyte stimulating

hormone) in human pituitary and tumor tissues. *J Clin Endocrinol Metab* 27:46, 1967.

166. Ratcliffe JG, Scott AP, Bennett HPJ, Lowry PJ, McMartin C, Strong JA, Walbaum PR: Production of a corticotrophin-like intermediate lobe peptide and of corticotrophin by a bronchial carcinoid tumour. *Clin Endocrinol* 2:51, 1973.

167. Shapiro M, Nicholson WE, Orth DN, Mitchell WM, Liddle GW: Differences between ectopic MSH and pituitary MSH. *J Clin Endocrinol Metab* 33:371, 1971.

168. Abe K, Nicholson WE, Liddle GW, Island DP, Orth DN: Radioimmunoassay of β-MSH in human plasma and tissues. *J Clin Invest* 46:1609, 1967.

169. Winkler AW, Crankshaw OF: Chloride depletion in conditions other than Addison's disease. *J Clin Invest* 17:1, 1938.

170. Schwartz WB, Bennett W, Curelop S, Bartter FC: A syndrome of renal sodium loss and hyponatremia probably resulting from inappropriate secretion of antidiuretic hormone. *Am J Med* 23:529, 1957.

171. Amatruda TT Jr, Mulrow PJ, Gallagher JC, Sawyer WH: Carcinoma of the lung with inappropriate antidiuresis. *N Engl J Med* 269:544, 1963.

172. Bartter FC, Schwartz WB: The syndrome of inappropriate secretion of antidiuretic hormone. *Am J Med* 42:790, 1967.

173. De Troyer A, Demanet JC: Clinical, biological and pathologic features of the syndrome of inappropriate secretion of antidiuretic hormone. *Q J Med* 180:521, 1976.

174. Vorherr H: Para-endocrine tumor activity with emphasis on ectopic ADH secretion. *Oncology* 29:382, 1974.

175. Hainsworth JD, Workman R, Greco FA: Management of the syndrome of inappropriate antidiuretic hormone secretion in small cell lung cancer. *Cancer* 51:161, 1983.

176. Østerlind K, Hansen M, Dombernowsky P: Hypouricemia and inappropriate secretion of antidiuretic hormone in small cell bronchogenic carcinoma. *Acta Med Scand* 209:289, 1981.

177. Land H, Schütz G, Schmale H, Richter D: Nucleotide sequence of cloned cDNA encoding bovine arginine vasopressin-neurophysin II precursor. *Nature* 295:299, 1982.

178. Yamaji T, Ishibashi M, Hori T: Propressophysin in human blood: A possible marker of ectopic vasopressin production. *J Clin Endocrinol Metab* 59:505, 1984.

179. Yamaji T, Ishibashi M, Yamada N, Kondo Y: Biosynthesis of the common precursor to vasopressin and neurophysin *in vitro* in transplantable human oat cell carcinoma of the lung with ectopic vasopressin production. *Endocrinol Jpn* 30:451, 1983.

180. Kondo Y, Mizumoto Y, Katayama S, Murase T, Yamaji T, Ohsawa N, Kosaka K: Inappropriate secretion of antidiuretic hormone in nude mice bearing a human bronchogenic oat cell carcinoma. *Cancer Res* 41:1545, 1981.

181. George JM, Capen CC, Phillips AS: Biosynthesis of vasopressin in vitro and ultrastructure of a bronchogenic carcinoma. *J Clin Invest* 51:141, 1972.

182. Vorherr H, Vorherr UF, McConnell TS, Goldberg NM, Kornfeld M, Jordan SW: Localization and origin of antidiuretic principle in para-endocrine-active malignant tumors. *Oncology* 29:201, 1974.

183. Pettengill OS, Faulkner CS, Wurster-Hill DH, Maurer LH, Sorenson GD, Robinson AG, Zimmerman EA: Isolation and characterization of a hormone-producing cell line from human small cell anaplastic carcinoma of the lung. *J Natl Cancer Inst* 58:511, 1977.

184. Spruce BA, Baylis PH: The regulation of vasopressin secretion in a patient with oat cell carcinoma of the bronchus. *Postgrad Med J* 59:246, 1983.

185. Russell JT, Brownstein MJ, Gainer H: Biosynthesis of vasopressin, oxytocin, and neurophysins: Isolation and characterization of two common precursors (propressophysin and prooxyphysin). *Endocrinology* 107:1880, 1980.

186. Wilson N, Ngsee J: Large oxytocin and antidiuretic hormone from bronchogenic carcinoma in man. *Horm Metab Res* 12:708, 1980.

187. Yamaji T, Ishibashi M, Katayama S: Nature of the immunoreactive neurophysins in ectopic vasopressin-producing oat cell carcinomas of the lung. *J Clin Invest* 68:388, 1981.

188. Marks LJ, Berde B, Klein LA, Roth J, Goonan SR, Blumen D, Nabseth DC: Inappropriate vasopressin secretion and carcinoma of the pancreas. *Am J Med* 45:967, 1968.

189. Legros JJ: The radioimmunoassay of human neurophysins: Contribution to the understanding of the physiopathology of neurohypophyseal function. *Ann NY Acad Sci* 248:281, 1975.

190. Decaux G, Unger J, Brimioulle S, Mockel J: Hyponatremia in the syndrome of inappropriate secretion of antidiuretic hormone: Rapid correction with urea, sodium chloride, and water restriction therapy. *JAMA* 247:471, 1982.

191. Wright PG, Laureno R, Victor M: Pontine and extrapontine myelinolysis. *Brain* 102:361, 1979.

192. Perks WH, Mohr P, Liversedge LA: Demeclocycline in inappropriate A.D.H. syndrome. *Lancet* 2:1414, 1976.

193. Decaux G, Waterlot Y, Genette F, Mockel J: Treatment of the syndrome of inappropriate secretion of antidiuretic hormone with furosemide. *N Engl J Med* 304:329, 1981.

194. Reeves RL, Tesluk H, Harrison CE: Precocious puberty associated with hepatoma. *J Clin Endocrinol Metab* 19:1651, 1959.

195. Masse SR, Dawson DT, Khaliq A: Ectopic gonadotropin in a case of anaplastic large-cell carcinoma of the lung. *Can Med Assoc J* 111:253, 1974.

196. Wilson TS, McDowell EM, McIntire R, Trump BF: Elaboration of human chorionic gonadotropin by lung tumors: An immunocytochemical study. *Arch Pathol Lab Med* 105:169, 1981.

197. Heitz PU, Kasper M, Klöppel G, Polak JM, Vaitukaitis JL: Glycoprotein-hormone alpha-chain production by pancreatic endocrine tumors: A specific marker for malignancy. *Cancer* 51:277, 1983.

198. Monteiro JCMP, Ferguson KM, McKinna JA, Greening WP, Neville AM: Ectopic production of human chorionic gonadotropin–like material by breast cancer. *Cancer* 53:957, 1984.

199. Blackman MR, Weintraub BD, Rosen SW, Kourides IA, Steinwascher K, Gail MH: Human placental and pituitary gonadotropin hormones and their subunits as tumor markers. A qualitative assessment. *J Natl Cancer Inst* 65:81, 1980.

200. Vaitukaitis JL: Secretion of human chorionic gonadotropin by tumors, in Lehmann FG (ed): *Carcino-embryonic Proteins: Chemistry, Biology, Clinical Applications.* New York, Elsevier/North-Holland, 1979, vol 1, pp 447–456.

201. Skrabanek P, Kirrane J, Powell D: A unifying concept of chorionic gonadotrophin production in malignancy. *Invest Cell Pathol* 2:75, 1979.

202. Nakagawara A, Ikeda K, Hayashida Y, Tsuneyoshi M, Enjoji M, Kawaoi A: Immunocytochemical identification of human chorionic gonadotropin- and alpha-fetoprotein-producing cells of hepatoblastoma associated with precocious puberty. *Virchows Arch [Pathol Anat]* 398:45, 1982.

203. Gadner H, Weber B, Riehm H: Adrenocortical carcinoma with ectopic LH production. *Z Kinderheilk* 118:63, 1974.

204. Kubo O, Yamasaki N, Kamijo Y, Amano K, Kitamura K, Demura R: Human chorionic gonadotropin produced by ectopic pinealoma in a girl with precocious puberty. *J Neurosurg* 47:101, 1977.

205. Kirschner MA, Cohen FB, Jespersen D: Estrogen production and its origin in men with gonadotropin-producing neoplasms. *J Clin Endocrinol Metab* 39:112, 1974.

206. Faiman C, Colwell JA, Ryan RJ, Hershman JM, Shields TW: Gonadotropin secretion from a bronchogenic carcinoma. *N Engl J Med* 277:1395, 1967.

207. Ghosh NK, Cox RP: Production of human chorionic gonadotropin in HeLa cell cultures. *Nature* 259:416, 1976.

208. Boothby M, Ruddon RW, Anderson C, McWilliams D, Boime I: A single gonadotropin α-subunit gene in normal tissue and tumor-derived cell lines. *J Biol Chem* 256:5121, 1981.
209. Sairam MR, Bhargavi GN: A role for glycosylation of the α subunit in transduction of biological signal in glycoprotein hormones. *Science* 229:65, 1985.
210. Masure HR, Jaffee WL, Sickel MA, Birken S, Canfield RE: Characterization of a small molecular size urinary immunoreactive human chorionic gonadotropin (hCG)–like substance produced by normal placenta and by hCG-secreting neoplasms. *J Clin Endocrinol Metab* 53:1014, 1981.
211. Cole LA, Birken S, Sutphen S, Hussa RO, Pattillo RA: Absence of the COOH-terminal peptide on ectopic human chorionic gonadotropin β-subunit (hCGβ). *Endocrinology* 110:2198, 1982.
212. Fein HG, Rosen SW, Weintraub BD: Increased glycosylation of serum human chorionic gonadotropin and subunits from eutopic and ectopic sources: Comparison with placental and urinary forms. *J Clin Endocrinol Metab* 50:1111, 1980.
212a. Nishimura R, Shin J, Ji I, Middaugh CR, Kruggel W, Lewis RV, Ji TH: A single amino acid substitution in an ectopic α subunit of a human chorionic gonadotropin. *J Biol Chem* 261:10475, 1986.
213. Yoshimoto Y, Wolfsen AR, Odell WD: Glycosylation, a variable in the production of hCG by cancers. *Am J Med* 67:414, 1979.
214. Cole LA, Hussa RO: Use of glycosidase digested human chorionic gonadotropin β-subunit to explain the partial binding of ectopic glycoprotein hormones to Con A. *Endocrinology* 109:2276, 1981.
214a. Hussa RO, Fein HG, Pattillo RA, Nagelberg SB, Rosen SW, Weintraub BD, Perini F, Ruddon RW, Cole LA: A distinctive form of human chorionic gonadotropin β-subunit-like material produced by cervical carcinoma cells. *Cancer Res* 46:1948, 1986.
214b. Nagelberg SB, Cole LA, Rosen SW: A novel form of ectopic human chorionic gonadotrophin β-subunit in the serum of a woman with epidermoid cancer. *J Endocrinol* 107:403, 1985.
215. Weintraub BD, Stannard BS, Rosen SW: Combination of ectopic and standard human glycoprotein hormone alpha with beta subunits: Discordance of immunologic and receptor-binding activity. *Endocrinology* 101:225, 1977.
216. Kuppermann HS, Epstein JA: Hormone changes in pregnancy, in Velardo JT (ed): *Essentials of Human Reproduction: Clinical Aspects, Normal and Abnormal.* New York, Oxford University Press, 1958, pp 88–100.
217. Hennen G, Pierce JG, Freychet P: Human chorionic thyrotropin: Further characterization and study of its secretion during pregnancy. *J Clin Endocrinol Metab* 29:581, 1969.
218. Odell WD, Bates RW, Rivlin RS, Lipsett MB, Hertz R: Increased thyroid function without clinical hyperthyroidism in patients with choriocarcinoma. *J Clin Endocrinol Metab* 23:658, 1963.
219. Cave WT Jr, Dunn JT: Choriocarcinoma with hyperthyroidism: Probable identity of the thyrotropin with human chorionic gonadotropin. *Ann Intern Med* 85:60, 1976.
220. Kenimer JG, Hershman JW, Higgins HP: The thyrotropin in hydatidiform moles is human chorionic gonadotropin. *J Clin Endocrinol Metab* 40:482, 1975.
221. Nisula BC, Ketelslegers J-M: Thyroid-stimulating activity and chorionic gonadotropin. *J Clin Invest* 54:494, 1974.
222. Pekonen F, Weintraub BD: Interaction of crude and pure chorionic gonadotropin with the thyrotropin receptor. *J Clin Endocrinol Metab* 50:280, 1980.
223. Ashitaka Y, Mochizuki M, Tojo S: Purification and properties of chorionic gonadotropin from the trophoblastic tissue of hydatidiform mole. *Endocrinology* 90:609, 1972.
224. Nadler WH, Wolfer JA: Hepatogenic hypoglycemia associated with primary liver carcinoma. *Arch Intern Med* 44:700, 1929.
225. Anderson N, Lokich JJ: Mesenchymal tumors associated with hypoglycemia. *Cancer* 44:785, 1979.
226. Steinke J: Hypoglycemia, in Marble A, White P, Bradley RF, Krall LP (eds): *Joslin's Diabetes Mellitus,* 11th ed. Philadelphia, Lea & Febiger, 1971, pp 797–817.
227. Shetty MR, Boghossian HM, Duffell D, Freel R, Gonzales JC: Tumor-induced hypoglycemia: A result of ectopic insulin production. *Cancer* 49:1920, 1982.
228. Smith NL, Janelli DE, Madariaga J: Hypoglycemia and Hodgkin's disease with hyperinsulinemia. *J Surg Oncol* 19:27, 1982.
229. Briselli MB, Mark EJ, Dickersin GR: Solitary fibrous tumors of the pleura: Eight new cases and review of 360 cases in the literature. *Cancer* 47:2678, 1981.
230. Honicky RE, dePapp EW: Mediastinal teratoma with endocrine function. *Am J Dis Child* 126:650, 1973.
231. Skrabanek P, Powell D: Ectopic insulin and Occam's razor: Reappraisal of the riddle of tumour hypoglycemia. *Clin Endocrinol* 9:141, 1978.
232. Nelson R, Burman SO, Kiani R, Chertow BS, Shah J, Cantave I: Hypoglycemic coma associated with benign pleural mesothelioma. *J Thorac Cardiovasc Surg* 69:306, 1975.
233. Rees LH, Ratcliffe JG: Ectopic hormone production by nonendocrine tumours. *Clin Endocrinol* 3:263, 1974.
234. Ha K, Ikeda T, Okada S, Inui K, Tagawa T, Takada K, Uchimura N, Kakudo K, Okada A, Yabuuchi H: Hypoglycemia in a child with hepatoblastoma. *Med Pediatr Oncol* 8:335, 1980.
235. Rosenzweig JL, Havrankova J, Lesniak MA, Brownstein M, Roth J: Insulin is ubiquitous in extrapancreatic tissues of rats and humans. *Proc Natl Acad Sci USA* 77:572, 1980.
236. Oelz O, Froesch ER, Bünzli HF, Humbel RE, Ritschard WJ: Antibody-suppressible and nonsuppressible insulin-like activities, in Steiner DF, Freinkel N (eds): *Handbook of Physiology.* Washington, American Physiological Society, 1972, sec 7, vol I, pp 685–702.
237. Field JB, Keen H, Johnson P: Insulin-like activity of nonpancreatic tumors associated with hypoglycemia. *J Clin Endocrinol Metab* 23:1229, 1963.
238. Gorden P, Hendricks CM, Kahn CR, Megyesi K, Roth J: Hypoglycemia associated with non-islet-cell tumor and insulin-like growth factors. *N Engl J Med* 305:1452, 1981.
239. Daughaday WH, Trivedi B, Kapadia M: Measurement of insulin-like growth factor II by a specific radioreceptor assay in serum of normal individuals, patients with abnormal growth hormone secretion and patients with tumor-associated hypoglycemia. *J Clin Endocrinol Metab* 53:289, 1981.
240. Froesch ER, Zapf J, Widmer U: Hypoglycemia associated with non-islet-cell tumor and insulin-like growth factors. *N Engl J Med* 306:1178, 1982.
241. Widmer U, Zapf J, Froesch ER: Is extrapancreatic tumor hypoglycemia associated with elevated levels of insulin-like growth factor II? *J Clin Endocrinol Metab* 55:833, 1982.
242. Yamanouchi T, Akanuma Y, Tsushima T, Shizume K, Mizoguchi H, Takaku F: New powerful insulin-like protein from human promyelocytic leukemia cells. *J Clin Endocrinol Metab* 114:1352, 1984.
242a. Stuart CA, Prince MJ, Peters EJ, Smith FE, Townsend CM III, Poffenbarger PL: Insulin receptor proliferation: A mechanism for tumor-associated hypoglycemia. *J Clin Endocrinol Metab* 63:879, 1986.
243. McCance RA: Osteomalacia with Looser's nodes (Milkman's syndrome) due to a raised resistance to vitamin D acquired about the age of 15 years. *Q J Med* 16:33, 1947.
244. Prader VA, Illig R, Uehlinger E, Stadler G: Rachitis infolge Knochentumors. *Helv Paediatr Acta* 14:554, 1959.
245. Ryan EA, Reiss E: Oncogenous osteomalacia: Review of the world literature of 42 cases and report of two new cases. *Am J Med* 77:501, 1984.
246. Lyles KW, Berry WR, Haussler M, Harrelson JM, Drezner

MK: Hypophosphatemic osteomalacia: Association with prostatic carcinoma. *Ann Intern Med* 93:275, 1980.

247. Taylor HA, Fallon MD, Velasco ME: Oncogenic osteomalacia and inappropriate antidiuretic hormone secretion due to oat-cell carcinoma. *Ann Intern Med* 101:786, 1984.

248. Saville PD, Nassim JR, Stevenson FH, Mulligan L, Carey M: Osteomalacia in Von Recklinghausen's neurofibromatosis. *Br Med J* 1:1311, 1955.

249. Aschinberg LC, Solomon LM, Zeis PM, Justice P, Rosenthal IM: Vitamin D–resistant rickets associated with epidermal nevus syndrome: Demonstration of a phosphaturic substance in the dermal lesions. *J Pediatr* 91:56, 1977.

249a. Seshadri MS, Cornish CJ, Mason RS, Posen S: Parathyroid hormone-like bioactivity in tumours from patients with oncogenic osteomalacia. *Clin Endocrinol* 23:689, 1985.

250. Milhaud G, Calmettes C, Raymond JP: Carcinoide sécrétant de la thyrocalcitonine. *C R Acad Sci [D] (Paris)* 270:2195, 1970.

251. Roos BA, Lindall AW, Baylin SB, O'Neil JA, Frelinger AL, Birnbaum RS, Lambert PW: Plasma immunoreactive calcitonin in lung cancer. *J Clin Endocrinol Metab* 50:659, 1980.

252. Schwartz KE, Wolfsen AR, Forster B, Odell WD: Calcitonin in nonthyroidal cancer. *J Clin Endocrinol Metab* 49:438, 1979.

253. Wallach SR, Royston I, Taetle R, Wohl H, Deftos LJ: Plasma calcitonin as a marker of disease activity in patients with small cell carcinoma of the lung. *J Clin Endocrinol Metab* 53:602, 1981.

254. Luster W, Gropp C, Sostmann H, Kalbfleisch H, Havemann K: Demonstration of immunoreactive calcitonin in sera and tissues of lung cancer patients. *Eur J Cancer Clin Oncol* 18:1275, 1982.

255. Becker KL, Nash DR, Silva OL, Snider RH, Moore CF: Urine calcitonin levels in patients with bronchogenic carcinoma. *JAMA* 243:670, 1980.

256. Samaan NA, Castillo S, Schultz PN, Khalil KG, Johnston DA: Serum calcitonin after pentagastrin stimulation in patients with bronchogenic and breast cancer compared to that in patients with medullary thyroid carcinoma. *J Clin Endocrinol Metab* 51:237, 1980.

257. Foa R, Oscier DG, Hillyard CJ, Incarbone E, McIntyre I: Production of immunoreactive calcitonin by myeloid leukaemia cells. *Br J Haematol* 50:215, 1982.

258. Pflüger K-H, Gropp C, Havemann K: Ectopically produced calcitonin in human hemoblastoses. *Klin Wochenschr* 60:667, 1982.

259. Zajac JD, Martin TJ, Hudson P, Niall H, Jacobs JW: Biosynthesis of calcitonin by human lung cancer cells. *Endocrinology* 116:749, 1985.

260. Greenberg PB, Beck C, Martin TJ, Burger HG: Synthesis and release of human growth hormone from lung carcinoma in cell culture. *Lancet* 1:350, 1972.

261. Melmed S, Ezrin C, Kovacs K, Goodman RS, Frohman LA: Acromegaly due to secretion of growth hormone by an ectopic pancreatic islet-cell tumor. *N Engl J Med* 312:9, 1985.

262. Kyle CV, Evans MC, Odell WD: Growth hormone–like material in normal human tissues. *J Clin Endocrinol Metab* 53:1138, 1981.

263. Dabek JT: Bronchial carcinoid tumor with acromegaly in two patients. *J Clin Endocrinol Metab* 38:329, 1974.

264. Sönksen PH, Ayres AB, Braimbridge M, Corrin B, Davies DR, Jeremiah GM, Oaten SW, Lowy C, West TET: Acromegaly caused by carcinoid tumours. *Clin Endocrinol* 5:503, 1976.

265. Zafar MS, Mellinger RC, Fine G, Szabo M, Frohman LA: Acromegaly associated with a bronchial carcinoid tumor: Evidence for ectopic production of growth hormone–releasing activity. *J Clin Endocrinol Metab* 44:66, 1979.

266. Shalet SM, Beardwell CG, MacFarlane IA, Ellison ML, Norman CM, Rees LH, Hughes M: Acromegaly due to production of a growth hormone releasing factor by a bronchial carcinoid tumour. *Clin Endocrinol* 10:61, 1979.

267. Leveston SA, McKeel DW Jr, Buckley PJ, Deschryver K, Greider MH, Jaffe BM, Daughaday WH: Acromegaly and Cushing's syndrome associated with a foregut carcinoid tumor. *J Clin Endocrinol Metab* 53:682, 1981.

268. Thorner MO, Perryman RL, Cronin MJ, Rogol AD, Draznin M, Johanson A, Vale W, Horvath E, Kovacs K: Somatotroph hyperplasia: Successful treatment of acromegaly by removal of a pancreatic islet cell tumor secreting a growth hormone–releasing factor. *J Clin Invest* 70:965, 1982.

269. Spero M, White EA: Resolution of acromegaly, amenorrhea-galactorrhea syndrome, and hypergastrinemia after resection of jejunal carcinoid. *J Clin Endocrinol Metab* 60:392, 1985.

270. Schulte HM, Benker G, Windek R, Olbricht T, Reinwein D: Failure to respond to growth hormone releasing hormone (GHRH) in acromegaly due to a GHRH secreting pancreatic tumor: Dynamics of multiple endocrine testing. *J Clin Endocrinol Metab* 61:585, 1985.

271. Thorner MO, Frohman LA, Leong DA, Thominet J, Downs T, Hellmann P, Chitwood J, Vaughan JM, Vale W: Extrahypothalamic growth hormone–releasing factor (GRF) secretion is a rare cause of acromegaly: Plasma GRF levels in 177 acromegalic patients. *J Clin Endocrinol Metab* 59:846, 1984.

272. Penny ES, Penman E, Price J, Rees LH, Sopwith AM, Wass JAH, Lytras N, Besser GM: Circulating growth hormone releasing factor concentrations in normal subjects and patients with acromegaly. *Br Med J* 289:453, 1984.

273. Mayo KE, Vale W, Rivier J, Rosenfeld MG, Evans RM: Expression-cloning and sequence of a cDNA encoding growth hormone–releasing factor. *Nature* 306:86, 1983.

274. Yamaguchi K, Abe K, Suzuki M, Adachi I, Kimura S, Shimada A, Ohno H, Kanai A, Kameya T: Production of immunoreactive pancreatic growth hormone–releasing factor in small cell carcinoma of the lung. *Gann* 74:814, 1983.

275. Asa SL, Kovacs K, Thorner MO, Leong DA, Rivier J, Vale W: Immunohistological localization of growth hormone–releasing hormone in human tumors. *J Clin Endocrinol Metab* 60:423, 1985.

276. Asa SL, Scheithauer BW, Bilbao JM, Horvath E, Ryan N, Kovacs K, Randall RV, Laws ER Jr, Singer W, Linfoot JA, Thorner MO, Vale W: A case of hypothalamic acromegaly: A clinicopathological study of six patients with hypothalamic gangliocytomas producing growth hormone–releasing factor. *J Clin Endocrinol Metab* 58:796, 1984.

277. Upton GV, Amatruda TT Jr: Evidence for the presence of tumor peptides with corticotropin-releasing factor–like activity in the ectopic ACTH syndrome. *N Engl J Med* 285:419, 1971.

278. Yamamoto H, Hirata Y, Matsukura S, Nakamura M, Tanaka A: Studies on ectopic ACTH-producing tumors: IV. CRF-like activity in tumor tissue. *Acta Endocrinol (Kbh)* 82:183, 1976.

279. Suda T, Demura H, Demura R, Wakabayashi I, Nomura K, Odagiri E, Shizume K: Corticotropin-releasing factor–like activity in ACTH producing tumors. *J Clin Endocrinol Metab* 44:440, 1977.

280. Carey RM, Varna SK, Drake CR, Thorner MO, Kovacs K, Rivier J, Vale W: Ectopic secretion of corticotropin-releasing factor as a cause of Cushing's syndrome. *N Engl J Med* 311:13, 1984.

281. Belsky JL, Cuello B, Swanson LW, Simmons DM, Jarrett RM, Braza F: Cushing's syndrome due to ectopic production of corticotropin-releasing factor. *J Clin Endocrinol Metab* 60:496, 1985.

281a. Zárate A, Kovacs K, Flores M, Morán C, Félix I: ACTH and CRF-producing bronchial carcinoid associated with Cushing's syndrome. *Clin Endocrinol* 24:523, 1986.

281b. Schteingart DE, Lloyd RV, Akil H, Chandler WF, Ibarra-Perez G, Rosen SG, Ogletree R: Cushing's syndrome secondary to ectopic corticotropin-releasing hormone-adrenocorticotropin secretion. *J Clin Endocrinol Metab* 63:770, 1986.

281c. Cunnah D, Jessop DS, Millar JGB, Neville E, Coates P, Doniach I, Hale AC, Besser GM, Rees LH: An adrenal medullary tumour presenting with Cushing's syndrome associated with elevated levels of human corticotrophin-releasing factor in plasma. *Endocrinology* 108(suppl):272, 1986.

282. Asa SL, Kovacs K, Tindall GT, Barrow DL, Horvath E, Vecsei P: Cushing's disease associated with an intrasellar gangliocytoma producing corticotrophin-releasing factor. *Ann Intern Med* 101:789, 1984.

283. Wilber JF, Spinella P: Identification of immunoreactive thyrotropin-releasing hormone in human neoplasia. *J Clin Endocrinol Metab* 59:432, 1984.

284. Szabo M, Berelowitz M, Pettengill OS, Sorenson GD, Frohman LA: Ectopic production of somatostatin-like immuno- and bioactivity by cultured human pulmonary small cell carcinoma. *J Clin Endocrinol Metab* 51:978, 1980.

285. Penman E, Wass JAH, Besser GM, Rees LH: Somatostatin secretion by lung and thymic tumours. *Clin Endocrinol* 13:613, 1980.

286. Spindel ER, Chin WW, Price J, Rees LH, Besser GM, Habener JF: Cloning and characterization of cDNAs encoding human gastrin-releasing peptide. *Proc Natl Acad Sci USA* 81:5699, 1984.

287. Tsutsumi Y, Osamura Y, Watanabe K, Yanaihara N: Immunohistochemical studies on gastrin-releasing peptide- and adrenocorticotropic hormone–containing cells in the human lung. *Lab Invest* 48:623, 1983.

288. Roth KA, Evans CJ, Weber E, Barchas JD, Bostwick DG, Bensch KG: Gastrin-releasing peptide-related peptides in a human malignant lung carcinoid tumor. *Cancer Res* 43:5411, 1983.

289. Bostwick DG, Roth KA, Barchas JD, Bensch KG: Gastrin-releasing peptide immunoreactivity in intestinal carcinoids. *Am J Clin Pathol* 82:428, 1984.

290. Howlett TA, Price J, Hale AC, Doniach I, Rees LH, Wass JAH, Besser GM: Pituitary ACTH dependent Cushing's syndrome due to ectopic production of a bombesin-like peptide by a medullary carcinoma of the thyroid. *Clin Endocrinol* 22:91, 1985.

290a. Sausville EA, Lebacq-Verheyden A-M, Spindel ER, Cuttitta F, Gazdar AF, Battey JF: Expression of the gastrin-releasing peptide gene in human small cell lung cancer. *J Biol Chem* 261:2451, 1986.

291. Hale AC, Price J, Ackland JF, Doniach I, Ratter S, Besser GM, Rees LH: Corticotrophin releasing factor–mediated ACTH release from rat anterior pituitary cells is potentiated by C-terminal gastrin releasing peptide. *J Endocrinol* 102:R1, 1984.

292. Moody TW, Bertness V, Carney DN: Bombesin-like peptides and receptors in human tumor cell lines. *Peptides* 4:683, 1983.

293. Willey JC, Lechner JF, Harris CC: Bombesin and the C-terminal tetradecapeptide of gastrin-releasing peptide are growth factors for normal human bronchial epithelial cells. *Exp Cell Res* 153:245, 1984.

294. Kameya T, Bessho T, Tsumuraya M, Yamaguchi K, Abe K, Shimosato Y, Yanaihara N: Production of gastrin releasing peptide by medullary carcinoma of the thyroid. *Virchows Arch [Pathol Anat]* 401:98, 1983.

295. Sorenson GD, Pettengill OS, Cate CC, Ghatei MA, Bloom SR: Modulation of bombesin and calcitonin secretion in cultures of small cell carcinoma of the lung, in Becker KL, Gazdar A (eds): *The Endocrine Lung in Health and Disease.* Philadelphia, Saunders, 1984, pp 596–602.

296. Hammond D, Winnick S: Paraneoplastic erythrocytosis and ectopic erythropoietins. *Ann NY Acad Sci* 230:219, 1974.

297. Wrigley PFM, Malpas JS, Turnbull AL, Jenkins GC, McArt A: Secondary polycythemia due to a uterine fibromyoma producing erythropoietin. *Br J Haematol* 21:551, 1971.

298. Ghio R, Haupt E, Ratti M, Boccaccio P: Erythrocytosis associated with a dermoid cyst of the ovary and erythropoietic activity of the tumour fluid. *Scand J Haematol* 27:70, 1981.

299. Montag TW, Murphy RE, Belinson JL: Virilizing malignant lipid cell tumor producing erythropoietin. *Gynecol Oncol* 19:98, 1984

300. Doll DC, Weiss RB: Neoplasia and the erythron. *J Clin Oncol* 3:429, 1985.

301. Golde DW, Hocking WG, Koeffler HP, Adamson JW: Polycythemia: Mechanisms and management. *Ann Intern Med* 95:71, 1981.

302. Jacobs K, Shoemaker C, Rudersdorf R, Neill SD, Kaufman RJ, Mufson A, Seehra J, Jones SS, Hewick R, Fritsch EF, Kawakita M, Shimizu T, Miyake T: Isolation and characterization of genomic and cDNA clones of human erythropoietin. *Nature* 313:806, 1985.

303. Jeffreys RV, Napier JAF, Reynolds SH: Erythropoietin levels in posterior fossa haemangioblastoma. *J Neurol Neurosurgy Psychiatry* 45:264, 1982.

304. Sytkowski AJ, Bicknell KA, Smith GM, Garcia JF: Secretion of erythropoietin-like activity by clones of human renal carcinoma cell line GKA. *Cancer Res* 44:51, 1984.

305. Hagiwara M, Chen I-L, McGonigle R, Beckman B, Kasten FH, Fisher JW: Erythropoietin production in a primary culture of human renal carcinoma cells maintained in nude mice. *Blood* 63:828, 1984.

306. Okabe T, Urabe A, Kato T, Chiba S, Takaku F: Production of erythropoietin-like activity by human renal and hepatic carcinomas in cell culture. *Cancer* 55:1918, 1985.

307. Ascensao JL, Gaylis F, Bronson D, Fraley EE, Zanjani ED: Erythropoietin production by a human testicular germ cell line. *Blood* 62:1132, 1983.

308. Saito T, Saito K, Trent DJ, Draganac PS, Andrews RB, Farkas WR, Dunn CDR, Etkin LD, Lange RD: Translation of messenger RNA from a renal tumor into a product with the biological properties of erythropoietin. *Exp Hematol* 13:23, 1985.

309. Murphy GP, Mirand EA, Staubitz WJ: The value of erythropoietin assay in the follow-up of Wilms' tumor patients. *Oncology* 33:154, 1976.

310. Napier JAF, Janowska-Wieczorek A: Erythropoietin measurements in the differential diagnosis of polycythaemia. *Br J Haematol* 48:393, 1981.

311. Koeffler HP, Goldwasser E: Erythropoietin radioimmunoassay in evaluating patients with polycythemia. *Ann Intern Med* 94:44, 1981.

312. Goldwasser E, Sherwood JB: Radioimmunoassay of erythropoietin. *Br J Haematol* 48:359, 1981.

313. Sue JM, Sytkowski AJ: Site-specific antibodies to human erythropoietin directed toward the NH_2-terminal region. *Proc Natl Acad Sci USA* 80:3651, 1983.

314. Fusco FD, Rosen SW: Gonadotropin-producing anaplastic large-cell carcinomas of the lung. *N Engl J Med* 275:507, 1966.

315. Weintraub BD, Rosen SW: Ectopic production of human chorionic somatomammotropin by nontrophoblastic cancers. *J Clin Endocrinol Metab* 32:94, 1971.

316. Rosen SW. Weintraub BD, Vaitukaitis JL, Sussman HH, Hershman JM, Muggia FM: Placental proteins and their subunits as tumor markers. *Ann Intern Med* 82:71, 1975.

317. Das S, Mukherjee K, Bhattacharya S, Chowdhury JR: Ectopic production of placental hormones (human chorionic gonadotropin and human placental lactogen) in carcinoma of the uterine cervix. *Cancer* 51:1854, 1983.

318. Sheth NA, Suraiya JN, Sheth AR, Ranadive KJ, Jussawalla DJ: Ectopic production of human placental lactogen by human breast tumors. *Cancer* 39:1693, 1977.

319. Horne CHW, Reid IN, Milne GD: Prognostic significance of inappropriate production of pregnancy proteins by breast cancers. *Lancet* 2:279, 1976.

320. Turkington RW: Ectopic production of prolactin. *N Engl J Med* 285:1455, 1971.

321. Rees LH, Bloomfield GA, Rees GM, Corrin B, Franks CM, Ratcliffe JG: Multiple hormones in a bronchial tumor. *J Clin Endocrinol Metab* 38:1090, 1974.

322. Purnell DM, Hillman EA, Heatfield BM, Trump BF: Immunoreactive prolactin in epithelial cells of normal and cancerous human breast and prostate detected by the unlabeled antibody peroxidase-antiperoxidase method. *Cancer Res* 42:2317, 1982.

323. Ganguly A, Gribble J, Tune B, Kempson RL, Luetscher JA: Renin-secreting Wilms' tumor with severe hypertension: Report of a case and brief review of the literature. *Ann Intern Med* 79:835, 1973.

324. Hollifield JW, Page DL, Smith C, Michelakis AM, Staab E, Rhamy R: Renin-secreting clear cell carcinoma of the kidney. *Arch Intern Med* 135:859, 1975.

325. Robertson PW, Klidjian A, Harding LK, Walters G, Lee MR, Robb-Smith AHT: Hypertension due to a renin-secreting renal tumour. *Am J Med* 43:963, 1967.

326. Pincoffs MC, Bradley JE: The association of adenosarcoma of the kidney (Wilms' tumor) with arterial hypertension. *Trans Assoc Am Physicians* 52:320, 1937.

327. Naruse K, Murakoshi M, Osamura RY, Naruse M, Toma H, Watanabe K, Demura H, Inagami T, Shizume K: Immunohistological evidence for renin in human endocrine tissues. *J Clin Endocrinol Metab* 61:172, 1985.

328. Hauger-Klevene JH: High plasma renin activity in an oat cell carcinoma: A renin-secreting carcinoma? *Cancer* 26:1112, 1970.

329. Genest J, Rojo-Ortega JM, Kuchel O, Boucher R, Nowaczynski W, Lefebvre R, Chrétien M, Cantin J, Granger P: Malignant hypertension with hypokalemia in a patient with renin-producing pulmonary carcinoma. *Trans Assoc Am Physicians* 88:192, 1975.

330. Aurell M, Rudin A, Tisell LE, Kindblom LG, Sandberg G: Captopril effect on hypertension in patient with renin-producing tumor. *Lancet* 2:149, 1979.

331. Atlas SA, Hesson TE, Sealey JE, Dharmgrongartama B, Laragh JH, Ruddy MC, Aurell M: Characterization of inactive renin ("prorenin") from renin-secreting tumors of nonrenal origin. *J Clin Invest* 73:437, 1984.

332. Ruddy MC, Atlas SA, Salerno FG: Hypertension associated with a renin-secreting adenocarcinoma of the pancreas. *N Engl J Med* 307:993, 1982.

333. Soubrier F, Devaux C, Galen FX, Skinner SL, Aurell M, Genest J, Menard J, Corvol P: Biochemical and immunological characterization of ectopic tumoral renin. *J Clin Endocrinol Metab* 54:139, 1982.

334. Guida PM, Todd JE, Moore SW, Beal JM: Zollinger-Ellison syndrome with interesting variations: Report of twelve cases including one of carcinoid tumor of the duodenum. *Am J Surg* 112:807, 1966.

335. Cassar J, Polak JM, Cooke WM: Possible parathyroid origin of gastrin in a patient with multiple endocrine adenopathy type I. *Br J Surg* 62:313, 1975.

336. Long TT III, Barton TK, Draffin R, Reeves WJ, McCarty KS Jr: Conservative management of the Zollinger-Ellison syndrome: Ectopic gastrin production by an ovarian cystadenoma. *JAMA* 243:1837, 1980.

337. Margolis RM, Jang N: Zollinger-Ellison syndrome associated with pancreatic cystadenocarcinoma. *N Engl J Med* 311:1380, 1984.

338. Wolfe MM, Alexander RW, McGuigan JE: Extrapancreatic extraintestinal gastrinoma: Effective treatment by surgery. *N Engl J Med* 306:1533, 1982.

339. Sporrong B, Alumets J, Clase L, Falkmer S, Håkanson R, Ljundberg O, Sundler F: Neurohormonal peptide in mucinous cystadenomas and cystadenocarcinomas of the ovary. *Virchows Arch [Pathol Anat]* 392:271, 1981.

340. Yang K, Ulich T, Cheng L, Lewin KJ: The neuroendocrine products of intestinal carcinoids: An immunoperoxidase study of 35 carcinoid tumors stained for serotonin and eight polypeptide hormones. *Cancer* 51:1918, 1983.

341. Trump DL, Livingston JN, Baylin SB: Watery diarrhea syndrome in an adult with ganglioneuroma-pheochromocytoma: Identification of vasoactive intestinal polypeptide, calcitonin, and catecholamines and assessment of their biologic activity. *Cancer* 40:1526, 1977.

342. Said SI, Faloona GR: Elevated plasma and tissue levels of vasoactive intestinal polypeptide in the watery-diarrhea syndrome due to pancreatic, bronchogenic and other tumors. *N Engl J Med* 293:155, 1975.

343. Going JJ, Harmer AJ, Gow IF, Edwards CRW: Hypersalivation and local pain associated with ectopic substance P production by a metastatic laryngeal carcinoid. *J Endocrinol* 104 (Suppl): 52, 1985 (abstract).

344. Emson PC, Gilbert RFT, Martensson H, Nobin A: Elevated concentrations of substance P and 5-HT in plasma in patients with carcinoid tumors. *Cancer* 54:715, 1984.

345. Wood JR, Wood SM, Lee YC, Bloom SR: Neurotensin-secreting carcinoma of the bronchus. *Postgrad Med J* 59:46, 1983.

346. Strodel WE, Vinik AI, Lloyd RV, Glaser B, Eckhauser FE, Fiddian-Green RG, Turcotte JG, Thompson NW: Pancreatic polypeptide-producing tumors: Silent lesions of the pancreas? *Arch Surg* 119:508, 1984.

347. Solt J, Kádas I, Polak JM, Németh A, Bloom SR, Rauth J, Horváth L: A pancreatic-polypeptide-producing tumor of the stomach. *Cancer* 54:1101, 1984.

348. Beutler B, Greenwald D, Hulmes JD, Chang M, Pan Y-CE, Mathison J, Ulevitch R, Cerami A: Identity of tumour necrosis factor and the macrophage-secreted factor cachectin. *Nature* 316:552, 1985.

349. Slungaard A, Ascensao J, Zanjani E, Jacob HS: Pulmonary carcinoma with eosinophilia: Demonstration of a tumor-derived eosinophilopoietic factor. *N Engl J Med* 309:778, 1983.

350. Greengard O, Head JF, Koss B, Manton M: Responses of bone marrow γ-glutamyltranspeptidase and alkaline phosphatase *in vitro* to tumor-elaborated granulocytopoietic factors. *Cancer Res* 44:472, 1984.

351. Simpson E, Harrod J, Eilon G, Jacobs JW, Mundy GR: Identification of a messenger ribonucleic acid fraction in human prostatic cancer cells coding for a novel osteoblast-stimulating factor. *J Clin Endocrinol Metab* 117:1615, 1985.

352. Mordes JP, Longcope C, Flatt JP, MacLean DB, Rossini AA: The rat LTW(m) Leydig cell tumor: Cancer anorexia due to estrogen. *Endocrinology* 115:167, 1984.

352a. Torti FM, Dieckmann B, Beutler B, Cerami A, Ringold GM: A macrophage factor inhibits adipocyte gene expression: An in vitro model of cachexia. *Science* 229:867, 1985.

353. Chawla SP, Buzdar AV, Hortobagyi GN, Blumenschein GR: Tumor-associated fever in breast cancer. *Cancer* 53:1596, 1984.

354. Samson MK, Buroker TR, Henderson MD, Baker LH, Vaitkevicius VK: Acquired hypertrichosis lanuginosa: Report of two new cases and review of the literature. *Cancer* 36:1519, 1975.

355. Nakanishi T, Sobue I, Toyokura Y: The Crow-Fukase syndrome: A study of 102 cases in Japan. *Neurology* 34:712, 1984.

356. Matsumine H: Accelerated conversion of androgen to estrogen in plasma-cell dyscrasia associated with polyneuropathy, anasarca, and skin pigmentation. *N Engl J Med* 313:1025, 1985.

356a. Schenkein DP, O'Neill WD, Shapiro J, Miller KB: Accelerated bone formation causing profound hypocalcemia in acute leukemia. *Ann Intern Med* 105:375, 1986.

357. Bagshawe KD: Tumour-associated antigens. *Br Med Bull* 30:68, 1974.

358. Moody TW, Pert CB, Gazdar AF, Carney DN, Minna JD: High levels of intracellular bombesin characterize human small-cell lung carcinoma. *Science* 214:1246, 1981.

359. Goldenberg DM, DeLand F, Kim E, Bennett S, Primus FJ, van Nagell JR, Estes N, De Simone P, Rayburn P: Use of radiolabeled antibodies to carcinoembryonic antigen for the detection and localization of diverse cancers by external photoscanning. *N Engl J Med* 298:1384, 1978.

360. Horne CHW, Reid IN, Milne GD: Prognostic significance of inappropriate production of pregnancy proteins by breast cancers. *Lancet* 2:279, 1976.

30

Hormone-Responsive Tumors

Jean-Claude Heuson
André Coune

There are multiple interrelationships between the endocrine system and cancer. Hormones are extensively involved in the regulation of cell growth and differentiation, factors critical for cancer. Recent studies with the animal retroviruses reveal that some of these either code for substances that are growth factors or else induce the expression of elements that participate in the cascade of growth factor action.[1] The findings that the retroviral gene *v-sis* codes for a protein with structural homology to platelet-derived growth factor and that another oncogene codes for a protein that resembles the epidermal growth factor receptor illustrate these interrelationships.[1]

In this context, it would not be surprising that endocrine events can influence the course of a number of tumors. These events can affect not only the induction, but also the maintenance of these tumors once established. The dependence of thyroid neoplasms on thyroid stimulating hormone discussed in Chap. 11 and the effects of cortisol on pituitary neoplasms discussed in Chap. 12 are examples. However, more common as a problem are the neoplasms that develop in the secondary sex organs, i.e., the breasts, prostate, and uterus; these are dealt with in this chapter.

Epidemiologic studies have indicated that, besides other risk factors such as geographic distribution and inheritance, endocrine events strongly affect the incidence of breast or uterine cancer. Therapeutically administered hormones (estrogens) are now recognized as having a promoting effect in the development of uterine and, possibly, breast carcinoma. Metabolic disorders such as obesity also seem to enhance distinctly the risk of developing these malignancies. The management of breast cancer in the advanced stage, as well as of uterine or prostatic carcinoma, has long relied essentially upon endocrine manipulations, whether ablative or additive. Efforts aimed at the refinement of these therapeutic measures have been aided by new insights into the physiology of endocrine glands, the metabolism of endogenously secreted hormones, and the mechanisms of hormone action, particularly the discovery of hormone receptors. The availability of new hormone-related compounds has also been a considerable stimulus.

BREAST CANCER

Incidence and Mortality in Western Countries

Carcinoma of the breast is the second most frequent cancer (after skin cancer) and the leading cause of cancer death among women in western countries.[2,2a] The highest registered incidence rates occur in the United States, among the white populations of Connecticut and the San Francisco Bay area in California; they ranged from 101.3 to 115.6 per 100,000 women for the period 1973 to 1977.[2]

Cutler et al.[3] analyzed the data from the Connecticut cancer registry and found that the reported incidence of breast cancer has been increasing steadily since the mid-1940s (Fig. 30-1). The age-adjusted rate shifted from 55 per 100,000 between 1940 and 1944 to 72 per 100,000 in the period 1965 to 1968. In contrast, over the same period, the mortality rate in Connecticut (and in the United States as a whole) did not change significantly, and the ratio of new cases to deaths occurring 5 years later increased from 2.1 to 2.4. A similar increase in ratio of incident cases to deaths was found in the province of Saskatchewan, Canada, which, like Connecticut, has a good cancer registry. The causes of these changes were not apparent from the available data, but they were probably minor. The data seem to indicate that, overall, breast cancer morbidity and mortality in the United States have remained fairly constant during the past three decades.[4]

It should be stressed that the difference between

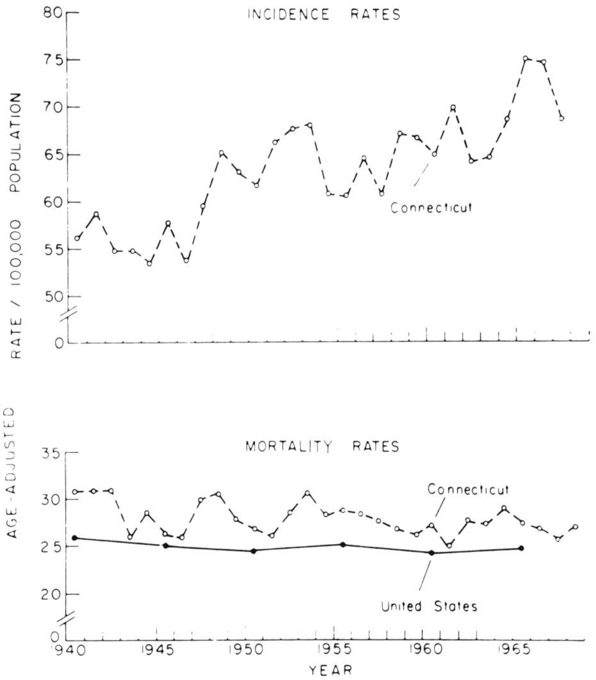

FIGURE 30-1 Breast cancer incidence and mortality in Connecticut, 1940–1968, and mortality in the United States, 1940–1965, age-adjusted to the 1950 total US population. (*From Cutler et al.*[3] *Courtesy of the authors and the publisher.*)

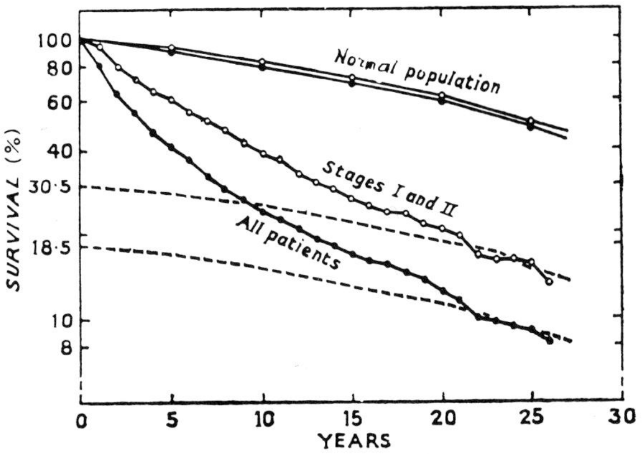

FIGURE 30-2 Survival rates after treatment in 704 cases of breast cancer compared with expected survival of normal populations of same age distribution. Interrupted lines show extrapolation back to zero time of the portion of the curves which are approximately parallel to those of the corresponding normal population. The intercepts on the vertical axis indicate the size of the cured groups. (*From Brinkley and Haybittle.*[6] *Courtesy of the authors and the publisher.*)

new cases and deaths due to breast cancer cannot be regarded as the number of *cures*, because many persons, still suffering from breast cancer, die of other causes. In cooperative studies reported by Mueller et al.[5] of 3225 women undergoing treatment for primary breast cancer, 914 died during the study, 705 of cancer of the breast and 209 of competing risks. Forces of mortality due to competing risks were greater in the older than the younger group.

Survival of breast cancer patients can be more accurately assessed in studies on the "curability" of breast cancer where large series of patients are subjected to a long-term follow-up. Brinkley and Haybittle[6] reported on such a study involving 704 women with breast cancer treated in England in 1947 to 1950 and followed for at least 22 years. Figure 30-2 shows the actuarial survival rates plotted on a logarithmic scale against years after treatment and compared with expected curves for the age-matched normal population. It is assumed that parallelism of the observed and expected curves indicates "cure." This state is reached after 21 years both for all patients (proportion cured approximately 18 percent) and for stages I and II combined (proportion cured approximately 30 percent). It is noteworthy that in the "cured" group, after 20 years of follow-up, 8 out of 23 deaths were still from cancer of the breast; this proportion is about 16 times higher than expected in the normal population. Other studies arrived at similar conclusions.[5,7] According to Baum, it seems that 20 to 30 percent of women treated for apparently localized breast cancer have a normal life expectancy, but doubt remains whether all patients diagnosed as suffering from the disease would ultimately die of it if they lived long enough.

Risk Factors and Etiology

SEX

Breast cancer occurs predominantly in women. Male breast carcinoma represents 0.8 to 1.0 percent of all breast carcinomas.

GEOGRAPHIC DISTRIBUTION AND AGE

Waterhouse et al. published extensive information on cancer incidence in five continents, including rates, age-standardized to a "world population."[2] Table 30-1 gives such rates in areas around the world, illustrating the extremes. The lowest are in Japan and Africa. Intermediate rates are found at sites in Europe, South America, and Asia. The highest rates occur in northwestern Europe and North America. The ratio of highest to lowest rates is about 5:1.

Besides differences in levels of breast cancer risk between different areas of the world, striking differences occur in age-specific incidence patterns (Fig. 30-3).[8] Where the risk is high, the rates increase

Table 30-1. Annual Incidence Rates for Breast Cancer in Women in Different Parts of the World*

Area	Rate per 100,000
Higher Incidence	
USA	65.7–80.3
UK	48.0–54.5
Scandinavia	44.4–52.4
Intermediate Incidence	
German Democratic Republic	33.4
Cali, Colombia	25.4
Bombay, India	20.1
Low Incidence	
Africa	13.8–15.3
Japan	12.1–16.6

*Age-standardized to world population, mostly around 1970
Source: Adapted from Waterhouse et al.[2]

throughout life, although the slope is flatter after menopausal ages. In Japan, where the risk is low, the slope becomes negative after the "menopausal break." de Waard[8] assumes that two types of human breast cancer exist, one largely confined to premenopausal ages and possibly related to ovarian function, the other mainly prevalent at and after menopause and possibly related to adrenocortical anomalies such as increased estrogen production brought about by affluence. The western (adrenal) type could be prevented by changing nutritional habits. However, MacMahon et al. reported that the risk reduction association with oophorectomy continues in the oldest age groups,[9] which suggests that a persistent role is played by ovarian factors even in postmenopausal women.

Differences in breast cancer rates of Asian and western populations are probably not genetically determined.[9] Evidence comes from studies of migrant populations. Thus, descendants of Japanese who have migrated to the United States have rates higher than women living in Japan, and descendants of Chinese in Hawaii have rates almost as high as those of Caucasian women. These findings suggest that a major part of the Asian-Caucasian difference in rates is due to environmental factors. However, such factors seem deeply ingrained in the parent culture and change only with the passage of generations.

Overnutrition has been proposed by de Waard as possibly being one of the environmental factors underlying the Asian-Caucasian difference.[8] The evidence, recently reviewed by Miller,[10] has come from two sources: animal experimentation and population correlation studies. Feeding rats a high-fat diet increases the incidence of mammary tumors. This effect is possibly mediated through prolactin. A correlation in the western world between animal fat intake and breast cancer incidence has been supported by data from Japan, where the incidence of breast cancer has recently been reported to be rising. de Waard has shown an association of breast cancer incidence with body height and weight in postmenopausal women. In fact, excessive weight per se may not be the factor involved, since after correction for height (Quetelet index = weight divided by the square of height), weight had no independent effect in a study of Dutch women. In differences between countries, weight and height seem involved. Thus, a comparison of Dutch women (tall and heavy on the average) with Japanese women (small and lean on the average) shows that the ratio of age-standardized breast cancer incidence rates of the two groups is 1:3.83 but that this difference is decreased by 37 or 51 percent, respectively, after correction for body weight or height.[11] In another study, an effect of height has not been found, but the effect of weight was confirmed in postmenopausal women. In still another study, of 524 patients, breast cancer was not related to height or

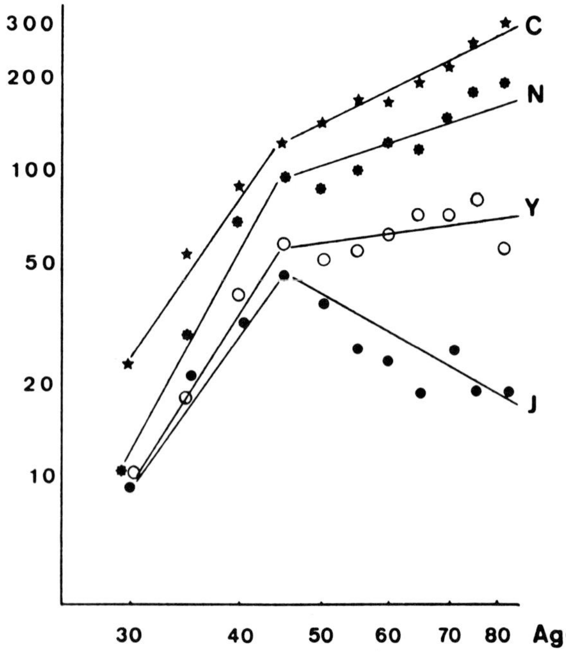

FIGURE 30-3 Age-specific incidence curves of breast cancer plotted on a logarithmic scale. Each of the curves, from Miyagi prefecture in Japan (J), Slovenia in Yugoslavia (Y), Norway (N), and Connecticut in the United States (C), seems to consist of two linear parts (drawn freehand), with the change in slope at about age 50. *(From de Waard.[8] Courtesy of the author and the publisher.)*

body weight.[12] A more direct assessment of the effect of diet was conducted by Miller et al. in a case-control study where a significant effect of high fat intake was disclosed.[10] Hill et al.[12a] have suggested that variation in the fat content of the diet influences gut bacteria and the subsequent production of possibly carcinogenic estrogens from biliary steroids present in the colon.[10]

AGE AS A PROGNOSTIC FACTOR

Besides increasing in incidence, breast cancer seems also to express its lethality more vigorously with advancing age. In a study on 3558 randomly chosen patients, Mueller et al. computed mortality rates for three age groups: 21 to 50 years at the time of diagnosis (1223 patients), 51 to 70 years (1556 patients), and 71 to 100 years (779 patients).[13] The "half-death time" for the youngest group was 13 years, for the middle group 8 years, and for the oldest group 5 years. This finding is contrary to the current wisdom that older women live longer with breast cancer than younger women. The authors suggest that a common factor (host-tumor relationship) increases breast cancer incidence and rate of dying with advancing age.

REPRODUCTIVE EXPERIENCE

The risk factors associated with reproductive experience have been thoroughly discussed in a review by MacMahon et al.,[9] to which the reader is referred for detailed information.

Pregnancy

Results of a collaborative study conducted in seven areas of the world having very different breast cancer incidence rates can be summarized as follows.[9] Breast cancer risk increases with increasing age at the time of first full-term pregnancy (approximately three times higher in women whose first full-term pregnancy came after age 35 compared to those whose first term pregnancy occurred before they were 18). To be protective, pregnancy must occur before age 30. However, the protective effect is essentially limited to the first birth and is exerted only by a full-term pregnancy, not by abortion. The protection conveyed by early first birth is manifested in all subsequent ages.

These findings suggest that etiologic factors are operating during the early period of reproductive life and that protection by a single full-term pregnancy is due either to a permanent change in the factors responsible for the high risk or to changes in the breast tissue that make it less susceptible to malignant transformation.

Lactation

Several studies carried out in both high- and low-risk areas failed to offer consistent evidence of a difference between patients and controls with regard to lactation experience when the lower parity of the patients was taken into account. Lactation therefore has little, if any, effect on breast cancer risk.[9]

Oophorectomy

After the initial observation by Lilienfeld in 1956, several authors have reported a lowered risk of breast cancer after surgical menopause, especially when the surgery is performed at younger ages.[13a–13c] From data collected by the Connecticut cancer registry, it appears that, overall, surgical menopause was associated with a 40 percent reduction of risk. The reduction of breast cancer risk in the decade after surgery was small, but thereafter the protective effect persisted for life.[13d] It is of interest that the protective effect of artificial menopause, when carried out before age 45, extends beyond age 70, like that of early pregnancy. In many studies, the data refer to "operative menopause" without specification as to the proportion of patients castrated. If the protective effect of operative menopause is indeed limited to women whose ovaries are removed, the effect of castration must be greater than the apparent effect seen in the overall operative menopause population.[9]

Age at Menarche

Association of increased breast cancer risk with early menarche has been reported in many case-control studies, although differences were small or absent in other reports.[9,13e–13h]

Age at Natural Menopause

In the opinion of McMahon et al.,[9] the weight of evidence suggests that women with late natural menopause have an increased breast cancer risk. These authors cite observations according to which women with natural menopause at age 55 or older had twice the risk of those whose menopause occurred naturally before age 45. The data point to a distinct role of ovarian function not only during the early reproductive years (early menarche, early first baby) but also during the second half of reproductive life (surgical menopause, late menopause). The mechanism may be different at different times, acting on initiation at early ages but on promotion later.[9]

ROLE OF INDIVIDUAL HORMONES

Extensive reviews on the role of hormones in breast cancer are available.[9,14,15,16]

Estrogens

A number of authors have reported that women with breast cancer, in comparison to those without cancer, excreted less estriol (E_3) than estrone (E_1) and estradiol (E_2). Other authors have observed that the urinary *estriol quotient* or *ratio* [$E_3/(E_1 + E_2)$] is higher in Asian than in American women, especially in the early reproductive years. The estriol-ratio, which is extremely high during pregnancy, could account for the protective effect of early pregnancy. The estriol hypothesis is based on the concept that E_3, which has weak estrogenic potency compared with E_2 and E_1, actually functions as a competitive inhibitor of the strong estrogens, thereby suppressing their postulated cancer-initiating and -promoting properties.

This theory has been challenged by Kirschner[14] and by others.[16a,16b] The diverse evidence against it can be summarized as follows. Breast cancer patients were found by several investigators to have elevated urinary estriol excretion and increased peripheral transformation of E_2 into E_3. In normal subjects and in women with breast cancer, circulating blood levels of estriol relative to E_1 and E_2 are extremely low and unlikely to compete with them significantly. In rodents, E_3 may be as carcinogenic as other estrogens. In vitro, in a human cancer cell line, estriol behaves as an estrogen and overcomes the antiestrogenic effect of the triphenylethylene tamoxifen. It was also shown that E_3 production rates and circulating levels are not significantly different in women with high urinary E_3 ratios and those with low ratios. An alternative to the estriol ratio hypothesis is that one of the factors influencing the distal metabolism and excretion of individual estrogens may be the risk factor rather than the estriol ratio itself.

Interest in the potential role of exogenous estrogens in the etiology of breast cancer has been much stimulated by recent reports implicating menopausal estrogen use with increased risk of endometrial cancer. Estrogens are widely used as a component of oral contraceptives and for the treatment of perimenopausal symptoms. Numerous epidemiologic studies on oral contraceptives failed to support a significant association of their use with subsequent development of breast cancer; on the contrary, there is evidence for a decreased risk of benign breast disease.[16c–16f] Most studies also failed to show an association of menopausal estrogen use with breast cancer risk, with the exception of the report by Hoover et al.,[16g] suggesting that breast cancer incidence rates increase after a latent period in excess of 10 years.[16h,16i] Moreover, an especially high risk was found to exist among women in whom benign disease developed after they had started taking conjugated estrogens. Clearly, more data are needed in this field.

Androgens

Interest has focused on androgens following the studies of Bulbrook,[16] who reported finding lower concentrations of androgen metabolites in women with breast cancer who failed to respond to endocrine treatments. A prospective study in Guernsey revealed below-normal urinary excretion of androgens in women who subsequently developed breast cancer, in unaffected sisters (aged 31 to 40 years) of women with breast cancer, and in women with benign breast disease.[16j] However, while there appears to be a reasonable correlation between risk and androgen levels in Caucasian women, this is totally reversed in Japanese women; their urinary and plasma androgen levels are significantly lower than those in western women, and rural Japanese women excrete less androgen metabolites than their urban counterparts, who have a greater incidence of breast cancer.[16] According to Bulbrook,[16] a relationship of breast cancer to urinary androgen metabolites might be better explained, rather than in terms of a hormonal effect on breast tissue, by the supposition that the androgens are correlated with other, more fundamental factors concerned with the development of breast cancer. Kirschner discussed this view further.[14]

Progesterone

Hormonal studies have led Sherman and Korenman to the conclusion that inadequate corpus luteum secretory function is one of the characteristic features of infertile and/or irregular menstrual cycles.[17] Reviewing the epidemiology of breast cancer in that light, these workers put forth the hypothesis that estrogenic stimulation in the absence of sufficient cyclic progesterone secretion may provide a setting favorable to the development of mammary carcinoma. Grattarola has provided evidence along this line by showing on endometrial biopsies an association of cystic disease of the breast or carcinoma of the breast before menopause with long-term estrogen stimulation unopposed by progesterone.[17a] The latter steroid also induces estradiol 17β-dehydrogenase in the endometrium and, possibly, in breast tissue, leading to accelerated conversion of estradiol into estrone and its exit out of the cell; moreover, the endometrial E_2 receptor level decreases during the luteal phase, possibly as an effect of the progesterone action.[15] Against this view, regular ovulation, with "normal progesterone protection," has been observed as commonly in premenopausal breast cancer patients as in normal controls, and no difference in plasma levels of progesterone was observed between Japanese and British women.[15,16] A protective role of progesterone against the development of breast cancer lacks supporting evidence and remains, therefore, purely hypothetical.

Prolactin

Prolactin plays a prominent part in the development and function of the normal mammary gland. It is known to stimulate growth of dimethylbenzanthracene-induced mammary carcinoma in the rat. Yet, epidemiologic studies failed to ascribe a distinct role to prolactin in the incidence of human breast cancer.[17b–d] There are no consistent data suggesting an association between the plasma prolactin level and the risk of breast cancer or the presence of an established breast cancer. Moreover, no significant correlation has been reported between the long-term use of potent prolactin stimulators, such as the rauwolfia derivatives, and the incidence of breast cancer.[14–16]

Conclusion

The following statement by Kirschner is probably acceptable to most scholars of breast cancer etiology:[14]

> Despite three decades of intensive investigation into the relationships between breast cancer and hormones, and despite the tantalizing associations that have been attempted from inconsistent data, there is as yet no clear-cut pattern of abnormal hormone production or abnormal hormone milieu found in women at increased risk for breast cancer.

FAMILIAL AGGREGATION

Female relatives of women with breast cancer have two to three times the risk of breast cancer as does the general population. This increased risk appears as great for paternal relatives as for those on the maternal side.[9] Recently, Anderson found evidence of genetic heterogeneity in breast cancer.[18] Thus, the risk for all women with a family history of breast cancer was increased 1.8 times. When the proband was premenopausal, the risk was threefold higher, but it was only 1.5 times greater if she was postmenopausal. Furthermore, when the proband had bilateral cancer and was premenopausal, the risk was increased ninefold, but it increased only fourfold if she was postmenopausal. Finally, Anderson identified a group of women whose risk for breast cancer was 47 times higher than that experienced by control women.[19] These very high risk women were sisters of patients whose mothers had breast cancer. The disease in women in these families developed before menopause and was often bilateral and was considered strongly heritable (30 percent risk in the daughters).

According to Anderson, another, less heritable form was identified in families comprising at least two affected sisters and an unaffected mother.[19] The risk in these families was threefold higher than that of controls, and the disease was primarily postmenopausal and unilateral. Besides these heritable forms, Anderson suggests that there may be a sporadic type of breast cancer not associated with a family history of the disorder.[18] Interestingly, younger familial patients (ages 20 to 44) had a threefold higher incidence of bilateral breast cancer than did older familial patients (ages 55 to 84), 15.5 vs. 4.8 percent; this trend did not exist in nonfamilial patients, in whom the incidences were 3.4 and 2.7 percent, respectively.

Human breast cancer appears to be a heterogeneous disease, the causes of which include a variety of interrelated genetic, environmental, societal, and physiological factors. Petrakis recently reviewed the evidence for a genetic role in susceptibility to breast cancer[20] and proposed a working hypothesis that indicates genetic-environmental interactions in breast cancer etiology and pathogenesis. In this model, the turnover rate of breast secretions is the primary determinant of the extent and duration of exposure of the breast epithelium to extrinsic and endogenous carcinogens.

VIRUSES

While viruses are known to be involved in mammary carcinogenesis in nonhuman animal species, especially rodents, the evidence that they might play a similar part in humans is still elusive. Morphological, biochemical, and immunological evidence exists for the presence of oncogenic RNA viruses in some human milk and breast cancer samples. These observations implicate oncogenic RNA viruses in the etiology of human breast cancer, although definitive proof of this etiology is at present lacking.[21] It is beyond the scope of this chapter to review and discuss the available evidence for a viral etiology of human breast cancer; moreover, such a discussion has no relevance to the present-day management of the disease.

Hormonal Regulation of Tumor Growth

The hormone dependence of human breast cancer was discovered at the turn of the century by Beatson, a Scottish surgeon who reported tumor regression in two patients after oophorectomy.[21a] Since then, adrenalectomy and hypophysectomy have been used to achieve similar results. As an alternative to these surgical ablative procedures, breast cancer regression can be produced by administering large doses of estrogen, androgen, progestin, or glucocorticoid.

The success of these therapeutic measures in 20 to 40 percent of breast cancer patients indicates that endogenous hormones are required for sustaining tumor growth in these patients and that administered hormones can interfere with it. Studies on hormone-dependent experimental models, particularly carcinogen-induced rat mammary tumors which regress after oophorectomy or hypophysectomy, have complemented clinical investigation to provide insight into the mechanisms underlying hormone responsiveness of tumors. The discovery of hormone receptors in breast tumors and the correlation of their presence with hormone responsiveness is the most significant and clinically relevant finding of recent years in this regard.

This section analyzes the role of hormones in the control of growth of breast cancer, both in animal models and in women. For a general review of these problems, the reader is referred to the excellent chapter by McGuire.[22]

MURINE MAMMARY TUMORS

Role of Hormones in Vivo

While hormones play a distinct role during induction of mammary tumors in the mouse, they usually lose this function once the tumor is established. In the rat, carcinogen-induced mammary carcinoma retains a high degree of hormone dependency. Thus, established tumors readily regress after oophorectomy or hypophysectomy. This tumor therefore represents an interesting model of human breast cancer. It has been successfully used as such for studying the mechanisms underlying hormone dependency of tumors and for screening new compounds with potential antitumor activity.[23,24]

Growth of established carcinogen-induced rat mammary tumors appears to be regulated by steroid and pituitary hormones. Oophorectomy of tumor-bearing rats results in a prompt and prolonged regression of most tumors. Concurrent enhancement of prolactin secretion by placement of median eminence hypothalamic lesions prevents this regression, although only temporarily. Daily injection of ovine prolactin or human placental lactogen effects similar results. For persistent growth of the tumors, however, the concurrent presence of ovarian steroids and especially estrogen is usually necessary. Tumor growth in intact animals is modified by changes in prolactin secretion. Thus, stimulation of prolactin by perphenazine or similar drugs of the phenothiazine class strongly enhances tumor growth, while selective inhibition of prolactin secretion and release by ergot derivatives significantly decreases tumor growth.

Prolactin can influence mammary tumor growth by a direct action on the tumor tissue. It may also have an indirect effect, via the ovaries; it is known that prolactin has both a luteolytic and a luteotrophic effect on the ovary. On the other hand, prolactin was found to enhance tumor growth in rats after oophorectomy-adrenalectomy or hypophysectomy[24a,24b] and to increase DNA and protein synthesis in vitro.[24c] In both cases, prolactin seemed to act by itself in the absence of steroids. Interestingly, there are two transplantable rat mammary tumors (R3230AC and 35-MT), the growth of which is inhibited, not enhanced, by increasing prolactin secretion. This effect may be due to a hormone-induced shift of the tumor tissue toward cell differentiation rather than division.

In oophorectomized-adrenalectomized rats, tumor regression is significantly prevented by physiological doses of estrogens. Increasing the dose to high, pharmacological levels abolishes this preventive effect. Likewise, large doses are inhibitory in intact tumor-bearing rats. While estrogens restore tumor growth after oophorectomy, they fail to do so when tumor regression is induced by hypophysectomy. Estrogens are therefore probably important, but not sufficient, for sustaining tumor growth in this animal model. It has been suggested that physiological doses of estrogens enhance the stimulating effect of prolactin and that pharmacological doses inhibit this action at the tissue site.[24]

The role of progesterone in the regulation of growth of the carcinogen-induced mammary cancer of the rat has been investigated. In intact rats, administration of progesterone accelerated the appearance of tumors, increased their number, and enhanced their growth rate. In oophorectomized rats, progesterone was initially found to largely prevent tumor regression,[24] but this finding could not be reproduced in later experiments. McCormick and Moon reported that administration of progesterone stimulated growth of half the tumors in nursing rats subjected to oophorectomy early in postpartum.[25] These data, some of which are not consistently reproducible, suggest that progesterone under various conditions can stimulate growth of these experimental mammary tumors. Conversely, progesterone has been reported to induce rat mammary tumor regression or prevent tumor appearance when combined with moderate to large doses of estrogens.

In Vitro Studies

Hormone action in breast cancer explants has been reviewed.[26] When carcinogen-induced rat mammary tumors were maintained in organ culture, individual tumors showed considerable difference in their hormonal requirements. Some were dependent upon insulin for their growth (i.e., for DNA synthesis), while others were totally autonomous of insulin, and were also uninfluenced by other hormones. In contrast, the insulin-dependent tumors were reactive to prolactin, progesterone, and estradiol in the presence of insulin. Twenty-five to fifty percent of them were stimulated by prolactin, an effect that was inhibited by estradiol. Progesterone had a stimulating effect of its own and acted synergistically with prolactin on growth in a majority of tumors.

Hormone Receptors

Further insight into the mechanism of hormone dependence of rat mammary tumors has evolved from studies of cellular hormone receptors.[22,23,27] Experimental mammary tumors of the rat contain plasma membrane–bound prolactin receptors, the concentration of which, in some cases, was found to be an indicator of the degree of hormone dependency. While small doses of estrogens are known to increase the number of prolactin-binding sites in the liver, their effect on prolactin receptors in mammary tumors has not been tested. High doses of estrogens decrease the number of tumor prolactin receptors;[27a] conversely, prolactin increases the estrogen receptor (ER) content of mammary tumors.[27b] These observations strengthen the concept of interrelations between prolactin and steroids in the control of tumor growth. These interactions may be explained on the basis of regulation of hormone receptors.

Cytoplasmic ER are present in all carcinogen-induced mammary carcinomas of intact rats, although the tissue content of receptors was found to be very variable.[27c] After oophorectomy, one-third of the remaining tumors contained no detectable ER, while the other two-thirds contained ER at significantly lower levels than in intact rats.[27] Presence of ER is therefore not a specific characteristic of hormone-dependent cancers in the rat, and loss of ER is not a prerequisite for acquisition of autonomy of growth from ovarian secretions. The finding of ER-containing rat tumors which do not respond to oophorectomy is similar to the situation in human breast cancer; this demands further study.[22] As already mentioned, prolactin increases ER concentration in rat mammary tumors.

Cytoplasmic progesterone receptors (PgR) were demonstrated to exist in carcinogen-induced rat mammary carcinomas using a tritiated synthetic progestin (R5020) as the ligand.[28] Like ER, PgR were present in a wide range of concentrations. ER and PgR concentrations were very significantly and positively correlated. After oophorectomy, ER concentration declined to approximately 50 percent of its pretreatment value, whereas PgR concentration fell to very low or undetectable levels. Estrogen administration to rats bearing regressed tumors induced a translocation of ER into the nuclei, but sharply increased the PgR levels. These data indicate that in rat mammary tumors PgR concentrations, as in normal target tissues, are estrogen-dependent.

General Conclusion

These complementary data from in vivo, in vitro (i.e., culture), and biochemical studies lead to several conclusions. The growth of the carcinogen-induced rat mammary tumor is regulated by the interplay of multiple hormonal factors, some of which are beginning to be understood. Most tumors are equipped with receptors for prolactin, estrogen, and progesterone. The concentrations of the individual hormone receptors vary and are influenced by the action of hormones. Estrogens are important but not sufficient by themselves. The in vivo data emphasize the prominent stimulating effect of prolactin; estrogens and prolactin appear to reinforce each other in a synergistic fashion, and both are required in many tumors. Synergism could conceivably result from mutual stimulation of the respective receptors, but other mechanisms could also be in operation. This synergism is in contradiction to the organ culture experiments, in which estrogens inhibit the prolactin-induced enhancement of DNA synthesis. There is no explanation for this contradiction. On the other hand, inhibition of tumor growth in vivo by pharmacological doses of estrogens could be the counterpart of the organ culture data and could partly be explained by the observed decrease in prolactin receptor content. Finally, progesterone stimulates tumor growth in intact rats, which is in keeping with the organ culture observations. Stimulating effects of progesterone in oophorectomized rats are inconsistent; they could result from disappearance of PgR after castration.

The foregoing analysis of the hormonal factors controlling growth of carcinogen-induced rat mammary tumors illustrates the way in which such intricate mechanisms can be approached by complementary experimental methods; it does not presume to suggest that similar mechanisms necessarily operate in human breast cancer (the relevance of the rat model to human breast cancer is discussed in the next section). The rat model is also interesting because of its usefulness in the screening of antitumor compounds, especially those acting through the endocrine system,[24] such as:

Bromocriptine, a potent inhibitor of prolactin release, successfully inhibits mammary tumor growth in the rat but not in patients with advanced breast cancer, thus illustrating differences in properties between these tumors.

Nafoxidine and tamoxifen, two nonsteroidal estrogen antagonists, are inhibitory in the rat and are also successful therapeutic agents in patients.

Compound A-43818, a synthetic analogue of gonadotropin-releasing hormone (GnRH), was found to induce tumor regression in the rat and is currently being subjected to a clinical trial in advanced breast cancer patients.

HUMAN BREAST CANCER

Clinical Evidence

For lack of experimental data, the role of individual hormones in the control of growth of human breast cancer is not well-known. Almost all the available information has been obtained from results of the various therapeutic endocrine measures currently used, most of which have been introduced empirically. The given rationale for their introduction still forms the background for interpreting their mechanisms of action. Some additional evidence has evolved from scanty in vitro experiments, but more progress has come from recent studies on hormone receptors in breast cancer tissue.

It has been known for a long time that partial or complete tumor regression is achieved in 20 to 40 percent of patients with advanced breast cancer by surgical ablation of the ovaries, the adrenals, or the pituitary.[22,29–31] Castration is assumed to achieve its therapeutic effect by removing the main source of endogenous estrogens. This interpretation is supported by the observation of Pearson et al., who showed that hypercalcemia (an indication of tumor activity) develops after administration of physiological doses of estrogens to oophorectomized patients in remission of skeletal metastases.[31a] Other direct evidence is lacking. Stoll, in a thoughtful article,[32] challenged this simple view and concluded that the explanation was unlikely to be a single hormonal relationship or unitary hypothesis.

The mechanism of the therapeutic effect of adrenalectomy in breast cancer is unknown. Estrogens have again been incriminated but without definitive evidence. Human adrenal cortical cells seem to produce extremely low amounts of estrogens, but adrenal steroids have been shown to be converted into active estrogens in the body; the conversion occurs especially in fatty tissues, but also in breast cancer tissue itself.

Surgical hypophysectomy is probably the most effective endocrine treatment of advanced breast cancer. Both retrospective and prospective controlled clinical trials have shown a definite advantage of hypophysectomy over adrenalectomy in terms of duration of remission and survival. This points to a significant role of one or several pituitary hormones in the maintenance of breast cancer tissue growth. Yet, it is unknown whether the role of these hormones is a direct one, exercised at the tumor tissue level, or is indirect, mediated by other endocrine glands, or both.[31] There is evidence, from calcium excretion studies in patients with osseous metastases, that administered estrogens, which "reactivate" tumor growth after oophorectomy, are unable to do so after successful hypophysectomy. This observation suggests that stimulation of tumor growth by estrogens requires the contemporaneous action of a hormonal factor from, or mediated by, the pituitary.[32a] Studies have been conducted in hypophysectomized patients wherein estrogen administration was complemented with human growth hormone (GH); other patients received ovine prolactin alone. In no case was there a significant modification of calcium metabolism, which would have been suggestive of reactivation of tumor growth. In another study, ovine prolactin was administered before hypophysectomy, i.e., at a time when endogenous estrogens are still present. An increase in calcium excretion occurred in patients who subsequently responded favorably to hypophysectomy, while no such elevation occurred in those who failed to respond. A puzzling observation is that sectioning the pituitary stalk induced tumor regression in concurrently lactating patients. Stalk section was associated with an elevation of blood prolactin levels but a decrease of GH concentration as well as concentrations of peripherally secreted hormones.

These endocrine studies suggest that hypophysectomy and stalk section induce breast cancer regression by a mechanism involving neither GH nor prolactin as the major factors. The results are consistent with the possibility that regression is due, in part, to a fall in adrenocorticotropin (ACTH) production and resultant decrease in the production of adrenal-derived estrogens. However, more than one factor probably needs to be invoked to explain the advantage of hypophysectomy over adrenalectomy. It is conceivable that synergism of some of the various stimulatory hormones, such as ACTH and prolactin, with estrogens is important. Another possible albeit unlikely explanation is that after stalk section the high prolactin levels induce differentiation and growth inhibition in the tumor tissue, as in the rat R3230AC tumor (see above). The failure of bromocriptine to provoke tumor regression, although it is a very effective prolactin suppressor, also suggests that prolactin may not play such an important part in human breast cancer as it does in the rat tumor.

In Vitro Studies

The hormonal effects on human breast cancer in organ culture have been reviewed.[26] It appears that survival during culture is not distinctly influenced by hormones, with only one exception: estradiol was found to improve considerably the survival of explants from scirrhous carcinomas. Estradiol seems to exert this action by inducing a collagen-degrading activity around the tumor cells which, by loosening the dense stroma, enhances the diffusion of oxygen and nutrients into the cultured cells and thereby improves their survival.

An interesting model is provided by the continuous cell line MCF-7, which is derived from a human breast cancer; this cell line displays interesting, hormone-sensitive properties.[33,34] Growth of this cell line is stimulated by estrogens at physiological concentrations. In contrast, growth is inhibited by tamoxifen or nafoxidine; this inhibition is reversed after concomitant addition of estrogen. Since MCF-7 contains receptors for estrogen (as well as for androgen, progestin, and glucocorticoids), this antagonist effect of antiestrogen and estrogen on growth is believed to be mediated through estrogen receptors. Dihydrotestosterone (DHT) was found also to stimulate MCF-7 cell growth, while corticosteroids but not progesterone are inhibitory. Interestingly, growth stimulation by DHT is mediated by the receptors for estrogens, not by those for androgens. A similar effect could conceivably exist in vivo and would then explain why hypercalcemia sometimes occurs at initiation of androgen (as well as estrogen) therapy of advanced breast cancer.

Another novel concept evolving from studies of the MCF-7 cell line is that ER might enhance cell growth by themselves in the absence of estrogen or another steroid. This concept is based on the observation that MCF-7 cells grow in the absence of estrogen, have a high ratio of nuclear to cytoplasmic ER (3:1), and are inhibited by antiestrogens in the absence of estrogens. This finding could explain, among other possible mechanisms, why some human breast cancers do not regress after endocrine ablations even though they contain ER. On the other hand, it was shown that MCF-7 PgR are inducible by estrogens, much like those in rat mammary tumors. Also, ovine and human prolactin increased twofold the level of ER in MCF-7.[35]

Hormone Receptors

Steroid hormone receptors in human breast cancer have been the subject of numerous studies, discussed in reviews;[22,27,28,36] much of the available basic information is presented in two books.[37,38] In the late 1950s, it was reported that radioactively labeled estrogen injected into experimental animals is concentrated and retained in those organs which either respond to estrogen or excrete it.[38a] Soon after, it was found that estrogen concentration is higher in breast cancer tissue of patients responding to adrenalectomy than in the tissue of those who failed to respond. The association is not sufficiently strong, however, to be useful for predicting response in individual patients. The ability of the estrogen target tissues to concentrate estrogen was ascribed to the presence of a high-affinity ER. In a clinical study of patients with advanced breast cancer, Jensen et al.[39] reported that adrenalectomy led to objective remission in most patients in whom tumor biopsy revealed ER, while those who were apparently ER-free usually failed to respond to therapy. This observation was largely confirmed in other laboratories, and studies were extended to androgen and progesterone receptors and to other forms of endocrine treatment.[39a,39b]

Revision was proposed of the concept that human breast cancers can be sharply distinguished on the basis of presence or absence of cytoplasmic ER.[27] Actually, most breast cancers (approximately 80 percent) contain detectable cytoplasmic ER, although at concentrations that are extremely variable (range 3 to 2000 fmol per milligram of tissue protein). The distribution of concentrations is continuous, with an increasing proportion toward the lower values. There is no clear-cut separation into two classes of tumors according to the presence or absence of receptors. Even so-called ER-negative tumors might contain trace amounts of ER that are not detectable by the methods available. However, it was found that the likelihood of inducing tumor regression by endocrine maneuvers is a function of the ER level in the tumor tissue.[27,34] These data suggest that most or all human breast cancers are hormone (estrogen?)-dependent, but to varying degrees that can be measured by the concentration of ER.

It was also proposed that some tumors containing substantial levels of ER and failing to respond to endocrine measures may have lesions distal to the receptor-binding step. Since PgR may be considered as an end product of estrogen action in several estrogen target tissues, including rat mammary tumors and the human MCF-7 cell line, it was proposed that PgR be tested as a marker of hormone dependency of human breast cancers.[28] Review of the recent literature indicates that frequency of response to endocrine therapies in patients whose tumors contain both ER and PgR is more than twice that in patients with tumors containing ER but not PgR (71 percent vs. 32 percent responders).[40] It is not entirely clear that this does not merely reflect higher ER levels in the former group, since the percentage of patients with PgR distinctly increases with ER concentration.[40] On the other hand, it is obvious that the detection of PgR in a tumor is not a prerequisite for a response to endocrine treatments.

Androgen receptors were found in 20 to 50 percent of the tumor samples examined. There was a correlation between presence of these receptors and response to some endocrine treatments.[36] Additional data are required to assess whether androgen receptors can be a guide to therapy.

It was only in the last decade that human breast cancer tissue was shown to bind with high affinity small amounts of human prolactin (20 percent of the samples) or GH (12 percent of the samples).[41] This opens a new and promising field of research in the hormone dependency of human breast cancer.

General Conclusions

Clinical evidence points to endogenous estrogen as the hormone primarily involved in the maintenance of breast cancer growth, since estrogen suppression causes tumor regression in 20 to 40 percent of patients. Prolactin, which is important in the rat mammary tumor model, appears of little importance, if any, and no clear-cut synergism with estrogen has been demonstrated. No other hormone from ovaries, adrenals, or pituitary has been shown or even suspected to act on human breast cancer growth. Yet, pituitary ablation studies suggest that some factor in addition to estrogen is contributory.

Evidence from in vitro experiments is especially scanty. Here again, the only hormone that appears influential is estrogen. There is, nevertheless, a hint that prolactin might be involved, since it enhances the level of ER. Hormone receptor studies also point to a prominent role of estrogens. They show that the presence of ER in a tumor is a prerequisite for its hormone dependency and that the ER level is correlated with the likelihood of success of endocrine therapy. A potential role of progesterone is less obvious. The presence of receptors for this hormone is associated with a higher rate of therapeutic success but is not a prerequisite for endocrine responsiveness. Finally, the recent finding of prolactin receptors in a small proportion of breast cancers and the correlation of their presence with the responsiveness of the tumor to estrogens suggests that measurements of the concentration of these receptors may be useful for assessing the potential response to therapy.

Therapy of Breast Cancer

PRIMARY BREAST CANCER

The concepts underlying the classic surgical approach to the treatment of "localized" breast cancer are being reconsidered. William S. Halsted maintained that cure would be the result of a carefully executed surgical procedure in which all local and regional disease was eliminated.[41a] Since breast cancer was believed to spread centrifugally via the lymphatics and along surface planes, preserving continuity with the original growth, the treatment consisted of en bloc dissection of the primary tumor in continuity with regional lymph nodes and all intervening and contiguous tissues. It is becoming widely accepted that breast cancer in most cases is a systemic disease at the time of diagnosis (see above). As a result, surgery alone is often a palliative procedure. Surgery should be redirected to the primary aim of reducing the tumor burden of the patient to a number of viable cells that are entirely destructible by (1) host immunological (and other) factors alone, (2) systematically administered anticancer agents, or (3) a combination of both. The surgical modalities are also being reconsidered and subjected to clinical trials. Surgery of primary breast cancer and systemic adjuvant therapy in primary breast cancer have been thoroughly discussed in two recent reviews.[42,43]

ADVANCED BREAST CANCER

Endocrine vs. Cytotoxic Therapy

Until the middle 1960s, various endocrine manipulations were usually the preferred treatment for advanced breast cancer, and chemotherapy was a second-line resource. This is explained by the low response rate and short duration of response to single-agent chemotherapy. Thus, cyclophosphamide, fluorouracil, and methotrexate were approximately equally effective, with response rates not exceeding 20 to 25 percent. Although endocrine treatments were not much more effective in terms of response rates, their side effects were usually less, and duration of response was about double.

The situation dramatically changed with the introduction of effective combination chemotherapy. Three- and four-drug chemotherapy regimens yield response frequencies of nearly 55 to 60 percent, with duration of response often reaching 9 to 12 months. Subsequent treatment with other combinations still produces response rates of 25 to 30 percent. Furthermore, combination chemotherapy proved effective in metastatic sites of dire prognosis (usually not responsive to endocrine therapy), such as visceral sites and especially the liver. Under these conditions, chemotherapy is a serious competitor of endocrine therapy; however, neither should be used as the first-line approach without careful consideration of prognostic variables and, especially, ER.

A detailed analysis of chemotherapy of advanced breast cancer is not the aim of this chapter (the reader is referred to a recent excellent review of the problem[44]). In this chapter the various modalities of endocrine therapy and the criteria used for selecting among them and between endocrine therapy and chemotherapy are discussed.

Criteria of Response

In order to assess the clinical effectiveness of cancer therapy, it is necessary first to define what "response" means. In patients with advanced breast cancer, metastatic tumors may be present at various sites. Assessment is difficult in such situations as pleural effusions, lung lymphangitis, lytic or blastic bone lesions, or even indistinct skin lesions. Lesions are therefore either clearly measurable in two dimensions, measurable in only one dimension, or evaluable only. Response is defined in terms of all the lesions that the patient has and is determined by means of serial measurements, x-rays, isotopic scans, or photographs. A time element is also added to response. Serial measurements are taken regularly, usually at least once every 4 weeks; the patient is completely reevaluated at regular intervals, usually 3 to 6 months, in order to ensure that lesions not only regress but that none progresses and no new lesion appears.

A protocol of evaluation and definition of response was elaborated by a committee of the International Union against Cancer (UICC) and published in 1977 in the major cancer journals in the world;[45] an amendment was added in 1978. The purpose of these documents was to propose uniform guidelines for use in investigation on breast cancer therapy. Categories of response are defined as follows:

1. Objective regression.
   a. Complete response. The disappearance of all lesions determined by two observations not less than 4 weeks apart.
   b. Partial response. Fifty percent or more decrease in measurable lesions and unequivocal improvement in evaluable but nonmeasurable lesions with no new lesions developing, determined by two observations not less than 4 weeks apart.
2. No change. Lesions unchanged (i.e., < 50 percent decrease or < 25 percent increase in the size of measurable lesions).
3. Progressive disease.
   a. Mixed. Some lesions regress, while others progress or new lesions appear.
   b. Failure. Progression of some or all lesions and/or appearance of new lesions. No lesions regress.
4. Duration of response.
   a. The period of *overall response* is from the date of start of treatment to the date of first observation of progressive disease.
   b. The period of *complete response* is from the date complete response was first recorded to the date of first observation of progressive disease.

It is essential to categorize a patient as having a regression at a stated time. It is also essential that *all* baseline studies should have been repeated at this time.

Modalities of Endocrine Therapy

CASTRATION Before "therapeutic" castration is addressed, it is worthwhile to review briefly the issue of "adjuvant" castration, i.e., castration performed at the time of primary treatment, because it is still often performed by surgeons or by radiotherapists. A review of the literature indicates that adjuvant castration may slightly lengthen the disease-free interval but does not affect survival.[45a] It is therefore quite clear that castration should be withheld until recurrence of the disease; then it should be performed if it is still indicated.

Therapeutic castration is the endocrine treatment of choice in patients with advanced breast cancer when they are premenopausal or within 1 year of natural menopause; it is largely ineffective afterward.[29] Castration is achieved either surgically or by irradiation. In the latter case, the most frequently used dose of 450 rads given as a single treatment is probably insufficient, since menstrual bleeding recurs in one-third of the patients younger than 40 and in 10 percent of those older than 40. Surgery results in a more rapid response and should probably be given priority unless it is contraindicated by the patient's status; objective remissions (complete or partial) are produced in about 40 percent of cases.[45b] In patients younger than 35 years old, the percentage of remissions seems smaller, on the order of 16 percent. Duration of remissions varies from 3 to 44 months. Recognition of a response to castration is of prime importance, since it has predictive value for subsequent major endocrine ablative procedures (see below). It should therefore always be especially carefully documented.

ADRENALECTOMY Bilateral surgical adrenalectomy is performed in pre- or in postmenopausal women. In the former (last menstrual period less than a year before, unless hysterectomy has been performed), either castration is carried out as a first step and, in responders, adrenalectomy is delayed until remission has come to an end (see below), or the two ablative procedures are performed in one step; the two-step procedure seems preferable since it spares adrenalectomy in about two-thirds of the cases. After menopause, it is acceptable not to remove the ovaries. Nevertheless, their ablation has been recommended, since they are a potential source of estrogen precursors. Adrenalectomized patients require lifelong corticosteroid substitution. In the absence of stress, the usual requirement is, on the average, 25 mg of cortisol daily and 0.1 mg of fludrocortisone every day or every other day. Any stress requires an immediate increase in dosage, up to 300 mg of cortisol daily, either orally or intravenously (IV) [intramuscular (IM) administration is unsuitable because the absorption may be slow; see Chap. 15].

Reported response rates have varied from 28 to 57 percent;[45c] this variability probably resulted from differences in patient selection or in criteria used for defining a remission. An overall response rate in unselected cases of about 30 percent appears to be a realistic figure, with an average survival in responders of about 21 months, compared with 9 months in nonresponders. Patients who respond to castration are more likely to benefit from adrenalectomy at the time of relapse than are nonresponders (40 vs. 0 to 27 percent);[45d] it has been stated that castration nonresponders *always* fail to respond to adrenalectomy,[45e] provided that accurate assessments of response have been obtained for each treatment.

HYPOPHYSECTOMY Hypophysectomy is performed by either the transfrontal or the transsphenoidal route, or by implantation of ^{90}Y into the sella turcica. The transsphenoidal ablative procedure is preferred on theoretical grounds. Substitution therapy (with ADH and thyroid and adrenal hormones) is required when the operation is complete. Retrospective studies demonstrated similar rates of remission with hypophysectomy or adrenalectomy. There was, however, one prospective randomized trial comparing these procedures; its results suggest that hypophysectomy is superior to oophorectomy-adrenalectomy (remission rates are 36 and 23 percent; mean survival 20.2 vs. 12.2 months, $p < 0.01$).[45f] This point should be confirmed before preference is given to one or the other procedure.

ESTROGEN ADMINISTRATION Estrogen administration is effective in postmenopausal patients, but much more so in patients at least 4 to 5 years after their menopause (remission rates 29 vs. 8 percent). "Withdrawal response" or "rebound regression" can occur in addition to the response during estrogen therapy. Withdrawal response consists of an objective remission after discontinuation of therapy, most often when the treatment was successful. In three series of cases, high frequencies of withdrawal response (9/14, 10/39, and 5/11) have been reported in responders.[30]

Diethylstilbestrol (DES) is usually given orally in a dosage of 15 mg daily or ethinyl estradiol at 3 mg daily. Four different doses of DES ranging from 1500 to 1.5 mg daily were tested in a large randomized trial.[46] The higher doses produced significantly higher regression rates (21 vs. 10 percent) and higher rates of severe digestive side effects (25 vs. 12 percent); the higher doses were also associated with higher rates of severe hypercalcemia (7.5 vs. 0 percent), edema (33 vs. 16 percent), and congestive failure (8 vs. 3 percent). Severe congestive heart failure was not dose-related (approximately 2 percent overall), and uterine bleeding was less frequent at the higher doses (7 vs. 22 percent).

ANDROGEN ADMINISTRATION Although effective in premenopausal women, androgen therapy is used almost exclusively after the menopause. Objective remission is achieved in 22 percent of patients and is more frequent with advancing age after menopause. Median duration of remission is 36 weeks. Median survival time of remitters is 23 months as compared with only 9 months in the total group. Withdrawal response is less frequent than with estrogen.[30]

The compound most used in the past for androgen therapy was testosterone propionate at a dosage of 100 mg IM three times per week. It has been practically abandoned because of its severe side effects, which are virilization (hoarseness, hirsutism, alopecia, dermatological changes, ruddy complexion), increased libido, extracellular fluid retention, and hypercalcemia. It may sometimes be useful, though, because of an early-occurring, beneficial side effect, a feeling of well-being.[46a] Not infrequently, patients bedridden by pain and debility, particularly from osseous lesions, are rehabilitated even in the absence of objective regression. Dromostanolone (17β-hydroxy-2α-methyl-5α-androstan-3-one), 100 mg IM three times weekly, allegedly has less androgenicity than testosterone propionate. Testolactone, a compound structurally related to androgens but devoid of significant hormonal properties or side effects, proved therapeutically as effective as other androgens; the optimum oral dose was 1000 mg daily. This drug was later found to be an inhibitor of peripheral aromatization of androstenedione to estrone (see below, Corticosteroids and Aminoglutethimide).

The Cooperative Breast Cancer Group compared androgen with estrogen therapy in randomized trials involving some 500 postmenopausal patients. The respective remission rates were 10 and 18 percent, establishing the superiority of estrogens over androgens.[46b,46c]

PROGESTINS Several synthetic compounds with potent progestational activity were found to induce essentially the same rate of remission as reference androgens. Medroxyprogesterone acetate was initially given orally at a daily dose of 266 mg and was found to be practically devoid of side effects. Much larger doses, up to 2000 mg, given either orally (PO) or IM have recently been tried. A dose-response relationship seemed to obtain: 250 mg IM twice weekly was less effective than 1000 mg IM five times a week. Optimal dosage seems to be about 500 mg IM daily for one month (loading dosage) followed by the same dose given twice weekly (maintenance dosage), or 900 mg daily PO. Response rates are on the order of 30 percent and remissions have been reported after failure of other endocrine treatments. Side effects are not negligible; they include gluteal abscesses (in 15 percent of patients with the higher IM dosages), weight gain (in 61 percent), moon face (in 14 percent), increased blood pressure, fine tremors, etc.[47] Megestrol acetate is another synthetic progestational agent which is therapeutically effective in advanced breast cancer.

ESTROGEN ANTAGONISTS Nafoxidine, tamoxifen, and clomiphene citrate are three related styrene derivatives which share the property of interfering with ER action in estrogen target tissues, including breast cancer. They are all antiestrogens and weak estrogens by various tests in several species. They were found effective in the treatment of advanced breast cancer in postmenopausal women. In a random trial, nafoxidine induced a remission in a higher proportion of recipients than ethinyl estradiol (31 vs. 14 percent, $p = 0.07$);[47a] side effects on skin and hair were prohibitive, although toxic reactions were otherwise much less severe than with estrogen. Tamoxifen is the antiestrogen currently most used because it is almost entirely devoid of serious side effects at the moderate doses usually employed, i.e., 20 to 40 mg daily PO. However, at higher doses (60 to 100 mg per square meter of body surface) given for more than a year, it produced superficial corneal opacities, visual defects and retinopathy in four patients so treated.[47b] A daily oral dose of 30 mg of tamoxifen seems as effective as the higher dose of 90 mg. Compared to pharmacological estrogens in two randomized trials in postmenopausal patients, tamoxifen induced as many responses as the estrogens with a much lower incidence of side effects. In a large series of selected postmenopausal patients, objective response was achieved in 50 percent with a mean duration of response of over 21 months and a mean survival of more than 40 months. Regressions occurred with an equal frequency in visceral, osseous, and soft tissue lesions. The response rate was higher in ER-containing cases than in those whose ER content was unknown, and more women who were late-menopausal (> 10 years) responded than those who recently reached menopause (< 10 years before). Tamoxifen was effective in premenopausal patients, and seemed to give rise to a similar rate and duration of remission as surgical oophorectomy.

Several studies of various other endocrine treatments after tamoxifen therapy indicate that a secondary response can be obtained, especially in those patients who had an initial response to the antiestrogen. The likelihood of a secondary response is low when the patient failed to respond to tamoxifen as the initial treatment. In premenopausal patients who initially responded to tamoxifen, oophorectomy appears to be the secondary treatment of choice; in postmenopausal patients, "medical adrenalectomy" with aminoglutethimide (see below) is the secondary treatment of choice. In addition to its effectiveness as a first-line endocrine treatment, tamoxifen is also effective when used as a secondary form of endocrine treatment, whether the first-line therapy was additive or ablative.[48]

CORTICOSTEROIDS AND AMINOGLUTETHIMIDE Corticosteroids have been widely used in the treatment of advanced breast cancer, either alone or in association with cytotoxic drugs in various recent modalities of combination chemotherapy. In the latter mode, their usefulness has not been clearly established.

Corticosteroids have been given to produce "medical adrenalectomy"; at physiological doses, similar to those administered as substitution therapy after surgical adrenalectomy, they are largely ineffective. At higher doses, i.e., cortisone, 100 mg PO daily, or prednisone, 20 mg PO daily in divided doses, mixed responses were observed. At still higher doses (prednisolone, 30 mg PO daily), objective responses of short duration were reported in some 10 percent of treated patients.[48a] Aside from achieving actual tumor regression, corticosteroids at these doses are said to produce "major clinical improvement" in many cases through a nonspecific anti-inflammatory effect.[45c] Favorable subjective or objective effects, which may be clinically useful although often of short duration, have been the following: sensation of well-being, increase in appetite and weight, sedation of bone pain, improvement of myelophthisic anemia, and decrease of lymphedema of the arm; painful enlargement of the liver from metastases and respiratory distress from neoplastic lymphangitis are also reduced. Corticosteroids are successfully used for the control of hypercalcemia. Dexamethasone, 6 to 10 mg daily, is often extremely effective in temporarily controlling the neurological manifestations of brain metastases.

While adrenal suppression by corticosteroids alone requires rather high doses, with resultant cushingoid side effects, effective suppression was obtained with near-physiological cortisol, 40 mg daily in three divided doses, provided that it was supplemented with aminoglutethimide, 1000 mg daily in four divided doses.[48b] This compound inhibits the cholesterol side chain cleavage and aromatase systems by blocking the terminal cytochrome P450s. Inhibition of the cholesterol side chain cleavage activity leads to medical adrenalectomy. Aromatase inhibition interferes with the conversion of androstenedione and testosterone into estrone and estradiol, respectively, in the peripheral tissues, which represents the main source of endogenous estrogens in postmenopausal women. Conversion of androgens into estrogens also occurs in the breast cancer tissue itself in many patients. The simultaneous administration of aminoglutethimide and cortisol to postmenopausal women lowers the circulating level of estrogens to a similar extent as does surgical adrenalectomy. The role of cortisol is to prevent adrenal cortical insufficiency and a reflex release of ACTH, which would overcome the blocking of the adrenal steroidogenesis. The efficacy of aminoglutethimide-cortisol administration as a treatment of postmenopausal patients with advanced breast cancer appears to be similar to that of surgical adrenalectomy or tamoxifen therapy, as shown by controlled clinical trials. A randomized trial comparing aminoglutethimide-cortisol and tamoxifen in a cross-over study revealed these regimens to be equally effective, both as first- and second-line therapies.[48c] Side effects are mild and often transient; they include lethargy and dizziness, allergic skin rashes and drug fever, pancytopenia (rare), and hyperadrenalism. Together with tamoxifen, aminoglutethimide-cortisol may be considered at present one of the best endocrine treatments of advanced breast cancer in postmenopausal patients.[49]

SELECTION AMONG ENDOCRINE TREATMENTS In premenopausal women, surgical castration is generally considered the first-line endocrine therapy for advanced breast cancer. There is probably no place for hormone administration in menstruating patients, although androgens are undoubtedly effective, as also are antiestrogens or huge doses of estrogens (i.e., 1000 mg of DES daily). In postmenopausal women, major ablative procedures have been claimed to be superior to hormone administration, but this has been substantiated by only one randomized study comparing adrenalectomy with androgen administration which showed an advantage of the former.[49a] It should be remembered that androgens are less effective than estrogens, and estrogens less effective than antiestrogens. The last group may currently be recommended as the first-line endocrine treatment in this category of patients.

Major ablative procedures may be specifically indicated when hormone administration induces hypercalcemia. In these cases, medical adrenalectomy with aminoglutethimide-cortisol may be equally effective. One important point is that one class of hormone may be successful when another has failed or when the remission has come to an end. It is known, however, that a secondary hormonal therapy is less often successful than a primary one. Hormone administration has produced occasional regression of reactivated tumors after oophorectomy or even major ablative procedures.

Aside from leading to objective remissions, hormones may at times be very useful in unresponsive patients, especially those who are bedridden and debilitated from bone pains. Androgens (testosterone, dromostanolone) are recommended in this situation (see Androgen Administration, above). Corticosteroids (prednisolone, 30 mg, then 15 to 20 mg daily) may also be beneficial in these patients under the specific circumstances described under Corticosteroids and Aminoglutethimide, above.

Choice between Endocrine Therapy and Chemotherapy

CLINICAL VARIABLES The predictive value of various clinical variables in regard to response to therapy, either endocrine or cytotoxic, has been reviewed.[50] The data are summarized here.

Disease-free interval distinctly influences survival after relapse, irrespective of treatment. Longer disease-free intervals are associated with longer survival, especially when cases with sites with dire prognoses (see below) are excluded. Length of free interval and slow rate of evolution are correlated with the success rate of endocrine therapy, but the reverse is true for single-agent chemotherapy.

The site of metastatic involvement greatly influences survival. Some sites have especially poor prognosis, such as liver, peritoneum, brain, or spinal cord. With involvement of these sites, patients had a median survival of only 6 months.[50a] In patients without such involvement, survival was inversely related to the number of disease sites. Response to therapy is also influenced by the anatomical site of metastatic deposits. Surgical ablative procedures are equally effective on soft tissue and osseous lesions, but decreasingly so in pleura or lung, liver, and brain, in that order. Osseous metastases respond less often to hormone administration than soft tissue lesions. Hypercalcemia is associated with low response rate. Massive liver infiltration almost never responds to endocrine therapy. In contrast, combination chemotherapy proved quite effective, and sometimes surprisingly so, in this situation. Bone lesions seem relatively less sensitive to chemotherapy than to endocrine ablative procedures. Brain metastases are notoriously resistant to endocrine and cytotoxic therapy; treatment for these employs dexamethasone and radiotherapy.

Age and menopausal status also influence prognosis and response to treatment. Survival and response to castration are lower under age 35. This may be related to a shorter average disease-free interval in this group.[50] In postmenopausal women, the response rate to endocrine treatments has consistently increased with advancing age after the menopause. In contrast, the highest response rates with chemotherapy occur within the first years of menopause.

HORMONE RECEPTORS As already indicated, receptors for estrogen, progestin, androgen, and prolactin have been identified in human breast cancer. Estrogen receptors have been thoroughly studied as predictors of response to endocrine therapy; the results are discussed here. More recently, substantial work has been devoted to PgR as predictors of hormone dependency. Their potential clinical usefulness[40] has already been discussed. It is recommended that both ER and PgR concentrations be measured when possible in order to predict as accurately as possible the likelihood of a response to endocrine therapy and to select an appropriate treatment, i.e., endocrine therapy vs. chemotherapy or a combination of both; the selection is based not only on receptor determinations but also on clinical prognostic factors (see below). Androgen and prolactin receptors have no definite clinical application so far.

Assays of specific ER proteins make use of the receptor's ability to bind tightly to ^{3}H-labeled estradiol. The dextran-coated charcoal (DCC) method is relatively easy, fast, and sensitive and does not require expensive equipment. A standard DCC assay has been proposed by the European Organization for Research on Treatment of Cancer (EORTC)[51] and is described below. The sucrose gradient technique is slow and expensive, but it does (in contrast to the DCC method) distinguish the molecular forms of the receptor. However, the potential advantage of this additional information remains to be established.[36] Other assay methods include agar gel electrophoresis, protamine sulfate precipitation, hydroxyapatite adsorption, and Sephadex gel filtration. At present, no one assay is ideal, but in terms of simplicity and cost, the DCC method is probably the best.

The potential use of ER for predicting response of advanced breast cancer to endocrine therapy was first suggested by Jensen et al.,[39] who reported that in most patients with ER-positive tumor biopsies objective remission was achieved with adrenalectomy while cases without ER did not proceed to remission. This relation was confirmed and extended to other forms of endocrine therapy. Large series, including an international review,[37] have shown that 55 to 60 percent of patients with ER-positive breast tumors respond to hormonal manipulation therapy. In contrast, only 8 to 16 percent of ER-free patients respond to similar treatment.

The predictive value of ER became weaker, however, when it was found that, with sensitive assays, as many as 80 percent of human breast cancers in fact contain ER.[51a] Quantitative interpretation of the results was therefore attempted. The findings were[27,52] that ER levels in positive tumors vary along a wide range, extending from 3 to 2000 fmol per milligram of tissue protein; the mean level is lower in pre- than in postmenopausal women. The ER concentration could be used to characterize individual patients, since assay values at different sites and with passing time are similar in a given patient. ER level is positively correlated with the probability of a response to endocrine therapy. Indeed, when compared with 11 clinical variables of known prognostic value, ER level is the most significant variable in predicting response.

The relationship between ER level and probability of response is shown in Fig. 30-4. The graph is a representation of Cox's linear logistic regression model applied to a set of data collected at one institution.[52] A similar relationship was found in another laboratory; the parameters of the model were not significantly different.[53] When such a relationship is available in a given laboratory, it enables the biologist to provide the clinician with an estimate of the probability of response in a patient, based on the patient's particular ER level. For the final therapeutic decision (endocrine vs. cytotoxic chemotherapy), the clinical variables of known significance in relation to response (see above) are taken into account, either empirically or by introducing them into an improved model.[52]

Additional information provided by Fig. 30-4 is that a continuous gradient of hormone dependency seems to exist among breast cancer patients. According to this view, some form of endocrine therapy should be given to all patients, even when concurrent chemotherapy is deemed necessary. Along this line, an EORTC clinical trial associating tamoxifen with combination chemotherapy has yielded promising results.[54] Further research is necessary, however, to determine if the effect is truly additive and if the concurrent use of endocrine therapy and chemotherapy is better than their sequential administration not only to induce remission but to prolong survival.[44]

Laboratory Procedure: Assay for Estrogen Receptors

Tumor tissue is obtained in the operating theater under local or general anesthesia. It should be a piece of primary tumor, involved axillary node, cutaneous nodule, deposit in the abdominal cavity, or involved bone (e.g., iliac crest). The minimum amount required is 300 mg. A small representative sample is saved for pathological section. Immediately after excision, the specimen for ER assay is dipped in ice-cold Krebs-Ringer-Henseleit solution and brought at once to the laboratory. It is washed three times in ice-cold "tris" buffer containing a reducing agent (β-mercaptoethanol or dithiothreitol) and either processed immediately or quickly frozen and stored in liquid nitrogen, dry ice, or a freezing cabinet kept at −60°C.[27] Care should be taken to avoid accidental thawing and refreezing.

The assay method is only outlined here; a detailed description has been given elsewhere.[36,51] After thawing, the sample is homogenized in an all-glass homogenizer, and extreme care is taken to avoid undue heating. The homogenate is centrifuged at high speed, and the supernate (cytosol) is used. Aliquots of the cytosol are incubated with increasing amounts of [^{3}H]estradiol. Unbound steroid is removed with DCC. Bound radioactivity is measured in a scintillation counter. Results are plotted in the coordinates of Scatchard. Calculation (computer analysis is used in some laboratories) yields an estimate of the dissociation constant (K_d) and number of binding sites. The latter is expressed as femtomoles per milligram of *tissue* protein, with blood serum-contaminating proteins taken into account. The data are interpreted as indicated above.

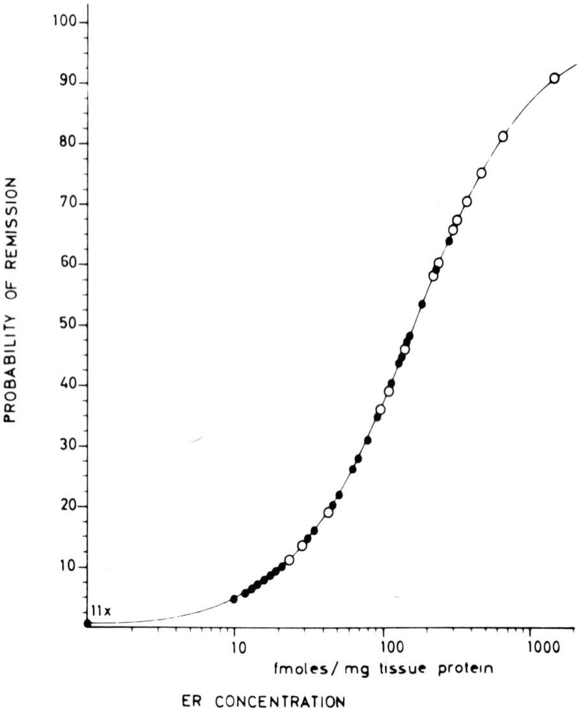

FIGURE 30-4 Relationship between the logarithm of estrogen receptor concentration and the probability of response to various endocrine treatments. [Data from 49 patients analyzed using Cox's linear logistic regression model; relationship is highly significant ($\chi^2 = 18.65$; $p = 0.000016$).] This relationship is represented in the figure by a sigmoid curve. Using the logistic model, the symbols on the curve give the *expected* probabilities of response calculated for each of the 49 patients from their receptor concentrations. The open circles (○) refer to the cases of remission, the filled circles (●) to those of failure. It is clear that remissions occurred along a wide range of probabilities extending from 11 to 91 percent. Their frequency increased, however, toward the right part of the curve. The model suggests that there exists a continuous gradient of hormone dependency among breast cancer patients. (*Modified and extended from Heuson et al.*[52] *Courtesy of the publisher.*)

False-positive results may be due to hyperplastic nonmalignant tissue contaminating the sample. Occasionally, nonbreast cancers (lymphomas, melanomas, and probably others) are positive. In both cases, ER levels are very low (approximately 10 fmol). *False-negative* results may occur after x-ray irradiation of the tissue, during or after systemic cytotoxic chemotherapy or endocrine therapy, or if tissue preparation is careless. Hormone administration, especially estrogens and antiestrogens, is likely to decrease the measured ER levels. After antiestrogen therapy, a delay of 6 to 8 weeks is probably required before meaningful results can be obtained.

ADENOCARCINOMA OF THE PROSTATE

Incidence

CLINICALLY MANIFEST CANCER

In American and European males, clinically manifest prostate adenocarcinoma is the second most common neoplasia, amounting to 16 percent of all malignant tumors in men. In the United States this carcinoma develops at a rate rising steadily with age, from 0.02 percent per year at age 50 to about 0.8 percent per year at age 80 in white males. Three American national surveys, spanning 34 years, show that the age-adjusted incidence rate of prostate adenocarcinoma for men below 75 years is much higher in the black population. During this period, a rise in incidence has been recorded in white and nonwhite persons, although the rate of increase has been much faster in the black population. For people older than 75 years, the peak incidence in black males is in the 80- to 84-year age group, followed by a drop at and above age 85 years, while the rate still increases with age, without any drop, in white males.[55]

The mortality rates are about one-third as great as the corresponding incidence rates. Although this cancer is considered the third most common cause of death in males older than 50 years, it must be stressed that intercurrent diseases are an important cause of death in the oldest patients, amounting to 45 percent of all deaths of prostate cancer patients older than 70 years.

INCIDENTAL CANCER

In several published series, prostatectomy specimens of men operated upon for a nonmalignant disease of the gland and prostates removed at postmortem examinations of men who died without a known prostate cancer were studied.[55a] These investigations revealed, in a variable percentage of cases, the presence of a microscopic prostate carcinoma; yet, in these cases there was no previously recognizable clinical or laboratory evidence of prostate cancer. The prevalence of this latent or incidental carcinoma also increases with age, as shown in several postmortem studies, ranging from 5 to 14 percent in the 50- to 59-year age group to 20 to 40 percent in the 70- to 79-year age group. As these values are much higher than the mortality rates from prostate cancer, it may be considered that most incidental carcinomas do not give rise later to clinically evident prostate cancers.

Risk Factors and Etiology

GEOGRAPHIC DISTRIBUTION

There is a wide geographic variation of mortality rates from prostate cancer. The rate is as high as 18 per 100,000 per year in Sweden and as low as 2 per 100,000 per year in Japan. However, males of Japanese origin living in the United States have a mortality rate from prostate cancer intermediate between the very low Japanese rate and the much higher rate of white males in the United States. Such an increase in mortality rates in immigrants occurs only after 20 or more years of living in the United States. As the prevalence of latent or incidental carcinoma is the same in the United States and in Japan, this indicates again that only a small fraction of the incidental cancers pursue an aggressive course.[56] There is, however, an important difference between the two populations: about 90 percent of the American latent carcinomas are of the proliferative type, while most of the latent carcinomas in Japan are of the silent type. Likewise, a comparison of a high-risk American black population with a low-risk Nigerian black population reveals that the age-adjusted incidences for latent carcinoma diagnosed at postmortem examination are approximately equal in both populations, although the incidence of invasive prostate adenocarcinoma is much higher in the American population.

SOCIOECONOMIC FACTORS

No epidemiologic study shows an association between the mortality rate or the incidence of prostate cancer and social class or number of years of education. The difference in incidence between nonwhite and white males in the United States cannot be explained by a difference in economic status. No consistent association of prostate cancer incidence with the site of residence, i.e., urban vs. rural, has been demonstrated. In patients older than 70, there seems to be an association between a low mortality rate from this cancer and Jewish ethnicity.

FAMILIAL AND GENETIC FACTORS

A positive correlation by country between mortality from carcinoma of the prostate and from carcinoma of the breast has been reported. Familial aggregation of cases of prostate carcinoma has been described. Nevertheless, no data are available suggesting a role of genetic determinants in this cancer. A retrospective study comparing the physical and demographic characteristics of young men who later died from prostate cancer with those of a control group did not reveal any special characteristic conferring a high risk for this tumor.[57] Some investigators report that the age-specific prostate cancer mortality is associated in white males with marital status, increasing in the order from single to married, widowed, and divorced, at all ages 65 and over; a similar pattern is suggested in black males. However, another well-controlled study does not show this association.[57a] The tumor seems to be more frequent in more fertile married males and in males with a greater sexual drive.[57b]

OCCUPATIONAL FACTORS

There is an excess frequency of prostate cancer in workers in the cadmium industry and an increased mortality from several cancers, including prostate carcinoma, in workers in the rubber industry. Although prostate cancer tissue is less rich in zinc ion than normal tissue, cadmium ion is known to compete for binding of zinc that may concentrate in prostate tissue. In rodents, cadmium compounds are known to induce neoplasia of the testis.

DIET

Data from several studies conducted among several ethnic and religious groups support the association between a high incidence of prostate carcinoma and the consumption of meat, milk, and eggs.

RELATION TO BENIGN HYPERTROPHY

Because of the high frequency in older men of both prostate carcinoma and benign prostate hyperplasia, a possible association between the two diseases has been investigated in two controlled studies.[58,59] In the first, a higher incidence of prostate carcinoma was found in patients with benign hypertrophy diagnosed by rectal examination, biopsy, or prostatectomy; in the second, which included a much larger number of cases, no higher incidence of prostate cancer was found in patients with benign hypertrophy diagnosed only on subtotal prostatectomy specimens. The populations of the two studies probably differed, and further investigations about this possible association are needed. In fact, benign hypertrophy cannot be considered as a histologic precursor of prostate cancer, but it may develop as a tissue response to some carcinogenic or endocrine stimulus that induces malignant transformation of the normal tissue.

ENDOCRINE FACTORS

The absence of prostate cancer and of benign prostate hypertrophy in prepubertal eunuchoid or true eunuchoid patients is sometimes considered as indicating that hormones play a role in the human prostate carcinogenesis process.[59a] Such an argument is probably not valid, since the absence of both pathological conditions in these patients is probably due to the lack of development of the prostate epithelium. In patients with prostate cancer and benign prostate hypertrophy, investigation of several urinary hormones and hormone metabolites has been performed. Using a linear discriminant function, coefficients can be attributed to each of these variables. These can provide an index score on which the cancer and hypertrophy patient groups are clearly separated. However, as these studies were performed when the disease was already clinically evident, they cannot provide reliable information on the possible endocrine changes that played a role at the time of induction of the tumor. No conclusion can be drawn from the hormone sensitivity of an established malignant tumor regarding the mechanisms of its induction or from the dependence of typical cell morphology on androgens in organ culture. Prolonged treatment with sex steroid hormones is not known to be associated with the development of prostate cancer in human beings. Aging in men is characterized by accelerated aromatization of androgens, a decrease in the apparent serum free testosterone concentration, and an increase in the serum estradiol/testosterone ratio. However, there is little evidence at present that modifications in the production rates, disposition, and catabolism of androgens and estrogens are causative factors in the development of prostate carcinoma in human beings. Although age is related to the incidence of prostate cancer, the mechanism of this relation remains still unclear.

POSSIBLE ROLE OF VIRUSES

A seroepidemiologic study showed that the serum of patients with benign prostate hypertrophy and those with prostate carcinoma contains antibodies against herpes simplex virus type 2, without any significant difference between the two groups.[59b] In a more recent study, an increased prevalence of antibody to herpes simplex virus type 2 has been found in the serum of patients with prostate carcinoma as compared to patients with benign hyperplasia; however there was some evidence that patients with cancer had had a larger number of sex partners. At present there is no substantial evidence for an etiologic relationship of any virus with human prostate adenocarcinoma.

INFORMATION FROM ANIMAL TUMOR MODELS

Spontaneous adenocarcinomas of the prostate occur, very infrequently, in several animal species; they usually occur in senescent individuals. In the AXC rat strain, a 70 percent frequency of spontaneous adenocarcinoma of the ventral prostate has been reported in aged (30- to 46-month-old) virgin males. The senescent ventral prostate in this rat strain is characterized by decrease in cytoplasmic and nuclear androgen receptor content, by decrease in 5α-DHT synthesis, and by increased capacity for the synthesis of 4-androstene-3,17-dione. As a different pattern of aging modifications is observed in the dorsal prostate, where no carcinoma develops, it is possible that the biochemical modifications occurring in the ventral prostate are related to the development of cancer in this organ.[60]

Adenocarcinomas of the prostate have also been reported in aged germ-free Wistar rats. As other prostate lesions and benign liver tumors are also present in the animals, it is possible they have been exposed to an unknown carcinogenic agent. Adenocarcinoma of the dorsal prostate is observed in Nb rats with an estrogen-induced Leydig cell carcinoma of the testes that induces marked secondary androgenization.

Whole-body irradiation of germ-free Wistar and Fisher rats is not associated with the development of prostate cancer, although several endocrine tumors and endocrine-sensitive breast tumors are induced. In some experimental animals carcinogenic hydrocarbons induce squamous cell prostate carcinomas that usually do not metastasize. In vitro malignant transformation of animal prostate cells by carcinogens or viruses, followed by retransplantation, leads to the development in the host of fibrosarcomas that are either hormone-insensitive or react to endocrine manipulations in a paradoxical way.

Hormonal Regulation of Tumor Growth

Despite the clinical effectiveness of endocrine manipulation in human prostate cancer, the hormonal factors that regulate the growth of this tumor are not well-known. Extrapolation to human beings of the numerous data from experiments performed in animal systems should be considered with the utmost caution. Indeed, the prostate gland is one of the very few organs that exhibit marked species-specific differences in embryogenesis, morphological structure, and function. These differences may explain the lack of availability of a suitable animal tumor model.

ANIMAL TUMORS

The normal canine prostate is more comparable to the human one than is the prostate of rodents, but unfortunately it cannot be considered to be the human gland's counterpart. The active androgen metabolite in the dog prostate probably is not 5α-DHT but 3α,17α-dihydroxy-5α-androstane; the only common prostate tumor in the dog is benign hypertrophy, which is still, unlike the human one, androgen-sensitive. Prostate carcinoma, although occurring spontaneously in senescent dogs and sharing many morphological, histochemical, and clinical similarities with the human cancer, has a low incidence and has not been known to show a clear-cut response to endocrine treatments.

The Dunning R3327H adenocarcinoma originating from the dorsal prostate of an old male Copenhagen rat can be transplanted subcutaneously in some types of rats. This tumor is known to contain 70 to 90 percent androgen-sensitive cells that have androgen receptors. The tumor undergoes partial involution with castration or antiandrogen or estrogen therapy, but, because of the unhampered growth of its hormone-insensitive cell population, a fraction ultimately relapses to a hormone-insensitive state. Several other tumor lines derived from the original Dunning tumor are anaplastic and androgen-insensitive. Tumors originating in aged germ-free Wistar rats, when transplanted, produce metastases to the viscera and bones. Although such metastatic spread is rather infrequent in most experimental tumor systems, the major drawback of this model is its paradoxical response to the administration of DES.

HUMAN TUMORS

As normal human prostate is less readily available than pathological tissues, most of the reported biochemical differences concern carcinomatous and benign hypertrophic tissues. No significant differences have been found in the plasma testosterone and DHT levels of patients with benign prostate hypertrophy and patients with prostate cancer. In vitro [^{3}H]testosterone uptake by both tissues is relatively similar, but there is much less conversion of testosterone to DHT in carcinomatous tissues, especially in metastatic lymph nodes in which the normal structure has been completely replaced with tumor cells.[61]

Xenografts of human prostate tumors in T-cell-deprived animals (nude mice) is a model of great potential, but is still in limited use.

ROLE OF HORMONES

In vitro techniques using incubation of tissue slices, constant-flow organ culture, and cell fractionation have provided some information about the effect of hormones on cell morphology and intracellular biochemical processes. All the present evidence suggests that the multiplication of normal prostate epithelial cells is dependent on the transformation in the cytoplasm of testosterone to DHT under the influence of the enzyme 5α-reductase, and subsequent incorporation of testosterone (as DHT) into the cell nucleus. The newly formed DHT is first bound to a specific high-affinity, low-capacity intracellular protein receptor with sedimentation coefficient 5 to 8 S. The steroid-receptor complex then binds to chromatin and leads to increases in the abundances of specific mRNAs. The magnitude of the response of the target cell is determined by the DHT-receptor complex concentration in the cell nucleus.

STEROID HORMONE RECEPTORS

Binding proteins for androgens have been characterized extensively in rat prostates. In humans, the investigation of androphilic macromolecules is complicated by the presence in prostate tissue samples of the plasma sex hormone–binding globulin (SHBG), which binds androgens with high affinity, and plasma albumin-steroid complexes. A high-affinity, low-capacity DHT receptor has been demonstrated in the primary human prostate tumor as well as in its metastatic lymph nodes.[62] Some tumor samples also contain estradiol receptors and perhaps PgR.

CLINICAL EVIDENCE

The reduced 5α-reductase activity and the variable concentration of macromolecules with affinity for DHT in carcinomatous human prostate tissue may indicate that this tissue has a diminished androgen sensitivity as compared with the normal gland. Interpretation of these data is rather difficult. For instance, human benign hypertrophic prostate tissue that has a much higher rate of DHT production than has carcinomatous tissue seems to be androgen-insensitive, and its growth rate is not modified by antiandrogenic treatments.[62a] The possibility that the prostate cancer cell uses testosterone instead of DHT for initiating the nuclear reactions, as in some other androgen-sensitive tissues, has not yet been investigated.

Observations of objective remissions induced by endocrine therapies are at present the only evidence of the hormone sensitivity of human prostate cancer. Bilateral orchiectomy results in a four- to eightfold decrease in plasma testosterone concentration.[62b] Although administration of testosterone to patients with prostate adenocarcinoma has, in a few cases, produced an obvious exacerbation of the disease, as indicated by an alteration of the clinical findings and an increase in the blood acid phosphatase activity, no correlation has been found among the levels of urinary androgen metabolites before orchiectomy, their fall after the operation, and the type of response to castration.[62c] In the same way, no correlation has been demonstrated in patients treated with DES in various dosages between the pretreatment plasma total testosterone levels and the clinical findings. In the Veterans Administration Cooperative Urological Research Group (VACURG) studies, there is no relation between the magnitude of the fall of the plasma total testosterone level induced by two different effective dosages of DES and the duration of the patients' survival. It should be added that in some rare cases administration of testosterone has been associated with both subjective and objective remission. Some of these tumors may have an estrogen dependence, as has been suggested by data showing an estrogen-like histologic pattern in some prostate cancers that had never been treated before with estrogenic compounds. The possible role of pituitary hormones, and especially of prolactin, has not been delineated in humans.

Natural History

PATHOLOGY

Hormone-sensitive prostate tumors are found only among the adenocarcinomas, which make up 95 percent or more of all prostate malignancies. Most of them arise from the acini, but a small proportion, about 2 percent, are of a distinctive ductal type. Although it is generally considered that most prostate adenocarcinomas originate in the posterior lobe of the gland, recent data show that they may arise anywhere in the gland.[56] Studies on prostatectomy specimens show that less than 10 percent of the tumors are single nodules; about 85 percent are multifocal or extensive at the time of diagnosis.

LOCAL EXTENSION AND DISSEMINATION

Some authors have proposed a histologic classification based on five different patterns, ranging from the very well differentiated tumor to the quite anaplastic tumor with little or no differentiation into glands.[62d]

However, as more than one pattern is present in many of the prostate carcinomas, these authors associate, for each tumor, a primary with a secondary histologic pattern. This enables them to classify the different cancers in a prognostic category. Nevertheless, other investigators have completely failed in attempting histologic grading of their cases, since several histologic patterns have been found in the same prostate tumor and even on the same slide.[63,63a]

About 84 percent of the tumors present with invasion of the perineural space, mainly located in the periphery of the gland near the junction of the lateral and posterior lobes. This phenomenon occurs early in the course of the disease and is not an unfavorable prognostic sign, since the perineural space is not, as was once thought, a lymphatic channel.

Local extension of the tumor results from invasion through the capsule of the gland; dissemination may occur by both the lymphatic and hematogenous routes. Lymph node metastases may occur very early in the course of the disease, but as the most common sites of involvement are the obturator, hypogastric, and iliac nodes, they are usually not detected by physical examination. Paraaortic lymph nodes are in most cases associated with pelvic nodes. Some rare cases have been reported in which cervical lymph nodes were the first clinical sign of the disease. The most frequent blood-borne metastases are the osseous ones, involving most frequently the pelvis, vertebrae, femurs, and ribs. Osteoblastic lesions are the most prominent. It has been reported that bone metastases are much more frequent in patients with anaplastic tumors, but, because of the difficulties of histologic grading, such an association is not firmly established. Pulmonary metastases are found in 25 percent of the cases at their terminal state, but visceral metastases may involve the liver, the adrenal glands, and even the brain, about 4 percent of the cases.

Clinical Staging and Diagnosis

CLASSIFICATION SYSTEMS

Two different staging systems are used. In the United States, a four-stage system is used, with each stage divided into two subgroups:

Stage A is represented by the incidental carcinoma found in tissue removed for a nonmalignant prostate disease. The subgroup A1 is defined as a well-differentiated, focal lesion; subgroup A2 is defined as a multifocal lesion, undifferentiated or not.

Stage B describes a tumor confined within the prostate capsule. If the tumor is less than 1.5 cm in diameter it is classified as subgroup B1; if the tumor is larger or is found in both prostate lobes it is classified as subgroup B2.

Stage C is a tumor that has spread to the periprostatic tissues. If the estimated weight of the tumor is less than 70 g it is classified as subgroup C1; if it weighs more than 70 g or has spread to the trigone, the bladder neck, or the seminal vesicles it is classified as subgroup C2.

Stage D describes a tumor with demonstrable metastases. If there is involvement of pelvic lymph nodes below the bifurcation of the common iliac artery or invasion of the adjacent organs it is classified as subgroup D1; if other lymph nodes are involved or if distal metastases are present, it is classified as subgroup D2.

In Europe, the TNM classification (T for primary tumor, N for lymph node, M for metastses) from the UICC is more frequently used. In this system each tumor is defined by the extension of the primary tumor, the involvement of regional lymph nodes, and the presence of distant metastases.

In the first VACURG study, the distribution of the patients at the time of admission was: stage A, 9 percent; stage B, 11 percent; stage C, 44 percent; and stage D, 36 percent. This indicates clearly that most cases are diagnosed at a rather advanced stage of the disease.

STAGING PROCEDURE

Digital rectal examination allows the delineation of an indurated area in the prostate and the detection of spread into the periprostatic tissues.

General physical examination may detect the presence of distant metastatic lymph nodes and painful bones suspected of harboring metastases.

Transrectal ultrasonography is now used for a more accurate delineation of the tumor areas in patients with localized prostate carcinoma.

Bipedal lymphangiography is considered of limited usefulness because of the difficulty of interpreting the node pictures. Computerized axial tomography (CT) is of value for the assessment of pelvic nodes if they are larger than 2 cm. Therefore, some centers resort to pelvic lymph node dissection for accurate staging.

Radioisotope bone scan is an extremely sensitive method for detecting the reactive bone formation accompanying osseous metastases. It is more sensitive but less specific than the x-ray skeletal survey, giving frequent false-positive results in older patients suffering from osteoarthritic disease. In less than 2 percent of patients with radiographic evidence of bone metastasis the bone scan is negative.

Radiographic skeletal survey discloses the type of bone involvement. In most cases the metastases are of the osteoblastic type with possible mixed osteolytic lesions. The pictures, although highly suggestive of disseminated prostate cancer, are not pathognomonic.

Bone biopsy is mandatory when the sole evidence of dissemination of the disease is a single "hot spot" on bone scan. In cases of multiple osseous involvement, it demonstrates that the radiographic pictures are due to prostate cancer metastasis. At the time of the biopsy, bone marrow may be taken in order to assess medullary cell distribution, which may be of great value if chemotherapy is planned. The value of the bone marrow acid phosphatase determination for the detection of osseous metastasis has not been established.

Intravenous urography or kidney ultrasonography is used to detect possible hydronephrosis due to ureteral obstruction.

Blood biochemical tests must include the determination of the serum creatinine concentration, alkaline phosphatase activity, which is increased in cases with osteoblastic lesions, and activities of acid phosphatase and its prostate fraction, increase of which probably indicates a disseminated stage of the disease.

X-ray of the chest may show lung and/or pleural involvement.

Evaluation of cardiac status is mandatory when estrogen therapy is planned.

DIAGNOSIS OF PATHOLOGY

Any suspicion of prostate carcinoma requires a histologic verification. Transrectal and transperineal needle biopsies are the most popular methods. The transrectal aspiration biopsy method using the equipment described by Franzen[63b] may be used as an office procedure because it produces little discomfort, is rather atraumatic, has a low rate of complications, and allows a reliable cytologic diagnosis of the disease to be made.[64]

Tumor Markers

ACID PHOSPHATASE

Although prostate carcinomatous tissue has a lower concentration of acid phosphatase than normal tissue, the serum acid phosphatase activity is increased in the majority of patients with disseminated prostate adenocarcinoma. This elevation correlates better with the extent of the disease than with the sites of metastases and is observed in 70 to 90 percent of the patients with bone involvement. Spurious increase in serum acid phosphatase activity may be observed if prostate massage or bladder catheterization has been performed in the preceding 24 h.

Several immunological methods for the determination of serum prostate acid phosphatase are now available. They are useful for monitoring the response to therapy, especially as, in some cases, these methods may detect an increase in activity that is not demonstrable by the usual enzymatic assay.[65]

OTHER TUMOR MARKERS

Prostate-specific antigen (PSA) is expressed by cancer cells independently from prostate acid phosphatase. An increase in serum PSA concentration has been demonstrated in 86 percent of stage D cases; PSA is a useful tumor marker for monitoring the response to therapy. Carcinoembryonic antigen concentration and ribonuclease activity are increased in the serum of some patients with prostate cancer. It has not yet been established that they are useful for the monitoring of the disease.[65]

STEROID RECEPTORS

Androgen and estrogen receptors, alone or in combination, have been described in human prostate adenocarcinoma. Because of the heterogeneity of the tumor, the lack of stability of some receptors, and the presence in tumor tissue of other binding proteins of plasma origin, this field is still far less developed than in human breast cancer. No definite information is available about the possible relation between the presence of these receptors and the type of response to endocrine manipulations.

Criteria for Prognosis

CLINICAL VARIABLES

As 45 percent of prostate cancer patients over age 70 die of intercurrent disease, the age of the patient is the first prognostic factor to be considered. The second variable is the clinical stage, as demonstrated by the 5-year survival rate of patients in the first VACURG study: 63 percent for stages A and B, with a very small number of deaths due to prostate cancer; 50 percent for stage C, with a 10 percent mortality rate due to cancer; and 23 percent for stage D, with a 42 percent mortality rate due to cancer.[65a] Some of these rates may be changing in the near future if staging laparotomy for the detection of involved regional lymph nodes is more extensively performed. However, it has been clearly demonstrated that the extension of the tumor in the prostate capsule and the seminal vesicles is determined accurately by rectal examination in about 80 percent of the cases. This is an important point, as shown by the differences in survival: 66.6 percent of the patients with normal seminal vesicles are living 7 years later, when only 32.2 percent of those with invasion of the vesicles are still living.[63] Stage C patients who develop evidence of metastasis have a different median survival according to the type of dissemination of the disease: 15 months with lymph node, lung, or liver involvement; 11 months with bone involvement; 10 months with a very high ($\geq$ 10 King-Armstrong units) serum acid phosphatase activity; and 8 months with upper urinary tract obstruction.[66] Another variable is related to the type of treatment: older age ($\geq$ 75 years) and anemia are highly significant risk factors in patients to be treated with estrogenic compounds, as these patients have been known to die of cardiovascular side effects of their treatment.

HISTOLOGIC AND ENDOCRINE VARIABLES

As stated above, there is much controversy about the value of histologic grading of prostate adenocarcinoma. In two studies, a high mortality rate was associated in advanced clinical stages with the less-differentiated tumors.[66a,66b]

No prognostic significance has been established for any endocrine parameter.

Evaluation of Response to Treatment

Duration of survival from the start of therapy has been used in several studies on prostate cancer as an objective criterion to evaluate the response. Unfortunately, this method is of no use for an adequate assessment of the remission rate produced by a given treatment. Moreover, it has several apparent drawbacks, such as the requirement for long-term studies because of the high percentage of cases which develop rather slowly, and interference in the interpretation of the mortality data by intercurrent diseases, which are fairly frequent among older patients. More recently, several clinical trials have been performed using some objective criteria:

Size of the primary prostate tumor, determined by rectal examination and transrectal ultrasonography. *Superficial lymph nodes* and cutaneous and subcutaneous *metastatic lesions,* although rather rare, are very useful; they are measured as in breast metastatic lesions. *Regional lymph nodes,* according to some authors, may be evaluated by lymphangiography; sufficiently large regional nodes can be assessed by CT. *Bone lesions,* frequently osteoblastic, lack sharp borders. Nevertheless, a quantitative analysis shows a correlation between the number of sites, the extent of involvement within each site, and patient survival. Bone radioisotope scan may also be used and quantified, provided that "hot spots" due to osteoarthritic lesions are not taken into account. *Nodular lung metastases, mediastinal lymph nodes,* and *liver involvement* are assessed as in breast cancer patients. Decrease in activity, or normalization of an elevated activity of, *serum prostate acid phosphatase* and/or decrease of an elevated *PSA concentration* may be indications of response. *Normalization of hemostatic parameters,* modified by acute or chronic disseminated intravascular coagulation, may also be informative. Decrease of *serum alkaline phosphatase activity* may be used, provided that its increase was due to the presence of osteoblastic metastases. *Degree of dilation of the upper urinary tract* can be an indicator of ureteral obstruction due to the disease.

The patient's physical state, even measured on a performance scale, is not an adequate criterion of response in older patients, because it is probably a better index of the impact of intercurrent diseases than of the prostate cancer. Pain, a subjective criterion, cannot be used alone for evaluation, because it may be modified by several factors different from tumor spreading.

Evaluation of the response to treatment must be based on arbitrary rules, using several parameters like a significant decrease in or disappearance of tumor masses, a decrease of at least 50 percent in or a normalization of the increased phosphatase activities, a recalcification of bone lytic lesions, or stabilization of disease or disappearance of bone sclerotic lesions. Appearance of a new metastatic focus must be considered evidence of progression.[67]

Treatment

TREATMENT OF STAGES A AND B

Despite the fact that a high number of therapeutic modalities are used all over the world to treat prostate cancer patients, only a few controlled, randomized therapeutic trials have been performed, making precise recommendation about treatment schedules difficult.[68] Although patients with incidental carcinoma (stage

A) were treated until recently by radical prostatectomy, there is now some evidence suggesting that stage A1 tumors may be reevaluated regularly and submitted to treatment if the disease becomes clinically manifest. Stage A2 tumors are much more aggressive; most authors consider that they must be treated at the time of diagnosis by radical prostatectomy or irradiation therapy. In stage B patients, preliminary data from VACURG suggest that regular observation is indicated, but in several hospitals the current practice is a staging laparotomy for assessment of the real stage of the disease. If the regional lymph nodes are not involved, a radical prostatectomy is performed or radiation therapy is started. Prostatectomy renders the patient sexually impotent and causes stress incontinence, at least temporarily; the rate of mortality from prostatectomy is about 1 percent. Megavoltage external beam irradiation is accompanied in about 12 percent of the cases by persistent severe gastrointestinal or genitourinary symptoms. Urethral stricture develops in about 4 percent of the patients, and sexual impotence is observed in at least 40 percent.

In a prospective randomized trial that compared the efficacy of surgery with that of irradiation, radical prostatectomy was found to be more effective than megavoltage irradiation. First evidence of treatment failure was used as the end point of the study.[69] These results have proved to be controversial. In cases with involvement of the regional lymph nodes, the irradiation fields are extended to include the pelvic nodes. Interstitial implantation of ^{125}I seeds into the prostate tumor and implantation of ^{198}Au grains combined with external irradiation are other therapeutic modalities not yet evaluated.

TREATMENT OF STAGES C AND D

In cases of periprostatic involvement (stage C), some physicians perform a staging laparotomy associated, as in stage B, with a radical prostatectomy or radiation therapy. The results of prostatectomy, however, are generally considered disappointing at this stage. In fact, in stage C patients, the most widely used therapeutic modality is endocrine treatment, as for stage D cases. It must be stressed that its remission rate has never been accurately established by adequate studies, but there is some evidence suggesting that it is efficient in at least 40 percent of the cases. VACURG studies have demonstrated that orchiectomy is somewhat less effective in preventing deaths from cancer than DES and that a combination regimen of orchiectomy followed by DES is not superior to the estrogen treatment alone.[69a] These studies have also shown that a 1-mg daily dose of DES is as effective as a 5-mg dose in reducing the death rate from cancer, despite the fact that it results in less lowering of the plasma testosterone level in stage D patients.[68] Many authors recommend a 3-mg daily dose of DES, although its toxicity has not yet been assessed. Chlorotrianisene, which is weakly estrogenic, does not lower the plasma testosterone level at dosages effective in prostate cancer. Its antineoplastic action may result from a direct effect on the tumor. The plasma testosterone level is actually rather low in patients with disseminated prostate cancer; there is no evidence of an elevated rate of testosterone production in these patients.

Estrogens may act both directly on the tumor and by a pituitary and testicular inhibition mechanism. Recent data suggest that even a 1-mg daily dose of DES may be associated with an increased risk of cardiovascular deaths in patients older than 75 years. Other side effects of estrogens are well-known, including GI intolerance, loss of libido, impotence, gynecomastia, coloration of the nipple (especially induced by DES), and changes in the concentrations of some of the plasma lipids and proteins. As the plasma corticosteroid-binding globulin level is increased by estrogens, patients who do not take the compound may be detected in the first period of treatment by failure of corticosteroid-binding globulin concentration to rise. There is no available evidence that DES diphosphoric esters, natural estrogens, and polyestradiol phosphate are superior to the cheap and stable DES. Although the proper timing of and indications for endocrine treatment remain matters of controversy, it is suggested that the treatment be started at the time of diagnosis only in patients with a progressing, large primary, or anaplastic tumor or pain due to metastasis.

A patient with a history of cardiovascular disease or who is in poor physical condition should not be treated with estrogens unless progression of the disease makes it mandatory. In such patients an alternative first therapy may be an orchiectomy, provided that there is no contraindication, or additive antiandrogen treatment. The first nonestrogenic androgen antagonists found to be active in patients with prostate carcinoma were pregnane derivatives such as progesterone, chlormadinone acetate, and medroxyprogesterone. These progestins are devoid of peripheral antiandrogen action; they inhibit the endocrine secretion of the hypophysis, inducing in this way a reduction of the testosterone synthesis rate. They are less effective than DES.

New antiandrogens that directly antagonize the action of androgen hormones at their target tissues have been synthesized. These compounds block the binding of the active androgens by the receptors. One of them, the steroidal compound cyproterone acetate, which has other endocrine properties, has been reported to be active in prostate cancer at a daily dosage of 200 to 300 mg.[70] Its side effects are malaise, flushing, dizziness, fluctuation in body weight, reversible loss of libido, gynecomastia, and a possible suppressive effect on ACTH secretion. Flutamide, a substituted anilide that is partially transformed in vivo into a more potent derivative, is active in human prostate cancer at a daily dosage of 750 to 1500 mg.[71] Although not yet (at the time of publication) approved by the U.S. Food and Drug Administration (FDA), it has been administered to patients, resulting, in most patients, in a rise in the 24-h mean plasma testosterone level; the elevation is due to increased testosterone production but is not accompanied by significant change in plasma DHT and luteinizing hormone levels. The plasma androsterone/etiocholanolone ratio is extremely elevated. Gynecomastia occurs as a side effect. No controlled trials have been conducted to evaluate the rate of objective remissions produced by these new drugs.

Interference with the hypophyseal secretion of prolactin by the use of an effective inhibitor, bromocriptine, has not resulted in objective remissions in prostate cancer patients.[72]

Conflicting results of the use of antiestrogens in advanced prostate cancer have been reported.

Recently, administration of gonadotropin releasing hormone (GnRH) analogues by the intranasal or the subcutaneous route has been shown to result in a reduction in plasma testosterone concentration to castrate levels. (GnRH analogues have not yet been approved by the FDA.) Preliminary reports suggest that these compounds have therapeutic efficacy in advanced prostate cancer.[72]

ENDOCRINE TREATMENT OF RESISTANT OR RELAPSING TUMORS

When resistance or relapse is observed in patients on endocrine treatment, the probability of a favorable response to a second endocrine therapy is rather low. Objective remissions have been reported with antiandrogen compounds in patients previously treated with estrogens. Surgical adrenalectomy and hypophysectomy have induced remissions of relatively short duration in a small number of patients. Aminoglutethimide at a 1-g daily dose, with cortisone replacement therapy, has been reported to be effective in a few cases.

CHEMOTHERAPY

Most authors consider that nonhormonal cytotoxic compounds should be tried in cases that are resistant to endocrine treatment. It should be stressed that most stage D patients probably have a reduced bone marrow reserve due to the extensive metastatic osseous involvement and, in some cases, the previous radiation therapy delivered to painful bone areas. Some of these patients also have reduced kidney function related to the ureteral obstruction. Moreover, most available compounds have not been adequately evaluated in prostate carcinoma. Only a few drugs seem to be active: fluorouracil, cyclophosphamide, doxorubicin (Adriamycin), mechlorethamine, and hydroxyurea; the objective response rate is about 20 to 30 percent.

Studies on combination chemotherapy have resulted in fairly high response rates. Unfortunately, lack of progression of the disease, a situation that probably reflects the natural history of the disease rather than the true impact of therapy, has been considered to constitute an objective response. In one study where stabilized cases were not taken into account, an objective remission rate of 48 percent was achieved by a combination of doxorubicin, mitomycin C and fluorouracil.[73]

Several reports have been published about estramustine, a conjugate of estradiol with an alkylating agent. This compound has been synthesized in the hope that the estradiol moiety would convey the alkylating agent to the carcinoma cells. It appears that about 20 percent of the compound is hydrolyzed in the liver; most of it is excreted in the bile, probably as an intact molecule. Estramustine, at an oral dosage of 15 mg per kilogram of body weight daily, is considered active in previously untreated patients as well as in patients refractory to an earlier endocrine treatment.[74] Strangely, this compound is not associated with myelosuppressive effects or clinical signs of estrogenic activity, and its mechanism of action is not well-understood, although its administration is associated with a lowering of the plasma testosterone level and it is split in vitro by prostate carcinomatous tissue into its constituents. There are no data indicating that this compound is more active than DES as a first treatment for stages C and D. In tumors relapsing after a previous regression induced by an endocrine therapy, estramustine may be used before chemotherapy with nonhormonal cytotoxic drugs is started.

ADJUVANT HORMONE TREATMENT AND CHEMOTHERAPY

Available information from the VACURG studies indicates that estrogen adjuvant endocrine therapy is associated in stage A and B patients with increased mortality. No information about the use of nonhormonal cytotoxic chemotherapy is available, but it should be remembered that even the efficiency of a surgical or radiation therapy of the disease at these stages has not yet been established.

Steroid Receptor Assay

As prostate carcinoma tissue samples are contaminated with SHBG, determination of the true steroid receptor concentration in this tissue is difficult. Therefore, it is suggested that the Scatchard plot method be used for the analysis of the DHT-binding capacity of the cytosolic receptor, once the receptors are separated from SHBG by protamine sulfate precipitation[75] or of the methyltrienolone-binding capacity of the prostate cytosol; methyltrienolone binds to the receptor but not to SHBG.[76] Tissue samples of about 500 mg, obtained by surgery, are required to perform a reliable analysis. They should be sent at once to the laboratory in ice-cold tris buffer.

Recent data suggest that quantitative determination of the nuclear androgen receptor concentration may be a more reliable parameter for predicting the response of the tumor to endocrine therapy.[77]

Therapeutic Prospects

There is now reasonable hope that evaluation of the more recent endocrine treatments and of combination chemotherapy in prostate cancer will be performed according to strict objective methods. This will allow the planning of a more efficient therapeutic strategy. Inhibitors of steroidogenesis such as GnRH analogues alone or in combination with antiandrogens will probably be used as first-line endocrine treatment, as they are able to induce "chemical castration." Further analysis of steroid receptors in prostate carcinoma cases will probably play an important role in the use of compounds such as the new steroidal alkylating agents. There is an urgent need for nonhormonal drugs with minimal bone marrow toxicity for cytotoxic chemotherapy. As prostate carcinoma consists of a heterogeneous population of cells, some of which are endocrine-insensitive from the outset, the value of combined endocrine and cytotoxic (or radiation) therapy from the start of treatment should be evaluated.[78]

ADENOCARCINOMA OF THE ENDOMETRIUM

Most cancers of the corpus uteri are adenocarcinomas arising from the endometrium. Several controversial matters concerning this hormone-sensitive tumor merit discussion.

Incidence

The annual incidence of endometrial adenocarcinoma is evaluated to be about 27 per 100,000 and is considered by some authors to have increased in the early 1970s.[78a] The incidence is higher in white women than in nonwhite women. Incidence seems to vary geographically in concert with breast and ovarian cancer.

However, it must be stressed that incidence data may be subject to several biases, as the reported rates are a function of (1) methods of detection, which have improved, and (2) reliability of the information conveyed to tumor registries. For instance, in nonwhite women there may be some uncertainty about the true endometrial origin of the reported cancers of the corpus uteri; about one-fourth of the tumors in these women are myometrial sarcomas. Rates of endometrial adenocarcinoma incidence start to increase sharply at about age 40, continuing through the late fifties; thereafter, the rates decline gradually. Despite its high incidence, endometrial adenocarcinoma is not a common cause of death; its annual mortality rate is less than 2 percent in the United States.

Risk Factors and Etiology

ENDOGENOUS ENDOCRINE FACTORS

There is an increased risk of endometrial adenocarcinoma in nulliparous women, those with early menarche, late menopause, or hypertension, and women who are obese, arthritic, or, perhaps, diabetic. There is also an association between risk for this cancer and higher socioeconomic status.[79] Some of these factors suggest the possible role of some endocrine aberration during the reproductive years. In fact, for many years, there has been widespread concern as to the potential role of estrogens in the pathogenesis of endometrial adenocarcinoma. It was known that administration of high doses of estrogens to rabbits was followed by development of endometrial cancer. The index of suspicion rose when it was demonstrated that aging, obesity, and hepatic disease, three factors known to be associated in human beings with a higher risk for this cancer, were characterized by a higher peripheral production rate of estrone from androstenedione of adrenal and ovarian origin. This strong correlation between constitutional features and metabolic modifications does not prove a causal relation; the association may be due to the identification of a population subset which is coincidentally at higher risk for the development of endometrial cancer.[80] Nevertheless, several ovarian abnormalities, like polycystic disease and endocrine and nonendocrine tumors, which are reported to be associated with a higher incidence of endometrial adenocarcinoma, are also characterized by an increased availability of androstenedione. In patients with this cancer, plasma estrone levels are three to five times higher than in normal postmenopausal women. Moreover, after menopause the estrogen stimulation of the target tissues is continuous and no longer modified by progesterone secretion.

EXOGENOUS FACTORS

It has been known for several years that long-duration estrogen treatment of patients with gonadal dysgenesis might be associated with the development of endometrial carcinoma, often of the adenosquamous type, which is known to have a poor prognosis. Several epidemiologic studies indicating a 5 to 14 times higher risk of appearance of endometrial adenocarcinoma in postmenopausal women previously treated with estrogens have been published.[81–84a] From one of these studies, it appears that women considered to be at low risk, i.e., those who are not obese and not hypertensive, are relatively more sensitive to the effects of exogenous estrogens. These investigations show that the risk of endometrial carcinoma is associated with all types of estrogen therapy and that the risk increases with larger doses and continuous administration of hormone.

The association of endometrial cancer and estrogen therapy has not been unanimously accepted because of many shortcomings in the studies. First, the investigations are retrospective. Information about past estrogen medication has been obtained in most of them from evaluation of the medical history and therefore might have been too limited. The appropriateness of the control population is doubtful: in one study women constituting the control population belonged, apparently, to another socioeconomic group; in two studies women who had had a hysterectomy were excluded. Other possible biases include the use of estrogen compounds for perimenopausal bleeding in patients with an unrecognized preexisting endometrial cancer; greater frequency of diagnostic examinations in women on estrogen therapy; relatively short interval (4 years in one case) between the start of the endocrine treatment and the detection of the cancer; and possible misinterpretation of atypical endometrial hyperplasia as carcinoma, as it is known that in a small number of cases such a distinction cannot be made with certainty. In one of the studies, the association of endometrial cancer with estrogen medication was shown to be valid if the analysis was restricted to patients with deep myometrial invasion, but there were few of these patients. The histology slides of the same study have been reviewed by three experts in the interpretation of endometrial pathology. They all agreed that the diagnosis was correct in 74 percent of the cases. Analysis restricted to these cases validates the original report.[85]

On the other hand, the results of a 10-year, prospective controlled study of estrogen replacement therapy with a placebo control show that none of the patients on endocrine treatment developed endometrial cancer while 2 of the 84 patients on placebo developed such a cancer.[86] It must be stressed that in this clinical trial all patients on estrogen medication were also treated for 7 days each month with medroxyprogesterone acetate, which may have had a protective effect.

In younger women, possible association of this type of cancer with the use of oral sequential contraceptive pills has been suggested. This contraceptive therapy was characterized by a high dose of estrogen followed by a weak progestogen for only 5 days. The present evidence for an association of unopposed estrogen stimulus with the development of endometrial cancer is highly presumptive and not conclusive.

STEROID RECEPTORS

Endometrial adenocarcinomas may contain cytoplasmic receptors for estradiol and progesterone. Investigation of a possible relation between the histologic grade of the tumor and the presence or absence of steroid receptors has given conflicting results.[87] Results from small series of patients suggest that there is a correlation between the presence of both ER and PgR and a good clinical response to progestational agents. However, the usefulness of steroid receptor concentration determinations in managing patients with endometrial carcinoma remains unestablished.

Treatment

There is a lack of accurate information about the treatment that should be performed in patients with a tumor that has not extended outside the uterus. A combination of surgical and radiation therapies is considered to give the best results.

ENDOCRINE TREATMENT

Progestational agents are widely used in the treatment of advanced or recurrent endometrial adenocarcinoma. This therapy is based on inducing endometrial atrophy in a normal uterus by administering continuous heavy doses of progesterone or other progestational compounds. The exact mechanism of action of these substances in endometrial cancer is not known; probably, they directly affect the carcinoma cells.

No controlled trials have been reported. Three different drugs are in current use. 17α-Hydroxyprogesterone caproate is given at a dosage of at least 1 g per week IM. Medroxyprogesterone is prescribed at a dosage of 200 to 800 mg daily by mouth, or the same dose once weekly IM. Medroxyprogesterone has also been used with success in some patients at a dosage of 400 to 800 mg IM monthly. Finally, medrogestone in a daily dose of 40 mg PO and megestrol acetate in a daily dose of 60 mg are also effective. The data collected from the literature show that each of these compounds induces an objective remission in about 35 percent of the patients adequately treated, with an average duration of response of about 26 months. Pulmonary metastases appear to respond much better than bulky pelvic and intraabdominal masses. In the latter situations, some physicians increase the dosage of the progestational compounds, using, for instance, 17α-hydroxyprogesterone caproate at a dosage of 3 to 5 g a week.

Studies of several small series of patients indicate that the antiestrogenic compound tamoxifen may be active in this type of tumor at a dosage of 20 to 40 mg daily.[88,89] At this dosage the compound induces an increase in the PgR content of endometrial adenocarcinomas with or without low receptor content. Tamoxifen may play a role in the future in combination or sequential treatment schedules. Use of these compounds as adjuvant therapy in primary treatment of this cancer does not seem to improve the prognosis of the patients.

CHEMOTHERAPY

Very little information is available about the value of nonhormonal cytotoxic chemotherapy in this type of cancer. Some compounds like fluorouracil, cyclophosphamide, and doxorubicin are active, but the induced rate of remission is low, about 20 to 30 percent. Evaluation of combination chemotherapy is still in progress.

REFERENCES

1. Bishop JM: Viral oncogenes. *Cell* 42:23, 1985.

2. Waterhouse J, Muir C, Shanmugaratnam K, Powell J, Peacham D, Whelan S: Cancer Incidence in Five Continents. *IARC Sci Publi:* No 42. Lyon, International Agency for Research on Cancer, 1982, vol IV.

2a. Segi M, Noye H, Segi R: *Age-Adjusted Death Rates for Cancer for Selected Sites (A-Classification) in 43 Countries in 1972.* Nagoya, Japan, Segi Institute of Cancer Epidemiology, 1977.

3. Cutler SJ, Christine B, Barclay THC: Increasing incidence and decreasing mortality rates for breast cancer. *Cancer* 28:1376, 1971.

4. Shimkin MB: Epidemiology of breast cancer, in Griem ML et al (eds): *Breast Cancer: A Challenging Problem.* Berlin, Springer-Verlag, 1973.

5. Mueller CB, Jeffries W: Cancer of the breast: Its outcome as measured by the rate of dying and causes of death. *Ann Surg* 182:334, 1975.

6. Brinkley D, Haybittle JL: The curability of breast cancer. *Lancet* 2:95, 1975.

7. Baum M: The curability of breast cancer, in Stoll BA (ed): *Breast Cancer Management, Early and Late.* London, Heinemann, 1977.

8. de Waard F: The epidemiology of breast cancer; review and prospects. *Int J Cancer* 4:577, 1969.

9. MacMahon BM, Cole P, Brown I: Etiology of human breast cancer: A review. *JNCI* 50:21, 1973.

10. Miller AB: Role of nutrition in the etiology of breast cancer. *Cancer* 39:2704, 1977.

11. de Waard F, Cornelis JP, Yoshida M: Breast cancer incidence according to weight and height in two cities of the Netherlands and in Aichi prefecture, Japan. *Cancer* 40:1269, 1977.

12. Holleb AI: Summary of the informal discussion of dietary factors and hormone-dependent cancers. *Cancer Res* 35:3387, 1975.

12a. Hill MJ, Goddard P, Williams REO: Gut bacteria and aetiology of cancer of the breast. *Lancet* 2:472, 1971.

13. Mueller CB, Ames F, Anderson CD: Breast cancer in 3558 women: Age as a significant determinant in the rate of dying and causes of death. *Surgery* 83:123, 1978.

13a. Lilienfeld AM: Relationship of cancer of the female breast to artificial menopause and marital status. *Cancer* 9:927, 1956.

13b. Kaplan SD, Acheson RM: A single etiological hypothesis for breast cancer? *J Chronic Dis* 19:1221, 1966.

13c. Feinleib M: Breast cancer and artificial menopause: A cohort study. *JNCI* 41:315, 1968.

13d. Trichopoulos D, MacMahon B, Cole P: The menopause and breast cancer risk. *JNCI* 48:605, 1972.

13e. Salber EJ, Trichopoulos D, MacMahon B: Lactation and reproductive histories of breast cancer patients in Boston, 1965–1966. *JNCI* 43:1013, 1969.

13f. Yuasa S, MacMahon B: Lactation and reproductive histories of breast cancer patients in Tokyo, Japan. *Bull WHO* 42:192, 1970.

13g. Ravnihar B, MacMahon B, Lindtner J: Epidemiologic features of breast cancer in Slovenia, 1965–1967. *Eur J Cancer* 7:295, 1971.

13h. Staszewski J: Age at menarche and breast cancer. *JNCI* 47: 935, 1971.

14. Kirschner MA: The role of hormones in the etiology of human breast cancer. *Cancer* 39:2716, 1977.

15. Vorherr H, Messer R: Breast cancer: Potentially predisposing and protecting factors. Role of pregnancy, lactation and endocrine status. *Am J Obstet Gynecol* 130:335, 1978.

16. Bulbrook RD: Endocrine status of women with enhanced risk of breast cancer, in Heuson JC, Mattheiem WH, Rozencweig M (eds): *Breast Cancer: Trends in Research and Treatment.* New York, Raven, 1976.

16a. Hellman L, Zumoff B, Fishman J, Gallagher TF: Peripheral metabolism of ^{3}H-estradiol and the excretion of endogenous estrone and estriol glucosiduronate in women with breast cancer. *J Clin Endocrinol Metab* 33:138, 1971.

16b. Rotti KJ, Stevens J, Watson D, Longscope C: Estriol concentrations in plasma of normal, non-pregnant women. *Steroids* 25:807, 1975.

16c. Arthes FG, Sartwell PE, Lewison EF: The pill, estrogens and the breast. Epidemiologic aspects. *Cancer* 28:1391, 1971.

16d. Boston Collaborative Drug Surveillance Programme: Oral contraceptives and venous thromboembolic disease, surgically confirmed gallbladder disease, and breast tumor. Lancet 1:1399, 1973.

16e. The Cancer and Steroid Hormone Study of the Centers for Disease Control and the National Institute of Child Health and Human Development. Oral-contraceptive use and the risk of breast cancer. *N Engl J Med* 315:405, 1986.

16f. Vessey M, Baron J, Doll R, McPherson K, Yeates D: Oral contraceptives and breast cancer: Final report of an epidemiological study. *Br J Cancer* 47:455, 1983.

16g. Hoover R, Gray LA Sr, Cole P, MacMahon B: Menopausal estrogens and breast cancer. *N Engl J Med* 295:401, 1976.

16h. Wallach S, Henneman PHH: Prolonged estrogen therapy in post-menopausal women. *JAMA* 171:1637, 1959.
16i. Lewison EF: Role of exogenous estrogens, in Stoll BA (ed): *Risk Factors in Breast Cancer. New Aspects of Breast Cancer.* London, Heinemann Medical Books Ltd, 1976.
16j. Bulbrook RD: Urinary androgen excretion and the etiology of breast cancer. *JNCI* 48:1039, 1972.
17. Sherman BM, Korenman SG: Inadequate corpus luteum function: A pathophysiological interpretation of human breast cancer epidemiology. *Cancer* 33:1306, 1974.
17a. Grattarola R: The premenstrual endometrial pattern of women with breast cancer. *Cancer* 17:1119, 1964.
17b. Franks S, Ralphs DNL, Seagroatt V, Jacob HS: Prolactin concentrations in patients with breast cancer. *Br Med J* 4:320, 1974.
17c. Kwa HG, De Jong-Bakker M, Engelsman E, Cleton FJ: Plasma-prolactin in human breast cancer. *Lancet* 1:433, 1974.
17d. Wilson RG, Buchan R, Roberts MM, Forrest APM, Boyns AR, Cole EN, Griffiths K: Plasma prolactin and breast cancer. *Cancer* 33:1325, 1974.
18. Anderson DE: A high risk group for breast cancer. *Cancer Bull* 25:23, 1973.
19. Anderson DE: Genetic study of breast cancer: Identification of a high risk group. *Cancer* 34:1090, 1974.
20. Petrakis NL: Genetic factors in the etiology of breast cancer. *Cancer* 39:2709, 1977.
21. Billiau A: Introduction: Virology, in Heuson JC, Mattheiem WH, Rozencweig M (eds): *Breast Cancer: Trends in Research and Treatment.* New York, Raven, 1976.
21a. Beatson GT: On the treatment of inoperable cases of carcinoma of the mamma: Suggestions for a new method of treatment with illustrative cases. *Lancet* 2:104, 1896.
22. McGuire WL: Physiological principles underlying therapy in breast cancer, in McGuire WL (ed): *Breast Cancer: Current Approaches to Therapy.* Edinburgh, Churchill Livingstone, 1977, vol 1.
23. Welsch CW, Nagasawa H: Prolactin and murine mammary tumorigenesis: A review. *Cancer Res* 37:951, 1977.
24. Heuson JC, Legros N, Heuson-Stiennon JA, Leclercq G, Pasteels JL: Hormone dependency of rat mammary tumors, in Heuson JC, Mattheiem WH, Rozencweig M (eds): *Breast Cancer: Trends in Research and Treatment.* New York, Raven, 1976.
24a. Nagasawa H, Yanai R: Effects of prolactin or growth hormone on growth of carcinogen-induced mammary tumors of adreno-ovariectomized rats. *Int J Cancer* 6:488, 1970.
24b. Pearson OH: Biological problems regarding hormonal surgery, in Dargent M, Romieu C (eds): *Major Endocrine Surgery for the Treatment of Cancer of the Breast in Advanced Stages,* Lyon, SIMEP, 1967.
24c. Welsch CW, Rivera EM: Differential effects of estrogen and prolactin on DNA synthesis in organ cultures of DMBA-induced rat mammary carcinoma. *Proc Soc Exp Biol Med* 139:623, 1972.
25. McCormick GM, Moon RC: Hormones influencing postpartum growth of 7,12-dimethylbenz(a)anthracene-induced rat mammary tumors. *Cancer Res* 26:626, 1967.
26. Legros N, Heuson JC: Hormone action in breast cancer explants, in Sharma RK, Criss WE (eds): *Endocrine Control in Neoplasia.* New York, Raven, 1978.
27. Leclercq G, Heuson JC: Quantitative aspects of estrogen receptors in relation with therapeutic response, in Lippman ME, Thomson EB (eds): *Steroid Receptors and the Management of Cancer.* Cleveland, CRC Press, 1979.
27a. Kledzik GS, Bradley CJ, Marshall S, Campbell GA, Meites J: Effects of high doses of estrogen on prolactin-binding activity and growth of carcinogen-induced mammary cancers in rats. *Cancer Res* 36:3265, 1976.
27b. Leung BS, Sasaki GH: On the mechanism of prolactin and estrogen action in 7,12-dimethylbenz(a)anthracene-induced mammary carcinoma in the rat. II. In vivo tumor responses and estrogen receptor. *Endocrinology* 97:564, 1975.
27c. DeSombre ER, Kledzik G, Marshall S, Meites J: Estrogen and prolactin receptor concentrations in rat mammary tumors and response to endocrine ablation. *Cancer Res* 36:354, 1976.
28. McGuire WL, Raynaud JP, Baulieu EE: Progesterone receptors: Introduction and overview, in McGuire WL et al (eds): *Progesterone Receptors in Normal and Neoplastic Tissues.* New York, Raven, 1977.
29. Stoll BA (ed): *Breast Cancer Management, Early and Late.* London, Heinemann, 1977.
30. Heuson JC: Hormones by administration, in Atkins H (ed): *The Treatment of Breast Cancer.* Lancaster, England, MTP, 1974.
31. Heuson JC: The role of prolactin inhibition in treatment, in Stoll BA (ed): *Mammary Cancer and Neuroendocrine Therapy.* London, Butterworth, 1974.
31a. Pearson OH, West CD, Hollander VP, Treves N: Evaluation of endocrine therapy for advanced breast cancer. *JAMA* 154:234, 1954.
32. Stoll BA: Hypothesis: Breast cancer regression under estrogen therapy. *Br Med J* 3:446, 1973.
32a. Pearson OH, Ray BS: Results of hypophysectomy in the treatment of metastatic mammary carcinoma. *Cancer* 12:85, 1959.
33. Lippman M: Hormone-responsive human breast cancer in continuous tissue culture, in Heuson JC, Mattheiem WH, Rozencweig M, (eds): *Breast Cancer: Trends in Research and Treatment.* New York, Raven, 1976.
34. McGuire WL, Zava DT, Horwitz KB, Garola RE, Chamnes GC: Receptors and breast cancer: Do we know it all? *J Steroid Biochem* 9:461, 1978.
35. Shafie S, Brooks SC: Effect of prolactin on growth and the estrogen receptor level of human breast cancer cells (MCF-7). *Cancer Res* 37:792, 1977.
36. Leclercq G, Heuson JC: Therapeutic significance of sex-steroid hormone receptors in the treatment of breast cancer. Perspectives in cancer research. *Eur J Cancer* 13:1205, 1977.
37. McGuire WL, Carbone PP, Vollmer EP (eds): *Estrogen Receptors in Human Breast Cancer.* New York, Raven, 1975.
38. McGuire WL, Raynaud JP, Baulieu EE (eds): *Progesterone Receptors in Normal and Neoplastic Tissues.* New York, Raven, 1977.
38a. Glascock RF, Hoeckstra WG: Selective accumulation of tritium-labelled hexoestrol by the reproductive organs of immature female goats and sheep. *Biochem J* 72:673, 1959.
39. Jensen EV, Block GE, Smith S, DeSombre ER: Estrogen receptors and breast cancer response to adrenalectomy. *Natl Cancer Inst Monogr* 34:55, 1971.
39a. Maass H: Oestrogen and androgen receptors in human breast cancer. *J Steroid Biochem* 6:XVII, 1975.
39b. Persijn JP, Korsten CB, Engelsman E: Oestrogen and androgen receptors in breast cancer and response to endocrine therapy. *Brit Med J* 4:503, 1975.
40. Clark GM, McGuire WL: Progesterone receptors and human breast cancer. *Breast Cancer Res Treat* 3:157, 1983.
41. Holdaway IM, Friesen HG: Hormone binding by human mammary carcinoma. *Cancer Res* 37:1946, 1977.
41a. Halsted WS: The results of operations for the cure of cancer of the breast performed at the Johns Hopkins Hospital from June 1889 to January 1894. *Ann Surg* 20:497, 1894.
42. Margolese RG: Choice for primary surgery, in Margolese RG (ed): *Breast Cancer.* New York, Churchill Livingstone, 1983.
43. Fisher B, Wickerham DL, Beazley R, Guzik J, Bornstein R, MacFarlane J, Deckers P, Paterson AHG, Dionne L, Spector J: The use of adjuvant therapy for primary breast cancer: An overview, in Margolese RG (ed): *Breast Cancer.* New York, Churchill Livingstone, 1983.
44. Aisner J: Chemotherapy in the treatment for advanced breast cancer, in Margolese RG (ed): *Breast Cancer.* New York, Churchill Livingstone, 1983.
45. Hayward JL, Carbone PP, Heuson JC, Kumaoka S, Segaloff A,

Rubens RD: Assessment of therapy in breast cancer. *Eur J Cancer* 13:89, 1977; *Br J Cancer* 35:292, 1977; *Cancer* 39:1289, 1977; *Jpn J Cancer Clin* 23:80, 1977; *Acta Oncol Brasileira* 1:37, 1977; *Turkish J Cancer* 7:1, 1977.

45a. Kennedy BJ, Mielke PW Jr, Fortuny IE: Therapeutic castration versus prophylactic castration in breast cancer. *Surg Gynecol Obstet* 118:524, 1964.

45b. MacDonald I: Endocrine ablation in disseminated mammary carcinoma. *Surg Gynecol Obstet* 115:215, 1962.

45c. Stoll BA: *Hormonal Management in Breast Cancer.* London, Pitman Medical Publishing Co Ltd, 1969.

45d. Silverstein MJ, Byron RL Jr, Yonemoto RH, Rühimaki DU, Schuster G: Bilateral adrenalectomy for advanced breast cancer; a 21 year experience. *Surgery* 77:825, 1975.

45e. Escher G: Panel discussion, in Segaloff A (ed): *Breast Cancer.* St. Louis, Mosby, 1958.

45f. Hayward JL, Atkins HJB, Falconer MA, MacLean KS, Salmon LFW, Schurr PH, Shaheen CH: Clinical trials comparing transfrontal hyphophysectomy with adrenalectomy and transethmoidal hyphophysectomy, in Joslin CAF, Gleave EN (eds): *The Clinical Management of Advanced Breast Cancer.* Cardiff, Alpha Omega Alpha Publishing, 1970.

46. Carter AC, Sedransk N, Kelley RM, Ansfield FJ, Ravdin RG, Talley RW, Potter NR: Diethylstilbestrol: Recommended dosages for different categories of breast cancer patients. Report of the Cooperative Breast Cancer Group. *JAMA* 237:2079, 1977.

46a. Kennedy BJ, Nathanson IT: Effects of intensive sex steroid therapy in advanced breast cancer, report to the Council of Pharmacy and Chemistry. *JAMA* 152:1135, 1953.

46b. Cooperative Breast Cancer Group: Progress report. Results of studies of the Cooperative Breast Cancer Group 1961–1963. *Cancer Chemother Rep* 41(suppl 1):1, 1964.

46c. Kennedy BJ: Diethylstilbestrol versus testosterone propionate therapy in advanced breast cancer. *Surg Gynecol Obstet* 120:1246, 1965.

47. Campio L, Robustelli Della Cuna G, Taylor RW (eds): *Role of Medroxyprogesterone in Endocrine-related Tumors.* New York, Raven, 1983, vol 2.

47a. Heuson JC, Engelsman E, Blonk-Van Der Wijst J, Maass H, Drochmans A, Michel J, Nowakowski H, Gorins A: Comparative trial of nafoxidine and ethinyl-oestradiol in advanced breast cancer: An EORTC Breast Cancer Cooperative Group Study. *Br Med J* 2:711, 1975.

47b. Kaiser-Kupfer MI, Lippman ME: Tamoxifen retinopathy. *Cancer Treat Rep* 62:315, 1978.

48. Pearson OH, Manni A, Arafah BM: Antiestrogen treatment of breast cancer: An overview. *Cancer Res* (suppl) 42:3424s, 1982.

48a. Stoll BA: Corticosteroids in the therapy of advanced mammary cancer. *Br Med J* 2:210, 1963.

48b. Santen RJ, Worgul TJ, Samojlik E, Interrante A, Boucher AE, Lipton A, Harvey HA, White DS, Smart E, Cox C, Wells SA: A randomized trial comparing surgical adrenalectomy with aminoglutethimide plus hydrocortisone in women with advanced breast cancer. *N Engl J Med* 305:545, 1981.

48c. Harvey HA, Lipton A, White DS, Santen RJ, Boucher AE, Shafik AS, Dixon RJ, and members of the Central Pennsylvania Oncology Group: Cross-over comparison of tamoxifen and aminoglutethimide in advanced breast cancer. *Cancer Res* 42:3451s, 1982.

49. Lipton A, Harvey HA, Santen RJ (eds): Aromatase: New Perspectives for Breast Cancer. *Cancer Res* (suppl) 42:3468s, 1982.

49a. Dao L, Nemoto T: An evaluation of adrenalectomy and androgen in disseminated mammary carcinoma. *Surg Gynecol Obstet* 121:1257, 1965.

50. Rozencweig M, Heuson JC: Breast cancer: Prognostic factors and clinical evaluation, in Staquet MJ (ed): *Cancer Therapy: Prognostic Factors and Criteria of Response.* New York, Raven, 1975.

50a. Cutler SJ, Black MM, Mork T, Harvei S, Freeman C: Further observations on prognostic factors in cancer of the female breast. *Cancer* 24:653, 1969.

51. EORTC Breast Cancer Cooperative Group: Standards for the assessment of estrogen receptors in human breast cancer. *Eur J Cancer* 9:379, 1973.

51a. Leclercq G, Heuson JC, Deboel MC, Mattheiem WH: Oestrogen receptors in breast cancer: a changing concept. *Br Med J* 1:185, 1975.

52. Heuson JC, Longeval R, Mattheiem WH, Deboel MC, Sylvester RJ, Leclercq C: Significance of quantitative estrogen receptors for endocrine therapy in advanced breast cancer. *Cancer* 39:1971, 1977.

53. Hähnel R: Personal communication, 1978.

54. Heuson JC: Current overview of EORTC clinical trials with tamoxifen. *Cancer Treat Rep* 60:1463, 1976.

55. Hutchison GB: Epidemiology of prostatic cancer. *Semin Oncol* 3:151, 1976.

55a. Whitmore WF Jr: The natural history of prostatic cancer. *Cancer* 32:1104, 1973.

56. Györkey F: Some aspects of cancer of the prostate gland, in Busch H (ed): *Methods in Cancer Research.* New York, Academic Press, 1973, vol 10.

57. Greenwald P, Damon A, Kirmss V, Polan AK: Physical and demographic features of men before developing cancer of the prostate. *JNCI* 53:341, 1974.

57a. Wynder EL, Mabuchi K, Whitmore WF Jr: Epidemiology of cancer of the prostate. *Cancer* 28:344, 1971.

57b. Steele R, Lees REM, Kraus AS, Rao C: Sexual factors in the epidemiology of cancer of the prostate. *J Chronic Dis* 24:29, 1971.

58. Armenian HK, Lilienfeld AM, Diamond EL, Bross IDJ: Relation between benign prostatic hyperplasia and cancer of the prostate. *Lancet* 2:115, 1974.

59. Greenwald P, Kirmss V, Polan AK, Dick VS: Cancer of the prostate among men with benign prostatic hypertrophy. *JNCI* 53:335, 1974.

59a. Franks LM: Etiology, epidemiology and pathology of prostate cancer. *Cancer* 32:1092, 1973.

59b. Herbert JT, Birkhoff JD, Feorino PM, Caldwell GG: Herpes simplex virus type 2 and cancer of the prostate. *J Urol* 116:611, 1976.

60. Shain SA, McCullough B, Nitchuk M, Boesel RW: Prostate carcinogenesis in the AXC rat. *Oncology* 34:114, 1977.

61. Kliman B, Prout GR Jr, MacLaughlin RA, Daly JJ, Griffin PP: Altered androgen metabolism in metastatic prostate cancer. *J Urol* 119:623, 1978.

62. Hawkins EF, Nijs M, Brassinne C: Steroid receptors in the human prostate. Detection of tissue-specific androgen binding in prostate cancer. *Clin Chim Acta* 75:303, 1977.

62a. Prout GR Jr, Kliman B, Daly JJ, MacLaughlin RA, Griffin PP: In vitro uptake of ^{3}H-testosterone and its conversion to dihydrotestosterone by prostatic carcinoma and other tissues. *J Urol* 116:603, 1976.

62b. Young HH, Kent JR: Plasma testosterone levels in patients with prostatic carcinoma before and after treatment. *J Urol* 99:788, 1968.

62c. Gallagher TF, Whitmore WF Jr, Zumoff B, Hellman L: Studies in prostate cancer before and after orchiectomy, in Vollmer EP (ed): *Workshop on the Biology of the Prostate and Related Tissues.* National Cancer Institute Monograph 12, 1963.

62d. Mellinger GT, Gleason D, Bailar J III: The histology and prognosis of prostatic cancer. *J Urol* 97:331, 1967.

63. Byar DP, Mostofi FK, Veterans Administration Cooperative Urological Research Group: Carcinoma of the prostate: Prognostic evaluation of certain pathologic features in 208 radical prostatectomies. *Cancer* 30:5, 1972.

63a. Terry R: Some questions raised by histologic study of RTOG

protocols 75-06 and 77-06 as illustrated by selected samples. *Prostate* 3:543, 1982.
63b. Franzen S, Giertz G, Zajicek J: Cytological diagnosis of prostate tumors by transrectal aspiration biopsy: a preliminary report. *Brit J Urol* 32:193, 1960.
64. Esposti PL, Elman A, Norlen H: Complications of transrectal aspiration biopsy of the prostate. *Scand J Urol Nephrol* 9:208, 1975.
65. Pontes JE: Biological markers in prostate cancer. *J Urol* 130:1037, 1983.
65a. Byar DP: Treatment of prostatic cancer: studies by the Veterans Administration Cooperative Urological Research Group. *Bull NY Acad Med* 48:751, 1972.
66. Veterans Administration Cooperative Urological Research Group: Factors in the prognosis of carcinoma of the prostate: A cooperative study. *J Urol* 100:59, 1968.
66a. Harada M, Mostofi FK, Corle DK, Byar DP, Trump BF: Preliminary studies of histologic prognosis in cancer of the prostate. *Cancer Treat Rep* 61:223, 1977.
66b. Brawn PN, Ayala AG, von Eschenbach AC, Hussey DH, Johnson DE: Histologic grading study of prostate adenocarcinoma: The development of a new system and comparison with other methods—A preliminary study. *Cancer* 49:525, 1982.
67. Coune A: Carcinoma of the prostate: Prognostic factors and criteria of response to therapy, in Staquet MJ (ed): *Cancer Therapy: Prognostic Factors and Criteria of Response.* New York, Raven, 1975.
68. Coune A: Carcinoma of the prostate, in Staquet MJ (ed): *Randomized Trials in Cancer: A Critical Review by Sites.* New York, Raven, 1978.
69. Paulson DF, Lin GH, Hinshaw W, Stephani S, the Uro-oncology Research Group: Radical surgery versus radiotherapy for adenocarcinoma of the prostate. *J Urol* 128:502, 1982.
69a. Jordan WP Jr, Blackard CE, Byar DP: Reconsideration of orchiectomy in the treatment of advanced prostatic carcinoma. *South Med J* 70:1411, 1977.
70. Schroeder FH, EORTC Urological Group: Treatment of prostatic cancer: The EORTC experience—preliminary results of prostatic carcinoma trials. *Prostate* 5:193, 1984.
71. Coune A, Smith P: Clinical trial of 2-bromo-α-ergocryptine (NSC-169774) in human prostatic cancer. *Cancer Chemother Rep* (part 1) 59:209, 1975.
72. Koutsilieris M, Tolis G: Gonadotropin-releasing hormone agonistic analogues in the treatment of advanced prostatic carcinoma. *Prostate* 4:569, 1983.
73. Logothetis CJ, Samuels ML, Von Eschenbach AC, Trindade A, Ogden S, Grant C, Johnson DE: Doxorubicin, mitomycin-C, and 5-fluorouracil (DMF) in the treatment of metastatic hormonal refractory adenocarcinoma of the prostate, with a note on the staging of metastatic prostate cancer. *J Clin Oncol* 1:368, 1983.
74. Müntzing J, Shukla SK, Chu TM, Mittelman A, Murphy GP: Pharmacoclinical study of oral estramustine phosphate (Estracyt) in advanced carcinoma of the prostate. *Invest Urol* 12:65, 1974.
75. Menon M, Tananis CE, McLoughlin MG, Lippman ME, Walsch PC: The measurement of androgen receptors in human prostatic tissue utilizing sucrose density centrifugation and a protamine precipitation assay. *J Urol* 117:309, 1977.
76. Snochowski M, Pousette A, Ekman P, Bression D, Andersson L, Högberg B, Gustafsson J-Å: Characterization and measurement of the androgen receptor in human benign prostatic hyperplasia and prostatic carcinoma. *J Clin Endocrinol Metab* 45:920, 1977.
77. Trachtenberg J, Walsch PC: Correlation of prostatic nuclear androgen receptor content with duration of response and survival following hormonal therapy in advanced prostatic cancer. *J Urol* 127:466, 1982.
78. Sinha AA, Blackard CE, Seal US: A critical analysis of tumor morphology and hormone treatments in the untreated and estrogen-treated responsive and refractory human prostatic carcinoma. *Cancer* 40:2836, 1977.
78a. Gusberg SB: Current concepts in cancer: The changing nature of endometrial cancer. *N Engl J Med* 302:729, 1980.
79. Elwood JM, Cole P, Rothman KJ, Kaplan SD: Epidemiology of endometrial cancer. *JNCI* 59:1055, 1977.
80. MacDonald PC, Siiteri PK: The relationship between the extraglandular production of estrone and the occurrence of endometrial neoplasia. *Gynecol Oncol* 2:259, 1974.
81. Smith DC, Prentice R, Thompson DJ, Herrmann WL: Association of exogenous estrogen and endometrial carcinoma. *N Engl J Med* 293:1164, 1975.
82. Ziel HK, Finkle WD: Increased risk of endometrial carcinoma among users of conjugated estrogens. *N Engl J Med* 293:1167, 1975.
83. Mack TM, Pike MC, Henderson BE, Pfeffer RI, Gerkins VR, Arthur M, Brown SE: Estrogens and endometrial cancer in a retirement community. *N Engl J Med* 294:1262, 1976.
84. McDonald TW, Annegers JF, O'Fallon WM, Dockerty MB, Malkasian GD Jr, Kurland LT: Exogenous estrogen and endometrial carcinoma: Case control and incidence study. *Am J Obstet Gynecol* 127:572, 1977.
84a. Shapiro S, Kelly JP, Rosenberg L, Kaufman DW, Helmrich SP, Rosenshein NB, Lewis JL Jr, Knapp RC, Stolley PD, Schottenfeld D: Risk of localized and widespread endometrial cancer in relation to recent and discontinued use of conjugated estrogens. *N Engl J Med* 313:969, 1985.
85. Gordon J, Reagan JW, Finkle WD, Ziel HK: Estrogen and endometrial carcinoma. An independent pathology review supporting original risk estimate. *N Engl J Med* 297:570, 1977.
86. Nachtigall LE, Nachtigall RH, Nachtigall RB, Beckman EM: Estrogens and endometrial carcinoma. *N Engl J Med* 294:848, 1976.
87. Gambrell RD Jr, Bagnell CA, Greenblatt RB: Role of estrogens and progesterone in the etiology and prevention of endometrial cancer: A Review. *Am J Obstet Gynecol* 146:696, 1983.
88. Swenerton KD, Shaw D, White GW, Boyes DA: Treatment of advanced endometrial cancer with tamoxifen. *N Engl J Med* 301:174, 1979.
89. Hald I: The use of tamoxifen in endometrial cancer. *Rev Endocr-Related Cancer* (suppl)8:9, 1981.

Prostaglandins, Kallikreins and Kinins, and Bartter's Syndrome

*Harry S. Margolius**
*Perry V. Halushka**
Jürgen C. Frölich†

PROSTAGLANDINS

HISTORICAL BACKGROUND

Before the turn of the century it was discovered that highly active biological material is present in seminal fluid. However, systematic scientific evaluation of this material only began when von Euler[1a] and Goldblatt[1b] showed, using pharmacological techniques, that this material was different from all the then-known autacoids. Von Euler named these substances *prostaglandins* (PGs) because he assumed that they were produced by the prostate. It is recognized now that the major portion of seminal fluid prostaglandins originates in the seminal vesicle. After the chemical identification of PGs by Bergström and Sjövall,[2] a new era in PG research began: it became possible to study pure compounds and to obtain information on their synthesis, release, and metabolism. Chemical synthesis of individual PGs and PG analogues also became possible. With the elucidation of their structures, research in the prostaglandin field virtually exploded. Indeed, this group of compounds has captured the interest of scientists from multiple and diverse areas of interest. Because these substances had initially been discovered in the male accessory genital glands, much of the initial effort was directed at elucidating the role of prostaglandins in reproduction. However, the discovery of PGs in other tissues raised the possibility that their role in cellular function might not be limited to reproduction. Subsequent research has shown that PGs are synthesized in virtually all cells of the mammalian organism except red blood cells and participate in many physiological functions. Prostaglandins play important roles in platelet aggregation, renal incretory and excretory function, pulmonary airway resistance, gastric secretion, parturition, inflammation, and fever (Table 31-1). This wide spectrum of activities is one of the reasons that prostaglandins are of such general interest. Because of the widespread occurrence of PGs and their involvement in such a multitude of activities, it is thought that they must act through a mechanism of fundamental importance, such as the cyclic nucleotide system or changes in intracellular free calcium concentrations. Efforts to link the PGs to the cyclic nucleotide system have been, however, only partially successful; additional mechanisms must be found to explain their function.

Understanding of the system was significantly advanced by the pioneering (and Nobel prize winning) work of Samuelsson, whose group elucidated the biosynthesis of PGs, thromboxanes (Tx's), and leukotrienes from arachidonic acid.[3] In addition, they established some of the methods for the quantification of concentrations of PGs and their metabolites. These scientists established that, under basal conditions, PGs do not occur in the circulation in biologically important amounts and, therefore, probably function physiologically as local mediators or modulators of hormone actions. In recent years much attention has been focused on their potential role in pathologic processes.

One of the major discoveries in the prostaglandin field was the finding, in Vane's laboratory, that aspirin and other nonsteroidal anti-inflammatory drugs have an inhibitory effect on PG biosynthesis.[4] This discovery provided an explanation for the effects and side effects of these drugs. Knowledge of their mode of action has already led to numerous new applications of these drugs in human therapy. Precise measure-

*Supported by National Institutes of Health Grants HL 29566 and HL 17705. P.V.H. is a Burroughs Wellcome Scholar in clinical pharmacology.

†Supported by the Robert Bosch Foundation, Stuttgart.

Table 31-1. Major Pharmacological Actions of Some Prostaglandins

Prostaglandin	Effect
Prostacyclin	Vasodilation
	Inhibition of platelet aggregation and ADP release
	Renin release
	Relaxation of uterine smooth muscle
	Bronchodilation
TxA_2	Platelet aggregation and ADP release
	Vasoconstriction
PGE_1	Inhibition of platelet aggregation
	Vasodilation
PGE_2	Vasodilation
	Contraction of uterine smooth muscle
	Increased gut motility
	Stimulation of renal Na^+ excretion
	Inhibition of renal ADH effect
	Bronchodilation
	Inhibition of gastric acid secretion
	Stimulation of erythropoietin secretion
	Sensitization to pain stimuli
	Fever
$PGF_{2\alpha}$	Uterine contraction
	Bronchoconstriction
	Increased gut motility

ments of PG, Tx, and leukotriene concentrations are technically difficult, and inhibition of PG synthesis by aspirin-like drugs has been a useful experimental tool for implicating the PG system in a variety of biological processes.

The first prostaglandins identified were PGE_2, $PGF_{2\alpha}$, and PGD_2. These prostaglandins are now referred to as the "classic" prostaglandins. In the course of studies on blood platelet PG synthesis, a potent vasoconstrictor substance with platelet-aggregating properties was discovered in 1975; it was named *thromboxane*.[5] The next exciting discovery was that of *prostacyclin* (PGI_2) in Vane's laboratory in 1976. Prostacyclin is a potent vasodilator and prevents platelet aggregation. Since it is formed by endothelial cells, its synthesis is a property of all vascularized tissues. The latest addition to the family tree of PGs, the *leukotrienes*, were described in 1979.[6] The name derives from the site of synthesis of these compounds, white blood cells (hence "leuko") and their triene structure.

NOMENCLATURE

Eicosanoids is the term that is used to refer to metabolites of eicosatrienoic, eicosatetraenoic, and eicosapentaenoic acids. PGs, Tx's and leukotrienes are considered to be eicosanoids. The term *prostaglandin*, in the chemically correct sense refers only to compounds derived from prostanoic acid, a chemical not found in nature. The classic prostaglandins PGA_2, PGB_2, PGC_2, PGD_2, PGE_2, and $PGF_{2\alpha}$ are all derived from prostanoic acid. They differ by virtue of functional groups on the cyclopentane ring (Fig. 31-1). They are further categorized as mono-, di-, or triunsaturated according to the number of carbon-carbon double bonds; the subscript 1 denotes a double bond between C_{13} and C_{14}, 2 denotes an additional double bond between C_5 and C_6, and 3 denotes a third double bond between C_{17} and C_{18}. The formulas for PGE_1, PGE_2, and PGE_3 are given in Fig. 31-2 as examples of this nomenclature. Thromboxane A_2 has a six-membered oxetane ring in place of the cyclopentane ring (Fig. 31-3). While many of the chemically feasible prostaglandins have been found in nature, there is considerable doubt as to the biosynthetic origin of PGA_2.

Leukotrienes are numbered 3 through 5 to denote the number of double bonds present in the fatty acid moiety of the molecule (Fig. 31-3). The letters C through F refer to the amino acid substitutents in the molecule; leukotrienes A and B do not have any amino acid substituents covalently linked to the fatty acid.

PROSTAGLANDINS AS TISSUE HORMONES

PGs could act by reaching target cells via the circulation like the classic hormones. However, this mode of action has not been shown to exist under basal conditions for any of the PGs. For substances such as bradykinin, serotonin, and prostaglandins the term *tissue*

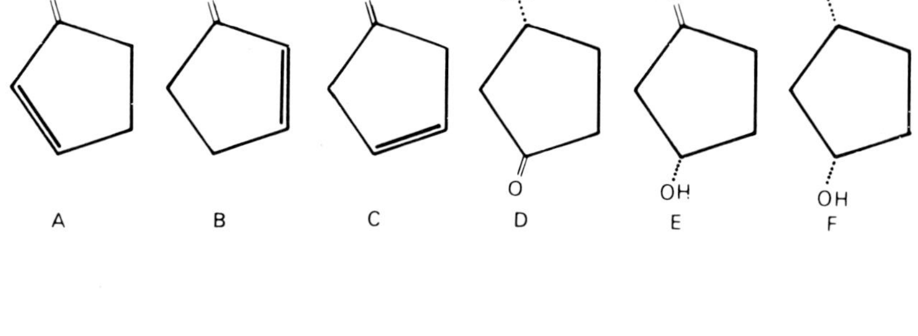

FIGURE 31-1 Structure of cyclopentane ring of various prostaglandins.

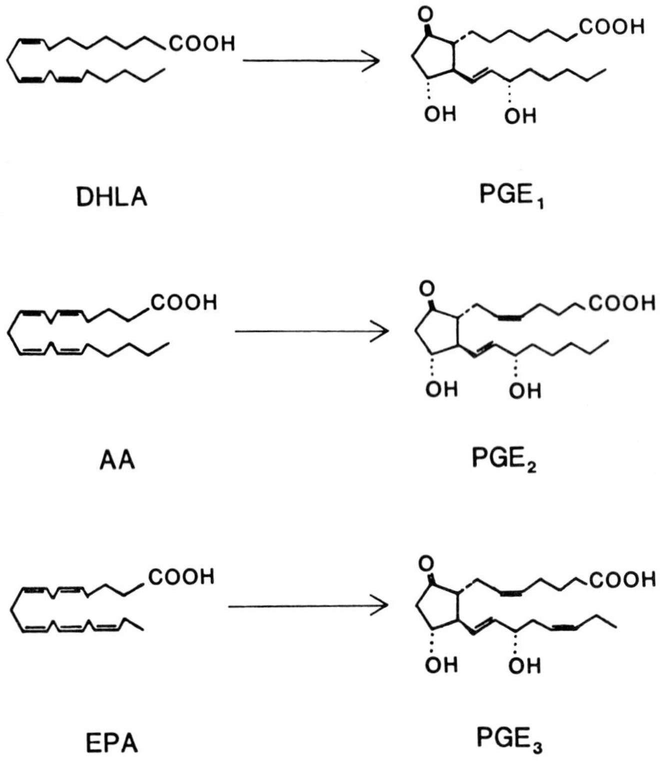

FIGURE 31-2 Structures of PGE_1, PGE_2, and PGE_3 and their precursor fatty acids.

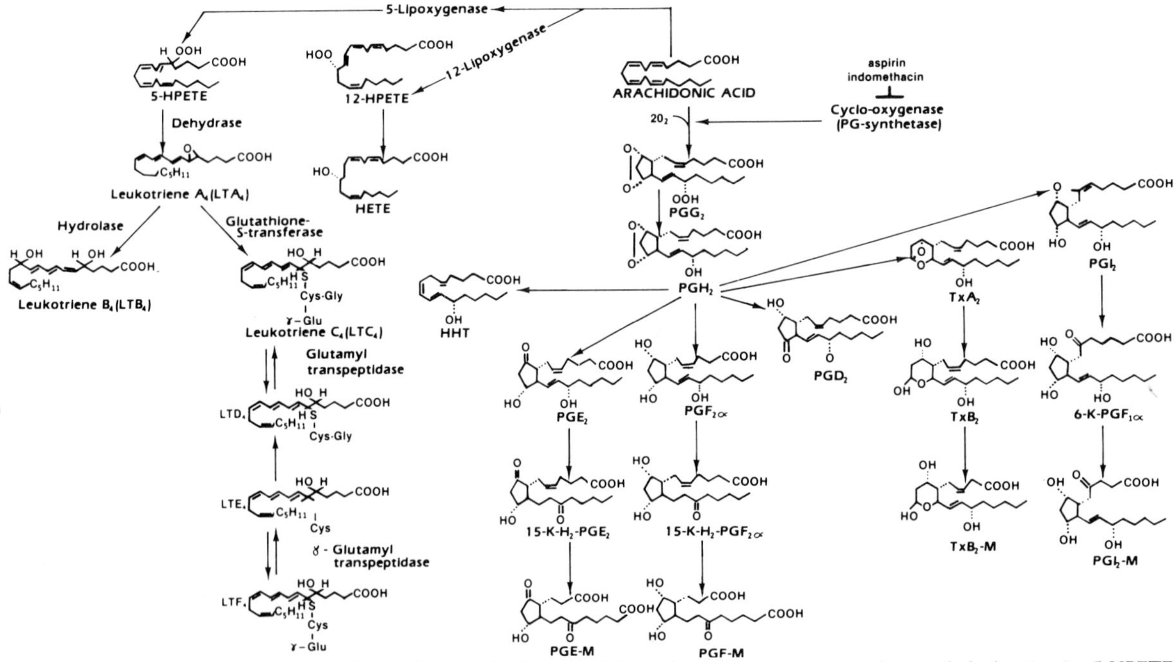

FIGURE 31-3 Synthesis and metabolism of prostaglandins (including thromboxane, prostacyclin, and leukotriene). 5-HPETE, 5-hydroperoxy-6,8,11,14-eicosatetraenoic acid; 12-HPETE, 12-hydroperoxy-5,8,11,14-eicosatetraenoic acid; HETE, 12-L-hydroxy-5,8,10,14-eicosatetraenoic acid; HHT, 12-hydroxy-5,8,10-heptadecatrienoic acid; 6-K-$PGF_{1\alpha}$, 6-keto-$PGF_{1\alpha}$; 15-K-H_2-PGE_2, 15-keto-13,14-dihydro-PGE_2; 15-K-$H_2PGF_{2\alpha}$, 15-keto-13,14-didhydro-$PGF_{2\alpha}$; PGE-M, 7α-hydroxy-5,11-diketotetranorprosta-1,16-dioic acid; PGF-M, 5α,7α-dihydroxy-11-ketotetranorprosta-1,16-dioic acid; TxB_2-M, dinor-TxB_2; PGI_2-M, dinor-6-keto-$PGF_{1\alpha}$.

hormone has been used. Tissue hormones are substances which exert their effects close to their place of synthesis. They are metabolized locally; the small amounts escaping local metabolism are removed by the lungs, preventing recirculation. They can be thought of as local mediators of functions such as tissue perfusion and tissue metabolism. Much of the understanding of the functional role of tissue hormones is fragmentary. The PGs provide a good model for studying tissue hormones because much of their basic biochemistry is now known

ACTIONS OF LEUKOTRIENES

The leukotrienes are believed to be involved in inflammatory processes (for review see Ref. 8). They are synthesized by leukocytes, macrophages, neutrophils, and lung tissue. Slow-reacting substance of anaphylaxis (SRS-A) is composed of a mixture of leukotrienes C_4, D_4, and E_4. Leukotriene B_4 is a very potent chemotactic substance for white blood cells. It also possesses calcium ionophoric actions and can activate neutrophils. Leukotrienes C_4 and D_4 increase capillary permeability to water and macromolecules, cause arteriolar vasoconstriction, and are also potent bronchoconstrictors. They are believed to be involved in asthma; however, there is no firm evidence for this at present.

Biochemistry

PROSTAGLANDIN SYNTHESIS AND METABOLISM

The quantities of naturally occurring PGs with differing degrees of unsaturation vary considerably; their abundances are influenced by dietary intake of the precursor fatty acids (listed below). The predominant precursor of the PGs is arachidonic acid, 5,8,11,14-eicosatetraenoic acid; it is converted to the dienoic PGs, i.e., PGs with two double bonds. The precursor of the monoenoic PGs, 8,11,14-eicosatrienoic acid, dihomogammalinolenic acid, and that of the trienoic prostaglandins, 5,8,11,14,17-eicosapentaenoic acid, are much less abundant. The major source of the latter fatty acid is marine animals.

8,11,14-Eicosatrienoic acid is the precursor of the 1 series PGs and thromboxanes. 5,8,11-Eicosatrienoic acid is the precursor for the 3 series leukotrienes. Arachidonic acid is the precursor of the 2 series PGs and thromboxanes and the 4 series leukotrienes. Eicosapentaenoic acid is the precursor of the 3 series PGs and Tx's and the 5 series leukotrienes.

Prostaglandins are not stored within cells; therefore, their release from a cell or tissue always denotes de novo synthesis. The conversion of the precursor fatty acid to a PG can only occur when the fatty acid is available in the free, nonesterified form.[9] The free levels of PG fatty acid precursors are extremely low in the cells. Thus, the rate-limiting step in eicosanoid synthesis is the liberation of substrate from its esterified form by the enzyme *phospholipase.* PG biosynthesis commences as soon as the free fatty acid becomes available.

There are large quantities of arachidonic acid available in the mammalian organism in biomembranes and in fat tissue. The phospholipids are the predominant precursor pool for PG biosynthesis.[10] Activation of phospholipase liberates fatty acids from these phospholipids and initiates PG biosynthesis; inhibition of phospholipase prevents it.[11] Phospholipase A_2 is inhibited by quinacrine, other antimalarials, and glucocorticosteroids. The loss of arachidonic acid from the various phospholipid pools following stimulation of PG biosynthesis has been measured and has been shown to occur in the phosphatidylcholine and phosphatidylinositol pools.[12] Once the arachidonic acid is available in free form, it is metabolized by one of several enzymes, *cyclooxygenase,* yielding the cyclic endoperoxides PGG_2 and PGH_2,[13] or *lipoxygenase,*[8] yielding, among other products, leukotrienes and a variety of hydroxy fatty acids (Fig. 31-3).

The cyclic endoperoxides can be further converted to PGs by isomerases or by spontaneous breakdown. The pathways of PG synthesis vary significantly depending on the individual tissue. The profile within a tissue may also change, depending on the physiological or pathologic state (see below). Thus platelets convert cyclooxygenase products predominantly to TxA_2 while the endothelium of blood vessels generates PGI_2 almost exclusively.

The various PGs have different and often opposing effects. This fact is important in understanding the pathophysiological role of PGs. For example, while the normal renal cortex synthesizes prostacyclin and PGE_2, which are both vasodilators, the hydronephrotic kidney acquires the capability to synthesize TxA_2, a potent vasoconstrictor.

The mechanisms which can initiate PG biosynthesis are numerous and not all have yet been recognized. Some of the well-documented stimuli are listed in Table 31-2, together with some of the PGs formed. A large number of stimuli can cause PG synthesis and release; usually, several PGs are released in response to a stimulus. PGs can be released very quickly: in the kidney, a 3000-fold increase of PGE_2 concentration has been observed within minutes after excision of the tissue.[14] In vivo the PG system in many tissues can respond in a similarly rapid fashion. For example, renal

Table 31-2. Release of Prostaglandins from Tissues

Tissue	Stimulus	Prostaglandin formed
Seminal vesicle	Androgens(?)	PGE_2, $PGF_{2\alpha}$, 19-OH-PGE_2
Platelet	Collagen Thrombin ADP Ca^{2+} ionophore	TxA_2, PGE_2, $PGF_{2\alpha}$, HHT*
Vasculature	Bradykinin	PGI_2, PGE_2
	Angiotensin Injury	PGI_2
Kidney	Angiotensin	PGI_2, PGE_2
	Bradykinin	PGI_2, PGE_2
	ADH	PGE_2 (medulla)
	Norepinephrine	PGE_2
	Ca^{2+} ionophore	PGE_2
	Ischemia	PGE_2, PGI_2
	Hydronephrosis	TxA_2
Lung	Antigen challenge	TxA_2
	Endotoxin	TxA_2
	Shock	PGE_2, TxA_2, PGI_2
Heart	Anaphylaxis Ischemia Bradykinin Catecholamines	PGI_2
CNS	Pyrogen	PGE_2
Uterus	Pregnancy	PGE_2, PGI_2
Leukocytes	Ca^{2+} ionophore	Leukotrienes, TxA_2

*HHT, 12-hydroxy-5,8,10-heptadecatrienoic acid.

ischemia can cause renal PG release within a few minutes.

Once released, the PGs generally have a short duration of action. Some are metabolized and others can be inactivated by spontaneous breakdown (e.g., prostacyclin, TxA_2). The metabolic fate of PGE_2 has been clearly delineated.[15] Infused PGE_2 disappears from the circulation with a half-life of about 18 seconds. The major metabolite of PGE_2 in the circulation is 15-keto-13,14-dihydro-PGE_2 (15-K-H_2-PGE_2, Fig. 31-3), while in urine 7α-hydroxy-5,11-diketotetranor-prosta-1,16-dioic acid (PGE-M, Fig. 31-3) is excreted. The formation of these metabolites proceeds via oxidation of the 15-hydroxyl moiety, reduction of the 13-14 double bond, and β oxidation of the carboxyl as well as the terminal methyl group. TxA_2 decomposes spontaneously and very rapidly to form TxB_2, a biologically inactive material. The major urinary metabolite of TxB_2 is excreted as dinor-TxB_2. Prostacyclin hydrolyzes to the inactive 6-keto-$PGF_{1\alpha}$ and is further metabolized to dinor-6-keto-$PGF_{1\alpha}$, which is its major urinary metabolite.[16] The major known metabolites of PGs in humans are shown in Fig. 31-3.

The location of metabolism is crucial to the function of the PG system. Local metabolism within the tissue of synthesis is a major pathway, and the enzymes responsible for C_{15} oxidation and dehydrogenation have been found in many tissues. Any PGs escaping local metabolism are removed by the lung, thus preventing the entry of PGs into the general circulation. Indeed, the appearance of large amounts of PGs in the general circulation might have disastrous effects, with TxA_2 causing generalized platelet aggregation and vasoconstriction or PGE_2 causing a fall in blood pressure, gut hypermobility, and uterine contraction. The administration of PGs for pharmacological effects always requires amounts that are several thousand times larger than the quantities synthesized endogenously. Prostacyclin may represent an exception to this rule, as its pulmonary metabolism is low.[17] Once a PG has been inactivated by the first metabolic step, metabolism proceeds at a somewhat slower rate, mainly by β and ω oxidation in the liver, and is followed by excretion in the urine.

On the basis of the excretion rate of the urinary metabolites of PGs and their half-life in the circulation, it has been calculated that plasma levels must be extremely low, on the order of 2 pg/ml for $PGF_{2\alpha}$, PGI_2, and PGE_2. Therefore, the numerous reports on measured circulating PG concentrations have to be viewed with great skepticism because the figures given are usually several orders of magnitude higher than would be expected on the basis of what is known about PG kinetics. Higher levels than those predicted may be measured because of generation of PGs from blood platelets or vascular endothelium during the sampling procedure. In addition, the methods used are often not sufficiently specific to distinguish between a PG and its closely related metabolites, which can be present in amounts which are 10-fold higher than the PG in question. Methods for measurement of PG metabolites have been developed and applied successfully to the determination of PG synthesis in humans.

SYNTHESIS AND METABOLISM OF LEUKOTRIENES

The initial step in the metabolism of arachidonic acid to leukotrienes is catalyzed by the enzyme 5-lipoxygenase (Fig. 31-3). The product of this reaction is 5-hydroperoxy-6,8,11,14-eicosatetraenoic acid, which is metabolized to leukotriene A_4 by a dehydrase. Leukotriene A_4 may be further metabolized enzymatically by a hydrolase to form leukotriene B_4 or by glutathione-S-transferase to leukotriene C_4. Leukotriene A_4 may also be converted nonenzymatically to several different hydroxy fatty acids. Leukotriene C_4 is further metabolized to leukotrienes D_4 and E_4 by the enzyme γ-glutamyl transpeptidase. Leukotriene C_4 is classified as a sulfidopeptide leukotriene because it is a conjugate of glutathione with leukotriene A_4. Glutathione is covalently linked to leukotriene A_4 at the 6 position of arachidonic acid through the sulfhydryl group of cysteine in glutathione. When the γ-glutamyl moiety of glutathione is removed by γ-glutamyl transpeptidase from leukotriene C_4, leukotriene D_4 is formed. Leukotriene E_4 is formed from leukotriene D_4 when the glycine residue is removed. Leukotriene F_4 is formed from leukotriene E_4 by the addition of a γ-glutamyl residue.

INHIBITION OF PROSTAGLANDIN BIOSYNTHESIS

One of the most useful tools in PG research became available when it was discovered that aspirin inhibits PG biosynthesis.[4] This finding was soon extended to include all other nonsteroidal anti-inflammatory drugs. Indeed, the finding of the inhibitory effect of these drugs has led to the formulation of a hypothesis positing that their effects and side effects are mediated by inhibition of cyclooxygenase. Evidence can now be cited in support of this claim.[18] During inflammation, sensitization of pain receptors occurs. This is probably due to the release of local substances. PGE_2 when injected into a joint or into the spleen, can produce pain that is not antagonized by aspirin. Furthermore, PGs can potentiate the pain response to bradykinin. Thus, PGs released during inflammation can sensitize pain receptors to other stimuli (e.g., bradykinin, mechanical effects). Fever can be evoked by injection of endotoxin or PGE. However, while endotoxin-induced fever can be blocked by aspirin or indomethacin, PGE-stimulated fever is unaffected. Also, endotoxin injected into the CSF causes an increase in CSF prostaglandin levels which can be blocked by aspirin.[19] (The role of PGs in fever and inflammation is not further covered here as it has limited relevance to endocrinology.)

Side effects of aspirin are gastric erosion, kidney damage, and delayed parturition. The exact mechanism of induction of the gastric lesion has not been elucidated, but it must depend on acid secretion and breakdown of cellular integrity. It has been found that indomethacin in the presence of gastrin causes a reduction of gastric blood flow and at the same time enhances acid output.[20] In the kidney, inhibitors of PG synthesis have been shown to induce reversable renal failure and other renal syndromes.[21] This side effect is particularly prominent in patients with underlying renal disease.

Organ Systems

REPRODUCTION

The discovery of the powerful contractile effect of PGs on the pregnant and nonpregnant myometrium in vitro has resulted in numerous investigations into the possible function of PGs in reproduction. While much of the early work was directed toward the elucidation of seminal PG function, the discovery of PGs in amniotic fluid and the finding that their levels increase with progression of labor has shifted the focus to investigation of uteroplacental PGs. It has now become apparent that PGs play a role in uterine contraction and indirectly figure in regulation of uterine blood flow in pregnancy and in ovulation. Application of the knowledge gained from these observations has led to the use of PGs to induce abortion and of PG synthesis inhibitors to prevent premature labor.

Uterine Prostaglandins

The uterus is contracted by PGE_2 and $PGF_{2\alpha}$, and PGI_2 reduces tonus and spontaneous contractions of the isolated myometrium. All these PGs are synthesized by the uterus, placenta, and amnion and can be found in amniotic fluid. Their levels increase during pregnancy, as reflected in uterine venous or peripheral plasma and urinary metabolite levels.[22]

Uterine PGs may play a role in delivery and menstruation. It has been suggested that dysmenorrhea is associated with excessive PG production leading to cramping.[23] Indeed, blockers of PG synthesis have been found useful in the treatment of dysmenorrhea.[24]

The role of PGs in uterine contraction can best be shown by the effects of inhibitors of PG synthesis, which prolong labor by reducing the frequency and force of contractions.[23] The broader use of these drugs as tocolytic agents has been prevented, in part, by fear of a reduction of uteroplacental blood flow and contraction of the ductus arteriosus. Animal studies have shown that indomethacin can reduce uteroplacental blood flow in dogs and rabbits. It now appears that uteroplacental blood flow is mostly regulated passively and reflects amniotic fluid pressure. Administration of indomethacin leads to a reduction of tonus of uterine muscles and thus reduces amniotic fluid pressure, which in turn increases uteroplacental blood flow.

During labor, PG levels in amniotic fluid and plasma levels of $PGF_{2\alpha}$ are increased about 20-fold above prelabor levels. Following delivery the levels decline within a few hours. The most convincing evidence that PGs have a role in uterine contractions at term comes from the observations on the effect of PG synthesis inhibitors in pregnant females. Delayed beginning of labor, prolonged labor, and increased blood loss have been observed in women taking aspirin.[25] Saline-induced abortion can be much delayed by indomethacin. Both of these observations indicate that PGs are important for uterine contractions and show that the common denominator for the similar action of both drugs is inhibition of PG biosynthesis.

The use of indomethacin as a tocolytic agent is under clinical investigation. While this therapy is probably efficacious, its safety has not been established and short- and long-term effects in the newborn are unknown.

Luteolysis

Luteolysis depends in some animal species on a factor released from the uterus. In sheep, it is likely that this factor is a PG traveling from the ipsilateral uterine horn to the ovary by transport from the uterine vein into the ovarian artery, because separation of these closely adjacent structures or administration of indomethacin prevents luteal regression in that species. However, in women no such mechanism can be postulated since women without a uterus do not have significant alterations in ovarian function. In addition, a role for PGs in luteal function in women is unlikely since neither infusions of large amounts of PGs nor administration of PG synthesis inhibitors has been shown to affect the human corpus luteum.

Ovulation

Luteinizing hormone (LH) can increase follicular PG synthesis, possibly by a cyclic nucleotide–mediated mechanism.[26] The production of PG has been shown to be of functional significance in ovulation: both indomethacin and antibodies to PGs can block ovulation in rats, rabbits, and primates.[27] No data are available for women. However, the fact that women who receive long-term treatment with high doses of aspirin can conceive[25] suggests that therapeutic doses of aspirin do not have a significant effect on ovulation.

Seminal Fluid Prostaglandins

The lumen of the seminal vesicles is the only place where PGs are stored. Fifteen PGs have been identified in seminal fluid; however, some of these may be artifacts generated in the process of analysis.[28] The predominant PGs of seminal fluid have been shown to be 19-hydroxy-PGE_2 and 19-hydroxy-PGE_1. Semen is the richest source of PGs known, although there are large species differences. Concentrations in men and rams range from 50 to 100 μg/ml; concentrations in bulls are much lower. Much effort has been spent trying to delineate a functional role for these PGs. It has been suggested that they affect sperm mobility and sperm penetration through the cervical mucus and that they decrease uterine motility, thus functioning as an exohormone.[29] The latter hypothesis receives some support from studies showing that the uterus responds to PGs with relaxation at the time of ovulation. However, none of these suggestions has been proved.

It has been found that infertile men have lower seminal PG levels than normal men.[29,30] There is some evidence that treatment with androgens can increase seminal PG levels. However, in infertile men whose PG concentrations were low, other factors known to be of importance for fertilization were also abnormal.[29,30]

RENAL PROSTAGLANDINS

The renal medulla exerts an antihypertensive effect that can be demonstrated by transplanting renal medullary tissue into anephric dogs.[31] This observation led to the search for a vasodepressor material synthesized in the renal medulla. PGE_2, $PGF_{2\alpha}$, and PGA_2 were isolated from this tissue;[32] PGA_2 was subsequently shown to be an artifact. Later, PGE_2, PGD_2, and PGI_2[33] were found to be synthesized in the renal cortex. The exact anatomic site of renal PG formation has not been determined. The vasculature of the renal cortex is capable of synthesizing PGI_2; interstitial cells and/or tubular cells in the medulla predominantly synthesize PGE_2. The in vitro rate of PG synthesis is about two times higher in the renal medulla than in the cortex. Nevertheless, cortical PGs play an important role in regulation of cortical renal function, including renal blood flow and renin release.

Both the cortex and the medulla can metabolize prostaglandins by Δ^{13} reduction and C_{15} dehydrogenation. The enzyme 9-ketoreductase can effect conversion of PGE_2 to $PGF_{2\alpha}$ in vitro; however, this has not been shown to be of significance in vivo.

Synthesis of PGs is stimulated in the kidney by ischemia, angiotensin, bradykinin, catecholamines, and antidiuretic hormone (ADH). It now appears that specific stimuli evoke specific PG responses; i.e., the type and location of PG synthesis depend on the stimulus. For example, ADH causes enhanced medullary PGE_2 synthesis, while some forms of renin release depend on cortical prostacyclin synthesis. These observations have led to a concept of compartmentalization of renal PG regulation.[34]

Renal Hemodynamics

Infusion of PGE_2, PGD_2, or PGI_2 increases renal blood flow. Infusion of arachidonic acid also increases renal blood flow, but, in contrast to the PGs, which increase flow to all zones of the renal cortex, arachidonic acid selectively increases flow to the juxtamedullary nephrons. This action of arachidonic acid can be blocked by indomethacin.

The renal effect resulting from inhibition of PG synthesis depends significantly on the conditions under which the inhibitor is given. Thus, in normal dogs at rest, indomethacin has no effect on renal blood flow, while in an anesthetized animal following surgery there is a significant reduction in blood flow. However, regardless of anesthesia, the renal response to stress is always affected by PGs. Hemorrhagic hypotension or angiotension infusion leads to a decrease of renal flow that is magnified when renal PG synthesis is blocked. Thus, renal PGs are thought to serve as a defense mechanism, protecting the kidney from excessive vasoconstrictor influences.

In situations of stress, renal blood flow is shifted toward the juxtamedullary nephrons. These nephrons provide the nutritive blood flow to the renal medulla. Inhibition of PG synthesis can prevent this shift. It has been speculated that under these conditions medullary blood flow could be reduced to a critical level, leading to papillary necrosis.

The glomerular filtration rate (GFR) also can be reduced by PG synthesis inhibitors. While this effect is hardly detectable in normal volunteers, in patients with reduced renal function the effect becomes clinically significant. Thus, in patients with advanced cirrhosis of the liver, nephrotic syndrome, or Bartter's syndrome, a pronounced reduction of GFR is noted when these drugs are given.

The source of the PGs that are important in the regulation of renal blood flow is not known. The most likely anatomical structure is the vasculature of the renal cortex, because the renal cortex is a rich source of prostacyclin[33] and arachidonic acid can increase renal blood flow even in the absence of glomerular filtration or urinary flow.[35] Thus, the effects of PGs on cortical blood flow can be explained without invoking transport of PGs from the medulla, the most active site of PG synthesis, to the cortex via tubular fluid, a mechanism postulated earlier.

Sodium

While infusion of the vasodilator prostaglandins E_2, I_2, and arachidonic acid causes natriuresis, the use of inhibitors of PG synthesis has not produced equally clear results. Indomethacin can cause natriuresis in some animals. In humans, however, indomethacin and other nonsteroidal anti-inflammatory drugs can cause significant sodium retention.[36] The mechanism of this sodium retention is not clear. A small reduction of GFR and possibly reduced renal blood flow under conditions of daily stress have been implicated. However, the possibility that distal tubular sodium reabsorption is involved was raised when it was found that PGE_2 can decrease sodium transport out of the isolated collecting duct.[37] These findings are consistent with a natriuretic function of endogenously synthesized renal PGs.

Renin

There is considerable evidence supporting a role of PGs in renin release.[34] Arachidonic acid can enhance renin release, an effect that can be prevented by the administration of indomethacin.[38] Infusion of PGs can also enhance renal renin release. Factors other than PG-induced vasodilation seem to be important, for in the presence of maximal vasodilation produced by papaverine, PGI_2 has been found to be more potent than PGE_2 in releasing renin.

The stimulators of renin release that can be blocked by indomethacin in animals include furosemide,[39] reduction of perfusion pressure by hemorrhage, and catecholamines.[40] Work on isolating the mechanism by which PGs influence renin release has shown that the mechanism in the macula densa depends on a PG for its proper function. Detailed analysis of the in vivo stimulation of renin release induced by arachidonic acid has revealed that the PG that is important in renin regulation may originate in the afferent arteriole.[41] Attempts to identify which PG might be involved in renin regulation have shown that PG-dependent renin release is not correlated with renal PGE_2 synthesis. The search for other PGs in the renal cortex revealed PGI_2 synthesis, which is now recognized to release renin in vitro with a potency similar to that of isoproterenol.[34] Indeed, it is now believed that PGI_2 is the renal PG primarily responsible for PG-induced renin release.

Studies in humans show that indomethacin can reduce plasma renin activity[42] and that this effect is independent of the sodium retention caused by this drug.[43] In rats, adrenergically mediated renin release can be blocked by indomethacin,[40] but this is not the case in humans.[43]

Antidiuretic Hormone

Studies in tissues thought to be useful as models of the medullary collecting duct with respect to the action of ADH have shown that PGE-type prostaglandins can prevent ADH action.[44] Thus, in the canine collecting duct and the toad bladder, PGE prevents ADH-induced water movement. In hypophysectomized, water-loaded dogs, indomethacin has been shown to enhance strikingly the hydrosmotic effect of exogenous ADH. Furthermore, the rate of PGE_2 synthesis in the renal medulla is enhanced by ADH in vitro and in vivo. From these observations the hypothesis has emerged that PGs function as negative feedback inhibitors of ADH action.[45]

In humans the importance of renal PGs in water metabolism has been demonstrated in studies comparing the effect of ADH in water-loaded normal volunteers before and after suppression of PG synthesis. Water loading in these experiments was carried out in order to suppress endogenous ADH synthesis. It was noted that indomethacin caused a significant augmentation of the effect of ADH on urinary concentration;[34,46] it thus appears that an antagonism between ADH and renal PGs also occurs in humans.

Erythropoietin

There is some evidence that erythropoietin release can be regulated by renal cortical PGs. Erythropoietin release stimulated by hypoxia and ischemia can be blocked by indomethacin; PGE_2, PGE_1, and arachidonic acid can enhance its release.[47] At present it is not known whether these effects are due to the influence of PGs on the erythropoietin-releasing cell or whether they are the results of changes in intrarenal blood flow distribution and oxygen tension.

GASTROINTESTINAL TRACT

Endogenous and exogenous PGs can significantly affect GI function. One of the important side effects of the administration of PGs for the induction of abortion is diarrhea. Small intestinal motility and secretion are enhanced by PGE_2 and $PGF_{2\alpha}$. Conversely, inhibition of PG synthesis can reduce some forms of diarrhea. In the stomach, PGE_2 and some chemical analogues have been found to reduce acid secretion and prevent mucosal lesions caused by aspirin.

Motility

The longitudinal muscles of the small intestine are exquisitely sensitive to stimulation by PGs. This property of the gut has been used to assay PGs. Diarrhea seen after the administration of a prostaglandin is probably not due to hypermotility per se but is a consequence of *enteropooling*. Enteropooling is the accumulation of intestinal fluid in the lumen; it has the effect of inducing intestinal hypermotility. Indomethacin can reduce peristalsis in animals, but this effect has not been shown to be a significant side effect of indomethacin in humans.

Secretion

Prostaglandins of the E and F types have been shown to inhibit water and electrolyte absorption across the wall of the small intestine and to increase their secretion. This effect is similar to that of cholera toxin, which has been linked to increased levels of cAMP.[48] Also, the mode of action of some cathartics, such as castor oil and bisacodyl, seems to involve PGs: they can stimulate intestinal PG synthesis and their pharmacological effect is much reduced in animals pretreated with indomethacin.

In certain diseases in which diarrhea is a prominent symptom, such as irradiation syndrome, Crohn's disease, Verner-Morrison syndrome, and medullary carcinoma of the thyroid, PGs have been implicated as causing or contributing to the diarrhea.[49] Diarrhea has been reduced by inhibiting PG synthesis in some patients, but this observation does not provide the basis for a therapeutic recommendation. That the use of inhibitors of PG synthesis is associated with reduced diarrhea in those syndromes does not constitute definite proof that PGs have a pathogenetic role in the diarrhea in each syndrome. Neither have the effects of PGs in other diarrheal states been carefully studied.

In the stomach, endogenous PGE_2 and PGI_2 can inhibit basal and gastrin- or histamine-stimulated acid secretion. This effect is coupled with an increase in gastric blood flow. Administraton of pentagastrin to dogs produces an increase in acid secretion; simultaneous administration of indomethacin causes a further increase in acid output and a reduction in gastric blood flow.[50] It is possible that this constellation of effects provides a partial explanation for the damaging effect of PG synthesis inhibitors on the gastric mucosa.

Cytoprotective Effect

The PGs which reduce gastric secretion can also prevent the formation of gastric ulcers produced experimentally in animals. Their effect is in part mediated by inhibition of acid secretion. However, in animals, indomethacin causes, in addition to the acute gastric ulcers, slowly developing multiple ulcers in the small intestine which are clearly not related to gastric acid secretion; these can also be prevented by PG administration. Thus, endogenous PGs are thought to exert a cytoprotective effect on the mucosa of the GI tract. The PGE analogues currently undergoing clinical trials for the treatment of peptic ulcer disease are also thought to exert a cytoprotective effect in the GI tract.

CARDIOVASCULAR SYSTEM

In recent years, the notion has been put forth that, to maintain vascular hemostasis and homeostasis, a dynamic balance exists between the vascular production of PGI_2 and the platelet production of TxA_2. It has been speculated that an imbalance between these two eicosanoids could favor a shift in either thrombotic potential or blood vessel tone within the vascular system.[51] An example of this altered balance has been demonstrated to occur during hydronephrosis induced by ureteral obstruction in rabbit kidneys.[52] The increased vascular resistance that occurs in this experimental model is accompanied by an overproduction of TxA_2. Both the increased vascular resistance and increased TxA_2 production are reduced by Tx synthetase inhibitors.[52]

The role of PGs in the regulation of vascular resistance has been studied by administering indomethacin to human subjects. In individuals under the stress of catheterization, indomethacin reduces mesenteric and renal blood flow.[53] Although the increase in muscle blood flow induced by exercise is not dependent on PG synthesis, postocclusive hyperemia in the arm and leg is markedly reduced by the drug.

In humans, the in vivo conversion of arachidonic acid to PGs has been found to be remarkably efficient. Infusion of arachidonic acid into muscle, kidney, and heart leads to synthesis of PGE_2, PGI_2, and PGD_2.[53] In view of the rapidity with which the arachidonic acid is converted to PGs, it is likely that most of this conversion occurs in the vasculature. The regulation of vascular PG synthesis has been studied intensively. Angiotensin II and catecholamines[54] increase PG synthesis, and their vasoconstrictor effect is in part antagonized by the released PGs. Thus, PGs are thought to play a local modulatory role to protect the tissue from the reduction of blood flow below a critical level. Bradykinin also releases PGs from blood vessels, lung, kidney, uterus, spleen, and heart;[55] this release is responsible for its vasodilating property in most instances. The type of PGs released depends on the system being stimulated. Thus, following bradykinin administration, PGE_2 is synthesized in the arteries.[56] Because PGE_2 is a vasodilator and $PGF_{2\alpha}$ is a vasoconstrictor, this finding has provided an explanation for the observation that bradykinin induces arterial dilatation and venous constriction. Thus, here, PG biosynthesis is tissue-specific although a single stimulus elicited the different effects. (The prostaglandin-kinin interaction is discussed in more detail in the second part of this chapter.)

CIRCULATING PROSTAGLANDINS

PGI_2 has been postulated to be a circulating hormone that is continuously released by either the lung and/or endothelial cells.[51] This notion was based in part on the observation that the metabolic clearance rate of PGI_2 is low. Subsequent evidence has convincingly shown that PGI_2 probably does not circulate in amounts sufficient to produce a significant physiological effect on platelet function.[57] However, a potential role of PGI_2 in modulating the thrombotic potential within the microcirculation has not been ruled out.

CIRCULATORY SHOCK

Prostaglandins and thromboxanes have been found to be elevated in several experimental models of circulatory shock.[58] Recently, central venous plasma TxB_2 and 6-keto-$PGF_{1\alpha}$ concentrations have been found to be elevated in patients in septic shock.[59] The role of the various eicosanoids in circulatory shock remains uncertain. Currently, evidence exists to support the following notions: (1) TxA_2 contributes to the increase in pulmonary artery pressure during endotoxemia, (2) PGI_2 and PGE_2 may contribute to hypotension associated with circulatory shock, and (3) fatty acid cyclooxygenase inhibitors may be beneficial in certain types of circulatory shock.[58] Clinical trials are currently under way, testing these notions in patients with septic shock. It has also been speculated that leukotrienes may be involved in the adult respiratory distress syndrome associated with various forms of circulatory shock.

BLOOD PRESSURE

Blood pressure in normal volunteers is not measurably affected by inhibition of PG synthesis. It is important to recall in this context that blood pressure is the result of both cardiac output and peripheral resistance. Thus, even when blood pressure remains unaltered, peripheral resistance may increase if there is a corresponding reduction in cardiac output. One of the classic studies of the role of PGs in the regulation of blood pressure in humans involved patients with Bartter's syndrome. These patients have a characteristic decrease in blood pressure responsiveness to the vasoconstrictor effect of angiotensin II. These patients have been shown to produce excessive amounts of vasodilator PGs, and indomethacin was found to normalize their blood pressure response to angiotensin and norepinephrine[60] (Fig. 31-4).

Indomethacin results in a modest increase in blood pressure in normal volunteers under moderate stress.[53] This effect is much more pronounced in cases of severe stress. In some models of hypertension, PG synthesis inhibition increases blood pressure. In spontaneously hypertensive rats and in rabbits with renal artery stenosis, PG synthesis inhibition increases blood pressure and may induce malignant hypertension.[61] It

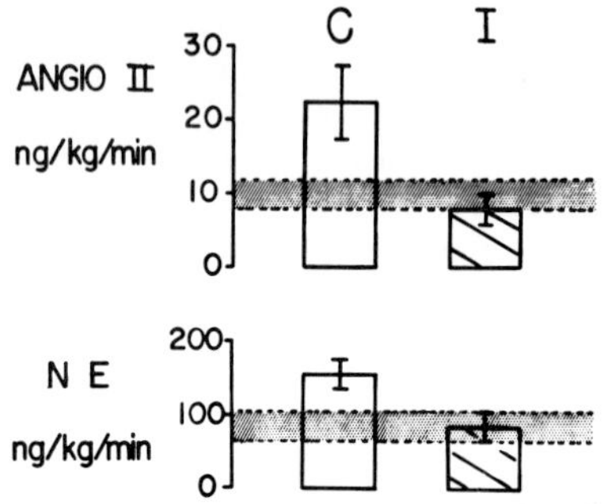

FIGURE 31-4 Effects of indomethacin on the blood pressure response to angiotensin II (angio II) and norepinephrine (NE) in patients with Bartter's syndrome. In the control phase (C) much larger amounts of these vasopressor agents were required to increase blood pressure by 20 mmHg than following blockade of prostaglandin synthesis by indomethacin (I). (*From Bartter et al.*[60])

is important to recognize that many factors have an important influence on vascular resistance. Angiotensin II plays a role in some forms of hypertension. While indomethacin can increase vascular resistance, it also lowers plasma renin activity and thereby decreases levels of angiotensin II. On the other hand, PGs can reduce adrenergic transmitter release from peripheral nerve endings,[62] and indomethacin can increase catecholamine release. The net effect of these various influences on blood pressure control in humans remains unclear.

CLINICALLY IMPORTANT CARDIOVASCULAR FUNCTIONS OF PROSTAGLANDINS

Antihypertensive Drugs

Although indomethacin has been shown to inhibit the effect of beta blockers, this inhibition cannot be demonstrated in patients on a low-sodium diet; this suggests that the sodium retention associated with indomethacin administration may be the basis of the apparent drug-drug interaction.[63] The vasodilating but not the antilipolytic effect of nicotinic acid can be blocked by indomethacin.

Ductus Arteriosus

The predominant PG of the ductus arteriosus is PGI_2.[64] It is possible that regulation of ductal PGI_2 synthesis is important in determining physiological closure at birth. It has been found that, in a large number of babies with persistent ductus arteriosus, closure can be effected by pharmacological inhibition of PG synthesis.[66] This therapy is not without hazard, as the immature kidney is particularly sensitive to these agents, and nephrotoxicity has been reported. PGE_1 or E_2 can be infused into the ductus arteriosus to prevent its closure. This effect is desirable in children with reduced pulmonary perfusion due to malformation of the pulmonary artery. By this means temporary improvement in oxygen saturation prior to surgery has been safely accomplished.[67]

Orthostatic Hypotension

Orthostatic hypotension in patients with parkinsonism or the Shy-Drager syndrome (primary orthostatic hypotension) has been shown to be improved by indomethacin.[68,69]

Blood Platelets

Among the prostaglandins are both platelet-aggregating (TxA_2, PGH_2) and antiaggregating (PGI_2, PGD_2, PGE_1) substances. When platelet aggregation is stimulated by ADP, epinephrine, thrombin, or collagen in platelet-rich plasma, the predominant product formed by the platelet cyclooxygenase is TxA_2. Aspirin given to normal volunteers or added to platelet-rich plasma in vitro prevents the second, generally irreversible wave of platelet aggregation induced by ADP, epinephrine, and low concentrations of thrombin or collagen. Arachidonic acid is stored esterified to phospholipids within the platelet membrane. In response to a variety of different aggregating agents, arachidonic acid is hydrolyzed from its storage sites by phospholipases A and C.[70] Once it is in the free acid form it is rapidly metabolized by fatty acid cyclooxygenase or is reesterified to membrane phospholipids. Early studies supported the hypothesis that the formation of TxA_2 was an absolute requirement in order for arachidonic acid to aggregate platelets. It has subsequently been shown that this is not the case; PGH_2 as well as TxA_2 can mediate arachidonic acid–induced platelet aggregation.[71]

This TxA_2 release by platelets can take place in vivo, and has been shown to have dramatic effects. In rabbits, intravenous (IV) injection of arachidonic acid causes sudden death, accompanied by the accumulation of platelet aggregates in the lungs. This effect of arachidonic acid can be blocked by aspirin, the selective TxA_2 synthesis inhibitor imidazole, or thromboxane receptor antagonists.[72] It is not clear whether the accumulation of the platelet aggregates or the powerful vasoconstrictor response to TxA_2 causes death. In other vascular beds, TxA_2 synthesized from platelets can cause vasoconstriction. For example, TxA_2 injected into the coronary artery of the rabbit and guinea pig can lead to spasm and subendocardial necrosis.

PGD_2 is formed in small amounts by human blood platelets on aggregation and has antiaggregatory properties.[73] Prostacyclin formed in the blood vessel wall is the most powerful endogenous antiaggregating substance known; it can prevent and even reverse TxA_2-induced platelet aggregation. In humans, infusion of PGI_2 causes an increase in bleeding time and a reduction in platelet aggregation in response to ADP.[74]

Aspirin blocks cyclooxygenase activity in a variety of tissues; the tissue cyclooxygenase inhibition is reversed within a short time after aspirin administration is stopped. In contrast, the blockade in platelets persists for a much longer time. In fact, contact of a platelet with aspirin causes covalent binding of the acetyl moiety of aspirin to platelet cyclooxygenase. The duration of the antiaggregatory effect of aspirin is not related to the brief half-life of aspirin but lasts for the entire life span of the platelet. This is due to the fact that the platelet cannot synthesize new cyclooxygenase. Only newly released platelets have normal function. It is at present not clear whether aspirin selectively blocks platelet cyclooxygenase in preference to the cyclooxygenase of vascular walls.[75] However, the antiaggregating properties of PG synthesis inhibitors are already being explored in the prevention of myocardial infarction,[76,77] thrombosis of dialysis shunts,[78] and cerebrovascular accidents.[79] What dose of aspirin should be used as an antithrombotic agent has been the subject of considerable investigation in recent years. Evidence is slowly accumulating that a low aspirin dosage (20 to 40 mg per day) may selectively inhibit platelet thromboxane formation while preserving vascular prostacyclin synthesis.[80] Further areas of investigation include the possible development of atherosclerosis as a consequence of endothelial damage produced by platelets[81] or by deficient vascular wall PGI_2 synthesis. Enhanced platelet TxA_2 synthesis has been demonstrated in vitro in diabetic subjects and has been linked to the angiopathy of diabetes.[82]

Lack of platelet PG synthesis due to the absence of cyclooxygenase has been described in a patient with a mild bleeding tendency.[83] This disorder is very rare and is characterized by the inability of platelets to synthesize TxA_2 and aggregate in response to ADP.[83]

LUNGS

Prostaglandins play a role in airway resistance and pulmonary vascular resistance. Inhalation of TxA_2, PGG_2, PGH_2, PGD_2, or $PGF_{2\alpha}$ causes bronchospasm,[84] while PGE_2 and PGI_2 cause bronchodilation.[85] It is notable that the sensitivity of asthmatic individuals to the bronchoconstricting effect of inhaled $PGF_{2\alpha}$ is enhanced several thousand times.[85] The possibility that endogenous PGs might modify airway resistance was raised by early observations showing a modest increase in the vital capacity and the forced expiratory volume in response to flufenamic acid, antipyrine, and aminopyrine in humans. Which of the several PGs might be involved is unclear. However, during asthmatic attacks, levels of the major circulating metabolite of $PGF_{2\alpha}$ were found to be elevated.[86] A more recent study on exercise and antigen-induced asthma in humans revealed no effect of indomethacin,[87] although in a single case aspirin, mefenamic acid, and ibuprofen were reported to be beneficial.[88]

There is a group of patients who respond to the administration of aspirin, indomethacin, phenylbutazone, and ibuprofen with a severe asthmatic attack. Such aspirin-sensitive asthmatic patients were formerly thought to suffer from an allergic reaction to the drug. However, the finding of sensitivity to all the drugs mentioned makes inhibition of cyclooxygenase more likely to be the actual effect of the drugs.[89] Inhibition of the synthesis of a bronchodilator PG in response to these drugs is not necessarily what causes the asthmatic attack. It is also possible that the inhibition of the cyclooxygenase pathway by these drugs leads to lipoxygenase pathway activity (Fig. 31-3), with increased levels of SRS-A and other products. The confusing and contradictory reports regarding the effects of the cyclooxygenase inhibitors on airway resistance require further study using well-characterized populations of asthmatic patients.

Pulmonary hypertension is seen in gram-negative sepsis and alveolar hypoxia. While indomethacin has no effect on the increase in pulmonary vascular resistance associated with hypoxia, it does block early pulmonary hypertension in response to endotoxin in animals. This response is associated with increased pulmonary synthesis of thromboxane; Tx may be responsible for some forms of pulmonary hypertension.[90]

METABOLIC EFFECTS

Lipolysis

Prostaglandins of the E series have been found to inhibit lipolysis in isolated fat cells stimulated by catecholamines, adrenocorticotropic hormone (ACTH), thyroid stimulating hormone, and glucagon.[91] The PG effect is probable due to inhibition of cAMP formation.[92] However, it has not been possible to show an effect of PG synthesis inhibition on lipolysis in vivo. In addition, nicotinic acid–induced lipolysis is not blocked by indomethacin in vivo.

Calcium Metabolism

Prostaglandins stimulate bone resorption in organ cultures;[93] PGE_2 is the most potent PG tested thus far in inducing bone resorption. Certain animal tumors produce large amounts of PGE_2, and it has been suggested that this PG is responsible for the hypercalcemia associated with these tumors.[94] The $HSDM_1$ tumor in the mouse and the VX_2 rabbit carcinoma have been found to cause hypercalcemia independently of bone metastases.[95] Cells from these tumors grown in tissue culture produce a factor which stimulates bone resorption and which has been found to be identical to PGE_2.[95] Levels of PGE_2 in blood draining the tumor and in the general circulation were found to be elevated, and the elevated PGE_2 levels coincided temporarily with the hypercalcemia. Both hypercalcemia and PGE_2 levels can be normalized by indomethacin.[95] All these studies lend support to the hypothesis that a tumor-produced most likely PG, PGE_2, can cause hypercalcemia.

A small subset of patients with hypercalcemia caused by carcinoma of the lung, uterine cervix, or pancreas has been identified in which indomethacin reduces plasma calcium levels.[96] Biochemical studies on levels of the PGE metabolite excreted in the urine revealed that only patients with an elevated level respond to PG suppression.[96] This is in contrast to patients with hypercalcemia associated with myeloma, malignant lymphoma, and lymphosarcoma, who have normal or even depressed PGE metabolite levels and whose hypercalcemia does not respond to inhibition of PG synthesis. The clinical value of treatment with PG synthesis inhibitors in responsive patients remains to be established, because these drugs can cause gastric ulceration and worsen renal failure, complications which are often already present in patients with hypercalcemia.

Diabetes

Prostaglandins may play a role in several aspects of diabetes. It was mentioned above that platelets of diabetic patients synthesize increased amounts of Tx compared to controls.[82] Vascular tissue from patients with juvenile-onset diabetes synthesizes abnormally small amounts of prostacyclin.[97] The combination of these effects could be responsible for increased formation of platelet aggregates and platelet deposits in vivo. These abnormalities may contribute to the accelerated atherosclerotic cardiovascular disease seen in diabetes mellitus.[98]

Insulin secretion may be in part influenced by PGs. Prostaglandins of the E series can reduce insulin release following glucose administration in dogs[99] and in humans.[100,101] Salicylic acid can increase basal and glucose-stimulated insulin release in normal and diabetic subjects and can reduce glucosuria in diabetic individuals. However, since these studies used salicylate, a PG synthesis inhibitor of doubtful efficacy, they will only become interpretable when supported by measurement of PG levels and the effects of other PG synthesis inhibitors.

Essential Fatty Acid Deficiency

Certain fatty acids are essential for normal growth, development, and function. These fatty acids are linoleic acid and arachidonic acid. Because linoleic acid is a precursor of arachidonic acid and arachidonic acid is converted to PGs, attempts have been made to correlate PG synthesis with levels of linoleic acid. It has been found that newborns are especially susceptible to the development of essential fatty acid deficiency. Within a few days of institution of parenteral nutrition that does not contain any of the essential fatty acids, newborns develop signs of essential fatty acid deficiency: prolonged bleeding time, abnormal resistance of platelets to aggregation by ADP,[102] delayed wound healing, and scaly skin lesions. Essential fatty acid deficiency is associated with a reduction in the concentration of a urinary metabolite of PGE, and he abnormalities can be corrected by replacing the essential fatty acid.[103] However, under certain conditions, the parenteral administration of linoleic acid during total parenteral alimentation may lead to an increase in linoleic acid levels in lipid pools but a decline of arachidonic acid levels and prostaglandin synthesis.[103] The mechanism responsible for this paradoxical response may be that, at high levels, linoleic acid competes with arachidonic acid for conversion to prostaglandins.

KALLIKREINS AND KININS

Over 75 years ago it was discovered that dog and human urine administered IV to experimental animals had hypotensive properties, but two decades passed before the material responsible for this phenomenon was found to be an enzyme. It was initially thought that this enzyme originated in the pancreas; the word *kallikrein* is derived from the Greek term for that organ. Interest in kallikrein was stimulated by the discovery and description of the pharmacology of the nonapeptide bradykinin, the product of the action of a kallikrein upon a circulating kininogen substrate. Since these early discoveries, many new findings have accelerated interest in kallikreins and kinins: (1) characterization of some of their biochemical properties and actions, (2) discovery of relations between these materials and other homeostatic systems, and (3) measurements of abnormal kallikrein and kinin levels in various pathophysiological states. Now, a marked increase in the rate of accumulation of knowledge is occurring because of recent exciting discoveries about the enzymes and peptides. These include (1) the description of a large family of tissue kallikrein genes, (2) location of tissue kallikreins in sites not known previously to contain the enzymes, e.g., brain, (3) descriptions of new enzymatic capabilities and actions, respectively, for kallikreins and kinins, and (4) discoveries of a new kinin and new kininogen, called *T-kinin* and *T-kininogen*. More comprehensive treatments of specific aspects of this subject can be found in selected recent reviews and symposia.[104–107a]

Biochemistry of the Systems

The kallikrein-kinin systems include enzymes, kallikrein inhibitors, kininogen substrates, kinins, and kininases. Kallikreins are serine-containing proteinases which liberate kinin peptides from kininogen substrates by limited proteolysis. The kinins are destroyed rapidly by enzymes called *kininases* (Fig. 31-5). There are two types of kallikreins, plasma and tissue (also called glandular) kallikreins. They differ in molecular weight and other physicochemical characteristics, are immunologically and enzymatically distinct, and are affected differently by protease inhibitors. They may be no more closely related than are other serine proteases, e.g., trypsin and thrombin, but they nevertheless carry the same name. Tissue kallikreins were considered until recently to have negligible lytic activity for other proteins, whereas plasma kallikrein is thought to activate neutrophils and participate in fibrinolysis.

The plasma kallikrein-kinin system has been studied more extensively than the tissue system. Plasma kallikrein exists in an inactive form, prekallikrein, a

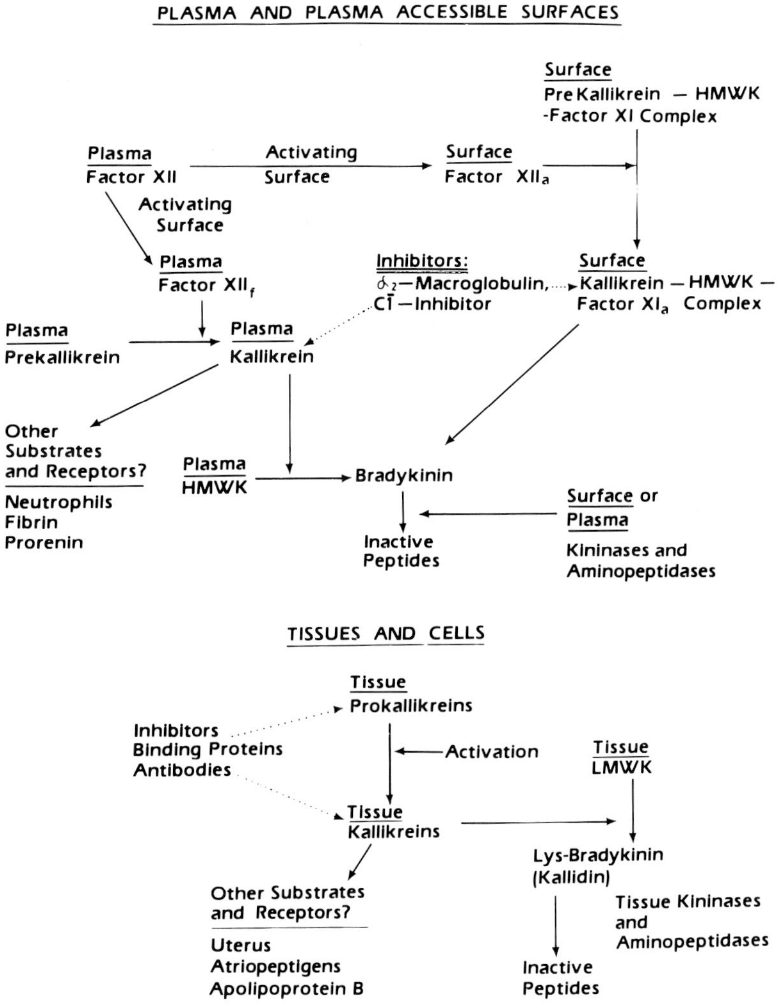

FIGURE 31-5 Kallikreins and kinin formation.

basic glycoprotein of relatively high molecular weight (88,000 M_r). When factor XII (Hageman factor) is activated by exposure to a negatively charged surface (e.g., subendothelial collagen), both the activated factor and a fragment thereof become available and, in turn, activate plasma prekallikrein or surface prekallikrein complexed with high-molecular-weight (HMW) kininogen and factor XI. The plasma kallikrein formed not only activates more factor XII in a positive feedback fashion but attacks kininogen to generate bradykinin. Thus, plasma kallikrein is not only involved in kinin generation but also in the intrinsic pathway of the blood coagulation cascade, fibrinolysis, and neutrophil activation. Plasma prekallikrein is also called *Fletcher factor*. Families whose members are deficient in this enzyme have been described; these individuals present with a prolonged clotting time. A kallikrein-like activity has also been described in basophils which is released after antigen-IgE interaction, in a fashion similar to the release of histamine and other mediators of the immediate hypersensitivity reaction.[108] Studies of patients with seasonal pollen allergies have shown that kallikrein-like activity appears with kinin and histamine in nasal secretions during local allergic reactions.[109]

Tissue kallikreins have been purified from many organs and secretions, such as the porcine pancreas, canine kidney, and human urine and saliva. They are acidic glycoproteins with reported molecular weights from 24,000 to 48,000. The pancreas, intestine, and urine contain a prekallikrein which can be activated by tryptic hydrolysis. In addition, the rat pancreas has been used to isolate and clone the mRNA for a pancreatic preprokallikrein. The mRNA sequence suggests that this tissue kallikrein is synthesized as a protein of 265 amino acids, including a putative secretory prepeptide and an activation peptide.[110] A mouse submaxillary gland complementary DNA (cDNA) clone, coding for a kallikrein, has been used to study kallikrein genes within the mouse genome. Surprisingly, evaluation of a genomic library revealed from 25 to 30 different kallikrein genes, suggesting that a large and closely related family of tissue kallikrein-like enzymes exists.[111] This work points to other proteins with structural similarity to tissue kallikreins [e.g., β-nerve growth factor (NGF)–endopeptidase, γ-NGF, epidermal growth factor binding protein, tonin] and the possibility that products of this gene family have functional roles unrelated to kinin generation, a possibility which had been considered previously.[106] Both polyclonal antisera and monoclonal antibodies have been raised against several purified tissue kallikreins; they are being used to measure tissue kallikrein synthesis rates and levels in various tissues using radioimmunoassays (RIAs) and also to localize kallikreins using immunohistochemistry.

Tissue kallikreins release the decapeptide *lysylbradykinin* (kallidin) from kininogens, whereas plasma kallikrein forms bradykinin (Fig. 31-6). The kallikreins can also hydrolyze substituted esters of arginine or lysine at a pH optimum of 8.5 to 9.0, and this "alkaline esterase" activity forms the basis for many convenient and sensitive assays of kallikrein-like activity. The techniques have limited specificity, since other proteases, such as trypsin or plasmin, if present in adequate amounts can cleave the substrates. In human urine, almost all esterase activity is kallikrein, and measurement of urinary kallikrein activity has allowed the discovery of phenomena which have stimulated interest in the system. Other assays which measure the kinin-generating capacity of kallikreins are available, as are the aforementioned new direct RIAs for kallikreins themselves.

There are at least four different plasma inhibitors of plasma kallikrein, α_2-macroglobulin, $C\bar{1}$ inactivator, α_1-antitrypsin, and antithrombin III. It is of interest that α_2-macroglobulin, which is believed to regulate kinin release by plasma kallikrein, does not bind to the tissue enzyme. A low-molecular-weight (4700 M_r) tissue kallikrein inhibitor is present in the rat kidney. Recently, the identification of tissue kallikrein autoantibodies as well as a unique high-molecular-weight (~52,000 M_r) binding protein has been reported. Other natural and synthetic kallikrein inhibitors, such as aprotinin, specific antibodies, isofluorphate analogues, and aromatic tris amidines, are now being used to assess the roles of kallikreins in organ function.

The plasma kininogen substrates for kallikreins are acidic glycoproteins. Kininogens are present in human renal distal tubular cells and urine, rat brain tissue, and some cultured mammalian cell lines of renal or neural origin. The HMW (69,896 M_r) kininogen is a good substrate for either plasma or tissue kallikreins, whereas the low-molecular-weight (LMW) form of 45,822 M_r is a preferred substrate for the tissue enzyme.

Several exciting advances in the study of kininogens have been made in the past few years. First, it is now known that bovine and human LMW and HMW kininogens are products of a single gene, the structure of which has been mapped completely.[112] This mechanism of biosynthesis is very similar to that of calcitonin and calcitonin gene–related peptide (see Chap. 23). Human kininogens are identical insofar as their NH_2-terminal heavy chains and the kinin moiety are concerned, but differ in the COOH-terminal light chain in both protein length and in some of the amino acids crucial for processing by kallikreins. For example, the short COOH-terminal light chain (of 38 amino acids) of LMW kininogen replaces the long (255-amino-acid), histidine-rich light chain of HMW kininogen. It is suggested these histidine-rich regions

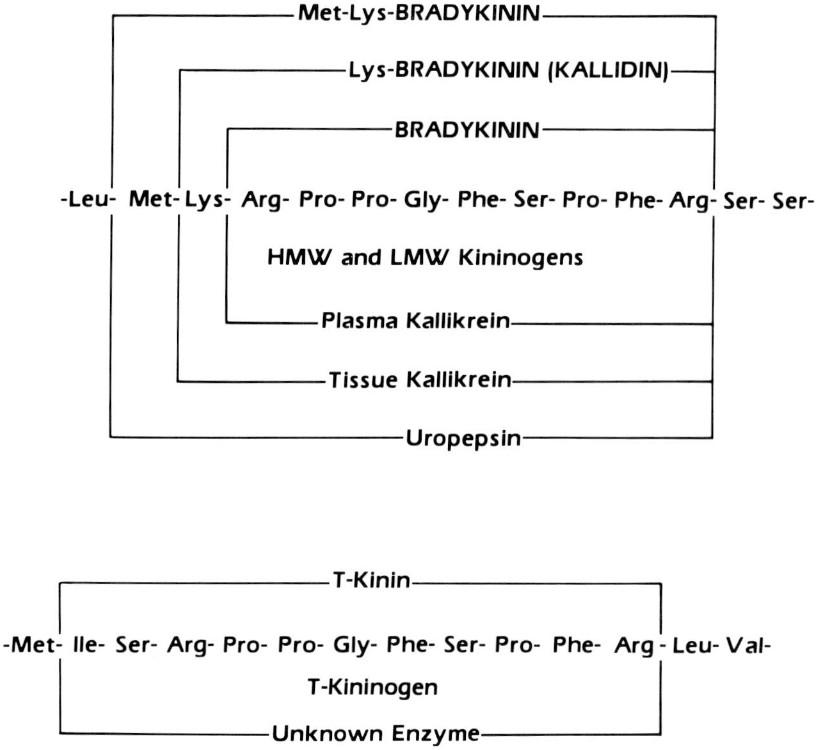

FIGURE 31-6 Sites of action of kinin-forming enzymes and the amino acid sequences of four mammalian kinins.

are important in the binding of HMW kininogen to the negatively charged surfaces necessary for the contact activation reactions in which LMW kininogens play no role. Furthermore, the light-chain sequence of human HMW kininogen possesses five arginine residues in substitution of other amino acids in the bovine HMW light chain. As a single arginine serves as a cleavage signal for kallikreins, it is possible that some of these arginine residues represent additional proteolytic cleavage sites. The biological significance of the resulting fragments remains to be evaluated.

Second, it has been established that the amino acid sequence deduced from a cDNA clone for the human α_2-thiol proteinase inhibitor, a protein known to inactivate several different thiol (cysteine)-containing proteases such as cathepsins, papain, or calpain, is identical to LMW kininogen.[113] Further work established that the binding site for these enzymes actually resides within the identical heavy chain of the LMW or HMW kininogens. These findings are thought-provoking when the role of this inhibitory capability and vasoactive kinin generation from the same molecule are considered in relation to inflammatory processes and diseases.

Third, a novel kininogen was discovered in rat plasma. Termed T-kininogen, it differs from the well-characterized HMW and LMW kininogens in that isoleucylserylbradykinin is present but lysylbradykinin is not.[114] High concentrations of trypsin release this T-kinin, but the actual enzyme responsible for proteolytic cleavage is still unknown. Most interestingly, the T-kininogen is structurally most similar to a protein known as α_1-MAP (major acute-phase protein), a glycoprotein whose concentration increases rapidly and greatly (about 20-fold) during acute inflammatory reactions in the rat. Further, it is now known that induced inflammatory states (e.g., by Freund's adjuvant intradermally, *Escherichia coli* lipopolysaccharide intraperitoneally) cause great increases in T-prekininogen mRNA levels in liver or T-kininogen levels in plasma, while the corresponding measurements for HMW or LMW kininogens exhibit no such changes. These discoveries are raising many questions about the supposed role of bradykinin in inflammation and the possible roles of T-kininogen and T-kinin.

The composition of the four mammalian kinins is shown in Fig. 31-6. Although T-kinin remains to be evaluated fully, the others possess widespread pharmacological activity; in microgram or smaller amounts, they cause vasodilatation, increased capillary permeability, edema, intense local pain, and contraction or relaxation of extravascular smooth muscles. Many other pharmacological properties have been described. The various physiological and biochemical effects which result from activation of tissue kallikrein are considered by most to be the result of the formation of bradykinin or lysylbradykinin. This may or may not be true; the issue probably will be unsettled, despite the discoveries of the tissue kallikrein gene family and of other in vitro processing capabilities for kallikreins, until the newly discovered kinin receptor blockers are used to define roles for tissue kallikreins and kinins. These competitive antagonists of synthetic or natural origin seem to be specific and reversible kinin inhibitors. Their evaluation is just beginning.[115,116]

Lysylbradykinin can be rapidly converted to bradykinin in plasma or urine by cleavage of its aminoterminal lysine residue through the action of an aminopeptidase. The significance of this conversion process is unclear. Hydrolysis of any one of the remaining peptide bonds in the kinins inactivates these substances. The enzymes with this hydrolytic capability are known as *kininase I* and *II*. Kininase I is a carboxypeptidase circulating in plasma. Kininase II (angiotensin I converting enzyme) is a peptidyl dipeptide hydrolase of much current interest since it cleaves either Phe_8-Arg_9 from bradykinin or His_9-Leu_{10} from angiotensin I. These actions result in destruction of biologically active kinin and formation of angiotensin II, respectively. During an investigation of the venom of the crotalid snake *Bothrops jararaca*, a pentapeptide which potentiated the effects of bradykinin was discovered. Subsequently, some larger peptide analogues were synthesized and found to inhibit kininase II and thus the formation of angiotensin II or the hydrolysis of bradykinin. Captopril is a mercaptopropanolyl derivative of proline which is not only more potent than earlier peptide inhibitors but is also orally active. The efficacy of this and other angiotensin I converting enzyme inhibitors in the treatment of hypertension and congestive heart failure is now well established, but no convincing evidence indicates a role for kinins in these therapeutic responses.

Another enzyme, called enkephalinase or neutral metalloendopeptidase (E.C.3.4.24.11), is found in human brain, kidney, and neutrophils and rapidly inactivates bradykinin by clearing the penultimate bond from the COOH-terminal end.[116a] This enzyme may be involved in renal and brain kinin catabolism.

Localization of System Components

Components of the plasma kallikrein-kinin system have been studied extensively because each component is present or can be activated in normal plasma. However, the discovery that kinin formation can still proceed in patients with Williams trait, who lack HMW kininogen, has drawn attention to alternative kinin-forming systems in the formed elements of blood. A kinin-like peptide can be generated in the presence of polymorphonuclear leukocytes and some neoplastic cells and, as mentioned above, by kallikrein release by basophils. A latent kallikrein-like enzyme exists in the red blood cell membrane, and tissue kallikrein mRNA and immunoreactive enzyme are present in the spleen.[117,118] In addition, it is now established that immunoreactive tissue kallikrein is present in human or rat plasma or serum.[119] It is complexed to a higher-molecular-weight entity by a new tissue kallikrein binding protein.[120] A tissue kallikrein similar to urinary kallikrein has been identified in the wall of rat tail arteries and veins.[121] The roles for these latent membrane-, or protein-bound kallikreins are unknown; speculation involves notions about local hemodynamics, membrane ion transport, and the catabolism of proteins or processing of prohormones.[107]

The tissue kallikreins present in secretions of the exocrine glands and the kidney are products of the organs themselves. With physiological,[122] biochemical,[123] and histochemical analyses,[124] the enzyme appears to be bound to membranes along ducts or duct cells and is particularly plentiful in the distal nephron and brain ventricular epithelium.[125] The enzyme and kinins gain access to urine and CSF from these sites. These findings support the idea that tissue kallikreins and locally produced kinins have a role in local membrane transport events. Another site of tissue kallikrein localization and synthesis is the anterior pituitary.[126] Its presence there and in certain hypothalamic nuclei, and the induction of kallikrein in the anterior pituitary by estrogen,[126a,127] have supported suggestions of direct or indirect participation in prohormone processing.

The kininases also seem to be widely distributed. Kininase II is present in the kidney in high concentration and has been located histochemically in glomeruli, along the proximal tubule, and in the vascular endothelium. Kininases are present in brain tissue; the extent of their distribution is just beginning to be determined.

Although plasma kininogens are synthesized in liver, a human renal kininogen has been found to be localized to tubular cells of the distal nephron.[128] Kininogen is also present in CSF, and authentic bradykinin has been identified in mammalian brain.[129]

Relations of Kallikreins and Kinins to Renin and Prostaglandins

How kallikreins and kinins are related to renin and PGs is the subject of widespread investigation. This is the result of the key observations that (1) angiotensin I converting enzyme and kininase II are the same entity; (2) kallikreins and kinins may have a role in the release of prorenin or its conversion to renin;[103] (3) kallikreins and kinins are potent stimulators of eicosanoid synthesis, and many responses to them seem to depend upon eicosanoid production; (4) abnormalities of all three systems are apparent in Bartter's syndrome.[130,132]

KALLIKREIN-KININ AND RENIN-ANGIOTENSIN RELATIONSHIPS

The discovery that angiotensin I converting enzyme and kininase II are the same entity did not receive the attention it deserved until other facts became apparent. First, abnormally reduced kallikrein excretion was noted in humans and animals with renovascular hypertension and high renin-angiotensin system activity. Second, the regulation of renal tissue kallikrein and kinin production was found to be affected by the same maneuvers or hormones which regulate renin and angiotensin (e.g., altered dietary electrolyte intake, aldosterone). Third, that kallikreins or kinins can release or convert prorenin to renin in vitro suggests that this could also occur in vivo. These and other findings, including the existence of a brain kallikrein-kinin system, suggest that there are important interrelations among components of these two systems, which are capable of releasing peptides having powerful and opposing effects upon systemic arterial pressure.

KALLIKREIN-KININ AND PROSTAGLANDINS

Bradykinin releases both arachidonic acid and PGs from various tissues, organs, and cells.[133] Prostaglandins of the E and F series, prostacyclin, and thromboxane can be elaborated. There is evidence that one or more PGs mediate some of the effects of kinins upon vascular smooth muscle, intestinal epithelia, or the kidney. In addition, pharmacological interference with PG synthesis reduces urinary kallikrein excretion.[131] The stimulation by aldosterone of renal and urinary kallikrein levels, stimulation of renal eicosanoid production by the renal kallikrein-kinin system, and PG stimulation of renin release from the kidney[134] suggest that many additional interactions and feedbacks probably remain to be described. The following discussions of some possible roles of the kallikreins and kinins must be considered in the context of what remains unknown about these interrelations.

The Roles of Kallikreins and Kinins

Comments here are limited to some areas of particular recent interest.

RENAL FUNCTION

It has long been known that pharmacological doses of kinins cause renal arteriolar vasodilatation. However, this does not mean that the renal kallikrein-kinin system performs this function in situ since, as affirmed by Nasjletti and Colina-Chourio, "probably no route of administration of kinins reproduces the effects evoked by release of kinins intrarenally."[135] Nevertheless, evidence is available which suggests that intrarenal kinin generation exerts some control over renal vascular resistance. Whether this regulation results from kinins generated along the vascular wall or in the interstitium is still uncertain. There is some clinical evidence which supports a direct correlation between the renal kallikrein-kinin system and renal blood flow. For example, Levy et al.[136] showed that urinary kallikrein excretion and renal blood flow were correlated in both normotensive and hypertensive men; the latter had both reduced kallikrein levels and reduced blood flow.

Whether the renal kallikrein-kinin system participates directly in the control of electrolyte and water excretion and, if so, acts as a natriuretic and diuretic or as an antinatriuretic, antidiuretic influence is still uncertain. However, there is information suggesting that the system has some sort of role in renal excretory function.

Administered kinins increase sodium and water excretion in humans and experimental animals; it has been suggested that PGs mediate some of the observed effects. Urinary kallikrein excretion is increased by low sodium or high potassium intake, fludrocortisone, or other mineralocorticoids, and is decreased by spironolactone, the specific aldosterone antagonist.[137] Most data suggest that kallikrein excretion is correlated with aldosterone activity, but recent work has shown that urinary kinin excretion varies in relation to ADH, suggesting a role for this hormone in the activation of the renal kallikrein-kinin system.[138]

A direct effect of kinins on epithelial ion transport has been discovered. That the peptides are very potent stimulators of net chloride secretion was first noted in intestine. The chloride stimulation occurs via a calcium-dependent mechanism.[139,140] In addition, inhibition by kinins of both chloride absorption and ADH-mediated water reabsorption has been shown recently in isolated perfused renal cortical collecting ducts,[141] and stimulation by bradykinin of sodium-potassium-chloride cotransport has been demonstrated in cultured vascular endothelial cells.[141a]

Despite these findings, the roles of kallikrein and kinins in renal function are unclear. However, the localization of system components along the nephron, the effects of kallikreins and kinins on renal hemodynamics, endocrine function, and tubular transporting events, and the regulation by aldosterone and ADH all serve to intensify present interest. This interest has also been stimulated by the discovery of abnormal kallikrein levels in various hypertensive states.

HYPERTENSION

In 1934, Elliot and Nuzum[142] discovered reduced urinary kallikrein excretion in humans with hypertension. They suggested that this could represent an important defect in a vasodilator mechanism, but their finding was ignored until reconfirmation was obtained later[143,144] (Fig. 31-7). In general, black patients with essential hypertension have been found to have the lowest levels of urinary kallikrein excretion, but studies in other populations (Japanese and Russian) have noted similarly reduced levels. Early studies did not account for effects of renal dysfunction and race, but many subsequent efforts have now described multiple abnormalities in components of kallikrein-kinin systems in human or experimental hypertension.[105-107] For example, urinary kinin excretion, kallikrein activation, and plasma LMW kininogen concentration have each been reported to be abnormal in humans or animal hypertensive models. Some interesting epidemiologic studies have examined urinary kallikrein excretion in normal children. Enzyme activity was found to be similar among family members, and enzyme levels in black children were lower than those in white children. An inverse relationship between measured blood pressure and urinary kallikrein excretion was found in these normotensive populations.[145]

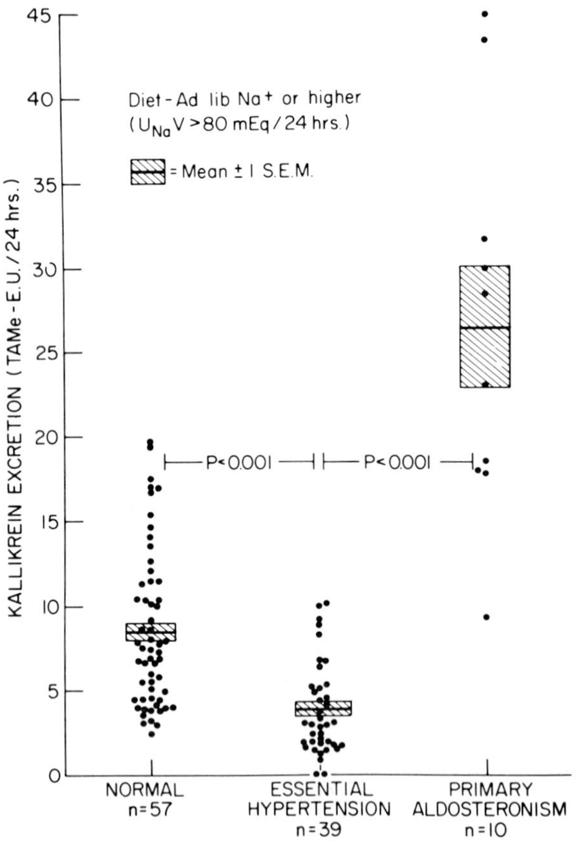

FIGURE 31-7 Kallikrein excretion in normal *subjects*, patients with essential hypertension, and patients with primary aldosteronism. (*From Margolius et al,*[144] *by permission of the American Heart Association, Inc.*)

The observation that kallikrein excretion is elevated in patients with primary aldosteronism (Fig. 31-7) led to the discovery of the relationship between kallikrein excretion and mineralocorticoid hormone activity. It has been suggested that localization of glandular kallikrein at sites where aldosterone is known to act (e.g., renal distal tubule, salivary ducts, sweat glands, colonic mucosa), along with the fact that enzyme activity is increased by aldosterone and decreased by spironolactone, might have meant that kallikrein is one of the aldosterone-induced proteins involved in ion translocation across cell membranes.[146] This hypothesis seems to have been disproved by recent studies, so the significance of the aldosterone-kallikrein relationship is unclear.

Patients with renovascular hypertension excrete less urinary kallikrein than normal, and some patients with pheochromocytoma excrete abnormally high amounts of kallikrein.

Various hypertensive animal models show abnormal kallikrein excretion, abnormal tissue kallikrein levels and activation in kidney and salivary glands, abnormal plasma kininogen concentration, and abnormal pharmacological responses to bradykinin. These data and the findings regarding human hypertension continue to stimulate research upon the role of the system in blood pressure regulation.

OTHER RENAL, CIRCULATORY, AND METABOLIC DISORDERS

Kallikrein excretion is extremely low in patients with renal parenchymal diseases, such as chronic glomerulonephritis or polycystic disease.[147] Transplanted human kidneys excrete kallikrein, but excretion rates are reduced with hypertension or episodes of rejection.[148]

In other disorders, components of the systems have been shown to be abnormally elevated, decreased, or, in some circumstances, absent, but the contributions of these abnormalities to pathogenesis is uncertain. Some examples include the following:

Elevated plasma kinin concentrations have been observed during acute asthmatic attacks; these may contribute to bronchoconstriction through formation of $PGF_{2\alpha}$.

Elevated central venous kinin concentrations have been noted during angina attacks and perhaps contribute to anginal pain.

Decreased plasma kininogen and prekallikrein concentrations have been measured in patients with septic shock accompanied by hypotension.

Diminished plasma kininogen and prekallikrein concentrations occur in the hepatorenal syndrome.

Increased plasma kinin concentration with decreased prekallikrein concentration has been observed in the postgastrectomy dumping syndrome.

These and other syndromes associated with kallikrein-kinin system abnormalities have been the subject of recent reviews and symposia.[105–107a]

BARTTER'S SYNDROME

Introduction

Bartter's syndrome is a renal and metabolic disorder characterized by hypokalemia, metabolic alkalosis, increased production and plasma levels of renin and aldosterone, and juxtaglomerular cell hyperplasia. Patients with this disorder are nevertheless normotensive and show diminished pressor responsiveness to either angiotensin II or norepinephrine.[149,150] Bartter's syndrome is now known to be accompanied by abnormalities in PG, kallikrein, and kinin concentrations. However, the etiology of the syndrome is still uncertain.

Clinical Presentation

Bartter's syndrome has been described in infants as well as in individuals in late middle age.[151] Most patients become symptomatic in the childhood years, although symptomatic presentation in early infancy has been reported.[152] Males and females are affected equally. Although the disorder has been described around the world in various racial groups, in the United States many more cases have been reported in black than in white children.[153] With appropriate treatment, the disorder can be controlled, perhaps throughout a normal life span, but if neglected this syndrome can lead to progressive renal failure and death.

The principal symptoms include muscle weakness and cramps; failure to thrive; polyuria, nocturia, and enuresis; anorexia, nausea, vomiting; constipation; and an increased appetite for salt. Rarely, the syndrome has been diagnosed in asymptomatic children being evaluated for other reasons. Signs associated with the disorder include proximal or truncal muscle weakness, mental retardation, and growth impairment, as well as short stature, positive Chvostek's and Trousseau's signs, carpopedal spasm, tetany, and, rarely, convulsions.

Gout appears to be a clinical complication of Bartter's syndrome.[154] In a series of 10 reported cases, 5 had hyperuricemia and 2 had gout that could not be explained by renal failure. This prevalence rate is much higher than that in the general population.

Whenever hypokalemia of unknown etiology is noted, the diagnosis of Bartter's syndrome should be considered. More common causes of decreased plasma potassium concentration (e.g., repeated vomiting, diarrhea with or without laxative abuse, surreptitious use of diuretics, primary aldosteronism, and disorders of glucocorticoid excess) should be ruled out. The presence of hypertension associated with hypokalemia, as in primary aldosteronism or renal parenchymal or vascular disease with secondary aldosteronism, eliminates the syndrome as a diagnostic possibility. Metabolic findings suggestive of Bartter's syndrome were noted in an infant with subsequently documented cystic fibrosis; measurement of excessive sweat sodium loss should be considered in suspected patients.[154a]

Biochemical, Histological, and Anatomical Findings

Hypokalemia, metabolic alkalosis, elevated plasma renin activity, and increased aldosterone concentration in plasma or urine are necessary for serious consideration of the diagnosis of Bartter's syndrome; other measures of adrenocortical function are normal. Urinary 17-hydroxy- and 17-ketosteroid excretion are normal and respond appropriately to ACTH infusion. Hypomagnesemia is a common but not universal finding that may be responsible for some of the symptoms. Hypercalcemia, hyponatremia, and carbohydrate intolerance have been noted in some cases, and hyperuricemia is common.

Abnormalities in red blood cells have been reported. Increased red cell Na^+, K^+-ATPase activity and intracellular sodium concentration are present. Alterations in red cell sodium efflux or influx may also occur.[155] Increases in red cell volume and number, as well as erythropoietin levels, have been noted. Renal concentrating ability is impaired with marked potassium and chloride loss. This is accompanied by resistance to the effects of ADH, inability to concentrate urine in response to fluid restriction, and polyuria and nocturia.

Abnormalities in PGs and the kallikrein-kinin system have been reported in patients with Bartter's syndrome.[130-132] Plasma bradykinin levels are elevated, while urinary kinin excretion is below normal. However, urinary kallikrein excretion is increased. Urinary PGE_2 excretion is abnormally increased. Furthermore, treatment with indomethacin or other PG synthesis inhibitors reverses all these abnormalities, decreases plasma renin activity and aldosterone concentration, and increases serum potassium concentration. These discoveries may provide insight into some other long-observed characteristics of the syndrome. For example, the relative insensitivity of patients with Bartter's syndrome to either angiotensin II or norepinephrine infusions has been found to be reversed by treatment with indomethacin.[156,157] Aprotinin, an inhibitor of tissue kallikreins, was also found to reduce the relative insensitivity to angiotensin II infusions in four recently studied patients with Bartter's syndrome.[157a]

Juxtaglomerular apparatus hyperplasia is characteristic of the syndrome (Fig. 31-8). Thickened and hyalinized periglomerular arterioles are also noted. However, this hyperplastic state is not pathognomonic of Bartter's syndrome; it can be seen in other disorders characterized by prolonged elevations of plasma renin activity (e.g., Addison's disease and laxative-induced hyperaldosteronism). Proximal tubules may be dilated and may contain hyaline droplets or vacuoles. Other distal tubular changes are variably present. Interstitial cell hyperplasia has also been observed, which is of interest because of the high PG-synthesizing capability and responsiveness to kinins at this site.

Growth retardation (e.g., retarded bone age, short stature) is most prominent in infancy and early childhood.[158] However, normal adolescent development subsequently occurs, sometimes even in the face of unsuccessful treatment. Mental retardation is not uniformly present and may only be a consequence of the metabolic abnormalities noted in infancy and childhood. Occasionally, nonspecific electroencephalographic abnormalities have been noted. Hydronephrosis and hydroureter, possibly due to the polyuria, have also been observed.[159]

Pathogenesis

Since the discovery of Bartter's syndrome, the search for a defect has ranged from a possible primary vascular site to the present view that the syndrome most likely represents a primary renal tubular disorder. Initially, Bartter et al.[149] hypothesized that impairment in the vascular response to angiotensin II could lead to decreased inhibition of renin production with a consequent increase in circulating plasma renin and angiotensin II activities and aldosterone concentration. The increase in aldosterone concentration was thought to be responsible for the hypokalemia, which in turn was regarded as the most likely cause for the majority of symptoms. This formulation has subsequently been shown to be unlikely, especially since total adrenalectomy fails to affect urinary potassium loss.[160]

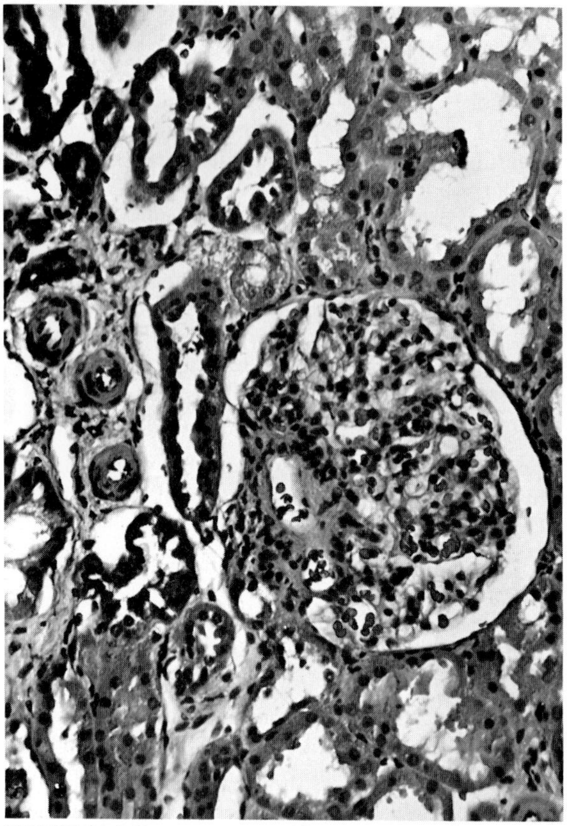

FIGURE 31-8 Percutaneous renal biopsy specimen showing characteristic glomerular changes with juxtaglomerular cell hyperplasia, hilar sclerosis, and mesangial cell proliferation. Prominent tubular vacuolization and some dilated tubules are seen. (*From Brackett NC Jr, Koppel M, Randall RE Jr, Nixon WP: Am J Med 44:803, 1968, by permission of the authors and the American Journal of Medicine.*)

Presently, attention is being directed to a defect in chloride reabsorption in the loop of Henle as the cause for the abnormalities of Bartter's syndrome.[161-163] This hypothesis is the result of a study in which defective distal chloride reabsorption was present in all of five patients with the syndrome. Furthermore, treatment of these patients with PG synthesis inhibitors, which is known to abolish all defects associated with the disorder, did not affect distal chloride reabsorption. It now seems possible that defective tubular chloride reabsorption could cause the hypokalemia by promoting an obligatory and excessive urinary potassium loss. The resultant hypokalemia, or reduced renomedullary interstitial potassium concentrations (already known to stimulate PGE_2 synthesis at this site[164]), stimulates PGE_2 production which, in turn, provokes the juxtaglomerular apparatus hyperplasia and increased renin secretion. This sequence leads to increased aldosterone elaboration from the adrenal cortex, which further enhances tubular potassium loss, produces the metabolic alkalosis, and is responsible for the increase in urinary kallikrein concentration. Finally, it is speculated that the hypokalemia results in excessive production of PGE_2 in the vascular walls, which is somehow also accompanied by high plasma bradykinin concentration, resulting in diminished pressor responsiveness to angiotensin II and norepinephrine. It is also known that the actions of ADH are antagonized by PGE_2, or maneuvers which increase its production, which might then lead to the renal concentrating defect. Additional work is necessary to confirm this proposal, especially since other reports are consistent with a salt-reabsorptive defect in more distal or even proximal nephron sites.[165,166,166a] However, it is clear that study of this disorder has provided a significant advance in the understanding of normal and abnormal renal-endocrine relationships.

Treatment

Supplementation of potassium intake, occasionally to an enormous degree, along with the administration of potassium-sparing diuretics such as spironolactone, triamterene, or, perhaps, amiloride, are the mainstay of present treatment. When dietary potassium supplements or potassium-sparing diuretics are used alone, results are not as satisfactory as they are when these methods of treatment are used together. With proper treatment, correction of hypokalemia and its attendant symptoms is usually observed, but improvement may not persist for prolonged periods. Additional improvement may be effected with the use of a high-sodium diet.[167]

Inhibition of PG synthesis has been useful in delineating PG abnormalities in Bartter's syndrome, as well as in producing short-term improvement. Aspirin has produced resolution of clinical symptoms and hypokalemia.[168] Ibuprofen or indomethacin[169] also correct the abnormalities, but results of treatment for longer than 1 year have not been reported. Complete resolution of negative potassium balance does not always occur with indomethacin treatment. A recent report documents progressive renal failure and associated focal, segmental glomerular sclerosis in a child receiving indomethacin for 1 year. Following renal transplantation, there was complete resolution of the symptoms and abnormal biochemical findings.[170]

There are several short reports on the use of the angiotensin converting enzyme inhibitor captopril in Bartter's syndrome. Some long-term (18 months) subjective improvement and an increased serum potassium concentration have been noted, but dosages were high and details of side effects or toxicities are unavailable.[171,172] Propranolol has been tried with little success. As noted previously, magnesium supplementation or attention to hyperuricemia may be required.

REFERENCES

1. Bergström S, Sjövall J: The isolation of prostaglandin E from sheep prostate glands. *Acta Chem Scand* 14:1071, 1960.

1a. von Euler US: On the specific vasodilating and plain muscle stimulating substances from accessory genital glands in man and certain animals (prostaglandin and vesiglandin). *J Physiol* 88:213, 1936.

1b. Goldblatt MW: Properties of human seminal plasma. *J Physiol* 84:208, 1955.

2. Bergström S, Sjövall J: The isolation of prostaglandin F from sheep prostate glands. *Acta Chem Scand* 14:693, 1960.

3. Samuelsson B, Goldyne M, Granström E, Hamberg M, Hammarström S, Malmsten C: Prostaglandins and thromboxanes. *Annu Rev Biochem* 47:997, 1978.

4. Vane JR: Inhibition of prostaglandin synthesis as a mechanism of action for aspirin-like drugs. *Nature (New Biol)* 231:232, 1971.

5. Hamberg M, Svensson J, Samuelsson B: Thromboxanes: A new group of biologically active compounds derived from prostaglandin endoperoxides. *Proc Natl Acad Sci USA* 72:2994, 1975.

6. Borgeat P, Samuelsson B: Transformation of arachidonic acid by rabbit polymorphonuclear leukocytes. *J Biol Chem* 254:2643, 1979.

7. Frölich JC, Sweetman BJ, Carr K, Hollifield JW, Oates JA: Assessment of the levels of PGA_2 in human plasma by gas chromatography–mass spectrometry. *Prostaglandins* 10:185, 1975.

8. Samuelsson B: Leukotrienes: Mediators of immediate hypersensitivity reactions and inflammation. *Science* 220:568, 1983.

9. Lands WEM, Samuelsson B: Phospholipid precursors of prostaglandins. *Biochim Biophys Acta* 164:426, 1968.

10. Kunze H, Vogt W: Significance of phospholipase A for prostaglandin formation. *Ann NY Acad Sci* 180:123, 1971.

11. Vargaftig BB, Dao Hai N: Selective inhibition by mepacrine of the release of "rabbit aorta contracting substance" evoked by the administration of bradykinin. *J Pharm Pharmacol* 24:159, 1972.

12. Bills TK, Smith JB, Silver MJ: Metabolism of arachidonic acid by human platelets. *Biochim Biophys Acta* 424:303, 1976.

13. Hamberg M, Svensson J, Samuelsson B: Prostaglandin endoperoxides: Novel transformations of arachidonic acid in human platelets. *Proc Natl Acad Sci USA* 71:3400, 1974.

14. Änggard E, Bohman SO, Griffin JE, Larsson C, Maunsbach AB: Subcellular localization of the prostaglandin system in the rabbit renal papilla. *Acta Physiol Scand* 84:231, 1972.

15. Hamberg M, Samuelsson B: On the metabolism of prostaglandins E_1 and E_2 in man. *J Biol Chem* 246:6713, 1971.

16. Rosenkranz B, Fischer C, Weimer KE, Frölich JC: Metabolism of prostacyclin and 6-keto-$PGF_{1\alpha}$ in man. *J Biol Chem* 233: 10194, 1980.

17. Armstrong JM, Chapple D, Dusting GJ, Hughes R, Moncada S, Vane JR: Cardiovascular actions of prostacyclin (PGI_2) in chloralose anaesthetized dogs. *Br J Pharmacol* 61:136P, 1977.

18. Vane JR, Ferreira SH (eds): *Handbook of Experimental Pharmacology: Anti-inflammatory Drugs*. New York, Springer-Verlag, 1979, vol 50/2.

19. Feldberg W, Milton AS: Prostaglandins and body temperature, in Vane JR, Ferreira SH (eds): *Handbook of Experimental Pharmacology: Inflammation*. New York, Springer-Verlag, 1978, vol 50/1, p 617.

20. Gerkens JC, Shand DG, Flexner C, Nies AS, Oates JA, Data JL: Effect of indomethacin and aspirin on gastric blood flow and acid secretion. *J Pharmacol Exp Ther* 203:646, 1977.

21. Clive DM, Stoff, JS: Renal syndromes associated with nonsteroidal anti-inflammatory drugs. *N Engl J Med* 310:563, 1984.

22. Green K, Bygdeman M, Toppozada M, Wiquist N: The role of prostaglandins in human parturition: Endogenous plasma levels of 15-keto-13,14-dihydro prostaglandin $F_{1\alpha}$ during labor. *Am J Obst Gynecol* 120:25, 1974.

23. Pickler VR, Hall WJ, Bert FA, Smith GN: Prostaglandins in endometrium and menstrual fluid from normal and dysmenorrhoeic subjects. *Br J Obstet Gynaecol* 72:185, 1965.

24. Chan WY: Prostaglandins and nonsteroidal antiinflammatory drugs in dysmenorrhea. *Annu Rev Pharmacol Toxicol* 23:131, 1983.

25. Lewis RB, Shulman SD: Influence of acetylsalicylic acid, an inhibitor of prostaglandin synthesis, on the duration of human gestation and labour. *Lancet* 2:1159, 1973.

26. Marsh JM, Yang NST, LeMaire WJ: Prostaglandin synthesis in rabbit graafian follicles in vitro: Effect of luteinizing hormone and cyclic AMP. *Prostaglandins* 7:269, 1974.

27. Wallach EE, de la Cruze A, Hunt J, Wright KH, Stevens VC: The effects of indomethacin on HMG-HCG induced ovulation in the rhesus monkey. *Prostaglandins* 9:645, 1975.

28. Jonsson HT Jr, Middleditch BS, Desiderio DM: Prostaglandins in human seminal fluid: Two novel compounds. *Science* 187:1093, 1975.

29. Bygdeman M, Fredericsson B, Svanborg K, Samuelsson B: The relation between fertility and prostaglandin content of seminal fluid in man. *Fertil Steril* 21:622, 1970.

30. Collier SG, Flower RJ, Stanton SL: Seminal prostaglandins in infertile men. *Fertil Steril* 4:57, 1973.

31. Muirhead EE, Jones F, Stirman JA: Antihypertensive property in renoprival hypertension of extract from renal medulla. *J Lab Clin Med* 56:167, 1960.

32. Larsson C, Änggard E: Mass spectrometric determination of prostaglandin E_2, $F_{2\alpha}$ and A_2 in cortex and medulla of the rabbit kidney. *Eur J Pharmacol* 28:326, 1976.

33. Whorton AR, Smigel M, Oates JA, Frölich JC: Regional differences in prostaglandin formation by the kidney: Prostacyclin is a major prostaglandin of renal cortex. *Biochim Biophys Acta* 529:176, 1978.

34. Frölich JC, Whorton AR, Walker L, Smigel M, Oates JA, France R, Hollifield JW, Data JL, Gerber JG, Nies AS, Williams W, Robertson GL: Renal prostaglandins: Regional differences in synthesis and role in renin release and ADH action. *Proceedings, Seventh International Congress of Nephrology*, Montreal, 1978. Basel, Karger, 1978, p 107.

35. Gerber JG, Data JL, Nies AS: Enhanced renal prostaglandin production in the dog: The effect of sodium arachidonate in the nonfiltering kidney. *Circ Res* 42:43, 1978.

36. Frölich JC, Hollifield JW, Dormois JC, Frölich BL, Seyberth HJ, Michelakis AM, Oates JA: Suppression of plasma renin activity by indomethacin in man. *Circ Res* 39:447, 1976.

37. Stokes JB, Kokko JP: Inhibition of sodium transport by prostaglandin E_2 across the isolated perfused rabbit collecting tubule. *J Clin Invest* 59:1099, 1977.

38. Larsson C, Weber P, Änggard E: Arachidonic acid increases and indomethacin decreases plasma renin activity in the rabbit. *Eur J Pharmacol* 28:391, 1974.

39. Romero JC, Dunlap CL, Strong CG: The effect of indomethacin and other anti-inflammatory drugs on the renin-angiotensin system. *J Clin Invest* 58:282, 1976.

40. Campbell WB, Graham RM, Jackson EK: Role of renal prostaglandins in sympathetically mediated renin release in the rat. *J Clin Invest* 64:448, 1979.

41. Seymour A, Zehr JE: Influence of renal prostaglandin synthesis on renin control mechanisms in the dog. *Circ Res* 45:13, 1979.

42. Donker AJM, Arisz L, Brentjens JRH, van der Hem GK, Hollemans HJG: The effect of indomethacin on kidney function and plasma renin activity in man. *Nephron* 17:288, 1976.

43. Frölich JC, Hollifield JW, Vesper BS, Shand DG, Wilson JP, Seyberth HJ, Frölich WH, Oates JA: Reducton of plasma renin activity by inhibition of the fatty acid cyclooxygenase: Independence of sodium retention. *Circ Res* 44:781, 1979.

44. Orioff J, Handler JS, Bergström S: Effect of prostaglandin (PGE_1) on the permeability response of toad bladder to vasopressin, theophylline and adenosine 3′,5′-monophosphate. *Nature* 205:397, 1965.

45. Zusman RM: Prostaglandins and water excretion. *Annu Rev Med* 32:359, 1981.

46. Berl T, Raz M, Walk H, Horowitz I, Czaczkes W: Prostaglandin synthesis inhibition and the action of ADH. Studies in man and rat. *Am J Physiol* 232:F529, 1977.

47. Fisher JW: Prostaglandins and kidney erythropoietin production. *Nephron* 24:111, 1979.

48. Kimberg DV, Field M, Johnson J, Henderson A, Gershon E: Stimulation of intestinal mucosal adenyl cyclase by cholera enterotoxin and prostaglandins. *J Clin Invest* 50:1218, 1971.

49. Rask-Madsen J, Bukhave K: Prostaglandins and chronic diarrhoea: Clinical aspects. *Scand J Gastroenterol* 14(suppl 53):73, 1979.

50. Gerkens JF, Shand DG, Flexner C, Nies AS, Oates JA, Data JL: Effect of indomethacin and aspirin on gastric blood flow and acid secretion. *J Pharmacol Exp Ther* 203:646, 1977.

51. Bunting S, Moncada S, Vane JR: The prostacyclin-thromboxane A_2 balance: Pathophysiological and therapeutic implications. *Br Med Bull* 39:271, 1983.

52. Currie MG, Needleman P: Renal arachidonic acid metabolism. *Annu Rev Physiol* 46:327, 1984.

53. Nowak J: Prostaglandins in the cardiovascular system in man. A biochemical and physiological study. *Acta Physiol Scand* (suppl) 467:1, 1979.

54. Malik KU: Prostaglandin-mediated inhibition of the vasoconstrictor responses of the isolated perfused rat splenic vasculature to adrenergic stimuli. *Circ Res* 43:225, 1978.

55. Nasjletti A, Malik KU: Relationships between the kallikrein-kinin and prostaglandin systems. *Life Sci* 25:99, 1979.

56. Terragno DA, Crowshaw, K, Terragno NA, McGiff JC: Prostaglandin synthesis by bovine mesenteric arteries and veins. *Circ Res* 37(suppl 1):76, 1975.

57. Blair IA, Barrow SE, Waddell KA, Lewis PJ, Dollery CT: Prostacyclin is not a circulating hormone in man. *Prostaglandins* 23:599, 1982.

58. Cook JA, Wise WC, Butler RR, Reines HD, Rambo W, Halushka PV: Potential role of thromboxane and prostacyclin in endotoxic and septic shock. *Am J Emerg Med* 2:28, 1984.

59. Reines HD, Halushka PV, Cook JA, Wise WC, Rambo W: Plasma thromboxane concentrations are raised in patients dying with septic shock. *Lancet* 2:174, 1982.

60. Bartter FC, Gill JR Jr, Frölich JC, Bowden RE, Hollifield JW, Radfar N, Keiser HR, Oates JA, Seyberth HW, Taylor AA: Prostaglandins are over-produced by the kidneys and mediate hyperreninemia in Bartter's syndrome. *Trans Assoc Am Physicians* 89:77, 1976.

61. Levy JV: Changes in systolic arterial blood pressure in normal and spontaneously hypertensive rats produced by acute adminis-

tration of inhibitors of prostaglandin biosynthesis. *Prostaglandins* 13:153, 1977.

62. Hedquist P, Starnje L, Wennmalm A: Facilitation of sympathetic neurotransmission in the cat spleen after inhibition of prostaglandin synthesis. *Acta Physiol Scand* 83:430, 1971.

63. Durao V, Prata MM, Concalves LMP: Modification of antihypertensive effect of β-adrenoceptor-blocking agents by inhibition of endogenous prostaglandin synthesis. *Lancet* 2:1005, 1977.

64. Pace-Asciak C, Rangaraj G: The 6-keto-$PGF_{1\alpha}$ pathway in the lamb ductus arteriosus. *Biochim Biophys Acta* 486:583, 1977.

65. Brash AR, Hickey DE, Graham TP, Stahlman MT, Oates JA, Cotton RB: Pharmacokinetics of indomethacin in the neonate. Relation of plasma indomethacin levels to response of the ductus arteriosus. *N Engl J Med* 305:67, 1981.

66. Gerseny WM, Peckham GJ, Ellison RC, Miettinen OS, Nadas AS: Effects of indomethacin in premature infants with patent ductus arteriosus: Results of a collaborative study. *J Pediatr* 102:895, 1983.

67. Neutze JB, Starling MB, Elliott RB, Barratt-Boyes BG: Palliation of cyanotic congenital heart disease in infancy with E-type prostaglandins. *Circ Res* 55:238, 1977.

68. Abate G, Polimeni RM, Cuccurullo F, Puddu P, Lenzi S: Effects of indomethacin on postural hypotension in parkinsonism. *Br Med J* 2:1466, 1979.

69. Kochar MS, Itskovitz HD: Treatment of idiopathic orthostatic hypotension (Shy-Drager syndrome) with indomethacin. *Lancet* 1:1011, 1978.

70. Lapetina E: Regulation of arachidonic acid production: Roles of phospholipases C and A_2. *Trends Pharmacol Sci* 3:115, 1982.

71. Grimm LJ, Knapp DR, Senator D, Halushka PV: Inhibition of platelet thromboxane synthesis by 7-(1-imidazolyl)-heptanoic acid: Dissociation from inhibition of aggregation. *Thromb Res* 24:307, 1981.

72. Lefer AM, Burke SE, Smith JB: Role of thromboxanes and prostaglandin endoperoxides in the pathogenesis of eicosanoid induced sudden death. *Thromb Res* 32:311, 1983.

73. Oelz O, Oelz R, Knapp HR, Sweetman BJ, Oates JA: Biosynthesis of prostaglandin D_2: Formation of PGD_2 by human platelets. *Prostaglandins* 13:225, 1977.

74. Whittle BJR, Moncada S: Pharmacological interactions between prostacyclin and thromboxanes. *Br Med Bull* 39:232, 1983.

75. Czervionke RL, Smith JB, Fry GL, Hoak JC, Haycraft DL: Inhibition of prostacyclin by treatment of endothelium with aspirin. *J Clin Invest* 63:1089, 1979.

76. Elwood PC, Cochrane AL, Burr ML, Sweetman PM, Williams G, Welsby E, Hughes SS, Kenton R: A randomized controlled trial of acetyl salicylic acid in the secondary prevention of mortality from myocardial infarction. *Br Med J* 1:436, 1974.

77. Veterans Administration Cooperative Study Group: Protective effects of aspirin against acute myocardial infarction and death in men with unstable angina. *N Engl J Med* 309:396, 1983.

78. Harter HR, Burch JW, Majerus PW, Stanford N, Delmez JA, Anderson CB, Weerts CA: Prevention of thrombosis in patients on hemodialysis by low-dose aspirin. *N Engl J Med* 301:577, 1979.

79. The Canadian Cooperative Study Group: A randomized trial of aspirin and sulfinpyrazone in threatened stroke. *N Engl J Med* 299:53, 1978.

80. Fitzgerald GA, Oates JA, Hawiger J, Maas RL, Roberts LJ II, Lawson JA, Brash AR: Endogenous biosynthesis of prostacyclin and thromboxane and platelet function using chronic administration of aspirin in man. *J Clin Invest* 71:676, 1983.

81. Mustard JF, Packham MA: The role of blood and platelets in atherosclerosis and the complications of atherosclerosis. *Thrombos Diathes Haemorrh* 33:444, 1975.

82. Halushka PV, Rogers C, Loadholt CB, Colwell JA: Increased platelet thromboxane synthesis in diabetes mellitus. *J Lab Clin Med* 97:87, 1981.

83. Malmsten C, Hamberg M, Svensson I, Samuelsson B: Physiological role of an endoperoxide in human platelets: Hemostatic defect due to platelet cyclooxygenase deficiency. *Proc Natl Acad Sci USA* 72:1446, 1975.

84. Hamberg M, Svensson J, Hedqvist P, Strandberg K, Samuelsson B: Involvement of endoperoxides and thromboxanes in anaphylactic reactions, in Samuelsson B, Paoletti R (eds): *Advances in Prostaglandin and Thromboxane Research.* New York, Raven, 1976, vol 2, p 495.

85. Smith AP, Cuthbert MF, Dunlop LS: Effects of inhaled prostaglandins E_1, E_2 and $F_{2\alpha}$ on the airways resistance of healthy and asthmatic man. *Clin Sci Mol Med* 48:421, 1975.

86. Green K, Hedqvist P, Svanborg N: Increased plasma levels of 15-keto-13,14-dihydro-prostaglandin $F_{2\alpha}$ after allergen-provoked asthma in man. *Lancet* 2:1419, 1974.

87. Smith AP: Effect of indomethacin in asthma: Evidence against a role for prostaglandins in its pathogenesis. *Br J Clin Pharmacol* 2:307, 1975.

88. Kordansky D, Adkinson NF, Norman PS, Rosenthal RR: Asthma improved by nonsteroidal anti-inflammatory drugs. *Ann Intern Med* 88:508, 1978.

89. Szczeklik A, Gryglewski RJ, Czerniawska-Mysik G, Zmuda A: Aspirin-induced asthma: Hypersensitivity to fenoprofen and ibuprofen in relation to their inhibitory action on prostaglandin generation by different microsomal enzymic preparations. *J Allergy Clin Immunol* 58:10, 1976.

90. Frölich JC, Ogletree M, Peskar BA, Brigham KL: Pulmonary hypertension correlated to pulmonary thromboxane synthesis, in Samuelsson B, Ramwell PW, Paoletti R (eds): *Advances in Prostaglandin and Thromboxane Research.* New York, Raven, 1980, vol 7, p 745.

91. Steinberg D, Vaughn M, Nestel PJ, Strand O, Bergström S: Effects of prostaglandin on hormone induced mobilization of free fatty acids. *J Clin Invest* 43:1533.

92. Butcher RW, Baird CE: Effects of prostaglandins on adenosine 3′,5′-monophosphate levels in fat and other tissues. *J Biol Chem* 243:1713, 1966.

93. Tashjian AH Jr, Tice JE, Slides K: Biological activities of prostaglandin analogues and metabolites on bone in organ culture. *Nature* 266:645, 1977.

94. Tashjian AH Jr, Voelkel EF, Levine L, Goldhaber P: Evidence that bone resorption stimulating factor produced by mouse fibrosarcoma cells is prostaglandin E_2: A new model for the hypercalcemia of cancer. *J Exp Med* 136:1329, 1972.

95. Voelkel EF, Tashjian AH Jr, Franklin R, Wasserman E, Levine L: Hypercalcemia and tumor prostaglandins: The VX_2 carcinoma model in the rabbit. *Metabolism* 24:973, 1975.

96. Seyberth HW, Segre GV, Morgan JL, Sweetman BJ, Potts JT, Oates JA: Prostaglandins as mediators of hypercalcemia associated with certain types of cancer. *N Engl J Med* 293:1278, 1975.

97. Silberbauer K, Schernthaner G, Sinzinger H, Piza-Katzer H, Winter M: Decreased vascular prostacyclin in juvenile-onset diabetes. *N Engl J Med* 7:336, 1979.

98. Colwell JA, Winocour PD, Lopes-Virella M, Halushka PV: New concepts about the pathogenesis of atherosclerosis in diabetes mellitus. *Am J Med* 67, 1983.

99. Robertson RP, Gavareski DJ, Porte D Jr, Bierman EL: Inhibition of in vivo insulin secretion by prostaglandin E_1. *J Clin Invest* 54:310, 1974.

100. Robertson RP, Chen M: A role for prostaglandin E defective insulin secretion and carbohydrate intolerance in diabetes mellitus. *J Clin Invest* 60:747, 1977.

101. Robertson RP: Prostaglandins, glucose homeostasis and diabetes. *Annu Rev Med* 34:1, 1983.

102. Lamberth EL Jr, Frölich JC: Essential fatty acids: Prostaglandins, in Meng HC, Wilmore D (eds): *Emulsions in Parenteral Nutrition.* Chicago, American Medical Association, 1976, p 14.

103. Friedman Z, Frölich JC: Essential fatty acids and the major urinary metabolites of the E prostaglandins in thriving neonates and in infants receiving parenteral fat emulsions. *Pediatr Res* 13:932, 1979.

104. Margolius HS: The kallikrein-kinin system and the kidney. *Annu Rev Physiol* 46:309, 1984.

105. Margolius HS: Kallikrein and kinins in hypertension, in Genest J, Kuchel O, Hamet P, Cantin M (eds): *Hypertension,* 2d ed. New York, McGraw-Hill, 1983.

106. Schacter M: Kallikreins (kininogenases)—a group of serine proteases with bioregulatory actions. *Pharmacol Rev* 31:1, 1980.

107. Fritz H, Back N, Dietze G, Haberland GL (eds): *Advances in Experimental Medicine and Biology,* vols 156A,B. Kinins-III. New York, Plenum, 1983.

107a. Greenbaum LM, Margolius HS (eds): *Advances in Experimental Medicine and Biology,* vols 198A,B. Kinins-IV. New York, Plenum, 1986.

108. Newball HH, Talamo RC, Lichtenstein LM: Anaphylactic release of a basophil kallikrein-like activity: II. A mediator of immediate hypersensitivity reactions. *J Clin Invest* 64:466, 1979.

109. Proud D, Togias A, Naclerio RM, Crush SA, Norman PS, Lichtenstein LM: Kinins are generated in vivo following nasal airway challenge of allergic individuals with allergen. *J Clin Invest* 72:1678, 1983.

110. Swift GH, Dagorn J-C, Ashley PL, Cummings SW, MacDonald RT: Rat pancreatic kallikrein mRNA: Nucleotide sequence and amino acid sequence of the encoded preproenzyme. *Proc Natl Acad Sci USA* 79:7263, 1982.

111. Mason AT, Evans BA, Cox DR, Shine J, Richards RI: Structure of mouse kallikrein gene family suggests a role in specific processing of biologically active peptides. *Nature* 303:300, 1983.

112. Kitamura N, Kitagawa H, Fukashima D, Takagaki Y, Miyata T, Nakanishi S: Structural organization of the human kininogen gene and a model for its evolution. *J Biol Chem* 260:8610, 1985.

113. Ohkubo I, Kurachi K, Takasawa T, Shiokawa H, Sasaki M: Isolation of a human cDNA for α_2-thiol proteinase inhibitor and its identity with low molecular weight kininogen. *Biochemistry* 23:5691, 1984.

114. Okamoto H, Greenbaum LM: Isolation and structure of T-kinin. *Biochem Biophys Res Commun* 112:701, 1983.

115. Vavrek RJ, Stewart JM: Competitive antagonists of bradykinin. *Peptides* 6:161, 1985.

116. Calixto TB, Nicolau M, Yunes RA: The selective antagonism of bradykinin action on rat isolated uterus by crude *Mandevilla velutina* extract. *Br J Pharmacol* 85:729, 1985.

116a. Connelly JC, Skidgel RA, Schulz WW, Johnson AR, Erdös EG: Neutral endopeptidase 24.11 in human neutrophils: Cleavage of chemotactic peptide. *Proc Natl Acad Sci USA* 82:8737, 1985.

117. Chao J, Chao L, Margolius HS: Identification of a kallikrein-like latent serine protease in human erythrocyte membranes. *Biochem Biophys Res Commun* 121:722, 1984.

118. Chao J, Chao L, Margolius HS: Isolation of tissue kallikrein in rat spleen by monoclonal antibody-affinity chromatography. *Biochim Biophys Acta* 801:244, 1984.

119. Shimamoto K, Margolius HS, Chao J, Mayfield RK, Stroud W, Kaplan AP: Immunoreactive glandular kallikrein in human serum. *J Lab Clin Med* 103:731, 1984.

120. Chao J, Tillman DM, Wang M, Margolius HS, Chao L: Identification of a new tissue kallikrein binding protein. *Biochem J* 239:325, 1986.

121. Nolly H, Scicli AG, Scicli G, Carretero OA: Characterization of a kininogenase from rat vascular tissue resembling tissue kallikrein. *Circ Res* 56:816, 1985.

122. Scicli AG, Carretero OA, Hampton A, Cortes P, Oza NB: Site of kininogenase secretion in the dog nephron. *Am J Physiol* 234:F36, 1978.

123. Yamada K, Erdös EG: Kallikrein and prekallikrein of the isolated basolateral membrane of rat kidney. *Kidney Int* 22:331, 1982.

124. Simson JAV, Spicer SS, Chao J, Grimm L, Margolius HS: Kallikrein localization in rodent salivary glands and kidney with the immune-peroxidase bridge technique. *J Histochem Cytochem* 27: 1567, 1979.

125. Simson JAV, Dom R, Chao J, Woodley C, Chao L, Margolius HS: Immunocytochemical localization of tissue kallikrein in brain ventricular epithelium and hypothalamic cell bodies. *J Histochem Cytochem* 33:951, 1985.

126. Fuller PJ, Clements JA, Whitfield PL, Funder JW: Kallikrein gene expression in the rat anterior pituitary. *Mol Cell Endocrinol* 39:99, 1985.

126a. Clements JA, Fuller PJ, McNally M, Nikolaidis I, Funder JW: Estrogen regulation of kallikrein gene expression in rat anterior pituitary. *Endocrinology* 119:268, 1986.

127. Chao J, Chao L, Swain C, Tsai J, Simson JAV, Margolius HS: Tissue kallikrein in rat brain II. Regional distribution and estrogen induction in the anterior pituitary. *Endocrinology,* in press, 1986.

128. Proud D, Perkins M, Pierce JV, Yates KN, Highet PF, Herring PL, Mangkornkanok/Mark M, Behu R, Carone F, Pisano JJ: Characterization and localization of human renal kininogen. *J Biol Chem* 256:10634, 1981.

129. Perry DC, Snyder SH: Identification of bradykinin in mammalian brain. *J Neurochem* 43:1072, 1984.

130. Vinci J, Gill JR, Bowden R, Pisano JJ, Izzo JL Jr, Radfar N, Taylor AA, Zusman RM, Bartter FC, Keiser HR: The kallikrein-kinin system in Bartter's syndrome and its response to prostaglandin synthetase inhibition. *J Clin Invest* 61:1671, 1978.

131. Halushka PV, Wohltmann H, Privitera PJ, Hurwitz G, Margolius HS: Bartter's syndrome: Urinary prostaglandin E-like material and kallikrein, indomethacin effects. *Ann Intern Med* 87:281, 1977.

132. Gill JR Jr, Frölich JC, Bowden RE, Taylor AA, Keiser HR, Seyberth HH, Oates JA, Bartter FC: Bartter's syndrome: A disorder characterized by high urinary prostaglandins and a dependence of hyperreninemia on prostaglandin synthesis. *Am J Med* 61:43, 1976.

133. Nasjletti A, Malik KU: Relationships between the kallikrein-kinin and prostaglandin systems. *Life Sci* 25:99, 1979.

134. Weber PC, Larsson C, Änggard E, Hamberg M, Corey EJ, Nicolaou KC, Samuelsson B: Stimulation of renin release from rabbit renal cortex by arachidonic acid and prostaglandin endoperoxides. *Circ Res* 39:869, 1976.

135. Nasjletti A, Colina-Chourio J: Interaction of mineralocorticoids, renal prostaglandins, and the renal kallikrein-kinin system. *Fed Proc* 35:189, 1976.

136. Levy SB, Lilley JJ, Frigon RP, Stone RA: Urinary kallikrein and plasma renin activity as determinants of renal blood flow. *J Clin Invest* 60:129, 1977.

137. Margolius HS, Horwitz D, Geller RG, Alexander RW, Gill JR Jr, Pisano JJ, Keiser HR: Urinary kallikrein excretion in normal man. Relationships to sodium intake and sodium-retaining steroids. *Circ Res* 35:812, 1974.

138. Kauker ML, Crofton JT, Share L, Nasjletti A: Role of vasopressin in regulation of renal kinin excretion in Long-Evans and diabetes insipidus rats. *J Clin Invest* 73:824, 1984.

139. Cuthbert AW, Margolius HS: Kinins stimulate net chloride secretion in the rat colon. *Br J Pharmacol* 75:587, 1982.

140. Cuthbert AW, Halushka PV, Margolius HS, Spayne JA: Role of calcium ions in kinin induced chloride secretion. *Br J Pharmacol* 82:587, 1984.

141. Shuster VL, Kokko JP, Jacobson HR: Interactions of lysyl-bradykinin and antidiuretic hormone in the rabbit cortical collecting tubule. *J Clin Invest* 73:1659, 1984.

141a. Brock TA, Brugnara C, Canessa M, Gimbrone MA Jr: Bradykinin and vasopressin stimulate Na^+-K^+-Cl^- cotransport in cultured endothelial cells. *Am J Physiol* 250:C888, 1986.

142. Elliot AH, Nuzum FR: Urinary excretion of a depressor substance (kallikrein of Frey and Kraut) in arterial hypertension. *Endocrinology* 18:462, 1934.

143. Margolius HS, Geller R, Pisano JJ, Sjoerdsma A: Altered urinary kallikrein excretion in human hypertension. *Lancet* 2:1063, 1971.

144. Margolius HS, Horwitz D, Pisano JJ, Keiser HR: Urinary kallikrein in hypertension. Relationship to sodium intake and sodium-retaining steroids. *Circ Res* 35:820, 1974.

145. Zinner SH, Margolius HS, Rosner B, Kass EH: Stability of blood pressure rank and urinary kallikrein concentration in childhood: An eight year follow-up. *Circulation* 58:908, 1978.

146. Margolius HS, Chao J, Kaizu T: The effects of aldosterone and spironolactone on renal kallikrein. *Clin Sci Mol Med* 51(suppl 3):279S, 1976.

147. Mitas JA, Levy SB, Holle R, Frigon RD, Stone RA: Urinary kallikrein activity in the hypertension of renal parenchymal disease. *N Engl J Med* 299:162, 1978.

148. O'Connor DT, Barg AP, Amend W, Vincenti F: Urinary kallikrein excretion after renal transplantation. Relationship to hypertension, graft source and renal function. *Am J Med* 73:475, 1982.

149. Bartter FC, Pronove J, Gill JR Jr, McCardle RC: Hyperplasia of the juxtaglomerular complex with hyperaldosteronism and hypokalemic alkalosis. *Am J Med* 33:811, 1962.

150. Gill JR Jr, Bartter FC: Hyperplasia of the juxtaglomerular complex with hyperaldosteronism and hypokalemic alkalosis, in de Graeff J, Leijnse B (eds): *Water and Electrolyte Metabolism.* Amsterdam, Elsevier, 1964, vol 3.

151. Bardgette JJ, Stein JH: Pathophysiology of Bartter's syndrome, in Brenner BM, Stein JH (eds) *Contemporary Issues in Nephrology: Acid-Base and Potassium Homeostasis.* New York, Churchill Livingstone, 1978, vol 2.

152. Wald MK, Perrin EV, Bolande RP: Bartter's syndrome in early infancy. *Pediatrics* 47:254, 1971.

153. Hall BD: Preponderance of Bartter's syndrome among blacks. *N Engl J Med* 285:581, 1971.

154. Meyer WJ III, Gill JR Jr, Bartter FC: Gout as a complication of Bartter's syndrome: A possible role for alkalosis in the decreased clearance of uric acid. *Ann Intern Med* 83:56, 1975.

154a. Davison AG, Snodgrass GJAI: Cystic fibrosis mimicking Bartter's syndrome. *Acta Paed Scand* 72:781, 1983.

155. Gardner JD, Simopoulos AP, Lapey A, Shibolet S: Altered membrane sodium transport in Bartter's syndrome. *J Clin Invest* 51:1565, 1972.

156. Bowden RD, Gill JR Jr, Radfar N, Taylor AA, Keiser HR: Prostaglandin synthetase inhibitors in Bartter's syndrome: Effect of immunoreactive prostaglandin E excretion. *JAMA* 239:117, 1978.

157. Silverberg AB, Mennes PA, Cryer PE: Resistance to endogenous norepinephrine in Bartter's syndrome. *Am J Med* 64:231, 1978.

157a. Rodriguez-Portales JA, Lopez-Moreno JM, Mahana D: Inhibition of the kallikrein-kinin system and vascular reactivity in Bartter's syndrome. *Hypertension* 7:1017, 1985.

158. Simopoulos AP, Bartter FC: Growth characteristics and factors influencing growth in Bartter's syndrome. *J Pediatr* 81:56, 1972.

159. Dehart HS, Bath NM, Glenn JF, Gunnels JC: Urologic considerations in Bartter's syndrome. *J Urol* 111:420, 1974.

160. Trygstad CW, Mangos JA, Bloodworth MD Jr, Lobeck CC: A sibship with Bartter's syndrome: Failure of total adrenalectomy to correct the potassium wasting. *Pediatrics* 44:234, 1969.

161. Gill JR Jr, Bartter FC: Evidence for a prostaglandin-independent defect in chloride reabsorption in the loop of Henle as a proximal cause of Bartter's syndrome. *Am J Med* 65:766, 1978.

162. Kurtzman NA, Gutierrez LF: The pathophysiology of Bartter's syndrome. *JAMA* 234:758, 1975.

163. Senta S, Konishi K, Saruta T, Ozawa Y, Kato E, Amagasaki Y, Nakata I: Hypokalemia and prostaglandin overproduction in Bartter's syndrome. *Nephron* 37:257, 1984.

164. Zusman RM, Keiser HR: Prostaglandin E_2 biosynthesis by rabbit renomedullary interstitial cells in tissue culture: Mechanism of stimulation by angiotenin II, bradykinin and arginine vasopressin. *J Biol Chem* 252:2069, 1977.

165. Zoccali C, Bartoli E, Curatola G, Maggiore Q: The renal tubular defect of Bartter's syndrome. *Nephron* 32:140, 1982.

166. Uribarri J, Alveranga D, Oh MS, Kukar NM, DelMonte ML, Carroll HJ: Bartter's syndrome due to a defect in salt reabsorption in the distal convoluted tubule. *Nephron* 40:52, 1985.

166a. Stein JH: The pathogenetic spectrum of Bartter's syndrome. *Kidney Int* 28:85, 1985.

167. Solomon RJ, Brown RS: Bartter's syndrome: New insights into pathogenesis and treatment. *Am J Med* 59:575, 1975.

168. Norby L, Lentz R, Flamenbaum W, Ramwell P: Prostaglandins and aspirin therapy in Bartter's syndrome. *Lancet* 2:604, 1976.

169. Verbeckmoes R, von Damme B, Clement J, Amery A, Michielsen P: Bartter's syndrome with hyperplasia of renomedullary cells: Successful treatment with indomethacin. *Kidney Int* 9:302, 1976.

170. Blethen SL, Van Wyk JJ, Lerentz WB, Jenrette JC: Reversal of Bartter's syndrome by renal transplantation in a child with focal, segmental glomerular sclerosis. *Am J Med Sci* 289:31, 1985.

171. Hené RJ, Koomans HA, Boer P, Dorhout Mees ET: Effect of captopril in Bartter's syndrome. *Nephron* 35:275, 1983.

172. Aurell M, Rudin A: Effect of captopril on blood pressure, renal function, the electrolyte balance and the renin-angiotensin system in Bartter's syndrome. *Nephron* 33:274, 1983.

Index

Abdominal pain, 27
hyperlipidemia and, 1270
hyperparathyroidism and, 1390
Abetalipoproteinemia, 1277–79
Absorption:
calcium, 1351–53, 1355, 1359
excessive, 1545–51
hyperparathyroidism and, 1383
laboratory studies, 1553
quantitation of, 1368–69
magnesium, 1362, 1440
oxalate, 1556, 1558–59
phosphorus, 1353–54, 1355
Acanthosis nigricans, 26
insulin resistance and, 1102–3
Acetaldehyde, 1196
Acetazolamide:
cystinuria and, 1515
nephrolithiasis induced by, 1525–26
Acetoacetate, 1059–60
diabetes mellitus and, 1149–54
norepinephrine and, 658
Acetoacetyl CoA, 1059, 1060
Acetohexamide, 1141, 1142
hypoglycemia induced by, 1194
Acetohydroxamic acid, 1524
Acetone, 1059
diabetes mellitus and, 1150, 1151
metabolism of, 1060
Acetylcholine. *See also* Neurotransmitters.
CRF control and, 194
pituitary effects of, 194, 195
receptors for, 91–92
vs. insulin receptors, 92
sympathetic nervous system and, 654
synthesis and metabolism, 196
Acetyl CoA:
cholesterol synthesis and, 69
diabetic ketoacidosis and, 1150
fat-carbohydrate interactions and, 1061
fatty acid oxidation and, 1057–58
fatty acid synthesis and, 1055–56
glucose-steroid relationship to, 10
insulin and, 1076
ketogenesis and, 1059–60
starvation and, 1050
tricarboxylic acid cycle and, 1052–53
Acetyl CoA carboxylase, 1055–56
Achilles tendonitis, hyperlipidemia and, 1260–61
Achondroplasia, 1611
α_1 Acid glycoprotein, 537
Acidification, urinary, 1524–25
Acid loading test, renal tubular acidosis and, 1526
Acidophils, pituitary, 250
Acidosis:
citrate and, 1565, 1566
diabetic (ketoacidosis). *See* Ketoacidosis, diabetic.
hypochloremic, hypoaldosteronism and, 598, 599
lactic, 1155
phenformin-induced, 1143
osteomalacia and, 1466
renal tubular:
hyperparathyroidism and, 1381–82
hypocitraturia and, 1566
nephrolithiasis and, 1525–27
prostate cancer and, 1758
Acne, 26
Acromegaly, 31, 300–306
in childhood, 1618–19
diabetes mellitus and, 302, 1164
differential diagnosis, 303
ectopic GH and, 1719
ectopic GRH and, 1719
hypothalamic disease and, 223, 229, 304–5
laboratory studies, 302–3
MEN 1 and, 1665
pathogenesis, 304–5
signs and symptoms, 300–302
therapy, 305–6
Acropachy, Graves' disease and, 420, 444
ACTH. *See* Adrenocorticotropic hormone.
Actin, 124
insulin secretion and, 1066
Activity. *See* Exercise.
Acyl CoA, 1058
diabetic ketoacidosis and, 1150
Addison's disease, 581–90. *See also* Adrenocortical insufficiency.
Adenine, 37
Adenohypophysis. *See* Pituitary gland, anterior *and specific hormones.*
Adenocarcinoma:
endometrial, 1762–64
prostate, 1753–62
Adenoma:
adrenal. *See* Adrenal glands, adenoma.
islet-cell, 1184. *See also* Islet cells, tumors of.
multiple endocrine. *See* Multiple endocrine neoplasia.
parathyroid, 1378–79. *See also* Parathyroid glands, adenoma.
pituitary, 287–88. *See also* Pituitary gland tumors.
thyroid, 423, 438
Adenosine diphosphate (ADP), tricarboxylic acid cycle and, 1052, 1053
Adenosine monophosphate, cyclic (cAMP), 111–12
ACTH and, 526
bacterial, 120–21
binding of, 11, 100, 120–21
calcium and, 127–28
evolution of, 10–11
glucagon and, 1085
glycogenolysis and, 118–19, 1047
glycogen synthase and, 1046
glycolysis and, 1048
hypercalciuria and, 1544, 1545
insulin and, 1068, 1080
lipolysis and, 119–20
nephrogenous, 1373–74, 1444
calcium tolerance test and, 1570
computation of, 1444
hypercalcemia and, 1403
hyperparathyroidism and, 1397
normal limits of, 1374
pseudohypoparathyroidism and, 1428, 1430
nuclear actions of, 121
parathyroid hormone and, 1373–74, 1443–44
phosphate transport and, 1334
phorphorylation and, 120–21
protein kinase and, 115–18
receptor protein (CRP), 120–21
second messenger hypothesis and, 110, 111
hormones involved in, 121–22
total excretion, 1373–74, 1443–44
TSH and, 402
vasopressin and, 350
Adenosine triphosphatase (ATPase):
diabetes mellitus and, 1127, 1128
Na^+,K^+-. *See* Na^+,K^+-ATPase.
sodium pump and, 715–16
thyroid hormone and, 398–99
Adenosine triphosphate (ATP):
aldosterone and, 566
glucose-alanine cycle and, 1063–64

Adenosine triphosphate (ATP) *(Cont.):*
glycolysis and, 1047–49
hypophosphatemia and, 1438
protein kinase and, 117
thyroid hormones and, 398–99
tricarboxylic acid cycle and, 1052–53
Adenosine triphosphate-citrate lyase, 1055
Adenylate cyclase, 112–15
adrenergic receptors and, 657
cholera toxin and, 112
desensitization of, 98
evolution of, 11
glycogenolysis and, 1047
GTP and, 95–96, 112, 114–15
hormone action and, 8
hypercalcemia and, malignancy-associated, 1407, 1408
Ns and Ni proteins and, 113–14
parathyroid hormone and, 1326
peptide hormones and, 87, 94–96, 112–15
pseudohypoparathyroidism and, 1428–29
PTH-like factor and, 1407, 1408
receptor coupling defect and, 157
receptor occupancy and, 100
regulation of, 112–15
hormone receptors and, 95–96, 113
stimulatory vs. inhibitory, 113–15
transduction and, 112
Adipoblasts, 1208, 1209
Adipose tissue. *See also* Fat.
basal state and, 1089
brown, 1216–17, 1219
diabetes mellitus and, 1106
distribution of fat and, 1230–31
lipoatrophic, 1163
eating behavior regulation and, 1214
excess. *See* Obesity.
fatty acid synthesis and, 1056
fuel storage and, 1088
growth and development of, 1208–10, 1222
hypercellularity, 1208–10, 1222
lipolysis in, 1056–57
measurement of, 1203
normal amount of, 1203–4
thermogenesis and, 1218–19
experimental, 1216–17
weight gain and, 25
Adrenal arteries, 513–14
Adrenalectomy:
adenoma and, 618
aldosteronism and, 762
breast cancer and, 1744, 1748
carcinoma and, 618
Cushing's disease and, 319, 603, 617–18, 1610
ectopic ACTH syndrome and, 1710–11
Nelson's syndrome and, 619
Adrenal glands, 511–631
accessory, 515
ACTH effects on, 525–27
adenoma:
aldosteronism and, 752–53, 759–64
biochemical parameters, 758
clinical picture, 609
CT scans of, 759–60
Cushing's syndrome and, 602, 604, 606, 618
DOC-producing, 766
vs. ectopic ACTH, 1707
vs. hyperplasia, 759–62
incidence, 600
MEN 1 and, 1665
pathologic findings, 764
treatment, 618, 762–63
anatomy, 513–14
androgens. *See* Androgens, adrenal.
antibodies to, 584–85, 1679–80
blood supply, 513–14
carcinoma:
aldosteronism and, 764
clinical picture, 609
Cushing's syndrome and, 602, 604, 606, 618
vs. ectopic ACTH, 1707
hypertension and, 767
incidence, 600
treatment of, 618
cortex, 511–631. *See also specific hormones.*
ACTH effects on, 515
chemistry, 515–17
congenital defects, 624–31
development of, 515
history of study of, 511–13
hyperfunction. *See* Adrenocortical hyperfunction; Cushing's syndrome.
hyperplasia. *See* hyperplasia *subentry below.*
inhibitors of, 521–22
insufficiency. *See* Adrenocortical insufficiency.
laboratory studies, 568–81
regulation of, 522–36
secretion rates, 520–21
steroids of, 517–22. *See also* Glucocorticoids; Mineralocorticoids; Steroid hormones; *and specific hormones.*
structure, 513–15
synthesis in, 71–73, 517–19
crisis, 589, 594–96
CT scans, 615, 616
aldosteronism and, 759–60
pheochromocytoma and, 670–71
fetal, 515, 520
hemorrhage, 585–86, 589
hyperplasia:
vs. adenoma, 759–62
aldosteronism and, 752, 753–55, 759–63
biochemical parameters, 758
congenital, 624–31, 765–66, 1020–30, 1614–16
corticosterone methyloxidase deficiency and, 630–31
Cushing's syndrome and, 601–2, 614
growth and, 1610, 1614–16
11β-hydroxylase deficiency and, 628, 1029–30
17α-hydroxylase deficiency and, 628–29
21-hydroxylase deficiency and, 624–28, 1021–29
3β-hydroxysteroid dehydrogenase deficiency and, 629–30, 1030
hypertension and, 752, 753–55, 759–63, 765–66
lipoid, 629, 1013
medullary, 1676
nodular, 602, 614
pituitary tumor (Cushing's disease) and, 315–20
sexual dimorphism and, 215–16
treatment, 1026–29
virilization and, 1020–30, 1614–16
innervation, 514
medulla, 652–59. *See also* Catecholamines.
MEN 2 and, 1676
pheochromocytoma, 667–72
physiology, 653–59
synthesis in, 652–53
nodules, 515, 602, 614
radionuclide studies, aldosteronoma and, 760–61
regenerative capacity, 515
tuberculosis, 581, 585
Adrenalitis, diffuse lymphocytic, 585
Adrenal veins, 513, 514
catheterization of, aldosteronism and, 760
Adrenarche, 1590
premature, 1617
Adrenergic nervous system. *See* Sympathetic nervous system.
Adrenergic receptors, 656–59
alpha, 657–59
agonists, 657, 676
antagonists, 657, 671
beta, 657–59
agonists, 657
antagonists, 657. *See also* Beta blocking agents.
antibodies to, 157
asthma and, 681
desensitization of, 98–99
glucocorticoids and, 558–59
kinase, 99
phospholipids and, 134
renin release and, 704
down regulation of, 657–58
glucose and, 1085
hyperglycemia and, 661
islet cell, 1071
Adrenocortical hyperfunction, 599–624. *See also* Cushing's syndrome.
aldosteronism and, 620–22
behavioral effects of, 213–14
ectopic ACTH syndrome and, 1706–11
hirsutism and virilism and, 622–24
Adrenocortical insufficiency, 581–99
ACTH deficiency and, 526, 590–91
ACTH stimulation tests and, 576–78
acute, 589, 594–95
amenorrhea and, 1683–84
anemia and, 583–84
autoimmunity and, 1678–84
behavioral effects of, 213
chronic, 587–89, 595–96
diabetes mellitus and, 583, 1682–83
diagnosis, 592–94
etiology, 581–82, 581–82, 590
evaluative scheme for, 593
heterogeneity of, 1680, 1681

Adrenocortical insufficiency *(Cont.)*:
  HLA typing and, 1686
  3β-HSD deficiency and, 1013–14
  hypercalcemia and, 1412
  hypoaldosteronism and, 597–99
  hypoparathyroidism and, 583, 1425, 1680–81
  hypotension and, 552
  hypovolemic hyponatremia and, 368
  idiopathic, 581–85, 1679–80, 1682
  laboratory studies, 589–90, 592
  ovarian failure and, 583
  pigmentation and, 587
  pluriglandular insufficiency and, 1678–84
  primary (Addison's disease), 581–90
    associated disorders, 582–84
    clinical features, 586–89
    genetic aspects, 585, 586
    hemorrhage and, 585–86, 589
    immunological aspects, 584–85
    incidence, 582
    invasive disorders and, 585
    pathology, 585–86
    pathophysiology, 586
  prognosis and survival, 552, 597
  Schmidt's syndrome and, 1682–83
  secondary, 590–92
    clinical features, 591–92
    pathophysiology, 590–91
  thyroid disease and, 583, 1682–83
  treatment, 594–97
  tuberculous, 1679
  vitiligo and, 583, 587
  withdrawl of steroid therapy and, 812–13
Adrenocorticotropic hormone (ACTH), 254–56
  actions, 254, 525–27
    nonadrenal, 525
  adrenal structural changes and, 515
  adrenal-inhibiting drugs and, 522
  adrenocortical insufficiency and, 526, 590–91
  aldosterone and, 533, 577, 755
  amino acid sequence of, 524, 525
  androgens and, adrenal, 535, 536
  antisera to, 571–72
  assays, 254–55, 571–72
    in children, 1622, 1623–24
    hypopituitarism and, 280–81
    in vivo, 169
    techniques for, 321–22
  behavioral effects of, 211–13
  big, 255
  biosynthesis, 64–65, 253
  biosynthetic capacity increased by, 74–75
  calcium and, 526
  cAMP and, 526
  cells secreting, 251–52
  chemistry, 252, 253
  cholesterol and, 526–27
  chronic disease and, 530
  circadian rhythm of, 219, 255, 527–30
    changes in, 529–30
  control of secretion of, 255–56, 523–24
  cortisol and, 255–56, 525–31
    ectopic syndrome and, 1706–11
    feedback inhibition by, 530–31
    measurement of, 280, 321, 322
    stimulation test, 576–78
  CRF and. *See* Corticotropin releasing factor.
  Cushing's syndrome and, 600. *See also* Cushing's disease.
  cytochemical assay, 255
  deficiency, 277, 525, 590–91
    diagnostic procedures, 280–81
    feedback and, 530–31
    glucocorticoid therapy including, 531, 811–12
    treatment of, 284–85
  depression (mental) and, 530
  dexamethasone test, 322, 574–75
  drugs affecting, 199
  ectopic, 1706–11
    vs. adrenal tumor, 1707
    clinical picture, 609, 1706–8
    vs. Cushing's disease, 1707–8
    Cushing's syndrome and, 604, 605–6, 618
    differential diagnosis, 612–14, 1706–8
    ectopic CRH and, 1719–20
    incidence, 600, 1696–97
    peptide products and, 1708–10
    prognosis, 620
    stress vs., 1708
    treatment of, 618, 1710–11
  extraadrenal effects, 254
  extrapituitary sources of, 257
  familial unresponsiveness to, 586
  feedback mechanism and, 187, 255–56, 530–31
    Cushing's disease and, 316, 318
    delayed, 531
    fast, 530–31
  fetal adrenal and, 520
  historical note on, 512
  11β-hydroxylase deficiency and, 628, 765
  21-hydroxylase deficiency and, 626, 627, 1022–23
  hypersecretion, 315–20, 602–5. *See also* Cushing's disease.
  hypoglycemia and, insulin-induced, 280–81, 321–22, 578
  hypopituitarism and, 277, 280–81, 284–85, 1610
  hypothalamic disease and, 226
  lipotropin vs., 256
  metabolism, 255, 524–25
  metyrapone test and, 281, 322
  morphine and, 212
  Nelson's syndrome and, 619
  neurotransmitter effects on, 195
  phospholipids and, 131, 133, 526
  pigmentation and, 254, 525
  pituitary content of, 255
  placental, 257
  plasma levels, 255, 321, 571–72
    adrenocortical insufficiency and, 592, 593
    Cushing's disease and, 316
    Cushing's syndrome and, 604, 612–13
  precursor, 64–65
  radioimmunoassay, 254
  radioreceptor assay, 255
  receptors for, 525
  spontaneous patterns of release, 527–30
  stimulation tests, 280–81, 576–78
    adrenocortical insufficiency and, 592
    in children, 1624
    glucocorticoid therapy and, 813
    rapid, 576–77
    techniques of, 321–22
    three-day, 577–78
  stress and, 256
  suppression tests, 322, 574–75
    in children, 1623
  therapeutic use of, 802–3, 812
  tumor secretion of:
    ectopic. *See* ectopic *subentry above.*
    pituitary, 315–20, 600–601. *See also* Cushing's disease.
  vasopressin and, 281, 523, 524
  venous sampling of, 615
Adrenodoxin, 70, 518
Adriamycin:
  carcinoid and, 1659
  prostate cancer and, 1761
  thyroid cancer and, 500
Affective function, hormones and, 213–14
Agglutination, tanned red cell, 408
Agonadism, 1010–11
Agranulocytosis, drug-induced, 434
Ahumada-Del Castillo syndrome, 306
Akee fruit, 1198
Alanine:
  diabetes mellitus and, 1105
  epinephrine and, 659
  glucose and, 1051, 1062–64
  hypoglycemia and, 1188
  insulin and, 1065, 1074–75
  norepinephrine and, 658
  protein feeding and, 1064
  release and uptake of, 1062, 1063
Alanine aminotransferase, 1051
Albers-Schönberg disease, 1477–78
Albright-McCune-Sternberg syndrome, 1482–83
Albright's fibrous dysplasia, 1482–83
Albright's hereditary osteodystrophy, 1427–30
Albumin:
  androgen binding by, 540
  cortisol binding by, 538
  gylcated, 1112, 1129
  steroid binding by, 135
  testosterone binding by, 840, 842
  thyroid hormone binding by, 78, 396, 397
    decreased levels of, 412
    familial disorder of, 411
Albuminuria, diabetes and, 1120
Alcohol:
  Cushing's syndrome and, 612
  fetal syndrome of, 1601
  gluconeogenesis and, 1051
  hyperlipidemia and, 1259, 1291–92
  hypoglycemia induced by, 1195–96
  hypophosphatemia and, 1436, 1437
  ketoacidosis and, 1151–52
  magnesium depletion and, 1440
  metabolism, 1196
  osteoporosis and, 1474

Alcohol dehydrogenase, 1196
Aldehyde dehydrogenase, 1196, 1656
Aldehyde oxidase, 653
Aldimine, 1054
Aldolase B, 1197
Aldose reductase, 1053, 1054
diabetes mellitus and, 1127
Aldosterone, 563–68
ACTH and, 533, 755
stimulation test, 577
actions, 563–65
agonists of, 567–68
angiotensin and, 532
hyperplasia and, 753, 754
antagonists of, 142–43, 567
ascites and, 621–22
assays, 728–30
ATP and, 566
atrial natriuretic factor and, 534, 722, 724
Bartter's syndrome and, 1788, 1789
binding of, 137, 539–40
biosynthesis, 519, 1012
pathway of, 71, 72
calcium and, 564
circadian rhythm of, 534, 761
Cushing's syndrome and, 605
deficiency, 597–99
ACTH deficiency and, 591
17α-hydroxylase deficiency and, 766
hypertension and, 768–69, 770
hypovolemic hyponatremia and, 368
dexamethasone and, 534, 754–55, 762
dopamine and, 533–34
edema and, 621–22
heart failure and, 621
historical note on, 512
11β-hydroxylase deficiency and, 628, 1029
21-hydroxylase deficiency and, 624, 626, 1024–25
18-hydroxylation defect and, 630
hypersecretion. *See* Aldosteronism.
inhibitors of, 522
kallikrein and, 564, 1786
kidney and, 563–66, 622
magnesium and, 564, 1440
menstrual cycle and, 620
metabolism, 542
variations in, 543, 544
molecular mechanisms, 565–67
Na^+,K^+-ATPase and, 566
pituitary gland and, 533
plasma levels, 729–30
postural changes in, 761
potassium and, 532–33, 564, 567
adenoma and, 752–53
diagnostic procedures, 755–57
hyperkalemia and, 597, 598
hyperplasia and, 753–54
pseudohypoaldosteronism and, 599
pregnancy and, 620–21
receptors for, 140, 565–66
regulation of, 531–35
renin and, 532
aldosteronism and, 752, 758
deficiency of, 597–98
excess of, 598–99
release patterns and, 534
secretion rate, 521
sodium and, 533, 563–67, 621–22
adenoma and, 752
diagnostic procedures, 756–58
pseudohypoaldosteronism and, 599
restriction of, 534, 535
spontaneous patterns of release, 534–35
stimulating factor (ASF), 754
structure, 136, 516
suppression tests, 729–30
thyroid disease and, 543
unresponsiveness to, 599
urinary, 728–29
Aldosteronism, 620–22, 751–64
adenoma and, 752–53, 759–64
adrenal vein catheterization and, 760
carcinoma and, 764
circadian changes and, 761
CT scanning and, 759–60
diagnosis, 755–62
etiologic determination, 759–62
initial, 755–58
glucocorticoid-remediable, 754–55, 762
history and physical findings, 755
18-hydroxycorticosterone and, 759, 761–62
hyperplasia and, 752, 753–55, 759–63, 1025
hypertension and, 724–25, 751–63
accelerated, 708
indeterminate, 754, 763
iodocholesterol scanning and, 760–61
magnesium and, 1440
occurrence and classification, 751–52
pathologic findings, 764
postural changes and, 761
primary, 751–64
saline infusion test, 761–62
secondary, 620–22
treatment, 762–63
types of, 752
Aldosteronoma, 752–53, 759–64
Alkaline phosphatase:
calcitonin therapy and, 1489
deficiency:
rickets and osteomalacia and, 1465–66
treatment of, 1467–68
disodium etidronate therapy and, 1490
hereditary increase in, 1480–81
hyperparathyroidism and, 1396
normal ranges, 1366
Paget's disease of bone and, 1486, 1488
serum activity, 1365–66
vitamin D and, 1354, 1355, 1481
Alkalinization:
for cystinuria, 1515
hypocitraturia and, 1566
renal tubular acidosis and, 1526–27
uric acid stones and, 1521
Alkalosis:
Bartter's syndrome and, 1787, 1789
citrate and, 1565
Cushing's syndrome and, 608
hypophosphatemia and, 1437
Allergy, insulin, 1138
Allopurinol, 1521, 1564
Allosterism, mathematical analysis and, 179
Allstrom-Hallgren syndrome, 233
Alopecia, 26
Alpha-adrenergic receptors. *See* Adrenergic receptors, alpha.
Alpha blocking agents, 657
pheochromocytoma and, 671
Alpha-fetoprotein. *See* α-Fetoprotein.
Alpha-lipoprotein. *See* Lipoprotein, high-density.
Alpha particle therapy, pituitary, 299
Cushing's disease and, 617
Alpha subunits, glycoprotein, 257
ectopic chorionic gonadotropin and, 1714
pituitary tumor secretion of, 321
Aluminum, renal osteodystrophy and, 1479
Amenorrhea, 29–30, 951–61
Addison's disease and, 583, 589, 1683–84
anorexia nervosa and, 234, 961
breast feeding and, 955–56
Cushing's syndrome and, 607–8
delayed puberty and, 953–54
flowchart for evaluating, 1034
exercise-related, 954, 961
galactorrhea and, 958
gonadal dysgenesis and, 951–52
hyperprolactinemia and, 230, 306–15, 958–60
hypogonadotropic hypogonadism (Kallmann) and, 953
hypopituitarism and, 952–53
hypothalamic hypogonadism and, 227
hypothyroidism and, 958
menopause and, 956
mosaicism and, 952
müllerian duct derivative abnormalities and, 954
nutritional, 954, 960–61
premature ovarian failure and, 956–58
primary, 951–55
secondary, 955–61
classification of, 956
testicular feminization and, 954
Turner's syndrome and, 951–52
virilization and, 954–55
weight loss and, 276–77, 960–61
Amiloride, aldosteronism and, 763
Amine precursor uptake and decarboxylation (APUD) cells:
ectopic hormone production and, 1700
MEN and, 1668
Aminergic system, 823. *See also* Dopamine; Norepinephrine; Serotonin.
Amines:
catechol-containing. *See* Catecholamines.
locally released, 85
Amino acid decarboxylase, 653
serotonin synthesis and, 1656
Amino acids. *See also specific type.*
ACTH sequence of, 524, 525
atrial natriuretic factor sequence of, 719
branched-chain, 1064
calcitonin gene-related peptide, 1340
cystinuria and, 1510–17
diabetes mellitus and, 1104–5
estrogen receptor, 139
gastrin, 1630, 1631
gastrointestinal hormone, 1639, 1645, 1656, 1650, 1651
glucocorticoids and, 140, 545–46

Amino acids *(Cont.)*:
gluconeogenesis and, 1049
hypophysiotropic hormone sequences of, 200
insulin and, 1070, 1075–76
composition of, 1064, 1065
kinin, 1783
oxytocin sequence of, 339, 340
parathyroid hormone, 1323
phosphorylation sites of, 118
protein meal and, 1064
sequence control of, 40–41
starvation and, 1183
synthesis and metabolism, 196, 1062–64
vasopressin sequence of, 339, 340
γ-Aminobutyric acid. *See* Gamma-aminobutyric acid.
Aminoglutethimide:
adrenal inhibition by, 521–22
breast cancer and, 1750
Cushing's disease and, 319, 618
prostate cancer and, 1761
Amiodarone, thyroid hormone and, 416
Ammonium chloride, aldosterone and, 533
Amphenone B, 522
Ampheramine, 199
Amphophils, 252
Amygdala, neurohypophysis and, 338
Amylase, diabetic ketoacidosis and, 1151
Amyloid, medullary thyroid carcinoma and, 502, 1670
Amyloglucosidase, 1046
Amyotrophy, diabetic, 1122
Anaphase lag, 985, 987
Androgen-binding protein (ABP), 841, 849
Androgens. *See also* Dihydrotestosterone; Testosterone.
adrenal, 840
actions, 568
binding of, 540
biosynthesis, 519
Cushing's syndrome and, 605, 606
regulation of, 535–36
antagonists of, 142
prostate cancer therapy and, 1760–61
assays, 579–81
behavioral effects of, 836
biosynthesis, 71–73, 519
breast cancer and, 1740, 1748–49
gender role and, 999–1000
growth and, 1589–90, 1609, 1615
hirsutism and virilism and, 30, 622–24, 965, 1615
17α-hydroxylase deficiency and, 629
imprinting and, 836
insensitivity to, 875, 1018–19
metabolism, 542–43
nuclear matrix and, 144
obesity and, 1233
osteoporosis and, 1472, 1473
ovarian, 925–26, 929
fetal, 941
recruitment of follicles and, 935
plasma levels, 580
polycystic ovary disease and, 962, 963
prostate cancer and, 1755, 1756, 1762
receptors for, 139–40
assay of, 1762
sexual differentiation and, 995–96
sexual dimorphism and, 215–16
structure of, 136
testicular, 838–40. *See also* Dihydrotestosterone; Testosterone.
Turner's syndrome and, 1612
urinary, 580
voice and, 27
Androstanediol, 542, 842
hirsutism and, 964
structure, 844
5α-Androstanedione, 542
Androstanes, 517
Androstenedione. *See also* Androgens.
ACTH and, 535, 536
actions, 568
adrenal hyperplasia and, congenital, 1025
binding of, 540
biosynthesis, 71, 73, 924–25, 1012
adrenal, 519
endometrial cancer and, 1762–63
17β-HSD deficiency and, 1015
21-hydroxylase deficiency and, 1022–23, 1025
metabolism, 75, 542–43, 926
ovarian follicle selection and, 936, 937
ovulation and, 944
regulation of, 535–36
secretion rate, 520, 521
structure, 516
testicular, 838
Androsterone, 516
structure, 844
Anemia, 27–28
hyperparathyroidism and, 28
hyperthyroidism and, 28, 427
hypopituitarism and, 27–28
hypothyroidism and, 28, 454
iron-deficiency, 28
pernicious:
Addison's disease and, 583–84, 590
autoimmunity and, 1685
Aneuploidy, 985–86
Aneurysms:
hypothalamic disorders and, 225
sellar region, 296, 297
ANF. *See* Atrial natriuretic factor.
Angina pectoris, hypothyroidism and, 453
Angiography:
digital subtraction, of kidney, 743–44
pancreaticoduodenal, 1186
parathyroid, 1399
Angioplasty, renal artery, 750
arteriogram of, 736
results, 751
Angiotensin, 701, 706–7
actions, 706–7
aldosterone and, 532
hyperplasia and, 753, 754
antagonists of, 707, 745
assay, 728
Bartter's syndrome and, 1788
blood pressure maintenance and, 707
in brain, 209
conversion of I to II, 702, 705
formation and metabolism, 702
forms (I, II, and III) of, 702, 706–7
glucocorticoids and, 553
glycogenolysis and, 119
hypertension and, 707–11, 728
low-renin essential, 771–72
kallikrein-kinin and, 1784–85
precursor, 65
prostaglandins and, 532
receptors for, 532, 706–7
disorders of, 155–56
renin and, 532, 703, 704. *See also* Renin.
plasma assays, 727
sodium and, 535, 706, 712
vasopressin and, 346–47
Angiotensin-converting enzyme, 705–6, 1784
inhibitors of, 705, 709
Bartter's syndrome and, 1789
renovascular hypertension and, 745, 748
Angiotensinogen, 705
renin and, 727
Anorexia, 27
Addison's disease and, 587
nervosa, 27, 234–35
amenorrhea and, 961
hypopituitarism vs., 279
tumors and, 1724
weight loss and, 25
Anosmia, 227, 864, 953
Anovulation, 30, 966–70. *See also* Ovulation.
Anoxemia, growth and, 1613
ANP. *See* Atrial natriuretic factor.
Antacids:
hypophosphatemia and, 1436
milk-alkali syndrome from, 1414
Antagonisms, hormone, 13
abnormal levels of, 17
Antibiotics, nephrolithiasis and, 1523–24
Antibodies:
adrenal, 584–85, 1679–80
adrenergic receptor, 157
antigen complex with, 168–71
calcitonin, salmon, 1488
circulating endogenous, 175
gastrin, 174
generation of, 171–72
H-Y, 990
islet cell, 1097–98, 1683, 1685
insulin, 97, 156–57, 1138, 1188
mathematical analysis (Scatchard plot) of hormone interaction with, 177–79
molecule of, 171
monoclonal, 172
to estrogen receptor, 139
ovarian, 584, 957, 1684
parathyroid, 1425
parietal cell, 584, 1685
polyclonal, 170, 173
radioimmunoassay and. *See* Radioimmunoassay.
receptor, 96–97, 156–157
second, 174–175
separation of hormone bound to, 174–76
sperm, 881
testicular, 584
thyroglobulin, 175, 408, 432, 1685
metastases and, 501

Antibodies *(Cont.)*:
thyroid, 408, 445, 1683, 1685
Addison's disease and, 584
titering of, 173
tumor markers and, 1726
Anticodon loop, 41
Antidiuretic hormone. *See also* Vasopressin.
assays, in vivo, 169
precursor, 64
syndrome of inappropriate secretion of (SIADH), 368–74
diagnosis, 373
etiology and pathophysiology, 368–72
neurologic disease and, 230
therapy, 373–74
tumors and, 1711–13
Antigen:
antibody complex with, 168–71
carcinoembryonic, 1725
HLA. *See* HLA system.
H-Y, 989-92. *See also* H-Y antigen.
prostate-specific, 1758
Antimüllerian hormone, 992–93
persistent müllerian ducts and, 1011
Antisera, generation of, 171–72
Antithyroid drugs, 432–36
hypothyroidism induced by, 449
Antitrypsin deficiency, hyperlipidemia and, 1259
Aorticorenal ganglion, 654
Apomorphine:
pituitary effects of, 199
schizophrenia and, 238
vasopressin and, 345, 346
Apoprotein, 1245–49
absence of (B), 1277–79
A-I deficiency, 1275, 1277
A-I Milano, 1276
biosynthesis, 1248
classification of lipoprotein and, 1245–46
C-II deficiency, 1270–72
C-III deficiency, 1275
function, 1248–49
structure, 1247–48
type III hyperlipoproteinemia and, 1268
Appetite, 27
control of, 232, 1212–13
drugs suppressing, 1238
hyperthyroidism and, 426
psychological factors and, 1222–23
Aprotinin, 1788
APUD cells:
ectopic hormone production and, 1700
MEN and, 1668
Arachidonic acid, 129–31
metabolism, 129–31, 973, 1770, 1771
platelets and, 1778
renal blood flow and, 1774–75
uterine, 972
Arcuate nucleus, 189, 190, 821
GnRH and, 832, 835
TRH and, 401
Arginine:
growth hormone and, 325, 1622
transport defect of, 1510–17
Aromatase, 73, 75
gynecomastia and, 888
hypothalamic activity of, 844, 847
luteinizing hormone and, 844, 847
luteolysis and, 931
ovarian, 926, 928
follicular selection and, 937, 938
Sertoli-Leydig cell interactions and, 851
testosterone metabolism and, 842, 851
Arrhythmias, 28
hyperthyroidism and, 426
pheochromocytoma and, 671
Arteriography, renal, 742–43
balloon angioplasty and, 736
digital subtraction, 743–44
Arterioles, hypertension and, 697, 699
Arteriovenous gradient, ectopic hormone and, 1694
Arthritis:
glucocorticoid therapy and, 794, 801
hyperparathyroidism and, 1391
obesity and, 1234
Paget's disease and, 1484
Arthropathy, neuropathic, 1122
Ascites:
aldosterone and, 621–22
hyponatremia and, 367
Ascorbic acid:
nephrolithiasis and, 1530
oxalate production and, 1556, 1558
Asparagine:
glycosylation and, 66
insulin and, 1065
Aspirin:
asthmatic attack from, 1779
hypercalcemia of malignancy and, 1705
platelets and, 1778, 1779
prostaglandin inhibition by, 1773
Assays, 19–21, 165–80. *See also under specific hormones.*
ACTH, 254–55, 280–81, 321–22, 571–72
aldosterone, 728–30
angiotensin, 728
antisera generation, 171–72
biological, 166–68
calcitonin, 1374–75
catecholamine, 662–64, 682–85
chemical, 20
in children, 1621–24
circulating endogenous antibody and, 175
competitive protein-binding, 19–20
cortisol, 569–71
cytochemical, 168
dose-response lines and. *See* Dose-response lines.
ectopic hormone, 1693–94
enzyme-linked immunosorbent, 177
free hormone, 20
FSH, 260–61, 281–83, 323–24
glucocorticoid, 569–79
gonadotropin, 281–83, 323–24
chorionic, 166, 167
growth hormone, 266, 283–84, 324–26
in children, 1608, 1621, 1622
immunoradiometric, 176–77
interpretation of, 20–21
in vitro, 167–68, 169
in vivo, 166–67, 169
iodination, 171
Leydig cell, 167
ligand, 168–76
luteinizing hormone, 166, 260–61, 281–83, 323–24, 837, 854–57
mathematical analysis of binding (Scatchard plot) and, 177–79
oxytocin, 348
parathyroid hormone, 1369–74, 1443–45
prolactin, 270–71, 284, 326–27
quality control of, 179–80
radioimmunologic, 168–76. *See also* Radioimmunoassay.
radioreceptor, 19–20, 176–79. *See also* Radioreceptor assay.
receptors and disease states and, 179
reference preparation and, 166, 176
renin, 727–28
sample handling in, 180
sensitivity of, 172–73
separation of bound and free hormone, 174–76
serum protein effect, 174
simultaneous, 21
specificity of, 173–74
stability of hormone and, 180
steroid, 175–76
symptoms and, 23–24
testosterone, 580, 855
thyroid hormone, 404–9
variables affecting, 409–10
thyrotropin, 258, 281, 323
validation of, 176
variation in, 179–80
vasopressin, 375
vitamin D, 1375–76
Assessment of endocrine status, 19–22
history and physical examination, 19
laboratory, 19–22
Association constants, 177–79
Asthma:
glucocorticoids and, 791, 802
prostaglandins and, 1779
sympathochromaffin system and, 681
Ataxia, hypogonadotropic, 868
Atherosclerosis, 1280–82
cholesterol and, 1261–62, 1280–82
diabetes mellitus and, 1107, 1114, 1123
glucocorticoid therapy and, 796
hypertension and, 699–700, 735–37
lipoprotein and, 1254
menopause and, 977–78
renal artery, 735–37, 739
natural history, 738–39
treatment, 746–51
Atrial natriuretic factor (peptide), 718–24
actions, 720–23
aldosterone and, 534, 722, 724
blood pressure and, 723
cardiac influences, 722–23
cGMP and, 723–24
circulation, 720
fluid balance and, 722, 724
kidney and, 720–22
molecular mechanisms, 723–24
receptors for, 723
regulation, 720
release, 719, 720

Atrial natriuretic factor (peptide) *(Cont.)*:
renin and, 722
sodium escape phenomenon and, 564
structure, 719
structure-activity considerations, 723
synthesis, 719–20
vascular effects, 722
vasopressin and, 722
water intake and, 723
Atromid-S. *See* Clofibrate.
Atropine, gastrin release and, 1632
Auriculin. *See* Atrial natriuretic factor.
Autocrine communication, 4
Autocrine secretion, 85
Autoimmunity (autoantibodies), 18
Addison's disease and, 581, 582, 584, 1678–84
diabetes mellitus and, 1097–98, 1683, 1685
hypoglycemia and, 1188
hypophysitis and, 1684–85
infertility and, 881
ovarian failure and, 957
pluriglandular, 1678–84
receptor disorders and, 156–57
tests for, 1678
thyroid, 418–20, 445–46, 1678, 1682–83
maternal, dysgenesis of thyroid and, 447
neonatal hyperthyroidism and, 440
tests for, 430
thyroxine-binding, 411
Turner's syndrome and, 1007
Autonomic nervous system, 651. *See also* Norepinephrine; Parasympathetic nervous system; Sympathetic nervous system.
dysfunction, 672–77
hypertension and, 697–98
indirect tests of function of, 685–86
neuropathy, 32
diabetic, 1122–23
Autophosphorylation, 101–2
protein kinase and, 117
Avogadro's number, 179
Axon terminals, adrenergic, 653–59
Azoospermia, 878–82
androgen resistance and, 875
autoimmunity and, 881
contraceptive induction of, 890–91
genetic disorders and, 881
idiopathic, 879–80
Klinefelter's syndrome and, 1001
obstructive vs. idiopathic, 853
varicocele and, 880
Azotemia, diabetic, 1120

B cells:
autoimmune thyroiditis and, 445
glucocorticoids and, 551
Graves' disease and, 419
Babinski-Froehlich syndrome, 233
Back pain:
osteoporosis and, 1468
Paget's disease and, 1484
Bacteria:
nephrolithiasis and, 1522
protein synthesis and, 51
recombinant DNA and, 44–45
Bacteriophage, cloning and, 49
Bantam syndrome, Seabright, 1426
Bardet-Biedl syndrome, 233
Baroreceptors:
hypertension and, 698
renal, 703
vasopressin and, 343, 344
Barr bodies, 988
Klinefelter's syndrome and, 872
testicular function and, 837
Bartter's syndrome, 622, 1787–89
biochemical, histological, and anatomical findings, 1787–88
clinical presentation, 1787
norepinephrine and, 679
pathogenesis, 1788–89
prostaglandins and, 1777, 1788, 1789
treatment, 1789
Basement membrane, diabetes and, 114–15, 1126
Basophils, pituitary, 250
adenoma and, 600–601
ACTH-secreting, 315
hypothalamic homografts and, 188
Bayes' theorem, thyroid cancer and, 491
Beckwith's syndrome, 1187
Beckwith-Wiedemann syndrome, 1621
Beclomethasone:
asthma and, 802
structure, 789
Behavior, 32, 211–16. *See also* Psychological factors.
ACTH and, 211–13
adrenocortical disorders and, 213–14
androgens and, 836
catecholamines and, 681
eating, 232, 234, 1212–15, 1222–23
glucocorticoids and, 555
GnRH and, 204
hyperparathyroidism and, 214
hypocalcemia and, 1423
hypothalamus and, 835–36
Klinefelter syndrome and, 870–71
menstrual cycle and, 214
modification therapy, obesity and, 1237–38
MSH and, 212
opioids and, 211, 212
pituitary hormones and, 211–13
prolactin and, 270
psychiatric illness and. *See* Psychiatric disorders.
sexual dimorphism and, 215–16
target gland hormones and, 213–14
TRH and, 202
vasopressin and, 213
XYY syndrome and, 873, 1003, 1619
Berardinelli-Seip syndrome, 1163
Beta-adrenergic receptors. *See* Adrenergic receptors, beta; Beta blocking agents.
Beta blocking agents, 657. *See also* Propranolol.
catecholamine clearance and, 664, 684
coronary heart disease and, 680
hyperlipidemia and, 1260
pheochromocytoma and, 671
postural hypotension and, 676
thyroid hormone and, 416, 435–36
Beta-lipoprotein. *See* Lipoprotein, low-density.
Betamethasone:
asthma and, 802
half-life and potency, 798
mineralocorticoid receptors and, 792
structure, 789
Beta subunits, glycoprotein, 257, 837
ectopic chorionic gonadotropin and, 1714
Bezafibrate, 1304
Bicarbonate:
atrial natriuretic factor and, 722
cystinuria and, 1515
diabetic ketoacidosis and, 1151, 1153
parathyroid hormone and, 1337
renal tubular acidosis and, 1525, 1526
uric acid stones and, 1521
Bicitra, cystinuria and, 1515
Biguanides, 1143–44
Bile acids:
deficiency of, 1284
sequestrants of, 1263, 1298–1300
Bile duct obstruction, hyperlipidemia and, 1259
Binding:
aldosterone, 137, 539–40
calcium, 123–26, 1320
intestinal, 1353
cAMP, 11, 100, 120–21
cellular response and, 88
competitive, 19–20, 137
cortisol assay and, 569, 571
conformational change caused by, 96–97
dissociation of, 104, 108
glucocorticoid, 536–39, 560
competitive, 569, 571
glucocorticoid regulatory element, 41–42
GTP influence on, 115
insulin, 1077–78, 1081
mathematical characterization, 177–79
oxytocin, 339
peptide receptor, 87–88
temperature and, 88
plasma, 6
steroid, 135–37
receptor, 3. *See also* Receptors.
altered affinity for, 155, 156
steroid, 75, 135–37
nuclear, 141, 143–44
termination of, 89, 104, 108
testosterone, 840–42
thyroid hormone, 78, 148–50, 395–98, 404–6, 410–12
tight (high-affinity), 104
steroid, 135
transcription of genes and, 61
transport protein vs. receptor, 82–83
vasopressin, 339
vitamin D, 1345, 1347
Bioassays, 166–68. *See also* Assays *and under specific hormones.*
cytochemical, 158
in vitro, 167–68, 169
in vivo, 166–67, 169
bone, 1456–58, 1758
diabetes mellitus and, 1126
endometrial, 970

Bioassays *(Cont.)*:
ovarian, 957
prostate, 1758
renal, 744
testicular, 852–53
thyroid, 490–92
Biorinil, 768
Biosynthesis of hormones, 59–79. *See also specific hormones.*
ACTH, 64–65, 253
adrenal steroid, 517–19
congenital enzyme defects and, 624–31
aldosterone, 71, 72, 519, 1012
androgen, 71–73, 519
atrial natriuretic factor, 719–20
calcitonin, 1339–40
catecholamine, 196, 652–53, 655
cholesterol, 106, 518, 1249–50
cortisol, 69, 71, 72, 518–19, 1012
11-deoxycortisol, 71, 518, 1012
ectopic hormone, 1698–1702
estrogen, 73
glucagon, 1082
glucocorticoid, 69, 71, 72
growth hormone, 264
genetic defects and, 16
insulin, 1065–67
lipotropin, 253
luteinizing hormone, 257
melatonin, 216
messenger RNA, 59–63
mineralocorticoid, 71, 72, 519, 1012
neurotransmitter, 194–96
ovarian hormone, 924–27
oxytocin, 339–40
parathyroid hormone, 1322–24
peptide hormone, 63–66
pineal principle, 216–18
progesterone, 71, 73, 1012
prolactin, 264
prostaglandin, 129–31, 1771–72
of receptors, peptide hormone, 102–4
steroid hormone, 68–75, 517–19, 924–27, 1012
testosterone, 72, 73, 838
thyroid hormone, 76–78, 392–95
defects in, 447–49
thyrotropin, 257
transcription of genes and, 60–61
vasopressin, 339–40
vitamin D, 73, 1345–51
Bisexuality, 1003–4
Bisphophonates, Paget's disease of bone and, 1489–90
Blindness, diabetes and, 1115, 1116, 1118
Blood-brain barrier, 187
osmoregulation and, 342–43
Blood pressure. *See also* Hypertension; Hypotension.
angiotensin and, 707
atrial natriuretic factor and, 723
classification of, 694
epinephrine and, 659, 660
glucocorticoids and, 552, 726
ions and, 711–18
measurement of, 732–33
norepinephrine and, 658, 668
posture and, 672–73
osmolality and, 345, 356
pheochromocytoma and, 667–72
physiology of control of, 697
prostaglandins and, 1777–78
vasopressin and, 343–45, 351–52, 356
Blood vessels. *See* Vasculature.
Blood volume. *See also* Hypervolemia; Hypovolemia.
osmolality and, 345, 356
vasopressin and, 343–45, 356
Blotting, hybridization and, 45
Body composition, fuel metabolism and, 1088–89
Body mass index, 1206
Body measurement, 1597
Bombesin, 1650
eating behavior and, 1213
Bone, 31, 1329–32, 1454–91
age determination, 1598
acromegaly and, 301
biopsy, 1456–58
prostate cancer and, 1758
brown tumors, 1385
calcitonin and, 1342–43
calcium and, 1332
cortical (compact), 1329, 1330
cysts, 1385
dysplasia, 1611
fibrous, 1482–83
formation, 1329, 1331
vitamin D and, 1356
GLA protein. *See* Osteocalcin.
glucocorticoids and, 554–55, 793–95
growth, 1591
growth factors, 1491
haversian, 1329
hungry, syndrome of, 1401, 1424, 1440
hypercalciuria and, 1551
hyperphosphatasia and, hereditary, 1481–82
hyperthyroidism and, 429, 1411
hypothyroidism and, 455
magnesium and, 1363
malignancy-related hypercalcemia and, 1403–11
marble, 1477–78
membrane (envelope), 1329
metabolism, 1330–32
clinical evaluation of, 1454–58
diseases of, 1454–91. *See also* Osteodystrophy; Osteomalacia; Osteopetrosis; Osteoporosis; Rickets.
local regulation of, 1491
morphogenetic protein, 1491
mosaic, 1486–87
Paget's disease of, 1483–91
pain in:
osteitis fibrosa cystica and, 1385
osteomalacia and, 1459
Paget's disease and, 1484
parathyroid hormone and, 1331–32
hyperparathyroidism and, 1384–88
metabolism of, 1328
responsiveness test, 1444–45
vitamin D potentiation of, 1356
quantitative histomorphometry and microradiography, 1457, 1470
radiology, 1456
fibrous dysplasia and, 1482, 1483
osteopetrosis and, 1478
osteoporosis and, 1468–69
Paget's disease and, 1484–85
radionuclide studies, 1456
Paget's disease and, 1484–85
prostate cancer and, 1757–58
remodeling, 1330–31
resorption, 1331. *See also* Osteolysis.
inhibition of, 1420–21
vitamin D and, 1356
testosterone and, 857
tetracycline test, 1458
trabecular (cancellous), 1329, 1330
vitamin D and, 1355–56
Bone marrow transplantation, osteopetrosis and, 1477–78
Bonnevie-Ullrich syndrome, 1005, 1611
Bradykinin:
angiotensin-converting enzyme and, 705
Bartter's syndrome and, 1788, 1789
carcinoid and, 1657
formation of, 1782
hydrolysis of, 1782
prostaglandins and, 1777, 1785
Brain. *See also* Hypothalamus; Nervous system; Pineal gland; Pituitary gland.
blood-brain barrier, 187, 342–43
as endocrine gland, 4
evolution of, 12
gigantism and, 237
glucocorticoids and, 555–56
glucose and:
consumption rate, 1090
deficiency of, 1180
growth of, 1581
hormone effects on, 211–16
hypertension and, 700
hyponatremia and, 371–72
pseudotumor cerebri, 237
sexual dimorphism and, 215–16
Brainstem, anatomic landmarks of, 822
Branchial dysembryogenesis, 1431
Branching enzyme, 1046
Breast:
cancer. *See separate entry below.*
hormones affecting, 886
male, 886. *See also* Gynecomastia.
prolactin and, 270
puberty and, 1593, 1595
testicular feminization and, 954
Breast cancer, 1736–52
adrenalectomy and, 1744, 1748
age and, 1737–39
androgens and, 1740, 1748–49
castration and, 1739, 1744, 1747–48
chemotherapy for, 1746–47, 1750–51
corticosteroids and, 1749–50
estrogens and, 179, 979, 1740, 1742–46, 1748–52
familial factors, 1741
geographic factors, 1737, 1738
hormonal regulation of, 1742–46
hypercalcemia and, 1360, 1403

Breast cancer *(Cont.)*:
hypophysectomy and, 1742, 1744–45, 1748
incidence and mortality, 1736–37
murine, 1742–44
progesterone and, 1740–41, 1743, 1746
prolactin and, 1741–44, 1746
receptors and, 1743, 1745–46, 1751–52
assays for, 179
reproductive experience and, 1739–40
risk factors and etiology, 1737–41
therapy, 1746–52
viruses and, 1741
Breast feeding:
amenorrhea and, 955–56
antithyroid drugs and, 439–40
Broad-beta disease, 1267–70
Bromocriptine:
acromegaly and, 306
breast cancer and, 1744
Cushing's disease and, 603, 617
growth hormone deficiency and, 229
hyperprolactinemia and, 230, 310, 312–15, 959–60
pituitary effects of, 199
Bronchi:
adenoma of, MEN 1 and, 1665
carcinoids of, 1658
Bronchoconstriction, carcinoid and, 1656
Brown tumors of bone, 1385
Bruits, abdominal renovascular hypertension and, 739
Brushite, nephrolithiasis and, 1507
Buffalo hump, 607
Bulimia, 234, 1223
Buserelin, 969
Bypass technique, renal artery, 749

C cells, thyroid. *See* Thyroid gland, C cells.
C peptide, 1065–66
diabetes mellitus and, 1099
hypoglycemia and:
autoimmune, 1188
factitious, 1194
insulinoma and, 1185
insulin precursor, 65
plasma levels, 1067
Cachectin, 1724
Cachexia:
diabetic, 1123
hypopituitarism and, 273
Caerulein, 1636
amino acid sequence of, 1631
Calciferol, 1344–46. *See also* Vitamin D.
for hypocalcemia, 1434–35
intestinal effects of, 1354
toxicity, 1413–14
Calcification:
pseudohypoparathyroidism and, 1428
renal. *See* Nephrocalcinosis.
sellar, 291
thyroid, medullary carcinoma and, 502, 1670
Calcineurin, 126
Calcitonin, 1337–44
actions, 1342–43
assays, 1374–75
biosynthesis, 1339–40
bone and, 1342–43
calcium and, 1340, 1341, 1672–73
gastrin and, 1343–44
renal excretion of, 1343
chemistry, 1338–39
D, 1338, 1341
ectopic, 1718
epinephrine and, 660
escape phenomenon, 1342–43
estrogen and, 1472
gastrin and, 1341, 1343–44
gene for, 40, 1339–40
organization of, 62
gene-related peptide (CGRP), 40, 63, 1337, 1339–40, 1672
structure of, 1340
glucagon and, 1673
historical note on, 1337
hypercalcemia and, 1421
immunochemical analysis of, 1673–74
kidney and, 1343
M, 1338
magnesium and, 1673
medullary thyroid carcinoma and, 502–3, 1670–74
metabolism, 1341
osteoporosis and, 977, 1470, 1476
Paget's disease of bone and, 1488–89
pentagastrin test for, 1672–73
phosphorus and, 1343
physiological significance of, 1343–44
plasma levels, 1375
provocative testing, 1672–73
radioimmunoassay, 1374–75
sample handling, 1443
regulation of, 1340–41
RNA and, 1337, 1339
salmon, 1338–39, 1476, 1488
antibodies to, 1488
secretion, 1340–41
as tumor marker, 1724
venous catheterization and, 1672, 1673
whiskey test for, 1673
Calcium, 122–28. *See also* Hypercalcemia; Hypocalcemia.
absorption, 1351–53, 1355, 1359
excessive, 1545–51
hyperparathyroidism and, 1383
laboratory studies, 1553
quantitation of, 1368–69
ACTH and, 526
aldosterone and, 564
balance, 1357
calculation of, 1369, 1370
hyperparathyroidism and, 1382
osteitis fibrosa cystica and, 1387
binding, 123–26, 1320
intestinal, 1353
bone and, 1332
calcitonin and, 1340, 1341, 1672–73
gastrin and, 1343–44
renal excretion and, 1343
calmodulin and, 123–26
cAMP and, 127–28
cGMP and, 128
chromaffin granule release and, 655
citrate binding of, 1564–65
creatinine and, 1443
deficiency. *See* Hypocalcemia.
dietary:
hypercalciuria and, 1532–35, 1538–40, 1547–52
hyperparathyroidism and, 1383
urinalysis and, 1367
distribution of, 1317, 1318
double-isotope techniques for, 1369
enzymes dependent on, 125–27
epinephrine and, 660
estrogen and, 1472
evolutionary development and, 1318
excess. *See* Hypercalcemia.
excretion rates, 1366–67, 1443
extracellular, 123, 1317, 1318, 1320–21
fecal, 1353, 1369
feedback system, 1358
free, 1364
functions of, 1319
glucocorticoids and, 554–55
osteoporosis and, 794–95
glycogenolysis and, 118–19
homeostasis, 1358–60, 1536
hormone action and, 8
hypertension and, 712–14
hyperthyroidism and, 429, 1411–12
hypothyroidism and, 455
inositol triphosphate and, 132–33
insulin release and, 1066, 1068–69
intracellular, 123, 1317, 1318
ionized, 1320–21, 1364
kidney and, 1335–37
hypercalcemia and, 1359–60, 1417
hypocalcemia and, 1431
leakage defect, 1352–45
vitamin D and, 1356–57
magnesium and, 1426, 1440
malabsorption, 1359
membrane passage of, 123
menopause and, 977
metabolism, 1318–21
muscle and, 1319
nephrolithiasis and, 1507–8, 1524–67. *See also* Calcium oxalate stones; Calcium phosphate stones; Hypercalciuria; Nephrolithiasis.
osteodystrophy and, renal, 1479, 1480
osteoporosis and, 977, 1470, 1472, 1473, 1475
parathyroid hormone and, 1320, 1326, 1358–60. *See also* Hyperparathyroidism.
bone metabolism and, 1332
renal transport and, 1336–37
secretion rate, 1324
sensors and, 1324
phosphatidylinositol and, 132
phospholipase and, 131, 132
potassium and, 533
pregnancy and, 1350
prostaglandins and, 1779–80
protein kinase C and, 126–27
pump, 123
pump-leak transport system, 1318–19
second messenger role of, 111, 123–27, 1319–20

Calcium *(Cont.)*:
serum levels, 1363–65
bone disease and, 1454–55
immunoreactive PTH and, 1372
maintenance of normal, 1358
normal range, 1364
state of, 1320, 1321
techniques for, 1363–64, 1442–43
ultrafilterable, 1364–65
sodium and, 718, 1335, 1336, 1538–40
somatostatin and, 204
stimulus-secretion hypothesis and, 122
stones. *See* Calcium oxalate stones; Calcium phosphate stones.
supplemental, 1433–35
hyperoxaluria and, 1561
osteoporosis and, 1475, 1476
tolerance test, 1369, 1553, 1569–70
flow diagram and data base for, 1569
hyperparathyroidism and, 1384, 1542
technique, 1569–70
total body, 1317
tubular maximum (TmCa) for, 1336
urinary, 1336, 1568. *See also* Hypercalciuria; Hypocalciuria.
balance data and, 1369
bone disease and, 1455
measurement, 1366–67, 1433
normal ranges, 1367
vascular smooth muscle and, 713
vitamin D and, 1348–49, 1358–60
absorptive role of, 1352–53, 1355
hydroxylase activity and, 1350
renal reabsorption and, 1356–57
Calcium channel blockers, aldosteronism and, 763
Calcium oxalate stones, 1527–67
activity product ratio and, 1508
dehydration and, 1531
diet and, 1527, 1531
family history and, 1529–30
formation product ratio and, 1508
frequency of, 1503, 1527
general considerations, 1527–29
hypercalciuria and, 1531–36
hyperoxaluria and, 1556–61
hyperuricosuria and, 1561–64
hypocitraturia and, 1564–66
idiopathic, 1566–67
medications and, 1530
pH and, 1530
recurrent, 1528
risk factors, 1528–29
solubility product and, 1504–05
Calcium phosphate stones, 1524–27
diagnosis, 1526
frequency, 1503
mixed, 1524, 1527
pathogenesis, 1505, 1524–25
risk populations, 1525–26
treatment, 1526–27
Call-Exner bodies, 912
Calmodulin, 123–27
functions of, 124–25
glycogenolysis and, 119
structure of, 125
Calories:
daily requirements of, by age, 1591
diabetes mellitus and, 1139–1140
hyperlipidemia and, 1290–91, 1294
restriction of, 1235–37
storage of, 1088–89
tabulation of, in food, 1295
Camalox, 1561
Campesterol, 1285
Cancer, 1736–64. *See also* Tumors *and specific sites and types.*
adrenal. *See* Adrenal glands, carcinoma.
breast, 1736–52
endometrial, 1762–64
genetic factors in, 55, 151. *See also* Oncogenes.
hypercalcemia and, 1403–11, 1702–6
hyperthyroidism and, 1715
parathyroid, 1379, 1391
prostate, 891, 1753–62
thyroid. *See* Medullary thyroid carcinoma; Thyroid glands, carcinoma.
vasopressin hypersecretion and, 371
Candidiasis, hypoparathyroidism and, 1681, 1682
Capping of mRNA, 60
Captopril, 705,1784
Bartter's syndrome and, 1789
renovascular hypertension and, 745, 748
Carbamazepine, vasopressin and, 348
Carbenoxolone, hypertension induced by, 768
Carbohydrates, 1045–55. *See also* Glucose; Glycogen.
diabetes mellitus and, 1104, 1105, 1139–40
dietary, 1139–40
hypoglycemia and, 1192
glucocorticoids and, 544–46
hyperlipidemia and, 1291
insulin and, 1068–70, 1073–75
metabolism, 1045–55
fat metabolism and, 1061–62
thyroid hormone and, 399
Carbon dioxide, tricarboxylic acid cycle and, 1052
Carboxyl proteinase, 68
Carcinoembryonic antigen, 1725
Carcinoid, 1652–59
acromegaly and, 303
age and sex and, 1654–55
anatomic distribution, 1654
bronchial, 1658
clinical features, 1655–56
diagnosis, 1657–58
dopamine and, 679
ectopic CRH and, 1719, 1720
gastric, 1658
histology, 1654
historical note on, 1652–53
malignancy and metastases, 1653, 1658–59
medullary thyroid carcinoma and, 1675
MEN 1 and, 1665
pathophysiology and chemistry, 1656–57
prevalence and size, 1653
secretory products of, 1655
treatment and prognosis, 1658–59
variants, 1658
Carcinoma. *See* Cancer; Tumors; *and specific sites.*
Cardiac output:
atrial natriuretic factor and, 722–23
hypertension and, 697, 698
Cardionatrin. *See* Atrial natriuretic factor.
Cardiovascular system, 28–29. *See also* Heart; Vasculature.
acromegaly and, 302
catecholamines and, 659–60, 680–81
glucocorticoids and, 552–53
hormones affecting, 14
hypertension and. *See* Hypertension.
hyperthyroidism and, 426
hypothyroidism and, 453
menopause and, 977–78
obesity and, 1232
prostaglandins and, 1777–79
vasopressin and, 343–45
Carnitine, 1058
hypoglycemia and, 1188
Carnitine acyltransferase, 1058
diabetic ketoacidosis and, 1150
Carpal tunnel syndrome, 32–33
Casein, hyperlipidemia and, 1292
Cassava, goiter and, 478–79, 482
Castrate syndrome, functional prepubertal, 873–74
Castration. *See also* Orchiectomy.
breast cancer and, 1739, 1744, 1747–48
Cataract, 33, 34
diabetes mellitus and, 1119
glucocorticoids and, 556, 793
hypoparathyroidism and, 1423
Catecholamines, 651–86. *See also* Dopamine; Epinephrine; Norepinephrine.
assays, 662–64, 682–85
sample handling, 683
behavioral disorders and, 681
biochemistry, 652
biologic effects of, 659–62
biosynthesis, 196, 652–53, 655
cardiovascular effects of, 659–60, 680–81
chromatography, 662, 683
clearance rates, 656, 662–64
clonidine suppression test, 670
conjugation of, 656
coronary heart disease and, 680
degradation, 196, 653
drugs affecting, 684
energy regulation and, 1087–88
fluorimetry, 682
gastrointestinal effects of, 681–82
glucocorticoids and, 556, 678
glucose and, 658, 659, 661, 1085
synergism and, 1092
glycogenolysis and, 119, 1047, 1085
gonadal disorders and, 678
gonadotropins and, 832–33
hypertension and, 680
hypoglycemia and, 677–78, 1086, 1180, 1190
inactivation of, 655–56
inhibitors of, 199
insulin and, 1071, 1085
kinetics, 662–64
Lesch-Nyhan syndrome and, 679

Catecholamines *(Cont.)*:
liver disease and, 681–82
mechanisms of action, 656–59
metabolic actions of, 661
migraine headache and, 681
mitral valve prolapse and, 680–81
myocardial infarction and, 680
obesity and, 679
ovaries and, 920
parathyroid hormone and, 1325
pheochromocytoma and, 667–72
pituitary disorders and, 678–79
plasma levels, 662–64, 682–84
metabolic effects and, 658–60
platelet, 669
porphyria and, 679
pulmonary disorders and, 681
receptors for, 656–59. *See also* Adrenergic receptors.
release (exocytosis) of, 655
renal disease and, 682
renin and, 704
seizures and, 681
single-isotope-derivative assay, 662, 663, 682–83
storage, 655
thyroid hormone and, 399, 678
urinary, 682
pheochromocytoma and, 669
sample handling, 684
Cathepsins, 703, 1326
Cation exchange resin, hypercalciuria and, 1555
Catechol-*O*-methyl transferase, 653, 656
diagnostic testing and, 682, 683
Celiac ganglion, 654
Cells:
adipose, 1208–10, 1222–22. *See also* Adipose tissue.
growth of, 1581, 1582
internalization by, 106–9
membrane of. *See* Membrane, cell.
neurosecretory. *See* Neurosecretory cells.
oncogenes and, 150–54
pituitary, 250–52, 338
protein pathway in, 65, 66
receptors within, 83–84
response of, 87, 88. *See also* Target cells.
occupancy of receptors and, 99–101
receptor regulation effect on, 104–6
Cerebral edema, diabetic ketoacidosis and, 1154
Cerebrospinal fluid:
pituitary hormones in, 295
rhinorrhea, postoperative, 298
vasopressin in, 349–50
Cervical ganglia, 654
Chalone, 1583
Charcot-Bouchard aneurysm, 700
Charcot's joint, 1122
Chase-Melson-Aurback test, 1444
Chemicals, goitrogenic, 484
Chemosis, hyperthyroidism and, 441, 443
Chemotherapy:
breast cancer and, 1746–47, 1750–51
carcinoid and, 1659
endometrial cancer and, 1764
prostate cancer and, 1761
thyroid carcinoma and, 500
Chenodeoxycholic acid deficiency, 1284
Chiari-Frommel syndrome, 306
Chief cells, parathyroid, 1321–22
hyperplasia of, 1378
pseudoadenomatous, 1379, 1393
Chimerism, 986
hermaphroditism and, 1004
Chloramine T, iodination and, 171
Chloride:
Bartter's syndrome and, 1787, 1788
phosphate ratio to, hypercalcemia and, 1396
water balance and, 353, 354
Chloroquine phosphate, hypercalcemia of malignancy and, 1705
Chlorpromazine, pituitary effects of, 199
Chlorpropamide, 1141–43
diabetes insipidus and, 365
hypoglycemia induced by, 1194
hyponatremia induced by, 1142
Chlorthalidone:
hypercalcemia induced by, 1413
for hypercalciuria, 1555
Cholecalciferol, 1344–46. *See also* Vitamin D.
Cholecystography, thyroid hormone and, 416, 435
Cholecystokinin, 1636–37
amino acid sequence of, 1631
chemistry, 1636
clinical use, 1637
distribution, release, and actions, 1637
eating behavior and, 1213
hypothalamic distribution of, 192
measurement, 1637
in vitro, 169
pituitary effects of, 199
Cholelithiasis. *See* Gallstones.
Cholera toxin, adenylate cyclase and, 112
Cholestanes, 517
Cholestanol accumulation, 1283–84
Cholesterol. *See also* Lipids.
abetalipoproteinemia and, 1278, 1279
ACTH and, 526–27
assays, 1306–7
atherosclerosis and, 1261–62, 1280–82
balance of, 1249
biosynthesis, 106, 518, 1249–50
cytochrome P450 and, 70
diabetes mellitus and, 1107, 1123
dietary, 1287–88, 1292–93
index of foods, 1294–96
drugs lowering, 1263–64, 1298–1305
elevated. *See* Hypercholesterolemia; Hyperlipidemia.
esters of, 69, 1250, 1251, 1281
storage disease, 1283
Tangier disease and, 1276–77
evolution of steriods and, 9–10
feedback inhibition of, 1250
hypertension and, 696
hyperthyroidism and, 428
hypothroidism and, 454
LDL, 69. *See also* Lipoprotein, low-density.
metabolism, 1249–50
obesity and, 1231–32, 1234
plasma levels:
age-related changes in, 1256, 1257
diet and, 1288, 1290, 1297
drug therapy and, 1299
familial increase in, 1262
increased. *See* Hypercholesterolemia; Hyperlipidemia.
normal values, 1256
thresholds for drug therapy and, 1265–66
protein complex with. *See* Lipoprotein.
side cleavage enzyme, 925
deficiency, 629, 1012–13
steroid hormone formation and, 68–69, 71
adrenal, 517–18
ovarian, 924–26
pregnenolone formation and, 516, 518
structure, 516
transport, 925
uptake of, 517–18
vitamin D synthesis and, 73
Cholesterol esterase, 69
Cholesterol ester hydrolase deficiency, 1283
Cholestyramine, 1298–99
hyperlipidemia and, 1263, 1298–99
indications and dosage, 1299
mechanism of action, 1298
side effects, 1298–99
Cholinergic fibers, 654. *See also* Acetylcholine.
Choloxin, 1303
Chondrocalcinosis, 31
hyperparathyroidism and, 1391
Chondrocytes, growth and, 1591
Chondrodystrophy, 1611
Chorea, Huntington's, 237
Choriocarcinoma, 892
hyperthyroidism and, 1715
Choristomas, 223
Chromaffin tissue (cells), 651
granules, 655
physiology, 655
synthesis in, 653
tumors of, 667–72
Chromatin, 37–38
sex, 988
steroid hormones and, 143–46
triiodothyronine receptors in, 397
Chromatography, 20
affinity, receptor purification by, 90
catecholamine, 662, 683
cortisol, 570
radioimmunoassay and, 174
vitamin D, 1375
Chromogranins, 655, 1672
Chromophobes, pituitary, 250, 287
ACTH-secreting tumors and, 315
GH-secreting tumors and, 300
MEN 1 and, 1664
Chromosomes:
anaphase lag of, 985, 987
aneuploidy, 985-86
banding, 985
deletion of, 986
duplications of, 986
growth disorders and, 1611–13, 1619

Chromosomes *(Cont.)*:
  mosaicism and. *See* Mosaicism.
  nondisjunction of, 985–86
  ovarian germ cell, 932
  ring, 986
  sex, 984
    anomalies of, 1000–1009
    dosage compensation and, 988
    growth and, 1582, 1611–12
    inactivation of, 988–89
    karyotype and, 985
    properties and functions of, 987–89
  spermatogenesis and, 827
  structural abnormalities, 986–87, 1004
  testicular function tests and, 857
  translocation of, 986
Chvostek's sign, 1422
Chylomicrons, 1246–47
  accumulation of, 1270–72
  atherosclerosis and, 1281–82
  diet and, 1288, 1293
  metabolism, 1251–52
Cilia:
  immotile, 880–81
  spermatozoan, 830
Cimetidine:
  gastrinoma and, 1636
  prolactinoma and, 308
Ciprofibrate, 1304
Circadian rhythms, 218–21
  ACTH and, 219, 255, 527–30
  aldosterone and, 534, 761
  corticosteroids and, 219
  cortisol and, 220, 255, 527–30
    Cushing's disease and, 316
  CRF and, 528
  Cushing's syndrome and, 316, 530
  glucocorticoid therapy and, 805–6
  luteinizing hormone and, 219
  melatonin and, 216–17
  suprachiasmatic nucleus and, 218–19
  synchronizers and, 218
  testosterone and, 840
Cirrhosis:
  glucose intolerance and, 1165
  hypogonadism and, 868–69
  vasopressin hypersecretion and, 367–68
Citrate, 1564–66
  acid-base status and, 1565
  fatty acid synthesis and, 1055
  glycolysis and, 1048
  hypocalcemia and, 1432
  nephrolithiasis and, 1565–66
  renal metabolism of, 1564–65
  renal tubular acidosis and, 1525, 1527
  steatorrhea and, 1559
Citrate synthase, 1052, 1053
Claudication, diabetes and, 1123
Climacteric, 974
  male, 874–75
  symptoms of, 976–77
Clinical manifestations of endocrine disease. *See* Symptoms of endocrine disease *and also under specific disease.*
Clinoid processes, 247
CLIP. *See* Corticotropin-like intermediate lobe peptide.
Clitoromegaly, 21-hydroxylase deficiency and, 1023
Clocks, body, 218–21. *See also* Circadian rhythms.
Clofibrate, 1301–2
  action and toxicity, 1301
  diabetes insipidus and, 366
  hyperlipidemia and, 1269, 1301–2
  indications and dosage, 1301–2
Clomiphene:
  azoospermia and, 880
  breast cancer and, 1749
  delayed puberty and, 866
  gonadotropins and, 283, 324–24, 855–56, 860
  luteal effects of, 931
  ovulation induced by, 967
    polycystic disease and, 963–64
  Prader-Willi syndrome and, 232, 233
  testicular stimulation by, 855–56
Clones, 44–45, 47–50
  chromosomal gene, 49
  estrogen receptor and, 139
  reverse transcription and, 48–49
  transfer of, into mammalian cells, 49–50
Clonidine:
  catecholamines and, 670
  growth hormone and, 283, 325, 1622
  postural hypotension and, 676
Coagulation, hypothyroidism and, 454–55
Coated-pit system, 106, 107–8
  LDL uptake and, 518
Cocaine, pupillary response to, 685
Codons, 40–41
  reverse transcription and, 48
Cognitive function, hormones and, 213–14
COLA transport defect, 1510–17
Cold pressor test, 685
Colestipol, 1298–99
  hyperlipidemia and, 1263, 1264, 1298–99
Collagen:
  bone, 1329
  fibromuscular dysplasia and, 737
  glucocorticoids and, 552
  glycation of, 1129
  hydroxyproline excretion and, 1455–56
Colloid, thyroid, 78, 390
  endocytosis by, 394
Colony stimulating factor, oncogenes and, 153
Coma:
  diabetic:
    ketotic, 1151, 1152
    nonketotic hyperosmolar, 1154–55
  hypoglycemic, 1152, 1181, 1195
  lactic acidosis, 1155
  myxedema, 460–61
Compactin, 1304–5
Computed tomography:
  adrenal, 615, 616
    aldosteronism and, 759–60
    pheochromocytoma and, 670–71
  orbital, 442
  pituitary, 291–93
    Cushing's disease and, 614
  renal, 742
Conalbumin, estrogen and, 145
Confusion, 32
Conjunctiva, 34
Connexin, 913
Constipation, 27
Contraceptive agents:
  endometrial cancer risk and, 1763
  estrogen therapy and, 285
  GnRH agonists and, 157
  hyperprolactinemia and, 959
  male, 890–91
  polycystic ovary disease and, 963
Contrast agents:
  iodinated, thyroid hormone and, 416, 435
  urographic, 741–42
Converting enzyme. *See* Angiotensin-converting enzyme.
Convulsions, 32
Coprosterol (coprostanol), 1250
Cori cycle, 1051
Cornea, 34
  HDL deficiency and, 1275
  hypercalcemia and, 1395
  hyperlipidemia and, 1282
  LCAT deficiency and, 1280
  mucosal neuromas and, 1677
Corona radiata, 915, 916, 932
Coronary artery disease:
  cholesterol and, 1261–62, 1280–82
  diabetes mellitus and, 1114, 1123
  HDL and, 1274
  hypertension and, 695–96
  menopause and, 978
  sympathochromaffin system and, 680
Corpus albicans, 906, 924
Corpus luteum, 921–24
  anatomy, 906
  degeneration (luteolysis), 923–24, 931
  differentiation, 929–31
  luteinization, 921–23, 930–31
  ovulation and, 944
  photomicrograph of, 922
  relaxin production by, 926
Cortexolone. *See* 11-Deoxycortisol.
Corticosteroid-binding globulin (CBG), 6, 75, 537–38
  aldosterone and, 539, 540
  competitive radioassay and, 569
  dissociation from, 539
  plasma levels, conditions affecting, 571
  properties, 537
  reservoir function of, 538–39
  steroid metabolism and, 539, 543
Corticosteroids. *See also* Glucocorticoids; Mineralocorticoids; Steroid hormones.
  circadian rhymicity of, 219
Corticosterone. *See also* Glucocorticoids.
  biosynthesis, 71, 1012
  18-hydroxylation defect and, 630–31
  metabolism, 542
  plasma levels, 731
  receptors for, 560
  secretion rate, 521
  structure, 516
Corticosterone methyl oxidase, 71
  deficiency of, 630–31
Corticotroph cells, 251–52

Corticotropin. *See* Adrenocorticotropic hormone (ACTH).
related peptides. *See* Endorphins; Lipotropin; Melanocyte-stimulating hormone.
Corticotropin-like intermediate lobe peptide (CLIP), 252
amino acid sequence of, 525
ectopic, 1710
Corticotropin releasing factor (CRF), 205–6, 423–24
ACTH stimulation test and, 280, 321
actions, 523–24
chemistry and effects, 205–6
circadian rhythm and, 528
cortisol and, 256
Cushing's disease and, 316, 317, 603, 604, 612
pathogenesis, 318
depression (mental) and, 530
ectopic, 1719–20
ectopic ACTH and, 1708
extrahypothalamic, 205
feedback mechanism and, 530–31
hypothalamic distribution of, 205
pituitary-adrenal testing with, 579
precursor of, 205
regulation, 194, 205–6
structure, 200, 205
vasopressin and, 352, 524
Cortisol, 522–31. *See also* Glucocorticoids; Hydrocortisone.
ACTH and, 255–56, 525–31
assay for, 280, 321, 322
ectopic, 1706–11
feedback inhibition of, 530–31
stimulation test, 576–78
actions, 544–61
androgens and, adrenal, 535–36
assays, 569–71
binding, 536–39
dissociation from, 539
biosynthesis, 69, 518–19, 1012
pathway of, 71, 72
blood pressure and, 552
cholesterol substrate for, 69
chromatography, 570
chronic disease and, 530
circadian rhythm of, 220, 255, 527–30
changes in, 529–30
Cushing's disease and, 316
clearance, 798
competitive protein-binding radioassay, 569, 571
CRF and, 256
Cushing's disease and. *See* Cushing's disease.
deficiency, 581–97. *See also* Adrenocortical insufficiency.
enzyme defects and, 624–30
familial, 586
depression (mental) and, 238, 530
dexamethasone test and, 322, 574–76
distribution of, in plasma, 536
drugs affecting, 544
energy regulation and, 1087–88
epinephrine and, 659
feedback mechanism, 527, 530–31
Cushing's disease and, 316
feeding and, 528–29, 1090
fetal, 520
fluorimetric assay, 570, 571
free, 570
CBG and, 539
urinary, 572
11β-hydroxylase deficiency and, 628
17α-hydroxylase deficiency and, 629
21-hydroxylase deficiency and, 624–28, 1022–23, 1027, 1614–15
hypersecretion, 599–620. *See also* Cushing's syndrome.
hypertension and, 726, 766–68
hyperthyroidism and, 428
hypoglycemia and, 1181
insulin-induced, 578, 810, 811
hypothyroidism and, 455
inhibitors of, 522
insulin and, 1086
hypoglycemia induced by, 578, 810, 811
insulin-like growth factor and, 1588
liver disease and, 543
metabolism, 75, 540–42
variations in, 543–44
metyrapone and, 579
mineralocorticoid activity of, 567, 792
myxedema coma and, 461
obesity and, 1215, 1233
plasma levels, 569–71
adrenal insufficiency and, 592
in children, 1623
Cushing's syndrome and, 610
dexamethasone suppression test and, 575
prednisone therapy and, 809–11
24-hour period, 528
plasma state of, 536–39
potency, 562
radioimmunossay, 570
radioreceptor assay, 570
receptors for, 559–61, 566
CBG and, 539
secretion rate, 520, 521, 573
Cushing's disease and, 604, 605
sleep and, 527
spontaneous patterns of release, 527–30
stress and, 529–30, 1092
structure, 136, 516, 789
surgery and, 529–30
therapeutic, 792, 798, 801. *See also* Glucocorticoids, therapeutic.
thyroid disease and, 428, 455, 543
transport, 75. *See also* Corticosteroid-binding globulin.
urinary, 541, 572–73
Cushing's syndrome and, 316, 610, 611
virilization and, 1020–21, 1614–15
Cortisone. *See also* Glucocorticoids.
ACTH deficiency and, 284
adrenal hyperplasia and, 1615
breast cancer and, 1749
chronic adrenal insufficiency and, 595
conversion of cortisol to, 540–41
historical note on, 512–13
21-hydroxylase deficiency and, 627
metabolism, 541–42, 797–98
structure, 789
surgical procedures and, 596–97
Cortoic acid, 541
Cortolonic acid, 541
Cosyntropin:
asthma and, 791
stimulation test with, 576–78
in children, 1624
Cotton wool spots, 1116–17
Counterregulatory hormones, 677, 1087–88, 1179, 1180
Covalent modification:
peptide hormone, 65–66
transcription of genes and, 61
Coxsackie virus, diabetes and, 1097
Cramps, hypocalcemia and, 1423
Craniopharyngioma, 288
growth hormone deficiency and, 1607
radiotherapy for, 299
surgery for, 298
Creatine phosphokinase, hypothyroidism and, 453
Creatinine:
calcium and, 1443
cAMP and, 1444
phosphorus and, 1368, 1443
Cremasteric muscles, 825
Cretinism, 478, 479
etiology, 478
historical note on, 473–74
sporadic nongoitrous, 447
Creutzfeldt-Jakob disease, hGH therapy and, 1609
Criminal behavior, XYY male and, 873, 1003, 1619
Crohn's disease, growth failure and, 1602
Crooke's changes, 252, 601
Cross-linking, receptor, 96–97
Cryptorchism, 883–86, 1020
vs. anorchia, 873–74
bilateral, 884
hypogonadism and, 884
Kallmann's syndrome and, 864, 865
müllerian duct persistence and, 1011
pathophysiology, 883–85
treatment, 885–86
tumors and, 885, 892
Crystalloid theory of nephrolithiasis, 1504–7
CTX syndrome, 1283–84
Cumulus granulosa cells, 915, 916, 933
ovulation and, 939, 940
Cushing's disease, 315–20. *See also* Cushing's syndrome.
adrenalectomy and, 603, 617–18
age and sex distribution, 600
behavioral effects, 213–14
clinical picture, 315–16, 609
CRF and, 316, 317, 603, 604, 612
definition, 599
dexamethasone test and, 322
differential diagnosis, 612–14
ectopic ACTH syndrome vs., 1707–8
endocrine abnormalities in, 602–3
erythrocytosis and, 28
etiology and pathogenesis, 317–18, 602–4
hypertension and, 767

Cushing's disease *(Cont.)*:
hypothalamic disease and, 226, 317–18, 603
hamartoma and, 223–24
laboratory findings, 316
pathology, 600–601
pathophysiology, 604–5
pituitary surgery and, 603, 615–17
prognosis, 620
radiology, 614
treatment, 318–20, 615–18, 1610
Cushing's syndrome, 599–620
ACTH and, 600. *See also* Cushing's disease.
ectopic, 604, 605–6, 618, 1706–11
adrenal hyperplasia and, 601–2, 614
adrenal tumors and, 602, 604, 606, 618
circadian rhythms and, 316, 530
classification and distribution, 600
clinical features, 606–9
by etiologic category, 608–9
dexamethasone suppression test and, 574, 610, 611, 613–14
diabetes mellitus and, 1164
diagnosis and differential diagnosis, 316–17, 609–15
etiologic determination in, 612–14
evaluative scheme for, 609
problems in, 611–12
tumor localization in, 614–15
etiology and pathogenesis, 602–4, 612–14
growth failure and, 1609–10
hypertension and, 552, 607, 766–68
iatrogenic, 792–96
laboratory studies, 608
MEN 1 and, 1665
Nelson's syndrome and, 619
obesity and, 606, 611, 1215, 1233
osteoporosis and, 608, 1473
pathology, 600–602
pathophysiology, 604–6
pituitary adenoma and, 600–601. *See also* Cushing's disease.
prognosis, 619–20
treatment, 615–18, 1610
Cyanide-nitroprusside test, 1514
Cyanoketone, 522
Cyclooxygenase:
arachidonic acid metabolism and, 1770, 1771
inhibition of, 1773, 1779
menorrhagia and, 974
pathway, 130, 973
uterine, 972
Cyclosporin A, diabetes and, 1098, 1148
Cyproheptadine:
aldosteronism and, 763
carcinoid and, 1659
Cushing's disease and, 320, 603–4, 617
pituitary effects of, 199
Cyproterone acetate, 1618
androgen antagonism and, 142
hirsutism and, 624
prostate cancer and, 1760–61
structure of, 136
Cystic fibrosis:
growth failure and, 1602
infertility and, 881
Cysteine:
EGF receptor, 92–93
insulin receptor, 94
Cystine stones, 1506, 1511–17
frequency of, 1503
Cystinosis, hypothyroidism and, 447
Cystinuria, 1510–17
diagnosis, 1514
genetics and occurrence, 1512
pathophysiology, 1512–14
treatment, 1515–17
Cytochemical assay, 168
ACTH and, 255
parathyroid hormone, 1373
TSH, 258
Cytochrome P450:
ACTH and, 526
cholesterol metabolism and, 1013
defective function of, 628, 629
17α-hydroxylase deficiency and, 1014
steroid synthesis and, 69–71
adrenal, 518
vitamin D hydroxylation and, 73
Cytoplasm, hormone action and, 84
Cytosine, 37

DAG. *See* Diacylglycerol.
Dawn phenomenon, glucose, 1137
DDAVP (Desmopressin), 339
amino acid sequence of, 340
comatose patient and, 366
diabetes insipidus and, 364–65
pituitary surgery and, 298
therapeutic trial of, 375
o,p'-DDD, 320, 1711
Deafness:
Paget's disease of bone and, 1484
Pendred's syndrome and, 448
Decidua basalis, capsularis and parietalis, 970
Dedifferentiation hypothesis of ectopic hormones, 1699
Deficiency syndromes, 15–17
Dehydration:
diabetes insipidus and, 358, 366
diabetic ketoacidosis and, 1150, 1151, 1153
hypercalcemia and, 1420
of malignancy, 1411
hypernatremia and, 361
hyperosmolar nonketotic coma and, 1155
nephrolithiasis and, 1520, 1531
osmolality and, 354
test, 374
thirst and, 352–53
WDHA syndrome and, 1640
7-Dehydrocholesterol, 73, 1345, 1346
Dehydroepiandrosterone (and DHEA-S). *See also* Androgens.
ACTH and, 535, 536
binding, 540
biosynthesis, 71–73, 519, 1012
fetal, 520
growth and, 1590
hirsutism and, 965
3β-hydroxysteroid dehydrogenase deficiency, and, 629, 630
metabolism, 542
plasma levels, 580
polycystic ovary disease and, 963
puberty and, 1593, 1594
regulation of, 535–36
secretion rate, 520, 521
structure, 516
3β-ol-Dehydrogenase isomerase, 925
Deiodinase, 78
Deiodination of thyroxine, 394–95, 403–4
decreased, 414
Demeclocycline, SIADH and, 374, 1713
De Morsier's syndrome, 1606
Demyelination, diabetes and, 1127
Densitometer, 168
Deoxycorticosterone:
adrenal adenoma and, 766
adrenal hyperplasia and, 765–66, 1615
assay, 730, 731
binding, 137, 540
biosynthesis, 71, 518, 519, 1012
Cushing's syndrome and, 606
historical note on, 512
11β-hydroxylase deficiency and, 628, 765, 1029–30
17α-hydroxylase deficiency and, 766
21-hydroxylase deficiency and, 624, 626, 1027
hypertension and, 724, 725, 764–66
aldosteronism and, 753
metabolism, 542
mineralocorticoid activity of, 567–68
receptors for, 565–66
regulation of, 531
secretion rate, 521
structure, 516
19-nor-Deoxycorticosterone, 519, 531
hypertension and, 726
11-Deoxycortisol:
biosynthesis, 71, 518, 1012
11β-hydroxylase deficiency and, 628, 1029–30
21-hydroxylase deficiency and, 624, 626
metabolism, 542
metyrapone and, 281, 322, 579
secretion rate, 521
structure, 136, 516
21-Deoxycortisol, 626
21-hydroxylase deficiency and, 1023
2-Deoxyglucose, vasopressin and, 346
Deoxyribonuclease, 38
Deoxyribonucleic acid. *See* DNA.
Depigmentation, 26
Depression (mental), 32, 213–14, 238
Cushing's syndrome and, 612
fatigue and, 24
glucocorticoids and, 238, 530, 555
Deprivation syndrome, 1613
de Quervain's thyroiditis, 461–62
Derepression hypothesis of ectopic hormones, 1698–99
Dermopathy:
diabetic, 1124
Graves', 444
Desamino-8-D-arginine vasopressin. *See* DDAVP.
Desensitization, target cell, 95, 97–99
GnRH agonists in, 157

Desmolase deficiency, 625, 1012–13, 1015
Desmopressin. *See* DDAVP.
Detergents, membrane dissolution by, 90
Dexamethasone:
ACTH test with, 322, 574–75
adrenal hyperplasia and, 1615
aldosterone and, 534, 754–55, 762
Cushing's disease and, 316, 319, 603
dose-response considerations, 804
gene expression and, 146
hirsutism and, 624
21-hydroxylase deficiency and, 627
hypertension and, 769–70
mineralocorticoid receptors and, 792
potency, 562, 797–99
receptors and, 140, 792
structure, 136, 789
suppression tests, 573–76
in children, 1623
Cushing's syndrome and, 574, 610, 611, 613–14
depression (mental) and, 238
high-dose, 574–76
low-dose, 573–74
Dextran-coated charcoal assay of estrogen receptors, 1751, 1752
Dextrothyroxine, hyperlipidemia and, 1264, 1303
DHC. *See* 11-Deoxycortisol.
DHT. *See* Dihydrotestosterone.
Diabetes insipidus, 356–67
DDAVP trial and, 375
diagnosis, 362–64
dipsogenic, 357, 361–62, 367
etiology, 356–57
familial, 356–57, 362
histiocytosis X and, 224
idiopathic, 356
immunologic disorders and, 224
nephrogenic, 357, 362, 367
neurogenic, 356, 358, 362–66
pathophysiology, 358–60
postoperative, 298
saline infusion test and, 375
therapy, 364–67
Diabetes mellitus, 1092–1165
acanthosis nigricans and, 1102–3
acromegaly and, 302, 1164
adrenocortical insufficiency and, 583, 1682–83
autoimmunity and, 1097–98, 1683, 1685
basement membrane changes and, 1114–15, 1126
biopsy studies, 1126
brittle, 1133, 1157
bronze, 1164
chemical (latent, subclinical), 1110
classification, 1093–94
clinical manifestations, 1115–25
coma and:
ketotic, 1151, 1152
nonketotic hyperosmolar, 1154–55
coronary artery disease and, 1114, 1123
Cushing's syndrome and, 1164
definition, 1093
diagnosis, 1108–12
criteria for, 1109–10
endocrine-associated, 1164–65
environmental agents and, 1096–97
epinephrine and, 677, 678
etiology, 1094–99
eye and, 33, 34, 1115, 1116–19
insulin therapy and, 1130
metabolic changes, 1127, 1128
fat tissue distribution and, 1230–31
fiber and, 1140
foot and, 1123–24
genetic factors, 54, 1094–96
complications and, 1125, 1130
GIP and, 1643
glucagon and, 1103, 1105, 1136–37, 1164–65
glucocorticoid therapy and, 808
glucose and, 1104
impaired tolerance to, 1094, 1110, 1165
laboratory studies, 1108–12
protein interactions with, 1105
growth hormone and, 1129, 1164
hemochromatosis and, 1164
historical note on, 1092–93
HLA antigens and, 1095, 1686
hyperlipidemia and, 1105–7, 1123, 1257–58, 1259
hypoglycemia as early manifestation of, 1192
hypopituitarism and, 278
infections and, 1125
insulin and, 1099–1103, 1131–39
complications (of diabetes) and, 1129–30
complications (of insulin) and, 1136–39
devices for delivery of, 1135–36
dosage adjustment, 1132–35
measurement of, 1111
pregnancy and, 1157–59, 1161–62
preparations of, 1131–32
secretion of, 1099–1101
receptors and, 1101–2
resistance to, 1101–3
treatment, 1131–39
insulin-dependent (type 1; juvenile), 1093–94
islet cells and, 1096, 1113
ketoacidosis and, 1149–54. *See also* Ketoacidosis, diabetic.
kidney and, 1114–15, 1119–21
biopsy studies, 1126
insulin therapy and, 1130
metabolic changes, 1127
lactic acidosis and, 1155
lipids and, 1105–7, 1123, 1163, 1257–58
ketoacidosis and, 1150
lipoatrophic, 1163
maturity-onset of young people (MODY), 1093, 1095
metabolic alterations, 1104–7, 1125–29
mortality, 1130
muscle and, 1122, 1126
neuropathy and, 32, 1115, 1121–23
metabolic changes and, 1127, 1128
non-insulin-dependent (type 2; maturity-onset), 1093, 1094
norepinephrine and, 677
nutrition and, 1098, 1139–40
obesity and, 1098, 1139, 1226–31, 1240
osteoporosis and, 1474
pancreoprival, 1163–64
pathogenesis, 1099–1104
of complications, 1125–30
pathology, 1113–15
pathophysiology, 1104–8
pheochromocytoma and, 1164
pluriglandular insufficiency and, 1165, 1682–83, 1684
pregnancy and, 1155–62
classification, 1158
congenital anomalies and, 1160
delivery and, 1162
diagnosis, 1158
effect of diabetes on pregnancy, 1159–61
effect of pregnancy on diabetes, 1158–59
gigantism in infant and, 1621
neonatal morbidity and, 1161
postnatal effects, 1161
postprandial hyperglycemia and, 1157
respiratory distress syndrome and, 1160
starvation and, accelerated, 1156–57
stillbirth and, 1160–61
treatment, 1161–62
prevalence, 1112–13
prostaglandins and, 1780
protein and, 1104–5
carbohydrate interactions with, 1105
urinary loss of, 1119–20
remission, transient, 1099
retinopathy and, 33, 34, 1115, 1116–19
insulin therapy and, 1130
secondary, 1093–94, 1163–65
skin changes in, 1124
somatomedins and, 1086
somatostatin and, 1149
stress and, 231
thyroiditis and, 1682–83, 1684
treatment, 1130–49
biguanides in, 1143–44
complications and, 1129–30
dietary, 1139–40, 1161
exercise and, 1144–47
future of, 1147–49
goals of, 1130–31, 1139
immunosuppressive,1147–48
insulin in, 1131–39. *See also* insulin *subentry above.*
oral hypoglycemic agents in, 1140–44
pregnancy and, 1161–62
sulfonylureas in, 1141–43
transplantation techniques, whole-pancreas and islet-cell, 1148–49
urinary symptoms, 29
vasculature and, 1114, 1123–24
viruses and, 1096–97
Diacylglycerol (DAG):
insulin and, 1080
phospholipids and, 131–33
protein kinase C and, 126, 127
Dialysis:
diabetic nephropathy and, 1121
hyperlipidemia and, 1258
hypophosphatemia and, 1465
renal osteodystrophy and, 1479
Diaphragma sellae, 192, 247
Diaphyseal dysplasia, 1611

Diapid, 364
Diarrhea, 27
 carcinoid and, 1656
 diabetic, 1123
 gastrinoma and, 1633
 MEN 2 and, 1677
 prostaglandins and, 1776
 WDHA syndrome and, 1640, 1641
Diazoxide, insulinoma and, 1186
Dibenzyline. *See* Phenoxybenzamine.
Dictyotene stage, 932, 933
Diencephalic syndrome of infancy, 233–34
Diet. *See also* Nutrition.
 anorexia nervosa and, 235
 cholesterol in, 1287–88, 1292–93
  index of foods, 1294–96
 diabetes mellitus and, 1139–40
  pregnancy and, 1161
 fat in, 1288–90, 1293
  index of foods, 1294–96
 fiber in. *See* Fiber, dietary.
 goiter and, 476–77, 482
 hypercalciuria and, 1532–35, 1538–40, 1547–52, 1568
 hyperlipidemia and, 1256–57
  therapy of, 1286–98
 hypoglycemia and, 1181, 1192
 iodine in, 76, 392, 476–77
 ketogenic, 1235–36
 liquid protein, 1236
 nephrolithiasis and, 1527, 1531
 obesity and, 1294–96
 oxalates in, 1555, 1556
 protein in. *See* Protein.
 protein-sparing, 1236
 sitosterolemia and, 1286
 uric acid stones and, 1521
Diethylstilbestrol (DES):
 breast cancer therapy with, 1748
 osteoporosis and, 1475
 prostate cancer and, 891, 1756, 1760
 pseudohermaphroditism and, 1019, 1030
Diffuse endocrine system, 1629
DiGeorge's syndrome, 1431
Diflunisal, 1074
Digital subtraction angiography, renal, 743–44
Dihydrocortisol, 540
Dihydroergotamine, hypotension and, 676
Dihydrotachysterol, 1346
 for hypocalcemia, 1433, 1434–35
 for osteomalacia and rickets, 1467
 structure, 1345
Dihydrotestosterone. *See also* Androgens.
 antagonists of, 142
 growth and, 1590
 LH and, 845, 846
 mechanisms of action of, 1016–17
 metabolism, 842
 ovarian, 926
 production of, 842, 1016–17
 prostate cancer and, 1755, 1756
 receptors for, 139–40
 5α-reductase deficiency and, 1017
 structure, 136, 844
 testicular secretion rate, 839
Dihydroxyacetone phosphate, 1056
16α,18-Dihydroxy-DOC, 725
1,25-Dihydroxyvitamin D, 1346
 bone and, 1355–56
 calcium and, 1349, 1350, 1358–60
  absorption of, 1352, 1355
 chemistry, 1345–46
 glucocorticoids and, 554, 555
 hormones affecting, 1350
 hyypercalcemia of malignancy and, 1405, 1410, 1705
 hypercalciuria and, 1383, 1384, 1541, 1543, 1545–50
 hyperparathyroidism and, 1383, 1397
 for hypocalcemia, 1433, 1434
 hypophosphatemia and, 1464
 intestinal effects of, 1354–55
  absorption and, 1352
 lymphoma and, 1410
 measurement, 1376
 metabolism, 1351
 osteomalacia and rickets and, 1463, 1467
 osetoporosis and, 1470, 1472, 1473, 1475
 phosphorus and, 1349–50, 1360–61
 plasma levels, hypercalcemia and, 1419
 pregnancy and, 1350
 production, 73, 1348–49
  disordered control of, 1548–50
 pseudohypoparathyroidism and, 1428
 renal osteodystrophy and, 1479, 1480
 sarcoidosis and, 1415–16
 structure, 1345
 suppression test, 1547
 transport, 75
24,25-Dihydroxyvitamin D, 1346
 bone and, 1356
 measurement, 1376
 metabolism, 1351
 osteomalacia and rickets and, 1460, 1463
 production, 1348–49
 renal osteodystrophy and, 1479, 1480
 structure, 1345
25,26-Dihydroxyvitamin D, 1351
Diiodothyronine, 392, 395
 structure, 391
Diiodotyrosine, 78, 394
 structure, 391
Dilantin. *See* Phenytoin.
Dimorphism, sexual, 984, 999–1000
Diphenylhydantoin. *See* Phenytoin.
Diplopia, 34
 hyperthyroidism and, 440, 443
Dipsogenic diabetes insipidus, 357, 361–62, 367
Dipsogens, 352–53
Disodium etidronate:
 osteomalacia induced by, 1465
 Paget's disease of bone and, 1489–90
Dissociation constants, 178
Dithiothreitol, 683
Diuresis:
 atrial natriuretic factor and, 720
 osmotic, diabetic ketoacidosis and, 1150
 solute, 350
 water, 350
Diuretics:
 Bartter's syndrome and, 1789
 diabetes insipidus and, 366, 367
 hypercalcemia induced by, 1413
 hypercalciuria and, 1554, 1555
 hyponatremia caused by, 368
 hypoparathyroidism and, 1435
 magnesium and, 714
 potassium and, 756–57
DKA. *See* Ketoacidosis, diabetic.
DNA (deoxyribonucleic acid), 35–55
 chromatin packaging of, 37–38
 complementary, 48–49
 ectopic hormones and, 1695–96
  variable state hypothesis and, 1700
 enhancers of, 42
 estrogen receptor and, 139
 5′-flanking, 39
 glucocorticoids and, 548
  action of, 41–42
  receptors for, 559–60
 libraries of, 48–49
 linker, 38, 48
 matrix-bound, 144
 mRNA synthesis and, 60–61
 oncogenes and, 151
 promoter region of, 39
  protein synthesis and, 51
 recombinant, 44–55
  chromosomal genes and, 49
  cloning, 44–45, 47–50, 139
  diagnostic use of, 53–54
  drug delivery systems and, 52–53
  ethical and biosafety considerations, 54
  hybridization, 45–46, 49
  impact of, on medicine, 55
  insulin produced by, 47–48, 52, 1066–67
  proteins produced by, 50–52
  reverse transcription of mRNA, 48–49
  sequencing, 46–47
  synthesis of DNA, 47–48
  therapeutic use of, 54
  transfer of cloned genes into mammalian cells, 49–50
  vaccine produced by, 52
 regulatory regions of, 60
 replication of, 37
 steroid binding and, 143–44
 structure of, 35–37, 143
 3′flanking, 39
 thyroid hormone and, 149
 transcription of, 38–40, 60–63
  enhancers of, 61
  gene expression and, 41–42
  reverse, 48–49
  sequences and, 61
  steroid hormones and, 145–46
DNase (deoxyribonuclease), 38
DOC. *See* Deoxycorticosterone.
Docking protein, 63
Docosahexaenoic acid, 1289
Dolichol, 66
Domperidone, TSH and, 402
Dopa, 652, 653
L-Dopa:
 for acromegaly, 306
 growth hormone and, 325, 1622
 prolactin and, 327
  tumor secretion of, 308

Dopamine. *See also* Catecholamines, Neurotransmitters.
agonists of, 199
aldosterone and, 533–34
antagonists of, 199
biosynthesis, 196, 652–53
carcinoid and, 679
cardiovascular effects of, 660
chemistry, 652
Cushing's disease and, 603–4
degradation, 196, 653
edema and, 679
growth hormone and, 1585
neuronal network distribution, 195, 823
opioids and, 208
Parkinson's disease and, 681
pituitary effects of, 194, 195
polycystic ovary disease and, 963
prolactin and, 194, 207, 271, 272
tumor secretion of, 308, 310, 311
receptors for, 658
schizophrenia and, 238
TSH and, 402
Dorsomedial nucleus, 189, 190
Dorsum sellae, 247
Dose-response lines, 166, 167
chorionic gonadotropin, 173
immunoradiometric assay and, 177
radioimmunoassay and, 169, 170
validation of assay and, 176
Double-antibody technique, 174–75
Double-isotope technique for calcium, 1369
Down regulation of receptors, 98–99, 104
adrenergic receptors and, 657–58
Down's syndrome, hypogonadism and, 873
Doxorubicin:
prostate cancer and, 1761
thyroid cancer and, 500
Dromostanolone, 1748–49
Drugs. *See also specific agents.*
antithyroid, 432–36
hypothyroidism induced by, 449
appetite suppressing, 1238
catecholamines and, 684
cortisol affected by, 544
glucose tolerance and, 1109
gynecomastia induced by, 888
hypercalcemia associated with, 1413–15
hyperlipoproteinemia induced by, 1259–60
hyperprolactinemia induced by, 309, 958
hypoglycemic, 1140–44, 1194, 1195
hyponatremia induced by, 230
lipid-lowering, 1263–64, 1298–1305
neurotransmitter-influencing, 195–97
tabulations of, 198, 199
pituitary hormones affected by, 199
pregnancy and, 1601
recombinant DNA and delivery of, 52–53
SIADH induced by, 369
thyroid hormone and, 412, 415–17
uricosuric, 1519–20
vasopressin-affecting, 347–48, 369
Ductus arteriosus, prostaglandins and, 1778
Duodenum:
gastrin production by, 1630–31
ulcer of. *See* Peptic ulcer.
Dwarfism:
Laron, 1606
psychosocial, 239, 1607, 1613
Dynamic testing, 21
Dynein, 830, 833, 881
Dynorphin, 209
Dysalbuminemic hyperthyroxinemia, familial, 411
Dysbetalipoproteinemia, 1267–70
Dysdifferentiation hypothesis of ectopic hormones, 1699
Dysgerminoma, ovarian, hypercalcemia and, 1410
Dysmenorrhea, 970–74
prostaglandins and, 1773
treatment, 974
Dysphagia, 27
Dyspnea:
hyperthyroidism and, 426
obesity and, 1233–34

Eating behavior, 232, 1212–15
anorexia nervosa and. *See* Anorexia nervosa.
psychological factors, 1222–23
Ecdysone, chromatin and, 146
Ectopic hormone production, 17, 1692–1726. *See also* Tumors *and under specific hormones.*
APUD cell hypothesis and, 1700
dedifferentiation hypothesis and, 1699
definition of, 1692
derepression hypothesis and, 1698–99
diagnostic criteria, 1693–96
DNA variable state hypothesis and, 1700
dysdifferentiation hypothesis and, 1699
growth factors and, 1701
hypercalcemia and, 1702–6
hyperthyroidism and, 1715
hypoglycemia and, 1716–17
incidence, 1696–98
mechanisms of, 1698–1702
oncogenes and, 1700–1701
osteomalacia and, 1717–18
RAN specific to, 1695–96
sponge hypothesis and, 1698
tumor markers and, 1724–26
Edema:
aldosterone and, 621–22
cerebral, diabetic ketoacidosis and, 1154
heart failure and, 29
hypervolemic hyponatremia and, 368, 372
idiopathic, 622, 679
insulin-induced, 1138–39
mucinous. *See* Myxedema.
periorbital, 33–34
hyperthyroidism and, 441, 443
hypothyroidism and, 451, 452
treatment, 373
weight gain and, 25
EDTA, hypercalcemia and, 1421
Edwards syndrome, 233
EGF. *See* Epidermal growth factor.
EGTA, catecholamine samples and, 683
EHDP, hypercalcemia and, 1421
Eicosanoids, 1769. *See also* Leukotrienes; Prostaglandins; Thromboxane.
glucocorticoids and, 549
Eicosapentaenoic acid, 1289
Eicosatetraenoic acid, 130, 1771
Electrocardiography:
hypertension and, 734
sympathetic function and, 686
Electrophoresis, lipoprotein, 1245, 1307
Electrostatic interactions, hormone-receptor, 88
Eledoisin, 1651
Ellsworth-Howard test, 1444
Embden-Meyerhof pathway, 1047
Embryonal cell carcinoma, testicular, 892
Emesis, vasopressin and, 345–46
Emiocytosis, 1066
Emotional deprivation, 239, 1613
Empty sella syndrome. *See* Sella turcica, empty.
Enalapril, 705
renovascular hypertension and, 748
Encephalopathy:
hepatic, 681
hypertensive, 700
Endarterectomy, renal artery, 749
Endochondrial ossification, 1591
Endocrine system:
assessment of, 19–22
history and physical examination, 19
laboratory, 19–22
definition of, 3
disorders of, 15–19
evolution of, 9–12
hyperfunction, 17
secondary, 18
hypofunction, 15–16
integration of, 12–13
treatment of diseases of, 22
Endocrinology, definitions and scope of, 3–5
Endocytosis, receptor, 103, 106–9
Endometrium, 970–74
anatomy and physiology, 970–72
biopsy, 970
cancer, 1762–64
incidence, 1762
risk factors and etiology, 1762–63
treatment, 1763–64
hyperplasia, 980
estrogen-induced, 979
menarcheal menorrhagia and, 955
prostaglandins of, 972–74
Endonucleases, restriction, 44
Endopeptidase, 68
Endoperoxides, 130
Endoplasmic reticulum:
calcium release from, 119
peptide hormone synthesis and, 63–64
protein pathway and, 66
receptor biosynthesis and, 102–3
steroid synthesis and, 70–71
Endorphins, 209–11, 256–57
behavior and, 212
biosynthesis, 1708, 1709
chemistry, 253, 254
Cushing's disease and, 315
eating behavior and, 1213
ectopic, 1710
ovarian, 927
pituitary effects of, 198–99, 208

Endosomes, 107–8
  insulin and, 1079
Endosteum, 1329
Energy:
  expenditure of, 1217–19
  hyperthyroidism and, 428
  obesity from imbalance of, 1210–11, 1214, 1216–19
  regulatory and counterregulatory hormones, 1087–88
  tricarboxylic acid cycle and, 1052–53
Enkephalinase, 1784
Enkephalins, 209–11, 256
  anatomy and, 822–23
  growth hormone and, 269–70
Enteroglucagon, 1082
Enuresis, 29
Enzyme-linked immunosorbent assay (ELISA), 177
Enzymes. *See also specific enzyme.*
  activation of, 87
  calcium-dependent, 125–27
  catecholamine synthesis, 652–53
  gluconeogenic, 1049–51
  glycogenic, 1045–47
  glycolytic, 1047–49
  hormone action and, 84
  lipoprotein metabolism, 1251
  oncogenes and, 152
  peptide hormones and, 64, 68, 87, 94–96, 112–18
  phosphorylation of, 120–21
  renin-angiotensin system, 703, 705–6
  restriction, 44
  reverse transcriptase, 48
  steroid synthesis, 70, 1012
    adrenal, congenital defects in, 624–31
    ovarian, 924–26
  thyroid hormone synthesis, 77, 78
  tricarboxylic acid cycle, 1052
  tropic hormone induction of, 74
Eosinophilic granuloma, 224
Eosinophils:
  glucocorticoids and, 550
  pituitary, GH-secreting tumors and, 300
Epidermal growth factor (EGF), 1583
  ectopic hormone production and, 1701
  fibroblast processing of, 107
  goiter and, 474
  hypercalcemia of malignancy and, 1407–9, 1704
  receptor for, 92–93
    vs. insulin receptor, 94
    linear structure of, 92
    oncogenes and, 153, 154
    phosphorylation of, 101, 102
    protein kinase C and, 127
  transcription of genes and, 61
  vaccinia virus and, 154
Epididymis, 830
  gross appearance of, 829
Epinephrine. *See also* Catecholamines; Neurotransmitters.
  actions, 659–62
  biosynthesis, 196, 652–53
  blood pressure and, 659, 660
  carcinoid flush and, 1657
  chemistry, 652
  degradation, 196, 653
  diabetes mellitus and, 677, 678
  fed state and, 1090
  glucagon and, 659, 661, 1085–86, 1092
  glucose and, 659, 661, 1085
    hyperglycemia and, 661, 1137
    hypoglycemia and, 677–78, 1180, 1190
    synergism and, 1092
  glycogenolysis and, 1047
  hormonal role of, 664–66
  insulin and, 659, 661, 1071, 1085
  melatonin and, 217
  neurotransmitter function of, 666
  parathyroid hormone and, 660, 679
  pheochromocytoma and, 668, 669
  plasma levels, 662–63, 682–84
    conditions affecting, 664, 665, 683–84
    metabolic effect and, 659, 662
    sample handling and, 683
  pupillary response and, 685
  receptors for, 657–59
  Somogyi phenomenon and, 1137
Epiphyses:
  bone age and, 1598
  dysplasia of, 1611
  endochondral ossification of, 1461
Episomes, 44
Epitaxy, 1505
Epithelium, glucocorticoids and, 551–52
erb gene, 151, 153
  EGF receptor and, 93
Ergocalciferol, 73, 1344–46. *See also* Vitamin D.
  for hypocalcemia, 1434
  structure, 1345
Ergotamine, hypotension and, 676
Erythroblastosis, oncogenes and, 151, 153
Erythrocytes, tanned, agglutination of, 408
Erythrocytosis:
  Cushing's disease and, 28
  tumor-associated, 1721–22
Erythropoiesis. *See* Hematopoiesis.
Erythropoietin, 28, 1721–22
  prostaglandins and, 1776
  recombinant DNA production of, 52
Escherichia coli:
  insulin synthesis by, 1066–67
  restriction enzyme of, 44
Estradiol. *See also* Estrogens.
  biosynthesis, 72, 73, 1012
  gynecomastia and, 886, 887, 889
  hyperthyroidism and, 428, 429
  Klinefelter's syndrome and, 871
  metabolism, 75
  neonatal, 997
  spermatogenesis and, 851
  structure, 136, 516
  testosterone conversion to, 842, 851
  therapeutic, 978, 980. *See also* Ethinyl estradiol.
Estramustine, prostate cancer and, 1761
Estranes, 517
Estriol. *See also* Estrogens.
  breast cancer and, 1740
  neonatal, 997
Estrodopaminergic neurons, 823
Estrogens:
  adrenal, 516, 519, 536
    actions, 568
  antagonists of, 141–42
    breast cancer therapy and, 1749
    hypercalcemia induced by, 1415
  biosynthesis, 73, 924–26
    adrenal, 516, 519
    control of, 931
    follicle selection and, 936–39, 943
    two-cell-two-gonadotropin concept of, 936, 937, 939
  breast cancer and, 179, 979, 1740, 1742–46, 1748–52
  calcitonin and, 1472
  calcium and, 1472
  EBG and, 537
  endometrial cancer and, 1762–63
  gene structure and, 147–48
  GnRH and, 846–47
  gonadotropins and, 261, 262, 844–48
    clomiphene test and, 283, 323–24
    receptors and, 838
  granulosa cell differentiation and, 927–28
  growth and, 1590–91
  17α-hydroxylase deficiency and, 629
  hypercalcemia induced by, 1415
  hyperprolactinemia and, 307, 958
  insulin and, 1157
  insulin-like growth factor and, 1588
  Klinefelter's syndrome and, 1002
  liver and, 543, 979
  luteolysis and, 931
  menarcheal menorrhagia and, 955
  menopause and deficiency of, 975, 977
  metrorrhagia and, 30
  mRNA and, 145
  nuclear matrix and, 144
  obesity and, 1233
  oocyte maturation and, 934
  osteoporosis and, 977, 979, 1472–73, 1475
  ovulation and, 943, 944
  placental, 520
  polycystic ovary disease and, 962
  premature ovarian failure with deficiency of, 956
  premenarche and, 941, 942
  prostaglandins and, endometrial, 972–73
  prostate cancer and, 1756, 1760
  proteins regulated by, 145
  receptors for, 137–39
    assays of, 179, 1751, 1752
    breast cancer and, 1743, 1745–46, 1751–52
    DCC method for, 1751, 1752
    monoclonal antibodies to, 139
  sexual dimorphism and, 215
  structure, 136
  TBG levels and, 411
  testosterone and, 844–45, 851
    ovarian follicle atresia and, 935–36
  therapeutic, 285, 978–80
    atherosclerosis and, 978
    breast cancer and, 979, 1748
    dosage, 978
    endometrial cancer risk and, 1763
    hyperlipidemia and, 1269, 1304

Estrogens, therapeutic *(Cont.)*:
hyperparathyroidism and, 1402
hyperprolactinemia induced by, 958
Marfan's syndrome and, 1620
menopause and, 977
osteoporosis and, 1475
ovarian failure and, 957
preparations used in, 978
prostate cancer and, 1760
risks of, 979–80
Turner's syndrome and, 951–52, 1612
virilization defect in fetus and, 1019
thyrotropin and, 259
Estrone. *See also* Estrogens.
biosynthesis, 73
neonatal, 997
structure, 516
Ethanol. *See also* Alcohol.
gluconeogenesis and, 1051
Ethinyl estradiol, 978
breast cancer and, 1748
gonadotropin deficiency and, 285
hyperlipidemia and, 1269
Marfan's syndrome and, 1620
menopause and, 977
osteoporosis and, 1475
tall stature therapy with, 1614
Turner's syndrome and, 951, 1009
Ethylenediaminetetraacetic acid (EDTA), hypercalcemia and, 1421
Ethylene glycol, 1558
Etidronic acid, hypercalcemia and, 1421
Etiocholanediol, 542
Etiocholanolone:
actions, 568
chemistry, 516
plasma levels, 521
structure, 844
Etomidate, 522
Eunuchoidal proportions, 870
Klinefelter's syndrome and, 1001
Eunuchoidism, hypogonadotropic, 863–67
Euphoria, glucocorticoid therapy and, 793
Eutopic hormone secretion, 1692
Evolution of endocrine system, 9–12
Excess syndromes, 17–18
Exercise:
amenorrhea and, 954, 961
diabetes mellitus and, 1144–47
fuel metabolism and, 1091
glucose and, 1091, 1144–46
hyperglycemia induced by, 1146
hypoglycemia induced by, 1145–46
insulin and, 1145, 1146–47
ketogenesis and, 1146
obesity and, 1221, 1237
water loss and, 354
Exocytosis:
catecholamine, 655
peptide hormone, 67
Exons, 39, 40
calcitonin, 62
calcitonin/CGRP, 1339–40
evolution and, 43
intron boundaries with, 61
mRNA synthesis and, 60, 61
steroid hormones and, 147
Exophthalmos, Graves', 34
Eye, 33–34. *See also* Vision
cotton wool spots of, 1116–17
Cushing's syndrome and, iatrogenic, 793
diabetes mellitus and, 33, 34, 1115, 1116–19
insulin therapy and, 1130
metabolic changes and, 1127, 1128
fish, 1275–76
glucocorticoids and, 556
hypercalcemia and, 1395
hyperthyroidism and, 425, 440–43
LCAT deficiency and, 1280
mucosal neuromas of, 1677
muscles, 34
pain in, 33
swellings about, 33–34
vascular changes in, 733–34
Eyebrow, loss of, 34
Eyelids, hyperthyroidism and, 425, 441

Face:
acromegaly and, 301
moon, Cushing's syndrome and, 606
Turner's syndrome and, 1005
Fajans-Conn criteria for diabetes, 1110
Fanconi syndrome, 1464
Fasting:
glucocorticoid release and, 528–29
glucose levels and, 1108
hypoglycemia and, 1182–88, 1200–1201
insulin-like growth factor and, 1588
in normal subjects, 1182–83
pregnancy and, 1157
protein-sparing, 1236
thyroid hormone and, 78
deficiency of, 414
Fat. *See also* Adipose tissue; Cholesterol; Fatty acids; Lipids.
dietary, 1288–90, 1293
index of foods, 1294–96
fuel storage and, 1088
reproductive capacity and, 960
saturated, 1288, 1290, 1294–96
unsaturated, 1288–90
weight gain and, 25
Fatigue, 24
hypothyroidism and, 451, 452
Fatty acids, 1055–62
carbohydrate metabolism and, 1061–62
diabetes mellitus and, 1105–7, 1150
ketoacidosis and, 1257
exercise and, 1091, 1144
glucose cycle with, 1049, 1062
hypoglycin ingestion and, 1198
insulin and, 1058, 1070–71, 1076
ketogenesis and, 1059–60, 1150, 1257
metabolism, 1254
mobilization of, 1056–57
omega-3 and omega-6, 1289, 1293–94
oxidation, 1057–59
prostaglandins and, 129–30, 1771, 1780
synthesis, 1055–56
thyroid hormone and, 399
Fatty acid synthase, 1055
Fatty acyl CoA, 1058
Feces:
calcium in, 1353, 1369
phosphorus in, 1353
WDHA syndrome and, 1640
Fed state, fuel metabolism and, 1090–91
Feedback mechanisms:
ACTH, 187, 255–56, 530–31
Cushing's disease and, 316, 318
calcium, 1358
cholesterol, 1250
cortisol, 527, 530–31
CRF, 530–31
gonadotropin, 262–63, 844–48, 850
gonadotropin releasing hormone, 1590
hypothalamic, 186–87
long-loop, 186–87
neuroendocrine system, 185–87
phosphorus, 1349
pituitary, 186–87
short-loop, 187
thyroid hormone, 78
TSH, 259–60
vasopressin, 348
Feeding center, 232
Feminization:
of genitalia, 994
testicular, 875, 954, 1018–19
incomplete, 1019
Fenofibrate, 1304
α-Fetoprotein:
sexual dimorphism of brain and, 215
as tumor marker, 1725
Fetus. *See also* Pregnancy.
ACTH and, 520
adrenal glands of, 515, 520
alcohol syndrome of, 1601
androgens of, 941
diabetic mother and, 1155–62
fuel metabolism and, 1156–57
genital development of, 992–97
glucocorticoids and, 520, 557–58
growth of, 1591–92, 1601
growth hormone and, 1588
infections of, 1601
insulin of, 1156, 1161, 1588
ovaries of, 908, 940–41, 997
interstitial cells of, 916, 917
sex steroids of, 994–96
testes of, 996–97
thyroid hormone and, 409–10, 1589
hyperthyroidism and, 439
virilization of, 1011–31
in female, 1020–31
in male, 1011–20
Fever, 25
adrenal crisis and, 589
Fiber, dietary:
diabetes mellitus and, 1140
hyperlipidemia and, 1291
obesity and, 1236
Fibric acid derivatives, 1304
Fibrin, menstrual blood flow and, 971–72
Fibroblasts:
EGF processing by, 107
glucocorticoids and, 551–52
growth factor and, 1583
multiplication factor of, 265
pneumonocyte factor of, 1583

Fibrogenesis imperfecta ossium, 1466
Fibromuscular dysplasia, 737–38
intimal, 737
medial, 737–38
natural history, 739
periarterial, 738
treatment, 746–51
Fish eye disease, 1275–76
Flavoprotein, steroid synthesis and, 70
Fletcher factor, 1782
Floating beta disease, 1267–70
Florinef. *see* 9α-Fluorocortisol.
Fludrocortisone:
adrenal hyperplasia and, 1615
hypertension induced by, 768
Fluids. *See also* Water.
atrial natriuretic factor and, 722, 724
diabetic ketoacidosis and, 1153
Fluocinolone:
mineralocorticoid receptors and, 792
myxedema and, localized, 444
structure, 789
Fluoride:
glucocorticoid therapy and, 795
for osteoporosis, 1476
rickets and osteomalacia induced by, 1465
Fluorimetry:
catecholamine, 682
cortisol, 570, 571
9α-Fluorocortisol (9α-fluorohydrocortisone):
chronic adrenal insufficiency and, 595, 596
ectopic ADH and, 1712
21-hydroxylase deficiency and, 628, 1027
hyporeninemic hypoaldosteronism and, 598
postural hypotension and, 676
structure of, 136
Fluorouracil, prostate cancer and, 1761
Fluoxymesterone:
delayed adolescence and, 1600
growth hormone deficiency and, 1609
hypogonadism and, 876
libido in female and, 285
testosterone deficiency and, 286
Turner's syndrome and, 1008, 1612
Fluphenazine, vasopressin and, 345
Flushes:
carcinoid, 1655–58
menopausal, 976
premature ovarian failure and, 956
Flutamide, 1761
antiandrogen effects of, 142
Fogarty Conference weight tables, 1205
Folic acid deficiency, 28
Follicle-stimulating hormone (FSH), 260–63
action, 260
amenorrhea and, 955, 956
assays, 260–61
in children, 1621
hypopituitarism and, 281–83
in vivo, 169
techniques, 323–24
cells secreting, 251, 825
chemistry, 253, 257, 848
circadian rhythm of, 220
clomiphene and, 283, 323–24, 856, 860
control of secretion of, 262–63
in male, 848–50
deficiency, 277–78, 862–69
diagnostic procedures, 281–83
treatment, 285–86
drugs affecting, 199
estrogen and, 261, 262
feedback effects, 262–63, 850
fetal gonadal function and, 997
GnRH and, 262–63. *See also* Gonadotropin releasing hormone.
stimulation test, 282, 323, 856
granulosa cell differentiation and, 927–29
growth and, 1589, 1590, 1609
hypersecretion, 882
in male, 872, 874, 878–79
premature ovarian failure and, 956, 957
hyperthyroidism and, 428–29
hypopituitarism and, 277–78, 281–83, 285–86, 1610
hypothalamic disease and, 226–28, 282–83
hypothyroidism and, 455
inhibin and, 263, 849, 850
Kallmann's syndrome and, 864–67
Klinefelter's syndrome and, 872, 1001, 1002
LH-Leydig cell interactions with, 850–51
LH ratio to, 848–49
luteinization and, 930–31
luteolysis and, 931
menopause and, 975, 976
metabolism, 261–62, 849
obesity and, 1233
ovarian follicle selection and, 936, 938, 943
ovarian hormone synthesis and, 926
ovulation and, 943, 944
therapeutic induction of, 967–69
pituitary levels of, 261
plasma levels, 261, 282, 323, 854–55, 857
polycystic ovary disease and, 962, 963
premenarche and, 941, 942
production rate, 849
puberty and, 1593, 1594
delayed, 865
in male, 858–60
radioimmunoassay, 260
receptors for:
granulosa cell, 927
testicular, 849
reference preparation, 260
releasing factor, 202. *See also* Gonadotropin releasing hormone.
secretion rate, 261–62
secretory pattern, 834, 835, 849
spermatogenesis and, 849–50
stimulation tests, 282, 323–24, 855–56
testosterone and, 263
tumor secretion of, pituitary, 320–21, 882
Turner's syndrome and, 1007–8
urinary, 260, 261, 854, 855, 857
delayed puberty and, 866
Follicular regulatory protein, 927
Foot, diabetic, 1123–24
Forbes-Albright syndrome, 306
Formation product, nephrolithiasis and, 1505, 1508
Fractures:
Milkman, 1460
osteoporosis and, 1469, 1472
Paget's disease and, 1484
Fructokinase, 1049, 1197, 1198
Fructose:
diabetes mellitus and, 1140
intolerance to, 1197–98
Fructose-1,6-diphosphatase, 1048
deficiency, 1197, 1198
Fructose-1,6-diphosphate, 1047–49
Fructose-2,6-diphosphate, 1047
insulin release and, 1068
Fructose-6-phosphate, 1047
Fructose-1-phosphate aldolase, 1197
Fructosuria, 1198
FSH. *See* Follicle-stimulating hormone.
Fuel metabolism, 1041–1308
amino acids and, 1062–64
availability (fed state) and, 1090–91
basal state and, 1089
body composition and, 1088–89
carbohydrates and, 1045–55
diabetes mellitus and, 1107
fats and, 1055–62
hormone interactions and, 1088–92
imbalances of, 1092
insulin and, 1064–82
maternal-fetal, 1156–57
need and, 1091
physiology of, 1043–92
regulatory and counterregulatory hormones, 1087–88
tricarboxylic acid cycle and, 1052–53
Fundus, optic, 733–34
diabetes mellitus and, 1116–17
Fungal infections:
diabetes mellitus and, 1125
hypoparathyroidism and, 1681, 1682
Furosemide:
calciuresis and, 1420
ectopic ADH and, 1712, 1713

G cells, 1630–31, 1635
electron micrograph of, 1632
G protein, 1085
pseudohypoparathyroidism and, 1428–29
Gaisböck's disease, 698
Galactorrhea, 30–31
amenorrhea and, 958
differential diagnosis, 309, 310
hyperprolactinemia and, 230, 306–15
normoprolactinemic, 310
Gallbladder:
cholecystokinin and, 1637
pancreatic polypeptide (PP) and, 1646
Gallium nitrate, hypercalcemia of malignancy and, 1706
Gallstones:
hyperparathyroidism and, 1390
obesity and, 1234
Gamma-aminobutyric acid. *See also* Neurotransmitters.
agonist of, 199
pituitary effects of, 195
synthesis and metabolism, 196
Gamma globulin, radioimmunoassay and, 171–72
Gangliocytoma, 223
Ganglioneuromatosis, MEN 2 and, 1677
Gangrene, diabetes and, 1123–24

Gastrectomy:
for gastrinoma, 1636
hypergastrinemia and, 1635
hypoglycemia after, 1191–92
Gastric inhibitory polypeptide (GIP), 1641–43
actions, 1642
amino acid sequence of, 1639
chemistry, 1641
diseases and, 1643
distribution, assay, and release, 1641–42
insulin and, 1070, 1642
Gastrinoma, 1630–36
actions and metabolism, 1632–33
antibodies to, separation technique for, 174–75
big, 1630, 1631
calcitonin and, 1341, 1343–44
chemistry, 1630
distribution, 1630–31
hyperparathyroidism and, 1389
inhibition of, 1632
measurement, 1631
pituitary effects of, 199
release, 1631–32
releasing peptide (GRP), 1640
ectopic, 1720–21
sample handling, 180
secretin test, 1634
somatostatin and, 1648, 1649
tumor secretion of. *See* Gastrinoma.
Zollinger-Ellison syndrome and, 1633–36
Gastrinoma, 1633–36, 1665
diagnosis, 1633–35
hyperparathyroidism and, 1389
MEN 1 and, 1663, 1664, 1669
nonpancreatic, 1723
symptoms and signs, 1633
therapy, 1636, 1669
Gastrointestinal system, 27. *See also* Intestine.
Addison's disease and, 587
carcinoid tumors of, 1652–59
catecholamines and, 681–82
diabetes mellitus and, 1123
endocrine disease and, 27
glucagon of, 1644
glucocorticoids and, 556–57
hormones of, 1629–52
hyperoxaluria and, 1558–59, 1561
hyperparathyroidism and, 1389–90
hyperthyroidism and, 426
hypothyroidism and, 454
insulin influences of, 1070, 1071
MEN 2 and, 1677
prostaglandins and, 1776
vitamin D effects on, 1354–55
absorption and, 1352–53, 1355
Gastroparesis diabeticorum, 1123
Gastroplasty, obesity and, 1239
Gemfibrozil, 1302
action and toxicity, 1302
hyperlipidemia and, 1264, 1274, 1302
indications and dosage, 1302
Gender role, 984, 999–1000. *See also* Sex assignment.
5α-reductase deficiency and, 1017, 1018
Genes, 33–55. *See also* Chromosomes; Genetic factors.
calcitonin, 40, 1339–40
organization of, 62
c-Ha-ras, 55
cloning of, 44–45, 49–50
coordinate induction of, 61
deletions of, 44
deregulation of, oncogenes and, 150–51
erb, 151, 153
EGF receptor and, 93
evolution of, 10, 11, 43–44
expression of, 39–43
protein production and, 51
regulation of, 41–43
RNA processing and, 42–43
steroids and, 146
thyroid hormone and, 150
transcription and, 41–42
transient assay of, 50
families of, 43
glucocorticoid, 41–42, 50, 146
growth hormone, 263
evolution of family of, 43
glucocorticoid regulatory element and, 42
21-hydroxylase, 1021–22
insulin, 54
kallikrein, 1782
lactogen, placental, 43
LDL receptor, 40
mRNA synthesis and, 60–63
myc, 151, 1701
neu, 153
nuclear matrix and, 144–45
ovalbumin, 147–48
polymorphisms of, 53–54
prolactin, 43
promoter region of, 39, 41–42
ras, 152–53
renin, 702
ros, 152
sis, 55, 154
src, 152
steroid hormones and, 145–48
therapeutic use of, 54
transcription of, 60–63. *See also* DNA, transcription of.
steroid hormone control of, 145–46
transfer techniques for, 49–50, 54
tumor-promoting, 55. *See also* Oncogenes.
upstream-downstream portions of, 35–37
viral transforming. *See* Oncogenes.
Genetic factors. *See also* Genes; Chromosomes.
abetalipoproteinemia and, 1278–79
Addison's disease and, 585, 586
cancer and, 55
breast, 1741
medullary, of thyroid, 501, 502
prostate, 1753–54
cystinuria and, 1512
diabetes insipidus and, 356–57
diabetes mellitus and, 54, 1094–96
complications and, 1125, 1130
diagnostic considerations, DNA in, 53–54
goiter and, 480–81
Graves' disease and, 420–21
growth and, 1582, 1599, 1611–14, 1619
growth hormone deficiency and, 1605–6
haploidy and, 984
hyperlipidemia and, 1263, 1265, 1268, 1271, 1273
hypertension and, 697
hypofunction of glands and, 16
hypogonadism and, 863, 867, 870–73
hypothyroidism and, 480–81
infertility and, 881
Klinefelter's syndrome and, 870–72
molecular mechanisms of disease and, 44
mosaicism and. *See* Mosaicism.
multiple endocrine neoplasia and, 1666, 1667–68
obesity and, 1211–12
ovarian failure and, 956–57
pluriglandular insufficiency and, 1686
sex determination and, 984, 985–89, 1000–1009
Genitals:
adrenal hyperplasia and, congenital, 1615
agonadism and, 1011
clinical approach to abnormalities of, in newborn, 1031–33
17,20-desmolase deficiency and, 1015
differentiation of, 992–96
androgens and, 995–96
external, 994
internal, 992–94
femininization of, 994
testicular, 954, 1018, 1019
flowchart for evaluation of, 1032
gonadal dysgenesis and, 1004, 1005
hermaphroditism and, 1004
17α-hydroxylase deficiency and, 1014
21-hydroxylase deficiency and, 627, 1023, 1029
3β-hydroxysteroid dehydrogenase deficiency and, 630, 1013
17β-hydroxysteroid dehydrogenase deficiency and, 1015
masculinization of, 955, 994, 995
multiple malformation syndromes and, 1020
plastic repair of, 1029, 1032
pseudohermaphroditism and, 1010
5α-reductase deficiency and, 1017
teratological malformations of, 1030–31
Germinal cells:
ovarian:
aging and, 911
differentiation of, 932–34
primordial, 932
sex determination and, 989, 992
testicular, 827–32
cryptorchism and, 885
failure of, 878–82. *See also* Azoospermia.
Leydig cell interactions with, 850–51
number determination, 852, 853
physiology, 848–51
stem cell renewal and differentiation pathways, 827, 830
tumors of, 892
Germinoma, pineal, 236

Gigantism, 301
  cerebral, 237, 1620
  in childhood, 1618–19
    diabetic mother and, 1621
  differential diagnosis, 303
  lipodystrophy and, 1621
Gilbert-Dreyfus syndrome, 1019
GIP. *See* Gastric inhibitory polypeptide.
GLA protein. *See* Osteocalcin.
Glaucoma, 34
  diabetes mellitus and, 1119
  glucocorticoids and, 556, 793
GLI (glucagon-like immunoreactants), 1082, 1644–45
Glicentin, 1082, 1645
Glioma, pineal gland, 236
Glipizide, 1141, 1142
Globulin. *See* Corticosteroid-binding globulin; Sex hormone-binding globulin; Thyroxine-binding globulin.
Globus hystericus, 483
Glomerular filtration rate:
  atrial natriuretic factor and, 720–21
  diabetes mellitus and, 1119
  glucocorticoids and, 553
  mineralocorticoids and, 564
  phosphorus and, 1361, 1367–68. *See also* Phosphorus, tubular maximum (TmP/GFR).
    threshold for, 1334
  prostaglandins and, 1775
Glomerulosclerosis, diabetic, 1114–15, 1120
Glucagon, 1082–85
  actions, 1083–85
  big plasma, 1082
  biosynthesis, 1082
  calcitonin and, 1673
  cAMP and, 1085
  chemistry, 1082
  circulating, 1082–83
    glucose and, 1068
  degradation, 1085
  diabetes mellitus and, 1103, 1105
    glucagonoma and, 1164–65
    hypoglycemia and, 1136–37
  energy regulation and, 1087–88
  epinephrine and, 659, 661, 1085–86, 1092
  exercise and, 1145
  fed state and, 1081, 1090
  gastrointestinal, 1644
  glucocorticoids and, 545
  glucose and, 1068, 1083–84, 1103
    hypoglycemia and, 677, 1136–37, 1180, 1190
    synergism and, 1092
  glycogenolysis and, 119
  growth hormone and, 1622
  insulin ratio to, 1083–84
  ketogenesis and, 1084–85
  MEN 1 and, 1664–65
  norepinephrine and, 658
  porcine, amino acid sequence of, 1639
  protein meal and, 1083, 1084
  receptors for, 1085
    hydrophobic interactions and, 89
  secretion, 1083
  somatostatin and, 1072, 1083
  stress and, 1092
  tumor secretion of, 1664–65
    diabetes mellitus and, 1164–65
Glucagon-like immunoreactants (GLI), 1082, 1644–45
Glucan transferase, 1046
Glucocorticoids, 522–31, 544–63. *See also* Cortisol.
  ACTH and, 255–56, 525–31
    ectopic, 1706–11
    glucocorticoid therapy and, 284–85, 531, 802–3, 811–12
    stimulation test, 576–78
  actions, 544–61, 790–91
  adrenergic receptors and, 558–59
  agonists, 561–62, 799
  angiotensin and, 553
  antagonists, 142, 561–62
  assays, 569–79
  behavioral effects, 555
  binding, 536–39
    activation step in, 560
    competitive, radioassay and, 569, 571
  biosynthesis, 69, 518–19, 1012
    pathway of, 71, 72
  blood pressure and, 552, 726
  bone and, 554–55, 793–95
  calcium and, 554–55
    osteoporosis and, 794–95
  carbohydrate metabolism and, 544–46
  cardiovascular system and, 552–53
  catecholamines and, 556, 678
  coverage for surgery (illness, or trauma), 596–97, 808, 814
    pituitary, for Cushing's disease, 616–17
  deficiency, 581–97. *See also* Adrenocortical insufficiency.
    enzyme defects and, 624–30
    familial, 586
  definition of, 563
  depression (mental) and, 238, 530, 555
  DNA and, 41–42, 50, 548
  eicosanoids and, 549
  epithelial tissue and, 551–52
  eye and, 556
  feedback mechanism and, 527, 530–31
  fibroblasts and, 551–52
  gastrointestinal effects, 556–57
  genes for, 41–42, 50, 146
    transcription of, 61
  glucagon and, 545
  glucose and, 544–46, 1086
    synergism and, 1092
  glycogen and, 546–47
  growth and development and, 557–58, 808–9
  hematopoiesis and, 551
  historical note on, 511–13
  hormonal interactions of, 558
  hypersecretion, 599–620. *See also* Cushing's syndrome.
  hypertension and, 726, 766–68
    insensitivity and, 769
  immune response and, 548–49, 790–91
  inflammatory response and, 548–49, 790, 801
  insulin and, 544, 546, 808, 1086
  integrated actions of, 13
  kidney and, 553, 566
  leukocytes and, 549–51
  lipids and, 547–48
  liver and, 544–45, 548
  luteinizing hormone and, 558
  metabolism, 540–42, 544–48, 797–99
    variations in, 543–44
  mineralocorticoid activity of, 539, 560, 565–67, 790, 792
  molecular mechanisms, 559–61, 791–92
  muscle and, 545, 548
  nervous system and, 555–56
  plasma state of, 536–39
  potassium and, 553–54
  prostaglandins and, 549, 553
  protein and, 145, 545–46, 548
  receptors for, 140, 559–61
    affinity enhancement and, 562–63
    gene expression and, 41–42
    heterogeneity of, 560
    mineralocorticoid receptors and, 539, 560, 565–67, 790, 792
    nuclear binding of, 143
    structure of, 559–60
    therapeutic effects and, 791–92, 800, 804
  regulation of, 522–31
  regulatory element (GRE), 41–42, 50, 143, 560
    gene expression and, 146
  renin and, 553
  resistance to, 769, 799–800
  RNA and, 145, 531, 548, 560–61, 792
  stress and, 559
  structure, 136, 516, 789
  structure-activity relations, 562–63
  synergisms, 558–59, 1092
  testosterone and, 558
  therapeutic, 788–814
    ACTH and, 284–85, 531, 802–3, 811–12
    addisonian crisis and, 594
    adjunctive therapy, 805
    adjusting dose of, 806
    adrenal hyperplasia and, 1615
    adverse effects, 791, 792–96, 805
    aerosol, 802
    agonist activity of, 799
    aldosteronism and, 754–55, 762
    alternate-day, 806–7
    asthma and, 791, 802
    atherosclerosis and, 796
    binding of, 538
    bioavailability of, 796–97
    bone necrosis from, 793
    breast cancer and, 1749–50
    chronic adrenal insufficiency and, 595
    circadin rhythm and, 805–6
    concentration at site of action, 799
    Cushing's syndrome induced by, 792–96
    diabetes mellitus and, 808
    distribution of, 797
    dose-response considerations, 796, 804
    empirical data for, 803
    eye changes and, 793
    hirsutism and, 965
    21-hydroxylase deficiency and, 627, 1027
    hypercalcemia and, 1421

Glucocorticoids, therapeutic *(Cont.)*:
hypothalamic-pituitary-adrenal axis suppression by, 806, 807, 809–14
indications, 789
infections complicating, 795
intraarticular, 801–2
intramuscular, 797
Kaposi's sarcoma and, 809
kinetic considerations, 792, 809–12
leukemia and, 790, 800, 804
metabolism and clearance of, 797–99
mineralocorticoid receptors and, 792
myopathy from, 795
objective criteria and, 805
oral, 800
osteoporosis and, 793–95, 1473, 1476
parenteral, 800–801
patient education and, 596
pediatric, 808–9
peptic ulcer and, 556–57, 808
physiological and pharmacological actions, 790–91
pituitary surgery and, 298
potency of, 562–63, 796–800
pregnancy and, 807–8
preparations used in, 800–803
psychiatric disorders and, 808
reversibility of effects of, 796
selection of patients for, 803
sensitivity to, 799–800, 803–4
short-term vs. long-term, 803
surgery and, 596–97, 616–17, 808, 814
thyroid storm and, 438
topical, 797, 802
withdrawal syndromes, 812–14
thyroid hormone and, 415, 543, 558
hyperthyroidism and, 428
hypothyroidism and, 455
thyrotropin and, 259, 402, 415
vitamin D and, osteoporosis and, 794–95
water balance and, 553
Glucokinase, 1045, 1047, 1074
Gluconeogenesis, 1049–51
alcohol and, 1196
diabetes mellitus and, 1104
exercise and, 1144–45
fat metabolism and, 1062
glucagon and, 1083
glucocorticoids and, 544–46
glycolysis integrated with, 1051–52
insulin and, 1074–75
starvation and, 1091, 1182, 1183
Glucose:
acetyl CoA and steroid relationship to, 10
alanine and, 1051, 1062–64
basal state and, 1089, 1909
catabolism, *See* Glycolysis.
catecholamines and, 658, 659, 661, 1085
synergism and, 1092
counterregulatory mechanisms, 677, 1087–88
dawn phenomenon and, 1137
deficiency, 1179–1201. *See also* Hypoglycemia.
diabetes mellitus and, 1104
impaired tolerance and, 1094, 1110, 1165
laboratory studies, 1108–12
protein interactions and, 1105
evolution of ligands and, 9, 10
excess. *See* Diabetes mellitus; Hyperglycemia.
exercise and, 1091, 1144–46
fasting and, 1108, 1182–83
fatty acid cycle with, 1062
fed state and, 1081, 1090
formation of, 1047. *See also* Gluconeogenesis.
GIP and, 1642
glucagon and, 1068, 1083–84, 1103
hypoglycemia and, 677, 1136–37, 1180, 1190
synergism and, 1092
glucocorticoids and, 544–46, 1086
synergism and, 1092
glycogenolysis and. *See* Glycogenolysis.
growth hormone and, 267–69, 325–26, 677, 1086, 1137
acromegaly and, 302–3
ingestion of, 1070, 1073–74, 1090
hypoglycemia and, 1181, 1190
insulin and:
biphasic response of, 1069
diabetes mellitus and, 1100–1102
metabolic actions of, 1073–75
obesity and, 1228–31
oral glucose ingestion and, 1070, 1073–74
stimulation of secretion of, 1068–70
metabolism, 1045–55
fat metabolism and, 1061–62
muscle and, 1144
pentose shunt and, 1053
phosphorylation of, 1045, 1074
plasma levels:
exercise and, 1144
fasting, 1108
glucose loading and, 1110
hypoglycemia definition and, 1180
hypoglycemic symptoms and, 1136
impaired tolerance and, 1110
insulin and, 1068
self-monitoring of, 1133–35
steady-state, 1101
polyol pathway and, 1053–54
pregnancy and, 1156–59
protein bonding of, 1054–55
starvation and, 1091, 1108
storage. *See* Glycogen.
synergism of hormones and, 13, 1092
thyroid hormones and, 399
hyperthyroidism and, 428
hypothyroidism and, 454
tolerance, 1108–9
cirrhosis or uremia and, 1165
impaired, 1094, 1110, 1165
obesity and, 1226, 1227
tolerance testing, 1108–11
flat curve and, 1110
hypoglycemia and, 1189–90, 1199
indications, 1110–11
intravenous, 1111
oral, 1108–11
pregnancy and, 1158
transport, 1080
receptor processing and, 109
tricarboxylic acid cycle and, 1052–53
tumor consumption of, 1187, 1716
urinary, 1111–12, 1116
monitoring of, 1132
vasopressin and, 342, 343, 346
WDHA syndrome and, 1640
Glucose-dependent insulinotropic polypeptide, 1642
Glucose-6-phosphatase, 1049, 1051
deficiency, uric acid stones and, 1519
Glucose-1-phosphate, 1047
Glucose-6-phosphate, 1045, 1047
Glucose-6-phosphate dehydrogenase, 1053
Glucuronide, corticosteroid metabolism and, 542
Glutamine:
cystinuria and, 1516
protein feeding and, 1064
release and uptake of, 1062, 1063
synthesis and metabolism, 196
Glutamyl transpeptidase, 1773
Glutathione:
catecholamine samples and, 683
leukotrienes and, 1773
Glyburide, 1141, 1142
Glycation:
lipoprotein, 1123
protein, 1054, 1112
diabetic complications and, 1128–29
Glyceric aciduria, 1557
Glycerol, 1055
epinephrine and, 659
gluconeogenesis and, 1050
norepinephrine and, 658
Glycerol kinase, 1056
Glycerol-3-phosphate, 1056, 1057
Glycerophosphate dehydrogenase, 1050
Glycine, production of, 1557
Glycogen, 1045–47
caloric value of, 1088
exercise and, 1091
glucocorticoids and, 546–47
insulin and, 1073–75
metabolism, 118–19. *See also* Glycogenolysis.
muscle, 1144
synthesis, 1045–47
Glycogenolysis, 118–19, 1047
catecholamines and, 119, 1047, 1085
exercise and, 1144
glucagon and, 119
insulin and, 1075
schema of, 120
starvation and, 1182, 1183
Glycogen phosphorylase, 118, 1046, 1047
Glycogen synthase, 119, 1046
glucocorticoids and, 547
Glycohemoglobin, 1054, 1112, 1113
diabetic complications and, 1128–29
Glycolic aciduria, 1557
Glycolysis, 1047–49
fat metabolism and, 1062
gluconeogenesis integrated with, 1051–52
insulin and, 1068, 1074
tricarboxylic acid cycle and, 1052

Glycoprotein:
  α_1 acid, 537
  ectopic, 1714–15
  metabolism of, 68
  pituitary hormones, 257–63. *See also* Follicle-stimulating hormone; Luteinizing hormone; Thyrotropin.
    classification, 253
  radioimmunoassay of, 173
  steroid hormone transport, 75
Glycosaminoglycans, hypothyroidism and, 451
Glycosuria, 1111–12, 1116
Glycosylation:
  peptide hormone, 65–66
  protein, 1054, 1055
Glycyrrhizic acid, 768
Glyoxalate, 1556–57
Goiter, 473–86
  age and, 475, 476, 480
  autoimmunity and, 445–46
  cancer and, 477, 483–84
  cassava and, 478–79, 482
  classification, 473, 474
  clinical presentation, 477, 483
  definition, 473
  diet and, 476–77, 482
  diffuse toxic, 418–21
  endemic, 476–79
    cretinism and, 478, 479
    development, 477
    prophylaxis, 479
  etiology, 474–76
  genetic factors, 480–81
  geography and, 476
  goitrogens, 478–79, 481–82
  historical overview, 473–74
  hyperthyroidism and, 422–23, 425–26, 437–38, 477, 484
  hypothyroidism and, 452
  incidence, 482–83
  iodide organification defect and, 448
  iodine deficiency and, 474, 476–78
  laboratory studies, 484
  malnutrition and, 479
  nontoxic, 482–86
  pregnancy and, 480
  sex and, 480
  sporadic, 479–82
  therapy, 484–86
  thyrotropin and, 474–76
  toxic multinodular, 422–23, 437–38
  toxic uninodular, 423
Goitrogens, 478–79, 481–82
Goldberg-Hogness box, 60
Goldblatt model of hypertension, 707
Golgi apparatus:
  endocytosis and, 107–8
  oligosaccharides and, 66
  peptide secretion and, 65, 66
  receptor biosynthesis and, 103
  transport proteins and, 109
Gonadarche, 1589–90
Gonadoblastoma, 1005
Gonadocrinins, 840
Gonadostat, 858, 860
Gonadotroph cells, 251, 825
Gonadotropin(s). *See also* Follicle-stimulating hormone; Luteinizing hormone.
  chorionic (hCG):
    anorchia and, 873
    assays, 166, 167
    chemistry, 253, 257
    corpus luteum and, 930–31
    cryptorchism and, 883, 886
    delayed adolescence and, 876, 1600
    desialylated, 167
    dose-response lines, 173
    ectopic, 1713–15
    fetal gonadal function and, 996, 997
    hyperthyroidism and, 424, 1715
    hypogonadism and, 876, 877
    infertility and, 286
    LH homology with, 173–74
    LH receptor suppression and, 838
    ovarian cytodifferentiation and, 929, 930–31
    testosterone and, 851, 857
    as tumor markers, 1724
  deficiency, 861–69, 877
  endocytosis of, 109
  inhibition of, 157–58
  neurotransmitter effects on, 195
  receptor regulation by, 104
Gonadotropin releasing hormone (GnRH), 202–4
  analogues of, 203–4. *See also* therapeutic *subentry below*.
    desensitization of pituitary by, 157
  anatomy and, 821–22
  anorexia nervosa and, 234
  assays, 835
  associated peptide (GAP), 271
  behavioral effects of, 204
  catecholamines and, 832–33
  chemistry and effects, 202–4
  deficiency, 862–64
  distribution, 191, 192, 202
    species differences in, 202, 203
  estrogen and, 203, 846–47
  fat tissue and, 960
  feedback mechanism, 1590
  fetal, 997
  FSH release and, 262–63, 848
    stimulation test, 282, 323, 856
  growth and, 1589, 1590, 1609
  hamartomas and, 223
  hypergonadism and, 228
  hyperprolactinemia and, 307, 862, 863
  hypogonadism and, 226–28
  Kallmann's syndrome and, 864–66, 953
  LH and, 262–63
    stimulation test, 282, 323, 856
  luteolysis and, 931
  neurotransmitters and, 195, 197, 204
  physiology, 832–35
  pituitary effects of, 836–37
  polycystic ovary disease and, 962, 963
  Prader-Willi syndrome and, 232, 233
  pulsatile release of, 203, 834–35
  structure, 200
  testicular germ cells and, 850–51
  testosterone and, 203, 845
  therapeutic, 157–58
    breast cancer and, 1744
    infertility and, 286
    ovulation induction and, 967, 969–70
    precocious puberty and, 228, 1618
    prostate cancer and, 891, 1761
Gonads. *See also* Ovaries; Testes.
  bisexual, 1003–4
  differentiation of, 989–92
  dysgenesis of, 1004–10
    Klinefelter's syndrome and, 870–72
    mixed, 1004–5
    mosaicism and, 952
    pseudohermaphroditism and, male, 1010
    short stature and, 1612
    Turner's syndrome and, 951–52, 1005–9
    XX, 1009
    XY (Swyer), 1009–10
  sex determination and, 984, 989–92
Gossypol, 891
Gout, 31
  Bartter's syndrome and, 1787
  hyperparathyroidism and, 1391
  nephrolithiasis and, 1517, 1518–19, 1561, 1562
Gpp(NH)p, adenylate cyclase activation and, 95–96, 112
Graafian follicle, 913–15
  artresia of, 935–36
  premenarche, 941, 942
Granuloma, eosinophilic, 224
Granulomatous diseases, hypercalcemia and, 1415–16, 1418
Granulosa cells, ovarian, 908, 911–16
  antibodies to, 1684
  antimüllerian hormone and, 993
  basal lamina of, 911, 912
  Call-Exner bodies and, 912
  cavitation and, 912–13
  degeneration of, 915–16, 935–36
  development of, 908, 911–15
  differentiation of, 927–29
  gap junction of, 913, 914
  graafian follicle and, 913–15
  heterogeneity in, 915, 929
  hormone synthesis and, 73, 924, 926
  luteinization and, 921–23
  luteolysis and, 923
  metabolism in, 926
  oocyte growth and, 932, 933
  premenarche, 941, 942
  receptor changes in, 927, 928
  recruitment of follicles and, 934
  selection of follicles and, 936, 938
  sexual differentiation and, 992
Gravel passage, 1502
Graves' disease, 418–21
  acropachy and, 420, 444
  clinical manifestations, 425–28, 440–44
  etiology and pathogenesis, 418–20
  euthyroid, 442–43
  genetic factors, 420–21
  myxedema and, localized, 420, 443–44
  ophthalmopathy, 33, 420, 440–43
  pathology, 421
  remissions, 421, 432
  treatment, 432–37

Growth, 31, 1581–1624
acromegaly and, 301, 1618–19. *See also* Acromegaly.
ACTH and, 1622, 1623–24
adipose tissue, 1208–10, 1222
adolescent, 1593–95
adrenal hyperplasia and, 1610, 1614–16
androgens and, 1589–90, 1609, 1615
anoxemia and, 1613
bone disorders and, 1458, 1611
brain, 1581
cellular, 1581, 1582
childhood (2 years to puberty), 1593
chromosomal abnormalities and, 1611–13, 1619
control of, 1582–91
curves, 1597–98
Cushing's syndrome and, 1609–10
emotional deprivation and, 239, 1613
endochondrial ossification and, 1591
estrogens and, 1590–91
excess, 1613–21. *See also* Acromegaly; Tall stature.
normal variants and, 1613–14
pathologic, 1614–21
genetic factors, 1582, 1599, 1611–14, 1619
gigantism and, 301. *See also* Gigantism.
cerebral, 237, 1620
glucocorticoids and, 557–58, 808–9
gonadotropins and, 1589, 1590, 1609
growth hormone and, 1584–89
assays, 1608, 1621, 1622
deficiency, 1604–9
excess, 1618–19
homocystinuria and, 1619–20
hormonal regulation of, 14, 15, 1583–91
hypopituitarism and, 861–62
infant (to 2 years), 1592
intrauterine, 1591–92, 1601
Klinefelter's syndrome and, 870, 1619
linear, 1591–93
Marfan's syndrome and, 1619–20
nutrition and, 1591, 1601–2
obesity and, 1620–21
physiology, 1591
precocious puberty and, 1610–11, 1616–18
prolactin and, 1623
pubertal, 1589–90, 1593–95
rickets and, 1458
short stature and, 1595–1613. *See also* Short stature.
Soto's syndrome and, 1620
stages of:
biologic, 1581
developmental, 1591–95
testing procedures for, 1621–24
thyroid hormone and, 460, 1589, 1602–4, 1619
thyrotropin (TSH) and, 1622
tissue-specific factors and, 1582–83. *See also* Growth factors.
Turner's syndrome and, 1008, 1612
vasopressin and, 1623
XYY genotype and, 1619
Growth factors, 1583
autocrine secretion and, 85
biosynthetic capacity and, 74–75
bone, 1491
colony-stimulating, oncogenes and, 153
ectopic hormone production and, 1701
epidermal. *See* Epidermal growth factor.
fibroblast, 1583
goiter and, 474
hypercalcemia of malignancy and, 1407–9, 1704
insulin-like. *See* Insulin-like growth factors.
nerve, 1583
oncogenes and, 153–54, 1701
platelet-derived. *See* Platelet-derived growth factors.
transforming. *See* Transforming growth factor.
tumor-derived, 1407–9, 1704
Growth hormone (GH), 264–70
action, 264–65, 1585–86
arginine infusion test, 325, 1622
assays, 324–26
in children, 1608, 1621, 1622
hypopituitarism and, 283–84
in vivo, 169
big, 264
biosynthesis, 264
breast cancer and, 1744
cells secreting, 250–51
chemistry, 253, 263
clonidine and, 283, 325, 1622
control of secretion of, 266–70, 1584
factors affecting, 268
Cushing's disease and, 317
deficiency, 278, 1604–9
causes, 1605
congenital, 1604–6
diagnosis, 283–84, 1608
genetic, 1605–6
hypothalamic disease and, 229
inflammatory disease and, 1607
isolated, 1605–6
radiation-induced, 1607
transient, 1607–8
trauma and, 1607
treatment, 286–87, 1608–9
tumors and, 1607
depression (mental) and, 238
diabetes mellitus and, 1129
acromegaly and, 1164
L-dopa and, 325, 1622
dopamine and, 1585
drugs affecting, 199
ectopic, 1718–19
emotional deprivation and, 239
energy regulation and, 1087–88
enkephalins and, 211, 269–70
epinephrine and, 659
fed state and, 1090
fetus and, 1588
genes for, 263
evolution of family of, 43
glucocorticoid regulatory element and, 42
glucose and, 267–69, 325–26, 677, 1086
acromegaly and, 302–3
dawn phenomenon and, 1137
growth and, 1584–89
assays and, 1608, 1621, 1622
excess, 1618–19
failure of, 1604–9
hormonal effects on, 269
hypersecretion, 300–306. *See also* Acromegaly.
hyperthyroidism and, 428
hypoglycemia and, 283, 324–25, 1181
in children, 1604, 1608, 1622
hypopituitarism and, 278, 283–84, 286–87
hypothyroidism and, 455, 1607–8
inactive, 1606
insulin and, 265, 1086
insulin hypoglycemia and, 283, 324–25, 1622
insulin-like growth factor and, 1585–89
metabolic changes and release of, 267–69, 1586
metabolism, 266
neural stimuli and, 267
neuropeptides and, 199
neurosecretory dysfunction and, 1606
neurotransmitters and, 195, 269
obesity and, 1215, 1233
opioid peptides and, 211, 269–70
pituitary levels, 266
plasma levels, 266, 283, 324
acromegaly and, 302
in children, 1608
puberty and, 1589, 1590
radioimmunoassay, 266
radioreceptor assay, 266
recombinant DNA production of, 52
release inhibiting hormone. *See* Somatostatin.
releasing hormone (GRH), 206–7, 266–67, 1584–85
acromegaly and, 229, 303, 304
chemistry and effects, 206–7
ectopic, 303, 304, 1719
hamartomas and, 223
regulation of, 1585
response test, 283, 284
structure of, 200
synthetic, 1585
therapeutic use of, 287
resistance to, 1606
schizophrenia and, 238
secretion rate, 266
secretory pattern, 220, 1585
secretory granules, 300
serotonin and, 1585
sleep-associated changes in, 220, 267, 268
somatostatin and. *See* Somatostatin.
stimulation tests, 283–84, 324–25
suppression test, 325–26
synthetic, 1608–9
therapeutic:
congenital deficiency and, 1604
Creutzfeldt-Jakob disease and, 1609
hypopituitary children and, 1608–9
short stature and, 1599
Turner's syndrome and, 1612
thryoid hormone and, 150, 428, 455, 1607–8
tibia test, 266

Growth hormone (GH) *(Cont.)*:
TRH and, 202
in acromegaly, 303
test, 325
tumor secretion of:
ectopic, 1718–19
pituitary, 300–306
Turner's syndrome and, 1008
Guanine, 37
Guanosine monophosphate, cyclic (cGMP), 122
atrial natriuretic factor and, 723–24
calcium and, 128
protein kinase and, 122
Guanosine triphosphatase (GTPase), 112
oncogenes and, 152–53
Guanosine triphosphate (GTP):
adenylate cyclase activation and, 95–96, 112, 114–15
oncogenes and, 152–53
Guanylate cyclase, 122
Gubernaculum, 883
Gut glucagon-like immunoreactants, 1644–45
Gynecomastia, 30, 886–89, 1595
causes, 887–88
drug-induced, 888
ectopic chorionic gonadotropin and, 1713
evaluation, 889
hyperthyroidism and, 429
Klinefelter's syndrome and, 870, 1001
pathologic, 887–89
physiologic, 887
treatment, 889

Hair:
increase of. *See* Hirsutism.
loss of, 26
Haloperidol:
pituitary effects of, 199
vasopressin and, 345
Hamartomas, hypothalamic, 223–24
HAM syndrome, 1425
Hand-Schüller-Christian disease, 224
hypothyroidism and, 449
Haploidy, 984
Haptens, 172
Harris lines, 1459
Hashimoto's thyroiditis, 445–46, 1678, 1682–83
Haversian system, 1329
Headache, 31–32
migraine, catecholamines and, 681
pituitary tumor and, 289
Head injuries, 225
hyperglycemia and, 231
Heart. *See also* Cardiovascular system.
ANF of. *See* Atrial natriuretic factor.
carcinoid and, 1656
coronary disease. *See* Coronary artery disease.
hypertension and, 695–96, 699
examination for, 734
output of. *See* Cardiac output.
size of, 29
Heart failure, 29
aldosterone and, 621
hyperthyroidism and, 426
hyponatremia and, 367
norepinephrine and, 680
Heat regulation, 235–36
obesity and, 1218–19
in animals, 1216–17
Heavy-particle therapy, pituitary tumors and, 299, 305–6
Height. *See also* Growth.
bone age and, 1598
chronologic age and, 1597–98
excess. *See* Tall stature.
measurement, 1597
short. *See* Short stature.
weight tables for, 1204–6
Hemagglutination, thyroid antibodies and, 408
Hematopoiesis, 27–28
glucocorticoids and, 551
hyperthyroidism and, 426–27
hypothyroidism and, 454–55
Hematuria, hypercalciuria and, 1530
Heme, steroid synthesis and, 70
Hemianopsia, pituitary tumor and, 289
Hemochromatosis:
diabetes mellitus and, 1164
hypogonadism and, 869
Hemoglobin, glycation of, 1054, 1112, 1113
diabetic complications and, 1128–29
Hemorrhage:
adrenal, 585–86, 589
pituitary, 275, 289
retinal, diabetes and, 1116, 1117–18
thyroid, 462
TSH stimulation and, 484
uterine, 30
menarcheal, 955
postmenopausal, 980
prostaglandins and, 973
Henle's loop:
Bartter's syndrome and, 1788
calcium reabsorption and, 1335
magnesium reabsorption in, 1362
vasopressin and, 350, 351
Heparin, aldosterone inhibition by, 522
Hermaphroditism, 1003–4
pseudo. *See* Pseudohermaphroditism.
Hexokinase, 1045, 1047, 1074
HHHO syndrome, 867
Hill plot, 179
Hilus cells, ovarian, 920–21
anatomy, 906
Hirsutism, 26, 964–66
adrenocortical hyperfunction and, 607, 622–24
assessment and investigation, 623, 964–65
21-hydroxylase deficiency and, 1023
idiopathic, 623, 964
polycystic ovary disease and, 623, 961, 964, 965
scoring system, 964, 965
testosterone and, 623
treatment, 623–24, 965–66
Histaminase, medullary thyroid carcinoma and, 502, 1675
Histamine:
carcinoid flush and, 1658
pituitary effects of, 195
prolactin and, 273
Histiocytosis X, hypothalamic, 224–25
Histones, 37–38, 143
History, 19
HLA system:
diabetes mellitus and, 1095, 1686
Graves' disease and, 419, 421
21-hydroxylase and, 1021–22
pluriglandular insufficiency and, 1686, 1687
HMG CoA reductase, 925, 1249
inhibitors of, 1304–5
HMG CoA synthase and lyase, 1059
Homatropine, pupillary response to, 685
Homocystinuria, 1619–20
vs. Marfan's syndrome, 1620
Hook effect, immunoradiometric assay and, 177
Hormones:
actions of, 8, 13–15, 82–158
classes of, 8–9, 83–84
general aspects of, 82–85
integrated, 12–13
local, 84–85
mobility of receptor and, 96–97
phospholipids and, 128–34
phosphorylation and, 101–2
termination of, 106–10
antagonisms of, 13
abnormal levels of, 17
assays of. *See* Assays *and also specific hormones.*
cardiovascular functions and, 14
circulation of, 4, 6
deficiency syndromes, 15–17
definition of, 3
development and, 15
diversification of, 11
evolution of, 9–10
excess syndromes, 17–18
gastrointestinal, 1629–52
glycoprotein, 257–63
ectopic, 1714–15
growth-affecting, 14, 15, 1583–91
hyporesponsiveness to, 16–17
interaction of receptor with, 59
internalization of, 7–8, 106–9
metabolism of, 6
mineral and water metabolism and, 14
peptide. *See* Peptide hormones.
receptors for. *See* Receptors.
regulation of. *See* Regulation *and also specific hormones.*
reproductive function and, 14–15
responsiveness of, 8
termination of, 13
stability of, 180
steroid. *See* Steroid hormones.
synergisms of, 13
therapeutic use of, 22
tropic, 14
types of, 5
Hormonosomes, 517
Hot flushes:
menopause and, 976
premature ovarian failure and, 956
Hungry bones syndrome, 1401, 1424, 1440

Hung-up reflexes, 33
Huntington's chorea, 237
Hyalinization:
  corticotroph, 252
  islet cell, 1113
  pituitary, 601
  seminiferous tubule, 879
Hyaluronic acid, hypothyroidism and, 451
H-Y antigen, 989–92
  hermaphroditism and, 1004
  XX males and, 1003
  XX gonadal dysgenesis (Swyer) and, 1009
Hybridization, nucleic acid, 45–46
  reverse transcription and, 49
Hydatidiform mole, hyperthyroidism and, 1715
Hydration, nephrolithiasis and, 1515, 1570–71
Hydrocephalus, hypothalamic disorders and, 225
Hydrocortisone. *See also* Cortisol; Glucocorticoids, therapeutic.
  absorption of, 797
  ACTH deficiency and, 284
  addisonian crisis and, 594
  adrenalectomy and, 1610
  adrenal hyperplasia and, 1615
  asthma and, 791
  binding of, 137
  breast cancer and, 1750
  growth failure and, 1604, 1608
  21-hydroxylase deficiency and, 1027
  hypercalcemia and, 1421
  pituitary surgery and, 298, 616–17
  sarcoidosis and, 1418
  surgical procedures and, 596
Hydrogen ion. *See also* pH.
  mineralocorticoids and, 564, 567
Hydroperoxyeicosatetraenoic acid (HPETE), 130, 1770
Hydrophobic interactions, hormone-receptor, 88–89
Hydroxyamphetamine, pupillary response and, 685
19-Hydroxyandrostenedione, 725
Hydroxyapatite, 1317
  nephrolithiasis and, 1507, 1524–27
β-Hydroxybutyrate, 1059–60
  diabetes mellitus and, 1149–54
  epinephrine and, 659
  norepinephrine and, 658
17-Hydroxycorticosteroids, urinary, 572–73
  ACTH stimulation test and, 577–78
  in children, 1623
  Cushing's syndrome and, 610
  dexamethasone suppression test and, 574, 575
  ectopic ACTH and, 1707
  obesity and, 1233
18-Hydroxycorticosterone:
  aldosteronism and, 759
    saline infusion and, 761–62
    17α-hydroxylase deficiency and, 766
    hypertension and, 725
    methyloxidase deficiency and, 630–31
  plasma levels, 730, 731
Hydroxycortisol, 541, 544
18-Hydroxydeoxycorticosterone, 725
25-Hydroxydihydrotachysterol, 1345
Hydroxyeicosatetraenoic acid (HETE), 130, 1770
5-Hydroxyindoleacetic acid:
  carcinoid and, 1656, 1657
  synthesis, 1656
  urinary, 1657
Hydroxyinfole-O-methyltransferase (HIOMT), 216
α-Hydroxy-β-ketoadipate, 1557
1-Hydroxylase, 1348, 1349
  regulation of, 1350
11β-Hydroxylase, 518
  deficiency, 628, 1029–30
    hypertension and, 765, 766
17α-Hydroxylase, 518
  deficiency, 625, 628–29, 873, 1014–15
    hypertension and, 765–66
  ovarian, 925–26
18-Hydroxylase defect, 625, 630–31
21-Hydroxylase, 518
  deficiency, 624–28, 1021–29
    biochemical defect, 624–25
    clinical features, 626–27
    diagnosis, 627, 1025–26
    genetic factors, 624–25
    incidence, 624
    pathogenesis, 1022–25
    pathology and pathophysiology, 626
    salt wasting and, 1022, 1023–25
    treatment, 627–28, 1026–29
    virilization and, 1021–29
  gene for, 1021–22
24-Hydroxylase, 1348, 1349, 1351
  regulation of, 1350
25-Hydroxylase, vitamin D metabolism and, 1347
Hydroxylation, steroid, 70, 71, 75
  adrenal, 518–19
  vitamin D, 73–74
Hydroxylysine, glycosylation and, 1054
3-Hydroxy-3-methylglutaryl coenzyme A. *See* HMG CoA reductase.
17-Hydroxypregnenolone, 518
  biosynthesis, 71, 1012
  3β-hydroxysteroid dehydrogenase deficiency and, 629–30, 1013
  21-hydroxylase deficiency and, 626
17-Hydroxyprogesterone:
  adrenal hyperplasia and, congenital, 1025
  biosynthesis, 72, 518, 1012
  endometrial cancer and, 1763–64
  genital evaluation and, 1031
  hirsutism and, 965
  21-hydroxylase deficiency and, 624, 626, 627, 1021–27
  LH receptor suppression and, 838
  neonatal, 997
  ovulation and, 944
  plasma levels, 521
    in infants, 1026
  structure, 516
  testicular secretion rate, 839
Hydroxyproline:
  bone dissolution and, 1332
  calcitonin therapy and, 1489
  Paget's disease of bone and, 1486, 1488
  urinary, 1443, 1455–56
3β-Hydroxysteroid dehydrogenase, 71
  adrenal steroid synthesis and, 518
  deficiency, 625, 629–30, 1013–14, 1030
  fetal adrenal, 520
  theca cell, ovarian, 916
17β-Hydroxysteroid dehydrogenase, 926
  deficiency, 1015–16
18-Hydroxysteroid dehydrogenase, 519
5-Hydroxytryptamine (5-HT). *See* Serotonin.
5-Hydroxytryptophan:
  carcinoid and, 1658
  synthesis, 1656
1α-Hydroxyvitamin D_3, 1346
  for hypocalcemia, 1434
  renal osteodystrophy and, 1480
  structure, 1345
25-Hydroxyvitamin D, 1346
  bone and, 1356
  for hypocalcemia, 1434
  measurement, 1375
  metabolism, 1347–48
  modification of, 73
  osteomalacia and rickets and, 1460, 1462, 1463
  production, 1347
  structure, 1345
  transport, 75, 1347
Hyperalbuminemia, hypercalcemia and, 1417
Hyperaldosteronism. *See* Aldosteronism.
Hyperalimentation:
  hypophosphatemia and, 1437
  osteomalacia and, 1466
Hyperalphalipoproteinemia, 1277
Hyperbetalipoproteinemia, 1260–64
Hypercalcemia, 1376–1422. *See also* Calcium.
  adrenal insufficiency and, 1412
  defense against, 1359–60
  diagnostic approach, 1396–98
  differential diagnosis, 1398, 1417–19
    tabulation of conditions, 1377
  diuretics and, 1413
  drug-associated, 1413–15
  endocrinopathies and, 1411–13
  estrogens and antiestrogens and, 1415
  familial, 1392–95
  glucocorticoids and, 554
  granulomatous diseases and, 1415–16, 1418
  hyperparathyroidism and, 1377–1402. *See also* Hyperparathyroidism.
  hyperthyroidism and, 429, 1411–12
  hypocalciuric, 1393–95
  idiopathic, of infancy, 1417
  immobilization and, 1416–17, 1420
  lithium and, 1414–15
  malignancy-associated, 1403–11, 1702–6
    breast cancer and, 1360
    clinical presentation, 1410, 1702–3
    differential diagnosis, 1318–19
    growth factors and, 1407–9, 1704
    humoral syndrome of, 1404–9, 1704
    local osteolytic, 1403
    lymphoma and, 1409–10. 1419
    mediators of, 1405–9
    parathyroid hormone and, 1407, 1410, 1703–4

Hypercalcemia, malignancy-associated
(Cont.):
pathophysiology, 1410
prostaglandins and, 1403, 1407, 1704–5
PTH-like factor and, 1407, 1408
treatment, 1411, 1705–6
uncommon variants of, 1410
vitamin D and, 1705
medical therapy, 1402, 1420–21
mild, 1397
milk-alkali syndrome and, 1414
moderate, 1397
pancreatitis and, 1390
pheochromocytoma and, 1412
prostaglandins and, 1403, 1407, 1704–5, 1780
protein abnormalities and, 1417
psychiatric symptoms and, 1388–89
renal failure and, 1417
renal transplants and, 1392
sarcoidosis and, 1415–16, 1418
serendipidity syndrome of, 1378
severe, 1397–98
VIP-oma and, 1412–13
vitamin A intoxication and, 1414
vitamin D and:
intoxication, 1413–14
malignancy and, 1705
Hypercalciuria, 1531–36
absorptive, 1545–55
bone involvement in, 1551
classification, 1536
constitutional, 1537–38, 1552
Cushing's syndrome and, 608
definition, detection, and incidence, 1532–35
diagnosis, 1367, 1551–53, 1569–70
diet and, 1532–35, 1547–50, 1568
dietary, 1538–40, 1551–52
family history and, 1529–30
hematuria and, 1530
hyperoxaluria and, 1559
hyperparathyroidism and, 1382–84, 1537, 1541–43, 1552
hyperuricosuria and, 1563, 1564
hypophosphatemia and, 1436, 1541, 1548
idiopathic, 1531, 1540–41
immobilization and, 1416, 1541
induction of, 1420
nephrolithiasis and, 1382–83, 1529, 1531–36
pathophysiology, 1535–36
pregnancy and, 1551
renal calcium leak and, 1542–45, 1553
renal tubular acidosis and, 1525
resorptive, 1540–41
sarcoidosis and, 1360, 1415–16
secondary, 1537
sodium and, 1538–40, 1544
treatment, 1553–56
vitamin D and, 1383, 1384, 1541, 1543, 1545–50
Hypercapnia, vasopressin and, 347
Hyperchloremia, hypoaldosteronism and, 598, 599
Hypercholesterolemia, 28, 1260–70. *See also* Hyperlipidemia.
atherosclerosis and, 1280–82
combined with hypertriglyceridemia, 1266–70
familial, 1264–65
coronary artery disease and, 1261–62
familial, 1260–65
clinical features, 1260–62, 1264–65
combined, 1264–65
genetics, 1263, 1265
laboratory features, 1262, 1265
obesity and, 1231–32
pathophysiology, 1262–63
treatment, 1263–64, 1265
sitosterolemia and, 1286
thresholds for drug treatment of, 1265–66
Hyperchylomicronemia, 1270–72
Hypercortisolism, 599–620. *See also* Adrenocortical hyperfunction; Cushing's syndrome.
ACTH-secreting tumors and, 1706–11
ectopic CRH and, 1719–20
Hyperesthesia, diabetes and, 1122
Hyperfunction syndromes, 17
secondary, 18
Hypergastrinemia, 1633–36
Hyperglycemia. *See also* Diabetes mellitus.
coma and, hyperosmolar nonketotic, 1154–55
complications from, 1125–29
Cushing's syndrome and, 608
dawn phenomenon, 1137
diagnosis, 1108–12
epinephrine-induced, 661
exercise-induced, 1146
glucocorticoids and, 544, 546
hepatic glucose balance and, 1075
hyperinsulinemia with, 1101
ketoacidosis and, 1150
neurologic disorders and, 231
pregnancy and, 1157
rebound, 1137
stress, 1092, 1165
symptoms, 1116
Hypergonadism, hypothalamic, 228–29
Hypergonadotropism, 870–78
treatment, 877–78
Hyperinsulinemia:
diabetes mellitus and, 1100
exercise and, 1147
fetal, 1161
hepatic glucose balance and, 1075
hyperglycemia with, 1101
hyperphagia and, 1230
hypertriglyceridemia and, 1106
hypoglycemia and, 1184–87. *See also* Hypoglycemia, insulin-induced.
islet-cell tumors and, 1184–87
obesity and, 1072–73, 1214–16, 1227–30
Hyperkalemia:
Addison's disease and, 590
diabetic neuropathy and, 1120
21-hydroxylase deficiency and, 1023
hypertension and, 770
hypoaldosteronism and, 597, 598
pseudohypoaldosteronism and, 599
Hyperlipidemia (hyperlipoproteinemia), 1255–74. *See also* Hypercholesterolemia; Lipoprotein; Hypertriglyceridemia.
alcohol and, 1259, 1291–92
alpha, 1277
beta, 1260–64
bile-duct obstruction and, 1259
classification, 1255
combined, 1266–70
familial, 1264–65
diabetes mellitus and, 1105–7, 1123, 1257–58, 1259
diagnostic criteria, 1255–56
diagnostic tests, 1306–8
dietary, 1256–57
dietary treatment, 1286–98
cholesterol-saturated fat index of foods and, 1294–96
phased approach to, 1296–98
single-diet concept for, 1292–96
specific nutrient effects and, 1287–92
drug-induced, 1259–60
drug therapy, 1266, 1298–1305
thresholds for, 1265–66
familial, 1260–65
combined, 1264–65
hepatic lipase deficiency and, 1270
hyperinsulinemia and, 1106
hypertension and, 1298
hypothyroidism and, 1258
obesity and, 1231–32, 1273, 1290–91, 1294–96
pregnancy and, 1297
protein and, 1292
renal disease and, 1258–59
secondary, 1256–60
surgical treatment, 1305–6
types I and V, 1270–72
clinical features, 1270–71
genetics, 1271
laboratory features, 1271–72
pathophysiology, 1272
treatment, 1272
types IIa and IIb, 1260–64
clinical features, 1260–62
genetics, 1263
laboratory features, 1262
pathophysiology, 1262–63
treatment, 1263–64
type III, 1267–70
clinical features, 1267–68
genetics, 1268
laboratory features, 1268
pathophysiology, 1268–69
treatment, 1269–70
type IV, 1272–74
clinical features, 1273
genetics, 1273
pathophysiology, 1273
treatment, 1273–74
Hypermagnesemia, 1442
Hypernatremia. *See also* Sodium.
differential diagnosis, 364
essential, 361
neurologic disease and, 230–31
osmoreceptor destruction and, 361, 364, 366–67
treatment, 366–67
Hyperosmolar nonketotic coma, 1154–55

Hyperoxaluria, 1556–61
classification, 1557–59
diagnosis, 1559–60
enteric, 1558, 1561
hypercalciuria and, 1559
hypocitraturia and, 1566
malabsorption and, 1558–59
treatment, 1560–61
Hyperparathyroidism, 1377–1402
acute, 1391
anemia and, 28
behavioral disorders and, 214
bone disease and, 1384–88
calcium absorption and, 1383
calcium balance and, 1382
chondrocalcinosis and, 1391
clinical presentation and pathophysiology, 1379–81
definitive diagnosis, 1396–98
differential diagnosis, 1418–19
familial, 1392–95
gastrointestinal system and, 1389–90
glucocorticoids and, 554
historical note on, 1377
hypercalciuria and, 1382–84, 1537, 1541–43, 1552
hypertension and, 1390
hypocalcemia and, 1431–32
hypophosphatemia and, 1465
incidence and natural history, 1377–78
joints and, 1390–91
laboratory studies, 1395–96
localization studies, 1398–1400
malignancies and, 1703–4
medical management, 1401–2, 1554
MEN 1 and, 1392–93, 1664, 1668
MEN 2 and, 1393, 1669, 1676–77
"moans" of, 1380
nephrolithiasis and, 1381–84, 1391, 1526
neuromuscular disorders and, 1388
normocalcemic, 1391
osteitis fibrosa cystica and, 1385–87
osteodystrophy and, renal, 1479–80
osteomalacia and, 1460, 1465
osteopenia and, 1387
osteoporosis and, 1469–70, 1473–74
pancreatitis and, 1389–90
pathology and etiology, 1378–79
pediatric, 1392
peptic ulcer and, 1389
pheochromocytoma and, 1393, 1412
physical findings, 1395
pregnancy and, 1391–92
primary, 1377–1402
psychiatric symptoms and, 1388–89
renal transplants and, 1392
spectrum of, 1380
subtle primary, 1541–42, 1552
treatment, 1553–54
surgical therapy, 1400–1401, 1553–54
tertiary, 1392
thyroid medullary carcinoma and, 1676–77
variants of, 1391–92
vitamin D and, 1383
Zollinger-Ellison syndrome and, 1389
Hyperphagia:
hyperinsulinemia and, 1230
hypothalamic role in, 1212–15
obesity and, 1210, 1219–21
psychological factors, 1222–23
Hyperphosphatasia, hereditary, 1481–82
Hyperphosphatemia, 1438–39. *See also* Phosphorus.
defense against, 1361
neonatal, 1431
pseudohypoparathyroidism and, 1428, 1430
treatment, 1439
Hyperpigmentation, 25–26. *See also* Pigmentation.
Hyperpituitarism, 300–321. *See also* Pituitary gland tumors.
posterior, 367–74
Hyperplasia, 17
Hyperprebetalipoproteinemia, 1272–74
Hyperprolactinemia, 306–15, 958–60
amenorrhea and, 958–60
differential diagnosis, 308–10
drug-induced, 309, 958
etiology, 958–59
gonadotropin deficiency and, 862–63
hypothalamic disease and, 229–30, 309, 310–11, 958
hamartoma and, 224
hypogonadism and, 227
idiopathic, 229–30, 310, 315, 959
impotence and, 890
laboratory studies, 308
pathogenesis, 310–11
renal disease and, 273
signs and symptoms, 307
therapy, 312–15, 959–60
Hyperpyrexia, 25
Hyperreninemia:
hypoaldosteronism and, 598–99
tumors and, 738
Hypersensitivity, target tissue, 18, 22
Hypertension, 28–29, 693–772
accelerated, 709
adrenal adenoma and, 752–53, 759–64
adrenal carcinoma and, 767
adrenal hyperplasia and, 752, 753–55, 759–63
congenital, 765–66
aldosterone and, 724–25. *See also* Aldosteronism.
deficiency of, 768–69, 770
angiotensin and, 707–11, 728
low renin and, 771–72
atherosclerosis and, 699–700, 735–37
atrial natriuretic factor and, 723
borderline, 698
brain effects, 695–96, 699
calcium and, 712–14
carbenoxolone-induced, 768
cardiac effects, 695–96, 699
catecholamines and, 680
complications, 698–701
coronary artery disease and, 695–96
Cushing's syndrome and, 552, 607, 766–68
deoxycorticosterone and, 724, 725, 764–66
aldosteronism and, 753
19-nor-deoxycorticosterone and, 726
dexamethasone-responsive, 769–70
diabetic nephropathy and, 1120, 1121
encephalopathy and, 700
environmental factors, 697
epidemiology, 694–96
essential, 693, 709–11
low-renin, 770–72
established (fixed), 698
evaluation of, 732–34
experimental, 707
fibromuscular dysplasia and, 737–38
general features, 694–701
genetic factors, 697
glucocorticoids and, 726, 766–68
insensitivity to, 769
Goldblatt model of, 707
hemodynamics, 698
18-hydroxycorticosterone and, 725
18-hydroxydeoxycorticosterone and, 725
11β-hydroxylase deficiency and, 765, 766
17α-hydroxylase deficiency and, 765–66
hyperlipidemia and, 1298
hyperparathyroidism and, 1390
iatrogenic, 768
intracranial, benign, 237
kallikrein-kinin system and, 1786
laboratory studies, 727–31, 734
licorice and, 768
magnesium and, 714
mineralocorticoids and, 724–25, 768. *See also* Aldosteronism.
unidentified, 769–70
obesity and, 1232
optic fundi and, 733–34
pheochromocytoma and, 667–72
physical examination, 732–34
potassium and, 714–15, 730, 755–57, 768–70
low renin and, 770
prostaglandins and, 1777–78
pseudohypoaldosteronism and, 770
renal effects of, 700–701
renin and, 707–11
essential hypertension and, 770–72
low, 710, 752, 758, 768–72
plasma determination, 744–45
renal vein, 745–46
tumor secretion of, 708, 738, 1722–23
renovascular, 708, 735–51
algorithm for evaluating, 747
anatomic causes, 737
clinical characteristics, 739
diagnostic studies, 740–46
experimental, 707
historical background, 735
medical therapy, 746–48
natural history, 738–39
pathologic etiology, 735–38
revascularization approaches to, 748–51
screening tests, 740, 746
secondary, 693–94, 732–70
clinical features suggesting, 733
types of, 695
sodium and, 710–12, 715–18
spironolactone and, 768–69
sympathetic activity and, 680, 697–98
vascular changes and, 697, 699
Hyperthermia:
hypothalamic disease and, 236
sympathetic function test using, 685

Hyperthyroidism, 417–44
acropachy and, 444
aldosterone and, 543
anemia and, 28
apathetic, 425
autoantibodies and, 418–20
bone and, 429, 1411
calcium and, 429, 1411–12
carcinoma and, 423, 1715
cardiovascular system and, 426
causes, 418–24
in childhood, 1619
clinical manifestations, 424–29, 440–44
tabulation of, 424
cortisol and, 428, 543
crisis (storm), 438
drug therapy for, 432–36
ectopic, 423
endocrine system and, 428–29
exogenous, 422
eyes and, 425, 440–43
factitious, 422
gastrointestinal system and, 426
general appearance and, 425
goiter and, 422–23, 425–26, 437–38, 477, 484
gonadotropins and, 428–29
chorionic, 424, 1715
Graves' disease and, 418–21, 432–37
hematopoietic system and, 426–27
hypercalcemia and, 1411–12
iatrogenic, 422
iodide-induced, 422
iodide therapy for, 435
laboratory diagnosis, 429–32
masked, 425
metabolism and, 428
myxedema and, 443–44
neonatal, 440
neuromuscular function and, 214, 427–28
nonthyroidal illness vs., 415
osteoporosis and, 1471, 1473
pathophysiology, 417–18
postpartum, 440
pregnancy and, 438–40
radionuclide studies, 430
radiotherapy for, 432–33, 436–37
remissions of, 421, 432
renal function and, 427
respiratory function and, 426
scheme for evaluating, 431
skin and, 425, 444
T_3 type, 418
T_4 type, 418
T_4/T_3 ratio and, 417–18
thyroidectomy for, 437
thyroiditis and, 421–22, 437
treatment, 432–38
trophoblastic, 423–24, 1715
TSH excess and, 423
Hyperthyroxinemia, 411, 415. *See also* Hyperthyroidism.
Hypertriglyceridemia, 1270–74. *See also* Hyperlipidemia.
carbohydrates and, 1291
combined with hypercholesterolemia, 1266–70
familial, 1264–65
diabetes mellitus and, 1106–7, 1123
obesity and, 1231, 1290–91
xanthomas and, 1124
Hyperuricosuria, 1506, 1561–64
calcium oxalate stones and, 1561–64
definition, 1561–62
diagnosis, 1563
drug-induced, 1519–20
hypercalciuria with, 1563, 1564
pathogenesis, 1562–63
treatment, 1563–64
uric acid stones and, 1517, 1519
Hyperventilation, hypophosphatemia and, 1437
Hypervitaminosis A, 1414
Hypervitaminosis D, 1413–14
Hypervolemia:
hyponatremia and, 367–68, 372, 373
vasopressin and, 345
Hypoalbuminemia:
hypocalcemia and, 1432
thyroxine deficiency and, 412
Hypoaldosteronism, 597–99. *See also* Aldosterone.
ACTH deficiency and, 591
hyperreninemic or normoreninemic, 598–99
hyporeninemic, 597–98
Hypoalphalipoproteinemia, 1276
Hypobetalipoproteinemia, 1279–80
Hypocalcemia, 1422–35. *See also* Calcium.
acute, 1433
chronic, 1433–35
citrated blood and, 1432
clinical manifestations, 1422–24
defense against, 1358–59
differential diagnosis, 1432–33
drug-induced, 1432
glucocorticoids and, 554
hyperparathyroidism and, 1431–32
hypoalbuminemia and, 1432
hypoparathyroidism and, 1424–31. *See also* Hypoparathyroidism.
hypophosphatemia and, 1432
neonatal, 1430–31
nonhypoparathyroid, 1422, 1431–32
osteomalacia and rickets and, 1431, 1465
pancreatitis and, 1431–32
postoperative, 437, 1401, 1424–25
pseudohypoparathyroidism and, 1428, 1430
renal insufficiency and, 1431
treatment, 1433–35
Hypocalciuria:
diuretics and, 1413
familial, 1393–95
pseudohypoparathyroidism and, 1430
Hypocitraturia, 1564–66
steatorrhea and, 1559
Hypofunction syndromes, 16
Hypoglycemia, 1179–1201
Addison's disease and, 587–89
alcohol-induced, 1195–96
alimentary, 1191–92
autoimmune, 1188
catecholamines and, 677–78, 1086, 1180, 1190
classification, 1182, 1184
coma and, 1152, 1181, 1195
cortisol and, 1181
counterregulatory mechanisms, 677, 1179, 1180
definition, 1179–80, 1189
diagnostic evaluation, 1199–1201
flowsheets for, 1199, 1200
drug-induced, 1142, 1194–95
early diabetes and, 1192
endocrine deficiency states and, 1187
episodic nature of, 1180–81
exercise-induced, 1145–46
factitious, 1194–95
fasting, 1182–88, 1200–1201
fructose intolerance and, 1197–98
fuel metabolism and, 1091
glucagon and, 677, 1136–37, 1180, 1190
glucose ingestion and, 1181, 1190
glucose tolerance test and, 1189–90, 1199
growth hormone and, 283, 324–25, 1181
in children, 1604, 1608, 1622
history and physical examination, 1199
hypoglycin and, 1198–99
idiopathic (functional), 1191
induced, 1193–99
insulin-induced, 1136–37, 1193–94
ACTH and, 280–81, 321–22, 578, 803
cortisol and, 578, 810, 811
diabetic therapy and, 1136–37, 1193–94
factitious, 1194
growth hormone and, 269, 283, 324–25, 1622
islet-cell tumors and, 1184–87
prolactin and, 326
insulin-like growth factor and, 1187
ketotic, 1188
laboratory studies, 1199–1201
leucine sensitivity and, 1196–97
leukemia cells and, promyelocytic, 1717
liver and, 1188, 1190–91
neonatal, 1161
nonhypoglycemia vs., 1181–82
norepinephrine and, 666–67
postprandial (reactive), 1188–93
classification, 1191–92
diagnosis, 1189, 1190, 1199–1200
pathophysiology, 1190–91
prevalence, 1189
treatment, 1192–93
pregnancy and, 1159
signs and symptoms, 1136, 1180–81, 1189
somatostatin and, 677
substrate deficiency and, 1188
treatment of, 1137, 1192–93
insulinoma and, 1186–87
tumors and, 1184–87
extrapancreatic, 1187, 1716–17
islet-cell, 1184–87
vasopressin and, 346
Hypoglycemic agents, 1140–44
biguanide, 1143–44
hypoglycemia induced by, 1142, 1194, 1195
sulfonylurea, 1141–43
Hypoglycin, 1198–99
Hypogonadism, 861–78
anorchia and, 873–74
classification, 862, 870

Hypogonadism *(Cont.)*:
- climacteric and, male, 874–75
- cryptorchism and, 884
- delayed puberty and, 869, 875–77
- Down's syndrome and, 873
- dysgenesis and. *See* Gonads, dysgenesis of.
- emotional disorders and, 868
- enzyme defects and, 874
- genetic disorders and, 870–73
- hemochromatosis and, 869
- hypergonadotropic, 870–78
- hyperprolactinemia and, 307, 862–63
- hypogonadotropic, 861–69, 877
- hypopituitarism and, 282, 861–62
- hypothalamic, 226–28
- Kallmann's syndrome and, 863–67, 953
- Klinefelter's syndrome and, 870–72, 1001–2
- Laurence-Moon-Biedl syndrome and, 867–68
- liver disease and, 868–69
- malnutrition and, 868
- mumps orchitis and, 874
- myotonic dystrophy and, 872
- pituitary tumor and, 320–21
- Prader-Labhart-Willi syndrome and, 867
- renal disease and, 869
- resistance to hormones and, 875
- spinal cord damage and, 869
- toxins and, 874
- treatment, 285–86, 875–78
- Turner's syndrome and, male, 872
- XX males and, 1003
- XYY syndrome and, 872–73

Hypogonadotropism, 861–69, 953
- treatment, 877

Hypokalemia. *See also* Potassium.
- aldosteronism and, 752–54
  - diagnostic procedures, 755–57
- Bartter's syndrome and, 1787, 1788–89
- Cushing's syndrome and, 608, 767
- hypertension and, 715, 730, 755–57, 768–70
- hypomagnesemia and, 1441
- hyponatremia and, 368, 372–73
- WDHA syndrome and, 1640

Hypomagnesemia, 1439–42. *See also* Magnesium.
- diagnosis, 1441
- hypoparathyroidism and, 1426, 1440
- neonatal, 1431
- pathogenesis, 1439–41
- symptoms, 1441
- treatment, 1441–42

Hyponatremia, 367–74. *See also* Sodium.
- adrenocortical insufficiency and, 590, 591
- cerebral, 230
- chlorpropamide-induced, 1142
- diagnosis, 372–73
- drug-induced, 230, 1142
- etiology and pathophysiology, 367–72
- euvolemic, 368–74
- hydration therapy and, 361
- 21-hydroxylase deficiency and, 1023–24
- hypervolemic, 367–368, 372, 373
- hypovolemic, 368, 372–73
- polydipsia and, 362
- SIADH and, 368–74
  - ectopic, 1711–13
- therapy, 373–74

Hypoparathyroidism, 1424–31
- adrenocortical insufficiency and, 583, 1425, 1680–81
- candidiasis and, 1681, 1682
- classification, 1422
- clinical manifestations, 1422–24
- DiGeorge's syndrome and, 1431
- eye findings in, 33, 34
- hypercalciuria and, 1543, 1545
- hypomagnesemia and, 1426, 1440
- idiopathic, 1425
- neonatal, 1430, 1431
- pluriglandular insufficiency and, 1680–82
- postoperative, 498, 1424–25
- pseudo, 1426–30. *See also* Pseudohypoparathyroidism.
- radiation and, 1425
- treatment, 1433–35

Hypophosphatasia:
- rickets and osteomalacia and, 1465–66
- treatment, 1467–68

Hypophosphatemia, 1435–38. *See also* Phosphorus.
- causes, 1436–37
- defense against, 1360–61
- dialysis and, 1465
- familial X-linked, 1464
- Fanconi syndrome and, 1464
- hypercalcemia and, malignancy-associated, 1404
- hypercalciuria and, 1436, 1541, 1548
- hyperparathyroidism and, 1396, 1465
- hypocalcemia and, 1432
- osteomalacia or rickets and, 1460, 1464–65, 1467
  - with hypercalciuria, 1548
- osteoporosis and, 1474
- pathogenesis, 1435–37
- pathophysiological consequences of, 1438
- time course of development of, 1436
- treatment, 1438, 1467
- tumor-associated, 1717–18
- vitamin D and, 1464

Hypophyseal arteries, 191, 248, 249, 824

Hypophysectomy. *See also* Pituitary gland surgery.
- aldosterone production and, 533
- breast cancer and, 1742, 1744–45, 1748
- Cushing's disease and, 615, 617
- diabetes insipidus and, 356

Hypophysiotropic hormones, 199–207. *See also specific hormone or factor, e.g.,* Corticotropin releasing factor; Gonadotropin releasing hormone.
- concept of, 187–90
- extrahypothalamic, 187
- hypothalamic distribution of, 191, 192
- neurotransmitter control of, 193–94
- structure of, 200

Hypophysis. *See* Pituitary gland.

Hypopituitarism, 273–87
- ACTH and, 277, 280–81, 284–85
- aldosterone and, 533
- amenorrhea and, 952–53
- anemia and, 27–28
- clinical features, 277–79
- diabetes insipidus and, 356–57
- diagnostic procedures, 279–84
- differential diagnosis, 279
- drug-induced, 276
- etiology, 273, 274
- familial, 275, 297
- general features, 278
- gonadotropins and, 277–78, 281–83, 285–86
- growth failure and, 1605–9
- growth hormone and, 278, 283–84, 286–87
- hypogonadism and, 282, 861–62
- hyponatremia and, 367–74
- hypothalamic disease and, 276, 279
- oxytocin and, 278
- postoperative, 299
- primary, 273–76
- prolactin and, 284, 287
- radiation-induced, 275, 299
- secondary, 276–77
- stalk lesions and, 276
- target organ disorder vs., 279
- transient, 1607
- treatment, 284–87, 1609, 1610
- TSH and, 277, 281, 285
- tumors and, 289
- vasopressin and, 278
  - SIADH and, 368–74
- weight loss and, 276–77, 279

Hyporeninemic hypoaldosteronism, 597–98

Hyporesponsiveness syndromes, 16–17, 22

Hyposmia, 227, 864, 953

Hypospadias:
- estrogen therapy in mother and, 1019
- isolated, 1020
- pseudovaginal perineoscrotal, 1017

Hypotension:
- adrenal insufficiency and, 552, 587, 589
- postural, 673–77
  - causes, 673, 674
  - diabetes mellitus and, 1122
  - hyperadrenergic vs. hypoadrenergic, 673–74
  - treatment, 676–77
- thirst and, 352–53
- vasopressin and, 345

Hypothalamic-pituitary-adrenal axis, 522–23
- ACTH therapy and, 803
- circadian rhythms and, 219
- glucocorticoid therapy and, 809–14
  - alternate-day, 806, 807
- testing, 569, 576–79, 813

Hypothalamic-pituitary-gonadal axis, 1590
- differentiation of, 994–97

Hypothalamic-pituitary-testes axis, 832–57
- anatomy, 821–25
- feedback interaction, 844–48
- germ cells and, 848–51
- germ cell–Leydig cell interactions and, 850–51
- Leydig cells and, 832–48
- physiology, 832–52

Hypothalamic-pituitary-thyroid axis, 400
- testing, 430–31

Hypothalamus, 221–36
acromegaly and, 223, 228, 304–5
ACTH and, 226. *See also* Corticotropin releasing factor.
acute vs. chronic lesions of, 221–22
afferent neural input, 832–34
aminergic system, 823
anatomy, 190–92, 821
landmarks of, 822
anorexia nervosa and, 234–35
behavioral centers, 835–36
Cushing's disease and, 226, 317–18, 603
diencephalic syndrome of infancy and, 233–34
etiology of diseases of, 222–25
feedback system, 186–87
gonadotropins and, 226–29, 282–83, 832–35. *See also* Gonadotropin releasing hormone.
grafts of pituitary tissue in, 187–88
growth hormone and, 229. *See also* Growth hormone releasing hormone.
hamartomas, 223–24
histiocytosis X, 224–25
hormones of, 187–90, 199–207. *See also* Hypophysiotropic hormones *and specific hormone or factor*.
hydrocephalus and, 225
hypergonadism and, 228–29
hyperprolactinemia and, 224, 227, 229–30, 309, 310–11, 958
hypogonadism and, 226–28
hypopituitarism and, 276, 279
hypothyroidism and, 226, 449–50
immunologic disorders, 224
medial basal, 821, 823–24
median eminence, 190, 821
neurohypophysis and, 338
neuronal-capillary relationship, 823, 824
portal system and, 191–92, 248
structural composition of, 191, 193
metabolic disorders and, 231–35
neural connections of, 190, 654, 832–34
neurosecretory cells of. *See* Neurosecretory cells.
nuclei of, 190
diagrams of, 189
obesity and, 232–33, 1212–15
peptidergic system of, 821–23
pituitary control by. *See* Hypophysiotropic hormones.
pituitary disturbances and, 225–31
portal system, 188, 191–92, 248, 824–25
precocious puberty and, 223, 228
pulse generator, 834–35
radiation damage to, 225
sarcoidosis, 224
steroid receptors of, 823
temperature regulation and, 235–36
thirst disorder and, 231
trauma, 225
TSH and, 226. *See also* Thyrotropin releasing hormone.
tumors, 222–24
adrenal insufficiency and, 590–91
vascular lesions, 225
vasopressin and, 230–31
Hypothermia, 25
hypoglycemia and, 1181
hypothalamic disease and, 235–36
hypothyroidism and, 460–61
Hypothyroidism, 444–61
adaptive, 444
aldosterone and, 543
amenorrhea and, 958
anemia and, 28
angina pectoris and, 453
autoimmune thyroiditis and, 445–46
biosynthetic defects and, 447–49
cardiovascular system and, 453
causes, 445–50
in childhood, 460, 1602–3
clinical manifestations, 450–56
tabulation of, 451
coma and, 460–61
congenital defects and, 447–48, 1602–3
cortisol and, 455, 543
cretinism and, 478
cystinosis and, 447
drug-induced, 449
dysgenesis of thyroid and, 447
endocrine system and, 455
euthyroid sick syndrome vs., 412
eye findings in, 33, 34
fluid and electrolytes and, 453–54
frequency, 444–45
gastrointestinal system and, 454
general appearance and, 451
genetic factors, 480–81
goiter and, 452, 474, 480–81
gonadal function and, 455
growth and, 460, 1589, 1602–4
growth hormone deficiency and, 1607–8
hematopoietic system and, 454–55
hyperlipidemia and, 1258
hypothalamic, 226, 449–50
hypothermia and, 460–61
hypothyrotropic, 449–50
iodide deficiency and, 448–49
iodide excess and, 449
laboratory diagnosis, 456–58
metabolism and, 454
musculoskeletal system and, 452–53
neonatal, 460, 1602–3
nervous system and, 214, 452
nonthyroidal illness and, 412–15, 444, 456
obesity and, 1215
pituitary, 277, 449
pluriglandular failure and, 1685–86
precocious puberty and, 297
prolactin and, 309
radiation-induced, 436–37, 446
renal function and, 453–54
resistance to hormone and, 450
respiratory function and, 453
scheme for evaluating, 457
skin and, 451–52
subclinical, 444, 446
treatment of, 459
surgery in patients with, 455
thyroidectomy-induced, 437, 446–47, 499–500
transient, 447
autoimmune, 446
treatment, 458–59
Hypothyroxinemia, 411–12, 414–15. *See also* Hypothyroidism.
Hypovolemia:
diabetic ketoacidosis and, 1151, 1154
hyponatremia and, 368, 372–73
thirst and, 352–53
vasopressin and, 343, 345
Hypoxanthine-guanine pyrophosphoribosyl transferase deficiency, 1519
Hypoxia, vasopressin and, 347

Iatrogenic disorders, 17
Ibuprofen, dysmenorrhea and, 974
IGF. *See* Insulin-like growth factors.
Ileal bypass:
hyperlipidemia and, 1264, 1305–6
nephrolithiasis and, 1558, 1559
obesity and, 1239
Imipramine, 199
Immobilization:
hypercalcemia and, 1416–17, 1420
hypercalciuria and, 1541
osteoporosis and, 1474
Immotile cilia syndrome, 880–81
Immune response. *See also* Antibodies; Autoimmunity.
Addison's disease and, 584–85
diabetes insipidus and, 224
glucocorticoids and, 548–49, 790–91
mechanisms of tissue injury, 1678
Immunization, 172
Immunoassay. *See* Radioimmunoassay.
Immunofluorescence, 1678
Immunogen, 171–72
Immunoglobulins. *See also* Antibodies.
glucocorticoids and, 551
molecule (schematic) of, 171
peptide hormone receptors and, 93, 94
radioassay of. *See* Radioimmunoassay.
thyroid-stimulating autoantibodies and, 419
Immunoradiometric assays (IRMAs), 176–77
Immunosorbent assay, enzyme-linked (ELISA), 177, 178
Immunosuppression, diabetes mellitus and, 1147–48
pancreatic transplants and, 1148, 1149
Impotence, 29, 889–90
diabetes mellitus and, 1122
diagnostic studies, 890
hyperprolactinemia and, 307, 862, 863, 890
prostatectomy and, 1760
psychogenic, 890
treatment, 890
Imprinting, androgen, 836
Incertohypothalamic system, 823
Incretin, 1070, 1642
Inderal. *See* Propranolol.
Indirect tests, 21–22
Indomethacin:
Bartter's syndrome and, 1789
blood pressure and, 1777–78
gastrointestinal effects of, 1776
hypercalcemia and, 1780
of malignancy, 1705
labor and, 1773, 1774
prostaglandin inhibition by, 1773

Indomethacin *(Cont.)*:
pulmonary function and, 1779
renin release and, 1775
Infections:
diabetes mellitus and, 1125
fetal, 1601
glucocorticoid therapy and, 795
nephrolithiasis and, 1507, 1521–24
testicular, 880
Infertility, 30
autoimmunity and, 881
cystic fibrosis and, 881
female, 966–70
genetic disorders and, 881
gonadotropin deficiency and, 286
hyperprolactinemia and, 307, 958–60
immotile cilia syndrome and, 880–81
infections and, 880
Klinefelter's syndrome and, 871
male, 878–82. *See also* Azoospermia.
approach to, 881–82
ovulation induction and, 966–70
polycystic ovary disease and, 963–64
prostaglandins and, 1774
sinopulmonary syndrome and, 880–81
weight loss and, 960, 961
Young's syndrome and, 881
Inflammation, glucocorticoids and, 548–49, 790, 801
Inflammatory bowel disease:
growth failure and, 1602
nephrolithiasis and, 1520, 1558
Infradian rhythms, 218
Infundibulum, pituitary, 248, 338
Inhibin:
FSH and, 263, 849, 850
FSH/LH ratio and, 848–49
germinal cell failure and, 879
ovary as source of, 927
polycystic ovary disease and, 963
spermatogenesis and, 850
Inositol phospholipids, 131–33
Inositol triphosphate, calcium and, 119, 132–33
Insulin, 1064–82
actions, 1073–77
alanine and, 1065, 1074–75
allergy to, 1138
amino acids and, 1070, 1075–76
compositional, 1064, 1065
antagonisms of, 13
antibodies to, 97, 156–57, 1138, 1188
bacterial synthesis of, 1066–67
basal state and, 1089
binding, 1077–78, 1081
biosynthesis, 1065–67
bovine, 1064, 1131, 1138
calcium and, 1066, 1068–69
cAMP and, 1068, 1080
chemistry, 1064–65
circadian rhythm of, 220
clamp technique, 1101, 1102, 1228
deficiency. *See* Diabetes mellitus.
degradation, 1082
devices for delivery of, 1135–36, 1161
diabetes mellitus and, 1099–1103, 1131–39
complications (of diabetes) and, 1129–30
complications (of insulin) and, 1136–39
dosage adjustment, 1132–35
measurement of, 1111
pregnancy and, 1157–59, 1161–62
secretion in, 1099–1101
resistance and, 1101–3
treatment, 1131–39
eating behavior and, 1213–14
edema induced by, 1138–39
energy regulation and, 1087–88
epinephrine and, 659, 661, 1071, 1085
estrogen and, 1157
excess. *See* Hyperinsulinemia.
exercise and, 1145, 1146–47
fats and, 1070–71, 1076
fatty acid oxidation and, 1058
fed state and, 1081, 1090
fetal, 1156, 1161, 1588
fish, 1185
gastric inhibitory polypeptide (GIP) and, 1070, 1642
gastrointestinal influences on, 1070, 1071
gene for, 54
glucagon ratio to, 1083–84
glucocorticoids and, 544, 546, 808, 1086
glucose and:
biphasic response to, 1069
diabetes mellitus and, 1100–1102
metabolism of, 1073–75
obesity and, 1228–31
oral ingestion of, 1070, 1073–74
stimulation of release by, 1068–70
glycogen and, 1073–75
glycolysis and, 1068, 1074
growth and, 1583–84
growth hormone and, 265, 1086
historical note on, 1064
hyperthyroidism and, 428
hypoglycemia induced by, 1136–37, 1193–94. *See also* Hypoglycemia, insulin-induced.
hypoglycemic agents and, 1141–44
intermediate-acting, 1131–33
internalization of, by target cell, 107
ketones and, 1070–71, 1076, 1150, 1151
therapy of, 1152–53
lente, 1131–33
lipodystrophy from, 1137–38
liver and, 1073–75
obesity and, 1228–29
long-acting, 1131, 1132
muscle effects of, 1075–76
nasal delivery of, 53
neural and neurohormonal regulation, 1071–72, 1085
norepinephrine and, 658, 1071, 1085
NPH, 1131–33
obesity and, 1072–73, 1214–16, 1227–31
resistance in, 1081, 1082, 1228–30
osmoregulation and, 343
plasma levels, 1067–68
glucose and, 1068, 1069
obesity and, 1227–28
porcine, 1064, 1065, 1131, 1138
portal vein levels, 1067, 1069
potassium and, 1076–77
precursor, 65
pregnancy and, 1157–59, 1161–62
preparations of, 1131–32
progesterone and, 1157
prostaglandins and, 1072, 1780
protein meal and, 1083, 1084
pumps for infusing, 1135–36
pregnancy and, 1161
rapid-acting, 1131–33
receptors for, 1077–80
ACh receptor vs., 92
antibodies to, 97, 156–57
diabetes mellitus and, 1101–2
disease states and, 179
down regulation of, 104
EGF receptor vs., 94
hydrophobic interactions and, 89
interactions of, 1077–78
obesity and, 1229–30
phosphorylation of, 102, 1079–80
postreceptor events and, 1080
structure and function, 93–94, 1077
turnover of, 1078–79
resistance to, 16, 1080–82, 1101–3, 1138
acanthosis nigricans and, 1102–3
aging and, 1109
factitius, 1138
lipoatrophic diabetes and, 1163
obesity and, 1228–30
types of, 1081
RNA and, 1066
secretion, 1067–73
diabetes mellitus and, 1099–1101
obesity and, 1231
semilente, 1131, 1132
sodium and, 1077
somatostatin and, 1072
Somogyi phenomenon and, 1137
starvation and, 1091, 1183
synthesis of, by recombinant DNA, 47–48, 52, 1066–67
tolerance test. *See* Hypoglycemia, insulin-induced.
triglycerides and, 1076
tumor secretion of, 1184–87, 1664, 1669
nonpancreatic, 1716
ultralente, 1131, 1132
zinc and, 1131
Insulin-like activity, nonsuppressible (NSILA), 265, 1086. *See also* Insulin-like growth factors.
Insulin-like growth factors (IGF), 265, 269, 1086–87, 1584
actions of, 1586–87
cortisol and, 1588
estrogen and, 1588
fasting and, 1588
fetus and, 1588
growth and, 1586–89
hypoglycemia and, 1187, 1716–17
vs. insulin properties, 1086
plasma levels, 1587
receptors for, 1086
structure of, 65
Insulinoma, 1184–87
diagnosis, 1185
MEN 1 and, 1664, 1669
treatment, 1186–87, 1669

Insulitis, 1096–97, 1113
Integration of endocrine system, 12–13
Interferon, glucocorticoids and, 551
Interleukin 1, testicular, 849
Interleukin 2, glucocorticoids and, 550
Internalization of hormones, 7–8, 106–10
International standard, 166
Interstitial cells:
  ovarian, 906, 916–21
    differentiation of, 929
  testicular. *See* Leydig cells.
Interstitial cell stimulating hormone. *See* Luteinizing hormone.
Intestine. *See also* Gastrointestinal system.
  calcium absorption by, 1351–53, 1355, 1359
    excessive, 1545–51
    laboratory studies, 1368–69, 1553
  inflammatory disease:
    growth failure and, 1602
    nephrolithiasis and, 1520, 1558
  magnesium absorption by, 1362
  oxalate absorption by, 1556, 1558–59
  phosphorus absorption by, 1353–54, 1355
  secretin and, 1643
  vasoactive peptide of. *See* Vasoactive intestinal polypeptide.
  vitamin D effects on, 1354–55
    absorption and, 1352–53, 1355
Intima, fibroplasia of, 737
Intravenous pyelography (urography), 740–42
  diabetes mellitus and, 1121
  nephrolithiasis and, 1568
Introns, 39–40
  evolution and, 43
  exon boundaries with, 61
  mRNA synthesis and, 60, 61
  steroid hormones and, 147–48
Inulin, excretion rate of, 1333
In vitro assays, 167–68, 169
In vitro fertilization:
  ovarian failure and, 957
  Turner's syndrome and, 952
In vivo assays, 166–67, 169
Iod-Basedow effect, 77, 473, 477
Iodination:
  contrast agent, thyroid hormone and, 416, 435
  radioimmunoassay and, 171
  radioreceptor assays and, 176
  thyroglobulin, 393
Iodine (iodide):
  antithyroid effects of, 403, 416
    hyperthyroidism and, 435
  balance, 76
  deficiency, 448–49
    cretinism and, 478
    goiter and, 474, 476–78
  dietary, 76, 392
    goiter and, 476–77
  economy of, 392–93
  excessive, 449
  hyperthyroidism induced by, 422
  metabolism of, 76–77
  organification defects, 448, 481
  perchlorate discharge test and, 448
  radioactive:
    adverse effects of, 436
    vs. antithyroid drugs, 433
    goiter treated by, 437–38
    hyperthyroidism and, 430, 432–33, 436–37
    hypothyroidism diagnosis and, 458
    hypothyroidism induced by, 446
    immunoassay and, 171
    receptor assays and, 176
    for thyroid cancer, 498–99, 500
    thyroid studies and, 408–9, 488
  supplemental, goiter and, 479
  thyroid hormone synthesis and, 393–95, 403
    defects in, 447–48
  for thyroid storm, 438
  transport, 393
    concentration defect, 447
  TSH and, 402–3
  urinary, 476
m-Iodobenzylguanidine, pheochromocytoma and, 671
Iodocholesterol scanning, adrenal, 760–61
Iodothyronines, 391–92, 395
  formation of, 393
  serum levels and production rates, 395
  structure, 391
Iodotyrosine, 77, 391–92
  deiodination of, 394
  defects in, 448, 481
Iodotyrosyl, 393
Ionophores, insulin release and, 1069
Iopanoic acid, 416
Ipodate, thyroid hormone and, 416, 435
Iron, steroid synthesis and, 70
Iron-deficiency anemia, 28
Islet cells (islets of Langerhans), 1043
  alpha, 1043, 1044
    glucagon synthesis by, 1082
    MEN 1 and, 1664–65
  antibodies to, 1097–98, 1683, 1685
  beta, 1043, 1044
    adrenergic receptors of, 1071
    degenerative changes in, 1113
    GIP and, 1642, 1643
    glucose effect on, 1068–70
    hyperplasia of, 1184
    insulin synthesis by, 1065–67
    MEN 1 and, 1664
    nesidioblastosis of, 1184
  delta (alpha$_2$), 1043, 1044
    MEN 1 and, 1664
    somatostatin of, 1072
  diabetes mellitus and, 1096, 1113
  electron micrograph of, 1044
  polypeptide of, 1087
  transplantation of, 1148–49
  tumors of:
    acromegaly and, 303
    gastrin-secreting, 1633–36, 1664, 1669
    glucagon-secreting, 1164–65, 1664–65
    insulin-secreting, 1184–87, 1664, 1669
    MEN 1 and, 1664–65, 1669
    somatostatin-secreting, 1649, 1664–65
    WDHA syndrome and, 1640, 1641
  viral infections and, 1096–97
Isocaproaldehyde, 72
Isocaproic acid, 925
Isochromosomes, 986
Isocitrate dehydrogenase, 1052, 1053
Isoleucine:
  diabetes mellitus and, 1105
  metabolism, 1062–63
  protein feeding and, 1064
Isosexual precocity:
  complete. *See* Puberty, precocious.
  incomplete, 228

Jejunoileal bypass. *See also* Ileal bypass.
  obesity and, 1239
Joints, 31
  Charcot's, 1122
  hyperparathyroidism and, 1390–91
  painful, Paget's disease and, 1484
Juxtaglomerular cells:
  hyperplasia of, 1788
  renin release and, 703

K cells, corpus luteum, 921, 923
K substance, 1651
Kallidin, 1782
Kallikreins, 1780–87
  aldosterone and, 564, 1786
  Bartter's syndrome and, 1788
  biochemistry, 1781–84
  carcinoid and, 1657
  genes for, 1782
  hypertension and, 1786
  inhibitors of, 1782
  localization of, 1784
  prostaglandins and, 1784
  renal function and, 1785–86
  renin-angiotensin system and, 1784–85
Kallmann's syndrome, 227, 863–67
Kaposi's sarcoma, glucocorticoid therapy and, 809
Karyotype:
  sexual differentiation and, 985
  testicular development and, 990
Kassinin, 1651
Katacalcin, 1340, 1672
Keratoconjunctivitis, 34
Keratopathy, 34
  hypercalcemia and, 1395
Ketimine, 1054
Ketoacidosis, diabetic, 1149–54
  clinical manifestations, 1151
  complications, 1154
  diagnosis, 1151–52
  exercise and, 1146
  hyperlipidemia and, 1257
  hypophosphatemia and, 1436, 1437
  magnesium depletion and, 1440
  pathogenesis, 1149–51
  pregnancy and, 1159
  treatment, 1152–54
Ketoamine, 1054
Ketaconazole, 522
  Cushing's disease and, 320
17-Ketogenic steroids, urinary, 572–73
  androgens and, 580
  in children, 1623
  ectopic ACTH and, 1707
  obesity and, 1233

Ketones, 1059–60
basal state and, 1089
carbohydrate metabolism and, 1061–62
diabetes mellitus and. *See* Ketoacidosis, diabetic.
dietary genesis of, 1235–36
glucagon and, 1084–85
hypoglycemia and, 1188
insulin and, 1070–71, 1076
pregnancy and, 1157–59
starvation and, 1183
utilization of, 1060
17-Ketosteroid reductase, 1015
deficiency, 873
Kidney:
acid production, 564, 567, 1524–25
aldosterone and, 563–66, 622
amino acid transport, 1513
AMP clearance and, 1373
atrial natriuretic factor and, 720–22
Bartter's syndrome and, 1787–89
biopsy, 744, 1126
calcification of. *See* Nephrocalcinosis.
calcitonin and, 1343
calcium and, 1335–37
hypercalcemia and, 1359–60, 1417
hypocalcemia and, 1431
leak of, 1542–45
vitamin D and, 1356–57
catecholamines and, 682
citrate and, 1564–65
CT scans, 742
cystinuria and, 1510–17
diabetes insipidus and, 357, 358, 362, 367
diabetes mellitus and, 1114–15, 1119–21
biopsy studies, 1126
insulin therapy and, 1130
metabolic changes, 1127
differentiation of, 992
function tests, divided, 744
GFR. *See* Glomerular filtration rate.
glucagon degradation by, 1085
glucocorticoids and, 553, 566
hyperlipidemia and, 1258–59
hypertension and, 700–701. *See also* Hypertension, renovascular.
hyperthyroidism and, 427
hypogonadism and, 869
hypothyroidism and, 453–54
insulin degradation by, 1082
kallikrein-kinin system and, 1785–86
magnesium and, 1362, 1440, 1442
medullary sponge, 1509–10
mineralocorticoids and, 563–66
osteodystrophy and, 1478–81
clinical presentation, 1478–79
pathogenesis, 1479–80
pathology, 1479
treatment, 1480–81
parathyroid hormone and, 1332–37
calcium transport and, 1336–37
metabolism of, 1328
phosphate transport and, 1334–35
phosphorus and, 1333–35, 1360–61
excess of, 1439
vitamin D and, 1356–57
wasting of, 1464–65
prolactin and, 273
prostaglandins and, 1774–76
pseudohermaphroditism and, 1010
radionuclide studies, 742
renin and, 703. *See also* Renin.
sodium and, 563–66
calcium reabsorption and, 1335, 1336
hyponatremia and, 367, 368
stones. *See* Nephrolithiasis.
transplantation:
diabetic nephropathy and, 1121
hyperparathyroidism and, 1392
osteodystrophy and, 1480
tubular acidosis, 1381–82
hypocitraturia and, 1566
nephrolithiasis and, 1525–27
prostate cancer and, 1758
ultrasonic duplex scanning, 742
uric acid and, 1517–18
vasopressin and, 350–51, 357, 362, 367
hyponatremia and, 367, 368
vitamin D and, 1356–57
metabolism of, 1348
water load test and, 375, 376
Kimmelstiel-Wilson lesions, 1114–15
Kininases, 705, 1781, 1784
Kininogens, 1782–83
Kinins, 1780–87
amino acid sequences of, 1783
Bartter's syndrome and, 1788
biochemistry, 1781–84
hypertension and, 1786
localization of, 1784
prostaglandins and, 1785
renal function and, 1785–86
renin-angiotensin system and, 1784–85
Kleine-Levin syndrome, 233
Klinefelter's syndrome, 870–72, 1000–1002, 1619
Korotkov technique, 733
Krebs cycle, 1052–53
Kultschitsky cells, ectopic hormones and, 1702
Kussmaul's breathing, diabetic ketoacidosis and, 1151

Labor, prostaglandins and, 1773
Laboratory testing, 19–22. *See also* Assays.
Lactate:
Cori cycle and, 1051
epinephrine and, 659
gluconeogenesis and, 1051–52
glycolysis and, 1047, 1049, 1051
ketosis and, 1060
norepinephrine and, 658
Lactate dehydrogenase, 1049
Lactation, 270
breast cancer and, 1739
nonpuerperal. *See* Galactorrhea.
Lactic acidosis, 1155
phenformin-induced, 1143
Lactogen, placental, 1157
chemistry, 253, 263
ectopic, 1722
gene for, 43
as tumor marker, 1726
Lactoperoxidase, iodination and, 171
Lactotroph cells, 251
Lagophthalmos, 34
Laron dwarfism, 1606
Laryngeal nerves:
anatomy, 390
parathyroidectomy and, 1401
thyroidectomy and, 498
Larynx, 26–27
Laser therapy, diabetic retinopathy and, 1118
Laurence-Moon syndrome, 233
Laurence-Moon-Biedl syndrome, 867–68, 1212
Lawrence syndrome, 1163
LCAT. *See* Lecithin:cholesterol acyltransferase.
Leanness, 1206
Learning, peptide hormones and, 211–13
Lecithin, 129
dietary, 1292
respiratory distress syndrome and, 1160
Lecithin:cholesterol acyltransferase (LCAT), 1251
deficiency, 1280
Lectins, receptor conformation and, 97
Lenticular opacities, 33, 34
Lentigenes, multiple, 868
Lesch-Nyhan syndrome, 1519
cathecholamines and, 679
Letterer-Siwe disease, 224
Leucine:
diabetes mellitus and, 1105
hypoglycemia induced by, 1196–97
metabolism, 1062–63
protein feeding and, 1064
Leukemia:
glucocorticoids and, 790, 800, 804
hypoglycemia and, 1717
Leukocytes, 28
glucocorticoids and, 549–51
hyperglycemia and, 1129
Leukotrienes:
actions, 1771
discovery of, 1769
nomenclature, 1769
synthesis and metabolism, 130, 973, 1770, 1772–73
uterine, 972
Levodopa, 199. *See also* L-Dopa.
Leydig cells, 825–27
assay, 167
differentiation of, 989
electron micrograph of, 828
germ cell interaction with, 850–51
hypoplasia, 1011
Kallmann's syndrome and, 867
Klinefelter's syndrome and, 872
ovarian hilus cells vs., 920
physiology, 837–40
postpuberty, 860
Sertoli cell interactions with, 851
Sertoli-cell-only syndrome and, 879
sexual differentiation and, 994, 996
synthetic pathway in, 838, 839
toxic damage to, 873
tumors of, 892

Libido, 29, 214
gonadotropin deficiency and, 285, 286
hyperprolactinemia and, 307
Licorice, hypertension and, 768
Ligands. *See also* Binding; Receptors.
assays of, 168–76
classes of action of, 83–84
desensitization to, 98–99
dissociation of, 104, 108
evolution of, 9–11
internalization of, 106–9
neurotransmitter vs. hormone use of, 4
oncogenes and, 152–53
phosphorylation dependent on, 101–2
regulatory, 9–11
temperature and, 88
Light, melatonin and, 216, 217
Limbic girdle, hypercalcemia and, 1395
Limbic system, 190
obesity and, 1212
Linoleic acid, 1254, 1289, 1292
prostaglandins and, 1780
Linolenic acid, 1289
Lipase:
hepatic, 1251
deficiency of, 1270
hormone-sensitive, 1056–57
lipoprotein, 1056, 1251
deficiency of, 1272
diabetes mellitus and, 1106
Lipemia retinalis, 1124, 1271
Lipids, 1244–1308. *See also* Cholesterol; Fat; Fatty acids; Hyperlipidemia; Lipoprotein; Triglycerides.
diabetes mellitus and, 1105–7, 1123, 1257–58
ketoacidosis and, 1150
lipoatrophy and, 1163
dietary effects on, 1287–92
drugs lowering, 1263–64, 1298–1305
glucocorticoids and, 547–48
homeostasis of, 1056
insulin and, 1070–71, 1076
metabolism, 1055–62, 1249–54
carbohydrate metabolism and, 1061–62
normal values for, 1256
protein complex with. *See* Lipoprotein.
storage diseases, 1280–86
synthesis, 1055–56
carbohydrates and, 1061
thyroid hormone and, 399–400
Lipoatrophic diabetes, 1163
Lipocortin, 52, 549
Lipodystrophy:
gigantism and, 1621
insulin, 1137–38
Lipohyalinosis, 700
Lipoid adrenal hyperplasia, 629, 1013
Lipolysis, 1056–57
cAMP and, 119–20
glucocorticoids and, 547
insulin and, 1076
obesity and, 1217
prostaglandins and, 1779
starvation and, 1183
Lipoma, MEN 1 and, 1665
Lipomodulin, regulatory defect of, 157
Lipooxygenase. *See* Lipoxygenase.
Lipoprotein, 1245–49. *See also* Hyperlipidemia.
abnormal, 1247
alpha. *See* high-density *below*.
apoprotein moieties of. *See* Apoprotein.
assays, 1306–8
atherogenicity of, 1254
beta. *See* low-density *below*.
classification, 1245–46
composition, 1246–47
dietary effects on, 1287–92
electrophoresis, 1245, 1307
glycation of, 1123
high-density (HDL), 1245, 1247
adrenal steroid synthesis and, 517–18
atherosclerosis and, 1274, 1281, 1282
coronary artery disease and, 1274
decreased levels of, 1274–77
disorders of, 1274–77
drug therapy and, 1300–1301
increased levels of, 1277
laboratory tests, 1306–7
metabolism, 1253–54
hypothyroidism and, 454
intermediate-density (IDL), 1245, 1267
lipase. *See* Lipase, lipoprotein.
low-density (LDL), 1245, 1247
absence of, 1278, 1279
adrenal steroid synthesis and, 517–18
atherosclerosis and, 1281
coated pits and, 518
decreased levels of, 1279–80
diet and, 1287, 1293
drug therapy and, 1298, 1300–1301, 1303
familial increase in, 1260–65
increased levels of, 1260–66. *See also* Hyperlipidemia.
internalization mechanism, 106
laboratory tests, 1306–7
metabolism, 1252–53
oncogenes and, 154
ovarian steroid synthesis and, 924–25
receptors for, 40, 69, 106, 154, 155, 1262–63
metabolism, 1251–54
normal values for, 1256
precipitation, 1307
structure, 1249
Tangier disease and, 1276–77
ultracentrifugation, 1245, 1307
very-low-density (VLDL), 1245, 1247
absence of, 1278, 1279
atherosclerosis and, 1281, 1282
diabetes mellitus and, 1105–6, 1123
drug therapy and, 1300
hepatic lipase deficiency and, 1270
increased levels of, 1264–65, 1266, 1268–69, 1273. *See also* Hyperlipidemia.
laboratory tests, 1307
lipoprotein lipase deficiency and, 1272
metabolism, 1252
obesity and, 1231
X, 1247, 1259
Lipostatic theory, 1214, 1222
Lipotropin, 256
vs. ACTH, 256
biosynthesis, 253, 1708
chemistry, 252–54
ectopic, 1709–10
opioids and, 209
pigmentation and, 254, 525
radioimmunoassay, 572
structure, 210
tumor secretion of, pituitary, 315
Lipoxygenase, 130, 973, 1770, 1771
uterine, 972
Lithium:
goitrogenesis of, 482
hypercalcemia induced by, 1414–15
hyponatremia and, 374
sodium transport and, 717
thyroid hormone and, 416
vasopressin and, 347
Lithotripsy, 1572
Lithotrite, ultrasound, 1571–72
Liver:
alcohol metabolism by, 1196
amino acid metabolism and, 1062
carcinoid and, 1655, 1658
catecholamines and, 681–82
diabetes mellitus and, 1115
encephalopathy and, 681
endocrine disease and, 27
estrogens and, 543, 979
fatty acid synthesis in, 1055
glucagon effects on, 1083–85
glucocorticoids and, 543, 544–45, 548
glucose and, 1049, 1190–91
exercise and, 1144–45
metabolism of, 1073–75
obesity and, 1228
hypoglycemia and, 1188, 1190–91
hypogonadism and, 868–69
insulin actions on, 1073–75
obesity and, 1228–29
ketogenesis and, 1059–60
osteomalacia and, 1462
parathyroid hormone and, 1328
testosterone metabolism and, 842
vitamin D metabolism and, 1347
Looser zones, 1460
Lopid. *See* Gemfibrozil.
Lorelco. *See* Probucol.
Lovastatin, 1264, 1304–5
Lubs syndrome, 1019
Lungs. *See also* Respiration.
cancer of:
acromegaly and, 303
ectopic ACTH and, 1706
ectopic GH and, 1718
ectopic vasopressin and, 1711
prostaglandins and, 1779
sympathochromaffin system and, 681
Luteinization, 921–23, 930–31
Luteinizing hormone (LH), 260–63
action, 260
aging and, in male, 860, 861
amenorrhea and, 955
anorexia nervosa and, 234, 235
assays, 260–61, 837, 854–57
in children, 1621
hypopituitarism and, 281–83
prostate weight, 166

Luteinizing hormone (LH), assays *(Cont.)*:
specificity of, 173–74
technique, 323–24
biosynthesis, 257
cells secreting, 251, 825
chemistry, 253, 257, 836–37
chorionic gonadotropin and, 838
clomiphene test and, 283, 323–24, 855–56, 860
corpus luteum differentiation and, 930–31
deficiency, 277–78, 862–69
cryptorchidism and, 883
diagnostic procedures, 281–83
treatment, 285–86
dihydrotestosterone and, 845, 846
drugs affecting, 199
estrogens and, 261, 262, 844–48
testing of, 283, 323–24
fat tissue and, 960
feedback interaction, 262–63, 844–48
fetal gonadal function and, 997
FSH-germ cell interactions with, 850–51
FSH ratio to, 848–49
glucocorticoids and, 558
GnRH, 262–63
stimulation test, 282, 323, 856
growth and, 1589, 1590, 1609
heterogeneity of, 257
hypersecretion, 870–78
Sertoli-cell-only syndrome and, 879
hyperthyroidism and, 428–29
hypopituitarism and, 277–78, 281–83, 285–86, 1610
hypothalamic disease and, 226–29, 282–83
hypothyroidism and, 455
Kallmann's syndrome and, 864–67
Klinefelter's syndrome and, 872, 1001, 1002
menopause and, 944, 975–76
metabolism, 261–62, 837
neuropeptides and, 199
obesity and, 1233
oocyte meiosis and, 933
opioids and, 208, 211, 834
ovarian follicle atresia and, 936
ovarian follicle selection and, 936
ovarian hormone synthesis and, 926, 929
ovulation and, 940, 944
phospholipids and, 134
pituitary levels, 261
plasma levels, 261, 282, 323, 854–57
polycystic ovaries and, 229, 962–63
Prader-Willi syndrome and, 232, 233
premenarche and, 941, 942
prepubertal, 858
production rate, 837
prostaglandins and, 940, 1774
puberty and, 1593, 1594
delayed, 865, 866, 876
in male, 858–60
radioimmunoassay, 260
receptors for, 837–38
down regulation of, 838
excess, 100
granulosa cell, 928
regulation of, 104
theca cell, 916–17
reference preparation, 260
regulation of, 262–63
in male, 832–48
releasing hormone. *See* Gonadotropin releasing hormone.
renal disease and, 869
resistance to, 875
secretion rate, 261–62
secretory pattern, 219–20, 836
episodic (pulsatile), 203, 834, 835, 837
sleep and, in puberty, 859
spermatogenesis and, 849, 850
stimulation tests, 282, 323–24, 855–57
structure of circulating, 837
testosterone and, 263, 844–46
concordance with, 840
tumor secretion of, pituitary, 320
urinary, 260, 261, 854, 855, 857
Kallmann's syndrome and, 865, 866
Luteinizing hormone releasing hormone. *See also* Gonadotropin releasing hormone.
degradation of, 68
Luteolysis, 923–24, 931
17,20-Lyase, 71, 519
ovarian, 925–26
ovulation and, 944
Lymphocytes. *See also* B cells; T cells.
adrenalitis and, 585
glucocorticoids and, 549–50
thyroid-stimulating autoantibodies and, 419–20
Lymphocytosis, 28
Lymphoma, hypercalcemia and, 1409–10, 1419
Lysine:
glycation of, 1129
transport defect, 1510–17
Lysolecithin, 1250–51
Lysophosphatidyl choline, 1251
Lysosomes:
endocytosis and, 108
insulin and, 1079
LDL uptake and, 518
lipid storage diseases and, 1283
receptor biosynthesis and, 103
receptor recycling and, 106
Lysylbradykinin, 1782, 1784

M kinase, 126
Macroadenoma, prolactin-secreting, 309, 312–14
Macrocortin, 52, 549
Macromastia, persistent pubertal, 887, 889
Macrophages:
corpus luteum, 921 923
glucocorticoids and, 550–51
hypertension and, 699
Macula densa, renin release and, 703
Maculopathy, diabetic, 1117
Magnesium, 1361–63, 1439–42
absorption of, 1362, 1440
alcoholism and, 1440
aldosterone and, 564, 753, 1440
balance, 1358
bone and, 1363
calcitonin and, 1673
calcium and, 1426, 1440
deficiency, 1439–42
diagnosis, 1441
pathogenesis, 1439–41
symptoms, 1441
treatment, 1441–42
diabetic ketoacidosis and, 1440
distribution, 1318
diuretics and, 714
epinephrine and, 660
evolutionary development and, 1318
excess, 1442
extracellular, 1318, 1320
homeostasis, 1361–63
hypertension and, 714
intracellular, 1318, 1321, 1362–63
kidney and, 1362, 1440, 1442
metabolism, 1320
neonatal, 1431
parathyroid hormone and, 1325, 1426, 1440
plasma levels, 1365
plasma state, 1321
potassium and, 1441
supplemental, 1441–42
nephrolithiasis and, 1560
total body, 1317, 1318
urinary, 1362, 1368, 1443
Magnesium ammonium phosphate stones, 1521–24
clinical manifestations, 1522–23
diagnosis, 1523
frequency, 1503, 1521
pathogenesis, 1506–7, 1522
risk populations, 1522
treatment, 1523–24
Magnesium sulfate, 1441–42
Magnetic resonance imaging (MRI):
pituitary, 291, 293
Cushing's disease and, 614–15
thyroid, 490
Malabsorption:
abetalipoproteinemia and, 1278
calcium, 1359
hyperoxaluria and, 1558–59
hypomagnesemia and, 1440
hypothyroidism and, 454
phosphorus, 1436, 1465
vitamin D, 1462, 1466
Malic enzyme, thyroid hormone and, 399
Malnutrition. *See also* Diet; Nutrition.
amenorrhea and, 954, 960–61
goiter and, 479
growth retardation and, 1591, 1601–2
hypogonadism and, 868
hypophosphatemic osteomalacia and, 1465
Malonyl CoA, 1055, 1056
diabetic ketoacidosis and, 1150
fatty acid oxidation and, 1058
insulin and, 1076
Mammillary nuclei, 190
Mania, 238
Mannitol:
hyponatremia and, 373
vasopressin and, 342
Mannose, peptide hormone, 66, 67
Marble bone disease, 1477–78

Marfan's syndrome, 1619–20
vs. homocystinuria, 1620
multiple mucosal neuromas and, 1677–78
Marijuana, adrenal inhibition by, 522
Masculinization. *See also* Virilization.
of genitalia, 994, 995
Mauriac syndrome, 1115
Maxam-Gilbert sequencing technique, 47
McCune-Albright syndrome, 228, 1617
McKenzie bioassay, 258
Media, fibromuscular dysplasia of, 737–38
Median eminence, hypothalamic, 190, 821
neurohypophysis and, 338
neuronal-capillary relationship, 823, 824
portal system and, 191–92, 248
structural composition of, 191, 193
Mediators, 8, 110–34
calcium, 123–28
cAMP, 121–22
cGMP, 122
evolution of, 10–11
hypercalcemia of malignancy and, 1405–9
peptide hormone, 87, 121–22
phospholipid, 128–34
Medrogesterone, endometrial cancer and, 1764
Medroxyprogesterone:
breast cancer and, 1749
endometrial cancer and, 1764
estrogen therapy and, 285, 979
menopause and, 977
menorrhagia and, 974
osteoporosis and, 1475
precocious puberty and, 1618
tall stature therapy with, 1614
Turner's syndrome and, 951, 1612
Medulla oblongata, sympathetic connections to, 653–54
Medullary thyroid carcinoma, 501–4, 1669–75
classification, 494
clinical course, 501–2
diagnosis, 502–3, 1671–75
embryology, 1670
hyperparathyroidism and, 1393, 1676–77
MEN 2 and, 1669–75
mucosal neuromas and, 1677
natural history, 501, 1671
occurrence, 1671
pathology, 1670–71
pheochromocytoma and, 1675–76
secretory products, 1671–75
therapy, 503–4
Mefenamic acid, menorrhagia and, 974
Megestrol, endometrial cancer and, 1764
Meiosis:
nondisjunction and, 985–86
oocyte, 908, 910, 932, 933–34
inhibitor (OMI) of, 933
sexual differentiation and, 992
spermatogenesis, 827, 832
Melanocyte-stimulating hormone (MSH), 256
actions, 525
Addison's disease and, 586
aldosteronism and, 754
amino acid sequence of, 525
behavioral effects of, 212
cells secreting, 251
chemistry, 252–54, 1708, 1709
ectopic, 1710
inhibiting factor, 207
oxytocin and, 207
precursor, 64
releasing factor, 207
Melanoma, malignant, hypercalcemia and, 1410
Melatonin, 216–18
action, 218
circadian variation in, 216–17
pinealoma and, 236
synthesis, 216
Membrana granulosa cells, 915, 916, 921, 933
Membrane, cell:
calcium permeability of, 123
components of, 94–96
detergent dissolution of, 90
oncogenes and, 152–53
phospholipids of. *See* Phospholipids.
receptors of, 84, 85–110. *See also* Receptors, peptide hormone; Receptors, surface.
steroid passage through, 137
structure of, 86, 91
Memory, peptide hormones and, 213
MEN. *See* Multiple endocrine neoplasia.
Menarche, 941, 951
delayed, 1600–1601
fat tissue and, 960
menorrhagia of, 955
premature, 1617
Menopause, 944, 974–80
amenorrhea and, 956
atherosclerosis and, 977–78
bleeding after, 980
breast cancer and, 1739–40
climacteric symptoms and, 976–77
estrogen therapy and, 977
osteoporosis and, 977, 1472, 1474–75
premature, 956–58
scheme of features of, 975
Menorrhagia, 970–74
menarcheal, 955
prostaglandins and, 973
treatment, 974
Menotropins, infertility and, 286
Menstrual cycle (menstruation), 29–30, 941–44
absent menses and. *See* Amenorrhea.
Addison's disease and, 1683–84
aldosterone and, 620
behavioral changes of, 214
blood loss of, 970–72
endocrine events in, diagram of, 943
endometrium and, 970–72
follicular phase of, 942–43
midfollicular phase of, 938
normal, 941–44
obesity and, 1232, 1233
pain and, 974
permanent cessation of. *See* Menopause.
polycystic ovary disease and, 961, 963
premenopause and, 975
premenstrual syndrome and, 974
prostaglandins and, 973, 1773, 1774
Mercaptopropionylglycine, 1516
Mesenchyme:
ovarian, 908, 916–17
sexual differentiation and, 989
Mesenteric ganglia, 654
Mesonephric ducts, 992–94
Mesovarium, 905, 906
Messengers, intracellular, 110–22. *See also* Adenosine monophosphate, cyclic.
Metabolism:
diabetes mellitus and, 1104–7, 1125–29
glucocorticoids and, 544–48
glycoprotein, 68
hormone, 6
hyperthyroidism and, 428
hypothalamic disorders and, 231–35
hypothyroidism and, 454
intermediary, 14
iodine, 76–77
mineral, 1317–21
obesity and, 1216–19
peptide hormone, 67–68
starvation and, 1182–83
steroid hormone, 75
thyroid hormone, 78–79
Metacarpal sign, pseudohypoparathyroidism and, 1428
Metanephrine, 653
plasma, 682
urinary, 682, 684
pheochromocytoma and, 669
Metaphyseal dysplasia, 1611
Meformin, 1143–44
Methimazole, 416
dosage, 433, 434
hyperthyroidism and, 433, 435
in pregnancy, 439
hypothyroidism induced by, 449
side effects of, 434–35
Methionine, protein synthesis and, 51
Methionyl-hGH, 287
Methoxyflurane, 1558
3-Methoxy-4-hydroxyphenylglycol (MHPG), 653
Methylation, phospholipid, 133–34
Methyldopa:
carcinoid and, 1659
catecholamines and, 684
pituitary effects of, 199
Methylenecyclopropylacetic acid, 1198
Methylglyoxal, 1060
Methylprednisolone. *See also* Glucocorticoids, therapeutic.
dose-response considerations, 804
half-life and potency of, 798
structure, 789
Methyltestosterone, hypogonadism and, 876
Methyltrienolone, receptor assay and, 1762
Methysergide, carcinoid and, 1659
Metoclopramide:
pituitary effects of, 199
prolactin and, 284, 326
Metoprolol, 657
Metropolitan Life weight tables, 1204–5
Metrorrhagia, 30
Metyrapone, 578–79
ACTH stimulation and, 281, 322
adrenal inhibition by, 522

Metyrapone *(Cont.)*:
adrenocortical insufficiency and, 592–94
cortisol and, 679
Cushing's disease and, 316, 319, 618
overnight test, 579
Mevastatin, 1304–5
Mevinolin, 1264, 1304–5
MIBG scans, pheochromocytoma and, 671
Microadenoma, prolactin-secreting, 309, 314–15
Microangiopathy, diabetic, 1114, 1116, 1119
pathogenesis, 1125, 1130
Microdensitometer, 168
Microsomal antigen, thyroid, antibodies to, 408
Microsurgery, renal artery, 749
Midodrine, postural hypotension and, 676
Migration inhibition factor:
autoimmune thyroiditis and, 445
Graves' disease and, 419
Milk, osteoporosis therapy and, 1476
Milk-alkali syndrome, 1414, 1526
Milkman fractures, 1460
Mineralocorticoids, 563–68. *See also* Aldosterone; Deoxycorticosterone.
actions, 563–65
agonists, 567–68
antagonists, 142–43, 567
biosynthesis, 71, 72, 519, 1012
definition of, 568
glucocorticoid activity as, 539, 560, 565–67, 790, 792
hypertension and, 723–25, 755, 768. *See also* Aldosteronism.
kidney and, 563–66
molecular mechanisms, 565–67
receptors for, 565–66
regulation, 531–35
structure, 136
therapeutic:
addisonian crisis and, 594
adrenal hyperplasia and, 1615
chronic adrenal insufficiency and, 595, 596
21-hydroxylase deficiency and, 627–28, 1027
hypertension induced by, 768
hyporeninemic hypoaldosteronism and, 598
postural hypotension and, 676
water balance and, 564
Minerals. *See also* Calcium; Magnesium; Phosphorus.
balance of, 1357–58, 1369
homeostasis of, 1357–63
metabolism of, 1317–21
Minipress, 671
Minisomatostatin, acromegaly and, 306
Minoxidil, 544
Mithramycin:
hyercalcemia and, 1411, 1420
Paget's disease of bone and, 1490
Mitochondria:
calcium metabolism and, 1319
citrate metabolism and, 1565
fatty acid transport into, 1058
steroid synthesis and, 70–71
Mitogen:
degradation of, 107
oncogenes and, 154
Mitomycin C, prostate cancer and, 1761
Mitotane:
adrenal function and, 522, 1711
Cushing's syndrome and, 618
Mitral valve prolapse, catecholamines and, 680–81
MMI. *See* Methimazole.
Molecular genetics. *See* DNA, recombinant.
Molecular mechanisms, 82–158
atrial natriuretic factor, 723–24
glucocorticoid, 559–61, 791–92
mineralocorticoid, 565–67
steroid hormone, 134–48
thyroid hormone, 148–50, 398
Moniliasis, hypoparathyroidism and, 1425
Monoamine oxidase, 653, 656
menstrual cycle and, 214
serotonin metabolism and, 1656
Monoaminergic neurons, 194, 195. *See also* Neurotransmitters.
drugs affecting, 198
Monoclonal antibodies, 172
to estrogen receptors, 139
Monocytes:
autoimmunity and, 1678
glucocorticoids and, 550, 551
Monoiodothyronine, 395
Monoiodotyrosine, 78, 394
structure, 391
Mononeuropathy, 32–33
diabetic, 1122
Monosomy, 985
Turner's syndrome and, 1005
Morphine, 198
ACTH and, 212
endogenous opioids and, 211
Morphogenetic protein, bone, 1491
Mosaicism, 986
gonadal dysgenesis and, 952, 1004, 1005
Klinefelter's syndrome and, 871–72
Turner's syndrome and, 1005, 1007
Motilin, 1652
Motor impairment, 33
Mouth, pigmentation of, 26
Mucosa, nasal, 26
Mucosal neuromas, multiple, 1677
Müllerian ducts, 992–93
amenorrhea and, 954
persistent, 1011
Multiglandular deficiencies. *See* Pluriglandular insufficiency syndromes.
Multiple endocrine neoplasia (MEN), 18, 1662–78
type 1 (MEN 1), 1662–69
clinical evaluation, 1666–67
components of, 1663–64
definition and history, 1662–63
epidemiology, 1667
gastrinoma and, 1663, 1664, 1669
glucagonoma and somatostatinoma and, 1664–65
hyperparathyroidism and, 1392–93, 1664, 1668
insulinoma and, 1664, 1669
management, 1668
other associated tumors, 1665–66
pathogenesis, 1667–68
pituitary tumors and, 1665, 1668–69
type 2 (MEN 2), 1669–78
hyperparathyroidism and, 1393, 1669, 1676–77
marfanoid habitus and, 1677–78
medullary thyroid carcinoma and, 1669–75
mucosal neuromas and, 1677
pheochromocytoma and, 667, 1669, 1675–76
Multiple myeloma, hypercalcemia and, 1403, 1406, 1417
Multiplication-stimulating activity, 1716. *See also* Insulin-like growth factors.
Mumps:
diabetes mellitus and, 1097
orchitis and, 874
Muscimol, 199
Muscle, 33
amino acid metabolism and, 1062–64, 1075–76
atrophy, 33
basal state and, 1089, 1090
calcium and, 1319
cramps, 1423
diabetes mellitus and, 1122, 1126
exercise and, fuel utilization in, 1091
eye, 34
fuel reserves and, 1088
glucocorticoids and, 545, 548, 795
glucose and, 1144
glycogen and, 1144
hyperparathyroidism and, 1388
hyperthyroidism and, 427–28
hypocalcemia and, 1422–23
hypomagnesemia and, 1441
hypothyroidism and, 452–53
insulin effects on, 1075–76
lactate production and, 1051
tetany, 1422–23
Mutation, 44
mRNA synthesis and, 60
oncogenes and, 151, 153
polymorphisms and, 53–54
two-hit, MEN and, 1667–68
myc gene, 151, 1701
Myelin, diabetes mellitus and, 1127, 1128
Myeloma, multiple, hypercalcemia and, 1403, 1406, 1417
Myocardial infarction, 28–29
diabetes mellitus and, 1123
familial hypercholesterolemia and, 1262
menopause and, 977–78
sympathochromaffin system and, 680
Myoinositol, 1053, 1127
neuronal metabolism of, 1127, 1128
Myopathy, 33
glucocorticoid-induced, 795
hyperparathyroidism and, 1388
hyperthyroidism and, 427–28
hypothyroidism and, 453
Myopia, 33
Myosin kinase, 126

Myotonic dystrophy, 872
Myxedema, 451
  coma, 460–61
  Graves' disease and, 420, 443–44
  madness, 452

N protein, pseudohypoparathyroidism and, 1428–29
NAD, NADH. *See* Nicotinamide adenine dinucleotide.
Nafoxidine, breast cancer and, 1744, 1745, 1749
Najjar syndrome, 1020
Na^+,K^+-ATPase, 715–16
  aldosterone and, 566
  diabetic complications and, 1127, 1128
  obesity and, 1216, 1218
  thyroid hormone and, 398–99
Naloxone, opioids and, 211
National Health and Nutrition Examination Survey (NHANES), 1205–6
Natriuresis:
  ANF and, 722
  hypercalcemia and, 1420
  prostaglandins and, 1775
  SIADH and, 371
Natriuretic factor, atrial. *See* Atrial natriuretic factor.
Nausea, vasopressin and, 345–46
Neck examination, 390
Necrobiosis lipoidica diabeticorum, 1124
Nelson's syndrome, 315, 619
Neomycin, hyperlipidemia and, 1302–3
Neonate:
  androgenization of, 215–16
  diabetic mother and, 1160, 1161, 1621
  genital abnormalities of. *See also* Genitals.
    clinical approach to, 1031–33
  hypercalcemia in, 1417
  hyperthyroidism in, 440
  hypocalcemia in, 1430–31
  hypoglycemia in, 1161
  hypothyroidism in, 460, 1602–3
  reproductive adaptations of, 997–99
  respiratory distress syndrome in, 1159
  size of, 1592
    diabetic mother and, 1621
Neovascularization, retinal, 1115, 1117–18
Nephrectomy, renovascular hypertension and, 749
Nephrocalcinosis, 29, 1381, 1501
  medullary, 1509
  renal tubular acidosis and, 1525, 1527
Nephrolithiasis, 29, 1500–1572
  acidosis and, renal tubular, 1381–82, 1525–27
  activity product ratio and, 1508
  age distribution by type of stone, 1503
  anatomical considerations, 1508–9
  bladder, 1501, 1522
  calcium oxalate, 1507–8, 1527–67. *See also* Calcium oxalate stones.
  calcium phosphate, 1507, 1524–27
  crystalloid theory of, 1504 -7
  Cushing's syndrome and, 608
  cystinuria and, 1506, 1510–17
  dehydration and, 1520, 1531
  diet and, 1527, 1531
  epitaxy and, 1505
  family history and, 1529–30
  formation product and, 1505, 1508
  frequency by composition, 1503
  general considerations, 1500–1503, 1527–29
  geographic factors, 1527
  gravel passage and, 1502
  hydration principles and, 1515, 1570–71
  hypercalciuria and, 1382–83, 1529, 1531–56
  hyperoxaluria and, 1556–61
  hyperparathyroidism and, 1381–84, 1391, 1526
  hyperuricosuria and, 1561–64
  hypocitraturia and, 1564–66
  idiopathic, 1566–67
  infection and, 1507, 1521–24
  inflammatory bowel disease and, 1520, 1558
  inhibitor theory of, 1504
  lithotripsy for, 1572
  magnesium ammonium phosphate, 1506–7, 1521–24
  matrix theory of, 1504, 1522
  medications and, 1530
  medullary sponge kidney and, 1509–10
  metabolic activity and, 1502, 1521
  mixed, 1502, 1507, 1527. *See also* Calcium oxalate stones.
  morbidity assessment, 1502
  nucleation and, 1505
  oxypurinol, 1520
  pain from, 1501
  pathogenesis, 1503–8
  pH and, 1506, 1507, 1524–27, 1530
  physical chemical aspects of, 1504–8
  precipitation-crystallization theory of, 1504–7
  Randall's plaque hypothesis of, 1501
  recurrent, 1508, 1528
  risk factors, 1518–19, 1522, 1525–26, 1528–29
  saturation-inhibition index and, 1508
  saturation zones of urine and, 1504–5
  solubility product and, 1504–5
  staghorn, 1500, 1502, 1514, 1522–23
  struvite, 1506–7, 1521–24
  surgical activity and, 1502
  testing, 1567–70
    initial evaluation, 1568
    oral calcium tolerance, 1569–70
    single stone event and, 1569
    subsequent evaluation, 1568–69
  theories of, 1504
  treatment, 1570–72
    hypercalciuria and, 1553–56
  ultrasound technique for, 1571–72
  urease and, 1522, 1523
  uric acid, 1506, 1517–21
  vitamin C and, 1530
  vitamin D and, 1383
  xanthine, 1520
Nephron:
  amino acid transport in, 1513
  calcium transport in, 1333, 1335, 1336
  magnesium reabsorption in, 1362
  phosphate transport in, 1333
  vasopressin and, 350–51
Nephropathy:
  diabetic, 1114–15, 1119–21
    biopsy studies, 1126
    insulin therapy and, 1130
    metabolic changes, 1127
  uric acid, 1517
Nephrotic syndrome:
  diabetic, 1120
  hyperlipidemia and, 1258
  hyponatremia and, 368
Nerve growth factor, 1583
Nervous system. *See also* Brain; Hypothalamus; Neuroendocrine system; Pituitary gland.
  adrenal gland innervation, 514
  autonomic. *See* Autonomic nervous system; Norepinephrine; Parasympathetic nervous system; Sympathetic nervous system.
  blood-brain barrier and, 187, 342–43
  catecholamines and, 681. *See also* Norepinephrine; Sympathetic nervous system.
  diabetes insipidus and, 356, 358, 362–66
  diabetes mellitus and, 1115, 1121–23
  endocrine disease and, 31–32
  evolution of, 12
  glucocorticoids and, 555–56
  hyperparathyroidism and, 1388
  hyperthyroidism and, 427
  hypocalcemia and, 1423
  hyponatremia and, 230, 371–72
  hypophosphatemia and, 1438
  hypopituitarism and, 276
  hypothyroidism and, 452
  insulin and, 1071–72, 1085
  obesity and, 1212–15
  ovaries and, 907–8, 920
  parasympathetic. *See* Parasympathetic nervous system.
  peptide hormone interactions with, 211–13
  pituitary supply from, 249
  rhythms and, 218–21
  sympathetic. *See* Catecholamines; Norepinephrine; Sympathetic nervous system.
Nesidioblastosis, 1184
  MEN and, 1667
neu oncogene, 153
Neuroblastoma, 672
Neuroendocrine system, 185–239. *See also* Hypothalamus; Nervous system; Neurotransmitters; Pituitary gland.
  anatomy, 190–93
  APUD cells and, 1700
  behavior and, 211–14
  disorders of, 221–38
  feedback and, 185–87
  hypophysiotropic concept and, 187–90. *See also* Hypophysiotropic hormones *and specific hormones*.
  paracrine secretion and, 85
  peptides of. *See* Neuropeptides *and also specific peptide*.
  pineal gland, 216–18
  rhythms of, 218–21

Neuroendocrine system *(Cont.)*:
  sympathochromaffin, 651–86. *See also* Catecholamines; Sympathetic nervous system.
Neuroendocrinology, 4
Neurofibromatosis, pheochromocytoma and, 667, 679–80
Neuroglycopenia, 1180
Neurohemal contact zone, 824
Neurohypophysis. *See* Pituitary gland, posterior *and specific hormones.*
Neurokinin K, 1651
Neuroleptics, prolactin and, 230
Neuromas:
  hyperparathyroidism and, 1393
  medullary thyroid carcinoma and, 501
  mucosal, multiple, 1677
Neuromodulators, 197
Neuromuscular disease, 32–33
Neuropathy, 32–33
  acromegaly and, 301–2
  diabetic, 32, 1115, 1121–23
    metabolic changes and, 1127, 1128
  hyperparathyroidism and, 1388
  pluriglandular insufficiency and, 1686
Neuropeptides, 197–99, 207–11. *See also specific peptide, e.g.,* Endorphins; Neurotensin; Substance P.
  behavior and, 211–13
  pituitary effects of, 197–99, 208
  synthesis of, 197
  Y, 1647
    amino acid sequence of, 1646
Neurophysins:
  action, 352
  ADH, 64
  biosynthesis, 340
  chemistry, 339
  ectopic, 1712
Neurosecretory cells, 185, 338
  loss of, diabetes insipidus and, 356
  neurotransmitter control of, 193–94
Neurotensin, 209
  actions, 199, 208, 1652
  chemistry, 1651–52
  distribution, 192, 1652
  measurement and release, 1652
Neurotransmitters, 4, 193–97. *See also* Acetylcholine; Dopamine; Epinephrine; Gamma-aminobutyric acid; Norepinephrine; Serotonin.
  biosynthesis and metabolism, 194–96
  drugs affecting, 195–97
    tabulations of, 198, 199
  GnRH and, 203
  growth hormone and, 269
  hypophysiotropic cell regulation by, 193–94
  peptide, 197–99
  pituitary function and, 188, 194, 195
  psychiatric disorders and, 237–38
  receptors for, 85–87
    drugs affecting, 198
  somatostatin and, 205
  TSH and, 195, 259–60
  vasopressin and, 213
Neutrophils, glucocorticoids and, 550, 551
NH_2-terminal peptide, 1708–9
Ni protein, 113–114, 133
Niacin. *See* Nicotinic acid.
Nicotinamide adenine dinucleotide (NAD, NADH, NADPH):
  adrenodoxin reductase and, 518
  alcohol metabolism and, 1196
  ethanol and, 1051
  fatty acid synthesis and, 1055
  ketosis and, 1060
  steroid synthesis and, 70, 71, 518
  tricarboxylic acid cycle and, 1052
Nicotinic acid:
  action and toxicity, 1300
  hyperlipidemia and, 1263, 1264, 1292, 1299–1300
  indications and dosage, 1300
Nifedipine, aldosteronism and, 763
Nitrogen:
  diabetes mellitus and, 1104–5
  protein feeding and, 1064
Nitroprusside test for cystinuria, 1514
Nocturia, 29
Nomifensine, prolactin and, 308
Nondisjunction, chromosomal, 985–86
Nonhypoglycemia, 1181–82
Non-(antibody-)suppressible insulin-like activity (NSILA), 265, 1086. *See also* Insulin-like growth factors.
Noonan's syndrome, 872, 1612–13
Norepinephrine. *See also* Catecholamines; Neurotransmitters.
  actions, 658, 660–62
  antagonists, 199
  axonal reuptake of, 656
  axonal secretion of, 655, 656
  Bartter's syndrome and, 679
  biosynthesis, 196, 652–53
  blood pressure and, 658, 668
    posture and, 672–76
  chemistry, 652
  degradation, 196, 653, 656
  diabetes mellitus and, 677
  glucose and, 658, 661
  heart failure and, 680
  hormonal function of, 666
  hypoglycemia and, 666–67, 1180
  inactivation of, 655–56
  infusion test, 685, 686
  insulin and, 658, 1071, 1085
  neuronal network distribution, 195, 823
  neurotransmitter function of, 666–67
  obesity and, 1212–13
  pheochromocytoma and, 668–70
  pineal gland and, 216, 217
  pituitary effects of, 195
  plasma levels, 662–64, 682–84
    conditions affecting, 664, 665, 683–84
    metabolic effect and, 658, 662
    sample handling and, 683
  postural hypotension and, 673–76
  potassium and, 714–15
  production rate, 664
  Raynaud's phenomenon and, 681
  receptors for, 657–59. *See also* Adrenergic receptors.
  renal disorders and, 682
  sodium and, 712
  storage and release, 655, 656
  sympathetic activity index and, 666–67
Norethindrone:
  estrogen therapy and, 979
  hyperlipidemia and, 1303–4
  menorrhagia and, 955, 974
  polycystic ovary disease and, 963
  tall stature therapy with, 1614
Norgestrel, 979
Normetanephrine, 653
  plasma, 682
  urinary, 682
Northern blotting, 46
  ectopic hormones and, 1696
Nose, 26
NSILA, 265, 1086. *See also* Insulin-like growth factors.
Ns protein, 113–14
NT peptide, 17–8–9
Nuclear magnetic resonance. *See* Magnetic resonance imaging.
Nucleation, nephrolithiasis and, 1505
Nucleic acid, 37
Nucleosides, 37
Nucleosomes, 37–38, 143
Nucleotides, 37. *See also* Adenosine monophosphate, cyclic; Guanosine monophosphate, cyclic.
Nucleus:
  hormone action and, 84, 144–45
  matrix of, 38
    organization and function of, 144
  oncogenes and, 151–52
  steroid receptors of, 137–38
    action of hormone and, 144–45
    binding by, 141, 143–44
  thyroid hormone receptors of, 149–50
Numbness, 32, 33
Nutrition. *See also* Diet.
  amenorrhea and, 954, 960–61
  diabetes mellitus and, 1098
  growth and, 1591, 1601–2
  obesity and, 1219–21, 1235–37, 1290–91, 1294–96
  parenteral:
    hypophosphatemia and, 1437
    osteomalacia and, 1466
  prostate cancer and, 1754
Nx protein, 133

Obesity, 25, 1203–40
  adipose cell hypothesis of, 1221–22
  arthritis and, 1234
  behavior modification for, 1237–38
  body mass index and, 1206
  cardiovascular system and, 1232
  catecholamines and, 679
  childhood, 1207, 1209, 1220–21, 1620–21
  classification of, 1224, 1225
  community involvement in, 1239–40
  cortisol and, 1215, 1233
  Cushing's syndrome and, 606, 611, 1215, 1233
  definition, 1203–6
  development of adipose tissue and, 1208–10, 1222

Obesity *(Cont.)*:
diabetes mellitus and, 1098, 1139, 1226–31, 1240
diet therapy for, 1235–37, 1294–96
drug therapy for, 1238–39
endocrine factors, 1215–16, 1232–33
energy imbalance and, 1210–11, 1214, 1216–19
etiology and pathogenesis, 1210–24
exercise and, 1221, 1237
Fogarty Conference tables and, 1205
gallstones and, 1234
genetic factors, 1211–12
growth hormone and, 1215, 1233
health consequences of, 1207–8, 1224–34, 1240
hirsutism and, 964
hyperlipidemia and, 1231–32, 1273, 1290–91, 1294–96
hypertension and, 1232
hypothalamic, 232–33, 1212–15
insulin and, 1072–73, 1214–16, 1227–31
resistance to, 1081, 1082, 1228–30
lipolytic defect and, 1217
metabolic factors, 1216–19
Metropolitan Life weight tables and, 1204–5
mortality, 1224–26
Na^+,K^+-ATPase activity and, 1216, 1218
NCHS tables and, 1205–6
neurologic factors, 1212–15
nutritional factors, 1219–21, 1235–37, 1290–91, 1294–96
polycystic ovary disease and, 961
Prader-Willi syndrome and, 232, 233
prevalence, 1206–7
psychological factors, 1222–23, 1238
pulmonary dysfunction and, 1233–34
resistance to weight loss and, 1208
sex steroids and, 1232–33
socioeconomic aspects, 1207, 1223–24
surgery for, 1239
thermogenesis and, 1218–19
experimental, 1216–17
thyroid hormones and, 1215, 1233
treatment of, 1234–40
18-OHB. *See* 18-Hydroxycorticosterone.
3β-ol-dehydrogenase isomerase, 925
Oleic acid, 1254, 1288, 1289
Olfaction, loss of, 26
Olfactory-genital dysplasia, 227
Oligomenorrhea, 29–30
hyperprolactinemia and, 307
Oligosaccharides:
peptide hormone, 65–66
structure of, 67
Oligospermia, 878
autoimmunity and, 881
genetic disorders and, 881
idiopathic, 879–80
varicocele and, 880
Omeprazole, 1636
Oncogenes, 55, 150–54
cytoplasmic, 152–54
ectopic hormone production and, 1700–1701
growth factors and, 153–54, 1701
MEN and, 1668
nuclear, 151–52
proto-, 55, 151–53
tyrosine phosphorylation and, 101
Onycholysis, 425
Oocytes, 908, 932–34
cavitation and, 912–13
degeneration of, 915, 916, 935
development of, 908, 911–13
dictyotene, 932, 933
fetal, 910
growth of, 932–33
in vitro fertilization of, 957
Turner's syndrome and, 952
maturation inhibitor, 927
meiosis of, 908, 910, 932, 933–34
inhibitor (OMI) of, 933
sexual differentiation and, 992
ovulation and, 939–40
Oogonia, 932
fetal, 910, 917
Oophorectomy, breast cancer and, 1739, 1742, 1744, 1747–48
o,p'-DDD, 320, 1711
Ophthalmic abnormalities. *See* Eyes; Vision.
Ophthalmopathy, Graves', 33, 420, 440–43
Ophthalmoplegia, 34
hyperthyroidism and, 427
Ophthalmoscopy, diabetes and, 1116–17
Opioids, 209–11
anatomy and, 822–23
behavioral effects of, 211, 212
gonadotropins and, 208, 211, 834
growth hormone and, 211
insulin and, 1072
pituitary effects of, 198–99, 208, 211
prolactin and, 211
receptors for, 209–10
vasopressin and, 208, 348
Optic chiasm:
pituitary tumor and, 289
vision studies and, 293–95
Optic nerve, 33
Graves' disease and, 442, 443
pituitary tumor and, 289
Orbit, CT scans and ultrasonography of, 442
Orchidometer, Prader, 852
Orchiectomy:
cryptorchism and, 885–86
prostate cancer and, 891, 1756, 1760
testicular femininization and, 1032
Orchiopexy, 885, 886
Orchitis, mumps, 874
Organum vasculosum of lamina terminalis, 821
Ornithine transport defect, 1510–17
Orthostatic hypotension. *See* Hypotension, postural.
Osmolality:
blood-brain barrier and, 342–43
blood volume or pressure and, 345, 356
hypernatremia and, 361, 364, 366
hyponatremia and, 369–72
sample handling for, 376
set point of, 341–42
hypernatremia and, 361
SIADH and, 370, 371
water load test and, 375, 376
sodium and, 354
thirst and, 352, 358, 359
urinary, 350, 355
diabetes insipidus and, 358–60, 362–63
vasopressin and, 341–43, 354–55
diabetes insipidus and, 358–60
SIADH and, 369–71
urinary, 350
water balance and, 353–56
Osmoreceptors, 341–43
ablation of, 357
dysfunctional, 360–61, 364
treatment, 366–67
thirst and, 352
water balance and, 354–56
Osmotic diuresis, diabetic ketoacidosis and, 1150
Ossification, endochondrial, 1591
Osteitis deformans, 1483–84, 1487
Osteitis fibrosa cystica, 1385–87
Osteoblasts, 1330
osteoclast stimulation by, 1332, 1491
osteoporosis and, 1470, 1472
Paget's disease and, 1484, 1486
parathyroid hormone and, 1332
vitamin D and, 1356
Osteocalcin, 1330
glucocorticoids and, 554
metabolic disease and, 1455
Osteoclasts, 1329–30, 1331
activating factor (OAF), 1403, 1491
hypercalcemia of malignancy and, 1705
breast cancer and, 1403
calcitonin and, 1342
glucocorticoids and, 554
hypercalcemia and, 1403, 1404, 1705
inclusions in, 1487
osteoblast stimulation of, 1332, 1491
osteopetrosis and, 1477, 1478
Paget's disease and, 1486, 1487
parathyroid hormone and, 1332, 1356
prostaglandins and, 1403
vitamin D and, 1356
Osteocytes, 1329, 1330
osteoid, 1330
osteolysis by, 1331
parathyroid hormone and, 1332
Osteodystrophy:
Albright's hereditary, 1427–30
renal, 1478–81
clinical presentation, 1478–79
pathogenesis, 1479–80
pathology, 1479
treatment, 1480–81
Osteogenesis imperfecta, 1471
Osteoid, 1330
osteomalacia and, 1461
Osteolysis, 1330, 1331
calcitonin and, 1342
glucocorticoids and, 554
malignancy-associated, 1403, 1404, 1703–5
Paget's disease and, 1484, 1486
vitamin D and, 1356
Osteomalacia, 31, 1458–68
classification, 1462
definition, 1458

Osteomalacia *(Cont.)*:
hypophosphatemia and, 1460, 1464–65, 1467
hypophosphatasia and, 1465–66
laboratory studies, 1460
pathogenesis, 1461–66
pathology, 1460–61
radiology and, 1459–60
renal osteodystrophy and, 1479
symptoms and signs, 1458–59
treatment, 1466–68
tumor-associated, 1717–18
vitamin D and, 1460, 1462–63
Osteonectin, 1330
Osteons, 1329
Osteopenia, 31, 1468, 1469
hyperparathyroidism and, 1387
hyperthyroidism and, 429
Osteopetrosis, 1477–78
Osteoporosis, 31, 1468–77
aging and, 1471–72
androgen deficiency and, 1472, 1473
circumscripta, 1484, 1485
classification, 1471
Cushing's syndrome and, 608, 1473
diabetes mellitus and, 1474
estrogens and, 977, 979, 1472–73, 1475
glucocorticoids and, 793–95, 1473, 1476
hyperparathyroidism and, 1469–70, 1473–74
hyperthyroidism and, 1471, 1473
immobilization and, 1474
juvenile, 1474, 1477
laboratory studies, 1469–70
menopause and, 977, 1472, 1474–75
pathogenesis, 1471–74
pathology, 1470–71
radiology, 1468–69
symptoms and signs, 1468
treatment, 1474–77
Osteosclerosis:
fragilis generalisata, 1477–78
renal osteodystrophy and, 1479, 1480
Osteotomy, tibial, Paget's disease and, 1490
Otitis media, 26
Ouabain, sodium transport and, 717, 718
Ovalbumin:
estrogen and, 145–48
gene for, 147–48
Ovaries, 905–80
Addison's disease and, 583
age-related changes in, 911, 940–44, 974–78
amenorrhea and, 951–61. *See also* Amenorrhea.
anatomy, 905–8
androgens of, 925–26, 929. *See also* Androgens.
fetal, 941
hirsutism and, 623
recruitment and, 935
antibodies to, 584, 957, 1684
biopsy, 957
blood supply, 906–7
follicular, 911–12
catecholamines and, 920
climacteric and, 976–77
clinical disorders of, 951–80
in middle age, 974–80
in teenagers, 951–55
in young adults, 955–74
corpora lutea, 921–24. *See also* Corpus luteum.
cortex of, 906
differentiation of, 927–34
sexual, 992
dysgenesis of, 951–52, 1009. *See also* Gonads, dysgenesis of.
dysmenorrhea and, 970–74
endocytosis in, 109
fetal, 908, 940–41, 997
interstitial cells of, 916, 917
follicles, 906, 908–16, 934–40
aging and, 908, 911
atretic, 915–16, 935–36
cavitation (antrum formation), 912–13
cellular events in development of, 910
classification and architecture, 909
control mechanisms, 934–40
gap junctions of, 913, 914
graafian, 913–15. *See also* Graafian follicle.
mesenchymal cell migration to, 911, 916
microenvironment (hormone concentration) of, 937
preovulatory, 939–40, 943
primary, 908
primordial, 908
recruitment of, 908, 934–35
regulatory protein, 927
secondary, 908–12
selection of, 936–39, 943
tertiary, 912–13
germ cells, 932–34
aging and, 911
differentiation of, 932–34
primordial, 932
granulosa cells. *See* Granulosa cells, ovarian.
hermaphroditism and, 1003–4
hilus cells, 906, 920–21
histology, 908–24
hormone replacement therapy and, 978–80
hormone synthesis by, 73, 924–27
cytodifferentiation and, 929, 930
protein, 926–27
steroid, 924–26. *See also* Androstenedione; Estradiol; Progesterone.
hyperprolactinemia and, 958–60
hypogonadotropic hypogonadism (Kallmann) and, 953
hypopituitarism and, 952–53
infertility and, 966–70
innervation, 907–8, 920
interstitial cells, 906, 916–21, 929
medulla of, 906
menarche and, 941
menopause and, 944, 974–80
menorrhagia and, 955, 970–74
menstrual cycle and, 941–44
neonatal, 999
ovulation and. *See* Ovulation.
physiology, 905–44
polycystic, 961–64
clinical features, 961
hirsutism and, 623, 961, 964, 965
hyperprolactinemia and, 958
hypothalamic disease and, 228–29
management, 963–64
pathophysiology, 962–63
premenarche vs., 941, 942
precocious pseudopuberty and, 1617
premature failure, 956–58
premenstrual syndrome and, 974
prostaglandins and, 929, 931
puberty and, 951–55
absent or minimal, 951–54
delayed, 953–54
normal, 951, 954
removal of, breast cancer and, 1739, 1742, 1744, 1747–48
struma ovarii (desmoid or teratoma), hyperthyroidism and, 423
theca cells. *See* Theca cells, ovarian.
virilization and, 954–55, 964–66
Overeating. *See* Hyperphagia.
Overweight, 1204, 1207. *See also* Obesity.
Ovotestis, 1004
Ovulation, 939–40
absent, 30, 966–70
endometrium and, 971
graafian follicle development and, 913–15
induction of, 966–70
agents for, 966
clomiphene, 967
GnRH, 967, 969–70
gonadotropic, 967–69
polycystic disease and, 963–64
luteal phase of, 942, 944
prostaglandins and, 1774
stigma and, 940
tests of, 966
time of, 942, 943
Oxalate, 1556–57
absorption of, 1556, 1558–59
dietary, 1555, 1556
metabolism, 1556–57
stones. *See* Calcium oxalate stones.
urinary, 1557, 1559–60. *See also* Hyperoxaluria.
Oxaloacetate, gluconeogenesis and, 1050
Oxalosis, 1558
Oxandrolone:
growth delay and, 1600
growth hormone deficiency and, 1609
hyperlipidemia and, 1303
Turner's syndrome and, 1008, 1612
Oxidases, mixed function, 924
19-Oxoandrostenedione, 725
18-Oxocortisol, aldosteronism and, 755
Oxygen, tricarboxylic acid cycle and, 1052
Oxyntmodulin, 1645
Oxyphil cells, parathyroid, 1322
Oxypurinol, uric acid stones and, 1520, 1521
Oxytocin, 338–41
actions, 352
amino acid sequence of, 339, 340
assays, 348
behavioral effects, 213
binding, 339
biosynthesis, 339–40
cells secreting, 338

Oxytocin *(Cont.)*:
chemistry, 338–39
corpus luteum function and, 931
deficiency, 278
distribution and clearance, 349
ectopic, 1712
MSH and, 207
ovarian, 926
regulation, 348–49

P substance. *See* Substance P.
Paget's disease of bone, 1483–91
clinical presentation, 1484–86
pathogenesis, 1487–88
pathology, 1486–87
treatment, 1488–91
Pain:
abdominal, 27
hyperlipidemia and, 1270
hyperparathyroidism and, 1390
back:
osteoporosis and, 1468
Paget's disease and, 1484
bone:
osteitis fibrosa cystica and, 1385
osteomalacia and, 1459
Paget's disease and, 1484
eye, 33
ureteral, stone and, 1501
Palmitic acid, 1254
Pampiniform plexus, 825
Pancreas, 1043
cholecystokinin action and, 1637
cholera of, 1640–41
islet cells of. *See* Islet cells.
polypeptide (PP) of, 1645–47
actions and metabolism, 1646–47
chemistry, 1645, 1646
diseases and, 1647
distribution, assay, and release, 1646
tumors and, 1723
transplantation of, 1148–49
Pancreatectomy:
diabetes mellitus after, 1163–64
insulinoma and, 1186
Pancreaticoduodenal angiography, 1186
Pancreatitis:
diabetes mellitus and, 1163–64
hyperlipidemia and, 1270–71
hyperparathyroidism and, 1389–90
hypocalcemia and, 1431–32
Panhypopituitarism, 277. *See also* Hypopituitarism.
Papilledema, 34
pituitary tumor and, 289
Parachlorophenylalanine, carcinoid and, 1659
Paracrine function, 4, 85
Parafascicular nuclei, 213
Paragangliomas, 667
Paralysis, hyperthyroidism and, 428
Paramesonephric ducts, 992–93
persistent, 1011
Paramethasone, 789
Paraneoplastic syndrome, 1692
Parasellar disease, 297
differential diagnosis, 296
Parasympathetic nervous system:
diabetes mellitus and, 1122–23
hypofunction, 675
indirect tests of function of, 686
ovaries and, 907
Parathyroidectomy, 1400–1401
hypoparathyroidism after, 1424
hypophosphatemia after, 1437
MEN and, 1668
Parathyroid glands, 1321–37. *See also* Parathyroid hormone.
adenoma, 1378–79
vs. hyperplasia, 1398
localization, 1398–1400
MEN and, 1392–93, 1664, 1676
anatomy and embryology, 1321
angiography, 1399
antibodies to, 1425
autotransplantation, 1400
carcinoma, 1379, 1391
chief cells, 1321–22
hyperplasia, 1378, 1379, 1393
crisis, 1391
exploration, 1400–1401
hyperfunction. *See* Hyperparathyroidism.
hyperplasia, 1378, 1379
vs. adenoma, 1398
localization, 1398–1400
MEN and, 1664, 1676
pseudoadenomatous, 1379, 1393
hypofunction. *See* Hypoparathyroidism.
infarction, 1392
oxyphil cells, 1322
Parathyroid hormone (parathormone, PTH), 1321–37
actions, 1328–37
adenylate cyclase and, 1326
analogues of, 1323–24
adenylate-cyclase-stimulating, hypercalcemia of malignancy and, 1407, 1408
antisera, 1371
assays, 1369–74, 1443–45
in vitro, 169
bicarbonate and, 1337
biosynthesis, 1322–24
bone and, 1331–32
hyperparathyroidism and, 1384–88
metabolic role of, 1328
responsiveness test, 1444–45
vitamin D potentiation and, 1356
calcium and, 1320, 1326, 1358–60. *See also* Hyperparathyroidism.
bone metabolism and, 1332
renal transport of, 1336–37
secretion rate (of PTH) and, 1324
sensors for, 1324
cAMP and, 1373–74, 1443–44
catecholamines and, 1325
circulating fragments, 1326–28
cytochemical assay, 1373
ectopic, 1703–4
epinephrine and, 660, 679
excess. *See* Hyperparathyroidism.
hypothyroidism and, 455
immunoreactive, 1326, 1371–73
calcium serum levels and, 1372
features of, 1327
hyperparathyroidism and, 1397
sample handling, 1443
kidney and, 1337
calcium transport and, 1336–37
metabolic role of, 1328
phosphate transport and, 1334–35
liver and, 1328
magnesium and, 1325, 1426, 1440
malignancy-associated hypercalcemia and, 1407, 1410
metabolism, 1326–28
phosphorus and, 1334–35, 1360–61
pseudohypoparathyroidism and, 1428, 1430
TmP/GFR and, 1370–71
recombinant DNA and, 52
regulation, 1324–26
resistance to, 1426–30
hypomagnesemia and, 1426
secretion, 1324–26
sodium and, 1337
stability of, 180
structure, 1322, 1323
sympathochromaffin system and, 679
vitamin D and, 1325, 1348–49, 1481
bone resorption and, 1356
hydroxylase activity and, 1350
Parathyroid secretory protein, 1324
Paraventricular nucleus, 189, 190, 338
Parenteral nutrition:
hypophosphatemia and, 1437
osteomalacia and, 1466
Paresthesias, hypocalcemia and, 1423
Parietal cell antibodies, 584, 1685
Parkinsonian multiple system atrophy, 674–75
Parkinson's disease, dopamine and, 681
Parvalbumin, 124
Patching, receptor, 107
PDGF. *See* Platelet-derived growth factor.
Pendred's syndrome, 448
Penicillamine, cystinuria and, 1516
Penis. *See also* Genitals.
differentiation of, 994
Pentagastrin, 1630, 1631
calcitonin test with, 1672–73
Pentose shunt, 1053
Pepsin, gastrin and, 1633
Peptic ulcer:
gastrinoma and, 1633, 1635, 1664
glucocorticoids and, 556–57, 808
hyperparathyroidism and, 1389
norepinephrine and, 682
prostaglandins and, 1776
Peptidase, 64, 68
Peptide C. *See* C peptide.
Peptide-histidine-isoleucine (PHI), 1640
Peptide hormones, 5, 59–68, 85–134. *See also specific hormone:* Glucagon; Insulin; *etc.*
actions of, 84
mediators of, 110–34
phosphorylation of receptor and, 101–2
adenylate cyclase and, 87, 94–96, 112–15
assays, biological, 169

Peptide hormones *(Cont.)*:
atrial natriuretic. *See* Atrial natriuretic factor.
binding of, 87–88
temperature and, 88
biosynthesis of, 63–66
mRNA and, 59–63
cAMP as second messenger of, 121–22
cellular pathway of, 65, 66
ectopic, 1708–15
endocytosis of, 106–9
enzymes and, 87, 94–96, 112–18
gastric inhibitory. *See* Gastric inhibitory polypeptide.
gastrin-releasing (GRP), 1650
glycogenolysis and, 119
glycosylation of, 65–66
hypophysiotropic. *See* Hypophysiotropic hormones *and also specific hormone or factor*.
hypothalamic, 192, 821–23
internalization of, 106–10
local regulation by, 85
metabolism of, 67–68
nervous system interactions of, 211–13
neurotransmitter functions of, 197–99
ovarian, 926–27
pancreatic, 1087. *See also* Pancreas, polypeptide of.
phospholipids and, 128–34
pituitary, 252–73
prostaglandins and, 129–31
receptors for, 85–110
antibodies to, 156–57
binding by, 87–88
biosynthesis and turnover of, 102–4
chemical and physical properties, 89–91
degradation of hormone and, 67–68
desensitization of target cell and, 97–99
general aspects of, 85–87
interactions of, with hormone, 88–89
membrane components and, 94–96
mobility of, 94–97
oncogenes and, 153, 154
structure of, 86, 91–94
secretion of, 65–66
target cells of, 85–87
transcription of genes and, 61
transport of, 68
vasoactive intestinal. *See* Vasoactive intestinal polypeptide.
YY, 1647
amino acid sequence of, 1646
Perchlorate discharge test, 448
Pergolide, acromegaly and, 306
Pergonal:
infertility and, 286
spermatogenesis and, 877
Periorbital edema, 33–34
hyperthyroidism and, 441, 443
hypothyroidism and, 451, 452
Periventricular nuclei, 190
Pertechnetate, thyroid gland and, 393, 409, 488–89
Petrosal sinus, ACTH sampling from, 615
PFK. *See* Phosphofructokinase.
pH;
citrate and, 1565
urinary, 564, 567
cystine and, 1515
nephrolithiasis and, 1506, 1507, 1524–27, 1530
uric acid and, 1506
Phagocytosis, diabetes mellitus and, 1125
Pharyngeal pouch syndrome, 1431
Phenformin, 1143
Phenothiazines, hyperprolactinemia induced by, 958
Phenoxybenzamine, pheochromocytoma and, 671
Phentolamine:
glucose and, 677
pituitary effects of, 199
Phenylalanine, catecholamine synthesis and, 652
Phenylethanolamine *N*-methyl transferase, 653
Phenytoin, thyroid hormone and, 416–17
Pheochromocytoma, 667–72, 1675–76
clinical manifestations, 668
diabetes mellitus and, 1164
diagnosis, 668–71
hyperparathyroidism and, 1393, 1412
medullary thyroid carcinoma and, 1675–76
MEN and, 667, 1669, 1675–76
neurofibromatosis and, 667, 679–80
origin and distribution, 667–68
screening, 671
treatment, 671–72
PHI (peptide-histidine; isoleucine), WDHA syndrome and, 1640
Phorbol esters, protein kinase C and, 126, 127
Phosphate. *See* Phosphorus.
Phosphatidylcholine, 129, 133–34, 1251
Phosphatidylinositol, 129, 131–33
angiotensin and, 532
diabetes mellitus and, 1128
oncogenes and, 152
peptide receptor, 89
Phosphaturia, 1334
osteomalacia and rickets and, 1464–65
tumor-associated, 1717
Phosphoenolpyruvate carboxykinase (PEPCK), 1049–51
Phosphofructokinase, 1047–49
fat metabolism and, 1062
insulin and, 1068, 1074, 1075
Phosphoglucomutase, 1047
Phosphoglycerate kinase, 1050
Phosphoinositides, 70, 131–33
Phosphokinase, 115. *See also* Protein kinase.
Phospholipase:
arachidonic acid metabolism and, 131
calcium and, 131, 132
glucocorticoids and, 549, 550
inositol triphosphate and, 132, 133
prostaglandin synthesis and, 1771
Phospholipids, 128–34
ACTH and, 526
arachidonic acid metabolism and, 129–31
calcium and, 131, 132
function of, 128–29
hormonal effects on, 129–34
inositol, 131–33
insulin and, 1080
metabolism of, 128–34, 1250–51
methylation of, 133–34
oncogenes and, 152
prostaglandin synthesis and, 1771
structure of, 128, 129
Phosphomethyltransferase, 133–34
Phosphoprotein phosphatase, 115, 1046
Phosphoribosyl pyrophosphate (PRPP) synthetase, uric acid stones and, 1519
Phosphorus (phosphate):
absorption, 1353–54, 1355
balance, 1357
calcitonin and, 1343
chloride ratio to, hypercalcemia and, 1396
creatinine and, 1368, 1443
deficiency. *See* Hypophosphatemia.
distribution, 1318
epinephrine and, 660
excess, 1438–39. *See also* Hyperphosphatemia.
extracellular, 1318, 1321
fecal, 1353
feedback mechanism, 1349
homeostasis, 1360–61
intracellular, 1318, 1320
kidney and, 1333–35, 1360–61
hyperphosphatemia and, 1439
vitamin D and, 1356–57
wastage by, 1464–65
malabsorption, 1436, 1465
metabolism, 1320
neonatal, 1431
osteoporosis and, 1470, 1474
parathyroid hormone and, 1334–35, 1360–61
resistance to, 1428, 1430
TmP/GFR and, 1370–71
pseudohypoparathyroidism and, 1444
serum levels, 1365, 1442
age and sex differences in, 1365
bone disease and, 1455
excretion rate and, 1333–34
maintenance of normal, 1360
state of, 1321
therapeutic, 1438
hypercalcemia and, 1402, 1421
hyperoxaluria and, 1561
hyperparathyroidism and, 1554, 1556
osteomalacia and rickets and, 1467
threshold, 1334
total body, 1317, 1318
tubular maximum (TmP/GFR), 1334, 1360–61, 1365
hypercalciuria and, 1548–50
hyperthyroidism and, 1411, 1412
measurement, 1367–68, 1443
nonogram for, 1368
parathyroid hormone and, 1370–71, 1396
vitamin D and, 1356–57
tubular reabsorption (TRP), 1368
urinary, 1333–34. *See also* tubular maximum *subentry above*.
measurement, 1367–68, 1443
osteomalacia and rickets and, 1464–65

Phosphorus (phosphate) *(Cont.)*:
vitamin D and, 1349–50, 1360–61
absorptive role of, 1355
renal reabsorption and, 1356–57
Phosphorylase:
glucocorticoids and, 547
glycogen metabolism and, 1046, 1047
Phosphorylase kinase, 118–19
glycogenolysis and, 1047
Phosphorylation:
amino acid sequences and, 118
calcium and, 126
cAMP action and, 120–21
cycle of dephosphorylation and, 115, 117
desensitization of target cells and, 98–99
EGF receptor, 92, 93
glucose, 1045, 1047
glycogenolysis and, 118–19, 1047
hormone action and, 101–2
insulin receptor, 102, 1079–80
lipolysis and, 119–20
oncogenes and, 152
phosphate transport and, 1334
protein kinase and, 115–18
Phosphotransferase, 116
Photocoagulation, diabetic retinopathy and, 1118
Physical examination, 19
Pickwickian syndrome, 1233
Pigmentation, 25–26
acanthosis nigricans and, 26
ACTH and, 254, 525
Addison's disease and, 587
Cushing's disease and, 315
fibrous dysplasia and, 1482
MSH and, 525
Nelson's syndrome and, 619
oral, 26
Pindolol, postural hypotension and, 676
Pineal gland, 216–18, 236–37
synthesis of principles of, 216–18
tumors, 236–37
Pitressin, 364. *See also* Vasopressin.
Pituitary gland, 247–376
adenomas, 287–88. *See also* tumors *subentry below*.
aldosteronism and, 754
anatomy, 192–93, 247–49, 825
landmarks of, 822
anterior, 247–327
anatomy, 193, 247–49, 825
hormones of, 252–73. *See also specific hormones*.
apoplexy, 275, 289
behavioral influences of, 211–13
blood supply, 248–49
catecholamines and, 678–79
cell types of, 250–52, 338
computed tomography, 291–93
Cushing's disease and, 614
craniopharyngioma, 288
CSF studies and, 295
drugs affecting, 199
embryology, 249–50
evolution of, 12
feedback mechanism, 186–87
GnRH effect on, 836–37. *See also* Follicle-stimulating hormone; Luteinizing hormone.
hemorrhage, 275, 289
hyperfunction, 300–321, 367–74. *See also* tumors *subentry below*.
hypofunction. *See* Hypopituitarism.
hypothalamic disease and, 225–31
hypothyroidism and, 449
infundibulum, 248, 338
ischemic necrosis of, 273–74
lazy, 1607
lymphocytic infiltration of, 1684–85
magnetic resonance imaging, 291, 293
nerve supply, 249
neuropeptides and, 197–99, 208
neurotransmitters and, 188, 194, 195
pars distalis, 193, 249
pars intermedia, 193, 249
pars nervosa, 338
pars tuberalis, 249
pharyngeal, 250
portal system, 188, 191–92, 248, 824–25
posterior, 338–76
anatomy, 338
hormones of. *See* Oxytocin; Vasopressin.
proton beam therapy, 299, 305–6, 319, 617
radiography, 290–93
radiotherapy, 298–99
adjunctive, 300
Cushing's disease and, 319, 617
GH deficiency induced by, 1607
GH-secreting tumor and, 305–6
hypopituitarism from, 275
prolactinoma and, 314
vs. surgery, 299–300
secretory granules, 250, 340
stellate cells, 193
surgery, 298
ACTH-secreting adenoma and, 319, 603, 615–17
advantages and disadvantages, 299
breast cancer and, 1742, 1744–45, 1748
complications, 617
diabetes insipidus and, 356
diabetic retinopathy and, 1119
GH-secreting tumor and, 305
MEN and, 1668–69
prolactinoma and, 314, 960
vs. radiotherapy, 299–300
stalk section, 276
testes and, 844–48. *See also* Luteinizing hormone.
transplants of, into hypothalamus, 187–88
tumors, 287–321
ACTH-secreting, 315–20, 600–601, 619. *See also* Cushing's disease.
adrenocortical insufficiency and, 590–91
alpha-subunit-secreting, 321
classification, 287–88
diagnostic procedures, 290–95
differential diagnosis, 295–97
GH-secreting, 300–306
gonadotropin-secreting, 320–21, 882
hypopituitarism and, 289
hypothyroidism and, 449
MEN 1 and, 1665, 1668–69
Nelson's syndrome and, 619
pregnancy and, 289–90
prolactin-secreting, 306–15, 958–60
signs and symptoms, 288–90
therapy, 298–300
TSH-secreting, 320, 423
vision and, 33, 289, 293–95
Placenta:
ACTH of, 257
fetal growth and, 1592, 1601
lactogen of. *See* Lactogen, placental.
steroid synthesis by, 520
Plasmacytoma, pluriglandular insufficiency and, 1686
Plasma membrane. *See* Membrane, cell.
Plasmids:
cloning and, 44–45
insulin synthesis and, 1067
protein synthesis and, 51
reverse transcription of mRNA and, 48–49
Plasmin, ovulation and, 940
Plasminogen activator, 927
ovulation and, 940
Platelet-derived growth factor, 1583
hypercalcemia of malignancy and, 1704
oncogenes and, 154, 1701
Platelets:
catecholamines in, 669
prostaglandins and, 1778–79
Plummer's disease, 477
Pluriglandular insufficiency syndromes, 1678–86
autoimmune, with Addison's disease, 1678–84
diabetes mellitus and, 1165, 1682–83, 1684
diagnosis, complications, and surveillance, 1685–86
genetics of, 1686
hypoparathyroidism and, 1680–82
nonautoimmune, 1686
Schmidt's syndrome and, 1682–83
thyroid disease and, 1682–83, 1684
POEMS syndrome, 1686
Poikilothermia, 236
Poly A tail, mRNA, 40, 48, 62
Polycitra, cystinuria and, 1515
Polycystic ovary disease, 961–64
clinical features, 961
hirsutism and, 623, 961, 964, 965
hyperprolactinemia and, 958
hypothalamic disease and, 228–29
infertility and, 963–64
management, 963–64
pathophysiology, 962–63
premenarche vs., 941, 942
Polycythemia, tumor-associated, 1721–22
Polydipsia, 357, 358, 361–62, 367
DDAVP trial and, 375
diabetes mellitus and, 1116
hyperthyroidism and, 427
saline infusion test and, 375
SIADH and, 369
treatment, 364–66
Polymorphisms, genetic, 53–54
Polyneuropathy, 32
diabetic, 1115, 1121–22

Polyol pathway, 1053–54
  diabetes mellitus and, 1127
Polypeptide hormones. *See* Peptide hormones.
Polysomy, 985, 989
Polyuria, 29, 350
  Cushing's syndrome and, 608
  diabetes insipidus and, 357, 358, 362, 367
  diabetes mellitus and, 1116
  differential diagnosis, 362–63
  fluid restriction test and, 374
  polydipsia and, 362, 367
  treatment, 364–67
  vasopressin-osmolality-thirst relations and, 358–60
Porphyria, catecholamines and, 679
Portal system:
  hepatic, insulin levels in, 1067, 1069
  hypothalamic-hypophyseal, 188, 191–92, 248, 824–25
Porter-Silber reaction, 573
Postpartum hyperthyroidism, 440
Postproline cleaving enzyme, 68
Postural hypotension. *See* Hypotension, postural.
Potassium. *See also* Hyperkalemia; Hypokalemia.
  aldosterone and, 532–33, 564, 567, 599
    adenoma secreting, 752–53
    deficiency of, 597, 598
    diagnostic procedures, 755–57
    hyperplasia and, 753–54
  assays, 730
  calcium and, 533
  Cushing's syndrome and, 767
  diabetic ketoacidosis and, 1153–54
  diuretics and, 756–57
  glucocorticoids and, 553–54
  hypertension and, 714–15, 730, 755–57, 768–70
    low-renin, 770
  insulin and, 1076–77
  magnesium and, 1441
  norepinephrine and, 714–15
  phosphate replacement and, 1438
  supplemental, Bartter's syndrome and, 1789
  transport, 715–17
Potassium citrate, hypocitraturia and, 1566
$pp60^{src}$, 152
Prader-Labhart-Willi syndrome, 867
Prader orchidometer, 852
Prader-Willi syndrome, 232, 233, 1212
Prasterone. *See* Dehydroepiandrosterone.
Prazosin, pheochromocytoma and, 671
Prealbumin, thyroxine-binding. *See* Thyroxine-binding prealbumin.
Precocious pseudopuberty, 883, 1617
Precocious puberty. *See* Puberty, precocious.
Prediabetes, 1112
Prednisolone. *See also* Glucocorticoids, therapeutic.
  breast cancer and, 1749–50
  distribution of, 797
  dose-response considerations, 804
  metabolism and clearance of, 797, 798
  mineralocorticoid receptors and, 792
  structure, 789
Prednisone. *See also* Glucocorticoids, therapeutic.
  ACTH deficiency and, 284
  alternate-day therapy with, 806, 807
  Graves' ophthalmopathy and, 443
  21-hydroxylase deficiency and, 627
  hypothalamic-pituitary-adrenal axis suppression and, 809–11
  metabolism of, 797–99
  potency of, 796, 797
  structure of, 789
  thyroiditis and, 462
  withdrawal protocol for, 813
Pregnancy:
  alcohol and, 1601
  aldosterone and, 620–21
  breast cancer and, 1739
  calcium and, 1350
  diabetes mellitus and, 1155–62
    classification, 1158–59
    congenital anomalies and, 1160
    delivery and, 1162
    diagnosis, 1158
    effect of diabetes on pregnancy, 1159–61
    effect of pregnancy on diabetes, 1158–59
    gigantism in infant and, 1621
    neonatal morbidity and, 1161
    postnatal effects, 1161
    postprandial hyperglycemia and, 1157–58
    respiratory distress syndrome and, 1160
    starvation and, accelerated, 1156–57
    stillbirth and, 1160–61
    treatment, 1161–62
  drugs during, 1601
  endometrial changes and, 970
  fuel metabolism and, 1156–58
  glucocorticoid therapy and, 807–8
  glucose and, 1156–59
  goiter and, 480
  hypercalciuria and, 1551
  hyperlipidemia and, 1297
  hyperparathyroidism and, 1391–92
  hyperthyroidism and, 438–40
  hypoglycemia and, 1159
  insulin and, 1157, 1159, 1161–62
  ketones and, 1157, 1159
  ovulation induction and, 968, 970
  pituitary tumors and, 289–90
  prolactin and, 270, 1158
    tumor secretion of, 312
  thyroid hormone and, 409
  toxemia of, renin-angiotensin-aldosterone axis and, 621
Pregnane, 516, 517
Pregnenolone:
  fetal, 941
  formation of, 69–70, 516, 518, 925, 926, 1012
    3β-hydroxysteroid dehydrogenase deficiency and, 629–30
  metabolism, 925–26
  modification of, 518
  steroid biosynthetic pathway and, 71, 72
  structure, 515–516
  testicular secretion rate, 839
Prekallikrein, 1781–82
Premarin, 978
  gonadotropin deficiency and, 285
  hyperlipidemia and, 1304
  menopause and, 977
Premenarche, 941
Premenstrual syndromes, 214, 974
Preoptic nucleus, 821
Preprocalcitonin, 1340
Preproenkephalin, 209, 210
Preproinsulin, 1065
Prepro-opiomelanocortin, schematic representation of, 210
Preproparathyroid hormone, 1322
Previtamin D_3, 1346
Pribnow box, 60
Probucol, 1300–1301
  action and toxicity, 1301
  hyperlipidemia and, 1263–64, 1300–1301
  indications and dosage, 1301
Progesterone:
  antagonists of, 142
  biosynthesis, 71, 73, 924–25, 1012
  breast cancer and, 1740–41, 1742
  cell surface actions of, 137
  endometrial cancer and, 1763
  21-hydroxylase deficiency and, 624, 626, 1021–23, 1025
  insulin and, 1157
  luteolysis and, 931
  menorrhagia and, 974
  neonatal, 997
  ovulation and, 940, 944
  plasma levels, 521
  proteins regulated by, 145
  receptors for, 139
    breast cancer and, 1743, 1746
    nuclear binding of, 143–44
  sexual dimorphism and, 215
  structure, 136, 516
  testicular secretion rate, 839
  therapeutic. *See also* Medroxyprogesterone.
    ovarian failure and, 957
    Turner's syndrome and, 951, 1612
    virilization defect in fetus and, 1019
  transport, 75
Progestins:
  androgen antagonism and, 142
  breast cancer and, 1749
  endometrial cancer and, 1763–64
  prostate cancer and, 1760
  sexual dimorphism of brain and, 215–16
  structure, 136
Progestogens:
  estrogen therapy and, 979
  menopause and, 977
  menorrhagia and, 955, 974
  polycystic ovary disease and, 963
  postmenopausal bleeding and, 980
  pseudohermaphroditism and, 1019
  withdrawal test, 966
Prohormones, 64–65
  impaired conversion of, 16
Proinsulin, 65, 1065–67
  discovery of, 1064
  insulinoma and, 1185

Proinsulin *(Cont.)*:
plasma levels, 1067
structure, 65
therapeutic, 1132
Prolactin, 270–73
action, 270
assays, 270–71, 284
in children, 1622
in vitro, 169
techniques for, 326–27
behavioral effects, 270
biosynthesis, 264
breast cancer and, 1741–44, 1746
cells secreting, 251
chemistry, 253, 263
circadian rhythm of, 220
control of secretion of, 271–73
factors affecting, 272
corpus luteum effects of, 930–31
Cushing's disease and, 317
deficiency, 284, 287
L-dopa test, 327
dopamine and, 194, 207, 271, 272
prolactinoma and, 308, 310, 311
drugs affecting, 199
gene for, 43
glycosylated, 264
gonadotropins and, 862–63
granulosa cell receptors for, 928
gynecomastia and, 886, 888
histamine and, 273
hypersecretion. *See* Hyperprolactinemia.
hypothalamic disease and, 224, 227, 229–30
hypothyroidism and, 309, 455
inhibiting factor, 207, 271
prolactinoma and, 311
insulin hypoglycemia and, 326
Kallmann's syndrome and, 866–67
lactation and, 270
metabolic clearance and secretion rate, 271
metoclopramide and, 284, 326
neuropeptides and, 199, 208
neurotransmitter effects on, 194, 195
opioid peptides and, 211
ovarian follicle selection and, 936, 938
pituitary levels, 271
plasma levels, 271, 326
hyperprolactinemia and, 308
polycystic ovary disease and, 963
pregnancy and, 270, 1158
radioimmunoassay, 270
radioreceptor assay, 270–71
releasing factor, 207
prolactinoma and, 310, 311
renal disease and, 273
secretory granules, 251
sleep-associated changes in, 268, 272
stimulation tests, 326
suppression tests, 326–27
testes and, 862–63
testosterone and, 851–52
TRH and, 201, 207, 271–72
prolactinoma and, 308
test, 282, 284, 326
tumor secretion of:
MEN 1 and, 1665
nonpituitary, 1722
pituitary, 306–15, 958–60
VIP and, 207
Promethazine, vasopressin and, 345
Pro-opiomelanocortin, 252, 524
Addison's disease and, 586
aldosterone and, 533, 754
behavioral effects of peptides derived from, 212, 213
hypertension and, 767
pre-POMC structure and, 210
processing, 1708, 1709
tumor production of, 1706, 1708–10
Proparathyroid hormone, 1322, 1323
Propranolol:
glucose and, 677
growth hormone and, 229, 1622
hypoglycemia and, 1193, 1195
parathyroid hormone and, 1325
pheochromocytoma and, 671
pituitary effects of, 199
renin release and, 704
thyroid hormone and, 416, 435–36
thyroiditis and, 462
thyroid storm and, 438
tremors and, 681
Propressophysin, 340
ectopic, 1711–12
Proptosis, 441–42
Propylthiouracil, 416
dosage, 433, 434
hyperthyroidism and, 433–35
in pregnancy, 439
hypothyroidism induced by, 449
side effects of, 434–35
thyroid storm and, 438
thyroxine-5′-deiodinase and, 394
Prorenin, 702–4
plasma concentration, 727
Prostacyclin:
actions, 1769
circulating, 1777
discovery of, 1769
ductus arteriosus and, 1778
function of, 130
platelet aggregation and, 1779
renal, 1774, 1775
renin release and, 1775
synthesis and metabolism, 130, 973, 1770, 1771–72
uterine, 972
Prostaglandins, 1768–80
actions, 1769
angiotensin and, 532, 704
Bartter's syndrome and, 1777, 1788, 1789
biosynthesis and metabolism, 130–31, 973, 1770, 1771–72
blood pressure and, 1777–78
calcium and, 1779–80
cardiovascular system and, 1777–79
chemistry, 1771–73
circulating, 1772, 1777
diabetes mellitus and, 1780
ductus arteriosus and, 1778
endometrial, 972–74
erythropoietin and, 1776
estrogen and, endometrial, 972–73
fatty acids and, 1771, 1780
gastrointestinal function and, 1776
glucocorticoids and, 549, 553
historical note on, 1768–69
hypercalcemia of malignancy and, 1403, 1407, 1704–5
inhibitors of, 1773. *See also* Aspirin; Indomethacin.
insulin and, 1072, 1780
kallikrein-kinin system and, 1785
lipolysis and, 1779
lungs and, 1779
luteinizing hormone and, 940
luteolysis and, 931, 1774
medullary thyroid carcinoma and, 1674–75
menorrhagia and, 973
metabolic effects of, 1779–80
nomenclature, 1769
osteoclasts and, 1403
ovarian cytodifferentiation and, 929, 931
ovulation and, 940, 1774
platelets and, 1778–79
release of, 1771–72
renal, 1774–76
renin and, 704, 1775
reproduction and, 1773–74
seminal fluid, 1774
shock and, 1777
sodium and, 1775
structure, 1769, 1770
as tissue hormones, 1769–71
uterine, 1773–74
vasopressin (ADH) and, 351, 1775–76
WDHA syndrome and, 1640
Prostaglandin synthetase, 130
Prostatectomy, 1760
Prostate gland:
antigen specific to (PSA), 1758
biopsy, 1758
cancer, 1753–62
hormonal regulation of, 1755–56
incidence, 1753
markers, 1758
natural history, 1756–57
prognosis, 1758–59
receptors and, 1756, 1758, 1762
risk factors and etiology, 1753–55
staging and diagnosis, 1757–58
treatment, 891, 1759–62
weight assay, 166
Prosterone, 71
Proteases, 68
radioimmunoassay and, 174
Protein:
androgen-binding (ABP), 841, 849
assay contamination by serum, 174
binding, vs. receptors, 82–83
calcitonin gene-related (CGRP), 40, 63, 1337, 1339–40, 1672
calcium-binding, 123–24, 1353
cAMP-binding (CAP), 11, 120–21
cellular pathway of, 65, 66
competitive binding assay, 19–20
diabetes mellitus and, 1104–5
carbohydrate interaction and, 1105
urinary loss in, 1119–20
dietary:
daily requirements, by age, 1591

Protein, dietary *(Cont.)*:
high content of, 1236
hyperlipidemia and, 1292
liquid, 1236
nephrolithiasis and, 1527, 1538
docking, 63
evolution of, 10–11
feeding of, 1064
diabetes mellitus and, 1103, 1105
gastrin release and, 1630–31
glucagon and, 1083, 1084, 1103
insulin and, 1083, 1084
fuel reserve and, 1089
fusion (hybrid), 47–48, 51
cDNA library and, 49
G, 1085
pseudohypoparathyroidism and, 1428–29
GLA. *See* Osteocalcin.
glucocorticoids and, 145, 545–46, 548
glycation of, 1054, 1112
diabetic complications and, 1128–29
glycosylation of, 1054, 1055
hormones. *See* Peptide hormones.
iodination of, 171
lipid complex with. *See* Lipoprotein.
N, pseudohypoparathyroidism and, 1428–29
Ns and Ni, adenylate cyclase and, 113–14
oncogene-encoded, 151–53
ovarian follicular, 936
parathyroid secretory, 1324
phosphokinase, 115. *See also* Protein kinase.
phosphorylation, 115–18. *See also* Phosphorylation.
precursor, 41, 63–65
RNA processing and, 62–63
receptor. *See* Receptors.
retinol-binding, 397
S-100, pituitary and, 193
starvation and, 1183
synthesis:
coding and, 40–41
hormone action and, 84
insulin and, 1075–76
by recombinant DNA techniques, 50–52
steroid hormones and, 145–46
thyroid hormone and, 150, 399
testosterone-binding, 840–42
thyroid hormone binding, 395–97, 404–6
abnormal, 411
transport, 6, 135–37
vitamin D-binding, 1346, 1347
Protein kinase, 115–18
binding by, 120–21
C, 126–27
calcium-calmodulin-dependent, 125
cAMP-dependent, 115–18
cGMP-dependent, 122
classification of, 115–16
EGF receptor, 92, 93
evolution of, 11
glycogenolysis and, 118–19
inositol triphosphate and, 132, 133
insulin receptor, 93, 1077, 1079–80
lipolysis and, 119–20
oncogenes and, 152
phosphate transport and, 1334
phosphorylation and, 101–2
properties of, 116–17
Proteinuria, diabetes mellitus and, 1119–20
Proteolysis:
hyperthyroidism and, 428
hypothyroidism and, 454
insulin and, 1076
peptide hormone synthesis and, 64
sites of cleavage, 68
thyroglobulin, 394
Proteus, nephrolithiasis and, 1522
Proton beam therapy, pituitary, 299, 305–6, 319
Cushing's disease and, 617
Proto-oncogenes, 55, 151–53
ectopic hormone production and, 1700–1701
Protoplasts, DNA transfer and, 49
Provitamin D, 1345, 1346
Provocative testing, 21
Psammoma bodies, 496
Pseudofractures, 1460
Pseudogout, 31
hyperparathyroidism and, 1391
Pseudohermaphroditism, 1011–31
female, 1020–31
adrenal hyperplasia and, 1020–30
environmental hormones and, 1030
teratological malformations and, 1030–31
male, 1011–20
androgen target tissue defects and, 1016–19
dysgentic, 1010
exogenous steroids and, 1019–20
Leydig cell hypoplasia and, 1011
testosterone synthesis defects and, 1011–16
of unknown etiology, 1020
Pseudohyperparathyroidism, 1702
Pseudohypoaldosteronism, 599
hypertension and, 770
Pseudohypoparathyroidism, 1426–30
clinical features, 1427–28
diagnosis, 1430
pathogenesis, 1428–30
receptor coupling defect and, 157
testing for, 1444–45
Pseudopseudohypoparathyroidism, 1426, 1428, 1430
Pseudotumor cerebri, 237
Psychiatric disorders, 32, 213–14, 237–39. *See also* Behavior; Psychological factors.
glucocorticoids and, 555, 808
hyperparathyroidism and, 1388–89
hypogonadism and, 868
hypopituitarism and, 278
polydipsia and, 357, 362, 369
Psychological factors. *See also* Behavior; Psychiatric disorders.
Cushing's syndrome and, 608
hypoglycemia and, 1181, 1191
impotence and, 890
menopause and, 976
obesity and, 1222–23, 1238
sexual differentiation and, 999–1000
short stature and, 1607, 1613
Psychoses, 32
Psychotropic agents, hyperprolactinemia induced by, 958
Puberty:
delayed, 869
diagnostic approach to, 1033, 1034
in female, 953–54
growth delay and, 1599–1601
Kallmann's syndrome and, 864–66
treatment, 875–77
female, 951–55
absent or minimal, 951–54
chronological age for events in, 1594
delayed, 953–54
normal, 951, 954
sequence of events in, 1593–94
growth and, 1589–90, 1593–95, 1599–1601
precocity and, 1610–11, 1616–18
gynecomastia and, 887
macromastia and, 887, 889
male, 858–60
chronological age for events in, 1595
sequence of events in, 1594–95
precocious, 30, 1616–18
classification, 1616
diagnosis, 1618
ectopic chorionic gonadotropin and, 1713
fibrous dysplasia and, 1482, 1483
heterosexual, 1617–18
hypothalamic disease and, 223, 228
hypothyroidism and, 297
idiopathic, 882, 1616, 1618
in male, 882–83
pineal tumor and, 236
pseudo, 883, 1617
short stature and, 1610–11, 1616
tall stature and, 1616–18
treatment, 883, 1618
Pulmonary disorders. *See* Lungs; Respiration.
Pulse, sympathetic function and, 686
Pupils, 34
sympathetic function and, 685
Purines:
DNA and, 37
hyperuricosuria and, 1562, 1563–64
metabolism, 1517, 1518
Pyelography, intravenous, 740–42
diabetes mellitus and, 1121
nephrolithiasis and, 1568
Pyelonephritis, diabetes mellitus and, 1125
Pygmies, 1606
Pyriodoxine deficiency, hyperoxaluria and, 1558, 1560
Pyrimidines, DNA and, 37
Pyriminil, diabetes mellitus and, 1097
Pyroglutamyl peptidase, 68
Pyruvaldehyde, 1060
Pyruvate:
alcohol metabolism and, 1196
fatty acid synthesis and, 1055
gluconeogenesis and, 1049, 1050
glycolysis and, 1047, 1049
norepinephrine and, 658
tricarboxylic acid cycle and, 1052–53
Pyruvate carboxylase, 1049, 1050

Pyruvate dehydrogenase, 1050
  tricarboxylic acid cycle and, 1052–53
Pyruvate kinase:
  gene for, 148
  glycolysis and, 1048, 1049
PYY, 1646, 1647

Questran. *See* Cholestyramine.

Radioenzymatic assay, catecholamine, 662, 663, 682–83
Radioimmunoassay, 19, 168–76
  ACTH, 254
  antisera generation for, 171–72
  atrial natriuretic factor, 719
  calcitonin, 1374–75
  circulating endogenous antibody and, 175
  cortisol, 570
  growth hormone, 266
  vs. immunoradiometric assay, 176–77
  iodination and, 171
  lipotropin, 572
  LH and FSH, 260
  parathyroid hormone, 1371–73
  prolactin, 270
  requisites for, 169–70
  sensitivity of, 171, 172–73
  separation of bound and free hormone for, 174–76
  serum protein effect and, 174
  specificity of, 173–74
  thyroid hormone, 404, 406
    autoantibodies and, 411
  thyrotropin, 258
  titering and, 173
Radioimmunolocalization, 1726
Radioiodine. *See* Iodine, radioactive.
Radiology:
  bone, 1456
    fibrous dysplasia and, 1482, 1483
    osteitis fibrosa cystica and, 1385, 1386
    osteomalacia and rickets and, 1459–60
    osteopetrosis and, 1478
    osteoporosis and, 1468–69
    Paget's disease and, 1484–85
  iodinated agents in, thyroid hormone and, 416, 435
  medullary sponge kidney and, 1509, 1510
  nephrolithiasis and, 1514, 1568–69
  pituitary gland, 290–93
  renovascular hypertension and, 736, 740–44
Radionuclide studies:
  adrenal, aldosteronoma and, 760–61
  bone, 1456
    Paget's disease and, 1484–85
    prostate cancer and, 1757–58
  double-isotope, calcium absorption and, 1369
  renal, 742
  thyroid gland, 393, 408–9
    cancer and, 486, 488–89
    hyperthyroidism and, 430
Radioreceptor assay, 19–20, 176–79
  ACTH, 255
  atrial natriuretic factor, 719
  cortisol, 570
  growth hormone, 266
  LH and FSH, 261
  prolactin, 270–71
Radiotherapy:
  goiter, 437–38
  hyperparathyroidism after, 1379
  hyperthyroidism, 432–33, 436–37
  hypoparathyroidism after, 1425
  hypothalamic damage from, 225
  hypothyroidism induced by, 436–37, 446
  implantation, in sella turcica, for Cushing's disease, 617
  pituitary, 298–99
    adjunctive, 300
    Cushing's disease and, 319, 617
    GH deficiency induced by, 1607
    GH-secreting tumor and, 305–6
    hypopituitarism from, 275
    prolactinoma and, 314
    proton beam, 299, 305–6, 319, 617
    vs. surgery, 299–300
  spermatogenic damage by, 873
  thyroid gland, 432–33, 436–37
    cancer induced by, 487, 495–96
    cancer treated by, 498–99, 500
  thyroiditis induced by, 422, 462
Ramus ovaricus, 906
Randall's plaque hypothesis, 1501
Ranitidine, gastrinoma and, 1636
ras genes, 152–53
Rathke's pouch, 249, 250
Raynaud's phenomenon, 681
Receptors:
  acetylcholine, 91–92
    vs. insulin receptor, 92
  ACTH, 525
  activation of, 83–84
  adenylate cyclase and, 95–96, 100, 113, 157
  adrenergic. *See* Adrenergic receptors.
  aggregation (clustering) of, 97, 107
  aldosterone, 140, 565–66
  androgen, 139–40
    assay of, 1762
  angiotensin, 532, 706–7
    disorders of, 155–56
  antibodies to, 96–97, 156–57
  atrial natriuretic factor, 723
  binding by, 3
    altered affinity for, 155, 156
    conformational change caused by, 96–97
    dissociation of, 104, 108
    GTP and, 115
    mathematical characterization of, 178–79
    tight (high-affinity), 104
  binding proteins vs., 82–83
  breast cancer and, 1743, 1745–46, 1751–52
  catecholamine, 656–59. *See also* Adrenergic receptors.
  classification of hormone action and, 9
  cross-linking of, 96–97
  deficiencies of, 155–56
  definition of, 3
  dihydrotestosterone, 139–40
  disease states and, 179
  disorders of, 154–58
  domains of, 83–84
  dopaminergic, 658
  effector coupling defect and, 157
  electrostatic interactions, 88
  endocytosis of, 103, 106–9
  endometrial cancer and, 1763
  epidermal growth factor, 92–93
    vs. insulin receptor, 94
    linear structure of, 92
    oncogenes and, 153, 154
    phosphorylation of, 101, 102
    protein kinase C and, 127
  estrogen, 137–39. *See also* Estrogens, receptors for.
  evolution of, 10–11
  fate of hormone complex with, 106–10
  floating, model of, 95
  FSH:
    granulosa cell, 927
    testicular, 849
  glucagon, 89, 1085
  glucocorticoid, 140, 559–61. *See also* Glucocorticoids, receptors for.
  hydrophobic interactions, 88–89
  hyporesponsiveness and, 16
  insulin, 1077–80. *See also* Insulin, receptors for.
  interactions of hormone with, 59, 88–89
  intracellular, 83–84
    thyroid hormone, 397–98
  LDL, 69, 1262–63
    decrease in, 155
    gene expression and, 40
    internalization mechanism, 106
    oncogenes and, 154
  LH, 837–38. *See also* Luteinizing hormone, receptors for.
  mechanisms of hormone action and, 8
  mineralocorticoid, 565–66
  neurotransmitter, 85–87
    drugs affecting, 198
  nuclear, 84
    steroid hormone, 137–38, 141, 143–45
    thyroid hormone, 149–50
  occupancy rate, 99–101, 144
    Scatchard plot and, 177–79
  oncogenes and, 152–54
  opioid, 209–10
  osmotic. *See* Osmoreceptors.
  overproduction of, 155
  patching of, 107
  peptide hormone, 85–110. *See also* Peptide hormones, receptors for.
    biosynthesis and turnover of, 102–4
    chemical and physical properties, 89–91
    degradation of hormone and, 67–68
    desensitization of target cell and, 97–99
    membrane components and, 94–96
    mobility of, 94–97
    structure of, 86, 91–94
  phosphorylation of, 101–2
  progesterone, 139, 143–44
    breast cancer and, 1743, 1746
  prolactin, granulosa cell, 928
  prostate cancer and, 1756, 1758, 1762
  purification of, 90–91
  radioassay of, 19–20, 176–79
  recycling of, 103, 106, 108

Receptors *(Cont.)*:
regulation of, 104–6
down (decrease in number), 98–99, 104, 155–56
increase in number, 104, 106–7, 155
in target cells, 104
saturation analysis of, 179
sequences of, 61
signal recognition particle, 63
somatomedin C, 93
spare (excess), 99–100
cellular response and, 105
steroid hormone, 137–41
activation of, 138, 141
agonists vs. antagonists and, 141
hypothalamic, 823
regulation of, 105
surface (membrane), 84, 85–110. *See also* Peptide hormones, receptors for.
effector systems and, 87
functional classes of, 109–10
internalization of, 106–9
recycling of, 103
structure of, 86
termination of interaction with, 89, 104, 108
testosterone and, 139–40, 843–44, 1017
thyroid hormone, 149–50, 397–98
TSH, 402
vitamin D, 1354, 1357, 1463
Receptosomes, 107–8
5α-Reductase, 75, 842
deficiency, 875, 1017–18
growth and, 1590
ovarian, 926
prolactin and, 852
sexual differentiation and, 996
sexual dimorphism of brain and, 215
Reference preparation, 166, 176
Reflexes, hung-up, 33
Refractoriness, target cell, 98
Regulation, 5, 7. *See also under specific hormones.*
ACTH, 255–56, 523–24
adenylate cyclase, 112–15
stimulatory vs. inhibitory, 113–15
adrenal steroid, 522–36
atrial natriuretic factor, 719
calcitonin, 1340–41
calcium, 123
domains of, 83–84
evolution of ligands and, 9–11
fuel metabolism, 1087–88
glucocorticoid, 522–31
gonadotropin, 262–63, 832–50
growth hormone, 266–70, 1584
hypophysiotropic hormone, 193–94
independent vs. complex network, 7
interrelated elements of (diagram), 7
local, 84–85
mineralocorticoid, 531–35
oncogenes and, 150–54
oxytocin, 348–49
parathyroid hormone, 1324–26
prolactin, 271–73
receptor, 98–99, 104–6, 155–56
of responsiveness of hormone, 8
simple and complex, 9
thyroid hormone, 400–404
thyrotropin, 150, 259–60, 400–402
Reifenstein syndrome, 1019
Reinke crystalloids, 827, 828
Relaxin, 926
Releasing factors. *See* Hypophysiotropic hormones *and also specific factor or hormone.*
Renal arteries:
atherosclerosis, 735–37
fibromuscular dysplasia, 737–38, 739
hypertension and. *See* Hypertension, renovascular.
natural history of lesions of, 738–39
revascularization procedures, 748–51
angioplastic, 750
results, 750–51
surgical, 749
thrombosis, 738
Renal arteriography, 742–43
balloon angioplasty and, 736
digital subtraction, 743–44
Renal tubular acidosis. *See* Acidosis, renal tubular.
Renal vein renin, 728, 745–46
Renin, 701–4
adrenal hyperplasia and, congenital, 1025
aldosterone and, 532, 534
deficiency of, 597–99
hypersecretion of, 752, 758
release patterns and, 534
angiotensin and, 532, 703, 704. *See also* Angiotensin.
plasma assays and, 727
angiotensinogen and, 727
ascites and, 621
assays, 727–28
in vitro, 169
atrial natriuretic factor and, 722
Bartter's syndrome and, 1788, 1789
catecholamines and, 704
chemistry, 702
circadian rhythm of, 220
Cushing's disease and, 767
deficiency, 597–98
excess, 598–99
gene for, 702
glucocorticoids and, 553
21-hydroxylase deficiency and, 1023, 1025, 1027
hypertension and, 707–11
essential, 770–72
low-renin, 710, 752, 758, 768–72
plasma determination, 744–45
renal vein determinations, 745–46
tumors and, 708, 738, 1722–23
kallikrein-kinin system and, 1784–85
menstrual cycle and, 620
plasma activity (PRA), 727–28
aldosteronism and, 758
experimental hypertension and, 707
normal values, 728
renovascular hypertension and, 744–45
saline infusion and, 731
sodium and, 709–10
tumors and, 708
plasma concentration (PRC), 727
essential hypertension and, 770
pregnancy and, 620, 621
production of, 702–3
prostaglandins and, 704, 1775
release of, 703–4
renal vein, 728, 745–46
sodium and, 709–10, 727
substrate, 705
sympathetic nerves and, 703–4
tumor secretion of, 708, 738, 1722–23
vasopressin and, 346–47
Renin-angiotensin system, 701–11. *See also* Angiotensin; Renin.
components of, 702–7
hypertension and, 707–11
Renke crystalloids, 920
Renogram, radioisotopic, 742
Reserpine, pituitary effects of, 199
Respiration:
diabetic ketoacidosis and, 1151, 1154
hyperthyroidism and, 426
hypothyroidism and, 453
obesity and, 1233–34
Respiratory distress syndrome, diabetes mellitus and, 1154
diabetic mother and, 1160
Responsiveness, hormone:
regulation of, 8
termination of, 13
Restriction enzymes (endonculeases), 44
Restriction fragment length polymorphisms (RFLP), 53–54
Retina, 33, 34
angioid streaks of, 1484
lipemia of, 1124, 1271
Retinol-binding protein, 397
Retinopathy, diabetic, 33, 34, 1115, 1116–19
insulin therapy and, 1130
metabolic changes and, 1127, 1128
Retroviruses, 55
oncogenic, 151. *See also* Oncogenes.
reverse transcription of mRNA and, 48
Revascularization, renal artery, 748–51
Reverse transcriptase, 48
Reyes syndrome, hypoglycemia and, 1188
Rhinorrhea, 26
CSF, pituitary surgery and, 298
Rhodopsin:
cGMP and, 122
phosphorylation of, 102
Rhodopsin kinase, 99, 102
Rhythms, 218–21. *See also* Circadian rhythms.
ultradian, 218, 219–20
Ribonucleic acid. *See* RNA.
Ribonucleoprotein (RNP), steroids and, 148
Ribophorins, 63–64
Ribosomes, 39
peptide hormone synthesis and, 63
receptor biosynthesis and, 102–3
Rickets, 1458–68
classification, 1462
definition, 1458
hypocalcemia and, 1431, 1465
hypophosphatasia and, 1465–66

Rickets *(Cont.)*:
hypophosphatemia and, 1460, 1464–65, 1467
with hypercalciuria, 1548
laboratory studies, 1460
pathogenesis, 1461–66
pathology, 1460–61
radiology and, 1459–60
symptoms and signs, 1458–59
treatment, 1466–68
vitamin D-deficient, 1461–62
vitamin D-dependent, 1463
vitamin D-resistant, 1464
RNA (ribonucleic acid), 38–49
glucocorticoids and, 145, 531, 548, 560–61, 792
hybridization, 45–46
messenger (mRNA), 39
biosynthesis of, 59–63
calcitonin and, 1337, 1339
capping of, 40, 60
ectopic hormone-specific, 1695–96
estrogen and, 145
5′-untreated region of, 51
gene expression and, 42–43
insulin synthesis and, 1066
peptid hormone synthesis and, 63
poly A tail of, 40, 48, 62
precursor, 39
precursor proteins and, 62–63
protein synthesis and, 40–41
reverse transcription of, 48–49
steroid hormones and, 145–48
3′-untranslated region of, 41
thyroid hormone and, 149, 150, 398, 399
transcript of, 39–40, 147–48
oocyte, 932
ribosomal (rRNA), 39
splicesomes and, 39
structure and function, 38–39
transfer (tRNA), 38–39
protein synthesis and, 41
RNA polymerase, 39
steroid hormones and, 146
transcription by, 60, 61
R 1881, structure of, 136
Rosewater syndrome, 1019
ros gene, 152
R 2956, structure of, 136
Rubella, diabetes mellitus and, 1097
Rud syndrome, 868
RU 486, 142
structure of, 136
RU 38486, 562

Salicylates. *See also* Aspirin.
hypoglycemia induced by, 1195
diabetic ketoacidosis and, 1153
hyponatremia and, 373, 374
SIADH and, 374
test, 375
thyroiditis and, 462
Saline infusion:
aldosteronism and, 761–62
calciuresis and, 1420
Salt craving, Addison's disease and, 587
Salt-wasting:
21-hydroxylase deficiency and, 626, 1022, 1023–25
pseudohypoaldosteronism and, 599
Sample handling, 180
Sanger chain termination technique, 47
Saralasin, 707
aldosteronism and, 761
renovascular hypertension and, 745
Sarcoidosis:
hypercalcemia and, 1415–16, 1418
hypercalciuria and, 1360
hypothalamic, 224
pituitary tumor vs., 297
vitamin D and, 1415–16
Sarcoma, Kaposi's, glucocorticoid therapy and, 809
Sarcoma virus, 151, 154
Satiety center, 232, 1212
Saturation analysis, receptor, 179
Saturation-inhibition index, 1508
Sauvagine, 205
Scans, radionuclide. *See* Radionuclide studies.
Scatchard plot, 178–79
insulin binding, 1078
Schizophrenia, 238–39
Schmidt's syndrome, 1682–83
diabetes mellitus and, 1165
Schmorl's node, 1469
Schwann cells, diabetes mellitus and, 1127
Seabright bantam syndrome, 1426
Second messengers, 8, 110–22
calcium, 123–27, 1319–20
cAMP. *See* Adenosine monophosphate, cyclic.
cGMP, 122
hypothesis of, 110–11, 121–22
Secosterols, 1344
Secretin, 1643–44
chemistry, 1639, 1643
discovery of, 1629, 1643
diseases and, 1643–44
distribution, assay, and release, 1643
gastric test with, 1634
metabolism and actions, 1643
Secretion. *See also specific hormones.*
autocrine, 85
calcitonin, 1340–41
episodic, 219
eutopic vs. ectopic, 1692
glucagon, 1083
insulin, 1067–73
paracrine, 85
parathyroid hormone, 1324–26
peptide hormone, 65–66
pituitary hormone, 250–52
posterior, 340–41
steroid hormone, 75
adrenal, 520–21
thyroid hormone, 78, 394
Secretory granules:
atrial natriuretic factor, 719
biosynthesis of peptide receptors and, 103
catecholamine, 655
gastrin, 1631, 1632
growth hormone, 300
insulin, 1065–66
islet cell, 1044
oxytocin, 340
peptide hormone, 67
pituitary, 250, 340
prolactin, 251
vasopressin, 340
Seizures (convulsions), 32
catecholamines and, 681
hypocalcemic, 1423
Seldinger technique, 743
Sella turcica, 192, 247
aneurysms and, 296, 297
calcification, 291
empty, 295–97
in children, 1606
CT scan of, 292
differential diagnosis, 296
hypopituitarism and, 275
primary, 295–97
enlarged, 297
differential diagnosis, 295, 296
symptoms and, 290
radioactive seed implantation in, 617
radiology, 290–91
shape and size of, 248
Semen analysis, 853–54, 878
Seminal vesicles:
prostaglandins and, 1774
prostate cancer and, 1759
Seminiferous tubules, 827
anatomic relationships, 827, 829
differentiation of, 989
failure of, 878–82
hyalinization of, 879
Klinefelter's syndrome and, 1001
spermatogenesis in, 830
Seminoma, 891
Sensitivity, radioimmunoassay, 171, 172–73
Sensory loss, diabetes and, 32
Septo-optic dysplasia, 1606
Serine:
glycosylation and, 1054
protein kinase and, 115, 118
phosphorylation and, insulin receptor, 1079–80
Serotonin. *See also* Neurotransmitters.
carcinoid and, 1655, 1656–57
CRF control and, 194
growth hormone and, 1585
inhibitors of, 199, 1659
medullary thyroid carcinoma and, 1675
melatonin and, 216
neuronal network distribution, 195, 823
pituitary effects of, 194, 195
synthesis and metabolism, 196, 1656
Sertoli cells, 827
antimüllerian hormone and, 992–93
differentiation of, 989
failure of, 878–82
FSH receptors of, 849
Leydig cell interactions with, 851
"only" syndrome and, 879
physiology, 849–50
tumors of, 892

Sex assignment, 984, 999–1000, 1031–33
hermaphroditism and, 1004
mixed gonadal dysgenesis and, 1005
5α-reductase deficiency and, 1017, 1018
testicular femininization and, 1018–19
Sex chromosomes. *See* Chromosomes, sex.
Sex determination, 983–1011. *See also* Sexual differentiation.
genetic sex and, 984, 985–89
gonadal sex and, 984, 989–92
historical note on, 983–84
hormonal sex and, 994–97
normal, 984–1000
Sex hormone-binding globulin (SHBG), 75
androgen excess and, 623
binding capacity, 580
fetal, 995
hyperthyroidism and, 428, 429
hypothyroidism and, 455
prostate cancer and, 1762
Sexual differentiation, 983–1033. *See also* Sex determination.
abnormal, 1000–1031
classification of, 1001
clinical features suggesting, 1000
clinical approach to disorders of, 1031–33
dimorphism and, 215–16, 984, 999–1000
errors of, 1011–31
gender role and, 999–1000. *See also* Sex determination.
hypothalamic-pituitary-gonadal axis and, 994–97
major determinants of, 991
normal, 984–1000
prenatal analysis of, 1031–32
Sexual function, 29–31. *See also* Impotence; Libido.
Sexual precocity. *See* Precocity, precocious.
Sheehan's syndrome, hypothyroidism and, 449
Shin spots, 1124
Shock:
diabetic ketoacidosis and, 1154
glucocorticoid therapy and, 804
prostaglandins and, 1777
Shohl's solution:
cystinuria and, 1515
renal tubular acidosis and, 1526–27
Shorr regimen, 1524
Short stature, 31, 1595–1613
anoxemia and, 1613
bone disorders and, 1611
causes, 1598–1613
chromosomal abnormalities and, 1611–13
clinical approach to, 1595–98
constitutional, 1599–1601
Cushing's syndrome and, 1609–10
deprivation syndromes and, 1613
differential diagnosis, 1596
endocrine causes of, 1602–10
genetic or familial, 1599
GH deficiency and, 1604–9
history, 1595, 1597
hypopituitarism and, 952–53
hypothyroidism and, 1602–4
idiopathic growth failure and, 1598
intrauterine factors and, 1501
malnutrition and, 1601–2
Noonan's syndrome and, 1612–13
normal, 1599–1601
pathologic, 1601–13
physical examination, 1597–98
precocious puberty and, 1610–11, 1616
pseudohypoparathyroidism and, 1427
radiography, 1598
Turner's syndrome and, 951–52, 1005, 1008, 1612
Shy-Drager syndrome, 674–76
Sialic acid, glycoproteins and, 257
Signal recognition particle, 38, 63
Sinopulmonary-infertility syndrome, 880–81
Sipple's syndrome, 1669. *See also* Multiple endocrine neoplasia, type 2.
sis oncogene, 154
Sitosterolemia, 1285–86
SKF 12185, 522
Skin, 25–26
acromegaly and, 300–301
coarse, dry, 26
Cushing's syndrome and, 607
diabetes mellitus and, 1124
endocrine disease and, 25–26
folds, obesity and, 1205–6
hyperthyroidism and, 425, 444
hypoparathyroidism and, 1423
hypopituitarism and, 278
hypothyroidism and, 451–52
pigmentation. *See* Pigmentation.
Sleep:
cortisol and, 527
growth hormone release and, 220, 267, 268
LH secretion and, 859
prolactin secretion and, 268, 272
rhythms and, 219, 220
testosterone secretion and, 858, 859
Smell disturbance, 26, 227, 864, 953
Smith-Lemli-Opitz syndrome, 1020
Sodium. *See also* Hypernatremia; Hyponatremia.
aldosterone and, 533, 563–67, 621–22
adrenal adenoma and, 752
diagnostic procedures, 757–58
restricted intake and, 534, 535
unresponsiveness to, 599
angiotensin and, 535, 706, 712
assays, 730
atrial natriuretic factor and, 722
calcium and, 718, 1335, 1336, 1538–40
cotransport (Na^+-K^+), 717
countertransport system (Na^+-Na^+ or Na^+-Li^+), 717
escape phenomenon, 563–64
glucocorticoids and, 553
21-hydroxylase deficiency and, 1023–25
hypercalciuria and, 1538–40, 1544
hypertension and, 710–12, 715–18
insulin and, 1077
-K^+,ATPase. *See* Na^+,K^+-ATPase.
kidney and, 563–66
calcium reabsorption and, 1335, 1336
hyponatremia and, 367, 368
norepinephrine and, 712
osmolality and, 354
parathyroid hormone and, 1337
prostaglandins and, 1775
pump, 715–16
thyroid hormone and, 398–99
renin and, 709–10
index, 727
restriction of, 534, 535, 711
sensitivity to, 710, 711–12
transport, 715–18
inhibitors of, 717–18
vasopressin and, 342
ectopic, 1711
renal reabsorption of, 350, 351
water balance and, 353–56
Sodium cellulose phosphate, 1555
Sodium ipodate and tyropanoate, 416, 435
Solubility product, nephrolithiasis and, 1504–5
Solute diuresis, 350
Somatomammotropic hormones, 263–73. *See also* Growth hormone; Lactogen, placental; Prolactin.
classification, 253
Somatomedin, 265, 1583, 1584. *See also* Insulin-like growth factors.
acromegaly and, 303
assays, 169
diabetes mellitus and, 1086
fetus and, 1588
growth and, 1586–89
receptor for, 93
testicular, 849
Somatostatin, 204–5, 266, 1584, 1647–49
acromegaly and, 304, 306
actions, 204–5, 1648
calcium and, 204
carcinoid and, 1657, 1659
chemistry, 204–5, 1647
clinical use, 1648–49
degradation of, 68
diabetes mellitus and, 1103, 1149
distribution of, 191, 192, 1647–48
eating behavior and, 1213
ectopic, 1720
extrahypothalamic, 204
gastrin and, 1648, 1649
glucagon and, 1072, 1083
hypoglycemia and, 677
hypothyroidism and, 450
inhibitory effects of, 1072, 1073
insulin and, 1072
measurement, 1647–48
metabolism, 68, 1648
neurotransmitters and, 205
release, 1648
TSH and, 259, 401, 450
Somatostatin-like immunoreactive substances, 1648, 1649
Somatostatinoma, 1649
MEN 1 and, 1664–65
Somatotroph cells, 250–51
Somogyi phenomenon, 1137
Sorbitol, 1053–54
diabetic complication and, 1127
Sotos's syndrome, 1620

Southern blotting, 46
SP. *See* Substance P.
Span measurement, 1597
Specificity, radioimmunoassay, 173–74
Spermatocytes, 827, 831
Spermatogenesis, 827–30
  aging and, 860–61
  contraceptive inhibition of, 890–91
  control of, 849–50
  evaluation of, 852–53
  failure of, 878–82. *See also* Azoospermia.
  Kallmann's syndrome and, 864
  maintenance of, 850
  radiotherapy and, 873
  stages of, 830, 833
Spermatogonia, 827, 831
Spermatozoa, 827–32
  analysis of, 853–54, 878
  antibodies to, 881
  capacitation of, 832
  diagrammatic representations of, 833
  fertilizing potential of, 854
  formation of, 827–30
  motility, 830
    defective, 880–81
  prostaglandins and, 1774
  release of, 830–32
  X-bearing vs. Y-bearing, 986–87
Spinal cord:
  hypogonadism and injury of, 869
  sympathetic connections to, 653–54
Spine:
  osteomalacia and, 1459
  osteopetrosis and, 1478
  osteoporosis and, 1468–69
  Paget's disease and, 1484
Spiral arteries, ovarian, 906–7
Spironolactone:
  aldosterone inhibition by, 142–43, 522
  aldosteronism and, 754, 762–63
  hirsutism and, 965
  hypertension and, 768–69
  structure of, 136
Splicesomes, 39
Spondyloepiphyseal dysplasia, 1611
Sponge hypothesis of ectopic hormones, 1698
src gene, 152
Standard, international, 166
Standard deviation, 1597
Starvation. *See also* Fasting.
  anorexia nervosa and, 234–35
  fuel metabolism and, 1090
  gluconeogenesis and, 1049–50, 1091
  obesity therapy by, 1236–37
  pregnancy and, 1156–57
  triiodothyronine deficiency and, 414
Stearic acid, 1254
Steatorrhea:
  abetalipoproteinemia and, 1278, 1279
  nephrolithiasis and, 1559, 1561
Stein-Leventhal disease. *See also* Polycystic ovary disease.
  hypothalamic disease and, 228–29
Stellate ganglia, 654
Steroid hormones, 68–75, 134–48. *See also* *specific hormone*.
  acetyl CoA and glucose relationship to, 10
  action of, 83–84, 134–48
    classes of, 134–35
    nuclear matrix role in, 144–45
    steps in, 138
  adrenal, 517–22. *See also* Aldosterone; Androgens; Cortisol; Glucocorticoids; Mineralocorticoids.
    biosynthesis, 517–19
    chemistry, 515–17
    congenital enzyme defects and, 624–31
    fetal, 520
    inhibitors of, 521–22
    nomenclature, 516–17
    regulation of, 522–36
  agonists of, 141
  antagonists of, 141–43
  binding of, 75
    nuclear, 141, 143–44
    plasma, 135–37
  biosynthesis, 68–75, 1012
    adrenal, 517–19
    cholesterol substrate for, 68–69
    pathway of, 71–74
    rate-controlling step in, 69–71
    tropic regulation of, 74–75
  chromatin and, 145–46
  evolution of, 9–10
  free, 75
  gene structure and, 147–48
  gene transcription and, 145–46
  gonadal. *See* Estrogens; Progesterone; Testosterone; *et al.*
  metabolism of, 75
  molecular mechanisms of, 134–48
  mRNA and, 145–48
  ovarian, 924–26. *See also* Androstenedione; Estrodiol; Progesterone.
  receptors for, 137–41
    activation of, 138, 141
    agonists vs. antagonists and, 141
    hypothalamic, 823
    regulation of, 105
  secretion of, 75
  separation of bound and free, 175–76
  sex. *See* Androgens; Estrogens; Progesterone; Testosterone.
  structures of, 136
  transport of, 75
  uptake of, by target cells, 137
Sterols:
  antirachitic, 1344–46
  storage diseases, 1280–86
Stigma, ovarian, 940
Stigmasterol, 1285
Stilbestrol, structure of, 136
Stimulus-secretion hypothesis, calcium and, 122
Stomach:
  acid output, 1633
  carcinoids of, 1658
  gastrin production by, 1630–31
Streptozotocin:
  carcinoid and, 1659
  insulinoma and, 1186–87
Stress:
  ACTH and, 256
    ectopic, 1708
  glucocorticoids and, 529–30, 559
  hyperglycemia and, 1092, 1165
  metabolic disorders and, 231
  vasopressin and, 347
Striae:
  Cushing's syndrome and, 607
Stroke, 28–29
  hypertension and, 696, 700
Struma ovarii, hyperthyroidism and, 423
Struvite stones, 1506–7, 1521–24
Substance K, 1651
Substance P, 1651
  actions, 199, 1651
  in brain, 192, 199, 208
  chemistry and release, 1651
  distribution, 192, 1651
  physiology and pathology, 1651
  tumor secretion of, 1723
Succinyl CoA, 1060
SU-8000 and SU-9055, 522
Sulfate storage shunt, 838
Sulfhydryls, cystinuria and, 1516
Sulfokinase, 519
Sulfonylureas, 1140–43
  hypoglycemia induced by, 1194, 1195
Suprachiasmatic nucleus, 189, 190, 821
  clock function of, 218–19
  vasopressin and, 338
Supraoptic nucleus, 189, 190, 338
  destruction of, 356
Supraopticohypophyseal tract, median eminence and, 192, 193
Surgery:
  adrenal. *See* Adrenalectomy.
  breast cancer, 1746, 1747–48
  carcinoid, 1658
  cortisol response to, 529–30
  craniopharyngioma, 298
  hyperlipidemia, 1264, 1305–6
  nephrolithiasis, 1524, 1571–72
  obesity treatment, 1239
  orchiectomy, 885–86, 891
  orchiopexy, 885, 886
  Paget's disease of bone and, 1490
  pancreatic, 1186
  parathyroid, 1400–1401. *See also* Parathyroidectomy.
  pheochromocytoma, 671–72
  pituitary, 298. *See also* Pituitary gland surgery.
  prostate gland, 1760
  renal artery revascularization, 749
  steroid coverage for, 596–97, 808, 814
  thyroid, *see* thyroidectomy
  transphenoidal, 298
  vitrectomy, 1119
Sutherland's concept of messengers, 85–86
Sweating, excessive, 26
Swyer syndrome, 1009–10
Sympathetic nervous system, 651–86. *See also* Catecholamines; Norepinephrine.
  activity index of, 666–67
  asthma and, 681

Sympathetic nervous system (*Cont.*):
coronary heart disease and, 680
diagnostic testing, 682–86
indirect methods of, 685–86
dysfunction, 672–76
ganglia of, 651, 654–55
pheochromocytoma and, 667
heart rate and, 686
hypertension and, 680
hypoglycemia and, 1180
melatonin and, 216, 217
organization, 653–55
ovaries and, 907–8, 920
pathophysiology, 667–82
physiology, 652–67
integrated, 662–64
postural reflex, 672–77
receptors. *See* Adrenergic receptors.
renin and, 703–4
stress and, 231
thyroid hormone and, 399
Sympathochromaffin system, 651–86. *See also* Catecholamines; Sympathetic nervous system.
diagnostic testing, 682–86
organization, 653–55
pathophysiology, 667–82
physiology, 652–67
integrated, 662–64
Symptoms of endocrine disease, 23–24
bone and joint, 31
cardiovascular, 28–29
gastrointestinal, 27
generalized, 24–25
hematopoietic, 27–28
nasal, 26
neurologic, 31–32
neuromuscular, 32–33
ophthalmic, 33–34
sexual, 29–31
skin, 25–26
temperature, 25
tongue, 26
urinary tract, 29
vocal, 26–27
weakness and fatigue, 24
weight gain, 25
weight loss, 24–25
Synacthen, 578
Syncytiotrophoblast, ectopic hormones and, 1701
Synergisms, hormone, 13
Synthesis of hormones. *See* Biosynthesis of hormones.

T cells:
autoimmunity and, 1678
thyroiditis and, 445
glucocorticoids and, 550, 551
Graves' disease and, 419–20
lymphoma, hypercalcemia and, 1410
Tachycardia, 28
Tachykinins, 1651
Tachyphylaxis, 98
Tall stature, 1613–21
acromegaly and, 1618–19. *See also* Acromegaly.
adrenal hyperplasia and, 1614–16
causes, 1614
chromosome abnormalities and, 1619
familial or constitutional, 1613–14
hyperthyroidism and, 1619
Klinefelter's syndrome and, 1000, 1619
miscellaneous syndromes of, 1619–21
precocious puberty and, 1616–18
XYY syndrome and, 872–73, 1619
Tamoxifen:
breast cancer and, 1744, 1745, 1749
endometrial cancer and, 1764
structure of, 136
Tancytes, 192, 823–24
Tangier disease, 1276–77
Target cells:
activation (response) of, 83–84
mediators of, 110–34
occupancy of receptors and, 99–101
peptide hormone, 87, 88
short-term vs. long-term, 110–11
desensitization of, 95, 97–99
effector systems of, 87
internalization by, 106–9
peptide hormone, 85–87
receptor regulation in, 104–6
steroid uptake by, 137
thyroid hormone, 149–50
hypersensitivity of, 18, 22
hyposensitivity of, 16–17
evaluation of, 22
TBG. *See* Thyroxine-binding globulin.
Temperature, 25
peptide hormone binding and, 88
regulation of, 235–36
thyroid hormones and, 398–99, 410
TSH and, 259
vasopressin and, 347
water loss and, 354
Tendonitis, hyperlipidemia and, 1260–61
Teprotide, 705
Teratoma, testicular, 892
Testes, 821–92
absent, 873–74, 1010, 1011
anatomy, 825–32
antibodies to, 881
Addison's disease and, 584
biopsy, 852–53
blood supply, 825
clinical disorders of, 861–92
clinical evaluation of, 852–57
contraception and, 890–91
differentiation of, 989–92
dysgenesis of, 1009–11. *See also* Gonads, dysgenesis of.
ectopic, 883–84
endocytosis in, 109
examination, 852
infertility and, 881–82
feminization syndrome, 875, 954, 1018–19
incomplete, 1019
fetal, 996–97
germinal cells, 827–32
cryptorchism and, 885
failure of, 878–82
Leydig cell interactions with, 850–51
number determination, 852, 853
physiology, 848–51
gonadotropin-producing tumors and, 882
hermaphroditism and, 1003–4
hypofunction, 861–78. *See also* Hypogonadism.
hypothalamic-pituitary axis with, 832–57. *See also* Hypothalamic-pituitary-testes axis.
impotence and, 889–90
infections, 880
infertility and, 878–82
Klinefelter's syndrome and, 1000–1001
Leydig cells. *See* Leydig cells.
mumps and, 874
physiology, 837–52
precocious pseudopuberty and, 1617
prolactin and, 862–63
puberty and, 858–60
delayed, 869
precocious, 882–83
regression of, 1010–11
removal of. *See* Orchiectomy.
retractile, 883, 84
rudimentary, 1010, 1011
seminiferous tubules. *See* Seminiferous tubules.
Sertoli cells. *See* Sertoli cells.
size assessment, 852
spermatogenesis by. *See* Spermatogenesis.
toxicosis syndrome, 883
toxins to, 874
tumors, 892
cryptorchism and, 885, 892
undescended, 883–86. *See also* Cryptorchism.
varicocele, 880
Testolactone, 1749
Testosterone, 838–48
actions, 842–44
mechanisms of, 1016–17
tabulation of, 845
adrenal, 568, 840
regulation of, 535–36
secretion rate, 521
synthesis, 516, 519
adrenal hyperplasia and, congenital, 1025
aging and, 860, 861
antagonists of, 142
assays, 580, 855
binding, 840–42
biosynthesis, 72, 73, 838, 839, 1012
adrenal, 516, 519
inborn errors of, 1011–16
ovarian, 73
bone age determination and, 857
chorionic gonadotropin and, 851
provocative test with, 857
circadian rhythm of, 220, 840
climacteric and, male, 874–75
contraception and, 890
Cushing's disease and, 605
deficiency, 862–78
estrogen and, 844–45, 851
ovarian follicle atresia and, 935–36

Testosterone *(Cont.)*:
fetal, 994–96
free, 580, 840, 842
FSH and, 263
glucocorticoids and, 558
GnRH and, 845
growth and, 1590
gynecomastia and, 886, 887, 889
hirsutism and, 623, 965
21-hydroxylase deficiency and, 1023, 1025, 1027
hypothyroidism and, 455
impotence and, 890
Kallmann's syndrome and, 864, 867
Klinefelter's syndrome and, 871, 872, 1001–2, 1619
LH and, 263, 844–46
concordance with, 840
libido in female and, 285
metabolism, 75, 542–43, 842
defective, 1017–18
structures of, 844
osteoporosis and, 1472, 1473
ovarian, 73, 926
ovarian follicle atresia and, 935–36
ovarian follicle recruitment and, 935
pituitary effects of, 844–48, 850
plasma levels, 521, 580, 840, 857
hypogonadism and, 877
polycystic ovary disease and, 963
prepubertal, 858
prolactin and, 851–52
prolactinoma and, 307
prostate cancer and, 891, 1755, 1756, 1760
puberty and, 858–60
delayed, 866, 876
receptors and, 139–40, 843–44, 1017
resistance to, 875, 1018–19
secretion, 838–40
sexual differentiation and, 993–96
sexual dimorphism and, 215
sleep and, 858, 859
spermatogenesis and, 849, 851
spinal cord damage and, 869
stimulation tests, 855–57
structure, 136, 516, 844
target tissue defects and, 1016–19
therapeutic, 286, 875–78
breast cancer and, 1748
delayed puberty and, 1600
dose-response profile, 878
growth failure and, 1609
Klinefelter's syndrome and, 1619
tall stature and, 1614
transport, 75, 840–42. *See also* Sex hormone-binding globulin.
XYY syndrome and, 873
Testosterone-estrogen-binding globulin (TeBG), 840–42
chemistry, 841
Tetany, 1422–23, 1432
hypomagnesemia and, 1441
pancreatitis and, 1431–32
postoperative, 1424
recalcification, 1401
treatment, 1433
Tetracosactrin, 576
Tetracycline, bone metabolism and, 1458
Tetradecanoylphorbol acetate (TPA), protein kinase C and, 126
Tetrahydrobiopterin, 652–53
Tetrahydrocannabinol, adrenal inhibition by, 522
Tetrahydrocortisol, 540
Tetraiodothyroacetic acid (tetrac), 392, 395
structure, 391
Tetraiodothyronine. *See* Thyroxine.
TGF. *See* Transforming growth factor.
Theca cells, ovarian:
antibodies to, 1684
biosynthesis in, 73
development of, 908
differentiated, 917, 918
graafian follicle and, 915
hormone synthesis and, 925, 926
hypertrophy of, 915, 917–19
interstitial, 913, 916–17
LH receptors of, 916–17
luteinization and, 921–23
luteolysis and, 923–24
ovulation and, 940, 944
premenarche, 941, 942
selection of follicles and, 936, 938
steroidogenesis and, 917
Thelarche, premature, 999, 1617
Therapeutic principles, 22
Thermoregulation, 235–36
obesity and, 1218–19
in animals, 1216–17
Thiazides:
diabetes insipidus and, 366, 367
hypercalcemia induced by, 1413
hypercalciuria and, 1552, 1554, 1555
hyponatremia caused by, 368
hypoparathyroidism and, 1435
Thiokinase, 1057
Thiolase, 1060
Thionamides, 433–34
Thiouracil, thyroid hemorrhage and, 484
Thirst, 352–53
blood volume and pressure and, 356
Cushing's syndrome and, 608
diabetes insipidus and, 358, 359, 362
hypernatremia and, 361, 364
hyponatremia and, 367
hypothalamic disorder and, 231
osmolality and, 358, 359
salt and water balance and, 354, 355
Thoracic ganglia, 654
Thrombosis, renal artery, 738
Thromboxane:
discovery of, 1769
platelets and, 1778–79
shock and, 1777
synthesis and metabolism, 130, 973, 1770, 1771–72
uterine, 972
Thymic hormone, 1583
Thymine, 37
Thyroglobulin, 77–78, 393–94
antibodies to, 175, 408, 432, 1685
metastases and, 501
carcinoma follow-up and, 500–501
hyperthyroidism and, 432
hypothyroidism and, 457–58
iodide inhibition of, 403
iodination of, 393
proteolysis of, 394
serum concentration, 408
synthesis, 393–94
defects in, 448, 481
Thyroglossal duct, 389
Thyroid-binding globulin. *See* Thyroxine-binding globulin.
Thyroid-binding prealbulin. *See* Thyroxine-binding prealbumin.
Thyroidectomy:
for cancer, 498, 499, 503
hypoparathyroidism after, 498, 1424–25
hypothyroidism induced by, 446–47
pregnancy and, 439
for solitary nodule, 494
subtotal, 437
Thyroid deiodinase, 78
Thyroid gland, 389–504
acromegaly and, 302
Addison's disease and, 583, 584
adenoma, 423, 438
MEN 1 and, 1665
MEN 2 and, 1671
anatomy, 389–90
anomalies, 389–90
antibodies to, 418–20, 445–46, 1683, 1685
Addison's disease and, 584
maternal, dysgenesis of thyroid and, 447
microsomal antigen and, 408
neonatal hyperthyroidism and, 440
tests for, 430
biopsy, 490–92
C cells (parafollicular cells), 391, 1338
adenoma, 1671
carcinoma. *See* Medullary thyroid carcinoma.
embryology, 1338, 1670
hyperplasia, 502–3, 1670–71
calcification, medullary carcinoma and, 502, 1670
calcitonin produced by, 1338–42
carcinoma, 494–504
age and, 487, 495, 496
anaplastic, 497, 500
classification, 494, 495
follicular, 490, 494, 497, 499–500
follow-up, 500–501
goiter and, 477, 483–84
hyperthyroidism and, 423
incidence, 495
laboratory studies, 488–92
medullary. *See* Medullary thyroid carcinoma.
natural history, 496–97
papillary, 491, 494–96, 498–99
predisposing factors, 486–88
probability of, by test results (Bayes' theorem), 490, 491
radiation and, 487, 495–96
radionuclide studies, 486, 488–89
recurrence rate, 498
sex and, 486–87, 496, 497
staging, 495
therapy, 497–500

Thyroid gland *(Cont.)*:
colloid, 78, 390
endocytosis by, 394
cysts, 489
dysgenesis, 447
embryology, 389, 1338, 1670
enlargement. *See* Goiter.
euthyroid sick syndrome and, 412
follicles, 390
hemorrhage, 462
TSH stimulation and, 484
histology, 390–91
hyperfunction. *See* Hyperthyroidism.
hypofunction. *See* Hypothyroidism.
lingual, 389
nodules, 486–94
adenomatous, 423
age and, 476, 487
cancer predisposition and, 486–88
cold, 486, 488, 493
goiter and, 477, 479–80, 482–85
hemorrhage in, 462
laboratory studies, 488–92
management, 492–93
physical characteristics, 487–88
nuclear magnetic resonance, 490
painful, 461–62
parafollicular cells. *See* C cells *subentry above.*
pertechnetate and, 393, 409, 488–89
physical examination, 390
radionuclide studies, 393, 408–9
cancer and, 486, 488–89
hyperthyroidism and, 430
radiotherapy, 432–33, 436–37, 498–99, 500
storm (crisis), 438
ultrasonography, 489–90
venous catheterization, 1399–1400
Thyroid hormone, 75–79, 391–462. *See also* Thyroxine; Triiodothyronine.
actions, 84, 150, 398–400
aging and, 410
amiodarone and, 416
assays, 404–9
variables affecting, 409–10
ATP and, 398–99
beta blocking agents and, 416, 435–36
binding, 78, 148–50, 395–98. *See also* Thyroxine-binding globulin.
autoantibodies, 411
capacity test, 405–6
cellular, 397–98
drugs affecting, 412
FDH syndrome and, 411
serum, 395–97, 404–6, 410–12
biosynthesis, 76–78, 392–95
defects in, 447–49, 481
iodine metabolism and, 76–77
pathway of, 77–78
catecholamines and, 399, 678
chemistry, 391–92
deficiency. *See* Hypothyroidism.
deiodination of, 394–95
drugs influencing, 412, 415–17, 432–36
ectopic, 423
environmental influences on, 410
excessive. *See* Hyperthyroidism.
fasting and, 78, 414
feedback mechanism and, 78
fetal, 409–10, 1589
free, index, 405–96
gene expression and, 150
glucocorticoids and, 415, 543, 558
hyperthyroidism and, 428
hypothyroidism and, 455
glucose and, 399
growth and, 1589, 1602–4, 1619
growth hormone and, 150, 428, 455, 1607–8
hypoalbuminemia and, 412
hypothalamic-pituitary-thyroid-peripheral axis and, 400
in infants and children, 410
inhibition of, 403–4
drugs for, 415–16, 432–36
iodide levels and, 403, 416
iodinated contrast agents and, 416, 435
lipid metabolism and, 399–400
lithium and, 416
metabolism 78–79, 394–95
methimazole and, 416, 433–35
molecular mechanisms, 148–50, 398
obesity and, 1215, 1233
phenytoin and, 416–17
pluriglandular failure and, 1685–86
precursors, 391–92
pregnancy and, 409
production rates, 394–95
propylthiouracil and, 416, 433–35
proteins regulated by, 150, 399
radioimmunoassay, 404, 406
autoantibodies and, 411
receptors for, 149–50, 397–98
regulation of, 400–404
replacement therapy, 458–59
in infants and children, 460
myxedema coma and, 461
preparations for, 458, 459
withdrawal of, 459–60
resistance to, 450
RNA and, 149, 150, 398, 399
secretion, 78, 394
serum concentration, 404–7
decreased, 411–12, 414–15, 456
free, 406
increased, 411, 415, 429–30
nonthyroidal illness and, 412–15
sex differences in, 410
sodium pump and, 398–99
stimulation of, 402–3
suppression test, 431
suppressive therapy, 484–86
cancer of thyroid and, 499
goiter and, 484–86
solitary nodule and, 493–94
sympathetic activity and, 399
thermogenesis and, 398–99
tissue action tests, 409
transport, 78, 395–97
TRH and. *See* Thyrotropin releasing hormone.
TSH and. *See* Thyrotropin.
Thyroiditis, 421–22, 437
adrenocortical insufficiency and, 1682–83
autoimmune (Hashimoto's), 445–46, 1678, 1682–83
diabetes mellitus and, 1682–83, 1684
painless, 421–22
pluriglandular insufficiency and, 1682–83, 1684
radiation, 422, 462
subacute (granulomatous, de Quervain's), 421, 461–62
suppurative, 462
Thyroid peroxidase, 77, 393
antithyroid drugs and, 433
hereditary defects in, 448
Thyroid-stimulating hormone. *See* Thyrotropin.
Thyronine, 391–92
structure, 391
Thyrotoxicosis. *See* Hyperthyroidism.
Thyrotroph cells, 251
Thyrotropin (thyroid-stimulating hormone, TSH), 78, 257–60, 400–403
actions, 257–58, 402–3
aging and, 410
amiodarone and, 416
assays, 258
biological, 169
hypopituitarism and, 281
techniques, 323
autoantibodies and, 418–20
biosynthesis, 257
cAMP and, 402
capillary rupture and, 484
cells seceting, 251
chemistry, 253, 257
circadian rhythm of, 220
deficiency, 277, 449
diagnostic procedures, 281
treatment, 285
dopamine and, 402
drugs affecting, 199
estrogen and, 259
excessive, 320, 423
feedback effects, 259–60
fetal, 410
glucocorticoids and, 259, 402, 415
goiter and, 474–76
hyperthyroidism and, 423
hypopituitarism and, 277, 281, 285, 1610
hypothalamic disease and, 226
hypothyroidism and, 449, 450, 456–57
insensitivity of thyroid and, 448
transient, 447
in infants and children, 410
inhibition of, 400–401
insensitivity to, 448
iodide and, 393, 402–3
metabolism 258–59
neurotransmitters and, 195, 259–60
nonthyroidal illness and, 415
pituitary levels, 258
pluriglandular insufficiency and, 1685, 1686
radioimmunoassay, 258
receptors for, 402
regulation of, 150, 259–60, 400–402
serum concentration, 258, 323, 407–8
hyperthyroidism and, 430
hypothyroidism and, 456–57

Thyrotropin (thyroid-stimulating hormone, TSH) (*Cont.*):
thyroxine replacement therapy and, 458–59
somatostatin and, 259, 401, 450
stimulation, 281, 323, 401–2, 407–8
in children, 1622
hyperthyroidism and, 430
hypothyroidism and, 456–57
suppression of, thyroid hormone therapy and, 484–86
cancer of thyroid and, 499
solitary nodule and, 493–94
temperature and, 259
TRH and. *See* Thyrotropin releasing hormone.
tumor secretion of:
pituitary, 320, 423
trophoblastic, 1715
Thyrotropin releasing hormone (TRH), 201–2, 401–2
behavioral effects, 202
chemistry and effects, 201–2
deficiency, 226, 449–50, 1610
degradation, 68
distribution, 191, 192, 501
eating behavior and, 1213
extrahypothalamic, 201
fetal, 410
goiter and, 474, 475
growth hormpone and, 202, 325
in acromegaly, 303
nonthyroidal illness and, 415
prolactin and, 201, 207, 271–72, 282, 284, 326
tumor secretion of, 308
structure, 200
TSH response test, 281, 323, 407–8
in children, 1622
hyperthyroidism and, 430
hypothyroidism and, 456–57
Thyroxine (T_4), 391–462. *See also* Thyroid hormone.
binding, 78, 148–50, 395–98. *See also* Thyroxine-binding globulin.
autoantibody, 411
biosynthesis, 76–78, 392–95
deficiency. *See* Hypothyroidism.
deiodination (conversion to T_3), 78, 148, 394–95, 403–4
decreased, 414
free, 396
index, 405–6
serum concentration, 406
hyperlipidemia and, 1303
increased levels. *See* Hyperthyroidism.
intracellular, 397
metabolism, 394–95
radioimmunoassay, 404
replacement therapy, 458–59
hyperthyroidism induced by, 422
in infants and children, 460, 1603, 1604
myxedema coma and, 461
schizophrenia and, 238–39
serum concentration, 404–5
decreased, 411–12, 414–15, 456
free, 406
increased, 411, 415, 429, 430
structure, 76, 391
suppressive therapy with, 485
cancer and, 499
solitary nodule and, 493
transport, 78
triiodothyronine ratio to, 417–18
TSH and. *See* Thyrotropin.
Thyroxine-binding globulin (TBG), 78, 148, 396, 404–6
capacity test, 405–6
conditions altering, 411
decreased levels of, 411–12
estrogen and, 411
increased levels of, 411
inherited defect of, 412
properties, 396
resin uptake test and, 405, 406
serum concentrations, 405, 410–12
sex differences in, 410
Thyroxine-binding prealbumin (TBPA), 78, 148–49, 397
decreased levels of, 412
increased affinity of, 411
properties, 396, 397
Thyroxine-5′-deiodinase, 394–95
conditions altering activity of, 403–4
decreased activity of, 414
Tibial osteotomy, Paget's disease and, 1490
Tibia test, growth hormone and, 266
Time-zone displacement, 220
Titering, antibody, 173
T-kinin and T-kininogen, 1781, 1783
Tolazamide, 1141, 1142
Tolbutamide, 1141
insulinoma test with, 1185
toxicity, 1143
Tongue, 26
Tonin, 703
Tonsils, cholesterol esters in, 1276
Torpedo californica, ACh receptor of, 91
Toxemia of pregnancy, renin-angiotensin-aldosterone axis and, 621
Transcortin. *See* Corticosteroid-binding globulin.
Transcription, gene, 60–63. *See also* DNA, transcription of.
Transducin:
adenylate cyclase regulation and, 113, 114
cGMP and, 122
Transduction, adenylate cyclase and, 112
Transforming genes. *See* Oncogenes.
Transforming growth factor (TGF), 850
ectopic hormone production and, 1701
hypercalcemia of malignancy and, 1704
oncogenes and, 154
phosphorylation and, 101
Transplantation:
bone marrow, osteopetrosis and, 1477–78
pancreatic, 1148–49
pituitary tissue, into hypothalamus, 187–88
renal:
diabetic nephropathy and, 1121
hyperparathyroidism and, 1392
osteodystrophy and, 1480
Transsphenoidal surgery, 298. *See also* Pituitary gland surgery.
Trauma, hypothalamic, 225
Tremor:
hyperthyroidism and, 427
propranolol and, 681
Triamcinolone:
absorption, 797
mineralocorticoid receptors and, 792
structure, 789
Triamterene, hypertension and, 769
Tricarboxylic acid cycle, 1052–53
Trichlormethiazide, hypercalciuria and, 1555
Triglycerides. *See also* Fatty acids; Lipids.
diabetes mellitus and, 1105–7
drugs lowering, 1299–1304
elevated. *See* Hyperlipidemia; Hypertriglyceridemia.
fuel reserves and, 1088
hyperthyroidism and, 428
insulin and, 1076
laboratory tests, 1307
obesity and, 1231, 1290–91
plasma levels, 1256
diet and, 1290
protein complex with. *See* Lipoprotein.
synthesis, 1055–56, 1250
1,24,25-Trihydroxyvitamin D, 1351
Triiodothyroacetic acid (triac), 392, 395
structure, 391
Triiodothyronine (T_3), 391–462. *See also* Thyroid hormone.
conversion of thyroxine to, 403–4
extrathyroidal production of, 394, 403–4
intracellular, 397–98
metabolism, 395
receptors for, 149–50
replacement therapy, hyperthyroidism induced by, 422
resin uptake test, 405–6
reverse, 392
caloric deficiency and, 414
formation of, 76, 78–79, 394, 395
metabolism, 395
serum concentration, 407
structure, 76, 391
serum concentration, 406–7
decreased, 414, 456
hyperthyroidism and, 429–30
structure, 76, 391
suppressive therapy with, goiter and, 485
thyroxine cOnversion to, 148, 394–95
decreased, 414
drugs inhibiting, 415–16, 435
thyroxine ratio to, 417–18
Trimethaphan, vasopressin and, 343
Triple phosphate stones, 1521–24
Trisomy, 985, 1003
Trophoblastic tumors, 1701
hyperthyroidism and, 423–24, 1715
Trophogene, ectopic hormones and, 1701
Tropic hormones, 14
Troponin C, 124
glycogenolysis and, 119
Trousseau's sign, 1422–23
Tryptophan, serotonin synthesis and, 1656

Tryptophan hydroxylase, 1656
TSH. *See* Thyrotropin.
Tuber cinereum, 190
Tuberculosis:
  Addison's disease and, 581, 585, 1679
  diabetes mellitus and, 1125
Tuberculum sellae, 247
Tuberohypophyseal pathway, 823
Tuberoinfundibular tract, 190
  terminals of, 193
Tubulin, 1066
Tumors. *See also* Adenoma; Cancer; *and specific organs and hormones involved.*
  ACTH secretion by, 315–20, 604, 605–6, 618, 1706–11
  adrenal. *See* Adrenal glands, *subentries* adenoma *and* carcinoma.
  brown, of bone, 1385
  calcitonin-secreting, 1718
  carcinoid. *See* Carcinoid.
  chorionic gonadotropin of, 1713–15
  chromaffin tissue, 667–72
  erythropoietin and, 1721–22
  gastrin releasing peptide and, 1720–21
  gastrin-secreting, 1633–36, 1664, 1669
  genes promoting, 55. *See also* Oncogenes.
  GH-secreting, 300–306, 1718–19
  glucagon-secreting, 1164–65, 1664–65
  glucose consumption by, 1187, 1716
  gonadotropin-secreting, 320–21
  GRH-secreting, 303, 304
  growth factors derived from, hypercalcemia and, 1407–9, 1704
  gut-brain peptides and, 1723
  hormone-responsive, 1736–64
  hormone secretion by, 1692–1726. *See also* Ectopic hormone production *and under specific hormones.*
  hyperthyroidism and, 423, 1715
  hypothalamic, 222–24
  hypothalamic releasing hormones secreted by, 1719–20
  insulin-secreting, 1184–87, 1664, 1669
  islet-cell. *See* Islet cells, tumors of.
  markers of, 1724–26
    prostate cancer and, 1758
    testicular neoplasia and, 892
  multiple endocrine. *See* Multiple endocrine neoplasia.
  necrosis factor of, 1724
  oncogenes and, 151. *See also* Oncogenes.
  osteomalacia and, 1717–18
  parasellar, 297
  parathyroid hormone secretion by, 1703–4
  pineal gland, 236–37
  pituitary. *See* Pituitary gland tumors.
  POMC peptides of, 1706, 1708–10
  prolactin-secreting, 306–15, 1722–23
  renin-secreting, 708, 738, 1722–23
  somatostatin-secreting, 1649, 1664–65
  sympathochromaffin system, 667–72
  testicular, 892
    cryptorchism and, 885, 892
  trophoblastic, 423–24, 1701, 1715
  TSH-secreting, 320, 423, 1715
  two-hit mutation model for, 1667–68
  vasopressin-secreting, 1711–13
Tunica albuginea, 825
  ovarian, 905
Tunica vaginalis, 825
Turner's syndrome, 951–52, 1005–9
  associated disorders, 1006–7
  clinical features, 1005–6
  diagnosis, 1007–8
  growth retardation and, 1612
  male, 872
  phenotype-karyotype correlations, 1007
  therapy, 1008–9
Tyramine:
  hepatic encephalopathy and, 681
  infusion test, 685
Tyrosine:
  catecholamine synthesis and, 652, 655
  phosphorylation of, 101–2
  thyroid hormones and, 392
  thyroid hormone synthesis and, 77–78
Tyrosine hydroxylase, 652, 653
Tyrosine kinase:
  autophosphorylation and, 101, 102
  epidermal growth factor and, 92
  insulin receptor, 1077, 1079–80
  oncogenes and, 152, 154
Tyrosyl, iodination and coupling of, 393–94

Ulcer:
  foot, diabetes and, 1123–24
  neuropathic, 1122
Ultimobranchial body, 1338
Ultimobranchial organ, 1670
Ultracentrifugation, lipoprotein, 1245, 1307
Ultradian rhythms, 218, 219–20
Ultrasonography:
  orbital, 442
  renal, 742
  thyroid, 489–90
Ultrasound destruction of stones, 1571–72
Ultraviolet light, vitamin D synthesis and, 73, 1346–47
Uracil, 38
Urea:
  vasopressin and, 342
  water balance and, 353, 354
Ureaplasma urealyticum, infertility and, 880
Urease, nephrolithiasis and, 1507, 1523, 1524
Uremia:
  diabetes mellitus and, 1120, 1121
  glucose intolerance and, 1165
  hyperlipidemia and, 1258
Ureteral colic, 1501
Uric acid:
  clearance of, 1517–18
  hyperparathyroidism and, 1391
  nephropathy, 1517
  pH and, 1506
  stones, 1517–21
    diagnosis, 1520
    frequency, 1503
    idiopathic, 1520
    mixed, 1561
    pathogenesis, 1506, 1518–20
    risk factors, 1518–19
    therapy, 1521
Uricase method, 1520
Uricosuria, 1517–18. *See also* Hyperuricosuria.
  drug-induced, 1519–20
Uridine diphosphate glucose (UDPG), 1046
Urinary tract, 29
  stones. *See* Nephrolithiasis.
Urine:
  acidification of, 1524–25
  aldosterone in, 728–29
  alkalinization, 1515, 1521
  androgens in, 580
  calcium in, 1336, 1568. *See also* Hypercalciuria; Hypocalciuria.
    balance data and, 1369
    bone disease and, 1455
    measurement, 1366–67, 1443
  cAMP in, 1373–74, 1443–44
  catecholamines in, 682, 684
    pheochromocytoma and, 669
  citrate in, 1564–66
  cortisol in, 541, 572–73
    Cushing's syndrome and, 316, 610, 611
  cystine in, 1510–17
  glucose in, 1111–12, 1116
    monitoring of, 1132
  gonadotropins in, 260, 261, 854, 855, 857
    Kallmann's syndrome and, 865, 866
  5-HIAA in, 1657
  17-hydroxycorticosteroids in, 572–73. *See also* 17-Hydroxycorticosteroids, urinary.
  hydroxyproline in, 1455–56
  hyponatremia and, 367, 368
  interpretation of assays, 21
  iodine in, 476
  17-ketogenic steroids in, 572–73. *See also* 17-Ketogenic steroids, urinary.
  magnesium in, 1362, 1368, 1443
  nephrolithiasis and. *See* Nephrolithiasis.
  osmolality of, 350, 355
    diabetes insipidus and, 358–60, 362–63
  oxalate in, 1557, 1559–60. *See also* Hyperoxaluria.
  pH of, 564, 567
    cystine and, 1515
    nephrolithiasis and, 1506, 1507, 1524–27, 1530
    uric acid and, 1506
  phosphate in, 1333–34
    measurement, 11367–38, 1443
    osteomalacia and rickets and, 1464–65
  protein in, diabetes mellitus and, 1119–20
  saturation zones of, 1504–5
  uric acid in, 1506, 1517–21, 1561–64
  vasopressin in, 349
  water loss and, 354, 355
Urogenital sinus, 994
Urography, intravenous, 740–42
Urotensin I, 205
Uterus:
  cancer, 1762–64
  differentiation of, 992
  dysfunctional bleeding of, 30
    menarcheal, 955
    postmenopausal, 980
    prostaglandins and, 973

Uterus (*Cont.*):
  prostaglandins and, 972–74, 1773–74
  vasculature of, 907

Vaccines, recombinant DNA production of, 52
Vaccinia virus, growth factors and, 154
Vacor, diabetes mellitus and, 1097, 1098
Vagina. *See also* Genitals.
  differentiation of, 994
  imperforate, 954
Valine:
  diabetes mellitus and, 1105
  metabolism, 1062–63
  protein feeding and, 1064
Valsalva maneuver, sympathetic function and, 685
Vanillylmandelic acid:
  formation of, 653
  urinary, 682, 684
    pheochromocytoma and, 669
Varicocele, 880
Vasculature. *See also* Cardiovascular system.
  adrenal, 513–14
  atherosclerosis of. *See* Atherosclerosis.
  atrial natriuretic factor and, 722, 724
  calcium and, 713
  catecholamines and, 659–60
  diabetes mellitus and, 1114, 1123–24
  fibromuscular dysplasia of, 737–38
  glucocorticoids and, 552–53
  hypertension and, 697, 699
  hypothalamic disorders and, 225
  ovarian, 906–7
    follicular, 911–12
  pituitary, 248–49
  prostaglandins and, 1777–78
  testicular, 825
    variocele and, 880
  thyroid, 390
  uterine, 907
Vas deferens, gross appearance of, 829
Vasectomy, 891
Vasoactive intestinal polypeptide (VIP), 1638–41
  actions, 197–98, 199, 208, 1639–40
  chemistry, 1638
  deficiency, 1641
  distribution, 192, 1638–39
  excess (WDHA syndrome), 1640–41
  hypercalcemia and, 1412–13
  measurement, 1638
  prolactin and, 207
  release and metabolism, 1639
  tumor secretion of, 1723
Vasoconstriction:
  angiotensin and, 706
  hypertension and, 697, 699
Vasodilatation, ANF and, 722, 724
Vasopressin (antidiuretic hormone), 338–76
  ACTH and, 281, 523, 524
  actions, 350–52
  amino acid sequence of, 339, 340
  assays, 375
    in children, 1623
    diabetes insipidus and, 359–60, 363–64
    SIADH and, 370
  atrial natriuretic factor and, 722
  behavioral effects, 213
  binding, 339
  biosynthesis, 339–40
  blood pressure and, 343–45, 351–52, 356
  blood volume and, 343–45, 356
  cells secreting, 338
  cerebrospinal fluid and, 349–50
  chemistry, 338–39
  corticotropin releasing factor and, 352, 524
  Cushing's disease and, 603
  deficiency, 278, 356–67, 1610
    diagnosis, 362–64
    etiology, 356–57
    pathophysiology, 358–62
    testing, 374–75
    therapy, 364–67
  diabetes insipidus and, 356–67
  distribution and clearance, 349
  drugs influencing, 347–48, 369
  ectopic, 1711–13
  emetic factors (nausea) and, 345–46
  extrahypophyseal pathways of, 349–56
  feedback effects on, 348
  glucose and, 342, 343, 346
  glycogenolysis and, 119
  half-life of, 349
  hypernatremia and, 361, 364, 366–67
  hypersecretion, 367–74
    diagnosis, 372–73
    etiology and pathophysiology, 367–72
    testing, 375
    treatment, 373–74
  hypoglycemia and, 346
  hyponatremia and, 367–74
    euvolemic, 368–74
    hypervolemic, 367–68, 372, 373
    hypovolemic, 368, 372–73
  hypoxia-hypercapnia and, 347
  kidney and, 350–51
    diabetes insipidus and, 357, 362, 367
    hyponatremia and, 367, 368
  neurologic disease and, 230–31
  neurotransmitters and, 213
  opioids and, 208
  osmolality and, 341–43, 354–55
    diabetes insipidus and, 358–60
    SIADH and, 369–71
    urinary, 350
  osmoreceptor dysfunction and, 357, 360–61, 364, 366–67
  ovarian, 926
  prostaglandins and, 351, 1775–76
  regulation of, 341–48
    variables influencing, 344
  renin-angiotensin system and, 346–47
  sodium and, 342
    ectopic syndrome and, 1711
    renal reabsorption of, 350, 351
  solutes and, 342–43
  stress and, 347
  syndrome of inappropriate secretion of (SIADH), 368–74
    diagnosis, 373
    etiology and pathophysiology, 368–72
    neurologic disease and, 230
    therapy, 373–74
    tumors and, 1711–13
  temperature and, 347
  thirst and, 352–53
  urinary, 349
  water and, 341, 354–56
    renal reabsorption of, 350, 351
    retention of, 367–74
vDAVP, amino acid sequence of, 340
Ventricular hypertrophy, hypertension and, 699, 734
Ventromedial nucleus, 189, 190
Verner-Morrison syndrome, 1640–41
VIP. *See* Vasoactive intestinal polypeptide.
VIP-oma, hypercalcemia and, 1412–13
Virilization, 30, 964–66
  adrenal hyperplasia and, 1020–30, 1614–16
  adrenocortical hyperfunction and, 622–24
  amenorrhea and, 954–55
  assessment and investigation, 964–65
  in childhood or adolescence, 1033
  fetal, 1011–31
    of female, 1020–31
    of male, 1011–20
  of genitalia, 955, 994, 995
  11β-hydroxylase deficiency and, 628, 1029–30
  21-hydroxylase deficiency and, 626–27, 1021–29
  incomplete, 1011–20
    androgen target tissue defects and, 1016–19
    exogenous steroids and, 1019–20
    gonadal dysgenesis and, 1010
    Leydig cell hypoplasia and, 1011
    testosterone synthesis defects and, 1011–16
    of unknown etiology, 1020
  management, 965–66
  neonatal androgenization and, 215–16
  tall stature and, 1614–16
  teratological malformations and, 1030–31
  Turner's syndrome and, 1007
Viruses:
  breast cancer and, 1741
  diabetes mellitus and, 1096–97
  mumps, orchitis and, 874
  oncogenes and, 55. *See also* Oncogenes.
  Paget's disease of bone and, 1487–88
  prostate cancer and, 1754–55
  sarcoma, 151, 154
  thyroiditis and, 461–62
  vaccinia, growth factors and, 154
Vision, 33–34. *See also* Eye.
  diabetes mellitus and, 33, 34, 1116, 1118
  evoked response, 294, 295
  field examination, 293, 295
  pituitary tumor and, 289, 293–95
Vitamin A:
  deficiency, 1278, 1279
  intoxication, 1414
Vitamin B_{12} deficiency, 28
Vitamin C:
  nephrolithiasis and, 1530
  oxalate production and, 1556, 1558
Vitamin D, 1344–57
  binding globulin (VDG), 75

Vitamin D *(Cont.)*:
binding, 1346, 1347
biological effects, 1351–57
biosynthesis, 73, 1346–47
bone and, 1355–56
calcium and, 1348–49, 1358–60
absorption of, 1352–53, 1355
hydroxylase activity and, 1350
renal reabsorption and, 1356–57
chemistry, 1344–46
deficiency, 1350
rickets and, 1461–62
glucocorticoid therapy and, 794–95
historical note on, 1344
hormones affecting, 1350
hydroxylation of, 73–74
hypercalcemia and, 1413–14
malignancy-associated, 1405, 1410, 1705
hypercalciuria and, 1383, 1384, 1541, 1543, 1545–50
hyperparathyroidism and, 1383, 1397
hypophosphatemia and, 1464
intestinal effects of, 1354–55
absorption and, 1352–53
intoxication, 1413–14, 1435
kidney and, 1356–57
metabolic role of, 1348
liver and, 1347
lymphoma and, 1410
malabsorption, 1462, 1466
mechanism of action, 1351–57
metabolic disorder of, 1462–63
metabolites of, 1346, 1347–51. *See also* 1,25-Dihydroxyvitamin D; 24,25-Dihydroxy vitamin D; 25-Hydroxyvitamin D.
nephrolithiasis and, 1383
osteodystrophy and, renal, 1479, 1480
osteomalacia and, 1460, 1462–63
osteoporosis and, 1470, 1472, 1473, 1475
parathyroid hormone and, 1325, 1348–49, 1481
bone resorption and, 1356
hydroxylase activity and, 1350
phosphorus and, 1349–50, 1360–61
absorption of, 1355
renal reabsorption and, 1356–57
plasma levels, 1375–76
hypercalcemia and, 1419
hyperparathyroidism and, 1397
potency, 1345–46
pregnancy and, 1350
pseudohypoparathyroidism and, 1428
receptors for, 1357, 1463
intestinal, 1354
resistance to, 1435, 1463
rickets and, 1460, 1461–64
sarcoidosis and, 1415–16
storage, 1347
structure, 1345
suppression test, 1547
therapeutic:
hypocalcemia and, 1433, 1434
osteodystrophy and, 1480
osteomalacia and rickets and, 1466–67
osteoporosis and, 1475, 1476
transport, 73, 1347
Vitamin D_2, 1344–46
assays, 1375
biosynthesis, 73
structure, 1345
Vitamin D_3, 1344–46
assays, 1375
biosynthesis, 73, 1346–47
structure, 1345
Vitamin E and K deficiency, 1278, 1279
Vitiligo, 26
Addison's disease and, 583, 587
pluriglandular insufficiency and, 1684
Vitrectomy, 1119
Voice, 26–27
Vomiting:
diabetic ketoacidosis and, 1151
vasopressin and, 345–46

Water, 353–56
DDAVP trial and, 375
diabetes insipidus and, 356–67
diuresis, 350
extracellular, 353, 354
glucocorticoids and, 553
hyperthyroidism and, 427
insensible loss of, 354, 355
intake of, 352, 354
atrial natriuretic factor and, 723
excessive, 357, 361–62, 367
SIADH and, 371, 373
intracellular, 353, 354
load test, 375, 376
mineralocorticoids and, 564
osmolality and, 353–56
restriction test, 374
retention of, hyponatremia and, 367–74
salt balance and, 353–56
thirst mechanism and, 352–53
urine output and, 354, 355
vasopressin and, 341, 354–56
impaired excretion and, 367–74
renal reabsorption and, 350, 351
Water supply, goitrogenic, 482
WDHA syndrome, 1640–41, 1723
diagnosis, 1640–41
treatment, 1641
Weakness, 24, 33
Addison's disease and, 587
Cushing's syndrome and, 608
episodic, 24, 33
generalized, 24
glucocorticoid therapy and, 795
hyperthyroidism and, 427–28
hypothyroidism and, 453
Weight:
chronologic age and, 1598
gain, 25
Cushing's syndrome and, 606
growth and, 1592–93
ideal, 1204
loss, 24–25
Addison's disease and, 587
amenorrhea and, 960–61
anorexia nervosa and, 234
diabetes mellitus and, 1116
diet for, 1235–37
hyperthyroidism and, 426
hypopituitarism and, 276–77, 279
infertility and, 960, 961
obesity therapy and, 1234–40
resistance to, in obesity, 1208
surgery for, 1239
standard tables for, 1204–06
Wermer's syndrome, 1663. *See also* Multiple endocrine neoplasia, type 1.
Whiskey test for calcitonin, 1673
Williams syndrome, 1417
Wolf-Chaikoff effect, 77
Wolffian ducts, 992–94
Wolman's disease, 1283
WR-2721, 1705

X chromosome, 984. *See also* Chromosomes, sex.
properties and function of, 988–89
Xanthelasma, 1261, 1282
Xanthine oxidase, 1518
Xanthinuria, 1520
Xanthomas, 1282–83
cerebrotendinous, 1283–84
diabetic, 1124
familial hypercholesterolemia and, 1260–61
HDL deficiency and, 1275
hyperchylomicronemia and, 1271
sitosterolemia and, 1285–86
striatum palmeris, 1267
tuberosum, 1267
type III hyperlipidemia and, 1267
XX males, 1003
XXY syndrome. *See* Klinefelter's syndrome.
XYY syndrome, 872–73, 1002–3, 1619

Y chromosome, 984. *See also* Chromosomes, sex.
properties and function of, 987–88
structural anomalies of, 1004
Yeasts:
cloning and, 49
protein synthesis and, 51
Yersinia, hyperthyroidism and, 419
Young's syndrome, infertility and, 881
YY peptide, 1647
amino acid sequence of, 1646

Zeitgeber, 218
Zimmerman reaction, 580
Zinc, insulin and, 1131
Zollinger-Ellison syndrome, 1633–36, 1664
diagnosis, 1633–35, 1666
historical note on, 1663
hyperparathyroidism and, 1389
nonpancreatic tumors and, 1723
symptoms and signs, 1633
therapy, 1636, 1669
Zona fasciculata, 514–15
hyperplasia, 602
synthesis in, 518, 519
Zona glomerulosa, 514
historical note on, 512
regulation of, 531–35
synthesis in, 71, 518, 519
Zona pellucida, 908, 932–33
Zona reticularis, 514–15
hyperplasia, 602